WHAT'S NEW?

PATHOPHYSIOLOGY

THE BIOLOGIC BASIS FOR DISEASE IN ADULTS AND CHILDREN

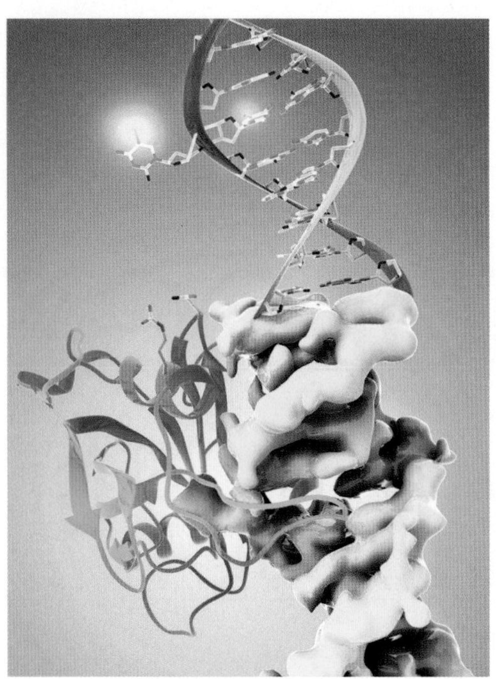

ABOUT THE COVER IMAGE

The cover image represents a stylized interface between genetics and epigenetics. Technological advances have changed our understanding of the genome and the role of transcriptional programs in the determination of cell fate and the response to environmental factors. We are beginning to understand how epigenetic modifications affect gene expression and alter cellular states without changing genomic DNA sequences. One analogy compares genetics to computer hardware with epigenetics as the software, software that may determine how the hardware behaves. Just as software can be tinkered with and erased, epigenetic marks may also be erasable, giving hope that we can intervene to change the landscape of the epigenome and prevent or cure disease. There is much to be learned and, over time, translated into clinical practice.

PATHOPHYSIOLOGY

THE BIOLOGIC BASIS FOR DISEASE IN ADULTS AND CHILDREN

SEVENTH EDITION

KATHRYN L. McCANCE, MSN, PhD
Professor Emeritus
College of Nursing
University of Utah
Salt Lake City, Utah

SUE E. HUETHER, MSN, PhD
Professor Emeritus
College of Nursing
University of Utah
Salt Lake City, Utah

SECTION EDITORS

Valentina L. Brashers, MD
Professor of Nursing and Woodard Clinical Scholar
Attending Physician in Internal Medicine
University of Virginia Health System
Charlottesville, Virginia

Neal S. Rote, PhD
Academic Vice-Chair and Director of Research
Department of Obstetrics and Gynecology
University Hospitals Case Medical Center
William H. Weir, MD. Professor of Reproductive Biology and Pathology
Case Western Reserve University School of Medicine
Cleveland, Ohio

ELSEVIER

with more than 1200 *illustrations*

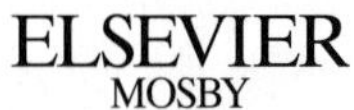

ELSEVIER
MOSBY

3251 Riverport Lane
St. Louis, Missouri 63043

PATHOPHYSIOLOGY: THE BIOLOGIC BASIS FOR DISEASE IN ADULTS AND CHILDREN, SEVENTH EDITION ISBN: 978-0-323-08854-1

Notices

Knowledge and best practice in this field are constantly changing. As new research and experience broaden our understanding, changes in research methods, professional practices, or medical treatment may become necessary.

Practitioners and researchers must always rely on their own experience and knowledge in evaluating and using any information, methods, compounds, or experiments described herein. In using such information or methods they should be mindful of their own safety and the safety of others, including parties for whom they have a professional responsibility.

With respect to any drug or pharmaceutical products identified, readers are advised to check the most current information provided (i) on procedures featured or (ii) by the manufacturer of each product to be administered, to verify the recommended dose or formula, the method and duration of administration, and contraindications. It is the responsibility of practitioners, relying on their own experience and knowledge of their patients, to make diagnoses, to determine dosages and the best treatment for each individual patient, and to take all appropriate safety precautions.

To the fullest extent of the law, neither the Publisher nor the authors, contributors, or editors assume any liability for any injury and/or damage to persons or property as a matter of products liability, negligence or otherwise, or from any use or operation of any methods, products, instructions, or ideas contained in the material herein.

Library of Congress Cataloging-in-Publication Data

Pathophysiology (McCance)
Pathophysiology: the biologic basis for disease in adults and children /[edited by] Kathryn L. McCance, Sue E. Huether; section editors, Valentina L. Brashers, Neal S. Rote. -- Seventh edition.
p. ; cm.
Preceded by Pathophysiology: the biologic basis for disease in adults and children / [edited by] Kathryn L. McCance, Sue E. Huether. 6th ed. c2010.
Includes bibliographical references.
ISBN 978-0-323-08854-1 (hardcover : alk. paper)
I. McCance, Kathryn L. II. Huether, Sue E. III. Title.
[DNLM: 1. Pathology--Nurses' Instruction. 2. Disease--Nurses' Instruction. 3. Physiological Phenomena--Nurses' Instruction. QZ 4]
RB113
616.07--dc23 2013033059

Senior Content Strategist: Sandra Clark
Senior Content Development Specialist: Karen C. Turner
Senior Content Coordinator: Brooke Kannady
Publishing Services Manager: Jeffrey Patterson
Senior Project Manager: Jeanne Genz
Design Direction: Amy Buxton
Multimedia Producer: Lisa Godoski

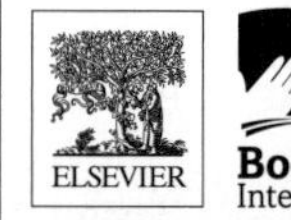

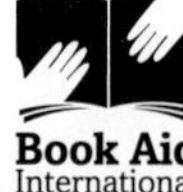

Printed in Canada

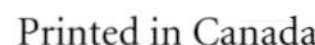

Last digit is the print number: 9 8 7 6 5 4 3 2

CONTRIBUTORS*

Rose Ann Urdiales Baker, PhD RN, PMHCNS-BC
Assistant Professor
College of Health Professions
The University of Akron
Akron, Ohio

Barbara Boss, PhD, APRN, FNP-BC, ANP-BC
Professor of Nursing and Director of DNP Program
University of Mississippi Medical Center
Jackson, Mississippi

Valentina L. Brashers, MD, FACP, FNAP
Professor of Nursing and Woodard Clinical Scholar
Attending Physician in Internal Medicine
University of Virginia Health System
Charlottesville, Virginia

Kristen Lee Carroll, MD
Associate Professor, Orthopedics
University of Utah
Salt Lake City, Utah
Shriner's Intermountain Unit
Shriner's Hospital for Children
Salt Lake City, Utah

Dennis Cheek, RN, PhD, FAHA
Abell-Hanger Professor of Gerontology Nursing
Harris College of Nursing and Health Sciences
Texas Christian University
Fort Worth, Texas

Margaret F. Clayton, PhD, APRN
Associate Professor, College of Nursing University of Utah
Salt Lake City, Utah

Christy L. Crowther-Radulewicz, MS, CRNP
Nurse Practitioner
Anne Arundel Orthopedic Surgeons
Annapolis, Maryland
Adjunct Faculty
Johns Hopkins University School of Nursing
Baltimore, Maryland

*The authors also would like to thank the previous edition contributors.

Susanna G. Cunningham, BSN, MA, PhD, FAAN, FAHA
Professor
School of Nursing
University of Washington
Seattle, Washington

Alexa K. Doig, PhD, RN
Associate Professor
College of Nursing
University of Utah
Salt Lake City, Utah

Todd C. Grey, MD
Chief Medical Examiner—State of Utah
Associate Clinical Professor
Department of Pathology
University of Utah School of Medicine
Salt Lake City, Utah

Mary Fran Hazinski, RN, MSN, FAAN, FAHA, FERC
Professor, Vanderbilt University School of Nursing
Assistant, Departments of Surgery and Pediatrics, Vanderbilt University School of Medicine
Clinical Nurse Specialist
Monroe Carell, Jr. Children's Hospital at Vanderbilt
Nashville, Tennessee

Robert E. Jones, MD, FACP, FACE
Professor of Medicine
University of Utah School of Medicine
Salt Lake City, Utah

Lynn B. Jorde, PhD
H.A. and Edna Benning Presidential Professor and Chair
Department of Human Genetics
University of Utah School of Medicine
Salt Lake City, Utah

Lynne M. Kerr, MD, PhD
Associate Professor
Departments of Pediatrics and Neurology
University of Utah Medical Center
Salt Lake City, Utah

Nancy E. Kline, PhD, RN, CPNP, FAAN
Director, Nursing Research, Medicine
Patient Services/Emergency Department
Boston Children's Hospital
Boston, Massachusetts

Gwen Latendresse, PhD, CNM
Assistant Professor
University of Utah College of Nursing
Salt Lake City, Utah

Linda L. Martin, DNP, RN, CFNP
Assistant Professor of Professional Practice
Texas Christian University
Harris College of Nursing and Health Sciences
Fort Worth, Texas

Sue A. McCann, MSN, RN, DNC
Programmatic Nurse Specialist
University of Pittsburgh Medical Center
Pittsburgh, Pennsylvania

Nancy L. McDaniel, MD
Associate Professor of Pediatrics
University of Virginia
Charlottesville, Virginia

Mary A. Mondozzi, MSN, RN
Burn Center Education/Outreach Coordinator
Akron Children's Hospital
The Paul and Carol David Foundation Burn Institute
Akron, Ohio

Stephen E. Morris, MD
Associate Professor of Surgery
Director, University of Utah Burn Center
Salt Lake City, Utah

Noreen Heer Nicol, PhD, RN, FNP, NEA-ABC
Associate Professor
University of Colorado, College of Nursing
Director, Children's Hospital Colorado
Denver, Colorado

Julia Phillippi, PhD, CNM, FACNM
Assistant Professor
Vanderbilt University School of Nursing
Nashville, Tennessee

Patricia Ring, RN, PNP-BC
Pediatric Nephrology Nurse Practitioner
Children's Hospital of Wisconsin
Milwaukee, Wisconsin

George W. Rodway, PhD, RN, ANP
Assistant Professor
Orvis School of Nursing
University of Nevada—Reno
Reno, Nevada

Neal S. Rote, PhD
Academic Vice-Chair and Director of Research
Department of Obstetrics and Gynecology
University Hospitals Case Medical Center
William H. Weir, MD. Professor of Reproductive Biology and Professor of Pathology
Case Western Reserve University School of Medicine
Cleveland, Ohio

Anna L. Schwartz, PhD, FNP-BC, FAAN
Associate Professor
School of Nursing
Northern Arizona University
Flagstaff, Arizona

Richard A. Sugerman, PhD
Professor of Anatomy, Emeritus
Director of Service Learning Projects
College of Osteopathic Medicine of the Pacific
Pomona, California

Lorey K. Takahashi, PhD
Professor of Psychology
University of Hawaii at Manoa
Honolulu, Hawaii

Gillian Tufts, DNP, FNP-C
Associate Professor
Clinical College of Nursing
University of Utah College of Nursing
Salt Lake City, Utah

REVIEWERS

Nancy M. Burruss, PhD, RN, CNE
Associate Professor
Bellin College
Green Bay, Wisconsin

David J. Derrico, RN, MSN
Clinical Assistant Professor
Adult and Elderly Department
University of Florida College of Nursing
Gainesville, Florida

Diane P. Genereux, PhD
Assistant Professor
Department of Biology
Westfield State University
Westfield, Massachusetts

Sandra L. Kaminski, MS, PA-C
Assistant Professor
School of Health and Medical Sciences
Seton Hall University
South Orange, New Jersey

Fei Li, PhD
Assistant Professor
Department of Biology
New York University
New York, New York

Carol Anne Marchetti, PhD, RN, CNS, NP
Assistant Professor
Bouve College of Health Sciences
School of Nursing
Northeastern University
Boston, Massachusetts

Denise Morita, MD
Assistant Professor
Department of Pediatrics
Division of Pediatric Neurology
University of Utah School of Medicine
Salt Lake City, Utah

Jason Mott, PhD, RN
Instructor of Nursing
Nursing Department
Bellin College
Green Bay, Wisconsin

Jane Cross Norman, PhD, RN, CNE
Masters of Science in Nursing
Program Director
Tennessee State University
Nashville, Tennessee

Abby Saunders, MS, PA-C
Physician Assistant
School of Health and Medical Sciences
Seton Hall University
South Orange, New Jersey

Lorna L. Schumann, PhD, NP-C, ACNS, BC, ACNP, BC, CCRN-R, FAANP
Associate Professor
College of Nursing
Washington State University
Spokane, Washington

Karin C. VanMeter, PhD
Lecturer
Department of Biomedical Sciences
College of Veterinary Medicine
Iowa State University
Ames, Iowa

PREFACE

Pathophysiology incorporates basic, translational, and clinical research to advance understandings of disease and dysfunction. The study of pathophysiology involves many biomedical sciences and a wide range of research activities. Multiple aspects of cellular physiology are progressing rapidly, generating vast amounts of data to understand. The information expansion involves a greater understanding of the behavior of individual cells, of their neighboring microenvironment, and of the molecules that not only make up those cells but also communicate with their surroundings. Importantly, the forward movement of biomedical sciences occurs within the context of social, economic, and political processes that determine how disease is defined, experienced, and treated.

Interdisciplinary research has led to significant advancements in genetics, epigenetics, cell signaling and communication, control of cell behavior, metabolism, and cell fate. Knowledge about normal cell structures and signaling pathways is at the forefront of translational science. Advancements in tools to observe cells have provided new understanding of cellular processes including migration of tumor cells, responses of the immune system, and influences of the microenvironment. Investigators are studying if or how early life events affect health and disease into adulthood and across generations. A wide range of research is centered on microbial mechanisms of pathogenesis, immune responses, epidemiology, and drug efficacy and resistance.

Although these advancements have created an ever-increasing state of excitement, they have also created the problem of how students, teachers, and clinicians can cope with the expanding new information. Compressing these data into simplified discussions for students and clinicians is challenging. Our approach in this book has been to present an organized, logical sequence of content based on current literature and research reports with understandable explanations and accompanied by illustrations and summary tables. The primary focus is on pathophysiology, and there is less emphasis on the evaluation and treatment that is found in clinical management textbooks. As in previous editions, the following is a list of our specific goals for the textbook:

- Draw attention to differences in etiology, epidemiology, pathophysiology, clinical manifestations, and treatment according to gender and age.
- Pay careful attention to presentations of emerging new data on controversial topics.
- Integrate health promotion and disease prevention by updating risk factors, explaining certain relationships between nutrition and disease, and referencing screening recommendations and other therapeutic approaches.

ORGANIZATION AND CONTENT: WHAT'S NEW IN THE SEVENTH EDITION

The book is organized into two parts. Part One presents the cellular and tissue responses common to disease. The pathophysiology of disease, organized by body systems, is presented in Part Two. All content has been reviewed and updated with extensive new references and two new chapters.

Part One: Central Concepts of Pathophysiology: Cells and Tissues

Part One begins with an in-depth study of the cell and progresses to cover the underlying processes of disease. Concepts covered include cell signaling and cell communication processes; genes and common genetic diseases; epigenetics and disease; fluid, electrolyte, and acid-base balance; inflammation, cytokines and their biologic functions, and normal and altered immunity; infection, stress, coping, and immunity; tumor biology, epidemiology of cancer, and cancer in children. Particularly important revisions and additions to Part One include the following:

- Updated content on cellular organelles, the plasma membrane, cell signaling, and communication (Chapter 1)
- Updated content on agents of cell injury, oxidative stress, apoptosis, autophagy, and aging (Chapter 2)
- A new chapter on epigenetics and disease (Chapter 6)
- Updated content on normal innate and adaptive immunity (Chapters 7 and 8)
- Updated content on alterations of immunity and inflammation (Chapter 9)
- Updated content on infection (Chapter 10)
- Reorganization and updated content on stress and disease (Chapter 11)
- Extensive revisions and reorganization of tumor biology and invasion and metastases (Chapter 12)
- Extensive revisions and reorganization of epidemiology of cancer (Chapter 13)

Part Two: Pathophysiologic Alterations: Organs and Systems

Part Two is a systematic survey of diseases within body systems. Each unit focuses on a specific body system and begins with an anatomy and physiology chapter to provide a basis of comparison for understanding the alterations created by disease. A brief summary of normal aging is included at the end of the section on anatomy and physiology. The discussion of each disease in the alterations' chapters is developed in a logical manner that begins with an introductory paragraph on etiology and epidemiology, followed by pathophysiology, clinical manifestations, and evaluation and treatment. Separate chapters are dedicated to pediatric pathophysiology, and sensitivity is paid to gender and age. Especially significant revisions and additions to Part Two include the following:

- Updated information on chronic pain syndromes and classification of sleep disorders (Chapter 16)
- Updated content on concepts of alterations in consciousness, memory, delirium syndromes, and dementia. New information related to motor neuron and movement disorders

including Parkinson disease and amyotrophic lateral sclerosis (Chapter 17)
- Updated information on traumatic brain and spinal cord injury, degenerative disorders of the spine, stroke and headache syndromes, and multiple sclerosis (Chapter 18)
- Updated content on schizophrenia, mood disorders, and anxiety (Chapter 19)
- Updates on childhood cerebrovascular disease, seizure disorders, and brain tumors (Chapter 20)
- Extensive updates on diabetes mellitus, insulin resistance, and thyroid and adrenal gland disorders (Chapter 22)
- Extensively rewritten material on female reproductive disorders including cancer, benign breast diseases, and breast cancer (Chapter 24)
- A separate chapter on male reproductive disorders and cancer with extensive updating and reorganization (Chapter 25)
- Extensive updating of sexually transmitted infections (Chapter 26)
- Updated content on normal blood cells, hemostasis, platelet function, and coagulation (Chapter 27)
- Revised and updated content on alterations of leukocyte, lymphoid, and hemostatic function (Chapter 29)
- Extensively rewritten chapter on the anatomy and physiology of the cardiovascular and lymphatic systems (Chapter 31)
- Extensively updated coverage of atherosclerosis, endothelial injury and dysfunction, coronary artery disease, myocardial infarction, and heart failure (Chapter 32)
- Major revisions to the immune mechanisms of asthma, chronic lung disease; and updates for respiratory tract infection, pulmonary hypertension, pulmonary embolism, and lung cancers (Chapters 35)
- Major updates for childhood asthma, respiratory distress syndrome, cystic fibrosis, lung infections, and sudden infant death syndrome (Chapter 36)
- Updates on kidney stones, urinary tract infection, glomerulopathies, chronic renal failure, and bladder and kidney tumors (Chapter 38)
- New information for urinary tract infection, glomerulonephritis, and renal failure in children (Chapter 39)
- Updates on gastroesophageal reflux disease, peptic ulcer disease, irritable bowel syndrome, inflammatory bowel disease, intestinal obstruction, obesity, colon cancer, and liver disease (Chapter 41)
- New information on gluten-sensitive enteropathy, necrotizing enterocolitis, bowel obstruction, infections of the intestine, and liver disease in children (Chapter 42)
- Updated content on alterations of the musculoskeletal system (Chapter 44)
- Updated content on pressure ulcers, dermatitis and psoriasis, vesicular disorder, scleroderma, and skin cancer (Chapter 46)
- Updated content on childhood atopic dermatitis, skin infections, and immune drug reactions (Chapter 47)
- Extensive updating and reorganization of content on septic shock, multiple organ dysfunction syndrome, and burns for adults and children (Chapters 48 and 49)

FEATURES TO PROMOTE LEARNING

Ease of learning has been enhanced by designing a number of features that guide and support understanding, including:

- Each chapter opener notes the corresponding module in the Online Review Course. The course is available as a separate purchase. Details of the course can be reviewed at www.us.elsevierhealth.com.
- *Chapter Outlines* for each chapter
- *Special Headings* to underscore the consistent treatment of each disease—Pathophysiology, Clinical Manifestations, and Evaluation and Treatment
- More than 85 *What's New?* boxes review the most current research and clinical developments; a list of these is included on the inside front cover
- *Nutrition & Disease* boxes to emphasize nutrition as a health promotion strategy that may alter disease risk or pathogenesis
- End-of-chapter *Summary Review* sections summarize the content in each chapter and serve as built-in content review guides
- Boldface *Key Terms* with end-of-chapter term lists and page numbers for rapid access
- A comprehensive *Glossary* with approximately 1000 terms helps students with the often-difficult terminology related to pathophysiology

ART PROGRAM

The art program was carefully crafted. It received as much attention as the narrative. Nearly 200 new or revised full-color illustrations were created and strategically placed throughout the textbook. Also included are many new high-quality, full-color photographs of clinical manifestations, pathologic specimens, and clinical imaging techniques. The combination of illustrations, algorithms, and photographs and the use of color for tables and boxes allow clarification for complex concepts and the emergence of easily recognized essential information.

ANCILLARIES

For Students

On **Evolve**, at http://evolve.elsevier.com/McCance/, students can access 550 review questions, 100 animations to help students master the text content, 28 case studies with questions and answers, and downloadable chapter Key Point documents for each chapter.

The newly rewritten **Study Guide** includes many different question types, aiming to help all different types of student learners. Question types include the following:

- Choose the Correct Words
- Complete These Sentences
- Categorize These Clinical Examples
- Explain the Pictures
- Teach These People about Pathophysiology
- Plus many more…

Answers are found in the back of the Study Guide for easy reference for students.

For Instructors

The **Evolve Instructor Resources** for this textbook provide the following teaching aids:

- Teach for Nurses instructor manual, broken down by chapter, detailing the resources available to instructors for their lesson planning, and including unique case studies and class activities they can share with students
- Test Bank in ExamView with approximately 1900 questions (in multiple choice, multiple response, and matching formats) with answers, rationales, and textbook page references
- Image Collection with all of the approximately 1200 figures from the text
- PowerPoint lecture slides for each chapter (approximately 3400 slides and 420 images total), including integrated Audience Response Questions in each chapter (218 total), and integrated case studies at the end of each unit (15 total)

Evolve is an Internet-based learning environment that works in coordination with the text. This resource enables you to publish your class syllabus, outline, and lecture notes; set up "virtual office hours" and e-mail communication; share important dates and information through the online class calendar; and encourage student participation through chat rooms and discussion boards. Free with qualified adoption. Contact your sales representative or visit http://evolve.elsevier.com for more information about integrating **Evolve** into your curriculum.

ACKNOWLEDGMENTS

The enormous task of keeping this book current and readable greatly depends on our contributors; several new writers have joined our team for this edition. We thank them for their knowledge and tremendous labor of reviewing relevant literature, synthesizing it, and writing and revising chapters to make them highly readable for others. This edition includes a new chapter on epigenetics and disease and separate chapters for female and male alterations of reproduction. Several chapters were completely rewritten for this edition. We have a special appreciation for Neal Rote and Tina Brashers, section editors, for their tireless editing, writing, and development of new art. Neal managed the immunity, infection, and hematology chapters. For this edition, he completely updated the tumor biology chapter. Neal also fully updated the glossary. Tina managed the endocrine, pulmonary, and cardiovascular alterations chapters. Both Neal and Tina have exceptional ability to integrate, simplify, and illustrate the complex content of pathophysiology. Always motivated to *really* help students and clinicians, we thank you both. In addition, Tina Brashers, Samantha Greed, Lori Kelly, Kathleen Whalen, Diane Young, and Linda Turchin developed modules for the Online Review Course. There were also many faculty and clinicians who provided reviews for content revision and we are grateful for their insight and recommendations.

We extend gratitude to those who contributed to the book supplements. Linda Felver has created an all new inventive and resourceful Study Guide. Thank you Linda for very astute edits. For the Student Evolve website, Blaine Winters and Gaye Ray wrote the review questions. For the Instructor Evolve website, Linda Turchin updated and revised the Test Bank. Joanna Cain and Stacy June Breedlove Shaffer created unique case studies for the Teach for Nurses Instructor's Manual and PowerPoints. Kim Webb fully updated the PowerPoint presentations and supplemental audience response questions. Former Content Development Specialist on our book, Charlene Ketchum, created the Teach for Nurses Instructor's Manual. Also thank you to freelancer Allison Smith, who aided in the update of the glossary. We would also like to acknowledge Nancy Blasdell, Diane Young, Margaret Clayton, Susan Frazier, and Linda Turchin for their previous contributions to the Evolve resources. Thank you all for your help.

The process of completing this book is dependent on the "behind the scenes work" of numerous people. Manuscript management and final word processing is a huge and complex effort and was completed by our "rock" Sue Meeks, who has worked with us for more than 30 years. Her extraordinary talent, unwavering dedication to excellence, and detail kept us sane and on track. Every edition is monumental work—and she retypes and recounts endlessly—and unruffled. As always, our deepest appreciation for your continuing skill and patience.

Our Senior Content Development Editor at Elsevier is Karen Turner. This job is key. Karen monitored closely with an eagle eye! Karen was especially helpful with illustrations and exacting surveillance necessary for staying consistent and clear. Her questions were thoughtful and critically timed. She is very organized and practical and kept this project on target. Thank you Karen. Senior Content Strategist Sandra Clark helped with the overall structure of the book and all the business needed for contributors, designers, artists, and other editors. This is a big job and Sandra made sure that we had all resources necessary to complete this book. Thank you, Sandra. Senior Content Coordinator Brooke Kannady, a delight to work with, coordinated all reviewer projects, was quick to respond to any of the production needs, and is very conscientious. Thank you, Brooke. To Sally Schrefer, endless thanks for constant inspiration over 24 years.

The project manager for a book of this size and complexity of content has an enormous responsibility. The Senior Project Manager was Jeanne Genz. From copy edit to final page proofs, she is exacting and a gem to work with. Thank you, Jeanne, especially for your early morning consultations. Our book designer was Amy Buxton and she did an outstanding job guiding the design of the interior portion of the book—we are especially pleased with the layout, dynamic colors, and presentation of pedagogy. She also coordinated the work that went into creating the striking cover design. Thank you, Amy.

The newly drawn and revised artwork for this edition was completed by George Barile of Accurate Art Inc. The art is key and challenging and our drawings are often pathetic, but George was persistent to get it right and creative. Thank you so much George for the conceptual arrangements, labels, and beautiful colors.

We thank Ramón Andrade Candelario at 3Dciencia for allowing us to use the beautiful cover image. We also thank the Department of Dermatology at the University of Utah School of Medicine, which provided numerous photos of skin lesions. Thanks to Dr. Arthur R. Brothman, University of Utah School of Medicine, for the *N-myc* gene amplification slides used to illustrate the discussion of neuroblastoma, and to Dr. John Hoffman for the PET scan images of non–small cell lung cancer.

We are grateful to the many colleagues and friends at the University of Utah Health Sciences Center for their assistance with references and consultation on content. Thanks for the outstanding extra help—Ruth Weinberg, your experience and editorial skill are exceptional.

Special thanks are given to students, particularly nursing and other health science students, for the e-mails and phone calls we receive. Your questions and suggestions are inspiring and guide us in our efforts to prepare a clear and up-to-date manuscript with much visual input.

Sincerely and with great affection we thank our families, especially John, Mae, and Dorothy. Although disentangling certain data is inconvenient at times, we thank those committed to "getting it right"—increasing patient-centered quality care, safety, and satisfaction.

INTRODUCTION TO PATHOPHYSIOLOGY

The word root "patho" is derived from the Greek word *pathos,* which means suffering. The Greek word root "logos" means discourse or, more commonly, system of formal study, and "physio" pertains to functions of organisms. Generally, pathophysiology is the systematic study of the functional changes in cells, tissues, and organs altered by disease and/or injury. Important, however, is the inextricable component of suffering.

Knowledge of cellular biology as well as anatomy and physiology and the various organ systems of the body is an essential foundation for the study of pathophysiology. To understand pathophysiology the student must also use principles, concepts, and basic knowledge from other fields of study, including biology, genetics, immunology, pathology, and epidemiology. A number of terms are used to focus the discussion of pathophysiology; they may be used interchangeably at times, but that does not necessarily indicate that they have the same meaning. These terms are reviewed in Table I-1.

Pathophysiology is one of the most important bridging sciences between preclinical and clinical courses for students in the health sciences and it requires in-depth study at an early stage in the curriculum. The definitions or conceptual models of pathophysiology that we carry in our minds influence what we do with our observations and the rationale that we provide for our actions. Therefore, the clinician must understand that although pathophysiology is a science, it also designates suffering in people; the clinician should never lose sight of this aspect of its definition.

TABLE I-1 TERMS AND DEFINITIONS RELATED TO PATHOPHYSIOLOGY

Term	Definition
Pathology	Study of structural alterations in cells, tissues, and organs that help to identify the cause of disease
Pathogenesis	Pattern of tissue changes associated with the development of disease
Etiology	Study of the cause(s) of disease and/or injury
Idiopathic	Diseases with no identifiable cause
Iatrogenic	Diseases and/or injury as a result of medical intervention
Clinical manifestations	Signs and symptoms
Nosocomial	Diseases acquired as a consequence of being in a hospital environment
Diagnosis	Naming or identification of a disease
Prognosis	Expected outcome of a disease
Acute disease	Sudden appearance of signs and symptoms lasting a short time
Chronic disease	Develops more slowly, lasting a long time or a lifetime
Remissions	Periods when clinical manifestations disappear or diminish significantly
Exacerbations	Periods when clinical manifestations become worse or more severe
Sequelae	Any abnormal conditions that follow and are the result of a disease, treatment, or injury

As students study clinically-related sciences, they learn to recognize and categorize disease. From the formulation of a differential diagnosis one understands the different *clinical manifestations,* the signs, and the symptoms of certain pathologies. These understandings structure further investigations, treatment plans, and evaluation. The interaction of these activities determines clinical outcomes and treatment success. Still, the concept of disease can be inherently ambiguous and elusive; many pathologies remain hidden and resist easy classification. One should appreciate that the naming and diagnosing of diseases involve evaluative judgments as well as scientific fact, and that the process is as much a social endeavor as it is a scientific one. Some diseases, such as tuberculosis, identify a highly specific causative or etiologic agent or process. Others, such as Alzheimer disease or arthritis, indicate pathologic changes of unclear cause. There is considerable need for more research to validate mental health diagnoses. In addition, syndromes and functional disorders simply describe multiple symptoms and signs that frequently occur together. Does commonality exist in all of these labels? The answer is "yes" and "no" and depends on our conception of health and disease. In the strictest sense, objective scientific facts help us know if an individual is healthy or suffering from disease. Critical to attaining health in the United States are nine domains particularly worrisome and include adverse birth outcomes, injuries and homicides, adolescent pregnancy and sexually transmitted infections, HIV and AIDS, drug-related mortality, obesity and diabetes, heart disease, chronic lung disease, and disability.[1]

An individual's conception of disease is based on personal beliefs and histories, professional and lay healers who interact with that individual, and society at large. Each idea or construct has the power to influence other ideas and constructs, and each relationship has the ability to shape the way disease is understood and experienced.[2] In short, defining and understanding disease are tremendously ambiguous. Although a discerning mind is key, perhaps an important trait for the new student of pathophysiology is an open and tolerant mind. To believe that science alone can overcome ignorance and that clinical training and technology can overcome ineptitude only encourages arrogance and undermines the scientific purpose.

Pathophysiology has had great success in explaining the mechanisms and clinical manifestations associated with infectious diseases. Syndromes of unclear etiology, such as headache and fibromyalgia, have proven to be troublesome. Even more difficult are multifactorial conditions, such as atherosclerosis or type 2 diabetes mellitus, in which several interacting factors contribute to the etiology. Learning how interacting factors relate to one another to increase morbidity or actually cause disease contributes to an appreciation of how emerging concepts revolutionize current understandings. One revolution in thought that has driven intensive research is that low levels of chronic inflammation cause or contribute to many diseases.

The language that clinicians use to discuss diseases and their manifestations is powerful. Lives are altered by a few words uttered by a clinician in a white coat or uniform. "AIDS," "cancer," and "heart attack" have become culturally ingrained symbols that portend an individual's future. Although some futures are determined by scientific evidence, others are determined by subjective experience.[3] For example, a person diagnosed with a familial disease may ask, "Will I suffer like my mother did?" This questioning influences individuals' suffering.

In conclusion, pathophysiology—the understanding of disease—requires descriptive evidence as well as an evaluative component regarding suffering and the language we use to describe it. Combining objective and subjective perspectives requires new conceptual models that take into account the complex interactions among the body, mind, environment, and spirit.

REFERENCES

1. Woolf SH, Aron L, editors: *Panel on understanding cross-national health differences among high-income countries,* Committee on Population, Division of Behavioral and Social Sciences and Education, National Research Council, Board on Population Health and Public Practice, Institute of Medicine, Bethesda, MD, 2013, Author.
2. Magid C: Developing tolerance for ambiguity, *JAMA* 285(1):88, 2001.
3. Goldstein J: In the twilight: life in the margins between sick and well, *JAMA* 285(1):92, 2001.

CONTENTS

PART TWO PATHOPHYSIOLOGIC ALTERATIONS: ORGANS AND SYSTEMS

UNIT V The Neurologic System

CHAPTER 1

Cellular Biology

Kathryn L. McCance

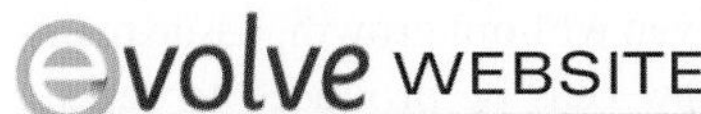

http://evolve.elsevier.com/McCance/
- Review Questions and Answers

CHAPTER OUTLINE

All body functions depend on the integrity of cells. Therefore, an understanding of cellular biology is intrinsically necessary for an understanding of disease. An overwhelming amount of information is revealing how cells behave as a multicellular "social" organism. At the heart of cellular biology is cellular communication ("cellular crosstalk")—how messages originate and are transmitted, received, interpreted, and used by the cell. Fossil records suggest that unicellular organisms resembling bacteria were present on earth 3.5 billion years ago, yet it took another 2.5 billion years for the first multicellular organisms to appear. This delay was seemingly slow because elaborate signaling mechanisms had to evolve that would allow cells to crosstalk. This streamlined conversation between, among, and within cells maintains cellular function and specialization. Intercellular signals allow each cell to determine its position and specialized role. Cells must demonstrate a "chemical fondness" for other cells and their surrounding environment to maintain the integrity of the entire organism. When they no longer tolerate this fondness, the conversation breaks down and cells either adapt (sometimes altering function) or become vulnerable to isolation, injury, or disease.

PROKARYOTES AND EUKARYOTES

Living cells generally are divided into two major classes—eukaryotes and prokaryotes. The cells of higher animals and plants are eukaryotes, as are the single-celled organisms fungi, protozoa, and most algae. Prokaryotes include cyanobacteria (blue-green algae), bacteria, and rickettsiae. Prokaryotes traditionally were studied as core subjects of molecular biology. Current emphasis is on the eukaryotic cell; much of its structure and function has no counterpart in bacterial cells.

Eukaryotes (*eu* = good; *karyon* = nucleus) are larger and have more extensive intracellular anatomy and organization than do prokaryotes. Eukaryotic cells have a characteristic set of membrane-bound intracellular compartments, called *organelles,* that includes a well-defined nucleus. **Prokaryotes** contain no organelles, and their nuclear material is not encased by a nuclear membrane. Prokaryotic cells are characterized by lack of a distinct nucleus.

Besides having structural differences, prokaryotic and eukaryotic cells differ in chemical composition and biochemical activity. The *nuclei* of prokaryotic cells carry genetic information in a single circular chromosome, and they lack a class of proteins called *histones,* which in eukaryotic cells bind with deoxyribonucleic acid (DNA) and are involved in the supercoiling of DNA (see Figure 1-2, p. 4). We now understand that the loops and coiling of DNA are important for many diseases (see Chapter 6). Eukaryotic cells have several chromosomes. Protein production, or synthesis, in the two classes of cells also differs because of major structural differences in ribonucleic acid (RNA)–protein complexes. Other distinctions include differences in mechanisms of transport across the outer cellular membrane and differences in enzyme content.

CELLULAR FUNCTIONS

Cells become specialized through the process of **differentiation,** or maturation, so that some cells eventually perform one kind of function and other cells perform other functions. Cells with a highly developed function, such as movement, often lack some other property, such as hormone production, which is more highly developed in some other type of specialized cell.

The eight chief cellular functions follow:

1. *Movement.* Muscle cells can generate forces that produce motion. Muscles that are attached to bones produce limb movements, whereas those that enclose hollow tubes or cavities move or empty contents when they contract. For example, the contraction of smooth muscle cells surrounding blood vessels changes the diameter of the vessels; the contraction of muscles in walls of the urinary bladder expels urine.
2. *Conductivity.* Conduction as a response to a stimulus is manifested by a wave of excitation, an electrical potential that passes along the surface of the cell to reach its other parts. Conductivity is the chief function of nerve cells.
3. *Metabolic absorption.* All cells take in and use nutrients and other substances from their surroundings. Cells of the intestine and the kidney are specialized to carry out absorption. Cells of the kidney tubules reabsorb fluids and synthesize proteins. Intestinal epithelial cells reabsorb fluids and synthesize protein enzymes.
4. *Secretion.* Certain cells, such as mucous gland cells, can synthesize new substances from substances they absorb and then secrete the new substances to serve as needed elsewhere. Cells of the adrenal gland, testis, and ovary can secrete hormonal steroids.
5. *Excretion.* All cells can rid themselves of waste products resulting from the metabolic breakdown of nutrients. Membrane-bound sacs (lysosomes) within cells contain enzymes that break down, or digest, large molecules, turning them into waste products that are released from the cell.
6. *Respiration.* Cells absorb oxygen, which is used to transform nutrients into energy in the form of adenosine triphosphate (ATP). Cellular respiration, or oxidation, occurs in organelles called *mitochondria.*
7. *Reproduction.* Tissue growth occurs as cells enlarge and reproduce themselves. Even without growth, tissue maintenance requires that new cells be produced to replace cells that are lost normally through cellular death. Not all cells are capable of continuous division (see Chapter 2).
8. *Communication.* Communication is vital for cells to survive as a society of cells. Pancreatic cells, for instance, secrete and release insulin necessary to signal muscle cells to absorb sugar from the blood for energy. Constant communication allows the maintenance of a dynamic steady state.

STRUCTURE AND FUNCTION OF CELLULAR COMPONENTS

Figure 1-1 shows a "typical" eukaryotic cell. It consists of three components: an outer membrane called the *plasma membrane,* or *plasmalemma;* a fluid filling called **cytoplasm;** and the intracellular "organs," or *organelles,* which are membrane bound and include the nucleus.

Nucleus

The **nucleus,** which is surrounded by the cytoplasm and generally is located in the center of the cell, is the largest membrane-bound organelle. Two membranes comprise the **nuclear envelope** (Figure 1-2, *A*). The outer membrane is continuous with membranes of the endoplasmic reticulum. The inner membrane encloses the neoplasm. The nucleus contains the **nucleolus,** a small dense structure composed largely of RNA; most of the cellular DNA; and the DNA-binding proteins, the histones, that regulate its activity. The DNA chain in eukaryotic cells is so extensive that the risk of breakage is high. Therefore, the histones that bind to DNA cause DNA to fold into chromosomes (Figure 1-2, *C*). The wrapping of DNA into tight packages of chromosomes is essential for cell division in eukaryotes.

The primary functions of the nucleus are cell division and control of genetic information. Other functions include the replication and repair of DNA and the transcription of the information stored in DNA. Genetic information is transcribed into RNA, which can be processed into messenger, transport,

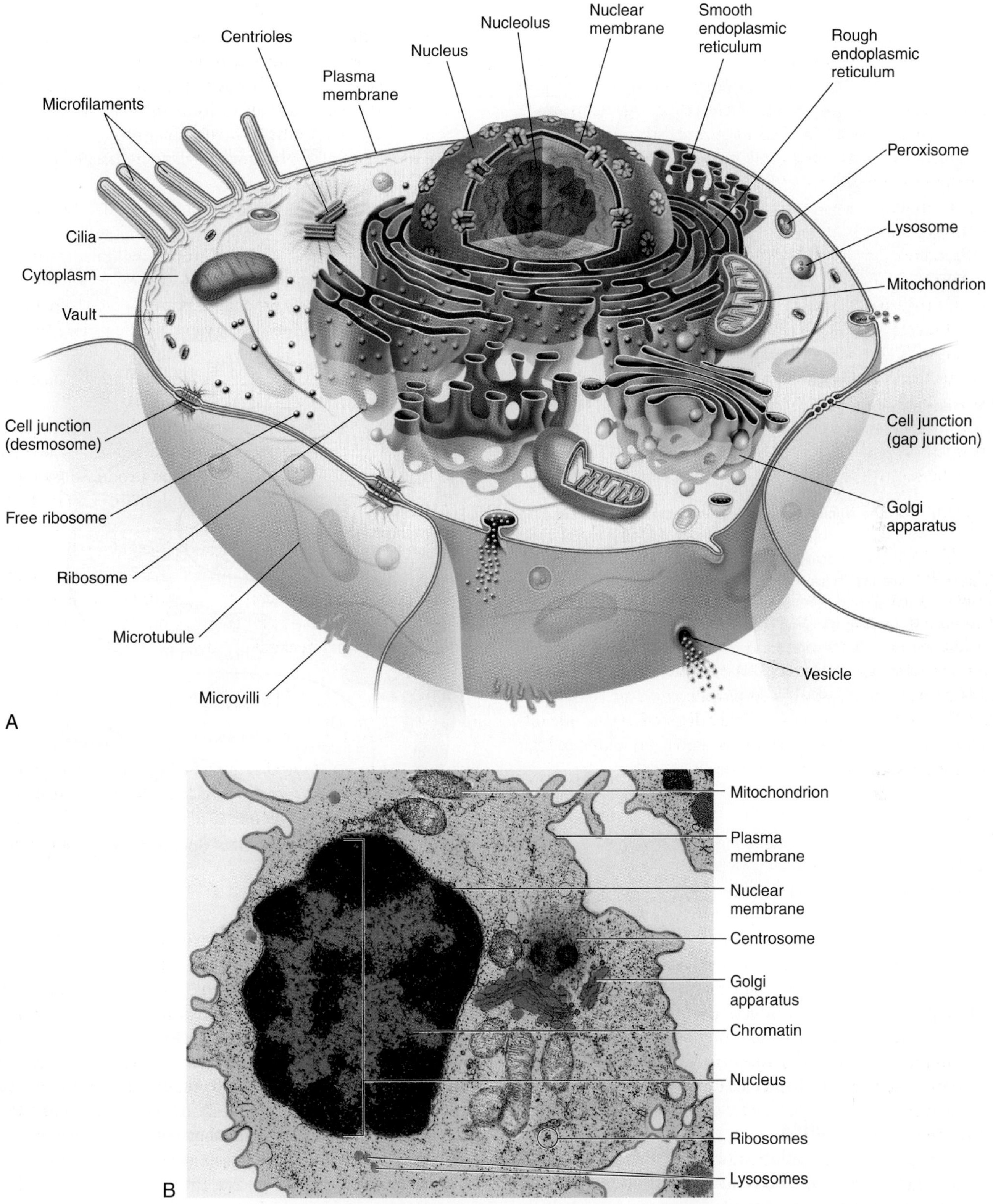

FIGURE 1-1 Typical or Composite Cell. **A,** Artist's interpretation of cell structure. **B,** Color-enhanced electron micrograph of a cell. Both show the many mitochondria known as the "power plants of the cell." Note, too, the innumerable dots bordering the endoplasmic reticulum. These are ribosomes, the cell's "protein factories." (**B** courtesy of A. Arlan Hinchee. From Patton KT, Thibodeau GA: *Anatomy & physiology,* ed 8, St Louis, 2013, Mosby.)

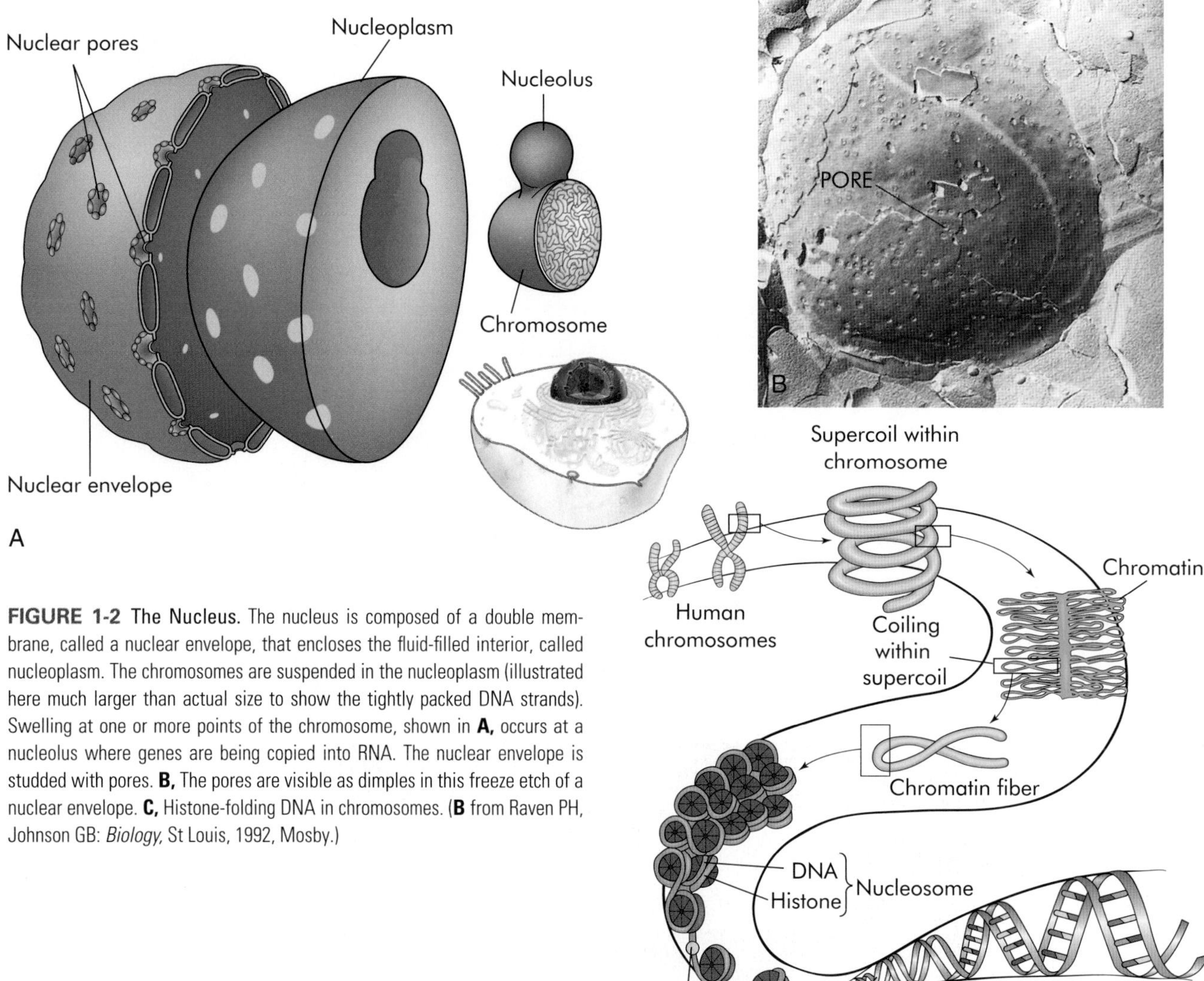

FIGURE 1-2 The Nucleus. The nucleus is composed of a double membrane, called a nuclear envelope, that encloses the fluid-filled interior, called nucleoplasm. The chromosomes are suspended in the nucleoplasm (illustrated here much larger than actual size to show the tightly packed DNA strands). Swelling at one or more points of the chromosome, shown in **A,** occurs at a nucleolus where genes are being copied into RNA. The nuclear envelope is studded with pores. **B,** The pores are visible as dimples in this freeze etch of a nuclear envelope. **C,** Histone-folding DNA in chromosomes. (**B** from Raven PH, Johnson GB: *Biology,* St Louis, 1992, Mosby.)

and ribosomal RNA and introduced into the cytoplasm, where it directs cellular activities. Most of the processing of RNA occurs in the nucleolus. (The role of DNA and RNA in protein synthesis is discussed in Chapter 4.)

Cytoplasmic Organelles

Cytoplasm is an aqueous solution (**cytosol**) that fills the **cytoplasmic matrix**—the space between the nuclear envelope and the plasma membrane. The cytosol represents about half the volume of a eukaryotic cell. It contains thousands of enzymes involved in intermediate metabolism and is crowded with ribosomes making proteins. Newly synthesized proteins remain in the cytosol if they lack a signal for transport to a cell organelle.[1] The organelles suspended in the cytoplasm are enclosed in biologic membranes, which enables them to simultaneously carry out functions that require different biochemical environments. These functions, many of which are directed by coded messages carried from the nucleus by RNA, include synthesis of proteins and hormones and their transport out of the cell, isolation and elimination of waste products from the cell, metabolic processes, breakdown and disposal of cellular debris and foreign proteins (antigens), and maintenance of cellular structure and motility. Also the cytosol functions as a storage unit for fat, carbohydrate, and secretory vesicles.

Ribosomes

Ribosomes are RNA-protein complexes (nucleoproteins) that are synthesized in the nucleolus and secreted into the cytoplasm through pores in the nuclear envelope called nuclear pore complexes (NPCs).[2] These tiny ribosomes may float free in the cytoplasm or attach themselves to the outer membranes of the endoplasmic reticulum (see Figure 1-1, *A*).

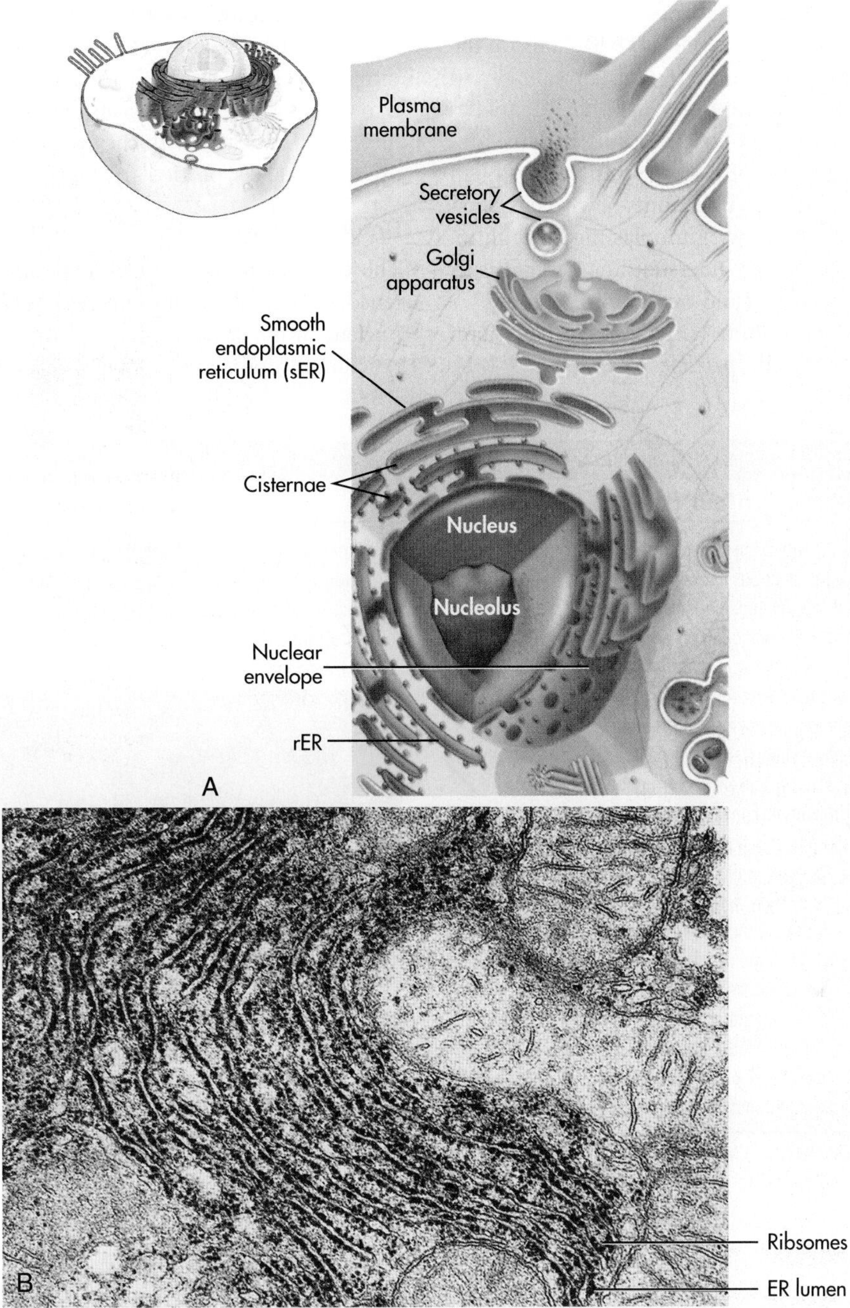

FIGURE 1-3 Endoplasmic Reticulum (ER). A, The ER consists of rough endoplasmic reticulum (rER) arranged into ribosome-coated cisternae and vesicles of smooth endoplasmic reticulum (sER). **B,** Electron micrograph of rough and smooth ER. (**B** courtesy Kelloes C, Farmer M, Center for Advanced Ultrastructural Research, University of Georgia. From Lindsay DT: *Functional human anatomy,* St Louis, 1996, Mosby.)

Their chief function is to provide sites for cellular protein synthesis. Newly formed ribosomes synthesize a "recognition sequence," or signal, like an address on a letter. Signal recognition particles (SRPs) in the cytosol bind to the ribosome after recognizing the SRP. Ribophorins, receiver proteins found on the rough sections of the endoplasmic reticulum (ER), act as the "address" site or binding site. The developing protein threads its way through the ER membrane into the lumen. The SRP is removed and the new protein chain is folded into its final conformation.

Endoplasmic Reticulum

The **endoplasmic reticulum (ER)** (*endo* = within; *plasma* = cytoplasm; *reticulum* = network) is a membrane factory that specializes in the synthesis and transport of the protein and lipid components of most of the cell's organelles. It consists of a network of tubular or saclike channels (cisternae) that extend throughout the cytoplasm and are continuous with the outer nuclear membrane (Figure 1-3). The folded membranes that form the cisternae of the endoplasmic reticulum may be *rough* (granular) or *smooth* (agranular). The **rough endoplasmic**

reticulum (rER) is rough because ribosomes and ribonucleoprotein particles are attached to it (see Figure 1-3). Some of the proteins synthesized by these ribosomes remain in the ER, and others are used to construct membranes of other organelles (the Golgi complex, lysosomes, peroxisomes, and nucleus) and of the cell itself. Importantly, the ER is responsible for much of a cell's protein synthesis and folding, and a new role is sensing cellular stress (see What's New? Endoplasmic Reticulum, Protein Folding, and ER Stress). Understanding mechanisms of cellular stress will aid diagnosis and treatment of disease.

Smooth endoplasmic reticulum (sER) does not contain ribosomes or ribonucleoprotein particles (see Figure 1-1). Rather, membranous surfaces of the smooth endoplasmic reticulum contain enzymes involved in the synthesis of steroid hormones and are responsible for a variety of reactions required to remove toxic substances from the cell. The endoplasmic reticulum communicates with the Golgi complex and interacts with other organelles, particularly lysosomes and peroxisomes.

Golgi Complex

The **Golgi complex** (or **Golgi apparatus**) is a network of flattened, smooth membranes and vesicles frequently located near the nucleus of the cell (Figure 1-4). Proteins from the endoplasmic reticulum are processed and packaged into small membrane-bound

WHAT'S NEW?

Endoplasmic Reticulum, Protein Folding, and ER Stress

Protein folding in the endoplasmic reticulum (ER) is critical for us. As the biologic workhorses, proteins perform vital functions in every cell. To do these tasks proteins must fold into complex three-dimensional structures (see figure at right). Most secreted proteins *fold* and are modified in an error-free manner, but ER or cell stress, mutations, or random (stochastic) errors during protein synthesis can decrease the folding amount or the rate of folding. Pathophysiologic processes, such as viral infections, environmental toxins, and mutant protein expression, can perturb the sensitive ER environment. Natural processes also can perturb the environment, such as the large protein-synthesizing load placed on the ER. These perturbations cause the accumulation of immature and abnormal proteins in cells, leading to **ER stress.** Fortunately, the ER is loaded with protective ways to help folding, for example, protein so-called *chaperones* that facilitate folding and prevent the formation of off-pathway types. Because specialized cells produce large amounts of secreted proteins, the movement or flux through the ER is tremendous. Therefore, misfolded proteins not repaired in the ER are observed in some diseases and can initiate apoptosis or cell death. It has recently been shown that the endoplasmic reticulum mediates intracellular signaling pathways in response to the accumulation of unfolded or misfolded proteins; collectively, the pathways are known as the **unfolded-protein response (UPR).** Investigators are studying UPR-associated inflammation and how the UPR is coupled to inflammation in health and disease. Specific diseases include Alzheimer disease, Parkinson disease, prion disease, amyotrophic lateral sclerosis, and diabetes mellitus. Additionally being studied is ER stress and how it may accelerate age-related dysfunction.

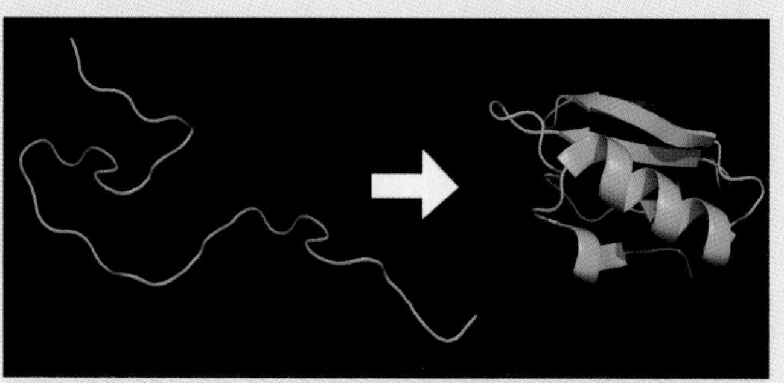

Protein Folding. Each protein exists as an unfolded polypeptide *(left)* or random coil after the process of translation from a sequence of mRNA to a linear string of amino acids. From amino acids interacting with each other they produce a three-dimensional structure called the folded protein *(right)* that is its native state.

Data from Brodsky J, Skach WR: *Curr Opin Cell Biol* 23:464-475, 2011; Jäger R et al: *Biol Cell,* Jan 23, 2012, [Epub ahead of print]; Ron D, Walter P: *Nat Rev Mol Cell Biol* 8:519–529, 2007.

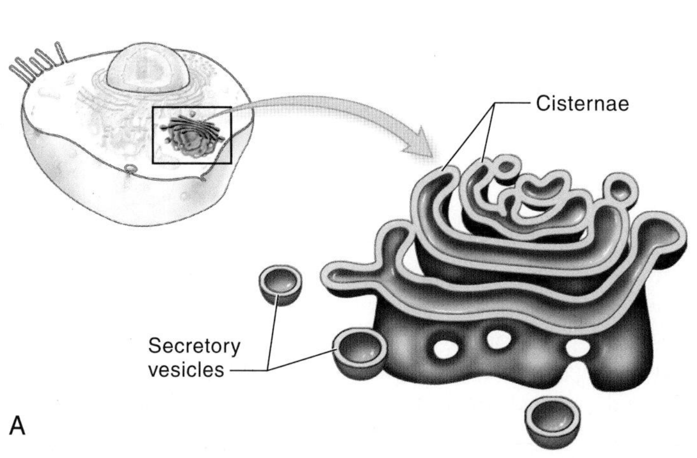

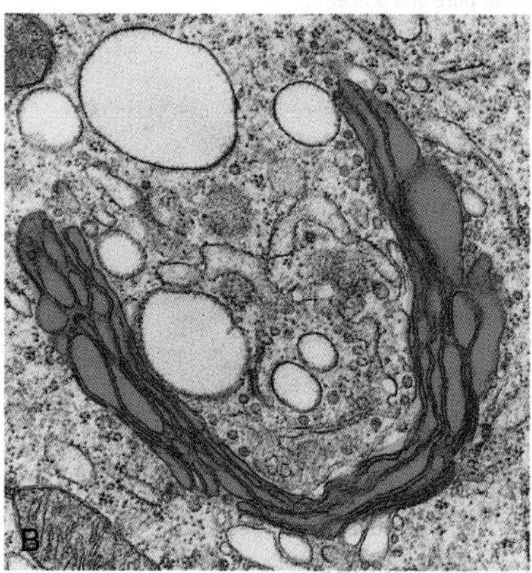

FIGURE 1-4 Golgi Complex. A, Schematic representation of the Golgi complex showing a stack of flattened sacs, or cisternae, and numerous small membranous bubbles, or secretory vesicles. **B,** Transmission electron micrograph showing the Golgi complex highlighted with color. (From Patton KT, Thibodeau GA: *Anatomy & physiology,* ed 8, St Louis, 2013, Mosby.)

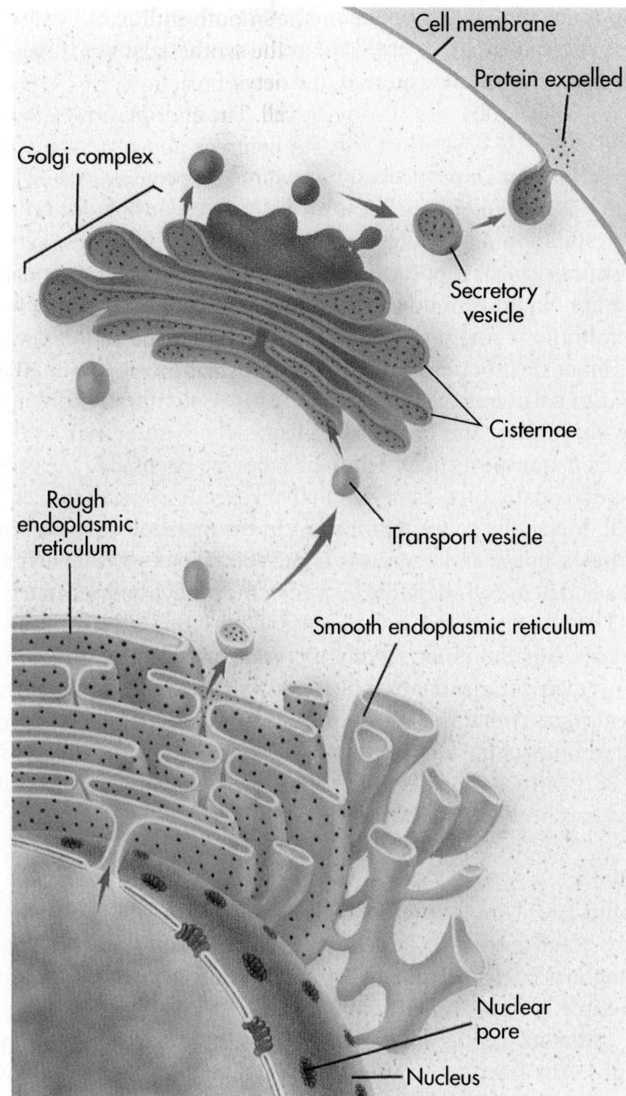

FIGURE 1-5 How the Internal Membrane System of a Cell Packages a Protein for Export. The instructions for making a protein that is destined for export from a cell, such as a digestive enzyme made by a pancreas cell, are first transcribed from DNA by RNA in the nucleus. The RNA then leaves the nucleus through a nuclear pore and proceeds to a ribosome located on the rough endoplasmic reticulum (rER). There it provides instructions for the correct sequence of amino acids for synthesizing that particular digestive enzyme. When enzyme synthesis is complete, the enzyme travels through the ER and is then encapsulated in a transport vesicle. The transport vesicle fuses with a Golgi body, releasing the enzyme. In the Golgi complex the enzyme is further modified and is then shunted to the flattened stacks, or cisternae. There the enzyme waits for a secretory vesicle, which will carry it to the perimeter of the cell, the cell membrane. The secretory vesicle membrane then fuses with the cell membrane, and the enzyme is released outside the cell. (From Raven PH, Johnson GB: *Understanding biology,* ed 3, Dubuque, IA, 1995, Brown.)

sacs or vesicles called **secretory vesicles,** which collect at the end of the membranous folds of the Golgi bodies—called **cisternae.** The secretory vesicles then break off from the Golgi complex and migrate to a variety of intracellular and extracellular destinations, including the plasma membrane. The vesicles fuse with the plasma membrane, and their contents are released from the cell. The best known vesicles are those that have coats made largely of the

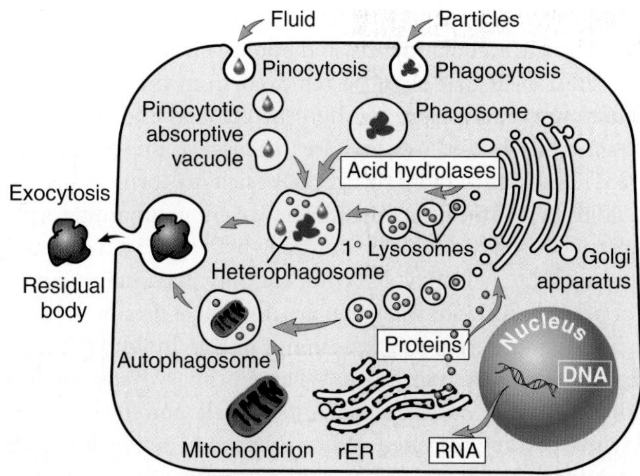

FIGURE 1-6 Lysosomes. Primary (1°) lysosomes, which originate from the Golgi apparatus, give rise to heterophagosomes and autophagosomes. Undigested material in phagosomes is extruded from the cell or remains in the cytoplasm as lipofuscin-rich residual bodies. rER, Rough endoplasmic reticulum. (From Damjanov I: *Pathology for the health professions,* ed 4, Philadelphia, 2012, Saunders.)

protein **clathrin** and are called *clathrin-coated vesicles.* They bud from the Golgi complex on the outward secretory pathway and from the plasma membrane on the inward endocytotic pathway (see p. 33). Many molecules, including lipids, proteins, glycoproteins, and enzymes of lysosomes, pass through the Golgi complex at some stage in their maturation. The Golgi complex is a refining plant and directs traffic (e.g., protein, polynucleotide, polysaccharide molecules) in the cell[1] (Figure 1-5).

Lysosomes

Lysosomes (*lyso* = dissolution; *soma* = body) are saclike structures that originate from the Golgi complex (see Figure 1-1, *A*). They contain more than 40 digestive enzymes called **hydrolases,** which catalyze bonds in proteins, lipids, nucleic acids, and carbohydrates. Lysosomes function as the intracellular digestive system (Figure 1-6). Lysosomal enzymes are capable of digesting most cellular constituents completely to their basic components, such as amino acids, fatty acids, and carbohydrates.

The lysosomal membrane acts as a protective shield between the powerful digestive enzymes within the lysosome and the cytoplasm, preventing their leakage into the cytoplasmic matrix. Disruption of the membrane by various treatments or cellular injury leads to a release of the lysosomal enzymes, which can then react with their specific substrates, causing *cellular self-digestion.* Lysosomal abnormalities are involved in a number of conditions that involve cellular injury and death.

Lysosomal storage diseases may be the result of a genetic defect or lack of one or more lysosomal enzymes. For example, the lack of lysosomal α-1,4-glucosidase leads to an accumulation of glycogen in lysosomes known as *Pompe disease.* Tay-Sachs disease is characterized by an accumulation of GM2 ganglioside (a lipid) in lysosomes as a result of the deficiency or absence of lysosomal hexosaminidase A. In gout, undigested uric acid accumulates within lysosomes, damaging the lysosomal membrane. Subsequent enzyme leakage results in cell death and tissue injury.

Lysosomes are necessary for normal digestion of cellular nutrients, intracellular debris, and potentially harmful extracellular substances that must be removed from the body. Extracellular substances are taken into the cell and encapsulated in a membrane-bound vesicle (see discussion on endocytosis, p. 33). Lysosomes merge with the vesicle to form a digestive vacuole. Lysosomes remain fully active by maintaining a low internal pH. They do this by pumping hydrogen ions into their interiors. The hydrolytic enzymes are only maximally active at acid pH values. Lysosomes that are not active do not maintain such an acid internal pH. Lysosomes in this "holding pattern" are called **primary lysosomes.** When a primary lysosome fuses with a vacuole or other organelle, its pH falls and the hydrolytic enzymes become activated. When it becomes active, it is called a **secondary lysosome,** or **heterophagosome.**

As cells complete their life span and die, lysosomes digest the resultant cellular debris. Lysosomes involved in this process, which is called **autodigestion,** are called **autolysosomes,** or **autophagosomes.** In living cells, cellular debris is encapsulated within a vesicle that reacts with a lysosome to complete its degradation. The degradation process, called **autophagy,** promotes homeostasis because it involves continuous biosynthesis and cell turnover. Recent data indicate that autophagy plays a crucial role in health and disease[3,4] (see Chapter 2).

Products of autophagy (and of phagocytosis, the ingestion of harmful foreign substances; see Chapter 7) pass out of the lysosome and are reused by the cell. Indigestible material is stored in vesicles called **residual bodies,** whose contents are actively expelled from the cell (see Figure 1-6). High concentrations of lipids may accumulate within the residual bodies and remain there for a long time. The lipids are eventually oxidized, and a pigmented substance containing polyunsaturated fatty acids and proteins accumulates in the cell. This pigmented substance, termed *lipofuscin,* is often called "age pigment" or "age spots," and is noted in older individuals (see Chapter 2).

Peroxisomes

Peroxisomes (microbodies) are membrane-bound organelles that contain several oxidative enzymes such as *catalase* and *urate oxidase.* These oxidative enzymes can detoxify compounds and fatty acids. Similar to lysosomes in microscopic appearance, peroxisomes are larger and oval or irregular in shape. Like mitochondria, peroxisomes are major sites of oxygen utilization. Peroxisomes are so named because they usually contain enzymes that use oxygen to remove hydrogen atoms from specific substrates in an oxidative reaction that produces hydrogen peroxide (H_2O_2). Hydrogen peroxide is a powerful oxidant, potentially destructive if it accumulates or escapes from peroxisomes. Catalase, an antioxidant enzyme, uses the H_2O_2 to oxidize a variety of other substrates—phenols, formic acid, formaldehyde, and alcohol—by the peroxidative reaction:

$$H_2O_2 + R^1H_2 \rightarrow R^1 + 2H_2O$$

Thus the breakdown of H_2O_2 yields H_2O and O_2 (see discussion of free radicals in Chapter 2). Peroxisomes also have an important role in the synthesis of specialized phospholipids necessary for nerve cell myelination. Such reactions are important in detoxifying various wastes within the cell or foreign components that enter the cell, such as ethanol. Impairment of peroxisomes can lead to disease.

Mitochondria

Mitochondria (*mito* = thread; *chondros* = granule), organelles found in large numbers in most cells, are responsible for cellular respiration and energy production (see p. 26). These cytoplasmic organelles appear as spheres, rods, or filamentous bodies that are bound by a double membrane (Figure 1-7). The **outer membrane** is smooth and surrounds the mitochondrion itself; the inner membrane is convoluted in the mitochondrial matrix to form partitions called **cristae.** The **inner membrane** contains the enzymes of the respiratory chain—the name given to the electron-transport chain. These enzymes are essential to the process of oxidative phosphorylation that generates most of the cell's ATP. Metabolic pathways involved in the metabolism of carbohydrates, lipids, and amino acids and special pathways involving urea and heme synthesis are located in the mitochondrial matrix.

The outer membrane is permeable (passable) to many substances, but the inner membrane is highly selective and contains many transmembranous transport systems. The inner membrane contains a transporter to move electrically charged calcium (calcium ions). (Membrane transport is discussed on p. 25.) Mitochondria contain their own DNA that codes for enzymes needed for oxidative phosphorylation.

Vaults

Vaults are cytoplasmic organelles, also called ribonucleoproteins, that are much larger than ribosomes and shaped like octagonal barrels (Figure 1-8). Their name comes from their multiple arches, which reminded their discoverers of vaulted or cathedral ceilings. A single cell can contain thousands of vaults. The function of vaults is not fully understood and may be related to their octagonal shape. Vaults have a large interior volume and can encapsulate proteins.[5] Similarly, the pores in the membrane surrounding the nucleus (see Figure 1-2, *B*) are also octagonally shaped and the same size as vaults, leading to speculation that vaults may be cellular "trucks." Further, vaults would dock at nuclear pores, pick up molecules synthesized in the nucleus, and deliver their load elsewhere in the cell. Because at any given time about 5% of the vaults are localized near the nuclear pores, it is thought that vaults may be carrying messenger RNA (mRNA) from the nucleus to the ribosomal sites of protein synthesis within the cytoplasm. Investigators suggest that vaults transport several copies of untranslated RNA and that they are transported along cytoskeletal-based cellular tracks—much like an assembly line.[6] Vault complexes are being exploited for the delivery of drugs to the inside of the cell, for example, in kidney diseases.

Cytosol

Cytosol is the gelatinous, semiliquid portion of the cytoplasm accounting for about 55% of the total cell volume. Functions of the cytosol include intermediary metabolism involving enzymatic biochemical reactions; ribosomal protein synthesis; and storage of carbohydrates, fat, and secretory vesicles.

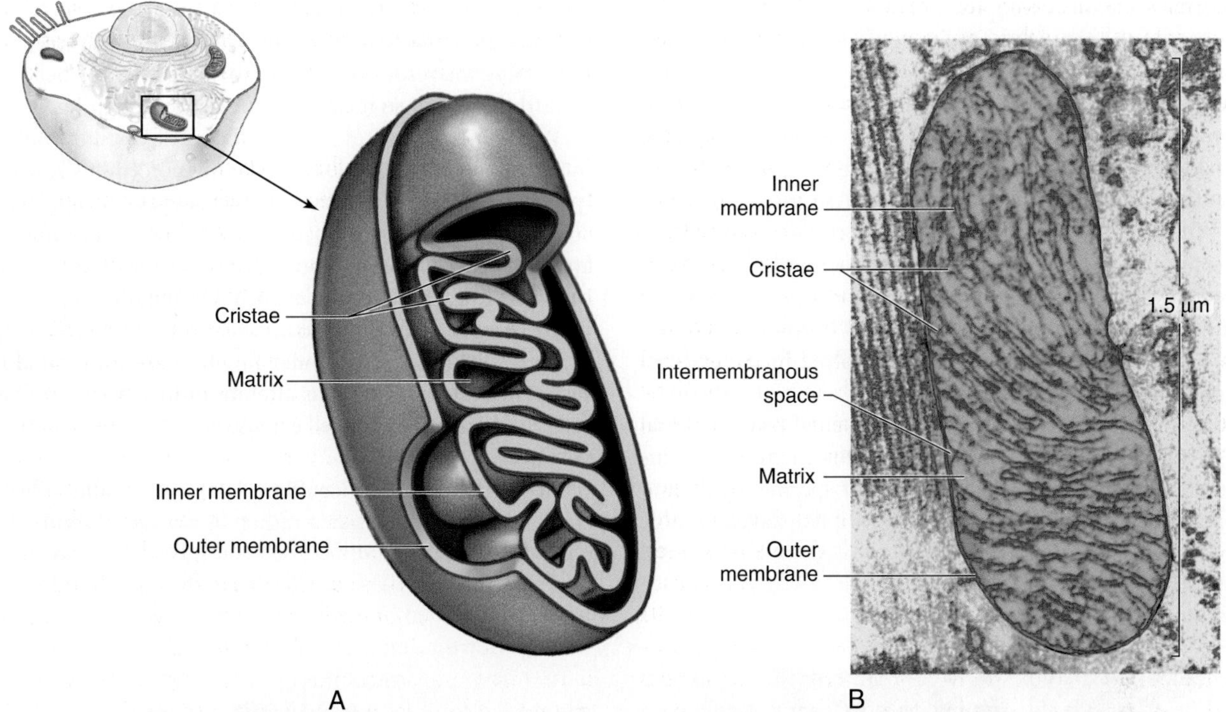

FIGURE 1-7 Mitochondrion. **A,** Cutaway sketch showing outer and inner membranes. Note the many folds (cristae) of the inner membrane. **B,** Transmission electron micrograph of a mitochondrion. Although some mitochondria have the capsule shape shown here, many are round or oval. (From Patton KT, Thibodeau GA: *Anatomy & physiology,* ed 8, St Louis, 2013, Mosby.)

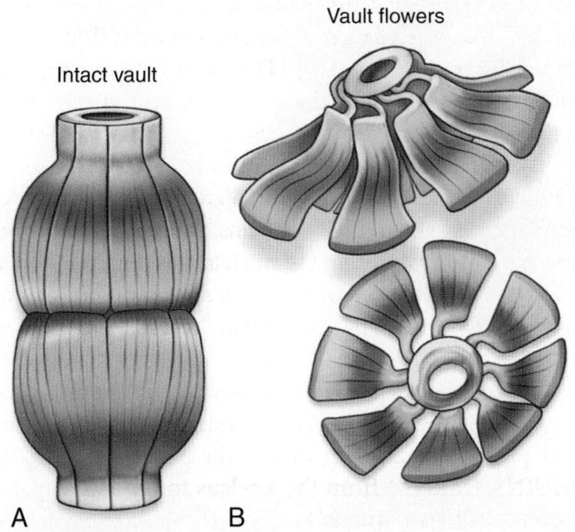

FIGURE 1-8 Vaults. **A,** Schematic three-dimensional representation of a vault, an octagonal barrel-shaped organelle believed to transport messenger RNA from the nucleus to the cytoplasmic ribosomes. **B,** Schematic representation of an opened vault, showing its octagonal structure.

Intermediary metabolism refers to the intracellular chemical reactions that include synthesis, degradation, and transformation of small organic molecules (e.g., simple sugars, fatty acids, and amino acids). All intermediary metabolism occurs in the cytoplasm or that portion of the cell interior not occupied by the nucleus—with most of the metabolism being accomplished in the cytosol. These reactions enable energy to be used for managing cellular activities and for providing substrates to maintain cell integrity.

Ribosomal protein synthesis takes place in free ribosomes in the cytosol. Cytosolic ribosomes that synthesize identical proteins are collected together in "factories" known as **polyribosomes.**

Excess stored nutrients not immediately used for ATP production are converted in the cytosol into storage forms; for example, excess glucose is stored as glycogen. These temporary masses are known as *inclusions* (see Chapter 2). Secretory vesicles that have been processed and packaged by the endoplasmic reticulum and Golgi complex also remain in the cytosol. By means of signaling, the vesicles transport and empty their contents outside the cell.

Cytoskeleton

All eukaryotic cells contain elaborate and specialized internal structures in the cytosol that provide the "bones and muscles" of the cell—the **cytoskeleton.** The cytoskeleton maintains the cell's shape and internal organization, and it permits movement of substances within the cell and movement of external projections (cilia or microvilli; flagella in sperm) outside the plasma membrane. The cytoskeleton is involved with the extracellular matrix and nuclear interior in force transmission (mechanical forces) called mechanotransduction. **Mechanotransduction** describes the cellular processes that translate mechanical stimuli into biochemical signals, allowing cells to adapt to their surroundings. Cell stresses, however, that involve alterations of mechanotransduction are associated with several diseases (see Chapter 2).[7,8]

The internal skeleton is composed of a network of protein filaments; two of the most important are microtubules and actin filaments, or microfilaments.

Microtubules are small, hollow, cylindrical, unbranched tubules made of protein. When found together, microtubules exhibit rigidity, unlike the rest of the cytoplasm. Microtubules thus add strength to the cell's structure (Figure 1-9, *A, B*). Within the cell, microtubules support and move organelles from one part of the cytoplasm to another, facilitate transport of impulses along nerve cells, and have roles in the inflammatory and immune responses and hormone secretion (Figure 1-9, *C*). Microtubules are also involved in the external movement, or motility, of some cells.

Microtubules are arranged in the thickened base, or basal body, of a protrusion from the cell's plasma membrane. This arrangement occurs in the basal bodies of sperm flagella and the cilia of certain other cells. The long, whiplike flagella enable the movement of sperm cells. Cilia usually move substances past the cell, which remains stationary. For example, cilia on cells lining the respiratory tract move together to "beat" mucus toward the throat so it can be removed by coughing.

While the cell is not in the process of division, only a few microtubules are assembled; cellular division (mitosis) or defense (phagocytosis) does, however, induce a cycle of rapid assembly and disassembly. Microtubules involved in cellular division are arranged in a **centriole.** Centrioles always consist of nine bundles containing three microtubules each. During division the pairs of centrioles split and migrate to opposite poles of the cell (see p. 37).

Alterations of microtubular function are implicated in disease processes. For example, alterations in actin microfilaments act as a driving force for cell extension during the dissemination of cancer.[9]

Actin filaments (microfilaments) are smaller fibrils that generally occur in bundles rather than singly (Figure 1-9, *B*).

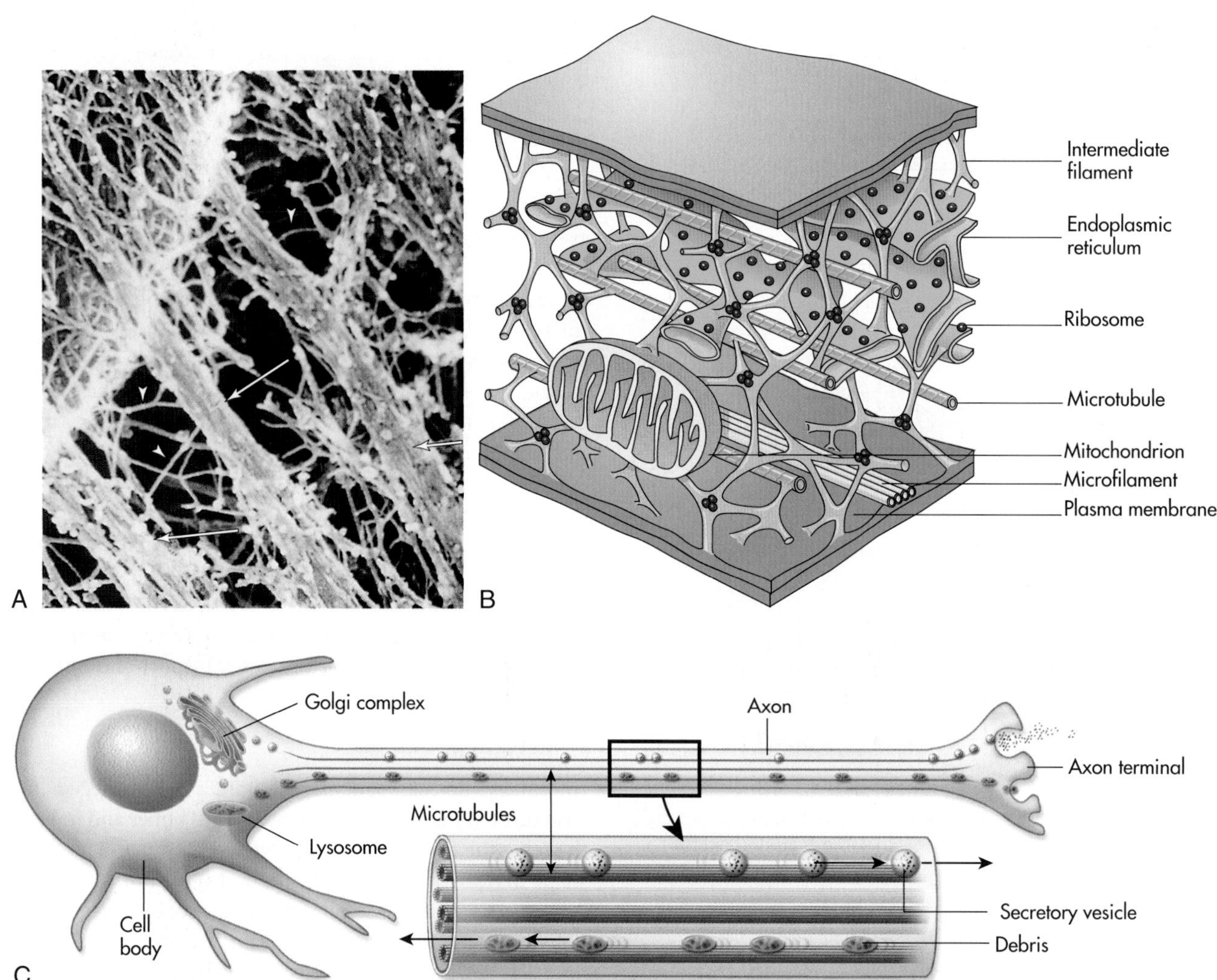

FIGURE 1-9 Cytoskeleton. **A,** Electron micrograph of a portion of the cell's internal framework. Arrowheads mark the intermediate filaments, and the complete arrows mark the microtubules. **B,** Artist's interpretation of the cell's internal framework. Note that the "free" ribosomes and other organelles are not really free at all. **C,** Microtubules are necessary for maintaining an asymmetric cell shape, such as that of a nerve cell. In addition, specific chemicals are released from the terminal end of the axon to influence neural transmission. (**A** and **B** from Patton KT, Thibodeau GA: *Anatomy & physiology,* ed 6, St Louis, 2007, Mosby.)

Like microtubules, actin filaments are associated with cellular locomotion and maintenance of cell and tissue shape.[9] Actin filaments link the interior of the cell to adjacent cells through cell junctions, for example, zonula adherens and zonula occludens (see p. 19).

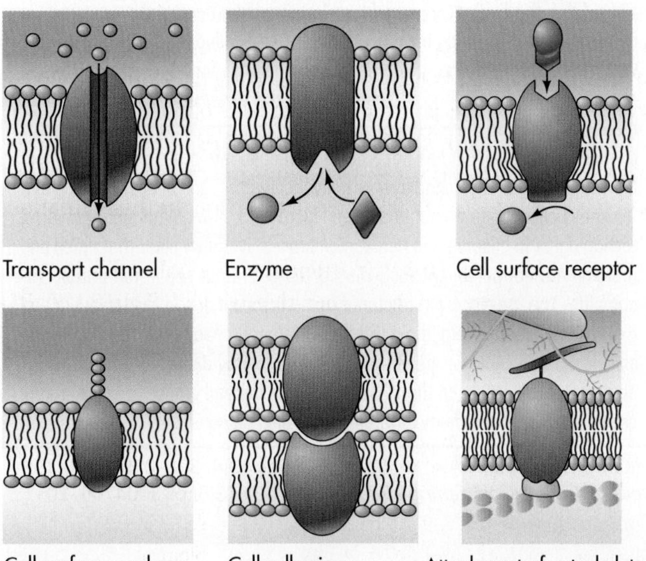

FIGURE 1-10 **Functions of Plasma Membrane Proteins.** The plasma membrane proteins illustrated here show a variety of functions performed by the different types of plasma membranes. (From Raven PH, Johnson GB: *Understanding biology*, ed 3, Dubuque, IA, 1995, Brown.)

In addition, microfilaments are necessary for regulating cell growth.[10] Cellular locomotion depends on contractile properties that involve both microtubules and actin filaments. The actin cytoskeleton in motile cells has recently been described as a "wave of excitation" that may account for the spontaneous migration of cells.[11] Anesthetic drugs can affect both microtubules and actin filaments, disrupting intracellular movement and cellular motility.

Plasma Membranes

Whether they surround the cell or enclose an intracellular organelle, membranes are exceedingly important to normal physiologic function because they control the composition of the space, or compartment, they enclose. Membranes can allow or exclude various molecules, and because of selective transport systems, they can move molecules into or out of the space (Figure 1-10). By controlling the movement of substances from one compartment to another, membranes exert a powerful influence on metabolic pathways. Directional transport is facilitated by polarized domains, distinct apical and basolateral domains. The direction of cells—**cell polarity**—maintains normal cell and tissue structure for numerous functions, most importantly transport of nutrients in and out of the cell, and becomes altered with diseases, for example, cancer (Figure 1-11). In addition to these functions, the plasma membrane has an important role in cell-to-cell recognition. For example, protein receptors for hormones and for other chemical signals are associated with the membrane and act as markers that identify a cell to its neighbors. Other functions of the

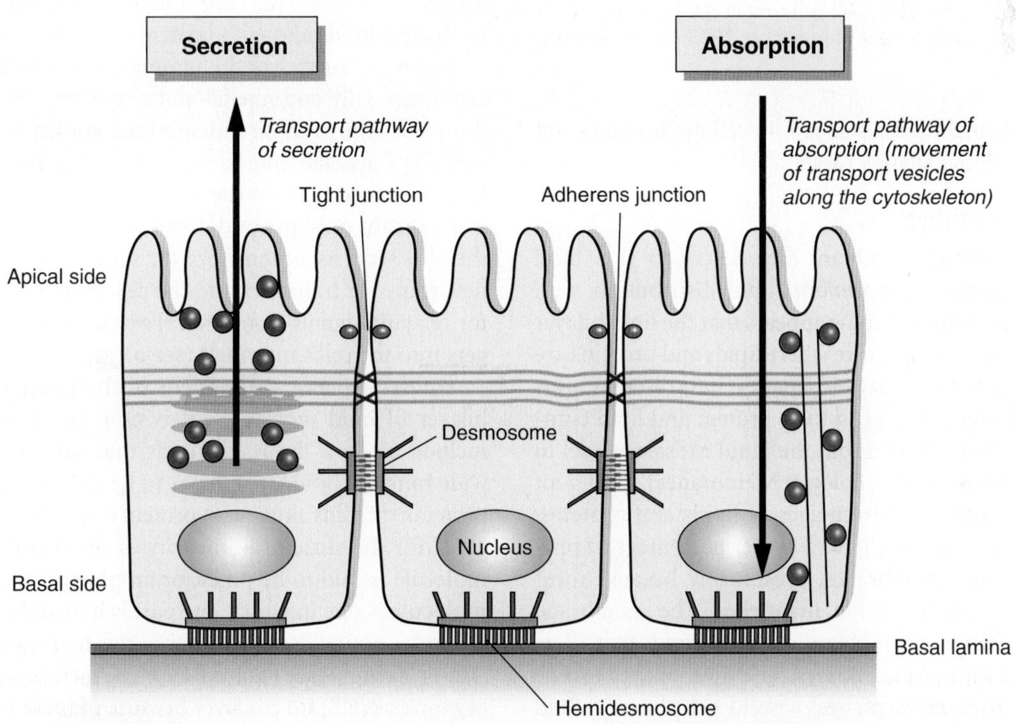

FIGURE 1-11 **Cell Polarity of Epithelial Cells.** A schematic of cell polarity (cell direction) of epithelial cells. Shown are the direction of the basal side and the apical side. Organelles and cytoskeleton are also arranged directionally to enable, for example, in an intestinal cell secretion and absorption. (Adapted from Life Science web textbook, The University of Tokyo.)

TABLE 1-1 PLASMA MEMBRANE FUNCTIONS

CELLULAR MECHANISM	MEMBRANE FUNCTIONS
Structure	Usually thicker than the membranes of intracellular organelles Containment of cellular organelles Maintenance of relationship with cytoskeleton, endoplasmic reticulum, and other organelles Outer surfaces in many cells are not smooth but are studded with cilia or even smaller cylindrical projections called microvilli; both are capable of movement; caveolae are also outer indentations Maintenance of fluid and electrolyte balance
Protection	Barrier to toxic molecules and macromolecules (proteins, nucleic acid, polysaccharides) Barrier to foreign organisms and cells
Activation of cell	Hormones (regulation of cellular activity) Mitogens (cellular division, see Chapter 4) Antigens (antibody synthesis, see Chapter 8) Growth factors (proliferation and differentiation)
Transport	Diffusion and exchange diffusion Endocytosis (pinocytosis and phagocytosis); receptor-mediated endocytosis Exocytosis (secretion) Active transport
Cell-to-cell interaction	Communication and attachment at junctional complexes Symbiotic nutritive relationships Release of enzymes and antibodies to extracellular environment Relationships with extracellular matrix

Modified from King DW, Fenoglio CM, Lefkowitch JH: *General pathology: principles and dynamics,* Philadelphia, 1983, Lea & Febiger.

plasma membrane include assistance with cellular mobility and maintenance of cellular shape (Table 1-1).

Membrane Composition

Historically, the plasma membrane was described as a fluid lipid bilayer composed of a *uniform* lipid distribution with inserted moving proteins.[12] It now appears that the lipid bilayer is a much more complex structure where lipids and proteins are not uniformly distributed but can separate into discrete units called microdomains, differing in their protein and lipid compositions[13] (see What's New? From the Fluid Mosaic Model to New Understandings about Biologic Membranes). Different membranes have different percentages of lipids and proteins. Intracellular membranes may have a higher percentage of proteins than do plasma membranes, presumably because most enzymatic activity occurs within organelles. The membrane organization is achieved through noncovalent bonds that allow different physical states called phases. The lipid bilayer can be structured into three main phases: a solid gel phase, a fluid liquid-crystalline (or liquid-disordered) phase, and a liquid-ordered phase (see Figure 1-13, p. 14). These phases can change under physiologic factors such as temperature and pressure alterations. The structure of a plasma membrane is shown in Figure 1-12 and Figure 1-13. Intracellular membranes have a higher percentage of proteins than do plasma membranes, presumably because most enzymatic activity occurs within organelles. Carbohydrates are mainly associated with plasma membranes, where they are chemically combined with lipids to form glycolipids and with proteins to form glycoproteins.

The outer surface of the plasma membrane in many types of cells, especially endothelial and adipocytes, is not smooth but dimpled with cavelike indentations known as caveolae ("tiny caves"). Caveolae and caveolae-like domains are structurally heterogeneous.[13] Caveolae were considered to be functionally insignificant until the mid-1990s, when evidence suggested that they (1) serve as a repository for some receptors, (2) provide a new route for transport into the cell, and (3) act as the initiator for relaying signals from several extracellular chemical messengers into the cell's interior[14] (see p. 20).

Lipids. A major component of the plasma membrane is a bilayer of lipid molecules. It is now known that membranes include up to a thousand lipids that vary in structure.[15] The wide range of lipids is thought to be the solvent for membrane proteins.[13] Lipids along with protein assemblies act as "molecular glue" for the structural integrity of the membrane. Each lipid molecule is said to be polar, or amphipathic. An **amphipathic molecule** is one in which one part is **hydrophobic** (uncharged, or "water hating") and another part is **hydrophilic** (charged, or "water loving") (see Figure 1-12). The membrane spontaneously organizes itself into a bilayer because of these two incompatible solubilities. The hydrophobic region (hydrophobic tail) of each lipid molecule is protected from water, whereas the hydrophilic region (hydrophilic head) is immersed in it. The

WHAT'S NEW?

From the Fluid Mosaic Model to New Understandings about Biologic Membranes

The understanding of biologic membranes has changed markedly, from the fluid mosaic model to the current model that lipids and proteins have the ability to separate into microdomains, differing in their protein and lipid compositions. From the fluid mosaic model in 1972, membranes were proposed as a homogeneous lipid fluid phase with proteins embedded. This model has been weak because it has not given us more decisive information on membrane structure and function and it deemphasizes the *dynamic* transitions in membrane proteins and the need for the bilayer to adapt to protein conformational changes. Specifically, it has not provided direction into protein assembly, lipid bilayer heterogeneity, monolayer or bilayer curvature, and bilayer bending and thickness changes or fluctuations (see Figure 1-13, *A-D*). With more powerful technologies to observe and define membranes, it is now clear that lipids and proteins are not homogeneously distributed but rather separated into microdomains. The presence of structured lipid microdomains in lipid bilayers and biologic membranes (e.g., lipid rafts) illustrates the need for a revision of the classic view of biologic membranes. This new view dispels the randomness and disordered nature of the classic view and instead emphasizes an orderly organization with the many different molecular components of the membrane.

Data from Bagatolli LA et al: *Prog Lipid Res* 49(4):378–389, 2010; Contreras FX et al: *Cold Spring Harb Perspect Biol* 3(6):pii a004705, 2011.

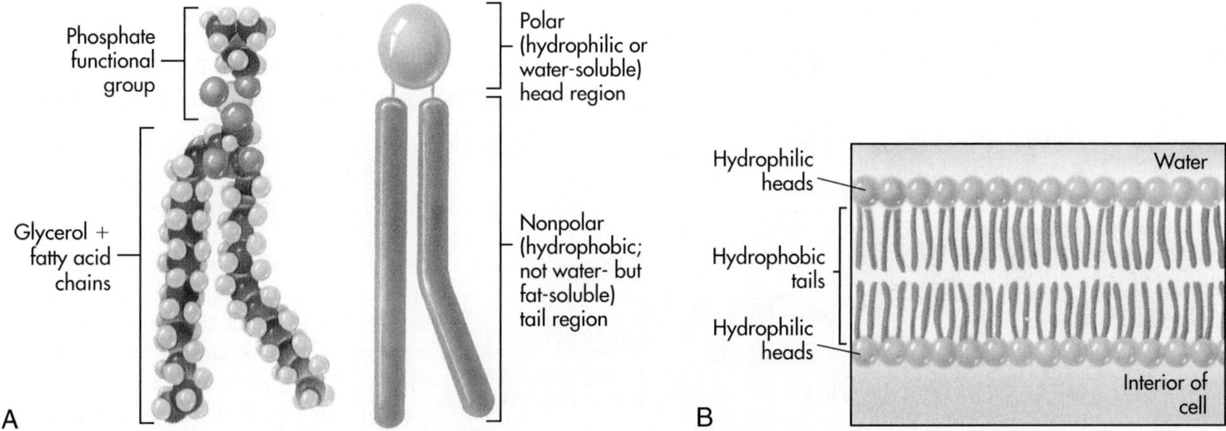

FIGURE 1-12 Structure of a Phospholipid Molecule. **A,** Each phospholipid molecule consists of a phosphate functional group and two fatty acid chains attached to a glycerol molecule. **B,** The fatty acid chains and glycerol form nonpolar, hydrophobic "tails," and the phosphate functional group forms the polar, hydrophilic "head" of the phospholipid molecule. When placed in water, the hydrophobic tails of the molecule face inward, away from the water, and the hydrophilic head faces outward, toward the water. (From Raven PH, Johnson GB: *Understanding biology,* ed 3, Dubuque, IA, 1995, Brown.)

bilayer's structure accounts for one of the essential functions of the plasma membrane: it is impermeable to most water-soluble molecules (molecules that dissolve in water) because they are insoluble in the oily core region. The bilayer serves as a barrier to the diffusion of water and hydrophilic substances while allowing lipid-soluble molecules, such as oxygen (O_2) and carbon dioxide (CO_2), to diffuse through it readily. Because the bilayer is fluid at temperatures above freezing, components of the cellular environment move slowly and selectively across the membrane all the time. (Components of the cellular environment are also discussed in Chapter 3.)

Some membranes contain certain lipids that organize into lipid rafts. **Lipid rafts** consist of cholesterol and sphingolipid-dependent microdomains that form a network of lipid-lipid, protein-protein, and protein-lipid interactions (Figure 1-13). Lipid rafts may have several functions including the segregation of signaling mechanisms and molecules, the control of cytoskeletal remodeling events, and the targeted movement of associated proteins.[16]

Proteins. A **protein** is made from a chain of amino acids, known as **polypeptides.** There are 20 types of amino acids in proteins and each type of protein has a unique sequence of amino acids. Proteins are the major workhorses of the cell. After translation of a protein, **posttranslational modifications (PTMs)** are the methods used to diversify the limited numbers of proteins generated. These modifications alter the activities and functions of proteins and have become very important in understanding diseases. Researchers have known for decades that pathogens interfere with the host's PTMs.[17] New approaches are being used to understand changes in proteins—a field called **proteomics** is the study of the **proteome** or entire set of proteins expressed by a genome from synthesis, translocation, and modification (e.g., folding) and their role in a staggering number of diseases (also see What's New? Endoplasmic Reticulum, Protein Folding, and ER Stress, p. 6).

Research suggests different ways to classify membrane proteins. One way is classification as peripheral or integral proteins. **Integral membrane proteins** are those embedded in the lipid bilayer and linked either to *phosphatidylinositol,* a minor phospholipid, or a fatty acid chain. The integral proteins can be removed from the membrane only by detergents that solubilize (dissolve) the liquid. **Peripheral membrane proteins** are not embedded in the bilayer but reside at one surface or the other, bound to an integral protein.

Although the classification of membrane proteins as peripheral or integral is commonly used, it does not describe how proteins are associated with the bilayer. Another mode of classification does so by taking into account the membrane-spanning, or transmembranous, nature of membrane proteins[1] (see Figure 1-13, *A*). According to this classification, proteins are associated with the lipid bilayer in four ways:

1. Some proteins, called **transmembrane proteins,** extend across the bilayer and are exposed to an aqueous environment on both sides.
2. Some intracellular proteins extend their polypeptide chain partially through the bilayer by means of a fatty acid chain.
3. Some cell surface proteins are attached to the bilayer by a covalent linkage (i.e., a specific oligosaccharide).
4. Some proteins do not extend even partially through the bilayer but are bound to the membrane by noncovalent linkages with other membrane proteins.

Proteins exist in densely folded molecular configurations rather than straight chains; so an excess of hydrophilic units is at the surface of the molecule and an excess of hydrophobic units is inside. Membrane proteins like other proteins are synthesized by the ribosome and then travel, called *trafficking,* to different membrane locations of a cell.[18] Trafficking places unique demands on membrane proteins for folding, translocation, and stability.[18] Thus, much research is now being done to understand misfolded proteins, for example, as a cause of disease (see What's New? Endoplasmic Reticulum, Protein Folding, and ER Stress, p. 6).

Proteins facilitate transport across membranes by serving as receptors, enzymes, or transporters. Proteins act as: (1) recognition and binding units (receptors) for substances moving in and

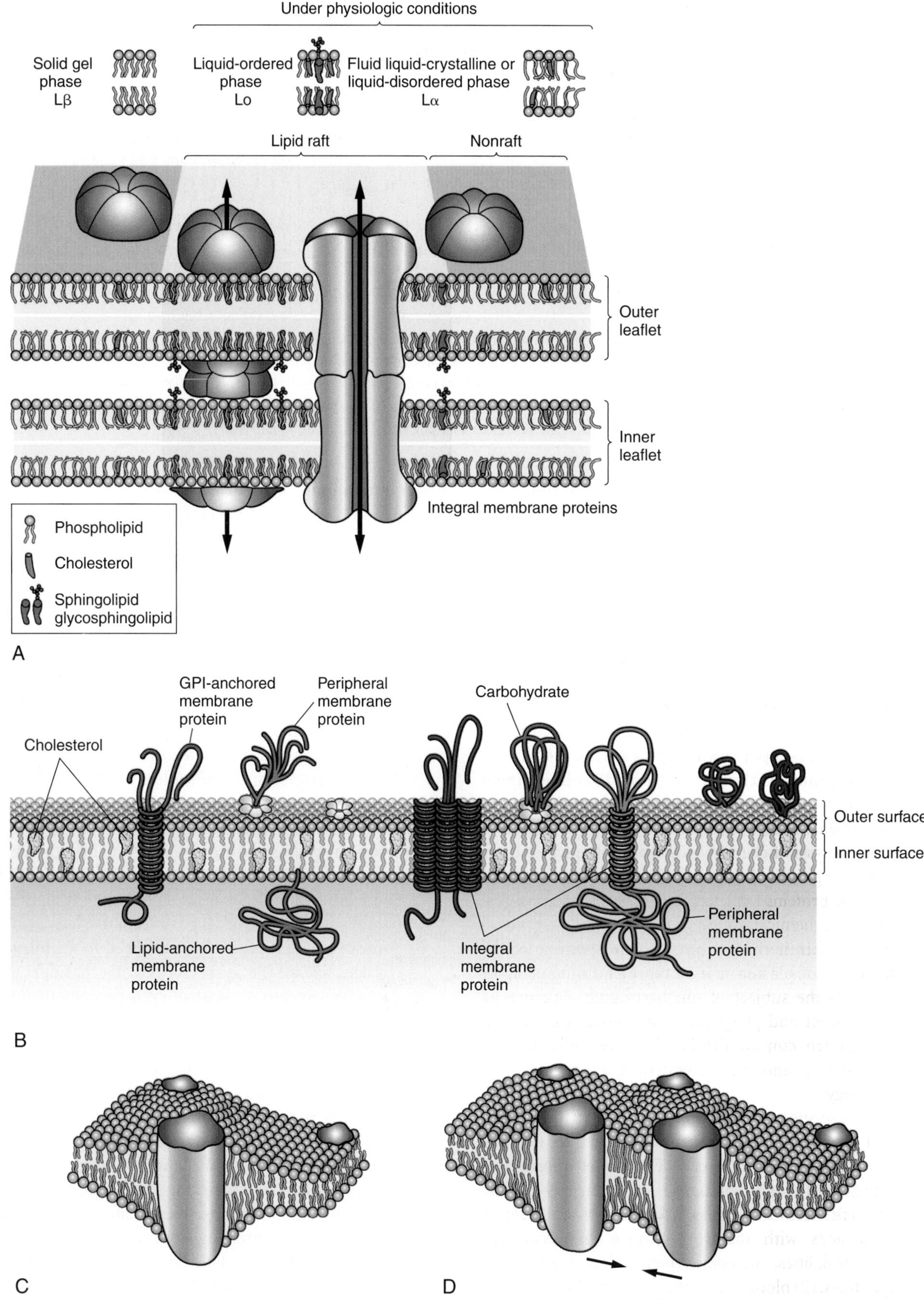
Under physiologic conditions
Solid gel phase Lβ
Liquid-ordered phase Lo
Fluid liquid-crystalline or liquid-disordered phase Lα
Lipid raft
Nonraft
Outer leaflet
Inner leaflet
Integral membrane proteins
Phospholipid
Cholesterol
Sphingolipid glycosphingolipid
A
GPI-anchored membrane protein
Peripheral membrane protein
Carbohydrate
Cholesterol
Outer surface
Inner surface
Peripheral membrane protein
Lipid-anchored membrane protein
Integral membrane protein
B
C
D

FIGURE 1-13

FIGURE 1-13 Lipid Bilayer Membranes. A, Concepts of biologic membranes have markedly changed in the last two decades, from the classic fluid mosaic model to the current model that lipids and proteins are not evenly distributed but can isolate into microdomains, differing in their protein and lipid composition. An example of a microdomain is lipid rafts (colored yellow). Rafts are dynamic domain structures composed of cholesterol, sphinogolipids, and membrane proteins important in different cellular processes. Various models exist to clarify the functions of domains. The three major phases of lipid bilayer organization include a solid gel phase (e.g., with low temperatures), a liquid-ordered phase (high temperatures), and a fluid liquid-crystalline (or liquid-disordered) phase. **B,** Some membrane-associated proteins are integrated into the lipid bilayer; other proteins are loosely attached to the outer and inner surfaces of the membrane. Transmembrane proteins protrude through the entire outer and inner surfaces of the membrane, and they can be attracted to microdomains through specific interactions with lipids. Interaction of the membrane proteins with distinct lipids depends on the hydrophobic thickness of the membrane, the lateral pressures of the membrane (mechanical force may shift protein channels from an open to closed state), the polarity or electrical charges at the lipid-protein interface, and the presence on the protein side of amino acid side chains. Important for pathophysiology is the proposal that protein-lipid interactions can be critical for correct insertion, folding, and orientation of membrane proteins. For example, diseases related to lipids that interfere with protein folding are becoming more prevalent. **C,** Investigators are studying the cooperative behavior of lipids, membrane fluctuations, and domains that influence protein organization and consequently protein function. Here a perturbed region develops around an integral protein. **D,** Two proteins are attracted because of the sharing of a perturbed region of the lipid bilayer. (Adapted from Bagatolli LA et al: *Prog Lipid Res* 49(4):378–389, 2010; Contreras F-X et al: *Cold Spring Harb Perspect Biol* 3(6):pii a004705, 2011; Cooper GM: *The cell—a molecular approach,* ed 2, Washington, DC, 2000; Defamie N, Mesnil M: *Biochim Biophys Acta*, 2011 Oct 2. [Epub ahead of print.].)

out of the cell; (2) pores or transport channels for various electrically charged particles called *ions* or *electrolytes* and specific carriers for amino acids and monosaccharides; (3) specific enzymes that drive active pumps that promote concentration of certain ions, particularly potassium (K^+), within the cell while keeping concentrations of other ions, for example, sodium (Na^+), below concentrations found in the extracellular environment; (4) cell surface markers, such as **glycoproteins** (proteins attached to carbohydrates) that identify a cell to its neighbor; (5) **cell adhesion molecules (CAMs),** or proteins that allow cells to hook together and form attachments to the cytoskeleton for maintaining cellular shape; and (6) catalysts of chemical reactions, for example, conversion of lactose to glucose. (Membrane transport is discussed on p. 28.) Membrane proteins are key components of energy transduction, converting chemical energy into electrical energy, or electrical energy into either mechanical energy or synthesis of ATP.[18]

The interaction of plasma membrane proteins with lipids is complex and is the subject of much research. The role of proteins in the onset and progression of disease is important because they govern communication between cells through enzymatic, transport, and recognition-receptor functions in cellular physiology.

Proteolytic Cascades. **Proteases** are enzymes that cause the breakdown of proteins. Certain proteases can be tethered to cell membranes. Proteases are involved in the physiologic regulation of essential processes by participating in a tightly orchestrated sequence of events termed a **proteolytic cascade.** Four major proteolytic cascades with disease relevance are candidates for treatment modalities, including (1) cell death or caspase-mediated apoptosis, (2) blood coagulation cascade, (3) degrading membrane enzymes or matrix metalloproteinase cascade, and (4) the complement cascade. Some proteases within a proteolytic cascade act as initiators; others are involved in amplification and propagation and execution (Figure 1-14). Understanding the various steps involved is crucial for designing drug interventions. Dysregulation of proteases features prominently in many human diseases, including cancer, autoimmunity, and neurodegenerative disorders.[19-21]

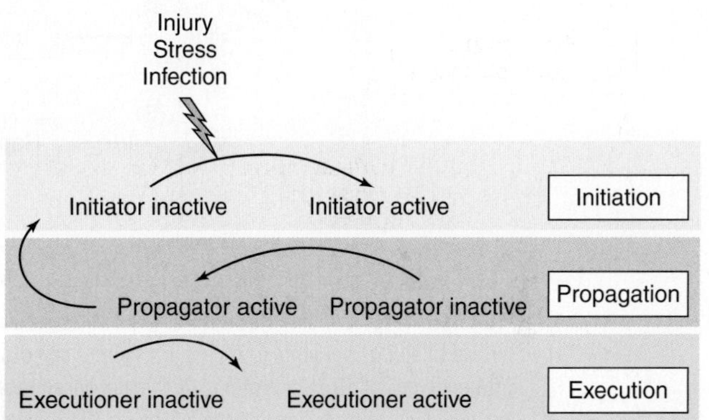

FIGURE 1-14 Schematic Representation of a Prototype Proteolytic Cascade. In the initiation phase, the cascade is triggered by an external stimulus, such as injury, stress, or infection. During the propagation phase, the initiator converts a downstream propagator into its active form by proteolysis. In the execution phase, the propagator will activate an executor. The process of coagulation is the best known proteolytic cascade. (Redrawn with permission from Amour A et al: *Biochem Soc Trans* 32:15–16, 2004. © The Biochemical Society.)

Carbohydrates. The carbohydrate (oligosaccharides) contained within the plasma membrane is generally bound to membrane proteins (glycoproteins) and lipids (glycolipids). Intercellular recognition, which is required for tissue formation, is an important function of membrane oligosaccharides.

Abnormal surface carbohydrate markers have been identified in certain tumor cells, leading investigators to claim that these

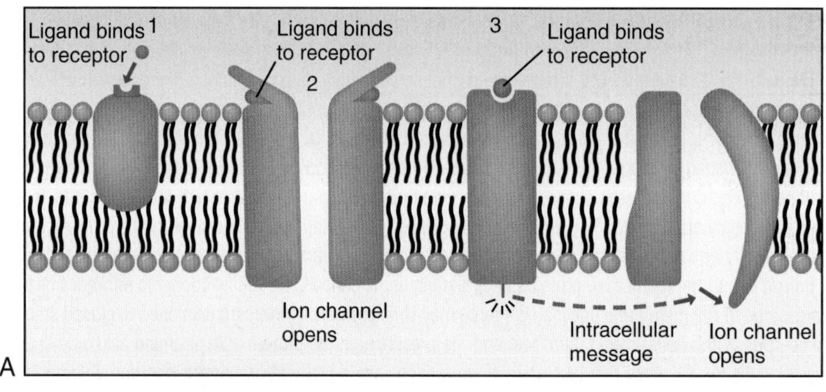

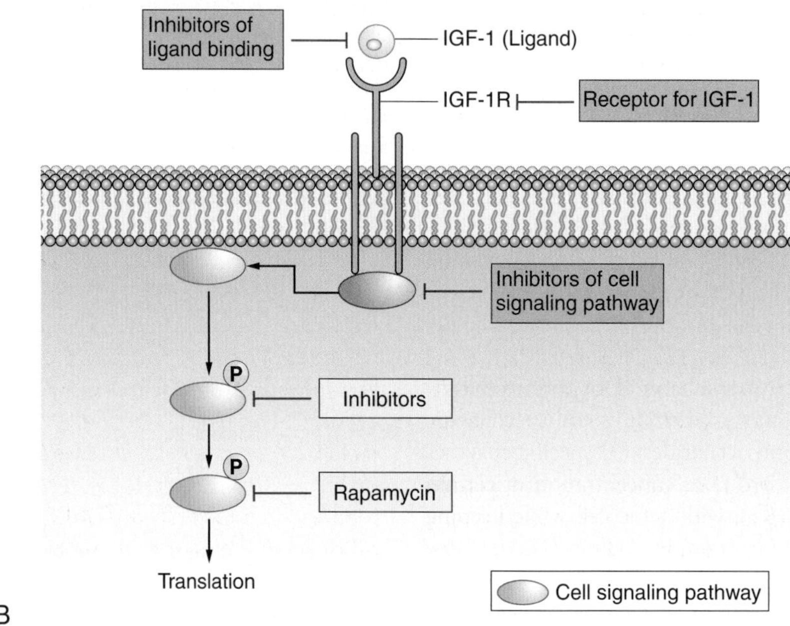

FIGURE 1-15 Cellular Receptors. **(A) 1,** Plasma membrane receptor for a ligand (here, a hormone molecule) on the surface of an integral protein. A neurotransmitter can exert its effect on a postsynaptic cell by means of two fundamentally different types of receptor proteins: **2,** channel-linked receptors, and **3,** non–channel-linked receptors. Channel-linked receptors are also known as ligand-gated channels. **(B)** Example of ligand-receptor interaction. Insulin-like growth factor 1 (IGF-1) is a ligand and binds to the insulin-like growth factor 1 receptor (IGF-1R). With binding at the cell membrane the intracellular signaling pathway is activated, causing translation of new proteins to act as intracellular communicators. This pathway is important for cancer growth. Researchers are developing pharmacologic strategies to reduce signaling at and downstream of the IGF-1R, hoping this will lead to compounds useful in cancer treatment.

markers are involved in tissue growth. Cells do not normally "trespass" their boundaries and overgrow their own territory.

Cellular Receptors

Cellular receptors are protein molecules (proteins are discussed on p. 13) on the plasma membrane, in the cytoplasm, or in the nucleus that are capable of recognizing and binding with specific smaller molecules called **ligands** (Figure 1-15). Hormones, for example, are ligands. Recognition and binding depend on the chemical configuration of the receptor and its smaller ligand, which must fit together somewhat like pieces of a jigsaw puzzle (see Chapter 21). Activation of a receptor also may depend on differences in *movement* and *binding* of the extracellular face of the receptor.[22]

Plasma membrane receptors are particularly important for cellular uptake of ligands (see Figure 1-15, *B*, and Table 1-2). They protrude from or are exposed at the external surface of the membrane and often are attached to integral proteins. Some of these recognition units have all the mobile properties related to membrane fluidity. The ligands that bind with membrane receptors include hormones, neurotransmitters, antigens, complement components, lipoproteins, infectious agents, drugs, and metabolites. The past several years have brought many new discoveries concerning the specific interactions of cellular receptors with their respective ligands. In many instances this information has provided a basis for understanding disease.

Although the chemical nature of both ligands and the receptors to which they bind differs, receptors are classified on the basis of their location and function (see Cellular Communication and Signal Transduction, p. 20). Cellular type determines overall cellular function, but plasma membrane receptors determine which ligands a cell will bind with and how the cell will

TABLE 1-2 CLASSES OF PLASMA MEMBRANE RECEPTORS

TYPE OF RECEPTOR	DESCRIPTION
Channel linked	Also called ligand-gated channels; involve rapid synaptic signaling between electrically excitable cells. Channels open and close briefly in response to neurotransmitters, changing ion permeability of plasma membrane of postsynaptic cell.
Catalytic	Once activated by ligands, function directly as enzymes. Composed of transmembrane proteins that function intracellularly as tyrosine-specific protein kinases.
G-protein linked	Indirectly activate or inactivate plasma membrane enzyme or ion channel; interaction mediated by guanosine triphosphate (GTP)–binding regulatory protein (G protein). When activated, a chain of reactions occurs that alters concentration of intracellular messengers, such as cyclic adenosine monophosphate (cAMP) and calcium, or signaling molecules. Behaviors of other target proteins are also altered. May also interact with inositol phospholipids, which are significant in cell signaling, and molecules involved in the inositol-phospholipid transduction pathway. A G-protein–linked receptor activates the enzyme phosphoinositide-specific phospholipase, which in turn generates two intracellular messengers: (1) inositol triphosphate (IP_3) releases Ca^{++}, and (2) diacylglycerol remains in the plasma membrane and activates protein kinase C. Protein kinase C further activates various cell proteins. Several different plasma membrane receptors are known to use the inositol-phospholipid transduction pathway.

Data from Alberts B et al: *Molecular biology of the cell,* ed 5, New York, 2008, Garland.

respond to binding with each. For example, the ability of a hormone or a neurotransmitter to stimulate a cell is regulated by the specificity and number of receptors present on the plasma membrane. Specific processes also control intracellular mechanisms. Hormone binding, for example, depends on special messenger molecules that regulate protein synthesis within the cell (see Chapter 21). Neurotransmitters (discussed in Chapter 15) also operate by causing special messengers to react with specific receptors.

Receptors for different drugs are found on the plasma membrane, in the cytoplasm, and in the nucleus. Membrane receptors have been found for certain anesthetics, opiates, endorphins, enkephalins, antibiotics, cancer chemotherapeutic agents, digitalis, and other drugs. Membrane receptors for endorphins, which are opiate-like peptides isolated from the pituitary gland, are found in large quantities in pain pathways of the nervous system (see Chapters 15 and 16). With binding, the endorphins (or drugs like morphine) change the cell's permeability to ions, increase the concentration of molecules that regulate intracellular protein synthesis, and initiate molecular events that modulate pain perception.

Receptors for infectious microorganisms, or antigen receptors, bind bacteria, viruses, and parasites. Antigen receptors on white blood cells (lymphocytes, monocytes, macrophages, granulocytes) recognize and bind with antigenic microorganisms and activate the immune and inflammatory responses (see Chapters 7 and 8).

CELL-TO-CELL ADHESIONS

Cells are small and squishy, not at all like bricks. They are enclosed by a flimsy membrane, yet the cell depends on the integrity of this membrane for its survival. How can cells be combined together strongly, with their membranes intact, to form a muscle that can lift this textbook? Plasma membranes not only serve as the outer boundaries of all cells but also allow groups of cells to be held together robustly, in **cell-to-cell adhesions,** to form tissues and organs. Once arranged, cells are held together by three different means: the extracellular matrix, cell adhesion molecules in the cell's plasma membrane, and specialized cell junctions.

Extracellular Matrix

Cells can be bound together by attachment to one another or via the **extracellular matrix** (also including the basement membrane), which the cells secrete around themselves. The extracellular matrix is an intricate meshwork of fibrous proteins embedded in a watery, gel-like substance composed of complex carbohydrates (Figure 1-16). The matrix is like glue; however, it does provide a pathway for diffusion of nutrients, wastes, and other water-soluble traffic between the blood and tissue cells. Interwoven within the matrix are three groups of **macromolecules:** (1) fibrous structural proteins, including collagen and elastin; (2) a diverse group of adhesive glycoproteins, such as fibronectin; and (3) proteoglycans and hyaluronic acid. The **basement membrane** is a thin layer of connective tissue underlying the epithelium of many organs and is also called the **basal lamina** (see Figure 1-16).

Collagen forms cable-like fibers or sheets that provide tensile strength or resistance to longitudinal stress. Collagen breakdown, such as occurs in osteoarthritis, destroys the fibrils that give cartilage its tensile strength.

Elastin is a rubber-like protein fiber most abundant in tissue that must be capable of stretching and recoiling, such as the lungs.

Fibronectin, a large glycoprotein, promotes cell adhesion and cell anchorage. Reduced amounts have been found in certain types of cancerous cells; this allows cancer cells to travel or metastasize to other parts of the body.

All of these macromolecules occur in intercellular junctions and cell surfaces and may assemble into two different components: interstitial matrix and basement membrane (BM)[23] (see Figure 1-16).

The extracellular matrix is secreted by **fibroblasts** ("fiber formers"), local cells that are present in the matrix. The matrix and the cells within it are known collectively as *connective tissue* because they connect cells together to form tissue and organs. Human connective tissues are enormously varied. They can be

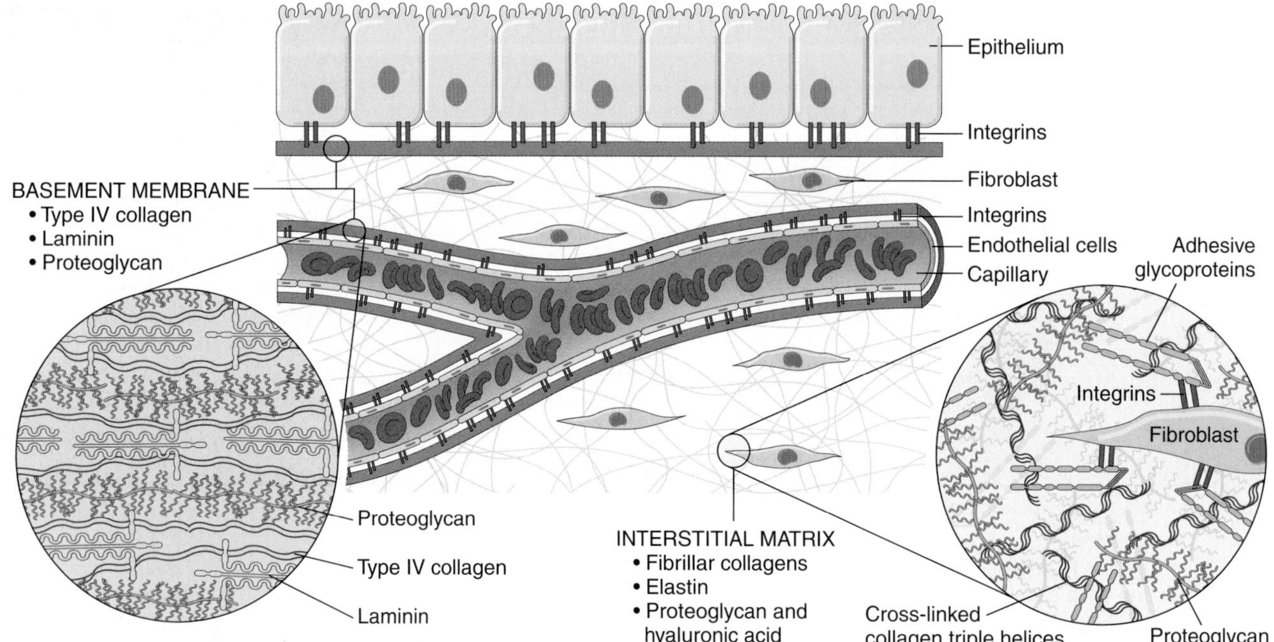

FIGURE 1-16 Extracellular Matrix. Tissues are not just cells but also extracellular space. The extracellular space is an intricate network of macromolecules called the *extracellular matrix (ECM)*. The macromolecules that constitute the ECM are secreted locally (by mostly fibroblasts) and assembled into a meshwork in close association with the surface of the cell that produced them. Two main classes of macromolecules include proteoglycans, which are bound to polysaccharide chains called glycosaminoglycans; and fibrous proteins (e.g., collagen, elastin, fibronectin, and laminin), which have structural and adhesive properties. Together the proteoglycan molecules form a gel-like ground substance in which the fibrous proteins are embedded. The gel permits rapid diffusion of nutrients, metabolites, and hormones between the blood and the tissue cells. Matrix proteins modulate cell-matrix interactions including normal tissue remodeling (which can become abnormal, for example, with chronic inflammation), embryogenesis, wound healing, and angiogenesis. Disruption of this balance results in serious diseases such as arthritis, tumor growth, and others. (From Kumar V et al: *Robbins & Cotran pathologic basis of disease,* ed 8, Philadelphia, 2010, Saunders.)

hard and dense, like bone; flexible, like tendons or the dermis of the skin; resilient and shock-absorbing, like cartilage; or soft and transparent, like the jelly-like substance that fills the eye. In all these examples, the majority of the tissue is composed of extracellular matrix, and the cells that produce the matrix are scattered within it like raisins in a pudding[24] (see Figure 1-16).

The matrix is not just passive scaffolding for cellular attachment; it also helps regulate the functions of the cells within which it interacts. The matrix helps regulate cell growth, movement, and differentiation.

Cell-Adhesion Molecules (CAMs)

Cell adhesion molecules (CAMs) are cell-surface proteins that bind the cell to an adjacent cell and to components of the extracellular matrix (ECM). CAMs include four protein families: the integrins, the cadherins, the selectins, and Ig (immunoglobulin) superfamily. **Integrins** are a major class of receptors within the ECM and regulate cell-ECM interactions with collagen, fibronectin, vitronectin, and fibrinogen. **Cadherins** are Ca^{+2} –dependent glycoproteins and have a unique pattern of tissue distribution, for example, epithelial (E-cadherin). **Selectins** are a family of proteins that bind certain carbohydrates, for example mucins. The **immunoglobulin superfamily CAMs (IgSF CAMs)** bind integrins or other IgSF CAMs.

Specialized Cell Junctions

Cells in direct physical contact with neighboring cells are often linked together at specialized regions of their plasma membranes called **cell junctions.** Cell junctions have two main functions: (1) to hold cells together and (2) to allow small molecules to pass from cell to cell, allowing coordination of the activities of cells that form tissues. The three main types of cell junctions are (1) desmosomes (adhering junctions, or macula adherens), (2) tight junctions (impermeable junctions, or zonula occludens), and (3) gap junctions (adhering [communicating] junctions) (Figure 1-17, *A*). Together they form the **junctional complex. Desmosomes** hold cells together by forming either continuous bands or belts of epithelial sheets or button-like points of contact. Desmosomes also act as a system of braces to maintain structural stability. **Tight junctions** are barriers to diffusion, prevent the movement of substances through transport proteins in the plasma membrane, and prevent the leakage of small molecules between the plasma membranes of adjacent cells. **Gap junctions** are clusters of communicating tunnels, **connexons,** that allow small ions and molecules to pass directly from the inside of one cell to the inside of another. Connexons are joining proteins that extend outward from each of the adjacent plasma membranes (see Figure 1-17, *C*). The integrity of connexons and dysregulation of intercellular ion movement

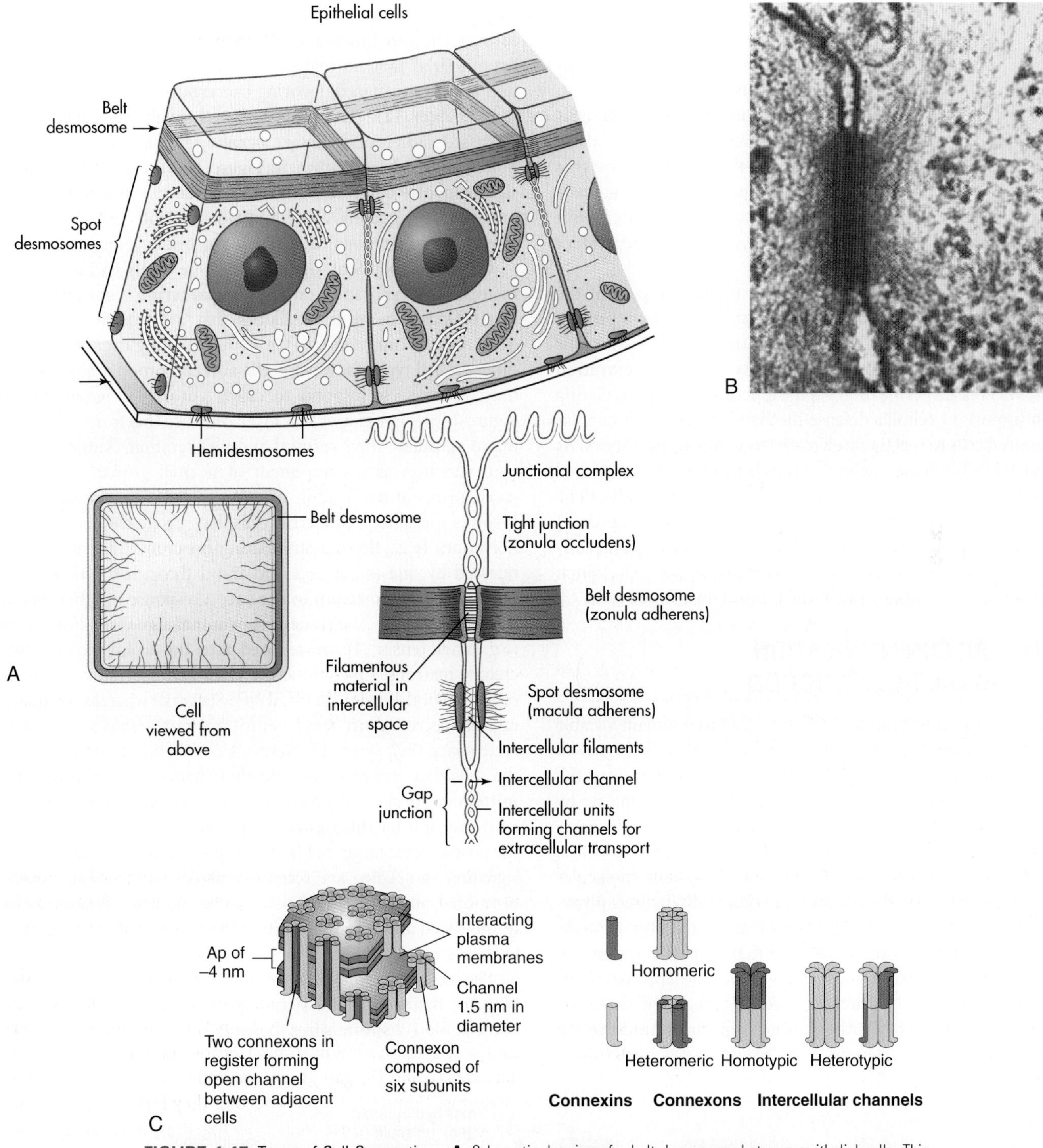

FIGURE 1-17 Types of Cell Connections. **A,** Schematic drawing of a belt desmosome between epithelial cells. This junction, also called *zonula adherens,* encircles each interacting cell. The spot desmosomes and hemidesmosomes, like the belt desmosomes, are adhering junctions. This tight junction is an impermeable junction that holds cells together but seals them in such a way that molecules cannot leak between them. The gap junction, as a communicating junction, mediates the passage of small molecules from one interacting cell to the other. **B,** Electron micrograph of desmosomes. **C,** Connexons. (**A, B** from Raven PH, Johnson GB: *Biology,* St Louis, 1992, Mosby. **C** from Alberts B et al: *Molecular biology of the cell,* ed 5, New York, 2008, Garland.)

has been linked to certain disorders, for example, atrial fibrillation.[25] Cells connected by gap junctions are considered ionically (electrically) and metabolically coupled. Gap junctions coordinate the activities of adjacent cells. They are important, for example, in synchronizing contractions of heart muscle cells through ionic coupling and in permitting action potentials to spread rapidly from cell to cell in neural tissues. The reason that gap junctions occur in tissues that are not electrically active is unknown. Although most gap junctions are associated with junctional complexes, they sometimes exist as independent structures.

The junctional complex is a highly permeable part of the plasma membrane. Its permeability is controlled by a process called **gating,** which depends on concentrations of calcium ions in the cytoplasm. Increased cytoplasmic calcium concentration causes decreased permeability at the junctional complex. Gating is an important cellular defense mechanism because it enables uninjured cells to seal themselves off from injured neighbors. As damaged cells release calcium, it travels through the junctional complex and increases calcium levels in neighboring cells. (The damaging effects of calcium influx are described in Chapter 2.) The increased calcium concentration decreases the permeability of the junctional complexes of the neighboring cells, which form a relatively impermeable wall around the injured area.

CELLULAR COMMUNICATION AND SIGNAL TRANSDUCTION

Cells need to communicate with each other to maintain a stable internal environment, or **homeostasis;** to regulate their growth and division and their development and organization into tissues; and to coordinate their functions. Cells communicate by using hundreds of kinds of signal molecules, for example, insulin (see Figure 1-15, *B*). Cells communicate in three main ways: (1) they display plasma membrane–bound signaling molecules (receptors) that affect the cell itself and other cells in direct physical contact (Figure 1-18, *A*); (2) they affect receptor proteins *inside* the target cell and the signal molecule has to enter the cell to bind to them (Figure 1-18, *B*); and (3) they form protein channels (gap junctions) that directly coordinate the activities of adjacent cells (Figure 1-18, *C*). Alterations in cellular communication affect disease onset and progression. In fact, if a cell is unable to perform gap junctional intercellular communication, it is hypothesized that normal growth control and cell differentiation are compromised, favoring cancerous tumor development (see Chapter 12). (Communication through gap junctions is discussed earlier, and contact signaling by plasma membrane–bound molecules is shown in Figure 1-18.) Secreted chemical signals involve communication at a distance. Primary modes of intercellular signaling are contact-dependent, paracrine, hormonal, neurohormonal, and neurotransmitter (Figure 1-19).

Contact-dependent signaling requires cells to be in close membrane-membrane contact. In **paracrine signaling,** cells secrete local chemical mediators that are quickly absorbed, destroyed, or immobilized. Paracrine signaling usually involves different cell types; however, cells also can produce signals that they, themselves, respond to called **autocrine signaling** (see Figure 1-19). For example, cancer cells use this form of signaling to stimulate their survival and proliferation. Autocrine circuits function as a component of normal growth-regulatory mechanisms in many adult tissue types.[26] **Hormonal signaling** involves specialized endocrine cells that secrete chemicals called hormones (e.g., thyroid-stimulating hormone); hormones are released by one set of cells and travel through the tissue and through the bloodstream to produce a response in other sets of cells (see Chapter 21). In **neurohormonal signaling,** hormones (e.g., angiotensin II) are released into the blood by neurosecretory neurons. Like endocrine cells, neurosecretory neurons release blood-borne chemical messengers, whereas ordinary neurons secrete short-range neurotransmitters into a small, discrete space (i.e., synapse). Neurons communicate directly with the cells they innervate by releasing chemicals or **neurotransmitters** at specialized junctions called **chemical synapses;** the neurotransmitter diffuses across the synaptic cleft and acts on the postsynaptic target cell (see Figure 1-20). Many of these same signaling molecules are receptors used in hormonal, neurohormonal, and paracrine signaling. The important differences lie in the speed and selectivity with which the signals are delivered to their targets.[1]

Plasma membrane receptors belong to one of three classes that are defined by the signaling (transduction) mechanism used. Table 1-2 summarizes these classes of receptors.

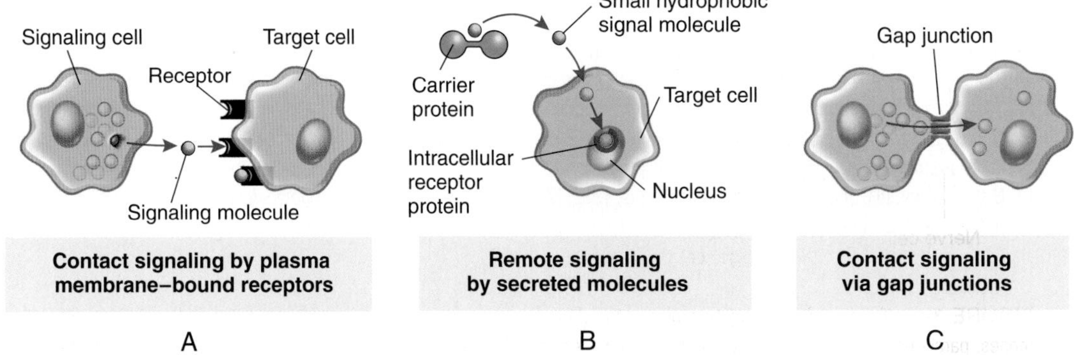

FIGURE 1-18 Cellular Communication. Three ways in which cells communicate with one another. (**B** adapted from Alberts B et al: *Molecular biology of the cell,* ed 5, New York, 2008, Garland.)

Signal Transduction

Signal transduction involves incoming signals or instructions from extracellular chemical messengers (ligands) that are conveyed to the cell's interior for execution. Cells respond to external stimuli by activating a variety of **signal transduction pathways,** which are communication pathways, or signaling cascades (Figure 1-20). Signals are passed between cells when a particular type of molecule is produced by one cell—the **signaling cell**—and received by another—the **target cell**—by means of a **receptor protein** that recognizes and responds specifically to the signal molecule (Figure 1-20, *A* and *B*). In turn, the signaling molecules activate a path of intracellular protein kinases that results in responses, such as grow and divide, survive, or differentiate (Figure 1-20, *C* and *D*). If deprived of appropriate signals, most cells undergo a form of cell suicide known as *programmed cell death,* or *apoptosis* (see p. 88).

Signal transduction pathways, or relay chains, of intercellular signaling molecules have several important functions (see Figure 1-20):

1. They physically *transfer* the signal from the place at which it is received to some other part of the cell where the response is expected.
2. They *amplify* the signal received, making it stronger; this is caused by a multiplying effect in the pathways; for example, binding of one ligand molecule to a receptor activates a number of adenylyl cyclase molecules.
3. They *distribute* the signal so that it influences several processes in parallel; at any step in the pathway, the signal can *diverge* and be relayed to several different intracellular targets, creating branches in the flow and causing a complex response (see Figure 1-20).
4. Last, the signal can be *modulated* by other interfering factors prevailing inside or outside the cell.

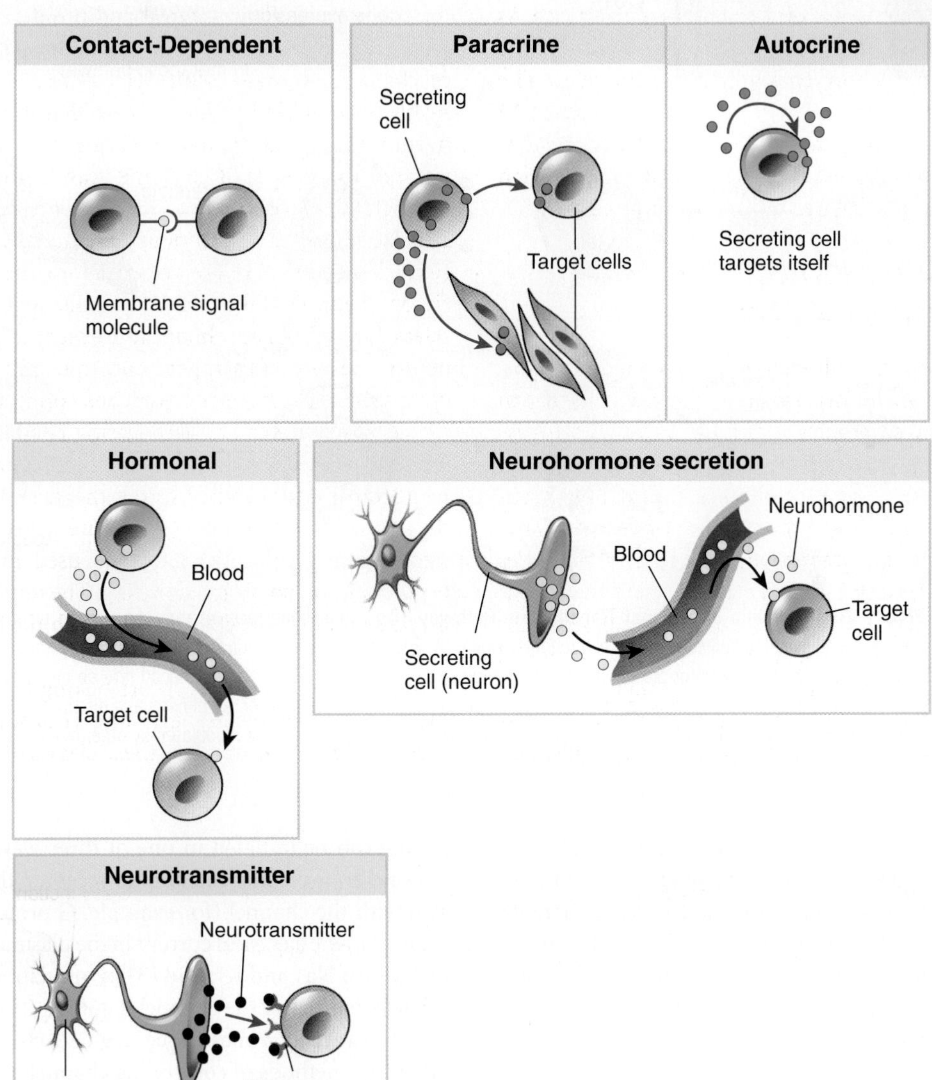

FIGURE 1-19 **Primary Modes of Chemical Signaling.** Five forms of signaling mediated by secreted molecules. Hormones, paracrines, neurotransmitters, and neurohormones are all intercellular messengers that accomplish communication between cells. Autocrines bind to receptors on the same cell. Not all neurotransmitters act in the strictly synaptic mode shown; some act in a contact-dependent mode as local chemical mediators that influence multiple target cells in the area.

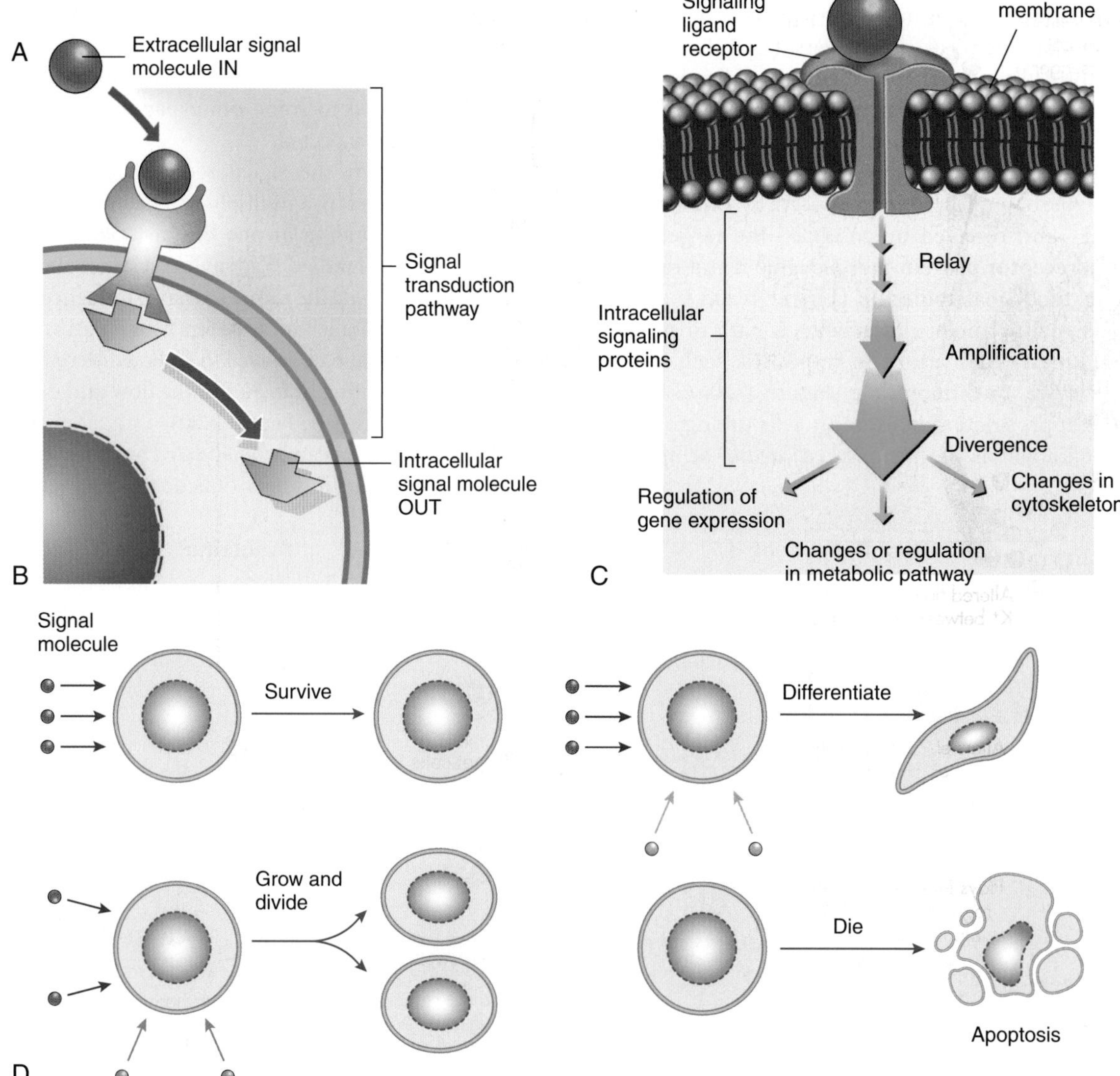

FIGURE 1-20 Schematic of a Signal Transduction Pathway. Like a telephone receiver that converts an electrical signal into a sound signal, a cell converts an extracellular signal, **A,** into an intracellular signal, **B. C,** An extracellular signal molecule (ligand) binds to a receptor protein located on the plasma membrane, where it is transduced into an intracellular signal. This process initiates a signaling cascade that relays the signal into the cell interior, amplifying and distributing it en route. Amplification is often achieved by stimulating enzymes. Steps in the cascade can be modulated by other events in the cell. **D,** Different cell behaviors rely on multiple extracellular signals.

Two general responses from binding of the extracellular signaling messenger (i.e., ligand), or **first messenger,** to the membrane receptors occur: (1) opening or closing specific channels in the membrane to regulate the movement of ions into or out of the cell, and (2) transferring the signal to an intracellular messenger, or **second messenger,** which in turn triggers a cascade of biochemical events within the cell.

Extracellular Messengers and Channel Regulation

Membrane channels, or "gates," can open and close depending on the circumstances of the first messenger. Opening and closing occur because of conformational changes (shaping) of the proteins that form the channels—blocking the channel (closing) or permitting passage through it (opening). Channel opening and closing can be initiated in one of three ways: (1) by binding of a ligand to a specific membrane receptor that is closely associated with the channel (for example, G proteins); (2) by making changes in the electrical current in the plasma membrane, altering the flow of Na^+ and K^+; and (3) by stretching or other mechanical deformation of the channel. Figure 1-21 summarizes ways by which extracellular messengers regulate channel function for the other two methods of controlling channels (see p. 23).

Second Messengers

Many ligands cannot enter their target cells to bring about the desired intracellular response. Instead, the first messengers, or ligands, issue orders by binding with receptors on the surface membrane, triggering a "pass it on" signal. Second messengers

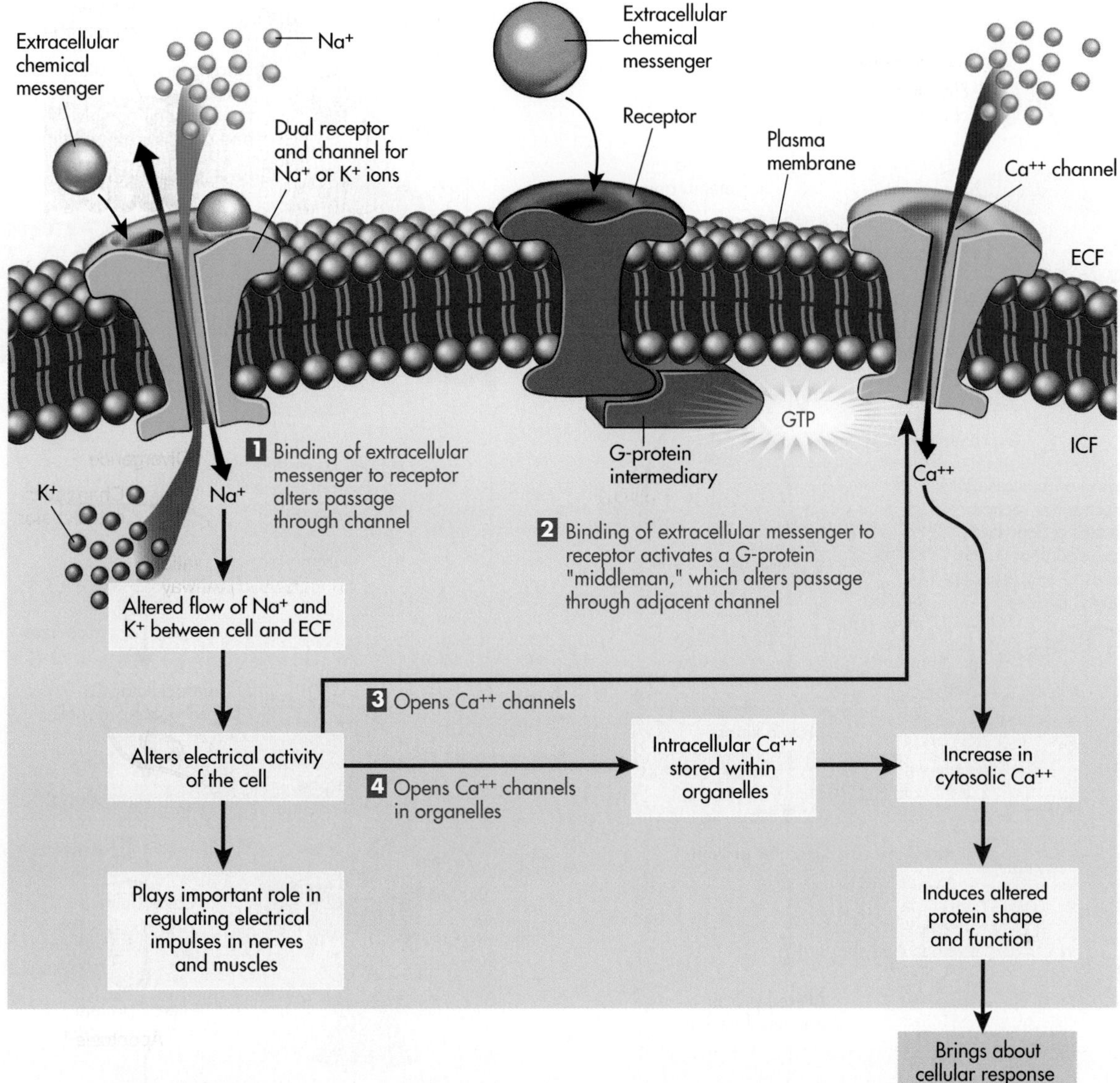

FIGURE 1-21 How Extracellular Messengers Regulate Channel Function. Binding of an extracellular messenger to a dual receptor/channel brings about a quick opening or closing of ion channels, such as Na^+ or K^+ channels, which generates electrical impulses **(1).** A transient opening of membrane Ca^{++} channels occurs when binding of an extracellular messenger to a receptor activates a G-protein intermediary, which alters a nearby ion channel, such as a Ca^{++} channel **(2).** A transient opening of Ca^{++} channels also occurs indirectly in response to electrical impulses produced by extracellular messenger-induced changes in Na^+ and K^+ channels **(3).** Release of Ca^{++} from intracellular stores results when Ca^{++} channels in organelles open in response to electrical impulses **(4).** An increase in cytosolic Ca^{++} concentration arising from pathways **2, 3,** or **4** causes change in the shape and function of specific intracellular proteins to produce the desired cellular response. *ECF,* Extracellular fluid; *GTP,* guanosine triphosphate; *ICF,* intracellular fluid. (Redrawn with permission from Sherwood L: *Human physiology,* ed 3. © 1997 Brooks/Cole, a part of Cengage Learning, Inc. Reproduced by permission. www.cengage.com/permissions.)

are generated in large numbers when the membrane-bound enzyme is activated, and they then rapidly diffuse away from their source, broadcasting the signal throughout the cell (Figure 1-22). Remember, most cell surface receptor proteins belong to one of three large classes: ion channel–linked receptors, G-protein–linked receptors, or enzyme-linked receptors.

The two major second messenger pathways are **cyclic adenosine monophosphate (cyclic AMP, cAMP)** and Ca^{++}. In the cAMP pathway, binding of the ligand to its surface receptor eventually activates the enzyme adenylyl cyclase on the inner surface of the membrane. A membrane-bound "middleman," a **G protein,** acts as an intermediary between the receptor and adenylyl cyclase. G proteins are named because they are bound to guanine nucleotides—**guanosine triphosphate (GTP)** or **guanosine diphosphate (GDP).** An unactivated G protein consists of a complex of alpha (α), beta (β), and gamma (γ) subunits, with a GDP molecule bound to the α subunit. The cAMP pathway with G proteins is summarized in Figure 1-22.

Instead of cAMP, some cells use Ca^{++} as a second messenger. In this pathway, binding of the first messenger to the surface

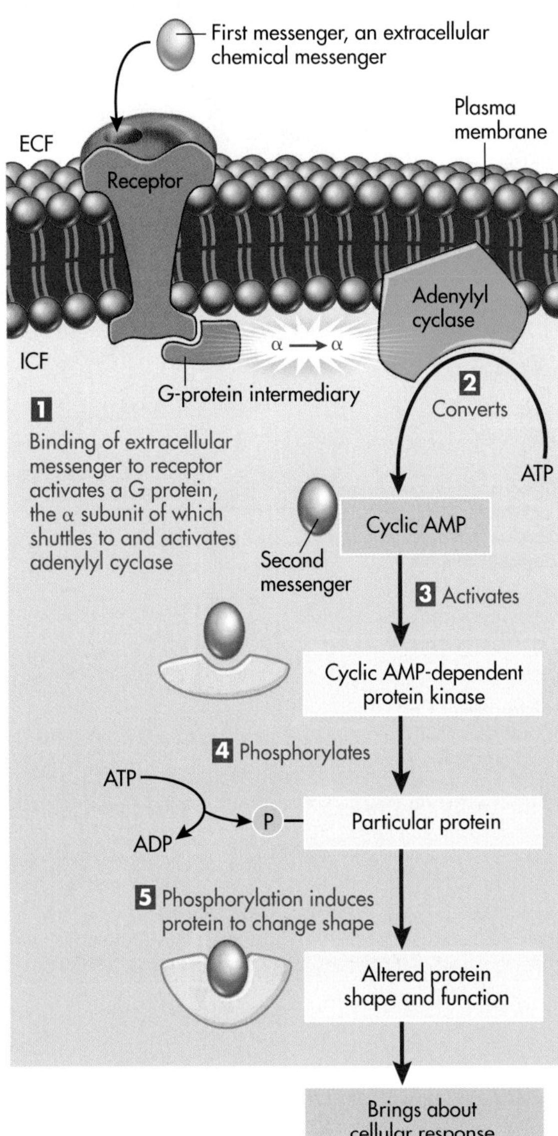

FIGURE 1-22 **Extracellular Messenger and Activation of the cAMP Second Messenger System.** The first messenger, or binding of an extracellular chemical messenger to a surface membrane receptor, activates the membrane-bound enzyme adenylyl cyclase by means of a G-protein intermediary **(1)**, which in turn converts intracellular ATP into cAMP **(2)**. cAMP is an intracellular second messenger, triggering the cellular response by activating the cAMP-dependent protein kinase **(3)**, which in turn phosphorylates **(4)**, and therefore modifies **(5)** a specific intracellular protein. The altered protein then directs the cellular response dictated by the extracellular messenger. *ADP,* Adenosine diphosphate; *AMP,* adenosine monophosphate; *ATP,* adenosine triphosphate; *ECF,* extracellular fluid; *ICF,* intracellular fluid. (Redrawn with permission from Sherwood L: *Human physiology,* ed 3, © 1997 Brooks/Cole, a part of Cengage Learning, Inc. Reproduced by permission. www.cengage.com/permissions.)

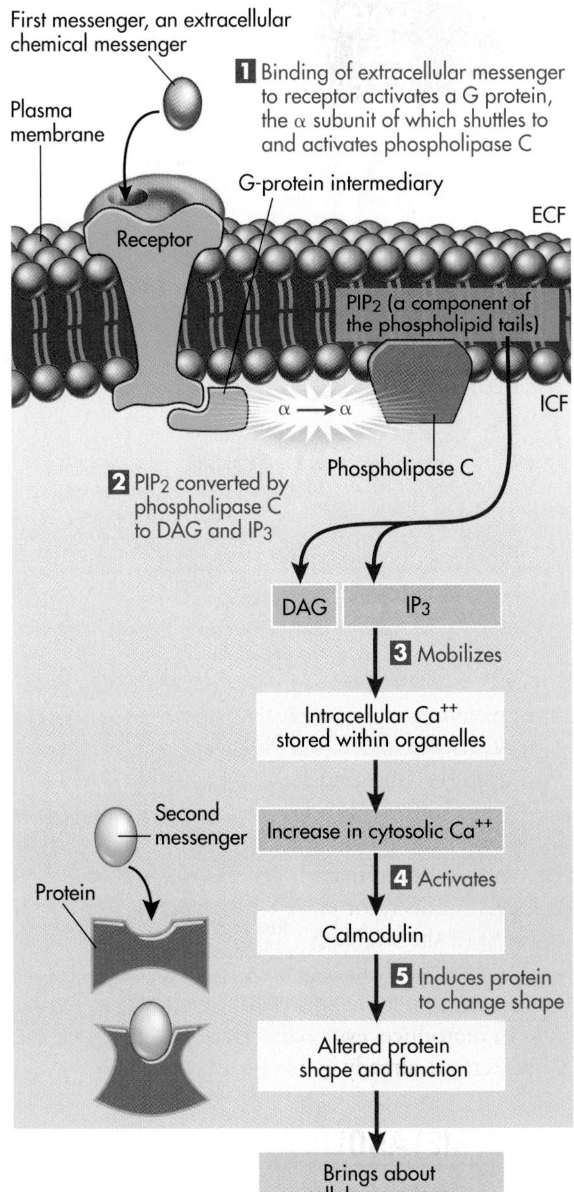

FIGURE 1-23 **Extracellular Messenger and Activation of the Calcium Second Messenger System.** Binding of an extracellular messenger to a membrane receptor activates the membrane-bound enzyme phospholipase C by means of a G-protein intermediary **(1)**. Phospholipase C converts phosphatidylinositol biphosphate *(PIP_2)* into diacylglycerol *(DAG)* and inositol triphosphate *(IP_3)* **(2)**. IP_3 then mobilizes Ca^{++} stored within organelles **(3)**. Ca^{++}, as a second messenger, activates calmodulin **(4)**, causing a change in the shape and function of a specific intracellular protein to produce the cellular response **(5)**. *ECF,* Extracellular fluid; ICF, intracellular fluid. (Redrawn with permission from Sherwood L: *Human physiology,* ed 3, © 1997 Brooks/Cole, a part of Cengage Learning, Inc. Reproduced by permission. www.cengage.com/permissions.)

receptor eventually leads, by means of G proteins, to activation of the enzyme phospholipase C, an enzyme protein effector (an ion channel for an enzyme) that is bound to the inner side of the membrane. Figure 1-23 summarizes the Ca^{++} second messenger pathway. The cAMP and Ca^{++} pathways frequently overlap in triggering a specific cellular response. For example, cAMP and Ca^{++} can influence each other. Calcium-activated calmodulin can regulate adenylyl cyclase and thus influence cAMP; conversely, cAMP-dependent kinase may phosphorylate and thereby change the activity of Ca^{++} channels or carriers. In some instances, both Ca^{++} and cAMP regulate the same intracellular protein. In a few cells, **cyclic guanosine monophosphate**

TABLE 1-3 HORMONE-INDUCED CELL RESPONSES MEDIATED BY cAMP

SIGNALING LIGANDS	TARGET TISSUE	MAJOR RESPONSE
Epinephrine	Heart	Increase in heart rate and force of contraction
Epinephrine, ACTH	Muscle	Glycogen breakdown
Glucagon	Fat	Fat breakdown
ACTH	Adrenal gland	Cortisol secretion
Antidiuretic hormone	Liver	Glycogen breakdown
Acetylcholine	Pancreas; smooth muscle	Amylase secretion; contraction
Antigen	Mast cells	Histamine secretion
Thrombin	Blood platelets	Serotonin and platelet-derived growth factor secretion; platelet aggregation

ACTH, Adrenocorticotropic hormone; *cAMP,* cyclic adenosine monophosphate.

(cyclic GMP, cGMP) serves as a second messenger similar to the cAMP pathway. For example, cGMP is the signal transduction pathway involved in vision. Some cellular responses mediated by cAMP and phospholipase C are summarized in Table 1-3. Major types of receptors and signal transduction pathways are contained in Table 1-4.

A large number of human disorders involve problematic signaling in cells. Cancer, for example, results from genetic mutations leading to the overactivity of proteins in signal relaying pathways that normally induce the cells to divide. Affected proteins cause cells to behave as if other cells were constantly telling them to reproduce, even when no such orders were sent.[27] Signal blockers are already in use against tumors.

TABLE 1-4 MAJOR TYPES OF RECEPTORS AND SIGNALING TRANSDUCTION PATHWAYS

RECEPTOR AND SIGNALING PATHWAY	LIGANDS
Receptors with Intrinsic Tyrosine Kinase Activity	
P13 kinase pathway, MAP-kinase pathway, IP_3 pathway	Signaling ligands include most growth factors (EGF, TGF-α, HGF, PDGF, VEGF, FGF), stem cell factor, insulin
Receptors Lacking Intrinsic Tyrosine Kinase Activity	
JAK/STAT pathway	Several cytokines including IL-2, IL-3, others; interferons α, β, and γ; erythropoietin; G-CSF; growth hormone; and prolactin
G-Protein–Coupled Receptors	
cAMP pathway	ADH, serotonin, histamine, epinephrine, norepinephrine, calcitonin, glucagon, parathyroid hormone, corticotropin, rhodopsin, and many drugs
Steroid Hormone Receptors	
Includes steroid hormone receptors as well as a group called peroxisome proliferator-activated receptors (PPARs)	Many steroid hormones, thyroid hormone, vitamin D, and retinoids

ADH, Antidiuretic hormone; *cAMP,* cyclic adenosine monophosphate; *EGF,* epidermal growth factor; *FGF,* fibroblast growth factor; *G-CSF,* granulocyte colony-stimulating factor; *HGF,* hepatocyte growth factor; IL-2, IL-3, interleukin-2 and interleukin-3; IP_3, inositol triphosphate; *JAK/STAT,* Janus kinase-signal transducers and activators of transcription; *MAP-kinase,* mitogen-activated protein kinase; *PDGF,* platelet-derived growth factor; *TGF-α,* transforming growth factor-alpha; *VEGF,* vascular endothelial growth factor.

CELLULAR METABOLISM

All the chemical tasks of maintaining essential cellular functions are referred to as **cellular metabolism.** The energy-using process of metabolism is called **anabolism** (*ana* = upward), and the energy-releasing process is known as **catabolism** (*cata* = downward). Metabolism provides the cell with the energy it needs to synthesize (produce) cellular structures.

Dietary proteins, fats, and starches are hydrolyzed in the intestinal tract into amino acids, fatty acids, and glucose, respectively. These constituents are then absorbed, circulated, and taken up by the cell, where they may be used for various vital cellular processes, including the production of ATP. The process by which ATP is produced is one example of a series of reactions called a **metabolic pathway.** A metabolic pathway involves several intermediate steps whose end products are not always detectable. A key feature of cellular metabolism is the directing of biochemical reactions by protein catalysts, or enzymes. Most biochemical reactions in a pathway are catalyzed by a specific enzyme. Each enzyme has a high affinity for a **substrate**—a specific substance that is converted to a product of the reaction.

Role of Adenosine Triphosphate

For a cell to function it must be able to extract and use the chemical energy contained within the structure of organic molecules. When 1 mole (mol) of glucose is metabolically broken down in the presence of oxygen into carbon dioxide (CO_2) and water (H_2O), 686 kilocalories (kcal) of energy are released. In a test tube this energy is released as heat. Because a cell cannot transform heat into work, chemical energy, rather than heat, is created by metabolism. The chemical energy lost by one molecule is transferred to the chemical structure of another molecule by an energy-carrying or transferring molecule, such as ATP. The energy stored in ATP can be used in a variety of energy-requiring reactions and in the process is generally converted to adenosine diphosphate (ADP) and inorganic phosphate (Pi). The energy available as a result of this reaction is about 7 kcal/mol of ATP. In addition to its use in synthesis (anabolism) of organic molecules, ATP is used by the cell for muscle contraction and active transport of molecules across cellular membranes. The function of ATP is not only to *store* energy but also to *transfer* it from one molecule to another. Energy is stored

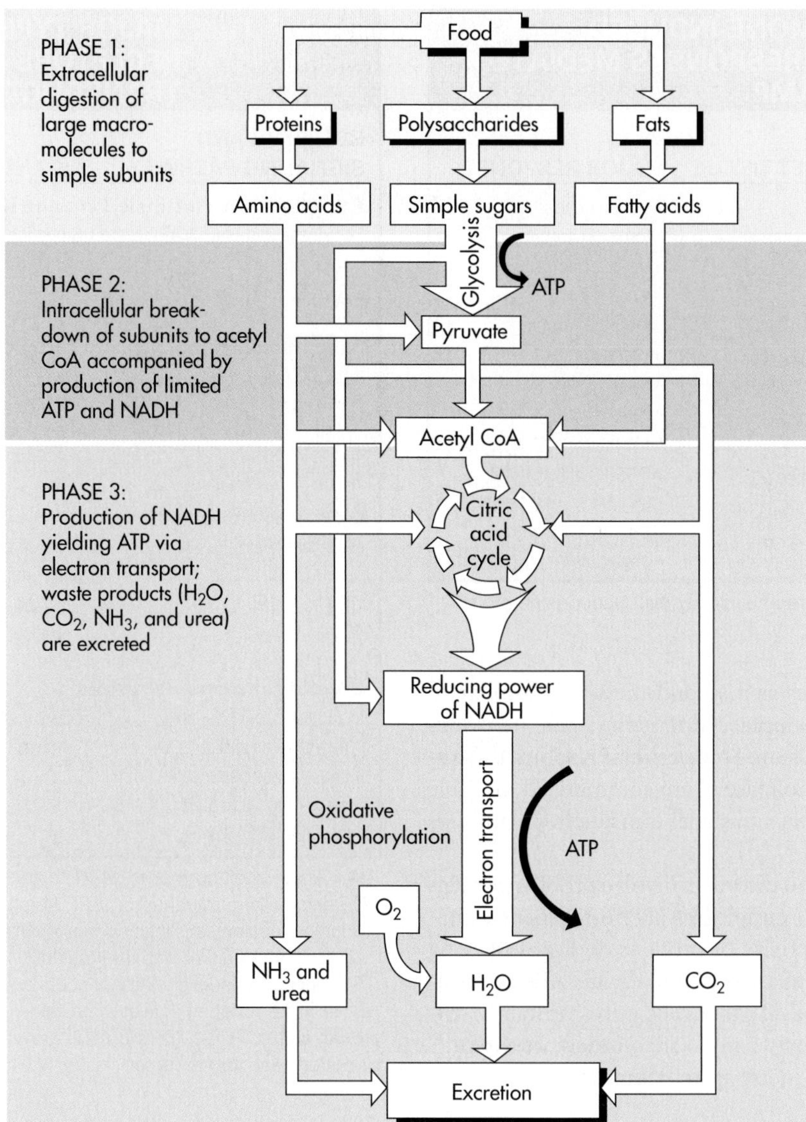

FIGURE 1-24 **Three Phases of Catabolism, Which Leads from Food to Waste Products.** These reactions produce ATP, which is used to drive other processes in the cell.

by molecules of carbohydrate, lipid, and protein, which, when catabolized, transfer energy to ATP.

Food and Production of Cellular Energy

The process of catabolism of the proteins, lipids, and polysaccharides found in food can be divided into the following three phases (Figure 1-24).

Phase 1: **Digestion.** Large molecules are broken down into their smaller subunits—proteins into amino acids, polysaccharides into simple sugars, and fats into fatty acids and glycerol. These processes occur outside the cell by the action of secreted enzymes.

Phase 2: **Glycolysis** and **oxidation.** The small molecules enter cells and are further broken down in the cytoplasm. Most of the sugars are converted into pyruvate. Pyruvate then enters mitochondria and is converted to the acetyl groups of acetyl coenzyme A (acetyl CoA). Acetyl CoA, like ATP, releases energy when it is hydrolyzed. The most important part of phase 2 is the lysis (splitting) of glucose, known as **glycolysis** (Figure 1-25). Glycolysis produces a net of two molecules of ATP per glucose molecule through the process of **oxidation,** or the removal and transfer of a pair of electrons. This process, often called **oxidative cellular metabolism,** involves 10 biochemical reactions. In reactions 1 through 5, glucose is converted to two, three-carbon aldehyde compounds (glyceraldehyde-3-phosphate [G3P]), which requires energy in the form of ATP. The next five reactions convert G3P molecules into pyruvate molecules and generate four molecules of ATP for each two molecules of G3P. In addition, two molecules of nicotinamide adenine dinucleotide (NAD) are further oxidized to produce four more molecules of ATP. After subtracting two molecules of ATP to drive the reactions, the net yield is six ATP molecules for each molecule of glucose.

Phase 3: **Citric acid cycle (Krebs cycle, tricarboxylic acid cycle).** Most of the ATP is generated during this final phase.

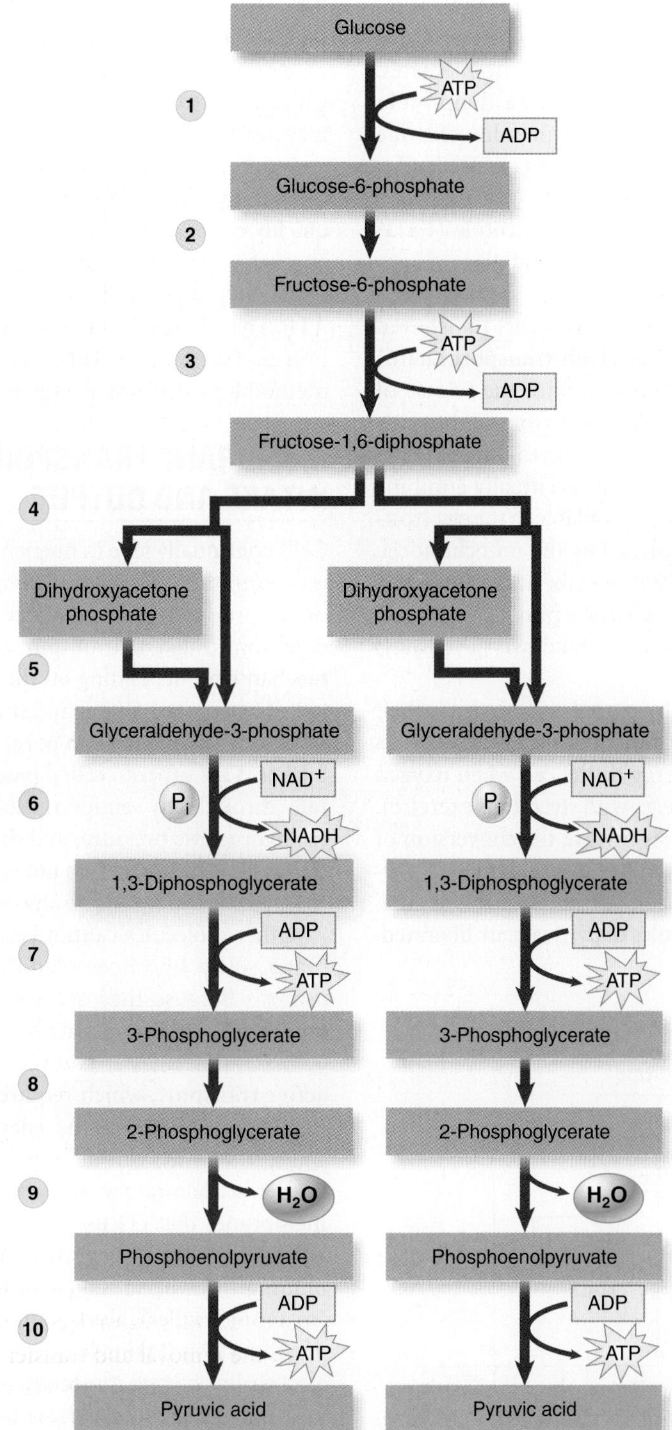

FIGURE 1-25 **Glycolysis.** Each of the numbered reactions is catalyzed by a different enzyme. At step **4,** a six-carbon sugar is broken down to give two, three-carbon sugars, so that the number of molecules at every step after this is doubled. Reactions **5** and **6** are the reactions responsible for the net synthesis of adenosine triphosphate *(ATP)* and reduced nicotinamide adenine dinucleotide *(NADH)* molecules. (From Patton KT, Thibodeau GA: *Anatomy & physiology,* ed 8, St Louis, 2013, Mosby.)

It begins with the citric acid cycle and ends with oxidative phosphorylation. About two thirds of the total oxidation of carbon compounds in most cells is accomplished during this phase. The major end products are carbon dioxide (CO_2) and two dinucleotides—reduced nicotinamide adenine dinucleotide (NADH) and the reduced form of flavin adenine dinucleotide ($FADH_2$)—which transfer their electrons into the electron-transport chain.

Oxidative Phosphorylation

Oxidative phosphorylation occurs in the mitochondria and is the mechanism by which the energy produced from carbohydrates, fats, and proteins is transferred to ATP. During the breakdown (catabolism) of foods, many of the reactions involve the removal of electrons from various intermediates. These reactions generally require a coenzyme (a nonprotein carrier molecule), such as nicotinamide adenine dinucleotide (NAD), to transfer the electrons and thus are called **transfer reactions.**

Molecules of NAD and flavin adenine dinucleotide (FAD) transfer electrons they have gained from the oxidation of substrates to molecular oxygen, O_2. The electrons from reduced NAD and FAD, NADH and $FADH_2$, respectively, are transferred to a series of carrier molecules (the **electron-transport chain**) on the inner surfaces of the mitochondria with the release of hydrogen ions. Some carrier molecules are a group of brightly colored iron-containing proteins known as **cytochromes** that accept a pair of electrons. These electrons eventually combine with molecular oxygen. If oxygen is not available to the electron-transport chain, ATP will not be formed by the mitochondria. Instead, an anaerobic (without oxygen) metabolic pathway synthesizes ATP. This process, called **substrate phosphorylation,** or **anaerobic glycolysis,** is linked to the breakdown (glycolysis) of carbohydrate (Figure 1-26).

Because glycolysis occurs in the cytoplasm of the cell, it provides energy for cells that lack mitochondria. However, as noted, glycolysis also provides energy to the cell when oxygen delivery is insufficient or delayed (e.g., with strenuous exercise). The reactions in anaerobic glycolysis involve the conversion of glucose to pyruvic acid (pyruvate) with the simultaneous production of ATP. With the glycolysis of one molecule of glucose, two ATP molecules and two molecules of pyruvate are liberated.

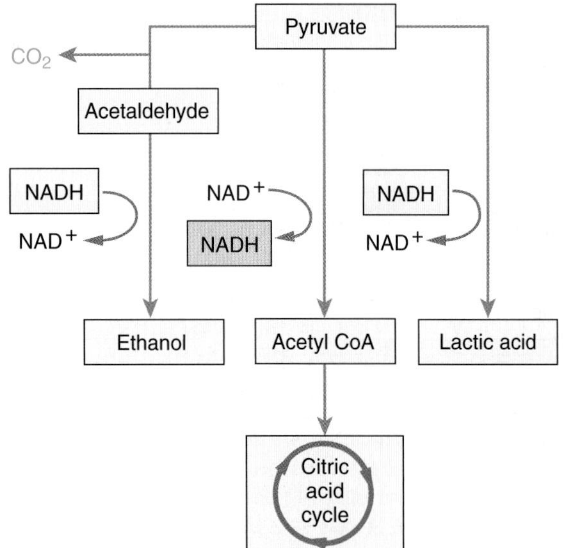

FIGURE 1-26 What Happens to Pyruvate, the Product of Glycolysis? In the presence of oxygen, pyruvate is oxidized to acetyl coenzyme A *(acetyl CoA)* and enters the citric acid cycle. In the absence of oxygen, pyruvate instead is reduced, accepting the electrons extracted during glycolysis and carried by reduced nicotinamide adenine dinucleotide *(NADH).* When pyruvate is reduced directly, as it is in muscle, the product is lactic acid. When CO_2 is first removed from pyruvate and the remainder reduced, as it is in yeasts, the product is ethanol.

If oxygen is present, the two molecules of pyruvate move into the mitochondria, where they enter the citric acid cycle.

If oxygen is absent, pyruvate is converted to lactic acid, which is released into the extracellular fluid (see Figure 1-26). Elevated lactate level is indicative of tissue hypoxia or low oxygen concentration. The conversion of pyruvic acid to lactic acid is reversible; therefore, once oxygen is restored, lactic acid is quickly converted back to either pyruvic acid or glucose. The anaerobic generation of ATP from glucose, through the reactions of glycolysis, is not as efficient as the aerobic generation of ATP. The addition of an oxygen-requiring stage to the catabolic process (stage 3) provides cells with a much more powerful method for extracting energy from food molecules.

MEMBRANE TRANSPORT: CELLULAR INTAKE AND OUTPUT

Cells continually take in nutrients, fluids, and chemical messengers from the extracellular environment and expel metabolites or the products of metabolism and end products of lysosomal digestion. Intake and output, or transport, occur by different mechanisms, depending on the characteristics of the substance to be transported. Water and small electrically uncharged molecules move easily through pores in the plasma membrane's lipid bilayer. This process, called **passive transport,** will occur naturally through any semipermeable barrier. It is driven by osmosis, hydrostatic pressure, and diffusion, all of which depend on the laws of physics and do not require life. The process is passive in that it does not require any expenditure of energy by the cell.

Other molecules cannot be driven across the plasma membrane solely by forces of diffusion, hydrostatic pressure, or osmosis because they are too large or are ligands that have bound with receptors on the cell's plasma membrane. Some of these molecules are moved into the cell by mechanisms of **active transport,** which requires life, biologic activity, and the expenditure of metabolic energy by the cell. Unlike passive transport, which can be duplicated across any semipermeable barrier in a laboratory, active transport occurs only across living membranes that (1) use energy generated by cellular metabolism and (2) have receptors that are capable of recognizing and binding with the substance to be transported. Large molecules (macromolecules), along with fluids, are transported by means of endocytosis (taking in) and exocytosis (expelling). Water and electrically charged molecules are transported by protein channels embedded in the plasma membrane. Ligands enter the cell by means of receptor-mediated endocytosis.

Movement of Water and Solutes

Cellular membranes are semipermeable and generally allow passage of water and small particles of dissolved substances called **solutes.** The movement of solute molecules through membranes is related to their size, solubility, electrical properties, and concentration on either side of the membrane (also see Chapter 3). Small lipid-soluble particles, such as oxygen, carbon dioxide, and urea, can readily pass through the lipid bilayers of the plasma membrane. Larger, water-soluble particles may pass through pores in the membranes. Although large protein molecules, such as albumin and globulin, pass through membranes by endocytosis, they influence the movement of water by exerting an osmotic effect (see p. 30).

Body fluids are composed of two types of solutes: **electrolytes,** which are electrically charged and dissociate into constituent **ions** when placed in solution; and nonelectrolytes, such as glucose, urea, and creatinine, which do not dissociate. Electrolytes account for approximately 95% of the solute molecules in body water. Electrolytes exhibit **polarity** by orienting themselves toward the positive or negative pole. Ions with a positive charge are known as **cations** and migrate toward the negative pole, or cathode, if an electrical current is passed through the electrolyte solution. **Anions** carry a negative charge and migrate toward the positive pole, or anode, in the presence of electrical current. Anions and cations are located in both the intracellular fluid (ICF) and extracellular fluid (ECF) compartments, although the concentration of particular ions varies depending on their location. (Fluid and electrolyte balance between body compartments is discussed in Chapter 3.) For example, Na^+ is the predominant extracellular cation, and K^+ is the principal intracellular cation. The difference in ICF and ECF concentrations of these ions is important to the transmission of electrical impulses across the plasma membranes of nerve and muscle cells.

Electrolytes are measured in milliequivalents per liter (mEq/L) or milligrams per deciliter (mg/dl). Milliequivalents per liter indicate the number of electrical charges per unit volume of fluid. The term *milliequivalent* thus indicates the chemical-combining activity of an ion, which depends on the electrical charge, or valence, of its ions. In abbreviations, valence is indicated by the number of plus or minus signs. Monovalent ions, or ions with one charge, include sodium (Na^+), chloride (Cl^-), and potassium (K^+). Divalent ions, which have two charges, include calcium (Ca^{++}) and magnesium (Mg^{++}). One milliequivalent of any cation can combine chemically with 1 mEq of any anion: one monovalent anion will combine with one monovalent cation. Divalent ions combine more strongly than monovalent ions. To maintain electrochemical balance, one divalent ion will combine with two monovalent ions (e.g., $Ca^{++} + 2\,Cl^- = CaCl_2$).

Passive Transport: Diffusion, Filtration, and Osmosis

Diffusion. **Diffusion** is the movement of a solute molecule from an area of greater solute concentration to an area of lesser solute concentration. This difference in concentration is known as a **concentration gradient.** Particles in a solution move randomly in any direction. If the concentration of particles in one part of the solution is greater than that in another part, the particles distribute themselves evenly throughout the solution. According to the same principle, if the concentration of particles is greater on one side of a *permeable membrane* than on the other side, the particles diffuse spontaneously from the area of greater concentration to the area of lesser concentration until equilibrium is reached. The higher the concentration on one side, the greater the diffusion rate. The overall effect of diffusion is the passive movement of particles "down" a concentration gradient, that is, from an area of high concentration to an area of low concentration.

The diffusion rate is influenced by differences of electrical potential across the membrane (see p. 36). Because the pores in the lipid bilayer are often linked with Ca^{++}, other cations (e.g., Na^+ and K^+) diffuse slowly because they are repelled by positive charges in the pores.

The rate of diffusion of a substance depends also on its size (diffusion coefficient) and its lipid solubility (Figure 1-27). Usually the smaller the molecule and the more soluble it is in oil, the more hydrophobic or nonpolar it is and the more rapidly it will diffuse across the bilayer. Oxygen, carbon dioxide, and the steroid hormones are all examples of nonpolar molecules. Water-soluble substances, such as sugars and inorganic ions, diffuse very slowly, whereas uncharged lipophilic ("lipid-loving") molecules, such as fatty acids and steroids, diffuse rapidly. Ions and other polar molecules generally diffuse across cellular membranes more slowly than lipid-soluble substances.

Water readily diffuses through biologic membranes because water molecules are small and uncharged. Although the mechanism is not known with certainty, the dipolar structure of water allows it to cross rapidly through the regions of the bilayer containing the lipid head groups. Lipid head groups constitute the two outer regions of the lipid bilayer.

Filtration: Hydrostatic Pressure. **Filtration** is the movement of water and solutes through a membrane because of a greater pushing pressure (force) on one side of the membrane than on the other side. **Hydrostatic pressure** is the mechanical force of water pushing against cellular membranes (Figure 1-28, *A*). In the vascular system, hydrostatic pressure is the *blood pressure* generated in vessels by the contraction of the heart. Blood

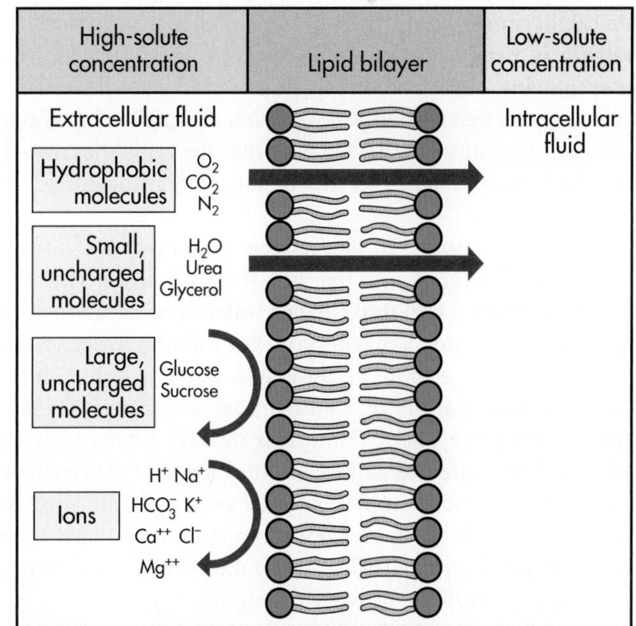

FIGURE 1-27 Passive Diffusion of Solute Molecules Across the Plasma Membrane. Oxygen, nitrogen, water, urea, glycerol, and carbon dioxide can diffuse readily down the concentration gradient. Macromolecules are too large to diffuse through pores in the plasma membrane. Ions may be repelled if the pores contain substances with identical charges. If the pores are lined with cations, for example, other cations will have difficulty diffusing because the positive charges will repel one another. Diffusion can still occur, but it occurs more slowly.

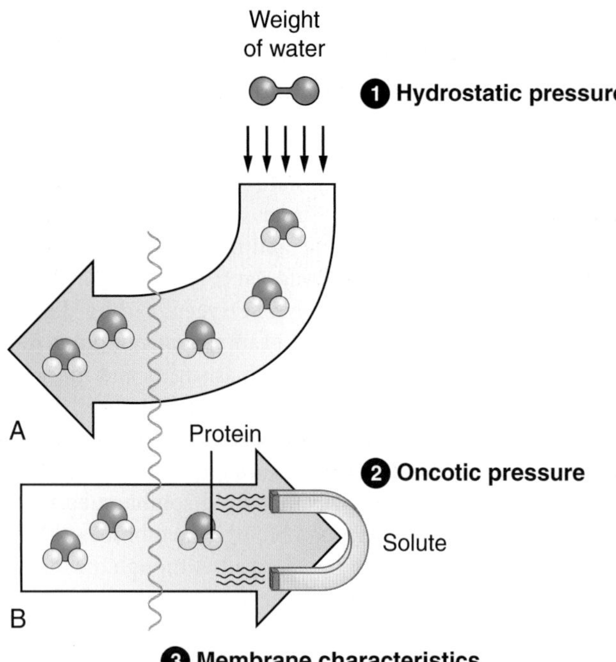

FIGURE 1-28 Hydrostatic Pressure and Oncotic Pressure in Plasma. **1,** Hydrostatic pressure in plasma. **2,** Oncotic pressure exerted by proteins in the plasma usually tends to *pull* water into the circulatory system. **3,** Individuals with low protein levels (e.g., starvation) are unable to maintain a normal oncotic pressure; therefore, water is not reabsorbed into the circulation and, instead, causes body edema.

reaching the capillary bed has a hydrostatic pressure of 25 to 30 mmHg, which is sufficient force to push water across the thin capillary membranes into the interstitial space. Hydrostatic pressure is partially balanced by osmotic pressure, whereby water moving *out* of the capillaries is partially balanced by osmotic forces that tend to *pull* water *into* the capillaries. Water that is not osmotically attracted back into the capillaries moves into the lymph system (see discussion of Starling forces in Chapter 3).

Osmosis. **Osmosis** is the movement of water "down" a concentration gradient, that is, across a semipermeable membrane from a region of higher water concentration to a region of lower water concentration. For osmosis to occur, the membrane must be more permeable to water than to solutes and the concentration of solutes must be greater so that water moves more easily. Osmosis is directly related to both hydrostatic pressure and solute concentration but *not* to particle size or weight. For example, particles of the plasma protein albumin are small but more concentrated in body fluids than the larger and heavier particles of globulin. Therefore, albumin exerts a greater osmotic force than globulin.

Osmolality controls distribution and movement of water between body compartments. The terms *osmolality* and *osmolarity* are often used interchangeably in reference to osmotic activity, but they define different measurements. **Osmolality** is a measure of the number of milliosmoles per kilogram (mOsm/kg) of water, or the concentration of molecules per *weight* of water. **Osmolarity** is a measure of the number of milliosmoles per liter (mOsm/L) of solution, or the concentration of molecules per *volume* of solution. When solute is added to water, the volume is expanded and includes the original liter of water plus the volume occupied by the solute particles. In measuring osmolarity, the volume of water is therefore reduced by an amount equal to the volume of added solute.

In solutions that contain only dissociable substances, such as Na^+ and Cl^-, the difference between the two measurements is negligible. In considering all the different solutes in plasma (e.g., proteins, glucose, lipids), however, the difference between osmolality and osmolarity becomes more significant. In plasma, less of the plasma weight is water and the overall concentration of particles is therefore greater. The osmolality will be greater than the osmolarity because of the smaller proportion of water. Osmolality is thus the preferred measure of osmotic activity in clinical assessment of individuals.

The normal osmolality of body fluids is 280 to 294 mOsm/kg. The osmolality of intracellular and extracellular fluid tends to equalize and so provides a measure of body fluid concentration and thus the body's hydration status (see Chapter 3). Hydration is also affected by hydrostatic pressure because the movement of water by osmosis can be opposed by an equal amount of hydrostatic pressure. The amount of hydrostatic pressure required to oppose the osmotic movement of water is called the **osmotic pressure** of the solution. Factors that determine osmotic pressure are the type and thickness of the plasma membrane, the size of the molecules, the concentration of molecules or the concentration gradient, and the solubility of molecules within the membrane. Examples of movement of water in relation to hydrostatic and osmotic forces occur in the glomerulus of the kidney (see Chapter 37) and in the capillaries of the microcirculation (see Chapter 31).

Effective osmolality is sustained osmotic activity and depends on the concentration of solutes remaining on one side of a permeable membrane. If the solutes penetrate the membrane and equilibrate with the solution on the other side of the membrane, the osmotic effect will be diminished or lost. For example, urea is a small solute that readily diffuses across cellular membranes. Solutions containing urea rapidly lose their effective osmolality because they rapidly equilibrate. Solutes too large to pass through the membrane thus sustain an effective osmolality, meaning that they enhance osmotic activity. Plasma proteins are examples of molecules that provide effective osmolality because they normally do not cross cellular membranes.

Plasma proteins also influence osmolality because they have a negative charge (see Figure 1-28, *B*). The principle by which the plasma protein charge influences osmolality is known as *Gibbs-Donnan equilibrium,* and it affects the distribution of ions across cellular membranes. Gibbs-Donnan equilibrium occurs when fluid in one compartment contains small, diffusible ions such as Na^+ and Cl^-, together with large, nondiffusible charged particles, such as plasma proteins. Because the body tends to maintain an electrical equilibrium, the nondiffusible protein molecules cause asymmetry in the distribution of small ions. Anions such as Cl^- are thus driven out of the cell or plasma, and cations such as Na^+ are attracted. The protein-containing compartment will maintain a state of electroneutrality, but the osmolality will be higher. The overall osmotic effect of colloids, such as plasma proteins, is called the **oncotic pressure,** or **colloid osmotic pressure.**

Tonicity describes the effective osmolality of a solution. (The terms *osmolality* and *tonicity* may be used interchangeably; also see Chapter 3.) Solutions, then, have relative degrees of tonicity. An **isotonic solution** (or isoosmotic solution) has the same osmolality or concentration of particles (285 mOsm/kg) as the ICF or ECF. Diarrhea, for example, is loss of isoosmotic fluid from the gastrointestinal tract. As a result, ECF volume decreases but there is no change in ECF osmolarity. Examples of isotonic solutions include 5% dextrose in water and normal (0.9%) saline solution. A **hypotonic solution** has a lower concentration and is thus more dilute than body fluids. Water is a hypotonic solution. Consequently, water is osmotically pulled into the cells, causing them to swell or burst. A **hypertonic solution** has a concentration of more than 285 to 294 mOsm/kg. An example of a hypertonic solution is 3% saline solution. Water can be pulled out of the cells by a hypertonic solution, so the cells shrink. The concept of tonicity is important when correcting water and solute imbalances by administering different types of replacement solutions.

Mediated and Active Transport

Mediated Transport. **Mediated transport** (passive and active) involves integral or transmembrane proteins with receptors having a high degree of specificity for the substance being transported. Inorganic anions and cations (e.g., Na^+, K^+, Ca^{++}, Cl^-, HCO^-_3) and charged and uncharged organic compounds (e.g., amino acids, sugars) require specific transport systems to facilitate movement through different cellular membranes. Rates at which substances are moved by mediated transport mechanisms have often been measured, yet the specific membrane proteins involved have not been identified. Mediated transport is much faster than simple diffusion.

A **transport protein** (carrier protein) is a transmembrane or integral protein that binds with and transfers a specific solute molecule across the lipid bilayer. (Proteins are discussed on p. 13.) Each transport protein, or transporter, has receptors for a specific solute. When the transporter is saturated—that is, when all receptor sites are occupied by solute molecules—the rate of transport is maximal. Solute binding can be blocked by **competitive inhibitors** that compete for the same receptor site and may or may not be transported by the transport protein. Noncompetitive inhibitors bind elsewhere but can alter the structure of the transporter.

The transporter protein is a multipass transmembrane protein; that is, its polypeptide chain crosses the lipid bilayer multiple times. This chain forms a continuous pathway enabling solutes to pass across the membrane without coming into direct contact with the hydrophobic interior of the lipid bilayer (Figure 1-29).

Another mechanism of mediated transport is the channel protein. The protein transporter creates a water-filled pore or channel across the bilayer through which specific ions can diffuse. These channels are sometimes called *ion channels,* and because they are permeable mainly to K^+, they are also called K^+ *leak channels* (Figure 1-30). The channel is controlled by a gate mechanism that determines which receptor-bound solutes can move into the channel that is created after receptor-solute contact. Binding stimulates conformational changes in the protein transporter that move the solute through the channel short distances at a time until it reaches the other side of the membrane. Ion channels are responsible for the electrical excitability of nerve and muscle cells and play a critical role in the membrane potential.

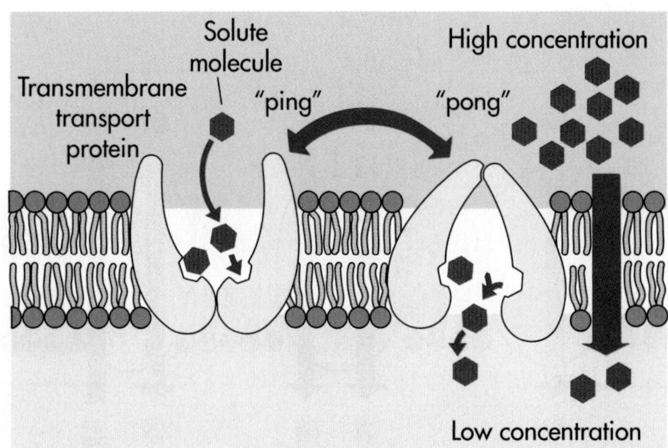

FIGURE 1-29 Conformational-Change Model of Mediated Transport (Facilitated Diffusion). The transporter protein has two states, "ping" and "pong." In the ping state, sites for molecules of a specific solute are exposed on the outside of the bilayer. In the pong state, the sites are exposed to the inner side of the bilayer.

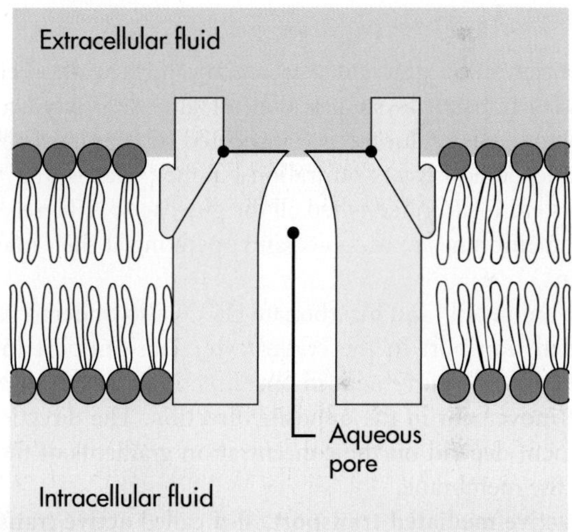

FIGURE 1-30 Channel Mode of Mediated Transport (Facilitated Diffusion). A channel protein forms a water-filled pore across the bilayer through which specific ions can diffuse.

Mediated transport systems can move solute molecules singly or two at a time. Two molecules can be moved simultaneously in one direction (a process called **symport**) or in opposite directions (called **antiport**), or a single molecule can be moved in one direction (called **uniport**) (Figure 1-31).

In **passive mediated transport,** also called **facilitated diffusion,** the protein transporter moves solute molecules through cellular membranes without expending metabolic energy. The direction of movement is the same as in simple diffusion—down

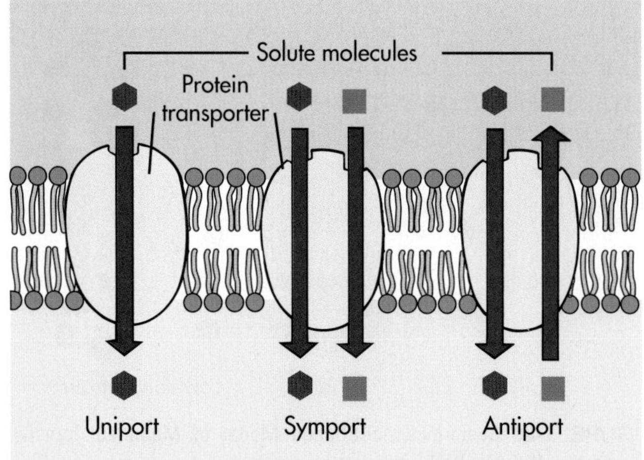

FIGURE 1-31 Mediated Transport. Simultaneous movement of a single solute molecule in one direction (uniport), of two different solute molecules in one direction (symport), and of two different solute molecules in opposite directions (antiport).

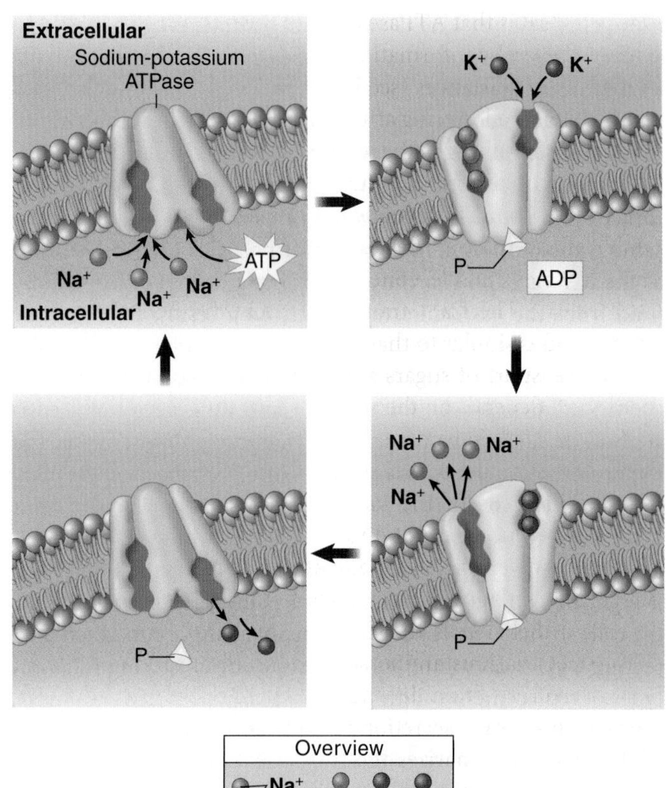

FIGURE 1-32 Active Transport and the Sodium-Potassium Pump. Three Na^+ ions bind to sodium-binding sites on the carrier's inner face. At the same time an energy-containing adenosine triphosphate (ATP) molecule produced by the cell's mitochondria binds to the carrier. The ATP breaks apart, transferring its stored energy to the carrier. The carrier then changes shape, releases the three Na^+ ions to the outside of the cell, and attracts two K^+ ions to its potassium-binding sites. The carrier then returns to its original shape, releasing the two K^+ ions and the remnant of the ATP molecule to the inside of the cell. The carrier is now ready for another pumping cycle. (From Patton KT, Thibodeau GA: *Anatomy & physiology,* ed 8, St Louis, 2013, Mosby.)

the concentration gradient. Perhaps the most widely referred to passive transport system is that for glucose in erythrocytes (red blood cells). Glucose is transported by a uniport mechanism and demonstrates saturation kinetics; that is, the transport system is saturated when all the glucose-specific receptors on the membrane are occupied and operating at their maximal capacity.

The anions Cl^- and bicarbonate HCO_3^- also undergo passive mediated transport in the erythrocyte. This antiport mechanism allows Cl^- movement in one direction and simultaneous HCO_3^- movement in the opposite direction. The directions of movement depend on the concentration gradients of the ions across the membrane.

In **active mediated transport,** also called **active transport,** the protein transporter moves molecules against, or up, the concentration gradient. Unlike passive mediated transport, active mediated transport requires the expenditure of energy. Many active mediated transport systems, or pumps, have ATP as their primary energy source, but not all. Some use the electrochemical gradient of Na^+ across the membrane (Figure 1-32). Energy in the form of ATP, however, is required for activation of the Na^+ gradient.

A "carrier" mechanism in the plasma membrane mediates the transport of ions, such as Na^+, K^+, H^+, Cl^-, and HCO_3^-, and of nutrients, such as glucose and amino acids. Energy supplied by ATP is required to pump ions against a concentration gradient. The best known pump is the Na^+– K^+–dependent ATPase pump. It continuously regulates the cell's volume by controlling leaks through pores or protein channels and maintains the ionic concentration gradient necessary for cellular excitation and membrane conductivity (see below). The maintenance of intracellular K^+ concentrations is also required for enzyme activity, including that of enzymes involved in protein synthesis.

Active Transport of Na^+ and K^+. The active transport system for Na^+ and K^+ is found in virtually all mammalian cells. The Na^+-K^+ antiport system (Na^+ moving out of and K^+ moving into the cell) uses the direct energy of ATP to move these cations. The transporter protein is an enzyme, adenosine triphosphatase (ATPase). ATPase has a requirement for Na^+, K^+, and Mg^{++} ions. The concentration of ATPase in plasma membranes is directly related to Na^+-K^+ transport activity. Approximately 60% to 70% of the ATP synthesized by cells, especially muscle and nerve cells, is used to maintain the Na^+-K^+ transport system. Excitable tissues (e.g., muscle and nerve tissues) have a high concentration of Na^+-K^+ ATPase, as do other tissues that transport significant amounts of Na^+, for example, kidneys and salivary glands. For every ATP molecule hydrolyzed, three molecules of Na^+ are transported out of the cell, whereas only two molecules of K^+ move into the cell. The process leads to an electrical potential and is called *electrogenic,* with the inside of the cell more negative than the outside. The exact mechanism for transport of Na^+ and K^+ across the membrane is uncertain.

One proposal is that ATPase induces the transporter protein to undergo several conformational changes, causing Na^+ and K^+ to move short distances (see Figure 1-32). The conformational change creates a lowering affinity for Na^+ and K^+ to the ATPase transporter, resulting in the release of the cations after transport.

The sarcoplasmic reticulum of heart muscle and skeletal muscle has an ATP-dependent Ca^{++} active transport system that regulates the Ca^{++} levels in the cell's cytoplasm, which in turn regulates muscle contraction and relaxation cycles (see Chapter 31). The Ca^{++} transport system depends on ATPase activity and is similar to that of Na^+-K^+ ATPase.

The transport of sugars and amino acids across the plasma membrane depends on the simultaneous movement (symport) of Na^+ or Na^+-dependent transport (see Figure 1-31). Na^+-dependent symport occurs primarily in the plasma membrane of epithelial cells of the kidney tubules and intestines. The transport of glucose is not directly dependent on the hydrolysis of ATP; however, the Na^+ gradient is ATP dependent, and thus ATP is indirectly involved in glucose transport.

The epithelial cells that line the intestines depend on Na^+ to transport various amino acids. Similarly, the uptake of Cl^- by the small intestine depends on Na^+ symport and antiport mechanisms for the secretion of Ca^{++} from the cell.

Table 1-5 summarizes the major mechanisms of transport through pores and protein transporters in the plasma membranes. Many disease states are caused or manifested by loss of these membrane transport systems.

TABLE 1-5 MAJOR TRANSPORT SYSTEMS IN MAMMALIAN CELLS*

SUBSTANCE TRANSPORTED	MECHANISM OF TRANSPORT	TISSUES
Sugars		
Glucose	Passive protein channel	Most tissues
Fructose	Active: symport with Na^+	Small intestines and renal tubular cells
	Passive	Intestines and liver
Amino Acids	Coupled channels	
Amino acid–specific transporters	Active: symport with Na^+	Intestines, kidney, and liver
All amino acids except proline	Active: group translocation	Liver
Specific amino acids	Passive	Small intestine
Other Organic Molecules		
Cholic acid, deoxycholic acid, and taurocholic acid	Active: symport with Na^+	Intestines
Organic anions (e.g., malate, α-ketoglutarate, glutamate)	Antiport with counter–organic anion	Mitochondria of liver cells
ATP-ADP	Antiport transport of nucleotides; can be active	Mitochondria of liver cells
Inorganic Ions		
Na^+	Passive	Distal renal tubular cells
Na^+/H^+	Active antiport, proton pump	Proximal renal tubular cells and small intestines
Na^+/K^+	Active: ATP driven, protein channel	Plasma membrane of most cells
Ca^{++}	Active: ATP driven, antiport with Na^+	All cells, antiporter in red cells
H^+/K^+	Active	Parietal cells of gastric cells secreting H^+
Cl^-/HCO_3^- (perhaps other anions)	Mediated: antiport (anion transporter–band 3 protein)	Erythrocytes and many other cells
Water	Osmosis passive	All tissues

Data from Alberts B et al: *Molecular biology of the cell,* ed 5, New York, 2008, Garland; Devlin TM, editor: *Textbook of biochemistry: with clinical correlations,* ed 3, New York, 1992, Wiley; Raven PH, Johnson GB: *Understanding biology,* ed 3, Dubuque, IA, 1995, Brown.

ADP, Adenosine diphosphate; *ATP,* adenosine triphosphate.

***Note:** The known transport systems are listed here; others have been proposed. Most transport systems have been studied in only a few tissues, and their sites of activity may be more limited than indicated.

Transport by Vesicle Formation

Endocytosis

Endocytosis is a cellular internalizing process where a section of the plasma membrane enfolds substances from outside the cell, invaginates (folds inward), and separates from the plasma membrane, forming a vesicle that moves into the inside of the cell (Figure 1-33, *A*). Endocytosis mediates cellular uptake of nutrients, regulates quantities of proteins in the plasma membrane, controls the signaling output of receptors, and is used by pathogens to gain entry into cells.[28] Thus endocytosis is important to counterbalance exocytosis and maintain homeostasis. Transport of nutrients involves the sequential formation and fission of membrane-bound vesicles.

Different mechanisms mediate endocytotic uptake of a large variety of distinctly sized cargoes, ranging from small molecules such as receptor ligands to large cargoes including viruses, bacteria, and extracellular aggregates.[29] Depending on the size of the cargoes and other factors binding of ligands on the cell surface activates appropriate intracellular mechanisms that then trigger changes in membrane shape to mediate their cell entry (Figure 1-34). Endocytosis can be subdivided into four different categories: (1) clathrin-mediated endocytosis, (2) caveolae-mediated endocytosis, (3) macropinocytosis, and (4) phagocytosis. Over time, however, these categories may change.

Because most cells continually ingest fluid and solutes by **pinocytosis,** the terms *pinocytosis* (cell ingestion of extracellular fluid and its contents) and *endocytosis* are often used interchangeably. **Micropinocytosis** is the taking up of specific macromolecules by invagination of the cell membrane, which is then pinched off, forming a small vesicle in the cytoplasm. In micropinocytosis the vesicle containing fluids, solutes, or both, fuses with a lysosome and lysosomal enzymes digest them for use by the cell. **Macropinocytosis** is when large droplets of fluid are trapped underneath the ruffles of the cell membrane.

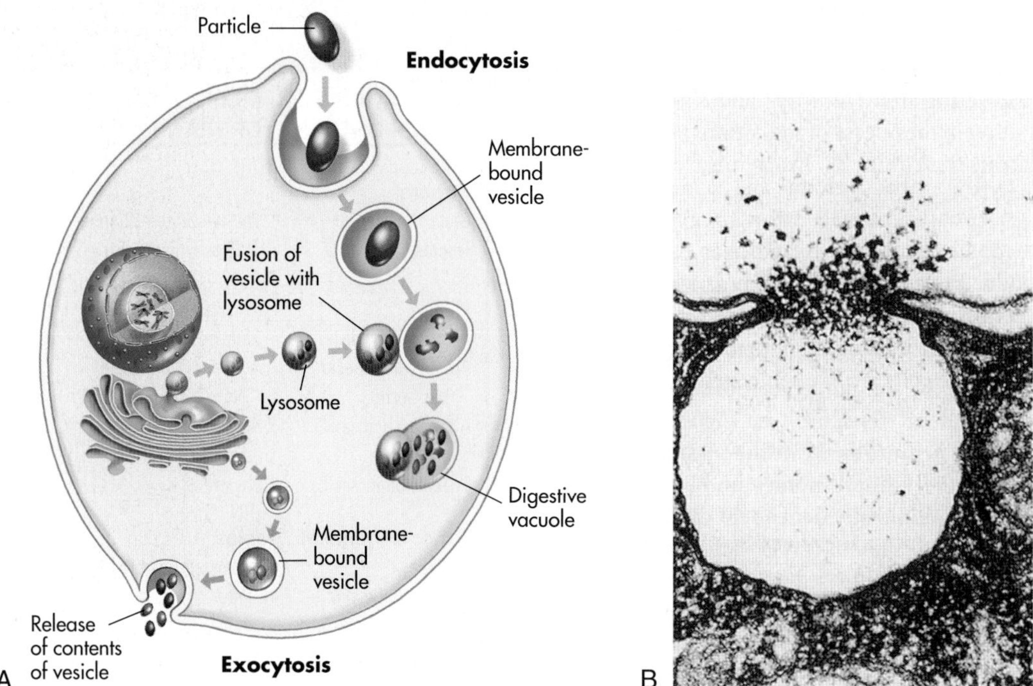

FIGURE 1-33 **Endocytosis and Exocytosis. A,** Endocytosis and fusion with lysosome and exocytosis. **B,** Electron micrograph of exocytosis. (**B** from Raven PH et al: *Biology,* ed 8, New York, 2008, McGraw-Hill.)

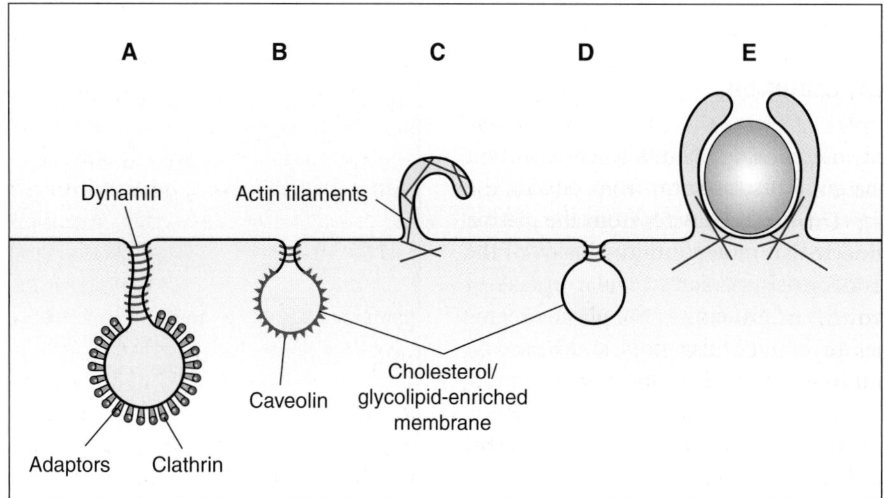

FIGURE 1-34 **Multiple Pathways of Endocytosis.** The pathways of endocytosis depend on the class of cargo (receptors, ligands, and lipid-associated molecules), the mechanism of vesicle formation (coats, GTPases, and dynamin), and the size of the endocytotic vesicle that eventually pinches off into the cytoplasm. **A,** *Clathrin-mediated endocytosis* (CME) uses adaptor proteins that link cargo proteins to the clathrin scaffold, forming the endocytotic vesicle. **B,** *Caveolae,* formed by caveolin proteins, are adorned in cholesterol, sphingolipids, and glycolipids believed concentrated in membrane microdomains. **C,** During *macropinocytosis* fluid-phase uptake is dependent on actin-driven membrane protrusions that enclose extracellular fluid and fuse with the plasma membrane. **D,** Some cargoes associate with membrane microdomains that eventually are internalized in a clathrin- and caveolin-independent manner. Different modes of internalization are distinguished by their dependence on dynamin, a membrane-remodeling GTPase. **E,** *Phagocytosis* mediates internalization by membrane protrusions formed around large, ligand-coated molecules. (Adapted from Krauss M, Haucke V: *Rev Physiol Biochem Pharmacol* 161:45–66, 2011.)

Macropinocytosis is an important pathway for antigen presentation by specialized antigen presenting cells.[30] In **phagocytosis** the large molecular substances are engulfed by the plasma membrane and enter the cell so that they can be isolated and destroyed by lysosomal enzymes (see Chapter 7). Substances that are not degraded by lysosomes are isolated in residual bodies and released by the cell by exocytosis. Both pinocytosis and phagocytosis require metabolic energy and often involve binding of the substance with plasma membrane receptors before membrane invagination and fusion with lysosomes in the cell.

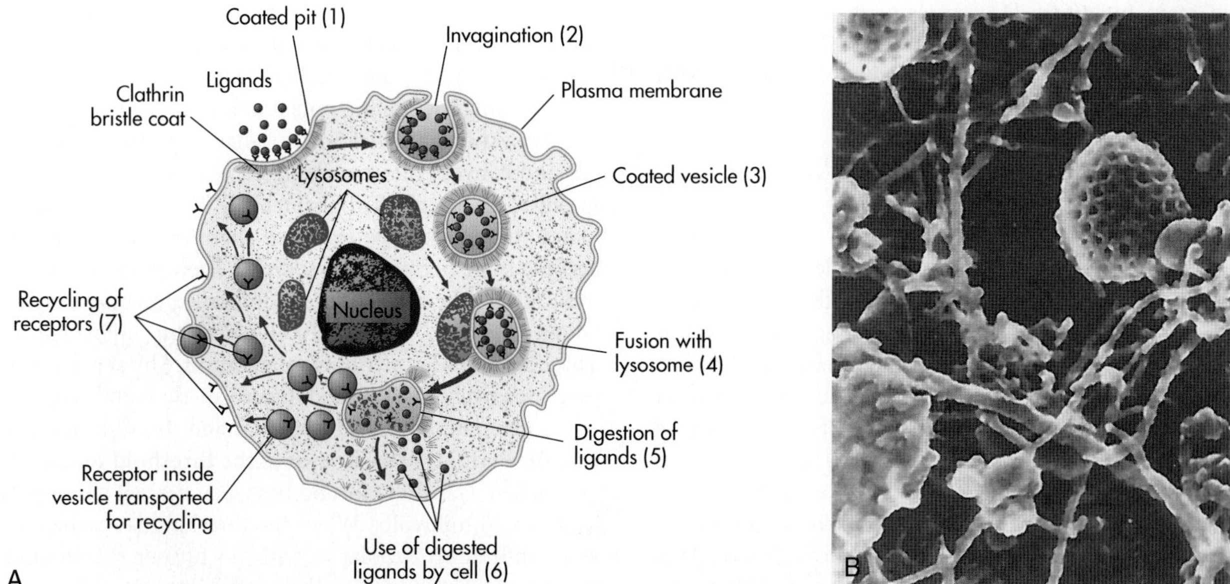

FIGURE 1-35 Ligand Internalization by Means of Receptor-Mediated Endocytosis. **A,** The ligand attaches to its surface receptor (through the bristle coat or clathrin coat) and, through receptor-mediated endocytosis, enters the cell **(1-3).** The ingested material fuses with a lysosome **(4)** and is processed by hydrolytic lysosomal enzymes **(5).** Processed molecules can then be transferred to other cellular components **(6)** or recycled **(7). B,** Electron micrograph of a coated pit showing different sizes of filaments (× 382,000). (**B** from Erlandsen SL, Magney JE: *Color atlas of histology,* St Louis, 1992, Mosby.)

Clathrin-Mediated Endocytosis. Ligand binding to *some* plasma membrane receptors leads to clustering, aggregation, and immobilization of the receptors in specialized areas of the membrane called **coated pits** (Figure 1-35). The pits, which are coated with a complex of proteins and cytosolic bristle-like structures (or clathrin), deepen and enfold (invaginate), internalizing ligand-receptor complexes and forming clathrin coated vesicles (CCVs). This internalization process, called **clathrin-mediated endocytosis,** is rapid and enables the cell to ingest large amounts of specific ligands, for example, low-density lipoprotein, growth factors, and antibodies, without ingesting large volumes of extracellular fluid. Additionally, clathrin is required for the internalization of pumps and transporters for ions and small nutrients to maintain homeostasis and synaptic transmission in neurons.[29] Inside the cell, the ingested material is processed by lysosomal enzymes.

Caveolae-Mediated Endocytosis. The outer surface of the plasma membrane is dimpled with tiny flask-shaped pits (cavelike) called caveolae. Caveolae are also called **microdomains. Caveolae** are cholesterol- and glycosphingolipid-rich microdomains where the protein caveolin is thought to be involved in several processes, including clathrin-independent endocytosis. Caveolae are present in most mammalian cell types and are abundant in endothelial and smooth muscle cells, adipocytes, and fibroblasts.[31] Although the role of caveolae in endocytic events is debated and still needs conclusive proof, caveolae-mediated endocytosis has been implicated in the endocytosis of simian virus 40 (SV40).[29] Additionally, evidence is accumulating that these microdomains are important in regulating endothelial cell functions mainly because they compartmentalize various signaling molecules.[31] Cavins have recently been found to be important in caveolae.[32,33]

Cavins are proteins present or isolated in caveolae and may be important for molecular organization of caveolae and certain protein degradations. Caveolae not only function as uptake vesicles but also are important sites for signal transduction (see p. 21). For example, strong evidence exists that plasma membrane estrogen receptors localize in caveolae and crosstalk with estradiol, causing several intracellular functions, including cell growth and survival, migration, and new blood vessel formation.[34-36]

Clathrin- and Caveolin-Independent Endocytosis. Some proteins or small molecules enter cells by clathrin- and caveolin-independent pathways (see Figure 1-34, *C* and *D*).[29] These routes are defined and classified by their requirements for dynamin during fission, and the regulatory roles of guanosinetriphosphatases (GTPases). The mechanism by which internalization occurs is not known but is thought to be dependent on cargo concentration and membrane curvature.

Exocytosis

In eukaryotic cells, secretion of macromolecules almost always occurs by exocytosis (see Figure 1-33, *B*). **Exocytosis** is the discharge or secretion of material from the intracellular vesicles at the cell surface. For example, to secrete macromolecules of insulin across plasma membranes, insulin-producing cells store and package insulin molecules in intracellular vesicles, which fuse with the plasma membrane and open to the extracellular space, or matrix, releasing the insulin. Not all secreted substances are secreted into the extracellular matrix. Some adhere to the plasma membrane and are thought to replace segments of the membrane lost through endocytosis or diffuse into the blood to nourish or signal other cells. Recent findings suggest membrane lipids may be a regulator of exocytosis.[37] Exocytosis has two main functions: (1) replacement of portions of the plasma membrane that have been removed by endocytosis, and (2) release of molecules synthesized by the cells into the extracellular matrix.

Movement of Electrical Impulses: Membrane Potentials

All body cells are electrically polarized, with the inside of the cell more negatively charged than the outside. The difference in electrical charge, or voltage, is known as the **resting membrane potential** and is about −70 to −85 millivolts. The difference in voltage across the plasma membrane is a result of the differences in ionic composition of ICF and ECF. Sodium ions have a greater concentration in the ECF, and potassium ions have a greater concentration in the ICF. The concentration difference is maintained by the active transport of Na^+ and K^+ (the sodium-potassium pump), which transports sodium outward and potassium inward (Figure 1-36). Because the resting plasma membrane is more permeable to K^+ than to Na^+, K^+ can diffuse easily from its area of higher concentration in the ICF to its area of lower concentration in the ECF. Because Na^+ and K^+ are both cations, the net result is an excess of anions inside the cell, resulting in the resting membrane potential.

Nerve and muscle cells are excitable and can change their resting membrane potential in response to electrochemical stimuli. Changes in resting membrane potential convey messages from cell to cell. When a nerve or muscle cell receives a stimulus that exceeds the membrane threshold value, there is a rapid change in the resting membrane potential known as the **action potential.** The action potential carries signals along the nerve or muscle cell and conveys information from one cell to another. (Nerve impulses are described in Chapter 15.) When a resting cell is stimulated through voltage-regulated channels, the cell membranes become more permeable to sodium. There is a net movement of sodium into the cell, and the membrane potential decreases, or "moves forward," from a negative value (in millivolts) to zero. This decrease is known as **depolarization.** The depolarized cell is more positively charged, and its polarity is neutralized.

To generate an action potential and the resulting depolarization, a critical value known as the **threshold potential** must be reached. Generally this occurs when the cell has depolarized by 15 to 20 millivolts. When the threshold is reached, the cell will continue to depolarize with no further stimulation. The sodium gates open, and sodium rushes into the cell, causing the membrane potential to reduce to zero and then become positive (depolarization). The rapid reversal in polarity results in the action potential.

During **repolarization** the negative polarity of the resting membrane potential is reestablished. As the voltage-gated sodium channels begin to close, voltage-gated potassium

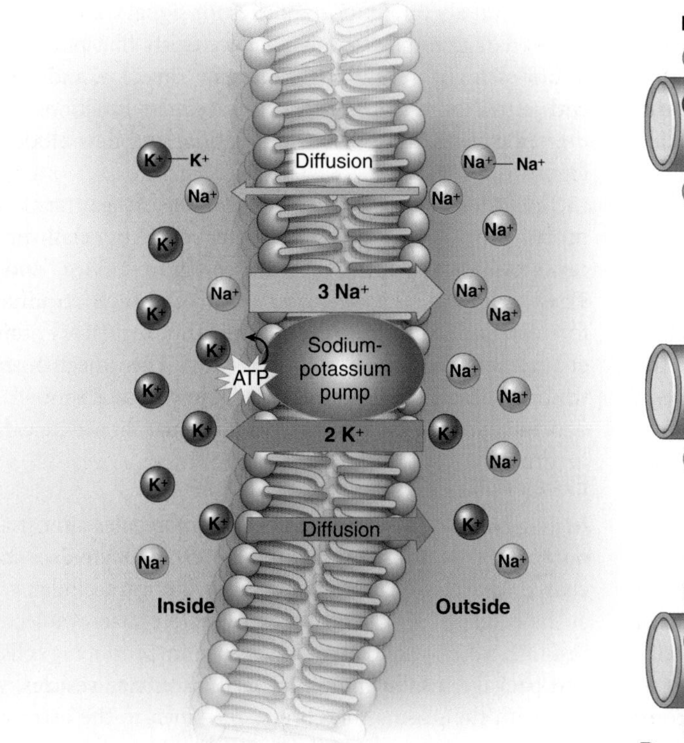

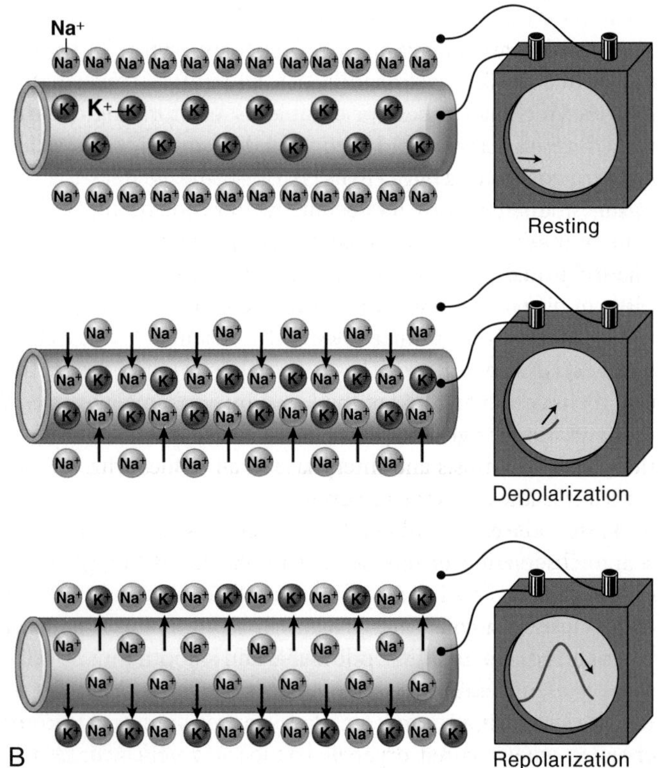

FIGURE 1-36 Sodium-Potassium Pump and Propagation of an Action Potential. **A,** Concentration difference of Na^+ and K^+ intracellularly and extracellularly. The direction of active transport by the sodium-potassium pump is also shown. **B,** Top diagram represents the polarized state of a neuronal membrane when at rest. The lower diagrams represent changes in sodium and potassium membrane permeabilities with depolarization and repolarization. (From Patton KT, Thibodeau GA: *Anatomy & physiology,* ed 8, St Louis, 2013, Mosby.)

channels open. Membrane permeability to sodium decreases, and potassium permeability increases, with an outward movement of potassium ions. The sodium gates close, and with the outward movement of potassium, the membrane potential becomes more negative. The Na^+-K^+ pump then returns the membrane to the resting potential by pumping potassium back into the cell and sodium out of the cell.

During most of the action potential, the plasma membrane cannot respond to an additional stimulus. This time is known as the **absolute refractory period** and is related to changes in permeability to sodium. During the latter phase of the action potential, when permeability to potassium increases, a stronger-than-normal stimulus can evoke an action potential, known as the **relative refractory period.**

When the membrane potential is more negative than normal, the cell is in a *hyperpolarized* (less excitable) state. A larger-than-normal stimulus is then required to reach the threshold potential and generate an action potential. When the membrane potential is more positive than normal, the cell is in a *hypopolarized* (more excitable than normal) state, and a smaller-than-normal stimulus is required to reach the threshold potential. Changes in the intracellular and extracellular concentration of ions or a change in membrane permeability can cause these alterations in membrane excitability. Understanding the mechanisms of ion movement and membrane excitability led to the discovery of calcium blocking agents for heart disease and migraine.

CELLULAR REPRODUCTION: THE CELL CYCLE

Human cells are subject to wear and tear, and most do not last for the lifetime of the individual. In almost all tissues, new cells are created as fast as old ones die. Cellular reproduction is therefore necessary for the maintenance of life. Reproduction of gametes (sperm and egg cells) occurs through a process called *meiosis,* described in Chapter 4. The reproduction, or division, of other body cells (somatic cells) involves two sequential phases: **mitosis,** or nuclear division, and **cytokinesis,** or cytoplasmic division. These two phases occur in close succession, with cytokinesis beginning toward the end of mitosis. Before a cell can divide, however, it must double its mass and duplicate all its contents. Most of the work of preparing for division occurs during the growth phase, called **interphase.** The alternation between mitosis and interphase in all tissues with cellular turnover is known as the **cell cycle.**

Most of the early work on the cell cycle was limited to microscopic observation of mitosis and cytokinesis. Interphase was considered the "resting stage" of the cell. With recent technologic advances a considerable amount has been learned about the interphase part of the cell cycle. During interphase many important processes are taking place as the cell produces DNA, RNA, protein, lipids, and other substances, and each pair of **chromosomes** (paired organelles that carry genetic information) makes exact copies of themselves.

The four designated phases of the cell cycle are (1) the G_1 phase (G = gap), which is the period between the M phase and the start of DNA synthesis; (2) the S phase (S = synthesis), in which DNA is synthesized in the cell nucleus; (3) the G_2 phase, in which RNA and protein synthesis occurs, the period between the completion of DNA synthesis and the next phase (M); and (4) the M phase (M = mitosis), which includes both nuclear and cytoplasmic division (Figure 1-37).

Phases of Mitosis and Cytokinesis

Interphase (the G_1, S, and G_2 phases) is the longest phase of the cell cycle. During interphase the chromatin consists of very long, slender rods that are jumbled together in the nucleus. Late in interphase, strands of **chromatin** (the substance that gives the nucleus its granular appearance) begin to coil, causing them to shorten and thicken.

The M phase of the cell cycle, mitosis and cytokinesis, begins with **prophase,** the first appearance of chromosomes. As the phase proceeds, each chromosome is seen as two identical halves called **chromatids,** which lie together and are attached at some point by a spindle attachment site called a **centromere.** (The two chromatids of each chromosome, which are genetically identical, are sometimes called *sister chromatids.*)

The nuclear membrane, which surrounds the nucleus, disappears. Spindle fibers are microtubules formed in the cytoplasm. **Spindle fibers** radiate from two centrioles located at opposite poles of the cell. The role of the spindle fibers is to pull the chromosomes to opposite sides of the cell.

During **metaphase,** the next phase of mitosis and cytokinesis, the spindle fibers begin to pull the centromeres of the chromosomes. The centromeres become aligned in the middle of the spindle, which is called the **equatorial plate** (or **metaphase plate**) of the cell. In this stage chromosomes are easiest to observe microscopically because they are highly condensed and arranged in a relatively organized fashion in the two-dimensional equatorial plate.

Anaphase begins when the centromeres split and the sister chromatids are pulled apart. The spindle fibers shorten, causing the sister chromatids to be pulled, centromere first, toward opposite sides of the cell. When the sister chromatids are separated, each is considered to be a chromosome. Thus the cell has 92 chromosomes during this stage. By the end of anaphase, 46 chromosomes are lying at each side of the cell. Barring mitotic errors, each of the two groups of 46 chromosomes is identical to the original 46 chromosomes present at the start of the cell cycle.

During **telophase,** the final stage, a new nuclear membrane is formed around each group of 46 chromosomes, the spindle fibers disappear, and the chromosomes begin to uncoil. Cytokinesis causes the cytoplasm to divide into roughly equal parts during this phase. At the end of telophase, two identical diploid cells, called *daughter cells,* have been formed from the original cell.

Rates of Cellular Division

Although the complete cell cycle lasts 12 to 24 hours, about 1 hour is generally required for the four stages of mitosis and cytokinesis. All types of cells undergo mitosis during formation of the embryo, but some adult cells, such as nerve cells, lens cells of the eye, and muscle cells, lose their ability to replicate and divide. The cells of other tissues, particularly epithelial cells (e.g., of the intestine, lung, skin), divide continuously and rapidly, completing the entire cell cycle in less than 10 hours.

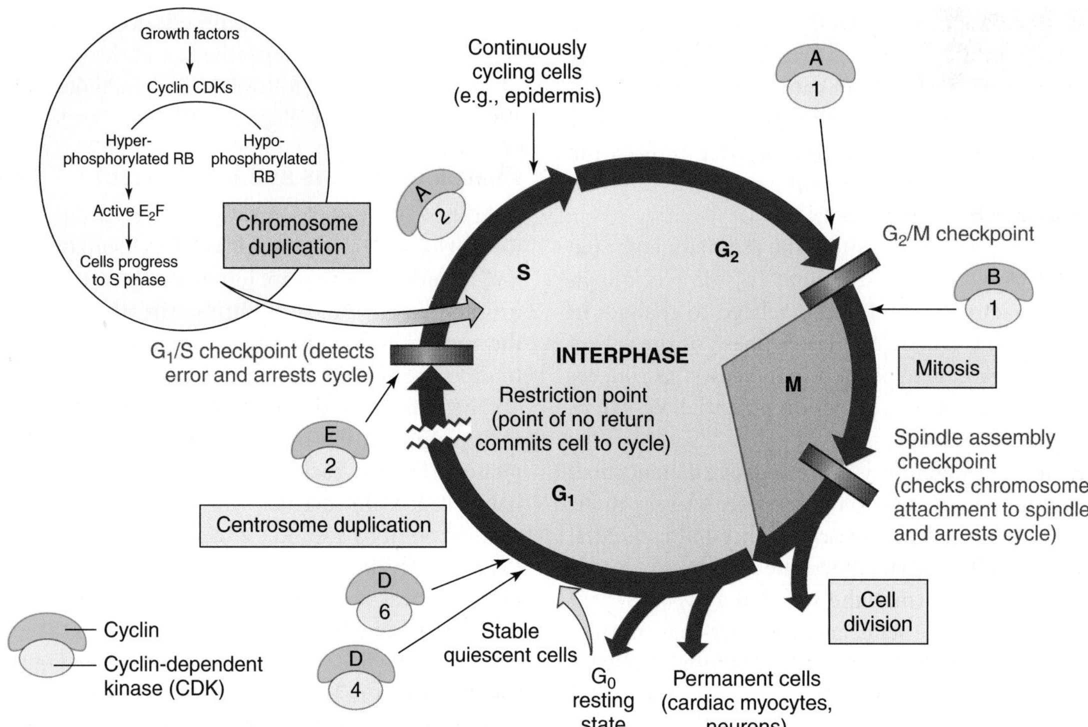

FIGURE 1-37 The Cell Cycle. The cell cycle consists of gap 1 (or G_1) (presynthesis), S (DNA synthesis), G_2 (premitotic), and M (mitotic) phases. Quiescent cells (quiet or resting state) are in the G_0 phase; however, most mature tissues have a combination of continuously dividing cells, terminally differentiated cells, stem cells, and some quiescent cells that infrequently enter the cell cycle. Continuously dividing cells replace those that are destroyed (e.g., epithelia of the oral cavity, skin). Quiescent or stable tissues exhibit a low level of replication; however, these cells can undergo rapid division in response to stimuli such as growth factors (e.g., EGF, TGF-α). Cyclins increase and activate cyclin-dependent protein kinase (CDK) complexes at the G_1/S restriction point, causing phosphorylation (addition of phosphate group) of the molecular ON-OFF switch, the retinoblastoma susceptibility protein (RB). In its hypophosphorylated state, RB prevents cells from replicating by forming a tight inactive complex with the transcription factor E_2F. Phosphorylation of RB eliminates the "brakes" to cell cycle progression and promotes cell replication. The orderly progression of cells through the phases of the cell cycle is regulated by cyclins, CDKs, and their inhibitors. Cyclin levels rise and fall (thus the name cyclin) during the cell cycle, periodically activating CDKs. Unless CDKs are bound to cyclins, they have no protein kinase activity. Cyclin-CDK complexes trigger cell cycle events. Each complex phosphorylates a different set of proteins that then promote advancement to the next phase (G_1, S, G_2, M, G_0). After completion of the task, cyclin levels decline rapidly. The activity of cyclin-CDK complexes is regulated by CDK inhibitors including Cip/Kip and 7NK4/ARF.

The difference between cells that divide slowly and cells that divide rapidly is the length of time spent in the G_1 phase of the cell cycle. Some cells that divide very slowly remain in the G_1 phase for days or even years. Once the S phase begins, however, progression through mitosis takes a relatively constant amount of time. Once a cell has progressed out of the G_1 phase, there is no turning back; it is committed to completing the S, G_2, and M phases. Times associated with the four successive phases differ.

The mechanisms that control cell division depend on the integrity of genetic, epigenetic (heritable changes in genome function that occur without alterations in the DNA sequence; see Chapters 6 and 12), and protein growth factors.[38] Individual cells are members of a complex cellular society in which survival of the *entire organism* is key and not survival or proliferation of just the *individual cells*. To grow and divide, a cell must receive specific positive signals from other cells. Many of these signals *are* protein growth factors that act by overriding intracellular negative controls that block progress of the cell cycle.[1]

When a need arises for new cells, as in repair of injured cells, previously nondividing cells must be rapidly triggered to reenter the cell cycle. With continual wear and tear, the cell birth rate and the cell death rate must be kept in balance. Therefore, cell-division controls must govern this balance. Protein growth factors governing the proliferation of different cell types and genes involved in the social control of cell division are being identified.[1]

The best model for understanding disruption of cell division and study of these genetic, epigenetic, and protein factors is tumor biology. Current emphasis in locating and identifying these genes is to study tumor cells that have presumably originated because of mutations to these genes, or proto-oncogenes (see Chapter 12).

Growth Factors

Growth factors, also called *cytokines,* are peptides that transmit signals within and between cells. They have a major role in the regulation of tissue growth and development (Table 1-6). Having nutrients is not enough for a cell to proliferate; it must

TABLE 1-6 **EXAMPLES OF GROWTH FACTORS AND THEIR ACTIONS**

GROWTH FACTOR	PHYSIOLOGIC ACTIONS
Platelet-derived growth factor (PDGF)	Stimulates proliferation of connective tissue cells and neuroglial cells
Epidermal growth factor (EGF)	Stimulates proliferation of epidermal cells and other cell types
Insulin-like growth factor 1 (IGF-1)	Collaborates with PDGF and EGF; stimulates proliferation of fat cells and connective tissue cells
Insulin-like growth factor 2 (IGF-2)	Collaborates with PDGF and EGF; stimulates proliferation of fat cells and connective tissue cells
Transforming growth factor-beta (TGF-β)	Stimulates or inhibits response of most cells to other growth factors; regulates differentiation of some cell types (e.g., cartilage)
Fibroblast growth factor (FGF)	Stimulates proliferation of fibroblasts, endothelial cells, myoblasts, and other cell types
Interleukin-2 (IL-2)	Stimulates proliferation of T lymphocytes
Nerve growth factor (NGF)	Promotes axon growth and survival of sympathetic and some sensory and CNS neurons
Hematopoietic cell growth factors (IL-3, GM-CSF, M-CSF, G-CSF, erythropoietin)	See Chapter 27

CNS, Central nervous system; *CSF,* colony-stimulating factor; *G,* granulocyte; *GM,* granulocyte-macrophage; *M,* macrophage.

also receive stimulatory chemical signals (growth factors) from other cells, usually its neighbors. These signals act to overcome intracellular braking mechanisms that tend to restrain cell growth and block progress through the cell cycle.

Different types of cells require different factors; for example, **platelet-derived growth factor (PDGF)** stimulates the production of connective tissue cells. Table 1-6 summarizes the most significant growth factors. Cells that respond to a particular growth factor have specific receptors for the growth factor in their plasma membrane. Recent evidence shows that some growth factors are also regulators of other cell processes, such as cellular differentiation. In addition to growth factors that stimulate cellular processes, there are factors that inhibit functions; these factors are not well understood. Cells that are starved of growth factors come to a halt after mitosis and enter the **arrested,** or **G_0, state** of the cell cycle[1] (see p. 37 for cell cycle). Certain growth factors can help move tumor cells from the G_0 state (resting) to the G_1 state, where they might be destroyed by chemotherapy or radiation.

TISSUES

The body is made up of four levels of organization: cells, tissues, organs, and systems. Cells of common structure and function are organized into **tissues,** of which there are four primary types: *muscle, neural, epithelial,* and *connective* tissue.

Tissue Formation

To form tissues, cells must exhibit intercellular recognition and adhesion. Specialized cells are thought to form a tissue in one of two ways. First and simplest is mitosis of one or more **founder cells** (the most basic precursor cell). Founder cells are prevented from "wandering away" by the presence of macromolecules in the extracellular matrix and by adherence to one another at specialized junctions on their plasma membranes. Mitosis of founder cells forms, for example, epithelial cell sheets (Figure 1-38, *A*).

The second way in which specialized cells form tissues involves their migration to and subsequent assembly at the site of tissue formation. During embryonic development, for example, cells from the neural crest migrate to several different regions, where they differentiate and assemble into a variety of tissues, including those of the peripheral nervous system. Migrant cells are thought to arrive at the site of tissue formation through chemotaxis or contact guidance. **Chemotaxis** is movement along a chemical gradient caused by chemical attraction (see Chapter 7). Cells at the migrant cells' destination secrete a chemical, called *chemotactic factor,* that attracts specific migrant cells. **Contact guidance** is movement along a pathway, or "pavement," in the extracellular matrix.[1]

Tissues are not randomly arranged into organs. No matter how tissue is formed, staying together in groups means that cells must recognize each other and remain distinct from the cells of surrounding tissues. Little is known about the mechanisms involved in these processes.

Stem cells are cells with the potential to develop into many different cell types during early development and growth. In many tissues, stem cells serve as an internal repair and maintenance system by dividing indefinitely. These cells can maintain themselves over very long periods of time, called **self-renewal,** and can generate all the differentiated cell types of the tissue, which is termed **multipotency.** This stem cell–driven tissue renewal is very evident in the epithelial lining of the intestine, stomach, and skin, which is continuously exposed to environmental factors.[39] There is growing evidence that stem cells self-renew through **asymmetric division,** where cellular contents and cell fates are distributed asymmetrically.[40] One daughter cell remains a stem cell and the other follows a pathway that ends in terminal differentiation. Differentiation occurs progressively as the offspring of stem cells commit to various cell lineages.

Types of Tissues

Epithelial Tissue

Epithelial tissue covers most internal and external surfaces of the body. Epithelial cells are closely joined and are attached to a basement membrane or lamina (extracellular matrix), which provides a supporting layer and separates the epithelium from underlying connective tissue (see Figure 1-15, p. 16). Because of its variety of locations, epithelial tissue has several diverse functions, including protection, absorption, secretion, and excretion. For example, the epidermis provides a protective barrier between the host and the outside environment, and the linings of the internal body organs help absorb substances into the body, excrete waste products, and secrete substances into body cavities.

Epithelial cell surfaces differ according to their location and function. Epithelial cells that line body cavities and blood vessels are smooth, whereas other epithelial cells have tiny cytoplasmic projections called **microvilli** on their free surfaces. Microvilli considerably increase a cell's surface area and are found on cells whose main functions are absorption and secretion, such as the epithelial cells lining the digestive tract. **Cilia,** which are hairlike projections that propel mucus, pus, and dust particles out of the body, characterize cells lining the respiratory passages.

Epithelial tissue is classified in two ways: (1) according to the number and arrangement of cell layers and (2) according to cell shape. Epithelium that is formed by a single layer of cells, all of which are in contact with the basement membrane, is called **simple epithelium. Stratified epithelium** has two or more layers of cells, and only the deepest layer is in contact with the basement membrane. Tissue that appears to consist of several cellular layers but is actually a single layer with all cells contacting the basement membrane is called **pseudostratified epithelium.**

Three basic cell shapes are found in epithelium: squamous, cuboidal, and columnar. **Squamous cells** are flat and thin; **cuboidal cells** are as high as they are wide and thus appear square in vertical sections; and **columnar cells** are taller than they are wide and appear rectangular in vertical sections. Overall classifications of epithelial tissue, which take into account both the number of cell layers and the cell shape, are summarized in Table 1-7.

Connective Tissue

Connective tissue varies considerably in structure and function but is most common as the framework on which epithelial cells cluster to form organs. Other functions include binding various tissues and organs together, supporting them in their locations, and serving as storage sites for excess nutrients.

In contrast to epithelial tissue, connective tissue is characterized by an abundant extracellular matrix that surrounds few cells. The extracellular matrix is composed of ground substance and fibers. **Ground substance** is a homogeneous mass that varies in consistency from fluid to semisolid gel. Fibers are produced by connective tissue cells (fibroblasts) found within the ground substance. The three types of fibers are collagenous (white), elastic (yellow), and reticular. **Collagenous fibers** are formed of bundles of smaller fibers appearing as wavy bands under the microscope. These fibers are composed of the protein collagen and are strong and inelastic. (Collagen synthesis by fibroblasts is described with respect to tissue repair in Chapter 7.) **Elastic fibers** are long, branching fibers composed of a protein called *elastin* that enables the fibers to return to

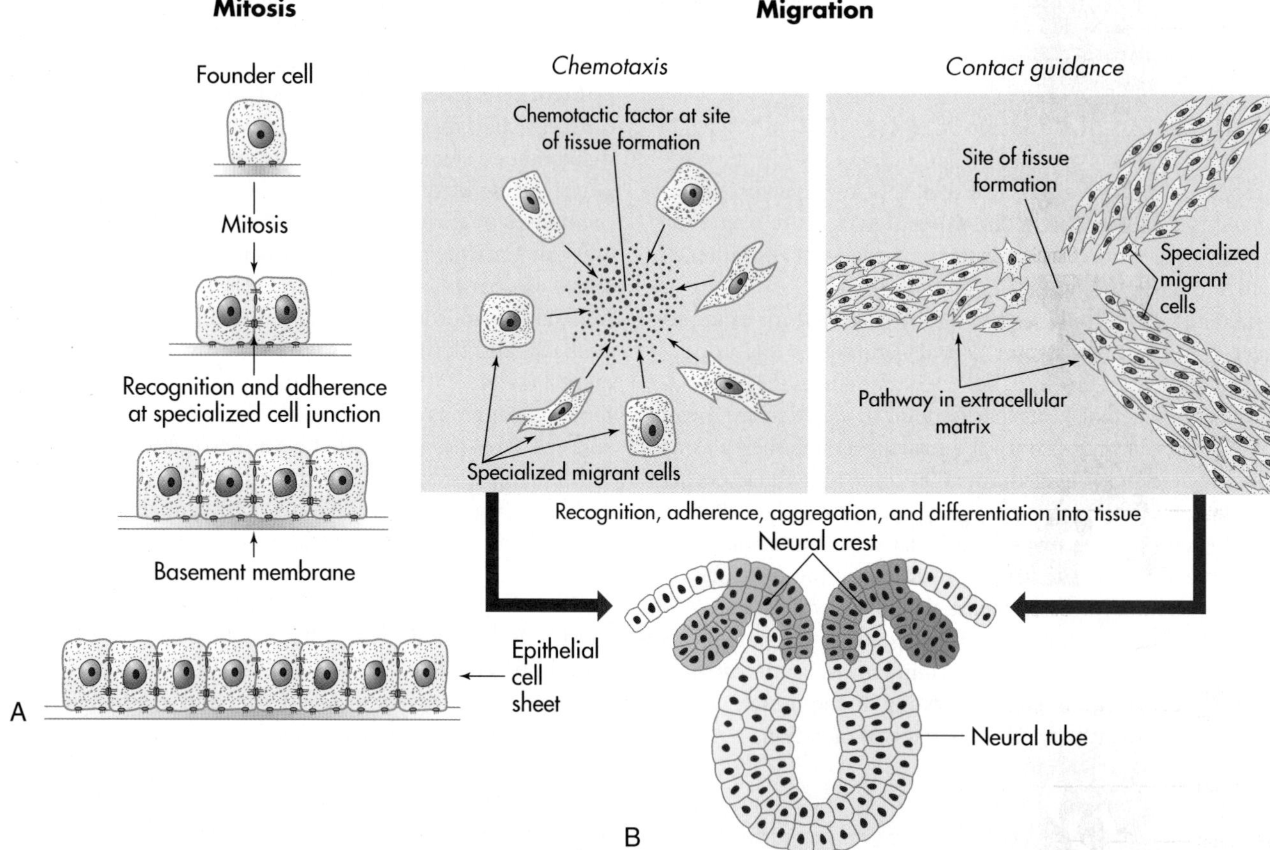

FIGURE 1-38 Tissue Formation by Mitosis and Migration. **A,** Tissue formation by mitosis. Founder cells are kept in place by extracellular matrix and recognition and adherence at cell junctions. **B,** Tissue formation by migration. Specialized cells are attracted to the site of tissue formation by chemotaxis or contact guidance; then they aggregate and differentiate into organized tissue.

their original length after stretching. Elastin occurs not only as fibers but also as membranes, particularly the membranes of blood vessels. **Reticular fibers** are thin, short, branching fibers that form an inelastic network made from a collagen-like protein called *reticulum*. Reticular fibers form the internal framework (stroma) to which the epithelial cells of glands are attached. They are found in loose connective tissue, generally in bone marrow and in the **parenchyma** (i.e., the essential substance of an organ rather than its framework) of the liver, spleen, and lymph nodes.

Connective tissues are classified according to the consistency (e.g., loose, dense) of the ground substance and the type and organization of the fibers within it. Table 1-8 summarizes the characteristics of connective tissues.

Muscle Tissue

Muscle tissue is composed of long, thin cells or fibers called *myocytes*. Myocytes are highly contractile. The three types of muscle tissues are skeletal, cardiac, and smooth (Table 1-9). (Muscles are discussed in detail in Chapter 43.)

Neural Tissue

Neural tissue is composed of highly specialized cells called *neurons*, which receive and transmit electrical impulses very rapidly across junctions called synapses. **Synapses** are points of functional contact between neurons. At synapses, impulses pass from neuron to neuron or from a neuron to a muscle cell while chemical messengers called *neurotransmitters* are released (see Chapter 15). The total number of neurons is fixed at birth, and replacement is impossible thereafter.

Different types of neurons have special characteristics that depend on their distribution and function within the nervous system. All neurons, however, are composed of the following parts: (1) a cell body, (2) a single axon, and (3) one or more dendrites (see Figure 15-1 on p. 449). The cell body contains special cytoplasmic structures, as well as microtubules, actin filaments, Golgi complex, lysosomes, and lipofuscin. The axons and dendrites can be very long. Generally, the axon conducts nerve impulses away from the cell body, and dendrites conduct nerve impulses toward the cell body. (Neuronal transmission is discussed in Chapter 15.)

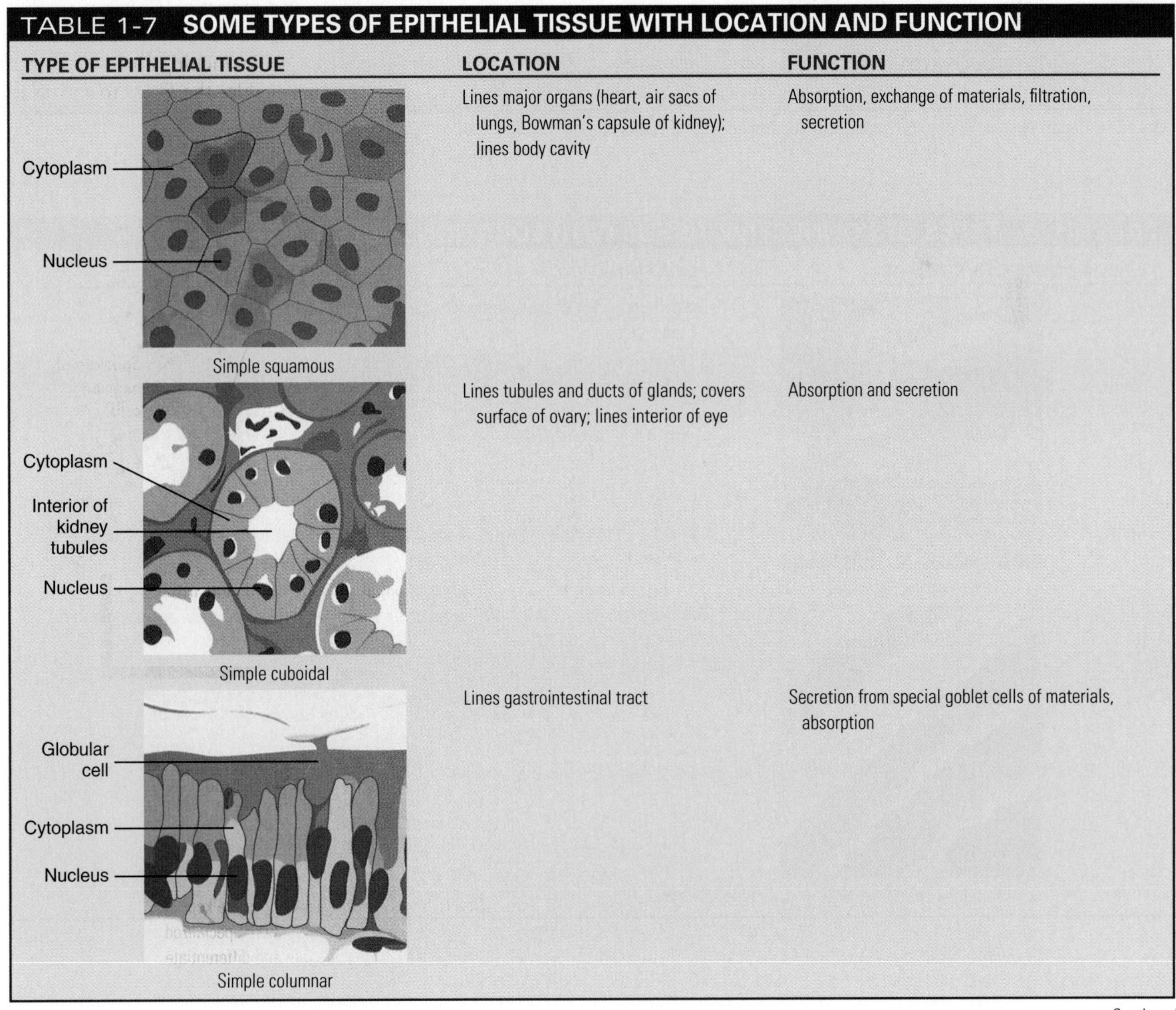

TABLE 1-7 SOME TYPES OF EPITHELIAL TISSUE WITH LOCATION AND FUNCTION

TYPE OF EPITHELIAL TISSUE	LOCATION	FUNCTION
Simple squamous	Lines major organs (heart, air sacs of lungs, Bowman's capsule of kidney); lines body cavity	Absorption, exchange of materials, filtration, secretion
Simple cuboidal	Lines tubules and ducts of glands; covers surface of ovary; lines interior of eye	Absorption and secretion
Simple columnar	Lines gastrointestinal tract	Secretion from special goblet cells of materials, absorption

Continued

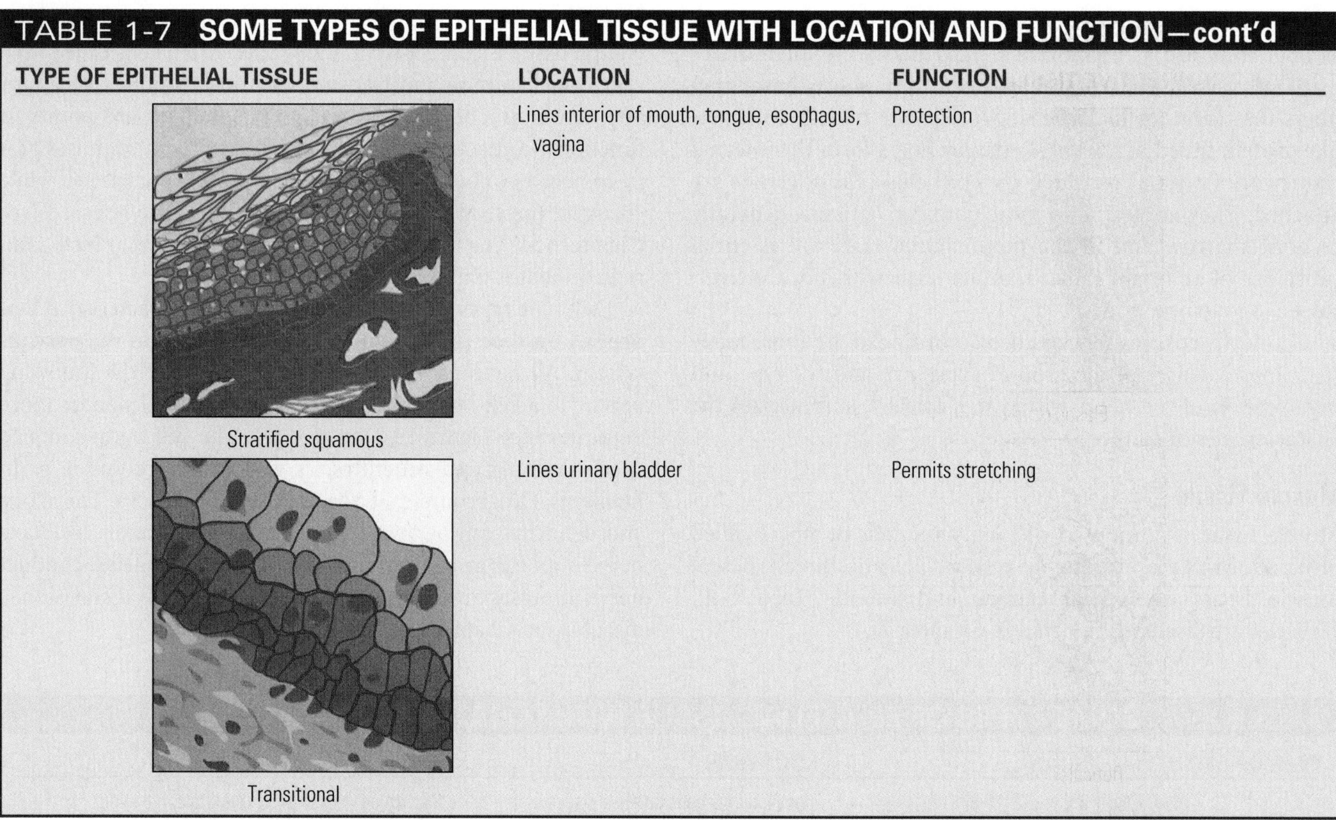

TABLE 1-7 SOME TYPES OF EPITHELIAL TISSUE WITH LOCATION AND FUNCTION—cont'd

TYPE OF EPITHELIAL TISSUE	LOCATION	FUNCTION
Stratified squamous	Lines interior of mouth, tongue, esophagus, vagina	Protection
Transitional	Lines urinary bladder	Permits stretching

Data from Raven PH, Johnson GB: *Understanding biology,* ed 3, Dubuque, IA, 1995, Brown.

TABLE 1-8 TYPES OF CONNECTIVE TISSUE WITH LOCATION AND FUNCTION

TYPE OF CONNECTIVE TISSUE	LOCATION	FUNCTION
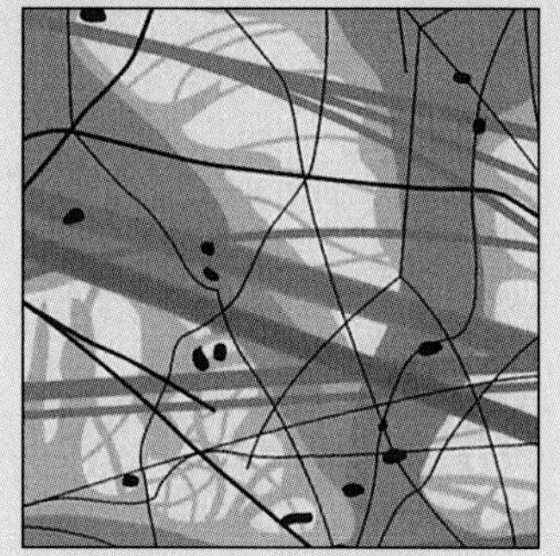 Loose connective tissue	Deep layers of skin, blood vessels, nerves, body organs	Support, elasticity
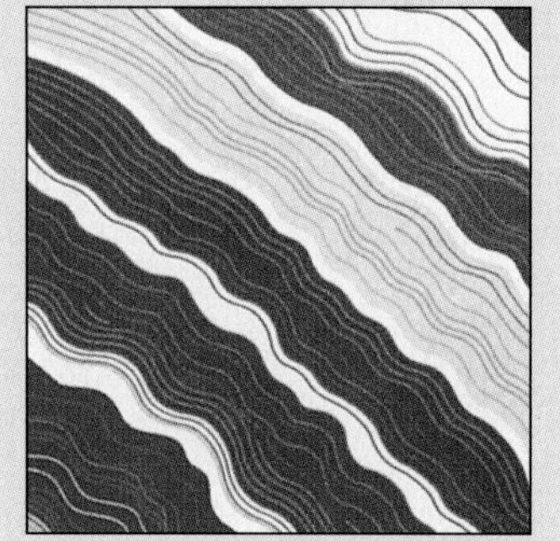 Dense connective tissue	Tendons, ligaments	Attaches structures to one another; provides great strength

TABLE 1-8 TYPES OF CONNECTIVE TISSUE WITH LOCATION AND FUNCTION—cont'd

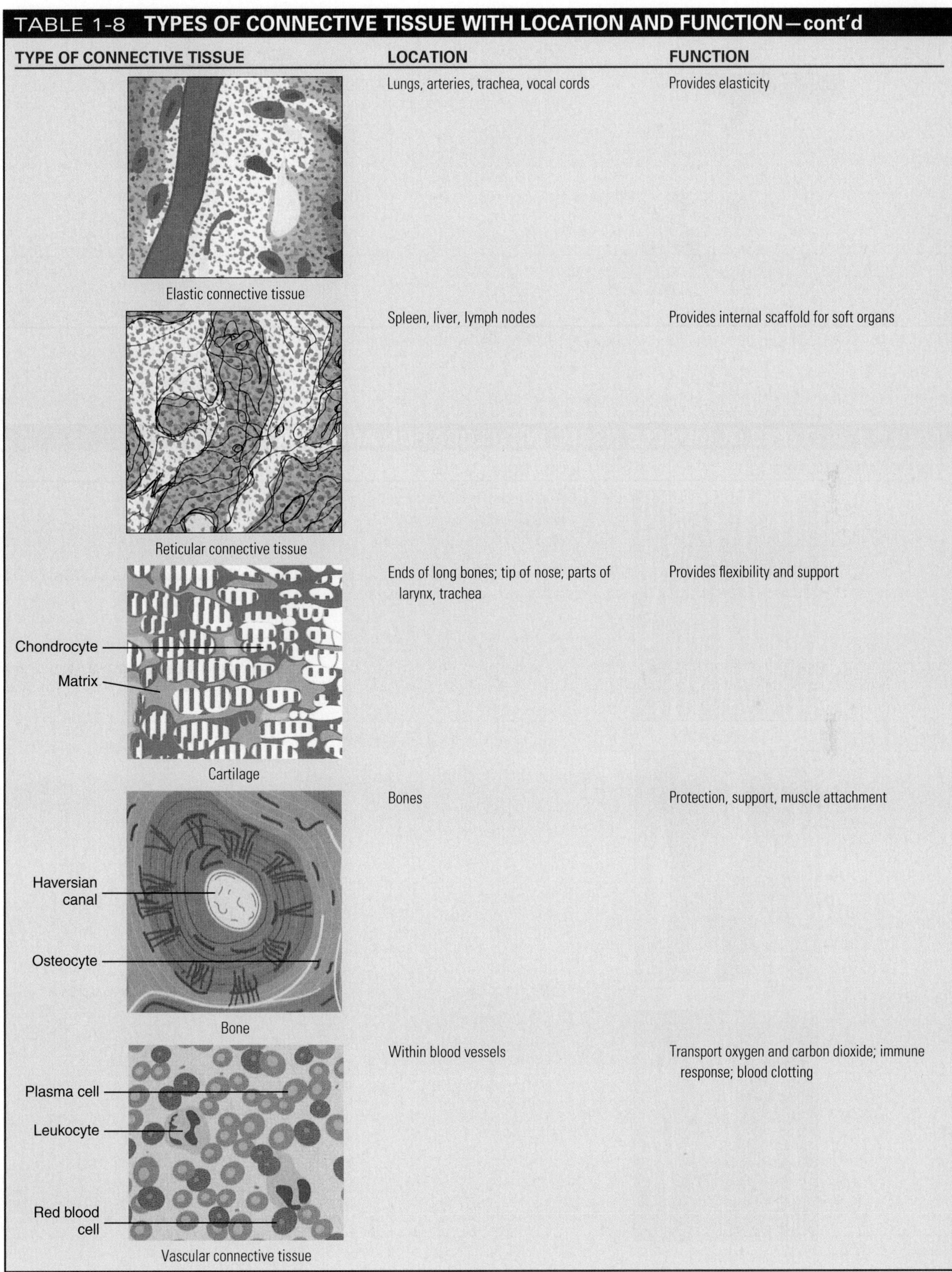

TYPE OF CONNECTIVE TISSUE	LOCATION	FUNCTION
Elastic connective tissue	Lungs, arteries, trachea, vocal cords	Provides elasticity
Reticular connective tissue	Spleen, liver, lymph nodes	Provides internal scaffold for soft organs
Cartilage	Ends of long bones; tip of nose; parts of larynx, trachea	Provides flexibility and support
Bone	Bones	Protection, support, muscle attachment
Vascular connective tissue	Within blood vessels	Transport oxygen and carbon dioxide; immune response; blood clotting

Continued

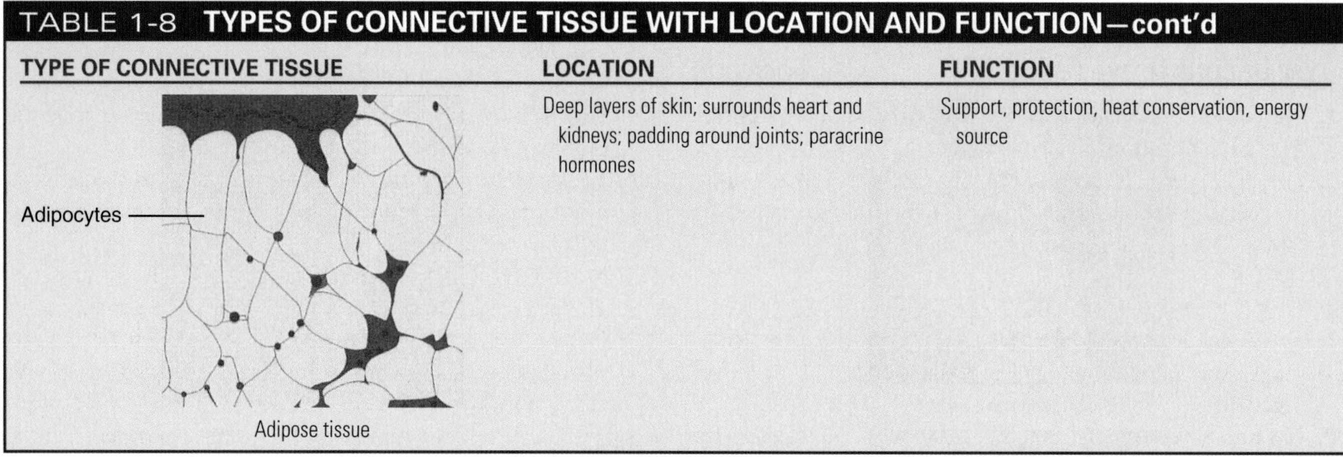

TABLE 1-8 TYPES OF CONNECTIVE TISSUE WITH LOCATION AND FUNCTION—cont'd

TYPE OF CONNECTIVE TISSUE	LOCATION	FUNCTION
Adipocytes Adipose tissue	Deep layers of skin; surrounds heart and kidneys; padding around joints; paracrine hormones	Support, protection, heat conservation, energy source

Data from Raven PH, Johnson GB: *Understanding biology,* ed 3, Dubuque, IA, 1995, Brown.

TABLE 1-9 TYPES OF MUSCLE TISSUE WITH LOCATION AND FUNCTION

TYPE OF MUSCLE TISSUE	LOCATION	FUNCTION
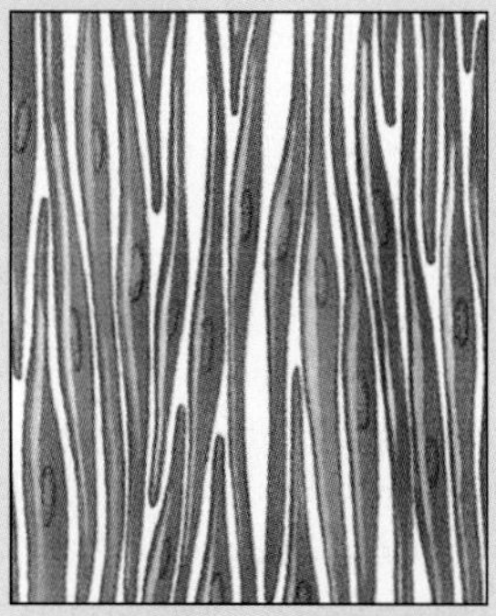 Smooth muscle	Gastrointestinal tract, uterus, urinary bladder, blood vessels	Propulsion of materials
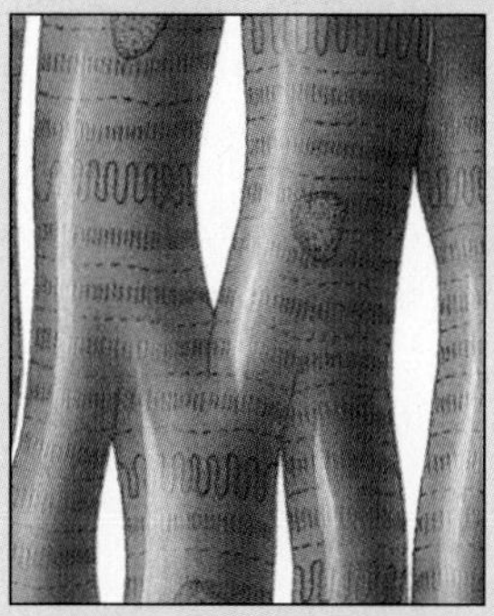 Cardiac muscle	Heart	Contraction
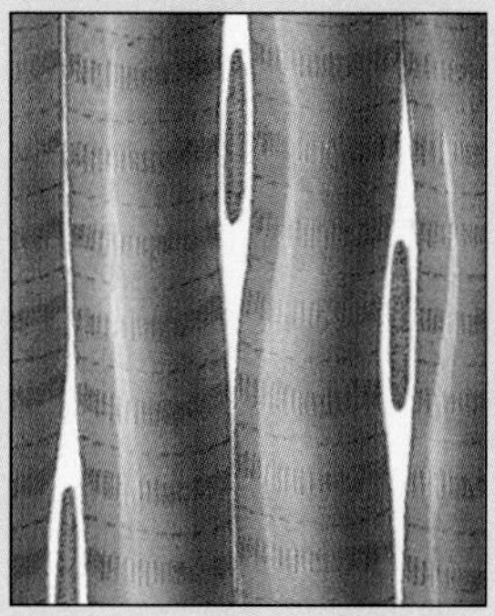 Skeletal muscle	Attached to bones	Movement

Data from Raven PH, Johnson GB: *Understanding biology,* ed 3, Dubuque, IA, 1995, Brown.

SUMMARY REVIEW

Cellular Functions

1. Cells become specialized through the process of differentiation, or maturation.
2. The eight specialized cellular functions are movement, conductivity, metabolic absorption, secretion, excretion, respiration, reproduction, and communication.

Structure and Function of Cellular Components

1. The eukaryotic cell consists of three general components: the plasma membrane, the cytoplasm, and the intracellular organelles.
2. The nucleus is the largest membrane-bound organelle and is usually found in the cell's center. The chief functions of the nucleus are cell division and control of genetic information.
3. Cytoplasm, or the cytoplasmic matrix, is an aqueous solution (cytosol) that fills the space between the nucleus and the plasma membrane.
4. The organelles are suspended in the cytoplasm and are enclosed in biologic membranes.
5. The endoplasmic reticulum (ER) is a network of tubular channels (cisternae) that extend throughout the outer nuclear membrane. It specializes in the synthesis and transport of protein and lipid components of most of the organelles. Importantly, the ER is responsible for protein folding and sensing cell stress.
6. The Golgi complex is a network of smooth membranes and vesicles located near the nucleus. The Golgi complex is responsible for processing and packaging proteins into secretory vesicles that break away from the Golgi complex and migrate to a variety of intracellular and extracellular destinations, including the plasma membrane.
7. Lysosomes are saclike structures that originate from the Golgi complex and contain digestive enzymes. These enzymes are responsible for digesting most cellular substances completely to their basic components, such as amino acids, fatty acids, and carbohydrates.
8. Cellular debris is encapsulated within a vesicle that reacts with a lysosome to complete its degradation, a process called autophagy. Autophagy plays a crucial role in health and disease.
9. Peroxisomes are similar to lysosomes but contain several oxidative enzymes, such as catalase and urate oxidase.
10. Mitochondria are found in great numbers in most cells and are responsible for cellular respiration and energy production. The enzymes of the respiratory chain (electron-transport chain), found in the inner membrane of the mitochondria, generate most of the cell's ATP.
11. Vaults are cytoplasmic organelles also called ribonucleoproteins. They are thought to function as cellular "trucks" carrying mRNA from the nucleus to the ribosomal sites of protein synthesis.
12. The cytoskeleton is the "bone and muscle" of the cell. The internal skeleton is composed of a network of protein filaments including microtubules and actin filaments (microfilaments).
13. The plasma membrane encloses the cell and, by controlling the movement of substances across it, exerts a powerful influence on metabolic pathways.
14. The plasma membrane is a bilayer of lipids and proteins not uniformly distributed but can separate into discrete units called microdomains.
15. Membrane functions are determined largely by proteins. These functions include (a) recognition and binding units (receptors) for substances moving in and out of the cell; (b) pores or transport channels; (c) enzymes that drive active pumps; (d) cell surface markers, such as glycoproteins; (e) cell adhesion molecules; and (f) catalysts of chemical reactions.
16. The information regarding concepts of biologic membranes has changed markedly in the last two decades.
17. A protein is made from a chain of amino acids known as polypeptides. Proteins are the major workhorses of the cell.
18. Cellular receptors are protein molecules on the plasma membrane, in the cytoplasm, or in the nucleus that are capable of recognizing and binding smaller molecules, called *ligands.*
19. The ligand-receptor complex initiates a series of protein interactions, causing adenylyl cyclase to catalyze the transformation of cellular ATP to messenger molecules that stimulate specific responses within the cell.
20. A field called *proteomics* is the study of the proteome or entire set of proteins expressed by a genome—from synthesis, translocation, and modification (e.g., folding) to their role in a staggering number of diseases.
21. The carbohydrate contained within the plasma membrane is generally bound to membrane proteins.

Cell-to-Cell Adhesions

1. Cell-to-cell adhesions are formed on plasma membranes, thereby allowing the formation of tissues and organs. Cells are held together by three different means: (a) the extracellular membrane, (b) cell adhesion molecules in the cell's plasma membrane, and (c) specialized cell junctions.
2. The extracellular matrix includes three types of protein fibers: collagen, elastin, and fibronectin. The matrix helps regulate cell growth and differentiation.
3. The basement membrane is a thin layer of connective tissue underlying the epithelium of many organs. It is also called the basal lamina.
4. The three main types of cell junctions are desmosomes, tight junctions, and gap junctions.

Cellular Communication and Signal Transduction

1. Cells communicate in three main ways: (a) they display plasma membrane–bound signaling molecules (receptors) that affect the cell itself and other cells in direct physical contact; (b) they activate receptor proteins inside the target cell, and the signal molecule has to enter the cell to bind to them; and (c) they form protein channels (gap junctions) that directly coordinate the activities of adjacent cells.

SUMMARY REVIEW—cont'd

2. Primary modes of intercellular signaling are contact-dependent, paracrine, hormonal, neurohormonal, and neurotransmitter.
3. Signal transduction involves signals or instructions from extracellular chemical messengers that are conveyed to the cell's interior for execution.
4. Signal transduction pathways (signaling cascades, relay chains) have several important functions, including physically transferring the signal around the cell, amplifying the signal, distributing the signal, and modulating the signal.
5. Two important second messenger pathways are cAMP and Ca^{++}.
6. G protein is an intermediary between the receptor and adenylyl cyclase.
7. Phospholipase C, an enzyme protein effector, is bound to the inner side of the membrane.

Cellular Metabolism

1. The chemical tasks of maintaining essential cellular functions are referred to as *cellular metabolism.* Anabolism is the energy-using process of metabolism, whereas catabolism is the energy-releasing process.
2. ATP functions as an energy-transferring molecule. Energy is stored by molecules of carbohydrate, lipid, and protein, which, when catabolized, transfer energy to ATP.
3. Oxidative phosphorylation occurs in the mitochondria and is the mechanism by which the energy produced from carbohydrates, fats, and proteins is transferred to ATP.

Membrane Transport: Cellular Intake and Output

1. Water and small, electrically uncharged molecules move through pores in the plasma membrane's lipid bilayer in the process called *passive transport.*
2. Passive transport does not require the expenditure of energy; rather, it is driven by the physical effects of osmosis, hydrostatic pressure, and diffusion.
3. Larger molecules and molecular complexes (e.g., ligand-receptor complexes) are moved into the cell by active transport, which requires expenditure of energy (by means of ATP) by the cell.
4. Endocytosis is a cellular internalizing process where a section of the plasma membrane enfolds substances from outside the cell, invaginates, and separates from the plasma membrane, forming a vesicle that moves inside the cell.
5. Endocytosis can be subdivided into four categories: (a) clathrin-mediated endocytosis, (b) caveolae-mediated endocytosis, (c) macropinocytosis, and (d) phagocytosis. Over time, however, these categories may change.
6. Two types of solutes exist in body fluids: electrolytes and nonelectrolytes. Electrolytes are electrically charged and dissociate into constituent ions when placed in solution. Nonelectrolytes do not dissociate when placed in solution.
7. Diffusion is the passive movement of a solute from an area of higher solute concentration to an area of lower solute concentration.
8. Hydrostatic pressure is the mechanical force of water pushing against cellular membranes.
9. Osmosis is the movement of water across a semipermeable membrane from a region of lower solute concentration to a region of higher solute concentration.
10. The amount of hydrostatic pressure required to oppose the osmotic movement of water is called the *osmotic pressure* of the solution.
11. The overall osmotic effect of colloids, such as plasma proteins, is called the *oncotic pressure* or *colloid osmotic pressure.*
12. Mediated transport can be passive or active. Mediated transport includes the movement of two molecules simultaneously in one direction (symport) or in opposite directions (antiport), or the movement of a single molecule in one direction (uniport).
13. Passive mediated transport is also called *facilitated diffusion.* It does not require the expenditure of metabolic energy.
14. Active mediated transport requires metabolic energy (ATP) to move molecules against the concentration gradient.
15. Active transport also occurs by endocytosis, or vesicle formation.
16. Pinocytosis is a type of endocytosis in which fluids and solute molecules are ingested through formation of small vesicles.
17. Phagocytosis is a type of endocytosis in which large particles, such as bacteria, are ingested through formation of large vesicles, called *vacuoles.*
18. All body cells are electrically polarized, with the inside of the cell more negatively charged than the outside. The difference in voltage across the plasma membrane is the resting membrane potential.
19. When an excitable (nerve or muscle) cell receives an electrochemical stimulus, cations enter the cell, causing a rapid change in the resting membrane potential known as the *action potential.* The action potential "moves" along the cell's plasma membrane and is transmitted to an adjacent cell. This is how electrochemical signals convey information from cell to cell.

Cellular Reproduction: The Cell Cycle

1. Cellular reproduction in body tissues involves mitosis (nuclear division) and cytokinesis (cytoplasmic division).
2. Only mature cells are capable of division. Maturation occurs during a stage of cellular life called *interphase* (growth phase).
3. The cell cycle is the reproductive process that begins after interphase in all tissues with cellular turnover. The four phases of the cell cycle are (a) the S phase, during which DNA synthesis takes place in the cell nucleus; (b) the G_2 phase, the period between the completion of DNA synthesis and the next phase (M); (c) the M phase, which involves both nuclear (mitotic) and cytoplasmic (cytokinetic) division; and (d) the G_1 phase (growth phase, or interphase), after which the cycle begins again.

SUMMARY REVIEW—cont'd

4. The M phase (mitosis) involves four stages: prophase, metaphase, anaphase, and telophase.
5. The mechanisms that control cell division depend on the integrity of genetic, epigenetic, and protein growth factors.
6. Cyclin–cyclin-dependent protein kinase (CDK) complexes trigger cell cycle events.

Tissues

1. Cells of one or more types are organized into tissues, and different types of tissues compose organs. Organs are organized to function as tracts or systems.
2. Specialized cells are thought to form tissue by mitosis of one or more founder cells or by migration of founder cells and their subsequent assembly at the site of tissue formation.
3. Stem cells are cells with the potential to develop into many different cell types during early development and growth.
4. The four basic types of tissues are epithelial, muscle, neural, and connective tissues.
5. Epithelial tissue covers most internal and external surfaces of the body. The functions of epithelial tissue include protection, absorption, secretion, and excretion.
6. Connective tissue binds various tissues and organs together, supporting them in their locations and serving as storage sites for excess nutrients.
7. Muscle tissue is composed of long, thin, highly contractile cells or fibers called *myocytes.* Muscle tissue that is attached to bones enables voluntary movement. Muscle tissues in internal organs enable involuntary movement, such as the heartbeat.
8. Neural tissue is composed of highly specialized cells called *neurons* that receive and transmit electrical impulses very rapidly across junctions called *synapses.*

KEY TERMS

Absolute refractory period, 37
Actin filament (microfilament), 10
Action potential, 36
Active mediated transport (active transport), 32
Active transport, 32
Amphipathic molecule, 12
Anabolism, 25
Anaerobic glycolysis, 28
Anaphase, 37
Anion, 29
Antiport, 31
Arrested (G_0) state, 39
Asymmetric division, 39
Autocrine signaling, 20
Autodigestion, 8
Autolysosome (autophagosome), 8
Autophagosomes, 8
Autophagy, 8
Basal lamina, 17
Basement membrane, 17
Cadherins, 18
Catabolism, 25
Cation, 29
Caveolae, 35
Cavin, 35
Cell adhesion molecule (CAM), 15, 18
Cell cycle, 37
Cell junction, 18
Cell polarity, 11
Cell-to-cell adhesion, 17
Cellular metabolism, 25
Cellular receptor, 16
Centriole, 10
Centromere, 37
Chemical synapse, 20
Chemotaxis, 39
Chromatid, 37
Chromatin, 37
Chromosome, 37
Cilia, 40
Cisternae, 7
Citric acid cycle (Krebs cycle, tricarboxylic acid cycle), 26
Clathrin, 7
Clathrin-mediated endocytosis, 35
Coated pit, 35
Collagen, 17
Collagenous fiber, 40
Colloid osmotic pressure, 31
Columnar cell, 40
Competitive inhibitor, 31
Concentration gradient, 29
Connexon, 18
Contact-dependent signaling, 20
Contact guidance, 40
Cristae, 8
Cuboidal cell, 40
Cyclic adenosine monophosphate (cyclic AMP, cAMP), 23
Cyclic guanosine monophosphate (cyclic GMP, cGMP), 24
Cytochrome, 28
Cytokinesis, 37
Cytoplasm, 2
Cytoplasmic matrix, 4
Cytoskeleton, 9
Cytosol, 4
Depolarization, 36
Desmosome, 18
Differentiation, 2
Diffusion, 29
Digestion, 26
Effective osmolality, 30
Elastic fiber, 40
Elastin, 17
Electrolyte, 29
Electron-transport chain, 28
Endocytosis, 12
Endoplasmic reticulum, 5
Equatorial plate (metaphase plate), 37
ER stress, 6
Eukaryote, 2
Exocytosis, 35
Extracellular matrix, 17
Facilitated diffusion, 31
Fibroblast, 17
Fibronectin, 17
Filtration, 29
First messenger, 22
Founder cell, 39
G protein, 23
Gap junction, 18
Gating, 20
Glycolysis, 26
Glycoprotein, 15
Golgi complex (Golgi apparatus), 6
Ground substance, 40
Growth factor, 38
Guanosine diphosphate (GDP), 23
Guanosine triphosphate (GTP), 23
Heterophagosome, 8
Homeostasis, 20
Hormonal signaling, 20
Hydrolases, 7
Hydrophilic, 12
Hydrophobic, 12
Hydrostatic pressure, 29
Hypertonic solution, 31
Hypotonic solution, 31
Immunoglobulin superfamily CAMs (IgSF CAMs), 18
Inner membrane, 8
Integral membrane protein, 13
Integrins, 18
Intermediary metabolism, 9
Interphase, 37
Ion, 29
Isotonic solution, 31
Junctional complex, 18
Ligand, 16
Lipid raft, 13
Lysosome, 7
Macromolecule, 17
Macropinocytosis, 33
Mechanotransduction, 9
Mediated transport, 31
Metabolic pathway, 25
Metaphase, 37
Microdomain, 35
Micropinocytosis, 33
Microtubule, 10
Microvilli, 40
Mitochondria, 8
Mitosis, 37
Multipotency, 39
Neurohormonal signaling, 20
Neurotransmitter, 20
Nuclear envelope, 2

KEY TERMS—cont'd

REFERENCES

1. Alberts B, et al: *Molecular biology of the cell*, ed 5, New York, 2008, Garland.
2. Mor A, Shav-Tal Y: Dynamics and kinetics of nucleo-cytoplasmic mRNA export, *Wiley Interdiscip Rev RNA* 1(3):388–401, 2010.
3. Lee J, Giordano S, Zhang J: Autophagy, mitochondria and oxidative stress: cross-talk and redox signaling, *Biochem J* 441(2):523–540, 2012.
4. Todde V, Veenhuis M, van der Klei IJ: Autophagy: principles and significance in health and disease, *Biochim Biophys Acta* 1792:3–13, 2009.
5. Yang J, et al: Vaults are dynamically unconstrained cytoplasmic nanoparticles capable of half vault exchange, *ACS Nano* 4(12):7229–7240, 2010.
6. van Zon A, et al: Vault mobility depends in part on microtubules and vaults can be recruited to the nuclear envelope, *Exp Cell Res* 312(3):245–255, 2006.
7. Hoffman BD, Grashoff C, Schwartz MA: Dynamic molecular processes mediate cellular mechanotransduction, *Nature* 475:316–323, 2011.
8. Jaalouk DE, Lammerding J: Mechanotransduction gone awry, *Nat Rev Mol Cell Biol* 10(1):63–73, 2009.
9. Mooney DJ, Mikos AG: Growing new organs, *Sci Am* 280(4):60–65, 1999.
10. Fasshauer M, Iwig M, Glaesser D: Synthesis of proto-oncogene proteins and cyclins depends on intact microfilaments, *Eur J Cell Biol* 77(3):188–195, 1998.
11. Iglesias PA, Devreotes PN: Biased excitable networks: how cells direct motion in response to gradients, *Curr Opin Cell Biol*, 2011 Dec 9. [Epub ahead of print.].
12. Defamie N, Mesnil M: The modulation of gap-junctional intercellular communication by lipid rafts, *Biochim Biophys Acta*, 2011 Oct 2. [Epub ahead of print.].
13. Contreras FX, et al: Specificity of intramembrane protein-lipid interactions, *Cold Spring Harb Perspect Biol* 3(6), pii a004705, 2011.
14. Lofthouse RA, et al: Identification of caveolae and detection of caveolin in normal human osteoblasts, *J Bone Joint Surg Br* 83(1):124–129, 2001.
15. van Meer G, Voelker DR, Feigenson GW: Membrane lipids: where they are and how they behave, *Nat Rev Mol Cell Biol* 9:112–124, 2008.
16. Simons K, Gerl MJ: Revitalizing membrane rafts: new tools and insights, *Nat Rev* 11:688–699, 2010.
17. Ribet D, Cossart P: Pathogen-mediated posttranslational modification: a re-emerging field, *Cell* 143:694–702, 2010.
18. Vinothkumar KR, Henderson R: Structures of membrane proteins, *Quart Rev Biophys* 43:65–158, 2012.
19. Amour A, et al: General considerations for proteolytic cascades, *Biochem Soc Trans* 32(Pt 1):15–16, 2004.
20. Logue SE, Martin SJ: Caspase activation cascades in apoptosis, *Biochem Soc Trans* 36(Pt 1):1–9, 2008.
21. Chang HY, Yang X: Proteases for cell suicide: functions and regulations of caspases, *Microbiol Mol Biol Rev* 64(4):821–846, 2000.
22. LaPorte SL, et al: Molecular and structural basis of cytokine receptor pleiotropy in the interleukin-4/13 system, *Cell* 132:259–272, 2008.
23. Kumar V, Abbas A, Fausto N: *Robbins & Cotran pathologic basis of disease*, ed 7, Philadelphia, 2005, Saunders.
24. Alberts B, et al: *Essential cell biology*, New York, 1998, Garland.
25. Friedrichs K, Klinke A, Baldus S: Inflammatory pathways underlying atrial fibrillation, *Trends Mol Med* 17(10):556–563, 2011.
26. Singh AB, Harris RC: Autocrine, paracrine, and juxtacrine signaling by EGFR ligands, *Cell Signal* 17(10):1183–1193, 2005.
27. Scott JD, Pawson T: Cell communication: the inside story, *Sci Am* 282(6):72–79, 2000.
28. Ferguson SM, De Camilli P: Dynamin, a membrane-remodelling GTPase, *Nat Rev Mol Cell Biol* 13:75–88, 2012.
29. Krauss M, Haucke V: Shaping membranes for endocytosis, *Rev Physiol Biochem Pharmacol* 161:45–66, 2012.
30. Gold S, et al: A clathrin independent macropinocytosis-like entry mechanism used by bluetongue virus-1 during infection of BHK cells, *PLoS One* 5(6), 2010.
31. Sowa G: Caveolae, caveolins, cavins, and endothelial cell function: new insights, *Front Physiol* 2:120, 2012.
32. Briand N, Dugail I, LeLay S: Cavin proteins: new players in the caveolae field, *Biochimie* 93(1):71–77, 2011.
33. Liu L, Pilch PF: A critical role of cavin (polymerase I and transcript release factor) in caveolae formation and organization, *J Biol Chem* 283:4314–4322, 2008.
34. Levin ER, Pietras RJ: Estrogen receptors outside the nucleus in breast cancer, *Breast Cancer Res Treat* 108(3):351–361, 2008.
35. Li L, Haynes MP, Bender JR: Plasma membrane localization and function of the estrogen receptor alpha variant (ER46) in human endothelial cells, *Proc Natl Acad Sci U S A* 100(8):4807–4812, 2003.
36. Mineo C, Shaul PW: Circulating cardiovascular disease risk factors and signaling in endothelial cell caveolae, *Cardiovasc Res* 70(1):31–41, 2006.
37. He B, et al: Exo 70 interacts with phospholipids and mediates the targeting of the exocyst to the plasma membrane, *EMBO J* 26(18):4053–4065, 2007.
38. Probst AV, Dunleavy E, Almouzni G: Epigenetic inheritance during the cell cycle, *Nat Rev Mol Cell Biol* 10:192–209, 2009.
39. Barker N, Bartfield S, Clevers H: Tissue-resident adult stem cell populations of rapidly self-renewing organs, *Cell Stem* 7:656–670, 2010.
40. Chang KC, Wang C, Wang H: Balancing self-renewal and differentiation by asymmetric division: insights from brain tumor suppressors in *Drosophila* neural stem cells, *Bioessays*, 2012 Jan 27. [Epub ahead of print.].

CHAPTER

2

Altered Cellular and Tissue Biology

Kathryn L. McCance, Todd Cameron Grey, and George Rodway

evolve WEBSITE

http://evolve.elsevier.com/McCance/

- Review Questions and Answers
- Animations
- Online Course: Module 1

CHAPTER OUTLINE

Injury to cells and their surrounding environment, called the extracellular matrix, leads to tissue and organ injury. Although the normal cell is restricted by a narrow range of structure and function, it can *adapt* to physiologic demands or stress to maintain a steady state called *homeostasis*. **Adaptation** is a reversible, structural, or functional response to both normal or physiologic conditions and adverse or pathologic conditions. For example, the uterus adapts to pregnancy—a normal physiologic state—by enlarging. Enlargement occurs because of an increase in the size and number of uterine cells. In an adverse condition, such as high blood pressure, myocardial cells are stimulated to enlarge by the increased work of pumping. Like most of the body's adaptive mechanisms, however, cellular adaptations to adverse conditions are usually only temporarily successful. Severe or long-term stressors overwhelm adaptive processes and cellular injury or death ensues. Altered cellular and tissue biology can result from adaptation, injury, neoplasia, accumulations, aging, or death. (Neoplasia is discussed in Chapters 12, 13, and 14.)

Knowledge of the structural and functional reactions of cells and tissues to injurious agents, including genetic defects, is key to understanding disease processes. Cellular injury can be caused by any factor that disrupts cellular structures or deprives the cell of oxygen and nutrients required for survival. Injury may be reversible *(sublethal)* or irreversible *(lethal)* and is classified broadly as chemical, hypoxic (lack of sufficient oxygen), free radical, unintentional or intentional, and immunologic or inflammatory. Cellular injuries from various causes have different clinical and pathophysiologic manifestations. Stresses from metabolic derangements may be associated with intracellular *accumulations* and include carbohydrates, proteins, and lipids. Sites of cellular death can cause accumulations of calcium resulting in *pathologic calcification.*

Cellular death is confirmed by structural changes seen when cells are stained and examined with a microscope. The most important changes are nuclear; clearly, without a healthy nucleus, the cell cannot survive.

Cellular aging causes structural and functional changes that eventually lead to cellular death or a decreased capacity to recover from injury. Mechanisms explaining how and why cells age are not known and distinguishing between pathologic changes and physiologic changes that occur with aging is often difficult. Aging clearly causes alterations in cellular structure and function, yet *senescence*—growing old—is both inevitable and normal.

CELLULAR ADAPTATION

Cells adapt to their environment to escape and protect themselves from injury. An adapted cell is neither normal nor injured—its condition lies somewhere between these two states. Cellular adaptations, however, are a common and central part of many disease states. In the early stages of a successful adaptive response, cells may have enhanced function; thus it is hard to differentiate a pathologic response from an extreme adaptation to an excessive functional demand. The most significant adaptive changes in cells include atrophy (decrease in cell size), hypertrophy (increase in cell size), hyperplasia (increase in cell number), and metaplasia (reversible replacement of one mature cell type by another less mature cell type). Dysplasia (deranged cellular growth) is not considered a true cellular adaptation but rather an atypical hyperplasia. These changes are shown in Figure 2-1.

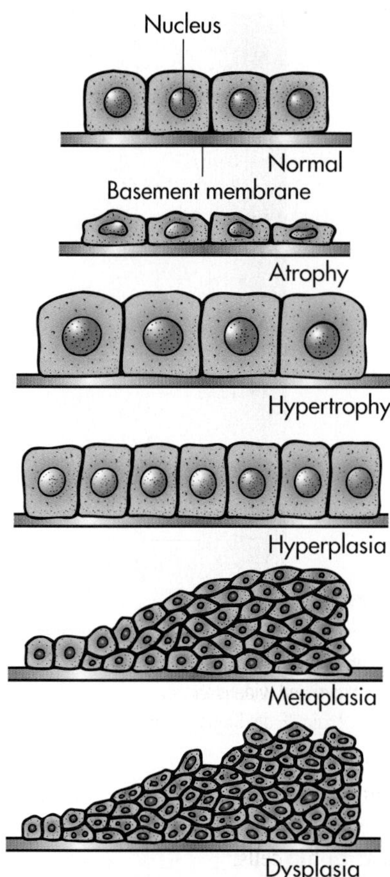

FIGURE 2-1 Adaptive Alterations in Simple Cuboidal Epithelial Cells. (From Lewis SM, Heitkemper MM, Dirksen SR: *Medical-surgical nursing: assessment and management of clinical problems,* ed 6, St Louis, 2004, Mosby.)

Atrophy

Atrophy is a decrease or shrinkage in cellular size. If atrophy occurs in a sufficient number of an organ's cells, the entire organ shrinks or becomes atrophic. Atrophy can affect any organ, but it is most common in skeletal muscle, the heart, secondary sex organs, and the brain (Figure 2-2). Atrophy can be classified as *physiologic* or *pathologic.* **Physiologic atrophy** occurs with early development. For example, the thymus gland undergoes physiologic atrophy during childhood. **Pathologic atrophy** occurs as a result of decreases in workload, use, pressure, blood supply, nutrition, hormonal stimulation, and nervous stimulation. Individuals immobilized in bed for a prolonged time exhibit a type of skeletal muscle atrophy called *disuse atrophy.* Aging causes brain cells to become atrophic and endocrine-dependent organs, such as the gonads, to shrink as hormonal stimulation decreases. Whether atrophy is caused by normal physiologic conditions or by pathologic conditions, atrophic cells exhibit the same basic changes.

The atrophic muscle cell contains less endoplasmic reticulum and fewer mitochondria and myofilaments (part of the muscle fiber that controls contraction) than does the normal cell. In muscular atrophy caused by nerve loss, oxygen consumption and amino acid uptake are rapidly reduced. The mechanisms probably include decreased protein synthesis, increased protein catabolism, or both. **Up-regulation of proteasome** (protein degrading complex) activity is characteristic of atrophic muscle changes.[1] The primary pathway of protein catabolism is the **ubiquitin-proteasome pathway.** Proteins degraded in this pathway are first conjugated to *ubiquitin* (another small protein) and then degraded by proteasomes.

Atrophy as a result of chronic malnutrition is often accompanied by a "self-eating" process called *autophagy* inducing **autophagic vacuoles.** These vacuoles are membrane-bound vesicles within the cell that contain cellular debris—small fragments of mitochondria and endoplasmic reticulum—and hydrolytic enzymes. Atrophic change causes a rapid increase in hydrolytic enzymes, which are isolated in autophagic vacuoles to prevent uncontrolled cellular destruction. Thus the vacuoles proliferate as needed to protect the uninjured organelles from the injured organelles and are eventually taken up and destroyed by lysosomes (see p. 7). Certain contents of the autophagic vacuole may resist destruction by lysosomal enzymes and persist in membrane-bound residual bodies. An example of this

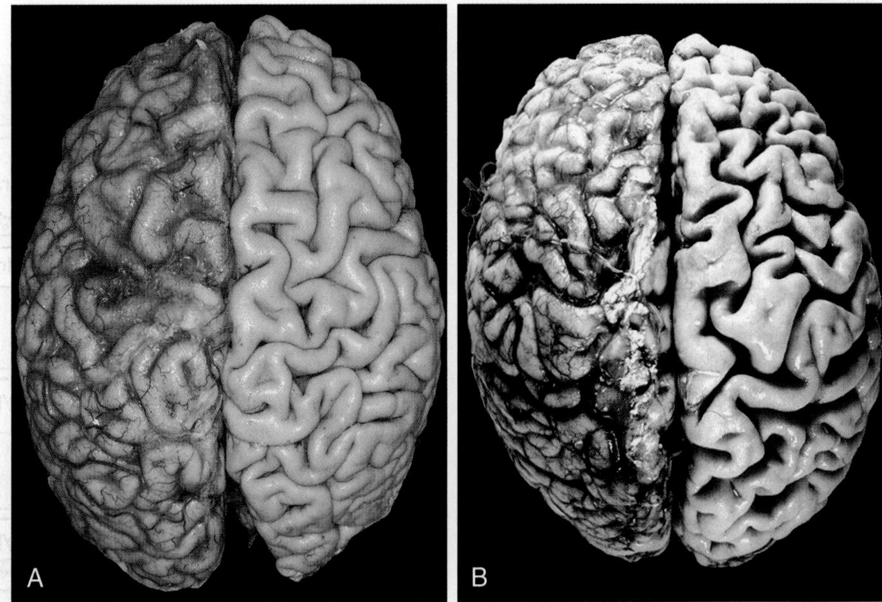

FIGURE 2-2 Atrophy. **A,** Normal brain of a young adult. **B,** Atrophy of the brain in an 82-year-old male with atherosclerotic disease. Atrophy of the brain is a result of aging and reduced blood supply. Note that loss of brain substance narrows the gyri and widens the sulci. The meninges have been stripped from the right half of each specimen to reveal the surface of the brain. (From Kumar V, Abbas A, Fausto N: *Robbins & Cotran pathologic basis of disease,* ed 8, Philadelphia, 2007, Saunders.)

is granules that contain **lipofuscin,** the yellow-brown age pigment. Lipofuscin accumulates primarily in liver cells, myocardial cells, and atrophic cells.

Hypertrophy

Hypertrophy is an increase in the size of cells and consequently in the size of the affected organ. The cells of the heart and kidneys are particularly responsive to enlargement. Hypertrophy, as an adaptive response (muscular enlargement), occurs in the striated muscle cells of both the heart and skeletal muscles. Physiologic hypertrophy in skeletal muscle occurs in response to heavy work. Muscular hypertrophy tends to diminish if the excessive workload diminishes.

The triggers for hypertrophy include two types of signals: *mechanical signals,* such as stretch, and *trophic signals,* such as growth factors and vasoactive agents. After removal of one kidney, the other kidney adapts to an increased demand for work with an increase in both the size and the number of cells. The major contribution to renal enlargement is hypertrophy.

Initial enlargement of the heart is caused by dilation of the cardiac chambers, is short-lived, and is followed by increased synthesis of cardiac muscle proteins, allowing muscle fibers to do more work. The nucleus also is hypertrophic and exhibits increased synthesis of deoxyribonucleic acid (DNA). The increase in cellular size is associated with an increased accumulation of protein in the cellular components (plasma membrane, endoplasmic reticulum, myofilaments, mitochondria) and *not* with an increase in the amount of cellular fluid. With time cardiac hypertrophy is characterized by extracellular matrix remodeling and increased growth of adult myocytes. The myocytes progressively increase in size and reach a limit beyond which no further hypertrophy can occur.[2] Although hypertrophy can be classified as *physiologic* or *pathologic,* time may be the critical factor or determinant of the transition from physiologic to pathologic cardiac hypertrophy. Pathologic hypertrophy in the heart is secondary to hypertension or valvular dysfunction. Eventually, however, advanced hypertrophy can lead to myocardial failure (Figure 2-3), suggesting that restrictions in myocyte growth are critical determinants of ventricular dysfunction[2] (see Chapter 32).

With physiologic hypertrophy, preservation of myocardial structure characterizes postnatal development, moderate endurance exercise training, pregnancy, and the early phases of increased pressure and volume loading on the adult human heart. This physiologic response is temporary, however, and aging, strenuous exercise, and sustained workload or stress lead to pathologic hypertrophy with structural and functional manifestations. A variety of intermediate signal-transduction pathways involved in myocardial growth have been reported using animal models.

Data for understanding myocyte hypertrophy have advanced; however, the reason the hypertrophied heart ultimately fails is not known. The molecular correlates that define decompensated (pathologic) hypertrophy remain obscure.[2] The fetal genes present in embryonic development, α-skeletal actin and β-myosin heavy chains, have been viewed as the hallmark of pathologic hypertrophy.[3]

Historically it was thought that myocardial cells could not adapt to increased metabolic demands by mitotic division and production of new cells to share the work. This is now being challenged (see What's New? Myocardial Hypertrophy, Stem Cells, Regeneration Controversy).

Hyperplasia

Hyperplasia is an increase in the number of cells resulting from an increased rate of cellular division. Hyperplasia as a response to injury occurs when the injury has been severe and prolonged.

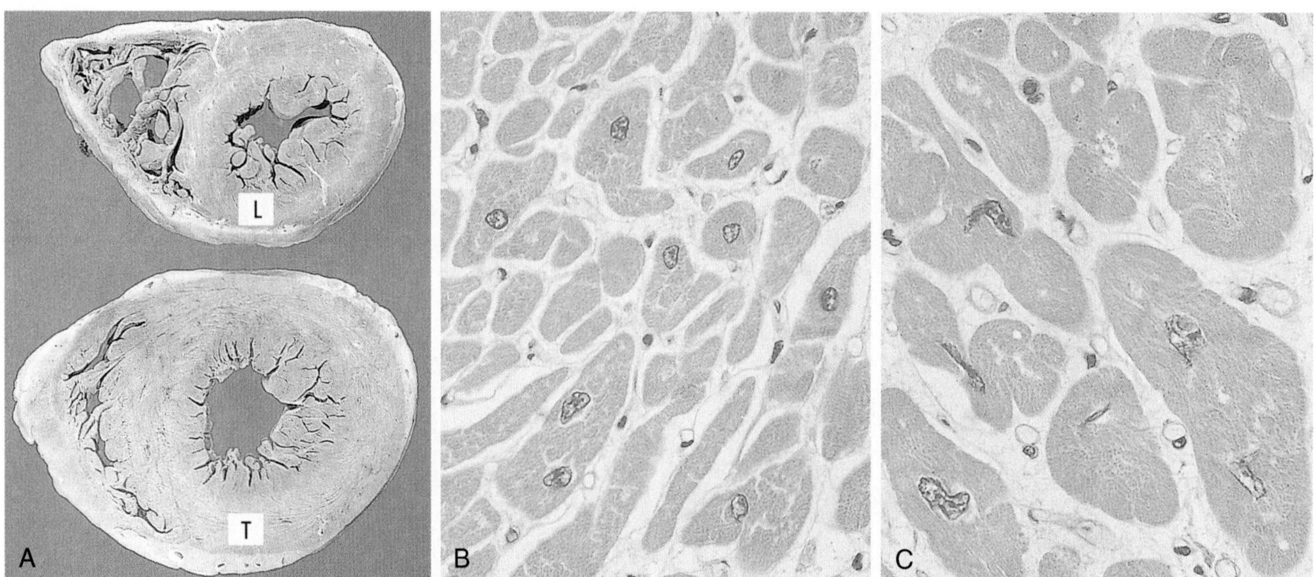

FIGURE 2-3 Hypertrophy of Cardiac Muscle in Response to Valve Disease. A, Transverse slices of a normal heart and a heart with hypertrophy of the left ventricle. (*L*, Normal thickness of left ventricular wall; *T*, thickened wall from heart in which severe narrowing of aortic valve caused resistance to systolic ventricular emptying.) **B,** Histology of cardiac muscle from a normal heart. **C,** Histology of cardiac muscle from a hypertrophied heart. (From Stevens A, Lowe JS, Scott I: *Core pathology,* ed 3, London, 2009, Mosby.)

WHAT'S NEW?

Myocardial Hypertrophy, Stem Cells, Regeneration Controversy

The human heart has been viewed as a terminally differentiated postmitotic organ where the number of cardiomyocytes is constant from birth, and these cells persist throughout the life span. The recent discovery that cardiac stem cells exist in the heart and differentiate into various cardiac cell lineages has changed the understanding of myocardial biology profoundly. So far, four potential sources of cells may account for new cardiomyocytes after birth: (1) adult cardiomyocytes may enter the cell cycle and divide, (2) bone marrow–derived cardiac stem cells or progenitor cells that have the ability to mature into cardiomyocytes may populate the heart after injury, (3) cells from the embryonic epicardium may be present, and (4) niches of cardiac or cardiac progenitor cells (CPCs) may give rise to cardiomyocytes.

From birth to adulthood and aging, the increase in myocardial mass was assumed to be regulated by a parallel increase in volume of cardiomyocytes and the changes in cell size were equal to the changes in heart weight. In the absence of cardiac disease, the number of myocytes was thought to remain constant throughout life. Hypertrophy was promoted as the exclusive mechanism used by the heart to increase its muscle mass. Myocytes increased their volume by turnover of their cytoplasmic proteins and mitochondrial organelles. Altogether, cardiomyocytes were regarded to live and function for nearly 100 years or longer. The assumption, although unstated, was that cardiomyocytes were basically immortal and died only by pathologic processes during one's life span. Myocytes, however, are formed postnatally and myocyte number decreases with aging. For example, investigators analyzed 74 normal human hearts of individuals 19 to 104 years of age and reported myocyte turnover in the female heart occurs at a rate of 10%, 14%, and 40% per year at 20, 60, and 100 years of age, respectively. The values were respectively 7%, 12%, and 32% per year in male hearts, demonstrating that myocyte growth involves a large and increasing number of cells with aging. However, the extent of myocyte turnover reported by different investigators varies substantially.

Ventricular dilation and wall thinning are the main structural aspects of heart failure. Understanding these structural aspects according to processes that modulate plasticity or regeneration and myocyte death will better define the cellular mechanisms of the failing heart. Cardiac stem cells or progenitor cells regulate myocyte turnover and this new novel information imposes a reconsideration of the mechanisms involved in myocardial aging and progression of myocardial hypertrophy to heart failure.

Data from Anversa P, Kajstura J, Leri A: Chapter 11: Cardiovascular regeneration and tissue engineering. In Bonow RO et al, editors: *Braunwald's heart disease: a textbook of cardiovascular medicine,* ed 9, St Louis, 2012, Elsevier Saunders; Leri A, Kajstura J, Amversa P: *Circ Res* 109:941–961, 2011; Kajstura J et al: *Circ Res* 107:305–315, 2010; Kajstura J et al: *Circ Res* 107:1374–1386, 2010; Olivetti G et al: *J Am Coll Cardiol* 26:1068–1079, 1995.

Loss of epithelial cells and cells of the liver and kidney triggers DNA synthesis and mitotic division. Increased cell growth is a multistep process involving the production of growth factors, which stimulate the remaining cells to synthesize new cell components and, ultimately, to divide. Hyperplasia and hypertrophy often occur together, although the specific mechanism is unknown. Both hyperplasia and hypertrophy take place if the cells are capable of synthesizing DNA.

Two types of normal, or physiologic, hyperplasia are compensatory hyperplasia and hormonal hyperplasia. **Compensatory hyperplasia** is an adaptive mechanism that enables certain organs to regenerate. For example, removal of part of the liver leads to hyperplasia of the remaining liver cells (hepatocytes) to compensate for the loss. Even with removal of 70% of the liver, regeneration is complete in about 2 weeks. The remarkable regenerating capacity of the liver was even

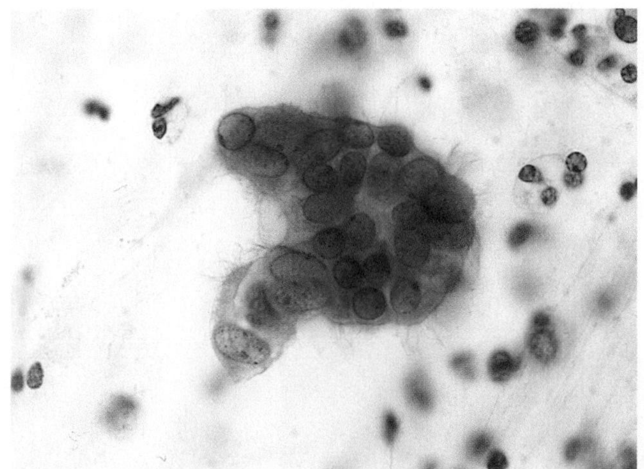

FIGURE 2-4 Hyperplasia of Bronchial Epithelium. (Bronchial Brush.) (From Damjanov I, Linder J: *Anderson's pathology,* ed 10, St Louis, 1996, Mosby.)

noted by the ancient Greeks. A protein, **hepatocyte growth factor (HGF),** is a mediator in vitro of liver regeneration. In addition, other in vitro growth factors and cytokines (cell-signaling proteins) that increase hepatic cell regeneration include transforming growth factor-alpha (TGF-α), epidermal growth factor (EGF), interleukin-6 (IL-6), and tumor necrosis factor-alpha (TNF-α).

Not all types of mature cells have the same capacity for compensatory hyperplastic growth. Nondividing tissues contain cells that can no longer (i.e., postnatally) go through the cell cycle and undergo mitotic division. These cells include neurons and skeletal and cardiac muscle cells. Destruction of neurons in the central nervous system is usually replaced by proliferation of the glial cells, the supportive structures. Recent data, however, have demonstrated neuron development from stem cells in adult brains.[4] Mature skeletal muscle cells do not divide but have been shown to have regenerative capacity from differentiation of satellite cells that are part of the endomysial sheaths. Additionally, large injury to cardiac muscle cells is followed by scar formation. However, laboratory experiments show cardiac muscle cells may have limited regenerative capacity.

Significant compensatory hyperplasia occurs in epidermal and intestinal epithelia, hepatocytes, bone marrow cells, and fibroblasts, and some hyperplasia is noted in bone, cartilage, and smooth muscle cells. An example of compensatory hyperplasia is a **callus,** or thickening, of the skin as a result of hyperplasia of epidermal cells in response to a mechanical stimulus. Another example is the response to wound healing as part of the inflammation process (see Chapter 7).

Hormonal hyperplasia occurs chiefly in estrogen-dependent organs, such as the uterus and breast. After ovulation, for example, estrogen stimulates the endometrium to grow and thicken for reception of the fertilized ovum. If pregnancy occurs, hormonal hyperplasia, as well as hypertrophy, enables the uterus to enlarge. (Hormone function is described in Chapters 21 and 22.)

Pathologic hyperplasia is the abnormal proliferation of normal cells and can occur as a response to excessive hormonal stimulation or the effects of growth factors on target cells (Figure 2-4). Hyperplastic cells are identified by pronounced enlargement of the nucleus, clumping of chromatin, and the presence of one or more enlarged nucleoli. The most common example is pathologic hyperplasia of the endometrium, which is caused by an imbalance between estrogen and progesterone secretion with oversecretion of estrogen (see Chapter 24). Pathologic endometrial hyperplasia, which causes excessive menstrual bleeding, is under the influence of regular growth-inhibition controls. If these controls fail, hyperplastic endometrial cells can undergo malignant transformation. (Malignant cell transformation is discussed in Chapter 12.)

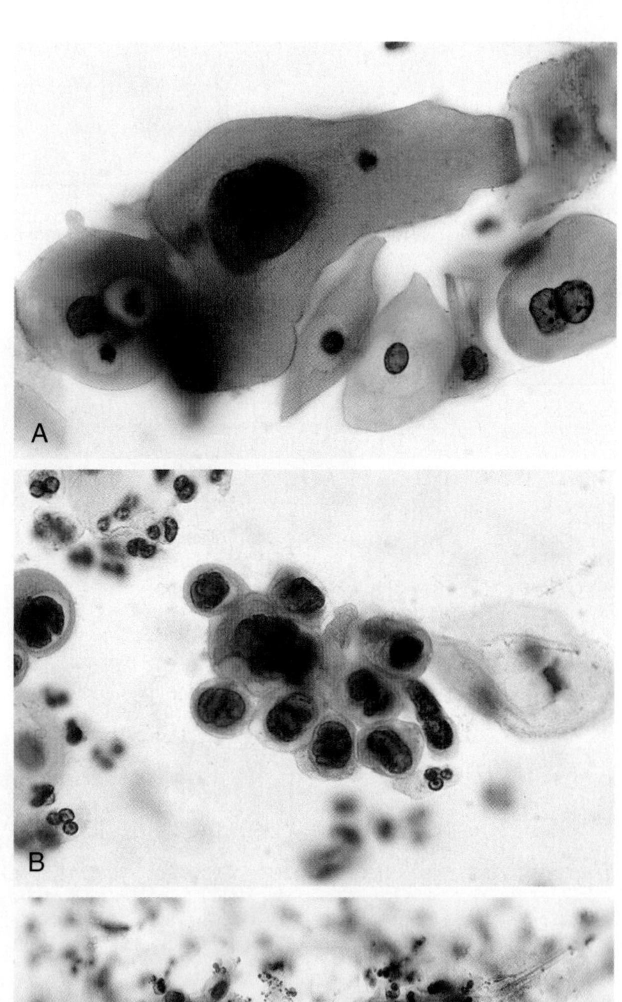

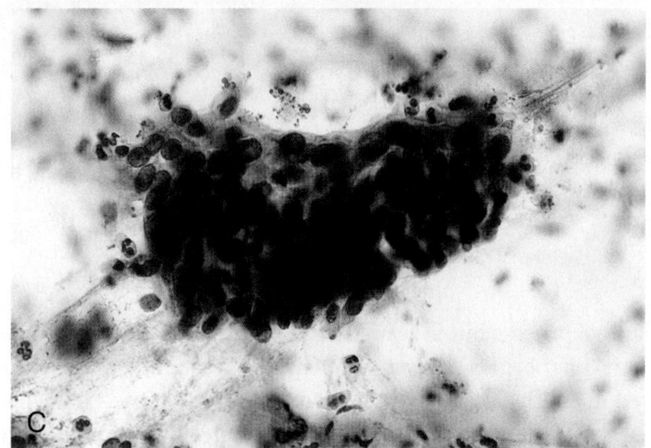

FIGURE 2-5 Dysplasia of Uterine Cervix. **A,** Mild dysplasia. **B,** Severe dysplasia. **C,** Carcinoma in situ (see Chapter 12). (From Damjanov I, Linder J: *Anderson's pathology,* ed 10, St Louis, 1996, Mosby.)

Dysplasia: Not a True Adaptive Change

Dysplasia refers to abnormal changes in the size, shape, and organization of mature cells. Dysplasia is not considered a true

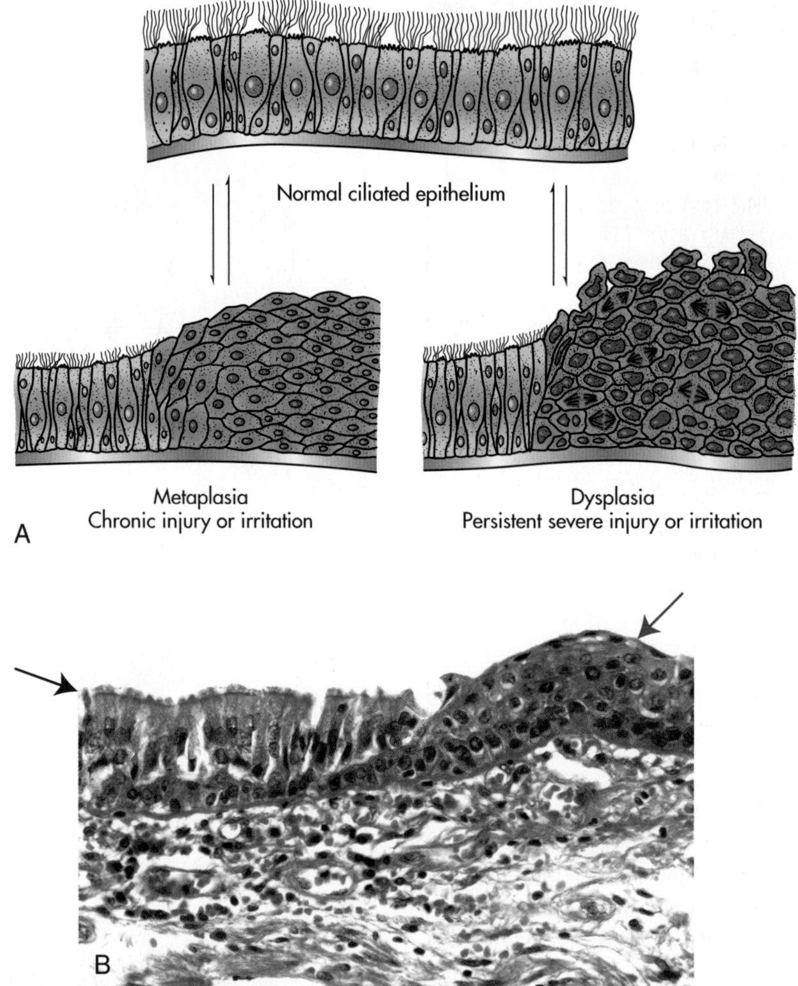

FIGURE 2-6 Reversible Changes in Cells Lining the Bronchi. A, Normal ciliated epithelium, metaplasia, and dysplasia. **B,** Histologic slide with upper left *(black arrow)* normal columnar epithelium and basement membrane, and upper right *(red arrow)* squamous metaplasia. (**B** from Kumar V, Abbas A, Fausto N: *Robbins & Cotran pathologic basis of disease,* ed 8, Philadelphia, 2007, Saunders.)

adaptive process but is related to hyperplasia and is often called **atypical hyperplasia.** Dysplastic changes frequently are encountered in epithelial tissue of the cervix and respiratory tract, where they are strongly associated with common neoplastic growths and often are found adjacent to cancerous cells. Importantly, the term *dysplasia* does *not* indicate cancer and may not progress to cancer.

Dysplasia is often classified as mild, moderate, or severe; however, this subjective scheme has prompted recommendations to use either "low grade" or "high grade," for example, of the female reproductive tract (i.e., Papanicolaou [Pap] test [discussed in Chapter 24]) (Figure 2-5). Data indicate that atypical hyperplasia is a strong predictor of breast cancer development.[5,6] If the inciting stimulus is removed, dysplastic changes often are reversible.

Metaplasia

Metaplasia is the reversible replacement of one mature cell by another, sometimes less differentiated, cell type. The best example of metaplasia is replacement of normal columnar ciliated epithelial cells of the bronchial (airway) lining by stratified squamous epithelial cells (Figure 2-6). The newly formed squamous epithelial cells do not secrete mucus or have cilia, causing loss of a vital protective mechanism.

Metaplasia is thought to develop from a reprogramming of stem cells existing in most epithelia or of undifferentiated **mesenchymal** (tissue from embryonic mesoderm) **cells** present in connective tissue. These precursor cells mature along a new pathway because of signals generated by cytokines and growth factors in the cell's environment.

Bronchial metaplasia can be reversed if the inducing stimulus, usually cigarette smoking, is removed. With prolonged exposure to the inducing stimulus, however, cancerous transformation can occur.

CELLULAR INJURY

Injury to cells and to extracellular matrix (ECM) leads to injury of tissues and organs ultimately determining the structural patterns of disease. Loss of function derives from cell and ECM injury and cell death. Cellular injury occurs if the cell is unable to maintain homeostasis—a normal or adaptive steady state—in the face of injurious stimuli or stress. Injured cells may recover (**reversible injury**) or

TABLE 2-1 PROGRESSIVE TYPES OF CELL INJURY AND RESPONSES

TYPE	RESPONSES
Adaptation	Atrophy, hypertrophy, hyperplasia, metaplasia
Active cell injury	Immediate response of "entire" cell
Reversible	Loss of adenosine triphosphate (ATP), swelling of cell, detachment of ribosomes, autophagy of lysosomes
Irreversible	"Point of no return" structurally when severe vacuolization of mitochondria occurs and Ca^{++} moves into the cell, including mitochondrial membrane damage
Necrosis	Common type of cell death with severe cell swelling and breakdown of organelles
Apoptosis, a type of programmed cell death	Cellular self-destruction for elimination of unwanted cell populations
Chronic cell injury (subcellular alterations)	Persistent stimuli response may involve only specific organelles or cytoskeleton (e.g., phagocytosis of bacteria)
Accumulations or infiltrations	Water, pigments, lipids, glycogen, proteins
Pathologic calcification	Dystrophic and metastatic calcification

die (**irreversible injury**). Injurious stimuli include chemical agents, lack of sufficient oxygen (hypoxia), free radicals, infectious agents, physical and mechanical factors, immunologic reactions, genetic factors, and nutritional imbalances. Types of cellular injury and their responses are summarized in Table 2-1 and Figure 2-7.

Cell injury and cell death often result from exposure to toxic chemicals, infections, and hypoxia. (Infections are discussed in Chapter 10.) The mechanisms causing chemical and hypoxic injury are perhaps the best understood. Both of these mechanisms can lead to disruption of selective permeability (i.e., transport mechanisms) of the plasma membrane; reduction or cessation of cellular metabolism; lack of protein synthesis; damage to lysosomal membranes with leakage of destructive enzymes into the cytoplasm; enzymatic destruction of cellular organelles; cellular death (exhibited by nuclear changes); and phagocytosis of the dead cell by cellular components of the acute inflammatory response (see Chapter 7). The extent of cellular injury depends on the type, state (including level of cell differentiation and increased susceptibility to fully differentiated cells), and adaptive processes of the cell, as well as the type, severity, and duration of the injurious stimulus. Two individuals exposed to an identical stimulus may incur varying degrees of cellular injury. Modifying factors, such as nutritional status, can profoundly influence the extent of injury. The precise "point of no return" that leads to cellular death is a biochemical puzzle, and the exact mechanisms responsible for the transition from reversible to irreversible cellular damage are being debated.

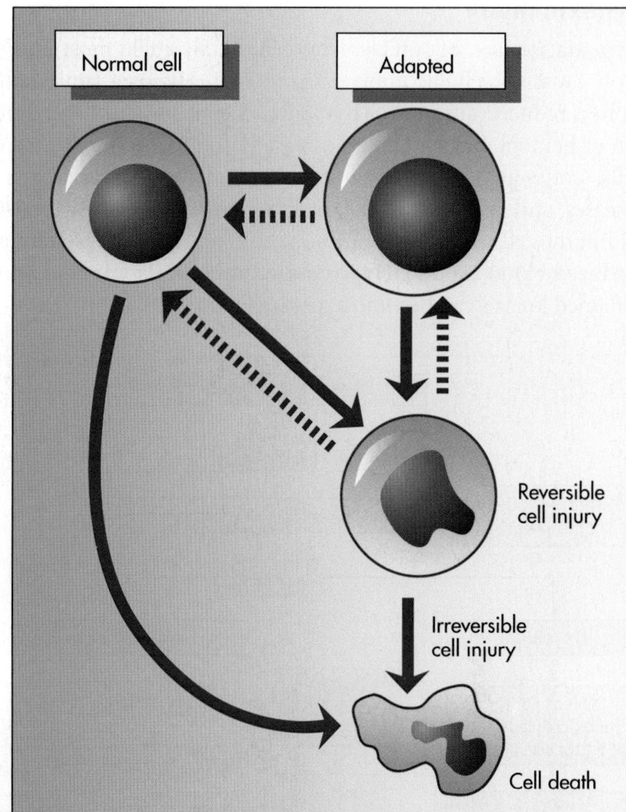

FIGURE 2-7 Cellular Injury and Responses. Depicted here is the relationship among normal, adapted (hypertrophy), and reversibly injured cells and cell death of myocardial cells.

TABLE 2-2 COMMON THEMES IN CELL INJURY AND CELL DEATH

THEME	COMMENTS
ATP depletion	Loss of mitochondrial ATP and decreased ATP synthesis; results include cellular swelling, decreased protein synthesis, decreased membrane transport, and lipogenesis, all changes that contribute to loss of integrity of plasma membrane (see text)
Oxygen and oxygen-derived free radicals	Lack of oxygen is key in progression of cell injury in ischemia (reduced blood supply); activated oxygen species (free radicals, H_2O_2, O_2^-, NO) cause destruction of cell membranes and cell structure
Intracellular calcium and loss of calcium steady state	Normally intracellular cytosolic calcium concentrations are very low; ischemia and certain chemicals cause an increase in cytosolic Ca^{++} concentrations; sustained levels of Ca^{++} continue to increase with damage to plasma membrane; Ca^{++} causes intracellular damage by activating a number of enzymes (see text)
Defects in membrane permeability	Early loss of selective membrane permeability found in all forms of cell injury (see text)

ATP, Adenosine triphosphate.

General Mechanisms of Cell Injury

Cells are complex units, and therefore the mechanisms responsible for cell injury leading to necrotic cell death are numerous and interrelated and depend on a delicate balance between intracellular and extracellular events. There are, however, common biochemical themes important to cell injury and cell death regardless of the injuring agent (Table 2-2). Examples of cell injury are: (1) hypoxic injury, (2) reactive oxygen species and free radical–induced injury, and (3) chemical injury.

Hypoxic Injury

Hypoxia, or lack of sufficient oxygen, is the single most common cause of cellular injury (Figure 2-8). Hypoxia can result from a reduced amount of oxygen in the air, loss of hemoglobin or hemoglobin function, decreased production of red blood cells, consequences of respiratory and cardiovascular system diseases, and poisoning of the oxidative enzymes (cytochromes) within the cells. The most common cause of hypoxia is **ischemia** (reduced blood supply). Hypoxia can induce inflammation and inflamed lesions can become hypoxic (Figure 2-9).

Ischemic injury is often caused by gradual narrowing of arteries (arteriosclerosis) and complete blockage by blood clots (thrombosis). Progressive hypoxia caused by gradual arterial obstruction is better tolerated than the sudden acute **anoxia** (total lack of oxygen) caused by a sudden obstruction, such as can occur with an embolus (a blood clot or other plug in the circulation). An acute obstruction in a coronary artery can cause myocardial cell death (infarction) within minutes if the blood supply is not restored, whereas the gradual onset of ischemia usually results in myocardial adaptation. Myocardial infarction and stroke, which

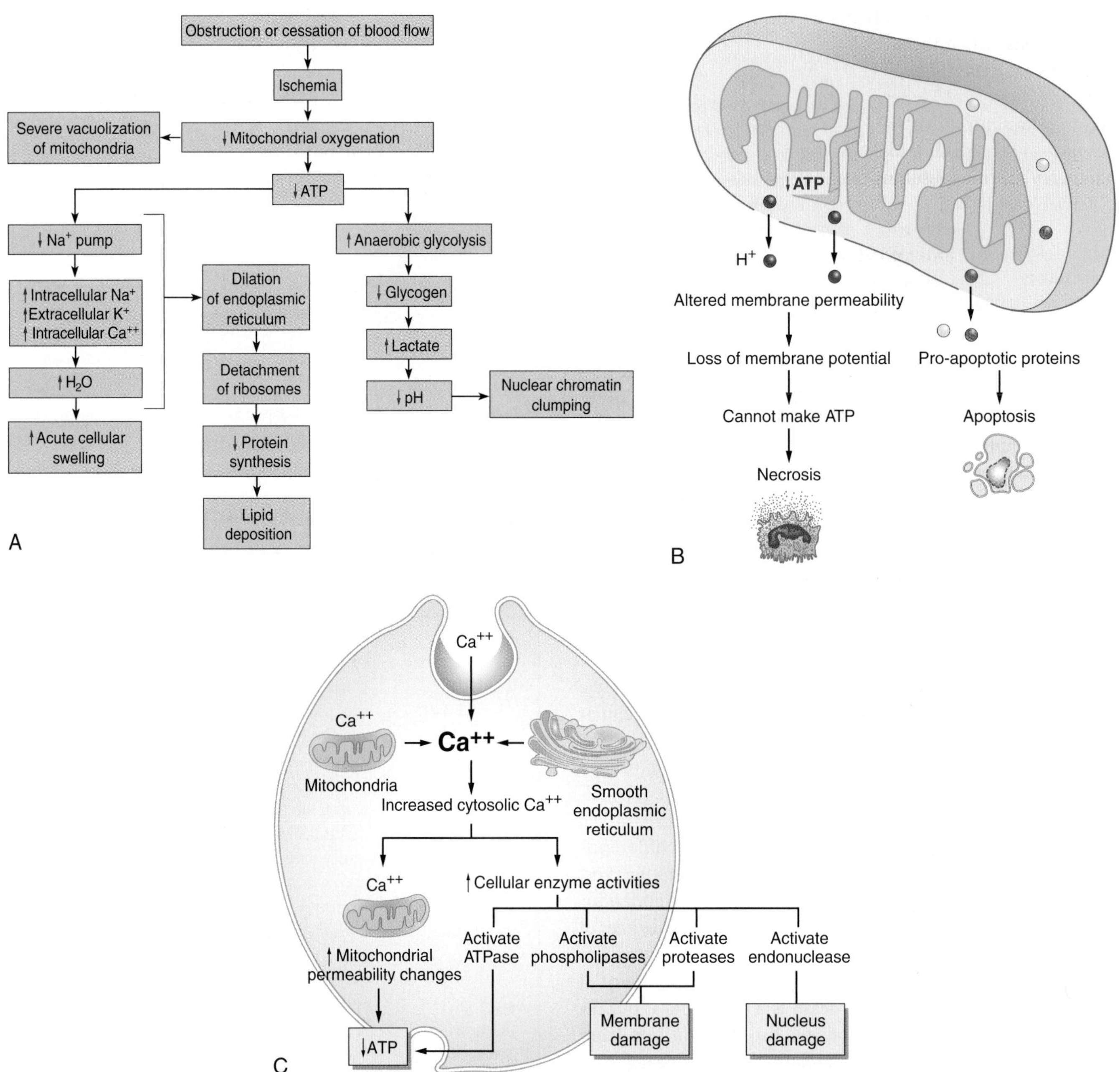

FIGURE 2-8 Hypoxic Injury Induced by Ischemia. A, Consequences of decreased oxygen delivery or ischemia with decreased ATP. The structural and physiologic changes are reversible if oxygen is delivered quickly. Significant decreases in ATP concentration result in cell death, mostly by necrosis. **B,** Mitochondrial damage can result in changes in membrane permeability, loss of membrane potential, and decreased ATP. Between the outer and inner membranes of the mitochondria are proteins that can activate the cell's suicide pathways, called apoptosis. **C,** Calcium ions are critical mediators of cell injury. Calcium ions are usually maintained at low concentrations in the cell's cytoplasm; thus ischemia and certain toxins can initially cause an increase in the release of Ca^{++} from intracellular stores and later an increased movement (influx) across the plasma membrane.

are common causes of death in the United States, generally result from atherosclerosis (a type of arteriosclerosis) and consequent ischemic injury. (Vascular obstruction is discussed in Chapter 32.)

Cellular responses to hypoxic injury in heart muscle have been extensively studied. Within 1 minute after blood supply to the myocardium is interrupted, the heart becomes pale and has difficulty contracting normally. Within 3 to 5 minutes the ischemic portion of the myocardium ceases to contract. The abrupt lack of contraction is caused by a rapid decrease in mitochondrial phosphorylation, which results in insufficient adenosine triphosphate (ATP) production. Lack of ATP leads to an increase in anaerobic metabolism, which generates ATP from glycogen when there is insufficient oxygen. When glycogen stores are depleted even anaerobic metabolism ceases.

A reduction in ATP levels causes the plasma membrane's sodium-potassium (Na^+-K^+) pump and sodium-calcium exchange to fail, which leads to an intracellular accumulation of sodium and calcium, resulting in cellular swelling and diffusion of potassium out of the cell. (The Na^+-K^+ pump is discussed in Chapter 1.) Because all cells are bathed in a fluid rich in calcium ions, cell membrane damage allows rapid movement of calcium intracellularly. The movement of water and ions into the cell causes early dilation of the endoplasmic reticulum. Dilation causes the ribosomes to detach from the rough endoplasmic reticulum, resulting in reduced protein synthesis. With continued hypoxia, the entire cell becomes markedly swollen, with increased concentrations of sodium, water, and chloride and decreased concentrations of potassium. These disruptions are reversible if oxygen is restored. If oxygen is not restored, however, there is **vacuolation** (formation of vacuoles or cytoplasmic small cavities) within the cytoplasm, swelling of lysosomes, and marked swelling of the mitochondria resulting from mitochondrial membrane damage. Continued hypoxic injury with accumulation of calcium subsequently activates multiple enzyme systems, including proteases, nitric oxide synthase, phospholipases, and endonuclease, resulting in cytoskeleton disruption, membrane damage, activation of inflammation, DNA

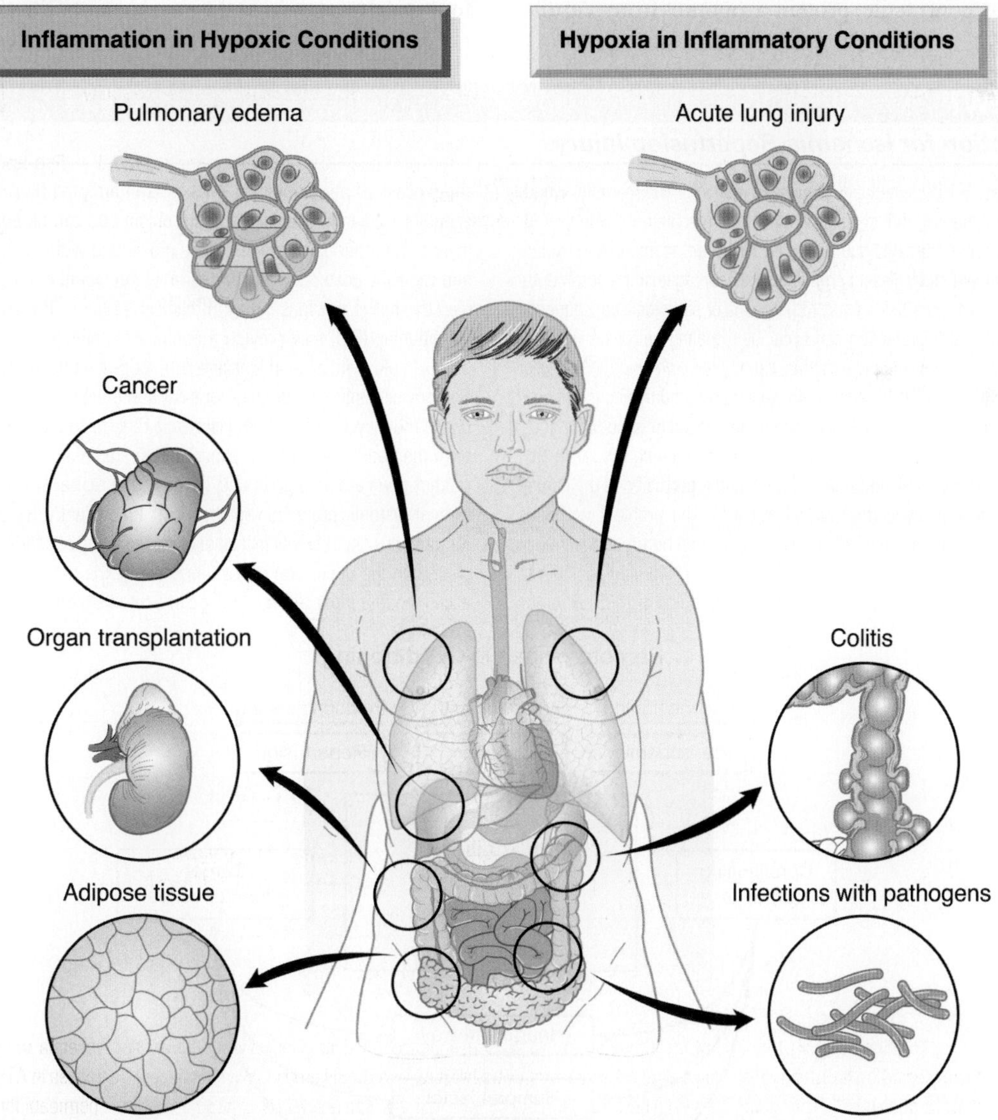

FIGURE 2-9 Hypoxia and Inflammation. Shown is a simplified drawing of clinical conditions characterized by tissue hypoxia that causes inflammatory changes *(left)* and inflammatory diseases that ultimately lead to hypoxia *(right)*. These diseases and conditions are discussed in more detail in their respective chapters. (Adapted from Eltzschig HK, Carmeliet P: *N Engl J Med* 364:656–665, 2011.)

and chromatin degradation, ATP depletion, and eventual cell death (see Figures 2-8 and 2-23 [p. 86]). Structurally, with plasma membrane damage, extracellular calcium readily moves into the cell and intracellular calcium stores are released.

Intracellular calcium results in the activation of enzymes that can further damage membranes, proteins, ATP, and nucleic acids. The increased permeability of the membrane causes continued loss of proteins, essential coenzymes, and ribonucleic acids. In addition, the substrates necessary to reconstitute ATP are lost. Increased intracellular calcium levels activate cell enzymes (caspases) that promote cell death by apoptosis (see Figure 2-26 [p. 89]). Continued ischemia causes irreversible injury that is associated structurally with severe swelling of the mitochondria, severe damage to plasma membranes, and swelling of lysosomes.

Acid hydrolases from leaking lysosomes are activated in the reduced pH of the injured cell and they digest cytoplasmic and nuclear components. Leakage of intracellular enzymes into the peripheral circulation provides a diagnostic tool for detecting tissue-specific cellular injury and death using blood samples; for example, the contractile protein troponin from cardiac muscle is found after myocardial injury and liver transaminases are found after hepatic injury.

Restoration of oxygen, however, can cause additional injury called **reperfusion (reoxygenation) injury.** Reperfusion injury results from the generation of highly reactive oxygen intermediates (oxidative stress), including hydroxyl radical (OH•), superoxide $O_2^{\overline{\cdot}}$, and hydrogen peroxide (H_2O_2) (see p. 59). These radicals can all cause further membrane damage and mitochondrial calcium overload. The white blood cells (neutrophils) are especially affected with reperfusion injury, including neutrophil adhesion to the endothelium.

Reperfusion is a serious complication and an important mechanism of injury in instances of tissue transplantation and in myocardial, hepatic, intestinal, cerebral, renal, and other ischemic syndromes, including stroke.[7] Xanthine dehydrogenase, an enzyme that normally uses oxidized nicotinamide adenine dinucleotide (NAD^+) as an electron acceptor, is converted during reperfusion with oxygen to xanthine oxidase. During the ischemic period, excessive ATP consumption leads to the accumulation of the purine catabolites hypoxanthine and

WHAT'S NEW?

Cardioprotection for Ischemia-Reperfusion Injury

Coronary heart disease (CHD) is the leading cause of morbidity and mortality worldwide. Despite optimal therapy and an amazing amount of research, individuals with CHD still suffer significant morbidity and mortality. Therefore, to improve individual outcomes novel treatment strategies for protecting the heart against the detrimental effects of acute ischemia-reperfusion injury (IRI), the major pathologic consequence of CHD, are required. Cardioprotection can occur by signaling pathways initiated before or at the beginning of sustained ischemia, called *preconditioning* (PC), and/or cardioprotection at the very start of reperfusion, called postconditioning (see figure below). *Perconditioning* is a term sometimes used for the period of ischemia.

Murray and colleagues first described ischemic preconditioning (IPC) in which the application of short cycles of nonlethal ischemia and reperfusion to the canine heart reduced subsequent myocardial infarct size (IS). The problem with this strategy is the requirement for the intervention to be applied before the ischemic event, which in the case of an acute myocardial infarction (MI) is impossible to predict. However, the introduction of ischemic postconditioning in 2003, whereby the process of myocardial reperfusion is interrupted by several short-lived episodes of ischemia, overcomes this problem and can be applied at the onset of myocardial reperfusion in individuals presenting with an acute MI. Yet, both IPC and ischemic postconditioning require an intervention to be applied to the heart directly that is not feasible in all clinical settings. Therefore, remote ischemic conditioning (RIC) may provide a noninvasive endogenous therapeutic strategy (for example, with a blood pressure cuff) for protecting the heart against acute IRI. Remote ischemic conditioning is the cardioprotective effect elicited from applying one or more cycles of nonlethal ischemia reperfusion to an organ or tissue remote from the heart. Furthermore, experimental studies found that it was possible to protect non-cardiac organs and tissues from acute IRI. Thus, RIC represents a form of systemic protection against acute IRI. Recently, it was discovered that the RIC stimulus could be noninvasively induced using a standard blood pressure cuff placed on the upper arm or leg. Importantly, the timing of the RIC stimulus can accommodate most clinical settings of acute IRI (see figure below).

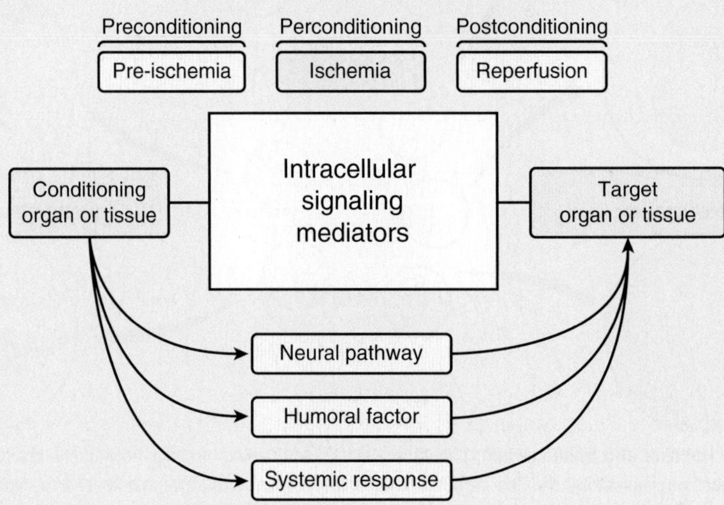

Data from Kharbanda RK et al: *Circulation* 106:2881–2883, 2002; Lim SY, Hausenloy DJ: *Front Physiol* 3:27, 2012.

xanthine, which upon subsequent reperfusion and influx of oxygen are metabolized by xanthine oxidase to make *massive* amounts of superoxide and hydrogen peroxide. These radicals can all cause membrane damage and mitochondrial calcium overload.[3] Cardiac ischemia and reperfusion injury cause excessive reactive oxygen species (ROS) and calcium overload of the mitochondria. These changes presumably lead to the opening of a large conductance pore on the mitochondrial membrane called the *mitochondrial permeability transition pore* (MPTP) with massive escape of ATP and solutes leading to cell death activation (apoptosis).[8] Cardioprotection from ischemia/reperfusion injury is an important focus of much research (see What's New? Cardioprotection for Ischemia-Reperfusion Injury). Other potential and current treatments include use of antioxidants, blockage of inflammatory mediators, and inhibition of apoptotic pathways.

Free Radicals and Reactive Oxygen Species—Oxidative Stress

An important mechanism of membrane damage is injury induced by free radicals, especially by excess ROS called **oxidative stress** (Figure 2-10). Oxidative stress occurs when *excess*

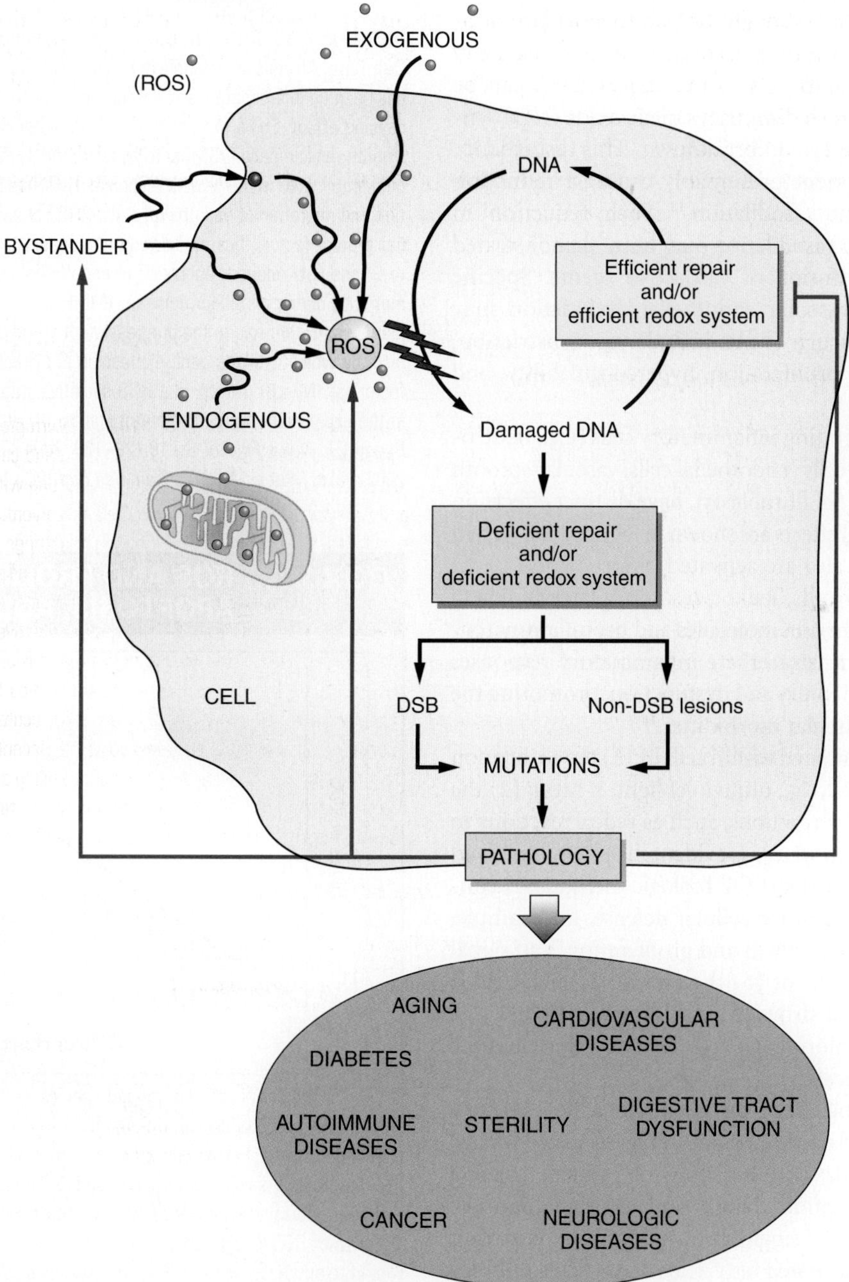

FIGURE 2-10 Oxidative Stress in Human Pathogenesis. Reactive oxygen species *(ROS)* have a role in a wide variety of diseases and age-related diseases including cancer, neurologic disease, type 2 diabetes, autoimmune and cardiovascular diseases, infertility, and normal aging. Chronic exposure to ROS and decreased DNA repair can result in persistent DNA mutations. Accumulation of DNA lesions can lead to DNA double strand breaks *(DSB)* and disease onset/progression. Diseased cells can in turn develop ROS and decrease the efficiency of the DNA repair mechanism. (Adapted from Sedelnikova OA et al: *Mutat Res* 704:152–159, 2010.)

ROS overwhelms endogenous antioxidant systems (Box 2-1). A **free radical** is an electrically uncharged atom or group of atoms having an unpaired electron. Having one unpaired electron makes the molecule unstable; thus to stabilize, it gives up an electron to another molecule or steals one. Therefore, it is capable of injurious chemical bond formation with proteins, lipids, and carbohydrates—key molecules in membranes and nucleic acids. Free radicals are difficult to control and initiate chain reactions. Emerging data indicate that ROS play major roles in the initiation and progression of cardiovascular alterations associated with hypertension, hyperlipidemia, diabetes mellitus, ischemic heart disease, chronic heart failure, and sleep apnea.[9,10] ROS generation is thought to lead to vascular endothelial injury and consequently atherosclerosis. Up-regulation of adhesion molecule production in the endothelium can be accomplished by ROS, which diminishes nitric oxide (NO) synthase activity and promotes NO breakdown. This disturbance of the vascular environment presumably causes a reduction of endothelial-dependent vasodilation.[11] Such reduction in endothelium-dependent vasodilation has been demonstrated through intra-arterial infusion of vasoactive agents. Specific mechanisms by which vascular endothelial dysfunction may lead to adverse cardiovascular events include vasoconstriction, vascular smooth muscle proliferation, hypercoagulability, and thrombosis.[12]

ROS produced by migrating inflammatory cells (e.g., neutrophils), as well as vascular cells (endothelial cells, vascular smooth muscle cells, and adventitial fibroblasts), have distinct effects on each cell type.[13] These cell effects are shown in Figure 2-11. When inflammatory responses also are activated, there is consequent activation of endothelial cells, leukocytes, and platelets. These activated cells express adhesion molecules and proinflammatory cytokines that may further exacerbate inflammatory responses and cause endothelial cell injury and dysfunction, promoting the development of cardiovascular morbidities.[14]

Free radicals may be initiated within cells by (1) the absorption of extreme energy sources (e.g., ultraviolet light, x-rays); (2) the occurrence of endogenous reactions, such as redox reactions in which oxygen is reduced to water, as evident in systems involved in electron and oxygen transport (all biologic membranes contain redox systems important for cellular defense, for example, inflammation, iron uptake, growth and proliferation, and signal transduction) (Figure 2-12); or (3) the enzymatic metabolism of exogenous chemicals or drugs (e.g., chloromethyl [$CCl_3^{\bullet}$], a product of carbon tetrachloride [CCl_4]). Table 2-3 describes the most significant free radicals.

Although wide-ranging effects can occur from these reactive species, three are particularly important in regard to cell injury: (1) peroxidation of lipids; (2) alterations of proteins causing fragmentation of polypeptide chains; and (3) alterations of DNA, including breakage of single strands. **Lipid peroxidation** is the destruction of unsaturated fatty acids. Fatty acids of lipids in membranes possess double bonds between some of the carbon atoms. Such bonds are vulnerable to attack by oxygen-derived free radicals, especially OH·. The lipid-radical interactions themselves yield peroxides. The peroxides instigate a chain reaction resulting in membrane, organelle, and cellular destruction.

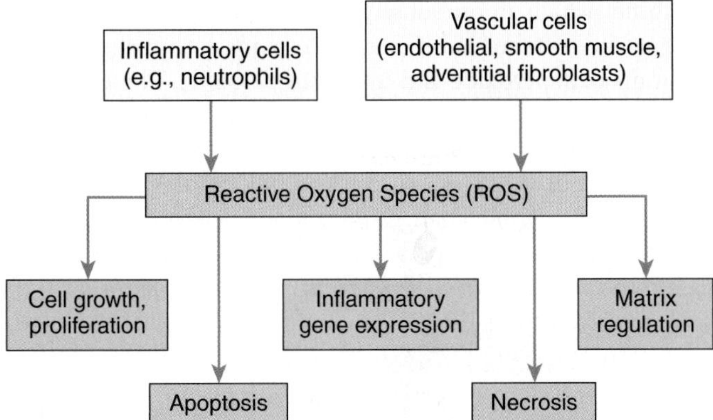

FIGURE 2-11 ROS Can Cause Distinct Functional Effects Depending on Cell Type. All cells are capable of making reactive oxygen species (ROS). Emphasis has been on inflammatory and vascular cells because of their widespread disease-causing effect. Some examples include angiotensin II, which can induce vascular smooth muscle cells (VSMCs) to hypertrophy; NAD(P)H oxidase–derived ROS has been implicated in the growth response; H_2O_2 has been shown to induce proliferation and migration of endothelial cells; ROS act as mediators of vascular endothelial growth factor, thus modulating angiogenesis; endothelial injury or exposure to O_2^- and H_2O_2 induces apoptosis of endothelial cells. Activity of the extracellular matrix by matrix metalloproteinases (MMPs) can be modulated by ROS. Cytokines play a significant role in the progression of vascular lesions. An important mechanism by which cytokine gene expression is increased is the activation of nuclear factor-κβ (NF-κβ). NF-κβ is a ROS-sensitive transcription factor and has a role in the expression of proinflammatory genes. (Data from Buetler TM, Krauskopf A, Ruegg UT: *News Physiol Sci* 19:120–123, 2004; Dröge W: *Physiol Rev* 82:47–95, 2002; Valko M et al: *Int J Biochem Cell Biol* 39[1]:44–84, 2007.) (Also see Box 2-1.)

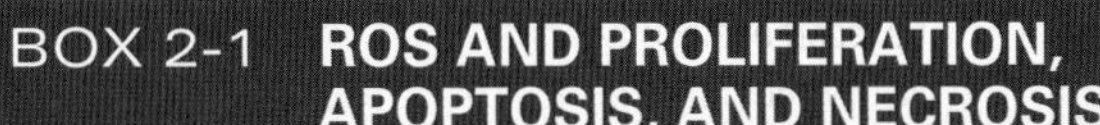

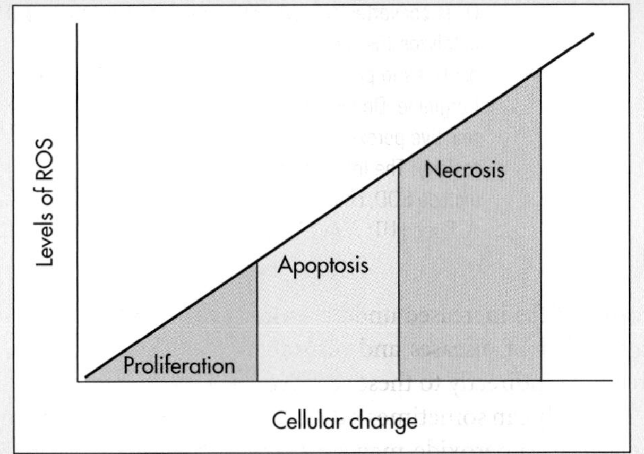

Cellular effects of reactive oxygen species (ROS) may depend on *concentration levels*. At low concentrations, ROS appear to exert a beneficial growth-stimulatory effect on a wide variety of cells and microorganisms. For example, bacteria such as *Escherichia coli* and *Salmonella typhimurium* need O_2^- for growth. Certain human cell lines also have shown this dependency in vitro. Yet when ROS levels increase, other signaling pathways may be activated that lead to apoptosis. When ROS levels rise even higher, a cell may die a sudden necrotic death. The apoptosis and necrosis modes are thought to be caused by oxidative stress. Thus the signaling functions of ROS are now appreciated.

Data from Buetler TM, Krauskopf A, Ruegg UT: *News Physiol Sci* 19:120–123, 2004; Valko M et al: *Int J Biochem Cell Biol* 39(1):44–84, 2007.

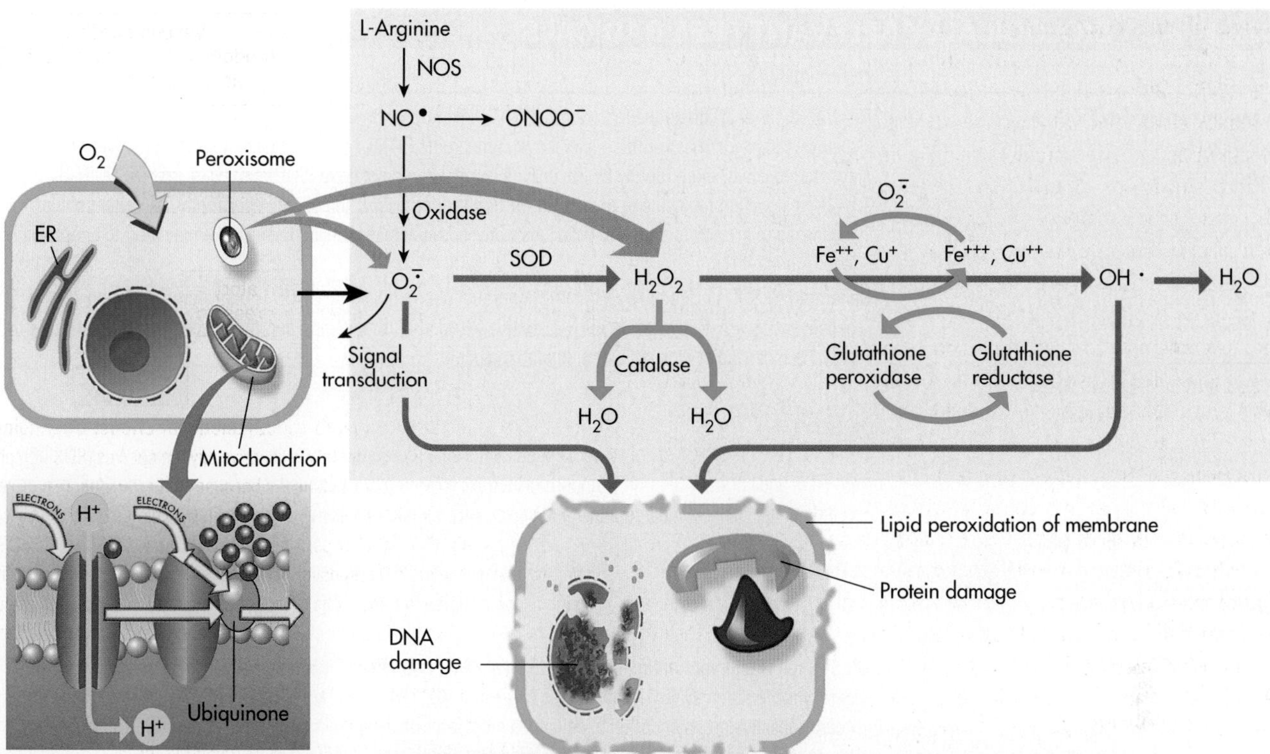

FIGURE 2-12 **Generation of Reactive Oxygen Species (ROS) and Antioxidant Mechanisms in Biologic Systems.** Mitochondria have four sites of entry for electrons coming into the electron-transport system: one for reduced nicotinamide adenine dinucleotide (NADH) and three for the reduced form of flavin adenine dinucleotide ($FADH_2$). These pathways meet at the small, lipophilic molecule ubiquinone (coenzyme Q), at the beginning of the common electron-transport pathway. Ubiquinone transfers electrons in the inner membrane, ultimately enabling their interaction with O_2 and H_2 to yield H_2O. In so doing, the transport allows free energy change and the synthesis of 1 mol of adenosine triphosphate (ATP). With the transport of electrons, free radicals are generated within the mitochondria. ROS (H_2O_2, OH•, and O_2^- and nitric oxide [NO]) act as physiologic modulators of some mitochondrial functions but also may cause cell damage. O_2 is converted to superoxide (O_2^-) by oxidative enzymes in the mitochondria, endoplasmic reticulum (ER), plasma membrane, peroxisomes, and cytosol. O_2 is converted to H_2O_2 by superoxide dismutase (SOD) and further to OH• by the Cu^{++}/Fe^{++} Fenton reaction. Superoxide catalyzes the reduction of Fe^{++} to Fe^{+++}, thus increasing OH• formation by the Fenton reaction. H_2O_2 is also derived from oxidases in peroxisomes. The NO• (radical) is produced by the oxidation of one of the terminal guanido-nitrogen atoms of l-arginine. Depending on the microenvironment, NO can be converted to other reactive nitrogen species including the highly reactive peroxynitrate ($ONOO^-$). Both OH• and $ONOO^-$ are very reactive and can modify cellular macromolecules and cause toxicity. The less reactive molecules O_2^- and H_2O_2 can serve as cellular signaling molecules. The major antioxidant enzymes include SOD, catalase, and glutathione peroxidase. (Data from Dröge W: *Physiol Rev* 82:47–95, 2002; Buetler TM, Krauskopf A, Ruegg UT: *News Physiol Sci* 19:120–123, 2004.)

Because of the increased understanding of free radicals, a growing number of diseases and disorders have been linked either directly or indirectly to these reactive species (Box 2-2).

The body can sometimes rid itself of free radicals. The oxygen free radical superoxide may spontaneously decay into oxygen and hydrogen peroxide. Table 2-4 summarizes other methods that contribute to inactivation or termination of free radicals. The toxicity of certain drugs and chemicals can be attributed to either the conversion of these chemicals to free radicals or the formation of oxygen-derived metabolites.[7] This process is discussed in Chemical Injury.

Mitochondria and ROS

During normal metabolism, the mitochondria are the greatest source and target of ROS. Usually ROS are reduced by intracellular antioxidant enzymes, including superoxide dismutase (SOD), glutathione peroxidase, and catalase, as well as antioxidant molecules, such as glutathione and vitamin E. These ROS, however, contribute to mitochondria dysfunction and are related to many human diseases and aging. In pathologic conditions, the large numbers of ROS overwhelm the balance by antioxidants. This inefficiency of antioxidants is even more serious in mitochondria because mitochondria in most cells lack catalase.[15] Consequently, the excessive production of hydrogen peroxide and eventually hydroxyl radicals (OH•) in mitochondria will damage lipid, proteins, and **mitochondrial DNA (mtDNA),** which then causes cells to die.[15-18] Mitochondrial oxidative stress has been implicated in heart disease, Alzheimer disease, Parkinson disease, prion diseases, and amyotrophic lateral sclerosis (ALS), as well as aging itself.[19-23] Accumulating evidence shows ROS important for cell proliferation and survival.[20] Dysfunction of autophagy may result in abnormal mitochondrial function

TABLE 2-3 BIOLOGICALLY RELEVANT FREE RADICALS

FREE RADICAL	COMMENTS
Reactive oxygen species (ROS) Superoxide O_2^- $O_2 \rightarrow$ oxidase O_2^-	Generated either (1) directly during autooxidation in mitochondria, or (2) enzymatically by enzymes in the cytoplasm, such as xanthine oxidase or cytochrome P-450; once produced, it can be inactivated spontaneously or more rapidly by the enzyme superoxide dismutase (SOD): $O_2^- + O_2^- + 2H^+ \rightarrow$ SOD $H_2O_2 +$ O_2^- O_2^-, a signaling molecule in growing or differentiating tissue, including hypertrophy, can alter cellular responses to growth factors and vasoconstrictor hormones; increasing levels of O_2^- may lead to apoptosis (see Figure 2-11)
Hydrogen peroxide (H_2O_2) $O_2^- + O_2^- + 2H \rightarrow$ SOD $H_2O_2 + O_2$ *or* Oxidases present in peroxisomes O_2 peroxisome $O_2^- \rightarrow$ SOD H_2O_2	Generated by SOD or directly by oxidases in intracellular peroxisomes; SOD is considered an antioxidant because it converts superoxide to $H_2O_2^-$, catalase (another antioxidant) can then decompose H_2O_2 to O_2 + H_2O; H_2O_2 can serve as a cellular signaling molecule
Hydroxyl radicals (OH•) $H_2O \rightarrow H• + OH•$ *or* $Fe^{++} + H_2O_2 \rightarrow Fe^{+++} + OH• + OH^-$ *or* $H_2O_2 + O_2^- \rightarrow OH• + OH^- + O_2$ Nitric oxide (NO)	Generated by the hydrolysis of water caused by ionizing radiation or by interaction with metals—especially iron (Fe) and copper (Cu); iron is important in toxic oxygen injury because it is required for maximal oxidative cell damage; OH• is highly reactive and can modify cellular macromolecules and cause toxicity
$NO• + O_2^- \rightarrow ONOO^- + H+$ ↑↓ $OH• + NO_2$ ONOOH $\rightarrow NO_3^-$	NO by itself is an important mediator that can act as a free radical; it can be converted to another radical—peroxynitrite anion (ONOO–), as well as NO_2• and NO_3^-. NO is formed in neuronal cells, where it modulates neurotransmission; in endothelial cells as a modulator of vessel relaxation; and in neutrophils and macrophages as a factor in vessel relaxation and inactivation of pathogens

Data from Kumar V et al: *Robbins & Cotran pathologic basis of disease,* ed 8, Philadelphia, 2010, Saunders; Buetler TM, Krauskopf A, Ruegg UT: *News Physiol Sci* 19:120–123, 2004.

BOX 2-2 DISEASES AND DISORDERS LINKED TO OXYGEN-DERIVED FREE RADICALS

- Deterioration noted in aging
- Atherosclerosis
  - Heart disease
  - Stroke
- Brain disorders
  - Ischemic brain injury
  - Aluminum toxicity
  - Alzheimer disease
  - Neurotoxins
- AIDS-associated dementia
- Cancer
- Cardiac myopathy
- Chronic granulomatous disease
- Diabetes mellitus
- Eye disorders
  - Macular degeneration
  - Cataracts
- Inflammatory disorders
- Other
- Iron overload
- Lung disorders
  - Asbestosis
  - Oxygen toxicity
  - Emphysema
- Nutritional deficiencies
- Radiation injury
- Reperfusion injury
- Rheumatoid arthritis
- Sleep apnea
- Skin disorders
  - Solar radiation
  - Burns
  - Contact dermatitis
  - Bloom syndrome
- Toxic states
  - Xenobiotics (CCl_4, paraquat, cigarette smoke, etc.)
  - Metal ions (Ni, Cu, Fe, etc.)
- Amyotrophic lateral sclerosis
- Huntington disease?
- Parkinson disease?

Data from Knight JA: *Ann Clin Lab Sci* 25(2):111, 1995; Bergendi L et al: *Life Sci* 65(18–19):1865, 1999; Maccarrone M, Ullrich V: *Cell Death Differ* 11:949–952, 2004.
AIDS, Acquired immunodeficiency syndrome.

TABLE 2-4 METHODS CONTRIBUTING TO INACTIVATION OR TERMINATION OF FREE RADICALS

METHOD	PROCESS
Antioxidants	Endogenous or exogenous; either blocks synthesis or inactivates (e.g., scavenges) free radicals; includes vitamin E, vitamin C, cysteine, glutathione, albumin, ceruloplasmin, transferrin
Enzymes	Superoxide dismutase,* which converts superoxide to H_2O_2; catalase* (in peroxisomes) decomposes H_2O_2; glutathione peroxidase* decomposes OH• and H_2O_2

*These enzymes are important in modulating the cellular destructive effects of free radicals, also released in inflammation.

and oxidative or nitrative (i.e., reactive nitrogen species) stress. Emerging investigations have provided new understanding of how autophagy of mitochondria (also known as mitophagy) is controlled, and the impact of autophagic dysfunction on cellular oxidative stress. Impaired mitochondrial function, oxidative stress, accumulation of protein aggregates, and autophagic stress are common in many diseases.[24] Additionally, investigators are trying to identify the polypeptides (i.e., proteomes) directly involved in diseases associated with mitochondrial dysfunction.

Chemical Injury

Mechanisms

Chemical injury begins with a biochemical interaction between a toxic substance and the cell's plasma membrane, which is ultimately damaged, leading to increased permeability. Not all the mechanisms causing chemically induced membrane destruction are known; however, the two general mechanisms include (1) direct toxicity by combining with a molecular component of the cell membrane or organelles and (2) reactive free radicals and lipid peroxidation.

Because it has been investigated extensively, carbon tetrachloride (CCl_4) injury is a useful example of chemical injury. Carbon tetrachloride, an agent formerly used in dry cleaning, harms cells because an enzyme system (P-450) in the smooth endoplasmic reticulum of liver cells converts it into chloromethyl ($CCl_3^{\bullet}$), a highly toxic free radical.

In CCl_4 injury, newly formed $CCl_3^{\bullet}$ rapidly destroys the endoplasmic reticulum of the liver cell by way of lipid peroxidation breaking down the reticulum's lipid component. The lipid molecules accumulate within the cytoplasm, starting within cisternae of the endoplasmic reticulum (Figure 2-13). Fatty liver develops because CCl_4 poisoning blocks the synthesis of **lipid-acceptor proteins (apoproteins)** that normally bind with triglycerides to form lipoproteins, which are transported out of the cell. Blockage of triglyceride (lipoprotein) secretion begins 10 to 15 minutes after CCl_4 exposure. Fat droplets that accumulate in cisternae of the endoplasmic reticulum combine to form larger droplets and fill vacuoles, which in turn fill the entire cytoplasm. Approximately 10 to 12 hours later the liver appears grossly enlarged and pale because of the accumulation of fat. (Accumulation of fat is discussed further on p. 84.)

During this process cellular swelling progresses because of alterations in the selective permeability of the plasma membrane. Cellular swelling becomes severe when the plasma membrane loses its ability to prevent the passive inward diffusion of sodium ions, water, and calcium. The most serious consequence of plasma membrane damage is, as in hypoxic injury, to the mitochondria. An influx of calcium ions from the extracellular compartment activates multiple enzyme systems resulting in cytoskeleton disruption, membrane damage, activation of inflammation, and eventually DNA degradation. Calcium ion accumulation in the mitochondria causes the mitochondria to swell, an occurrence that is associated with irreversible cellular injury. The injured mitochondria can no longer generate ATP, but they do continue to accumulate calcium ions. The influx of calcium into the mitochondria interferes with oxidative metabolism (by uncoupling oxidative phosphorylation).

Decreasing cellular pH (caused by the loss of oxidative phosphorylation and ATP-stimulating glycolysis), together with fluid and electrolyte imbalances (increased levels of sodium, calcium, and water and decreased concentration of potassium), leads to lysosomal membrane injury, causing a leakage of lysosomal enzymes into the cytoplasm. Enzymatic digestion of cellular organelles, including the nucleus and nucleolus, ensues, halting synthesis of deoxyribonucleic acid (DNA) and ribonucleic acid (RNA). The leakage of lysosomal enzymes apparently occurs late in chemical injury, well after irreversible lipid accumulation, mitochondrial swelling, and ATP loss.

Chemical Agents Including Drugs

Numerous chemical agents cause cellular injury. Minute amounts of some, such as arsenic and cyanide, can rapidly destroy enough cells to cause death of the individual. Long-term exposure to air pollutants, insecticides, and herbicides can cause cellular injury (Figure 2-14). Carbon monoxide, carbon tetrachloride, and social drugs, such as alcohol, can significantly alter cellular function and injure cellular structures. Over-the-counter and prescribed drugs also may cause cellular injury, sometimes leading to death. The leading cause of child poisoning is medications (see What's New? The Percentage of Child Medication–Related Poisoning Deaths Is Increasing). Acetaminophen (known as paracetamol outside the United States), commonly used as an analgesic, is one of the most common causes of poisoning

WHAT'S NEW?

The Percentage of Child Medication–Related Poisoning Deaths Is Increasing

Today, the leading cause of child poisoning is medications. Each year, more than 500,000 children, ages 5 and younger, experience a potential poisoning related to medications. More than 60,000 children are treated in emergency departments because of accidental medication exposure or overdose. One of every 150 2-year-olds is being sent to the emergency department for an unintentional medication overdose. Among children younger than age 5, 95% of emergency room visits are caused by unsupervised accidental ingestions and about 5% from dosing errors made by clinicians.

Importantly, investigators analyzed records from the American Association of Poison Control Centers' National Poison Data System (NPDS), an electronic database of all calls to the 61 poison control centers across the United States. Their analysis included all calls for children age 5 years or younger who were seen in a hospital emergency department between 2001 and 2008 for either unintentional self-exposure to a single drug (prescription or over-the-counter [OTC]) or unintentional therapeutic error for a single drug (prescription or OTC). The number of such calls during this 8-year period totaled 453,559. Medication-related poisoning deaths among children 5 years and younger now most frequently involve exposures to opioid analgesics and cardiovascular medications. About half of all poisoning-related deaths involve analgesics, antihistamines, and sedatives.

Development of new medications also has led to more of them being available in American homes. With aging, more adults are taking OTC and prescription medications as well as multiple medications. Oxycodone, morphine, and methadone prescriptions have increased between 159% and 559%, depending on the drug; the number of prescribed cardiovascular drugs (e.g., metoprolol) has increased about fivefold. Additionally, more medications, such as those utilized for attention-deficit disorder and diabetes, are being prescribed to younger adults and children.

How can we increase the safety of children exposed to so many medications? Safe storage is the *most* important solution and safe dosing from clinicians will reduce dosing errors. Additionally, improvements are continuing through improved packaging and labeling of medications as well as education of parents and consumers on dosing information.

Data from Bond GR, Woodward RW, Ho M: *J Pediatr* 160(2):265–270, 2011; Bronstein AC et al: *Clin Toxicol* 49:910–941, 2011; Budnitz DS, Lovegrove MC: *J Pediatr* 160(2):190–192, 2012; Bunitz DS, Salis S: *Pediatrics* 127(6):e1597–e1599, 2011; Centers for Disease Control and Prevention: Available at www.cdc.gov/features/medication storage/. Accessed February 9, 2012.

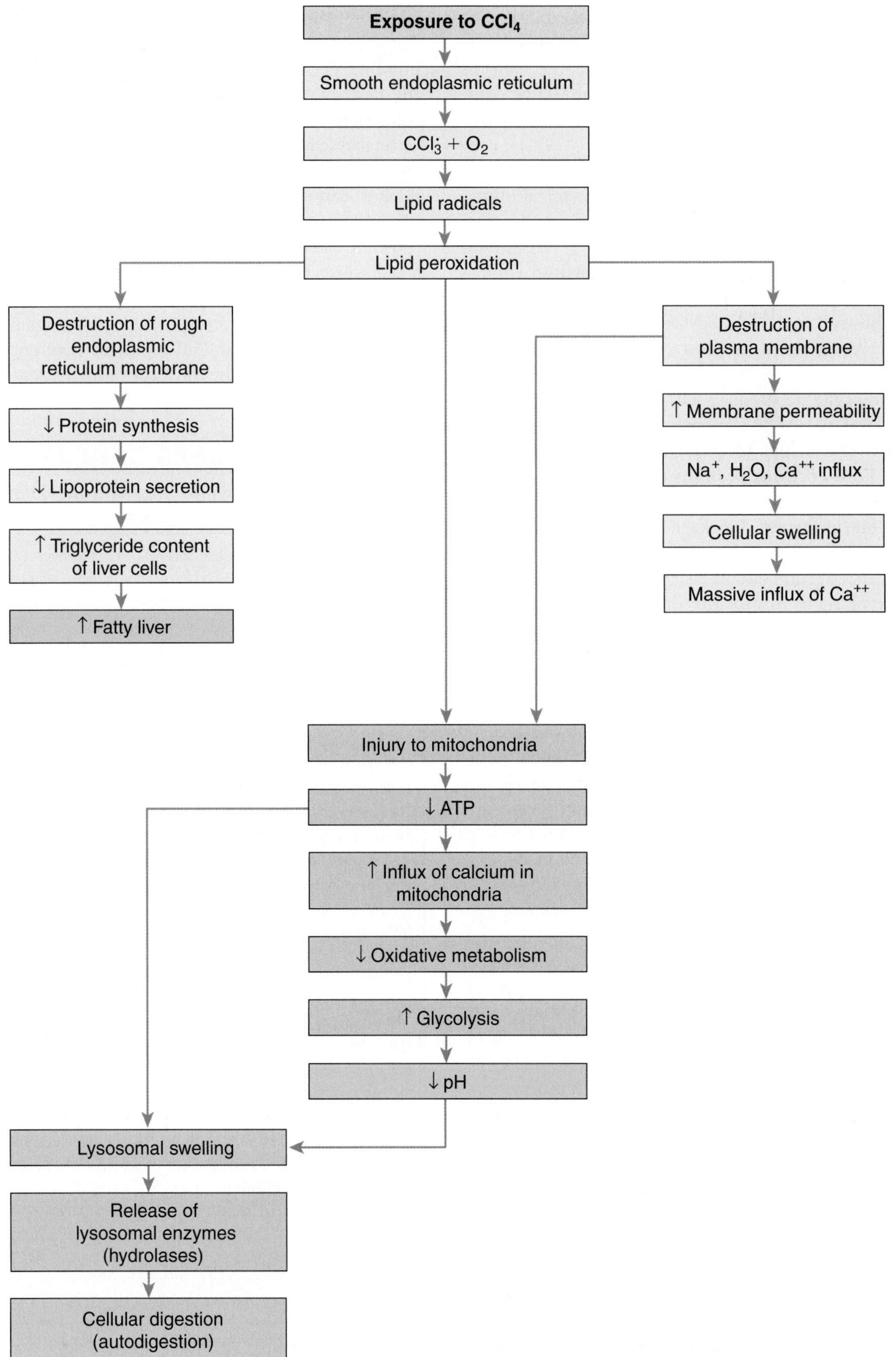

FIGURE 2-13 Chemical Injury of Liver Cells Induced by Carbon Tetrachloride (CCl_4) Poisoning. *Light blue boxes* are mechanisms unique to chemical injury; *purple boxes* involve hypoxic injury. *Green boxes* are clinical manifestations.

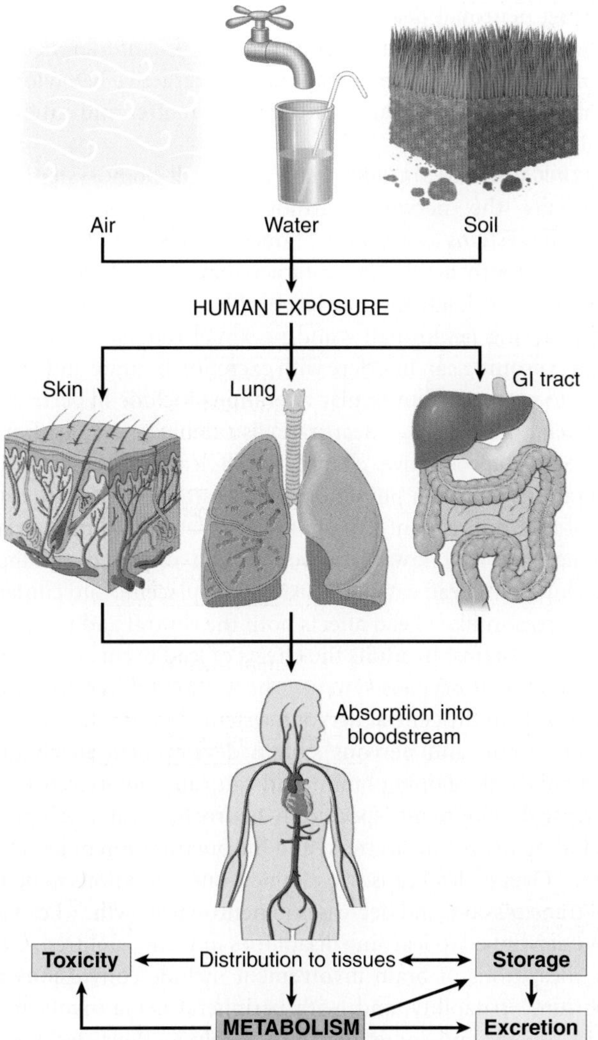

FIGURE 2-14 **Human Exposure to Pollutants.** Pollutants contained in air, water, and soil are absorbed through the lungs, gastrointestinal tract, and skin. In the body they may act at the site of absorption but are generally transported through the bloodstream to various organs where they can be stored or metabolized. Metabolism of xenobiotics may result in the formation of water-soluble compounds that are excreted, or a toxic metabolite may be created by activation of the agent. (From Kumar V et al, editors: *Robbins & Cotran pathologic basis of disease,* ed 8, St Louis, 2010, Saunders.)

worldwide. Drug-induced acute liver failure accounts for about 20% of liver failure in children and a higher percentage in adults[25] (see What's New? in Chapter 41). Accidental or suicidal poisonings by chemical agents cause numerous deaths. The injurious effects of some of these agents—lead, carbon monoxide, ethyl alcohol, and mercury—exemplify common cellular injuries.

Lead. **Lead** is a heavy toxic metal ubiquitous in older homes, the environment, and the workplace. In the United States, despite efforts to reduce exposure by passing government regulations, discontinuing the production of leaded gasoline, and banning the use of lead paint, excessive lead exposure still persists in homes, the environment, and the workplace for many people and lead toxicity is still a primary hazard to children (see What's New? Low Level Lead Exposure Harms Children: A Renewed Call for Primary Prevention). Lead exposure also remains an important safety and health concern worldwide. On a scale unprecedented in decades, for example, lead-contaminated gold ore in Nigeria caused significant childhood poisoning and deaths.[26] Worrisome is lead exposure to the fetus during pregnancy because the developing nervous system is especially vulnerable. Compared to adults, developing fetuses and young children absorb lead more easily;[27] however, the exact transport mechanisms have not yet been elucidated. Exposure to lead during neurologic development has significant effects on neurobehavioral and intellectual performance, resulting in learning disorders, hyperactivity, and attention problems.[27]

The most common source of childhood lead exposure is old paint containing lead. Homes built before 1978 are likely to contain lead paint.[28] Lead-based paint has a sweet taste and is often ingested by children when they have access to surfaces painted with it. Children also may play in lead-contaminated soil. Other sources of lead in daily life include toys, jewelry, imported candies, foods, supplements, cosmetics (tiro, surma, kajal in Asia and kohl in the Middle East),[29] dust and soil found in inner-city urban and possibly rural areas, debris from household renovations, baby formula mixed with lead-contaminated tap water, newsprint, water that flows through lead pipes, hair dyes, food stored in soldered tin cans or eaten off of pottery made with lead-based glazes, and contamination from leaded gasoline. If nutrition is compromised, especially if dietary intake of iron, calcium, zinc, and vitamin D is insufficient, lead's toxic effects are enhanced.

Occupational exposure is a common cause of lead poisoning in adults. Approximately 95% of all elevated blood lead levels (BLLs) reported among adults in the United States are work related.[30,31] Industries with the highest number of lead-exposed workers are battery manufacturing, secondary smelting and

WHAT'S NEW?

Low Level Lead Exposure Harms Children: A Renewed Call for Primary Prevention

An advisory committee of the CDC recently suggested that the current threshold for harmful lead exposure in children should be cut in half because even lower levels cause irreversible harm. The report noted that studies have found reduced intelligence quotients (IQs) and behavioral problems in children with exposure levels less than 10 mcg/dl and that such low levels have effects on cardiovascular, endocrine, and immunologic systems. Based on these data, the panel recommended reducing the threshold for harmful levels of lead in the blood to 5 mcg/dl. Despite progress in reducing blood lead levels (BLLs), racial and income disparities persist. An internal review process from both the Centers for Disease Control and Prevention and the U.S. Department of Health and Human Services will determine how to implement any accepted recommendations. This is a very important process because BLLs appear to be irreversible, underscoring the need for primary prevention.

Data from Advisory Committee on Childhood Lead Poisoning Prevention of the Centers for Disease Control and Prevention: *Low level lead exposure harms children: a renewed call for primary prevention,* 2012. Available at www.cdc.gov/nceh/lead/ACCLPP/Final_Document_030712.pdf. Accessed September 24, 2012.

refining of nonferrous metals, and painting and paper hanging. The most common nonoccupational exposures of lead are shooting firearms, remodeling buildings, renovating, painting, possessing retained bullets in the body (gunshot wounds, especially retained bullet in joints), and lead casting.[31]

The organ systems affected by lead include the nervous, hematopoietic (tissues that produce blood cells), reproductive, gastrointestinal, cardiovascular, and musculoskeletal systems as well as the kidneys.

PATHOPHYSIOLOGY. Exposure occurs through inhalation, ingestion, and uncommonly skin contact. Lead is taken in through direct contact with the mouth, nose, and eyes (i.e., mucous membranes); and through cuts in the skin. Tetraethyl lead, still used in aviation fuel, can pass through skin but inorganic lead, found in the most common sources of paint, food, and consumer products, is only minimally absorbable through skin.[32,33] Absorption of inorganic lead is primarily from ingestion and inhalation.[32] In adults, 95% of inhaled lead dust passes into the bloodstream and 35% to 40% is deposited in the lungs.[32] Usually about 15% of ingested lead is absorbed, but these rates are higher in children, pregnant women, and those with deficiencies in calcium, zinc, or iron.[34] The main tissues that store lead are the blood, soft tissues, and bone. The persistence of lead or half-life in these tissues is weeks for blood, months for soft tissue, and years for bone.[34] In adults, 94% of absorbed lead is deposited in the bones and teeth. Children store about 70% of absorbed lead in their bones and teeth; thus, other tissues in children are more greatly affected compared to adults.[35] The estimated half-life of lead in bone is 20 to 30 years, and lead can move from bone to the bloodstream years after the initial exposure.[33] Lead can be reintroduced continuously to the blood from bone remodeling.[35] Other tissues can store lead including the brain, spleen, kidneys, liver, and lungs, however, not at the levels found in blood, bone, and teeth.[36]

A primary cause of lead's toxicity is its ability to bind to sulfhydryl groups found on many enzymes.[37] Lead can mimic other metals (calcium, iron, zinc) in biologic processes because it acts as a cofactor in several enzymatic reactions.[36] Lead's role as a cofactor interferes with the enzyme's ability to catalyze reactions. A primary cause of pathology is lead's interference with a main enzyme called δ-aminolevulinic acid dehydratase, or ALAD, important in the synthesis of heme in hemoglobin.[33] Lead can interfere with another heme enzyme called ferrochelatase. Ferrochelatase catalyzes the reaction of protoporphyrin and Fe^{+} to form heme. Interference with the formation of heme causes the production of zinc protoporphyrin and the development of anemia. A significant manifestation of lead toxicity is anemia caused by lysis of red blood cells (hemolysis). Lead interferes with the release of glutamate, a neurotransmitter involved in many functions, including learning, by blocking *N*-methyl-D-aspartate (NMDA) receptors.[38] Overall, lead interferes with mitochondrial oxidative phosphorylation, ATPases, and calcium-dependent messengers; increases intracellular oxidation; and results in cell death by apoptosis. Lead appears to have its greatest effects during the later stages of brain development, possibly by altering development of synaptic connections (i.e., trimming/pruning) and causing neuronal death (apoptosis).[27] Alterations in calcium concentration may play a crucial role in the interference with neurotransmitters, which may cause hyperactive behavior and proliferation of capillaries of the white matter and intercerebral arteries.[27,39]

CLINICAL MANIFESTATIONS. Lead affects all body systems and especially the nervous, cardiovascular, reproductive, and immune systems as well as the bones, kidneys, and teeth. Hearing loss, tooth decay, and cataracts have been linked to lead exposure.[40,41] High and low levels of lead can damage the kidneys causing nephropathy and proximal tubular dysfunction. Lead poisoning can interfere with excretion of urate and predispose to gout. Cardiovascular alterations include hypertension, coronary heart disease, heart rate disturbances, and death from stroke.[42] Reproductive changes from lead exposure include alterations in sperm physiology and anatomy. High blood levels of lead in pregnant women are associated with miscarriage, premature birth, low birth weight, and impaired childhood development. Lead can pass through the placenta and contaminate breast milk.[36] Lead affects both the central and peripheral nervous systems. In adults the effects of lead occur primarily in the peripheral nervous system, whereas in children the effects are mostly in the central nervous system.[43] Lead interferes with normal brain and nervous system development in children. In a child's developing brain, lead can cause interference with synapse development (specifically neurochemical development including neurotransmitters) and the organization of ion channels.[44] Overall, lead causes loss of neurons, alterations in neuronal transmission, and decreases in neuronal growth.[37] Lead also has been linked to learning disabilities in young children. Other manifestations of brain involvement include convulsions and delirium, irritability, and, with peripheral nerve involvement, wrist, finger, and sometimes foot paralysis. Renal lesions can cause tubular dysfunction resulting in glycosuria (glucose in the urine), aminoaciduria (amino acids in the urine), and hyperphosphaturia (excess phosphate in the urine). Gastrointestinal symptoms are less severe and include nausea, loss of appetite, weight loss, and abdominal cramping.

EVALUATION, PREVENTION, AND TREATMENT. Diagnosis involves the medical history and clinical signs and determination of routes of exposure. The main method of evaluation is laboratory analysis of the blood lead level (BLL). The current acceptable BLL in healthy persons with excessive exposure to environmental sources of lead is less than 10 micrograms/deciliter (mcg/dl) for children and less than 25 mcg/dl for adults. In 2012 there was a recommendation to reduce the value for children to 5 mcg/dl. Because 95% to 99% of lead in blood is sequestered in red blood cells, lead needs to be measured in whole blood, not serum.[45] Lead in bones may be measured noninvasively by K x-ray fluorescence (KXRF); however; this method is not widely available.

The most important strategy for lowering exposures to lead is prevention. Prevention methods include individual and family, preventive medicine, and public health. There is an urgent need to focus on preventive strategies, especially for fetal development and the developing child. The key for adults is prevention of exposures at the workplace and home. The main methods of treatment are removal of the source of exposure and, for those with high blood levels, chelation therapy. Additionally, treatment may include correcting deficiencies of iron, calcium, and zinc; irrigating the bowel; removing strategic bullets or shrapnel; and administering medications for control of seizures.

Carbon Monoxide. Gaseous substances can be classified according to their ability to asphyxiate (interrupt respiration) or irritate. Toxic asphyxiants, such as carbon monoxide, hydrogen cyanide, and hydrogen sulfide, directly interfere with cellular respiration. Carbon monoxide is widely available.

Carbon monoxide (CO), a gas, is odorless, colorless, and undetectable unless it is mixed with a visible or odorous pollutant. It is produced by the incomplete combustion of such fuels as gasoline. In dense urban environments, CO produced by incomplete combustion from motor vehicles increases air pollution. CO is a leading cause of unintentional poisoning deaths in the United States with more than 50,000 emergency department visits per year (68,316 exposures reported between 2000 and 2009) and about 500 deaths per year.[46] Those who (1) breathe air polluted by gasoline engines or defective furnaces and appliances; (2) work in occupations such as coal mining, firefighting, welding,[47] or engine repair; and (3) smoke cigarettes, cigars, or pipes are at risk for CO exposure. At highest risk for CO poisoning are unborn babies, infants, and people with chronic heart disease, respiratory disease, and anemia. Fatalities are highest for those 65 years and older.

The pathophysiology of carbon monoxide poisoning is not completely understood. Although CO is a chemical agent, the ultimate injury it produces is a hypoxic injury, namely, oxygen deprivation. It directly reduces the oxygen-carrying capacity of blood and promotes tissue hypoxia because it shifts the oxyhemoglobin curve to the left (see Chapter 34). Normally, oxygen molecules are carried to tissues bound to hemoglobin in red blood cells (see Chapter 31). Because CO's affinity for hemoglobin is 200 times greater than that of oxygen, it quickly binds with the hemoglobin, preventing oxygen molecules from doing so. Minute amounts of CO can produce significant percentages of **carboxyhemoglobin** (carbon monoxide bound with hemoglobin, COHb). CO also is an anesthetic agent and causes loss of airway capacity in animal studies. Other mechanisms may include disruption of cellular oxidative processes, binding to myoglobin and hepatic cytochromes, and lipid peroxidation of brain lipids.[48]

Although COHb levels on hospital admission may not reflect the severity of the CO poisoning, minor doses may be asymptomatic and include headache, giddiness, tinnitus (ringing in the ears), nausea, weakness, and vomiting. Higher doses may appear as confusion, poor concentration, loss of short-term memory, seizures, and loss of consciousness. Poor outcomes are noted with individuals older than 35 years, exposure greater than 24 hours, acidosis, and loss of consciousness.[48]

Ethanol. Alcohol (*ethanol*) is the number one mood-altering drug used in the United States. It is estimated there are more than 10 million chronic alcoholics in the United States. Alcohol contributes to more than 100,000 deaths annually with 50% of these deaths from drunk driving accidents, alcohol-related homicides, and suicides.[49] A blood alcohol concentration of 80 mg/dl is the legal definition of drunk driving in the United States. This level of alcohol in an average person may be reached after consumption of three drinks (three 12-ounce bottles of beer, 15 ounces of wine, and 4 to 5 ounces of distilled liquor). The effects of alcohol vary by age, gender, and percentage body fat; the rate of metabolism affects the blood alcohol level. Importantly, alcohol-related problems include family violence and workplace disabilities. Because alcohol is not only a psychoactive drug but also a food, it is considered part of the basic food supply in many societies.

A large intake of alcohol has enormous effects on nutritional status. Major nutritional deficiencies include magnesium, vitamin B_6, thiamine, and phosphorus. Chronic intake of alcohol and vitamin deficiencies may adversely affect the brain and peripheral nerves (e.g., Wernicke encephalopathy, peripheral neuropathy, Korsakoff pyschosis). Folic acid deficiency is a common problem in chronic alcoholic populations. Ethanol alters folic acid (folate) homeostasis by decreasing intestinal absorption of folate, increases liver retention of folate, and increases the loss of folate through urinary and fecal excretion.[25] Folic acid deficiency becomes especially serious in pregnant women who consume alcohol and may contribute to fetal alcohol syndrome (see p. 68).

Most of the alcohol in blood is metabolized to *acetaldehyde* in the liver by three enzyme systems: alcohol dehydrogenase (ADH), the microsomal ethanol-oxidizing system (MEOS; CYP2E1), and catalase (Figure 2-15).

The major pathway involves ADH, an enzyme located in the cytosol of hepatocytes. The microsomal ethanol-oxidizing system (MEOS) depends on cytochrome P-450 (CYP2E1), an enzyme needed for cellular oxidation. Activation of CYP2E1 requires a high ethanol concentration and thus is thought to be important in the accelerated ethanol metabolism (i.e., tolerance) noted in persons with chronic alcoholism. Acetaldehyde has many toxic tissue effects and is responsible for some of the acute effects of alcohol and for development of oral cancers.[50]

After ingestion, alcohol is absorbed, unaltered, into the stomach and small intestine from which it is transported to the liver. Fatty foods and milk slow absorption. Alcohol then is distributed to all tissues and fluids of the body in direct proportion to the blood concentration. Individuals differ in their capability to metabolize alcohol. Genetic differences in metabolism of liver alcohol, including aldehyde dehydrogenases, have been identified. People with chronic alcoholism develop certain levels of tolerance because of enzyme induction, leading to an increased rate of metabolism (e.g., P-450).

Studies conducted since 1997 have contributed to our understanding of the association between alcohol consumption and cardiovascular disease. Consistent results validate the so-called *J-shaped inverse association* between alcohol and cardiovascular disease mortality and morbidity. That is, moderate drinkers exhibit a decreased risk compared with both heavy drinkers and nondrinkers. Surprisingly, consistent epidemiologic studies show that daily light to moderate alcohol intake reduces the risk of coronary heart disease (CHD) as compared with those who do not drink alcoholic beverages at all. The suggested mechanisms for cardioprotection include increased levels of high-density lipoprotein–cholesterol (HDL-C), prevention of clot formation, reduced platelet aggregation, and increased clot degradation (fibrinolysis). Alcohol also may increase insulin sensitivity.[51] Limited data suggest that the level for optimal

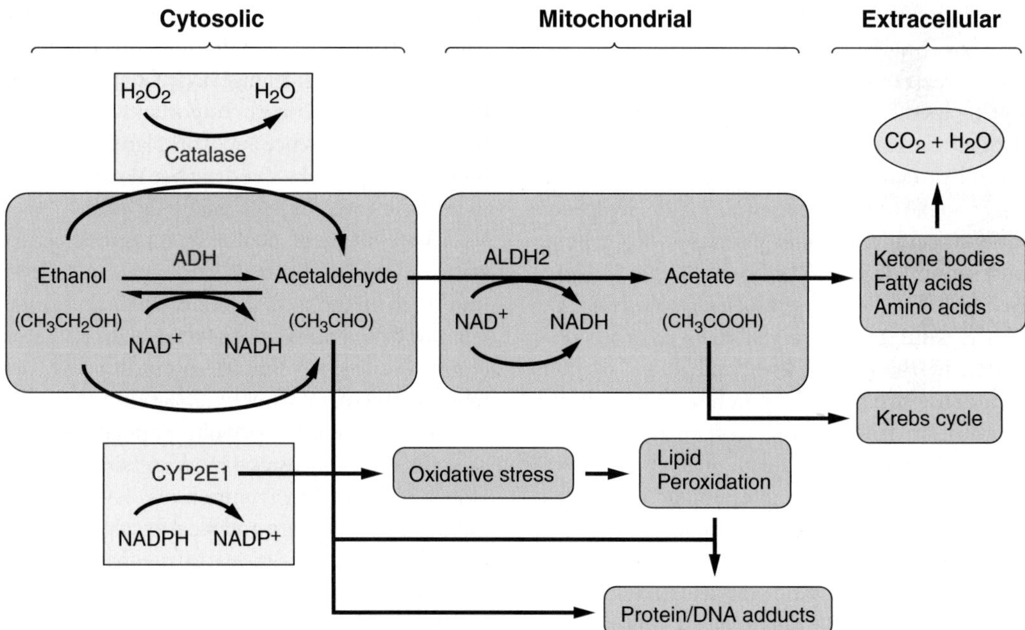

FIGURE 2-15 Ethanol Metabolism Pathway. Ethanol is metabolized into acetaldehyde through the cytosolic enzyme alcohol dehydrogenase (ADH), the microsomal enzyme cytochrome P-450 2E1 (CYP2E1), and the peroxisomal enzyme catalase. The ADH enzyme reaction is the main ethanol metabolic pathway involving an intermediate carrier of electrons, namely, nicotinamide adenine dinucleotide (NAD^+), which is reduced by two electrons to form NADH. Acetaldehyde is metabolized mainly by aldehyde dehydrogenase 2 (ALDH2) in the mitochondria to acetate and NADH before being cleared into the systemic circulation. (Adapted from Zhang Y, Ren J: *Pharmacol Ther* 132[1]:86–92, 2011.)

benefit may be slightly lower for women; therefore, the American Heart Association recommends no more than two drinks per day for men and one drink per day for women. Individuals who do not consume alcohol should not be encouraged to start regular drinking.

The major effects of *acute alcoholism* (drunkenness) involve the central nervous system (CNS). Alcohol intoxication causes CNS depression. Depending on the amount consumed, depression is associated with sedation, drowsiness, loss of motor coordination, delirium, altered behavior, loss of consciousness, and, with toxic amounts (300 to 400 mg/dl), lethal coma or respiratory arrest because of medullary center depression. Much investigation is under way to determine the extent of the relationship between alcohol level and snoring and obstructive sleep apnea (cessation of breathing).[52,53] Acute alcoholism may induce reversible hepatic and gastric changes.

Chronic alcoholism causes structural alterations in practically all organs and tissues in the body, especially the liver and stomach. The most significant alterations occur in the liver, a condition called alcohol-induced liver disease (ALD). ALD includes fatty liver, alcoholic hepatitis, and cirrhosis. ALD may eventually develop into hepatocellular carcinoma. Reactive oxygen and nitrogen species (ROS/RNS) and dysregulated redox signaling pathways are associated with alcohol consumption and provide insight into the molecular basis of hepatic cell dysfunction, destruction, and remodeled tissue or fibrosis.[54] Oxidative stress is associated with cell membrane phospholipid depletion, which alters the fluidity and function of cell membranes as well as intercellular transport. The initial liver histologic changes are characterized by accumulation of inflammatory cells and matrix deposition around the portal vein.[55] With ALD and hepatitis C virus (HCV), liver fibrosis is defined as the abnormal accumulation of extracellular matrix (ECM).[56,57] Inflammation plays a crucial role in ALD.[57]

Cirrhosis is associated with portal hypertension and an increased risk for hepatocellular carcinoma.[49] Acute gastritis is a direct toxic effect and chronic use can lead to acute and chronic pancreatitis. Oxidative stress is associated with cell membrane phospholipid depletion, which alters the fluidity and function of cell membranes as well as intercellular transport. Chronic alcoholism is related to several disorders, including injury to the myocardium (alcoholic cardiomyopathy), increased tendency to hypertension, and regressive changes in skeletal muscle (see Chapter 35). Ethanol is implicated in the onset of a variety of immune defects, including effects on the production of cytokines involved in inflammatory responses.

The activation of methionine, an essential amino acid, to *S*-adenosyl-l-methionine (SAMe) is decreased in those with alcoholism.[58] Oxidative stress is associated with phospholipid depletion. The replacement of polyenylphosphatidylcholine (PPC) has been studied in both baboons and para-null mice.[58]

Prenatal alcohol exposure causes **fetal alcohol syndrome (FAS).** Alcohol crosses the placenta, reaching the fetus rapidly.[59] Research has demonstrated an unimpeded bidirectional movement of alcohol between the fetus and the mother. The fetus may completely depend on maternal hepatic detoxification because the activity of alcohol dehydrogenase (ADH) in fetal liver is less than 10% of that of the adult liver. Additionally, the amniotic fluid acts as a reservoir for alcohol, prolonging fetal exposure.[59] The specific mechanisms of injury are unknown; however, acetaldehyde can alter fetal development by disrupting

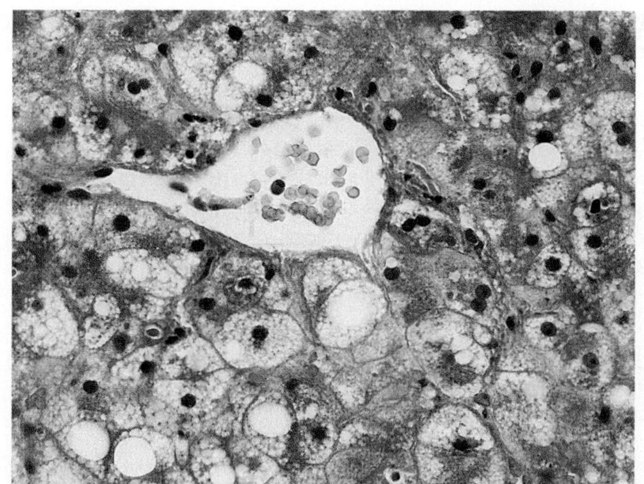

FIGURE 2-16 Alcoholic Hepatitis. Chicken-wire fibrosis extending between hepatocytes. (Mallory trichrome stain.) (From Damjanov I, Linder J: *Anderson's pathology,* ed 10, St Louis, 1996, Mosby.)

differentiation and growth; DNA and protein synthesis; modification of carbohydrates, proteins, and fats; and the flow of nutrients across the placenta.[59,60] Additionally, alcohol may cause fetal disturbances, even preconceptual effects, epigenetically.[61]

FAS can lead to growth retardation, cognitive impairment, facial anomalies, and ocular disturbances.[62] In some cases, full-blown FAS may not be indicated but CNS defects may *still* be present and are classified as alcohol-related birth defects (ARBDs) and alcohol-related neurodevelopmental disorders (ARNDs).

Autopsies of children with FAS have revealed widespread severe damage, including failure of certain brain regions to develop, malformations of brain tissue, and failure of certain cells to migrate to their necessary location during development. Imaging studies reveal that in addition to an overall reduction in brain size, the corpus callosum is reduced in size or missing, the cerebellum is significantly reduced in size, and the basal ganglia and caudate nucleus are significantly reduced.

Additionally, ethanol has been shown to increase apoptotic cell death.[63] Whatever the cause, people with chronic alcoholism have a significantly shortened life span related mainly to damage to the liver, stomach, brain, and heart (Figure 2-16).

Mercury. Mercury has been used medically and commercially for centuries.[64] In the past it was a common component in medications. Mercury is still present in some thermometers and blood pressure cuffs and in batteries, switches, and fluorescent light bulbs. Large amounts of mercury exist as part of the electrodes formed in the electrolytic production of chlorine and sodium hydroxide from saline. Today people are exposed to mercury from two major sources: fish consumption and dental amalgams. Since 2001 no vaccine contains **thimerosal** (a preservative in multidose vials of vaccines containing ethyl mercury) except inactivated influenza vaccines. All of these uses give rise to possible accidental and occupational exposures.[64]

Dental Amalgams. Dental amalgams have been used for more than 150 years. They are believed to be more durable and easier to use than other types of fillings, as well as being relatively inexpensive. Amalgams consist of about 50% mercury amalgamated or combined with other metals, such as silver and copper. The controversies and heated debates concerning amalgams peaked in the 1970s with the discovery that amalgams can release mercury vapors into the mouth in concentrations that are higher than those deemed safe by occupational health guidelines.

Since then it was realized that the actual inhaled dose was small because of the small volume of the oral cavity.[64] Yet, brain, blood, and urinary mercury concentrations correlate with the number of amalgam surfaces present in a person. Removal of amalgam fillings also can cause temporary elevations in blood mercury concentration because the removal transiently increases the amount of mercury vapor inhaled.

Current health risk concerns arise from claims that long-term exposure to low concentrations of mercury vapor either causes or worsens degenerative diseases, such as amyotrophic lateral sclerosis, Alzheimer disease, multiple sclerosis, and Parkinson disease. Concern about the effect of mercury vapor in relation to Alzheimer disease was intensified for a time after a report that the brains of individuals with Alzheimer disease had elevated mercury concentrations. Several epidemiologic investigations, however, failed to provide evidence of a role of dental amalgams in these degenerative diseases; these include a long-term Swedish study, an ongoing Swedish study, and a study of 129 nuns 75 to 102 years of age. Recently, a randomized prospective trial of 507 children failed to show exposure to mercury from amalgams is linked to neurobehavioral or neurologic effects.[65] A difficult problem is that mercury can inhibit various biochemical processes in vitro without having the same effects in vivo. Thus, at present it is unknown whether removal of amalgams reduces risk of certain diseases, especially because removal itself affects blood concentrations of mercury vapor, which will rise before they eventually decline, thereby adding to the controversy.

Fish Consumption. The major source of exposure to methyl mercury is the consumption of fish and sea mammals. Clinical reports of mercury poisoning from fish consumption are those from Japan in the 1950s and 1960s. Environmental Protection Agency (EPA) guidelines are derived from reports of neuropsychologic changes noted in the Faeroe Islands study, in which subjects had been inadvertently exposed to methyl mercury mainly from whale consumption. A similar study in the United States shows methyl mercury levels to be slightly higher than the EPA guideline for safe consumption.[64] The health risk posed by exposure to mercury from fish consumption is being debated. The U.S. Food and Drug Administration (FDA) has, however, recommended that pregnant women, nursing mothers, and young children avoid eating fish with a high mercury content (>1 part per million [ppm]), such as shark, swordfish, tile fish, king mackerel, and whale meat.[64] Other advocates, however, have published more extensive lists including fish with the lowest levels, e.g., blue crab, croaker, fish sticks, flounder, haddock, trout, salmon (wild), and shrimp.[66]

Social or Street Drugs. The social or "recreational" use of psychoactive drugs is widespread in many parts of the world. Most popular and dangerous are the drugs methamphetamine ("meth"), marijuana, cocaine, and heroin. Although the prevalence of cocaine use in the general population decreased

TABLE 2-5 SOCIAL OR STREET DRUGS AND THEIR EFFECTS

TYPE OF DRUG	DESCRIPTION AND EFFECTS
Marijuana	Active substance: δ-9-tetrahydrocannabinol (THC), found in resin of the *Cannabis sativa* plant
	With smoking (e.g., "joints"), about 50% is absorbed through the lungs; when ingested, only 10% is absorbed; with heavy use the following adverse effects have been reported: alterations of sensory perceptions, cognitive and psychomotor impairment (e.g., inability to judge time, speed, distance); smoking 3 or 4/day is similar to smoking 20 cigarettes/day in regard to frequency of chronic bronchitis and may contribute to lung cancer; data, from animal studies only, indicate reproductive changes including reduced fertility, decreased sperm motility, and decreased circulatory testosterone level; fetal abnormalities including low birth weight and increased frequency of childhood leukemia; increased frequency of infectious illness is thought to be the result of depressed cell-mediated and humoral immunity
Methamphetamine (meth)	Amine derivation of amphetamine ($C_{10}H_{15}N$) used as crystalline hydrochloride
	CNS stimulant; in large doses causes irritability, aggressive (violent) behavior, anxiety, excitement, auditory hallucinations, and paranoia (delusions and psychosis); mood changes are common and the abuser can swiftly change from friendly to hostile; paranoiac swings can result in suspiciousness, hyperactive behavior, and dramatic mood swings
	Appeals to abusers because body's metabolism is increased and produces euphoria, alertness, and perception of increased energy
	Stages:
	Low intensity: user is not psychologically addicted and uses methamphetamine by swallowing or snorting
	Binge and high intensity: user has psychologic addiction and smokes or injects to achieve a faster, stronger high
	Tweaking: most dangerous stage; user is continually under the influence, not sleeping for 3 to 15 days, extremely irritated, and paranoid
Cocaine and crack	Extracted from the leaves of the coca plant and sold as a water-soluble powder (cocaine hydrochloride) liberally diluted with talcum powder or other white powders; extraction of pure alkaloid from cocaine hydrochloride is "free-base" called crack because it "cracks" when heated
	Crack is more potent than cocaine; cocaine is widely used as an anesthetic, usually in procedures involving the oral cavity; it is a potent CNS stimulant, blocking reuptake of the neurotransmitters norepinephrine, dopamine, and serotonin; also increases synthesis of norepinephrine and dopamine; dopamine induces a sense of euphoria, and norepinephrine causes adrenergic potentiation, including hypertension, tachycardia, and vasoconstriction; cocaine can therefore cause severe coronary artery narrowing and ischemia; not clear why cocaine increases thrombus formation; other cardiovascular effects include arrhythmias, sudden death, dilated cardiomyopathy, rupture of descending aorta (i.e., secondary to hypertension); effects on the fetus include premature labor, retarded fetal development, stillbirth, hyperirritability
Heroin	Opiate closely related to morphine, methadone, and codeine
	Highly addictive, and withdrawal causes intense fear ("I'll die without it"); sold "cut" with similar-looking white powder; dissolved in water it is often highly contaminated; feeling of tranquility and sedation lasts only a few hours and thus encourages repeated intravenous or subcutaneous injections; acts on the receptors enkephalins, endorphins, and dynorphins, which are widely distributed throughout the body with high affinity for the CNS; effects can include infectious complications, especially *Staphylococcus aureus,* granulomas of the lung, septic embolism, and pulmonary edema—in addition, viral infections from casual exchange of needles and HIV; sudden death is related to overdosage secondary to respiratory depression, decreased cardiac output, and severe pulmonary edema

Data from Cotran RS, Kumar V, Collins T: *Robbins pathologic basis of disease,* ed 7, Philadelphia, 2005, Saunders; Nahas G, Sutin K, Bennett WM: *N Engl J Med* 343(7):514, 2000.
CNS, Central nervous system; *HIV,* human immunodeficiency virus.

in 1986, morbidity and mortality related to cocaine increased sharply in the 1990s. Illicit use of drugs is a prevalent risk behavior among adolescents. Table 2-5 summarizes the effects of these drugs.

Unintentional and Intentional Injuries

Unintentional and intentional injuries are an important health problem in the United States. Death due to injury is significantly more common for men than women; the overall rate for men is 84.38/100,000 vs. 34.31/100,000 for women. Significant racial differences exist in the death rate, too: whites at 59.59/100,000, blacks at 65.15/100,000, and other racial groups at a combined rate of 35.12/100,000. A bimodal age distribution for injury-related deaths also has been noted, with peaks in the young adult and older adult groups. Unintentional injury is the leading cause of death for people between the ages of 1 and 34 years, with intentional injury (suicide, homicide) ranking between the second and fourth leading causes of death in this age group (see Table 2-6). Firearm injury in the United States has averaged 32,300 deaths annually between 1980 and 2007.[67] Firearm injury is the second leading cause of injury after motor vehicle crashes.[67] There are an average of five nonfatal firearm injuries for every two firearm deaths; in 2008 there were 78,622 nonfatal firearm injuries in the United States.[68] Of those injuries, 73% were the result of interpersonal violence.[67] Among the leading causes of death for ages 15 to 24, homicide ranks second and suicide ranks third with the number of firearm-related homicides and suicides outnumbering the next leading causes of death (i.e., cancer, heart disease, congenital disorders, cerebrovascular, influenza and pneumonia, and combined [complicated pregnancy, HIV, and septicemia]).[67] Unintentional injury ranks fifth in the United States for cause of death including falls, motor vehicle traffic deaths, and poisonings.[69] Deaths from all causes and deaths from injuries compares the United States with summary estimates of mortality for WHO member states for the year 2008 (Figure 2-17). The more common terms used to describe and classify unintentional and intentional injuries and brief descriptions of important features of these are discussed in Table 2-6.

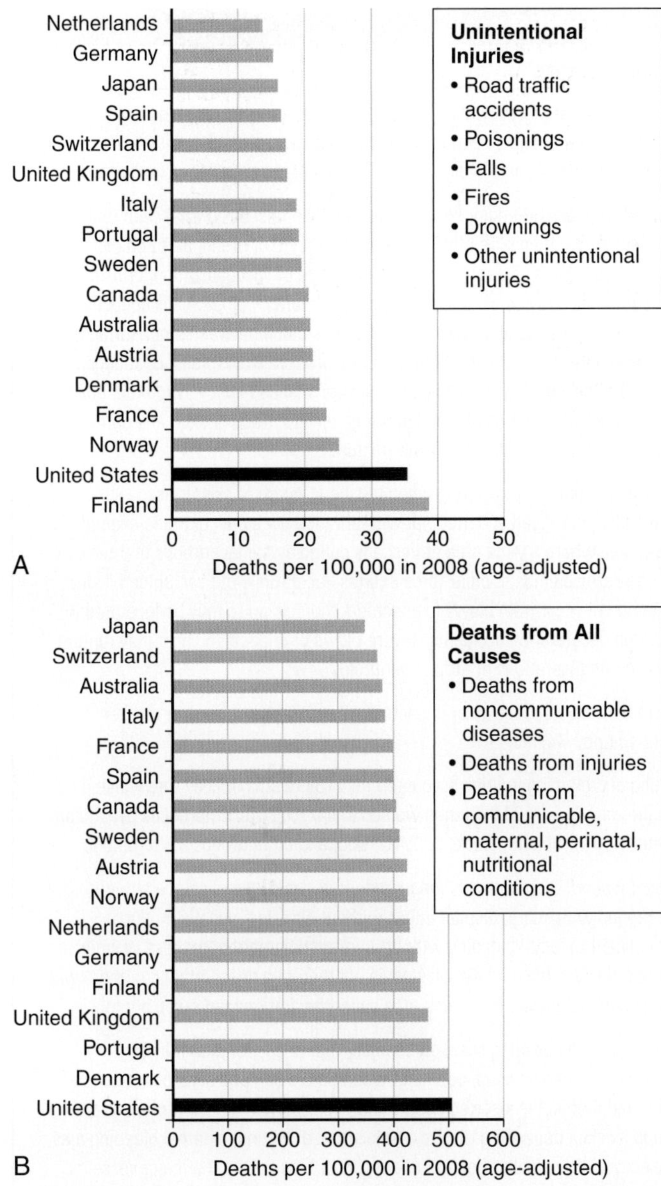

FIGURE 2-17 Global Health Data for Deaths from Unintentional Injury and from All Causes. Summary estimates of mortality for WHO member states for the year 2008. The age-adjusted death rates and the relative ranking of countries in relation to others vary from year to year. **A,** Unintentional injuries and **B,** death from all causes. (Data from World Health Statistics, 2011. World Health Organization, World Press, Geneva, Switzerland.)

Additionally, each year many unnecessary deaths occur in hospitals as a result of errors by healthcare professionals (see below). An accurate account is a tremendous challenge because of disagreements over reported statistics.[70] Statistics on nonfatal injuries are harder to document accurately, but they are known to be a significant cause of morbidity and disability and to cost society billions of dollars annually (see p. 70).

Injury from Errors in Health Care

Errors in health care (collectively called medical errors) are an unintended event, no matter how trivial or commonplace. They are errors that could or did harm individuals. A number of global and regional initiatives have been instituted to improve the safety of care, for example, the WHO 2008 Safe Surgery Saves Lives campaign extended the concept of a checklist,[71] and researchers from the United States found that it can reduce mortality and morbidity.[72] The use of the checklist strategy has exploded into many facets of patient care and now a call for it in nonsurgical, interventional specialties, for example, endoscopy, cardiac catherization and interventional radiology.[73] During the years 1999 to 2009, rates of death from complications of medical and surgical care declined among all age groups for persons ≧45 years. The *rate* of decline was lower among adults from 45 to 64 years compared with the rates of decline for all older age groups.[74]

Although progress is being made, medical errors are a concern as a cause of death and injury in the United States.[75] Studies have shown that in a single month an estimated 1.5% of Medicare beneficiaries experienced an event that contributed to their deaths, which projects to 15,000 individuals. An additional 13.5% of Medicare beneficiaries experienced events during their hospital stays that resulted in temporary harm.[76] According to the Institute of Medicine (IOM), many of the errors in health care result from a culture and system that is fragmented, and remedy of this major problem will require extensive foundation or infrastructure building. Errors involve medicines, surgery, diagnosis (i.e., wrong, overdiagnosis [is widespread in the United States, as well as overtreatment], underdiagnosis), equipment, and laboratory reports.[77] A 2006 follow-up to the IOM 1999 study found that medication errors are among the most common medical mistakes, harming at least 1.5 million people every year. According to this study, 400,000 preventable drug-related injuries occur each year in hospitals, 800,000 in long-term care settings, and approximately 530,000 among Medicare recipients in outpatient clinics.[78] Errors can occur anywhere in the healthcare system including hospitals, clinics, outpatient surgery centers, physician offices, nurse practitioner offices, pharmacies, and an individual's home. Errors in health care are associated with inexperienced physicians and nurses, new procedures, start of new clinician rotations, extremes of age, and complex care and urgent care. Additionally, financial incentives may be one reason.[79] Contributors to the problem are documentation errors, illegible handwriting, inadequate nurse-to-patient ratios, similarly named medications, and poor communication (language barriers). *The Joint Commission's Annual Report on Quality and Safety 2007* found that inadequate communication between healthcare providers, or between providers and the individual and family members, was the main cause of more than half of the serious adverse events in accredited hospitals.[80] Actions by patients also may contribute significantly to medical errors.[81]

More is known about errors in hospitals than in other healthcare delivery settings. Medication-related error has been studied for several reasons: (1) it is the most common type of error, (2) substantial numbers of people are affected, and (3) it accounts for a large increase in healthcare costs. Medication errors are methodologically easier to study because the drug-prescribing process provides documentation of medical decisions, administration of drugs is recorded, supplying drugs are documented, and deaths attributable to medication errors are recorded on death certificates.

TABLE 2-6 UNINTENTIONAL AND INTENTIONAL INJURIES

TYPE OF INJURY	DESCRIPTION
Blunt-Force Injuries	Mechanical injury to body resulting in tearing, shearing, or crushing; most common type of injury seen in healthcare settings; caused by blows or impacts; motor vehicle accidents and falls most common cause (see photo)
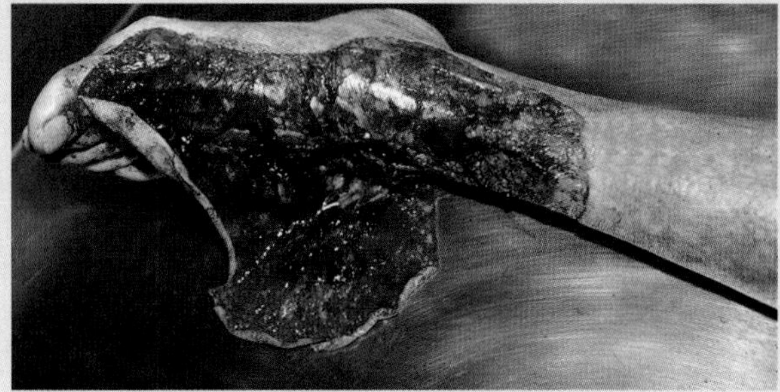	*Contusion (bruise):* Bleeding into skin or underlying tissues; initial color will be red-purple, then blue-black, then yellow-brown or green; duration of bruise depends on extent, location, and degree of vascularization; bruising of soft tissue may be confined to deeper structures; *hematoma* is collection of blood in soft tissue; *subdural hematoma* is blood between inner surface of dura mater and surface of brain; can result from blows, falls, or sudden acceleration/deceleration of head as occurs in *shaken baby syndrome; epidural hematoma* is collection of blood between inner surface of skull and dura; is most often associated with a skull fracture
	Laceration: Tear or rip resulting when tensile strength of skin or tissue is exceeded; is ragged and irregular with abraded edges; an extreme example is *avulsion,* where a wide area of tissue is pulled away; lacerations of internal organs are common in blunt-force injuries; lacerations of liver, spleen, kidneys, and bowel occur from blows to abdomen; thoracic aorta may be lacerated in sudden deceleration accidents; severe blows or impacts to chest may rupture heart with lacerations of atria or ventricles
	Fracture: Blunt-force blows or impacts can cause bone to break or shatter (see Chapter 44)
Sharp-Force Injuries	Cutting and piercing injuries accounted for 2734 deaths in 2007; men have a higher rate (1.37/100,000) than women (0.44/100,000); differences by race are whites 0.71/100,000, blacks 2.12/100,000, and other groups 0.80/100,000
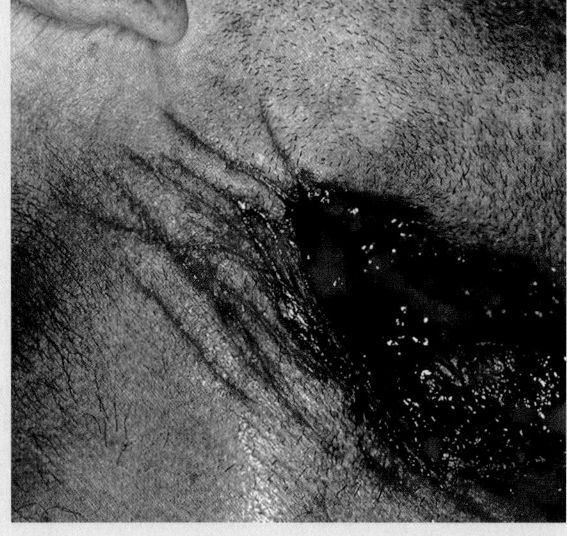	*Incised wound:* Wound that is *longer* than it is *deep;* wound can be straight or jagged with sharp, distinct edges without abrasion; usually produces significant external bleeding with little internal hemorrhage; these wounds are noted in sharp-force injury suicides; in addition to a deep, lethal cut, there will be superficial incisions in same area called *hesitation marks* (see photo)
	Stab wound: Penetrating sharp-force injury that is *deeper* than it is *long;* if a sharp instrument is used, depths of wound are clean and distinct but can be abraded if object is inserted deeply and wider portion (e.g., hilt of a knife) impacts skin; depending on size and location of wound, external bleeding may be surprisingly small; after an initial spurt of blood, even if a major vessel or heart is struck, wound may be almost completely closed by tissue pressure, thus allowing only a trickle of visible blood despite copious internal bleeding
	Puncture wound: Instruments or objects with sharp points but without sharp edges produce puncture wounds; classic example is wound of foot after stepping on a nail; wounds are prone to infection, have abrasion of edges, and can be very deep
	Chopping wound: Heavy, edged instruments (axes, hatchets, propeller blades) produce wounds with a combination of sharp- and blunt-force characteristics

TABLE 2-6 **UNINTENTIONAL AND INTENTIONAL INJURIES—cont'd**

TYPE OF INJURY	DESCRIPTION
Gunshot Wounds	Accounted for more than 31,224 deaths in the United States in 2007; men more likely to die than women (18.16 vs. 2.73/100,000); black men between ages of 15 and 24 have greatest death rate (86.95/100,000); gunshot wounds are either penetrating (bullet remains in body) or perforating (bullet exits body); bullet also can fragment; most important factors or appearances are whether it is an entrance or exit wound and range of fire *Entrance wound:* All wounds share some common features; overall appearance is most affected by range of fire
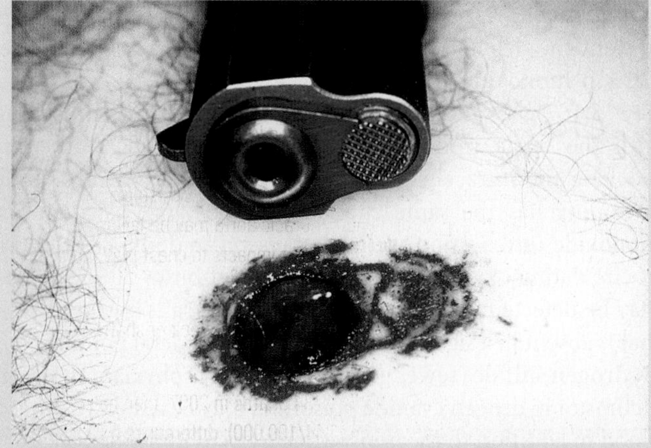	*Contact range entrance wound:* Distinctive type of wound when gun is held so muzzle rests on or presses into skin surface; there is searing of edges of wound from flame and soot or smoke on edges of wound in addition to hole; hard contact wounds of head cause severe tearing and disruption of tissue (because of thin layer of skin and muscle overlying bone); wound is gaping and jagged, known as *blow back;* can produce a patterned abrasion that mirrors weapon used (see photo)
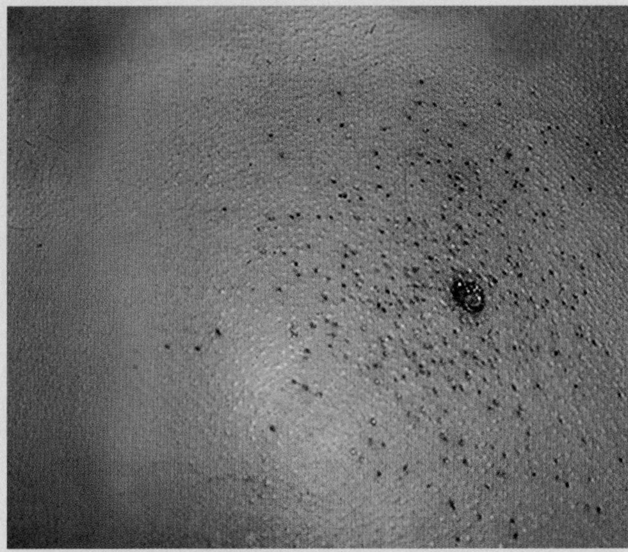	*Intermediate (distance) range entrance wound:* Surrounded by gunpowder tattooing or stippling; *tattooing* results from fragments of burning or unburned pieces of gunpowder exiting barrel and forcefully striking skin; *stippling* results when gunpowder abrades but does not penetrate skin (see photo) *Indeterminate range entrance wound:* Occurs when flame, soot, or gunpowder does not reach skin surface but bullet does; *indeterminate* is used rather than *distant* because appearance may be same regardless of distance; for example, if an individual is shot at close range through multiple layers of clothing the wound may look the same as if the shooting occurred at a distance *Exit wound:* Has the same appearance regardless of range of fire; most important factors are speed of projectile and degree of deformation; size cannot be used to determine if hole is an exit or entrance wound; usually has clean edges that can often be reapproximated to cover defect; skin is one of toughest structures for a bullet to penetrate; thus it is not uncommon for a bullet to pass entirely through body but stopped just beneath skin on "exit" side
	Wounding potential of bullets: Most damage done by a bullet is a result of amount of energy transferred to tissue impacted; speed of bullet has much greater effect than increased size; some bullets are designed to expand or fragment when striking an object, for example, *hollow-point* ammunition; lethality of a wound depends on what structures are damaged; wounds of brain may not be lethal; however, they are usually immediately incapacitating and lead to significant long-term disability; a person with a "lethal" injury (wound of heart or aorta) also may not be immediately incapacitated

The IOM report has galvanized a national movement to improve client safety and eliminate healthcare errors. "Errors and excess mortality can be eliminated but only if concern and attention is shifted away from individuals and toward the error-prone systems in which clinicians work."[82]

Asphyxial Injuries

Asphyxial injuries are caused by a failure of cells to receive or use oxygen. Deprivation of oxygen may be partial *(hypoxia)* or total *(anoxia)*. Asphyxial injuries can be grouped into four general categories: suffocation, strangulation, chemical asphyxiants, and drowning.

Suffocation. **Suffocation,** or oxygen failing to reach the blood, can result from a lack of oxygen in the environment (entrapment in an enclosed space or filling the environment with a suffocating gas) or blockage of the external airways. Classic examples of these types of asphyxial injuries are a child who is trapped in an abandoned refrigerator or a person who commits suicide by putting a plastic bag over the head. A reduction in the ambient oxygen level to 16% (normal is 21%) is immediately dangerous. If the level is below 5%, death can ensue within a matter of minutes. The diagnosis of these types of asphyxial injuries depends on the history of the injury, because there will be no specific physical findings.

Diagnosis and treatment in **choking asphyxiation** (obstruction of the internal airways) depend on locating and removing the obstructing material. Injury or disease also may cause swelling of the soft tissues of the airway, leading to partial or complete obstruction and subsequent asphyxiation. Suffocation also may result from compression of the chest or abdomen (mechanical or compressional asphyxia), preventing normal respiratory movements. Usual signs and symptoms include florid facial congestion and petechiae (pinpoint hemorrhages) of the eyes and face.

Strangulation. **Strangulation** is caused by compression and closure of the blood vessels and air passages resulting from external pressure on the neck. This causes cerebral hypoxia or anoxia secondary to the alteration or cessation of blood flow to and from the brain. It is important to remember that the amount of force needed to close the jugular veins (2 kg [4.5 lb]) or carotid arteries (5 kg [11 lb]) is significantly less than that required to crush the trachea (15 kg [33 lb]). It is the alteration of cerebral blood flow in most types of strangulation that causes injury or death—not the lack of airflow. With complete blockage of the carotid arteries, unconsciousness can occur within 10 to 15 seconds.

A noose is placed around the neck, and the weight of the body is used to cause constriction of the noose and compression of the neck in **hanging strangulations.** The body does not need to be completely suspended to produce severe injury or death. Depending on the type of ligature used, there usually is a distinct mark on the neck, an inverted V with the base of the V pointing toward the point of suspension. Internal injuries of the neck are actually quite rare in hangings, and only in judicial hangings, in which the body is weighted and dropped, is significant soft tissue or cervical spinal trauma seen. Petechiae of the eyes or face may be seen, but they are rare.

In **ligature strangulation,** the mark on the neck is horizontal, without the inverted V pattern seen in hangings. Petechiae may be more common because intermittent opening and closure of the blood vessels may occur as a result of the victim's struggles. Internal injuries of the neck are rare.

Variable amounts of external trauma on the neck with contusions and abrasions are noted in **manual strangulation** caused either by the assailant or by the victim clawing at one's own neck in an attempt to remove the assailant's hands. Internal damage can be quite severe, with bruising of deep structures and even fractures of the hyoid bone and tracheal and cricoid cartilages. Petechiae are common.

Chemical Asphyxiants. **Chemical asphyxiants** either prevent the delivery of oxygen to the tissues or block its use. Carbon monoxide is the most common chemical asphyxiant (see p. 67). **Cyanide** acts as an asphyxiant by combining with the ferric iron atom in cytochrome oxidase, thereby blocking the intracellular use of oxygen. A victim of cyanide poisoning has the same cherry-red appearance as a carbon monoxide intoxication victim because cyanide blocks the use of circulating oxyhemoglobin. An odor of bitter almonds also may be detected. (The ability to smell cyanide is a genetic trait that is absent in a significant portion of the general population.) **Hydrogen sulfide (sewer gas)** is a chemical asphyxiant in which victims of hydrogen cyanide poisoning may have brown-tinged blood in addition to the nonspecific signs of asphyxiation.

Drowning. **Drowning** is an alteration of oxygen delivery to tissues resulting from the breathing in of fluid, usually water. Each year there are thousands of drowning deaths in the United States. Although research done in the 1940s and 1950s indicated that changes in blood electrolyte levels and volume as a result of absorption of fluid from the lungs may be an important factor in some drownings, the major mechanism of injury is hypoxemia (low blood oxygen levels). Even in freshwater drownings, where large amounts of water can pass through the alveolar-capillary interface, there is no evidence that increases in blood volume cause significant electrolyte disturbances or hemolysis, or that the amount of fluid loading is beyond the compensatory capabilities of the kidneys and heart. Airway obstruction is the more important pathologic abnormality, underscored by the fact that in up to 15% of drownings, little or no water enters the lungs because of vagal nerve–mediated laryngospasms. This phenomenon is called *dry-lung drowning.*

No matter what mechanism is involved, cerebral hypoxia leads to unconsciousness in a matter of minutes. Whether this progresses to death depends on a number of factors, including the age and health of the individual. One of the most important factors is the temperature of the water. Irreversible injury develops much more rapidly in warm water than it does in cold water. Submersion times of up to 1 hour with subsequent survival have been reported in children retrieved from very cold water. Complete submersion is not necessary for a person to drown. An incapacitated or helpless individual (such as a person with epilepsy or alcoholism, or an infant) may drown in only a few inches of water.

It is important to remember that there are no specific or diagnostic findings to *prove* that a person recovered from the water is actually a drowning victim. In cases in which water has entered the lung, there may be large amounts of foam coming from the nose and mouth, although this also can be seen in certain types of drug overdoses. A body recovered from water with signs of prolonged immersion could just as easily be a victim of some other type of injury who has been put in the water to obscure the actual cause of death. When working with a living victim recovered from water, it is essential to keep in mind that an underlying condition may have led to the person's becoming incapacitated and submersed—a condition that also may need to be treated or corrected while correcting hypoxemia and dealing with its sequelae.

Infectious Injury

The pathogenicity (virulence) of microorganisms lies in their ability to survive and proliferate in the human body, where they injure cells and tissues. The disease-producing potential of a microorganism depends on its ability to (1) invade and destroy cells, (2) produce toxins, and (3) produce damaging hypersensitivity reactions (see Chapter 9 for further discussion).

Immunologic and Inflammatory Injury

Cellular membranes are injured by direct contact with cellular and chemical components of the immune and inflammatory responses, such as phagocytic cells (lymphocytes, macrophages) and substances such as histamine, antibodies, lymphokines, complement, and proteases (see Chapter 7). Complement is responsible for many of the membrane alterations that occur during immunologic injury. Membrane alterations are associated with rapid leakage of potassium (K^+) out of the cell and rapid influx of water. Antibodies can interfere with membrane function by binding to and occupying receptor molecules on the plasma membrane. This type of injury is found in certain forms of diabetes mellitus and in myasthenia gravis. Antibodies also can block or destroy cellular junctions, interfering with intercellular communication (see Chapters 8 and 9).

Injurious Genetic/Epigenetic Factors

Genetic disorders may be the result of genetic factors that alter the cell's nucleus and the plasma membrane's structure, shape, receptors, or transport mechanisms. For example, enzymatic genetic defects can lead to abnormalities in membrane transport. Genetic disorders can cause structural alterations of the red blood cell (for example, sickle cell anemia). (Mechanisms causing genetic abnormalities are discussed in Unit II.) Certain human diseases, for example, cancer, can occur because of misregulation of gene expression linked to alterations of epigenetic patterning (see Chapters 6, 12, and 13).

Injurious Nutritional Imbalances

Essential nutrients—proteins, carbohydrates, lipids (fats), vitamins, and minerals—are required for cells to function normally. If these nutrients are not consumed in the diet and transported to the body's cells or if excessive amounts of nutrients are consumed and transported, pathophysiologic cellular effects develop.

Proteins, which consist of chains of amino acids, are the major structural units of the cell and participate in many enzymatic and hormonal functions. Protein deficiency causes a decrease in the intestinal mucosal mass, decreasing the absorptive function. The integrity of the pancreas is also affected, resulting in diminished exocrine secretion. With starvation or malnutrition, the lowered levels of plasma proteins, particularly albumin, cause fluid to move into the interstitium (edema). Protein-calorie malnutrition (PCM) is the predominant worldwide type of malnutrition. Malnourished children are very susceptible to disease and often die of infectious diseases. Even with adequate protein intake, cellular injury can occur if amino acid transport mechanisms fail or are defective. In Fanconi syndrome, for example, renal tubular cells may contain accumulated protein droplets that have been absorbed but cannot be transported.

Glucose is the major carbohydrate obtained from the breakdown of starch (see Chapter 1). **Hyperglycemia** (excessive glucose in the blood) caused by excessive carbohydrate intake may lead to obesity. Deficiencies of glucose result from starvation or from lack of use, as in diabetes. In both conditions the body compensates by metabolizing fat (lipids). (For details on diabetes, see Chapter 22.)

In lipid deficiency, or **hypolipidemia,** the body compensates by mobilizing fatty acids from adipose tissue. This causes an increase in the production and circulation of ketone bodies, which are acidic byproducts of lipid metabolism. The excretion of ketone bodies results in loss of water and electrolytes and causes dehydration and thirst. Severe increases in the concentration of ketone bodies cause ketoacidosis, coma, and death. **Hyperlipidemia,** or an increase in the levels of lipoproteins in the blood, results in deposits of fat in the heart, liver, and muscle.

Vitamins are not sources of energy but are necessary for maintaining normal cellular functions. Adequate vitamin intake is necessary because most vitamins are not synthesized by the body. Research from the 1990s resulted in the identification of 13 vitamins as being essential for humans. These include 8 B vitamins (thiamine, niacin, riboflavin, folate, vitamin B_6, vitamin B_{12}, biotin, and pantothenic acid), vitamin C or ascorbic acid, and the fat-soluble vitamins A, D, E, and K. (Minerals are discussed in Chapter 3.) Vitamins are involved in numerous reactions, including metabolism of visual pigments (vitamin A), calcium and phosphate metabolism (vitamin D), prothrombin synthesis (vitamin K), and antioxidation reactions (vitamins E and C). Pyridoxal (vitamin B_6) affects amino acid transfer reactions; flavin adenine dinucleotide (FAD), flavin mononucleotide (FMN), and nicotinamide adenine dinucleotide (NAD) help transfer electrons in various reactions (see Chapter 1).

Injurious Physical Agents

Injurious physical agents include temperature extremes, atmospheric pressure changes, radiation, illumination, mechanical factors, noise, and prolonged vibration. Physical injury can result from excessive exposure to many environmental agents, as well as to agents used for the diagnosis and treatment of illness.

Temperature Extremes and Climate Change

Much research is occurring to elucidate linkages between climate change and epidemics. Climate change is affecting human health including: (1) an increase in heat- and pollution-related deaths with cardiovascular, cerebrovascular, and respiratory diseases; (2) an increase in gastroenteritis and infectious disease epidemics because of water and food contamination as a result of flooding, lack of clean water, and sewage treatment; (3) an increase in vector-borne infectious diseases (for example, malaria, West Nile virus infection, hantavirus pulmonary syndrome); and (4) an increase in the number of people affected by malnutrition because of food crop disruptions.[49,83,84] Climate change is just one of several factors impacting the incidence of disease. Chilling or freezing of cells causes **hypothermic injury.** Hypothermia has proved to be strongly injurious to a variety of cells. *Accidental hypothermia* is an unintentional drop in core body temperature below 35° C (95° F). At these temperatures, the compensatory mechanisms that conserve temperature start to fail. **Primary accidental hypothermia** is the physiologic result of a previously healthy person to the changes that occur with cold. The mortality rate is higher in those who develop **secondary hypothermia** as a consequence of a serious systemic disorder, for example, endocrine disorders. Primary accidental hypothermia is a worldwide problem with most cases evident in the winter months. Surprisingly, however, it commonly occurs in warmer regions. The highest risks are to the elderly and neonates. The elderly have diminished thermal perception and regulation and are susceptible because of increased likelihood of immobility, impaired nutritional status, the presence of coexisting diseases, and the impact of economic factors. Neonates have high rates of heat loss because of their increased surface-to-mass ratio and lack of shivering and other behavioral responses. Individuals at increased risks for hypothermia include those with occupations or hobbies that have extensive cold weather exposure, such as people in the military, hunters, sailors, skiers, swimmers, and climbers. Prolonged exposure to low ambient temperature is a common risk factor found in homeless persons. Some causes of secondary hypothermia include hypothyroidism, hypoglycemia, adrenal insufficiency, metabolic alterations associated with uremia, neurologic injury, extensive burns, acute myocardial infarction (can be reversed with resuscitation), skin diseases, and hepatic failure.[85]

Submersion in cold water can induce a high incidence of cardiac arrhythmias in healthy volunteers.[86] Immersion in cold water is a common cause of death in children and in adults.[87] Deaths caused by cold water have historically been ascribed to hypothermia; however, reports of two newer antagonistic responses are emerging—they are called the *cold shock response* and the *diving response* (see What's New? Cold Water Immersion and Cold Shock Response and the Diving Response).

Hypothermic injury has long been attributed to disturbances of cellular ion balance or homeostasis, especially of sodium balance (i.e., increased intracellular sodium levels). Hypothermia increases the level of intracellular Ca^{++} by slowing Na^+-K^+-ATPase pump activity, leading to Na^+ accumulation intracellularly.[88] In recent years, however, a role for ROS has gained importance.[89] In animal studies, hypothermia resulted in cell damage caused by formation of ROS.[90,91] Hypothermic perfusion of the heart increased superoxide

WHAT'S NEW?

Cold Water Immersion and Cold Shock Response and the Diving Response

Submersion and breath-holding in cold water can activate two antagonistic responses called the *cold-shock response* and the *diving response.* The cold-shock response triggers tachycardia from activation of the sympathetic nervous system. Sympathetic activation affects the sinoatrial (SA) and atrioventricular (AV) nodes of the heart and the myocardium. The release of breath-holding may be involved, with many arrhythmias occurring within 10 seconds of stopping breath-holding. Paradoxically, the diving response promotes a parasympathetically mediated brachycardia. The simultaneous activation of both the sympathetic and parasympathetic branches of the autonomic nervous system is sometimes called "autonomic conflict."

Certain individuals may have vulnerable risk factors including ischemic heart disease, myocardial hypertrophy, acquired (drug-induced) long QT syndrome (LQTS), QT interval mismatch to heart rate, atherosclerosis, and conduction pathologies (e.g., LQTS). There is a strong association between sudden cardiac arrest and swimming in children with LQTS. Certain drugs also may prolong QT interval (e.g., antihistamines, antibiotics, class Ia anti-arrhythmics, gastrointestinal prokinetics, and antipsychotics). The actual number of immersion-related deaths because of "autonomic conflict" is unknown and may be undiagnosed because of drowning.

Data from Patton JF et al: *Brain Res Brain Res Rev* 49:399–404, 2010; Tipton MJ et al: *Aviat Space Environ Med* 81:399–404, 2010; Shattock MJ, Tipton MJ: *J Physiol,* April 2012. [Epub ahead of print.]

(O_2^-) concentration (see Table 2-3); in turn, O_2^- reacted with nitric oxide (NO) to form another radical peroxynitrate anion ($ONOO^-$).[88] In some cell types, such as hepatocytes and liver endothelial cells, hypothermia can cause pronounced cell injury mediated by ROS. During the body's exposure to cold, injury is inhibited by hypoxia and by a number of antioxidants, especially iron chelators.

Indirect forms of injury occur because of changes in small blood vessels (the microcirculation). Slow chilling can cause vasoconstriction followed by paralysis of vasomotor control, resulting in vasodilation and increased membrane permeability causing cellular and tissue swelling. With an abrupt drop in temperature, vasoconstriction and increased viscosity of the blood cause ischemic injury—infarction and necrosis (cellular death) in affected tissues. With continued exposure to freezing temperatures, vasodilation produces severe swelling that causes degenerative changes in the myelin sheath that surrounds peripheral nerves, resulting in sensory and motor disturbances. Thrombosis also can occur and may lead to gangrene of the affected part. (Gangrene is discussed on p. 91.) These conditions often are called *frostbite.*

Therapeutically, hypothermia is widely used to protect cells and tissues against injurious processes. Therapeutic hypothermia (TH) has been used clinically to preserve the heart during surgery and to preserve organs before transplantation.[92] TH in animals to protect the heart against acute infarction has had positive results; however, studies in humans are limited.

Hyperthermia is an uncontrolled increase in body temperature that exceeds the body's ability to lose heat. **Hyperthermic**

injury (injury caused by excessive heat) is common and varies depending on the nature, intensity, and extent of the injury. Three types of hyperthermic injury include heat cramps, heat exhaustion (illness), and heat stroke. (For more detail see Chapter 16.)

Heat cramps (cramping of voluntary muscles) are usually a result of vigorous exercise that causes a loss of salt and water as a consequence of sweat. Treatment is salt replacement.

Heat exhaustion occurs when sufficient salt and water loss results in hemoconcentration. Hypotension occurs secondary to fluid loss (hypovolemia), and the individual feels weak, is nauseated, and can suddenly collapse. Collapsing results from a failure of the cardiovascular system to compensate for hypovolemia. Heat exhaustion is probably the most common heat-related injury.

Heat stroke is a life-threatening condition associated with high environmental temperatures and humidity. Core body temperature rises as a result of thermoregulatory failures. Clinically, a rectal temperature of 106° F (41° C) is considered a life-threatening sign. Generalized peripheral vasodilation and decreased circulating blood volume are significant. At risk are older adults, athletes, military recruits, and people with cardiovascular disorders.

Malignant hyperthermia occurs in individuals with an inherited disorder (e.g., ryanodine receptor intracellular calcium release channel) of skeletal muscle sarcoplasmic reticulum in response to inhalational anesthetics or to succinylcholine.[93] This rare condition is often fatal. The condition includes elevated temperature, increased muscle metabolism, muscle rigidity, rhabdomyolysis, acidosis, and cardiovascular alterations within minutes.

Drug-induced hyperthermia has become increasingly common because of the increase in abuse of psychotropic drugs and illicit drugs. Examples of drugs include amphetamines, cocaine, phencyclidine (PCP), methylenedioxymethamphetamine (MDMA; ecstasy), lysergic acid diethylamide (LSD), salicylates, lithium, anticholinergics, and sympathomimetics.

Neuroleptic malignant syndrome is hyperthermia caused by the administration of neuroleptic drugs (antipsychotics, phenothiazines, haloperidol, prochlorperazine, metoclopramide) or the withdrawal of dopaminergic drugs and is characterized by lead-pipe muscle rigidity, autonomic dysregulation, hyperthermia, and extrapyramidal side effects.[94]

Burns are caused by local heat injury. A *full-thickness burn* is an open wound involving skin layers—epidermis, dermis, and subcutaneous layers—and causing extensive loss of fluids and plasma proteins. Cellular regeneration is not possible; therefore, skin from a donor or from the host must be grafted to the site. *Partial-thickness burns* result in reddening of the area as a result of dilation of small blood vessels and increased permeability of cellular membranes, with loss of protein-rich fluid, resulting in the typical "burn blister." In surface epithelial cells, membrane permeability increases, causing both cytoplasmic and nuclear swelling. Temperature-sensitive enzymes within certain cells respond to heat by increasing cellular metabolism, with detrimental effects. Intense heat also damages the vascular endothelium and causes coagulation of the blood vessels. (Burns are discussed further in Chapter 48.)

Epidemiologic investigators have reported a positive relationship between overheating in infants (that is, overdressing infants in the winter) and the prevalence of sudden infant deaths. Studies suggest interactions between body temperature and respiratory responses to hypoxia or increased carbon dioxide concentration (hypercapnia). The hypoxia/*hypo*thermia interaction depresses breathing, reducing the ventilatory response to hypercapnia. The effects of *hyper*thermia seem to be a significant problem only when it accompanies an infection and fever and alters or depresses the breathing responses. (Temperature changes are also discussed in Chapter 16.) Recent recommendations to reduce the risk of all sleep-related infant deaths include positioning the infant supine, using a firm sleep surface, breast-feeding, room-sharing without bed-sharing, performing routine immunizations, considering use of a pacifier, and avoiding soft bedding, overheating, and exposure to tobacco smoke, alcohol, and illicit drugs. *(Policy Statement—Sudden Infant Death Syndrome and Other Sleep-Related Infant Deaths: Expansion of Recommendations for a Safe Infant Sleeping Environment).*[95]

Changes in Atmospheric Pressure

Sudden increases or decreases in atmospheric pressure cause **blast injury,** which can be transmitted by either air (air blast) or water (immersion blast). With sudden increases in pressure, tissue injury is caused by compressive waves of air impingeing on the body, followed by a sudden wave of decreased pressure. The pressure changes may collapse the thorax, rupture internal solid organs, and cause widespread hemorrhage. In increased pressure caused by immersion blast, water pressure is applied suddenly to all sides of the body, forcing the body up out of water. The positive pressure compresses the abdomen and ruptures hollow internal organs, such as the spleen, kidneys, and liver.

Decompression Sickness. **Decompression sickness (DCS)** (diver disease, the bends, or caisson disease) is a condition arising with sudden decreases in pressure; carbon dioxide and nitrogen that are normally dissolved in the blood come out of solution and form tiny bubbles called *gas emboli.* Deep-sea divers and underwater construction workers who return to the surface too quickly develop decompression sickness. Oxygen is quickly redissolved, but nitrogen bubbles may persist and obstruct blood vessels. Ischemia resulting from gas emboli causes cellular hypoxia, particularly in the muscles, joints, and tendons. Emboli and interstitial gas accumulate around the joints and skeletal muscles, causing the individual to bend in pain. Tissues of the heart and brain also may be affected by emboli, causing necrosis. The gases can be promptly redissolved in blood by raising the atmospheric pressure. This is accomplished by placing the individual in a decompression chamber and increasing the pressure until it approximates pressure at the depth to which the diver had descended. This redissolves the gas bubbles in the blood. Pressure is then decreased gradually until it equals pressure at the surface of the water. This slows the release of gas bubbles out of solution.

Nitrogen concentrations can have a crippling anesthetic effect on the brain. This narcosis has been referred to as "rapture of the deep," where both physical and cognitive abilities may be seriously impaired.[96] Thus, when diving to great depths, both the volume of nitrogen and the volume of oxygen must be decreased. This is accomplished by the addition of an "inert" gas (one that has no metabolic activity within the body). It has been suggested that problems associated with deep, long-duration dives could be avoided by replacing the nitrogen in a diver's gas supply with helium, an inert gas and nature's second lightest gas.[97] Helium's great advantage is that it does not lead to nitrogen narcosis—it is less soluble in blood and fat than nitrogen.

Decompression sickness can happen with very rapid ascent to high altitude in an aircraft that is not properly pressurized.[98] Although decompression sickness is not a concern when people ascend slowly (e.g., on foot) to a low atmospheric pressure environment, such as altitudes above 10,000 feet, there is a significant decrease in available oxygen because of decreased partial pressure of the inspired gases. The hypoxemia that occurs may result in pathologic conditions unique to the hypoxic environment at high altitude.

High Altitude Illness: HAPE, HACE, AMS. High altitude illness, in the form of high altitude pulmonary edema (HAPE) or high altitude cerebral edema (HACE), is potentially fatal. Both conditions, in addition to a less serious, more common form, are known as acute mountain sickness (AMS). Several factors, including rate of ascent to altitude, final altitude reached, altitude at which a person sleeps, and individual physiologic differences, are believed to influence development of these conditions.[99] Additional risk factors include certain preexisting cardiopulmonary conditions, residence at low altitude, prior history of high altitude illness, and the level of exertion at altitude.[100]

Acute mountain sickness (AMS) is defined as the presence of a combination of nonspecific symptoms that appear within a few hours after ascent to altitude, and may include headache, loss of appetite, nausea, vomiting, weakness, lassitude, dizziness, and difficulty sleeping.[101] Symptoms are usually most noticeable during the first few days at altitude, but may reappear on further ascent to a higher altitude. AMS is usually a relatively benign, self-limited condition and does not include abnormal neurologic symptoms or signs. An increase in severity of symptoms or signs of neurologic dysfunction, such as ataxia or altered consciousness, indicates transition to **high altitude cerebral edema (HACE).** HACE is a clinical diagnosis defined as the onset of ataxia, altered consciousness (including confusion, impaired mentation, stupor, and coma), and severe lassitude. Severe headache, nausea, and vomiting are frequently present. In both AMS and HACE, headache is most likely initially produced by hypoxemia-induced cerebral vasodilation and a significant increase in blood flow. In addition, recent magnetic resonance imaging (MRI) studies suggest that in persons ascending to high altitudes and suffering moderate to severe AMS, some degree of cerebral edema occurs. However, in milder forms of AMS (a subjective distinction), brain edema is present in some MRI studies, but not in all.[101] The cerebral edema may be either cytotoxic or vasogenic in nature (see Chapter 17).

As potentially lethal as HACE can be, HAPE is actually thought to account for most deaths from high altitude illness.[101]

High altitude pulmonary edema (HAPE) is a noncardiogenic pulmonary edema associated with pulmonary hypertension and elevated capillary pressure. The incidence of HAPE also is related to rate of ascent, the ultimate altitude reached, and individual susceptibility. Victims of HAPE have a relatively exaggerated pulmonary hypertensive response on ascent to altitude as a result of augmented hypoxic pulmonary vasoconstriction. Heightened sympathetic nervous system activity, vascular endothelial dysfunction, and hypoxemia resulting from a suboptimal ventilatory response to hypoxia are responsible for the pulmonary vasoconstriction and subsequent pulmonary hypertension. Recent evidence suggests HAPE-prone individuals are characterized by a genetic defect in the transepithelial sodium and water transport mechanism that may impair alveolar fluid clearance.[102] Persons with congenital or acquired pulmonary circulation abnormalities are more susceptible to HAPE, supporting the suggestion that edema results from overperfusion in a restricted pulmonary vascular bed. Another proposed explanation for elevated pulmonary capillary pressure is uneven hypoxic pulmonary vasoconstriction.[103] It is now generally accepted that HAPE is initiated as a noninflammatory unidirectional dysfunction of the alveolar-capillary barrier that is essentially a form of hydrostatic pulmonary edema (i.e., there is an increase in pulmonary capillary pressure, but no elevation in left atrial pressure) (see Chapter 35).

Ionizing Radiation

Ionizing radiation (IR) is any form of radiation capable of removing orbital electrons from atoms, resulting in the production of negatively charged free electrons and positively charged ionized atoms. Ionizing radiation is emitted by x-rays, γ-rays, and alpha and beta particles (which are emitted from atomic nuclei in the process of radioactive decay) and from neutrons, deuterons, protons, and pions. Ionizing radiation of three types (x-radiation, gamma radiation, and neutrons) was classified as a carcinogen in 2004.

An important source of exposure to ionizing radiation is the environment. This source includes emission from radioactive material inside the body, cosmic rays from outer space, and radiation emitted from such substances as soil and building materials. Environmental radioactivity is emitted primarily by uranium, thorium, and potassium. Other sources are from medical procedures (e.g., x-rays, computed tomography [CT] scans) used for medical diagnosis and treatment, uranium and thorium mines, nuclear weapons, and nuclear reactors that generate electricity. Medical radiation now comprises about 48% to 50% of the per capita radiation doses compared with 15% in the 1980s; since 1980 medical radiation exposure has increased 600% in the U.S. population (Figure 2-18). Table 2-7 includes types of ionizing radiation and their magnitude of tissue penetration.

Cellular damage from IR in the absence of effective repair involves two types of damage: (1) deterministic and (2) stochastic. *Deterministic effects* are thought to occur above a threshold dose and have dose-related increasing risks. Deterministic effects include induced dermatitis, erythema, and generation of cataracts. Recent human and lab studies suggest a lower dose

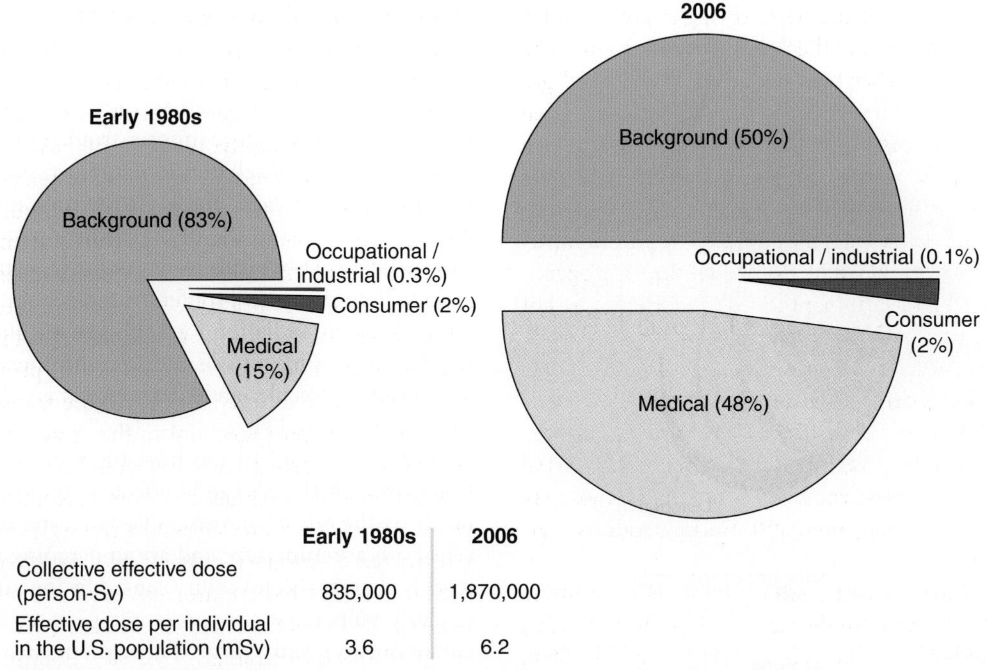

	Early 1980s	2006
Collective effective dose (person-Sv)	835,000	1,870,000
Effective dose per individual in the U.S. population (mSv)	3.6	6.2

FIGURE 2-18 Ionizing Radiation Exposure of the Population of the United States. (National Council on Radiation Protection & Measurements: *Ionizing radiation exposure of the population of the United States, NCRP report 160,* Bethesda, MD: Author.)

TABLE 2-7 TYPES OF IONIZING RADIATION AND THEIR TISSUE PENETRATION

TYPE	TISSUE PENETRATION
X-rays	High
Gamma (γ) rays	High
Beta (β) particles	Low
Alpha (α) particles	Very low
Protons	Intermediate between α and β
Neutrons	High

Data from Damjanov I, Linder J, editors: *Anderson's pathology,* ed 10, St Louis, 1996, Mosby.

(0.5 gray [Gy]) than previously reported (2 Gy for acute radiation, 4 Gy fractionated doses) or no threshold for cataracts.[104] *Stochastic effects* include cell generation or hereditary effects and cancer. Although not completely clear, the probability of a stochastic effect increases with dose probably with no threshold (an assumption based on molecular studies, because a very small x-ray dose can cause a base change in DNA), but importantly, the severity of the outcome is *not* related to dose but rather the entire tissue and stress response (see below).[105,106] Historically, radiation dose–related cancer risks at low doses were estimated from data of the atomic-bomb survivors and of individuals treated with moderate- to high-dose radiation.[106] The effects of low doses were mathematically extrapolated from high doses. After review from national and international expert committees and publications from 2005 to 2008, the available biologic and biophysical data support a linear no-threshold risk model for cancer.[106] Additionally, this understanding combined with an uncertain dose and dose rate effectiveness factor for extrapolation from high doses is considered a conservative estimate for radiation protection for low doses and low dose rates.[106] Complicating these standards, however, has been the emerging data from radiobiology suggesting a much more complex understanding regarding low dose and low dose rates because of nontargeted effects of low dose radiation (e.g., effects in nonirradiated cells near and distant from irradiated cells.[107] The **nontargeted effects** of ionizing radiation include bystander effects and genomic instability. **Bystander effects,** or effects on cells not directly in the radiated field, are affected by the radiation and show high levels of mutations, chromosomal aberrations, and membrane signaling changes leading to what some call "horizontal transmission." **Genomic instability** is where generations of cells derived from an irradiated progenitor cell appear normal but time-lethal (i.e., irreversible) and nonlethal mutations appear in distant progeny, sometimes called "vertical transmission."[108] Importantly, a new paradigm shift of the effects of IR or radiobiology is occurring. These effects represent a tissue response or cell stress response from IR. The current theory that all radiation damage results from energy deposition in those cells' DNA was challenged by four key lines of evidence reported from 1986 to 1996 and includes: (1) new lethal mutations could occur in cells that had recovered from irradiation and continued dividing for several generations,[109] (2) a delayed appearance of new chromosome aberrations was demonstrated in bone marrow stem cell lines from irradiated stem cells,[110] (3) a very low dose exposure of alpha radiation resulted in more cells with chromosome damage than would have been predicted mathematically,[111] and (4) the cell medium from irradiated cells was found to cause similar levels of clonogenic genomic instability and cell death as cells *directly* irradiated.[112] Thus, from newer evidence are

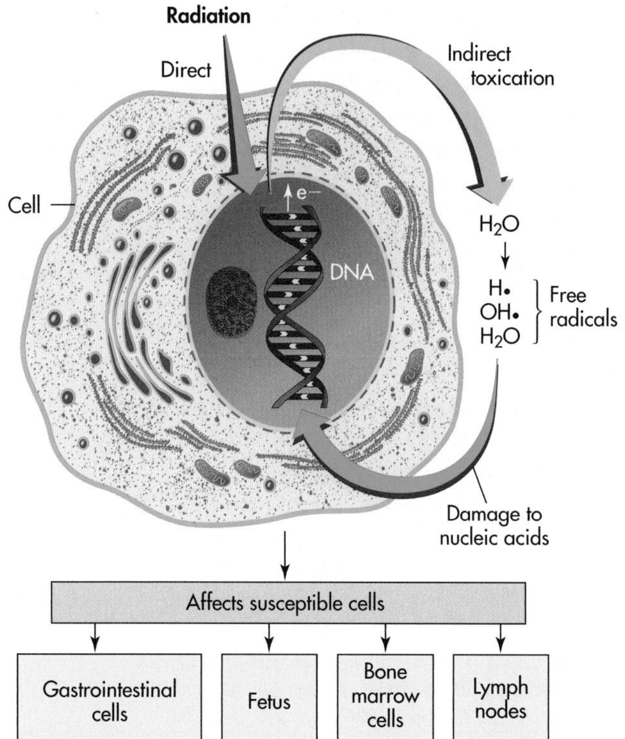

FIGURE 2-19 Cellular Damage Caused by Ionizing Radiation. Radiation can damage macromolecules in two ways: (1) directly, in which the micromolecules are ionized; and (2) indirectly, in which water is ionized and produces free radicals that in turn damage macromolecules. Cells that are particularly susceptible to damage are those of the gastrointestinal tract, bone marrow, lymph nodes, fetus, and ovarian follicles (also see Chapter 19).

radiobiologic understandings for low dose radiation, yet many biologic questions remain.[108] Importantly, many teams of investigators studying radiation effects have consisted of both physicists *and* biologists. Additionally, much research is now involved concerning the effects of radiation on epigenetics and the entire tissue and organismic "stress" response, including the role of the microenvironment.

Ionizing radiation (IR; x-radiation and γ-rays) causes a large spectrum of genetic changes including gene mutations, mini–satellite mutations (altered numbers of tandem repeats of DNA sequences), micronucleus formation (sign of chromosome damage or loss), chromosomal aberrations (structural or number), ploidy changes (number of sets of chromosomes), DNA strand breaks, and chromosomal instability. DNA may be damaged *directly* or *indirectly* by interaction with reactive products (i.e., free electrons, hydroxyl radicals, hydrogen free radicals) from the degradation of water (Figure 2-19). Because IR has many multicellular effects, their interactions with the cells and cellular products that comprise the microenvironment will affect tissue and determine the overall response.[113] Epigenetic mechanisms (a change in gene *expression* and not in the DNA sequence) that damage genes are involved in radiation-induced tumor formation. These mechanisms include genomic instability; mutations by irradiation of the cytoplasm (includes ROS, inflammatory cell signaling pathways, extracellular matrix alterations); "bystander effects" induction of genetic damage in innocent or cells not *directly* irradiated, possibly through cellular gap junctions; and persistent signaling pathways (see Chapter 13).

All phases of the cell cycle can be affected by ionizing radiation. Sensitivity of the cell appears to be greatest in G_2, that gap of the cell just before mitosis; irradiation during this phase retards the onset of cell division. Radio-resistance is greatest in the latter part of the S phase. At the time of therapeutic irradiation those cells in the most sensitive parts of the cell cycle will be killed. Those cells in the radio-resistant part of the cell cycle will continue to proliferate and repopulate the tumor—requiring more radiation for a therapeutic effect or cell killing. Irradiation during mitosis induces chromosomal aberrations. Membrane molecules and enzymes also are damaged by radiation (see Chapter 13).

Not all cells and tissues have the same sensitivity to radiation, although all cells can be affected. Radiosensitivity depends partly on the rate of mitosis and cellular maturity. Because fetal cells both are immature and are undergoing rapid cycling, the fetus is at great risk for injury caused by ionizing radiation. Particularly vulnerable are embryonic germ cells, which are precursors of ova and sperm. Throughout life, cells of the bone marrow, intestinal mucosa, testicular seminiferous epithelium, and ovarian follicles are susceptible to injury because they are always undergoing mitosis, which ensures the presence of vulnerable, immature daughter cells. Exposure to x-radiation and γ-radiation is most strongly correlated with leukemia and cancers of the thyroid, breast, and lung; these correlates have been reported at absorbed low levels, less than 0.2 gray Gy. The risk of developing these cancers may to some extent depend on age at exposure. The Life Span Study, which had a wide range in age at exposure and a wide dose range (from less than 0.005 Gy to 2-4 Gy), was evidence of a linear dose response for all solid tumors with significant radiation-associated excess risks observed in most, but not all, types of solid tumors. In utero radiation exposure from the bombings was associated with an increased adult-onset risk of solid tumors.[114] The studies of diagnostic x-rays in utero and risk of pediatric leukemia and other cancers are characterized by uncertainties, especially a lack of dose measurement data.[106] Ultrasound replaced abdominal x-rays and measurements of the pelvis several decades ago in pregnant women; however, there recently have been reports of increasing levels of radiologic imaging in pregnant women.[115] Many organizations have specific papers on safety and imaging pregnant women, including the American College of Radiology, American Congress of Obstetricians and Gynecologists, and internationally, for example, Health & Safety Executive from Great Britain and the International Commission on Radiological Protection Publication (ICRP). Radiation exposure to children may increase the incidence of lymphomas, leukemias, melanomas, breast cancers, and others. The increased frequency of pediatric CT exams in the United States is mainly because of the increased use of fast helical CT, which reduces the need for sedation.[116]

Radiation-induced cancers are found in the "cancer-prone" ages (usually 50 to 80 years of age), independent of age at exposure; therefore, the latency period between radiation exposure and the potential appearance of a cancer decreases significantly with increasing age at exposure.[117] From these effects, more recent analyses of cancer incidence among atomic-bomb (A-bomb) survivors suggest that the lifetime risk of radiation-induced cancer is not so different for exposure at age 5 years vs. exposure at age 55 years.[114,118]

Studies of A-bomb survivors have found increased mortality from noncancer diseases.[119] The majority of radiation-induced noncancer deaths are cardiovascular problems (i.e., myocardial infarction and stroke). Individuals exposed to radiation at less than 40 years of age revealed an excess relative risk of myocardial infarction of 0.25. In addition, radiation exposure was significantly related to hypertension and elevated total cholesterol level. Risk estimates for heart disease and stroke indicated higher susceptibility in women.[120] Studies of the late effects of radiation in A-bomb survivors reveal elevated levels of mediators of inflammation (interleukin-6 [IL-6] and C-reactive protein [CRP]). Persistent elevations were documented of leukocyte counts, erythrocyte sedimentation rates, immunoglobulins, and sialic acid with radiation exposure. Also elevated were other inflammatory markers (tumor necrosis factor-alpha [TNF-α], IL-10, immunoglobulin [Ig], IgM, IgA, and interferon-gamma [IFN-γ]). The elevations of autoantibodies and T-cell–immune alterations is important because they may activate prolonged inflammation, which is a key contributor to cardiovascular effects.[120] The bone marrow and thymus gland are both radiosensitive, and documented immunologic effects measured from 40 to 50 years after radiation exposure suggest permanent genetic damage to lymphocyte progenitor cells.[120] A recent meta-analysis supports an association between circulatory disease mortality and low and moderate doses of ionizing radiation.[121] In Japanese atomic-bomb survivors, respiratory and digestive diseases also were increased.[119]

The effects of ionizing radiation may be acute or delayed. Acute effects of high doses, such as skin redness, skin damage, or chromosomal aberrations, occur within hours, days, or months. The delayed effects of low doses may not be evident for years.

Illumination and Luminance: Light Is Electromagnetic Radiation

Light is electromagnetic radiation visible in the adult human eye in the range of 380 to 780 nanometers (nm). All radiations like light carry energy, with the shorter wavelengths being the most energetic.[122] Luminance (radiance, measured in watts per square meter per steradian, $W\ m^{-2}\ sr^{-1}$), formerly called brightness, is measured in candela per square meter (cd/m^2) and illuminance (irradiance, W/m^2) is the light flux density on a receiving surface measured in lux. Consequently, the smaller the emitting surface the more concentrated the flux in the viewing direction and the higher the luminance.[122] The optical system images everything on the retina, a highly specialized sense organ, and most relevant for retinal illumination is the luminance of the viewed objects. The mechanisms of light-induced damage include (1) heat or thermal damage; (2) photochemical damage, thought to come mainly from oxidative stress by forming ROS, known as photosensitizers; and (3) thermoacoustic damage from light (e.g., laser) pulses shorter than ≈1 ns.[122-125] Thermal damage occurs from absorption of heat. The absorption rate (W/m^3) is the important factor for causing damage of the radiant energy (heat). The depth of penetration of the radiant energy depends on the incident wavelength and the primary absorbers—melanin and hemoglobin or oxyhemoglobin.[122] Photochemical damage occurs at short visible wavelengths and for exposure longer than ≈1 ns; it is thought to be the result of light absorption to the chromophore, the most sensitive molecule that absorbs the radiation (light leads to the production of ROS and oxidative stress; the retina is very sensitive to oxidative stress).[122] Thermoacoustic (photomechanical) damage occurs with light pulses shorter than ≈1 ns and when the light energy is deposited faster than mechanical relaxation can occur. Tissue is disrupted by shear forces or cavitation (i.e., production of a cavity). Photomechanical damage can be produced from sources such as intense pulsed lasers.[122]

Ocular exposures are accidental and intended (for example, in ophthalmic applications). Adherence to standards for ocular safety is a main concern for protection of the eye from laser exposures and light exposures from ophthalmic instruments. Additionally, to improve the energy performances of artificial light sources and to protect the environment, new light sources are available, such as compact fluorescent lamps or light-emitting diodes (LEDs). The potential risks of these new light sources need safety evaluation to determine health risks, especially hazards to the eye (see What's New? Health Risks Related to Use of LED Lighting Systems).

Focused light rays can increase oxidative stress, which can be prevented by a wide array of retinal antioxidant mechanisms.[126] Antioxidant mechanisms can, however, be overwhelmed by excessive light exposure, particularly of short-wavelength, high-frequency blue light, and of ultraviolet light. Since fluorescent lighting was introduced to the workplace, complaints of headaches, eyestrain, and eye discomfort have increased.[66] The

WHAT'S NEW?

Health Risks Related to Use of LED Lighting Systems

The number of light-emitting diodes (LEDs) is increasing in the marketplace because they produce light with low energy consumption. In the European Union, LEDs will become the major domestic sources of light by 2016. Therefore, safety standards, especially for exposures to children, need careful study. Rodent studies may not be the best models because rodents are mostly nocturnal and have rod-rich retina without macula. The French Agency for Food, Environmental and Occupational Health & Safety (ANSES) recommends that consumer information about health risks from LED lighting systems be made available immediately after conclusive testing. ANSES recommends (1) avoiding the use of light sources emitting cold-white light (light with a strong blue component) in places frequented by children or in the objects children use (e.g., toys, electronic devices, game consoles, joysticks, night lights); (2) ensuring high-quality controls from manufacturers of LEDs and qualifying their products according to different risk groups; and (3) using a clear labeling system for consumers with a mandatory label of the photobiologic safety information with risk groups listed on the packaging for all types of lighting. White LEDs expose the retina to violet, indigo, and blue light at higher levels than in previous light sources. This is the first time that the population will be exposed to substantial amounts of blue light.

Data from Behar-Cohen F et al: *Prog Retinal Eye Res* 30:239–257, 2011.

rapid modulation of light from fluorescent lamps is responsible for eyestrain and headaches. The modulation can be reduced by wearing tinted glasses. The shorter wavelengths in radiant energy in environmental lighting influence the absorption, scattering, and fluorescence, thus obscuring vision.[127]

Vision is obstructed at night by decreased illumination and by disabling glare from oncoming vehicle headlights. High-intensity discharge (HID) headlamps project light farther down roads, thus improving the driver's safety. However, oncoming glare, which is proportional to headlamp brightness, is *not* good for any drivers of oncoming vehicles and even worse for older drivers.[128] Older drivers experience more intraocular light scattering, increased glare sensitivity, and longer recovery time in reaction to photo stress.[129]

Mechanical Stresses

Mechanical stimulation of body tissues and cells is constant. These stresses and strains are from the external environment and internal physiologic conditions. For example, gravity as an external force and the pumping of the heart as an internal force are continual. Mechanical stimuli can cause cells to respond in a variety of ways, for example, **compression** is a perpendicular-acting force, **tension** is a stretching force, and **torsion** is a twisting force. Fluid **shear forces** or layers rubbing against each other, for example, endothelial cells can activate hormone release and intracellular signaling, as well as stiffen the cells by inducing rearrangement of the cytoskeleton. Mechanical compression of chondrocytes can modulate proteoglycan synthesis, and tensile stretching of cell structures can alter cell motility and orientation. Mechanical signals or signaling, called **mechanotransduction,** are eventually converted to biologic and chemical responses in the cell. Understanding molecular mechanisms driving cell shape changes is an important topic in cell and tissue structure. For example, achieving cell division successfully has led to the study of cytokinesis as a function of mechanical factors.[130]

Acutely mechanical forces elicit adaptive responses (to rapidly alter function) chronically; however, the responses may induce tissue remodeling to accommodate load-bearing capabilities.[131] When the mechanical forces exceed unknown thresholds, injury results.[131] Injury can initiate more reparative responses, transient or continuous dysfunction, or progressive degenerative changes that incorporate nearby and surrounding tissue. Cellularly, the structural responses to deformation and strain (e.g., biomechanical) are causing investigators to focus on the cell membrane. Disruption of cell membranes, or mechanoporation, is central to the biologic progression. Mechanical injury can progress to cell death involving both cell necrosis and delayed apoptosis.[131] The heterogeneous distribution of atherosclerosis in the vasculature is possibly related to biomechanical factors; that is, certain arteries (e.g., coronary and carotid arteries) are more susceptible to plaque formation than others.[132] Biomechanical forces probably are not systemic and vary with location. Mechanical stimuli include *shear forces* because of blood flow, **strain** from pressure distention of the vessel walls, and strain from **tethering** to a surrounding tissue area (e.g., the heart).[132]

The major focus of occupational biomechanics is the response of tissue to mechanical stress, especially the prevention of overexertion disorders of the lower back and upper extremities. Many mechanical stresses can cause overt injuries (e.g., a head injury when a worker is struck in the head with a dropped object). Most stresses, however, are subtle and can cause *accumulative* injuries and disorders. Table 2-8 summarizes common types of occupational mechanical stresses and associated types of injury. More realistic mechanical models of living cells will contribute greatly to the study of mechanotransduction in humans.

Noise

Noise is sound that has the potential for inflicting harm to the body. The most common pathophysiologic effect of noise is hearing impairment. Noise trauma can be caused by acute loud noise, as well as by the cumulative effects of various intensities, frequencies, and durations of noise. Common irritating noise is caused by numerous sources, including lawn care machinery; wood and metal working with electrical equipment; gun target practice; hunting; snowmobiles; outboard motors; chain saws; and high-decibel, low-frequency speakers. According to the National Institutes of Health, more than 10 million Americans suffer some permanent noise-associated hearing loss, and

TABLE 2-8 COMMON TYPES OF OCCUPATIONAL MECHANICAL STRESSES AND ASSOCIATED TYPES OF INJURY

MECHANICAL STRESSES	TYPE OF INJURY
Forceful exertions (e.g., lifting, pushing, pulling of heavy loads)	Low back pain
Awkward trunk postures (e.g., flexion, lateral bending, axial twisting, prolonged sitting)	Low back pain
Whole body vibration (e.g., vibrating seat or platform)	Low back pain; bone deformities; alterations in nerve conduction (carpal tunnel syndrome)
Repetitive or prolonged exposure (e.g., to any of the above)	Low back pain; numbness and tingling of wrists and hands
Extreme reaching Low temperatures (e.g., exposure to cold air, tools, materials) Vibration (segmental and whole) Forceful exertions (e.g., friction, balance, posture, pace, use of heavy objects) Ulnar deviation of the wrist	Trauma disorders of upper arms (synovitis, Raynaud phenomenon, bursitis, tendinitis)
Repetitive functions (e.g., walking, climbing stairs, carrying, shoveling, pushing, lifting objects, computer use)	Localized and/or whole body fatigue (shortness of breath, general weakness, hypoxic injury)

20 million are exposed to hazardous noise in work environments.[133] The largest increase in hearing loss from noise occurs in people 45 to 64 years old. Noise pollution is now considered a public health threat. Some evidence exists that noise in hospitals is associated with negative outcomes in patients, both psychologically and physiologically.[134]

Two types of hearing loss are associated with noise: (1) acoustic trauma, or instantaneous damage caused by a single sharply rising wave of sound (e.g., gunfire); and (2) noise-induced hearing loss, the more common type, which is the result of prolonged exposure to intense sound (e.g., noise associated with the workplace and leisure-time activities). Acoustic trauma can rupture the eardrum, displace the ossicles of the middle ear, and damage the organ of Corti in the inner ear.

If the offending noise has not been too loud or the exposure to it too long, hearing will return to its original level, a type of hearing loss called a *temporary threshold shift* (TTS). If the noise is louder than a certain value or the exposure time is long, the hearing threshold never returns to its original value, causing a *permanent threshold shift* (PTS). Structural changes associated with TTS, although not fully established, include intracellular changes in the sensory cells (hair cells) and swelling of the auditory nerve endings. With PTS, cochlear blood flow may be impaired and hair cells are damaged with each exposure. Noise-induced hearing loss is gradual and painless. Symptoms of noise-induced hearing loss include loudness recruitment and tinnitus. In loudness recruitment, soft sounds are not heard but loud sounds are heard normally. Tinnitus is a constant high-pitched ringing that annoys the individual and contributes to loss of sleep. The Occupational Safety and Health Administration (OSHA) requires industries to protect workers when the exposure is over an 8-hour period and averages 85 decibels.

MANIFESTATIONS OF CELLULAR INJURY

Cellular Manifestations: Accumulations

An important manifestation of cell injury is the resultant metabolic disturbances of intracellular accumulation of abnormal amounts of various substances. **Cellular accumulations,** also known as **infiltrations,** occur as a result of not only sublethal injury sustained by cells but also normal (but inefficient) cell function. Two categories of substances can cause accumulations: (1) *a normal cellular substance,* such as water, proteins, lipids, and carbohydrate excesses; or (2) an *abnormal substance,* either endogenous, such as a product of abnormal metabolism or synthesis, or exogenous, for example, infectious agents or a mineral. These products can accumulate transiently or permanently and can be toxic or harmless. Most accumulations are attributed to four types of mechanisms, all abnormal (Figure 2-20). Abnormal accumulations of these substances can occur in the cytoplasm (frequently in the lysosomes) or in the nucleus if (1) the normal, endogenous substance is produced in excess or at an increased rate; (2) an abnormal substance, often the result of a mutated gene, accumulates because of defects in protein folding, transport, or abnormal degradation; (3) an endogenous substance (normal or abnormal) is not effectively catabolized, usually because of lack of a vital lysosomal enzyme; or (4) harmful exogenous materials, such as heavy metals, mineral dusts, or microorganisms, accumulate because of inhalation, ingestion, or infection.

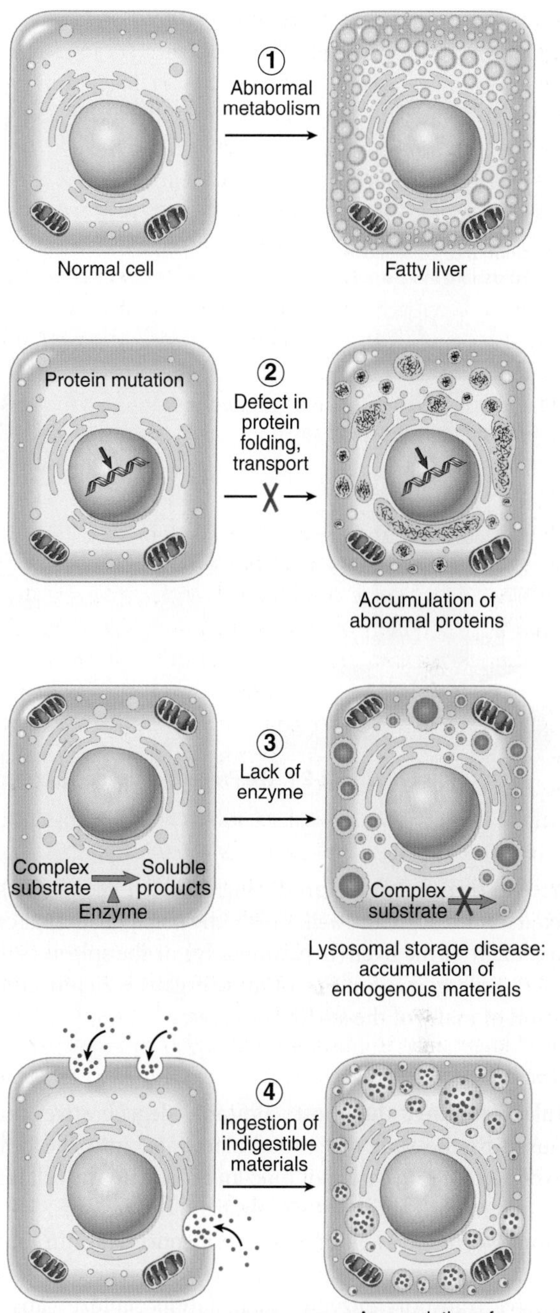

FIGURE 2-20 Mechanisms of Intracellular Accumulations. (From Kumar V et al: Cellular responses to stress and toxic insults: adaptation, injury, and death. In Kumar V et al, editors: *Robbins & Cotran pathologic basis of disease,* ed 8, St Louis, 2010, Saunders.)

In all storage diseases the cells attempt to digest, or catabolize, the "stored" substances. As a result, excessive amounts of metabolites (products of catabolism) accumulate in the cells and are expelled into the extracellular matrix, where they are taken up by phagocytic cells called *macrophages* (see Chapter 7). Some of these scavenger cells circulate throughout the body, whereas others remain fixed in certain tissues, such as the liver or spleen. As more and more macrophages and other phagocytes

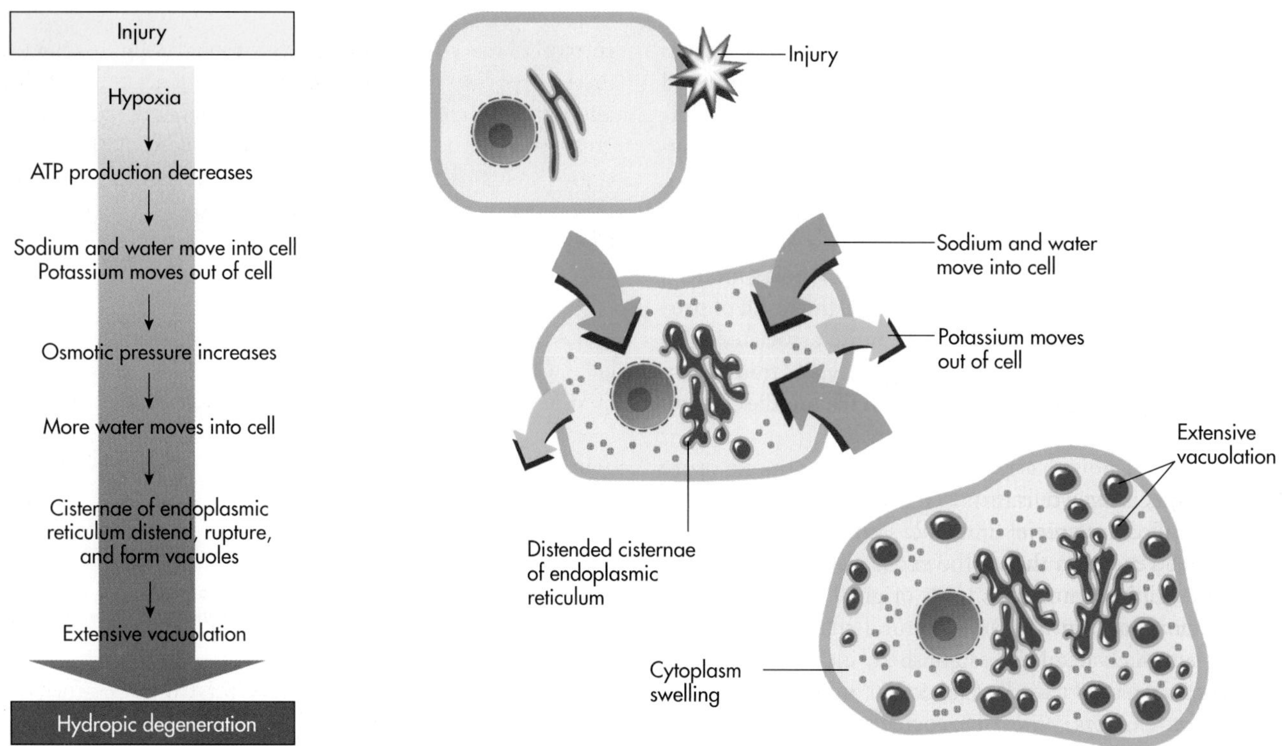

FIGURE 2-21 The Process of Oncosis (Formerly Known as Hydropic Degeneration). *ATP,* Adenosine triphosphate.

migrate to tissues that are producing excessive metabolites, the affected tissues begin to swell. This is the mechanism that causes enlargement of the liver (hepatomegaly) or the spleen (splenomegaly). Enlargement of one of these organs is a clinical manifestation of many of the storage diseases.

Water

Cellular swelling, the most common degenerative change, is caused by the shift of extracellular water into the cells. In hypoxic injury, movement of fluid and ions into the cell is associated with acute failure of metabolism and loss of ATP production. Normally, the pump that transports sodium ions out of the cell is maintained by the presence of ATP and ATPase, the active transport enzyme. In metabolic failure caused by hypoxia, reduced levels of ATP and ATPase permit sodium to accumulate in the cell, whereas potassium diffuses outward. The increase of intracellular sodium concentration increases osmotic pressure, which draws more water into the cell (transport mechanisms are described in Chapter 1). The cisternae of the endoplasmic reticulum become distended, rupture, and coalesce to form large vacuoles that isolate the water from the cytoplasm, a process called *vacuolation.* Progressive vacuolation results in cytoplasmic swelling called **oncosis** (which has replaced the old term *hydropic [water] degeneration*) or **vacuolar degeneration** (Figure 2-21). If cellular swelling affects all cells in an organ, the organ increases in weight and becomes distended and pale.

Cellular swelling is reversible and is considered to be sublethal. It is, in fact, an early manifestation of almost all types of cellular injury, including severe or lethal cell injury. It is also associated with high fever, hypokalemia (abnormally low concentrations of potassium in the blood; see Chapter 3), and certain infections.

Lipids and Carbohydrates

Certain metabolic disorders result in the abnormal intracellular accumulation of carbohydrates and lipids. The accumulations are caused by inherited disorders with insufficient enzymes or ineffective forms of enzymes. Carbohydrate excess disorders are called **mucopolysaccharidoses (MPSs)** and accumulations of both carbohydrates and lipids are called **mucolipidoses (MLs).** MPSs and MLs are classified as **lysosomal storage diseases** because they involve increased storage of carbohydrates or lipids, or both, in lysosomes. Substrate accumulation leads to lysosomal distortion with significant pathologic consequences. These substances may accumulate throughout the body but are found primarily in the cells of the spleen, liver, and central nervous system (CNS). Several of the most prevalent disorders include Tay-Sachs disease, Fabry disease, Gaucher disease, Niemann-Pick disease, the mucopolysaccharidoses, and Pompe disease. Accumulations in cells of the CNS can cause neurologic dysfunction and severe mental retardation. The mucopolysaccharidoses are progressive disorders that usually involve multiple organs, including the liver, spleen, heart, and blood vessels. The accumulated mucopolysaccharides are found in reticuloendothelial cells, endothelial cells, intimal smooth muscle cells, and fibroblasts throughout the body. These carbohydrate accumulations can cause corneal clouding, joint stiffness, and mental retardation.

Although lipids sometimes accumulate in heart and kidney cells, the most common site of intracellular lipid accumulation,

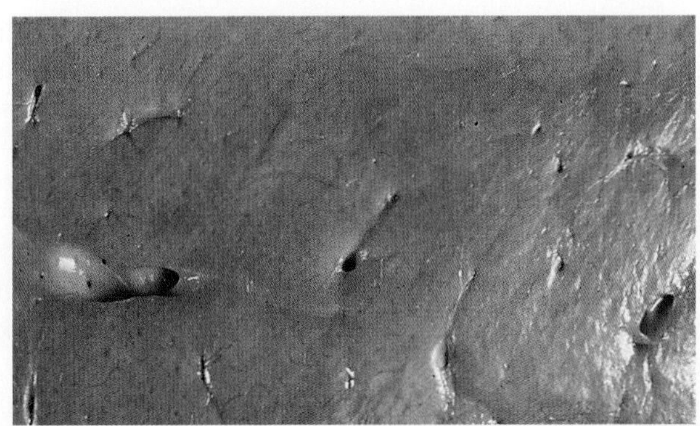

FIGURE 2-22 Fatty Liver. The liver appears yellow. (From Damjanov I, Linder J: *Pathology: a color atlas,* St Louis, 2000, Mosby.)

or **fatty change,** is liver cells. Because hepatic metabolism and secretion of lipids are crucial to proper body function, imbalances and deficiencies in these processes lead to major pathologic changes. Lipid accumulation in liver cells causes an organic condition known as *fatty liver,* or *fatty change* (Figure 2-22). As lipids fill the cells, vacuolation pushes the nucleus and other organelles aside. Grossly, the liver looks yellowish and greasy.

Lipid accumulation in liver cells occurs after cellular injury sets one or more of the following mechanisms in motion:

1. Increased movement of free fatty acids into the liver (starvation, for example, increases breakdown of triglycerides in adipose tissue, releasing fatty acids that subsequently enter liver cells)
2. Failure of the metabolic process that converts fatty acids to phospholipids, resulting in the preferential conversion of the fatty acids to triglycerides
3. Increased synthesis of triglycerides from fatty acids (increases in amounts of the enzyme α-glycerophosphatase, which can accelerate triglyceride synthesis)
4. Decreased synthesis of apoproteins (lipid-acceptor proteins)
5. Failure of lipids to bind with apoproteins and form lipoproteins
6. Failure of mechanisms that transport lipoproteins out of the cell
7. Direct damage to the endoplasmic reticulum by free radicals released by alcohol's toxic effects

Alcohol abuse is one of the most common causes of fatty liver (see Chapter 41). Fatty change caused by alcohol can lead to a form of liver fibrosis called *cirrhosis.* If alcohol intake ceases, the cirrhotic liver can return to a normal size and function. Fatty change from other causes, notably carbon tetrachloride poisoning, is often irreversible.

Cholesterol and cholesterol esters can accumulate and is noted in many pathologic states. These states include atherosclerosis, in which atherosclerotic plaques, smooth muscle cells, and macrophages within the intimal layer of the aorta and large arteries are filled with lipid-rich vacuoles of cholesterol and cholesterol esters. Other states include cholesterol-rich deposits in the gallbladder and Niemann-Pick disease (type C), which involve genetic mutations of an enzyme affecting cholesterol transport.

Glycogen

Intracellular accumulations of glycogen are seen in genetic disorders called *glycogen storage diseases* and in disorders of glucose and glycogen metabolism. Like water and lipid accumulation, glycogen accumulation results in excessive vacuolation of the cytoplasm. The most common cause of glycogen accumulation is diabetes mellitus, a disorder of glucose metabolism (see Chapter 22).

Proteins

Proteins provide cellular structure and constitute most of the cell's dry weight. They are synthesized on ribosomes in the cytoplasm from the essential amino acids lysine, threonine, leucine, isoleucine, methionine, tryptophan, valine, phenylalanine, and histidine. Protein accumulation probably damages cells in two ways. First, metabolites (enzymes) produced when the cell attempts to digest some proteins can damage cellular organelles when released from lysosomes. Second, excessive amounts of protein in the cytoplasm push against cellular organelles, disrupting organelle function and intracellular communication.

Protein excess accumulates primarily in the epithelial cells of the renal convoluted tubule and in the antibody-forming plasma cells (B lymphocytes) of the immune system. Several types of renal disorders cause excessive excretion of protein molecules in the urine (proteinuria). Normally, little or no protein is present in the urine, and its presence in significant amounts indicates cellular injury and altered cellular function in the glomerular membrane.

Accumulations of protein in B lymphocytes can occur during active synthesis of antibodies in the immune response. The excess aggregates of protein are called *Russell bodies.* Russell bodies have been identified in multiple myeloma (plasma cell tumor) (see Chapter 29).

Mutations in protein can slow protein folding, resulting in the accumulation of partially folded intermediates. An example is α_1-antitrypsin deficiency, which can cause emphysema. Certain types of cell injury are associated with the accumulation of cytoskeletal proteins. For example, the *neurofibrillary tangle* found in the brain in Alzheimer disease contains cytoskeletal protein fibrils.

Pigments

Pigment accumulations may be normal or abnormal, endogenous (produced within the body) or exogenous (produced outside the body). Endogenous pigments are derived, for example, from amino acids (e.g., tyrosine, tryptophan). They include melanin and the blood proteins—porphyrins, hemoglobin, and hemosiderin (ferritin). Lipid-rich pigments such as lipofuscin (the aging pigment or spots) give a yellow-brown color to cells undergoing slow, regressive, and often atrophic changes. Exogenous pigments include mineral dusts containing silica and iron particles, lead, silver salts, and dyes for tattoos.

Melanin. **Melanin** accumulates in epithelial cells (keratinocytes) of the skin and retina. It is an extremely important pigment because it protects the skin against long exposure to sunlight and is considered an essential factor in the prevention of skin

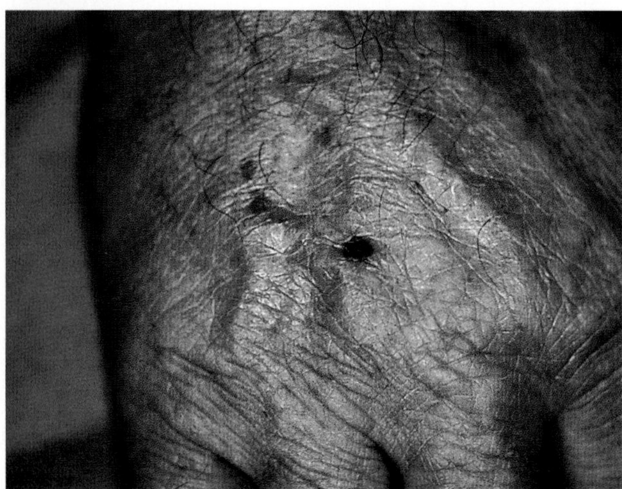

FIGURE 2-23 Blue Nevus, Common Type. Nevus is dark blue-black, small, and symmetric. (From Damjanov I, Linder J: *Anderson's pathology,* ed 10, St Louis, 1996, Mosby.)

cancer (see Chapters 13 and 46). Ultraviolet light (e.g., sunlight) stimulates the synthesis of melanin, which probably absorbs ultraviolet rays during subsequent exposure. Melanin also may protect the skin by trapping the injurious free radicals produced by the action of ultraviolet light on skin.

Melanin is a brown-black pigment derived from the amino acid tyrosine. It is synthesized by epidermal cells called *melanocytes* and is stored in membrane-bound cytoplasmic vesicles called *melanosomes.* Melanosomes are particularly abundant in projections of melanocytic cytoplasm, called *dendrites,* from which they are transmitted to neighboring keratinocytes, where melanin accumulation occurs. (Keratinocytes, which constitute 95% of epidermal cells, are discussed with other skin components in Chapter 46.) The dendritic melanocytes form bridges between neighboring keratinocytes and inject melanosomes into the keratinocytes by an unknown mechanism.

Melanin also can accumulate in melanophores (melanin-containing pigment cells), macrophages, or other phagocytic cells in the dermis. Presumably these cells acquire the melanin from nearby melanocytes or from pigment that has been extruded from dying epidermal cells. This is the mechanism that causes freckles.

Although rare, melanin accumulation occurs in the skin of individuals with Addison disease (adrenocortical insufficiency resulting from disorders of the adrenal cortex; see Chapter 22). The increased melaninogenesis (melanin production) seen in Addison disease is caused by the loss of feedback control of adrenocorticotropic hormone (ACTH). Decreased hormonal secretion from the adrenal gland causes increased release of ACTH from the pituitary gland. In Addison disease the increase in melanin production occurs presumably because a segment of the ACTH molecule contains the melanin-stimulating hormone (MSH).

An increase in melanin concentration also occurs in the benign form of "pigmented moles" called *nevi* (Figure 2-23) (see Chapter 46). Malignant melanoma is a cancerous skin tumor that contains melanin and invades normal tissue early and widely and often leads to death.

A decrease in melanin production occurs in the inherited disorder of melanin metabolism called *albinism.* Albinism is often diffuse, involving all the skin, the eyes, and the hair. Albinism is also related to phenylalanine metabolism. In classic forms of this disease, the person with albinism is unable to convert tyrosine to dopa (3,4-dihydroxyphenylalanine), an intermediary in melanin biosynthesis. Melanin-producing cells are present in normal numbers, but they are unable to make melanin. Individuals with albinism are very sensitive to sunlight and quickly become sunburned. They are also at high risk for skin cancer.

Hemoproteins. **Hemoproteins** are among the most essential of the normal endogenous pigments. They include hemoglobin and the oxidative enzymes—the cytochromes. Knowledge of iron uptake, metabolism, excretion, and storage is central to an understanding of disorders involving these pigments (see Chapter 27). Hemoprotein accumulations in cells are caused by excessive storage of iron, which is transferred to the cells from the bloodstream. Iron enters the blood from three primary sources: (1) tissue stores, (2) the intestinal mucosa, and (3) macrophages that remove and destroy dead or defective red blood cells. The amount of iron in blood plasma also depends on the metabolism of the major iron-transport protein, *transferrin.*

Iron is stored in tissue cells in two forms: as ferritin and, when greater levels of iron are present, as hemosiderin. **Hemosiderin** is a yellow-brown pigment derived from hemoglobin. With pathologic states, excesses of iron cause hemosiderin to accumulate within cells. Accumulation of hemosiderin often occurs in areas of bruising and hemorrhage and in the lungs and spleen after congestion caused by heart failure. With a local hemorrhage, the skin first appears red-blue and then lysis of the escaped red blood cells occurs, causing the hemoglobin to be transformed to hemosiderin. The color changes noted in bruising reflect this transformation.

Hemosiderosis is a condition in which excess iron is stored as hemosiderin in the cells of many organs and tissues. This condition is common in individuals who have received repeated blood transfusions or prolonged parenteral administration of iron. Hemosiderosis is also associated with increased absorption of dietary iron, conditions in which iron storage and transport are impaired, and hemolytic anemia. Excessive alcohol ingestion also can lead to hemosiderosis. Normally, absorption of excessive dietary iron is prevented by an iron absorption process in the intestines. Failure of this process can lead to total-body iron accumulations in the range of 60 to 80 grams (g), compared with normal iron stores of 4.5 to 5 g. Excessive accumulations of iron, such as occur in hemochromatosis (a genetic disorder of iron metabolism and the most severe example of iron overload), are associated with liver and pancreatic cell damage.

Bilirubin is a normal yellow-to-green pigment of bile derived from the porphyrin structure of hemoglobin. Excesses of bilirubin within cells and tissues cause jaundice (icterus), or yellowing of the skin. Jaundice occurs when the bilirubin level exceeds 1.5 to 2 mg/dl of plasma, compared with the normal values of 0.4 to 1 mg/dl. Hyperbilirubinemia occurs with (1) destruction of red blood cells (erythrocytes), such as in hemolytic jaundice; (2) diseases affecting the metabolism and excretion of bilirubin in the liver; and (3) diseases that cause

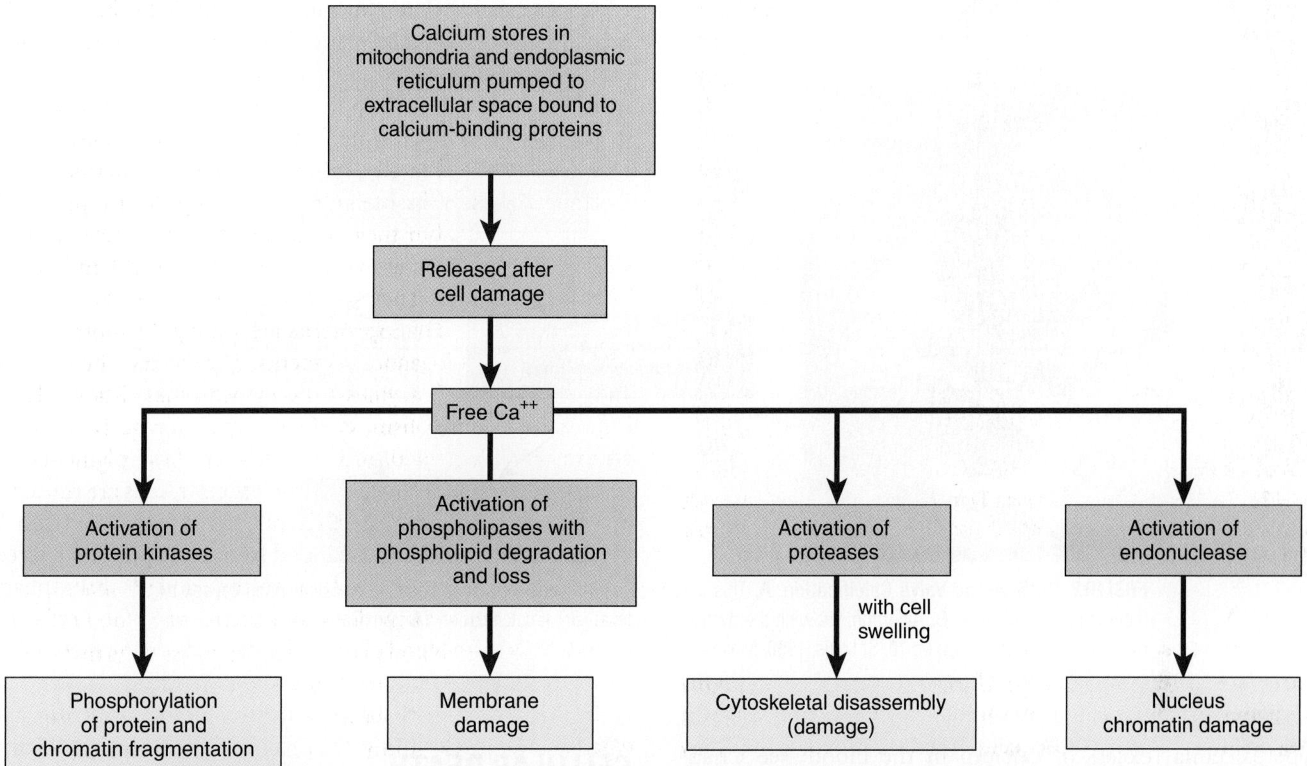

FIGURE 2-24 Free Cytosolic Calcium: A Destructive Agent. Calcium is normally removed from the cytosol by adenosine triphosphate (ATP)–dependent calcium pumps. In normal cells, calcium is bound to buffering proteins, such as calbindin or paralbumin, and is contained in the endoplasmic reticulum and the mitochondria. If there is abnormal permeability of calcium ion channels, direct damage to membranes, or depletion of ATP (i.e., hypoxic injury), calcium level increases in the cytosol. If the free calcium cannot be buffered or pumped out of cells, uncontrolled enzyme activation takes place, causing further damage. Uncontrolled entry of calcium into the cytosol is an important final pathway in many causes of cell death.

obstruction of the common bile duct, such as gallstones or pancreatic tumors. (For a detailed description of these diseases, see Chapter 41.) Certain drugs, specifically chlorpromazine and other phenothiazine derivatives, estrogenic hormones, and halothane (an anesthetic), can cause the obstruction of normal bile flow through the liver.

Because unconjugated bilirubin is lipid soluble, it can injure the lipid components of the plasma membrane. Albumin, a plasma protein, provides significant protection by binding unconjugated bilirubin in plasma. Unconjugated bilirubin causes two cellular effects: uncoupling of oxidative phosphorylation and loss of cellular proteins. These two effects could cause structural injury to the various membranes of the cell.

Calcium

Calcium salts accumulate in both injured and dead tissues (Figure 2-24). An important mechanism of cellular calcification is the influx of extracellular calcium in injured mitochondria (see p. 56). Another mechanism that causes calcium accumulation in alveoli (gas-exchange airways of the lungs), gastric epithelium, and renal tubules is the excretion of acid at these sites, leading to the local production of hydroxyl ions. Hydroxyl ions result in precipitation of calcium hydroxide ($Ca[OH]_2$) and hydroxyapatite ($3Ca_3[PO_4]_2Ca[OH]_2$), a mixed salt. Damage occurs when calcium salts clump and harden, interfering with normal cellular structure and function.

Pathologic calcification can be dystrophic or metastatic. **Dystrophic calcification** is the calcification of dying and dead tissues and occurs in chronic tuberculosis of the lungs and lymph nodes, in arteries with advanced atherosclerosis (narrowing as a result of plaque accumulation), and often in injured heart valves (Figure 2-25). Calcification of the heart valves interferes with opening and closing of the valves, causing heart murmurs (see Chapter 32). Calcification of the coronary arteries predisposes them to severe narrowing and thrombosis, which can lead to myocardial infarction. Another site of dystrophic calcification is the center of tumors. Over time, the center is deprived of oxygen supply, dies, and becomes calcified. The calcium salts appear as gritty, clumped granules that can become hard as stone. When several layers clump together, they resemble grains of sand and are called **psammoma bodies.**

The exact pathogenic mechanisms responsible for dystrophic calcification are unknown. A popular hypothesis is that with progressive deterioration of dead cells, the exposed denatured (changed) proteins preferentially bind with phosphate ions. The phosphate ions then react with calcium ions to form deposits of phosphate carbonate precipitates and, sometimes, crystalline formations of calcium phosphate. Dystrophic calcification develops slowly and is an explicit marker for the site of dead cells.

Metastatic calcification consists of mineral deposits that occur in undamaged normal tissues as the result of

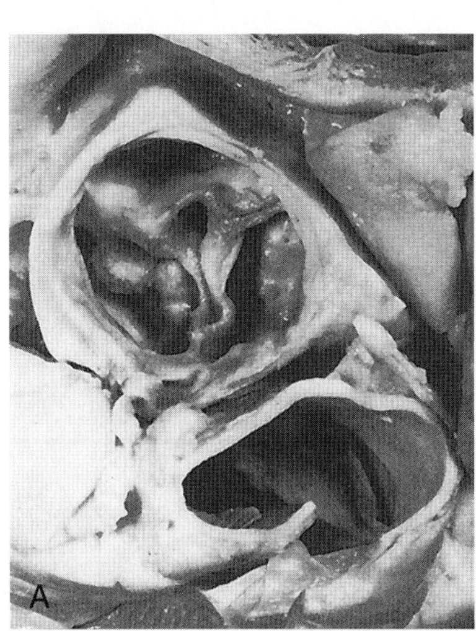

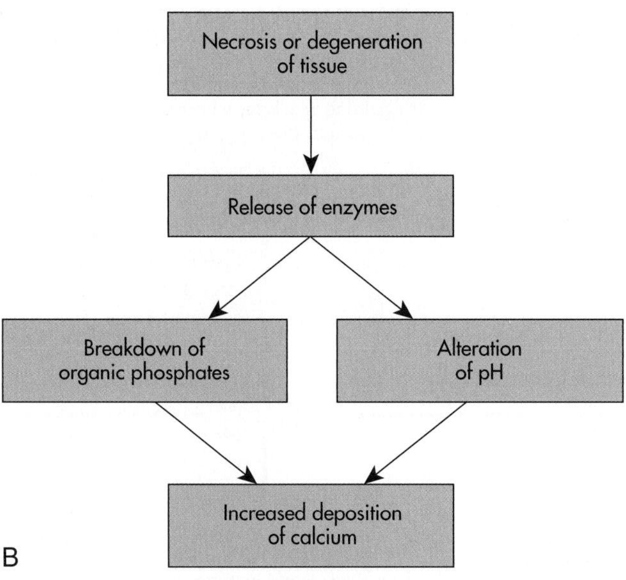

FIGURE 2-25 **Aortic Valve Calcification. A,** This aortic valve was unable to close because of calcification caused by rheumatic heart disease. **B,** Algorithm showing the dystrophic mechanism of calcification. (**A** from Damjanov I, Linder J, editors: *Anderson's pathology,* ed 10, St Louis, 1996, Mosby.)

hypercalcemia (excess of calcium in the blood; see Chapter 3). Conditions that cause hypercalcemia include hyperparathyroidism, toxic levels of vitamin D, hyperthyroidism, idiopathic hypercalcemia of infancy, Addison disease (adrenocortical insufficiency), systemic sarcoidosis, milk-alkali syndrome, and the increased bone demineralization that results from bone tumors, leukemia, and disseminated cancers. Hypercalcemia also can occur in some instances of advanced renal failure with phosphate retention, resulting in hyperparathyroidism.

Urate

In humans, uric acid (**urate**) is the major end product of purine catabolism because of the absence of the enzyme urate oxidase. Serum urate concentration is, in general, stable: approximately 5 mg/dl in postpubertal males and 4.1 mg/dl in postpubertal females. Disturbances in maintaining serum urate levels result in hyperuricemia and deposition of sodium urate crystals in the tissues, leading to painful disorders collectively called *gout.* These disorders include acute arthritis, chronic gouty arthritis, tophus (firm nodular subcutaneous deposits of urate crystals surrounded by fibrosis), and nephritis (inflammation of the nephron). Chronic hyperuricemia results in the deposition of urate in tissues, cell injury, and inflammation. Because urate crystals are not degraded by lysosomal enzymes, they persist in dead cells.

Systemic Manifestations

Systemic manifestations of cellular injury include a general sense of fatigue and malaise, a loss of well-being, and altered appetite. Fever is frequently present because of biochemicals produced during the inflammatory response (see Chapter 7). Table 2-9 summarizes the most significant systemic manifestations of cellular injury.

CELLULAR DEATH

Cell death has historically been classified as necrosis and apoptosis. **Necrosis** is characterized by rapid loss of the plasma membrane structure, organelle swelling, mitochondrial dysfunction, and the lack of typical features of apoptosis.[135] Apoptosis is known as a regulated or programmed cell process characterized by the "dropping off" of cellular fragments called apoptotic bodies. Until recently, only necrosis was considered passive or accidental, occurring after severe and sudden injury. It is the main outcome in several common injuries including ischemia, toxin exposure, certain infections, and trauma. It has now been proposed that under certain conditions, such as activation of death proteases, necrosis may be *regulated* or *programmed* in a well-orchestrated way as a back-up for apoptosis (apoptosis may progress to necrosis).[136,137] Hence, the new term used is **programmed necrosis,** or **necroptosis.** Historically, programmed cell death only referred to apoptosis. Now programmed cell death can be divided into several categories: type I apoptosis; type II autophagy (self-eating); and others include necrosis, senescence, and mitotic catastrophe.[138] Figure 2-26 illustrates the structural changes in cell injury resulting in necrosis or apoptosis. Table 2-10 compares the unique features of necrosis and apoptosis. Other forms of cell loss include autophagy (see p. 92).

Necrosis

Cellular death eventually leads to cellular dissolution, or necrosis. Necrosis is the sum of cellular changes after local cell death and the process of cellular self-digestion, known as autodigestion or **autolysis** (see Figure 2-26). Cells die long before any necrotic changes are noted by light microscopy.[139] The structural signs that indicate irreversible injury and progression

TABLE 2-9 SYSTEMIC MANIFESTATIONS OF CELLULAR INJURY

MANIFESTATION	CAUSE
Fever	Release of endogenous pyrogens (interleukin-1, tumor necrosis factor-alpha [TNF-α], prostaglandins) from bacteria or macrophages; acute inflammatory response
Increased heart rate	Increase in oxidative metabolic processes resulting from fever
Increase in number of leukocytes (leukocytosis)	Increase in total number of white blood cells because of infection; normal is 5000-9000/mm^3 (increase is directly related to the severity of the infection)
Pain	Various mechanisms, such as release of bradykinins, obstruction, pressure
Presence of cellular enzymes in extracellular fluid	Release of enzymes from cells of tissue*
Lactate dehydrogenase (LDH) (LDH isoenzymes)	Release from red blood cells, liver, kidney, skeletal muscle
Creatine kinase (CK) (CK isoenzymes)	Release from skeletal muscle, brain, heart
Aspartate aminotransferase (AST; SGOT)	Release from heart, liver, skeletal muscle, kidney, pancreas
Alanine aminotransferase (ALT; SGPT)	Release from liver, kidney, heart
Alkaline phosphatase (ALP)	Release from liver, bone
Amylase	Release from pancreas
Aldolase	Release from skeletal muscle, heart

*The rapidity of enzyme transfer is a function of the weight of the enzyme and the concentration gradient across the cellular membrane. The specific metabolic and excretory rates of the enzymes determine how long levels of enzymes remain elevated.

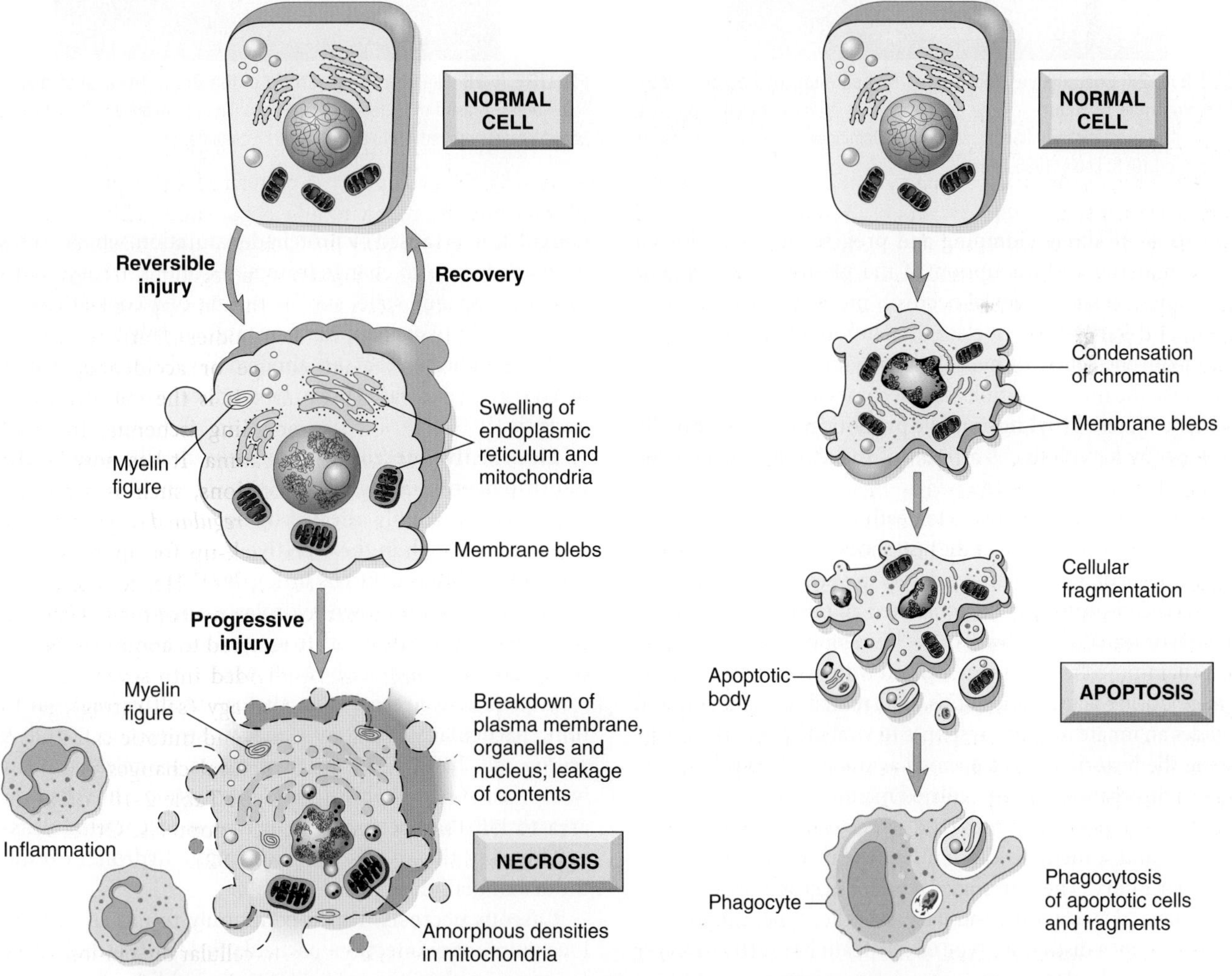

FIGURE 2-26 Schematic Illustration of The Morphologic Changes in Cell Injury Culminating in Necrosis or Apoptosis. Myelin figures come from degenerating cellular membranes and are noted within the cytoplasm or extracellularly. (From Kumar V et al: Cellular responses to stress and toxic insults: adaptation, injury, and death. In Kumar V et al, editors: *Robbins & Cotran pathologic basis of disease,* ed 8, St Louis, 2010, Saunders.)

TABLE 2-10 FEATURES OF NECROSIS AND APOPTOSIS

FEATURE	NECROSIS	APOPTOSIS
Cell size	Enlarged (swelling)	Reduced (shrinkage)
Nucleus	Pyknosis → karyorrhexis → karyolysis	Fragmentation into nucleosome-size fragments
Plasma membrane	Disrupted	Intact; altered structure, especially orientation of lipids
Cellular contents	Enzymatic digestion; may leak out of cell	Intact; may be released in apoptotic bodies
Adjacent inflammation	Frequent	No
Physiologic or pathologic role	Invariably pathologic (culmination of irreversible cell injury)	Often physiologic, means of eliminating unwanted cells; may be pathologic after some forms of cell injury, especially DNA damage

From Kumar V et al: Cellular responses to stress and toxic insults: adaptation, injury, and death. In Kumar V et al, editors: *Robbins & Cotran pathologic basis of disease,* ed 8, St Louis, 2010, Saunders.

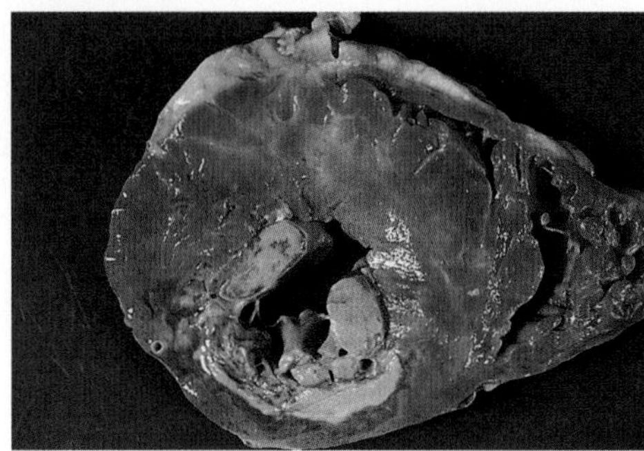

FIGURE 2-27 Coagulative Necrosis of Myocardium of Posterior Wall of Left Ventricle of Heart. A large anemic *(white)* infarct is readily apparent; note also the necrosis of papillary muscle. (From Damjanov I, Linder J: *Anderson's pathology,* ed 10, St Louis, 1996, Mosby.)

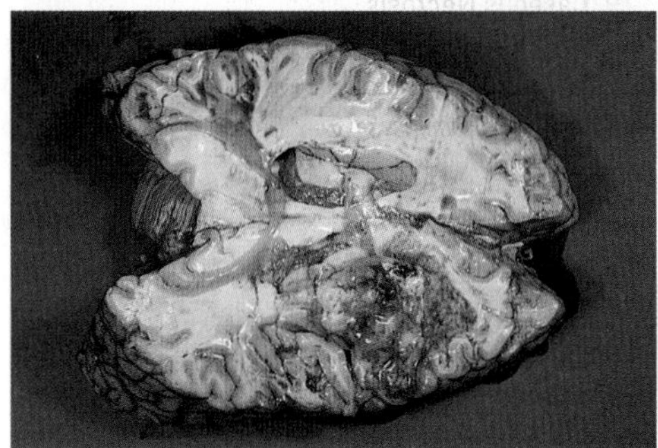

FIGURE 2-28 Liquefactive Necrosis of the Brain. The area of infarction is softened as a result of liquefactive necrosis. (From Damjanov I: *Pathology for the health professions,* ed 4, Philadelphia, 2012, Saunders.)

to necrosis are dense clumping and progressive disruption of genetic material and disruption of the plasma and organelle membranes. In later stages of necrosis, most organelles are disrupted, and **karyolysis** (nuclear dissolution and lysis of chromatin from the action of hydrolytic enzymes) is under way. In some cells, the nucleus shrinks and becomes a small, dense mass of genetic material **(pyknosis).** The pyknotic nucleus eventually dissolves (by karyolysis) as a result of the action of hydrolytic lysosomal enzymes on DNA.

Although necrosis still refers to death induced by nonspecific trauma or injury (cell stress or the heat shock response), the recent identification of molecular regulators governing programmed necrosis (necroptosis) has demonstrated an interconnected large network of signaling pathways.[137,140] Emerging evidence shows that programmed necrosis is associated with development, tissue damage during acute pancreatitis, and retinal detachment; and provides an innate immune response to viral infection, thus challenging the historic view of necrosis as passive cell death occurring in a disorganized or unregulated manner.[137,140]

Different types of necroses tend to occur in different organs or tissues and sometimes can indicate the mechanism or cause of cellular injury. The four major types of necroses are coagulative, liquefactive, caseous, and fatty. Another type, gangrenous necrosis, is *not* a distinctive type of cell death but refers to larger areas of tissue death.

Coagulative necrosis, which occurs primarily in the kidneys, heart, and adrenal glands, commonly results from hypoxia caused by severe ischemia or hypoxia caused by chemical injury, especially ingestion of mercuric chloride (Figure 2-27). Coagulation is caused by protein denaturation, which causes the protein albumin to change from a gelatinous, transparent state to a firm, opaque state, similar to that of a cooked egg white. The necrotic tissues appear firm and slightly swollen. Recent evidence indicates that an abnormality in intracellular levels of Ca^{++} (e.g., increased) may be a critical event in coagulation necrosis.[141]

Liquefactive necrosis commonly results from ischemic injury to neurons and glial cells in the brain (Figure 2-28). Dead brain tissue is readily affected by liquefactive necrosis because brain cells are rich in the digestive hydrolytic enzymes and lipids, and the brain contains little connective tissue. As the cells are digested by their own hydrolases, the tissue becomes soft, liquefies, and is walled off from healthy tissue, forming cysts. (Cyst formation is described in Chapter 7.)

Liquefactive necrosis can also result from bacterial infection, particularly by staphylococci, streptococci, and *Escherichia coli.* In this case the hydrolases are released from the lysosomes of neutrophils (phagocytes attracted to the infected area to kill the bacteria). Liquefaction of bacterial cells and neighboring tissue cells by neutrophilic hydrolases results in the accumulation of pus.

Caseous necrosis, which commonly results from tuberculous pulmonary infection, particularly *Mycobacterium tuberculosis,* is a combination of coagulative and liquefactive necrosis (Figure 2-29). The dead cells disintegrate, but the debris is not digested completely by hydrolases. Tissues appear soft and granular and resemble clumped cheese, hence its name. A granulomatous inflammatory wall encloses areas of caseous necrosis.

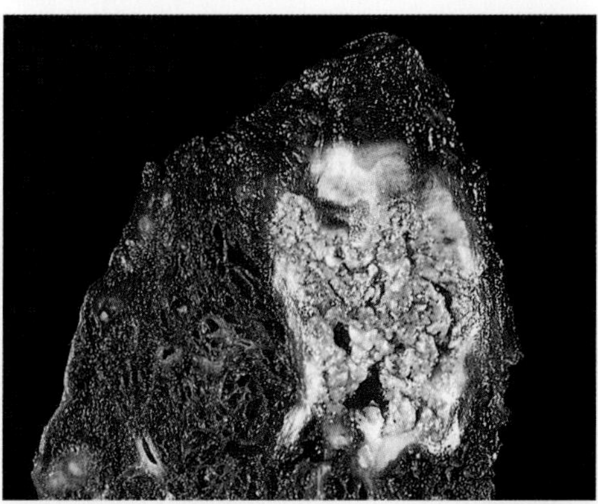

FIGURE 2-29 Caseous Necrosis. Tuberculosis of the lung, with a large area of caseous necrosis containing yellow-white and cheesy debris. (From Kumar V et al: Cellular responses to stress and toxic insults: adaptation, injury, and death. In Kumar V et al, editors: *Robbins & Cotran pathologic basis of disease,* ed 8, St Louis, 2010, Saunders.)

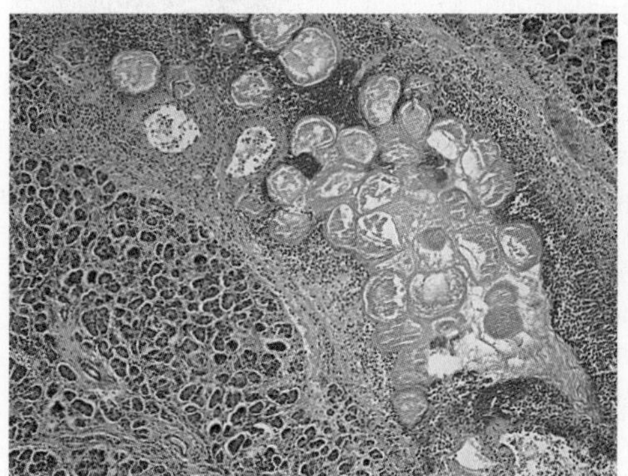

FIGURE 2-30 Fat Necrosis of Pancreas. Interlobular adipocytes are necrotic; these are surrounded by acute inflammatory cells. (From Damjanov I, Linder J: *Anderson's pathology,* ed 10, St Louis, 1996, Mosby.)

Fat necrosis, which occurs in the breast, pancreas, and other abdominal structures, is cellular dissolution caused by powerful enzymes called *lipases* (Figure 2-30). Lipases break down triglycerides, releasing free fatty acids, which then combine with calcium, magnesium, and sodium ions, creating soaps (a process known as *saponification*). The necrotic tissue appears opaque and chalk white.

Gangrenous necrosis, a term commonly used in surgical clinical practice, refers to death of tissue and results from severe hypoxic injury, commonly occurring because of arteriosclerosis, or blockage, of major arteries, especially in the lower leg. With hypoxia and subsequent bacterial invasion, the tissues can undergo necrosis. **Dry gangrene** is usually the result of coagulative necrosis. The skin becomes very dry and shrinks, resulting in wrinkles, and its color changes to dark brown or black (Figure 2-31). **Wet gangrene** develops when neutrophils invade the site, causing liquefactive necrosis. This usually occurs in internal organs, causing the site to become cold, swollen, and black. A foul odor is present, produced by pus, and if systemic symptoms become severe, death can ensue.

Gas gangrene, a special type of gangrene, is caused by infection of injured tissue by one of many species of *Clostridium.*

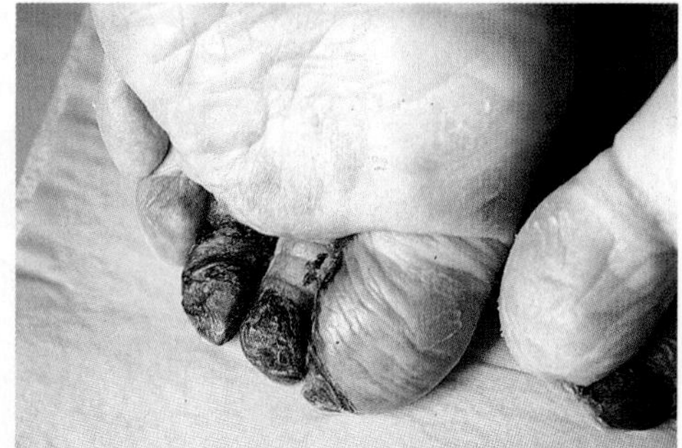

FIGURE 2-31 Gangrene of Toes. Dry gangrene. (From Damjanov I: *Pathology for the health professions,* ed 4, Philadelphia, 2012, Saunders.)

These anaerobic bacteria produce hydrolytic enzymes and toxins that destroy connective tissue and cellular membranes and cause bubbles of gas to form in muscle cells. Gas gangrene can be fatal if enzymes lyse the membranes of red blood cells, destroying their oxygen-carrying capacity. Death is the result of shock. The condition is treated with antitoxins and supplemental oxygen delivered in a hyperbaric (pressurized) chamber.

Apoptosis

Apoptosis ("dropping off") is an important distinct type of cell death that differs from necrosis in several ways (see Figure 2-26 and Table 2-10). Apoptosis is an active process of cellular self-destruction—called *programmed cell death (type I)*—in both normal and pathologic tissue changes. It depends on a tightly regulated cellular program for its initiation and execution.[142] The average adult may create 10 billion new cells every day and destroy the same number.[143] Normal physiologic death by apoptosis occurs during embryogenesis; involution of hormone-dependent tissue after hormone withdrawal, such as involution of the lactating breast after weaning; cell loss in proliferating cell populations, such as immature lymphocytes in the bone marrow or thymus that do not express appropriate receptors; and elimination of possibly harmful lymphocytes that may be self-reactive and cause death of cells after they perform useful functions (for example, neutrophils after an acute inflammatory reaction). Death by apoptosis causes loss of cells in many pathologic states including the following:

- *Severe cell injury.* When cell injury exceeds repair mechanisms, the cell triggers apoptosis. DNA damage can result either directly or indirectly from production of free radicals.
- *Accumulation of misfolded proteins.* This may result from genetic mutations or free radicals. Excessive accumulation of misfolded proteins in the endoplasmic reticulum (ER) leads to a condition known as **endoplasmic reticulum stress (ER stress).** ER stress results in apoptotic cell death. This mechanism has been linked to several degenerative diseases of the CNS and other organs.
- *Infections (particularly viral).* Apoptosis may be the result of the virus directly or indirectly by the host immune response. Cytotoxic T lymphocytes respond to viral infections by inducing apoptosis and, therefore, eliminating the infectious cells. This process can cause tissue damage and it is the same for cell death in tumors and rejection of tissue transplants.

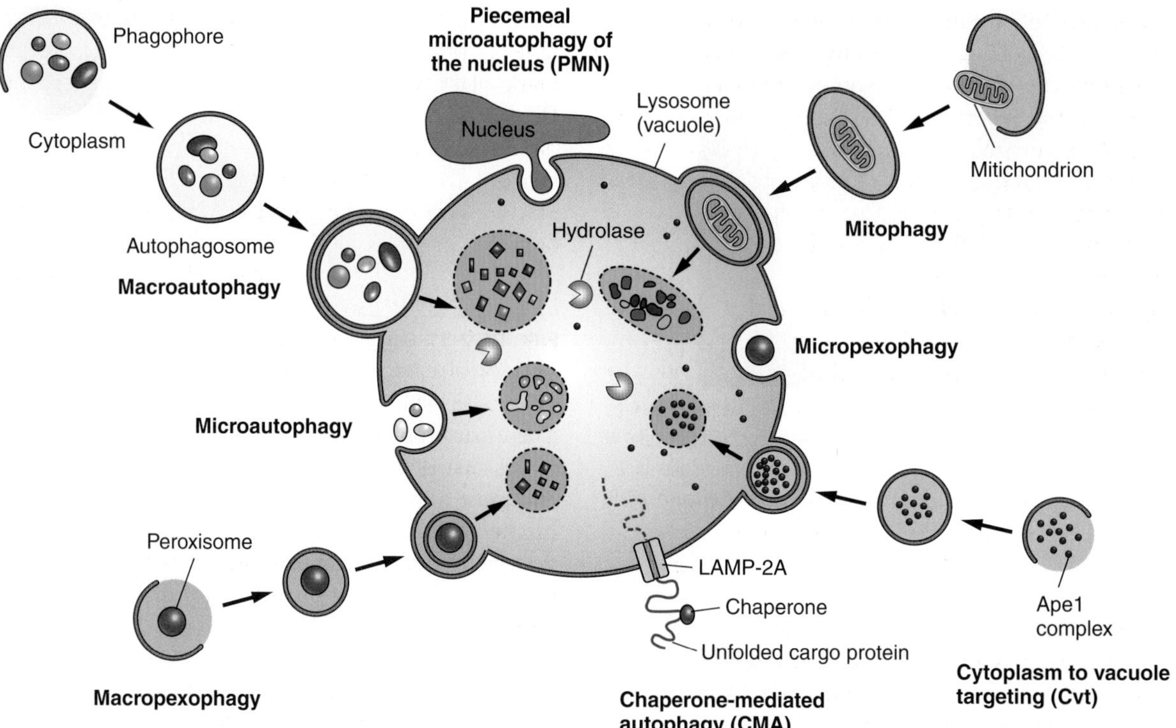

FIGURE 2-32 Autophagy. Three primary modes of autophagy include macrophagy, microphagy, and chaperone-mediated autophagy. Macrophagy is the formation of an autophagosome, a vacuole of nonlysosomal origin; microphagy involves direct uptake of cytosol, inclusions (e.g., glycogen), and organelles (e.g., ribosomes, peroxisomes at the lysosome vacuole); and chaperone-mediated autophagy (CMA) is a translocation process facilitated by certain proteins that are transported across the lysosomal membrane and degraded. Depending on the cargoes, autophagy can be selective or nonselective. During nonselective autophagy, a part of the cytoplasm is confiscated into a double-membrane autophagosome; it then fuses with the lysosome/vacuole. Specific degradation of peroxisomes can be achieved by either macroautophagy (macropexophagy) or microautophagy (micropexophagy). Piecemeal microautophagy of the nucleus causes degradation of a portion of the nucleus. Mitophagy, or degradation of the mitochondria, also occurs. (From Yen WL, Klionsky DJ: *Pathophysiology [Bethesda]* 23(5):248–262, 2008.)

- *Obstruction in tissue ducts.* In organs with duct obstruction, including the pancreas, kidney, and parotid gland, apoptosis causes pathologic atrophy.

Excessive or insufficient apoptosis is known as *dysregulated apoptosis.* A low rate of apoptosis can permit the survival of abnormal cells, for example, mutated cells that can increase cancer risk. Defective apoptosis may not eliminate lymphocytes that react against host tissue (self-antigens) leading to autoimmune disorders. Increased apoptosis is known to occur in several neurodegenerative diseases, ischemic injury (such as myocardial infarction and stroke), and death of virus-infected cells in many viral infections.

Autophagy: Death but Also Survival

The term **autophagy** is Greek, meaning "eating of self" (Figure 2-32). Autophagy, as a "recycling factory," is a self-destructive process and a survival mechanism. It is now considered important in diverse processes such as development, cell proliferation, remodeling, aging, tumor suppression, neurodegeneration, antigen presentation, innate immunity, regulation of organismal life span, and cell death.[144] When cells are starved or nutrient deprived, the autophagic process institutes cannibalization and recycles the digested contents.[145,146] Autophagy can maintain cellular metabolism under starvation conditions and remove damaged organelles and misfolded proteins under stress conditions, improving the survival of cells.

With metabolic stress, autophagy provides ATP and other macromolecules as energy sources to enable cell survival; if, however, the stress is excessive, cells may progress to autophagic programmed cell death, which is distinct from apoptosis.[138,147] Autophagic cell death **(type II programmed cell death)** is characterized by double- or multiple-membrane cytoplasmic vesicles engulfing bulk cytoplasm/cytoplasmic organelles, such as mitochondria and ER. However, in **type I programmed cell death** apoptosis is largely the result of caspase activation and destruction of the cellular components (see p. 91). It should be noted that several studies have failed to show a direct causal link between cell death and autophagy; thus autophagy may not be an executor of cell death but is required with other prodeath signals.[138] Research has shown cells undergoing autophagic cell death were engulfed by macrophages as well as targeted cells.[148]

Autophagy has been highlighted in cancer. It is controversial whether autophagy kills cancer cells or enables their survival under conditions of cell stress (for example, hypoxia). Some reports support that autophagy promotes cancer cell survival after chemotherapy or radiation therapy.[138,149] A causative link between autophagy inhibition and increased tumor formation is the persistent DNA damage induced by ROS associated with dysfunctional mitochondria found in autophagic-deficient tissue.[150] These data and others have led investigators to hypothesize that autophagy probably functions to prevent cancer initially, but once a tumor develops the cancer cells can use autophagy for their own survival. Autophagy and apoptosis may be interconnected and possibly simultaneously regulated by the same trigger in tumor cells.[138]

Investigators are excited about the prospect of autophagy for the development of cancer and other therapeutic strategies. As a critical garbage-collecting and recycling process in healthy cells, the process of autophagy decelerates and may become less discriminating as the cell ages. Consequently, harmful agents accumulate in cells, damaging them and leading to aging. For example, failure to clear protein products in neurons of the CNS causing dementia and failure to clear ROS-producing mitochondria lead to nuclear DNA mutations and cancer. Thus, these processes may even partially define aging. Therefore, normal autophagy may potentially rejuvenate an organism and prevent cancer development as well as other degenerative diseases.[151] Autophagy also may be the last immune defense against infectious microorganisms that penetrate intracellularly.[152]

AGING AND ALTERED CELLULAR AND TISSUE BIOLOGY

The terms aging and life span tend to be used synonymously; however, they are not equivalent. *Aging* is usually defined as a normal physiologic process that is universal and inevitable, whereas *life span* is the time from birth to death and has been used to study the aging process.[153] Aging is associated with a gradual loss of homeostatic mechanisms whose underlying cause is perplexing,[154] and is a complex process because of a multiplicity of factors. Investigators are focused on genetic, epigenetic, inflammatory, oxidative stress, and metabolic origins of aging, including the study of genetic signatures in humans with exceptional longevity; the identification and recent discovery of epigenetic mechanisms that modulate gene expression; the role of intrauterine environment and lifelong patterns of health; personality, behavior, and social support; insulin/insulin-like growth factor 1 (IGF-1) signaling; and the contributions of cellular dysfunction and senescence to an inflammatory microenvironment that leads to chronic disease, frailty, and decreased life span. A major challenge of aging research has been to separate the causes of cell and tissue aging from the vast changes that accompany it.[154] Public health issues related to healthy aging require understanding of the nature of aging and the factors that predict healthy aging and delayed transition to increasing vulnerability and frailty.

Aging traditionally has not been considered a disease because it is "normal"; disease is usually considered "abnormal." Conceptually, this distinction seems clear until the concept of "injury" or "damage" is introduced; disease has been defined by some pathologists as the result of injury. *Chronologic aging* has been defined as the time-dependent loss of structure and function that proceeds very slowly and in such small increments that it appears to be the result of the accumulation of small, imperceptible injuries—a gradual result of wear and tear. One of the hallmarks of aging is the accumulation of damaged macromolecules. DNA damage can lead to cellular dysfunction both directly and indirectly as a consequence of cellular responses to damage that can lead to altered gene expression.[155,156] Age-related changes to macromolecules for long-lived cells, such as neurons and myofibers, lead to gradual loss of structure and function.

Replicative aging is the accumulation of cellular damage in continuously dividing cells, for example, epithelia of the skin or gastrointestinal tract. Replicative aging and chronologic aging are particularly important for adult stem cells because they divide throughout life.[157] As mutations increase with age, cell fates include apoptosis, malignant transformation, cell cycle arrest, or senescence.[158]

Despite the fact that aging and death are inevitable, life span, on the other hand, can be experimentally changed.[154] Genetic and environmental interventions have extended the life span of model organisms, such as the nematode worm *Caenorhabditis elegans (C. elegans),* the fruit fly *Drosophilia melanogaster,* and mice.[159,160] Extending life span, however, is not equivalent to delaying aging![154] For example, treatment of an acute infection can prevent death but the fundamental *rate* of aging continues. Yet, investigators will study and try to isolate, manipulate, and reset so-called longevity genes to slow the rate of aging.

Recent advances in stem cell biology have begun to reveal the molecular mechanisms behind reprogramming events that occur during fertilization and when the nucleus of a mature somatic cell is transferred to an enucleated oocyte. Called somatic cell nuclear transfer (SCNT), this process gave rise to the first cloned mammal, Dolly the sheep, and led to the explosion of research in cloning.[154] SCNT is important in terms of demonstrating the ability of the oocyte cytoplasm to reprogram the donor nucleus. These reprogramming events have led to the process to create induced pluripotent stem cells (iPSCs).[161] The major emphasis of reprogramming research is the reversal of the differentiated program and attainment of a pluripotent state (differentiated cells in all three germ layers of the embryo) and not the reversal of aging.[154,162] Nevertheless, each of these processes is discussed in the context of resetting the aging clock.

Restoration of youthfulness to aged cells and tissues has created so-called rejuvenating interventions. Experiments to test whether cells and tissues from an old animal can be restored to a younger self include the approach called heterochronic (i.e., young-to-old or old-to-young) transplantations and heterochronic parabiosis, when the systemic circulations of two animals are joined. The systemic environment may become more youthful with restoration of protein components in the blood and tissues, especially chemokines and cytokines.[163]

Pharmacologic interventions may restore youthfulness at cellular and biochemical levels. The enzyme mammalian target of rapamycin (mTOR) senses cellular nutrient levels, thus regulating rates of protein synthesis and energy utilization.[154] Administration of the drug rapamycin, an mTOR inhibitor, can extend the life span of mice.[164] These and future studies may not just change differentiation programs of cells and tissue, but possibly alter the aging clock. Although the accumulation of nuclear and mitochondrial DNA mutations has been correlated with aging and increasing the burden of mitochondrial DNA mutations can shorten life span, there is no direct evidence—yet—that a reduction in DNA mutations will increase life span. Observations in *C. elegans* suggest strongly that the causes of aging may be largely epigenetic.[154,165]

Normal Life Span and Life Expectancy

The **maximal life span** of humans is between 80 and 100 years and does not vary significantly among populations. In primitive societies, few individuals reach the maximal life span. However, in societies with improved sanitation, housing, nutrition, and health care, many individuals attain the maximal life span. **Life expectancy** is the average number of years of life remaining at a given age. Although a slow but steady rise in life expectancy has occurred generally in the United States, disparities exist among various counties. A surprising government-sponsored study by Harvard researchers found life expectancy actually *declined* in a number of counties (e.g., smallest unit of analysis) from 1983 to 1999 (see What's New? Decline in Life Expectancy in Some U.S. Counties).

Life Expectancy Differences Across America

Although maximal life span has not changed significantly over time, improved public health strategies and health advances in the United States during the last century added about 30 years to life expectancy between 1900 and 2000. This increase in life expectancy has not affected all Americans. In each successive age group from 65 years and older, women outnumber men; thus women have a greater life expectancy than men. Increases in life expectancy have resulted in a larger older adult population and, for some, inherent problems of disability, disease, and socioeconomic hardship.

Longevity in the United States has recently been the subject of several reports.[166-168] Although U.S. spending on health care far exceeds that of other developed countries, life expectancy and key measures of health lag behind other high-income countries[169] (Table 2-11).

In the United States, chronic health conditions associated with modifiable risk factors, such as smoking, nutrition, weight, and physical activity, represent 6 of the 10 costliest medical conditions.[170] These preventable conditions lead to diseases and injuries and cause soaring medical and labor costs that saddle U.S. employers and bankrupt families. All of these conditions are highly amendable to population-based preventive strategies, which have been slow to develop; 20% of adults still smoke and 50% of adults and 20% of children are overweight or obese.[171] It is estimated that one third of American adults will develop diabetes by 2050 (up from one tenth today).[172] The current generation of children and young adults in the United States could

WHAT'S NEW?

Decline in Life Expectancy in Some U.S. Counties

Continuing rise in life expectancy for *all* Americans is not happening. Long-term analysis of county trends has revealed startling data.

Between 1961 and 1999, the *average* life expectancy in the United States increased from 73.5 to 79.6 years for women and from 66.9 to 74.1 years for men. However, the differences in mortality by county between the most disadvantaged populations and those with the most advantages began to *widen* in the early 1980s. Life expectancy between 1961 and 1999 in the male advantaged population (best-off group) rose from 70.5 to 78.7 years and from 76.9 to 83 years for females. In the female disadvantaged populations (worst-off group) starting in the early 1980s, life expectancy remained relatively stable (68.7 years in 1961, 74.5 years in 1983, and only 75.5 years in 1999). The worst-off men had a decline, rising again in the 1990s.

The gains made, particularly for cardiovascular disease, began to plateau in the 1980s because of rising mortality from lung cancer, chronic obstructive pulmonary disease, and diabetes. A major contributor, which peaked later for women than for men, is smoking. Smoking is thought to be a significant contributor for women, as well as overweight, obesity, and hypertension. The worst-off counties also showed a rise in the prevalence of HIV/AIDS and homicide in men.

Statistically significant declines for women occurred in 180 of 3141 counties and in 11 counties for men. In addition, 783 counties showed life expectancy declines for women whereas 48 counties showed declines for men, but this was not statistically significant. Life expectancy was worse in all southwestern Virginia counties, with a drop over the 16-year period of about 6 years in women and 2.5 years in men. The greatest improvements occurred in western desert counties, where life expectancy rose almost 5 years for women and about 7 years for men.

The life expectancy "gap" is *increasing* between rich and poor and between high and low educational attainment. This increase is occurring despite the gap between men and women and between blacks and whites. In addition, other indices include geography and community assets.

The analysis of county data demonstrates that the 1980s and 1990s were the beginning of the era of increased inequalities in mortality in the United States. Dividing the United States into "eight Americas," it is now evident that disparities in mortality affect millions of Americans. The gap is enormous. The "eight Americas" analysis revealed the highest levels of life expectancy on record, which were for U.S.-born Asian females (America 1), 3 years higher than that of females in Japan. The next highest group was low-income, white rural populations in Minnesota, the Dakotas, Iowa, Montana, and Nebraska (America 2), with a life expectancy of 76.2 years for males and 81.8 years for females. Blacks living in high-risk urban areas (America 8) had the lowest life expectancy, with almost 4 times as many of these individuals likely to die before age 60 and 3.8 and 4.7 times (females and males, respectively) more likely to die before age 45 (compared to the America 1 [Asian] group)! The excess young and middle-aged deaths in America 8 were observed to be caused by injuries, cardiovascular disease, liver cirrhosis, diabetes, HIV, and homicide.

In summary, large disparities in life expectancy exist across America because of differences in the prevalence of chronic diseases and injuries with known risk factors, including alcohol use, tobacco smoking, overweight and obesity, elevated blood pressure, elevated cholesterol level, and poor glucose control.

Data from Ezzati M et al: *PLoS Med* 5(4):e66, doi: 10.1371/journal.pmed.0050066; Murray CJL et al: *PLoS Med* 3(9):e260, doi:10.1371/journal.pmed.0030260.

AIDS, Acquired immunodeficiency syndrome; *HIV,* human immunodeficiency virus.

TABLE 2-11 U.S. HEALTH RANKINGS FOR LIFE EXPECTANCY, INFANT MORTALITY, AND MATERNAL MORTALITY

	U.S. RANKING (U.S./TOTAL OTHER COUNTRIES)		
SOURCE	**LIFE EXPECTANCY**	**INFANT MORTALITY**	**MATERNAL MORTALITY**
UN	28/146 (2005-2010 data)	32/146 (2005-2010 data)	n/a
OECD	26/34	30/34 (2008 data)	25/34 (2007 data)
CIA	50/221 (2011 estimated data; in 2010 data, US ranked 49th)	47/222 (2011 estimated data)	52/176 (2011 estimated data)

Data from Central Intelligence Agency: *World factbook,* Washington, DC, 2011, Author; National Research Council: *Explaining divergent levels of longevity in high-income countries,* Washington, DC, 2011, National Academies Press; Organization for Economic Cooperation and Development: *Doing better for children,* Paris, France, 2009, OECD Publishing.
n/a, Not available.

become the first generation to have shorter life spans, multiple medical conditions, and fewer healthy years of life than those of their parents.[173]

Aging: Degenerative Extracellular Changes

Extracellular factors that affect the aging process include the binding of collagen; the increase in free radicals' effects on cells; the structural alterations of fascia, tendons, ligaments, bones, and joints; and the development of peripheral vascular disease, particularly arteriosclerosis (see Chapter 32).

Aging affects the extracellular matrix with increased cross-linking, decreased synthesis and increased degradation of collagen. These changes, together with the disappearance of elastin and changes in proteoglycans and plasma proteins, cause disorders that result in dehydration and wrinkling of the skin (see Chapter 46). Other age-related defects in the extracellular matrix include skeletal muscle alterations (e.g., atrophy, decreased tone, loss of contractility), cataracts, diverticula, hernias, and rupture of intervertebral disks.

Free radicals of oxygen (see p. 59) that result from oxidative stress (e.g., respiratory chain, phagocytosis, prostaglandin synthesis) are known to damage tissues during the aging process. These oxygen products are extremely reactive and can damage nucleic acids, destroy polysaccharides, oxidize proteins, peroxidize unsaturated fatty acids, and kill and lyse cells. Oxidant effects on target cells can lead to malignant transformation, presumably through DNA damage. That progressive and cumulative damage from oxygen radicals may lead to harmful alterations in cellular function is consistent with those alterations of aging. This hypothesis is founded on the wear-and-tear theory of aging, which states that damages accumulate with time, decreasing the organism's ability to maintain a steady state. Because these oxygen-reactive species not only can permanently damage cells but also may lead to cell death, there is new support for their role in the aging process.

Of much interest is the relationship between aging and the disappearance or alteration of extracellular substances important for blood vessel integrity. Advancing age is an important risk factor for the development of cardiovascular diseases. Vascular oxidative stress increases with age without a compensatory

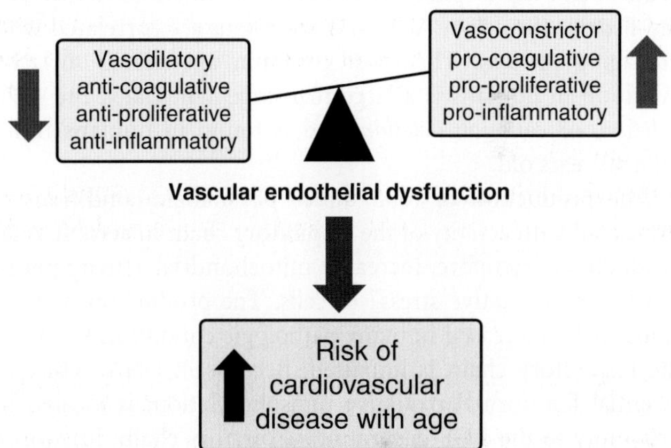

FIGURE 2-33 Vascular Endothelial Function and Increased Risk of Cardiovascular Diseases. Endothelial dysfunction is characterized by a shift from a vasodilatory, anti-coagulative, anti-proliferative, and anti-inflammatory state to a pro-proliferative and pro-inflammatory state, leading to an increased risk of cardiovascular disease with aging. (Adapted from Seals DR, Jablonski KL, Donato AJ: *Clin Sci* 120:357–375, 2011.)

increase in antioxidant defenses.[174] Vascular endothelial dysfunction is characterized by a shift from a vasodilatory, anti-coagulative, anti-proliferative, and anti-inflammatory state to a pro-inflammatory, pro-proliferative, and pro-coagulative state with consequent increased risk for cardiovascular events and diseases (Figure 2-33).

Oxidative stress plays an important role in initial atherosclerotic lesion formation: its progression and destabilization.[175] With aging, lipid, calcium, and plasma proteins are deposited in vessel walls. These depositions cause basement membrane thickening and alterations in smooth muscle functioning, resulting in arteriosclerosis (a progressive disease that causes serious problems in the aged, including stroke, myocardial infarction, renal disease, and peripheral vascular disease).

Cellular Aging

Cellular changes characteristic of aging include atrophy, decreased function, and loss of cells, possibly by apoptosis.

Loss of cellular function from any of these causes initiates the compensatory mechanisms of hypertrophy and hyperplasia of remaining cells, which can lead to metaplasia, dysplasia, and neoplasia. All these changes can alter receptor placement and function, nutrient pathways, secretion of cellular products, and neuroendocrine control mechanisms. In the aged cell, DNA, RNA, cellular proteins, and membranes are most susceptible to injurious stimuli. DNA is particularly vulnerable to such injuries as breaks, deletions, and additions. Although it can repair itself with time, the aged cell's capacity for DNA repair is decreased. Lack of DNA repair increases the cell's susceptibility to mutations that may be lethal or may promote the development of neoplasia.

Mitochondria are the organelles responsible for the generation of most of the energy used by eukaryotic cells. Mitochondrial DNA (mtDNA) encodes some of the proteins of the electron transfer chain, the system necessary for the conversion of adenosine diphosphate (ADP) to ATP. Mutations in mtDNA can deprive the cell of ATP, and mutations are correlated with the aging process. The most common age-related mtDNA mutation in humans is a large rearrangement called the *4977 deletion,* or *common deletion,* and is found in humans more than 40 years old.

The production of ROS under physiologic conditions is associated with activity of the respiratory chain in aerobic ATP production. Therefore, increased mitochondrial activity per se can be an "oxidative stress" to cells. The production of ROS is markedly increased in many pathologic conditions in which the respiratory chain is impaired. Because mtDNA, which is essential for normal oxidative phosphorylation, is located in proximity to the ROS-generating respiratory chain, it is more oxidatively damaged than is nuclear DNA. Cumulative damage of mtDNA is implicated in the aging process as well as in the progression of such common diseases as diabetes, cancer, and heart failure.

Tissue and Systemic Aging

It is probably safe to say that every physiologic process can be shown to function less efficiently with increasing age. The most characteristic tissue change with age is a progressive stiffness or rigidity that affects many systems, including the arterial, pulmonary, and musculoskeletal systems. A consequence of blood vessel and organ stiffness is a progressive increase in peripheral resistance to blood flow. The movement of intracellular and extracellular substances also usually decreases with age as does the diffusion capacity of the lung. Blood flow through organs decreases; for example, renal plasma flow decreases.

Changes in the endocrine and immune systems include thymus atrophy. Although this occurs at puberty, it causes a decreased immune response to T-dependent antigens (foreign proteins), increased formation of autoantibodies and immune complexes (antibodies bound to antigen), and an overall decrease in the immunologic tolerance for the host's own cells, which further diminishes the effectiveness of the immune system later in life. The reproductive system loses ova in women, and spermatogenesis in men is decreased. Responsiveness to hormones decreases in the breast and endometrium.

The stomach experiences decreases in the rate of emptying and secretion of hormones and hydrochloric acid. Muscular atrophy diminishes mobility by decreasing motor tone and contractility. **Sarcopenia,** the loss of muscle mass and strength, can occur into old age. The skin of the aged individual is affected by atrophy and wrinkling of the epidermis and by alterations in underlying dermis, fat, and muscle.

Total body changes include a decrease in height; a reduction in circumference of the neck, thighs, and arms; widening of the pelvis; and lengthening of the nose and ears. Several of these changes are the result of tissue atrophy and decreased bone mass caused by osteoporosis and osteoarthritis. Some body composition changes include an increase in body weight, which begins in middle age (men gain until 50 years of age and women until 70 years), and an increase in fat mass followed by a decrease in stature, weight, **fat-free mass (FFM),** and body cell mass at older ages. FFM includes all minerals, proteins, and water plus all other constituents except lipids. As the amount of fat increases, the percentage of total body water decreases. Increased body fat and centralized fat distribution (abdominal) are associated with non–insulin-dependent diabetes and heart disease. Total body potassium concentration also decreases because of decreased cellular mass. An increased sodium/potassium ratio suggests that the decreased cellular mass is accompanied by an increased extracellular compartment.

Although some of these alterations are probably inherent in aging, others represent consequences of aging. Advanced age increases susceptibility to disease, and death occurs after an injury or insult because of diminished cellular, tissue, and organic function. To determine that an individual "died of old age" would be a monumental if not impossible task.

Frailty

Frailty is a common clinical syndrome in older adults, leaving a person vulnerable to falls, functional decline, disability, disease, and death. Recently, investigators hypothesized that the clinical manifestations of frailty include a cycle of negative energy balance, sarcopenia, and diminished strength and tolerance for exertion.[176,177] For research and clinical purposes, the criteria indicating compromised energetics include low grip strength, slowed walking speed, low physical activity, and unintentional weight loss.[177] The syndrome is complex, involving oxidative stress, dysregulation of inflammatory cytokines and hormones, malnutrition, physical inactivity, and muscle apoptosis (see review).[177] Additionally, the clinical condition of frailty includes decreased lean body mass (sarcopenia), osteopenia, cognitive impairment, and anemia.[178] Several physiologic gender differences may explain differing levels of frailty: (1) higher baseline levels of muscle mass for men may be protective against frailty, (2) testosterone and growth hormone can provide advantages in muscle mass maintenance, (3) cortisol is more dysregulated in older women than older men, (4) alterations in immune function and immune responsiveness to sex steroids make men more vulnerable to sepsis and infection and women vulnerable to chronic inflammatory conditions and muscle mass loss, and (5) lower levels of activity and caloric intake may influence greater susceptibility to frailty in women.

SOMATIC DEATH

Somatic death is death of the entire person. Unlike the changes that follow cellular death in a live body, **postmortem change** is diffuse and does not involve components of the inflammatory response. Within minutes of death, manifestations of postmortem change appear, eliminating any difficulty in determining that death has occurred. The most notable manifestations are complete cessation of respiration and circulation. The surface of the skin usually becomes pale and yellowish; however, the lifelike color of the cheeks and lips may persist after death from causes such as carbon monoxide poisoning, drowning, and chloroform poisoning.

Body temperature falls gradually immediately after death and then more rapidly (approximately 1.0° to 1.5° F/hr) until, after 24 hours, body temperature equals that of the environment. After death caused by certain infective diseases, body temperature may continue to rise for a short time. Postmortem reduction of body temperature is called **algor mortis.**

Blood pressure within the retinal vessels decreases, causing muscle tension to decrease and the pupils to become dilated. The face, nose, and chin begin to look "sharp" or "peaked" as blood and fluids drain from these areas. Gravity causes blood to settle in the most dependent, or lowest, tissues, which develop a purple discoloration called **livor mortis.** Incisions at this time usually fail to cause bleeding. The skin loses its elasticity and transparency.

Within 6 hours after death, acidic compounds accumulate within the muscles because of the breakdown of carbohydrate and the depletion of ATP. This interferes with ATP-dependent detachment of myosin from actin (contractile proteins), and muscle stiffening, or **rigor mortis,** develops. The smaller muscles are usually affected first, particularly the muscles of the jaw. Within 12 to 14 hours, rigor mortis usually affects the entire body. Rigor mortis gradually diminishes and the body becomes flaccid in 12 to 14 hours.

Signs of putrefaction—state of decay with foul-smelling odor—are generally obvious about 24 to 48 hours after death. Putrefactive changes vary depending on the temperature of the environment. The most visible is greenish discoloration of the skin, particularly on the abdomen. The discoloration is thought to be related to the diffusion of hemolyzed blood into the tissues and the production of sulfhemoglobin. Slippage or loosening of the skin from underlying tissues occurs at the same time. After this, swelling or bloating of the body and liquefactive changes occur, sometimes causing opening of the body cavities. At a microscopic level, putrefactive changes are associated with the release of enzymes and lytic dissolution called **postmortem autolysis.**

SUMMARY REVIEW

Cellular Adaptation

1. Injury to cells and their surrounding environment, called the extracellular matrix, leads to tissue and organ injury. Cellular adaptation is an alteration that enables the cell to maintain a steady state despite adverse conditions.
2. Atrophy is a decrease in cellular size. The mechanisms probably include decreased protein synthesis, increased protein catabolism, or both.
3. Physiologic atrophy occurs with early development; for example, the thymus gland involutes and atrophies. Pathologic atrophy occurs as a result of decreases in workload, use, pressure, blood supply, nutrition, hormonal stimulation, and nervous stimulation.
4. Aging causes brain cells and endocrine-dependent organs, such as the gonads, to become atrophic.
5. Hypertrophy is an increase in the size of cells caused by increased work demands or hormonal stimulation. Hypertrophy can be physiologic or pathologic. Amounts of protein in the plasma membrane, endoplasmic reticulum, microfilaments, and mitochondria are increased.
6. Hyperplasia is an increase in the number of cells caused by an increased rate of cellular division. Compensatory hyperplasia enables certain organs to regenerate. Hormonal hyperplasia is stimulated by hormones to replace lost tissue or support new growth, such as during pregnancy.
7. Pathologic hyperplasia is the abnormal proliferation of normal cells in response to excessive hormonal stimulation of growth factors on target cells.
8. Dysplasia, or atypical hyperplasia, is an abnormal change in the size, shape, and organization of mature tissue cells.
9. Metaplasia is the reversible replacement of one mature cell type by another less mature cell type. Metaplasia is thought to develop from a reprogramming of stem cells existing in most epithelia or of undifferentiated mesenchymal cells in connective tissue.

Cellular Injury

1. Injury to cells and to the extracellular matrix (ECM) leads to injury of tissues and organs, ultimately determining the structural patterns of disease. Injured cells may recover (reversible injury) or die (irreversible injury).
2. Cellular injury is caused by a lack of oxygen (hypoxia), free radicals, caustic or toxic chemicals, infectious agents, unintentional and intentional injury, inflammatory and immune responses, genetic factors, insufficient nutrients, or physical trauma from many causes. Injurious stimuli cause cell stress.
3. Cell injury can be acute or chronic, and it can be reversible or irreversible. It can involve necrosis, apoptosis, autophagy, accumulation, or pathologic calcification.
4. Four biochemical themes are important to cell injury: (a) depletion of ATP, (b) decreased levels of oxygen and increased levels of oxygen-derived free radicals, (c) increased concentration of intracellular calcium and loss of calcium steady state, and (d) defects in membrane permeability.

SUMMARY REVIEW—cont'd

5. The sequence of events leading to cell death is commonly decreased ATP production, failure of active transport mechanisms (the Na^+-K^+ pump), cellular swelling, detachment of ribosomes from the endoplasmic reticulum, cessation of protein synthesis, mitochondrial swelling as a result of calcium accumulation, vacuolation, leakage of digestive enzymes from lysosomes, autodigestion of intracellular structures, lysis of the plasma membrane, and death.
6. The initial insult in hypoxic injury is usually ischemia—the cessation of blood flow into vessels that supply the cell with oxygen and nutrients.
7. An important mechanism of membrane damage is injury caused by free radicals, including oxidative stress. Free radicals are difficult to control and initiate chain reactions.
8. Free radicals can cause (a) lipid peroxidation or the destruction of unsaturated fatty acids, (b) alterations of proteins, and (c) alterations in DNA.
9. The initial insult in chemical injury is damage or destruction of the plasma membrane. Examples of chemical agents that cause cellular injury include lead, carbon monoxide, ethanol, mercury, and social or street drugs. The leading cause of child poisoning is medications.
10. Unintentional and intentional injuries are an important health problem in the United States. Death caused by injuries is more common in men than women and more prevalent among blacks vs. whites and other racial groups.
11. Injuries by blunt force are the result of the application of mechanical energy to the body resulting in tearing, shearing, or crushing of tissues. The most common types of blunt-force injuries include motor vehicle accidents and falls.
12. Asphyxial injuries are caused by a failure of cells to receive or use oxygen. These injuries can be grouped into four general categories: suffocation, strangulation, chemical asphyxiants, and drowning.
13. Injury from microorganisms lies in their ability to survive and proliferate in the human body. Injury depends on the microorganisms' ability to invade and destroy cells, produce toxins, and produce damaging hypersensitivity reactions.
14. A leading cause of errors in health care is medication errors.
15. Activation of inflammation and immunity, which occurs after cellular injury or infection, involves powerful biochemicals and proteins capable of damaging normal (uninjured and uninfected) cells.
16. Genetic disorders injure cells by altering the nucleus and the plasma membrane's structure, shape, receptors, or transport mechanisms.
17. Deprivation of essential nutrients (proteins, carbohydrates, lipids, vitamins) can cause cellular injury by altering cellular structure and function, particularly of transport mechanisms, chromosomes, the nucleus, and DNA.
18. Injurious physical agents include temperature extremes and climate change, changes in atmospheric pressure, ionizing radiation, illumination, mechanical stresses (e.g., repetitive body movements), and noise.

Manifestations of Cellular Injury

1. Manifestations of cellular injury include accumulations of water, lipids, carbohydrates, glycogen, proteins, pigments, hemosiderin, bilirubin, calcium, and urate.
2. Accumulations harm cells by "crowding" the organelles and by causing excessive (and sometimes harmful) metabolites to be produced during their catabolism. The metabolites are released into the cytoplasm or expelled into the extracellular matrix.
3. Cellular swelling, the accumulation of excessive water in the cell, is caused by the failure of transport mechanisms and is a sign of many types of cellular injury.
4. Accumulations of organic substances—lipids, carbohydrates, glycogen, proteins, and pigments—are caused by disorders in which (a) cellular uptake of the substance exceeds the cell's capacity to catabolize (digest) or use it or (b) cellular anabolism (synthesis) of the substance exceeds the cell's capacity to use or secrete it.
5. Dystrophic calcification (accumulation of calcium salts) is always a sign of pathologic change because it occurs only in injured or dead cells. Free calcium in the cytosol can cause activation of protein kinases, activation of phospholipases and membrane damage, and damage or disassembly of the cytoskeleton. Metastatic calcification, however, can occur in uninjured cells in individuals with hypercalcemia.
6. Disturbances in urate metabolism can result in hyperuricemia and deposition of sodium urate crystals in tissue, leading to a painful disorder called *gout.*
7. Systemic manifestations of cellular injury include fever, leukocytosis, increased heart rate, pain, and serum elevations of enzymes in the plasma.

Cellular Death

1. Two main types of cell death are necrosis and apoptosis. Type I cell death (e.g., caspases) is often referred to as apoptosis, whereas type II is called autophagic cell death.
2. Necrosis is the sum of the changes after local cell death and includes the processes of inflammation and cellular lysis.
3. The four major types of necrosis are coagulative, liquefactive, caseous, and fat. Different types of necrosis occur in different tissues.
4. Structural signs that indicate irreversible injury and progression to necrosis are the dense clumping and disruption of genetic material and the disruption of the plasma and organelle membranes.
5. Gangrenous necrosis, or gangrene, is tissue necrosis caused by hypoxia and subsequent bacterial invasion.
6. Apoptosis, a different type of cellular death, is a process of selective cellular self-destruction called programmed cell death. Other forms of programmed cell death (type II) include autophagic ("eat oneself") cell death.

Aging

1. It is difficult to determine the physiologic (normal) from the pathologic changes of aging. One of the hallmarks of aging is

SUMMARY REVIEW—cont'd

the accumulation of damaged macromolecules. Life span can be experimentally changed.

2. Humans have an inherent maximal life span (80 to 100 years) that is dictated by currently unknown intrinsic mechanisms.
3. Although the maximal life span has not changed significantly over time, the average life span, or life expectancy, has increased. However, this increase in life expectancy in the United States is not experienced by all Americans.
4. The emerging focus in the biology of aging includes epigenetic and genetic changes, inflammatory response, oxidative stress, metabolic and endocrine regulation, intrauterine and lifelong patterns of health, decline in cell renewal by adult stem cells, and accumulated cell damage related to cancer and aging.
5. Frailty is a common clinical syndrome in older adults, leaving a person vulnerable to falls, functional decline, disability, disease, and death. The syndrome is complex, involving oxidative stress, dysregulation of inflammatory cytokines and hormones, malnutrition, physical inactivity, and muscle apoptosis. Women have a higher risk of frailty than men.

Somatic Death

1. Somatic death is death of the entire organism. Postmortem change is diffuse and does not involve the inflammatory response.
2. Manifestations of somatic death include cessation of respiration and circulation, gradual lowering of body temperature, dilation of pupils, loss of elasticity and transparency in the skin, stiffening of muscles (rigor mortis), and discoloration of the skin (livor mortis). Signs of putrefaction are obvious about 24 to 48 hours after death.

KEY TERMS

REFERENCES

1. Dahlmann B: Role of proteasomes in disease, *BMC Biochem* 8(Suppl): S3, 2007.
2. Leri A, Kajstura J, Amversa P: Role of cardiac stem cells in cardiac pathophysiology: a paradigm shift in human myocardial biology, *Circ Res* 109:941–961, 2011.
3. Murphy E, Steenbergen C: Mechanisms underlying acute protection from cardiac ischemia—reperfusion injury, *Physiol Rev* 88(2):581–609, 2008.
4. Song HJ, Stevens CF, Gage FH: Neural stem cells from adult hippocampus develop essential properties of functional CNS neurons, *Nat Neurosci* 5:438–445, 2002.
5. Degnim AC, et al: Stratification of breast cancer risk in women with atypia: a Mayo cohort study, *J Clin Oncol* 25(19):2672–2677, 2007.
6. Reis-Filho JS, Lakhani SR: The diagnosis and management of pre-invasive breast disease: genetic alterations in pre-invasive lesions, *Breast Cancer Res* 5:313–319, 2004.
7. Valko M, et al: Free radicals and antioxidants in normal physiological functions and human disease, *Int J Biochem Cell Biol* 39(1):44–84, 2007.
8. Murphy E, Steenbergen C: What makes the mitochondria a killer? Can we condition them to be less destructive? *Biochim Biophys Acta* 1813:1302–1308, 2011.
9. Eltzschig HK, Eckle T: Ischemia and reperfusion—from mechanism to translation, *Nat Med* 17:1391–1401, 2011.
10. Lavie L: Oxidative stress inflammation and endothelial dysfunction in obstructive sleep apnea, *Front Biosci (Elite ed)* 4:1391–1403, 2012.
11. Kvietys PR, Granger DN: Role of reactive oxygen and nitrogen species in the vascular responses to inflammation, *Free Radic Biol Med* 52:556–592, 2012.
12. Davignon J, Ganz P: Role of endothelial dysfunction in atherosclerosis, *Circulation* 109:27–32, 2004.
13. Papaharalambus CA: Basic mechanisms of oxidative stress and reactive oxygen species in cardiovascular injury, *Trends Cardiovasc Med* 17(2):48–54, 2007.
14. Lavie L: Intermittent hypoxia: the culprit of oxidative stress, vascular inflammation and dyslipidemia in obstructive sleep apnea, *Exp Rev Respir Med* 2:75–84, 2008.
15. Bai J, Cederbaum AI: Mitochondrial catalase and oxidative injury, *Biol Signals Recept* 10(3-4):189–199, 2001.
16. Bayir H, Kagan VE: Bench to bedside review: mitochondrial injury, oxidative stress and apoptosis—there is nothing more practical than a good theory, *Crit Care* 12:206, 2008.
17. Lee HC, Wei YH: Mitochondrial biogenesis and mitochondrial DNA maintenance of mammalian cells under oxidative stress, *Int J Biochem Cell Biol* 37(4):822–834, 2005.
18. Samper E, Nicholls DG, Melov S: Mitochondrial oxidative stress causes chromosomal instability of mouse embryonic fibroblasts, *Aging Cell* 2(5):277–285, 2003.
19. Lenaz G, et al: Role of mitochondria in oxidative stress and aging, *Ann N Y Acad Sci* 959:99–213, 2002.
20. Ray PD, et al: Reactive oxygen species (ROS) homeostasis and redox regulation in cellular signaling, *Cell Signal* 24:981–990, 2012.
21. Robb EL, Page MM, Stuart JA: Mitochondria, cellular stress resistance, somatic cell depletion and lifespan, *Curr Aging Sci* 2(1):12–27, 2009. review.
22. Young KJ, Bennett JP: The mitochondrial secret(ase) of Alzheimer's disease, *J Alzheimers Dis*, 2010. [Epub ahead of print.].
23. Zhang K: Integration of ER stress, oxidative stress and the inflammatory response in health and disease, *Int J Exp Med* 3(1):33–40, 2010.
24. Lee J, Giordano S, Zhang J: Autophagy, mitochondria and oxidative stress: cross-talk and redox signaling, *Biochem J* 441(2):523–540, 2012.
25. Murray KF, et al: Drug-associated hepatotoxicity and acute liver failure, *J Pediatr Gastroenterol Nutr* 47(5):395–405, 2008.
26. Dooyema CA, et al: Outbreak of fatal childhood lead poisoning related to artisan gold mining in Northwestern Nigeria, *Environ Health Perspect* 120(4):601–607, 2010.
27. Markel H: Getting the lead out: the Rhode Island Lead Pain Trials and their impact on children's health, *JAMA* 297(24):2773–2775, 2007.
28. Kuehn BM: Panel advises tougher limits on lead exposure, *JAMA* 307(5):445, 2012.
29. Centers for Disease Control and Prevention (CDC): Infant lead poisoning associated with use of tiro, an eye cosmetic from Nigeria—Boston, MA, 2011, *MMWR Morb Mortal Wkly Rep* 61(30):574–576, 2012.
30. Centers for Disease Control and Prevention (CDC): Adult blood level epidemiology and surveillance—United States, 2003-2004, *MMWR Morb Mortal Wkly Rep* 55(32):876–879, 2006.
31. National Institute for Occupational Safety and Health: *Adult blood lead epidemiology & surveillance (ABLES)*, Atlanta, GA, 2012, U.S. Department of Health and Human Services, CDC, National Institute for Occupational Safety and Health. Accessed April 9, 2012. Available at www.sdc.gov/niosh/topics/ables/ables.
32. Merrill JC, Morton JJP, Soileau SD: Metals. In Hayes AW, editor: *Principles and methods of toxicology*, ed 5, Milton Park, UK, 2007, Taylor & Francis UK, CRC Press, p 860.
33. Patrick L: Lead toxicity, a review of the literature. Part I: exposure, evaluation, and treatment, *Altern Med Rev* 11(1):2–22, 2006.
34. Karri SK, Saper RB, Kales SN: Lead encephalopathy due to traditional medicines, *Curr Drug Safety* 3(1):54–59, 2008.
35. Barbosa F Jr, et al: A critical review of biomarkers used for monitoring human exposure to lead: advantages, limitations, and future needs, *Environ Health Perspect* 113(12):1669–1674, 2005.
36. Dart RC, Hurlbut KM, Boyer-Hassen LV: Lead. In Dart RC, editor: *Medical toxicology*, ed 3, Philadelphia, 2004, Lippincott Williams & Wilkins, p 1426.
37. Pearson HA, Schonfeld DJ: Lead. In Rudolph CD, editor: *Rudolph's pediatrics*, ed 21, Philadelphia, 2003, McGraw-Hill Professional, p 369.
38. Xu J, et al: Effects of lead exposure on hippocampal metabotripic glutamate receptor subtype 3 and 7 in developmental rats, *J Negat Results Biomed* 8:5, 2009.
39. Sadakata T, Furuichi T: Ca(2+)-dependent activator protein for secretion 2 and autistic-like phenotypes, *Neurosci Res* 67(3):197–202, 2010.
40. Lanphear BP, et al: Low-level environmental lead exposure and children's intellectual function: an international pooled analysis, *Environ Health Perspect* 113(7):894–899, 2005.
41. Pokras MA, Kneeland MR: Lead poisoning: using transdisciplinary approaches to solve an ancient problem, *EcoHealth* 5(3):379–385, 2008.
42. Navas-Acien A, et al: Lead exposure and cardiovascular disease—a systematic review, *Environ Health Perspect* 115(3):472–482, 2007.
43. Sanders T, et al: Neurotoxic effects and biomarkers of lead exposure: a review, *Rev Environ Health* 24(1):15–45, 2009.
44. Mycyk M, Hryhorczuk D, Amitai Y: Lead. In Erickson TB, et al, editors: *Pediatric toxicology: diagnosis and management of the poisoned child*, Philadelphia, 2005, McGraw-Hill Professional, p 462.
45. Longo DL, et al: *Harrison's principles of internal medicine*, ed 18, New York, 2012, McGraw-Hill.
46. Centers for Disease Control and Prevention (CDC): Carbon monoxide exposures, *MMWR Morb Mortal Wkly Rep* 60(30):1014–1017, 2011.
47. Meo SA, Al-Khlawi T: Health hazards of welding fumes, *Saudi Med J* 24(11):1176–1182, 2003.
48. Bennett MH, Mitchell SJ: Hyperbaric and diving medicine. In Longo DL, et al, editors: *Harrison's principles of internal medicine*, ed 18, New York, 2012, McGraw-Hill Medical, chap e52.
49. Kumar V, et al: Environmental and nutritional diseases. In Kumar V, et al, editors: *Robbins & Cotran pathologic basis of disease*, ed 8, St Louis, 2010, Saunders/Elsevier.
50. Heard KJ: Acetylcysteine for acetaminophen poisoning, *N Engl J Med* 359(3):285–292, 2008.
51. Romanoff R, et al: Acute ethanol exposure inhibits renal folate transport, but repeated exposure upregulates folate transport proteins in rats and human cells, *J Nutr* 137:1260–1265, 2007.
52. Guilleminault A, Abad VC: Obstructive sleep apnea syndromes, *Med Clin North Am* 88(3):611–630, 2004.
53. Punjabi NM: The epidemiology of adult obstructive sleep apnea, *Proc Am Thorac Soc* 5(2):136–143, 2008.
54. Zhu H, et al: Oxidative stress and redox signaling mechanisms of alcoholic liver disease: updated experimental and clinical evidence, *J Dig Dis* 13(3):133–142, 2012.
55. Bataller R, Brenner DA: Liver fibrosis, *J Clin Invest* 115(2): 209–218, 2005.
56. Guyot C, et al: Hepatic fibrosis and cirrhosis: the (myo) fibroblastic cell subpopulations involved, *Int J Biochem Cell Biol* 38(2):135–151, 2006.
57. Neuman MG, et al: Markers of inflammation and fibrosis in alcoholic hepatitis and viral hepatitis, *Int J Hepatol* 2012:231210, 2012.
58. Lieber CS: Metabolism of alcohol, *Clin Liver Dis* 9(1):1–35, 2005.
59. Vaux KK, Chambers C: *Fetal alcohol syndrome*, 2009. Available at emedicine.medscape.com/article/974016-overview.
60. Gutierrez C, et al: An experimental study on the effects of ethanol and folic acid deficiency, alone or in combination, on pregnant Swiss mice, *Pathology* 39(5):495–503, 2007.

61. Haycock PC: Fetal alcohol spectrum disorders: the epigenetic perspective, *Biol Reprod* 81(4):607–617, 2009.
62. Saito M, et al: Ethanol alters lipid profiles and phosphorylation status of AMP-activated protein kinase in the neonatal mouse brain, *J Neurochem* 103(3):1208–1218, 2007.
63. Donohue TM Jr, et al: Role of the proteasome in ethanol-induced liver pathology, *Alcohol Clin Exp Res* 31(9):1446–1459, 2007.
64. Clarkson TW, Magos L, Myers GI: The toxicology of mercury—current exposures and clinical manifestations, *N Engl J Med* 349(18):1731–1737, 2003.
65. Lauterbach M, et al: Neurological outcomes in children with and without amalgam-related mercury exposure: seven years of longitudinal observations in a randomized trial, *J Am Dent Assoc* 139(2):138–145, 2008.
66. Environmental Working Group (EWG): *Health/toxics: mercury*, 2008. Available at www.ewg.org/mercury. Accessed.
67. U.S. Centers for Disease Control and Prevention: *WISQUARS database*, 2013. Available at www.cdc.gov/ncipc/wisqars. Accessed.
68. Annest JL, et al: National estimates of nonfatal firearm-related injuries: beyond the tip of the iceberg, *JAMA* 273(22):1749–1754, 1995.
69. Kochanek D, et al: Deaths: preliminary data for 2009, *Natl Vital Stat Rep* 59(4), 2011.
70. Kopec D, et al: The state-of-the-art in the reduction of medical errors, *Stud Health Technol Inform* 121:126–137, 2006.
71. Gawande A: *The checklist manifesto; how to get things right*, New York, 2009, Picado.
72. Haynes AB, et al: Changes in safety attitude and relationship to decreased postoperative morbidity and mortality following implementation of a checklist-based surgical safety intervention, *BMJ Qual Saf* 20(1):102–107, 2011.
73. Marjot T, Maruthappu M, Shalhoub J: Checklists for invasive procedures, *N Engl J Med* 368(3):293–294, 2013.
74. Centers for Disease Control and Prevention: National vital statistics system, *MMWR Morb Mortal Wkly Rep* 61(37):750, 2012.
75. Agency for Healthcare Research and Quality (AHRQ): *20 tips to help prevent medical error in children*. Pub No. 02P034 , September 2002. Available at www.ahrq.gov.
76. Levinson DR: *Adverse events in hospitals: national incidence among Medicare beneficiaries*, Washington, DC, 2010, U.S. Department of Health and Human Services.
77. Hoffman JR, Cooper RJ: Overdiagnosis of disease: a modern epidemic, *Arch Intern Med* 172(15):1123–1124, 2012.
78. National Academy of Science: *Medication errors injure 1.5 million people and cost billions of dollars annually*, Washington, DC, 2006, Author.
79. Brawley OW (with Goldberg P): *How we do harm: a doctor breaks ranks about being sick in America*, New York, 2001, St. Martins Press.
80. The Joint Commission: *The Joint Commission's annual report on quality and safety 2007: improving America's hospitals*. Accessed September 9, 2008. Available at www.jointcommissionreport.org.
81. Palmieri PA, et al: The anatomy and physiology of error in adverse healthcare events, *Adv Health Care Manag* 7:33–68, 2008.
82. Leape LL: Institute of Medicine medical errors figures are not exaggerated, *N Engl J Med* 342:1123–1125, 2000.
83. Cann KF, et al: Extreme water-related weather events and waterborne disease, *Epidemiol Infect* 9:1–16, 2012. [Epub ahead of print.].
84. Grasso M, et al: The health effects of climate change: a survey of recent quantitative research, *Int J Environ Res Public Health* 9(5):1523–1547, 2012.
85. Danzi D: Hypothermia and frostbite. In Longo DL, et al, editors: *Harrison's principles of internal medicine*, ed 18, New York, 2012, McGraw-Hill.
86. Shattock MJ, Tipton MJ: Autonomic conflict: a different way to die during cold water immersion, *J Physiol*, April 2012. [Epub ahead of print.].
87. Bierens JJ, Knape JT, Gelissen HP: Drowning, *Curr Opin Crit Care* 8:578–586, 2002.
88. Camara AK, et al: Hypothermia augments reactive oxygen species detected in the guinea pig isolated perfused heart, *Am J Physiol Heart Circ Physiol* 286(4):H1289–H1299, 2004.
89. Rauen U, de Groot H: Mammalian cell injury induced by hypothermia—the emerging role for reactive oxygen species, *Biol Chem* 383 (3-4):477–488, 2002.
90. Bartels-Stringer M, et al: Preserved vascular reactivity of rat renal arteries after cold storage, *Cryobiology* 48(1):95–98, 2004.
91. Osorio RA, et al: Reactive oxygen species in pregnant rats: effects of exercise and thermal stress, *Comp Biochem Physiol C Toxicol Pharmacol* 135(1):89–95, 2003.
92. Schwartz BG, et al: Therapeutic hypothermia for acute myocardial infarction and cardiac arrest, *Am J Cardiol*, April 2012. [Epub ahead of print.].
93. Lanner JT: Ryanodine receptor physiology and its role in disease. In Islam MS, editor: *Calcium signaling, advances in experimental medicine and biology*, Karolinska Institute, New York, 2012, Springer.
94. Dinarello CA, Porat R: Fever and hypothermia. In Longo DL, et al, editors: *Harrison's principles of internal medicine*, ed 18, New York, 2012, McGraw-Hill.
95. Task Force on Sudden Infant Death Syndrome, Moon RY: SIDS and other sleep-related infant deaths: expansion of recommendations for a safe infant sleeping environment, *Pediatrics* 128(5):1030–1039, 2011.
96. Lynch JH, Bove AA: Diving medicine: a review of current evidence, *J Spec Oper Med* 9:72–79, 2009.
97. NOAA: *NOAA diving manual: diving for science and technology*, ed 4, Palm Beach Gardens, FL, 2010, Best Publishing.
98. Webb JT, Pilmanis AA: Fifty years of decompression sickness research at Brooks AFB, TX: 1960-2010, *Aviat Space Environ Med* 82(Suppl):A1–25, 2011.
99. Luks AM, et al: Wilderness Medical Society consensus guidelines for the prevention and treatment of acute altitude illness, *Wilderness Environ Med* 21:146–155, 2010.
100. Schoene RB: Illnesses at high altitude, *Chest* 134:402–416, 2008.
101. Imray C, et al: Acute mountain sickness: pathophysiology, prevention, and treatment, *Prog Cardiovasc Dis* 52:467–484, 2010.
102. Scherrer U, et al: New insights in the pathogenesis of high-altitude pulmonary edema, *Prog Cardiovasc Dis* 52:485–492, 2010.
103. Stream JO, Grissom CK: Update on high-altitude pulmonary edema: pathogenesis, prevention, and treatment, *Wilderness Environ Med* 19:293–303, 2008.
104. Ainsbury EA, et al: Radiation cataractogenesis: a review of recent studies, *Radiat Res* 172:1–9, 2009.
105. Hall E, Giaccia AJ: Milestones in the radiation sciences. In Hall E, Giaccia AJ, editors: *Radiobiology for the radiologist*, ed 6, Philadelphia, 2006, Lippincott Williams & Wilkins, pp 1–4.
106. Linet S, et al: Cancer risks associated with external radiation from diagnostic imaging procedures, *CA Cancer J Clin* 62:75–100, 2012.
107. Dauer LT, et al: Review and evaluation of updated research on the health effects associated with low-doses of ionizing radiation, *Radiat Prot Dosimetry* 140:103–136, 2010.
108. Mothersill C, Seymour C: Are epigenetic mechanisms involved in radiation-induced bystander effects? *Front Genet* 3:74, 2012.
109. Seymour CB, Mothersill C, Alper T: High yields of lethal mutations in somatic mammalian cells that survive ionizing radiation, *Int J Radiat Biol Rel Stud Phys Chem Med* 50:167–179, 1986.
110. Kadhim MA, et al: Transmission of chromosomal instability after plutonium alpha-particle irradiation, *Nature* 355:738–740, 1992.
111. Nagasawa H, Little JB: Induction of sister chromatid exchanges by extremely low doses of alpha-particles, *Cancer Res* 52: 6394–6396, 1992.
112. Mothersill C, Seymour C: Medium from irradiated human epithelial cells but not human fibroblasts reduces the clonogenic survival of unirradiated cells, *Int J Radiat Biol* 71:421–427, 1997.
113. Barcellos-Hoff MH, Park C, Wright EG: Radiation and the microenvironment—tumorigenesis and therapy, *Nat Rev Cancer* 5:867–875, 2005.
114. Preston DL, et al: Solid cancer incidence in atomic bomb survivors: 1958-1998, *Radiat Res* 168:1–64, 2007.
115. Lazarus E, et al: Utilization of imaging in pregnant patients: 10 year review of 5270 examinations in 3285 patients—1997-2006, *Radiology* 251(2):517–524, 2009.
116. Brenner DJ, et al: Estimated risks of radiation-induced fatal cancer from pediatric CT, *AJR Am J Roentgenol* 176:289–296, 2001.
117. Brenner DJ, Shuryak I, Einstein AJ: Impact of reduced patient life expectancy on potential cancer risks, *Imaging Radiol* 261(1):193–198, 2011.
118. Shuryak I, Sachs RK, Brenner DJ: Cancer risks after radiation exposure in middle age, *J Natl Cancer Inst* 102(12):1628–1636, 2012.
119. Preston DL, Shimizu Y, Pierce DA: Studies of mortality of atomic bomb survivors. Report 13: solid cancer and noncancer disease mortality, *Radiat Res* 160:381–407, 2003.
120. Hoel DG: Ionizing radiation and cardiovascular disease, *Ann N Y Acad Sci* 1076:309–317, 2006.
121. Little MP, et al: Systematic review and meta-analysis of circulatory disease from exposure to low-level ionizing radiation and estimates of potential population mortality risks, *Environ Health Perspect*, 2012 June 22. [Epub ahead of print.].

122. Behar-Cohen F, et al: Light-emitting diodes (LED) for domestic lighting: any risks for the eye? *Prog Retinal Eye Res* 30:239–257, 2011.
123. Delori FC, et al: Maximum permissible exposures (ANSI 2000) for ocular safety with emphasis on ophthalmic devices, *J Opt Soc Am A Opt Image Sci Vis* 24(5):1250–1265, 2007.
124. Organisciak DT, Vaughan DK: Retinal light damage: mechanisms and protection, *Prog Retinal Eye Res* 29(2):113–134, 2011.
125. Youssef PN, Sheibani N, Albert DM: Retinal light toxicity, *Eye (London)* 25(1):1–14, 2011.
126. Siu TL, Morley JW, Coroneo MT: Toxicology of the retina: advances in understanding the defence mechanisms and pathogenesis of drug- and light-induced retinopathy, *Clin Exp Ophthalmol* 36(2):176–185, 2008.
127. Wilkins AJ, Wilkinson P: A tint to reduce eye-strain from fluorescent lighting? Preliminary observations, *Ophthalmic Physiol Opt* 11(2): 172–175, 1991.
128. Rubin GS, et al: A prospective, population-based study of the role of visual impairment in motor vehicle crashes among older drivers: the SEE study, *Invest Ophthalmol Vis Sci* 48(4):1483–1491, 2007.
129. Mainster MA, Timberlake GT: Why HID headlights bother older drivers, *Br J Ophthalmol* 87(1):113–117, 2003.
130. Mohan K, et al: Separation anxiety: stress, tension and cytokinesis, *Exp Cell Res*, 2012. [Epub ahead of print.].
131. Barbee KA: Mechanical cell injury, *Ann N Y Acad Sci* 1066: 67–84, 2005.
132. Van Epps JS, Vorp DA: Mechanopathobiology of atherogenesis: a review, *J Surg Res* 142(1):202–217, 2007.
133. National Institute on Deafness and Other Communication Disorders (NIDCD): *Statistics about hearing disorders, ear infections, and deafness.* Washington, DC, 2005, National Institutes of Health. Available at www.nidcd.nih.gov/health/statistics/nearing.asp.
134. Ryherd E, West J, Ljungkvist L: Characterizing noise and perceived work environments in a neurological intensive care unit, *J Accoust Soc* 123:747–756, 2008.
135. Cho YS, et al: Physiological consequences of programmed necrosis, an alternative form of cell demise, *Mol Cells* 29(4):327–332, 2010.
136. Majno G, Joris I: Apoptosis, oncosis, and necrosis: an overview of cell death, *Am J Pathol* 146(1):3–15, 1995.
137. Moquin D, Chan F: The molecular regulation of programmed necrotic cell injury, *Trends Biochem Sci* 35(8):434–441, 2010.
138. Rikiishi H: Novel insights into the interplay between apoptosis and autophagy, *Int J Cell Biol*, 2012. [Epub ahead of print.].
139. Raloff J: Coming to terms with death: accurate descriptions of a cell's demise may offer clues to diseases and treatments, *Sci News* 159: 378–380, 2001.
140. Wang Z, et al: The mitochondrial phosphatase PGAM5 functions at the convergence point of multiple necrotic death pathways, *Cell* 148: 228–243, 2012.
141. Bicknell KA, Coxon CH, Brooks G: Can the cardiomyocyte cell cycle be reprogrammed? *J Mol Cell Cardiol* 42(4):706–721, 2007.
142. Glick D, Barth S, MacLeod KF: Autophagy: cellular and molecular mechanisms, *J Pathol* 221(1):3–12, 2010.
143. Wyllie AH, Kerr JFR, Currie AR: Cell death: the significance of apoptosis, *Int Rev Cytol* 68:251–306, 1980.
144. Shintani T, Klionsky DJ: Autophagy in health and disease: a double-edged sword, *Science* 306(5698):990–995, 2004.
145. Marshall L, et al: Identifying and managing adverse environmental health effects. 1. Taking an exposure history, *CMAJ* 166(8):1049–1055, 2002.
146. Mizushima N: Autophagy: process and function, *Genes Dev* 21(22): 2861–2873, 2007. review.
147. Kepp O, et al: Cell death assays for drug discovery, *Nat Rev Drug Discov* 10(3):221–237, 2012.
148. Petrovski G, et al: Clearance of dying autophagic cells of different origin by professional and non-professional phagocytes, *Cell Death Differ* 14(6):1117–1128, 2007.
149. Apel A, et al: Blocked autophagy sensitizes resistant carcinoma cells to radiation therapy, *Cancer Res* 68(5):1485–1494, 2008.
150. Mathew R, et al: Role of autophagy in cancer, *Nat Rev Cancer* 7(12): 961–967, 2007.
151. Johnson HA: Is aging physiological or pathological? In Johnson HA, editor: *Relation between normal aging and disease*, New York, 1985, Raven.
152. Hayflick L: Biological aging is no longer an unsolved problem, *Ann N Y Acad Sci* 1100:1–13, 2007. review.
153. Tissenbaum HA: Genetics, life span, health span, and the aging process in Caenorhabditis elegans, *J Gerontol A Biol Sci Med Sci* 67A(5):503–510, 2012.
154. Rando TA, Chang HY: Aging rejuvenation, and epigenetic reprogramming: resetting the aging clock, *Cell* 148:46–57, 2012.
155. Campisi J, Vijg J: Does damage to DNA and other macromolecules play a role in aging? If so, how? *J Gerontol A Biol Sci Med Sci* 64:175–178, 2009.
156. Seviour EG, Lin SY: The DNA damage response: balancing the scale between cancer and ageing, *Aging (Albany, NY)* 2:900–907, 2010.
157. Charville GW, Rando TA: Stem cell ageing and non-random chromosome segregation, *Philos Trans R Soc Lond B Biol Sci* 366:85–93, 2011.
158. Kuilman T, et al: The essence of senescence, *Genes Dev* 24: 2463–2479, 2010.
159. Fontana L, Partridge L, Longo VD: Extending healthy life span—from yeast to humans, *Science* 328:321–326, 2010.
160. Kenyon CJ: The genetics of ageing, *Nature* 464:504–512, 2010.
161. Takahashi K, Yamanaka S: Induction of pluripotent stem cells from mouse embryonic and adult fibroblast cultures by defined factors, *Cell* 126:663–676, 2006.
162. Hanna JH, Saha K, Jaenisch R: Pluripotency and cellular reprogramming: facts, hypotheses, unresolved issues, *Cell* 143:508–525, 2010.
163. Villeda SA, et al: Age-related changes in the systemic milieu regulate adult neurogenesis, *Nature* 477:90–94, 2011.
164. Harrison DE, et al: Rapamycin fed late in life extends lifespan in genetically heterogeneous mice, *Nature* 460:392–395, 2009.
165. Greer EL, et al: Transgenerational epigenetic inheritance of longevity in *Caenorhabditis elegans, Nature* 479:365–371, 2011.
166. Central Intelligence Agency: *World factbook*, Washington, DC, 2011, Author.
167. National Research Council: *Explaining divergent levels of longevity in high-income countries*, Washington, DC, 2011, National Academies Press.
168. Organization for Economic Cooperation and Development: *Doing better for children*, Paris, France, 2009, OECD Publishing.
169. Darzi A, et al: *The five bad habits of healthcare. How new thinking about behaviour could reduce health spending*, Geneva, Switzerland, 2011, World Economic Forum and Imperial College Vlaev.
170. Institute of Medicine (IOM): *For the public's health: investing in a healthier future*, Washington, DC, 2012, The National Academies Press.
171. Cory SA, et al: Prevalence of selected risk behaviors and chronic diseases and conditions—steps communities, United States, 2006-2007, *MMWR Surveill Summ* 59(8):1–37, 2010.
172. Boyle J, et al: Projection of the year 2050 burden of diabetes in the US population: dynamic modeling of incidence, mortality, and prediabetes prevalence, *Popul Health Metr* 8(1):29, 2010.
173. Olshansky SJ, et al: A potential decline in life expectancy in the United States in the 21st century, *N Engl J Med* 352(11):1138–1145, 2005.
174. Seals DR, Jablonski KL, Donato AJ: Aging and vascular endothelial function in humans, *Clin Sci* 120:357–375, 2011.
175. Higashi Y, et al: IGF-1, oxidative stress, and atheroprotection, *Trends Endocrinol Metab* 21(4):245–254, 2011.
176. Fried LP, et al: Frailty in older adults: evidence for a phenotype, *J Gerontol A Biol Sci Med Sci* 56(3):M146–M156, 2001.
177. Walston JD: Frailty. Preface, *Clin Geriatr Med* 27(1):xi, 2011.
178. Gillick M: Pinning down frailty, *J Gerontol A Biol Sci Med Sci* 56(3):M134–M135, 2001.

CHAPTER

3

The Cellular Environment: Fluids and Electrolytes, Acids and Bases

Alexa K. Doig and Sue E. Huether

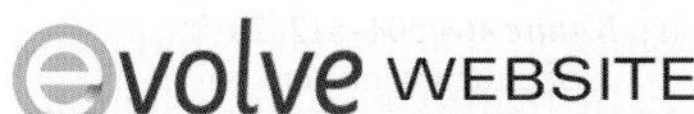

http://evolve.elsevier.com/McCance/
- Review Questions and Answers
- Animations
- Online Course: Module 2

CHAPTER OUTLINE

The cells of the body live in a fluid environment that requires electrolyte and acid-base concentrations maintained within a very narrow range. A balance is maintained by an integration of renal, hormonal, and neural functions. Changes in the composition of electrolytes affect electrical potentials of excitatory cells and cause shifts of fluid from one compartment to another that can affect cell function. Fluid fluctuations also affect blood volume and therefore blood pressure. Alterations in pH (measure of the acidity or alkalinity of a solution) disrupt the cellular function of enzyme systems and can cause cell injury. Disturbances in fluid and electrolyte or acid-base balance are common and can be life threatening. Understanding how alterations occur and the body's ability to compensate or correct the disturbance is important for comprehending many pathophysiologic conditions.

DISTRIBUTION OF BODY FLUIDS

The fluids of the body are distributed among functional compartments, or spaces, and provide a transport medium for cellular and tissue function. Water moves freely among body compartments and is distributed by osmotic and hydrostatic forces. Two thirds of the body's water is **intracellular fluid** (ICF) and one third is in the **extracellular fluid** (ECF) compartments.

The two main ECF compartments are the **interstitial fluid** and the **intravascular fluid,** the latter being the blood plasma. Other ECF compartments include the lymph and the transcellular fluids, such as the saliva, intestinal, biliary, hepatic, pancreatic, and cerebrospinal fluids; sweat; urine; and pleural, synovial, peritoneal, pericardial, and intraocular fluids (Table 3-1).

The sum of fluids within all compartments constitutes the **total body water (TBW)** (Table 3-2). The volume of TBW is usually expressed as a percentage of body weight in kilograms. The standard value for TBW is 60% of the weight of a 70-kg adult male, which is equivalent to 42 L of fluid (Table 3-3). The rest of the body weight is composed of fat and fat-free solids, particularly bone.

Although daily fluid intake may fluctuate widely, the body regulates water volume within a relatively narrow range. The primary sources of body water are drinking of fluids, ingestion of water in food, and derivation of water from oxidative metabolism. Normally, the largest amounts of water are lost through renal excretion. Lesser amounts are eliminated through the stool and through vaporization from the skin and lungs (insensible water loss) (Table 3-4).

Although the amount of fluid within the various compartments is relatively constant, exchange of solutes (e.g., salts) and water occurs between compartments to maintain their unique compositions. The percentage of TBW varies with the amount of body fat and age. Because fat is water repelling (hydrophobic), very little water is contained in adipose cells. Individuals with more body fat have proportionately less TBW and tend to be more susceptible to fluid imbalances that cause dehydration.

AGING AND DISTRIBUTION OF BODY FLUIDS

The distribution and amount of TBW change with age (see Table 3-3). In newborn infants, TBW is about 75% to 80% of body weight because infants store less fat. In the immediate postnatal period, a physiologic loss of body water occurs, equivalent to about 5% of body weight as the infant adjusts to a new environment. Infants are particularly susceptible to significant changes in TBW because of their high metabolic rate and potential for evaporative fluid loss attributable to their greater body surface area in proportion to total body size. Loss of fluids from diarrhea can represent a significant proportion of body weight in infants. Renal mechanisms that regulate fluid and electrolyte conservation may not be mature enough to counter the losses, so dehydration can develop rapidly.

During childhood, TBW slowly decreases to 60% to 65% of body weight. At adolescence the percentage of TBW approaches adult proportions, and gender differences begin to appear. Males eventually have a greater percentage of body water as a function of increasing muscle mass. Females have more body fat and less muscle as a function of estrogens and therefore have less body water.

With increasing age the percentage of TBW declines further still. The decrease is caused in part by an increased amount of fat

TABLE 3-1 APPROXIMATE CONCENTRATIONS OF ELECTROLYTES IN TRANSCELLULAR FLUIDS

FLUID	NA+ (mEq/L)	K+ (mEq/L)	CL− (mEq/L)	HCO_3^- (mEq/L)
Saliva	33	20	34	40
Gastric juice*	60	9	84	0
Bile	149	5	101	45
Pancreatic juice	141	5	77	92
Ileal fluid	129	11	116	29
Cecal fluid	80	21	48	22
Cerebrospinal fluid	141	3	127	23
Sweat	45	5	58	0

*The Cl^- concentration exceeds the Na^+, K^+ concentration by 15 mEq/L in gastric juice. This largely represents the secretions of hydrochloric acid by parietal cells.

TABLE 3-2 DISTRIBUTION OF BODY WATER

	PERCENTAGE OF BODY WEIGHT	VOLUME (L)
Intracellular fluid (ICF)	40	28
Extracellular fluid (ECF)	20	14
Interstitial	(15)	(11)
Intravascular	(5)	(3)
Total body water (TBW)	60	42

TABLE 3-3 TOTAL BODY WATER* IN RELATION TO BODY WEIGHT

BODY BUILD	TBW (%) ADULT MALE	TBW (%) ADULT FEMALE	TBW (%) INFANT
Normal	60	50	70
Lean	70	60	80
Obese	50	42	60

*NOTE: TBW (total body water) is a percentage of body weight.

TABLE 3-4 NORMAL WATER GAINS AND LOSSES (70-KG MAN)

	DAILY INTAKE (ML)		DAILY OUTPUT (ML)
Drinking ≈60%	1400-1800	Urine ≈60%	1400-1800
Water in food ≈30%	700-1000	Stool ≈2%	100
Water of oxidation ≈10%	300-400	Skin ≈10%	300-500
		Lungs ≈28%	600-800
TOTAL	2400-3200		2400-3200

and a decreased amount of muscle and by a reduced ability to regulate sodium and water balance. With older age the kidneys becomes less efficient at conserving sodium and therefore have difficulty concentrating the urine. Insensible water loss through the skin may increase and thirst perception may be impaired. The normal reduction of TBW in older adults becomes clinically important when the body is under stress, such as development of fever or dehydration; loss of body fluids at such times can be severe and life threatening.[1]

Water Movement Between ICF and ECF

The movement of water between ICF and ECF compartments is primarily a function of osmotic forces. (Osmosis and other mechanisms of passive transport are discussed in Chapter 1.) Water moves freely by diffusion through the lipid bilayer cell membrane and through **aquaporins,** a family of water channel proteins that provide permeability to water.[2] The osmolality (number of osmoles of solute per kilogram of fluid [Osm/kg]) of TBW is normally at equilibrium. Sodium is responsible for the osmotic balance of the ECF space. Potassium maintains the osmotic balance of the ICF space. The osmotic force of ICF proteins and other nondiffusible substances is balanced by the active transport of ions out of the cell. Water crosses cell membranes freely so the osmolality of TBW is normally at equilibrium. Normally the ICF is not subject to rapid changes in osmolality but when ECF osmolality changes, water moves from one compartment to another until osmotic equilibrium is reestablished (see Figure 3-6, p. 110).

Water Movement Between Plasma and Interstitial Fluid

The distribution of water and the movement of nutrients and waste products between the plasma in the tissue capillaries and interstitial spaces occur as a result of changes in hydrostatic pressure and osmotic forces at the arterial and venous ends of the capillary. Water, sodium, and glucose move readily across the capillary membrane. The plasma proteins maintain the effective osmolality (concentration of solutes per kilogram of solution), do not cross the capillary membrane, and generate plasma oncotic pressure. Albumin is the plasma protein that is primarily responsible for the plasma oncotic pressure because it has the highest concentration. Osmotic forces within the capillary are balanced by the hydrostatic pressure, which is primarily determined by blood pressure and blood volume.

As plasma flows from the arterial to the venous end of the capillary, four forces determine if fluid moves out of the capillary and into the interstitial space (filtration) or if fluid moves back into the capillary from the interstitial space (reabsorption):

1. **Capillary hydrostatic pressure (blood pressure)** facilitates the outward movement of water from the capillary to the interstitial space.
2. **Capillary (plasma) oncotic pressure** osmotically attracts water from the interstitial space back into the capillary.
3. **Interstitial hydrostatic pressure** facilitates the inward movement of water from the interstitial space into the capillary.
4. **Interstitial oncotic pressure** osmotically attracts water from the capillary into the interstitial space.

The movement of fluid back and forth across the capillary wall is called **net filtration** and is best described by the **Starling hypothesis:**

Net filtration = (Forces favoring filtration) − (Forces opposing filtration)

Forces favoring filtration = Capillary hydrostatic pressure and interstitial oncotic pressure

Forces opposing filtration = Capillary oncotic pressure and interstitial hydrostatic pressure

Normally the interstitial forces are negligible because only a very small percentage of plasma proteins crosses the capillary membrane and interstitial fluid moves into cells or is drawn back into the plasma. Thus the major forces for filtration are within the capillary.

As the plasma flows from the arterial to the venous end of the capillary, the force of hydrostatic pressure facilitates the movement of water across the capillary membrane. Oncotic pressure remains fairly constant because plasma proteins normally do not cross the capillary membrane. At the arterial end of the capillary, hydrostatic pressure is greater than capillary oncotic pressure and water filters into the interstitial space. Because of oncotic forces, some water moves back into the capillary, but the net effect is loss of water from the capillary. This loss of water from the plasma decreases the hydrostatic pressure within the capillary; thus at the venous end of the capillary, oncotic pressure exceeds hydrostatic pressure. Fluids then are attracted back into the circulation, balancing the movement of fluids between the plasma and the interstitial space. The overall effect is filtration at the arterial end and reabsorption at the venous end (Figure 3-1). Interstitial hydrostatic pressure promotes the movement of about 10% of the interstitial fluid along with small amounts of protein into the lymphatics, which eventually returns to the circulation.

An important factor in capillary filtration of fluid is the integrity of the capillary membrane. Changes in membrane permeability may permit the escape of plasma proteins into the interstitial space. The normal relationship defined by the Starling hypothesis is altered with the osmotic movement of water into the interstitial space, causing tissue edema.

ALTERATIONS IN WATER MOVEMENT

Edema

Edema is the excessive accumulation of fluid within the interstitial spaces. It is often a problem of fluid distribution and does not necessarily indicate a fluid excess. In some conditions, sequestered fluids can cause both edema and intravascular dehydration. The pathophysiologic process of edema is related to an increase in the forces favoring fluid filtration from the capillaries or lymphatic channels into the tissues. The four most common mechanisms are:

1. Increased capillary hydrostatic pressure
2. Decreased plasma oncotic pressure
3. Increased capillary membrane permeability
4. Lymphatic obstruction (Figure 3-2)

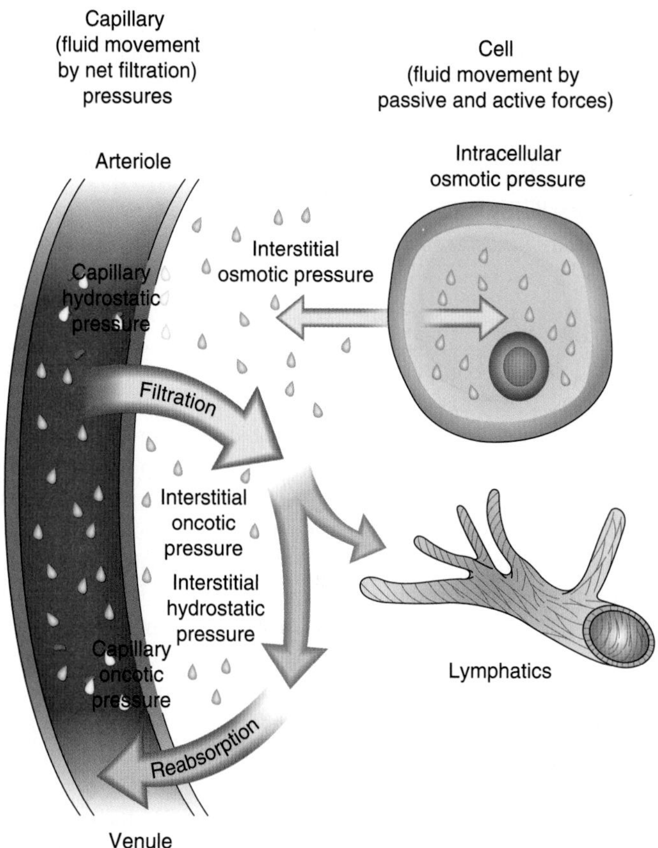

Arterial Capillary Pressures	
Capillary hydrostatic pressure	35 mmHg
Interstitial fluid hydrostatic pressure	2 mmHg
Net hydrostatic pressure	**33 mmHg**
Capillary oncotic pressure	24 mmHg
Interstitial fluid oncotic pressure	0 mmHg
Net oncotic pressure	**24 mmHg**
Net filtration pressure	**+9 mmHg**

Venous Capillary Pressures	
Capillary hydrostatic pressure	18 mmHg
Interstitial fluid hydrostatic pressure	1 mmHg
Net hydrostatic pressure	**17 mmHg**
Capillary oncotic pressure	25 mmHg
Interstitial fluid oncotic pressure	0 mmHg
Net oncotic pressure	**25 mmHg**
Net filtration pressure	**–8 mmHg**

FIGURE 3-1 Capillary Filtration Forces. Water, electrolytes, and small molecules exchange freely between the vascular compartment and the interstitial space at the site of capillaries and small venules. The rate and amount of exchange are driven by the physical forces of hydrostatic and oncotic pressures and the permeability and surface area of the capillary membranes. The two opposing hydrostatic pressures are capillary hydrostatic pressure and interstitial hydrostatic pressure. The two opposing oncotic pressures are capillary oncotic pressure and interstitial oncotic pressure. The *forces that favor filtration* from the capillary are capillary hydrostatic pressure and interstitial oncotic pressure, and the *forces that oppose filtration* are capillary oncotic pressure and interstitial hydrostatic pressure. The sum of their effects is known as *net filtration pressure* (NFP). In the example of normal exchange illustrated here, a small amount of fluid moves to the lymph vessels, which accounts for the net filtration difference between the arterial and venous ends of the capillary.

PATHOPHYSIOLOGY. Increased capillary hydrostatic pressure can result from venous obstruction or sodium and water retention. Venous obstruction causes hydrostatic pressure to increase behind the obstruction, pushing fluid from the capillaries into the interstitial spaces. Venous blood clots, hepatic obstruction, right heart failure, tight clothing around the extremities, and prolonged standing are common causes of venous obstruction. Right congestive heart failure, renal failure, and cirrhosis of the liver are conditions associated with excessive sodium and water retention, which in turn cause volume overload, increased venous pressure, and edema.

Decreased plasma oncotic pressure results from *losses or diminished production of plasma albumin.* Decreased oncotic

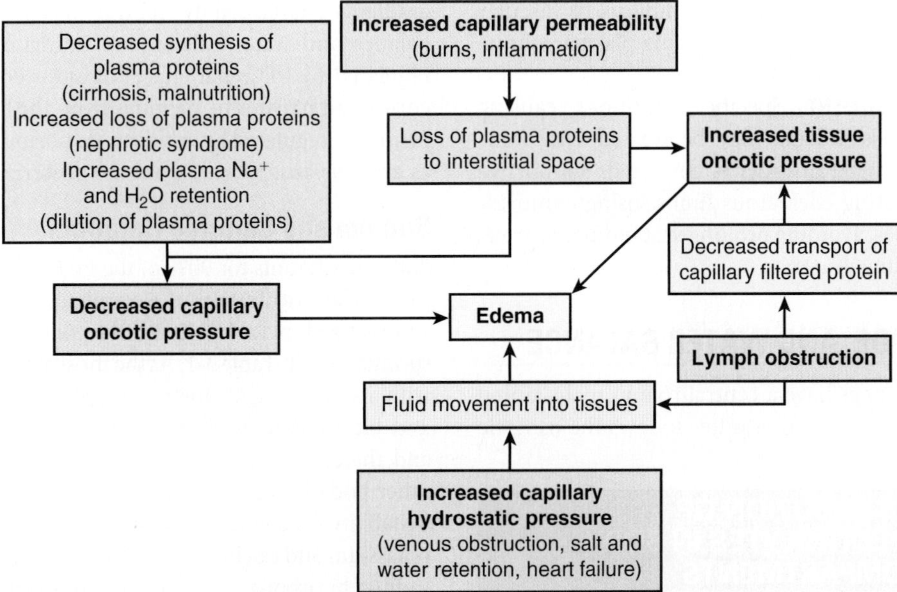

FIGURE 3-2 Mechanisms of Edema Formation.

attraction of fluid within the capillary causes fluid to move into the interstitial space, resulting in edema. Decreased synthesis of plasma protein and decreased oncotic pressure may occur with liver disease or protein malnutrition. Losses of plasma proteins occur with glomerular diseases of the kidney (nephrotic syndrome), hemorrhage, and serous drainage from open wounds or burns.

Increased capillary permeability is usually associated with *inflammation and the immune response.* (Immunity is discussed in Chapters 7, 8, and 9; inflammation is discussed in Chapters 7 and 9.) These responses are often the result of trauma such as burns or crushing injuries, neoplastic disease, allergic reactions, and infection. Excess amounts of fluid escape from the plasma to the interstitial space and produce edema. This type of edema is often very severe because of loss of proteins from the vascular space, which decreases capillary oncotic pressure and increases interstitial oncotic pressure.

Lymphatic obstruction occurs when the *lymphatic channels are blocked* because of infection or tumor. Proteins and fluids are not reabsorbed and accumulate in the interstitial space, causing **lymphedema.** Lymphedema of the arm or leg also can occur after surgical removal of axillary or femoral lymph nodes, respectively, for treatment of cancer.[3]

CLINICAL MANIFESTATIONS. Edema may be localized or generalized. Some *localized edema* is usually limited to the site of tissue injury, as in a sprained joint. Local edema can also occur within particular organs, causing, for example, cerebral edema in the brain and pulmonary edema in the lungs. Edema of specific organs, such as the brain, lung, or larynx, can be life threatening.

Generalized edema is manifested by a more uniform distribution of fluid in interstitial spaces throughout the body. *Dependent edema,* in which fluid accumulates in gravity-dependent areas of the body, might appear in the feet and legs when standing and in the sacral area and buttocks when supine. Dependent edema can be identified by using the fingers to press away

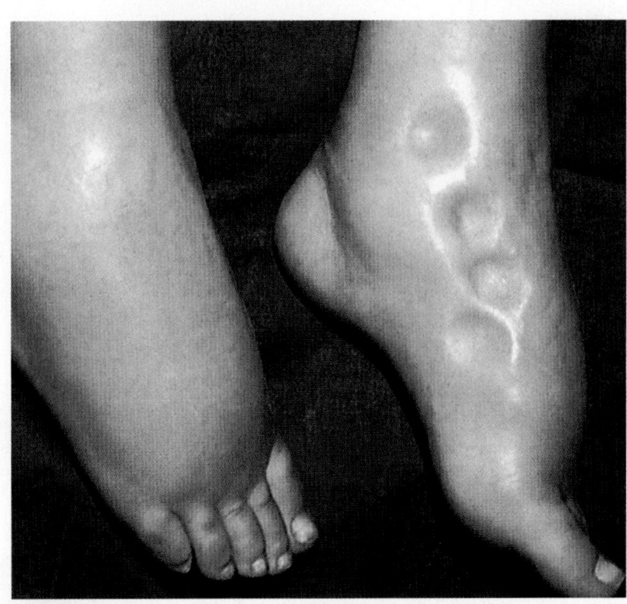

FIGURE 3-3 Pitting Edema. (From Bloom A, Ireland J: *Color atlas of diabetes,* ed 2, St Louis, 1992, Mosby.)

edematous fluid in tissues overlying bony prominences. A pit will be left in the skin; hence the term *pitting edema* (Figure 3-3).

Edema is usually associated with swelling and puffiness, tight-fitting clothes and shoes, and limited movement of the affected area. Weight gain can be significant. The accumulation of fluid increases the distance required for nutrients, oxygen, and wastes to move between capillaries and cells in the tissues. Increased tissue pressure also may diminish capillary blood flow, leading to ischemia. Therefore, wounds heal more slowly and formation of pressure sores increases (see Chapter 46).

As edematous fluid accumulates, it is trapped in a "third space" (i.e., the interstitial space) and dehydration can develop as a result of this sequestering of fluid. Such sequestration occurs with severe burns, in which large amounts of vascular fluid are lost to the interstitial spaces, reducing plasma volume and causing shock (see Chapter 48).

EVALUATION AND TREATMENT. Specific conditions causing edema require diagnosis. Edema may be treated symptomatically until the underlying disorder is corrected. Supportive measures include elevating edematous limbs, using compression stockings or devices, avoiding prolonged standing, restricting salt intake, and taking diuretics.

SODIUM, CHLORIDE, AND WATER BALANCE

The kidneys and hormones have a central role in maintaining sodium and water balance. Because water follows the osmotic gradients established by changes in salt concentration, sodium balance and water balance are intimately related. Sodium is regulated by the renal effects of aldosterone from the adrenal cortex and natriuretic peptides from the heart. Water balance is primarily regulated by antidiuretic hormone (ADH; also known as *arginine-vasopressin*) from the posterior pituitary.

TABLE 3-5 DISTRIBUTION OF ELECTROLYTES IN BODY COMPARTMENTS

	EXTRACELLULAR FLUID (mEq/L)	INTRACELLULAR FLUID (mEq/L)
Cations		
Sodium	142	10
Potassium	5	156
Calcium	5	4
Magnesium	2	26
TOTAL	154	196
Anions		
Bicarbonate	24	12
Chloride	104	4
Phosphate	2	40-95
Proteins	16	54
Other anions	8	31-86
TOTAL	154	196 (average)

Sodium and Chloride Balance

Sodium accounts for 90% of the ECF cations (positively charged ions). The distribution of electrolytes in body compartments is summarized in Table 3-5 and the concentration of electrolytes is summarized in Table 3-1. As the most abundant ECF cation, along with its constituent anions (negatively charged ions) chloride and bicarbonate, sodium regulates extracellular osmotic forces and therefore regulates water balance. Sodium is important in other body functions, including maintenance of neuromuscular irritability for conduction of nerve impulses (in conjunction with potassium and calcium), regulation of acid-base balance (through sodium bicarbonate and sodium phosphate), participation in cellular chemical reactions, and transport of substances across the cellular membrane (see Chapter 1).

The kidney, in conjunction with neural and hormonal mediators, maintains normal serum sodium concentration within a narrow range (135 to 145 mEq/L) primarily through renal tubular reabsorption. The average dietary intake of sodium ranges from 5 to 6 g/day; the minimal daily requirement of sodium is 500 mg. Sweating depletes sodium and water volume and increases the body's sodium requirement.

Hormonal regulation of sodium balance is mediated by **aldosterone,** a mineralocorticoid (steroid) synthesized and secreted from the adrenal cortex as the end product of the renin-angiotensin-aldosterone system (Figure 3-4) (also see Chapters 21 and 37). When circulating blood pressure and renal blood flow, or serum sodium concentrations, are reduced, **renin,** an enzyme secreted by the juxtaglomerular cells of the kidney, is released. Renin stimulates the formation of **angiotensin I,** an

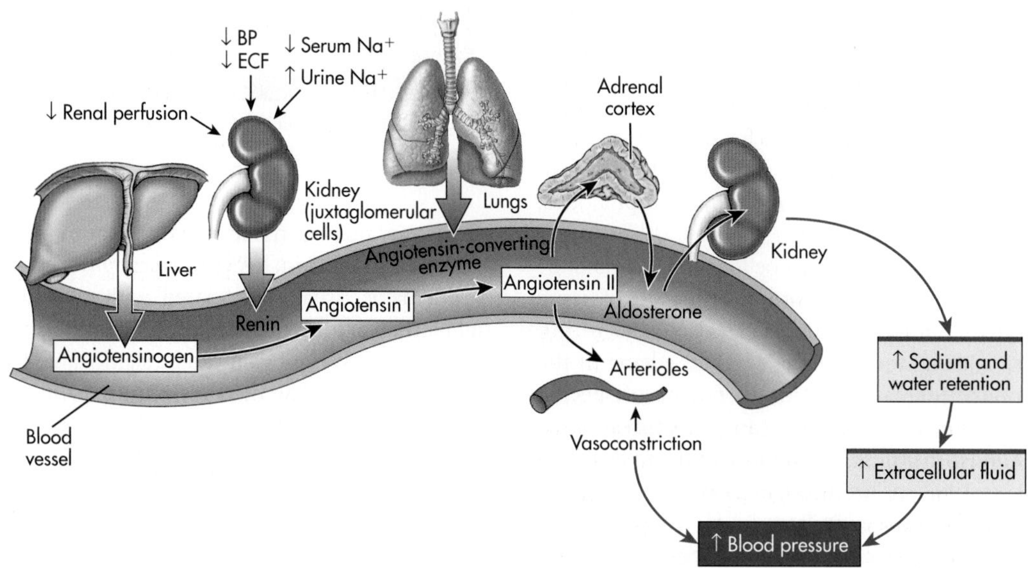

FIGURE 3-4 The Renin-Angiotensin-Aldosterone System. *BP,* Blood pressure; *ECF,* extracellular fluid; *Na,* sodium. (From Lewis et al: *Medical-surgical nursing: assessment and management of clinical problems,* ed 8, St. Louis, 2011, Mosby.)

inactive polypeptide. Angiotensin-converting enzyme (ACE) in pulmonary vessels converts angiotensin I to angiotensin II. **Angiotensin II** has two major functions: it causes vasoconstriction, which elevates systemic blood pressure, and it stimulates the secretion of aldosterone. Aldosterone promotes sodium and water reabsorption by the proximal tubules of the kidneys, thus conserving sodium, blood volume, and blood pressure. Aldosterone also stimulates secretion (and therefore excretion) of potassium by the distal tubule of the kidney, reducing potassium concentrations in the ECF. The restoration of sodium levels, blood volume, and renal perfusion then inhibits further release of renin.

Natriuretic peptides are hormones that include atrial natriuretic peptide (ANP) produced by myoendocrine atrial cells, brain natriuretic peptide (BNP—named brain since it was first discovered in porcine brain) produced by myoendocrine ventricular cells, and urodilatin (an ANP analog) synthesized within the kidney. ANP and BNP are released when there is an increase in transmural atrial pressure caused by increased intra-atrial volume as may occur with heart failure.[4] ANP and BNP increase sodium and water excretion by the kidneys, which lowers blood volume and pressure. Urodilatin is released from distal tubular kidney cells when there is increased arterial pressure and increased renal blood flow. These hormones are natural antagonists to the renin-angiotensin-aldosterone system. The restoration of lower atrial pressure then inhibits further release of ANP and BNP.

Chloride is the major anion in the ECF and provides electroneutrality, particularly in relation to sodium. Chloride transport is generally passive and follows the active transport of sodium so that increases or decreases in chloride are proportional to changes in sodium. Chloride concentration tends to vary inversely with changes in the concentration of bicarbonate (HCO_3^-), the other major ECF anion.

Water Balance

One manner by which water balance is regulated is through the perception of thirst. Thirst is a sensation that stimulates water-drinking behavior. Thirst is experienced when water loss equals 2% of an individual's body weight or when there is an increase in osmolality. Dry mouth, hyperosmolality, and plasma volume depletion activate hypothalamic **osmoreceptors.** The action of the osmoreceptors then causes thirst. Drinking water restores plasma volume and dilutes the ECF osmolality.

Water balance also is directly regulated by **antidiuretic hormone (arginine-vasopressin),** which is secreted when plasma osmolality increases or circulating blood volume decreases and blood pressure drops (Figure 3-5). Increased plasma osmolality occurs with a water deficit or sodium excess in relation to water. The increased osmolality stimulates hypothalamic osmoreceptors. In addition to causing thirst, the stimulated osmoreceptors signal the posterior pituitary to release ADH. The action of ADH is to increase the permeability of renal tubular cells to water, increasing water reabsorption and promoting the restoration of plasma volume and blood pressure. Urine concentration increases, and the reabsorbed water decreases plasma osmolality, returning it toward normal. Like most hormones, ADH is regulated by a feedback mechanism. The restoration of plasma osmolality, blood volume, and blood pressure then inhibits ADH secretion.

With fluid loss (dehydration) (e.g., from vomiting, diarrhea, or excessive sweating), a decrease in blood volume and blood pressure often occurs. **Baroreceptors (volume/pressure sensitive receptors)** (stretch receptors that are sensitive to changes in arterial volume and pressure) also stimulate the release of ADH. Baroreceptors are located in the right and left atria and large veins, and in the aorta, pulmonary arteries, and carotid sinus. When arterial and atrial pressure drops baroreceptors signal the hypothalamus to release ADH. The reabsorption of water mediated by ADH then promotes the restoration of plasma volume and blood pressure (see Figure 3-5). ADH also stimulates arterial vasoconstriction.

ALTERATIONS IN SODIUM, CHLORIDE, AND WATER BALANCE

Alterations in sodium and water balance are closely related. Water imbalances may develop because of changes in osmotic gradients caused by gain or loss of salt. Likewise, sodium imbalances occur with alterations in body water volume. Generally the alterations can be classified as changes in tonicity, or the change in concentration of electrolytes in relation to water (see Chapter 1). Alterations can therefore be classified as isotonic, hypertonic, or hypotonic (Table 3-6 and Figure 3-6).

Isotonic Alterations

The term **isotonic** refers to a solution that has the same concentration of solutes as the plasma. Isotonic alterations occur when changes in TBW are accompanied by proportional changes

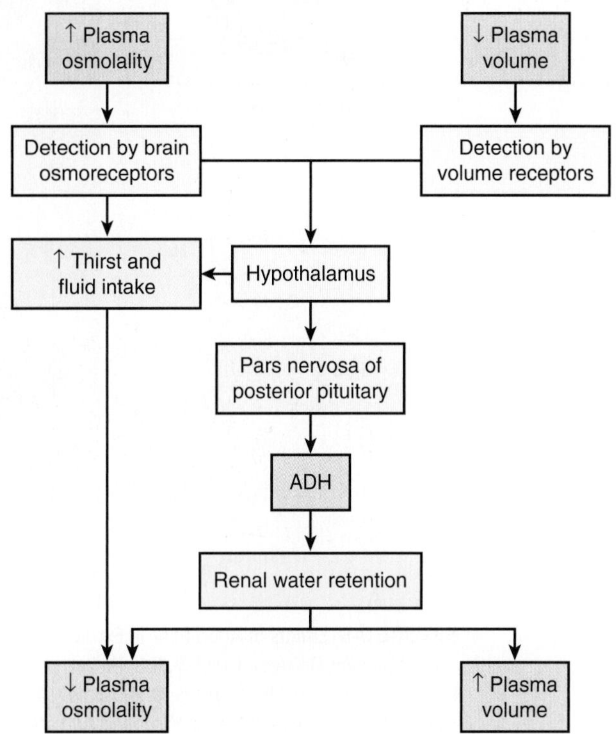

FIGURE 3-5 The Antidiuretic Hormone (ADH) System.

in the amounts of electrolytes and water. For example, if an individual loses pure plasma or ECF, fluid volume is depleted but the number and type of electrolytes (e.g., sodium) and the osmolality remain within a normal range. Excessive amounts of isotonic body fluids can result from excessive administration of intravenous normal saline (0.9% NaCl) or oversecretion of aldosterone with renal retention of both sodium and water. *Isotonic fluid loss* results in hypovolemia. Causes include hemorrhage, severe wound drainage, and excessive diaphoresis (sweating). Loss of extracellular volume results in weight loss, dryness of skin and mucous membranes, decreased urine output, increased hematocrit value, and symptoms of hypovolemia. Indicators of hypovolemia include a rapid heart rate and flattened neck veins, and can present with a normal or decreased blood pressure. In severe states, hypovolemic shock (severe hypotension) can occur (see Chapter 48).

Isotonic fluid excesses result in hypervolemia. Causes include excessive administration of intravenous fluids, hypersecretion of aldosterone, the effects of drugs such as cortisone, or renal failure. Weight gain and a decrease in hematocrit level and plasma protein concentration caused by the diluting effect of excess plasma volume will occur. The neck veins may distend, and the blood pressure increases. Increased capillary hydrostatic pressure leads to edema formation. If the plasma volume is great enough, pulmonary edema and heart failure develop.

TABLE 3-6 WATER AND SOLUTE IMBALANCES

TONICITY	MECHANISM
Isotonic (isoosmolar) imbalance	Gain or loss of extracellular fluid (ECF) resulting in a concentration equivalent to a 0.9% sodium chloride (salt) solution (normal saline); no shrinking or swelling of cells
Hypertonic (hyperosmolar) imbalance	Imbalance that results in an ECF concentration >0.9% salt solution; that is, water loss or solute gain; cells shrink in a hypertonic fluid
Hypotonic (hypoosmolar) imbalance	Imbalance that results in an ECF <0.9% salt solution; that is, water gain or solute loss; cells swell in a hypotonic fluid

Hypertonic Alterations

Hypertonic fluid alterations develop when the osmolality of the ECF is elevated above normal (greater than 294 mOsm). The most common causes are an increased concentration of ECF sodium (hypernatremia) or a deficit of ECF free water. In both instances the hypertonicity of the ECF attracts water from the intracellular space, causing ICF dehydration. A primary increase

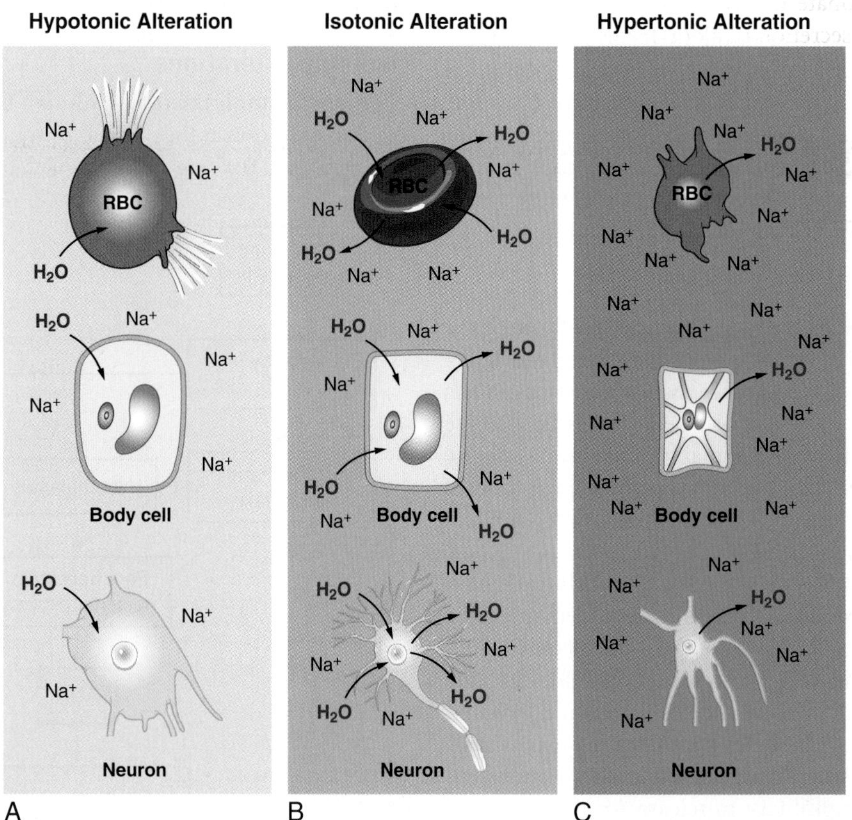

FIGURE 3-6 Effects of Alterations in Extracellular Sodium Concentration in RBC, Body Cell, and Neuron. **A,** *Hypotonic Alteration:* Decrease in ECF sodium (Na) concentration (hyponatremia) results in ICF osmotic attraction of water with swelling and potential busting of cells. **B,** *Isotonic Alteration:* Normal concentration of sodium in the ECF and no change in shifts of fluid in or out of cells. **C,** *Hypertonic Alteration:* An increase in ECF sodium concentration (hypernatremia) results in osmotic attraction of water out of cells with cell shrinkage. *RBC,* Red blood cell.

in the amount of ECF sodium causes an osmotic attraction of water and symptoms of *hypervolemia*. In contrast, a hypertonic state caused primarily by free water loss leads to *hypovolemia* (Table 3-7).

Hypernatremia

PATHOPHYSIOLOGY. **Hypernatremia** occurs when serum sodium levels exceed 147 mEq/L. Increased serum sodium concentration may be caused by loss of water (most common) or an acute gain in sodium. With water loss, both ICF dehydration and ECF dehydration occur. Hyperosmolality is a common result of hypernatremia. Because sodium is largely in the ECF, increases in the concentration of sodium cause intracellular dehydration and hypervolemia (see Table 3-7 and Figure 3-6, *C*).

Increased sodium concentration caused by water deprivation or water loss is associated with fever or respiratory tract infections, which increase the respiratory rate and enhance water loss from the lungs. Diabetes insipidus (deficiency of ADH), polyuria (frequent urination), profuse sweating, and diarrhea cause water loss in relation to sodium concentration. Infants with severe diarrhea are particularly vulnerable. Insufficient water intake also can cause hypernatremia (e.g., individuals who are immobilized or receiving gastric feedings, those who are comatose or confused, or infants because they cannot communicate thirst).

Increased sodium retention occurs because of (1) inappropriate administration of hypertonic saline solution (e.g., as sodium bicarbonate for treatment of acidosis during cardiac arrest); (2) oversecretion of aldosterone (as in primary hyperaldosteronism), where sodium reabsorption exceeds water reabsorption; or (3) Cushing syndrome (caused by excess secretion of adrenocorticotropic hormone [ACTH], which also causes increased secretion of aldosterone). High amounts of dietary sodium rarely cause hypernatremia in a healthy individual because the sodium is eliminated by the kidneys. However, increased amounts of dietary sodium (greater than 5 grams per day) is associated with cardiovascular disease (see Chapter 32).

CLINICAL MANIFESTATIONS. Water is redistributed to the extracellular space, and intracellular dehydration ensues. Thirst, fever, dry mucous membranes, hypotension, tachycardia, low jugular venous pressure, and restlessness are associated with hypernatremia as a result of water loss. Pulmonary edema occurs when water shifts from the ICF to the interstitial space. Central nervous system symptoms are the most serious and are related to alterations in membrane potentials and shrinking of brain cells. Symptoms include muscle twitching and hyperreflexia (hyperactive reflexes), confusion, coma, convulsions, and cerebral hemorrhage from stretching of veins.

EVALUATION AND TREATMENT. The serum sodium level is usually more than 147 mEq/L. If there is water loss, urine specific gravity will be greater than 1.030 and the levels of hematocrit and plasma proteins will be elevated. The treatment of hypernatremia is to give an isotonic salt-free fluid (5% dextrose in water) until the serum sodium level returns to normal.[5] Fluid replacement must be given slowly to prevent cerebral edema and serum sodium levels need to be closely monitored. Hypervolemia and hypovolemia require treatment of the underlying clinical condition.

TABLE 3-7 CAUSES AND CONSEQUENCES OF HYPERTONIC IMBALANCES

CAUSATIVE FACTOR	MECHANISM	ECF EFFECTS	ICF EFFECTS
Increased sodium (hypernatremia)	Excessive hypertonic salt solutions Intravenous hypertonic sodium Saline-induced abortions Selected infant formulas Hyperaldosteronism Cushing syndrome	Hypervolemia Weight gain Bounding pulse Increased blood pressure Edema Venous distention Neuromuscular symptoms Muscle weakness Seizures	Intracellular dehydration Thirst Fever Decreased urine output Shrinkage of brain cells Confusion Coma Cerebral hemorrhage
Water deficit	Water deprivation Confusion or coma Inability to communicate Loss of thirst Water loss Watery diarrhea Diabetes insipidus Excessive diuresis Excessive diaphoresis	Hypovolemia Weight loss Weak pulses Postural hypotension Tachycardia	Intracellular dehydration See above
Other factors	Hyperglycemia	Initial dilutional hyponatremia Polyuria Polydipsia Weight loss Hypovolemia Late hypernatremia	Intracellular dehydration See above

ECF, Extracellular fluid; *ICF*, intracellular fluid.

TABLE 3-8 CAUSES AND CONSEQUENCES OF HYPOTONIC IMBALANCES

CAUSATIVE FACTOR	MECHANISM	ECF EFFECTS	ICF EFFECTS
Decreased sodium (hyponatremia)	Inadequate intake Hypoaldosteronism Excessive diuretic therapy Furosemide Ethacrynic acid Thiazides	Extracellular volume contraction and hypovolemia (but may not if there is water excess)	Increased intracellular water; edema Brain cell swelling, irritability, depression, confusion Systemic cellular edema, including weakness, anorexia, nausea, and diarrhea
Water excess	Excessive pure water intake Excessive administration of hypotonic intravenous solutions Drinking water to replace isotonic fluid losses Tap water enemas Psychogenic polydipsia Renal water retention Syndrome of inappropriate secretion of antidiuretic hormone (SIADH)	Extracellular volume expands with hypervolemia (but may not if fluid is trapped in intracellular space)	Edema (see above)
Other factors	Isotonic dehydration treated with intravenous D_5W; glucose in D_5W solution is metabolized to water, contributing to hyponatremia Nephrotic syndrome Cirrhosis Cardiac failure	Hypervolemia or hypovolemia	Edema (see above)

D_5W, Dextrose 5% in water; *ECF,* extracellular fluid; *ICF,* intracellular fluid.

Hyperchloremia

Because chloride follows sodium, **hyperchloremia** (elevation of serum chloride concentration greater than 105 mEq/L) often accompanies hypernatremia, as well as plasma bicarbonate deficits, as in hyperchloremic metabolic acidosis (see p. 126). There are no specific symptoms or treatment for chloride excess and treatment is related to management of the underlying disorder.

Water Deficit

PATHOPHYSIOLOGY. **Dehydration** refers to water deficit, but also is commonly used to indicate both sodium and water loss (isotonic or isoosmolar dehydration). **Pure water deficits** (hyperosmolar or hypertonic dehydration) are rare because most people have access to water. Individuals who are comatose or paralyzed continue insensible water losses through the skin and lungs with a minimal obligatory formation of urine. Hyperventilation caused by fever also may precipitate water deficit. The most common cause of water loss is increased renal clearance of free water as a result of impaired tubular function or inability to concentrate the urine, as with diabetes insipidus (decreased or absent ADH) (see Table 3-7 and Chapter 22).

CLINICAL MANIFESTATIONS. Marked water deficit is manifested by symptoms of dehydration: headache, thirst, dry skin and mucous membranes, weight loss, decreased urine output, and concentrated urine (with the exception of diabetes insipidus). Skin turgor may be normal or decreased. Symptoms of hypovolemia, including tachycardia, weak pulses, and postural hypotension, may be present.

EVALUATION AND TREATMENT. Elevated levels of hematocrit, serum sodium concentration, urine and serum osmolality, and urine specific gravity are associated with moderate water loss.

Treatment is to give water and stop fluid loss. Fluid replacement must be given slowly enough to prevent rapid movement of water into brain cells, which causes cerebral edema, seizures, brain injury, and death. When intravenous replacement is required, hypotonic saline solutions or 5% dextrose in water is used because pure water lyses red blood cells.

Hypotonic Alterations

Hypotonic fluid imbalances occur when the osmolality of the ECF is less than normal (less than 280 mOsm). The most common causes are sodium deficit (hyponatremia) or free water excess (water intoxication). Both causes lead to an intracellular overhydration (cellular edema) and cell swelling when water moves into the cell, where the osmotic pressure is greater (see Figure 3-6, *A*). Cerebral and pulmonary edema occur in conjunction with these fluid shifts.[6] With hyponatremia, the plasma volume then decreases, leading to symptoms of hypovolemia. With free water excess, the ECF volume is elevated, causing symptoms of hypervolemia (Table 3-8).

Hyponatremia

PATHOPHYSIOLOGY. **Hyponatremia** develops when the serum sodium concentration decreases to less than 135 mEq/L. It is the most common electrolyte disorder in hospitalized individuals.[7] Hyponatremia may be caused by sodium loss, inadequate sodium intake, or dilution of the body's sodium level. Clinical syndromes

WHAT'S NEW?

Hyponatremia and Hospitalization

Hyponatremia (serum sodium concentration <135 mmol/L) and severe hyponatremia (serum sodium concentration <120 mmol/L) are the most common electrolyte abnormalities among hospitalized individuals with risk for severe morbidity and mortality. Hyponatremia can be difficult to diagnose because it can develop with euvolemia, hypervolemia, or hypovolemia. In addition to older adults, children and premenopausal women are at particular risk as well as those receiving treatment in intensive care units and persons with cirrhosis with ascites, heart failure syndromes, brain injury, sepsis, or multiple organ failure. Death or brain damage may range from 50% to 83% and is related to cerebral edema, increased intracranial pressure, and cerebral hypoxemia, with symptoms of seizure, respiratory arrest, coma, and death. Use of thiazide diuretics is a common cause of hyponatremia and can occur within 2 weeks of initiation of treatment. Postoperative hyponatremia is caused by administration of hypotonic fluids and dysregulation of the secretion of antidiuretic hormone (arginine-vasopressin). Treatment with fluid restriction, diuretic treatment, sodium replacement, and urea administration is effective in less severe cases. Hypertonic sodium chloride is usually safe with acute hyponatremia. Brain myelinolysis is a risk if treatment is given too rapidly. Arginine-vasopressin receptor antagonists (vaptans) can provide effective treatment and they work by increasing blood flow to the kidney with increased urine formation without loss of electrolytes. Vaptans are contraindicated in hypovolemic hyponatremia. Frequent monitoring with attention to subtle symptoms and early treatment lead to improved outcomes.

Data from Aperis G, Alivanis P: *Rev Recent Clin Trials* 6(2):177–188, 2011; Chawla A et al: *Clin J Am Soc Nephrol* 6(5):960–965, 2011; Elhassan EA, Schrier RW: *Exp Opin Investig Drugs* 20(3):373–380, 2011; Human T: *Pharmacother* 31(5 Suppl):18S–24S, 2011; Robertson GL: *Nat Rev Endocrinol* 7(3):151–161, 2011; Pfennig CL, Slovis CM: *Emerg Med Pract* 14(10):1–26, 2012; Vaishya R et al: *J Indian Med Assoc* 110(2):94–97, 2012; Konishi M et al: *J Card Fail* 18(8):620–625, 2012; Lindner G, Schwarz C: *Minerva Med* 103(4):279–291, 2012.

that may cause hyponatremia include syndrome of inappropriate secretion of antidiuretic hormone (SIADH, excess ADH) or failure of the distal tubules to reabsorb sodium. Sodium deficits usually cause hypoosmolality and water moves into cells, resulting in cell swelling (see Figure 3-6, *A*, and What's New? Hyponatremia and Hospitalization).

Pure sodium deficits are usually caused by diuretics[8] and extrarenal losses such as vomiting, diarrhea, gastrointestinal suctioning, or burns. **Inadequate intake of dietary sodium** is rare but can occur in individuals consuming low-sodium diets, particularly among those taking diuretics. **Dilutional hyponatremias** occur when there is an excess of TBW in relation to total body sodium or a shift of water from the ICF to the ECF space (e.g., administration of mannitol). Replacement of fluid loss with intravenous 5% dextrose in water also can cause a dilutional hyponatremia because once the glucose is metabolized, a hypotonic solution remains with a diluting effect. Use of excess hypotonic saline (e.g., 0.45% NaCl) may also result in dilution. In addition, excessive sweating may stimulate thirst and intake of large amounts of water, which dilute sodium; this condition may be associated with endurance exercise in which there is only pure water replacement.

Hyponatremia may cause hypotonic or hypertonic alterations. During acute oliguric renal failure, severe congestive heart failure, or cirrhosis, renal excretion of water is impaired. Both TBW and sodium levels are increased, but TBW level exceeds the increase in sodium level, producing a **hypotonic hyponatremia. Hypertonic hyponatremia** develops with the shift of water from the ICF to the ECF as occurs with hyperglycemia, hyperlipidemia, and hyperproteinemia. The osmotic fluid shift to the ECF in turn dilutes the concentration of sodium and other electrolytes.

CLINICAL MANIFESTATIONS. Cellular swelling and deficits of intracellular sodium alter the ability of cells to depolarize and repolarize normally (see Chapter 1). Neurologic changes characteristic of hyponatremia include lethargy, headache, confusion, apprehension, seizures, and coma. Pure sodium losses may be accompanied by loss of ECF, causing hypovolemia with symptoms of hypotension, tachycardia, and decreased urine output. Dilutional hyponatremia is accompanied by weight gain, edema, ascites, and jugular vein distention. Cerebral edema can be a life-threatening complication of hypervolemic hyponatremia caused by increases in intracranial pressure.

EVALUATION AND TREATMENT. In hyponatremic states, serum sodium concentration falls to less than 135 mEq/L. With pure sodium deficits, the hematocrit and plasma protein levels may be elevated. Urine specific gravity is less than 1.010 when renal function is normal because sodium is maximally conserved.

Treatment of hyponatremia is related to the contributing disorder. Losses of sodium and water volume are calculated from the clinical evaluation, and appropriate solutions then are selected for replacement. Restriction of water intake is required in most cases of dilutional hyponatremia because body sodium levels may be normal or increased even though serum concentrations are low. Hypertonic saline solutions are used cautiously with severe hyponatremia or the presence of symptoms such as seizures.[9]

Hypochloremia

Hypochloremia, a low level of serum chloride (less than 97 mEq/L), usually occurs with hyponatremia or an elevated bicarbonate concentration, as in metabolic alkalosis (see p. 128). Sodium deficit related to restricted intake, use of diuretics, and vomiting are accompanied by chloride deficiency. Cystic fibrosis is a genetic disease characterized by hypochloremia (see Chapters 36 and 42). In all cases, treatment of the underlying cause is required.

Water Excess

PATHOPHYSIOLOGY. When the body is functioning normally, it is almost impossible to produce an excess of TBW since water balance is regulated by the kidneys. However, some individuals with psychogenic disorders develop **water intoxication** from compulsive water drinking. Intensive exercise with replacement of large volumes of electrolyte-free water also causes overhydration. Acute renal failure, severe congestive heart failure, and cirrhosis are clinical conditions that can precipitate water excess. **Decreased urine formation** from renal disease or decreased renal blood flow contributes to water excess. The overall effect is dilution of the ECF with the movement of water to the intracellular space by osmosis. The syndrome of inappropriate secretion of ADH (SIADH), also known as vasopressin dysregulation, enhances water retention because ADH levels are elevated (see Chapter 22, p. 718). Water excess is usually accompanied by hyponatremia.

CLINICAL MANIFESTATIONS. The symptoms of water excess are related to the rate at which water loading has occurred. Acute excesses cause cerebral edema with confusion and convulsions. Weakness, nausea, muscle twitching, headache, and weight gain are common symptoms of chronic water accumulation.

EVALUATION AND TREATMENT. Serum sodium concentration can be decreased, but this also can occur with a pure sodium deficit. Serum and urine osmolalities are decreased because water concentration will be in excess of sodium concentration. Urine sodium concentration will be reduced. The hematocrit value is reduced from the dilutional effect of water excess.

Fluid restriction for 24 hours is an effective treatment if there are no severe neurologic symptoms or convulsions. Small amounts of intravenous hypertonic sodium chloride (i.e., 3% sodium chloride) can be given when neurologic symptoms are severe.

ALTERATIONS IN POTASSIUM, CALCIUM, PHOSPHATE, AND MAGNESIUM BALANCE

Potassium

Potassium (K^+) is the major intracellular electrolyte and is found in most body fluids (see Table 3-5, p. 108). The ICF concentration of K^+ is 150 to 160 mEq/L; the ECF concentration is 3.5 to 5.0 mEq/L. Total body potassium content is about 4000 mEq, with most of it located in the cells. Daily dietary intake of potassium is 40 to 150 mEq/day, with an average of 1.5 mEq/kg body weight.

Potassium balance is maintained by renal excretion of K^+ absorbed from the gastrointestinal tract. Absorbed dietary K^+ moves rapidly into cells. However, the distribution of K^+ between intracellular and extracellular fluids can fluctuate and is influenced by several factors. Aldosterone, insulin, epinephrine (β-adrenergic stimulation), and alkalosis facilitate the shift of K^+ into cells. Insulin deficiency, aldosterone deficiency, acidosis, and strenuous exercise facilitate the shift of K^+ out of cells. α-Adrenergics impair K^+ entry into cells. Glucagon blocks entry of K^+ into cells, and glucocorticoids promote K^+ excretion. Potassium also will move out of cells along with water when there is increased ECF osmolarity (number of osmoles of solute per liter of fluid). If cells lyse, they release their intracellular K^+ into the ECF, which can cause an acute rise in plasma K^+ levels.

Besides acting to conserve sodium, *aldosterone is a major factor in potassium regulation.* Elevated plasma K^+ concentration causes adrenal secretion of aldosterone. Aldosterone then stimulates the release of K^+ into the urine by the distal renal tubules.

Insulin contributes to the regulation of plasma potassium levels by stimulating the Na^+-K^+-ATPase pump, thereby promoting the movement of K^+ into liver and muscle cells simultaneously with glucose transport. The intracellular movement of K^+ prevents an acute hyperkalemia related to food intake. Insulin also can be used to treat hyperkalemia. However, dangerously low levels of plasma K^+ can result from the administration of insulin when K^+ levels are depressed. Potassium balance is especially significant in the treatment of conditions requiring insulin administration, such as insulin-dependent diabetes mellitus (type 1).

The difference in the K^+ intracellular to extracellular concentration is maintained by a sodium-potassium active transport system (Na^+-K^+-ATPase pump). The ratio of ICF K^+ concentration to ECF K^+ concentration is the major determinant of the resting membrane potential, which is necessary for the transmission and conduction of nervous impulses, maintenance of normal cardiac rhythms, and contraction of skeletal and smooth muscles (see Figure 1-35, p. 35). The constant diffusion of positively charged K^+ out of the cell (i.e., down its concentration gradient) makes the interior of cells electronegative in relation to the ECF. Changes in the ratio of ICF to ECF potassium are responsible for many of the symptoms associated with K^+ imbalance.

As the predominant ICF ion, K^+ exerts a major influence on the regulation of ICF osmolality and fluid balance, as well as on intracellular electrical neutrality in relation to hydrogen (H^+) and Na^+ levels. Potassium is also necessary for a variety of metabolic functions and is required for glycogen deposition in liver and skeletal muscle cells.

The kidney provides the most efficient regulation of K^+ level balance over time. The amount of K^+ excreted varies in proportion to the dietary intake (40 to 120 mEq/day). Potassium is freely filtered by the renal glomerulus, and 90% is reabsorbed by the proximal tubule and loop of Henle. **Principal cells** in the collecting duct secrete K^+ and **intercalated cells** in the collecting duct reabsorb K^+. Dietary K^+ intake, aldosterone level, and distal tubule urine flow determine the amount of K^+ excreted from the body. Unlike sodium, the renal mechanism for conserving K^+ is weak, even when total body K^+ stores are depleted. The gut also may sense the amount of K^+ ingested and stimulate renal K^+ excretion.[10] However, a low K^+ intake also suppresses renal K^+ excretion.

Renal regulation of potassium level includes:

1. The concentration gradient for K^+ at the distal tubule and collecting duct
2. The distal tubule flow rate and distal tubule sodium delivery
3. The action of aldosterone
4. Changes in pH (causing acidosis or alkalosis)

The concentration of K^+ in the distal tubular cells is determined primarily by the plasma concentration in the peritubular capillaries. When plasma K^+ concentration increases because of increased dietary intake or shifts from the ICF to the ECF occur, K^+ is secreted into the urine by principal cells in the collecting ducts. Decreased levels of plasma K^+ result in decreased collecting duct secretion and reabsorption by intercalated cells, although K^+ losses of approximately 5 to 15 mEq/day will continue.

Changes in distal tubule flow rate and distal tubule sodium delivery also influence the concentration gradient for K^+ secretion. When the flow rate and sodium delivery are high, as occurs with the administration of diuretics, the concentration of K^+ in the distal tubular urine is lower, favoring the secretion of K^+ into the tubule. Potassium secretion decreases when distal tubule flow rate and sodium delivery are low. However, aldosterone stimulates K^+ secretion by the distal tubule and serves to preserve K^+ secretion and K^+ balance during dehydration and extracellular volume depletion, when tubular delivery of Na^+ and flow rate are reduced.

Changes in pH and thus in hydrogen ion concentration also affect K^+ balance.[11] Hydrogen ions move from the ECF to the ICF during states of acidosis. When hydrogen is moving into the cell, K^+ shifts out of the cell to the ECF to maintain a balance of cations across the cell membrane. This occurs in part because of a decrease in Na^+-K^+-ATPase pump activity. The decreased ICF K^+ level in the distal tubular cells results in decreased secretion of K^+ into the urine, contributing to hyperkalemia (hyperkalemic acidosis), although total body K^+ level may not change. In contrast, intracellular fluid levels of hydrogen are diminished during states of alkalosis. Alkalosis causes K^+ to shift into the cell, so the distal tubular cells increase their secretion of K^+ into the urine, contributing to hypokalemia (hypokalemic alkalosis). The management of alterations associated with acid-base imbalances requires that the acid-base imbalances must be treated before or concurrently with treatment of changes in K^+ concentration.

Potassium adaptation is the ability of the body to adapt to increased levels of K^+ intake over time. A sudden increase in K^+ level may be fatal, but if the intake is slowly increased by amounts of more than 120 mEq/day, the kidney can increase the urinary excretion of K^+ and maintain K^+ concentration balance.

Hypokalemia

PATHOPHYSIOLOGY. Potassium deficiency, or **hypokalemia,** develops when the serum K^+ concentration decreases to less than 3.5 mEq/L. Because intracellular and total body stores of K^+ are difficult to measure, changes in K^+ balance are described by the plasma concentration, although changes in total body K^+ level are not always reflected in the plasma K^+ concentration. Generally, lowered serum K^+ level indicates a loss of total body K^+. Because K^+ is lost from the ECF, the change in the concentration gradient favors movement of K^+ from the cell to the ECF. The ICF/ECF concentration ratio is maintained, but the amount of total body K^+ is depleted.[12]

Factors contributing to the development of hypokalemia include *reduced intake of potassium,* increased entry of K^+ into cells, and increased losses of body K^+. Dietary deficiency of K^+ is a rare cause but may occur in elderly individuals with both low protein intake (meat) and inadequate intake of fruits and vegetables, and in individuals with alcoholism or anorexia nervosa. Reduced K^+ intake generally becomes a problem when combined with other causes of K^+ depletion.

ECF hypokalemia can develop without losses of total body K^+ when K^+ is redistributed between the ECF and ICF. Alkalosis, particularly respiratory alkalosis, is the most common clinical cause of these shifts. In alkalosis, ECF hydrogen moves out of the cell to correct the alkalosis, which causes K^+ to move into the cell to maintain an ionic balance. Insulin also promotes cellular uptake of K^+ and can cause an ECF potassium deficit, particularly with the intake of high carbohydrate loads. Severe, even fatal, hypokalemia may occur if insulin is administered without also providing K^+ supplements.

Treatment of pernicious anemia with vitamin B_{12} or folate also may precipitate hypokalemia if the formation of new red blood cells causes enough K^+ uptake to effect an extracellular decrease in K^+ concentration. **Familial hypokalemic periodic paralysis** is a rare genetically transmitted disease that also causes K^+ to shift into the intracellular space.

Hypokalemia also can occur when K^+ shifts from the ICF to the ECF, as occurs in conjunction with renal losses. For example, in diabetic ketoacidosis, the increased hydrogen ion concentration in the ECF causes H^+ to shift into the cell in exchange for K^+ at the same time diuresis is occurring. A normal level of K^+ is maintained in the plasma, but K^+ continues to be lost in the urine, causing a deficit in the amount of total body potassium. Total body K^+ depletion becomes evident when insulin treatment and rehydration therapy are initiated.

Potassium loss also occurs through normal body functions, but without causing hypokalemia. Average daily losses of K^+ are as follows:

Location	Daily Loss (mEq/L)
Stool	5-10
Sweat	0-20
Urine	40-120

Losses of K^+ from body stores are most commonly caused by gastrointestinal and renal disorders. Diarrhea (from any cause), intestinal drainage tubes or fistulae, and laxative abuse also may result in hypokalemia. Normally, only 5 to 10 mEq of potassium and 100 to 150 ml of water are excreted in the stool each day. With diarrhea, fluid and electrolyte losses can be voluminous, with several liters of fluid and 100 to 200 mEq of K^+ lost per day. Vomiting or applying continuous nasogastric suction frequently is associated with K^+ depletion, partly because of the K^+ lost from the gastric fluid but principally because of renal compensation for volume depletion and the metabolic alkalosis (elevated bicarbonate levels) that occurs from sodium, chloride, and hydrogen ion losses. The loss of fluid and sodium stimulates the secretion of aldosterone and ADH, which in turn causes renal loss of K^+. The elevated flow of bicarbonate at the distal tubule contributes to renal excretion of K^+ because of increased tubular lumen electronegativity.

Renal losses of K^+ are related to increased secretion of K^+ by the distal tubule. Use of diuretics, excessive aldosterone secretion, increased distal tubular flow rate, and low plasma magnesium concentration all may contribute to urinary losses of K^+. Many diuretics, including thiazides, furosemide, ethacrynic acid, and osmotic diuretics, inhibit the reabsorption of sodium chloride, causing the diuretic effect. The distal tubular flow rate then increases, promoting K^+ excretion. If sodium loss is severe, the compensating aldosterone secretion (which causes secondary hyperaldosteronism) may further deplete K^+ stores. Primary hyperaldosteronism with excessive secretion of aldosterone from an adrenal adenoma also causes K^+ wasting. Many kidney diseases result in a reduced ability to conserve sodium. The disordered

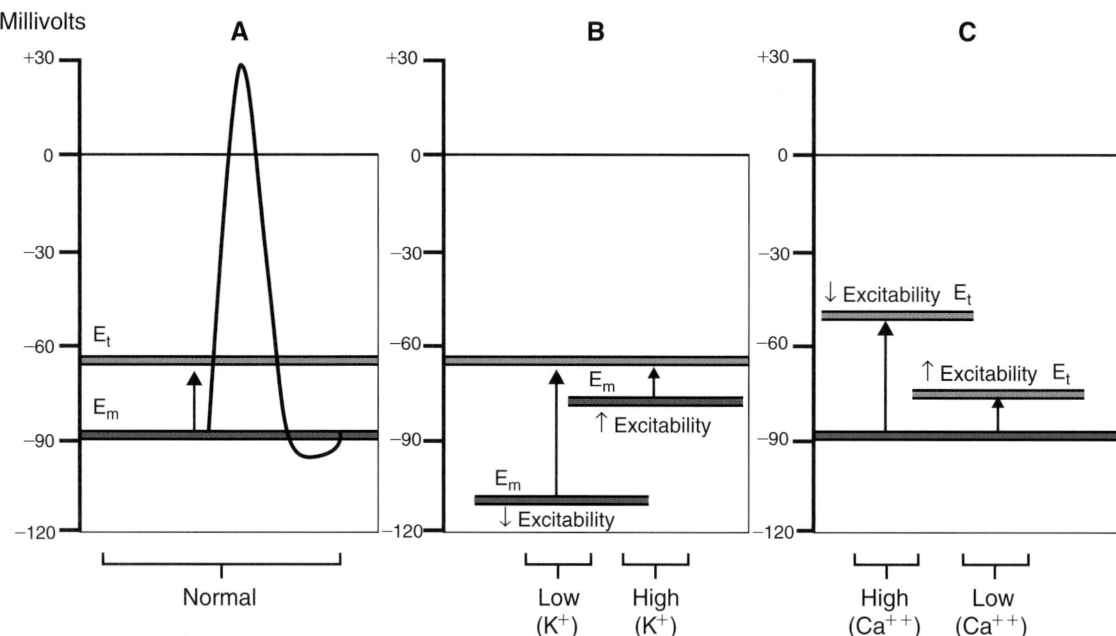

FIGURE 3-7 Effects of Potassium (K^+) and Calcium (Ca^{++}) on Membrane Excitability. **A,** Normal membrane excitability: Potassium affects resting membrane potential (E_m), and calcium affects threshold potential (E_t). **B,** Effects of potassium (K^+) changes on membrane potential. **C,** Effect of calcium (Ca^{++}) on threshold potential. **NOTE:** *Hyperpolarization* can be caused by either hypokalemia (E_m more negative) or hypercalcemia (E_t less negative)–distance between E_m and E_t is increased (decreased excitability); and *hypopolarization* can be caused by either hyperkalemia (E_m less negative) or hypocalcemia (E_t more negative)—distance between E_m and E_t is decreased (increased excitabillity).

sodium reabsorption produces a diuretic effect, and the increased distal tubule flow rate favors the secretion of K^+. Magnesium deficits stimulate renin release and hyperaldosteronism, causing hypokalemia. Several antibiotics, including amphotericin B, gentamicin, and carbenicillin, are known to cause hypokalemia.

CLINICAL MANIFESTATIONS. Mild losses of K^+ are usually asymptomatic. A wide range of dysfunctions may result from severe hypokalemia (<2.5 mEq/L). *Neuromuscular and cardiac effects* of hypokalemia produce the most common symptoms.[13] Neuromuscular excitability is decreased, causing skeletal muscle weakness, smooth muscle atony, and cardiac dysrhythmias. As Chapter 1 describes, the resting membrane potential (E_m) is determined by the *ratio* of extracellular to intracellular K^+ ion concentration. Because the concentration of K^+ in the ECF is small, only small changes in ECF potassium level are required to influence the resting membrane potential and affect neuromuscular excitability (the difference between resting membrane and threshold potentials)[1] (Figure 3-7, *A*). When extracellular K^+ levels decrease rapidly, intracellular K^+ diffuses more readily out of the cell and the resting membrane potential becomes more negative (i.e., from −90 to −100 millivolts). If the threshold potential (E_t) remains stable, the difference between resting membrane potential and threshold potential increases and the cell membrane becomes **hyperpolarized,** requiring a stronger stimulus (decreased excitability) to initiate depolarization and an action potential (Figure 3-7, *B* [low K^+]).

The *cardiac effects of hypokalemia* are related to decreased membrane excitability (see Figure 3-7, *B*). Because K^+ contributes to the repolarization phase of the action potential, hypokalemia delays ventricular repolarization and the frequency of action potentials. The membrane potential remains partially depolarized with slowed conduction and abnormal pacemaker activity. A variety of dysrhythmias may occur, including sinus bradycardia, atrioventricular block, and paroxysmal atrial tachycardia. The characteristic changes in the electrocardiogram reflect delayed repolarization. For instance, the amplitude of the T wave is decreased, the amplitude of the U wave is increased, and the ST segment is depressed (Figure 3-8). In severe states of hypokalemia, P waves peak and the QRS complex is prolonged. Hypokalemia also increases the risk of digitalis toxicity by slowing the sodium-potassium pump, which augments the action of digitalis in cardiac muscle by excessively increasing intracellular calcium and sodium concentrations.

Plasma calcium concentration also contributes to changes in neuromuscular excitability associated with hypokalemia. Increases in ECF calcium concentration tend to make the threshold potential (E_t) less negative and decrease membrane excitability, potentiating hyperpolarization, decreased excitability, and the neuromuscular effects of hypokalemia (Figure 3-7, *C*).

Carbohydrate metabolism is affected because hypokalemia depresses insulin secretion and alters hepatic and skeletal muscle glycogen synthesis. Renal function is impaired, with a decreased ability to concentrate urine. Polyuria (increased urine) and polydipsia (increased thirst) are associated with decreased responsiveness to ADH. Chronic potassium deficits lasting more than 1 month may damage renal tissue, with resulting interstitial fibrosis and tubular atrophy.

The onset of symptoms is related to the *rate of potassium depletion.* Because the body can accommodate slow losses of K^+, the decrease in ECF concentration may be slow enough to allow K^+ to shift from the intracellular space. The extracellular to intracellular K^+ concentration gradient then is restored toward normal,

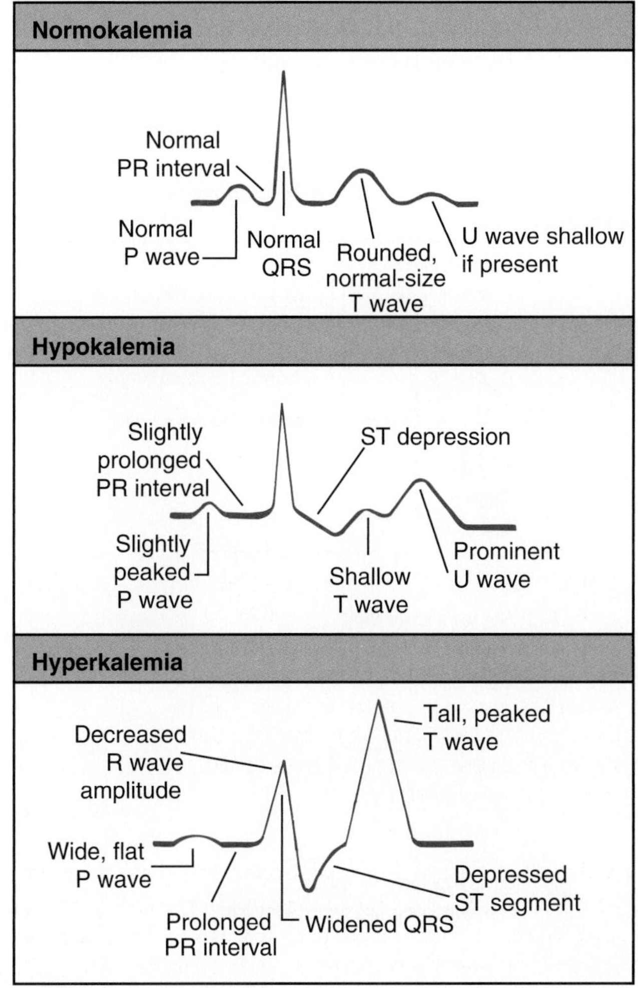

FIGURE 3-8 Electrocardiogram (ECG) Changes with Potassium Imbalance.

with less severe neuromuscular changes. With acute losses of K^+, changes in neuromuscular excitability are more profound. Skeletal muscle weakness initially occurs in the larger muscles of the legs and arms and ultimately affects the diaphragm and depresses ventilation. Paralysis and respiratory arrest then can occur. Loss of smooth muscle tone is manifested by orthostatic hypotension, constipation, intestinal distention, anorexia, nausea, vomiting, and paralytic ileus. Table 3-9 contains a summary of K^+ alterations.

EVALUATION AND TREATMENT. The diagnosis of hypokalemia is based on serum K^+ levels; however, it is important to examine the medical history and identify disorders associated with K^+ loss or shifts of extracellular K^+ to the intracellular space. Treatment involves an estimation of total body K^+ losses and correction of acid-base imbalances. Further losses of K^+ should be prevented, and the individual should be encouraged to eat foods rich in K^+. Potassium replacement is instituted cautiously to prevent hyperkalemia. The maximal rate of oral replacement is 40 to 80 mEq/day if renal function is normal. A maximal safe rate of intravenous replacement is 20 mEq/hr for adults. Because K^+ is irritating to blood vessels, a maximal concentration of 40 mEq/100 ml should be used. Serum K^+ values can be monitored until normokalemia is achieved.

Hyperkalemia

PATHOPHYSIOLOGY. An elevation of ECF potassium concentration *above 5.5 mEq/L* constitutes **hyperkalemia.** Because of efficient renal excretion, excesses of total body potassium are relatively rare. Acute increases in serum K^+ concentration are handled quickly through an increase in cellular uptake and renal excretion of body K^+ excesses.

Excesses of serum K^+ may be caused by *excessive intake,* a *shift of potassium from the ICF to the ECF,* or *decreased renal excretion.*[14] If renal function is normal, slow, long-term increases in K^+ intake are usually well tolerated through K^+ adaptation, although acute K^+ loading can exceed renal excretion rates. Use of stored whole blood, administration of intravenous boluses of penicillin G, or replacement of K^+ can precipitate hyperkalemia, particularly if renal function is impaired. Dietary excesses of K^+ are uncommon, but accidental ingestion of K^+ salt substitutes can cause toxicity.

Potassium shifts from the ICF to the ECF occur with a *change in cell membrane permeability* (e.g., from cell hypoxia, acidosis, or insulin deficiency). Burns, massive crush injuries, and extensive surgeries can cause cell trauma and loss of ICF potassium to the ECF. If renal function is sustained, K^+ will be excreted. As cell repair begins, hypokalemia develops if the excreted K^+ is not replaced.

Hypoxia can lead to hyperkalemia by diminishing the efficiency of cell membrane active transport, resulting in the escape of K^+ to the ECF. In states of *acidosis,* hydrogen ions shift into the cells in exchange for ICF potassium; hyperkalemia and acidosis therefore often occur together. Because insulin promotes cellular entry of K^+, *insulin deficits,* which occur with conditions such as diabetic ketoacidosis, are accompanied by hyperkalemia. *Digitalis overdose* may cause hyperkalemia by inhibiting the Na^+-K^+-ATPase pump. This pump normally maintains intracellular K^+ concentration and moves sodium and calcium to the ECF (see Chapter 1).

Decreased renal excretion of potassium is commonly associated with hyperkalemia. Renal failure that results in oliguria (urine output <30 ml/hr) is accompanied by elevations of serum K^+ concentration. The severity of hyperkalemia is related to the severity of renal dysfunction, the amount of K^+ intake, and the degree of acidosis from the renal failure. In acute renal failure K^+ levels rise more rapidly with more serious consequences than the slower rises associated with chronic renal failure. Hypoaldosteronism also can cause decreases in the urinary excretion of K^+. For example, Addison disease results in decreased production and secretion of aldosterone and thus contributes to hyperkalemia. Drugs that decrease renal potassium excretion (i.e., ACE inhibitors, angiotensin receptor blockers, and aldosterone antagonists) also may contribute to hyperkalemia. Frequently, however, these drugs are used in combination with diuretics that cause K^+ wasting in an attempt to balance renal K^+ gains and losses.

CLINICAL MANIFESTATIONS. Symptoms of hyperkalemia vary, but common characteristics are muscle weakness or paralysis and dysrhythmias with changes in the electrocardiogram. During mild attacks, increased neuromuscular irritability may be manifested as tingling of lips and fingers, restlessness, intestinal

TABLE 3-9 POTASSIUM ALTERATIONS

CAUSES	HYPOKALEMIA <3.5 mEq/L	HYPERKALEMIA >5.0 mEq/L
Intake	Decreased intake: starvation or anorexia nervosa, inadequate replacement	Excess dietary or intravenous intake
Loss	Increased renal loss: renal tubular failure, K^+-losing diuretics, hyperaldosteronism, vomiting, diarrhea, use of selected antibiotics	Decreased renal loss: renal failure, K^+-sparing diuretics, hypoaldosteronism
Cellular shifts	Shift from ECF to ICF: metabolic alkalosis, insulin administration	Shift from ICF to ECF: metabolic acidosis, cell injury
ORGAN SYSTEM MANIFESTATIONS		
Cardiovascular	Postural hypotension Dysrhythmias ECG changes (flattened T waves, U waves, ST depression, peaked P wave, prolonged QT interval) Weak, irregular pulse rate Ventricular fibrillation Cardiac arrest	Dysrhythmias ECG changes (peaked T waves, prolonged PR interval, absent P wave with widened QRS complex) Bradycardia Heart block Cardiac arrest
Nervous	Lethargy Fatigue Confusion Paresthesias Decreased tendon reflexes	Anxiety Tingling Numbness
Gastrointestinal	Nausea and vomiting Decreased motility Distention Decreased bowel sounds Ileus	Nausea and vomiting Diarrhea Colicky pain
Kidney	Inability to concentrate urine Water loss Thirst Kidney damage	Oliguria Kidney damage
Skeletal and smooth muscle	Weakness Flaccid paralysis Respiratory arrest Constipation Bladder dysfunction	Early: hyperactive muscles Late: weakness and flaccid paralysis

cramping, and diarrhea. Severe hyperkalemia causes muscle weakness, loss of muscle tone, and paralysis. In mild states of hyperkalemia, the more rapid repolarization is reflected in the electrocardiogram as narrow and taller T waves with a shortened QT interval. Severe hyperkalemia (serum levels ≥6 mEq/L) depresses the ST segment, prolongs the PR interval, and widens the QRS complex (loss of atrial activity) (see Figure 3-8). Delayed conduction and bradydysrhythmias are common in hyperkalemia, with alterations in cardiac conduction causing ventricular fibrillation or cardiac arrest.

As with hypokalemia, changes in the ratio of intracellular to extracellular K^+ concentration contribute to the symptoms of hyperkalemia. If extracellular K^+ concentration increases without a significant change in intracellular K^+ concentration, the resting membrane potential becomes more positive (i.e., changes from −90 to −80 millivolts) and the cell membrane is **hypopolarized** (the inside of the cell becomes less negative or partially depolarized [increased excitability]) (see Figure 3-7, *B*). (Electrical properties of cells are discussed in Chapter 1.) With relatively mild elevations in extracellular K^+ concentration, the cell more rapidly repolarizes and becomes more irritable (peaked T waves). An action potential then is initiated more rapidly because the distance between the resting membrane potential and the threshold potential has been shortened. With more severe hyperkalemia, the resting membrane potential approaches or exceeds the threshold potential (wide QRS merging with T wave). In this case the cell is not able to repolarize and therefore does not respond to excitation stimuli. The most serious consequence is cardiac standstill.

Like the effects of hypokalemia, the neuromuscular effects of hyperkalemia are related to the rate of increase in the ECF potassium concentration and the presence of other contributing factors, such as acidosis and calcium balance. Long-term increases in ECF potassium concentration result in shifts of K^+ into the cell because the tendency is to maintain a normal ratio of intracellular/extracellular potassium concentrations. Acute elevations of extracellular K^+ concentration affect neuromuscular irritability because this ratio is disrupted.

Because calcium influences the threshold potential, changes in extracellular fluid calcium concentration can augment or override the effects of hyperkalemia. With hypocalcemia the threshold potential becomes more negative, enhancing the neuromuscular effects of hyperkalemia. Hypercalcemia causes the threshold potential to become less negative, counteracting the effects of hyperkalemia on resting membrane potential (see Figure 3-7, *C*). See Table 3-9 for a summary of potassium alteration.

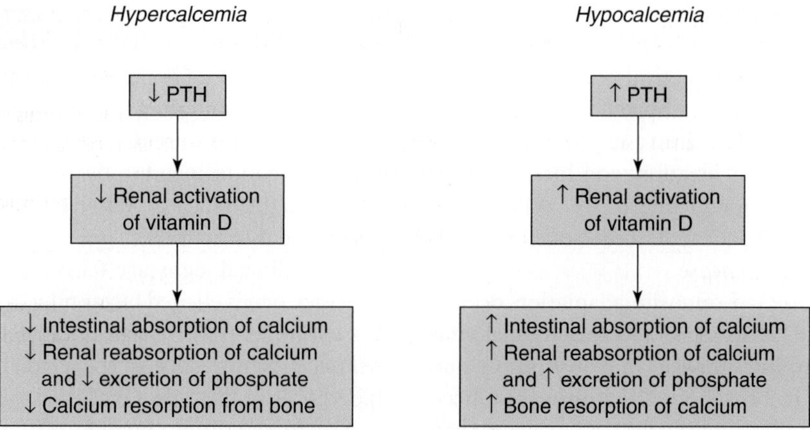

FIGURE 3-9 Hormonal Regulation of Calcium Balance. *PTH,* Parathyroid hormone.

EVALUATION AND TREATMENT. Hyperkalemia should be investigated when there is a history of renal disease, massive trauma, insulin deficiency, Addison disease, use of potassium salt substitutes, or metabolic acidosis. The acuity of the onset of symptoms may be related to the underlying cause.

Management of hyperkalemia is related to treating the contributing causes and correcting the potassium excess. Normalizing the extracellular potassium concentration can be achieved with a variety of methods; the treatment chosen is related to the cause and severity of the problem. Calcium gluconate can be administered to restore normal neuromuscular irritability when serum potassium levels are dangerously high. Administration of glucose, which readily stimulates insulin secretion, or administration of glucose and insulin for those with diabetes, facilitates cellular entry of potassium. Buffered solutions correct metabolic acidosis and lower serum potassium level. Oral or rectal administration of cation exchange resins, which exchange sodium for potassium in the intestine, can be effective. Dialysis effectively removes potassium when renal failure has occurred.

Calcium and Phosphate

The total body content of calcium is about 1200 g. Most calcium (99%) is located in bone as hydroxyapatite (an inorganic compound that contributes to bone rigidity), and the remainder is in the plasma and body cells. The total fraction of calcium circulating in the blood is small (9.0 to 10.5 mg/dl) and about 50% is bound to plasma proteins, primarily albumin. About 40% is in the free or ionized form (5.5 to 5.6 mg/dl). Ionized calcium has the most important physiologic functions.

Calcium (Ca^{++}) is a necessary ion for many fundamental metabolic processes. It is the major cation associated with the structure of bones and teeth. It serves as an enzymatic cofactor for blood clotting and is required for hormone secretion and the function of cell receptors. Plasma membrane stability and permeability are directly related to calcium ions, as is the transmission of nerve impulses and the contraction of muscles. Intracellular calcium is located primarily in the mitochondria.

Phosphate ($HPO_4^=$) is found primarily in bone (85%), with smaller amounts found within the intracellular and extracellular spaces. In the plasma, phosphate exists in phospholipids and phosphate esters and as inorganic phosphate, which is the ionized form. The normal serum levels of inorganic phosphate range from 2.5 to 4.5 mg/dl and may be as high as 6.0 to 7.0 mg/dl in infants and young children. Intracellular phosphate has many metabolic forms, including the high-energy structures creatine phosphate and adenosine triphosphate (ATP). Phosphate acts as an intracellular and extracellular anion buffer in the regulation of acid-base balance; in the form of ATP it provides energy for muscle contraction.

Calcium and phosphate concentrations are rigidly controlled. They are related by the product of calcium (Ca^{++}) and phosphate ($HPO_4^=$), which is a constant (K) [$Ca^{++} \times HPO_4^= = K$]. Thus, if the concentration of one ion increases or decreases, that of the other increases or decreases.

Calcium and phosphate balance is regulated by three hormones: parathyroid hormone (PTH), vitamin D, and calcitonin. Acting together, these substances determine the amount of dietary calcium and phosphate absorbed from the intestine, the deposition and absorption of calcium and phosphate from bone, and the renal reabsorption and excretion of calcium and phosphate by the kidney.

The parathyroid glands secrete PTH in response to low levels of serum calcium. (The specific actions of PTH in relation to calcium and phosphate are described in Chapter 21.) **Parathyroid hormone** controls levels of ionized calcium and phosphate in the blood and other extracellular fluids. The renal regulation of calcium and phosphate balance requires PTH. PTH stimulates reabsorption of calcium along the distal tubule of the nephron and inhibits phosphate reabsorption by the proximal tubule of the nephron. The net result is an increase in serum calcium concentration and increased urinary excretion of phosphate. Figure 3-9 summarizes hormonal regulation of calcium.

Another compound important to calcium and phosphate regulation is vitamin D. **Vitamin D** (cholecalciferol) is a fat-soluble steroid ingested in food or synthesized in the skin in the presence of ultraviolet light. Several steps of activation are required before vitamin D can act on target tissues. The first step occurs in the liver; final activation is in the kidney. The renal activation of vitamin D begins when the serum calcium level decreases and stimulates secretion of PTH. PTH then acts to increase calcium reabsorption and enhance renal excretion of phosphate, producing decreased phosphate levels. The combination of low calcium level and increased PTH secretion causes the renal activation of vitamin D. The activated vitamin D (vitamin D_3—calcitriol) then circulates as a hormone in the plasma and acts to increase absorption of calcium and phosphate in the small intestine, enhance bone calcification, and increase renal tubular reabsorption of calcium and phosphate. When renal failure occurs, vitamin D is not activated; serum calcium levels decrease; and phosphate levels increase.

As calcium levels increase, an opposite adaptation occurs, leading to suppression of PTH secretion, decreased renal vitamin D activation, decreased intestinal calcium absorption, and increased renal phosphate reabsorption. **Calcitonin** (produced by C cells of the thyroid gland) primarily decreases calcium levels by inhibiting osteoclastic activity in bone.

The fractions of serum calcium that are freely ionized or bound to plasma proteins are influenced by pH. In states of acidosis, levels of ionized calcium increase. When alkalosis develops, with an increase in pH, the amount of protein-bound calcium increases and the physiologically active, ionized calcium level decreases. The decreased concentration of ionized calcium may be great enough to cause symptoms of hypocalcemia, such as tetany.

Hypocalcemia

PATHOPHYSIOLOGY. **Hypocalcemia** occurs when serum total calcium concentrations are less than 8.5 mg/dl and ionized levels are less than 4.0 mg/dl. In general, deficits in calcium are related to inadequate intestinal absorption, decreases in levels of PTH and vitamin D, or deposition of ionized calcium into bone or soft tissue.

Nutritional deficiencies of calcium can occur in the instance of inadequate sources of dairy products or green, leafy vegetables. Excessive amounts of dietary phosphorus also bind with calcium, so neither mineral is absorbed when such an excess occurs. Removal of the parathyroid glands (e.g., during total thyroidectomy) with the resulting loss of PTH also causes hypocalcemia. Vitamin D deficiency, which can result from inadequate intake or avoidance of sunlight, causes decreased intestinal absorption of calcium. Malabsorption of fat, including fat-soluble vitamin D, also may contribute to calcium deficiency. Neoplastic bone metastases tend to inhibit bone resorption and increase calcium deposition into bone, thereby decreasing serum calcium levels.

Blood transfusions are also a common cause of hypocalcemia because the citrate solution used in storing whole blood binds with calcium and makes it unavailable to the tissues. Pancreatitis causes release of lipases into soft tissue spaces, so the free fatty acids that are formed bind calcium, causing a decrease in the concentration of ionized calcium. Metabolic or respiratory alkalosis causes symptoms of hypocalcemia because the change in pH enhances protein binding of ionized calcium. Hypoalbuminemia lowers total serum calcium levels by decreasing the amount of bound calcium in the plasma.

CLINICAL MANIFESTATIONS. The clinical manifestations of hypocalcemia are caused primarily by an increase in neuromuscular excitability. Calcium deficits cause partial depolarization of nerves and muscle as the threshold potential becomes more negative and approaches the resting membrane potential (hypopolarization) (see Figure 3-7, *C*). Therefore, a smaller stimulus is required for initiating the action potential. The symptoms are related to neuromuscular irritability and include paresthesias around the mouth and in the digits, carpopedal spasm (muscle spasms in the hands and feet), laryngospasm, hyperreflexia, seizures, and dysrhythmias.

Two clinical signs are Chvostek sign and Trousseau sign. *Chvostek sign* is elicited by tapping on the facial nerve just below the temple. A positive sign is a twitch of the nose or lip. *Trousseau sign* is contraction of the hand and fingers when the arterial blood flow in the arm is occluded for 5 minutes.

Severe symptoms include convulsions and *tetany,* a continuous severe muscle spasm that can interfere with breathing and cause death. The characteristic electrocardiogram (ECG) change is a prolonged QT interval, indicating prolonged ventricular depolarization and decreased cardiac contractility. Intestinal cramping and hyperactive bowel sounds also may be present because hypocalcemia affects the smooth muscles of the gastrointestinal tract. Table 3-10 contains a summary of the manifestations of calcium level alterations.

EVALUATION AND TREATMENT. The health history may signify underlying pathologic conditions that require further evaluation and treatment. Severe symptoms of hypocalcemia require emergency treatment with intravenous 10% calcium gluconate. Oral calcium replacement should be initiated, and serum calcium levels should be monitored. Decreasing phosphate intake facilitates long-term management of hypocalcemia.[14a]

Hypercalcemia

PATHOPHYSIOLOGY. **Hypercalcemia** with total serum calcium concentrations exceeding 12 mg/dl can be caused by a number of diseases. The most common among these are hyperparathyroidism; bone metastases with calcium resorption from breast, prostate, or cervical cancer, or hematologic malignancy; sarcoidosis; and excess vitamin D. Many tumors produce PTH and elevate the serum calcium levels. Sarcoidosis appears to increase vitamin D levels. Prolonged immobilization can also lead to hypercalcemia from enhanced bone resorption and decreased calcium deposition into bone. Acidosis decreases serum binding of calcium to albumin, increasing ionized calcium levels.

CLINICAL MANIFESTATIONS. Many symptoms of hypercalcemia are nonspecific. Because serum calcium levels are increased, a greater amount of calcium is also contained inside the cells. The threshold potential becomes more positive (hyperpolarized) (e.g., moves from −60 to −50 millivolts) and the cell membrane becomes refractory to depolarization (decreased excitability) because there is a greater difference between threshold potential and resting membrane potential (see Figure 3-7, *C*). Thus many of the symptoms are related to loss of cell membrane excitability. (Membrane potentials and membrane excitability are discussed in Chapter 1.) Fatigue, weakness, lethargy, anorexia, nausea, and constipation are common.

Mental status changes and confusion may occur. Impaired renal function frequently develops, and kidney stones form as precipitates of calcium salts. A shortened QT segment and

TABLE 3-10 ALTERATIONS IN CALCIUM, PHOSPHATE, AND MAGNESIUM LEVELS

CAUSES	MANIFESTATIONS
Hypocalcemia (<8.5 mg/dl)	
Inadequate intestinal absorption, deposition of ionized calcium into bone or soft tissue, blood administration, or decreases in PTH and vitamin D levels; nutritional deficiencies occur with inadequate sources of dairy products or green, leafy vegetables; alkalosis, elevated calcitonin level	Increased neuromuscular excitability; tingling, muscle spasms (particularly in hands, feet, and facial muscles), intestinal cramping, hyperactive bowel sounds; osteoporosis and fractures; severe cases show convulsions and tetany; prolonged QT interval, cardiac arrest
Hypercalcemia (>10-12 mg/dl)	
Hyperparathyroidism; bone metastases with calcium resorption from breast, prostate, renal, and cervical cancer; sarcoidosis; excess vitamin D; many tumors that produce PTH; calcium-containing antacids	Many nonspecific; fatigue, weakness, lethargy, anorexia, nausea, constipation; impaired renal function, kidney stones; dysrhythmias, bradycardia, cardiac arrest; bone pain, osteoporosis, fractures
Hypophosphatemia (<2.0 mg/dl)	
Intestinal malabsorption related to vitamin D deficiency, use of magnesium- and aluminum-containing antacids, long-term alcohol abuse, and malabsorption syndromes; respiratory alkalosis; increased renal excretion of phosphate associated with hyperparathyroidism	Conditions related to reduced capacity for oxygen transport by red blood cells and disturbed energy metabolism; leukocyte and platelet dysfunction; deranged nerve and muscle function; in severe cases, irritability, confusion, numbness, coma, convulsions; possibly respiratory failure (because of muscle weakness), cardiomyopathies, bone resorption (leading to rickets or osteomalacia)
Hyperphosphatemia (>4.7 mg/dl)	
Acute or chronic renal failure with significant loss of glomerular filtration; treatment of metastatic tumors with chemotherapy that releases large amounts of phosphate into serum; long-term use of laxatives or enemas containing phosphates; hypoparathyroidism	Symptoms primarily related to low serum calcium levels (caused by high phosphate levels) similar to symptoms of hypocalcemia; when prolonged, calcification of soft tissues in lungs, kidneys, joints
Hypomagnesemia (<1.5 mEq/L)	
Malnutrition, malabsorption syndromes, alcoholism, urinary losses (renal tubular dysfunction, loop diuretics)	Behavioral changes, irritability, increased reflexes, muscle cramps, ataxia, nystagmus, tetany, convulsions, tachycardia, hypotension
Hypermagnesemia (>3.0 mEq/L)	
Usually renal insufficiency or failure; also excessive intake of magnesium-containing antacids, adrenal insufficiency	Lethargy, drowsiness; loss of deep tendon reflexes; nausea and vomiting; muscle weakness; hypotension; bradycardia; respiratory distress; heart block, cardiac arrest

PTH, Parathyroid hormone.

depressed widened T waves also may be observed on the ECG, with bradycardia and varying degrees of heart block.

EVALUATION AND TREATMENT. With elevated serum calcium levels, often a reciprocal decrease in serum phosphate values occurs. Specific diagnostic procedures to identify the contributing pathologic condition are required.

Treatment is related to the severity of symptoms and the underlying disease. When renal function is normal, oral phosphate administration is effective. When acute illness and high calcium levels are present, treatment options include intravenous administration of large amounts of normal saline to enhance renal excretion of calcium, administration of bisphosphonates in the absence of renal failure, and administration of calcitonin. Corticosteroids and the cytotoxic drug mithramycin (blocks osteoclastic function) also are used to treat hypercalcemia. Ultimately, the underlying pathologic condition must be treated. (Table 3-10 contains a summary of the manifestations of alterations in calcium levels.)

Hypophosphatemia

PATHOPHYSIOLOGY. **Hypophosphatemia** is a serum phosphate level less than 2.5 mg/dl and is usually an indication of phosphate deficiency. In some conditions, total body phosphate is normal but serum concentrations are low. The most common causes are intestinal malabsorption and increased renal excretion of phosphate. Inadequate absorption is associated with vitamin D deficiency, use of magnesium- and aluminum-containing antacids (which bind with phosphorus), long-term alcohol abuse, and malabsorption syndromes. Respiratory alkalosis can cause severe hypophosphatemia because of cellular use of phosphorus for accelerated glycolysis (ATP) formation. Increased renal excretion of phosphorus is associated with hyperparathyroidism.

CLINICAL MANIFESTATIONS. The consequences of phosphate deficiency are not clinically evident until hypophosphatemia is severe. There is reduced capacity for oxygen transport by red blood cells and disturbed energy metabolism. Transport and release of oxygen are associated with 2,3-diphosphoglycerate (2,3-DPG) and ATP levels. When phosphate is depleted, 2,3-DPG and ATP levels become low and diminish release of oxygen to the tissues. The oxyhemoglobin curve shifts to the left (see Chapter 34), and hypoxia can occur with bradycardia and varying degrees of heart block.

Leukocyte and platelet dysfunctions also are associated with hypophosphatemia. There is a greater risk of infection and blood-clotting impairment, with potential for hemorrhage. Nerve and muscle function can be affected because of derangement in energy metabolism. Muscle weakness may become serious enough to cause respiratory failure, and cardiomyopathies also can develop. Irritability, confusion, numbness, coma, and convulsions develop with severe phosphate losses. In response to low phosphate levels, bone resorption occurs and may lead to rickets or osteomalacia. (Table 3-10 contains a summary of the manifestations of phosphate level alterations.)

EVALUATION AND TREATMENT. To correct the condition, the underlying cause must be identified and treated. The rate and amount of replacement are determined by the cause and presenting symptoms.[15] (Table 3-10 contains a summary of the manifestations of alterations in phosphate levels.)

Hyperphosphatemia

PATHOPHYSIOLOGY. Hyperphosphatemia, or an elevated serum phosphate level of more than 4.5 mg/dl, develops with exogenous or endogenous addition of phosphorus to the ECF or with significant loss of glomerular filtration.[16] Because most phosphate is located in cells, the cell destruction associated with treatment of metastatic tumors with chemotherapy can release large amounts of phosphate into the ECF. Long-term use of phosphate-containing enemas or laxatives also may lead to hyperphosphatemia. Hypoparathyroidism can cause elevated phosphate levels by increasing renal tubular reabsorption of phosphate.

High levels of serum phosphate also lower serum calcium levels, and increased amounts of phosphate and calcium are deposited in bone and soft tissues. Serum calcium levels may become low enough to cause symptoms of hypocalcemia, including tetany.

CLINICAL MANIFESTATIONS. Symptoms of hyperphosphatemia are related primarily to low serum calcium levels and thus are comparable to symptoms of hypocalcemia. With prolonged hyperphosphatemia, calcification of soft tissues occurs in the lungs, kidneys, and joints.

EVALUATION AND TREATMENT. To correct hyperphosphatemia, the underlying pathologic condition must be identified and treated. Aluminum hydroxide may be administered because it binds phosphate in the gastrointestinal tract and is then eliminated; however, aluminum can be toxic, causing encephalopathy and osteomalacia. Non-aluminum and non–calcium phosphate binders (lanthanum carbonate or sevelamer) are being evaluated but cost and toxicity are concerns.[17] Dialysis is required for management of renal failure. (Table 3-10 contains a summary of the manifestations of alterations in phosphate concentration.)

Magnesium

Magnesium (Mg^{++}) is a major intracellular cation, second to potassium. About 40% to 60% is stored in muscle and bone with 30% in the cells. A small amount (1%) is in the serum. Plasma concentration is 1.8 to 2.4 mg/dl with about one third bound to plasma proteins and the rest in ionized form. Regulation of magnesium metabolism is balanced by the small intestine and kidney. Low serum levels cause renal conservation of magnesium. Magnesium is a cofactor in intracellular enzymatic reactions, protein synthesis, nucleic acid stability, and neuromuscular excitability. Calcium and magnesium often interact in reactions at the cellular level.[18]

Hypomagnesemia occurs when serum magnesium concentration is less than 1.5 mEq/L and increases in neuromuscular excitability and tetany are present. Malnutrition, malabsorption syndromes, alcoholism, renal tubular dysfunction, metabolic acidosis, and use of loop and thiazide diuretics can cause magnesium losses. Hypomagnesemia is associated with insulin resistance, diabetes mellitus, left ventricular hypertrophy, systemic inflammation, hypoalbuminemia, and osteoporosis.[19] Because magnesium inhibits potassium channels, loss of magnesium results in movement of potassium out of the cell, with renal excretion resulting in hypokalemia. Signs and symptoms of hypomagnesemia are similar to those of hypocalcemia. Depression, confusion, irritability, increased reflexes, muscle weakness, ataxia, nystagmus, tetany, convulsions, and tachydysrhythmias may be observed.[20] Treatment is intramuscular or intravenous administration of magnesium sulfate.

Magnesium supplements have several benefits including improved myocardial metabolism and cell function; improved vascular smooth muscle tone and peripheral vascular resistance, afterload, and cardiac output; reduced cardiac dysrhythmias; and improved lipid and glucose metabolism. Magnesium also reduces vulnerability to oxygen-derived free radicals and systemic inflammation, improves human endothelial function, and inhibits platelet function, including platelet aggregation and adhesion.[19,20]

Hypermagnesemia, in which magnesium concentration is greater than 2.5 mEq/L, is rare and usually is caused by renal failure.[21] Magnesium-containing antacids (e.g., Gaviscon, Gelusil) can potentiate excess magnesium. Excess magnesium depresses skeletal muscle contraction and nerve function. Signs and symptoms include nausea and vomiting, muscle weakness, hypotension, bradycardia, and respiratory depression. Treatment is avoidance of magnesium-containing substances and removal of magnesium by dialysis. (Table 3-10 contains a summary of the manifestations of magnesium level alterations.)

ACID-BASE BALANCE

Acid-base balance and hydrogen ion concentration must be regulated within a narrow range for the body to function normally. Slight changes in amounts of hydrogen can significantly alter biologic processes in cells and tissues. Hydrogen ion is necessary to maintain membrane integrity and the speed of enzymatic reactions. Most pathologic conditions disturb acid-base balance, and the degree of severity may be more harmful than the disease process.

Hydrogen Ion and pH

The hydrogen ion concentration, $[H^+]$, is commonly expressed as the pH, the negative logarithm of hydrogen ions in solution. The symbol **pH** represents the acidity or alkalinity of a solution. The logarithmic value means that as the pH changes 1 unit (e.g., from 7.0 to 6.0), the $[H^+]$ changes tenfold (i.e., from 0.0000001 to 0.000001). The relationship is commonly expressed as follows:

$$\text{pH} = \log \frac{1}{[H^+]} \text{ or pH } = -\log_{10}[H^+]$$

As the [H^+] increases, the pH decreases; likewise, as the [H^+] decreases, the pH increases. The greater the [H^+], the more acidic the solution and the lower the pH. The lower the [H^+], the more basic the solution and the higher the pH. In biologic fluids, a pH of less than 7.4 is defined as acidic and a pH greater than 7.4 is defined as basic.

Different body fluids have different pH values as follows:

Body Fluid	pH
Gastric juices	1.0-3.0
Urine	5.0-6.0
Arterial blood	7.38-7.42
Venous blood	7.32-7.36
Cerebrospinal fluid	7.28-7.32
Pancreatic fluid	7.8-8.0

Body acids are formed as end products of cellular metabolism. The average person generates 50 to 100 mEq/day of acid from the metabolism of protein, carbohydrates, and fats and from loss of alkaline fluids in the stools. To maintain a normal pH, an equal amount of acid therefore must be neutralized or excreted. The lungs, kidneys, and bone are the major organs involved in the regulation of acid-base balance. The systems are interrelated and work together to regulate short- or long-term changes in acid-base status. Body acids exist in two forms: **volatile** (respiratory acids—eliminated as carbon dioxide [CO_2] gas) and **nonvolatile** (metabolic acids—eliminated by the kidney or metabolized by the liver). The volatile acid is carbonic acid (H_2CO_3), which is formed from the hydration of carbon dioxide:

Regulated by lung — Regulated by kidney

$$CO_2 + H_2O \leftrightarrow H_2CO_3 \quad \leftrightarrow \quad HCO_3^- + H^+$$

Carbonic acid is a weak acid, and in the presence of carbonic anhydrase, it readily dissociates into carbon dioxide and water. CO_2 is produced as an end product of oxidative metabolism. The more oxygen that is consumed, the more CO_2 is produced. The carbon dioxide is then eliminated by pulmonary ventilation. Sulfuric, phosphoric, and other metabolic acids (lactic acid, pyruvic acid, and keto acids [such as acetoacetic acid and β-hydroxybutyric acid, associated with diabetes mellitus]) are nonvolatile strong acids produced from the incomplete metabolism of proteins, carbohydrates, and fats. (Strong acids are those that readily give up their hydrogen; weak acids do not.) Nonvolatile acids are eliminated by the renal tubules in conjunction with the regulation of the concentration of HCO_3^-. Thus the lungs and kidneys, with the help of body buffer systems, are the prime regulators of acid-base balance.

Buffer Systems

Buffering occurs in response to changes in acid-base status. **Buffers** can absorb excessive H^+ (acid) or OH^- (base) to minimize fluctuations in pH. The buffer systems are located in both the ICF and ECF compartments, and they function at different rates. Buffer systems exist as buffer pairs, consisting of a weak acid and its conjugate base (Table 3-11). The most important plasma buffer systems are bicarbonate–carbonic acid and hemoglobin. Phosphate and protein are the most important intracellular buffers. Ammonia and phosphate are important renal buffers.

An important factor for effective buffering is a function known as the *pK value,* which represents the pH at which a buffer pair is half dissociated. Buffer pairs can associate and dissociate (see Table 3-11).

The pK provides a rate constant for the chemical reaction. A buffer system is most effective when the pK for the buffer is close to the pH of the fluid in which the buffer is acting. There is an equal concentration of acid and its conjugate base when pK equals pH. For the bicarbonate–carbonic acid buffer system, the pK is 6.1. This value is not as high as the pK for other buffer systems (see Table 3-11), but this buffer system is still very effective because carbon dioxide is rapidly removed from the blood by the lungs.

The pK value is also a term in the equation used to determine pH. The relationships among pH, pK, and the ratio of bicarbonate to carbonic acid can be expressed as follows by the *Henderson-Hasselbalch equation:*

$$pH = pK + \log\frac{[HCO_3^-]}{[H_2CO_3]}$$

TABLE 3-11 BUFFER SYSTEMS

BUFFER PAIRS	BUFFER SYSTEM	PK VALUES	REACTION	RATE
HCO_3^-/H_2CO_3	Bicarbonate	6.1	$H^+ + HCO_3^- \rightleftharpoons H_2O + CO_2$	Instantaneous
Hb^-/HHb	Hemoglobin	7.3	$HHb \rightleftharpoons H^+ + Hb^-$	Instantaneous
$HPO_4^=/H_2PO_4^-$	Phosphate	6.8	$HPO^-_4 + H^+ \rightleftharpoons H_2PO_4^-$	Instantaneous
Pr^-/HPr	Plasma proteins	6.7	$HPr \rightleftharpoons H^+ + Pr^-$	Instantaneous
ORGANS	**MECHANISM**			**RATE**
Lungs	Regulates retention or elimination of CO_2 and therefore H_2CO_3 concentration			Minutes to hours
Ionic shifts	Exchange of intracellular potassium and sodium for hydrogen			2-4 hours
Kidneys	Bicarbonate reabsorption and regeneration, ammonia formation, phosphate buffering			Hours to days
Bone	Exchanges of calcium and phosphate, release of carbonate			Hours to days

H^+, Hydrogen ion; *HCO_3^-,* bicarbonate; *H_2CO_3,* carbonic acid; *Hb^-,* hemoglobin; *$H_2PO_4^-$,* monobasic phosphate; *$HPO_4^=$,* dibasic phosphate; *HPr,* hydrogenated protein; *HHb,* hydrogenated hemoglobin; *Pr^-,* protein.

The pH then can be determined when specific values are included in the equation:

$$\begin{aligned} pH &= pK + \log\frac{[HCO_3^-]}{[H_2CO_3]} \\ &= 6.1 + \log\frac{24}{1.2} \\ &= 6.1 + \log\frac{20}{1} \\ &= 6.1 + 1.3 \\ &= 7.40 \end{aligned}$$

Bicarbonate Buffering–Carbonic Acid

The bicarbonate–carbonic acid buffer pair operates in both the lung and the kidney. The greater the carbon dioxide partial pressure (Pco_2), the more carbonic acid is formed. The relationship that exists between carbonic acid concentration ($[H_2CO_3]$) and carbon dioxide partial pressure (Pco_2) can be expressed as follows:

$$[H_2CO_3] = 0.03 \times PCO_2 \text{ (mmHg)}$$

The 0.03 represents the solubility coefficient for carbon dioxide in water. The Pco_2 of arterial blood ($Paco_2$) is normally about 40 mmHg. Therefore the amount of H_2CO_3 is equal to about 1.2 mmol/L (0.03 × 40). As the amount of carbon dioxide increases or decreases, the amount of H_2CO_3 changes in the same direction.

The relationship between the levels of bicarbonate and carbonic acid is usually expressed as a ratio. When the pH is 7.40, this ratio is 20:1 (bicarbonate/carbonic acid) (Figure 3-10). The ratio is defined by the amount of bicarbonate and carbon dioxide (carbonic acid) in the arterial blood. Bicarbonate concentration ($[HCO_3^-]$) is normally about 24 mEq/L. Therefore, the 20:1 ratio can be developed as follows:

$$\frac{[HCO_3^-] = 24 \text{ mEq/L}}{[H_2CO_3] = (0.03 \times 40 \text{ mmHg})} = \frac{24}{1.2} = \frac{20}{1}$$

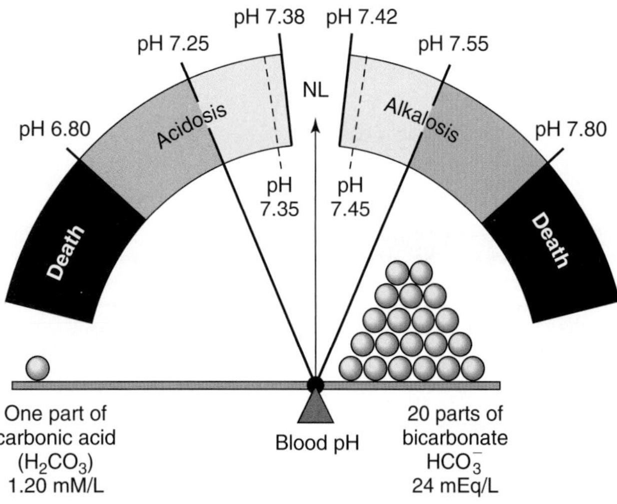

FIGURE 3-10 **Ratio of Carbonic Acid and Bicarbonate Concentration in Maintaining pH within Normal Limits.** An increase in H_2CO_3 or decrease in HCO_3^- concentration causes acidosis. A decrease in H_2CO_3 or increase in HCO_3^- concentration causes alkalosis. *NL,* Normal. (From Monahan FD et al: *Medical-surgical nursing: health and illness perspectives,* ed 8, St Louis, 2007, Mosby.)

The values for $[HCO_3^-]$ and $Paco_2$ ($[H_2CO_3]$) can increase or decrease proportionately, but the 20:1 ratio is maintained.

The lungs can decrease the amount of carbonic acid by exhaling CO_2 and leaving water. The kidneys can reabsorb bicarbonate or regenerate new bicarbonate from CO_2 and water. The renal mechanism does not act as rapidly as the lungs, but the two systems are very effective together because acid concentration can be rapidly adjusted by the lungs and bicarbonate is easily reabsorbed or regenerated by the kidneys. The pH equation can be symbolically expressed as follows:

$$pH = \frac{\text{Base}}{\text{Acid}} \text{ or } pH = \frac{\text{Renal regulation (slow)}}{\text{Pulmonary regulation (fast)}}$$

or

$$pH = \frac{\text{Metabolic acid-base function}}{\text{Respiratory acid-base function}}$$

Changes in either the numerator or the denominator will change the pH. For example, if the amount of bicarbonate is decreased, the pH also decreases, causing a state of acidosis. The pH can be returned to a normal range if the value of the denominator or the amount of carbonic acid also decreases. When a disease process causes an alteration in the bicarbonate/carbonic acid ratio, the kidneys or lungs (i.e., the organ not responsible for causing the alteration) respond to restore the ratio and maintain

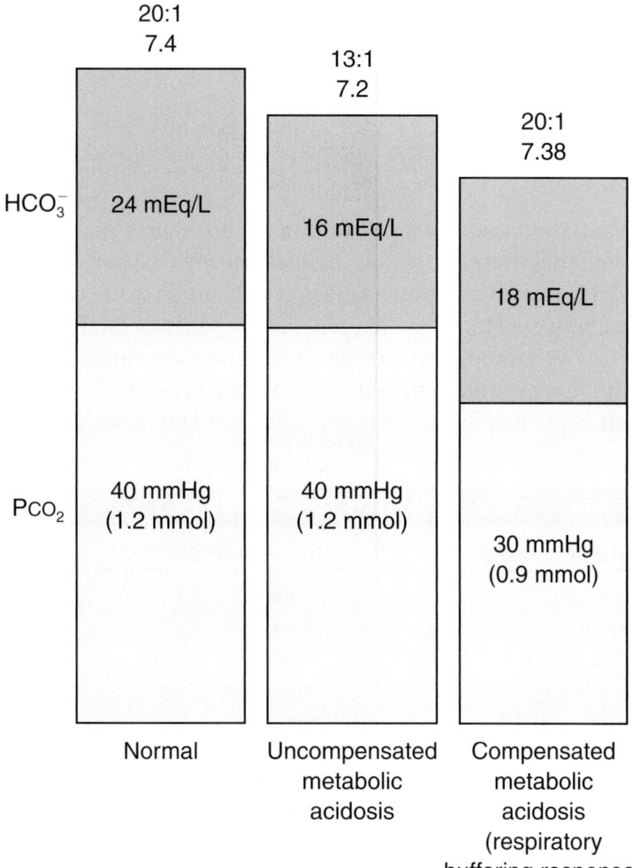

FIGURE 3-11 **Compensated Maintenance of $[HCO_3^-]/Pco_2$ (H_2CO_3) Ratio in Metabolic Acidosis.**

a normal pH. Renal and respiratory adjustments to *primary* changes in pH are known as **compensation.** With compensation, a 20:1 ratio may be achieved, but the actual values for HCO_3^- and H_2CO_3 concentrations are not normal. The respiratory system compensates for changes in pH by increasing or decreasing ventilation, a rapid response occurring within minutes to hours. The renal system compensates by producing more acidic or more alkaline urine, which may take hours to days. **Correction** occurs when the values for both components of the buffer pair ratio (bicarbonate and carbonic acid) return to normal (Figure 3-11).

Protein Buffering

Both intracellular and extracellular proteins have negative charges and can serve as buffers for H^+, but because most proteins are inside cells, they are primarily an intracellular buffer system. Hemoglobin (Hb) is an excellent intracellular blood buffer because of its ability to bind with H^+ (forming HHb) and carbon dioxide (forming $HHbCO_2$). Hemoglobin bound to H^+ becomes a weak acid. Less saturated hemoglobin (venous blood) is a better buffer than hemoglobin saturated with oxygen (arterial blood). The pH control system is illustrated in Figure 3-12.

Respiratory and Renal Buffering

The respiratory system regulates acid-base balance by controlling the rate of ventilation when there is metabolic acidosis or alkalosis. Central chemoreceptors sense increases or decreases in pH and $Paco_2$ (see Figure 32-11). When acidemia exists, the respiratory rate increases (eliminating CO_2 and reducing

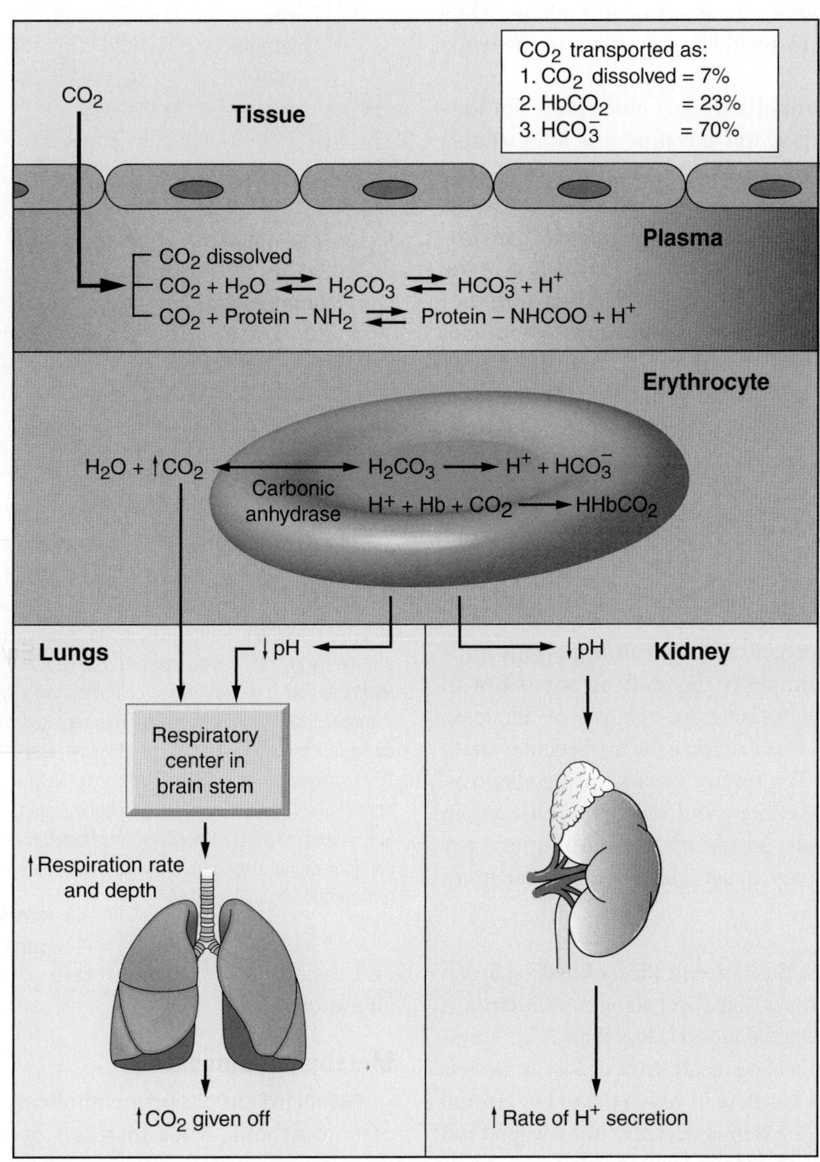

FIGURE 3-12 Integration of pH Control Mechanisms. CO_2 is produced in tissue cells and diffuses to plasma, where it is transported as dissolved CO_2, or it combines with water to form carbonic acid (H_2CO_3), or it combines with protein from which hydrogen has been released. Most of the CO_2 diffuses into the red blood cells and combines with water to form H_2CO_3. The H_2CO_3 dissociates to form hydrogen ion (H^+) and bicarbonate (HCO_3^-). Hydrogen ion combines with hemoglobin that has released its oxygen to form HHb, which buffers the hydrogen ion and makes venous blood slightly more acidic than arterial blood. The increase in H^+ concentration coupled with elevated CO_2 levels results in $HHbCO_3$ and an increase in the respiratory rate (eliminates CO_2) and secretion of H^+ by the kidneys.

carbonic acid concentration) (see Figure 3-12). When alkalemia occurs, the respiratory rate decreases (retaining CO_2 and increasing carbonic acid concentration).

The distal tubule of the kidney regulates acid-base balance by secreting hydrogen into the urine and regenerating bicarbonate with a maximum urine acidity of about pH 4.4 to 4.7. Buffers in the tubular fluid combine with hydrogen ions, allowing more H^+ to be secreted before the limiting pH value is reached. Dibasic phosphate ($HPO_4^=$) and ammonia (NH_3) are two important renal buffers. Dibasic phosphate is filtered at the glomerulus. About 75% is reabsorbed, and the remainder is available for buffering H^+. Secreted H^+ combines with $HPO_4^=$ to form monobasic phosphate ($H_2PO_4^-$). The remaining negative charge on the molecule makes it lipid insoluble, preventing it from diffusing back across the tubular cells and into the blood. Thus the $H_2PO_4^-$ containing the secreted H^+ is excreted in the urine (Figure 3-13).

Ammonia (NH_3) is an important renal buffer; it is not ionized (does not carry a charge), and therefore it is lipid soluble and can cross the tubular cell membrane. The presence of NH_3 in the tubular cells creates a concentration gradient, and it diffuses into the renal tubular fluid, where it combines with hydrogen to form ammonium ion (NH_4^+), which is eliminated in the urine (see Figure 3-13). NH_4^+ is lipid insoluble and does not readily diffuse back into the tubular cells. The renal buffering of hydrogen ions requires the use of CO_2 and H_2O to form H_2CO_3. The enzyme carbonic anhydrase catalyzes the formation of $H^+ + HCO_3^-$. The hydrogen is secreted from the tubular cell and buffered in the lumen by phosphate and ammonia. The bicarbonate is reabsorbed. The end effect is the addition of new bicarbonate, which contributes to the alkalinity of the plasma, because the hydrogen ion is excreted from the body (see Figure 3-13).

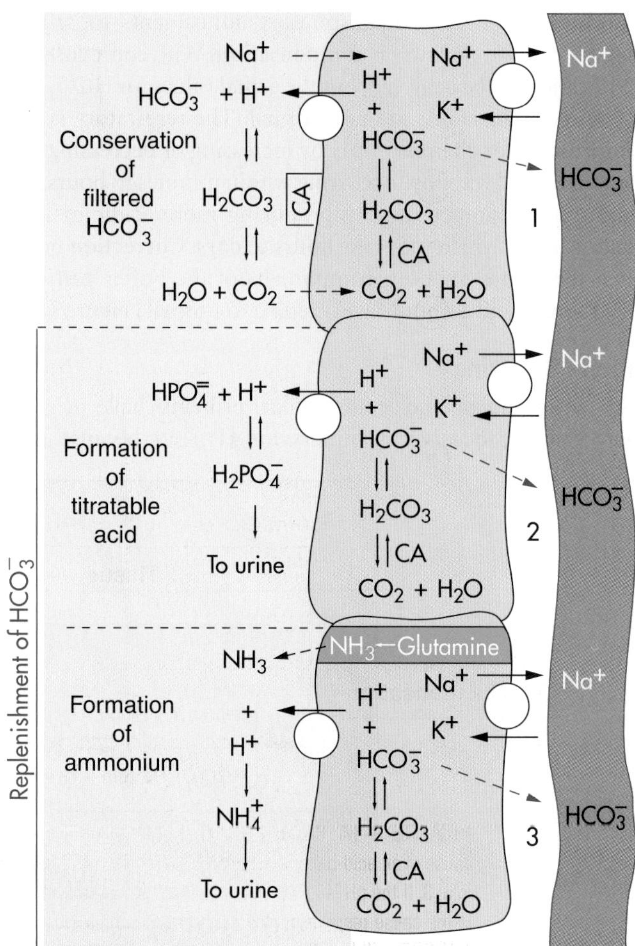

FIGURE 3-13 Renal excretion of acid. **1,** *Conservation of Filtered Bicarbonate.* Filtered bicarbonate combines with secreted hydrogen ion in the presence of carbon anhydrase *(CA)* to form carbonic acid (H_2CO_3), which then dissociates to water (H_2O) and carbon dioxide (CO_2); both diffuse into the epithelial cell. The CO_2 and H_2O combine to form H_2CO_3 in the presence of CA, and the resulting bicarbonate ion (HCO_3^-) is reabsorbed into the capillary. **2,** *Formation of Titratable Acid.* Hydrogen ion is secreted and combines with dibasic phosphate ($HPO_4^=$) to form monobasic phosphate ($H_2PO_4^-$). The secreted hydrogen ion is formed from the dissociation of H_2CO_3, and the remaining HCO_3^- is reabsorbed into the capillary. **3,** *Formation of Ammonium.* Ammonia (NH_3) is produced from glutamine in the epithelial cell and diffuses to the tubular lumen, where it combines with H^+ to form ammonium ion (NH_4^+). Once NH_4^+ has been formed, it cannot return to the epithelial cell (diffusional trapping), and the bicarbonate remaining in the epithelial cell is reabsorbed into the capillary.

Other Buffers

A cellular ion exchange mechanism is also an important buffering system. The best example is the shift of potassium in exchange for hydrogen during states of acidosis or alkalosis. During acidosis, potassium tends to leave the intracellular space in exchange for hydrogen. The reverse occurs during alkalosis. Although the ionic shifts facilitate buffering, the changes in intracellular or extracellular potassium concentrations may have serious consequences (e.g., hyperkalemia or hypokalemia).

Acid-Base Imbalances

Pathophysiologic changes in the concentration of hydrogen ion or base in the blood lead to acid-base imbalances. **Acidemia** is a state in which the pH of arterial blood is less than 7.35. A systemic increase in hydrogen ion concentration or loss of base is termed **acidosis. Alkalemia** is a state in which the pH of arterial blood is greater than 7.45. A systemic decrease in hydrogen ion concentration or an excess of base is termed **alkalosis.** Acid-base imbalances may have a metabolic or respiratory etiology or may be of mixed etiology. Acid-base imbalances are assessed using a measurement of arterial blood gases that includes the reporting of pH, $Paco_2$, and HCO_3^- concentration. The medical history is important to determining the cause of the disorder. Figure 3-14 summarizes the relationships among pH, $Paco_2$, and bicarbonate concentration during different acid-base alterations.

Metabolic Acidosis

PATHOPHYSIOLOGY. In **metabolic acidosis,** the concentration of non-carbonic acids increases or bicarbonate (base) is lost from the extracellular fluid or cannot be regenerated by the kidney (Table 3-12). This can occur quickly, as in lactic acidosis from poor perfusion or hypoxemia, or more slowly, as in renal failure (failure to excrete acid) or diabetic ketoacidosis (excess production of keto acids from lack of insulin) (see Chapter 23).

The buffer systems compensate for the excess acid and attempt to maintain the arterial pH within a normal range.

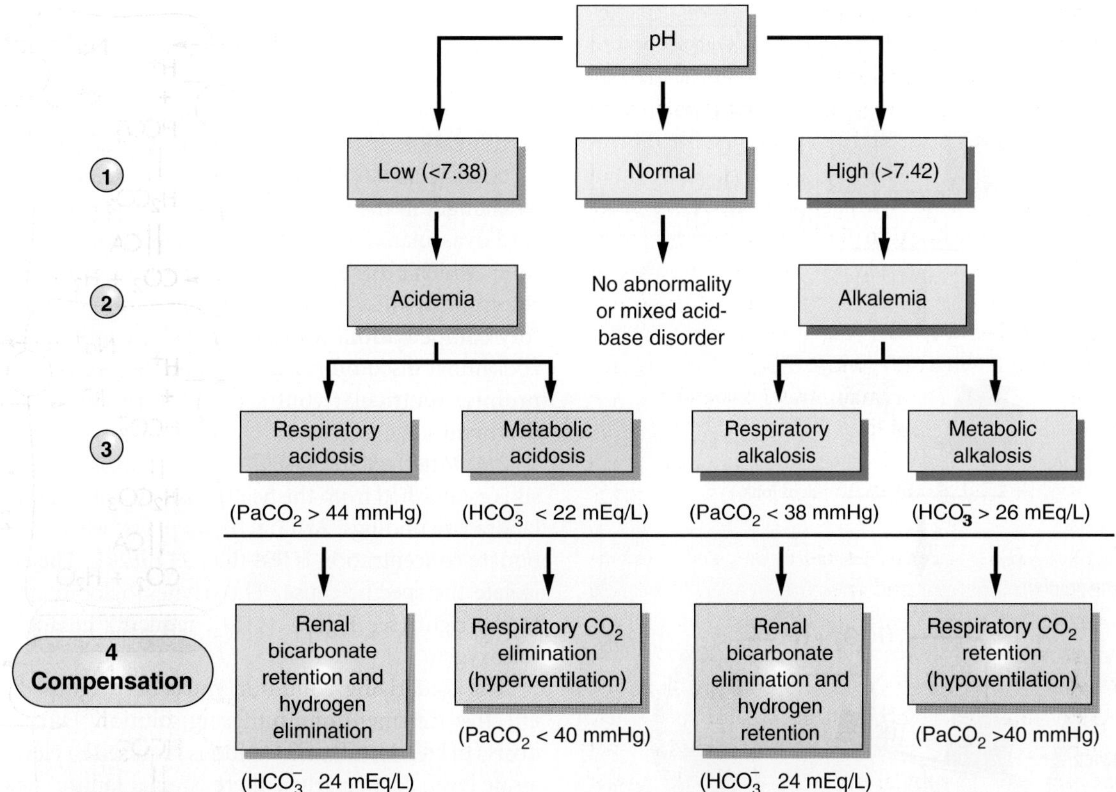

FIGURE 3-14 Primary and Compensatory Acid-base Changes. A systematic approach can be used to interpret the cause of an acid-base imbalance. **1,** Is the pH low or high? **2,** If the pH is low there is acidemia; if the pH is high there is alkalemia. **3,** If the pH is low (acidemia), is the cause respiratory (high $Paco_2$) or metabolic (low HCO_3^-)? If the pH is high (alkalemia), is the cause respiratory (low $Paco_2$) or metabolic (high HCO_3^-)? **4,** Is there compensation for the primary acid-base disorder? *(a)* HCO_3^- will be ≥24 mEq/L if there is renal compensation for a primary respiratory acidosis; *(b)* $Paco_2$ will be <40 mmHg if there is respiratory compensation of a primary metabolic acidosis; *(c)* HCO_3^- will ≤24 mEq/L if there is renal compensation for primary respiratory alkalosis; *(d)* $Paco_2$ will be >40 mmHg if there is respiratory compensation for primary metabolic alkalosis. **NOTE:** Examine the pH first. Then examine the changes in HCO_3^- and $Paco_2$. HCO_3^- will be elevated when there is primary metabolic alkalosis or renal compensation for primary respiratory acidosis. HCO_3^- will be decreased when there is primary metabolic acidosis or renal compensation for primary respiratory alkalosis. $Paco_2$ will be elevated when there is primary respiratory acidosis or respiratory compensation for primary metabolic alkalosis. $Paco_2$ will be decreased when there is primary respiratory alkalosis or respiratory compensation for metabolic acidosis.

TABLE 3-12 CAUSES OF METABOLIC ACIDOSIS

INCREASED NON–CARBONIC ACIDS (ELEVATED ANION GAP)	BICARBONATE LOSS (NORMAL ANION GAP)
Increased H^+ load	Diarrhea
Ketoacidosis (e.g., diabetes mellitus, starvation)	Ureterosigmoidoscopy
Lactic acidosis (e.g., shock)	Renal failure
Ingestions (e.g., ammonium chloride, ethylene glycol, methanol, salicylates, paraldehyde)	Proximal renal tubule acidosis
Decreased H^+ excretion	
Uremia	
Distal renal tubule acidosis	

Hydrogen ions will move to the intracellular space, and potassium will move to the extracellular space to maintain an ionic balance (see p. 115). Buffering by bicarbonate lowers the serum value of hydrogen ions and increases the pH. The respiratory system compensates for a metabolic acidosis as the reduced pH stimulates hyperventilation, lowering the $Paco_2$ and the amount of H_2CO_3 circulating in the blood. The kidneys excrete the excess acid as NH_4^+ and titratable acid ($H_2PO_4^-$). When acidosis is severe, buffers become depleted and cannot compensate for the increasing H^+ load and the pH continues to decrease. The ratio of bicarbonate to carbonic acid decreases to less than 20:1 (Figure 3-15). In states of metabolic acidosis, potassium is redistributed from the intracellular to the extracellular space, and is reabsorbed at the apical membrane of the renal collecting tubule (see p. 114). There is also an increase in the levels of ionized calcium because acidosis decreases the amount of calcium bound to albumin (see p. 114).

The evaluation of the **anion gap** can be helpful when used cautiously to distinguish different types of metabolic acidosis.[22]

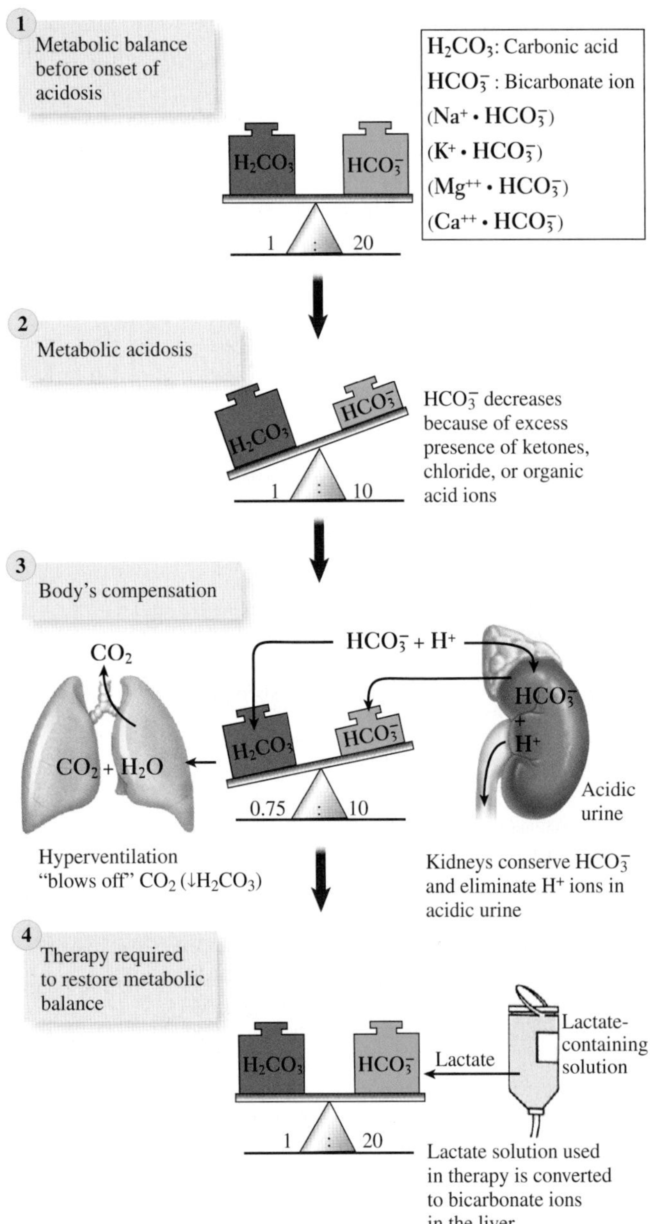

FIGURE 3-15 Metabolic Acidosis with Compensation and Correction. See text for abbreviations. (From Patton KT, Thibodeau GA: *Anatomy & physiology,* ed 8, St Louis, 2013, Mosby.)

Normally, the concentrations of cations and anions in the plasma are equivalent. Some anions, such as protein, sulfates, phosphates, and organic acids, however, are not measured in the common laboratory evaluations of the blood. Therefore the normal anion gap represents these unmeasured negative ions (sulfate, phosphate, lactate, keto acids, albumin). A convenient measure of the anion gap is the difference between the sum of Na^+ and K^+ and the sum of HCO_3^- and Cl^-, or about 10 to 12 mEq/L:

$$\text{Anion gap} = [Na^+ (140) + K^+ (4.0)] - [HCO_3^- (24) + Cl^- (110)] = 10-12 \text{ mEq/L}$$

In metabolic acidosis a **normal anion gap** is characteristic of conditions related to bicarbonate loss with retention of chloride to maintain an ionic balance. This is called **hyperchloremic metabolic acidosis** and it occurs with renal failure, diabetic ketoacidosis, or prolonged diarrhea with bicarbonate loss. An elevated anion gap is characteristic of acidosis associated with accumulation of anions other than chloride (see Table 3-12).

CLINICAL MANIFESTATIONS. Metabolic acidosis is manifested by changes in the neurologic, respiratory, gastrointestinal, and cardiovascular systems. Headache and lethargy are early symptoms, which progress to coma with severe acidosis. Deep, rapid respirations (Kussmaul respirations) are indicative of respiratory compensation. Anorexia, nausea, vomiting, diarrhea, and abdominal discomfort are common. Severe acidosis can compromise ventricular contraction and produce life-threatening dysrhythmias.

EVALUATION AND TREATMENT. The diagnosis of metabolic acidosis is established from the health history, clinical symptoms, and laboratory findings. Arterial blood pH is below 7.35, and bicarbonate concentration is less than 24 mEq/L. The anion gap can isolate the specific cause. The oxyhemoglobin curve is shifted to the right (see Figure 34-18), reducing hemoglobin affinity for oxygen.

The underlying condition must be diagnosed to establish effective treatment of a buffering solution. During severe acidosis (pH ≤7.1), administration is required to elevate the pH to a safe level, particularly if there is renal failure. Accompanying sodium and water deficits must also be corrected.[22]

Metabolic Alkalosis

PATHOPHYSIOLOGY. Metabolic alkalosis occurs when bicarbonate concentration is increased, usually caused by excessive loss of metabolic acids. Conditions that can result in metabolic alkalosis are prolonged vomiting, gastric suctioning, excessive bicarbonate intake, hyperaldosteronism with hypokalemia, and diuretic therapy.[23]

Respiratory compensation for metabolic alkalosis occurs when the elevated pH inhibits the respiratory center. The rate and depth of ventilation are decreased, causing retention of carbon dioxide. The ratio of HCO_3^- concentration to H_2CO_3 concentration is reduced toward normal. Respiratory compensation is not very efficient, however, and chronic or severe metabolic alkalosis requires therapeutic intervention (Figure 3-16).

Hypochloremic metabolic alkalosis occurs when acid loss is caused by vomiting or gastric suctioning with depletion of ECF sodium, chloride, and potassium. Renal compensation is not very effective because the volume depletion and loss of electrolytes stimulate a paradoxical response by the kidneys. The kidneys increase bicarbonate reabsorption to maintain an anionic balance because the ECF chloride concentration is decreased. The resulting excretion of H^+ and reabsorption of bicarbonate prevent correction of the alkalosis (Figure 3-17). The kidneys also increase sodium reabsorption. When potassium concentration is depleted, hydrogen ion moves to the intracellular space and is excreted to maintain an electrochemical balance.

With alkalemia, hydrogen ions are redistributed from the intracellular to the extracellular space and potassium moves to the intracellular space to preserve electroneutrality. With hyperaldosteronism, the excess aldosterone causes sodium retention and loss of hydrogen and potassium ions. Mild volume expansion ensues, and bicarbonate is retained along with the sodium, thereby causing alkalosis. Diuretics, such as thiazides, ethacrynic acid, and furosemide, produce mild alkalosis by enhancing sodium, potassium, and chloride excretion more than bicarbonate excretion.

CLINICAL MANIFESTATIONS. Because of the many causes of metabolic alkalosis, the symptoms vary. Some common symptoms, such as weakness, muscle cramps, and hyperactive reflexes, are related to volume depletion and electrolyte losses. Because alkalosis increases binding of Ca^{++} to plasma proteins (albumin), ionized calcium concentration decreases, causing excitable cells to become hypopolarized, which initiates an action potential more easily. Paresthesias (especially numbness/tingling of the fingertips and perioral area), tetany, and seizures may develop (see Hypocalcemia, p. 120).

Respirations are slow and shallow to increase carbon dioxide retention. Confusion and convulsions occur with severe alkalosis. Atrial tachycardia is a potential problem. The oxyhemoglobin curve is shifted to the left (see Figure 34-18), decreasing the dissociation of oxyhemoglobin and increasing the risk of dysrhythmias.

EVALUATION AND TREATMENT. The health history provides significant clues to the diagnosis of metabolic alkalosis. The arterial pH is greater than 7.45, and bicarbonate levels exceed 26 mEq/L. With respiratory compensation, the $Paco_2$ rises above 40 mmHg. With hypochloremic metabolic alkalosis, serum chloride values are below normal. Serum potassium levels are usually depleted because hydrogen is released from the cells in exchange for potassium to help regulate the pH level. The potassium is then secreted from renal distal tubule cells into the urine.

With hypochloremic alkalosis or contraction alkalosis with volume depletion, a sodium chloride solution is required for *correction*. The renal stimulus to increase ECF volume by retaining Na^+ is diminished, and HCO_3^- can be excreted as $NaHCO_3$ in the urine. The administration of potassium corrects alkalosis caused by hyperaldosteronism or hypokalemia. The potassium causes hydrogen to move back into the ECF and decreases loss of hydrogen from the distal tubule.

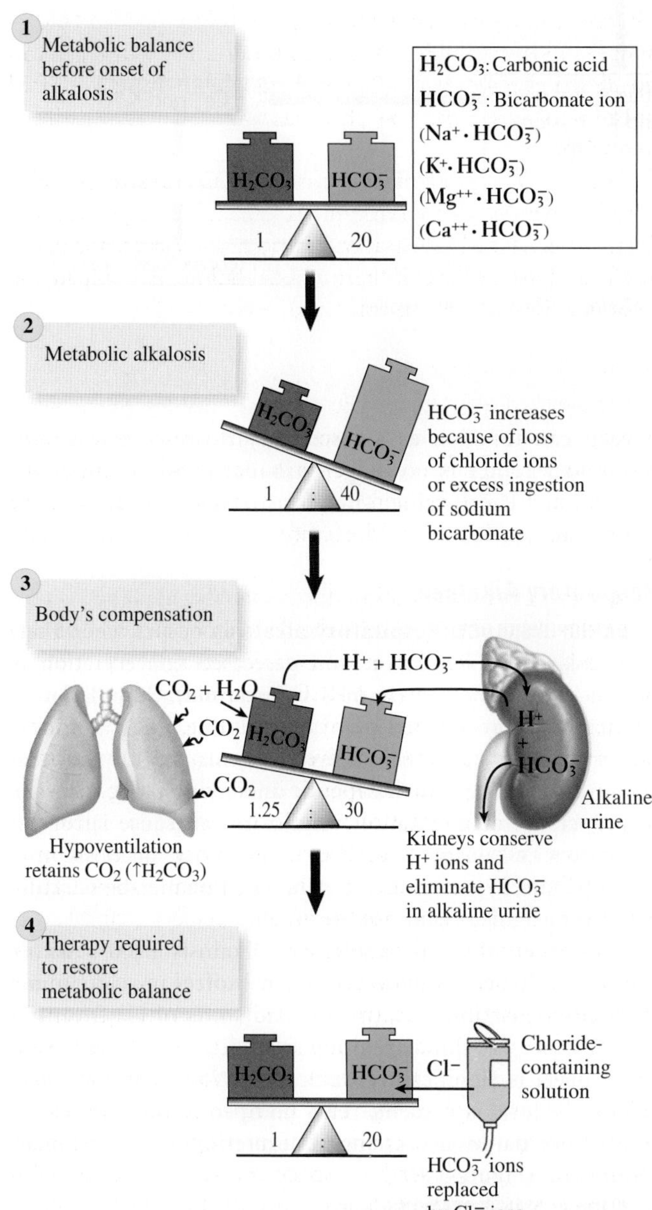

FIGURE 3-16 Metabolic Alkalosis with Compensation and Correction. See text for abbreviations. (From Patton KT, Thibodeau GA: *Anatomy & physiology*, ed 8, St Louis, 2013, Mosby.)

Respiratory Acidosis

PATHOPHYSIOLOGY. Respiratory disorders of acid-base balance are caused by increases or decreases of alveolar ventilation in relation to the metabolic production of carbon dioxide. **Respiratory acidosis** occurs when there is alveolar hypoventilation. Carbon dioxide is retained, increasing $[H^+]$ (as H_2CO_3) and producing acidosis. Carbon dioxide excess in the blood is called **hypercapnia.** The common causes include depression of the respiratory center (brainstem trauma, oversedation), paralysis of the respiratory muscles, disorders of the chest wall (kyphoscoliosis, pickwickian syndrome, flail chest), and disorders of the lung parenchyma (pneumonitis, pulmonary edema, emphysema, asthma, bronchitis).

Respiratory acidosis may be acute or chronic. Airway obstruction is the most common cause of acute respiratory acidosis. Acute compensation for respiratory acidosis is not effective because the renal buffer mechanism takes time to function. Further, the protein buffers provide marginal compensation, and HCO_3^- is not a good buffer for CO_2. Acute uncompensated respiratory acidosis is characterized by decreased arterial pH, elevated $Paco_2$, and normal or slightly increased bicarbonate concentration.

Chronic respiratory acidosis is commonly associated with chronic obstructive pulmonary disease and deformities of the chest wall or neuromuscular disorders. Renal compensation is effective and is established over several days. The acidosis produced from CO_2 retention stimulates the kidney to secrete hydrogen ions and regenerate bicarbonate. Serum bicarbonate and $Paco_2$ levels are elevated, and pH is restored toward normal (Figure 3-18).

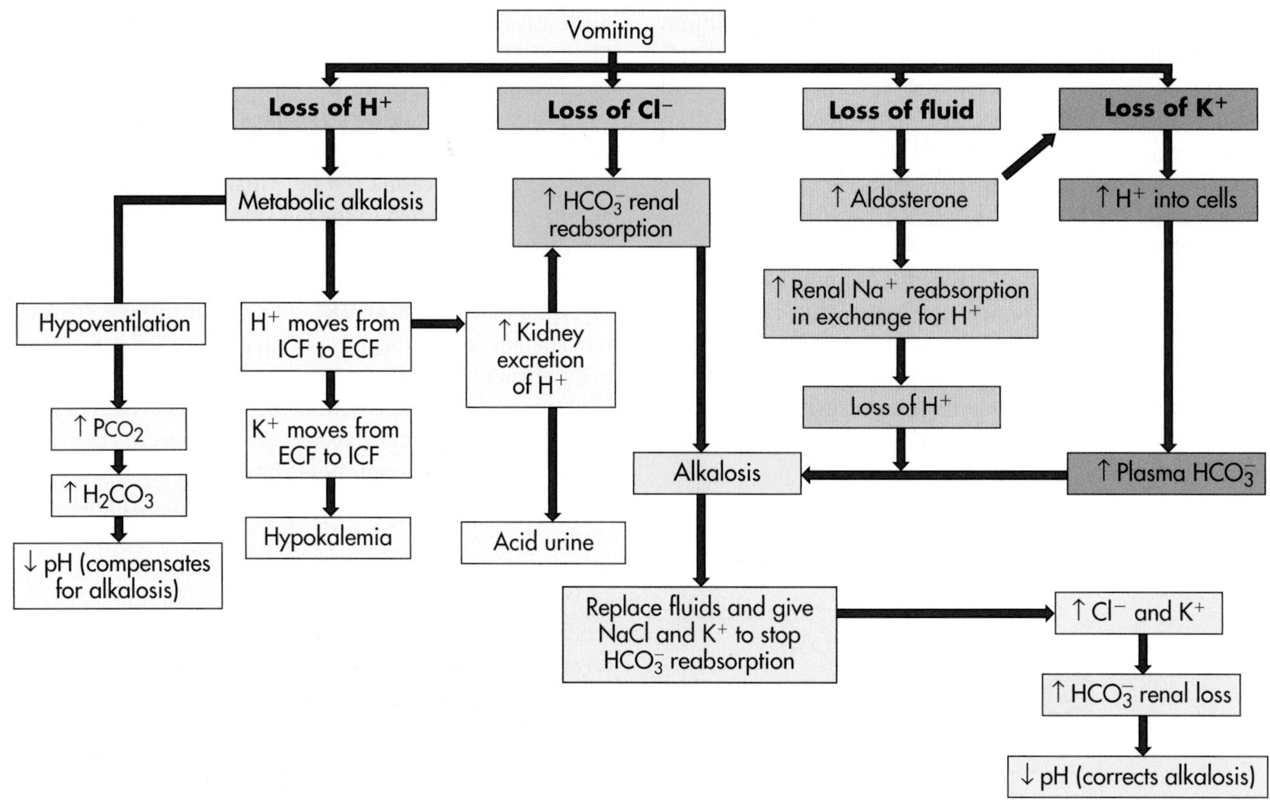

FIGURE 3-17 Hypochloremic Metabolic Alkalosis. See text for abbreviations.

CLINICAL MANIFESTATIONS. The symptoms of respiratory acidosis are related to acuity of onset and severity of $Paco_2$ retention. Initial symptoms include headache, restlessness, blurred vision, and apprehension followed by lethargy, muscle twitching, tremors, convulsions, and coma. Neurologic symptoms are caused by a decrease in the pH of cerebrospinal fluid and vasodilation because CO_2 readily crosses the blood-brain barrier. The respiratory rate is rapid at first and gradually becomes depressed because over time, the respiratory center adapts to increasing levels of CO_2. Cyanosis does not occur unless there is an accompanying hypoxemia, and the skin may instead be pink from vasodilation caused by the elevated CO_2 level.

EVALUATION AND TREATMENT. The primary diagnostic indicators are an arterial pH less than 7.35 and hypercapnia. Acute respiratory acidosis must be distinguished from chronic acidosis; the health history and clinical laboratory data are therefore helpful.

In many cases, restoration of adequate alveolar ventilation removes excess CO_2. If alveolar ventilation cannot be maintained spontaneously because of drug overdose or neuromuscular disorders, mechanical ventilation is required. When the hypercapnea is caused by alterations in gas diffusion at the alveolar-capillary membrane, ventilation may not be effective. The values of arterial pH, Pco_2, Po_2, and HCO_3^- must be carefully monitored. Rapid reduction of $Paco_2$ can cause respiratory alkalosis with seizures and death.

The underlying diseases are treated to achieve maximal ventilation. In the presence of hypoxemia and hypercapnia, oxygen can function as a respiratory depressant when the respiratory center is no longer stimulated by the lower pH and elevated $Paco_2$ value. Therefore, oxygen should be given cautiously.

Respiratory Alkalosis

PATHOPHYSIOLOGY. Respiratory alkalosis occurs when there is alveolar hyperventilation and decreased concentration of plasma carbon dioxide (termed **hypocapnia**). Stimulation of ventilation is precipitated by hypoxemia (i.e., high altitudes); hypermetabolic states such as fever, anemia, and thyrotoxicosis; early salicylate intoxication; or anxiety or panic disorder. Improper use of mechanical ventilators can cause iatrogenic respiratory alkalosis. Secondary respiratory alkalosis may develop from hyperventilation stimulated by metabolic acidosis, causing a mixed acid-base disorder.

The onset of acute respiratory alkalosis occurs within minutes of hyperventilation. Cellular buffers provide immediate compensation (i.e., protein and shifts of H^+ from ICF to ECF). The H^+ shifts are not very effective, however, if the $Paco_2$ level is significantly decreased. When chronic respiratory alkalosis is present, renal compensation restores pH toward normal by decreasing H^+ excretion and bicarbonate absorption (Figure 3-19).

CLINICAL MANIFESTATIONS. Respiratory alkalosis, like metabolic alkalosis, is irritating to the central and peripheral nervous systems. Symptoms include dizziness, confusion, tingling of extremities (paresthesias), convulsions, and coma. Carpopedal

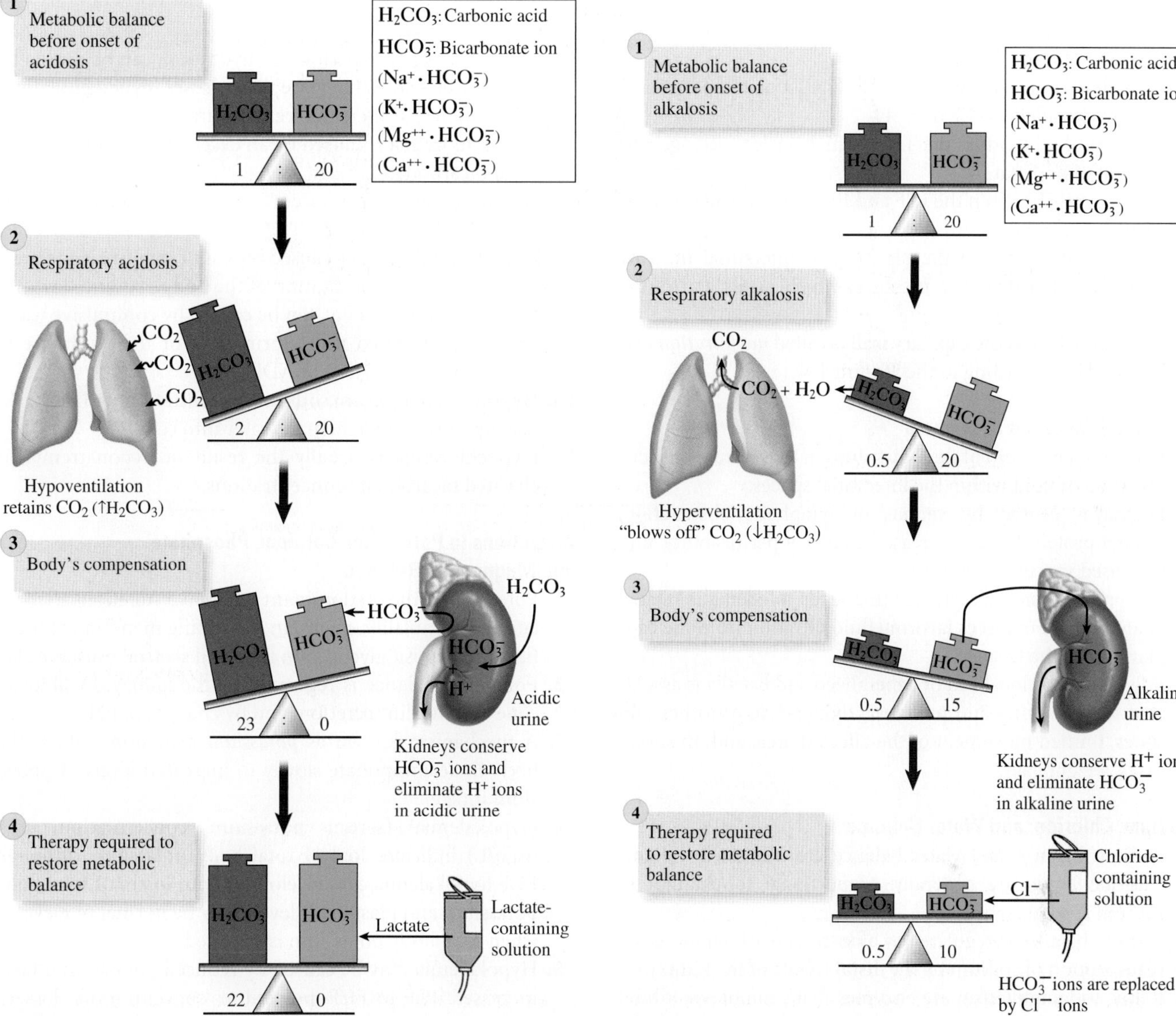

FIGURE 3-18 Respiratory Acidosis with Compensation and Correction. See text for abbreviations. (From Patton KT, Thibodeau GA: *Anatomy & physiology,* ed 8, St Louis, 2013, Mosby.)

FIGURE 3-19 Respiratory Alkalosis with Compensation and Correction. See text for abbreviations. (From Patton KT, Thibodeau GA: *Anatomy & physiology,* ed 8, St Louis, 2013, Mosby.)

spasm and other symptoms of hypocalcemia are similar to those of metabolic alkalosis (see p. 128). Deep and rapid respirations (tachypnea) are primary symptoms of the disorders that cause respiratory alkalosis.

EVALUATION AND TREATMENT. The underlying disturbance must be identified. The arterial pH is greater than 7.45, and the $Pa{CO_2}$ is less than 38 mmHg. In acute states, bicarbonate levels are normal. With chronic respiratory alkalosis, a compensatory decrease in the bicarbonate level occurs and the pH is closer to normal.

Treating the underlying disturbance is the most effective treatment. Hypoxemia must be corrected and hypermetabolic states reversed. Symptoms from hysterical hyperventilation can be corrected by rebreathing from a paper bag, which increases the concentration of inspired carbon dioxide and reverses the respiratory alkalosis.

SUMMARY REVIEW

Distribution of Body Fluids

1. Body fluids are distributed among functional compartments and are classified as ICF or ECF.
2. The sum of all fluids is the TBW, which varies with age and amount of body fat.
3. Water moves between the ICF and ECF compartments principally by osmosis.
4. Water moves between the plasma and interstitial fluid by osmosis and hydrostatic pressure, which occur across the capillary membrane.
5. Movement across the capillary wall is called *net filtration* and is described according to the Starling law.

Alterations in Water Movement

1. Edema is a problem of fluid distribution that results in accumulation of fluid within the interstitial spaces.
2. Edema is caused by venous or lymphatic obstruction, plasma protein losses, increased capillary permeability, and increased vascular volume.
3. The pathophysiologic process that leads to edema is related to an increase in forces favoring fluid filtration from the capillaries into the tissues.
4. Edema may be localized or generalized and usually is associated with swelling and puffiness, tighter-fitting clothes and shoes, limited movement of the affected area, and, in severe cases, weight gain.

Sodium, Chloride, and Water Balance

1. Sodium balance and water balance are intimately related; chloride levels are generally proportional to changes in sodium levels.
2. Sodium balance is regulated by aldosterone, which increases reabsorption of sodium by the distal tubule of the kidney.
3. Renin and angiotensin are enzymes that promote or inhibit secretion of aldosterone and thus regulate sodium and water balance.
4. Atrial natriuretic hormone is also involved in decreasing tubular resorption and promoting urinary excretion of sodium.
5. Water balance is regulated by the sensation of thirst and by the level of antidiuretic hormone, which is initiated by an increase in plasma osmolality or a decrease in circulating blood volume.

Alterations in Sodium, Chloride, and Water Balance

1. Alterations in water balance may be classified as isotonic, hypertonic, or hypotonic.
2. Isotonic alterations occur when changes in TBW are accompanied by proportional changes in concentrations of electrolytes.
3. Hypertonic alterations develop when the osmolality of the ECF is elevated above normal, usually because of an increased concentration of ECF sodium or a deficit of ECF water.
4. Hypernatremia (sodium levels >147 mEq/L) may be caused by an acute increase in sodium level or a loss of water.
5. Water deficit, or hypertonic dehydration, can be caused by lack of access to water, pure water losses, hyperventilation, arid climates, or increased renal clearance.
6. Hyperchloremia is caused by an excess of sodium or a deficit of bicarbonate.
7. Hypotonic alterations occur when the osmolality of the ECF is less than normal.
8. Hyponatremia may be caused by loss of sodium, inadequate intake of sodium, or dilution of the body's sodium level.
9. Water excess is rare but can be caused by compulsive water drinking, decreased urine formation, or the syndrome of inappropriate secretion of ADH.
10. Hyponatremia (serum sodium concentration <135 mEq/L) usually causes movement of water into cells.
11. Hypochloremia is usually the result of hyponatremia or elevated bicarbonate concentrations.

Alterations in Potassium, Calcium, Phosphate, and Magnesium Balance

1. Potassium is the predominant ICF ion; it functions to regulate ICF osmolality, maintain the resting membrane potential, and deposit glycogen in liver and skeletal muscle cells.
2. Potassium balance is regulated by the kidney, by aldosterone and insulin secretion, and by changes in pH.
3. A mechanism known as *potassium adaptation* allows the body to accommodate slowly to increased levels of potassium intake.
4. Hypokalemia (serum potassium concentration <3.5 mEq/L) indicates loss of total body potassium, although ECF hypokalemia can develop without losses of total body potassium and plasma K^+ levels may be normal or elevated when total body potassium is depleted.
5. Hypokalemia may be caused by reduced potassium intake, increased ICF-to-ECF potassium concentration, loss of potassium from body stores, increased aldosterone secretion (e.g., caused by hypernatremia), and increased renal excretion.
6. Hyperkalemia (potassium levels >5.5 mEq/L) may be caused by increased potassium intake, a shift from ICF to ECF potassium, or decreased renal excretion.
7. Calcium is a necessary ion in the structure of bones and teeth, in blood clotting, in hormone secretion and the function of cell receptors, and in membrane stability.
8. Phosphate acts as a buffer in acid-base regulation and provides energy for muscle contraction.
9. Calcium and phosphate concentrations are rigidly controlled by PTH, vitamin D, and calcitonin.
10. Hypocalcemia (serum calcium concentration <8.5 mg/dl) is related to inadequate intestinal absorption, deposition of ionized calcium into bone or soft tissue, blood administration, or decreased PTH and vitamin D levels.
11. Hypercalcemia (serum calcium concentration >12 mg/dl) can be caused by a number of diseases, including hyperparathyroidism, bone metastases, sarcoidosis, and excess vitamin D.

SUMMARY REVIEW—cont'd

12. Hypophosphatemia is usually caused by intestinal malabsorption and increased renal excretion of phosphate.
13. Hyperphosphatemia develops with acute or chronic renal failure with significant loss of glomerular filtration.
14. Magnesium is a major intracellular cation and is principally regulated by PTH.
15. Magnesium functions in enzymatic reactions and often interacts with calcium at the cellular level.
16. Hypomagnesemia (serum magnesium concentrations <1.5 mEq/L) may be caused by malabsorption syndromes.
17. Hypermagnesemia (serum magnesium concentrations >2.5 mEq/L) is rare and is usually caused by renal failure.

Acid-Base Balance

1. Hydrogen ions, which maintain membrane integrity and the speed of enzymatic reactions, must be concentrated within a narrow range if the body is to function normally.
2. Hydrogen ion concentration is expressed as pH, which represents the negative logarithm of hydrogen ions in solution.
3. Different body fluids have different pH values.
4. The renal and respiratory systems, together with the body's buffer systems, are the principal regulators of acid-base balance.
5. Buffers are substances that can absorb excessive acid or base to minimize fluctuations in pH.
6. Buffers exist as acid-base pairs; the principal plasma buffers are bicarbonate, protein (hemoglobin), and phosphate.
7. Buffer pairs can associate and dissociate; the pK value is the pH at which a buffer pair is half dissociated.
8. The lungs and kidneys act to compensate for changes in pH by increasing or decreasing ventilation and by producing more acidic or more alkaline urine.
9. Correction is a process different from compensation; correction occurs when the values for both components of the buffer pair are returned to normal.
10. Acid-base imbalances are caused by changes in the concentration of H^+ in the blood; an increase causes acidosis, and a decrease causes alkalosis.
11. An abnormal increase or decrease in bicarbonate concentration causes metabolic acidosis or metabolic alkalosis; changes in the rate of alveolar ventilation produce respiratory acidosis or respiratory alkalosis.
12. Metabolic acidosis is caused by an increase in the concentrations of non-carbonic acids or by loss of bicarbonate from the extracellular fluid.
13. Metabolic alkalosis occurs with an increase in bicarbonate concentration usually caused by loss of metabolic acids from conditions such as vomiting, gastrointestinal suctioning, excessive bicarbonate intake, hyperaldosteronism, and diuretic therapy.
14. Respiratory acidosis occurs with a decrease of alveolar ventilation and an increase in levels of carbon dioxide, or hypercapnia.
15. Respiratory alkalosis occurs with alveolar hyperventilation and excessive reduction of carbon dioxide concentration, or hypocapnia.

KEY TERMS

Acidemia, 126
Acidosis, 126
Aldosterone, 108
Alkalemia, 126
Alkalosis, 126
Angiotensin I, 108
Angiotensin II, 109
Anion gap, 127
Antidiuretic hormone (arginine-vasopressin), 109
Aquaporin, 105
Baroreceptor (volume/pressure sensitive receptor), 109
Buffer, 123
Buffering, 123
Calcitonin, 120
Calcium (Ca^{++}), 119
Capillary hydrostatic pressure (blood pressure), 105
Capillary (plasma) oncotic pressure, 105
Chloride, 109
Compensation, 125
Correction, 125
Decreased plasma oncotic pressure, 106
Decreased urine formation, 113
Dehydration, 112
Dilutional hyponatremia, 113
Edema, 105
Extracellular fluid (ECF), 103
Familial hypokalemic periodic paralysis, 115
Hypercalcemia, 120
Hypercapnia, 129
Hyperchloremia, 112
Hyperchloremic metabolic acidosis, 128
Hyperkalemia, 117
Hypermagnesemia, 122
Hypernatremia, 111
Hyperphosphatemia, 122
Hyperpolarized, 116
Hypertonic fluid, 110
Hypertonic hyponatremia, 113
Hypocalcemia, 120
Hypocapnia, 130
Hypochloremia, 113
Hypochloremic metabolic alkalosis, 128
Hypokalemia, 115
Hypomagnesemia, 122
Hyponatremia, 112
Hypophosphatemia, 121
Hypopolarized, 108
Hypotonic fluid, 112
Hypotonic hyponatremia, 113
Inadequate intake of dietary sodium, 113
Increased capillary hydrostatic pressure, 106
Increased capillary permeability, 107
Intercalated cell, 114
Interstitial fluid, 104
Interstitial hydrostatic pressure, 105
Interstitial oncotic pressure, 105
Intracellular fluid (ICF), 103
Intravascular fluid, 104
Isotonic, 109
Lymphatic obstruction, 107
Lymphedema, 107
Magnesium (Mg^{++}), 122
Metabolic acidosis, 126
Metabolic alkalosis, 128
Natriuretic peptide, 109
Net filtration, 105
Nonvolatile, 123
Normal anion gap, 128
Osmoreceptor, 109
Parathyroid hormone (PTH), 119
pH, 122
Phosphate ($HPO_4^{=}$), 119
Principal cell, 114
Potassium adaptation, 115
Pure sodium deficit, 113
Pure water deficit, 112
Renin, 108
Respiratory acidosis, 129
Respiratory alkalosis, 130
Sodium, 108
Starling hypothesis, 105
Total body water (TBW), 104
Vitamin D, 119
Volatile, 123
Water intoxication, 113

REFERENCES

1. Maughan RJ: Hydration, morbidity, and mortality in vulnerable populations, *Nutr Rev* 70(Suppl 2):S152–S155, 2012.
2. Verkman AS: Aquaporins in clinical medicine, *Annu Rev Med* 63:303–316, 2012.
3. Paskett ED et al: Cancer-related lymphedema risk factors, diagnosis, treatment, and impact: a review, *J Clin Oncol* 30(30):3726–3733, 2012.
4. Nishikimi T, Kuwahara K, Nakao K: Current biochemistry, molecular biology, and clinical relevance of natriuretic peptides, *J Cardiol* 57(2):131–140, 2011.
5. Sam R, Feizi I: Understanding hypernatremia, *Am J Nephrol* 36(1):97–104, 2012.
6. Agrawal V et al: Hyponatremia and hypernatremia: disorders of water balance, *J Assoc Physicians India* 56:956–964, 2008.
7. Waikar SS, Mount DB, Curhan GC: Mortality after hospitalization with mild, moderate, and severe hyponatremia, *Am J Med* 122(9):857–865, 2009.
8. Egom EE, Chirico D, Clark AL: A review of thiazide-induced hyponatraemia, *Clin Med* 11(5):448–451, 2011.
9. Lindner G, Schwarz C: An update on the current management of hyponatremia, *Minerva Med* 103(4):279–291, 2012.
10. Youn JH, McDonough AA: Recent advances in understanding integrative control of potassium homeostasis, *Annu Rev Physiol* 71:381–401, 2009.
11. Aronson PS, Giebisch G: Effects of pH on potassium: new explanations for old observations, *J Am Soc Nephrol* 22(11):1981–1989, 2011.
12. Unwin RJ, Luft FC, Shirley DG: Pathophysiology and management of hypokalemia: a clinical perspective, *Nat Rev Nephrol* 7(2):75–84, 2011.
13. Osadchii OE: Mechanisms of hypokalemia-induced ventricular arrhythmogenicity, *Fundam Clin Pharmacol* 24(5):547–559, 2010.
14. Pepin J, Shields C: Advances in the diagnosis and management of hypokalemic and hyperkalemie emergencies, *Emerg Med Pract* 14(2):1–17, 2012.

14a. Fong J, Khan A: Hypocalcemia: updates in diagnosis and management for primary care, *Can Fam Physician* 58(2):158–162, 2012.

15. Felsenfeld AJ, Levine BS: Approach to treatment of hypophosphatemia, *Am J Kidney Dis* 60(4):655–661, 2012.
16. Cirillo M, Bilancio G, Marcarelli F: Ageing and changes in phosphate transport: clinical implications, *J Nephrol* 23(Suppl 16):S152–S157, 2010.
17. Hutchison AJ, Smith CP, Brenchley PE: Pharmacology, efficacy and safety of oral phosphate binders, *Nat Rev Nephrol* 7(10):578–589, 2011.
18. Romani AM: Cellular magnesium homeostasis, *Arch Biochem Biophys* 512(1):1–23, 2011.
19. Rosanoff A, Weaver CM, Rude RK: Suboptimal magnesium status in the United States: are the health consequences underestimated? *Nutr Rev* 70(3):153–164, 2012.
20. Shechter M: Magnesium and cardiovascular system, *Magnes Res* 23(2):60–72, 2011.
21. Spiegel DM: Magnesium in chronic kidney disease: unanswered questions, *Blood Purif* 31(1-3):172–176, 2011.
22. Kraut JA, Madias NE: Metabolic acidosis: pathophysiology, diagnosis and management, *Nat Rev Nephrol* 6(5):274–285, 2010.
23. Gennari FJ: Pathophysiology of metabolic alkalosis: a new classification based on the centrality of stimulated collecting duct ion transport, *Am J Kidney Dis* 58(4):626–636, 2011.

CHAPTER

4

Genes and Genetic Diseases

Lynn B. Jorde

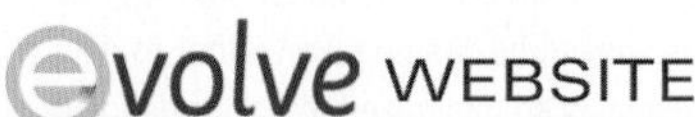

http://evolve.elsevier.com/McCance/

- Review Questions and Answers
- Animations
- Online Course: Module 3

CHAPTER OUTLINE

In the nineteenth century, microscopic studies of cells led scientists to suspect that the nucleus of the cell contained the important mechanisms of inheritance. Scientists found that chromatin, the substance that gives the nucleus a granular appearance, is observable in nondividing cells (also see Chapter 6). Just before the cell divides, the chromatin condenses to form microscopically observable, threadlike structures called chromosomes. (Cell division and chromosomes are discussed in Chapter 1.) With the rediscovery of Gregor Mendel's important breeding experiments at the turn of the twentieth century, it soon became apparent that the chromosomes contained **genes,** the basic units of inheritance. Genes are composed of sequences of **deoxyribonucleic acid (DNA),** a primary constituent of chromosomes; the other primary constituent consists of proteins, such as histones, that cause the DNA to coil into a highly compressed structure (Figure 1-2, Chapter 1). By serving as the blueprints of proteins in the body, genes ultimately influence all aspects of body structure and function. Humans have approximately 20,000 to 25,000 genes. An error in one of these genes can lead to a recognizable genetic disease. The composition of genes at a given locus is known as the ***genotype.*** The outward appearance of an individual, which is the result of both genotype and environment, is the ***phenotype*** (p. 151).

To date, more than 21,000 human genetic traits have been identified and cataloged.[1] About one third of pediatric inpatients are children with genetic diseases.[2] In addition, many common diseases that affect primarily adults, such as hypertension, coronary heart disease, diabetes, and cancer, are now known to have important genetic components. (These diseases are also affected by environmental factors. The interaction between genetic and environmental components is discussed in Chapter 5.)

BOX 4-1 GENETIC TESTING

The genetic causes of several thousand different diseases have now been identified and the pace of discovery is accelerating. Consequently, it is now possible to perform genetic tests to help determine whether an individual carries specific disease-causing mutations. Chromosome disorders, such as trisomy 21, are routinely detected using karyotypes or other, more automated approaches. More than 2700 diseases can now be diagnosed by testing for specific mutations (www.ncbi.nlm.nih.gov/sites/GeneTests/). In addition, genetic tests have been developed to help predict susceptibility for a number of common, genetically complex diseases.

Genetic testing can be applied in a variety of contexts, including:

1. *Carrier screening.* Genetic tests can identify heterozygous carriers for many recessive diseases, such as cystic fibrosis, sickle cell disease, and Tay-Sachs disease. It is becoming increasingly common for couples to undergo carrier screening to help make reproductive decisions, especially in populations in which specific diseases are relatively common (e.g., Tay-Sachs disease in the Ashkenazi Jewish population, β-thalassemia in Mediterranean populations). As a result, the prevalence of some of these diseases has declined dramatically in the past two decades.
2. *Prenatal diagnosis.* Several forms of prenatal genetic diagnosis are available, including:
   a. *Amniocentesis.* This procedure, which is usually carried out at about 16 weeks' gestation, involves the withdrawal of a small amount of amniotic fluid from the uterus. This fluid contains fetal cells, which can be cultured and karyotyped to detect chromosome abnormalities. In addition, genetic testing for single-gene disorders can be undertaken using DNA from these cells. Neural tube defects (spina bifida and anencephaly) can be detected as an elevation of α-fetoprotein level in amniotic fluid. Because there is a risk of fetal loss as a result of this procedure (estimated to be less than 1/200 above the background loss rate), it is usually recommended for women whose age is greater than 30 to 35 years or for couples who have a known increased risk of a specific genetic disease.
   b. *Chorionic villus sampling (CVS).* Carried out at 10 to 12 weeks' gestation, CVS is performed by extracting a small amount of villous tissue directly from the chorion. This procedure does not require in vitro culturing of cells for chromosome analysis because sufficient numbers are directly available in the extracted tissue. Chorionic villus sampling involves a slightly higher fetal loss rate (approximately 1%) than that of amniocentesis.
   c. *Preimplantation genetic diagnosis (PGD).* This relatively new procedure is carried out on early embryos (typically 8 to 12 cells) created by in vitro fertilization. One or two cells are removed from the embryo (which causes no damage), and these cells can be tested for chromosome abnormalities or single-gene disorders. If a genetic disorder is found in the cell, the embryo is not implanted in the mother's uterus.
   d. *Analysis of fetal DNA in maternal circulation.* By approximately 6 to 8 weeks' gestation, fetal cells can be found in the mother's bloodstream and these cells (or cell-free fetal DNA) can be tested for some disease-causing mutations. This approach is still largely experimental, but it is developing rapidly and has the advantages of early diagnosis and minimal risk to the mother and fetus. In addition to these diagnostic procedures, prenatal screening is now routinely carried out by measuring various analytes in maternal serum samples to assess the risk of conditions, such as trisomy 21, 13, and 18, and neural tube defects. Newborn screening also is commonly performed for a variety of genetic conditions such as PKU and galactosemia. A positive screening result is an indication for a subsequent diagnostic test (e.g., amniocentesis for a positive prenatal screening result or DNA sequencing for a positive newborn screening result).
3. *Presymptomatic diagnosis.* Many hereditary diseases, such as familial breast or colon cancer, can be tested genetically before an individual develops the disease. For some of these conditions, measures can be taken either to diagnose the disease early (e.g., colonoscopy) or to minimize the risk of developing the disease.
4. *Testing for drug efficacy or sensitivity.* A number of genes are now known to be associated with sensitivity to specific therapeutic drugs, and people are sometimes tested for variants in these genes to help guide drug treatment. For example, abacavir, an antiviral drug used in treating human immunodeficiency virus (HIV) infection, can cause severe adverse reactions in those who have a specific HLA-B variant (HLA-B*57:01), and the FDA now recommends testing for this variant before administering abacavir. For other drugs, such as warfarin, genetic testing for variants in specific genes (*CYP2C9* and *VKORC1*) may help to guide drug dosage.

Although genetic testing can be very informative, it also has limitations. Genetic testing usually reveals the presence or absence of a disease-causing mutation, but many genetic diseases have incomplete penetrance. For example, a woman who carries a mutation in the *BRCA1* or *BRCA2* genes has a lifetime breast cancer risk of approximately 70% to 80% (but not 100%). In addition, the absence of a disease-causing mutation does not guarantee that the disease in question will not occur (e.g., a woman who does not have a *BRCA1* or *BRCA2* mutation still has nearly the same risk of developing breast cancer as do other women because these genes account for only a few percent of all cases of breast cancer). Individuals and families should be advised of these and other limitations of genetic testing.

Data from Harper JC, Sengupta SB: *Hum Genet* 131(2):175–186, 2012; South ST et al: *Clin Obstet Gynecol* 51(1):62–73, 2008.

Great progress is being made in the diagnosis of genetic diseases and the understanding of genetic mechanisms underlying them. Genetic testing is used increasingly to guide drug choice and dosage, and gene therapy—the direct alteration of genes in cells—is now carried out effectively for some diseases. Genetics is now one of the most rapidly advancing fields of medicine (Boxes 4-1 and 4-2).

DNA, RNA, AND PROTEINS: HEREDITY AT THE MOLECULAR LEVEL

DNA

Composition and Structure

Genes are composed of DNA and the most important constituent of DNA is four types of nitrogenous bases (Figure 4-1). The four bases, **adenine, cytosine, guanine,** and **thymine,** are commonly represented by their first letters: A, C, G, and T, respectively.

In the early 1950s, James Watson and Francis Crick determined the physical structure of DNA. They proposed the now-famous **double-helix** model, in which DNA can be envisioned as a twisted ladder with chemical bonds as its rungs (see Figure 4-1). Projecting from each side of the ladder, at regular intervals, are the nitrogenous bases. The base projecting from one side is bound to the base projecting from the other by a weak hydrogen bond. Therefore, the nitrogenous bases form the rungs of the ladder; adenine pairs with thymine, and guanine pairs with cytosine. Each DNA subunit—consisting of one deoxyribose molecule, one phosphate group, and one base (see Figure 4-1)—is called a **nucleotide.**

BOX 4-2 GENE THERAPY

Gene therapy, in which the harmful effects of a disease-causing mutation are corrected by altering the person's DNA, has been a long-sought goal in human genetics. Hundreds of individuals are currently enrolled in dozens of clinical trials of gene therapy. Many technical challenges have arisen, but gene therapy is now beginning to yield positive therapeutic results.

In somatic cell gene therapy, the DNA of a specific set of an individual's somatic cells is altered (it is also possible to perform germline therapy, which affects all cells, including reproductive cells; however, for technical and ethical reasons, this is not being pursued in humans). Most commonly, somatic cell therapy is used for conditions in which a mutation has caused the absence of a gene product in a cell (e.g., adenosine deaminase in T cells, which leads to immunodeficiency). A "vector" is used to carry a normal copy of the mutated gene into the individual's cells. These vectors are usually viruses, such as retroviruses or adenoviruses, which have been genetically modified so that they contain the normal human gene and cannot make copies of themselves (otherwise they could cause a viral infection). Once inside the individual's cells, the normal human gene begins to encode the missing gene product.

This approach faces a number of technical hurdles, including immune responses against the vector and difficulties in producing sufficient quantities of the desired gene product. In one case, an immune response against an adenoviral vector proved fatal, and several cases of leukemia have resulted from the insertion of a modified retrovirus near an oncogene. Nevertheless, gene therapy has now been successful in treating a number of inherited conditions, including two forms of severe combined immunodeficiency (SCID), β-thalassemia, and X-linked adrenoleukodystrophy. In some cases, symptoms have been completely reversed through gene therapy. In addition to the treatment of hereditary diseases, gene therapy is being used to alter tumor cells in the treatment of various types of cancer. It is hoped that further research will lead to safe, efficient, and cost-effective treatment of many human diseases through gene therapy.

Data from Kay MA: *Nat Rev Genet* 12(5):316–328, 2011.

DNA as the Genetic Code

To serve as the basis of genetic inheritance DNA must be able to provide a code for all the body's proteins. Proteins are composed of one or more **polypeptides** (intermediate protein compounds), which are in turn composed of sequences of **amino acids** (organic acids containing NH_2). The body contains 20 different types of amino acids, and the amino acid sequences that make up polypeptides must in some way be specified by the DNA molecule.

Because there are 20 possible amino acids and only four bases, each single nucleotide cannot specify an amino acid. Similarly, the amino acids cannot be specified by couplets of bases (e.g., adenine-guanine, thymine-guanine, guanine-cytosine) because there are only 4 × 4, or 16, possible couplets. If series of 3 bases are translated into amino acids, however, there are 4 × 4 × 4, or 64, possible combinations—more than enough to specify each different amino acid. By manufacturing synthetic nucleotide sequences and allowing them to direct the formation of amino acids in the laboratory, it was proved that amino acids were specified by these triplets of bases, or **codons.**

Of the 64 possible codons, three signal the end of a gene and are known as **termination,** or **nonsense, codons.** The remaining 61 all specify amino acids, which means that most amino acids can be specified by more than one codon. The genetic code is thus said to be redundant, although each codon can specify only one amino acid.

Another significant feature of the genetic code is that it is nearly universal: with the exception of ciliated protozoa and some plants, all organisms use precisely the same DNA codes to specify proteins. An important general exception to this rule occurs in mitochondria—cytoplasmic organelles that are the sites of cellular respiration (see Chapter 1). The mitochondria have their own extranuclear DNA. Several codons of mitochondrial DNA encode different amino acids than do the same nuclear DNA codons.

Replication

In addition to having the ability to specify amino acid sequences, DNA must be able to replicate itself accurately during cell division if it is to serve as the basic genetic material. DNA replication consists of the breaking of the weak hydrogen bonds between the bases, leaving a single strand with each base unpaired. The consistent pairing of adenine with thymine and of guanine with cytosine, known as **complementary base pairing,** is the key to accurate replication. The principle of complementary base pairing dictates that the unpaired base will attract a free nucleotide only if the nucleotide has the proper complementary base. Thus a portion of a single strand with a sequence of bases labeled ATTGCT will bond with a series of free nucleotides with the bases TAACGA. When replication is complete, a new double-stranded molecule identical to the original is formed (Figure 4-2, *A*). The single strand is said to be a **template (guide),** or molecule on which a complementary molecule is built, and is the basis for synthesizing the new double strand.

Several different proteins are involved in DNA replication. One protein unwinds the double helix, one holds the strands apart, and others perform different distinct functions. The most important of these proteins is the enzyme known as **DNA polymerase.** This enzyme travels along the single DNA strand, adding the correct nucleotides to the free end of the new strand (see Figure 4-2, *B*). Besides adding the new nucleotides, the DNA polymerase performs a proofreading procedure. After the new nucleotide has been added to the chain, the DNA polymerase checks to make sure that its base is actually complementary to the template base. If it is not, the incorrect nucleotide is excised and replaced with a correct one. This procedure, one of the mechanisms of DNA repair, substantially enhances the accuracy of DNA replication.

Mutation

A **mutation** is any inherited alteration of genetic material. Microscopically observable alterations of chromosome number or structure are examples of mutations. Some mutations are much too small to be observed under a microscope. An example is the **base pair substitution,** in which one base pair is replaced by another. This mutation is sometimes called **missense mutation** because the "sense" of the codon produced after transcription of the mutant gene is altered (Figure 4-3). This substitution sometimes results in a change in amino acid sequence, but because of the redundancy of the genetic code, it may have no consequence. Profound consequences can result

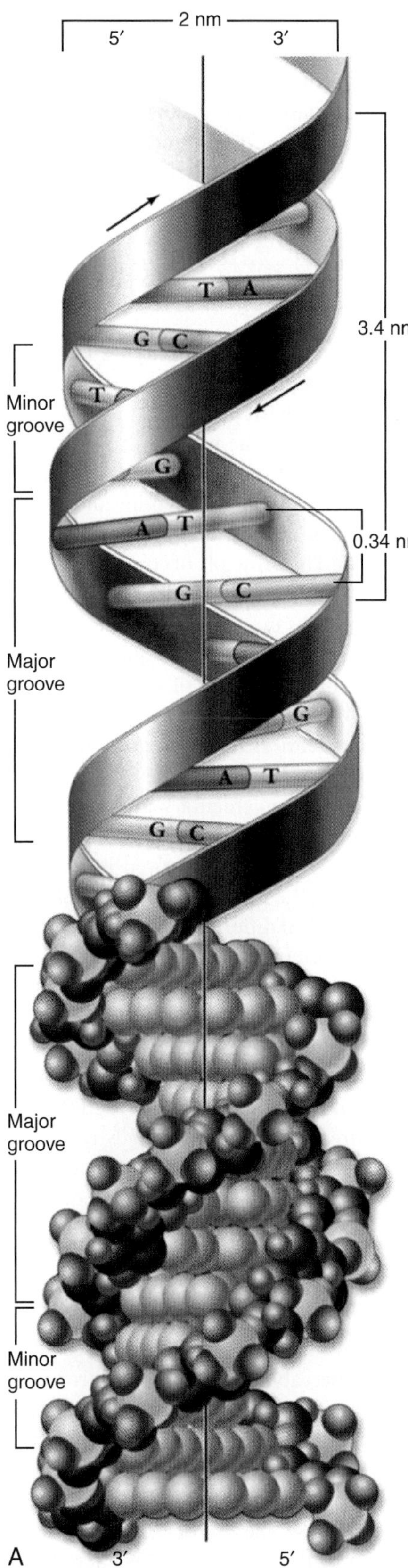

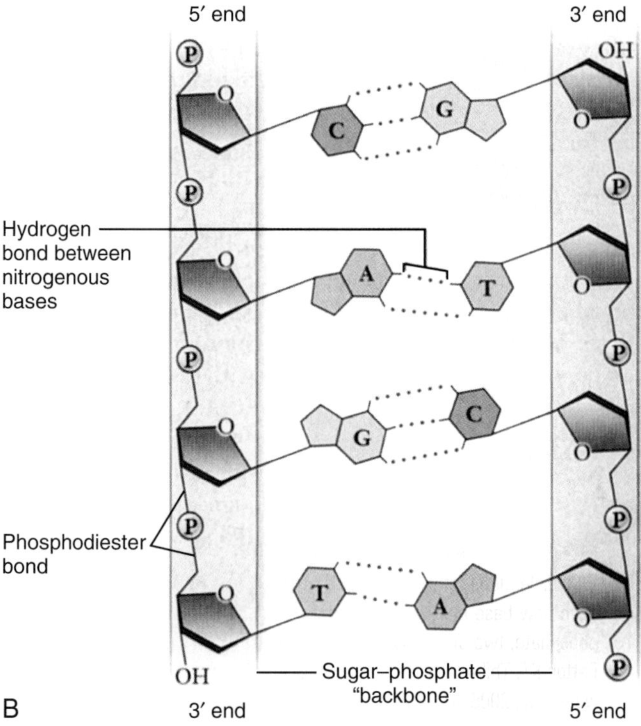

FIGURE 4-1 Structure of DNA. **A,** Double helix. Shown with the phosphodiester backbone as a ribbon on top and a space-filling model on the bottom. The bases protrude into the interior of the helix where they hold it together by base pairing. The backbone forms two grooves, the larger major groove and the smaller minor groove. **B,** Base pairing holds strands together. The H-bonds that form between A and T and between G and C are shown with dashed lines. These produce AT and GC base pairs that hold the two strands together. This always pairs a purine with a pyrimidine, keeping the diameter of the double helix constant. *A,* Adenine; *C,* cytosine; *G,* guanine; *T,* thymine. (From Raven PH et al: *Biology,* ed 8, New York, 2008, McGraw-Hill.)

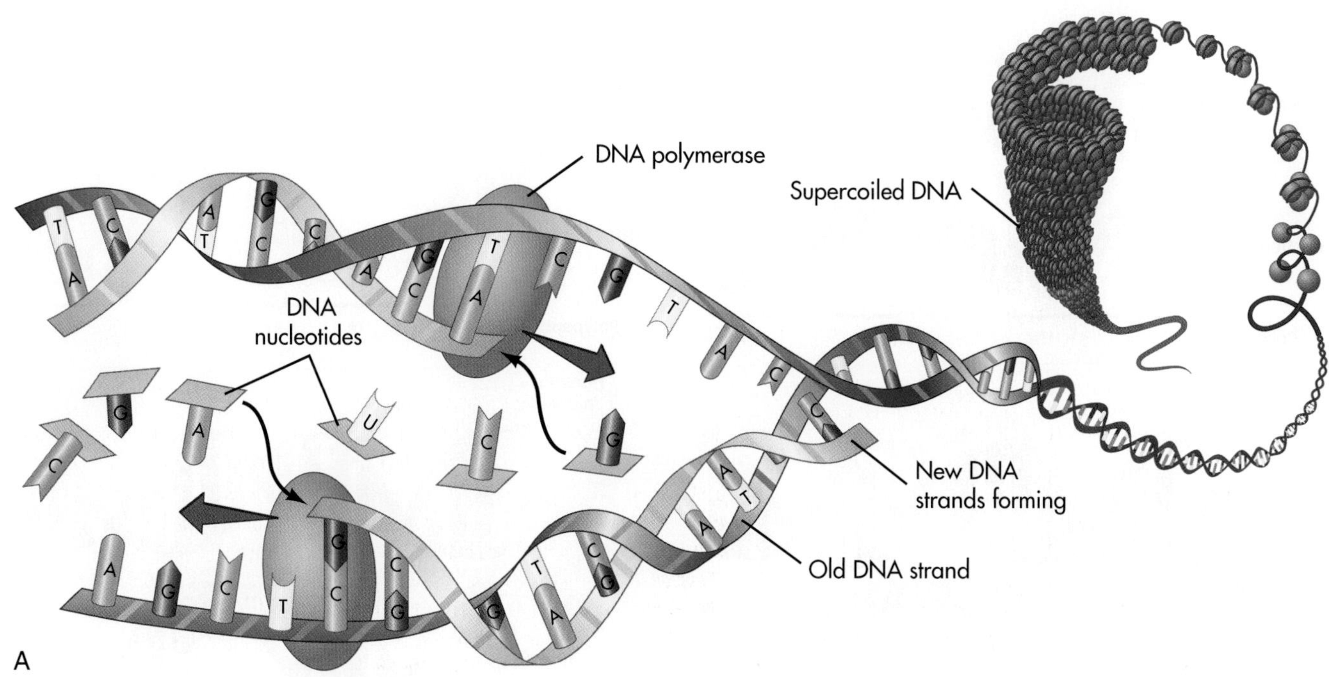

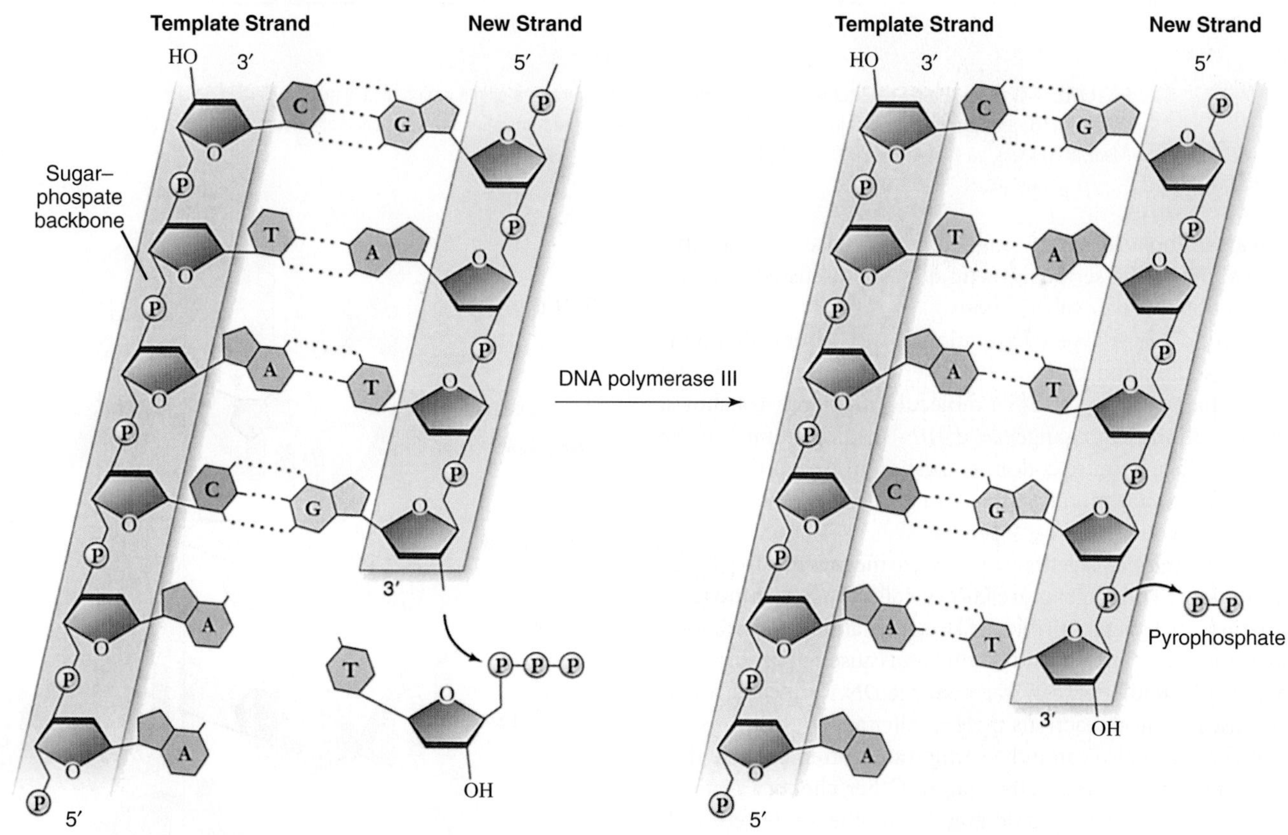

FIGURE 4-2 Replication and Action of DNA. **A,** Replication of DNA. **B,** Action of DNA polymerase. DNA polymerases add nucleotides to the 3′ end of a growing chain. The nucleotide added depends on the base that is in the template strand. Each new base must be complementary to the base in the template strand. With the addition of each new nucleotide, triphosphate, two of its phosphates are cleaved off as pyrophosphate. *A,* Adenine; *T,* thymine; *G,* guanine; *C,* cytosine. (**A** from Patton KT, Thibodeau GA: *Anatomy & physiology,* ed 8, St Louis, 2013, Mosby; **B** adapted from Raven PH et al: *Biology,* ed 8, New York, 2008, McGraw-Hill.)

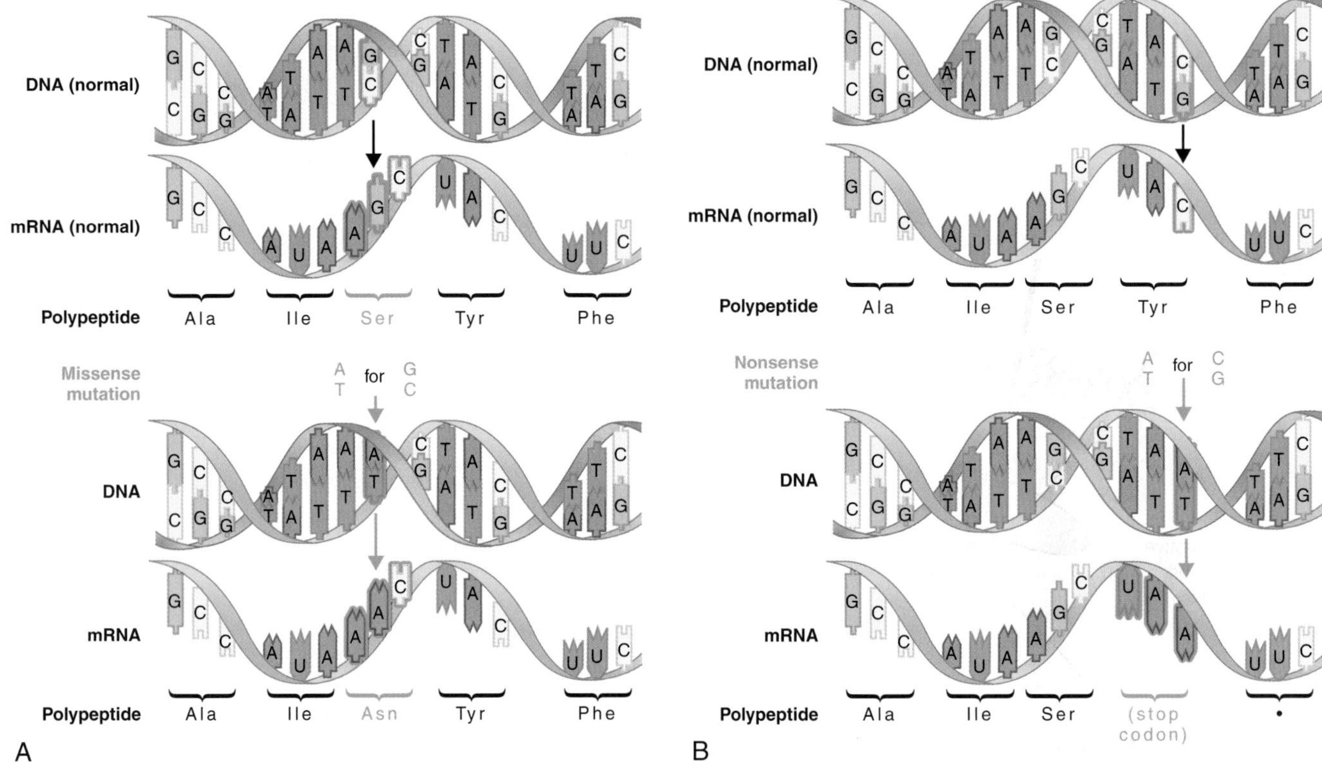

FIGURE 4-3 Base Pair Substitution. Missense mutations **(A)** produce a single amino acid change, whereas nonsense mutations **(B)** produce a stop codon in the mRNA. Stop codons terminate translation of the polypeptide. (From Jorde LB et al: *Medical genetics,* ed 4, St Louis, 2010, Mosby.)

when an amino acid sequence is altered by a base pair substitution. (Many of the serious genetic diseases discussed later are the result of base pair substitutions.)

A second major type of mutation is the **frameshift mutation.** This alteration involves the insertion or deletion of one or more base pairs to the DNA molecule. As Figure 4-4 shows, these mutations can change the entire "reading frame" of the DNA sequence because codons consist of groups of three base pairs. A frameshift mutation thus can greatly alter the resulting amino acid sequence.

A large number of agents are known to increase the frequency of mutations. These agents are known collectively as **mutagens.** Radiation, such as that produced by x-rays and nuclear fallout, is an important mutagen and is known to cause cell damage (see Chapter 12). Radiation can fragment the DNA molecule and it can cause chemical reactions that can alter a DNA base. A variety of chemicals also can induce mutations, often because they are chemically similar to DNA bases. Other chemicals mimic the effects of ionizing radiation, and still others interfere with the process of base pairing. Hundreds of chemicals are now known to be mutagenic in humans or laboratory animals, such as nitrogen mustard, vinyl chloride, alkylating agents, formaldehyde, and sodium nitrite. Some of these chemicals, however, are much more potent mutagens than others. Nitrogen mustard, for example, is extremely mutagenic, whereas sodium nitrate is a weak mutagen.

Measurement of the mutation rate in humans is difficult, in part because mutations are very rare events. Current estimates

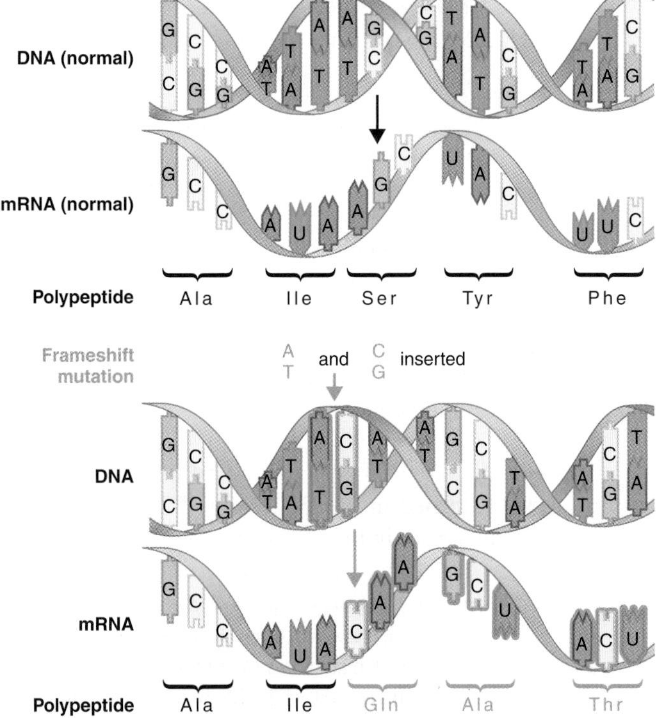

FIGURE 4-4 Frameshift Mutations. Frameshift mutations result from the addition or deletion of a number of bases that is not a multiple of 3. This mutation alters all of the codons downstream from the site of insertion or deletion. (From Jorde LB et al: *Medical genetics,* ed 4, St Louis, 2010, Mosby.)

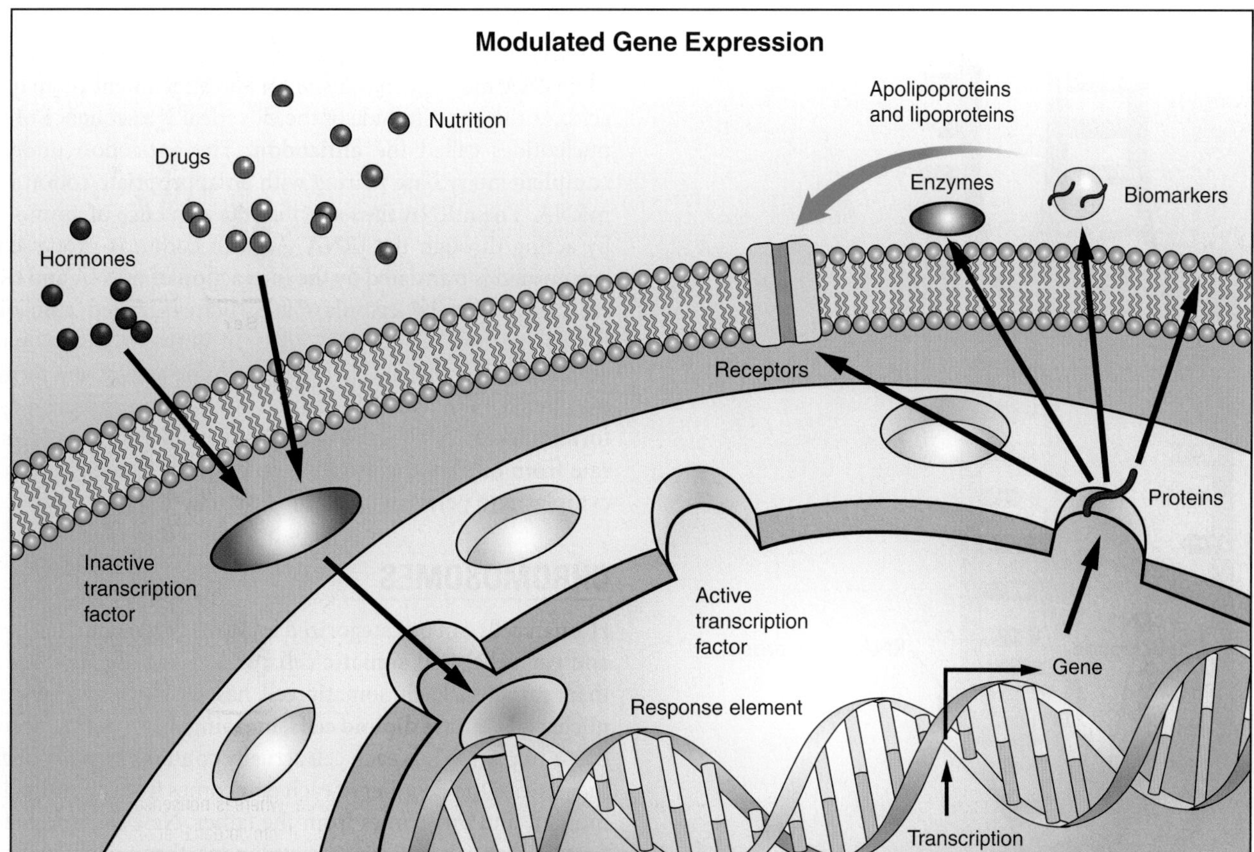

FIGURE 4-5 Transcription Factors and Simplified Schematic of Gene Expression. Transcription factors are proteins and bind to specific sites on DNA. They read and interpret the genetic blueprint of the DNA thereby controlling transcription or the flow of genetic information from DNA to mRNA. Transcription factors are essential for gene expression; for example, proteins that function as receptors, enzymes, or biomarkers. Environmental stimuli: for example, hormones involve signaling cascades that can involve transcription factors. Transcription factors can alter gene expression to promote pathophysiology.

are that the **mutation rate** in humans is about 10^{-4} to 10^{-7} per gene per generation. This rate appears to vary from one gene to another, with greater mutation rates for larger genes. At the nucleotide level, the human mutation rate is approximately 10^{-8} per nucleotide per generation. Certain DNA sequences have particularly high mutation rates and are known as **mutational hot spots.** In particular, sequences consisting of a cytosine base followed by a guanine base (CG) are highly susceptible to mutation and are known to account for a disproportionately large percentage of disease-causing mutations.[3]

From Genes to Proteins

Whereas DNA is formed and replicated in the cell nucleus, protein synthesis takes place in the cytoplasm. The transport of the DNA code from nucleus to cytoplasm and the subsequent protein formation involve two basic processes: transcription and translation. Both of these processes are mediated by **ribonucleic acid (RNA),** a type of nucleic acid that is chemically very similar to DNA. RNA differs from DNA in that uracil rather than thymine is one of the four nitrogenous bases. The other bases of RNA, as in DNA, are adenine, cytosine, and guanine. Uracil is structurally very similar to thymine, so it also can pair with adenine. Whereas DNA usually occurs as a double strand, RNA usually occurs as a single strand.

Transcription

Transcription is the process by which RNA is synthesized from a DNA template. The result is the formation of **messenger RNA (mRNA)** from the base sequence specified by the DNA molecule. Transcription of a gene begins when an enzyme called **RNA polymerase** binds to a **promoter site** on the DNA. A promoter site is a sequence of DNA that specifies the beginning of a gene. In addition to RNA polymerase, proteins called **transcription factors** bind to DNA sequences called **transcription factor binding sites** near genes to regulate the timing of transcription, as well as the specific tissues in which genes are actively transcribed (e.g., clotting factor VIII primarily in hepatocytes) (Figure 4-5). Transcription factors can either activate or repress the expression of genes. In addition, transcription is sometimes up-regulated by the binding of nearby DNA sequences called **enhancers.** The RNA polymerase pulls a portion of the DNA strands apart from one another, allowing unattached DNA bases to be exposed. One of the DNA strands then provides the template for the sequence of mRNA nucleotides.

The sequence of bases in the mRNA is thus complementary to that of the template strand, and with the exception of the presence of uracil instead of thymine, the mRNA sequence is identical to that of the other DNA strand. Transcription continues until a DNA sequence called a **termination sequence** is

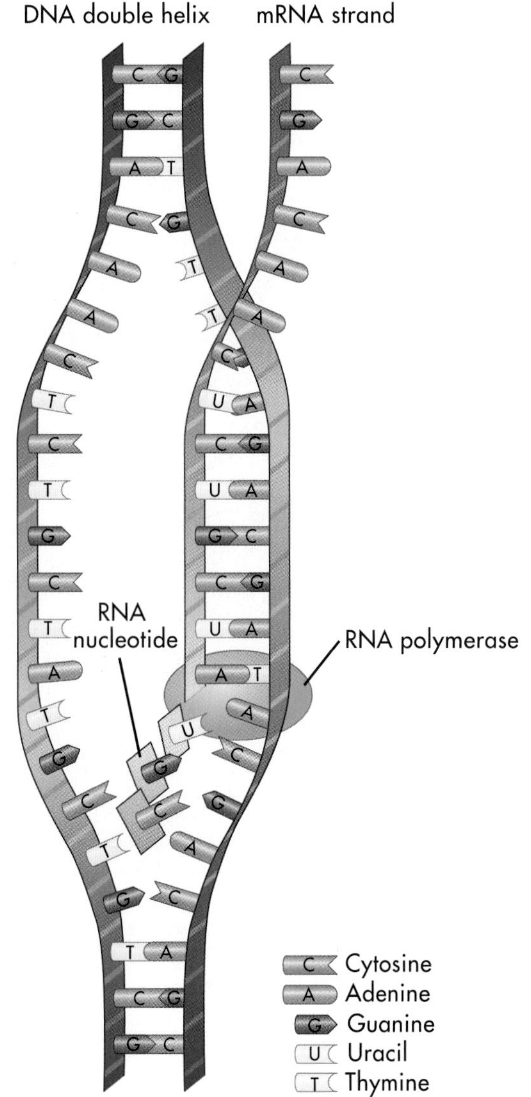

FIGURE 4-6 **General Scheme of RNA Transcription.** See text for explanation. (From Patton KT, Thibodeau GA: *Anatomy & physiology,* ed 8, St Louis, 2013, Mosby.)

reached. Then the RNA polymerase detaches from the DNA, and the transcribed mRNA is freed to move out of the nucleus and into the cytoplasm. Figure 4-6 summarizes the process of transcription.

RNA Splicing

After the mRNA first has been transcribed from the DNA template, it reflects exactly the base sequence of the DNA. In eukaryotes an important step takes place before this RNA leaves the nucleus. Many of the RNA sequences are removed and the remaining sequences are spliced together to form the functional mRNA that will migrate to the cytoplasm. The excised sequences are called **introns,** and the sequences that are left to code for proteins are called **exons.** The functions of most introns remain poorly understood.

Translation

Translation is the process by which RNA directs the synthesis of a polypeptide (Figure 4-7). However, mRNA cannot code directly for amino acids. Instead, it interacts with **transfer RNA (tRNA),** a cloverleaf-shaped strand of about 80 nucleotides. The tRNA molecule has a site for the attachment of an amino acid. At the opposite side of the cloverleaf is a sequence of three nucleotides called the **anticodon.** The anticodon undergoes complementary base pairing with an appropriate codon in the mRNA. The mRNA thus specifies the sequence of amino acids by acting through the tRNA. As each codon is processed, an amino acid is translated by the interaction of mRNA and tRNA, which is aided by cytoplasmic structures called **ribosomes.** Bonds are formed between adjacent amino acids to make a growing polypeptide. When the ribosome arrives at a termination signal on the mRNA sequence, translation and polypeptide formation cease. The mRNA, ribosome, and polypeptide separate from one another and the polypeptide is released into the cytoplasm to perform its required function.

CHROMOSOMES

Human cells can be categorized into two types: **gametes** (sperm and egg cells) and **somatic cells,** which include all cells other than gametes. Each somatic cell has 46 chromosomes in its nucleus. These are **diploid cells,** meaning that the chromosomes occur in pairs. Thus each cell actually contains 23 pairs of chromosomes. One member of each pair comes from an individual's mother, and one comes from the father. New somatic cells are formed through mitosis and cytokinesis, through which the cell nucleus and cytoplasm are replicated. (The division process that creates new copies of somatic cells is described in Chapter 1.) Gametes are **haploid cells:** they have only one member of each chromosome pair, giving them a total of 23 chromosomes. The process by which these haploid cells are formed from diploid cells is called **meiosis** (Figure 4-8).

In 22 of the 23 chromosome pairs, the two members of each pair are virtually identical in microscopic appearance and DNA sequence and are thus said to be **homologous** to one another. These 22 chromosome pairs are homologous in both males and females and are termed **autosomes.** The remaining pair of chromosomes, the **sex chromosomes,** consists of two homologous X chromosomes in females and a nonhomologous pair, X and Y, in males.

Figure 4-9, *A,* illustrates a **metaphase spread,** which is a photograph of the chromosomes as they appear in the nucleus of a somatic cell during metaphase. (Chromosomes are easiest to visualize during this stage of mitosis.) A **karyotype** is an ordered display of chromosomes. In Figure 4-9, *B,* the chromosomes are arranged according to size, with the **homologous chromosomes** paired. The 22 autosomes are numbered according to length, with chromosome 1 as the longest and chromosome 22 as the shortest. Some natural variation in relative chromosome length can be expected from person to person, however, so it is not always possible to distinguish each chromosome by its length. Therefore, the position of the centromere is also used to classify the chromosomes (Figure 4-10).

The chromosomes in Figure 4-9, *A,* were stained with a substance that binds preferentially to certain areas of chromosomes. The resulting distinctive **chromosome bands** are

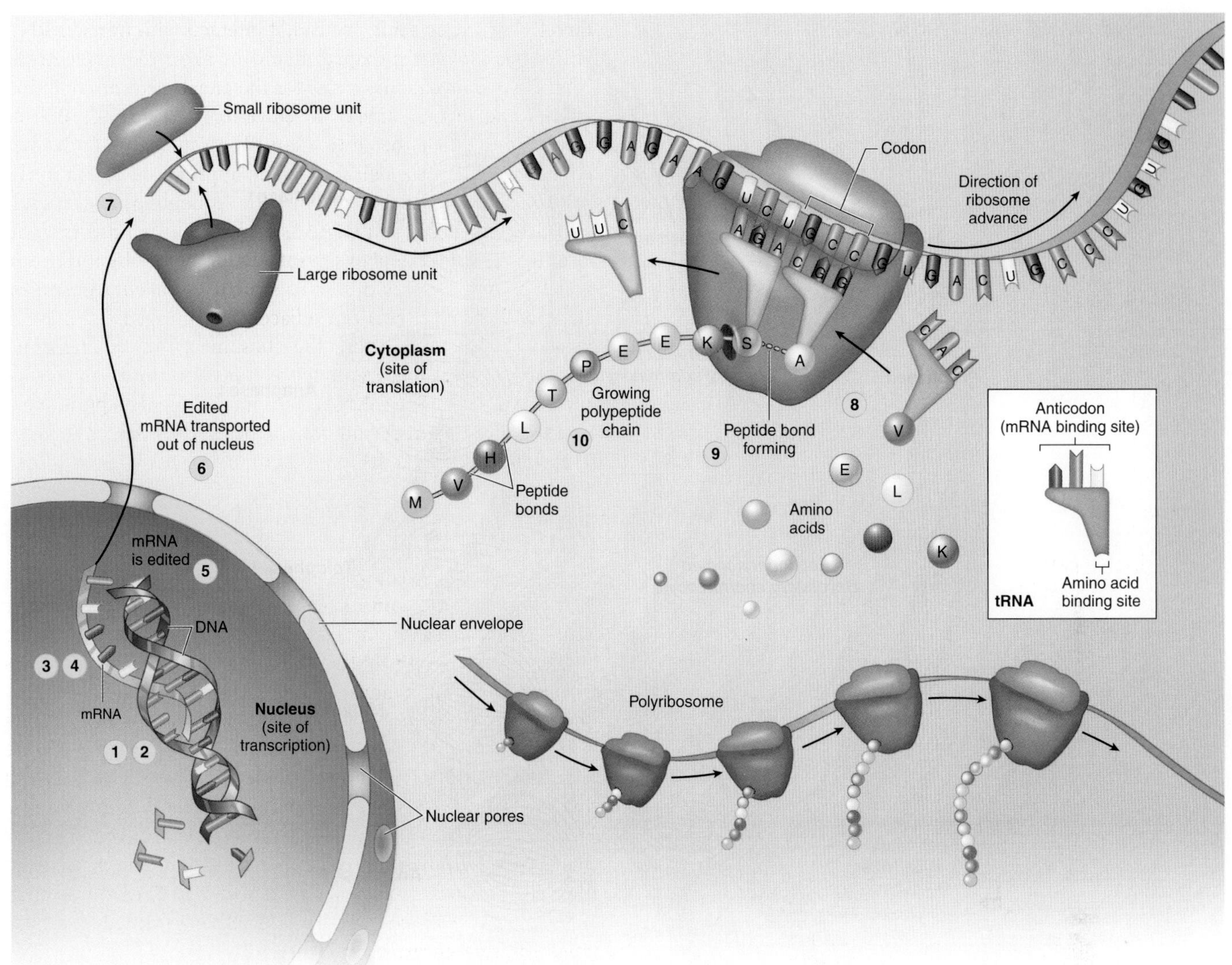

FIGURE 4-7 **Protein Synthesis.** Protein synthesis begins with *transcription,* a process in which an mRNA molecule forms along one gene sequence of a DNA molecule within the cell's nucleus **(1-3).** As it is formed, the mRNA molecule separates from the DNA molecule **(4),** is edited **(5),** and leaves the nucleus through the large nuclear pores **(6).** Outside the nucleus, ribosome subunits attach to the beginning of the mRNA molecule and begin the process of *translation* **(7).** In translation, transfer RNA (tRNA) molecules bring specific amino acids—encoded by each mRNA codon—into place at the ribosome site **(8).** As the amino acids are brought into the proper sequence, they are joined together by peptide bonds **(9)** to form long strands called *polypeptides* **(10).** Several polypeptide chains may be needed to make a complete protein molecule. *A,* Adenine; *C,* cytosine; *G,* guanine; *U,* uracil. (From Patton KT, Thibodeau GA: *Anatomy & physiology,* ed 8, St Louis, 2013, Mosby.)

evident in various patterns in the different chromosomes so that each chromosome can be distinguished easily. One of the most commonly used stains is **Giemsa stain.** By using banding techniques, chromosomes can be unambiguously numbered, and individual variation in chromosome composition can be studied. Missing or duplicated portions of chromosomes, which often result in serious diseases, also can be readily identified.

Chromosome Aberrations and Associated Diseases

Chromosome abnormalities are the leading known cause of mental retardation and miscarriage. A major chromosome aberration occurs in more than half of conceptions. Most of these fetuses do not survive to term; in fact, about 50% of all recovered first-trimester spontaneous abortuses have major chromosomal aberrations.[4] About 1 in 150 live births has a major diagnosable chromosome abnormality.[5]

Polyploidy

Cells that have a multiple of the normal number of chromosomes are said to be **euploid cells** (Greek *eu* = good or true). Because normal gametes are haploid and most normal somatic cells are diploid, they are both euploid forms. When a euploid

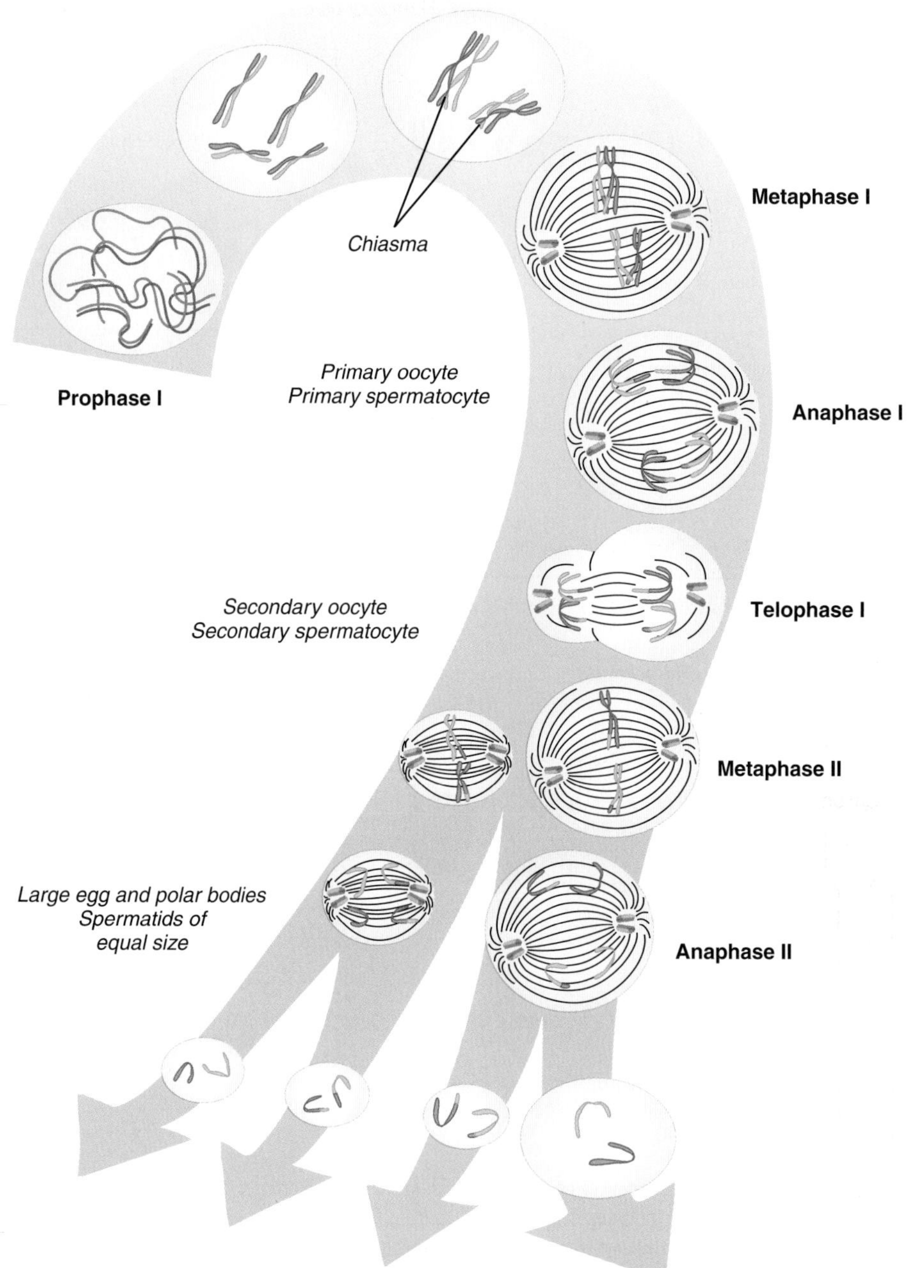

FIGURE 4-8 Stages of Meiosis. From these stages, haploid gametes are formed from a diploid stem cell. For brevity, prophase II and telophase II are not shown. Note the relationship between meiosis and spermatogenesis and oogenesis. (From Jorde LB et al: *Medical genetics,* ed 4, St Louis, 2010, Mosby.)

cell has more than the diploid number of chromosomes, it is said to be a **polyploid cell.** Several types of body tissues, including some liver, bronchial, and epithelial tissues, are normally polyploid. A zygote having three copies of each chromosome, rather than the usual two, has a form of polyploidy called **triploidy. Tetraploidy,** a condition in which euploid cells have 92 chromosomes, also has been observed. Nearly all triploid and tetraploid conceptions are spontaneously aborted or stillborn, and the small proportion that survive to term die shortly after birth. Triploidy and tetraploidy are relatively common conditions at conception, accounting for approximately 10% of all known miscarriages.[4]

Aneuploidy

Aneuploid cells are defined as those that do not contain a multiple of 23 chromosomes. An aneuploid cell containing three copies of one chromosome is said to be trisomic (a condition termed **trisomy**). **Monosomy,** the presence of only one copy of a given chromosome in a diploid cell, is the other common form of aneuploidy. Among the autosomes, monosomy of any chromosome is lethal, but newborns with trisomy of chromosomes 13, 18, or 21 can survive. This difference illustrates an important principle: loss of chromosome material has more serious consequences than duplication of chromosome material.

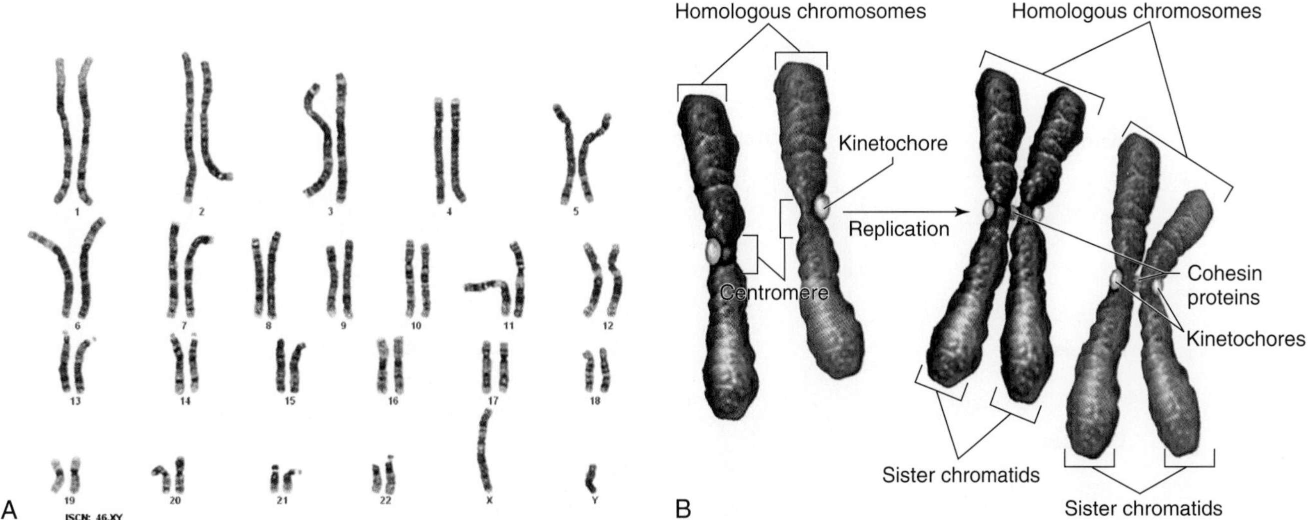

FIGURE 4-9 Karyotype of Chromosomes. **A,** Human karyotype. **B,** Homologous chromosomes and sister chromatids. (**A** courtesy of the Clinical Cytogenetics Section, Laboratory of Pathology, National Cancer Institute, National Institutes of Health, Bethesda, MD. **B** from Raven PH et al: *Biology,* ed 8, New York, 2008, McGraw-Hill.)

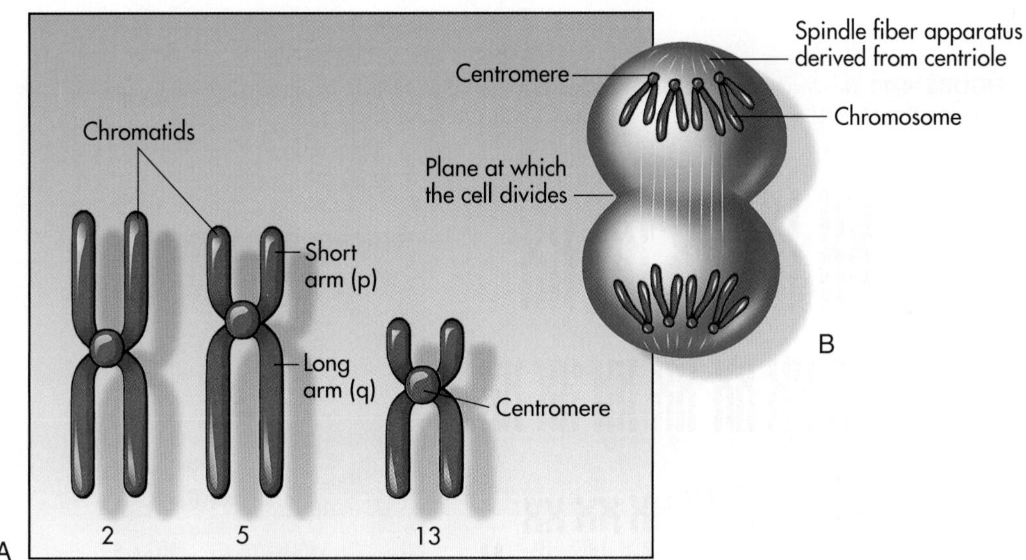

FIGURE 4-10 Structure of Chromosomes. **A,** Human chromosomes 2, 5, and 13. Each is replicated and consists of two chromatids. Chromosome 2 is a metacentric chromosome because the centromere is close to middle; chromosome 5 is submetacentric because the centromere is set off from the middle; chromosome 13 is acrocentric because the centromere is at or very near the end. **B,** During mitosis, the centromere divides and chromosomes move to opposite poles of the cell. At the time of centromere division, the chromatids are designated chromosomes.

Aneuploidy of the sex chromosomes is usually less serious than that of the autosomes. For the Y chromosome, this is true because very little genetic material is located on this chromosome. For the X chromosome, inactivation of extra chromosomes largely diminishes their effect. A zygote bearing *no* X chromosome, however, will not survive.

Aneuploidy is usually the result of **nondisjunction,** an error in which homologous chromosomes or sister chromatids fail to separate normally during meiosis or mitosis (Figure 4-11). Nondisjunction during either stage of meiosis produces some gametes that have two copies of a given chromosome and others that have no copies of the chromosome. When such gametes unite with normal haploid gametes, the resulting zygote is monosomic or trisomic for that chromosome.

Autosomal Aneuploidy. Trisomy can occur for any chromosome at conception, but the only forms seen with an appreciable frequency in live births are trisomies of the thirteenth, eighteenth, or twenty-first chromosome. Fetuses with most other chromosomal trisomies do not survive to term. Trisomy 16, for example, is the most commonly known trisomy among abortuses, but it is not seen in live births.[4]

Partial trisomy, in which only an extra portion of a chromosome is present in each cell, also can occur. The consequences of partial trisomies are not as severe as those of complete

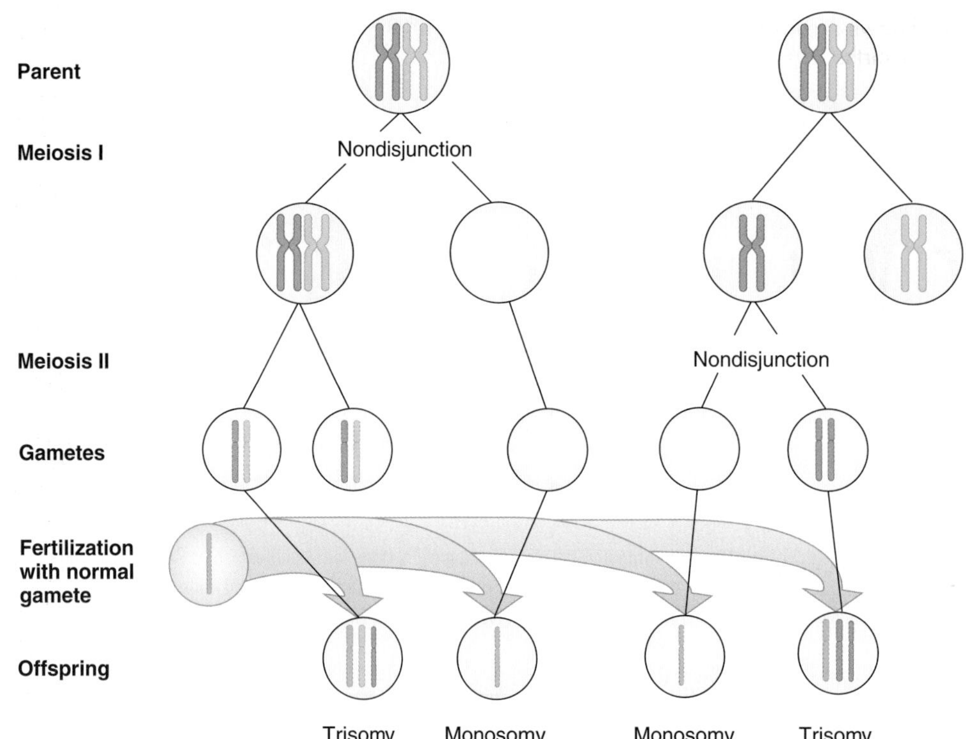

FIGURE 4-11 Nondisjunction Causes Aneuploidy When Chromosomes or Sister Chromatids Fail to Divide Properly. (From Jorde LB et al: *Medical genetics*, ed 4, St Louis, 2010, Mosby.)

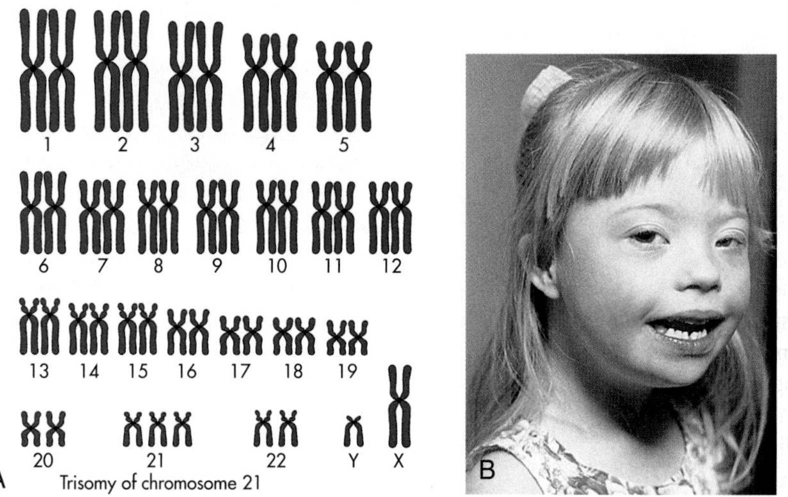

FIGURE 4-12 Down Syndrome. **A,** The karyotype of Down syndrome consists of 47 chromosomes and shows trisomy 21. **B,** A child with Down syndrome. (**A** from Damjanov I: *Pathology for the health professions*, ed 4, Philadelphia, 2012, Saunders; **B** courtesy Olney A, MacDonald M, University of Nebraska Medical Center, Omaha.)

trisomies. Trisomies also may occur in only some cells of the body. Individuals thus affected are said to be **chromosomal mosaics,** meaning that the body has two or more different cell lines, each of which has a different karyotype. Mosaics are usually formed by early mitotic nondisjunction occurring in one embryonic cell but not in others.

The most well-known example of aneuploidy in an autosome is trisomy of the twenty-first chromosome, which causes **Down syndrome** (named after J. Langdon Down, who first described the disease in 1866). Down syndrome was formerly called *mongolism,* but this inappropriate term is no longer used. Down syndrome is seen in 1 in 800 live births.[4] Individuals with this disease typically have intelligence quotients (IQs) between 25 and 70. The facial appearance is distinctive (Figure 4-12), with a low nasal bridge, epicanthal folds, protruding tongue, and flat, low-set ears. Poor muscle tone (hypotonia) and short stature are both characteristic. Congenital heart defects affect about one third to one half of liveborn children with Down syndrome; a reduced ability to fight respiratory tract infections and an increased susceptibility

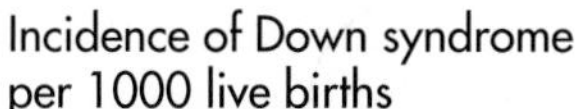

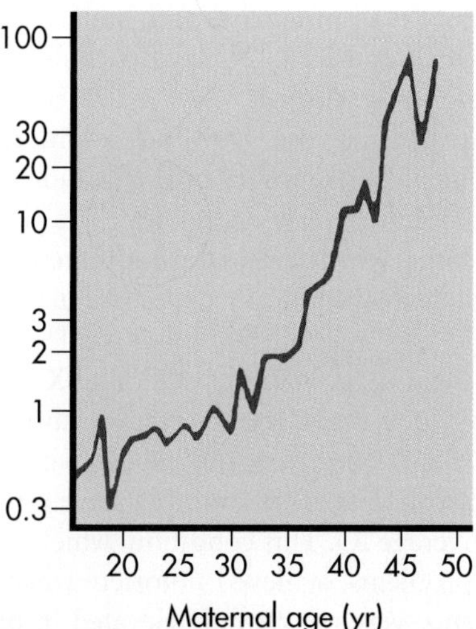

FIGURE 4-13 Down Syndrome Incidence Increases with Maternal Age. Rate is per 1000 live births related to maternal age.

to leukemia also contribute to reduced survival rate. By 40 years of age, individuals with Down syndrome virtually always develop symptoms that are nearly identical to those of Alzheimer disease because one of the genes that can cause Alzheimer disease is located on chromosome 21. About three fourths of fetuses known to have Down syndrome are spontaneously aborted or stillborn. About 20% of infants born with Down syndrome die during their first 10 years of life. For those who survive beyond 10 years, average life expectancy is now about 60 years.

About 97% of Down syndrome cases are caused by nondisjunction during the formation of one of the parent's gametes or during early embryonic development. The remaining 3% result from translocations (discussed later). In approximately 90% to 95% of cases, the nondisjunction occurs in the formation of the mother's egg cell. Paternal nondisjunction is responsible for the remaining cases. Among individuals with Down syndrome, about 1% are known to be mosaics. Because mosaics have a large number of normal cells, the effects of the trisomic cells are attenuated and symptoms are sometimes less severe.

The risk of having a child with Down syndrome increases greatly with maternal age. As Figure 4-13 demonstrates, women younger than 30 years have a risk ranging from about 1 in 1000 births to 1 in 2000 births. The risk begins to rise substantially after 35 years of age, and it reaches 3% to 5% for women older than 45 years of age. This dramatic increase in risk is a consequence of the age of maternal egg cells, which are held in an arrested state of prophase I from the time they are formed in the female embryo until they are shed in ovulation. Thus an egg cell formed by a 45-year-old woman is itself 45 years old. This long suspended state may allow for the accumulation of errors leading to nondisjunction. The risk of Down syndrome, as well as other trisomies, does not appear to increase with paternal age.[6]

Sex Chromosome Aneuploidy. Among live births, about 1 in 400 males and 1 in 650 females have a form of sex chromosome aneuploidy.[7] Because these conditions are generally less severe than autosomal aneuploidies, all forms except complete absence of an X chromosome allow at least some individuals to survive.

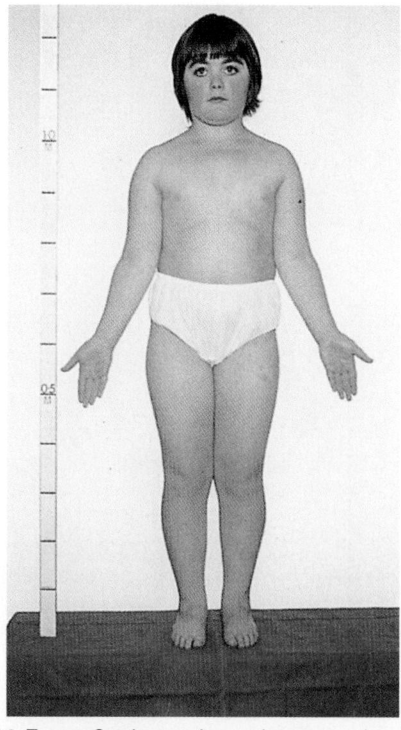

FIGURE 4-14 **Turner Syndrome.** A sex chromosome is missing, and the person's chromosomes are 45,X. Characteristic signs are short stature, female genitalia abnormality, webbed neck, shieldlike chest with underdeveloped breasts and widely spaced nipples, and imperfectly developed ovaries. (From Patton KT, Thibodeau GA: *Anatomy & physiology*, ed 8, St Louis, 2013, Mosby.)

One of the most common sex chromosome aneuploidies, affecting about 1 in 1000 newborn females, is trisomy X. Instead of two X chromosomes, these females have three X chromosomes in each cell. Most of them have no overt physical abnormalities, although sterility, menstrual irregularity, or cognitive deficits are sometimes seen. A very small proportion of females have four or even five X chromosomes, and their mental function is more severely compromised. Another sex chromosome aneuploidy is the presence of a single X chromosome and no homologous X or Y chromosome, resulting in a total of 45 chromosomes. The karyotype is designated 45,X, and it causes a set of symptoms known as **Turner syndrome** (Figure 4-14). Because they have no Y chromosome, only females are affected by Turner syndrome. They are usually sterile, however, and have gonadal streaks rather than ovaries. These streaks of connective tissue are susceptible to cancer in mosaics who have some cells containing a Y chromosome. Other features of the disorder include short stature, webbing of the neck in about half of cases, widely spaced nipples, coarctation (narrowing) of the aorta (in 15% to 20% of cases), edema of the feet in newborns, and sparse body hair. Their IQs are typically in the normal range, although they often have some impairment of spatial and mathematical reasoning ability. About three fourths of recognized 45,X conceptions inherit their X chromosome from the mother. Thus most cases are caused by a loss of the paternal X chromosome.

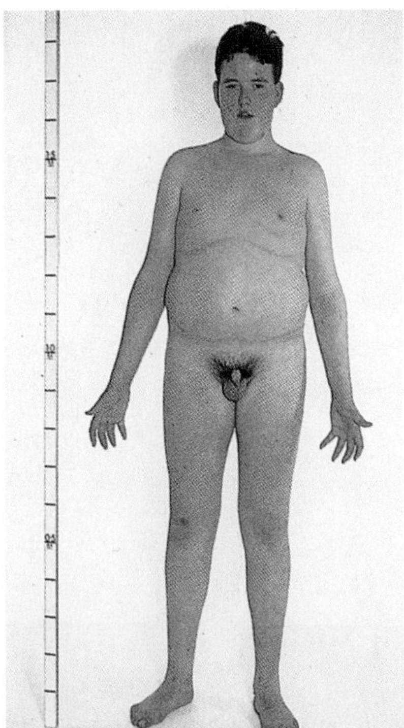

FIGURE 4-15 Klinefelter Syndrome. This young man exhibits many characteristics of Klinefelter syndrome: small testes, some development of the breasts, sparse body hair, and long limbs. This syndrome results from the presence of two or more X chromosomes with one Y chromosome (genotypes XXY or XXXY, for example). (From Patton KT, Thibodeau GA: *Anatomy & physiology*, ed 8, St Louis, 2013, Mosby.)

The frequency of Turner syndrome is low compared with that of other sex chromosome aneuploidies: only about 1 in 2500 newborn females is affected.[8] The 45,X karyotype is more common among conceptions, however, and about 15% to 20% of spontaneous abortions with chromosome abnormalities have this karyotype, making it one of the most common single-chromosome aberrations. Thus the condition is highly lethal during gestation: less than 1% of 45,X conceptions survive to term. Most fetuses that survive to term are mosaics, with combinations of 45,X cells and XX, XXX, or XY cells. It is likely that the presence of some normal cells in mosaic fetuses enhances fetal survival.

Teenagers with Turner syndrome are typically treated with estrogen to promote the development of secondary sexual characteristics. The dose is then continued at a reduced level to maintain these characteristics and to help avoid osteoporosis. Human growth hormone is sometimes administered to increase stature.

Individuals with at least two X chromosomes and a Y chromosome in each cell (47,XXY karyotype) have a disorder known as **Klinefelter syndrome** (Figure 4-15). Because of the presence of a Y chromosome, these individuals have a male appearance, but they are usually sterile, and about half develop female-like breasts (a condition called *gynecomastia*). The testes are small, body hair is sparse, the voice is often somewhat high pitched, stature is elevated, and a moderate degree of mental impairment may be present. Klinefelter syndrome is found in about 1 in 1000 male births. About two thirds of the cases are caused by nondisjunction of the X chromosomes in the mother, and the frequency of the disorder rises with maternal age. Individuals with the XXXY and XXXXY karyotypes also are considered to have Klinefelter syndrome, and the degree of physical and mental impairment increases with each additional X chromosome. Regardless of the number of X chromosomes, however, these individuals have a male appearance. The presence of a single Y chromosome, which causes the undifferentiated gonads to become testes, always produces a male. Mosaicism is sometimes seen in Klinefelter syndrome and results in less severe disease; the most prevalent combination is XXY and XY cells.

About 1 in 1000 males has an extra Y chromosome, producing the 47,XYY karyotype. Individuals with this karyotype tend to be taller than average, and they have a 10- to 15-point reduction in average IQ. This condition, which causes few serious physical problems, achieved notoriety when it was found that its incidence was significantly elevated in prison populations. This discovery led to the suggestion that this chromosome might predispose affected individuals to violent, criminal behavior. Several dozen studies have addressed this issue, and they have shown that 47,XYY males are not inclined to commit violent crimes. However, even after adjusting for the effects of decreased IQ, some evidence exists for an increased incidence of behavioral disorders.

Abnormalities of Chromosome Structure

In addition to the loss or gain of whole chromosomes, parts of chromosomes can be lost or duplicated as gametes are formed, and the arrangement of genes on chromosomes can be altered. Unlike aneuploidy and polyploidy, these changes sometimes do not have serious consequences for an individual's health. Some of them can even remain entirely unnoticed, especially when very small pieces of chromosomes are involved. Nevertheless, abnormalities of chromosome structure also can produce serious disease in individuals or their offspring.

During meiosis and mitosis, chromosomes usually maintain their structural integrity very well, but **chromosome breakage** occasionally does occur. Mechanisms exist to "heal" these breaks, and generally the break is repaired perfectly with no damage resulting to the daughter cell. Sometimes, however, the breaks remain, or they heal in a fashion that alters the structure of the chromosome. Chromosome breakage occurs spontaneously, but it also can be caused by ionizing radiation, some viral infections, and certain chemicals.

Deletions. Broken chromosomes and loss of DNA cause **deletions** (Figure 4-16, *A*). Usually a gamete with a deletion unites with a normal gamete to form a zygote. The zygote thus has one chromosome with the normal complement of genes and one with some missing genes. Because a fairly large number of genes can be lost in a deletion, serious consequences can result even though one copy of the chromosome is normal. An often cited example of a disease caused by a chromosomal deletion is the **cri du chat syndrome** (Figure 4-17). The term, which literally means "cry of the cat," describes the characteristic cry of the affected child. Other symptoms include low birth weight, severe mental retardation, microcephaly (smaller than normal

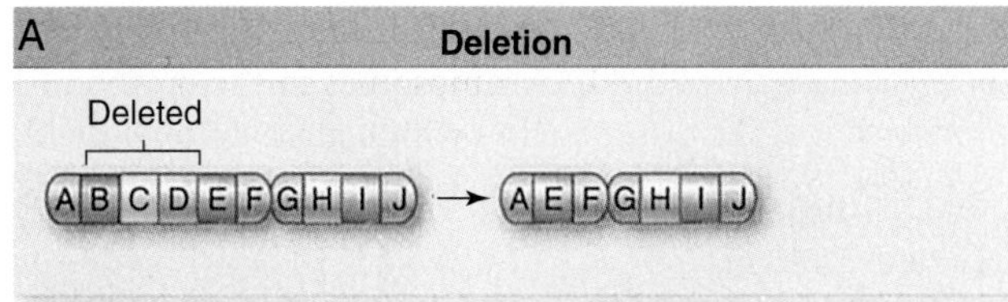

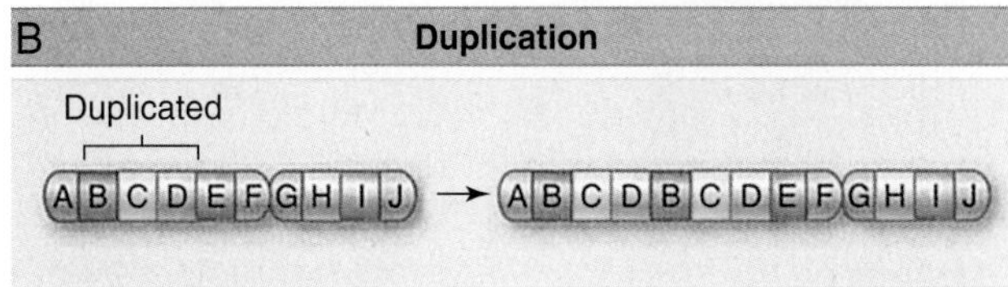

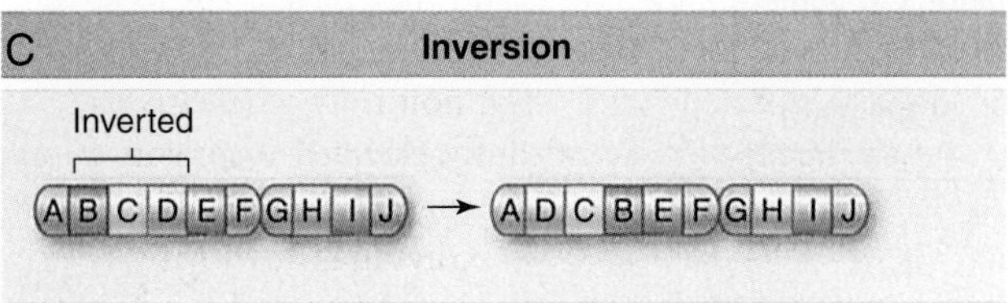

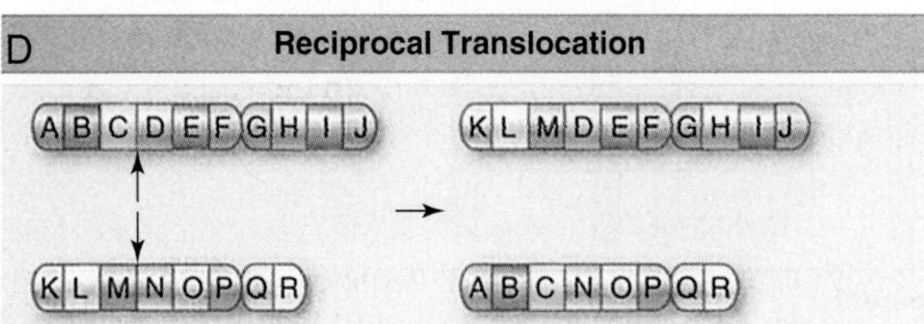

FIGURE 4-16 **Chromosomal Mutations.** Larger-scale changes in chromosomes are also possible. Material can be deleted **(A)**, duplicated **(B)**, and inverted **(C)**. Translocations occur when one chromosome is broken and becomes part of another chromosome. This often occurs where both chromosomes are broken and exchange material, an event called a reciprocal translocation **(D)**. (From Raven PH et al: *Biology,* ed 8, New York, 2008, McGraw-Hill.)

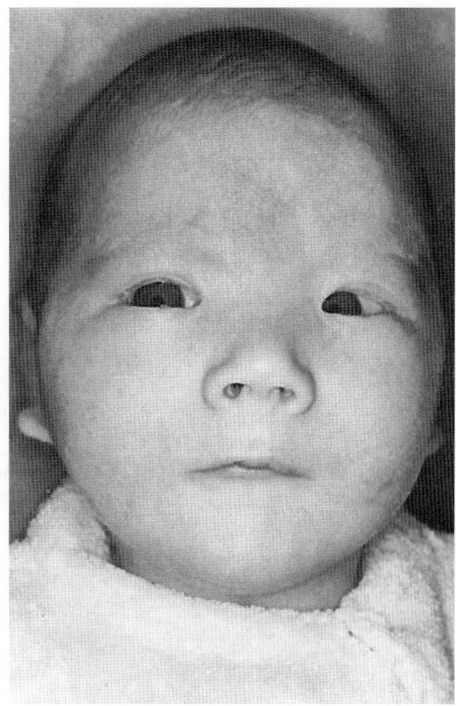

FIGURE 4-17 **Infant with Cri Du Chat Syndrome.** This syndrome is caused by deletion of part of the short arm of chromosome 5. (From Nussbaum RL, McInnes RR, Willard HF: *Thompson & Thompson genetics in medicine,* ed 7, Philadelphia, 2007, Saunders.)

head size), heart defects, and the typical facial appearance shown in Figure 4-17. The disease is caused by a deletion of part of the short arm of chromosome 5.

Duplications. **Duplications** of chromosome material are, like deletions, a form of chromosome aberration (see Figure 4-16, *B*). Because a deficiency of genetic material is more harmful than an excess, duplications usually have less serious consequences than deletions. For example, a deletion of a region of chromosome 5 causes cri du chat syndrome, but a duplication of the same region causes less severe disease.

Inversions. An **inversion** is the occurrence of two breaks on a chromosome, followed by the reinsertion of the missing fragment at its original site but in inverted order (see Figure 4-16, *C*). Thus a chromosome symbolized as ABCDEFG might become ABEDCFG after an inversion.

Unlike deletions and duplications, inversions result in no loss or gain of genetic material. They are thus said to be a "balanced" alteration of chromosome structure, and they often have no apparent physical effect. Genes are sometimes influenced by neighboring DNA sequences, however, and this **position effect,** a change in a gene's expression caused by its position, does sometimes result in disease in persons with inversions.

The serious problems caused by inversions usually occur in the offspring of individuals carrying the inversion. Because chromosomes must line up in perfect order during prophase I, a chromosome with an inversion must form a loop to align with its normal homolog. Crossing over within this loop can result in duplications or deletions in the chromosomes of daughter cells. Thus the offspring of individuals who carry inversions often have chromosome deletions or duplications.

Translocations. The interchanging of genetic material between nonhomologous chromosomes is called **translocation,** and the most clinically significant type of translocation is termed a **Robertsonian translocation.** In this translocation the long arms of two nonhomologous chromosomes fuse at the centromere, forming a single chromosome (Figure 4-18). Robertsonian translocations are confined to chromosomes 13, 14, 15, 21, and 22 because the short arms of these chromosomes are very small and contain no essential genetic material. When a Robertsonian translocation takes place, the short arms are usually lost during subsequent cell divisions. Because the carriers of Robertsonian translocations (about 1 in 500 individuals) lose no important genetic material, they are normal, although they have only 45 chromosomes in each cell. Their offspring, however, may have serious deletions or duplications (see Figure 4-18). For example, a common Robertsonian translocation involves the fusion of the long arms of chromosomes 21 and 14. An offspring who inherits a gamete carrying the fused chromosome receives an extra copy of the long arm of chromosome 21 and thus develops Down syndrome. Robertsonian translocations are responsible

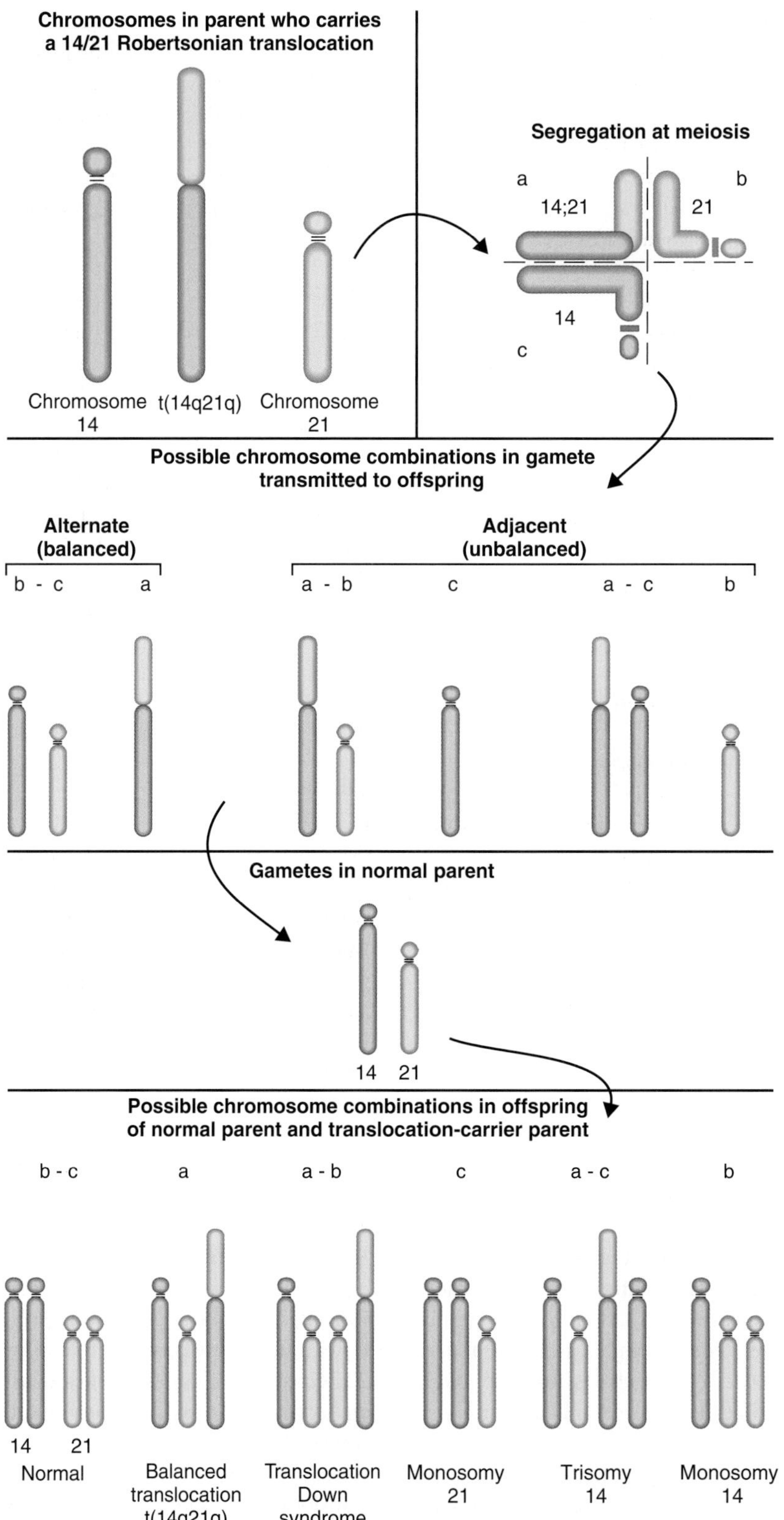

FIGURE 4-18 Possible Segregation Patterns for the Gametes Formed by a Carrier of a Robertsonian Translocation. Alternate segregation (quadrant a alone, or quadrant b with quadrant c) produces either a normal chromosome constitution or a translocation carrier with a normal phenotype. Adjacent segregation (quadrant a with b, quadrant c alone, quadrant a with c, or quadrant b alone) produces unbalanced gametes and results in conceptions with translocation Down syndrome, monosomy 21, trisomy 14, or monosomy 14, respectively. For example, monosomy 14 is produced when the parent who carries the translocation transmits a copy of chromosome 21 but does not transmit a copy of chromosome 14 (as in the lower right corner). (From Jorde LB et al: *Medical genetics,* ed 4, St Louis, 2010, Mosby.)

for approximately 3% to 5% of Down syndrome cases. Parents who carry a Robertsonian translocation involving chromosome 21 have an increased risk for producing multiple offspring with Down syndrome.

A **reciprocal translocation** occurs when breaks take place in two different chromosomes and the material is exchanged (see Figure 4-16, *D*). As with Robertsonian translocations, the carrier of a reciprocal translocation is usually normal because the individual has a normal complement of genetic material. However, the carrier's gametes can be normal, can carry the translocation, or can have duplications and deletions.

Fragile Sites. For reasons not yet fully understood, a number of areas on chromosomes develop microscopically observable breaks and gaps when the cells are cultured in a folate-deficient medium. Most of these **fragile sites** have no apparent relationship to disease. However, one fragile site, located on the long arm of the X chromosome, is associated with a disorder of considerable importance, both clinically and genetically. This disorder is known as *fragile X syndrome,* and it is associated with substantial cognitive impairment. With a relatively high population prevalence (affecting approximately 1 in 4000 males and 1 in 8000 females), fragile X syndrome is the second most common genetic cause of mental retardation (after Down syndrome).[9]

Fragile X syndrome is usually caused by an elevated number (more than about 200) of repeated DNA sequences in the first exon of the fragile X gene. These "repeats" consist of CGG sequences that are duplicated many times. Most individuals have fewer than 50 of these repeats, but those who have 50 to 200 are more likely to produce affected offspring because DNA replication becomes unstable.[9] An increase in the number of these repeated sequences in successive generations can lead to expression of fragile X syndrome. More than 20 other genetic diseases also are caused by this mechanism.[10,11]

ELEMENTS OF FORMAL GENETICS

The mechanisms by which an individual's set of paired chromosomes produces traits are the principles of genetic inheritance. Mendel's work with garden peas first defined these principles. Later geneticists have refined Mendel's work to explain patterns of inheritance for traits and diseases that appear in families.

Many traits can be attributed primarily to single genes and are often called *mendelian traits* (after Gregor Mendel). Each gene occupies a position along a chromosome known as a **locus.** The genes at a particular locus can take different forms (i.e., they can be composed of different nucleotide sequences) called **alleles.** For example, most people have a type of hemoglobin known as *hemoglobin A.* A few individuals have an alternative form of hemoglobin, termed *hemoglobin S,* which differs from hemoglobin A by a single amino acid substitution in the β-globin component of the molecule. The β-globin locus thus has two different alleles, one that encodes hemoglobin A and another that encodes hemoglobin S. A locus containing two or more alleles that each occur with an appreciable frequency in a population is said to be **polymorphic** or a **polymorphism.**

Because humans are diploid organisms, each chromosome is represented twice, with one member of the chromosome pair contributed by the father and one by the mother. At a given locus an individual has one gene whose origin is paternal and one whose origin is maternal. When the two genes are identical, the individual is **homozygous** at that locus. When the genes are not identical, the individual is **heterozygous** at the locus.

Phenotype and Genotype

The composition of genes at a given locus is known as the **genotype.** The outward appearance of an individual, which is the result of both genotype and environment, is the **phenotype** (see also Chapter 6, epigenetics). For example, an infant who is born with an inability to metabolize the amino acid phenylalanine has the single-gene disorder known as *phenylketonuria (PKU)* and thus has the PKU genotype. If the condition is left untreated, abnormal metabolites of phenylalanine will begin to accumulate in the infant's brain and irreversible mental retardation will occur. Mental retardation is thus one aspect of the PKU phenotype. By imposing dietary restrictions to limit the intake of food containing phenylalanine, however, retardation can be prevented. Although the child still has the PKU genotype, a modification of the environment (in this case the child's diet) produces an outwardly normal phenotype.

Dominance and Recessiveness

In many loci the effects of one allele mask those of another when the two are found together in a **heterozygote.** The allele whose effects are observable is said to be **dominant.** The allele whose effects are hidden is said to be **recessive** (from the Latin root for "hiding"). Traditionally, for loci having two alleles, the dominant allele is denoted by an uppercase letter and the recessive allele is denoted by a lowercase letter. When one allele is dominant over another, the heterozygote genotype *Aa* has the same phenotype as the dominant homozygote *AA.* For the recessive allele to be expressed, it must exist in the **homozygote** form, *aa.*

When the heterozygote is distinguishable from both homozygotes, the locus is said to exhibit **codominance.** For example, in the MN blood group, both alleles, *M* and *N,* of the heterozygote are detectable and therefore codominant. Another example is the ABO blood group, in which heterozygotes having the *A* and *B* alleles express both of them as A and B antigens on their red cells (forming blood group AB).

A **carrier** is an individual who has a disease-causing allele but is phenotypically normal. Most recessive disease-causing alleles occur in heterozygotes who carry one copy of the allele but do not express the disease. Because many recessive alleles are lethal in the homozygous state, they are eliminated from the population when they occur in homozygotes. By "hiding" in carriers, however, most recessive alleles survive to be passed on to the next generation.

TRANSMISSION OF GENETIC DISEASES

An important aspect of a genetic disease is the pattern in which it is inherited through the generations of a family, or its **mode of inheritance.** Once the mode of inheritance is known, much can be learned about the disease-causing gene itself, and reliable genetic counseling can be given to members of families in which the disease is present.

Modes of inheritance were systematically studied by Mendel, who formulated two basic laws of inheritance. His **principle of segregation** states that homologous genes separate from one another during reproduction and that each reproductive cell carries only one of the homologous genes. Mendel's second law, the **principle of independent assortment,** states that the hereditary transmission of one gene has no effect on the transmission of another. Mendel discovered these laws in the mid-nineteenth century by performing breeding experiments with garden peas. He had no knowledge of chromosomes. Early in the twentieth century geneticists found that the behavior of chromosomes does essentially correspond to Mendel's laws, which now form the basis for the **chromosome theory of inheritance.**

The known single-gene diseases can be classified into four major modes of inheritance: autosomal dominant, autosomal recessive, X-linked dominant, and X-linked recessive. The first two types involve genes known to occur on the 22 pairs of autosomes. The last two types occur on the X chromosome; only a few disease-causing genes, primarily affecting male fertility, are found on the Y chromosome. The number of diseases assigned to each category is growing rapidly. Current catalogs of single-gene traits, which include disease-producing and nonclinical traits (e.g., attached earlobes), list nearly 20,000 known autosomal traits and nearly 1200 X-linked traits.[1]

An important tool in the analysis of modes of inheritance is the **pedigree** chart. It summarizes family relationships and shows which members of a family are affected by a genetic disease (Figure 4-19). Generally, the pedigree begins with one individual in the family, the **proband,** also termed the **propositus** (male) or **proposita** (female). This individual is usually the first person in the family diagnosed or seen in a clinic.

Autosomal Dominant Inheritance

Characteristics of Pedigrees

Diseases caused by autosomal dominant genes are rare. The most common occur in fewer than 1 in 500 individuals, so it is uncommon for two individuals both affected by the same autosomal dominant disease to produce offspring together. Figure 4-20, *A*, illustrates this unusual pattern. More often, affected offspring are produced by the union of a normal parent with an affected heterozygous parent. The diagram (Punnett square) in Figure 4-20, *B*, illustrates this mating. The affected parent can pass either a disease gene or a normal gene to his or her children. Each event has a probability of 0.5; thus on average, half of the children will be heterozygous and will express the disease, and half will be normal.

Figure 4-21, *A*, is a typical pedigree showing the transmission of an autosomal dominant gene. The gene shown here causes achondroplasia (Figure 4-21, *B*). Several important characteristics of this pedigree support the conclusion that the trait is caused by an autosomal dominant gene:

1. The two sexes exhibit the trait in approximately equal proportions, and males and females are equally likely to transmit the trait to their offspring.
2. There is no skipping of generations. If an individual has achondroplasia, one parent must also have it. If neither parent has the trait, none of the children has it (with the exception of new mutations, as discussed later).
3. Affected heterozygous individuals transmit the trait to approximately half of their children, but because gamete transmission is subject to chance fluctuations, it is possible that all or none of the children of an affected parent may have the trait. When large numbers of matings of this type are studied, however, the proportion of affected children will closely approach one half.

Recurrence Risks

Parents at risk for producing children with a genetic disease nearly always ask the question, "What is the *chance* that our child will have this disease?" The probability that a family member

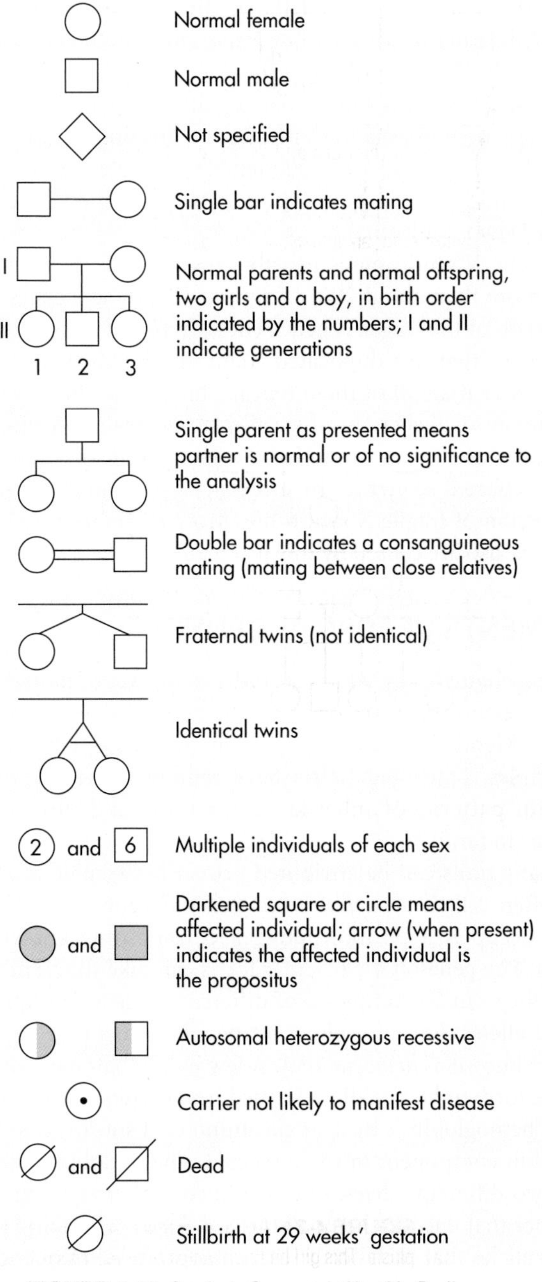

FIGURE 4-19 Symbols Commonly Used in Pedigrees.

will have a genetic disease is termed the **recurrence risk.** When one parent is affected by an autosomal dominant disease (and is a heterozygote) and the other is normal, the recurrence risks for each child are one half.

An important principle is that each birth is an independent event, much like a coin toss. Thus, even though parents may already have had a child with the disease, their recurrence risk remains one half. If they have had several children, all affected (or all unaffected) by the disease, the law of independence dictates that the probability that their next child will have the disease is still one half. Parents' misunderstanding of this principle is a common problem encountered in genetic counseling.

If a child has been born with an autosomal dominant disease and there is no history of the disease in the family, the child is probably the product of a new mutation. The gene transmitted by one of the parents has thus undergone a mutation from a normal to a disease-causing allele. The genes at this locus in most of the parent's other germ cells would still be normal. In this situation the recurrence risk for the parent's subsequent offspring is not greater than that of the general population. The offspring of the affected child, however, will have a recurrence risk of one half. Because these diseases often reduce the potential for reproduction, a large proportion of the observed cases of many autosomal dominant diseases are the result of new mutations. For example, approximately seven eighths of all cases of achondroplasia are caused by new mutations.

A

Affected parent		Affected parent: D	Affected parent: d
	D	DD Homozygous affected (usually rare)	Dd Heterozygous affected
	d	Dd Heterozygous affected	dd Homozygous normal

B

Affected parent		Normal parent: d	Normal parent: d
	D	Dd Heterozygous affected	Dd Heterozygous affected
	d	dd Homozygous normal	dd Homozygous normal

FIGURE 4-20 Punnett Square and Autosomal Dominant Traits. **A,** Punnett square for the mating of two individuals with an autosomal dominant gene. Here both parents are affected by the trait. **B,** Punnett square for the mating of a normal individual with a carrier for an autosomal dominant gene.

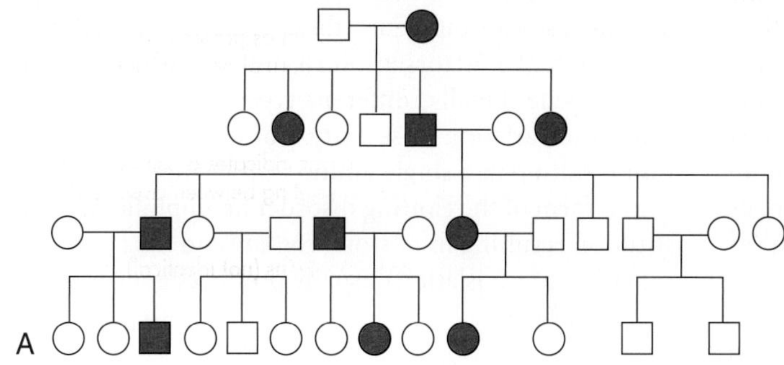

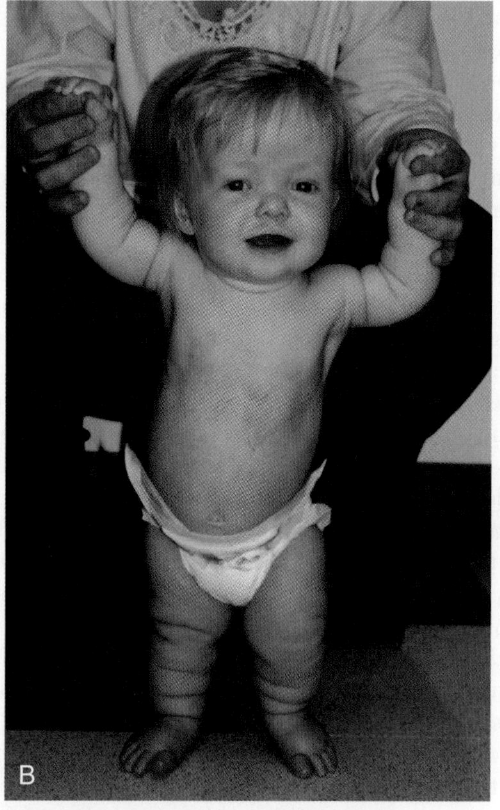

FIGURE 4-21 Achondroplasia. **A,** Pedigree showing the transmission of an autosomal dominant disease. **B,** Achondroplasia. This girl has short limbs relative to trunk length. She also has a prominent forehead, low nasal root, and redundant skin folds in the arms and legs. (**B** from Jorde LB et al: *Medical genetics,* ed 4, St Louis, 2010, Mosby.)

Occasionally, two or more offspring will present symptoms of an autosomal dominant disease when there is no family history of the disease. Because mutation is a rare event, it is unlikely that this disease would be a result of multiple mutations in the same family. The mechanism most likely to be responsible is termed **germline mosaicism.** During the embryonic development of one of the parents, a mutation occurred that affected all or part of the germline but few or none of the somatic cells of the embryo. Thus the parent carries the mutation in his or her germline but does not actually express the disease. As a result, the unaffected parent can transmit the mutation to multiple offspring. This phenomenon, although relatively rare, can have significant effects on recurrence risks.[12]

Penetrance and Expressivity

An important variation seen in some genetic diseases is incomplete penetrance. The **penetrance** of a trait is the percentage of individuals with a specific genotype who also exhibit the expected phenotype. Incomplete penetrance means that individuals who have a disease-causing allele may not exhibit the disease phenotype at all, even though the allele and the associated disease may be transmitted to the next generation. A pedigree illustrating the transmission of an autosomal dominant allele with incomplete penetrance is given in Figure 4-22. Retinoblastoma, the most common malignant eye tumor affecting children, typically exhibits incomplete penetrance. About 10% of the individuals who are **obligate carriers** of the allele (i.e., those who have an affected parent and affected children and therefore must themselves carry the allele) do not have the disease. The penetrance of the disease-causing genotype is then said to be 90%.

The gene responsible for retinoblastoma encodes a **tumor-suppressor gene:** the normal function of its protein product is to regulate the cell cycle so that cells do not divide in an uncontrollable manner. When a mutation alters the protein, its tumor-suppressing capacity is lost and a tumor can form[13,14] (see Chapters 12 and 20).

Huntington disease is another well-known autosomal dominant condition and its main features are progressive dementia and increasingly uncontrollable movements of the limbs (discussed further in Chapter 18). The latter is known as chorea (Greek *khoreia* = dance; the disease is sometimes called *Huntington chorea*).

One of the key features of this disease is that symptoms are not usually seen until age 40 years or later, a pattern known as **age-dependent penetrance.** Thus people who develop the disease often have had children before they are aware that they have the disease-causing allele. If the disease were present at birth, nearly all those affected would die before reaching reproductive age, and the occurrence of the allele in the population would be much lower. An individual whose parent has the disease has a 50% chance of developing it during middle age. He or she is thus confronted with a torturous question: "Should I have children, knowing that there is a 50-50 chance that I may have this disease gene and pass it to half my children?" Age-dependent penetrance characterizes a number of important genetic diseases, including familial breast cancer, hemochromatosis, and polycystic kidney disease.

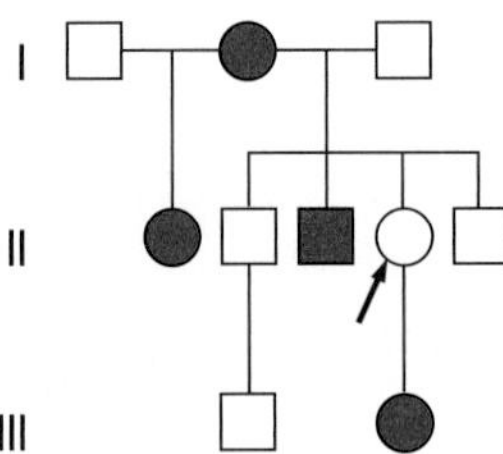

FIGURE 4-22 Pedigree for Retinoblastoma Showing Incomplete Penetrance. The female with marked arrow in line II must be heterozygous, but she does not express the trait.

Most genetic diseases exhibit variable expressivity. **Expressivity** is the extent of variation in phenotype associated with a particular genotype. If the expressivity of a disease is variable, the penetrance may be complete but the severity of the disease can vary greatly. A well-known example of variable expressivity in an autosomal dominant disease is type 1 neurofibromatosis, or von Recklinghausen disease. Like the retinoblastoma gene, the neurofibromatosis gene normally encodes a tumor suppressor.[15] The expression of this gene can vary from a few harmless café-au-lait spots ("coffee with milk," describing the light brown color) on the skin to malignant tumors, scoliosis, seizures, gliomas, hypertension, learning disabilities, and neuromas (Figure 4-23). A parent with mild expression of the disease—so mild that he or she is not aware of it—can transmit the gene to a child, who can then exhibit severe expression of the disease. Several factors can cause variation in expressivity. Genes at other loci can sometimes modify the expression of a disease-causing gene (these are termed *modifier genes*). Environmental factors also can influence the expression of a disease gene. Finally, different types of mutations at a locus can cause variation in severity. For example, a base substitution resulting in a single amino acid change usually produces a mild form of the clotting disorder hemophilia A. A base substitution resulting in a "stop" codon (and thus premature termination of translation) usually produces a more severe form of hemophilia A.

Autosomal Recessive Inheritance

Characteristics of Pedigrees

Like autosomal dominant diseases, those caused by autosomal recessive alleles are rare in populations, although the number of carriers for recessive diseases can be high. The most common lethal recessive disease in white children, cystic fibrosis, occurs in about 1 in 2500 births. Approximately 1 in 25 whites carries one copy of an allele that can cause cystic fibrosis (see Chapter 36). Because an individual must be homozygous for a recessive allele to express the disease, the carriers are phenotypically normal. Because most recessive alleles are maintained in normal carriers, they are able to survive in the population from one generation to the next. As with many autosomal dominant diseases, many autosomal recessive diseases are characterized by delayed age of onset, incomplete penetrance, and variable expressivity.

Figure 4-24 shows a pedigree for cystic fibrosis. The cystic fibrosis gene encodes a protein product that forms chloride

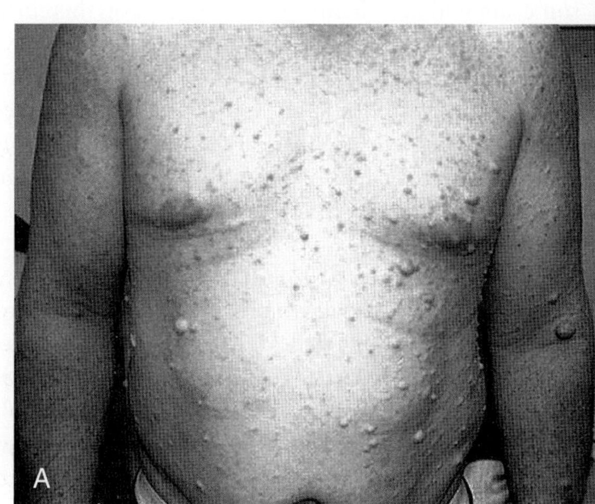

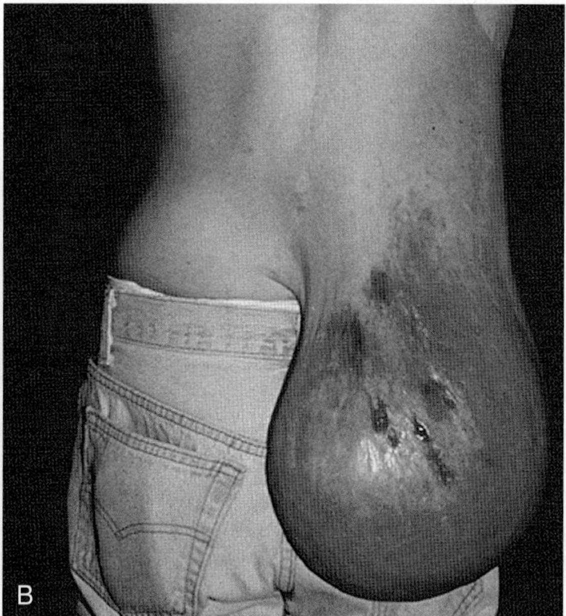

FIGURE 4-23 Neurofibromatosis. **A,** Young adult with multiple dermal neurofibromas of the trunk. **B,** Individual has a large plexiform neurofibroma hanging from lower right back, causing considerable inconvenience and discomfort (substantially improved by surgical removal of tumor). (**A** from Jorde LB et al: *Medical genetics,* ed 3, St Louis, 2003, Mosby. **B** courtesy Dr. D. Viskochil, University of Utah Health Sciences Center, Salt Lake City.)

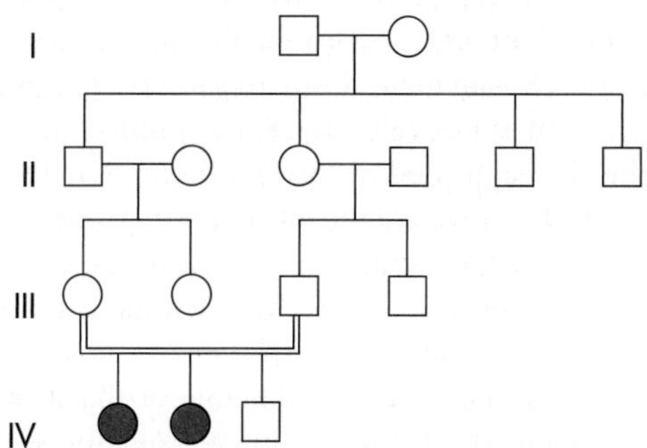

FIGURE 4-24 Pedigree for Cystic Fibrosis.

	D	d
D	DD Homozygous normal	Dd Heterozygous carrier
d	Dd Heterozygous carrier	dd Homozygous affected

FIGURE 4-25 Punnett Square for the Mating of Heterozygous Carriers. This is typical of most cases of recessive disease.

channels in the membranes of specialized epithelial cells.[16] Defective transport of chloride ions leads to a salt imbalance that results in secretions of abnormally thick, dehydrated mucus. Some of the digestive organs, particularly the pancreas, become obstructed, causing malnutrition, and the lungs become clogged with mucus, making them highly susceptible to bacterial infections (especially *Pseudomonas*). Death from lung disease or heart failure occurs on average by about 40 years of age. In the pedigree shown, the two affected individuals are the offspring of the marriage of two first cousins. Marriage between related individuals, termed **consanguinity** (from the Latin root meaning "with blood"), is often a factor in producing children with recessive diseases because related individuals are more likely to share the same recessive genes. Consanguinity is seen most often in rare recessive diseases because carriers of common recessive diseases (such as cystic fibrosis) have a fairly high probability of encountering one another just by chance.

Important criteria for discerning autosomal recessive inheritance include the following:

1. Males and females are affected in equal proportions.
2. Consanguinity is sometimes present.
3. The disease is seen in siblings but usually not in their parents.
4. On the average, one fourth of the offspring of carrier parents will be affected.

Recurrence Risks

In most cases of recessive disease, both parents of affected individuals are heterozygous carriers. On the average, one fourth of their offspring will be normal homozygotes, one half will be phenotypically normal carrier heterozygotes, and one fourth will be homozygotes with the disease (Figure 4-25). Thus the recurrence risk for the offspring of carrier parents is 25%. In any given family, chance fluctuations are likely, but a study of a large number of families would yield figures close to these proportions.

If two parents have a recessive disease, they each must be homozygous for the disease. Therefore, when two parents are affected by a recessive disease, all their children also must be affected. This observation helps to distinguish recessive from dominant inheritance, because two parents both affected by a dominant gene are nearly always both heterozygotes, and thus one fourth of their children will be unaffected.

Because carrier parents usually are unaware that they both carry the same recessive gene, they often produce an affected child before realization of their condition. **Carrier detection tests** can identify heterozygotes by measuring the reduced amount of a critical enzyme available. The critical enzyme is lacking in a homozygous recessive individual, but an essentially normal phenotype is seen when it is present in a reduced quantity in the carrier. Often carriers can be detected by direct examination of the disease locus for a mutation. Such testing is especially valuable for siblings of known carriers, who may themselves be carriers. Genetic testing is now available for more than 2000 diseases.

Consanguinity

Consanguinity and **inbreeding** are related concepts. *Consanguinity* refers to the mating of two related individuals, and the offspring of such matings are said to be *inbred.* Consanguinity is often an important characteristic of pedigrees for recessive diseases because relatives share a certain proportion of genes received from a common ancestor. The proportion of shared genes depends on the closeness of their biologic relationship. For example, siblings share one half of their DNA, on average, because of their descent from the same parents. With each decreasing degree of relationship, this proportion is reduced by one half. Uncles share one fourth of their DNA with nephews and nieces; first cousins share one eighth; first cousins once removed* share one sixteenth; second cousins share one thirty-second; and so on. With consanguineous matings, recessive disorders are significantly increased. Most empirical studies show that the proportion of offspring of marriages of first cousins who are affected by genetic diseases is approximately double that of the general population.[17] Marriages between first cousins are prohibited in most states of the United States. Marriages between closer relatives (except between double first cousins†) are prohibited throughout the United States.

X-Linked Inheritance

Not all genetic diseases are caused by genes located on the 22 autosomes. Some conditions are instead caused by genes located on the sex chromosomes, and that mode of inheritance is referred to as **sex-linked.** The Y chromosome contains only a few dozen genes, so most sex-linked traits are located on the X chromosome and are said to be X-linked. Only a few diseases are known to be inherited as X-linked dominant traits. Because these diseases are so seldom encountered, only the much more common X-linked recessive diseases are discussed here.

*First cousins once removed are the offspring of one's own first cousins.
†Double first cousins share both sets of grandparents; ordinarily, first cousins share just one set of grandparents.

Females receive two X chromosomes, one from the father and one from the mother, so they can be homozygous for a disease allele at a given locus, homozygous for the normal allele at the locus, or heterozygous. Males, having only one X chromosome, are said to be **hemizygous** for genes on this chromosome. A male who inherits a recessive disease gene on the X chromosome will be affected by the disease because the Y chromosome does not carry a normal allele to counteract the effects of the disease-causing allele. Males are more frequently affected by X-linked recessive diseases, with the difference becoming more pronounced as the disease becomes rarer.

X Inactivation

In the late 1950s Mary Lyon proposed that one X chromosome in the somatic cells of females is permanently inactivated, a process termed *X inactivation.*[18] This explains why most gene products coded by the X chromosome are present in equal amounts in males and females, even though males have only one X chromosome and females have two X chromosomes. This phenomenon is called **dosage compensation.** The inactivated X chromosomes are observable in many interphase cells as highly condensed chromatin bodies, termed **Barr bodies** (after Barr and Bertram, who discovered them in the late 1940s). Normal females have one Barr body in each somatic cell, whereas normal males have no Barr bodies.

The actual process of inactivation occurs very early in embryonic development—approximately 7 to 14 days after fertilization. In each somatic cell one of the two X chromosomes is inactivated. In some cells the X chromosome contributed by the father is inactivated; in others the maternal X chromosome is inactivated. Because the inactivation process is random, the maternal X chromosome is inactivated in approximately half the cells and the paternal X chromosome is inactivated in approximately half the cells. Once the X chromosome has been inactivated in a cell, all the descendants of that cell have the same chromosome inactivated. Thus inactivation is said to be *random* but *fixed.*

Some individuals do not have the normal number of X chromosomes in their somatic cells. For example, males with Klinefelter syndrome typically have two X chromosomes and one Y chromosome and they have one Barr body in each cell. Females whose cell nuclei have three X chromosomes have two Barr bodies in each cell, and females whose cell nuclei have four X chromosomes have three Barr bodies in each cell. Females with Turner syndrome have only one X chromosome and no Barr bodies. Thus the number of Barr bodies is always one less than the number of X chromosomes in the cell. All but one X chromosome are always inactivated.

People with abnormal numbers of X chromosomes, such as those with Turner syndrome or Klinefelter syndrome, are not physically normal. This situation presents a puzzle because they presumably have only one active X chromosome, the same as individuals with normal numbers of chromosomes. However, the distal portions of the short and long arms of the X chromosome, as well as several other regions on the chromosome, are not inactivated. Thus X inactivation is also known to be *incomplete.*

Although the mechanism underlying X inactivation is still incompletely understood, the gene responsible for initiating X inactivation, *XIST,* has been located.[19] This gene encodes an mRNA that coats one of the X chromosomes, which is then inactivated. Methylation of X chromosome DNA, a process in which DNA is inactivated when cytosine bases are enzymatically converted to 5-methylcytosine, occurs on the inactivated X chromosome. Inactive X chromosomes can be at least partially reactivated in vitro by administering 5-azacytidine, a demethylating agent.

Sex Determination

The process of sexual differentiation, in which the embryonic gonads become either testes or ovaries, begins during the sixth week of gestation. A key principle of sex determination in mammals is that one copy of the Y chromosome is sufficient to initiate the process of gonadal differentiation that produces a male fetus (Figure 4-26, *A*). The number of X chromosomes does not alter this process. For example, an individual with two X chromosomes and one Y chromosome in each cell is still phenotypically a male. Thus it is logical that the Y chromosome must contain a gene that begins the process of male gonadal development.

This gene, termed *SRY* (for "sex-determining region on the Y"), has been located on the short arm of the Y chromosome.[20,21] The *SRY* gene lies immediately proximal to the distal tip of the Y chromosome, known as the **pseudoautosomal** region (Figure 4-26, *B*). This portion of the Y chromosome is so named because it pairs with the distal tip of the short arm of the X chromosome during meiosis and exchanges genetic material with it (crossover), just as autosomes do. The DNA sequences of these regions on the X and Y chromosomes are highly similar. The remainder of the X and Y chromosomes, however, do not exchange material and are not similar in DNA sequence. An important piece of evidence that supports *SRY* as the male-determining gene is that female mouse embryos injected with this gene develop as phenotypic males.

Although the *SRY* gene is located on the Y chromosome, the other genes that contribute to male differentiation are located on other chromosomes. Thus *SRY* appears to act as a trigger that initiates the action of genes on other chromosomes (e.g., those that control Sertoli cell differentiation or secretion of müllerian-inhibiting substance). This concept is supported by the fact that the *SRY* gene is similar in sequence to other genes that are known to regulate the transcription of DNA (i.e., they turn other genes on and off).

Occasionally the crossover between X and Y occurs closer to the centromere than it should, placing the *SRY* gene on the X chromosome after crossover. This variation can result in offspring with an apparently normal XX karyotype but a male phenotype. Such XX males are seen in about 1 in 20,000 live births and closely resemble males with Klinefelter syndrome, although their stature is normal. Conversely, it is possible to inherit a Y chromosome that has lost the *SRY* gene (because of either a crossover error or a deletion of the gene). This situation produces an XY female. Such females have gonadal streaks rather than ovaries and have poorly developed secondary sex characteristics.

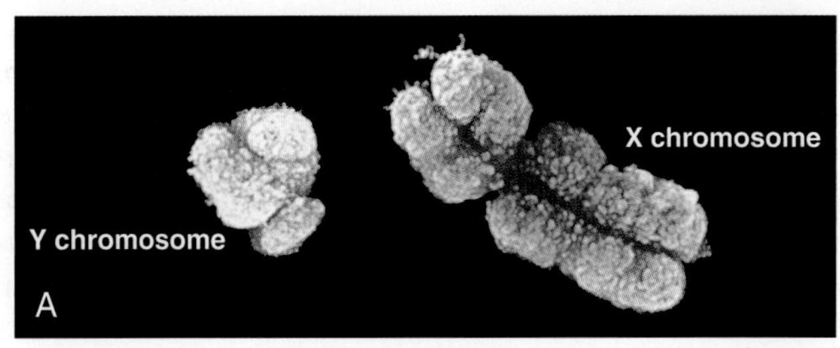

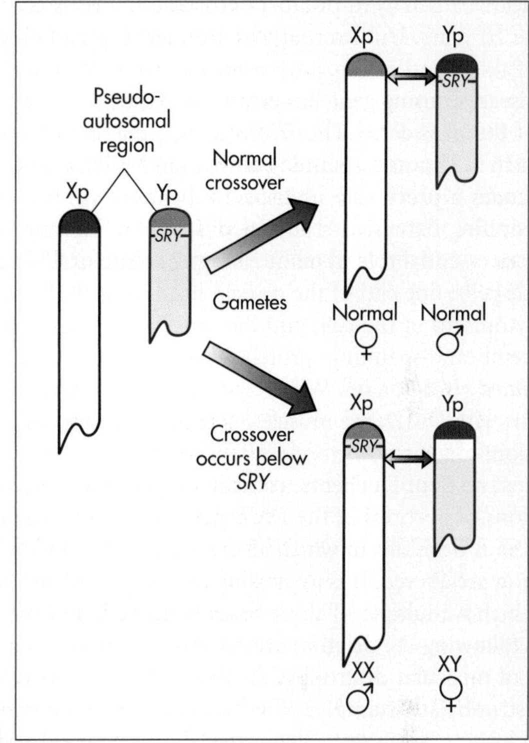

FIGURE 4-26 **The Distal Short Arms of the X and Y Chromosomes Exchange Material During Meiosis in the Male. A,** X and Y chromosomes. **B,** The region of the Y chromosome in which this crossover occurs is called the *pseudoautosomal region.* (Xp and Yp refer to the short arms of each chromosome.) The *SRY* gene, which triggers the process leading to male gonadal differentiation, is located just outside the pseudoautosomal region. Occasionally, the crossover occurs on the centromeric side of the *SRY* gene, causing it to lie on an X chromosome instead of a Y chromosome. An offspring receiving this X chromosome will be an XX male, and an offspring receiving the Y chromosome will be an XY female. (**A** from Raven PH et al: *Biology,* ed 8, New York, 2008, McGraw-Hill. **B** from Jorde LB et al: *Medical genetics,* ed 3, St Louis, 2003, Mosby.)

Characteristics of Pedigrees

Pedigrees for X-linked recessive conditions show the following distinctive features:

1. The trait is seen much more often in males than in females because females must inherit two copies of the recessive allele (one from each parent) to express the disease, while males need only inherit one copy (from their mother) to express the disease.
2. Because a father can give a son only a Y chromosome, the trait is never transmitted from father to son.
3. The gene can be transmitted through a series of carrier females, causing the appearance of a "skipped generation."

4. The gene is passed from an affected father to all his daughters, who, as phenotypically normal carriers, transmit it to approximately half their sons, who are affected.

The most common and severe of all X-linked recessive disorders is Duchenne muscular dystrophy (DMD), which affects approximately 1 in 3500 males. As its name suggests, this disorder is characterized by progressive muscle degeneration. Affected individuals are usually unable to walk by 10 to 12 years of age. The disease affects the heart and respiratory muscles, and death caused by respiratory or cardiac failure usually occurs before 20 years. Until recently, the underlying pathologic origin of this disorder was a mystery. However, identification of the disease-causing gene has greatly increased our understanding of the disorder.[22] The *DMD* gene is the largest gene ever found in the human, spanning more than 2 million DNA bases. It encodes a previously undiscovered muscle protein, termed **dystrophin.** Extensive study of dystrophin indicates that it plays an essential role in maintaining the structural integrity of muscle cells: one end of the protein binds to actin filaments in the cytoplasm of the cell, and the other end binds to a group of membrane-spanning proteins known as the *dystrophin-associated glycoproteins.* When dystrophin is absent, as in individuals with DMD, the muscle cell cannot survive, and muscle deterioration ensues.

Most cases of Duchenne muscular dystrophy are caused by deletions of portions of the *DMD* gene. They generally involve frameshift deletions in which all the amino acids following the deletion are altered. It is interesting that an "in frame" deletion (in which a multiple of three bases is deleted, and the amino acids following the deletion are not altered) produces a milder form of muscular dystrophy, the Becker type. These two types of dystrophy are examples of a disease in which different types of mutations at the same locus produce variable expression of the disease.

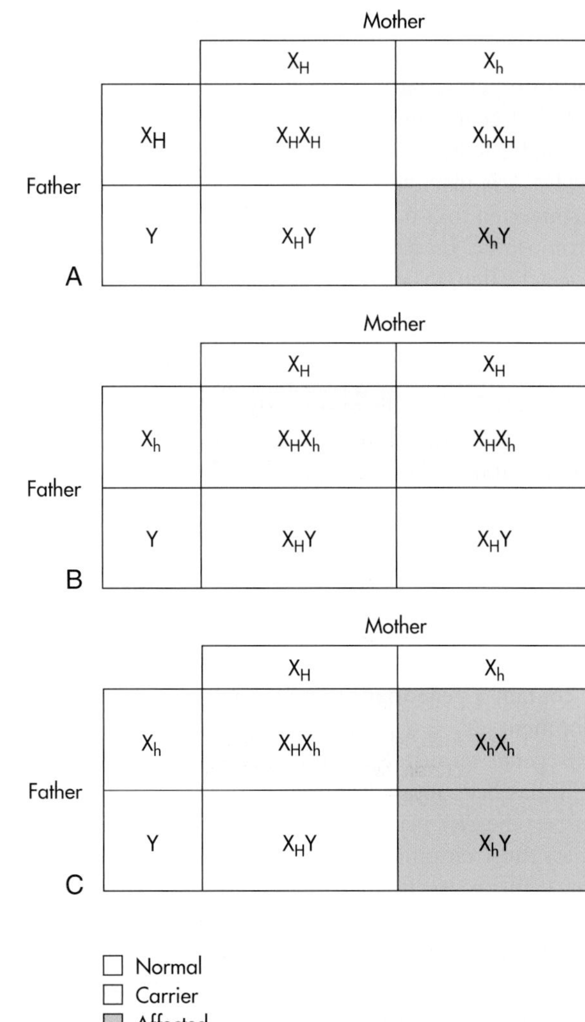

FIGURE 4-27 Punnett Square and X-linked Recessive Traits. **A,** Punnett square for the mating of a normal male (X_HY) and a female carrier of an X-linked recessive gene (X_HX_h). **B,** Punnett square for the mating of a normal female (X_HX_H) with a male affected by an X-linked recessive disease (X_hY). **C,** Punnett square for the mating of a female who carries an X-linked recessive gene (X_HX_h) with a male who is affected with the disease caused by the gene (X_hY).

Recurrence Risks

The most common mating type involving X-linked recessive genes is the combination of a carrier female and a normal male. On the average, the carrier mother will transmit the disease-causing allele to half her sons and half her daughters. As Figure 4-27, *A*, shows, half the daughters in such a mating will be carriers, whereas half will be normal. Half the sons will be normal, on the average, whereas half will have the disease.

The other common mating type is an affected father and a normal mother (see Figure 4-27, *B*). In this situation all the sons must be normal because the father can transmit only his Y chromosome to them. Because all the daughters must receive the father's X chromosome, they will all be heterozygous carriers. Because the sons *must* receive the Y chromosome and the daughters *must* receive the X with the disease gene, these are predictions and not probabilities. None of the children will express the disease.

The final mating pattern, less common than the other two, involves an affected father and a carrier mother (see Figure 4-27, *C*). With this pattern, on average, half the daughters will be heterozygous carriers and half will be homozygous for the disease allele and thus affected. Half the sons will be normal, and half will be affected. Some X-linked recessive diseases, such as DMD, are fatal or incapacitating before the affected individual reaches reproductive age, and therefore affected fathers are rare or nonexistent.

Sex-Limited and Sex-Influenced Traits

Confusion sometimes exists regarding the difference between traits that are sex-linked and those that are sex-limited or sex-influenced. A **sex-limited trait** is one that can occur in only one of the sexes, often because of anatomic differences. Inherited uterine and testicular defects are two obvious examples.

A **sex-influenced trait** is one that occurs much more often in one sex than in the other. A good example of a sex-influenced trait is male-pattern baldness, which occurs in both males and females but is much more common in males. Another example is breast cancer, which is approximately 70 times more common in females than males.

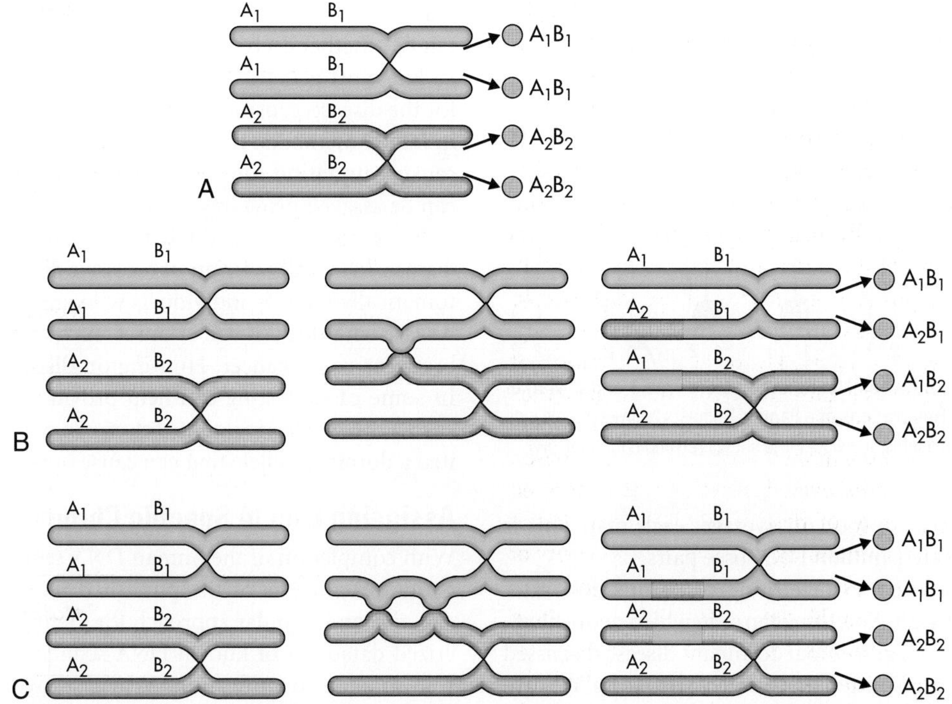

FIGURE 4-28 The Genetic Results of Crossing Over. A, No crossing over: A_1 and B_1 remain together after meiosis. **B,** Crossing over between A and B results in a recombination: A_1 and B_2 are inherited together on one chromosome, and A_2 and B_1 are inherited together on another chromosome. **C,** A double crossover between A and B results in no recombination of alleles.

Evaluation of Pedigrees

With complications such as incomplete penetrance, variable expressivity, delayed age of onset, and sex-influenced traits, it is not always possible simply to look at a disease pedigree and determine the mode of inheritance. A sophisticated statistical approach has evolved to deal with such complications. Incorporated into computer programs, these statistical techniques assess the probability of observing a certain pedigree if a particular mode of inheritance (e.g., autosomal dominant with incomplete penetrance) is in effect.

LINKAGE ANALYSIS AND GENE IDENTIFICATION

Locating the positions of genes on chromosomes has been one of the most important endeavors in human genetics. It is an important first step in identifying a disease-causing gene and can be used to predict the likelihood that certain individuals will develop a genetic disease.

Classic Pedigree Analysis

Mendel's second law, the principle of independent assortment, states that an individual's genes will be transmitted to the next generation independently of one another. This law is only partly true, however, because genes located close together on the same chromosome *do* tend to be transmitted together to the offspring. Thus Mendel's principle of independent assortment holds true for most pairs of genes but not those that occupy the same region of a chromosome. Such loci demonstrate **linkage** and are said to be linked.

During the first meiotic stage, the arms of homologous chromosome pairs intertwine and sometimes exchange portions of their DNA (Figure 4-28) in a process known as **crossing over.** During crossing over, new combinations of alleles can be formed. For example, two loci on a chromosome have alleles *A* and *a* and alleles *B* and *b*. Alleles *A* and *B* are located together on one chromosome arm, and alleles *a* and *b* are located on the other arm. The genotype of this individual is denoted as *AB/ab*.

As Figure 4-28, *A*, shows, the allele pairs *AB* and *ab* would be transmitted together when no crossing over occurs. However, when crossing over does occur (see Figure 4-28, *B*), all four possible pairs of alleles can be transmitted to the offspring: *AB*, *aB*, *Ab*, and *ab*. The process of forming such new arrangements of alleles is called **recombination.** Crossing over does not necessarily lead to recombination, however, because double crossing over between two loci can result in no actual recombination of the alleles at the loci (see Figure 4-28, *C*).

The rate of crossing over can be used to infer the distance between two loci on a chromosome because the probability of crossovers occurring between two loci increases as the loci become more distant. For example, if an individual with genotype *AB/ab* produces recombinant offspring gametes (composition of *Ab* and *aB)* 2% of the time, it is said that the two loci are two map units apart. One **map unit** equals a 1% recombination rate between two loci. When loci on the same chromosome are 50 or more map units apart, they are considered unlinked because their recombination frequency is just as great as it would be if they were on different chromosomes (where the probability of being transmitted together must equal one half). Recombination frequencies provide a good estimate of actual

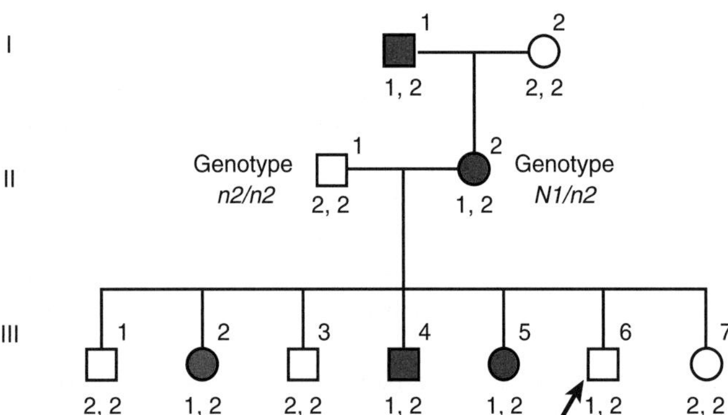

FIGURE 4-29 Linkage between Neurofibromatosis Type 1 and a Marker Polymorphism in Three Generations of a Family. Numbers below symbols indicate marker polymorphism alleles. Individual III-6 shows recombination *(arrow)*.

physical distance between loci: on average, each map unit is equal to approximately 1 million DNA base pairs.

Pedigrees can be used to determine recombination rates between loci. Figure 4-29 shows a pedigree in which neurofibromatosis type 1 (NF1), an autosomal dominant disease discussed previously, is being transmitted in a family. The NF1 alleles are labeled *N* (the dominant disease-causing allele) and *n* (the normal allele). The individuals in this pedigree have been typed for a **marker polymorphism,** a small DNA sequence whose chromosome location is known and can be typed in the laboratory. The alleles of the marker polymorphism are labeled 1 and 2. Examination of generations I and II shows that the NF1 locus must be on the same chromosome as marker allele 1 because the mother, whose marker genotype was 2,2, was unaffected with the disease. The daughter's genotype would then be *N1/n2,* in which *N* indicates the disease allele and *n* indicates the normal allele. The daughter's husband (individual II-1) must have the genotype *n2/2n2.* If the marker locus and NF1 are linked, the children of this union who are affected with NF12 should have marker allele 1; those who are unaffected should have the marker genotype 2,2 (i.e., they inherited a copy of the normal chromosome from their affected mother). In six of seven cases we find this to be true. In one case a recombination occurred (individual III-6), indicating a recombination rate of 1 in 7, or 14%. The two loci are therefore 14 map units apart. In practice, a much larger sample of families would be used to ensure against statistical artifacts.

Once a close linkage has been established between a disease locus and a **marker polymorphism** and once the alleles of the two loci that are inherited together within a family have been determined, reliable predictions of whether a member of a family will develop the disease can be made. If, for example, the recombination rate between a disease locus and a marker polymorphism is less than 1%, family members can simply have the marker locus assayed to determine, with 99% or greater certainty, whether each member carries the disease-causing allele.

For most genetic diseases, it is now possible to test directly for the disease-causing mutation, often by sequencing the DNA in family members. In some cases, however, the actual disease-causing mutation cannot be identified, but linked marker loci can be assayed providing an indirect genetic test. These genetic tests are now used routinely to confirm diagnosis of a genetic disease, to identify carriers of recessive diseases, and to presymptomatically identify individuals who are at risk for inheriting a disease with delayed age of onset, such as autosomal dominant breast or colon cancer, Huntington disease, and many others. In some cases, testing can help provide preventive treatment, such as prophylactic oophorectomy in women who have inherited a dominant allele that can cause breast or ovarian cancer.

Assigning Loci to Specific Chromosomes

With completion of the human DNA sequence (see following), computer analysis of the published sequence has become an effective and popular approach for identifying genes. Computerized databases of known DNA sequences play an important role in gene identification. When studying a specific region of DNA to find a gene, it is common to search for similarity between DNA sequences from the region and DNA sequences in the database. The sequences in the database may derive from genes with known function or tissue-specific expression patterns. Suppose, for example, that we have used linkage analysis to identify a region containing a gene that causes a developmental disorder such as a limb malformation. As we evaluate DNA sequences in the region, we would look for similarity between a DNA sequence from this region and a plausible sequence from the database (e.g., sequence from a gene that encodes a protein involved in bone development, such as a fibroblast growth factor). Because genes that encode similar protein products usually have similar DNA sequences, a match between the sequence from our region and a sequence in the database could be a vital clue that this particular DNA sequence is actually part of the gene that causes the limb malformation.

As the cost of sequencing whole human genomes has declined, it is now common to search for a disease-causing mutation in an individual or a family by evaluating their entire DNA sequence. Their sequences are compared with those of unaffected individuals, and statistical methods are used to determine which, if any, of their DNA variants cause disease. Linkage results, as discussed previously, can help to define a specific chromosome region that contains a disease-causing variant in a family. Currently, the genetic causes of about 3000 mendelian conditions have been determined, enabling genetic testing, more accurate diagnosis, and in some cases more effective treatment of disease.

SUMMARY REVIEW

DNA, RNA, and Proteins: Heredity at the Molecular Level

1. Genes, the basic units of inheritance, are composed of DNA and are located on the chromosomes.
2. The most important constituent of DNA is the four types of nitrogenous bases, labeled A, C, G, and T. The physical structure of DNA is a double helix.
3. The DNA bases code for amino acids, which in turn make up proteins. The amino acids are specified by triplet codons of nitrogenous bases.
4. DNA replication is based on complementary base pairing, in which a single strand of DNA serves as the template for attracting bases that form a new strand of DNA.
5. DNA polymerase is the primary enzyme involved in replication. It adds bases to the new DNA strand and performs "proofreading" functions.
6. A mutation is an inherited alteration of genetic material (i.e., DNA).
7. Substances that cause mutations are called mutagens.
8. The mutation rate in humans varies from locus to locus and ranges from 10^{-4} to 10^{-7} per gene per generation.
9. Transcription and translation, the two basic processes in which proteins are specified by DNA, both involve RNA. RNA is chemically similar to DNA, but it is single stranded and has uracil rather than thymine as one of its four nitrogenous bases.
10. Transcription is the process by which DNA specifies a sequence of mRNA.
11. Much of the RNA sequence is spliced from the mRNA before the mRNA leaves the nucleus. The excised sequences are called introns, and those that remain to code for proteins are called exons.
12. Transcription factors bind to DNA sequences called transcription factor binding sites near genes to regulate the timing of transcription, as well as the specific tissues in which genes are actively transcribed.
13. Translation is the process by which RNA directs the synthesis of polypeptides. This process takes place in the ribosomes.
14. During translation, mRNA interacts with tRNA, a molecule that has an attachment site for a specific amino acid.

Chromosomes

1. Human cells consist of diploid somatic cells (body cells) and haploid gametes (sperm and egg cells).
2. Humans have 23 pairs of chromosomes: 22 of these pairs are autosomes. The remaining pair consists of the sex chromosomes. Females have two homologous X chromosomes as their sex chromosomes; males have an X and a Y chromosome.
3. A karyotype is an ordered display of chromosomes arranged according to length and the location of the centromere.
4. Various types of stains can be used to make chromosome bands more visible.
5. About 1 in 150 live births has a major diagnosable chromosome abnormality. Chromosome abnormalities are the leading known cause of mental retardation and miscarriage.
6. Polyploidy is a condition in which a euploid cell has some multiple of the normal number of chromosomes. Humans have been observed to have triploidy (three copies of each chromosome) and tetraploidy (four copies of each chromosome); both conditions are lethal.
7. Somatic cells that do not have a multiple of 23 chromosomes are aneuploid. Aneuploidy is usually the result of nondisjunction.
8. Trisomy is a type of aneuploidy in which one chromosome is present in three copies in somatic cells. A partial trisomy is one in which only part of a chromosome is present in three copies.
9. Monosomy is a type of aneuploidy in which one chromosome is present in only one copy in somatic cells.
10. In general, monosomies cause more severe physical defects than do trisomies, illustrating the principle that the loss of chromosome material has more severe consequences than the duplication of chromosome material.
11. Down syndrome, a trisomy of chromosome 21, is the most well-known disease caused by a chromosome aberration. It affects 1 in 800 live births and is much more likely to occur in the offspring of women older than 35 years of age.
12. Most aneuploidies of the sex chromosomes have less severe consequences than those of the autosomes.
13. The most commonly observed sex chromosome aneuploidies are the 47,XXX karyotype, 45,X karyotype (Turner syndrome); 47,XXY karyotype (Klinefelter syndrome); and 47,XYY karyotype.
14. Abnormalities of chromosome structure include deletions, duplications, inversions, and translocations.

Elements of Formal Genetics

1. Mendelian traits are caused by single genes, each of which occupies a position, or locus, on a chromosome.
2. Alleles are different forms of genes located at the same locus on the chromosome.
3. At any given locus in a somatic cell, an individual has two genes, one from each parent. An individual may be homozygous or heterozygous for a locus.
4. An individual's genotype is his or her genetic makeup, and the phenotype reflects the interaction of genotype and environment.
5. At a heterozygous locus, a dominant gene's effects mask those of a recessive gene. The recessive gene is expressed only when it is present in two copies.

Transmission of Genetic Diseases

1. Genetic diseases caused by single genes usually follow autosomal dominant, autosomal recessive, or X-linked recessive modes of inheritance.
2. Pedigree charts are an important tool in the analysis of modes of inheritance.
3. Recurrence risks specify the probability that future offspring will inherit a genetic disease. For single-gene diseases, recurrence risks remain the same for each offspring, regardless of the number of affected or unaffected offspring.

SUMMARY REVIEW—cont'd

4. The recurrence risk for autosomal dominant diseases is usually 50%.
5. Germline mosaicism can alter recurrence risks for genetic diseases because unaffected parents can produce multiple affected offspring. This situation occurs because the germline of one parent is affected by a mutation but the parent's somatic cells are unaffected.
6. Skipped generations are not seen in classic autosomal dominant pedigrees.
7. Males and females are equally likely to exhibit autosomal dominant diseases and to pass them on to their offspring.
8. A gene that is not always expressed phenotypically is said to have incomplete penetrance.
9. Penetrance may be age-dependent, as in Huntington disease and familial breast cancer.
10. Variable expressivity is a characteristic of many genetic diseases.
11. Most commonly, parents of children with autosomal recessive diseases are both heterozygous carriers of the disease gene. In this case, the recurrence risk for autosomal recessive diseases is 25%.
12. Males and females are equally likely to be affected by autosomal recessive diseases.
13. Consanguinity is sometimes present in families with autosomal recessive diseases, and it becomes more prevalent with rarer recessive diseases.
14. Carrier detection tests for an increasing number of autosomal recessive diseases are available.
15. The frequency of genetic diseases approximately doubles in the offspring of first-cousin matings.
16. In each normal female somatic cell, one of the two X chromosomes is inactivated early in embryogenesis.
17. X inactivation is random, fixed, and incomplete (i.e., only part of the chromosome is actually inactivated). It may involve methylation.
18. Gender is determined embryonically by the presence of the *SRY* gene on the Y chromosome. Embryos that have a Y chromosome (and thus the *SRY* gene) become males, whereas those lacking the Y chromosome become females. When the Y chromosome lacks the *SRY* gene, an XY female can be produced. Similarly, an X chromosome that contains the *SRY* gene can produce an XX male.
19. X-linked genes are those that are located on the X chromosome. Nearly all known X-linked diseases are caused by X-linked recessive genes.
20. Males are hemizygous for genes on the X chromosome.
21. X-linked recessive diseases are seen much more often in males than in females because males need only one copy of the gene to express the disease.
22. Fathers cannot pass X-linked genes to their sons.
23. Skipped generations are often seen in X-linked recessive disease pedigrees because the gene can be transmitted through carrier females.
24. Recurrence risks for X-linked recessive diseases depend on the carrier and affected status of the mother and father.
25. A sex-limited trait is one that occurs in only one of the sexes.
26. A sex-influenced trait is one that occurs more often in one sex than in the other.

Linkage Analysis and Gene Identification

1. During meiosis I, crossing over occurs and can cause recombinations of alleles located on the same chromosome.
2. The frequency of recombinations can be used to infer the map distance between loci on the same chromosome.
3. A marker locus, when closely linked to a disease-gene locus, can be used to predict whether an individual will develop a genetic disease.
4. The complete human genome sequence will facilitate gene identification, diagnosis, and disease treatment.

KEY TERMS

Adenine, 136
Age-dependent penetrance, 154
Allele, 151
Amino acid, 137
Aneuploid cell, 144
Anticodon, 142
Autosome, 142
Barr body, 156
Base pair substitution, 137
Carrier, 151
Carrier detection test, 156
Chromosomal mosaic, 146
Chromosome band, 142
Chromosome breakage, 148
Chromosome theory of inheritance, 152
Codominance, 151
Codon, 137
Complementary base pairing, 137
Consanguinity, 155
Cri du chat syndrome, 148
Crossing over, 159
Cytosine, 136
Deletion, 148
Deoxyribonucleic acid (DNA), 135
Diploid cell, 141
DNA polymerase, 137
Dominant, 151
Dosage compensation, 156
Double helix, 136
Down syndrome, 146
Duplication, 149
Dystrophin, 158
Enhancers, 141
Euploid cell, 143
Exon, 142
Expressivity, 154
Fragile site, 151
Frameshift mutation, 140
Gamete, 142
Gene, 135
Genotype, 135
Germline mosaicism, 154
Giemsa stain, 143
Guanine, 136
Haploid cell, 142
Hemizygous, 156
Heterozygote, 151
Heterozygous, 151
Homologous, 142
Homologous chromosome, 142
Homozygote, 151
Homozygous, 151
Inbreeding, 156
Intron, 142
Inversion, 149
Karyotype, 142
Klinefelter syndrome, 148
Linkage, 159
Locus, 151
Map unit, 159
Marker polymorphism, 160
Meiosis, 142
Messenger RNA (mRNA), 141
Metaphase spread, 142
Missense mutation, 137
Mode of inheritance, 151

KEY TERMS – cont'd

REFERENCES

1. Online: *Mendelian inheritance in man.* Available at www.omim.org.
2. Hall JG et al: The frequency and financial burden of genetic disease in a pediatric hospital, *Am J Med Genet* 1(1):417–436, 1978.
3. Crow JF: The origins, patterns and implications of human spontaneous mutation, *Nat Rev Genet* 1:40–47, 2000.
4. Hall H, Hunt P, Hassold T: Meiosis and sex chromosome aneuploidy: how meiotic errors cause aneupolidy; how aneuploidy causes meiotic errors, *Curr Opin Genet Dev* 16(3):323–329, 2006.
5. Tolie JL, MacFayden U et al: Clinical genetics of common autosomal trisomies. In Rimoin DL, editor: *Emery and Rimoin's principles and practice of medical genetics*, ed 5, Philadelphia, 2007, Churchill Livingstone, pp 1015–1037.
6. Antonarakis SE, Epstein CJ: The challenge of Down syndrome, *Trends Mol Med* 12(10):473–479, 2006.
7. Jorde LB, et al: *Medical genetics*, ed 4, St Louis, 2010, Mosby.
8. Graham GE, Allanson JE, Gerritsen JA: Sex chromosome abnormalities. In Rimoin DL, et al: *Emery and Rimoin's principles and practice of medical genetics*, ed 5, Philadelphia, 2007, Churchill Livingstone, pp 1038–1057.
9. Garber KB, Visootsak J, Warren ST: Fragile X syndrome, *Eur J Hum Genet* 16(6):666–672, 2008.
10. Ranum NL, Cooper TA: RNA-mediated neuromuscular disorders, *Annu Rev Neurosci* 29:259–277, 2006.
11. Orr HT, Zoghbi HY: Trinucleotide repeat disorders, *Annu Rev Neurosci* 30:575–621, 2007.
12. Zlotogora J: Germ line mosaicism, *Hum Mol Genet* 102(4):381–386, 1998.
13. McDermott U, Downing JR, Stratton MR: Genomics and the continuum of cancer care, *N Engl J Med* 364:340–350, 2011.
14. Knudson AG: Cancer genetics, *Am J Med Genet* 111(1):96–102, 2002.
15. Jett K, Friedman JM: Clinical and genetic aspects of neurofibromatosis 1, *Genet Med* 12:1–11, 2010.
16. Mogayzel PJ Jr, Flume PA: Update in cystic fibrosis 2009, *Am J Respir Crit Care Med* 181:539–544, 2010.
17. Jorde LB: Inbreeding in human populations. In Dulbecco R, editor: *Encyclopedia of human biology*, vol. 5, New York, 1997, Academic Press.
18. Lyon MF: Sex chromatin and gene action in the mammalian X-chromosome, *Am J Hum Genet* 14:135–148, 1962.
19. Chow J, Heard E: X inactivation and the complexities of silencing a sex chromosome, *Curr Opin Cell Biol* 21:359–366, 2009.
20. Fleming A, Vilain E: The endless quest for sex determination genes, *Clin Genet* 67(1):15–25, 2005.
21. Bushby K et al: Diagnosis and management of Duchenne muscular dystrophy, part 1: diagnosis, and pharmacological and psychosocial management, *Lancet Neurol* 9:77–93, 2010.
22. Lander ES: Initial impact of the sequencing of the human genome, *Nature* 470:187–197, 2011.

CHAPTER

5

Genes, Environment-Lifestyle, and Common Diseases

Lynn B. Jorde

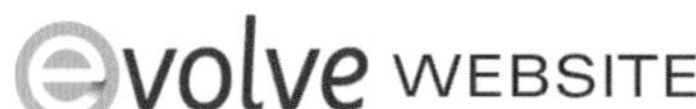

http://evolve.elsevier.com/McCance/

- Review Questions and Answers
- Online Course: Module 3

CHAPTER OUTLINE

Chapter 4 focuses on diseases that are caused by single genes or by abnormalities of single chromosomes. Much progress has been made in identifying specific mutations that cause these diseases, leading to better risk estimates and, in some cases, more effective treatment of the disease. However, these conditions form only a small portion of the total burden of human genetic disease. Most congenital malformations are not caused by single genes or chromosome defects. Many common adult diseases, such as cancer, heart disease, and diabetes, have genetic components, but again they are usually not caused by single genes or by chromosomal abnormalities.[1] These diseases, whose treatment collectively occupies the attention of most healthcare practitioners, are the result of a complex interplay of multiple genetic and environmental* factors.

*In human genetics, it is common practice to use the term "environment" to designate all nongeneric factors, such as diet and lifestyle.

FACTORS INFLUENCING INCIDENCE OF DISEASE IN POPULATIONS

Concepts of Incidence and Prevalence

How common is a given disease, such as diabetes, in a population? Well-established measures are used to answer this question.[2] The **incidence rate** is the number of new cases of a disease reported during a specific period (typically 1 year) divided by the number of individuals in the population. The denominator is often expressed as *person-years.* The incidence rate can be contrasted with the **prevalence rate,** which is the proportion of the population affected by a disease at a specific point in time. Prevalence is thus determined by both the incidence rate and the length of the survival period in affected individuals. For example, the prevalence rate of acquired immunodeficiency syndrome (AIDS) is larger than the yearly incidence rate because most people with AIDS survive for at least several years after diagnosis.

Many diseases vary in prevalence from one population to another. Cystic fibrosis is relatively common among Europeans, occurring about once in every 2500 births. In contrast, it is quite rare in Asians, occurring only once in every 90,000 births. Similarly, sickle cell disease affects approximately 1 in 600 American blacks, but it is seen much less frequently in whites. Both of these diseases are single-gene disorders, and they vary among populations because disease-causing mutations are more or less common in different populations. (This is in turn the result of differences in the evolutionary history of these populations.) Nongenetic (environmental) factors have little influence on the current prevalence of these diseases.

The picture often becomes more complex with the common diseases of adulthood. For example, colon cancer was until recently relatively rare in Japan, but it is the second most common cancer in the United States. Stomach cancer, on the other hand, is common in Japan but relatively rare in the United States. These statistics, in themselves, cannot distinguish environmental from genetic influences in the two populations. However, because large numbers of Japanese emigrated first to Hawaii and then to the U.S. mainland, we can observe what happens to the rates of stomach and colon cancer among the migrants. It is important that the Japanese émigrés maintained a genetic identity, marrying largely among themselves. Among first-generation Japanese in Hawaii, the frequency of colon cancer rose several-fold—not yet as high as in the U.S. mainland but higher than that in Japan. Among second-generation Japanese on the U.S. mainland, colon cancer rates rose to 5%, equal to the U.S. average. At the same time, stomach cancer has become relatively rare among Japanese-Americans.

These observations strongly indicate an important role for environmental factors in the etiology of cancers of the colon and stomach. In each case, diet is a likely culprit—a high-fat, low-fiber diet in the United States is thought to increase the risk of colon cancer, whereas techniques used to preserve and season the fish commonly eaten in Japan are thought to increase the risk of stomach cancer. It is interesting that the incidence of colon cancer in Japan has increased dramatically during the past several decades as the Japanese population has adopted a more "Western" diet. These results do not, however, rule out the potential contribution of genetic factors in common cancers. Genes also play a role in the etiology of colon and other cancers.

Analysis of Risk Factors

The comparison just discussed is one example of the analysis of risk factors (in this case, diet) and their influence on the prevalence of disease in populations. A common measure of the effect of a specific risk factor is the **relative risk.** This quantity is expressed as a ratio:

$$\frac{\text{Increased rate of the disease among individuals exposed to a risk factor}}{\text{Incidence rate of the disease among individuals } \textit{not} \text{ exposed to a risk factor}}$$

A classic example of a relative risk analysis was carried out in a sample of more than 40,000 British physicians to determine the relationship between cigarette smoking and lung cancer. This study compared the incidence of death from lung cancer in physicians who smoked with those who did not. The incidence of death from lung cancer was 1.66 (per 1000 person-years) in heavy smokers (more than 25 cigarettes daily), but it was only 0.07 in the nonsmokers. The ratio of these two incidence rates is 1.66/0.07, which yields a relative risk of 23.7 deaths. Thus, it is concluded that the risk of dying from lung cancer increased by about 24-fold in heavy smokers compared with nonsmokers. Many other studies have obtained similar risk figures.

Although cigarette smoking clearly increases one's risk of developing lung cancer (as well as heart disease, as we will see later), it is equally clear that *most* smokers do not develop lung cancer. Other lifestyle factors are likely to contribute to one's risk of developing this disease (e.g., exposure to cancer-causing substances in the air, such as asbestos fibers). In addition, differences in genetic background may be involved. Smokers who have variants in genes, such as *CYP1A1* and *GSTM1,* that are involved in the metabolism of components of tobacco smoke are at significantly increased risk of developing lung cancer.

Many factors can influence the risk of acquiring a common disease such as cancer, diabetes, or high blood pressure. These include age, gender, diet, amount of exercise, and family history of the disease. Usually, complex interactions occur among these genetic and nongenetic factors. The effects of each factor can be quantified in terms of relative risks. The following discussion demonstrates how genetic and environmental factors contribute to the risk of developing common diseases.

PRINCIPLES OF MULTIFACTORIAL INHERITANCE

Basic Model

Traits in which variation is thought to be caused by the combined effects of multiple genes are **polygenic** ("many genes"). When environmental factors are also believed to cause variation in the trait, which is usually the case, the term **multifactorial trait** is used.[3] Many **quantitative traits** (those, such as blood pressure, that are measured on a continuous numeric scale) are multifactorial. Because they are caused by the additive effects of many genetic and environmental factors, these traits tend to follow a normal, or bell-shaped, distribution in populations.

An example illustrates this concept. To begin with the simplest case, suppose (unrealistically) that height is determined by a single gene with two alleles, *A* and *a.* Allele *A* tends to make people tall, whereas allele *a* tends to make them short. If there is no dominance at this locus, then the three possible genotypes (*AA, Aa, aa*) will produce three phenotypes: tall, intermediate, and short, respectively. Assume that the gene frequencies of *A* and *a* are each 0.50. If we look at a population of individuals, we will observe the height distribution depicted in Figure 5-1, *A.*

Now suppose, a bit more realistically, that height is determined by two loci instead of one. The second locus also has two alleles, *B* (tall) and *b* (short), and they affect height in exactly the same way as alleles *A* and *a.* There are now nine possible genotypes in our population: *aabb, aaBb, aaBB, Aabb, AaBb, AaBB, AAbb, AABb,* and *AABB.* An individual may have zero, one,

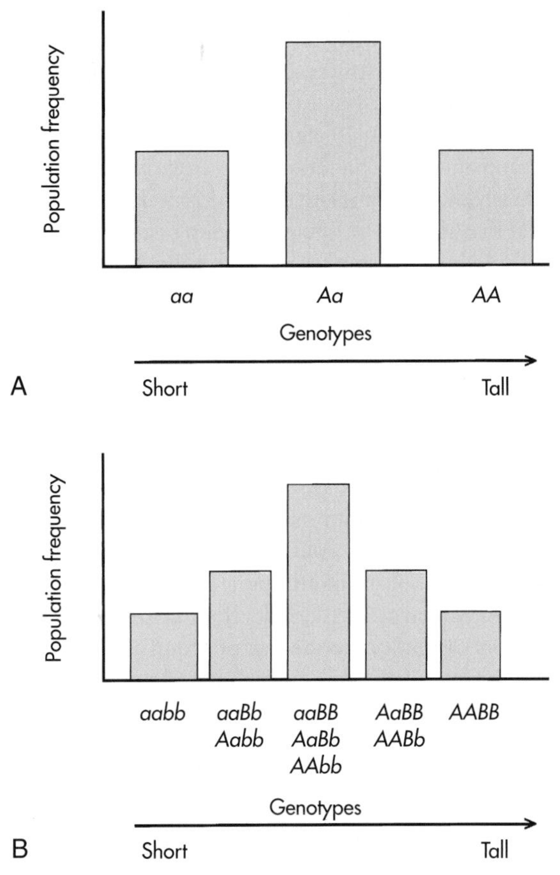

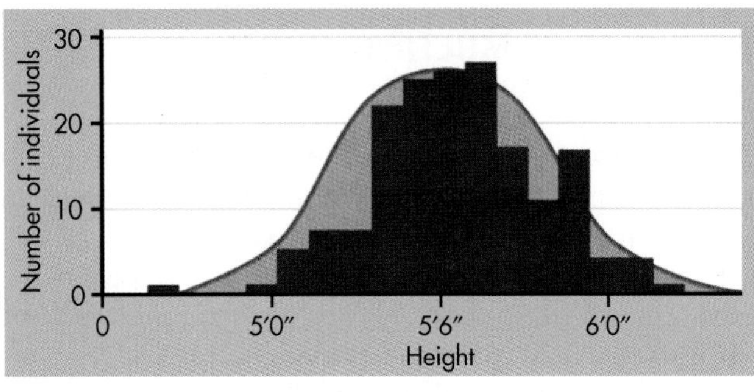

C

FIGURE 5-1 Distribution of Height. A, Distribution of height in a population, assuming that height is controlled by a single locus with genotypes *AA, Aa,* and *aa.* **B,** Distribution of height, assuming that height is controlled by two loci. Five distinct genotypes are shown instead of three, and the distribution begins to look more like the normal distribution. **C,** Height is portrayed, realistically, as a trait with a continuous statistical distribution. Because many genes contribute to height and tend to segregate independently of one another, the cumulative contribution of different combinations of alleles to height forms a continuous distribution of possible heights, in which the extremes are much rarer than the intermediate values. Variation also can be due to environmental factors such as nutrition. (**A** and **B** adapted from Jorde LB et al: *Medical genetics,* ed 4, St Louis, 2010, Mosby; **C** from Raven PH et al: *Biology,* ed 8, New York, 2008, McGraw-Hill.)

two, three, or four "tall" alleles, so now five distinct phenotypes are possible (see Figure 5-1, *B*). Although the height distribution in our fictional population is still not normal compared with an actual population, it approaches a normal distribution more closely than in the single-gene case just described.

From extension of this example, *many* genes and environmental factors influence height, each having a small effect. Then many phenotypes are possible, each differing slightly from the others, and the height distribution of the population approaches the bell-shaped curve shown in Figure 5-1, *C.*

It should be emphasized that the individual genes underlying a multifactorial trait such as height follow the mendelian principles of segregation and independent assortment, just like any other gene. The only difference is that many of them *act together* to influence the trait. More than 100 genes have now been shown to be associated with variation in human height.

Blood pressure is another example of a multifactorial trait. A correlation exists between parents' blood pressures (systolic and diastolic) and those of their children. The evidence is good that this correlation is partially caused by genes, but blood pressure is also influenced by environmental factors, such as diet, exercise, and stress. Two goals of genetic research are the identification and measurement of the relative roles of genes and environment in the causation of multifactorial diseases.

Threshold Model

A number of diseases do not follow the bell-shaped distribution. Instead, they appear to be either present or absent in individuals, yet they do not follow the inheritance patterns expected of single-gene diseases. A commonly used explanation for such diseases is that there is an underlying **liability distribution** for the disease in a population (Figure 5-2). Those individuals who are on the "low" end of the distribution have little chance of developing the disease in question (i.e., they have few of the alleles or environmental factors that would cause the disease). Individuals who are closer to the "high" end of the distribution have more of the disease-causing genes and environmental factors and are more likely to develop the disease. For diseases that are either present or absent, it is thought that a **threshold of liability** must be crossed before the disease is expressed. Below the threshold, an individual appears normal; above it, he or she is affected by the disease.

A disease that is thought to correspond to this threshold model is *pyloric stenosis,* a disorder that presents shortly after birth and is caused by a narrowing or obstruction of the pylorus, the area between the stomach and intestine. Chronic vomiting, constipation, weight loss, and imbalance of electrolyte levels result from the condition, but it sometimes resolves spontaneously or can be corrected by surgery. The prevalence of pyloric stenosis is about 3 per 1000 live births in whites. It is much more common in males than females, affecting 1 of 200 males and 1 of 1000 females. It is thought that this difference in prevalence reflects two thresholds in the liability distribution—a lower one in males and a higher one in females (see Figure 5-2). A lower male threshold implies that fewer disease-causing factors are required to generate the disorder in males.

The liability threshold concept may explain the pattern of recurrence risks for pyloric stenosis seen in Table 5-1. Note that males, having a lower threshold, always have a higher risk than females. However, the sibling risk also depends on the gender of the proband (i.e., the individual from which the pedigree begins). It is higher when the proband is female than when the

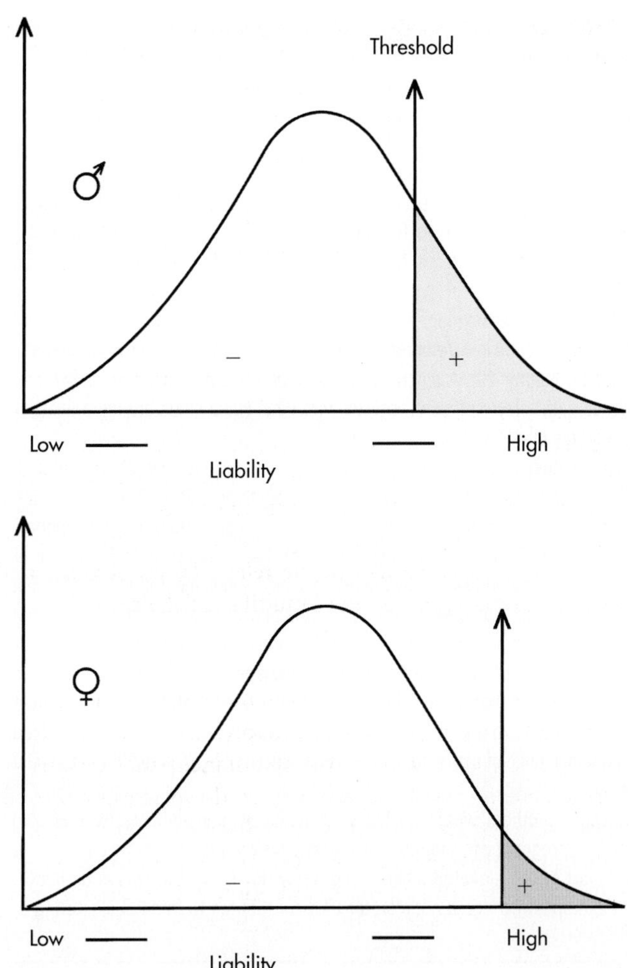

FIGURE 5-2 A Liability Distribution in a Population for a Multifactorial Disease. To be affected with the disease, an individual must exceed the threshold on the liability distribution. This figure shows two thresholds, a lower one for males and a higher one for females (as in pyloric stenosis; see text). (From Jorde LB et al: *Medical genetics,* ed 4, St Louis, 2010, Mosby.)

proband is male. This reflects the concept that females, having a higher liability threshold, must be exposed to more disease-causing factors than males to develop the disease. Thus a family with an affected female must have more genetic and environmental risk factors, producing a higher recurrence risk for pyloric stenosis in future offspring. It would be expected that the highest risk category would be *male* relatives of *female* probands; Table 5-1 shows that this is the case.

A similar pattern has been observed in a study of *autism,* a behavioral disorder in which the male/female ratio is approximately 4:1. As expected for a multifactorial disorder, the recurrence risks for siblings of male probands (3.5%) is substantially lower than that of siblings of female probands (7%). When the sex ratio for a disease is reversed (i.e., more affected females than males), one would expect a higher recurrence risk when the proband is male.

A number of other congenital malformations are thought to correspond to this model. They include isolated *cleft lip and/or cleft palate (CL/P), neural tube defects (anencephaly, spina bifida), clubfoot (talipes),* and some forms of congenital heart

TABLE 5-1 RECURRENCE RISKS (%) FOR PYLORIC STENOSIS, SUBDIVIDED BY GENDERS OF AFFECTED PROBANDS AND RELATIVES

	MALE PROBANDS		FEMALE PROBANDS	
RELATIVES	**LONDON**	**BELFAST**	**LONDON**	**BELFAST**
Brothers	3.8	9.6	9.2	12.5
Sisters	2.7	3.0	3.8	3.8

Data from Carter CO: *Br Med Bull* 32(1):21–26, 1976.
Note that the risks differ somewhat between the two populations.

disease. In this context, isolated means that this is the only observed disease feature (i.e., the feature is not part of a larger constellation of findings, as in CL/P secondary to trisomy 13). In addition, many common adult diseases, such as *hypertension, coronary heart disease, stroke, diabetes mellitus* (types 1 and 2), and some cancers, are caused by complex genetic and environmental factors and can thus be considered multifactorial diseases.

Recurrence Risks and Transmission Patterns

Whereas recurrence risks can be given with confidence for single-gene diseases (e.g., 50% for typical autosomal dominant diseases, 25% for autosomal recessive diseases), the situation is more complicated for multifactorial diseases. This is because the number of genes contributing to the disease is usually not known, the precise allelic constitution of the parents is not known, and the extent of environmental effects can vary substantially. For most multifactorial diseases, **empirical risks** (i.e., risks based on direct observation of data) have been derived. To estimate empirical risks, a large series of families is examined in which one child has developed the disease (the proband). Then the siblings of each proband are surveyed to calculate the percentage of siblings who also have developed the disease. For example, in the United States about 3% of siblings of individuals with neural tube defects also have neural tube defects (Box 5-1). Thus the recurrence risk for parents who have had one child with a neural tube defect is 3% in the United States. For conditions such as CL/P that are not lethal or severely debilitating, recurrence risks also can be estimated for the offspring of affected parents. Empirical recurrence risks are, of course, specific for each multifactorial disease.

In contrast to most single-gene diseases, recurrence risks for multifactorial diseases can change substantially from one population to another because gene frequencies as well as environmental factors can differ among populations (note the differences between the London and Belfast populations in Table 5-1).

It is sometimes difficult to distinguish polygenic or multifactorial diseases from single-gene diseases that have reduced penetrance or variable expression. Large data sets and good epidemiologic data are necessary to make the distinction. Several criteria are commonly used to define multifactorial inheritance.

BOX 5-1 NEURAL TUBE DEFECTS

Neural tube defects (NTDs), which include *anencephaly, spina bifida,* and *encephalocele* (as well as several other less common forms), are one of the most important classes of birth defects, and they are seen in 0.5 to 2 of 1000 pregnancies.[4] The prevalence of NTDs among different populations varies considerably, with an especially high rate among some northern Chinese populations (as high as 6 or more per 1000 births). The prevalence of NTDs has been decreasing in many parts of the United States and Europe during the past three decades, partly because of dietary changes.

Normally the neural tube closes at about the fourth week of gestation. A defect in closure, or a subsequent reopening of the neural tube, results in a neural tube defect. Spina bifida (Figure 5-3, *A*) is the most commonly observed NTD and consists of a protrusion of spinal tissue through the vertebral column (the tissue usually includes meninges, spinal cord, and nerve roots). About 75% of individuals with spina bifida have secondary hydrocephalus, which sometimes in turn produces mental retardation. Paralysis or muscle weakness, lack of sphincter control, and clubfeet are often observed. A study conducted in British Columbia showed that survival rates for people with spina bifida have improved dramatically over the past several decades. Less than 30% of people born between 1952 and 1969 survived to 10 years of age, whereas 65% of those born between 1970 and 1986 survived to this age. Anencephaly (see Figure 5-3, *B*) is characterized by partial or complete absence of the cranial vault and calvarium and partial or complete absence of the cerebral hemispheres. At least two thirds of newborns with anencephaly are stillborn; term deliveries do not survive more than a few hours or days.

NTDs are thought to arise from a combination of genetic and environmental factors. In most populations surveyed thus far, empirical recurrence risks for siblings of affected people range from 2% to 5%. Consistent with a multifactorial model, the recurrence risk increases with additional affected siblings. Studies conducted in Great Britain showed that the sibling recurrence risk was approximately 5% when one sibling was affected and 10% when two were affected. A Hungarian study showed that the overall prevalence of NTDs was 1 in 300 births and that the sibling recurrence risks were 3%, 12%, and 25% after one, two, and three affected offspring, respectively. Recurrence risks tend to be slightly lower in populations with lower NTD prevalence rates, as predicted by the multifactorial model. Recurrence risk data support the idea that the major forms of NTDs are caused by similar factors. An anencephalic conception increases the recurrence risk for subsequent spina bifida conceptions, and vice versa.

NTDs can usually be diagnosed prenatally, sometimes by ultrasound and usually by an elevation in α-fetoprotein (AFP) level in the maternal serum or amniotic fluid (see Chapter 20). A spina bifida lesion can be either open or closed (i.e., covered with a layer of skin). Fetuses with open spina bifida are more likely to be detected by AFP assays.

A major epidemiologic finding is that mothers who supplement their diet with folic acid at the time of conception are less likely to produce children with NTDs. This result has been replicated in several different populations and thus appears to be well confirmed. It has been estimated that as many as 50% to 70% of NTDs can be avoided simply by dietary folic acid supplementation.[5] (Traditional prenatal vitamin supplements have little effect because administration does not usually begin until well after the time that the neural tube closes.) It is now recommended that all women of reproductive age supplement their diet with 0.4 mg of folic acid each day; many foods in the United States are supplemented with folic acid. Consequently, average folate levels in U.S. females have doubled and the incidence of neural tube defects has declined by 30% to 50% in the past decade.

Because mothers would be likely to ingest similar amounts of folic acid from one pregnancy to the next, folic acid deficiency could well account for at least part of the elevated sibling recurrence risk for NTDs. This is an important example of a *nongenetic* factor that contributes to familial clustering of a disease.

First, *the recurrence risk becomes higher if more than one family member is affected.* For example, the sibling recurrence risk for a *ventricular septal defect* (VSD, a type of congenital heart defect) is 3% if one sibling has been affected by a VSD but increases to approximately 10% if two siblings have been diagnosed with VSDs.[6] In contrast, the recurrence risk for single-gene diseases remains the same regardless of the number of affected siblings. It should be emphasized that this increase does not mean that the family's risk has actually *changed.* Rather, it means that there is more information about the family's true risk; because they have had two affected children, they are probably located higher on the liability distribution than a family with only one affected child. In other words, they have more risk factors (genetic or environmental) and are more likely to produce an affected child.

Second, *if the expression of the disease in the proband is more severe, the recurrence risk is higher.* This is again consistent with the liability model because a more severe expression indicates that the affected individual is at the extreme tail end of the liability distribution (see Figure 5-2). His or her relatives are thus at a higher risk for inheriting disease genes. For example, the occurrence of a bilateral (both sides) CL/P confers a higher recurrence risk on family members than does the occurrence of a unilateral (one side) cleft.

Third, *the recurrence risk is higher if the proband is of the less commonly affected gender* (see the preceding discussion of pyloric stenosis). This is because an affected individual of the less susceptible gender is usually at a more extreme position on the liability distribution.

Fourth, *the recurrence risk for the disease usually decreases rapidly in more remotely related relatives* (Table 5-2). Whereas the recurrence risk for single-gene diseases decreases by 50% with each degree of relationship (e.g., an autosomal dominant disease has a 50% recurrence risk for siblings, 25% for uncle-nephew relationships, 12.5% for first cousins), it decreases much more quickly for multifactorial diseases. This reflects the fact that many genes and environmental factors must combine to produce a trait. All the necessary risk factors are unlikely to be present in less closely related family members.

Finally, *if the prevalence of the disease in a population is f, the risk for offspring and siblings of probands is approximately* $\sqrt{f}$. This does not hold true for single-gene traits because their recurrence risks are independent of population prevalence. It is not an absolute rule for multifactorial traits either, but many such diseases tend to conform to this prediction. Examination of the risks given in Table 5-2 shows that the first three diseases follow the prediction fairly well. However, the observed sibling risk for the fourth disease, infantile autism, is substantially higher than that predicted by $\sqrt{f}$.

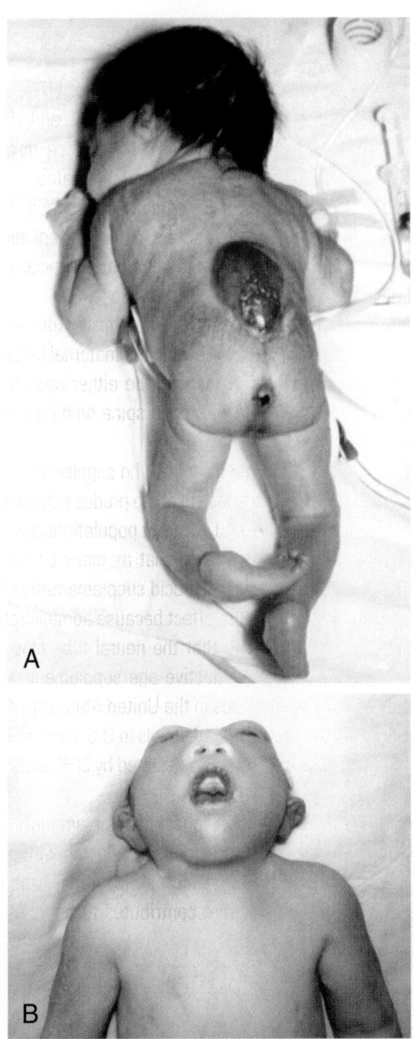

FIGURE 5-3 Spina Bifida and Anencephaly. **A,** Spina bifida in a newborn. **B,** Anencephaly, showing the absence of the cranial vault. (From Jones KL: *Smith's recognizable patterns of human malformation,* ed 6, Philadelphia, Saunders, 2006, p. 705.)

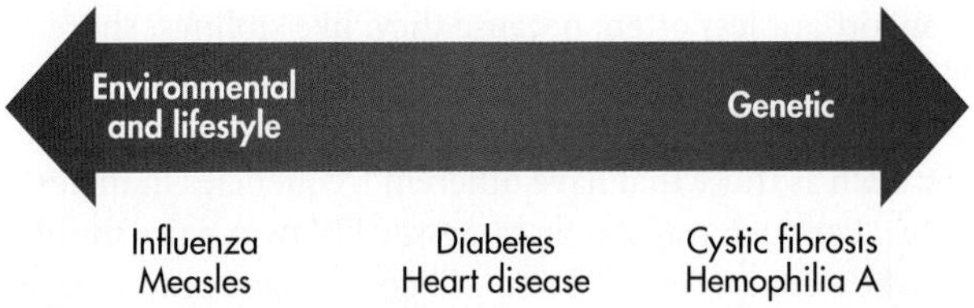

NATURE AND NURTURE: DISENTANGLING THE EFFECTS OF GENES AND ENVIRONMENT

Family members share genes and a common environment. Family resemblance in traits such as blood pressure reflects both genes (nature) and environment (nurture). For centuries people have debated the relative importance of these two types of factors. It is a mistake, of course, to view them as mutually exclusive. Few traits are influenced only by genes or only by environmental factors. Most are influenced by both. It is useful to try to determine the *relative* influence of genetic and environmental factors (Figure 5-4). This can lead to a better understanding of disease etiology. It can also help in planning public health strategies. A disease in which the genetic influence is relatively small, such as lung cancer, may be prevented most effectively through emphasis on lifestyle changes (avoidance of tobacco). When a disease has a relatively larger genetic component, as in breast cancer, examination of family history should be emphasized in addition to lifestyle modification.

Environmental and lifestyle — Genetic

Influenza, Measles — Diabetes, Heart disease — Cystic fibrosis, Hemophilia A

FIGURE 5-4 Continuum of Genetic Diseases. Some diseases (e.g., cystic fibrosis) are strongly determined by genes, whereas others (e.g., infectious diseases) are strongly determined by environmental factors. (Adapted from Jorde LB et al: *Medical genetics,* ed 4, St Louis, 2010, Mosby.)

TABLE 5-2 RECURRENCE RISKS (%) FOR FIRST-, SECOND-, AND THIRD-DEGREE RELATIVES

	RISK			
DEGREE	FIRST DEGREE	SECOND DEGREE	THIRD DEGREE	GENERAL POPULATION
Cleft lip/palate	4	0.7	0.3	0.1
Clubfoot	2.5	0.5	0.2	0.1
Congenital hip dislocation	5	0.6	0.4	0.2

Here, two research strategies are reviewed that often are used to estimate the relative influence of genes and environment: twin studies and adoption studies.

Twin Studies

Twins occur with a frequency of about 1 in 100 births in white populations. They are a bit more common in blacks and a bit less common among Asians. **Monozygotic (MZ, identical) twins** originate when, for unknown reasons, the developing embryo divides to form two separate but identical embryos. Because they are genetically identical, MZ twins are an example of natural clones. **Dizygotic (DZ, fraternal) twins** are the result of a double ovulation followed by the fertilization of each egg by a different sperm. Thus dizygotic twins are genetically no more similar than siblings. Because two different sperm cells are required to fertilize the two eggs, it is possible for each DZ twin to have a different father. Whereas MZ twinning rates are constant across populations, DZ twinning rates vary somewhat. DZ twinning increases with maternal age until about 40 years, after which it declines.

Because MZ twins are genetically identical, any differences between them should be caused only by environmental effects.[7] MZ twins should thus resemble one another very closely for traits that are strongly influenced by genes. DZ twins provide a convenient comparison because their environmental differences should be similar to those of MZ twins, but their genetic differences are as great as those between siblings. Twin studies thus usually consist of comparisons between MZ and DZ twins.[8] If both members of a twin pair share a trait (e.g., a cleft lip), it is said to be a **concordant trait.** If they do not share the trait, it is a **discordant trait.** For a trait determined totally by genes, MZ twins should always be concordant, whereas DZ twins should be concordant less often, because they, like siblings, share only 50% of their genes. Concordance rates may differ between opposite-sex DZ twin pairs and same-sex DZ pairs for some traits, such as those that have different frequencies in males and females. For such traits, only same-sex DZ twin pairs should be used when comparing MZ and DZ concordance rates, because MZ twins are necessarily of the same sex.

TABLE 5-3 CONCORDANCE RATES IN MZ AND DZ TWINS FOR SELECTED TRAITS AND DISEASES*

	CONCORDANCE RATE		
TRAIT OR DISEASE	**MZ TWINS**	**DZ TWINS**	**HERITABILITY**
Affective disorder (bipolar)	0.79	0.24	>1*
Affective disorder (unipolar)	0.54	0.19	0.7
Alcoholism	>0.6	<0.3	0.6
Autism	0.92	0	>1
Blood pressure (diastolic)†	0.58	0.27	0.62
Blood pressure (systolic)†	0.55	0.25	0.6
Body fat percentage†	0.73	0.22	>1
Body mass index†	0.95	0.53	0.84
Cleft lip/palate	0.38	0.08	0.6
Clubfoot	0.32	0.03	0.58
Dermatoglyphics (finger ridge count)†	0.95	0.49	0.92
Diabetes mellitus	0.45-0.96	0.03-0.37	>1
Diabetes mellitus (type 1)	0.55	—	—
Diabetes mellitus (type 2)	0.9	—	—
Epilepsy (idiopathic)	0.69	0.14	>1
Height†	0.94	0.44	1
Intelligence quotient (IQ)†	0.76	0.51	0.5
Measles	0.95	0.87	0.16
Multiple sclerosis	0.28	0.03	0.5
Myocardial infarction (males)	0.39	0.26	0.26
Myocardial infarction (females)	0.44	0.14	0.6
Schizophrenia	0.47	0.12	0.7
Spina bifida	0.72	0.33	0.78

***Note:** Heritability, which is defined as the proportion of the variation in a trait that is due to genetic factors, can be measured as $2(C_{MZ} - C_{DZ})$, where C_{MZ} and C_{DZ} are the concordance rates for MZ twins and DZ twins, respectively. These figures were compiled from a large variety of sources and represent primarily European and U.S. populations.
†Several heritability estimates exceed 1. Because it is impossible for >100% of the variance of a trait to be genetically determined, these values indicate that other factors, such as shared environmental factors, must be operating.
‡Because these are quantitative traits, correlation coefficients are given rather than concordance rates.
DZ, Dizygotic; *MZ,* monozygotic.

Table 5-3 gives concordance rates for a number of traits. Note that the concordance rates for contagious diseases such as measles are quite similar in MZ and DZ twins. This is expected because a contagious disease is unlikely to be influenced markedly by genes. On the other hand, the concordance rates are quite dissimilar for *schizophrenia* and *bipolar affective disorder,* suggesting a sizable genetic component for these diseases. The MZ correlations for dermatoglyphics (fingerprints), which are determined almost entirely by genes, are close to 1.0.

At one time, twins were thought to provide a perfect "natural laboratory" in which to determine the relative influences of genetics and environment, but several difficulties arose. One of the most important is the assumption that the environments of MZ and DZ twins are equally similar. As one would expect, MZ twins are often treated more similarly than DZ twins. A greater similarity in environment can make MZ twins more concordant for a trait, inflating the apparent influence of genes. In addition, MZ twins may be more likely to seek the same type of environment, further reinforcing environmental similarity. On the other hand, it has been suggested that MZ twins tend to develop personality differences in an attempt to assert their individuality.

Adoption Studies

Studies of adopted children also are used to estimate the genetic contribution to a multifactorial trait. Children born to parents who have a disease but are then subsequently adopted by parents lacking the disease can be studied to find out whether these children develop the disease. In some cases such children develop the disease more often than a comparative control population (i.e., adopted children who were born to parents who do *not* have the disease). This provides some evidence that genes may be involved in the causation of the disease, because the adopted children do not share an environment with their affected natural parents. For example, about 8% to 10% of adopted children of a schizophrenic parent develop *schizophrenia,* whereas only 1% of adopted children of normal parents develop schizophrenia.

As with twin studies, several precautions must be exercised in interpreting the results of adoption studies. First, prenatal environmental influences could have long-lasting effects on an adopted child. Second, children are sometimes adopted after they are several years old, ensuring that some environmental influence would have been imparted by the natural parents. Finally, adoption agencies sometimes try to match the adoptive parents with the natural parents in terms of background, socioeconomic status, and so on. All of these factors could exaggerate the apparent influence of biologic inheritance.

These reservations, as well as those summarized for twin studies, underscore the need for caution in basing conclusions on twin and adoption studies. These approaches do not provide definitive measures of the role of genes in multifactorial disease nor can they identify specific genes responsible for disease. Instead, they serve a useful purpose in providing a preliminary indication of the extent to which a multifactorial disease may be caused by genetic factors. Sophisticated molecular techniques are being used to identify the specific genes that underlie predisposition to multifactorial diseases.

BOX 5-2 α_1-ANTITRYPSIN DEFICIENCY: THE INTERACTION OF GENES AND ENVIRONMENT-LIFESTYLE

α_1-Antitrypsin (α_1-AT) deficiency is one of the most common autosomal recessive disorders among whites, affecting approximately 1 in 2500 members of this ethnic group. α_1-AT, synthesized primarily in the liver, is a serine protease inhibitor. It does bind trypsin, as its name suggests. However, α_1-AT binds much more strongly to neutrophil elastase, a protease that is produced by neutrophils (a type of leukocyte) in response to infections and irritants. It carries out its binding and inhibitory role primarily in the lower respiratory tract, where it prevents elastase from digesting the alveolar septi of the lung.

Individuals with less than 10% to 15% of the normal level of α_1-AT activity will experience significant lung damage and typically develop emphysema during their 30s, 40s, or 50s. In addition, at least 10% develop liver cirrhosis as a result of the accumulation of variant α_1-AT molecules in the liver; α_1-AT deficiency accounts for nearly 20% of all nonalcoholic liver cirrhosis cases in the United States. An important feature of this disease is that cigarette smokers with α_1-AT deficiency develop emphysema much earlier than do nonsmokers. This is because cigarette smoke irritates lung tissue, increasing secretion of neutrophil elastase. At the same time it inactivates α_1-AT, so there is also less inhibition of elastase. One study showed that the median age of survival of nonsmokers with α_1-AT deficiency was 62 years, whereas it was only 40 years for smokers with this disease. Because the combination of cigarette smoking (an environmental factor) and the α_1-AT mutation (a genetic factor) produces more severe disease than either factor alone, it is an example of a gene-environment interaction.

This discussion should make clear that most common diseases are not the result of either genetics *or* environment. Instead, genetic and nongenetic factors usually interact to influence one's likelihood of developing a common disease. In some cases a genetic predisposition may interact with an environmental factor to increase the risk of disease acquisition to a much higher level than would either factor acting alone. A good example of a **gene-environment interaction** is given by α_1-antitrypsin deficiency, a genetic condition that causes pulmonary emphysema and is greatly exacerbated by cigarette smoking (Box 5-2).

GENETICS OF COMMON DISEASES

Some common multifactorial disorders, the congenital malformations, are by definition present at birth. Others, including heart disease, cancer, diabetes, and most psychiatric disorders, are seen primarily in adolescents and adults. Because these disorders are complex, unraveling their genetics is a daunting task. Nonetheless, significant progress is being made.

Congenital Malformations

Congenital diseases are present at birth. Approximately 2% of newborns present with a congenital malformation; most of these are multifactorial in etiology. Table 5-4 lists some more common congenital malformations. In general, sibling recurrence risks for most of these disorders range from 1% to 5%.

Some congenital malformations, such as CL/P and pyloric stenosis, are relatively easy to repair and thus are not considered to be serious problems. Others, such as the neural tube defects, usually have more severe consequences. Although some cases of congenital malformations occur in the absence of any other problems, it is quite common for them to be associated with other disorders. For example, hydrocephaly and clubfoot are often seen secondary to spina bifida, CL/P is often seen in babies with trisomy 13, and congenital heart defects are seen in children with many other disorders, including Down syndrome.

TABLE 5-4 PREVALENCE RATES OF COMMON CONGENITAL MALFORMATIONS IN WHITES

DISORDER	PREVALENCE PER 1000 BIRTHS (APPROXIMATE)
Cleft lip/palate	1
Clubfoot	1
Congenital heart defects	4-8
Hydrocephaly	0.5-2.5
Isolated cleft palate	0.4
Neural tube defects	1-3
Pyloric stenosis	3

Environmental factors also cause some congenital malformations. An example is thalidomide, a sedative used during pregnancy in the early 1960s. When ingested during early pregnancy this drug often caused **phocomelia** (severely shortened limbs) in babies. Maternal exposure to retinoic acid, which is used to treat acne, can cause congenital defects of the heart, ear, and central nervous system. Maternal rubella infection can cause congenital heart defects.

Multifactorial Disorders in the Adult Population

Until quite recently, very little was known about specific genes responsible for common adult diseases. With the more powerful laboratory and analytic techniques now available, this situation is changing. This section reviews recent progress in understanding the genetics of the major common adult diseases. Table 5-5 gives approximate prevalence figures for these disorders in the United States.

Coronary Heart Disease

It is well-known that coronary heart disease (CHD) is the leading killer of Americans, accounting for approximately 25% of all deaths in the United States. It is caused by *atherosclerosis* (narrowing as a result of the formation of lipid-laden lesions) of the coronary arteries. This narrowing impedes blood flow to the heart and can eventually result in a *myocardial infarction* (destruction of heart tissue caused by an inadequate supply of oxygen). When atherosclerosis occurs in arteries supplying blood to the brain, a *stroke* can result. Many risk factors for heart disease have been identified, including obesity, cigarette smoking, hypertension, elevated cholesterol level, and positive family history (usually defined as having one affected first-degree relative). Many studies have examined the role of family history in CHD, and they show that an individual with a positive family history is two to seven times more likely to have heart disease than is an individual with no family history (this would be the relative risk of heart disease as a result of a positive

TABLE 5-5 PREVALENCE OF COMMON ADULT DISEASES IN THE UNITED STATES

DISEASE	NUMBER AFFECTED (APPROXIMATE)
Alcoholism	14 million
Alzheimer disease	4 million
Arthritis	43 million
Asthma	17 million
Cancer	8 million
Cardiovascular disease (all forms)	
Coronary artery disease	13 million
Congestive heart failure	5 million
Congenital defects	1 million
Hypertension	50 million
Stroke	5 million
Depression and bipolar disorder	17 million
Diabetes (type 1)	1 million
Diabetes (type 2)	15 million
Epilepsy	2.5 million
Multiple sclerosis	350,000
Obesity*	60 million
Parkinson disease	500,000
Psoriasis	3-5 million
Schizophrenia	2 million

Data from National Center for Chronic Disease Prevention and Health Promotion; American Heart Association (2002 Heart and Stroke Statistical Update); National Institute on Alcohol Abuse and Alcoholism; Office of the U.S. Surgeon General; American Academy of Allergy, Asthma and Immunology; Cown WM, Kandel ER: *JAMA* 285:594–600, 2001; Flegal et al: *JAMA* 288:1723–1727, 2002.
*Body mass index >30.

family history). Generally, these studies also show that the risk increases if (1) there are more affected relatives; (2) the affected relative or relatives are female (the less commonly affected sex) rather than male; and (3) the age of onset in the affected relative is early (before 55 years). For example, one study showed that men between the ages of 20 and 39 years had a relative risk of 3 for CHD if they had one affected first-degree relative. The relative risk increased to 13 if two first-degree relatives were affected with CHD before 55 years of age.[11]

What part do genes play in the familial clustering of heart disease? Because of the key role of lipids in atherosclerosis, many studies are focusing on the genetic determination of various lipoproteins.[12] An important advance in this area has been the isolation and cloning of the gene for the low-density lipoprotein (LDL)–receptor defects that cause *familial hypercholesterolemia* (Box 5-3). Many other genes involved in lipid variation, coagulation, and hypertension have been identified, including several genes encoding apolipoproteins (the protein components of lipoproteins) (Table 5-6).[13] Functional analysis of these genes is leading to an increased understanding, and eventually more effective treatment, of CHD.

Environmental factors, many of which are easily modified, are also important causes of CHD. Abundant epidemiologic evidence shows that cigarette smoking and obesity increase the risk of CHD, whereas exercise and a diet low in saturated fats decrease the risk. Indeed, the approximate 50% decline in CHD prevalence in the United States during the past 40 years is usually attributed to a decrease in the proportion of adults who smoke cigarettes, a decreased consumption of saturated fats, and an increased emphasis on exercise and a generally healthier lifestyle.

Hypertension

Systemic hypertension, which has a worldwide prevalence of approximately 25% to 30%, is a key risk factor for heart disease, stroke, and kidney disease. Studies of blood pressure correlations within families indicate that about 20% to 40% of the variation in both systolic and diastolic blood pressure is caused by genetic factors. The fact that this figure is substantially less than 100% indicates that environmental factors also must be important causes of blood pressure variation. The most important environmental risk factors for hypertension are increased sodium intake, decreased physical activity, psychosocial stress, and obesity (but, as discussed later, the latter factor is itself influenced by both genes and environment).

Blood pressure regulation is a highly complex process that is influenced by many physiologic systems, including various aspects of kidney function, cellular ion transport, and heart function.[14] Because of this complexity, much research is now focused on specific components that may influence blood pressure variation, such as the renin-angiotensin system (involved in sodium reabsorption and vasoconstriction), vasodilators such as nitric oxide and the kallikrein-kinin system, and ion-transport systems such as adducin and sodium-lithium countertransport (Figure 5-7). These individual factors are more likely to be under the control of smaller numbers of genes than is blood pressure itself, simplifying the task of identifying these genes and their role in blood pressure regulation. For example, linkage and association studies have implicated several genes involved in the renin-angiotensin system (e.g., the genes that encode angiotensinogen, angiotensin-converting enzyme, type 1 and angiotensin II type 1 receptor) in the causation of hypertension.

Cancer

Cancer is the second leading cause of death in the United States. It is well established that many major types of cancer (e.g., breast, colon, prostate, ovarian) cluster strongly in families. This is caused by both shared genes and shared environmental factors. Although numerous cancer genes are being isolated,[15] environmental factors also play an important role in causing cancer. In particular, tobacco use is estimated to account for one third of all cancer cases in the United States, making it the most important known cause of cancer.[16]

Breast Cancer. Breast cancer is the most common cancer among women, affecting approximately 12% of American women who live to 85 years or more. Formerly the leading cause of cancer death among women, it has been surpassed by lung cancer. Breast cancer aggregates strongly in families. If a woman has one affected first-degree relative, her risk of developing breast cancer doubles. This risk increases if the age of onset in

BOX 5-3 FAMILIAL HYPERCHOLESTEROLEMIA

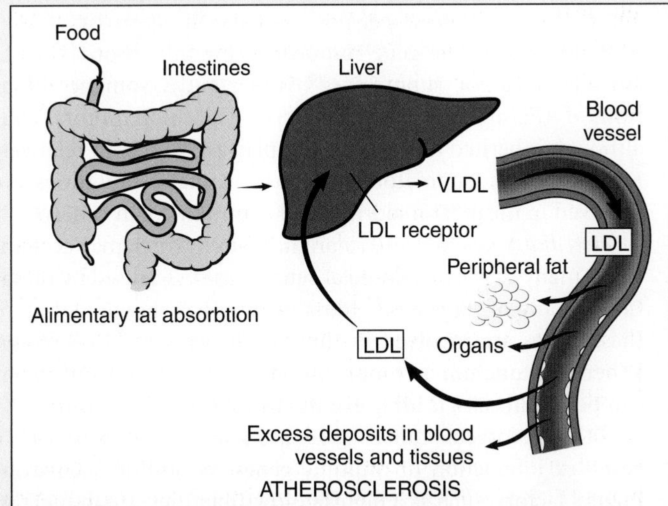

Autosomal dominant familial hypercholesterolemia (FH) is an important cause of heart disease, accounting for approximately 5% of myocardial infarctions in individuals less than 60 years of age.[9] FH is one of the most common autosomal dominant disorders: in most populations surveyed to date, about 1 in 500 people is a heterozygote. Plasma cholesterol levels are approximately twice as high as normal (i.e., about 300 to 400 mg/dl), resulting in substantially accelerated atherosclerosis and distinctive cholesterol deposits in skin and tendons (*xanthomas* [see Figure 5-5]). Data compiled from five studies showed that approximately 75% of men with FH developed coronary disease and 50% had a fatal myocardial infarction by 60 years. The corresponding percentages for women were lower (45% and 15%) because women generally develop heart disease at a later age than men.

Consistent with Hardy-Weinberg predictions, about 1 in 1 million births is homozygous for the FH gene. Homozygotes are much more severely affected, with cholesterol levels ranging from 600 to 1200 mg/dl. Most experience myocardial infarctions before 20 years of age, and a myocardial infarction at 18 months of age has been reported. If untreated, most FH homozygotes die before 30 years of age.

All cells require cholesterol as a component of their plasma membrane. They can either synthesize their own cholesterol or, preferably, obtain it from the extracellular environment, where it is carried primarily by low-density lipoprotein (LDL). In a process known as *endocytosis,* LDL-bound cholesterol is taken into the cell via LDL receptors on the cell's surface (see Figure 5-6). FH is most commonly caused by a reduction in the number of functional LDL receptors on cell surfaces. Lacking the normal number of LDL receptors, cellular cholesterol uptake is reduced and circulating cholesterol levels increase.

Much of what we know about endocytosis has been learned through the study of LDL receptors. The process of endocytosis and the processing of LDL in the cell are described in detail in Figure 5-6 (endocytosis is discussed in Chapter 1). These processes result in a fine-tuned regulation of cholesterol levels within cells, and they influence the level of circulating cholesterol as well.

The identification of the LDL receptor gene in 1984 was critical in understanding exactly how LDL receptor defects cause FH. More than 1000 different mutations, including missense and nonsense substitutions as well as insertions and deletions, have been identified in the LDL receptor gene. These can be grouped into five broad classes according to their effects on the activity of the receptor.[10] Class 1 mutations result in no detectable protein product. Thus heterozygotes would produce only half the normal number of LDL receptors. Class 2 mutations in the LDL receptor gene result in production of the LDL receptor, but it is altered such that it cannot leave the endoplasmic reticulum. It is eventually degraded. Class 3 mutations produce an LDL receptor that is capable of migrating to the cell surface but incapable of normal binding to LDL. Class 4 mutations, which are comparatively rare, produce receptors that are normal except that they do not migrate specifically to coated pits and thus cannot carry LDL into the cell. The final group of mutations, class 5, produces an LDL receptor that cannot dissociate from the LDL particle after entry into the cell. The receptor cannot return to the cell surface and is degraded. Each class of mutations reduces the number of effective LDL receptors, resulting in decreased LDL uptake and hence elevated levels of circulating cholesterol. The number of effective receptors is reduced by about half in FH heterozygotes, and homozygotes have virtually no functional LDL receptors.

Understanding the defects that lead to FH has helped to develop effective therapies for the disorder. Dietary reduction of cholesterol (primarily through the reduced intake of saturated fats) has only modest effects on cholesterol levels in FH heterozygotes. Because cholesterol is reabsorbed into the gut and then recycled through the liver (where most cholesterol synthesis takes place), serum cholesterol levels can be reduced by the administration of bile acid–absorbing resins, such as cholestyramine. The absorbed cholesterol is then excreted. It is interesting that reduced recirculation from the gut causes the liver cells to form additional LDL receptors, lowering circulating cholesterol levels. However, the decrease in the concentration of intracellular cholesterol also stimulates cholesterol synthesis by liver cells, so the overall reduction in plasma LDL level is only about 15% to 20%. This treatment is much more effective when combined with agents that reduce cholesterol synthesis by inhibiting 3-hydroxy-3-methylglutaryl coenzyme A (HMG-CoA) reductase (the "statin" class of drugs). Decreased synthesis leads to further production of LDL receptors. When these therapies are used in combination, serum cholesterol levels in FH heterozygotes can be reduced to approximately normal levels.

The picture is less encouraging for FH homozygotes. The therapies just discussed can enhance cholesterol elimination and reduce its synthesis, but they are largely ineffective because homozygotes have few or no LDL receptors. Liver transplants, which provide hepatocytes that have normal LDL receptors, have been successful in some cases, but this option is often limited by a lack of donors. Plasma exchange, carried out every 1 to 2 weeks, in combination with drug therapy, can reduce cholesterol levels by about 50%. However, this therapy is difficult to continue for long periods. Somatic cell gene therapy, in which hepatocytes carrying normal LDL receptor genes are introduced into the portal circulation, is now being tested. It may eventually prove to be an effective treatment for FH homozygotes.

The FH story illustrates how medical research has made important contributions both to our understanding of basic cell biology and to advances in clinical therapy. The process of receptor-mediated endocytosis, elucidated largely by research on the LDL receptor defects, is of fundamental significance for cellular processes throughout the body. Equally important is that this research, by clarifying how cholesterol synthesis and uptake can be modified, has led to significant improvements in therapy for this important cause of heart disease.

Illustration from Damjanov I: *Pathology for the health professions,* ed 4, Philadelphia, 2012, Saunders.

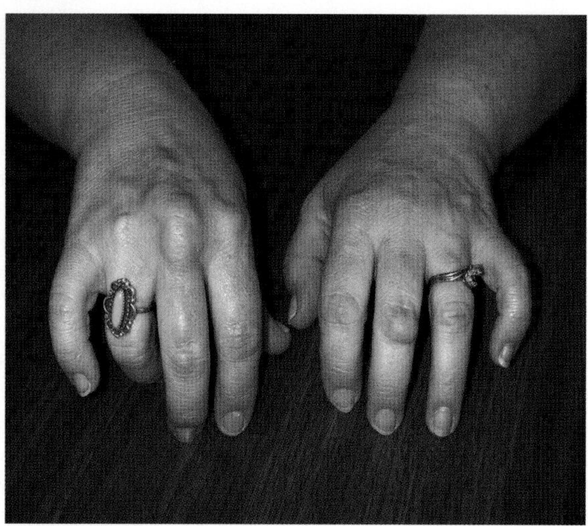

FIGURE 5-5 **Xanthoma.** Fatty deposits, referred to as xanthomas as seen here on the knuckles, are often noted in individuals with familial hypercholesterolemia. (From Jorde LB et al: *Medical genetics,* ed 4, St Louis, 2010, Mosby.)

the affected relative is early and if the cancer is bilateral (tumors in both breasts).

An autosomal dominant form of breast cancer accounts for approximately 5% of breast cancer cases in the United States. Genes responsible for this form of breast cancer have been mapped to chromosomes 17 *(BRCA1)* and 13 *(BRCA2).* It is possible to test each of these genes for inherited cancer-causing mutations.[17] Women who inherit a mutation in *BRCA1* or *BRCA2* experience a 50% to 80% lifetime risk of developing breast cancer. *BRCA1* mutations also increase the risk of ovarian cancer among women (20% to 50% lifetime risk), and they confer a modestly increased risk of prostate and colon cancers. *BRCA2* mutations also confer an increased risk of ovarian cancer (10% to 20% lifetime prevalence). Approximately 6% of males who inherit a *BRCA2* mutation will develop breast cancer; this represents a 100-fold increase over the risk in the general male population. The evaluation of the *BRCA1* and *BRCA2* gene products, which are both involved in deoxyribonucleic acid (DNA) repair, is yielding valuable evidence on the etiology of breast cancer in general.

Although *BRCA1* and *BRCA2* mutations are the most common known causes of inherited breast cancer, this disease also can be caused by inherited mutations in several other tumor-suppressor genes (e.g., the *CHK2* and *TP53* genes). Germline mutations in a tumor-suppressor gene called *PTEN* are responsible for Cowden disease, which is characterized by multiple benign tumors and an increased susceptibility to breast cancer.

Colorectal Cancer. Colorectal cancer is second only to lung cancer in the number of cases occurring annually in the United States, with approximately 143,000 new cases (and 52,000 deaths) estimated in 2012.[18] Approximately 1 in 20 Americans will develop colorectal cancer. Like breast cancer, it clusters in families (in fact, familial clustering of this form of cancer was reported in the medical literature as early as 1881). The risk of colorectal cancer in people with one affected first-degree relative is two to three times higher than that in the general population.

This familial aggregation is caused in part by subsets of colorectal cancer cases that are inherited as single-gene traits. *Familial adenomatous polyposis* occurs in approximately 1 in 8000 whites. The gene responsible for this disorder, *APC,* encodes a tumor suppressor.[19] Importantly, somatic mutations of *APC* are found in at least 85% of all colon tumors. Thus although inherited *APC* mutations play a vital role in relatively rare familial adenomatous polyposis, somatic mutations are involved in the great majority of all common colon cancers.

Hereditary nonpolyposis colorectal cancer, which may account for as many as 5% of colorectal cancer cases, is caused by mutations in any of six genes.[20] Identification has shown that all of these genes are involved in the vital process of DNA repair. When this function is compromised, cancer-causing mutations can persist in cells, leading eventually to growth of a tumor.

Other colorectal cancer cases are likely to be caused by a complex interaction of multiple genes. In addition, environmental factors, such as a high-fat, low-fiber diet, are thought to increase the risk of colorectal cancer.

Other Cancers. The genetic basis of various other cancers, including retinoblastoma, has been discussed. Although each of these cancers is relatively rare, study of the causative genes has provided many important insights into the nature of carcinogenesis in general. This will lead to more effective treatment and prevention of all cancers.

Diabetes Mellitus

Like the other disorders discussed in this chapter, the etiology of diabetes mellitus is complex and not fully understood. Nevertheless, progress is being made in understanding the genetic basis of this disorder, which is a leading cause of blindness, heart disease, and kidney failure.[21,22] An important advance has been the recognition that diabetes is actually a heterogeneous group of disorders, all characterized by elevated blood glucose level. The focus here is on the two major types of diabetes: type 1 (insulin-dependent diabetes mellitus [IDDM]) and type 2 (non–insulin-dependent diabetes mellitus [NIDDM]).

Type 1 Diabetes. Type 1 diabetes, which is characterized by T-cell infiltration of the pancreas and destruction of the insulin-producing beta cells, usually (though not always) presents before age 40. Individuals with type 1 diabetes must receive exogenous insulin to survive. In addition to T-cell infiltration of the pancreas, autoantibodies are formed against pancreatic cells; the latter can be observed long before clinical symptoms occur. These findings, along with a strong association between type 1 diabetes and the presence of several human leukocyte antigen (HLA) class II alleles, indicate that this is an autoimmune disease.

Siblings of individuals with type 1 diabetes face a substantial elevation in risk: approximately 6%, as opposed to a risk of about 0.3% to 0.5% in the general population. The recurrence risk is also elevated when there is a diabetic parent, although this risk varies with the sex of the affected parent. The risk for offspring of diabetic mothers is only 1% to 3%, whereas it is 4% to 6% for the offspring of diabetic fathers (because type 1 diabetes affects males and females in roughly equal proportions in the general population, this risk difference is inconsistent

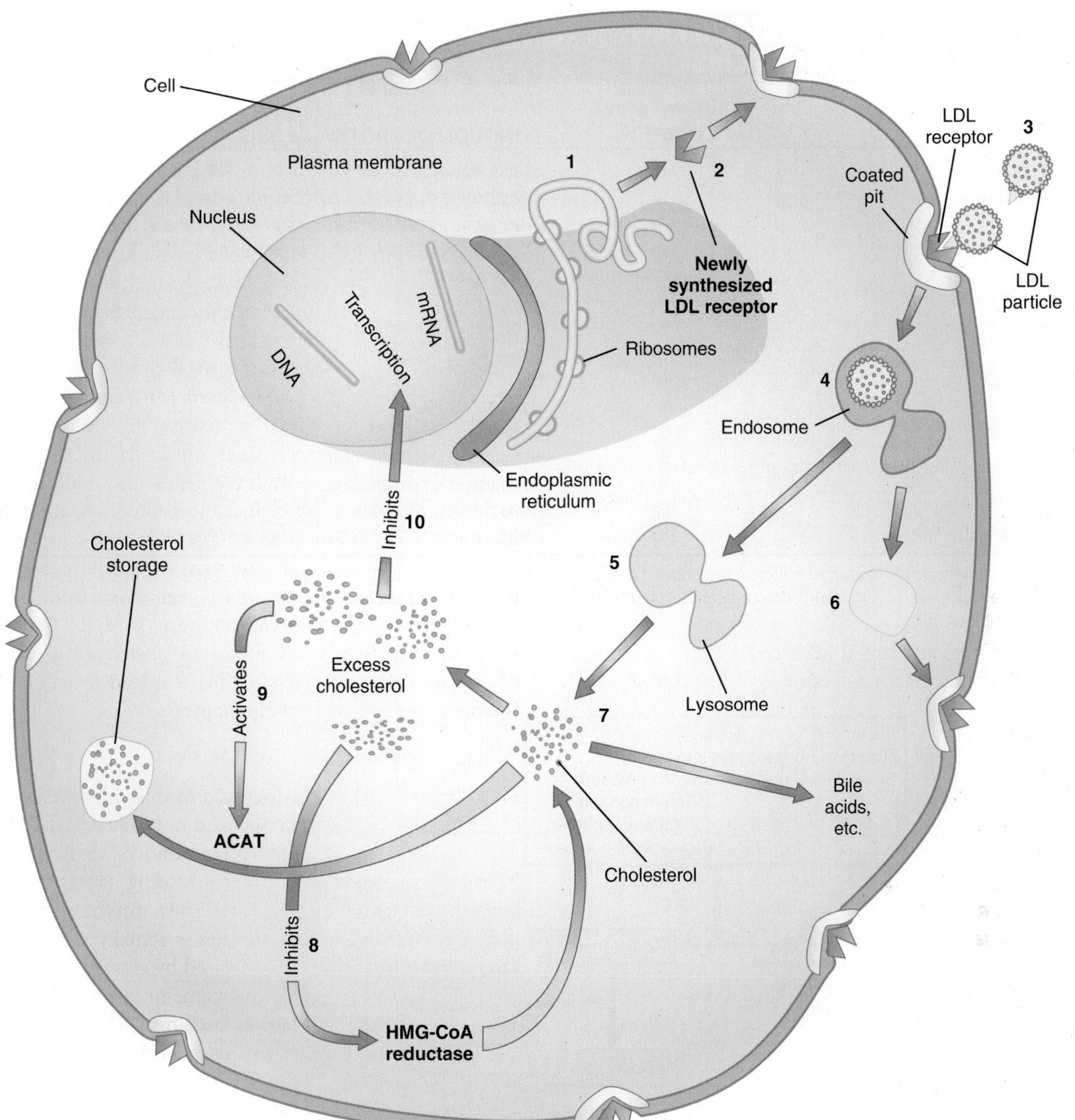

FIGURE 5-6 **Process of Receptor-Mediated Endocytosis.** Numbers in parentheses correspond to numbers shown in the figure. **(1)** The low-density lipoprotein (LDL) receptors, which are glycoproteins, are synthesized in the endoplasmic reticulum of the cell. **(2)** From here, they pass through the Golgi apparatus to the cell surface, where part of the receptor protrudes outside the cell. **(3)** The circulating LDL particle is bound by the LDL receptor and localized in cell surface depressions called *coated pits* (so named because they are coated with a protein called clathrin). **(4)** The coated pit invaginates, bringing the LDL particle inside the cell. **(5)** Once inside the cell, the LDL particle is separated from the receptor, taken into a lysosome, and broken down into its constituents by lysosomal enzymes. **(6)** The LDL receptor is recirculated to the cell surface to bind another LDL particle (each LDL receptor goes through this cycle approximately once every 10 minutes even if it is not occupied by an LDL particle). **(7)** Free cholesterol is released from the lysosome for incorporation into cell membranes or metabolism into bile acids or steroids. Excess cholesterol can be stored in the cell as a cholesterol ester or removed from the cell by associating with high-density lipoprotein (HDL). **(8)** As cholesterol levels in the cell rise, cellular cholesterol synthesis is reduced by inhibition of the rate-limiting enzyme HMG-CoA (3-hydroxy-3-methylglutaryl coenzyme A) reductase. **(9)** Rising cholesterol levels also increase the activity of acyl coenzyme A (acyl CoA): cholesterol acyltransferase (ACAT), an enzyme that modifies cholesterol for storage as cholesterol esters. **(10)** In addition, the number of LDL receptors is decreased by lowering the transcription rate of the LDL receptor gene itself. This decreases cholesterol uptake. (From Jorde LB et al: *Medical genetics,* ed 4, St Louis, 2010, Mosby.)

TABLE 5-6 LIPOPROTEIN GENES KNOWN TO CONTRIBUTE TO CORONARY ARTERY DISEASE RISK

GENE	CHROMOSOME LOCATION	FUNCTION OF PROTEIN PRODUCT
Apolipoprotein A-I	11q	HDL component; LCAT cofactor
Apolipoprotein A-IV	11q	Component of chylomicrons and HDL; may influence HDL metabolism
Apolipoprotein C-III	11q	Allelic variation associated with hypertriglyceridemia
Apolipoprotein B	2p	Ligand for LDL receptor; involved in formation of VLDL, LDL, IDL, and chylomicrons
Apolipoprotein D	2p	HDL component
Apolipoprotein C-I	19q	LCAT activation
Apolipoprotein C-II	19q	Lipoprotein lipase activation
Apolipoprotein E	19q	Ligand for LDL receptor
Apolipoprotein A-II	1p	HDL component
LDL receptor	19p	Uptake of circulating LDL particles
Lipoprotein (a)	6q	Cholesterol transport
Lipoprotein lipase	8p	Hydrolysis of lipoprotein lipids
Hepatic triglyceride lipase	15q	Hydrolysis of lipoprotein lipids
LCAT	16q	Cholesterol esterification
Cholesterol ester transfer protein	16q	Facilitates transfer of cholesterol esters and phospholipids between lipoproteins

Adapted in part from King RA, Rotter JI, editors: *The genetic basis of common diseases*, ed 2, New York, 2002, Oxford University Press.
HDL, High-density lipoprotein; IDL, intermediate-density lipoprotein; *LCAT,* lecithin cholesterol acyltransferase; *LDL,* low-density lipoprotein; *VLDL,* very-low-density lipoprotein.

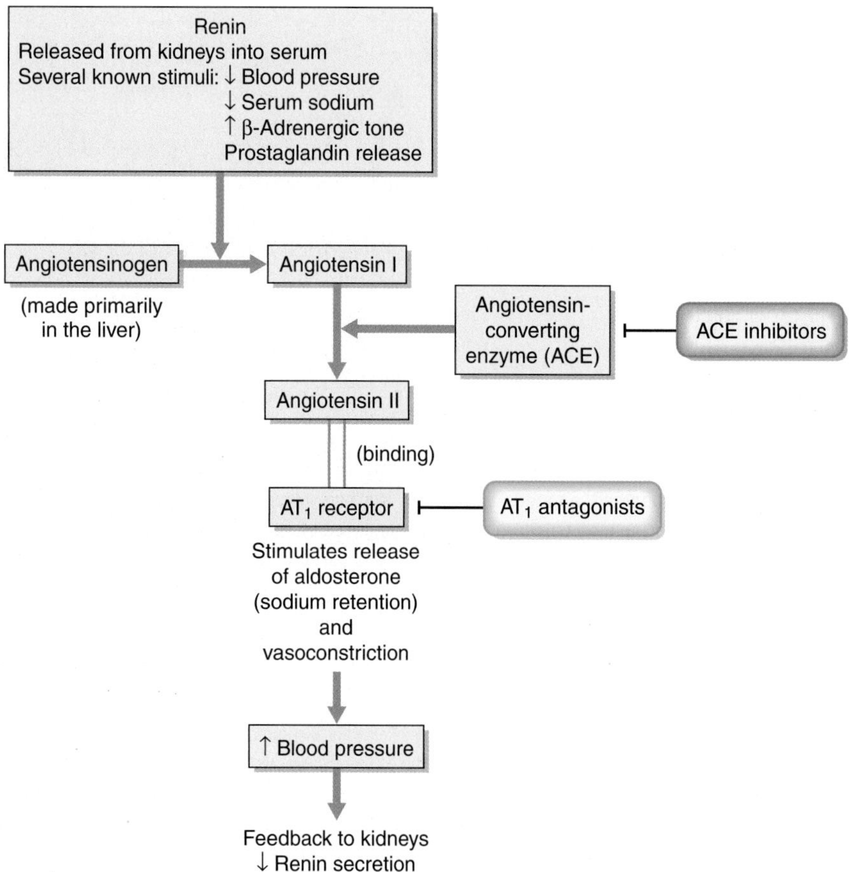

FIGURE 5-7 **Renin-Angiotensin-Aldosterone System.** (Modified from King RA, Rotter JI, Motulsky AG (eds): The genetic basis of common diseases, New York, Oxford University Press, 1992. In Jorde LB et al: *Medical genetics,* ed 4, St. Louis, 2010, Mosby.)

with the sex-specific threshold model for multifactorial traits). Twin studies show that the empirical risks for identical twins of people with type 1 diabetes range from 30% to 50%. In contrast, the concordance rates for dizygotic twins are 5% to 10%. The fact that type 1 diabetes is not 100% concordant among identical twins indicates that genetic factors are not solely responsible for the disorder. There is good evidence that specific viral infections contribute to the causation of type 1 diabetes in at least some individuals, possibly by activating an autoimmune response.

The association of specific HLA class II alleles (see Chapter 22) and type 1 diabetes has been studied extensively, and it is estimated that the HLA system accounts for about 40% of the familial clustering of type 1 diabetes. Approximately 95% of whites with type 1 diabetes have the HLA DR3 and/or DR4 alleles, whereas only about 50% of the general white population has either of these alleles. If an affected proband and a sibling are heterozygous for the DR3 and DR4 alleles, the sibling's risk of developing type 1 diabetes is nearly 20% (i.e., about 40 times higher than the risk in the general population). In addition, the presence of aspartic acid at position 57 of the DQ chain is strongly associated with resistance to type 1 diabetes. In fact, those who do not have this amino acid at position 57 (and instead are homozygous for a different amino acid) are 100 times more likely to develop type 1 diabetes. The aspartic acid substitution alters the shape of the HLA class II molecule and thus its ability to bind and present peptides to T cells. Altered T-cell recognition may help protect individuals with the aspartic acid substitution from an autoimmune episode.

The insulin gene, which is located on the short arm of chromosome 11, is another logical candidate for type 1 diabetes susceptibility. Polymorphisms within and near this gene have been tested for association with type 1 diabetes. It is estimated that inherited genetic variation in the insulin region accounts for approximately 10% of the familial clustering of type 1 diabetes.

Within the past several years, additional genes have been shown to be associated with susceptibility to type 1 diabetes. The most significant of these are cytotoxic lymphocyte associated-4 *(CTLA4)*, which encodes a protein involved in the regulation of T-cell proliferation, and *PTPN22*, which encodes a lymphoid-specific tyrosine phosphatase that negatively regulates T-cell activation. It is interesting that variation in the latter gene has been associated with several other autoimmune diseases, including systemic lupus erythematosus (SLE), rheumatoid arthritis, and autoimmune thyroid disease.

Type 2 Diabetes. Type 2 diabetes accounts for more than 90% of all diabetes cases and affects 10% to 20% of the adult populations of many developed countries. A number of features distinguish it from type 1 diabetes. There is nearly always some endogenous insulin production in people with type 2 diabetes, and the disease can often be treated successfully with dietary modification and/or oral drugs. People with type 2 diabetes suffer from insulin resistance (i.e., their cells have difficulty in using insulin). This disease typically occurs among people older than age 40 and, in contrast to type 1 diabetes, is seen more commonly among the obese. The incidence of type 2 diabetes is rising dramatically among adolescents and young adults in developed countries, however, and is strongly correlated with an increased incidence of obesity. Neither HLA associations nor autoantibodies are seen commonly in this form of diabetes. Monozygotic twin concordance rates are substantially higher than those seen in type 1 diabetes, often exceeding 90% (because of age dependence, the concordance rate increases if older subjects are studied). The empirical recurrence risks for first-degree relatives of type 2 diabetes cases are higher than those for type 1, generally ranging from 15% to 40%. The differences between type 1 and type 2 diabetes are summarized in Table 5-7.

TABLE 5-7 COMPARISON OF MAJOR FEATURES OF TYPES 1 AND 2 DIABETES

FEATURE	TYPE 1 DIABETES	TYPE 2 DIABETES
Age of onset	Usually <40 yr	Usually >40 yr (except maturity-onset diabetes of the young [MODY])
Insulin production	None	Partial
Insulin resistance	No	Yes
Autoimmunity	Yes	No
Obesity	Not common	Common
Monozygotic (MZ) twin concordance	0.55	0.90
Sibling recurrence risk	1-6%	10-15%

Hundreds of studies have been undertaken to identify genes that may contribute to type 2 diabetes susceptibility. The most significant gene identified thus far is *TCF7L2*, which encodes a transcription factor involved in the secretion of insulin. A variant of *TCF7L2* is associated with a 50% increased risk of developing type 2 diabetes. A significant association has also been observed between type 2 diabetes and a common allele of the gene that encodes peroxisome proliferator–activated receptor-gamma (PPAR-γ), a transcription factor that is involved in adipocyte differentiation and glucose metabolism. Although this allele confers only a 25% increase in the risk of developing type 2 diabetes, it is found in more than 75% of individuals of European descent and thus helps to account for a significant proportion of type 2 diabetes cases. Variation in *KCNJ11*, which encodes a potassium channel necessary for glucose-stimulated insulin secretion, confers an additional 20% increase in type 2 diabetes susceptibility. The associations between diabetes susceptibility and each of these genes have been widely replicated in multiple populations.

The two most important risk factors for type 2 diabetes are positive family history and obesity; the latter increases insulin resistance. The disease tends to rise in prevalence when populations adopt a diet and exercise pattern typical of U.S. and European populations. Increases have been seen, for example, among Japanese immigrants to the United States and among some native populations of the South Pacific, Australia, and the Americas. Several studies, conducted on male and female subjects, have shown that regular exercise can substantially lower one's risk of developing type 2 diabetes, even among individuals with a family history of the disease. This is partly because exercise reduces obesity. However, even in the absence of weight loss, exercise increases insulin sensitivity and improves glucose tolerance.

Because of the dramatic increase in obesity in the United States and other developed countries, the prevalence of type 2 diabetes is also rising rapidly, and the average age of onset is decreasing. A small proportion of type 2 diabetes cases occurs early in life, typically before 25 years of age, and typically exhibits autosomal dominant inheritance (unlike most type 2 diabetes cases). This subset is termed *maturity-onset diabetes of the young* (MODY). Studies of MODY pedigrees have shown that about half of cases of the disease are caused by mutations in the glucokinase gene. Glucokinase converts glucose to glucose-6-phosphate in the pancreas. In addition to the glucokinase gene, five other genes, all of which are involved in pancreatic development or regulation of insulin levels, have now been shown to be causes of MODY.

Obesity

Obesity is most commonly defined as a body mass index (BMI) greater than 30.* Using this criterion, approximately one third of American adults are obese, and an additional one third are overweight (BMI greater than 25 but less than 30). The proportion of obese adults and children continues to increase rapidly. Although obesity itself is not a "disease," it is an important risk factor for several common diseases, including heart disease, stroke, hypertension, and type 2 diabetes.

As one might expect, there is a strong correlation between obesity in parents and their children. This could easily be ascribed to common environmental effects: parents and children usually share similar dietary and exercise habits. However, there is good evidence for genetic components as well. Four adoption studies each showed that the body weights of adopted individuals correlated significantly with their natural parents' body weights but not with those of their adoptive parents. Twin studies also provide evidence for a genetic effect on body weight, with most studies yielding heritability estimates between 0.60 and 0.80.

Research, aided substantially by mouse models, has shown that several genes each play a role in human obesity. Important among these are the genes that encode leptin (Greek, "thin") and its receptor. The leptin hormone is secreted by adipocytes (fat storage cells) and binds to receptors in the hypothalamus, the site of the body's appetite control center. Cloning of the human leptin gene and its receptor led to optimistic predictions that leptin could be a key to weight loss in humans (without the perceived unpleasantness of dieting and exercise). Although mutations in the human leptin gene and its receptor have been identified in a few humans with severe obesity (BMI >40), they both appear to be extremely rare. Clinical trials using recombinant leptin have demonstrated moderate weight loss in a subset of obese individuals. In addition, leptin participates in important interactions with other components of appetite control, such as neuropeptide Y and α-melanocyte-stimulating hormone and its receptor, the melanocortin-4 receptor (MC4R). Mutations in the gene that encodes MC4R have been found in 3% to 5% of severely obese individuals. Recently, homozygosity for a DNA variant in the *FTO* gene (which is seen in 16% of whites) has been associated with 40% and 70% increases in the risks of overweight and obesity, respectively. Identification of these human genes is leading to a better understanding of natural weight control in the human, and it could eventually lead to effective treatments for some cases of obesity.

*BMI is defined as W/H^2, in which W is weight in kilograms and H is height in meters.

Alzheimer Disease

Alzheimer disease (AD), which is responsible for 60% to 70% of cases of progressive cognitive impairment among older adults, affects approximately 5% to 10% of the population older than 65 years of age and 40% of the population older than 85 years of age. Because of the aging of the population, the number of Americans with AD is predicted to increase substantially during the coming decade. AD is characterized by progressive dementia and memory loss and by the formation of amyloid plaques and neurofibrillary tangles in the brain, particularly in the cerebral cortex and hippocampus. The plaques and tangles lead to progressive neuronal loss, and death usually occurs within 7 to 10 years after the first appearance of symptoms.

The risk of developing AD doubles in individuals who have an affected first-degree relative. Although most cases do not appear to be caused by single loci, approximately 10% follow an autosomal dominant mode of transmission. About 3% to 5% of AD cases occur before age 65 and are considered early onset; these are much more likely to be inherited in autosomal dominant fashion.[23]

AD is a genetically heterogeneous disorder. Approximately half of early-onset cases can be attributed to mutations in any of three genes, all of which affect amyloid-β deposition.[24] Two of the genes, presenilin 1 *(PS1)* and presenilin 2 *(PS2)*, are very similar to one another, and their protein products are involved in cleavage of the amyloid-β precursor protein (APP). When APP is not cleaved normally, a long form of it accumulates excessively and is deposited in the brain. This is thought to be a primary cause of AD. Mutations in *PS1* typically result in especially early onset of AD, with the first occurrence of symptoms in the fifth decade of life.

A small number of cases of early-onset AD are caused by mutations of the gene that encodes APP itself, which is located on chromosome 21. These mutations disrupt normal cleavage sites in APP, again leading to the accumulation of the longer protein product. It is interesting that this gene is present in three copies in trisomy 21 individuals, in which the extra gene copy leads to amyloid deposition and the occurrence of AD in those with Down syndrome (see Chapter 4).

An important risk factor for the more common late-onset form of AD is allelic variation in the apolipoprotein E *(APOE)* locus, which has three major alleles: *ε2, ε3,* and *ε4.* Studies conducted in diverse populations have shown that persons who have one copy of the $\varepsilon 4$ allele are at least 2 to 5 times more likely to develop AD, whereas those with two copies of this allele are at least 5 to 10 times more likely to develop AD. The risk varies somewhat by population, with higher $\varepsilon 4$-associated risks in Europeans and Japanese and relatively lower risks in Hispanics and blacks. Despite the strong association between $\varepsilon 4$ and AD, approximately half of individuals who develop late-onset AD do not have a copy of the $\varepsilon 4$ allele, and many who are homozygous for $\varepsilon 4$ remain free of AD even at advanced age. The apolipoprotein E protein product is not involved in cleavage of APP but instead appears to be associated with clearance of amyloid from the brain.

Alcoholism

At some point, alcoholism is diagnosed in approximately 10% of adult males and 3% to 5% of adult females in the United States. The national cost of alcoholism, in terms of lost productivity and direct medical costs, is approximately $200 billion per year. More than 100 studies have shown that this disease clusters in families.[25] The risk of developing alcoholism among individuals with one affected parent is three to five times higher than for those with unaffected parents.

Most twin studies have yielded concordance rates for DZ twins less than 30% and concordance rates for MZ twins in excess of 60%. Adoption studies have shown that the offspring of an alcoholic parent, even when raised by nonalcoholic parents, have a fourfold increased risk of developing the disorder. To control for possible prenatal effects in an alcoholic mother, some studies have included only the offspring of alcoholic fathers. The results have remained the same. One study showed that the offspring of nonalcoholic parents, when reared by alcoholics, did *not* have an increased risk of developing alcoholism. These data argue that there may be genes that predispose some people to alcoholism.

It has long been known that an individual's physiologic response to alcohol can be influenced by variation in the key enzymes responsible for alcohol metabolism: alcohol dehydrogenases (ADHs), which convert ethanol to acetaldehyde; and aldehyde dehydrogenases (ALDHs), which convert acetaldehyde to acetate. In particular, an allele of the *ALDH2* gene *(ALDH2*2)* results in excessive accumulation of acetaldehyde and thus in facial flushing, nausea, palpitations, and lightheadedness. Because of these unpleasant effects, individuals who have the *ALDH2*2* allele are much less likely to become alcoholics. This "protective" allele is common in some Asian populations but is rare in other populations.

A number of other genes are associated with susceptibility to alcohol addiction, including genes that encode components of gamma-aminobutyric acid (GABA) receptors. This finding is biologically plausible, because the GABA neurotransmitter system inhibits excitatory signals in neurons, exerting a calming effect. Alcohol has been shown to increase GABA release, and allelic variation in GABA receptor genes may modulate this effect.

It should be underscored that genes may increase one's *susceptibility* to alcoholism. Obviously this is a disease that requires an environmental component, regardless of genetic constitution.

TABLE 5-8 RECURRENCE RISKS FOR RELATIVES OF SCHIZOPHRENIC PROBANDS

RELATIONSHIP TO PROBAND	RECURRENCE RISK (%)
Monozygotic twin	44.3
Dizygotic twin	12.1
Offspring	9.4
Sibling	7.3
Niece/nephew	2.7
Grandchild	2.8
First cousin	1.6
Spouse	1

Data from McGue M, Gottesman II, Rao DC: *Behav Genet* 16(1):75–87, 1986.
Figures are based on multiple studies of Western European populations.

Psychiatric Disorders

The major psychiatric diseases, schizophrenia and affective disorder, have been the subjects of numerous genetic studies.[26] Twin, adoption, and family studies have shown that both disorders aggregate in families.

Schizophrenia. *Schizophrenia* is a severe emotional disorder characterized by delusions, hallucinations, retreat from reality, and bizarre, withdrawn, or inappropriate behavior. (Contrary to popular belief, schizophrenia is not a "split personality" disorder.) The lifetime recurrence risk for schizophrenia among the offspring of one affected parent is approximately 8% to 10%, which is about 10 times higher than the risk in the general population.[27] As one might expect, the empirical risks increase when more relatives are affected. For example, an individual with an affected sibling and an affected parent has a risk of about 17%, and an individual with two affected parents has a risk of 46%. The risks decrease when the affected family member is a second- or third-degree relative. Details are given in Table 5-8. On inspection of Table 5-8, it may seem puzzling that the proportion of schizophrenic probands who have a schizophrenic parent is only about 5%, which is substantially lower than the risk for other first-degree relatives (e.g., siblings, affected parents and their offspring). This can be explained by the fact that people with schizophrenia are less likely to marry and produce children than are other individuals. Thus substantial selection against schizophrenia occurs in the population.

Twin and adoption studies also indicate that genetic factors are likely to be involved in schizophrenia. Data pooled from five different twin studies show a 47% concordance rate for MZ twins, compared with a concordance rate of only 12% for DZ twins. When the offspring of a schizophrenic parent are adopted by normal parents, their risk of developing the disease is about 10%, which is approximately the same as the risk when raised by a schizophrenic biologic parent. Recent studies have identified promising associations between schizophrenia and several brain-expressed genes whose products interact with glutamate receptors. These include dysbindin (*DTNBP1;* chromosome 6p), neuregulin 1 (*NRG1;* chromosome 8p), and D-amino acid oxidase activator (*G30;* chromosome 13q). Another susceptibility gene is *DISC1* (Disrupted-in-Schizophrenia-1), which was originally identified by its consistent translocation in affected members of a large schizophrenia pedigree. Each of these associations has been replicated in multiple populations. However, the precise mechanisms through which mutations in these genes contribute to schizophrenia susceptibility are not yet known.

Bipolar Disorder. *Bipolar disorder,* also known as *manic-depressive disorder,* is a form of psychosis with extreme mood swings and emotional instability. The incidence of the disorder in the general population is approximately 0.5%, but it rises to 5% to 10% among those with an affected first-degree relative. A study using the Danish twin registry yielded concordance rates of 79% and 24% for MZ and DZ twins, respectively.[28] The corresponding concordance rates for unipolar disorder (major depression) were 54% and 19%. In general, it appears that bipolar disorder is more strongly influenced by genetic factors than is unipolar disorder.

As with schizophrenia, many large-scale studies have been undertaken to identify genes associated with susceptibility to bipolar disorder. Some of these loci were identified because their products are involved in neurotransmitter systems that are targets of drugs used to treat the disease (e.g., the serotonin, dopamine, and noradrenaline systems). Examples of these genes include those that encode monoamine oxidase A (MAOA), the serotonin transporter (5HTT), and catechol-*O*-methyltransferase (COMT), a gene that has also been associated with schizophrenia susceptibility. In addition, the *NRG1* and *DISC1* genes, which were discussed previously because of their association with schizophrenia, have been shown in some studies to be associated with susceptibility to bipolar disorder.

Comments on Psychiatric Disorders. Large-scale linkage studies involving hundreds of polymorphisms throughout the genome have been carried out for both schizophrenia and bipolar affective disorder. Most of these studies have produced negative results, although a few recent large-scale studies have yielded promising findings. A number of candidate genes have been tested for linkage or association with both diseases. Most of these candidates were chosen on the basis of the known involvement of certain neurotransmitters, receptors, or neurotransmitter-related enzymes in each disease (e.g., schizophrenia can be treated by drugs that block dopamine receptors, and bipolar affective disorder is sometimes treated with lithium). None of the candidate genes tested thus far, including those for sodium-lithium countertransport, various components of the dopaminergic system, and several neurotransmitter-related enzymes (e.g., monoamine oxidase, dopamine-β-hydroxylase, tyrosine hydroxylase), have been shown unequivocally to be linked or associated with either disease.

These results reflect some of the difficulties encountered in conducting genetic studies of psychiatric disorders. These disorders are undoubtedly heterogeneous, reflecting the influence of numerous genetic and environmental factors. Also, definition of the phenotype is not always straightforward and it may change through time, significantly complicating genetic analysis.

Other Complex Disorders

The disorders discussed in this chapter represent some of the most common multifactorial disorders and those for which significant progress has been made in identifying genes. Many other multifactorial disorders are being studied as well, and in some cases specific susceptibility genes have been identified. These include, for example, Parkinson disease, hearing loss, multiple sclerosis, amyotrophic lateral sclerosis, epilepsy, asthma, inflammatory bowel disease, and some forms of blindness.

Some General Principles and Conclusions

Some general principles can be deduced from the results obtained thus far on the genetics of complex disorders. First, the more strongly inherited forms of complex disorders generally have an earlier age of onset (e.g., breast cancer, AD, heart disease). Often these represent subsets of cases in which there is single-gene inheritance. Second, when laterality is a component, the bilateral forms are more likely to cluster strongly in families (e.g., breast cancer, CL/P). Third, although the sex-specific threshold model fits some of the complex disorders (e.g., pyloric stenosis, CL/P, autism, heart disease), it fails to fit others (e.g., type 1 diabetes).

A tendency exists, particularly among the lay public, to assume that the presence of a genetic component means that the course of a disease cannot be altered. *This is incorrect.* Most of the diseases discussed in this chapter have both genetic and environmental components. Thus lifestyle modification (e.g., diet, exercise, stress reduction) often can reduce risk significantly. Such modification may be especially important for individuals with a family history of a disease because they are likely to develop the disease earlier in life. Those with a family history of heart disease, for example, can often add many years of productive living with relatively minor lifestyle alterations. By targeting those who can benefit most from intervention, genetics helps to serve the goal of preventive medicine.

In addition, it should be stressed that the identification of a specific genetic lesion can lead to more effective prevention and treatment of the disease. Identification of mutations that cause autosomal dominant breast cancer may enable early screening and prevention of metastasis. Pinpointing a gene responsible for a neurotransmitter defect in a behavioral disorder such as schizophrenia could lead to the development of more effective drug treatments. In some cases, such as those with familial hypercholesterolemia, gene therapy may prove to be useful in treating the disease. It is important for healthcare practitioners to help individuals understand these facts.

Although the genetics of common disorders is complex and often confusing, the community health effect of these diseases, together with the evidence for hereditary factors in their etiology, demands that genetic studies be pursued. Substantial progress is already being made. The next decade will undoubtedly witness many further advances in the understanding and treatment of these disorders.

SUMMARY REVIEW

Factors Influencing Incidence of Disease in Populations

1. The incidence rate is the number of new cases of a disease reported during a specific period (typically 1 year) divided by the number of individuals in the population.
2. The prevalence rate is the proportion of the population affected by a disease at a specific point in time. This rate, and the incidence rate, can be used to compare population variations in disease frequency.
3. Relative risk is a common measure of the effect of a specific risk factor. It is expressed as a ratio of the incidence rate of the disease among individuals exposed to a risk factor divided by the incidence of the disease among individuals *not* exposed to a risk factor.
4. Many factors can influence the risk of acquiring a common disease, such as cancer, diabetes, or hypertension. The factors can include age, gender, diet, exercise, and family history of the disease.

Principles of Multifactorial Inheritance

1. Traits in which variation is thought to be caused by the combined effects of multiple genes are polygenic.
2. The term *multifactorial* is used when environmental factors also are believed to cause variation in the trait.
3. Many quantitative traits (e.g., blood pressure) are multifactorial.
4. Because traits are caused by the additive effects of many genetic and environmental factors, they tend to follow a normal or bell-shaped distribution in populations.
5. Those diseases, however, that do not follow a bell-shaped distribution appear to be either present or absent in individuals. They do not follow the inheritance patterns of single-gene disease. Instead, such diseases may follow an underlying liability distribution. It is thought that a threshold of liability must be crossed before the disease is expressed.
6. Examples of diseases that correspond to the liability model include pyloric stenosis, neural tube defects, CL/P, and some forms of congenital heart disease.
7. Many of the common adult diseases, such as hypertension, coronary heart disease, stroke, diabetes mellitus (types 1 and 2), and some cancers, are caused by complex genetic and environmental factors and are thus multifactorial diseases.
8. For most multifactorial diseases, empirical risks (risks based on direct observation of data) have been derived.
9. In contrast to most single-gene diseases, recurrence risks for multifactorial diseases can change significantly from one population to another because gene frequencies, as well as environmental factors, can differ among populations.
10. Several criteria are used to define multifactorial inheritance: (a) the recurrence risk becomes higher if more than one family member is affected; (b) if the expression of the disease in a proband is more severe, the recurrence risk is higher; (c) the recurrence risk is higher if the proband is of the less commonly affected sex; (d) the recurrence risk for the disease usually decreases rapidly in more remotely related relatives; and (e) if the prevalence of the disease in a population is f, the risk for offspring and siblings of probands is approximately $\sqrt{f}$.

Nature and Nurture: Disentangling the Effects of Genes and Environment

1. Family members share genes and a common environment; therefore, resemblance in traits, such as high blood pressure, reflects both genetic and environmental factors (nature and nurture, respectively).
2. Few traits are influenced *only* by genes or *only* by environment. Most are influenced by both.
3. When a disease has a relatively larger genetic component, as in breast cancer, examination of family history should be emphasized in addition to lifestyle modification.
4. Two research strategies often are used to estimate the relative influence of genes and environment-lifestyle: twin studies and adoption studies.
5. Monozygotic twins originate when the developing embryo divides to form two separate but identical embryos.
6. Dizygotic twins are the result of a double ovulation followed by the fertilization of each egg by a different sperm.
7. If both members of a twin pair share a trait, they are said to be *concordant.* If they do not share the same trait, they are *discordant.*
8. Studies of adopted children also are used to estimate the genetic contribution to a multifactorial trait.
9. A genetic predisposition may interact with an environmental-lifestyle factor to increase the risk of disease; this is called a *gene-environment interaction.*

Genetics of Common Diseases

1. Congenital diseases are those present at birth. Most of these diseases are multifactorial in etiology.
2. Multifactorial diseases in adults include coronary heart disease, hypertension, breast cancer, colon cancer, diabetes mellitus, obesity, AD, alcoholism, schizophrenia, and bipolar affective disorder.
3. It is incorrect to assume that the presence of a genetic component means that the course of a disease cannot be altered—most diseases have *both* genetic and environmental aspects.

KEY TERMS

Concordant trait, 169
Congenital disease, 171
Discordant trait, 169
Dizygotic (DZ, fraternal) twin, 169
Empirical risk, 167
Gene-environment interaction, 171
Incidence rate, 164
Liability distribution, 166
Monozygotic (MZ, identical) twin, 169
Multifactorial trait, 165
Phocomelia, 171
Polygenic, 165
Prevalence rate, 164
Quantitative trait, 165
Relative risk, 165
Threshold of liability, 166

REFERENCES

1. King RA, Rotter JI, Motulsky AG: *The genetic basis of common diseases*, ed 2, Oxford, 2002, Oxford University Press.
2. Rothman KJ: *Modern epidemiology*, New York, 1998, Lippincott.
3. Tiwari HK et al: Multifactorial inheritance and complex diseases. In Rimoin DL, et al, editor: *Emery and Rimoin's principles and practice of medical genetics*, ed 5, Philadelphia, 2007, Churchill Livingstone, pp 299–306.
4. Greene ND et al: Genetics of human neural tube defects, *Hum Mol Genet* 18(R2):R113–R129, 2009.
5. Daly LE et al: Folate levels and neural tube defects: implications for prevention, *JAMA* 274(21):1698–1702, 1995.
6. Harper PS: *Practical genetic counseling*, ed 7, London, 2010, Hodder Arnold.
7. Boomsma D, Busjahn A, Peltonen L: Classical twin studies and beyond, *Nat Rev Genet* 3(11):872–882, 2002.
8. Kaprio J, Silventoinen K: Advanced methods in twin studies, *Methods Mol Biol* 713:143–152, 2011.
9. Marks D et al: A review on the diagnosis, natural history, and treatment of familial hypercholesterolaemia, *Atherosclerosis* 168(1):1–14, 2003.
10. Varret MM et al: Genetic heterogeneity of autosomal dominant hypercholesterolemia, *Clin Genet* 73(1):1–13, 2008.
11. Hunt SC, Williams RR, Barlow GK: A comparison of positive family history definitions for defining risk of future disease, *J Chronic Dis* 39(10):809–821, 1986.
12. Libby P et al: Progress and challenges in translating the biology of atherosclerosis, *Nature* 473(7347):317–325, 2011.
13. O'Donnell CJ, Nabel EG: Genomics of cardiovascular disease, *N Engl J Med* 365(22):2098–2109, 2011.
14. Jeunemaitre X et al: Molecular basis of human hypertension. In Rimoin DL, et al, editor: *Emery and Rimoin's principles and practice of medical genetics*, ed 5, Philadelphia, 2007, Churchill Livingstone, pp 1283–1300.
15. Vogelstein B, Kinzler KW: *The genetic basis of human cancer*, ed 2, New York, 2002, McGraw-Hill.
16. Peto J: Cancer epidemiology in the last century and the next decade, *Nature* 411(6835):390–395, 2001.
17. Robson M, Offit K: Management of an inherited predisposition to breast cancer, *N Engl J Med* 357(2):154–162, 2007.
18. National Cancer Institute: www.cancer.gov/cancertopics/types/colon-and-rectal.
19. Galiatsatos P, Foulkes WD: Familial adenomatous polyposis, *Am J Gastroenterol* 101(2):385–398, 2006.
20. Markowitz SD, Bertagnolli MM: Molecular basis of colorectal cancer, *N Engl J Med* 361(25):2449–2460, 2009.
21. Feero WG et al: Genomics, type 2 diabetes, and obesity, *N Engl J Med* 363(24):2339–2350, 2010.
22. Concannon P et al: Genetics of type 1 diabetes, *N Engl J Med* 360(16):1646–1654, 2009.
23. Bertram L et al: The genetics of Alzheimer disease: back to the future, *Neuron* 68(2):270–281, 2010.
24. Blennow K, de Leon MJ, Zetterberg H: Alzheimer's disease, *Lancet* 368(9533):387–403, 2006.
25. Gelernter J, Kranzler HR: Genetics of alcohol dependence, *Hum Genet* 126(1):91–99, 2009.
26. Burmeister M et al: Psychiatric genetics: progress amid controversy, *Nat Rev Genet* 9(7):527–540, 2008.
27. Gejman PV et al: Genetics of schizophrenia: new findings and challenges, *Annu Rev Genom Hum Genet* 12(1):121–144, 2011.
28. Bertelsen A, Harvald B, Hauge MA: Danish twin study of manic-depressive disorders, *Br J Psychiatry* 130:330–351, 1977.

CHAPTER

6

Epigenetics and Disease

Lynn B. Jorde

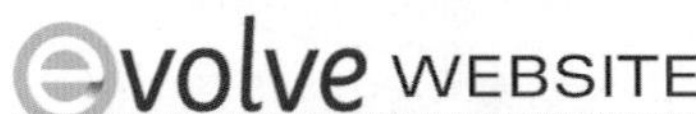

http://evolve.elsevier.com/McCance/

- Review Questions and Answers

CHAPTER OUTLINE

The traditional focus of human genetics has been on the ways in which alterations of DNA sequences can lead to disease (Chapter 4). In some cases, diseases and other phenotypic variation are caused by mechanisms *other* than changes in the DNA sequences—termed epigenetics ("upon genetics").[1] **Epigenetics** is the study of heritable changes in gene expression or phenotype caused by mechanisms other than changes in DNA sequences. Epigenetic modifications can cause individuals with the same DNA sequences (such as identical twins) to have different disease profiles. There are three major types of epigenetic modifications (Figure 6-1):

1. **DNA methylation:** The attachment of a methyl group to a cytosine base is followed by a guanine base (a "CpG dinucleotide") (Figures 6-1 and 6-2).[2] DNA methylation causes a gene to become transcriptionally inactive or silent.[3] When the DNA sequence in the promoter region of a gene becomes heavily methylated, the DNA is less likely to be transcribed into mRNA. Methylation along with histone hypoacetylation (the acetyl group consists of a methyl group single-bonded to a carbonyl) and condensation of chromatin together inhibit the binding of transcription-binding factors (see Chapter 4) that regulate transcription. In other words, the gene becomes transcriptionally inactive. Aberrant methylation can lead to silencing of tumor-suppressor genes in the development of cancer (see Chapter 12 and Figure 6-1). DNA methylation is a key component of X-inactivation, the transcriptional silencing of genes on the X chromosome, discussed in Chapter 4. As with X-inactivation, epigenetic modifications are maintained in successive mitotic cell divisions, but most are erased from the genome when new gametes (sperm or egg cells) are formed.
2. **Histone modification** (e.g., histone acetylation and deacetylation, alterations in chromatin): Chromatin compaction and organization help to regulate gene expression, determining and maintaining cell identity. Chromatin structure must

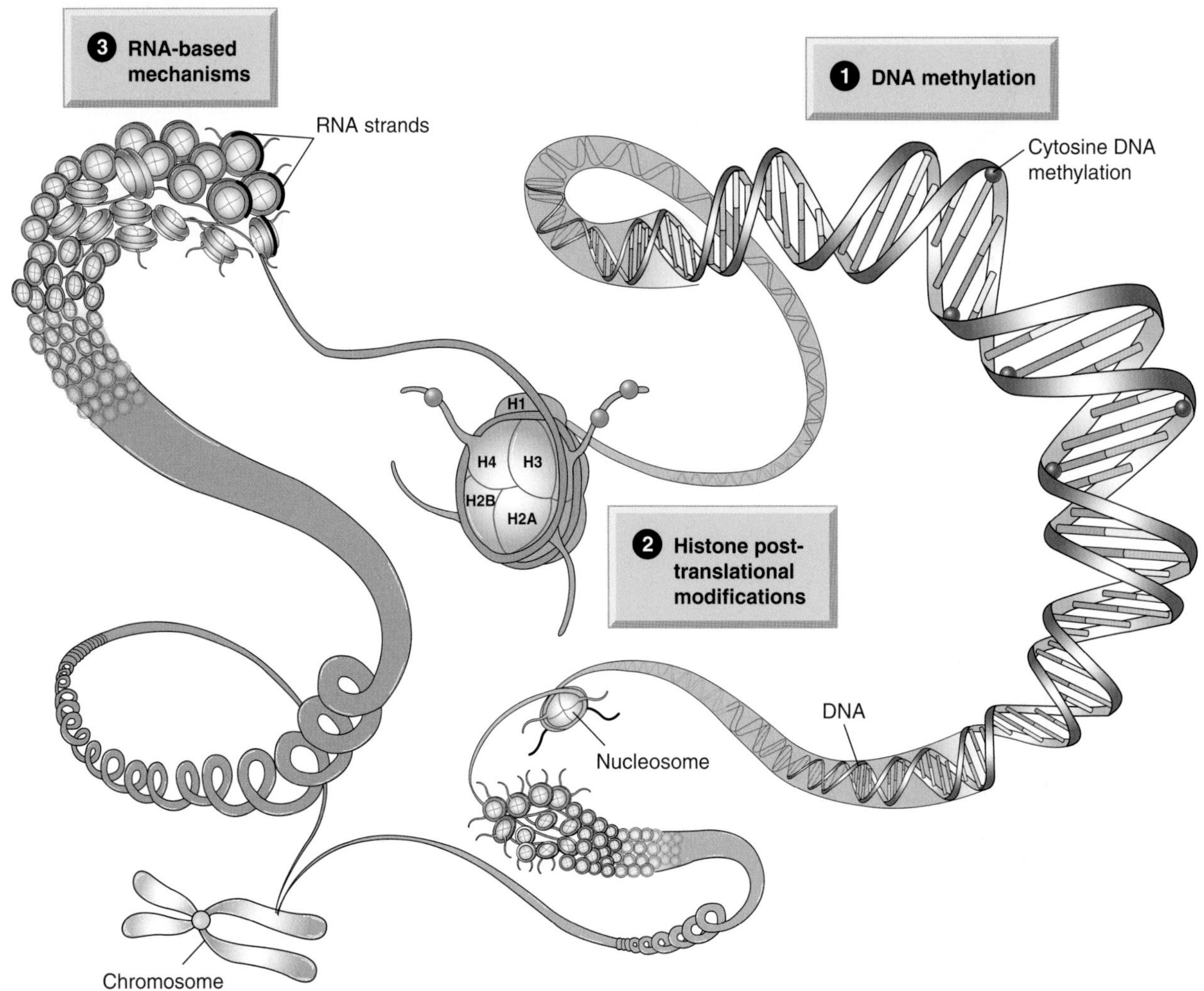

FIGURE 6-1 Three Major Types of Epigenetic Processes. Investigators are studying the following epigenetic mechanisms: **(1)** DNA methylation, **(2)** histone modifications, and **(3)** RNA based-mechanisms. See text for discussion.

be controlled in self-renewing and differentiated cells in cell renewal systems. For example, there are differences in chromatin structure in stem cells and terminally differentiated cells.[4]

3. **Micro-ribonucleic acids (miRNAs or miRs):** These RNAs are encoded by short DNA sequences (approximately 22 nucleotides) located in introns of genes or transcribed from noncoding DNA located between genes. Gene expression networks can be regulated by changes in miRNAs and other noncoding RNAs. **Noncoding RNAs (ncRNAs)** have been shown to regulate gene expression by novel mechanisms such as RNA interference, gene cosuppression, gene silencing, imprinting (see p. 187), and DNA demethylation. It is becoming clear that these novel RNAs perform critical functions during development and cell differentiation. MicroRNAs regulate diverse signaling pathways, and those that stimulate cancer development and progression are called **oncomirs.** For example, miRNAs have been linked to carcinogenesis because they can act as either oncogenes or tumor-suppressor genes (see Chapter 12).

EPIGENETICS AND DEVELOPMENT

Early in embryonic development, all cells of the embryo have the potential to become any type of cell in the fetus or adult. These **embryonic stem cells** are said to be pluripotent. A key event in early embryogenesis is the differential epigenetic modification (including extensive methylation) of specific DNA nucleotide sequences in these cells. This modification helps to determine the fate of each cell (i.e., the type of cell it becomes, such as a myocyte, neuron, or fibroblast) by helping to ensure that specific genes are expressed only in the cells and tissue types in which their gene products are needed (e.g., factor VIII expression primarily in hepatocytes, or dopamine receptor expression in neurons). Thus, even though nearly all cells have the same DNA sequence, the transcriptional activity of most genes varies substantially and depends on cell and tissue type. A small percentage of genes, termed **housekeeping genes,** are necessary for the function and maintenance of all cells. These genes escape the methylation process and remain transcriptionally active in all cells.

Much remains to be learned about factors that cause epigenetic modifications. Findings so far indicate that specific

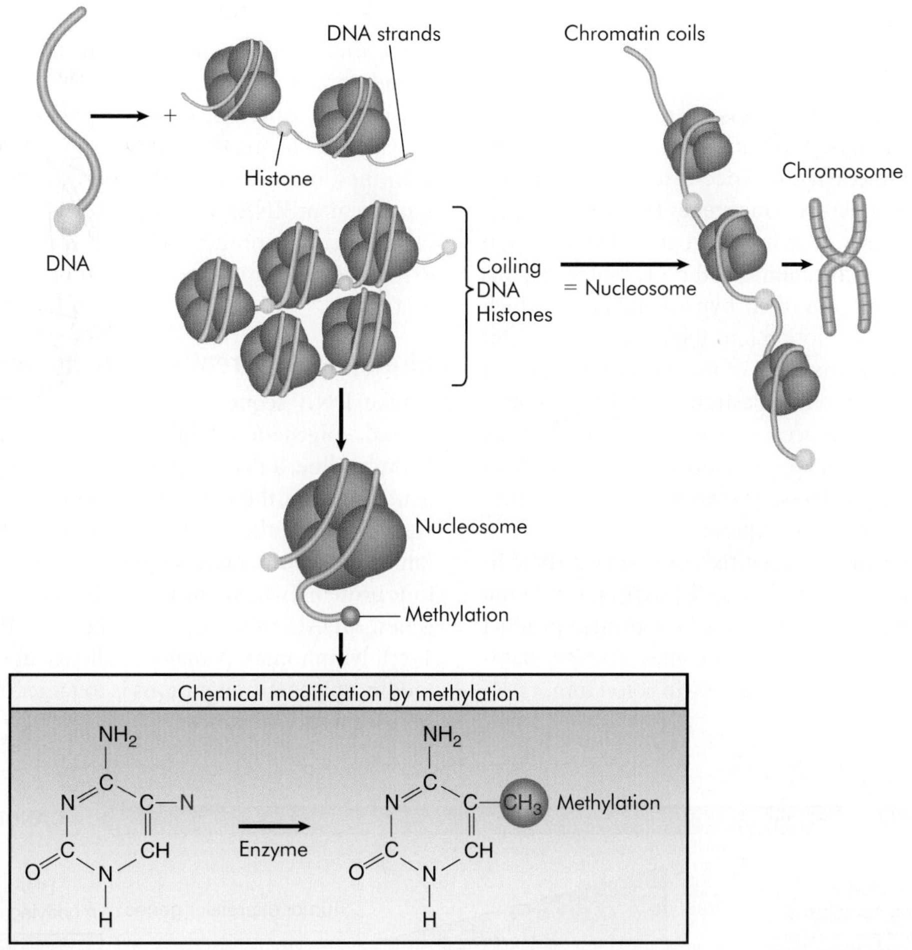

FIGURE 6-2 Epigenetic Modifications. Because DNA is a long molecule, it needs packaging to fit in the tiny nucleus. Packaging involves *coiling* of the DNA in a "left-handed" spiral around spools, made of four pairs of proteins individually known as histones and collectively as the histone octamer. The entire spool is called a nucleosome (also see Figure 1-2). Nucleosomes are organized into chromatin, the repeating building blocks of a chromosome. Histone modifications are correlated with methylation, are reversible, and occur at multiple sites. Methylation occurs at the 5 position of cytosine and provides a "footprint" or signature as a unique epigenetic alteration *(red).* When genes are expressed, chromatin is open or active; however, when chromatin is condensed because of methylation and histone modification, genes are inactivated.

environmental or nongenetic factors, such as diet and exposure to certain chemicals, can drive such modifications. For example, alcohol has been shown to affect methylation patterns in animal models,[5] so the harmful effects of fetal alcohol exposure may be mediated through epigenetic mechanisms. Maternal dietary deficiency during pregnancy may cause epigenetic modifications of fetal genes, leading to an increased risk of obesity and diabetes in the offspring later in life.[6] In some animal models, the insulin-like growth factor 2 gene *(IGF2)* is a target of these epigenetic modifications. Although the observed changes in methylation status of CpG sequences in these genes are typically small, it is possible that they affect phenotypic development. The hereditary transmission of epigenetic changes to successive generations has been termed **epigenetic transgenerational inheritance.** If demonstrated to occur in humans, transgenerational inheritance could have important implications for disease and disease prevention.

Twin Studies Provide Insights on Epigenetic Modification

A powerful means to test for epigenetic effects is to compare methylation and other signatures of epigenetic modification in identical (monozygotic) twin pairs, whose DNA sequences are essentially the same. As twins age, they demonstrate increasing differences in methylation patterns of the DNA sequences of their somatic cells; these changes are reflected in increasing numbers of phenotypic differences.[7] Twins with significant lifestyle differences (e.g., smoking vs. nonsmoking) accumulated larger numbers of differences in their methylation patterns. The twins, despite having identical DNA sequences, become more and more different as a result of epigenetic changes, which in turn affect the expression of genes. These results, along with findings generated in animal studies, suggest that changes in epigenetic patterns may be an important part of the aging process.[8]

EPIGENETICS AND CANCER

DNA Methylation and Cancer

The best evidence for epigenetic effects on disease risk comes from studies of human cancer (Figure 6-3).[9,10] Tumor cells typically exhibit hypomethylation (decreased methylation), which can increase the activity of oncogenes (see Chapter 12). Hypomethylation increases as tumors progress from benign neoplasms to malignancy. In addition, the promoter regions of tumor-suppressor genes are often hypermethylated, which decreases their rate of transcription and their ability to inhibit tumor formation. Hypermethylation of the promoter region of the *RB1* gene is often seen in retinoblastoma,[11] and hypermethylation of the *BRCA1* gene is seen in some cases of inherited breast cancer.[12] Similarly, von Hippel-Lindau disease, in which renal cell carcinomas frequently occur, can be caused by hypermethylation of the *VHL* promoter region.

A major cause of one form of inherited colon cancer (hereditary nonpolyposis colorectal cancer [HNPCC]) is the methylation of the promoter region of a gene, *MLH1*, whose protein product repairs damaged DNA. When *MLH1* becomes inactive, damaged DNA accumulates, eventually resulting in colon tumors[13,14] (see Figure 41-28).

miRNAs and Cancer

Hypermethylation also is seen in miRNA genes, which encode small (22 base pair) RNA molecules that bind to the ends of mRNAs, degrading them and preventing their translation. More than 1000 miRNA sequences have been identified in humans, and hypermethylation of specific subgroups of miRNAs is associated with tumorigenesis. When miRNA genes are methylated, their mRNA targets are over-expressed, and this over-expression has been associated with metastasis.[9]

Strategies for Treating Epigenetic Disease

Unlike DNA sequence mutations, which cannot be directly altered, epigenetic modifications can be reversed. For example, 5-azacytidine, a demethylating agent, has been used as a therapeutic drug in the treatment of leukemia and myelodysplastic syndrome. Another class of drugs, histone deacetylase (HDAC) inhibitors, counteracts the removal of acetyl groups from histone proteins, which can silence the activity of tumor-suppressor genes. HDAC inhibitors have been used in the treatment of T-cell lymphomas. A major challenge in developing drugs that modify epigenetic alterations is to target only the genes responsible for a specific cancer.

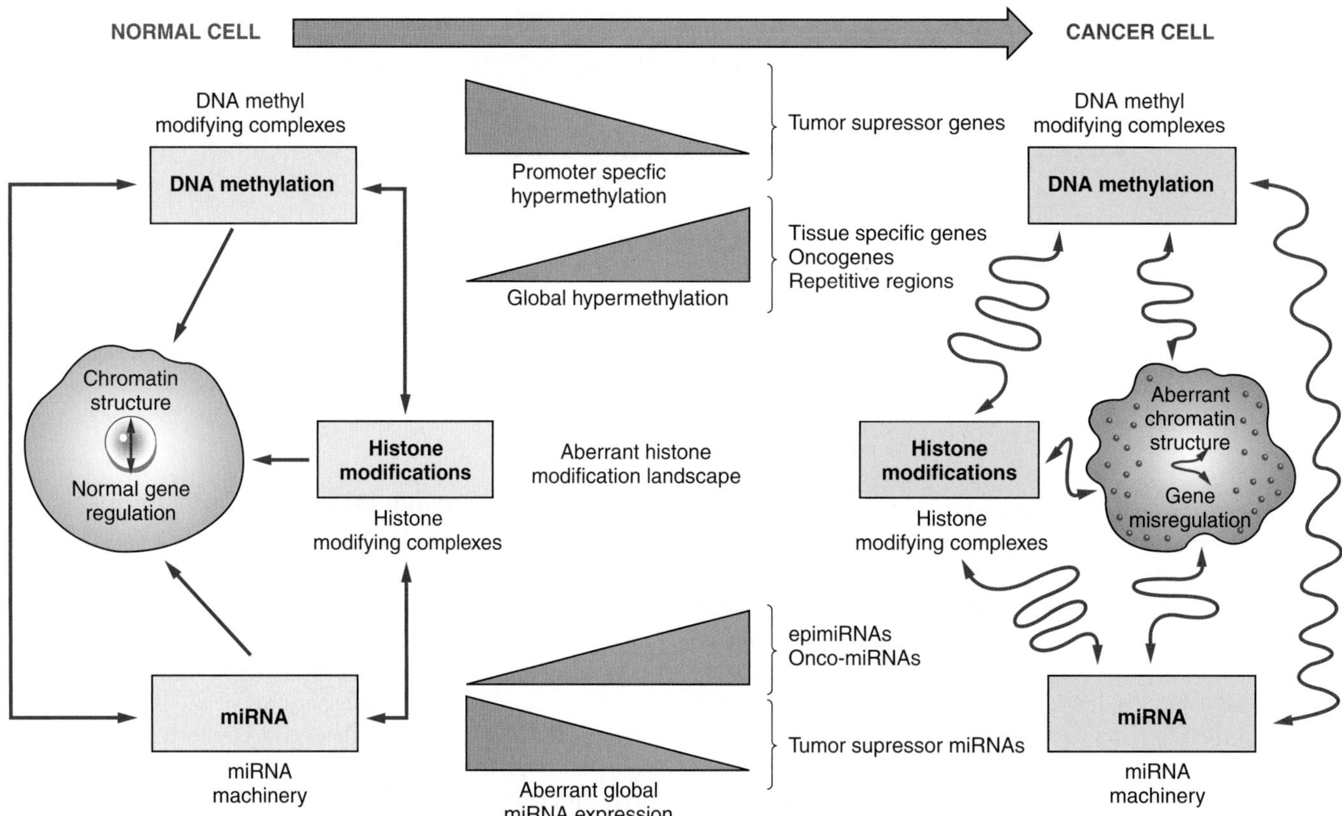

FIGURE 6-3 **Global Epigenomic Alterations and Cancer.** Oncogenesis involves accumulated genetic alterations combined with the epigenetic changes: DNA methylation, histone modifications, and miRNAs. In cancer cells, tumor-suppressor genes become hypermethylated and with histone modifications cause abnormal gene silencing. The gene silencing of tumor-suppressor genes results in tumor progression. Global hypomethylation leads to chromosomal instability and fragility. Additionally, these modifications create abnormal mRNA and miRNA expression, which leads to activation of oncogenes and silencing of tumor-suppressor genes. (Adapted from Sandoval J, Esteller M: *Curr Opin Genet Dev* 22:50–55, 2012.)

GENOMIC IMPRINTING

Gregor Mendel's nineteenth century experiments with garden peas indicated that the phenotype is typically the same whether a given allele is inherited from the mother or the father. It is now clear that this principle, which has long been part of the central dogma of genetics, does not always hold. For some human genes, the gene is transcriptionally active on only one copy of a chromosome (e.g., the copy inherited from the father). On the other copy of the chromosome (in this example, the one inherited from the mother), the gene is transcriptionally inactive. This process of gene silencing, in which genes are predictably silenced depending on which parent transmits them, is known as *imprinting,* and the transcriptionally silenced genes are then said to be "imprinted." Approximately 100 human genes are thought to be imprinted. Imprinted genes are usually heavily methylated (in contrast to the nonimprinted copy of the allele, which is typically not methylated). Next we describe some important human diseases that can be caused by abnormal imprinting patterns.

Prader-Willi and Angelman Syndromes

A well-known disease example of imprinting is associated with a deletion of about 4 million base pairs (Mb) of the long arm of chromosome 15. When this deletion is inherited from the father, the child manifests **Prader-Willi syndrome,** whose features include short stature, hypotonia, small hands and feet, obesity, mild to moderate mental retardation, and hypogonadism (Figure 6-4, *A*).[15] The same 4-Mb deletion, when inherited from the mother, causes **Angelman syndrome,** which is characterized by severe mental retardation, seizures, and an ataxic gait (Figure 6-4, *B*).[16] These diseases are each seen in about 1 of every 15,000 live births, and chromosome deletions are responsible for about 70% of cases of both diseases. The deletions that cause Prader-Willi and Angelman syndromes are indistinguishable at the DNA sequence level and affect the same group of genes.

For several decades, it was unclear how the same deletion could produce such disparate results in different persons. Further analysis showed that the 4-Mb deletion (the *critical region*) contains several genes that are normally transcribed only on the copy of chromosome 15 that is inherited from the father.[17] These genes are transcriptionally inactive (imprinted) on the copy of chromosome 15 inherited from the mother. Similarly, other genes in the critical region are transcriptionally active only on the chromosome copy inherited from the mother and are inactive on the chromosome inherited from the father. Thus, several genes in this region are normally active on only one chromosome copy (Figure 6-5). If the single active copy of one of these genes is lost because of a chromosome deletion, then no gene product is produced at all, resulting in disease.

Molecular analysis has revealed much about genes in this critical region of chromosome 15.[17,18] The gene responsible for Angelman syndrome encodes a ligase involved in protein

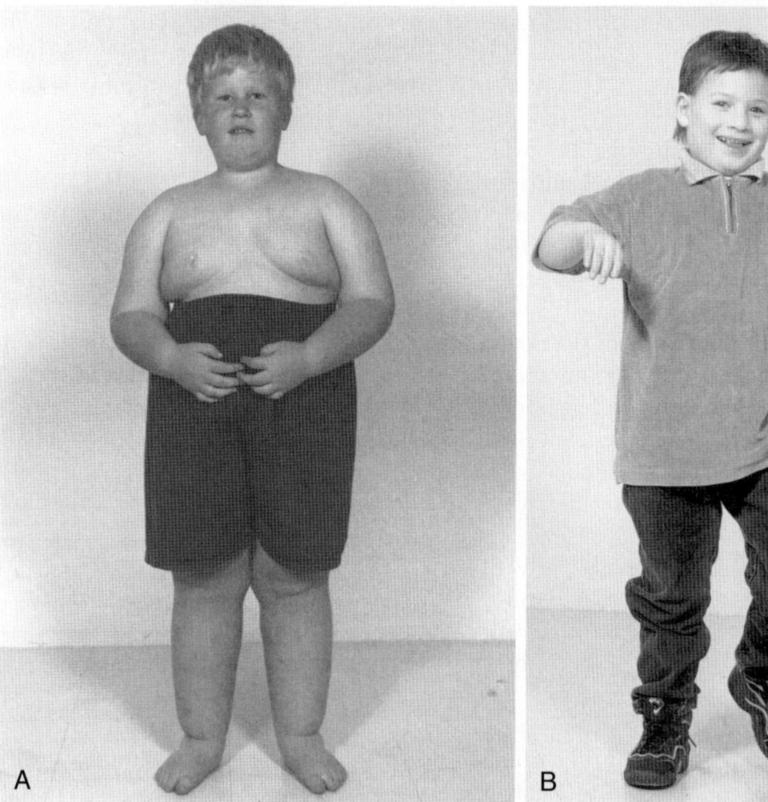

FIGURE 6-4 Prader-Willi and Angelman Syndromes. **A,** A child with Prader-Willi syndrome (truncal obesity, small hands and feet, inverted V-shaped upper lip). **B,** A child with Angelman syndrome (characteristic posture, ataxic gait, bouts of uncontrolled laughter). (From Jorde LB, Carey JC, Bamshad MJ: *Medical genetics,* ed 4, Philadelphia, 2010, Mosby.)

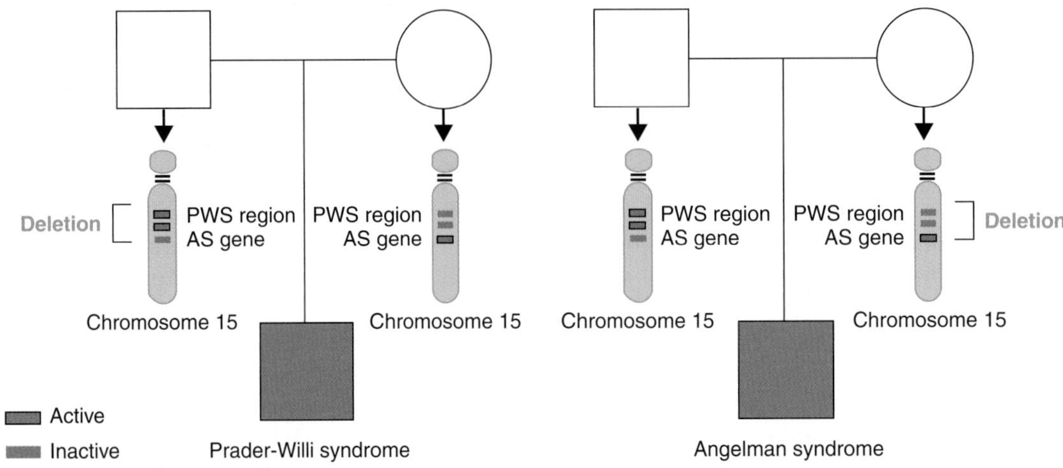

FIGURE 6-5 **Prader-Willi Syndrome and Angelman Syndrome Pedigrees.** These pedigrees illustrate the inheritance patterns of Prader-Willi syndrome, which can be caused by a 4-Mb deletion of chromosome 15q when inherited from the father. In contrast, Angelman syndrome can be caused by the same deletion but only when it is inherited from the mother. The reason for this difference is that different genes in this region are normally imprinted (inactivated) in the copies of 15q transmitted by the mother and the father. (From Jorde LB, Carey JC, Bamshad MJ: *Medical genetics*, ed 4, Philadelphia, 2010, Mosby.)

degradation during brain development (consistent with the mental retardation and ataxia observed in this disorder). In brain tissue, this gene is active only on the chromosome copy inherited from the mother. Consequently, a maternally transmitted deletion removes the single active copy of this gene. Several genes in the critical region are associated with Prader-Willi syndrome, and they are transcribed only on the chromosome transmitted by the father. A paternally transmitted deletion removes the only active copies of these genes, producing the features of Prader-Willi syndrome.

Beckwith-Wiedemann Syndrome

Another well-known example of imprinting is Beckwith-Wiedemann syndrome, an overgrowth condition accompanied by an increased predisposition to cancer. **Beckwith-Wiedemann syndrome** is usually identifiable at birth because of large size for gestational age, neonatal hypoglycemia, a large tongue, creases on the earlobe, and omphalocele.[19] Children with Beckwith-Wiedemann syndrome have an increased risk of developing Wilms tumor or hepatoblastoma. Both of these tumors can be treated effectively if they are detected early, so screening at regular intervals is an important part of management. Some children with Beckwith-Wiedemann syndrome also develop asymmetric overgrowth of a limb or one side of the face or trunk (hemihyperplasia).

As with Angelman syndrome, a minority of Beckwith-Wiedemann syndrome cases (about 20% to 30%) are caused by the inheritance of two copies of a chromosome from the father and no copy of the chromosome from the mother (uniparental disomy, in this case affecting chromosome 11). Several genes on the short arm of chromosome 11 are imprinted on either the paternally or the maternally transmitted chromosome. These genes are found in two separate, differentially methylated regions (DMRs). In DMR1, the gene that encodes insulin-like growth factor 2 *(IGF2)* is inactive on the maternally transmitted chromosome but active on the paternally transmitted chromosome. Thus, a normal individual has only one active copy of *IGF2*. When two copies of the paternal chromosome are inherited (i.e., paternal uniparental disomy) or there is loss of imprinting on the maternal copy of *IGF2*, an active *IGF2* gene is present in double dose. This produces increased levels of insulin-like growth factor 2 during fetal development, contributing to the overgrowth features of Beckwith-Wiedemann syndrome. (Note that, in contrast to Prader-Willi and Angelman syndromes, which are produced by a missing gene product, Beckwith-Wiedemann syndrome is caused, in part, by overexpression of a gene product.)

Russell-Silver Syndrome

Russell-Silver syndrome is characterized by growth retardation, proportionate short stature, leg length discrepancy, and a small, triangular-shaped face. About one third of Russell-Silver syndrome cases are caused by imprinting abnormalities of chromosome 11p15.5 that lead to down-regulation of *IGF2* and therefore diminished growth. Another 10% of cases of Russell-Silver syndrome are caused by maternal uniparental disomy. Thus, while up-regulation, or extra copies, of active *IGF2* causes overgrowth in Beckwith-Wiedemann syndrome, down-regulation of *IGF2* causes the diminished growth seen in Russell-Silver syndrome.

FUTURE DIRECTIONS

Robust experimental observations are clarifying the roles of epigenetic states in determining cell fates and disease phenotypes. The well-documented involvement of epigenetic abnormalities in carcinogenesis and the mounting evidence for these epigenetic changes in other common diseases (discussed in other chapters) will likely elucidate possibilities for reversing the epigenetic abnormalities and preventing their establishment in utero.

SUMMARY REVIEW

Epigenetics and Development

1. Epigenetics bridges DNA information and function by modifying gene expression without any alteration in DNA sequence. These often heritable chemical modifications of DNA sequence are collectively termed epigenetics.
2. Investigators are studying three major types of epigenetic processes: (a) DNA methylation, which results from attachment of a methyl group to a cytosine base that is followed by a guanine base (a "CpG dinucleotide"); (b) histone modification, which includes histone acetylation and alterations in chromatin; and (c) micro-ribonucleic acids (miRNAs or miRs), short nucleotides derived from introns of protein coding genes or transcribed as independent genes from regions of the genome whose functions, if any, remain poorly understood. MiRNAs regulate diverse signaling pathways.
3. DNA methylation is, at present, the best-studied epigenetic process. When a gene becomes heavily methylated the DNA is less likely to be transcribed into mRNA.
4. Methylation, along with histone hypoacetylation and condensation of chromatin, inhibits the binding of proteins that promote transcription, such that the gene becomes transcriptionally inactive.
5. Environmental factors, such as diet and exposure to certain chemicals, may cause epigenetic modifications.
6. The heritable transmission to future generations of epigenetic modifications is called transgenerational inheritance.
7. As twins age, they demonstrate increasing differences in methylation patterns of their DNA sequences, causing increasing numbers of phenotypic differences.
8. In studies of twins with significant lifestyle differences (e.g., smoking vs. nonsmoking) large numbers of differences in their methylation patterns are observed to accrue over time.

Epigenetics and Cancer

1. The best evidence for epigenetic effects on disease risk comes from studies of human cancer.
2. Methylation densities decline as tumors progress, which can increase the activity of oncogenes, causing tumors to progress from benign neoplasms to malignancy. Additionally, the promoter regions of tumor-suppressor genes are often hypermethylated. These elevated methylation levels decrease their rate of transcription at these critical genes, thus reducing the ability to inhibit tumor formation.
3. Hypermethylation also is seen in miRNA genes and is associated with tumorigenesis.
4. Unlike DNA sequence mutations, epigenetic modifications can be reversed through pharmaceutical intervention. For example, 5-azacytidine, a demethylating agent, has been used as a therapeutic drug in the treatment of leukemia and myelodysplastic syndrome.

Genomic Imprinting

1. Gregor Mendel's experiments with garden peas demonstrated that the phenotype is the same whether a given allele is inherited from the mother or the father. This principle, which has long been part of the central dogma of genetics, does not always hold. For some human genes, a given gene is transcriptionally active on only one copy of a chromosome (e.g., the copy inherited from the father). On the other copy of the chromosome (the one inherited from the mother), the gene is transcriptionally inactive. This process of gene silencing, in which genes are silenced depending on which parent transmits them, is known as *imprinting,* and the transcriptionally silenced genes are said to be "imprinted."
2. When an allele is imprinted, it typically has heavy methylation. By contrast, the nonimprinted allele is typically not methylated.
3. A well-known disease example of imprinting is associated with a deletion of about 4 million base pairs (Mb) of the long arm of chromosome 15. When this deletion is inherited from the father, the child manifests Prader-Willi syndrome.
4. The same 4-Mb deletion, when inherited from the mother, causes Angelman syndrome.
5. Another well-known example of imprinting is Beckwith-Wiedemann syndrome, an overgrowth condition accompanied by an increased predisposition to cancer.
6. Although up-regulation, or extra copies, of active *IGF2* causes overgrowth in Beckwith-Wiedemann syndrome, down-regulation of *IGF2* causes the diminished growth seen in Russell-Silver syndrome.

Future Directions

1. Robust experimental observations are defining the roles of epigenetic states in shaping cell fates.
2. The well-documented involvement of epigenetic abnormalities in carcinogenesis and the mounting evidence for these epigenetic changes in other common diseases (discussed throughout the text) will likely elucidate new therapies with the possibilities of reversing the epigenetic abnormalities.

KEY TERMS

REFERENCES

1. Esteller M: *An introduction to epigenetics: epigenetics in biology and medicine*, Boca Raton, FL, 2009, CRC Press Taylor & Francis Group.
2. Robertson KD: DNA methylation and human disease, *Nat Rev Genet* 6:597–610, 2005.
3. Cedar H, Bergman Y: Programming of DNA methylation patterns, *Annu Rev Biochem* 81:97–117, 2012.
4. Johnstone SE, Baylin SB: Stress and the epigenetic landscape: a link to the pathobiology of human diseases? *Nat Rev Genet* 11:806–812, 2010.
5. Kaminen-Ahola N et al: Maternal ethanol consumption alters the epigenotype and the phenotype of offspring in a mouse model, *PLoS Genet* 6(1):e1000811, 2010.
6. Feil R, Fraga MF: Epigenetics and the environment: emerging patterns and implications, *Nat Rev Genet* 13:97–109, 2011.
7. Fraga MF et al: Epigenetic differences arise during the lifetime of monozygotic twins, *Proc Natl Acad Sci U S A* 102:10604–10609, 2005.
8. Berdasco M, Esteller M: Hot topics in epigenetic mechanisms of aging: 2011, *Aging Cell* 11(2):181–186, 2012.
9. Esteller M: Epigenetics in cancer, *N Engl J Med* 358:1148–1159, 2008.
10. Sandoval J, Esteller M: Cancer epigenomics: beyond genomics, *Curr Opin Genet Dev* 22:50–55, 2012.
11. Giacinti C, Giordano A: RB and cell cycle progression, *Oncogene* 25(38):5220–5227, 2006.
12. Hansmann T et al: Constitutive promoter methylation of *BRCA1* and *RAD51C* in patients with familial ovarian cancer and early-onset sporadic breast cancer, *Hum Mol Genet* 21(21):4669–4679, 2012.
13. Lynch HT, de la Chapelle A: Hereditary colorectal cancer, *N Engl J Med* 348:919–932, 2003.
14. Pino MS, Chung DC: Microsatellite instability in the management of colorectal cancer, *Expert Rev Gastroenterol Hepatol* 5(3):385–399, 2011.
15. Cassidy SB et al: Prader-Willi syndrome, *Genet Med* 14:10–26, 2012.
16. Williams CA, et al: Angelman syndrome 2005: updated consensus for diagnostic criteria, *Am J Med Genet A* 140A:413–418, 2006.
17. Horsthemke B, Wagstaff J: Mechanisms of imprinting of the Prader-Willi/Angelman region, *Am J Med Genet A* 146A:2041–2052, 2008.
18. Jiang Y-H, Bressler J, Beaudet AL: Epigenetics and human disease, *Annu Rev Genom Hum Genet* 5:479–510, 2004.
19. Weksberg R, Shuman C, Smith AC: Beckwith-Wiedemann syndrome, *Am J Med Genet C Semin Med Genet* 137:12–23, 2005.

CHAPTER

7

Innate Immunity: Inflammation

Neal S. Rote, Sue E. Huether, and Kathryn L. McCance

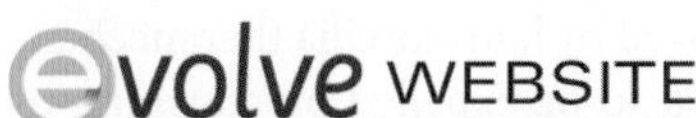

http://evolve.elsevier.com/McCance/

- Review Questions and Answers
- Animations
- Online Course: Module 4

CHAPTER OUTLINE

People are exposed daily to an environment containing a large variety of toxic substances and potentially infectious and disease-causing microorganisms. Without an efficient system of protection most individuals would succumb to these hazards early in life. That system consists of multiple complementary and interdependent layers. An outer layer of specialized epithelium, including the skin and mucosal surfaces, is relatively resistant to most environmental hazards and resists infection with disease-causing microorganisms.[1] If the epithelial barrier is damaged, a highly efficient local and systemic response (**inflammation**) is mobilized to limit the extent of damage, protect against infection, and initiate repair of the damaged tissue. The natural epithelial barrier and inflammation confer innate resistance and protection, commonly referred to as **innate, native,** or **natural immunity.** Inflammation associated with infection usually initiates an adaptive process that results in a long-term and very effective immunity to the infecting microorganism, referred to as **adaptive, acquired,** or **specific immunity.** Adaptive immunity is relatively slow to develop but has memory and more rapidly targets and eradicates a second infection with a particular disease-causing microorganism.

The information presented in this chapter introduces the components and processes of innate immunity and sets the stage for Chapter 8, which discusses adaptive immunity. Although inflammation and adaptive immunity provide protection, either genetic or acquired aberrations in these processes can lead to disease. Diminution of innate or adaptive immunity may lead to critically decreased resistance to infection. Excessive inflammation or adaptive immunity may lead to damage to normal tissue or organs. Both may result in severe and potentially fatal disease, examples of which are discussed in Chapter 9. Many microorganisms that cause disease have developed methods of bypassing our protective systems. These are discussed in Chapter 10. Each chapter is designed to render an overview and is not intended to be all-inclusive. Protective mechanisms consist of a very large number of soluble factors and cells and would require many more pages to discuss in adequate detail. Different classes or groups of molecules and cells will be discussed, but only a few examples will be described in detail. Some components directly participate in the protective response, whereas others are designed to limit the extent of the response.

HUMAN DEFENSE MECHANISMS

Innate immunity includes two lines of defense: natural barriers and inflammation (Table 7-1). **Natural barriers** are physical, mechanical, and biochemical barriers at the body's surfaces and are in place at birth to prevent damage by substances in the environment and thwart infection by pathogenic microorganisms. If the surface barriers are breached, the second line of defense, the **inflammatory response,** is activated to protect the body from further injury, prevent infection of the injured tissue, and promote healing. The inflammatory response is a rapid activation of biochemical and cellular processes that is relatively nonspecific, with similar responses being initiated against a wide variety of causes of tissue damage.

FIRST LINE OF DEFENSE: PHYSICAL, MECHANICAL, AND BIOCHEMICAL BARRIERS

Physical and Mechanical Barriers

The physical barriers that protect against damage and infection are composed of tightly associated epithelial cells including those of the skin and of the membranous sheets lining the gastrointestinal, genitourinary, and respiratory tracts (Figure 7-1). The mucosal epithelial cells are highly interconnected junctions that prohibit the passage of microorganisms into the underlying tissue.[2] The normal turnover of the cells in these sites as well as mechanisms for "washing" the surfaces may mechanically remove many infectious microorganisms and prevent their residence on the epithelial surfaces. For instance, the routine sloughing off and replacement of dead skin cells also removes adherent bacteria. Mechanical cleansing of the surfaces includes vomiting and urination. Goblet cells of the upper respiratory tract produce mucus that coats the epithelial surface and traps microorganisms that are removed by hairlike cilia that mechanically move the mucus upward to be expelled by coughing or sneezing. Additionally, the low temperature on the skin generally inhibits microorganisms, most of which prefer temperatures near 37° C for more efficient growth.

Biochemical Barriers

Epithelial surfaces also provide biochemical barriers by synthesizing and secreting substances meant to trap or destroy microorganisms. Mucus, perspiration (or sweat), saliva, tears, and earwax are all examples of biochemical secretions that can trap and kill potential disease-causing microorganisms. Sebaceous

TABLE 7-1 OVERVIEW OF HUMAN DEFENSES

	INNATE IMMUNITY		
CHARACTERISTICS	BARRIERS	INFLAMMATORY RESPONSE	ADAPTIVE (ACQUIRED) IMMUNITY
Level of defense	First line of defense against infection and tissue injury	Second line of defense; occurs as a response to tissue injury or infection	Third line of defense; initiated when innate immune system signals the cells of adaptive immunity
Timing of defense	Constant	Immediate response	Delay between primary exposure to antigen and maximum response; immediate against secondary exposure to antigen
Specificity	Broadly specific	Broadly specific	Response is very specific toward "antigen"
Cells	Epithelial cells	Mast cells, granulocytes (neutrophils, eosinophils, basophils), monocytes/macrophages, natural killer (NK) cells, platelets, endothelial cells	T lymphocytes, B lymphocytes, macrophages, dendritic cells
Memory	No memory involved	No memory involved	Specific immunologic memory by T and B lymphocytes
Peptides	Defensins, cathelicidins, collectins, lactoferrin, bacterial toxins	Complement, clotting factors, kinins	Antibodies, complement
Protection	Protection includes anatomic barriers (i.e., skin and mucous membranes), cells and secretory molecules or cytokines (e.g., lysozymes, low pH of stomach and urine), and ciliary activity	Protection includes vascular responses, cellular components (e.g., mast cells, neutrophils, macrophages), secretory molecules or cytokines, and activation of plasma protein systems	Protection includes activated T and B lymphocytes, cytokines, and antibodies

glands in the skin secrete antibacterial and antifungal fatty acids and lactic acid. Perspiration, tears, and saliva contain an enzyme (lysozyme) that attacks the cell walls of gram-positive bacteria. These glandular secretions result in an acidic skin surface (pH 3 to 5), which is an inhospitable environment for most bacteria.

Epithelial-Derived Chemicals

The epithelial surfaces of the body secrete a complex array of proteins that destroy potential pathogens. Epithelial cells secrete small-molecular-weight **antimicrobial peptides.**[3] These are generally positively charged polypeptides of approximately 15 to 95 amino acids and can be divided into two classes—cathelicidins and defensins—based on their 3-dimensional structures. Both classes are in very high local concentrations and are toxic to several bacteria, fungi, and viruses. **Cathelicidins** have a linear α-helical shape, and only one is currently known to function in humans. In contrast, about 50 different defensins have been identified thus far. All are triple-stranded β-sheet structures. **Defensin** molecules contain 3 intrachain disulfide bonds and can be further subdivided into α (at least 6 identified in humans) and β types (at least 10 identified, but perhaps up to 40 different molecules), depending on how the cysteine residues are connected during formation of the disulfide linkages.[4] The α-defensins often require activation by proteolytic enzymes, whereas the β-defensins are synthesized in active forms. Bacteria have cholesterol-free cell membranes, which may allow cathelicidins to insert into and disrupt their membranes. Given the similarity in their chemical charges, defensins may kill bacteria in the same way. These same chemicals also may contribute to other means of protection because they are also produced by monocytes, macrophages, and neutrophils, which are components of the inflammatory response. Cathelicidin is stored in neutrophils, mast cells, and a variety of epithelial cells. The α-defensins are particularly rich in the granules of neutrophils and may contribute to the killing of bacteria by those cells. They are also found in Paneth cells lining the small intestine, where they protect against a variety of disease-causing microorganisms. The β-defensins are found in a variety of epithelial cells lining the respiratory, urinary, and intestinal tracts, as well as in the skin. In addition to antibacterial properties, β-defensins may also help protect epithelial surfaces from human immunodeficiency virus (HIV) infection. Both classes of antimicrobial peptides also can activate cells of innate and adaptive immunity.

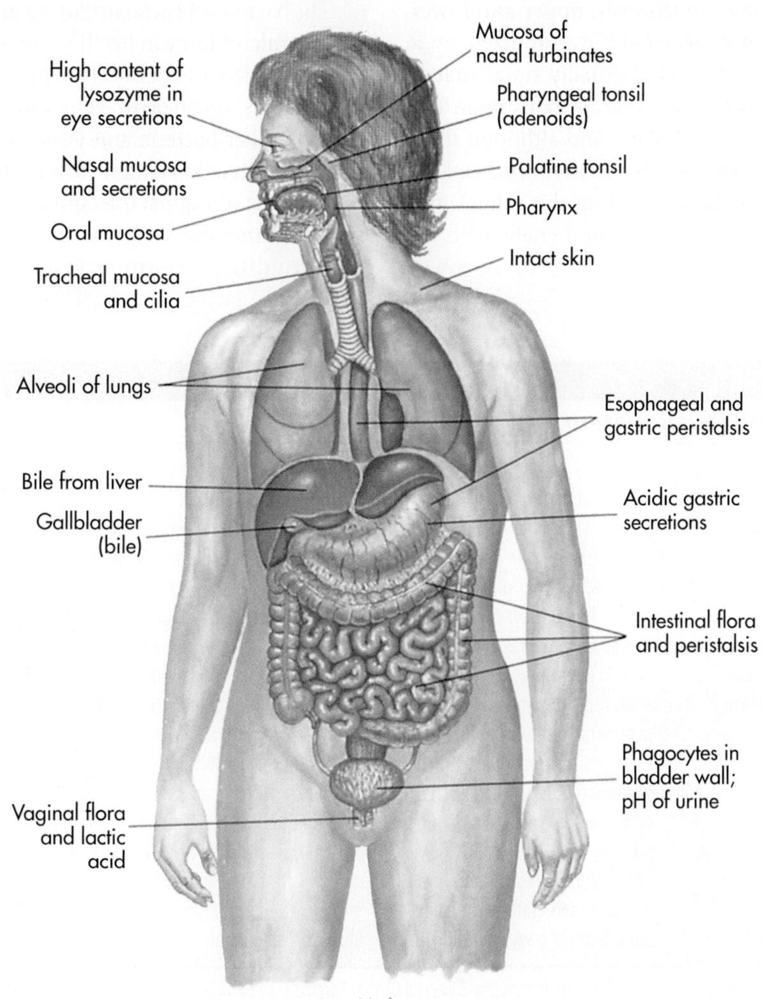

FIGURE 7-1 The Closed Barrier. The digestive, respiratory, and genitourinary tracts and the skin form closed barriers between the internal organs and the environment. (From Grimes DE: *Infectious diseases,* St Louis, 1991, Mosby.)

The lung also produces and secretes a family of glycoproteins, **collectins,** which includes surfactant proteins A through D and mannose-binding lectin. The binding site of each collectin reacts with different affinities to a range of monosaccharides, enabling collectins to recognize a wide array of pathogenic microorganisms. Collectin binding facilitates recognition of the microorganism by macrophages, enhancing macrophage attachment, phagocytosis, and killing. Collectins play a major role in protection against respiratory tract infections.

Other *epithelial antimicrobials* include resistin-like molecule β, bactericidal/permeability-inducing protein, and antimicrobial lectins. **Resistin-like molecule** β is found in the intestinal goblet cells, where it appears to protect against helminth infections. **Bactericidal/permeability-inducing (BPI) protein** is stored in neutrophils and intestinal epithelium. BPI protein specifically reacts with lipopolysaccharide on the surface of gram-negative bacteria, resulting in bacterial lysis. **Antimicrobial lectins** are carbohydrates that are found in intestinal epithelium and have activity against gram-positive bacteria.

Bacteria-Derived Chemicals

The body's surfaces are colonized with a spectrum of microorganisms, the **normal microbiome.** Each surface, including the skin and the mucous membranes of the eyes, upper and lower gastrointestinal tracts, urethra, and vagina, is colonized by a combination of mostly bacteria and occasionally fungi that is unique to the particular location. The microorganisms in the microbiome do not normally cause disease, and although their relationship with humans has been referred to as *commensal* (to the benefit of one organism without affecting the other), the relationship may be more *mutualistic* (to the benefit of both organisms). Using the colon for an example, at birth the lower gut is relatively sterile but colonization with bacteria begins quickly, with the number, diversity, and concentration increasing progressively during the first year of life. To the benefit of humans, many of these microorganisms help digest fatty acids, large polysaccharides, and other dietary substances; produce biotin and vitamin K; and assist in the absorption of various ions, such as calcium, iron, and magnesium.[5]

These bacteria contribute to our innate protection against pathogenic microorganisms in the colon. They compete with pathogens for nutrients and block attachment to the epithelium. Members of the normal microbiome also produce chemicals (ammonia, phenols, indoles, and other toxic materials) and toxic proteins *(bacteriocins)* that inhibit colonization by pathogenic microorganisms. Prolonged treatment with broad-spectrum antibiotics can alter the normal intestinal microbiome, decreasing its protective activity, and lead to an overgrowth of pathogenic microorganisms, such as the yeast *Candida albicans* or the bacteria *Clostridium difficile* (overgrowth can cause pseudomembranous colitis, an infection of the colon). Additionally, the normal microbiome of the gut help train the adaptive immune system by inducing the growth of gut-associated lymphoid tissue (where cells of the adaptive immune system reside) and the development of both local and systemic adaptive immune systems.[6]

The bacterium *Lactobacillus* is a major constituent of the normal vaginal microbiome in healthy women.[7] This microorganism produces a variety of chemicals (e.g., hydrogen peroxide, lactic acid, bacteriocins) that help prevent infections of the vagina and urinary tract by other bacteria and yeast. Prolonged antibiotic treatment can diminish colonization with *Lactobacillus* and increase the risk for urologic or vaginal infections, such as vaginosis.

Some members of the normal bacterial microbiome are opportunistic; opportunistic microorganisms can cause disease

NUTRITION & DISEASE

Essential Fatty Acids and Inflammation

Both omega-3 and omega-6 polyunsaturated fatty acids are essential fatty acids available only in the diet. They are essential because human physiologic processes cannot add the necessary double bonds to the carbon chains. Omega-6 fatty acids are contained in vegetable oils, and most are linolenic acid. Omega-3 essential fatty acids, which are mostly alpha-linolenic acid, are found in green leafy vegetables, walnuts, flaxseed, and canola oil. The metabolic products of alpha-linolenic acid are eicosapentaenoic acid (EPA) and docosahexaenoic acid (DHA), and the richest source of these acids is in the oils of deep-sea cold-water fish. Both the omega-3 and omega-6 fatty acids use the same enzymes to produce their metabolic products, and they compete for this enzyme, delta-5-desaturase. *Delta-5-desaturase* converts EPA into anti-inflammatory prostaglandins (PGs) of the PGE_3 series. The omega-6 fatty acid dihomogamma-linolenic acid (DGLA) can be converted to either anti-inflammatory PG_1 or arachidonic acid (AA), a precursor of inflammatory PG_2 and leukotrienes. Conversion of DGLA into PG_1 does not require any enzymes, but conversion of DGLA into AA requires the enzymes delta-6- and delta-5-desaturase. When the diet is high in omega-3 fatty acids, most of the delta-5-desaturase will be used in the omega-3 pathway and the production of anti-inflammatory prostaglandins. Little delta-5-desaturase will be available to convert DGLA into arachidonic acid, and subsequent inflammatory mediators. DGLA ends up being converted into the anti-inflammatory PG_1, and, overall, inflammation is decreased. The resulting anti-inflammatory effects of omega-3 essential fatty acids decrease the risk for cardiovascular disease, cancer, and other conditions associated with inflammation. Omega-3 fatty acids have been shown to decrease blood triglyceride concentrations; decrease production of chemoattractants, growth factors, and adhesion molecules; lower blood pressure; increase nitric oxide production and endothelial relaxation and vascular compliance; decrease thrombosis and cardiac dysrhythmias; and stabilize atherosclerotic plaque. The American diet tends to be high in saturated and omega-6 fatty acids and deficient in omega-3 fatty acids, with a ratio estimated at about 15:1. The Mediterranean-style diet has more whole grains, fish, olive oil, fresh fruits and vegetables, and a more balanced ratio of omega-6 to omega-3 fatty acids estimated at about (3-4):1. Increasing omega-3 fatty acids in the diet may significantly improve health and reduce the risk of cardiovascular disease and cancer.

Data from Abeywardena MY, Patten GS: *Endocr Metab Immune Disord Drug Targets* 11(3):232–246, 2011; Berquin IM et al: *Cancer Lett* 269(2):363–377, 2008; Calder PC: *Clin Sci (Lond)* 107(1):1–11, 2004; Chrysohoou C et al: *J Am Coll Cardiol* 44(1):152–158, 2004; Das UN: *Lipids Health Dis* 7:37, 2008; Esposito K et al: *JAMA* 292(12):1440–1446, 2004; Manson JE et al: *Contemp Clin Trials* 33(1):159–171, 2012; Pottala JV et al: *Circ Cardiovasc Qual Outcomes* (4):406–412, 2010; Sijben JW, Calder PC: *Proc Nutr Soc* 66(2):237–259, 2007.

if the individual's defenses are compromised. These microorganisms are normally controlled by the innate and adaptive immune systems and contribute to our defenses. For example, *Pseudomonas aeruginosa* is a member of the normal microbiome of the skin and produces a toxin that protects against infections with staphylococcal and other bacteria. However, severe burns compromise the integrity of the skin and may lead to life-threatening systemic pseudomonal infections.

SECOND LINE OF DEFENSE: THE INFLAMMATORY RESPONSE

If cells and tissues are damaged the **inflammatory response** is usually activated (Figure 7-2). Injury can have a variety of causes including infection, mechanical damage, oxygen deprivation (ischemia), nutrient deprivation, genetic or immune defects, chemical agents, temperature extremes, or ionizing radiation. Inflammation (1) depends on the activity of both *cellular and chemical components*, and (2) is *nonspecific*, meaning that it takes place in approximately the same way regardless of the type of stimulus or whether exposure to the same stimulus has occurred in the past.

Vascular Response

Inflammation occurs in tissue that has a blood supply (vascularized) and results in a group of easily observable characteristics: *redness, heat, swelling,* and *pain.* This tetrad represents the "cardinal signs of inflammation" and was identified in the first century by a Roman writer, Celsus. Microscopically, inflammatory changes occur at the vascular level (Figure 7-3). The three characteristic changes in the microcirculation (arterioles, capillaries, and venules) near the site of an injury include the following:

1. Blood vessel dilation (vasodilation)
2. Increased vascular permeability and leakage of fluid out of the vessel
3. White blood cell adherence to the inner walls of vessels and their migration through vessel walls to the site of injury (diapedesis)

The effects of inflammation are visible within seconds. First, arterioles near the site of infection or injury constrict briefly. Vasodilation then causes slower blood velocity and increases local blood flow to the injured site. The increased flow and capillary permeability result in leakage of plasma from the vessels, causing swelling (edema) in the surrounding tissue. As plasma moves outward, blood remaining in the microcirculation flows more slowly and becomes more viscous. The increased blood flow and increasing concentration of red cells at the site of inflammation cause locally increased warmth and redness. Leukocytes adhere to vessel walls. At the same time, biochemical mediators (e.g., histamine, bradykinins, leukotrienes, prostaglandins) stimulate the endothelial cells that line capillaries and venules to retract, creating spaces at junctions between the cells,

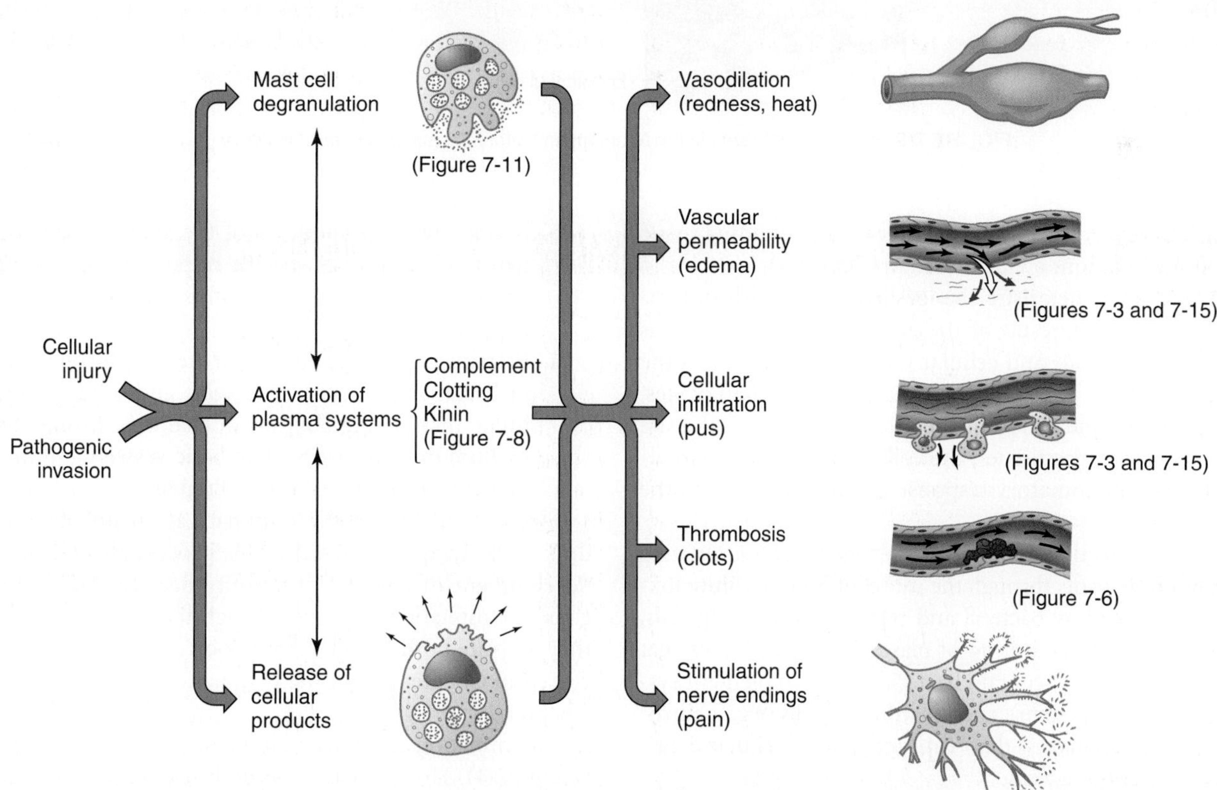

FIGURE 7-2 Acute Inflammatory Response. Inflammation is usually initiated by cellular injury, which results in mast cell degranulation, the activation of three plasma systems, and the release of subcellular components from the damaged cells. These systems are interdependent, so that induction of one (e.g., mast cell degranulation) can result in activation of the other two. The result is the development of microscopic changes in the inflamed site, as well as characteristic clinical manifestations. The figure numbers refer to those in which more detailed information may be found on that portion of the response.

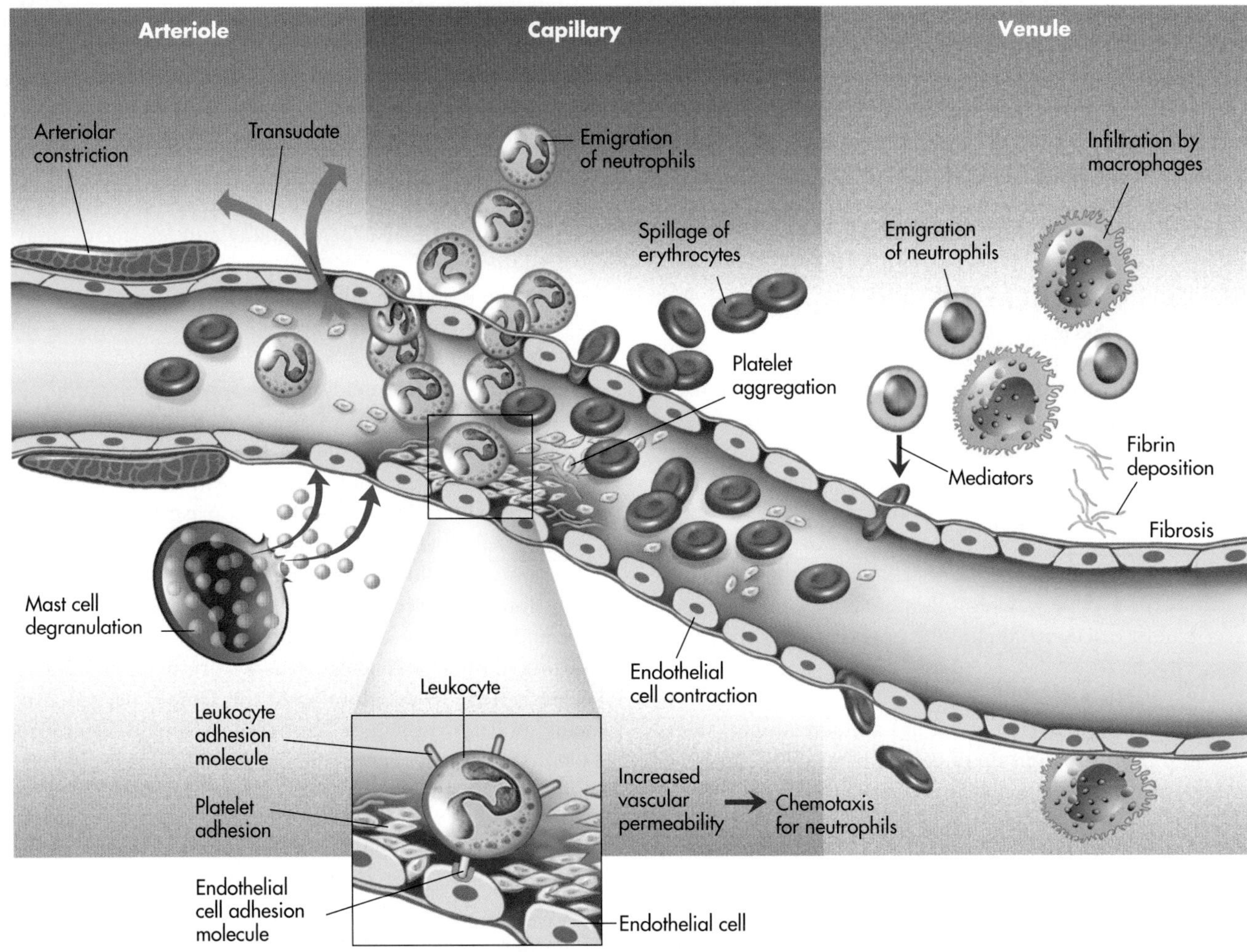

FIGURE 7-3 Sequence of Events in the Acute Inflammatory Response. See text for details.

allowing leukocytes and plasma to enter the surrounding tissue (intercellular junctions are described in Chapter 1).

Each of the characteristic changes associated with inflammation is the direct result of the activities and interactions of a host of chemicals and cellular components found in the blood and tissues. The vascular changes deliver leukocytes, plasma proteins, and other biochemical mediators to the site of injury. Once in the tissues, the cells and chemicals associated with the inflammatory response act in concert to do the following:

1. Prevent infection and further damage by contaminating microorganisms through the influx of fluid to dilute toxins produced by bacteria and released from dying cells, the influx and activation of plasma protein systems that help destroy and contain bacteria (e.g., complement system, clotting system), and the influx of cells (e.g., neutrophils, macrophages) that "eat" and destroy cellular debris and infectious agents.
2. Limit and control the inflammatory process through the influx of plasma protein systems (e.g., clotting system), plasma enzymes, and cells (e.g., eosinophils) that prevent the inflammatory response from spreading to areas of healthy tissue.
3. Interact with components of the adaptive immune system to elicit a more specific response to contaminating pathogen(s) through the influx of macrophages and lymphocytes.[8]
4. Prepare the area of injury for healing through removal of bacterial products, dead cells, and other products of inflammation (e.g., by way of channels through the epithelium or drainage by lymphatic vessels) and initiation of mechanisms of healing and repair.

Fluid and debris that accumulate at an inflamed site are drained by lymphatic vessels. This process also facilitates the development of adaptive immunity because microbial antigens in lymphatic fluid pass through the lymph nodes, where they activate both B and T lymphocytes. (This process is discussed in Chapter 8, and the lymphatic system is described in Chapter 27.)

Inflammation and repair can be divided into several phases (Figure 7-4). The characteristics of the early (i.e., acute) inflammatory response differ from those of the later (i.e., chronic) response, and each phase involves different biochemical mediators and cells that function together. The acute inflammatory response is of short duration; that is, it continues only until the immediate threat to the host is eliminated. This usually takes

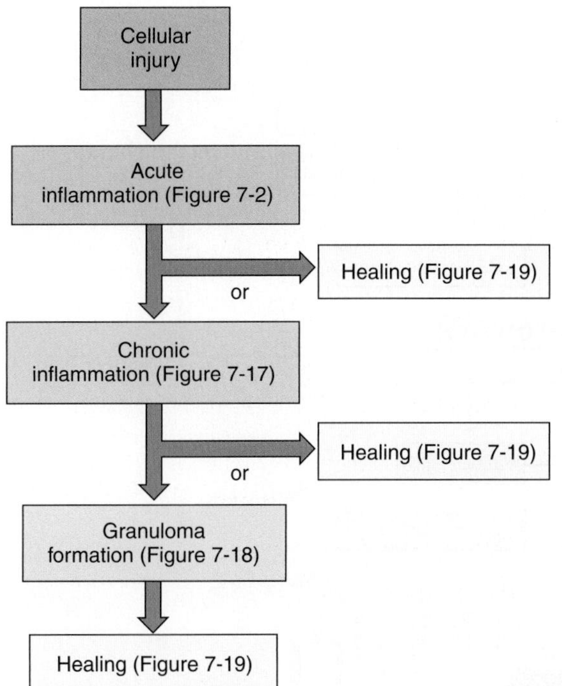

FIGURE 7-4 Inflammatory Phases. Cellular injury leads to acute inflammation and may result in resolution and healing of the injured site or may progress into chronic inflammation. Chronic inflammation in turn may result in healing or progress to development of a granuloma. The final step of the inflammatory process is usually healing and reconstruction of the damaged tissue. The figure numbers refer to those in which more detailed information on that portion of the process may be found.

8 to 10 days from onset to healing. The acute inflammatory response begins immediately after cellular injury or infection occurs and involves a vascular response, activation of plasma protein systems, and activation of a variety of cells. (Mechanisms of cellular injury are described in Chapter 2.)

Plasma Protein Systems

Three key **plasma protein systems** are essential to an effective inflammatory response. These are the complement system, the clotting system, and the kinin system (Figures 7-5, 7-6, and 7-7, respectively). Although each system has a unique role in inflammation, they also have many similarities. Each system consists of multiple proteins in the blood. To prevent activation in unnecessary situations, each protein is normally in an inactive form. Several of the proteins are enzymes that circulate in inactive forms as **proenzymes.** Each system contains a few proteins that can be activated by products of tissue damage or infection. Activation of the first component of a system results in sequential activation of other components, leading to a biologic function that helps protect the individual. This sequential activation is referred to as a *cascade*. Thus, we refer to the complement cascade, the clotting cascade, or the kinin cascade. In some cases, activation of a protein may require that it be enzymatically cut into two pieces or fragments of different size. Usually the larger fragment continues the cascade by activating the next component, and the smaller fragment frequently has potent biologic activities to promote inflammation.

Complement System

The complement system consists of several plasma proteins (sometimes called *complement components*) that together constitute about 10% of the total circulating serum protein. The complement system is extremely important because activation of the **complement cascade** may destroy pathogens directly and can activate or collaborate with virtually every other component of the inflammatory response. Proteins of the complement system are among the body's most potent defenders, particularly against bacterial infection.

Activation of the complement system can be accomplished in three different pathways, all of which converge at the third component (C3) of the pathway:

1. **Classical pathway:** activated by proteins of the adaptive immune system (antibodies) bound to their specific targets (antigen)
2. **Lectin pathway:** activated by mannose-containing bacterial carbohydrates
3. **Alternative pathway:** activated by gram-negative bacterial and fungal cell wall polysaccharides

The principal routes by which the complement cascade may be activated are shown in Figure 7-5.

Activation of the *classical pathway* begins with the activation of complement protein C1 and is preceded by formation of a complex between an antigen and an antibody to form an **antigen-antibody complex (immune complex)** (discussed in Chapter 8). The antigen may be a unique chemical component of the surface of a bacterium or other microorganism. Most pathogens express multiple antigens; therefore, multiple antibodies are usually bound in the complex. The first component of the classical complement cascade, C1, has six sites that can bind to antibodies, and efficient activation of the complement cascade usually requires concurrent binding of C1 to at least two antibody molecules. The complex formed by antigen-antibody-complement binding is shown in Figure 7-5. C1 is a macromolecular complex consisting of C1q and two molecules each of C1r and C1s. A conformational change in C1 results in an enzymatically active molecule whose substrates are C4 and C2. The resultant complex formed by the interaction of C1, C4, and C2 uses C3 as a substrate, resulting in the production of C3a and C3b. A complex that has C3 as a substrate is generally referred to as a **C3 convertase.** The addition of C3b to the complex changes the substrate specificity to C5, resulting in the conversion of C5 to C5a and C5b. A complex that has C5 as a substrate is generally called a **C5 convertase.** Thus activation of C1 initiates the sequential enzymatic activation of all other components of the classical pathway, ultimately resulting in the activation of C5. The classical pathway also can be activated to a lesser degree by biologic molecules other than antibody, including heparin (a charged molecule that prevents clotting), deoxyribonucleic acid (DNA) or ribonucleic acid (RNA), and C-reactive protein, which is increased in the blood during inflammation.

Even under normal conditions small amounts of circulating C3 are spontaneously broken down into C3b and C3a by a number of naturally occurring enzymes in the blood. The rate of C3 spontaneous activation is generally very low, and C3b is readily inactivated by complement regulator proteins in the

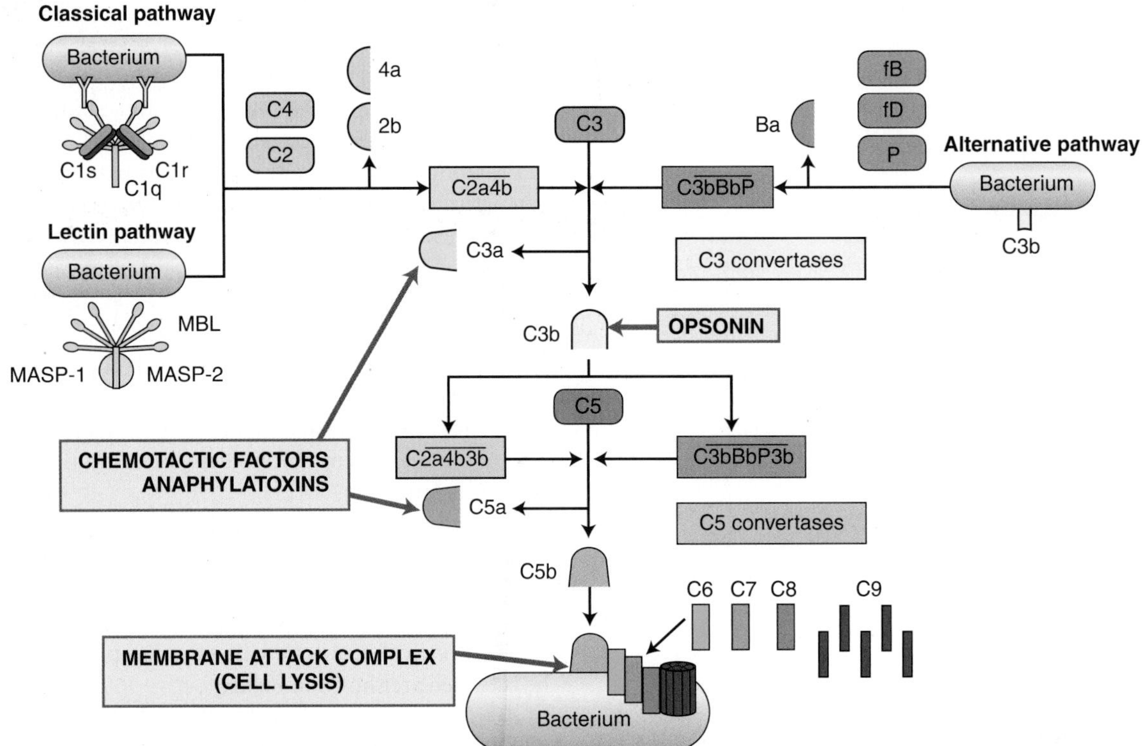

FIGURE 7-5 **Pathways of Complement Cascade Activation.** The complement system is activated by three pathways: the classical pathway, the lectin pathway, and the alternative pathway. During activation, many complement components are cleaved into fragments (2b, 4a, Ba, C3a, and C5a). The smaller fragments frequently have potent biologic activities and may serve as chemotactic factors and anaphylatoxins. The larger activated fragments are usually converted into active enzymes (indicated by the bar above the names) and form complexes with additional components in the cascade. The classical pathway is usually activated by antigen-antibody complexes through component C1, which consists of C1q and two C1r and C1s molecules. As indicated, the C1q must simultaneously bind to two antibody molecules (indicated by Y-shaped structures). The lectin pathway is activated by mannose-binding lectin (MBL), which binds to two mannose-rich pathogen-associated molecular patterns on the surface of a bacterium. MBL contains two associated enzymes, MASP-1 and MASP-2, and functions in a manner similar to C1. C1 and MBL each activate complement components C4 and C2. The alternative pathway is activated by many agents, such as bacterial polysaccharides, which bind and stabilize C3b, which is produced by normal breakdown of C3 in the blood. The C3b forms the site of binding of factor B (fB), which is activated by factor D (fD) into Bb and the small fragment Ba. Properdin (P) helps stabilize the complex. Each pathway produces C3 and C5 convertases, which are enzymatically active complexes that activate C3 and C5, respectively. C3b produced by the C3 convertase can function as an opsonin. C5b initiates assemblage of the membrane attack complex (MAC), which results in multiple C9 molecules forming a pore in the bacterial membrane.

blood (e.g., factor H and factor I). However, materials produced by some infectious microorganisms (e.g., lipopolysaccharides [endotoxins] on the bacterial surface, yeast cell wall carbohydrates [zymosans]) can bind the naturally produced C3b and protect it from inactivation. This will initiate activation of the *alternative complement pathway*. The C3b bound to bacterial products can react with another normally occurring component, factor B. The complex of C3b and factor B is recognized by an enzyme, factor D, which activates factor B, producing factor Bb. The resultant C3b/Bb complex is very unstable unless it binds to properdin (P). The C3b/Bb/P complex is a C3 convertase that produces further C3b, resulting in a C3b/Bb/P/C3b complex that is a C5 convertase, which activates C5.

The *lectin pathway* is similar to the classical pathway but is antibody independent. It is activated by a plasma protein called *mannose-binding lectin (MBL)*. MBL is similar to C1q and binds to bacterial polysaccharides containing the carbohydrate mannose. MBL-associated serine proteases (MASP-1 and MASP-2) substitute for C1r and C1s and activate C4 and C2 to create a C3 convertase.

After activation of C5, the cascade continues through the terminal components C6, C7, C8, and C9. Components C5b through C9 assemble to form complexes *(membrane attack complex,* or *MAC)* capable of creating pores in cell membranes and permitting the influx of water and ions and may ultimately result in **cell lysis.**

The most important result of complement activation is the production of fragments during the activation of C4, C2, C3, and C5. The fragments C4a, C2b, C3a, and C5a are soluble and of low-molecular-weight that contribute in other ways to the inflammatory response. C2b affects smooth muscle, causing vasodilation and increased vascular permeability. C3a and C5a, and to a limited extent C4a, are **anaphylatoxins;** that is, they induce rapid **mast cell degranulation** (release of granular

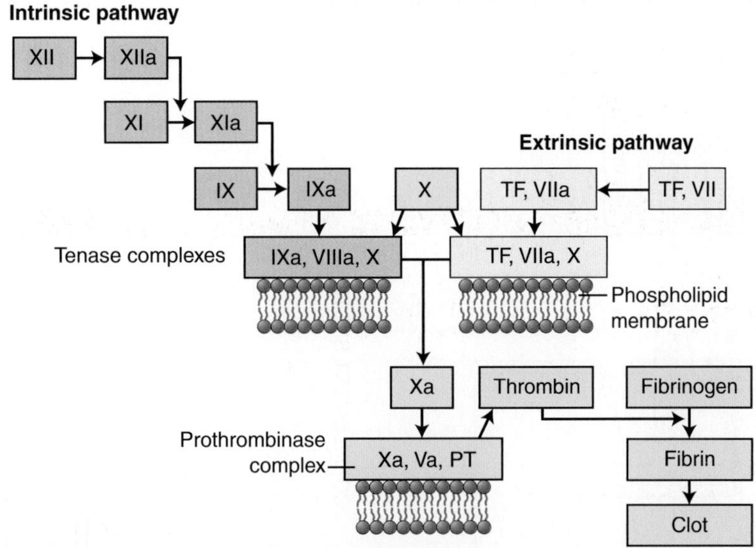

FIGURE 7-6 **Coagulation Cascade.** Clotting is activated through two pathways: the intrinsic pathway and the extrinsic pathway. The intrinsic pathway is initiated by the activation of Hageman factor (XII) into XIIa (activated factors are enzymes and are indicated by a lowercase a). The sequential activation of other intrinsic pathway components results in formation of a complex of IXa, VIIIa, and X. The extrinsic pathway is activated by exposure of tissue factor (TF) during tissue damage. TF complexes with factor VII, which is activated (VIIa) and forms a complex with factor X (TF, VIIa, X). Both the intrinsic and the extrinsic pathway complexes are dependent on calcium, form on phospholipid membranes that are rich in phosphatidylserine, and have "tenase" activity (can activate factor X into Xa). Factor X begins a common pathway in which Xa complexes with Va and prothrombin (PT), with calcium and phospholipid membranes, to form an active prothrombinase (activates prothrombin into thrombin). Thrombin is an enzyme that cuts high-molecular-weight fibrinogen into fibrin molecules. Fibrin polymerizes to form a clot.

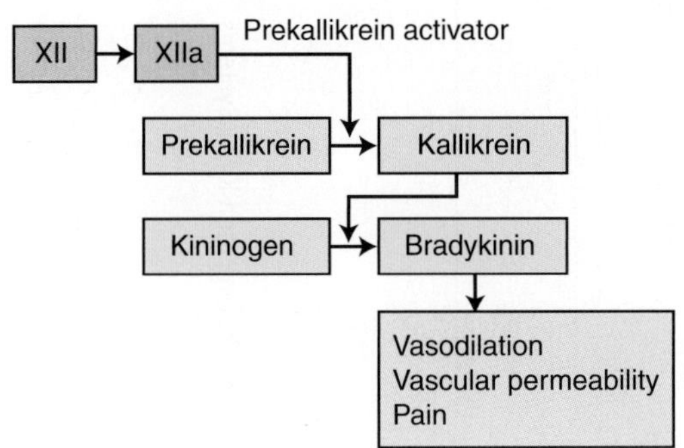

FIGURE 7-7 **Plasma Kinin Cascade.** The kinin pathway is activated by factor XIIa from the clotting system, which functions as an enzyme (prekallikrein activator) to convert prekallikrein into kallikrein. Enzymatically active kallikrein converts kininogen into bradykinin.

contents) and the release of histamine (see Figure 7-11, p. 206), causing vasodilation and increased capillary permeability.[9] C5a is the major chemotactic factor for neutrophils. C3a is approximately 100 times less potent in chemotactic and anaphylatoxic activity. A **chemotactic factor** is a biochemical substance that attracts leukocytes to the site of inflammation.

The dual functions of a chemotactic factor and an anaphylatoxin are not needed simultaneously or to the same degree. Anaphylatoxic activity is necessary early in inflammation and occurs close to the inflammatory site to induce local mast cell degranulation and to increase the number of soluble mediators available to enhance vascular permeability and vasodilation. Chemotactic activity, on the other hand, is required for a much longer period and occurs distal to the inflammatory site to attract leukocytes from the circulation. Thus it is beneficial to an effective inflammatory response to limit the range of anaphylatoxic activity while allowing widespread chemotactic activity. A plasma enzyme, a **carboxypeptidase,** removes a terminal arginine on both C3a and C5a peptides, thereby producing "C3a desArg" and "C5a desArg," which are inactive as anaphylatoxins but retain chemotactic activity. Thus chemotactic activity is retained, while not inducing distal mast cell degranulation that would result in considerable enlargement of the inflammatory response to the detriment of surrounding healthy tissue.

C3b adheres to the surface of a pathogenic microorganism and serves as an efficient opsonin. **Opsonins** are molecules that "tag" microorganisms for destruction by cells of the inflammatory system (primarily neutrophils and macrophages [see pp. 208 and 209]). C3b on the cell surface also can be broken down by several enzymes in the blood into inactive fragments (e.g., iC3b), which retain opsonic activity.

In summary, the complement cascade can be activated by at least three different means, and its products have four functions: (1) anaphylatoxic activity resulting in mast cell degranulation, (2) leukocyte chemotaxis, (3) opsonization, and (4) cell lysis.

Clotting System

The clotting (coagulation) system is a group of plasma proteins that form a fibrinous meshwork at an injured or inflamed site. This (1) prevents the spread of infection to adjacent tissues, (2) traps microorganisms and foreign bodies at the site of inflammation for removal by infiltrating cells (e.g., neutrophils and macrophages), (3) forms a clot that stops bleeding, and (4) provides

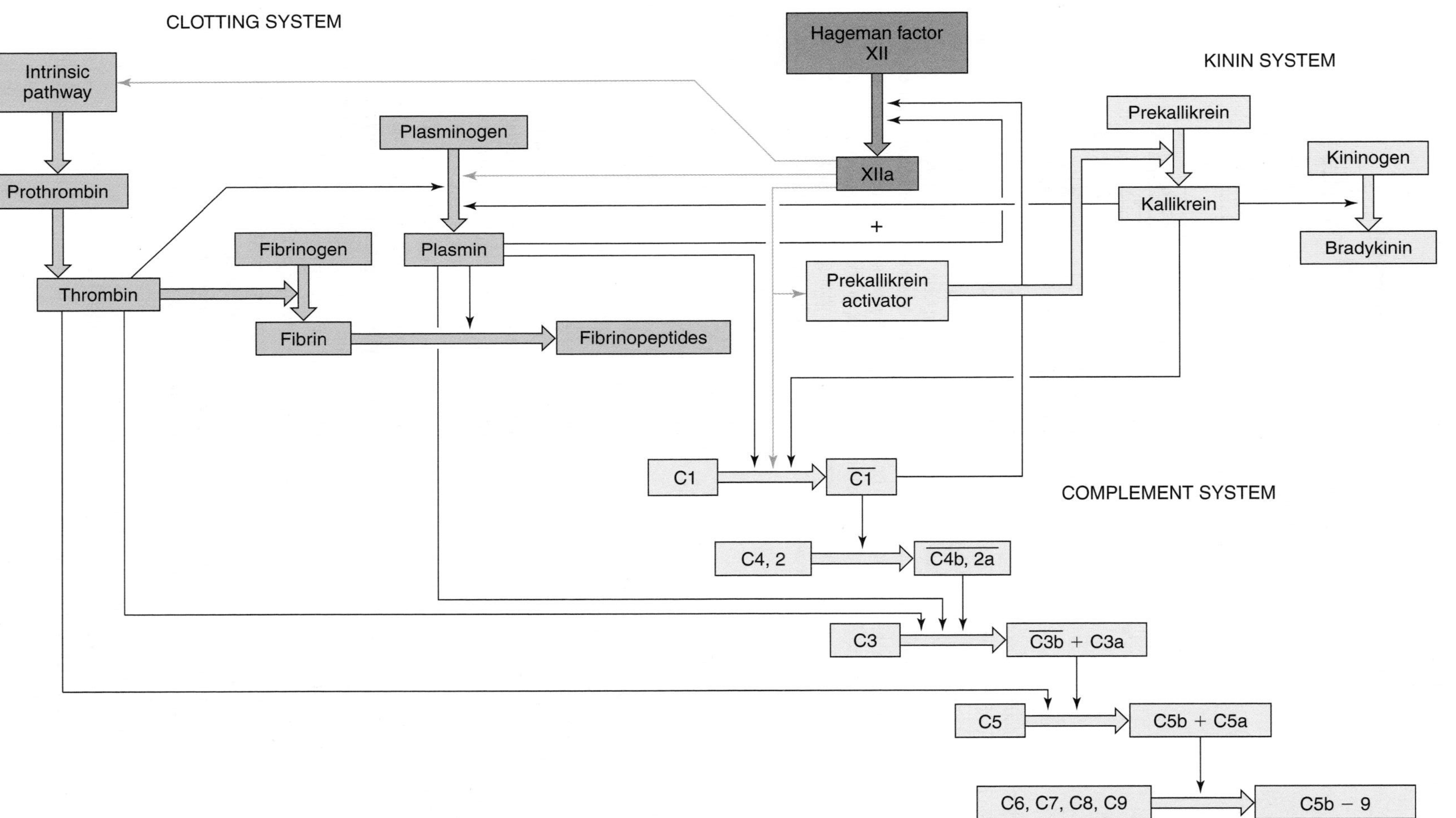

FIGURE 7-8 **Interactions Between the Complement, Clotting, and Kinin Systems.** *Thick colored arrows* denote the activation of factors within a system. *Thin arrows* denote where a particular factor activates another system.

a framework for future repair and healing. The main substance in this fibrinous mesh is an insoluble protein called *fibrin* that is the end product of the **coagulation cascade.**

The clotting system can be activated by many substances that are released during tissue injury and infection, including collagen, proteinases, kallikrein, and plasmin, as well as by bacterial products such as endotoxins. Like the complement cascade, the coagulation cascade can be activated through different convergent pathways (see Figure 7-6). The tissue factor (extrinsic) pathway is activated by tissue factor (TF) (also called tissue thromboplastin) that is released by damaged endothelial cells in blood vessels and reacts with activated factor VII (VIIa). The contact activation (intrinsic) pathway is activated when the vessel wall is damaged and Hageman factor (factor XII) in plasma contacts negatively charged subendothelial substances. The pathways converge at factor X. Activation of factor X begins a common pathway leading to activation of fibrin that polymerizes to form a fibrin clot. The coagulation system is discussed in more detail and illustrated again in Chapter 27.

As with the complement system, activation of the clotting system produces fragments that enhance the inflammatory response. Two low-molecular-weight fibrinopeptides, A and B, are released from fibrinogen when fibrin is produced. Both fibrinopeptides (especially fibrinopeptide B) are chemotactic for neutrophils and increase vascular permeability by enhancing the effects of bradykinin (formed from the kinin system).

Kinin System

The third plasma protein system, the **kinin system,** augments inflammation in several ways. The primary kinin produced from the kinin system is **bradykinin,** which causes dilation of blood vessels, acts with prostaglandins to stimulate nerve endings and induce pain, causes smooth muscle cell contraction, increases vascular permeability, and may increase leukocyte chemotaxis (see Figure 7-2). Bradykinin induces smooth muscle contraction more slowly than histamine and, along with prostaglandins of the E series, is probably responsible for endothelial cell retraction and increased vascular permeability in the later phases of inflammation (endothelial cell retraction is shown in Figures 7-3 and 7-15).

The kinin system is activated by stimulation of the **plasma kinin cascade** (see Figure 7-7). The conversion of plasma prekallikrein to kallikrein is induced by *prekallikrein activator,* which is identical to factor XIIa (the product that results from activation of Hageman factor—factor XII) of the clotting cascade. Kallikrein then converts kininogen to bradykinin. Although the plasma kinin cascade is one pathway that leads to the production of bradykinin, tissue kallikreins in saliva, sweat, tears, urine, and feces provide other sources for this inflammatory mediator. These tissue kallikreins convert serum kininogens to kallidin, also known as *Lys-bradykinin,* which may be converted to bradykinin by plasma aminopeptidase. In order to limit the extent of inflammation, kinins are rapidly degraded by **kininases,** enzymes present in plasma and tissues.

Interactions Among the Plasma Protein Systems

The three plasma protein systems are highly interactive so that activation of one system results in the production of a large number of very potent, biologically active substances that further activate the other systems (Figure 7-8). Very tight control of these processes is essential for two reasons:

1. The inflammatory process is critical for an individual's survival; thus, efficient activation must be guaranteed regardless of the cause of tissue injury.
2. The biochemical mediators generated during these processes are so potent and potentially detrimental to the host itself that their actions must be strictly confined to injured or infected tissues only.

Therefore, multiple mechanisms are available to either *activate* or *inactivate (regulate)* these plasma protein systems. As an example, **plasmin** regulates clot formation by degrading fibrin and fibrinogen, and it can activate the complement cascade through components C1, C3, and C5. Plasmin can activate the plasma kinin cascade as well by activating **Hageman factor (factor XII)** and producing prekallikrein activator. This activation of Hageman factor has four effects that impact all three of the plasma protein systems:

1. Activation of the clotting cascade through factor XI
2. Control of clotting through conversion of plasminogen proactivator to plasminogen activator, resulting in the generation of plasmin
3. Activation of the kinin system by activated Hageman factor (prekallikrein activator)
4. Activation of C1 in the complement cascade

The activity of plasmin itself is also regulated because it is synthesized as a proenzyme, plasminogen. Plasminogen is converted to plasmin by several factors, including plasminogen activator generated from the kallikrein system, thrombin generated from the clotting system, bacterial factors such as streptokinase produced by hemolytic streptococci, plasminogen activators produced by endothelial cells, and several cellular enzymes released during tissue destruction.

Many enzymes from the plasma regulate the activity of these pathways, such as carboxypeptidase that inactivates the anaphylatoxic activities of C3a and C5a, and kininases that degrade kinins. Many other natural inhibitors are present, including enzymes that degrade histamine (histaminase), activated complement components, kallikrein, and plasmin. Another example of a common regulator is **C1-esterase inhibitor (C1-inh).**[10] C1-inh inhibits complement activation through reactivity with C1 (classical pathway), MASP-2 (lectin pathway), and C3b (alternative pathway). It is also a major inhibitor of the clotting and kinin pathways (e.g., kallikrein, activated Hageman factor XIIa). A genetic defect in C1-inh (C1-inh deficiency) results in **hereditary angioedema,** which is a self-limiting edema of cutaneous and mucosal layers resulting from stress, illness, or relative minor or unapparent trauma. The disease is characterized by hyperactivation of all three plasma protein systems, although excessive production of bradykinin appears to be the principal cause of increased vascular permeability.

Cellular Mediators of Inflammation

Inflammation is a process in vascular tissue; thus the cellular components of inflammation are found in the blood and in the tissue surrounding the blood vessels. The vessels are lined with endothelial cells, which under normal conditions actively maintain normal blood flow. During inflammation the vascular endothelium becomes a principal coordinator of blood clotting and the passage of cells and fluid into the tissue. The tissue close to the vessels contains mast cells, which are probably the most important activators of inflammation. The tissue also contains dendritic cells, which connect the innate and adaptive immune responses. The blood contains a complex mixture of cells (see Figure 7-3). Blood cells are divided into erythrocytes (red blood cells), platelets, and leukocytes (white blood cells). Erythrocytes carry oxygen to the tissues, and platelets are small cell fragments involved in blood clotting. Leukocytes are subdivided into **granulocytes** (containing many enzyme-filled cytoplasmic granules), monocytes, and lymphocytes. Granulocytes are the most common leukocytes and are classified by the type of stains needed to visualize their granules (basophils, eosinophils, and neutrophils). Monocytes are precursors of macrophages that are found in the tissues. Various forms of lymphocytes participate in the innate (natural killer [NK] cells) and the adaptive immune response (B and T cells).

The cells of the inflammatory system secrete and respond to biochemical mediators. Thus most of these cells are recruited and activated by products of the plasma protein systems and by biochemicals released during cell destruction, secreted by other inflammatory cells, or produced by microbes. These inflammatory cells and protein systems, along with the substances they produce, preferably act at the site of tissue injury to confine the extent of damage, kill microorganisms, and remove the debris of "battle" in preparation for healing: tissue regeneration or repair (processes known as *resolution*).

Cellular Receptors

Cells of both innate and adaptive immunity must recognize and respond to their environment, whether to products of damaged cells or to potential pathogenic microorganisms. Each cell has receptors on the cell surface that specifically bind soluble substances (ligands) produced during tissue damage or infection. The binding of a ligand to its receptor results in activation of intracellular signaling pathways and activation of the cell. As will be discussed in Chapter 8, B and T lymphocytes of the adaptive immune system have evolved surface receptors (i.e., the T-cell receptor, or TCR, and the B-cell receptor, or BCR) that bind a large spectrum of antigens. Cells involved in innate resistance have evolved a different set of receptors that recognize a much more limited array of specific molecules. These are referred to as **pattern recognition receptors (PRRs),** and they recognize molecular "patterns" on infectious agents or their products **(pathogen-associated molecular patterns,** or **PAMPs),** or products of cellular damage (necrosis or apoptosis; **damage-associated molecular patterns,** or **DAMPs**). PRRs are generally found on cells at the interface of the host and environment (i.e., skin, respiratory tract, gastrointestinal tract, genitourinary tract), where they monitor for products of cellular damage and potentially infectious microorganisms. Although most PRRs are on the cell surface, some are secreted or intracellular.[11] An example of a secreted PRR is mannose-binding lectin of the lectin pathway of complement activation. Cellular PRRs include Toll-like receptors, complement receptors (CRs), scavenger receptors, glucan receptors, and mannose receptors. A group of intracellular protein complexes, called **inflammasomes,** function as PRRs within cells.[12] Inflammasomes primarily bind cellular stress–related molecules, a type of DAMPs, and control the production of interleukin-1β (IL-1β).[13]

In humans, at least 11 different **Toll-like receptors (TLRs)** have been described, 10 of which are functional.[14] They are expressed on the surface of many cells that have direct and early contact with potential pathogenic microorganisms. These include mucosal epithelial cells, mast cells, neutrophils, macrophages, dendritic cells, and some subpopulations of lymphocytes. (Dendritic cells are found in the skin, mucosa, and lymphoid tissues, where they have developed from Langerhans cells and function as highly specialized initiators of the adaptive immune response.) TLRs recognize a large variety of PAMPs located on the microorganism's cell wall or surface (e.g., bacterial lipopolysaccharide [LPS], peptidoglycans, and lipoproteins, yeast zymosan, viral coat proteins), other surface structures (e.g., bacterial flagellin), or microbial nucleic acid (e.g., bacterial DNA, viral double-stranded RNA). Some TLRs recognize host factors that are produced by "stressed" or damaged cells (e.g., breakdown products of extracellular matrix proteins, chromatin). Interactions between PAMPs and TLRs, with the collaboration of other cellular receptors (e.g., CD14), can result in activation of the cell and the release of soluble products (e.g., cytokines) that increase local resistance to the pathogenic microorganism. TLRs are also one of the bridges between innate resistance and the adaptive immune response through the induction of cytokines that increase the response of lymphocytes to foreign antigens on the pathogens. Genetic polymorphisms in TLRs may explain some observed differences among individuals' resistance and susceptibility to infections. Information on each of the TLRs found in humans is shown in Table 7-2.

Complement receptors are found on many cells of the innate and adaptive immune responses (e.g., granulocytes, monocytes/macrophages, lymphocytes, mast cells, erythrocytes, platelets), as well as some epithelial cells. They recognize several fragments produced through activation of the complement system. Under a variety of normal and disease-related conditions, immune complexes of antibody, antigen, and complement form in the blood and are removed by cells expressing surface complement receptor-1 (CR1), which binds to C4b, C3b, and C3b breakdown products (e.g., iC3b). CR2 is found on B lymphocytes, as well as dendritic cells and some epithelial cells, and recognizes C3b breakdown products (particularly iC3b). CR2 appears to facilitate B-cell function and antibody production. Both CR3 and CR4 are integrins that primarily recognize C3b breakdown products (particularly iC3b). CR3 (integrin αMβ2, also called CD11b/CD18) facilitates phagocytosis by neutrophils and monocytes/macrophages. CR4 (αXβ2, also called CD11c/CD18) is found primarily on platelets. (**Integrins** are cell surface receptors that have a role in cell adhesion and attachment and mediate intracellular signaling within the extracellular matrix [see Figure 1-14, p. 15].)

Scavenger receptors are primarily expressed on macrophages and facilitate recognition and phagocytosis of bacterial

TABLE 7-2 CELLULAR SOURCE AND MICROBIAL TARGET FOR EACH TOLL-LIKE RECEPTOR (TLR)

RECEPTOR	CELLULAR EXPRESSION PATTERN	PAMP RECOGNITION
TLR1	Cell surface (ubiquitous): neutrophils, monocytes/macrophages, dendritic cells, T cells, B cells, NK cells	Fungal, bacterial, viral; forms heterodimer with TLR2 (see TLR2 recognition)
TLR2	Cell surface: neutrophils, monocytes/macrophages, dendritic cells	Fungal (yeast zymosan), bacterial (gram-positive bacterial peptidoglycan, lipoproteins), viral (lipoproteins)
TLR3	Intracellular: monocytes/macrophages, dendritic cells, T cells, NK cells, epithelial cells	Double-stranded RNA produced by many viruses
TLR4	Cell surface: granulocytes, monocytes/macrophages, dendritic cells, T cells, B cells, epithelial cells	Bacterial (primarily gram-negative bacterial LPS, lipoteichoic acids), viral (RSV F protein, hepatitis C)
TLR5	Cell surface: granulocytes, monocytes/macrophages, dendritic cells, NK cells, epithelial cells	Bacterial (flagellin); forms heterodimer with TLR4
TLR6	Cell surface: monocytes/macrophages, dendritic cells, B cells, NK cells	Fungal, bacterial, viral; forms heterodimer with TLR2 (see TLR2 recognition)
TLR7	Intracellular: monocytes/macrophages, dendritic cells, B cells	Natural ligand uncertain; may bind viral single-strand RNA
TLR8	Cell surface: monocytes/macrophages, dendritic cells, NK cells	Natural ligand uncertain; may bind fungal PAMPs or viral single-stranded RNA
TLR9	Intracellular: monocytes/macrophages, dendritic cells, B cells	Bacterial (unmethylated DNA [CpG dinucleotides])
TLR10	Cell surface: monocytes/macrophages, dendritic cells, B cells	Natural ligand uncertain; may form heterodimers with TLR2
TLR11	TLR11 gene does not code a full length protein in humans	No known immune response

DNA, Deoxyribonucleic acid; *LPS,* lipopolysaccharide; *NK,* natural killer; *PAMPs,* pathogen-associated molecular patterns; *RNA,* ribonucleic acid; *RSV,* respiratory syncytial virus.

pathogens, as well as damaged cells and altered soluble lipoproteins associated with vascular damage (e.g., high-density lipoprotein [HDL], acetylated low-density lipoprotein [LDL], oxidized LDL). More than eight receptors have been identified. Some scavenger receptors (e.g., SR-PSOX) recognize the cell membrane phospholipid phosphatidylserine (PS). PS is normally sequestered on the cytoplasmic surface of the cell membrane, but is externalized under a very limited variety of conditions, including erythrocyte senescence and cellular apoptosis. Thus macrophages, through this receptor, can identify and remove old red blood cells and cells undergoing apoptosis. Another important scavenger receptor is CD14, which recognizes the complex of LPS and LPS-binding protein. LPS-binding protein is up-regulated during inflammation by the cytokines interleukin-6 (IL-6) and IL-1 and helps remove bacterial LPS (endotoxin) from the circulation.

Cellular Products

To elicit an effective inflammatory (or adaptive immune) response, it is necessary that many different kinds of cells cooperate. Many cells secrete soluble factors that contribute to the regulation of innate or adaptive resistance by affecting other neighboring cells (Figure 7-9). These factors are referred to as *chemokines* or **cytokines** and are either *proinflammatory* or *anti-inflammatory* in nature, depending on whether they respectively tend to induce or inhibit the inflammatory response. These molecules usually diffuse over short distances, bind to the appropriate target cells, and affect the function of the target cell. Some effects occur over long distances, such as the systemic induction of fever by some cytokines (i.e., endogenous pyrogens) that are produced at an inflammatory site. The binding of chemokines or cytokines to a target cell often induces synthesis of additional cellular products. For example, binding of the cytokine tumor necrosis factor-alpha (TNF-α) to a cell may result in synthesis and release of IL-1. Chemokine and cytokine binding is mediated through specific cell surface receptors that are themselves sometimes under the regulation of secreted cellular products.

The actions of chemokines and cytokines are *pleiotropic,* indicating that the same molecule may have a large variety of different biologic activities depending on the particular target cell to which it binds. In addition, the same molecule may be produced by a large spectrum of cells, many of which are not part of inflammation or the immune system. These molecules may be *synergistic,* so that their combined activity exceeds the sum of their individual activities, or have *antagonistic* properties that cause them to inhibit each other.[15] (A partial list of relevant cytokines is provided in Chapter 8, Table 8-5.)

Cytokines. The majority of important cytokines are classified as interleukins or interferons. Other critical cytokines, however, are not classified as either. Many of these same cytokines are produced by cells of the acquired immune system in response to specific antigens and are discussed further in Chapter 8.

The **interleukins (ILs)** are biochemical messengers produced predominantly by macrophages and lymphocytes in response to their recognition of a microorganism or stimulation by other products of inflammation. One important function of this class of cytokines is enhancement of the adaptive immune response against pathogenic microorganisms and other foreign substances. Interleukins, however, are both produced by and have effects on a large variety of cells, often independent of infection.

Two major proinflammatory cytokines are IL-1 and IL-6. IL-1 is produced mainly by macrophages that have been stimulated by substances associated with infection, including many of the PAMPs discussed earlier in this chapter, as well as by other cytokines. IL-1 is synthesized in two forms, α and β, that often elicit the same biologic responses. IL-1 is an endogenous pyrogen (i.e., fever-causing cytokine) that reacts with receptors on

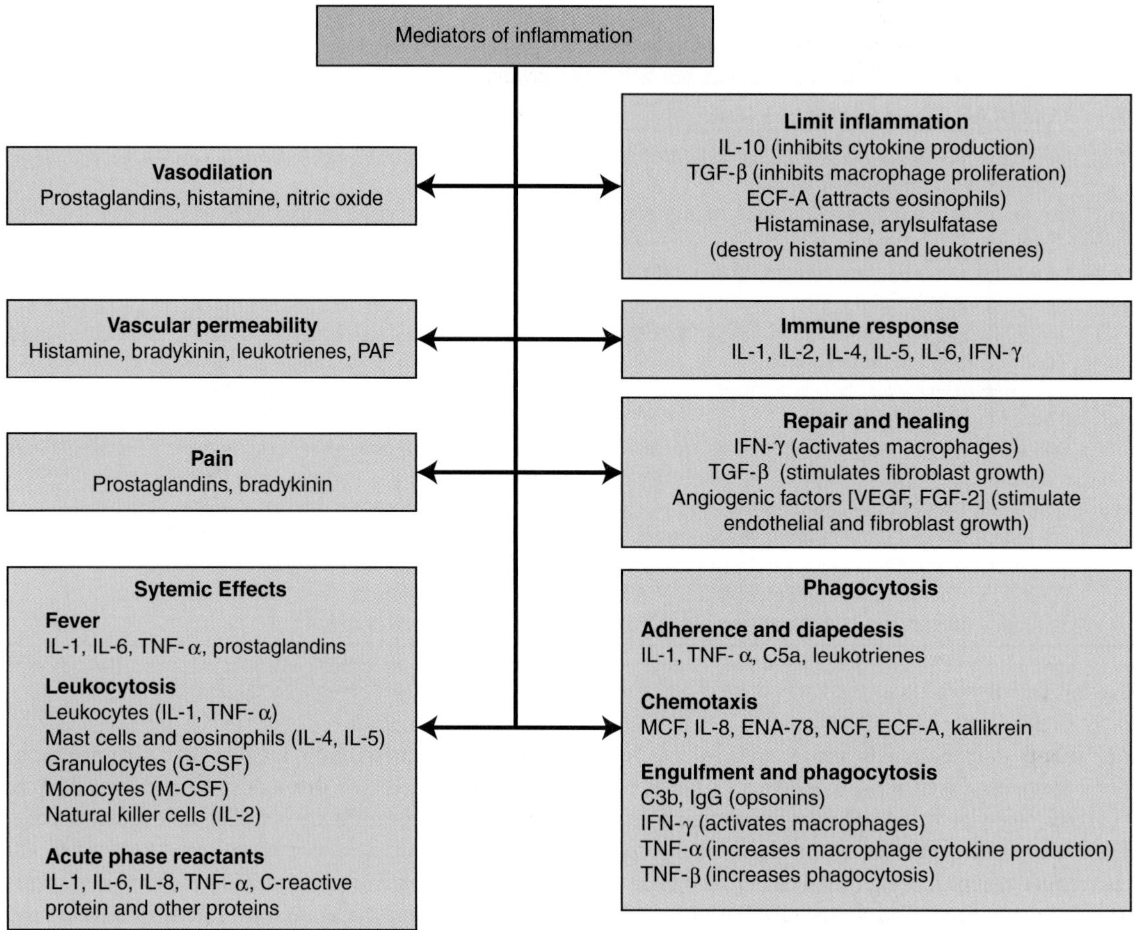

FIGURE 7-9 **Principal Mediators of Inflammation.** *C3b,* Large fragment produced from complement component C3; *C5a,* small fragment produced from complement component C5; *ECF-A,* eosinophil chemotactic factor of anaphylaxis; *ENA,* epithelial-dermoid neutrophil attractant; *FGF,* fibroblast growth factor; *G-CSF,* granulocyte colony-stimulating factor; *IFN,* interferon; *IgG,* immunoglobulin G (predominant class of antibody in the blood); *IL,* interleukin; *MCF,* monocyte chemotactic factor; *M-CSF,* monocyte colony-stimulating factor; *NCF,* neutrophil chemotactic factor; *PAF,* platelet-activating factor; *TGF,* T-cell growth factor; *TNF,* tumor necrosis factor; *VEGF,* vascular endothelial growth factor.

cells of the hypothalamus and affects the body's thermostat. It also activates phagocytes and lymphocytes, thereby enhancing both innate and adaptive immunity, and acts as a growth factor for many cells. It has several effects on neutrophils, including induction of proliferation (resulting in an increase in the number of circulating neutrophils), chemotaxis, increased cellular respiration, and increased lysosomal enzyme activity. IL-6 is produced by macrophages, lymphocytes, fibroblasts, and other cells. IL-6 directly induces hepatocytes (liver cells) to produce many of the proteins needed in inflammation (acute-phase reactants, discussed later in this chapter). IL-6 also stimulates growth and differentiation of blood cells in the bone marrow and the growth of fibroblasts (required for wound healing).

Some cytokines are anti-inflammatory and diminish the inflammatory response. The most important are IL-10 and transforming growth factor-beta (TGF-β). IL-10 is primarily produced by lymphocytes and suppresses the growth of lymphocytes and the production of proinflammatory cytokines by macrophages, leading to the down-regulation of both inflammation and the adaptive immune response. TGF-β and other transforming growth factors are produced by many types of cells in response to inflammation and induce differentiation of other cell types, such as immature blood cells.

More than 30 human interleukins have been identified, although the functions of several have not yet been defined. Their varied effects include the following:

1. Alteration of adhesion molecule expression on many types of cells
2. Induction of leukocyte chemotaxis
3. Induction of proliferation and maturation of leukocytes in the bone marrow
4. General enhancement or suppression of inflammation (see Table 8-5)

Interferons (IFNs) are low-molecular-weight proteins that primarily protect against viral infections and modulate the inflammatory response. (Mechanisms of viral infection are described in Chapter 10.) IFNs are produced and released by virally infected cells in response to viral double-stranded RNA and other viral PAMPs. Different kinds of IFNs are produced by different types of cells—macrophages are the primary producers of type I interferons (IFN-α and IFN-β), whereas T lymphocytes release type II interferon (IFN-γ). These IFNs do not kill

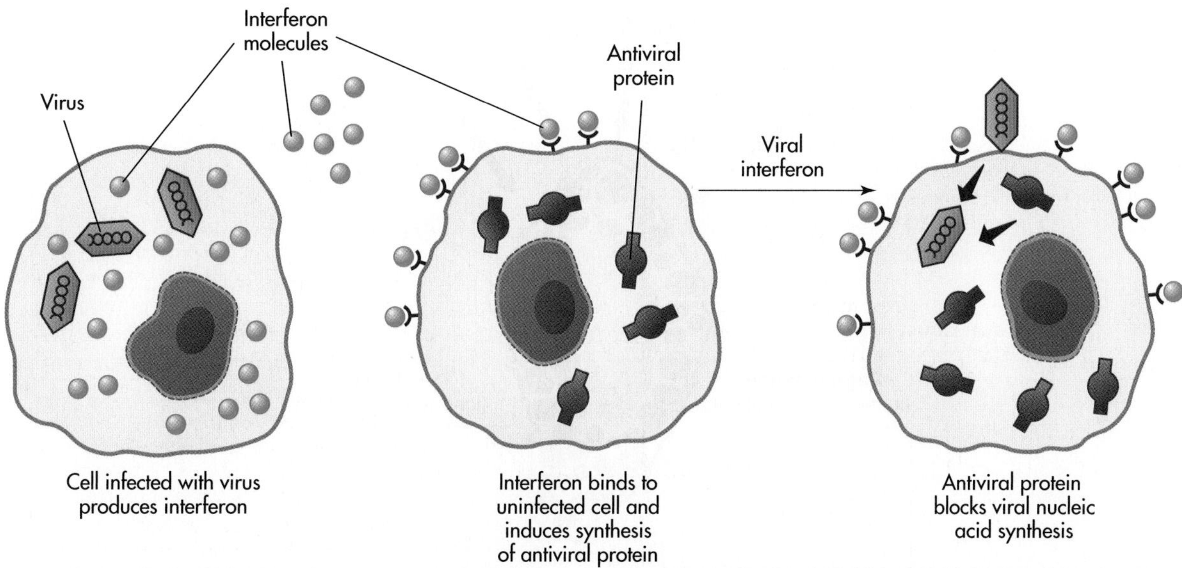

FIGURE 7-10 The Action of Interferon.

viruses directly but instead prevent them from infecting additional healthy cells.[16] Interferons also enhance the efficiency of developing an adaptive immune response.[17]

IFN-α and IFN-β induce production of antiviral proteins, thereby conferring protection on uninfected cells. IFN-α or IFN-β is released from virally infected cells, attaches to a receptor on a neighboring cell, and, if the neighboring cell is uninfected, stimulates the production of a variety of antiviral proteins that will interfere with transcription of viral nucleic acids or with viral replication[18] (Figure 7-10). These interferons have no effect on cells that have already been virally infected. IFN-γ enhances the inflammatory response by increasing the microbicidal activity of macrophages. This cytokine also facilitates development of the adaptive immune response against viral antigens on infected cells. Interferons are species specific, meaning that human interferon is effective only in humans; however, these cytokines are not virus specific, meaning that they are effective against almost all viruses.

Despite the numerous interleukins and interferons, other essential cytokines are needed to mount an efficient inflammatory response. One of the most important of these is **tumor necrosis factor-alpha (TNF-α).**[19] Macrophages secrete TNF-α in response to recognition of PAMPs by TLRs. Other cells, such as mast cells, are additional and crucial sources of this proinflammatory cytokine. TNF-α is initially synthesized as a membrane-spanning protein, which is cleaved into a soluble form by a membrane-associated protease, TNF-converting enzyme (TACE). Soluble TNF-α induces a multitude of proinflammatory effects, including enhancement of endothelial cell adhesion molecule expression and induction of chemokine production by both endothelial cells and macrophages. When secreted in large amounts, TNF-α has systemic effects as well:

1. Induces fever by acting as an endogenous pyrogen
2. Causes increased synthesis of proinflammatory proteins by the liver
3. Causes muscle wasting (cachexia) and intravascular thrombosis as a consequence of prolonged production in cases of severe infection or cancer
4. Probably responsible for fatalities from shock caused by gram-negative bacterial infections

Chemokines. **Chemokines** are members of a family of low-molecular-weight (8 to 10 kDa) peptides that function primarily to induce leukocyte chemotaxis. This response can be elicited either by soluble chemokines or by chemokines that are bound to extracellular glycosaminoglycan carbohydrates. Chemokines can be synthesized by multiple cell types, including macrophages, fibroblasts, and endothelial cells, in response to proinflammatory cytokines. Macrophages can be stimulated to produce chemokines by recognition of either infectious microorganisms or a β-defensin (both through TLR4). To date, more than 40 different human chemokines have been described, the vast majority of which are classified as either CC-chemokines (β-chemokines) or CXC-chemokines (α-chemokines), depending on the arrangement of cysteine amino acids in the protein. This amino acid arrangement also determines which target cell(s) will respond to a given chemokine. CC-chemokines affect mainly monocytes, lymphocytes, and eosinophils, whereas CXC-chemokines generally affect neutrophils. Examples of CC-chemokines include RANTES (regulated on activation, normal T expressed and secreted), monocyte/macrophage chemotactic proteins (MCP-1, MCP-2, and MCP-3), and macrophage inflammatory proteins (MIP-1α and MIP-1β). CXC-chemokines include IL-8 and epithelial-dermoid neutrophil attractant (ENA-78).

Mast Cells

A central cell in inflammation is the mast cell. **Mast cells,** first described by Paul Ehrlich[20] in 1877, are cellular bags of granules located in the loose connective tissues close to blood vessels (Figure 7-11). They are found in large numbers in areas directly exposed to the environment including the skin and the linings of the gastrointestinal and respiratory tracts. A great number of stimuli cause mast cells to become activated, resulting in initiation of the inflammatory response.[21] Typical causes of mast cell activation include (1) physical injury (e.g., heat,

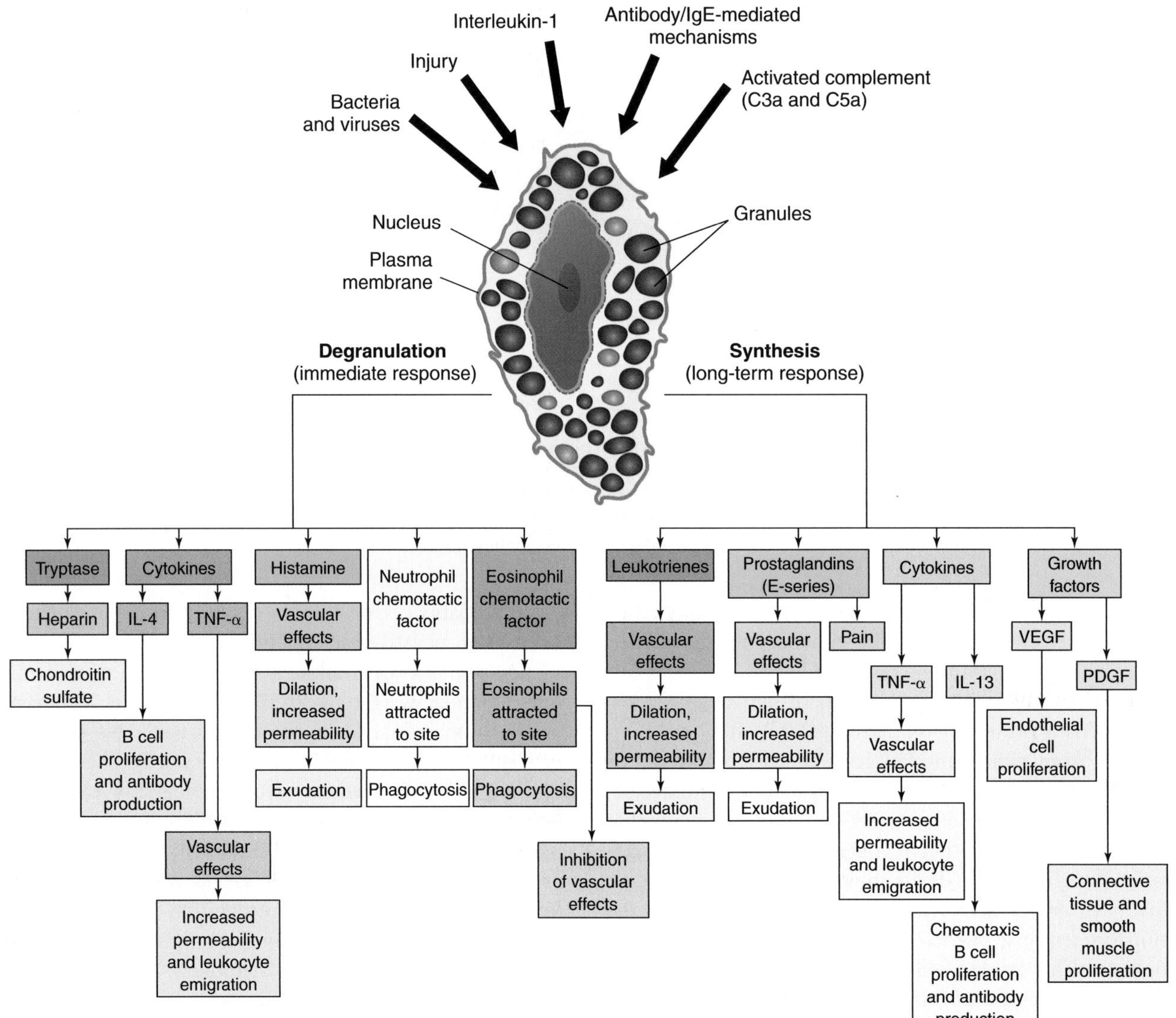

FIGURE 7-11 Effects of Degranulation *(left)* and Synthesis *(right)* by Mast Cells. The depiction of a tissue mast cell shows darkly stained granules in the cytoplasm. *IL-4,* Interleukin-4; *IL-13,* interleukin-13; *PDGF,* platelet-derived growth factor; *TNF-α,* tumor necrosis factor-alpha; *VEGF,* vascular endothelial growth factor.

mechanical trauma, ultraviolet light, and x-rays), (2) chemical agents (e.g., toxins, snake and bee venoms, proteolytic enzymes, and antimicrobial peptides), (3) immunologic means (e.g., anaphylatoxins released during activation of complement components or particular types of antibody [e.g., immunoglobulin E (IgE)] produced by cells of the adaptive immune response [see Chapter 8]), and (4) activation of TLRs by bacteria and viruses. Soluble and extremely potent chemicals from the mast cell are responsible for its effects on inflammation. These are released in two ways: by release of the contents of their preformed granules *(degranulation)* and by new synthesis of lipid-derived inflammatory mediators. Mast cells are also involved in initiating many allergic responses (discussed in Chapters 8 and 9).

Mast Cell Degranulation. In response to a stimulus, biochemical mediators in the mast cell granules, including histamine, chemotactic factors (e.g., neutrophil chemotactic factor, **eosinophil chemotactic factor of anaphylaxis** or **ECF-A**), and cytokines (e.g., TNF-α, IL-4), are released within seconds and exert their effects immediately (see Figure 7-11).

Histamine is a vasoactive amine that causes temporary, rapid constriction of the large vessel walls and dilation of the postcapillary venules, both of which result in increased blood flow into the microcirculation. Histamine also causes increased vascular permeability resulting from retraction of endothelial cells lining the capillaries (see Figure 7-3). The pharmacologic effects of histamine are partially determined by histamine receptors on the person's target cells. Two main histamine receptors are the H1 and H2 receptors (Figure 7-12), and two other receptors, H3 and H4, have been described. Binding of histamine to the *H1 receptor* is essentially proinflammatory; that is, it promotes inflammation. On the other hand, binding to the *H2 receptor* is generally anti-inflammatory because it results in suppression of leukocyte function. The H1 receptor is present on smooth muscle cells, especially those of the bronchi, and causes bronchial smooth

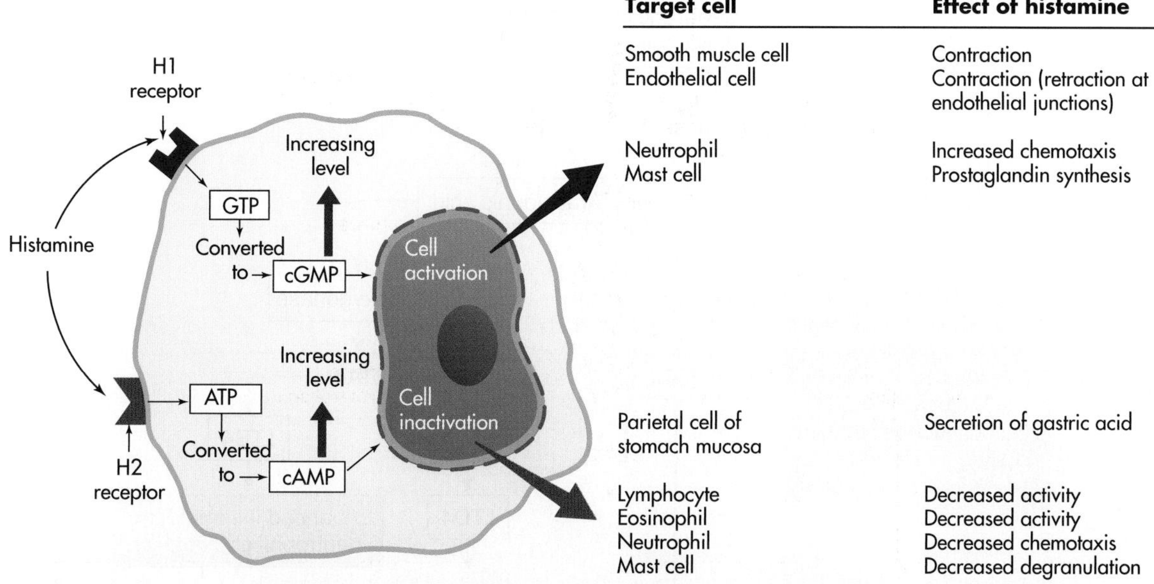

FIGURE 7-12 Effects of Histamine Through H1 and H2 Receptors. Effects depend on (1) density and affinity of H1 or H2 receptors on the target cell, and (2) the identity of the target cell. *ATP,* Adenosine triphosphate; *cAMP,* cyclic adenosine monophosphate; *cGMP,* cyclic guanosine monophosphate; *GTP,* guanosine triphosphate.

muscle to contract (bronchoconstriction) when stimulated. Both types of receptors are distributed among many different cells and are often present on the same cells and may act in an antagonistic fashion. For instance, neutrophils express both types of receptors, with stimulation of H1 receptors resulting in the augmentation of neutrophil chemotaxis, and H2 stimulation resulting in its inhibition. The H2 receptor is especially abundant on parietal cells of the stomach mucosa and induces the secretion of gastric acid as part of the normal physiology of the stomach. The role of H1 and H2 receptors is discussed further in Chapter 9.

Two chemotactic factors, neutrophil chemotactic factor and ECF-A, are also released during mast cell degranulation. **Chemotaxis** is directional movement of cells along a chemical gradient formed by a chemotactic factor (see Figure 7-3). **Neutrophil chemotactic factor** attracts neutrophils, and ECF-A attracts eosinophils to the site of inflammation. Neutrophils are the predominant leukocytes at work during the early phases of acute inflammation, and eosinophils have several functions in the inflammatory process; both of these important inflammatory cells are discussed in more detail later in this chapter.

Mast Cell Synthesis of Mediators. Activated mast cells begin new synthesis of other mediators of inflammation, including those derived from plasma membrane lipids, cytokines (TNF-α, various interleukins), and factors that stimulate cell growth and angiogenesis. Leukotrienes, prostaglandins, and platelet-activating factor are lipid-derived products that are synthesized during mast cell activation (Figure 7-13). Leukotrienes are a product of another lipid, arachidonic acid, which is released from mast cell membranes by an intracellular phospholipase that acts on membrane phospholipids.[22] **Leukotrienes** are acidic, sulfur-containing lipids that produce effects similar to those of histamine, namely, smooth muscle contraction, increased vascular permeability, and perhaps neutrophil and eosinophil chemotaxis. Leukotrienes appear to be important in the later stages of the inflammatory response because they stimulate slower and more prolonged responses than do histamines.[23]

The mast cell also synthesizes **prostaglandins,** which, like leukotrienes, are a product of arachidonic acid and cause increased vascular permeability and neutrophil chemotaxis. Prostaglandins also induce pain. They are long-chain unsaturated fatty acids produced by the action of the enzyme *cyclooxygenase* and are classified into groups (E, D, A, F, and B) according to their structure. Prostaglandins E_1 and E_2 cause increased vascular permeability and smooth muscle contraction, apparently acting directly on postcapillary venules.[24] They can inhibit some aspects of inflammation by suppressing both the release of histamine from mast cells and the release of lysosomal enzymes (enzymes responsible for killing and digesting microorganisms) from neutrophils. Enhancement or suppression of the inflammatory response may be related to the concentration of prostaglandins. Aspirin and some other nonsteroidal anti-inflammatory drugs (NSAIDs) block the synthesis of prostaglandins of the E series and other arachidonic acid derivatives, thereby inhibiting inflammation.

Platelet-activating factor (PAF), another mast cell–derived lipid, is produced by removal of a fatty acid from the plasma membrane phospholipid phosphatidylcholine by phospholipase A_2. Although mast cells are a major source of PAF, this molecule also can be produced during inflammation by neutrophils, monocytes, endothelial cells, and platelets. The biologic activity of PAF is virtually identical to that of leukotrienes, namely, causing endothelial cell retraction to increase vascular permeability, leukocyte adhesion to endothelial cells, and platelet activation.

Endothelium

The blood vessel walls consist of a layer of endothelial cells that adhere to an underlying matrix of connective tissue that

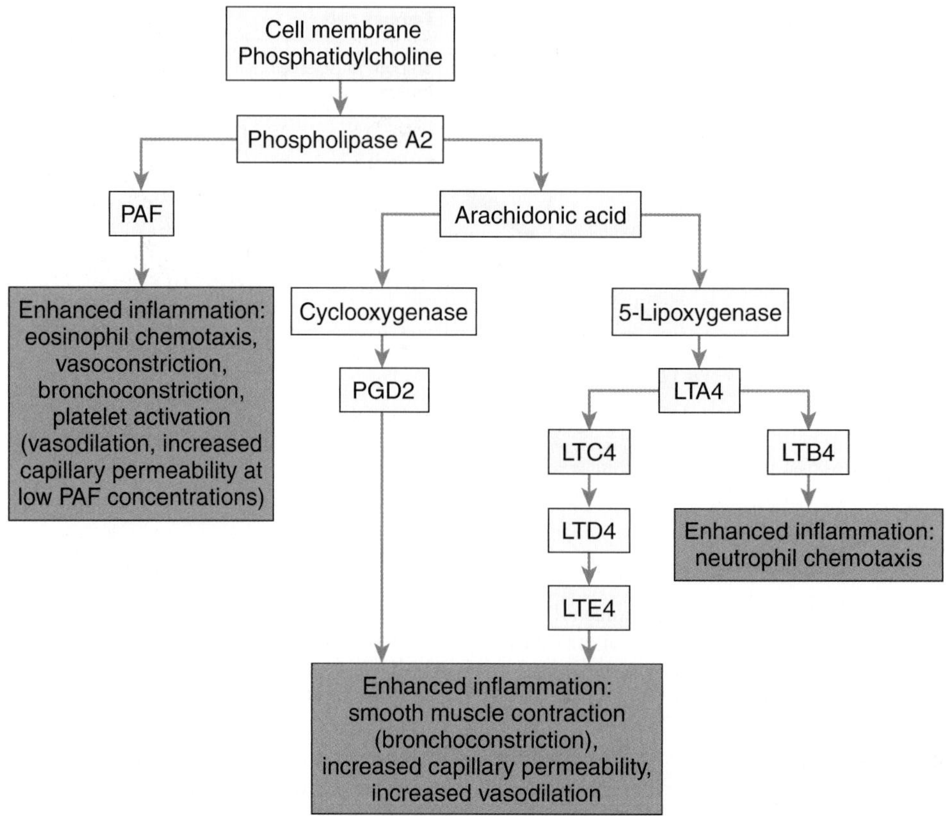

FIGURE 7-13 Production of Lipid Vasoactive Substances by Mast Cells. *LTA4, LTC4, LTD4, LTE4, LTB4,* Various leukotriene molecules; *PAF,* platelet-activating factor; *PGD2,* prostaglandin D2.

contains a variety of proteins, including collagen, fibronectin, and laminins. Circulating cells and platelets and components of plasma protein systems continually contact endothelial cells, which contribute to regulation of normal blood flow by preventing spontaneous activation of platelets and members of the clotting system. Endothelial cells produce nitric oxide (NO) from arginine and prostacyclin (PGI_2) from arachidonic acid. Both NO and PGI_2 maintain blood flow and pressure and inhibit platelet activation. PGI_2 and NO are synergistic. NO is released continually to relax vascular smooth muscle and suppress the effects of low levels of cytokines, thus maintaining vascular tone. PGI_2 production varies a great deal and is increased when additional regulation is needed.

Damage to the endothelial cell lining of the vessel exposes the subendothelial connective tissue matrix, which is prothrombogenic, and initiates platelet activation and formation of clots (the contact activation [intrinsic] clotting pathway). Proinflammatory cytokines affect the endothelium, resulting in adherence of leukocytes to the vessel surface, invasion of leukocytes into the tissue, and efflux of plasma from the vessel.

Platelets

Platelets (thrombocytes) are cellular fragments formed from megakaryocytes. They circulate in the bloodstream until vascular injury occurs, after which platelets can be activated by many products of both the innate and the adaptive immune responses, including collagen, thrombin, thromboxane, PAF, and antigen-antibody complexes.[25] Activation results in (1) the interaction of platelets with components of the coagulation cascade to stop bleeding, and (2) degranulation. Platelets contain alpha (α) granules and dense granules. *Alpha granules* generally contain polypeptides that affect inflammation, including coagulation proteins (e.g., fibrinogen, factor V), soluble adhesion molecules (e.g., von Willebrand factor, vitronectin), growth factors (e.g., platelet-derived growth factor, epidermal growth factor), protease inhibitors (e.g., plasminogen activator inhibitor-1, α_2-antiplasmin), and membrane adhesion molecules (e.g., P-selectin, αIIbβ3). *Dense granules* contain several small molecules, including adenosine diphosphate (ADP), serotonin, calcium, and magnesium. Serotonin is a vasoactive amine with vascular effects similar to those of histamine. (Platelet function is described in detail in Chapter 27.)

Phagocytes

The primary role of most granulocytes (neutrophils, eosinophils, basophils) and monocytes/macrophages is **phagocytosis;** the process by which a cell ingests and disposes of damaged cells and foreign material, including microorganisms.

Neutrophils. The **neutrophil,** or **polymorphonuclear neutrophil (PMN),** is a member of the granulocytic series named for the characteristic staining pattern of its granules as well as its multilobed nucleus. Neutrophils are the predominant **phagocytes** in the early inflammatory site, arriving within 6 to 12 hours after the initial injury, where they ingest (phagocytose) bacteria, dead cells, and cellular debris. Several inflammatory mediators (e.g., some bacterial proteins, complement fragments

C3a and C5a, and mast cell neutrophil chemotactic factor) specifically attract neutrophils from the circulation and activate them. Macrophages and lymphocytes, on the other hand, enter the site later, usually after 24 hours, and gradually replace the neutrophils.

Because the neutrophil is a mature cell incapable of division and sensitive to the acidic environment of inflammatory lesions, it is short-lived at the inflammatory site and becomes a component of the purulent exudate, or *pus,* which is removed from the body through the epithelium or through the lymphatic system. (The lymphatic system is described in Chapter 27.) The primary roles of the neutrophil are removal of debris in sterile lesions, such as burns, and phagocytosis of bacteria in nonsterile lesions.

Eosinophils. Another population of granulocytes is the **eosinophil.** Eosinophils have two specific functions: (1) they serve as the body's primary defense against parasites and (2) they help regulate vascular mediators released from mast cells. Their role in resistance to parasites occurs in collaboration with specific antibodies produced by the adaptive immune system and will be discussed in Chapter 8.

The second function, regulation of mast cell–derived inflammatory mediators, is a critical function of eosinophils. As with most defense systems of the body, the acute inflammatory response is usually needed only in a circumscribed area and for a limited time. Therefore, control mechanisms are necessary to prevent biochemical mediators from evoking more inflammation than is needed. Mast cells produce ECF-A, which attracts eosinophils to the site of inflammation. Eosinophil lysosomes contain several enzymes that degrade vasoactive molecules, thereby controlling the vascular effects of inflammation. These enzymes include histaminase, which mediates the degradation of histamine, and arylsulfatase B, which mediates the degradation of some of the lipid-derived mediators produced by mast cells.

Basophils. The **basophil** is the least prevalent granulocyte in the blood. It is very similar to mast cells in the content of its granules and, in addition, is an important source of the cytokine IL-4, which is a key regulator of the adaptive immune response. Although often associated with allergies and asthma, its primary role is yet unknown.

Monocytes and Macrophages. **Monocytes** are the largest normal blood cells (14 to 20 μm in diameter) and have a nucleus that is often indented, or horseshoe shaped. Monocytes are produced in the bone marrow, enter the circulation, and migrate to the inflammatory site where they develop into macrophages. Monocytes also appear to be the precursors of macrophages that are found in tissues (tissue macrophages, discussed in Chapter 8), including Kupffer's cells in the liver, alveolar macrophages in the lungs, and microglia in the brain.[26] **Macrophages** are generally larger (20 to 40 μm) and are more active as phagocytes than their monocytic precursors. Macrophages, particularly those residing in the tissues, are often important cellular initiators of the inflammatory response (Figure 7-14).

Phagocytosis. Because most phagocytes are circulating in the blood, they must leave the bloodstream and migrate to the site of inflammation before initiating phagocytosis (Figure 7-15). Under normal conditions, the circulation in the capillaries and venules is rapidly moving with red blood cells in the main stream and neutrophils and other leukocytes tending to flow more slowly along the vessel's periphery. Many of the biochemical products produced early at inflammatory sites (e.g., histamine, TNF-α, bradykinin, leukotrienes, prostaglandins) diffuse to the vessels and affect both leukocytes and endothelial cells. Both cell populations respond by producing new **adhesion molecules** (selectins and integrins) on their surfaces (Table 7-3) (see p. 202 for integrins). **Selectins** are adhesion molecules that bind carbohydrate ligands. The reciprocal change in adhesion molecules on leukocytes, as well as platelets, promotes their interaction with the endothelial cells. The initial change of surface molecules increases the adhesion, or stickiness, between leukocytes and endothelial cells, causing the leukocytes to adhere more avidly to the walls of the capillaries and venules in a process called **margination,** or **pavementing.** Adhesion molecules that are expressed later lead to **diapedesis,** or emigration of the cells through the endothelial junctions that have retracted in response to the same mediators. The leukocytes digest the basement membrane and migrate into the surrounding tissues.

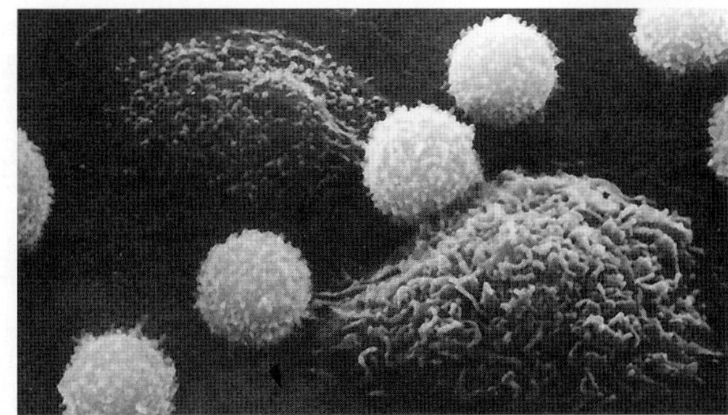

FIGURE 7-14 Scanning Electron Micrograph of Lymphocytes and Macrophages. The lymphocytes are small and spherical; the macrophages are larger and more irregular in shape. (From Raven PH, Johnson GB: *Biology,* St Louis, 1992, Mosby.)

Additionally, **endothelial cells** release NO, a gas that under normal conditions maintains vascular tone. Inflammation induces additional endothelial nitric oxide synthase, increasing the amount of NO production. Effects of NO on inflammation include vasodilation by inducing relaxation of vascular smooth muscle, a response that is local and short-lived, and suppression of mast cell function as well as platelet adhesion and aggregation.

Once inside the connective tissue in the perivascular space, leukocytes migrate to the inflammatory site by means of chemotaxis. They detect chemotactic factors in the environment through chemoreceptors at multiple locations on their plasma membranes and migrate in the direction of highest concentration (see Figure 7-15). The primary chemotactic factors include many bacterial products, complement fragments C3a and C5a, kallikrein, plasminogen activator, products of fibrin degradation (fibrinopeptides), and chemokines. Eosinophils and neutrophils also respond to chemotactic factors

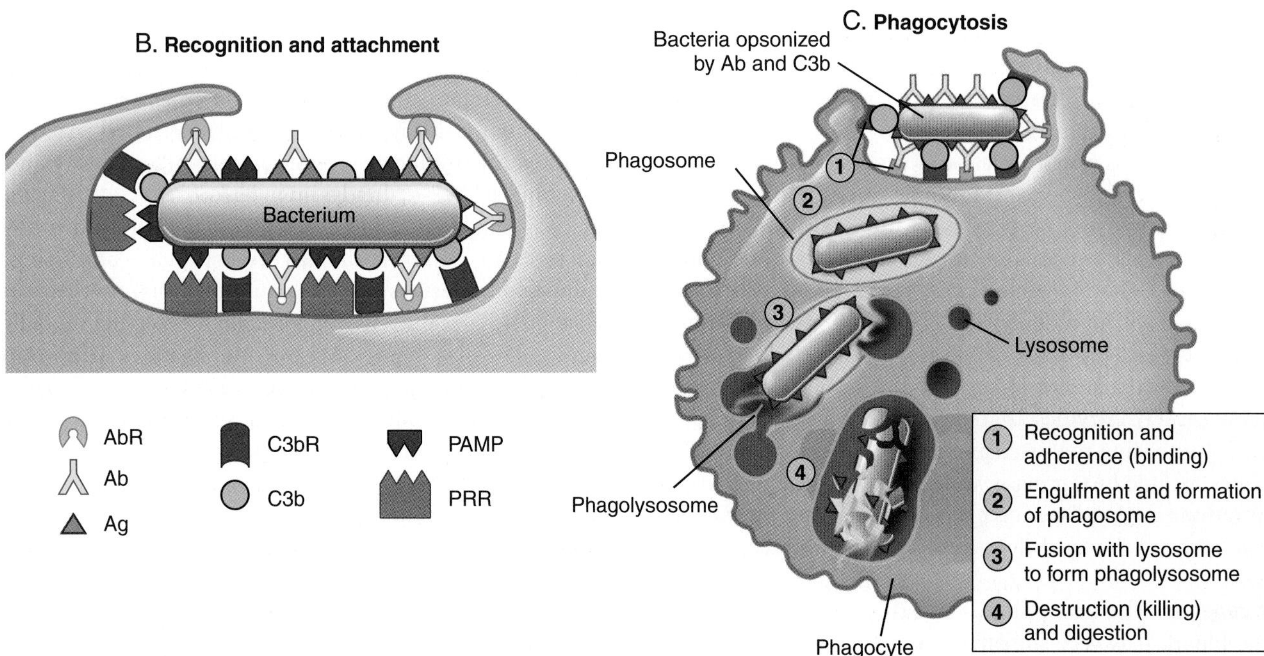

FIGURE 7-15 Process of Phagocytosis. The process that results in phagocytosis is characterized by three interrelated steps: adherence and diapedesis, tissue invasion by chemotaxis, and phagocytosis. **A, Tissue damage.** *Adherence, margination, and diapedesis:* The primary phagocyte in the blood is the neutrophil, which usually moves freely within the vessel **(1).** At sites of inflammation, the neutrophil progressively develops increased adherence to the endothelium, leading to accumulation along the vessel wall (margination or pavementing) **(2).** At sites of endothelial cell retraction the neutrophil exits the blood by means of diapedesis **(3).** *Chemotaxis:* In the tissues, the neutrophil detects chemotactic factor gradients through surface receptors **(1)** and migrates towards higher concentrations of the factors **(2).** The high concentration of chemotactic factors at the site of inflammation immobilizes the neutrophil **(3).** **B, Recognition and attachment.** *Specific receptors and ligands for recognition and attachment.* **C, Phagocytosis. (1)** Opsonized microorganisms bind to the surface of a phagocyte through specific receptors. **(2)** The microorganism is engulfed (ingested) into a phagocytic vacuole, or phagosome. **(3)** Lysosomes fuse with the phagosome, resulting in the formation of a phagolysosome. During this process the microorganism is exposed to products of the lysosomes, including a variety of enzymes and products of the hexose-monophosphate shunt (e.g., H_2O_2, O_2^-). **(4)** The microorganism is killed and digested. *Ab,* Antibody; *AbR,* antibody receptor; *Ag,* antigen; *C3b,* complement component C3b; *C3bR,* complement C3b receptor; *PAMP,* pathogen-associated molecular pattern; *PRR,* pattern recognition receptor.

released from mast cells (ECF-A, neutrophil chemotactic factor [NCF]). Monocytes are attracted toward a factor (monocyte chemotactic factor) that has been released by neutrophils already at the site of injury. And although histamine is not itself chemotactic, it may facilitate the chemotactic effects of other factors.

Once the phagocytic cell enters the inflammatory site, the process of phagocytosis involves four steps: (1) *opsonization (recognition* of the target and *adherence* of the phagocyte to it); (2) *engulfment* (ingestion or endocytosis) and *formation of phagosome;* (3) *fusion* with lysosomal granules within the phagocyte (phagolysosome); and (4) *destruction* of the target

TABLE 7-3 EXAMPLES OF CELLULAR ADHESION MOLECULES (CAMS) INVOLVED IN LEUKOCYTE INTERACTION WITH ENDOTHELIAL CELLS

	ACTIVITY OF LEUKOCYTE		
	"ROLLING" LOW AFFINITY	"MARGINATION" FIRM ATTACHMENT	"DIAPEDESIS"
Leukocyte adhesion molecule	L-selectin	Integrin α4β1 (VLA-4) Integrin α4β7	Integrin αLβ2 (LFA-1) Integrin αMβ2 (MAC-1) PCAM-1
Endothelial adhesion molecule	P-selectin E-selectin	VCAM-1	ICAM-1 ICAM-2 PCAM-1

Selectins (lectin-like molecules): *L-selectin,* leukocyte selectin; *P-selectin,* platelet selectin; *E-selectin,* endothelial selectin.
Integrins (noncovalent heterodimers of alpha [α] and beta [β] subunits): *VLA-4,* very late antigen-4; *LFA-1,* lymphocyte function antigen-1; *MAC-1,* macrophage antigen-1.
Immunoglobulin-like molecules: VCAM-1, vascular cell adhesion molecule-1; *ICAM-1, ICAM-2,* immunoglobulin-like molecules-1 and -2; *PCAM-1,* platelet-endothelial cell adhesion molecule-1.

(see Figure 7-15, *C*) (lysosomes are described in Chapter 1). Throughout the process, both the target and the digestive enzymes are isolated within membrane-bound vesicles. Isolation protects the phagocyte itself from the harmful effects of the target microorganisms, as well as its own enzymes.

Most phagocytes can trap and engulf bacteria using cellular PRRs and PAMPs normally expressed on the bacterial surface (see Figure 7-15, *B*). However, that process is slow and inefficient. Opsonization, usually by antibody or complement component C3b, greatly enhances both recognition and adherence. Phagocytosis of an opsonized (antibody and/or complement-protein coated) red blood cell is illustrated in Figure 7-16. Opsonins function as "glue" between the phagocyte and the target cell because receptors on the phagocyte are specific for sites on the opsonin (Fc receptors for antibody, C3b receptors for C3b). This enables the phagocyte to bind an opsonized target very tightly to its surface. Antibody forms a stronger attachment, but C3b facilitates phagocytosis to a greater extent.

Although the inflammatory response is considered to be nonspecific, opsonins and other recognition molecules add a degree of specificity to efficient phagocytosis. Antibodies on the surface of bacteria are directed against antigens that are highly specific to that particular microorganism. If the complement fragment C3b serves as an opsonin, those bacteria with certain polysaccharide coatings are particularly sensitive to activation of the alternative and lectin pathways of complement activation.

Engulfment (endocytosis) is carried out by small pseudopods that extend from the plasma membrane and surround the adherent microorganism (see Figures 7-15 and 7-16), forming an intracellular phagocytic vacuole, or **phagosome.** The membrane that surrounds the phagosome consists of inverted plasma membrane. After the formation of the phagosome, lysosomes converge, fuse with the phagosome, and discharge their contents, creating a **phagolysosome.** The **primary lysosomal granules** *(azurophilic granules)* contain a variety of bactericidal molecules, including myeloperoxidase, lysozyme, defensins, acid hydrolases, elastase, and others. Most phagocytes also contain **secondary granules** *(specific granules)* with molecules that are bactericidal and involved in remodeling the surrounding tissue, including lysozyme, collagenase, lactoferrin, and other proteases. Destruction of the bacterium takes place within the phagolysosome and is accomplished by both oxygen-dependent and oxygen-independent mechanisms.

Phagocytosis is accompanied by a burst of oxygen uptake by the phagocyte, termed the "respiratory burst," which results from a shift in much of the cell's glucose metabolism to the hexose-monophosphate shunt. The nicotinamide adenine dinucleotide phosphate (NADPH) that is produced because of this shift is used by a membrane-associated enzyme, NADPH oxidase, to generate superoxide, a reactive oxygen intermediate that is converted to hydrogen peroxide and other reactive oxygen species. These steps comprise the *oxygen-dependent killing mechanism.* Many of the reactive oxygen species are directly toxic to the microorganism. Hydrogen peroxide also can collaborate with the lysosomal enzyme *myeloperoxidase* and halide anions (Cl^- and Br^-) to form acids, such as hypochlorous (HClO) and hypobromous (HBrO) acids.[27] These acids probably kill bacteria and fungi by adding Cl^- or Br^- to the surface of these cells. *Oxygen-independent mechanisms* of microbial killing are likely the result of (1) the acidic pH (3.5 to 4.0) of the phagolysosome caused by lactic acid production; (2) the presence of cationic proteins, such as defensins and cathelicidins, that bind to and damage target cell membranes; (3) enzymatic attack of the mucopeptides in the target cell wall by lysozyme and elastase; and (4) inhibition of bacterial growth by lactoferrin binding of iron.

When a phagocyte dies at an inflammatory site, it frequently lyses (breaks open) and releases its cytoplasmic contents, including the lysosomal enzymes, into the tissue. Enzymes released from lysosomes can digest the connective tissue matrix, causing much of the tissue destruction associated with inflammation. The destructive effects of many enzymes released by dying phagocytes are minimized by natural inhibitors found in the blood, such as **α_1-antitrypsin,** a plasma protein produced by the liver. An inherited deficiency of α_1-antitrypsin often results in chronic lung damage and emphysema as a result of inflammation. (The pulmonary effects of α_1-antitrypsin deficiency are described in Chapter 35.) Released lysosomal products also may contribute to inflammation by increasing vascular permeability, attracting additional monocytes, and activating the complement and kinin systems.

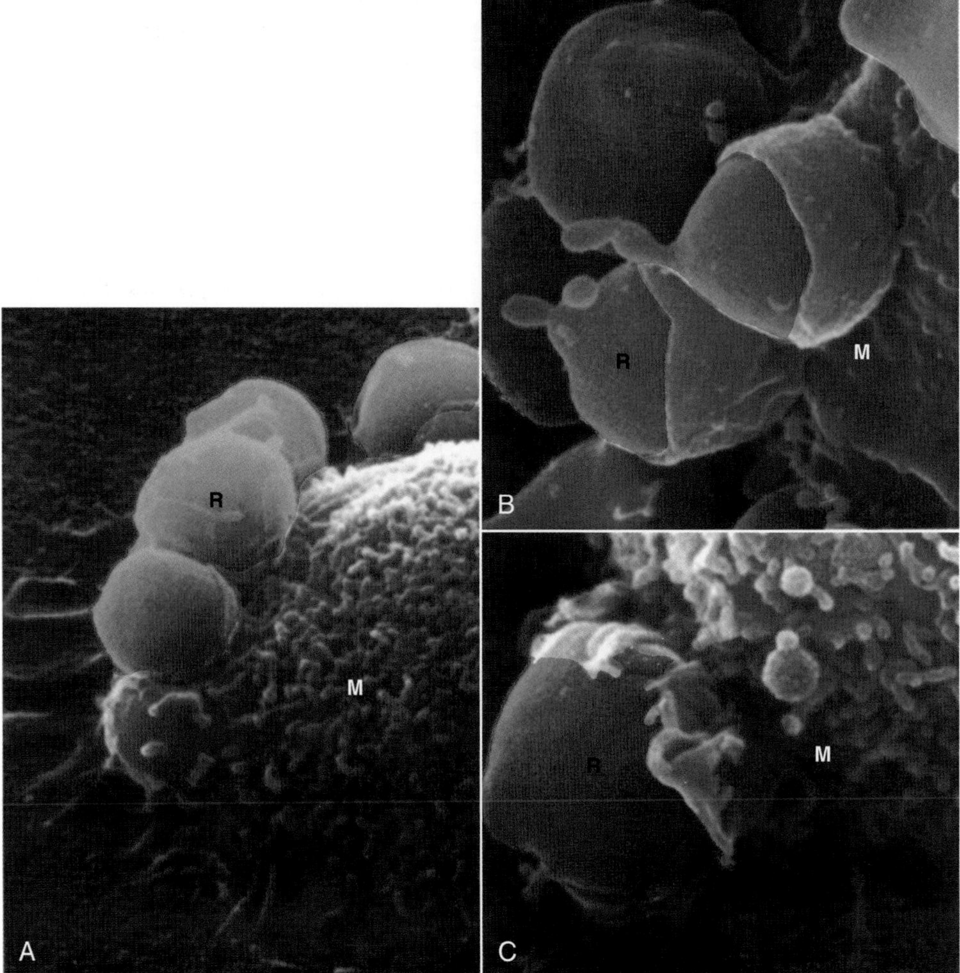

FIGURE 7-16 **Steps in Phagocytosis.** This scanning electron micrograph shows the progressive steps in phagocytosis. **A,** Red blood cells *(R)* attach to the surface of a macrophage *(M)*. **B,** Part of the macrophage *(M)* membrane starts to enclose the red cell *(R)*. **C,** The red blood cells are almost totally engulfed by the macrophage. (From King DW, Fenoglio CM, Lefwitch JH: *General pathology: principles and dynamics,* Philadelphia, 1983, Lea & Febiger.)

Monocyte-derived macrophages from the circulation may appear at the inflammatory site as soon as 24 hours after the initial neutrophil infiltration, but usually arrive 3 to 7 days later. They migrate to the site more slowly than neutrophils because they move more sluggishly and also because many of the chemotactic factors that attract them, such as macrophage chemotactic factor, must first be released by neutrophils.[28] Macrophages are better suited than neutrophils to long-term defense against infectious agents because macrophages can survive and divide in the acidic inflammatory site or where there is low oxygen tension.

Neutrophils and monocytes/macrophages differ chiefly in the following ways:

1. *Speed:* Neutrophils arrive at the injury site first.
2. *Active life span:* Macrophages survive and divide in the inflammatory site, whereas neutrophils cannot.
3. *Chemotactic factors:* Neutrophils and macrophages are not attracted by the same factors.
4. *Enzymatic content of their lysosomes, or digestive vacuoles, differs.*
5. *Role in the immune response:* Macrophages, but not neutrophils, are involved in activation of the adaptive immune system.
6. *Role in wound repair:* Macrophages are the primary cells that infiltrate tissue in wounds, remove cells and cellular debris, and produce cytokines that suppress further inflammation and initiate healing.

Macrophage Activation. Several bacteria are resistant to killing by granulocytes and can even survive inside macrophages. Microorganisms such as *Mycobacterium tuberculosis* (tuberculosis), *Mycobacterium leprae* (leprosy), *Salmonella typhi* (typhoid fever), *Brucella abortus* (brucellosis), and *Listeria monocytogenes* (listeriosis) can remain dormant or even multiply inside the phagolysosomes of macrophages. However, the bactericidal activity of macrophages can be markedly increased with the help of inflammatory **cytokines** produced by cells of the adaptive immune system (subsets of T lymphocytes) or cells activated through Toll-like receptors (TLRs). (Cytokines were discussed in detail earlier in this chapter [see p. 203]) Macrophages have cell surface receptors for these cytokines and are further activated to become more effective killers of infectious microorganisms.

Macrophage activation results in increased (1) phagocytic activity, (2) size, (3) plasma membrane area, (4) glucose metabolism, and (5) number of lysosomes. Activated macrophages also secrete factors that stimulate the growth, differentiation, and activation of additional inflammatory cells as well as control the initiation of healing processes. These include granulocyte colony-stimulating factor (G-CSF), interferon-gamma (IFN-γ), interleukin-1β (IL-1β), angiogenic factor, fibroblast activating factor, and growth factors that promote regrowth of damaged tissues. Macrophages are also the primary cells that infiltrate wounds to remove cellular debris and initiate the regenerative process. In some cases, inadequate macrophage activation results from defects in the adaptive immune responses and deficits in the production of appropriate cytokines. For example, a form of leprosy called *lepromatous leprosy* is characterized by the survival of phagocytosed *M. leprae* bacteria in macrophage phagolysosomes. In individuals with lepromatous leprosy, cells of the adaptive immune system have failed to secrete the cytokines necessary to transform macrophages into highly efficient killing cells.

Natural Killer Cells and Lymphocytes

The main function of **natural killer (NK) cells** is recognition and elimination of cells infected with viruses, although they are also somewhat effective at elimination of other abnormal host cells, specifically cancer cells. NK cells seem to be more efficient in this role when they encounter an infected cell within the circulatory system as opposed to within tissues.[29] Along with TLRs, NK cells have additional inhibitory and activating receptors that allow differentiation between infected or tumor cells and normal cells. If the NK cell binds to a target cell through activating receptors, it produces several cytokines and toxic molecules that can kill the target. NK cells and lymphocytes, which are the principal cells of the adaptive immune response, will be discussed in much more detail in Chapter 8.

LOCAL MANIFESTATIONS OF INFLAMMATION

The cells and plasma protein systems described previously interact to produce all the characteristics of inflammation, whether local or systemic, as well as determine the duration of inflammation, either acute or chronic. Local inflammation accompanies all types of cellular and tissue injury, whether infected or sterile, from fractures or strains of the musculoskeletal system to burn injuries (see Chapter 2), and is responsible for initiating healing.

All the *local* manifestations of acute inflammation (i.e., swelling, pain, heat, and redness) result from vascular changes and the subsequent leakage of circulating components into the tissue. **Heat** and **redness** are the result of vasodilation and increased blood flow through the injured site. **Swelling** occurs as exudate (fluid and cells) accumulates. Swelling is usually accompanied by **pain** caused by pressure exerted by exudate accumulation, as well as the presence of soluble biochemical mediators such as prostaglandins and bradykinin. Loss of function may be associated with these manifestations.

Exudate varies in composition, depending on the stage of the inflammatory response and, to some extent, the injurious stimulus. In early or mild inflammation, the exudate is watery **(serous)** with very few plasma proteins or leukocytes. An example of serous exudate is the fluid in a blister. In more severe or advanced inflammation, the exudate may be thick and clotted **(fibrinous exudate),** such as in the lungs of individuals with pneumonia. If a large number of leukocytes accumulate, as in persistent bacterial infections, the exudate consists of pus and is called a **purulent (suppurative) exudate.** Purulent exudate is characteristic of walled-off lesions (**cysts** or **abscesses**). If bleeding occurs, the exudate is filled with erythrocytes and is described as a **hemorrhagic exudate.**

Although the local manifestations of inflammation can affect all vascularized tissues, lesions vary depending on the organ or tissue involved. The lesion resulting from widespread cellular death (necrosis), for example, differs in myocardial (heart muscle), brain, and hepatic (liver) tissues. Cellular death resulting from myocardial infarction (deprivation of oxygen caused by cessation of blood flow) causes a response that proceeds to replacement of the dead tissue with a fibrinous scar. The same injury to brain tissue is more likely to result in the formation of an abscess filled with necrotic tissue (types of necrosis are described in Chapter 2). Destruction of liver tissue stimulates the regrowth, or regeneration, of liver cells.

SYSTEMIC MANIFESTATIONS OF ACUTE INFLAMMATION

The three primary *systemic* changes associated with the acute inflammatory response are fever, leukocytosis (a transient increase in the levels of circulating leukocytes), and plasma protein synthesis (increased levels of circulating plasma proteins).

Fever

An early systemic response is **fever,** which is partially induced by specific cytokines, for example, IL-1 released from neutrophils and macrophages. These fever-causing cytokines are known as **endogenous pyrogens** to differentiate them from pathogen-produced *exogenous pyrogens.* Pyrogens act directly on the hypothalamus, the portion of the brain that controls the body's thermostat. The release of endogenous pyrogens by inflammatory cells occurs after phagocytosis, after exposure to bacterial endotoxins, or after exposure to antigen-antibody complexes. (Mechanisms of temperature regulation are discussed in Chapter 16.)

The generation of a febrile response can be beneficial because the microorganisms that cause some conditions (e.g., syphilis, gonococcal urethritis) are highly sensitive to small increases in body temperature. On the other hand, fever may have some harmful side effects because it may enhance the person's susceptibility to the effects of endotoxins associated with gram-negative bacterial infections (bacterial toxins are described in Chapter 2).

Leukocytosis

Another systemic change associated with acute inflammation is **leukocytosis.** During many infections, the numbers of

TABLE 7-4 CIRCULATING LEVELS OF ACUTE-PHASE REACTANTS DURING INFLAMMATION

FUNCTION	INCREASED	DECREASED
Coagulation components	Fibrinogen Prothrombin Factor VIII Plasminogen	None
Protease inhibitors	α_1-Antitrypsin α_1-Antichymotrypsin	Inter-α-antitrypsin
Transport proteins	Haptoglobin Hemopexin Ceruloplasmin Ferritin	Transferrin
Complement components	C1s, C2, C3, C4, C5, C9, factor B, C1 inhibitor	Properdin
Miscellaneous proteins	α_1-Acid glycoprotein Fibronectin Serum amyloid A (SAA) C-reactive protein (CRP)	Albumin Prealbumin α_1-Lipoprotein β-Lipoprotein

circulating leukocytes, primarily neutrophils, increase. This increase is usually accompanied by a “left shift” in the ratio of immature to mature neutrophils, so that the more immature forms of neutrophils, such as band cells, metamyelocytes, and occasionally myelocytes, are present in relatively greater than normal proportions. (Chapter 27 discusses the development and maturation of blood cells.) Production of immature leukocytes increases primarily because proliferation and release of granulocyte and monocyte precursors in the bone marrow are stimulated by several products of inflammation, including complement product C3a and G-CSF.

Plasma Protein Synthesis

The synthesis of many plasma proteins, most of which are products of the liver, is increased during the primary stages of inflammation. These proteins, which can be either proinflammatory or anti-inflammatory in nature, are referred to as **acute-phase reactants** (Table 7-4). Acute-phase reactants reach maximal circulating levels within 10 to 40 hours of initial infection. In addition to inducing fever, IL-1 also indirectly induces the synthesis of acute-phase reactants. IL-1 up-regulates release of IL-6, which then increases synthesis of acute-phase reactants directly by stimulating liver cells. Administration of IL-1 into animals leads to fever and elevation of most acute-phase reactants, including fibrinogen, C-reactive protein, haptoglobin, amyloid A, α_1-antitrypsin, and ceruloplasmin.

Acute inflammation can be verified by a series of hematologic tests, which are described in detail in Chapter 27. For example, an increase in blood levels of acute-phase reactants, primarily fibrinogen, is usually associated with an increased erythrocyte sedimentation rate. The alteration in plasma proteins probably leads to an enhanced erythrocyte rouleaux formation (stacking of erythrocytes, as in a stack of coins) and thereby an increased rate of sedimentation. Although increased erythrocyte sedimentation is a nonspecific reaction, it is considered a good indicator of an acute inflammatory response. Other symptoms of acute inflammation include somnolence (drowsiness), malaise (generalized feeling of discomfort or illness), anorexia (lack of desire to eat), and muscle aching.

CHRONIC INFLAMMATION

Superficially, the difference between acute and chronic inflammation is purely one of duration, in that chronic inflammation lasts 2 weeks or longer, regardless of cause. Characteristic histologic and mechanistic differences also may be present (Figure 7-17). Chronic inflammation is sometimes preceded by an unsuccessful acute inflammatory response. For example, if bacterial contamination or foreign objects (e.g., dirt, wood splinters, glass) persist in a traumatic wound, an acute response may be prolonged beyond 2 weeks. Pus formation, suppuration (purulent discharge), and incomplete wound healing may characterize this type of chronic inflammation.

Chronic inflammation can occur also as a distinct process without much previous acute inflammation. Some microorganisms (e.g., mycobacteria that cause tuberculosis) have cell walls with a very high lipid and wax content, making them relatively insensitive to degradation by phagocytes and therefore relatively resistant to clearance in an acute inflammatory response. Other microorganisms, such as those that cause leprosy, syphilis, and brucellosis, can survive within the macrophage and thereby also avoid clearance by the acute inflammatory response. In addition, some microorganisms produce toxins that stimulate tissue-damaging reactions even after they themselves are killed. Persistent inflammation can result from prolonged irritation by these toxins. Finally, chemicals, particulate matter, or physical irritants (e.g., inhaled dusts, wood splinters, and suture material) also can cause an inflammatory response that lasts longer than 2 weeks.

Chronic inflammation is characterized by a dense infiltration of lymphocytes and macrophages. If macrophages are unable to limit the tissue damage or infection, the body attempts to wall off and isolate the infected area, thus forming a **granuloma** (Figure 7-18).[30] Granulomas may form if neutrophils and macrophages are unable to destroy microorganisms during the acute inflammatory response. For example, infections caused by some bacteria (*Listeria* sp., *Brucella* sp.), fungi (histoplasmosis, coccidioidomycosis), and parasites (leishmaniasis, schistosomiasis, toxoplasmosis) can result in granuloma formation. Large antigen-antibody complexes such as those present in rheumatoid arthritis also can result in the formation of these structures. The process of granuloma formation begins when some of the macrophages differentiate into large **epithelioid cells,** cells that are incapable of phagocytosing large bacteria but are capable of taking up debris and other small particles. Other macrophages fuse into multinucleated **giant cells,** which are active phagocytes that can engulf very large particles—larger than those that can be engulfed by a single macrophage. These two types of differentiated macrophages form the center of the granuloma, which is surrounded by a wall of lymphocytes. The granuloma itself is also often encapsulated by fibrous deposits of collagen and may become cartilaginous or possibly calcified by deposits of calcium carbonate and calcium phosphate.

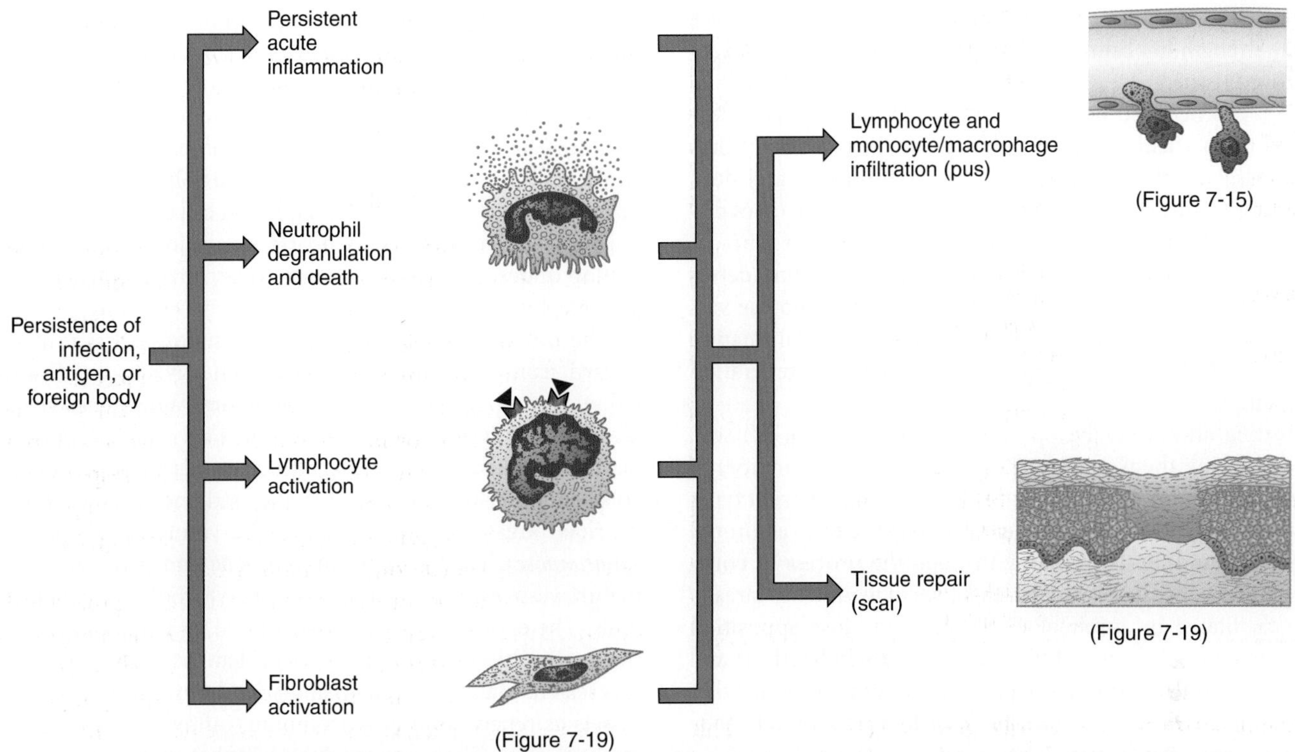

FIGURE 7-17 The Chronic Inflammatory Response. Inflammation usually becomes chronic because of the persistence of an infection, an antibody, or a foreign body in the wound. Chronic inflammation is characterized by the persistence of many of the processes of acute inflammation. In addition, the presence of large amounts of neutrophil degranulation and death, the activation of lymphocytes, and the concurrent activation of fibroblasts result in the release of mediators that induce the infiltration of more lymphocytes and monocytes/macrophages and the beginning of wound healing and tissue repair.

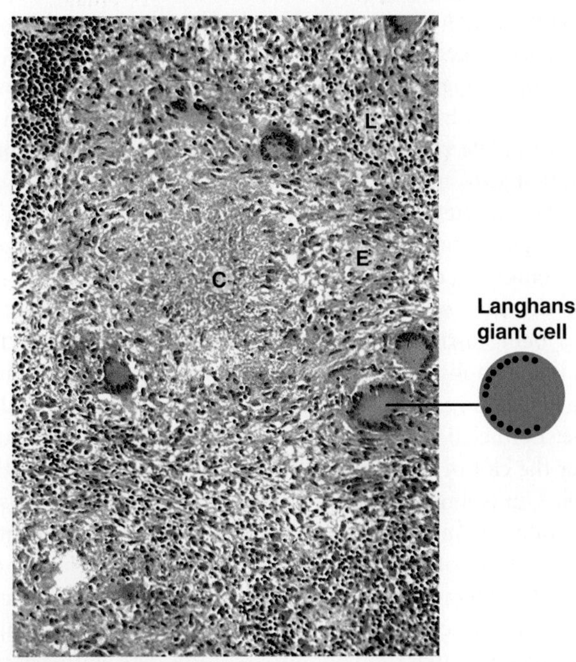

FIGURE 7-18 Tuberculous Granuloma. A central area of amorphous caseous necrosis *(C)* is surrounded by a zone of lymphocytes *(L)* and enlarged epithelioid cells *(E)*. Activated macrophages frequently fuse to form multinucleated cells (Langhans giant cells). In tuberculoid granulomas the nuclei of the giant cells move to the cellular margins in a horseshoe-like formation.

The classic granuloma associated with tuberculosis is characterized by a wall of epithelioid cells surrounding a center of dead and decaying tissue (caseous necrosis, see Chapter 2) and mycobacteria. Decay of cells within the granuloma results in the release of acids and the enzymatic contents of lysosomes from dead phagocytes. In this inhospitable environment, the cellular debris is broken down and a clear fluid remains (liquefaction necrosis, see Chapter 2). Eventually this fluid diffuses out and leaves a hollow, thick-walled structure in the tissue that may remain for the life of the individual.

RESOLUTION AND REPAIR

Destruction of tissue is followed by a period of healing that begins during acute inflammation and may not be complete for as long as 2 years. The most favorable outcome of healing is tissue **regeneration** with complete return to normal structure and function. This is an ideal that is often not possible, particularly in adults. If damage is minor, no complications occur, and destroyed tissues are capable of regeneration, it is possible to return injured tissues to an approximation of their original structure and physiologic function. This restoration is called **resolution.** If extensive damage is present, injury occurs in tissues not capable of regeneration, infection results in abscess or granuloma formation, or fibrin persists in the lesion, resolution is not possible and repair takes place instead. **Repair** is the replacement of destroyed tissue with scar tissue. **Scar tissue** is composed primarily of collagen that seals the lesion and restores tensile strength but cannot execute the physiologic functions of destroyed tissue.

Both regeneration and repair actually begin with phagocytosis of the particulate matter found at the site of injury (fibrin from dissolved clots, microorganisms, erythrocytes, and dead tissue cells). This cleanup of the lesion, which also involves dissolution of fibrin clots (or scabs) by fibrinolytic enzymes, is called **débridement.** After débridement, the remaining debris is drained away by blood vessels and lymphatics, and the vascular dilation and permeability associated with inflammation are reversed, thus preparing the lesion for either regeneration or repair.

Healing always involves processes that (1) fill in, (2) seal, and (3) shrink the wound.[31] These common denominators of healing vary in importance and duration among different types of wounds. A clean incision, such as a paper cut or a sutured surgical wound, heals primarily through the process of collagen synthesis. Because sealing of this type of wound has already been facilitated by minimal tissue loss and close apposition of the wound edges, very little sealing (**epithelialization**) and shrinkage (**contraction**) are required for healing. Wounds that heal under conditions of minimal tissue loss are said to heal by **primary intention** (Figure 7-19).

Other wounds do not heal so neatly and easily. Healing of an open wound, such as a stage IV pressure sore (decubitus ulcer), requires a great deal more tissue replacement than healing of a sutured surgical incision. With an open wound, epithelialization, scar formation, and contraction take longer and healing occurs through **secondary intention** (see Figure 7-19). Healing by either primary or secondary intention may occur at different rates for different types of tissue injury.

Both resolution and repair occur in two overlapping phases. The first phase, called the **reconstructive phase,** begins 3 to 4 days after the initial injury and continues for as long as 2 weeks. During this phase the lesion is characterized by fibroblast (connective tissue cell) proliferation, followed by collagen synthesis by the fibroblasts, epithelialization, contraction of the wound, and cellular differentiation. The second phase, the **maturation phase,** begins several weeks after injury and is normally complete within 2 years. During this phase cellular differentiation, scar formation, and scar remodeling continue.

Reconstructive Phase

Because surgical wounds exhibit both the reconstructive and the maturation phases, they are useful models of both normal and abnormal (dysfunctional) healing. Such wounds are initially sealed off by a blood clot containing fibrin and trapped cells. The cross-linked mesh of fibrin is created by activation of the coagulation cascade and initially traps platelets to form a platelet plug that further seals damaged vessels (see Chapter 27). Most surgical wounds are completely sealed with platelet plugs within hours after closure. This sealing helps unite the wound edges and acts to create a physical barrier to bacterial invasion, although pathogenic invasion is not always prevented. The fibrin mesh ultimately acts as a scaffold for the collagen or regenerated tissue cells that ultimately fill the wound.

For healing to proceed, the fibrin clot must be dissolved and then replaced by normal tissue (for resolution) or scar tissue (for repair). Enzymatic digestion of the clot usually occurs after activation of the plasma fibrinolytic system (plasmin generation, see Chapter 27) or release of lysosomal enzymes from dead neutrophils. Macrophages invade the dissolving clot and, by phagocytosis, clear away debris and dead cells. Débridement by macrophages and remaining neutrophils is followed by regeneration of destroyed cells (resolution) or, if regeneration is not possible, by repair (see Figure 7-19).

The process of healing begins as **granulation tissue** grows inward from surrounding healthy connective tissue. Granulation tissue is filled with new capillaries (angiogenesis) that give it a red, granular appearance and is surrounded by fibroblasts and macrophages. First, capillary buds sprout from vascular endothelial cells around the wound and extend into the débrided areas. Loops form when the young capillaries join *(anastomose).* The loops are more fragile and permeable than mature vessels, resulting in leakage of erythrocytes and neutrophils. The erythrocytes are phagocytosed by macrophages and the neutrophils assist in further débridement of the inflammatory lesion. Many of the new capillaries differentiate into larger vessels as repair continues promoting influx of nutrients and removal of metabolic wastes. New lymphatic vessels also grow into the granulation tissue by a similar process.

In addition to their role in débriding, macrophages at the site of injury secrete several biochemical mediators and cytokines that orchestrate and promote healing. The following are some examples of these mediators:

1. **Transforming growth factor-beta (TGF-β)** stimulates fibroblasts entering the lesion to synthesize and secrete the collagen precursor **procollagen.**
2. **Angiogenesis factors,** such as vascular endothelial growth factor (VEGF) and fibroblast growth factor-2 (FGF-2), stimulate vascular endothelial cells to form capillary buds that grow into the wound.
3. **Matrix metalloproteinases (MMPs)** may function in the degradation and remodeling of extracellular matrix proteins (e.g., collagen and fibrin) at the site of injury.

As the clot or scab is being dissolved and granulation tissue is being formed, the healing wound must be protected. This is accomplished by epithelialization, the process by which epithelial cells grow into the wound from surrounding healthy tissue. Epithelial cells migrate through the collagenous matrix under the clot or scab using MMPs to unravel collagen as they travel. Unraveling the collagen enables the epithelial cells to move rather than remain immobile (see Figure 7-19); the intact collagen ahead of them provides a pathway on which they can maneuver forward. Eventually the migrating epithelial cells contact similar cells from all sides of the wound and seal it, thereby halting migration and proliferation. The epithelial cells undergo differentiation to give rise to the various epidermal layers (see Chapter 46). Epithelialization of a skin wound can be hastened if the wound is kept moist, preventing the fibrin clot from becoming a scab.

Fibroblasts are the most important cells during the reconstructive phase of wound healing because they synthesize and

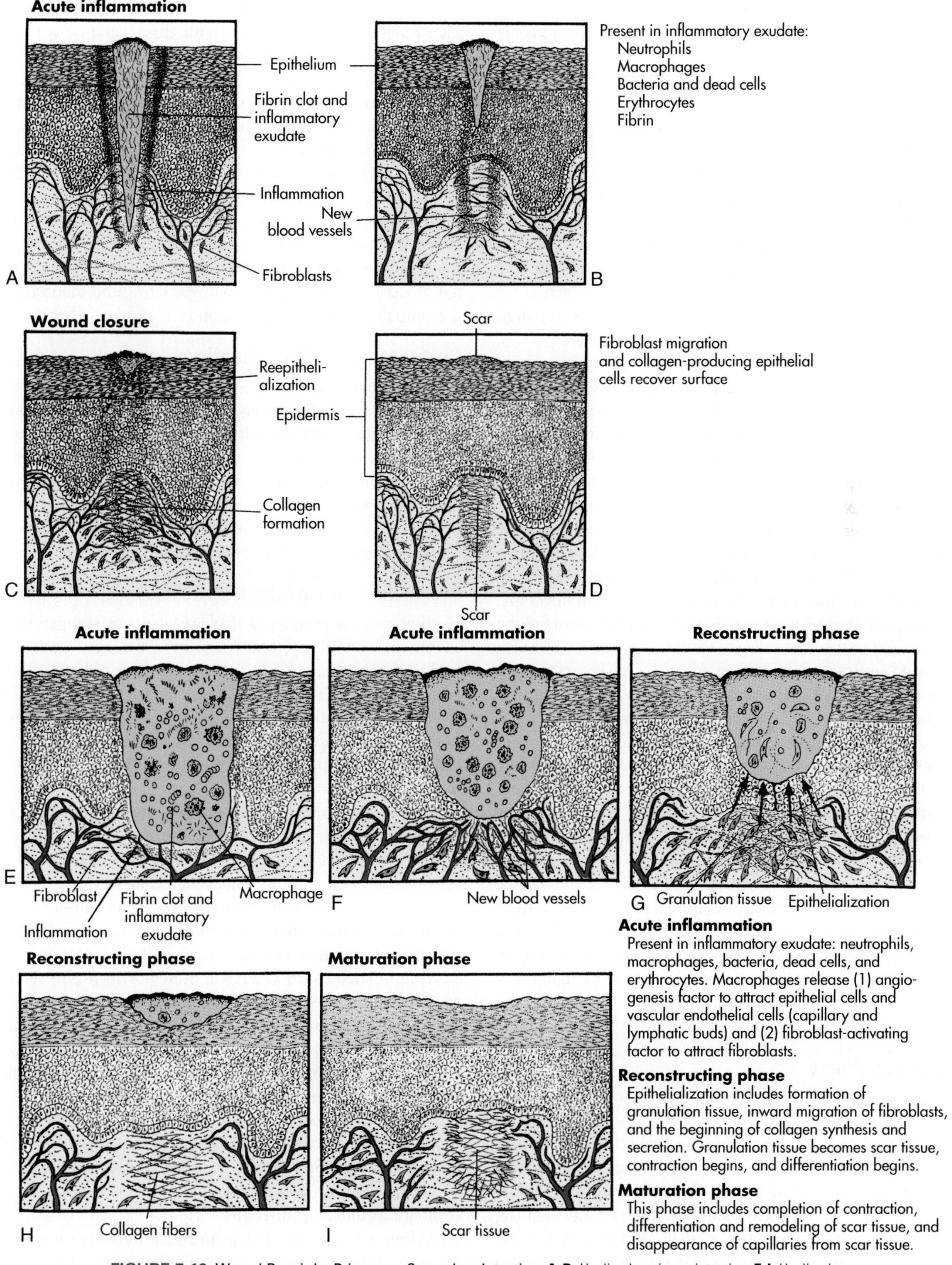

Acute inflammation
Present in inflammatory exudate: neutrophils, macrophages, bacteria, dead cells, and erythrocytes. Macrophages release (1) angiogenesis factor to attract epithelial cells and vascular endothelial cells (capillary and lymphatic buds) and (2) fibroblast-activating factor to attract fibroblasts.

Reconstructing phase
Epithelialization includes formation of granulation tissue, inward migration of fibroblasts, and the beginning of collagen synthesis and secretion. Granulation tissue becomes scar tissue, contraction begins, and differentiation begins.

Maturation phase
This phase includes completion of contraction, differentiation and remodeling of scar tissue, and disappearance of capillaries from scar tissue.

FIGURE 7-19 Wound Repair by Primary or Secondary Intention. **A-D,** Healing by primary intention. **E-I,** Healing by secondary intention.

secrete collagen and other connective tissue proteins. Fibroblasts are stimulated by macrophage-derived TGF-β to proliferate, enter the lesion, and produce these proteins. The collagen and connective tissue proteins produced by fibroblasts are deposited in débrided areas about 6 days after the fibroblasts have entered the lesion. **Collagen** is the most abundant protein in the body. It contains high concentrations of the amino acids glycine, proline, and lysine, although many of the proline and lysine amino acids are enzymatically modified as the protein is being synthesized. Modification of these amino acids requires several cofactors and is absolutely necessary for proper collagen polymerization and function. The required cofactors include iron, ascorbic acid (vitamin C), and molecular oxygen (O_2); the absence of any of these results in incomplete or impaired wound healing.

Immature collagen (i.e., procollagen) is secreted by fibroblasts as a complex of three polypeptide chains cross-linked by intermolecular bonds. Procollagen is converted to mature collagen by the proteolytic removal of small polypeptide sequences at both ends of the trimer. As healing progresses, collagen molecules are cross-linked by intramolecular covalent bonds to form collagen fibrils that are further cross-linked to form collagen fibers. The process of complete collagen matrix assembly takes several months because collagen is initially deposited randomly but then is remodeled by repeated dissolution (by MMPs) and reassembly. During this remodeling period, collagen fibers orient along the lines of mechanical stress; further cross-linking adds strength to the final collagen matrix.

Wound contraction is the final process of the reconstructive phase of healing. It is necessary for closure of all wounds, but especially those that heal by secondary intention. Contraction is noticeable 6 to 12 days after injury and may amount to inward movement of the wound edge by approximately 0.5 mm/day in normal healing. The granulation tissue of a healing wound contains **myofibroblasts**—specialized cells that are likely responsible for wound contraction. As their name implies, myofibroblasts have features of both smooth muscle cells and fibroblasts. They appear microscopically similar to fibroblasts, but differ in that their cytoplasm contains bundles of parallel fibers similar to those found in smooth muscle cells. Wound contraction occurs as extensions from the plasma membrane of myofibroblasts establish connections between neighboring cells, contract their fibers, and exert tension on the neighboring cells while anchoring themselves to the wound bed.

Maturation Phase

Collagen matrix assembly, tissue regeneration, and wound contraction all *begin* during the reconstructive phase but are not yet completed when the reconstructive phase ends, about 2 weeks after injury. Therefore, these processes continue into the **maturation phase**—a phase that can persist for years. During the maturation phase scar tissue is remodeled and capillaries disappear, leaving the scar avascular. Within 2 to 3 weeks after maturation has begun, the scar tissue has gained about two thirds of its eventual maximal strength.

Neither epidermal wounds that heal by secondary intention nor unsutured internal lesions are completely restored by healing. At best, repaired tissue regains 80% of its original tensile strength. Only epithelial, hepatic (liver), and bone marrow cells are capable of the complete mitotic regeneration known as *compensatory hyperplasia* (hyperplasia is described in Chapter 2). In fibrous connective tissue such as joints and ligaments, normal healing results in replacement of the original tissue with new tissue that does not have exactly the same structure or function as that of the original tissue. Some tissues heal without replacement of cells. For example, damage resulting from myocardial infarction heals with a scar composed of fibrous tissue rather than with cardiac muscle cell replacement.[32] Although the composition of various healed tissues may differ, the healing process—reconstruction followed by wound maturation—is essentially the same for all wounds.

Dysfunctional Wound Healing

Dysfunctional wound healing may occur if any of the involved processes occurs abnormally. This can include abnormalities in the inflammatory response itself, insufficient or excessive repair, or reinfection of the wound. Abnormalities may result from a predisposing disease, such as diabetes mellitus, or from an adaptive condition, such as hypoxemia (insufficient oxygen concentration in arterial blood). Numerous drugs and nutritional deficiencies can affect wound healing as well.[33]

Dysfunction During Inflammatory Response

Healing may be prolonged if bleeding is not stopped during acute inflammation. *Hemorrhage* in a damaged area delays healing for several reasons. Initially the excess blood cells that accumulate at the site of injury must be cleared—a process that requires additional time. In addition to the cellular accumulation caused by excessive bleeding, formation of a clot increases the amount of space that granulation tissue has to fill and serves as a mechanical barrier to oxygen diffusion. The great amount of fibrin that is released during hemorrhage also must eventually be reabsorbed in order to prevent its organization into *fibrous adhesions.* Once formed, these **adhesions** can bind organs together by fibrous bands; with time, shrinkage of these bands can distort or strangulate nearby organs. This is clinically significant, particularly if they form within the pleural, pericardial, or abdominal cavities.

Accumulated blood as a result of hemorrhage also serves as an excellent culture medium for bacteria, promoting continued *infection* and prolonging inflammation by increasing purulent exudate formation. Prolonged infection can promote *excess scar formation* or even prevent healing completely. Continued infection of a wound, termed *wound sepsis,* can be clinically treated in several ways. Most important is the débridement of necrotic tissue and foreign bodies. This removal is accomplished either through surgery or through the use of absorbent dressings. Wound irrigation and antibiotic therapy also may assist in combating continued infection.

Although local hemorrhage during the inflammatory process can pose a huge impediment to healing, many additional factors, both physiologic and pharmacologic, also may adversely affect the healing of an inflamed tissue. *Hypovolemia*—decreased blood volume—hinders inflammation. The physiologic response to hypovolemia is vessel constriction rather than the dilation required to deliver inflammatory cells to the site of injury. Optimal nutrition is important during all phases of healing because metabolic needs are increased. The most essential nutrients for healing are glucose, oxygen, and amino acids. Because leukocytes need glucose to produce the energy needed for chemotaxis, phagocytosis, and intercellular killing, the wounds of persons with diabetes who receive insufficient insulin heal poorly, mainly attributable to a prolonging of the infection. Persons with diabetes are also at risk for ischemic wounds because they are likely to have both small-vessel diseases that impair the microcirculation and altered (glycosylated) hemoglobin, which has an increased affinity for oxygen and thus does not readily release oxygen in tissues. (Hemoglobin's function as the oxygen-carrying component of blood is described in Chapter 27.) Oxygen delivery is also compromised by hypoxemic states because ischemic tissue is susceptible to infection. *Hypoproteinemia* prolongs inflammation because the associated decrease in available amino acids is an impediment to fibroblast proliferation. Finally, anti-inflammatory steroids can have an impact upon wound healing. These drugs prevent macrophages from migrating to the site of injury and inhibit their release of collagenase and plasminogen activator. *Anti-inflammatory steroids* also inhibit fibroblast migration into the wound during the reconstructive phase of healing and impair angiogenesis, wound contraction, and reepithelialization.

Dysfunction During Reconstructive Phase of Healing

Three of the essential processes that occur during the reconstructive phase are assembly and remodeling of the collagen matrix, epithelialization of the wound bed, and contraction of the wound. Dysfunctional wound healing can result from the impairment of any of these processes.

Impaired Collagen Matrix Assembly. A number of factors may interfere with the production of collagen in healing tissues, most being nutritional. Scurvy, for example, is a condition caused by a deficiency in ascorbic acid, one of the cofactors required for the amino acid modification that is necessary for proper collagen matrix assembly. The complication of scurvy is a poorly formed collagen matrix and, therefore, greatly impaired wound healing. Other nutrients, including iron, copper, and calcium, play additional roles in the enzymatic reactions required for collagen modification and assembly. Usually, however, such minute amounts of these substances are required that deficiencies are not clinically significant. Nutritionally, appropriate protein intake is also essential for collagen synthesis. The amino acid methionine that is found in proteins is converted to cysteine, the role of which in collagen synthesis is twofold: (1) it functions as an important cofactor in the enzymatic reactions required for collagen synthesis; and (2) it contains sulfur, which contributes to formation of the strong covalent bonds in cross-linked collagen fibrils.

Dysfunctional healing also may result from excessive production of collagen. Overproduction of collagen causes surface overhealing, which is manifested in the skin by formation of a keloid or a hypertrophic scar (Figure 7-20). A **keloid** is a raised scar that extends beyond the original boundaries of the wound.

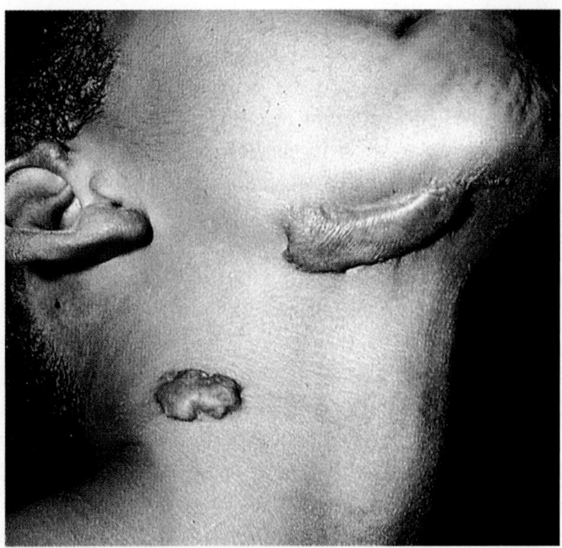

FIGURE 7-20 Keloids. (From Damjanov I, Linder J: *Anderson's pathology,* ed 10, St Louis, 1996, Mosby.)

It invades surrounding tissue and is likely to recur after surgical removal. A familial tendency toward keloid formation has been observed, with a greater incidence in blacks relative to whites. Similar to a keloid, a **hypertrophic scar** is also raised but differs in that it remains within the original boundaries of the wound. Hypertrophic scars tend to regress over time, whereas keloids do not. Both keloids and hypertrophic scars are caused by an imbalance between collagen synthesis and collagen degradation in which synthesis is increased relative to degradation. Although the precise mechanism of this imbalance is unknown, recent evidence suggests that keloid fibroblasts have lower rates of apoptosis and an inability to respond to normal suppressive feedback.

Impaired Epithelialization. The process of **epithelialization** is suppressed by anti-inflammatory steroids, hypoxemia, and nutritional deficiencies. Anti-inflammatory steroids inhibit phagocyte production of the biochemical mediators required for epithelialization, hypoxemia deprives cells of the energy required for the process, and dietary zinc is necessary for the MMP activity that is crucial to cellular migration.

Wound care techniques also may greatly influence epithelial cell migration. External wounds that are draining or healing by secondary intention often are clinically débrided and protected with dressings.[34] The ideal dressing is one that absorbs some drainage without being incorporated into the clot or granulation tissue. Because epithelial cells must migrate across the wound during healing, dressings that débride healthy epithelial cells along with necrotic tissue prolong epithelialization. Many solutions that traditionally have been used to clean or irrigate wounds are now known to be deleterious to the fragile new cells in the wound bed. Normal saline is the most innocuous solution that can be used to cleanse or irrigate a wound that is healing primarily by epithelialization. Solutions such as povidone-iodine and hydrogen peroxide are desiccating (drying) and, as such, inhibit rather than promote epithelial cell migration.

Impaired Contraction

Excessive wound contraction may result in a deformity or **contracture.** Burn wounds are especially susceptible to the development of contractures. Internal contractures may occur as well, and are common in cirrhosis of the liver. Internally, scar tissue that becomes contracted constricts blood flow that may contribute to the development of portal hypertension and esophageal varices. Other types of internal contraction deformity include duodenal strictures caused by dysfunctional healing of an ulcer and esophageal strictures caused by chemical burns.

Proper positioning and range-of-motion exercises, as well as surgery, are among the physical means used to overcome the excessive myofibroblast-derived tension that results in contractures. Clinical use of pharmacologic methods for control of wound contracture is still largely experimental, but includes control of myofibroblast contraction by the administration of smooth muscle cell inhibitors such as colchicine and inhibition of proper collagen matrix assembly with drugs that prevent either collagen cross-linking or MMP activity. These latter treatments are based on the knowledge that myofibroblast binding to collagen can "lock" contracted cells into position.

Wound Disruption

Finally, a potential complication in the healing of wounds that are sutured closed is **dehiscence,** in which the wound pulls apart at the suture line. The greatest incidence of dehiscence occurs 5 to 12 days after suturing, paradoxically at the time when collagen synthesis is at its peak. Approximately 50% of dehiscence occurrences are associated with wound sepsis, although dehiscence also may occur when sutures break as a result of excessive strain. Obesity increases the risk of suture breakage because adipose tissue is difficult to suture. Wound dehiscence usually is heralded by an increase in serous drainage from the wound. In addition, patients may report a feeling that "something gave way." Prompt surgical attention is required.

PEDIATRICS AND MECHANISMS OF SELF-DEFENSE

Neonates commonly have transiently depressed inflammatory and immune function. For example, neutrophils and perhaps monocytes may not be capable of efficient chemotaxis. Insufficient response to chemotactic factors appears to be caused by lack of fluidity in the phagocyte's plasma membrane so that pseudopod formation and migration are impaired. Neonates are prone to infections associated with chemotactic defects, including cutaneous abscesses caused by staphylococci and cutaneous candidiasis. Further, neutrophils in neonates who were stressed by in utero infection or respiratory insufficiency have diminished oxidative and bacterial responses. (Acquired phagocytic defects, which may be induced by a variety of infections, metabolic disorders, nutrition deficiencies, or drugs, are described in Chapter 9.)

Neonates also are partially deficient in complement, especially components of the alternative pathway. They tend to have a relative deficiency of factor B and to develop severe, overwhelming sepsis and meningitis when infected with bacteria against which there is no transferred maternal antibody. Low levels of mannose-binding lectin increase the risk for neonatal hospital-acquired sepsis.[35] Neonates also may be deficient in some of the collectins and collectin-like proteins. This is especially true of preterm neonates. Some preterm infants with respiratory distress syndrome are deficient in at least one collectin, which provides innate defense against respiratory tract infections.

AGING AND MECHANISMS OF SELF-DEFENSE

The older adult population is also at risk for impaired inflammation and wound healing. In some cases, impaired healing is not directly associated with aging in general but can instead be linked to a chronic illness such as cardiovascular disease or diabetes mellitus. In addition, many older adults require medications such as anti-inflammatory steroids that can interfere with the healing process.

Older adults have increased susceptibility to bacterial infections of the lungs, urinary tract, and skin. Because of impaired sensation or mobility and physiologic changes in the skin, older adults are at increased risk for sustaining various wounds. With aging, subcutaneous fat is lost, diminishing a layer of protection. Collagen fibers become thicker and a certain percentage of elastin is lost, further contributing to loss of protection. The regenerative capability of the skin is maintained with aging, but the epidermis undergoes age-associated changes that include atrophy of the underlying capillaries. The consequent decrease of perfusion makes older adults more susceptible than younger people to the adverse effects of hypoxia in the wound bed. In addition, aging fibroblasts may have a slower rate of proliferation, and therefore wound healing is attenuated.

Infections of other organ systems in older adults may be due to a diminished natural ability to ward off infection. Several cellular components of innate resistance are deficient in number (e.g., alveolar macrophages) or have diminished activity (e.g., neutrophil chemotaxis, degranulation, and phagocytosis). One explanation for this diminished inflammatory cellular activity is an age-related decrease in expression and function of several, if not all, TLRs.

SUMMARY REVIEW

Human Defense Mechanisms

1. There are two types of human defense mechanisms: innate resistance or immunity conferred by natural barriers and the inflammatory response; and the adaptive (acquired) immune system.

First Line of Defense: Physical, Mechanical, and Biochemical Barriers

1. Physical and mechanical barriers are the first lines of defense encountered by invading pathogens; these include the skin and mucous membranes.
2. Antibacterial peptides in mucous secretions, perspiration, saliva, tears, and other secretions provide a biochemical barrier against invading pathogens in the extracellular space.
3. Cathelicidins and defensins are two classes of antimicrobial peptides produced by epithelial cells.
4. The normal microbiome provides protection by inhibiting colonization by pathogens and by releasing chemicals that prevent infection.

Second Line of Defense: The Inflammatory Response

1. The inflammatory response, our body's second line of defense against invading microorganisms, is nonspecific, is rapidly initiated, and has no memory cells.
2. The vascular response in acute inflammation includes vasodilation, increased capillary permeability, and white blood cell adherence to inner vessel walls and their migration through vessel walls.
3. Three plasma protein systems provide a biochemical barrier against invading pathogens in the circulation. These include the complement system, the clotting system, and the kinin system.
4. The plasma protein systems work with each other as well as with antimicrobial peptides and the cellular component of the innate immune system to prevent microbial infection.
5. The complement proteins can be activated in three pathways: the classical pathway, the alternative pathway, and the lectin pathway.
6. Activation of the complement pathways results in opsonization, anaphylatoxin activation, cell lysis, and leukocyte chemotaxis.
7. The clotting (coagulation) cascade prevents spread of microorganisms, contains microorganisms and foreign bodies at the site of greatest inflammatory cell activity, and provides a framework for repair and healing.
8. The kinin system proteins promote vasodilation and increased capillary permeability and induce pain.
9. Plasmin and Hageman factor (factor XII) interact to activate the clotting cascade, the complement system, and the kinin proteins.
10. The plasma proteins are finely regulated to prevent injury to host tissue and to guarantee activation when needed. Some of the inhibitors in the plasma protein systems include carboxypeptidase, histaminases, kinases, and C1 esterase inhibitor.
11. Many different types of cells are involved in the inflammatory process including mast cells, granulocytes (neutrophils, eosinophils, basophils), monocytes/macrophages, NK cells and lymphocytes, and cellular fragments (platelets).
12. The cells of the innate immune system secrete many biochemical mediators that are responsible for the vascular changes associated with inflammation and for modulating the localization and activities of other inflammatory cells. The mediators include histamine, chemotactic factors, leukotrienes, prostaglandins, and platelet-activating factor.
13. The inflammatory response is initiated upon tissue injury or when PAMPs are recognized by PRRs on cells of the innate immune system.
14. The PRRs include TLRs, complement, scavenger, glycan, and mannose receptors.
15. TLRs recognize PAMPs, complement receptors recognize complement fragments, and scavenger receptors promote phagocytosis.
16. Cytokines are soluble factors that regulate the inflammatory response and include interleukins, interferons, and tumor necrosis factor.
17. ILs are biochemical messengers primarily produced by macrophages and lymphocytes and significantly help regulate the inflammatory response.
18. IFNs provide protection from viral infection in uninfected cells.
19. Tumor necrosis factor is primarily produced by macrophages and promotes inflammation with both local and systemic effects.
20. Chemokines are synthesized by a number of different cells and induce leukocyte chemotaxis, and are classified as either CC or CXC, depending on their amino acid arrangement. CC chemokines affect monocytes, lymphocytes, and eosinophils. CXC chemokines generally affect neutrophils.
21. Mast cells are central cells of inflammation and release histamine, chemotactic factors, cytokines, leukotrienes, prostaglandins, growth factors, and other mediators.
22. H1-histamine receptors promote inflammation, and H2-histamine receptors inhibit the inflammatory response.
23. Endothelial cells line the circulatory system (vascular endothelium) and maintain normal blood flow by preventing spontaneous activation of platelets and clotting.
24. During inflammation the endothelium expresses receptors that help leukocytes leave the circulation and retract to allow fluid to pass into the tissues.
25. Platelets interact with the coagulation cascade to stop bleeding and release a number of mediators that promote and control inflammation.
26. Neutrophils are the predominant phagocyte of early inflammation. They are attracted to the inflammatory site by chemotactic factors.
27. Eosinophils help control mast cell vascular mediators and defend against parasite infection.
28. Basophils are granulocytes that are very similar to mast cells.

SUMMARY REVIEW—cont'd

29. The monocyte/macrophage is the predominant phagocyte in the late inflammatory response, is highly phagocytic, is responsive to cytokines, and promotes wound healing.
30. Phagocytosis is the destruction of microorganisms and cellular debris.
31. The stages of phagocytosis include recognition and adherence, engulfment, lysosomal fusion, and destruction.
32. Opsonins, such as antibody and complement component C3b, coat microorganisms and make them more susceptible to phagocytosis.
33. Phagocytic killing can be oxygen-dependent with the production of reactive oxygen intermediates or oxygen-independent with lysosomal enzymes.
34. Monocytes and macrophages arrive at the inflammatory site later than neutrophils and remain longer to clean up debris and promote wound healing.
35. NK cells recognize and eliminate viruses, cancer cells, and other abnormal cells.

Local Manifestations of Inflammation

1. Local manifestations of inflammation are the result of the vascular changes associated with the inflammatory process, including vasodilation and increased capillary permeability. The symptoms include redness, heat, swelling, and pain.
2. The functions of the vascular changes are to dilute toxins, carry plasma proteins and leukocytes to the injury site, and carry bacterial toxins and debris away from the site.

Systemic Manifestations of Acute Inflammation

1. The three primary systemic effects of inflammation are fever, leukocytosis, and increase in levels of circulating plasma proteins.
2. Acute-phase reactants are proteins produced by the liver during acute inflammation and include fibrinogen, C-reactive protein, haptoglobin, amyloid A, α_1-antitrypsin, and ceruloplasmin.

Chronic Inflammation

1. Chronic inflammation can be a continuation of acute inflammation that lasts 2 weeks or longer. It also can occur as a distinct process without much preceding acute inflammation.
2. Chronic inflammation is characterized by a dense infiltration of lymphocytes and macrophages. The body may wall off and isolate the infection to protect against tissue damage by formation of a granuloma.

Resolution and Repair

1. Resolution (regeneration) is the return of tissue to nearly normal structure and function. Repair is healing by scar tissue formation.
2. Inflammatory lesions proceed to resolution, meaning that original tissue structure and function have been restored if little tissue has been lost or injured tissue is capable of regeneration. This is called *healing by primary intention.*
3. Inflammatory lesions that involve extensive damage or tissues incapable of regeneration heal by the process of repair that results in the formation of a scar. This is called *healing by secondary intention.*
4. Resolution and repair occur in two separate phases: the *reconstructive phase,* in which the wound begins to heal, and the *maturation phase,* in which the healed wound is remodeled.
5. Dysfunctional wound healing can occur as a result of abnormalities in either the inflammatory response or the reconstructive phase of resolution and repair.

Pediatrics and Mechanisms of Self-Defense

1. Neonates commonly have transiently depressed inflammatory function.
2. Infants often have deficiencies in complement and in a number of collectins, making them more susceptible to bacterial infection.

Aging and Mechanisms of Self-Defense

1. Older adults are at risk for impaired wound healing, often because of underlying illnesses.
2. Diminished immune function may interfere with an older adult's natural ability to ward off infection.

KEY TERMS

α_1-Antitrypsin, 211
Abscess, 213
Acquired immunity, 191
Acute-phase reactant, 214
Adaptive immunity, 191
Adhesion, 218
Adhesion molecule, 209
Alternative pathway, 197
Anaphylatoxin, 198
Angiogenesis factor, 216
Antigen-antibody complex (immune complex), 197
Antimicrobial lectin, 194
Antimicrobial peptide, 193
Bactericidal/permeability-inducing (BPI) protein, 194
Basophil, 209
Bradykinin, 201
C1 esterase inhibitor (C1-inh), 201
C3 convertase, 197
C5 convertase, 197
Carboxypeptidase, 201
Cathelicidin, 193
Cell lysis, 198
Chemokine, 205
Chemotactic factor, 199
Chemotaxis, 207
Classical pathway, 197
Coagulation cascade, 201
Collagen, 218
Collectin, 194
Complement cascade, 197
Complement receptor, 202
Contraction, 216
Contracture, 220
Cyst, 213
Cytokine, 203
Damage-associated molecular pattern (DAMP), 202
Débridement, 216
Defensin, 193
Dehiscence, 220

KEY TERMS—cont'd

REFERENCES

1. Duerr CU, Hornef MW: The mammalian intestinal epithelium as integral player in the establishment and maintenance of host-microbial homeostasis, *Semin Immunol* 24(1):25–35, 2012.
2. Goto Y, Kiyono H: Epithelial barrier: an interface for the cross-communication between gut flora and immune system, *Immunol Rev* 245(1):147–163, 2012.
3. Nakatsuji T, Gallo RL: Antimicrobial peptides: old molecules with new ideas, *Soc Invest Dermatol* 132(3 Pt 2):887–895, 2012.
4. Lehrer RI, Lu W: α-defensins in human innate immunity, *Immunol Rev* 245(1):84–112, 2012.
5. Fagundes CT et al: Adapting to environmental stresses: the role of the microbiota in controlling innate immunity and behavioral responses, *Immunol Rev* 245(1):250–264, 2012.
6. Renz H, Brandtzaeg P, Hornef M: The impact of perinatal immune development on mucosal homeostasis and chronic inflammation, *Nat Rev Immunol* 12(1):9–23, 2012.
7. Ursell LK et al: The interpersonal and intrapersonal diversity of human-associated microbiota in key body sites, *J Allergy Clin Immunol* 129(5):1204–1208, 2012.
8. Dempsey PW, Vaidya SA, Cheng G: The art of war: innate and adaptive immune responses, *Cell Mol Life Sci* 60(12):2604–2621, 2003.
9. Holst B et al: Complement takes its Toll: an inflammatory crosstalk between Toll-like receptors and the receptors for complement anaphylatoxin C5a, *Anaesthesia* 67(1):60–64, 2012.
10. Longhurst H, Cicardi M: Hereditary angio-oedema, *Lancet* 379(9814):474–481, 2012.
11. Clarke TB, Weiser JN: Intracellular sensors of extracellular bacteria, *Immunol Rev* 243(1):9–25, 2011.
12. Strowig T et al: Inflammasomes in health and disease, *Nature* 481(7381):278–286, 2012.
13. Blander JM, Sander LE: Beyond pattern recognition: five immune checkpoints for scaling the microbial threat, *Nat Rev Immunol* 12(3):215–225, 2012.
14. Lee CC, Avalos AM, Ploegh HL: Accessory molecules for Toll-like receptors and their function, *Nat Rev Immunol* 12(3):168–179, 2012.
15. Delgoffe GM, Murray PJ, Vignali AA: Interpreting mixed signals: the cell's cytokine conundrum, *Curr Opin Immunol* 23(5):632–638, 2011.
16. Kotenko SV: IFN-λs, *Curr Opin Immunol* 23(5):583–590, 2011.
17. MacMicking JD: Interferon-inducible effector mechanisms in cell-autonomous immunity, *Nat Rev Immunol* 12(5):367–382, 2012.
18. Wang BX, Fish EN: The yin and yang of viruses and interferons, *Trends Immunol* 33(4):190–197, 2012.
19. Croft M et al: TNF superfamily in inflammatory disease: translating basic insights, *Trends Immunol* 33(3):144–152, 2012.
20. Ehrlich P: Dietbage zur Kenntnis der Anilinsfarb und Ihrer Verwendung nin ungen der Mikroskopichen technik, *Arch Mikr Anat* 13:263, 1877.
21. Amin K: The role of mast cells in allergic inflammation, *Respir Med* 106(1):9–14, 2012.
22. Astudillo AM et al: Dynamics of arachidonic acid mobilization by inflammatory cells, *Biochim Biophys Acta* 1821(2):249–256, 2012.
23. Barnes PJ: Pathophysiology of allergic inflammation, *Immunol Rev* 242(1):31–50, 2011.
24. Kalinski P: Regulation of immune responses by prostaglandin E_2, *J Immunol* 188(1):21–28, 2012.
25. Reitsma PH, Versteeg HH, Middeldorp S: Mechanistic view of risk factors for venous thromboembolism, *Arterioscler Thromb Vasc Biol* 32(3):563–568, 2012.
26. Murray PJ, Wynn TA: Protective and pathogenic functions of macrophage subsets, *Nat Rev Immunol* 11(11):723–737, 2011.
27. Prokopowicz Z et al: Neutrophil myeloperoxidase: soldier and statesman, *Arch Immunol Ther Exp (Warsz)* 60(1):43–54, 2012.
28. Shi C, Pamer EG: Monocyte recruitment during infection and inflammation, *Nat Rev Immunol* 11(11):762–774, 2011.
29. Sun JC, Lanier LL: NK cell development, homeostasis and function: parallels with CD8+ T cells, *Nat Rev Immunol* 11(10):645–657, 2011.
30. Ramakrishnan L: Revisiting the role of the granuloma in tuberculosis, *Nat Rev Immunol* 12(5):352–366, 2012.
31. Porfyris C, Tziotzios C, Vale ID: Cutaneous scarring: pathophysiology, molecular mechanisms, and scar reduction therapeutics. Part I. The molecular basis of scar formation, *J Am Acad Dermatol* 66(1):1–10, 2012.
32. Frangogiannis NG: Regulation of the inflammatory response in cardiac repair, *Circ Res* 110(1):159–173, 2012.
33. Hayes GL et al: Nutritional supplements in critical illness, *AACN Adv Crit Care* 22(4):301–316, 2011.
34. Tziotzios C, Profyris C, Sterling J: Cutaneous scarring: pathophysiology, molecular mechanisms, and scar reduction therapeutics. Part II. Strategies to reduce scar formation after dermatologic procedures, *J Am Acad Dermatol* 66(1):13–24, 2012.
35. de Benedetti F et al: Low serum levels of mannose binding lectin are a risk for neonatal sepsis, *Pediatr Res* 61(3):325–328, 2007.

CHAPTER

8

Adaptive Immunity

Neal S. Rote and Kathryn L. McCance

evolve WEBSITE

http://evolve.elsevier.com/McCance/

- Review Questions and Answers
- Animations
- Online Course: Module 5

CHAPTER OUTLINE

The third line of defense in the human body is **adaptive (acquired) immunity,** often called the immune response or **immunity.**[1] Once external barriers have been compromised and inflammation (see Chapter 7) has been activated, the adaptive immune response is called into action. The molecules and cells of the immune response are closely integrated with those of the innate response. Both systems are essential for complete protection against infectious disease: inflammation is relatively rapid, nonspecific, and short-lived, whereas adaptive immunity is slower acting, specific, and very long-lived. Thus, inflammation is the "first responder" that contains the initial injury and slows spread of infection, whereas adaptive immunity slowly augments the initial defenses against infection and provides long-term security against reinfection. The collaborative and beneficial nature of inflammation and adaptive immunity can, on occasion, fail. Chapter 9 discusses these medically relevant aberrations in both inflammation and immunity, including allergies, diseases that involve unwanted immunologic destruction of healthy tissue, and diseases that are caused by a deficiency in the normal immune or inflammatory responses. Chapter 10 presents an overview of infection and Chapter 11 discusses the connection between stress and

TABLE 8-1 CLINICAL USE OF ANTIGEN OR ANTIBODY

ANTIGEN SOURCE	PROTECTION: COMBAT ACTIVE DISEASE	PROTECTION: VACCINATION	DIAGNOSIS	THERAPY
Infectious agents	Neutralize or destroy pathogenic microorganisms (e.g., antibody response against viral infections)	Induce safe and protective immune response (e.g., recommended childhood vaccines)	Measure circulating antigen from infectious agent or antibody (e.g., diagnosis of hepatitis B infection)	Passive treatment with antibody to treat or prevent infection (e.g., administration of antibody against hepatitis A)
Cancers	Prevent tumor growth or spread (e.g., immune surveillance to prevent early cancers)	Prevent cancer growth or spread (e.g., vaccination with cancer antigens)	Measure circulating antigen (e.g., circulating PSA for diagnosis of prostate cancer)	Immunotherapy (e.g., treatment of cancer with antibodies against cancer antigens)
Environmental substances	Prevent entrance into body (e.g., secretory IgA limits systemic exposure to potential allergens)	No clear example	Measure circulating antigen or antibody (e.g., diagnosis of allergy by measuring circulating IgE)	Immunotherapy (e.g., administration of antigen for desensitization of individuals with severe allergies)
Self-antigens	Immune system tolerance to self-antigens, which may be altered by an infectious agent leading to autoimmune disease (see Chapter 9)	Some cases of vaccination alter tolerance to self-antigens leading to autoimmune disease	Measure circulating antibody against self-antigen for diagnosis of autoimmune disease (see Chapter 9)	No clear example

PSA, Prostate-specific antigen.

disease and the interrelatedness of the immune, nervous, and endocrine systems.

GENERAL CHARACTERISTICS OF ADAPTIVE IMMUNITY

The immune system of the normal adult is continually challenged by a spectrum of substances that it may recognize as foreign, or "non-self." These substances, called foreign **antigens,** are often associated with pathogens such as viruses, bacteria, fungi, or parasites, although they are also found on noninfectious environmental agents such as pollens, foods, and bee venom, and still others are associated with clinically derived drugs, vaccines, transfusions, and transplanted tissues (Table 8-1). Unlike inflammation, which is nonspecifically activated by damage to cells as well as by the action of pathogenic microorganisms, the immune response is primarily designed to afford long-term specific protection (i.e., immunity) against particular invading microorganisms; that is, it has a "memory" function. The products of the adaptive immune response include a type of serum protein—**immunoglobulins,** or **antibodies**—and a type of blood cell—**lymphocytes** (Figure 8-1).

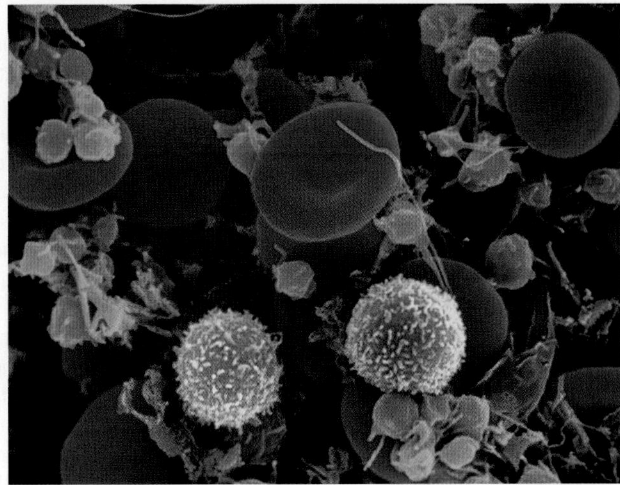

FIGURE 8-1 Scanning Electron Micrograph Showing Lymphocytes (Yellow), Red Blood Cells, and Platelets. (Copyright Dennis Kunkel Microscopy, Inc.)

Specificity and memory are the primary characteristics that differentiate the immune response from other protective mechanisms. This chapter first discusses the nature of that specificity by defining the various types of antigens that may be seen by the immune system, the ways in which they are recognized by antibodies and lymphocytes, and the specific intercellular recognition molecules that are necessary for effective immune responses. After the recognition molecules are defined, the development of the immune response is discussed. An immune response can be divided into two phases (Figure 8-2). Before birth, humans produce a large population of **T lymphocytes (T cells)** and **B lymphocytes (B cells)** that have the capacity to recognize almost any foreign antigen found in the environment. Each individual T or B cell, however, specifically recognizes only one particular antigen, but the sum of the population of lymphocyte specificities may represent millions of foreign antigens. This process is called the *generation of clonal diversity* and occurs in specialized (primary) lymphoid organs—the thymus for T cells and the bone marrow for B cells. While passing through these tissues, the lymphocytes mature and undergo changes that commit them to becoming either B or T cells. Lymphocytes are released from these organs into the circulation as immature cells that have the capacity to react with antigen (**immunocompetent**). These cells migrate to other (secondary) lymphoid organs in the body in preparation for exposure to antigen (Figure 8-3).

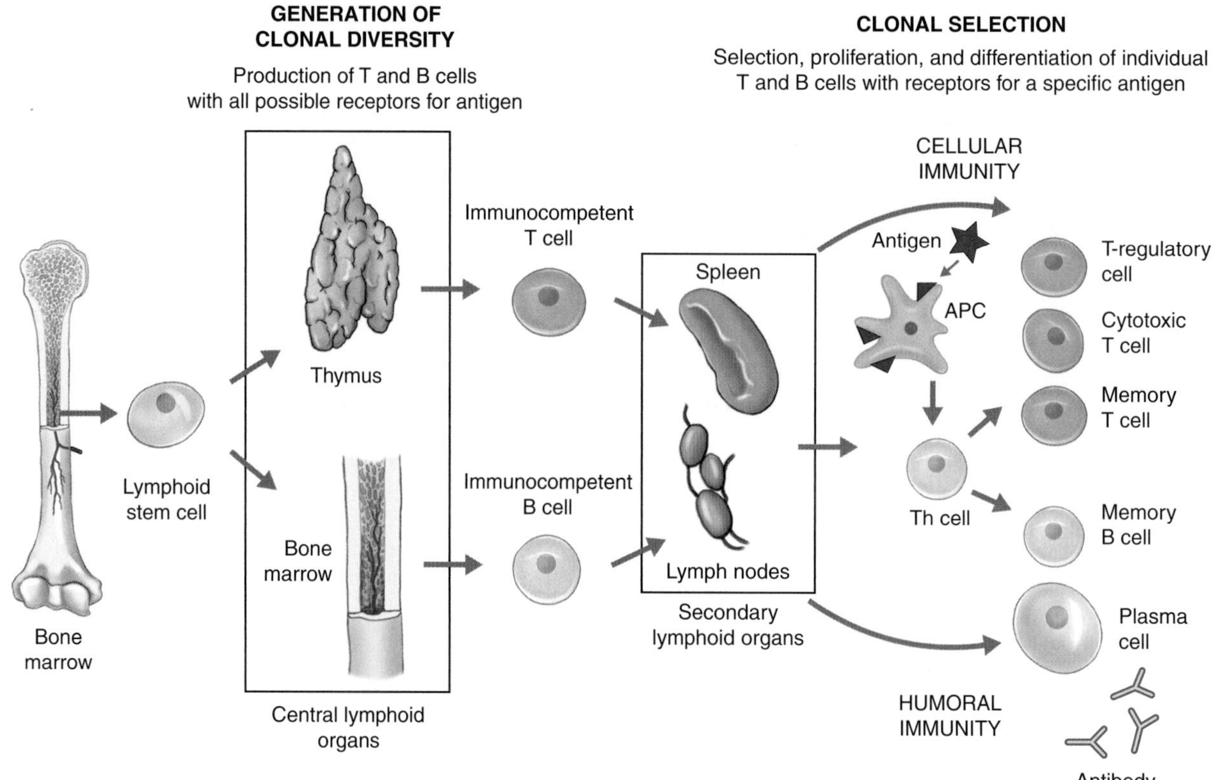

FIGURE 8-2 Overview of Immune Response. The immune response can be separated into two phases: the *generation of clonal diversity* and *clonal selection.* During the generation of clonal diversity, lymphoid stem cells from the bone marrow migrate to the central lymphoid organs (the thymus or regions of the bone marrow), where they undergo a series of cellular division and differentiation stages resulting in either immunocompetent T cells from the thymus or immunocompetent B cells from the bone marrow. (This process is outlined in more detail in Figures 8-10 and 8-12.) These cells are still naïve in that they have never encountered foreign antigen. The immunocompetent cells enter the circulation and migrate to the secondary lymphoid organs (e.g., spleen and lymph nodes), where they take up residence in B- and T-cell–rich areas. The clonal selection phase is initiated by exposure to foreign antigen. The antigen is usually processed by antigen-presenting cells (APCs) for presentation to helper T cells (Th cells) (more detail in Figure 8-16). The intercellular cooperation among APCs, Th cells, and immunocompetent T and B cells results in a second stage of cellular proliferation and differentiation (more details in Figures 8-19 and 8-22). Because antigen has "selected" those T and B cells with compatible antigen receptors, only a small population of T and B cells undergo this process at one time. The result is an active cellular immunity or humoral immunity, or both. Cellular immunity is mediated by a population of "effector" T cells that can kill targets (cytotoxic T cells) or regulate the immune response (T-regulatory cells), as well as a population of memory cells (memory T cells) that can respond more quickly to a second challenge with the same antigen. Humoral immunity is mediated by a population of soluble proteins (antibodies) produced by plasma cells and by a population of memory B cells that can produce more antibody rapidly to a second challenge with the same antigen.

The lymphocytes remain dormant until antigen initiates the second phase of the immune response, *clonal selection*. This process involves a complex interaction among cells. To initiate an effective immune response, most antigens must be "processed" because they cannot react directly with cells of the immune system but must be shown or "presented" to the immune cells in a very specific manner. This is the job of antigen-processing (antigen-presenting) cells, generally referred to as APCs. In general, three groups of cells must cooperate to make an immune response. The APCs interact with subpopulations of T cells that facilitate immune responses (T-helper cells), and immunocompetent B or T cells, resulting in differentiation of B cells into active antibody-producing cells (plasma cells) and T cells into effector cells, such as T-cytotoxic cells. The last portion of this chapter discusses how these products (antibody and T cells) protect against infection, including how they interact with components of the inflammatory process.

Humoral and Cell-Mediated Immunity

The immune response has two arms: antibody and T cells, both of which protect against infection.[2] Antibody circulates in the blood and binds to antigens on infectious agents. This interaction can result in direct inactivation of the microorganism or activation of a variety of inflammatory mediators (e.g., complement, phagocytes) that will destroy the pathogen. Antibody is primarily responsible for protection against many bacteria and viruses. This arm of the immune response is termed **humoral immunity.**

T cells also undergo differentiation during an immune response and develop into several subpopulations of cells that

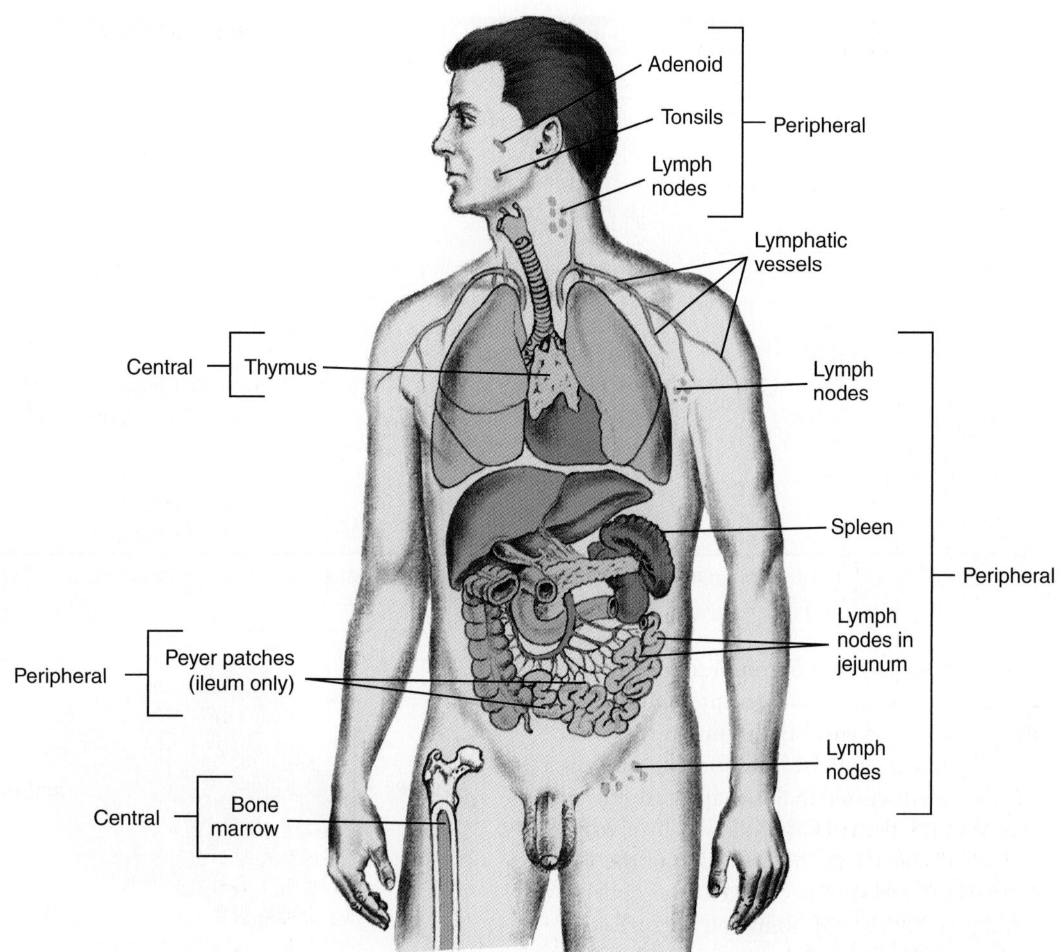

FIGURE 8-3 **Lymphoid Tissues: Sites of B-Cell and T-Cell Differentiation.** Immature lymphocytes migrate through central (primary) lymphoid tissues: the bone marrow (central lymphoid tissue for B lymphocytes) and the thymus (central lymphoid tissue for T lymphocytes). Mature lymphocytes later reside in the T and B lymphocyte–rich areas of the peripheral (secondary) lymphoid tissues.

react directly with antigen on the surface of infectious agents. Some develop into T cells that can stimulate the activities of other leukocytes via cell-to-cell contact or through the secretion of cytokines. Others develop into T-cytotoxic cells (Tc cells) that attack and kill targets directly. Targets for Tc cells include cells infected by a variety of viruses, as well as cells that have become cancerous. This arm of the immune response is termed **cellular immunity.** As discussed in this chapter, the humoral and cellular immune responses are interdependent at many levels. In the end, the success of an acquired immune response depends on the functions of both the humoral and the cellular responses, as well as the appropriate interactions between them. Additionally, both arms produce specialized subpopulations of **memory cells** that are long-lived and capable of "remembering" the antigen and responding more rapidly and efficiently on subsequent exposure to the same antigen. On reexposure, memory cells do not require much further differentiation and will therefore rapidly become new plasma cells or effector T cells.

Active vs. Passive Immunity

Adaptive immunity can be either active or passive, depending on whether the antibodies or T cells are produced by the individual in response to antigen or are administered directly. **Active acquired immunity (active immunity)** is produced by an individual either after natural exposure to an antigen or after immunization, whereas **passive acquired immunity (passive immunity)** does not involve the host's immune response at all. Rather, passive immunity occurs when preformed antibodies or T lymphocytes are transferred from a donor to the recipient. This can occur naturally, as in the passage of maternal antibodies across the placenta to the fetus, or artificially, as in a clinic using immunotherapy for a specific disease. Unvaccinated individuals who are exposed to particular infectious agents (e.g., hepatitis A virus, rabies virus) often will be given immunoglobulins that are prepared from individuals who already have antibodies against that particular pathogen. Whereas active acquired immunity is long-lived, passive immunity is only temporary because the donor's antibodies or T cells are eventually destroyed.

RECOGNITION AND RESPONSE

The foundation of any successful immune response is the specific recognition of antigen by antibody or receptors on the

TABLE 8-2 SELECT CD MOLECULES AND THEIR FUNCTIONS

CD MOLECULES	PRIMARY LOCATION	FUNCTIONS
CD1	APCs	Presents lipid antigens
CD2	All T cells, NK cells	T-cell marker; adhesion molecule that binds to CD58 (LFA-3) and provides a co-stimulatory signal
CD3	All T cells	Associated with TCR and provides intracellular signaling
CD4	Th cells	Binds to MHC class II as co-receptor with the TCR
CD8	Tc cells	Binds to MHC class I as co-receptor with the TCR
CD19	B cells	Complexes with CD21 to form a co-receptor for B cells
CD20	B cells	Major regulator of B-cell function
CD21	B cells	Receptor for complement that complexes with CD19 to form a co-receptor for B cells
CD25	Activated T cells	α-Chain of IL-2 receptor
CD28	T cells	Adhesion molecule that binds to CD80 to provide co-stimulatory signal for Tc cells
CD40	B cells, macrophages	Adhesion molecule that binds to CD154 to provide co-stimulatory signal for B cells
CD45	All lymphocytes	Has multiple types; augments antigen signal
CD58 (LFA-3)	Most cells	Adhesion molecule that binds to CD2 to provide a co-stimulatory signal
CD80 (B7-1)	APCs	Adhesion molecule that binds to CD28 to provide a co-stimulatory signal
CD154 (CD40L)	Th2 cells	Adhesion molecule that binds to CD40 to provide a co-stimulatory signal

APCs, Antigen-presenting cells; *IL,* interleukin; *MHC,* major histocompatibility complex; *NK,* natural killer; *Tc,* cytotoxic cell; *TCR,* T-cell receptor; *Th,* helper T cell.

surface of B or T cells, followed by a set of complex intercellular communications among a variety of antigen-presenting cells and lymphocytes. To fully understand the immune response, it is necessary to initially understand the basis for that recognition. Many of the molecules discussed in this chapter are part of a nomenclature that uses the prefix "CD" followed by a number (e.g., CD1 or CD2) (Table 8-2). The definition of the **CD (cluster of differentiation)** format has changed over time. It was originally used to describe proteins found on the surface of lymphocytes. Currently, CD is the accepted format for labeling a very large family of proteins found on the surface of many cells. Many have alternative names, which may be used in this chapter. The list of identified molecules is constantly increasing (the number of molecules with a CD designation is probably in excess of 250). In a similar fashion, the list of known cytokines is continually growing, with more than 100 having been identified so far. A large number of CD molecules and cytokines contribute to the acquired immune response. We have attempted to focus on a small number of highly important examples to illustrate the immensely complicated, but highly effective, interactions that take place to produce a protective immune response.

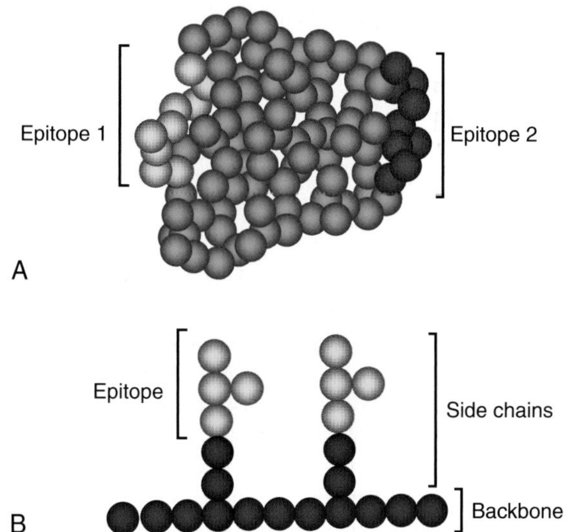

FIGURE 8-4 Antigenic Determinants (Epitopes). Shown are generic examples of epitopes on protein **(A)** and polysaccharide **(B)** molecules. In **A,** an antigenic protein may have multiple different epitopes (epitopes 1 and 2) that react with different antibodies. Each sphere represents an amino acid with the yellow spheres representing epitope 1 and the red spheres representing epitope 2. Individual epitopes may consist of eight or nine amino acids. In **B,** a polysaccharide is constructed of a backbone with branched side chains. Each sphere represents an individual carbohydrate with the yellow spheres representing the carbohydrates that form the epitope. In this example, two identical epitopes are shown that would bind two identical antibodies.

Antigens and Immunogens

An **antigen** is a molecule that can *react with* antibodies or antigen receptors on B and T cells. Most, but not all, antigens are also **immunogens.** An antigen that is **immunogenic** will induce an immune response resulting in the production of antibodies or functional T cells. Although the terms *antigen* and *immunogen* commonly are used as synonyms, there are some differences between the two, so a substance may be antigenic yet not be immunogenic.

To function as an antigen, at least a portion of a molecule's chemical structure must be recognized by and bound to an antibody and/or to specific receptors on a lymphocyte. The precise portion of the antigen that is configured for recognition and binding is called its **antigenic determinant,** or **epitope.** The matching portion on the antibody or the lymphocyte receptor is sometimes referred to as the *antigen-binding site,* or **paratope.** The size of an antigenic determinant is relatively small, perhaps just a few amino acids or carbohydrate residues on the surface of a large molecule (Figure 8-4). Therefore, macromolecules (e.g., proteins, polysaccharides, nucleic acids) usually contain multiple and diverse antigenic determinants, and the immune response against the macromolecule will usually consist of a mixture of specific antibodies against several of these determinants.

Certain criteria influence the degree to which an antigen is immunogenic. These include: (1) being foreign to the host, (2) being appropriate in size, (3) having an adequate chemical complexity, and (4) being present in a sufficient quantity.

Foremost among the criteria for immunogenicity is the antigen's foreignness. A **self-antigen** that fulfills all these criteria *except* foreignness does not normally elicit an immune response. Thus most individuals are tolerant to their own antigens. The immune system has an exquisite ability to distinguish self (self-antigens) from non-self (foreign antigens). **Tolerance,** once thought to be a state of nonresponsiveness in which the immune system passively allowed self-antigens to persist, is now known to have a variety of mechanisms. In some cases, a state of **central tolerance** exists, in which lymphocytes with receptors against self-antigens have been eliminated. In other cases, tolerance is **peripheral tolerance** and part of the adaptive immune response. Rather than merely tolerating some self-antigens, the immune system actively prevents their recognition by lymphocytes and antibodies. The response to self-antigens may be actively regulated by specialized T lymphocytes called *T-regulatory (Treg) cells* (see Figure 8-2). Some pathogens have a survival advantage by their capacity to mimic self-antigens and avoid inducing an immune response.

Molecular size also contributes to an antigen's immunogenicity. In general, large molecules (those bigger than 10,000 daltons), such as proteins, polysaccharides, and nucleic acids, are most immunogenic. Low-molecular-weight molecules, such as amino acids, monosaccharides, fatty acids, and the purine and pyrimidine bases, tend to be unable to induce an immune response. Many small molecules can function as **haptens:** antigens that are too small to be immunogens by themselves but become immunogenic in combination with larger molecules that function as **carriers** for the hapten. For example, the antigens of penicillin and poison ivy are haptens, but they initiate allergic responses only after binding to large-molecular-weight proteins in the allergic individual's blood or skin. Antigens that induce an allergic response are also called **allergens.**

Chemical complexity affects immunogenicity. The best immunogens contain a diversity of chemically different components. For instance, a large synthetic protein consisting only of alanine amino acids would not be very immunogenic, despite its size and foreignness. However, if other amino acids, such as tyrosine, tryptophan, or phenylalanine, were inserted into the structure, the degree of immunogenicity would increase greatly.

Finally, antigens that are present in extremely small or large quantities may be unable to elicit an immune response and therefore by definition are also nonimmunogenic. In many cases, high or low extremes of antigen quantities may induce a state of tolerance rather than immunity.

Even if an antigen fulfills all these criteria, the quality and intensity of the immune response may still be affected by a variety of additional factors. For example, the route and vehicle of antigenic entry or administration are critical to the immunogenicity of some antigens. This has important clinical implications. The most common routes for clinical administration of antigen, such as vaccines, are intravenous, intraperitoneal, subcutaneous, intranasal, and oral. Each route preferentially stimulates a different set of lymphocyte-containing (lymphoid) tissues and therefore results in the induction of different types of cell-mediated or humoral immune responses. For some vaccines, the route may affect the protectiveness of the immune response so that the individual is protected if immunized by one route, but may remain susceptible to infection if administered through a different route. Immunogenicity of an antigen also may be altered by being delivered along with substances that stimulate the immune response; these substances are known as *adjuvants.* Finally, the genetic makeup of a host can play a critical role in the immune system's ability to respond to many antigens; some individuals appear to be unable to respond to immunization with a particular antigen, whereas they respond well to other antigens. For instance, a small percentage of the population fails to produce a measurable immune response to the most common vaccines, despite multiple injections. Many other factors can modulate the immune response. These include the individual's age, nutritional status, genetic background, and reproductive status, as well as exposure to traumatic injury, concurrent disease, or the use of immunosuppressive medications.

Molecules That Recognize Antigen

Antigen is directly recognized by three molecules: circulating antibody and antigen receptors on the surface of B lymphocytes (**B-cell receptor,** or **BCR**) and T lymphocytes (**T-cell receptor,** or **TCR**) (Figure 8-5).

Antibody

An **antibody,** or immunoglobulin, is a serum glycoprotein produced by plasma cells in response to a challenge by an immunogen. The term *immunoglobulin* is used to denote all molecules that are known to have specificity for antigen, whereas the term *antibody* is generally used to denote one particular set of immunoglobulins with specificity against a known antigen. There are five molecular classes of immunoglobulins (IgG, IgA, IgM, IgE, and IgD) that are characterized by antigenic, structural, and functional differences (Figure 8-6). Within two of the immunoglobulin classes are several distinct subclasses including four subclasses of IgG and two subclasses of IgA.

Classes. IgG is the most abundant class of immunoglobulins; they constitute 80% to 85% of those circulating in the body and account for most of the protective activity against infections (Tables 8-3 and 8-4). As a result of selective transport across the placenta, maternal IgG is also the major class of antibody found in blood of the fetus and newborn. Four subclasses of IgG have been described: IgG1, IgG2, IgG3, and IgG4.

IgA can be divided into two subclasses, IgA1 and IgA2. IgA1 molecules are found predominantly in the blood, whereas IgA2 is the predominant class of antibody found in normal body secretions. The IgA molecules found in bodily secretions are dimers anchored together through a J chain and "secretory piece." This secretory piece is attached to the IgAs inside mucosal epithelial cells and may function to protect these immunoglobulins against degradation by enzymes also found in the secretions.

IgM is the largest of the immunoglobulins and usually exists as a pentamer that is stabilized by a J (joining) chain. It is the

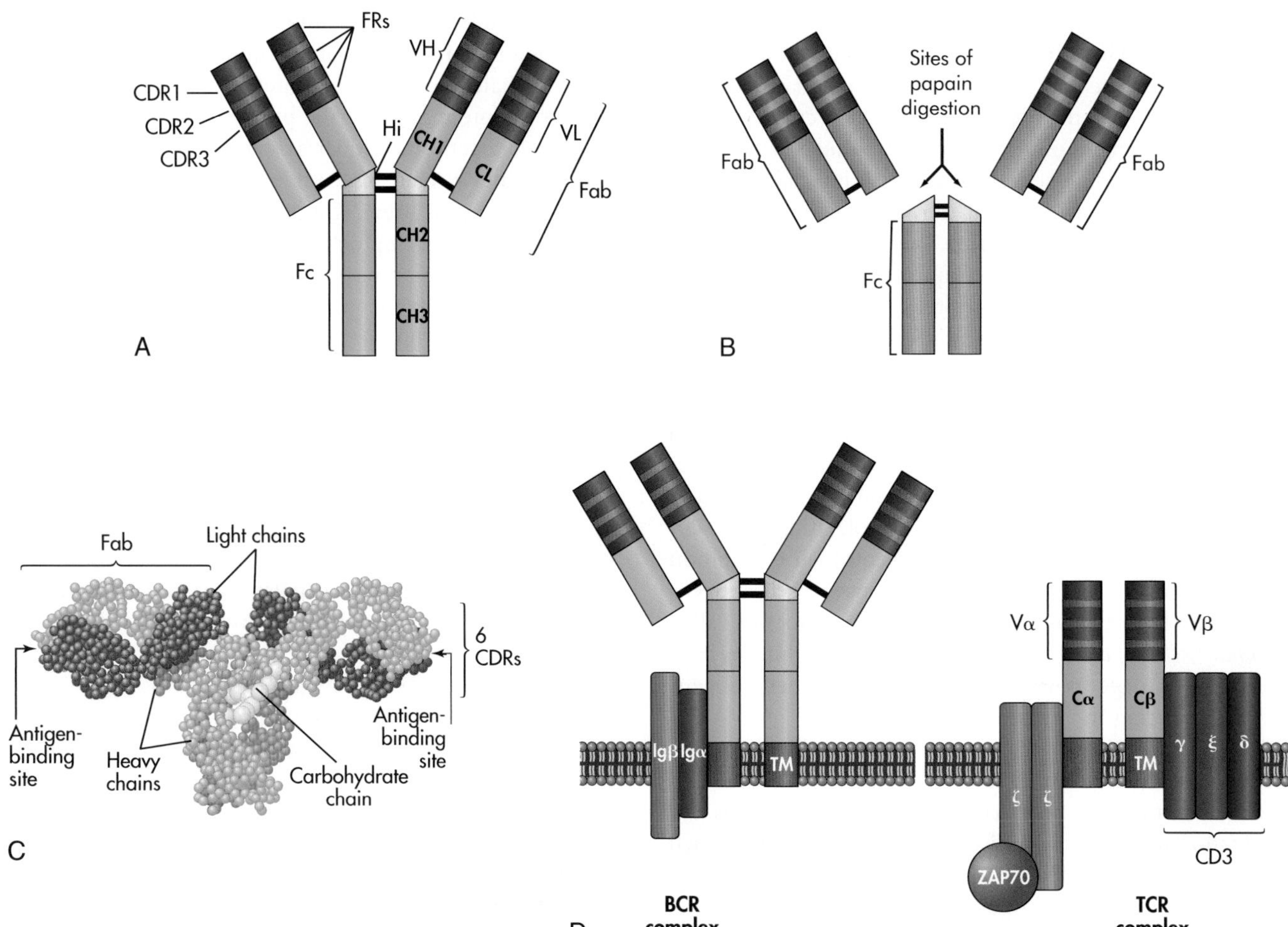

FIGURE 8-5 **Antigen-Binding Molecules.** Antigen-binding molecules include soluble antibody **(A, B, C)** and cell surface receptors **(D)**. **A,** The typical antibody molecule consists of two identical heavy chains and two identical light chains connected by interchain disulfide bonds (– between chains in the figure). Each heavy chain is divided into three regions with relatively constant amino acid sequences (CH1, CH2, and CH3) and a region with a variable amino acid sequence (VH). Each light chain is divided into a constant region (CL) and a variable region (VL). The hinge region (Hi) provides flexibility in some classes of antibody. Within each variable region are three highly variable complementary-determining regions (CDR1, CDR2, CDR3) separated by relatively constant framework regions (FRs). **B,** Fragmentation of the antibody molecule by limited digestion with the enzyme papain has identified three important portions of the molecule: an Fc and two identical Fab fragments. Both Fab fragments bind antigen. As the antibody folds **(C)**, the CDRs are placed in proximity to form the antigen-binding site. **D,** The antigen receptor on the surface of B cells (BCR complex) is a monomeric antibody with a structure similar to that of circulating antibody, with an additional hydrophobic transmembrane region (TM) that anchors the molecule to the cell surface. The active BCR complex contains molecules (Igα and Igβ) that are responsible for intracellular signaling after the receptor has bound antigen. The T-cell receptor (TCR) consists of an α-chain and a β-chain joined by a disulfide bond. Each chain consists of a constant region (Cα and Cβ) and a variable region (Vα and Vβ). Each variable region contains CDRs and FRs in a structure similar to that of antibody. The active TCR is associated with several molecules that are responsible for intracellular signaling. These include CD3, which is a complex of γ (gamma), ε (epsilon), and δ (delta) subunits, and a complex of two ζ (zeta) molecules. The ζ molecules are attached to a cytoplasmic protein kinase (ZAP70) that is critical to intracellular signaling. (**C** from Patton KT, Thibodeau GA: *Anatomy & physiology,* ed 8, St Louis, 2012, Mosby.)

first antibody produced during the initial, or primary, response to antigen. IgM is synthesized early in neonatal life, and its synthesis may be increased as a response to infection in utero.

Information on the role of IgD is limited. This class of immunoglobulins is found in very low concentrations in the blood, where they do not appear to have a known function. IgD is located primarily on the surface of developing B lymphocytes, where they function as one type of B-cell antigen receptor.

IgE is the least concentrated of any of the immunoglobulin classes in the circulation. It appears to have very specialized functions as a mediator of many common allergic responses (see Chapter 9) and in the defense against parasitic infections.

Molecular Structure. Structural analysis of immunoglobulins began with Porter's early studies on the effects of the enzyme papain on IgG.[3] The nomenclature of antibody structure originated from that work. Limited digestion with the enzyme papain cleaved IgG into three fragments, two of which were

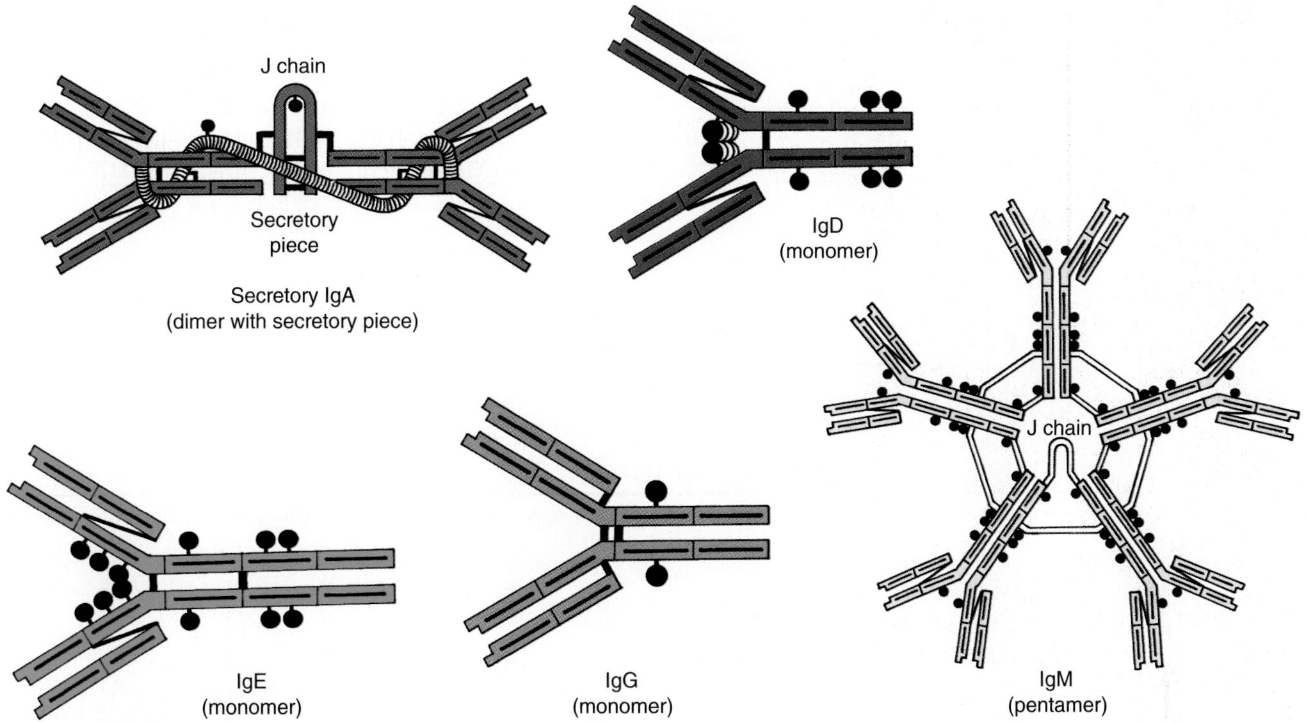

FIGURE 8-6 Structure of Different Immunoglobulins. Secretory IgA, IgD, IgE, IgG, and IgM. The black circles attached to each molecule represent carbohydrate residues.

TABLE 8-3 PHYSICOCHEMICAL PROPERTIES OF IMMUNOGLOBULINS

CLASS	SUBCLASS	HEAVY CHAIN	MOLECULAR WEIGHT (DALTONS)	ADULT SERUM LEVELS (mg/dl)
IgG	IgG1	(γ_1)	146,000	800-900
	IgG2	(γ_2)	146,000	280-300
	IgG3	(γ_3)	165,000	90-100
	IgG4	(γ_4)	146,000	50
IgM	IgM	(μ)	970,000	120-150
IgA	IgA1	(α_1)	160,000	280-300
	IgA2	(α_2)		50
	sIgA	(α_1, α_2)	385,000	5
IgD	IgD	(δ)	184,000	3
IgE	IgE	(ε)	190,000	0.03

Ig, Immunoglobulin; *s,* secretory.

identical. The two identical fragments were found to retain the ability to bind antigen, and each was termed an **antigen-binding fragment (Fab).**[4] The third fragment crystallized when separated from the Fab portions and was termed the **crystalline fragment (Fc)** (see Figure 8-5).

What Porter learned about the structure of IgG still applies not only to this class of immunoglobulins but also to each of the other classes. The Fab portions of an immunoglobulin contain the recognition sites (receptors) for antigenic determinants and confer the molecule's specificity toward a particular antigen. The Fc portion is responsible for most of the biologic functions of antibodies, including activation of the complement cascade and opsonization by binding to Fc receptors on the surface of the cells of the innate immune system.

The basic structure of the antibody molecule consists of four polypeptide chains—two identical light (L) chains and two identical heavy (H) chains (see Figure 8-5). Within the same molecule, the two heavy chains are identical and the two light chains are identical. The class of antibody is determined by which heavy chain is used: gamma (IgG), mu (IgM), alpha (IgA), epsilon (IgE), or delta (IgD). The light chains of an antibody molecule are of either the kappa (κ) or the lambda (λ) type. The light and heavy chains are held together by two major forces: noncovalent bonds and disulfide linkages. A set of disulfide linkages between the heavy chains occurs in the **hinge region** and in some instances lends a degree of molecular flexibility at that site so that the Fab regions can move.

Light and heavy chains are further subdivided into constant (C) and variable (V) regions. The constant regions have relatively stable amino acid sequences within a particular immunoglobulin class or subclass. Thus the amino acid sequence of the constant region of one IgG1 should be almost identical with the sequence of the same region of another IgG1, even if they react with different antigens. Conversely, among different antibodies, the sequences of the variable regions are characterized by a large number of amino acid differences. Therefore, two IgG1 molecules against different antigens may have many differences in the amino acid sequence of their variable regions. The variable region can be further subdivided because most of the region's variability in amino acid sequence is localized in three areas of the variable region. These three areas were once called *hypervariable regions,* but are now called **complementary-determining**

TABLE 8-4 BIOLOGIC PROPERTIES OF IMMUNOGLOBULINS

	COMPLEMENT ACTIVATION		BINDING TO FC RECEPTORS ON						
SUBCLASS	CLASSICAL	ALTERNATIVE	MACROPHAGES	PMNS	MAST CELLS	PLATELETS	PLACENTAL TRANSFER	PRESENCE IN SECRETIONS	INDUCTION OF AGGLUTINATION
IgG1	++	–	+	+	–	+	+++	±	+
IgG2	+	–	–	–	–	+	+	±	+
IgG3	+++	–	+	+	–	+	+++	±	+
IgG4	–	–	–	±	+	+	++	±	
IgM	++++	–	–	–	–	–	–	+	+++
IgA1	–	+	–	±	–	–	–	+	–
IgA2	–	+	–	±	–	–	–	+	–
sIgA	–	–	–	–	–	–	–	++++	–
IgD	–	±	–	–	–	–	–	–	–
IgE	–	±	?	–	+++	–	–	+	–

Fc, Crystalline fragment; *Ig*, immunoglobulin; *PMN*, polymorphonuclear neutrophil; *sIgA*, secretory immunoglobulin A; –, lack of activity; +, relative degree of activity.

regions (CDRs). The four regions separating the CDRs have relatively stable amino acid sequences and are called **framework regions (FRs).**

Antigen Binding

The combined amino acid sequences of the variable regions of both the heavy (V_H) and light (V_L) chains determine the conformation of the antigen-binding site and therefore the antigenic specificity of the immunoglobulin molecule. Most proteins will naturally fold and take on secondary or tertiary structures. As the immunoglobulin molecules fold, the FRs control the accuracy of folding in the variable region, and the CDRs in both variable regions are moved into proximity, resulting in an antigen-binding site formed by the three CDRs of the heavy chain and the three CDRs of the light chain. The chemical nature of the particular amino acids in those sites, as well as the topography of the site, determines the specificity toward a particular antigen. The antigen that will bind most strongly must have complementary chemistry and topography with the binding site formed by the antibody. The antigen fits into this binding site with the specificity of a key into a lock and is held there by noncovalent chemical interactions (Figure 8-7). In some cases the substitution of a single critical amino acid in a CDR may have a significant effect on the shape of the binding site and thus the specificity of the antibody molecule.

Because the heavy and light chains are identical within the same antibody molecule, the two binding sites are also identical and have specificity for the same antigen. The number of functional binding sites is called the antibody's **valence.** Most antibody classes (i.e., IgG, IgE, IgD, and circulating IgA) have a valence of 2, but secretory IgA has a valence of 4. IgM, being a pentamer, has a theoretical valence of 10, but can simultaneously use only about five binding sites because a large antigen binding to one site blocks antigen binding to another site.

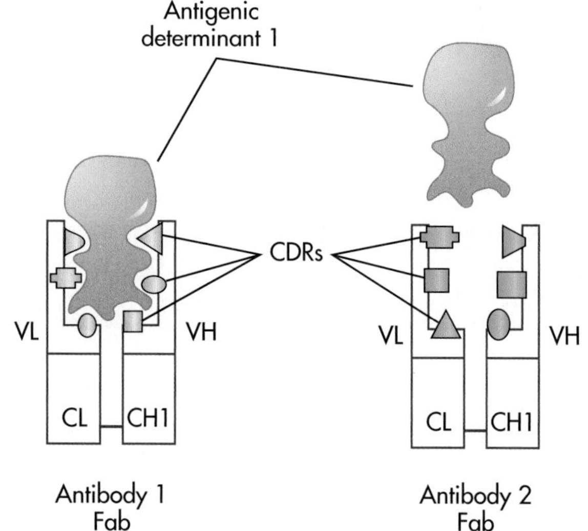

FIGURE 8-7 Antigen-Antibody Binding. The specificity required for antibody binding with an antigen is determined by the shape and chemistry of the six complementary-determining regions (CDRs) in the combining site on the variable region of the antibody. This figure indicates two different antibodies (Fab portions of antibody 1 and antibody 2) that have different sets of CDRs and therefore different specificities. As indicated, the antigenic determinant that reacts well with antibody 1 is unable to react with antibody 2 because of differences in the antibody combining site. *C*, Constant; *CH*, constant region of the heavy chain; *CL*, constant region of the light chain; *Fab*, antigen-binding fragment, *V*, variable; *VH*, variable heavy chain, *VL*, variable light chain.

B-Cell Receptor Complex

The **B-cell receptor (BCR) complex** is located on the surface of B lymphocytes (see Figure 8-5). Its role is to recognize antigen, but unlike circulating antibody, the receptor must communicate that information to the cell's nucleus. Therefore, the BCR complex consists of antigen-recognition molecules and accessory molecules involved in intracellular signaling (Igα and Igβ). BCRs on the surface of immunocompetent B cells are membrane-associated IgM (mIgM) and IgD (mIgD) immunoglobulins that are produced from the same genes that are used by plasma cells to produce soluble antibodies. As a BCR, however, mIgM is a monomer rather than the pentamer primarily found in the blood.

The BCR signaling complex consists of two Igα and Igβ heterodimers that are closely associated with the BCR and contain tyrosine kinase signaling activity. The antibody portion of the BCR complex is responsible for recognition and binding to an antigen, but by itself cannot provide the intracellular signals required to activate the B cell and complete its maturation and the production of antibodies. That message is conveyed by the Igα and Igβ heterodimers.

T-Cell Receptor Complex

T lymphocytes use a similar but distinct array of proteins in their recognition and response to antigens. The **T-cell receptor (TCR) complex** is composed of an antibody-like transmembrane protein (TCR) and a group of accessory proteins (collectively referred to as CD3) that are involved in intracellular signaling (see Figure 8-5). Similar to activation of the B lymphocyte, the TCR is responsible for recognition and binding to the antigen, whereas the accessory proteins are responsible for the intracellular signaling necessary for activation and differentiation of the T cell. Each of the individual components of the TCR complex is important, and several severe defects in the T-cell immune response have been related to mutations in individual components of the complex (see Chapter 9).

Molecules That Present Antigen

For an effective immune response, most antigens must be processed within cells and expressed on the surface of those cells in a very specific manner. Some types of antigen are managed only by highly specialized cells: **antigen-presenting cells,** or **APCs.** Other types of antigens can be processed and presented by almost any type of cell. Several sets of cell surface molecules have the responsibility for appropriately presenting antigen. These molecules are described below.

Major Histocompatibility Complex

An essential set of recognition molecules are members of the **major histocompatibility complex (MHC).** Most antibody and cellular immune responses are dependent on antigen presentation by APCs. Additionally, the role of T-cytotoxic cells in killing virally infected cells depends on presentation of the viral antigen on the infected cell's surface. **Antigen presentation** is the primary role of molecules of the MHC.

MHC molecules are glycoproteins found on the surface of all human cells except red blood cells. They are divided into two general classes, class I and class II, based on their molecular structure, distribution among cell populations, and function in antigen presentation. MHC class I molecules are heterodimers composed of a large α-chain along with a smaller chain called *β2-microglobulin.* MHC class II molecules are also heterodimers with both α- and β-chains. The general properties of each of the MHC classes are summarized in Figure 8-8.

Molecules of the two MHC classes are encoded from different genetic loci that are located as a large complex of genes on the short arm of human chromosome 6 (see Figure 8-8). The MHC also contains other genes that control the quality and quantity of an immune response, which are commonly referred to as class III MHC genes. The primary **MHC class I genes** consist of three closely linked loci on this chromosome labeled A, B, and C. The primary **MHC class II genes** are located within the D region, which actually consists of three separate and independent loci: DR, DP, and DQ.

The class I and class II MHC loci are the most genetically diverse (polymorphic) of any human genetic loci. Within the human population, the number of possible different alleles (i.e., forms of the gene) expressed by each locus is astounding: 649 at the A locus, 1029 at the B locus, 350 at the C locus, 643 at the DR locus (α and β), 125 at the DQ locus (α and β), and 154 at the DP locus (α and β). These numbers are based on the polymorphism of observed DNA sequences and may not reflect differences in function. Clearly, not every allele is expressed in the same individual. Humans have two copies of each MHC locus (one inherited from each parent) that are codominant so that molecules encoded by each parent's genes are expressed on the cell surface. Within an individual, each locus will be expressing only one allele. For instance, each person will have only two different A proteins (one from each parent). However, with the tremendous number of possible alleles that can be expressed, it is likely that any two unrelated individuals will have different sets of MHC molecules on their cell surfaces so that each of us is distinct.

Transplantation. The diversity of MHC molecules becomes clinically relevant during organ transplantation. Cells in transplanted tissue or organs from one individual will have a different set of MHC surface antigens than those of the recipient; therefore, the recipient can mount an immune response against the foreign MHC antigens, resulting in rejection of the transplanted tissue. As a result of studies of transplantation, the human MHC molecules are also referred to as **human leukocyte antigens (HLAs),** and the different MHC genetic loci are commonly called HLA-A, HLA-B, HLA-C, HLA-DR, HLA-DQ, and HLA-DP. To minimize the chance of tissue rejection, the donor and recipient are often *tissue typed* beforehand to identify differences in HLA antigens. The more similar two individuals are in their HLA tissue type, the more likely a transplant from one to the other will be successful.

Although a large number of alleles exist at the molecular level, the diversity is considerably less at the antigenic level: there are approximately 67 different HLA-A antigens, 149 HLA-B antigens, and 39 HLA-C antigens. Because of the large number of different alleles, it is highly unlikely that a perfect "match" can be found in the general population between a potential donor and the recipient.

The specific combination of alleles at the six major HLA loci on one chromosome (A, B, C, DR, DQ, and DP) is termed a **haplotype.** Each individual has two HLA haplotypes, one from the paternal chromosome 6 and another from the maternal chromosome. Because the different HLA loci within the MHC are in such close proximity to one another, haplotypes are not *usually* disrupted by recombination and are thus inherited intact. Each parent passes on one HLA haplotype to each of his or her offspring, meaning that children usually share one haplotype with each parent (Figure 8-9). Odds dictate that children will share one haplotype with half of their siblings and either no haplotypes or both haplotypes with a quarter of their siblings.

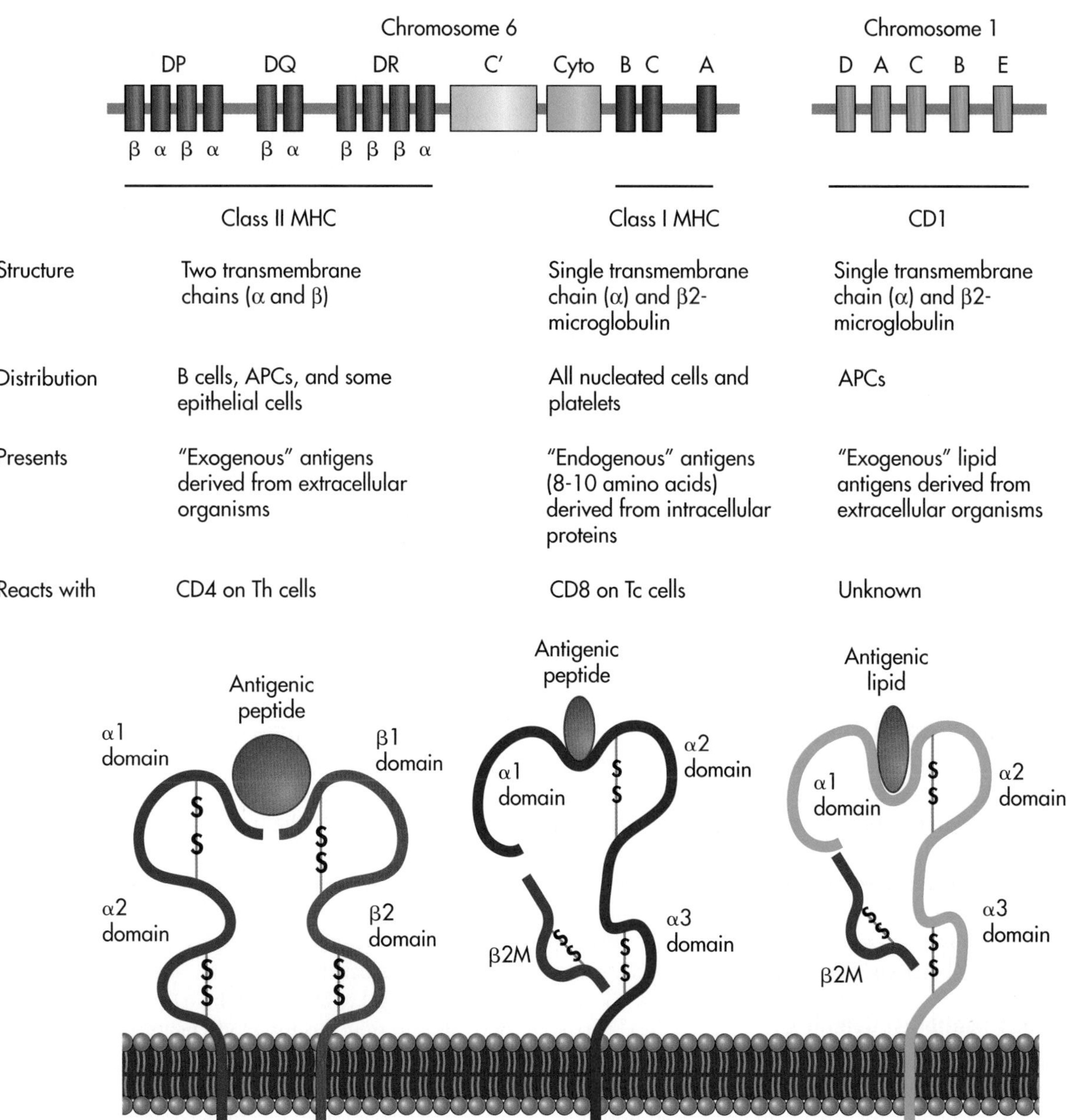

FIGURE 8-8 Genetics and Structure of Antigen-Presenting Molecules. Three sets of molecules are primarily responsible for antigen presentation: MHC class I, MHC class II, and CD1. The MHC molecules are encoded from the MHC region on chromosome 6, which contains information for class I and class II molecules, as well as for several other molecules that participate in the innate or immune responses. These include several complement proteins (C′) and cytokines (Cyto), which are referred to as MHC class III molecules. Three principal class I molecules, HLA-A, HLA-B, and HLA-C, are presented here, but this region contains information for the α-chains of several other molecules, including HLA-E, HLA-F, and HLA-G. The MHC class I products complex with β2-microglobulin, which is encoded by a gene on chromosome 15. The MHC class I molecules present small peptide antigens in a pocket formed by the α1 and α2 domains of the α-chain. The conformation of the molecule is stabilized by β2-microglobulin (β2M) as well as by intrachain disulfide bonds (-S-S-). The α- and β-chains of class II molecules are also encoded in this region: HLA-DR, HLA-DP, and HLA-DQ. In some cases, multiple genes for α- and β-chains are available. The MHC class II molecules present peptide antigens in a pocket formed by the α1 domain of the α-chain and the β1 domain of the β-chain. The genes for CD1 molecules are encoded on chromosome 1, which contains genes for five α-chains (CD1A-E), and the α-chains complex with β2-microglobulin to present lipid antigens in a pocket formed by the α1 and α2 domains. All three sets of antigen-presenting molecules are anchored to the plasma membrane by hydrophobic regions on the ends of the α- and β-chains. *MHC,* Major histocompatibility complex.

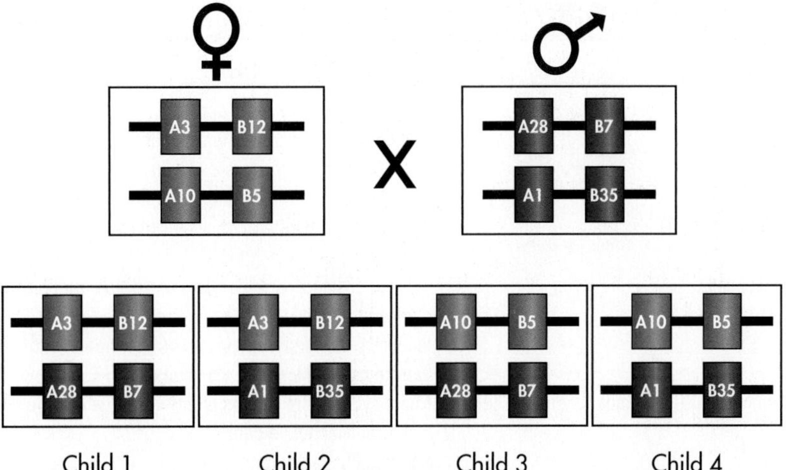

FIGURE 8-9 **Inheritance of HLA.** HLA alleles are inherited in a codominant fashion so that both maternal and paternal antigens are expressed. Specific HLA alleles are commonly given numbers to indicate different antigens. In this example, the mother has linked genes for HLA-A3 and HLA-B12 on one chromosome 6 and genes for HLA-A10 and HLA-B5 on the second chromosome 6. The father has HLA-A28 and HLA-B7 on one chromosome and HLA-A1 and HLA-B35 on the second chromosome. On one particular chromosome, the HLA antigens are firmly linked, with crossovers occurring in only 1% of individuals. The children from this pairing may have one of four possible combinations of maternal and paternal HLA. *HLA,* Human leukocyte antigen.

Thus the chance of finding a match among siblings is much higher (25%) than that from the general population.

It should be noted, however, that although HLA alleles are the primary contributor to rejection of a transplant, a number of other antigens also have a role in determining tissue compatibility. Some of these are encoded on other chromosomes and are inherited independently of HLA antigens. This means that although two people have the same HLA makeup, a graft or transplant still may be rejected because of differences between other antigens. It is preferable to obtain a graft or transplant from a closely related individual, such as a sibling, because the chance of sharing both the same HLA antigens and other undetermined antigenic differences encoded outside the MHC is much greater.

CD1

Another set of antigen-presenting molecules are members of the CD1 group. CD1 molecules have very low genetic polymorphism, a structure similar to MHC class I, and are found primarily on APCs and cells in the thymus. Unlike MHC molecules that present proteins, the CD1 molecules appear to specialize in presenting lipid antigens contained in lipoproteins, glycolipids, and other molecules. These antigens are commonly important factors in infections with bacteria of the *Mycobacterium* spp. (e.g., *Mycobacterium tuberculosis* that causes tuberculosis and *Mycobacterium leprae* that causes leprosy), which have a very large amount of lipid in their cell membranes.

Molecules That Hold Cells Together

The efficient development of an immune response requires several antigen-independent interactions between cells. The interactions between specific cellular receptors and their ligands result in intracellular signaling events that are independent of the TCR or BCR complexes but are necessary complements to the antigen-specific signal. Several of these molecules are listed in Box 8-1.

BOX 8-1 IMPORTANT ADHESION MOLECULE PAIRINGS

Th-cell CD4	⇔	MHC class II on APC
Tc-cell CD8	⇔	MHC class I on APC
Tc-cell CD2	⇔	CD58 (LFA-3) on APC
Tc-cell CD28	⇔	CD80 (B7-1) on APC
Tc-cell LFA-1	⇔	ICAM-1 on APC
Th-cell CD40L (CD154)	⇔	CD40 on B cell
Th-cell CD40L (CD154)	⇔	CD40 on APC

APC, Antigen-presenting cell; *ICAM,* intercellular adhesion molecule; *LFA,* lymphocyte function associated antigen; *MHC,* major histocompatibility complex; *Tc,* cytotoxic cell; *Th,* helper T cell.

Cytokines and Their Receptors

As discussed in Chapter 7, cytokines are low-molecular-weight proteins, or glycoproteins, that function as chemical signals between cells. A large number of cytokines are secreted by APCs and lymphocytes and provide both positive and negative regulation of the immune response. The effects of particular cytokines depend on binding to specific cellular receptors, which are linked to intracellular signaling pathways. The lymphocyte may respond in many ways. One of the most common responses is an increase in the production of proteins, many of which are other cytokines or cytokine receptors. Many cytokines also cause a lymphocyte to proliferate and differentiate. The participation of cytokines is essential to the development of an adequate immune response, and in general, the precise combination of cytokines influences the ultimate response of

TABLE 8-5 KEY CYTOKINES AND RECEPTORS THAT INFLUENCE THE IMMUNE RESPONSE

CYTOKINE	PRIMARY SOURCE	PRIMARY FUNCTION
Interleukin (IL)		
IL-1	APCs	Stimulates T cells to proliferation and differentiation; induces acute-phase proteins in inflammatory response; endogenous pyrogen
IL-2	Th1 cells, NK cells	Stimulates proliferation and differentiation of T cells and NK cells
IL-4	Th2 cells, mast cells	Induces B-cell proliferation and differentiation; up-regulates MHC class II expression; induces class-switch to IgE
IL-5	Th2 cells, mast cells	Induces eosinophil proliferation and differentiation; induces B-cell proliferation and differentiation
IL-6	Th2 cells, APCs	Induces B-cell proliferation and differentiation into plasma cells; induces acute-phase proteins in inflammatory response
IL-7	Thymic epithelial cells, bone marrow stromal cells	Major cytokine for induction of B- and T-cell proliferation and differentiation in central lymphoid organs
IL-8	Macrophages	Chemotactic factor for neutrophils
IL-10	Th cells, B cells	Inhibits cytokine production; activator of B cells
IL-12	B cells, APCs	Induces NK-cell proliferation; increases production of IFN-γ
IL-13	Th2 cells	IL-4–like properties; decreases inflammatory responses
IL-17	Th17 cells	Increases inflammation; increased influx of neutrophils and macrophages; increased epithelial cell chemokine production
IL-22	Th17 cells	Increases inflammation; increased epithelial cell production of antimicrobial peptides
Interferon (IFN)		
IFN-α, IFN-β	Macrophages, some virally infected cells	Antiviral; increases expression of MHC class I; activates NK cells
IFN-γ	Th1 cells, NK cells, Tc cells	Increases expression of MHC class II; activates macrophages and NK cells
Tumor Necrosis Factor (TNF)		
TNF-α (cachectin)	Macrophages	IL-1–like properties; induces cellular proliferation
TNF-β (lymphotoxin)	Tc cells	Kills some cells; increases phagocytosis by macrophages and neutrophils
Transforming Growth Factor (TGF)		
TGF-β	Lymphocytes, macrophages, fibroblasts	Chemotactic for macrophages; increases macrophage IL-1 production; stimulates wound healing

CYTOKINE RECEPTORS	LIGAND	ADDITIONAL INFORMATION
Class I receptor dimers (α- and β-chains)	IL-3, IL-5, IL-6, IL-11, IL-12, IL-13	IL-3 and IL-5 share a common α-chain; IL-6 and IL-11 share a common β-chain
Trimers (α-, β-, and γ-chains)	IL-2, IL-4, IL-7, IL-9, IL-15	All share a common γ-chain
Class II receptors	IFN-α, -β, and -γ	Two chains
TNF receptors	TNF-α, TNF-β, CD40, Fas	Single chain
Immunoglobulin-like receptors	IL-1	Single chain with immunoglobulin-like characteristics

APCs, Antigen-presenting cells; *MHC,* major histocompatibility complex; *NK,* natural killer; *Tc,* cytotoxic cells; *Th,* helper T cells.

a given cell. Specific deficiencies in the immune response that result from genetic mutations that lead to defective cytokine production or defective cytokine receptors are discussed in Chapter 9. Table 8-5 provides information about key cytokines and receptors that are known to influence the immune response.

GENERATION OF CLONAL DIVERSITY

It has been suggested that more than 10^8 different antigenic determinants may be recognized by receptors on an individual's immunocompetent B cells. A similar number may be recognized by T-cell receptors. However, each T or B cell has only a single receptor specificity that recognizes only one antigen, and each is present before that individual is ever exposed to foreign antigen. Thus before the individual is exposed to any foreign antigen, millions of different T- and B-cell antigen receptors must be constructed to recognize *any* potential antigenic determinant.

Several theories were proposed to explain how such a great diversity of recognition could be produced. The process occurs in two phases: the **generation of clonal diversity,** during which all the necessary receptor specificities are produced; and **clonal selection,** during which antigen selects those lymphocytes with compatible receptors, expands their population, and causes differentiation into antibody-secreting plasma cells or mature T cells (Table 8-6).[5,6] The generation of clonal diversity takes place in the **primary (central) lymphoid organs** (i.e., thymus

TABLE 8-6 GENERATION OF CLONAL DIVERSITY VS. CLONAL SELECTION

	GENERATION OF CLONAL DIVERSITY	CLONAL SELECTION
Purpose?	To produce large numbers of T and B lymphocytes with the maximum diversity of antigen receptors	Select, expand, and differentiate clones of T and B cells against a specific antigen
When does it occur?	Primarily in the fetus	Primarily after birth and throughout life
Where does it occur?	Central lymphoid organs: thymus for T cells, bone marrow for B cells	Peripheral lymphoid organs, including lymph nodes, spleen, and other lymphoid tissues
Is foreign antigen involved?	No	Yes; antigen determines which clones of cells will be selected
What hormones/cytokines are involved?	Thymic hormones, IL-7, others	Many cytokines produced by Th cells and APCs
Is tolerance induced?	Central tolerance induced as autoreactive cells are deleted	Peripheral tolerance induced as autoreactive cells are regulated
Final product?	Immunocompetent T and B cells that can react with antigen but have not seen antigen, and migrate to the secondary lymphoid organs	Plasma cells that produce antibody, effector T cells that help (Th), kill targets (Tc), or regulate immune responses (Treg); memory B and T cells

APCs, Antigen-presenting cells; *IL,* interleukin; *Tc,* cytotoxic T cells; *Th,* helper T cells; *Treg,* regulatory T cells.

and bone marrow), is driven by hormones, does not require foreign antigen, and results in the generation of immature but immunocompetent T and B cells with receptors that can recognize virtually any antigenic molecule. Both T and B cells are derived from common precursor cells **(lymphoid stem cells)** that arise either in the liver (in the fetus) or in the bone marrow (of a child or adult). These precursor cells are distinct from the precursor cells that give rise to cells of the innate immune system. The immunocompetent T and B cells migrate from the primary lymphoid organs to **secondary (peripheral) lymphoid organs** (e.g., spleen, lymph nodes, adenoids, tonsils, Peyer patches), where they await antigen. Clonal selection is initiated by antigen and results in a mature and specific immune response against that antigen.

Although generation of clonal diversity primarily occurs in the fetus, it probably continues to a low degree throughout most of adult life. Clonal selection usually begins at birth and proceeds throughout the life of the individual as new antigens are encountered, although it can begin as early as the eighth week of gestation in humans.

As a result of this process, T and B lymphocytes have the capacity to react against virtually any antigen found in nature. This endless array of possible antibodies and TCRs certainly cannot be constructed from the amount of deoxyribonucleic acid (DNA) that is in the nucleus of a human lymphocyte. The enormous repertoire of specificities is instead made possible by rearrangement of existing DNA during T- and B-cell development in the primary lymphoid organs. Loci in the DNA that encode for the variable regions of immunoglobulins and TCRs are recombined in a unique way to generate receptors that collectively can recognize and bind to any possible antigen. The DNA in the nucleus of a developing T and B cell is actually cut and spliced (repaired), a process known as **somatic recombination,** so that after this manipulation, the progeny of a single lymphocyte will synthesize identical immunoglobulins or TCRs. Those variable regions, however, are cut and spliced differently from those of another lymphocyte, making each cell unique and therefore able to react with different antigens. The particular process for B and T cells is discussed next.

T-Cell Maturation

Central Lymphoid Organ

The central lymphoid organ for T-cell development is the thymus, which is an organ located near the heart. Precursor cells (lymphoid stem cells) arise in early embryonic life from the yolk sac and fetal liver and later from the bone marrow. They migrate to the thymus and enter the subcapsular region. As the cells move through the thymic cortex to the medulla, they are instructed by interactions with various thymic cells (epithelial cells, macrophages, and dendritic cells) and thymic hormones to undergo proliferation and progressive development of the characteristics of immunocompetent T cells[7] (Figure 8-10). Changes include development of the T-cell receptor complex and expression of characteristic surface molecules. Many T cells randomly develop TCRs against self-antigens, but are deleted during this process. The final antigen-reactive T cells are released into the blood and take up residence in the secondary lymphoid organs to await antigen.

Production of the T-Cell Receptor

Like antibody, the TCR reacts with antigen (see Figure 8-5). Although the structure of the TCR closely resembles a Fab portion of antibody, the TCR uses different protein chains than are used for antibody. The most common TCR contains α- and β-chains, each of which has a variable region and a constant region. Within each variable region are three CDR regions separated by FR regions.

The great amount of variable region diversity necessary for identifying the huge number of antigens found in nature is produced by random recombination of multiple genes to encode the variable regions of both the α- and β-chains. In the germline genes, the information for the amino acid sequence of the α-chain variable region is found on chromosome 14 in two separated, but closely associated, locations: a set of *V* region genes and a set of *J* region genes (Figure 8-11). The TCR α-chain locus has multiple (at least 50) *V* genes and multiple (at least 50) *J* genes. During somatic recombination in a developing T cell, one of the possible *V* genes is randomly selected and spliced to one of the *J* genes, with the intervening DNA being removed. This DNA rearrangement process is controlled by two enzymes

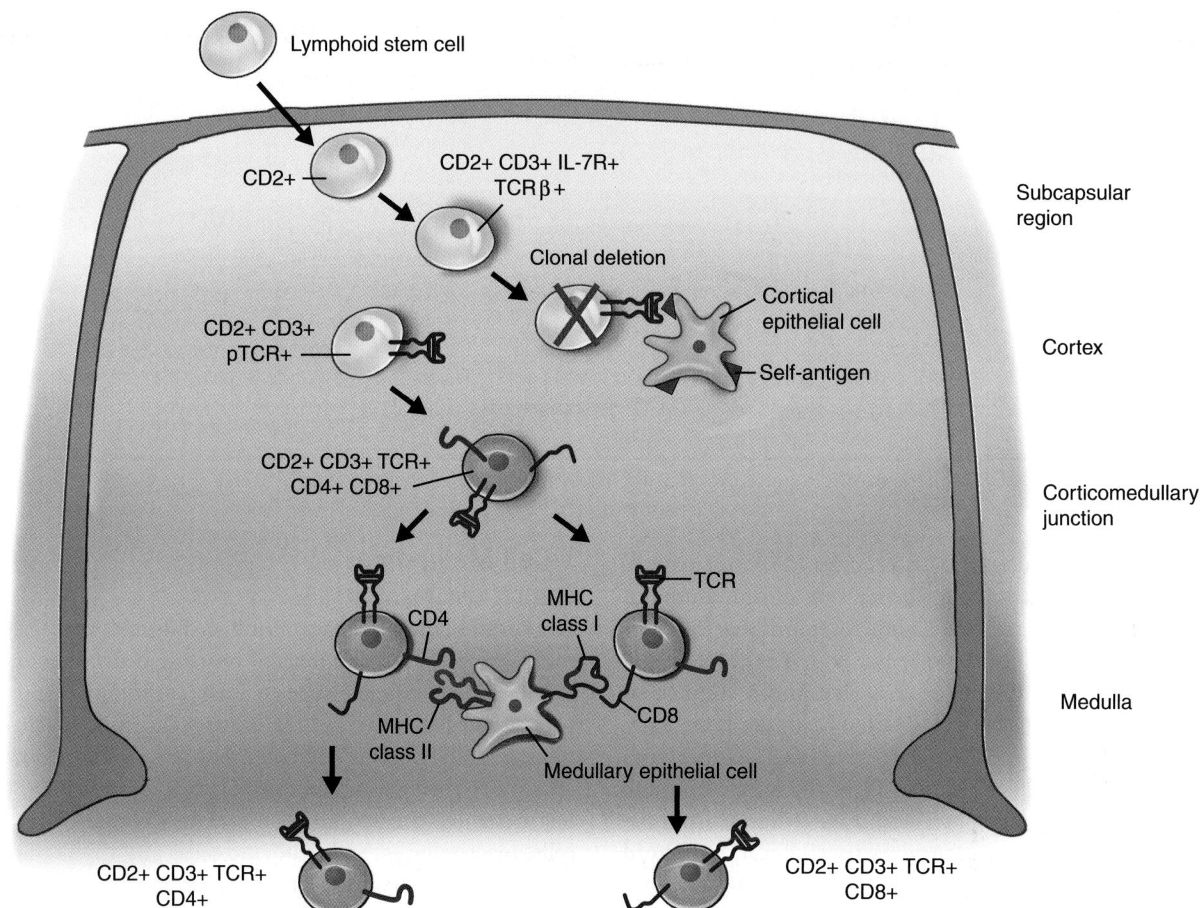

FIGURE 8-10 T-Cell Development in the Thymus. During the generation of clonal diversity in the fetus, lymphoid stem cells undergo several stages of cellular division and differentiation in a central lymphoid organ (the thymus) under the control of hormones but without the influence of foreign antigen. A simplified scheme for that process is presented here. The differentiation process is characterized by the up-regulation of many important surface molecules (only some of which are shown) and the random development of a huge number of different T-cell receptors against all possible antigens that the adult may encounter. The lymphoid stem cell enters the subcapsular region of the thymus, where it begins to undergo differentiation. One of the first surface changes is the appearance of the molecule CD2, which is a marker for all T cells. In the cortex of the thymus, the developing cell encounters epithelial cells that guide most of the early differentiation process. The pre–T cell begins expressing the surface receptor for the cytokine IL-7, which is produced by the epithelial cell along with other thymic hormones to drive the T-cell differentiation process. At this stage the T cell begins constructing the T-cell receptor (TCR) by first rearranging and expressing the TCR β-chain (more detail is provided in Figure 8-11) and expressing CD3 molecules. Although the TCR α-chain has not yet been produced, the β-chain is expressed on the surface as a pre-TCR (pTCR) using a protein that acts as a surrogate for the α-chain. Because of the randomness of the process, some pTCRs are produced with specificities toward self-antigens. Many of these undergo negative selection and are deleted (clonal deletion) by apoptosis induced through interactions with self-antigens presented by the epithelial cells. Survivors of negative selection move toward the thymic cortex and begin expressing the TCR α-chain, the normal TCR, and both CD4 and CD8 on their surfaces. These CD4+, CD8+ "double-positive" cells encounter medullary epithelial cells that express both MHC class I and MHC class II molecules. The phenotype of the developing T cell is positively selected so that interaction between CD4 and MHC class II selects for retention of CD4 expression, whereas interaction between CD8 and MHC class I favors the CD8 phenotype. Thus two populations of "single-positive" immunocompetent T cells leave the thymus: one cell is CD4+, CD8– (destined to be a helper T [Th] cell) and the other is CD4–, CD8+ (destined to be a cytotoxic T [Tc] cell).

produced by genes *RAG-1* and *RAG-2* (recombination activating genes). These enzymes cut double-stranded DNA at specific recognition sites (recombinant signal sequences) and then repair the break, resulting in excision of the DNA between the selected *V* and *J* genes. At transcription, the genetic information for the α-chain variable region is still separated from the gene for the α-chain constant region. This product is transcribed into messenger ribonucleic acid (mRNA) that contains information for the variable region *(VJ)* separated by a span of RNA from the information for the α-chain constant region. An RNA-processing step removes the intervening span, bringing the message for the variable and constant regions together into a final mRNA product that is translated into the intact α-chain protein. The random selection and pairing of 50 *V* and 50 *J*

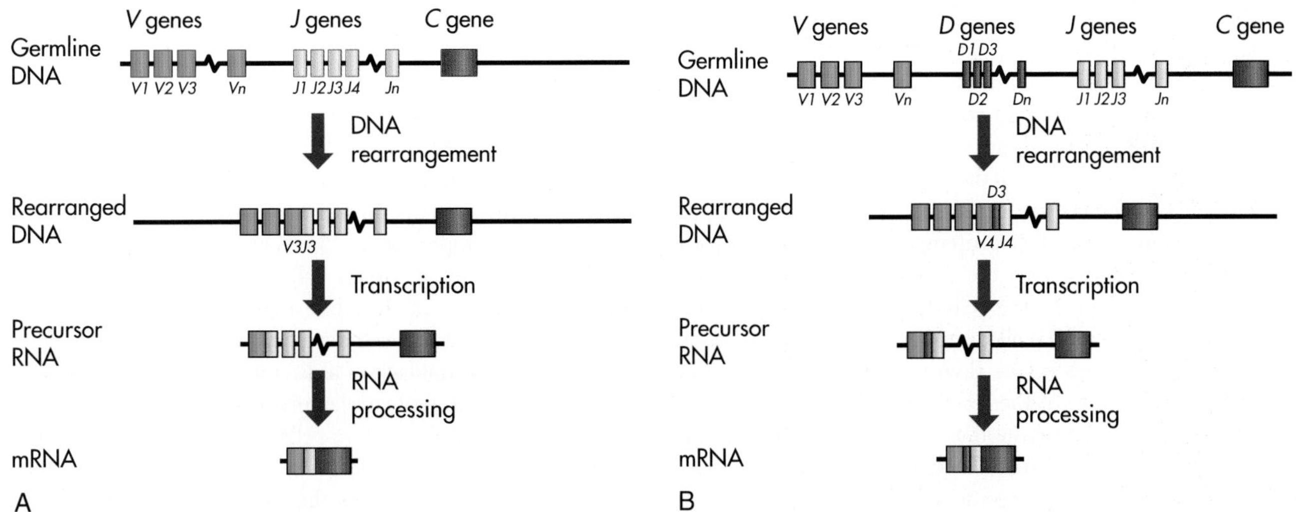

FIGURE 8-11 DNA Rearrangement of Genes for Antigen-Binding Molecules. During the generation of clonal diversity, a tremendous number of different antigen-binding molecules are produced. These include the B-cell receptor (BCR), which consists of a membrane-bound antibody molecule, and the T-cell receptor (TCR). The process by which receptor diversity is created is identical for all antigen-binding molecules and is summarized in this figure. Maximum diversity with minimum use of DNA is accomplished by random rearrangement of sets of genes that encode different portions of the variable regions. **A,** The variable regions of the light chain of antibody and the α-chain of the TCR independently rearrange two sets of genes: *V* region genes and *J* region genes. The light chain uses its own set of genes, and the α-chain uses a completely different set. In neither case is the exact number of *V* or *J* region genes known; therefore, in this figure they are numbered from 1 to an unknown value *(n)*. In a particular cell's DNA, one *V* gene is randomly selected and moved to a position immediately adjacent to a randomly selected *J* gene. In this example, *V3* and *J3* were selected. The DNA between the selected genes is enzymatically removed and the DNA repaired, so that the rearranged DNA in this example is missing the portion found in the germline DNA between *V3* and *J3*. This product is transcribed into a precursor ribonucleic acid (RNA) that contains information for the rearranged *VJ* pair, a span containing other unselected *J* regions, and information for the appropriate constant region (*C* gene) of the molecule. The RNA between the *VJ* and the *C* regions is not translated; therefore, it is removed by RNA processing to produce a messenger RNA (mRNA) that is translated. **B,** The variable region of the antibody heavy chain and the TCR β-chain results from a similar DNA rearrangement, with the added diversity contributed by a group of *D* region genes. The joining of *D* and *J* occurs first, with the removal of intervening DNA. In this example, *D3* and *J4* were chosen. This is followed by rearrangement of the *V* gene (e.g., *V4*) and formation of a *VDJ* region in the rearranged DNA. The precursor RNA contains information for the *VDJ*, the intervening portion of DNA, and the appropriate constant region. After RNA processing, an mRNA is formed for the intact antibody heavy chain or the TCR β-chain. Once the DNA is rearranged and spliced in a given B or T cell, all of the antigen receptors produced by that cell employ the same *V, D,* and *J* segments and have the same specificity.

genes by a large number of developing T cells can result in more than 2500 possible α-chains.

In a similar fashion, the TCR β-chain locus on chromosome 7 has three sets of genes that rearrange to encode the variable region of that chain: at least 20 *V* genes, 13 *J* genes, and 2 intervening and relatively short *D* genes that add further diversity. Using the RAG-1 and RAG-2 enzymes, a developing T cell randomly selects a set of *V, D,* and *J* genes for DNA recombination. The *VDJ* rearranged segment is transcribed with a β-chain constant region, the intervening RNA is removed during processing, and the final mRNA is translated into an intact β-chain.[8]

The α- and β-chains are joined by that cell and inserted into the membrane to make an antigen-specific TCR. The enormous number of possible combinations of α-chain *V* and *J* regions along with the β-chain *V, D,* and *J* regions enables the generation of a population of T cells with a large diversity of TCRs (estimated at 1.3×10^5 possible combinations). For both chains, the *V* region genes encode the amino acid sequences that include CDR1 and CDR2 and their appropriate FR regions. The *J* regions contain information for CDR3 and FR4. The TCR β-chain *D* regions encode a short amino acid sequence found in the CDR3 and greatly increases the diversity of the β-chain CDR3. Imprecise joining increases the diversity of the CDR3 regions of both the α- and β-chains even further. For example, the sites of *VJ* and *VDJ* joining may shift slightly resulting in an amino acid being inserted or deleted from the protein.

Although the αβ TCR is the preferred antigen receptor, some T cells use alternative genes: gamma (γ) (chromosome 7) and delta (δ) (chromosome 14, in the middle of α-chain genes). T cells with γδ TCRs appear to migrate to unique areas of the body (the epithelial areas in the skin, reproductive tract, intestine, respiratory tract) and have different and less well understood functions than the T cells with αβ TCRs.

Changes in Characteristic Surface Markers

Differentiation of T cells in the thymus also results in changes in a variety of important surface molecules. As the developing T cells move through the thymic cortex, they initiate the expression of the molecule CD2 on the cell surface. CD2 is a marker for T cells and is expressed on virtually every subpopulation of cells that have undergone development in the thymus. Within the cortex, the cells begin rearranging the variable region genes necessary for forming a functional T-cell receptor. The T-cell receptor undergoes several stepwise changes until the final αβ TCR is formed. Concurrently, the TCR accessory molecules (collectively called CD3) are expressed. The cell also begins making two important surface proteins, CD4 and CD8, which are concurrently expressed on the developing cell's surface at this stage.[9] These CD4+, CD8+ cells are often called "double-positive" cells. Much of T-cell development is controlled by hormones and cytokines in the thymus, and an early step in maturation is expression of the receptor for interleukin-7 (IL-7R), which is a major cytokine that drives the differentiation process. After entering the medulla of the thymus, the double-positive cells become "single-positive." That is, some of the cells suppress production of the CD8 molecule and remain only CD4+, whereas others suppress CD4 production and remain CD8+.[10] This branch in the differentiation pathway leads to two groups of cells with different functional characteristics: CD4 cells tend to recognize antigen presented by MHC class II molecules and develop into helpers in the later clonal selection process (T-helper cells), whereas CD8 cells recognize antigen presented by MHC class I molecules and become mediators of cell-mediated immunity and kill other cells directly (T-cytotoxic cells).[11]

Central Tolerance

During the random rearrangement of *VJ* and *VDJ* genes to produce the T-cell receptor, some combinations result in specificities that recognize self-antigens. If some of these *autoreactive* T cells were allowed to progress further in development and leave the thymus, a severe immunologic reaction against the individual's own tissues could result. One stage at which tolerance for self-antigens is maintained is the deletion of autoreactive T cells in the thymus, which is referred to as central tolerance.

A variety of self-antigens are expressed by thymic cells. Many thymic cells express MHC class I or MHC class II molecules. During the T-cell's double-positive stage, if a TCR strongly reacts with MHC class I or class II, the T cell will undergo apoptosis, referred to as *clonal deletion*. A large spectrum of other self-antigens is expressed on the surface of thymic macrophages, dendritic cells, and especially epithelial cells.[12] If a developing T-cell's TCR binds strongly with a self-antigen, it is deleted. Although this process of *negative selection* induces more than 95% of T cells to undergo apoptosis in the thymus, a limited number of autoreactive clones persist and must be controlled by other means in the peripheral lymphoid organs (**peripheral tolerance**).

The destiny of the double-positive cells with TCRs specific for foreign antigens (which are not expressed in the thymus) is determined by their interaction in the thymus with MHC antigens. If their surface CD4 molecules bind to MHC class II molecules on the thymic cells, the T cell will become CD4 single-positive. However, if their surface CD8 reacts with MHC class I molecules, the cells will become CD8 single-positive. This *positive selection* process results in about 60% of immunocompetent T cells being CD4+ and 40% being CD8+ when they leave the thymus.[13]

B-Cell Maturation

Central Lymphoid Organ

Although the thymus is the central lymphoid organ for T-cell development, humans do not appear to have a discrete organ for B-cell development. In chickens, B lymphocytes undergo differentiation in an organ called the *bursa of Fabricius*. In humans, portions of the bone marrow function as a bursal-equivalent tissue for B-cell development.[14]

Regardless of the lack of a discrete organ, B-cell differentiation undergoes a very similar process to that described above for T cells.[15] Lymphoid stem cells in the bone marrow interact with stromal cells through a variety of intercellular adhesion molecules (Figure 8-12). As the stem cell begins to mature, it progressively develops a variety of necessary surface markers, the earliest being CD45R and the IL-7 receptor. IL-7, produced by the stromal cells, is critical in driving the further differentiation and proliferation of the B cell. The next stage in development is formation of the B-cell receptor.

Production of the B-Cell Receptor

The BCR is an antibody that is anchored to the plasma membrane. The process by which BCR diversity is generated is virtually identical to the process in T cells and also requires the genetic rearrangement of *V*, *D*, and *J* genes. The segments of DNA that encode either kappa (κ) (chromosome 2) or lambda (λ) (chromosome 22) light chains contain about 70 *V* and 5 *J* segments, whereas the heavy-chain locus on chromosome 14 contains about 80 *V*, 30 *D*, and 6 *J* regions. The locus for the antibody heavy chain also contains multiple sequential regions for different constant regions, with the gene for the mu (μ) constant region being closest to the *VDJ* region, and the delta (δ) constant region gene being next in sequence (Figure 8-13). These are followed by the constant region genes for other classes and subclasses. In the developing B cell, the initial RNA transcript contains information for the *VDJ* recombination, the μ constant region, and the δ constant region. Transcription is signaled to stop immediately after the δ constant region. During the following RNA processing step to form a final mRNA product, the cell can alternatively process some mRNAs to retain the μ constant region only or process other mRNA molecules to remove the μ constant region and retain the δ constant region. Thus one cell can use multiple mRNA molecules and alternative RNA processing to simultaneously produce two different heavy chains, μ and δ, both of which have the same variable region.

The developing B cell rearranges and expresses the heavy chain, which is followed by the rearrangement of either the κ or the λ light chain so that only one type is produced. The light chains are assembled with two μ heavy chains to form a monomeric IgM antibody or with two δ-chains to form an IgD antibody. Because each heavy chain used the same *VDJ* rearrangement and the same light chain, the variable regions and therefore the specificities of the IgM and IgD are identical. At this stage of B-cell development, both antibodies have hydrophobic, or sticky, "tails" that result in insertion into the plasma

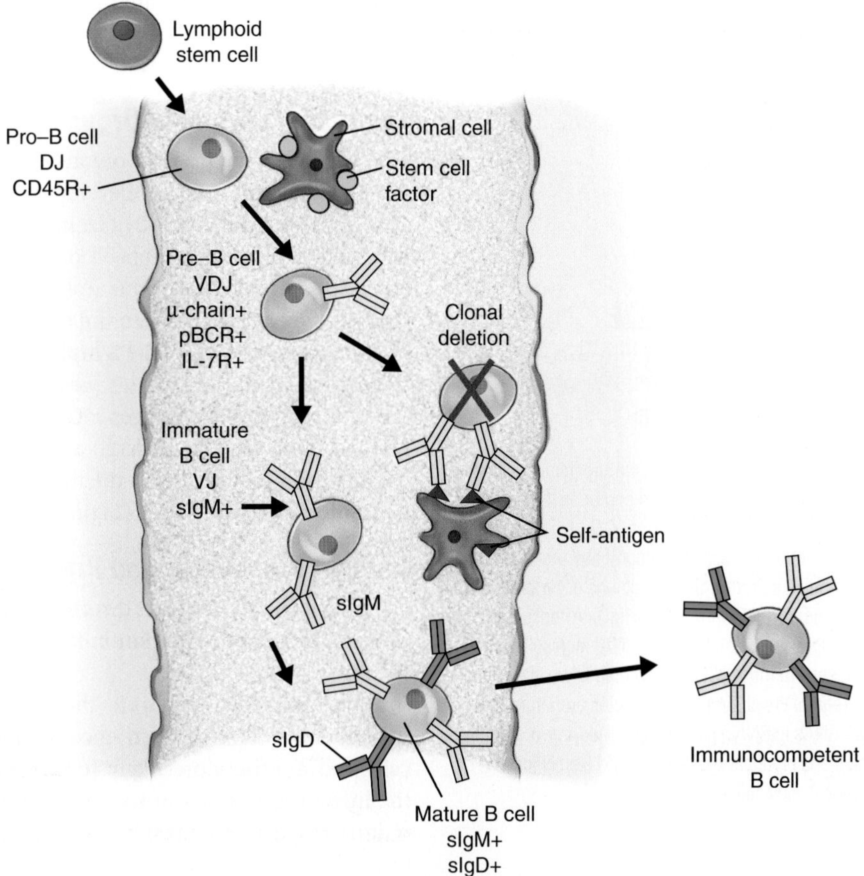

FIGURE 8-12 B-Cell Development in the Bone Marrow. During the generation of clonal diversity, lymphoid stem cells enter portions of the bone marrow that serve as the central lymph organ for B-cell development. Interactions with a series of bone marrow stromal cells guide the proliferation and differentiation process through direct cell-to-cell contact and the production of cytokines and hormones by the stromal cells, but without the presence of foreign antigen. A simplified scheme for that process is presented here. As with T-cell development, the differentiation process of B cells is characterized by the up-regulation of many important surface molecules (only some of which are shown) and the random development of a huge number of different B-cell receptors. The early B cell (pro–B cell) binds to a membrane-bound cytokine (stem cell factor) on the stromal cell and initiates expression of the surface molecule CD45R and begins to rearrange the *DJ* regions of the antibody heavy-chain gene. As the cell progresses to the pre–B-cell stage, it concludes DNA rearrangement of the heavy chain *(VDJ)* and begins expressing cytoplasmic mu (μ) heavy chain. The μ- chain is incorporated into a pre–B-cell receptor (pBCR) using a surrogate protein in place of the light chain. The cell also up-regulates the IL-7 receptor (IL-7R), which interacts with IL-7 produced by the stromal cells to drive the remaining steps in differentiation. Some pBCRs have specificities toward self-antigen. Many of these encounter self-antigen expressed on the stromal cells and undergo negative selection (clonal deletion). The surviving cells (immature B cells) rearrange the light-chain DNA *(VJ)* and express a BCR consisting of light chain and the μ-heavy chain (surface IgM [sIgM]). In the mature B cell, changes in processing of the heavy-chain precursor RNA result in co-expression of sIgM and IgD (sIgD) (see Figure 8-13 for more details).

membrane and the co-expression of IgM and IgD receptors on the cell surface.

Changes in Characteristic Surface Markers

As with T cells, B-cell differentiation is also characterized by the development of a variety of important surface molecules. These include CD21 (a complement receptor) and CD40 (adhesion molecule required for later interactions with Th).

Central Tolerance

During the very earliest stages of formation of the BCR in the bone marrow, a large number of autoreactive B cells are eliminated if exposed to self-antigen.[16] It is estimated that more than 90% of developing B cells are induced to undergo apoptosis.

INDUCTION OF AN IMMUNE RESPONSE: CLONAL SELECTION

As described in the previous chapter, successful invasion by a pathogen will initially elicit an inflammatory response as a host attempts to destroy and clear the invading microorganism. In addition to carrying out their roles as inflammatory effector cells, some of the cells involved in innate immunity are responsible for communicating with immature B and T lymphocytes to initiate specific and longer-acting acquired immunity. This

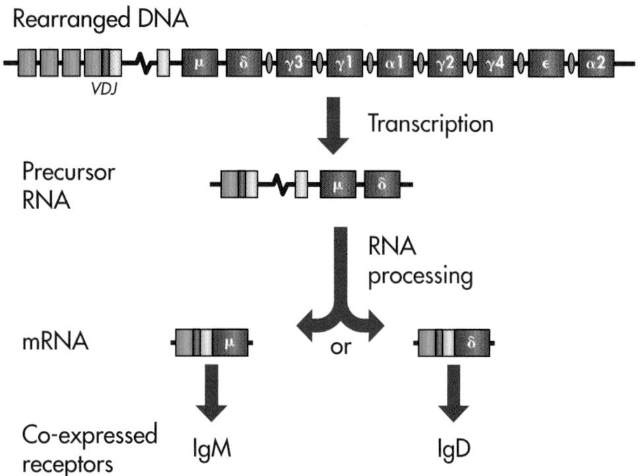

FIGURE 8-13 Genetics of the B-Cell Receptor. Most mature immunocompetent B cells express both surface IgM and IgD as the B-cell receptor. In the germline DNA, the heavy-chain gene complex consists of a series of *V, D, J,* and constant region genes. In humans, each class and subclass of antibody has a unique constant region gene arranged in the indicated order. Switch regions occur preceding every constant region gene, except mu (μ) (IgM) and delta (δ) (IgD). After successful DNA rearrangement of the *VDJ* regions, a ribonucleic acid (RNA) molecule is transcribed that contains the information from the *VDJ,* intervening DNA, the μ constant region, and the δ constant region. Precursor RNA molecules are alternatively processed to produce messenger RNAs (mRNAs) containing either μ or δ. Initially, RNA processing favors the μ chain and production of surface IgM (see Figure 8-12), but as the B cell matures, both mRNA molecules are produced.

intercellular communication occurs via direct cellular contact in peripheral lymphoid tissues and is essential for the specificity of the adaptive immune response.

Secondary Lymphoid Organs

The secondary lymphoid organs include the spleen, lymph nodes, adenoids, tonsils, Peyer patches (intestines), and the appendix (see Figure 8-3). Immunocompetent lymphocytes enter the secondary lymphoid organs through the blood and enter specialized small veins, called **high endothelial venules (HEVs),** where they bind to the endothelium through a family of adhesion molecules. The lymphocytes migrate from the vessels into the lymphoid tissues, which contain B- and T-cell–rich areas. B lymphocytes that encounter antigen in the secondary lymph organs usually undergo a process of differentiation and proliferation that results in the formation of specialized germinal centers in these organs (Figure 8-14).[17]

Antigen Processing and Presentation

Most antigens do not react directly with T or B cells, but require processing and presentation in the appropriate fashion. This is the duty of APCs.

Pathogens that penetrate the external barriers and enter the tissues or bloodstream encounter a variety of phagocytic cells and are therefore likely to be ingested and destroyed. If the infectious agent is in the tissues, they may elicit an inflammatory response that results in the infiltration of macrophages

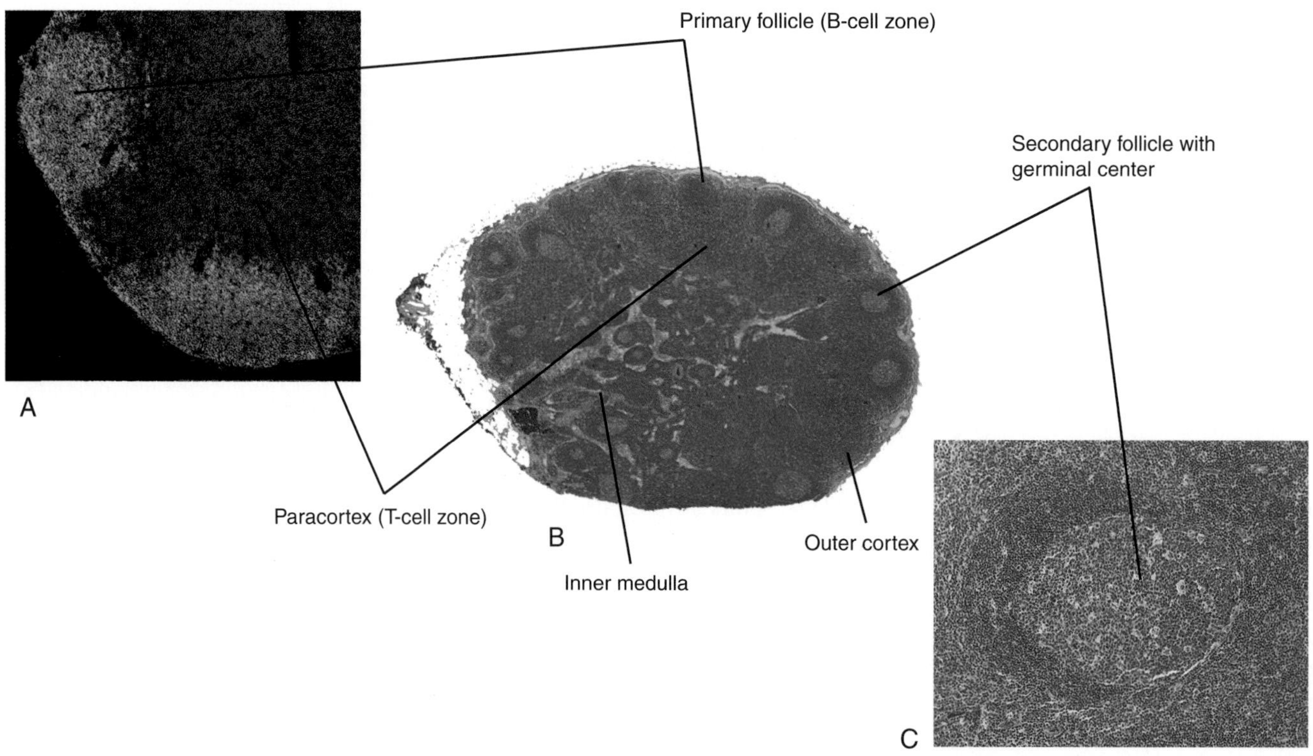

FIGURE 8-14 Histology of a Secondary Lymphoid Organ. A, The lymph node contains areas (primary follicles) that are rich in immunocompetent B cells *(stained green),* and T cells *(stained red)* in the paracortex. **B,** A lymph node is organized into an outer cortex and an inner medulla. **C,** In response to antigen, B cells undergo proliferation, resulting in the formation of secondary follicles with germinal centers. (Modified from Kumar V et al: *Robbins & Cotran pathologic basis of disease,* ed 8, Philadelphia, 2010, Saunders.)

into the site. Additionally, the infectious agent or fragments of the microorganism may be removed by the lymphatics, which drain to the lymph nodes. The lymph nodes are extremely rich in dendritic cells and macrophages, which phagocytose the material and function as APCs for T and B lymphocytes in the lymph nodes. Pathogens entering through the bloodstream may be removed by phagocytic cells in the spleen and other lymphoid tissues. In either case, the phagocytic cells that digest invading pathogens are also responsible for processing antigens from the pathogen and displaying or presenting those antigens on the phagocyte's surface to neighboring lymphocytes in order to initiate the adaptive immune response against that specific pathogen.

Many cells have the capacity to present antigen to some degree, but dendritic cells, macrophages, and B lymphocytes are so efficient at antigen presentation that they are considered "professional" APCs. Each of these three APCs is responsible for the presentation of antigens of different types and from different sources. B cells present antigen to Th cells that facilitate development of the humoral immune response. Macrophages are very effective in presenting antigen to memory Th cells in order to initiate a rapid response to antigens (i.e., secondary immune response). The dendritic cells are perhaps the most effective in presenting antigen to naïve immunocompetent Th cells. Dendritic cells develop from bone marrow precursor cells, either of myeloid or of lymphoid lineage (at least two populations of dendritic cells have been described). They migrate to the peripheral tissues (e.g., skin, intestinal tract) and to the secondary lymphoid organs. Immature dendritic cells at a site of inflammation function as phagocytes, and the process of phagocytosis can initiate differentiation and directed migration to the secondary lymphoid organs, particularly the lymph nodes (Figure 8-15).[18] Thus dendritic cells can carry processed antigen from a site of inflammation to the T-cell–rich areas of the lymph nodes.

Both antigen processing and presentation are necessary for an adaptive immune response to occur. Although B and T

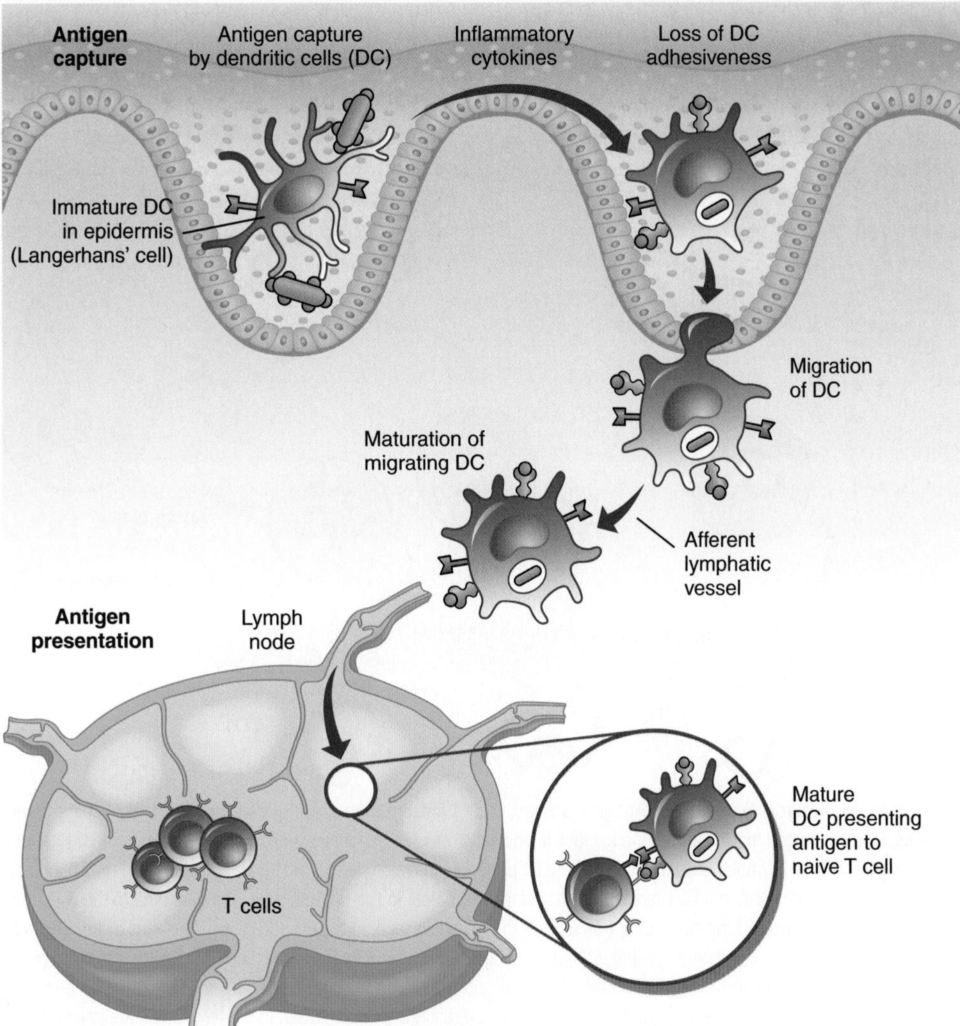

FIGURE 8-15 The Role of the Dendritic Cell in Capturing Antigen. Immature dendritic cells in the tissues encounter and phagocytose antigen, which results in the production of inflammatory cytokines and a loss of adhesive interactions with neighboring cells. The maturing dendritic cell migrates through the lymphatic vessels to a regional lymph node, where it presents the antigen to immunocompetent T cells to initiate the clonal selection process. (Redrawn from Kumar V, Abbas A, Fausto N: *Robbins & Cotran pathologic basis of disease,* ed 8, Philadelphia, 2010, Saunders.)

lymphocytes are immunocompetent before they have "seen" an antigen on the surface of an APC, they are considered "naive" until they have actually done so. The processing and presentation of antigens to naïve lymphocytes result in activation of an acquired immune response only if (1) the antigen is of the appropriate type; (2) the lymphocytes are prepared to recognize the presented antigen; and (3) the antigen is presented appropriately.

Pathways of Antigen Processing

In general, the immune system responds to two types of antigens: exogenous and endogenous. Using infection as a model, exogenous antigens are carried on microorganisms that are trapped and killed by phagocytic cells; therefore, they come from outside the cell. Endogenous antigens are synthesized within a cell. These include viral antigens because viruses infect cells and use the normal cellular protein-synthesizing machinery to translate the viral genes into viral proteins. Endogenous antigens also may include those uniquely produced by cancerous cells. When many cells undergo malignant change, they begin producing unique proteins that are specific to cancer cells and are presented as foreign antigens on the cell surface.

Exogenous and endogenous antigens are preferentially presented by different classes of MHC molecules: class I MHC molecules generally present endogenous antigens, and class II molecules prefer exogenous antigens (Figure 8-16).[19] Because class I MHC molecules are expressed on all cells, except red blood cells, any change in that cell attributable to viral infection or malignancy may result in foreign antigen being presented by MHC class I on that cell's surface. Class II MHC molecules are co-expressed with MHC class I molecules on a more limited number of cells that have APC function, including

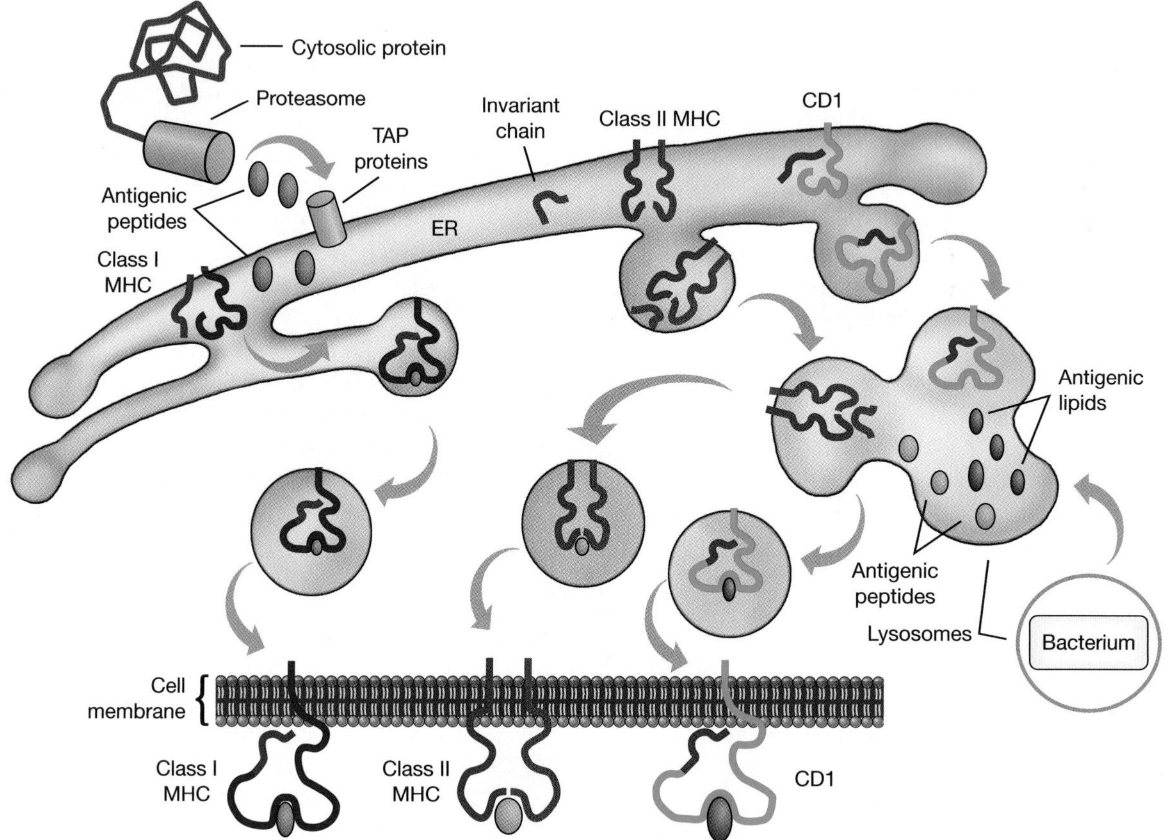

FIGURE 8-16 Antigen Processing. Antigen processing and presentation are required for initiation of most immune responses. Foreign antigen may be either endogenous (cytosolic protein) or exogenous (e.g., bacterium). Endogenous antigenic determinants (antigenic peptides) are produced by cellular proteasomes and transported by TAP proteins into the endoplasmic reticulum (ER) where the MHC and CD1 molecules are being assembled. In the ER, antigenic peptides bind to the α-chains of the MHC class I molecule, and the complex is transported to the cell surface. In the ER, the α- and β-chains of the MHC class II molecules are also being assembled, but the antigen-binding site is blocked by a small molecule (invariant chain) to prevent interactions with endogenous antigenic peptides. The MHC class II–invariant chain complex is transported to lysosomes, where exogenous antigenic fragments have been generated as a result of phagocytosis. In the lysosomes the invariant chain is digested and replaced by exogenous antigenic peptides, after which the MHC class II–antigen complex is inserted into the cell membrane. CD1 is also assembled in the ER, but its antigen-binding site is specific for lipid antigenic determinants and does not bind endogenous antigenic peptides. The CD1 molecule is transported to the lysosomes and may encounter and bind antigenic lipids produced by phagocytic digestion of engulfed bacteria. The CD1-antigen complex is transported to the cell membrane and presents lipid antigens. *MHC,* Major histocompatibility complex; *TAP,* transporter associated with antigen processing.

macrophages, dendritic cells, B lymphocytes, activated T lymphocytes, and some endothelial cells.

Thus, the term **antigen processing** relates to the process by which exogenous and endogenous antigens are linked with the appropriate MHC molecules. Endogenous antigens are usually components of proteins synthesized in the cytosol. They are degraded in the cytosol by proteasomes into small peptides and transported by TAP (transporter associated with antigen processing) proteins (TAP-1 and TAP-2) into the endoplasmic reticulum, where MHC class I and class II molecules are assembled.[20] The class I MHC molecules have open antigen-binding sites so that antigen, the class I MHC α-chain, and a β2-microglobulin molecule form a stable complex that is transported through the Golgi apparatus to the plasma membrane. The antigenic peptides presented by class I MHC molecules are usually very small, 8 to 10 amino acids in length.

MHC class II molecules are also assembled in the endoplasmic reticulum but do not bind with endogenous antigen because the antigen-binding site is blocked by a small protein called **invariant chain.** Exogenous antigens are internalized by phagocytosis and small antigenic molecules produced by digestion in the lysosomes. The MHC class II complexes of the class II α- and β-chains, with invariant chain, are transported to the lysosomes containing exogenous antigens. In the lysosomal environment, the invariant chain is digested and replaced by antigenic molecules that are usually slightly larger (in excess of 12 amino acids in length) than those presented by MHC class I molecules.

CD1 presents a variety of lipid-containing antigens that are usually derived from phagocytosis and digestion of infectious microorganisms with very high lipid content in their cell membranes. Therefore, CD1 complexes with antigen in the lysosomes, in a fashion similar to MHC class II. The "pocket" that holds antigen for presentation by CD1 is generally more narrow and deeper than that described for MHC molecules, and it is lined with many hydrophobic amino acids that interact with lipid.

T-Helper Lymphocytes

Regardless of whether an antigen primarily induces a cellular or humoral immune response, a subpopulation of T lymphocytes, **T-helper cells (Th cells),** is usually necessary for the process. As indicated by the name, this group of T cells *helps* the antigen-driven maturation of both B and T cells. They perform this task by facilitating and magnifying the interaction between APCs and the immunocompetent lymphocytes. This extremely important role involves three distinct steps: (1) the Th cell directly interacts with the APC through a variety of antigen-specific and antigen-independent receptors; (2) the Th cell undergoes a differentiation process during which a variety of cytokine genes are activated; and (3) depending on the pattern of cytokines expressed, the mature Th cell interacts with either immunocompetent B or T cells to enhance their response to antigen, which results in differentiation into either plasma cells or effector T cells, such as T-cytotoxic cells. Th cells are critical to most immune responses, and a variety of major Th-cell defects that lead to severely diminished immune responses are discussed in later chapters.

APC-Th Cooperation

Cells that are destined to become Th cells emerge from the thymus with characteristic cell surface markers. They have a functional αβ TCR complex and express the surface molecule CD4 and lack CD8. These are generally referred to as precursor Th cells, or sometimes Thp cells (Figure 8-17). As described previously, the TCR recognizes antigen and the CD4 molecule confines antigen presentation to MHC class II molecules; thus CD4+ cells are *class II restricted.* In order to undergo maturation, the Th cell must receive three independent signals: (1) antigen binding through the combined interaction of the TCR complex and CD4, (2) co-stimulatory signals through a variety of intercellular adhesion molecules, and (3) activation of specific cytokine receptors. If the appropriate signaling pathways are activated, the cell will differentiate through multiple intermediate stages into functional Th cells.

The complex of an antigenic peptide presented by an MHC class II molecule is recognized by multiple molecules on the Th-cell surface. The TCR binds directly to the antigen, whereas CD4 independently binds to a different site on the MHC class II β-chain. This co-recognition of the MHC-antigen complex by the TCR and CD4 brings CD4 into proximity with the CD3 components of the TCR complex, which initiates a series of enzymatic interactions among other molecules associated with the cytoplasmic portions of CD3 and CD4, such as the protein kinases $p56^{lck}$ and ZAP70. These molecules activate a signaling pathway from the TCR to the Th-cell nucleus.

The antigenic signal alone is inadequate and may even inactivate the Th cell if co-stimulatory signals are not present.[21] Co-stimulatory molecules are necessary for proper differentiation to occur. A variety of molecular interactions have been described, but the most critical appears to involve B7 on the APC and CD28 on the Th cell. Other interactions occur between CD48 on the APC and CD2 on the Th cell and between a variety of other adhesion molecules. In each case, the Th-cell molecule sends an activation signal to the nucleus. An additional signal is provided by cytokine. At this early stage of Th-cell differentiation, IL-1 secreted by the APC provides this signal through interaction with the IL-1 receptor on the Th cell.[22]

The initial differentiation response by the Th cell includes the production of the cytokine IL-2 and up-regulation of IL-2 receptors. IL-2 is secreted and acts in an autocrine (self-stimulating) fashion to induce further maturation and proliferation of the Th cell. Without IL-2 production, the Th cell cannot efficiently mature into a functional helper cell.[23] At this point, Th cells undergo one of several different differentiation pathways into Th subsets.

Th Subsets

The most clearly characterized Th-cell subsets are **Th1** and **Th2 cells,** and the newly described **Th17 cells** (see Figure 8-17). These subsets have different functions: Th1 cells help develop cellular immunity, Th2 cells help develop humoral immunity, and Th17 cells increase the inflammatory response. A fourth

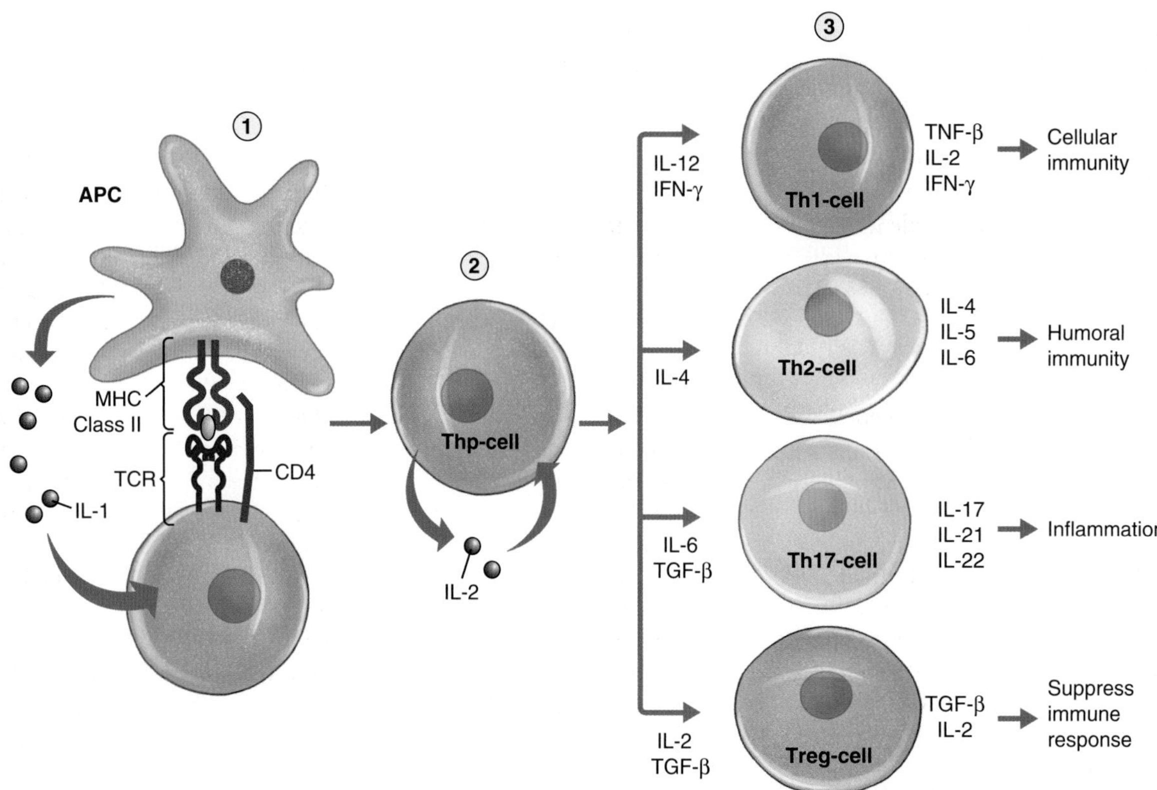

FIGURE 8-17 Development of T-Cell Subsets. The most important step in clonal selection is the production of populations of helper T (Th) cells (Th1, Th2, and Th17) and regulatory T (Treg) cells that are necessary for the development of cellular and humoral immune responses. In this model, APCs (probably multiple populations) may influence whether a precursor Th cell (Thp cell) will differentiate into a Th1, Th2, Th17, or Treg cell. Differentiation of the Thp cell is initiated by three signaling events. **(1)** The antigen signal is produced by the interaction of the T-cell receptor (TCR) and CD4 with antigen presented by MHC class II molecules. A set of co-stimulatory signals is produced from interactions between adhesion molecules (e.g., CD80 and CD28) (not shown). A third signal is produced by the interactions of cytokines (particularly interleukin-1 [IL-1]) with appropriate cytokine receptors (IL-1R) on the Thp cell. **(2)** The Thp cell up-regulates IL-2 production and expression of the IL-2 receptor (IL-2R), which act in an autocrine fashion to accelerate Thp-cell differentiation and proliferation. **(3)** Commitment to a particular phenotype results from the relative concentrations of other cytokines. IL-12 and IFN-γ produced by some populations of APCs favor differentiation into the Th1-cell phenotype; IL-4, which is produced by a variety of cells, favors differentiation into the Th2-cell phenotype; IL-6 and TGF-β (T-cell growth factor) facilitate differentiation into Th17 cells; IL-2 and TGF-β induce differentiation into Treg cells. The Th1 cell is characterized by the production of cytokines that assist in the differentiation of cytotoxic T (Tc) cells, leading to cellular immunity, whereas the Th2 cell produces cytokines that favor B-cell differentiation and humoral immunity. Th1 and Th2 cells affect each other through the production of inhibitory cytokines: IFN-γ will inhibit the development of Th2 cells, and IL-4 will inhibit the development of Th1 cells. Th17 cells produce cytokines that affect phagocytes and increase inflammation. Treg cells produce immunosuppressive cytokines that prevent the immune response from being excessive. *APC,* Antigen-presenting cell; *IFN,* interferon; *MHC,* major histocompatibility complex; *TGF,* transforming growth factor.

subset, Treg cells, is discussed later in this chapter. The Th subsets differ considerably in the spectrum of cytokines produced by each, as well as the expression of surface cytokine receptors and intercellular adhesion molecules. Th1 cells produce IL-2, tumor necrosis factor-beta (TNF-β), and interferon-gamma (IFN-γ);[24] Th2 cells produce IL-4, IL-5, IL-6, and IL-13,[25] and Th17 cells produce IL-17, IL-21, and IL-22.[26] As will be seen in the next portions of this chapter, the Th1 cytokines affect Tc-cell development, and the Th2 cytokines are needed for B-cell maturation, including class-switch. Th17-cell cytokines affect inflammatory responses, particularly infiltration of neutrophils and macrophages and production of antimicrobial proteins and chemokines by epithelial cells. Members of the IL-17 cytokine family induce epithelial cell chemokines and neutrophil infiltration, and IL-22 more specifically affects epithelial cell antimicrobial protein production.[27] Thus Th17 cells control many aspects of inflammation, including chronic inflammation.[28] Th1, Th2, and Th17 cells also have different cytokine receptors, so that IFN-γ produced by Th1 cells will bind to receptors on Th2 and Th17 cells and suppress their function. Likewise, Th2 cells produce IL-4, which suppresses Th1 and Th17 cells through their IL-4 receptors. Thus in some instances the immune response favors antibody formation, with suppression of a cell-mediated response, whereas in other instances the opposite is true. For example, antigens derived from viral or bacterial pathogens and those derived from cancer cells are hypothesized to induce a greater number of Th1 cells relative to Th2 cells, whereas antigens derived from multicellular parasites and allergens are hypothesized to result in production of more Th2 cells. Many antigens (e.g., tetanus vaccine), however, produce excellent humoral and cell-mediated responses simultaneously.

How a Th cell is guided into becoming a Th1, Th2, or Th17 cell is not fully known. Some evidence indicates that different subpopulations of APCs influence the choice by secreting different profiles of cytokines that may favor one route of differentiation over another (see Figure 8-17).

B-Cell Activation: The Humoral Immune Response

When an immunocompetent B cell encounters an antigen for the first time, only those cells with specific BCRs complementary to that antigen's determinant sites are stimulated to proliferate and differentiate (clonal selection), resulting in multiple copies of that particular B cell. The differentiated B cell becomes a **plasma cell** and can be found in the blood, secondary lymphoid organs (primarily spleen and lymph nodes), and some inflammatory sites. Each plasma cell is a factory for antibody production and is dedicated to the secretion of a single class or subclass of antibody with one variable region and therefore specificity against one antigenic determinant.

Primary and Secondary Immune Responses

The immune response to antigenic challenge has classically been divided into two phases—the primary and secondary responses—that can be most easily demonstrated by serologic tests that measure plasma concentrations of antibody over time (Figure 8-18). On initial exposure to most antigens, there is a latent period, or lag phase, during which B-cell differentiation and proliferation occur. After approximately 5 to 7 days, IgM antibody specific for that antigen can be detected in the circulation. The lag phase is a result of the time necessary for clonal selection, including processing and presentation of antigens, induction of Th cells, interactions between immunocompetent B cells and Th cells, and maturation and proliferation of the B cells into plasma cells and memory cells.

This is the initial response, or **primary immune response.** Typically, IgM will be produced first, followed by IgG against the same antigen. The quantity of IgG produced may be about equal to or less than the amount of IgM production. If no further exposure to the antigen occurs, the circulating antibody is catabolized (broken down) and measurable quantities fall. The individual's immune system, however, has been primed. A second challenge by the same antigen results in the **secondary (anamnestic) immune response,** which is characterized by the more rapid production of a larger amount of antibody than that produced by the primary response. The rapidity of the secondary immune response is the result of the presence of memory cells that do not require further differentiation. IgM may be transiently produced in the secondary response and the quantity may be about the same as that produced in the primary response. IgG production is increased considerably, making it the predominant antibody class of the secondary response. It is often present in concentrations several times larger than those of IgM, and levels of circulating IgG specific for that antigen may remain elevated for an extended period of time. If the antigenic challenge is in the form of a vaccine or occurs through natural infection, the level of protective IgG may remain elevated for decades.

The existence of a prolonged and protective secondary immune response explains how vaccinations provide protection against certain pathogenic microorganisms. Edward Jenner, an English physician of the late eighteenth century, performed the first well-documented vaccine trial.[29,30] Although some of the stories about Jenner's experiments are fanciful, it is known that Jenner recognized that milkmaids were protected from the deadly smallpox virus if they had previously developed cowpox, a bovine equivalent of smallpox that causes only mild disease

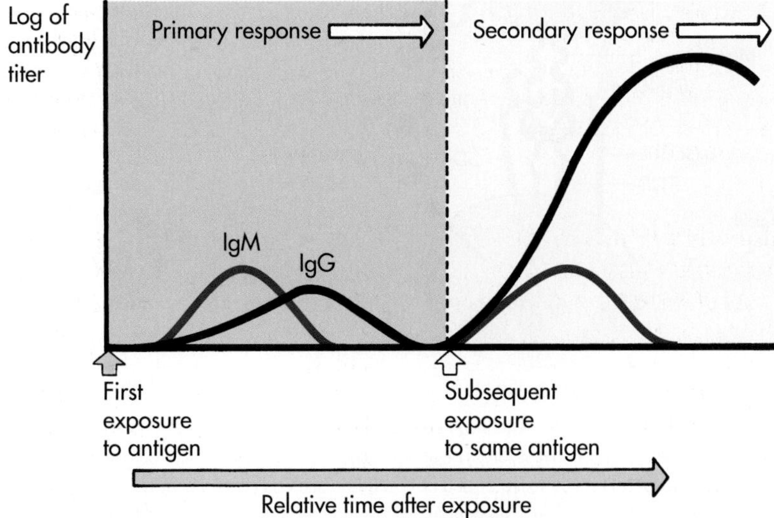

FIGURE 8-18 Primary and Secondary Immune Responses. Antigen responses are dominated by two classes of immunoglobulins, IgM and IgG. IgM predominates on initial exposure to the antigen in the primary response, with IgG appearing later. After the host's immune system is primed, another challenge by the same antigen induces the secondary response in which some IgM and larger amounts of IgG are produced.

in humans. Jenner took material from a cowpox pustule on the hand of an infected milkmaid and injected it into the arm of an 8-year-old boy. After the boy's initial inflammatory reaction to the injection subsided, Jenner injected the boy again, this time with material from a smallpox pustule. Fortunately, the experiment was a success because Jenner is reported to have reinjected smallpox virus into the boy at least 20 times without the child becoming ill. In Jenner's experiment, the antigens on the cowpox virus and the smallpox virus were sufficiently similar that the cowpox antigen functioned as an altered or attenuated smallpox antigen. The antibodies and lymphocytes that recognized and destroyed cowpox also were able to recognize the smallpox virus, thereby protecting the immunized child against smallpox. In 1798, Jenner used the term *vaccination* (*vacca* = cow) to describe his technique.

Cellular Interactions

As with most aspects of immunity, a sequence of cellular interactions is required to produce an effective antibody response (Figure 8-19). The immunocompetent B cell is also an APC and expresses surface IgM and IgD BCRs. Unlike the T-cell receptor that can only "see" processed and presented antigen, the BCR can react with soluble antigen. Antigen binding to the BCR complex activates intracellular kinases, in a fashion similar to the TCR receptor complex. In many instances, circulating antigen, either on macromolecules or on the surface of a pathogen, will have activated the complement system through the alternative or lectin pathways. Thus complement receptors on the B cell, such as CD19 and CD21, act as co-receptors to bind antigen.[31] As a result of signaling from the BCR complex and other surface co-receptors, the antigen-bearing macromolecule internalizes, degrades in the lysosomes, and complexes with MHC class II molecules for presentation on the cell surface, where it is recognized by a Th2 cell through the TCR and CD4. The intercellular bridge created through antigen induces the Th2 cell to up-regulate additional surface receptors and secrete cytokines. Direct interaction between CD40 on the B-cell surface and the CD40 ligand (CD40L, also called *CD154*) on the Th2 cell, as well as the interaction of B7 on the B cell and CD28 on the Th cell, and exposure of the B cell to Th2-cell cytokines (particularly IL-4) induce proliferation of the B cell and maturation into a plasma cell.[32] A major component of maturation is class-switch.

Class-Switch

The immunocompetent B cell uses IgM and IgD as receptors. During the clonal selection process, however, each B cell has the option of changing the class of antibody to a secreted form of one of the four IgG subclasses, one of the two IgA subclasses, or IgE, or continuing to produce IgM but changing to a secreted form, usually a pentamer. This process is called **class-** or **isotype-switch.** During this process the variable region of the antibody heavy chain is conserved, and the light chain remains

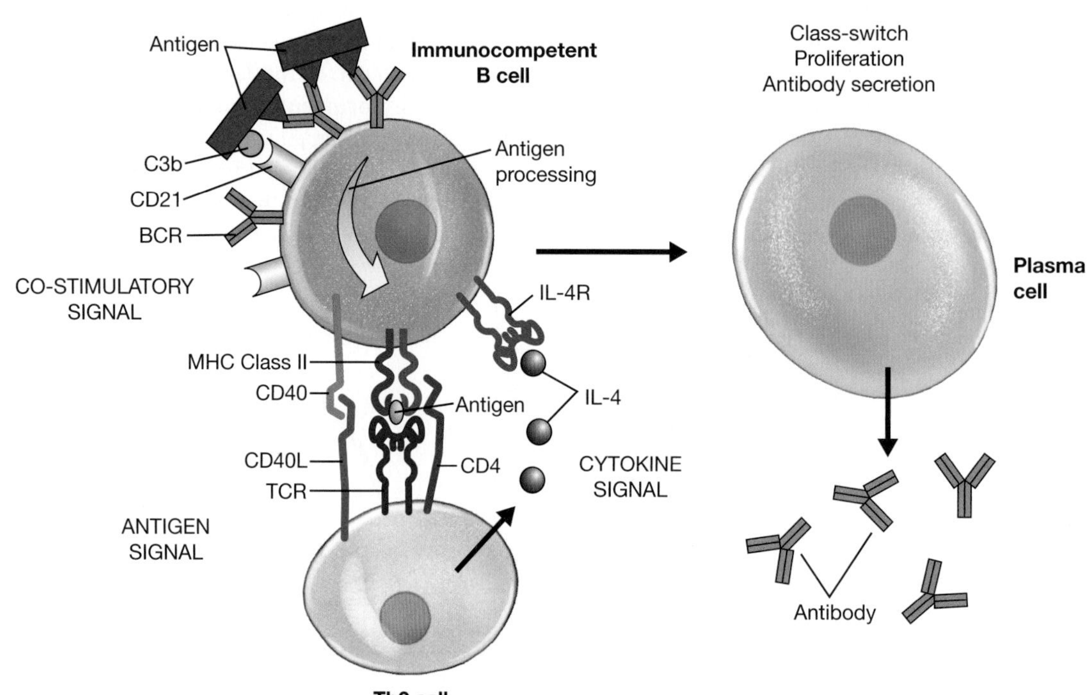

FIGURE 8-19 B-Cell Clonal Selection. Immunocompetent B cells undergo proliferation and differentiation into antibody-secreting plasma cells. Three signals are necessary. The antigen signal is provided by the B cell itself. A B cell can recognize soluble antigen directly through the B-cell receptor and co-receptors, such as complement receptors (CD21), which usually involve accessory molecules such as CD19 (not shown). Antigen is internalized and processed for presentation by MHC class II molecules, which interact with the T-cell receptor (TCR) and CD4 on Th2 cells. Co-stimulatory signals are provided through adhesion molecules, particularly CD40 and CD40L (CD154). The cytokine signal is provided by Th2 cytokines (particularly IL-4) binding to appropriate cytokine receptors (IL-4R) on the B cell. Additional cytokines influence switch to particular classes or subclasses of antibody. *MHC,* Major histocompatibility complex.

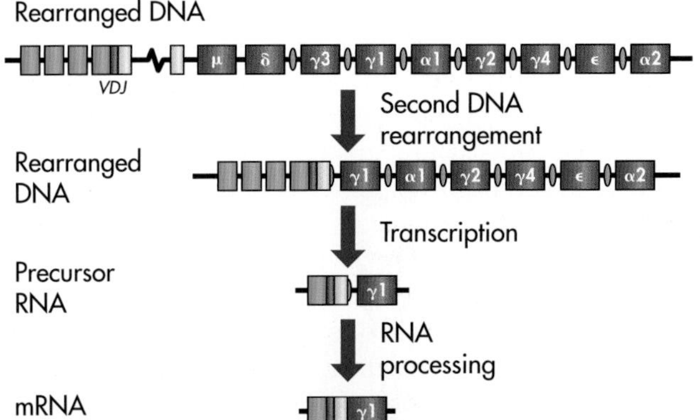

FIGURE 8-20 **Genetics of Class-Switch.** During clonal selection, most B cells switch from expression of surface IgM and IgD to a different class or subclass of antibody. A first set of DNA rearrangements during the generation of clonal diversity resulted in formation of the *VDJ* region. The class-switch process involves a second DNA rearrangement during which the *VDJ* region is moved to a switch region *(orange ovals)* immediately preceding the new class/subclass of antibody. In this example, the B cell undergoes class-switch to a γ1 heavy chain and secretion of an IgG1 antibody. The intervening DNA between the *VDJ* and the selected switch region is excised, and the DNA is repaired (DNA after second rearrangement) and transcribed into a precursor ribonucleic acid (RNA). The RNA is processed to a messenger RNA (mRNA) with information for the new heavy chain.

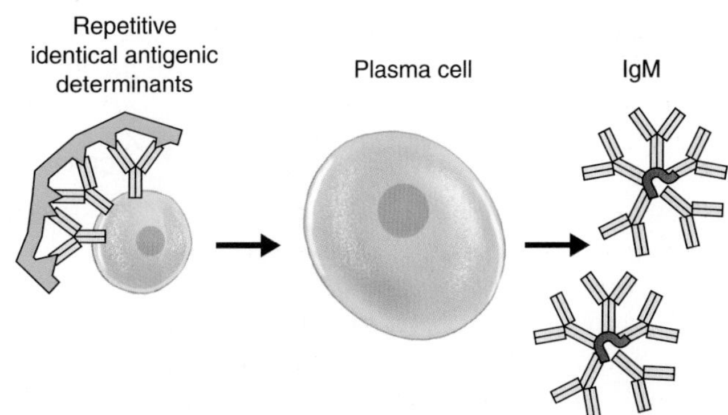

FIGURE 8-21 **Activation of a B Cell by a T-Cell–Independent Antigen.** Molecules containing repeating identical antigenic determinants may interact simultaneously with several receptors on the surface of the B cell and induce the proliferation and production of immunoglobulins, mainly IgM.

unchanged from that used in the BCR; therefore, the antigenic specificity also remains unchanged.

The mechanism of class-switch involves another DNA rearrangement, during which the *VDJ* region encoding the heavy-chain's variable region is moved to another site on the DNA that is adjacent to the gene for a different constant region under the control of activation-induced cytidine deaminase (AICD) (Figure 8-20). The DNA is cut and mended with removal of the DNA that was between the *VDJ* site and the new constant region. Specific recognition sites (switch regions) precede each constant region gene, and the particular constant region chosen for class-switch appears to be, at least partially, under the control of specific Th2 cytokines. For instance, IL-4 and IL-13 appear to preferentially stimulate switch to IgE, and transforming growth factor-beta (TGF-β) and IL-5 appear to play major roles in class-switch to IgA.

A few antigens can bypass the need for Th cells and can directly stimulate B-cell maturation and proliferation. These are called *T-independent antigens* (Figure 8-21). They are mostly bacterial products that are large and are likely to have repeating antigenic determinants (multiple identical antigenic determinant sites) that bind and cross-link several B-cell receptors. The accumulated intracellular signal is adequate to induce differentiation to a plasma cell but is not adequate to induce class-switch. The CD40-CD40L interaction is a necessary component of the signal that leads to class-switch. Therefore, T-independent antigens usually induce a relatively pure IgM primary and secondary immune response.

Cellular Differentiation

During the clonal selection process, B cells differentiate into antibody-producing plasma cells and into a set of long-lived memory cells. During the differentiation of B cells into plasma cells, the CDR portions of the antibody variable region are prone to somatic point mutations that lead to changes in single amino acids. Some of these changes produce better antibodies that bind more strongly (higher affinity) to the antigen. The presence of antigen creates a positive selective pressure toward the developing B cells that express the higher-affinity antibody, which results in a process called *affinity maturation,* in which the quality of the circulating antibody improves over time. Plasma cells may migrate to special regions of the spleen, lymph nodes, and mucosal-associated lymphoid tissues that support the plasma cell's long-term survival and function so that an adequate level of protective antibody is available in the circulation for decades after vaccination or resolution of infection.[33]

The memory cells remain inactive until subsequent exposure to the same antigen.[34] On reexposure, these memory cells do not require much further differentiation and will therefore differentiate rapidly into new plasma cells.

T-Cell Activation: The Cellular Immune Response

Activation of the cell-mediated arm of the immune response begins with the binding of antigen to specific T-cell receptors. Through a variety of intercellular collaborations that are mediated by specific cellular receptors and cytokines, the naïve T cell proliferates and differentiates into a functional (effector) T cell. The two main effector functions of activated T cells are (1) direct killing of foreign and/or abnormal cells and (2) assistance and/or activation of other cells, such as macrophages. The first function is carried out by a subclass of T cells, termed T-cytotoxic lymphocytes (Tc cells, or CTLs). Activation of macrophages is performed by a special subset of Th cells. Additional T cells develop into cells that regulate the immune response in order to avoid inadvertently attacking self-antigens or to avoid overactivation of the immune response. This mixed population of cells is termed **T-regulatory (Treg) cells.** Finally, **T-memory cells** are also produced to help induce secondary cell-mediated immune responses.[35]

Cellular Interactions

During the clonal selection phase of the cell-mediated immune response, immunocompetent T cells in the peripheral lymphoid

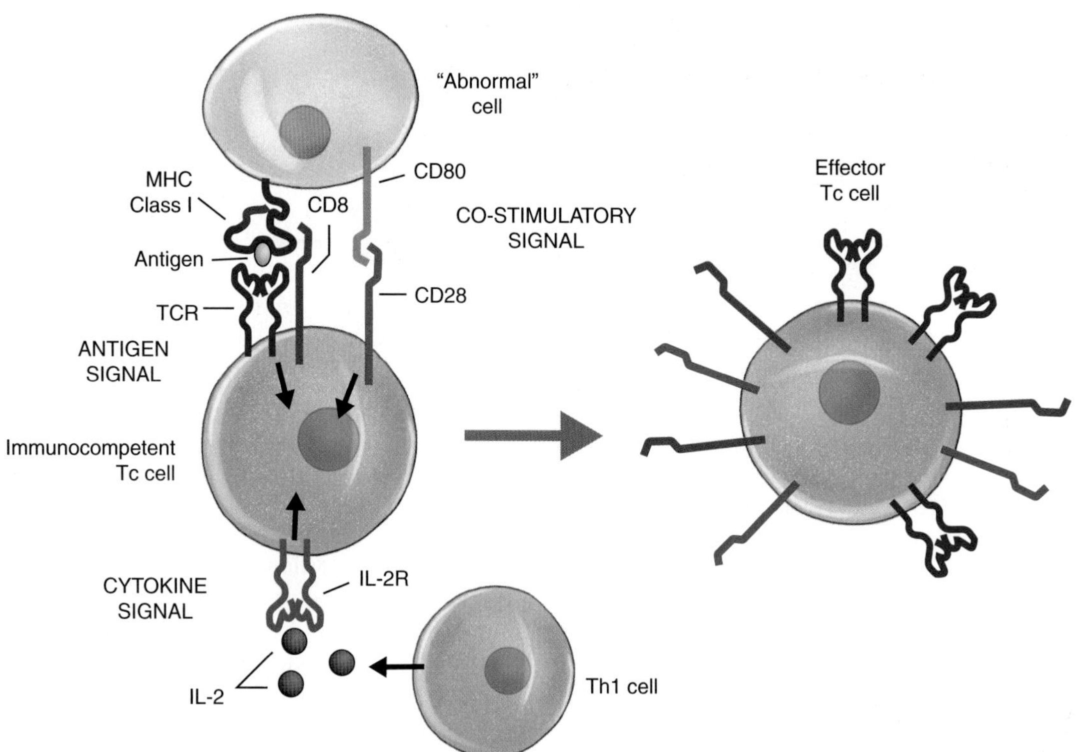

FIGURE 8-22 **Tc-Cell Clonal Selection.** The development of effector cytotoxic T (Tc) cells during clonal selection results from three cooperative signaling events provided by antigen, co-stimulatory adhesion molecules, and cytokines. The immunocompetent Tc cell "sees" antigen presented by MHC class I molecules on the surface of a virally infected or cancerous "abnormal" cell. The antigen–MHC class I complex is recognized simultaneously by the T-cell receptor (TCR), which binds to antigen, and CD8, which binds to the MHC class I molecule. The proximity of signaling molecules associated with the cytoplasmic portions of CD8 and the TCR result in intracellular signaling. A separate signal results from the interaction of several groups of adhesion molecules (e.g., CD80 and CD28 in this example). The third signal is provided by the interaction of cytokine, particularly IL-2 from Th1 cells, and the appropriate receptor. *MHC,* Major histocompatibility complex.

organs must recognize antigen that has been processed and presented by MHC class I molecules (Figure 8-22). The antigen is usually an endogenous antigen expressed on the surface of cells infected with a virus or cells that have become malignant. The T cells have a functional αβ TCR complex and express the surface molecule CD8, rather than CD4. The presence of the CD8 molecule confines antigen recognition to MHC class I molecules; therefore, CD8+ T cells are *class I restricted.* The TCR binds directly to the antigenic peptide, whereas CD8 independently binds to a different site on the MHC class I α-chain. This co-recognition of the MHC-antigen complex by the TCR and CD8 brings CD8 into proximity with the CD3 components of the TCR complex, which initiates a series of enzymatic interactions among other molecules associated with the cytoplasmic portions of CD3 and CD4, as was described for Th-cell activation. These molecules activate a signaling pathway from the TCR to the T-cell nucleus.

To undergo maturation, the T cell must receive independent signals from a variety of co-stimulatory intercellular adhesion molecules and specific cytokine receptors. If the appropriate signaling pathways are activated, the cell will proliferate and differentiate through multiple intermediate stages into functional Tc cells. The co-stimulatory signals for Tc-cell maturation are virtually the same as has been described for Th-cell maturation: B7 on the cell-presenting antigen and CD28 on the T cell, CD48 on the antigen-presenting cell and CD2 on the T cell, and a variety of other adhesion molecules. Development of Tc cells also requires cytokines, especially IL-2, produced by the Th1 cell.

Cellular Differentiation

The result of these cellular interactions is the production of active Tc cells with the capacity to identify antigens on the surface of infected or malignant cells and then to destroy those cells. As with B cells, some of the T cells that become activated in response to antigen presentation will not become effectors that destroy infected targets, but instead develop into a population of T-memory cells. These cells have the capacity to rapidly respond to further exposure to the same antigen.

Superantigens

A group of molecules has the ability to bind the variable portion of the TCR β-chain outside of its normal antigen-specific binding site, as well as the α-chain of MHC class II molecules outside of their antigen-presentation sites (Figure 8-23). Thus these molecules are not digested and processed by an APC to be presented to an immune cell. This binding results in adherence of the TCR and MHC class II molecules, independent of antigen recognition, and provides an activation signal for Th-cell

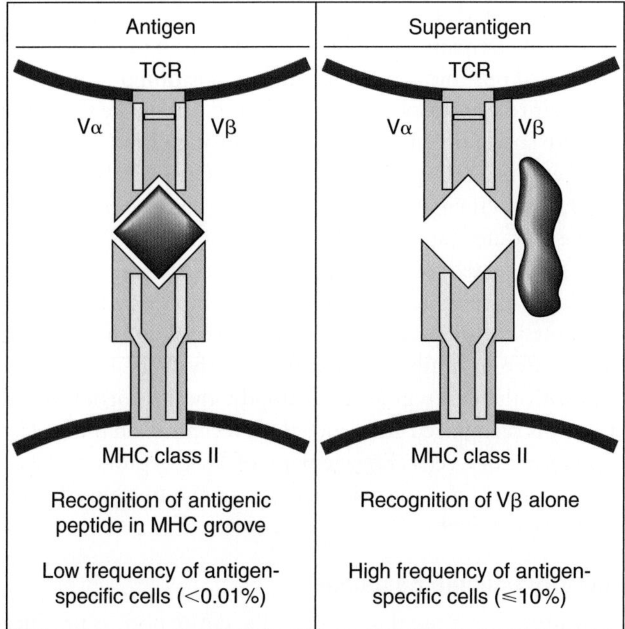

FIGURE 8-23 Superantigens. The T-cell receptor (TCR) and an MHC class II molecule normally simultaneously interact with a processed antigen to induce T-cell differentiation. Superantigens, such as some bacterial toxins, bind directly to the TCR and the MHC class II molecules. Superantigens activate Th cells independently of TCR antigen specificity. *MHC,* Major histocompatibility complex; *V,* variable; *Vα,* variable region of the α-chain; *Vβ,* variable region of the β-chain.

activation and proliferation. The normal antigen-specific recognition between Th cells and APCs results in activation of relatively few cells: only those cells with specific TCRs against that antigen. The type of binding described here results in activation of large populations of T lymphocytes, regardless of antigen specificity. Thus these molecules have been referred to as **superantigens (SAGs).**

SAGs induce an excessive production of cytokines, including IL-2, IFN-γ, and TNF-α. The overproduction of inflammatory cytokines results in symptoms of a systemic inflammatory reaction, including fever, low blood pressure, and, potentially, fatal shock. Some examples of SAGs are the bacterial toxins produced by *Staphylococcus aureus* and *Streptococcus pyogenes* (including the superantigens that cause toxic shock syndrome and food poisoning).[36] Some viruses are also able to produce superantigens, although the exact nature of these antigens is unclear.

EFFECTOR MECHANISMS

Antibody Function

Protection Against Infection

The chief function of circulating antibodies is to protect the host from infection. Protection can be afforded by antibody in several ways, either directly or indirectly (Figure 8-24). Directly, antibody can cause **neutralization** (inactivating or blocking the binding of an antigen to a receptor), **agglutination** (clumping insoluble particles that are in suspension), or **precipitation**

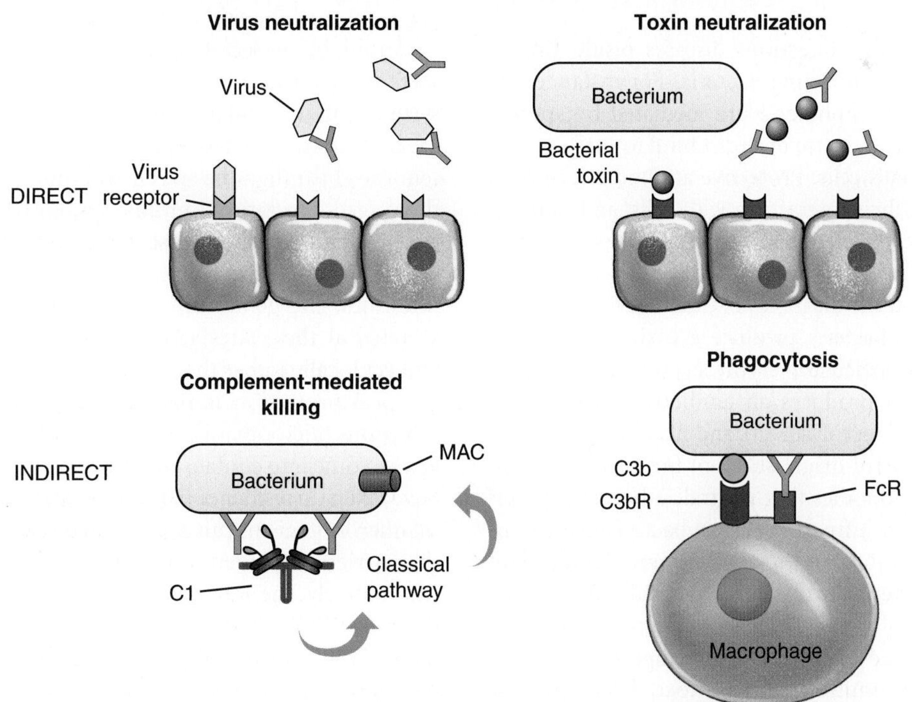

FIGURE 8-24 Direct and Indirect Functions of Antibody. Protective activities of antibodies can be direct (through the action of antibody alone) or indirect (requiring activation of other components of the innate immune response, usually through the Fc region). Direct means include neutralization of viruses or bacterial toxins before they bind to receptors on the surface of the host's cells. Indirect means include activation of the classical complement pathway through C1, resulting in formation of the membrane attack complex (MAC), or by increased phagocytosis of bacteria opsonized with antibody and complement components bound to appropriate surface receptors (FcR and C3bR).

(making a soluble antigen into an insoluble precipitate) of infectious agents or their toxic products. Indirectly, antibodies activate several components of innate immunity, including complement and phagocytes.

Direct Effects. To cause infection, many pathogens must attach to specific receptors on the host's cells. For instance, viruses that cause the common cold or the influenza virus must attach to specific receptors on epithelial cells. Some bacteria, such as *Neisseria gonorrhoeae* that causes gonorrhea, must attach to specific sites on epithelial cells. Antibodies may protect the host against infection by covering the portions of the microorganism that it needs to bind to the host cell. Neutralization, or prevention of attachment to the host cell, thereby prevents infection of the host.

Protection against many viral infections can be elicited effectively by vaccination with inactivated or **attenuated** (weakened) **viruses** to induce neutralizing antibody production at the site of typical viral entrance into the body. A good indication of the degree of protection against viral infection is the level of circulating antibodies found in the blood. The level of circulating antibodies is referred to as an **antibody titer.** However, many viruses (e.g., measles, herpes) are inaccessible to antibodies after initial infection because they do not circulate in the bloodstream but instead remain inside infected cells, spreading by direct cell-to-cell contact. Neutralizing antibodies against this type of virus are most effective in preventing the initial infection. Other viruses, such as polio and influenza, spread through the blood, are more susceptible to the effects of circulating antibodies, and can be controlled by antibodies even after the initial infection.

The symptoms of some infectious diseases result directly from toxins produced by infecting bacteria. For instance, the symptoms of tetanus or diphtheria are mediated by specific toxins. To cause disease, most toxins must bind to surface molecules on the individual's cells. Protective antibodies can bind to the toxins, prevent their interaction with cells, and neutralize their biologic effects. Detection of the presence of an antibody response against a specific toxin (antibodies referred to as *antitoxins*) can aid in the diagnosis of diseases. For example, group A streptococcal bacteria produce a toxin, streptolysin O, that destroys cells, particularly erythrocytes and leukocytes. The infected individual produces an antibody that can neutralize this toxin (antistreptolysin O) and also be detected in laboratory tests as a useful diagnostic tool for group A streptococcal infections. Antibodies that neutralize bacterial toxins can be induced to confer immunity against bacterial pathogens by means of immunization. To prevent harming the recipient of immunization, bacterial toxins are chemically inactivated to destroy their harmful properties but still retain immunogenicity. These are referred to as *toxoids*. Examples of bacterial pathogens for which immunization with toxoids can provide immunologic protection include those that cause diphtheria and tetanus.

Indirect Effects. Antibody can be protective by interacting with or activating components of nonspecific inflammation. Indirect effects are mediated by the Fc portion of the antibody molecule and include opsonic activity resulting in enhanced phagocytosis and activation of the complement system that may lead to complement-mediated destruction of the pathogen or increased opsonic activity through deposition of C3b.

In their role as **opsonins,** antibody and C3b make the pathogen more susceptible to phagocytosis through binding to Fc or C3b receptors on the phagocyte's surface. **Opsonization** is often necessary for efficient bacterial clearance because many bacteria have an outer capsule that deters recognition by phagocytes unless it is coated with an antibody or complement protein. Bacterial surface molecules are usually complex and have multiple accessible antigenic determinants, enabling them to bind several different antibodies simultaneously. When an antigen reacts with the Fab regions of antibody, the Fc portion of that antibody is recognized and binds to Fc receptors on the surfaces of inflammatory cells. Engagement of Fc receptors results in their activation, making phagocytosis of the opsonized bacterium more efficient.

Secretory Immune Response

The immune response that protects the entire body is produced by the **systemic immune system.** A distinct set of lymphoid tissues makes up another, partially independent, immune system at the external surfaces of the body. This system is called the **secretory (mucosal) immune system** (Figure 8-25). Most humoral immune responses occur when antibodies or B cells encounter antigens in the blood, but sometimes this encounter occurs in other body fluids. Antibodies are present in bodily secretions such as tears, sweat, saliva, mucus, and breast milk, where they can protect the body against antigens that have not yet penetrated the skin or mucous membranes.

Antibodies in secretions are produced by plasma cells of the secretory (mucosal) immune system. The B cells of these two systems follow a different pattern of migration after they leave the bone marrow.[37] B lymphocytes of the systemic immune system travel through the spleen and most lymph nodes, whereas those of the secretory immune system travel through a different group of lymphoid tissues including the lacrimal and salivary glands and the lymphoid tissues of the breasts, bronchi, intestines, and genitourinary tract. Immunoglobulins that are secreted at these sites are called **secretory immunoglobulins** and act locally rather than systemically.

Local protection is necessary to combat antigens (chiefly infectious microorganisms) that are inhaled, swallowed, or otherwise come into contact with external body surfaces. Once they have taken up residence in the external layers of the body, harmful microorganisms can cause local disease or possibly penetrate the barriers described in Chapter 7 to cause systemic disease. Alternatively, the microorganisms may fail to cause disease in the individual, either because the microorganisms are passed out of the body without any ill effects or because the infection is thwarted by the systemic immune system. In the latter case the individual may continue to "carry" the infectious agent in the mucosal areas, thereby enabling its spread to other individuals. The major function of the secretory immune system is to halt viral and bacterial invasion before local or systemic disease can develop and to prevent a carrier state that may result in spread of the infection to others.

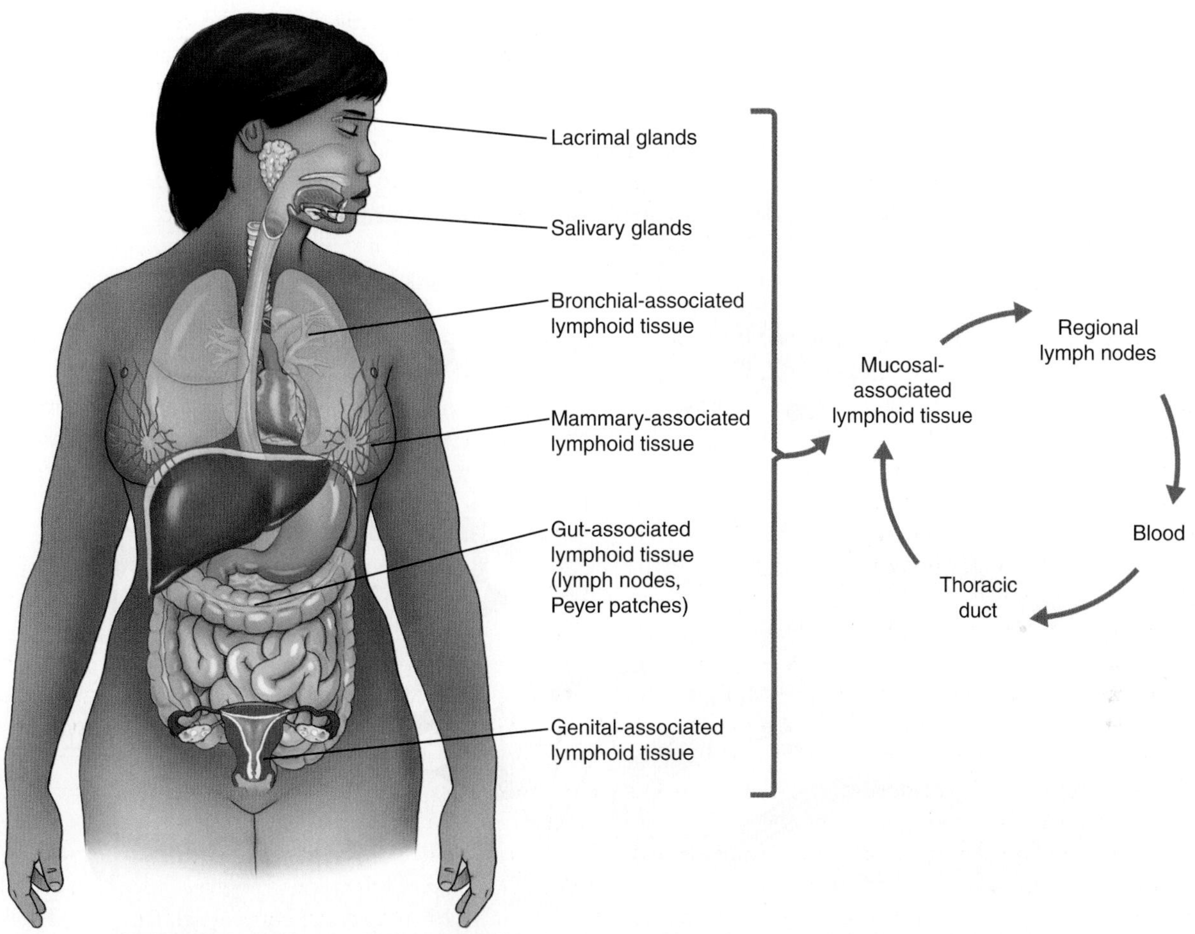

FIGURE 8-25 **Secretory Immune System.** Lymphocytes from the mucosal-associated lymphoid tissues circulate throughout the body in a pattern separate from other lymphocytes. For example, lymphocytes from the gut-associated lymphoid tissue circulate through the regional lymph nodes, the thoracic duct, and the blood and return to other mucosal-associated lymphoid tissues rather than to lymphoid tissue of the systemic immune system.

IgA is the dominant secretory immunoglobulin, although IgM and IgG also are present in secretions.[38] The primary role of IgA is to prevent the attachment and invasion of pathogens through mucosal membranes, such as those of the gastrointestinal, pulmonary, and genitourinary tracts.[39] To induce protective immunity against some pathogens that enter through these routes, local immunization seems to be preferable to inducing only systemic immunity. For instance, two different vaccines have been used against polio. The Sabin vaccine was administered orally as an attenuated (i.e., inactivated so as to render relatively harmless) live virus. This route caused a transient, limited infection and induced effective systemic immunity and secretory immunity, preventing both the disease and the establishment of a carrier state. The Salk vaccine, on the other hand, consisted of killed viruses that were administered intradermally. It induced adequate systemic protection but did not generally prevent an intestinal carrier state.

Because B lymphocytes of the secretory/mucosal immune system travel through breast-associated lymphoid tissue, most antigens to which the mother has been exposed gastrointestinally (e.g., poliovirus) induce secretion of specific IgAs, IgMs, and IgGs into the breast milk. Antibodies in the milk may provide protection against these infectious disease agents to the nursing newborn. Although colostral antibodies (i.e., found in colostrum of breast milk) provide the newborn with passive immunity against gastrointestinal infections, they do not provide systemic immunity because they do not cross the newborn's gut into the bloodstream after the first 24 hours of life. Passive systemic immunity is provided by maternal antibodies that passed across the placenta into the fetus before birth.

The mechanisms and functions of antigen-antibody binding are the same in the secretory immune system as they are in the systemic immune systems; that is, binding neutralizes or opsonizes the antigen, preventing it from harming the host. The major differences between the two systems include (1) the order of utilization—the secretory immune response is part of the body's first-line defense, whereas the systemic response is the body's final defense; (2) the lymphocytes of each system follow different paths of migration and pass through different secondary lymphoid tissues; and (3) the secretory response occurs locally and externally (in body secretions), whereas the systemic response occurs systemically and internally (in blood and tissues).

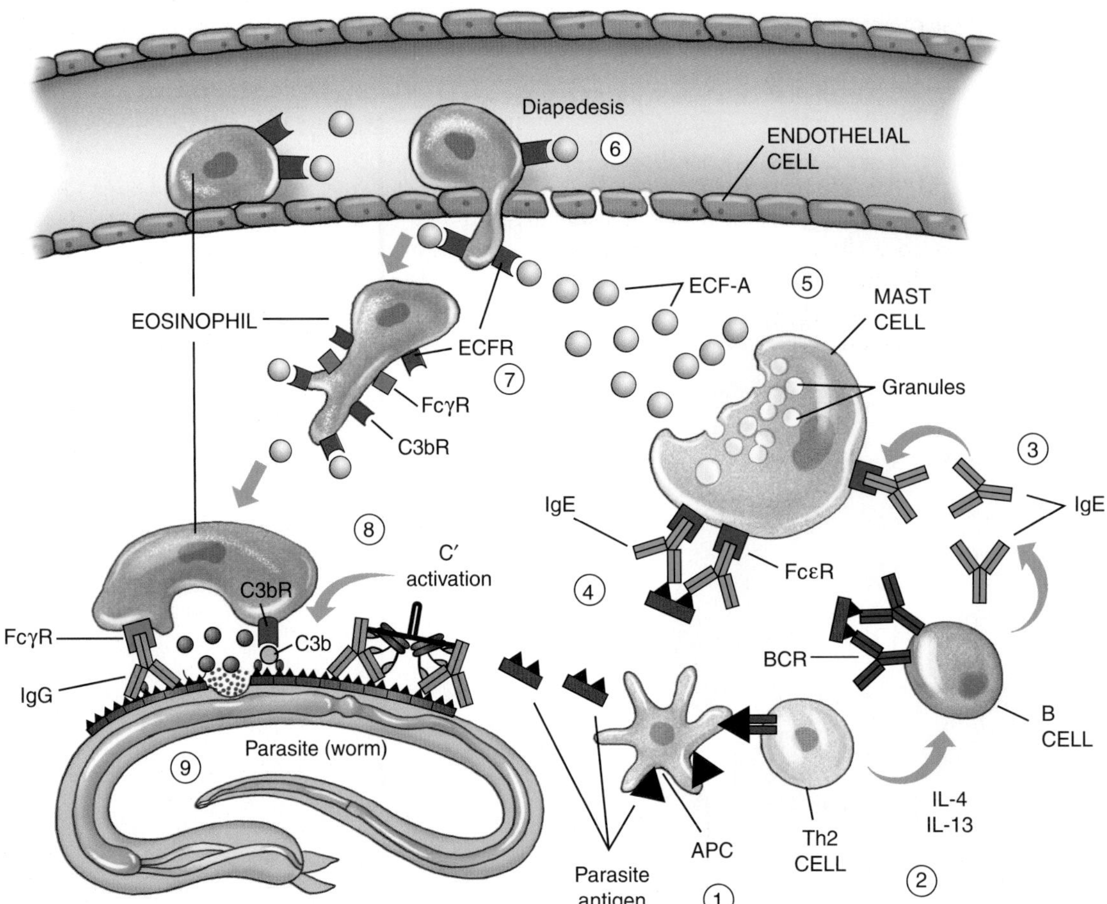

FIGURE 8-26 **IgE Function.** Soluble antigens from a parasitic infection are processed by local antigen-presenting cells (APCs) and presented to Th2 cells **(1)**, which respond by producing cytokines that favor class-switch to IgE production **(2)**. B cells bind soluble parasite antigen, and some switch to producing IgG, whereas others switch to IgE. The secreted IgE molecules bind to IgE-specific receptors (FcεR) on the mast cell surface **(3)**. Additional soluble parasite antigen cross-links IgE-FcεR complexes on the mast cell surface **(4)**, leading to mast cell degranulation and release of many proinflammatory products, including eosinophil chemotactic factor of anaphylaxis (ECF-A) **(5)**. Eosinophils have receptors for ECF-A (ECFR) and are stimulated to increase adherence to the vessel walls and initiate diapedesis **(6)** and invasion of the surrounding tissue. The eosinophil also responds by increasing the density of surface receptors for IgG (FcγR) and complement component C3b (C3bR) **(7)**. IgG had previously attached to the antigens on the parasite's surface and activated the complement cascade (C′ activation) in a failed attempt to damage the parasite. The eosinophil attaches to the parasite's surface through Fc and C3b receptors **(8)**. Once bound to the parasite, the eosinophil releases its lysosomal enzymes onto the parasite, damaging its outer membrane **(9)**.

IgE

IgE is a special class of antibody that is designed to help protect the individual from infection with large parasitic worms. However, when IgE is produced against relatively innocuous environmental antigens, it is also the primary cause of common allergies (e.g., hay fever, dust allergies, bee stings). The role of IgE in allergies is discussed in Chapter 9.

Large multicellular parasites usually invade mucosal tissues (Figure 8-26). In response to parasitic antigens, a variety of different antibody classes are produced with many B cells class-switching to IgE-secreting plasma cells under the direction of Th2 cells primarily producing IL-4 and IL-13.[40] IgG, IgM, and IgA bind to the surface of parasites, activate complement, generate chemotactic factors for neutrophils and macrophages, and serve as opsonins for those phagocytic cells. The influx of neutrophils and macrophages progressively leads to development of a granulomatous response around the parasite. Unique to parasitic infections, the eosinophil is a primary cell in the granuloma. The influx of eosinophils results from IgE-triggered mast cell degranulation. Mast cells in the tissues have very high affinity Fc receptors for IgE, which rapidly bind IgE to the mast cell surface.[41] Soluble macromolecules with multiple antigenic determinants are released from the parasite, react with the IgE-Fc receptors, and initiate mast cell degranulation (see Chapter 7). Eosinophil chemotactic factor of anaphylaxis (ECF-A) is released from mast cell granules and attracts eosinophils to the site of infection, as well as up-regulates surface receptors for IgG and complement component C3b. Eosinophil attachment to the parasite results in degranulation, releasing a variety of very toxic proteins that are at unusually high concentrations in eosinophilic granules, *major basic protein* (binds to heparin sulfate proteoglycans), *eosinophil cationic protein* (a member of the RNase

A family), and others. These can cause extensive damage to the parasite if an adequate number of eosinophils are involved.

T-Lymphocyte Function

Killing Abnormal Cells

T-Cytotoxic Lymphocytes. **T-cytotoxic lymphocytes (Tc cells)** are responsible for the cell-mediated destruction of such targets as tumor cells or cells infected with viruses. To perform this function, the Tc cell must directly adhere to the target cell through antigen presentation in association with MHC class I molecules and appropriate adhesion molecules (Figure 8-27). Most Tc-cell killing requires the αβ TCR complex and CD8 and is therefore *class I restricted.* Because of the cellular distribution of MHC class I molecules, Tc cells can recognize antigen on the surface of almost any type of cell that has been infected by a virus or has become cancerous.

After attachment to a target cell, killing can occur by at least two different mechanisms that induce apoptosis: through the actions of perforin and granzyme or by direct receptor interactions. Perforins and granzymes are contained in the Tc-cell lysosomal granules, which are released onto the surface of the target cell. Perforin acts in a fashion similar to C9 of the complement

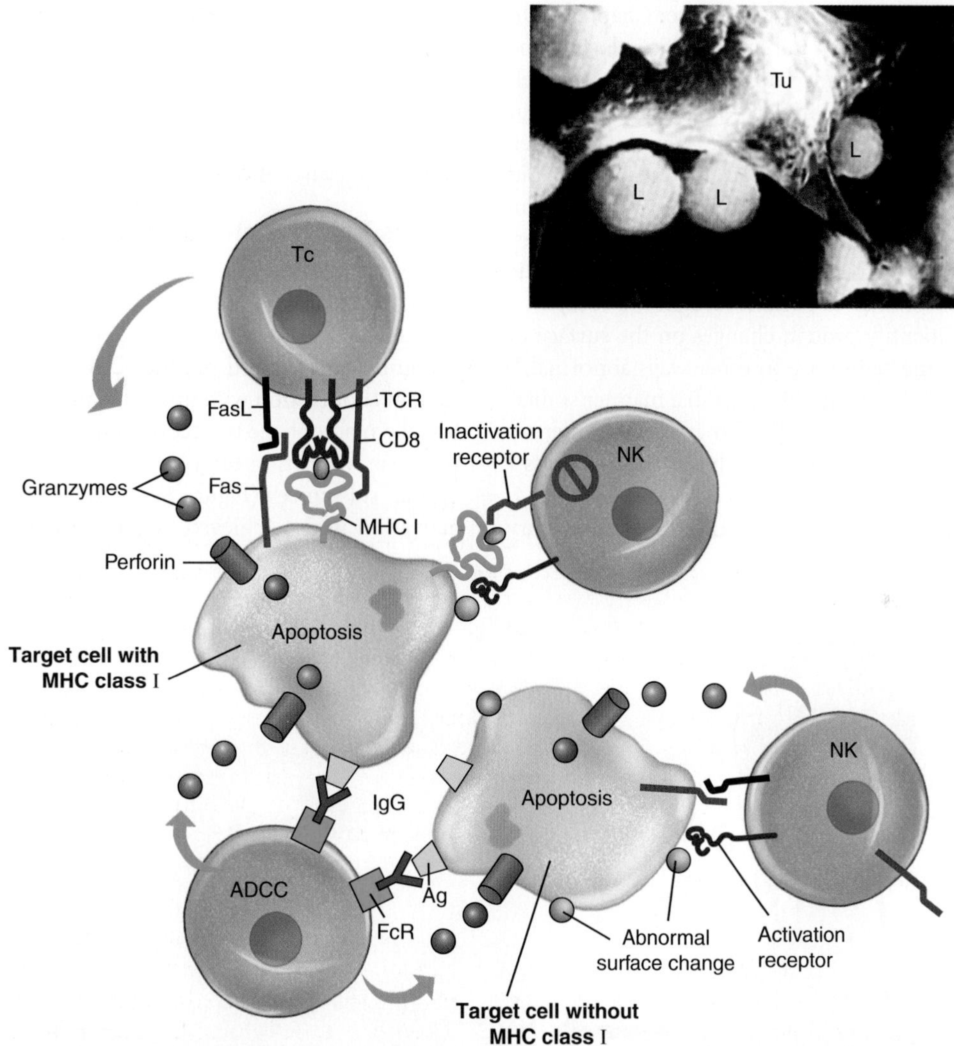

FIGURE 8-27 Cell Killing Mechanisms. Several cells have the capacity to kill abnormal (e.g., virally infected, cancerous) target cells. Cytotoxic T (Tc) cells recognized endogenous antigen presented by MHC class I molecules *(cell on upper left).* The intercellular interaction is enhanced through a variety of co-stimulatory adhesion molecules (not shown). The Tc cell mobilizes multiple killing mechanisms that induce apoptosis of the target cell, including the secretion of perforin that creates pores for the entrance of granzymes into the target cell and stimulation of Fas molecules on the target cell surface by Fas ligand (FasL) on the Tc cell. Natural killer (NK) cells *(cells on right)* use the same mechanisms to kill target cells through activation receptors that recognize "abnormal surface changes." NK cells specifically kill targets that have down-regulated expression of surface MHC class I molecules. Targets expressing MHC class I molecules inactivate NK cells through a variety of inactivation receptors *(cell on upper right).* Several cells, including macrophages and NK cells, can kill by antibody-dependent cellular cytotoxicity (ADCC). IgG antibody binds to foreign antigen on the target cell. Cells involved in ADCC *(cell on lower left)* bind IgG through Fc receptors (FcRs) and initiate killing. The insert is a scanning electron microscopic view of Tc cells *(L)* attacking a much larger tumor cell *(Tu). MHC,* Major histocompatibility complex. (Insert from Abbas A, Lichtman A: *Cellular and molecular immunology,* ed 5, Philadelphia, 2003, Saunders.)

cascade and penetrates, polymerizes, and forms pores in the target cell's plasma membrane. The granzymes enter the target cell through the perforin-lined pores and activate cellular enzymes (caspases) that are involved in apoptosis, resulting in death of the target. Additionally, target cell apoptosis can be induced directly through the stimulation of specific receptors on the cell surface. For instance, Tc cells express a surface molecule called *Fas ligand*, which is very similar to TNF-α and reacts with a protein called *Fas* (CD95) on the target cell surface. Activation of Fas signals the target cell to undergo apoptosis.

Other Cells That Kill Abnormal Cells. A variety of other cells kill targets in a fashion similar to Tc lymphocytes. Prominent among these cells are natural killer (NK) cells (see Chapter 7). In many ways, NK cells complement the effects of Tc cells. In some instances, a virally infected or cancerous cell will "protect" itself by down-regulating MHC class I molecule expression. Without surface MHC class I molecules, a cell becomes resistant to Tc-cell recognition and killing. NK cells are a special group of lymphoid cells that are similar to T cells but do not undergo maturation in the thymus and lack antigen-specific receptors. Instead, they express Fc receptors (CD16) for IgG and a variety of NK-specific cell surface receptors (similar to pattern recognition receptors, see Chapter 7) that identify protein changes on the surface of cells that have been infected or are in other ways abnormal.[42] After attachment, the NK cell kills its target in a manner similar to that of Tc cells. However, NK cells also express another set of receptors, inhibitory receptors, which bind to MHC class I molecules.[43] If the target cell continues to express MHC class I, the NK cell will bind to the class I molecule, and an inhibitory signal will result. Thus NK cells do not inadvertently kill MHC class I–bearing cells. If these cells are infected or malignant, yet still express MHC class I, they remain sensitive to Tc-cell killing. Thus Tc cells kill abnormal cells that continue to express MHC class I, whereas NK cells kill abnormal cells that have suppressed MHC class I expression.

NK cells, as well as some macrophages, can specifically kill targets through use of antibody. These cells express Fc receptors on their surface. If a pathogen or abnormal cell expresses a foreign antigen that elicits IgG antibody, which binds to the antigen, the NK cell can attach to the IgG through Fc receptors and activate its normal killing mechanisms. This is referred to as **antibody-dependent cell-mediated cytotoxicity (ADCC)** (see Figure 8-27).

Another population of NK-like cells has been identified, NK-T cells.[44] NK-T cells are produced in the thymus and more closely resemble Tc cells. However, they express TCRs that have very limited variability and recognize antigens presented by CD1.

T Cells That Activate Macrophages

Under conditions of chronic inflammation, T cells produce cytokines that activate macrophages (see Chapter 7). Macrophage activation is usually accomplished by Th1 cells that recognize antigen and produce cytokines (particularly IFN-γ) that, in cooperation with microbial products (e.g., LPS), stimulate the macrophage to become a more efficient phagocyte and increase production of proteolytic enzymes and other antimicrobial substances (Figure 8-28). IFN-γ–induced macrophage activation is also achieved by NK cells and CD8+ T-cytotoxic

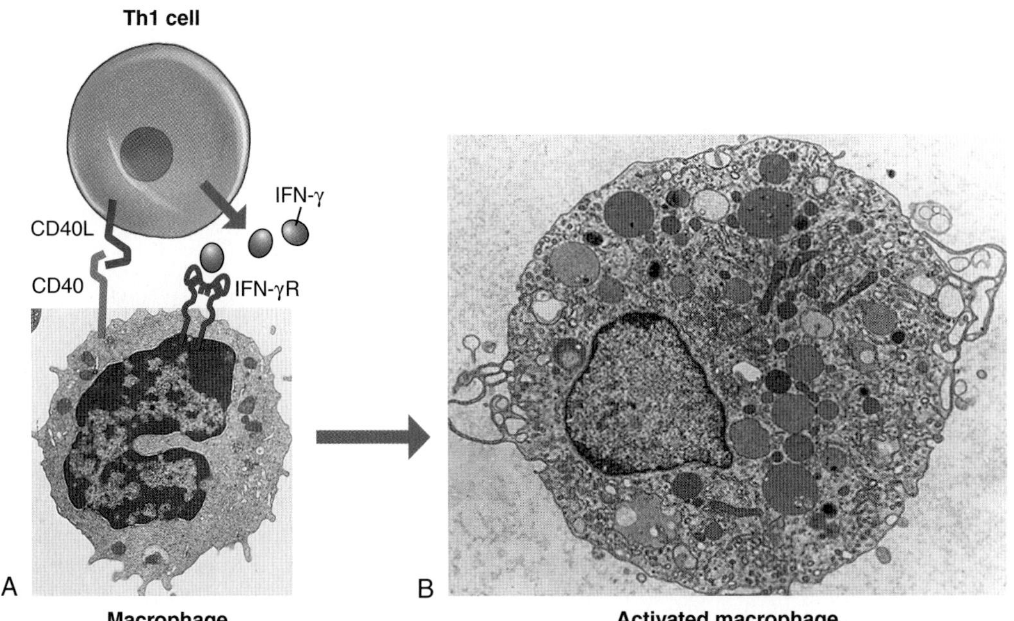

FIGURE 8-28 Activation of a Macrophage by a T Cell. A population of T cells that helps immune and inflammatory responses (helper T cells or Th1 cells) produces cytokines that activate macrophages. Optimal macrophage activation also requires close contact among the cells, which is mediated by a variety of adhesion molecules expressed on the surface of each cell (CD40L and CD40 shown here). *CD40L,* CD40 ligand; *IFN-γ,* interferon-gamma; *IFN-γR,* receptor for interferon gamma. (Micrograph in **A** courtesy Dr. Noel Weidner, Department of Pathology, University of California, San Diego. **B** from Fawcett DW: *Bloom and Fawcett: a textbook of histology,* ed 12, New York, 1994, Chapman & Hall. With kind permission of Springer Science and Business Media.)

cells. Additional signals (e.g., the CXC chemokine macrophage migration inhibitory factor) retain macrophages at inflammatory sites and increase intercellular adhesion between the Th1 cell (CD40L) and the macrophage (CD40).

T-Regulatory Lymphocytes

One form of peripheral tolerance to self-antigens occurs in Treg cells, a subpopulation of CD4+ T cells (see Figure 8-17).[45] As with Th cells, Treg cells are activated by antigen presented in the context of class II MHC and differentiation under the control of specific cytokines, primarily TGF-β and IL-2, during which they express CD25 (the α-chain of the IL-2 receptor) and are frequently designated CD4+, CD25+ Treg cells.[46] The role of Treg cells is to control or limit the immune response to protect the host's own tissues against autoimmune reactions. Treg cells produce very high levels of TGF-β and IL-10, an immunosuppressive cytokine, which generally decrease Th1 and Th2 activity and suppress antigen recognition and Th-cell proliferation. The role of Treg cells and other regulatory cells (e.g., CD25 cells, CD8+ regulatory cells, and Breg cells) is under intense investigation to determine the degree of their heterogeneity of derivation, function, and specificity.

FETAL AND NEONATAL IMMUNE FUNCTION

The normal human infant is immunologically immature at birth. Although cell-mediated immunologic capabilities begin developing early in gestation and probably are completely functional at birth, antibody production is clearly deficient. In the last trimester, the fetus appears capable of producing a primary immune response (almost entirely IgM) to antigenic challenge in utero but is unable to produce a significant IgG response. Although some IgA can be detected, the capacity to produce IgA is underdeveloped.

To protect the child against infectious agents both in utero and during the first few postnatal months, a system of active transport facilitates the passage of maternal antibodies into the fetal circulation (Figure 8-29). In the placenta, maternal and fetal blood is separated by a layer of specialized cells termed *trophoblasts*. Immunoglobulins are too large to diffuse across this cellular layer so the trophoblastic cells actively transport immunoglobulins from the maternal to the fetal circulation. Active transport of maternal IgG is mediated by surface receptors that are specific for the Fc portion of free IgG but not for IgM, IgE, or IgA. Active transport sometimes results in higher antibody titers in umbilical cord blood than in maternal blood. (Active transport mechanisms are discussed in Chapter 1.)

At birth, total IgG levels in the umbilical cord are near adult levels (Figure 8-30). When the source of maternal antibodies is severed at birth, antibody titers in the newborn begin to drop as maternal antibody is catabolized. Thus antibody titers drop rapidly as the neonate's production of IgG is beginning to rise. The rate of catabolism is usually more rapid than the rate of production so that the total immunoglobulin levels reach a minimum at 5 to 6 months in the normal child, occasionally causing transient hypogammaglobulinemia (insufficient quantities of circulating immunoglobulins). Many normal infants experience recurrent mild respiratory tract infections at this age.

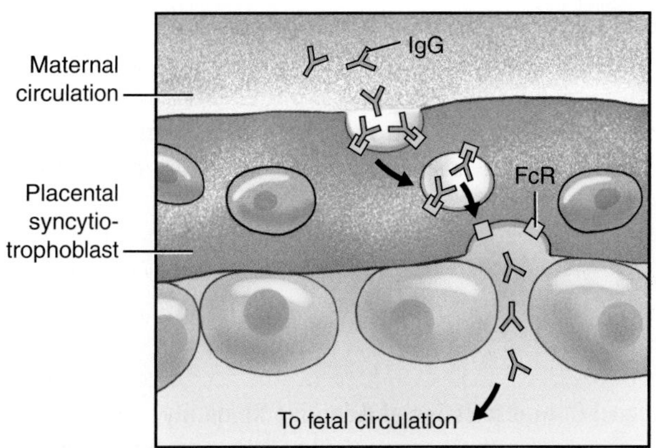

FIGURE 8-29 Transport of IgG Across the Syncytiotrophoblast. The human placenta is covered with a specialized multinucleated cell, the syncytiotrophoblast. Transport of maternal IgG across the syncytiotrophoblast and into the fetal circulation is an active process. Maternal IgG binds to Fc receptors on the surface of the syncytiotrophoblast and is internalized by the process of endocytosis. Receptors on the syncytiotrophoblast are specific for the Fc portion of IgG and do not bind other classes of immunoglobulins. Interaction of IgG with Fc receptors protects the antibody from lysosomal digestion during transport of the vacuole across the cell (i.e., transcytosis). On the fetal side of the syncytiotrophoblast, IgG is released by exocytosis (see Chapter 1).

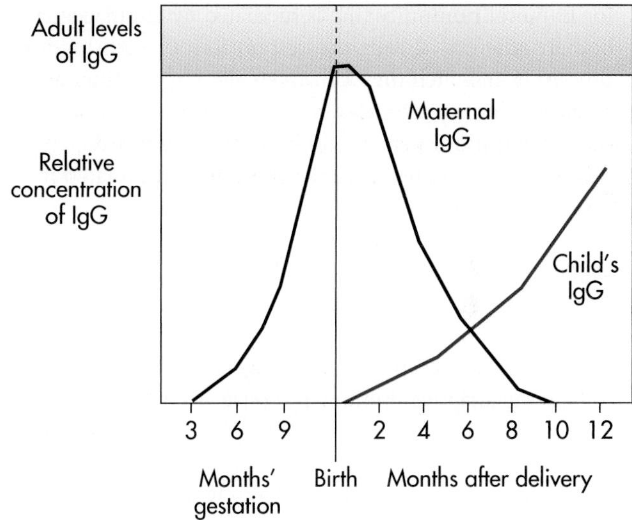

FIGURE 8-30 Antibody Levels in Umbilical Cord Blood and in Neonatal Circulation. Early in gestation maternal IgG begins crossing the placenta and enters the fetal circulation as shown in Figure 8-29. At birth, the fetal circulation may contain nearly adult levels of IgG, which is almost exclusively from the maternal source. The fetal immune system has the capacity to produce IgM and small amounts of IgA before birth (not shown). After delivery, maternal IgG is rapidly catabolized and neonatal IgG production increases.

AGING AND IMMUNE FUNCTION

Immune function decreases in old age as a result of changes in both lymphocyte function and relative lymphocyte populations. Individuals older than 60 years of age generally exhibit decreased T-cell activity as demonstrated by laboratory assays of T-cell function, as well as in vivo reductions in cell-mediated responses to infections. The thymus, where T cells begin their development, reaches its maximum size at sexual maturity and then begins involuting until thymic size is only 15% of its maximum by middle age. Thymic capacity to mediate T-cell differentiation decreases with this atrophy.[47] Although the total number of circulating T cells does not decrease with age, there is a shift in the populations of T-cell subtypes.[48]

B-cell function is also altered with age as shown by decreases in specific antibody production in response to antigenic challenge, with concomitant increases in circulating immune complexes and in circulating autoantibodies (antibodies against self-antigens). A decrease in the number of circulating memory B cells is also observed.

SUMMARY REVIEW

General Characteristics of Adaptive Immunity

1. Compared with the innate inflammatory response, the adaptive immune response is slower, is specific (rather than nonspecific or general), and has "memory" that makes it much longer lived.
2. The adaptive immune response is most often initiated by cells of the innate system. These cells process and present portions of invading pathogens (i.e., antigens) to lymphocytes in peripheral lymphoid tissue.
3. The adaptive immune response is mediated by two different types of lymphocytes—B lymphocytes and T lymphocytes. Each has distinct functions. B cells are responsible for humoral immunity that is mediated by circulating antibodies, whereas T cells are responsible for cell-mediated immunity, in which they kill targets directly or stimulate the activity of other leukocytes.
4. Adaptive immunity can be either active or passive depending on whether immune response components originated in the host or came from a donor.

Recognition and Response

1. Antigens are the molecules that can react with components of the adaptive immune system, including antibodies and lymphocyte surface receptors. Immunogens are antigens that can initiate the adaptive immune response. To be immunogenic, an antigen must be of the correct type, size, and complexity and be present in sufficient quantities. Haptens are small-molecular-weight antigens that are not themselves immunogenic.
2. Both B and T lymphocytes bind antigen through cognate receptor complexes on their surfaces. These receptor complexes (i.e., the BCR and TCR complexes, respectively) work in conjunction with accessory proteins to produce lymphocyte activation.
3. The antigen-binding molecule of the BCR is antibody. Antibodies are composed of four polypeptide chains—two identical heavy chains and two identical light chains—held together by disulfide bonds. Each heavy chain has a variable region and a large constant region. Each light chain has a variable region and a short constant region. The class of antibody is determined by which constant regions make up their heavy chains, giving each class a slightly different molecular structure. The classes include IgG (the most prevalent), IgA (mostly in secretions), IgE (the most rare), IgD, and IgM (the first and largest immunoglobulin produced). The parts of antibody that bind antigen are called the Fab, and the part that reacts with cells and molecules of the innate system is called the Fc. Antigen binds to hypervariable regions (complementary-determining regions, or CDRs) of both the heavy and the light chains.
4. For most antigens to elicit an immune response, they must be presented to lymphocytes by molecules on the surface of antigen-presenting cells. Endogenous protein antigens are presented by class I molecules of MHC. Exogenous protein antigens are presented by class II MHC molecules. Lipid antigens are presented by CD1.
5. The MHC is a cluster of genes found on human chromosome 6. The products of these genes are also called *HLA antigens.* The MHC genes are highly polymorphic, having many different possible alleles. An individual will carry only two alleles at each locus, one from each parent. The particular combination of alleles a given individual carries defines his or her MHC haplotype.
6. For an immune response to develop, a variety of cells must interact through surface adhesion molecules.
7. During their interactions, cells must communicate with each other through soluble cytokines. In addition to their roles in the innate immune response, cytokines have multiple functions in the adaptive immune response including both positive and negative regulation of B-cell and T-cell maturation. In general, it is the precise combination of cytokines influencing a given cell that ultimately determines that cell's response.

Generation of Clonal Diversity

1. The generation of clonal diversity occurs in the primary lymphoid organs (thymus for T cells, bone marrow for B cells) in the fetus.
2. An individual's population of T cells and B cells has the collective ability to respond to virtually any antigen. This ability results from genetic rearrangement of various genes to form the variable regions for the TCR and BCR. Rearrangement of *V* and *J* genes results in the variable regions of the TCR α-chain and the BCR light chain, and rearrangement of *V, D,* and *J* genes result in the variable regions of the TCR β-chain and the BCR heavy chain.
3. Differentiation of B cells and T cells in the primary lymphoid organs results in expression of several characteristic surface markers, such as CD4 on helper T cells, CD8 on cytotoxic T cells, and CD21 and CD40 on B cells.
4. During generation of clonal diversity, B cells and T cells that produce receptors against self-antigens are eliminated by a process of central tolerance.

SUMMARY REVIEW—cont'd

5. Cells leaving the primary lymphoid organs are immunocompetent (capable of reacting to antigen) and enter the circulation and secondary lymphoid organs.

Induction of an Immune Response: Clonal Selection

1. Clonal selection is the process by which antigen selects lymphocytes with complementary TCRs or BCRs and induces an immune response with the production of specific antibody or cytotoxic T cells, or both.
2. For lymphocyte activation, most antigens must be processed and presented by an APC in the context of the appropriate molecule, either MHC class I, MHC class II, or CD1 molecules.
3. Most immune responses require helper T cells (Th cells). Precursor Th cells interact with APCs through the TCR-CD4 complex, a variety of adhesion molecules, and cytokines, especially IL-1, and develop into either Th1 or Th2 subsets. Th1 cells are responsible for helping to activate macrophages and cytotoxic T cells, whereas Th2 cells are responsible for helping to activate B cells.
4. Another set of Th cells, Th17 cells, provides help in developing inflammation, particularly attraction of neutrophils and macrophages and induction of chemokine and antimicrobial protein production by epithelial cells.
5. B-cell activation results from recognition of soluble antigen by the BCR, processing of the antigen, and presentation by MHC class II antigens to Th2 cells. Interactions between the B cells and Th2 cells through adhesion molecules (e.g., CD40 and CD40L) are also required. Depending on the particular combination of cytokines produced by the Th2 cell, the B cells can undergo class-switch from making IgM antibody to making and secreting either IgA, IgE, or IgG.
6. The humoral immune response is divided into two phases, primary and secondary. These differ in the relative amounts of IgG produced—the secondary response having a much higher proportion of IgG relative to IgM. The two responses also differ in the speed with which each occurs after antigen challenge—the secondary response being much more rapid than the primary response because of the presence of memory cells in the secondary phase.
7. B cells become activated upon recognition of a particular antigen to proliferate and differentiate either into plasma cells that function as factories for the synthesis of large amounts of antibody that is specific for the recognized antigen or into memory B cells.
8. T-cell activation results from recognition by the TCR and CD8 of antigen presented by MHC class I. Appropriate intercellular adhesion molecules and cytokines, such as IL-2 from Th1 cells, are also necessary for efficient differentiation. T cells become CTLs or memory T cells.
9. Superantigens are molecules produced by infectious agents that can bind to the TCR of the Th cell outside the normal antigen-binding site and to class II MHC on the APCs, resulting in activation of a large number of Th cells and excessive production of proinflammatory cytokines that may cause shock and death of the patient. Examples of these antigens, called *superantigens,* include the bacterial toxins that can cause toxic shock syndrome and food poisoning.

Effector Mechanisms

1. The antibodies that are produced by B cells affect antigens by several different mechanisms that can be categorized as either direct or indirect. Direct mechanisms are mediated by the antigen-binding portions of antibodies (the Fab portions containing the variable regions). This binding results in neutralization of the biologic activity of antigens and possibly removal of the antigen by agglutination or precipitation. Indirect mechanisms depend on both the Fab and the non–antigen-binding portion of antibodies (the Fc portions containing the constant regions), which interact with components of innate immunity.
2. Antibodies of the systemic immune system function throughout the body, whereas antibodies of the secretory (mucosal) immune system—primarily immunoglobulins of the IgA class—are associated with bodily secretions and function to prevent pathogenic infection on epithelial surfaces.
3. Cytotoxic T cells (Tc cells) adhere directly to antigen presented by MHC class I on target cells (virus-infected cells or cancer cells) through the TCR, CD8, and a variety of adhesion proteins. This contact results in killing of the target by apoptosis through the release of perforin and granzymes and/or direct stimulation of apoptotic receptors on the target (e.g., Fas).
4. NK cells kill targets in a fashion similar to that of Tc cells. However, NK cells recognize target cells that do not express MHC class I.
5. With infections that are resistant to cells of innate immunity, some Th1 cells produce cytokines that activate macrophages to become more efficient phagocytes.
6. Treg cells control (suppress) immune responses and prevent overreaction against foreign and self-antigens.

Fetal and Neonatal Immune Function

1. The human neonate has a poorly developed immune response, particularly in the production of IgG. The fetus and neonate are protected in utero and during the first few postnatal months by maternal antibody that was actively transported across the placenta.
2. The maternal antibodies are slowly catabolized after birth until they disappear altogether by about 10 months of age. The neonate begins producing IgG at birth, and the child's antibodies reach protective levels after about 6 months of age.

Aging and Immune Function

1. T-cell activity is deficient in older adults, and a shift in the balance of T-cell subsets is observed. These changes may result in increased susceptibility to infection.
2. Antibody production to specific antigens is inferior, although older adults tend to have increased levels of circulating autoantibodies.

KEY TERMS

Active acquired immunity (active immunity), 227
Adaptive (acquired) immunity, 224
Agglutination, 251
Allergen, 229
Antibody, 229
Antibody-dependent cell-mediated cytotoxicity (ADCC), 256
Antibody titer, 252
Antigen, 225, 228
Antigen-binding fragment (Fab), 227
Antigen presentation, 233
Antigen-presenting cell (APC), 233
Antigen processing, 245
Antigenic determinant, 228
Attenuated virus, 252
B lymphocyte (B cell), 225
B-cell receptor (BCR), 232
B-cell receptor (BCR) complex, 232
Carrier, 229
CD (cluster of differentiation), 228
Cellular immunity, 227
Central tolerance, 229
Class-switch, 248
Clonal selection, 236
Complementary-determining region (CDR), 231
Crystalline fragment (Fc), 231
Epitope, 228
Framework region (FR), 232
Generation of clonal diversity, 236
Haplotype, 233
Hapten, 229
Hinge region, 231
High endothelial venule (HEV), 242
Human leukocyte antigen (HLA), 233
Humoral immunity, 226
Immunity, 224
Immunocompetent, 225
Immunogen, 228
Immunogenic, 228
Immunoglobulin, 225
Invariant chain, 245
Isotype-switch, 248
Lymphocyte, 225
Lymphoid stem cell, 237
Major histocompatibility complex (MHC), 233
MHC class I gene, 233
MHC class II gene, 233
Memory cell, 227
Neutralization, 251
Opsonin, 252
Opsonization, 251
Paratope, 228
Passive acquired immunity (passive immunity), 227
Plasma cell, 247
Peripheral tolerance, 229, 240
Precipitation, 251
Primary (central) lymphoid organ, 236
Primary immune response, 247
Secondary (anamnestic) immune response, 247
Secondary (peripheral) lymphoid organ, 237
Secretory (mucosal) immune system, 252
Secretory immunoglobulin, 252
Self-antigen, 229
Somatic recombination, 237
Superantigen (SAG), 251
Systemic immune system, 252
T-cell receptor (TCR), 229
T-cell receptor (TCR) complex, 233
T-cytotoxic lymphocyte (Tc cell), 249
Th1 cell, 245
Th2 cell, 245
Th17 cell, 245
T-helper cell (Th cell), 245
T lymphocyte (T cell), 225
T-memory cell, 249
T-regulatory (Treg) cells, 249
Tolerance, 229
Valence, 232

REFERENCES

1. Bonilla FA, Oettgen HC: Adaptive immunity, *J Allergy Clin Immunol* 125(2):S33–S40, 2010.
2. Chaplin DD: Overview of the immune response, *J Allergy Clin Immunol* 125(2):S3–S23, 2010.
3. Porter RR: The hydrolysis of rabbit γ-globulin and antibodies with crystalline papain, *Biochem J* 73:119–126, 1959.
4. Schroeder HW Jr, Cavacini L: Structure and function of immunoglobulins, *J Allergy Clin Immunol* 125(2 Suppl 2):S41–S52, 2010.
5. Burnet FM: *The clonal selection theory of acquired immunity*, London, 1959, Cambridge University Press.
6. Jerne NK: The natural-selection theory of antibody formation, *Proc Natl Acad Sci U S A* 41:849–857, 1955.
7. He R, Geha RS: Thymic stromal lymphopoietin, *Ann N Y Acad Sci* 1183(1):13–24, 2010.
8. Chaumeil J, Skok JA: The role of CTCF in regulating V(D)J recombination, *Curr Opin Immunol* 24(2):153–159, 2012.
9. Xiong Y, Bosselut R: CD4-CD8 differentiation in the thymus: connecting circuits and building memories, *Curr Opin Immunol* 24(2):139–145, 2012.
10. Wang L, Xiong Y, Bosselut R: Maintaining CD4-CD8 lineage integrity in T cells: where plasticity serves versatility, *Semin Immunol* 23(5):360–367, 2011.
11. Klein L, Jovanovic K: Regulatory T cell lineage commitment in the thymus, *Semin Immunol* 23(6):401–409, 2011.
12. Guerder S et al: Differential processing of self-antigens by subsets of thymic stromal cells, *Curr Opin Immunol* 24(1):99–104, 2012.
13. Hsieh C-S, Lee H-M, Lio C-WJ: Selection of regulatory T cells in the thymus, *Nat Rev Immunol* 12(3):157–167, 2012.
14. Mercier FE, Ragu C, Scadden DT: The bone marrow at the crossroads of blood and immunity, *Nat Rev Immunol* 12(1):49–60, 2012.
15. Nutt SL et al: The genetic network controlling plasma cell differentiation, *Semin Immunol* 23(5):341–349, 2011.
16. Pillai S, Mattoo H, Cariappa A: B cells and autoimmunity, *Curr Opin Immunol* 23(6):721–731, 2011.
17. Shlomchik MJ, Weisel F: Germinal center selection and the development of memory B and plasma cells, *Immunol Rev* 247(1):52–63, 2012.
18. Bennett CL, Chakraverty R: Dendritic cells in tissues: in situ stimulation of immunity and immunopathology, *Trends Immunol* 33(1):8–13, 2012.
19. Neefjes J et al: Towards a systems understanding of MHC class I and MHC class II antigen presentation, *Nat Rev Immunol* 11(12):823–836, 2011.
20. Krüger E, Kloetzel P- M: Immunoproteasomes at the interface of innate and adaptive immune responses: two faces of one enzyme, *Curr Opin Immunol* 24(1):77–83, 2012.
21. Gascoigne NR et al: Co-receptors and recognition of self at the immunological synapse, *Curr Top Microbiol Immunol* 340(1):171–189, 2010.
22. Sims JE, Smith DE: The IL-1 family: regulators of immunity, *Nat Rev Immunol* 10(2):89–102, 2010.
23. Liao W, Lin J-X, Leonard WJ: IL-2 family cytokines: new insights into the complex roles of IL-2 as a broad regulator of T helper cell differentiation, *Curr Opin Immunol* 23(5):598–604, 2011.
24. Oestreich KJ, Weinmann AS: Transcriptional mechanisms that regulate T helper 1 cell differentiation, *Curr Opin Immunol* 24(2):191–195, 2012.
25. Paul WE, Zhu J: How are T_H2-type immune responses initiated and amplified? *Nat Rev Immunol* 10(4):225–235, 2010.
26. Rutz S, Ouyang W: Regulation of interleukin-10 and interleukin-22 expression in T helper cells, *Curr Opin Immunol* 23(5):605–612, 2011.
27. Gaffen SL: Recent advances in the IL-17 cytokine family, *Curr Opin Immunol* 23(5):613–619, 2011.
28. Milner JD: IL-17 producing cells in host defense and atopy, *Curr Opin Immunol* 23(6):784–788, 2011.
29. Eyler JM: Smallpox in history: the birth, death, and impact of a dread disease, *J Lab Clin Med* 142(4):216–220, 2003.
30. Jenner E: *An inquiry into the causes and effects of the variolae vaccinae: a disease discovered in some of the western counties of England, particularly Gloucestershire, and known by the name of the cow pox*, London, 1798, Sampson Low.
31. Rawlings DJ et al: Integration of B cell responses through Toll-like receptors and antigen receptors, *Nat Rev Immunol* 12(4):282–294, 2012.
32. Welinder E, Ahsberg J, Sigvardsson M: B-lymphocyte commitment: identifying the point of no return, *Semin Immunol* 23(5):335–340, 2011.
33. Tangye SG: Staying alive: regulation of plasma cell survival, *Trends Immunol* 32(12):595–602, 2011.
34. McHeyzer-Williams M et al: Molecular programming of B cell memory, *Nat Rev Immunol* 12(1):24–34, 2012.
35. Weng N-P, Araki Y, Subedi K: The molecular basis of the memory T cell response: differential gene expression and its epigenetic regulation, *Nat Rev Immunol* 12(4):306–315, 2012.

36. Brosnahan AJ, Schlievert PM: Gram-positive bacterial superantigen outside-in signaling causes toxic shock syndrome, *FEBS J* 278(23):4649–4667, 2011.
37. Macpherson AJ, Geuking MB, McCoy KD: Homeland security: IgA immunity at the frontiers of the body, *Trends Immunol* 33(4):160–167, 2012.
38. Cerutti A et al: Regulation of mucosal IgA responses: lessons from primary immunodeficiencies, *Ann N Y Acad Sci* 1238:132–144, 2011.
39. Geuking MB, McCoy KD, Macpherson AJ: The function of secretory IgA in the context of the intestinal continuum of adaptive immune response in host-microbial mutualism, *Semin Immunol* 24(1):36–42, 2012.
40. Taylor MD, van der Werf N, Maizels RM: T cells in helminth infection: the regulators and the regulated, *Trends Immunol* 33(4):181–189, 2012.
41. Danilowicz-Luebert E et al: Modulation of specific and allergy-related immune responses by helminthes, *J Biomed Biotechnol* 2011:1–18, 2011.
42. Elliott JM, Yokoyama WM: Unifying concepts of MHC-dependent natural killer cell education, *Trends Immunol* 32(8):364–372, 2011.
43. Thielens A, Vivier E, Romagne E: NK cell MHC class I specific receptors (KIR): from biology to clinical intervention, *Curr Opin Immunol* 24(2):239–245, 2012.
44. Engel I, Kronenberg M: Making memory at birth: understanding the differentiation of natural killer T cells, *Curr Opin Immunol* 24(2):184–190, 2012.
45. Ding Y, Xu J, Bromberg JS: Regulatory T cell migration during an immune response, *Trends Immunol* 33(4):174–180, 2012.
46. Hall BM et al: Distinct regulatory CD4$^+$T cell subsets; differences between naïve and antigen specific T regulatory cells, *Curr Opin Immunol* 23(5):641–647, 2011.
47. Buchholz VR, Neuenhahn M, Busch DH: CD8+ T cell differentiation in the aging immune system: until the last clone standing, *Curr Opin Immunol* 23(4):549–554, 2011.
48. Blackman MA, Wookland DL: The narrowing of the CD8 T cell repertoire in old age, *Curr Opin Immunol* 23(4):537–542, 2011.

CHAPTER

9

Alterations in Immunity and Inflammation

Neal S. Rote and Kathryn L. McCance

evolve WEBSITE

http://evolve.elsevier.com/McCance/

- Review Questions and Answers
- Online Course: Module 6

CHAPTER OUTLINE

The immune system is a finely tuned network that protects the host against foreign antigens, particularly infectious agents. Sometimes this network breaks down, causing the immune system to react inappropriately. Inappropriate immune responses may be (1) exaggerated against environmental antigens (allergy); (2) misdirected against the host's own cells (autoimmunity); (3) directed against beneficial foreign tissues, such as transfusions or transplants (alloimmunity); or (4) insufficient to protect the host (immune deficiency). All of these can be serious or life threatening. Exaggerated immune responses (allergy) are the most common, but usually the least life threatening.

HYPERSENSITIVITY: ALLERGY, AUTOIMMUNITY, AND ALLOIMMUNITY

Hypersensitivity is an altered immunologic response to an antigen that results in disease or damage to the host. *Hypersensitivity reactions* can be classified in two ways: by the source of the antigen that the immune system is attacking (allergy, autoimmunity, alloimmunity; Table 9-1) and by the mechanism that causes disease (types I, II, III, and IV; see Table 9-3). The term **allergy** originally denoted both facets of the immune response: immunity, which is beneficial, and hypersensitivity, which is harmful. Allergy has now come to mean the deleterious effects of hypersensitivity to environmental antigens, and immunity means the protective responses to antigens expressed by disease-causing agents.

Autoimmunity is a disturbance in the immunologic tolerance of self-antigens. The immune system normally does not strongly recognize the individual's own antigens. Healthy individuals of all ages, but particularly older adults, may produce low quantities of antibodies against their own antigens *(autoantibodies)*, without development of overt autoimmune disease. Therefore, the presence of low quantities of autoantibodies does not necessarily indicate a disease state. Autoimmune diseases occur when the immune system reacts against self-antigens to

TABLE 9-1 RELATIVE INCIDENCES AND EXAMPLES OF HYPERSENSITIVITY REACTIONS*

	MECHANISM			
TARGET ANTIGEN	TYPE I (IMMUNOGLOBULIN E–[IGE] MEDIATED)	TYPE II (TISSUE SPECIFIC)	TYPE III (IMMUNE COMPLEX)	TYPE IV (CELL MEDIATED)
Allergy	++++	+	+	++
Environmental antigens	Hay fever	Hemolysis in drug allergies	Gluten (wheat) allergy	Poison ivy allergy
Autoimmunity	±	++	+++	+
Self-antigens	May contribute to some type III reactions	Autoimmune thrombocytopenia	Systemic lupus erythematosus	Hashimoto thyroiditis
Alloimmunity	±	++	+	++
Another person's antigens	May contribute to some type III reactions	Hemolytic disease of the newborn	Anaphylaxis to IgA in IV gamma globulin	Graft rejection

*The frequency of each reaction is indicated in a range from rare (±) to very common (++++). An example of each reaction is given.

such a degree that the person's own tissues are damaged by autoantibodies or autoreactive T cells. Many clinical disorders are associated with autoimmunity and are collectively referred to as **autoimmune diseases** (Table 9-2).

Alloimmunity (also termed *isoimmunity*) occurs when the immune system of one individual produces an immunologic reaction against tissues of another individual. Alloimmunity can be observed during immunologic reactions against transfusions, transplanted tissue, or the fetus during pregnancy.

The mechanism that initiates the onset of hypersensitivity, whether it consists of allergy, autoimmunity, or alloimmunity, is not completely understood. It is generally accepted that genetic, infectious, and possibly environmental factors contribute to hypersensitivity. Most diseases caused by hypersensitivity develop because of the interactions of at least three variables: (1) an original "insult," which alters **immunologic homeostasis** (a steady state of tolerance to self-antigens or lack of immune reaction against environmental antigens); (2) the individual's genetic makeup, which determines the degree of the resultant immune response from the effects of the insult; and (3) an immunologic process that causes the symptoms of the disease.

Mechanisms of Hypersensitivity

Diseases caused by hypersensitivity reactions can be characterized also by the particular immune mechanism that results in the disease (see Table 9-1). These mechanisms are apparent in most hypersensitivity reactions and have been divided into four distinct types: **type I (immunoglobulin E [IgE]–mediated) hypersensitivity reactions, type II (tissue-specific) hypersensitivity reactions, type III (immune complex–mediated) hypersensitivity reactions,** and **type IV (cell-mediated) hypersensitivity reactions** (Table 9-3).[1] This classification is artificial and seldom is a particular disease associated with only a single mechanism. The four mechanisms are interrelated, and in most hypersensitivity reactions, several mechanisms can be at work simultaneously or sequentially. Some of the mechanisms are secondary to the disease and not directly involved in the pathologic process, whereas others are the primary cause of tissue destruction.

Hypersensitivity reactions require *sensitization* against a particular antigen that results in primary and secondary immune responses. An individual is sensitized when an adequate amount of antibodies or T cells is available to cause a noticeable reaction on reexposure to the antigen. Some individuals become sensitized quite rapidly (after an apparent single exposure to the antigen), whereas others require multiple exposures that may occur over years. After sensitization has been achieved, hypersensitivity reactions can be immediate or delayed, depending on the time between reexposure to the antigen and the onset of clinical symptoms. Reactions that occur within minutes to a few hours are termed **immediate hypersensitivity reactions. Delayed hypersensitivity reactions** may take several hours to appear and are at maximum severity days after reexposure to the antigen.

The most rapid and severe immediate hypersensitivity reaction is **anaphylaxis.**[2] Anaphylaxis occurs within minutes of reexposure to the antigen and can be either systemic (generalized) or cutaneous (localized).[3] Symptoms of systemic anaphylaxis include itching, erythema, headaches, vomiting, abdominal cramps, diarrhea, and breathing difficulties. In severe cases, contraction of bronchial smooth muscle, laryngeal edema, and vascular collapse may result in respiratory distress, decreased blood pressure, shock, and death. Examples of systemic anaphylaxis are allergic reactions to bee stings, peanuts, and fish. Cutaneous anaphylaxis causes the less severe symptom of local inflammation.

Type I: IgE-Mediated Hypersensitivity Reactions

Type I reactions are mediated by antigen-specific IgE and the products of tissue mast cells[4] (Figure 9-1). Most common allergies (e.g., pollen allergies) are type I reactions. In addition, most type I reactions occur against environmental antigens and are therefore allergic. Because of this strong association, many healthcare professionals use the term *allergy* to indicate only IgE-mediated reactions. However, IgE can contribute to a few autoimmune and alloimmune diseases, and many common allergies (e.g., poison ivy) are not mediated by IgE.

In some individuals, exposure to an environmental antigen causes primarily IgE production. Repeated exposure to the antigen usually is required to elicit enough IgE so that the person becomes "sensitized." IgE has a relatively short life span in the blood because it rapidly binds to very-high-affinity Fc receptors

TABLE 9-2 **DISORDERS ASSOCIATED WITH AUTOIMMUNITY**

SYSTEM DISEASE	ORGAN OR TISSUE	PROBABLE SELF-ANTIGEN
Endocrine System		
Hyperthyroidism (Graves disease)	Thyroid gland	Receptors for thyroid-stimulating hormone on plasma membrane of thyroid cells
Autoimmune thyroiditis	Thyroid gland	Thyroglobulin; microsomes
Primary myxedema	Thyroid gland	Microsomes
Insulin-dependent diabetes	Pancreas	Islet cells, insulin, insulin receptors on pancreatic cells
Addison disease	Adrenal gland	Surface antigens on steroid-producing cells; microsomes of adrenal cortex
Premature gonadal failure	Ovary	Interstitial cells; corpus luteum
Male infertility	Testis	Surface antigens on spermatozoa
Orchitis	Testis	Germinal epithelium
Female infertility	Ovary	Zona pellucida
Idiopathic hypoparathyroidism	Parathyroid gland	Surface antigens on chief cells (epithelial cells of gland)
Partial pituitary deficiency	Pituitary gland	Prolactin-producing cells; growth hormone–producing cells
Skin		
Pemphigus vulgaris	Skin	Intercellular substances in stratified squamous epithelium
Bullous pemphigoid	Skin	Basement membrane
Dermatitis herpetiformis	Skin	Basement membrane (immunoglobulin A [IgA])
Vitiligo	Skin	Surface antigens on melanocytes (melanin-producing cells)
Neuromuscular Tissue		
Polymyositis (dermatomyositis)	Muscle	Nuclear materials; myosin
Multiple sclerosis	Neural tissue	Unknown
Myasthenia gravis	Neuromuscular junction	Acetylcholine receptors; striations of skeletal and cardiac muscle
Polyneuritis	Nerve cell	Peripheral myelin
Rheumatic fever	Heart	Cardiac tissue (subsarcolemmal membrane); cross reaction with group A streptococcal antigen
Cardiomyopathy	Heart	Cardiac muscle
Postvaccinal or postinfectious encephalitis	Central nervous system	Central nervous system myelin or basic protein
Gastrointestinal System		
Celiac disease (gluten-sensitive enteropathy)	Intestine	Gluten
Ulcerative colitis	Colon	Mucosal cells
Crohn disease	Ileum	Unknown
Pernicious anemia	Stomach	Surface antigens of parietal cells; intrinsic factor
Atrophic gastritis	Stomach	Parietal cells
Primary biliary cirrhosis	Liver	Mitochondria; cells of bile duct
Chronic active hepatitis	Liver	Surface antigens, nuclei, microsomes, mitochondria or hepatocytes; smooth muscle
Eye		
Sjögren syndrome	Lacrimal gland	Antigens of lacrimal gland, salivary gland, thyroid, and nuclei of cells; immunoglobulin G (IgG)
Uveitis	Uveal structures	Antigens of the iris, ciliary body, and choroid
Connective Tissue		
Ankylosing spondylitis	Joints	Sacroiliac and spinal apophyseal joint
Rheumatoid arthritis	Joints	IgG, collagen
Systemic lupus erythematosus	Multiple sites	Numerous antigens in nuclei, organelles, and extracellular matrix
Mixed connective tissue disease	Multiple sites	Ribonucleoprotein and numerous other nucleoproteins
Polyarteritis nodosa (necrotizing vasculitis)	Arterioles (small arteries)	Unknown
Scleroderma (progressive systemic sclerosis)	Multiple organs	Nuclear antigens; IgG
Felty syndrome	Joints	IgG
Antiphospholipid antibody syndrome	Platelets, endothelial cells, trophoblast of placenta	Membrane phospholipids, especially phosphatidylserine
Renal System		
Immune complex glomerulonephritis	Kidney	Numerous immune complexes
Goodpasture syndrome	Kidney	Glomerular basement membrane

TABLE 9-2 DISORDERS ASSOCIATED WITH AUTOIMMUNITY—cont'd

SYSTEM DISEASE	ORGAN OR TISSUE	PROBABLE SELF-ANTIGEN
Hematologic System		
Idiopathic neutropenia	Neutrophil	Surface antigens on polymorphonuclear neutrophils
Idiopathic lymphopenia	Lymphocytes	Surface antigens on lymphocytes
Autoimmune hemolytic anemia	Erythrocytes	Surface antigens on erythrocytes
Autoimmune thrombocytopenic purpura	Platelets	Surface antigens on platelets
Respiratory System		
Goodpasture syndrome	Lung	Septal membrane of alveolus

TABLE 9-3 IMMUNOLOGIC MECHANISMS OF TISSUE DESTRUCTION

TYPE	NAME	RATE OF DEVELOPMENT	CLASS OF ANTIBODY INVOLVED	PRINCIPAL EFFECTOR CELLS INVOLVED	COMPLEMENT PARTICIPATION	EXAMPLES OF DISORDERS
I	IgE-mediated reaction	Immediate	IgE	Mast cells	No	Seasonal allergic rhinitis
II	Tissue-specific reaction	Immediate	IgG IgM	Macrophages in tissues	Frequently	Autoimmune thrombocytopenic purpura, Graves disease, autoimmune hemolytic anemia
III	Immune complex–mediated reaction	Immediate	IgG IgM	Neutrophils	Yes	Systemic lupus erythematosus
IV	Cell-mediated reaction	Delayed	None	Lymphocytes, macrophages	No	Contact sensitivity to poison ivy and metals (jewelry)

Ig, Immunoglobulin.

on the plasma membranes of mast cells (see Figure 9-1). The subclass IgG4 also has specific receptors on the mast cell and may contribute to the type I mechanism. Antibody that binds to mast cells is termed **cytotropic antibody** (able to bind to cell surfaces) or **reagin** (skin-sensitizing antibody). Unlike Fc receptors on phagocytes, which bind IgG that has reacted with antigen, the Fc receptors on mast cells bind with IgE that has not previously interacted with antigen.

If further exposure of a sensitized individual to the antigen occurs, one molecule of antigen may bind simultaneously to two molecules of IgE-Fc receptor complexes on the mast cell's surface (cross-link) resulting in activation of intracellular signaling pathways and mast cell degranulation (see Figure 9-1, *B,* and Chapter 7). The antigen that triggers cross-linking must have at least two antigenic determinants on the same molecule. Sometimes an IgE-mediated response is beneficial to the host, as is the case of some immune reactions against parasites. (This mechanism is described in Chapter 8 and illustrated in Figure 8-26.)

The products of mast cell degranulation can modulate almost all aspects of an acute inflammatory response. (The effects of biochemical mediators released by mast cells are illustrated in Figure 7-11). The most potent mediator is histamine, which affects several key target cells. Acting through the H1 receptors, histamine contracts bronchial smooth muscles, causing bronchial constriction; increases vascular permeability, causing edema; and causes vasodilation, increasing blood flow into the affected area (see Figures 7-3 and 7-12). The interaction of histamine with H2 receptors results in increased gastric acid secretion and a decrease of histamine released from mast cells and basophils. The action of histamine through H2 receptors suggests an important negative-feedback mechanism that stops degranulation. That is, the released histamine inhibits release of additional histamine by interacting with H2 receptors on the mast cells. Histamine also may affect control of the immune response through H2 receptors on most cells of the immune system. Another important activity of histamine is enhancement of the chemotactic activity of other factors, such as eosinophil chemotactic factor of anaphylaxis (ECF-A), which attracts eosinophils into sites of allergic inflammatory reactions and prevents them from migrating out of the inflammatory site. (The role of the eosinophil in inflammation is discussed in Chapter 7.)

Type II: Tissue-Specific Hypersensitivity Reactions

Type II hypersensitivity reactions are generally characterized by a specific cell or tissue being the target of an immune response. In addition to major histocompatibility locus antigens (HLAs; discussed in Chapter 8), most cells have other antigens on their surfaces. Some of these other antigens are called **tissue-specific antigens** because they are expressed on the plasma membranes of only certain cells in specific tissues. Platelets, for example, have groups of antigens that are found on no other cells of the body. The symptoms of many type II diseases are determined by which tissue or organ expresses the particular antigen. Environmental antigens (e.g., drugs or their metabolites) may bind to the plasma membranes of specific cells (especially erythrocytes and platelets) and function as targets of type II reactions.

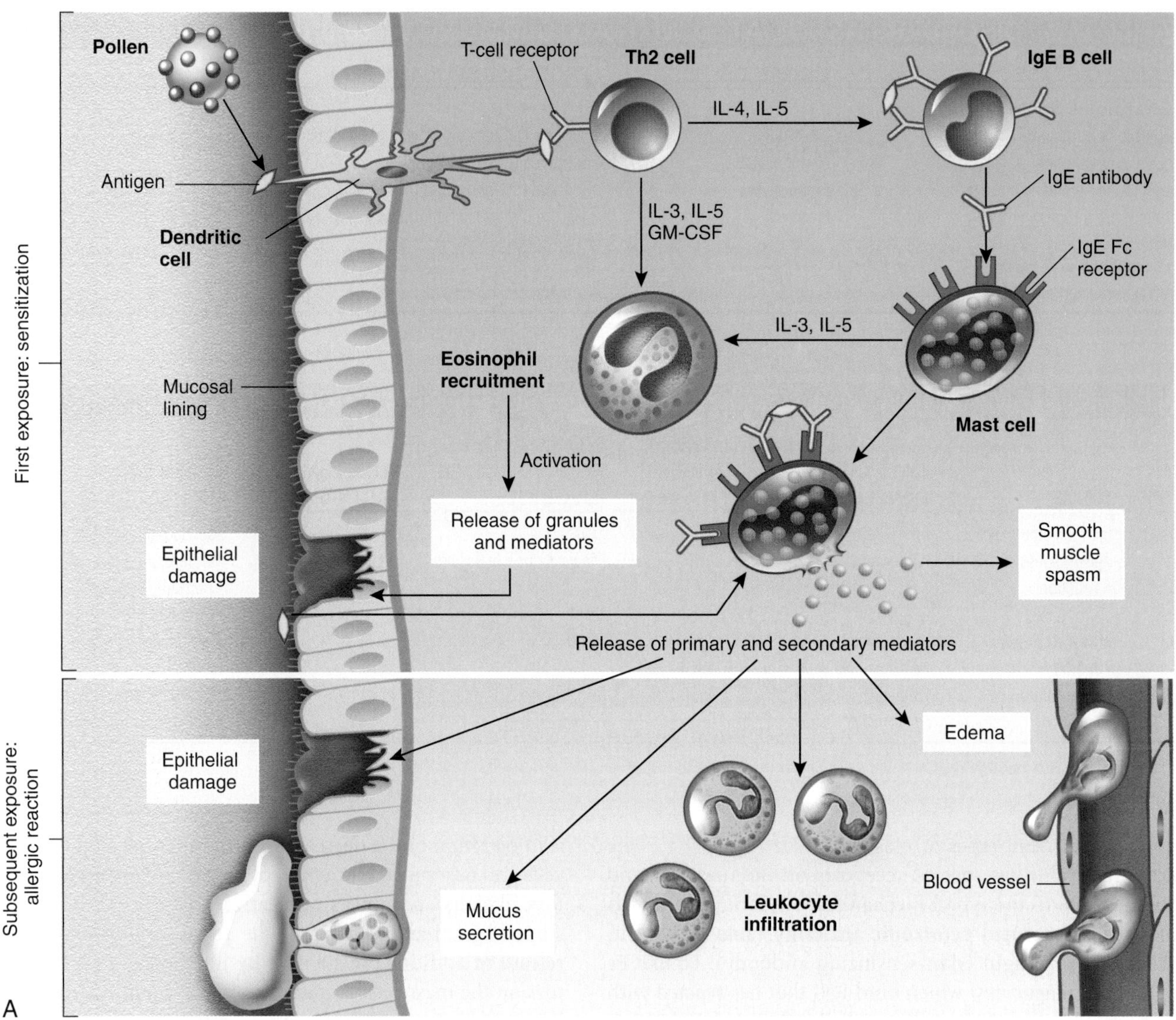

FIGURE 9-1 **Mechanism of Type I IgE–Mediated Reactions. A,** Th2 cells are activated by antigen-presenting dendritic cells to produce cytokines, including IL-3, IL-4, IL-5, and granulocyte-macrophage colony-stimulating factor (GM-CSF). IL-3, IL-5, and GM-CSF attract and promote the survival of eosinophils. Other cytokines (e.g., IL-4) induce B cells to class-switch to IgE-producing plasma cells. The IgE coats the surface of the mast cell by binding with IgE-specific Fc receptors on the mast cell's plasma membrane (sensitization). Further exposure to the same allergen cross-links the surface-bound IgE and activates signals from the cytoplasmic portion of the IgE Fc receptors. These signals initiate two parallel and interdependent processes: mast cell degranulation and discharge of preformed mediators (e.g., histamine, eosinophil-chemotactic factor of anaphylaxis) and production of newly formed mediators such as arachidonic metabolites (leukotrienes, prostaglandins). Many local type I hypersensitivity reactions have two well-defined phases. The initial phase is characterized by vasodilation, vascular leakage, and, depending on the location, smooth muscle spasm or glandular secretions. These changes usually become evident within 5 to 30 minutes after exposure to the antigen. The late phase occurs 2 to 8 hours later without additional exposure to the antigen. The late phase has more intense infiltration of tissues with eosinophils, neutrophils, basophils, monocytes, and Th cells and tissue destruction in the form of mucosal epithelial cell damage.

The five general mechanisms by which type II hypersensitivity reactions can affect cells are shown in Figure 9-2. All of these mechanisms begin with antibody binding to tissue-specific antigens or antigens that have attached to particular tissues. First, the cell can be destroyed by antibody (IgG or IgM) and activation of the complement cascade through the classical pathway. Formation of the membrane attack complex (C5-9) damages the membrane and may result in lysis of the cell (see Figure 9-2, *A*). For example, erythrocytes are destroyed by complement-mediated lysis in individuals with autoimmune hemolytic anemia (see Chapter 28) or as a result of an alloimmune reaction to ABO-mismatched transfused blood cells.

Second, antibody may cause cell destruction through phagocytosis by macrophages. IgG and also C3b of the complement system are opsonins that bind to receptors on the macrophage (see Figure 9-2, *B*). Phagocytosis of the target cell follows.

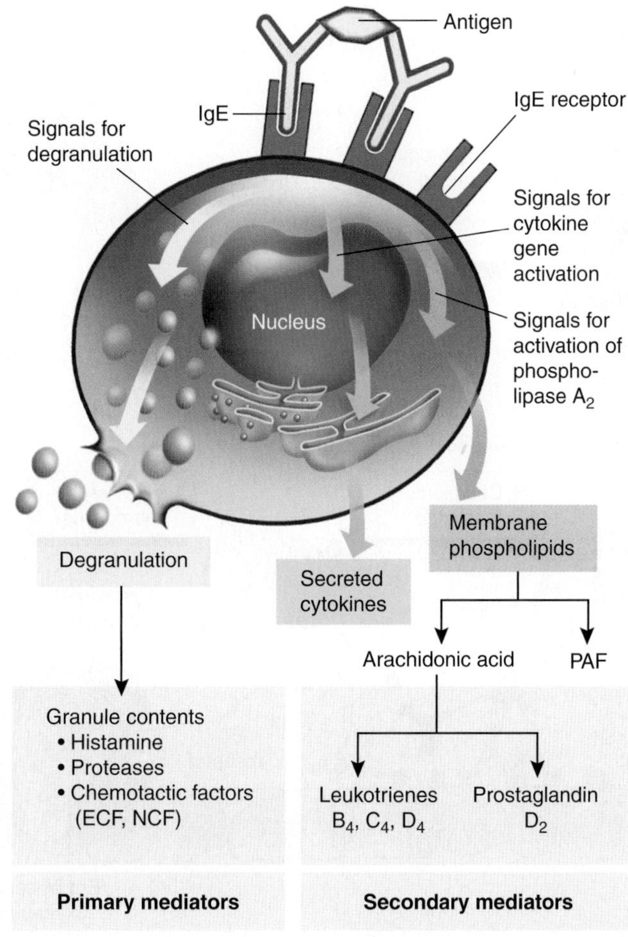

FIGURE 9-1, cont'd B, Activation of mast cells leading to degranulation of preformed mediators (primary mediators) and synthesis of newly formed (de novo) mediators (secondary mediators). *ECF,* Eosinophilic chemotactic factor; *NCF,* neutrophil chemotactic factor; *PAF,* platelet-activating factor.

(Phagocytosis is illustrated in Figures 7-15 and 7-16.) For example, antibodies against platelet-specific antigens or against red blood cell antigens of the Rh system coat those cells at low density, resulting in their preferential removal by phagocytosis in the spleen, rather than by complement-mediated lysis.

Third, antibody and complement may attract neutrophils. Either antigen expressed normally on the vessel walls or soluble antigen in the circulation (e.g., released from cells within the body or from infectious agents or by way of drugs or medications) that has been deposited on the surface of endothelial cells may bind antibody (see Figure 9-2, *C*). The antibody initiates the complement cascade, resulting in the release of C3a and C5a, which are chemotactic for neutrophils, and deposition of complement component C3b. Neutrophils bind to the tissues through receptors for the Fc portion of antibody (Fc receptor) or for C3b and attempt to phagocytose the tissue. Because the tissue is large, phagocytosis cannot be completed; even so, neutrophils release their granules onto the healthy tissue. The components of neutrophil granules, as well as the several toxic oxygen products produced by these cells, will damage the tissue.

The fourth mechanism is **antibody-dependent cell-mediated cytotoxicity (ADCC)** (see Figure 9-2, *D*). This mechanism involves a subpopulation of cytotoxic cells that are not antigen specific (natural killer [NK] cells). Antibody on the target cell is recognized by Fc receptors on the NK cells, which release toxic substances that destroy the target cell.

The fifth mechanism does not destroy the target cell, but rather causes it to malfunction. In this mechanism of type II injury, the antibody is usually directed against antigenic determinants associated with specific cell surface receptors, and the symptoms of the disease are a result of a direct effect of antibody binding alone (see Figure 9-2, *E*). The antibody reacts with the receptors on the target cell surface and modulates the function of the receptor by preventing interactions with their normal ligands, replacing the ligand and inappropriately stimulating the receptor, or destroying the receptor. For example, in the hyperthyroidism (excessive thyroid activity) of Graves disease, autoantibody binds to and activates receptors for thyroid-stimulating hormone (TSH) (a pituitary hormone that controls the production of the hormone *thyroxine* by the thyroid). In this way the antibody stimulates the thyroid cells to produce thyroxine.[5] Under normal conditions, the increasing levels of thyroxine in the blood would signal the pituitary to decrease TSH production, which would result in less stimulation of the TSH receptor in the thyroid and a concomitant decrease in thyroxine production. Because the level of anti-TSH receptor

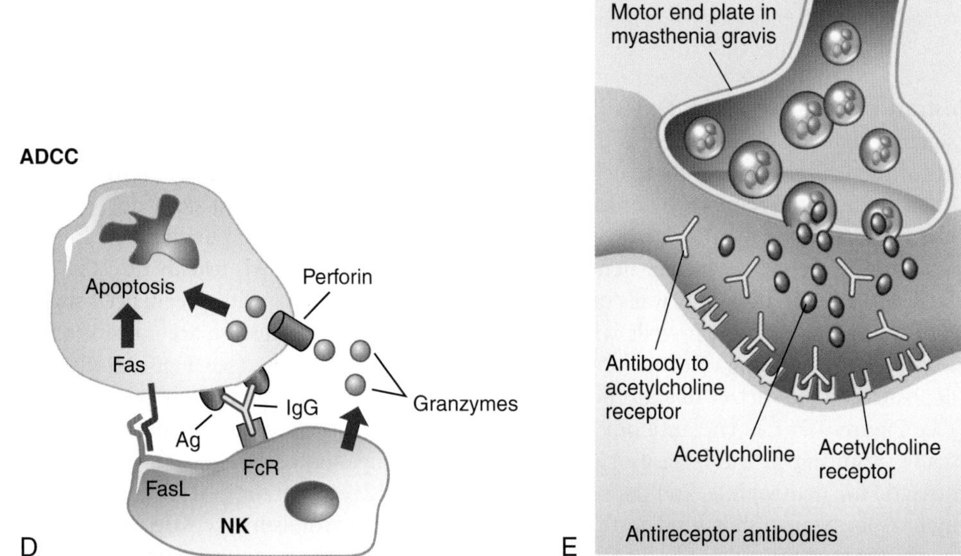

FIGURE 9-2 **Mechanisms of Type II, Tissue-Specific, Reactions.** Antigens on the target cell bind with antibody and are destroyed or prevented from functioning by **A,** complement-mediated lysis (an erythrocyte target is illustrated here); **B,** clearance (phagocytosis) by macrophages in the tissue; **C,** neutrophil-mediated immune destruction; **D,** antibody-dependent cell-mediated cytotoxicity (ADCC) (apoptosis of target cells is induced by granzymes and perforin produced by natural killer [NK] cells and interactions of Fas ligand [FasL] on the surface of NK cells with Fas on the surface of target cells); or **E,** modulation or blocking the normal function of receptors by antireceptor antibody. This example of mechanism **E** depicts myasthenia gravis in which acetylcholine receptor antibodies block acetylcholine from attaching to its receptors on the motor end plates of skeletal muscle, thereby impairing neuromuscular transmission and causing muscle weakness. *C1,* Complement component C1; *C3b,* complement fragment produced from C3, which acts as an opsonin; *C5a,* complement fragment produced from C5, which acts as a chemotactic factor for neutrophils; *Fcγ receptor,* cellular receptor for the Fc portion of IgG; *FcR,* Fc receptor.

antibody is not controlled by the pituitary, increasing amounts of thyroxine in the blood have no effect on antibody levels, and thyroxine production continues to increase despite decreasing amounts of TSH (see Chapter 22).

Type III: Immune Complex–Mediated Hypersensitivity Reactions

Mechanisms of Type III Hypersensitivity. Most type III hypersensitivity diseases are caused by antigen-antibody (immune) complexes that are formed in the circulation and deposited later in vessel walls or extravascular tissues (Figure 9-3). The primary difference between type II and type III mechanisms is that in type II hypersensitivity antibody binds to the antigen on the cell surface, whereas in type III the antibody binds to soluble antigen that was released into the blood or body fluids, and the complex is then deposited in the tissues. Type III reactions are not organ specific, and symptoms have little to do with the particular antigenic target of the antibody. The harmful effects of immune complex deposition are caused by complement activation, particularly through the generation of chemotactic factors for neutrophils. The neutrophils bind to antibody and C3b contained in the complexes and attempt to ingest the immune complexes.

They are often unsuccessful because the complexes are bound to large areas of tissue. During the attempted phagocytosis, large quantities of lysosomal enzymes are released into the inflammatory site instead of into phagolysosomes. The attraction of neutrophils and the subsequent release of lysosomal enzymes cause most of the resulting tissue damage.

Immune complexes can be of various sizes, depending on the relative amounts of antigen and antibody. Fairly large immune complexes are cleared rapidly from the circulation by tissue macrophages, whereas very small complexes eventually are filtered from blood through the kidneys, without any pathologic consequences. Intermediate-sized immune complexes (formed at a ratio of antigen to antibody that has a slight excess of antigen) are likely to be deposited in certain target tissues, where they have severe pathologic consequences, such as inflammation in the kidneys (glomerulonephritis), the vessels (vasculitis), or the joints (arthritis or degenerative joint disease).

Immune Complex Disease. The nature of the immune complexes may change during the progression of the disease, with resultant changes in the severity of the symptoms. Immune complex formation is dynamic as variations in the ratio of antigen to antibody, the class and subclass of antibody, and the quantity and quality of circulating antigen occur. Thus complexes formed early in a disease process may differ from those formed later, and several types of immune complexes may be present simultaneously. With the tremendous potential heterogeneity of immune complexes, it is not surprising that immune complex diseases are characterized by a variety of symptoms and periods of remission or exacerbation of symptoms.

Because many immune complexes activate complement very effectively, complement levels in the blood may decrease during active disease. At times the individual's blood may become **hypocomplementemic** (i.e., contains below normal amounts of complement activity). During type I, II, or IV hypersensitivity

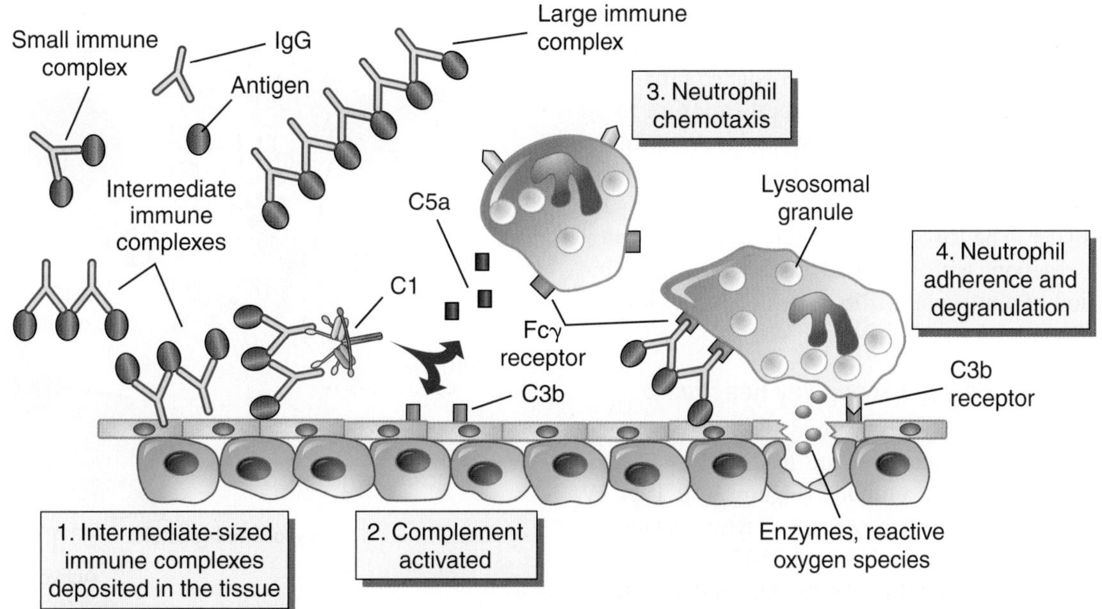

FIGURE 9-3 Mechanism of Type III, Immune Complex–Mediated, Reactions. Immune complexes form in the blood from circulating antigen and antibody. Both small and large immune complexes are removed successfully from the circulation and do not cause tissue damage. Intermediate-sized complexes are deposited in certain target tissues in which the circulation is slow or filtration of the blood occurs. The complexes activate the complement cascade through C1 and generate fragments including C5a and C3b. C5a is chemotactic for neutrophils, which migrate into the inflamed area and attach to the IgG and C3b in the immune complexes. The neutrophils attempt unsuccessfully to phagocytose the tissue and in the process release a variety of degradative enzymes that destroy the healthy tissues. Fcγ receptor is the cellular receptor for the Fc portion of IgG.

reactions, complement levels are unaffected, or some components of the complement cascade, such as C3, may even be increased.

Two prototypic models of type III hypersensitivity help explain the variety of diseases in this category. Serum sickness is a model of systemic type III hypersensitivities, and the Arthus reaction is a model of localized or cutaneous reactions.

Serum Sickness. The systemic prototype of immune complex–mediated disease is called **serum sickness** because it was initially described as being caused by the therapeutic administration of foreign serum, such as horse serum that contained antibody against tetanus toxin.[6] Foreign serum generally is not administered to individuals today, although serum sickness reactions can be caused by the repeated intravenous administration of other antigens, such as drugs, and the characteristics of serum sickness are observed in systemic type III autoimmune diseases. Serum sickness–type reactions are caused by the formation of immune complexes in the blood and their subsequent generalized deposition in target tissues. Typically affected tissues are the blood vessels, joints, and kidneys. Other symptoms include fever, enlarged lymph nodes, rash, and pain at sites of inflammation.

A form of serum sickness is **Raynaud phenomenon,** a condition caused by the temperature-dependent deposition of immune complexes in the capillary beds of the peripheral circulation. Certain immune complexes precipitate at temperatures below normal body temperature, particularly in the tips of the fingers, toes, and nose, and are called **cryoglobulins.** The precipitates block the circulation and cause localized pallor and numbness, followed by cyanosis (a bluish tinge resulting from oxygen deprivation) and eventually gangrene if the circulation is not restored.

Arthus Reaction. An **Arthus reaction** is the prototypic example of a localized immune complex–mediated inflammatory response.[7] It is caused by repeated local exposure to an antigen that reacts with preformed antibody and forms immune complexes in the walls of the local blood vessels. Symptoms of an Arthus reaction begin within 1 hour of exposure and peak 6 to 12 hours later. The lesions are characterized by a typical inflammatory reaction, with increased vascular permeability, an accumulation of neutrophils, edema, hemorrhage, clotting, and tissue damage.

Type IV: Cell-Mediated Hypersensitivity Reactions

Whereas types I, II, and III hypersensitivity reactions are mediated by antibody, type IV reactions are mediated by T lymphocytes and do not involve antibody (Figure 9-4). Type IV mechanisms occur through either cytotoxic T lymphocytes (Tc cells) or lymphokine-producing Th1 and Th17 cells. Tc cells attack and destroy cellular targets directly. Th1 and Th17 cells produce cytokines that recruit and activate phagocytic cells, especially macrophages. Destruction of the tissue is usually caused by direct killing by toxins from Tc cells or by the release of soluble factors, such as lysosomal enzymes and toxic reactive oxygen species (ROS), from activated macrophages.

Clinical examples of type IV hypersensitivity reactions include graft rejection and allergic reactions resulting from contact with such substances as poison ivy and metals. A type IV component also may be present in many autoimmune diseases. For example, T cells against type II collagen (a protein present in joint tissues) contribute to the destruction of joints in rheumatoid arthritis; T cells against a thyroid cell surface antigen contribute to the destruction of the thyroid in autoimmune thyroiditis (Hashimoto disease); and T cells against an antigen on the surface of pancreatic beta cells (the cell that normally produces insulin) are responsible for beta-cell destruction in insulin-dependent (type 1) diabetes mellitus.[8]

A type IV hypersensitivity reaction in the skin was thoroughly described first by Ehrlich in 1891 and led to the development of a diagnostic skin test for tuberculosis.[9] The reaction follows an intradermal injection of tuberculin antigen into a suitably sensitized individual and is called a *delayed hypersensitivity skin test* because of its slow onset—24 to 72 hours to reach maximum intensity. The reaction site is infiltrated with T lymphocytes and macrophages, resulting in a clear hard center (induration) and a reddish surrounding area (erythema).

Antigenic Targets of Hypersensitivity Reactions

Allergy

Allergy is a hypersensitivity response against an environmental antigen **(allergen).** Although the most common allergies are type I hypersensitivities, any of the other three mechanisms may cause allergic responses.[10]

Typical allergens that induce type I hypersensitivity include pollens (e.g., ragweed), molds and fungi (e.g., *Penicillium notatum*), foods (e.g., milk, eggs, fish), animals (e.g., cat dander, dog dander), cigarette smoke, components of house dust (e.g., fecal pellets of house mites), and almost anything else we

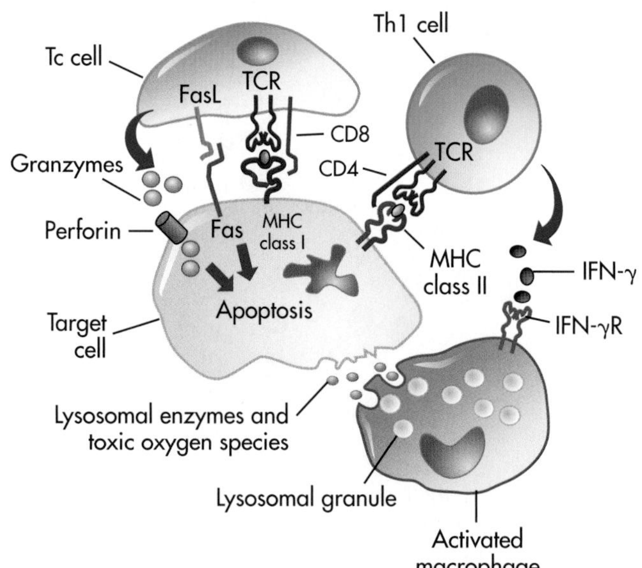

FIGURE 9-4 **Mechanism of Type IV, Cell-Mediated, Reactions.** Antigens from target cells stimulate T cells to differentiate into cytotoxic T cells (Tc cells), which have direct cytotoxic activity, and helper T cells (Th1 cells) involved in delayed hypersensitivity. The Th1 cells produce lymphokines (especially interferon-gamma [IFN-γ]) that activate the macrophage through specific receptors (e.g., IFN-γ receptor [IFN-γR]). The macrophages can attach to targets and release enzymes and reactive oxygen species that are responsible for most of the tissue destruction.

may encounter in our environment. Allergens that primarily elicit type IV allergic hypersensitivities include plant resins (e.g., poison ivy, poison oak), metals (e.g., nickel, chromium), acetylates, and chemicals in rubber, cosmetics, detergents, and topical antibiotics (e.g., neomycin). Type II and type III allergic hypersensitivities are relatively rare but may include antibiotics (e.g., penicillin, sulfonamides) and soluble antigens produced by infectious agents (e.g., hepatitis B).

Usually a sensitization process involving multiple exposures to the allergen occurs before adequate amounts of antibody or T cells are available to elicit a hypersensitivity response. In some instances, exposure to a particular allergen may not be apparent in the case of allergens that are drugs, additives, or preservatives in food. For example, an individual may become sensitized by drinking milk that contains trace amounts of penicillin used for treating cows for mastitis. Thus, the first therapeutic exposure to penicillin may cause an unexpected hypersensitivity reaction. Additionally, penicillin shares a β-lactam structure with cephalosporin, so that one antibiotic may be sensitive against another.

Genetic Predisposition. Certain individuals are genetically predisposed to develop allergies, particularly type I allergies, and are called **atopic.**[11] In families in which one parent has an allergy, allergies develop in about 40% of the offspring. If both parents have allergies, the incidence in the offspring may be as high as 80%. (Principles of genetic inheritance are discussed in Chapter 4.)

Atopic individuals tend to produce higher quantities of IgE and to have more Fc receptors for IgE on their mast cells. The airways and the skin of atopic individuals are also more responsive to a wide variety of both specific and nonspecific stimuli than are the airways and skin of individuals who are not atopic. Multiple genes have been associated with the atopic state, including polymorphisms in a large variety of cytokines that regulate IgE synthesis (e.g., interleukin [IL]-4, IL-5, IL-12, IL-13) and cellular receptors.

Clinical Symptoms of Type I Allergies

The clinical manifestations of type I reactions are attributable mostly to the biologic effects of histamine. Tissues most commonly affected contain large numbers of mast cells and are sensitive to the effects of histamine released from them. These tissues are found in the gastrointestinal tract, the skin, and the respiratory tract (Figure 9-5 and Table 9-4). The particular symptoms frequently reflect the main portal of entry for the allergen. For instance, pollens and other airborne allergens usually cause respiratory symptoms.

Effects of allergens on the mucosa of the eyes, nose, and respiratory tract include conjunctivitis (inflammation of the membranes lining the eyelids), rhinitis (inflammation of the mucous membranes of the nose), and asthma (constriction of the bronchi).[12] Symptoms are caused by vasodilation, hypersecretion of mucus, edema, and swelling of the respiratory mucosa. Because

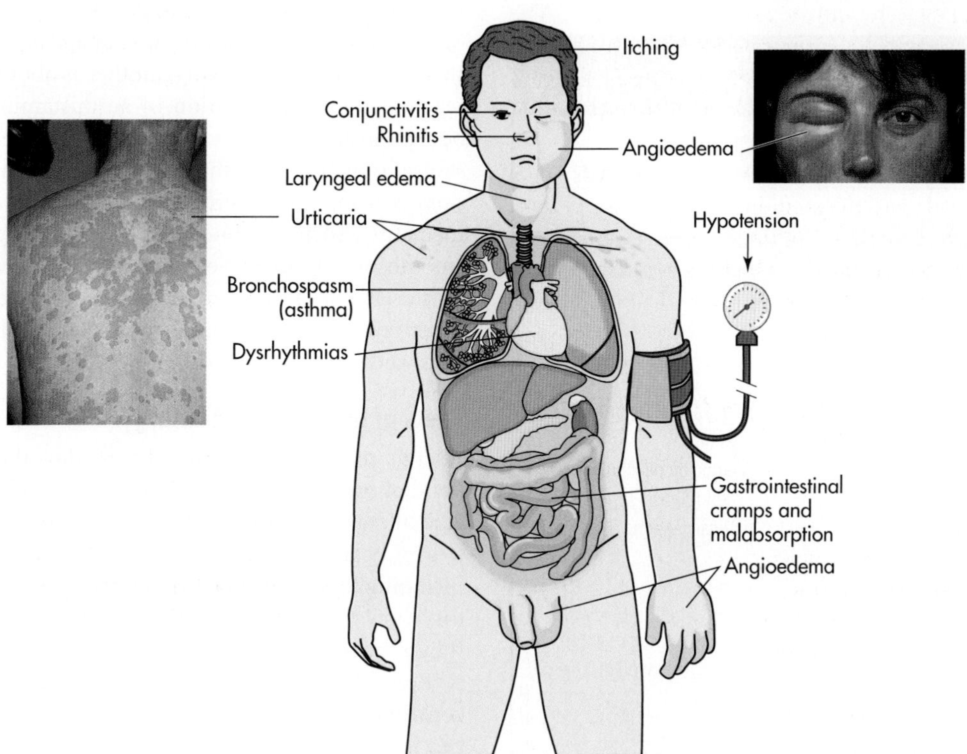

FIGURE 9-5 Type I Hypersensitivity Reactions. Manifestations of allergic reactions as a result of type I hypersensitivity include itching, angioedema (swelling caused by exudation), edema of the larynx, urticaria (hives), bronchospasm (constriction of airways in the lungs), hypotension (low blood pressure), and dysrhythmias (irregular heartbeat) because of anaphylactic shock, and gastrointestinal cramping caused by inflammation of the gastrointestinal mucosa. Photographic inserts show a diffuse allergic-like eye and skin reaction on an individual. The skin lesions have raised edges and develop within minutes or hours, with resolution occurring after about 12 hours. (Inserts from Male D et al: *Immunology,* ed 8, St Louis, 2013, Mosby.)

the mucous membranes lining the respiratory tract (accessory sinuses, nasopharynx, and upper and lower respiratory tracts) are continuous, they are all adversely affected. The degree to which each is affected determines the symptoms of the disease.

Gastrointestinal allergies are caused primarily by allergens that enter through the mouth—usually foods or medicines. Symptoms include vomiting, diarrhea, or abdominal pain and may be severe enough to result in malabsorption or protein-losing enteropathy, if the reactions are prolonged or recurrent. Foods most often implicated in gastrointestinal allergies are milk, chocolate, citrus fruits, eggs, wheat, nuts, peanut butter, and fish.[13] When food is the allergen, the active immunogen may be a product of food breakdown by digestive enzymes.

Urticaria, or **hives,** is a dermal (skin) manifestation of type I allergic reactions (see Figure 9-5). The underlying mechanism is the localized release of histamine and increased vascular permeability, resulting in limited areas of edema. Urticaria is characterized by white fluid-filled blisters (wheals) surrounded by areas of redness (flares). The **wheal and flare reaction** is usually accompanied by itching. Not all urticarial symptoms are caused by allergic (immunologic) reactions. Some, termed *nonimmunologic urticaria,* result from exposure to cold temperatures, emotional stress, medications, systemic diseases, hyperthyroidism, or malignancies (e.g., lymphomas).

If possible, avoidance of the allergen is the best method to limit allergic responses. Approximately 30% of laboratory animal handlers have allergies to animal dander and must use face masks or other devices to avoid contact.

Although some type I allergic responses can be controlled by blocking histamine receptors with antihistamines, the primary mechanism of control is the autonomic nervous system. The autonomic nervous system includes biochemical mediators (e.g., epinephrine, acetylcholine) that, like the mediators of the inflammatory response, have profound effects on cells. These mediators bind to appropriate receptors on mast cells and the target cells of inflammation (e.g., smooth muscle), thereby controlling (1) the release of inflammatory mediators from mast cells and (2) the degree to which target cells respond to inflammatory mediators (see Chapter 7).

TABLE 9-4 CAUSES OF CLINICAL MANIFESTATIONS OF ALLERGY

TYPICAL ALLERGEN	MECHANISM OF HYPERSENSITIVITY	CLINICAL MANIFESTATION
Ingestants		
Foods	Type I	Gastrointestinal allergy
Drugs	Types I, II, III	Urticaria, immediate drug reaction, hemolytic anemia, serum sickness
Inhalants		
Pollens, dust, molds	Type I	Allergic rhinitis, bronchial asthma
Aspergillus fumigatus	Types I, III	Allergic bronchopulmonary aspergillosis
Thermophilic actinomycetes*	Types III, IV	Extrinsic allergic alveolitis
Injectants		
Drugs	Types I, II, III	Immediate drug reaction, hemolytic anemia, serum sickness
Bee venom	Type I	Anaphylaxis
Vaccines	Type III	Localized Arthus reaction
Serum	Types I, III	Anaphylaxis, serum sickness
Contactants		
Poison ivy, metals	Type IV	Contact dermatitis

*An order of fungi that is stimulated by warmth to grow and proliferate.
Modified from Bellanti JA: *Immunology III,* Philadelphia, 1985, Saunders.

Allergic Disease: Bee Sting Allergy

An example of a life-threatening allergy is an anaphylactic reaction to a bee sting. Bee venoms contain a mixture of enzymes and other proteins that may serve as allergens. About 1% of children may have an anaphylactic reaction to bee venom. Within minutes they may develop excessive swelling (edema) at the bee sting site, followed by generalized hives, itching, and swelling in areas distal from the sting (e.g., eyes, lips), and other systemic symptoms including flushing, sweating, dizziness, and headache. The most severe symptoms may include gastrointestinal (e.g., stomach cramps, vomiting), respiratory (e.g., tightness in the throat, wheezing, difficulties breathing), and vascular (e.g., low blood pressure, shock) reactions. Severe respiratory and vascular reactions may lead to death.

If a child has had a previous anaphylactic reaction to bee stings, the chance of having another is about 60%. During the reaction the administration of antihistamines has little effect because histamine has already bound H1 receptors and initiated severe bronchial smooth muscle contraction. Most individuals carry self-injectable epinephrine. Autonomic nervous system mediators, such as epinephrine, bind to specific receptors on smooth muscle and reverse the effects of histamine and result in muscle relaxation. Similar anaphylactic reactions have been described against peanuts and other nuts, shellfish, fish, milk, eggs, and some medications.

Tests of IgE-Mediated Allergy

Allergic reactions can be life threatening; therefore, it is essential that severely allergic individuals be made aware of the specific allergen against which they are sensitized and instructed to avoid contact with that material.[14] Several tests are available, including food challenges, skin tests with allergens, and laboratory tests for measurements of total IgE and allergen-specific IgE in the blood.[15]

Reactivity to a particular food allergen may be tested by controlled administration of small doses of the suspected allergen in order to evoke a mild allergic response. This approach can be dangerous if the individual has a history of anaphylactic responses. A safer approach is injection of an allergen into (intradermal) or onto (epicutaneous or prick test) the skin. If the individual is allergic to a particular allergen, a local wheal and flare reaction may occur within a few minutes at the site of injection. The diameter of the flare reaction is usually indicative of the individual's degree of sensitivity to that allergen. In the most severely allergic individuals, even the extremely small amounts of allergen used for the skin test may evoke a systemic anaphylaxis. Skin test is also contraindicated if the individual is using medications that may affect the test or has diffuse dermatitis, which would make the reaction difficult to interpret.

A variety of laboratory tests can detect IgE antibodies in serum. These assays have various commercial acronyms, depending on whether they are radioimmunoassays (RIAs; reactivity detected by measuring a radioactive reagent) or enzyme immunoassays (EIAs or ELISA [enzyme-linked immunosorbent assay]; reactivity detected by measuring a color change caused by an enzyme-labeled reagent). One set of assays measures circulating levels of total IgE, with atopic individuals usually having elevated levels. Other assays are capable of measuring circulating levels of specific IgE antibodies against selected allergens. The amount of IgE against a specific allergen correlates well with the degree of skin test reactivity and the severity of clinical symptoms related to the same allergen, although the laboratory text is less sensitive.

Desensitization. Clinical **desensitization** to allergens can be achieved in some individuals. Minute quantities of the allergen are injected in increasing doses over a prolonged period. The procedure may reduce the severity of the allergic reaction in the treated individual. However, this form of therapy is associated with a risk of systemic anaphylaxis, which can be severe and life threatening. This approach works best for routine respiratory allergens[16] and biting insect allergies (80% to 90% rate of desensitization over 5 years of treatment). Food allergies have been very difficult to suppress, but some promising trials are underway to evaluate desensitization by oral or sublingual administration of increasing amounts of allergen.[17]

The mechanisms by which desensitization occurs may be several, one of which is the production of large amounts of so-called blocking antibodies, usually circulating IgG. A **blocking antibody** presumably competes in the tissues or in the circulation for binding with antigenic determinants on the allergen so that the allergen is "neutralized" and is unable to bind with IgE on mast cells. Sublingual desensitization (another approach that works best with some food allergies) produces sIgA and circulating IgG that may prevent the allergen from accessing mast cells. Desensitization injections also may stimulate the generation of clones of T-regulatory lymphocytes, which inhibit hypersensitivity by suppressing the production of IgE or modifying the Th1/Th2 interactions in favor of production of anti-inflammatory cytokines.

Other approaches to suppressing type I allergic responses have been tested, with some preliminary success. An example is injection of anti-IgE antibody directed against the Fc portion of the IgE in order to decrease binding of IgE to mast cells.

Type IV Allergic Hypersensitivities. The allergens that induce a type IV allergic reaction are mostly haptens that react with normal self-proteins in the skin. When presented in this fashion, these antigens are recognized by pattern recognition receptors (PRRs) on antigen-presenting cells in the skin and induce a cell-mediated response.[18] (Pattern recognition receptors are discussed in Chapter 7.) The primary result is an allergic **contact dermatitis** that is confined to the area of contact with the allergen. The best-known example is poison ivy (Figure 9-6). The antigen in that instance is a plant catechol, *urushiol,* that reacts with normal skin proteins and evokes a cell-mediated immune response.

As noted, type I hypersensitivity reactions may result in a skin reaction (e.g., hives formed during an allergic reaction to a particular food). The distribution of the lesions may suggest whether the reaction is caused by immediate (type I) or delayed (type IV) hypersensitivity mechanisms.[19] Immediate hypersensitivity reactions, termed **atopic dermatitis,** are usually characterized by widely distributed lesions, whereas contact dermatitis (delayed hypersensitivity) consists of lesions only at the site of contact with the allergen, such as a metal allergy to jewelry (see Figure 9-6).

Types II and III Allergic Hypersensitivities. Type II allergic hypersensitivities are usually against allergic haptens that bind to the surface of cells and elicit an IgG or IgM response. For instance, allergic reactions against many drugs (e.g., penicillin, sulfonamides) occur after the drug binds to proteins on the plasma membranes of a person's cells and becomes immunogenic.[20] The immune system attacks the allergen on the cell membrane and destroys the cell as well. In allergic reactions to penicillin, the immunogenic antigen is a metabolite of penicillin catabolism that binds to the plasma membranes of erythrocytes or platelets and induces an antibody response that destroys the cells (type II hypersensitivity), causing anemia or thrombocytopenia. Type II allergic reactions also can occur against antigens of infectious diseases. For instance, encephalitis secondary to a rubella infection may result from damage to cells of the nervous system by an immune response against rubella virus antigen on the cell's plasma membrane.

Type III allergic reactions occur after the formation of immune complexes containing soluble allergens. For instance, Arthus reactions may be observed after injection, ingestion, or inhalation of allergens. Skin reactions can follow subcutaneous or intradermal inoculation with drugs, fungal extracts, or antigens used in skin tests. Gastrointestinal reactions, such as gluten-sensitive enteropathy (celiac disease), follow ingestion of antigen, usually gluten from wheat products (see Chapter 41). Allergic alveolitis is a type III acute hemorrhagic inflammation of the air sacs (alveoli) of the lungs resulting from inhalation of fungal antigens, usually particles from moldy hay (farmer's lung) or pigeon feces (pigeon breeder's disease)[21] (see Chapter 35). Circulating drugs (e.g., penicillin) or antigens produced from infectious diseases (e.g., hepatitis B, streptococcal infection) may form circulating immune complexes that are deposited in the circulation (vasculitis) or the kidneys (glomerulonephritis).

Autoimmunity

Breakdown of Tolerance. Self-antigens are usually in a state of tolerance, or immunologic homeostasis, with the host's own immune system. *Central tolerance* develops in humans during the embryonic period as autoreactive lymphocytes are either eliminated or suppressed in the primary lymphoid organs during differentiation and proliferation of immature T or B lymphocytes (see Figures 8-10 and 8-12). Clones of cells with antigen receptors

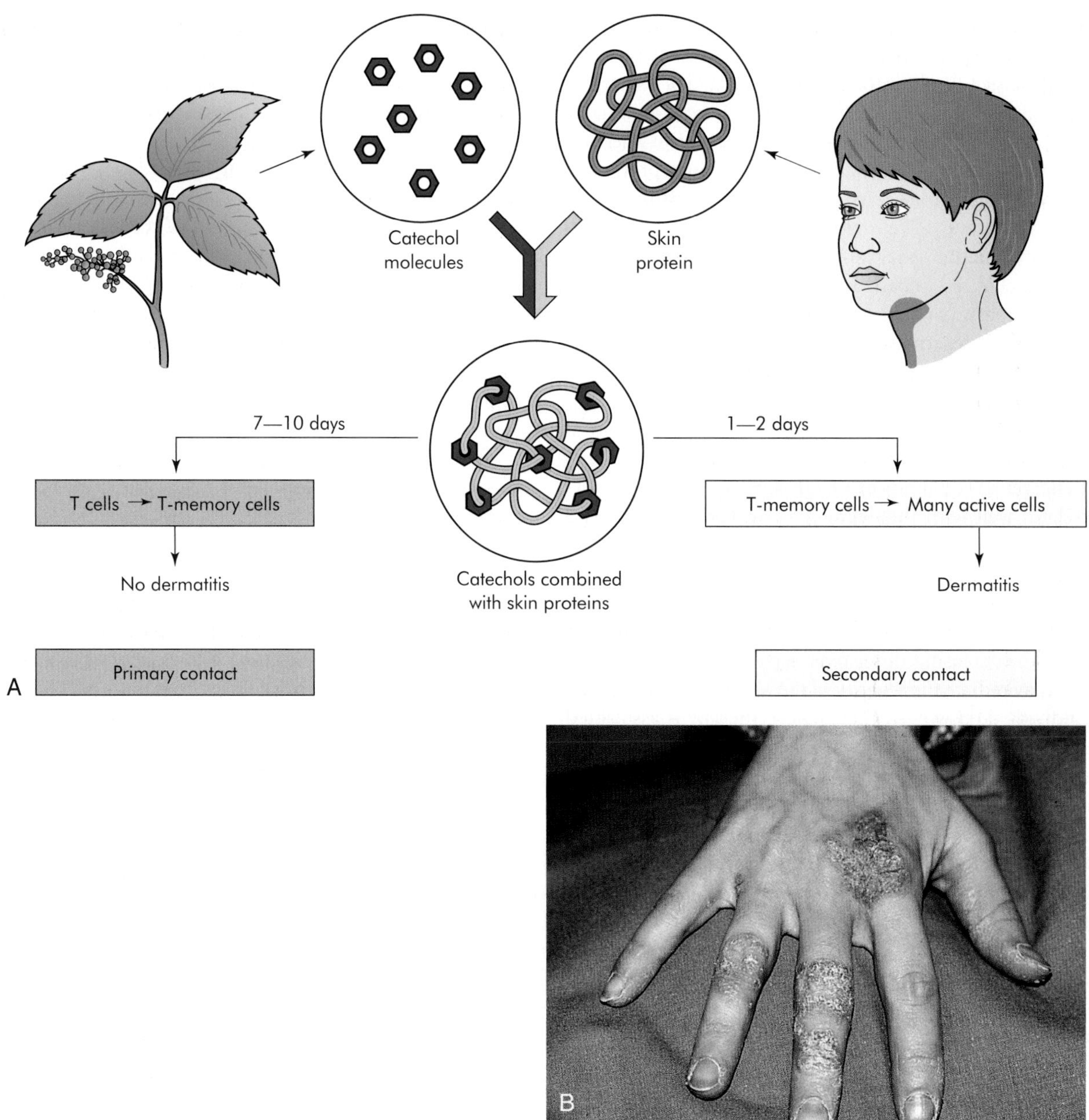

FIGURE 9-6 **Development of Allergic Contact Dermatitis, a Delayed Hypersensitivity Reaction. A,** Shown here is the development of allergy to catechols from poison ivy. No dermatitis results from the primary contact because the antigens (catechols) are sensitizing the immune response and producing memory T cells. Secondary contact, however, quickly activates a type IV, cell-mediated reaction that causes dermatitis. **B,** This contact dermatitis was caused by a delayed hypersensitivity reaction that led to vesicles and scaling at the sites of contact. (From Damjanov I, Linder J: *Anderson's pathology,* ed 10, St Louis, 1996, Mosby.)

for self-antigens are deleted. *Peripheral tolerance* is maintained in the secondary lymphoid organs through the action of T-regulatory lymphocytes or antigen-presenting dendritic cells. **Autoimmunity** is a breakdown of tolerance in which the body's immune system begins to recognize self-antigens as foreign. In most autoimmune conditions the mechanism of tolerance breakdown is unknown, although several potential mechanisms have been suggested.

Sequestered Antigen. The induction of central tolerance requires that the self-antigen be present in the fetus and exposed to the developing fetal immune system. Some self-antigens may not normally encounter the immune system in either fetal or adult life, but are sequestered or hidden from the immune system in **immunologically privileged sites,** so named because foreign tissues can be transplanted into these sites with less chance of immunologic rejection. For example, several sites (e.g., anterior chamber of the eye, the brain) are separated from the circulation by barriers (blood-ocular and blood-brain barriers) that offer protection against many immune cells and lead to relatively poor lymphatic drainage. Lymphocytes that enter these sites encounter tissue that expresses Fas ligand (FasL) and tumor necrosis factor (TNF)–related apoptosis-inducing ligand (TRAIL).

These molecules induce the lymphocytes to undergo apoptosis, thus protecting the tissue. Self-antigens in these sites are not normally seen by the immune system and are therefore not immunogenic. However, if the barriers are damaged, antigenic sensitization can occur, and the resultant antibodies and lymphocytes can enter the site and cause additional damage to the tissue. For instance, physical trauma to one eye may result in release of sequestered antigen into the blood or lymphatics, resulting in immunologic injury to the other eye (sympathetic uveitis).

Infectious Disease. A long-standing hypothesis is that foreign antigens from infectious microorganisms can initiate autoimmune disease through a process of **molecular mimicry.** Some antigens of infectious agents so closely resemble (mimic) a particular self-antigen that antibodies or T cells produced to protect against the infection also recognize the self-antigen as foreign (**cross-reactive antibody** or **T cell**). The relationship between many autoimmune diseases and predisposing infections, such as enterovirus infection and type 1 diabetes, is being investigated.[22] However, the only clearly defined example so far is acute rheumatic fever that may occur after a group A streptococcal sore throat (see following).

Neoantigen. In certain situations a neoantigen that induces an allergic reaction may also lead to autoimmunity. Many **neoantigens** (new antigens) are haptens that become immunogenic after binding to self-proteins. The immune reaction against the neoantigen may lead to an immunologic reaction against normal antigenic determinants on the protein. Other new antigenic determinants may result from posttranslational modifications of a normal protein so that one or more amino acids are chemically altered (e.g., addition or removal of amino acid side groups, phosphorylation) without affecting the protein's function.[23] Many experimental autoimmune diseases (e.g., experimental autoimmune thyroiditis) can be initiated by immunization with molecules containing neoantigenic determinants.

Forbidden Clone. During differentiation and proliferation of lymphoid stem cells into immature T and B lymphocytes (see Figures 8-10 and 8-12), some lymphocytes produce receptors that react with self-antigens. Many autoreactive lymphocytes interact with self-antigens and other co-stimulatory molecules on the surface of thymic epithelial cells and are induced to undergo clonal deletion by a process of apoptosis. Thus lymphocytes reactive against self-antigen are prevented, or "forbidden," from maturing. Autoimmunity may result from the survival of a forbidden clone and its proliferation later in life.

Defective Peripheral Tolerance. Tolerance to some self-antigens is controlled in the secondary lymphoid organs. This process is controlled by a variety of cells, including antigen-presenting dendritic cells and members of a family of T-regulatory lymphocytes (Treg cells) that normally suppress immune responses against self. Defects in particular regulatory cells may result in expansion of clones of autoreactive cells and the development of autoimmune disease. Systemic lupus erythematosus, which is characterized by the production of a large array of autoantibodies, may be caused by a general breakdown in the regulatory network.

Original Insult. Although many theories exist, the initial cause of most autoimmune diseases is unknown (see What's New? Maternal Microchimerism and Autoimmune Disease).

WHAT'S NEW?

Maternal/Fetal Microchimerism and Autoimmune Disease

A rapidly growing body of evidence suggests that we are in a state of **microchimerism (Mc);** possessing a small number of cells originating from another individual.[1] The placenta, which was once considered a cellular "barrier," is more porous than suspected and routinely allows bidirectional passage of both maternal and fetal cells. Passage results during normal pregnancy, as well as spontaneous miscarriages and elective terminations,[2] and includes a broad spectrum of cells, ranging from erythrocytes and mature white blood cells, to stem cells at various stages of differentiation. Most gravid women (having been pregnant) have detectable fetal cells (fetal Mc) in their blood and many organs (e.g., white blood cells, hepatocytes, kidney tubular epithelium, neurons and glia, cardiomyocytes, endothelial cells, thyrocytes, intestinal epithelium, and islet β cells), which apparently originated as fetal stem cells that differentiated in the maternal tissues. As early as 6 weeks gestation, maternal Mc is apparent in fetal blood and tissues (e.g., thymus, lung, heart, pancreas, liver, spleen, kidney, adrenal gland, ovary, testis, and brain).[3] Maternal Mc originates predominately from maternal cells, but may also include cells from one's grandmother, a non-identical twin, or older siblings, all of which were harbored in the mother's blood and tissues. Both maternal and fetal Mc persists for decades after pregnancy.

The long-term implications of Mc may include both detrimental and beneficial effects. Fetal cells express both maternal and paternal **HLA** antigens and are recognized as partially foreign by maternal immune cells. Most studies of maternal Mc use assays for the presence of the Y chromosome in maternal blood or organs. Many autoimmune diseases are associated with increased numbers of male cells in the diseased organs (e.g., scleroderma, dermatomyositis, Sjögren syndrome, thyroiditis, primary biliary cirrhosis, hyper- and hypothyroidism, and systemic lupus erythematosus) suggesting that Mc may contribute to the etiology of these diseases.[1] Maternal Mc in the offspring also may affect their risk for autoimmune disease. Increased levels of maternal cells in the child's blood have been reported in cases of juvenile inflammatory myopathy, neonatal lupus syndrome, type 1 diabetes, and biliary atresia. Maternal cells were found as myocytes in the myocardium of infants with fatal neonatal lupus-associated heart block and as insulin-producing cells in the pancreas of diabetics.[1] It cannot yet be determined whether the foreign cells are initiators of autoimmune damage or whether injury to the tissue results in increased proliferation. Thus these observations remain intriguing but of unknown significance.

Beneficial effects of Mc are also observed. Treg cells may control immunologic tolerance to maternal cells. A significantly greater success rate of liver transplantation was observed with maternal or sibling donors than paternal donors.[4] Thus Mc may modulate the immune response and minimize rejection of organs from selected donors. Fetal Mc occurs in several regions of the brain, but at a significantly lower incidence and concentration in women with Alzheimer's disease than those without neurologic disease.[5] Whether Mc is protective or not remains unknown.

References

1. Nelson JL: *Trends Immunol* 33(8):421–427, 2012.
2. Peterson SE et al: *Human Reprod* 27(9):2607–2612, 2012.
3. Boyon C et al: *Eur J Obset Gynecol Reprod Biol* 158(2):148–152, 2011.
4. Nijagal A, Fleck S, Mackenzie TC: *Chimerism* 3(2):37–39, 2012.
5. Chan WFN et al: *Plos ONE* 7(9):e45592. doi:10.1371/journal.pone.0045592, 2012.

It is suspected that some autoimmune diseases are initiated by infections that have resolved without leaving evidence that would lead to identification of the particular infectious agent. The evidence for an infectious causation is clear for only one autoimmune disease: acute rheumatic fever. In a small number of individuals with group A streptococcal sore throats, the M proteins in the bacterial capsule induce antibodies that also react with proteins in the heart valve, damaging the valve.

Additionally, some streptococcal skin or throat infections result in the release of bacterial antigens into the blood and the formation of circulating immune complexes. The complexes may deposit in the kidneys and initiate an immune complex glomerulonephritis (inflammation of the kidney). Thus capsular antigens of the group A *Streptococcus* may mimic *(antigenic mimicry)* normal heart antigens resulting in a type II autoimmune hypersensitivity (rheumatic fever), whereas in another person this infection may release bacterial antigen (an environmental antigen) into the blood, resulting in a type III allergic hypersensitivity (poststreptococcal glomerulonephritis).

Genetic Factors. Genetic factors that contribute to autoimmunity are easier to identify than the original insult that initiates the disease. It is fairly well established that autoimmune diseases can be familial. Affected family members may not all develop the same disease, but several members may have different disorders characterized by a variety of hypersensitivity reactions, including autoimmune and allergic.

Associations with particular autoimmune diseases have been identified for a variety of major histocompatibility complex (MHC) alleles (see Chapter 8) or non-MHC genes. The specific HLA alleles of susceptible and resistant individuals have been analyzed for almost every known disease, and almost universally individuals with certain diseases are more likely than the general population to have a specific HLA allele or set of alleles. Some associations are strong; others are more tenuous (Table 9-5). The reason some HLA alleles are associated with inappropriate immune function is unclear, but it may directly involve the ability of particular HLA molecules to present antigen or the use of particular HLAs as receptors for disease-causing microorganisms. These genes may determine an individual's susceptibility to specific infectious agents or the capacity of that individual to mount an immune response against specific antigens. Therefore, an individual of a specific HLA type may have inappropriate or exaggerated immune responses against a microorganism, resulting in a hypersensitivity reaction.

A large variety of non-MHC genes also have been identified as risk factors for the development of specific autoimmune diseases. Most of these genes encode for inflammatory cytokines or co-stimulatory molecules found on the cell surface.

Alloimmunity

Alloimmunity occurs when an individual's immune system reacts against antigens on the tissues of other members of the same species. The two clinically relevant examples of this reactivity are (1) several transient neonatal diseases (in which the maternal immune system becomes sensitized against antigens expressed by the fetus) and (2) transplant rejection and transfusion reactions (in which the immune system of a recipient of an organ transplant or blood transfusion reacts against antigens on the donor cells).

Transient Neonatal Alloimmunity. Because the fetus is a hybrid between the mother and father, it expresses paternal antigens that are not found in the mother. Occasionally these fetal antigens cross the placenta and elicit an immune response in the mother (e.g., production of alloantibodies against the fetal antigens). The maternal alloantibody may be transported across the placenta into the fetal circulation, bind to the fetal cells, and produce alloimmune disease in the fetus and neonate. The mother's immune system produces the antibody, but because her cells do not express the target antigen, she has no symptoms of the disease.

Neonatal alloimmune disease may be secondary to maternal autoimmune diseases in which the mother produces an IgG autoantibody specific for maternal self-antigens that are found on fetal cells as well. Therefore, symptoms of the same autoimmune disease may affect mother and child, even though the autoantibody is being produced only by the mother's immune system. This form of disease usually occurs only in association with type II (tissue-specific) hypersensitivity reactions. It does not occur in association with IgE-mediated (type I) reactions, immune complex–mediated (type III) reactions, or cell-mediated (type IV) reactions because the immunologic factors (IgE, immune complexes, T cells) that cause these reactions do not readily cross the placenta and enter the fetal circulation in sufficient quantity.

TABLE 9-5 EXAMPLES OF ASSOCIATIONS BETWEEN SPECIFIC HLA ALLELES AND DISEASE

DISEASE	HLA ALLELE	RR
Acute anterior uveitis	B27	14
Addison disease	DR3	6
Ankylosing spondylitis	B27	90
Behçet syndrome	B51	4
Celiac disease	DR3	11
Chronic active hepatitis	DR3	13
Dermatitis herpetiformis	DR3	16
Diabetes (type 1)	DR3	5
	DR4	6
	DR3/DR4	20
Goodpasture syndrome	DR2	16
Graves disease	DR3	4
Hashimoto disease	DR11	3
Multiple sclerosis	DR2	4
Myasthenia gravis	DR3	3
Pemphigus vulgaris	DR4	13
Postgonococcal arthritis	B27	14
Reiter syndrome	B27	37
Rheumatoid arthritis	DR4	4
Sjögren syndrome	DR3	9
Systemic lupus erythematosus	DR3	6

HLA, Human leukocyte antigen; *RR,* the approximate relative risk, which is the frequency of a disease in individuals with the particular HLA allele compared with individuals without that allele.

Symptoms of the alloimmune disease may be present in utero or immediately after birth and may be fatal to the fetus or neonate. At birth, maternal circulating antibody can no longer enter the child, and if symptoms are successfully treated, the disease will disappear as the maternal antibody is catabolized. Examples of maternal immunologic hypersensitivity diseases in which the child can be affected include the following antibody-mediated diseases:

1. Graves disease—an autoimmune disease in which maternal antibody against the receptor for TSH causes neonatal hyperthyroidism
2. Myasthenia gravis—an autoimmune disease in which maternal antibody binds with receptors for neural transmitters on muscle cells (acetylcholine receptors), causing neonatal muscular weakness (see Chapter 18)
3. Immune thrombocytopenic purpura—both autoimmune and alloimmune variants in which maternal antiplatelet antibody destroys platelets in the fetus and neonate (see Chapter 29)
4. Alloimmune neutropenia—in which maternal antibody against neutrophils destroys neutrophils in the neonate
5. Systemic lupus erythematosus—autoimmune disease in which diverse maternal autoantibodies induce anomalies (e.g., congenital heart defects) in the fetus or cause pregnancy loss
6. Rh and ABO alloimmunization (e.g., erythroblastosis fetalis)—in which maternal antibody against erythrocyte antigens induces anemia in the child (see Chapter 30)

Autoimmune and Alloimmune Diseases

Many examples of autoimmune or **alloimmune diseases** have been described. Several basic principles are exemplified by two examples: systemic lupus erythematosus (an autoimmune disease) and tissue rejection (i.e., transplant rejection or transfusion reaction) (an alloimmune phenomenon). Most of the classic autoimmune diseases, including disorders of the endocrine system (autoimmune thyroiditis and Graves disease), hematologic system (the hemolytic and pernicious anemias), nervous system (myasthenia gravis), and connective tissue in joints (rheumatoid arthritis), are discussed in Unit II of this book.

Systemic Lupus Erythematosus

Systemic lupus erythematosus (SLE) is a chronic, multisystem, inflammatory disease and is one of the most common, complex, and serious of the autoimmune disorders.[24] SLE is characterized by the production of a large variety of autoantibodies against nucleic acids, erythrocytes, coagulation proteins, phospholipids, lymphocytes, platelets, and many other self-components. The most characteristic autoantibodies produced in SLE are against nucleic acids (e.g., single-stranded deoxyribonucleic acid [DNA], double-stranded DNA), histones, ribonucleoproteins, and other nuclear materials.

Deposition of circulating immune complexes containing antibody against DNA produces tissue damage in individuals with SLE. DNA and DNA-containing immune complexes have a high affinity for glomerular basement membranes and therefore may be selectively deposited in the glomerulus (Figure 9-7). (Kidney structures are described in Chapter 37.) The presence of DNA in the circulation increases from cellular damage in response to trauma, drugs, or infections and is usually removed in the liver. Removal of circulating DNA is slowed in the presence of immune complexes, thereby increasing the potential for deposition in the kidney. (The liver's role in removing waste products from the blood is discussed in Chapter 40.) Deposition of immune complexes composed of DNA and antibody also causes inflammatory lesions in the renal tubular basement membranes, brain (choroid plexus), heart, spleen, lung, gastrointestinal tract, skin (see Figure 9-7), and peritoneum.

SLE, as with most autoimmune diseases, occurs more often in women (approximately a 10:1 predominance of females), especially in the 20- to 40-year-old age group. Blacks are affected more often than whites (about an eightfold increased risk). A genetic predisposition for the disease has been implicated on the basis of increased incidence in twins and the existence of autoimmune disease in the families of individuals with SLE.

A transient lupus-like syndrome that is indistinguishable both clinically and in the laboratory from spontaneously occurring SLE can develop from the prolonged use of medications, particularly hydralazine (an antihypertensive agent) and

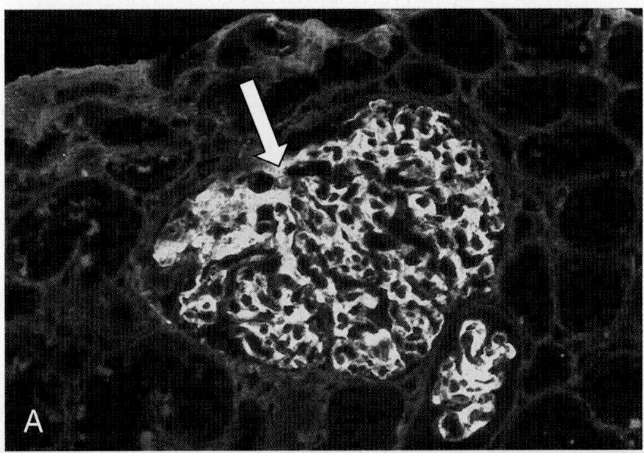

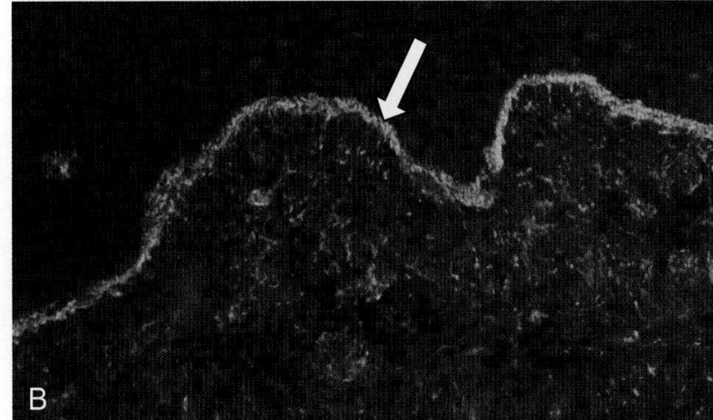

FIGURE 9-7 Deposition of IgG in the Kidney and Skin of Individuals with Lupus. These photographs of tissue were obtained from individuals with lupus and stained with fluorescent anti-IgG. **A,** Section from a kidney showing a glomerulus with deposits of IgG (*arrow,* indicating bright areas of staining). **B,** Section of the skin showing deposition of IgG along the dermal-epidermal junction (*arrow,* indicating bright green staining). (**A** courtesy Dr. Helmut Rennke, Department of Pathology, Brigham and Women's Hospital, Boston; **B** courtesy Dr. Richard Sontheimer, Department of Dermatology, University of Texas Southwestern Medical School, Dallas.)

procainamide (an antidysrhythmic drug). In genetically susceptible individuals, certain environmental agents, such as ultraviolet light, and several infectious agents may trigger lupus-like immune reactions.

Clinical manifestations of SLE include arthralgias or arthritis (90% of individuals), vasculitis and rash (70% to 80% of individuals), renal disease (40% to 50% of individuals), hematologic abnormalities (50% of individuals, with anemia being the most common complication), and cardiovascular diseases (30% to 50% of individuals). As with most autoimmune diseases, the disease process develops slowly (up to 10 years from occurrence of the first autoantibody until diagnosis)[25] and is characterized by frequent remissions and exacerbations. Because the signs and symptoms affect almost every body system and tend to be intermittent, SLE is extremely difficult to diagnose. This has led to the development of a list of 11 common clinical findings. The serial or simultaneous presence of at least four of them indicates that the individual has SLE[26]:

1. Facial rash confined to the cheeks (malar rash)
2. Discoid rash (raised patches, scaling)
3. Photosensitivity (skin rash developed as a result of exposure to sunlight)
4. Oral or nasopharyngeal ulcers
5. Nonerosive arthritis of at least two peripheral joints
6. Serositis (pleurisy, pericarditis)
7. Renal disorder (proteinuria of 0.5 g/day or cellular casts)
8. Neurologic disorders (seizures or psychosis)
9. Hematologic disorders (hemolytic anemia, leukopenia, lymphopenia, or thrombocytopenia)
10. Immunologic disorders (positive lupus erythematosus [LE] cell preparation, anti–double-stranded DNA, anti-Smith [Sm] antigen, false-positive serologic test for syphilis, or antiphospholipid antibodies [anticardiolipin antibody or lupus anticoagulant])
11. Presence of antinuclear antibody (ANA)

There is no cure for SLE or most other autoimmune diseases. The goals of treatment are to control symptoms and prevent further damage by suppressing the autoimmune response. Nonsteroidal anti-inflammatory drugs, such as aspirin, ibuprofen, or naproxen, reduce inflammation and relieve pain. Corticosteroids are often prescribed for more serious active disease. Immunosuppressive drugs (e.g., methotrexate, azathioprine, or cyclophosphamide) are used to treat severe symptoms involving internal organs. Ultraviolet light can worsen symptoms (known as flares), and protection from sun exposure is helpful. Prolonged use of certain drugs can cause transient SLE-like symptoms, and the medication history is important for diagnostic evaluation.

Other therapeutic approaches have been attempted for SLE and other autoimmune diseases. Several decades ago preparations of intravenous immune globulin (IVIg), which was routinely used to replenish antibodies in persons with antibody deficiencies, were administered to children with autoimmune thrombocytopenia (an autoimmune disease in which platelets were destroyed by an autoantibody).[27] IVIg therapy resulted in a rebound of platelet levels and temporary resolution of the thrombocytopenia. IVIg is currently being used for a variety of autoimmune diseases, including SLE. More recently, monoclonal antibodies and other reagents have specifically targeted and suppressed B and T cells that are participating in autoimmune responses.[28] This approach has been somewhat successful in SLE, rheumatoid arthritis, and other autoimmune diseases. Improved outcomes may be available in the future with the continued advances in medical research and the use of stem cell treatments.

Transfusion Reactions

Red blood cells (erythrocytes) express several important surface antigens, known collectively as the **blood group antigens,** which can be targets of alloimmune reactions. More than 80 different red cell antigens are grouped into several dozen blood group systems, each determined by a different locus or set of loci. The most important of these, because they provoke the strongest humoral alloimmune response, are the ABO and Rh systems.

ABO System. Human blood transfusions were carried out as early as 1818, but they were often unsuccessful. Sometimes after a transfusion, the recipient's red blood cells would clump together, thereby blocking the capillaries and causing death in some instances. In 1901, Karl Landsteiner reported that this reaction was related to the ABO antigens located on the surface of erythrocytes.

The **ABO blood group** consists of two major carbohydrate antigens, labeled A and B (Figure 9-8). These two carbohydrate antigens are codominant, which means that both A and B can be simultaneously expressed, resulting in an individual having any one of four different blood types. The erythrocytes of persons with blood type A have the type A carbohydrate antigen (i.e., carry the A antigen), those with blood type B carry the B antigen, those with blood type AB carry both A and B antigens, and those of blood type O carry neither the A nor the B antigen. A person with type A blood also has circulating antibodies to the B carbohydrate antigen. If this person receives blood containing B antigens (i.e., blood from a type AB or B individual), a severe transfusion reaction occurs and the transfused erythrocytes are destroyed by agglutination (Figure 9-9) or complement-mediated lysis. Similarly, a type B individual (whose blood contains anti-A antibodies) cannot receive blood from a type A or AB donor. Type O individuals, who have neither A nor B antigen but have both anti-A and anti-B antibodies, cannot accept blood from any of the other three types. These naturally occurring antibodies, called **isohemagglutinins,** are immunoglobulins of the IgM class and are induced by similar antigens expressed on naturally occurring bacteria in the intestinal tract.

Because individuals with type O blood lack both types of antigens, they are considered **universal donors,** meaning that anyone can accept their red blood cells. Similarly, type AB individuals are considered **universal recipients** because they lack both anti-A and anti-B antibodies and can be transfused with any ABO blood type. When large volumes of *whole blood* (i.e., cells plus plasma) are transfused, however, antibodies in the *donor's* blood can bind to antigenic determinants on the *recipient's* erythrocytes, causing agglutination of the recipient's own cells. Agglutination and lysis cause harmful transfusion

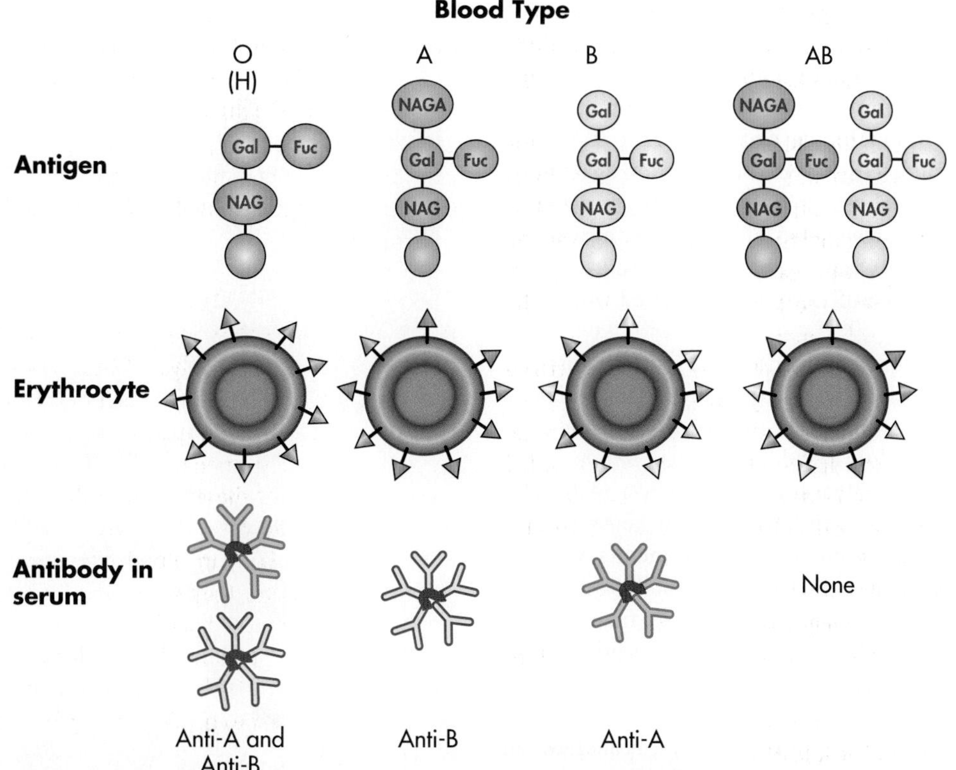

FIGURE 9-8 **ABO Blood Types.** This figure shows the antigens and antibodies associated with the ABO blood groups. The surfaces of erythrocytes of individuals with blood group O have the core H antigenic carbohydrate. Their sera contain IgM antibodies against both A and B carbohydrates. In individuals of the blood group A, some of the H antigens have been modified into A antigens by the addition of *N*-acetylgalactosamine (NAGA). The sera of these individuals have IgM antibodies against the B antigen. In individuals with blood group B, some of the H antigens have been modified into B antigens by the addition of galactose (Gal). These individuals have IgM antibodies against the A antigen in their sera. In individuals of the blood group AB, some of the H antigens have been modified into both the A and B antigens. These individuals do not have antibody to either A or B antigens. *Fuc,* Fucose; *NAGA, N*-acetylgalactosamine.

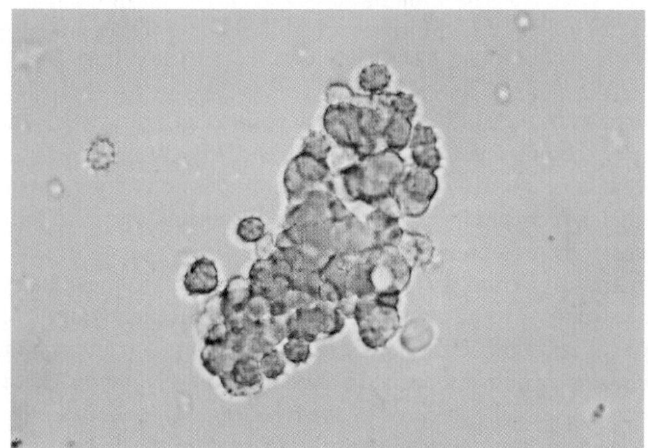

FIGURE 9-9 **Mismatched Transfused Blood Cells.** Agglutination of erythrocytes caused by anti-A blood-typing serum. (Copyright Ed Reschke.)

reactions that can be prevented only by complete and careful ABO matching between donor and recipient.

Rh System. The **Rh blood group** is the most polymorphic system of red cell antigens, consisting of at least 50 separate antigens. At least five major antigens and a large number of rare variants have been identified and are expressed primarily on erythrocytes. The major antigens are contained on two proteins encoded from two closely linked genes, *RHD* and *RHCE.* The RhD protein expresses the dominant antigen, which determines whether an individual is Rh-positive or Rh-negative. Individuals who express the D antigen on the RhD protein are Rh-positive, whereas individuals who do not express the D antigen are Rh-negative. The letter *d* is used to indicate lack of D. Rh-positive individuals can have either a *DD* or a *Dd* genotype, whereas Rh-negative individuals have the *dd* genotype. About 15% of North American whites are Rh-negative, whereas the Rh-negative genotype is much less common among members of other ethnic groups. Rh-negative individuals can make anti-D if exposed to Rh-positive erythrocytes, but because the letter *d* is used to indicate the lack of the D antigen and does not represent a different antigen, Rh-positive individuals do not produce an antibody against *d.* The second protein, RhCE, expresses two different antigens, C and E, each of which has two different alleles (*C* or *c, E* or *e*). Therefore, four potential haplotypes of C and E antigens are commonly observed: *CE, Ce, cE,* and *ce.*

IgG anti-D alloantibody produced by Rh-negative mothers against erythrocytes of their Rh-positive fetuses was the primary cause of Rh maternal-fetal incompatibility and the resulting hemolytic disease of the newborn (see Chapter 30). However, over the past several decades, the incidence of mothers with high titers of anti-D antibody has decreased dramatically because of the use of prophylactic anti-D immunoglobulin. By mechanisms that are still not completely understood, administration of anti-D antibody within a few days of exposure to RhD-positive erythrocytes completely prevents sensitization against the D antigen. Because hemolytic disease of the newborn related to the D antigen has been controlled, alloantibodies against the other Rh antigens (usually C, c, or E) have become more important. In general, these alloantibodies are associated with a less severe hemolytic disease.

A form of autoimmune hemolytic anemia is often caused by autoantibodies against Rh antigens, especially e. This variant is caused by IgG antibodies that react with erythrocytes at normal body temperature (thus called *warm autoimmune hemolytic anemia*) and increase phagocytic destruction of the red blood cell. This characteristic differentiates the warm variant from another form of autoimmune hemolytic anemia, which is caused by IgM autoantibodies that react optimally with erythrocytes in the cooler portions of the body (e.g., fingers, toes) and is referred to as *cold autoimmune hemolytic anemia*.

Graft Rejection

Transplantation of organs commonly is complicated by an immune response against antigens—primarily HLA—on the donated tissue. Most of our knowledge on the transplantation of organs is based on renal transplant studies. The primary mechanism of the rejection of transplanted organs is a type IV cell-mediated reaction. Two randomly chosen individuals are almost certainly antigenically different to some degree. Organ transplants between them could be rejected in approximately 2 weeks without the extensive use of immunosuppressive drugs.

After the donor and recipient are matched for ABO antigens, antigens of the HLA system are the principal targets of the rejection reaction; HLA matching of donor and recipient enhances the probability of acceptance of the graft. Not all HLA loci are equally important; matching at the HLA-DR locus appears to be the most critical for graft acceptance, and matching at HLA-A and HLA-B of slightly lesser importance. (These loci are discussed in Chapter 8.)

Transplant rejection may be classified as hyperacute, acute, or chronic, depending on the amount of time that elapses between transplantation and rejection. **Hyperacute rejection** is immediate and rare. When the circulation is reestablished to the grafted area, the graft may immediately turn white (the so-called *white graft*) instead of a normal pink. Hyperacute rejection usually occurs in recipients with preexisting antibody to antigens in the graft. The antibodies may have resulted from rejection of a previous graft or from prior blood transfusions that contained platelets and white blood cells with foreign HLA. Additionally, about half of women who have had multiple pregnancies have circulating antibodies against their husband's HLA antigens. As the circulation to the graft is established, antibodies bind to the vascular endothelial cells in the grafted tissue and activate the inflammatory response, including the coagulation cascade, which results in stasis of blood flow into the tissue (Figure 9-10). (Coagulation is described in Chapters 7 and 27.)

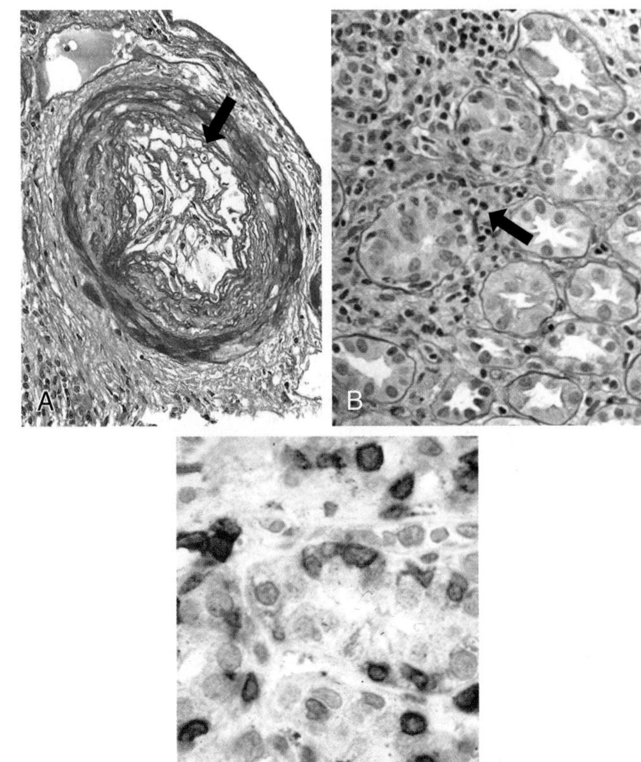

FIGURE 9-10 Examples of Hyperacute and Acute Rejection of Renal Allografts. A, Hyperacute antibody-mediated damage to the blood vessel of a renal allograft. The blood vessel is thickened, and the lumen *(arrow)* is obstructed by proliferating fibroblasts and macrophages. **B,** Acute cellular rejection of a renal allograft with intense mononuclear cell infiltrate *(arrow)*. **C,** Acute cellular rejection stained with immunoperoxidase reagent *(brown)* against T cells, which are infiltrating the tissue. (**A** courtesy Dr. Ihsan Housini, Department of Pathology, University of Texas Southwestern Medical School, Dallas; **B** and **C** courtesy Dr. Robert Colvin, Department of Pathology, Massachusetts General Hospital, Boston.)

Biopsies of the graft often show deposits of antibody (IgG and IgM), complement, and neutrophils. This condition is rare because of effective pretransplantation cross-matching during which a recipient is tested for antibodies against the HLA antigens of the potential donor.

Acute rejection is primarily a cell-mediated immune response that occurs within days to months after transplantation. This type of rejection occurs when the recipient develops an immune response against unmatched HLAs after transplantation. Sensitization is usually initiated by the recipient's lymphocytes interacting with the donor's dendritic cells within the transplanted tissue, resulting in induction of recipient Th1 and Tc cells against the donor's antigens. The Th1 cells release cytokines that activate infiltrating macrophages, and the Tc cells directly attack the endothelial cells in the transplanted tissue. A biopsy of the rejected organ usually shows an infiltration of lymphocytes and macrophages characteristic of a type IV reaction. Immunosuppressive drugs may delay or lessen the intensity of acute rejection.

Another form of acute rejection, *acute antibody-mediated rejection*, has recently been recognized and accounts for about

10% of acute rejections. This form of rejection is mediated by antibody and complement.[29] The predominant antibodies are against HLA antigens or, on occasion, autoantigens in the graft (e.g., vimentin, angiotensin receptor), but, unlike those antibodies that cause hyperacute rejection, are not present at the time of transplantation. Sensitization takes 2 weeks or longer and results in the accumulation of antibody, complement, neutrophils, and thrombi in the vasculature of the graft (a type II hypersensitivity reaction).

Chronic rejection may occur after a period of months or years of normal function. It is characterized by slow, progressive organ failure. Chronic rejection may be caused by inflammatory damage to endothelial cells lining blood vessels as a result of a weak cell-mediated immunologic reaction against minor histocompatibility antigens on the grafted tissue.[30] Antibodies against HLA and other antigens also may cause chronic rejection through activation of complement or antibody-dependent cellular cytotoxicity (ADCC) with NK cells.[31]

DEFICIENCIES IN IMMUNITY

Disorders resulting from immune deficiency are the clinical sequelae (results) of impaired function of one or more components of the immune or inflammatory response, including B cells, T cells, phagocytes, and complement (Table 9-6). An **immune deficiency** is the failure of these mechanisms of self-defense to function at their normal capacity, resulting in increased susceptibility to infections. **Primary (congenital) immune deficiency** is caused by a genetic anomaly, whereas **secondary (acquired) immune deficiency** is caused by another illness, such as cancer or viral infection, or by normal physiologic changes, such as aging. Acquired forms of immune deficiency are far more common than the congenital forms.

Initial Clinical Presentation

The clinical hallmark of immune deficiency is a tendency to develop unusual or recurrent, severe infections. Preschool and school-age children normally may have 6 to 12 infections per year, of which 3 or 4 are ear infections, and adults may have 2 to 4 infections per year. Most of these are not severe and are limited to viral infections of the upper respiratory tract, recurrent streptococcal pharyngitis, or mild otitis media.

Potential immune deficiencies are considered if the individual has had severe, documented bouts of pneumonia, otitis media, sinusitis, bronchitis, septicemia, or meningitis or infections with opportunistic microorganisms that normally are not pathogenic or usually confined to one site (e.g., *Pneumocystis jirovecii,* disseminated *Candida* infection, cytomegalovirus [CMV]).[32] Infections are generally recurrent with only short intervals of relative health, and multiple simultaneous infections are common. Individuals with primary immune deficiencies often have eight or more ear infections, two or more serious sinus infections, and two or more pneumonias, recurrent abscesses or infections in unusual sites, or persistent fungal infections (particularly thrush in an individual at least 1 year old) within a year. Recurrent internal infections, such as meningitis, osteomyelitis, or sepsis, are common. Prolonged antibiotic use is commonly ineffective by oral or injected routes and may necessitate intravenous administration. Additional symptoms may include failure to thrive and chronic diarrhea. A familial history of immune deficiency may be found in some types of primary deficiency.

The type of recurrent infections that manifest may indicate the type of immune defect. Deficiencies in T-cell immune responses are suggested when recurrent infections are caused by certain viruses (e.g., varicella, vaccinia, herpes, cytomegalovirus), fungi and yeasts (e.g., *Candida, Histoplasma*), or certain atypical microorganisms (e.g., *P. jirovecii*). B-cell deficiencies and phagocyte deficiencies, however, are suggested if the individual has documented, recurrent infections with microorganisms that require opsonization (e.g., encapsulated bacteria) or viruses against which humoral immunity is normally effective (e.g., rubella). Some complement deficiencies resemble defects in antibody or phagocyte function, but others are commonly associated with disseminated infections with bacteria of the genus *Neisseria (Neisseria meningitidis* and *Neisseria gonorrhoeae).*

Much of our current understanding of the development of the immune system and the interactions of the cells in the immune response was developed by studying congenital and acquired immune deficiencies or, as they have been called, "experiments of nature." Many immune deficiencies result from selective alteration or removal of one component of the immune system. We can understand the importance of that component by observing the effect of its removal on the remainder of the immune response.

Primary Immune Deficiencies

Most primary immune deficiencies are the result of a single gene defect[33] (Figure 9-11). Generally, the mutations are sporadic and not inherited: a family history exists in only about 25% of individuals. The sporadic mutations occur before birth, but the onset of symptoms may be early or later, depending on the particular syndrome. In approximately 60% of the cases symptoms of immune deficiency appear within the first 2 years of life, whereas other immune deficiencies are progressive, with the onset of symptoms appearing in the second or third decade of life. The most common symptoms include sinusitis (68% of individuals), pneumonia (51%), ear infections (51%), diarrhea (30%), and bronchitis (55%), with the incidence varying depending on the specific syndrome.

Many immune deficiencies also are associated with other characteristic defects, some of which appear to be unrelated to the immune system yet may be inherently life threatening. Examples include eczema and thrombocytopenia (in Wiskott-Aldrich syndrome); cardiac anomalies, low levels of calcium in the blood, and structural anomalies of the face (in DiGeorge syndrome); or a severe lack of muscular coordination and dilation of the small blood vessels (in ataxia-telangiectasia). These associated symptoms can be useful diagnostically. For instance, the principal immunologic defect in **DiGeorge syndrome** is the partial or complete absence of T-cell immunity. However, this syndrome is also characterized by severe congenital structural defects of the heart and low levels of calcium, which may result in seizures.

TABLE 9-6 **CLASSES OF PRIMARY IMMUNE DEFICIENCIES**

CLASSIFICATION	EXAMPLE	MUTATION	IMMUNE DEFICIENCY
B-Cell Defects			
B-cell receptor signaling	Bruton's/X-linked agammaglobulinemia	Btk	Little or no B-cell maturation or antibody
	Autosomal agammaglobulinemia	IgM μ-chain	
Class-switch: hyper-IgM	X-linked hyper-IgM syndrome	CD40 ligand	Little or no class-switch to IgG or IgA, with overproduction of IgM
	Autosomal hyper-IgM syndrome	CD40	
	AICD deficiency	AICD	
Class-switch: selective	IgG subclass deficiency	Unknown	Defective switch to an IgG subclass
	Selective IgA deficiency	Unknown	Defective switch to IgA
	Common variable immune deficiency	Multiple	Defective switch to ≥1 antibody class
T-Cell Defects			
Defective primary lymphoid organ for T-cell development	DiGeorge syndrome	Development of 3rd and 4th pharyngeal pouches	Little or no T-cell maturation
Antigen specific response	Chronic mucocutaneous candidiasis	Unknown	Little or no response to *Candida*
Combined T- and B-Cell Defects			
SCID: No WBC stem cells	Reticular dysgenesis	Unknown	Complete; lack of white blood cells
SCID: Enzyme defects	Adenosine deaminase deficiency	ADA	Complete; few or no T, B, or NK cells
	Purine nucleoside phosphorylase deficiency	PNP	Partial; few T or NK cells
SCID: Cytokine receptor defects	X-linked SCID	IL-2Rγ	Partial; little or no maturation of Th or NK cells
	IL-7 receptor deficiency	IL-7Rα	
	JAK3 deficiency	JAK3	
SCID: TCR/BCR defects	RAG-1 or RAG-2 deficiency	RAG-1/RAG-2	Complete; little or no maturation of T or B cells; normal NK cells
SCID: TCR defects	CD45 deficiency	CD45	Partial; incomplete T-cell maturation, normal B and NK cells
	CD3 deficiency	CD3 γ-, δ-, or ε-chains	
	ZAP-70 deficiency	ZAP-70	
Antigen presentation defects	MHC class I deficiency	TAP1 or TAP2	Abnormal cytotoxic T-cell activity
	MHC class II deficiency	Multiple	Abnormal helper T-cell activity
Cytoskeletal defect	Wiskott-Aldrich syndrome	WASP	Altered T and B cells; decreased IgM
DNA repair defect	Ataxia-telangiectasia	ATM	Altered T and B cells; absent IgA
Complement Defects			
Classical pathway	C1q,r,s, C4, or C2 deficiency	C1q,r, or s, C4, or C2	Defective classical pathway, intact alternative pathway
Lectin pathway	Mannose-binding lectin deficiency	MBL	Defective lectin pathway
Alternative pathway	Properdin, factor D or B deficiency	Properdin, factor D or B	Defective alternative pathway
	Factor H, factor I deficiency	Factor H, factor I	Secondary C3 deficiency
C3	C3 deficiency	C3	Entire complement cascade blocked
Terminal pathway	C5, C6, C7, C8, or C9 deficiency	C5, C6, C7, C8, or C9	Membrane attack complex blocked, normal opsonization and chemotaxis
Phagocyte Defects			
Quantitative defects	Severe congenital neutropenia	ELA2, WASP	Inadequate numbers of neutrophils
	Cyclic neutropenia	ELA2	
Adhesion defects	Leukocyte adhesion defect-1 (LAD-1)	CD18	Decreased phagocyte adhesion to endothelium
	LAD-2	Transport enzymes for fucose	
Phagocytosis defects	C3 receptor deficiency	C3R	Defective opsonization
Bacterial killing defects	Chédiak-Higashi syndrome	CHS1	Defective lysosomal granules
	Myeloperoxidase deficiency	MPO	Lack of myeloperoxidase
	Chronic granulomatous disease	NADPH oxidase	Defective production of H_2O_2

AICD, Activation-induced cytidine deaminase; *MHC,* major histocompatibility complex; *NADPH,* nicotinamide adenine dinucleotide phosphate; *NK,* natural killer; *RAG,* recombination activating gene; *SCID,* severe combined immune deficiency; *TCR/BCR,* T-cell receptor/B-cell receptor; *ZAP,* zeta-chain associated protein.

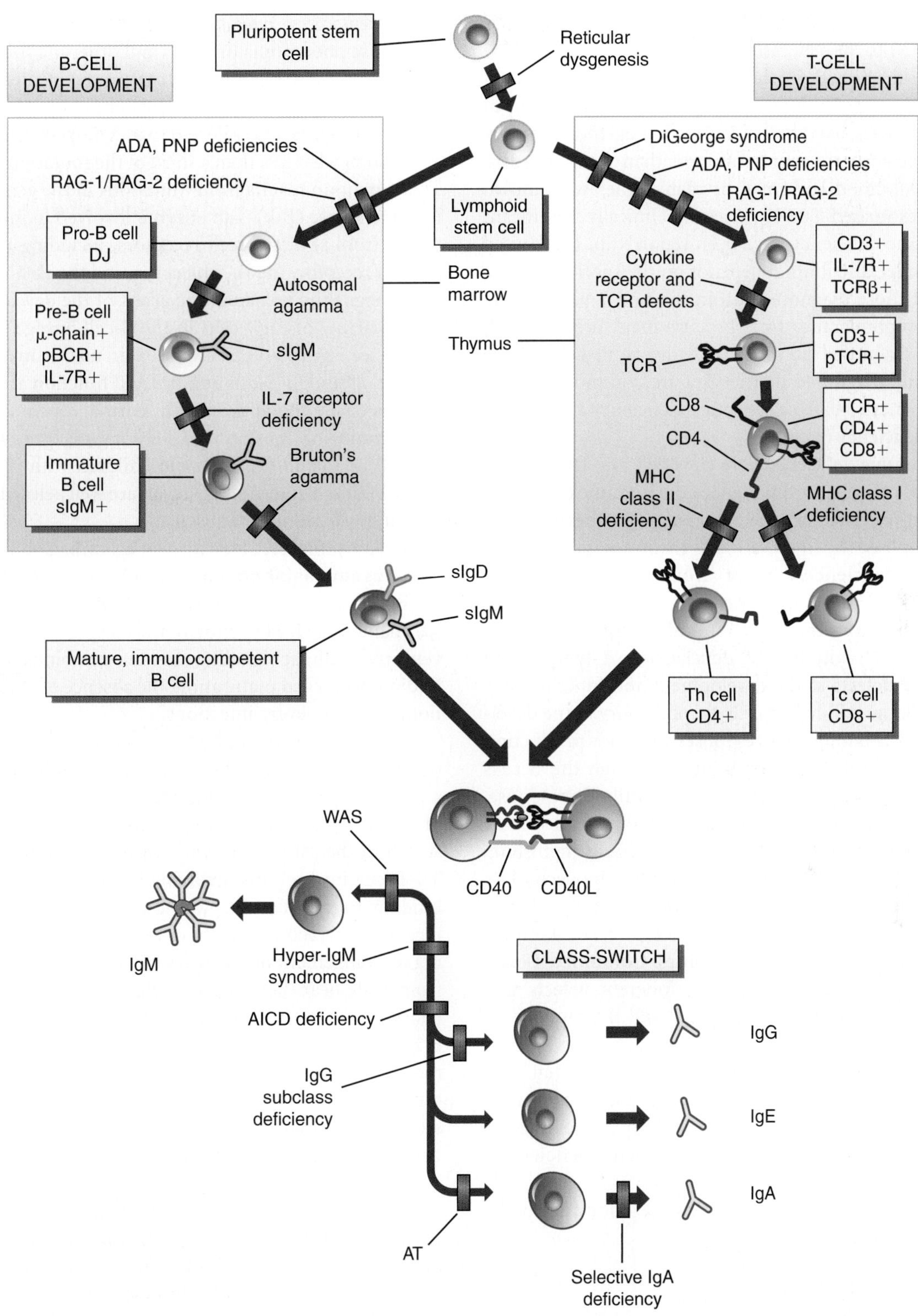

FIGURE 9-11 Lymphocyte Development Defects. This diagram shows defects in lymphocyte development that may account for congenital (primary) immune deficiencies. See the text and refer to Figures 8-10 through 8-12 for more detailed information. Pluripotent stem cell indicates the common stem cells for lymphocytic, granulocytic, and monocytic lineages. Cytokine receptor defects include X-linked severe combined immunodeficiency (SCID) (IL-2 receptor defect), JAK3 defects, and IL-7 receptor defects. T-cell receptor (TCR) defects include defects in CD3, CD45, and ZAP-70. Neither common variable immune deficiency nor chronic mucocutaneous candidiasis is included in this figure because the cause of these defects remains unknown. See Table 9-6 for further information on each defect. *ADA,* Adenosine deaminase deficiency; *agamma,* agammaglobulinemia; *AICD deficiency,* activation-induced cytidine deaminase deficiency; *AT,* ataxia-telangiectasia; *PNP,* purine nucleoside phosphorylase deficiency; *sIgM and sIgD,* surface IgM and IgD, respectively; *WAS,* Wiskott-Aldrich syndrome.

Individual primary immune deficiencies are very rare. For instance, only 30 to 50 new cases of severe combined immune deficiency are diagnosed in the United States yearly. However, approximately 150 different genetic defects resulting in immune deficiencies have been identified. Together, primary immune deficiencies are more common than cystic fibrosis, hemophilia, childhood leukemia, or many other well-known diseases. An estimated 50,000 cases of clinically significant primary immune deficiency have been reported in the United States. The gender distribution depends on the specific disease, but in general those diagnosed within the first 2 years of life have a male preponderance (5:1) because many are X-linked, whereas those diagnosed later are evenly distributed. The three most commonly diagnosed deficiencies are common variable immune deficiency (34%), selective IgA deficiency (24%), and IgG subclass deficiency (17%).

Primary immune deficiencies are classified into five groups, based on which principal component of the immune or inflammatory systems is defective. This chapter uses the five classifications proposed by the National Institutes of Health.[34] **B-lymphocyte deficiencies** result from defects in B-cell immune responses. T-cell immunity rarely depends on competent B-cell responses; thus T-cell immune responses are not affected in pure B-lymphocyte deficiencies. **T-lymphocyte deficiencies** are defects in the development and function of T lymphocytes. Because T-helper cells are obligatory in the development of many B-lymphocyte responses, antibody production is often diminished in these conditions, although the B cells are fully capable of producing an adequate antibody response. Many textbooks disagree on the classification of several specific immune deficiencies because of the difficulty in distinguishing between primary B-cell defects and those that are secondary to a primary T-cell defect. The classifications described below define T-cell defects as those with a clear defect in T-cell immunity, with normal B-cell immune responses. **Combined T- and B-lymphocyte deficiencies** result from inherent defects that directly affect the development of both T and B lymphocytes. Some combined deficiencies result in major defects in both T- and B-cell immune responses, whereas others are "partial" and more adversely affect T cells than B cells. The partial combined deficiencies include many conditions that may be classified as T-cell defects in other textbooks. **Complement deficiencies** and **phagocytic deficiencies** frequently present like antibody deficiencies because of the close interactions among antibody, complement, and phagocytes.

B-Lymphocyte Deficiencies

A defect in B-cell development results in lower levels of circulating immunoglobulins and increased susceptibility to infections in which antibodies are the primary protective mechanism.[35] The condition in which immunoglobulin levels are lower than normal is termed **hypogammaglobulinemia.** The condition in which they are totally or almost totally absent is termed **agammaglobulinemia.** (Normal lymphocyte development is discussed in Chapter 8.) Recurrent infections range from life threatening to mild, depending on the severity of the deficiency. Characteristic infections include encapsulated bacteria (e.g., *Streptococcus pneumoniae* or *Haemophilus influenzae*) that may cause pneumonia or sepsis and other microorganisms that cause infections of the sinuses, ears, and gastrointestinal tract.

The most severe B-lymphocyte deficiency is **Bruton's agammaglobulinemia,** also referred to as X-linked agammaglobulinemia. Somewhat less than a third of the mutations are sporadic. This condition results from mutations in the gene for Bruton's tyrosine kinase (Btk)—an enzyme involved in intracellular signaling from several B-cell receptors, including the IgM B-cell antigen receptor, the IL-5 receptor, and the IL-6 receptor. Ineffective signaling results in the arrest of the development in the bone marrow of early cells in the B-cell lineage into mature B cells[36] (see Figure 9-11). Few or no circulating mature B cells are present, although T-cell number and function are normal. At 6 months of life the approximate normal serum concentrations of immunoglobulins are IgG, 400 mg/dl; IgM, 40 mg/dl; and IgA, 30 mg/dl. In 6-month-old children with Bruton's agammaglobulinemia, serum IgG levels are well below 100 mg/dl and IgM and IgA are almost absent.

An autosomal recessive form of agammaglobulinemia (**autosomal agammaglobulinemia**) results from other mutations in the B-cell receptor. The most common is a mutation of the mu (μ) chain of the IgM portion of the receptor. This mutation prevents intracellular signaling after antigen binds to the receptor, leading to blocked maturation, the absence of antibody production, and very severe infections.

Several defects in antibody class-switch have been identified (see Figure 9-11). **X-linked hyper-IgM syndrome** results from a mutation in CD40 ligand, which is expressed on the surface of T-helper (Th) cells. Th cells stimulate B cells to undergo a switch in the class of antibody they produce through multiple Th–B-cell interactions involving ligands expressed on one cell binding to specific receptors on the other cell. The ligand-receptor interaction results in an intracellular signal facilitating rearrangement of the genes for the antibody variable region from a site near the constant region gene for the μ chain to the constant region for a different antibody H chain (see Figure 8-20). A critical ligand-receptor interaction occurs between the receptor CD40 on the B cell and its ligand (CD154 or CD40L) on the Th cell. A mutation in CD40L results in **defective class-switch,** decreased or absent production of IgG and IgA, poor development of memory B cells, and overproduction of IgM. T-cell immunity is not affected.

Defects in other components of the Th–B-cell interaction result in **autosomal hyper-IgM syndrome.** Mutations in CD40 on B cells result in a similar effect to that described previously. A defect in a DNA editing enzyme (activation-induced cytidine deaminase; AICD) also inhibits class-switch. During class-switch and movement of the H chain genetic information for the variable region to a different constant region gene, the double-stranded DNA must be cut and mended. This enzyme is responsible for cutting and mending the DNA.

Deficiencies in certain subclasses of antibody (**IgG subclass deficiency**), particularly IgG2, may result from a defect in switch to a particular subclass constant region (see Figure 9-11). The level of IgG2 subclass is often increased in response to polysaccharide antigens such as those on the surface of encapsulated bacteria. Low levels of IgG2 may be responsible for recurrent risk for pneumonias caused by these bacteria. Whether IgG subclass deficiencies are unique immune deficiency conditions is unclear because many are apparently early indications of the development of common variable immune deficiency (see following) or are secondary to selective IgA deficiency.

One of the most common primary immune deficiencies is a **selective IgA deficiency.** Because many affected individuals are asymptomatic, the true incidence is uncertain, although estimates ranging from 1 person in 300 to 1 in 3000 have been made. Individuals with selective IgA deficiency are able to produce other classes of immunoglobulins but fail to produce IgA (see Figure 9-11). Many will have B cells that have undergone class-switch to IgA, but for unknown reasons, cannot undergo the terminal steps of differentiation to IgA-secreting plasma cells. Although many individuals are asymptomatic, others present with a history of severe recurring sinus, lung, and gastrointestinal infections. They commonly also have chronic intestinal candidiasis (infection with *Candida albicans*). (The secretory, or mucosal, immune system is described in Chapter 8.)

Complications of IgA deficiency include severe atopic disease and autoimmune diseases; selective IgA deficiency is two or three times more common in atopic individuals than in others. Secretory IgA normally may prevent the uptake of allergens from the environment so that IgA deficiency may lead to increased allergen uptake and a more intense challenge to the immune system because of prolonged exposure to environmental antigens. One of the most severe complications of IgA deficiency is an anaphylactic reaction that can follow administration of blood products that contain IgA. Serious anaphylactic reactions can occur in individuals totally lacking IgA because the immune system recognizes donor IgA as a foreign antigen. Initial sensitization can occur in fetal life through exposure to maternal IgA that leaks across the placenta or later through the ingestion of maternal IgA in breast milk or bovine IgA in cow's milk. Sensitization also can occur with initial administration of blood products containing IgA. The individual's primed immune system then acts against donor IgA on subsequent exposure.

Common variable immune deficiency is the most commonly diagnosed immune deficiency. As the name implies, the presentation is very heterogeneous. It is characterized by hypogammaglobulinemia, but the particular class of antibody that is decreased varies: most have low amounts of IgG, which may or may not be accompanied by decreased levels of IgA or IgM, or both, with normal numbers of B cells. Some may have accompanying T-cell defects. Multiple genetic defects in terminal differentiation account for this condition, although the specific defects have not been identified in most people. The age of onset of symptoms, such as recurrent bacterial respiratory tract infections, is generally later than most primary immune deficiencies (late twenties). Secondary complications include arthritis (infectious and noninfectious), gastrointestinal symptoms (malabsorption, chronic diarrhea), autoimmune disease (anemia, thrombocytopenia, endocrine diseases), and cancer (of the lymphoid system, skin, and gastrointestinal tract).

T-Lymphocyte Deficiencies

Two well-studied examples of T-lymphocyte defects that represent different ends of the T-cell differentiation process include DiGeorge syndrome and chronic mucocutaneous candidiasis. Lymphoid stem cells begin maturing into functional T lymphocytes in the thymus. DiGeorge syndrome (congenital thymic aplasia or hypoplasia) is caused by the lack, or more commonly partial lack, of the thymus, resulting in greatly decreased T-cell numbers and function and in life-threatening viral, fungal, and intracellular bacterial infections[37] (see Figure 9-11). The defect is attributed usually to deletions on chromosome 22 (some deletions also have been identified on chromosome 10),[38] about 25% of which are inherited. The deleted region encodes information for formation of organs that originate from the third and fourth pharyngeal pouches during the twelfth week of gestation. In addition to the lack of thymus development, the individual may present with a partial or complete absence of the parathyroid gland (resulting in decreased blood calcium levels), major structural defects in the heart and the aorta (resulting in inadequate blood flow and inadequate oxygenation of the tissues), and abnormal facial characteristics (e.g., underdeveloped chin, low-set ears, shortened structure of the upper lip) (Figure 9-12).

Chronic mucocutaneous candidiasis is a primary defect of T lymphocytes in response to a specific infectious agent, the yeast *C. albicans.* At least seven variants of this condition have been described. All are characterized by mild to extremely severe chronic mucocutaneous candidiasis: *Candida* infections that involve the mucous membranes, nails, and skin. Invasive candidiasis is extremely rare. Although most B- and T-cell immune responses may be normal, most individuals with this defect cannot react to antigens from *Candida.* The cause of this defect is unknown.

Combined T- and B-Lymphocyte Deficiencies

The most severe deficiencies usually occur when both the B- and T-cell immune responses are affected. A great deal of knowledge about the evolution of bone marrow stem cells into functional B- and T-cell effectors came from studying children with the

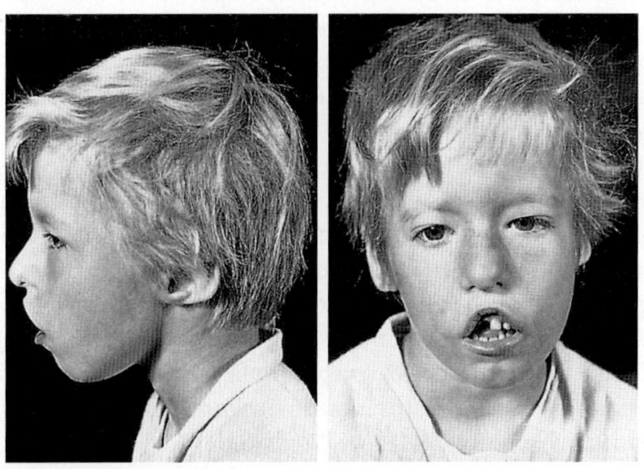

FIGURE 9-12 Facial Anomalies Associated with DiGeorge Syndrome. Note the wide-set eyes, low-set ears, and shortened structure of the upper lip. (From Roitt I, Brostoff J, Male D: *Immunology,* ed 6, St Louis, 2001, Mosby.)

most severe immune deficiency, **severe combined immune deficiency (SCID).** The most severe form of SCID is **reticular dysgenesis** (failure of blood cells to develop), in which a common stem cell for all white blood cells is absent; therefore, T cells, B cells, and phagocytic cells never develop (see Figure 9-11). Most children with reticular dysgenesis die in utero or very soon after birth. More typically, a defect occurs after some stem cells become committed to developing into lymphocytes (lymphoid stem cells); therefore, most individuals with SCID are deficient in lymphocyte development, but have normal numbers of all other white blood cells. SCID often results in few or absent T and B lymphocytes in the circulation and secondary lymphoid organs (spleen, lymph nodes). The thymus is usually hypoplastic (underdeveloped) because of the absence of T cells. Immunoglobulin levels, especially of IgM and IgA, are absent or greatly reduced, although IgG levels may be almost normal in the first months of life because of the presence of maternal antibodies. In the most severe defects, death occurs at about 1 year of life.

At least 20 different forms of SCID have been identified. Depending on the specific genetic mutation, the defect may involve T cells, B cells, and NK cells or may suppress more severely the function of one cell type, with relatively minor effects on the others. All three cells are adversely affected (T−, B−, NK−) in SCID resulting from a deficiency of adenosine deaminase **(adenosine deaminase [ADA] deficiency),** which is an enzyme involved in purine metabolism (see Figure 9-11). This defect is autosomal recessive and results in the accumulation of toxic purine metabolites to which rapidly dividing cells, such as lymphocytes, are especially sensitive. ADA deficiency accounts for about 16% of all persons with SCID. The development of T cells, B cells, and NK cells is arrested very early, and very few lymphocytic cells are found in the blood. In some forms of SCID, the defect resides in receptors for cytokines that are necessary for maturation of lymphocytes (see Figure 9-11). T cells and NK cells are preferentially affected (T−, B+, NK−), but often the defect results in the production of immature B cells that cannot respond well to antigen because of the lack of Th cells. The most common (44% of those with SCID) is an **X-linked SCID** resulting from a defect in the IL-2 receptor gamma (γ)-chain (IL-2Rγ). This protein is a component of several receptors for cytokines, including IL-2, IL-4, IL-7, IL-9, IL-15, and IL-21. These cytokines participate in the early development of immunocytes, particularly T and NK cells. Defective IL-2Rγ results in arrested maturation of T and NK cells and the production of immature B cells. A similar deficiency occurs with mutation in JAK3 **(JAK3 deficiency),** which is an enzyme (a tyrosine kinase) that associates with IL-2Rγ in normal cells and communicates information from the receptor to the nucleus. Thus cells with defects in JAK3 cannot respond to cytokines that bind to these receptors on the cell surface. An autosomal form results from mutations of one of the protein chains (α-chain) of the IL-7 receptor **(IL-7 receptor deficiency).** IL-7 appears to be necessary for the maturation of T cells, so that this deficiency has relatively normal levels of B cells and NK cells.

Mutations in another purine metabolism enzyme, purine nucleoside phosphorylase **(purine nucleoside phosphorylase [PNP] deficiency),** are less severe than ADA deficiency (see Figure 9-11). T cells and NK cells appear to be more susceptible to mutations in PNP so that B-cell function can be relatively normal.

Another form of SCID preferentially affects T cells and B cells (T−, B−, NK+). T and B lymphocytes possess receptors for antigen, whereas NK cells do not. Those receptors result from a process of genetic rearrangement of *V* and *J* genes to form the variable regions of the L chain (B-cell receptor [BCR]) and the α-chain (T-cell receptor [TCR]) and the *V, D,* and *J* genes to form the variable regions of the H chain (BCR) and the β-chain (TCR). Successful rearrangement is controlled by two recombination activating enzymes (RAG-1 and RAG-2). RAG enzymes cut and repair double-stranded breaks in DNA that are necessary for genetic rearrangement. **RAG-1** or **RAG-2 deficiencies** are autosomal recessive and result in arrested lymphocyte development from blocked recombination of variable regions of B-cell and T-cell receptors (see Figure 9-11).

Forms of partial SCID, with the defect being primarily of T cells, arise from mutations in several components of the TCR complex (see Figure 9-11). Defects in the TCR result in inadequate maturation of T cells, with normal B and NK cells. Antibody production may be depressed because of the lack of Th cells. The TCR is a complex organization of proteins that react with antigen (α- and β-chains), and then provide an intracellular signal to the nucleus (γ-, δ-, and ε-chains [collectively called CD3] and the associated molecules CD45 and ZAP-70). Examples of these deficiencies include mutations in CD3, CD45, or ZAP-70. The T-cell defect in each can range from mild to severe in nature, with normal B lymphocytes.

Even if nearly adequate numbers of B and T cells are produced, their ability to process and present antigen may be defective. The **bare lymphocyte syndrome** is a group of immune deficiencies characterized by an inability of lymphocytes and macrophages to present antigen because of defects in class I or class II MHC antigen expression (see Figure 9-11). **MHC class I deficiency** results from mutations in the genes for TAP1 or TAP2, which control the transport of antigenic protein fragments across the endoplasmic reticulum and the formation of MHC class I/antigen complexes for transportation to the cell surface (see Figure 8-16). Because MHC class I molecules preferentially present antigen to CD8+ Tc cells, the resultant deficiency is of CD8+ cytotoxic cells, with normal levels of CD4+ helper cells and normal antibody production. **MHC class II deficiency** is more severe. A variety of mutations prevent normal production of MHC class II molecules, which present antigen to CD4+ helper cells. Because of defective recruitment of T-helper cells, normal antibody responses are greatly suppressed. Children with this deficiency develop life-threatening infections and usually die before age 5 years.

Some combined immune deficiencies are secondary to mutations that affect a variety of cells other than immunocytes. For instance, **Wiskott-Aldrich syndrome** (WAS; an X-linked recessive disorder) results from sporadic mutations in the WAS protein (WASP), which is involved in intracellular signaling and regulation of the organization of the cell's actin cytoskeleton (see Figure 9-11). The defects in the cytoskeleton lead to the classic symptoms of thrombocytopenia (with resultant bleeding disorders), scaly eczema, and defective T and B cells. IgA and IgG levels are usually normal, but IgM responses are highly depressed. Antibody responses against antigens that elicit primarily an IgM response, such as polysaccharide antigens from bacterial cell walls (e.g., of *Pseudomonas aeruginosa, S. pneumoniae, H. influenzae,* and other microorganisms with polysaccharide outer capsules), are deficient. Persons with WAS have a very high risk of lymphoid malignancies (leukemias and lymphomas).

Ataxia-telangiectasia (AT) is an autosomal recessive disorder resulting from a large variety of sporadic mutations in the *ATM* gene, which encodes a protein involved in repair of double-stranded breaks in DNA. Affected infants often develop ataxia (unsteady gait), which usually becomes apparent when the child is learning to walk. The neurologic defect may eventually lead to confinement in a wheelchair. Telangiectasia (dilation of capillaries) can occur in the eyes and skin, especially on the ears, neck, and extremities. Both B and T cells are variably affected and unrepaired double-stranded DNA breaks are commonly observed in the regions encoding the T-cell and B-cell receptors. About 70% of those with AT are IgA deficient, occasionally accompanied by deficiencies in IgG (see Figure 9-11). Individuals with AT are at high risk for developing leukemias and lymphomas.

Complement Deficiencies

Complement activation is a necessary component of protection against many infectious agents. IgG and complement components, such as C3b, are opsonins and facilitate phagocytosis by neutrophils and macrophages. Defects in the complement cascade often resemble antibody deficiencies, with recurrent infections with encapsulated bacteria (e.g., *H. influenzae* and *S. pneumoniae*) that are highly sensitive to opsonin-assisted phagocytosis. In addition to recurrent infections, deficiencies in the classical pathway commonly lead to a SLE-like syndrome. As noted previously, excessive levels of circulating complexes of antibody, antigen, and complement may lead to type III hypersensitivity diseases (immune complex diseases). However, healthy individuals release small amounts of soluble intracellular antigens into the blood during normal cell turnover. Low levels of naturally occurring autoantibodies and limited activation of the classical pathway of the complement system through C3 facilitate the removal of this debris by phagocytes. Some complement defects may slow the clearance from the blood of natural immune complexes, leading to SLE-like symptoms.

C3 deficiency is the most severe complement defect (Figure 9-13). C3 is the component that unites all pathways of complement activation, and complement component C3b is a major opsonin. Persons with C3 deficiency are at risk for recurrent life-threatening infections with encapsulated bacteria at an early age, as well as a SLE-like syndrome that may be complicated by kidney disease (glomerulonephritis). **C2 deficiency,** more so than **C1** or **C4 deficiencies,** also has an increased risk for recurrent respiratory tract infections with encapsulated bacteria (e.g., *S. pneumoniae, H. influenzae*).

Mannose-binding lectin (MBL) deficiency is the primary defect of the lectin pathway of complement activation.

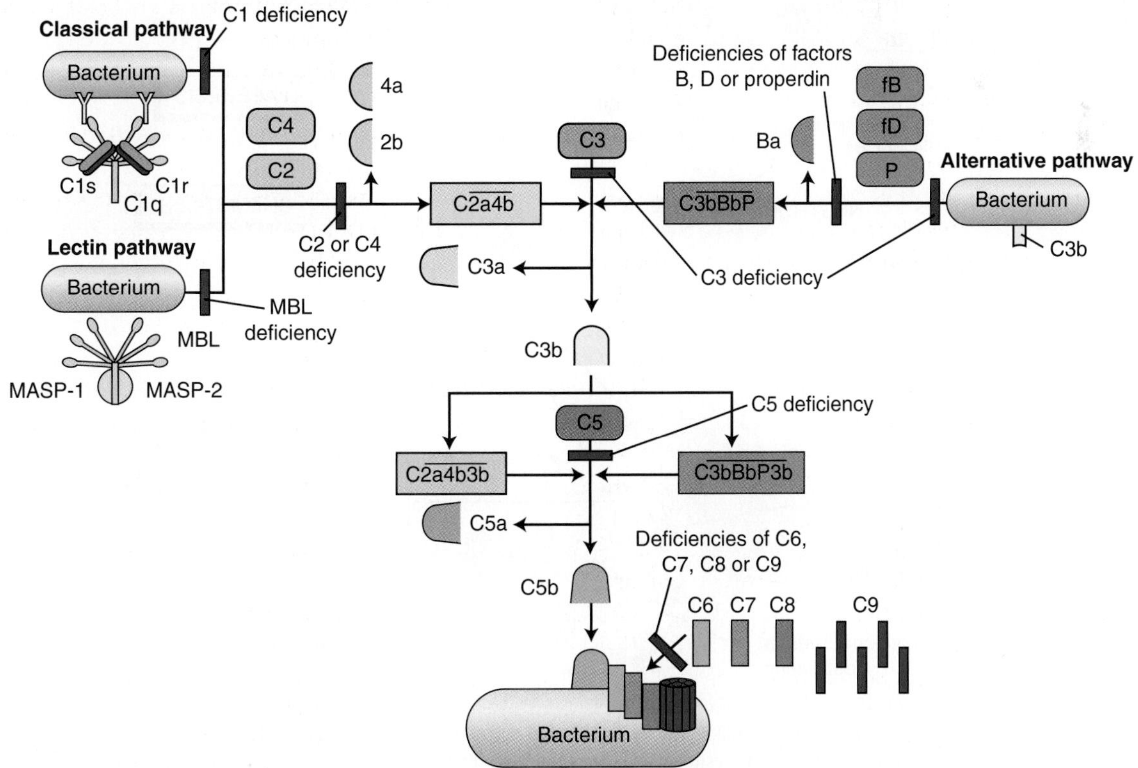

FIGURE 9-13 Complement Defects. The complement cascade is initiated through three pathways: the classical pathway, the lectin pathway, and the alternative pathway. Each of the three pathways produces a C3 convertase, which activates C3 leading to the formation of a C5 convertase. The activation of C5 initiates formation of the membrane attack complex (MAC). For more details, see the text and Figure 7-5. The most severe defect is a C3 deficiency because it blocks all three pathways. *MASP,* MBL-associated serine protease; *MBL,* mannose-binding lectin.

The defect results in increased risk of infection with microorganisms that have polysaccharide capsules rich in mannose, particularly the yeast *Saccharomyces cerevisiae* and encapsulated bacteria such as *N. meningitidis* and *S. pneumoniae.*

Deficiencies in the alternative pathway also result in recurrent infections with encapsulated bacteria. **Properdin deficiency** is associated with recurrent meningococcal infections and is X-linked, whereas all other complement deficiencies are autosomal recessive. Symptoms generally appear in the second decade of life. Factor I and factor H are major regulators of the complement cascade and control the level of spontaneous activation of C3. **Factor I deficiency** and **factor H deficiency** can be severe because they lead to increased spontaneous destruction of C3 and a secondary C3 deficiency.

Deficiencies of components of the terminal portion of the complement cascade (C5, C6, C7, C8, or C9 deficiencies) are associated with increased infections with only one group of bacteria—those of the genus *Neisseria (N. meningitidis* or *N. gonorrhoeae). Neisseria* usually cause localized infections (meningitis or gonorrhea), but those individuals with terminal pathway defects have more than an 8000-fold increased risk for systemic infections with atypical strains of these microorganisms. **C9 deficiency** is the most common terminal pathway defect, appears primarily in Japanese populations, and is generally asymptomatic. The other deficiencies of the terminal pathway are extremely rare, but are characterized by more aggressive infections. The risk for systemic infections with *Neisseria* is also increased in those with deficiencies of C2, factor D, factor B, and properdin.

Phagocytic Deficiencies

Phagocytosis is generally aided by bacterial opsonization with IgG or C3b; therefore, defects in phagocytic killing usually result in recurrent infections with the same group of microorganisms (encapsulated bacteria) associated with antibody and complement deficiencies. Phagocytosis is a multistep process that involves initial adhesion between circulating phagocytes and the endothelial cells lining the circulation (see Figure 7-15). The phagocytes exit the circulation and move to a site of infection by a chemotactic process in response to soluble chemotactic factors released by the infection. The process of phagocytosis itself begins with attachment of the phagocyte to the targeted bacteria through the interaction of opsonins on the microorganism and matched receptors on the phagocyte's surface. Phagocytic engulfment results in internalization of the infectious agent and activation of a variety of oxygen-dependent and oxygen-independent killing mechanisms. Deficiencies can arise from mutations that affect one or more of these steps (Figure 9-14).

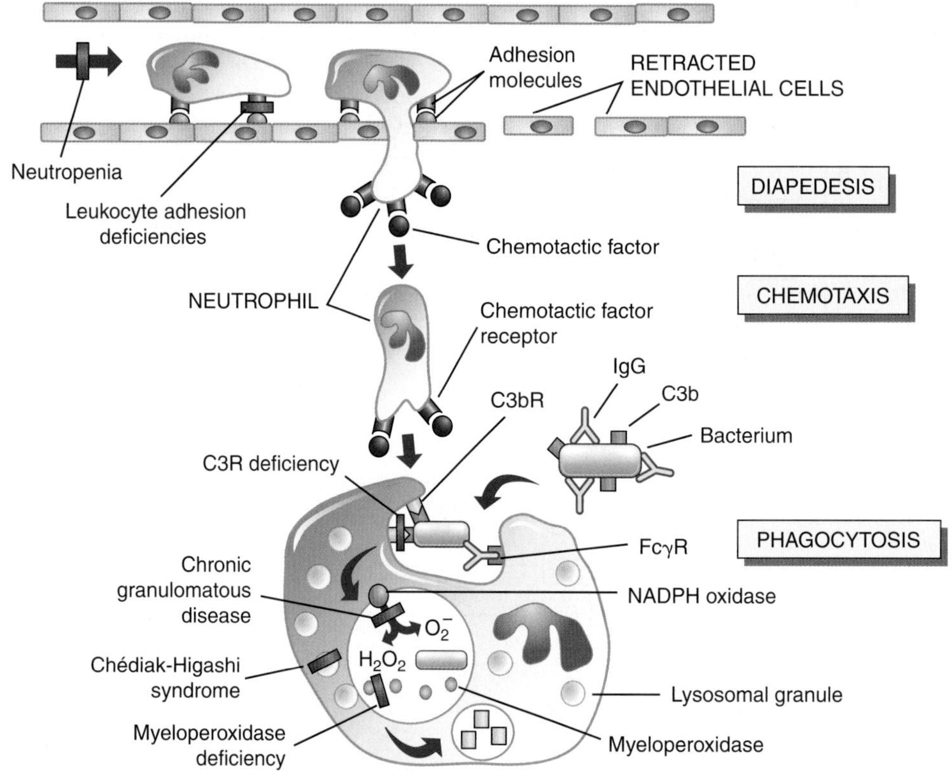

FIGURE 9-14 Phagocytic Defects. Several genetic defects in the process leading up to and including phagocytosis result in increased susceptibility to bacterial infections. See the text and refer to Figure 7-15 and Table 7-3 for more detailed information. The phagocyte leaves the bloodstream and enters the tissue through interactions between leukocyte and endothelial adhesion molecules and the process of diapedesis. The cell is attracted to the inflammatory site by chemotaxis, where it encounters opsonized bacteria, and attaches to and engulfs the microorganism. Inside the phagocyte the bacteria are killed and broken down by the combination of lysosomal granule constituents and reactive oxygen products of the hexose-monophosphate shunt and nicotinamide adenine dinucleotide phosphate (NADPH) oxidase. *C3R,* C3 receptor, which includes the C3b receptor *(C3bR); FcγR,* receptor for the Fc portion of IgG; *H_2O_2,* hydrogen peroxide; O_2^-, reactive oxygen.

Inadequate numbers of phagocytes, particularly neutrophils **(severe congenital neutropenias),** result in a variety of recurrent and severe bacterial infections beginning early in life. Approximately 50% of these individuals have a mutation in the neutrophil elastase gene *(ELA2)*. Other mutations have been identified (e.g., *WAS* gene) in the other 50%. A milder form, **cyclic neutropenia,** is autosomal dominant with almost 100% of affected individuals having a mutation in the *ELA2* gene. Changes in neutrophil levels are cyclic and may remain at or near normal for 2 to 3 weeks, followed by periods of neutropenia lasting a few days to weeks. During the neutropenia, the individual has increased susceptibility to recurrent bacterial infections.

Near sites of inflammation, soluble mediators diffuse into the circulation and induce expression of a variety of adhesion molecules on the phagocyte surface, which interact with complementary molecules on the endothelial cells to increase adherence between the phagocyte and the vessel wall and allow for margination and diapedesis to occur. **Leukocyte adhesion deficiencies (LADs)** result from mutations in various phagocyte adhesion molecules (see Table 7-3). Leukocyte adhesion deficiency, type 1 (LAD-1) results from an autosomal recessive mutation in CD18, which is a β_2-integrin chain that is shared by several different receptors. LAD-2 results from a defect in adding the monosaccharide fucose to carbohydrates on the phagocyte surface. Surface carbohydrates with fucose are ligands for selectins on the endothelial and leukocyte. These and other defects in leukocyte adhesion molecules usually result in increased levels of neutrophils in the blood (leukocytosis) because they cannot leave the circulation and in increased recurrent bacterial and fungal infections.

Additional deficiencies diminish the leukocyte's recognition of opsonins of the complement cascade (e.g., C3b). Deficiencies in the complement receptor for C3 **(C3 receptor deficiency)** result in recurrent bacterial infections, particularly of the skin.

A variety of defects in killing of microorganisms have been described. **Chédiak-Higashi syndrome** results from a defect in cytoplasmic granules from an autosomal recessive mutation in the lysosomal trafficking regulator gene *(CHS1)*. The CHS1 protein helps control movement of granules to cellular membranes in preparation for degranulation. As a result of these mutations, the granules remain in the cytoplasm and form large aggregates that are readily apparent microscopically. Leukocytes from individuals with Chédiak-Higashi syndrome have decreased chemotaxis, granular fusion, and bacterial killing. Platelet granules also may be affected, resulting in prolonged bleeding, and partial albinism can occur because of defects in melanocyte granules. Affected children develop recurrent infections of the skin, respiratory tract, and mucous membranes, especially with gram-positive bacteria.

The enzyme myeloperoxidase participates in a major mechanism of bacterial killing in phagocytes. Myeloperoxidase is found in primary granules and catalyzes the formation of acids from halides (e.g., chloride ion) and hydrogen peroxide (H_2O_2). As a result of phagocytosis, neutrophils and other phagocytes switch much of their glucose metabolism to the hexose-monophosphate shunt. A byproduct of this pathway is the conversion of molecular oxygen by nicotinamide adenine dinucleotide phosphate (NADPH) oxidase and other enzymes into highly reactive and toxic oxygen derivatives, including hydrogen peroxide. Two deficiencies in the myeloperoxidase–hydrogen peroxide killing process have been extensively studied. **Myeloperoxidase deficiency** is a relatively mild disorder characterized by a complete or partial deficiency in myeloperoxidase. Individuals do not have severe recurrent infections because most infectious bacteria are sensitive to direct killing by many of the toxic oxygen molecules produced by NADPH oxidase. The exception is the person with concurrent diabetes, who may have recurrent disseminated candidiasis.

Chronic granulomatous disease (CGD) is a more severe defect in the myeloperoxidase–hydrogen peroxide system.[39] Several forms of the disease have been characterized, both X-linked (about 70% of the individuals) and autosomal recessive, with the X-linked form being more severe. CGD occurs from a variety of mutations (at least four have been identified) in portions of the NADPH oxidase complex, resulting in deficiencies in the production of hydrogen peroxide and other oxygen products. Thus individuals have adequate myeloperoxidase and chloride but lack the necessary hydrogen peroxide. Individuals with CGD have recurrent severe pneumonias; tumor-like granulomas in lungs, skin, and bones; and other infections with some normally relative innocuous microorganisms, such as *Staphylococcus aureus, Serratia marcescens, Aspergillus* spp., and others. These are catalase-positive microorganisms. Infections with more virulent, but catalase-negative, microorganisms (e.g., *S. pneumoniae*) are rare. Most microorganisms produce their own hydrogen peroxide as a byproduct, which accumulates in the phagocytic vacuole and can be used by the phagocyte's myeloperoxidase to kill the microorganism. Some microorganisms also produce the enzyme catalase, which breaks down hydrogen peroxide. Thus catalase-negative microorganisms donate hydrogen peroxide to the phagocyte's myeloperoxidase, leading to their own death. Catalase-positive microorganisms, however, destroy the bacterial hydrogen peroxide and survive and cause infection.

Secondary Immune Deficiencies

Secondary, or acquired, immune and inflammatory deficiencies are far more common than primary deficiencies.[40] These deficiencies are not related to genetic defects, but are complications of other physiologic or pathophysiologic conditions. Some conditions that are known to be associated with acquired deficiencies include:

- Normal physiologic conditions
  - Pregnancy
  - Infancy
  - Aging
- Psychologic stress
  - Emotional trauma
  - Eating disorders
- Dietary insufficiencies
  - Malnutrition caused by insufficient intake of large categories of nutrients, such as protein or calories
  - Insufficient intake of specific nutrients, such as vitamins, iron, or zinc

- Malignancies
  - Malignancies of lymphoid tissues, such as Hodgkin disease, acute or chronic leukemia, or myeloma
  - Malignancies of nonlymphoid tissues, such as sarcomas and carcinomas
- Metabolic diseases or genetic syndromes
  - Diabetes
  - Cystic fibrosis
  - Alcoholic cirrhosis
  - Sickle cell disease
  - SLE
  - Chromosome abnormalities, such as trisomy 21 (Down syndrome)
- Environmental agents
  - Ultraviolet (UV) light
  - Ionizing radiation
  - Chronic hypoxia
- Physical trauma
  - Burns
- Medical treatments
  - Stress caused by surgery
  - Anesthesia
  - Immunosuppressive treatment with corticosteroids or antilymphocyte antibodies
  - Splenectomy
  - Cancer treatment with cytotoxic drugs or ionizing radiation
- Infections
  - Congenital infections, such as rubella, cytomegalovirus, hepatitis B
  - Acquired infections, such as acquired immunodeficiency syndrome (AIDS)

Although secondary deficiencies are common, many are not clinically relevant. In many cases, the degree of the immune deficiency is relatively minor and without any apparent increased susceptibility to infection. Alternatively, the immune system may be substantially suppressed, but only for a short duration, thus minimizing the incidence of clinically relevant infections. Some secondary immune deficiencies, however, are extremely severe and may result in recurrent life-threatening infections.

Normal Physiologic Conditions

The competence of an individual's immune system varies throughout life. Pregnancy itself is considered by many to be an immunocompromised condition. Pregnant women may have decreased reactivity or altered results in several tests of the immune system, including skin tests against various antigens, circulating numbers of T lymphocytes, and other very general tests. Pregnancy itself, however, is not associated with a marked change in infections, suggesting that the mother's immune system is not severely altered.

The newborn child is immunologically immature. Although T-cell immune responses may be normal or near normal, other components of the immune system (especially antibody production) are just beginning to mature. Beginning at about 32 weeks of pregnancy, the placenta transports maternal antibodies into the fetal blood to protect the child during the first months of life (see Figure 8-30). After the delivery, the level of the mother's antibodies slowly decreases in the newborn so that maternal antibodies no longer protect the child by about 6 months of life. By 6 to 8 months, the newborn should be efficiently protected by antibodies produced by its own B cells. In some infants, the development of antibody production is delayed, and a transient low level of antibody may persist for several months **(transient hypogammaglobulinemia of infancy),** during which the child has increased susceptibility to infections. Premature infants are particularly immunologically immature and are at increased risk for neonatal infections. The blood of infants born before 32 weeks' gestation is generally devoid of maternal antibody.

Aging is also associated with a progressive depression in immune responses. Older adults generally have more severe bacterial and fungal infections, greater difficulty resolving those infections, and lower responses to vaccination.

Several meaningful changes occur during aging, although variations in the degree of change and a corresponding increased susceptibility to infection can be considerable among individuals. The thymus involutes over time, resulting in decreased production of fresh T cells. A concurrent depletion of T-memory cells results in depressed responses to both new and "recall" antigens. A shift toward Th2 cells also may occur with a resultant decrease in Th1 cytokines. Total numbers of B cells may decrease. Numbers of NK cells may remain normal, although their activity is decreased. Similarly, neutrophil numbers may remain normal, with decreased phagocytosis and killing.

Psychologic Stress

The relationship between emotional stress and depressed immune function has become an area of intense clinical and research interest. For many decades anecdotal reports have suggested that increased incidences of infection and malignancy are associated with periods of both intense stress (e.g., the loss of a loved one, divorce) and relatively minor stress (e.g., final examination periods at colleges and universities). In addition, early studies showed that immune function, as demonstrated by delayed hypersensitivity skin test results, could be depressed through posthypnotic suggestion.

We are now beginning to understand the mechanisms of the relationship between emotional stress and the immune system. Many lymphoid organs are innervated and can be affected by nerve stimulation. In addition, lymphocytes have receptors for many hormones (e.g., sex hormones, neurotransmitters, and neuropeptides) and can respond to changing levels of these chemicals with increased or decreased function. For instance, stress-induced catecholamines affect the expression of adhesion molecules and the movement of lymphocytes among lymphoid organs. (Further discussion of the effects of stress on susceptibility to disease is the subject of Chapter 11.)

Dietary Insufficiencies

Nutritional status can have a profound effect on immune function, and malnutrition is the predominant cause of secondary immune deficiencies worldwide. Severe deficits in calorie or protein intake lead to deficiencies in T-cell function and numbers. The humoral immune response is less affected by starvation, although complement activity, neutrophil chemotaxis, and bacterial killing within neutrophils often are depressed, resulting in infections with microorganisms that are normally destroyed by opsonization and phagocytosis.

Deficient zinc intake can profoundly depress both T- and B-cell function. Zinc is required as a cofactor for at least 70 different enzymes, some of which are found in lymphocytes and are necessary for their function. Secondary zinc deficiencies may be associated with malabsorption syndrome (failure to absorb zinc), chronic renal disease (loss of zinc in the urine), chronic diarrhea (loss of zinc through the gut), or burns or severe psoriasis (loss of zinc through the skin). Deficiencies of other enzyme cofactors, such as vitamins (e.g., pyridoxine, pantothenic acid, folic acid, and vitamins A, C, E, and B_{12}), also may result in severe depressions of B- and T-cell function, phagocytosis, and complement activity.

Malignancies

Many malignancies are complicated by a wasting syndrome (cachexia) in the later stages, which can suppress the immune system secondary to the resultant malnutrition. Additionally, a very close relationship exists between the immune system and the development of malignancies. It is generally accepted that successful malignancies have developed mechanisms to avoid rejection by the individual's immune system. Persons with primary immune deficiencies are usually at greater risk for developing malignancies, particularly malignancies of lymphoid tissues, such as leukemias or lymphomas. Malignancies aggressively depress the individual's immune system. The effect is commonly nonspecific, resulting in a generalized deficiency of the immune response and a greatly increased susceptibility to developing life-threatening infections. In fact, many people with malignancies die from infection rather than from direct effects of the tumor.

Malignancies of lymphoid tissues, such as Hodgkin disease, acute or chronic leukemia, or myeloma, result in depletion of normal lymphocytes and their replacement by the malignant cells. Thus the number of B or T cells capable of responding to infections is depleted. Many malignancies, even those of non–lymphoid tissues, produce cytokines (e.g., transforming growth factor-beta [TGF-β] and vascular endothelial growth factor [VEGF]) that nonspecifically suppress the immune responses.

Metabolic Diseases or Genetic Syndromes

Diabetes suppresses many aspects of the immune and inflammatory responses, including phagocytosis and chemotaxis, lymphocyte proliferation, and glucose metabolism. The effects of trisomy 21 are less severe, but primarily include diminished neutrophil function. People with cystic fibrosis have decreased airway clearance of bacteria, thus increasing the probability of major respiratory tract infections.

Environmental Agents

Individuals are constantly exposed to environmental agents that affect the immune system. UV light from sun exposure or tanning salons induces apoptosis of lymphoid stem cells, increases production of Treg cells that suppress defenses against cancer, and increases production of anti-inflammatory cytokines. Ionizing radiation affects rapidly dividing cells, including those of the immune system. At very high doses, the entire immune system can be depleted.

Physical Trauma

Trauma that compromises the epithelial barrier also predisposes an individual to infection. Burn victims are susceptible to severe bacterial infections. Thermal burns appear to be associated with suppressed neutrophil function (especially chemotaxis), complement levels, cell-mediated immunity, and primary humoral responses, although secondary humoral responses are normal. The mechanism of this immunosuppression may be twofold. Blood from burned individuals contains nonspecific immunosuppressive factors (all immune responses are suppressed, regardless of the antigen involved). In addition, burn victims also have increased regulatory T-cell function, which may increase antigen-specific suppression.

Medical Treatments

Medical treatments themselves may produce suppression of immune responses. Depression of B- and T-cell formation is manifested as a progressive increase in infections with opportunistic microorganisms (especially *P. jirovecii*, cytomegalovirus, *C. albicans*, and other fungi), the extent and location of which are unusual.

Many drugs that are used to fight cancer (e.g., cancer chemotherapeutic agents) are not specific for cancer cells, but are designed to attack cells in susceptible stages in their cell cycles or rapidly proliferating cells, which includes cells of the immune system as well as malignant cells. The immunosuppressive effects of chemotherapeutic drugs are exacerbated by concurrent treatment with ionizing radiation (x-rays), which also affect cells that are rapidly making new DNA. Therefore, a person's immune response can be profoundly depressed as a result of the therapy. Other drugs, such as corticosteroids, are intentionally used to suppress the immune system and control hypersensitivity diseases (especially autoimmune disease) or prevent rejection of transplants. Because of their nonspecific activity, however, immune responses against infectious agents also can be suppressed, increasing an individual's susceptibility to infection. The list of drugs that affect the immune response is ever increasing and includes analgesics, antithyroid medications, anticonvulsants, antihistamines, antimicrobial agents, antilymphocyte antibodies, and tranquilizers.

Surgery and anesthesia also can suppress T- and B-cell function. Transient, severe lymphopenia is a common postoperative condition that can last as long as 1 month. Surgery to remove the spleen (splenectomy) can result in a depressed humoral response against encapsulated bacteria (especially *S. pneumoniae, H. influenzae, S. aureus,* group A streptococci, and *N. meningitidis*), depressed serum IgM levels, and decreased levels of opsonins.

Infections

Many infectious microorganisms are successful at invading the human body because they have evolved mechanisms for fighting off specific immune/inflammatory responses against themselves (discussed in Chapter 10). However, some infectious agents (e.g., human immunodeficiency virus [HIV], Epstein-Barr virus [EBV], CMV, herpes simplex virus type 6, measles) can generally suppress the immune response. HIV is one of the few microorganisms that directly attacks the central processes involved in the development of an immune response (discussed in detail in Chapter 10). It infects and destroys the T-helper cell, which is necessary to provide help for the maturation of both plasma cells and T-cytotoxic cells.[41] Therefore, HIV suppresses the immune response against itself and secondarily creates a generalized immune deficiency by suppressing the development of immune responses against other pathogens and opportunistic microorganisms.

Several viruses (e.g., hepatitis B, rubella, CMV) can establish congenital infections through transmission from an infected mother to her child at birth when the child's immune system is immature. These children may have suppressed immune responses, although the degree of the deficiency is not usually severe; however, as the child's immune system develops, the viral antigens may be partially seen as "self" so that a chronic infection is established.

Evaluation and Care of Those with Immune Deficiency

Routine care of individuals with immune deficiencies must be tempered with the knowledge that the immune system may be totally ineffective. Administration of conventional immunizing agents or blood products to these individuals may be unsafe because of the risk that the immunizing agent will cause an uncontrolled infection. Attenuated vaccines contain live but weakened microorganisms (e.g., live polio vaccine; vaccines against measles, mumps, and rubella) that can cause disseminated infection. Although the vaccine virus is attenuated enough to be destroyed by a normal immune system, it can survive, multiply, and cause severe disease in an immune-deficient recipient. Additionally, even healthy recipients of vaccines containing live microorganisms can shed those microorganisms for a short time, increasing the risk of infection to family members or other close associates who are immune deficient. Even simple procedures, such as penetrating the skin for routine blood tests, may lead to fatal septicemia (bacterial infection of the blood) in the immune-deficient person.

Individuals with immune deficiencies are also at risk for **graft-versus-host disease (GVHD)**. Mature T cells in a transplanted graft (e.g., transfused blood) are capable of a destructive cell-mediated reaction against unmatched histocompatibility antigens on the tissues in the graft recipient. Symptoms of an acute graft-versus-host reaction usually appear within 10 to 30 days after the transplant. The primary targets for GVHD are the skin (e.g., rash, loss or increase of pigment, thickening of skin), liver (e.g., damage to bile duct, hepatomegaly), mouth (e.g., dry mouth, ulcers, infections), eyes (e.g., burning, irritation, dryness), and gastrointestinal tract (e.g., severe diarrhea) and may lead to death from infections.

GVHD is not a problem when the recipient is immunocompetent, that is, has an immune system that can control the donor's lymphocytes. If, however, the recipient's immune system is deficient, the grafted T cells remain unchecked and attack the recipient's tissues. Most GVHD is prevented by treating whole blood with irradiation to kill white blood cells before transfusion.

The most common presenting symptom of immune deficiencies is recurrent severe infections. Significant information concerning the nature of the specific immune deficiency can be obtained by noting the types of infection, as well as certain characteristics of the affected individual, including gender, age of disease onset, the presence of any associated anomalies, family history, and risk factors associated with secondary immune deficiencies. Humoral deficiencies are generally characterized by recurrent sinopulmonary infections with encapsulated bacteria, gastrointestinal malabsorption, and poor growth. T-cell defects generally present with failure to thrive, chronic diarrhea, persistent thrush, and opportunistic infections (e.g., *Mycobacterium, Pneumocystis, Candida,* and certain viruses). Phagocytic defects are usually associated with recurrent abscesses, oral ulcers, and infections with specific bacteria (e.g., catalase-positive bacteria). Complement defects may be linked to SLE-like disease and recurrent and disseminated infections with *Neisseria* spp.

A variety of laboratory tests are available to evaluate specific immune deficiencies[42] (Table 9-7). The choice of which particular tests to perform is determined on the characteristics described previously. A basic screening test is a **complete blood count (CBC)** with a differential. The CBC provides information on the numbers of red cells, white cells, and platelets, and the differential indicates the quantities of lymphocytes, granulocytes, and monocytes in the blood. Quantitative determination of immunoglobulins (IgG, IgM, IgA) is a screening test for antibody production, and an assay for total complement (total hemolytic complement, CH_{50}) is useful if a complement defect is suspected.

If the nature of the immune deficiency remains uncertain after the screening tests, additional relatively common tests can be performed. For instance, subpopulations of lymphocytes (T or B) can be quantified using characteristic surface markers, such as surface immunoglobulin for B cells and CD3 for T cells. T-cell populations can be further subdivided using additional surface markers, such as CD4 (T-helper cells) or CD8 (T-cytotoxic cells). For antibodies, routine assays are available to quantify subclasses of IgG, such as IgG2.

An additional level of testing would include determination of immune responses against specific antigens. Determination of isohemagglutinins is informative about antigen-specific IgM production. Antibody responses to vaccines (e.g., tetanus, pertussis, measles, diphtheria, hepatitis B) are usually indicative of IgG responses. T-cell immunity against specific antigens can be measured by skin tests against antigens to which the individual had been exposed: "recall antigens." These include antigens from vaccines (e.g., mumps, tetanus) or from microorganisms with which the person had a previous active infection (e.g., *Candida*). An adequate T-cell immunity results in a positive delayed hypersensitivity skin test reaction.

If the tests do not identify the immune deficiency, more esoteric tests are offered by reference laboratories or research

TABLE 9-7 LABORATORY EVALUATION OF IMMUNODEFICIENCIES

FUNCTION TESTED	LABORATORY TEST	INTERPRETATION OF TEST
Tests of Humoral Immune Function		
Antibody production	Total immunoglobulin levels	Presence of antibody-producing B cells
	Levels of isohemagglutinins	Capacity to produce specific IgM antibodies
	Levels of antibodies against vaccines—especially diphtheria and tetanus toxoids	Capacity to produce specific IgG antibodies
B-cell numbers	Numbers of lymphocytes with surface immunoglobulin	Presence of circulating B cells
Tests of Cellular Immune Function		
Delayed hypersensitivity	Skin test reaction against previously encountered antigens—especially *Candida albicans* or tetanus toxoid	Presence of antigen-responsive T cells and skin test cellular interactions (e.g., lymphokine activity and macrophage function)
T-cell numbers	Numbers of T cells forming rosettes with sheep erythrocytes or expressing membrane CD3 or CD11 antigen	Presence of circulating T cells
T-cell proliferation in vitro	Proliferative response to nonspecific mitogens (e.g., phytohemagglutinin)	Capacity of all T cells to divide in response to nonspecific stimulation (mitogens)
	Proliferative response to antigens (e.g., tetanus toxoid)	Capacity of antigen-reactive T cells to respond to antigen

laboratories. These include quantification of individual complement components, in vitro proliferation (mitogenic response) of T or B cells to antigens or nonspecific mitogens, and a variety of tests of phagocyte function (e.g., nitroblue tetrazolium test [NBT] for hexose-monophosphate shunt activity, specific tests for phagocytosis, chemotaxis, or bacterial killing).

Replacement Therapies for Immune Deficiencies

Gamma-Globulin Therapy

Individuals with B-cell deficiencies that cause hypogammaglobulinemia or agammaglobulinemia usually can be treated successfully with administration of gamma globulins, which are antibody-rich fractions prepared from plasma pooled from large numbers of donors. Administration of gamma globulin temporarily replaces the individual's antibodies. Antibodies from these preparations are removed slowly from the person's blood, with half of the antibodies being removed by 3 to 4 weeks. Thus individuals must be treated repeatedly to maintain a protective level of antibodies in the blood.

Commercial gamma-globulin preparations are usually administered intramuscularly or by intravenous (IV) infusion. The dosage varies among individuals and is primarily determined by body weight. The schedule and dosage are also determined according to titers of circulating immunoglobulins and the incidence of infections in the individual. Commercial gamma-globulin preparations usually contain small amounts of IgM and IgA. Individuals with selective IgA deficiency occasionally develop allergic reactions to IgA in gamma-globulin preparations.[43]

Individuals who need larger amounts of IgM or IgA can be given fresh frozen plasma in monthly IV infusions. Complications associated with plasma therapy include the potential transmission of hepatitis or AIDS. The plasma is irradiated to destroy immunocompetent T cells and to avoid GVHD in individuals with accompanying T-cell deficiencies. Administration of fresh frozen plasma is successful in individuals with WAS (IgM deficient), AT (IgA deficient), or complement component deficiencies.

Transplantation and Transfusion

Several primary immune deficiencies originate from defects in lymphoid stem cells that interfere with their development in the primary lymphoid organs. Some of these (e.g., SCID, WAS, leukocyte adhesion defect) have benefited from replacement of stem cells through transplantation of bone marrow, umbilical cord cells, or other cell populations that are rich in stem cells.

The source of donor cells, particularly bone marrow, may contain a mixed population of stem cells and more mature T lymphocytes. In order to avoid GVHD, the preferred donor would be matched with the recipient for HLA antigens. Several other diseases involving depletion of the bone marrow (i.e., aplastic anemia, leukemia requiring eradication of tumor cells in the marrow) also are treated by bone marrow transplantation. At least 75% of bone marrow transplants between individuals who are matched for HLA-A, HLA-B, HLA-C, and HLA-DR are accepted. In immunocompetent recipients, most rejections of HLA-matched transplants occur because of recognition of minor histocompatibility antigens by individuals who have received multiple blood transfusions and are, as a result, sensitized against those antigens, which are not evaluated in tissue typing. For stem cell transplants, differences in minor histocompatibility antigens may lead to GVHD. Because HLA antigens are inherited in a codominant fashion, the preferred donor would be a relative, especially a sibling. Although the donor is not tested for minor histocompatibility antigens, the use of a close relative also would minimize differences at those loci.

Chronic GVHD appears in 30% to 50% of transplants between HLA-matched siblings and 60% to 70% of transplants between unrelated donors. Symptoms may appear about 4 to 7 months after the transplant, but may begin much earlier or later. Depletion of T cells from bone marrow before transplantation significantly lowers the incidence of both acute and chronic GVHD. One method of doing this is to infuse the graft with monoclonal antibody against plasma membrane antigens found only on mature T cells. Another method is to use fetal tissue as the graft. For example, fetal liver, which contains stem cells but not immunocompetent lymphocytes, is sometimes grafted in place of bone marrow if an HLA-matched donor cannot be found.

Steroids are commonly used to suppress GVHD in recipients of bone marrow transplants performed to treat certain malignancies or primary immune deficiencies. In cases where steroids are ineffective, promising new data support the use of **mesenchymal stem cells (MSCs)**.[44] Stem cells are relatively undifferentiated cells and can be obtained from a variety of sources (e.g., embryos, bone marrow, adult tissues). MSCs are present in all adult tissues. These particular stem cells undergo differentiation into other cell types and, more importantly, have potent immunosuppressive properties. Several recent clinical trials have demonstrated complete suppression of GVHD in a large number of recipients of MSCs.[45]

One therapy for deficiency diseases in which the individual lacks a thymus or thymic function (e.g., DiGeorge syndrome, ataxia-telangiectasia, or chronic mucocutaneous candidiasis) is reconstitution of thymic function. The procedure involves transplantation of fetal thymic tissue, which lacks immunocompetent T cells, or thymic epithelial cells (the cells that produce the thymic hormones) from which mature T cells have been removed. In some individuals transplantation increases the number of circulating mature T cells, but in most cases improvement is only temporary.

Enzymatic defects that cause SCID (e.g., adenosine deaminase deficiency) have been treated successfully with transfusions of glycerol frozen-packed erythrocytes. The donor erythrocytes contain the needed enzyme and can, at least temporarily, provide sufficient enzyme for normal lymphocyte function. An alternative method is administration of purified adenosine deaminase that has been stabilized with polyethylene glycol (PEG).

Treatment with Soluble Immune Modulators

The administration of soluble materials that affect lymphocyte function can restore T-cell function, especially in individuals with WAS or chronic mucocutaneous candidiasis. Successful for some individuals is the use of transfer factor, a low-molecular-weight nucleoprotein prepared from lymphocyte lysates, which can confer specific reactivity against certain antigens. Thymosin, a thymic hormone, also has been used, although with limited success. Cytokine therapy also has been effective in some cases of chronic granulomatous disease.

Gene Therapy

The first successful therapeutic replacement of defective genes was performed in two girls with SCID caused by an ADA deficiency.[46] The normal gene for ADA was cloned and inserted into a retroviral vector.[47] The gene for ADA replaced some retroviral genes, resulting in a virus that carried the normal human gene but did not cause disease. The virus was used to infect bone marrow stem cells from these children. The retrovirus inserted the normal ADA gene into the individuals' genetic material. The genetically altered stem cells were infused into the children, resulting in reconstitution of their immune systems. Gene therapy has now been used to successfully reconstitute the immune systems in individuals with ADA deficiency, X-linked SCID, and WAS.[48] However, the treatment trials have not been without some major complications, such as leukemia, that raise questions concerning the use of retroviral vectors for the insertion of new genes.

SUMMARY REVIEW

Hypersensitivity: Allergy, Autoimmunity, and Alloimmunity

1. Inappropriate immune responses are misdirected responses against the host's own tissues (autoimmunity); directed responses against beneficial foreign tissues, such as transfusions or transplants (alloimmunity); exaggerated responses against environmental antigens (allergy); or insufficient responses to protect the host (immune deficiency).
2. Allergy, autoimmunity, and alloimmunity are collectively known as hypersensitivity reactions.
3. Mechanisms of hypersensitivity are classified as type I (IgE-mediated) reactions, type II (tissue-specific) reactions, type III (immune complex–mediated) reactions, and type IV (cell-mediated) reactions.
4. Hypersensitivity reactions can be immediate (developing within minutes to a few hours) or delayed (developing within several hours or days).
5. Anaphylaxis, the most rapid immediate hypersensitivity reaction, is an explosive reaction that occurs within minutes of reexposure to the antigen and can lead to cardiovascular shock.
6. Allergens are antigens that cause allergic responses.
7. Type I (IgE-mediated) reactions are mediated through the binding of IgE to Fc receptors on mast cells and cross-linking of IgE by antigens that bind to the Fab portions of IgE. Cross-linking causes mast cell degranulation and the release of histamine (the most potent mediator) and other inflammatory substances.
8. Histamine enhances the chemotaxis of eosinophils into sites of type I allergic reactions.
9. Atopic individuals tend to produce higher quantities of IgE and to have more Fc receptors for IgE on their mast cells.
10. Type II (tissue-specific) reactions are caused by five possible mechanisms: complement-mediated lysis, opsonization and phagocytosis, neutrophil-mediated tissue damage, antibody-dependent cell-mediated cytotoxicity, and modulation of cellular function.
11. Type III (immune complex–mediated) reactions are caused by the formation of immune complexes that are deposited in target tissues, where they activate the complement cascade, generating chemotactic fragments that attract neutrophils into the inflammatory site. Neutrophils release lysosomal enzymes that result in tissue damage.

SUMMARY REVIEW—cont'd

12. Intermediate-sized immune complexes are the most likely to have severe pathologic consequences.
13. Immune complex disease can be a systemic reaction, such as serum sickness, or a localized response, such as the Arthus reaction.
14. Type IV (cell-mediated) reactions are caused by either cytotoxic T lymphocytes (Tc cells) or lymphokine-producing Th1 cells.
15. Typical allergens include pollen, molds and fungi, certain foods (milk, eggs, fish), animals, certain drugs, cigarette smoke, and house dust.
16. Clinical manifestations of allergic reactions usually are confined to the areas of initial intake or contact with the allergen. Ingested allergens induce gastrointestinal symptoms, airborne allergens induce respiratory tract or skin manifestations, and contact allergens induce allergic responses at the site of contact.
17. Autoimmunity is a breakdown of immunologic homeostasis, the immune system's tolerance of self-antigens. Central tolerance develops during the embryonic period. Peripheral tolerance is maintained in secondary lymphoid organs by regulatory T lymphocytes or antigen-presenting dendritic cells.
18. Autoimmune disease can be caused by the exposure of a previously sequestered antigen, the development of a neoantigen, the complications of infectious disease, the emergence of a forbidden clone of lymphocytes, or the consequence of ineffective peripheral tolerance.
19. Alloimmunity is the immune system's reaction against antigens on the tissues of other members of the same species.
20. Alloimmune disorders include transient neonatal disease, in which the maternal immune system becomes sensitized against antigens expressed by the fetus; transplant rejection; and transfusion reactions, in which the immune system of the recipient of an organ transplant or blood transfusion reacts against foreign antigens on the donor's cells.
21. SLE is a chronic, multisystem, inflammatory disease and is one of the most serious of the autoimmune disorders. SLE is characterized by the production of a large variety of autoantibodies.
22. Hyperacute graft rejection (preexisting antibody) is immediate and rare, acute rejection is cell mediated and occurs days to months after transplantation, and chronic rejection is caused by inflammatory damage to endothelial cells as a result of a weak cell-mediated reaction.
23. Red blood cell antigens may be the targets of autoimmune or alloimmune reactions. The most important of these, because they provoke the strongest humoral immune response, are the ABO and Rh systems.

Deficiencies in Immunity

1. Disorders resulting from immune deficiency are the clinical sequelae of impaired function of components of the immune or inflammatory response, phagocytes, or complement.
2. Immune deficiency is the failure of mechanisms of self-defense to function in their normal capacity.
3. Immune deficiencies are either congenital (primary) or acquired (secondary). Primary immune deficiencies are caused by genetic defects that disrupt lymphocyte development, whereas secondary immune deficiencies are secondary to disease or other physiologic alterations.
4. The clinical hallmark of immune deficiency is a propensity to unusual or recurrent severe infections. The type of infection usually reflects the immune system defect.
5. The most common infections in individuals with defects of the cell-mediated immune response are fungal and viral, whereas infections in individuals with defects of the humoral immune response or complement function are primarily bacterial.
6. Defects in B-cell function are diverse, ranging from a complete lack of the human bursal equivalent function, the lymphoid organs required for B-cell maturation (as in Bruton's agammaglobulinemia), to deficiencies in a single class of immunoglobulins (e.g., selective IgA deficiency).
7. DiGeorge syndrome (congenital thymic aplasia or hypoplasia) is characterized by complete or partial lack of the thymus (resulting in depressed T-cell immunity) and the parathyroid glands (resulting in hypocalcemia) and the presence of cardiac anomalies.
8. SCID is a total lack of T-cell function and a severe (either partial or total) lack of B-cell function. SCID can result from mutations in critical enzymes (ADA deficiency, PNP deficiency), in cytokine receptors (X-linked SCID, JAK3 deficiency, IL-7 receptor deficiency), or in antigen receptors (RAG-1/RAG-2 deficiencies, CD45 deficiency, CD3 deficiency, ZAP-70 deficiency). Other combined defects may result from deficiencies in antigen-presenting molecules (bare lymphocyte syndrome), cytoskeletal proteins (WAS), or DNA repair (ataxia-telangiectasia).
9. Almost any portion of the complement cascade may be defective. The most severe defect is C3 deficiency, which results in recurrent life-threatening bacterial infections. Defects in proteins of the membrane attack complex usually result in unusual disseminated infections with bacteria of the *Neisseria* spp.
10. Defects in phagocyte function, which include insufficient numbers of phagocytes or defects of chemotaxis, phagocytosis, or killing, can result in recurrent life-threatening infections such as septicemia and disseminated pyogenic lesions.
11. Acquired immunodeficiencies are caused by superimposed conditions, such as aging, malnutrition, infections, malignancies, physical or psychologic trauma, environmental factors, some medical treatments, or other diseases.
12. Deficiencies in immunity usually are treated by replacement therapy. Deficient antibody production is treated by replacement of missing immunoglobulins with commercial gamma-globulin preparations. Lymphocyte deficiencies are treated with the replacement of host lymphocytes with transplants of bone marrow, fetal liver, or fetal thymus from a donor.

KEY TERMS

ABO blood group, 278
Acute rejection, 280
Adenosine deaminase (ADA) deficiency, 286
Agammaglobulinemia, 284
Allergen, 270
Allergy, 262
Alloimmune disease, 277
Alloimmunity, 263, 276
Anaphylaxis, 263
Antibody-dependent cell-mediated cytotoxicity (ADCC), 267
Arthus reaction, 270
Ataxia-telangiectasia (AT), 287
Atopic, 271
Atopic dermatitis, 273
Autoimmune disease, 263
Autoimmunity, 262
Autosomal agammaglobulinemia, 284
Autosomal hyper-IgM syndrome, 284
Bare lymphocyte syndrome, 286
Blocking antibody, 273
Blood group antigen, 278
B-lymphocyte deficiency, 284
Bruton's agammaglobulinemia, 284
C1 deficiency, 287
C2 deficiency, 287
C3 deficiency, 287
C4 deficiency, 287
C9 deficiency, 288
C3 receptor deficiency, 289
Chédiak-Higashi syndrome, 289
Chronic granulomatous disease (CGD), 289
Chronic mucocutaneous candidiasis, 285
Chronic rejection, 281
Combined T- and B-lymphocyte deficiency, 284
Common variable immune deficiency, 285
Complement deficiency, 284
Complete blood count (CBC), 292
Contact dermatitis, 273
Cross-reactive antibody (T cell), 275
Cryoglobulin, 270
Cyclic neutropenia, 289
Cytotropic antibody, 265
Defective class-switch, 284
Delayed hypersensitivity reaction, 263
Desensitization, 273
DiGeorge syndrome, 281
Factor H deficiency, 288
Factor I deficiency, 288
Graft-versus-host disease (GVHD), 292
Hyperacute rejection, 280
Hypersensitivity, 262
Hypocomplemententemic, 269
Hypogammaglobulinemia, 284
IgG subclass deficiency, 284
IL-7 receptor deficiency, 286
Immediate hypersensitivity reaction, 263
Immune deficiency, 281
Immunologic homeostasis, 263
Immunologically privileged site, 274
Isohemagglutinin, 278
JAK3 deficiency, 286
Leukocyte adhesion deficiency (LAD), 289
Mannose-binding lectin (MBL) deficiency, 287
Mesenchymal stem cell (MSC), 294
MHC class I deficiency, 286
MHC class II deficiency, 286
Microchimerism, 275
Molecular mimicry, 275
Myeloperoxidase deficiency, 289
Neoantigen, 275
Phagocytic deficiency, 284
Primary (congenital) immune deficiency, 281
Properdin deficiency, 288
Purine nucleoside phosphorylase (PNP) deficiency, 286
RAG-1 deficiency, 286
RAG-2 deficiency, 286
Raynaud phenomenon, 270
Reagin, 265
Reticular dysgenesis, 286
Rh blood group, 279
Secondary (acquired) immune deficiency, 281
Selective IgA deficiency, 285
Serum sickness, 270
Severe combined immune deficiency (SCID), 286
Severe congenital neutropenia, 289
Systemic lupus erythematosus (SLE), 277
Tissue-specific antigen, 265
T-lymphocyte deficiency, 284
Transient hypogammaglobulinemia of infancy, 290
Type I (immunoglobulin E [IgE]–mediated) hypersensitivity reactions, 263
Type II (tissue-specific) hypersensitivity reaction, 263
Type III (immune complex–mediated) hypersensitivity reaction, 263
Type IV (cell-mediated) hypersensitivity reaction, 263
Universal donor, 278
Universal recipient, 278
Urticaria (hives), 272
Wheal and flare reaction, 272
Wiskott-Aldrich syndrome (WAS), 286
X-linked hyper-IgM syndrome, 284
X-linked SCID, 286

REFERENCES

1. Gell PGH, Coombs RRA, Lachman PT: *Clinical aspects of immunology*, Oxford, England, 1975, Blackwell Scientific.
2. Simons FER: Anaphylaxis, *J Allergy Clin Immunol* 125(2):S161–S181, 2010.
3. Portier P, Richet C: De l'action anaphylactique de certains venins, *Comptes Rendus Societie Biologie (Paris)* 54:170, 1902.
4. Stone KD, Prussin C, Metcalfe DD: IgE, mast cells, basophils, and eosinophils, *J Allergy Clin Immunol* 125(2):S73–S80, 2010.
5. Franklyn JA, Boelaert K: Thyrotoxicosis, *Lancet* 379(9821):1155–1166, 2012.
6. Pirquet C, Schick B: *Serum sickness*, Leipzig, Germany, 1905, Franz Denticke.
7. Arthus M, Breton M: Lésions cutanées produites par les injections de sérum, *Compt Rendus Soc Biol* 55:817, 1903.
8. Roep BO, Peakman M: Diabetogenic T lymphocytes in human type 1 diabetes, *Curr Opin Immunol* 23(6):746–753, 2011.
9. Koch R: Fortsetzung der mitteilungen, ber ein heilmittel gegen tuberkulose, *Deutsche Med Wochenschr* 9:101, 1891.
10. Lambrecht BN, Leung DYM: Initiation and maintenance of allergic inflammation: team work at the interface of innate and adaptive immunity, *Curr Opin Immunol* 23(6):769–771, 2011.
11. Holloway JW, Yang IA, Holgate ST: Genetics of allergic disease, *J Allergy Clin Immunol* 125(2):S81–S94, 2010.
12. Dykewicz MS, Hamilos DL: Rhinitis and sinusitis, *J Allergy Clin Immunol* 125(2):S103–S115, 2010.
13. Burks AW et al: ICON: food allergy, *J Allergy Clin Immunol* 129(4): 906–920, 2012.
14. Mousallem T, Burks AW: Immunology in the Clinic Review Series; focus on allergies: immunotherapy for food allergy, *Clin Exp Immunol* 167(1):26–31, 2011.
15. Hamilton RG: Clinical laboratory assessment of immediate-type hypersensitivity, *J Allergy Clin Immunol* 125(2):S284–S296, 2010.
16. Stokes JR, Casale TB: Allergic rhinitis and asthma: celebrating 100 years of immunotherapy, *Curr Opin Immunol* 23(6):808–813, 2011.
17. Berin MC, Sicherer S: Food allergy: mechanisms and therapeutics, *Curr Opin Immunol* 23(6):794–800, 2011.
18. Kaplan DH, Igyârtô BZ, Gaspari AA: Early immune events in the induction of allergic contact dermatitis, *Nat Rev Immunol* 12(2):114–124, 2012.
19. Novak N, Leung DYM: Advances in atopic dermatitis, *Curr Opin Immunol* 23(6):778–783, 2011.
20. Khan DA, Solensky R: Drug allergy, *J Allergy Clin Immunol* 125(2): S126–S137, 2010.
21. Peden D, Reed CE: Environmental and occupational allergies, *J Allergy Clin Immunol* 125(2):S150–S160, 2010.
22. Coppieters KT, et al: Immunology in the clinic review series: focus on type 1 diabetes and viruses: the role of viruses in type 1 diabetes: a difficult dilemma, *Clin Exp Immunol* 168(1):5–11, 2011.
23. Doyle HA, Mamula MJ: Autoantigenesis: the evolution of protein modifications in autoimmune disease, *Curr Opin Immunol* 24(1): 112–118, 2012.
24. Tsokos GC: Systemic lupus erythematosus, *N Engl J Med* 365(22):2110–2121, 2011.
25. Arbuckle MR et al: Development of autoantibodies before the clinical onset of systemic lupus erythematosus, *N Engl J Med* 349(16):1526–1533, 2003.
26. American College of Rheumatology: *Systemic lupus erythematosus*, 2012 Available at www.rheumatology.org/practice/clinical/patients/diseases_and_conditions/lupus.asp.
27. Lux A et al: The pro and anti-inflammatory activities of immunoglobulin G, *Ann Rheum Dis* 69(Suppl 1):i92–i96, 2010.
28. Lee S, Ballow M: Monoclonal antibodies and fusion proteins and their complications: targeting B cells in autoimmune diseases, *J Allergy Clin Immunol* 125(2):S814–S820, 2010.
29. Levine MH, Abt PL: Treatment options and strategies for antibody mediated rejection after renal transplantation, *Semin Immunol* 24(2):136–142, 2012.

30. Issa F, Chandrasekharan D, Wood KJ: Regulatory T cells as modulators of chronic allograft dysfunction, *Curr Opin Immunol* 23(5):648–654, 2011.
31. Smith RN, Colvin RB: Chronic alloantibody mediated rejection, *Semin Immunol* 24(2):115–121, 2012.
32. Arkwright PD, Gennery AR: Ten warning signs of primary immunodeficiency: a new paradigm is needed for the 21st century, *Ann N Y Acad Sci* 1238:7–14, 2011.
33. Notarangelo LD: Primary immunodeficiencies, *J Allergy Clin Immunol* 125(2):S182–S194, 2010.
34. National Institute of Child Health and Human Development, NIH, DHHS: *Primary immunodeficiency*Washington, DC, 2003, Government Printing Office. Available at www.nichd.nih.gov/publications/pubs/primary_immuo.cfm. Updated 04/07/2008.
35. Vale AM, Schroeder HW Jr: Clinical consequences of defects in B-cell development, *J Allergy Clin Immunol* 125(4):778–787, 2010.
36. Bruton OC: Agammaglobulinemia, *Pediatrics* 9(6):722–728, 1952.
37. DiGeorge AM: Congenital absence of the thymus and its immunologic consequences. In Bergsma D, McKusick FA, editors: *Immunologic deficiency diseases in man, National Foundation—March of Dimes original article series*, Baltimore, 1968, Williams & Wilkins.
38. Demczuk S, Aurias A: DiGeorge syndrome and related syndromes associated with 22q11.2 deletions, *Ann Genet* 38:59, 1995.
39. Kuijpers T, Lutter R: Inflammation and repeated infections in CGD: two sides of a coin, *Cell Mol Life Sci* 69(1):7–15, 2012.
40. Chinen J, Shearer WT: Secondary immunodeficiencies, including HIV infection, *J Allergy Clin Immunol* 125(2):S195–S203, 2010.
41. Cohen MS, et al: Acute HIV-1 infection, *N Engl J Med* 364(20): 1943–1954, 2011.
42. Oliveira JB, Fleisher TA: Laboratory evaluation of primary immunodeficiencies, *J Allergy Clin Immunol* 125(2):S297–S305, 2010.
43. Rachid R, Bonilla FA: The role of anti-IgA antibodies in causing adverse reactions to gamma globulin infusion in immunodeficient patients: a comprehensive review of the literature, *J Allergy Clin Immunol* 129(3):628–634, 2012.
44. Brignier AC, Gerwirtz AM: Embryonic and adult stem cell therapy, *J Allergy Clin Immunol* 125(2):S336–S344, 2010.
45. Toubai T et al: Mesenchymal stem cells for treatment and prevention of graft-versus-host disease after allogeneic hematopoietic cell transplantation, *Curr Stem Cell Res Therapy* 4(4):252–259, 2009.
46. Blaese RM: Development of gene therapy for immunodeficiency: adenosine deaminase deficiency, *Pediatr Res* 33(Suppl 1):S49–S53, 1993.
47. Onodera M et al: Gene therapy for severe combined immunodeficiency caused by adenosine deaminase deficiency: improved retroviral vectors for clinical trials, *Acta Haematol* 101(2):89–96, 1999.
48. Fischer A, Hacein-Bey-Abina S, Cavazzana-Calvo M: Gene therapy for primary adaptive immune deficiencies, *J Allergy Clin Immunol* 127(6):1356–1359, 2011.

CHAPTER

10

Infection

Neal S. Rote and Sue E. Huether

evolve WEBSITE

http://evolve.elsevier.com/McCance/

- Review Questions and Answers
- Animations
- Online Course: Module 7

CHAPTER OUTLINE

For most of human history infectious disease was the primary disease-related cause of death; bubonic/pneumonic plague (The Black Death) of the 14th century killed more than 50 million people worldwide, the Spanish influenza of 1918 to 1919 killed between 50 and 100 million people within 2 years, and it was not uncommon for frequent regional outbreaks of diseases such as smallpox or cholera to kill hundreds of thousands of people.[1] Modern health care has shown great progress in preventing and treating infectious diseases through the success of public health initiatives, vaccination programs, and the use of antibiotics. The greatest progress has occurred in developed countries where death from infections is most common among those with debilitating diseases, nutritional deficiencies, or immunosuppression. Death from influenza and pneumonia was the eighth leading cause of death in the United States in 2011.[2] As a result of these initiatives, smallpox has been eradicated from the globe (the last reported case was in 1975 in Somalia), measles is almost eradicated in the Western Hemisphere, and many diseases, such as tuberculosis and polio, are on the decline. Although the advent of sanitary living conditions, clean water, uncontaminated food, vaccinations, and antimicrobials had improved the health in many countries, infectious disease remains a significant threat to life in many parts of the world, including India, Africa, and Southeast Asia. The impact of differences in economic prosperity is significant.[2a] The leading causes of death in high-income countries were heart disease, stroke, and other cerebrovascular diseases; cancers of the respiratory tract; and Alzheimer disease and other dementias, with lower respiratory tract infections (influenza and pneumonia) the sole infectious cause in the top 10. In low-income countries, where the implementation of

TABLE 10-1 EXAMPLES OF EMERGENT INFECTIONS

YEAR	DISEASE	CAUSATIVE AGENT	SITE OF DISCOVERY
1955	Orally transmitted non-A, non-B infectious hepatitis	Hepatitis E virus	India
1967	Viral hemorrhagic fever	Marburg virus	Germany
1969	Lassa fever	Lassa virus	Nigeria
1976	Ebola hemorrhagic fever	Ebola virus	Zaire and Sudan
1976	Legionnaires disease	*Legionella pneumophila*	United States
1978	Toxic shock syndrome	Toxin-producing strains of *Staphylococcus* spp.	United States
1981	Acquired immunodeficiency syndrome (AIDS)	Human immunodeficiency virus	United States
1982	Lyme disease	*Borrelia burgdorferi*	Northeast United States
1982	Hemolytic-uremic syndrome, bloody diarrhea	*Escherichia coli* 0157:H7	United States, Japan
1983	Peptic ulcer disease	*Helicobacter pylori*	Australia
1986	Roseola	Human herpesvirus 6	United States
1989	Non-A, non-B infectious hepatitis, hepatocellular carcinoma	Hepatitis C virus	United States
1992	Cholera	*Vibrio cholerae* 0139	Indonesia
1993	Hemorrhagic fever with renal syndrome	Hantavirus	Korea
1994	Kaposi sarcoma	Human herpesvirus 8	United States
1994	Encephalitis transmitted from horses to humans	Hendra virus	Australia
1995	Bovine spongiform encephalopathy (BSE or "mad cow" disease)	Prion, variant of Creutzfeldt-Jakob disease agent	United Kingdom
1999	Encephalitis transmitted from pigs to humans	Nipah virus	Malaysia
2003	SARS (severe acute respiratory syndrome)	SARS-associated coronavirus	China
2006	Lymph node infection in individuals with chronic granulomatous disease	*Granulobacter bethesdensis*	United States
2007	New strain of Ebola hemorrhagic fever	*Bundidugyo ebolavirus*	Uganda
2007	Encephalitis and myocarditis	Saffold virus	United States
2013	Influenza A strain	Avian virus	China

programs to prevent infection has been less effective, 6 of the top 10 causes of death are caused by infection: lower respiratory tract infections (#1), diarrheal diseases (#2), HIV/AIDS (#3), malaria (#5), tuberculosis (#7), and neonatal infections (#10).

Despite the widespread implementation of progressive public health and immunization policies, infectious disease remains a significant cause of morbidity and mortality because of the emergence of previously unknown infections, the reemergence and spread of old infections that were thought to be under control, and the development of infectious agents that are resistant to multiple antibiotics. The causes for these occurrences are numerous and include the following:

- Vast and rapid urbanization in many areas of the world, resulting in a breakdown in public health programs and a more rapid spread of infection
- Poverty and social inequality
- War and famine
- Global travel, allowing more rapid spread of disease from isolated areas to virtually any point around the world in a few hours
- Globalization of the food supply
- Human encroachment into wilderness areas, resulting in contact with previously sequestered infectious agents
- Practice of prescribing antibiotics excessively or not taking antibiotics for a complete course of therapy, or, even when appropriately used, facilitates emergence of antibiotic-resistant microorganisms
- Decreases in federal research budgets to study infectious disease
- Denial of a problem by governments, allowing infections to spread in an uncontrolled way
- Diminished use of effective insecticides
- Increased global warming, allowing insect vectors to spread into and breed in areas that were previously too cool for them

EMERGING INFECTIONS

The emergence of previously unknown infections is not a new event in human history. However, the current rate may be unprecedented.[3] Within 1 generation, more than 40 previously unknown infections have arisen, and some examples are presented in Table 10-1. Several have extremely high mortality rates of more than 50% including severe acute respiratory syndrome (SARS) (in those older than 65 years), Ebola virus, Marburg virus, "mad cow" disease, Nipah virus (up to 75%), and acquired immunodeficiency syndrome (AIDS) (almost 100% in untreated persons). However, most either spread very slowly (e.g., AIDS) or initially appear in relatively isolated areas and are effectively controlled by quarantine (e.g., Ebola virus). Although none of these infections has developed into the worldwide scourges portrayed in the Hollywood movies *Andromeda Strain* and *I Am Legend*, the potential of reversion to more rapidly spreading variants is a concern of public health agencies worldwide.

Concurrently, the incidence and spread of at least 20 previously known infections are increasing. A new strain of cholera that arose in Indonesia in 1961 has spread to Africa and in 1991 to South America. Malaria, dengue fever, and yellow fever are reemerging in areas where they had been eliminated or were unknown. The incidence of tuberculosis is increasing in countries that had reported declines and has risen by almost 33% between the mid-1980s and early 1990s. Diphtheria has reemerged as a major health issue in Russia. In 1994 plague was reported in India after being dormant for a generation. War has led to outbreaks of Marburg hemorrhagic fever during civil war in Angola during 1975 to 2002 and cholera in the Democratic Republic of the Congo among Rwandan refugees in 1994; about 50,000 refugees died from a combination of cholera and shigella dysentery. The spread of cholera, yellow fever, and epidemic meningococcal disease has rebounded. Decreased insect control programs that were previously successful have led to spread of vector-borne diseases: African trypanosomiasis, dengue hemorrhagic fever, and malaria. Although the United States is relatively free of most of these diseases, the effects of global warming and relaxed control of vectors may result in resurgence. It should not be forgotten that in 1793 a yellow fever outbreak in Philadelphia killed 2000 of the city's 55,000 inhabitants and forced the U.S. government to abandon the city until the outbreak ceased. To date, outbreaks of locally acquired malaria in the United States have been rare. However, West Nile Virus, also spread by mosquitoes, appeared initially in the Western Hemisphere in 1999 in the New York City area and has spread throughout the continental United States, Canada, and Mexico.[4]

Many common and reemerging infections have become antibiotic and drug resistant. *Streptococcus pneumoniae,* a common cause of otitis media, pneumonia, and bacteremia, has been treated routinely and successfully with penicillin. Now at least 25% of isolates are penicillin resistant, and some are resistant to multiple antibiotics. Multiple antibiotic-resistant forms of *Staphylococcus aureus,* a primary cause of infections of wounds, surgical incisions, and catheter insertion, are endemic in some hospitals. Some forms of this microorganism once were sensitive only to a single antibiotic, vancomycin, and now have become vancomycin-resistant. Antimicrobial resistance is now routinely observed in tuberculosis, diarrheal diseases, hospital-acquired infections, malaria, meningitis, respiratory tract infections, sexually transmitted infections (STIs), and human immunodeficiency virus (HIV).

Added to this collage of microbiologic dangers is the rising risk of bioterrorism. Agents such as smallpox, anthrax, and plague are continuing threats to public health and safety. All healthcare providers should have information about the characteristics and clinical manifestations of these biologic agents. The theoretical threat of bioterrorism became real in 2001 when letters containing anthrax were mailed; 22 individuals became infected and 5 died.

MICROORGANISMS AND HUMANS: A DYNAMIC RELATIONSHIP

For many microorganisms the human body is a hospitable site in which to grow and flourish because of its sufficient nutrients and appropriate conditions of temperature and humidity. In many cases a symbiotic relationship exists, in which both humans and microorganisms benefit (Box 10-1). These microorganisms make up the *normal microbiome*—the resident microorganisms found in different parts of the body, including the skin, mouth, gastrointestinal tract, respiratory tract, and genital tract[5] (see Chapter 7). For instance, the normal bacterial microbiome of the human gut is provided with nutrients from ingested food and in exchange produce enzymes that facilitate the digestion and use of many of the more complex molecules found in the human diet, produce antibacterial factors (e.g., bacteriocins, colicins) that prevent colonization by pathogenic microorganisms, and produce usable metabolites (e.g., vitamin K, B vitamins). This beneficial homeostasis is normally maintained through the physical integrity of the gut and other mechanisms that sequester these microorganisms on the mucosal surface.

BOX 10-1 THE MANY RELATIONSHIPS BETWEEN HUMANS AND MICROORGANISMS

Symbiosis: Benefits only the human; no harm to the microorganism
Mutualism: Benefits the human and the microorganism
Commensalism: Benefits only the microorganism; no harm to the human
Pathogenicity: Benefits the microorganism; harms the human
Opportunism: A situation in which benign microorganisms become pathogenic because of decreased human host resistance

MICROORGANISMS AND INFECTIONS

Process of Infection

The symbiotic relationship with the normal flora can be breached as a result of injury that compromises the physical protective barriers. Damage to the intestinal tract releases intestinal bacteria into the bloodstream, potentially leading to sepsis, shock, and death. Cuts in the skin may allow normally noninfectious bacteria (e.g., *S. aureus*) to cause local infections (e.g., abscesses, boils) and invade further and infect various organs. Symbiosis is also maintained by the immune and inflammatory systems. If those systems are compromised, many microorganisms will leave their normal sites and cause infection elsewhere in the body. Individuals with immune deficiencies easily become infected with *opportunistic microorganisms,* which normally would not cause disease but seize the opportunity to do so when a person's defensive systems are weakened or suppressed (see Chapter 9).

Unlike opportunistic infectious agents, *true pathogens* have devised means to circumvent the individual's defenses (discussed in Chapters 7 and 8) and directly cause infection. Successful infection with these agents is usually dependent on adequate numbers of microorganisms rather than compromise of the host's defenses.

From the perspective of the microorganisms that cause disease, the infectious process undergoes four separate stages of progression: colonization, invasion, multiplication, and spread.

Colonization

Infectious microorganisms usually exist in reservoirs, such as the environment (e.g., contaminated water, soil), animals, or another human who is infected or in a noninfectious state within the individual's normal microbiome. An individual may obtain an infectious microorganism from a reservoir by several means.

Infections contracted from animal reservoirs (zoonotic infections) may be transmitted by direct contact (e.g., transmission of the rabies virus through bites) or indirectly by means of vectors (e.g., insects). Mechanical vectors (e.g., housefly) passively transfer microorganisms from a contaminated site to an individual. Biologic vectors (e.g., fleas, lice, mosquitoes, ticks) transmit infectious microorganisms through bites and stings. Individuals can also become infected by direct exposure to contaminated materials, such as fecal-oral transmission through food or water (e.g., salmonella food poisoning, cholera, hepatitis A infection, polio, rotavirus infection) or soil (e.g., tetanus).

Human-to-human transmission may occur through aerosolized microorganisms in droplets (e.g., produced by coughing or sneezing), which is the primary means of transmission for respiratory tract infections (e.g., agents that cause the common cold, influenza, streptococcal sore throat, bacterial meningitis). Other infectious agents require physical contact (e.g., sexual contact, blood transfusion, direct contact with contaminated clothes or bandages, entrance through wounds or openings in the skin). Direct contact is usually required for transmission of sexually transmitted infections (STIs), hepatitis B virus, cytomegalovirus (CMV), herpes simplex virus, or warts. Some microorganisms have the capacity to spread from mother to child across the placenta (e.g., *Treponema pallidum, Listeria monocytogenes,* CMV, *Toxoplasma gondii*), ascending the birth canal or during delivery (e.g., group B *Streptococcus, Escherichia coli, Chlamydia trachomatis, Neisseria gonorrhoeae,* hepatitis B virus, HIV, *Candida albicans*), or through the breast milk (e.g., *S. aureus*). This is classified as *vertical transmission,* whereas spread from one person to another is *horizontal transmission.* In a very few instances, the infectious agent may develop airborne transmission. Effective *airborne transmission* may occur by the prolonged presence of aerosolized droplets released by respiration, exercise, or other body activity and has been observed with SARS, tuberculosis, norovirus, and smallpox.

After deposition in receptive environments for colonization, the microorganism stabilizes the adherence to the tissue through specific surface receptors. For instance, infectious agents that cause respiratory tract infections specifically bind to molecules found on respiratory epithelium. Adherence helps protect the microorganism from removal by mechanical nonspecific forces, such as coughing of respiratory mucus. The specificity of adherence results in a particular microorganism being limited to the locations where infections can occur **(tissue tropism),** such as the confinement of common cold viruses to producing respiratory tract infections.

Invasion

Once colonization has occurred the infectious agent can invade the surrounding tissue and, in many cases, other sites in the individual. Successful infectious agents have developed mechanisms to penetrate the tissues and evade the host's nonspecific and specific defenses (inflammation and immunity). Many of these are discussed throughout this chapter.

Multiplication

Within the warm and nutrient-filled environment of human tissue, most microorganisms undergo rapid multiplication with production of many new infectious progeny. Viral pathogens replicate within infected cells, and some bacteria are intracellular pathogens and replicate in macrophages and other cells.

Spread

Many successful pathogens produce localized infections without spread to other regions of the body (e.g., *Vibrio cholerae*). Others, however, are highly invasive and may enter the lymphatics, blood, and internal organs. Successful spread relies on a variety of virulence factors, including adhesion molecules, toxins, and protection against the individual's inflammatory and immune systems. Fungi, in particular, are opportunistic. In an individual with an intact immune system, the microorganism remains localized, whereas the infection may rapidly spread if the individual's immune or inflammatory systems are compromised.

Clinical Infectious Disease

From the perspective of the individual who is infected, the clinical process occurs in the following four distinct stages:

- *Incubation period*—the period from initial exposure to the infectious agent and the onset of the first symptoms, during which the microorganism has entered the individual, undergone initial colonization, and begun multiplying, but is yet in insufficient numbers to cause symptoms; this period may last from several hours to years
- *Prodromal stage*—the occurrence of initial symptoms, which are often very mild and include a feeling of discomfort and tiredness
- *Invasion period*—the pathogen is multiplying rapidly, invading farther and affecting the tissues at the site of initial colonization as well as other areas; the immune and inflammatory responses are being triggered; development of symptoms specifically related to the pathogen and symptoms related to the ongoing protective inflammatory response
- *Convalescence*—in most instances, the individual's immune and inflammatory systems have successfully removed the infectious agent, and symptoms decline; alternatively, the disease may be fatal or may enter a latency phase with resolution of symptoms until reactivation at a later time

Clinical manifestations of infectious disease vary, depending on the pathogen, the organ system affected, and the severity. Effects of infection may be acute, chronic, secondary to the immune and inflammatory responses, or a consequence of bacterial toxins or viral injury. Manifestations can arise directly from the infecting microorganism or its products; however, the majority of manifestations result from the host's inflammatory and immune responses. Infectious diseases typically begin with the nonspecific or general symptoms of fatigue, malaise, weakness, and loss of concentration. Generalized aching and loss of appetite are common complaints. However, the hallmark of most infectious diseases is fever.

Fever is not failure of the body to regulate temperature; rather, body temperature is being regulated at a higher level than

TABLE 10-2 HISTORIC EXAMPLES OF PANDEMICS

YEAR	CAUSE	SITE	ESTIMATED DEATHS
1347-1352	Bubonic plague (black death) (70% mortality rate)	Europe (worldwide)	50 million (a third of Europe's population); up to 100 million worldwide
1775-1782	Smallpox (35% mortality rate)	North America	>150,000
1829-1851	Cholera	Europe	Several hundred thousands
1914-1918	Typhus *(Rickettsia prowazekii)*, spread by body lice, 40% mortality rate	Europe during WWI	9 million
1916	Polio	United States	6000
1918-1919	Influenza (Spanish flu)	United States, became worldwide	20-40 million
1981-?	AIDS	Worldwide	>25 million
2009	Influenza H1N1	Worldwide	284,000

normal. Body temperature is regulated by nervous system feedback to the hypothalamus, which functions as a central thermostat (see Chapter 16). A large number of agents (pyrogens) can produce fever. In current classification, those pyrogens derived from outside the host are termed **exogenous pyrogens** and those produced by the individual are termed **endogenous pyrogens.** There is little evidence that exogenous pyrogens cause fever directly. Such pyrogens indirectly affect the hypothalamus through endogenous pyrogens released by cells of the host. A number of cytokines have been identified as endogenous pyrogens. They are interleukin-1 and interleukin-6 (IL-1 and IL-6, respectively), interferon (IFN), tumor necrosis factor (TNF), and others (see Figure 16-8). These cytokines seem to raise the thermoregulatory set point through stimulation of prostaglandin synthesis and turnover in both thermoregulatory (brain) and nonthermoregulatory (peripheral) tissue. Although it is generally believed that fever has a beneficial value in infection, the molecular mechanism behind the beneficial effects has not been established. Many investigators, however, consider fever as an adaptive host-defense response.

Several factors influence the capacity of a pathogen to cause disease.

- *Communicability:* The ability to spread from one individual to others and cause disease: measles and pertussis spread very easily; HIV is of lower communicability
- *Immunogenicity:* The ability of pathogens to induce an immune response
- *Infectivity:* The ability of the pathogen to invade and multiply in the host
- *Mechanism of action:* How the microorganism damages tissue
- *Pathogenicity:* The ability of an agent to produce disease—success depends on communicability, infectivity, extent of tissue damage, and virulence
- *Portal of entry:* The route by which a pathogenic microorganism infects the host: direct contact, inhalation, ingestion, or bites of an animal or insect
- *Toxigenicity:* The ability to produce soluble toxins or endotoxins, factors that greatly influence the pathogen's degree of virulence
- *Virulence:* The capacity of a pathogen to cause severe disease—for example, measles virus is of low virulence; rabies virus is highly virulent

Infectious diseases are also classified by their prevalence and spread within the community.

- *Endemic:* Diseases with relatively high, but constant, rates of infection in a particular population
- *Epidemic:* The number of new infections in a particular population greatly exceeds the number usually observed
- *Pandemic:* An epidemic that spreads over a large area, such as a continent or worldwide (Table 10-2)

Classes of Infectious Microorganisms

Infectious disease can be caused by microorganisms that range in size from 20 nm (poliovirus) to 10 m (tapeworm). Classes of pathogenic microorganisms and their characteristics are summarized in Table 10-3 and discussed in detail in the following sections.

Bacterial Infection

Bacteria are prokaryotic unicellular microorganisms with no nuclei, mitochondria, or membrane-bound organelles. They are generally divided into several groups.

- *"True bacteria"* divide by binary fission and may have a variety of morphologies, including cocci (spherical), bacilli (rod shaped), vibrios (comma-shaped rods), or spirilla (twisted, rod shaped). Most disease-causing bacteria fall into this classification.
- *Filamentous bacteria* may have branching, mycelium-like structures that resemble fungi. Examples include the mycobacteria *Mycobacterium tuberculosis* and *Mycobacterium leprae* that respectively cause tuberculosis and leprosy.
- *Spirochetes* are flexible spiral filaments that are motile. Most are anaerobic. Pertinent examples include *Borrelia recurrentis* (relapsing fever), *T. pallidum* (syphilis), and *Borrelia burgdorferi* (Lyme disease).
- *Mycoplasma* lack a rigid cell wall and are small and pleomorphic. They are the smallest and most simple members of the bacteria. *Mycoplasma pneumoniae* causes atypical pneumonia, and *Mycoplasma genitalium* is a suspected cause of urethritis and pelvic inflammatory disease.
- *Rickettsia* are strict intracellular parasites that can be rod-shaped, spherical, or pleomorphic. They are typically spread by insect vectors and cause Rocky Mountain spotted fever *(Rickettsia rickettsii)* and typhus *(Rickettsia prowazekii)*.

TABLE 10-3 CLASSES OF ORGANISMS INFECTIOUS TO HUMANS

CLASS	SIZE	SITE OF REPRODUCTION	EXAMPLE
Virus	20-300 nm	Intracellular	Poliomyelitis
Chlamydiae	200-1000 nm	Intracellular	Urethritis
Rickettsiae	300-1200 nm	Intracellular	Rocky Mountain spotted fever
Mycoplasma	125-350 nm	Extracellular	Atypical pneumonia
Bacteria	0.8-15 mcg	Skin	Staphylococcal wound infection
		Mucous membranes	Cholera
		Extracellular	Streptococcal pneumonia
		Intracellular	Tuberculosis
Fungi	2-200 mcg	Skin	Tinea pedis (athlete's foot)
		Mucous membranes	Candida (e.g., thrush)
		Extracellular	Sporotrichosis
		Intracellular	Histoplasmosis
Protozoa	1-50 mm	Mucosal	Giardiasis
		Extracellular	Sleeping sickness
Helminths	3 mm to 10 m	Intracellular	Trichinosis
		Extracellular	Filariasis

- *Chlamydia* are also strict intracellular parasites, but with more complex intracellular life cycles. The primary chlamydial pathogen is *Chlamydia trachomatis,* which causes the most common bacterial sexually transmitted infection (pelvic inflammatory disease) and eye infections (conjunctivitis).

Bacteria are also categorized as gram-negative or gram-positive. Gram-negative bacteria do not retain crystal violet dye in the Gram-staining process whereas gram-positive bacteria do retain crystal violet dye. Gram-negative bacteria also have a lipopolysaccharide (LPS) coat in the outer membrane, which consists of lipid A, a core polysaccharide, and O antigen. The LPS coat is also known as endotoxin (see Figure 10-1 and further discussion on p. 306). Common bacterial pathogens are listed in Table 10-4.

Transmission and Colonization. Transmission of bacterial infections occurs through the same routes generally described previously. Many pathogenic bacteria normally reside in humans without causing disease, for instance, *Streptococcus pyogenes* (pharyngitis), *S. pneumoniae* (pneumonia, meningitis), *Neisseria meningitidis* (meningitis), and *Haemophilus influenzae* type b (meningitis). In most cases they either are present in inadequate numbers to cause disease or are effectively controlled by local protective mechanisms. Others reside in nature and cause infection after being ingested or entering wounds (e.g., *V. cholerae* [cholera] in contaminated water or *Clostridium tetani* [tetanus] in contaminated soil).

A large number require human-to-human contact, including several that are unstable on environmental surfaces (e.g., *Bordetella pertussis* [whooping cough], *N. gonorrhoeae* [gonorrhea], *T. pallidum* [syphilis]). Even the human-to-human spread of infectious bacteria contracted initially from environmental reservoirs can be facilitated by certain aspects of the disease (e.g., the explosive diarrhea of cholera). Chlamydia, which may be contracted as an STI, can spread from the mother to child during childbirth and may establish long-term intracellular persistence in the newborn.

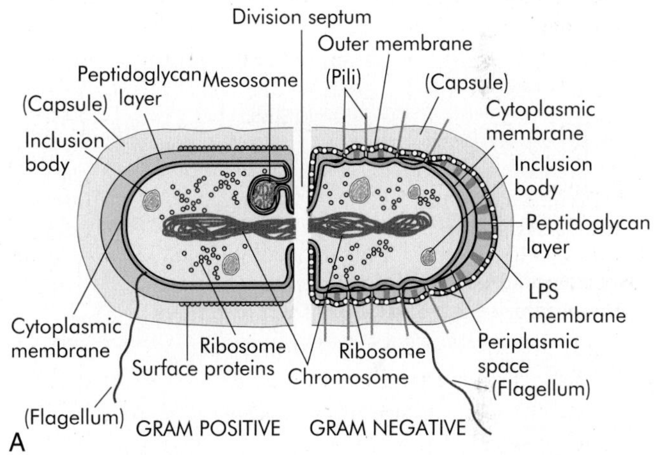

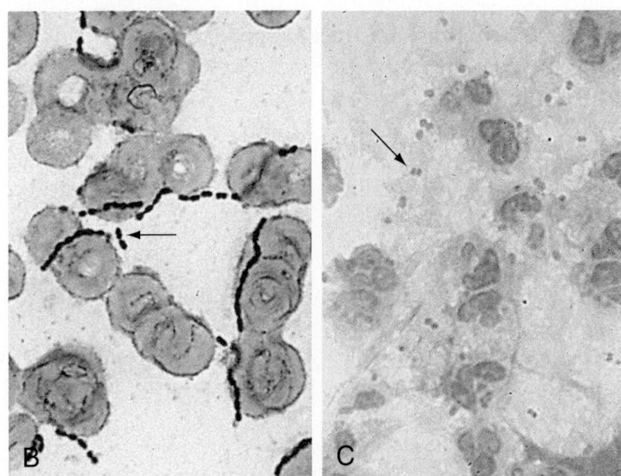

FIGURE 10-1 Gram-Positive and Gram-Negative Bacteria. A, The structure of the bacterial cell wall determines its staining characteristics with Gram stain. Gram-positive bacteria have a thick layer of peptidoglycan *(left).* Gram-negative bacteria have a thin peptidoglycan layer and an outer membrane of lipopolysaccharide (LPS) *(right).* **B,** Example of a gram-positive (darkly stained microorganisms, *arrow*) group A *Streptococcus.* This microorganism consists of cocci that frequently form chains. **C,** Example of a gram-negative (pink microorganisms, *arrow*) *Neisseria meningitidis* in cerebrospinal fluid. *Neisseria* form complexes of two cocci (diplococci).

TABLE 10-4 COMMON BACTERIAL INFECTIONS

MICROORGANISM	GRAM STAIN	RESPIRATORY PATHWAY	INTRACELLULAR OR EXTRACELLULAR
Respiratory Tract Infections			
Upper Respiratory Tract Infections			
Corynebacterium diphtheriae (diphtheria)	Gram +	Facultative anaerobic	Extracellular
Haemophilus influenzae	Gram –	Facultative anaerobic	Extracellular
Streptococcus pyogenes (group A)	Gram +	Facultative anaerobic	Extracellular
Otitis Media			
Haemophilus influenzae	Gram –	Facultative anaerobic	Extracellular
Moraxella catarrhalis	Gram –	Aerobic	Extracellular
Streptococcus pneumoniae	Gram +	Facultative anaerobic	Extracellular
Lower Respiratory Tract Infections			
Bacillus anthracis (pulmonary anthrax)	Gram +	Facultative anaerobic	Extracellular
Bordetella pertussis (whooping cough)	Gram –	Aerobic	Extracellular
Chlamydia pneumoniae	Not stainable	Aerobic	Obligate intracellular
Escherichia coli	Gram –	Facultative anaerobic	Extracellular
Haemophilus influenzae	Gram –	Facultative anaerobic	Extracellular
Klebsiella pneumoniae	Gram –	Facultative anaerobic	Extracellular
Legionella pneumophila	Gram –	Aerobic	Facultative intracellular
Mycobacterium tuberculosis	Weak gram +	Aerobic	Extracellular
Mycoplasma pneumoniae	Not stainable	Aerobic	Extracellular
Neisseria meningitidis (develops into meningitis)	Gram –	Aerobic	Extracellular
Pseudomonas aeruginosa	Gram –	Aerobic	Extracellular
Streptococcus agalactiae (group B; develops into meningitis)	Gram +	Facultative anaerobic	Extracellular
Streptococcus pneumoniae	Gram +	Facultative anaerobic	Extracellular
Yersinia pestis (plague)	Gram –	Facultative anaerobic	Extracellular
Gastrointestinal Tract Infections			
Inflammatory Gastrointestinal Tract Infections			
Bacillus anthracis (gastrointestinal anthrax)	Gram +	Facultative anaerobic	Extracellular
Clostridium difficile	Gram +	Anaerobic	Extracellular
Escherichia coli 0157:H7	Gram –	Facultative anaerobic	Extracellular
Vibrio cholerae	Gram –	Facultative anaerobic	Extracellular
Vibrio parahaemolyticus	Gram –	Facultative anaerobic	Extracellular
Invasive Gastrointestinal Tract Infections			
Brucella abortus (brucellosis, undulant fever leading to sepsis, heart infection)	Gram –	Aerobic	Intracellular
Campylobacter jejuni	Gram –	Microaerophilic	Extracellular
Francisella tularensis	Gram –	Strict anaerobic	Facultative intracellular
Helicobacter pylori (gastritis and peptic ulcers)	Gram –	Microaerophilic	Extracellular
Listeria monocytogenes (leading to sepsis and meningitis)	Gram +	Aerobic	Intracellular
Salmonella typhi (typhoid fever)	Gram –	Anaerobic	Extracellular
Shigella sonnei	Gram –	Facultative anaerobic	Extracellular
Food Poisoning			
Bacillus cereus	Gram +	Facultative anaerobic	Extracellular
Clostridium botulinum	Gram +	Anaerobic	Extracellular
Clostridium perfringens	Gram +	Anaerobic	Extracellular
Staphylococcus aureus	Gram +	Facultative anaerobic	Extracellular
Sexually Transmitted Infections			
Chlamydia trachomatis (pelvic inflammatory disease)	Not stainable	Aerobic	Intracellular
Neisseria gonorrhoeae (urethritis)	Gram –	Aerobic	Facultative intracellular
Treponema pallidum (spirochete; syphilis)	Gram –	Aerobic	Extracellular
Skin and Wound Infections			
Bacillus anthracis (cutaneous anthrax)	Gram +	Facultative anaerobic	Extracellular
Borrelia burgdorferi (Lyme disease; spirochete)	Gram –	Aerobic	Extracellular

TABLE 10-4 COMMON BACTERIAL INFECTIONS—cont'd

MICROORGANISM	GRAM STAIN	RESPIRATORY PATHWAY	INTRACELLULAR OR EXTRACELLULAR
Clostridium tetani (tetanus)	Gram +	Anaerobic	Extracellular
Clostridium perfringens (gas gangrene)	Gram +	Anaerobic	Extracellular
Mycobaterium leprae (leprosy)	Gram + (weakly)	Aerobic	Extracellular
Pseudomonas aeruginosa	Gram –	Aerobic	Extracellular
Rickettsia prowazekii (rickettsia; typhus)	Gram –	Aerobic	Obligate intracellular
Staphylococcus aureus	Gram +	Facultative anaerobic	Extracellular
Streptococcus pyogenes (group A)	Gram +	Facultative anaerobic	Extracellular
Eye Infections			
Chlamydia trachomatis (conjunctivitis)	Not stainable	Aerobic	Obligate intracellular
Haemophilus aegyptus (pink eye)	Gram –	Facultative anaerobic	Extracellular
Zoonotic Infections			
Bacillus anthracis (anthrax)	Gram +	Facultative anaerobic	Extracellular
Brucella abortus (brucellosis, also called undulant fever)	Gram –	Aerobic	Intracellular
Borrelia burgdorferi (spirochete; Lyme disease)	Gram –	Aerobic	Extracellular
Listeria monocytogenes	Gram +	Aerobic	Intracellular
Rickettsia rickettsii (rickettsia; Rocky Mountain spotted fever)	Gram –	Aerobic	Obligate intracellular
Rickettsia prowazekii (rickettsia; typhus)	Gram –	Aerobic	Obligate intracellular
Yersinia pestis (plague)	Gram –	Facultative anaerobic	Extracellular
Nosocomial Infections			
Enterococcus faecalis	Gram +	Facultative anaerobic	Extracellular
Enterococcus faecium	Gram +	Facultative anaerobic	Extracellular
Escherichia coli (cystitis)	Gram –	Facultative anaerobic	Extracellular
Pseudomonas aeruginosa	Gram –	Obligate anaerobic	Extracellular
Staphylococcus aureus	Gram +	Facultative anaerobic	Extracellular
Staphylococcus epidermidis	Gram +	Facultative anaerobic	Extracellular

The establishment of stable colonization requires adhesion. Many bacteria attach through **pili** (also called **fimbriae**), which are thin rod-like projections from the bacterial surface (see Figures 10-1 and 10-2). Pathogenic strains of *Escherichia coli* involved in urinary tract infections have a variety of different specific pili-associated adhesion molecules, including mannose-binding protein that binds with glycoproteins specifically expressed on the bladder epithelium and PapG (pyelonephritis-associated protein) adhesin that binds to galactoses of the human P blood group. PapG is a specific adhesion for urinary tract epithelium, but PapG variants are specific for other cell types so that the particular PapG expressed will determine the preferred site of infection with *E. coli*. The particular adhesin may vary depending on growth conditions under which bacteria may undergo a "phase change" and shift from one type to another.

Neisseria spp. bind to urinary tract epithelial cell membrane–associated cofactor protein (CD46), which is a receptor that regulates complement and protects cells by helping inactivate C3b and C4b. Several other microorganisms (e.g., *B. pertussis, Legionella pneumophila, Mycobacterium tuberculosis*) bind to the CR3 complement receptor (a receptor for C3b and C3b breakdown products) on the surface of monocytes/macrophages. *B. pertussis* expresses a surface hemagglutinin that recognizes CR3, whereas *L. pneumophila* and *M. tuberculosis* initially absorb inactivated C3b (C3bi) for use as an adhesin for CR3.

A variety of proteins and carbohydrates not associated with pili function as adhesion molecules. Flagella (used for motion) act as adhesions in *V. cholerae*. Hemagglutinins on *B. pertussis, Salmonella* spp., and *Helicobacter pylori* bind to erythrocyte surface molecules. Fibronectin is a common component of mucosal cell surfaces and is frequently used as a receptor. Several bacteria *(S. pyogenes, S. aureus, T. pallidum)* have developed specific adhesion molecules that recognize a particular amino acid sequence (Arg-Gly-Asp) in fibronectin. Many other bacteria have developed adhesion molecules that bind to collagen, laminin, and vitronectin, which are plentiful in connective tissue. A surface polysaccharide (poly-*N*-acetylglucosamine) is on nonencapsulated *Staphylococcus* spp., *E. coli* that infect the urinary system. *Yersinia pestis,* which causes plague, mediates adherence to the material in catheters and prosthetic devices, thus increasing the risk of infection of joint replacements and other implanted materials.

Although discussions of infectious diseases generally focus on single microorganisms that can be isolated and identified as part of the diagnostic workup, the microorganism frequently exists in the individual as part of complex multicellular masses called **biofilms.**[6] Biofilms consist of mixed species of microorganisms, including bacteria, fungi, and viruses.[7] Growth of bacteria in biofilms offers survival advantage by protection from the host's protective responses and exposure to antibiotics.[8] These structures are associated with chronic and recurrent infections

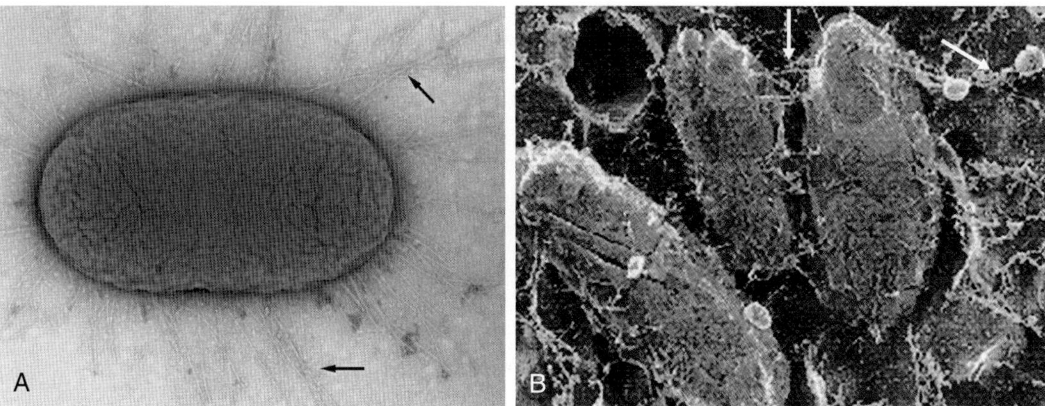

FIGURE 10-2 Attachment of *Escherichia coli* Through Pili. **A,** Transmission electron micrograph showing pili *(arrows)* of pathogenic *E. coli.* **B,** Scanning electron micrograph of *E. coli (orange)* attached by pili *(arrows)* to bladder epithelium *(blue).* (**A** courtesy Eric Buckles and Paula J. Fernandes; **B** modified from Wein A et al: *Campbell-Walsh urology,* ed 9, Philadelphia, 2007, Saunders.)

associated with persistent nasopharyngeal colonization with staphylococci; otitis media; urinary tract infections secondary to indwelling catheters; foot ulcers in diabetic persons; infected burn wounds; vaginitis; osteomyelitis; pneumonia secondary to cystic fibrosis; and diseases of the oral cavity related to dental plaque, such as dental caries and periodontitis.[9,10]

Invasion and Evasion. Invasion results in direct confrontation with the individual's primary defense mechanisms against bacteria, which include the complement system, antibodies, and phagocytes, such as neutrophils and macrophages (see Chapters 7, 8, and 9). Bacterial survival and growth depend on the effectiveness of the body's defenses and on the bacterium's capacity to resist those defenses and obtain nutrients and multiply. Evasion of the body's defense mechanisms may result in infectious microorganisms being transported in the blood (**bacteremia**) to infect other organs or even multiplying in the blood (**sepsis**).

Efficient pathogens produce a variety of toxic molecules that may kill the individual's cells, disrupt the tissue, and protect against inflammation. **Exotoxins** are proteins released during bacterial growth. They are usually enzymes and have highly specific effects; they include cytotoxins, neurotoxins, pneumotoxins, enterotoxins, and hemolysins. Exotoxins can damage cell membranes, activate second messengers, and inhibit protein synthesis. For instance, a key component of invasion by *N. meningitidis* is a toxin that weakens intercellular adhesion between epithelial cells, thus allowing penetration into the underlying tissue. Pathogenic strains of streptococci and staphylococci produce hyaluronidase, lipases, and hemolysins that break down cells and intercellular matrix. Exotoxins are immunogenic and elicit the production of antibodies known as **antitoxins.** Consequently, vaccines are available for many of the exotoxins (i.e., tetanus, diphtheria, and pertussis).

Endotoxins are **lipopolysaccharides (LPSs)** contained in the cell walls of gram-negative bacteria and released during lysis (or destruction) of the bacteria (see Figure 10-1). The innermost part of the lipopolysaccharide, *lipid A,* is made of polysaccharides and fatty acids and is responsible for the substance's toxic effects. Bacteria that produce endotoxins are called *pyrogenic bacteria* because they stimulate the release of inflammatory mediators and produce fever and the local and systemic effects of inflammation including septic shock and damage to multiple organs (Figure 10-3).[11] Endotoxin also may be released from the membrane of the bacteria, either during bacterial growth or during treatment with antibiotics. Therefore, antibiotics cannot prevent the toxic effects of the endotoxin. Evasion of the individual's immune and inflammatory systems is multifaceted, and the most successful pathogens incorporate several mechanisms (Table 10-5).[12]

Rapid Division. Because the primary immune response may take 3 to 5 days to reach protective levels, some pathogens proliferate at rates that surpass the development of the immune system. Cholera causes severe vomiting and watery diarrhea, has a 60% mortality rate, and develops within 2 to 3 days of ingestion of the bacteria. Some strains of toxin-producing group A streptococci cause destructive skin infections and pneumonia that may kill an individual within 2 days. Group B streptococci from the maternal vagina may ascend the birth canal, penetrate fetal membranes, and infect the fluid surrounding the fetus. This microorganism may have already established an active infection of the child's lungs by the time of birth, resulting in a pneumonia (50% mortality rate in newborns) that is too advanced to be treated successfully by antibiotics.

Intracellular Survival. Bacteria may hide from the immune response by growth in sites that are relatively poorly protected by immune cells, for example, *V. cholerae* in the gastrointestinal (GI) tract and *Salmonella typhi* in the intestinal tract and biliary tract (gallbladder). Even asymptomatic people may undergo prolonged local colonization and shed infectious microorganisms in urine and feces, thus creating a *carrier state.*

Survival within cells *(intracellular bacteria)* affords a distinct advantage to some bacteria. Many intracellular bacteria can survive and even multiply in macrophages *(Brucella, Listeria, M. leprae, M. tuberculosis)* or in other cells *(Yersinia, Shigella, Listeria, E. coli).*[13] Normally a macrophage would efficiently kill bacteria by fusing lysosomal granules with the phagosome to produce a phagolysosome and using oxygen-dependent and oxygen-independent mechanisms. Successful

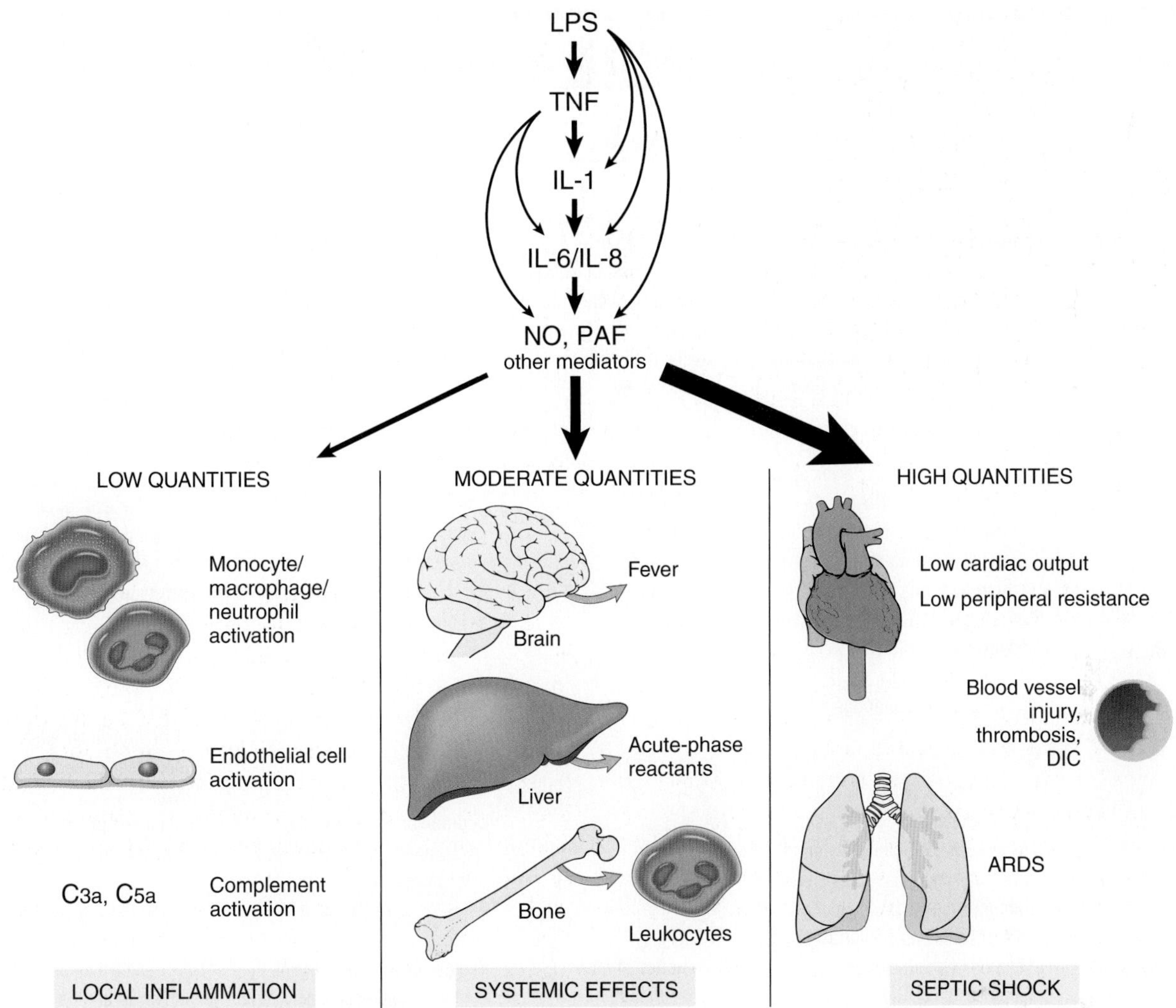

FIGURE 10-3 **The Many Activities of Lipopolysaccharide (LPS).** Bacterial endotoxin *(LPS)* activates almost every aspect of inflammation. The release of LPS from gram-negative bacteria triggers successive waves of cytokine production, including tumor necrosis factor *(TNF)*, interleukin-1 *(IL-1)*, interleukin-6 *(IL-6)*, and interleukin-8 *(IL-8)*, and secondary mediators of inflammation, such as nitric oxide *(NO)* and platelet-activating factor *(PAF)*. At low levels of LPS the effect is local. Moderate levels of LPS cause more systemic inflammatory responses. High levels of LPS may lead to septic shock and death. *ARDS*, Acute respiratory distress syndrome; *DIC*, disseminated intravascular coagulation. (From Kumar V, Abbas A, Fausto N: *Robbins & Cotran pathologic basis of disease*, ed 7, Philadelphia, 2005, Saunders; Modified from Abbas AK et al: *Cellular and molecular immunology*, ed 4, Philadelphia, 2000, WB Saunders.)

intracellular bacteria may block killing in several ways. Several microorganisms are resistant to killing and survive in the phagolysosome.

Species of *Salmonella* secrete products that alter the environment of the phagolysosome. Production of catalase and superoxide dismutase *(N. gonorrhoeae, Brucella abortus, S. aureus)* destroys toxic oxygen products produced by the hexose-monophosphate shunt.[14] *S. aureus* also produces a cell-bound pigment (carotenoid) that "quenches" singlet oxygen. A second means of avoiding killing is escape from the phagosome. Several bacteria secrete lysins (e.g., hemolysin of *Shigella*, listeriolysin O and phospholipase C of *L. monocytogenes*, phospholipase A of *Rickettsia* spp.) that break down the phagosome membrane, and the bacteria are released into the cytoplasm, where they multiply.[15] A third means of avoiding killing is by prevention of phagosome-lysosome fusion. *M. tuberculosis* and *T. gondii* produce toxins that prevent fusion so that the environment in the phagosome remains relatively nontoxic.

Protection Against Phagocytosis. Bacteria produce a large variety of toxins and extracellular enzymes, some of which kill phagocytic cells (e.g., *Pseudomonas aeruginosa* exotoxin A). Staphylococcal hemolysins and toxins from *Bacillus anthracis* and *B. pertussis* decrease phagocytic and chemotactic activities and may be toxic. Streptococcal products, such as streptolysin O, bind to cholesterol in the phagocyte's plasma membrane and initiate destruction through the internal release of enzymes in lysosomal granules.

Antiphagocytic **capsules** are expressed by most bacterial pathogens involved in pneumonia and meningitis (Figure 10-4). Capsules are mostly polysaccharide, although some very important proteins may be capsular components, which inhibit complement activation and phagocytosis. Such coatings inhibit

TABLE 10-5 MECHANISMS USED BY MICROORGANISMS TO DEFEND AGAINST INFLAMMATION AND IMMUNITY

STRATEGY	BACTERIAL MECHANISM	FUNGAL MECHANISM	PARASITE/PROTOZOAL MECHANISM	VIRAL MECHANISM
Rapid division	Initial proliferation in protective environment	NA	NA	Rapid proliferation of viruses with small genomes
Intracellular survival	Intracellular bacteria block granule fusion, survive in phagolysosomes, enter and multiply in cytoplasm	Multiplication in phagosomes, inhibition of lysosomal enzymes	Resistance to lysosomal enzymes, block granule fusion, enter and multiply in cytoplasm	Obligative intracellular life cycle, latency (e.g., herpes simplex virus in dorsal root ganglia)
Protection against phagocytosis	Capsules with antiphagocytic and anticomplement activities, toxins to kill phagocytes (e.g., α-toxin and leukocidin)	Polysaccharide capsule, toxins that inhibit phagocytosis	Glycocalyx, toxins that inhibit phagocytosis	NA
Coating with self	Adsorption of fibronectin or IgG (e.g., protein A), sialic acid capsule	NA	Adsorption of IgG by Fc receptor	Enveloped viruses with plasma membrane
Antigenic variation	Large diversity of surface molecules, phase changes in pili or membrane proteins, strain-to-strain serotype differences	Changes in surface antigens	Changing morphologic forms during life cycle, antigen switching	Viral enzymes that produce translational errors, antigen shift and drift, diversity of serotypes
Degrade immune molecules	Proteases for IgA and IgG, degrade complement, defensins, and cathelicidins	NA	IgG and IgA proteases	
Neutralization of immune molecules	Shedding of surface antigens	NA	Shedding of surface antigens	Secretion of viral proteins to neutralize antibody, molecules to neutralize cytokines
Complement evasion	Proteases degrade complement (e.g., C3b, C5a), capsules that prevent complement deposition, inhibitors of complement components and convertases	NA	Degrade or inactivate C3b, C3a, and C5a; break down C3 convertase	Cellular complement inhibitors in envelope
Immune suppression	Induction of anergy, direct suppression of Th cell development	Stimulation of anti-inflammatory cytokines, inhibition of proinflammatory cytokines	Release of soluble antigens that induce "tolerance," polyclonal B-cell activation, induction of anti-inflammatory cytokines, cytotoxic molecules	Infect and kill immune cells, inhibit Tc and natural killer (NK) recognition of major histocompatibility complex (MHC), inhibit antigen presentation

NA, Not applicable.

phagocytosis and include the thick polysaccharide covering of the pneumococcus *(S. pneumoniae),* the waxy capsule surrounding the tubercle bacillus *(M. tuberculosis),* the polysaccharide "slime" capsule of *P. aeruginosa,* and the M protein of *S. pyogenes.* The M protein binds fibrinogen and fibrin and functions as an adhesin.

Coating with Self-Protein. Some bacterial surface proteins (e.g., protein G of *S. pyogenes*) bind the Fc portion of the individual's antibody, thus forming a protective coat of "self" protein. Binding through the Fc holds the antibody in an orientation that does not allow complement activation or phagocytosis. *T. pallidum* coats itself with fibronectin. Capsules are produced that contain sialic acid (*E. coli* K-12), which closely resembles the sialic acid on the surface of most human cells, and hyaluronic acid (group A streptococci), which is the basic substance in connective tissue.

Antigenic Variation. Antigenic variation allows the pathogen to alter surface molecules that express antigens that are the targets of protective immune responses. Thus as the individual develops protective levels of antibodies, the pathogen responds by changing antigens and becoming resistant. The three primary mechanisms of antigenic variation are *mutation, recombination,* and *gene switching.* Antigenic variation can occur during the course of an infection in the host or during the spread of infection through the environment.

Neisseria use pili to adhere to epithelium, and antibody against these antigens can abrogate adherence. *Neisseria* undergoes *phase shifts* during which pilar antigens are changed by progressive silencing of 1 set of 10 or 11 available pili genes and activation of others that express different antigens. The spirochete *B. recurrentis* (relapsing fever) repeatedly relapses with spiking fevers as a result of as many as 10 episodes of antigenic changes over weeks or months. Many other bacteria have a large number of different antigenic types (serotypes) across the species. At least 80 different strains of group A *S. pyogenes* express different serotypes of the capsular M protein. *S. pneumoniae* has

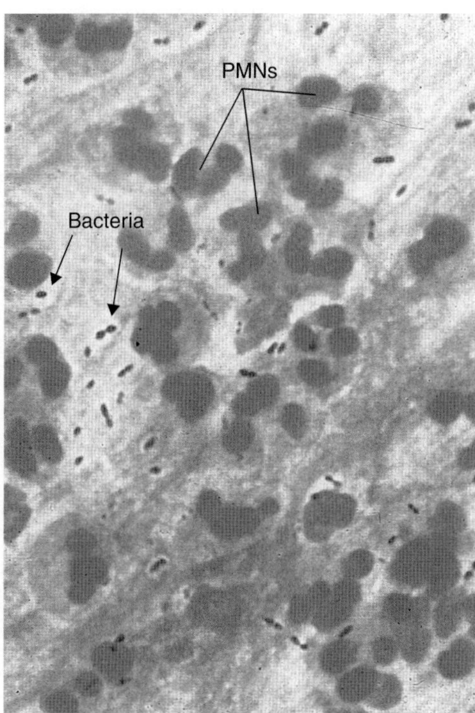

FIGURE 10-4 Bacterial Capsule. Gram stain of a sputum sample from an individual with pneumococcal pneumonia (× 1000 magnification). The sputum is rich in polymorphonuclear *(PMN)* cells and slightly elongated, gram-negative cocci *(Streptococcus pneumoniae)*. Clear areas *(arrows)* around the bacteria indicate capsules. (Modified from Mandell G, Bennett J, Dolin R: *Principles and practice of infectious diseases*, ed 7, Philadelphia, 2010, Churchill Livingstone.)

at least 100 different serotypes based on capsular polysaccharides. Multiple serotypes are also found in *V. cholerae, S. aureus, E. coli, N. gonorrhoeae,* and others. Although the particular serotype is stable on that bacterium, an immune response against one serotype will result in increased growth of a different serotype. Some gram-negative bacteria can revert to "rough" forms in which serotype-specific carbohydrates are deleted, thus becoming resistant to antibody and activation of complement.

Degradation of Immune Molecules. Protection is afforded by the breakdown of molecules of the immune or inflammatory system. An **IgA protease** produced by meningitis-causing microorganisms and other related bacteria *(N. gonorrhoeae, N. meningitidis, H. influenzae, S. pneumoniae)* cleaves IgA at the hinge region into ineffective Fc and Fab′$_2$ regions.[16] A staphylokinase produced by *Staphylococcus* spp. activates plasmin (resulting in the breakdown of clots) and degrades IgG and C3b of the complement system. *Pseudomonas* produces elastase (breakdown C3 of the complement system) and a 56-kDa protease (breaks down C5a).

Salmonella membrane protease degrades nonspecific antimicrobial molecules like defensins and cathelicidins. *Salmonella* can also alter surface lipid A by changing its fatty acid content to become resistant to small-molecular-weight antimicrobials.

Neutralization of Immune Molecules. Bacteria may spontaneously release surface molecules that bind to and neutralize antibody. These include endotoxin from gram-negative bacteria, capsular antigens from *S. pneumoniae* and *N. meningitidis,* and protein A from *S. aureus.* During infection the blood may contain high levels of complexes between antibody and bacterial antigen. At certain antigen/antibody ratios the complexes will deposit in the kidney, joints, and other target organs and initiate type III hypersensitivity reactions (see Chapter 9).

Complement Evasion. Complement is a major component of the defense against bacterial infection through production of opsonin (C3b) and chemotactic factors (C3a, C5a) for neutrophils. Teichoic acid in the Gram-positive cell wall provides resistance against complement-mediated lysis. Bacterial regulatory proteins (e.g., *Borrelia* complement-regulator-acquiring protein, *Neisseria* porins, and members of the *Streptococcus* M protein family) affect complement activation, including destabilization of the C3 convertase complex or degradation of the opsonin C3b.[17]

Immune Suppression. Although more prominent in viral infections, some bacterial pathogens can broadly suppress immune responses against their own antigens as well as other antigens unrelated to the infectious agent. Chronic bacterial infections, like leprosy *(M. leprae)* and tuberculosis *(M. tuberculosis),* induce anergy (suppressed response to multiple antigens) in infected hosts. *H. pylori* can release LPS that binds to dendritic cells and blocks development of Th1 cells, as well as produce toxins that block the T-cell IL-2 receptor signaling pathway, thus inhibiting maturation of Th cells. *N. gonorrhoeae* pili antigens bind to adhesion molecules on CD4+ cells and prevent their activation.

Tissue Damage. Bacterial infections damage tissue either directly by means of bacterial products or indirectly as a result of inflammation. Many toxins break down tissue directly. These include a large variety of proteases, lipases, hyaluronidases, hemolysins, and many others discussed previously. Some bacterial diseases arise completely from the systemic effects of toxins. Diphtheria is a respiratory tract infection *(Corynebacterium diphtheriae)* with systemic complications caused by toxin that inhibits messenger ribonucleic acid (mRNA) translation and causes low blood pressure, necrosis in the heart and liver, degeneration of myelin sheaths, and death. Gastrointestinal pathogens *(V. cholerae, Salmonella, Shigella, E. coli)* may produce enterotoxins that are cytotoxic and alter the permeability of intestinal cells leading to diarrheal diseases.

Necrotizing fasciitis, commonly called flesh-eating disease, is an unusual rapidly progressing bacterial infection of the soft tissue. Group A *Streptococcus* is the primary cause of this disease, although mixed infections with other bacterial microorganisms may cause similar soft tissue damage. The microorganisms usually invade the subcutaneous tissue from a minor wound infection. Severe and rapid tissue destruction proceeds from the combined effects of bacterial toxins and enzymes released from damaged cells. Rapid surgical débridement is absolutely necessary to limit morbidity and prevent the individual's death.

Clostridia are anaerobic bacteria that produce some of the most powerful toxins known. One type of food poisoning is caused by *Clostridium botulinum* that produces a paralytic neurotoxin (botulinum toxin) that blocks the release of acetylcholine at nerve-muscle synapses and results in flaccid paralysis. Infection of deep wounds with *C. tetani* results in release of a neurotoxin that causes severe muscle spasms, spastic paralysis of the voluntary muscles, and potentially death. *C. perfringens* produces multiple toxins that cause gas gangrene. One of these, alpha toxin, is a lecithinase that destroys the infected tissue by digesting cellular plasma membranes. Infection of the colon with *Clostridium difficile* results in watery diarrhea from toxins that damage the mucosa.

Bacterial superantigens are toxins that increase the adherence between major histocompatibility complex (MHC) class II proteins on antigen-presenting cells and the T-cell receptor. Because the effect is independent of antigen, a large population of T cells is activated and overproduces proinflammatory cytokines, such as IL-1, IL-6, and TNF-α. Superantigens are responsible for several diseases, including food poisoning (enterotoxins of *S. aureus* and *C. perfringens*), toxic shock syndrome (toxic shock syndrome toxin [TSST] of *S. aureus*), and scarlet fever (erythrogenic toxin of *S. pyogenes*).

Inflammation is the body's initial response to the presence of the bacteria. Vascular permeability is increased, allowing blood-borne substances (e.g., the complement system) involved in bacterial destruction to access the site of infection. The release of anaphylatoxins (C5a and C3a) of the complement cascade may increase the inflammatory response and lead to an increase in capillary permeability sufficient to permit the escape of large volumes of plasma, contributing to hypotension and, in severe cases, cardiovascular shock (see Chapter 48). Many persistent bacterial infections (e.g., *M. tuberculosis*) may lead to formation of *granulomas,* which diminishes the function of the affected organ (e.g., the lung).

The release of a sufficient amount of endotoxin can lead to fatal **endotoxic shock (septic shock),** which is one of the leading causes of death in intensive care units. The usual cause is proliferation of gram-negative bacteria, although shock may be caused by a few gram-positive bacteria and fungi. Once in the blood, endotoxins cause the release of vasoactive peptides and cytokines that affect blood vessels, producing vasodilation, which reduces blood pressure, causes decreased oxygen delivery, and produces subsequent cardiovascular shock (see Figure 10-3 and Chapter 48). Endotoxin can activate the coagulation cascade, leading to the syndrome of disseminated (or diffuse) intravascular coagulation (see Chapter 27). Additionally, endotoxin induces the release of TNF-α (cachectin) by macrophages. TNF is a potent proinflammatory cytokine that is also called *cachectin* because of its role in promoting cachexia in individuals with cancer. (Cachexia is discussed in Chapter 12; cytokines are discussed in Chapters 7 and 8.)

Example of Bacterial Pathogenesis. *S. aureus* has become a major cause of hospital-acquired (nosocomial) infections. This microorganism is a common commensal inhabitant of normal skin and nasal passages (about 30% of individuals are nasal carriers) and can be transmitted by direct skin-to-skin contact or by contact with shared items or surfaces that have become contaminated from another person's infection (e.g., towels, used bandages).[9]

Skin infections may occur at sites of trauma, such as cuts and abrasions, and at areas of the body covered by hair (e.g., back of neck, groin, buttock, armpit, beard area of men). Most infections are relatively mild and localized, appearing as red and swollen pustules on the skin, containing pus or other drainage (Figure 10-5). They can develop into abscesses, boils, carbuncles, cellulitis, or furunculosis. Invasive disease may originate from wound infections (e.g., trauma, surgical wounds, indwelling medical devices, prosthetic joints) and lead to fatal septicemia and abscesses in internal organs (e.g., lungs, kidney, bones, skeletal muscle, meninges, or heart).[18]

Adherence to tissue is mediated by surface proteins that attach to connective tissue (laminin, fibrin, fibronectin) and endothelium. Attachment to collagen occurs in osteomyelitis and septic arthritis–causing strains, and capsular polysaccharide mediates attachment to prosthetic devices.

Staphylococci also produce very effective polysaccharide capsules that protect against phagocytosis as well as surface protein A that binds IgG by the Fc portion and a surface coagulase that induces fibrin clotting on the bacterial surface; both processes mask bacterial antigens under a surface of self-proteins. Staphylococcal protein A, as well as a protein called staphylococcal binder of immunoglobulin, is also secreted and binds and neutralizes IgG.[19] *Staphylococcus* produces proteins that inhibit complement activity, including C3 and C5 convertases, C5, C2, and the C5a receptor that mediates complement-induced chemotaxis.[20] Many pathogenic strains have increased resistance to intracellular oxidative killing when engulfed by a phagocyte.

Invasion is mediated by a variety of toxins, including membrane-damaging toxins (α-toxin, which forms pores in membranes; hemolysin, which destroys erythrocytes; β-toxin, which is a sphingomyelinase; δ-toxin, a detergent-like toxin; leukocidin, which lyses phagocytes), coagulase (causes clots), staphylokinase (breaks down clots), exfoliative toxins (causes separation of epidermis resulting in scalded skin syndrome), lipase (degrades lipids on skin surface; facilitates abscess formation), and a variety of enterotoxins. Many of the enterotoxins are superantigens that are responsible for staphylococcal food poisoning with diarrhea and vomiting and toxic shock syndrome. Each infectious strain of *S. aureus* produces a few of these toxins so that strains may differ in their capacities to cause particular diseases; thus, different strains can cause purulent dermal infections, food poisoning, or toxic shock syndrome.

Antibiotic resistance has become a major problem with *S. aureus.* For several decades pathogenic strains have commonly produced **β-lactamase,** an enzyme that destroys penicillin. More recently staphylococci have developed resistance (methicillin-resistant *Staphylococcus aureus* [MRSA]) to broad-spectrum antibiotics, including methicillin-like antibiotics, which were widely used to treat penicillin-resistant microorganisms.

Fungal Infections

Fungi are eukaryotic microorganisms with thick rigid cell walls and the capacity to form a variety of complex structures (Figure 10-6). Fungi may grow as a **mold** with branched filaments or as a meshwork mycelium structure (e.g., *Aspergillus* spp., causing aspergillosis), **yeast** with ovoid or spherical shapes (*C. albicans,* which causes candidiasis), or **dimorphic** with a yeastlike appearance in tissue and mycelium in culture (e.g., *Histoplasma capsulatum,* which causes histoplasmosis, a systemic respiratory disease). The cell wall is composed of polysaccharides that differ from the peptidoglycans of bacteria and are thus are resistant to bacterial cell wall inhibitors such as penicillin and cephalosporin. In contrast to bacteria, the cytosol of fungi contains organelles: mitochondria, Golgi apparatus, microtubules, microvesicles, endoplasmic reticulum, and nuclei. Molds are aerobic, and yeasts are facultative anaerobes. Common pathologic fungi are summarized in Table 10-6.

Fungi are diagnosed by microscopic observation of specimens treated with potassium hydroxide and stained to enhance visualization of spheres and filaments. Specimens also can be cultured. Skin tests are available for species of *Aspergillus.* Many of the antifungal drugs (e.g., amphotericin B, ketoconazole, fluconazole) used to treat deep or systemic infections are toxic to the host because the fungal cell composition is similar to the human cell.

Transmission and Colonization. Infection with a fungus is called **mycosis.** Most pathogenic fungi (e.g., *H. capsulatum, Coccidioides immitis, Blastomyces dermatitidis*) grow as saprophytes in the environment and are transmitted by inhalation or contamination of wounds. The majority of medically relevant fungi either exist as human commensals or cause relatively mild infections (superficial mycoses) of the skin, nails, hair, and mucous membranes of the mouth and vagina. These include dermatophytes (e.g., tineas, which refers to several skin mycoses including ringworm, athlete's foot, and others) and yeasts (e.g., *Candida, Aspergillus, Cryptococcus*).

Human-to-human transmission is only a concern with dermatophyte infections. Systemic mycosis caused by pathogenic fungi generally results from inhalation of spores present in a

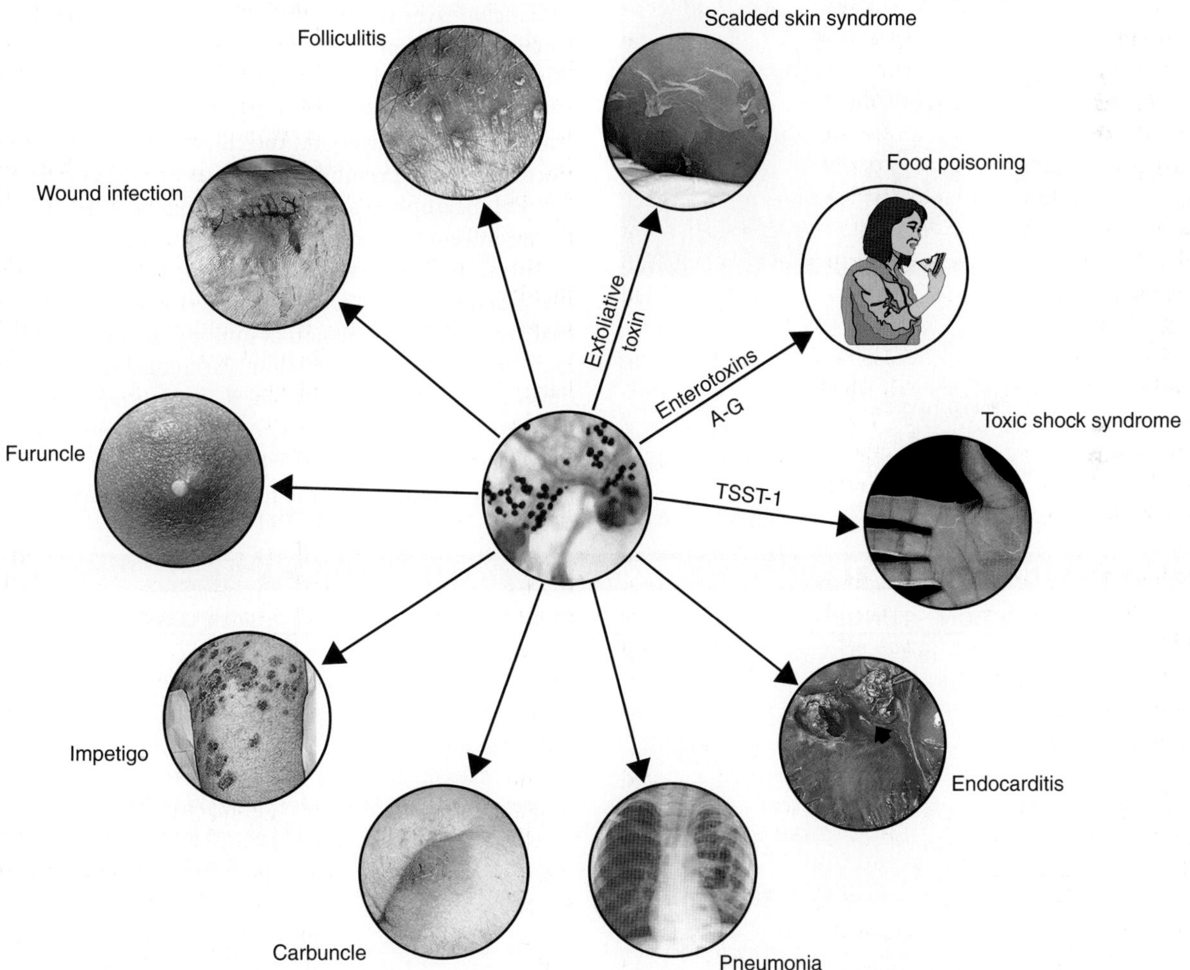

FIGURE 10-5 ***Staphylococcus aureus*** **Infections.** Different strains of *S. aureus* (gram-positive cocci in sputum from an individual with pneumonia *[center photograph]*) cause a variety of infections. The particular infection may depend on the toxin produced: exfoliative toxin (scalded skin syndrome), enterotoxins A-G (food poisoning), or toxic shock syndrome toxin-1 *(TSST-1).* (Toxic shock syndrome, carbuncle, impetigo, and wound infection photos from Cohen J, Powderly WG: *Infectious diseases,* ed 3, St Louis, 2010, Mosby. Folliculitis photo from Goldman L, Ausiello D: *Cecil medicine,* ed 24, Philadelphia, 2012, Saunders. Center photo and photos of food poisoning and endocarditis from Kumar V et al: *Robbins & Cotran pathologic basis of disease,* ed 8, Philadelphia, 2010, Saunders. Furuncle photo from Long S et al: *Principles and practice of pediatric infectious diseases,* ed 4, Philadelphia, 2012, Saunders. Scalded skin syndrome and pneumonia photos from Mandell G et al: *Principles and practice of infectious diseases,* ed 7, Philadelphia, 2010, Churchill Livingstone.)

contaminated environment and initially presents as a pulmonary infection. Infection that disseminates to other organs can be life threatening. Systemic mycosis caused by opportunistic fungi is usually secondary to immunosuppression caused by genetic defects, infections such as HIV, cancer, and drugs used to prevent transplant rejection.

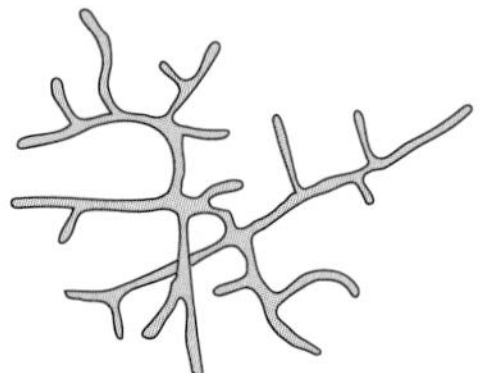

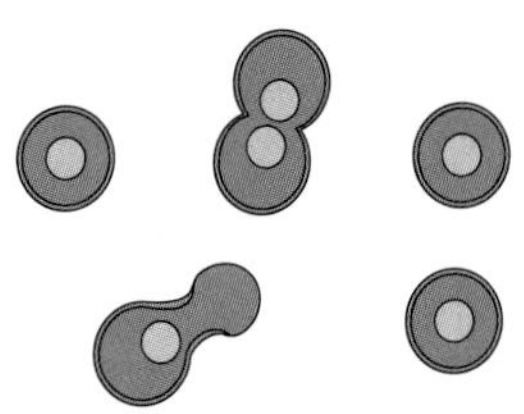

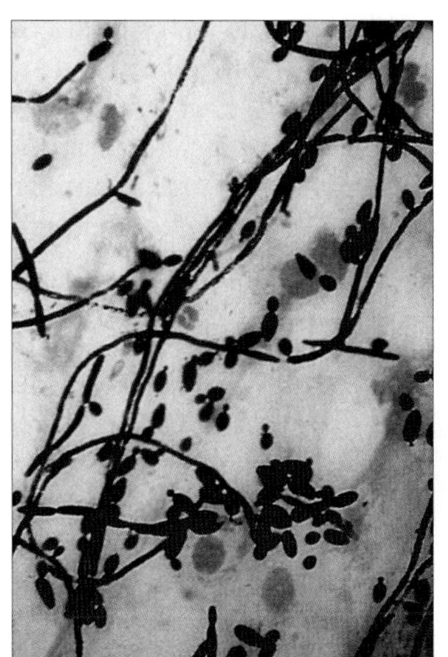

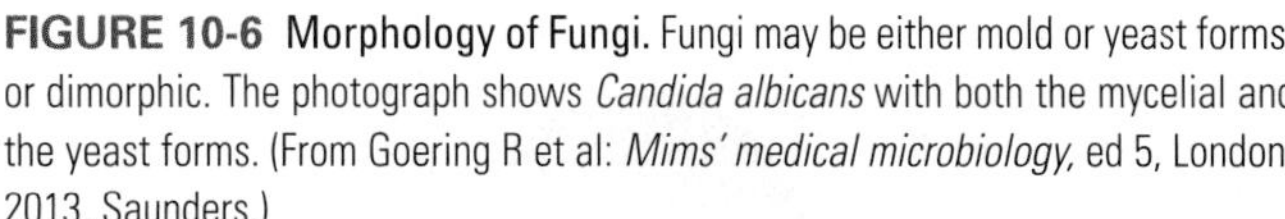

FIGURE 10-6 Morphology of Fungi. Fungi may be either mold or yeast forms, or dimorphic. The photograph shows *Candida albicans* with both the mycelial and the yeast forms. (From Goering R et al: *Mims' medical microbiology*, ed 5, London, 2013, Saunders.)

Specific adherence to the epithelium is provided by several polysaccharides on the fungal surface. Glucan, mannan, glycoprotein, and chitin molecules adhere with host receptors, including Toll-like receptors (TLRs), mannose receptors, dectin-1, and cadherins, respectively. A cell wall adhesion molecule, agglutinin-like sequence 3 (ALS3), on several fungi (e.g., *C. albicans*) promotes adherence to epithelial cells as well as silicone, thus facilitating infection of implants and other medical devices.

In 2006 the opportunist pathogen *Pneumocystis carinii* was reclassified as a fungus, and the specific variant that infects humans was renamed *Pneumocystis jiroveci*.[21] Despite the official change in nomenclature, much of the literature will continue to use *P. carinii* for some time. As with many fungi and protozoa, *Pneumocystis* has two life-cycle forms: a trophic form and the cyst form. Two surface proteins, glycoprotein A (gpA) and major surface glycoprotein (MSG), mediate attachment to alveolar epithelial cells.

Invasion and Evasion. The host defense against fungal infection includes the fungistatic properties of neutrophils and macrophages. T lymphocytes are crucial in limiting the extent of infection and producing cytokines to further activate macrophages. Human host defense against the inhaled spores begins with the mucous layer and the ciliary action in the respiratory tract, which then remove the fungus or facilitate phagocytosis by local macrophages. Pathogenic fungi have developed means to circumvent these mechanisms (see Table 10-5).[22]

Intracellular Survival. Fungal virulence and resistance to the individual's protective mechanisms is a complex process that requires the expression of multiple genes at different stages and different sites of infection. Pathologic fungi are generally dimorphic (e.g., *H. capsulatum, B. dermatitidis, C. immitis*) and readily adapt to the host environment, responding to temperature variations, low oxygen environment, more alkaline pH, and other conditions in the host tissue by undergoing changes

TABLE 10-6 COMMON PATHOGENIC FUNGI

PRIMARY SITE OF INFECTION	FUNGUS	DISEASE (PRIMARY)	SYMPTOMS
Superficial (no tissue invasion, little inflammation)	*Malassezia furfur*	Tinea versicolor, seborrheic dermatitis, dandruff	Red rash on body
Cutaneous (no tissue invasion, inflammatory response)	Dermatophytes		
	Trichophyton mentagrophytes	Tinea pedis (athlete's foot)	Scaling, fissures, itching
	Trichophyton rubrum	Tinea cruris (jock itch)	Rash, itching
	Microsporum canis	Tinea corporis (ringworm)	Lesion, raised border, scaling
	Candida albicans	Cutaneous candidiasis	Lesions in most areas of skin, mucous membranes, thrush, vaginal infection
Subcutaneous (tissue invasion)	*Sporothrix schenckii*	Sporotrichosis	Ulcers or abscesses on skin and other organ systems
Systemic (dimorphic; causes disease in healthy individuals)	*Stachybotrys chartarum* or "black mold"	Black mold disease	Rash, headaches, nausea, pains
	Coccidioides immitis	Coccidioidomycosis	Valley fever, flulike symptoms
	Histoplasma capsulatum	Histoplasmosis	Lung, flulike symptoms, disseminates to multiple organs, eye
	Blastomyces dermatitidis	Blastomycosis	Flulike symptoms, chest pains
Systemic (opportunistic)	*Aspergillus fumigatus, Aspergillus flavus*	Aspergillosis	Invasive to lungs and other organs
	Pneumocystis jiroveci	Pneumocystis pneumonia (PCP)	Pneumonia
	Cryptococcus neoformans	Cryptococcosis	Pneumonia-like illness, skin lesions, disseminates to brain, meningitis
	Candidia albicans	Systemic candidiasis	Sepsis, endocarditis, meningitis

in morphology and switching from avirulent mold forms to virulent yeast forms. Similar conditions also trigger yeasts (e.g., *C. albicans*) to switch from the yeast form to its more virulent hyphal form.

The more virulent morphologies allow fungi to survive in macrophages after phagocytosis. After phagocytosis by macrophages, the yeast form of *Histoplasma* replicates in phagosomes and phagolysosomes. Some yeast may produce proteins that inhibit the activity of lysosomal proteases. The macrophage either may be destroyed as a result of membrane modification by the fungus or, in the case of fungi like *Histoplasma,* may harbor the fungus in granulomas. Breakdown of the granulomas over time may result in release of viable fungi and recurrence of the infection.

Protection Against Phagocytosis. Encapsulated yeast cells (e.g., *Cryptococcus neoformans*) are more resistant to phagocytosis than unencapsulated yeast. The cryptococcal polysaccharide capsule is antiphagocytic by blocking recognition by macrophages and may also be immunosuppressive by inhibiting migration of leukocytes into the site of fungal infection. *Aspergillus fumigatus* and many other fungi produce toxic metabolites (e.g., gliotoxin) that inhibit macrophage and neutrophil phagocytosis. Molecules like gliotoxin may also be immunosuppressive, including suppression of mast cell activation, degranulation, and secretion of leukotrienes and cytokines.

Antigenic Variation. Altered antigen expression affords protection against the developing immune responses, although this defense strategy is rarely used by fungal pathogens. *Pneumocystis* contains approximately 80 different gpA and MSG genes, only 1 of which is expressed at a time. Modulation of these antigens may provide resistance against immune destruction.

Immune Suppression. Several yeasts stimulate the production of immunosuppressive cytokines, resulting in downregulation of some aspects of the host's immune response. The yeast *C. neoformans* suppresses inflammation by inhibiting production of the proinflammatory cytokines TNF-α and IL-12 and inducing production of the anti-inflammatory cytokine IL-10. The overall result is suppression of macrophage function and protection against killing.

Tissue Damage. Fungal infections damage tissue directly by secretion of enzymes and indirectly by initiation of an inflammatory response. Secreted enzymes, such as proteases, phospholipases, and elastases, damage cells and intercellular matrix, leading to necrosis. Many molds secrete mycotoxins when grown in environmental locations, such as on nuts, beans, and grains. Ingestion of this toxin affects muscle coordination, causes tremors, and may be fatal. Some fungal toxins may cause cancer; aflatoxins produced by some *Aspergillus* are especially carcinogenic.

The typical immune and inflammatory reaction against fungal infections involves a cell-mediated response with infiltration of T cells and macrophages, as well as neutrophils. The inflammatory site is rich in proinflammatory cytokines. Fungal infections can be very difficult for these systems to eradicate, leading to progressively increasing production of cytokines. Thus, as the host's response increases so do the destructive effects on surrounding healthy tissue. In cases of persistent infection, granulomas form and compromise the normal function of the infected tissue.

Example of Fungal Pathogenesis. *Candida albicans* is the most common cause of fungal infections in humans. It is an opportunistic yeast that is a commensal in the normal microbiome of many healthy individuals, residing in the skin, gastrointestinal tract, mouth (30% to 55% of healthy individuals), and vagina (20% of healthy women) and normally under the control of local defense mechanisms, including members of the bacterial microbiome that produce antifungal agents. In healthy individuals, particularly those whose normal microbiome has been disturbed by antibiotic therapy (e.g., diminished levels of *Lactobacillus* in the vaginal microbiome), *Candida* overgrowth may occur resulting in vaginitis or oropharyngeal infection (thrush). In those with an intact immune system the infection remains localized.

In immunocompromised individuals, particularly those with diminished levels of neutrophils (neutropenia), disseminated infection may occur. *Candida* is the most common fungal infection in people with cancer (particularly acute leukemia and other hematologic cancers), transplantation (bone marrow and solid organ), and HIV/AIDS. Almost 90% of people with AIDS have *Candida* at least one time during the disease, although infection is usually contained locally (thrush or vaginitis) because of adequate numbers of neutrophils (Figure 10-7). Invasive candidiasis may also be secondary to indwelling

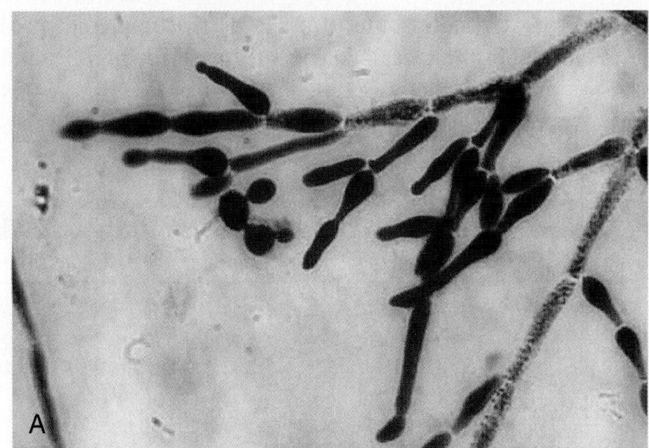

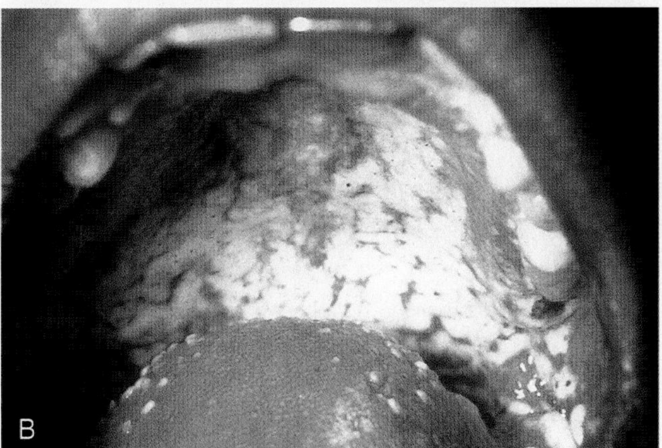

FIGURE 10-7 ***Candida albicans.*** **A,** Gram stain of sputum showing chains of elongated budding yeasts of *C. albicans* producing pseudohyphae (×1000). **B,** Oral candidiasis (thrush). (**A** from McPherson R, Pincus M: *Henry's clinical diagnosis and management by laboratory methods,* ed 22, Philadelphia, 2012, Saunders; **B** courtesy Dr. Stephen Raffanti.)

catheters, intravenous lines, or peritoneal dialysis, which provides direct entrance into the blood.

Disseminated candidiasis may involve several internal organs, including abscesses in the kidney, brain, liver, and heart, and is characterized by persistent or recurrent fever, gram-negative shock-like symptoms (hypotension, tachycardia), disseminated intravascular coagulation (DIC), and death. The mortality rates of sepsis or disseminated candidiasis are in the range of 30% to 40%.[23]

Like most pathogenic yeasts, *Candida* undergoes morphologic changes from unicellular yeast to filamentous hyphal forms under conditions of neutral to alkaline pH, elevated temperature, and changes in host serum factors. Switching of morphology results in altered profiles of surface antigens and increased resistance to immunologic destruction as well as altered tissue adhesion specificity.[24] *Candida* expresses diverse surface adhesion molecules that permit adherence to materials in implants, epithelium, extracellular matrix (fibronectin, laminin, collagen), and leukocytes and facilitate invasion into tissue. One surface adherence molecule is a glycoprotein, INT1p (integrator complex subunit 1), which specifically binds to integrins. EAP1 (enhanced adhesion to plastic) is a glycoprotein that permits *Candida* to bind to epithelial cells and a variety of synthetic materials found in implants.

Candida secretes several enzymes that function as virulence factors and contribute to tissue destruction. Acid proteases and phospholipases damage the cell membrane and enhance invasive capacity. Secreted aspartic proteinases (Saps) increase the virulence of *Candida* by destroying cell membranes and removing surface molecules, including from cells of the immune and inflammatory systems.

Candida may suppress the host's immune system. Production of the cytokine granulocyte-monocyte colony-stimulating factor (GM-CSF) suppresses monocyte/macrophage function, including the production of components of the complement cascade. Decreased production of C3 results in less opsonization (C3b) and production of chemotactic activity (C3a) for phagocytes.

Parasitic and Protozoal Infections

Parasitic organisms establish symbiosis with another species in which the parasite benefits at the expense of the other species. Parasites range from unicellular protozoal to large worms. Parasitic worms (helminths) include intestinal and tissue nematodes (e.g., hookworm, roundworm), flukes (e.g., liver fluke, lung fluke), and tapeworms. A protozoan is a eukaryotic, unicellular microorganism with a nucleus and cytoplasm. Pathogenic protozoa include malaria *(Plasmodium)*, amoebae (e.g., *Entamoeba histolytica*, which causes amoebic dysentery), and flagellates (e.g., *Giardia lamblia*, which causes diarrhea; *Trypanosoma*, which causes sleeping sickness). Although less common in the United States, parasites and protozoa are common causes of infections worldwide, with a significant effect on the mortality and morbidity of individuals in developing countries. Important parasites of humans are listed in Table 10-7.

Transmission and Colonization. Parasitic and protozoal infections are rarely transmitted from human to human. The predominant means is through vectors in which the organism

TABLE 10-7 PARASITES THAT ARE IMPORTANT IN HUMANS

CATEGORY	SUBGROUP	SPECIES	DISEASE	ORGANS AFFECTED/SYMPTOMS
Protozoa	Amoeboid	*Entamoeba histolytica*	Amebiasis	Dysentery, liver abscess
	Flagellate	*Giardia lamblia*	Giardiasis*	Diarrhea
		Leishmania donovani, L. tropica	Leishmaniasis	Sores on skin, progression to liver, spleen
		Trichomonas vaginalis	Trichomoniasis	Inflammation of reproductive organs
		Trypanosoma cruzi, T. brucei	Chagas disease: African sleeping sickness	Generalized, blood, lymph nodes, progressing to cardiac and central nervous system (CNS)
	Ciliate	*Balantidium coli*	Balantidiasis	Small intestines, invasion of colon, diarrhea
	Sporozoa (nonmotile)	*Cryptosporidium parvum, C. hominis*	Cryptosporidiosis*	Intestine, diarrhea
		Plasmodium spp.	Malaria	Blood, liver
		Toxoplasma gondii	Toxoplasmosis*	Intestine, eyes, blood, heart, liver
Helminths	Flukes (trematodes)	*Fasciola hepatica*	Fasciolosis	Liver destruction
		Paragonimus westermani	Lung fluke disease	Granuloma in lung, spinal cord
		Schistosoma mansoni	Schistosomiasis	Blood, diarrhea, bladder, generalized symptoms
	Tapeworms (cestodes)	*Taenia solium*	Pork tapeworm	Encysts in muscle, brain, liver
	Roundworms (nematodes)	*Ascaris lumbricoides*	Ascariasis	Intestinal obstruction, bile duct obstruction
		Necator americanus (hookworm)	Hookworm disease	Intestinal parasite
		Trichuris trichiura (whipworm)	Trichuriasis	Diarrhea
		Trichinella spiralis	Trichinosis*	Intestine, diarrhea, muscle, CNS, death
		Wuchereria bancrofti	Filariasis, elephantiasis	Lymphatics
		Enterobius vermicularis (pinworm)	Pinworm infection	Intestines
		Strongyloides stercoralis (threadworm)	Strongyloidiasis	Intestinal parasite, skin infection
		Onchocerca volvulus	Onchocerciasis	Blindness, dermatitis

*Most common in the United States.

spends part of its life cycle. Examples include the transmission of malaria (*Plasmodium* spp.) by mosquitoes, trypanosomes (*Trypanosoma cruzi,* which causes Chagas disease in South America; *Trypanosoma brucei,* which causes sleeping sickness in Africa) by the tsetse fly, and *Leishmania* spp. by sand fleas. Many of the protozoal infectious agents (e.g., *E. histolytica, G. lamblia*) are encountered in contaminated water or food and transmission is by ingestion.

The initial attachment depends on whether the microorganism is injected into the bloodstream by a vector or whether entrance is through the gastrointestinal tract. Microorganisms in the bloodstream frequently have surface lectins that react with carbohydrates on specific cells. Malarial parasites attach to erythrocytes that express Duffy blood group antigens. Thus Duffy-negative individuals are resistant to malaria. *T. cruzi* can infect both CD4-negative and CD8-positive T cells through a T-cell surface receptor. Several parasites express surface glycoproteins that facilitate preferential entrance into monocytes/macrophages using various receptors, including the receptors for complement component C3b (*Leishmania* spp.). *Leishmania* expresses a surface glycoprotein (gp63) that is necessary for its entrance into macrophages. The gp63 molecule binds complement components (C3b, C3bi) and uses the macrophage complement receptors. *E. histolytica* expresses two surface proteins that react with the disaccharide galactose/*N*-acetylgalactosamine on epithelium.

Invasion and Evasion. An effective immune response varies depending on the particular parasite or protozoa. Intercellular pathogens are susceptible to cell-mediated immunity and activation of macrophages by T cells. Other organisms are more sensitive to antibody, particularly used in antibody-dependent cell-mediated cytotoxicity (ADCC) by macrophages and natural killer (NK) cells. Many helminth infections are sensitive to damage by eosinophils, which are attracted by IgE-mediated mast cell degranulation and release of eosinophil chemotactic factor of anaphylaxis (ECF-A). Evasion of the individual's defenses is accomplished by several means (see Table 10-5).[25]

Intracellular Survival. *Leishmania* spp. are obligative intracellular parasites of monocytes/macrophages. They are protected from being killed in the phagosome and phagolysosome in which they multiply. Protection may be afforded by a surface protein that inhibits fusion of lysosomes to the phagosome, thus decreasing the amount of degradative enzymes within the phagolysosome. *Toxoplasma* spp. may be protected by entrance into a variety of cells, including macrophages. The probability of survival is increased by inhibiting fusion of lysosomes with the phagosome. Many of the intracellular organisms are sensitive to macrophage activation by T cells. *T. cruzi* bypasses the effects of macrophage activation by escaping from the phagosome and growing in the macrophage cytoplasm.

Protection Against Phagocytosis. Because many unicellular parasites survive within macrophages, the development of antiphagocytic capsules does not seem to be a major protective strategy. In some cases, a surface glycocalyx may function in a similar fashion as capsules to mask surface antigens from binding antibody. Some organisms produce toxins to protect themselves against phagocytosis; *E. histolytica* releases phospholipase and pore-forming proteins that disrupt the phagocyte's plasma membrane.

Coating with Self-Proteins. Pathogens that coat themselves with human proteins may be disguised and "fool" the immune system. Schistosomes and trypanosomes mask their antigens by absorbing IgG by the Fc portion of the molecule.

Antigenic Variation. In general, those organisms that undergo part of their life cycle in humans or may assume multiple morphologic forms will also undergo antigenic changes related to the stage in the life cycle or morphology. Some protozoa have developed very complex alterations in surface antigens using **gene switching.** Infection with African trypanosomes may lead to fatal neurologic disease. During infection protective antibody is produced against surface antigens called variable surface glycoproteins (VSGs). The parasite remains extracellular and an IgG or IgM response will successfully kill most of the microorganisms. However, a small percentage will undergo a gene shift that results in a change in VSG.[26] The existing antibodies will not recognize the new VSG, and the level of schistosomes will rebound, causing recurrent disease. The schistosome has genetic information (about 10% of the genome) for hundreds of variations in VSG, which are expressed one at a time. Thus the organism undergoes periodic shifts in VSG expression, resulting in periodicity of parasites in the blood. A similar process occurs in some helminths *(Trichinella spiralis).*

Degradation of Immune Molecules. If a microorganism is sensitive to a particular component of the immune or inflammatory system, a survival advantage is obtained by production of enzymes that specifically degrade that component. Schistosomes secrete an enzyme that diminishes the effectiveness of IgG by specifically removing a critical peptide. *E. histolytica* secretes a protease that can degrade IgG and IgA.

Neutralization of Immune Molecules. Large parasitic organisms may release a large amount of soluble antigen to neutralize antibody.

Complement Evasion. Complement activation is effective against several parasites. Some parasites (e.g., *Echinococcus* spp., *Leishmania* spp.) produce complement regulatory proteins that affect complement function by destabilizing C3 convertase or promoting degradation of C3b. Trypanosomes produce complement regulatory factors, including a surface gp63-like molecule, that confer resistance to complement. *E. histolytica* produces complement regulatory factors that inactivate C3a and C5a, thus inhibiting phagocyte chemotaxis activity.

Immune Suppression. Parasites may produce both pathogen-specific and nonspecific immune suppression. The release of large amounts of soluble antigen may induce specific tolerance to the pathogen as well as induce dysfunctional macrophage antigen processing. The function of immune cells is directly blocked by secretion of cytotoxic molecules *(T. spiralis),* selective inhibitors of T-cell function (schistosomes), or inducers of polyclonal B-cell activation (B-cell mitogen released by trypanosomes).

E. histolytica induces T-cell hyporesponsiveness by induction of IL-4 and IL-10 that down-regulate maturation of Th cells. The VSG molecules of African trypanosomes stimulate macrophages to overproduce TNF-α and CD8-positive cells to secrete high levels of interferon-gamma (IFN-γ), which impairs T-cell responses.[27] *Leishmania* has developed an interesting approach to circumventing antigen processing by macrophages. This pathogen adsorbs IgG, which binds to the macrophage Fc receptor, resulting in the hyperproduction of IL-10 and suppression of IL-12 from infected macrophages. IL-10 prevents macrophage responses to IFN-γ, allowing the parasites to survive even in the immunologically intact individual.

Tissue Damage. Tissue damage may result directly by parasitic infestation in the tissue or be secondary to the individual's immune and inflammatory responses. The particular process depends a great deal on burden of parasites infesting the site and sensitivity of the particular site to damage. Large infestations may lead to physical loss of function in a tissue or organ. For instance, a large number of intestinal parasites (e.g., the roundworm *Ascaris lumbricoides,* tapeworms, *Giardia* spp.) compete for and prevent uptake of nutrients, leading to various forms of malabsorption, blocked uptake of fats, or anemia from malabsorption of B_{12} or from large amounts of blood loss. Filarial parasites (e.g., *Wuchereria bancrofti* and *Brugia malayi,* which causes elephantiasis) block the lymphatics and cause accumulation of lymph in tissues. The larvae of tapeworms (e.g., *Taenia solium*) encyst in and prevent normal function of organs (e.g., muscle, liver, eye), which is particularly dangerous in the human brain.

Toxins released from parasites may cause significant irreversible organ damage. Proteolytic enzymes from *E. histolytica* are very cytolytic, leading to ulceration of intestinal walls, bloody diarrhea, amoebic dysentery, dehydration, and death in infants and young children. *T. cruzi* (causes Chagas disease) secretes proteases and phospholipases that damage the myocardium and intestinal smooth muscle and secretes a small-molecular –weight neurotoxin that affects the anatomic nervous system and causes fever.

The infected individual's immune and inflammatory responses result in considerable histopathology. Schistosomiasis results in the deposition of eggs in organs (e.g., the liver), which leads to formation of granulomas and tissue destruction through fibrosis. Some parasitic products (*T. brucei,* malarial parasites) activate macrophages to overproduce cytokines, which leads to exacerbated inflammation. The IgE produced against parasitic worms is protective, but can also stimulate excessive degranulation of mast cells and even anaphylactic shock. Polyclonal B-cell activation leads to the production of a broad spectrum of autoantibodies that may precipitate autoimmune diseases. Overproduction of antigens by some pathogens (e.g., malaria, trypanosomiasis, schistosomiasis) may lead to excessive levels of pathogenic circulating immune complexes and initiation of type III hypersensitivity reactions (see Chapter 9) in the kidneys and vasculature.

Example of Parasitic Pathogenesis. Malaria is one of the most common infections worldwide. The World Health Organization (WHO) estimated in 2010 that there were 219 million cases of malaria worldwide and that malaria accounted for an estimated 666,000 deaths, 90% of which are in Africa, mostly among children.[28] Malaria is caused by four species of *Plasmodium* parasites that infect humans: *Plasmodium falciparum* (accounts for most fatalities), *Plasmodium vivax and Plasmodium ovale* (both of which are more benign), and *Plasmodium malariae.* The four strains differ in disease severity and incidence of fever. Infection with *P. falciparum,* the most severe form, results in severe chills, high fever, sweating, headache, muscle pains, vomiting, severe anemia, pulmonary edema, and many other complications. Neurologic complications may result from infected red blood cells (RBCs) adhering to endothelium in capillaries of the brain. The individual may develop cardiovascular collapse, shock, coma, and death.

Transmission is through the bite of an infected female *Anopheles* mosquito, where the microorganism grows in the salivary gland. The infectious form enters the bloodstream, survives in the liver, and invades parenchymal cells. After several rounds of division, the liver cell ruptures, and several thousand parasites enter the blood, where they infect red blood cells (Figure 10-8). Multiplication occurs in RBCs, resulting in the release of daughter parasites that reinfect other erythrocytes.

P. vivax and *P. ovale* malaria can remain dormant in the liver for years, protected from the immune system by intracellular residence. The parasite in the blood avoids destruction by phagocytes in the spleen by expressing adhesion proteins that cause adherence and sequestration along the walls of the small vessels. Additionally, *P. falciparum* undergoes gene switching among about 60 different antigenic variants of antigens expressed on the surface of infected erythrocytes (*P. falciparum*

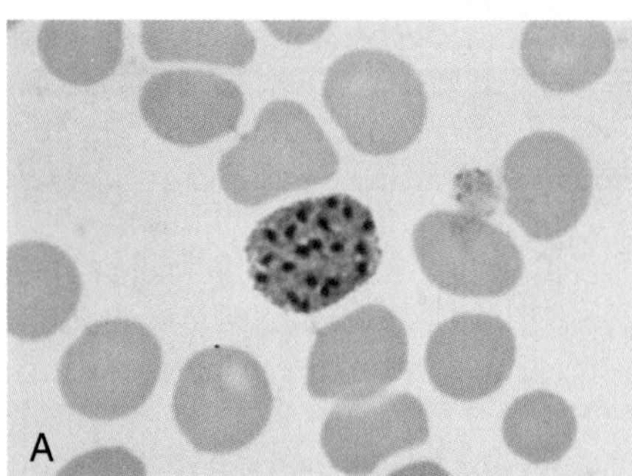

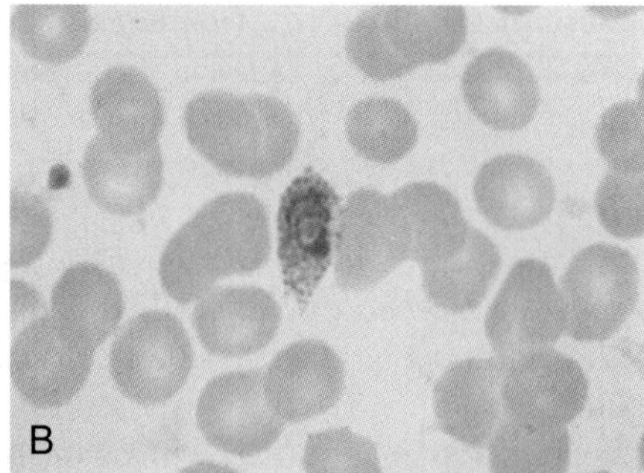

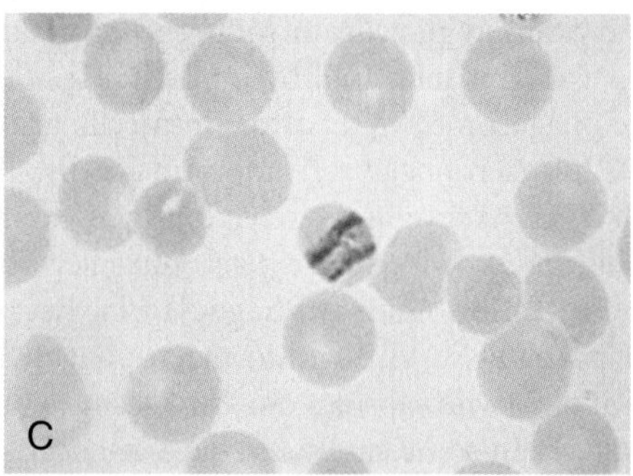

FIGURE 10-8 Malaria. Giemsa-stained smears. **A,** *Plasmodium vivax* schizont. **B,** *Plasmodium ovale* trophozoite. **C,** Characteristic band from trophozoite of *Plasmodium malariae* containing intracellular pigment hemozoin. (From Kliegman R et al: *Nelson textbook of pediatrics,* ed 19, St Louis, 2011, Saunders.)

erythrocyte membrane protein, *Pf*EMP). Malaria induces a form of immune suppression. Numbers of CD4 and CD8 T cells are diminished and lymphocytes from individuals infected with *P. falciparum* do not proliferate in the presence of *Pf*EMP antigen in vitro.

Malarial parasites have developed broad drug resistance including chloroquine, the previous mainstay of the preventive and therapeutic arsenal of antimalarial drugs.[29] Most resistance originates from mutations in the target genes (antigenic variation). Resistance to drugs that cause cellular damage appear to result from increased activity, or even novel development, of drug transporters that eliminate the drugs from the parasitic organism.

Viral Infection and Injury

Viruses are extremely simple microorganisms and do not possess any of the metabolic organelles found in prokaryotes (e.g., bacteria) or eukaryotes (e.g., human cells). The basic viral structure (virion) consists of nucleic acid protected by a protein shell, the capsid. The capsid may take many characteristic shapes: helical, icosahedral, or large pleiomorphic (poxvirus) (Figure 10-9). Some viruses also have a protective envelope surrounding the capsid, which consists of the plasma membrane from the previously infected cell.

Viruses are classified by the format of nucleic acid in the virion, which may be RNA or deoxyribonucleic acid (DNA) and either single-stranded (ss) or double-stranded (ds), and by whether the virus uses the enzyme reverse transcriptase (RT) for replication. Thus seven classifications are used: dsDNA (e.g., herpesvirus, smallpox virus), ssDNA (parvovirus), dsRNA (rotavirus), ssRNA +sense (+sense functions as mRNA) (e.g., hepatitis A and C viruses, SARS virus, poliovirus, rhinovirus), ssRNA−sense (e.g., Ebola virus, Marburg virus, Nipah virus, influenza virus, and viruses that cause measles, mumps, and rabies, hantavirus, Lassa virus), ssRNA +sense with RT (e.g., HIV), and dsDNA with RT (e.g., hepatitis B virus).

Viral diseases are the most common afflictions of humans and include the common cold, the "cold sore" of herpes simplex virus, several forms of hepatitis, HIV, and several types of cancer. Examples of human diseases caused by specific viruses are listed in Table 10-8.

Transmission and Colonization. Viruses are obligatory intracellular parasites; thus transmission is usually from one infected individual to an uninfected individual or from an animal reservoir (**zoonotic infection**). Transmission may be direct or through a vector, such as mosquitoes. Human-to-human transmission may take many forms, including aerosols of respiratory fluids, contact with infected blood, or sexual contact.

The viral life cycle is completely intracellular and involves several steps: *attachment* to the target cell (determines host range and tropism), *penetration* (by endocytosis or membrane

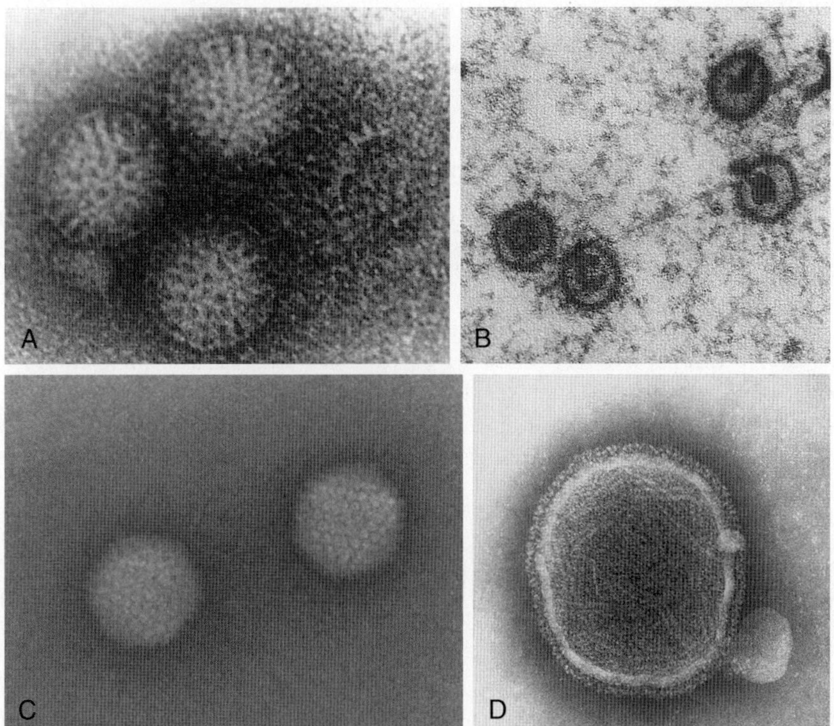

FIGURE 10-9 Electron Micrographs of Representative Viral Structures. A, Rotavirus: particles with a double shell and a characteristic "wheel-and-spoke" appearance. **B,** Epstein-Barr virus: icosahedral enveloped DNA virus. **C,** Adenovirus: particles with characteristic icosahedral structures. **D,** Paramyxovirus: spherical enveloped RNA virus. RNA is seen spilling out of the disrupted virus. (**A** from Long S, Pickering L, Prober C: *Principles and practice of pediatric infectious diseases,* ed 3, Philadelphia, 2005, Saunders; **B** and **D** photos courtesy Science Source; © Photo Researchers, Inc., New York, NY; **C** from Mandell GL, Bennett JE, Dolin R: *Mandell, Douglas, and Bennett's principles and practice of infectious diseases,* ed 7, Philadelphia, 2010, Churchill Livingstone.)

fusion), *uncoating* (release of viral nucleic acid from the viral capsid by viral or host enzymes), *replication* (synthesis of viral proteins and mRNA), *assembly* (formation of new virions), and *release* (by lysis, budding) (Figure 10-10).

Attachment involves specific interactions between surface proteins on the virus and receptors on the cell to be infected. The specificity of the virus for these receptors and the distribution of receptors throughout the individual's tissues dictate the range of host cells that a particular virus can infect. For example, HIV has a glycoprotein (gp120) that attaches to the CD4 molecule expressed on helper T cells, monocytes, and microglia. Rotavirus recognizes sialic acid and other constituents of epithelial junctions. Epstein-Barr virus (EBV, which causes mononucleosis) binds to complement receptor 2 (CR2) on B lymphocytes.

Once bound, the virion penetrates the plasma membrane by receptor-mediated endocytosis, by envelope fusion with the plasma membrane, or by directly crossing the plasma membrane. Within the cytoplasm the virus uncoats the protective

TABLE 10-8 HUMAN DISEASES CAUSED BY SPECIFIC VIRUSES

BALTIMORE CLASSIFICATION	FAMILY	VIRUS	ENVELOPE	MAIN ROUTE OF TRANSMISSION	DISEASE
dsDNA	Adenoviruses	Adenovirus	No	Droplet contact	Acute febrile pharyngitis
	Herpesviruses	Herpes simplex type 1 (HSV-1)	Yes	Direct contact with saliva or lesions	Lesions in mouth, pharynx, conjunctivitis
		Herpes simplex type 2 (HSV-2)	Yes	Sexually, contact with lesions during birth	Sores on labia, meningitis in children
		Herpes simplex type 8 (HSV-8)	Yes	Sexually?, body fluids	Kaposi sarcoma
		Epstein-Barr virus (EBV)	Yes	Saliva	Mononucleosis, Burkitt lymphoma
		Cytomegalovirus (CMV)	Yes	Body fluids, mother's milk, transplacental	Mononucleosis, congenital infection
		Varicella-zoster virus (VZV)	Yes	Droplet contact	Chickenpox, shingles
ssDNA	Papovaviruses	Papillomavirus	No	Direct contact	Warts, cervical carcinoma
dsRNA	Reoviruses	Rotavirus	No	Fecal-oral	Severe diarrhea
ssRNA+	Picornaviruses	Coxsackievirus	No	Fecal-oral, droplet contact	Nonspecific febrile illness, conjunctivitis, meningitis
		Hepatitis A virus	No	Fecal-oral	Acute hepatitis
		Poliovirus	No	Fecal-oral	Poliomyelitis
		Rhinovirus	No	Droplet contact	Common cold
	Flaviviruses	Hepatitis C virus	Yes	Blood, sexually	Acute or chronic hepatitis, hepatocellular carcinoma
		Yellow fever virus	Yes	Mosquito vector	Yellow fever
		Dengue virus	Yes	Mosquito vector	Dengue fever
		West Nile virus	Yes	Mosquito vector	Meningitis, encephalitis
	Togaviruses	Rubella virus	Yes	Droplet contact, transplacental	Acute or congenital rubella
	Coronaviruses	SARS	Yes	Droplets in aerosol or direct contact	Severe respiratory disease
	Caliciviruses	Norovirus	No	Fecal-oral	Gastroenteritis
ssRNA–	Orthomyxoviruses	Influenza virus	Yes	Droplet contact	Influenza
	Paramyxoviruses	Measles virus	Yes	Droplet contact	Measles
		Mumps virus	Yes	Droplet contact	Mumps
		Parainfluenza virus	Yes	Droplet contact	Croup, pneumonia, common cold
		Respiratory syncytial virus (RSV)	Yes	Droplet contact, hand-to-mouth	Pneumonia, influenza-like syndrome
	Rhabdoviruses	Rabies virus	Yes	Animal bite, droplet contact	Rabies
	Bunyaviruses	Hantavirus	Yes	Aerosolized animal fecal material	Viral hemorrhagic fever
	Filoviruses	Ebola virus	Yes	Direct contact with body fluids	Viral hemorrhagic fever
		Marburg virus	Yes	Direct contact with body fluids	Viral hemorrhagic fever
	Arenavirus	Lassa virus	Yes	Aerosolized animal fecal material	Viral hemorrhagic fever
ssRNA+ with RT	Retroviruses	HIV	Yes	Sexually, blood products	AIDS
dsDNA with RT	Hepadnaviruses	Hepatitis B virus	Yes	All body fluids	Acute or chronic hepatitis, hepatocellular carcinoma

AIDS, Acquired immunodeficiency syndrome; *DNA,* deoxyribonucleic acid; *ds,* double-stranded; *HIV,* human immunodeficiency virus; *RNA,* ribonucleic acid; *RT,* reverse transcriptase; *SARS,* severe acute respiratory syndrome; *ss*; single-stranded.

nucleocapsid and releases viral genetic information. Most RNA viruses directly produce mRNA, which is translated into viral proteins, and genomic RNA, which is eventually packaged into new viruses. One particular family of viruses, retroviruses (e.g., HIV), carries the enzyme *reverse transcriptase* that creates a double-stranded DNA version of the virus. The DNA "provirus" enters the cell's nucleus, where it becomes integrated into the host cell's chromosomal DNA. DNA viruses also enter the nucleus and are transcribed into mRNA before protein translation. Some DNA viruses also may integrate into the infected cell's chromosomal DNA.

The translation of viral-specific mRNA results in viral proteins that self-assemble. New virions are released from the cell for transmission of the viral infection to neighboring uninfected cells. Enveloped viruses are released through *budding,* in which shed viral particles are enveloped in the plasma membrane from the surface of the infected cell. Nonenveloped viruses commonly are released in large numbers concurrent with the destruction of the cell. Viral DNA that has become integrated with host DNA is transmitted to the daughter cells during mitosis. By this process, viral genes can become part of the genetic information of the cell and its progeny.

Invasion and Evasion. The primary defense mechanisms against viruses include antibody that prevents viral entrance into a cell and cellular immunity that recognizes antigenic changes on the surface of infected cells. Nonspecific defense includes production of α- and β-interferons that block intracellular viral replication. However, many viruses are highly successful pathogens and have developed a variety of mechanisms for bypassing immune rejection (see Table 10-5, p. 308).

Rapid Division. Some viruses, particularly those with small genomes, rapidly proliferate after the initial infection and by doing so produce a large number of virions more quickly than the immune system can develop. Norovirus and rotavirus (causes of severe diarrhea and vomiting) and Ebola virus, Marburg virus, and hantavirus (causes of hemorrhagic fever) have very short incubation periods. By the development of an effective adaptive immune response in 4 or 5 days, the virus has spread and caused severe clinical disease.

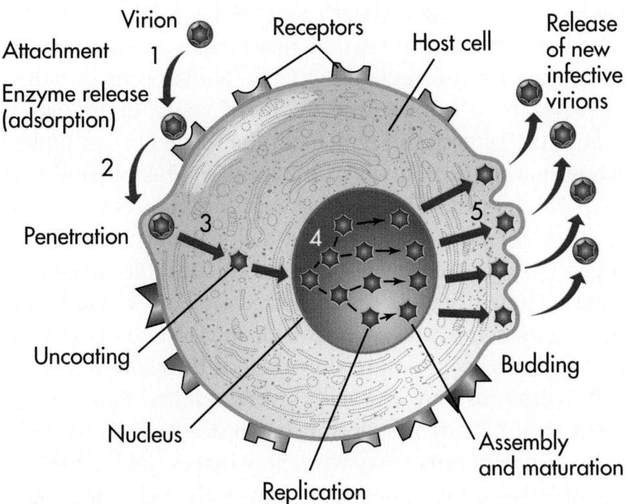

FIGURE 10-10 Stages of Viral Infection of an Infected Cell.

Intracellular Survival. As obligative intracellular pathogens, viruses hide within cells and away from normal inflammatory or immune responses. Viral agents that spread from cell to cell after the initial infection must encounter the immune response, which in most cases cures the infection. Thus most viral infections are self-limiting.

If a symbiotic relationship is maintained between the cell and the virus, persistent unapparent infection may result (latency). The infected cell will be functional, and the virus persists until it is activated to replicate (e.g., the recurrent coldsores of herpes simplex virus infection).[30] Latent viruses usually possess latency-associated transcript (LAT) genes that control persistence indefinitely. Reactivation usually results from expression of lytic genes that lead to increased viral expression and destruction of the infected cell. Latency is characteristic of several chronic viral infections (e.g., HIV, hepatitis B and C viruses).

The interferon response is particularly effective against many viral infections, and viral survival mechanisms have evolved to mitigate the antiviral effects of interferon. The V and P proteins of the measles virus may function as regulators of transcription and prevent the synthesis of interferon, as well as the induction of protective genes by interferon.[31] In a similar fashion, the influenza virus produces a family of viral proteins that inhibit the pathways leading to the production of interferon and to activation of interferon-activated protective genes.[32]

Coat with Self-Proteins. Enveloped viruses are the prime examples of how this mechanism may succeed. The viral capsid is completely surrounded by a cellular plasma membrane that is highly similar to that of an uninfected cell. Only a few critical differences exist. In order to infect another cell the viron expresses envelope proteins (SU and TM proteins) that are critical for the intercellular fusion process. These proteins are virus-specific and targets for protective immune responses. Other viruses, such as the hepatitis C virus, bind on their surface normal proteins from the infected host, such as lipoproteins, that mask the viral epitopes from circulating antibody.[33]

Antigenic Variation. One of the classic examples of antigenic variation is influenza. This virus undergoes frequent antigen shifts and drifts, which are described in detail within the following section titled Example of Viral Pathogenesis. Other viruses (e.g., HIV) add antigenic diversity by incorporating frequent functional translational errors. Some viral enzymes are designed to create small errors in reading mRNA leading to minor changes in the viral proteins. These changes are not at functionally critical sites, but may provide resistance to specific and nonspecific defense mechanisms.

In a manner similar to bacteria, some viruses have multiple stable antigenic serotypes. A person who recovers from an infection with one serotype may not have protective immunity against other serotypes of the same virus. At least 100 serotypes of rhinovirus can cause the "common cold," which explains why individuals can catch many colds throughout their lives. HIV and hepatitis C virus also have multiple serotypes.

Neutralization of Immune Molecules. As with other pathogens, the secretion of large amounts of soluble viral antigen may lead to neutralization of antibody and formation of immune complexes. With infections such as hepatitis B significant levels of circulating immune complexes may form and be deposited in target tissues, such as the kidneys.

Some viruses also have the capacity to neutralize cytokines, such as IL-1 and TNF-α. Cells infected with vaccinia virus produce a protein that can bind to IL-1. These molecules are frequently called cytokine decoys.

Complement Evasion. Several viruses induce expression of regulators of complement activation. Cellular complement inhibitors are incorporated into the envelope of some viruses (e.g., HIV-1, vaccinia). Cytomegalovirus (CMV) induces complement inhibitors on the surface of infected cells. Herpes simplex virus expresses a cell surface protein (glycoprotein C-1) that binds and inhibits C3b, as well blocks the membrane attack complex.

Immune Suppression. HIV and other viruses have developed the capacity to infect and kill immune cells, thus protecting themselves, but also leading to a broad immunosuppression against other antigens. This process is discussed more thoroughly in the section on AIDS.

Some viruses have developed mechanisms for interfering with antigen processing and presentation by major histocompatibility complex (MHC) class I molecules. Endogenous antigens, such as viral antigens, are normally degraded by proteasomes, transported by transporters with antigen processing (TAP) proteins into the endoplasmic reticulum, and complexed with MHC class I molecules for expression on the cell surface and presentation to appropriate cells of the immune response (see Chapter 8). Many of the herpesviruses and retroviruses prevent steps in this process. For instance, Epstein-Barr virus inhibits degradation by the proteasomes. Herpes simplex virus can prevent binding of the antigenic peptide to MHC class I. Inhibition of antigen presentation by MHC class I prevents the generation of effective T-cell immune responses.

Human CMV has developed a unique modification of affecting MHC processing. NK cells are the principal defenders against tumor cells or virally infected cells that have down-regulated MHC expression and are therefore not recognized by T-cytotoxic cells. NK cell function is suppressed by targets with surface class I MHC molecules. CMV is capable of preventing antigen presentation by MHC class I and stimulates the expression of a MHC-like molecule that cannot present antigen but is recognized as a suppression signal by NK cells. Thus CMV-infected cells are protected from both T-cytotoxic cells and NK cell killing.

Tissue Damage. Once inside the infected cell, viruses may have many harmful effects, including the following:

- Cytopathic effects resulting from inhibition of cellular DNA, RNA, or protein synthesis, disruption of lysosomal membranes, resulting in release of "digestive" lysosomal enzymes that can kill the cell (cell lysis)
- Promotion of apoptosis of the cell
- Fusion of infected, adjacent cells, thereby producing **multinucleated giant cells** (herpesviruses and paramyxoviruses [measles virus, mumps virus, respiratory syncytial virus])
- Transformation of infected cell into cancerous cells, resulting in uninhibited and unregulated growth
- Alteration of the antigenic properties, or "identity," of the infected cell, causing the immune system to attack the cell as if it were foreign

Example of Viral Pathogenesis. Influenza is an ssRNA (−strand) with a segmented genome (seven or eight pieces of ssRNA) (Figure 10-11). It is transmitted through aerosols or body fluids and is highly infectious. The virions attach to respiratory epithelial cells and enter by endocytosis. Symptoms begin 1 to 4 days after infection and may include chills, fever, sore throat, muscle aches, severe headaches, coughing, weakness, generalized discomfort, nausea, and vomiting, and may lead to pneumonia; it can be fatal, particularly in young children and older adults. The normal rate of infectivity is about 5% to 15%, with a mortality rate of about 0.1%, and in most cases recovery occurs in 1 to 2 weeks. Yearly seasonal influenza outbreaks result in about 250,000 to 500,000 deaths worldwide.

The influenza virion expresses two surface proteins that are essential to virulence. The hemagglutinin (HA) protein is a glycoprotein that is necessary for entrance into cells by binding to glycan receptors, which are richly expressed on the surface of respiratory epithelium.[34] The surface neuraminidase (NA) is an enzyme that is necessary for release of new virions from infected cells by cleaving cellular sialic acids (a common component of mammalian cell membranes).

Antibodies against the HA and NA antigens are responsible for protection against influenza infection. Infections are seasonal and protection gained from 1 year's infection does not totally protect against influenza in the following year because the HA and NA antigens undergo yearly change. Usually antigenic variation is relatively minor (**antigenic drift**) and results from **mutations.** Individuals frequently have partial protection resulting from the previous year's infection, which lessens the effects of the disease. Two groups of influenza virus, influenza A and influenza B, infect humans, and the yearly vaccine against influenza virus is a trivalent mixture of inactivated proteins from two influenza A subtypes and one influenza B subtype. Influenza B almost exclusively infects humans, mutates at a much lower rate than influenza A, and has reduced rate of antigenic change. Influenza B, however, has antigenically distinct subtypes based on HA (16 forms) and NA (9 forms) antigens and is infectious to birds and mammals. Currently subtypes H1N1, H1N2, and H3N2 are the primary causes of influenza worldwide. Information regarding subtype H5N1 (avian influenza) is summarized in What's New? Avian Influenza.

Periodically influenza A undergoes major antigenic changes (**antigenic shifts**) (see Figure 10-11). Shifts occur in animals coinfected by a human and an avian strain of influenza.[35] Because the genome is segmented, the segments can undergo **recombination** during which the human virus obtains a new HA or NA antigen. When such changes occur, previous protection may not exist, resulting in a major pandemic and much more severe disease. In 1918 an antigenic shift occurred in the western United States (first reported in Fort Riley, Kansas) resulting in an influenza A virus with an H1N1 serotype (called Spanish flu). The virus spread worldwide throughout 1918 and 1919. Symptoms were unusually severe, resulted from excessive production of cytokines, and included deaths from secondary bacterial pneumonia, massive hemorrhages, and pulmonary edema. Spanish flu possessed an extremely high rate of infectivity (up to 50%) and mortality (killed 20% or more of those

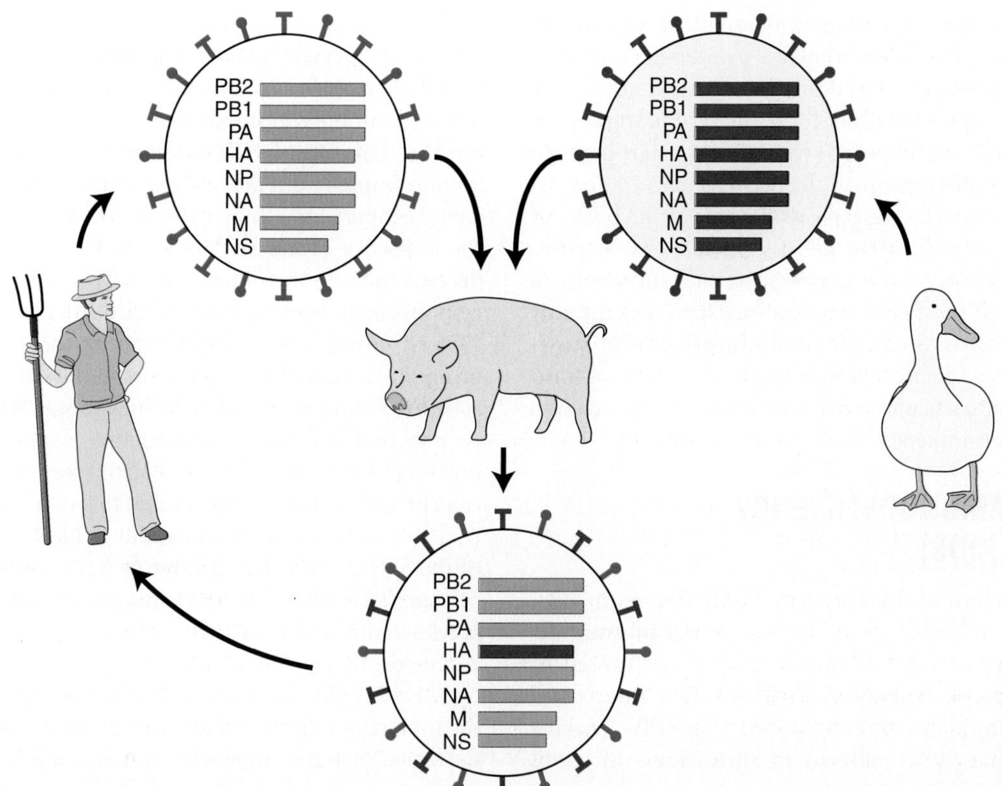

FIGURE 10-11 **Antigenic Shifts in Influenza Virus.** One theory proposes that antigenic shifts occur when a human influenza virus *(blue)* and an avian influenza virus *(red)* coinfect a species that is permissive for both. The eight ssRNA strands are co-expressed in the same infected cell, resulting in mixing of the strands so that a hybrid virus can be produced. The hybrid virus indicated here contains all the genetic information of the original virus that infected humans, but contains a new hemagglutinin *(HA)*-containing stand from the avian virus. This virus expresses a new HA antigen and will be less susceptible to residual immunity that normally provides partial protection against yearly influenza infections.

WHAT'S NEW?

Avian Influenza

Influenza viruses infect a wide variety of species, including humans, different strains of birds, and swine. The species specificity of a particular variant of influenza is determined by the amino acid sequence of the hemagglutinin (HA) molecule on the viral surface. Influenza viruses have a relatively high mutation rate that can result in minor changes in the HA and change the species specificity. As a result, an influenza virus strain that primarily infects birds may, after a mutation, become efficiently infectious for humans.

Various strains of a highly pathogenic avian influenza A (H5N1) have arisen in the past few years. These strains were first reported in 1996 in China. The most pathogenic variants have a near 100% mortality rate in domestic poultry and have spread globally, killing tens of millions of birds. The global spread may be a result of collateral nonfatal infection of wild migrating birds, such as ducks and geese.

In 1997, the first human infections with the H5N1 avian virus were reported in Hong Kong involving 18 cases, 6 of whom died. From 2003 through 2012, the WHO has reported a total of 608 confirmed H5N1 cases and 359 deaths across 15 countries worldwide. So far, human infections occur primarily in those individuals who have been in close contact with infected birds (especially those who have handled sick, dead, or frozen poultry). Human-to-human transmission is rare. No cases have been identified among short-term travelers visiting countries affected by outbreaks. The H5N1 strain infects the lungs and targets type 2 alveolar pneumocytes and macrophages. It also passes throughout the body to the gastrointestinal tract, brain, liver, and blood cells and can be transmitted transplacentally from the mother to the fetus. Symptoms include fever, cough, sore throat, muscle aches, eye infections (conjunctivitis), pneumonia, acute respiratory distress, and other severe and life-threatening complications. Diagnosis is made by detection of viral ribonucleic acid (RNA) obtained through throat swabs. The mortality rate in human infections is about 60%. Host immunogenic variation may play a role in the outcome of the immune response.

The concern is that further mutations may lead to a strain that spreads and infects humans more efficiently, resulting in a rapid pandemic. These concerns are not unfounded. Highly pathogenic H5N1 strains have undergone continued evolution and expansion of host range with increasing mortality rates among wild birds and infectivity for other mammals, including dogs and cats. In 2007, a H5N1 strain was clearly transmitted from an infected individual to six other members of the same Indonesian family group. The virus was further transmitted from one of those six, an infected child, to the child's caregiver. Seven of the eight individuals died.

Whether highly pathogenic variants of H5N1 avian influenza virus eventually mutate into a major human pathogen remains to be seen. Prevention efforts rely on the development, distribution, and use of vaccines. Antiviral agents are used for active infection and prophylaxis of those who have been exposed to the virus. Candidate genes influencing susceptibility are being identified.

Data from Chmielewski R, Swayne DE: *Annu Rev Food Sci Technol* 2:37–57, 2011; Juno J, Fowke KR, Keynan Y: *Clin Dev Immunol* 2012:797180, 2012; Steel J: *BioDrugs* 25(5):285–298, 2011; Van Kerkhove MD et al: *PLoS One* 6(1):e14582, 2011, review, erratum in *PLoS One* 7(1), 2012; Watanabe Y et al: *Trends Microbiol* 20(1):11–20, 2012; World Health Organization: *Cumulative number of confirmed human cases of avian influenza/(H5N1) Reported to WHO,* 2012. Available at www.who.int/influenza/human_animal_interface/H5N1_cumulative_table_archives/en/index.html.

infected) and resulted in an estimated 40 million deaths worldwide. A unique aspect of this influenza pandemic concerned the age of the most susceptible populations.[36] Most mortalities secondary to influenza generally occur in the very young or very old. Although those two age groups were at risk, a startling high mortality rate was observed in adults between ages 20 and 39. Strain variations caused by antigenic drift occur within both HA and NA, and some may further affect virulence of that virus. The 1918 H1N1 serotype also possessed several mutations in the HA that resulted in a far greater virulence than the currently circulating H1N1 type. Studies have demonstrated that survivors of the 1918 pandemic still have protective levels of antibodies against that particular virus, confirming that protection against a particular influenza strain may be lifelong.

ACQUIRED IMMUNODEFICIENCY SYNDROME (AIDS)

The most notable form of secondary or acquired immune deficiency caused by an infectious agent is **acquired immunodeficiency syndrome (AIDS).** AIDS is a viral disease caused by the **human immunodeficiency virus (HIV).** HIV infects and depletes a portion of the immune system (Th cells), making individuals extremely susceptible to life-threatening infections and malignancies.

Despite major efforts by healthcare agencies around the world, HIV/AIDS remains the major cause of worldwide morbidity and mortality. Although aggressive antiretroviral therapy and public health campaigns have stabilized the number of new cases and deaths in the United States from HIV/AIDS, the number of cases and deaths continues to increase rapidly worldwide. Surveillance reports from the Centers for Disease Control and Prevention (CDC) estimates that more than a million (1,148,200) adults and adolescents were living with HIV infection in the United States in 2010, of whom 18% were undiagnosed, and that approximately 50,000 new HIV infections occur yearly.[37] Most new infections (61%) occurred in gay or bisexual men. The number of new AIDS diagnoses in the United States increases by more than 30,000 per year (estimated at about 35,000 in 2011). The estimated number of AIDS-related deaths in 2010 was 15,529. Cumulatively since 1981 more than a million individuals (1,155,792) have been diagnosed with AIDS in the United States, of which almost 636,000 have died as a result, and more than 490,000 are still living with AIDS. In the United States, AIDS is predominantly related to a history of male-to-male sexual contact: about 50% of the newly diagnosed cases were attributed to male-to-male sexual contact, 30% to high-risk heterosexual contact, and 14% to injected drug abuse. About 25% of new cases were diagnosed in females, primarily (74%) contracted through high-risk heterosexual contact.

Sub-Saharan Africa is still the epicenter of the AIDS pandemic. In 2009, the World Health Organization (WHO) estimated that 22.5 million people living with HIV infection (68% of the global total) resided in sub-Saharan Africa. South Africa continues to have the largest estimated number of infected individuals (5.6 million), and Swaziland has the highest adult prevalence (26%) of HIV infection in the world.[38] Women remain at greatest risk of infection: of all women infected with HIV globally, 76% of them reside in sub-Saharan Africa. Throughout the region, women, especially those aged 15 to 19, are the majority of HIV-infected individuals. HIV infection among women aged 20 to 24 in South Africa is approximately 21%, compared to 7% in age-matched men. It is estimated that the incidence of new HIV infections in women in the region exceeds those in men by 1.3 times. It is estimated that AIDS is responsible for almost 50% of all deaths in South Africa and 71% of deaths among individuals in the 15- to 40-year age group. It is the leading cause of maternal deaths and is responsible for 35% of deaths in children younger than 5 years of age. As a result, the average life expectancy is now 54 years, whereas it would be at least 64 without AIDS. More than half of the current 15-year-olds are not expected to live to age 60.

The outlook for the future is not all bleak. Through the work of the WHO and other groups, as well as the implementation of aggressive AIDS awareness programs and greatly increased access to antiretroviral therapy in many sub-Saharan African countries, the incidence of HIV infection and death caused by AIDS is falling across the region. The HIV infection rate in the total region fell by more than 25% between 2001 and 2009. Between 2004 and 2009, the number of AIDS-related deaths decreased by 20%.

Transmission

HIV is a blood-borne pathogen present in body fluids (e.g., blood, vaginal fluid, semen, breast milk) with the typical routes of transmission: blood or blood products, intravenous drug abuse, heterosexual and homosexual activity, and maternal-child transmission before or during birth. As of 2009, an estimated 8640 children in the United States developed AIDS after contracting HIV infection from their mothers across the placenta, through contact with infected blood during delivery, or through the milk during breast-feeding. Without treatment, symptoms usually develop within 6 months of life, and life expectancy is generally less than 3 years. However, adequate use of prenatal antiviral therapy has reduced maternal-child transmission dramatically; only 12 new cases were reported in 2009.

As with all blood-borne infections, healthcare providers are at increased risk of contracting the infection from an individual's blood.[39] The first reported case of occupational HIV infection was an emergency department nurse who became infected in 1986. The route of infection was probably through cuts in her hand that came into contact with contaminated blood through a gauze pad she was holding on a person's open wound. The infectivity of HIV is relatively low compared to other major blood-borne contaminants; from a single needle stick of contaminated blood the probability of acquiring an HIV infection is 0.3%, compared to 3% for hepatitis C and 30% for hepatitis B.[40] Tens of thousands of healthcare workers have become infected with HIV, but as of May 2011, only 57 cases of confirmed HIV infection and 143 possible cases were contracted by occupational exposure, and no new cases of occupational HIV infection have been identified since 1999.[41] Since initiation of widespread educational programs on universal precautions published by the

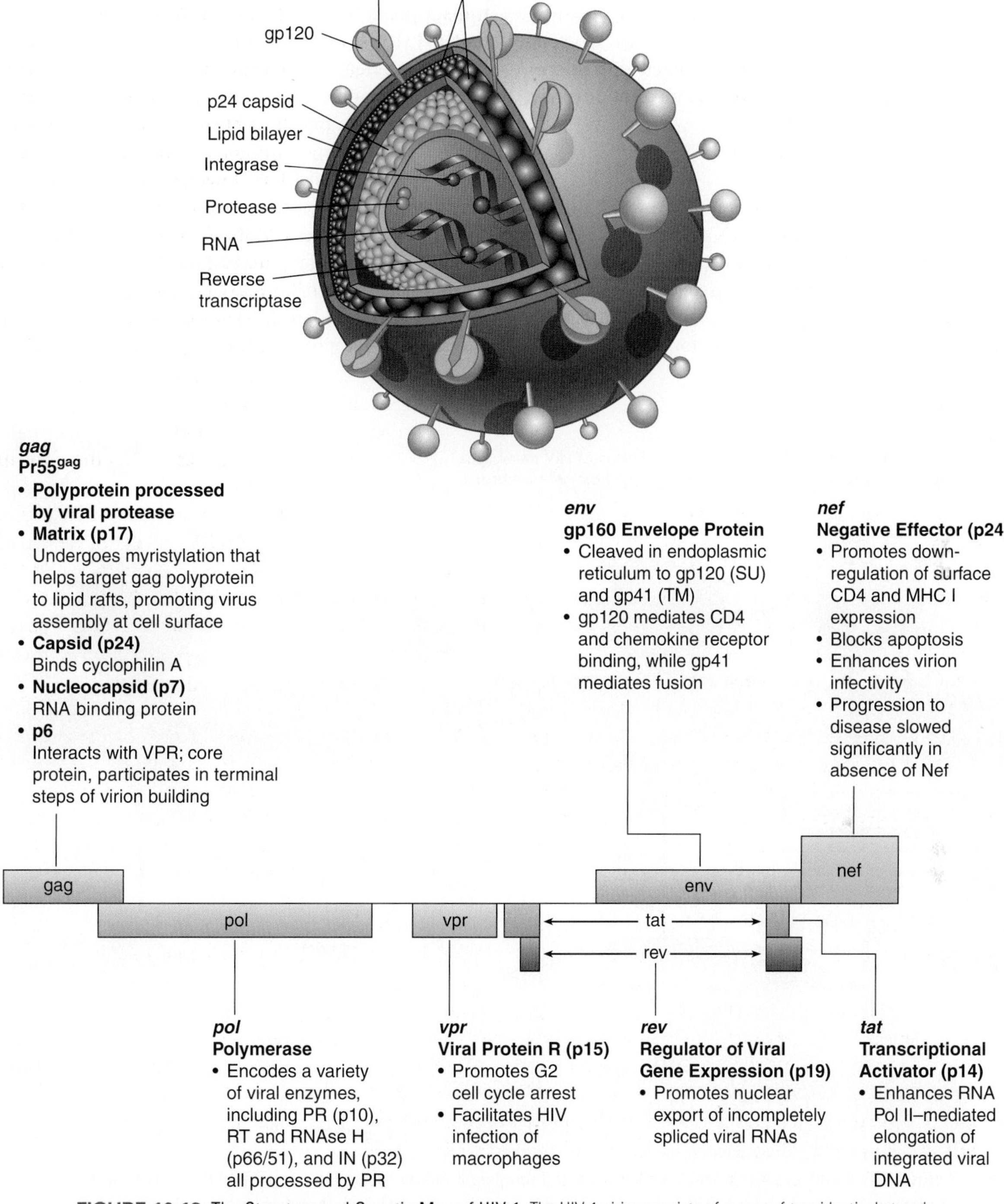

FIGURE 10-12 The Structure and Genetic Map of HIV-1. The HIV-1 virion consists of a core of two identical strands of viral RNA molecules of viral enzymes (reverse transcriptase [RT], protease [PR], integrase [IN]) encoated in a core capsid structure consisting primarily of the structural viral protein p24. The capsid is further encased in a matrix consisting primarily of a viral protein, p17. The outer surface is an envelope consisting of the plasma membrane of the cell from which the virus budded (lipid bilayer) and two viral glycoproteins: a transmembrane gp41 and a noncovalently attached surface protein, gp120. The HIV-1 genome contains regions that encode the structural proteins *(gag)*, the viral enzymes *(pol)*, and the envelope proteins *(env)*. The *gag* region is translated into a large precursor ($Pr55^{gag}$) that is cut by the HIV protease into smaller proteins that construct the capsid and matrix. The *env* region is translated into a gp160 precursor protein that is cut by a host-cell protease into the gp120 and gp41 envelope proteins. The genome of complex retroviruses, like HIV-1, often contains a variety of small regions that regulate expression of the virus. (Modified from Kumar V et al: *Robbins & Cotran pathologic basis of disease,* ed 8, Philadelphia, 2010, Saunders.)

CDC only 3 new cases have been reported. Nurses (42% of total cases) and clinical laboratory technicians (28% of cases) are by far the most commonly exposed healthcare workers. In the event of occupational exposure to HIV-contaminated specimens, post-exposure prophylaxis with antiretroviral medications may be appropriate.[42,43]

Pathogenesis

HIV-1 was initially isolated by researchers at the Pasteur Institute as the lymphadenopathy/AIDS virus (LAV), a discovery for which they received the 2008 Nobel Prize in Medicine.[44] A second major and less virulent variant, HIV-2, was identified later and is found mostly in western Africa. HIV is a member of the retrovirus family, which carries genetic information in the form of two copies of RNA (Figure 10-12). Retroviruses use a viral enzyme, **reverse transcriptase,** to convert RNA into double-stranded DNA (Figure 10-13). Using a second viral enzyme, an **integrase,** the new DNA is inserted into the infected cell's genetic material, where it may remain dormant. If the cell is activated, translation of the viral information may be initiated, resulting in the formation of new virions, lysis and death of the infected cell, and shedding of infectious HIV particles. If, however, the cell remains relatively dormant, the viral genetic material may remain latent for years, and is probably present for the life of the individual.

The primary surface receptor on HIV is the envelope glycoprotein gp120, which binds to the molecule CD4, found primarily on the surface of helper T cells (see Figure 10-13).[45] Several other necessary co-receptors have been identified on the target cells,

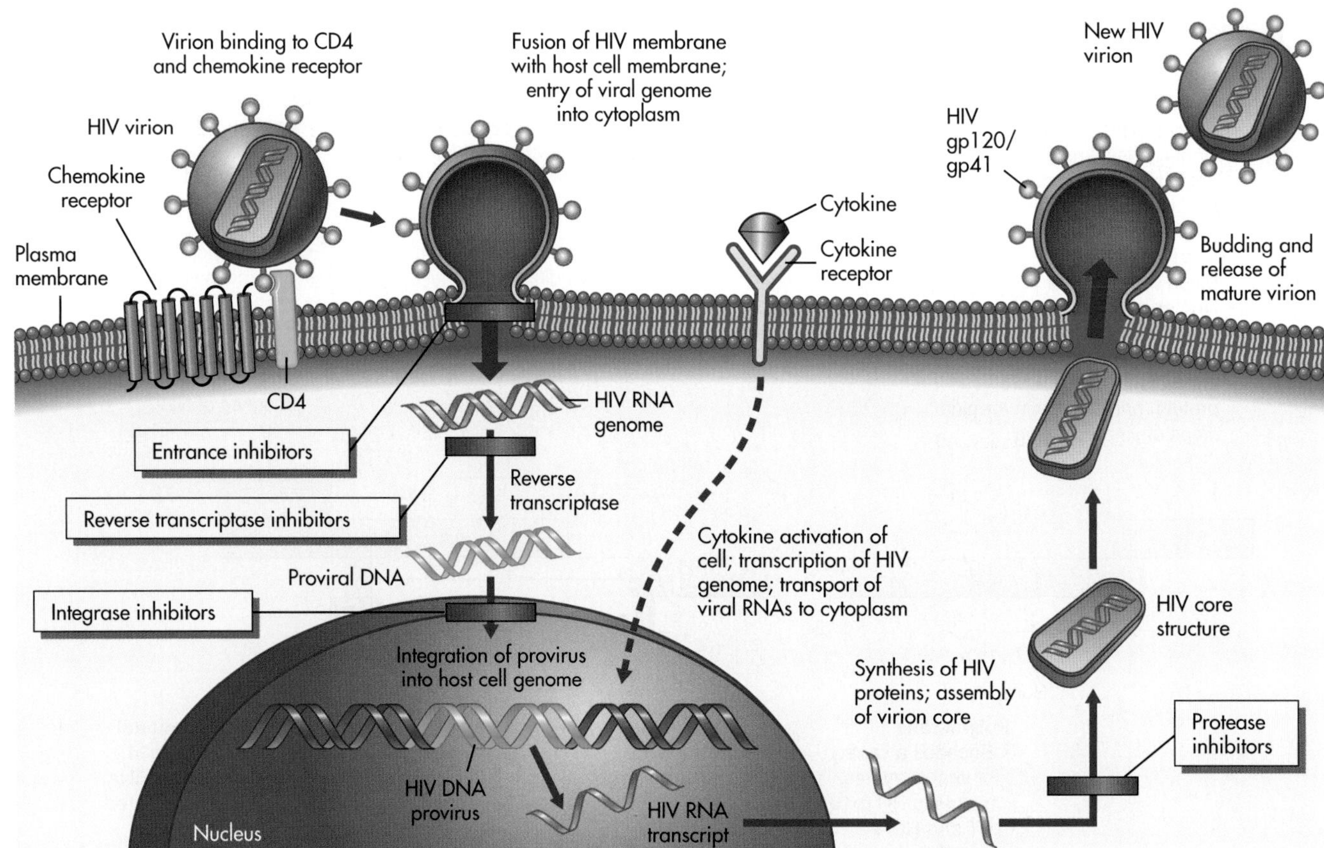

FIGURE 10-13 Life Cycle and Possible Sites of Therapeutic Intervention of HIV-1. HIV infection begins when a virion, or virus particle, binds to CD4 and chemokine co-receptors on a susceptible cell. The HIV virion has viral proteins gp41 and gp120 on its surface (envelope), which interact with CD4 and the CCR5 co-receptor and initiate fusion between the viral envelope and the plasma membrane, resulting in the core of the virus being injected into the cytoplasm. Uncoating occurs in the cytoplasm, during which the core proteins are removed, and the viral RNA is released into the infected cell's cytoplasm. The viral RNA is converted to a double-stranded DNA provirus by the action of the viral reverse transcriptase. The provirus migrates into the nucleus and is integrated into the cell's own DNA. The provirus may remain latent. If the infected cell is activated (e.g., by cytokines), the provirus may be transcribed and translated into viral protein precursors. The precursor proteins are modified by viral (gag proteins) and cellular (env proteins) proteases into smaller proteins that are used to package the viral RNA into new virions that bud from the cell. The HIV-1 life cycle is susceptible to blockage at several sites. Some agents could block the attachment and entrance of the virus (entrance inhibitors). Reverse transcriptase inhibitors (e.g., azidothymidine [AZT]) prevent the reverse transcription of viral RNA into DNA. Drugs also may be able to inhibit the viral integrase (integrase inhibitors) and prevent insertion of the provirus into the host's chromosomes. Protease inhibitors specifically inhibit the viral protease and prevent the processing of the gp160 into viral capsid and matrix proteins. (Modified from Kumar V, Abbas A, Fausto N: *Robbins & Cotran pathologic basis of disease,* ed 7, Philadelphia, 2005, Saunders.)

particularly the chemokine receptors CXCR4 and CCR5. Different strains of HIV-1 are selective for the CXCR4 or CCR5 co-receptors, which influences the tropism for different target cells. Strains that prefer the CXCR4 co-receptor tend to be T-cell tropic, usually found later in an infection, and cause infected cells to fuse and form a multinucleate **syncytium.** Strains that react better with the co-receptor CCR5 are macrophage-tropic, usually cause the primary HIV infection, and do not cause syncytium formation.

The primary cellular targets for HIV include the following:

- CD4-positive Th cells
- Dendritic cells (depending on the level of chemokine receptors the cell expresses)
- Macrophages (express low levels of CD4, but high amounts of heparin sulfate proteoglycans [syndecan] and other molecules [CCR5] that bind to gp120 and adsorb HIV)
- CD8-positive Tc cells (low rate of infection, but CD4 can be expressed by activated CD8-positive Tc cells)
- Double positive thymic cells (express CD4 and CD8 simultaneously)
- NK cells (some are CD4+, CCR5+)
- Neural cells of monocyte origin (macrophages and microglial cells)

Initially, the lymphoid areas of the mucosal surfaces are the primary sites of infection (Figure 10-14). Dendritic cells and mucosal T cells probably spread the infection to other peripheral lymphoid organs (especially follicular dendritic cells in the lymph nodes, which infect T cells).[46] Infection also may involve the thymus and bone marrow, including the bone marrow stromal cells. Cells in the central nervous system (e.g., astrocytes and monocytes), the gastrointestinal tract (particularly in the rectum and ileum), and other anatomic sites act as reservoirs in which HIV can be relatively protected from antiviral drugs.[47] The virus is also found in T cells and macrophages in semen and in the renal epithelium.

The major immunologic finding in AIDS is the striking decrease in the number of CD4+ Th cells (Figure 10-15). Individuals who are not HIV infected typically have 800 to 1000 CD4+ cells/μL of blood, with a range from 600 to 1200/μL. Numbers of CD8+ Tc cells are usually normal or slightly elevated. The decrease in CD4+ cell numbers results in a reversal of the normal CD4/CD8 T-cell ratio (normally about 1.9) to lower than 0.9 and often near zero.

HIV causes destruction of Th cells by a variety of means. Production of new HIV virions can be directly cytopathic to the infected cell, causing lysis (breakdown of the cell) or inducing

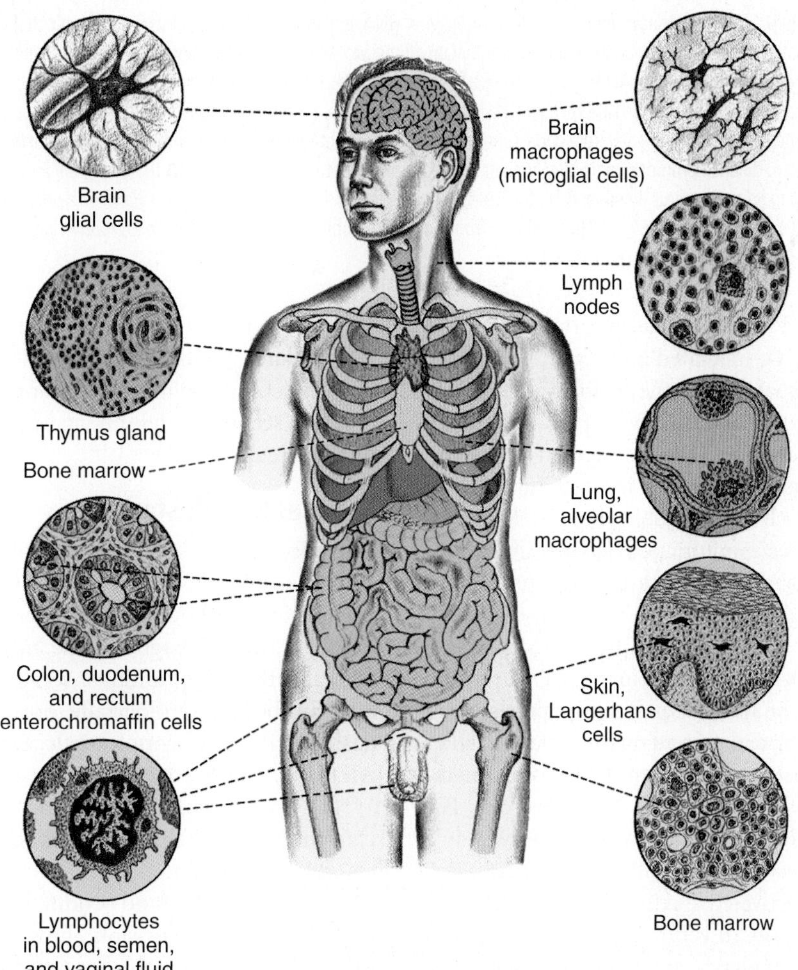

FIGURE 10-14 **Distribution of Tissues That Can Be Infected by HIV.** Infection is closely linked to the presence of CD4 receptors or chemokine co-receptors on host tissue, particularly T cells and macrophages. (Modified from Weber JN, Weiss RA: *HIV infection: the cellular picture, in the science of AIDS: readings from Scientific American,* New York, 1989, Freeman.)

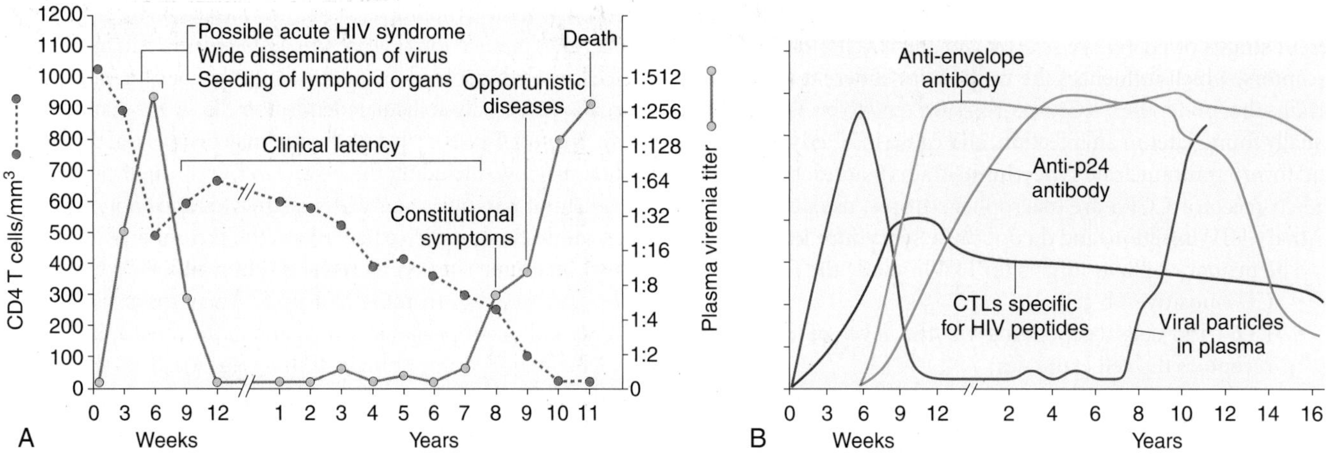

FIGURE 10-15 Typical Course of Progression from HIV Infection to AIDS in Untreated Persons. **A,** Within weeks after infection, the person may experience symptoms of acute HIV syndrome. During this early period the virus progressively infects mucosal T cells and dendritic cells, propagates, and spreads to the lymphoid organs, with a sharp decrease in the number of circulating CD4+ Th cells. The resulting immune response usually induces a period of clinical latency, during which viral replication and T-cell destruction continue in the lymph nodes, although the individual is generally asymptomatic. As the disease progresses, the person may develop HIV-related disease (constitutional symptoms)—a variety of symptoms of acute viral infection that do not involve opportunistic infections or malignancies. When the number of CD4+ cells is critically suppressed, the person becomes susceptible to a variety of opportunistic infections and cancers. The length of time for progression from HIV infection to AIDS may vary considerably from person to person. **B,** Antibody and Tc cell (cytotoxic T lymphocytes [CTLs]) levels change during the progression to AIDS. During the initial phase antibodies against HIV-1 are not yet detectable (window period), but viral products, including p24 antigen, viral RNA, and infectious virus, may be detectable in the blood a few weeks after infection. Most antibodies produced against envelope proteins in the early phase are absorbed onto viral particles in the blood and are not detectable by most routine assays. During the latent phase of infection antibody levels against p24 and other viral proteins, as well as HIV-specific CTLs, generally increase, then remain constant until the development of AIDS. As the immune system becomes severely depressed and excess viral antigen is released into the blood, measurable antibody levels decrease. Disease progression usually ends in the death of the untreated individual. (**A** redrawn from Fauci AS, Lane HC: Human immunodeficiency virus disease: AIDS and related conditions. In Fauci AS et al, editors: *Harrison's principles of internal medicine,* ed 14, New York, 1997, McGraw-Hill; **B** from Kumar V, Abbas A, Fausto N: *Robbins & Cotran pathologic basis of disease,* ed 8, Philadelphia, 2010, Saunders.)

apoptosis. Additionally, HIV-infected cells express new surface antigens and are targets for Tc-mediated lysis.

However, it is not unusual for a large majority (>98%) of peripheral CD4+ Th cells to *not* be infected with HIV-1, although a significant amount (10% to 50%) show signs of apoptosis. Therefore, HIV-1 killing is probably an indirect rather than direct effect. HIV-infected cells shed soluble viral envelope protein, gp120, which can induce apoptotic cell death of uninfected T lymphocytes, neurons, and monocytes through interaction with cell surface receptors. The interaction between viral envelope protein on the surface of infected cells and its receptors on neighboring uninfected cells also can result in intercellular fusion and syncytium formation. The syncytia undergo apoptosis after a phase of latency. Envelope protein present on the surface of HIV-1–infected cells also can create partial fusion (hemifusion, membrane damage) that results in death of the uninfected cell. The presence of HIV virions and soluble viral antigen can result in a chronic activation of uninfected T cells with HIV-specific T-cell receptors (TCRs). Because activated T cells more efficiently support HIV replication, the most susceptible cells are those with TCRs against HIV, which undergo antigen-driven activation and infection. This observation may not bode well for successful vaccine development if the induced and supposedly protective CD4+ cells are also the most susceptible targets for HIV.

As a result of these processes the level of T cells decreases (particularly T-memory cells, which seem more susceptible to HIV infection), thymic production of new T cells is decreased, and the secondary lymphoid organs (particularly the lymph nodes) are damaged.

Clinical Manifestations

Depletion of CD4+ cells has a profound effect on the immune system, causing a severely diminished response to a wide array of infectious pathogens and malignant tumors (Box 10-2).

At the time of diagnosis, the individual may manifest one of several different conditions: serologically negative (no detectable antibody), serologically positive (positive for antibody against HIV) but asymptomatic, early stages of HIV disease, or AIDS (see Figure 10-15).

The presence of circulating antibody against the HIV indicates infection by the virus, although many of these individuals are asymptomatic. Antibody appears rather rapidly after infection through blood products, usually within 4 to 7 weeks. After sexual transmission, however, the individual can be infected yet seronegative for 6 to 14 months or, in at least one case, for years. In addition, in the late stages of the disease, some individuals become seronegative because of a deficient immune system.

BOX 10-2 AIDS-DEFINING OPPORTUNISTIC INFECTIONS AND NEOPLASMS FOUND IN INDIVIDUALS WITH HIV INFECTION

Protozoal and Helminthic Infections

Cryptosporidiosis or isosporiasis (enteritis)
Toxoplasmosis (pneumonia or central nervous system [CNS] infection)

Fungal Infections

Pneumocystosis (pneumonia or disseminated infection)
Candidiasis (esophageal, tracheal, or pulmonary)
Cryptococcosis (CNS infection)
Coccidioidomycosis (disseminated)
Histoplasmosis (disseminated)

Bacterial Infections

Mycobacteriosis (atypical, e.g., *Mycobacterium avium-intracellulare*, disseminated or extrapulmonary; *Mycobacterium tuberculosis*, pulmonary or extrapulmonary)
Nocardiosis (pneumonia, meningitis, disseminated)
Salmonella infections (disseminated)

Viral infections

Cytomegalovirus (pulmonary, intestinal, retinitis, or CNS infections)
Herpes simplex virus (localized or disseminated)
Varicella-zoster virus (localized or disseminated)
Progressive multifocal (leukoencephalopathy)

Neoplasms

Kaposi sarcoma
B-cell non-Hodgkin lymphomas
Primary lymphoma of the brain
Invasive cancer of the uterine cervix

Adapted from Kumar V et al: *Robbins & Cotran pathologic basis of disease,* ed 8, Philadelphia, 2010, Saunders.

The period between infection and the appearance of antibody is referred to as the **window period** (see Figure 10-15). Although the individual may not have antibody, he or she may have virus growing, have virus in the blood and body fluids, and be infectious to others. Early symptoms are relatively nonspecific to HIV and include fatigue, fever, muscle aches, and headaches.

Those with the early stages of HIV disease *(early stage disease* or *clinical latency)* are usually asymptomatic. The early stage may last as long as 10 years in untreated people, during which viral load increases and numbers of CD4+ cells progressively decrease. Some estimates are that approximately 99% of untreated HIV-infected individuals would eventually progress to AIDS.

The currently accepted definition of AIDS relies on both laboratory tests and clinical symptoms. The most common laboratory test is for antibodies against HIV proteins (particularly p24). If the individual is seropositive, the diagnosis of AIDS is made in association with various clinical symptoms (see Box 10-2). The symptoms include atypical or opportunistic infections and cancers, as well as indications of debilitating chronic disease (e.g., wasting syndrome, recurrent fevers) (Figure 10-16). Most commonly, new cases of AIDS are diagnosed initially by decreased CD4+ T-cell numbers at or below 200 cells/μL.

Treatment and Prevention

The current regimen of **antiretroviral therapy (ART)** for treatment of HIV infection is a combination of drugs.[48] As of 2012, more than 20 antiretroviral drugs that fell into 6 different mechanisms were available for ART. Classes of antiretroviral agents included inhibitors of the enzyme reverse transcriptase (nucleoside reverse transcriptase inhibitors [NRTIs] and non-nucleoside reverse transcriptase inhibitors [NNRTIs]), inhibitors of the viral protease (protease inhibitors [PIs]), inhibitors of fusion between HIV and the cell membrane (fusion inhibitors), inhibitors of HIV binding to CCR3 (CCR5 antagonists), and inhibitors of the viral integrase enzyme (integrase strand transfer inhibitors [INSTIs]). Several preferred and alternative therapeutic regimens are recommended, depending on the particular individual. In general, the combination includes at least three drugs: two NRTIs and one from another class (NNRTI, PI, INSTI, or CCR5 antagonist) (see Figure 10-13). Death from AIDS-related diseases has been reduced significantly since the introduction of ART; without treatment an individual may live only 9 to 10 months after diagnosis of AIDS, whereas those who respond well to ART may survive for several decades. However, many people do not respond to ART therapy, those who do respond are not "cured," and resistant variants to these drugs have been identified. Many individuals who initiate antiretroviral therapy will still have a shortened life expectancy secondary to HIV-associated persistent immune activation. Although the capacity of the immune system to respond to specific pathogens is greatly diminished, HIV infection nonspecifically activates T cells and monocytes resulting in greatly increased production of inflammatory cytokines and an increased risk for developing chronic and potentially fatal morbidities, such as cardiovascular disease, renal disease, diabetes, and liver disease.[49]

Drug therapy for AIDS is difficult because, like most retroviruses, the AIDS virus incorporates into the genetic material of the host and may never be removed by antimicrobial therapy. Therefore, drug administration to control the virus may have to continue for the lifetime of the individual. Additionally, HIV may persist in regions where the antiviral drugs are not as effective, such as the central nervous system (CNS).

To date, the development of an effective vaccine is the only hope for preventing the spread of HIV infection. Most common antiviral vaccines (e.g., rubella, mumps, influenza) induce protective antibodies that block the initial infection. Only one vaccine (rabies) is used after the infection has occurred. That approach is successful because the rabies virus proliferates and spreads very slowly. Whether an HIV vaccine would be effective in either preventing or treating HIV infection is problematic, and the results of recent vaccine trials have for the moment dampened enthusiasm. The USPSTF recommends that clinicians screen adolescents and adults aged 15 to 65 years for HIV infection. Those younger or older who are at increased risk should also be screened.[49a]

Pediatric AIDS and Central Nervous System Involvement

The clinical diagnosis of HIV in children is very often a difficult task (Box 10-3). The presence of passive maternal antibody limits the use of HIV antibody testing in infants in the high-risk

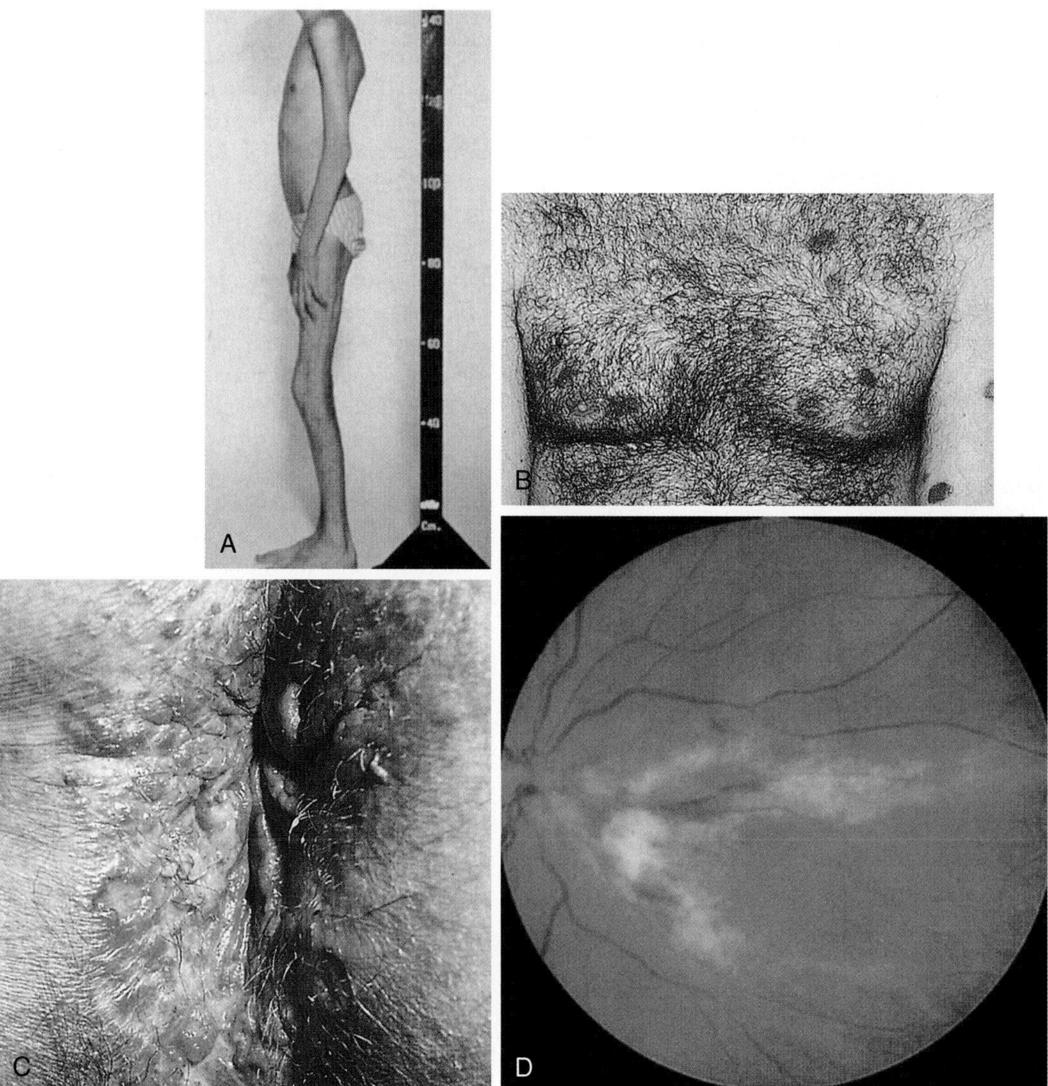

FIGURE 10-16 Clinical Symptoms of AIDS. **A,** Severe weight loss and anorexia. **B,** Biopsy-proven Kaposi sarcoma lesions. **C,** Perianal vesicular and ulcerative lesions of herpes simplex infection. **D,** Deterioration of vision from cytomegalovirus retinitis leading to areas of infection; unless treated the progressive impairment will lead to blindness. (**A** and **D** from Taylor PK: *Diagnostic picture tests in sexually transmitted diseases,* London, 1995, Mosby; **B** and **C** from Morse SA, Holmes KK, Ballard RC, editors: *Atlas of sexually transmitted diseases and AIDS,* ed 4, London, 2011, Saunders.)

category up to 18 months of age. In this age group, diagnosis of HIV infection must be made by assays to measure viral DNA or RNA in the blood. For children older than 18 months, the diagnosis of HIV infection is confirmed by the presence of specific antibodies to the virus.

HIV directly invades most major organ systems, including the CNS. Therefore, the clinical manifestations vary greatly from child to child. The initial signs and symptoms may be nonspecific and subtle, and they may progress slowly or rapidly to an acute, life-threatening condition. A definite diagnosis of HIV is made by obtaining a personal history, performing virologic testing, and assessing clinical manifestations. Monitoring CD8+ T lymphocytes and monocytes, in addition to CD4+ Th lymphocytes, has been suggested for predicting risk for progressive encephalopathy. Decreases in the number of CD8+ Tc lymphocytes diminish defenses against viral infection and facilitate infected monocytes to cross the blood-brain barrier.

A particularly vulnerable site of HIV infection in infants and children is the CNS. HIV encephalopathy is more common in the advanced stages. Because survival of children with HIV has been prolonged with effective treatment, the incidence of progressive encephalopathy has increased. The 1994 classification from the CDC requires one of the following progressing findings to be present for at least 2 months, in the absence of a concurrent illness other than HIV that could explain the following findings:

- Failure to attain or loss of developmental milestones, or loss of intellectual ability, verified by standard developmental scale or neuropsychologic tests
- Impaired brain growth or acquired microcephaly demonstrated by head circumference measurements or brain atrophy demonstrated by computed tomography (CT) or magnetic resonance imaging (MRI) with serial imaging required in children less than 2 years of age

BOX 10-3 PEDIATRIC HUMAN IMMUNODEFICIENCY VIRUS (HIV) CLASSIFICATION

IMMUNOLOGIC CATEGORIES	N: NO SIGNS/ SYMPTOMS	A: MILD SIGNS/ SYMPTOMS	B: MODERATE SIGNS/ SYMPTOMS	C: SEVERE SIGNS/ SYMPTOMS
1. No evidence	N1	A1	B1	C1
2. Evidence of moderate suppression	N2	A2	B2	C2
3. Severe suppression	N3	A3	B3	C3

Clinical Categories for Children with HIV Infection

Category N: Not symptomatic

Children who have no signs or symptoms considered to be the result of HIV infection or who have only one of the conditions listed in Category A

Category A: Mildly symptomatic

Children with two or more of the conditions listed below but none of the conditions listed in Category B or C:

Lymphadenopathy
Hepatomegaly
Splenomegaly
Dermatitis
Parotitis
Recurrent or persistent upper respiratory tract infection, sinusitis, or otitis media

Category B: Moderately symptomatic

Children who have symptomatic conditions other than those listed for Category A or C that are attributed to HIV infection; examples of conditions in clinical Category B include but are not limited to:

Anemia (≤8 g/dl), neutropenia (≤1000 mm^3), or thrombocytopenia (≤100,000 mm^3) persisting ≥30 days
Bacterial meningitis, pneumonia, or sepsis (single episode)
Candidiasis or oropharyngeal infection (thrush) persisting (≥2 months) in children ≥6 months of age
Cardiomyopathy
Cytomegalovirus infection with onset before 1 month of age
Diarrhea, recurrent or chronic
Hepatitis
Herpes simplex virus (HSV), recurrent stomatitis (more than two episodes within 1 year)
HSV bronchitis, pneumonitis, or esophagitis with onset before 1 month of age
Herpes zoster (shingles) involving at least two distinct episodes or more than 1 dermatome
Leiomyosarcoma
Lymphoid interstitial pneumonia (LIP) or pulmonary lymphoid hyperplasia complex
Neuropathy
Nocardiosis
Persistent fever (lasting ≥1 month)
Toxoplasmosis, onset before 1 month of age
Varicella, disseminated (complicated chickenpox)

Category C: Severely symptomatic

Children who have any condition listed in the 1987 surveillance case definition of acquired immunodeficiency with the exception of LIP

Data from Centers for Disease Control and Prevention: *MMWR Morb Mortal Wkly Rep* 43(12):1, 1994.

- Acquired symmetric motor deficits manifested by affecting a child 1 month of age or older
- The onset of progressive encephalopathy may be a prognostic indicator of a poor outcome.

It may be difficult to completely differentiate the effect of HIV infection on the CNS from the effect of prenatal and perinatal exposure. In addition, other insults may accompany HIV in a young child and affect growth and development, such as drug exposure, prematurity, chronic illness, and a chaotic social atmosphere. The pathogenesis of HIV encephalopathy in children is poorly understood, but the presence of inflammatory mediators may be a contributing factor.

A growing number of investigational protocols are available for treatment of children with HIV. In general, treatment is focused on the preservation and maintenance of the immune system, aggressive response to opportunistic infections, and support and relief of symptomatic occurrences and administration of ART.[50]

COUNTERMEASURES AGAINST PATHOGENS

An extremely effective means of countering infectious microorganisms is rigorous use of environmental infection control measures, including control of insect vector populations, establishment of modern sanitation facilities, provision of clean water and uncontaminated food supplies, and other measures. Additionally, prophylactic or interventive procedures have been developed to prevent pathogens from initiating disease (vaccines) or to subdue the pathogen once the disease process has started (antimicrobials). Vaccine development has focused successfully on preventing the most severe and common infections (Table 10-9). With the initial success of antibiotic therapy, there was no perceived need for vaccination against many common and non–life-threatening infections. The increasing problem of antibiotic-resistant pathogens, however, forced a reappraisal of that strategy, and a greater emphasis is being placed on the development of new vaccines.

Infection Control Measures

Although effective means of safeguarding populations from exposure to infectious disease are well-known, lack of implementation or breakdowns in application of these initiatives has led to the reemergence of some infectious diseases.

John Snow, a British physician, is considered the "father of epidemiology."[51] Industrialization in England in the nineteenth century resulted in rapid expansion of London's population that outgrew city services. An outbreak of cholera in the Soho area of London in 1854 resulted in more than 600 deaths. Snow discovered that the outbreak centered around one particular public water pump, which got water from a well that had been

TABLE 10-9 REDUCTION IN VACCINE-PREVENTABLE DISEASES IN THE UNITED STATES

DISEASE	BASELINE 20TH CENTURY ANNUAL CASES*	2008 CASES	% REDUCTION
Diphtheria	175,885	0	100.0
Measles	503,282	55	99.9
Mumps	152,209	454	95.7
Pertussis	147,271	10,735	92.7
Smallpox	48,164	0	100.0
Polio	16,316	0	100.0
Rubella	47,745	11	99.9
Tetanus	1,314	19	98.6
Haemophilus influenzae type b, invasive	20,000	30	99.9

From National Institute of Allergy and Infectious Disease, National Institutes of Health: Vaccine, Vaccine Benefits, Updated May 11, 2010 available at http://www.niaid.nih.gov/topics/vaccines/understanding/pages/vaccinebenefits.aspx. Accessed February 25, 2013.
*Average number of reported cases over multiple years before initiation of vaccine (Centers for Disease Control and Prevention: *MMWR Morb Mortal Wkly Rep* 48[12]:243–248, 1999, *Morb Mortal Wkly Rep* 57[11]:289–291, 2008).

dug 3 feet from a cesspool (open sewage was common in London at that time). After the pump was closed, the rate of new cholera cases rapidly diminished. Snow's observation stimulated the development of the construction of clean water supplies and sewers throughout the city.

Sewage removal and other public health initiatives (e.g., routine trash collection, disposal of garbage by incineration or in landfills) are now the expected norm in developed countries. The quality of water and food, as well as disposal of human and animal waste, remains poor in many developing countries. Rapid urbanization as well as other problems (e.g., poverty, overcrowding, mass relocation of people because of war, rapid destruction of forests) has put pressure on already inadequate systems.[52] A 1991 outbreak of cholera in Peru resulted in an estimated 10,000 deaths and was attributed to inadequate sanitation.

Additionally, previously successful programs designed to control the breeding of insect vectors have been reversed. Despite an international emphasis on draining standing water that provides breeding grounds for mosquitoes, large unmanaged areas still abound. A very successful international mosquito eradication program resulted in decreasing incidence of mosquito-borne diseases. Some regions were declared "free" of mosquito-borne diseases. However, since the international ban on DDT (dichlorodiphenyltrichloroethane) for agricultural work and limitation of its use for control of disease vectors, mosquitoes and mosquito-related diseases have rebounded in previously disease-free areas. In northern India, heavy rains in the 1990s resulted in an increase in standing water that was not drained because of the lack of government-provided public health information and inadequate insecticides to control mosquitoes. Since 1996, recurrent and increasingly severe outbreaks of dengue fever (caused by dengue virus, which is related to yellow fever virus and West Nile virus) have occurred in this region. In the 2006 outbreak 10,344 cases were reported, with 162 deaths. This problem is exacerbated by the development of insecticide-resistant mosquitoes.

Antimicrobials

Since the first use of penicillin during World War II, antibiotics have had the greatest effect on controlling infection. Antibiotics are natural products of fungi, bacteria, and related microorganisms and kill or inhibit the growth of other microorganisms. Numerous chemicals or antimicrobials have been identified that either prevent the growth of microorganisms or directly destroy them. Antibiotics generally act by preventing the function of enzymes or cell structures that are unique to the infecting agent. Because viruses use the enzymes of the host's cells, there has been far less success in developing antiviral antibiotics.

Immediately after antibiotics became widely used, antibiotic-resistant microorganisms were observed.[53] By 1944 an adequate supply of penicillin allowed its widespread use to treat infections. In 1946 a hospital in Britain reported that 14% of all *S. aureus* infections were penicillin resistant. By 1950 the same hospital reported an increase to 59% and to greater than 89% in the 1990s. Over the past few decades healthcare providers have observed increasing incidences of drug-resistant malaria, tuberculosis, gonorrhea, salmonellosis, shigellosis, and staphylococcal infections (see What's New? Drug-Resistant Tuberculosis). *S. pneumoniae,* which causes pneumonia, meningitis, and acute otitis media (ear infections), was once routinely susceptible to penicillin. Since the 1980s, however, the incidence of penicillin-resistant microorganisms has risen to greater than 30% in some populations.

The goal of antibiotic therapy is elimination of the pathogenic microorganism. Some antibacterial antibiotics are **bactericidal** (kill the organism), whereas others are **bacteriostatic** (inhibit growth until the organism is destroyed by the individual's own protective mechanisms). The mechanisms of action of most antibiotics are (1) inhibition of the function or production of the cell wall, (2) prevention of protein synthesis, (3) blockage of DNA replication, or (4) interference with folic acid metabolism.

Antibiotic resistance is usually a result of one of four general mechanisms resulting from genetic mutations that can be transmitted directly to neighboring microorganisms by plasmid exchange.[54] One mechanism microorganisms commonly develop is the capacity to inactivate antibiotics. For example, resistance to penicillin, cephalosporins, and other β-lactam-containing antibiotics results from the production of an enzyme (β-lactamase) that breaks down the structure of the antibiotic.[55] Other forms of resistance result from modification of the target molecule. Azidothymidine (AZT) is a family of antivirals that suppresses the enzymatic activity of reverse transcriptase, a viral-specific enzyme responsible for the replication of viral RNA and the production of a DNA copy. HIV frequently mutates and produces an AZT-resistant reverse transcriptase. Some bacteria have gained the capacity to produce penicillin-binding proteins

WHAT'S NEW?

Drug-Resistant Tuberculosis

Tuberculosis (TB) is one of the oldest known human diseases. Evidence of molecular biomarkers of infection with the etiologic agent of TB, the bacterium *Mycobacterium tuberculosis,* dates to the earliest Egyptian dynastic period (about 3500-2650 BCE) and even earlier. *M. tuberculosis* was not discovered as the cause of TB until 1882 by Robert Koch, who won the 1905 Nobel Prize for his work.

The bacterium primarily attacks the lungs and spreads from person to person through droplets, released into the air during coughing or sneezing. Few individuals (approximately 10%) with adequate immune responses develop overt disease; however, most will not completely destroy the microorganisms and will develop a chronic asymptomatic infection that can be activated if the immune system is suppressed, such as associated with aging, progressive genetic immunodeficiency, immunosuppressive medication, HIV infection, and other conditions. If the individual is immunocompromised upon initial exposure to *M. tuberculosis,* the probability of developing clinical, rather than chronic, TB is near 50%.

For centuries TB was a major cause of death throughout the world. The spread of the disease was limited by the recognition in the 19th century that TB was caused by a contagion, which led to separation of infected individuals in isolation wards and sanatoriums. The advent of antibiotic use after World War II increased optimism that TB could be controlled. The rapid spread of AIDS in the 1980s, however, resulted in a rebound in the incidence of TB. The World Health Organization (WHO) estimated that in 2010 8.8 million individuals (1.1 million of whom were HIV-infected) contracted TB and 1.4 million (350,000 of whom were HIV-infected) died of TB. Most deaths from TB occurred in Southeast Asia, Africa, and the Western Pacific.

In 1993, the WHO declared a TB "global emergency" and initiated a global TB control program. Although the number of new cases of TB has declined slowly, the global incidence decreased by 1% to 3% annually since 2002; since 1990, deaths fell by 40% globally; and record low rates of TB have been achieved in the United States and most of Western Europe. However, the goals of the program will not be met. *M. tuberculosis* developed resistance to the limited battery of available anti-tuberculosis drugs. Development of drug resistance has been increased in many countries by provision of incomplete or erratic therapy by poorly trained physicians, substandard quality of real or counterfeit medications, lack of expert testing for drug-resistant strains, and other inadequacies in healthcare systems.

Drug resistance has been classified as multidrug-resistant (MDR) TB and extensively drug-resistant (XDR) TB. MDR TB is defined as resistance to the two first-line drugs isoniazid and rifampicin. XDR TB is defined as MDR TB that is also resistant to second-line drugs, including all fluoroquinolones and at least one of three injectable drugs (capreomycin, kanamycin, or amikacin). Both classes of drug resistance occur in individuals with untreated TB who were infected from others with a drug-resistant strain or those who were poorly treated initially and developed recurrence with a drug-resistant strain. In most countries, accurate estimates of drug resistance are difficult to obtain because of inadequate laboratory testing facilities. In Azerbaijan, a careful study reported that 22.3% of new and 55.8% of previously treated TB cases were MDR. A recent study from China, where an estimated 1 million new cases of TB occur yearly, estimated that 1 in 10 infected persons have MDR TB and 1 in 120 have XDR TB. Drug-resistant TB is difficult to treat because anti-tuberculosis drugs are expensive and have several side effects and because MDR TB may require up to 2 years of treatment with success rates of 70% or less; XDR TB may be incurable in many individuals.

The situation has become worse. Reports from India of 12 individuals with TB that is resistant to all approved first- and second-line drugs have sparked concern in both the medical and lay communities. These reports are not the first of such cases; earlier reports of similar broadly resistant TB had occurred in 15 cases in Iran in 2009 and in two cases in Italy in 2007. The term *totally drug-resistant (TDR) TB* has been used unofficially to describe this disease. Will TDR TB become a predominant form in the future, and how will it be contained? Many new anti-tuberculosis drugs are in the developmental pipeline, but efficacy, side effects, cost, and other important considerations remain unknown. An effective vaccine would be the ideal solution, but only one vaccine is currently available. The bacille Calmette-Guérin (BCG) vaccine was developed a century ago using an attenuated strain of the bovine form of TB *(Mycobacterium bovis)* and is administered to children in many countries. Although it protects against disseminated infection and death in children, there is no protection against chronic infection or pulmonary TB in adults. At least a dozen new vaccines are in development, but will take years to be approved, even if one is found to be effective.

Data from Arya SC, Agarwal N: *Int J Tuberc Lung Dis* 16(6):852, 2012; Brennan MJ, Thole J: *Tuberculosis* 92(Suppl 1):S6–S13, 2012; Chaisson RE, Nuermberger EL: *N Engl J Med* 366(23):2223–2224, 2012; Donoghue HD: *Clin Microbiol Infect* 17(6):821–829, 2011; Loewenberg S: *Lancet* 379(9812):205, 2012; Migliori GB et al: *Clin Infect Dis* 54(9):1379–1380, 2012; Rappuoli R, Aderem A: *Nature* 473(7348):463–469, 2011; Raviglione M et al: *Lancet* 379(9829):1902–1913, 2012; Udwadia ZF et al: *Clin Infect Dis* 54(4):579–581, 2012; Zumla A et al: *J Infect Dis* 205(Suppl 2):S228–S240, 2012; Zumia A et al: *Nat Rev Drug Disc* 11(3):171–172, 2012.

that block penicillin from binding to sites in the bacterial cell wall, and other bacteria have modified antibiotic-sensitive binding sites on the ribosomes and developed resistance to antibiotics that interfere with protein synthesis. A third mechanism of resistance results from alteration of metabolic pathways that may be sensitive to antibiotics to alternative, more antibiotic-resistant pathways. Some bacteria have gained resistance to sulfonamide by converting from use of environmental *para*-aminobenzoic acid for conversion to folic acid, which is an antibiotic-sensitive step in nucleic acid synthesis, to the direct use of environmental folic acid. A fourth mechanism is mediated by multidrug transporters in the microorganism's membrane. These transporters affect the rate of intracellular accumulation of the antimicrobial by preventing entrance or, more commonly, increasing active efflux of the antibiotic. Antibiotic-resistant strains of *M. tuberculosis* are protected from aminoglycosides and tetracycline by the transporters with antigen processing (TAP) protein (a mycobacterial multidrug efflux pump).

Many microorganisms are now resistant to multiple antibiotics. **Methicillin-resistant *Staphylococcus aureus* (MRSA)** incorporates several different mechanisms of resistance. MRSA produces a β-lactamase (penicillinase). Penicillinase-resistant antibiotics (e.g., methicillin) can be used as a substitute, but MRSA carrying the gene *mecA* is also methicillin resistant because of a lower affinity for β-lactams. Resistance to the glycopeptide antibiotic vancomycin is controlled by the gene *vanA,* which results in alterations in peptidoglycans and loss of the vancomycin-binding site.

Why have multiple antibiotic–resistant microorganisms appeared? Overuse of antibiotics can lead to the destruction of the normal microbiome, allowing the selective overgrowth of antibiotic-resistant strains or pathogens that had previously been kept under control. For example, after treatment with the antibiotic clindamycin, the normal intestinal microbiome can become compromised, allowing the overgrowth of *Clostridium difficile* and the development of pseudomembranous colitis.[56] Also, lack of compliance concerning the necessity of completing the therapeutic regimen with antibiotics allows the selective resurgence of microorganisms that are more relatively resistant to the antibiotic.

With the development of multiple antibiotic–resistant strains, creativity in addressing this challenge must be rekindled. Antibiotics should no longer be used for minor infections, such as mild to moderate sinusitis.[57] New antibiotics may solve a portion of the problem or may exacerbate it further as pathogens develop resistance to new antibiotics as well. Available antibiotics that prove to be no longer effective must be replaced with alternative forms of therapy, including the increased development and use of vaccines and other therapies.

Active Immunization: Vaccines

Contracting and surviving an infectious disease is the most effective means of developing lifelong immunity against a particular pathogen. However, some infections cause a great deal of morbidity and mortality. The purpose of vaccination is to induce active immunologic protection before exposure to the risks of infection. For each vaccine an initial immunization protocol is developed to produce large numbers of memory cells and a sustained protective secondary immune response in the greatest number of individuals. In general, vaccine-induced protection does not persist as long as infection-induced immunity; thus, booster injections may be necessary to maintain protection throughout life. The Centers for Disease Control and Prevention maintain the most current immunization schedules for people of all ages. The schedules can be reviewed at www.cdc.gov/vaccines/recs/schedules/default.htm.

Mass vaccination programs have led to major changes in the health of the world's population. In the early 1950s an estimated 50 million cases of smallpox occurred each year, with about 15 million deaths. The World Health Organization (WHO) conducted a smallpox immunization campaign from 1967 to 1977 that resulted in the global eradication of smallpox by 1979. The 1988 immunization initiative against polio resulted in a 99% decrease in that disease. In 1960, 2525 cases of paralytic polio were reported in the United States, but no cases of naturally acquired polio have been reported since 1979. In 1994, polio was declared officially eradicated in all the Americas. The goal of the WHO is to eradicate polio worldwide by 2022.[58] Similar trends occurred for each disease against which an effective vaccine has been developed.

Development of a successful vaccine depends on many factors. These include characterizing the desired protective immune response (e.g., antibody, T cell), identifying the appropriate antigen to induce that response (i.e., immune responses against some antigens on an infectious agent are ineffective or even increase the risk for infection), determining the most effective route of administration (e.g., injected, oral, inhaled), optimizing the number and timing of vaccine doses to induce protective immunity in a large proportion of the at-risk population, and deciding the most effective, yet safe, form in which to administer the vaccine. For instance, most vaccines against viral infections (e.g., measles, mumps, rubella, varicella [chickenpox], rotavirus) contain live viruses that are weakened (**attenuated**) to continue expressing the appropriate antigens but are unable to establish more than a limited and easily controlled infection. The limited proliferative capacity of attenuated live viruses appears to afford better long-term protection than using purified viral antigen. Two exceptions are the vaccines against hepatitis B, which uses a recombinant viral protein, and hepatitis A, which is an inactivated (killed) virus.

Even attenuated viruses can, however, establish life-threatening infections in vaccine recipients whose immune system is congenitally deficient or suppressed (see Chapter 9). Two different vaccines were developed against polio. The Sabin vaccine is an attenuated virus that is administered orally (oral polio vaccine [OPV]). It provides systemic protection and induces a secretory immune response to prevent growth of the poliovirus in the intestinal tract. The live attenuated vaccine causes polio in some children who have unsuspected immune deficiencies (about 1 case in 2.4 million doses). The Salk vaccine is a completely inactivated virus administered by injection (inactivated polio vaccine [IPV]). It induces protective systemic immunity but does not provide adequate secretory immunity. Therefore, even if the individual is protected from systemic infection the "wild-type" poliovirus can transiently infect the intestinal mucosa, be shed, and spread to others.[59] When polio was epidemic, the live oral vaccine was preferred; however, about eight cases of paralytic polio per year in the United States resulted from the vaccine strain proliferating in individuals with inadequate immune systems. As a result, the CDC currently recommends vaccination with the killed virus.

Some common bacterial vaccines are killed microorganisms or extracts of bacterial antigens. The vaccine against pneumococcal pneumonia consists of a mixture of capsular polysaccharides from 10 strains of *S. pneumoniae.* Of the more than 90 known strains of this microorganism, only these 10 cause the most severe illnesses. However, the capsular vaccine is not very immunogenic in young children. A "conjugated" vaccine is available that contains capsular polysaccharides from seven strains that are conjugated to carrier proteins in order to increase immunogenicity. A similar vaccine is available for *Haemophilus influenzae* type B (Hib).

Some bacterial diseases are caused by potent toxins that act locally or systemically. These include diphtheria, cholera, and tetanus. Vaccination against the toxins is achieved using **toxoids**—purified toxins that have been chemically detoxified without loss of immunogenicity. Pertussis (whooping cough) vaccine was changed from a killed whole cell vaccine to an acellular vaccine that contained the pertussis toxin and additional bacterial antigens.

With so many available vaccines there has been an effort to mix vaccines in order to minimize the number of required injections. One of the first licensed vaccine mixtures was DPT, which now usually contains diphtheria (D) and tetanus (T) toxoids and acellular pertussis vaccine (aP). More recent mixtures include DTaP with inactivated poliovirus, either with Hib conjugate to tetanus toxoid or with hepatitis B vaccine.

Common problems include access to vaccination programs in less developed countries or compliance of the susceptible population even when vaccination programs are available.[60] Depending on the microorganism, a certain percentage of the population (usually about 85%) should be immunized in order to achieve protection of the total population. This is referred to as *herd immunity*. If this level of immunization is not achieved, outbreaks of infection can occur. For instance, an effective measles (rubeola) vaccine was made available in 1963 and resulted in a dramatic decrease in the number of measles cases.[61] Many parents became complacent and did not obtain measles vaccination for their preschool children. As a result, a large increase in the number of cases and deaths in 1989 and 1990 occurred, which initiated a reemphasis on complete immunization before children could start school. More recently resistance to immunization with measles has increased, and in early 2008 the number of measles cases in the United States increased by about fourfold. In several European countries immunization programs have been disrupted by anti-vaccine groups. As a result the incidence of pertussis (whooping cough) increased by 10 to 100 times compared with neighboring countries that maintained a high incidence of immunization.

The refusal to vaccinate has generally been based on potential vaccine dangers. As with any medicine, complications can arise. In the case of vaccines, these include pain and redness at the injection site, fever, allergic reactions to vaccine ingredients, infection associated with attenuated viruses in immunodeficient individuals, and others. For instance, rotavirus is the most common cause of diarrheal disease in children globally, and more than 500,000 children die each year from severe acute diarrhea.[62] A rotavirus vaccine approved more than a decade ago was found to increase the risk for a life-threatening bowel obstruction resulting from twisting of the intestines, and the vaccine was recalled.[63] New rotavirus vaccines are available that are safe from adverse events.[63a] A commonly discussed fear is related to the presence of the preservative thimerosal in vaccines. Thimerosal is a mercury-containing compound that has been used as a preservative since the 1930s. Although no cases of mercury toxicity have been reported secondary to vaccination, thimerosal was removed from all vaccines in 2001, with the exception of inactivated influenza vaccines.[64] In 2003, groups in northern Nigeria claimed that the oral polio vaccine was unsafe, which led to suspension of polio immunization in two states and reduction of immunization in other states. The result was a 36% increase in cases of polio and thousands of cases of paralysis, including in previously polio-free areas.

Passive Immunotherapy

Passive immunotherapy is a form of countermeasure against pathogens in which preformed antibodies are given to the individual. This form of therapy has been used for decades. Horse serum–containing antibodies were given to treat diphtheria, pneumococcal pneumonia, tetanus, and other diseases in the early twentieth century. However, because of foreign proteins in the serum, many individuals developed an immune reaction against the horse proteins and an immune complex–mediated serum sickness. Passive immunotherapy with **human immunoglobulin** has been approved for several infections, including hepatitis B and hepatitis A. Treatment of potential rabies infection after a bite combines passive and active immunization. The rabies virus proliferates very slowly. Individuals who have been bitten receive a onetime injection with human rabies immunoglobulin, or more recently with monoclonal antibody, to further slow viral proliferation, followed by multiple injections with a killed viral vaccine to induce greater protective immunity.[65] For several other diseases more specific therapy with monoclonal antibodies is being evaluated, and a monoclonal antibody against respiratory syncytial virus has been approved for therapy.[66]

In the past, vaccines and therapeutic antibodies were developed for only the most deadly pathogens. With the increase in antibiotic-resistant microorganisms, the development and widespread use of new vaccines and antibodies against these microorganisms must be considered. For example, otitis media, a purulent ear infection, is caused primarily by *Streptococcus*, *Haemophilus*, and *Staphylococcus*. This infection routinely has been treated successfully with antibiotics; however, the increase in multiple antibiotic–resistant microorganisms may force a reevaluation of the use of childhood immunization as an alternative to preventing this disease. Other vaccines used now only to a limited degree may be used more widely in the future, and others may be developed soon, including vaccines against cholera, typhoid, malaria, West Nile virus, hantavirus, SARS, and several other diseases.

SUMMARY REVIEW

Emerging Infections

1. Deaths from infections are the eighth (influenza and pneumonia) and tenth (sepsis) leading causes of death in the United States and account for about one third of deaths worldwide.
2. Infectious disease is a significant cause of death and morbidity because of the reemergence of old infections thought to be controlled, the emergence of previously unknown infections, and the development of infections resistant to multiple antibiotics.
3. The current rate of emergence of previously unknown infections may be unprecedented. More than 40 unknown infections have arisen within 1 generation.
4. Although most infections are controlled, some uncontrolled infections have high mortality rates including SARS, Ebola virus, Marburg virus, "mad cow disease," Nipah virus, and AIDS.
5. Many common and reemerging infections have become antibiotic and drug resistant. At least 25% of *S. pneumoniae* infections are penicillin resistant and some are resistant to multiple antibiotics.

SUMMARY REVIEW—cont'd

6. Resistant forms of *S. aureus,* a primary cause of infections of wounds, surgical incisions, and catheters, are endemic in some hospitals.
7. Antimicrobial resistance is routinely observed in tuberculosis, diarrheal diseases, hospital-acquired infections, malaria, meningitis, respiratory tract infections, STIs, and HIV.

Microorganisms and Humans: A Dynamic Relationship

1. The human body is a hospitable site for microorganisms to grow and flourish. These microorganisms make up the *normal microbiome* of the body.
2. The beneficial homeostasis between humans and microorganisms is maintained through the physical integrity of the gut and other mechanisms that sequester these microorganisms on the mucosal surface.

Microorganisms and Infections

1. The symbiotic relationship with the normal microbiome can be altered by injury, compromising protective barriers.
2. Cuts in the skin and compromised immunity can increase infections.
3. Damage to the intestinal tract releases intestinal bacteria into the bloodstream, potentially leading to sepsis, shock, and death.
4. When an individual's immune system is deficient, the person can become infected with opportunistic infections.
5. Unlike opportunistic infectious agents, true pathogens can circumvent an individual's defenses and directly cause infection. Successful infection with these agents usually requires adequate numbers of microorganisms rather than compromised immune defenses.
6. The process of infection includes colonization, invasion, multiplication, and spread.
7. Infectious microorganisms usually exist in reservoirs (e.g., contaminated soil, contaminated water, breast milk), animals, or another human.
8. As part of colonization, the microorganism stabilizes the adherence to tissue through surface receptors. Once colonization occurs, the infectious agent can invade surrounding tissue.
9. Because tissue is warm and nutrient rich, most microorganisms undergo *rapid* multiplication. Viral pathogens replicate within infected cells, and some bacteria are intracellular pathogens and replicate in macrophages and other cells.
10. Many pathogens produce only localized infections. Others are, however, highly invasive.
11. Successful spreading requires a variety of virulence factors, including adhesion molecules, toxins, and the ability to evade immunity.
12. Clinical infectious disease occurs in four distinct stages: (a) incubation period, (b) prodromal state, (c) invasion period, and (d) convalescence.
13. The hallmark of most infectious diseases is fever. Body temperature is regulated at a higher than normal level.
14. A large number of agents (pyrogens) can produce fever. Current classifications include endogenous (e.g., cytokines) and exogenous agents. However, the evidence for exogenous agents is limited and they indirectly affect the hypothalamus through endogenous pyrogens.
15. Several factors influence the capacity of a pathogen to cause disease, including communicability, immunogenicity, infectivity, mechanisms of action, pathogenicity, entry portal, toxigenicity, and virulence.
16. Infectious diseases also are classified by their prevalence and spread as endemic, epidemic, and pandemic.
17. Classes of infectious microorganisms include bacterial, fungal, parasitic, protozoal, and viral.
18. Bacteria are divided into several groups: "true bacteria," filamentous, spirochetes, mycoplasma, rickettsia, and chlamydia.
19. Stable colonization of bacteria requires adhesion. Many bacteria attach through pili, also called fimbriae.
20. Invasion by bacteria results in direct confrontation with an individual's defense mechanisms, including complement, antibodies, and phagocytes (neutrophils, macrophages). Evasion of these defenses can result in bacteremia and sepsis.
21. Efficient pathogens can produce a variety of toxic molecules that may kill the individual's cells, disrupt tissue, and protect themselves against inflammation. Exotoxins are released by bacteria during bacterial growth and can damage cell membranes, activate second messengers, and inhibit protein synthesis.
22. Endotoxins are contained in the cell walls of gram-negative bacteria and released during lysis of the bacteria. Bacteria that produce endotoxins are called *pyrogenic bacteria* because they activate inflammation and produce fever.
23. Bacteria can protect against phagocytosis by producing toxins and extracellular enzymes that destroy phagocytic cells.
24. Some bacteria can coat the Fc portion of an individual's antibody, preventing complement activation or phagocytosis.
25. Antigenic variation allows the pathogen to alter surface molecules that express antigens that are the targets of protective immune responses. The pathogen thus becomes resistant.
26. Other self-protective mechanisms for bacteria and other pathogens include degradation of immune molecules, neutralization of immune molecules, complement evasion, and immune suppression.
27. Tissue damage from bacterial infections is either directly by bacterial products or indirectly from infection.
28. *S. aureus* has become a major cause of hospital-acquired (nosocomial) infections. Antibiotic resistance also has become a major problem with *S. aureus.*
29. Fungal infection is called mycosis. Most pathologic fungi are from the environment and transmitted by inhalation or contamination of wounds.
30. In 2006, the opportunistic pathogen *P. carinii* was reclassified as a fungus and the specific variant that infects humans was renamed *P. jiroveci.*
31. *C. albicans* is the most common cause of fungal infections in humans. It resides in the skin, gastrointestinal tract, mouth, and vagina. Local defense mechanisms, including members of the bacterial microbiome, produce antifungal

SUMMARY REVIEW—cont'd

agents. The infection remains localized in individuals with an intact immune system.

32. Parasitic organisms establish a symbiosis with another species, whereby the parasite benefits. They range from unicellular protozoa to large worms. Although less common in the United States, parasites and protozoa are common causes of infection worldwide.
33. Parasitic and protozoal infections are rarely transmitted from human to human. Infection mainly spreads through vectors and includes malaria by mosquito bites, trypanosomes by the tsetse fly, and *Leishmania* spp. by sand fleas. Others are found in contaminated water or food (e.g., *G. lamblia*).
34. Malaria is one of the most common infections worldwide. It is transmitted through the bite of an infected *Anopheles* mosquito. The parasite enters the bloodstream, survives in the liver, and invades parenchymal cells. After several rounds of division, the liver cell ruptures and thousands of parasites enter the blood, infecting red blood cells.
35. Viruses are classified by the format of nucleic acid in the virion (RNA or DNA), either single stranded (ss) or double stranded (ds), and whether it uses the enzyme RT for replication.
36. Viral diseases are the most common affliction of humans and include the common cold, the "coldsore," hepatitis, HIV, and several types of cancer.
37. Viruses are intracellular parasites. The viral life cycle is completely intracellular and involves several stages: attachment, penetration, uncoating, replication, assembly, and release. New virions are released from the cell for transmission of the viral infection to neighboring, uninfected cells.
38. The primary defense mechanisms against viruses include antibody and cellular immunity. Nonspecific defenses include α- and β-interferons that block intracellular replication.
39. Successful viruses use a variety of mechanisms for bypassing immune rejection, including rapid division, intracellular survival, coating with self-proteins, antigenic variation, neutralization, complement evasion, and immune suppression.
40. Viruses inside the infected cell have several harmful effects, including inhibition of DNA, RNA, or protein synthesis; disruption of lysosomal membranes, resulting in lytic enzyme release; promotion of cell apoptosis; fusion of adjacent cells (i.e., giant cells); transformation into a neoplastic cell; and alteration of antigenic properties (i.e., decreasing immune effectiveness).

Acquired Immunodeficiency Syndrome (AIDS)

1. AIDS is a viral disease caused by HIV.
2. HIV infects and depletes a portion of the immune system (Th cells), making individuals susceptible to life-threatening infections and malignancies.
3. HIV/AIDS remains a major cause of death worldwide.
4. Aggressive antiretroviral therapy and public health campaigns have stabilized the number of new cases and deaths in the United States from HIV/AIDS, but the cases and deaths continue to increase rapidly worldwide.
5. In 2009, 50% of newly diagnosed cases of AIDS in the United States were attributed to male-to-male sexual contact, 30% to high-risk heterosexual contact, and 14% to injected drug abuse. About 25% of newly diagnosed cases were female, with about 74% contracted through high-risk heterosexual contact.
6. The epicenter of the AIDS pandemic is sub-Saharan Africa. Women have the highest risk of infection. Because of AIDS, the average life expectancy in South Africa has dropped from 64 years to 54 years.
7. HIV is a blood-borne pathogen present in body fluids (e.g., blood, vaginal fluid, semen, breast milk) with typical routes of transmission: blood or blood products, intravenous drug abuse, heterosexual and homosexual activity, and maternal-child transmission before or during birth.
8. At the end of 2009, an estimated 8640 children in the United States developed AIDS after contracting HIV infection from their mothers (e.g., across the placenta, through contact with infected blood during delivery, or through ingestion of infected breast milk).
9. Healthcare providers are at increased risk of contracting infections from another person's blood. However, as of May 2011, only 57 cases of confirmed HIV infection and 143 possible cases were contracted by occupational exposure.
10. HIV is a member of the *retrovirus* family, which carries genetic information in the form of two copies of RNA. An enzyme, reverse transcriptase (RT), converts RNA into a double-stranded DNA. Another enzyme, an *integrase,* inserts the new DNA into the infected cell's genetic material. On activation, translation of the viral information may be initiated, forming new virions, resulting in lysis and death of the infected cell, and shedding infectious HIV particles.
11. The primary surface receptor on HIV is the envelope glycoprotein gp120, which binds to the CD4 molecule found mostly on the surface of T-helper cells. Several other important co-receptors have been identified.
12. The major immunologic finding in AIDS is the striking decrease in the number of CD4 Th cells.
13. The presence of circulating antibody against HIV indicates infection by the virus, although many individuals are asymptomatic.
14. The current treatment for HIV infection is a combination of drugs called antiretroviral therapy (ART).

Countermeasures Against Pathogens

1. Effective means of countering infectious microorganisms are rigorous use of environmental infection control measures, including control of insect vector populations, establishment of modern sanitation facilities, and provision of clean water and uncontaminated food supplies. Prophylactic or interventive procedures include vaccines and antimicrobials.
2. With antibiotic-resistant pathogens, a greater emphasis is placed on the development of new vaccines.

KEY TERMS

Acquired immunodeficiency syndrome (AIDS), 322
Antibiotic resistance, 310
Antigenic drift, 320
Antigenic shift, 320
Antigenic variation, 308
Antiretroviral therapy (ART), 327
Antitoxin, 306
Attenuated, 332
Bacteremia, 306
Bacterial superantigens, 310
Bactericidal, 330
Bacteriostatic, 330
β-Lactamase, 310
Biofilms, 305
Capsule, 307
Dimorphic, 310
Endogenous pyrogen, 302
Endotoxic shock (septic shock), 310
Endotoxin, 306
Exogenous pyrogen, 302
Exotoxin, 306
Fever, 301
Gene switching, 315
Human immunodeficiency virus (HIV), 322
Human immunoglobulin, 333
IgA protease, 309
Integrase, 324
Lipopolysaccharide (LPS), 306
Methicillin-resistant *Staphylococcus aureus* (MRSA), 331
Mold, 310
Multinucleated giant cell, 320
Mutation, 320
Mycosis, 311
Passive immunotherapy, 333
Pili (fimbriae), 305
Recombination, 320
Reverse transcriptase, 324
Sepsis, 306
Syncytium, 325
Tissue tropism, 301
Toxoid, 332
Window period, 327
Yeast, 310
Zoonotic infection, 317

REFERENCES

1. Morens DM, Folkers GK, Fauci AS: Emerging infections: a perpetual challenge, *Lancet Infect Dis* 8(11):710–719, 2008.
2. Hoyert DL, Xu J: Preliminary Data for 2011, *National Vital Statistics Report* 61(6):1–7, 2012. Available at http://www.cdc.gov/nchs/fastats/lcod.htm/.

2a. World Health Organization (WHO): *The top 10 causes of death, fact sheet #310 (updated June 2011)*. Available at www.who.int/mediacentre/factsheets/fs310/en/index.html.

3. Fauci AS, Morens DM: The perpetual challenge of infectious diseases, *N Engl J Med* 366(5):454–461, 2012.
4. National Institute of Allergy and Infectious Diseases: *West Nile Virus* (updated November, 2012). Available at www.niaid.nih.gov/topics/westnile/Pages/default/aspx.
5. Clemente JC et al: The impact of the gut microbiota on human health: an integrative view, *Cell* 148(6):1258–1270, 2012.
6. Johnjulio W et al: Introduction to biofilms in family medicine, *South Med J* 105(1):24–29, 2012.
7. Peters BM et al: Polymicrobial interactions: impact on pathogenesis and human disease, *Clin Microbiol Rev* 25(1):193–213, 2012.
8. Otto M: Molecular basis of *Staphylococcus epidermidis* infections, *Semin Immunopathol* 34(2):201–214, 2012.
9. Edwards AM, Massey RC, Clarke SR: Molecular mechanisms of *Staphylococcus aureus* nasopharyngeal colonization, *Mol Oral Microbiol* 27(1):1–10, 2012.
10. Stafford G et al: Sialic acid, periodontal pathogens, and *Tannerella forsythia*: stick around and enjoy the feast!, *Mol Oral Microbiol* 27(1):11–22, 2012.
11. Fry DE: Sepsis, systemic inflammatory response, and multiple organ dysfunction: the mystery continues, *Am Surg* 78(1):1–8, 2012.
12. Bardoel BW, van Strijp AG: Molecular battle between host and bacterium: recognition in innate immunity, *J Mol Recognit* 24(6):1077–1086, 2011.
13. Lam GY et al: Interactions of *Listeria monocytogenes* with the autophagy system of host cells, *Adv Immunol* 113:7–18, 2012.
14. Criss AK, Seifert HS: A bacterial siren song: intimate interactions between *Neisseria* and neutrophils, *Nat Rev Microbiol* 10(3):178–190, 2012.
15. Camejo A, et al: The arsenal of virulence factors deployed by *Listeria monocytogenes* to promote its cell infection cycle, *Virulence* 2(5):379–394, 2011.
16. Woof JM, Russell MW: Structure and function relationships in IgA, *Mucosal Immunol* 4(6):590–597, 2011.
17. Sarma JV, Ward PA: The complement system, *Cell Tissue Res* 343(1):227–235, 2011.
18. Lobdell KW, Stamou S, Sanchez JA: Hospital-acquired infections, *Surg Clin North Am* 92(1):65–77, 2012.
19. Kim HK et al: Recurrent infections and immune evasion strategies of Staphylococcus aureus, *Curr Opin Microbiol* 15(1):92–99, 2012.
20. Garcia BL et al: Advances in understanding the structure, function, and mechanism of the SCIN and Efb families of staphylococcal immune evasion proteins, *Adv Exp Med Biol* 946:113–133, 2012.
21. D'Avignon LC, Schofield CM, Hospenthal DR: Pneumocystis pneumonia, *Semin Respir Crit Care Med* 29(2):132–140, 2008.
22. Collette JR, Lorenz MC: Mechanisms of immune evasion in fungal pathogens, *Curr Opin Microbiol* 14(6):668–675, 2011.
23. Cheng S-C et al: Interplay between *Candida albicans* and the mammalian innate host defense, *Infect Immun* 80(4):1304–1313, 2012.
24. Gow NAR et al: *Candida albicans* morphogenesis and host defense: discriminating invasion from colonization, *Nat Rev Microbiol* 10(2):112–122, 2011.
25. Danilowicz-Luebert E et al: Modulation of specific and allergy-related immune responses by helminthes, *J Biomed Biotechnol* 1–18, 2011. 2011.
26. MacGregor P et al: Trypanosomal immune evasion, chronicity and transmission: an elegant balancing act, *Nat Rev Microbiol* 10(6):431–438, 2012.
27. Namangala B: How the African trypanosomes evade host immune killing, *Parasite Immunol* 33(8):430–437, 2011.
28. World Health Organization (WHO): *Fact sheet #24: malaria, April, 2012*:1–7. Available at www.who.int/mediacentre/factsheets/fs094/en/index.html.
29. Goldberg DE, Siliciano RF, Jacobs WR Jr: Outwitting evolution: fighting drug-resistant TB, malaria, and HIV, *Cell* 148(6):1271–1283, 2012.
30. Laing KJ et al: Immunology in the clinic review series; focus on host responses: T cell responses to herpes simplex viruses, *Clin Exp Immunol* 167(1):47–58, 2011.
31. Rima BK, Duprex WP: New concepts in measles virus replication: getting in and out in vivo and modulating the host cell environment, *Virus Res* 182(1-2):47–62, 2011.
32. Garcia-Sastre A: Induction and evasion of type 1 interferon responses by influenza viruses, *Virus Res* 162(1-2):12–18, 2011.
33. Di Lorenzo C, Angus AGN, Patel AH: Hepatitis C virus evasion mechanisms from neutralizing antibodies, *Viruses* 3(11):2280–2300, 2011.
34. Yan N, Chen ZJ: Intrinsic antiviral immunity, *Nat Immunol* 13(3):214–222, 2012.
35. Centers for Disease Control and Prevention (CDC): *Transmission of avian influenza A viruses between animals and people (last reviewed November 25, 2011)*. Available at www.cdc.gov/flu/avianflu/virus-transmission.htm.
36. Shanks GD, Brundage JF: Pathogenic responses among young adults during the 1918 influenza pandemic, *Emerg Infect Dis* 18(2):201–207, 2012.
37. Centers for Disease Control and Prevention (CDC): *Monitoring selected national HIV prevention and care objectives by using HIV surveillance data—United States and 6 U.S. dependent areas—2010.* HIV Surveillance Supplemental Report 2012: 17(No. 3, part A). Available at: http://www.cdc.gov/hiv/surveillance/resources/reports/2010supp_vol17no3/index.htm. Published June 2012.
38. Joint United Nations Programme on HIV/AIDS (UNAIDS): *World AIDS day report, 2011*Geneva, Switzerland, 2011, UNAIDS. Available at www.unaids.org/en/media/unaids/contentassets/documents/unaidspublication/2011/JC2216_WorldAIDSday_report_2011_en.pdf.
39. Deuffic-Burban S, et al: Blood-borne viruses in health care workers: prevention and management, *J Clin Virol* 52(1):4–10, 2011.
40. Petroll AE, Hare CB, Pinkerton SD: The essentials of HIV: a review for nurses, *J Infus Nurs* 31(4):228–235, 2008.
41. Centers for Disease Control and Prevention (CDC): *Surveillance of occupationally acquired HIV/AIDS in healthcare personnel, as of December 2010 (updated May, 2011)*. Available at www.cdc.gov/HAI/organisms/hiv/Surveillance-Occupationally-Acquired-HIV-AIDS.html.
42. Rey D. Post-exposure prophylaxis for HIV infection, *Expert Rev Anti Infect Ther* 9(4):431–442, 2011.

43. Tolle MA, Schwarzwald H: Postexposure prophylaxis against human immunodeficiency virus, *Am Fam Physician* 82(2):161–166, 2010.
44. Barre-Sinoussi F et al: Isolation of a T-lymphotropic retrovirus from a patient at risk for acquired immune deficiency syndrome (AIDS), *Science* 220(4599):868–871, 1983.
45. Engelman A, Cherepanov P: The structural biology of HIV-1: mechanistic and therapeutic insights, *Nat Rev Microbiol* 10(4):279–290, 2012.
46. Cohen MS et al: Acute HIV-1 infection, *N Engl J Med* 364(20):1943–1954, 2011.
47. Smith MZ, Wightman F, Lewin SR: HIV reservoirs and strategies for eradication, *Curr HIV/AIDS Rep* 9(1):5–15, 2012.
48. Department of Health and Human Services (DHHS) Panel on Antiretroviral Guidelines for Adults and Adolescents: *Guidelines for the use of antiretroviral agents in HIV-1-infected adults and adolescents.* Available at http://aidsinfo.nih.gov/ContentFiles/AdultandAdolescentGL.pdf. Accessed April 15, 2013.
49. Hunt PW: HIV and inflammation: mechanisms and consequences, *Curr HIV/AIDS Rep* 9(2):139–147, 2012.
49a. Moyer VA: Screening for HIV: U.S. Preventative Task Force Recommendation Statement. *Ann Intern Med*, April 30, 2013. doi: 10.7326/0003-4819-159-1-201307020-00645.
50. Department of Health and Human Services (DHHS) Panel on Antiretroviral Therapy and Medical Management of HIV-Infected Children. *Guidelines for the use of antiretroviral agents in pediatric HIV infection.* Available at http://aidsinfo.nih.gov/contentfile/lvguidelines/pediatric guideline.pdf. Accessed April 15, 2013.
51. Snow SJ: John Snow: the making of a hero? *Lancet* 372(9632):22–23, 2008.
52. de Waal A: On famine crimes and tragedies, *Lancet* 372(9649):1538–1539, 2008.
53. Hawkey PM: The growing burden of antimicrobial resistance, *J Antimicrob Chemother* 62(Suppl 1):i1–i9, 2008.
54. Barie PS: Multidrug-resistant organisms and antibiotic management, *Surg Clin North Am* 92(2):345–391, 2012.
55. Rice LB: Mechanisms of resistance and clinical relevance of resistance to β-lactams, glycopeptides, and fluoroquinolones, *Mayo Clin Proc* 87(2):198–208, 2012.
56. Cohen SH et al: Clinical practice guidelines for *Clostridium difficile* infection in adults, *Infect Control Hosp Epidemiol* 31(5):431–455, 2010.
57. Smith SR, Montgomery LG, Williams JW Jr: Treatment of mild to moderate sinusitis, *Arch Intern Med* 172(6):510–513, 2012.
58. World Health Organization: *Poliomyelitis fact sheet no. 114*, October 2012. Available at www.who.int/mediacentre/factsheets/fs114/en/.
59. Okayasu H et al: Mucosal immunity and poliovirus vaccines: impact on wild poliovirus infection and transmission, *Vaccine* 29(46):8205–8214, 2011.
60. Rainey JJ et al: Reasons related to non-vaccination and under-vaccination of children in low and middle income countries: findings from a systemic review of the published literature, 1999-2009, *Vaccine* 29(46):8215–8221, 2011.
61. Moss WJ, Griffin DE: Measles, *Lancet* 379(9811):153–164, 2012.
62. Denehy PH: Effects of vaccine on rotavirus disease in the pediatric population, *Curr Opin Pediatr* 24(1):76–84, 2012.
63. Centers for Disease Control and Prevention (CDC): Intussusception among recipients of rotavirus vaccine—United States, 1998-1999, *MMWR Morb Mortal Wkly Rep* 48(27):577–581, 1999.
63a. Soares-Weiser K et al: Vaccines for preventing rotavirus diarrhoea: vaccines in use, *Cochrane Database Syst Rev* 11:CD008521, 2012.
64. Sadanand S: Vaccination: the present and the future, *Yale J Biol Med* 84(4):353–359, 2011.
65. Both L et al: Passive immunity in prevention of rabies, *Lancet Infect Dis* 12(5):397–407, 2012.
66. Geevarghese B, Simoes EA: Antibodies for prevention and treatment of respiratory syncytial virus infections in children, *Antivir Ther* 17 (1 Pt B):201–211, 2012.

CHAPTER

11

Stress and Disease

Margaret F. Clayton and Kathryn L. McCance

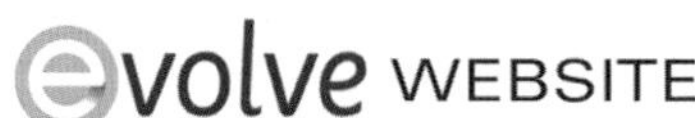

http://evolve.elsevier.com/McCance/

- Review Questions and Answers

CHAPTER OUTLINE

To observe the obvious, modern society is full of stress. As a culture, Westerners are champions of the work ethic, a Protestant philosophy originating in the sixteenth century that views idleness as taboo. Stressful experiences include daily hassles, major life events (e.g., loss of family member, loss of job), abuse, trauma, work-life balance, and many other events. For example, the pressure to remain in contact despite illness, travel, vacation, and other events that used to provide socially acceptable temporary absences is now customary in the American, and indeed global, culture. This prevalent assumption of constant availability is a newly identified stressor contributing to the more global and better studied stressors of work-related and relationship stressors. When added to other well-identified stressors such as financial problems, the result may be potential suffering from the so-called *stress-related disorders.*

When thinking about stress, one must consider the factors producing a perception of stress. Stress begins with a stimulus that the brain perceives as stressful, which in turn promotes adaptational and survival-related physiologic responses. These responses can become dysregulated and cause pathophysiologic conditions.[1] Another way to think about stress involves short- or long-term stressors and a discussion of the physiologic responses to these different types of events. Today most researchers feel that acute stress is considered to be immunoenhancing (protective) while chronic stress is now thought to be immunosuppressive (destructive).[1]

HISTORICAL BACKGROUND AND GENERAL CONCEPTS

Walter B. Cannon used the term *stress* to encompass both physiologic and psychologic ideas as early as 1914.[2] He applied the engineering concept of stress and strain in a physiologic context and believed that emotional stimuli also were capable of causing stress. In 1946, Hans Selye popularized these same findings, viewing stress as a biologic phenomenon.[3] Originally, Selye inadvertently discovered the biologic syndrome of stress while he was attempting to discover a new sex hormone by injecting crude ovarian extracts into rats.[3] He repeatedly found that three structural changes occurred: (1) enlargement of the cortex of the

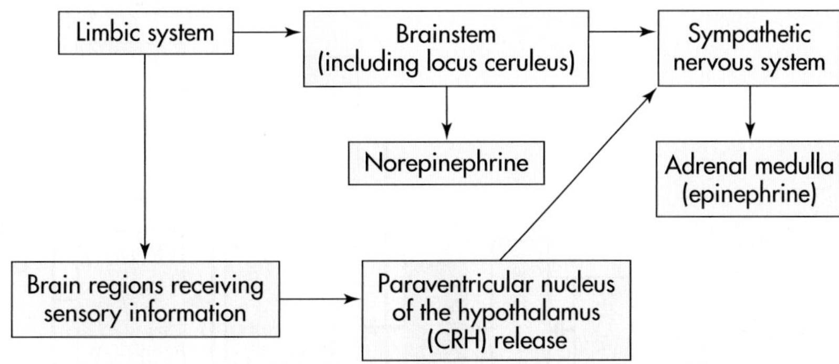

FIGURE 11-1 Neural Recognition and Response to Real or Predicted Stressors.

adrenal gland, (2) atrophy of the thymus gland and other lymphoid structures, and (3) development of bleeding ulcers in the stomach and duodenal lining. Selye soon discovered that these manifestations were not specific to injected ovarian extracts but also occurred after he exposed the rats to other noxious stimuli, such as cold, surgical injury, and restraint. He called these stimuli stressors. Selye concluded that this triad or syndrome of manifestations represented a nonspecific response to noxious stimuli, naming it the **general adaptation syndrome (GAS).** He identified three successive stages of the GAS: (1) the alarm stage or reaction, in which the central nervous system (CNS) is aroused and the body's defenses are mobilized (e.g., "fight or flight") (Figure 11-1); (2) the stage of resistance or adaptation, during which mobilization contributes to "fight or flight"; and (3) the stage of exhaustion, where continuous stress causes the progressive breakdown of compensatory mechanisms (acquired adaptations) and homeostasis. Exhaustion marks the onset of certain diseases (diseases of adaptation).

Initially one becomes alarmed by a stressor that activates the hypothalamus and sympathetic nervous system (see Figures 11-1 and 11-2). The resistance or adaptation phase begins with the actions of the hormones cortisol, norepinephrine, and epinephrine. Exhaustion (also known as allostatic overload; discussed later) occurs if stress continues and adaptation is not successful, ultimately causing impairment of the immune response, heart failure, and kidney failure, leading to death.

From a physiologic perspective, what is emerging across the disciplines involved—molecular biology, immunology, neurology, endocrinology, and behavioral science—is a more holistic and complex model that involves biochemical relationships of the CNS, autonomic nervous system (ANS), endocrine system, and immune system that cause the stress responses identified by Selye. More simply, these relationships are often cited together as the **hypothalamic-pituitary-adrenal (HPA) axis** (Figure 11-3). The reader may find it helpful to become familiar with the ANS function content in Chapter 15, p. 470.

In sequence, the hypothalamus secretes **corticotropin-releasing hormone (CRH),** which binds to specific receptors on pituitary cells that, in turn, produce **adrenocorticotropic hormone (ACTH).** ACTH is then transported through the blood to the adrenal glands located on the top of the kidneys. After binding to specific receptors on the adrenal glands, the glucocorticoid hormones (primarily cortisol; from the adrenal cortex) are released. Cortisol initiates a series of metabolic changes discussed in the section Glucocorticoids: Cortisol; however, overall, these hormones are thought to enhance immunity during acute stress and suppress immunity during chronic stress because of prolonged exposure and increased concentration.[1]

CONCEPTS OF STRESS

Selye believed that stressors cause a general or nonspecific response. However, research in the past 50 years has shown the remarkable sensitivity of the central nervous system and endocrine system to psychologic influences (emotion is included in psychologic and social stress and acts through psychologic mechanisms). Thus, although Selye's identification of the GAS is regarded as tremendously important and the cornerstone of stress research, the idea that stress is a purely physiologic response is vastly oversimplified. In the mid-1950s, studies showed that activation of the adrenal cortex occurred in humans in response to psychologic stressors,[4] in monkeys with conditioned emotional responses,[5] and in humans subjected to a stressful interview technique.[6] In the early 1960s, researchers found that plasma cortisol levels in groups of subjects increased while they watched war movies and decreased while they viewed Disney nature films.[7,8] Mason later demonstrated that the initiation of the GAS depended on psychologic factors surrounding the stressors.[9] He also showed that various factors, such as degrees of discomfort or unpleasantness or suddenness of the stress, could account for the presence or absence of physiologic stress responses.[9]

The term *stress* has been used persistently and widely across many disciplines despite numerous disagreements over its definition. Nevertheless, in recent years **stress** has been more usefully defined as a *transactional* or *interactional concept.* Transactionally, stress is viewed as the state of affairs arising when a person relates to (i.e., interacts or transacts with) situations in certain ways. People are not disturbed by situations per se but by the ways they appraise and react to situations. In general, a person experiences stress when a demand *exceeds* a person's coping abilities, resulting in reactions such as disturbances of cognition, emotion, and behavior that can adversely affect well-being. Moreover, psychologic stressors can elicit reactive or anticipatory stress responses. The **reactive response** is a physiologic response derived from psychologic stressors. For example, the stress of an examination may

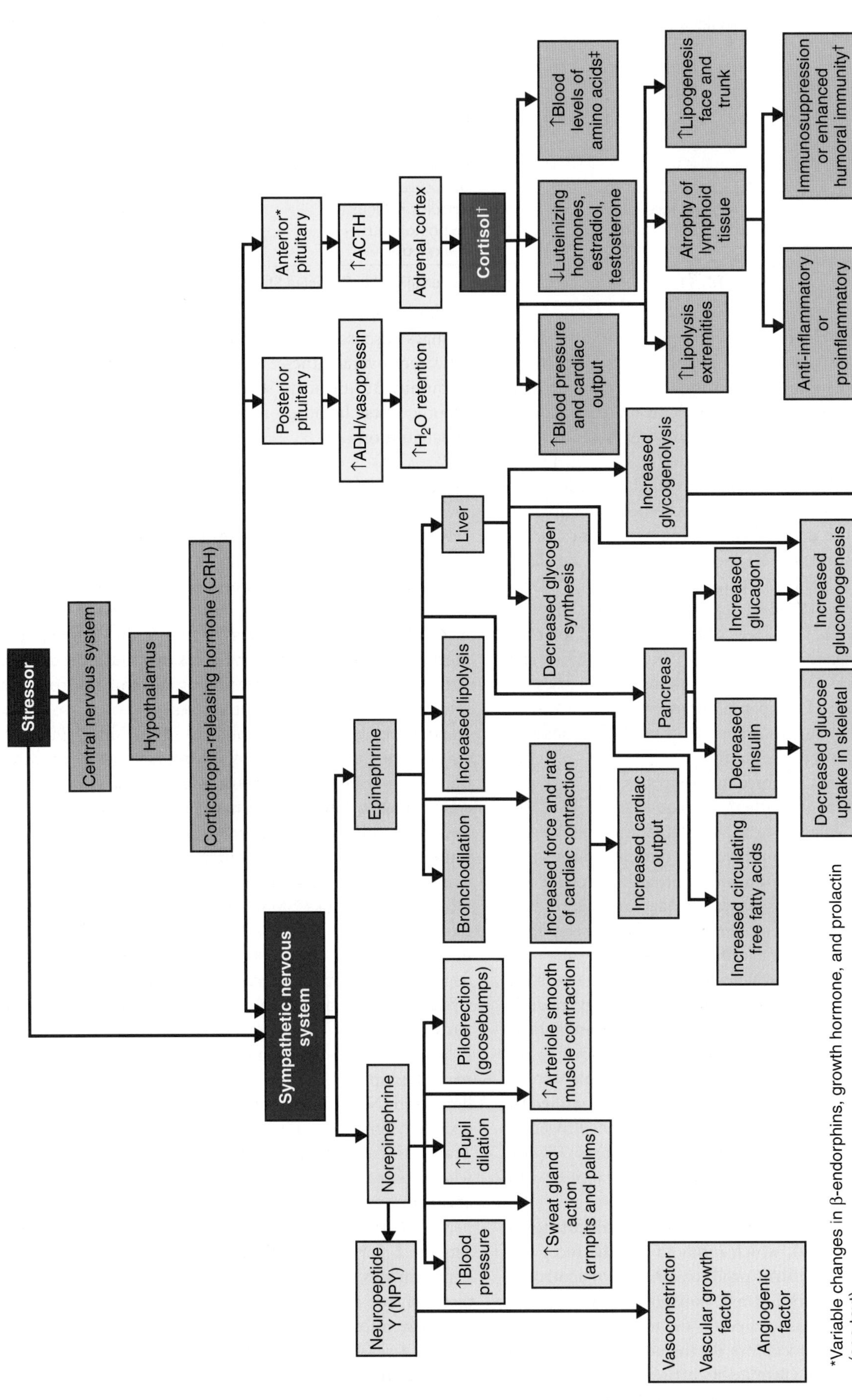

*Variable changes in β-endorphins, growth hormone, and prolactin (see text).
†Effects may be dependent on *amount* of cortisol and nature of the stressor.
‡Caused by protein catabolism in muscle, adipose tissue, skin, bones, lymphoid tissue.
ADH, Antidiuretic hormone; *ACTH*, adrenocorticotropic hormone.

FIGURE 11-2 The Stress Response.

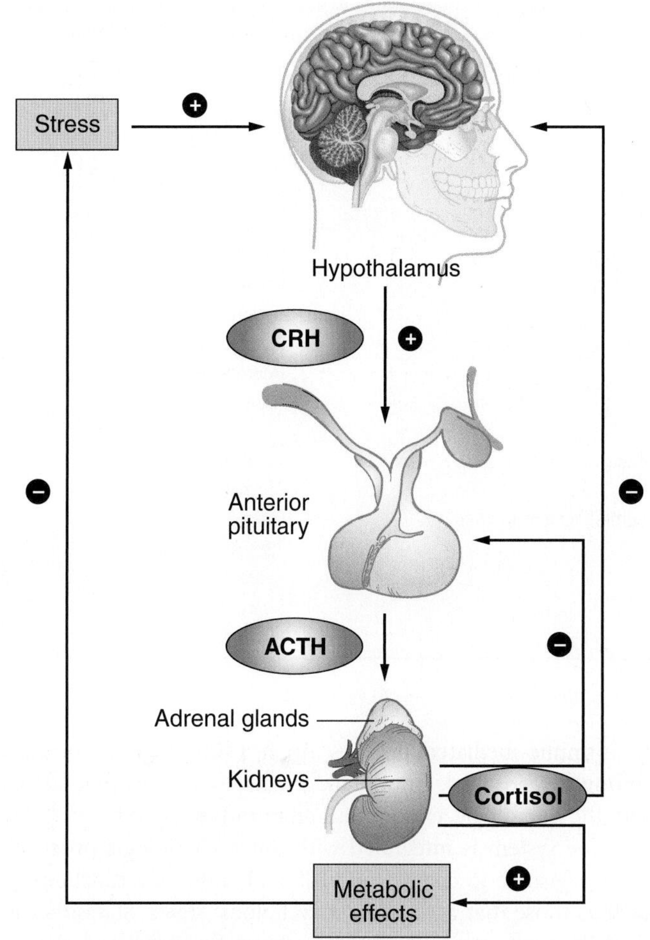

FIGURE 11-3 Hypothalamic-Pituitary-Adrenal (HPA) Axis. The response to stress begins in the brain. The hypothalamus is the control center in the brain for many hormones including corticotropin-releasing hormone (CRH). *ACTH, Adrenocorticotropic hormone.*

produce an increased heart rate and dry mouth in the unprepared student. The **anticipatory response** occurs when physiologic responses develop in anticipation of disruption of the optimal steady-state, also known as **homeostasis.** These anticipatory responses can be generated either by species-specific innate programs, such as reacting to the presence of predators and unfamiliar situations, or by experience-dependent memory programs created by conditioning.[10] Anticipatory responses are learned responses under fine control by regions located in the brain's limbic system. These regions are those most frequently associated with learning and memory and include the hippocampus, amygdala, and prefrontal cortex. In order for these regions to elicit a stress response, the paraventricular nucleus (PVN) of the hypothalamus must be stimulated. The limbic structures rarely interact directly with the PVN and are believed to influence the stress response through intermediary neurons, some of which are primarily used for the reactive response.

In a **conditional response** one learns that specific stimuli (i.e., objects or situational context) are associated with danger, and as such anticipation of subsequent encounters with the stimulus produces a physiologic stress response. For example, a child that is abused by a parent may experience a physiologic stress response in anticipation of further abuse when the parent enters the room. Under some circumstances these memory programs may become so strong that psychologic disorders, such as phobias, develop. In a similar fashion, some persons develop **posttraumatic stress disorder (PTSD)** in response to the memory, as opposed to the anticipation of traumatic events. PTSD is characterized by flashback memories, sleep disturbances, depression, and other symptoms. These symptoms have the potential to greatly interfere with normal activities such as employment and frequently disrupt personal relationships and quality of life.

Today there is evidence implicating stress as a precipitating factor for some diseases and conditions and as an exacerbating factor, worsening symptoms and outcomes, in others, such as atherosclerosis, irritable bowel syndrome, ulcers, asthma, autoimmune disorders, anxiety, delayed wound healing, chronic pain and fatigue syndromes, reproductive dysfunction, diabetes, and depression.[9-11] In addition, evidence published since 2000 generally supports a relationship between stress and human immunodeficiency virus (HIV) progression.[12]

Psychologic stress may cause or exacerbate (worsen) several disease states, including many of the diseases implicated as the leading causes of death in the United States (Table 11-1). For example, stress-induced chronic inflammation is suggested as being important in the functional decline that leads to frailty, disability, and untimely death; cardiovascular disease; and infectious diseases.[12-16] Additionally, important effects of acute emotional stress, such as the death of a loved one, on the heart muscle include three areas: (1) left ventricular contractile dysfunction, (2) myocardial ischemia, and (3) disturbances of heart rhythm (see What's New? Acute Emotional Stress and Adverse Heart Effects). Other examples include research linking stress to the recurrence of genital herpes virus in women with HIV.[13] As evidence has mounted concerning the important role that stress plays in certain disease processes, research has focused on the mechanisms responsible for these mind-body interactions. Along with a greater understanding of the relationship between the human stress response and disease, new strategies for treatment of stress-related disorders are emerging. It has recently been demonstrated that the interactions among social, psychologic, biologic, and behavioral factors are inherent in the causes and courses of many diseases. Molecular biologists, immunologists, neurologists, clinicians, and behavioral scientists are now exploring the role of the other half of the mind-body (dualistic) model—that is, the mind. What is emerging is a more holistic and complex model of health and disease states. This model involves the biochemical relationships of the central and autonomic nervous systems, the endocrine system, and the immune system and their relationships to stress-elicited coping behaviors, such as smoking and poor diet, that can also modify the integrity of the immune system. Discoveries of these complex links have led to the creation of the field of psychoneuroimmunology.

TABLE 11-1 **EXAMPLES OF STRESS-RELATED DISEASES AND CONDITIONS**

TARGET ORGAN OR SYSTEM	DISEASE OR CONDITION	TARGET ORGAN OR SYSTEM	DISEASE OR CONDITION
Cardiovascular system	Coronary artery disease Hypertension Stroke Disturbances of heart rhythm	Gastrointestinal system	Ulcer Irritable bowel syndrome Diarrhea Nausea and vomiting Ulcerative colitis
Muscle	Tension headaches Muscle contraction backache	Genitourinary system	Diuresis Impotence Frigidity
Connective tissues	Rheumatoid arthritis (autoimmune disease) Related inflammatory diseases of connective tissue	Skin	Eczema Neurodermatitis Acne
Pulmonary system	Asthma (hypersensitivity reaction) Hay fever (hypersensitivity reactions)	Endocrine system	Type 2 diabetes mellitus Amenorrhea
Immune system	Immunosuppression or deficiency Autoimmune diseases	Central nervous system	Fatigue and lethargy Type A behavior Overeating Depression Insomnia

WHAT'S NEW?

Acute Emotional Stress and Adverse Heart Effects

Myocardial Ischemia

- Individuals with coronary heart disease may develop myocardial ischemia during mental or acute emotional stress even though their exercise results are negative.
- Systemic vascular resistance increases during periods of mental or acute emotional stress with concomitant increased myocardial oxygen demand.

Left Ventricular Dysfunction

- This condition is more evident in older women.
- After acute emotional stress or trauma, there is an increase in sudden chest pain and shortness of breath.
- Left ventricular dysfunction is more common in the cardiac apex.
- Alterations occur possibly because of increases in the levels of catecholamines. Increased stress in daily life is associated with enhanced HPA axis response, a higher cortisol awakening response, and higher mean day and evening cortisol levels.

Ventricular Dysrhythmias

- Intense or unusual acute stress precipitates about 20% of serious ventricular dysrhythmias or sudden cardiac death.
- Altered brain activity may lead to changes in ventricular repolarization and electrical instability of the cardiac muscle.

Data from Critchley HD et al: *Brain* 128(Pt 1):75–85, 2005; Ramachandruni S et al: *J Am Coll Cardiol* 47(5):987–991, 2006; Soufer R: *Circulation* 110(13):1710–1713, 2004; Wittstein IS et al: *N Engl J Med* 352(6):539–548, 2005; Ziegelstein RC: *JAMA* 298(3):324–329, 2007. Kumari M et al: *Psychoneuroendocrinology*, 35(7):1091–1099, 2010.

Psychoneuroimmunologic Mediators of Stress

Psychoneuroimmunology (PNI) is the study of how the consciousness *(psycho)*, brain and spinal cord *(neuro)*, and the body's defenses against infection and abnormal cell division *(immunology)* interact. Psychoneuroimmunology assumes that all immune-mediated diseases result from interrelationships among psychosocial, emotional, genetic, and behavioral factors with the neurologic, endocrine, and immune systems.[11,17,18] The immune system is integrated with other physiologic processes and is sensitive to changes in CNS and endocrine functioning, such as those that accompany psychologic states. Stressors can elicit the stress response or stress system through the action of the nervous and endocrine systems. Stressors include infection, noise, decreased oxygen supply, pain, malnutrition, heat, cold, trauma, prolonged exertion, radiation, responses to life events (including anxiety, depression, anger, fear, loss, and excitement), obesity, old age, drugs, disease, surgery, and medical treatment.

Although the field of PNI is relatively new, and a body of scientific literature is present, the subject of PNI has caused strenuous scientific debate, especially with respect to the causal role of personality in cancer mortality and morbidity.[19] For example, mouse models suggest a strong link between stress and breast cancer progression, yet this effect has not been consistently found in humans.[19,20] What is certain, however, is that hormones released by the stress response influence many metabolic systems and corresponding physiologic events, even if the mechanisms and subsequent physiologic events are yet to be fully understood. Further, sufficient data now exist to conclude that immune modulation by psychosocial stressors or interventions leads directly to health outcomes.[21-37] The strongest support to date for the link between psychosocial stressors and health outcomes remains in studies of infectious disease and wound healing.[38-43] However, a very recent meta-analysis of 10 studies conducted among persons living in England found that any level of psychologic distress is associated with increased mortality and increased risk of death from cardiovascular disease, external causes, and cancer (albeit only at higher levels of distress); 68,000 persons were used in this study and personal factors, such as age, smoking, and alcohol use, were adjusted accordingly.[44]

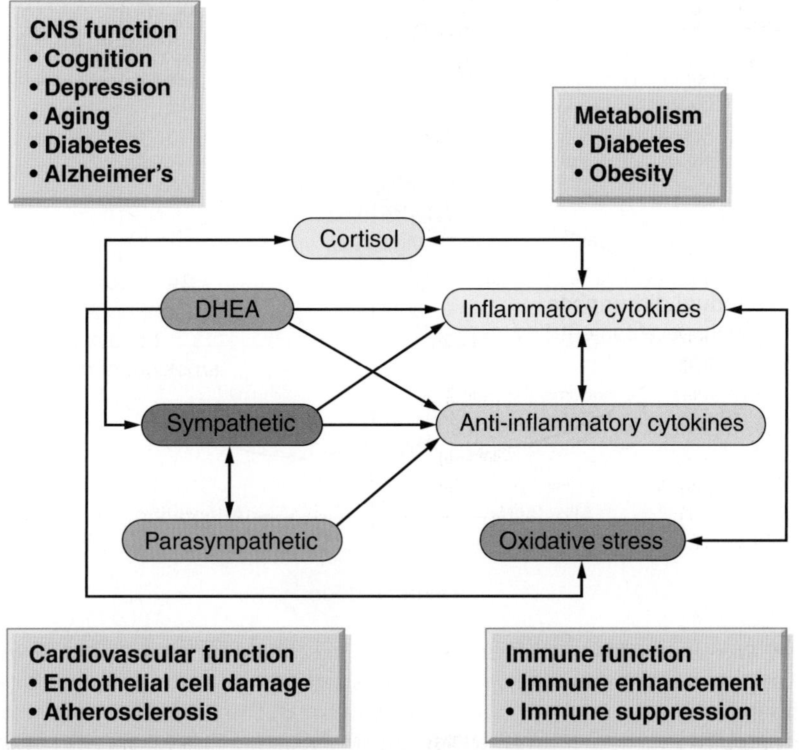

FIGURE 11-4 Stress Interactions Are Nonlinear and Complex. Nonlinearity means that when one mediator is increased or decreased, the subsequent compensatory changes in other mediators depend on time and level of change, causing multiple interacting variables. The inevitable consequences from adapting to daily life over time include changes in behavioral responses. For example, these changes include sleeping patterns, tobacco use, alcohol consumption, physical activity, and social interactions. These behavioral patterns are a part of the allostatic overload with chronic elevations in cortisol level, sympathetic activity, and proinflammatory cytokines, and a decrease in parasympathetic activity. (From McEwen BS: *Eur J Pharmacol* 583[2-3]:174–185, 2008.) *DHEA,* Dehydroepiandrosterone.

STRESS RESPONSE

The **stress response** is initiated by the central nervous system and endocrine system (see Figure 11-1). Specifically, **corticotropin-releasing hormone (CRH)** is released from the hypothalamus, and influences the sympathetic nervous system, the pituitary gland, and the adrenal gland (see Figure 11-2). CRH is also released peripherally at inflammatory sites called **peripheral**, or **immune, CRH.** The activation of these systems redirects adaptive energy to the CNS and stressed body sites.

Where the stress response begins depends on whether the stressor is perceived or real. Perceived stressors elicit an anticipatory response that usually begins in the limbic system of the brain, the area responsible for emotions and cognition. The limbic system indirectly elicits both an endocrine stress response by stimulating neural pathways responsible for receiving sensory information and a central stress response by directly stimulating the locus ceruleus (LC) to release norepinephrine (see Figure 11-1). Norepinephrine release promotes arousal, increased vigilance, increased anxiety, and other protective emotional responses. Real stressors elicit a reactive response that can begin either in the limbic system or in regions of the brain receiving specific sensory information (see Figure 11-1). This information is then relayed to the PVN. The PVN stimulates the LC and both central and endocrine stress responses.

Central Stress Response

Better understanding is emerging regarding the physiology involved in meeting the demands and challenges of daily life. Some refer to these challenges as "stressors," and the chronically stressed person may use the term "stressed out." The physiology is complex, involving both protection and damage. As previously mentioned, glucocorticoids from the adrenal cortex in response to ACTH from the pituitary gland (see Figure 11-3) comprise the major stress hormones along with the catecholamines epinephrine and norepinephrine. Other central hormones/mediators also play a role including the proinflammatory and anti-inflammatory cytokines that are regulated by glucocorticoids and catecholamines (Figure 11-4).[21]

Catecholamines can increase proinflammatory cytokine production, causing, for example, increased heart rate and blood pressure. Glucocorticoids are known to inhibit this proinflammatory production; however, inhibition depends on dose and cell or tissue type.[30] More simply, glucocorticoids can also promote inflammation depending on dose and cell type.[31] The increased understanding of these effects suggests the possibility that chronic and dysfunctional HPA axis stimulation (as may

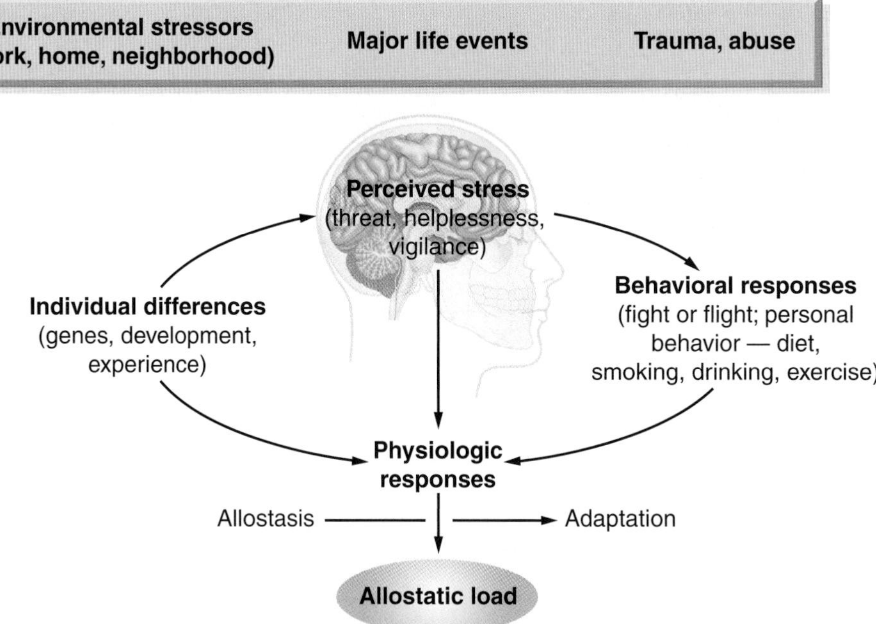

FIGURE 11-5 **Physiologic and Behavioral Stress Responses.** Stress processes arise from bidirectional communication patterns between the brain and other physiologic systems (autonomic, immune, neural, and endocrine). Importantly, these bidirectional mechanisms are protective, promoting short-term adaptation (allostasis). Chronic stress mechanisms, however, can lead to long-term dysregulation and promote behavioral responses and physiologic responses that lead to stress-induced disorders/diseases (allostatic load) that compromise health. (From McEwen BS: *Eur J Pharmacol* 583[2-3]:174–185, 2008.)

occur during chronic inflammation) increases inflammation in the brain and other tissue, possibly contributing to other diseases including osteoporosis, metabolic disease (diabetes, obesity), and cardiovascular disease.[32] Additionally, these interactions are nonlinear and are very complex.

Parasympathetic System

The parasympathetic system balances the sympathetic nervous system and, thus, also influences adaptation or maladaptation to stressful events. The parasympathetic system also has anti-inflammatory effects. The parasympathetic system opposes the sympathetic (catecholamine) responses, for example, by slowing the heart rate.[31] Researchers evaluate the relative balance of the parasympathetic and sympathetic nervous systems using a technique known as heart rate variability (the measurement of R wave variability from heartbeat to heartbeat).

Allostasis is considered an adaptive physiologic response to stressful events (e.g., fight or flight).[21] Chronic or dysregulated **allostasis** (long-term or chronic exaggerated responses to stress) can lead to disease. **Allostatic load** (Figure 11-5) is the individualized cumulative amounts of stressors that exist in our lives and that influence our physiologic responses. Allostatic load includes our genetic makeup, our lifestyle (including damaging health behaviors), daily events, and dramatic events (such as disasters).[21,45] Over time this load exacts a toll on our bodies (i.e., "wear and tear"). Because the brain is a key player in deciding what is stressful, it is influential in determining when we have reached allostatic overload. Moreover, these responses are individualized in that what would be considered normal for one person is considered extremely stressful for another.[45] Under conditions of allostatic overload, the parasympathetic system may decrease its restraint of the sympathetic system, resulting in increased or prolonged inflammatory responses.[21,31] Physiologically, in response to acute and chronic stress some regions of the brain (the hippocampus, amygdala, and prefrontal cortex) may respond by undergoing structural remodeling, which can alter behavioral and physiologic responses (such as cognitive impairment or depression).[21] Key mediators involved in **allostatic overload** (exaggerated pathophysiologic responses to stress) include the glucocorticoid cortisol, catecholamines (released from sympathetic nervous system activation), and proinflammatory cytokines; in addition, there is a decline in parasympathetic activity. A prevalent example is sleep deprivation resulting from excessive stress. Sleep deprivation has significant damaging effects including elevated evening cortisol level; elevated insulin and blood glucose levels; increased blood pressure; reduced parasympathetic activity; increased levels of proinflammatory cytokines; and increased concentrations of the gut hormone ghrelin, which increases appetite. Altogether, these alterations can lead to increased caloric intake, depressed mood, cognitive problems, and a host of other responses from insomnia.[34]

Neuroendocrine Regulation

The sympathetic nervous system (SNS) is aroused during the stress response and causes the medulla of the adrenal gland to release catecholamines (80% epinephrine and 20% norepinephrine) into the bloodstream. The adrenal medulla is actually an extension of the SNS because preganglionic fibers from the splanchnic nerve terminate in the medulla, where they innervate

TABLE 11-2 PHYSIOLOGIC EFFECTS OF CATECHOLAMINES*

ORGAN/TISSUE	PROCESS OR RESULT
Brain	Increased blood flow; increased glucose metabolism
Cardiovascular system	Increased rate and force of contraction
	Peripheral vasoconstriction
Pulmonary system	Bronchodilation
Skeletal muscle	Increased glycogenolysis
	Increased contraction
	Increased dilation of muscle vasculature
	Decreased glucose uptake and utilization (decreases insulin release)
Liver	Increased glucose production
	Increased glycogenolysis
Adipose tissue	Increased lipolysis
	Decreased glucose uptake
Skin	Decreased blood flow
Gastrointestinal and genitourinary tracts	Decreased protein synthesis
	Decreased smooth muscle contraction
	Increased renin release
	Increased gastrointestinal sphincter tone
Lymphoid tissue	Acute and chronic stress inhibits several components of innate immunity, particularly decreasing number of natural killer cells
Macrophages	Inhibit and stimulate macrophage activity
	Depend on availability of type 1/ proinflammatory cytokines, presence or absence of antigenic stressors, and peripheral corticotropin-releasing hormone (CRH)

Data from Elenkov IJ, Chrousos GP: *Ann N Y Acad Sci* 966:290–303, 2002; Granner DK: Hormones of the adrenal medulla. In Murray RK et al, editors: *Harper's biochemistry*, ed 25, New York, 2000.
*Some of these responses require glucocorticoids (e.g., cortisol) for maximal activity (see text for explanation).

the chromaffin cells that produce the catecholamine hormones. Simultaneously, hypothalamic CRH stimulates the pituitary gland to release a variety of hormones, including antidiuretic hormone and oxytocin from the posterior pituitary gland, and prolactin, endorphins, growth hormone (GH), and adrenocorticotropic hormone (ACTH) from the anterior pituitary gland. ACTH stimulates the cortex of the adrenal gland to release cortisol (see Figure 11-2).

Catecholamines

Circulating catecholamines essentially mimic direct sympathetic stimulation. Catecholamines cannot cross the blood-brain barrier and are synthesized locally in the brain. In response to stress, the chromaffin cells of the adrenal medulla produce large quantities of epinephrine and small amounts of norepinephrine. Once released, catecholamines circulate bound to the plasma protein albumin. The physiologic effects of the catecholamines on organs and tissues are summarized in Table 11-2. Norepinephrine regulates blood pressure by constricting smooth muscle in all blood vessels. During stress, norepinephrine raises blood pressure by constricting peripheral vessels; it dilates the pupils of the eye, causes piloerection, and increases sweat gland action in the armpits and palms (see Figure 11-2).

TABLE 11-3 PHYSIOLOGIC ACTIONS OF α- AND β-ADRENERGIC RECEPTORS

RECEPTOR	PHYSIOLOGIC ACTIONS
α_1	Increased glycogenolysis; smooth muscle contraction (blood vessels, genitourinary tract)
α_2	Smooth muscle relaxation (gastrointestinal tract); smooth muscle contraction (some vascular beds); inhibition of lipolysis, renin release, platelet aggregation, and insulin secretion
β_1	Stimulation of lipolysis; myocardial contraction (increased rate, increased force of contraction)
β_2	Increased hepatic gluconeogenesis; increased hepatic glycogenolysis; increased muscle glycogenolysis; increased release of insulin, glucagon, and renin; smooth muscle relaxation (bronchi, blood vessels, genitourinary tract, gastrointestinal tract)

Epinephrine is rapidly transported to and acts on several organs, but it is metabolized quickly, making it short-acting. Metabolically, epinephrine causes transient hyperglycemia (high blood glucose level), decreases glucose uptake in the muscles and other organs, and decreases insulin release from the pancreas. This is accomplished by activating enzymes whose actions promote glucose formation (gluconeogenesis) and glycogen breakdown (glycogenolysis) in the liver, while inhibiting glycogen formation. This prevents glucose from being taken up by peripheral tissue and preserves it for the CNS. Further, very little adrenal norepinephrine reaches distal tissue; thus, the effects caused by norepinephrine during the stress response are primarily elicited from the SNS.[46,47]

Epinephrine has a greater influence on cardiac action and is the principal catecholamine involved in metabolic regulation. Epinephrine enhances myocardial contractility (inotropic effect), increases the heart rate (chronotropic effect), and increases venous return to the heart, all of which increase cardiac output and blood pressure. Epinephrine dilates blood vessels of skeletal muscle, allowing for greater oxygenation. Epinephrine in the liver and skeletal muscles is rapidly metabolized and dilates blood vessels supplying skeletal muscles, allowing for more oxygenation. Epinephrine also mobilizes free fatty acids and cholesterol by stimulating lipolysis, freeing triglycerides and fatty acids from fat stores, and by inhibiting the degradation of circulating cholesterol to bile acids. The metabolic actions of epinephrine aid the metabolic actions of cortisol, which are similar.

Table 11-2 summarizes other well-known effects of adrenal catecholamines. All of these effects prepare the body to take physical action: to fight or flee. Stressors commonly associated with catecholamine release by the adrenal medulla include exercise, thermal changes, and acute emotional states.

The catecholamines stimulate two major classes of receptors: α-adrenergic receptors and β-adrenergic receptors. These two classes are divided further into two subclasses: (1) α_1 and α_2 and (2) β_1 and β_2. Table 11-3 summarizes the actions of the two subclasses of adrenergic receptors. Epinephrine binds to and

TABLE 11-4 PHYSIOLOGIC EFFECTS OF CORTISOL

FUNCTIONS AFFECTED	PHYSIOLOGIC EFFECTS
Carbohydrate and lipid metabolism	Diminishes peripheral uptake and utilization of glucose; promotes gluconeogenesis in liver metabolism cells; enhances gluconeogenic response to other hormones; promotes lipolysis in adipose tissue
Protein metabolism	Increases protein synthesis in liver and decreases protein synthesis (including immunoglobulin synthesis) in muscle, lymphoid tissue, adipose tissue, skin, and bone; increases plasma level of amino acids; stimulates deamination in liver
Anti-inflammatory effects (systemic effects)	High levels of cortisol used in drug therapy suppress inflammatory response; inhibit proinflammatory activity of many growth factors and cytokines; however, over time some individuals may develop tolerance to glucocorticoids, causing an increased susceptibility to both inflammatory and autoimmune disease
Proinflammatory effects (possible local effects)	Cortisol levels released during stress response may increase proinflammatory effects
Lipid metabolism	Lipolysis in extremities and lipogenesis in face and trunk
Immune effects	*Treatment* levels of glucocorticoids are immunosuppressive; thus, they are valuable agents used in numerous diseases; the T-cell or innate immunity system is particularly affected by these larger doses of glucocorticoids with suppression of Th1 function or innate immunity; *stress* can cause a different pattern of immune response; these nontherapeutic levels can suppress innate (Th1) and increase adaptive (Th2) immunity—the so-called Th1 to Th2 shift; several factors influence this complex physiology and include long-term adaptations, reproductive hormones (i.e., overall, androgens suppress and estrogens stimulate immune responses), defects of hypothalamic-pituitary-adrenal axis, histamine-generated responses, and acute vs. chronic stress; thus stress seems to cause a Th2 shift *systemically* whereas *locally*, under certain conditions, it can induce proinflammatory activities and by these mechanisms may influence onset or course of infections and autoimmune/inflammatory, allergic, and neoplastic diseases
Digestive function	Promotes gastric secretion
Urinary function	Enhances excretion of calcium
Connective tissue function	Decreases proliferation of fibroblasts in connective tissue (thus delaying healing)
Muscle function	Maintains normal contractility and maximal work output for skeletal and cardiac muscle
Bone function	Decreases bone formation
Vascular system/myocardial function	Maintains normal blood pressure; permits increased responsiveness of arterioles to constrictive action of adrenergic stimulation; optimizes myocardial performance
Central nervous system function	Somehow modulates perceptual and emotional functioning; essential for normal arousal and initiation of daytime activity
Possible synergism with estrogen in pregnancy?	Suppresses maternal immune system to prevent rejection of fetus?

activates both α- and β-adrenergic receptors. Norepinephrine at physiologic concentrations binds primarily to α-adrenergic receptors.[48]

Catecholamines can modify the numbers of cells of the immune system circulating in the blood.[49] Injection of epinephrine into healthy human subjects is associated with a transient increase of the number of lymphocytes (e.g., T cells and natural killer [NK] cells) in the peripheral blood. Specifically, the levels of T cytotoxic and NK cells increase, whereas little change occurs in B lymphocytes. The main change involves the NK cells.[49] Qualitatively, lymphocyte responsiveness of T and B lymphocytes is reduced. Similar quantitative and qualitative changes are found 5 to 6 minutes after exposure to a psychologic or physical stressor.[50] However, the effects of acute elevation of catecholamine levels on the alteration of lymphocyte function are short-lived, lasting only about 2 hours.[51]

Glucocorticoids: Cortisol

The adrenal cortex is activated during stress by ACTH (see Figure 11-2), which increases adrenocortical secretion of glucocorticoid hormones, primarily cortisol (*hydrocortisone* is a synthetically produced but chemically identical version of cortisol). These steroid molecules reach *all* tissues, including the brain, easily penetrate cell membranes, and react with numerous intracellular glucocorticoid receptors. Because they spare almost no tissue or organ and influence a large proportion of the human genome, they exert significant diverse biologic actions.[22] The feedback mechanisms of the HPA axis sense and determine the circulating glucocorticoid levels, whereas other tissues passively accept the actions of circulating glucocorticoids.[22] Chronic dysregulation of the HPA axis, especially elevated cortisol level, has been linked to a wide variety of disorders including obesity, sleep deprivation, lipid abnormalities, hypertension, diabetes, atherosclerosis, loss of bone density, hippocampal atrophy, and cognitive impairment.[45]

Cortisol circulates in the plasma, both protein bound and free. The main plasma-binding protein is called **transcortin** or **corticosteroid-binding globulin.** The unbound, or free, fraction is approximately 8% of the total plasma cortisol and is biologically active.[48] Cortisol mobilizes substances needed for cellular metabolism. One of the primary effects of cortisol is the stimulation of gluconeogenesis, or the formation of glucose from noncarbohydrate sources, such as amino acids or free fatty acids in the liver. In addition, cortisol enhances the elevation of blood glucose level promoted by other hormones, such as epinephrine, glucagon, and growth hormone. This action by cortisol is said to be *permissive* for the actions of other hormones. Cortisol also inhibits the uptake and oxidation of glucose by many body cells. The overall action of cortisol increases blood glucose concentration, thereby enabling the body to combat the stressor. The physiologic effects of cortisol are summarized in Table 11-4.

Cortisol also affects protein metabolism. It has an anabolic effect; that is, it increases the rate of synthesis of proteins and ribonucleic acid (RNA) in the liver. The anabolic effect of cortisol, however, is countered by its catabolic effect on protein

BOX 11-1 GLUCOCORTICOIDS, INSULIN, INFLAMMATION, AND OBESITY

The signs and symptoms of Cushing syndrome (e.g., excess glucocorticoids [GCs]) include truncal obesity, relatively thin extremities, a "moon face," and a "buffalo [neck] hump." In such individuals the possibility of associated hypertension is high as well as increased risk of infection and metabolic syndrome or frank type 2 diabetes. In addition, the likelihood of an elevated ratio of intra-abdominal subcutaneous fat mass to nonabdominal fat mass is high because the glucocorticoids mediate the redistribution of stored calories into the abdominal region. The specific increase in abdominal fat stores is a consequence of elevated levels of glucocorticoids combined with increased insulin action. However, the increased levels of glucocorticoids need not be present in the circulation, but can be generated locally in fat by conversion of inactive cortisone to active cortisol through the action of the isoenzyme 11-β-hydroxysteroid dehydrogenase (11-β-HSD) type-1. This conversion is referred to as "pre-receptor" metabolism of cortisol. The active steroid is secreted directly to the liver through the portal vein. In vitro insulin synthesis and secretion from the pancreas are inhibited by the glucocorticoids. However, increasing levels of glucocorticoids in vivo are associated with increasing insulin secretion possibly because of an anti-insulin effect on the liver, which appears to be vulnerable to the negative effects of glucocorticoids on insulin action. Hepatic insulin resistance is strongly associated with abdominal obesity.

Recent data reveal that the plasma concentration of inflammatory mediators, such as tumor necrosis factor-alpha (TNF-α) and interleukin-6 (IL-6), is increased in the insulin-resistant states of obesity and type 2 diabetes. Two mechanisms might be involved in the pathogenesis of inflammation: (1) glucose and macronutrient intake (i.e., which can be mediated through chronic stress) causes oxidative stress; and (2) the increased concentrations of TNF-α and IL-6 associated with obesity and type 2 diabetes might interfere with insulin signal transduction. This interference might promote inflammation. Chronic overnutrition (obesity) might thus be a proinflammatory state with oxidative stress.

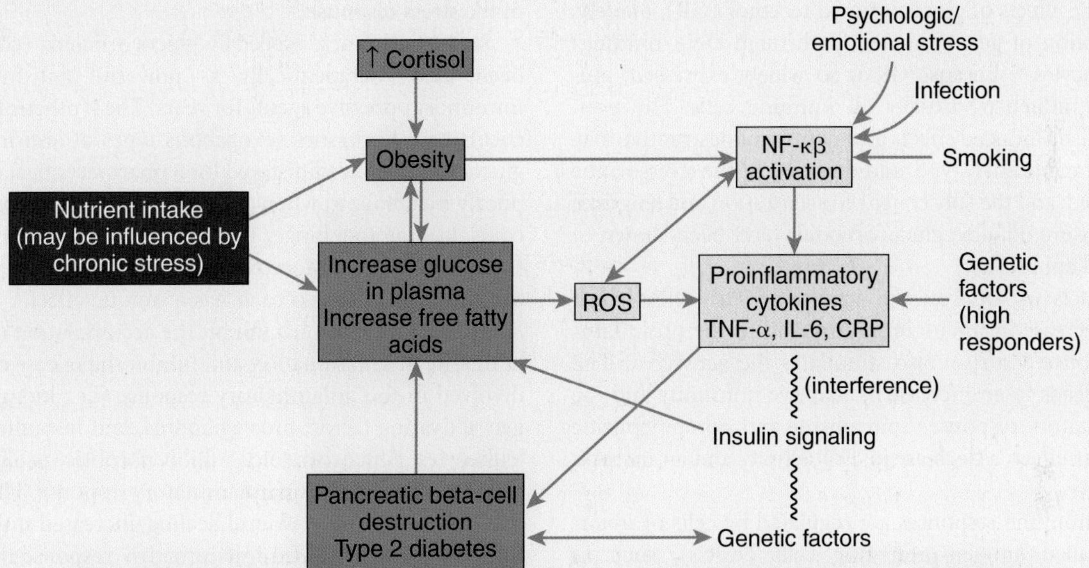

Stress, Inflammation, Obesity, and Type 2 Diabetes. The induction of reactive oxygen species (ROS) generation and inflammation through the proinflammatory transcription factor, NF-kβ, activates most proinflammatory genes. Macronutrient intake, obesity, free fatty acids, infection, smoking, psychologic stress, and genetic factors increase the production of ROS. Interference with insulin signaling (insulin resistance) leads to hyperglycemia and proinflammatory changes. Proinflammatory changes increase the levels of TNF-α and IL-6, and also lead to the inhibition of insulin signaling and insulin resistance. Inflammation in pancreatic beta cells leads to beta-cell dysfunction, which in combination with insulin resistance leads to type 2 diabetes. *CRP,* C-reactive protein.

Data from Dallman MF et al: *Endocrinology* 145(6):2633–2638, 2004; Dandona P, Aljada A, Brandyopadhyay A: *Trends Immunol* 25(1):4–7, 2004; Kim SP et al: *Diabetes* 52:2453–2460, 2003; Masuzaki H et al: *Science* 94:2166–2170, 2001; Padgett DA, Glaser R: *Trends Immunol* 24(8):444–448, 2003; Spencer SJ, Tilbrook A: *Stress* 14(3), 2011.

stores in other tissues. Protein catabolism acts to increase levels of circulating amino acids, and chronic exposure to excess cortisol can severely deplete protein stores in muscle, bone, connective tissue, and skin. Further, cortisol acts to reduce protein synthesis in nonhepatic tissues, a loss for which dietary protein cannot compensate. Some evidence suggests that cortisol depresses transport of amino acids into muscle cells while enhancing their uptake into the liver. Finally, cortisol promotes gastric secretion in the stomach and intestines, potentially causing gastric ulcers. This could account for the gastrointestinal ulceration observed by Selye. This is in opposition to norepinephrine, which reduces gastric secretion.

Cortisol also has a powerful effect that reverses the insulin-induced suppression of hepatic gluconeogenesis, as well as basal levels of cortisol that stimulate the activity of hepatic enzymes responsible for glycogen and glucose production. The increased amino acid uptake into liver and the increased levels of glucose-producing enzymes favor the production of glucose. Although diseases of excess cortisol secretion, such as Cushing disease, produce characteristics of type 2 (non–insulin-dependent) diabetes mellitus, recent studies found that chronic stress also may facilitate the development of type 2 diabetes.[52,53] Glucocorticoids contribute to the development of metabolic syndrome and the pathogenesis of obesity (Box 11-1). The mechanism for this action is under investigation, but it is believed that the development of diabetes is secondary to cortisol-induced obesity. Cortisol promotes lipogenesis in certain regions of the body and to a lesser extent promotes lipolysis in other regions by increasing the actions of lipolytic hormones, such as catecholamines and growth hormone. Chronic cortisol excess induces lipogenesis in the abdomen, trunk, and face, resulting in central obesity. Finally, glucocorticoids may affect fetal programming of the HPA axis by causing an adverse intrauterine environment because of alterations in cortisol secretion during pregnancy.[54]

Cortisol and the Immune System

Cortisol secretion during stress exerts beneficial effects by inhibiting initial inflammatory effects, for example, vasodilation and increased capillary permeability.[32] Cortisol also promotes resolution and repair. These actions are mainly accomplished by facilitating the effects of glucocorticoid receptor (GR), namely, the transcription of genetic material (through DNA binding) within leukocytes.[32] Because GR is so widely expressed, glucocorticoids influence virtually all immune cells. However, whether cortisol-induced effects are adaptive or destructive may depend on the intensity, type, and duration of the stressor; the tissue involved; and the subsequent concentration and length of cortisol exposure. Finally, glucocorticoids have been shown to induce T-cell apoptosis.[32]

Cortisol acts to suppress the activity of Th1 cells, which leads to a decrease in innate immunity and to the proinflammatory response. Cortisol also stimulates the activity of Th2 cells, which leads to an increase in adaptive immunity and the anti-inflammatory response. Epinephrine and norepinephrine have a similar effect: a decrease in Th1 activity and an increase in Th2 activity.

Initially, immune responses are regulated by cells of *innate immunity* called antigen-presenting cells (APCs), such as monocytes/macrophages, dendritic cells, and other phagocytic cells, and by Th1 and Th2 lymphocytes (cells involved in *adaptive immunity*). These cells secrete chemical messengers, called *cytokines,* that regulate innate and adaptive immune responses. Cytokines are a group of chemicals such as interferons, interleukins, and tumor necrosis factors that can stimulate or inhibit various components of the immune system. Antigen-presenting cells also release cytokines that induce T cells to differentiate into Th1 cells. Th1 cells and APC cytokines work together to stimulate the activity of cytotoxic T cells, natural killer cells, and activated macrophages—the major components of innate immunity. These cytokines also stimulate the synthesis of nitric oxide and other inflammatory mediators that increase chronic delayed-type inflammatory responses. Because of this effect, these cytokines are sometimes referred to as proinflammatory cytokines.

The cytokines secreted by the Th2 cells act to inhibit Th1 cells and can promote adaptive immunity by stimulating the growth and activation of mast cells and eosinophils, as well as the differentiation of B-cell immunoglobulins. Thus, these cytokines are sometimes referred to as anti-inflammatory cytokines[55] (Figure 11-6). Moreover, cytokines can act synergistically, antagonistically, or reciprocally. However, the roles of cytokines are highly complex and much remains unknown. Regardless, the decrease in Th1 activity and increase in Th2 activity is sometimes called a **Th1 to Th2 shift.** Individuals experiencing a Th1 to Th2 shift are more likely to experience allergic responses, infections, and temporary worsening of autoimmune conditions such as arthritis.

The preceding description of the effect of stress hormones on the Th1-Th2 balance may not be accurate for certain local responses.[55,56] It has been documented that the release of catecholamines (epinephrine and norepinephrine) can cause certain epithelial cells of the lung to release cytokines that promote recruitment of leukocytes, potentially enhancing inflammation and worsening lung function. This paradoxical stress-induced potentiation of inflammation in the lungs may explain why "acute respiratory distress syndrome" often develops in individuals with major infections associated with profound activity of the stress response.[57]

Stress hormones, especially glucocorticoids (cortisol), have been used therapeutically as powerful anti-inflammatory/immunosuppressive agents for years. The synthetic forms of glucocorticoid hormones (exogenous types of anti-inflammatory glucocorticoids administered for a pharmaceutical reaction) are poorly metabolized when compared to endogenous glucocorticoids, leading to a longer half-life and no circadian rhythm for these compounds. Moreover, these synthetic compounds bind to different targets, so each has a unique effect.[31] Therapeutic levels of glucocorticoids inhibit the accumulation of leukocytes at the site of inflammation and inhibit the release of substances involved in the inflammatory response (i.e., kinins, plasminogen-activating factor, prostaglandins, and histamine) from the leukocytes. Glucocorticoids inhibit fibroblast proliferation and function at the site of an inflammatory response. This inhibition accounts for the poor wound healing, increased susceptibility to infection, and decreased inflammatory response that often are noted in individuals with chronic glucocorticoid excess.

Paradoxically, elevated levels of glucocorticoids and catecholamines (epinephrine and norepinephrine)—both endogenous and exogenously administered—may decrease innate immunity and increase autoimmune responses. These effects can accentuate inflammation in general and potentially increase neuronal death (e.g., in stroke victims).[31] This may help explain the seemingly contradictory stress response of immunosuppression and increased risk of infection (decreased innate immunity) with a heightened antibody response and autoimmune disease (increased adaptive immunity).

Corticotropin-releasing hormone (CRH) influences the immune system indirectly by the activation of cortisol (glucocorticoids) and catecholamines. CRH is secreted by the hypothalamus and also peripherally at inflammatory sites (called peripheral or immune CRH).[25,55] Peripheral (immune) CRH is proinflammatory, causing an increase in vasodilation and vascular permeability.[58] Therefore, it appears that mast cells are the target of peripheral CRH. Mast cells release histamine, which is a well-known mediator of acute inflammation and allergic reactions (see Figure 11-6). Recent evidence has indicated that immune cells may have histamine receptors and that

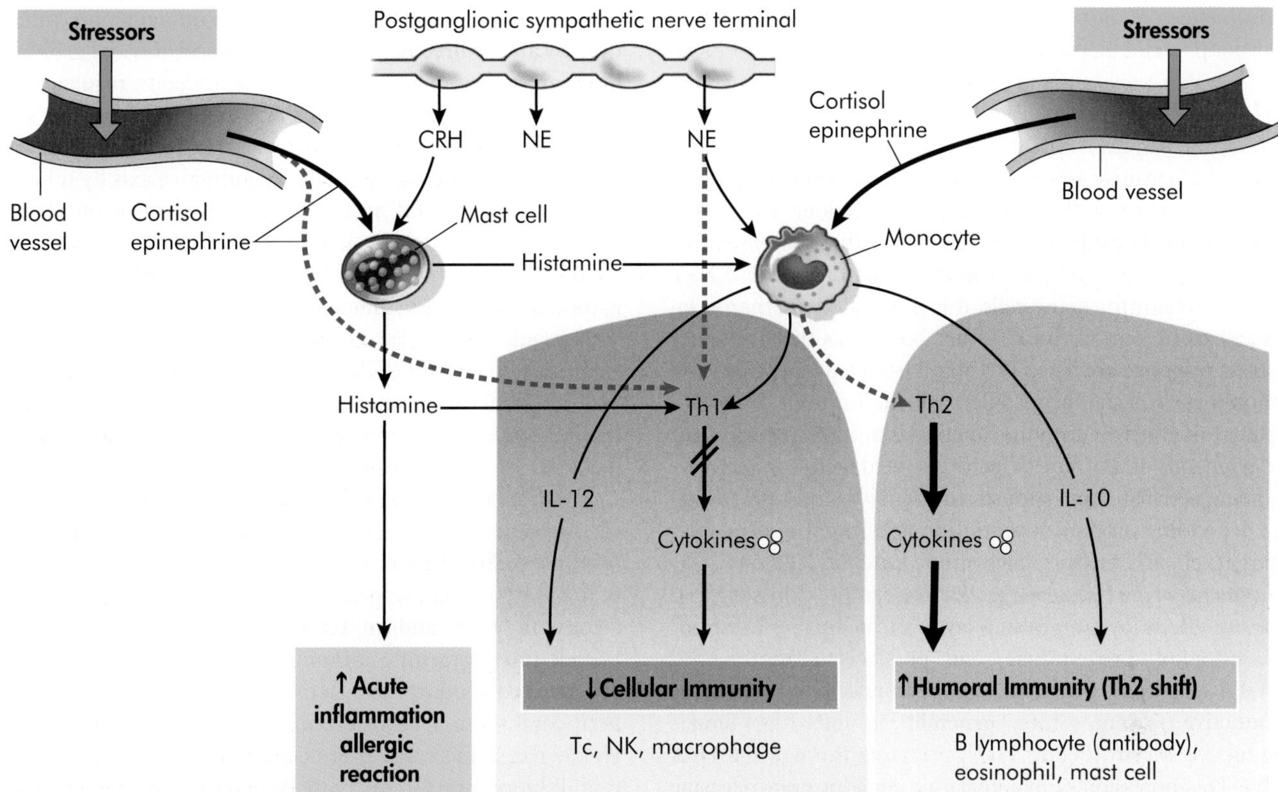

FIGURE 11-6 Effect of Corticotropin-Releasing Hormone (CRH)—Mast Cell—Histamine Axis, Cortisol, and Catecholamines on the Th1/Th2 Balance—Innate and Adaptive Immunity. Adaptive immunity provides protection against multicellular parasites, extracellular bacteria, some viruses, soluble toxins, and allergens. Innate immunity provides protection against intracellular bacteria, fungi, protozoa, and several viruses. Type 1 cytokines or proinflammatory cytokines include IL-12, interferon-gamma (IFN-γ), and tumor necrosis factor-alpha (TNF-α). Type 2 cytokines or anti-inflammatory cytokines include IL-10 and IL-4. Solid lines *(black)* represent stimulation, whereas dashed lines *(blue)* represent inhibition (i.e., Th1 and Th2 are mutually inhibitory, IL-12 and IFN-γ inhibit Th2, and vice versa; IL-4 and IL-10 inhibit Th1 responses). Stress and CRH modulate inflammatory/immune and allergic responses by stimulating cortisol (glucocorticoid), catecholamines, and peripheral (immune) CRH secretion and by changing the production of regulatory cytokines and histamines. *CRH* (peripheral, immune), Corticotropin-releasing hormone; *IL,* interleukin; *NE,* norepinephrine; *NK,* natural killer cell; *Tc,* cytotoxic T cell; *Th,* helper T cell; *dashed lines,* decreased (inhibited); *solid lines,* increased (stimulation). (Redrawn from Elenkov IJ, Chrousos GP: *Trends Endocrinol Metab* 10[9]:359–368, 1999.)

histamine may have an effect similar to catecholamines. This finding suggests that histamine induces acute inflammation and allergic reactions while suppressing Th1 activity (decreasing innate immunity) and promoting Th2 activity (increasing adaptive immunity).[57-59] A number of stress factors initiate CRH production, including high levels of interleukin-1 (IL-1) and IL-6. Increased CRH secretion results in an increase in cortisol secretion. Cortisol in turn inhibits further cytokine release by macrophages and monocytes. The observation that IL-1 can elicit changes in the nervous and endocrine systems by stimulating CRH production in the hypothalamus is part of a growing body of evidence demonstrating immune-induced regulation of the CNS. The release of the immune inflammatory mediators IL-6, tumor necrosis factor-alpha (TNF-α), and interferon is triggered by bacterial or viral infections, cancer, and tissue injury that in turn initiate a stress response through the HPA pathway. Enhanced systemic production of these cytokines also induces other CNS and behavior changes seen frequently during the acute phase of an infectious episode, acting either directly in a distant, systemic "endocrine" way or indirectly through the mediation of neuropeptides. These effects include pyrogenesis (fever), induction of slow-wave sleep, and anorexia, all of which are adaptive responses to infection and possibly cancer. Slow-wave sleep is associated with enhanced release of growth hormone (GH) and a reduction in levels of cortisol, which is beneficial for tissue repair and enhanced immune response.

In summary, stress can activate an excessive immune response and, through cortisol and catecholamines, suppress the Th1 response, causing a Th1 to Th2 shift. Locally, stress can exert proinflammatory or anti-inflammatory effects depending on the chemicals that are released in the local environment and the way that the cells of the local environment respond to those chemicals. Moreover, different types of stressors may have variable effects on the immune response. Thus *systemic responses to stress* may cause a decrease in innate immunity and enhance adaptive immunity, whereas *local responses to stress,* under certain conditions, can induce proinflammatory activities that may influence the onset and cause of infectious, autoimmune/inflammatory, allergic, and neoplastic diseases.

Other Hormones

The immune system is integrated with other physiologic processes and is sensitive to changes in CNS and endocrine functioning, such as those that accompany psychologic states. For example, **neuropeptide Y (NPY),** a sympathetic neurotransmitter, has been shown to be a stress mediator. Because NPY is a growth factor for many cells, it is implicated in atherosclerosis and tissue remodeling.[49] Other hormones that influence the stress response are listed in Table 11-5. Neuropeptides and hormones have a significant effect on the immune response. Whether this effect on immune function is suppressive or potentiating depends on the type of factor secreted, with some factors enhancing activity, some suppressing activity, and some doing both, depending on the concentration and length of exposure, the target cell, and the specific immune function studied.

Hormones of the Female Reproductive System. Cortisol exerts inhibiting effects by suppressing levels of luteinizing hormone (LH), estradiol, progesterone, and possibly testosterone.[60,61] The HPA axis exerts powerful, multilevel effects on the female reproductive system. Stress generally inhibits the female reproductive system (Figure 11-7), primarily through the HPA axis by (1) suppression of hypothalamic gonadotropin-releasing hormone (GnRH) secretion by CRH and CRH stimulation of β-endorphin release; (2) inhibition of GnRH, pituitary LH, and ovarian estradiol (E_2) secretion by cortisol; and (3) cortisol-induced target tissue resistance by estradiol.[62,63] The locus ceruleus–norepinephrine (LC/NE) system provides positive input to the reproductive system, which is frequently altered by the stress-activated HPA axis. Sexual stimulation and GnRH neuron activation, however, may cause the gonadal axis to be resistant to suppression by the HPA axis. Through estradiol, the reproductive system provides positive input to both components of the stress system by stimulating CRH secretion and inhibiting reuptake and catabolism of catecholamines. Table 11-6 presents potential pathologic effects of central and peripheral CRH in women.

Estrogen stimulates the HPA axis. In addition, HPA axis responsiveness is greater in women than that in men.[63] Estrogen directly stimulates the CRH gene promoter and the central noradrenergic (norepinephrine) system, which may help explain adult women's slight hypercortisolism, increases in affective anxiety and eating disorders, mood cycles, and vulnerability to autoimmune and inflammatory disease, all of which follow estradiol concentration fluctuations. Estradiol down-regulates glucocorticoid receptor binding in the anterior pituitary, hypothalamus, and hippocampus—this tends to *increase* HPA activity by interfering with glucocorticoid-negative feedback, whereas progesterone opposes these effects.[64] Thus alterations in estradiol levels during normal menses, perimenopause (including increases as well as decreases), and menopause alter the regulatory feedback loop, and adaptations over time develop as a new equilibrium is established in the relationship (see Figure 11-7). Over time, these changes increase the incidence of mood alterations, eating disorders, anxiety, depression, weight alterations, and inflammatory and immune disorders.

The adipocyte-derived peptide hormone leptin interacts directly and indirectly with the adrenal and gonadal axes; leptin levels are higher in women than in men. Leptin regulates appetite (satiety) and energy balance. It also inhibits the HPA axis at both hypothalamic and adrenocortical levels. In addition, leptin positively influences the female reproductive axis by inhibition of the HPA axis and arcuate proopiomelanocortin (POMC) neuronal system and through activation of the LC/NE system. By promoting satiety and sympathetic system outflow, leptin is thought to provide the peripheral signal to a central mechanism regulating the size of body fat stores.[65] Thus leptin may be significant in control of the onset of puberty because of its relationship to the amount of fat mass, in the adaptive activation of the HPA axis, and in inhibition of gonadal function that takes place in cases of starvation and anorexia nervosa.[66-68]

Endorphins and Enkephalins. Endorphins and enkephalins (endogenous opiates) are released into the blood as part of the response to stressful stimuli. They are proteins found in the brain that have pain-relieving capabilities. Stressful stimuli include traumatic injury and an acute, intense stress situation, such as first-time parachute jumping. In inflamed tissue, immune cell–derived endorphins activate endorphin receptors on peripheral sensory nerves, leading to pain relief or analgesia.[69] Hemorrhage increases β-endorphin levels, which appear to inhibit blood pressure increase or delay compensatory changes that would increase blood pressure.[70] Thus endogenous opiates modulate blood pressure instability and neuroendocrine and cytokine responses to blood losses.[71,72]

In a number of conditions or activities in which endogenous opiate activity is increased, subjects not only experience insensitivity to pain but also report increased feelings of excitement, positive well-being, or euphoria. In addition, cells of the immune system synthesize and release opioids when the lymphoid cells are activated.[73] T and B lymphocytes and mononuclear phagocytic cells have receptors for opioids. Endorphins may play a role in the excitement and exhilaration produced by dancing, contact sports, and combat. There is little direct evidence, however, documenting the endorphin system in most of these activities.

Growth Hormone (Somatotropin). Growth hormone (GH) is released from the anterior pituitary gland and is produced by lymphocytes and mononuclear phagocytic cells.[74] GH affects protein, lipid, and carbohydrate metabolism and counters the effects of insulin. It is involved in tissue repair and may participate in the growth and function of the immune system. Receptors for GH are present on lymphoid cells.[75] This finding suggests a role for GH in regulating phagocytic function and possibly antigen presentation. GH levels increase in the blood after a variety of acutely stressful stimuli, such as cardiac catheterization, electroshock therapy, gastroscopy, surgery, fever, and physical exercise. Psychologic stimuli associated with increased levels of GH include taking examinations, viewing violent or sexually arousing films, anticipating exhausting exercise, and performing certain psychologic tests. However, prolonged activation of the stress response (chronic stress) leads to suppression of GH and other growth factor effects on target tissues.[76] (This is not to be confused with a congenital

TABLE 11-5 OTHER HORMONES THAT INFLUENCE THE STRESS RESPONSE

HORMONE	SOURCE	ACTION
β-Endorphins (endogenous opiates)	Pituitary and hypothalamus	Activates endorphin (opiate) receptors on peripheral sensory nerves, leading to pain relief or analgesia Hemorrhage increases levels to inhibit blood pressure or delay compensatory changes that would increase blood pressure[1]
Growth hormone (GH, somatotropin)	Anterior pituitary gland	Affects protein, lipid, and carbohydrate metabolism Counters effects of insulin Involved in tissue repair May participate in growth and function of immune system[2] Levels increase after a variety of stressful stimuli (cardiac catheterization, electroshock therapy, gastroscopy, surgery, fever, physical exercise) Increased levels associated with psychologic stimuli (taking examinations, viewing violent or sexually arousing films, certain psychologic performance tests) Prolonged stress (chronic stress) suppresses growth hormone
Prolactin	Anterior pituitary gland; numerous extrapituitary tissue sites	Increases in response to many stressful stimuli (including procedures such as gastroscopy, proctoscopy, pelvic examination, and surgery)[3] Requires more intense stimuli than those leading to increases in catecholamine or cortisol levels Levels show little change after exercise
Oxytocin	Hypothalamus	Promotes bonding and social attachment In animals associated with reduced hypothalamic-pituitary-adrenal (HPA) activation levels and reduced anxiety[4]
Testosterone	Leydig cells in testes	Regulates male secondary sex characteristics and libido Levels decrease after stressful stimuli (anesthesia, surgery, marathon running, mountain climbing)[5] Decreased by psychologic stimuli; however, some data indicate that psychologic stress associated with competition (e.g., pistol shooting) increases both testosterone and cortisol levels, especially in athletes older than 45 years[6] Markedly reduced in individuals with respiratory failure, burns, and congestive heart failure[7] Decreased levels occur during aging and are associated with a lower cortisol responsiveness to stress-induced inflammation[8]
Estrogen	Ovaries	Works in concert with oxytocin, exerting a calming effect during stressful situations[9]
Melatonin	Produced by pineal gland	Increases during stress response; release is suppressed by light and increased in the dark; receptors have been identified on lymphoid cells, possibly higher density of receptors on T cells than B cells; suppression of lymphocyte function by trauma was reversed by melatonin[10]
Somatostatin (SOM)	Produced by sensory nerve terminals found in and released from lymphoid cells and hypothalamus	Natural killer (NK) function and immunoglobulin synthesis are decreased by SOM; growth hormone secretion decreased by SOM
Vasoactive intestinal peptide (VIP)	Found in neurons of central nervous system (CNS) and in peripheral nerves	VIP increases during stress; VIP-containing nerves are located in both primary and secondary lymphoid tissues, around blood vessels, and in gastrointestinal tract; VIP receptors are on both T and B cells; VIP may influence lymphocyte maturation; cytokine production by T cells is modified by VIP; B cells and antibody production are influenced by VIP
Calcitonin gene–related peptide (CGRP)	Found in spinal cord motor neurons and in sensory neurons near dendritic cells of skin and in primary and secondary lymphoid tissues	CGRP receptors are present on T and B lymphocytes; thus it is likely that CGRP can modulate immune function; CGRP may enhance acute inflammatory response because it is a vasodilator; maturation of immune B lymphocytes is inhibited by CGRP; IL-1 is inhibited by CGRP, which is important for activation of T cells; it has been shown to interfere with lymphocyte activation
Neuropeptide Y (NPY)	Present in neurons of CNS and in neurons throughout body; co-localized in nerve terminals in lymphatic tissues with norepinephrine	Lymphocytes have receptors for NPY and thus may modulate their function;[11] several lines of evidence suggest that NPY is a neurotransmitter and neurohormone involved in stress response; increased levels of NPY occur in plasma in response to severe or prolonged stress; it may be responsible for stress-induced regional vasoconstriction (splanchnic, coronary, and cerebral); it may also increase platelet aggregation[2]
Substance P (SP)	Produced by a neuropeptide classified as tachykinin (increases heart rate subsequent to lowering blood pressure) found in brain, as well as nerves innervating secondary lymphoid tissues	SP increases in response to stress; receptors for SP are found on membranes of both T and B cells, mononuclear phagocytic cells, and mast cells; proinflammatory activity induces release of histamine from mast cells during stress response; causes smooth muscle contraction, causes macrophages and T cells to release cytokines, and increases antibody production

References

1. Amico JA et al: *J Neuroendocrinol* 16(4):319–324, 2004.
2. Rabin BS: The nervous system—immune system connection. In *Stress, immune function, and health: the connection,* New York, 1999, Wiley-Liss.
3. Rohleder N et al: *J Neuroimmunol* 126(1-2):69–77, 2002.
4. Marucha PT, Kiecolt-Glaser JK, Favagehi M: *Psychosom Med* 60(3):362–365, 1998.
5. Chesnokova V, Melmed S: *Endocrinology* 143(5):1571–1574, 2002.
6. Guezennec CY et al: *Int J Sports Med* 16(6):368–372, 1995.
7. Bauer-Wu SM: *Clin J Oncol Nurs* 6(3):167–170, 2002.
8. Bauer-Wu SM: *Clin J Oncol Nurs* 6(4):243–246, 2002.
9. Repka-Ramirez MS, Baraniuk JN: *Clin Allergy Immunol* 17:1–17, 2002.
10. Maestroni GJ: *Adv Exp Med Biol* 460:396, 1999.
11. Petito JM, Huang Z, McCarthy DB: *J Neuroimmunol* 54:81, 1994.

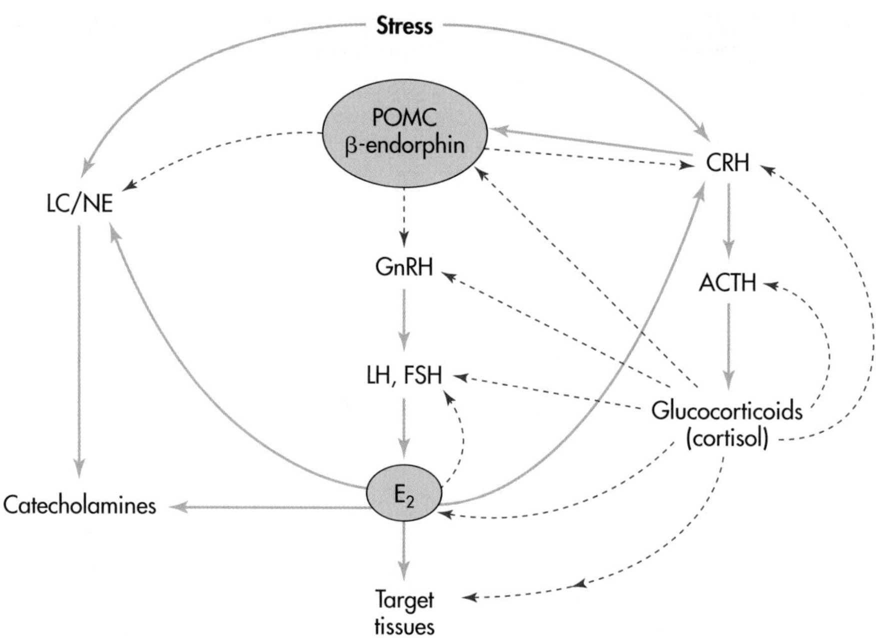

FIGURE 11-7 Stress and the Female Reproductive System. Interactions of the reproductive system with the hypothalamic-pituitary-adrenal (HPA) axis and locus ceruleus–norepinephrine system (LC/NE). Corticotropic cells of the pituitary gland express proopiomelanocortin (POMC) peptides. Stress generally inhibits the female reproductive system primarily through the HPA by (1) suppressing hypothalamic gonadotropin-releasing hormone (GnRH) secretion by corticotropin-releasing hormone (CRH) and CRH-induced β-endorphins; (2) inhibiting GnRH, pituitary luteinizing hormone (LH), and ovarian estradiol (E_2) secretion by cortisol; and (3) enhancing cortisol-induced target tissue resistance to estradiol. The LC/NE system provides positive input to the reproductive system, which can be overridden by the stress-activated HPA. Estradiol can cause the reproductive system to stimulate the stress system by stimulating CRH secretion and inhibiting reuptake and catabolism of catecholamines. *ACTH,* Adrenocorticotropic hormone; *FSH,* follicle-stimulating hormone. Dashed lines refer to inhibitory pathways. Solid lines refer to direct stimulatory pathways. (Adapted from Chrousos GP et al: *Ann Intern Med* 129[3]:229–240, 1998.)

GH deficiency, which leads to short stature, decreased muscular strength, and bone density pathology.) When under stress, chronic glucocorticoid stimulation decreases the release of GH from the pituitary gland, resulting in potentially decreased skeletal muscle, increased bone catabolism, reduced oxygen uptake, increased fat production, worsening sleep patterns, decreased force of cardiac contractions, decreased thyroid function, and poorer mood state. In other words, glucocorticoids antagonize the beneficial actions of GH.[77]

Prolactin. Prolactin is released from the anterior pituitary gland as well as numerous extrapituitary tissue sites. It is necessary for lactation and breast development. Prolactin receptors are present in many different tissues, including the liver, kidney, intestine, and adrenals. Prolactin is also produced by lymphoid cells.[78] Prolactin levels in plasma increase as a result of a variety of stressful stimuli, including gastroscopy, proctoscopy, pelvic examination, and surgery. The level of prolactin also rises during parachute jumping, during motion sickness, after taking examinations, and after receiving various sexual stimuli, for example, stimulation of the nipple or areola in women. Unlike GH, prolactin levels show little change after exercise. Like GH, however, a prolactin level increase appears to require more intense stimuli than those leading to increases in catecholamine or cortisol levels. Immune cells also are influenced by prolactin. Prolactin acts as a second messenger for IL-2 and is known to have a positive influence on B-cell activation and differentiation. Several classes of lymphocytes have receptors for prolactin, suggesting a direct effect of prolactin on immune function.

Oxytocin. Oxytocin is well known as a hormone produced in high levels by the hypothalamus during childbirth and lactation. It is also produced during orgasm in both sexes and has been shown to promote bonding and social attachment. Oxytocin also has antistress properties, as has been shown in animal experiments in which elevations in endogenous oxytocin level were associated with reduced HPA activation levels and reduced anxiety.[79] Oxytocin in some tissues works in concert with estrogen; these two hormones have a calming effect during stressful situations.[80] In contrast, another hormone closely resembling oxytocin, vasopressin, acts in concert with testosterone to increase blood pressure and heart rate, thus enhancing the “fight or flight” stress response. Thus different effects of stress on males and females may be explained, in part, by gender-related hormonal profiles that dictate to some extent the characteristics, quality, and outcomes of the stress response.

Testosterone. Testosterone, a hormone secreted by Leydig cells, regulates male secondary sex characteristics and libido. Testosterone levels decrease after stressful stimuli. This decrease in testosterone level occurs after stimuli such as ether or anesthetic administration, surgery, marathon running,

TABLE 11-6 **POTENTIAL PATHOLOGIC EFFECTS OF CENTRAL AND PERIPHERAL CORTICOTROPIN-RELEASING HORMONE (CRH) IN WOMEN**

CHANGES	ALTERATIONS
Central CRH	
Increased secretion	Hypercortisolism
	Melancholic depression
	Eating disorders
	Chronic active alcoholism
	Chronic active exercise
	Consequences: osteoporosis, visceral obesity, infertility
	Tau protein misfolding-Alzheimer disease?*
Decreased secretion	Atypical depression
	Seasonal affective disorder
	Chronic fatigue and fibromyalgia syndromes
	Rheumatoid arthritis
	Postpartum blues, depression, and autoimmunity
	Premenstrual tension syndrome
	Menopausal depression
Peripheral CRH	
Increased secretion of immune CRH	Inflammatory disorders
Increased secretion of placental CRH	Premature labor
Decreased secretion of placental CRH	Delayed labor
Decreased secretion of ovarian CRH	Ovarian dysfunction
	Anovulation
	Defective corpus luteum function
Increased secretion of ovarian CRH	Early menopause
Decreased secretion of endometrial CRH	Infertility
	Early spontaneous abortion

Data from Chrousos GP et al: *Ann Intern Med* 129(3):229–240; Kalantaridou SN et al: *J Reprod Immunol* 62(1-2):61–68, 2004.
*New line of investigation: Filipcik P et al: *Cell Mol Neurobiol* 32(5): 837–845, 2012.

and mountain climbing. The mechanism causing decreased levels of testosterone is thought to be exerted by cortisol and β-endorphin.

Psychologic stimuli also lead to a decrease in testosterone levels. Men engaged in rigorous combat training and those engaged in the first several weeks of officer candidate school experience significant drops in testosterone levels.[81,82] However, other data have shown that the psychologic stress associated with some types of competition (e.g., pistol shooting) *increases* both testosterone and cortisol levels, especially in athletes older than 45 years.[83] Moreover, individuals with acute illness, such as respiratory failure, burns, and congestive heart failure, show a marked reduction in plasma testosterone level.[84]

The direct immunologic effects of sex hormones contribute to the sexual dimorphism seen in the incidence of autoimmune disease[85] and the greater susceptibility to sepsis and mortality in males following injury.[86] Estrogens generally are associated with a depression of T-cell–dependent immune function and an enhancement of B-cell functions, and androgens suppress both T- and B-cell responses.[84] In injury, however, males produce greater amounts of proinflammatory cytokines, a profile that is associated with poor outcome.[87] Additionally, androgens appear to induce a greater degree of immune cell apoptosis following injury, a mechanism that may elicit a greater immunosuppression in injured males vs. females.[88] (A list of other hormones, including melatonin, substance P, neuropeptide Y, calcitonin gene–related peptide, somatostatin, and vasoactive intestinal peptide, is contained in Table 11-5.)

Stress and the Immune System

Many immune-related conditions and diseases are associated with stress. Several conditions with variable pathophysiologic characteristics appear to have a common origin[89,90] relating to chronic inflammatory processes. These conditions include cardiovascular disease, osteoporosis, arthritis, type 2 diabetes mellitus, chronic obstructive pulmonary disease (COPD), other diseases associated with aging, and some cancers; all are characterized by the prolonged presence of proinflammatory cytokines.[89,91] It is important to remember that inflammation is associated with impairment of normal tissue function. Athough inflammation is a normal response and considered beneficial, an excessive inflammatory response can damage tissue. Stress and negative emotions are associated directly with the production of increased levels of proinflammatory cytokines, providing a possible link between stress, immune function, and disease.[92,93] Stress and negative emotions are associated directly with the production of increased levels of proinflammatory cytokines, providing a possible link between stress, immune function, and disease (see What's New? Psychosocial Stress and Progression to Coronary Heart Disease). Research is now focused on the regulatory interactions between the immune system and the nervous and endocrine systems, which may represent mechanistic pathways for stress-associated immune-mediated diseases. The immune, nervous, and endocrine systems communicate through similar pathways using hormones, neurotransmitters, neuropeptides, and immune cell products.[32] The complexity of this system can be daunting. Various components of immune system responses can be affected by neuroendocrine-produced factors involved in the stress reaction. Conversely, immune cell–derived cytokines and other products affect neurocrine and endocrine cells.[94]

The immune, nervous, and endocrine systems communicate through similar pathways involving hormones, neurotransmitters, neuropeptides, and immune cell products. Immune system responses are potentially affected by all known neuroendocrine-produced factors involved in the stress reaction. Conversely, immune cell–derived cytokines and other products have effects on neurocrine and endocrine cells. Several pathways regulate communication among these systems with both direct and indirect patterned effects (Figure 11-8).

The stress response directly influences the immune system through hypothalamic and pituitary peptides and through products of the sympathetic branch of the ANS. These factors include CRH, ACTH, endorphins, substance P, epinephrine, norepinephrine, dopamine, serotonin, histamine, GH,

WHAT'S NEW?

Psychosocial Stress and Progression to Coronary Heart Disease

The link between stress and coronary heart disease was proposed as early as the 1970s; however, it was only recently that evidence and proposed mechanisms for development of the disease were identified. Much work continues to focus on elucidating the interaction between stress and cardiovascular disease.

Studies show that persons with highly reactive personality types and who experience high levels of anxiety with stress are much more likely to progress from prehypertension to hypertension and then to develop cardiac disease, specifically coronary heart disease, than those who have better coping abilities. Further long-term psychologic stress, such as that experienced in a strained marriage or an unhappy work environment, not only was shown to speed the progression of hypertension and coronary heart disease but also is correlated with higher mortality rates from coronary heart disease.

Trait anger, defined as a stable personality trait characterized by frequency, intensity, and duration of anger, also was shown to be a factor in the development of coronary heart disease at higher rates than in the general population. Individuals with trait anger also experienced more strokes. Hostile individuals with advanced cardiovascular disease may be particularly susceptible to stress-induced increases in sympathetic activity and inflammation.

One popular mechanism for the interaction between psychosocial stress and cardiovascular disease suggests that stress triggers an inflammatory response that, over time, increases the chances of developing coronary heart disease. The primary mechanisms proposed are chronically elevated cortisol levels and dysregulation of the circadian rhythm for cortisol release. Further, chronic stress alters hypothalamic-pituitary-adrenal (HPA) function, resulting in an abnormal stress response pattern. This alteration in HPA activity was found in persons with coronary heart disease along with increased levels of inflammatory markers. The elevation in levels of inflammatory markers seen with chronic stress is important because these markers were shown to interact with lipids, specifically low-density lipoprotein (LDL), to increase the production of atherosclerotic plaques.

Because coronary heart disease is one of the major causes of death in industrialized countries, development of successful interventional programs is of high priority. Programs in which dietary changes, exercise, stress management, and positive support systems are implemented continue to show positive results for slowing the progression of heart disease and decreasing the risk factors for disease development. Further, individuals in these programs experience improvement in depression, stress, and overall mental health.

Data from Brydon L et al: *J Psychosom Res* 68(2):109–116, 2010; Chida Y, Steptoe A: *Hypertension* 55:1026–1032, 2010; Davidson KW: *Cleve Clin J Med* 75(Suppl 2):S15–S19, 2008; Richardson S et al: *Am J Cardiol* 110(12):1711–1716, 2012; Shamaei-Tousi A et al: *Cell Stress Chaperones* 12(4):384–392, 2007; Steptoe A, Brydon L: *Neurosci Biobehav Rev* 33:63–70, 2009; Vizza J et al: *J Cardiopulm Rehabil Prev* 27(6):376–383, 2007.

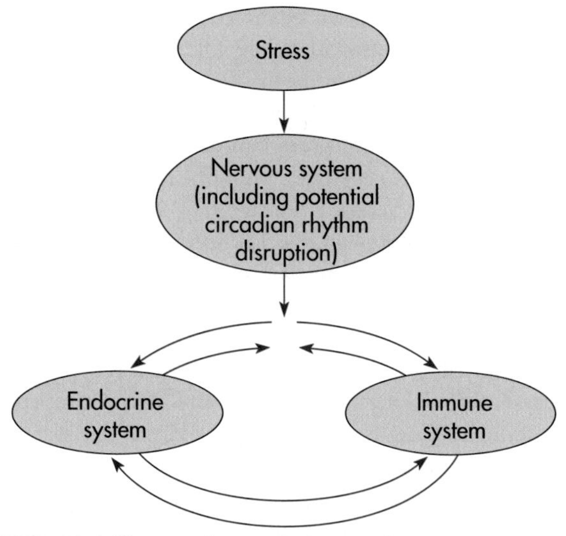

FIGURE 11-8 Nervous System–Endocrine System–Immune System Interactions. Interconnections of pathways of communication among the immune, nervous, and endocrine systems.

vasoactive intestinal polypeptide (VIP), β-endorphin, methionine-enkephalin, leucine-enkephalin, and somatostatin. Direct suppressive effects of CRH have also been reported on two immune cell types possessing CRH receptors—the monocyte/macrophage and CD4 (T helper) lymphocyte.[95] Release of endogenous opiates occurs during stress, and these peptides are known to have concentration-dependent, enhancing or suppressive effects on various immune cells.[96] Immune cells have been shown to have surface receptors for epinephrine, serotonin, ACTH, CRH, endorphins, GH, and prolactin, as well as intracellular steroid receptors.

Products of the sympathetic branch of the ANS also influence immune cell behavior. There is direct innervation of the thymus, spleen, lymph nodes, and bone marrow,[97] and histochemical studies have verified the presence of cholinergic and adrenergic nerve terminals in the lymphoid organs and tissues. There is evidence for the interaction of norepinephrine released from nerve endings with lymphocytes and macrophages in the spleen. This finding implicates the presence of a route of communication between the ANS and immune system through direct delivery of chemical mediators that alter immune cell behavior in a paracrine (cell to adjacent cell) fashion in the microenvironment of the lymphoid organ.

The pineal gland regulates the immune response and mediates the apparent effects of the circadian rhythm on immunity. Blockage of production of melatonin (by continuous light or by pharmacologic means) results in suppression of the immune response, whereas administration of melatonin reverses these effects. This immunomodulation pathway may affect immune changes found with dysregulation of circadian rhythm, a common occurrence among older adults, acutely ill persons, and stressed individuals.[98] Melatonin also modulates seasonal changes in immune function and affects tumor development.[99]

In summary, stress-induced immune changes affect many immune cell functions, including decreased natural killer cell and T-cell cytotoxicity and impaired B-cell function.[11] These impairments in immune function may have health consequences for stressed individuals, including increased risk of infection and some types of cancer.[100,101] The complex and bidirectional communication among systems involves common use of signal molecules and their receptors, which in turn regulates the behavior of cells in each system. Thus the most recent findings are that (1) there are direct effects of CNS neuropeptides on immune cells; (2) stress-induced endocrine products influence immune cell and neurologic cell function; and (3) immune cell products (cytokines) affect nervous and endocrine cell function through direct and indirect pathways.

STRESS, PERSONALITY, COPING, AND ILLNESS

It is not entirely clear why cortisol secretion during stress is beneficial. It has been suggested that gluconeogenesis prompted by cortisol ensures an adequate source of glucose (energy) for body tissues, and nerve cells in particular. The pooling of amino acids from catabolized proteins may ensure amino acid availability for protein synthesis in certain cells. The redistribution of protein to sites where replacement is critical, such as muscle or cells of damaged tissue, would be beneficial. Short-term, cortisol-induced alterations in immune cell distribution (e.g., traffic) patterns may be adaptive, with a decrease in peripheral blood cell numbers as effector cells locate to sites of injury or inflammation. In addition, decreased immune cell activity by cortisol may be beneficial in some situations because it prevents immune-mediated tissue damage by prolonged cell exposure to high levels of certain cytokines. Whether cortisol-induced effects are adaptive or destructive may depend on the intensity, type, and duration of the stressor, and the subsequent concentration and length of cortisol exposure that target cells of the individual experience.

Extreme physiologic stressors, such as severe burn injury, represent a predictable stimulus for the stress responses described previously. A less severe and defined event or situation, however, can be a stressor for one person and not for another. Many stressors, such as fasting or temperature changes, do not necessarily cause a physiologic stress response if psychologic factors are minimized. Stress itself is not an independent entity but a system of interdependent processes that are moderated by the nature, intensity, and duration of the stressor and the perception, appraisal, and coping efficacy of the affected individual, all of which in turn mediate the psychologic and physiologic response to stress. Further, adjustment to repetitive stressors is known to be individualized, based on a person's appraisal of a situation.[102] Illustrating the influence of an individualized stress appraisal on physiologic processes, a meta-analysis of the relationships between stressors and immunity found that a higher *perception* of stress was associated with reduced T-cytotoxic (Tc) cell cytotoxicity although not with levels of circulating Th or Tc lymphocytes.[103]

Psychosocial distress may be predictive of psychologic and physical health outcomes. In **psychologic distress** the individual feels a general state of unpleasant arousal after life events that manifests as physiologic, emotional, cognitive, and behavioral changes. Periods of depression and emotional upheaval often are associated with adverse life events and place the affected individual at risk for immunologic deficits, increasing the risk of ill health.[104] An older meta-analysis of studies demonstrates the longstanding relationship between depression and reduction in lymphocyte proliferation and NK cell activity.[105] Multiple moderating factors may be important in immune modulation in depressed individuals, including comorbidities such as alcoholism. Examples of triggering mechanisms include bereavement, academic and job-related pressures, life events (positive and negative changes), and aging. Adverse life events having the most negative effect on immunity are characterized as uncontrollable, undesirable, and overtaxing the individual's ability to cope.

Studies have strengthened the association of stress with potential for illness in humans (see What's New? Telomeres, Disease, and Childhood Stress). One study examined medical students who were immunized with hepatitis B vaccine on the third day of a stressful examination period; the time to seroconversion and level of antibody titer to the vaccine were measured later. The students with the most rapid seroconversion and the highest titers also reported being less stressed and had a good social support system (which may reduce stress).[106] Even more convincing is a study in which the psychologic stress status was determined in healthy individuals after experimentally controlled exposure to a respiratory tract virus by nasal inoculation. Individuals reporting more stress had an increased incidence of clinical cold and respiratory symptoms compared with subjects reporting less stress, and other infections, including HIV, were shown to be potentially influenced by psychosocial factors.[107-110]

Animal studies have found that stress contributes to the initiation, growth, and metastasis of certain tumors.[111] Studies of mechanisms in humans reveal stress affects important processes in cancer including antiviral responses, deoxyribonucleic acid

WHAT'S NEW?

Telomeres, Disease, and Childhood Stress

Shortening of the tips of chromosomes, or telomeres, is a potential physiologic mechanism linked to stress, cellular aging, and disease mortality. In experimental animal studies, telomere-deficient mice have been used to study telomere loss and shortening and associated tissue atrophy, stem cell depletion, organ system failure, and impaired tissue injury responses. Accumulating evidence reveals telomere damage as a stimulus for age-associated organ damage and disease risk. In humans, an emerging field is the discovery of mechanisms that mediate the effects of childhood stress on late-life disease, morbidity, and mortality. For example, recent evidence from the Environmental-Risk Longitudinal Twin Study found that children who experienced two or more kinds of violence exposure (i.e., maternal domestic violence, frequent bullying victimization, physical maltreatment by an adult) showed significantly more telomere erosion between age 5 at baseline and age 10 at follow-up measurements. This was observed even after adjusting for gender, socioeconomic status, and body mass index. In addition, investigators in 2004 compared telomere lengths in white blood cells of mothers of chronically ill children compared to those from mothers of healthy children. The longer the mother was a care provider for her child, the shorter were her telomeres. For mothers with the most self-reported stress, telomere shortening was equivalent to at least a decade of aging. In addition, a study of 4441 women aged 41 to 80 provided support for an association between adverse experiences during childhood and shorter telomere length in adulthood.

Data from Armanios M, Blackburn EH: *Nat Rev Genet* 13(10):693–704, 2012; Blackburn EH, Epel ES: *Nature* 490(7419):169–171, 2012; Epel ES et al: *Proc Natl Acad Sci U S A* 101(49):17312–17315, 2004; Jaskelioff M et al: *Nature* 469(7328):102–106, 2011; Shalev I et al: *Mol Psychiatry* 2012 Apr 24 [Epub ahead of print]; Surtees PG et al: *J Gerontol A Biol Sci Med Sci* 66(11):1152–1162, 2011.

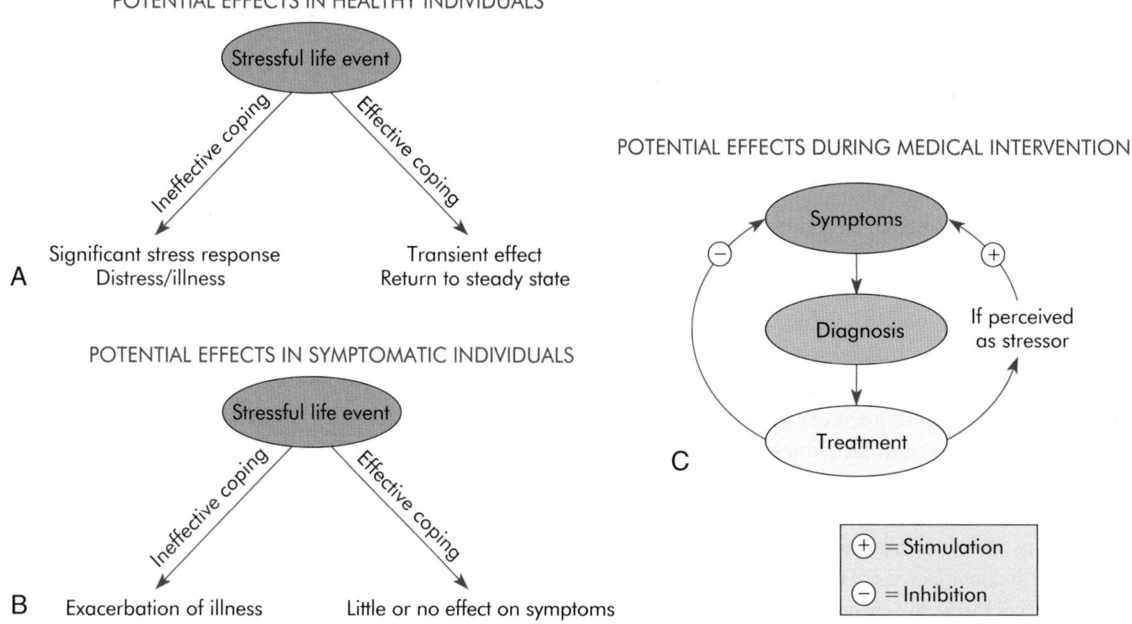

FIGURE 11-9 Health Outcome Determination in Stressful Life Situations Is Moderated by Numerous Factors. Whether an individual experiences distress or illness depends on the subject's appraisal of the event and the coping strategies used during the stressful period. Models **A** and **B** reflect possible outcomes in stressed healthy and symptomatic individuals. Model **C** illustrates the dynamic clinical setting in which the diagnosis of a serious illness and subsequent medical interventions may be perceived as stressful challenges and have potentially detrimental influences on physical outcome.

(DNA) repair, and aspects of cellular aging.[111] The role of epigenetics and stress is a new and developing field with strong implications for the intersection between stress and disease. A very recent study suggests that breast cancer bone metastases may be influenced by chronic stress by increasing the levels of Receptor Activator of Nuclear Factor κB Ligand (RANKL) that are expressed by osteoblasts, a known chemoattractant for RANK-expressing breast cancer cells.[112] However, the overall evidence is mixed from prospective studies linking stress with cancer incidence and progression. Stress may be more likely to influence progression and recurrence of cancer; however, the critical prospective studies have been mostly unsupportive.[12] Studies examining impairments in antiviral immunity and chronic activation of hormonal responses (e.g., HIV-related tumors, hepatocellular carcinoma, and cervical cancer) may be more successful designs for defining the stress-related mechanisms.[111]

Previous and current evidence is showing a relationship between immune stimulation and heart disease.[113] The relationship between stress and cardiovascular health may be mediated by stress-induced changes in immune function, which may potentiate proinflammatory processes and permit alterations that lead to heart disease[114] (see What's New? Acute Emotional Stress and Adverse Heart Effects [p. 342] and What's New? Psychosocial Stress and Progression to Coronary Heart Disease [p. 354]). A new study of heart disease and inflammation demonstrates that monocytes and splenic macrophages invade atherosclerotic plaques after an initial myocardial infarction (heart attack), rendering them unstable and as such contribute to secondary heart attacks.[115]

In the past decade a significant amount of evidence has accumulated linking severe psychosocial stress resulting from negative life events to a chronic syndrome with mental and physical consequences. Posttraumatic stress disorder (PTSD) has been described in many populations.[116-118] A cascade model has been proposed to describe the pathogenesis and clinical course illustrating the clinical, epidemiologic, neurobiologic, and psychosocial components of PTSD.[119] The study of PTSD has contributed to the knowledge concerning mechanisms involved in the chronic stress and disease relationship. Recently an appreciation of the association of chronic stress with high levels of cortisol production and paradoxical biounavailability (i.e., bound to plasma protein and therefore not bioavailable) of cortisol has been gained.[120]

The interaction with healthcare providers in a clinical setting, the diagnosis of a major illness, and the execution of various clinical procedures (e.g., blood draws, injections, examinations, surgical procedures) also may represent significant negative life events to many individuals (Figure 11-9) (for example, mammography and the activation of the HPA axis).

The influence of repetitive but episodic stress on cancer survivors demonstrates a connection between events such as mammography and activation of the HPA axis. Early research with breast cancer survivors by Cordova and colleagues[121] demonstrated a link between sympathetic activity and HPA axis activation, noting that some women reported symptoms of PTSD (heart palpitations, panic, shakiness, nausea) during thoughts of recurrence triggered by events such as finding themselves near the hospital where they received initial treatment.[121] HPA axis activation also influences organs and tissues that enable bidirectional communication processes (feedback loops) between neuroendocrine and immune processes.[94] For example, among breast cancer survivors 3 to 5 years post diagnosis, elevated baseline cortisol levels and blunted cortisol reactivity were reported in response to the anticipation of a real, regularly scheduled mammogram, and alterations in cortisol level and heart rate variability were reported in women simulating the threat of cancer with a controlled laboratory stressor.[122,123] Further, Ma and colleagues[122] reported that the threat of cancer recurrence (using a simulated mammography event as a stressor to elicit thoughts of cancer recurrence) elicited greater alterations in heart rate variability when compared with another simulated controlled stressor. These studies suggest activation of the autonomic nervous system to events, such as mammography, that occur repeatedly throughout breast cancer survivorship, although the timing of onset of these autonomic activation responses to a stressor is unclear. Similar ANS activation may occur in association with events particular to the management of many other types of chronic illnesses as well as interactions with the healthcare system.

These additional stresses may affect the course of illness as well as interfere with the efficacy of the medical intervention. Identifying and reducing stress in the clinical setting have particular applicability in both disease prevention and illness management. In addition to medical procedures, patient-provider communication also provides an important area for future research. Recent studies of cancer communication and patient-provider interaction have demonstrated a link between communication events and emotional outcomes, such as uncertainty and mood state in breast cancer survivors.[124,125] Although a logical extension, it remains to be seen if these emotional outcomes affect physiologically based health outcomes caused by activation of the HPA axis and subsequent immune processes.

Coping

Personality characteristics are associated with individual differences in appraisal and response to stressors.[126] The coping response of individuals may exaggerate or moderate physical consequences of the stress response. **Coping** is defined as the process of managing stressful demands and challenges that are appraised as taxing or exceeding the resources of the person.[127] One response may be a negative change in behavior resulting in potentially adverse health effects (e.g., increased smoking, change in eating habits). Serious disturbances of the sleep-wake cycle are observed in many people under stress and in many clinical settings. Further, sleep disturbances may exacerbate the pathophysiologic status of certain patient populations.[128-130] Investigators have reported that sleep deprivation and circadian disruption, even in young, otherwise healthy individuals, have detrimental influences on respiratory and immune system function. Even partial sleep deprivation was associated with reduced NK cell activity in healthy subjects, and only recently have seriously ill patients been assessed for adequacy and structure of sleep during recovery.[128]

Coping can be considered as adaptive or maladaptive. Adaptive coping strategies, especially those that are problem focused and those that encourage seeking social support, are beneficial during stressful experiences. The extent to which an individual responds to distress, using effective positive coping strategies, determines the degree of successful moderation of the stress challenge. Conversely, ineffective negative coping attempts may exacerbate the effects of distress on health, thus augmenting the potential for illness. Mediating factors that may influence stress susceptibility or resilience include age, socioeconomic status, gender, social support status, personality and lifestyle, self-esteem, genetics, life events, past experiences, and current health status.[131] Evidence suggests that effective intervention may result in greater stress resilience and improved psychologic and physiologic outcomes. In a study of nursing home residents randomly assigned to control or social support intervention groups, improved psychologic measures and immune function (NK cell activity) were observed in the experimental group at 6 weeks.[132] In another study, women with recurrent metastatic breast cancer were given either routine follow-up (routine care) or weekly support group sessions. Survival in the support treatment group was an average of 19 months longer than in the routine care group, suggesting a mediating influence of additional support for these women.[25,133]

The importance of social support for seriously ill individuals has focused attention on the health and well-being of family members who function as caregivers (see What's New? Partner's Survival and Spouse's Hospitalizations and/or Death). Significant stress manifested as depression, anxiety, and fatigue has been noted in family caregivers of those with cancer, Alzheimer disease, and burn trauma.[134] Individuals and caretakers exhibited suppression of various measures of immune function, with improved function associated with better perceived social support.[135-137] Gender-based coping differences may be attributed, in part, to the hormonal milieu of the individual, with females more likely to offer social support, a behavior with an oxytocin/estrogen association.[73]

WHAT'S NEW?

Partner's Survival and Spouse's Hospitalizations and/or Death

A Harvard study shows that a spouse's chances of dying increase not only when the partner dies but also when that partner becomes seriously ill. The 9-year follow-up study consisted of 518,240 elderly couples. Mortality after the partner's hospitalization varied according to the spouse's diagnosis. For elderly people whose spouse had been hospitalized, the short-term risk of dying approaches that of an elderly person after his or her spouse's death. A wife's hospitalization increased her husband's chances of dying within 1 month by 35%; a husband's hospitalization increased his wife's chances of dying by 44%. Likewise, a wife's death increased her partner's 1-month mortality risk by 53%, and a husband's death raised his partner's risk by 61%. The researchers commented that a spouse's illness or death can increase a partner's mortality by causing severe stress and removing a primary source of emotional, psychologic, practical, and financial support.

From a recent review, longitudinal studies put the long-term excess risk of death associated with widowhood compared to marriage at about 15%, and estimates of short-term effects during the first few months immediately post-bereavement range from 50% to 90%. However, there is substantial heterogeneity in the magnitude of effects reported in different studies.

Data from Christakis NA, Allison PD: *N Engl J Med* 354(7):719–730, 2006; Moon JR et al: *PLoS One* 6(8):e23465, 2011.

Interventions to prevent or manage stress-related psychologic or physical problems include both short- and long-term coping strategies. Stress management consists of educational components specific to the individual's problems and relaxation techniques, which may include meditation, imagery, massage, and biofeedback. These approaches may be used on an individual or a support group basis. Incorporation of these approaches into clinical training facilitates their use in the clinical arena. Research should focus on the efficacy of such approaches with various populations.

AGING AND STRESS: STRESS-AGE SYNDROME

A set of neurohormonal and immune alterations, as well as tissue and cellular changes, sometimes develops with aging. These changes, which recently have been defined as stress-age syndrome, include the following:[131,138]

- Alterations in the excitability of structures of the limbic system and hypothalamus
- Increase of the blood concentrations of catecholamines, antidiuretic hormone (ADH), ACTH, and cortisol
- Decrease of the concentrations of testosterone, thyroxine, and others
- Alterations of opioid peptide concentration
- Immunodepression and pattern of chronic inflammation
- Alterations in lipoproteins
- Hypercoagulation of the blood
- Free radical damage of cells

Some of the alterations are adaptational, whereas others are potentially damaging. These stress-related alterations of aging can influence the course of developing stress reactions and lower adaptive reserve and coping.[139]

Interventions to potentially prevent or manage stress-related psychologic or physical problems include both short- and long-term coping strategies. Educational components are specific to the individual's problems. Relaxation techniques may include meditation, mindfulness, imagery, massage, yoga, and biofeedback. These approaches may be used on an individual or group basis. Incorporation of these approaches into clinical training facilitates their use in the clinical arena. Future research should focus on the efficacy of such approaches with various populations.

In summary, it is clear that the mind and body are connected through a multitude of complex physical and emotional interactions. Understanding the complexity of these interactions is a challenge for many researchers. Areas of promise include investigating relationships between the potential for illness with respect to stressors, as well as developing effective stress management techniques and approaches that can be easily and cost-effectively employed.

SUMMARY REVIEW

Historical Background and General Concepts

1. Modern society is full of stress.
2. In general, a person experiences stress when a demand exceeds a person's coping abilities.
3. Hans Selye identified three structural changes in rats subjected repeatedly to noxious stimuli (stressors): enlargement of the cortex of the adrenal gland, atrophy of the thymus gland and other lymphoid tissues, and ulceration of the gastrointestinal tract.
4. Selye believed that the three changes were caused by a nonspecific physiologic response to any long-term stressor. He called this response the general adaptation syndrome (GAS).
5. The GAS occurs in three stages: the alarm stage, the stage of resistance or adaptation, and the stage of exhaustion. Diseases of adaptation develop if the stage of resistance or adaptation does not restore homeostasis.
6. Selye identified three components of physiologic stress: the stressor, the physiologic or chemical disturbance produced by the stressor, and the body's adaptational response to the stressor.
7. We now know that, while important, the physiologic view of stress as outlined in the GAS is an oversimplified model of stress responses. We currently view the stress response as the product of the interaction of the mind and body.

Concepts of Stress

1. Psychologic stress may cause or exacerbate (worsen) several disease states. Stress is related to the severity of symptoms and the outcomes of diseases and conditions. Research is focused on the mechanisms responsible for these mind-body interactions.
2. Stress has been defined as the state of affairs arising when a person relates to (i.e., interacts or transacts with) situations in a certain way. The way a person appraises and reacts to situations has a profound impact on stress.
3. The nonspecific physiologic response consists of interaction among the sympathetic branch of the autonomic nervous system (ANS) and other neural signals that activate the endocrine system, known as the HPA axis.
4. The nonspecific physiologic response is a common residual response and can be elicited with diverse agents such as cold, heat, x-rays, adrenaline, insulin, tubercle bacilli, and muscular exercise. Although the reactions of these stages are nonspecific, evidence supports the coexistence of highly specific, adaptive reactions to any of these agents.
5. As with a physically mediated stress response, psychologic stressors can elicit a reactive stress response; that is, a physiologic response can be derived from psychologic stressors.
6. Another type of psychologic-mediated stress response is the anticipatory response.
7. In a conditioned response, the organism learns that specific stimuli are associated with danger and anticipation of subsequent encounters with that particular stimulus produces a physiologic stress response (e.g., PTSD).
8. Psychoneuroimmunology (PNI) is the study of the interaction of consciousness *(psycho)*, the brain and spinal cord *(neuro)*, and the body's defense against external infection and abnormal cell division *(immunology)*.

SUMMARY REVIEW—cont'd

9. Psychoneuroimmunology assumes that all immune-related disease is multifactorial. The immune system is integrated with other physiologic processes and is sensitive to changes in CNS and endocrine functioning, such as those that accompany psychologic states.
10. CRH is released centrally from the brain and peripherally at inflammatory sites.

Stress Response

1. The stress response is initiated by the CNS and endocrine system. Where the stress response begins depends on whether the stressor is perceived or real.
2. Perceived stressors elicit an anticipatory response that usually begins in the limbic system of the brain. The limbic system elicits an endocrine stress response indirectly by stimulating neural pathways responsible for receiving sensory information and elicits a central response directly by stimulating the LC to release LC/NE.
3. Real stressors elicit a reactive response that can begin either in the limbic system or in the brain in response to specific sensory information. This information is then relayed to the PVN. The PVN stimulates the LC and both central and endocrine stress responses.
4. The neuroendocrine response to stress consists of sympathetic stimulation of the adrenal medulla to secrete catecholamines (norepinephrine and epinephrine) and stressor-induced stimulation of the hypothalamus to secrete CRH, which in turn stimulates the pituitary to secrete ACTH, which then stimulates the adrenal cortex to secrete steroid hormones, particularly cortisol.
5. In general, the catecholamines prepare the body to act, and cortisol mobilizes energy stores (e.g., glucose) and other substances needed to fuel the action.
6. Epinephrine exerts its chief effects on the cardiovascular system. Epinephrine increases cardiac output and increases blood flow to the heart, brain, and skeletal muscles by dilating vessels that supply these organs. It also dilates the airways, thereby increasing delivery of oxygen to the bloodstream.
7. Norepinephrine's chief effects complement those of epinephrine. Norepinephrine constricts blood vessels of the viscera and skin; this has the effect of shifting blood flow to the vessels dilated by epinephrine. Norepinephrine also increases mental alertness.
8. CRH influences the immune system indirectly by the activation of glucocorticoids (cortisol) and catecholamines. Peripheral CRH is proinflammatory, causing vasodilation and vascular permeability. It appears that the mast cells are the target of peripheral CRH.
9. Cortisol's chief effects involve metabolic processes. By inhibiting the use of metabolic substances while promoting their formation, cortisol mobilizes glucose, amino acids, lipids, and fatty acids and delivers them to the bloodstream. Cortisol's effect on the immune system is concentration and location dependent and may include either stimulation or inhibition of the immune system.
10. The nervous, endocrine, and immune systems communicate through the common use of signal molecules and their receptors, which in turn regulate the behavior of cells in each system during stress challenge.
11. There are direct and indirect pathways of influence among the nervous, endocrine, and immune systems. Neuropeptides have direct effects on immune cells, as well as indirect influences through neuromediated endocrine modulation of immune function. Endocrine products (cortisol) also influence nerve cell behavior. Immune cell products affect both nerve and endocrine cell function, reflecting an adaptive role for the immune system as a "signal" organ to alert other systems of threatening stimuli.
12. Other hormones are affected by the stress response and include increased circulating levels of β-endorphins, growth hormone, and prolactin and a decrease in antidiuretic hormone level with extreme stress. Concentrations of luteinizing hormone, estradiol, progesterone, and possibly testosterone decrease during the stress response.

Stress, Personality, Coping, and Illness

1. Stress is a system of interdependent processes that are moderated by the nature, intensity, and duration of the stressor and the coping efficacy of the affected individual, all of which in turn mediate the psychologic and physiologic response to stress.
2. Many studies have linked psychologic distress with altered immune function, and evidence strengthens the association of stress with potential for illness in humans.
3. Adaptive coping strategies, especially those that are problem focused and those that encourage seeking social support, are beneficial during stressful experiences.

Aging and Stress: Stress-Age Syndrome

1. With aging, sometimes a set of neurohormonal and immune alterations develop; these changes have been defined recently as stress-age syndrome.
2. These stress-related alterations of aging can influence the course of developing stress reactions and lower adaptive reserve and coping.

KEY TERMS

Adrenocorticotropic hormone (ACTH), 339
Allostasis, 344
Allostatic load, 344
Allostatic overload, 344
Anticipatory response, 341
Conditional response, 341
Coping, 357
Corticosteroid-binding globulin, 346
Corticotropin-releasing hormone (CRH), 339, 343
General adaptation syndrome (GAS), 339
Homeostasis, 341
Hypothalamic-pituitary-adrenal (HPA) axis, 339
Neuropeptide Y (NPY), 350
Peripheral (immune) CRH, 348
Posttraumatic stress disorder (PTSD), 341
Psychologic distress, 355
Psychoneuroimmunology (PNI), 342
Reactive response, 339
Stress, 339
Stress response, 343
Th1 to Th2 shift, 348
Transcortin, 346

REFERENCES

1. Dhabhar FS, McEwen BS: Enhancing versus suppressive effects of stress hormones on skin immune function, *Proc Natl Acad Sci U S A* 96(3):1059–1064, 1999.
2. Cannon WB, Bringer CAL, Fritz R: Experimental hyperthyroidism, *Am J Physiol* 36:363, 1914.
3. Selye H: The general adaptation syndrome and the diseases of adaptation, *J Clin Endocrinol* 6:117–230, 1946.
4. Hill SR et al: Studies on adrenocortical and psychological responses to stress in man, *Arch Intern Med* 97:269, 1956.
5. Mason JW, Brady JV: Plasma 17-hydroxycortico-steroid changes related to reserpine effects on emotional behaviors, *Science* 124:983, 1956.
6. Hetzel BS et al: Changes in urinary 17-hydroxycorticosteroid excretion during stressful life experiences in man, *J Clin Endocrinol Metab* 15(9):1057–1068, 1955.
7. Handlon JH et al: Psychological factors lowering plasma 17-hydroxycorticosteroid concentration, *Psychosom Med* 24:535–541, 1962.
8. Wadeson RW et al: Plasma and urinary 17-OHCS responses to motion pictures, *Arch Gen Psychiatry* 14:146–156, 1963.
9. Mason JW: Organization of psychoendocrine mechanisms: a review and reconsideration of research. In Greenfield NS, Steinbach RA, editors: *Handbook of psychophysiology*, New York, 1972, Holt, Rinehart, & Winston.
10. Herman JP et al: Central mechanisms of stress integration: hierarchical circuitry controlling hypothalamo-pituitary-adrenocortical responsiveness, *Front Neuroendocrinol* 24(3):151–158, 2003.
11. Kiecolt-Glaser JK et al: Psychoneuroimmunology: psychological influences on immune function and health, *J Consult Clin Psychol* 70(3): 537–547, 2002.
12. Vedhara K, Irwin M, editors: *Human pyschoimmunology*, Oxford, England, 2005, Oxford University Press.
13. Pereira DB et al: Stress as a predictor of symptomatic genital herpes virus recurrence in women with human immunodeficiency virus, *J Psychosom Res* 54(3):237–244, 2003.
14. Hamerman D: Toward an understanding of frailty, *Ann Intern Med* 130(11):945–950, 1999.
15. Taaffe DR et al: Cross-sectional and prospective relationships of interleukin-6 and C-reactive protein with physical performance in elderly persons: MacArthur studies of successful aging, *J Gerontol A Biol Sci Med Sci* 55(12):M709–M715, 2000.
16. Black PH, Garbutt LD: Stress, inflammation and cardiovascular disease, *J Psychosom Res* 52(1):1–23, 2002.
17. Bauer-Wu SM: Psychoneuroimmunology. Part I: Physiology, *Clin J Oncol Nurs* 6(3):167–170, 2002.
18. Bauer-Wu SM: Psychoneuroimmunology. Part II: Mind-body interventions, *Clin J Oncol Nurs* 6(4):243–246, 2002.
19. Ranchor AV, Sanderman R, Coyne JC: Invited commentary: personality as a causal factor in cancer risk and mortality—time to retire a hypothesis? *Am J Epidemiol* 172(4):386–388, 2010.
20. Sloan EK et al: The sympathetic nervous system induces a metastatic switch in primary breast cancer, *Cancer Res* 70(18):7042–7052, 2010.
21. McEwen BS: Central effects of stress hormones in health and disease: understanding the protective and damaging effects of stress and stress mediators, *Eur J Pharmacol* 583(2-3):174–185, 2008.
22. Chrousos GP, Kino T: Glucocorticoid signaling in the cell: expanding clinical complications to complex human behavioral and somatic disorders, *Ann N Y Acad Sci* 1179:153–166, 2009.
23. Liu LY et al: School examinations enhance airway inflammation to antigen challenge, *Am J Respir Crit Care Med* 165(8):1062–1067, 2002.
24. Cacioppo JT et al: Autonomic, neuroendocrine, and immune responses to psychological stress: the reactivity hypothesis, *Ann N Y Acad Sci* 840:664–673, 1998.
25. Calcagni E, Elenkov I: Stress system activity, innate and T helper cytokines, and susceptibility to immune-related diseases (review), *Ann N Y Acad Sci* 1069:62–76, 2006.
26. Maier SF, Watkins LR: Cytokines for psychologists: implications of bidirectional immune-to-brain communication for understanding behavior, mood, and cognition, *Psychol Rev* 105(1):83–107, 1998.
27. Charmandari E, Tsigos C, Chrousos G: Endocrinology of the stress response (review), *Annu Rev Physiol* 67:259–284, 2005.
28. Carrillo-Vico A et al: A review of the multiple actions of melatonin on the immune system (review), *Endocrine* 27(2):189–200, 2005.
29. Bruunsgard H, Pedersen BK: Age-related inflammatory cytokines and disease, *Immunol Allergy Clin North Am* 23(1):15–39, 2003.
30. MacPherson A, Dinkel K, Sapolsky R: Glucocorticoids worsen excitoxin-induced expression of proiinflammatory cytokines in hippocampal cultures, *Exp Neurol* 194(2):376–383, 2005.
31. Sorrells SF et al: The stressed CNS: when glucocorticoids aggravate inflammation (review), *Neuron* 64(1):33–39, 2009.
32. Coutinho AE, Chapman KE: The anti-inflammatory and immunosuppressive effects of glucocorticoids, recent developments and mechanistic insights, *Mol Cell Endocrinol* 335(1):2–13, 2010.
33. Thayer JF, Lane RD: A model of neurovisceral integration in emotion regulation and dysregulation, *J Affective Dis* 61:201–216, 2000.
34. McEwen BS: Sleep deprivation as neurobiologic and physiologic stressor, allostasis and allostatic load, *Metabolism* 55:S20–S23, 2006.
35. Alevizaki M et al: High anticipatory stress plasma cortisol levels and sensitivity to glucocorticoids predict severity of coronary artery disease in subjects undergoing coronary angiography, *Metabolism* 56:222–226, 2007.
36. Kajantie E et al: Body size at birth predicts hypothalamic-pituitary-adrenal axis response to psychosocial stress at 60 to 70 years, *J Clin Endocrinol Metab* 92(11):4094–4100, 2007.
37. Elenkov IJ et al: Cytokine dysregulation, inflammation, and well-being, *Neuroimmunomodulation* 12(5):255–269, 2005.
38. Cohen S et al: Types of stressors that increase susceptibility to the common cold in healthy adults, *Health Psychol* 17(3):214–223, 1998.
39. McCain NL et al: A randomized clinical trial of alternative stress management interventions in persons with HIV infection, *J Consult Clin Psychol* 76(3):431–441, 2008.
40. Glaser R et al: Chronic stress modulates the immune response to a pneumococcal pneumonia vaccine, *Psychosom Med* 62(6):804–807, 2000.
41. Marucha PT, Kiecolt-Glaser JK, Favagehi M: Mucosal wound healing is impaired by examination stress, *Psychosom Med* 60(3):362–365, 1998.
42. Pacak K et al: Heterogeneous neurochemical responses to different stressors: a test of Selye's doctrine of nonspecificity, *Am J Physiol* 275 (4 Pt 2):R1247–R1255, 1998.
43. Repka-Ramirez MS, Baraniuk JN: Histamine in health and disease, *Clin Allergy Immunol* 17:1–25, 2002.
44. Russ TC et al: Association between psychological distress and mortality: individual participant pooled analysis of 10 prospective cohort studies, *BMJ* 345:e4933, 2012.
45. Seeman T et al: Socio-economic differentials in peripheral biology: cumulative allostatic load, *Ann N Y Acad Sci* 1186:223–239, 2010.
46. Dimsdale JE, Ziegler MG: What do plasma and urinary measures of catecholamines tell us about human response to stressors? *Circulation* 83(4 Suppl):II36–II42, 1991.
47. Herd JA: Cardiovascular response to stress, *Physiol Rev* 71(1):305–330, 1991.

48. Sapolsky RM, Romero LM, Munck AU: How do glucocorticoids influence stress responses? Integrating permissive, suppressive, stimulatory, and preparative actions, *Endocr Rev* 21(1):55–89, 2000.
49. Rabin BS: The nervous system—immune system connection. In Rabin BS, editor: *Stress, immune function, and health: the connection*, New York, 1999, Wiley-Liss.
50. Moyna NM et al: The effects of incremental submaximal exercise on circulating leukocytes in physically active and sedentary males and females, *Eur J Appl Physiol Occup Physiol* 74(3):211–218, 1996.
51. Kapcala LP et al: The protective role of the hypothalamic-pituitary-adrenal axis against lethality produced by immune, infections, and inflammatory stress, *Ann N Y Acad Sci* 771:419–437, 1995.
52. Drapeau V et al: Is visceral obesity a physiological adaptation to stress? *Panminerva Med* 45(3):189–195, 2003.
53. Rosmond R: Stress induced disturbances of the HPA axis: a pathway to type 2 diabetes? *Med Sci Monit* 9(2):RA35–RA39, 2003.
54. Kajantie E et al: Body size at birth predicts hypothalamic-pituitary-adrenal axis response to psychosocial stress at 60 to 70 years, *J Clin Endocrinol Metab* 92(11):4094–4100, 2007.
55. Elenkov IJ, Chrousos GP: Stress hormones, proinflammatory and antiinflammatory cytokines, and autoimmunity, *Ann N Y Acad Sci* 966:290–303, 2002.
56. Elenkov IJ: Glucocorticoids and the Th1/Th2 balance, *Ann N Y Acad Sci* 1024:138–146, 2004. review.
57. Meduri GU, Chrousos GP: Duration of glucocorticoid treatment and outcome in sepsis: is the right drug used the wrong way? *Chest* 114(2):355–360, 1998.
58. Chrousos GP, Elenkov IJ: Interactions of the endocrine and immune systems. In DeGroot LG, Jameson JL, editors: *Endocrinology*, ed 4, Philadelphia, 2001, Saunders.
59. Rocklin RE, editor: *Histamine and H_2 antagonists in inflammation and immunodeficiency*, New York, 1990, Marcel Dekker.
60. Chrousos GP, Gold PW: The concepts of stress and stress system disorders: overview of physical and behavioral homeostasis, *JAMA* 267(9):1244–1252, 1992.
61. Chrousos GP et al: Interactions between the hypothalamic-pituitary-adrenal axis and the female reproductive system, *Ann Intern Med* 129(3):229–240, 1998.
62. Kalantaridou SN et al: Stress and the female reproductive system. Review, *J Reprod Immunol* 62(1-2):61–68, 2004.
63. Gallucci WT et al: Sex differences in sensitivity of the hypothalamic-pituitary-adrenal axis, *Health Psychol* 12(5):420–425, 1993.
64. Peiffer A, Lapointe B, Barden H: Hormonal regulation of type II glucocorticoid receptor messenger ribonucleic acid in rat brain, *Endocrinology* 129(4):2166–2174, 1991.
65. Caro JF et al: Leptin: the tale of an obesity gene, *Diabetes* 45(11):1455–1462, 1996.
66. Ahima RS et al: Role of leptin in the neuroendocrine response to fasting, *Nature* 382(6588):250–252, 1996.
67. Boden G et al: Effect of fasting on serum leptin in normal human subjects, *J Clin Endocrinol Metab* 81(9):3419–3423, 1996.
68. Grinspoon S et al: Serum leptin levels in women with anorexia nervosa, *J Clin Endocrinol Metab* 81(11):3861–3863, 1996.
69. Machelska H et al: Opioid control of inflammatory pain regulated by intercellular adhesion molecule-1, *J Neurosci* 22(13):5588–5596, 2002.
70. Molina PE: Stress-specific opioid modulation of haemodynamic counter-regulation, *Clin Exp Pharmacol Physiol* 29(3):248–253, 2002.
71. Jochem J, Josko J, Gwozdz B: Endogenous opioid peptides system in haemorrhagic shock—central cardiovascular regulation, *Med Sci Monit* 7(3):545–549, 2001.
72. Molina PE: Opiate modulation of hemodynamic, hormonal, and cytokine responses to hemorrhage, *Shock* 15(6):471–478, 2001.
73. Cabot PJ et al: Immune cell-derived beta-endorphin: production, release, and control of inflammatory pain in rats, *J Clin Invest* 100(1):142–148, 1997.
74. Weigent DA et al: Characterization of the promoter-directing expression of growth hormone in a monocyte cell line, *Neuroimmunomodulation* 7(3):126–134, 2000.
75. Kelly PA et al: The prolactin/growth hormone receptor family, *Endocr Rev* 12(3):235–251, 1991.
76. Burguera B et al: Dual and selective actions of glucocorticoid upon basal and stimulated growth hormone release in man, *Neuroendocrinology* 51(1):51–58, 1990.
77. Tsigos C, Chrousos GP: Hypothalamic-pituitary-adrenal axis, neuroendocrine factors and stress, *J Psychosom Res* 53(4):865–871, 2002.
78. Van De Weerdt C et al: Far upstream sequences regulate the human prolactin promoter transcription, *Neuroendocrinology* 71(2):124–137, 2000.
79. Neumann ID: Alterations in behavioral and neuroendocrine stress coping strategies in pregnant, parturient, and lactating rats, *Prog Brain Res* 133:143–152, 2001.
80. Liu Y et al: Differential expression of vasopressin, oxytocin, and corticotrophin-releasing hormone messenger RNA in the paraventricular nucleus of the prairie vole brain following stress, *J Neuroendocrinol* 13(12):1059–1065, 2001.
81. Aakvaag A et al: Testosterone and testosterone-binding globulin (TeBG) in young men during prolonged stress, *Int J Androl* 1:22, 1978.
82. Kreuz LE, Rose RM, Jennings JR: Suppression of plasma testosterone levels and psychological stress: a longitudinal study of young men in Officer Candidate School, *Arch Gen Psychiatry* 26(5):479–482, 1972.
83. Guezennec CY et al: Effect of competition stress on tests used to assess testosterone administration in athletes, *Int J Sports Med* 16(6):368–372, 1995.
84. Rose RM: Psychoendocrinology. In Wilson JD, Foster DW, editors: *Williams textbook of endocrinology*, ed 7, Philadelphia, 1985, Saunders.
85. Da Silva JA: Sex hormones and glucocorticoids: interactions with the immune system, *Ann N Y Acad Sci* 876:102–117, 1999.
86. Offner PJ, Moore EE, Biffl WL: Male gender is a risk factor for major infections after surgery, *Arch Surg* 134(9):935–938, 1999.
87. Angele MK et al: Sex steroids regulate pro- and anti-inflammatory cytokine release by macrophages after trauma-hemorrhage, *Am J Physiol* 277(1 Pt 1):C35–C42, 1999.
88. Angele MK et al: Gender dimorphism in trauma-hemorrhage–induced thymocyte apoptosis, *Shock* 12(4):316–322, 1999.
89. Rohleder N et al: Age and sex steroid-related changes in glucocorticoid sensitivity of proinflammatory cytokine production after psychosocial stress, *J Neuroimmunol* 126(1-2):69–77, 2002.
90. Bone RC: Toward an epidemiology and natural history of SIRS (systemic inflammatory response syndrome), *JAMA* 268(24):3452–3455, 1992.
91. Poynter ME, Daynes RA: Peroxisome proliferator–activated receptor alpha activation modulates cellular redox status, represses nuclear factor-kappaB signaling, and reduces inflammatory cytokine production in aging, *J Biol Chem* 273(49):32833–32841, 1998.
92. Kopnisky KL, Stoff DM, Rausch DM: Workshop report: the effects of psychological variables on the progression of HIV-1 disease, *Brain Behav Immun* 18(3):246–261, 2004.
93. Wellen KE, Hotamisligil GS: Inflammation, stress, and diabetes, *J Clin Invest* 115(5):1111–1119, 2005.
94. Reiche EMV, Nunes SOV, Morimoto HK: Stress, depression, the immune system, and cancer (review), *Lancet Oncol* 5(10):617–625, 2004.
95. Jain R et al: Corticotropin-releasing factor modulating the immune response to stress in the rat, *Endocrinology* 128(3):1329–1336, 1991.
96. Dunn AJ: Psychoneuroimmunology for the psychoneuroendocrinologist: a review of animal studies of nervous system-immune system interactions, *Psychoneuroendocrinology* 14(4):251–274, 1989.
97. Rabin BS et al: Bidirectional interaction between the central nervous system and the immune system, *Clin Rev Immunol* 9(4):279–312, 1989.
98. Schwab RJ: Disturbances of sleep in the intensive care unit, *Crit Care Clin* 10(4):681–694, 1994.
99. Nelson RJ, Drazen DL: Melatonin mediates seasonal adjustment in immune function, *Reprod Nutr Dev* 39(3):383–398, 1999.
100. Imia K et al: Natural cytotoxic activity of peripheral-blood lymphocytes and cancer incidence: an 11-year follow-up study of a general population, *Lancet* 356(9244):1795–1799, 2000.
101. Teicher MH et al: Developmental neurobiology of childhood stress and trauma, *Psych Clin North Am* 25(2):297–426, 2002, vii-viii.
102. McEwen BS: Protective and damaging effects of stress mediators, *N Engl J Med* 338(3):171–179, 1998.
103. Segerstrom SC, Miller GE: Psychological stress and the human immune system: a meta-analytic study of 30 years of inquiry, *Psychol Bull* 130(4):601–630, 2004.
104. Rozlog LA et al: Stress and immunity: implications for viral disease and wound healing, *J Periodontol* 70(7):786–792, 1999.
105. Irwin M: Immune correlates of depression, *Adv Exp Med Biol* 461:1–24, 1999.
106. Glaser R et al: Stress-induced modulation of the immune response to recombinant hepatitis B vaccine, *Psychosom Med* 54(1):22–29, 1992.
107. Cohen S: Psychosocial stress and susceptibility to upper respiratory infections, *Am J Respir Crit Care Med* 152(4 Pt 2):S53–S58, 1995.

108. Evans DL et al: Stress-associated reductions of cytotoxic T lymphocytes and natural killer cells in asymptomatic HIV infection, *Am J Psychiatry* 152(4):543–550, 1995.
109. Nott KH, Vedhara K, Spickett GP: Psychology, immunology and HIV, *Psychoneuroendocrinology* 20(5):451–474, 1995.
110. Sheridan JF et al: Psychoneuroimmunology: stress effects on pathogenesis and immunity during infection, *Clin Microbiol Rev* 7(2):200–212, 1994.
111. Antoni MH et al: The influence of bio-behavioral factors on tumor biology: pathways and mechanisms, *Nat Rev Cancer* 6(3):240–248, 2006.
112. Campbell JP et al: Stimulation of host bone marrow stromal cells by sympathetic nerves promotes breast cancer bone metastasis in mice, *PLoS Biol* 10(7), 2012, e1001363.
113. Sharma R, Coats AJ, Anker SD: The role of inflammatory mediators in chronic heart failure: cytokines, nitric oxide, and endothelin-1, *Int J Cardiol* 72(2):175–186, 2000.
114. Sher L: Effects of psychological factors on the development of cardiovascular pathology: role of the immune system and infection, *Med Hypotheses* 53(2):112–113, 1999.
115. Dutta P et al: Myocardial infarction accelerates atherosclerosis, *Nature* 487(7407):325–329, 2012.
116. Bremner JD et al: Neural correlates of memories of childhood sexual abuse in women with and without posttraumatic stress disorder, *Am J Psychiatry* 156(11):1787–1795, 1999.
117. Clohessy S, Ehlers A: PTSD symptoms, response to intrusive memories and coping in ambulance service workers, *Br J Clin Psychol* 38(Pt 3): 251–265, 1999.
118. Donnelly CL, Amaya-Jackson L, March JS: Psychopharmacology of pediatric posttraumatic stress disorder, *J Child Adolesc Psychopharmacol* 9(3):203–220, 1999.
119. Heim C, Ehlert U, Hellhammer DH: The potential role of hypocortisolism in the pathophysiology of stress-related bodily disorders, *Psychoneuroendocrinology* 25(1):1–35, 2000.
120. Alarcon RD, Glover SG, Deering CG: The cascade model: an alternative to comorbidity in the pathogenesis of posttraumatic stress disorder, *Psychiatry* 62(2):114–124, 1999.
121. Cordova MJ et al: Frequency and correlates of posttraumatic-stress-disorder-like symptoms after treatment for breast cancer, *J Consult Clin Psychol* 63(6):981–986, 1995.
122. Ma Z, Faber A, Dube L: Exploring women's psychoneuroendocrine responses to cancer threat: insights from a computer-based guided imagery task, *Can J Nurs Res* 39(1):98–115, 2007.
123. Porter LS et al: Cortisol levels and responses to mammography screening in breast cancer survivors: a pilot study, *Psychosom Med* 65(5): 842–848, 2003.
124. Clayton MF, Dudley WN, Musters A: Communication with breast cancer survivors, *Health Commun* 23(3):207–221, 2008.
125. Clayton MF, Mishel MH, Belyea M: Testing a model of symptoms, communication, uncertainty, and well-being, in older breast cancer survivors, *Res Nurs Health* 29(1):18–39, 2006.
126. Kiecolt-Glaser JK et al: Psychoneuroimmunology and psychosomatic medicine: back to the future, *Psychosom Med* 64(1):15–28, 2002. (Review).
127. Folkman S, Lazarus RS: The relationship between coping and emotion: implications for theory and research, *Soc Sci Med* 26(3):309–317, 1988.
128. Irwin M et al: Partial sleep deprivation reduces natural killer cell activity in humans, *Psychosom Med* 56(6):493–498, 1994.
129. Pollmacher T et al: Influence of host defense activation on sleep in humans, *Adv Neuroimmunol* 5(2):155–169, 1995.
130. White D et al: Sleep deprivation and the control of ventilation, *Am Rev Respir Dis* 128(6):984–986, 1983.
131. Frolkis VV: Stress-age syndrome, *Mech Ageing Dev* 69(1-2):93–107, 1993.
132. Kiecolt-Glaser J et al: Psychosocial enhancement of immunocompetence in a geriatric population, *Health Psychol* 4(1):25–41, 1985.
133. Spiegel D: Psychosocial intervention in cancer, *J Natl Cancer Inst* 85(15):1198–1205, 1993.
134. Pinquart M, Sörensen S: Differences between caregivers and noncaregivers in psychological health and physical health: a meta-analysis, *Psychol Aging* 18(2):250–267, 2003.
135. Baron RS et al: Social support and immune function among spouses of cancer patients, *J Pers Soc Psychol* 59(2):344–352, 1990.
136. Kiecolt-Glaser J et al: Chronic stress and immune function in family caregivers of Alzheimer's disease victims, *Psychosom Med* 45(5):523, 1987.
137. Shelby J et al: Severe burn injury: effects on psychologic and immunologic function in noninjured close relatives, *J Burn Care Rehabil* 13(1):58–63, 1992.
138. Mazzeo RS: Aging, immune function, and exercise: hormonal regulation, *Int J Sports Med* 21(Suppl 1):S10–S13, 2000. (Review).
139. Frolkis W: Stress-age syndrome, *Mech Ageing Dev* 69(1-2):93–107, 1993.

CHAPTER

12

Cancer Biology

*Neal S. Rote and David M. Virshup**

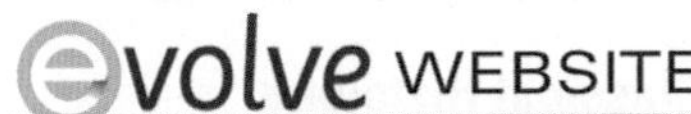

WEBSITE

http://evolve.elsevier.com/McCance/

- Review Questions and Answers
- Animations
- Online Course: Module 8

CHAPTER OUTLINE

Cancer is a leading disease, cause of death, and source of morbidity of adults in the Western world. The incidence of cancer increases markedly with advancing age and is strongly affected by gender, lifestyle, ethnicity, infection, and genetics. Over the past 35 years intensive research has led to a significantly enhanced understanding of this complex and frightening disease. We now understand that cancer is a collection of more than 100 different diseases, caused by an accumulation of genetic and epigenetic alterations. Environment, heredity, and behavior interact to modify the risk of developing cancer and the response to treatment. Improvements in treatment strategies and supportive care, coupled with new, often individualized therapies based on advances in our fundamental understanding of the basic pathophysiology of malignancy, have contributed to an increasing number of effective options for these diverse, often lethal, disorders collectively called *cancer.*

CANCER CHARACTERISTICS AND TERMINOLOGY

Any discussion of cancer must start with a definition of what it is and what it is not. Although most readers may have an intuitive understanding of this disorder, composing an exact definition that encompasses this broad category is more challenging. In general, a **tumor** is an abnormal growth resulting from uncontrolled proliferation and serves no physiologic function.

*Dr. Virshup contributed to the previous edition.

TABLE 12-1 CHARACTERISTICS OF BENIGN VS. MALIGNANT TUMORS

BENIGN TUMORS	MALIGNANT TUMORS
Grow slowly	Grow rapidly
Have a well-defined capsule	Are not encapsulated
Are not invasive	Invade local structures and tissues
Are well differentiated; look like the tissue from which they arose	Are poorly differentiated; may not be able to determine tissue of origin
Have a low mitotic index; dividing cells are rare	High mitotic index; many dividing cells
Do not metastasize	Can spread distantly, often through blood vessels and lymphatics

The term *cancer* derives from the Greek word for crab, *karkinoma,* which the physician Hippocrates used to describe the appendage-like projections extending from tumors. The word tumor originally referred to any swelling that was caused by inflammation, but is now generally reserved for describing a new growth, or **neoplasm.** Not all tumors or neoplasms, however, are cancer. The term **cancer** refers to a *malignant* tumor and is not used to refer to *benign* growths, such as lipomas or hypertrophy of an organ. Yet it is important to recognize that benign neoplasms also can be life threatening if they enlarge in critical locations. For example, a benign meningioma at the base of the skull may cause symptoms by compressing adjacent normal brain tissue. The definitions of benign vs. malignant are presented in the following text and in Table 12-1.

Tumor Classification and Nomenclature

Proper identification of a cancer is important for many reasons. Different lesions will have different causes, different rates and patterns of progression, and different responses to treatment. Cancer classification starts with knowing the site of origin and microscopic appearance of the lesion, but can extend to a detailed description of critical genetic changes in the cancer.

Benign tumors, which are not referred to as cancers, are usually encapsulated and well differentiated. They retain some normal tissue structure and do not invade the capsules surrounding them or spread to regional lymph nodes or distant locations. Benign tumors are generally named according to the tissues from which they arise, and include the suffix "-oma." For example, a benign tumor of the smooth muscle of the uterus is a *leiomyoma,* and a benign tumor of fat cells is a *lipoma.*

Some tumors initially described as benign can progress to cancer and then are referred to as **malignant tumors.** These tumors are distinguished from benign tumors by their more rapid growth rates and specific microscopic alterations, including loss of differentiation and absence of normal tissue organization. One of the hallmarks of cancer cells, as seen under the microscope, is **anaplasia,** the loss of cellular differentiation, irregularities of the size and shape of the nucleus, and the loss of normal tissue structure. Malignant tumors may present with different degrees of encapsulation; some lack a capsule, and even if a capsule is apparent, its integrity has been compromised so that tumor cells can grow to invade nearby blood vessels, lymphatics, and surrounding structures. The most important and most deadly characteristic of malignant tumors is their ability to spread far beyond the tissue of origin, a process known as *metastasis* (Figures 12-1 and 12-2; see Table 12-1).

In general, cancers are named according to the cell type from which they originate. Cancers arising in epithelial tissue are called **carcinomas,** and if they arise from or form ductal or glandular structures are named **adenocarcinomas.** Hence, a malignant tumor arising from breast glandular tissue is a mammary adenocarcinoma. Cancers arising from connective tissue usually have the suffix **sarcoma.** For example, malignant cancers of skeletal muscle are known as rhabdomyosarcomas. Cancers of lymphatic tissue are called **lymphomas,** whereas cancers of blood-forming cells are called **leukemias.** However, many cancers, such as Hodgkin disease and Ewing sarcoma, are named for historical reasons that do not follow this naming convention. Table 12-2 presents the nomenclature and classification of selected tumors.

Classification of Tumors—Classical Histology and Modern Genetics

Carcinoma in situ (often abbreviated **CIS**) refers to preinvasive epithelial malignant tumors of glandular or squamous cell origin. Cancers develop incrementally, as they accumulate specific genetic lesions. Careful surveillance for cancer often detects abnormal growths in epithelial tissues that have atypical cells and an increased proliferation rate compared with normal surrounding tissues. These early stage cancers are localized to the epithelium and have not penetrated the local basement membrane or invaded the surrounding stroma (see Figure 12-1). Based on these characteristics, they are not malignant but are often called **carcinoma in situ (CIS).** CIS is recognized in a number of sites, including the cervix, skin, oral cavity, esophagus, and bronchus. In glandular epithelium, in situ lesions occur in the stomach, endometrium, breast, and large bowel. In the breast, ductal carcinoma in situ (DCIS) fills the mammary ducts but has not progressed to local tissue invasion. DCIS lesions are readily treatable, although the optimal therapeutic approach is controversial. CIS lesions can have one of the following three fates: they can remain stable for a long time, they can progress to invasive and metastatic cancers, or they can regress and disappear. CIS can vary from low-grade to high-grade dysplasia, with the high-grade lesions having the highest likelihood of becoming invasive cancers. The time that such preinvasive lesions remain in situ before becoming invasive is unknown.[1] Some carcinomas of the cervix appear as preinvasive lesions in situ for several years before they progress to invasive carcinoma and metastatic tumors (see Figure 12-1). Knowing how to best treat low-grade CIS lesions is challenging because the proportion that progress to cancer vs. the proportion that will never cause clinical problems is usually not known. Although most persons prefer removal of any CIS as opposed to "watchful waiting," this topic continues to be a source of great debate.

Because our knowledge about the molecular alterations in cancer can influence the choices of therapy, it becomes increasingly important for clinicians to accurately molecularly classify each cancer. The classification, and hence the treatment

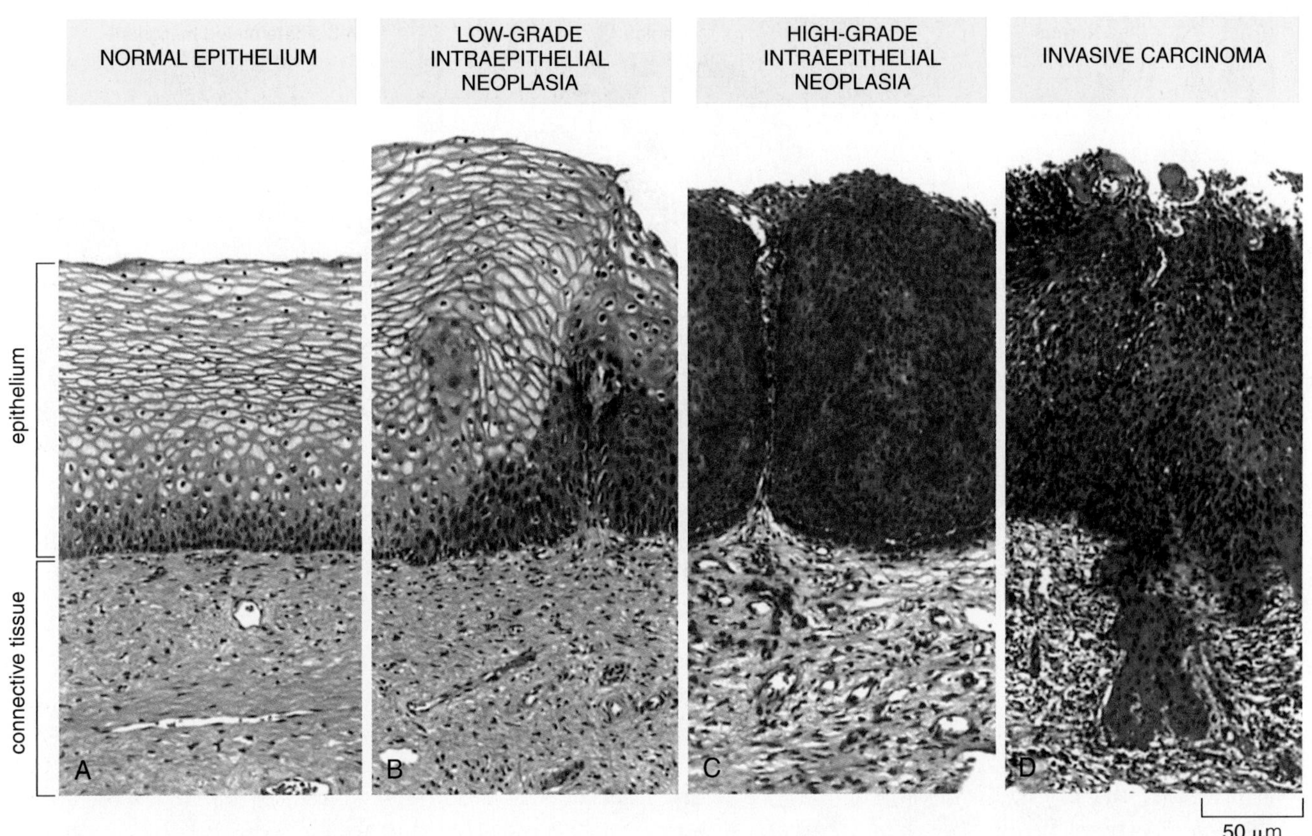

FIGURE 12-1 Progression from Normal to Neoplasm in the Uterine Cervix. A sequence of cellular and tissue changes progressing from low-grade to high-grade intraepithelial neoplasms (also called carcinoma in situ) and then to invasive cancer is seen often in the development of cancer. In this example of the early stages of cervical neoplastic changes, the presence of anaplastic cells and the loss of normal tissue architecture signify the development of cancer. The high rate of cell division and the presence of local mutagens and inflammatory mediators all contribute to the accumulation of genetic abnormalities that lead to cancer. (From Alberts B et al: *Molecular biology of the cell,* ed 5, New York, 2002, Garland.)

decisions, of cancers was originally based on gross and light microscopic appearance and is now commonly accompanied by immunohistochemical analysis of protein expression. Increasingly, this is supplemented by a more extensive molecular analysis of the tumors. Sometimes a single gene is examined (for example, to determine if there is a characteristic chromosomal translocation diagnostic of chronic myelogenous leukemia [CML]), and sometimes a panel of genes and proteins are examined (e.g., in breast cancer) to determine if the tumor expresses estrogen receptor, progesterone receptor, and the epidermal growth factor (EGF) receptor HER2, or if there are mutations in specific genes that include response to therapy. In a research setting, and increasingly in clinical settings, expression and mutation analysis of a large number of genes can be measured using polymerase chain reaction (PCR), microarray, or advanced DNA sequencing technology. These analyses can be used to classify tumors more precisely and may predict the most effective therapy. This detailed analysis of each tumor is a form of **personalized medicine** that offers therapy based on a very detailed knowledge of each individual's characteristics and their specific cancer.[2] This enhanced molecular characterization subdivides cancers into therapeutically and prognostically relevant smaller groups. As an example, breast cancers can now be subclassified into more than four types (luminal A, luminal B, basal-like, and others) based on their expression of specific markers, such as estrogen receptor, HER2/Neu, and other specific genes and proteins. Each subtype has a different response to therapy and a different prognosis (Figure 12-3).

Tumor Markers

During surveillance or diagnosis of cancer as well as following therapy, specific biochemical markers of tumors have proven to be helpful. These **tumor markers** are substances produced by both benign and malignant cells that either are present in or on tumor cells or are found in blood, spinal fluid, or urine (Table 12-3). Some tumor markers have been known for many decades. For diseases associated with a tumor marker, there is indeed a "blood test for cancer." Tumor markers include hormones, enzymes, genes, antigens, and antibodies. Liver and germ cell tumors secrete a protein known as *alpha fetoprotein (AFP)* into the blood, and prostate tumors secrete *prostate specific antigen (PSA)* into the blood. If the tumor marker itself has biologic activity, then it can cause symptoms, a phenomenon known as a **paraneoplastic syndrome.** For example, the adrenal medulla normally secretes the catecholamine epinephrine (adrenaline). Benign tumors of the adrenal medulla (pheochromocytoma) can produce catecholamines (e.g., adrenaline) in vast excess, leading to rapid pulse rate, high blood

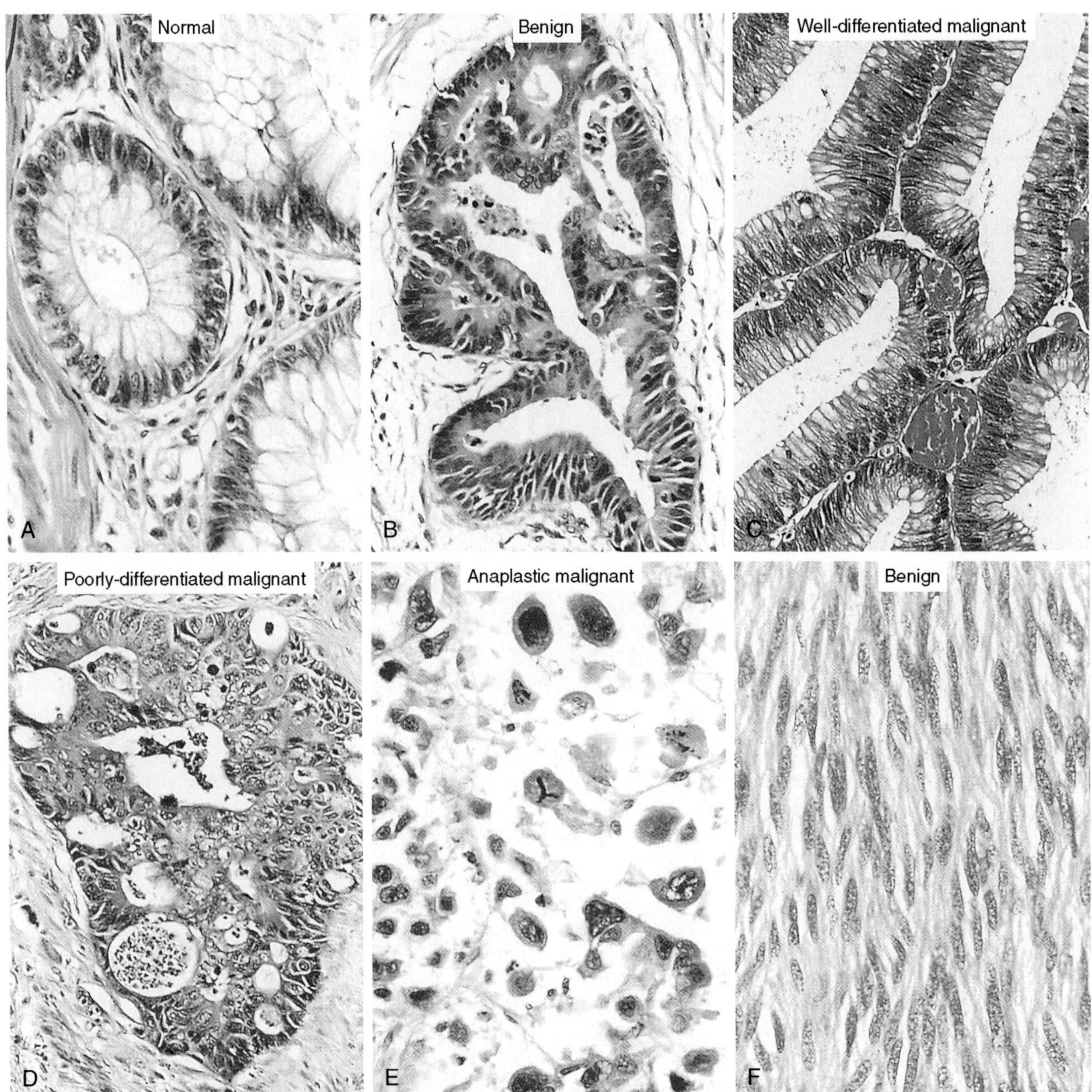

FIGURE 12-2 Loss of Cellular and Tissue Differentiation During the Development of Cancer. The cells of a benign neoplasm **(B)** resemble those of the normal colonic epithelium **(A),** in that they are columnar and have an orderly arrangement. Loss of some degree of differentiation is evident in that the neoplastic cells do not show much mucin vacuolization. Cells of the well-differentiated malignant neoplasm **(C)** of the colon have a haphazard arrangement and although gland lumina are formed, they are architecturally abnormal and irregular. Nuclei vary in shape and size, especially when compared with those in **A.** Cells in the poorly differentiated malignant neoplasm **(D)** have an even more haphazard arrangement, with very poor formation of gland lumina. Nuclei show greater variation in shape and size compared with the well-differentiated malignant neoplasm in **C.** Cells in anaplastic malignant neoplasms **(E)** bear no relation to the normal epithelium, with no recognizable gland formation. Tremendous variation is found in the size of cells and their nuclei, with very intense staining (hyperchromatic nuclei). Not knowing the site of origin would make it impossible to classify this tumor by microscopic appearance alone. Well-differentiated tumors often resemble their cell of origin, as shown in the example of a benign tumor of smooth muscles **(F).** (From Stevens A, Lowe J: *Pathology,* ed 2, London, 2000, Mosby.)

pressure, diaphoresis (i.e., sweating), and tremors. Detection of elevated blood or urine levels of catecholamines helps to confirm the diagnosis, and treatment of the disease relieves the symptoms. Tumor markers can be used in three ways: (1) to screen and identify individuals at high risk for cancer; (2) to help diagnose the specific type of tumor in individuals with clinical manifestations relating to their tumor, as in adrenal tumors or enlarged liver or prostate; and (3) to follow the clinical course of a tumor. For example, a falling PSA level after radiation or surgical therapy for prostate cancer indicates successful treatment, and a later rise in the PSA level may indicate a recurrence.

TABLE 12-2 NOMENCLATURE AND CLASSIFICATION OF BENIGN AND MALIGNANT TUMORS*

CELL OR TISSUE OF ORIGIN	BENIGN TUMOR	MALIGNANT TUMOR
Tumors of Epithelial Origin		
Squamous cells	Squamous cell papilloma	Squamous cell carcinoma
Basal cells	—	Basal cell carcinoma
Glandular or ductal epithelium	Adenoma	Adenocarcinoma
	Cystadenoma	Cystadenocarcinoma
Transitional cells	Transitional cell papilloma	Transitional cell carcinoma
Bile duct	Bile duct adenoma	Bile duct carcinoma (cholangiocarcinoma)
Liver cells	Hepatocellular adenoma	Hepatocellular carcinoma
Melanocytes	Nevus	Malignant melanoma
Renal epithelium	Renal tubular adenoma	Renal cell carcinoma
Skin adnexal glands		
Sweat glands	Sweat gland adenoma	Sweat gland carcinoma
Sebaceous glands	Sebaceous gland adenoma	Sebaceous gland carcinoma
Germ cells (testis and ovary)	—	Seminoma (dysgerminoma)
		Embryonal carcinoma, yolk sac carcinoma
Tumors of Mesenchymal Origin		
Hematopoietic/lymphoid tissue		
Leukocytes		Leukemias
Granular leukocytes and precursors		Granulocytic leukemia
		Myelocytic leukemias
		Myelogenous leukemias
Plasma cells		Multiple myeloma
Lymphoid		
Nongranular leukocytes and prelymphocytes		Lymphomas
Proliferating lymphocytes and monocytes		Lymphocytic leukemia
Proliferating immature precursor monocytes		Lymphoblastic leukemia
Solid tumors of lymph tissue (thymus, spleen, lymph nodes)		Lymphoma or lymphosarcoma
Neural and retinal tissue		
Nerve sheath	Neurilemoma, neurofibroma	Malignant peripheral nerve sheath tumor
Nerve cells	Ganglioneuroma	Neuroblastoma
Retinal cells (cones)	—	Retinoblastoma
Connective tissue		
Fibrous tissue	Fibromatosis (desmoid)	Fibrosarcoma
Fat	Lipoma	Liposarcoma
Bone	Osteoma	Osteogenic sarcoma
Cartilage	Chondroma	Chrondrosarcoma
Muscle		
Smooth muscle	Leiomyoma	Leiomyosarcoma
Striated muscle	Rhabdomyoma	Rhabdomyosarcoma
Endothelial and related tissues		
Blood vessels	Hemangioma	Angiosarcoma
		Kaposi sarcoma
Lymph vessels	Lymphangioma	Lymphangiosarcoma
Synovium	—	Synovial sarcoma
Mesothelium	—	Malignant mesothelioma
Meninges	Meningioma	Malignant meningioma
Tumors of Uncertain Origin	—	Ewing tumor

Modified from Murphy GP et al: *American Cancer Society's textbook of clinical oncology,* ed 2, New York, 1995, American Cancer Society.

***Note:** This list is intended to provide only an introduction to tumor nomenclature.

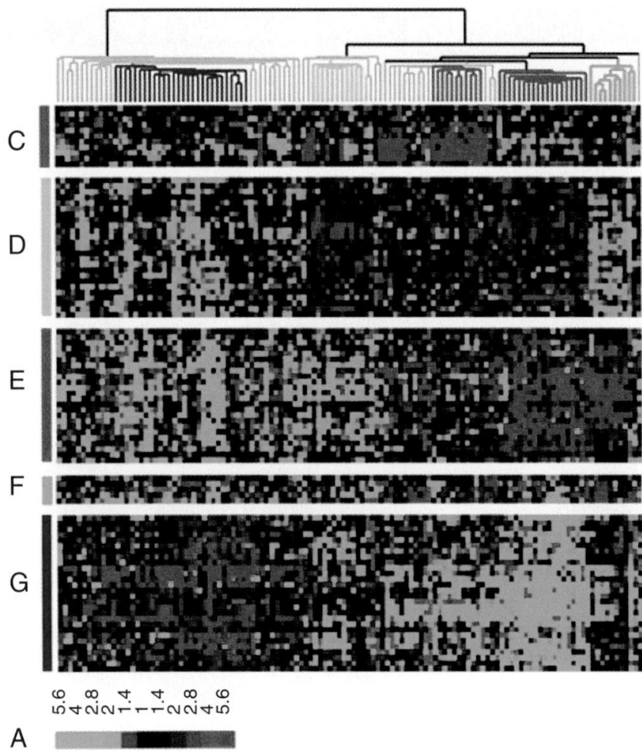

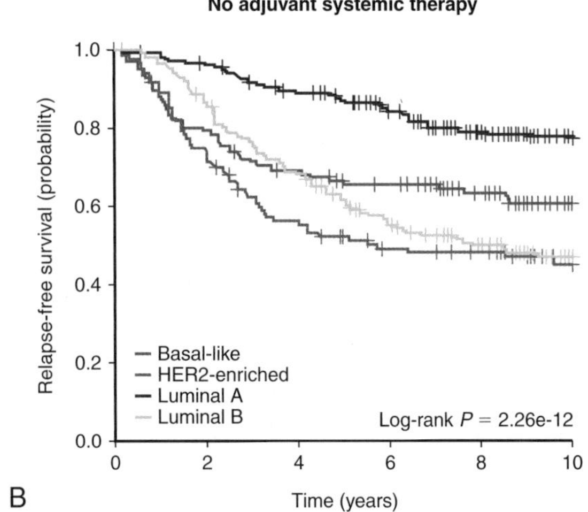

FIGURE 12-3 Molecular Markers Aid in Cancer Classification and Treatment Choices. **A,** Cancers can be classified based on gene expression patterns. In this breast cancer study, gene expression was measured in tumors from 115 patients. Each row is a different gene, and each column is a different patient sample. Red denotes high gene expression; green signifies low gene expression. Using this molecular subtyping method, breast cancer can be subdivided into at least four molecular subtypes—luminal A, luminal B, HER2, and basal. The group on the far right is normal breast tissue. **B,** Molecular classification predicts overall survival. In this group of women, breast cancer molecular subtypes were determined by gene expression profiles in a group of women with similar stage tumors, as in **(A)**. The molecular subtype is a good predictor of response to chemotherapy and survival. This molecular subtyping method can help select the best therapy for women. (**A** from Sorlie T et al: *Proc Natl Acad Sci U S A* 100[14]:8418–8423, 2003; **B** from Parker JS et al: *J Clin Oncol* 27[8]:1160–1167, 2009.)

There are several significant problems in using tumor marker assays to screen populations of healthy individuals for cancer. Testing large populations will always detect a few normal individuals with test results at the high end of the normal distribution (the "false positives"), which can lead to expensive and invasive additional tests, and unnecessary concern. Similarly, some individuals with disease will have test results in the normal range ("false negatives"). Furthermore, some nonmalignant conditions also can produce tumor markers. The presence of an elevated tumor marker therefore may suggest a specific diagnosis, but it is not used alone as a definitive diagnostic test. Identification of ideal sensitive and specific tumor markers that are elevated early in the course of common cancers remains a high priority because the early detection of cancer often improves the treatment outcome.

The Biology of Cancer Cells

Transformation and Differentiation

Cancer cells behave differently than normal cells in several important ways. **Transformation** refers to the process by which a normal cell becomes a cancer cell. **Autonomy** refers to the cancer cell's independence from normal cellular controls and is part of the transformational process. These differences are most readily seen in specialized laboratory assays, especially those examining the growth patterns of normal and cancerous cells in laboratory incubators. Transformed cells lack many of the normal "social controls" seen in nontransformed cells. They often have markedly decreased requirements for external growth factors. Normal cells cease to divide when they fill a petri (or tissue culture) dish. Transformed cells, unlike normal cells, lack **contact inhibition** and continue to crowd, eventually piling up on each other (Figure 12-4). Normal cells usually will not grow unless they are attached to a firm surface (like a petri dish). However, cancer cells are often **anchorage independent;** that is, they continue to divide even when suspended in a soft agar gel. Normal cells have a limited life span in the laboratory; they may divide in a petri dish 10 or 50 times, but then they cease growing. Cancer cells usually are **immortal** in that they seem to have an unlimited life span and will continue to divide for years under appropriate laboratory conditions. One of the most commonly used laboratory cell lines, HeLa cells, was derived from a cervical cancer specimen obtained in 1951 that continues to grow and divide in laboratories around the world.[3] Cancerous cells can be assayed in mice as well; when normal human cells are injected into a special type of mouse (genetically engineered to lack an immune system to prevent rejection of human cells) they will not grow. However, cancerous cells from humans can continue to grow and even metastasize in these mice.

Cancer cells often show defects in the normal process of differentiation; that is, the process of acquiring a specialized function and organization, such as evolving into a muscle cell (see Chapter 43) or a nerve cell (see Chapter 15). **Anaplasia** is the absence of differentiation (see Figure 12-2) and means literally "without form." In clinical specimens, *anaplasia* is recognized by a loss of organization and a marked increase in nuclear size with evidence of ongoing proliferation. In

TABLE 12-3 **EXAMPLES OF TUMOR MARKERS**

MARKER NAME	NATURE	TYPE OF CANCER
Alpha fetoprotein (AFP)	70-kDa protein	Hepatic, germ cell
Carcinoembryonic antigen (CEA)	200-kDa glycoprotein	GI, pancreas, lung, breast, etc.
β-Human chorionic gonadotropin (β-hCG)	Glycopeptide hormone β-chain	Germ cell
Prostate-specific antigen (PSA)	33-kDa glycoprotein	Prostate
Catecholamines	Epinephrine and precursors	Pheochromocytoma (adrenal medulla)
Homovanillic acid/vanillylmandelic acid (HVA/VMA)	Catecholamine metabolites	Neuroblastoma
Urinary Bence Jones protein	Ig light chain	Multiple myeloma
Adrenocorticotropic hormone (ACTH)	Peptide hormone	Pituitary adenomas

GI, Gastrointestinal; *Ig,* immunoglobulin; *kDa,* kilodalton.

A

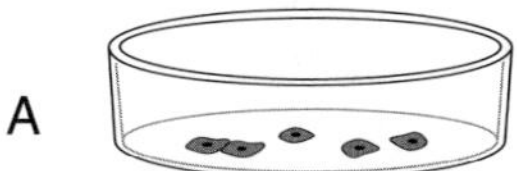

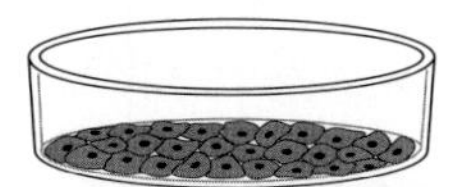

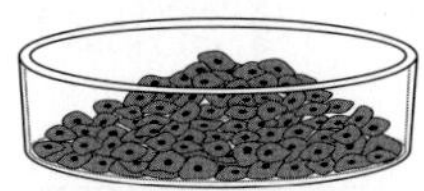
Cancer cells do not exhibit contact inhibition, and continue to divide, piling up on each other.

B

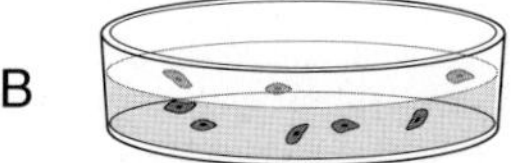

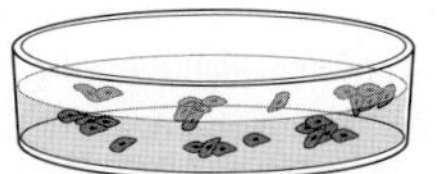

FIGURE 12-4 Cancerous Cells Show Abnormal Growth in the Laboratory. Cancer cells, unlike most normal cells **(A),** usually continue to grow and pile on top of one another after they have formed a confluent monolayer in culture (loss of contact inhibition) and **(B)** can grow without being attached to a surface, called anchorage independence.

contrast to normal cells, which are uniform in size and shape, *anaplastic* cells are of variable size and shape, or **pleomorphic.** For example, a benign muscle tumor (benign myoma) will retain the ability to make muscle, whereas in a malignant muscle tumor (rhabdomyosarcoma), new muscle formation is seen only rarely, and even then appears highly disorganized. Thus the muscle cancer cells appear undifferentiated. The most malignant tumors tend to have the most *anaplasia* and be the least differentiated.

Cancer Metabolism

Cancer cells live in a distinct milieu from normal cells and have different nutritional requirements from nonproliferating cells. The successful cancer cell divides rapidly, with the consequent requirement for the building blocks of new cells. Cancers often must grow in a hypoxic and acidic environment. Cancers also are parasites, able to selectively extract nutrients from the bloodstream without any evolutionary pressure for balanced metabolism. Nonmalignant cells in the presence of adequate oxygen normally generate adenosine triphosphate (ATP) by mitochondrial oxidative phosphorylation (OXPHOS), generating 36 ATP molecules from each glucose molecule that is broken down to water and carbon dioxide. Only in the absence of sufficient oxygen do normal cells perform anaerobic glycolysis, generating only two ATP molecules per molecule of glucose, with lactic acid as a byproduct. However, even in the presence of oxygen, cancer cells perform glycolysis, not OXPHOS[4] (Figure 12-5). Although this aerobic glycolysis was originally postulated as some form of cancer-specific mitochondrial dysfunction, it is now apparent that this is instead a highly regulated and beneficial adaptation for cancer cells. This shift from OXPHOS to glycolysis allows lactate and its metabolites to be used for the more efficient production of lipids and other molecular building blocks needed for rapid cell growth. Furthermore, many cancer genes promote this switch to aerobic glycolysis. Alterations in a number of cancer genes, including receptor tyrosine kinases, *AKT, PTEN, TP53,* and *MYC,* inhibit OXPHOS and promote the activity of glycolytic and related metabolic pathways that support the rapid growth of cancers.[4,5]

Clinically the high glucose utilization of a cancer can be exploited for its detection. ^{18}F-Fluorodeoxyglucose (FDG) is incorporated into cells in the same way as glucose, with two key differences. Because it is missing a key hydroxyl group it cannot be broken down by glycolysis and, thus, FDG accumulates in cells. Because it is tagged with ^{18}F, it can be imaged by positron emission tomography (a PET scan). Small metastatic tumor masses that are consuming huge amounts of glucose can readily be detected with this imaging method (Figure 12-6).

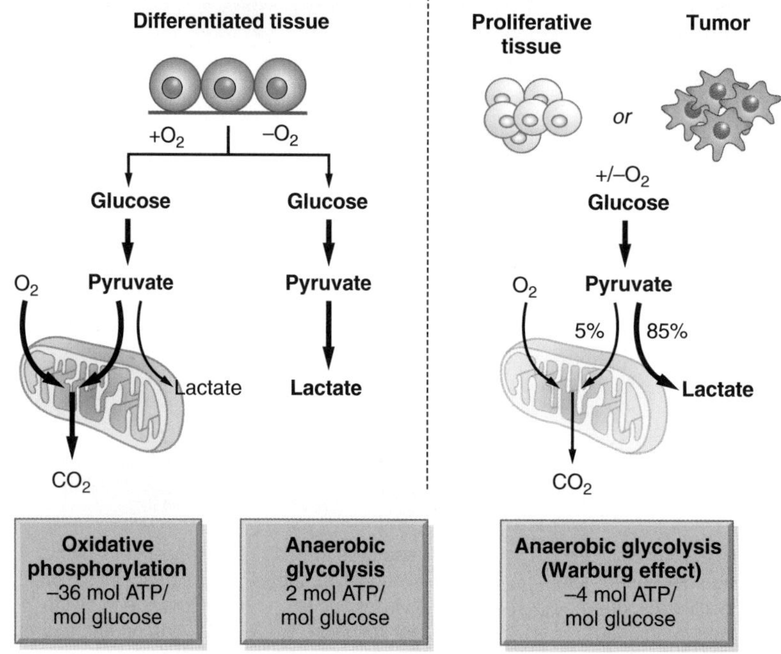

FIGURE 12-5 Cancers Have Altered Metabolism. Normal tissues use oxidative phosphorylation (OXPHOS) to turn glucose into CO_2 and energy (in the form of ATP). Cancers take a different approach; even in the presence of oxygen, they do not use OXPHOS. Instead, they consume large quantities of glucose to make cellular building blocks, supporting rapid proliferation. *ATP,* Adenosine triphosphate. (From Van der Heiden MG, Cantley LC, Thompson CB: *Science* 324:1029–1033, 2009.)

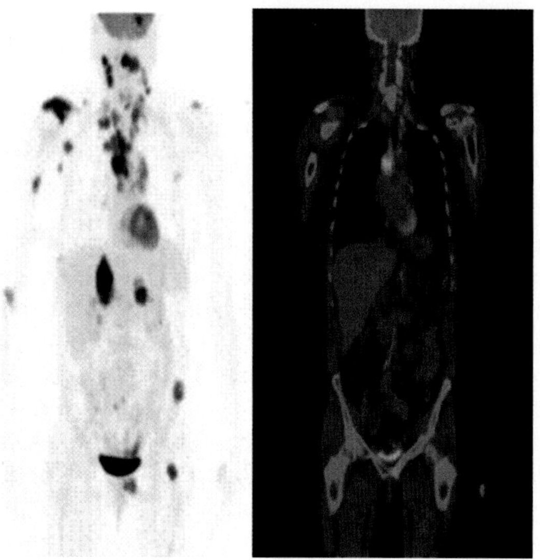

FIGURE 12-6 Intense Glucose Requirement Aids in Diagnosis of Metastatic Non–Small Cell Lung Cancer. This 54-year-old woman had a non–small cell lung cancer (NSCLC) resected from the left upper lobe. Five years later, these studies were obtained. The positron emission tomography (PET) scan using 18-fluorodeoxyglucose (FDG) shows metastatic lesions in the brain, right shoulder, and mediastinal and cervical lymph nodes, as well as in the liver, left pelvis, and proximal femur. *PET whole-body image (left):* Representative coronal image from the whole-body FDG-PET/CT–fused image of the same patient *(right).* The fused image consists of the computed tomography (CT) image with the metabolic information superimposed in color. The pattern of spread is most likely from the primary tumor to the large mediastinal lymph nodes, followed by lymphatic spread to cervical nodes. Blood-borne dissemination produced the bone, brain, and liver metastases. Normally, only the heart, brain, and bladder show a strong signal in PET scans. (Images courtesy John Hoffman, MD, Huntsman Cancer Institute, Salt Lake City, UT.)

Cancer Stem Cells

Many tissues, most notably the skin, intestines, and blood-forming cells, continuously renew themselves. The human gut sheds and replaces hundreds of grams of cells each day. This ongoing proliferation of these tissues with a high turnover rate depends on their regeneration from a small fraction of cells known as **adult stem cells.** Adult stem cells have two essential characteristics: first, they self-renew (that is, some fraction of the cell divisions creates new stem cells); and second, they are **multipotent,** or have the ability to differentiate into multiple different cell types. In the bone marrow, it is estimated that only 0.05% (1 in 20,000) of the blood-forming cells are stem cells, yet this small pool of stem cells can be stimulated to divide and to repopulate all the mature bone marrow–derived cells in approximately 2 weeks after bone marrow transplantation. As few as 10 stem cells are sufficient to entirely repopulate the entire bone marrow of a mouse in bone marrow transplantation experiments. Similarly, the absorptive and goblet cells lining the intestine have a life span of less than 1 week, after which they undergo cell death, or apoptosis, and slough into the intestinal lumen. They too must be replenished by ongoing proliferation of intestinal stem cells. A key feature of stem cells is that they can divide asymmetrically (i.e., during division, the cytoplasmic contents are unevenly distributed between the daughter cells); they can give rise to another stem cell and one daughter cell that ultimately terminally differentiates into diverse cell types, depending on the needs of the tissue (Figure 12-7). Multipotent bone marrow stem cells can self-renew and differentiate into all types of bone marrow–derived cells, such as red cells, lymphocytes, and neutrophils. Certain adult stem cells have a broader range of potential fates. For example, mesenchymal stem cells

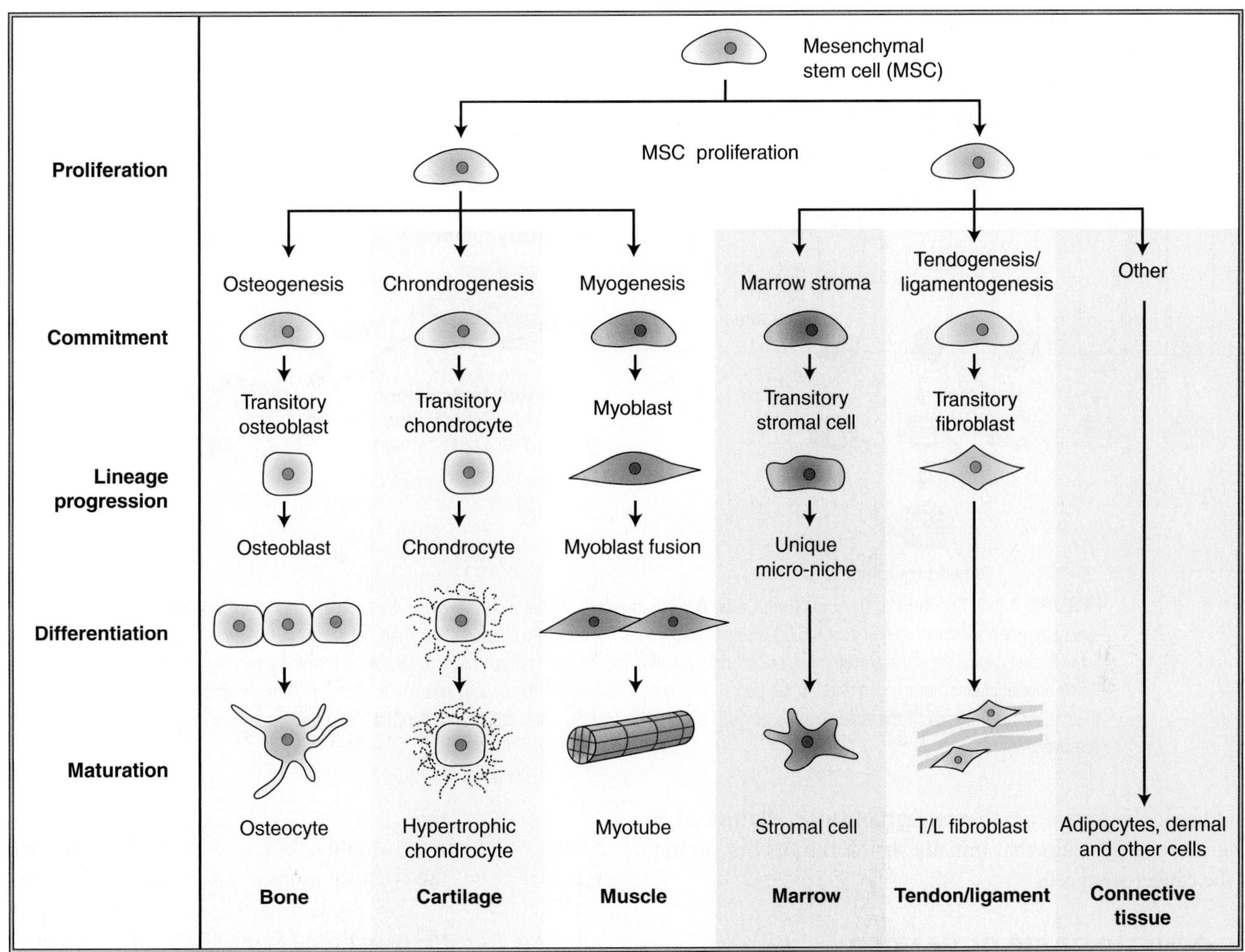

FIGURE 12-7 **Postulated Multiple Lineage–Specific Differentiation of Mesenchymal Stem Cells.** Differentiation occurs progressively as the offspring of stem cells commit to various lineages. Mesenchymal stem cells can renew themselves and give rise to multiple tissue types. (Modified from Caplan A, Bruder S: *Trends Mol Med* 7[6]:259–264, 2001.)

are able to differentiate into multiple types of cells, such as blood vessels, neurons, and muscle cells. Theoretically, such a stem cell might be able to give rise to all cell types in the body, and as such, could be useful in regeneration of diseased tissues.

Many cancers, like normal tissues, are heterogeneous, with differences in cell shape, size, behavior, and protein expression. There are two models to explain this heterogeneity within tumors. In the clonal evolution model, all the cancer cells divide regularly, and heterogeneity arises from proliferation, mutation, epigenetic changes, differences in local environment, and natural differentiation of cells. In this model, most of these cells are still robust cancer cells, capable of forming complex tumors in experimental animals. In contrast, in the cancer stem cell model, heterogeneity arises because there is a rare cancer stem cell whose offspring do not have stem cell properties, but undergo a limited number of divisions while generating heterogeneity through epigenetic and environmental alterations. However, similar to the adult tissue stem cells, only the cancer stem cell, if transplanted, is postulated to be capable of forming complex and heterogeneous tumors. The typical cancer stem cell experiment separates cancer cells into different pools depending on some measurable characteristic such as cell surface proteins, and then assays how many cells must be injected into an experimental mouse to form a cancer. In some cases, these tumor-initiating cells are very rare, with only 1 in 10,000 human colon cancer cells able to re-form a complex and heterogeneous colon cancer in mice (Figure 12-8).[6] However, these tumor-initiating cells are not always rare; in human melanomas, one in four cells can initiate a complex tumor in the appropriate mouse model.[7] This is an experimentally difficult area of research, because human cancers are examined in mice where there are multiple barriers to transplantation, including immune responses, as well as species differences in the various growth factors, cytokines, and microenvironment that can all influence the results. Therefore most progress is likely to be made by studying cancer stem cells arising in mouse tumors rather than human tumors.

Enthusiasm for the cancer stem cell model arises, in part, from its therapeutic potential. Most of the drugs now used in treating cancer can kill a large fraction of cancer cells but may not touch the cancer stem cell. If less than 1 in 100,000 cells in a cancer is responsible for perpetuating a cancer, then perhaps we

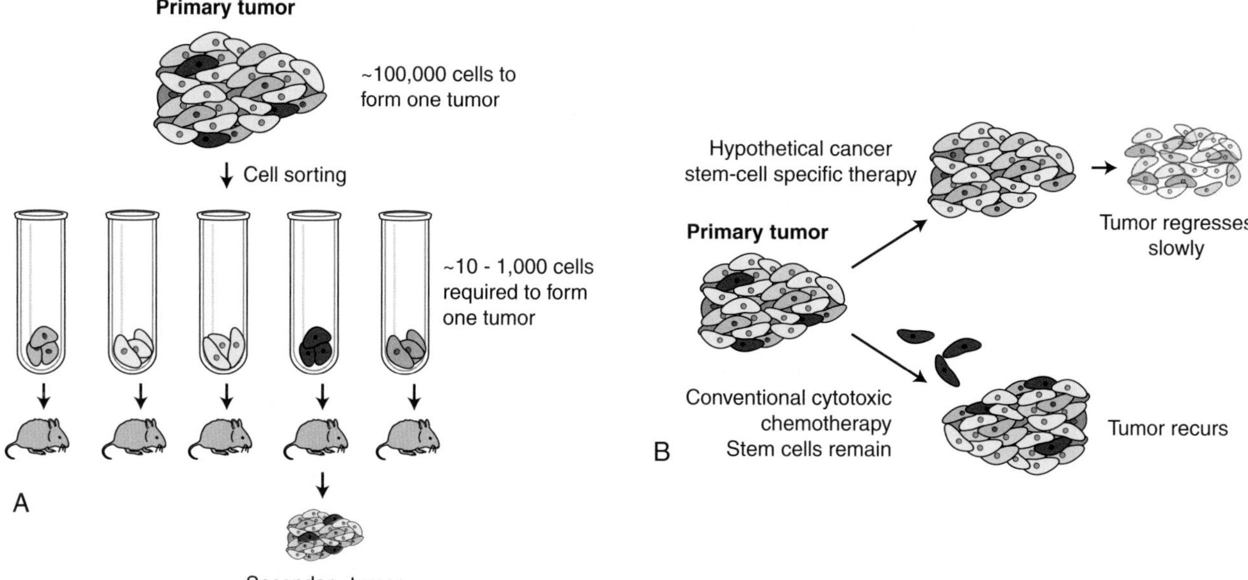

FIGURE 12-8 **Concept of Cancer Stem Cells. A,** Only rare cells within a cancer can initiate cancer regrowth. In laboratory experiments it takes as many as 100,000 breast cancer cells injected into a mouse mammary fat pad to form a new cancer. If the breast cancer cells are sorted, one rare subtype *(shown here in red)* is much more proficient at forming new cancers. **B,** Conventional chemotherapy can destroy the bulk of a cancer. However, if the cancer stem cells *(red cells)* are not destroyed, the cancer may regrow. If therapies can be devised that kill the cancer stem cells, then durable long-term responses may be achieved.

should be looking for drugs that target those rare cells instead of using more toxic drugs that initially shrink tumors but do not kill the cancer stem cells.

THE GENETIC BASIS OF CANCER

Cancer-Causing Mutations in Genes

Before the advent of modern molecular biology, many different causes of cancer were postulated, based on epidemiologic studies as well as investigations of specific carcinogens and viruses. We now understand that changes in the genes of the cancer cell cause the cell to become cancerous. As our knowledge of cancer biology continues to increase so too does our understanding of the many ways that heritable changes in cells can contribute to cancer. These changes include deoxyribonucleic acid (DNA) mutations, but also include changes in DNA and histone chemical modification (epigenetic changes), and, most recently recognized, changes in non–coding microribonucleic acid (miRNA) expression (also see Chapters 4, 6, and 13). Although the word *mutation* is used extensively here, it can also refer to heritable changes in gene and non–coding RNA expression (**epigenetics**) that do not involve changes in DNA sequence.

Cancer is predominantly a disease of aging. Perhaps the most revealing epidemiologic data are presented in Figure 12-9. The incidence of most cancer, that is, the fraction of individuals in each age group who develop cancer, increases dramatically with age. The best explanation for these epidemiologic data is that each individual acquires a number of genetic "hits" or mutations over time. When sufficient mutations have occurred, cancer develops. These epidemiologic data are consistent with the

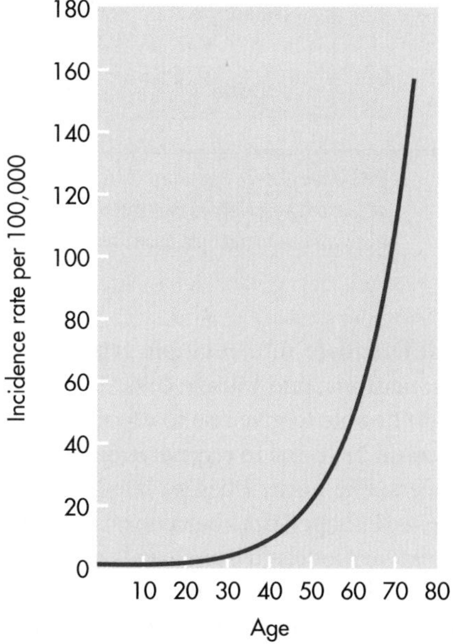

FIGURE 12-9 **Marked Increases in Cancer with Age.** The graph depicts the number of cases of colon cancer diagnosed per 100,000 women in England and Wales in 1 year. The incidence of cancer increases dramatically with advancing age. These data suggest that accumulation of genetic and epigenetic alterations over time increases the risk of developing cancer. The slope of the curve suggests that five to seven mutations must occur before full-blown cancer develops. (Modified from Alberts B et al: *Molecular biology of the cell,* ed 4, New York, 2002, Garland.)

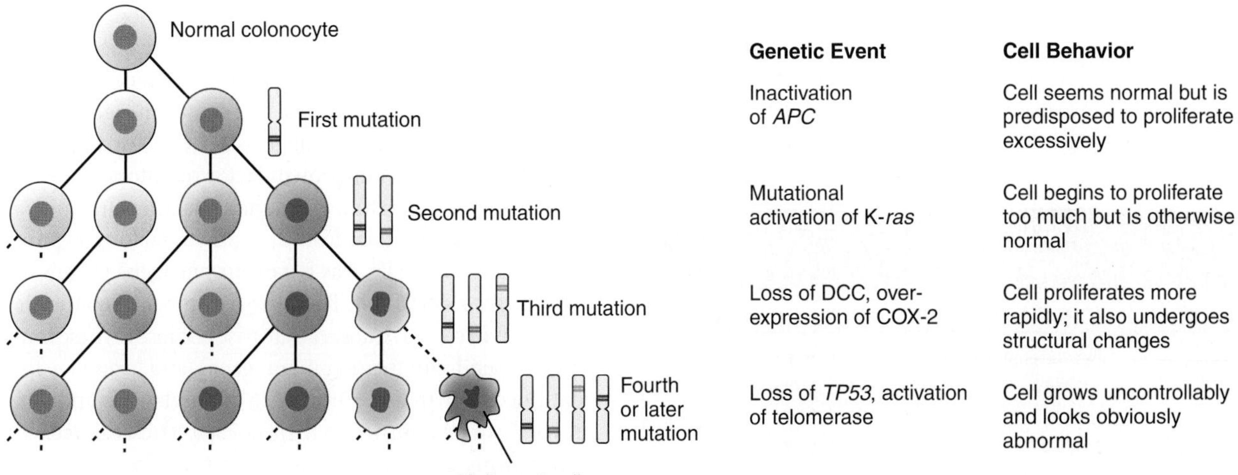

FIGURE 12-10 Clonal Proliferation Model of Neoplastic Progression. During clonal proliferation, progressively altered populations of cells arise over time. As genetic and epigenetic changes occur, different subclones (indicated by different color cells) coexist for a time. Clones that grow the fastest out-compete other clones, producing increasingly more malignant, and abnormal-appearing, growths. The sequential accumulation of mutations has been well studied in the progression from a normal colon cell to a benign intestinal polyp to a malignant colon cancer. One of the earliest mutations in colon cancer is loss of the tumor-suppressor gene *APC*. Additional mutations, often in the oncogene *ras*, activation of COX-2, and loss of the tumor suppressors DCC and *TP53* occur as the lesion progresses from a benign polyp to an invasive carcinoma. *APC*, Adenomatous polyposis coli; *COX-2*, cyclooxygenase-2; *DCC*, deleted in colon cancer. (Modified from Mendelsohn I et al: *The molecular basis of cancer*, ed 2, Philadelphia, 2001, Saunders; Kumar V, Cotran RS, Robbins SL: *Basic pathology*, ed 6, Philadelphia, 1997, Saunders.)

observation of mutations in early and advanced cancers and with data obtained from the study of experimental cancers created in the laboratory—the accumulation of four to seven specific hits over time is required to cause a full-blown cancer.[8]

Clonal Selection

As a cell accumulates specific mutations, it can acquire, step-by-step, the characteristics of a cancer cell, for example, anchorage-independent growth, lack of contact inhibition, and immortality. That mutant cell may then have a selective advantage over its neighbors; its progeny can accumulate faster than its nonmutant neighbors. This is referred to as **clonal proliferation** or **clonal expansion** (Figure 12-10). As a clone with a mutation proliferates, it may become an early stage tumor, for example, a carcinoma in situ or a benign colonic polyp. Additional heritable changes can occur in these early lesions that permit progression to more advanced tumors. The process of tumor development is a form of darwinian evolution; cells with a genetic change that confers a survival advantage out-compete their neighbors. The progressive accumulation of distinct advantageous (from the point of view of the cancer cell, not the individual!) mutations leads from normal cells to fully malignant cancers.

One organ in which this correlation of genetic and clinical progression has been especially well studied is the colon.[9] The colon is accessible to inspection with a colonoscope, and so neoplastic lesions of varying size can readily be detected and removed. Intestinal polyps are benign neoplasms and the first stage in development of colon cancer. Small polyps tend to have only a few detectable mutations. Large polyps have more mutations, whereas frank colon cancers have even more mutations. This type of genetic information provided the framework for the now widely accepted concept that it is the *stepwise accumulation* of alterations in specific genes that is required for the development of cancer (see Figure 12-10).

Oncogenes and Tumor-Suppressor Genes: Accelerators and Brakes

Passengers and Drivers

The previous discussion refers to the heritable changes in cells as being key in the development of cancer. New technologies that provide massive amounts of information about chromosome and gene structure allow us to see multiple alterations in cancer cells. These methods include massively parallel high-throughput DNA sequencing (the process by which the sequence of nucleotides along a strand of DNA is determined), high-density single-nucleotide polymorphism (SNP), and chromosome copy number analysis (CNA). These approaches confirm that there are a small number of very common genetic alterations in cancer and a very large number of alterations that individually are rare.[10] It is clear that some mutations can contribute to cancer progression (e.g., mutations in *p53* or *RAS*). These mutations are **driver mutations;** they drive the progression of cancer. Conversely, not all mutations in cancer contribute to the malignant phenotype. Some are just random events, and are referred to as **passenger mutations;** they are just along for the ride. The increasing amount of cancer genome analysis data poses the following question: how do we determine which mutations are drivers and which are passengers?

What Are the Driver Mutations? To understand how genetic mutations cause cancer, first it is important to distinguish between oncogenes and tumor-suppressor genes. Table 12-4 compares the two types of cancer genes. **Oncogenes** are mutant genes that in their normal nonmutant state direct synthesis of proteins that positively regulate (accelerate) proliferation. Conversely, **tumor-suppressor genes** encode proteins that in their normal state negatively regulate (halt, or "put the brakes on") proliferation. Hence, they also have been referred to as anti-oncogenes.

TABLE 12-4 COMPARISON OF CANCER GENE TYPES

GENE TYPE	NORMAL FUNCTION	MUTATION EFFECT
Caretaker	DNA and chromosome stability	Chromosome instability and increased rates of mutation
Dominant oncogenes*	Encode proteins that promote growth (e.g., growth factors)	Overexpression or amplification causes gain of function
Tumor suppressors (recessive oncogenes)	Encode proteins that inhibit proliferation and prevent or repair mutations	Requires loss of function of both alleles to increase cancer risk

*Nonmutant state referred to as proto-oncogene.

In its normal, nonmutant state, an oncogene is referred to as a **proto-oncogene.** An example of a proto-oncogene would be a growth factor (e.g., epidermal growth factor) or a growth factor receptor (e.g., epidermal growth factor receptor). Other positive regulators of proliferation are in the signal transduction pathway that transmits the signal from the growth factor receptor to the cell nucleus. Normally, Ras is a proto-oncogene (Figure 12-11).

Oncogene Addiction. There are a number of common driver mutations in cancer. Cancers that arise because of these mutations often depend on these mutant genes and proteins for their continued growth and survival. If the mutations and abnormal proteins can be returned to their normal states, the cancers often stop growing and even regress. The cancers are addicted to their mutant cancer genes, a concept known as **oncogene addiction.** This also provides a key example of how targeted cancer therapy can work—for example, if the oncogene is a protein kinase (e.g., BCR-ABL, EGFR, HER2, or BRAF) that can be inhibited by a drug, then the cancer can be deprived of the function of the oncogene. Treating the addiction treats the cancer.[11]

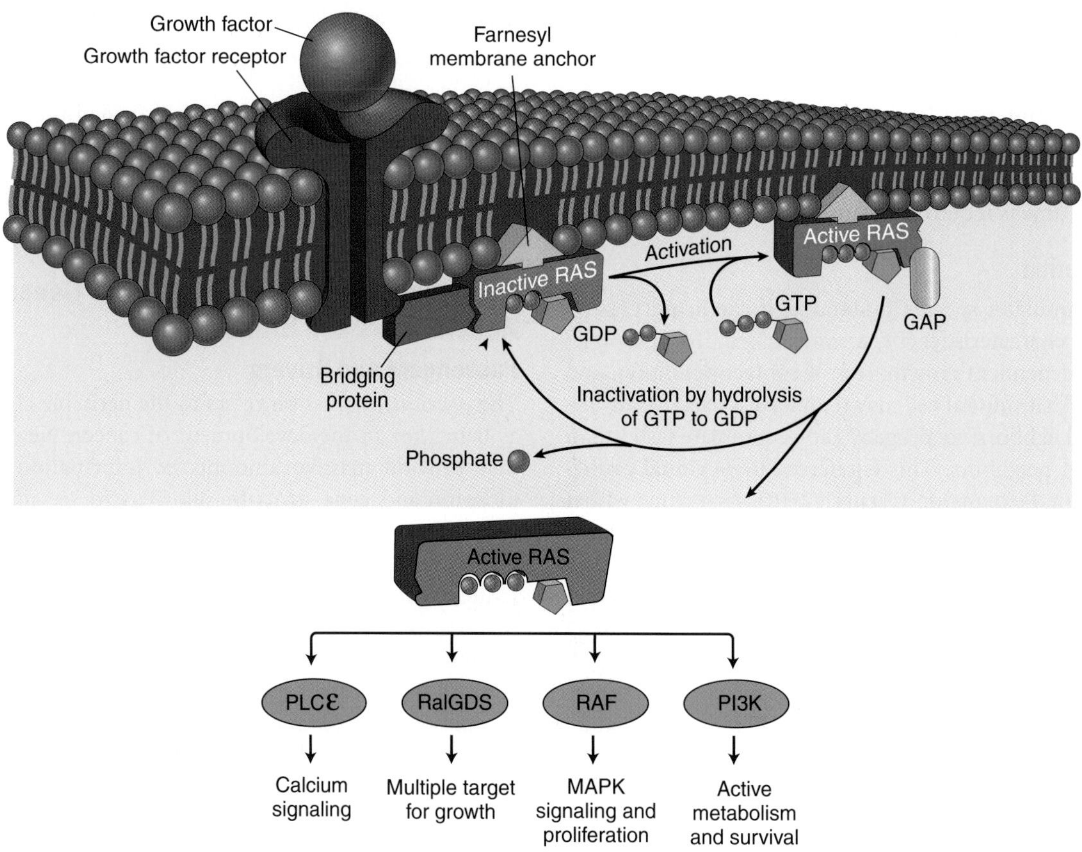

FIGURE 12-11 Many Growth Factors Signal Through the RAS Protein. When a normal cell is stimulated through a growth factor binding to its receptor, inactive RAS exchanges GDP for GTP, becoming active. Active (GTP-bound) RAS sends growth signals throughout the cell by interacting with a number of signaling proteins, including RalGDS, RAF, PLCε, and PI3K. RAS is normally inactivated when it hydrolyzes GTP to GDP. Oncogenic Ras has a mutation that blocks hydrolysis of GTP, thereby locking RAS in the active configuration. *GDP,* Guanosine diphosphate; *GAP,* guanosine triphosphate-activating protein; *GTP,* guanosine triphosphate; *MAPK,* mitogen-activated protein kinase; *PI3K,* phosphoinositide 3-kinase; *PLCε,* phospholipase C-epsilon; *RAF,* serine/threonine-specific protein kinase; *RalGDS,* Ral guanine nucleotide dissociation stimulator; *Ras,* RAS protein. (Adapted from Kumar V, Abbas AK, Aster J: *Robbins basic pathology,* ed 9, Philadelphia, 2013, Saunders.)

Gene Changes That Occur in Cancer

The activation and inactivation of various genes is key in the development of cancer. The following three types of DNA changes occur in cancer: small DNA changes, large DNA changes, and epigenetic changes.

Mutation of Normal Genes into Oncogenes

Point Mutations. Several types of genetic events can activate oncogenes (Box 12-1 and Figure 12-12). Perhaps the most common events are small-scale changes in DNA such as **point mutations,** the alteration of one or a few nucleotide base pairs (see Chapter 4). This type of mutation can have profound effects on the activity of proteins. A point mutation in the *ras* gene converts it from a regulated proto-oncogene to an unregulated oncogene, an accelerator of cellular proliferation. Activating point mutations in *ras* are found in many cancers, especially pancreatic and colorectal cancer.[12] Specialized tests, such as direct DNA sequencing, can detect such point mutations in clinical samples.

BOX 12-1 TYPES OF GENETIC LESIONS IN CANCER

1. Point mutations
2. Subtle alterations (insertions, deletions)
3. Chromosome changes (aneuploidy and loss of heterozygosity)
4. Amplifications
5. Gene silencing (DNA methylation, histone modification, microRNAs)
6. Exogenous sequences (tumor viruses)

Chromosome Translocations and Copy Number Variation. **Chromosome translocations** are large changes in chromosome structure in which a piece of one chromosome is translocated to another chromosome. Translocations can activate oncogenes in one of two distinct mechanisms. First, a translocation can cause excess and inappropriate production of a proliferation factor. One of the best examples is the t(8;14) translocation found in many Burkitt lymphomas;[13] t(8;14) designates a chromosome that has a piece of chromosome 8 fused to a piece of chromosome 14 (see Chapter 29). Burkitt lymphoma is an aggressive cancer of B lymphocytes. The *myc* proto-oncogene found on chromosome 8 is normally activated at low levels in proliferating lymphocytes and is deactivated in mature lymphocytes. The **MYC protein** is part of the positive signal for cell proliferation. If accidental formation of the t(8;14) translocation occurs, the *myc* gene is aberrantly placed under the control of a B-cell immunoglobulin gene *(Ig)* present on chromosome 14. The *Ig* gene is very active in maturing B lymphocytes. The t(8;14) translocation alters the control of *myc;* its normal low level is switched to high levels, as directed by an *Ig* gene promoter. MYC protein, when inappropriately high, drives proliferation and blocks

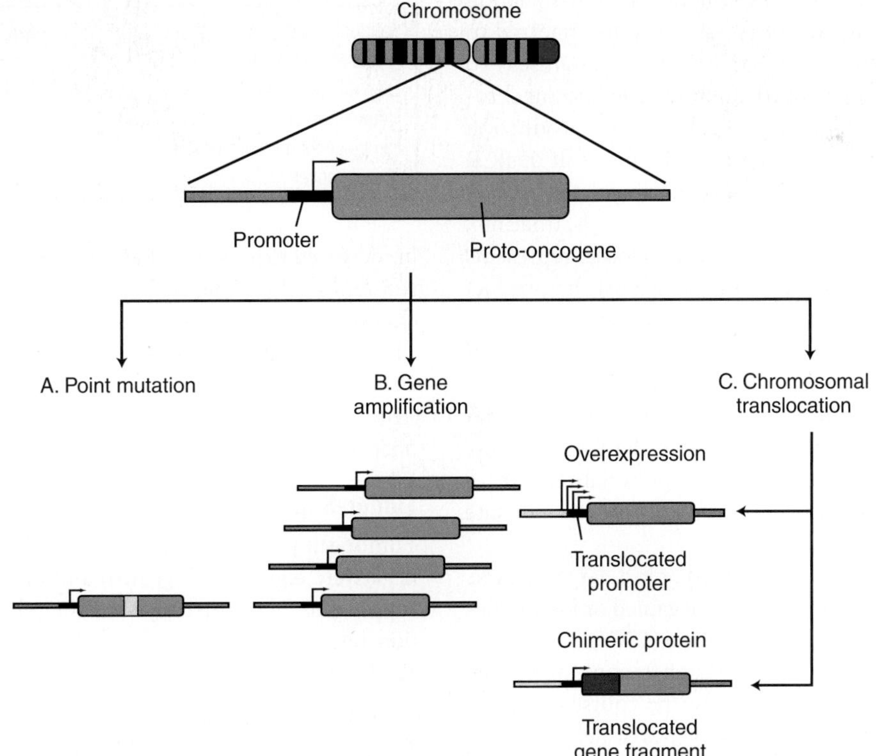

FIGURE 12-12 Oncogene Activation Mechanisms. Cellular genes may become cancerous oncogenes as a result of **(A)** point mutations that alter one or a few nucleotide base pairs, causing the production of a protein that is activated as a result of the altered sequence (e.g., *ras*); **(B)** amplification of the cellular gene, resulting in higher levels of protein expression (e.g., *N-myc* in neuroblastoma); or **(C)** chromosomal translocations that either lead to the juxtaposition of a strong promoter, causing increased protein expression (*c-myc* in Burkitt lymphoma), or produce a novel fusion protein that is derived from gene fragments normally present on different chromosomes (*Bcr-Abl* in chronic myeloid leukemia). (From Haber DA: *Molecular genetics of cancer.* In *ACP medicine,* Danbury, CT, 2004, WebMD.)

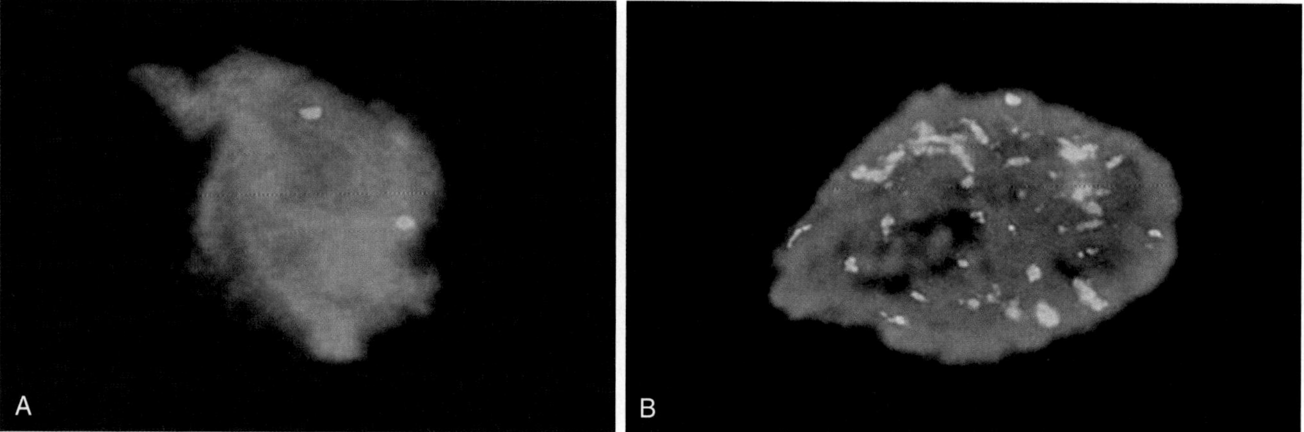

FIGURE 12-13 ***N-myc*** **Gene Amplification in Neuroblastoma.** The *N-myc* gene is detected in human neuroblastoma cells using a technique called FISH (fluorescent in situ hybridization). **A,** A single pair of *N-myc* genes are detected in normal cells and in low-grade neuroblastoma. **B,** Multiple, amplified copies of the *N-myc* gene are detected in some cases of neuroblastoma. Amplification of the *N-myc* gene is strongly associated with a poor prognosis in childhood neuroblastoma. (Courtesy Arthur R. Brothman, PhD, FACMG, University of Utah School of Medicine, Salt Lake City, UT.)

differentiation. Hence, the t(8;14) translocation causes cancer of maturing B cells (see Figure 12-12, *C*).

Second, chromosome translocations also can lead to production of novel proteins with growth-promoting properties. In a different type of leukemia, chronic myeloid leukemia (CML), a specific chromosome translocation is almost always present. This translocation, t(9;22), was first identified in association with CML in Philadelphia in 1960 and so is often referred to as the Philadelphia chromosome.[14] This translocation fuses two chromosomes in the middle of two different genes, *bcr* on chromosome 9 and *abl* on chromosome 22. The result is production of a BCR-ABL fusion protein containing the first half of BCR and the second half of ABL. BCR-ABL is a misregulated protein tyrosine kinase that promotes growth of myeloid cells. Imatinib, a drug that specifically targets this tyrosine kinase, represents the first successful chemotherapy targeted against the product of a specific oncogenic mutation. Imatinib and related tyrosine kinase inhibitors (TKIs) are highly effective in the treatment of CML and, because of their specificity, lack the toxic side effects noted with nonspecific anticancer drugs.[15] However, imatinib is not effective in cancers that do not have the t(9;22) translocation or related mutations. In modern personalized cancer therapy, knowledge of the specific genetic alteration can dictate the optimal drugs for the individual.

Just as single nucleotides can be gained or lost, larger regions of DNA encompassing entire genes can be gained or lost, a phenomenon known as **copy number variation (CNV).**[16] CNV can be inherited and accounts for a significant fraction of human genetic diversity. CNV also can occur in the course of cancer development, where it can amplify oncogenes or delete tumor-suppressor genes.

Gene Amplification. Another type of genetic abnormality that can activate oncogenes is **gene amplification** (see Figures 12-12, *B*, and 12-13). Amplifications are the result of duplication of a small piece of a chromosome over and over again, so that instead of the normal two copies of a gene, tens or even hundreds of copies are present (see Chapter 4). Gene amplification results in increased expression of an oncogene, or in some cases, drug resistance genes. The *N-myc* oncogene is amplified in 25% of childhood neuroblastoma cases and confers a poor prognosis.[17] The epidermal growth factor receptor *erbB2* is amplified in 20% of breast cancers.[18] Individuals whose cancers have *erbB2* amplification respond well to drugs specifically targeted to this oncogene.[19]

TABLE 12-5 SOME FAMILIAL CANCER SYNDROMES CAUSED BY LOSS OF TUMOR-SUPPRESSOR GENE FUNCTION

SYNDROME	GENE
Retinoblastoma	*RB1*
Li-Fraumeni syndrome	*p53 (TP53)*
Familial melanoma	*$p16^{INK4a}$* (CDKN2A)
Neurofibromatosis	*Neurofibromin (NF1)*
Familial adenomatous polyps	*APC*
Breast cancer	*BRCA1*

Tumor-Suppressor Genes

Tumor-suppressor genes are genes whose major function is to negatively regulate cell growth and prevent mutations. Tumor suppressors may normally slow the cell cycle, inhibit proliferation resulting from growth signals, or stop cell division when cells are damaged. Examples of several tumor suppressors are given in Table 12-5. One of the first discovered tumor-suppressor genes, the **retinoblastoma *(Rb)* gene,** normally strongly inhibits the cell division cycle (see Chapter 1). When it is inactivated, the cell division cycle can proceed unchecked. *Rb* is mutated in childhood retinoblastoma, and in many lung, breast, and bone cancers as well.

Whereas oncogenes are activated in cancers, tumor suppressors must be inactivated to allow cancer to occur (see Table 12-5 and Figure 12-14). A single genetic event can activate an

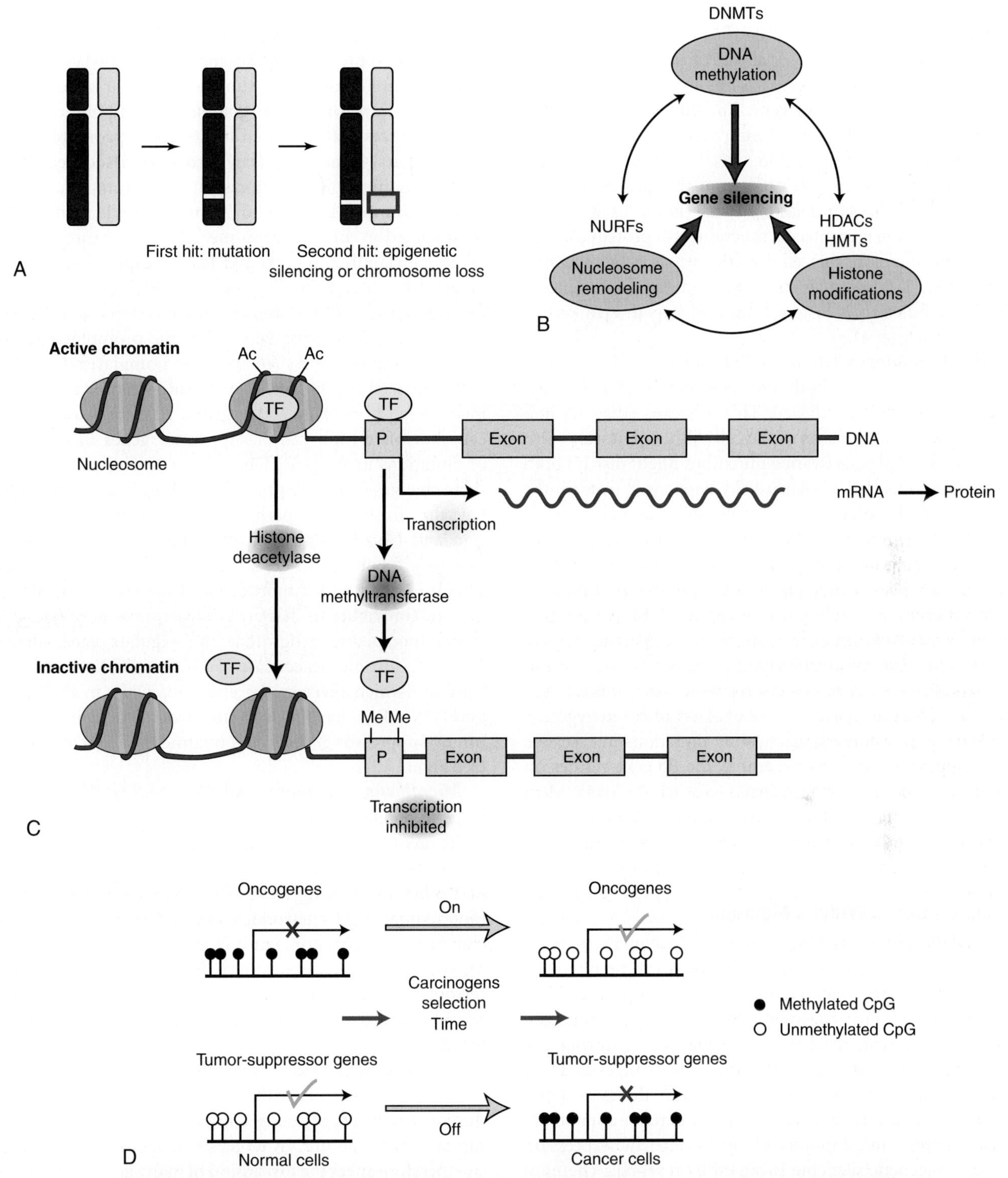

FIGURE 12-14 **Silencing Tumor-Suppressor Genes by Epigenetic Alterations.** Tumor-suppressor genes can be turned off by a variety of mechanisms. **A,** In this example, the first hit is a point mutation in a tumor-suppressor gene *(white box),* followed by either epigenetic silencing or chromosome loss of the second allele *(red box).* **B,** Genes can normally be silenced by a variety of interacting processes including DNA methylation, histone modifications, nucleosome remodeling, and microRNAs (not shown). A number of cellular enzymes contribute to these modifications, including DNA methyltransferases *(DNMTs),* histone deacetylases *(HDACs),* histone methyltransferases *(HMTs),* and complex nucleosomal remodeling factors *(NURFs).* Gene silencing is essential for normal development and differentiation. **C,** Histone modification and promoter methylation regulate gene expression. Genes are transcribed when chromatin is modified by addition of acetyl *(Ac)* groups to specific lysine groups in histones. Gene expression can be turned off when specific acetyl groups are removed by HDACs or when the CpG-rich promoter regions of genes are modified by direct DNA methylation (by DNA methyltransferase). In addition, small endogenous RNA molecules (microRNAs or miRNA) can bind to mRNA and reduce gene expression. **D,** Changes in promoter methylation turn cancer genes off and on. Oncogenes can be turned on by promoter hypomethylation, and tumor-suppressor genes can be turned off by promoter hypermethylation. Each of these changes can produce selective growth and survival advantage for the cancer cell. (**B** adapted from Jones PA, Baylin SB: *Cell* 128:683–692, 2007; **C** from Gluckman PD et al: *N Engl J Med* 359[1]:66, 2008; **D** from Shames DS, Minna JF, Gazdar AF: *Curr Mol Med* 7:85–102, 2007.)

oncogene because it can act in a dominant manner in the cell. However, we have two copies, or alleles, of each gene, one from each parent. It therefore takes two hits to inactivate the two alleles of a tumor-suppressor gene. The first allele of a tumor suppressor is often inactivated by point mutations. For example, the *Rb* gene may be inactivated on one chromosome by a point mutation (e.g., the copy inherited from the father). Because the other copy of the retinoblastoma gene (in this example, the one from the mother) is intact, a functional RB protein can still be made and therefore the cell division cycle can be regulated appropriately. If the remaining gene is mutated or silenced, then all RB function is lost and another step toward cancer occurs (see Chapter 4).

Loss of Heterozygosity. For the function of a tumor suppressor to be lost, both chromosomal copies (alleles) of the gene must be inactivated. This is because they act in a recessive manner at the level of the cell. Although it may seem intuitive that simple inactivating mutations might disrupt both alleles, in fact this is not what usually happens.[20] Instead, the first allele (in the preceding example, the paternal copy) is inactivated by simple mutation, but the second allele (in this example, the maternal copy) is lost because entire regions of the maternal chromosome are epigenetically silenced or a piece of the chromosome is simply lost (see Figure 12-14, *A*). Because humans have two chromosomes, one from each parent, they are always *heterozygous* for nearby multiple genetic markers; loss of one copy (allele) of a chromosome region in a tumor is referred to as **loss of heterozygosity,** or **LOH.** Loss of heterozygosity, like silencing, can unmask inactivating mutations in recessive tumor-suppressor genes. For example, the *Rb* gene resides on chromosome 13, in a region referred to as q14 (13q14). Most individuals with *Rb* mutations have a subtle mutation in one allele and have lost the other copy of *Rb* through loss of the 13q14 chromosome region on the other chromosome.

Turning Off Genes Without Mutation

Epigenetic Silencing. Abnormal gene silencing is emerging as a major cause of cancer. Gene expression can be regulated in a heritable manner (i.e., passed from a parent to a child or from a single cell to its progeny) by an "epigenetic" mechanism called **silencing.** Inheritance of silencing occurs during cell division and does not require mutations or changes in DNA sequence (also see Chapter 6). More simply, the same DNA sequence can produce dramatically different phenotypes depending on chemical modifications that alter the expression of genes. Epigenetic silencing is caused by reversible chemical modification (methylation [addition of a methyl group] or acetylation [addition of an acetyl group]) of histones and related chromatin components, as well as methylation of cytosine residues in DNA (known as **DNA methylation**) (see Figure 12-14, Figures 6-2, 6-3, and Chapter 16). Whole regions of chromosomes are normally shut off by silencing, so that the pattern of gene expression is different than that seen in other cells with the same genes. In this way, the progeny of liver cells remain liver cells, and skin cells remain skin cells. Notably, *global* changes in epigenetic silencing can turn these cells back into stem cells.[21]

Changes in gene silencing contribute to the development of cancer.[22] Many cancers have increased methylation of DNA in the promoter region of tumor-suppressor genes (in CpG islands or C-cytosine and G-guanine, p-phosphodiester bond, rich sequences that are often located near promoter regions; see Chapters 4 and 13). They also have associated changes in the modification of histones in the chromatin, including methylation of lysines 9 and 27 in histone H3. In addition, overexpression of chromosome silencing proteins known as the polycomb complex, and loss of expression of histone deacetylases (enzymes that remove acetyl groups from histone proteins) SIRT1 is seen in human cancers. These changes in chromatin-modifying genes alter the promoter regions of genes leading to their silencing. The boundaries of the normally silenced regions can also spread in cancer cells, thereby inactivating previously active genes. In either case, silencing can shut off critical tumor-suppressor genes in the absence of mutations in the gene. Early in the development of cancer, these changes in gene expression can lead to a selective advantage for affected cells, perhaps leading to their immortalization and clonal expansion. Silencing of tumor suppressors may be a faster way to create cancer cells than mutational or genetic loss of tumor suppressors.[23] Conversely, loss of silencing can contribute to inappropriate expression of oncogenes. Chemotherapeutic drugs that can regulate gene silencing, including histone deacetylase (HDAC) inhibitors and 5-azacytidine (which reverses the effects of DNA methyltransferases [DNMTs]), have proven effective in reactivating silenced tumor-suppressor genes in the treatment of selected cancers[24] (see Figure 12-14).

MicroRNAs, Oncomirs, and Non–coding RNAs. Changes in gene regulation can affect not just single genes, but also entire networks of signaling. Gene expression networks can be regulated by changes in **microRNAs (miRNAs,** or **miRs)** and other non–coding RNAs (ncRNAs). miRNAs are short (approximately 22 nucleotides) RNAs derived from introns of protein coding genes or transcribed as independent genes from regions of the genome previously believed to have no function (erroneously called junk DNA). The human genome encodes more than 1000 miRs. miRs regulate diverse signaling pathways; the miRs that stimulate cancer development and progression are termed **oncomirs.** miRs decrease the stability and expression of other genes by pairing with mRNA in a process that involves the RNA-induced silencing complex, or RISC. A single miR can have multiple mRNA targets. Changes in miR abundance can therefore affect the expression of many genes, making miRs both powerful regulators and challenging subjects to study.[25] Beyond miRs, longer RNAs without apparent protein coding capacity also are implicated in cellular regulation with an emerging appreciation of their role in cancer.[26]

miRs can play both positive and negative roles in cancer. The importance of miRs in cancer was first shown in chronic lymphocytic leukemia (CLL), where a chromosome region encoding miR15 and miR16 was found to be deleted in a large number of individuals. Decreased expression of these two miRs is seen in many cases of CLL, as well as in prostate and several other cancers, and results in increased expression of a number of oncogenes. Conversely, increased expression of a cluster of miRs (17-18-19-20-92) is seen in some lymphomas and solid tumors, causing the decreased expression of a number of tumor-suppressor genes. miR expression can be easily assessed with microarray technology, leading to the realization that substantial changes in miR expression are seen in many cancers.

Guardians of the Genome

The previous discussion of mutations leads naturally to the question of how mutations occur in the first place. The integrity of genetic information can be compromised at several points: during each round of DNA synthesis, during each mitosis when chromosomes are segregated to daughter cells, and when external mutagens (e.g., chemicals and radiation) alter or disrupt DNA. Multiple mechanisms have evolved to protect and repair the genome.[27] These repair mechanisms are directed by **caretaker genes,** genes that are responsible for the maintenance of genomic integrity. Caretaker genes encode proteins that are involved in repairing damaged DNA, such as occurs with errors in DNA replication, mutations caused by ultraviolet or ionizing radiation, and mutations caused by chemicals and drugs. Loss of function of caretaker genes leads to increased mutation rates. If DNA damage is severe, the cell undergoes programmed cell death, or apoptosis, rather than simply dividing with damaged DNA.

Inherited mutations can disrupt the caretaker genes that protect the integrity of the genome. Examples include the disorder xeroderma pigmentosum (XP); affected individuals have defects in the repair of ultraviolet light–induced DNA damage and should avoid direct sunlight exposure. They have a very high incidence of skin cancer. Hereditary nonpolyposis colorectal cancer (HNPCC) results from an inherited defect in repairing DNA base pair mismatches that occur occasionally during DNA replication. Affected individuals have an increased rate of small insertions and deletions in DNA, leading to a high rate of colon and other cancers.[28] Finally, there are inherited mutations that threaten the integrity of entire chromosomes. Bloom syndrome, caused by mutations in a DNA helicase, and Fanconi aplastic anemia, caused by loss of function of a multiprotein complex required for repair of DNA double-stranded breaks, are autosomal recessive disorders in which affected individuals demonstrate marked chromosomal instability. Chromosome breaks, aberrant fusions, and chromosome loss are common. As a consequence, these individuals have a high risk of developing cancer at an early age.

The rate of individual gene mutation is probably too low to account for the acquisition of many new mutations during the evolution of a malignant cancer clone. In addition to abnormal epigenetic silencing, **chromosome instability** (often referred to as CIN) also appears to be increased in malignant cells.[29] The underlying mechanism of this instability is not clear but may be caused by malfunctions in the cellular machinery that regulates chromosome segregation at mitosis.[30] Chromosome instability results in a high rate of chromosome loss, as well as loss of heterozygosity and chromosome amplification. Each of these events can accelerate the loss of tumor-suppressor genes and the overexpression of oncogenes.

Genetics and Cancer-Prone Families

Genetic events are the primary basis of carcinogenesis. Most of the genetic and epigenetic alterations that cause cancer occur within the somatic tissues during the lifetime of the individual. As previously discussed, the frequency of genetic changes can be increased by exposure to **mutagens,** that is, agents causing mutations, and by defects in DNA repair. Because these genetic events occur in somatic cells as opposed to germ cells, they are not transmitted to future generations. Even though they are genetic events they are not inherited! It is possible, however, for cancer-predisposing mutations to occur in germline cells (cells that produce gametes). Mutations present in germline cells result in the transmission of cancer-causing genes from one generation to the next, producing families with a high incidence of specific cancers. These inherited mutations that predispose to cancer are almost invariably found in tumor-suppressor genes (see Table 12-5).

Although rare, such "cancer families" demonstrate that inheritance of a mutated gene can cause cancer (Figure 12-15).

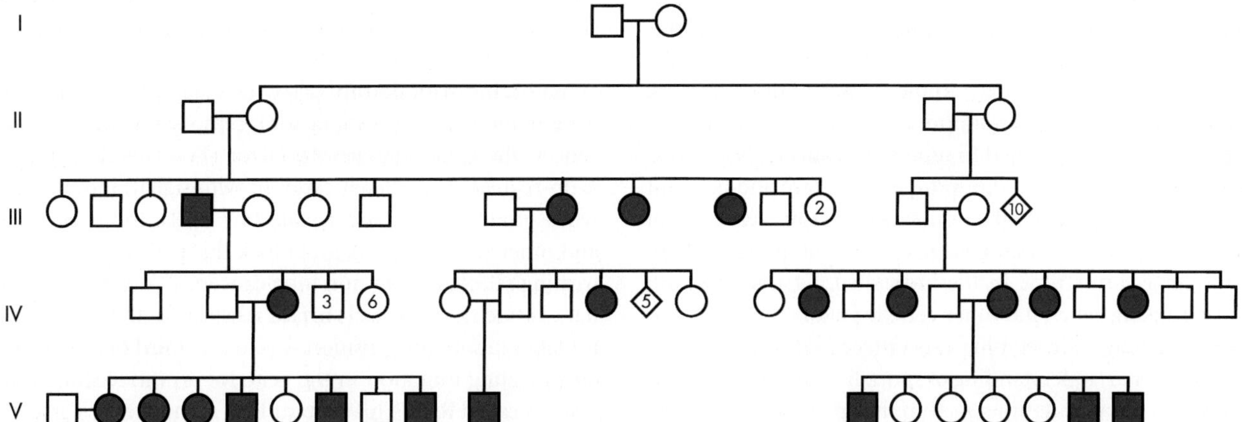

FIGURE 12-15 Familial Colon Cancer Pedigree. Darkened symbols represent individuals diagnosed with colon cancer. One of the individuals in the first generation must have carried a mutation in the *APC* gene. (From Jorde LB et al: *Medical genetics,* ed 4, St Louis, 2010, Mosby.)

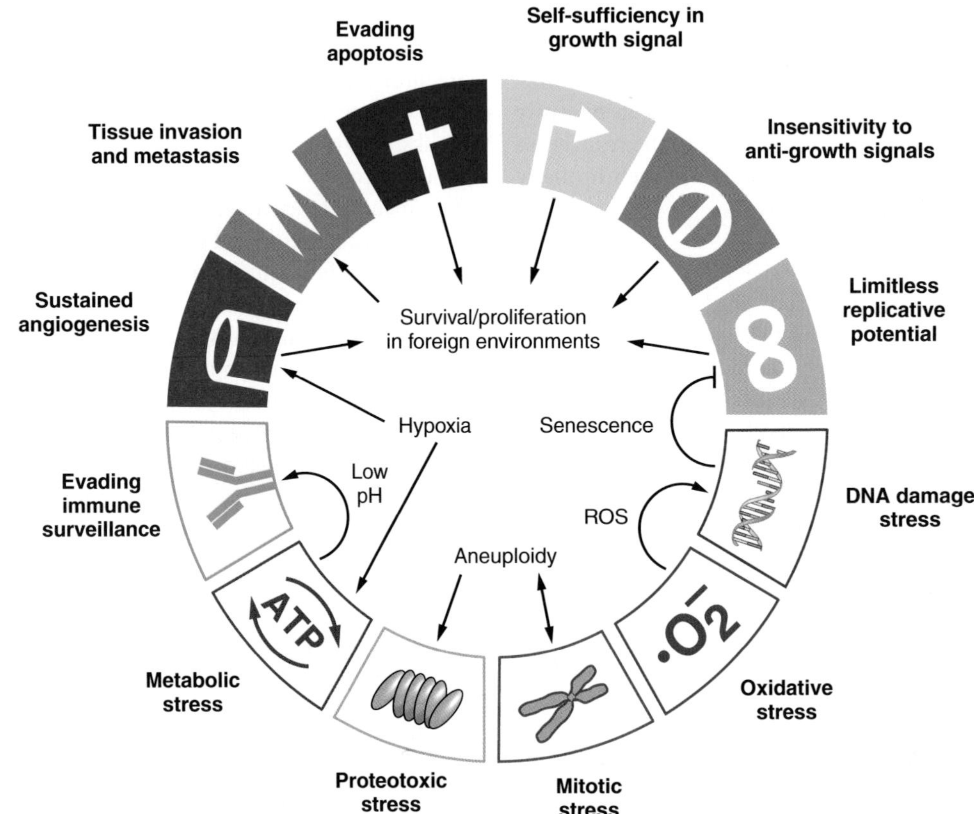

FIGURE 12-16 **Hallmarks of Cancer.** Cancers acquire alterations in specific pathways during their evolution. The six key pathways that must be altered are shown at the top of the circle, and supporting pathways are shown at the bottom of the circle. Mutation in key genes often alters several pathways; for example, *p53* mutations alter both angiogenesis and evasion of apoptosis. ⌒ = Inhibits. (From Luo J, Solimini NL, Elledge SJ: *Cell* 136:823–837, 2009.)

Inheritance of one mutant allele in these families predisposes a person to a specific form of cancer.[31] Individuals who inherit the germline mutant allele will inevitably suffer loss of the normal allele by loss of heterozygosity (LOH) or **epigenetic silencing** (see Figure 12-14) in some cells and eventually develop the tumor. Examples of human cancers that can be inherited are retinoblastoma, a childhood cancer of the eye that can be caused by germline mutations in one allele of the *Rb* gene; Wilms tumor, a childhood cancer of the kidney *(Wt1);* neurofibromatosis *(Nf1);* inherited breast cancer *(BRCA1);* and familial polyposis coli or adenomas of the colon *(APC).* A specific tumor-suppressor gene has been found in each of these cancers. In many cases, these tumor-suppressor genes also are inactivated in sporadic (as opposed to inherited) cancers. For example, inherited mutations in the *APC* gene are rare and account for only a few percent of all colon cancers. However, 85% of sporadic colon cancers also have acquired mutations of *APC,* which occurred over time in the individual. Characterization of cancer-causing genes and other genetic factors helps identify individuals prone to developing cancer (see Figure 12-15) and contributes to our understanding of sporadic cancers. Individuals known to carry mutations in tumor-suppressor genes (for example, women with a germline *BRCA1* mutation) are offered targeted cancer screening to facilitate early cancer detection and therapy.[32]

Types of Genes Misregulated in Cancer

Alterations in Progrowth and Antigrowth Signals

We now understand that multiple genetic hits are required for the evolution of full-blown cancer. One key question is, what types of genes must be altered to cause a cancer? In 2000, a highly influential paper by Hanahan and Weinberg[33] proposed six specific pathways that must be misregulated for cancer to develop (see Figures 12-10, 12-11, and 12-16). First, cancer cells must have mutations that enable them to proliferate in the absence of external growth signals. To achieve this, some cancers acquire the ability to secrete growth factors that stimulate their own growth, a process known as **autocrine stimulation** (also see Chapter 1). Other cancers have an increase in growth factor receptors; for example, in breast cancer, the epidermal growth factor (EGF) receptor HER2/neu is up-regulated, and likely sends growth signals into the cell even when growth factors are at very low levels. Inhibitors of HER2 and other EGF receptors that block this pathway are effective in treating selected breast and lung cancers.[34] Alternatively, the signal cascade from the cell surface receptor to the nucleus may be mutated in the "on" position. Up to one third of all cancers have an activating mutation in the gene for an intracellular signaling protein called **RAS.** This mutant RAS stimulates cell growth even when growth factors are missing (see Figure 12-11).

Cells also usually receive diverse "antigrowth" signals from their normal milieu. Contact with other cells, with basement

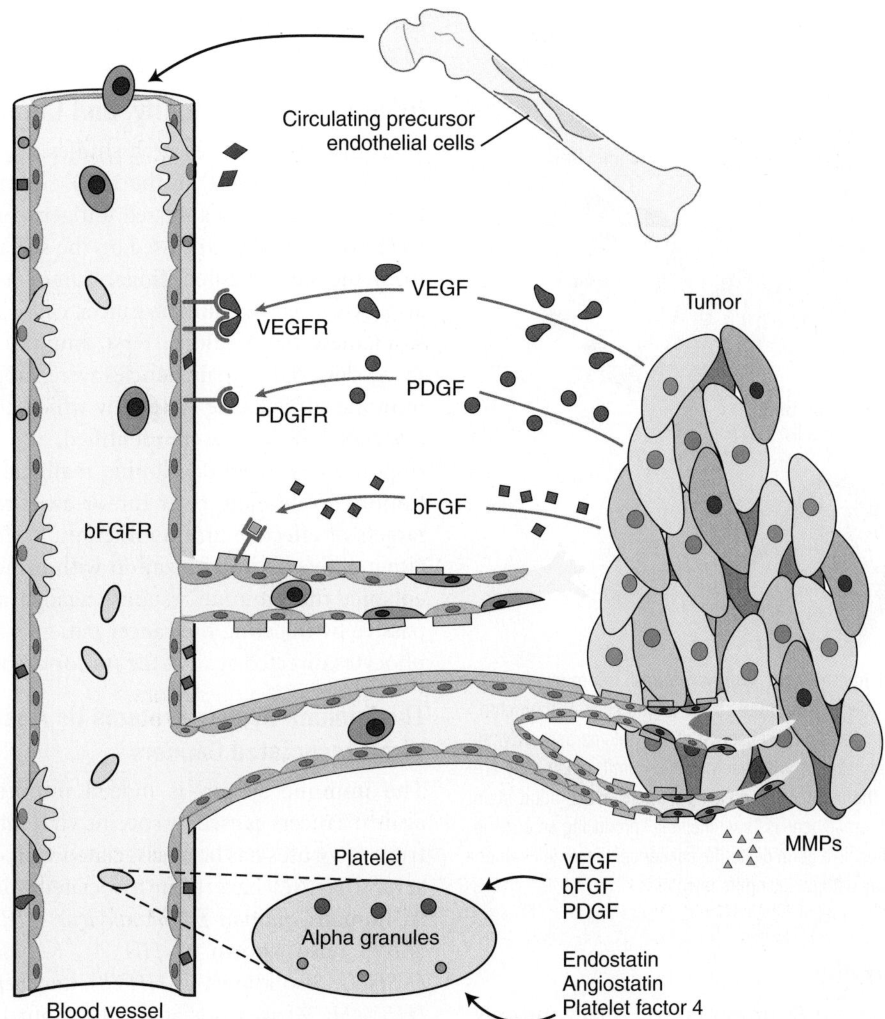

FIGURE 12-17 Tumor-Induced Angiogenesis. Malignant tumors secrete angiogenic factors and tissue-remodeling matrix metalloproteinases *(MMPs)* that actively induce formation of new blood vessels. New blood vessels are formed from both local endothelial cells and circulating precursor cells recruited from the bone marrow. Circulating platelets can also release regulatory proteins into the tumor. *bFGF* and *bFGFR,* Basic fibroblast growth factor and its receptor, respectively; *PDGF* and *PDGFR,* platelet-derived growth factor and its receptor, respectively; *VEGF* and *VEGFR,* vascular endothelial growth factor and its receptor, respectively. (Adapted from Folkman J: *Nat Rev Drug Discov* 6[4]:273–286, 2007.)

membranes, and with soluble factors all normally signal cells to stop proliferating. These mechanisms can put a halt to unregulated cell growth. In addition, this normal antigrowth signal must be inactivated or ignored. Common mutations that subvert the antigrowth signal include inactivation of the tumor-suppressor *retinoblastoma* or, conversely, activation of the protein kinases that drive the cell cycle, the *cyclin-dependent kinases* (see Chapter 1). Next, cells have a mechanism that causes them to self-destruct when growth is excessive and cell cycle checkpoints have been ignored. This self-destruct mechanism, called **apoptosis,** is triggered by diverse stimuli, including normal development and excessive growth (see Chapter 2). The pathway to apoptosis is disabled in advanced cancers. The most common mutations conferring resistance to apoptosis occur in the *TP53* gene.

Angiogenesis

If cancers are to grow larger than a millimeter in diameter, they need their own blood supply to deliver oxygen and nutrients. However, in adults new blood vessel growth is normally limited to areas of wound healing and to the uterus during the proliferative phase of the menstrual cycle. Tiny cancers lack the ability to grow new blood vessels and may never grow larger than a grain of sand. More advanced cancers can, however, secrete multiple factors that stimulate new blood vessel growth (called neovascularization or **angiogenesis**). The **angiogenic factors,** such as *vascular endothelial growth factor (VEGF), platelet-derived growth factor (PDGF),* and *basic fibroblast growth factor (bFGF),* by recruiting new vascular endothelial cells and initiating the proliferation of existing blood vessel cells, allow small cancers to become large cancers.[35] Therapies directed against new vessel growth are in clinical use; these agents include bevacizumab, a monoclonal antibody that inhibits VEGF; erlotinib, sorafenib, and sunitinib, inhibitors of the VEGF and PDGF receptor tyrosine kinases; and thalidomide, which decreases vascular proliferation[36] (Figure 12-17).

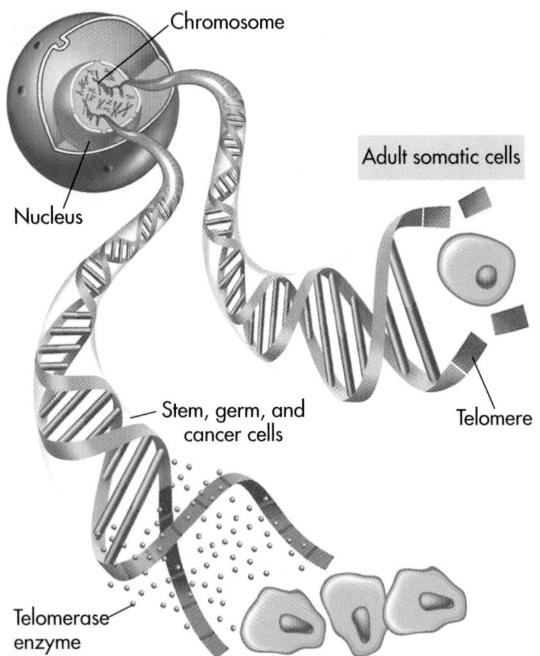

FIGURE 12-18 Control of Immortality: Telomeres and Telomerase. Normal adult somatic cells cannot divide indefinitely because the ends of their chromosomes are capped by telomeres. In the absence of the telomerase enzyme, telomeres become progressively shorter with each division until, when they are critically short, they signal to the cell to stop dividing. In germ cells, adult stem cells, and cancer cells the telomerase gene is "switched on," producing an enzyme that rebuilds the telomeres. Thus, like germ cells, the cancer cell becomes immortal and able to divide indefinitely without losing its telomeres.

Telomeres and Immortality

A hallmark of cancer cells is their immortality. Usually the only cells in the body that are "immortal" are germ cells (those that generate sperm and eggs) and stem cells. Other cells in the body are not immortal and can divide only a limited number of times (known as the Hayflick limit) before they cease dividing. One major block to unlimited cell division (i.e., immortality) is the size of a specialized structure called the *telomere.* **Telomeres** are protective ends, or caps, on each chromosome and are placed and maintained by a specialized enzyme called **telomerase** (Figure 12-18). As you might expect, telomerase is usually active only in germ cells (in ovaries and testes) and in stem cells. All other cells of the body lack telomerase. Therefore, when non–germ cells begin to proliferate abnormally, their telomere caps become smaller and smaller with each cell division. Short telomeres normally signal the cell to cease cell division. If the telomeres become critically small, the chromosomes become unstable and fragment, and then the cells die. Cancer cells, when they reach a critical age, activate telomerase somehow in order to restore and maintain their telomeres and thereby make it possible to divide over and over again.[37] Because telomerase is specifically activated in cancer cells, and potentially in cancer stem cells, it is an attractive therapeutic target.[38]

Finally, it appears genetic differences exist between cells that successfully metastasize and those that do not.[39] Specific genes regulate the ability to metastasize. Decreased cell-to-cell adhesion, the secretion of various proteases that digest surrounding barriers, and the ability to grow in new locations all contribute to successful metastasis[40] (discussed later in this chapter).

Inflammation, Immunity, and Cancer

With the advent of research studies on cancer in inbred mice (genetically identical) in the 1950s, immunologists recognized that many cancers expressed antigens on the cell surface that were not normally expressed on the surface of non–cancer cells from the same tissue. Similar tumor-associated antigens are also expressed on human cancer cells. Two hypotheses arose from these observations. First, immunologists predicted that many developing malignancies were suppressed by an efficient immune surveillance system by which cells expressing tumor-associated antigens were identified, and the resultant immune response destroyed developing malignant cells. Second, when tumors do develop, their tumor-associated antigens could be targets of effective immunotherapy. Immunotherapy could be either active by immunization with tumor antigens to elicit or enhance the immune response against a particular cancer, or passive by injecting the cancer patient with antibodies or lymphocytes directed against the tumor-associated antigens.

The Immune System Protects Us Against Viral-Associated Cancers

The immune system is indeed important in protecting us against cancers caused by specific viral infections. A broad spectrum of viruses has been associated with cancer in animals, and several viruses have been associated with human cancer.[41,42] In humans, *human papillomavirus (HPV), Epstein-Barr virus (EBV)* (also known as *HHV4*), *Kaposi sarcoma herpesvirus (KSHV)* (also known as *HHV8*), and *hepatitis B* and *C viruses (HBV, HCV)* are associated with about 15% of all human cancers worldwide (Table 12-6). Cancer of the cervix and hepatocellular carcinoma account for approximately 80% of the cases of virus-linked cancer.

Virtually all cervical cancer is caused by infection with specific types of HPV, which infects basal skin cells and commonly causes warts. There are more than 120 HPV types, but only about 40 can infect human mucosal tissue, and only a few (HPV16, -18, -31, and -45) are associated with the highest risk for developing cervical, anogenital, and penile cancer (see Chapters 10 and 26). Most HPV infection is handled effectively and rapidly by the immune system and does not cause cancer. Cancer is more common in people with prolonged infection with HPV (a decade or more), during which the viral DNA becomes integrated into the genomic DNA of the infected basal cell of the cervix and directs the persistent production of viral oncogenes. Early oncogenic HPV infection is readily detected by the Papanicolaou (Pap) test, an examination of cervical epithelial scrapings. Early detection of cellular atypia in a Pap test alerts healthcare providers to the possibility of cervical carcinoma in situ, which can be effectively treated. The Pap test is probably the most effective cancer screening test developed to date. Vaccines protecting against the common oncogenic HPV types (HPV16 and HPV18 [types that cause 70% of cervical cancers] and HPV6 and HPV11 [types that cause 90% of genital warts]) were approved for clinical use beginning in

TABLE 12-6 HUMAN VIRUSES ASSOCIATED WITH CANCER

VIRUS FAMILY	TYPE	HUMAN CANCER	COFACTORS
Hepatitis viruses	Hepatitis B	Hepatocellular carcinoma	Alcohol, smoking, aflatoxins
	Hepatitis C	Hepatocellular carcinoma	Alcohol
Herpesviruses	Epstein-Barr	Burkitt lymphoma, nasopharyngeal carcinoma	Malaria
	KSHV/HHV8 immunodeficiency	Kaposi sarcoma	
Papillomaviruses	HPV16, HPV18, HPV31, HPV33, others	Cervical, anogenital	Smoking, oral contraceptives
Retroviruses	HTLV-1	Adult T-cell leukemia/lymphoma	Unknown

Modified from Mendelsohn J et al, editors: *The molecular basis of cancer,* ed 2, Philadelphia, 2001, Saunders.
KSHV/HHV8, Kaposi sarcoma–associated herpesvirus/human herpesvirus-8; *HPV,* human papillomavirus; *HTLV-1,* human T-cell lymphotropic virus type 1.

2006; if these vaccines are administered to young women and men before an initial HPV infection, this is likely to prevent many cases of cervical cancer.[43]

EBV and HHV8 are members of the Herpesviridae family.[44] More than 90% of adults have been infected with EBV, usually as children and without symptoms. EBV infection during adolescence may cause infectious mononucleosis. The virus infects B lymphocytes and stimulates their proliferation; the infection usually remains latent throughout the individual's life. In individuals who are immunosuppressed because of HIV infection or because of drugs given for an organ transplant, persistent EBV infection can lead to the development of B-cell lymphomas. Development of B-cell lymphomas in persons with organ transplants is known as **post-transplant lymphoproliferative disorder (PTLD).**[45] One effective therapy for PTLD is, if possible, to decrease or stop the administration of immunosuppressant drugs and allow the immune system to attack the virus. EBV infection also is associated with Burkitt lymphoma in areas of endemic malaria and with nasopharyngeal carcinoma, a cancer endemic in Chinese populations in Southeast Asia.[46,47] HHV8 is linked to the development of Kaposi sarcoma, a cancer that was once seen primarily in older men but now occurs in a markedly more virulent form in immunocompromised individuals, especially those with acquired immunodeficiency syndrome (AIDS).[48] HHV8 also has been linked to several rare lymphomas.

Human T-cell lymphotropic virus type 1 (HTLV-1) is an oncogenic retrovirus linked to the development of adult T-cell leukemia and lymphoma (ATLL).[49] HTLV is transmitted vertically (that is, inherited by children from infected parents) and horizontally (e.g., by breast-feeding, sexual intercourse, blood transfusions, and exposure to infected needles). Infection with HTLV may be asymptomatic, and only a small fraction of infected individuals develop ATLL, often many years after acquiring the virus.

Chronic hepatitis B infections are common in parts of Asia and sub-Saharan Africa and confer up to a 200-fold increased risk of developing liver cancer. Chronic hepatitis C infections have become increasingly recognized in Western countries. Up to 80% of liver cancer cases worldwide are associated with chronic hepatitis caused either by HBV or by HCV. The initial infection with hepatitis B or C is not associated with cancer; instead, it is acquisition of a chronic viral hepatitis that markedly increases cancer risk.[50] In both cases, it appears that a lifetime of chronic liver inflammation predisposes to the development of hepatocellular carcinoma. Widespread use of the HBV vaccine is expected to significantly decrease the incidence of chronic hepatitis B and hence hepatocellular carcinoma. Unfortunately, a vaccine for HCV is not yet available.

The immune surveillance hypothesis would predict that compromise of the immune system, either by administration of immunosuppressive drugs or by development of genetic or acquired immunodeficiencies, would result in increased incidences of all types of cancer. However, defective immune responses generally only increase the risk for lymphoid cancers, many of which are associated with viral infections.[51] For instance, individuals taking chronic powerful immunosuppressive drugs, such as those given for kidney, heart, or liver transplant, have a much higher risk of developing viral-associated cancers, with a 10-fold increased risk of non-Hodgkin lymphoma (caused by Epstein-Barr virus) and up to a 1000-fold increased risk of Kaposi sarcoma (caused by human herpesvirus 8 [HHV8]). The same immunosuppressed individuals, however, have only a slight increase in the risk of common cancers such as lung and colon cancer (and this could well be because of increased inflammation at those sites), and no increase in the risk of breast or prostate cancer.[52,53] Although the immune system is indeed important in protecting us against cancers caused by specific viral infections, it does *not* effectively protect us against most common cancers.

Inflammation as a Cause of Cancer

Although the immune surveillance theory remains controversial the general opinion remained that an immune or inflammatory response to malignancy is a detrimental condition that successful tumors have evolved methods of evading. We now realize that the relationship between a cancer and the immune and inflammatory systems is much more complex. Inflammatory and immune responses may create a local environment in which cells can develop into a malignant phenotype and may even benefit progression and spread of malignancies.[54] In fact, chronic inflammation has been recognized for close to 150 years as being an important factor in the development of cancer.[55] Epidemiologic studies strongly support the conclusion that chronic inflammation predisposes to cancer. Chronic inflammations may result from many causes; for example, solar irradiation, asbestos exposure (mesothelioma), pancreatitis, and infection (Table 12-7). Additionally, some organs appear to

TABLE 12-7 **CHRONIC INFLAMMATORY CONDITIONS AND INFECTIOUS AGENTS ASSOCIATED WITH NEOPLASMS**

INFLAMMATORY CONDITION	ASSOCIATED NEOPLASM(S)
Asbestosis, silicosis	Mesothelioma, lung carcinoma
Bronchitis	Lung carcinoma
Cystitis, bladder inflammation	Bladder carcinoma
Gingivitis, lichen planus	Oral squamous cell carcinoma
Inflammatory bowel disease, Crohn disease, chronic ulcerative colitis	Colorectal carcinoma
Lichen sclerosus	Vulvar squamous cell carcinoma
Chronic pancreatitis, hereditary pancreatitis	Pancreatic carcinoma
Reflux esophagitis, Barrett esophagus	Esophageal carcinoma
Sialadenitis	Salivary gland carcinoma
Sjögren syndrome, Hashimoto thyroiditis	MALT lymphoma
Skin inflammation	Melanoma
INFECTIOUS AGENT	**ASSOCIATED NEOPLASM(S)**
AIDS (HIV, herpesvirus type 8)	Non-Hodgkin lymphoma, squamous cell carcinomas, Kaposi sarcoma
Chronic cholecystitis	Gallbladder cancer
Chronic cystitis (schistosomiasis)	Bladder, liver, rectal carcinoma; follicular lymphoma of the spleen
Gastritis, gastric ulcers *(Helicobacter pylori)*	Gastric adenocarcinoma, MALT
Hepatitis	Liver carcinoma
Mononucleosis (Epstein-Barr virus)	B-cell non-Hodgkin lymphoma, Burkitt lymphoma
Opisthorchis, cholangitis (liver flukes, bile acids)	Cholangiosarcoma, colon carcinoma
Osteomyelitis	Skin carcinoma in draining sinuses
Pelvic inflammatory disease, chronic cervicitis (HPV, gonorrhea, chlamydia)	Ovarian carcinoma, cervical/anal carcinoma

Modified from Coussens LM, Werb Z: *Nature* 420(6917):860–867, 2002; Dalgleish AG, O'Byrne KJ: *Adv Cancer Res* 84:231–276, 2002; Shacter E, Weitzman SA: *Oncology* 16(2):217–226, 229, 2002.
HIV, Human immunodeficiency virus; *HPV,* human papillomavirus; *MALT,* mucosa-associated lymphoid tissue.

be more susceptible to the oncogenic effects of chronic inflammation; for example, the gastrointestinal (GI) tract, prostate, thyroid gland, pancreas, urinary bladder, pleura, and skin.

Individuals who have suffered with ulcerative colitis for 10 years or more have up to a 30-fold increase in the risk of developing colon cancer. Chronic viral hepatitis caused by hepatitis B virus (HBV) or hepatitis C virus (HCV) infection markedly increases the risk of liver cancer. One large study found a 66% increase in the risk of lung cancer among women with chronic asthma, an inflammatory disease of the airways (see Chapter 35).

Inflammation and cancer have much in common.[56] In both cancer and inflammation (e.g., after injury and during infection), inflammatory cells, including neutrophils, lymphocytes, and macrophages, migrate to the site of injury and release cytokines and growth and survival factors that stimulate local cell proliferation and new blood vessel growth to promote wound healing by tissue remodeling (Figure 12-19) (see Chapter 5). These factors combine in chronic inflammation to promote continued proliferation.[57] In addition, inflammatory cells release compounds such as reactive oxygen species (ROS) and other reactive molecules that can promote mutations and block the cellular response to DNA damage. Notably, an increased abundance of the enzyme cyclooxygenase-2 (COX-2), which generates prostaglandins during acute inflammation, has been associated with colon and some other cancers. Meta-analyses of multiple clinical studies have concluded that long-term high-dose use of nonsteroidal anti-inflammatory drugs (NSAIDs), such as aspirin, that inhibit COX-2 can reduce the risk of colon cancer by as much as 20% (see Chapter 5).[58]

A specific example is the association between gastric inflammation induced by infection with the bacterium *Helicobacter pylori (H. pylori)* and the risk for gastric cancer. *H. pylori* is a bacterium that infects more than half of the world's population. Chronic infection with *H. pylori* is an important cause of peptic ulcer disease and is strongly associated with gastric carcinoma, a leading cause of cancer deaths worldwide. It is also associated with a less common cancer, gastric mucosa–associated lymphoid tissue (MALT) lymphomas. *H. pylori* infection is often acquired in childhood and disproportionately affects lower socioeconomic classes. Although most infections are asymptomatic, prolonged chronic inflammation can lead to increased gastric acid secretion, atrophic gastritis, and duodenal ulcers, or to benign cellular proliferation that can, in a small fraction of individuals, progress to dysplastic changes and finally frank gastric adenocarcinoma. *H. pylori* infection can both directly and indirectly produce genetic and epigenetic changes in infected stomachs, including mutations in *p53* and alterations in the methylation of specific genes.[59,60] Eradication of *H. pylori* from infected individuals before the development of dysplasia may prevent the development of cancer.[61] However, there is no expert consensus on the value of population screening and treatment strategies.

Inflammation, Immunity, and Progression of Cancer

Once cells with malignant phenotypes have developed, additional complex interactions occur between the tumor and the

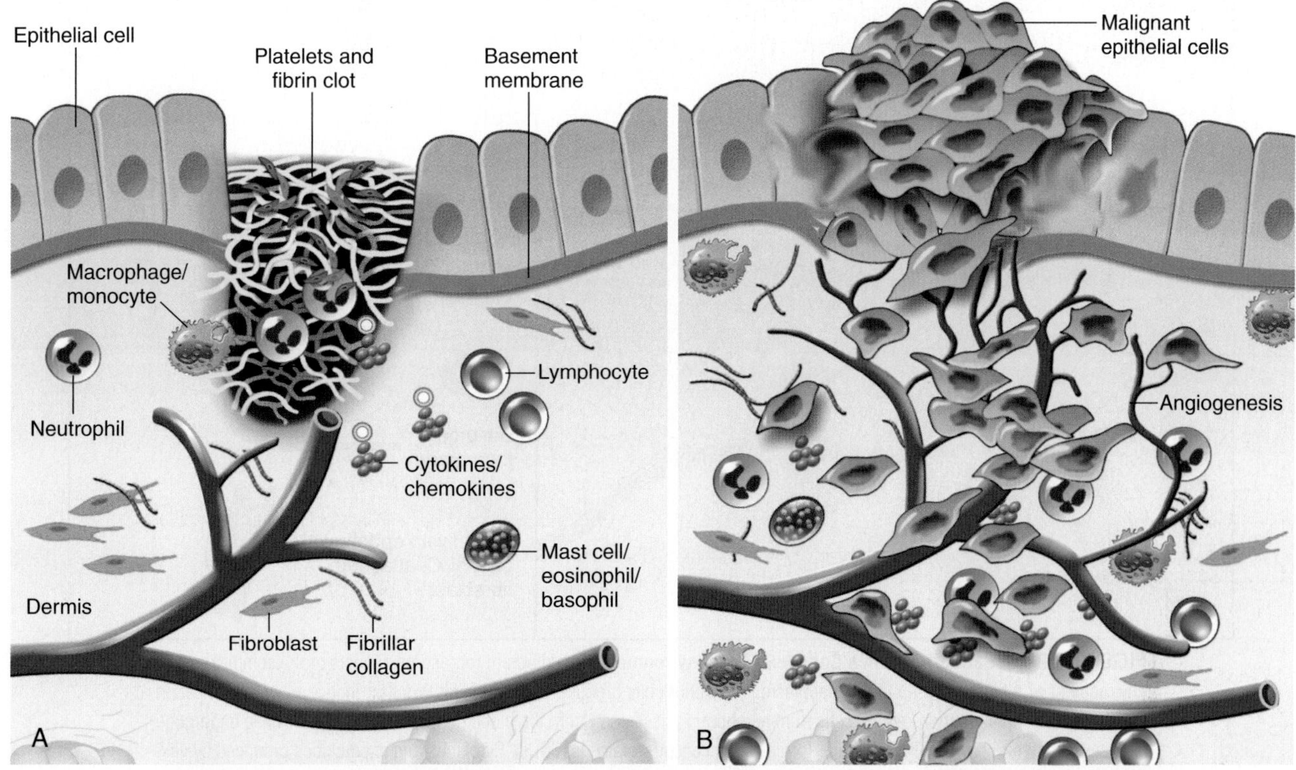

FIGURE 12-19 **Wound Healing vs. Invasive Tumor Growth. A,** Wounds simulate a local inflammatory response. With tissue injury, a blood clot with activated platelets forms, releasing multiple factors that stimulate wound healing. Chemotactic factors such as transforming growth factor-beta and platelet-derived growth factor, derived from activated platelets, initiate granulation tissue formation, activation of fibroblasts, and secretion of proteolytic enzymes (including matrix metalloproteinases) necessary for remodeling of the extracellular matrix. Signaling from many cell types in the wound, including stromal cells, facilitates healing. Once the wound is healed, the signals presumably stop. **B,** Invasive carcinomas act as disorganized wounds. Neoplastic cells produce angiogenic factors, cytokines, and chemokines that are mitogenic and/or chemoattractants for numerous cells. In return, activated fibroblasts and infiltrating inflammatory cells also secrete proteolytic enzymes, cytokines, and chemokines, which are mitogenic for neoplastic cells as well as for endothelial cells involved in neoangiogenesis. These factors, which in the normal situation promote wound healing, now can stimulate tumor growth and angiogenesis, induce fibroblast migration and maturation, and promote metastatic spread through the venous or lymphatic networks. (Adapted from Coussens LM, Werb Z: *Nature* 420[6917]:860–867, 2002.)

surrounding stroma and cells of the immune and inflammatory systems (Figure 12-20). Normal tissues contain a complex mixture of cell types, including fibroblasts, vascular cells, adipocytes, mesenchymal cells (including mesenchymal stem cells), inflammatory cells, and immune cells, and a supporting extracellular matrix. Cancers disrupt this environment, initiate or enhance inflammation, and in turn recruit local and distant cells (macrophages, lymphocytes, and other cellular components of inflammation). The acute inflammatory response related to infection, instead of cancer, undergoes several phases; the initial phase is protective and focused on destruction of the contaminating infectious agents, whereas the later phases are focused on the initiation and progression of healing, as well as preventing the development of autoimmune responses against the normal cellular debris of tissue destruction and regeneration (see Chapter 7). Successful tumors appear capable of manipulating cells of the inflammatory and immune responses towards the phenotypes associated with wound healing and tissue regeneration, which is a process that includes induction of cellular proliferation, neovascularization, and local immune suppression. These activities benefit cancer progression, as well as increase resistance to chemotherapeutic agents.[62]

One of the key cells that promote tumor survival is the tumor-associated macrophage, or TAM.[63] Many tumors produce cytokines and chemokines that are chemotactic factors for monocytes/macrophages (for example, colony-stimulating factor-1 [CSF-1; also known as macrophage colony stimulating factor or M-CSF], vascular endothelial growth factor [VEGF], the chemokine ligand 2 [CCL2; also known as monocyte chemotactic protein-1 or MCP-1]). These chemotactic factors, especially CCL2, are commonly expressed by human tumors (for example, levels of CCL2 in human breast and cancers of the esophagus are related to the degree of macrophage infiltration and progression of the tumor). Thus monocytes are attracted from the blood and into the tumor, where they mature into macrophages. Monocytes have the capacity to differentiate into several macrophage phenotypes, depending upon the conditions in the microenvironment. The classical pro-inflammatory macrophage (M1) is the primary macrophage in the acute inflammatory response and is responsible for removal and

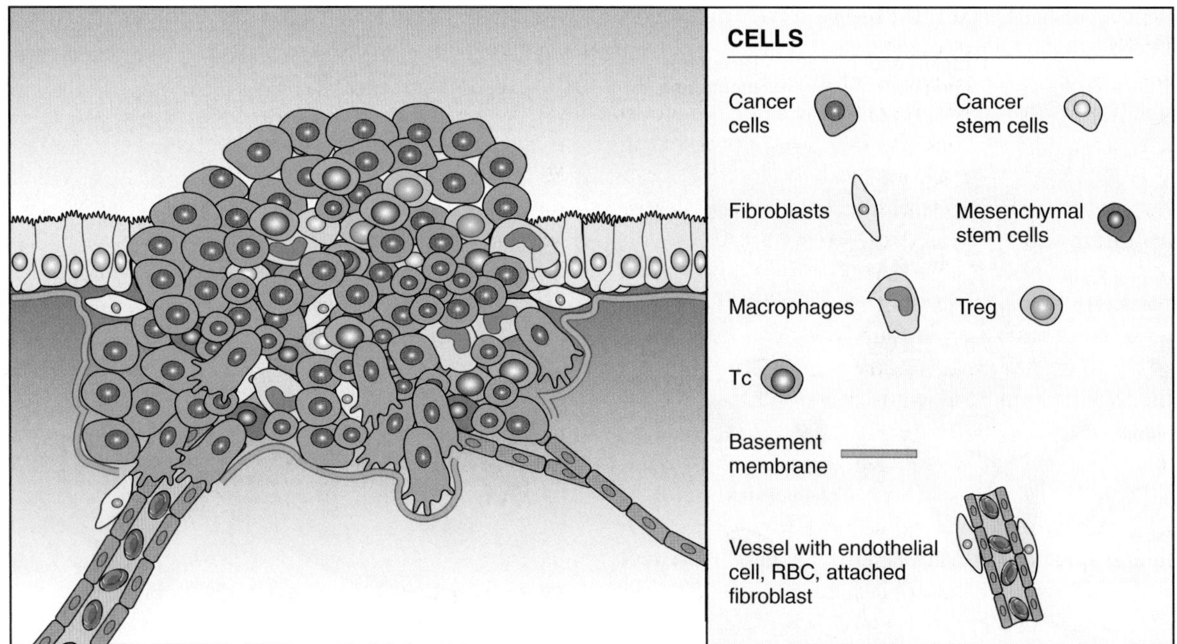

FIGURE 12-20 Cancers Live in a Complex Microenvironment. This diagram represents aspects of the complex microenvironment of a high-grade epithelial neoplasm. The tumor cells produce angiogenic factors that induce neovascularization and invasion by inflammation-related cells from neighboring tissue and from the blood. Individual cancer cells have undergone diverse phenotypic changes, including the formation of cancer stem cells (CSCs). Cytokines and chemokines produced by vascular endothelial cells (ECs) directly affect the proliferation and spread of cancer cells. Cancer-associated fibroblasts originate from fibroblasts associated with blood vessels or invasion from surrounding tissues and produce factors that primarily affect tumor cell proliferation and breakdown of the underlying extracellular matrix. Circulating monocytes invade the tumor and differentiate into tumor-associated macrophages (macrophages) (TAMs) of the M2 phenotype. TAMs produce factors that affect most other cells in the microenvironment. T lymphocytes infiltrate the tumor in the form of CD8+ cytotoxic cells (Tc) and CD4+ regulatory cells (Treg). The Tc cells are suppressed through the combined effect of cytokines and chemokines produced by Treg cell, TAMs, and tumor cells.

destruction of infectious agents. During healing, however, a different phenotype (M2) produces anti-inflammatory mediators to suppress ongoing inflammation and induce cellular proliferation, angiogenesis, and wound healing.[64] TAMs appear to phenotypically mimic the M2 phenotype. The transition to the M2 phenotype is under control of Th2 cytokines (for example, tumor necrosis factor-alpha [TNF-α], colony-stimulating factor-2 [CSF2; also known as granulocyte/macrophage colony stimulating factor or GM-CSF], interleukin-4 [IL-4], IL-10, IL-13).

TAMs have diminished cytotoxic response, and develop the capacity to block cytotoxic T-cell and NK cell functions and produce cytokines that are advantageous for tumor growth and spread. TAMs secrete cellular growth factors (for example, TGF-β and fibroblast growth factor [FGF-2]) that favor tumor cell proliferation, angiogenesis, and tissue remodeling, similar to their activities in wound healing. They also secrete angiogenesis factors (for example, VEGF) that induce neovascularization and matrix metalloproteinase (MMP) that degrade intercellular matrix. The overall effect is increased tumor growth, increased oxygen delivered to the tumor, invasion of the blood vessels, and invasion through the degraded matrix into the local tissue. Most tumors have large numbers of TAMs, whose presence frequently correlates with reduced survival (for instance, in individuals with breast cancer, some forms of lung cancer, and Hodgkin lymphoma). Therapies targeting the nonmalignant TAMs are effective at slowing cancer progression.[65]

Many tumors also have an abundance of tumor-infiltrating lymphocytes. Although the immune cells frequently found in tumors were once thought to be futile attempts at an antitumor response, instead it appears that cancers actively recruit an immune and stromal response to assist in remodeling of tissues, formation of new blood vessels, and promotion of metastasis[66] (see Figure 12-20) cells are generally in low amounts in tumors. The predominant lymphocytes are regulatory T (Treg) cells.[67] Treg cells are CD4+ cells that differentiate under the control of specific cytokines, primarily TGF-β, and express CD25 (the α-chain of the IL-2 receptor) and are thus frequently designated CD4+, CD25+ Treg cells. The role of Treg cells during wound healing is to control or limit the immune response to protect the host's own tissues against autoimmune reactions. Their role in tumors is manipulated to prevent a destructive antitumor immune response and provide cytokines that facilitate tumor cell proliferation and spread.[68] Treg cells and TAMs, as well as stromal cells, produce very high levels of TGF-β and IL-10, an immunosuppressive cytokine, which generally decrease Th1 and Th2 activity, suppress antigen recognition and cell proliferation by Th cells, and suppress the capacity of CD8+ cytotoxic T (Tc) cells to recognize, proliferate in response to antigen, and kill tumor cells. Increased levels of Treg cells in blood and lymph nodes and also infiltrating the tumor correlate with poor outcomes in breast and GI tumors.[69]

In several conditions the release of immunosuppressive factors into the tumor microenvironment increases resistance of the tumor to chemotherapy and radiotherapy.[70] In advanced non–small cell lung cancer an elevated ratio of Treg to Tc cells is related to a poor response to platinum-based chemotherapy. Other cytokines appear to increase the cancer cells' resistance to apoptosis. For example, the Th2 cytokine IL-4 increases the resistance of thyroid cancer to chemotherapy; IL-6 produced by adipocytes and fibroblasts activates survival pathways in breast cancer leading to resistance to radiotherapy; and adipocytes enhance the transcription of the anti-apoptotic factor Bcl-2 in leukemia cells.[71]

A major component of wound healing is angiogenesis—the process of establishing new blood vessels within the tissue undergoing repair. Access to a blood supply is a major benefit to the growth and spread of cancer. Vascular endothelial growth factor (VEGF), an extremely potent inducer of angiogenesis, is secreted by most cells in the tumor microenvironment, including tumor-infiltrating monocytes, endothelial cells, adipocytes, cancer-associated fibroblasts, and some tumor cells. Tumor cells may also have VEGF receptors. VEGF may, thus, induce increased resistance to chemotherapy. For instance, in soft tissue sarcomas VEGF induces increased expression of anti-apoptotic proteins (survivin, Bcl-2) and activation of Pi3K/Akt-mediated survival pathways. The use of angiogenic inhibitors targeting VEGF signaling can inhibit angiogenesis and diminish tumor growth.

Tumor growth and progression is enhanced by, and perhaps is dependent upon, interactions with cells in the microenvironment. Suppression of tumor-enhancing inflammatory/immune responses may provide powerful adjunctive approaches to traditional antitumor therapeutic regimens, such as chemotherapy and radiation therapy.[72] Tumor-infiltrating cells, such as TAM and Treg cells, express cell-specific surface markers. Antibodies directed against those markers can induce apoptosis of these cells. Additionally, the effects of specific cytokines, chemokines, and other tumor-enhancing mediators produced in the tumor microenvironment may be neutralized by specific antagonists.[73] These are also usually in the form of monoclonal antibodies. For instance, TNF-α antagonist has been used effectively in rheumatoid arthritis to inhibit production and neutralize the effects of TNF-α, including reduction of angiogenesis, leukocyte infiltration, and production of metalloproteinases. Trials are currently underway to assess the effects of TNF-α antagonists on the progress of cancer. Other antagonists are under investigation, including those against IL-1β, TGF-β, CSF-1 (M-CSF), VEGF, IL-6, IL-10, and metalloproteinases. Chemokine antagonists are also under development. A potential complication of adjunctive therapy directed against cellular or molecular products of inflammation concerns the importance of these constituents in normal inflammatory/immune responses. If the proposed antagonists were administered systemically, suppression of responses elsewhere in the body may increase the individual's susceptibility to infection. Delivery systems that concentrate the antagonists proximal to the tumor environment may be the most effective means of administration.

CANCER INVASION AND METASTASIS

Metastasis is the spread of cancer cells from the site of the original tumor to distant tissues and organs through the body. Metastasis is a defining characteristic of cancer, contributes significantly to the pain and suffering from cancer, and is the major cause of death from cancer. Cancer that has not metastasized can often be cured by a combination of surgery, chemotherapy, and radiation. These same therapies are frequently ineffective against cancer that has metastasized. For example, in appropriately treated women with low-stage breast cancer, the 5-year survival rate is often greater than 90%.[74] Tragically, less than 30% of women with metastatic breast cancer are alive 5 years after diagnosis.[75] A growing body of basic and clinical research is defining the biologic principles of metastasis, with the hope that this improved understanding will lead to novel diagnostic approaches and better therapies to prevent and treat metastatic cancers.[76]

Invasion, or local spread, is a prerequisite for metastasis and is the first step in the metastatic process. In its earliest stages local invasion may occur by direct tumor extension. Eventually, however, cells migrate away from the primary tumor and invade the surrounding tissues. Mechanisms important in local invasion include recruitment of macrophages and other cell types to the primary tumor, where they promote digestion of connective tissue capsules and other structural barriers by secreted proteases; changes in cell-to-cell adhesion, often by changes in the expression of cell adhesion molecules such as cadherins and integrins, making the cancer cells more slippery and mobile; and increased motility of individual tumor cells[77] (Figure 12-21). Tumors that are encased in a capsule, such as breast ductal carcinoma, must breakdown the capsule in order to initiate local spread.[78] The capsule consists of layers of epithelial cells and myoepithelial cells in contact to the tumor and contained by a basement membrane (see Figure 24-43). The myoepithelial cells may be tumor suppressive; they produce proteins that are tumor suppressors (e.g., TGF-α, IL-6), as well as angiogenesis inhibitors and proteinase inhibitors.[79] The mechanism of capsular dissolution is unclear, but may result from production of enzymes by the tumor or the influx of leukocytes.[80] Information about mechanical stress and associated tumor cell response is contained in What's New? Mechanical Stress and Tumors.

To transition from local to distant metastasis, the cancer cells must also be able to invade local blood and lymphatic vessels, a task facilitated by stimulation of neoangiogenesis and lymphangiogenesis by factors such as VEGF. Finally, a successful metastatic cell must be able to survive in the circulation, attach in an appropriate new microenvironment, and multiply to produce an entire new tumor, similar to the characteristics of a cancer stem cell. Different cancers have different patterns of spread, determined by a combination of factors. Cancers often spread first to regional lymph nodes through the lymphatics and then to distant organs through the bloodstream. A cancer's ability

WHAT'S NEW?

Mechanical Stress and Tumors

Cells, whether in isolation or in tissues, often face and respond to a wide variety of external stimuli. These environmentally induced changes, called *perturbations,* can be chemical or physical and responses can be physiologic, such as cellular homeostatic activities or tissue development movements, or pathologic, such as malignant transformation or inflammation. Cellular responses to chemical signals have been studied in great detail, but the elements involved in the recognition of physical stresses (e.g., hypoxia, osmotic shock, ionizing radiation, or mechanical stretching) and the mechanisms related to cell responses to these stimuli remain barely analyzed. These responses include a variety of conserved adaptive behaviors, such as wound healing, cell migration, extravasation, secretion, and necrotic or apoptotic death.[1]

Mechanical stress is a key physical stimulus sensed by cells. At the cellular level, mechanical cues or stressors can modulate almost all aspects of cell behavior, including growth, differentiation, migration, gene expression, protein synthesis, and apoptosis,[2] many of them of important clinical interest (e.g., cancer metastasis, stem cell proliferation, and differentiation and wound healing). Mechanical cues control specific physiologic processes, such as sound sensation, by cells of the inner ear or blood flow across the endothelium.[2] Importantly in some cases, organs and tissues adapt their structures and functions in response to acute or chronic mechanical stress (e.g., pressure overload causes cardiovascular hypertrophy and muscle disuse results in atrophy).

For tumor biology, the cell surface integrin family act as critical mechanosensors.[3] Integrin-mediated cell adhesion and signaling are crucial events for numerous cell fates and include morphogenesis, differentiation, cell growth, the immune response, and cell survival.[4] *Integrins* function as noncovalent transmembrane receptors that are organized in focal adhesions (FAs) and link the extracellular matrix (ECM) to the actin cytoskeleton; they do not directly interact with actin filaments. A number of actin-binding proteins, including talin, α-actinin, and filamin, have been identified as intermediates.[5] Integrins can mediate the sensing of mechanical properties of the ECM by changing their affinity, conformation, clustering, and recruitment and by transducing these signals to the activation of downstream signaling cascades. The molecular architecture of FAs suggests that mechanical force is, itself, essential for focal adhesion formation and maintenance. From stretch-induced recruitment, talin may serve as a molecular ruler that specifies focal adhesion molecular architecture.[6]

Investigators are studying the relationships of cues from the microenvironment and tumor behavior. For example, recent work showed the mechanical tone of nontumorigenic host epithelium directs the phenotype of tumor cells.[7] Investigators established a three-dimensional ex vivo model of both normal and malignant mammary epithelial growth to test the importance of the ECM in regulating local migration of tumor cells and dissemination.[8] From their studies, they determined that breaks in the basement membrane could induce invasion and dissemination from the resulting direct contact between cancer cells and collagen I.[8] Uncontrolled growth in a confined space generates compressive forces. To understand how this may affect tumor behavior, investigators from various fields, including chemical engineering and radiation oncology, found that compressive stress accumulated during tumor growth can enable coordinated migration of cancer cells by stimulating formation of leader cells and enhancing cell–substrate adhesion.[9] This novel mechanism represents a potential target for the prevention of cancer cell migration and invasion. Overall, the research on mechanical stress and associated tumor cell response is just beginning.

References

1. Gillespie PG, Walker RG: *Nature* 413:194–202, 2001.
2. Ingber DE: *Circ Res* 91:877–887, 2002.
3. Baker EL, Zaman MH: *J Biomech* 43:38–44, 2010.
4. Shimaoka M, Springer TA: *Nat Rev Drug Discov* 2:703–716, 2003.
5. Tremuth L et al: *J Biol Chem* 279:22258–22266, 2004.
6. Yu H, Mouw JK, Weaver VM: *Trends Cell Biol* 21:47–56, 2011.
7. Boghaert E et al: *Proc Natl Acad Sci U S A* 109(48):19632–19637, 2012.
8. Nguyen-Nqoc KV et al: *Proc Natl Acad Sci U S A* 109(39):E2595–E2604, 2012.
9. Tse JM et al: *Proc Natl Acad Sci U S A* 109(3):911–916, 2012.

to establish a metastatic lesion in a new location requires that the cancer both attach to specific receptors and survive in the specific environment. Because metastasis requires successful completion of each and every step, there may be many opportunities to interrupt this potentially lethal pathway.

Only Rare Cells in a Cancer Are Able to Metastasize

Metastasis is a highly inefficient process. A landmark clinical review examined a group of women with advanced ovarian cancer.[81] These unfortunate women had accumulated a large amount of peritoneal fluid filled with malignant ovarian cancer cells (malignant ascites). To relieve the pressure caused by the ascites, the fluid was surgically shunted into the venous circulation. This palliative procedure relieved the abdominal pressure but had the side effect of moving millions of ovarian cancer cells an hour directly into the bloodstream. Despite this direct injection of billions of cancer cells into the circulation, these women unexpectedly had no increased number of metastases when they died. The conclusion from this clinical study is that most cancer cells cannot successfully cause metastases, a conclusion that has been supported by many other clinical and laboratory studies.[82] The reason lies both in the seed and in the soil. Cancer cells (the seeds) must surmount multiple physical and physiologic barriers in order to spread, survive, and proliferate in distant locations, and the destination (the soil) must be receptive to the growth of the cancer. It has been suggested that the metastatic cell must, like a decathlon champion, be successful in every event to allow a cancer to spread.[82]

How do cancer cells develop the ability to metastasize? The same heritable changes that occur to cause the primary cancer, including gene mutations, deletions, translocations, epigenetic silencing, and changes in miRNA expression, all work to provide genetic heterogeneity in the tumor cells as they proliferate. As this diversity increases, this increases the number of cells in the cancer mass with new abilities that can facilitate metastasis.

Detachment and Invasion

In order for cells to move away from their normal niche, they must be able to detach from the stroma and migrate. Cells are normally attached to extracellular matrix (ECM). To facilitate cancer spread, many tumors and their associated inflammatory cells secrete proteases and protease activators, such as the matrix metalloproteinases (MMPs) and plasminogen activators. Active proteases digest the extracellular matrix and basement membranes, creating pathways through which cells can move, while releasing bioactive peptides as digestion products that further

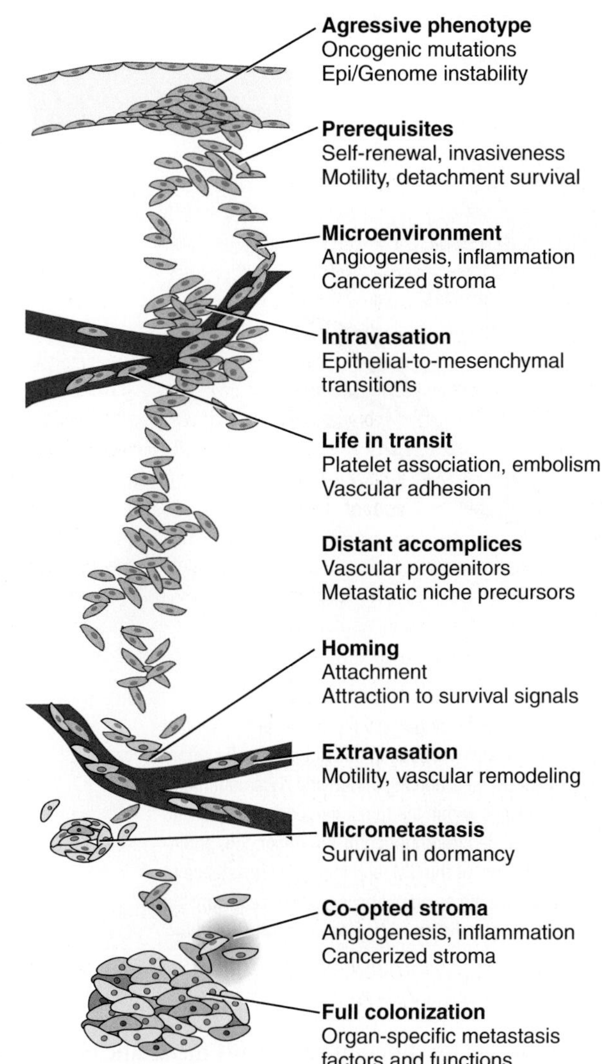

FIGURE 12-21 Multistep Nature of Metastasis. (From Gupta GP, Massagué J: *Cell* 127[4]:697–708, 2006.)

stimulate tumor growth and mobility. However, the production of metalloproteinases alone is inadequate to explain the metastatic process.

The process by which neoplastic cells dissociate from the primary tumor, spread into the lymphatics and blood vessels, and establish macrometastases in foreign microenvironments is a fascinating, and yet not fully understood, utilization of pathways that are more commonly observed in embryonic and fetal development. Carcinomas originate from highly differentiated and polarized epithelial cells that form structured sheets stabilized by multiple adherences to neighboring cells and to a basement membrane (an extracellular meshwork of collagens and other connective tissue proteins) along the cells' basal surface. Although the degree of malignant transformation resulting in a primary tumor may be adequate for local expansion of the tumor, neoplastic cells in the primary carcinoma usually retain some epithelial-like characteristics that prevent dissociation from the extracellular matrix and preclude successful metastasis to distal sites. A greater degree of cellular "dedifferentiation" is necessary to produce the "seeds" that can separate from the primary tumor and flourish in a potentially hostile secondary site. This results from a programmed transition of the still partially epithelial-like carcinoma to a more undifferentiated mesenchymal-like phenotype (**epithelial-mesenchymal transition [EMT]**) (Figure 12-22).[83] A similar process occurs with tumors of endothelial origin (endothelial-mesenchymal transition).[84]

EMT is a process that occurs normally in embryonic development (for example, cell movement related to morphogenesis during gastrulation and neural crest formation) and implantation, as well as wound healing and tissue repair. Generally, cells that have transitioned into a mesenchymal-like phenotype have suppressed expression of adhesion molecules with a loss of polarity, increased migratory capacity, elevated resistance to apoptosis, and the potential to redifferentiate into other cell types. These properties permit the tumor cells to dissociate from the primary tumor and be transported to a distal site. The degree of dedifferentiation may be variable, but most cells undergoing EMT acquire stem cell traits that facilitate initial growth in a new microenvironment.[85] The EMT is not a stable transition; the metastatic tumor tends to regain some characteristics of the primary tumor, thus reverting to some extent to its epithelial origins.

The transition to a mesenchymal-like phenotype is, in most cases, driven by cytokines and chemokines produced within the tumor microenvironment (see Figure 12-22). IL-8 is an effective driver of carcinoma cells into EMT. TGF-β induces loss of E-cadherin (an integral component of tight junctions) and β_4-integrin in mammary gland tumor cells. The loss of E-cadherin in particular allows cells to detach from extracellular matrix and migrate more readily.

Genetic changes associated with the EMT are under the control of a variety of transcription factors, for example, Snail, Slug, and Twist.[86] Most are repressors of transcription, so that expression of adhesion molecules such as E-cadherin is greatly diminished. The translational factor Slug also represses transcription of Bcl-2 antagonists, resulting in increased Bcl-2 expression and increased resistance to apoptosis.

Survival and Spread in the Circulation

Normal cells, when separated from their ECM, undergo *anoikis*, a form of apoptosis (see Chapter 2). The process of EMT frequently results in increased resistance to apoptosis. In addition, tumor cells that have already adapted to a hypoxic environment have already been selected for resistance to apoptosis, often by loss of normal cell death pathways. For example, neuroblastomas with loss of the pro-apoptotic caspase-8 genes are able to avoid apoptosis after loss of integrins, and are more able to metastasize than the same cells with normal levels of caspase-8. Accordingly, individuals whose neuroblastomas have low levels of caspase-8 have a poor prognosis[87] (see Chapter 2).

Selective Adherence in Favorable Sites

After release from the ECM and digestion of basement membranes, cancer cells gain access to the circulation through new tumor-associated blood vessel growth or angiogenesis (described earlier), also known as neovascularization. Mobile tumor cells are able to enter the circulation, perhaps facilitated

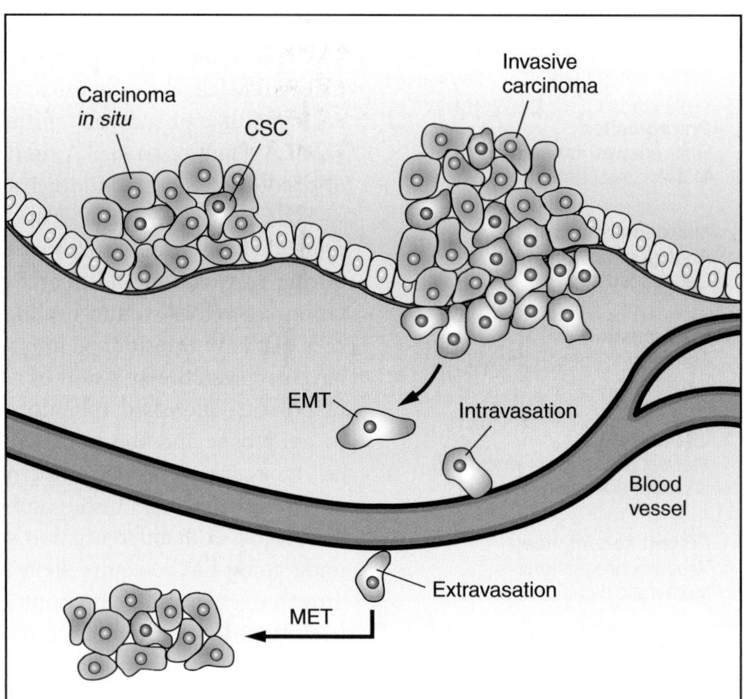

FIGURE 12-22 Epithelial-Mesenchymal Transition (EMT). Tumors of epithelial origin usually retain epithelial-like characteristics that preclude spread into adjacent tissues and metastasis to distal sites. As seen in this diagram, cells within carcinoma in situ or non-invasive carcinoma (not shown) retain adhesion to adjacent cells and the underlying basement membrane (BM). The process of transition to mesenchymal-like cells is driven by cytokines within the tumor microenvironment and induction of a family of EMT-inducing transcription factors. The outcome included dedifferentiation of the tumor cell, potentially to a cancer stem cell phenotype, loss of adhesion-related molecules, breakdown of the BM, and increased resistance to apoptosis, which result in a locally invasive carcinoma and release into the bloodstream or lymphatic vessels of cells capable of relocalization, redifferentiation (potentially through a reverse mesenchymal-to-epithelial transition process; MET), and formation of a metastasis. *CSC,* Cancer stem cell. (From Craene BD, Berx G: *Nat Rev Cancer* 13[2]:97–110, 2012.)

by the leaky newly made vessels and attraction of the cells because of chemoattractants coming from these new vessels. Once in the circulation, metastatic cells must be able to withstand the physiologic stresses of travel in the blood and lymphatic circulation, including high shear rates and exposure to immune cells. One mechanism is for tumor cells to bind to blood platelets, giving them a protective coat of nonmalignant blood cells that both shields the tumor cells and creates a small tumor embolus, or cancer clot, that can promote cancer cell survival in distant locations.

The patterns of metastasis are dictated by the interaction between the cancer cells and the microenvironments in which they land. Two distinct mechanisms give rise to patterns of distant spread. First, cancer cells spread through vascular and lymphatic pathways, as well as natural tissue planes. The **neovascularization** of a cancer offers malignant cells direct access into the venous blood, and draining lymphatics can carry malignant cells to regional lymph nodes. Single cells, clumps, and even tumor fragments can disseminate by these routes. Anatomic patterns of lymphatic and venous blood flow help determine how colon cancers spread to the liver, liver cancers spread through the portal vein to the lungs, lung cancers spread through the systemic circulation to the brain, and breast cancer spreads through lymphatics to axillary lymph nodes (Figure 12-23). There is also a major yet poorly understood selectivity of different cancers for different sites. Thus metastatic breast cancer often spreads through the bloodstream to bones but rarely to kidney or spleen, whereas lymphomas often spread to the spleen but uncommonly spread to bone. In a key study, Schackert and Fidler[88] injected different types of cancer cells into the carotid artery of mice. Despite identical blood flow–mediated distribution of the cancer cells, each cancer cell type produced cancers in very different parts of the brain. This tissue selectivity is likely caused by specific interactions between the cancer cells and specific receptors on the small blood vessels in different organs (Table 12-8). Experimental metastasis studies in mice are beginning to reveal additional molecular reasons for this tissue specificity (Figure 12-24). Examples include interaction between $\alpha3\beta1$ integrins binding to laminin-5 receptors in the lung, and the chemokine receptor CXCR4 on breast cancer cells promoting homing to lung tissues expressing the ligand CXCL12.[89]

Escape from the Circulation and Development of a New Microenvironment

As the study with women with ovarian cancer illustrates, pumping millions of cancer cells in the bloodstream does not necessarily cause metastatic disease. Cancer cells may arrive in a new location and survive but not proliferate to form a clinically relevant metastasis. The tumor cells that do not make the transition from simple survival to robust proliferation in a new

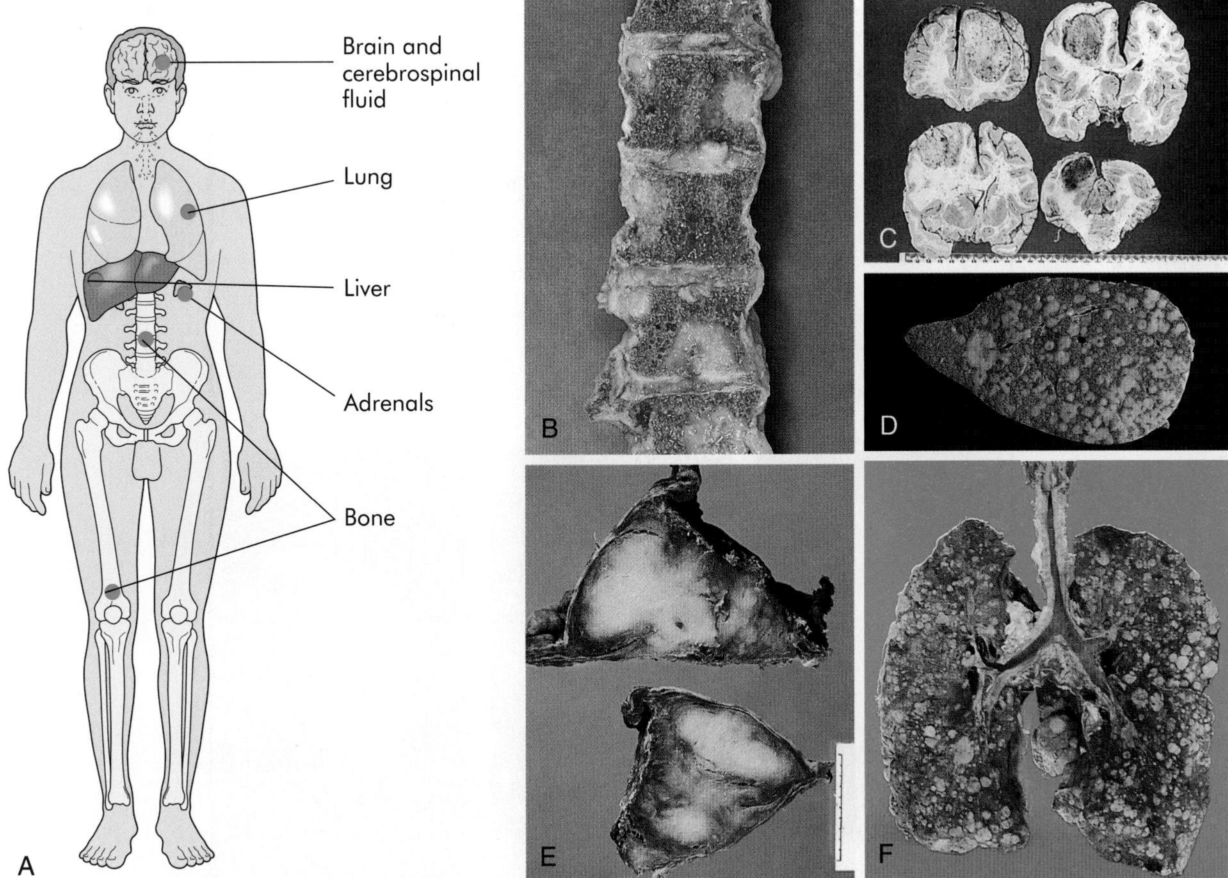

FIGURE 12-23 Patterns of Metastatic Spread. **A,** Sites of hematogenous metastasis. Blood-borne tumor metastasis leads to growth of secondary tumors in several main sites. The macroscopic appearance of bone metastasis is shown in **B,** where lesions are seen in vertebrae. **C,** Numerous metastases from a neoplasm of the stomach are seen in the brain. **D,** The liver is the most common site for metastases from tumors in the gastrointestinal tract that arose from a colonic neoplasm. **E,** Metastatic tumor has replaced both adrenal glands, as is commonly seen with spread from lung and breast tumors. **F,** The lung is the most common site for blood-borne metastases from tumors outside the spinal tract, particularly mesenchymal tumors.

TABLE 12-8 COMMON SITES OF METASTASIS

PRIMARY TUMOR	MAJOR ANATOMIC PATHWAY	COMMON SITE OF DISTANT METASTASIS
Lung	Pulmonary vein, left ventricle	Multiple organs, including brain
Colorectal	Mesenteric lymphatics, portal venous system	Liver
	Inferior vena cava, right ventricle, pulmonary artery	Lungs
Testicular	Lymphatics to periaortic area to subclavian veins to right ventricle	Lungs, liver, brain
Prostate	Regional lymphatics and veins, which drain to Batson plexus of presacral veins	Bones (especially lumbar spine), liver
Breast	Axillary, transpectoral, and internal mammary lymphatics	Bones, lung, brain, liver
Head and neck	Direct extension	Lymphatics, liver, bones
Ovarian	Direct extension, peritoneal seeding, mesenteric veins	Peritoneal surfaces, diaphragm, omentum, liver
Sarcoma (extremity)	Inferior vena cava, right ventricle, pulmonary artery	Lungs
Melanoma	Regional lymphatics	In transit lymphatics, lung, liver, brain, gastrointestinal tract

location are said to be in a state of *dormancy*. This dormancy may account for the observation that solitary tumor cells can be detected in the blood years after a complete clinical remission in individuals, and that many people with detectable micrometastases will not develop clinically obvious metastases.[88,90] One of the factors that allow proliferation of cancer cells in the new environment may be cancer's recruitment of normal cells from local and circulating bone marrow stem cells. One developing concept is that successful metastatic tumor cells secrete factors that recruit circulating mesenchymal stem cells to the metastatic

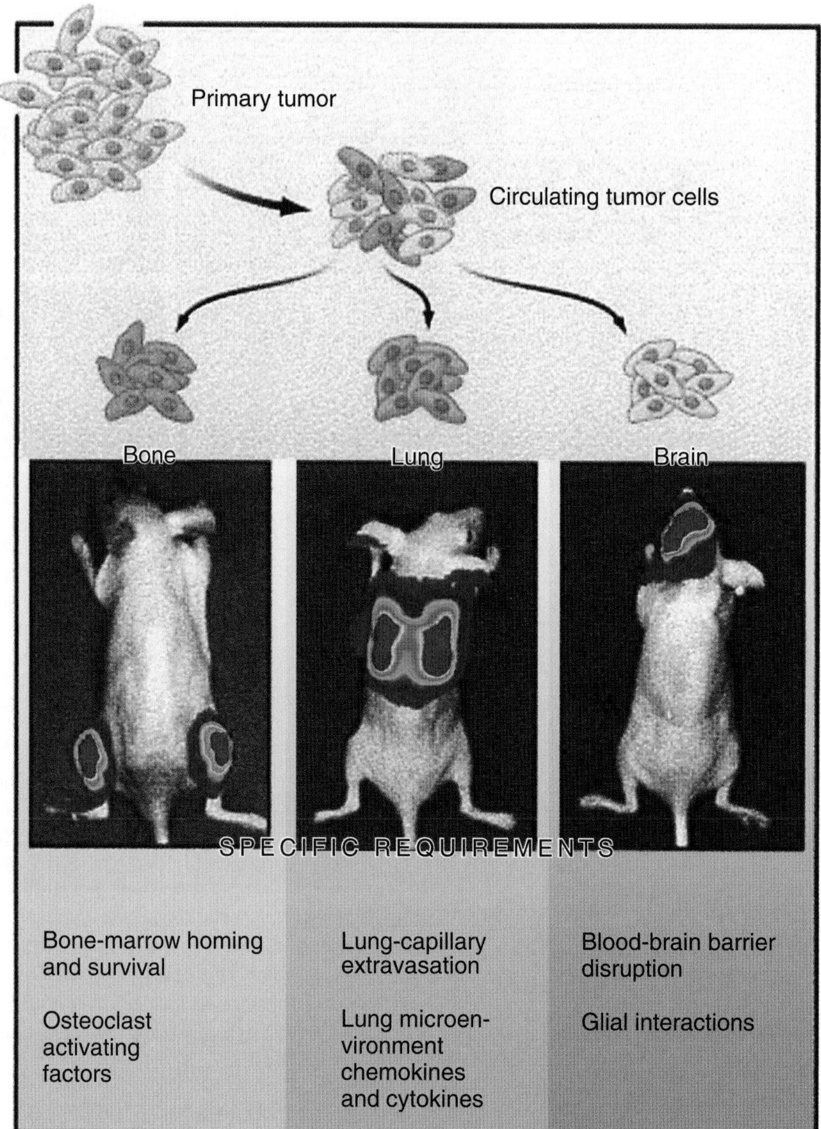

FIGURE 12-24 Clues Regarding How the Patterns of Metastatic Spread Are Determined. Different cancer cells from the same cancer can spread to different locations. This is because tumors are heterogeneous mixtures of cells, with variations in the genes that are turned on and off. Different anatomic locations favor different types of cells. Studies with mice illustrated here show that expression of specific factors such as adhesion molecules, chemokines, and host factors such as blood-brain barrier disruption can favor the spread of specific cancer cells to different locations. In this example, cancer cells were visualized by genetically tagging cells with firefly luciferase for bioluminescent imaging. (From Gupta GP, Massagué J: *Cell* 127[4]:679–695, 2006.)

site (see Figure 12-17). These newly recruited stem cells then differentiate into tumor-supporting stroma and new blood vessels. One area of research is aimed at understanding why some micrometastases remain dormant; new therapies might block their progression to clinically important disease.

CLINICAL MANIFESTATIONS AND TREATMENT OF CANCER

Clinical Manifestations of Cancer

Diagnosis and Staging

Cancer can be discovered in many ways: after screening tests, from routine exams, and after investigation of symptoms (see What's New? Screening Mammography: Why It Has Not Lived Up to Expectations). The symptoms a cancer produces are as diverse as the types of cancer. The location of the cancer can determine symptoms by physical pressure, obstruction, and loss of normal function, or a cancer can cause problems far away from its source by pressing on nerves or secreting bioactive compounds. Whatever the initial complaint, once the diagnosis is suspected and a tumor has been identified, it is essential that tumor tissue be obtained to establish a definitive diagnosis and correctly classify the disease. Various methods of obtaining tissue are described in Table 12-9.

Once tissue is obtained, it is examined microscopically by the pathologist for the histologic hallmarks of cancer detailed

WHAT'S NEW?

Screening Mammography: Why It Has Not Lived Up to Expectations

Screening mammograms illustrate many of the difficulties that arise from population-based screening tests. The goal of screening tests is early and accurate detection of a treatable disease without causing false alarms (a low false-positive rate) or missing a diagnosable disease (a low false-negative rate). We also do not want to detect disease or conditions that are insignificant and do not require treatment, known as overdiagnosis. Recently, investigators examined the extent of overdiagnosis of breast cancer. Various databases were examined to study breast cancer trends between 1976 (just before screening mammography was introduced) and 2008. During this interval the incidence of ductal carcinoma in situ (DCIS) and localized disease (early stage cancers) doubled from 112 to 234 per 100,000 women, an increase of 122 cases per 100,000 women.[1] During the same interval, the annual incidence of late stage cancers decreased minimally from 102 to 94 per 100,000 women, a decrease of 8 per 100,000 women. The higher increase in early stage cases compared to late stage cases (112 vs. 8 per 100,000) suggests substantial overdiagnosis.[2] The investigators estimate that, as a result of breast cancer overdiagnosis, more than 1 million U.S. women have been presumably treated unnecessarily (overtreatment) with approaches including surgery, radiotherapy, and chemotherapy during the last 30 years.[1] These authors also conclude that the improvement in breast cancer mortality during those years is mainly because of treatment and not screening. This question, however, is debated. The Cochrane reviewers analyzed tumor sizes and stages and reported that screening has not lowered the rate of advanced cancers and recent observational studies of breast cancer mortality have failed to find an effect related to mammography screening.[3] Results from the Norwegian screening program found 15% to 25% of cases of breast cancer are overdiagnosed.[4] The Nordic Cochrane Center found that 13 years of breast screening had no measurable effect on breast cancer mortality in Norway.[5] An independent expert panel in the United Kingdom estimated the risks and benefits of screening for breast cancer in women 50 to 70 years of age invited for mammography every 3 years in the UK. They found for every 180 women who are screened, 1 life is saved but 3 women are diagnosed and treated for cancer that would not otherwise have become apparent in their lifetimes.[6] A study involving women from 30 European countries showed that the mean decrease in breast cancer mortality between 1989 and 2005 among women less than 50 years of age was 37%; the corresponding decrease was 21% among women aged 50 to 69 years.[7] The declines in mortality, however, began before the start of organized screening programs in many countries and may possibly be the result of tamoxifen treatment.[3] Another study compared three pairs of similar neighboring countries where screening was introduced 10 to 15 years apart.[8] The pairs were Northern Ireland and the Republic of Ireland, the Netherlands and Belgium, and Sweden and Norway. There was no relationship between the start of screening mammography and reduction in breast cancer mortality.[8]

Authors state that most publications on mammography screening have examined the effects on mortality separately from harms, such as overtreatment.[9] The Canadian Task Force on Preventive Health Care has new recommendations for screening for breast cancer in women at average risk aged 40 to 74 years.[10] These new guidelines are cautious, advising against routine screening in women aged 40 to 49 years. This Task Force recommends screening women aged 50 to 69 years every 2 to 3 years, admitting that this is a weak recommendation based on moderate-quality evidence, and screening women aged 70 to 74 years on the same schedule based on low-quality evidence.[11] This Task Force suggested that women who do not place a high value on a small reduction in breast cancer mortality from screening and those who are concerned about false-positives on mammography and overdiagnosis may decline screening.[10] The United States Preventive Services Task Force (USPSTF) recommendations include the following:

- The USPSTF recommends biennial screening mammography for women aged 50 to 74 years.
  Grade: B Recommendation
- The decision to start regular, biennial screening mammography before the age of 50 years should be an individual one and take the woman's context into account, including the woman's values regarding specific benefits and harms.
  Grade: C Recommendation
- The USPSTF concludes that the current evidence is insufficient to assess the additional benefits and harms of screening mammography in women 75 years or older.
  Grade: I Statement
- The USPSTF recommends against teaching breast self-examination (BSE).
  Grade: D Recommendation
- The USPSTF concludes that the current evidence is sufficient to assess the additional benefits and harms of clinical breast examination (CBE) beyond screening mammography in women 40 years or older.
  Grade: I Statement
- The USPSTF concludes that the current evidence is insufficient to assess the additional benefits and harms of either digital mammography or magnetic resonance imaging (MRI) instead of film mammography as screening modalities for breast cancer.
  Grade: I Statement
- Overall, considering benefits, overdiagnosis, overtreatment, and potential harms, including unnecessary surgery, radiotherapy, increased number of biopsies, and administration of toxic drugs, *all* of which may contribute to the biology of breast carcinogenesis, there will be continued debate regarding the role of screening mammography in decreasing breast cancer mortality.

References

1. Bleyer A, Welch HG: *N Engl J Med* 1998:367, 2012.
2. Brett AS: *J Watch General Med* Nov 29, 2012.
3. Gøtzsche PC et al: *Cancer Causes Control* 23(1):15–21, 2012.
4. Kalager M et al: *Ann Intern Med* 156(3):491–499, 2012.
5. Jørgensen KJ, Brodersen J, Gøtzsche PC: *Int J Cancer* 132(7):1725–1726, 2013.
6. *BMJ* 345:e7460, 2012.
7. Autier P et al: *BMJ* 341:c3620, 2010.
8. Autier P et al: *BMJ* 343:d4411, 2011.
9. Hackshaw A: *BMJ* 344:d8279, 2012.
10. Canadian Task Force on Preventive Health Care et al: *CMAJ* 183(17):1991–2001, 2011.
11. Gøtzsche PC: *CMAJ* 183(17):1957–1958, 2011.

in the beginning of this chapter. The classification of the cancer can be further facilitated by a variety of clinically available tests, including immunohistochemical stains, flow cytometry, electron microscopy, chromosome analysis, and nucleic acid–based molecular studies.

If the diagnosis of cancer is established, it is critical to determine if the cancer has spread, known as the **stage** of the cancer. Staging initially involves determining the size of the tumor, the degree to which it has locally invaded, and the extent to which it has spread (metastasized) (Figure 12-25). Specific molecular

TABLE 12-9 OBTAINING TISSUE—THE BIOPSY

PROCEDURE	PURPOSE	EXAMPLE
Excisional biopsy	Complete removal, usually with a margin of normal tissue	Full resection (e.g., mastectomy, partial colectomy)
Incisional biopsy	Removal of a portion of a lesion	Lymph node biopsy, muscle mass biopsy
Core needle biopsy	Often performed with direct vision, or guided with ultrasound or computed tomography (CT)	Needle biopsy of prostate or liver mass
Fine needle aspiration	Obtains dissociated cells for cytologic study but does not preserve tissue structure	Thyroid, breast mass
Exfoliative cytology	Cells shed from the surface, for example, from cervix, sputum (lung) or urine	Brushings from lung or colon endoscopy

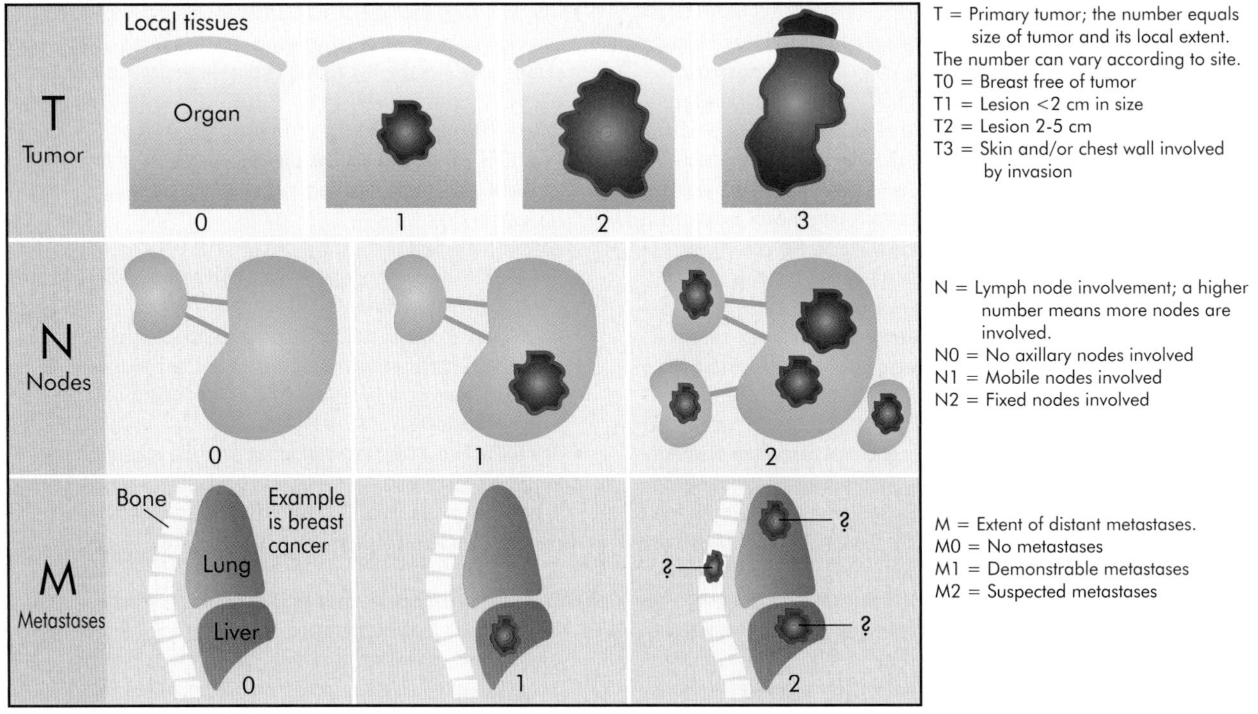

FIGURE 12-25 Tumor Staging by the TNM System. Example of staging for breast cancer.

tests are increasingly used in staging as well. Diverse schemes are used for staging different tumors. In general, a four-stage system is used, with carcinoma in situ regarded as a special case. Cancer confined to the organ of origin is stage 1; cancer that is locally invasive is stage 2; cancer that has spread to regional structures, such as lymph nodes, is stage 3; and cancer that has spread to distant sites, such as a liver cancer spreading to the lung or a prostate cancer spreading to bone, is stage 4. One common scheme for standardizing staging is the World Health Organization's TNM system: *T* indicates tumor spread, *N* indicates node involvement, and *M* indicates the presence of distant metastasis (see Figure 12-25). The prognosis generally worsens with increasing tumor size, lymph node involvement, and metastasis (Table 12-10). Staging also may alter the choice of therapy, with more aggressive therapy being delivered to more invasive disease.

TABLE 12-10 CANCER SURVIVAL DEPENDS ON TUMOR TYPE AND STAGE OF DISEASE

	STAGE			
DISEASE	**I**	**II**	**III**	**IV**
Colon cancer	>90	75	50	<10
Hodgkin disease	99	95	85	70
Pancreatic cancer	37	26	10	1

Comment: Estimated percentage of individuals surviving 5 years for selected tumors, by stage at diagnosis. Additional factors such as age, molecular lesions, histologic subtypes, and type of treatment modify the outcome as well.

Paraneoplastic Syndromes

Paraneoplastic syndromes are symptom complexes that are triggered by a cancer but are not caused by direct local effects of the tumor mass. They are most commonly caused by biologic substances released from the tumor (e.g., hormones) or by an immune response triggered by the tumor. For example, a small fraction of carcinoid tumors release hormones, including serotonin, into the bloodstream that cause flushing, diarrhea,

TABLE 12-11 PARANEOPLASTIC SYNDROMES

CLINICAL SYNDROMES	MAJOR FORMS OF UNDERLYING CANCER	CAUSAL MECHANISM
Endocrinopathies		
Cushing syndrome	Small cell carcinoma of lung Pancreatic carcinoma Neural tumors	ACTH or ACTH-like substance
Syndrome of inappropriate antidiuretic hormone (SIADH) secretion	Small cell carcinoma of lung; intracranial neoplasms	Antidiuretic hormone or atrial natriuretic hormones
Hypercalcemia	Squamous cell carcinoma of lung Breast carcinoma Renal carcinoma Adult T-cell leukemia/lymphoma Ovarian carcinoma	Parathyroid hormone–related protein (PTHRP), TGF-α, TNF, IL-1
Hypoglycemia	Fibrosarcoma Other mesenchymal sarcomas Hepatocellular carcinoma	Insulin or insulin-like substance
Carcinoid syndrome	Bronchial adenoma (carcinoid) Pancreatic carcinoma Gastric carcinoma	Serotonin, bradykinin
Polycythemia	Renal carcinoma Cerebellar hemangioma Hepatocellular carcinoma	Erythropoietin
Nerve and Muscle Syndrome		
Myasthenia	Bronchogenic carcinoma	Immunologic
Disorders of central and peripheral nervous systems	Breast carcinoma	
Dermatologic Disorders		
Acanthosis nigricans	Gastric carcinoma Lung carcinoma Uterine carcinoma	Immunologic; secretion of epidermal growth factor
Dermatomyositis	Bronchogenic, breast carcinoma	Immunologic
Osseous, Articular, and Soft Tissue Changes		
Hypertrophic osteoarthropathy and clubbing of the fingers	Bronchogenic carcinoma	Unknown
Vascular and Hematologic Changes		
Venous thrombosis (Trousseau phenomenon)	Pancreatic carcinoma Bronchogenic carcinoma Other cancers	Tumor products (mucins that activate clotting)
Nonbacterial thrombotic endocarditis	Advanced cancers	Hypercoagulability
Anemia	Thymic neoplasms	Unknown
Others		
Nephrotic syndrome	Various cancers	Tumor antigens, immune complexes

From Kumar V, Abbas AK, Fausto N: *Pathologic basis of disease*, ed 7, Philadelphia, 2005, Saunders.
ACTH, Adrenocorticotropic hormone; *IL*, interleukin; *TGF*, transforming growth factor; *TNF*, tumor necrosis factor.

wheezing, and rapid heartbeat. A number of cancers trigger an antibody response that attacks the nervous system, causing a variety of neurologic disorders that can precede other symptoms of cancer by months.[91]

Although infrequent, paraneoplastic syndromes are significant because they may be the earliest symptom of an unknown cancer and, in affected individuals, can be serious, often irreversible, and sometimes life-threatening. Table 12-11 presents the classifications of paraneoplastic syndromes. Other clinical manifestations of cancer are summarized in Box 12-2.

Cancer Treatment

The diagnosis of cancer has a profound effect on individuals and their families. Responses range from depression to resigned fatalism to an aggressive no-holds-barred pursuit of therapy. The choice of therapy should be based on a full consideration of the individual's diagnosis, prognosis, and therapeutic options by the individual, the family, and the medical team. Many types of cancer can be effectively treated with chemotherapy, radiotherapy, surgery, and combinations of these modalities. Caregivers must recognize that many individuals seek additional

BOX 12-2 SUMMARY OF OTHER CLINICAL MANIFESTATIONS OF CANCER

Pain: There is little or no pain during the early stages of malignant disease. Significant pain can occur in many individuals who are terminally ill with cancer. Direct pressure, obstruction, invasion of a sensitive structure, stretching of visceral surfaces, tissue destruction, infection, and inflammation all can cause pain.

Fatigue: The most frequently reported symptom of cancer and cancer treatment. The exact mechanisms that produce fatigue are poorly understood. Suggested causes include sleep disturbances, various biochemical changes secondary to disease and treatment, numerous psychosocial factors, level of activity, nutritional status, and other environmental and physical factors.

Cachexia: A syndrome that includes many symptoms including anorexia, early satiety (filling), weight loss, anemia, asthenia (marked weakness), taste alterations, and altered protein, lipid, and carbohydrate metabolism. It is the most severe form of malnutrition associated with cancer and results in wasting, emaciation, and decreased quality of life. Cytokines and metabolites from the tumor may contribute to cachexia.

Anemia: Commonly associated with malignancy, with 20% of persons diagnosed with cancer having hemoglobin concentrations less than 9 g/dl (normal value = 15 g/dl). Mechanisms of anemia include chronic bleeding (resulting in iron deficiency), severe malnutrition, cytotoxic chemotherapy, and malignancy in blood-forming organs. Chronic bleeding and iron deficiency can accompany colorectal or genitourinary malignancy. Iron also is malabsorbed in individuals with gastric, pancreatic, or upper intestinal cancer.

Leukopenia and Thrombocytopenia: Causes can include many chemotherapeutic drugs because they are toxic to the bone marrow, often causing granulocytopenia and thrombocytopenia. Granulocytopenia also can result from radiation therapy if it encompasses significant areas of the bone marrow. Thrombocytopenia is a major cause of hemorrhage in people with cancer and is often treated with platelet transfusions. Thrombocytopenia is a disorder of disseminated intravascular coagulation that occurs in individuals with acute promyelocytic leukemia and severe infections.

Infection: The most significant cause of complications and death in patients with malignant disease. When the absolute granulocyte count falls below 500 cells per μL, the risk of serious microbial (bacterial and fungal) infection increases. Advanced disease can predispose to infection and immunosuppression from the underlying cancer and the radiotherapy and chemotherapy used to treat it. (Factors that predispose individuals with cancer to infection are summarized in Table 12-12.) The prevalence of hospital-acquired (nosocomial) infections increases because of indwelling medical devices, inadequate wound care, and the introduction of microorganisms from visitors and other individuals.

Gastrointestinal Tract (GI): The GI tract relies on rapidly growing cells to produce an effective barrier to trauma and infection and to provide an absorptive surface for nutrients. Chemotherapy and radiation therapy may cause a decreased cell turnover, thereby leading to oral ulcers (stomatitis), malabsorption, and diarrhea. The disruption of barrier defenses also increases the risk for infection, especially invasion by a person's own GI flora.

Hair Loss (Alopecia) and Skin: Results from chemotherapy effects on hair follicles. It is usually temporary, although hair may regrow with a different texture initially. Not all chemotherapeutic agents cause alopecia. Decreased renewal rates of the epidermal layers in the skin may lead to skin breakdown and dryness, altering the normal barrier protection against infection. Radiation therapy may cause skin erythema (redness) and contribute to breakdown.

Data from Miller AH et al: *J Clin Oncol* 26(6):971–982, 2008; Pachman DR et al: *J Clin Oncol* 30(30):3687–3695, 2012.

non–science-based explanations and therapies and often use alternative therapies, either concurrently or sequentially. Alternative therapies can be biologically harmless or harmful; rarely is there any evidence they are medically effective and in the worst cases they can be expensive, delay the use of effective therapies, and produce unknown side effects. A challenge for the medical team is to provide the same level of psychosocial comfort and support that alternative therapies can provide, while also providing scientifically rational evidence-based therapies.

Chemotherapy

The era of modern chemotherapy began with the observation in World War II that mustard gas exposure caused suppression of the bone marrow. Related compounds, such as nitrogen mustard and cyclophosphamide, were then tested and produced clinical responses in hematologic malignancies, including lymphomas. Also in the late 1940s, based on the remarkable clinical observation that the vitamin folic acid could *increase* leukemia growth, anti–folate drugs were developed (leading ultimately to methotrexate) that produced remissions in previously untreatable leukemias.[92]

All chemotherapeutic agents take advantage of specific vulnerabilities in target cancer cells. Antimetabolites, such as methotrexate and L-asparaginase, block normal growth pathways in all cells, but leukemia and other cancer cells are exquisitely sensitive to folic acid and asparagine deprivation, whereas nonmalignant cells are far less sensitive. Similarly, some cancer cells are highly sensitive to DNA-damaging agents, such as cyclophosphamide and anthracyclines, because of the oncogenic mutations that accelerate the cell cycle and DNA synthesis. Cellular checkpoints prevent normal cells treated with microtubule-directed drugs, such as vincristine and the taxanes, from undergoing mitosis, whereas cancer cells treated with these agents lack normal checkpoints, continue through mitosis, and undergo mitotic catastrophe (see Chapter 1).

Single chemotherapeutic agents often shrink cancers, but these drugs given alone rarely if ever provide a cure. Hence, chemotherapy drugs are usually given in combinations designed to attack a cancer from many different weaknesses at the same time and to limit the dose and therefore the toxicity of any single agent. Cancers contain a very large number of cells, and commonly a small fraction of those cells may be resistant to a particular drug. However, those cells are likely to be sensitive to the second or third drug in a chemotherapy cocktail. Scheduling of drug administration is also very important, with many studies showing cancers are more likely to develop drug resistance if there are significant delays between planned courses of chemotherapy.

The newest highly targeted agents used to treat cancer exploit specific vulnerabilities uncovered by molecular analysis in specific diseases. These new drugs are still used in combination with conventional chemotherapy and to be effective they must be used in diseases in which the molecular target is present. For example, imatinib is a competitive inhibitor of

TABLE 12-12 FACTORS PREDISPOSING INDIVIDUALS WITH CANCER TO INFECTION

FACTOR	BASIS
Age	Many common malignancies occur mostly in older age. Immunologic functions decline with age. General debility reduces immunocompetence. Immobility predisposes to infection. Far-advanced cancer often results in immobility and general debility that worsens with age. Elderly persons are predisposed to nutritional inadequacies. Malnutrition impairs immunocompetence.
Tumor	Nutritional derangements can result. Sites and circumstances favorable to growth of microorganisms (obstruction, serous or blood effusion, ulceration) can be created. Far-advanced disease predisposes patients to debility and immobility. Humoral or cellular immune defects may result. Metastasis to bone marrow may cause leukopenia or other defects in immunity.
Leukemias	Inadequate granulocyte production (impaired phagocytosis) results. Thrombocytopenia (bleeding, breaks in skin integrity) can occur. Late effect: Chronic lung disease from *Pneumocystis jiroveci* pneumonia can develop during therapy.
Lymphomas and other mononuclear phagocyte malignancies	Humoral and cellular immune defects (anergy, altered immunoglobulin production) result. Late effect: Splenectomy in children can cause increased susceptibility to infection.
Surgical treatment	Invasive procedure interrupts first lines of defense. Radical nature of surgery (removal of large blocks of tissue in lengthy procedures) causes hemorrhage, decreased tissue perfusion, creation of dead spaces, devitalization of tissues. Procedure may be "dirty" surgery (bowel, infected or contaminated areas). Surgery patients are often older and at poor risk. Long preoperative hospitalization often precedes surgery. Patients may have received previous adrenocorticosteroid therapy. Patients may have infections at sites remote from operative area. Nutritional derangements (especially important in head and neck surgery) may result. Lymph node dissection may predispose patient to local infection and impair containment to area. Gynecologic surgery may result in fistulae. Lung surgery may cause bronchopleural fistulae. Debility and immobility may result.

Data from Donovan MI, Girton SF: *Cancer care nursing,* ed 2, New York, 1984, Appleton-Century-Crofts; Murphy GP, Lawrence W, Lenhard RE: *Clinical oncology,* ed 2, New York, 1994, American Cancer Society.

tyrosine kinases, primarily the BCR-ABL tyrosine kinase. It is highly effective in treating CML and gastrointestinal stromal tumor (GIST) but ineffective in virtually all other cancers. Several monoclonal antibodies directed against cellular receptors or cell surface antigens are in use or being evaluated. These include antibodies against the CD20 antigen expressed on some B-cell lymphomas, the epidermal growth factor (EGF) receptor on colon cancers and head and neck cancers, and the HER2 EGF receptor on breast cancer. Fortunately, because these drugs are so tightly targeted they have much less toxicity than conventional chemotherapies that have targets in virtually all cells.

Chemotherapy can be used for several distinct purposes. **Induction chemotherapy** seeks to cause shrinkage or disappearance of tumors. In Hodgkin disease, for example, chemotherapy alone can be used in some cases to cure the disease. In other settings, chemotherapy may shrink the tumor and improve symptoms without ultimately providing a cure. **Adjuvant chemotherapy** is given after surgical excision of a cancer with the goal of eliminating micrometastases. **Neoadjuvant chemotherapy** is given before localized (surgical or radiation) treatment of a cancer. As with induction chemotherapy, the effectiveness, or lack thereof, of neoadjuvant therapy can be measured (for example, with follow-up scans). Neoadjuvant therapy can shrink a cancer so that surgery may spare more normal tissue. For example, in the bone cancer *osteogenic sarcoma,* neoadjuvant therapy often converts a large tumor mass into a much smaller mass, allowing the surgeon to perform a limb-sparing excision rather than an amputation.

Radiation Therapy

Radiation therapy is used to kill cancer cells while minimizing damage to normal structures. Ionizing radiation damages cells by imparting enough energy to cause molecular damage, especially to DNA. The damage may be lethal, in which the cell is killed by radiation; potentially lethal, in which the cell is so severely affected by radiation that modifications in its environment will cause it to die; or sublethal, in which the cell can subsequently repair itself. Cellular compartments with rapidly renewing cells are, in general, more radiosensitive. Effective cell killing by radiation also requires good local delivery of oxygen, something not always present in large cancers. Radiation produces slow changes in most cancers and irreversible changes in normal tissues as well. Because of these irreversible changes, each tissue has a maximum lifetime dose of radiation it can tolerate. Radiation is well suited to treat localized disease in areas that are hard to reach surgically, for example, in the brain and pelvis. A number of radiation delivery methods are available, with external beam being the most common. Radiation sources, such as small ^{125}I-labeled capsules (also called seeds), can also be temporarily placed into body cavities, a delivery method termed **brachytherapy.** Brachytherapy is useful in the treatment of cervical, prostate, and head and neck cancers.

Radiation therapy and chemotherapy may affect the gametes, leading to varying degrees of decreased fertility and premature menopause. These effects are dose and age dependent, with the prepubertal gonad thought to be more resistant to damage. The potential for harm also is dependent on the agent used, with the alkylating category of chemotherapies carrying the greatest risk. Craniospinal irradiation for central nervous system tumors also may affect the hypothalamus or pituitary gland, with subsequent secondary gonadal failure because of lack of production of gonadotropin-releasing hormone, luteinizing hormone, and follicle-stimulating hormone. The potential for reproductive harm should be addressed before therapy, if possible, with provisions made for sperm or embryo banking.

Surgery

Surgery plays many roles in the care of individuals with cancer. The multiple approaches to obtaining tissue for diagnosis have been discussed. Surgery is often the definitive treatment of cancers that do not spread beyond the limits of surgical excision. It is also indicated for the relief of symptoms, such as those caused by tumor mass obstruction. In selected high-risk diseases, surgery plays a role in the prevention of cancer. For example, individuals with familial adenomatous polyposis because of germline mutations of the *APC* gene have close to a 100% lifetime risk of colon cancer, so a prophylactic colectomy is indicated. Similarly, women with *BRCA1/2* mutations have a markedly increased risk of breast and ovarian cancer, and often choose prophylactic mastectomy or bilateral salpingo-oophorectomy (removal of ovaries and fallopian tubes), or both.[93]

Key principles apply specifically to cancer surgery, including obtaining adequate surgical margins during a resection to prevent local recurrences, placing needle tracks and biopsy incision scars (that may be contaminated with cancer cells) carefully so they can be removed in subsequent incisions, avoiding the spread of cancer cells during surgical procedures through careful technique, and paying attention to obtaining adequate tissue specimens during biopsies so that the pathologist can be confident of the diagnosis. Additionally, the surgeon provides critical staging information by inspection, sampling, and removal of local and regional lymph nodes during procedures.

SUMMARY REVIEW

Cancer Characteristics and Terminology

1. Benign tumors are usually encapsulated and well differentiated and do not spread to distant locations.
2. Malignant tumors, compared with benign tumors, have more rapid growth rates, specific microscopic alterations (anaplasia, loss of differentiation), absence of normal tissue organization, and no capsule; they invade blood vessels and lymphatics and have distant spread.
3. Carcinomas arise from epithelial tissue, and leukemias are cancers of blood-forming cells. CIS refers to preinvasive epithelial tumors of glandular or squamous cell origin.
4. Localized cancer is considered low stage, whereas cancer that has spread regionally and distantly is termed stage 3 and stage 4, respectively.
5. Cancer cells are characterized by anaplasia, or loss of differentiation, and autonomy, or independence, from normal cellular controls.
6. In the adult, undifferentiated cells not committed to a specific function are known as pluripotent cells, precursor cells, or adult stem cells. Cancerous growth depends on derangements of cell differentiation.
7. Tumor markers are substances (i.e., hormones, enzymes, genes, antigens, antibodies) found in cancer cells and in blood, spinal fluid, or urine. They are used to screen and identify individuals at high risk for cancer, to help diagnose specific types of tumors, and to follow the clinical course of cancer.

The Genetic Basis of Cancer

1. Genetic events are the primary basis of carcinogenesis. Mutations in cancer-causing genes accumulate with age, causing the increasing risk of cancer with advanced age.
2. Epidemiologic and molecular data suggest it takes five or six distinct mutations in different signaling pathways to produce cancer. Mutations activate growth-promotion pathways, block antigrowth signals, prevent apoptosis, turn on telomerase and new blood vessel growth, and allow tissue invasion and distant metastasis.
3. In rare families, cancer is inherited in an autosomal dominant fashion as a result of mutations in tumor-suppressor genes such as *TP53, RB1,* and *BRCA1.*
4. Proto-oncogenes encode for growth factors (e.g., PDGF), growth factor receptors (e.g., HER2), signal transducers (e.g., RAS), and nuclear growth–promoting proteins (e.g., MYC).
5. Three key genetic mechanisms have a role in human carcinogenesis: (a) activation of proto-oncogenes resulting in hyperactivity of growth-related gene products (such genes are called *oncogenes*); (b) mutation of genes resulting in loss or inactivity of gene products that normally would inhibit growth (such genes are called *tumor-suppressor genes*); and (c) mutation of genes resulting in overexpression of products that prevent normal cell death, or apoptosis, thus allowing continued growth of tumors.
6. Tumor-suppressor genes encode for proteins that act as inhibitors of growth factor stimulation. Tumor-suppressor gene proteins block specific phases of the cell cycle, induce

SUMMARY REVIEW—cont'd

end-stage (e.g., terminal) differentiation, and stimulate cell senescence or death.

7. Carcinogenesis, or the development of cancer, involves both inactivation of tumor-suppressor genes (usually by loss of heterozygosity, or by "silencing") and activation of oncogenes.
8. Epigenetic changes in genes by DNA methylation and covalent histone modification can mimic mutation by heritably inactivating tumor-suppressor genes.
9. Like many normal adult tissues, cancers can contain rare stem cells. To fully eradicate a cancer, it may be necessary to target the cancer stem cell.
10. Caretaker genes are responsible for maintaining genomic integrity. Inherited mutations can disrupt caretaker genes and cause chromosome instability.
11. A number of viruses can cause cancer. Human cervical cancer is caused by papillomavirus infection. Kaposi sarcoma is caused by infection with HHV8, a member of the Herpesviridae family. Chronic hepatitis infection with HBV or HCV is the leading cause of liver cancer.
12. Defects in the immune system increase the risk of viral-associated cancers but have a minimal effect on the risk of other cancers.
13. Active inflammation predisposes to cancer by stimulating a wound-healing response that includes proliferation and new blood vessel growth.
14. Vaccinations can prevent hepatitis B–associated liver cancer and many human papillomavirus-caused cervical cancers.
15. Chronic *H. pylori–associated inflammation* causes stomach cancer and a rare lymphoma.
16. Metastasis is the major cause of death from cancer.
17. Cancers metastasize by several routes, including direct invasion and spread through lymphatics and veins.
18. Metastasis is a complex process that requires cells to have many new abilities, including the ability to invade, survive, and proliferate in a new environment and recruit new blood vessel growth.
19. Carcinomas undergo a process of epithelial-mesenchymal transition (EMT) during which many epithelial-like characteristics are lost (e.g., polarity, adhesion to basement membrane) resulting in increased migratory capacity, increased resistance to apoptosis, and dedifferentiation to a stem cell–like state that favors growth in foreign microenvironments and establishment of metastatic disease.

Clinical Manifestations

1. Clinical manifestations of cancer include fatigue, pain, cachexia, anemia, leukopenia, thrombocytopenia, and infection.
2. Paraneoplastic syndromes are rare symptom complexes often caused by release of active substances from or stimulation of an immune response by a cancer that causes symptoms not directly produced by the local effects of the cancer.
3. Pain is generally associated with the late stages of cancer. It can be caused by pressure, obstruction, invasion of a structure sensitive to pain, stretching, tissue destruction, and inflammation.
4. Fatigue is the most frequently reported symptom of cancer and cancer treatment.
5. Cachexia (loss of appetite, early satiety, weakness, inability to maintain weight, taste alterations, altered metabolism) leads to protein-calorie malnutrition and progressive wasting.
6. Anemia associated with cancer usually occurs because of malnutrition, chronic bleeding and resultant iron deficiency, chemotherapy, radiation, and malignancies in the blood-forming organs.
7. Leukopenia is usually a result of chemotherapy (which is toxic to bone marrow) or radiation.
8. Infection may be caused by leukopenia, immunosuppression, or debility associated with advanced disease. It is the most significant cause of complications and death.

Cancer Treatment

1. Cancer is treated with surgery, radiation therapy, chemotherapy, and combinations of these modalities.
2. The theoretic basis of chemotherapy is the vulnerability of tumor cells in various stages of the cell cycle. The goal of chemotherapy is to eradicate enough tumor cells so the body's natural defenses can eradicate remaining cells.
3. Modern chemotherapy uses combinations of drugs with different targets and different toxicities.
4. A new generation of specific targeted drugs attacks targets identified by the molecular analysis of cancers.
5. Ionizing radiation causes cell damage, so the goal of radiation therapy is to damage the tumor without causing excessive toxicity or damage to undiseased structures.
6. Surgical therapy is used for nonmetastatic disease, for which cure is possible by removing the tumor, and as a palliative measure to alleviate symptoms.

KEY TERMS

Adenocarcinoma, 364
Adjuvant chemotherapy, 397
Adult stem cell, 370
Anaplasia, 364, 368
Anchorage independent, 368
Angiogenesis, 381
Angiogenic factor, 381
Apoptosis, 381
Autocrine stimulation, 380
Autonomy, 368
Benign tumor, 364
Brachytherapy, 398
Cancer, 364
Carcinoma, 364
Carcinoma in situ (CIS), 364
Caretaker gene, 379
Chromosome instability, 379
Chromosome translocation, 375
Clonal expansion, 373
Clonal proliferation, 373
Contact inhibition, 368
Copy number variation (CNV), 376
DNA methylation, 378
Driver mutation, 373
Epigenetic silencing, 380
Epigenetics, 372
Epithelial-mesenchymal transition (EMT), 389
Gene amplification, 376
Human T-cell lymphotropic virus type 1 (HTLV-1), 383
Immortal, 368
Induction chemotherapy, 397
Leukemia, 364

KEY TERMS—cont'd

Loss of heterozygosity (LOH), 378
Lymphoma, 364
Malignant tumor, 364
Metastasis, 387
MicroRNA (miRNA, miR), 378
Multipotent, 370
Mutagen, 379
MYC protein, 375
Neoadjuvant chemotherapy, 397
Neoplasm, 364
Neovascularization, 390
Oncogene, 374
Oncogene addiction, 374
Oncomir, 378
Paraneoplastic syndrome, 365, 394
Passenger mutations, 373
Personalized medicine, 365
Pleomorphic, 369
Point mutation, 375
Post-transplant lymphoproliferative disorder (PTLD), 383
Proto-oncogene, 374
RAS, 380
Retinoblastoma *(Rb)* gene, 376
Sarcoma, 399
Silencing, 378
Stage, 393
Telomerase, 382
Telomere, 382
Transformation, 368
Tumor marker, 365
Tumor-suppressor gene, 374

REFERENCES

1. Allegra CJ et al: National Institutes of Health State-of-the-Science Conference statement: diagnosis and management of ductal carcinoma in situ September 22-24, 2009, *J Natl Cancer Inst* 102:161–169, 2010.
2. Weng L et al: Pharmacogenetics and pharmacogenomics: a bridge to individualized cancer therapy, *Pharmacogenomics* 14(3):315–324, 2013.
3. Skloot R: *Immortal life of Henrietta Lacks*, New York, 2010, Crown Publishing Group, Division of Random House, Inc.
4. Wu CA et al: Nutrient deprivation induces the Warburg effect through ROS/AMPK-dependent activation of pyruvate dehydrogenase kinase, *Biochim Biophys Acta*, 2013 Jan 31. [Epub ahead of print.].
5. Teicher BA, Linehan WM, Helman LJ: Targeting cancer metabolism, *Clin Cancer Res* 18(20):5537–5545, 2012.
6. O'Brien CA, Kreso A, Jamieson CHM: Cancer stem cells and self-renewal, *Clin Cancer Res* 16:3113–3120, 2010.
7. Shackleton M et al: Heterogeneity in cancer: cancer stem cells versus clonal evolution, *Cell* 138:822–829, 2009.
8. Armitage P, Doll R: The age distribution of cancer and a multi-stage theory of carcinogenesis, *Br J Cancer* 91(12):1983–1989, 2004.
9. Kinzler KW, Vogelstein B: Lessons from hereditary colorectal cancer, *Cell* 87(2):159–170, 1996.
10. Dawson SJ et al: A new genome-driven integrated classification of breast cancer and its implications, *EMBO J*, 2013 Feb 8. [Epub ahead of print.].
11. Bellovin DI, Das B, Felsher DW: Tumor dormancy, oncogene addiction, cellular senescence, and self-renewal programs, *Adv Exp Med Biol* 734:91–107, 2013.
12. Takashima A, Faller DV: Targeting the RAS oncogene, *Expert Opin Ther Targets*, 2012 Jan 30. [Epub ahead of print.].
13. Peker D et al: Burkitt lymphoma arising from lymphoplasmacytic lymphoma following acquisition of MYC translocation and loss of the ETV6 tumor suppressor gene, *Arch Pathol Lab Med* 137(1):130–133, 2013.
14. Nowell P, Hungerford D: A minute chromosome in human granulocytic leukemia, *Science* 132:1497, 1960.
15. Druker BJ: Translation of the Philadelphia chromosome into therapy for CML, *Blood* 112:4808–4817, 2008.
16. Schrider DR et al: Gene copy-number polymorphism caused by retrotransposition in humans, *PLoS Genet* 9(1):e1003242, 2013.
17. Sridhar S et al: New insights into the genetics of neuroblastoma: implications for diagnosis and therapy, *Mol Diagn Ther*, 2013 Jan 18. [Epub ahead of print.].
18. Hampton T: Genetics studies provide new insights into breast cancer biology and treatment, *JAMA* 309(5):427–429, 2013.
19. Ciardiello F, Tortora G: EGFR antagonists in cancer treatment, *N Engl J Med* 358(11):1160–1174, 2008.
20. Bakhoum SF, Compton DA: Chromosomal instability and cancer: a complex relationship with therapeutic potential, *J Clin Invest* 122(4):1138–1143, 2012.
21. Biran A, Meshorer E: Concise review: chromatin and genome organization in reprogramming, *Stem Cells* 30(9):1793–1799, 2012.
22. Dawson MA, Kouzarides T: Cancer epigenetics: from mechanism to therapy, *Cell* 150(1):12–27, 2012.
23. van Vlerken LE, Hurt EM, Hollingsworth RE: The role of epigenetic regulation in stem cell and cancer biology, *J Mol Med (Berlin)* 90(7): 791–801, 2012.
24. Lane AA, Chabner BA: Histone deacetylase inhibitors in cancer therapy, *J Clin Oncol* 27:5459–5468, 2009.
25. Nana-Sinkam SP, Croce CM: Clinical applications for microRNAs in cancer, *Clin Pharmacol Ther* 93(1):98–104, 2013.
26. Guil S, Esteller M: Cis-acting noncoding RNAs: friends or foes, *Nat Struct Mol Biol* 19(11):1068–1075, 2012.
27. Basu B et al: Targeting the DNA damage response in oncology: past, present and future perspectives, *Curr Opin Oncol* 24(3):316–324, 2012.
28. Lynch PM: Current approaches in hereditary nonpolyposis colorectal cancer, *J Natl Compr Canc Netw* 10(8):961–967, 2012.
29. Tanaka H et al: Telomere fusions in early human breast carcinoma, *Proc Natl Acad Sci U S A* 109(35):14098–14103, 2012.
30. Casper AM, Rosen DM, Rajula KD: Sites of genetic instability in mitosis and cancer, *Ann N Y Acad Sci* 1276:24–30, 2012.
31. Albright F et al: Significant evidence for a heritable contribution to cancer predisposition: a review of cancer familiality by site, *BMC Cancer* 12:1–7, 2012.
32. Gopie JP, Vasen HF, Tibben A: Surveillance for hereditary cancer: does the benefit outweigh the psychological burden? A systemic review, *Crit Rev Oncol Hematol* 83(3):329–340, 2012.
33. Hanahan D, Weinberg RA: The hallmarks of cancer, *Cell* 100(1):57–70, 2000.
34. LoRusso PM: Mammalian target for rapamycin as a rational therapeutic target for breast cancer treatment, *Oncology* 84(1):43–56, 2013.
35. Kubota Y: Tumor angiogenesis and anti-angiogenic therapy, *Keio J Med* 61(2):47–56, 2012.
36. Wu JM, Staton CA: Anti-angiogenic drug discovery: lessons from the past and thoughts for the future, *Expert Opin Drug Discov* 7(8):723–743, 2012.
37. Shay JW, Wright WE: Role of telomeres and telomerase in cancer, *Semin Cancer Biol* 21(6):349–353, 2011.
38. Podlevsky JD, Chen JJ: It all comes together at the ends: telomerase structure, function, and biogenesis, *Mutat Res* 730(1-2):3–11, 2012.
39. Trapé AP, Gonzalez-Angulo AM: Breast cancer and metastasis: on the way toward individualized therapy, *Cancer Genomics Proteomics* 9(5):297–310, 2012.
40. Comen EA: Tracking the seed and tending the soil: evolving concepts in metastatic breast cancer, *Discov Med* 14(75):97–104, 2012.
41. Butt AQ, Miggin SM: Cancer and viruses: a double-edged sword, *Proteomics* 12(13):2127–2138, 2012.
42. Harford JB: Viral infections and human cancers: the legacy of Denis Burkitt, *Br J Haematol* 156(6):709–718, 2012.
43. Goldstone SE, Vuocolo S: A prophylactic quadrivalent vaccine for the prevention of infection and disease related to HPV-6, -11, -16 and -18, *Expert Rev Vaccines* 11(4):395–406, 2012.
44. Carbone A, De Paoli P: Cancers related to viral agents that have a direct role in carcinogenesis: pathological and diagnostic techniques, *J Clin Pathol* 65(8):680–686, 2012.
45. Murukesan V, Mukherjee S: Managing post-transplant lymphoproliferative disorders in solid-organ transplant recipients: a review of immunosuppressant regimens, *Drugs* 72(12):1631–1643, 2012.
46. Yang XR et al: Evaluation of risk factors for nasopharyngeal carcinoma in high-risk nasopharyngeal carcinoma families in Taiwan, *Cancer Epidemiol Biomarkers Prev* 14(4):900–905, 2005.
47. Raab-Traub N: Novel mechanisms of EBV-induced oncogenesis, *Curr Opin Virol* 2(4):453–458, 2012.
48. Mesri EA, Cesarman E, Boshoff C: Kaposi's sarcoma and its associated herpesvirus, *Nat Rev Cancer* 10(10):707–719, 2010.
49. Cook LB et al: HTLV-1: persistence and pathogenesis, *Virology* 435(1):131–140, 2013.

50. Stauffer JK et al: Chronic inflammation, immune escape, and oncogenesis in the liver: a unique neighborhood for novel interactions, *Hepatology* 56(4):1567–1574, 2012.
51. Rosenzweig SD, Holland SM: Recent insights into the pathobiology of innate immune deficiencies, *Curr Allergy Asthma Rep* 11(5):369–377, 2011.
52. Alberu J: Clinical insights for cancer outcomes in renal transplant patients, *Transplant Proc* 42(9 Suppl):S36–S40, 2010.
53. Villeneuve PJ et al: Cancer incidence among Canadian kidney transplant recipients, *Am J Transplant* 7:941–948, 2007.
54. Kundu JK, Surh Y- J: Emerging avenues linking inflammation and cancer, *Free Radic Biol Med* 52(9):2013–2037, 2012.
55. Fitzpatrick FA: Inflammation, carcinogenesis and cancer, *Int Immunopharmacol* 1(9-10):1651–1667, 2001.
56. Mantovani A et al: Tumour immunity: effector response to tumour and role of the microenvironment, *Lancet* 371:771–783, 2008.
57. Hanahan D, Weinberg RA: Hallmarks of cancer: the next generation, *Cell* 144(5):646–674, 2011.
58. Dubé C et al: The use of aspirin for primary prevention of colorectal cancer: a systematic review prepared for the U.S. Preventive Services Task Force, *Ann Intern Med* 146(5):365–375, 2007.
59. Ruggiero P: *Helicobacter pylori* infection: what's new, *Curr Opin Infect Dis* 25(3):337–344, 2012.
60. Zhao C, Bu X: Promoter methylation of tumor-related genes in gastric carcinogenesis, *Histol Histopathol* 27(10):1271–1282, 2012.
61. Kato M, Asaka M: Recent development of gastric cancer prevention, *Jpn J Clin Oncol* 42(11):987–994, 2012.
62. Balkwill FR, Mantovani A: Cancer-related inflammation: common themes and therapeutic opportunities, *Semin Cancer Biol* 22(1):33–40, 2012.
63. Hao N-B et al: Macrophages in tumor microenvironments and the progression of tumors, *Clin Dev Immunol* 2012:1–11, 2012.
64. Porta C et al: Macrophages in cancer and infectious diseases: the 'good' and the 'bad', *Immunotherapy* 3(10):1185–1202, 2011.
65. Mitchem JB et al: Targeting tumor-infiltrating macrophages decreases tumor-initiating cells, relieves immunosuppression, and improves chemotherapeutic responses, *Cancer Res* 73(3):1128–1141, 2013.
66. Hanahan D, Coussens LM: Accessories to crime: functions of cells recruited to the tumor microenvironment, *Cancer Cell* 21(3):309–322, 2012.
67. Tan W et al: Tumour-infiltrating regulatory T cells stimulate mammary cancer metastasis through RANKL-RANK signalling, *Nature* 470(7335):548–553, 2011.
68. Ruffell B et al: Lymphocytes in cancer development: polarization towards pro-tumor immunity, *Cytokine Growth Factor Rev* 21(1):3–10, 2010.
69. DeNardo DG et al: Leukocyte complexity predicts breast cancer survival and functionally regulates response to chemotherapy, *Cancer Discov* 1(1):54–67, 2011.
70. Demaria S et al: Cancer and inflammation: promise for biological therapy, *J Immunother* 33(4):335–351, 2010.
71. Castells M et al: Implication of tumor microenvironment in chemoresistance: tumor-associated stromal cells protect tumor cells from cell death, *Int J Mol Sci* 13(8):9545–9571, 2012.
72. Shiao SL et al: Immune microenvironments in solid tumors: new targets for therapy, *Genes Dev* 25(24):2559–2572, 2011.
73. Wang K, Grivennikov SI, Karin M: Implications of anti-cytokine therapy in colorectal cancer and autoimmune diseases, *Ann Rheum Dis*, 2012 Dec 19. [Epub ahead of print.].
74. Fyles AW et al: Tamoxifen with or without breast irradiation in women 50 years of age or older with early breast cancer, *N Engl J Med* 351: 963–970, 2004.
75. Carrick S et al: Single agent versus combination chemotherapy for metastatic breast cancer, *Cochrane Database Syst Rev*(2):CD003372, 2005.
76. Valastyan S, Weinberg RA: Tumor metastasis: molecular insights and evolving paradigms, *Cell* 147(2):275–292, 2011.
77. Talmadge JE, Fidler IJ: AACR centennial series: the biology of cancer metastasis: historical perspective, *Cancer Res* 70:5649–5669, 2010.
78. Man Y-G: Tumor cell budding from focally disrupted tumor capsules: a common pathway for all breast cancer subtype derived invasion? *J Cancer* 1:32–37, 2010.
79. Khamis ZI, Sahab ZJ, Sang Q-XA: Active roles of tumor stroma in breast cancer metastasis, *Int J Breast Cancer* 1-10:2012, 2012.
80. Man Y-G et al: Tumor-infiltrating immune cells promoting tumor invasion and metastasis: existing theories, *J Cancer* 4(1):84–95, 2013.
81. Tarin D et al: Clinicopathological observations on metastasis in man studied in patients treated with peritoneovenous shunts, *BMJ* 288(6419):749–751, 1984.
82. Mendoza M, Khanna C: Revisiting the seed and soil in cancer metastasis, *Int J Biochem Cell Biol* 41(7):1452–1462, 2009.
83. Craene BD, Berx G: Regulatory networks defining EMT during cancer initiation and progression, *Nat Rev Cancer* 13(2):97–110, 2012.
84. Medici D, Kalluri R: Endothelial-mesenchymal transition and its contribution to the emergence of stem cell phenotype, *Semin Cancer Biol* 22(5-6):379–384, 2012.
85. Scheel C, Weinberg RA: Cancer stem cells and epithelial-mesenchymal transition: concepts and molecular links, *Semin Cancer Biol* 22(5-6): 396–403, 2012.
86. Nieto MA, Cano A: The epithelial-mesenchymal transition under control: global programs to regulate epithelial plasticity, *Semin Cancer Biol* 22(5-6):361–368, 2012.
87. Kiss NB et al: Quantitative global and gene-specific promoter methylation in relation to biological properties of neuroblastomas, *BMC Med Genet* 13:83, 2012.
88. Schackert G, Fidler IJ: Site-specific metastasis of mouse melanomas and a fibrosarcoma in the brain or meninges of syngeneic animals, *Cancer Res* 48:3478–3484, 1998.
89. Gupta GP, Massagué J: Cancer metastasis: building a framework, *Cell* 127(4):697–708, 2006.
90. Aguirre-Ghiso JA: Models, mechanisms and clinical evidence for cancer dormancy, *Nat Rev Cancer* 7(11):834–846, 2007.
91. Sharp L, Vernino S: Paraneoplastic neuromuscular disorders, *Muscle Nerve* 46(6):841–850, 2012.
92. Spain PD, Kadan-Lottick N: Observations of unprecedented remissions following novel treatment for acute leukemia in children in 1948, *J R Soc Med* 105(4):177–181, 2012.
93. Ballinger LL: Hereditary gynecologic cancers: risk assessment, counseling, testing and management, *Obstet Gynecol Clin North Am* 39(2):165–181, 2012.

CHAPTER

13

Cancer Epidemiology

Kathryn L. McCance

evolve WEBSITE

http://evolve.elsevier.com/McCance/

- Review Questions and Answers
- Animations
- Online Course: Module 8

CHAPTER OUTLINE

Although cancer arises from a complicated and an interacting web of multiple etiologies, avoiding high-risk behaviors and exposure to individual **carcinogens,** or cancer-causing substances, will prevent many types of cancer (Figure 13-1).[1-3] Research has shown that lifestyle behaviors, dietary and environmental factors (such as exposure to ultraviolet radiation and infections), and occupational exposure contribute to the number of cancer cases and deaths.[4-6] In this context, any of the following factors can contribute to the development of cancer[7-9]:

- Lifestyle choices, such as nutritional intake, smoking, or alcohol use
- Environmental conditions, including exposure to sunlight, natural and medical radiation, workplace exposures, and involuntary or unknown exposures
- Lack of physical exercise and overweight/obesity
- Sexual practices
- Prescribed and illicit medications
- Socioeconomic factors that affect exposures and susceptibility
- Carcinogenic substances present in air, water, and soil

The question of estimating the environmentally attributable risk for cancer is deceptive because such estimates vary tremendously as a result of the definition of the environment used. Therefore, another way of examining what portion of cancer risk is attributable to the environment involves asking, "What is not attributable to the environment?"[10] In this context, it is usually those cancers caused by highly penetrant genes; inherited mutations very rarely predispose us to cancer.[11-14] The International Agency for Research on Cancer (IARC) completed a review of the more than 100 chemicals, occupations, physical

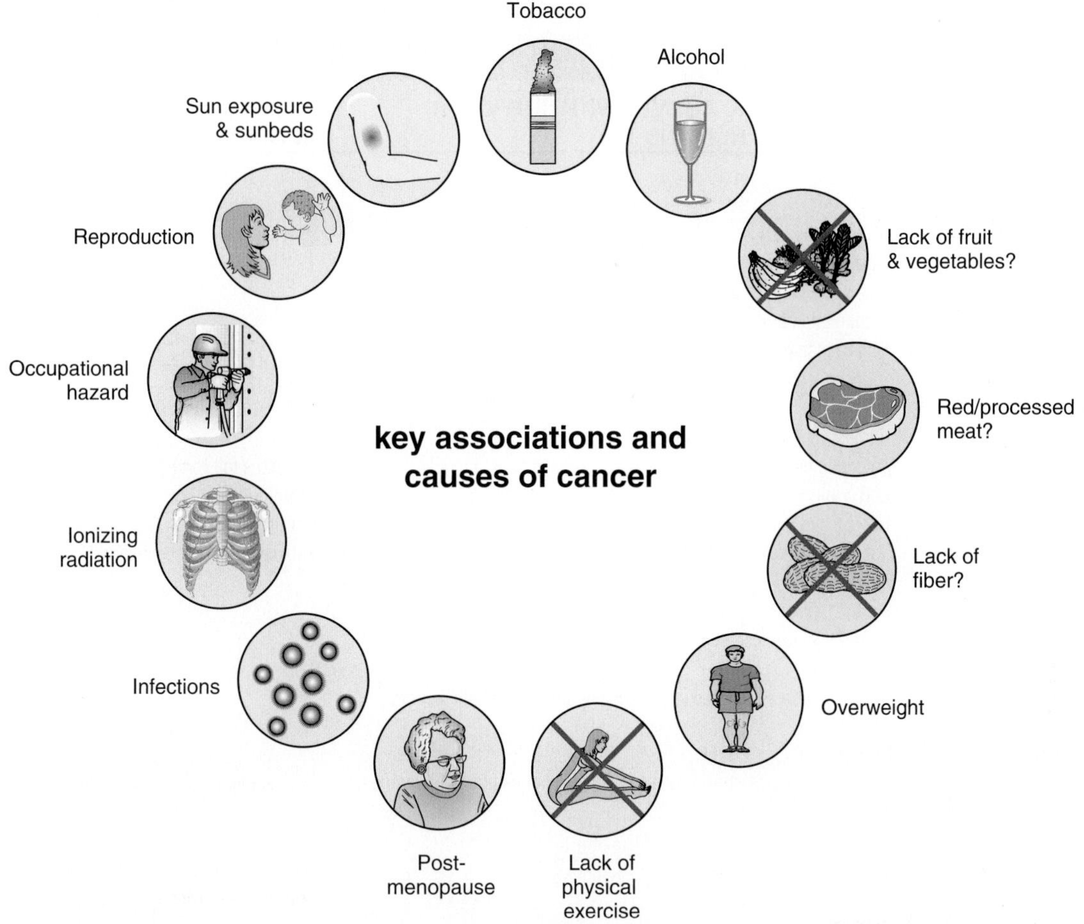

FIGURE 13-1 Key Associations and Causes of Cancer. Tobacco, alcohol, obesity, lack of physical activity, hormones, infections, ionizing radiation, occupational hazards, reproductive factors, and ultraviolet light are key associations and causes of cancer. Studies of diet are ongoing.

agents, biologic agents, and other agents classified as carcinogenic to humans.[7] Simplified tables with a list of classifications by cancer sites with sufficient or limited evidence in humans are contained in Table 13-1.

GENETICS, EPIGENETICS, AND TISSUE

Cancers are caused by environmental-lifestyle behaviors and by exposures and genetic factors. Cancer is driven by genetic alterations and epigenetic abnormalities (see Chapter 12).[15-18] These changes are mitotically and meiotically heritable[19,20] (see Chapter 4). Although driver and passenger genetic alterations are key, a wealth of data now indicate the importance of epigenetic processes, especially those with resultant gene silencing (not broken, but mute) of key regulatory genes (see Chapters 6 and 12 and Figure 13-2).

There has been intense scrutiny of the biology of aberrant gene silencing and associated environmental factors. Much research has focused on the abnormal appearance of an epigenetic alteration—DNA methylation (the addition of a methyl group [CH_3])—in the proximal promoter regions of associated genes (see Figure 13-2, *B*). Some of these genes are known as key tumor-suppressor genes.[15-18,21] The promoter DNA hypermethylation and gene silencing (i.e., epigenetic alterations) cause a loss of function and this loss facilitates tumor initiation and progression.[15-18,21]

Cancer development and progression involves the tissue microenvironment or stroma (see Chapter 12). The microenvironment participates in a complex signaling process that facilitates tumor promotion and metastasis because stromal tissue has various immune cells. Extensive clinical and experimental evidence shows that infiltrating immune cells cause chronic inflammation and, therefore, create a permissive tumor-progressing environment. Chronic inflammation also can *precede* and presumably initiate malignant change, as for example in inflammation-induced colon cancer.[22] It is well documented that chronic inflammation induced by bacteria, viruses, autoimmune processes, and toxins promotes common types of cancer, including colon, liver, and lung cancer. Inflammation can be caused by numerous environmental factors, for example, inhaling tobacco smoke, asbestos fibers, or fine particles in the air from diesel engine exhaust and industrial sources. These sources are major factors in lung and other respiratory tract cancers.[23,24] Cancer development in the presence of chronic inflammation involves the continuous presence of cytokines, chemokines, reactive oxygen species (ROS), oncogenes, cyclooxgenase-2 (COX-2), 5-lipoxygenase (5-LOX), and matrix metalloproteinases (MMPs) as well as the activation of essential transcription factors, such as nuclear factor κB (NF-κB).

Text continued on p. 408

TABLE 13-1 LIST OF CLASSIFICATIONS BY CANCER SITES WITH SUFFICIENT OR LIMITED EVIDENCE IN HUMANS

CANCER SITE	CARCINOGENIC AGENTS WITH SUFFICIENT EVIDENCE IN HUMANS	AGENTS WITH LIMITED EVIDENCE IN HUMANS
Lip, Oral Cavity, and Pharynx		
Lip		Solar radiation
Oral cavity	Alcoholic beverages	
	Betel quid with tobacco	
	Betel quid without tobacco	
	Human papillomavirus type 16	
	Tobacco, smokeless	
	Tobacco smoking	
Salivary gland	X-radiation, γ-radiation	Radioiodines, including iodine-131
Tonsil	Human papillomavirus type 16	
Pharynx	Alcoholic beverages	Asbestos (all forms)
	Betel quid with tobacco	Mate drinking, hot
	Human papillomavirus type 16	Printing presses
	Tobacco smoking	Tobacco smoke, secondhand
Nasopharynx	Epstein-Barr virus	
	Formaldehyde	
	Salted fish, Chinese-style	
	Wood dust	
Digestive tract, upper	Acetaldehyde associated with consumption of alcoholic beverages	
Digestive Organs		
Esophagus	Acetaldehyde associated with consumption of alcoholic beverages	Dry cleaning
	Alcoholic beverages	Mate drinking, hot
	Betel quid with tobacco	Pickled vegetables (traditional Asian)
	Betel quid without tobacco	Rubber production industry
	Tobacco, smokeless	Tetrachloroethylene
	Tobacco smoking	
	X-radiation, γ-radiation	
Stomach	*Helicobacter pylori*	Asbestos (all forms)
	Rubber production industry	Epstein-Barr virus
	Tobacco smoking	Lead compounds, inorganic
	X-radiation, γ-radiation	Nitrate or nitrite (ingested) under conditions that result in endogenous nitrosation
		Pickled vegetables (traditional Asian)
		Salted fish (Chinese style)
Colon and rectum	Alcoholic beverages	Asbestos (all forms)
	Tobacco smoking	*Schistosoma japonicum*
	X-radiation, γ-radiation	
Anus	Human immunodeficiency virus type 1	Human papillomavirus types 18, 33
	Human papillomavirus type 16	
Liver and bile duct	Aflatoxins	Androgenic (anabolic) steroids
	Alcoholic beverages	Arsenic and inorganic arsenic compounds
	Clonorchis sinensis	Betel quid without tobacco
	Estrogen-progestogen contraceptives	Human immunodeficiency virus type 1
	Hepatitis B virus	Polychlorinated biphenyls
	Hepatitis C virus	*Schistosoma japonicum*
	Opisthorchis viverrini	Trichloroethylene
	Plutonium	X-radiation, γ-radiation
	Thorium-232 and its decay products	
	Tobacco smoking (in smokers and in smokers' children)	
	Vinyl chloride	
Gallbladder	Thorium-232 and its decay products	
Pancreas	Tobacco, smokeless	Alcoholic beverages
	Tobacco smoking	Thorium-232 and its decay products
		X-radiation, γ-radiation
Digestive tract, unspecified		Radioiodines, including iodine-131

TABLE 13-1 LIST OF CLASSIFICATIONS BY CANCER SITES WITH SUFFICIENT OR LIMITED EVIDENCE IN HUMANS—cont'd

CANCER SITE	CARCINOGENIC AGENTS WITH SUFFICIENT EVIDENCE IN HUMANS	AGENTS WITH LIMITED EVIDENCE IN HUMANS
Respiratory Organs		
Nasal cavity and paranasal sinus	Isopropyl alcohol production	Carpentry and joinery
	Leather dust	Chromium (VI) compounds
	Nickel compounds	Formaldehyde
	Radium-226 and its decay products	Textile manufacturing
	Radium-228 and its decay products	
	Tobacco smoking	
	Wood dust	
Larynx	Acid mists, strong inorganic	Human papillomavirus type 16
	Alcoholic beverages	Mate drinking, hot
	Asbestos (all forms)	Rubber production industry
	Tobacco smoking	Sulfur mustard
		Tobacco smoke, secondhand
Lung	Aluminum production	Acid mists, strong inorganic
	Arsenic and inorganic arsenic compounds	Art glass, glass containers, and pressed ware (manufacture of)
	Beryllium and beryllium products	Biomass fuel (primarily wood), indoor emissions from household combustion of
	Bis(chloromethyl) ether; chloromethyl methyl ether (technical grade)	Bitumens, oxidized, and their emissions during roofing
	Cadmium and cadmium compounds	Bitumens, hard, and their emissions during mastic asphalt work
	Chromium (VI) compounds	Carbon electrode manufacture
	Coal, indoor emissions from household combustion	α-Chlorinated toluenes and benzyl chloride (combined exposure)
	Coal gasification	Cobalt metal with tungsten carbide
	Coal-tar pitch	Creosotes
	Coke production	Engine exhaust, diesel
	Hematite mining (underground)	Frying, emissions from high-temperature
	Iron and steel founding	Insecticides, nonarsenical (occupational exposures in spraying and application)
	MOPP (vincristine-prednisone-nitrogen mustard-procarbazine mixture)	Printing processes
	Nickel compounds	2,3,7,8-Tetrachlorodibenzo-*para*-dioxin
	Painting	Welding fumes
	Plutonium	
	Radon-222 and its decay products	
	Rubber production industry	
	Silica dust, crystalline	
	Soot	
	Sulfur mustard	
	Tobacco smoke, secondhand	
	Tobacco smoking	
	X-radiation, γ-radiation	
Bone, Skin, and Mesothelium, Endothelium, and Soft Tissue		
Bone	Plutonium	Radioiodines, including iodine-131
	Radium-224 and its decay products	
	Radium-226 and its decay products	
	Radium-228 and its decay products	
	X-radiation, γ-radiation	
Skin (melanoma)	Solar radiation	
	Ultraviolet-emitting tanning devices	
Skin (other malignant neoplasms)	Arsenic and inorganic arsenic compounds	Creosotes
	Azathioprine	Human immunodeficiency virus type 1
	Coal-tar distillation	Human papillomavirus types 5 and 8 (in individuals with epidermodysplasia verruciformis)
	Coal-tar pitch	Nitrogen mustard
	Cyclosporine	Petroleum refining (occupational exposures)
	Methoxsalen plus ultraviolet A	Ultraviolet-emitting tanning devices
	Mineral oils, untreated or mildly treated	Merkel cell polyomavirus (MCV)
	Shale oils	
	Solar radiation	
	Soot	
	X-radiation, γ-radiation	

Continued

TABLE 13-1 LIST OF CLASSIFICATIONS BY CANCER SITES WITH SUFFICIENT OR LIMITED EVIDENCE IN HUMANS—cont'd

CANCER SITE	CARCINOGENIC AGENTS WITH SUFFICIENT EVIDENCE IN HUMANS	AGENTS WITH LIMITED EVIDENCE IN HUMANS
Mesothelium (pleura and peritoneum)	Asbestos (all forms) Erionite Painting	
Endothelium (Kaposi sarcoma)	Human immunodeficiency virus type 1 Kaposi sarcoma herpesvirus	
Soft tissue		Polychlorophenols or their sodium salts (combined exposures) Radioiodines, including iodine-131 2,3,7,8-Tetrachlorodibenzo-*para*-dioxin
Breast and Female Genital Organs		
Breast	Alcoholic beverages Diethylstilbestrol Estrogen-progestogen contraceptives Estrogen-progestogen menopausal therapy X-radiation, γ-radiation	Estrogen menopausal therapy Ethylene oxide Shiftwork that involves circadian disruption Tobacco smoking
Vulva	Human papillomavirus 16	Human immunodeficiency virus type 1
Vagina	Diethylstilbestrol (exposure in utero) Human papillomavirus 16	Human immunodeficiency virus type 1
Uterine cervix	Diethylstilbestrol (exposure in utero) Estrogen-progestogen contraceptives Human immunodeficiency virus type 1 Human papillomavirus types 16, 18, 31, 33, 35, 39, 45, 51, 52, 56, 58, 59 Tobacco smoking	Human papillomavirus types 26, 53, 66, 67, 68, 70, 73, 82 Tetrachloroethylene
Endometrium	Estrogen menopausal therapy Estrogen-progestogen menopausal therapy Tamoxifen	Diethylstilbestrol
Ovary	Asbestos (all forms) Estrogen menopausal therapy Tobacco smoking	Talc-based body powder (perineal use) X-radiation, γ-radiation
Male Genital Organs		
Penis	Human papillomavirus type 16	Human immunodeficiency virus type 1 Human papillomavirus type 18
Prostrate		Androgenic (anabolic) steroids Arsenic and inorganic arsenic compounds Cadmium and cadmium compounds Rubber production industry Thorium-232 and its decay products X-radiation, γ-radiation
Testis		Diethylstilbestrol exposure in utero
Urinary Tract		
Kidney	Tobacco smoking X-radiation, γ-radiation	Arsenic and inorganic arsenic compounds Cadmium and cadmium compounds Printing processes
Renal pelvis and ureter	Aristolochic acids, plants containing phenacetin Phenacetin, analgesic mixtures containing Tobacco smoking	Aristolochic acids
Urinary bladder	Aluminum production 4-Aminobiphenyl Arsenic and inorganic arsenic compounds Auramine production Benzidine Chlornaphazine Cyclophosphamide Magenta production 2-Naphthylamine	4-Chloro-*ortho*-toluidine Coal-tar pitch Coffee Dry cleaning Engine exhaust, diesel Hairdressers and barbers (occupational exposure) Printing processes Soot Textile manufacturing

TABLE 13-1 LIST OF CLASSIFICATIONS BY CANCER SITES WITH SUFFICIENT OR LIMITED EVIDENCE IN HUMANS—cont'd

CANCER SITE	CARCINOGENIC AGENTS WITH SUFFICIENT EVIDENCE IN HUMANS	AGENTS WITH LIMITED EVIDENCE IN HUMANS
	Painting	
	Rubber production industry	
	Schistosoma haematobium	
	Tobacco smoking	
	ortho-Toluidine	
	X-radiation, γ-radiation	
Eye, Brain, and Central Nervous System		
Eye	Human immunodeficiency virus type 1	Solar radiation
	Ultraviolet-emitting tanning devices	
	Welding	
Brain and central nervous system	X-radiation, γ-radiation	Radiofrequency electromagnetic fields (including from wireless phones)
Endocrine Glands		
Thyroid	Radioiodines, including iodine-131	
	X-radiation, γ-radiation	
Lymphoid, Hematopoietic, and Related Tissue		
Leukemia and/or lymphoma	Azathioprine	Bis(chloroethyl)nitrosourea (BBCNU)
	Benzene	Chloramphenicol
	Busulfan	Ethylene oxide
	1,3-Butadiene	Etoposide
	Chlorambucil	Hepatitis B virus
	Cyclophosphamide	Magnetic fields, extremely low frequency (childhood leukemia)
	Cyclosporine	Mitoxantrone
	Epstein-Barr virus	Nitrogen mustard
	Etoposide with cisplatin and bleomycin	Painting (childhood leukemia from maternal exposure)
	Fission products, including strontium-90	Petroleum refining (occupational exposures)
	Formaldehyde	Polychlorophenols or their sodium salts (combined exposures)
	Helicobacter pylori	Radioiodines, including iodine-131
	Hepatitis C virus	Radon-222 and its decay products
	Human immunodeficiency virus type 1	Styrene
	Human T-cell lymphotropic virus type 1	Teniposide
	Kaposi sarcoma herpesvirus	Tetrachloroethylene
	Melphalan	Trichloroethylene
	MOPP (vincristine-prednisone-nitrogen mustard-procarbazine mixture)	2,3,7,8-Tetrachlorodibenzo-*para*-dioxin
	Phosphorus-32	Tobacco smoking (childhood leukemia in smokers' children)
	Rubber production industry	Malaria (caused by infection with *Plasmodium falciparum* in holoendemic areas)
	Semustine (methyl-CCNU)	
	Thiotepa	
	Thorium-23 and its decay products	
	Tobacco smoking	
	Treosulfan	
	X-radiation, γ-radiation	
Multiple or Unspecific Sites		
Multiple sites (unspecified)	Cyclosporine	Chlorophenoxy herbicides
	Fission products, including strontium-90	Plutonium
	X-radiation, γ-radiation (exposure in utero)	
All cancer sites (combined)	2,3,7,8-Tetrachlorodibenzo-*para*-dioxin	

Adapted from Cogliano VJ et al: *J Natl Cancer Inst* 103:1–13, 2011. Available at http://jnci.oxfordjournals.org/content/early/2011/12/11/jnci.djr483.short?rss=1.

Note: This table does not include factors not covered in the IARC Monographs, notably genetic traits, reproductive status, and some nutritional factors.

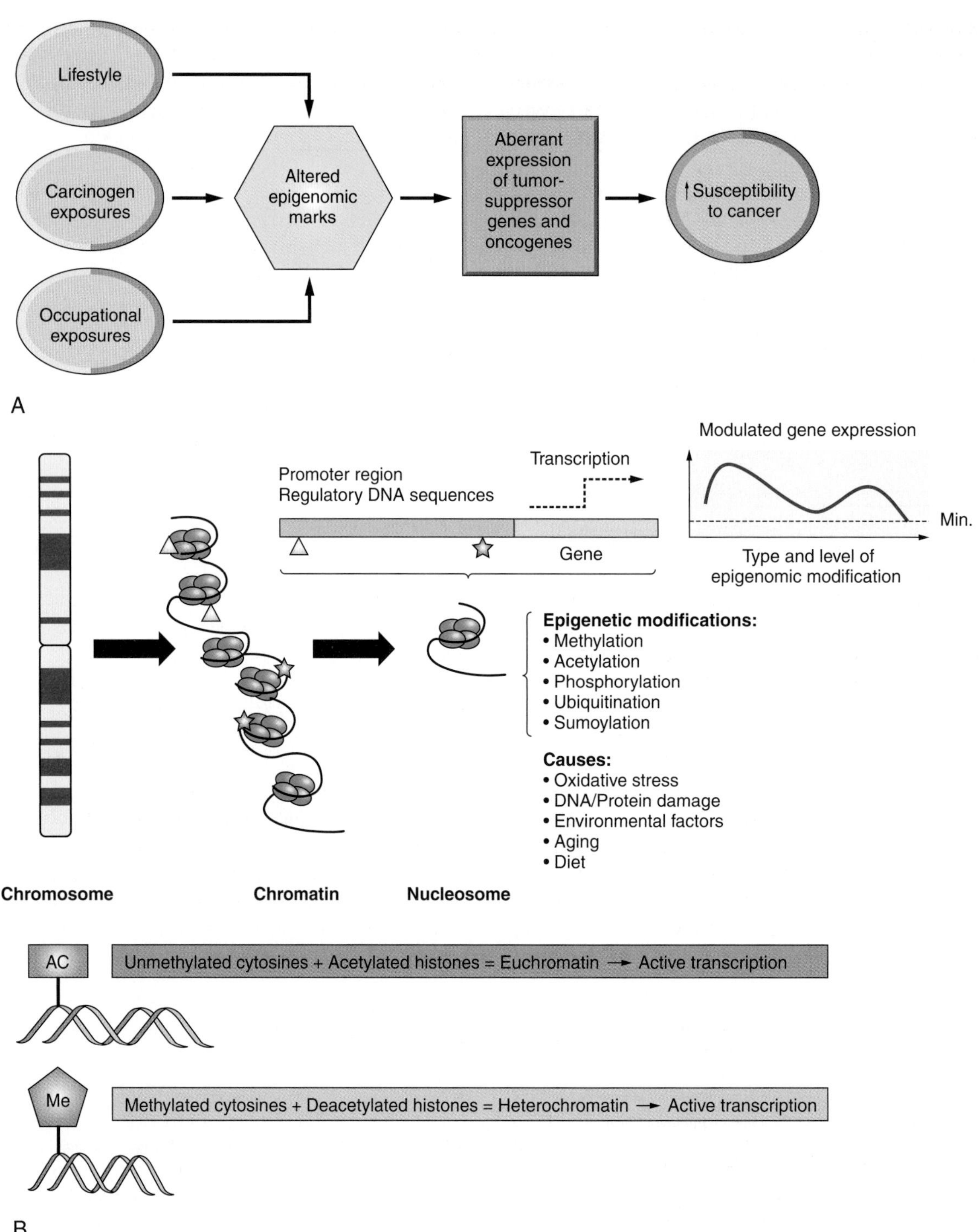

FIGURE 13-2 Epigenetic Modulation and Modifications. **A,** Overview of the potential role of epigenetic modulation by dietary and other environmental factors in cancer development. **B,** Epigenetic modulations' model according to current knowledge. The different types of chemical modifications, such as methylation or acetylation, of promoter regions and/or other regulatory DNA sequences outside the gene can have severe impact on gene transcription and translation and a resultant high modulation of gene expression and product (protein) functionality. (From World Cancer Research Fund/American Institute for Cancer Research: *Food, nutrition, physical activity, and the prevention of cancer: a global perspective,* Washington, DC, 2007, AICR.)

Investigators are working hard to understand and connect the complex and intricate relationships between genotype, phenotype, and the environment in order to understand a person's chances of developing cancer (see Figure 13-2, *A* and *B*). The root cause of cancer is more than inherited or acquired genetic mutations and involves epigenetic changes that frequently precede and induce cancer-causing genetic mutations.[25] The past decade has highlighted the major role epigenetic processes play in cancer initiation, progression, and treatment.[25] Additionally, if these early epigenetic alterations can be detected and reversed, cancer may be prevented. In the 1980s, cancer biologist Stephen Baylin hypothesized that if a tumor-suppressor gene is hypermethylated its activity would decrease or stop entirely. Firm evidence came in 1994 when Baylin and oncologist James Herman showed that 20% of the individuals with the noninherited form of renal cell carcinoma (RCC) did not have a mutation in von Hippel-Lindau and their genes were silenced not by a mutation but rather by epigenetic hypermethylation.[26] These and many other investigators' stunning experiments and observations have changed the biology of cancer dramatically! *The paradigm shift from a genetic to an epigenetic model is critical for prevention strategies because these changes are potentially reversible and may precede genetic mutations.* Investigators are linking epigenetic abnormalities to mutations in genes that control DNA methylation, the packaging and the function of DNA in chromatin, and metabolism[25] (see Chapter 12). We know that environmental contaminants can damage the immune system, altering signaling processes that facilitate tumor proliferation. At the interface of environment and genetics is chronic inflammation. Inflammation has been linked with increased DNA methylation, an epigenetic alteration. A notable example is found in persons with ulcerative colitis, who can develop colon cancer at an age younger than the 60- to 70-year average. The epigenetic changes that occur in colon cancer, including DNA hypermethylation and gene silencing, are accelerated and appear in the inflamed tissue before the actual cancer.[27-29]

INCIDENCE AND MORTALITY TRENDS

Incidence Trends

Cancer is reported to become a major cause of morbidity and mortality in the coming decades in all regions of the world (What's New? Global Cancer Transitions).[30] In the National Cancer Institute's 2011 annual report to the nation, trends were reported for all cancers combined, for childhood cancers, and for the top 15 cancers for each of the major racial and ethnic groups by gender.[31] The report also presents incidence of malignant and nonmalignant brain tumors in children and adults by race, gender, age group, and histologic type. Overall, cancer incidence rates for all racial and ethnic groups combined decreased by 0.8% per year during the most recent study period, 2003 to 2007. A significant decrease of 0.6% per year was noted in women and a nonsignificant decrease of 0.8% per year was noted in men influenced by a nonsignificant increase in prostate cancer incidence (2005 to 2007).[31] The most frequently diagnosed cancers, prostate and breast, showed possible changing trends. Cancer of the prostate showed a nonsignificant annual increase of 3.0% for the period 2005 to 2007 after a significant decrease for the period 2001 to 2005. Breast cancer showed a decrease from 1999 to 2007 after a sharp decrease in 2002 to 2003; the lower rates thereafter remained stable. The cancer rates among children (from birth to age 19 years) showed an increase of 0.6% per year for the entire period of 1992 to 2007. The long-term increase in cancer incidence rates in children is possibly related to increases in lymphoid leukemias and a smaller increase in other childhood cancers[31] (see Chapter 14).

From the period 2003 to 2007, 5 of the 15 most common cancers among men—lung and bronchus (lung), colorectal, oral and pharynx (oral), stomach, and malignant brain tumors—showed a significant decrease. Significant increases among men in the period 2003 to 2007 included melanoma of the skin, kidney and renal pelvis (kidney), pancreas, and liver and intrahepatic bile duct (liver). Cancers that had neither an increase nor a decrease in the period 2003 to 2007 included prostate (see preceding paragraph), bladder, esophageal cancers, leukemia, myeloma, and non-Hodgkin lymphoma.

Significant, increasing trends among women were noted in three of the four cancers increasing in men (kidney, pancreas, and melanoma of the skin); leukemia and thyroid cancer also increased.[31] Significant decreasing trends occurred with cancers

WHAT'S NEW?

Global Cancer Transitions

The United Nations has estimated that the global population will reach 7 billion by 2012 and 8.3 billion by 2030. Population aging and growth will be greatest in low- and middle-income countries. Researchers used four levels of a Human Development Index [HDI] (low, medium, high, and very high), as an indicator of life expectancy, education, and gross domestic product per head, to present an overview of global patterns of cancer incidence and mortality. This important report is the first of its kind to present this global overview. These statistics may translate to a global incidence of 20.3 million new cancer cases by 2030 (compared with an estimated 12.7 million cases in 2008) and a predicted 13.2 million cancer-related deaths worldwide by 2030, an increase from the 7.6 million cancer-related deaths in 2008. In both high HDI and very high HDI regions, four cancers (female breast, lung, colorectal, and prostate cancers) explain almost half of the overall cancer burden. In medium HDI regions, lung and female breast cancers are the most common types of cancer along with stomach and liver cancers. In low HDI regions, female breast and liver cancers also are common, as well as the infection-related cancers cervical cancer and Kaposi sarcoma. In these low HDI regions, cervical cancer was more common than both breast cancer and liver cancer. Across 184 countries, 9 different cancers were most commonly diagnosed in men, including the 3 most common—prostate, lung, and liver cancers. Breast and cervical cancers were the most common in women. In medium HDI and high HDI settings, the decreases in incidence of cervical and stomach cancers seem to be offset by the rising increases in incidence of female breast, prostate, and colorectal cancers. The reduction in infection-related cancers appears to be offset by simultaneous increases in cancers related to the "western lifestyle" and changes in tobacco consumption and the effect on lung and other cancers.

Targeted interventions can substantially reduce the incidences of cancers worldwide and include primary prevention strategies to decrease or eliminate certain lifestyle factors—including tobacco avoidance and cessation of smoking, reduction in the number of obese individuals, reduction in alcohol intake, increase in physical activity, and implementation of vaccination programs for liver and cervical cancer as well as effective early detection programs for colorectal, breast, and cervical cancer. Reductions in mortality could be implemented that increase access to curative treatment because provision of palliative care for those individuals dying of cancer will help to reduce population inequities.

Data from Bray F et al: *Lancet Oncol* 13(8):790–801, 2012; Ferlay J et al: *Int J Cancer* 127:2893–2917, 2010.

of the breast, lung, colon or rectum, uterus, cervix, bladder, and oral cavity. No significant trends were observed in non-Hodgkin lymphoma, ovarian cancer, and malignant brain tumors.[31]

This current analysis shows the relative stability of long-term trends of malignant brain tumors of the neuroepithelial tissue. From the period 1980 to 2007, brain tumors increased 1.9% per year during 1980 to 1987 followed by a decrease of 0.4% per year during the remaining 20 years. Yet, marked differences occurred for histologic groups of brain tumors because of changing diagnostic methods, pathologic coding schemes, and classifications. Better classifications have enabled progress in understanding the pathogenesis of malignant gliomas.[31] The trends in nonmalignant tumors are not now known because they only became reportable on a national level in 2004.[31]

Mortality Trends

Since the mid-1970s, cancer death rates have decreased for children. Long-term (1975 to 2007) trends in death rates continued to decrease in children, although at a slower rate in the recent decade[31] (see Chapter 14). Death rates from the periods 1998 to 2007 and from 2003 to 2007 continued to decrease for 7 of the top 15 cancer types in both men and women (colorectal, brain, stomach, and kidney cancers; non-Hodgkin lymphoma; leukemia; and myeloma).[31] Decreasing death rates for men also included lung, prostate, and oral cavity, and for women breast and bladder cancers. Overall, however, death rates continued to increase for cancers of the liver and pancreas among men and women, for uterine cancer in women, and for melanoma of the skin in men.[31] Importantly, lung cancer death rates in women showed a significant decrease during the period 2003 to 2007, following long-term increases during the period 1975 to 2003.

IN UTERO AND EARLY LIFE CONDITIONS

From studies of the etiology of certain cancers, it is widely accepted that a long latency period precedes the onset of adult cancers. Accumulating data suggest early life events influence later susceptibility to certain chronic diseases.[32] Throughout in utero development, the placenta plays a major role in controlling growth and development.[33] Because the placenta is a regulator of the intrauterine environment and can be influenced by exposures throughout pregnancy,[33] much research is being done with DNA methylation linking environmental cues to placental pathologies and adult life (Figure 13-3).

Children may be affected by prenatal exposures, parental exposures before conception, and exposure to breast milk. **Developmental plasticity** is the degree to which an organism's development is contingent on its environment. It requires stable gene expression that in part appears to be modulated by epigenetic processes such as DNA methylation and histone modification (Figure 13-4).[32] Sensitivity to environmental-lifestyle factors influences the mature phenotype and is dependent on the interactions of both the genome and the epigenome. Abnormal DNA hypermethylation in cancer is noted in many genes important to embryonic development.[25] Although the developing embryo is protected from the physical and chemical toxins or dangers of the outside environment by the uterine environment, elements of the maternal diet, drugs, or accidentally ingested and/or inhaled toxins can be delivered to the embryo through the maternal circulation.[34] Known environmental effects include drugs, such as valproic acid (VPA, an anti-epileptic),[35] or the effects of high maternal alcohol consumption.[36,37]

Perhaps one of the best examples of early life events and future cancer is the chemical exposure to diethylstilbestrol (DES), a synthetic estrogen. This medication was prescribed between 1938 and 1971 to attempt to prevent multiple pregnancy-related problems, such as miscarriage, premature birth, and abnormal bleeding.[38] By the 1950s it became clear that DES interfered with the *development* of the reproductive system in the fetus and it did not prevent miscarriage. Recent data suggest that DES-associated increase in clear cell adenocarcinoma is elevated throughout a woman's reproductive years.[39] More recent studies have revealed that daughters of women who took DES during pregnancy may have a slightly increased risk of breast cancer before age 40 (i.e., 1.9 times the risk compared with unexposed women at age 40).[40] For every 1000 DES-exposed women ages 45 to 49 it is estimated that 4 will be diagnosed with breast cancer.

Research from animal studies has demonstrated a relationship between DES exposure and an increased rate of a rare type of testicular cancer (rete testis) and prostate cancer.[41,42] In terms of in utero exposures, testicular cancer has been linked to exposure to abnormal levels of estrogen,[43] and testicular cancer is a risk factor for men with undescended testicles, a factor in some studies correlated with DES exposure. However, studies in humans determining the risk of testicular or prostate cancer and DES exposure are unclear and continuing.[44]

Additionally, investigators are studying diet during pregnancy. Recently, a striking experiment in mice demonstrated how extra vitamin doses during pregnancy in the mother's diet changed the fur color of her pups.[45] This was the first study to show maternal nutrition and subsequent phenotype changes. The nutrients (B_{12}, folic acid, choline, and betaine) silenced the gene that rendered mice fat and yellow but did not alter its DNA sequence. Silencing, or switching the gene off, linked prenatal diet to such diseases as diabetes, obesity, and cancer. These concepts, called the developmental basis of health and disease, are defining the hypothesis of disease onset. Subsequently, the focus of disease prevention and intervention needs to include the decades before onset—that is, during the in utero and neonatal periods.

In summary, epidemiologic and animal studies reveal that small changes in the developmental environment can alter phenotypic changes, resulting in individual responses in adulthood. Continuing evidence indicates that epigenetic mechanisms are responsible for tissue-specific gene expression during cellular differentiation and that these mechanisms modulate developmental phenotypic changes. The phenotypic effects of epigenetic modifications during development may need long latency periods, such as in cancer, thus manifesting later in life. In addition, epigenetic effects may help explain transgenerational effects (Tables 13-2 and 13-3).

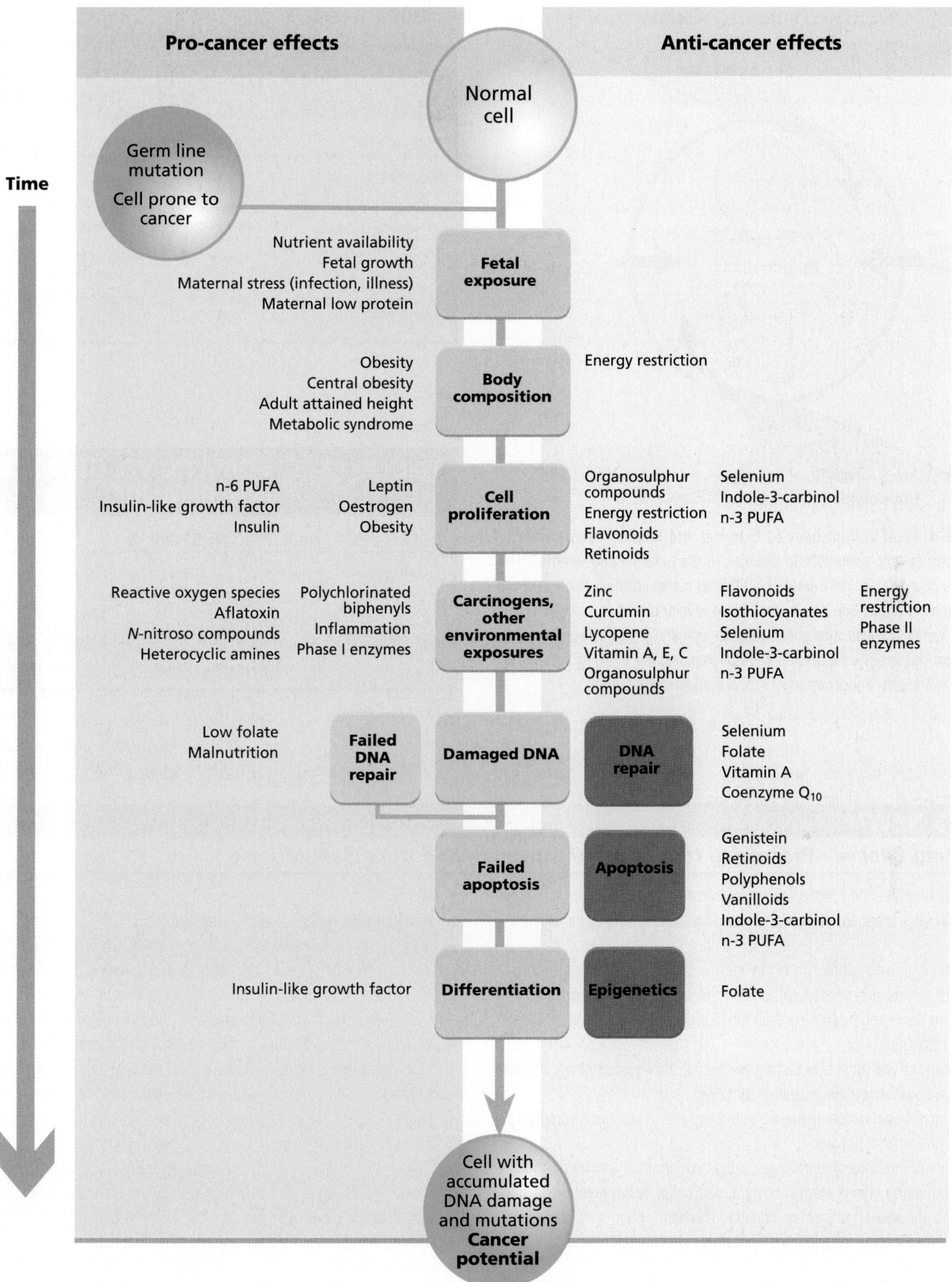

FIGURE 13-3 Pro- and Anti-Cancer Effects. (From World Cancer Research Fund/American Institute for Cancer Research: *Food, nutrition, physical activity, and the prevention of cancer: a global perspective,* Washington, DC, 2007, AICR.)

It should be noted that lifestyle habits are modifiable and that changing them can translate to reduced cancer risk, but a critical question is whether we are intervening early enough in life to achieve benefits.[1] Protective measures in very young and young people—for example, avoiding sun exposure during peak hours (10 AM to 3 PM) and covering the skin whenever possible, increasing physical exercise, and avoiding high-risk sexual practices, will reduce cancer incidence. Understanding that it takes years to develop tumors, cancer prevention beginning early in life will help reduce the burden of cancer on individuals and society[1] (see What's New? Preventing Cancer—Protecting the Health of Current and Future Generations).

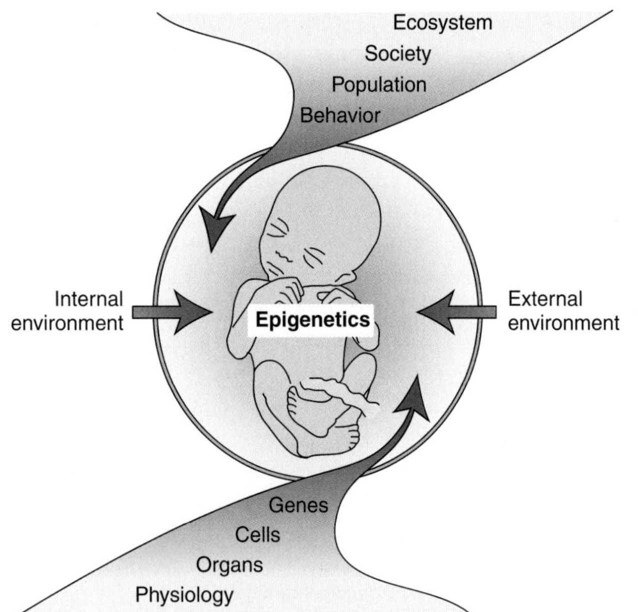

FIGURE 13-4 Fetal Vulnerability to External and Internal Environments. The fetus is particularly vulnerable to changes in the external and internal environments, which can have immediate and lifelong consequences. Such environmentally induced changes can occur at multiple levels, including molecular and behavioral. Ultimately these alterations may be epigenetic, inducing mitotically heritable alterations in gene expression without changing the DNA. (Adapted from Crews E, McLachlan JA: *Endocrinology* 147[6 Suppl]:S4–S10, 2006.)

TABLE 13-2 DIFFERENCES BETWEEN MULTIGENERATIONAL AND TRANSGENERATIONAL PHENOTYPES

PHENOTYPE	EXPOSURE	DEFINITION
Multigenerational	Direct	Simultaneous exposure of multiple generations to an environmental factor
Transgenerational	Initial germline exposure (ancestral)	Transgenerational phenotype is transmitted to future generations through germline inheritance

TABLE 13-3 SOMATIC VS. GERM CELL INHERITANCE

CELL TYPE	BIOLOGIC RESPONSE
Somatic cells	Critical for adult-onset disease in exposed individual; not transmitted to future generations as transgenerational effect
Germ cells	Allow transmission between generations; promote transgenerational phenotype

WHAT'S NEW?

Preventing Cancer—Protecting the Health of Current and Future Generations

- Essentials for preventing cancer include eliminating smoking, decreasing obesity, promoting exercise, eliminating infections, and avoiding an unhealthy diet.
- Interventions targeting lifestyle behaviors for cancer prevention are crucial. Continued efforts are needed to educate students and clinicians to target high-risk patients and promote prevention in pregnant women and in women, men, and children.
- Additionally, efforts must also focus more broadly than just smoking, lifestyle behaviors, and chemopreventive interventions.
- Establish a national cancer prevention strategy and redirect accordingly both research and policy agendas.
- Create a more integrated, coordinated, and transparent system for promulgating and enforcing environmental contaminant policy and regulations, driven by science and free of political or industry influence.
- Set tangible goals for reducing or eliminating toxic environmental exposures in cancer causation.
- The Kids Safe Chemical Act is an important first step toward a precautionary chemicals' management policy.
- Shift the burden of proving safety to chemical manufacturers before new chemical approval.
- Thoroughly assess workplace chemicals and other exposures. Previous occupational risks are outdated.*
- Increase concordance of exposure measures and standards to facilitate interagency and international regulatory policy and enforcement.
- Increase information sharing among the public, researchers, regulatory agencies, industry, and other appropriate groups.
- Involve environmental and public health advocates in developing environmental cancer research, policy agendas, and information dissemination.
- Strengthen research on workplace exposures and on the impact of in utero and childhood exposures that appear to have multigenerational effects.
- Accelerate the development of new research models and endpoints to better quantify exposures at individual, occupational, and population levels.
- Scientists disagree about cancer risk attributable to various environmental exposures. The unequal burden of exposure to known and suspected carcinogens must be addressed.
- Cancer risk should include geographic areas and vulnerable populations (including, but not limited to, children, migrant and other farm workers, cancer "hotspots," socioeconomic differences).
- Actions to minimize radiation exposure from medical sources include the education of healthcare providers, radiology technicians, and the public about the extent of radiation exposure from commonly used imaging and nuclear medicine examinations. Radiation dose–lowering techniques and inspection of radiation-emitting equipment must be implemented.
- Healthcare providers, especially physicians, nurse practitioners, and physicians' assistants, should routinely query patients about their previous and current workplace and home environments.
- Public health messages need development and dissemination to raise awareness of environmental cancer risks.

*Data from 2008-2009 Annual Report, President's Cancer Panel: *Reducing environmental cancer risk. What we can do now* (Suzanne H. Reuben for the President's Cancer Panel), U.S. Department of Health and Human Services, NIH, NCI, April 2010.

ENVIRONMENTAL-LIFESTYLE FACTORS

Tobacco Use

Cigarette smoking is carcinogenic and remains the most important cause of cancer. Tobacco accounts for nearly one in five deaths,[46] yet it is the single most preventable cause of death and disease in the United States.[47] The risk is greatest in those who begin to smoke when young and continue throughout life. Globally, tobacco use accounts for 80% of the worldwide lung cancer burden in males and about 50% in females.[48,49] Male lung cancer death rates are decreasing in most Western countries and increasing in China and several other Asian and African countries. However, the highest lung cancer incidence rates are still found in North America, Northern Europe, and Australia/New Zealand.[50] Rates in females are increasing in many countries including Spain, France, Belgium, and the Netherlands and are now plateauing in the United States, Canada, and the United Kingdom. Overall, lung cancer rates in females lag behind males where females started smoking later than males.[50] Half of all long-term smokers die prematurely from smoking-related causes, and for every person who dies from tobacco use another 20 people suffer with at least 1 serious tobacco-related illness.[51] The prevalence of current smoking among U.S. adults declined from 24.7% in 1997 to 18.9% in 2011.[52] Non-Hispanic white adults were the most likely to be current smokers followed by non-Hispanic black adults and Hispanic adults.[52]

Forms of tobacco used in the United States include cigarettes, cigars, pipes, and imported nonconventional cigarettes (e.g., bidis and clove cigarettes). Besides lung cancer, tobacco use increases the risk for cancers of the mouth, lips, nasal cavity and sinuses, larynx, pharynx, esophagus, stomach, pancreas, kidney, bladder, uterus, cervix, colorectum, and ovaries as well as acute leukemia.[46] The relationship between breast cancer and smoking has been the subject of much controversy and conflicting epidemiologic reports published since 2002, partially from confounding with alcohol use. Reanalyses of evidence from recent cohort studies suggest an increased risk of breast cancer related to smoking independent of alcohol use.[53] In younger premenopausal women an increased risk of breast cancer was related to exposure to passive smoke.[53] Biologic mechanistic studies also support a positive association between cigarette smoking and breast cancer.[53] A 2009 Report from the Canadian Expert Panel on Tobacco Smoke and Breast Cancer Risk concluded from epidemiologic and toxicologic studies and biologic understandings that both pre- and postmenopausal breast cancers are consistent with causality.[54] In addition, smoking causes *even more* deaths from vascular diseases (e.g., coronary heart disease, peripheral vascular disease, abdominal aortic aneurysm), respiratory diseases (e.g., emphysema, bronchitis, airway obstruction), and other diseases than from cancer.

Secondhand smoke, also called **environmental tobacco smoke (ETS),** is the combination of sidestream smoke (burning end of a cigarette, cigar, or pipe) and mainstream smoke (smoke exhaled by the smoker). More than 4000 chemicals have been identified in mainstream tobacco smoke (250 chemicals as toxic),[55] of which 60 are considered carcinogenic.[56] Nonsmokers who live with smokers are at greatest risk for lung cancer as well as numerous noncancerous conditions.[57] One in vitro study supported a relationship between nicotine and genotoxic effects in fetal cells.[58] Other studies are emerging on the relationship of both maternal and paternal smoking and in utero effects. Smoking during pregnancy causes lower birth rates, an increased incidence of spontaneous abortion and preterm birth, increased placental pathology, and increased stillbirth rates.[59]

Cigar or pipe smoking, or both, is strongly and causally related to cancers of the oral cavity, oropharynx, hypopharynx, larynx, esophagus, lung, and probably the pancreas.[60] Pipe smokers have an increased risk of dying from cancers of the lung, throat, esophagus, larynx, pancreas, and colorectum.[61] Smoking bidi, a small amount of tobacco wrapped in the leaf of another plant (used in South Asia), delivers higher amounts of nicotine per gram of tobacco and comparable or greater amounts of tar compared with cigarettes.[62] Bidi smokers have the same risks of cancers and higher risks of heart attacks and chronic bronchitis than those found in nonsmokers.[62] Several types of cancers have been linked to hookah or water pipe smoking.[62]

United Kingdom researchers reported for the first time that starting smoking results in epigenetic changes associated with the development of cancer.[63] These researchers showed that smoking increased DNA methylation. Figure 13-5 illustrates a working model of carcinogenesis by cigarette smoke. Measures

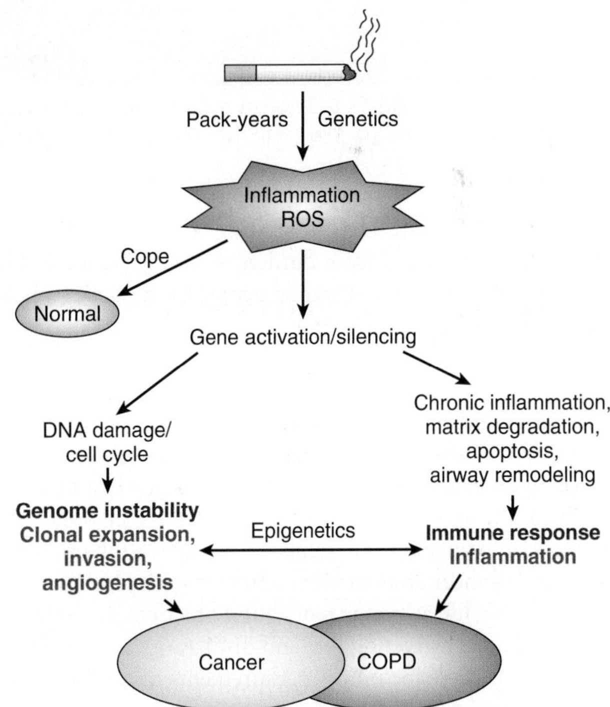

FIGURE 13-5 Working Model of Carcinogenesis by Cigarette Smoke. The major inducer of both lung cancer and COPD is cigarette smoke. Nonsmokers may develop these diseases caused by other environmental or genetic/epigenetic factors. Cigarette smoke induces an inflammatory response and causes an increase in reactive oxygen species (ROS), causing oxidative stress. Oxidative stress is a risk factor for many diseases because it can alter many cellular proteins. A combination of immune-inflammatory signals and epigenetic events may increase the risk for individuals with COPD developing lung cancer. (From Adcock IM et al: *Respiration* 81[4]:265–284, 2011.)

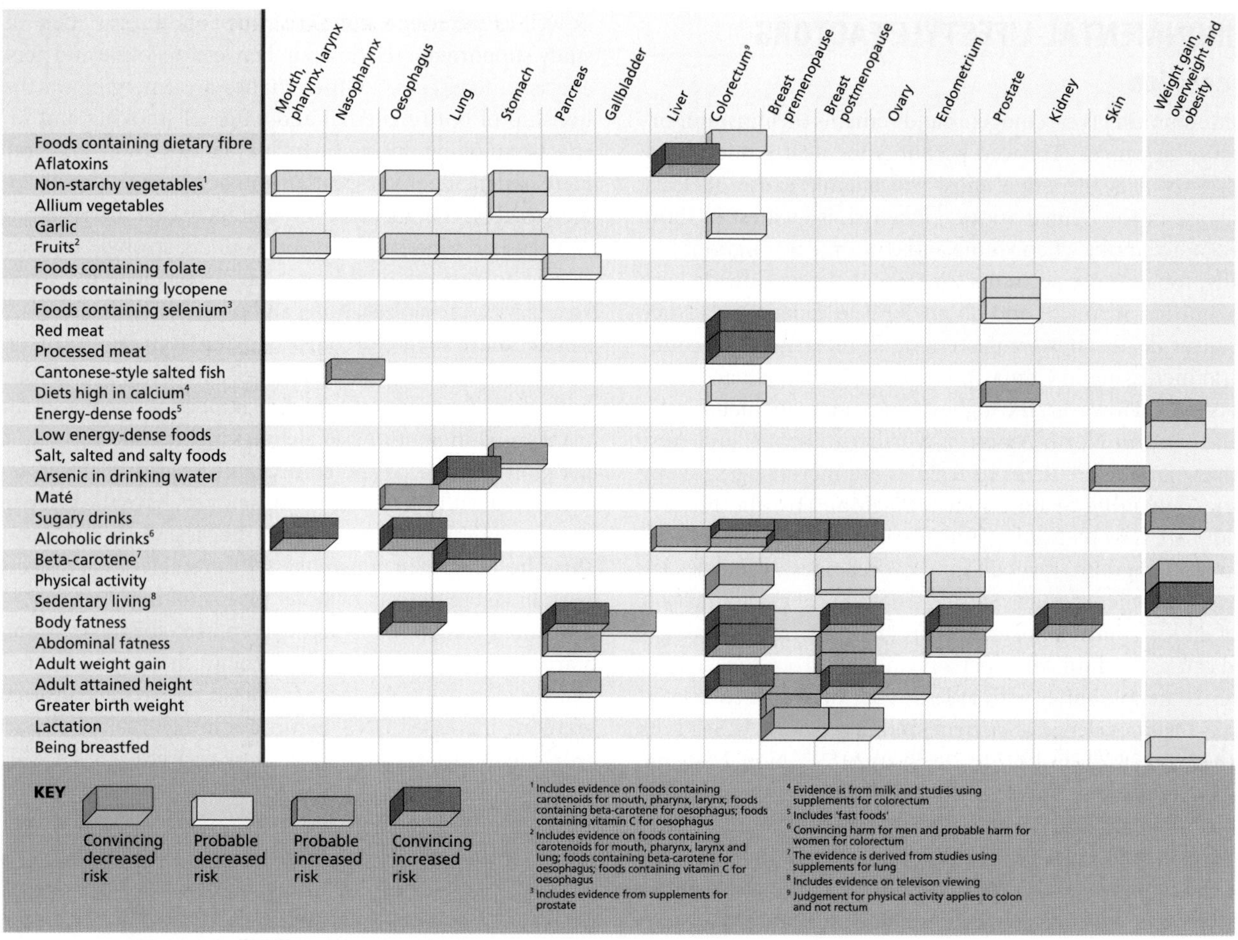

Mouth, pharynx, larynx
Nasopharynx
Oesophagus
Lung
Stomach
Pancreas
Gallbladder
Liver
Colorectum9
Breast premenopause
Breast postmenopause
Ovary
Endometrium
Prostate
Kidney
Skin
Weight gain, overweight and obesity
Foods containing dietary fibre
Aflatoxins
Non-starchy vegetables1
Allium vegetables
Garlic
Fruits2
Foods containing folate
Foods containing lycopene
Foods containing selenium3
Red meat
Processed meat
Cantonese-style salted fish
Diets high in calcium4
Energy-dense foods5
Low energy-dense foods
Salt, salted and salty foods
Arsenic in drinking water
Maté
Sugary drinks
Alcoholic drinks6
Beta-carotene7
Physical activity
Sedentary living8
Body fatness
Abdominal fatness
Adult weight gain
Adult attained height
Greater birth weight
Lactation
Being breastfed
KEY
Convincing decreased risk
Probable decreased risk
Probable increased risk
Convincing increased risk
1 Includes evidence on foods containing carotenoids for mouth, pharynx, larynx; foods containing beta-carotene for oesophagus; foods containing vitamin C for oesophagus
2 Includes evidence on foods containing carotenoids for mouth, pharynx, larynx and lung; foods containing beta-carotene for oesophagus; foods containing vitamin C for oesophagus
3 Includes evidence from supplements for prostate
4 Evidence is from milk and studies using supplements for colorectum
5 Includes 'fast foods'
6 Convincing harm for men and probable harm for women for colorectum
7 The evidence is derived from studies using supplements for lung
8 Includes evidence on televison viewing
9 Judgement for physical activity applies to colon and not rectum

FIGURE 13-6 **Summary of Convincing and Probable Judgments.** (From World Cancer Research Fund/American Institute for Cancer Research: *Food, nutrition, physical activity, and the prevention of cancer: a global perspective,* Washington, DC, 2007, AICR.)

that prevent young adults from starting smoking would substantially avoid future disease burden. A strong public health approach is one that *prevents* young people from *starting* smoking and helps others *stop* smoking.

Diet

Understanding dietary factors that increase the risk for cancer can be difficult. The ways in which diet affects one's likelihood of developing cancer are complicated by the variety of foods consumed, the many constituents of foods, the metabolic consequences of eating, and the temporal changes in the patterns of food use. Cancer risks in older adults may depend as much on diet in early life as on current eating practices. In addition, studies in humans targeting diet and disease associations face a variety of challenges including measurements of specific nutrients, food types, and dietary patterns.

Dietary sources of carcinogenic substances include compounds produced in the cooking of fat, meat, or protein, and naturally occurring carcinogens associated with plant food substances, such as alkaloids or mold byproducts.[64] Figure 13-6 is a summary of convincing and probable judgments related to food and physical activity risk factors and the prevention of cancer.[64] Dietary components can act directly as mutagens or interfere with mutagen elimination. Abundant evidence exists

Nutrigenomics
Food, nutrition, obesity, physical activity, and gene expression
Nutrigenetics
DNA
RNA
Protein
Metabolite
Genomics
Epigenomics
Transcriptomics
Proteomics
Metabolomics

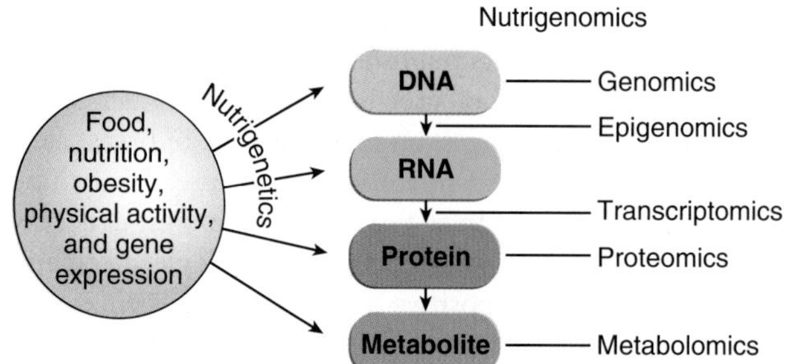

FIGURE 13-7 **Basis for the Study of Food, Nutrition, Obesity, Physical Activity, and the Cancer Process.** The genetic message in the DNA code is translated to RNA, and then into protein synthesis, and so determines metabolic processes. Research methods, called "-omics," address these different stages. (Adapted from World Cancer Research Fund/American Institute for Cancer Research: *Food, nutrition, physical activity, and the prevention of cancer: a global perspective,* Washington, DC, 2007, AICR.)

that nutritional factors in many processes are related to cancer development (Figure 13-7).

Research is ongoing to understand the complexity of genomics, epigenomics, transcription factors (transcriptomics), proteomics, and metabolic factors (metabolomics) and the way that modifying any one, or more, influences cancer risk. **Nutrigenomics** is the study of nutrition on the phenotypic variability

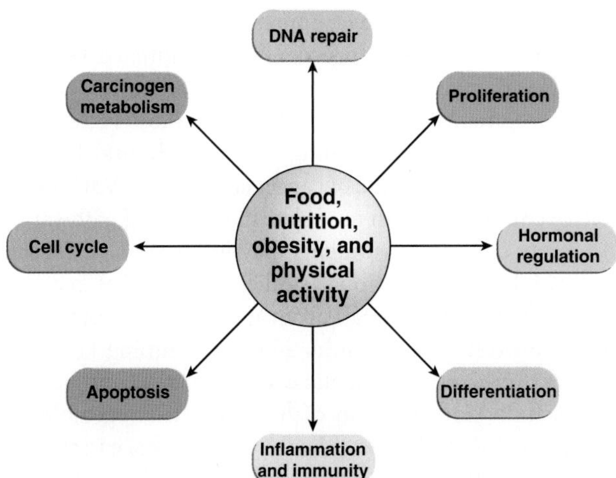

FIGURE 13-8 Food, Nutrition, Obesity, Physical Activity, and Cellular Processes Linked to Cancer. Food, nutrition, and physical activity can influence fundamental processes shown here, which may promote or inhibit cancer development and progression. (Adapted from World Cancer Research Fund/American Institute for Cancer Research: *Food, nutrition, physical activity, and the prevention of cancer: a global perspective,* Washington, DC, 2007, AICR.)

of individuals based on genomic differences (see Figure 13-7). Investigators are focusing on the sequence and functions of genes, single nucleotide polymorphisms (SNPs), and amplifications and deletions within the DNA sequences as modifiers of the response to foods and drinks and their components.[64]

Nutrition, Obesity, Alcohol Consumption, and Physical Activity: Impacts on Cancer

What we eat, how much we weigh, and how much we move influence our risks of developing cancer. Mounting evidence is clear—everyday *choices* impact our chances of getting or preventing cancer. Ongoing tedious and comprehensive investigative work is linking diet, body weight, and exercise to risk of specific cancers.

Nutrition. Important cellular processes affected by nutrition include the cell cycle; the balance between cell proliferation and cell death (e.g., apoptosis); cell differentiation; genes, including oncogenes and tumor-suppressor genes; cell signaling; gene expression; cellular microenvironment that influences gene expression; epigenetic regulation; hormonal regulation; DNA damage and repair; carcinogen metabolism; and inflammation and immunity (Figure 13-8).

Gene expression is influenced by epigenetic processes like DNA methylation or acetylation (addition of an acetyl group) (see Chapters 6 and 12). Dietary sources of methyl groups including folate, methionine, betaine, serine, and choline are primary potential donors as modulators of DNA methylation[65] (Figure 13-9).

B vitamins, coenzymes in one-carbon metabolism (vitamins B_2, B_6, B_{12}), also are modulators of DNA methylation.[66] To date there are limited human studies of the effects of methyl donor supply on methylation of specific genomic sequences.[65] However, a recent study[67] found that periconceptional maternal supplementation with 400 micrograms (mcg) of folic acid/day was associated with increased methylation in offspring aged

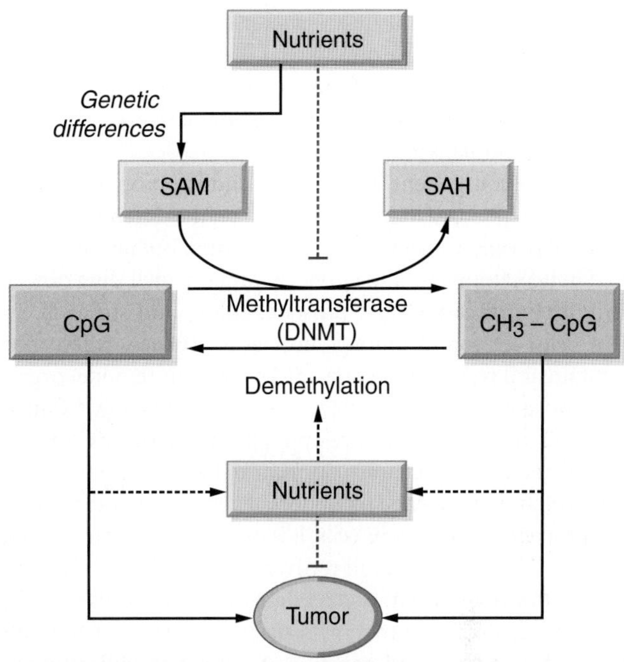

FIGURE 13-9 Dietary Factors, DNA Methylation, and Cancer. Certain dietary factors (see Table 13-5) may supply methyl groups (+CH3) that can be donated through *S*-adenosylmethionine (*SAM)* to many acceptors in the cell (DNA, proteins, lipids, and metabolites). Donation and removal (demethylation) are affected by numerous enzymes, including DNA methyltransferase *(DNMT).* Increased DNMT activity occurs in many tumor cells. Hypermethylation can inhibit or silence tumor-suppressor genes (see Chapter 12), and DNA methylation inhibitors as anticancer agents can block DNMT, thus reactivating tumor-suppressor genes. DNA hypomethylation can reactivate and mutate genes, including cancer-causing oncogenes. *SAH, S*-Adenosylhomocysteine.

17 months. In the Waterland study, methylation effects were found to be similar in all tissues examined, suggesting that the mechanism may alter markings in stem cells early in embryogenesis before tissue differentiation, and persist into adult life.[45] Choline deficiency in pregnancy results in hypermethylation of genomic DNA and of the *IGF2* gene.[68] Several studies have reported that severe folate deficiency (which increases risk of hepatocellular cancer) induces hypomethylation of the *p53* tumor-suppressor gene.[69] In vitro studies have shown that several bioactive food components, including tea polyphenols and bioflavonoids, inhibit DNA methyltransferase (DNMT-1)-mediated DNA methylation in a dose-dependent manner[70] (see Figure 13-9). Acetylation and deacetylation are mediated by enzyme histones (see Figure 6-1), histone acetyl transferase (HAT), and histone deacetylation (HDAC). Dietary components have been identified that act as regulators of gene expression by epigenetic mechanisms.[71] For example, there is strong evidence for the epigenetic effects of organosulfur compounds from garlic and of isothiocyanates from cruciferous vegetables.[71] Interest in reservatrol is growing because of its demonstrable role in possibly delaying age-related diseases, including cancers.[72] Butyrate produced in the colon by bacterial fermentation of non-starch polysaccharide (fiber), diallyl disulfide from garlic and other allium vegetables, and sulforaphane from

cruciferous vegetables can act as histone deacetylase inhibitors to maintain DNA stability or modify transcription.[64]

MicroRNAs (miRNAs) expression in response to diet may be involved in several cancers.[64] Several dietary factors, including macronutrients (fat, protein, and alcohol) and micronutrients (folate and vitamin E), alter the expression of many miRNAs in animals and humans[65] (see Chapter 12).

Bioactive components have a profound effect on differentiation and a major area of investigation is on the differentiation of cancer stem cells. Cancer stem cells have been isolated and identified in hematopoietic and epithelial cancers, including cancers of the brain, breast, ovary, prostate, colon, and stomach.[64,73] Stem cells are found among most adult tissues, where they maintain and regenerate tissues. Stem cells can remodel organs in response to physiologic triggers—*adaptive resizing*.[74] Cancer stem cells utilize several developmental mechanisms for self-renewal and these mechanisms appear to be fundamental to the initiation and recurrence of tumors. Even if chemotherapy or radiation eliminates cancer cells, it is only when the cancer stem cells are destroyed that a full recovery is achievable.[73] Repopulation with radioresistant or chemoresistant stem cells may significantly contribute to therapy resistance. Evidence from both drug and bioactive food constituents shows modifications in cancer stem cell self-renewal capabilities; for example, retinoic acid may promote differentiation of breast cancer stem cells.[75] Adequate consumption of specific food compounds, including vitamins A and D, genistein, green tea, epigallocatechin gallate (EGCG), sulforaphane, theanine, curcumin, choline, and possibly many others, may suppress cancer stem renewal.[73] Uncontrolled self-renewal process may be initiated by abnormal developmental signals that come from the extracellular microenvironment known as "niches." The loss of regulation in self-renewal signals, including Wnt, Notch, and hedgehog pathways, is a characteristic of cancer stem cells.[73] Various food bioactive components can modulate the signaling pathway.

A variety of food constituents may influence DNA repair[64] (Figure 13-10). Observational studies suggest that malnutrition can reduce DNA repair from damage.[76] In vivo studies have demonstrated that healthy adults consuming kiwi fruits, cooked carrots, or supplemental coenzyme Q_{10} improved their DNA repair.[64] Consumption of lycopene-rich vegetable juice was associated with significantly decreased damage to the DNA of lung epithelial cells in healthy adults.[77]

Humans are constantly exposed to a variety of compounds termed **xenobiotics** (Greek *xenos,* "foreign"; *bios,* "life") that include toxic, mutagenic, and carcinogenic chemicals. Many of these chemicals are found in the human diet. Most xenobiotics are transported in the blood by lipoproteins and penetrate lipid membranes. These chemicals can react with cellular macromolecules, such as proteins and DNA, or can react directly with cell structures to cause cell damage.[78] The body has two main defense systems for counteracting these effects: (1) detoxification enzymes and (2) antioxidant systems (see Chapter 2). Enzymes that activate xenobiotics are called **phase I activation enzymes** and are represented by the multigene cytochrome P-450 family, aldehyde oxidase, xanthine oxidases, and

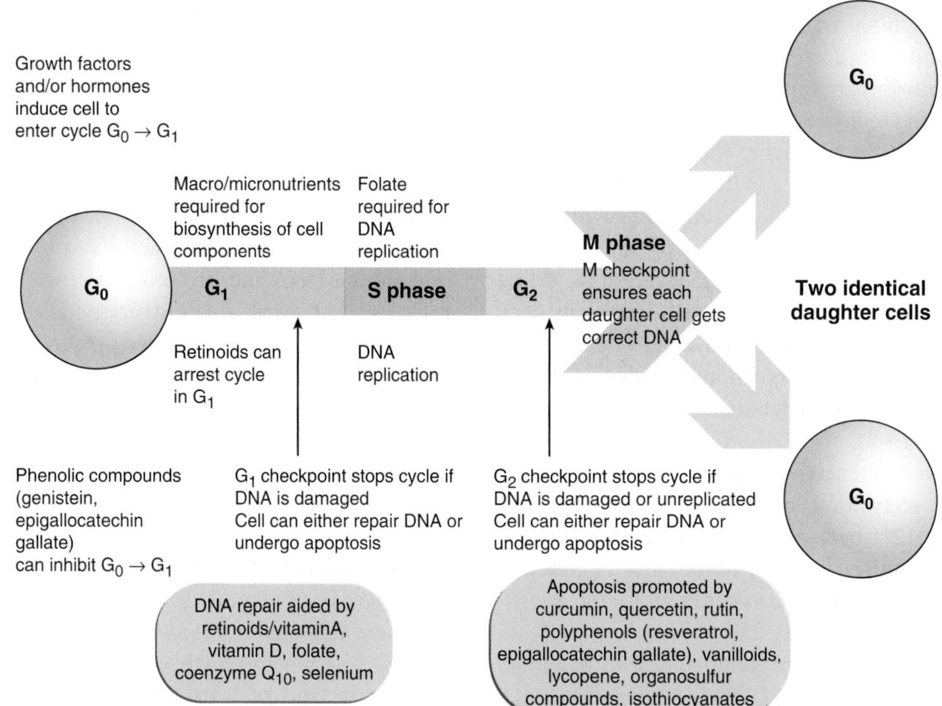

FIGURE 13-10 Cell Cycle and Nutrition Regulation. Nutrition may influence the regulation of the normal cell cycle, which ensures correct DNA replication. G_0 represents the resting phase, G_1 the growth and preparation of the chromosome for replication, S the synthesis of DNA, G_2 the preparation of the cell for division, and M mitosis. (Adapted from World Cancer Research Fund/American Institute for Cancer Research: *Food, nutrition, physical activity, and the prevention of cancer: a global perspective,* Washington, DC, 2007, AICR.)

peroxidases. **Phase II detoxification enzymes** then protect further against a large array of reactive intermediates and nonactivated xenobiotics.[64] These enzymes are located predominantly in the liver and provide clearance of compounds through the portal circulation, thereby preventing the potentially carcinogenic agent(s) from entering the body through the gastrointestinal tract and portal circulation. They also occur in the skin epithelia and can be induced in other extrahepatic tissue, such as the lung. They represent a potential target to influence carcinogen metabolism. Isothiocyanates from cruciferous vegetables induce the expression of phase II detoxification enzymes. Food and nutrition modify carcinogen metabolism and may modify carcinogenesis. Some examples include selenium, allyl sulfur, sulforaphane, and isoflavonoids. The enzyme CYP3A4 is involved in the metabolism of many drugs and is sensitive to foods.[64] Interactions, for example, have been reported for grapefruit juice, red wine, garlic, and drugs.

Glutathione-*S*-transferases (GSTs) are enzyme housekeepers involved in the metabolism of environmental carcinogens and reactive oxygen species. Individuals who lack these enzymes may be at higher risk for cancers because of decreased capacity to dispose of activated carcinogens. For example, the fungi that produce aflatoxins can grow on certain crops like peanuts and certain cereal (grains) are carcinogens activated by phase I enzymes in the liver that can produce DNA adducts. Individuals lacking these enzymes are at higher risk of colon cancer. Diets high in isothiocyanates (from cruciferous vegetables) may decrease this risk.[79] Individuals who consume diets high in red meat and processed meat and who carry certain genetic polymorphisms have an increased risk of developing colorectal cancer.[64,80] Processed meats include those preserved by preservatives or by smoking, curing, or salting. The European Prospective Investigation into Cancer and Nutrition (EPIC) study, which included 478,040 people from 10 countries, reports that the most convincing data are from meats, including sausages, bratwursts, frankfurters, and hot dogs, all of which have nitrites, nitrates, or other preservatives. These *N*-nitroso compounds can increase nitrogenous residues in the colon and cause DNA damage.[64,81] Dietary components either can be activated into potential carcinogens through metabolic processes or can be inactivated and prevent DNA damage.[64] High intake of red meat may result in the synthesis of higher levels of heme iron; iron can activate oxidative stress and inflammation in the colon. A new report suggests meat may have certain thermoresistant oncogenic bovine viruses (e.g., polyoma-papilloma) or possible single-stranded DNA viruses.[82] Certain single nucleotide polymorphisms (SNPs) in the *N*-acetyltransferase gene alter the activity of the enzyme involved in the activation of heterocyclic amines from cooking meat at high temperatures and may increase the risk of colon cancer.[64]

Other foods that alter the metabolism of carcinogens and induce GSTs include cruciferous vegetables, especially brussels sprouts and red cabbage. Red cabbage leads to changes in meat-derived mutagens in urine.[64] Flavonoids found in plants may alter carcinogen metabolism, and dietary indole-3-carbinol inhibited spontaneous occurrence of endometrial adenocarcinomas in rats.[64]

Chronic inflammation and immune function may help explain patterns of cancer around the world. People who are undernourished or live in poverty may have impaired immune status, which can be a factor in cancers caused by infectious agents, for example, cancers of the liver and cervix.[64] Undernutrition can include deficiencies in vitamin A, riboflavin, vitamin B_{12}, folic acid, vitamin C, selenium, and zinc, and these nutrient deficiencies may be related to chronic inflammation and immune alterations.[64] The cytokine interleukin-6 (IL-6) can act as either a proinflammatory or an anti-inflammatory cytokine; consequently, it can enhance both innate and adaptive immunity as well as stimulate or suppress tumor growth.

In summary, epidemiologic and laboratory evidence suggests that diet has important consequences for cancer development and perhaps its rate of progression.[21,83] Diet affects many pathways to cancer including cell cycle control, differentiation, DNA repair, gene silencing, inflammation, apoptosis, and carcinogen metabolism. Many of these processes are likely influenced, if not regulated, by DNA methylation, an epigenetic mechanism that affects gene function. As illustrated in Figure 13-2, it is possible that many environmental factors interact with the genome to produce altered epigenetic markers that change the expression of cancer-causing genes, tumor-suppressor genes, and oncogenes. Future research is needed to define robust biomarkers of cancer risk.

Obesity. Obesity in most developed countries (and in urban areas of many developing countries) has been increasing rapidly over the past 20 years. Obesity in the United States is an epidemic and constitutes a startling setback to major improvements in other areas of health during the past century.[84] Childhood obesity also is increasing. Numerous health conditions are linked to obesity and physical inactivity. The substantial suffering and long-term human and societal costs of obesity underlie the urgency to accelerate progress in obesity prevention.[84] This will require a comprehensive approach including the involvement of knowledgeable healthcare personnel, the provision of appropriate education from schools, the access to healthy food and beverage choices, and the promotion of physical activity.

Studies have significantly improved the understanding of the relationship between overweight/obesity, energy balance and cancer risk, cancer recurrence, and survival (Figure 13-11).[64,85-87] Consensus now exists that obesity is a risk factor for cancers of the endometrium, colorectum, kidney, esophagus, breast (postmenopausal), and pancreas. Evidence is evolving of the association between obesity and cancers of the thyroid, gallbladder, liver, and ovary as well as aggressive types of prostate cancer and non-Hodgkin lymphoma.[64,85,87] Importantly, obesity is recognized as a poor prognostic factor for several cancers.[88-90] Worrisome are the effects of obesity on incidence and the poor outcomes in individuals with cancer because of the rising obesity epidemic.[91]

The only globally accepted criteria for overweightness and obesity are based on body mass index (BMI). Widely accepted standards based on BMI criteria for overweightness and obesity are recommended by the WHO[92] and supported by other panels and federal agencies (WHO classifications are shown in Table 13-4).

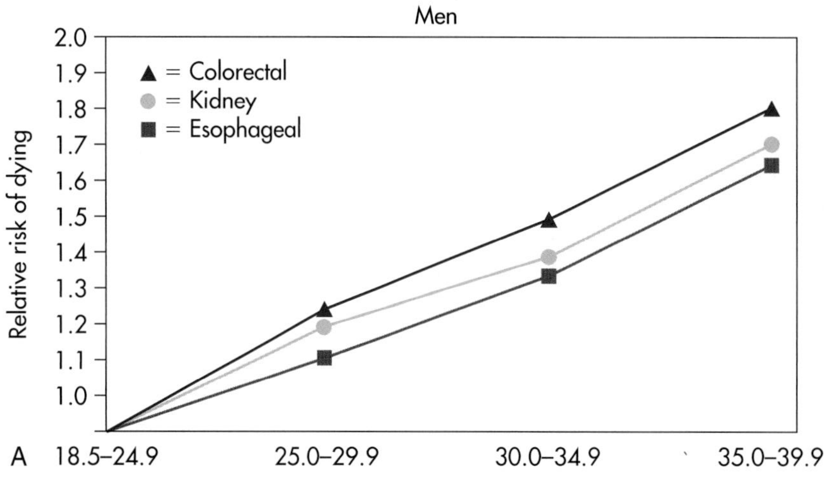

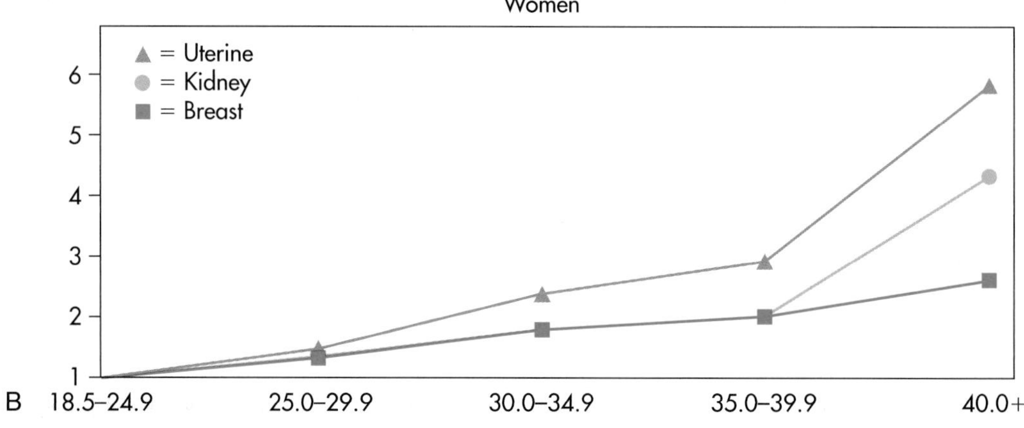

FIGURE 13-11 Weight and Risk of Dying from Cancer. **A,** As a man's body mass index (BMI) rises above the normal range (18.5 to 24.9), his risk of dying of colorectal, esophageal, kidney, and other cancers also rises. For example, the risk of dying from colorectal cancer is 10% higher for men who are overweight (BMI 25 to 29.9) than for men of normal or lower BMI. For the most obese men (BMI 35 or higher) the risk is almost double (84%). **B,** As a woman's BMI rises above the normal range (18.5 to 24.9), her risk of dying of breast, kidney, uterine, and other cancers rises. For example, the risk of dying from breast cancer is 34% higher for women who are overweight. For the most obese women (BMI >40), the risk of dying from breast cancer is double. The risk of kidney disease is almost five times higher, and the risk of uterine cancer is six times higher. (Data from Calle EE et al: *N Engl J Med* 348:1625–1638, 2003.)

TABLE 13-4 WHO* CLASSIFICATION OF BODY MASS INDEX (BMI)

BMI (kg/mM²)*	WHO CLASSIFICATION	OTHER DESCRIPTIONS
<18.5	Underweight	Thin
18.5-24.9	Normal range	"Healthy," "normal," or "acceptable" weight
25-29.9	Grade 1 overweight	Overweight
30-39.9	Grade 2 overweight	Obese
≥40	Grade 3 overweight	Morbidly overweight

*The cutoffs are somewhat arbitrary, although they are derived from epidemiologic studies of BMI and overall mortality. It is important to understand that within each category of BMI there can be substantial individual variation in total and visceral adiposity and in related metabolic factors. These variations are also true for the normal range BMI. *WHO,* World Health Organization.

Worldwide estimates are 1.5 billion adults are overweight (BMI ≥25 to 29.9 kg/m^2) and 500 million are obese (BMI ≥30 kg/m^2).[93] There is considerable concern for children with early onset of obesity.

Mechanisms Associated with Energy Balance and Obesity. The IOM and National Cancer Policy Forum convened to discuss mechanisms of obesity and cancer, cancer recurrence and mortality, research needs, and future directions.[94] A simple model based on energy balance and energy expenditure was utilized. **Energy balance** measures intake-absorbable energy against the energy demands of the body. Energy expenditure is comprised of: (1) the resting metabolic rate (RMR), the energy required for normal body functions, which constitutes the majority of energy needs; (2) the thermic effect of food, or the amount of energy needed to digest and metabolize food; and (3) physical activity, a moderate and modifiable part of energy expenditure. This model does not include body composition (i.e., lean tissue, adipose tissue) or the dynamic state of body

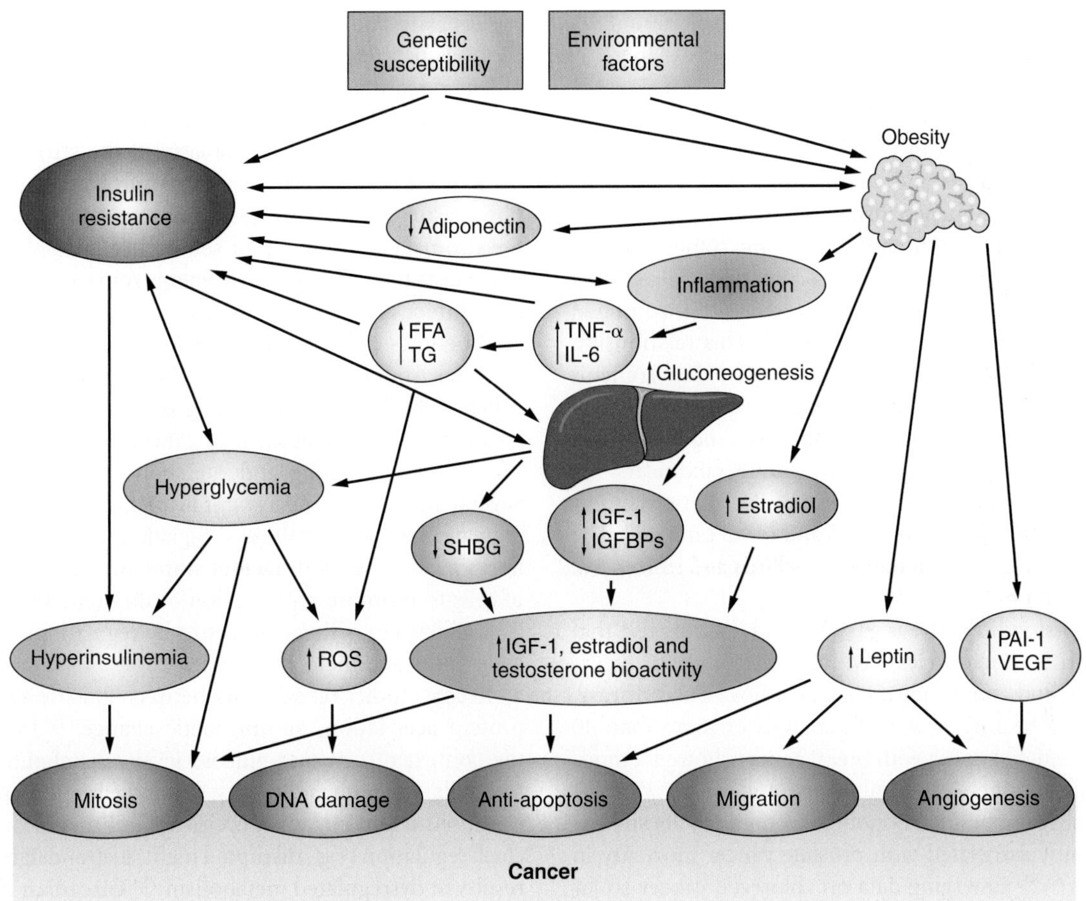

FIGURE 13-12 Obesity, Insulin Resistance, Inflammation, and Cancer. A proposed model of the role of insulin resistance, obesity, genetic susceptibility, and environmental factors and cancer. This model suggests insulin resistance and inflammation as driving forces for cancer development. *FFA,* Free fatty acids; *IGFBPs,* IGF-binding proteins; *IL-6,* interleukin-6; *PAI-1,* plasminogen activator inhibitor 1; *ROS,* reactive oxygen species; *SHBG,* sex hormone–binding globulin; *TG,* triglycerides; *TNF-α,* tumor necrosis factor-alpha; *VEGF,* vascular endothelial growth factor. (Adapted from Arcidacono B et al: *Exp Diabetes Res* 789174, 2012.)

composition. Because lean mass determines resting metabolic rate it is unknown whether obesity itself drives cancer progression or whether components of energy balance (i.e., too much consumed or too little expended) have a greater impact, and therefore it is uncertain which factors hold more promise for cancer control and prevention.[85]

Overall, the putative mechanisms whereby obesity drives the progression of cancer are not completely known and the process is complex. Earlier studies linked levels of circulating free hormones (e.g., estradiol) and hormonally driven cancers as an important mechanism. (Chapters 22 and 24 contain discussions on hormones and cancer risk.) Research now includes other mechanisms whereby energy balance may affect: (1) genomic instability, (2) dysregulated growth signaling and cellular energetics, (3) inhibition of apoptosis and immune surveillance, and (4) angiogenesis. Additionally, numerous signaling pathways and factors are involved in the acceleration of cancer. Data now exist for several factors including energy-driven signaling from insulin, insulin-like growth factor 1 (IGF-1), phosphatidylinositol 3-kinase, and AMP-activated protein kinase and many others.[85] These pathogenic effects of insulin might be mediated by insulin receptors in the preneoplastic or neoplastic target cells, or could be caused by alterations in endogenous hormone metabolism secondary to hyperinsulinemia. Insulin resistance increases with body fatness, particularly with abdominal fatness, and the pancreas compensates by increasing insulin production. Hyperinsulinemia is associated with a risk of cancers of the colon, endometrium, and possibly kidney and pancreas.[64] Like sex steroids, leptin produced by adipose cells also can stimulate premalignant and malignant cell types.[64]

Insulin promotes the synthesis and biologic activity of **insulin-like growth factor 1 (IGF-1),** a peptide hormone that has mitotic and anti-apoptotic effects.[95] Intense investigation is ongoing on the relationship between IGF-1 and the development of certain cancers (Figure 13-12). For example, a pooled reanalysis of world-wide prospective data showed IGF-1 is associated with an increased risk for prostate cancer.[96] Insulin also can promote the synthesis and biologic availability of the male and female sex hormones, including estrogens, progesterone, and androgens[97] (see Figure 13-6).

Parts of the insulin resistance syndrome have been well studied in both breast and colon cancer.[96] As an example, in individuals with nondiabetic breast cancer, higher levels of fasting insulin were associated with a twofold to threefold increase in risk of mortality.[98,99] One biologic basis for this effect is the overexpression of insulin receptors, especially the fetal insulin receptor (IRα) on breast cancer cells.[100] Similar findings are reported for colon cancer and suggest that adiposity, physical activity, and diet influence insulin and IGF levels that can stimulate growth and inhibit apoptosis of micrometastases—possibly a cause of recurrence.[101] It has recently been reported that postmenopausal diabetic women treated with insulin had a significantly higher risk of lung cancer.[102] This relationship needs much further investigation. Additionally, the Women's Health Initiative (WHI) investigators report that diabetes severity assessed by duration or need of pharmacologic care had stronger links to risk of liver, pancreatic, and rectal cancer.[103] A first review of epidemiologic studies revealed diabetes mellitus as an independent risk factor for colon and rectal cancer.[104] The biologic mechanisms between diabetes mellitus and cancer risk are currently unknown.

The survivorship literature is growing and data suggest that increasing BMI is related to less favorable outcomes for recurrence, survival, and comorbidities (e.g., cardiovascular disease, diabetes, wound healing).[85] A meta-analysis of more than 40 studies of women diagnosed with breast cancer showed a modest but significant increase in all-cause and breast cancer–specific mortality in obese vs. nonobese women.[105] Obesity has been consistently associated with prostate cancer mortality in cohort studies.[85,106] Emerging data on colorectal cancer so far show mixed findings.

Adipose tissue can have greater effects on the physiology of other tissue (see Chapter 41). The metabolic function of adipose tissue is derived in part because it can secrete many proteins, collectively called **adipokines.**[107] Adipose tissue is a source of inflammatory modulators, and increasing evidence indicates that obesity is casually linked to inflammation (Figure 13-13).[108,109]

The adipokine leptin enhances the production of inflammatory factors and tumor necrosis factor-alpha (TNF-α).[85] These inflammatory factors also are modulated by sex hormones (e.g., estradiol and testosterone) and growth factors, especially vascular endothelial growth factor (VEGF). Importantly, increased adiposity is correlated with *lower* levels of adiponectin that normally induces apoptosis, thus increasing cell proliferation.[85] Lower levels of adiponectin also give rise to insulin resistance—a state characterized by the reduced metabolic response of tissues to insulin and to compensatory hyperinsulinemia.

Adipokines have both proinflammatory and anti-inflammatory activities and their balance can contribute to the initiation and progression of obesity-induced metabolic changes that can affect other organs (including the brain, heart, vasculature, liver, and muscle) and increase the risk of cancer, cardiovascular disease, and metabolic disturbances.[107]

Cancers have altered metabolism. Normal tissues use oxidative phosphorylation (OXPHOS) to convert glucose into CO_2 and energy (i.e., ATP). Some cancers use a different approach; they consume large quantities of glucose—*aerobic glycolysis*—to make cellular building blocks **(Warburg effect)**, supporting rapid proliferation[110,111] (see Chapter 12). However, this concept has been challenged because some tumors use oxidative phosphorylation.[112] New research reveals that cancer cells can use *oxidative* stress as a "weapon" to extract recycled nutrients from cancer-associated fibroblasts in the stromal tissue. The oxidative stress changes the normal fibroblast cancer-associated fibroblasts (CAFs). This transition seems to cause the aging of the stromal environment, or senescence. Autophagic senescent fibroblasts then produce high-energy nutrients resulting in anabolic tumor growth. This two-compartment tumor metabolism is sometimes called the **Reverse Warburg effect.** It is possible that this simple model of metabolism by the cancer could explain why chronological aging is one of the most important factors for the development of cancer. Emerging data indicate that cellular signaling and metabolism are tightly linked.[111] Several signaling pathways implicated in cell proliferation also regulate metabolic pathways. Signaling pathways activated by hormones and growth factors stimulate the metabolic activity of cells to promote proliferation or differentiation.[111] Metabolism affects key cellular processes by regulating signaling, gene expression, and metabolic processes.[111]

Recent studies reveal a link between glucose availability and protein acetylation, an epigenetic change.[111] Importantly, in the context of constant glucose levels, metabolite levels seem to oscillate in a circadian way within cells and tissues.[111] Food metabolism and circadian cycles are linked and impairment of clock regulation (e.g., disrupted night sleep and light; shift work) results in dysregulated metabolism.[113] **Circadian rhythms** pervade mammalian biology (Figure 13-14). They manifest and permeate temporal organization in behavioral, physiologic, cellular, and neuronal processes.[114] This ancient timekeeper interacts with multiple cell systems, including signaling mechanisms, and the cell cycle, thus impacting disease. Evidence is emerging that circadian mechanisms are linked to cell proliferation and its control at the DNA (epigenetic), RNA, and protein levels. Circadian disruption accelerates malignant growth.[114] In addition to nutrient levels oscillating metabolically, circadian rhythms appear to affect detox cycles.[113,114] Mutations in internal clock genes alter glucose and lipid metabolism and affect the function of the kidney.[115]

Alcohol Consumption. Alcohol is classified by the International Agency for Cancer Research as a human carcinogen. Excessive alcohol plays a contributory role in several common cancers.[65] Overall, there are strong data describing alcohol as a cause of cancers of the mouth, pharynx, larynx, esophagus, liver, colorectum, and breast (Table 13-5).[64,65,116] The evidence does not show any "safe limit" of intake, and the effect is from ethanol regardless of the type of drink.[64]

Animal studies show chronic alcohol intake is associated with reduced genomic DNA methylation in the colon.[117] Alcohol and cancers of the esophagus and liver also involve epigenetic alterations.[118,119] The molecular actions of ethanol are believed to include site-specific changes to histone modifications and alterations of one-carbon metabolism causing methylation changes.[65] MicroRNA expression has recently been linked to alcohol consumption in a case-control study of head and neck cancer (i.e., head and neck squamous cell carcinoma

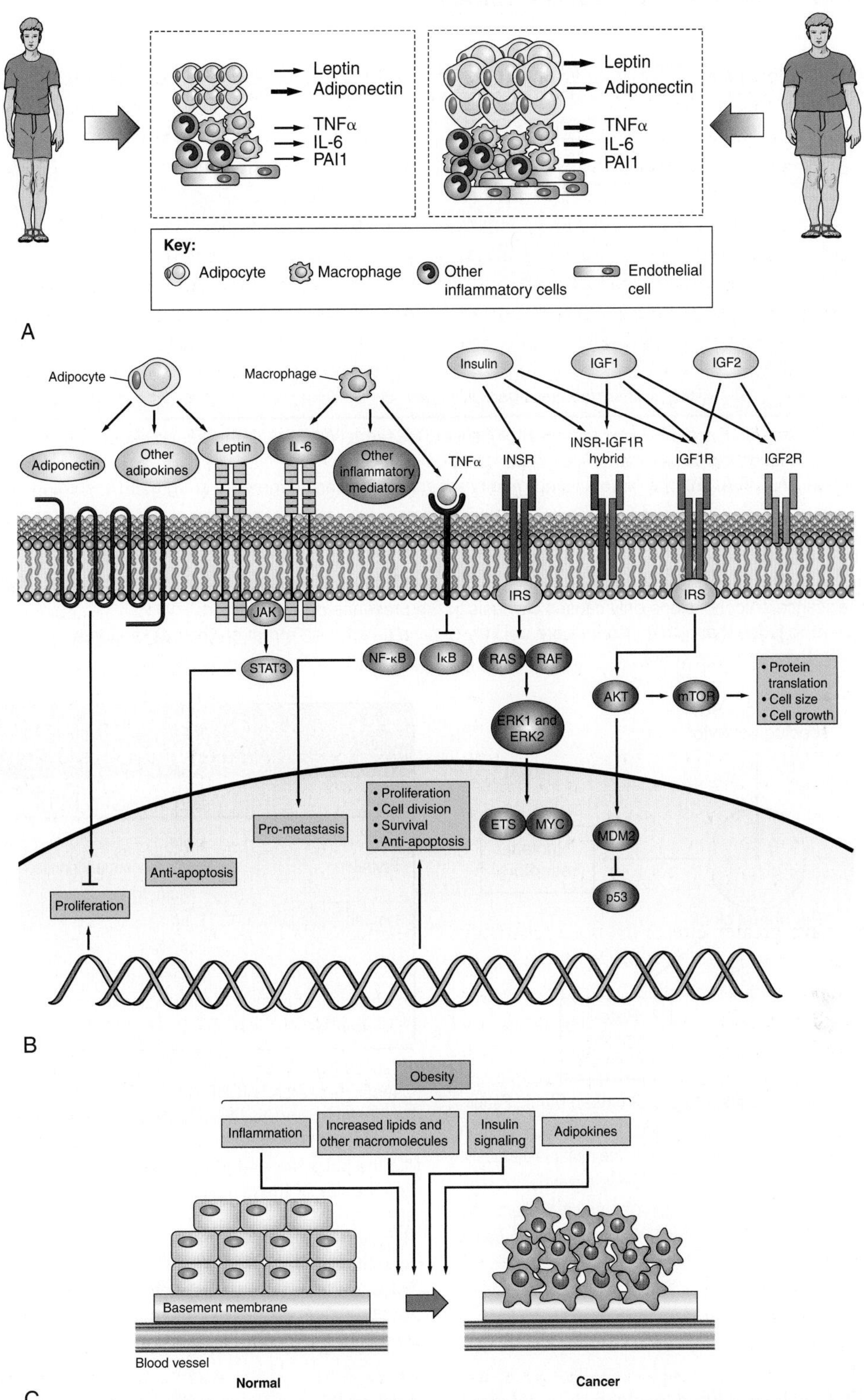

FIGURE 13-13 **Adipose Tissue, Obesity, Inflammation, Insulin, and Cancer.** **A,** Changes in adipose tissue and obesity. Adipose tissue is composed of adipocytes and stromal-vascular tissue (pre-adipocytes, macrophages, other inflammatory cells, endothelial cells). With obesity there is an increase in the size and number of adipocytes and increases in the inflammatory and vascular compartment (endothelial). **B,** Adipokine and inflammatory signaling in obesity. Overall, adiponectin inhibits proliferation and metastasis. Circulating leptin can bind to the leptin receptor or IL-6 and activate JAK signaling and STAT signaling. STAT3 can function as an oncogenic transcription factor. Inflammatory cells in adipose tissue produce IL-6 and TNFα as well as other cytokines. IL-6 activates JAK-STAT signaling which promotes proliferation and metastasis. TNFα activates NF-κB through the degradation of the inhibitor of κB kinase (IκB). NF-κB is now free to translocate to the nucleus where it inhibits apoptosis and promotes proliferation and metastasis. Obesity increases circulating insulin and possibly IGF-1 and IGF-2. Binding of insulin, IGF-1 and IGF-2 results in phosphorylation of IRS proteins that can activate downstream signaling, such as ERK pathways. The oncogenic pathways MYC (oncogene) and ETS (oncogene) are activated by ERK. Activation of PI3K pathways causes AKT (serine/threonine protein kinase) phosphorylation and mTOR activation promoting protein synthesis and cell growth. AKT also activates MDM2 that degrades p53 preventing cell cycle checkpoints and apoptosis. **C,** A summary of increased inflammation, increased availability of lipids and other macromolecules, insulin, and changes in adipokine signaling may contribute to the conversion of normal epithelial cells to an invasive tumor. *ERK,* extracellular signal-regulated kinase; *IGF,* insulin-like growth factor; *IL-6,* interleukin-6; *IRS,* insulin receptor substrate; *JAK,* Janus tyrosine kinase; *mTOR,* mammalian target of rapamycin; *MDM2,* mouse double minute2 homolog; mammalian target of rapamycin; *NF-κB,* nuclear factor κB; *PAI1,* plasminogen activator inhibitor-1; *PI3K,* phosphoinositide 3-kinase; *STAT,* activator of transcription signaling; *TNFα,* tumor necrosis factor alpha. (Adapted from Kandekar MJ et al: Molecular mechanism of cancer development in obesity, *Nat Rev Cancer* 11[12]:886-895, 2011.)

TABLE 13-5 ALCOHOLIC DRINKS AND RISK OF CANCER*

	DECREASES RISK		INCREASES RISK	
	EXPOSURE	CANCER SITE	EXPOSURE	CANCER SITE
Convincing			Alcoholic drinks	Mouth, pharynx and larynx, esophagus Colorectum (men)† Breast (pre- and postmenopause)
Probable			Alcoholic drinks	Liver‡ Colorectum (women)†
Limited—suggestive				
Substantial effect on risk unlikely	Alcoholic drinks (adverse effect): kidney§			

Adapted from World Cancer Research Fund/American Institute for Cancer Research (WCRF/AICR): *Second expert report: food, nutrition, physical activity, and the prevention of cancer: a global perspective,* London, 2007, Author.
*In the judgment of the Panel (WCRF/AICR), the factors listed modify the risk of cancer. Judgments are graded according to the strength of the evidence.
†The judgments for men and women are different because there are fewer data for women. Increased risk is only apparent above a threshold of 30 g/day of ethanol for both genders.
‡Cirrhosis is an essential precursor of liver cancer caused by alcohol. The International Agency for Research on Cancer has graded alcohol as a class 1 carcinogen for liver cancer. Alcohol alone only causes cirrhosis in the presence of other factors.
§The evidence was sufficient to judge that alcoholic drinks are unlikely to have an adverse effect on the risk of kidney cancer; it was inadequate to draw a conclusion regarding the protective effect.

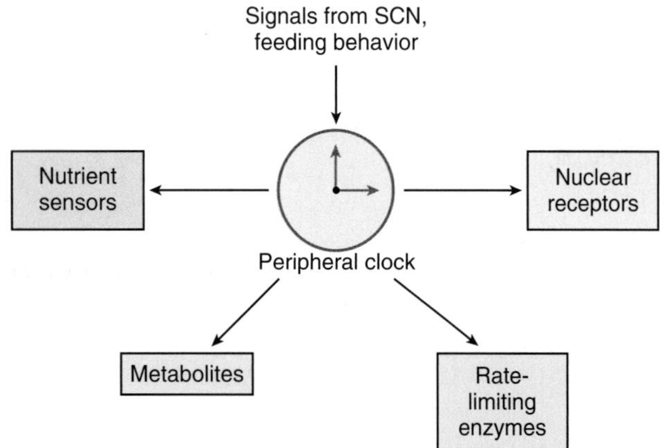

FIGURE 13-14 Regulation of Metabolism by the Circadian Clock. Peripheral clocks, such as that in the liver, are regulated by the master clock present in the suprachiasmatic nucleus *(SCN).* The liver clock can regulate multiple metabolic pathways by various mechanisms. These mechanisms include regulation of rate-limiting steps, control of metabolite levels, interaction of nutrient sensors, and modulation of nuclear sensors. (Adapted from Sahar S, Sassone-Corsi P: *Trends Endocrinol Metab* 23[1]:1–8, 2011.)

TABLE 13-6 PHYSICAL ACTIVITY AND RISK OF CANCER*,†

	DECREASES RISK	INCREASES RISK
Convincing	Colon‡	
Probable	Breast (postmenopausal) Endometrium	
Limited—suggestive	Lung Pancreas Breast (premenopausal)	
Substantial effect on risk unlikely	None identified	

Adapted from World Cancer Research Fund/American Institute for Cancer Research (WCRF/AICR): *Second expert report: food, nutrition, physical activity, and the prevention of cancer: a global perspective,* London, 2007, Author.
*In the judgment of the Panel (WCRF/AICR), physical activity† modifies the risk of the cancers. Judgments are graded according to the strength of the evidence.
†Physical activity of all types: occupational, household, transport, and recreational.
‡Much of the evidence grouped colon cancer and rectal cancer is together categorized as "colorectal cancer." The Panel judges that the evidence is stronger for colon cancer than for rectal cancer.

[HNSCC]).[120] The risk may be modified by alcohol dehydrogenase genes.[121] Alcohol is now an established risk factor for breast cancer in women and has been linked to genome-wide leukocyte DNA hypomethylation.[122] Alcohol interacts with smoke, increasing the risk of malignant tumors, possibly by acting as a solvent for the carcinogenic chemicals in smoke products.

Other mechanisms involved in alcohol-related carcinogenesis include the effect of acetaldehyde, the first metabolite of ethanol oxidation; the induction of cytochrome P-450 2E1 (genetic variant CYP2E1) leading to the generation of reactive oxygen species (ROS); the development of increased procarcinogen activation (e.g., nitrosamines) and the modulation of cellular regeneration (cell cycle); and the manifestation of nutritional deficiencies (e.g., retinol, retinyl esters, folic acid, other vitamins). Nutritional deficiencies may result in altered mucosal integrity, enzyme and metabolic dysfunction, and other structural abnormalities.

Physical Activity. Studies suggest that regular exercise decreases the risk of breast cancer, colon cancer, and endometrial cancer, independent of weight changes. The World Cancer Research Fund summarized the effects as *convincing* for cancers of the colon and *probable* for postmenopausal breast cancer and endometrial cancer[64] (Table 13-6).

The effect of physical activity on the risk of rectal cancer is much less certain,[87,123] and one study shows an inverse

TABLE 13-7 NUMBER OF NEW CANCER CASES* IN 2008 ATTRIBUTABLE TO INFECTION, BY INFECTIOUS AGENT, AND DEVELOPMENT STATUS†

	LESS DEVELOPED REGIONS	MORE DEVELOPED REGIONS	WORLD
Hepatitis B and C viruses	520,000 (32.0%)	80,000 (19.4%)	600,000 (29.5%)
Human papillomavirus	490,000 (30.2%)	120,000 (29.2%)	610,000 (30.0%)
Helicobacter pylori	470,000 (28.9%)	190,000 (46.2%)	660,000 (32.5%)
Epstein-Barr virus	96,000 (5.9%)	16,000 (3.9%)	110,000 (5.4%)
Human herpesvirus type 8	39,000 (2.4%)	4,100 (1.0%)	43,000 (2.1%)
Human T-cell lymphotropic virus type 1	660 (0.0%)	1,500 (0.4%)	2,100 (0.1%)
Opisthorchis viverrini and *Clonorchis sinensis*	2,000 (0.1%)	0 (0.0%)	2,000 (0.1%)
Schistosoma haematobium	6,000 (0.4%)	0 (0.0%)	6,000 (0.3%)
TOTAL	**1,600,000 (100.0%)**	**410,000 (100.0%)**	**2,000,000 (100.0%)**

Data from de Martel C et al: *Lancet Oncol* 13(6):607–615, 2012.
*Numbers are rounded to two significant digits.
†Data are number of new cancer cases attributed to a particular infectious agent (proportion of the total number of new cases attributed to infection that is attributable to a specific agent).

relationship.[124] Evidence of a reduction in breast cancer risk in postmenopausal women was associated with higher levels of activity (dose-response effect).[64,125] A recent meta-analysis concluded that physical activity seems to be related to a reduction in the risk of endometrial cancer independent of body weight.[126] Several biologic mechanisms suggest physical activity may protect against cancers of the breast and endometrium, by decreasing insulin and IGF levels, decreasing obesity, altering inflammatory mediators, decreasing levels of circulating sex hormones and metabolic hormones, improving immune function, and enhancing cytochrome P-450 activity, thus modifying carcinogen activation.[64,127-130] For colon cancer, physical activity increases gut motility, which reduces the length of transit time that the bowel lining is exposed to potential mutagens.[129] Other mechanisms of protection may include a reduction in insulin resistance, reduced body fatness, and changes in steroid hormone metabolism.[64] A randomized trial found that after 12 months of moderate-intensity exercise, postmenopausal women had significantly decreased levels of serum estrogens.[131] Physical activity also helps prevent type 2 diabetes, which has been associated with risk of cancer of the colon and pancreas.[129,132] However, evidence that physical activity protects against pancreatic cancer is limited.

Many questions are unanswered regarding frequency, intensity, and duration of exercise. Much of the literature suggests that between 3.5 and 4 hours of vigorous activity per week are necessary to optimize protection for colon cancer.[130] There is likely a dose-response relationship for colon cancer and breast cancer, and 30 to 60 minutes per day of moderate to vigorous intensity is proposed to decrease breast cancer risk.[133] A recent 12-month randomly controlled trial supported the Institute of Medicine and Department of Agriculture guidelines of 60 minutes per day of moderate to vigorous physical activity for decreasing weight, BMI, and amounts of body fat and intra-abdominal fat.[134] Several reports suggest that physical activity after a cancer diagnosis is associated with better cancer-specific sequelae and improved overall survival time with early-stage breast, prostate, and colorectal cancers.[85] Further research is needed on cancer outcomes and physical activity.

Infection, Sexual and Reproductive Behavior, Human Papillomaviruses

Infection is an important contributor to cancer worldwide and the population attributable fraction (PAF) indicated that 16.1% of cancers diagnosed in 2008 were caused by infection, or about 2 million new cases.[135] Infection and cancer rates vary widely by region: with a 7.4% rate for more developed regions and a 22.9% rate for less developed regions.[135] The highest PAF is for sub-Saharan Africa with a rate of 32.7%. Agents classified by the IARC were used in this report because the strength of published evidence is controversial.[135] The four top notable infections and new cancer cases include human papillomavirus (HPV), *Helicobacter pylori (H. pylori)*, hepatitis B virus (HBV), and hepatitis C virus (HCV) (Table 13-7). According to the investigators these results probably are conservative and underestimate the true burden of infection-associated cancers.[135] Most of the following discussion will be about human papillomavirus (HPV); however, hepatitis B and hepatitis C can infect the liver and together account for the large majority of liver cancer cases (see Chapter 41). It has been estimated that *H. pylori* accounts for about 75% of all stomach cancers.[136] Epstein-Barr virus (EBV) is linked to cancers of the nasopharynx, Hodgkin disease, and non-Hodgkin lymphoma. Human herpesvirus type 8 is linked to Kaposi sarcoma and human T-cell lymphotropic virus type 1 is linked to leukemia and lymphoma.

Human papillomavirus (HPV) is the most common sexually transmitted virus in the United States. At least 50% of sexually active people will have genital HPV at some time in their lives.[137] HPVs are a group of more than 150 related viruses. More than 40 of these viruses can easily spread from direct skin contact or through vaginal, rectal, or oral sex.[138] *Low-risk HPVs* do not cause cancer but can cause skin warts, called condylomata acuminata. *High-risk*, or oncogenic, *HPVs* can cause cancer. Even though about a dozen HPVs are identified, HPV types 16 and 18 are responsible for the majority of cancers.[138] However, most high-risk HPV infections may cause cytologic abnormalities or abnormal cell changes that disappear unexpectedly. Persistence of infection with high-risk HPV is a prerequisite for the development of cervical intraepithelial neoplasia (CIN) (see

Figure 24-19), lesions, and invasive cervical cancers.[139] Almost all cervical cancers are caused by HPV infections, with HPV types 16 and 18 responsible for about 70% of all cases.[140,141] HPV can cause anal cancer, with about 85% of all cases caused by HPV-16.[138] HPV types 16 and 18 also have been found to be responsible for almost half of vaginal, vulvar, and penile cancers.[142] Recently, HPV infections have been found to cause cancer of the oropharynx (soft palate, base of the tongue, tonsils).[138] More than half of the oropharyngeal cancers diagnosed in the United States are linked to HPV-16.[143] The incidence of HPV-associated oropharyngeal cancer has increased during the past 20 years, especially among men, and it has been estimated that by 2020 HPV will cause more oropharyngeal cancers than cervical cancers in the United States.[144] Factors that may increase the risk of developing cancer following a high-risk HPV infection include smoking, decreased immunity, having many children (for increased risk of cervical cancer), long-term oral contraceptive use (for increased risk of cervical cancer), poor oral hygiene (for increased risk of oropharyngeal cancer), and chronic inflammation.[141]

HPVs infect epithelial cells that cover the inside and outside surfaces of the body, including the skin, throat, genital tract, and anus. Because HPVs are not thought to enter the bloodstream, having an HPV infection in one part of the body should not cause an infection in another part of the body.[138] Once an HPV virus enters an epithelial cell, the virus begins to make proteins that can interfere with normal functions in the cell, enabling the cell to grow in an uncontrolled manner, and to avoid apoptosis.[138] These infected cells are often recognized by the immune system and eliminated. Sometimes, however, infected cells are not destroyed and a persistent infection results. As the persistently infected cells continue to grow, they may develop mutations that promote even more cell growth, leading to the formation of a high-grade lesion and, ultimately, a tumor.[138] Investigators believe that it can take between 10 and 20 years from the time of an initial HPV infection until tumor formation. However, even high-grade lesions do not always lead to cancer.[138]

Other Viruses and Microorganisms

A discussion of the relationship between viruses, bacteria, and cancer is contained in Chapter 12 and appropriate chapters in Unit II. Other microorganisms involved in carcinogenesis include parasites such as *Opisthorchis viverrini* and *Schistosoma haematobium*. Their specific roles in carcinogenesis are thought to be related to cofactors or carcinogens, or both.

Ionizing Radiation

Much of the knowledge of the effects of ionizing radiation (IR) on human cancer has stemmed from observations of the Hiroshima and Nagasaki atomic bomb (A-bomb) exposures, particularly the Life Span Study. These data provide estimates of human cancer risk over the dose range from 20 to 250 centigray (cGy) for low linear energy transfer (LET) radiation, such as x-rays or γ-rays. Other evidence is derived from groups exposed for medical reasons, underground miners exposed to radon gas, and other occupational exposures (Table 13-8). The atomic bomb exposures in Japan caused acute leukemias in adults and children and increased frequencies of thyroid and breast carcinomas. Lung, stomach, colon, esophageal, and urinary tract cancers and multiple myeloma have been added to the list. At Nagasaki and Hiroshima, leukemia incidence in individuals 15 years or younger reached its peak 6 to 7 years after the explosions and has steadily declined since 1952. People 45 years and older at the time of exposure had a latent period of 20 years before developing acute leukemia.

TABLE 13-8 CANCER ASSOCIATED WITH EXPOSURE TO IONIZING RADIATION

CANCER TYPE	AB	AS	PM	TC	TH	RP	UM	RD
Leukemia	X	X			X			X
Thyroid	X			X				
Breast	X		X					
Lung	X	X			X		X	
Bone						X		
Stomach	X	X						
Esophagus	X	X						
Lymphoma	X	X						X
Brain			X				X	
Liver				X				
Skin				X			X	X

Data from Jones JA, Casey RC, Karouia F: Ionizing radiation as a carcinogen. In McQueen E, editor: *CA comprehensive toxicology,* ed 2, St Louis, 2010, Elsevier.

AB, Atomic bomb survivors; *AS*, ankylosing spondylitis patients; *PM*, postpartum mastitis patients; *TC*, tinea capitis patients; *TH*, individuals receiving thorotrast; *RP*, radium dial painters; *UM*, underground miners; *RD*, radiologists.

Recently, standard models and evaluations of age of exposure to radiation and radiation-induced cancer risks have been questioned.[145-148] Epidemiologic data from Japanese atomic bomb survivors and from children exposed to radiation for medical intervention suggest that excess relative risks (ERRs) for radiation-induced cancers at a given age are exceptionally higher for individuals exposed during childhood than for those exposed at older ages.[149] These data also are published by the International Commission on Radiological Protection (ICRP) and the National Academy of Sciences Committee on the Biological Effects of Ionizing Radiation (BEIR Committee).[150] What is at question is the ERRs of radiation exposure in adulthood and radiation-induced cancer risk. Recent analyses of Japanese bomb survivors suggest that the ERR for cancer induction decreases with increasing age at exposure only until exposure ages of 30 to 40 years; with radiation exposure at older ages, the ERR does not decrease further and for many individual cancer sites (liver, colon, lung, stomach, and bladder) the ERR may actually increase in all solid cancers combined.[146,148,149,151] These new data present a challenge to our conceptual understanding of the mechanisms of cancer induction.[148] Biologic models of cancer development all predict that ERRs should decrease continuously with increasing age of radiation exposure. Recent models, however, of radiation carcinogenesis show IR acts not only as an initiator of premalignant cell clones but also

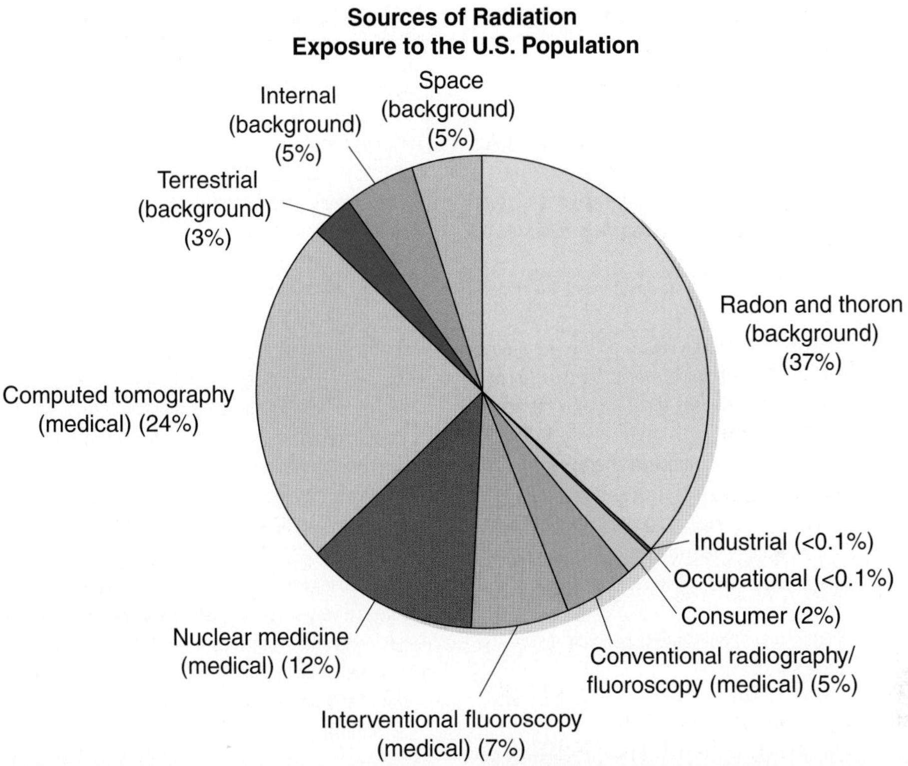

Sources of Radiation
Exposure to the U.S. Population

Internal (background) (5%)
Space (background) (5%)
Terrestrial (background) (3%)
Radon and thoron (background) (37%)
Computed tomography (medical) (24%)
Industrial (<0.1%)
Occupational (<0.1%)
Consumer (2%)
Nuclear medicine (medical) (12%)
Conventional radiography/ fluoroscopy (medical) (5%)
Interventional fluoroscopy (medical) (7%)

FIGURE 13-15 **Pie Chart Showing Sources of Exposure to Ionizing Radiation.** Percent contribution of various sources of exposure to the total collective effective dose (1,870,000 person-Sv) and the total effective dose per individual in the U.S. population (6.2 mSv) for 2006. Percent values have been rounded to the nearest 1%, except those <1%. *Sv,* Sievert. (From NCRP: *2009 Ionizing radiation exposure of the population of the United States,* NCRP Report No. 160, Bethesda, Md, Author.)

as a promoter of preexisting premalignant cell alterations.[146,148,151] Promotion is used here to mean the process by which an initiated cell clonally expands. Therefore promotional processes from radiation can result in increasing excess lifetime cancer risks with increasing age at exposure. From these new data investigators propose that radiation-induced cancer risks after exposure in middle age may be almost twice as high as previously estimated.[148]

Human exposure to IR includes emissions from x-rays, radioisotopes, and other radioactive sources (Figure 13-15). Health risks involve not only neoplastic diseases but also cardiovascular disease and stroke following high doses in therapeutic medicine and lower doses in A-bomb survivors (BEIR VII).[152,153] Late effects of radiation in A-bomb survivors show persistent elevations in the levels of inflammatory markers, implying immunologic damage may be the cause of later cardiovascular effects.[154] Investigators for the first time using a model of umbilical vein endothelial cells showed that low doses (0.05 Gy) of x-rays induce DNA damage and apoptosis in endothelial cells. These data will need continued research.[154a] Cardiac and blood vessel damage may manifest years after completion of radiation therapy.[155] Other risks include somatic mutations that may contribute to other diseases (e.g., respiratory diseases, birth defects, and eye maladies) and, from animal studies, inherited mutations that may affect the incidence of diseases in future generations. An important summary point in BEIR VII[152] is the concern from medical exposure, for example, computed tomography (CT) (see What's New? CT Scans and Issues). In 2009 the National Council on Radiation Protection and Measurements[156] reported Americans were exposed to more than seven times as much IR from medical procedures compared to the 1980s (Figure 13-16). In Europe, 20 millisieverts (mSv) is the annual allowable occupational exposure of radiation, and in the United States the annual allowable occupational exposure is 50 mSv.[157] The increase in imaging is likely driven by several factors, including improvements in the technology, that have led to increased clinical applications, patient demand, physician demand, defensive medical practices, and medical uncertainty.[158,159]

Evidence, usually epidemiologic, shows cancer associated with exposure to IR (see Table 13-8). Evidence includes animal models and in vitro studies as well as exposed groups including atomic/nuclear survivors, survivors of industrial accidents and the Techa River basin in Siberia, and medical diagnostic/therapeutic data. The studies of exposed groups are large enough to allow epidemiologists to derive detail concerning the dose and quality, age at exposure, and other factors on cancer incidence in a large variety of organs.[160] From data collected over several decades, exposed cohorts reveal that IR is a potent carcinogen.[160] Additionally, reports of occupational exposures may have increased the incidence of certain types of cancer, for example, underground miners and lung cancer.[161] Certain medical conditions, especially those with a genetic basis, predispose individuals to ionizing radiation–induced injury.[160] The most well-known condition is ataxia-telangiectasia (AT), a rare (1 in 300,000 people) condition in which individuals have a strong sensitivity to IR. Additionally, individuals with *BRCA1/BRCA2* pathway mutations have increased radiosensitivity caused by insufficient DNA repair and cell cycle control mechanisms.[162]

WHAT'S NEW?

CT Scans and Issues

Radiation: General Issues

- Many uncertainties exist about low-dose radiation and harmless and harmful effects.
- Currently, almost all of the available epidemiologic data are generated from people exposed to background radiation, such as the Japanese survivors of the atomic bombs.
- Biologic data, especially for low-dose radiation, are insufficient for understanding both harmless and harmful effects.
- The effects of low-dose radiation (LDR) are mainly based on the linear non-threshold (LNT) hypothesis and include the following *overestimated effects*[1]:
  1. No injurious effects are detected at a dose less than 100 mSv for adults and less than 50 mSv for children.
  2. Exposure to LDR has adaptive and hormesis protective effects.
  3. The progression of carcinogenesis is not linear.
  4. Cancer may not develop until there is accumulated genetic damage.
- The LNT hypothesis includes the following *underestimated effects:*
  1. The bystander effect and associated chromosomal effects have not been fully studied.
  2. Amplification of damaged chromosomes could lead to genomic instability.
  3. Some people are hypersensitive to radiation.
- Carcinogenesis is considered the most serious consequence of LDR and it affects other tissues, for example, blood vessels.[2-4]
- The hereditary effect is the variation of damage that could occur in germ cells. Recent epidemiologic studies showed no direct connection between LDR and the hereditary effect.[3] The ICRP estimated the hereditary effect as 0.2%/Sv. Biologic studies are needed.
- Approximately 5% to 10% of individuals are hypersensitive to radiation, for example, those with the ataxia-telangiectasia mutated *(ATM)* gene. *ATM* plays a major role in the response to ionizing radiation.[5]
- The accumulative effects of LDR from repeated CT scans may lead to buildup of radiation doses.[6]
- The proportion of annual CT scans in some developed countries increased from 6.1% (1970-1979) to 48% (1991-1996). In the last 25 years, usage of CT has increased 12 times in the United Kingdom and more than 20 times in the United States.[7]
- Calculations from nuclear industry personnel of 15 different countries are in the range of low-dose radiation and CT. About 0.6% and 1.5% of the cumulative cancer risk could be attributed to diagnostic x-rays in England and Germany, respectively. About 3.2% of new cancer cases in Japan are considered the result of two examinations every year. It is estimated that about 29,000 cancers could be related to CT scans in the United States every year; scans of the abdomen and pelvis are the most common.[8,13] Other estimates indicate that CT scan–induced cancer risk is about 0.7%,[9] CT angiography risk is about 0.13%,[10] and CT colonoscopy cancer risk is 0.15%.[11,12] The carcinogenic risk of low doses and low dose rates of radiation from CT is estimated at 5%/Sv.[1] The mathematical extrapolation of LNT to LDR may not be accurate because of the biology of LDR.
- CT scans can save lives, improve diagnostic accuracy, limit medical procedures, and save healthcare dollars.
- Researchers report that certain CT scans are unnecessary and a survey revealed that about 77% of lumbar spine, 36% of head, 37% of abdomen, 20% of nasal sinuses, and 3% of cervical spine CT scans should have been MRI scans instead.[1]
- It is probable that at least 25% of CT scans are not clinically warranted.

Biology and CT Radiation

- Radiation from CT scans can activate antioxidants, such as superoxide dismutase (SOD), DNA repair mechanisms, and the immune system, to recognize mutated cells.[14]
- Repeated CT scanning can alter the balance between antioxidant and oxidant systems and increase the number of ROS.
- ROS can lead to DNA single- and double-strand breaks, DNA interstrand cross-linking, and eventually the formation of apurinic and apyrimidinic sites.[15]
- A quantitative marker of LDR-induced double-strand breaks is a member of the histone H2A family, H2AX, which becomes phosphorylated within 1 to 3 minutes of DNA damage and forms foci at the break sites.[16,17]
- Continuous DNA damage can lead to chromosomal aberration, chromosomal damage in cell progeny, and elevated levels of γ-H2AX. Such alterations might lead to genomic instability and currently there are reported increases in the number of cases of non-Hodgkin lymphoma and breast cancer.[18-20]
- With the increase in multi-slice CT (MSCT), the radiation dose is gradually increasing. The 64-slice CT to do heart scanning included exposures of other tissues: heart, 32.4 mSv; breast, 39.1 mSv; lung, 33.2 mSv; and spinal cord, 29.8 mSv.[21,22]
- Organ doses relevant to most CT usage are between 5 and 100 mSV; the exposure is a very small but well-established individual cancer risk, particularly for patients without significantly reduced life expectancy.[23-26]
- Epigenetics including DNA methylation and miRNA expression could be especially helpful in understanding the biology of radiation-induced genomic instability (RIGI).

Children

- About 600,000 children under the age of 15 have abdominal and head CT scans in the United States every year, and it is estimated that about 500 children might eventually die from CT-induced cancer.[5]
- Children are more sensitive to radiation and their carcinogenic risks are about 4 times those of an adults' risk (a 1-year-old infant is 10 to 15 times more prone to develop cancer than an adult).[27]
- CT-induced cancer risks were 3% (10 years old) and 2% (15 years old) in children who received abdominal and pelvic CT scans for renal calculi detection.[28]
- German investigators have planned to conduct a historic cohort study to investigate cancer incidence from CT exposure in children younger than age 15.[29]

Confusion for Healthcare Providers and Patients

- Surveys are being done to understand the radiation knowledge of patients and healthcare workers.
- A survey reported more than 70% of patients underestimated the radiation dose from CT scans and had very limited understanding of radiation-induced cancer risks.[30]
- Another survey revealed about 7% of patients were informed about the benefits and risks before having a CT scan and 53% of radiologists and 91% of emergency department physicians believed CT scans would not increase cancer risks.[31]
- About 43% of hospital imaging departments made technologic adjustments for pediatric patients.[32]
- About 33% of CT imaging departments indicated they had adjusted the tube current down to less than 100 milliamperes (mA) when they performed helical CT scans of the chest on 4-year-old children.[33]
- A German study revealed physicians overestimated the radiation exposure from conventional x-rays but underestimated the exposures from CT scans.[34]

References

1. Shumei MA et al: *Int J Radiat Biol*, December 2012. [Epub ahead of print.].
2. Dauer LT et al: *Radiat Prot Dosimetry* 140(2):103–136, 2010.
3. Hall EJ: *Pediatr Radiol* 39(Suppl 1):S57–S64, 2009.
4. Lee PJ, Mallik R: *Cardiol Rev* 13(2):80–86, 2005.

WHAT'S NEW?

CT Scans and Issues—cont'd

5. Pauwels EK, Bourgignon M: *Acta Radiol* 52(7):767–773, 2011.
6. Brenner DJ, Elliston EJ: *Radiology* 232(3):735–738, 2004.
7. Hall EJ: *J Radiol Prot* 29(2A):A171–A184, 2009.
8. Berrington de Gonzalez A, Darby S: *Lancet* 363(9406):345–351, 2004.
9. Sodickson A et al: *Radiology* 251(1):175–184, 2009.
10. Huda W et al: *AJR Am J Roentgenol* 196(2):W159–165, 2011.
11. Berrington de Gonzalez A et al: *Gastrointest Endosc Clin North Am* 20(2):279–291, 2010.
12. Berrington de Gonzalez A: *AJR Am J Roentgenol* 196(4):816–823, 2011.
13. Berrington de Gonzalez A et al: *Arch Intern Med* 169(22):2071–2077, 2009.
14. Gori T, Munzel T: *Eur Heart J* 33(3):292–295, 2012.
15. Feinendegen LE, Pollycove M, Sondhaus CA: *Toxicol Med* 2(3):143–171, 2004.
16. Sharma A, Singh K, Almasan A: *Methods Mol Biol* 920:613–626, 2012.
17. Wu CY et al: *J Biol Chem* 286(35):30806–30815, 2011.
18. Lu J et al: *Breast Cancer Res Treat* 110(2):357–366, 2008.
19. Novik KL et al: *Cancer Epidemiol Biomarkers Prev* 16(6):1098–1106, 2007.
20. Streffer C: *Mutat Res* 568(1):79–87, 2004.
21. Meer AB et al: *J Am Coll Radiol* 9(4):245–250, 2012.
22. Smith-Bindman R et al: *Arch Intern Med* 169(22):2078–2086, 2009.
23. Brenner DJ, Shuryak I, Einstein AJ: *Radiology* 261:193–198, 2011.
24. Brenner DJ, Hall EJ: *N Engl J Med* 357:2277–2284, 2007.
25. Pearce MS et al: *Lancet*, 2012 Jun 7. [Epub ahead of print.]
26. Hall EJ, Brenner DJ: *BRJ Radiol* 81:362–378, 2008.
27. Schweitzer T et al: *Childs Nerv Syst* 28(7):1077–1082, 2012.
28. Kuhns LR et al: *Pediatr Emerg Care* 27(4):345–350, 2011.
29. Krille L et al: *Radiat Environ Biophys* 51(2):103–111, 2012.
30. Baumann BM et al: *Ann Emerg Med* 58(1):1–7e2, 2011.
31. Lee CI et al: *Radiology* 231(2):393–398, 2004.
32. Linton O, Mettler FA: *AJR Am J Roentgenol* 181(2):321–329, 2003.
33. Sodickson A et al: *Radiology* 251(1):175–184, 2009.
34. Merzenich H et al: *BMC Health Serv Res* 12:47, 2012.

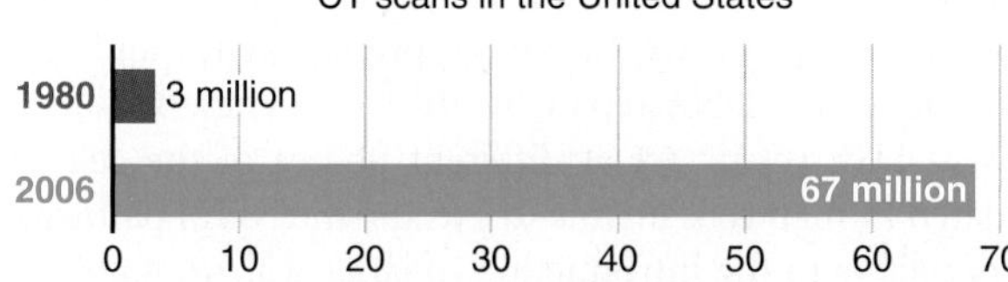

MEDIAN EFFECTIVE RADIATION DOSE FOR EACH TYPE OF CT STUDY			
ANATOMIC AREA, STUDY TYPE	MEDIAN (mSv)	RANGE (mSv)	DOSE EQUIVALENT (NO. OF CHEST X-RAYS)
Head and Neck			
Routine head	2	0.3-6	30
Routine neck	4	0.7-9	55
Suspected stroke	14	4-56	199
Chest			
Chest, no contrast	8	2-24	117
Chest, with contrast	8	2-19	119
Suspected pulmonary embolus	10	2-30	137
Coronary angiogram	22	7-39	309
Abdomen-Pelvis			
Routine abdomen-pelvis, no contrast	15	3-43	220
Routine abdomen-pelvis, with contrast	16	4-45	234
Multiphase abdomen pelvis	31	6-90	442
Suspected aneurysm or dissection	24	4-68	347

FIGURE 13-16 **CT Scans in the United States.** NCRP estimates that 67 million CT scans (compared to 3 million in 1980), 18 million nuclear medicine procedures, and 17 million interventional fluoroscopy procedures were performed in the United States in 2006. (From NCRP: *2009 Ionizing radiation exposure of the population of the United States,* NCRP Report No. 160, Bethesda, Md, Author.)

Studies conducted jointly by the U.S. Air Force and NASA from 1963 to 1969 studied the relative biologic effectiveness (RBE) of different types of radiation exposures on rhesus monkeys and mice.[160] Long-term follow-up studies of the exposed animals showed an induction of solid tumors and leukemia and the extent of life-shortening depended on dose and not on proton energy level.[163] The general characteristics of radiation carcinogenesis were determined from studies done after World War II, mainly from rats and mice.[160] However, together with epidemiologic studies of humans, these animal studies elucidated radiation carcinogenesis.[164,165] The BEIR VII report that focused on low-level radiation determined that the radiation-induced life shortening observed in mice is reflective in humans of radiation-induced cancer mortality.[166] These studies are important because they show that IR is universally carcinogenic to animals and humans and that there are wide differences in radiation responses according to species, organ, and radiation distribution.[160]

The universal nature of radiation as a carcinogen relates to its ability to penetrate cells and deposit energy in tissues at random. By the 1980s, using in vitro models, the *general* characteristics of IR-induced carcinogenesis were well established.[167] The past two decades have focused on *specific* cellular and molecular mechanisms that relate to the induction of cancer, including dose-response relationships for chromosome aberrations, cell transformation, gene expression (genetic and epigenetic), alternative targets, mutagenesis in somatic cells, and the biologic effects that occur in nonirradiated cells (i.e., **nontargeted effects**) and effects on the microenvironment.[160] Through much of the twentieth century, radiobiology was thought to be a relatively simple science and was dominated by physicists. Now, with biologists entering the field, it has become apparent that radiobiology is not so simple and involves much more understanding beyond a DNA-centric model, including alternative targets, such as membranes, repair, and rescue within a biologic system.[168] Because models and underlying assumptions are incomplete, investigators are working hard to understand induced repair, adaptive responses, hormesis, low-dose hypersensitivity,

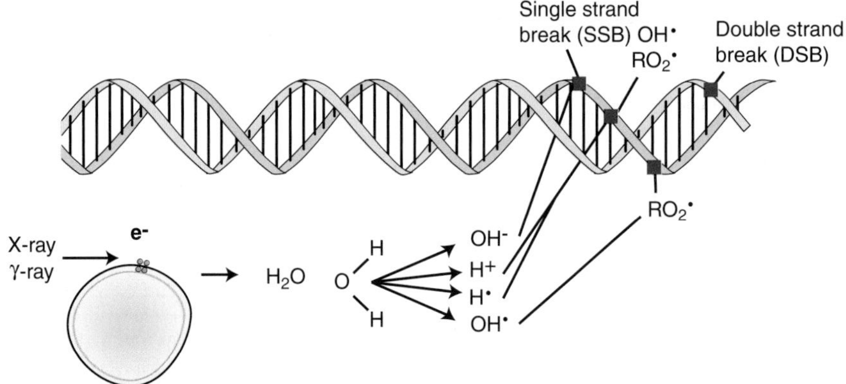

FIGURE 13-17 **Free Radicals.** Free radicals formed by water nearby and around DNA cause indirect effects. These effects have a short life of single free radicals. Oxygen can modify the reaction, enabling longer lifetimes of oxidative free radicals.

nontargeted effects, signaling, exosomes, and long-term persistence of radiation damage and clonal heterogeneity.[168]

Oncogenes and Tumor-Suppressor Genes

Part of the biologic response of radiation-induced cancer is oncogene activation. Although evidence suggests that interindividual differences in radiation responses may be attributed to certain genes, IR can activate oncogenes, resulting in uncontrolled cell growth[160] (see Chapter 12). **Tumor-suppressor genes** also are sensitive to IR. Several tumor-suppressor genes have been identified that are deactivated by IR that promotes carcinogenesis.[160] Recent research has shown that cells can detect and respond epigenetically, altering gene expression after low doses of radiation.[160] Gene expression can change as a function of radiation dose and radiation type.[160]

Chromosomal Aberrations

IR is a mutagen and carcinogen; it can penetrate cells and tissues and deposit energy in tissues at random in the form of ionizations (e.g., removal of an electron from the target atom). Importantly, arising from IR is the localized release of large amounts of energy that can break a chemical bond (electron volts [eV] is the energy per ionizing event). Damage from IR can occur either *directly* from biologic macromolecules (e.g., DNA) or *indirectly*, in the medium from which organelles are suspended in mostly water, and *irreversibly* from ionizations that can attack by water-based free radicals (e.g., H•, OH•) (radiolysis).[169] Electromagnetic radiations, such as x-rays and γ-rays, damage by reactive species produced by ionizations elsewhere in the cell and thus have indirect action. The biologic effects of indirect action include cell killing (days), mutation (generation), and carcinogenesis (years). IR affects many cell processes, including gene expression, mitochondrial function disruption, cell cycle arrest, and cell death. IR is a potent DNA-damaging agent, causing cross-linking, nucleotide base damage, and single (SSBs)- and double-strand breaks (DSBs) (Figure 13-17). Damage to DNA and disrupted cellular regulation processes can lead to carcinogenesis.[170-172] The **double-strand break (DSB)** is considered the important lesion in the induction of both chromosomal abnormalities and gene mutations. Repair of radiation-induced DNA double-strand breaks in human fibroblasts is consistent with a continuous spectrum of repair probability[173-175] (Figure 13-18). The misrepair of DSBs could lead to substantial chromosomal instability.[176] Importantly, DSBs are probably repaired by the nonhomologous end-joining (NHEJ) pathway.[150] Another pathway is by homologous recombination (HR); for example, *BRCA1* and *BRCA2* are tumor-suppressor genes and one of their functions is DNA repair by HR.[177,178] These two mechanisms of DSB repair act at different phases of the cell cycle. Irradiated human cells unable to execute the NHEJ pathway are supersensitive to the introduction of large-scale mutations and chromosomal aberrations.[169]

Cell Transformation

Cell transformation describes the total changes associated with loss of normal homeostatic control.[160] The majority of studies on cell transformation in vitro have been quantitative, using rodent-derived models. Few human-derived assays have been conducted. Overall, the exposure to high-LET radiation results in a higher transformation frequency than exposure to low-LET radiation.[160] There is no tendency, however, for the response per unit dose to decrease at low doses or low dose rates, and a number of studies have shown an enhanced effect.[160]

Nontargeted Effects

A long-held assumption is that cellular alterations—mutations and malignant transformation—occur only in cells directly radiated. There is clear evidence indicating that cells not directly traversed by a radiation particle, but in the vicinity of a cell that has been exposed to or received signals from irradiated cells, can participate in the damage response.[179] The **DNA damage response (DDR)** is a coordinated series of events that allows DNA damage detection, signaling that includes cell cycle checkpoint activation, and repair.[180,181] Emerging and important data indicate that the DDR should be considered not only at the DNA level but also in the chromatin of cell nuclei where DNA envelopes histone proteins.[182] Additionally, the importance of the plasticity of the microenvironment is becoming integrated into the radiation response.

It is now known that cells not directly exposed to radiation, but instead the progeny of cells that were irradiated many cell divisions previously, may express a high level of gene

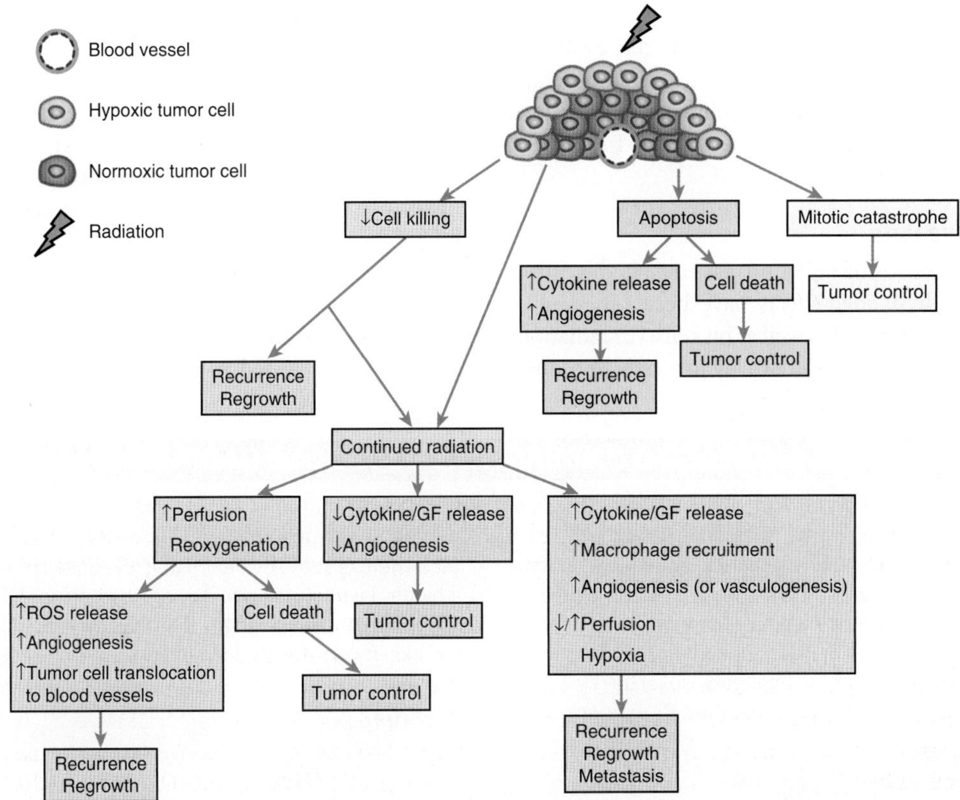

FIGURE 13-18 Simplified Model of the Effects of Radiation on Tumor Microenvironment. Tumor cells that are not hypoxic cells (i.e., called normoxic) are more sensitive to radiation and hence more susceptible to cell death (apoptosis) and mitotic catastrophe or destruction. In some cases, however, pro-apoptotic mechanisms can cause the release of cytokines that promote tumor regrowth and recurrence. Hypoxic cells are resistant to radiation therapy and more likely lead to tumor recurrence. Continuous radiation (especially fractionated) can lead to reoxygenation, which can improve radiation-induced cell killing or promote release of reactive oxygen species (ROS) and angiogenesis and/or induce tumor cell movement to blood vessels; both mechanisms can result in tumor regrowth and recurrence. Decreased cytokine production and destruction of blood vessels from continued administration of high doses of radiation can increase tumor cell killing. In certain situations, however, irradiation is associated with the production of an aggressive phenotype of the remaining cells that survive radiation therapy. This failure is caused by the release of protective cytokines and/or growth factors (GF), recruitment of macrophages, altered perfusion of blood, and hypoxia that increase angiogenesis or blood vessel growth, resulting in tumor regrowth and recurrence and/or metastasis. Importantly, the effects of radiation on tumor microenvironment depend on many factors. (Adapted from Fokas E, McKenna WG, Muschel RJ: The impact of tumor microenvironment on cancer treatment and its modulation by direct and indirect antivascular strategies, *Cancer Metastasis Rev* 31(3-4):823–842, 2012. [Epub ahead of print.])

mutations, cell lethality, and chromosomal aberration. Altogether these effects are called **genomic instability.** Effects in the distant progeny are also called transgeneration inheritance or effects (see p. 410). The directly irradiated cells also can lead to genetic effects in so-called bystander cells or innocent cells (called **bystander effects**) even though they themselves received no direct radiation exposure.[179] The bystander effect has been demonstrated in three-dimensional human tissues[183] and recently in whole animal organisms.[184] Signaling communication is thought to occur from direct physical connection between cells or gap junctions, called gap junctional intercellular communication (GJIC). Other mechanisms, however, may be involved. Numerous intercellular and intracellular signaling pathways are implicated in the bystander response and these effects have been shown to be transmitted to their descendents. The bystander and genomic instability effects also have been termed nontargeted effects.

Acute, Latent, and Microenvironmental Effects

IR causes acute and persistent short- and long-term effects.[185-188] Acute exposure to IR can cause damage to several organ systems, especially those with highly proliferative cells such as the hematopoietic system, the skin, and the gastrointestinal system[189] (see Chapter 2). Investigators have postulated that radiation's carcinogenic potential persists because of nontargeted radiation effects that alter cell and tissue signaling and change the microenvironment.[190,191] Figure 13-18 provides a simplified model of the effects of radiation on tumor microenvironment. With improvement in cancer survival the long-term risks of a second cancer from treatment become more important.[192]

Radiation-induced cancer in humans has latent periods, usually 5 to 10 years but can be decades.[160,193] British investigators reported the following results: for solid cancers, radiation-related excess risk starts to appear about 5 years after exposure in therapeutically irradiated groups, and for leukemia, it starts to appear within 5 years of exposure.[194] Using U.S. Surveillance Epidemiology and End Results (SEER) data, the estimated excess of second cancers that could be related to radiotherapy is about 8%; data from the United Kingdom, which included diagnostic procedures and excluded therapeutic irradiation, yielded an estimation of 15%.[192,194]

Low Dose and Dose Rate

New studies on low doses of radiation have resulted in three paradigm shifts: (1) bystander effects have been observed in which nonhit cells may respond as well as hit cells; (2) radiation-induced changes in gene expression at very low radiation doses alter response pathways, some of which appear to involve adaptive or protective responses; and (3) early changes in the initiation phase of radiation-induced cancer were thought to be induced by gene mutation and chromosomal aberrations only; however, it is now understood that genomic instability that leads to the loss of genetic control appears to have a major role in the development of cancer.[195] Constant debate involves risk estimates for human exposure at low-dose, low-LET ionizing radiation (0 to 100 mSv or less than 0.1 Gy). Accurate measurements of risks from low doses and low dose rates of radiation are statistically difficult because they require such large populations that theoretic models are used to estimate response curves (Box 13-1).

BOX 13-1 THEORETIC MODELS TO UNDERSTAND LOW-DOSE RADIATION

Several models include the linear no-threshold (LNT) relationship, in which any dose, including very low doses, has the potential to cause mutations (see **A**). Another model, the linear-quadratic relationship, proposes there is a risk mathematical term that is directly proportional to the dose (linear term) and another term proportional to the square of the dose (quadratic term) (see **B**). The threshold model proposes a threshold dose below which radiation may not cause cancer in humans (see **C**). Proponents of this model argue that such thresholds are derived, for example, from the ability to repair damage caused by lower doses of radiation. There is some evidence that low doses may actually produce a higher level of risk per unit of dose, which is called the supralinear hypothesis (see **D**). **E,** Stochastic or random probability is a major model for understanding low-dose radiation. Currently, the shape of the response curve for the low-dose region is really unknown.

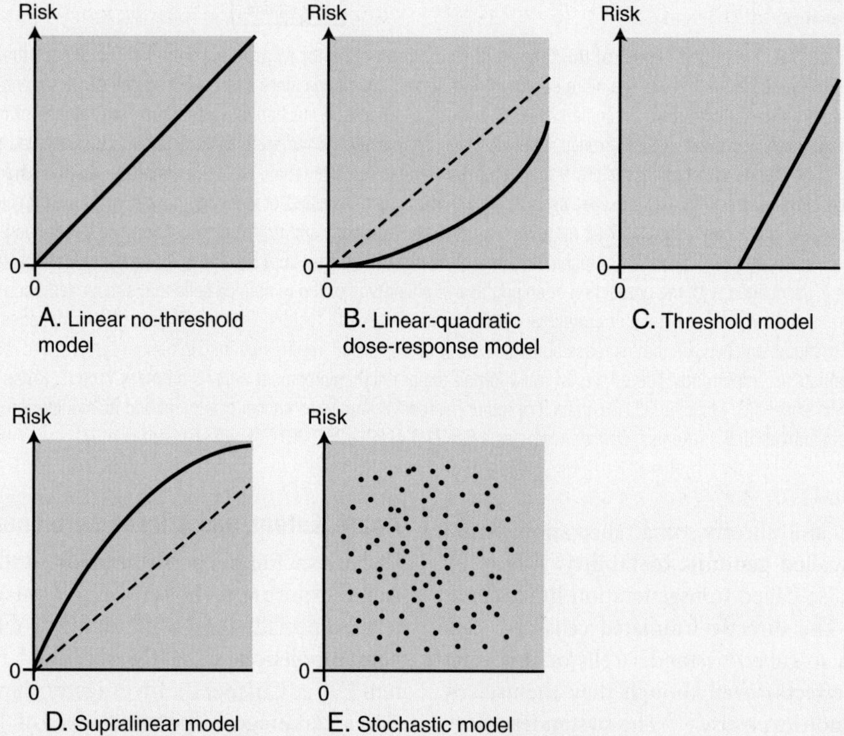

Theoretic Models for Estimating Risk of Low-Dose Ionizing Radiation. Collective population dose is expressed as a person-rem (roentgen equivalent, man). Estimating a collective dose then enables an application of a "constant risk factor" to obtain a statistical estimate of the number of additional cancers (above background radiation) from that exposure. These computations apply to low doses–low dose rates only **(A).** Many propose the best fit is the linear no-threshold (LNT) model **(B).** The most common alternative to the LNT model is the linear-quadratic model. The quadratic term is the square of the dose. The linear term is equal to zero **(C).** The threshold model is a threshold below which there is *no* increase in cancer risk. Proponents of this model argue that because some toxic chemicals/materials exhibit such thresholds, radiation must also have a threshold. Their arguments are related to repair of the radiation damage caused by lower doses of radiation **(D).** Some evidence exists that low levels of radiation produce a higher level of risk per unit dose, which is called the supralinear model. The stochastic model is where effects are random and the events cannot be predicted **(E).** (Adapted from Makhijani A, Smith B, Thorne MC: *Science for the vulnerable: setting radiation and multiple exposure environmental health standards to protect those at most risk,* Takoma Park, Md, 2006, Institute for Energy and Environmental Research.)

Data from Hoel DG: *Ann N Y Acad Sci* 1076:309–331, 2006; Preston DL et al: *Radiat Res* 160:381–407, 2003.

Extrapolations from high dose or high dose rate down to very low doses and very low dose rates using these mathematical models may underestimate or overestimate cancer risks at low doses. Consequently, animal studies are also ongoing to experimentally understand the biology of low-dose radiation and low dose rates of radiation. The risks of low doses of radiation are controversial and the uncertainties associated with the best estimates are great.[196] The risk of neoplastic transformation in bystander cells remains unclear.

Ultraviolet Radiation

Ultraviolet sunlight *causes* basal cell carcinoma and squamous cell carcinoma (i.e., photocarcinogenesis), two common skin cancers found in white individuals (see following discussion about melanoma). Exposure to ultraviolet radiation (UVR) can emanate from natural and artificial sources; however, the principal source of exposure for most people is sunlight. With further depletion of the stratospheric ozone layer, people and the environment will be exposed to higher intensities of UVR. The degree of damage in skin depends on the intensity and wavelength content (i.e., ultraviolet A [UVA] or ultraviolet B [UVB]; ultraviolet C possess the highest energy but does not penetrate the atmosphere) and the depth of penetration. UV radiation is known to cause specific gene mutations; for example, squamous cell carcinoma involves mutation in the *TP53* gene, basal cell carcinoma in the *patched* gene, and melanoma in the CDKN2A/*p16* gene.[197] In addition, UV light induces the release of TNF-α in the epidermis, which may reduce immune surveillance against skin cancer.[198]

Skin exposure to UVR and ionizing radiation, as well as chemical (xenobiotic) agents/drugs, produces ROS in large quantities that can overwhelm tissue antioxidants and other oxygen-degrading pathways.[199] Uncontrolled release of ROS is an important contributor to skin carcinogenesis.[199] Healthy genes are needed to coordinate the levels of antioxidants and decrease harmful ROS. Imbalances in ROS and antioxidants can lead to oxidative stress, tissue injury, and direct DNA damage. ROS can induce a number of transcription factors (e.g., activator protein 1 [AP-1] and NF-κB)[200] and increase regulating genes that induce inflammation.[201,202] Inflammation is a critical component of tumor progression. The pathophysiology of skin carcinogenesis is discussed further in Chapter 46.

Basal cell carcinoma (BCC) commonly occurs on the head and neck. Individuals with these tumors generally have fair complexions, light-colored eyes, and fair hair. They tend to sunburn rather than tan and live in areas of high sunlight exposure. Usually these cancers arise on areas of the body that receive the greatest sun exposure, although they are not necessarily restricted to these skin sites. Squamous cell carcinoma (SCC) is found more commonly in men who work outdoors. These tumors are distributed over the head, neck, and exposed areas of the upper extremities (see Chapter 46).

The incidence of melanoma in the United States (from the most recent SEER data) has been increasing annually at a rate of about 2.8% from 1981 to 2008.[203] Because mortality rates have not risen as rapidly, however, controversy exists as to whether the incidence increase is a true increase in clinically significant melanoma or is a result of overdiagnosis.[204] Overdiagnosis may include lesions that are histologically malignant but biologically benign.[205] Melanomas most commonly affect whites, and the lower incidence of melanoma in darker-skinned individuals is thought to be the result of higher melanin densities in these individuals.[206] Established risk factors for melanoma are genetic and phenotypic traits; increasing age; fair skin and hair color; the presence of >20 nevi, ≥3 atypical nevi, or freckling; an increased likelihood of burning with sun exposure; a history of immunosuppression, previous psoralen UVA treatment, solar keratoses, squamous cell carcinoma, or xeroderma pigmentosum; and a family history of dysplastic nevi or melanoma.[207,208]

Environmental exposures important in melanoma include history of three or more episodes of sunburn, periodic excessive sunlight exposure (e.g., vacations with intense exposure), possibly long-term continuous sunlight exposure,[209] and UV exposure at tanning salons.[207] Other environmental factors, such as ozone depletion and latitudes closer to the equator, also may be related.[207] Sun exposure and the risk of melanoma remain complex. Melanomas can appear suddenly without warning but can arise from or near a mole (melanocytic nevus). When detected in the early stages, melanoma is highly curable.[210] About 20% of melanomas, however, are diagnosed at nonlocalized and advanced stages.[210] According to Sekulic and colleagues,[211] the failure of current diagnostic methods to accurately predict individual risk of disease progression and outcome challenges the ability to diagnose melanoma in early stages. Recent progress in understanding the molecular alterations in melanoma will likely advance its diagnosis, prognosis, and treatment.

Until 1998 a direct causal relationship between UVB light and melanoma in humans had not been established. Grafted newborn human foreskin (xenograft) onto RAG-1–immunodeficient mice showed such a relationship.[212] Melanocytic hyperplasia occurred in 73% of UVB-treated xenografts. One graft treated with 9,10-dimethylbenz[*a*]anthracene (DMBA) and UVB light developed a human malignant melanoma. This was the first experiment to show that exposure to both UVB light and an exogenous carcinogen could result in a new malignant melanoma. Recent evidence shows UV signature mutations in human melanoma.[213,214] (For further specific pathophysiology discussion, see Chapter 46.)

Increased understanding of the intricate cellular interactions in melanoma will further our knowledge of melanoma etiology and pathogenesis. This knowledge is essential for early detection and treatment.

Electromagnetic Radiation

Health risks associated with **radiofrequency electromagnetic radiation (RF-EMR)** are very controversial. RF-EMR is in the frequency range of 30 kHz to 300 GHz. Electromagnetic fields (EMFs) generated by RF sources couple with the body and result in induced electric and magnetic fields with associated currents inside tissue.[215] Exposure to electric and magnetic fields is widespread. Electric fields are shielded or weakened by walls and other objects; however, magnetic fields are not.[216] EMRs are a type of nonionizing, low-frequency radiation without enough energy to pull electrons from their orbits around atoms and ionize (charge) the atoms. Microwaves, radar, mobile and cell phones, mobile phone base stations, appliances, power frequency radiation associated with electricity and radio waves, fluorescent lights, computers, and other electric equipment create EMRs of varying strength. The major debate for more than four decades has focused on the association of exposure to EMR and resultant health consequences, including cancer. Scientific evidence is accumulating although hampered by the availability of methods to accurately measure exposure, the lack of a clear dose-response relationship, and the difficulty in reproducing effects. In addition, with competing priorities such as convenience, financial interest, and health necessity, a consensus of the risk/benefit ratio of EMR exposure may be difficult to achieve, and safety standards significantly vary, up to 1000 times among countries.[217,218] In 1998, the National Institute of Environmental Health Sciences Electric and Magnetic Fields Working Group[219] recommended that low-frequency electromagnetic fields (EMFs) be classified as possible carcinogens. Overall, there is limited evidence that magnetic fields cause childhood leukemia[216] (see Chapter 14). Studies of magnetic field exposure from power lines and electric blankets in adults reveal little evidence of an association with leukemia, brain tumors, or breast cancer.[216]

Most exposure to EMF from occupational sources comes from near-field sources; the highest exposure to the general population comes from transmitters close to the body, such as hand-held devices like mobile telephones.[215] Epidemiologic evidence for an association between EMF and cancer has been derived from case-control, cohort, and time-trend studies. The most extensively studied exposure is from use of wireless telephones (mobile and cordless); other exposures include occupational settings and sources from the general environment[215] (also see Chapter 14). The one cohort study and five case-control studies judged by the WHO International Agency for Research on Cancer Monograph Working Group to offer potentially useful information about associations between wireless phones and glioma, with time-trend analyses, did not show an increased rate of brain tumors after the increase in mobile phone use. However, these studies had limitations because most of the analyses examined trends only in the early 2000s.[215] The INTERPHONE study,[220] a multicenter case-control study, is the largest study so far that studies the relationship between mobile phone use and brain tumors—glioma, acoustic neuroma, and meningioma. The pooled analyses included 2708 glioma cases and 2972 controls. The odds ratios (ORs) in terms of time spent on the phone showed that the highest time spent on the phone (>1640 hours of use) was related to glioma risk (OR 1.40; 95% confidence interval [CI] 1.03-1.89). There was a suggestion of increased risk of tumors on the same side of the head as the phone use (ipsilateral exposure) in the temporal lobe, where radiofrequency (RF) EMF exposure is highest.[215] The OR for glioma increased with increasing RF dose for exposure 7 years or more before diagnosis, and there was no association with estimated dose for exposure less than 7 years before diagnosis.[215] A Swedish investigative group performed a pooled analysis of two similar studies between the relationship of glioma, acoustic neuroma, and meningioma manifestation and mobile and cordless phone use.[221] Study participants who used a mobile phone for more than 1 year had an OR for glioma of 1.3 (95% CI 1.1-1.6). The OR increased with increasing time since first use and with total call time, 3.2 (2.0-5.1) for more than 2000 hours of use.[215] Ipsilateral use of the phone was associated with higher risk.[215] Similar findings were reported for cordless phones.[215] Although the INTERPHONE and Swedish studies were judged susceptible to bias, the Working Group concluded that the findings could not be dismissed because of bias alone and a causal relationship between phones and glioma is possible.[215] The Working Group concluded there is "limited evidence in humans" for the carcinogenicity of RF-EMF based on associations between glioma and acoustic neuroma and exposure to RF-EMF from wireless phones.[215] The Working Group reviewed animal studies and concluded there is "limited evidence" in experimental animals for the carcinogenicity of RF-EMF.[215]

The Working Group also reviewed numerous studies' endpoints relevant to mechanisms of carcinogenicity from RF-EMF.[215] The mechanisms included genotoxicity, effects on immune function, gene and protein expression, cell signaling, oxidative stress, and apoptosis. Additionally, studies on the possible effects of RF-EMF on the blood-brain barrier were analyzed. Overall, the Working Group reported there was evidence of RF-EMF on some of these endpoints, but they provided weak mechanistic evidence of RF-EMF–induced cancer in humans.[215] The outcome of the Working Group was to classify RF-EMF as "possibly carcinogenic to humans" (Group 2B).

There are no studies of adults who have used cell phones as children or adolescents. Concern is for children in whom the effects may be compounded because of increased vulnerability to radiation and their longer use of cell phones into adulthood. Ongoing unbiased research is desperately needed. Absolute proof of causation may be hindered because of the ethical questions of exposing individuals to potentially harmful interventions.[222] Chapter 14 discusses cancer in children.

Chemicals and Occupational Hazards as Carcinogens

An estimated 80,000 synthetic chemicals are used in the United States. Of those, only about 7% have been tested for their health effects.[223] It is disturbing that another 1000 are manufactured each year. Exposure to chemicals occurs every day—they are present in air, soil, food, water, household products, toys, personal care products, workplaces, and homes. The number of known carcinogens in experimental animals is large. It is suspected that most of these chemical carcinogens are potentially carcinogenic in humans but documentation is lacking. Table 13-1 provides a summary of the chemicals according to sufficient or limited evidence in humans by cancer site. Known and probable carcinogenic agents are updated by the International Agency for Research on Cancer (IARC). Chemical carcinogenesis involves the classical genotoxic mechanisms and exposure to genotoxic carcinogens might also involve a variety of nongenotoxic effects in cells.[224] Recently, a number of studies reported that the carcinogenic effects induced by several chemicals, including 2-acetylaminofluorene, tamoxifen, trichloroethylene, aflatoxin B_1, ochratoxin, nickel, and chromium, do not follow a classic genotoxic carcinogenesis model, but rather involve a spectrum of cellular alterations encompassing epigenetic alterations.[225] These epigenetically reprogrammed cells show an epigenetic profile similar to that frequently observed in cancer cells, including altered histone patterns, hypomethylation of DNA repetitive elements, alterations in proto-oncogenes, and hypermethylation of tumor-suppressor genes. Altered epigenetic status confers genome instability and loss of controlled growth signals, typically observed in cancer cells.[226]

A substantial percentage of cancers of the upper respiratory passages, lung, bladder, and peritoneum are attributed to occupational factors; however, fewer studies of nonsmokers exist.[227] One notable occupational factor is **asbestos,** which increases the risk of mesothelioma and lung cancer. Asbestos was used in homes and buildings built before the 1970s to insulate ceiling tiles, flooring, and pipe covers. In Western Europe, the epidemic of mesothelioma in building workers and other workers born after 1940 did not become apparent until the 1990s because of long latency. No exposure to asbestos is without risk and a large number of countries still use, export, and import asbestos-containing products (see Table 13-1).

Carcinoma of the bladder has been linked with the manufacture of dyes, rubber, paint, and aromatic amines, especially β-naphthylamine and benzidine. Benzol inhalation is linked to leukemia in shoemakers and in workers in the rubber cement, explosives, and dyeing industries. Other notable occupational hazards include heavy metals (e.g., high-nickel alloy, chromium VI compounds, inorganic arsenic), silica, polycyclic aromatic hydrocarbons, sulfuric acid, and chloromethyl ether. Studies of occupational exposure to diesel exhaust indicate an increased risk of lung cancer.[228] Disentangling data related to lung cancer, air pollution, and occupational risks is complex, especially in combination with active and passive smoking and the interplay of environmental factors and genetic polymorphisms at multiple loci.

Air Pollution

In the United States, two types of air pollution are most important and widespread: ozone and particle pollution.[229] Other important air pollutants include carbon monoxide, lead, nitrogen dioxide, sulfur dioxide, mercury, arsenic, benzene, formaldehyde, and acid gases.[229] Ozone is an extremely reactive gas molecule composed of three oxygen atoms. It is the main ingredient in smog air pollution. The ozone layer found in the upper atmosphere (the stratosphere) is called ozone (O_3), or good ozone, and protects life on earth by absorbing UV radiation emitted from the sun. The heavy use of propellants, such as aerosols, has decreased the size of the good ozone layer, leading to the banning of chlorofluorocarbons. The accumulating ozone at the lower atmospheric level or ground level is a toxic air pollutant. This ground-level ozone is a gas formed by reactions with nitrogen oxides, volatile organic compounds (VOCs), and sunlight. This gas mixture is emitted from motor vehicle exhausts and industrial emissions. Nasty combinations of mixtures cause damage (i.e., ROS and inflammation) to lung tissue, especially in people with preexisting lung diseases. These mixtures can also affect healthy people when combined with other air pollutants, such as sulfur dioxide. Sulfur dioxide is produced by power plants burning oil and coal, copper smelting, and paper mills. Fine or ultrafine particles, those less than 10 micrometers in diameter, are considered the most harmful. Fine or ultrafine particles are easily absorbed by the lungs and phagocytosed by macrophages and neutrophils that release tissue-damaging inflammatory mediators. Acute exposure to diesel exhaust that contains fine particles is linked to lung, throat, and eye irritations; asthma attacks; and myocardial ischemia.[230] Importantly, according to the WHO diesel exhaust is carcinogenic and causes lung cancer.[231] Long-term exposure to other sources of air pollution may cause lung cancer.[232] Evidence for cancers, other than lung cancer and childhood cancer, is inconsistent.[233]

Indoor pollution generally is considered worse than outdoor pollution, partly because of cigarette smoke. Environmental tobacco smoke (ETS; passive smoking) can cause the formation of reactive oxygen free radicals and thus DNA damage. The IARC has classified ETS as a human carcinogen. Another significant indoor air pollutant is radon gas. **Radon** is a natural radioactive gas derived from the radioactive decay of uranium that is ubiquitous in rock and soil; it can become trapped in houses and gives rise to radioactive decay products known to be carcinogenic to humans. The most hazardous houses can be identified by testing and then by being modified to prevent further radon contamination. Exposure levels are greater from underground mines than from houses. Most of the lung cancers associated with radon are bronchogenic; however, small cell carcinoma does occur with greater frequency in underground miners. Radon increases the risk of lung cancer in underground miners whether they smoke or not.

In China, some regions report very high levels of lung cancer in women who spend much of their time indoors. Exposures from heating and cooking combustion sources (e.g., oil vapors, volatile toxicants) are identified as risk factors for lung cancer.[234,235] In addition, domestic coal use and ETS increase the risk of lung cancer in women and men.[236]

Inorganic arsenic (known as a carcinogen since the late 1960s), found principally in underground water (from 1000 to 4000 mcg/L), is found in many regions of the world. According to the IARC, strong evidence indicates an increased risk of bladder, skin, and lung cancers following consumption of water with high levels of arsenic (generally greater than 200 mcg/L).[237] Evidence for cancers of the liver, colon, and kidney is weaker. Other sources of inorganic arsenic are related to occupational exposures.

The central hypothesis, based on rat studies, for the mechanisms related to particle-induced lung carcinogenesis is that insoluble particles cause pulmonary inflammation (e.g., cytokine release, ROS), which leads to oxidative stress and oxidation of DNA, proliferative response, and tissue remodeling progressing toward fibrosis and tumor development. Additional research is needed to understand the surface chemistry and lung tissue remodeling in relation to insoluble particles, lung carcinogenesis, and other respiratory problems.

SUMMARY REVIEW

Genes, Epigenetics, Tissue

1. Cancer arises from a complicated and an interacting web of multiple causes. Avoiding high-risk behaviors and exposures to individual carcinogens, or cancer-causing substances, will prevent many types of cancer.
2. Lifestyle behaviors, dietary choices, and environmental factors, such as exposure to ultraviolet radiation and occupational carcinogens, contribute to the number of cancer cases and deaths.
3. Investigators are connecting the intricate web between genotype, phenotype, high-risk lifestyle behaviors, the environment, and carcinogenesis. The root cause of cancer is more than inherited or acquired genetic mutations and involves epigenetic changes that frequently precede and induce cancer-causing genetic mutations.
4. Cancer development and progression involves the tissue microenvironment or stroma.
5. The microenvironment participates in a complex signaling process that facilitates tumor promotion and metastases because stromal tissue has immune cells. Chronic inflammation from infiltrating immune cells can be caused by numerous environmental factors, for example, inhaling tobacco smoke.

Incidence and Mortality Trends

1. Cancer is reported to become a major cause of morbidity and mortality in the coming decades in all regions of the world.
2. Overall, cancer incidence rates in the United States for all racial and ethnic groups combined decreased by 0.8% per year during the most recent study period, 2003 to 2007.
3. Death rates from the periods 1998 to 2007 and 2003 to 2007 continued to decrease for 7 of the top 15 cancer types in both men and women (colorectal, brain, stomach, and kidney cancers; non-Hodgkin lymphoma; leukemia; and myeloma). Decreasing death rates for men also included lung, prostate, and the oral cavity, and for women breast and bladder cancers. Death rates continued to increase for cancers of the liver and pancreas among men and women, uterine cancer in women, and melanoma of the skin in men.

In Utero and Early Life Conditions

1. Accumulating data suggest early life events influence later susceptibility to certain chronic conditions, including cancer.
2. Developmental plasticity is the degree to which an organism's development is contingent on its environment. It requires stable gene expression that in part appears to be modulated by epigenetic processes such as DNA methylation, histone modification, and microRNAs.
3. Epidemiologic and animal studies reveal that small changes in the developmental environment can alter phenotypic changes, resulting in individual responses in adulthood.

Tobacco Use

1. Cigarette smoking is carcinogenic and the most important cause of cancer. The risk is greatest in those who begin to smoke when young and continue throughout life.
2. Cigarette smoking accounts for one of every five deaths each year in the United States. Yet it is the single most preventable cause of death and disease.
3. In addition, smoking causes even more deaths from vascular, respiratory, and other diseases than from cancer.
4. Smoking tobacco is linked to cancers of the lung, lower urinary tract, upper aerodigestive tract, liver, kidney, pancreas, cervix, and uterus and to myeloid leukemia.
5. Environmental tobacco smoke (ETS) is the combination of sidestream and mainstream smoke.
6. More than 60 chemicals in tobacco smoke are considered carcinogenic. Nonsmokers who live with smokers are at greatest risk for lung cancer, as well as other noncancerous conditions. In utero effects from maternal or paternal smoking and subsequent disease are being investigated.
7. Cigar or pipe smoking is strongly and causally related to cancers of the oral cavity, oropharynx, hypopharynx, larynx, esophagus, lung, and possibly the pancreas. Bidi smoking can cause cancers of the respiratory and digestive tracts and also increase the risk of heart attacks and chronic bronchitis.

Diet

1. Dietary sources of carcinogenic substances include compounds produced in the cooking of fat, meat, or protein, and naturally occurring carcinogens associated with plant food substances, such as alkaloids or mold byproducts.
2. Research is ongoing to understand the complexity of nutrition and genomics, epigenomics, transcription factors (transcriptomics), proteomics, and metabolic factors (metabolomics) and the effect on cancer risk of modifying one or more of these factors.
3. Nutrition directly influences epigenetic factors that silence genes that should be active or activate genes that should be silent. The expression of microRNAs in response to diet may be involved in several cancers.
4. Dietary components can act directly as mutagens or interfere with the elimination of mutagens.
5. Dietary factors may affect the cell cycle, differentiation, DNA damage and repair, stem cell renewal, hormonal axes, the balance of cellular proliferation and cell death, the microenvironment, cell signaling, inflammation, and immunity.
6. Xenobiotics that include toxic, mutagenic, and carcinogenic chemicals are found in the human diet.
7. Food and nutrition modify carcinogen metabolism and include the examples selenium, allyl sulfur, sulforaphane, and isoflavonoids.
8. *N*-Nitroso compounds can increase nitrogenous residues in the colon and cause DNA damage.
9. Undernutrition can be a factor in cancers caused by infectious agents, for example, cancers of the liver and cervix.
10. Future research is needed to define robust biomarkers of cancer risk.

SUMMARY REVIEW—cont'd

Obesity

1. Obesity has been increasing in most developed countries and in urban areas of developing countries.
2. Childhood obesity has been increasing. There is considerable concern for children with early onset of obesity.
3. The substantial suffering and long-term human and societal costs of obesity underlie the urgency to accelerate progress in obesity prevention.
4. Studies have significantly improved the understanding of the relationship between overweight/obesity, energy balance and cancer risk, cancer recurrence, and survival.
5. Consensus now exists that obesity is a risk factor for cancers of the endometrium, colorectum, kidney, esophagus, breast (postmenopausal), and pancreas. Evidence is evolving of the association of obesity with cancers of the thyroid, gallbladder, liver, and ovary and also with aggressive types of prostate cancer and non-Hodgkin lymphoma.
6. Obesity is recognized as a poor prognostic factor for several cancers.
7. Overall, the putative mechanisms whereby obesity drives the progression of cancer are not completely known and the process is complex.
8. Earlier studies centered on mostly hormonal effects; however, research now includes other mechanisms whereby energy balance may affect (a) genomic instability, (b) dysregulated growth signaling and cellular energetics, (c) inhibition of apoptosis and immune surveillance, and (d) angiogenesis.
9. Numerous signaling pathways and factors are involved in the acceleration of carcinogenesis. Data now exist for several factors, including energy-driven signaling from insulin, insulin-like growth factor 1 (IGF-1), phosphatidylinositol 3-kinase, and AMP-activated protein kinase and many others.
10. Adipose tissue is a source of inflammatory modulators and increasing evidence indicates that obesity is causally linked to inflammation
11. Cancers have altered metabolism. Tumors consume large quantities of glucose to make cellular building blocks, called the Warburg Effect. Yet, some tumors do use oxidative stress as a weapon to extract recycled nutrients from cancer-associated fibroblasts in stromal tissue (Reverse Warburg Effect).
12. Food metabolism and circadian cycles are linked and impairment of inner clock regulation results in dysregulated metabolism.
13. Overall, there are strong data supporting alcohol as a cause of cancers of the mouth, pharynx, larynx, esophagus, liver, colorectum, and breast.

Infection, Sexual and Reproductive Behavior, Human Papillomaviruses

1. Infection is an important contributor to cancer worldwide and the population attributable fraction (PAF) was 16.1% of cancers diagnosed in 2008 were caused by infection, or about 2 million new cases.
2. Infection and cancer rates vary widely by region, with a 7.4% rate for more developed regions and 22.9% rate for less developed regions. The highest PAF is for sub-Saharan Africa with a rate of 32.7%.
3. The four top notable infections and new cancer cases include HPV, *Helicobacter pylori (H. pylori),* hepatitis B virus, and hepatitis C virus.
4. Hepatitis B and C can infect the liver and together account for the large majority of liver cancer diagnoses.
5. It has been estimated that *H. pylori* accounts for about 75% of all stomach cancers.
6. *High-risk,* or oncogenic, *HPVs* can cause cancer. High-risk types of HPV are required for the development of most cervical cancers. HPV types 16 and 18 cause the majority of cancers.
7. HPV types 16 and 18 also have been found to cause almost half of vaginal, vulvar, and penile cancers. Recently, HPV infections have been found to cause cancer of the oropharynx (soft palate, base of the tongue, tonsils).
8. Factors that may increase the risk of developing cancer following a high-risk HPV infection include smoking, decreased immunity, having many children (for increased risk of cervical cancer), long-term oral contraceptive use (for increased risk of cervical cancer), poor oral hygiene (for increased risk of oropharyngeal cancer), and chronic inflammation.
9. HPVs infect epithelial cells that cover the inside and outside surfaces of the body, including the skin, throat, genital tract, and anus.

Physical Activity

1. Physical activity reduces the risk for breast cancer, colon cancer, and endometrial cancer, independent of weight changes.
2. Biologic mechanisms for the protective effects of exercise include decreasing insulin and IGF levels, decreasing obesity, increasing free-radical scavenger systems, changing inflammatory mediators, decreasing the levels of circulating sex hormones and metabolic hormones, improving immune function, and enhancing cytochrome P-450 function, thus modifying carcinogen activation and increasing gut motility.
3. Several reports suggest that implementing a physical activity program after a cancer diagnosis is associated with better cancer-specific outcomes and overall survival with early-stage breast, prostate, and colorectal cancers.
4. Many unanswered questions remain regarding the frequency, intensity, and duration of exercise required for optimal health benefits.

Ionizing Radiation

1. Much of the knowledge of the effects of ionizing radiation (IR) on human cancer has stemmed from observations of the Hiroshima and Nagasaki atomic bomb exposures, particularly the Life Span Study. Other evidence is derived from groups exposed for medical reasons, underground miners exposed to radon gas, and other occupational exposures.

SUMMARY REVIEW—cont'd

2. The atomic bomb exposures in Japan caused acute leukemias in adults and children and increased frequencies of thyroid and breast carcinomas. Lung, stomach, colon, esophageal, and urinary tract cancers and multiple myeloma have been added to the list.
3. Recent models of radiation carcinogenesis show ionizing radiation (IR) acts not only as an initiator of premalignant cell clones but also as a promoter of preexisting premalignant cell alterations.
4. Health risks from IR involve cancers, cardiovascular diseases, respiratory diseases, birth defects, and eye maladies.
5. In 2009 the National Council on Radiation Protection and Measurements reported Americans were exposed to more than seven times as much IR from medical procedures compared to IR exposure in the 1980s.
6. Ionizing radiation is a mutagen and carcinogen and can penetrate cells and tissues and deposit energy in tissues at random in the form of ionizations.
7. The past two decades have focused on cellular and molecular mechanisms that relate to the induction of cancer, including dose-response relationships for chromosome aberrations and for cell transformation; gene expression (genetic and epigenetic); alternative targets, such as membranes; mutagenesis in somatic cells; the biologic effects that occur in nonirradiated cells (i.e., nontargeted effects); and effects on the microenvironment.
8. Because models and underlying assumptions of IR and cell damage are incomplete, investigators are working hard to understand induced repair, adaptive responses, hormesis, low-dose hypersensitivity, nontargeted effects, signaling, exosomes, and long-term persistence of radiation damage and clonal heterogeneity.
9. A long held assumption is that cellular alterations—mutations and malignant transformation—occur only in cells directly radiated. It is now known that radiation may induce a type of genomic instability to the progeny of the directly irradiated cells over many cell generations and can affect so-called innocent bystander cells.
10. Epigenetic events after radiation include alterations in pathways affecting cell adhesion, extracellular matrix interactions, and cell-to-cell communication.

Ultraviolet Radiation

1. Ultraviolet radiation (UVR) causes basal cell carcinoma and squamous cell carcinoma. The principal source of UVR is sunlight.
2. The degree of damage in skin depends on the intensity and wavelength content—ultraviolet A (UVA) or ultraviolet B (UVB).
3. UVR is known to cause specific gene mutations; for example, squamous cell carcinoma involves mutation in the TP53 gene, basal cell carcinoma in the patched gene, and melanoma in the p16 gene.
4. Skin exposure to UVR produces ROS in large quantities that can overwhelm tissue antioxidants and other oxygen-degrading pathways. Imbalances in ROS can lead to oxidative stress, tissue injury, and direct DNA damage.
5. ROS can induce a number of transcription factors (e.g., activator protein 1 [AP-1] and NF-κB) and increase the levels of regulating genes that induce inflammation. Inflammation is a critical component of tumor progression.
6. The incidence of melanoma in the United States has been increasing annually at a rate of about 2.8% from 1981 to 2008. Because mortality rates have not risen as rapidly, however, controversy exists as to whether the incidence increase is a true increase in clinically significant melanoma or is a result of overdiagnosis.
7. The relationship between sun exposure and the risk of melanoma remains complex.
8. Increased understanding of the intricate cellular interactions in melanoma will enhance knowledge of melanoma etiology and pathogenesis. This knowledge is essential for early detection and treatment.

Electromagnetic Radiation

1. Health risks associated with electromagnetic radiation (EMR) are controversial. Exposure to electric and magnetic fields is widespread. EMRs are a type of nonionizing and low-frequency radiation.
2. EMRs generated by radiofrequency sources couple with the body and result in induced electric and magnetic fields with associated currents inside tissue.
3. Microwaves, radar, mobile and cell phones, mobile phone base stations, appliances, power frequency radiation associated with electricity and radio waves, fluorescent lights, computers, and other electric equipment create EMRs of varying strength.
4. Data measuring the relationships between EMR exposure and cancer are limited because of inadequate methods to accurately measure exposure, lack of clear dose-response relationships and reproduction of effects, financial interests, and other priorities such as convenience.
5. Most exposure to EMFs from occupational sources comes from near-field sources; the highest exposure to the general population comes from transmitters close to the body, such as hand-held devices like mobile telephones.
6. The WHO International Agency for Research on Cancer Monograph Working Group reported that the INTERPHONE and Swedish studies were judged susceptible to bias, the findings could not be dismissed because of bias alone, and a causal relationship between phones and glioma is possible.
7. The outcome of the Working Group was to classify RF-EMF as "possibly carcinogenic to humans" (Group 2B). The mechanisms included genotoxicity, effects on immune function, gene and protein expression, cell signaling, oxidative stress, apoptosis, and, possibly, the blood-brain barrier.
8. There are no studies of adults who have used cell phones as children or adolescents. Concern is for children in whom the effects may be compounded because of increased vulnerability to radiation and their longer use of cell phones into adulthood.

SUMMARY REVIEW—cont'd

Chemicals and Occupational Hazards

1. An estimated 80,000 synthetic chemicals are used in the United States. Of those, only about 7% have been tested for their health effects and another 1000 are synthesized each year.
2. Chemicals are present in air, soil, food, water, personal care products, toys, household products, medications, workplaces, and homes.
3. Known and probable carcinogenic agents are updated by the International Agency for Research on Cancer (IARC).
4. The number of known carcinogens in experimental animals is large. It is suspected that most of these chemical carcinogens are potentially carcinogenic in humans but documentation is lacking.
5. Chemical carcinogenesis involves the classic genotoxic mechanisms, and exposure to genotoxic carcinogens also might involve a variety of nongenotoxic effects, including epigenetic alterations in cells.
6. A number of studies reported that the carcinogenic effects induced by several chemicals do not follow a classic genotoxic carcinogenesis model, but rather involve a spectrum of cellular alterations encompassing epigenetic alterations.
7. A substantial percentage of cancers of the upper respiratory passages, lung, bladder, and peritoneum are attributed to occupational factors; however, fewer studies of nonsmokers exist.
8. Disentangling data related to lung cancer, air pollution, and occupational factors is complex, especially in combination with active and passive smoking, environmental factors, and multiple interacting genes.

Air Pollution

1. In the United States, two types of air pollution are most important and widespread: ozone and particle pollution. Other important air pollutants include carbon monoxide, lead, nitrogen dioxide, sulfur dioxide, mercury, arsenic, benzene, formaldehyde, and acid gases.
2. Ozone is the main ingredient in smog air pollution.
3. Ground-level ozone is a gas formed by reactions with nitrogen oxides, volatile organic compounds (VOCs), and sunlight. This gas mixture is emitted from motor vehicle exhausts and industrial emissions.
4. Fine or ultrafine particles are easily absorbed by the lungs and phagocytosed by macrophages and neutrophils that release tissue-damaging inflammatory mediators.
5. The indoor air pollution environmental tobacco smoke (ETS; passive smoking) can cause the formation of reactive oxygen free radicals and thus DNA damage. The IARC has classified ETS as a human carcinogen.
6. Strong evidence indicates an increased risk of bladder, skin, and lung cancers following consumption of water with high levels of arsenic (generally greater than 200 mcg/L).

KEY TERMS

REFERENCES

1. Colditz GA, Wolin KY, Gehlert S: Applying what we know to accelerate cancer prevention, *Sci Transl Med* 4(127): 127rv4, 2012.
2. National Cancer Institute (NCI): *2008-2009 Annual Report President's Cancer Panel: Reducing environmental cancer risk. What we can do now*, Washington, DC, 2010, U.S. Department of Health and Human Services.
3. Parkin DM, Boyd L, Walker LC: The fraction of cancer attributable to lifestyle and environmental factors in the UK in 2010, *Br J Cancer* 105(Suppl 2):S77–S81, 2011.
4. Clapp RW et al: Environmental and occupational causes of cancer; new evidence 2005-2007, *Rev Environ Health* 23(1):1–37, 2008.
5. Clapp RW, Howe GK, Jacobs MM: Environmental and occupational causes of cancer: a call to act on what we know, *Biomed Pharmacother* 61(10):631–639, 2007.
6. National Cancer Institute (NCI): *Cancer and the environment: what you need to know, what you can do,* Washington, DC, 2004, U.S. Department of Health and Human Services. Available at www.nci.nih.gov/newscenter/benchmarks-vol4-issue3.
7. Cogliano VJ et al: Preventable exposures associated with cancers, *J Natl Cancer Inst* 103:1–13, 2011.
8. Institute of Medicine (IOM): *Rebuilding the unity of health and the environment: a new vision of environmental health for the 21st century. Workshop summary*, Washington, DC, 2001, National Academies Press.
9. National Toxicology Program: *Report on carcinogens*, ed 12, Washington, DC, 2011, U.S. Department of Health and Human Services.
10. McGuinn LA et al: Cancer and environment: definitions and misconceptions, *Environ Res* 112:230–234, 2012.
11. Kaiser J: Profile: Bert Vogelstein. Cancer genetics with an edge, *Science* 337(6092):282–284, 2012.
12. Vogelstein B, Kinzler KW: *The genetic basis of human cancer*, New York, 1998, McGraw-Hill.
13. Vineis P: A self-fulfilling prophecy: are we underestimating the role of the environment in gene–environment interaction research? *Int J Epidemiol* 33(5):945–946, 2004.
14. Vineis P: Individual susceptibility to carcinogens, *Oncogene* 23(38):6477–6483, 2004.
15. Esteller M: Epigenetics in cancer, *N Engl J Med* 358:1148–1159, 2008.
16. Feinberg AP, Tycko B: The history of cancer epigenetics, *Nat Rev Cancer* 4:143–153, 2004.
17. Herman JG, Baylin SB: Gene silencing in cancer in association with promoter hypermethylation, *N Engl J Med* 349:2042–2054, 2003.
18. Jones PA, Baylin SB: The epigenomics of cancer, *Cell* 128:683–692, 2007.

19. Chuang JC, Jones PA: Epigenetics and microRNAs, *Pediatr Res* 61(5 Pt 2):24R–29R, 2007.
20. Sasaki H, Matsui Y: Epigenetic events in mammalian germ-cell development: reprogramming and beyond, *Nat Rev Genet* 9(2):129–140, 2008.
21. Baylin SB, Ohm JE: Epigenetic gene silencing in cancer—a mechanism for early oncogenic pathway addiction, *Nat Rev Cancer* 6(2):107–116, 2006.
22. O'Hagan HM et al: Oxidative damage targets complexes containing DNA methyltransferases, SIRT1, and polycomb members to promoter CpG islands, *Cancer Cell* 20(5):606–619, 2011.
23. International Agency for Research on Cancer (IARC): *Special report: policy—a review of human carcinogens—part C: metals, arsenic, dusts, and fibres*, 2012. Available at http://monographs.iarc.fr/ENG/Monographs/vol100C/index.php. Accessed July 2012.
24. Straif K et al: A review of human carcinogens—part C: metals, arsenic, dusts, and fibres, *Lancet Oncol* 10(5):453–454, 2009.
25. Baylin SB, Jones PA: A decade of exploring the cancer epigenome—biological and translational implications, *Nat Rev Cancer* 11(10):726–734, 2011.
26. Herman JG et al: Silencing of the VHL tumor-suppressor gene by DNA methylation in renal carcinoma, *Proc Natl Acad Sci U S A* 91:9700–9704, 1994.
27. Koizumi K et al: Array-based identification of common DNA methylation alterations in ulcerative colitis, *Int J Oncol* 40(4):983–994, 2012.
28. Pozza A et al: Colonic carcinogenesis in IBD: molecular events, *Ann Ital Chir* 82(1):19–28, 2011.
29. Ullman TA, Itzkowitz SH: Intestinal inflammation and cancer, *Gastroenterology* 140(6):1807–1816, 2011.
30. Bray F et al: Global cancer transitions according to the Human Development Index (2008-2030): a population-based study, *Lancet Oncol* 13(8):790–801, 2012.
31. Kohler BA et al: Annual report to the nation on the status of cancer, 1975-2007, featuring tumors of the brain and other nervous system, *J Natl Cancer Inst* 103(9):1–23, 2011.
32. Gluckman PD et al: Effect of in utero and early-life conditions on adult health and disease, *N Engl J Med* 359(1):61–73, 2008.
33. Koukoura O, Sifakis S, Spandidos D: DNA methylation in the human placenta and fetal growth, *Mol Med Rep* 5:883–889, 2012.
34. Turner BM: Epigenetic responses to environmental change and their evolutionary implications, *Philos Trans R Soc Lond B Biol Sci* 364(1524):3403–3418, 2009.
35. Duncan S: Teratogenesis of sodium valproate, *Curr Opin Neurol* 20:175–180, 2007.
36. Disney ER et al: Strengthening the case: prenatal alcohol exposure is associated with increased risk for conduct disorder, *Pediatrics* 122(6):e1225–e1230, 2008.
37. Chiaffarino F et al: Alcohol drinking and risk of small for gestational age birth, *Eur J Clin Nutr* 60:1062–1066, 2006.
38. Rubin MM: Antenatal exposure to DES: lesions learned…future concerns, *Obstet Gynecol Surv* 62(8):548–555, 2007.
39. Triosi R, Potischman N, Hoover RN: Exploring the underlying hormonal mechanisms of prenatal risk factors for breast cancer: a review and commentary, *Cancer Epidemiol Biomarkers Prev* 16(9):1700–1712, 2007.
40. Palmer JR et al: Prenatal diethylstilbestrol exposure and risk of breast cancer, *Cancer Epidemiol Biomarkers Prev* 15(8):1509–1514, 2006.
41. McLachlan JA: Commentary: prenatal exposure to diethylstilbestrol (DES): a continuing story, *Int J Epidemiol* 35(4):868–870, 2006.
42. Newbold RR et al: Proliferative lesions and reproductive tract tumors in male descendents of mice exposed developmentally to diethylstilbestrol, *Carcinogenesis* 21:1355–1363, 2000.
43. Petridou E et al: Baldness and other correlates of sex hormones in relation to testicular cancer, *Int J Cancer* 71(6):982–985, 1997.
44. Strohsnitter WC et al: Cancer risk in men exposed in utero to diethylstilbestrol, *J Natl Cancer Inst* 93(7):545–551, 2001.
45. Waterland RA, Jirtle RL: Transposable elements: targets for early nutritional effects on epigenetic gene regulation, *Mol Cell Biol* 23:5293–5300, 2003.
46. American Cancer Society (ACS): Tobacco-related cancers fact sheet. In American Cancer Society, editor: *Cancer facts and figures, 2012*, Atlanta, 2012, Author.
47. Centers for Disease Control and Prevention (CDC): *Smoking and secondhand smoke.* Available at www.cancer.gov/cancer/lung. Accessed July 2010.
48. Jemal A et al: Cancer statistics, 2009, *CA Cancer J Clin* 59:225–249, 2009.
49. Mackay J et al: *The cancer atlas*, Atlanta, 2006, American Cancer Society.
50. International Agency for Research on Cancer (IARC): *GLOBOCAN: cancer incidence, mortality and prevalence worldwide in 2008*, Lyon, France, 2010, Author.
51. Centers for Disease Control and Prevention (CDC): Cigarette smoking—attributable morbidity—United States, 2000, *MMWR Morb Mortal Wkly Rep* 52(35):842–844, 2003.
52. Centers for Disease Control and Prevention (CDC): *Early release of selected estimates based on data from the 2011 National Health Interview Survey*. Available at www.cdc.gov/nchs/nhis/releases.htm. Accessed June 2012.
53. Luo J et al: Association of active and passive smoking with risk of breast cancer among postmenopausal women: a prospective cohort study, *BMJ* 342:d1016, 2011.
54. Collishaw NE et al: Canadian expert panel on tobacco smoke and breast cancer risk. *Ontario Tobacco Research Unit (OTRU): Special report series*, Toronto, Ontario, April 2009, Canada.
55. Centers for Disease Control and Prevention: *Smoking and tobacco use, fact sheet*, September 2006. Available at www.cdc.gov/tobacco/data_statistics/factsheets/secondhandsmoke.htm.
56. National Cancer Institute: *Secondhand smoke: questions and answers*, 2005. Available at www.cancer.gov/cancertopics/factsheet/tobacco/ETS. Accessed July 2008.
57. Centers for Disease Control and Prevention (CDC): *CDC's Tobacco Laboratory, Division of Laboratory Sciences, National Center for Environmental Health 2008-2009: Smoking and tobacco use*, Atlanta, 2012, Author.
58. Demirhan O et al: The genotoxic effect of nicotine on chromosomes of human fetal cells: the first report described as an important study, *Inhal Toxicol* 23(11):829–834, 2011.
59. Prins JR et al: Smoking during pregnancy influences the maternal immune response in mice and humans, *Am J Obstet Gynecol* 207(1):76e1–76e14, 2012.
60. American Cancer Society (ACS): *Cancer facts and figures, 2012*, Atlanta, 2012, Author.
61. American Cancer Society: *What are the health effects of smoking pipes or cigars?* Atlanta, 2011, Author.
62. American Cancer Society: *What about exotic forms of smoking tobacco, such as clove cigarettes, bidis, and hookahs?* Atlanta, 2011, Author.
63. Ma YT et al: Smoking initiation is followed by the early acquisition of epigenetic change in cervical epithelium: a longitudinal study, *BMJ* 104(9):1500–1504, 2011.
64. World Cancer Research Fund/American Institute for Cancer Research (WCRF/AICR): *Second expert report: food, nutrition, physical activity, and the prevention of cancer: a global perspective*, London, 2007, Author.
65. Mathers JC, Strathdee G, Relton CL: Induction of epigenetic alterations by dietary and other environmental factors, *Adv Genet* 71:3–39, 2010.
66. Choi S-W, Corrocher R, Friso S: Nutrients and DNA methylation. In Choi S-W, Frisco S, editors: *Nutrients and epigenetics*, Boca Raton, FL, 2009, CRC Press Taylor & Francis Group, pp 105–126.
67. Steegers-Theunissen RP et al: Periconceptional maternal folic acid use of 4000 microg per day is related to increased methylation of the IGF2 gene in the very young child, *PLoS One* 4(11):e7845, 2009.
68. Kovacheva VP et al: Gestational choline deficiency causes global and Igf2 gene DNA hypermethylation by up-regulation of Dnmt1 expression, *J Biol Chem* 282(43):31777–31788, 2007.
69. Kim YI et al: Folate deficiency in rats induces DNA strand breaks and hypomethylation within the p53 tumor suppressor gene, *Am J Clin Nutr* 65(1):46–52, 1997.
70. Lee WJ, Shim JY, Zhu BT: Mechanisms for the inhibition of DNA methyltransferases by tea catechins and bioflavonoids, *Mol Pharmacol* 68(4):1018–1030, 2005.
71. Delage B, Dashwood RH: Dietary manipulation of histone structure and function, *Annu Rev Nutr* 28:347–366, 2008.
72. Baur JA, Sinclair DA: Therapeutic potential of resveratrol: the in vivo evidence, *Nat Rev Drug Discov* 5(6):493–506, 2006.
73. Kim YS et al: Cancer stem cells: potential target for bioactive food components, *J Nutr Biochem* 23:691–698, 2012.
74. O'Brien LE et al: Altered modes of stem cell division drive adaptive intestinal growth, *Cell* 147:603–614, 2011.
75. Ginestier C et al: Retinoid signaling regulates breast cancer stem cell differentiation, *Cell Cycle* 8:3297–3302, 2009.
76. Gonzalez C et al: Hydrogen peroxide-induced DNA damage and DNA repair in lymphocytes from malnourished children? *Environ Mol Mutagen* 39:33–42, 2002.

77. Arab L, Steck-Scott S, Fleishauer AT: Lycopene and the lung, *Exp Biol Med (Maywood)* 227:894–899, 2002.
78. Omiecinski CJ et al: Xenobiotic metabolism, disposition, and regulation by receptors: from biochemical phenomenon to predictors of major toxicities, *Toxicol Sci* 120(Suppl 1):S49–S75, 2011.
79. Yang G et al: Isothiocyanate exposure, glutathione S-transferase polymorphisms, and colon cancer risk, *Am J Nutr* 91(3):704–711, 2010.
80. Eicholzer M et al: Polymorphisms in heterocyclic aromatic amines metabolism-related genes are associated with colorectal adenoma risk, *Int J Mol Epidemiol Genet* 3(2):96–106, 2012.
81. Norat T et al: Meat, fish, and colorectal cancer risk: the European prospective investigation into cancer and nutrition [see comment], *J Natl Cancer Inst* 97(12):906–916, 2005.
82. zur Hausen H: Red meat consumption and cancer: reasons to suspect involvement of bovine infectious factors in colorectal cancer, *Int J Cancer* 130(11):2475–2483, 2012.
83. Feinberg AP, Ohlsson R, Henikoff S: The epigenetic progenitor origin of human cancer, *Nat Rev Genet* 7(1):21–33, 2006.
84. Glickman D et al: *Accelerating progress in obesity prevention: solving the weight of the nation*, Washington, DC, 2012, The National Academies Press.
85. Demark-Wahnefried W et al: The role of obesity in cancer survival and recurrence, *Cancer Epidemiol Biomarkers Prev*, 2012. [Epub ahead of print.].
86. Haslam D: Obesity: a medical history, *Obes Rev* 8(Suppl 1):31–36, 2007.
87. International Agency for Research on Cancer (IARC): *Handbook of cancer prevention, vol 6: weight control and physical activity*, Lyon, France, 2002, Author.
88. Cao Y, Ma J: Body mass index, prostate cancer-specific mortality, and biochemical recurrence: a systematic review and meta-analysis, *Cancer Prev Res (Phila)* 4:486–501, 2011.
89. Ewertz M et al: Effect of obesity on prognosis after early-stage breast cancer, *J Clin Oncol* 29:25–31, 2011.
90. Sinicrope FA et al: Obesity is an independent prognostic variable in colon cancer survivors, *Clin Cancer Res* 16:1884–1893, 2010.
91. Flegal KM et al: Prevalence of obesity and trends in the distribution of body mass index among US adults, 1999-2010, *JAMA* 307(5):491–497, 2012.
92. World Health Organization (WHO): *Global strategy on diet, physical activity, and health (online)*, 2004. Available at www.who.int/dietphysical activity/strategy/eb11344/en/.
93. World Health Organization (WHO): *Obesity and overweight fact sheet n311*, February 2011. Available at www.who.int/mediacentre/factsheets/fs311/en/.
94. Institute of Medicine (IOM): *The role of obesity in cancer survival and recurrence: workshop summary*, Washington, DC, 2012, The National Academies Press.
95. Patel AV et al: IGF-1, IGFBP-1, and IGFBP-3 polymorphisms predict circulating IGF levels but not breast cancer risk: findings from the Breast and Prostate Cancer Cohort Consortium (BPC3), *PLoS One* 3(7):e2578, 2008.
96. Price AJ et al: Insulin-like growth factor-1 concentration and risk of prostate cancer: results from the European Prospective Investigation into Cancer and Nutrition, *Cancer Epidemiol Biomarkers Prev*, July 2012. [Epub ahead of print.].
97. Calle EE, Kaaks R: Overweight, obesity and cancer: epidemiological evidence and proposed mechanisms, *Nat Rev Cancer* 4(8):579–591, 2004.
98. Duggan C et al: Associations of insulin resistance and adiponectin and mortality in women with breast cancer, *J Clin Oncol* 29:32–39, 2011.
99. Goodwin PJ et al: Fasting insulin and outcome in early-stage breast cancer: results of a prospective cohort study, *J Clin Oncol* 20:42–51, 2002.
100. Law JH et al: Phosphorylated insulin-like growth factor-insulin receptor is present in all breast cancer subtypes and is related to poor survival, *Cancer Res* 68:10238–10246, 2008.
101. Wolpin BM et al: Insulin, the insulin-like growth factor axis, and mortality in patients with nonmetastatic colorectal cancer, *J Clin Oncol* 27:176–185, 2009.
102. Luo J et al: Diabetes and lung cancer among postmenopausal women, *Diabetes Care* 35(7):1485–1491, 2012.
103. Luo J et al: Diabetes mellitus as a risk for gastrointestinal cancers among postmenopausal women, *Cancer Causes Control*, May 2012. [Epub ahead of print.].
104. Yuhara H et al: Is diabetes mellitus an independent risk factor for colon cancer and rectal cancer? *Am J Gastroenterol* 106(11):1911–1921, 2011.
105. Protani MW, Nagle CM, Webb PM: Obesity and ovarian cancer survival: a systematic review and meta-analysis, *Cancer Prev Res (Phila)*, 2012. [Epub ahead of print.].
106. Calle EE et al: Overweight, obesity, and mortality from cancer in a prospectively studies cohort of U.S. adults, *N Engl J Med* 348:1625–1638, 2003.
107. Ouchi N et al: Adipokines in inflammation and metabolic disease, *Nat Rev Immunol* 11:85–97, 2011.
108. Hotamisligil GS: Inflammation and metabolic disorders, *Nature* 444:860–867, 2006.
109. Shoelson SE, Lee J, Goldfine AB: Inflammation and insulin resistance, *J Clin Invest* 116:1793–1801, 2006.
110. Vander Heiden MG, Cantley LC: Thompson CB: Understanding the Warburg Effect: the metabolic requirements of cell proliferation, *Science* 324(5930):1029–1033, 2009.
111. Wellen KE, Thompson CB: A two-way street: reciprocal regulation of metabolism and signaling, *Nat Rev Mol Cell Biol* 13:270–276, 2012.
112. Diaz-Ruiz R et al: Tumor cell energy metabolism and its common features with yeast metabolism, *Biochim Biophys Acta* 1796:252–265, 2009.
113. Asher G, Schibler U: Crosstalk between components of circadian and metabolic cycles in mammals, *Cell Metab* 13:125–137, 2011.
114. Reddy AB, O'Neill JS: Health clocks, healthy body, healthy mind, *Trends Cell Biol* 20(1):36–44, 2010.
115. Sahar S, Sassone-Corsi P: Regulation of metabolism: the circadian clock dictates the time, *Trends Endocrinol Metab* 23(1):1–8, 2011.
116. American Cancer Society (ACS): *Cancer treatment and survivorship facts & figures 2012-2013*, Atlanta, 2012, Author.
117. Sauer J et al: Ageing, chronic alcohol consumption and folate are determinants of genomic DNA methylation, p16 promoter methylation and the expression of p16 in mouse colon, *Br J Nutr* 104:24–30, 2010.
118. Hernandez-Vargas H et al: Hepatocellular carcinoma displays distinct DNA methylation signatures with potential as clinical predictors, *PLoS One* 5(3):e9749, 2010.
119. Toh Y et al: Alcohol drinking, cigarette smoking, and the development of squamous cell carcinoma of the esophagus: molecular mechanisms of carcinogenesis, *Int J Clin Oncol* 15:135–144, 2010.
120. Avissar M et al: Micro RNA expression in head and neck cancer associates with alcohol consumption and survival, *Carcinogenesis* 30:2059–2063, 2009.
121. Chang JS, Strif K, Guha N: The role of alcohol dehydrogenase genes in head and neck cancers: a systematic review and meta-analysis of ADH1B and ADH1C, *Mutagenesis* 27(3):275–286, 2012.
122. Choi YJ et al: Association between global DNA hypomethylation in leukocytes and risk of breast cancer, *Carcinogenesis* 30:1889–1897, 2009.
123. Friendenreich C et al: Physical activity and risk of colon and rectal cancers: the European perspective investigation into cancer and nutrition, *Cancer Epidemiol Biomarkers Prev* 15:2398–2407, 2006.
124. Slattery ML et al: Physical activity and colorectal cancer, *Am J Epidemiol* 158:214–224, 2003.
125. Parkin DM: Cancers attributable to inadequate physical exercise in the UK in 2010, *Br J Cancer* 105:S38–S41, 2011.
126. Voskuil DW et al: Task force physical activity and cancer. Physical activity and endometrial cancer risk, a systematic review of current evidence, *Cancer Epidemiol Biomarkers Prev* 16:639–648, 2007.
127. McTiernan A: Mechanisms linking physical activity with cancer, *Nat Rev Cancer* 8(3):205–211, 2008.
128. Rogers CJ et al: Physical activity and cancer prevention: pathways and targets for intervention, *Sports Med* 38(4):271–296, 2008.
129. Slattery ML: Physical activity and colorectal cancer, *Sports Med* 34(4):239–252, 2004.
130. McTiernan A et al: Physical activity and cancer etiology: associations and mechanisms, *Cancer Causes Control* 9(5):487–509, 1998, review.
131. McTiernan A et al: Effect of exercise on serum estrogens in postmenopausal women: a 12-month randomized clinical trial, *Cancer Res* 64(8):2923–2928, 2004.
132. Calle EE et al: Diabetes mellitus and pancreatic cancer mortality in a prospective cohort of United States adults, *Cancer Causes Control* 9(4):403–410, 1998.
133. Lee IM: Physical activity and cancer prevention…data from epidemiologic studies, *Med Sci Sports Exerc* 35(11):1823–1827, 2003.
134. McTiernan A et al: Exercise effect on weight and body fat in men and women, *Obesity* 15(6):1496–1512, 2007.
135. de Martel C et al: Global burden of cancers attributable to infections in 2008: a review and synthetic analysis, *Lancet Oncol* 13(6):607–615, 2012.

136. Dart H, Wolin KY, Colditz GA: Commentary: eight ways to prevent cancer: a framework for effective prevention messages for the public, *Cancer Causes Control* 23(4):601–608, 2012.
137. Centers for Disease Control and Prevention (CDC): *Human papillomavirus (HPV)*, Atlanta, 2012, Author.
138. National Cancer Institute (NCI): *HPV and cancer*, Washington, DC, 2012, Author.
139. Bosch FX, de Sanjose S: Human papillomavirus and cervical cancer—burden and assessment of causality, *J Natl Cancer Inst Monogr* 31:3–13, 2003.
140. Muñoz N et al: Against which human papillomavirus types shall we vaccinate and screen? The international perspective, *Int J Cancer* 111(2):278–285, 2004.
141. Schiffman M et al: Human papillomavirus and cervical cancer, *Lancet* 370(9590):890–907, 2007.
142. Watson M et al: Using population-based cancer registry data to assess the burden of human papillomavirus-associated cancers in the United States: overview of methods, *Cancer* 113(Suppl 10):2841–2854, 2008.
143. Jayaprakash V et al: Human papillomavirus types 16 and 18 in epithelial dysplasia of oral cavity and oropharynx: a meta-analysis, 1985-2010, *Oral Oncol* 47(11):1048–1054, 2011.
144. Chaturvedi AK et al: Human papillomavirus and rising oropharyngeal cancer incidence in the United States, *J Clin Oncol* 29(32):4294–4301, 2011.
145. Heidenreich WF et al: Promoting action of radiation in the atomic bomb survivor carcinogenesis data? *Radiat Res* 168(6):750–756, 2007.
146. Little MP: Heterogeneity of variation of relative risk by age at exposure in the Japanese atomic bomb survivors, *Radiat Environ Biophys* 48(3):253–262, 2009.
147. Shuryak I et al: A new view of radiation-induced cancer: integrating short- and long-processes. Part l: Approach, *Radiat Environ Biophys* 48(3):263–274, 2009.
148. Shuryak I, Sachs RK, Brenner DJ: Cancer risks after radiation exposure in middle age, *J Natl Cancer Inst* 102(21):1606–1609, 2010.
149. Preston DL et al: Solid cancer incidence in atomic bomb survivors: 1958-1998, *Radiat Res* 168(1):1–64, 2007.
150. Committee on the Biological Effects of Ionizing Radiation: *Health risks from exposure to low levels of ionizing radiation, BEIR VII Phase 2, Washington, DC*, 2006, National Academies Press.
151. Walsh L: Heterogeneity of variation of relative risk by age at exposure in Japanese atomic bomb survivors, *Radiat Environ Biophys* 48(3):345–347, 2009.
152. Committee on the Biological Effects of Ionizing Radiation: *Health risks from exposure to low levels of ionizing radiation, BEIR VII Phase 2*, Washington, DC, 2006, National Academies Press.
153. Preston DL et al: Studies of mortality of atomic bomb survivors. Report 13: solid cancer and noncancer disease mortality: 1950-1997, *Radiat Res* 160:381–407, 2003.
154. Hoel DG: Ionizing radiation and cardiovascular disease, *Ann N Y Acad Sci* 1076:309–317, 2006.
154a. Rombouts C et al: Differential response to acute low dose radiation in primary and immortalized endothelial cells, *Int J Radiat Biol*, June 21, 2013. doi:10.3109/09553002.2013.806831.
155. Yusuf SW, Sami S, Daher IN: Radiation-induced heart disease: a clinical update, *Cardiol Res Pract* 317659:2011, 2011.
156. National Council on Radiation Protection & Measurements (NCRP): *1929-2009: Medical radiation exposure of the U.S. population greatly increased since the early 1980s*, Bethesda, Md, March 2009, Author.
157. U.S. Nuclear Regulatory Commission: *NRC regulations (10 CFR) part 20: standards for protection against radiation: subpart C—occupational dose limits.* Available at www.nrc.gov/reading-rm/doc-collections/cfr/part020 /part020–1201.html. Accessed September 27, 2011.
158. Smith-Bendman R et al: Use of diagnostic imaging studies and associated radiation exposure for patients enrolled in large integrated health care system, 1996-2010, *JAMA* 307(22):2400–2409, 2012.
159. Studdert DM et al: Defensive medicine among high-risk specialist physicians in a volatile malpractice environment, *JAMA* 293(21):2609–2617, 2005.
160. Jones JA, Casey RC, Karouia F: Ionizing radiation as a carcinogen. In McQueen CA, editor: *Comprehensive toxicology*, ed 2, St Louis, 2010, Elsevier.
161. Lubin JH et al: Lung cancer in radon-exposed miners and estimation of risk from indoor exposure, *J Natl Cancer Inst* 87(11):817–827, 1995.
162. Ernestos B et al: Increased chromosomal radiosensitivity in women carrying BRCA1/BRCA2 mutations assessed with the G2 assay, *Int J Oncol Biol Phys* 76(4):1199–1205, 2010.
163. Dalrymple GV et al: A review of the USAF/NASA proton bioeffects project: rationale and acute effects, *Radiat Res* 126(2):117–119, 1991.
164. United Nations Scientific Committee on the Effects of Atomic Radiation (UNSCEAR): *Report to the general assembly, with scientific annexes*, New York, 1993, Author.
165. United Nations Scientific Committee on the Effects of Atomic Radiation (UNSCEAR): *Sources and effects of ionizing radiation. Report to the general assembly with scientific annexes B exposure from natural radiation sources 9*, New York, 1998, Author.
166. Committee on the Biological Effects of Ionizing Radiation: *Health risks from exposure to low levels of ionizing radiation, BEIR VII Phase 2*, Washington, DC, 2006, The National Academies Press.
167. Little JB: Radiation carcinogenesis, *Carcinogenesis* 21(3):397–404, 2000.
168. Mothersill C, Seymour C: *Changing paradigms in radiobiology* 750(2):85–95, 2012.
169. Little JB: Cellular radiation effects and the bystander response, *Mutat Res* 597:113–118, 2006.
170. Barcellos-Hoff MH: Integrative radiation carcinogenesis: interactions between cell and tissue responses to DNA damage, *Semin Cancer Biol* 15:138–148, 2005.
171. Kovalchuk O, Baulch JE: Epigenetic changes and nontargeted radiation effects—is there a link? *Environ Mol Mutagen* 49(1):16–25, 2008.
172. Sowa M et al: Effects of ionizing radiation on cellular structures, induced instability and carcinogenesis, *EXS* 96:293–301, 2006.
173. Foray N et al: Repair of radiation-induced DNA double-strand breaks in human fibroblasts is consistent with a continuous spectrum of repair probability, *Int J Radiat Biol* 74(5):551–560, 1998.
174. Milligan JR et al: DNA repair by thiols in air shows two radicals make a double-strand break, *Radiat Res* 143(3):273–280, 1995.
175. Ward JF: DNA damage produced by ionizing radiation in mammalian cells: identities, mechanisms of formation, and repairability, *Prog Nucl Acid Res Mol Biol* 35:95–125, 1988.
176. Jeggo PA, Lobrich M: Contribution of DNA repair and cell cycle checkpoint arrest to the maintenance of genomic stability, *DNA Repair (Amst)* 5:1192–1198, 2006.
177. Pellegrini L et al: Insights into DNA recombination from the structure of a RAD51-BRCA2 complex, *Nature* 420:287–293, 2002.
178. Tutt A, Ashworth A: The relationship between the roles of BRCA genes in DNA repair and cancer predisposition, *Trends Mol Med* 8:571–576, 2002.
179. Hei TK et al: Radiation induced non-targeted response: mechanism and potential clinical implications, *Curr Mol Pharmacol* 4:96–105, 2011.
180. Ciccia A, Elledge SJ: The DNA damage response: making it safe to play with knives, *Mol Cell* 40:179–204, 2010.
181. Giglia-Mari G, Zotter A, Vermeulen W: DNA damage response, *Cold Spring Harb Perspect Biol* 3(1), 2011.
182. Soria G, Polo SE, Almouzni G: Prime, repair, restore: the active role of chromatin in the DNA response, *Mol Cell* 46(6):722–734, 2012.
183. Belyako OV et al: Biological effects in unirradiated human tissue induced by radiation damage up to 1 mm away, *Proc Natl Acad Sci U S A* 102:14203–14208, 2005.
184. Bertucci A et al: Microbeam irradiation of the *C. elegans* nematode, *J Radiat Res* 50:A49–A54, 2009.
185. Amundson S et al: Fluorescent cDNA microarray hybridization reveals complexity and heterogeneity of cellular genotoxic stress responses, *Oncogene* 18:3666–3672, 1999.
186. Mancuso M et al: Oncogeneic bystander radiation effects in patched heterozygous mouse cerebellum, *Proc Natl Acad Sci U S A* 105(34):12445–12450, 2008.
187. Nguyen DH et al: Radiation acts on the microenvironment to affect breast carcinogenesis by distinct mechanisms that decrease cancer latency and affect tumor type, *Cancer Cell* 19:640–651, 2011.
188. Ojima M et al: Persistence of DNA double-strand breaks in normal human cells induced by radiation-induced bystander effect, *Radiat Res* 175:90–96, 2011.
189. Chute JP: To survive radiation injury, remember you're a PCs, *Nat Med* 18(7):1013–1014, 2012.
190. Barcellos-Hoff MH, Nguyen DH: Radiation carcinogenesis in context: how do irradiated tissues become tumors? *Health Phys* 97(5):446–457, 2009.
191. Wright EG: Manifestations and mechanisms of non-targeted effects of ionizing radiation, *Mutat Res* 687(1-2):28–33, 2010.
192. Barrington de Gonzalez A et al: Proportion of second cancers attributable to radiotherapy treatment in adults: a prospective cohort study in the US SEER cancer registries, *Lancet Oncol* 12(4):353–360, 2011.

193. Nakashima M et al: Foci formation of P53-binding protein 1 in thyroid tumors: activation of genomic instability during thyroid carcinogenesis, *Int J Cancer* 122(5):1082–1088, 2008.
194. Parkin DM, Darby SC: Cancers in 2010 attributable to ionising radiation exposure in the UK, *Br J Cancer* 105:S57–S65, 2011.
195. Brooks AL: Paradigm shifts in radiation biology: their impact on intervention for radiation-induced disease, *Radiat Res* 164(4 Pt 2):454–461, 2005.
196. Brenner DJ: We don't know enough about low-dose radiation risk, *Nature News*, 2011. doi:10.1038/news.2011.206.
197. Cleaver JE, Crowley E: UV damage, DNA repair, and skin carcinogenesis, *Front Biosci* 7:d1024–d1043, 2002.
198. Streilein JW et al: Immune surveillance and sunlight-induced skin cancer, *Immunol Today* 15(4):174–179, 1994.
199. Bickers DR, Ather M: Oxidative stress in the pathogenesis of skin disease, *J Invest Dermatol* 126:2562–2575, 2006.
200. Bickers DR, Ather M: Oxidative stress in the pathogenesis of skin disease, *J Invest Dermatol* 126:2562–2575, 2006.
201. Streilein JW et al: Immune surveillance and sunlight-induced skin cancer, *Immunol Today* 15(4):174–179, 1994.
202. Dhar A, Young MR, Colburn NH: The role of AP-1, NF-kappaB, and ROS/NOS in skin carcinogenesis: the JB6 model is predictive, *Mol Cell Biochem* 234(1-2):185–193, 2002.
203. Howlader N et al: *SEER cancer statistics review, 1975-2008*, Bethesda, Md, 2011, National Cancer Institute.
204. Welch HG, Black WC: Overdiagnosis in cancer, *J Natl Cancer Inst* 102:605–613, 2010.
205. Glusac EJ: The melanoma "epidemic": lessons from prostate cancer, *J Cutan Pathol* 39(1):17–20, 2012.
206. Wu X-C et al: Racial and ethnic variations in incidence and survival of cutaneous melanoma in the United States, 1999-2006, *J Am Acad Dermatol* 65(5):S26–S37, 2011.
207. Little EG, Eide MJ: Update on the current state of melanoma incidence, *Dermatol Clin* 30(3):355–361, 2012.
208. Reyes-Ortiz CA, Goodwin JS, Freeman JL: The effect of socioeconomic factors on incidence, stage at diagnosis and survival of cutaneous melanoma, *Med Sci Monit* 11(5):RA163–RA172, 2005.
209. Fernandez AA et al: Recent advances in sunlight-induced carcinogenesis using the *Xiphophorus* melanoma model, *Comp Biochem Physiol C Toxicol Pharmacol* 155(1):64–70, 2012.
210. Heymann WR: Screening for melanoma, *J Am Acad Dermatol* 56(1):144–145, 2007.
211. Sekulic A et al: Malignant melanoma in the 21st century: the emerging molecular landscape, *Mayo Clin Proc* 83(7): 825–846, 2008.
212. Berking C et al: Basic fibroblast growth factor and ultraviolet B transform melanocytes in human skin, *Am J Pathol* 158(3):943–953, 1998.
213. Pleasance ED et al: A comprehensive catalogue of somatic mutations from a human cancer genome, *Nature* 463:191–196, 2010.
214. Wang H-T, Choi B, Tang M- S: Melanocyte are deficient in repair of oxidative DNA damage and UV-induced photoproducts, *Proc Natl Acad Sci U S A* 107:12180–12185, 2010.
215. Baan R et al: Carcinogenicity of radiofrequency electromagnetic fields, *Lancet Oncol* 12(7):624–626, 2011.
216. National Cancer Institute (NCI): *Fact sheet: magnetic field exposure and cancer*, Washington, DC, 2005, National Institutes of Health, National Cancer Institute. Available at www.cancer.gov/cancertopics/factsheet/Risk/magnetic-fields. Accessed July 2012.
217. Belyaev IY: Dependence of non-thermal biological effects of microwaves on physical and biological variables: implications for reproducibility and safety standards, *Eur J Oncol Library* 5:187–219, 2010.
218. Genuis SJ: Fielding a current idea: exploring the public health impact of electromagnetic radiation, *Public Health* 122(2):113–124, 2008.
219. National Institute of Environmental Health Sciences (NIEHS) Working Group Report: *Assessment of health effects from exposure to power-line frequency electric and magnetic fields*, Washington, DC, 1998, U.S. Government Printing Office.
220. INTERPHONE Study Group: Brain tumour risk in relation to mobile telephone use: results of the INTERPHONE International Case-control Study, *Int J Epidemiol* 39:675–694, 2010.
221. Hardell L, Carlberg M, Mild K: Pooled analysis of case-control studies on malignant brain tumours and the use of mobile and cordless phones including living and deceased subjects, *Int J Oncol* 38:1465–1474, 2011.
222. Li G, Satayamoorthy K, Herlyn M: N-cadherin-mediated intercellular interactions promote survival and migration of melanoma cells, *Cancer Res* 61(9):3819–3825, 2001.
223. Gray J: *State of the evidence 2008: the connection between breast cancer and the environment*, San Francisco, Breast Cancer Fund.
224. Tryndyak VP et al: Effect of long-term tamoxifen exposure on genotoxic and epigenetic changes in rat liver: implications for tamoxifen-induced hepatocarcinogenesis, *Carcinogenesis* 27:1713–1720, 2006.
225. Karpinets TV, Foy BD: Tumorigenesis: the adaptation of mammalian cells to sustained stress environment by epigenetic alterations and succeeding matched mutations, *Carcinogenesis* 26:1323–1334, 2005.
226. Tabish AM et al: Epigenetic factors in cancer risk: effect of chemical carcinogens on global DNA methylation pattern in human TK6 cells, *PLoS One* 7(4):e34674, 2012.
227. Neuberger JS, Field RW: Occupation and lung cancer in nonsmokers, *Rev Environ Health* 18(4):251–267, 2003, review.
228. Vineis P et al: Outdoor air pollution and lung cancer: recent epidemiologic evidence, *Int J Cancer* 111(5):647–652, 2004.
229. American Lung Association: *State of the air report 2012*, Washington, DC, 2011, Author.
230. Puett RC et al: Chronic fine and course particulate exposure, mortality, and coronary heart disease in the Nurses' Health Study, *Environ Health Perspect* 117(11):1697–1701, 2009.
231. Gulland A: Diesel engine exhaust causes lung cancer, says WHO, *BMJ* 344:e4174, 2012.
232. Demetriou CA et al: Biomarkers of ambient air pollution and lung cancer: a systematic review, *Occup Environ Med*, July 2012. [Epub ahead of print.].
233. Boffetta P et al: Mortality among workers employed in the titanium dioxide production industry in Europe, *Cancer Causes Control* 15(7):697–706, 2004.
234. Boffetta P: Involuntary smoking and lung cancer, *Scand J Work Environ Health* 28(Suppl 2):30–40, 2002.
235. Hecht SS et al: Elevated levels of volatile organic carcinogen and toxicant biomarkers in Chinese women who regularly cook at home, *Cancer Epidemiol Biomarkers Prev* 19(5):1185–1192, 2010.
236. Zhao Y et al: Air pollution and lung cancer risks in China—meta-analysis, *Sci Total Environ* 366(2-3):500–513, 2006.
237. Borm PJ, Schins RP, Albrecht C: Inhaled particles and lung cancer, part B: paradigms and risk assessment, *Int J Cancer* 110(1):3–14, 2004.

CHAPTER

14

Cancer in Children

Nancy E. Kline

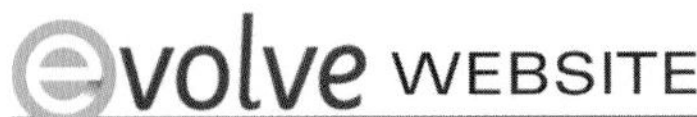

http://evolve.elsevier.com/McCance/

- Review Questions and Answers

CHAPTER OUTLINE

Cancer in children is rare, but it is still the leading cause of death from disease in this patient population. The 5-year survival rates in children with cancer have improved from 59% in the 1970s to 83% today.[1] Some of the factors leading to improved cure rates in children with cancer include the use of combination chemotherapy, the utilization of immunotherapy, and the participation of many subjects in clinical trials.

INCIDENCE AND TYPES OF CANCER

In 2012, approximately 12,060 children (from birth to 14 years of age) in the United States will be diagnosed with cancer, and approximately 1340 will die from the disease, one third of these from leukemia.[1]

The types of malignancies in children are vastly different from those that affect adults. The most common types of cancer among adults include prostate, breast, lung, and colon. Children (birth to 14 years of age) with leukemias and brain tumors account for 61% of childhood cancers; neuroblastoma and soft tissue or bone sarcomas are less common. Although many adult cancers have associated lifestyle factors that could theoretically be avoided, such as smoking and lifetime exposure to sun, very few environmental factors have been linked to pediatric malignancies. Yet more data are emerging that the developing child may be affected by parental exposures before conception, exposures in utero, and the contents of breast milk.[2,3]

The incidence of cancer among adolescents and young adults represents only 2% of all invasive cancers. However, the malignancy rate in this age group (15- to 39-year-olds) is three times higher than that in children younger than 15 years. Each year about 70,000 adolescents and young adults will be diagnosed with cancer. The following are the most common cancers diagnosed among the 15- to 39-year-old population in the United States[3] (these cancers are discussed in the appropriate chapters):

- Hodgkin lymphoma
- Leukemia
- Germ cell tumors (particularly testicular)
- Central nervous system (CNS) tumors
- Non-Hodgkin lymphoma
- Thyroid cancer
- Melanoma
- Sarcomas
- Breast, cervical, liver, and colorectal cancers

Most childhood cancers originate from the **mesodermal germ layer** that gives rise to connective tissue, bone, cartilage, muscle, blood, blood vessels, gonads, kidney, and the lymphatic system. Thus the more common childhood cancers are leukemias, sarcomas, and embryonic tumors. **Embryonic tumors** originate during intrauterine life. These tumors contain abnormal cells that appear to be immature embryonic tissue, unable to mature or differentiate into fully developed functional cells. Embryonic tumors are diagnosed early in life (usually before 5 years of age). Embryonic tumors often contain the term **blast cell** in their name, which refers to the immature nature of the cells.

Leukemia is the most common malignancy in children and the most common type of leukemia is acute lymphoblastic leukemia (ALL), which represents approximately 75% of all pediatric leukemia cases. Although the presenting signs of the various types of leukemia may be similar, the treatment and response to treatment of childhood leukemias vary greatly (see Chapter 30).

CNS tumors are the most common types of solid tumors in children and account for 27% of all childhood cancers[1] (see Chapter 20). Not all brain tumors are diagnosed malignant by histologic studies, but even a benign tumor can have devastating effects, depending on the anatomic location. The treatment for brain tumors in children often presents difficulties because therapies, such as radiation, may have debilitating effects on the developing brain, particularly in children younger than 3 years of age.

Lymphoma, including non-Hodgkin lymphoma and Hodgkin lymphoma, is a malignancy that occurs in children and adults. However, the subtypes of lymphoma and treatments in the two populations often differ (see Chapter 30).

Many pediatric solid tumors usually develop only in children but in very rare instances may occur in adults. These tumors include neuroblastoma, Wilms tumor, rhabdomyosarcoma, retinoblastoma, osteosarcoma, and Ewing sarcoma.

Childhood cancers are most often diagnosed during peak times of physical growth. In general, they are extremely fast growing, with 80% having distant spread (metastases) at diagnosis. Overall, cancer is 10% to 25% more common in white than in black children. Boys are more likely to develop cancer than girls.

ETIOLOGY

The causes of cancer in children are largely unknown. A few environmental factors are known to predispose a child to cancer, but causal factors have not been established for most childhood cancers. A number of host factors, many of which are genetic risk factors or congenital conditions, have been implicated in the development of childhood cancer (Table 14-1). It is most likely the interaction of many factors that produces cancer, a concept referred to as multiple causation or **multifactorial etiology.** According to this premise, cancer develops because of the predisposing characteristics of the person and the interaction with environmental causes.

The **multiple causation** concept is useful when the results of epidemiologic studies are interpreted. For example, laboratory and epidemiologic studies may indicate that exposure to a certain chemical can cause leukemia, but not all children exposed to that chemical will develop leukemia. Additional studies will be needed to determine what other factors must interact with chemical exposure to cause the disease.

TABLE 14-1 CONGENITAL FACTORS ASSOCIATED WITH CHILDHOOD CANCER

SYNDROME	ASSOCIATED CHILDHOOD CANCER
Chromosomal Alterations	
Down syndrome	Acute leukemia
13q syndrome	Retinoblastoma
Chromosomal Instability	
Ataxia-telangiectasia	Lymphoma
Bloom syndrome	Acute leukemia, lymphoma, Wilms tumor
Fanconi anemia	Nonlymphocytic leukemia, myelodysplastic syndrome, hepatic tumors
Hereditary Syndromes	
Beckwith-Wiedemann syndrome	Wilms tumor, sarcoma, brain tumors, neuroblastoma, hepatoblastoma
Neurofibromatosis type 1	Brain tumors, sarcomas, neuroblastomas, Wilms tumor, nonlymphocytic leukemia
Neurofibromatosis type 2	Meningioma (malignant or benign), acoustic neuroma/schwannoma, gliomas, ependymomas
Tuberous sclerosis	Glial tumors
Li-Fraumeni syndrome	Sarcoma, adrenocortical carcinoma
von Hippel-Lindau disease	Cerebellar hemangioblastoma, retinal angioma, renal cell carcinoma, pheochromocytomas
Ataxia-telangiectasia	Leukemia, lymphoma, brain tumors
Gorlin syndrome	Medulloblastoma, skin tumors
Immune Deficiency Disorders	
Congenital	
Agammaglobulinemia	Lymphoma, leukemia, brain tumors
Immunoglobulin A (IgA) deficiency	Lymphoma, leukemia, brain tumors
Wiskott-Aldrich syndrome	Leukemia, lymphoma
Acquired	
Aplastic anemia	Leukemia
Organ transplantation	Leukemia, lymphoma
Congenital Malformation Syndromes	
Aniridia, hemihypertrophy, hamartoma, genitourinary anomalies	Wilms tumor
Cryptorchidism	Testicular tumor
Gonadal dysgenesis	Gonadoblastoma
Family Susceptibility	
Twin or sibling with leukemia	Leukemia

TABLE 14-2 SELECTED ONCOGENES AND TUMOR-SUPPRESSOR GENES ASSOCIATED WITH CHILDHOOD CANCER

GENE	ASSOCIATED PEDIATRIC TUMOR
Oncogenes	
bcr-abl	Acute lymphoblastic leukemia
N-myc	Neuroblastoma
c-myb	Neural tumors, leukemia, lymphoma, rhabdomyosarcoma, Wilms tumor, neuroblastoma
erb B	Glioblastomas
N-ras	Neuroblastoma, leukemia
H/K-ras	Neuroblastoma, rhabdomyosarcoma, leukemia
ATM	Lymphoma, leukemia
Tumor-Suppressor Genes	
Rb1	Retinoblastoma, sarcoma
WT1, WT2	Wilms tumor, leukemia
WTC	Wilms tumor
NF-1	Sarcoma, primitive neuroectodermal tumor, juvenile chronic myelocytic leukemia
NF-2	Brain tumors, melanoma, meningiomas
p16	Brain tumors, leukemia
TP53	Sarcoma, leukemia, brain tumors, lymphoma
DCC	Ewing sarcoma, rhabdomyosarcoma
$p16^{INK4a}$	Glioma, leukemia
$p15^{ARF}$	Glioblastoma, T-cell ALL
CDC2L1	Non-Hodgkin lymphoma, neuroblastoma

Data from Dome JS, Coppes MS: *Curr Opin Pediatr* 14(1):5–11, 2002; Linblom A, Nordenskjold M: *Semin Cancer Biol* 10(4):251–254, 2000; Tischkowitz M, Rosser E: *Eur J Cancer* 40:2459–2470, 2004; Look A, Kirsch IR: Molecular basis of childhood cancer. In Pizzo PA, Poplack DG, editors: *Principles and practices of pediatric oncology,* ed 6, Philadelphia, 2011, Lippincott Williams & Wilkins.
ALL, Acute lymphocytic leukemia.

Genetic Factors

Oncogenes and tumor-suppressor genes are associated with the development of childhood cancer (Table 14-2; also see Chapter 12). **Proto-oncogenes** code for proteins that help to regulate normal cell growth and differentiation. If mutated, proto-oncogenes become oncogenes that help to turn normal cells into cancer cells. Changes produced by specific oncogenes cause the cell cycle to become dysregulated. An example of an oncogene identified in pediatric cancer is *N-myc,* which is involved in neuroblastoma and glioblastoma. Tumor-suppressor genes arise from genes that normally suppress cancer cell proliferation but have lost their suppressor function, thus leading to uncontrolled growth. Some childhood cancers identified with tumor-suppressor genes include osteosarcoma, leukemia, rhabdomyosarcoma, retinoblastoma, and Wilms tumor.[4]

Other genetic factors involve chromosomal aberrations or single-gene defects. These chromosomal abnormalities include aneuploidy, amplifications, deletions, translocations, and susceptibility to breakage, known as fragility. A well-known chromosomal abnormality is the Philadelphia chromosome found in chronic and acute myelogenous leukemias.[5] Chromosomal deletions are often observed in retinoblastoma and osteosarcoma.

WHAT'S NEW?

Far Fewer Genetic Mutations in Pediatric Cancer

A collaborative study conducted at 20 different centers in the United States examined how DNA in medulloblastoma in children differs from the DNA in adult cancers. The investigators found that the tumors in children had 5 to 10 times fewer mutations than the tumors in adults. However, although the tumors in the children had fewer mutations, more than one third were known to disrupt gene function, which is a much higher percentage than that found in adult tumors.

The findings from this study suggest that childhood cancer is very different than adult cancers. As scientists better understand which genes are most important for causing and preventing cancer, they will be able to more readily identify the type of cancer a person has and also develop targeted therapies.

Data from Parsons DW et al: *Science* 331(6016):435–439, 2011.

Some chromosomal defects and congenital malformations are associated with the development of pediatric cancer. Trisomy 21 (Down syndrome) is the most common genetic defect linked to the development of acute leukemia. Children with Down syndrome have a 10- to 20-fold increased risk of developing acute lymphoblastic and myelogenous leukemias and a higher risk for developing acute megakaryocytic leukemia. The risk is highest between 1 and 4 years of age.[6] Wilms tumor is associated with several congenital syndromes: aniridia, or congenital absence of the iris of the eye; ambiguous genitalia and mental retardation (AGR), neurofibromatosis, and Beckwith-Wiedemann syndrome.[7] Retinoblastoma, a malignant embryonic tumor of the eye, occurs as an inherited defect or as an acquired mutation (see Chapter 20).

Several single-gene defects have been associated with the subsequent development of childhood cancers. Fanconi anemia and Bloom syndrome, two autosomal recessive conditions, are risk factors for the development of acute lymphocytic leukemia (ALL) (see Chapter 30).

Although not determined to be genetically transmitted, a child who has a sibling with leukemia has a risk for the development of leukemia that is two to four times greater than that for children with healthy siblings. The occurrence of leukemia in monozygous twins is estimated as being as high as 25%.

In families with a history of Li-Fraumeni syndrome (LFS) (an autosomal dominant disorder involving the *p53* tumor-suppressor gene), the risk of developing cancer as a child or adult is significantly higher than that seen in the unaffected population. Children and adults in these families are at risk for soft tissue sarcoma, breast cancer, leukemia, osteosarcoma, melanoma, and cancer of the colon, pancreas, adrenal cortex, and brain. Individuals with LFS are at increased risk for developing multiple primary cancers.[8] Overall, cancers in children are very different than adult cancers and are associated with far fewer genetic mutations (see What's New? Far Fewer Genetic Mutations in Pediatric Cancer).

Environmental Factors

Although many adult cancers are associated with environmental agents, few childhood tumors share a similar strong association. Because of the lengthy latency period required between

TABLE 14-3 DRUGS THAT MAY INCREASE RISK OF CHILDHOOD CANCER

DRUG CLASS	USES	CANCER RISK
Anabolic androgenic steroids	Stimulate bone growth and appetite Induce puberty Increase muscle mass and physical strength	Hepatocellular carcinoma Brain tumors
Cytotoxic chemotherapy	Used in cancer treatment	Leukemia
Immunosuppressive agents	Prevent organ rejection following transplantation surgery	Lymphoma

exposure and development of cancer, presumably early exposure to carcinogens does not result in cancer until the child is an adult. A recent meta-analysis of 1426 cases of neuroblastoma failed to show an association between paternal occupational exposure to pesticide and development of disease.[9]

Prenatal Exposure

Prenatal exposure to some drugs and pesticides has been linked to childhood cancers. The most well-described drug is diethylstilbestrol (DES), which was prescribed by physicians to prevent spontaneous miscarriage (in women with previous miscarriage). In 1971, DES was identified as a transplacental chemical carcinogen because a small percentage of the daughters of the women who took DES developed adenocarcinomas of the vagina and cervix. Since then, other studies have attempted to identify drugs taken by pregnant women that may cause cancer in their offspring, but no other drugs have been found. Prior research suggested an association between antenatal x-ray exposure and childhood cancer, but studies have not been replicated or supported in recent literature. In 2006 the Office of the U.S. Surgeon General suggested evidence of a causal relationship between childhood leukemia, lymphoma, and brain tumors and prenatal or postnatal environmental tobacco smoke exposure; the results have suggested an association between parental exposure to pesticides before or during pregnancy.[2] A recent study suggested that the risk of leukemia and lymphoma increased when the mother was exposed to pesticides in the prenatal period and the risk of brain tumors was correlated with paternal exposure (occupational or household use) either before or after birth.[10]

Childhood Exposure

Childhood exposure to ionizing radiation, drugs, or viruses has been associated with the risk of developing cancer. Retrospective research has shown a significant correlation between radiation-induced malignancies from radiotherapy (cancer treatment) or from radiation exposure from diagnostic imaging.[11] Few studies have followed children for a long enough period of time to determine whether there is an increased risk of cancer in adulthood, although there are current studies with more rigorous methodology to assess this risk[12] (see What's New? CT Scans in Childhood Appear to Increase Cancer Risk). In addition to the drug and environmental agents that are known to cause cancer in adults and therefore also are risks for exposure during childhood, a few drugs may particularly increase cancer risk during childhood (Table 14-3). Exposures during childhood to unspecified residential pesticides and insecticides have been associated with childhood leukemia.[13]

WHAT'S NEW?

CT Scans in Childhood Appear to Increase Cancer Risk

The findings from a recent study of 176,587 children suggest that those who had 2 or 3 computed tomography (CT) scans of the head before age 22 years were 3 times as likely to develop brain cancer as those in the general population, and the risk of developing leukemia was 3 times as great in those who received 5 to 10 CT scans. Previous studies have speculated that there may be increased risk from repeated CT scans, but this large study was the first to provide direct evidence. Although the risk remains low, it amounts to 1 additional case of brain cancer for every 30,000 children scanned or to 1 additional case of leukemia for every 10,000 persons who were scanned. Although it remains important for children to receive CT scans to detect head injuries, the results of this study suggest that children should only be scanned when necessary and also with the lowest dose of radiation possible.

Pearce MS et al: *The Lancet* 380(9840):499–505, 2012.

The relationship between childhood cancer and exposure to radon[14] and electromagnetic fields has been the focus of many epidemiologic studies, yet no conclusive evidence has been observed. In 2007 a task group of scientific experts convened by the World Health Organization (WHO) reported that it could not confirm the existence of any health consequences from exposure to low-level magnetic fields.[15]

The strongest association between viruses and the development of cancer in children has been the relationship between exposure to Epstein-Barr virus (EBV) and development of Burkitt lymphoma, nasopharyngeal carcinoma, and Hodgkin disease. Children with acquired immunodeficiency syndrome (AIDS) have an increased risk of developing non-Hodgkin lymphoma and Kaposi sarcoma. However, with the use of highly active antiretroviral therapy in the developed world, the incidence of AIDS-related malignancies has declined dramatically[16] (see Chapter 10).

PROGNOSIS

More than 80% of children diagnosed with cancer are cured. Mortality rates have declined from 6.5 per 100,000 in 1969 to 2.2 per 100,000 in 2008, largely because of advances in treatment and increased participation in clinical trials.[1]

Some of the factors leading to improved cure rates in pediatric oncology include the use of combination chemotherapy and multimodal treatment for childhood solid tumors. Additionally, development of research centers for comprehensive childhood cancer treatment, cooperation among treatment institutions, and development of cooperative study groups enable the most efficient advancement of treatment regimens. Currently, clinical trials are being conducted by the Children's Oncology Group (COG) at more than 180 hospitals across the United States and are funded by the National Cancer Institute through CureSearch® for Children's Cancer. Side effects of treatment are better managed as a result of improvements in nursing and supportive care, recognition of the psychologic effects of cancer treatment, and continued follow-up to track trends in the late effects of cancer treatment. Young children are particularly prone to long-term sequelae of cancer therapy. Clinical trials are continually focusing on more effective, targeted therapies with fewer side effects.

SUMMARY REVIEW

Incidence and Types

1. Cancer in children is rare, but is still the leading cause of death from disease in this population.
2. Leukemias and brain tumors account for 61% of cancer in children from birth to 14 years of age, with neuroblastoma and soft tissue or bone sarcomas less common.
3. The most common cancers among the adolescent and young adult populations (15 to 39 years of age) are Hodgkin lymphoma, leukemia, germ cell tumors (particularly testicular), central nervous system (CNS) tumors, non-Hodgkin lymphoma, thyroid cancer, melanoma, sarcomas, and breast, cervical, liver, and colorectal cancers.

Etiology

1. It is most likely the interaction of many factors produces cancer in children, a concept referred to as multiple causation or multifactorial etiology.
2. Oncogenes and tumor-suppressor genes have been associated with childhood malignancies.
3. Chromosomal aberrations or single-gene defects including aneuploidy, amplifications, deletions, translocations, and fragility are associated with the development of childhood cancer.
4. Wilms tumor and retinoblastoma are pediatric malignancies that are linked in a familial manner.
5. Childhood exposure to ionizing radiation, drugs, or viruses has been associated with the risk of developing cancer.

Prognosis

1. More than 80% of children diagnosed with cancer are cured.
2. Mortality rates have declined significantly in the past 40 years largely because of advances in treatment and increased participation in clinical trials.
3. Young children are particularly prone to long-term sequelae of cancer therapy. It is imperative that more effective, targeted therapies with fewer side effects be found.

KEY TERMS

Blast cell, 443
Embryonic tumors, 443
Mesodermal germ layer, 443
Multifactorial etiology, 443
Multiple causation, 443
Proto-oncogenes, 444

REFERENCES

1. American Cancer Society: *Cancer facts and figures 2012*, Atlanta, 2012, Author.
2. Wigle DT et al: Epidemiologic evidence of relationships between reproductive and child health outcomes and environmental chemical contaminants, *J Toxicol Environ Health B Crit Rev* 11(5-6): 373–517, 2008.
3. National Cancer Institute: *Adolescents and young adults with cancer.* Available at www.cancer.gov/cancertopics/aya/types. Retrieved July 29, 2012.
4. Plon SE, Malkin D: Childhood cancer and heredity. In Pizzo PA, Poplack DG, editors: *Principles and practice of pediatric oncology*, ed 6, Philadelphia, 2011, Lippincott Williams & Wilkins, pp 17–37.
5. Alvarnez JC et al: Acute lymphoblastic leukemia, *J Natl Comp Canc Netw* 10(7):858–914, 2012.
6. Margolin JF et al: Acute lymphoblastic leukemia. In Pizzo PA, Poplack DG, editors: *Principles and practice of pediatric oncology*, ed 6, Philadelphia, 2011, Lippincott Williams & Wilkins, pp 518–565.
7. Fernandez C et al: Renal tumors. In Pizzo PA, Poplack DG, editors: *Principles and practice of pediatric oncology*, ed 6, Philadelphia, 2011, Lippincott Williams & Wilkins, pp 861–885.
8. Tabori U, Malkin D: Risk stratification in cancer predisposition syndromes: lessons learned from novel molecular developments in Li-Fraumeni syndrome, *Cancer Res* 68(7):2053–2057, 2008.
9. Moore A, Enquobahrie DA: Paternal occupational exposure to pesticides and risk of neuroblastoma among children: a meta analysis, *Cancer Causes Control* 22(11):1529–1536, 2011.
10. Vinson F et al: Exposure to pesticides and risk of childhood cancer: a meta analysis of recent epidemiological studies, *Occup Environ Med* 68(9):694–702, 2011.
11. Buka I et al: Trends in childhood cancer incidence: review of environmental linkages, *Pediatr Clin North Am* 54(1):177–203, 2007.
12. Linet MS et al: Cancer risks associated with external radiation from diagnostic imaging procedures, *CA Cancer J Clin* 62:75–100, 2012.
13. Turner MC, Wigle DT, Krewski D: Residential pesticides and childhood leukemia: a systematic review and meta-analysis, *Environ Health Perspect* 118(1):33–41, 2010.
14. Tong J et al: Environmental radon exposure and childhood leukemia, *J Toxicol Environ Health B Crit Rev* 15(5):332–347, 2012.
15. Repacholi M: Concern that "EMF" magnetic fields from power lines causes cancer, *Sci Total Environ* 426:454–458, 2012.
16. Pajand O et al: Detection of Epstein-Barr virus DNA in plasma and lymph node biopsy samples in pediatric and adult patients with Hodgkin lymphoma, *Pediatr Hematol Oncol* 28(1):10–15, 2011.

CHAPTER

15

Structure and Function of the Neurologic System

Richard A. Sugerman

evolve WEBSITE

http://evolve.elsevier.com/McCance/
- Review Questions and Answers
- Animations

CHAPTER OUTLINE

The human nervous system is a remarkable structure that is responsible for the body's ability both to interact with the environment and to regulate activities involving our internal organs, muscles, and glands. The nervous system *drives* the other systems of the body. It is a network composed of complex structures that transmit electrical and chemical signals between the body's many organs and tissues and the brain.

OVERVIEW AND ORGANIZATION OF THE NERVOUS SYSTEM

Although the nervous system functions as a unified whole, structures and functions of the nervous system have been divided to facilitate comprehension. Structurally, the nervous system is divided into the central nervous system and the peripheral nervous system. The **central nervous system (CNS)** consists of the brain and spinal cord, enclosed within the protective cranial vault and vertebrae, respectively. The **peripheral nervous system (PNS)** is composed of the **cranial nerves,** which project from the brain and pass through foramina (openings) in the skull, and the **spinal nerves,** which project from the spinal cord and pass through intervertebral foramina of the vertebrae. Peripheral nerve pathways are differentiated into **afferent pathways (ascending pathways)** that carry sensory impulses toward the CNS and **efferent pathways (descending pathways)** that innervate **effector organs,** such as skeletal, cardiac, and smooth muscle, as well as glands, by transmitting motor impulses away from the CNS. Organs innervated by specific components of the nervous system are called *effector organs.* Cranial nerves are viewed most correctly as modified spinal nerves. Some cranial nerves function similarly to spinal nerves, whereas others have specialized sensory tasks, such as smell, taste, sight, and hearing.

Functionally, the PNS can be divided into the somatic nervous system and the autonomic nervous system. The **somatic nervous system** consists of motor and sensory pathways regulating voluntary motor control of skeletal muscle. The **autonomic nervous system (ANS)** also consists of motor and sensory components and is involved with regulation of the body's internal environment (viscera) through involuntary control of organ systems. The ANS is further divided into sympathetic and parasympathetic divisions. Today we understand that some aspects of the ANS can be controlled through mental practice with or without biofeedback techniques.

CELLS OF THE NERVOUS SYSTEM

The two basic types of cells that comprise nervous tissue are neurons and neuroglial cells. The neuron is the primary information/communication cell of the nervous system. Working in parallel systems, neurons can scan the environment, integrate many systems at higher cognitive levels, and initiate body responses to maintain homeostasis. The **neuroglial cells** are found in the CNS and PNS and can provide structural support and nutrition for neurons, remove debris, increase the speed of nerve impulses, and play a significant role, along with neurons, in processing and storing information (i.e., memory).[1]

Neurons

Neuronal structure varies considerably throughout the CNS. Neurons vary in size from micrometers to several meters long and have from one to many cell processes. Even the shapes and complexity of the processes can vary considerably. **Neurons** are specialized cells that share many of the same metabolic activities and constituents as other types of cells. The fuel source for the neuron is predominantly glucose; insulin, however, is not required for cellular glucose uptake in the CNS. Neurons contain many cellular constituents, namely, neurotubules, neurofilaments, neurofibrils, and Nissl substances. **Neurofilaments** and **neurofibrils** are composed of structural proteins and are responsible for structural support within the cell and movement of neuron processes, as seen in amoebae and white blood cells. **Microtubules** also are made of protein and are believed to be involved in the transport of cellular products. **Nissl substances** consist of endoplasmic reticulum and ribosomes and are involved in protein synthesis. The CNS is formed with more neurons than it needs, and those neurons that do not become involved in functional systems die. Some neurons continue to divide after birth. Olfactory neurons in the nose continue to divide throughout life.

A neuron (Figure 15-1) has three components: a cell body (soma) and the thin processes of the cell—the dendrites and axons. Most cell bodies are located within the CNS. Dense, packed cell bodies in the CNS are called **nuclei.** Cell bodies in the PNS are usually found in groups called **ganglia** or **plexuses.** The **dendrites** are extensions that carry nerve impulses *toward* the cell body. The **dendritic zone** is the receptive portion of a neuron that receives a stimulus and continues further conduction. **Axons** are long, conductive projections from the cell body that carry nerve impulses *away* from the cell body. The **axon hillock** is the cone-shaped, organelle-free area where the axon leaves the cell body. In large nerves, axons are bundled together as **fascicles.** The initial segment of the axon has the lowest threshold for stimulation, and as a result, action potentials begin there.

A typical neuron has only one axon, which may be covered with a segmented layer of lipid material called **myelin,** which acts as an insulating substance. This entire membrane is referred to as the **myelin sheath;** the thin membrane between the myelin sheath and the **endoneurium,** a delicate connective tissue around each axon in the PNS (see Figure 15-1, *C*), is the **neurilemma (Schwann sheath).** The neurilemma and the myelin sheath are interrupted at regular intervals by the **nodes of Ranvier.** Myelin acts as an insulator that allows ions to flow between segments rather than along the entire length of the membrane, resulting in increased velocity of neuronal conduction. This mechanism is referred to as **saltatory conduction.** If the Schwann cells are loosely wrapped around the axon, it is referred to as *unmyelinated,* and conduction velocity is not increased. Axons are capable of extensive branching, which occurs at the nodes of Ranvier. Two major principles of information processing in the nervous system are *divergence* and *convergence.* **Divergence** refers to the ability of these branching axons to influence many different neurons. **Convergence** is the term applied to branches of numerous neurons converging on and influencing one or a few neurons. Disorders of the myelin sheath (demyelinating diseases), such as multiple sclerosis and Guillain-Barré syndrome, demonstrate the important role myelin plays in nerve function (see Chapter 18). Besides depending on the myelin coating, conduction velocities also are influenced by the diameter of the axon. Larger axons transmit impulses at a faster rate.

Neurons are structurally classified on the basis of the number of processes (projections) extending from the cell body. There are four basic types of cell configuration: (1) unipolar, (2) pseudounipolar, (3) bipolar, and (4) multipolar (Figure 15-2). **Unipolar neurons** have one process that branches shortly after leaving the cell body. One example is found in the retina.

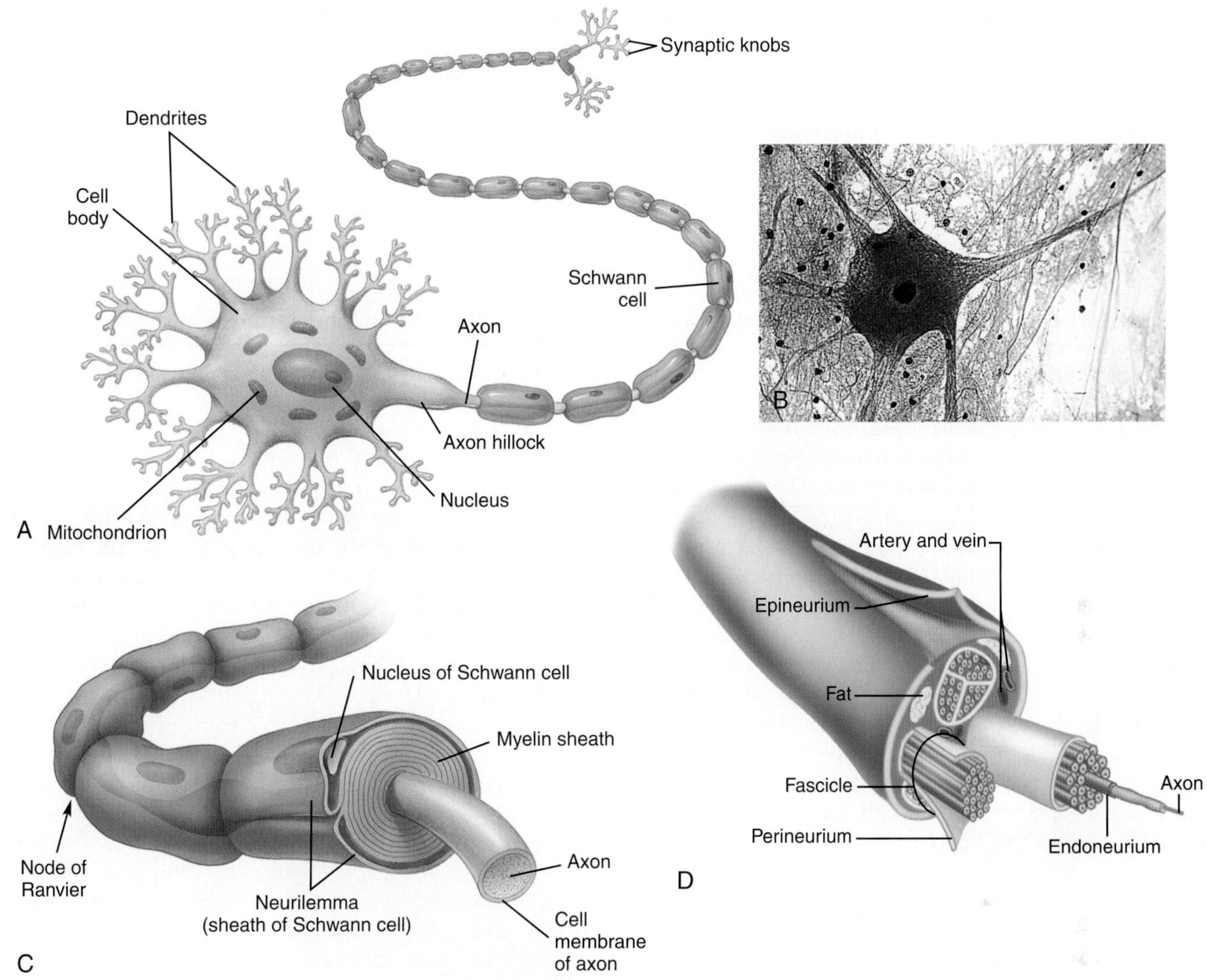

FIGURE 15-1 Structure of a Typical Neuron. **A,** Many dendrites carry nerve impulses to the cell body, and from the cell body the nerve impulses are conducted along a single, long axon. Long axons are encased at intervals by a myelin sheath. **B,** Photomicrograph of a neuron. **C,** A segment of myelinated fiber in cross section, showing myelin sheath composed of several layers of myelin, which insulate the axon. **D,** Axons bundled into fascicles. (**A** and **C** from Thibodeau GA, Patton KT: *Structure and function of the human body,* ed 12, St Louis, 2004, Mosby; **B,** copyright Edward Reschke; **D** from Patton KT, Thibodeau GA: *Anatomy & physiology,* ed 8, St Louis, 2013, Mosby.)

Pseudounipolar neurons (some authors call them *unipolar*) have one process that has its dendritic portion extending away from the CNS and its axon portion projecting into the CNS (see Figure 15-2, *C*). The configuration is typical of sensory neurons in both cranial and spinal nerves. **Bipolar neurons** have two distinct processes arising from the cell body. This type of neuron connects to rod and cone cells of the retina. **Multipolar neurons** are the most common and have multiple dendrites and a single axon. A motor neuron is typically multipolar.

Functionally, there are three types of neurons (with their direction of transmission and typical configuration noted in parentheses): (1) sensory (afferent, mostly pseudounipolar), (2) associational (interneurons, multipolar), and (3) motor (efferent, multipolar). **Sensory neurons** carry impulses from peripheral sensory receptors to the CNS (Box 15-1). **Association neurons (interneurons)** transmit impulses from neuron to neuron, for example, from sensory to motor neurons, and are also involved in cognitive function. **Motor neurons** transmit impulses away from the CNS to an effector organ. In skeletal muscle the end processes form a complex neuromuscular (myoneural) junction.

Neuroglia and Schwann Cells

Neuroglia comprise the general classification of cells that support the neurons of the CNS. They make up approximately half of the total brain and spinal cord volume and are 5 to 10 times more numerous than neurons. Different types of neuroglia serve different functions. **Astrocytes,** for example, fill the spaces between neurons and surround blood vessels in the CNS (see What's New? Astrocytes). **Oligodendrocytes** function to deposit myelin within the CNS. Oligodendroglia are the CNS counterpart of the Schwann cells. **Ependymal cells** line the cerebrospinal fluid (CSF)–filled cavities of the CNS. **Microglia** remove debris (phagocytosis) in the CNS. Characteristics and

WHAT'S NEW?

Astrocytes

Neuroglial (glia) cells have been considered the *glue* that exists between or around neurons. Until recently, neurons have been considered the major players in the nervous system and glia just minor support cells. Astrocytes, the most abundant glial cells in the nervous system, were believed to be simple nutrient support "housekeeping" cells for neurons, and it was thought they helped form the blood-brain barrier. Recent reports on astrocytes portray a "partnership" with glial cells. Astrocytes (1) can be a source for new neurons; (2) build a structural framework around neurons, forming glia-vascular units to provide the specific blood flow (nutrients) that a neuron requires; (3) may regulate synaptic formation and maintenance, which helps consolidate memories; and (4) have a two-way interaction with neurons at synapses through the release of glial neurotransmitters that could facilitate either excitation or inhibition of neuron activity at the pre- and postsynaptic membranes. Alterations in astrocyte function play a significant role in brain malfunctions including hepatic encephalopathy, seizures, Alzheimer disease, and brain tumor invasiveness.

Data from Parpura V et al: *J Neurochem* 21(1):4–27, 2012; Ranson BR, Ransom CB: *Methods Mol Biol* 814:3–7, 2012; Stantello M, Cali C, Bezzi P: *Adv Exp Med Biol* 970:307–331, 2012; Steindler DA: *Methods Mol Biol* 814:9–22, 2012.

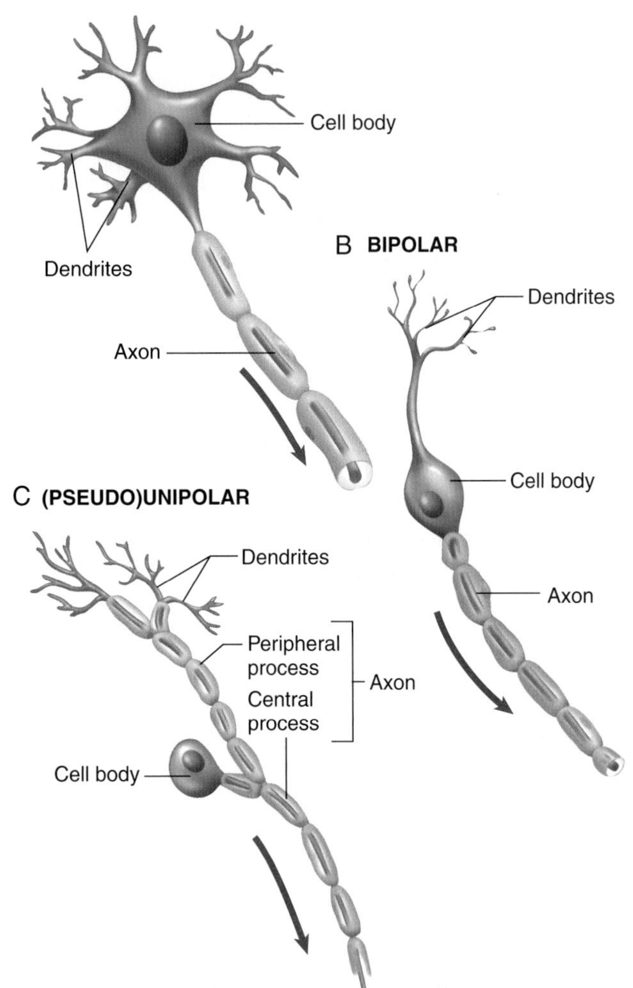

FIGURE 15-2 Structural Classification of Neurons. (From Patton KT, Thibodeau GA: *Anatomy & physiology*, ed 8, St Louis, 2013, Mosby.)

BOX 15-1 MAJOR TYPES OF SENSORY RECEPTORS

Nociceptors (pain)
Mechanoreceptors (touch, pressure, and mechanical deformation or encapsulated endings)
Photochemical (light on the retina)
Chemoreceptors (flavors, odors, oxygen levels, osmolarity of body fluids, and carbon dioxide levels in the blood)
Thermoreceptors (heat and cold)
Proprioception (sensing location of body parts)
Audition and balance (sound and positional movement)

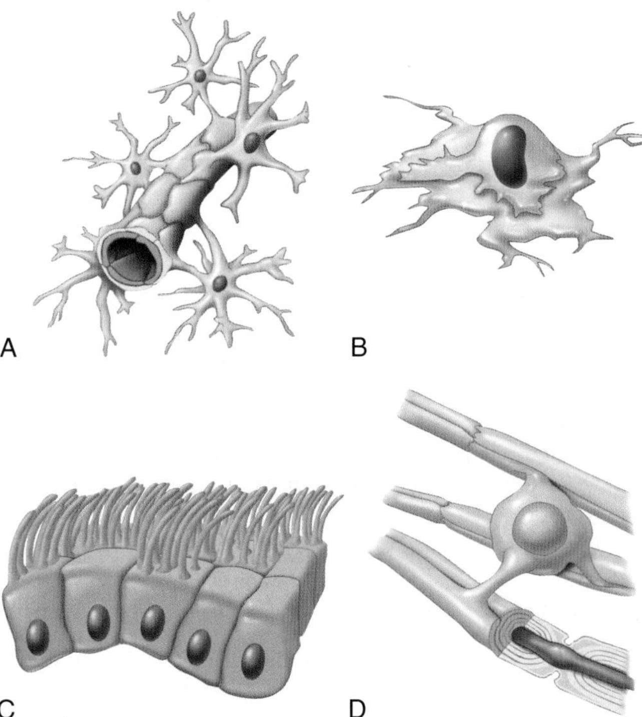

FIGURE 15-3 Types of Neuroglial Cells. **A,** Astrocyte attached to brain capillary; **B,** microglial cell; **C,** ependymal cells that form sheets to line fluid cavities in brain; **D,** oligodendrocyte wrapped around CNS nerve fiber forming myelin. (From Patton KT, Thibodeau GA: *Anatomy & physiology*, ed 8, St Louis, 2013, Mosby.)

functions of neuroglia and Schwann cells are summarized in Figure 15-3 and Table 15-1.

The **Schwann cell,** or **neurolemmocyte,** is a glial cell that wraps around and covers axons in the peripheral nervous system. Schwann cells form and maintain the myelin sheath, and the nodes of Ranvier form the spaces on either side of the Schwann cell. If the myelin layer is tightly wrapped many times around the axon forming nodes of Ranvier, it increases conduction velocity and the neuron is referred to as *myelinated* (see Figure 15-1).

Nerve Injury and Regeneration

When an axon is severed, a typical sequence of events, known as **wallerian degeneration**, occurs. In the axon distal to the cut, the myelin sheath shrinks and disintegrates and this axon portion degenerates and disappears. The myelin sheaths re-form

TABLE 15-1 SUPPORT CELLS OF THE NERVOUS SYSTEM

CELL TYPE	PRIMARY FUNCTIONS
Astrocytes	Form specialized contacts between neuronal surfaces and blood vessels Provide rapid transport for nutrients and metabolites Believed to form an essential component of the blood-brain barrier Appear to be the scar-forming cells of the CNS, which may be the foci for seizures Appear to work with neurons in processing information and memory storage
Oligodendroglia (oligodendrocytes)	Formation of myelin sheath and neurilemma in the CNS
Schwann cells	Formation of myelin sheath and neurilemma in the PNS
Microglia	Responsible for clearing cellular debris (phagocytic properties)
Ependymal cells	Serve as a lining for ventricles and choroid plexuses involved in production of cerebrospinal fluid

CNS, Central nervous system; *PNS,* peripheral nervous system.

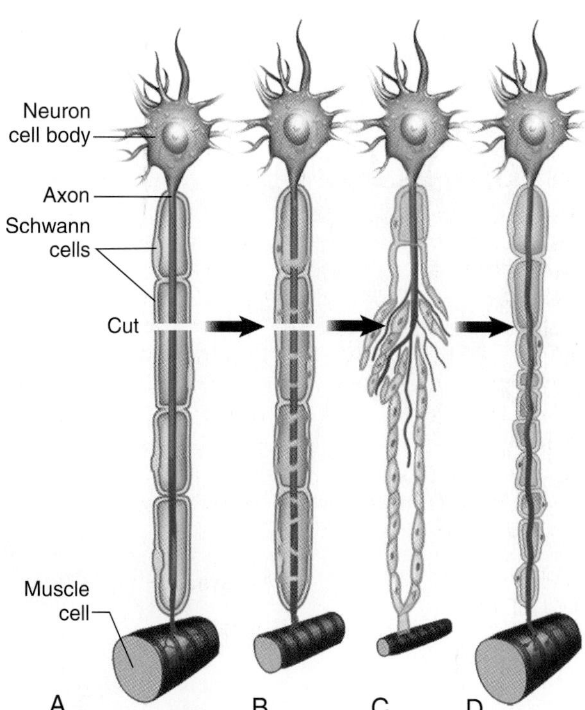

FIGURE 15-4 Repair of a Peripheral Nerve Fiber. When cut, a damaged motor axon can regrow to its distal connection only if the neurilemma remains intact (to form a guiding tunnel) and if scar tissue does not block its pathway. (From Patton KT, Thibodeau GA: *Anatomy & physiology,* ed 8, St Louis, 2013, Mosby.)

into Schwann cells that align in a column between the cut and the effector organ.

At the proximal end of the injured axon, similar changes occur, but only back as far as the next node of Ranvier. The cell body responds to trauma by swelling and then dispersing the Nissl substance (chromatolysis). During the repair process the cell increases metabolic activity, protein synthesis, and mitochondrial activity. Approximately 7 to 14 days after the injury, new terminal sprouts project from the proximal segment and may enter the remaining Schwann cell pathway. (Figure 15-4 contains a representation of these events.) This process, however, is limited to myelinated fibers and generally occurs only in the PNS. The regeneration of axonal constituents in the CNS is limited by increased scar formation and the different nature of myelin formation by the oligodendrocyte.

Nerve regeneration depends on many factors, such as location of the injury, the type of injury, the inflammatory responses, and the process of scarring. The closer the injury is to the cell body of the nerve, the greater the chances that the nerve cell will die and not regenerate. A crushing injury allows recovery more fully than does a cut injury. Crushed nerves sometimes recover fully, whereas cut nerves often form connective tissue scars that block or slow regenerating axonal branches.

NERVE IMPULSE

Neurons generate and conduct electrical and chemical impulses by selectively changing the electrical portion of their plasma membranes and influencing other nearby neurons by the release of chemicals (neurotransmitters). A neuron in its unexcited state maintains a resting membrane potential (see Chapter 1). When the membrane potential is raised sufficiently, an action potential is generated (see Figure 1-35), and the nerve impulse then flows to all parts of the neuron. The action potential response occurs only when the stimulus has sufficient strength; if it is too weak, the membrane remains unexcited. This property is sometimes termed the *all-or-none response.*

Synapses

Neurons are not physically continuous with one another. The region between adjacent neurons is called a **synapse.** Impulses are transmitted across the synapse by chemical (see Figures 15-5 and 15-14) and electrical conduction (Chapter 1); only chemical conduction is discussed here. The neurons that conduct a nerve impulse are named according to whether they relay impulses *toward* the synapse **(presynaptic neurons)** or *away* from the synapse **(postsynaptic neurons).** Four basic types of connections occur in regions of contact between the presynaptic and postsynaptic neurons. These are between axons (axo-axonic), from axon to cell body (axo-somatic), from axon to dendrite (axo-dendritic), and from dendrite to dendrite (dendro-dendritic).

Impulses are transmitted across the synapse by chemical conduction. The conducting substance is called a **neurotransmitter** and it is often formed in the neuron, transported to the **synaptic knobs (boutons)** of the presynaptic neuron's axon, and stored in synaptic vesicles within the knobs. Action potentials in the presynaptic neuron cause the synaptic vesicles to release their neurotransmitter(s) through the plasma membrane into the **synaptic cleft** (the space between the neurons), where they bind to specific neurotransmitter (protein) receptor sites on the plasma membrane of the postsynaptic neuron

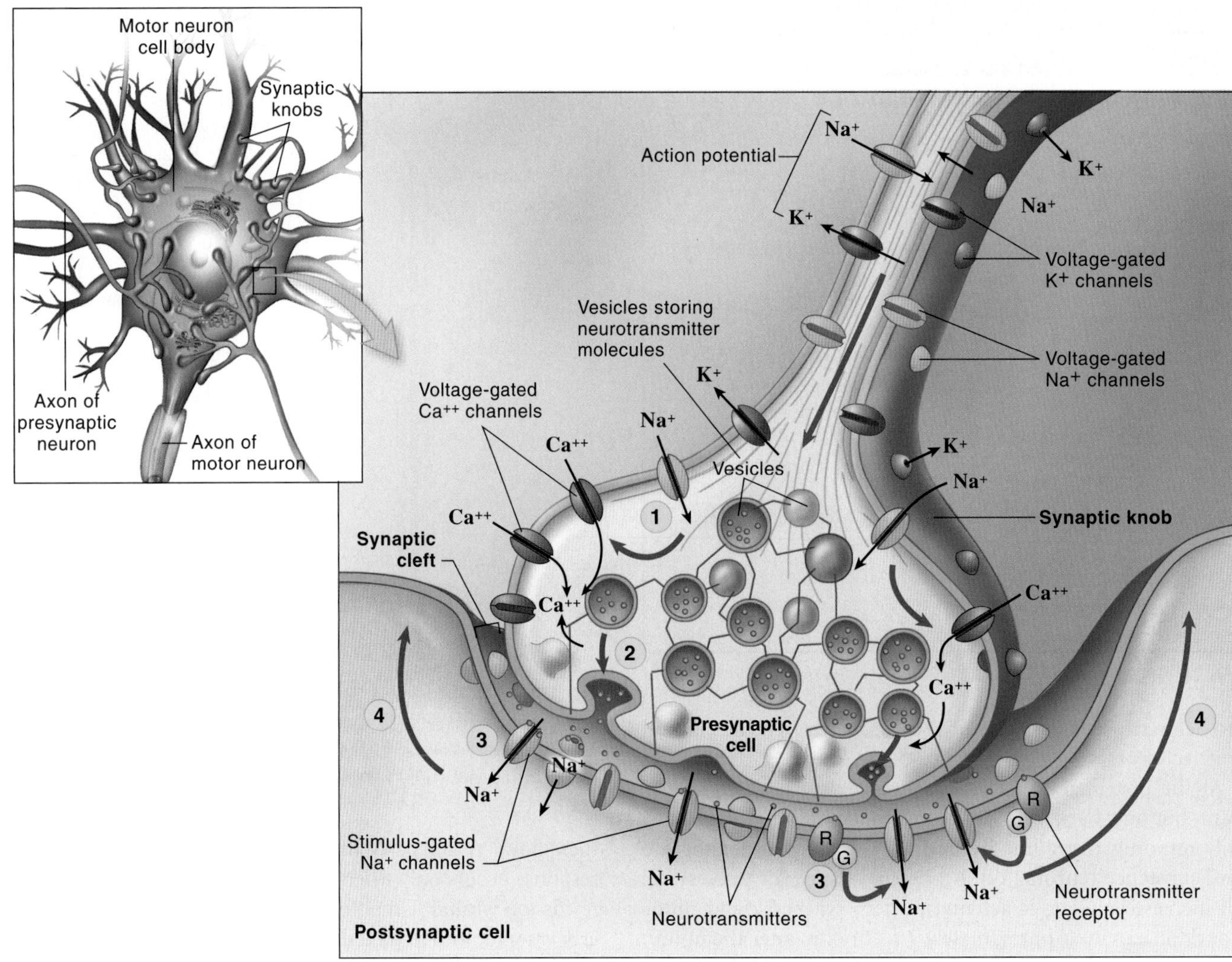

FIGURE 15-5 Neuronal Transmission and Synaptic Cleft. The electrical impulse travels along the axon of the first neuron to synapse at synaptic knobs. The chemical transmitter is secreted into the synaptic space to depolarize the membrane (dendrite or cell body) of the next neuron in the pathway. Details illustrate the synaptic knob (axon terminal) of a presynaptic neuron, the plasma membrane of a postsynaptic neuron, and a synaptic cleft. At step **(1)**—the arrival of an action potential at the synaptic knob—voltage-gated Ca^{++} channels open and allow extracellular Ca^{++} to diffuse into the presynaptic cell. At step **(2)** the Ca^{++} triggers the rapid exocytosis of neurotransmitter molecules from vesicles in the knob. At step **(3)** neurotransmitter diffuses into the synaptic cleft and binds to receptor molecules in the plasma membrane of the postsynaptic neuron. The postsynaptic receptors directly or indirectly trigger the opening of stimulus-gated ion channels, initiating a local potential in the postsynaptic neuron. At step **(4)** the local potential may move toward the axon, where an action potential may begin. (From Patton KT, Thibodeau GA: *Anatomy & physiology*, ed 8, St Louis, 2013, Mosby.)

(see Figure 15-5). Neurons can synthesize more than one neurotransmitter, and postsynaptic membranes can contain more than one type of transmitter-specific receptor.

Neurotransmitters

A neurotransmitter is defined as a chemical that "must be synthesized in the neuron, become localized in the presynaptic terminal (synaptic bouton), be released into the synaptic cleft, bind to a receptor site (binding site) on the postsynaptic membrane of another neuron or effector where it affects ion channels, and last, be removed by a specific mechanism from its site of action." More than 46 neurotransmitters, including norepinephrine, acetylcholine, dopamine, histamine, gamma-aminobutyric acid (GABA), and serotonin, have been identified.[2,3] Many of these transmitters have more than one function. For example, norepinephrine in the brain probably helps regulate mood, functions in dream sleep, and maintains arousal. Several neurotransmitters are amino acids, including GABA, glutamic acid, and aspartic acid. Small chains of amino acids, such as enkephalins and endorphins, also function as neurotransmitters. They (neuropeptides) are involved in the perception and integration of pain, as well as in emotional experiences. Neurotransmitter and neuromodulator substances are listed in Table 15-2.

Because the neurotransmitter is normally stored on one side of the synaptic cleft and the receptor sites are on the other side,

TABLE 15-2 SUBSTANCES THAT ARE NEUROTRANSMITTERS OR NEUROMODULATORS

SUBSTANCE	LOCATION	EFFECT	CLINICAL EXAMPLE
Acetylcholine	Many parts of the brain, spinal cord, neuromuscular junction of skeletal muscle, and many ANS synapses	Excitatory or inhibitory	Alzheimer disease (a type of dementia) is associated with a decrease in the number of acetylcholine-secreting neurons. Myasthenia gravis (weakness of skeletal muscles) results from a reduction in the number of acetylcholine receptors.
Monoamines			
Norepinephrine	Many areas of the brain and spinal cord; also in some ANS synapses	Excitatory or inhibitory	Cocaine and amphetamines* result in overstimulation of postsynaptic neurons.
Serotonin	Many areas of the brain and spinal cord	Generally inhibitory	Is involved with mood, anxiety, and sleep induction. Levels of serotonin are elevated in schizophrenia (delusions, hallucinations, withdrawal).
Dopamine	Some areas of the brain and ANS synapses	Generally excitatory	Parkinson disease (depression of voluntary motor control) results from destruction of dopamine-secreting neurons. Drugs used to increase dopamine production induce vomiting and schizophrenia.
Histamine	Posterior hypothalamus	Excitatory (H1 and H2 receptors) and inhibitory (H3 receptors)	There is no clear indication of histamine-associated pathologic conditions. Histamine is involved with arousal and attention and links to other brain transmitter systems.
Amino Acids			
Gamma-aminobutyric acid (GABA)	Most neurons of the CNS have GABA receptors	Majority of postsynaptic inhibition in the brain	Drugs that increase GABA function have been used to treat epilepsy by inhibiting excessive discharge of neurons.
Glycine	Spinal cord	Most postsynaptic inhibition in the spinal cord	Glycine receptors are inhibited by strychnine.
Glutamate and aspartate	Widespread in brain and spinal cord	Excitatory	Drugs that block glutamate or aspartate, such as riluzole, are used to treat amyotrophic lateral sclerosis. These drugs might prevent overexcitation from seizures and neural degeneration.
Neuropeptides			
Endorphins and enkephalins	Widely distributed in the CNS and PNS	Generally inhibitory	Morphine and heroin bind to endorphin and enkephalin receptors on presynaptic neurons and reduce pain by blocking the release of neurotransmitter.
Substance P	Spinal cord, brain, and sensory neurons associated with pain, GI tract	Generally excitatory	Substance P is a neurotransmitter involved in pain transmission pathways. Blocking release of substance P by morphine reduces pain.

From Seeley R, Stephens TD, Tate P: Anatomy and physiology, ed 7, New York, 2006, McGraw-Hill.
ANS, Autonomic nervous system; *CNS,* central nervous system; *GI,* gastrointestinal; *PNS,* peripheral nervous system.
*Increase the release and block the reuptake of norepinephrine.

chemical synapses operate in one direction. Therefore, action potentials are transmitted along a multineuronal pathway in one direction. The binding of the neurotransmitter at the receptor site changes the permeability of the postsynaptic neuron and, consequently, its membrane potential. Two possible scenarios can then follow: (1) the postsynaptic neuron may be excited (depolarized; **excitatory postsynaptic potentials [EPSPs]**), or (2) the postsynaptic neuron's plasma membrane may be inhibited (hyperpolarized; **inhibitory postsynaptic potentials [IPSPs]**). Cannabinoid transmitters are released from postsynaptic neurons that modulate neurotransmitter release from presynaptic neurons.[4,5] (Chapter 1 contains a review of electrical impulses and membrane potentials.)

Usually, a single EPSP cannot induce a neuron's action potential and the propagation of the nerve impulse. Whether an action potential occurs depends on the number and frequency of potentials the postsynaptic neuron receives—a concept known as **summation. Temporal summation** (time relationship) refers to the effects of successive, rapid impulses received from a single neuron on the same synapse. **Spatial summation** (spacing effect) is the combined effects of impulses from a number of neurons on a single synapse at the same time. **Facilitation** refers to the effect of EPSPs on the plasma membrane potential. The plasma membrane is facilitated when summation brings the membrane closer to the threshold potential and decreases the stimulus required to induce an action potential. The effect that a neurotransmitter has on the plasma membrane potential depends on the balance of these effects. The mechanisms of convergence, divergence, summation, and facilitation allow for the integrative processes of the nervous system.

Two points could be helpful in understanding the complexity of brain physiology. First, the aforementioned neuromodulators appear to function to raise or lower the membrane potentials of neurons. These chemicals facilitate or inhibit the effect of neurotransmitters. Second, reciprocal synapses between dendrites—that is, one dendrite being able to depolarize or hyperpolarize the membrane potential of another dendrite through the use of neurotransmitters—demonstrate that the interactions between neurons are far more complicated than postulated by simple on-off models of brain function.

TABLE 15-3 DIVISIONS OF THE CENTRAL NERVOUS SYSTEM

PRIMARY VESICLES	SECONDARY VESICLES	ASSOCIATED STRUCTURES
Forebrain (prosencephalon)	Telencephalon	Cerebral hemispheres
		Cerebral cortex
		Rhinencephalon
		Basal ganglia
	Diencephalon	Epithalamus
		Thalamus
		Hypothalamus
		Subthalamus
Midbrain (mesencephalon)	Mesencephalon	Corpora quadrigemina (tectum)
		Cerebral peduncles
		Tegmentum
		Red nucleus
		Substantia nigra
		Basis pedunculi
Hindbrain (rhombencephalon)	Metencephalon	Cerebellum
		Pons
	Myelencephalon	Medulla oblongata
Spinal cord	Spinal cord	Spinal cord

CENTRAL NERVOUS SYSTEM

Brain

The human brain enables individuals to reason, function intellectually, express personality and mood, and interact with the environment. The brain is a pinkish gray organ that weighs approximately 3 pounds and has the consistency of tofu or custard. It receives approximately 15% to 20% of the total cardiac output. The three major divisions of the brain, based on embryologic origin, are: (1) the forebrain, formed by the two cerebral hemispheres; (2) the midbrain, which includes the corpora quadrigemina, tegmentum, and cerebral peduncles; and (3) the hindbrain, which includes the cerebellum, pons, and medulla (Table 15-3). The midbrain, medulla oblongata, and pons make up the **brainstem,** which connects the hemispheres of the brain, cerebellum, and spinal cord. A collection of nuclei (nerve cell bodies) within the brainstem collectively constitute the **reticular formation** (Figure 15-6). The reticular formation is a large network of connected tissue nuclei that regulate vital reflexes, such as cardiovascular function and respiration. The reticular formation is essential for maintaining wakefulness and in conjunction with the cerebral cortex is referred to as the **reticular activating system.** Some nuclei within the reticular formation are involved in motor movements.[1]

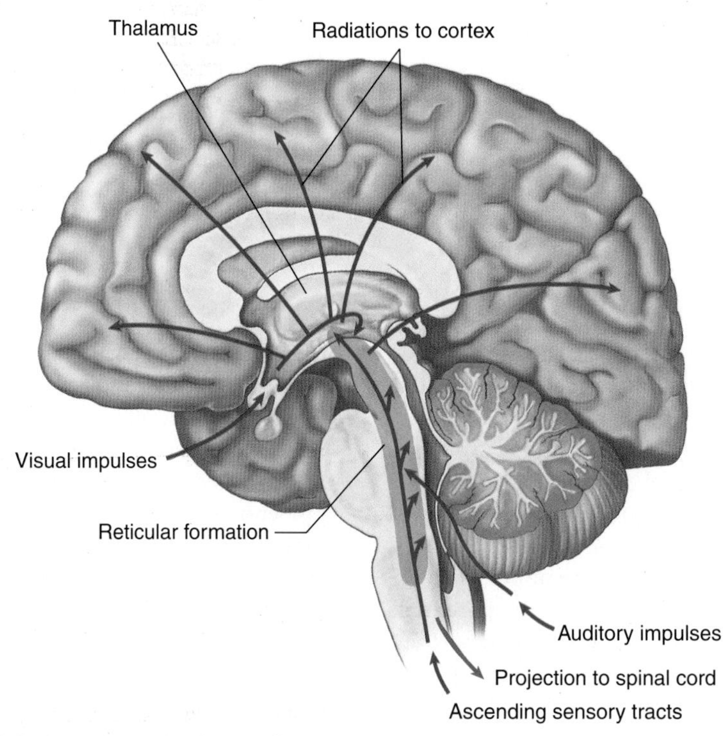

FIGURE 15-6 Reticular Activating System. System consists of nuclei in the brainstem reticular formation plus fibers (axons) that conduct to the nuclei from below and fibers that conduct from the nuclei to widespread areas of the cerebral cortex. Functioning of the reticular activating system is essential for consciousness. (From Patton KT, Thibodeau GA: *Anatomy & physiology,* ed 8, St Louis, 2013, Mosby.)

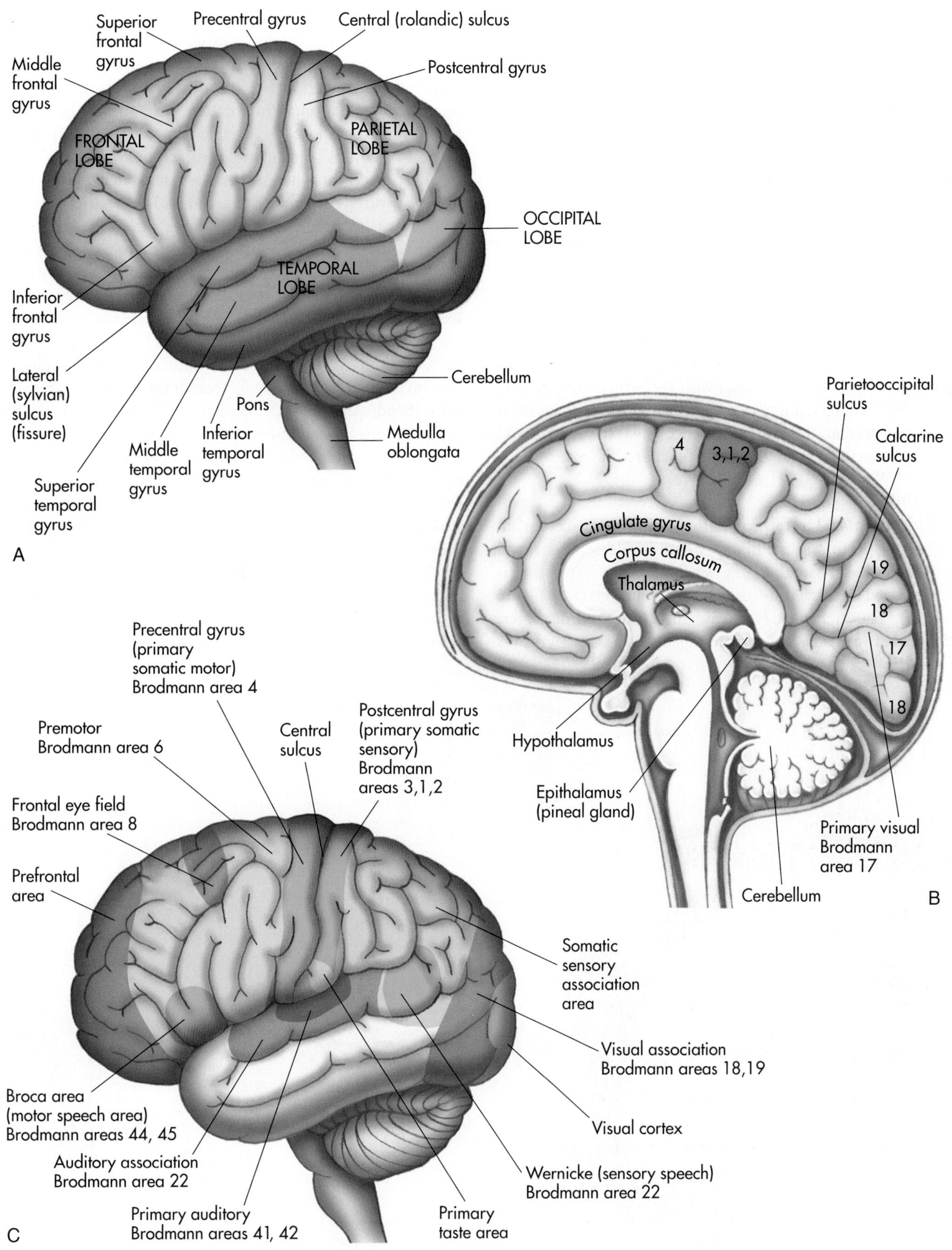

FIGURE 15-7 Cerebral Hemispheres. **A,** Left hemisphere of cerebrum *(lateral view)*. **B,** Functional areas of the cerebral cortex *(midsagittal view)*. **C,** Functional areas of the cerebral cortex *(lateral view)*.

In general, many major divisions of the brain are associated with specific functions, such as the occipital lobe and vision, but attributing specific functions to definite regions of the brain is not entirely accurate. Many activities, such as motor movements and memory, may actually be performed in several regions. Understanding functional specificity is very useful to clinical personnel, especially when attempting to localize pathologic conditions in the nervous system. A neurologist often can localize the site of a tumor, stroke, or bullet wound in an individual just by performing a neurologic examination.

Many attempts have been made to ascribe function to various regions of the cerebral cortex. (Figure 15-7, *B* and *C*, illustrates these regions and identifies some functional areas.) Another basic CNS principle, **plasticity,** holds that the CNS is capable of change. For example, children with brain damage may experience "relocation" of some functional areas to other parts of the brain. This propensity for plasticity decreases with age, which explains why older individuals tend not to recover from brain injuries as well as younger individuals. This varying balance between specificity and plasticity makes understanding brain functions difficult.

Forebrain

Telencephalon. The **telencephalon** consists of the **cerebrum** (the largest portion of the brain), which includes the cerebral cortex and **basal ganglia.** The surface of the cerebrum is characterized by numerous convolutions called *gyri* (see Figure 15-7, *A*). The gyri greatly increase the cortical surface area. Grooves between adjacent gyri are called **sulci.** Deeper grooves are referred to as **fissures.** The **cerebral cortex** contains the cell bodies and dendrites of neurons, which often are referred to as **gray matter.** Gray matter is organized into columns perpendicular to the surface that receive, integrate, store, and transmit information. **White matter** lies beneath the cerebral cortex and is composed of myelinated nerve fibers, which send neuron "messages" throughout the nervous system and body.

The two cerebral hemispheres are separated by the longitudinal fissure. The surface of each hemisphere is divided into lobes that take their names from the region of the skull under which each of them lies. The posterior margin of the **frontal lobe** is the **central sulcus (fissure of Rolando,** central fissure); it borders inferiorly on the **lateral sulcus (sylvian fissure, lateral fissure)** (see Figure 15-7, *A*). The **prefrontal area** is responsible for goal-oriented behavior (i.e., ability to concentrate), short-term or recall memory, and elaboration of thought and inhibition on the limbic (emotional) areas of the CNS. The **premotor area** (Brodmann area 6) (see Figure 15-7, *C*) is involved in programming motor movements. This area also contains the neurons that contribute to the **basal ganglia system** (extrapyramidal system—efferent pathways outside the pyramids of the medulla oblongata). The frontal eye fields (the lower portion of Brodmann area 8), which are involved in controlling eye movements, are located in the middle frontal gyrus.

The **primary motor area** (Brodmann area 4) is located along the **precentral gyrus** forming the **primary voluntary motor area,** which has a somatotopic organization that often is referred to as a *homunculus* (little man) (Figure 15-8). Electrical

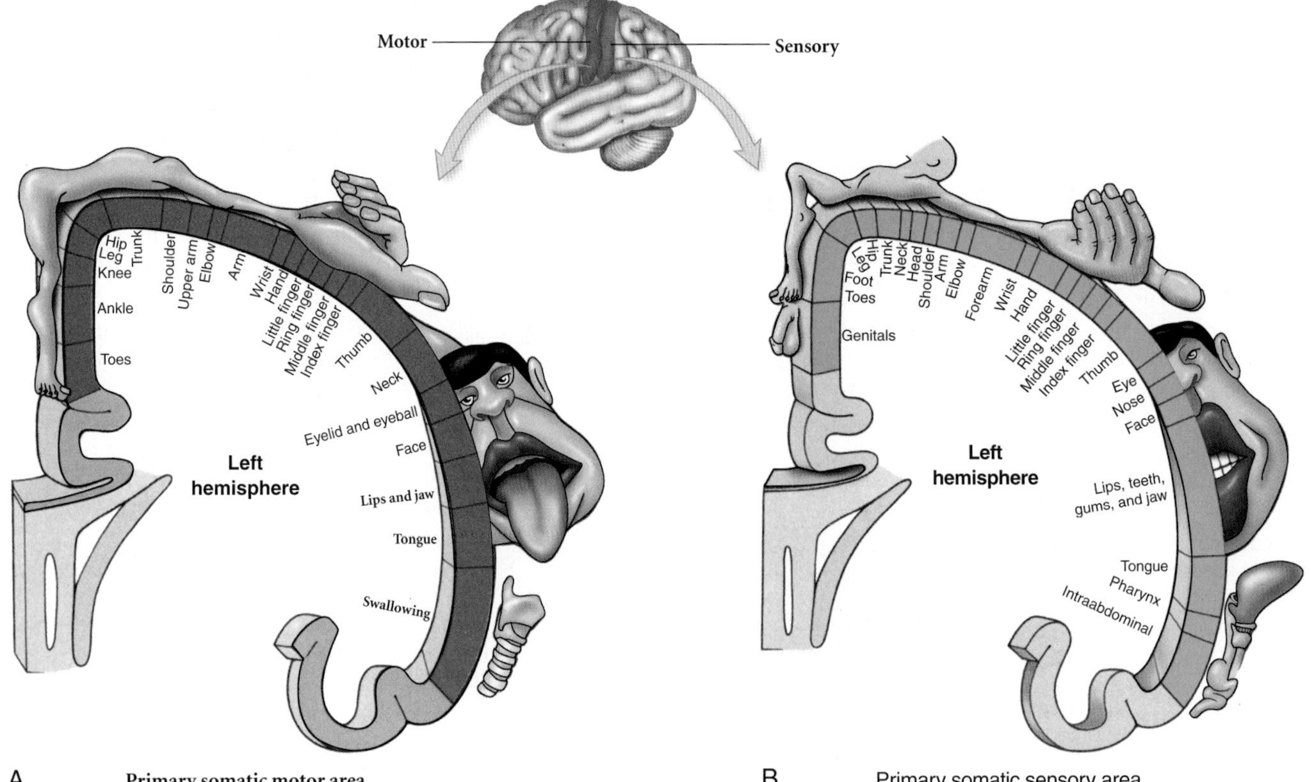

FIGURE 15-8 Primary Somatic Sensory **(A)** and Motor **(B)** Areas of the Cortex. (From Patton KT, Thibodeau GA: *Anatomy & physiology,* ed 8, St Louis, 2013, Mosby.)

stimulation of specific areas of this cortex causes specific muscles of the body to move. The medial part of the cortex in the **longitudinal fissure** (midline space between the two cerebral hemispheres) affects the lower limb and foot, whereas on the lateral surface, the superior third controls the torso and arm, the middle third the hand, and the lowest third the face and mouth/throat. The axons traveling from the cell bodies in and on either side of this gyrus project fibers (axons) that form the **corticospinal tracts** (pyramidal system) that descend down the spinal cord. Cerebral impulses control function on the opposite side of the body, a phenomenon called **contralateral control** (Figure 15-9, *A*). The **Broca speech area** (Brodmann areas 44, 45) is rostral to the inferior edge of the premotor area (Brodmann area 6) on the inferior frontal gyrus. It is usually on the left hemisphere and is responsible for the motor aspects of speech. Damage to this area, commonly as a result of a cerebrovascular accident (stroke), results in the inability to form, or difficulty in forming, words (expressive aphasia or dysphasia) (see Chapter 18).

The **parietal lobe** lies within the borders of the central, parietooccipital, and lateral sulci. This lobe contains the major area for somatic sensory input, located primarily along the **postcentral gyrus** (Brodmann areas 3, 1, 2), which is adjacent to the primary motor area. Communication between the motor and sensory areas (and among other regions in the cortex) is provided by **association fibers** (i.e., axons from association fibers). Much of this region is involved in sensory association (storage, analysis, and interpretation of stimuli). (Figure 15-8 shows the distribution of functions associated with both the primary motor area and the primary sensory area of the cerebral cortex.)

The **occipital lobe** lies caudal to the parietooccipital sulci and superior to the cerebellum. The primary visual cortex (Brodmann area 17) is located in this region and receives input from the retinas. Much of the remainder of this lobe is involved in visual association (Brodmann areas 18, 19). The **temporal lobe** lies inferior to the lateral sulcus and is composed of the superior, middle, and inferior temporal gyri. The primary auditory cortex (Brodmann area 41) and its related association area (Brodmann area 42) lie deep within the lateral sulcus on the superior temporal gyrus. The **Wernicke area** (posterior portion of Brodmann area 22) is located on the superior temporal gyrus. This area is responsible for reception and interpretation of speech, and dysfunction may result in receptive aphasia or dysphasia. The Wernicke area, along with adjacent portions of the parietal lobe, constitutes a *sensory speech area*. The temporal lobe also is involved as a major area for long-term memory and secondary functions, such as balance, taste, and smell.

Another cerebral area, the **insula,** lies hidden from view deep in the lateral sulcus. Lying directly beneath the longitudinal fissure is a massive white matter pathway called the **corpus callosum (commissural fibers).** The corpus callosum connects the two cerebral hemispheres and is essential in the coordination of activities between hemispheres, especially specific tasks that may be present in only one hemisphere (see Figures 15-7, *C*, and 15-15). As a last resort, part or all of the corpus callosum is cut to prevent the spread of epileptic loci (site of seizure activity) through the corpus callosum to the opposite cerebral hemisphere. Epileptic loci often are found in the temporal lobe (see Chapters 17 and 20). This procedure, evolved in the well-known split-brain studies, results initially in temporary aphasia and paralysis.

Inside the cerebrum are numerous tracts (white matter) and nuclei (gray matter). The major **cerebral nuclei** are called *basal ganglia* and include the corpus striatum and **amygdala.** The **corpus striatum** consists of the **lentiform nucleus** (lens shaped), the putamen and globus pallidus, and the ram's horn–shaped caudate nucleus. The **internal capsule** is a thick white-matter region in which afferent and efferent pathways, to and from the cerebral cortex, pass through the center of the cerebral hemispheres. The corpus striatum appears striped because of the rostral connections between its gray matter and the white matter of the internal capsule.

Functionally, the basal ganglia include, in addition to the corpus striatum, the subthalamic nucleus of the diencephalon and the substantia nigra of the mesencephalon. The basal ganglia plus their interconnections with the thalamus, premotor cortex, red nucleus, reticular formation, and spinal cord are part of the basal ganglia system (extrapyramidal system). The basal ganglia system is believed to exert a fine-tuning effect on motor movements. Parkinson disease and Huntington disease are conditions associated with defects of the basal ganglia (Box 15-2). They are characterized by various involuntary or exaggerated motor movements (see Chapter 17).

The **limbic system,** first described in 1878 by Broca, is composed of the **Papez circuit** (amygdala, parahippocampal gyrus, **hippocampus,** fornix, mamillary body of the hypothalamus, thalamus, and cingulate gyrus), septal area, habenula, nucleus accumbens, and other portions of the hypothalamus, and related autonomic nuclei. It is an extension or modification of the olfactory system (rhinencephalon). Its principal effects are believed to be involved with primitive behavioral responses, visceral reaction to emotion, feeding behaviors, biologic rhythms, and the sense of smell. Expression of affect (emotional and behavioral states) is mediated by extensive connections with the limbic system and prefrontal cortex. The limbic system has as one of its major functions the consolidation of memory through a reverberating circuit (see Chapter 17 and Figure 17-9).

Diencephalon. The **diencephalon,** surrounded by the cerebrum, is made up of four divisions: **epithalamus, thalamus, hypothalamus,** and **subthalamus** (see Table 15-3 and Figure 15-7, *B*). The epithalamus forms the roof of the third ventricle (a brain cavity) and composes the most superior portion of the diencephalon. It has connections between the limbic system and other parts of the brain. The pineal body (a component of the epithalamus) secretes melatonin, which maintains circadian rhythms and the sleep-wake cycle (see Chapters 16 and 21). The largest component of the diencephalon is the thalamus. It is approximately the size and volume of the thumb from the tip to the first joint. It borders and surrounds the third ventricle, and it is a major integrating center for afferent impulses to the cerebral cortex, except for olfaction. The perception of various sensations occurs at this level but requires cortical processing for interpretation. The thalamus also serves as a relay center for sensory aspects of motor information from the basal ganglia

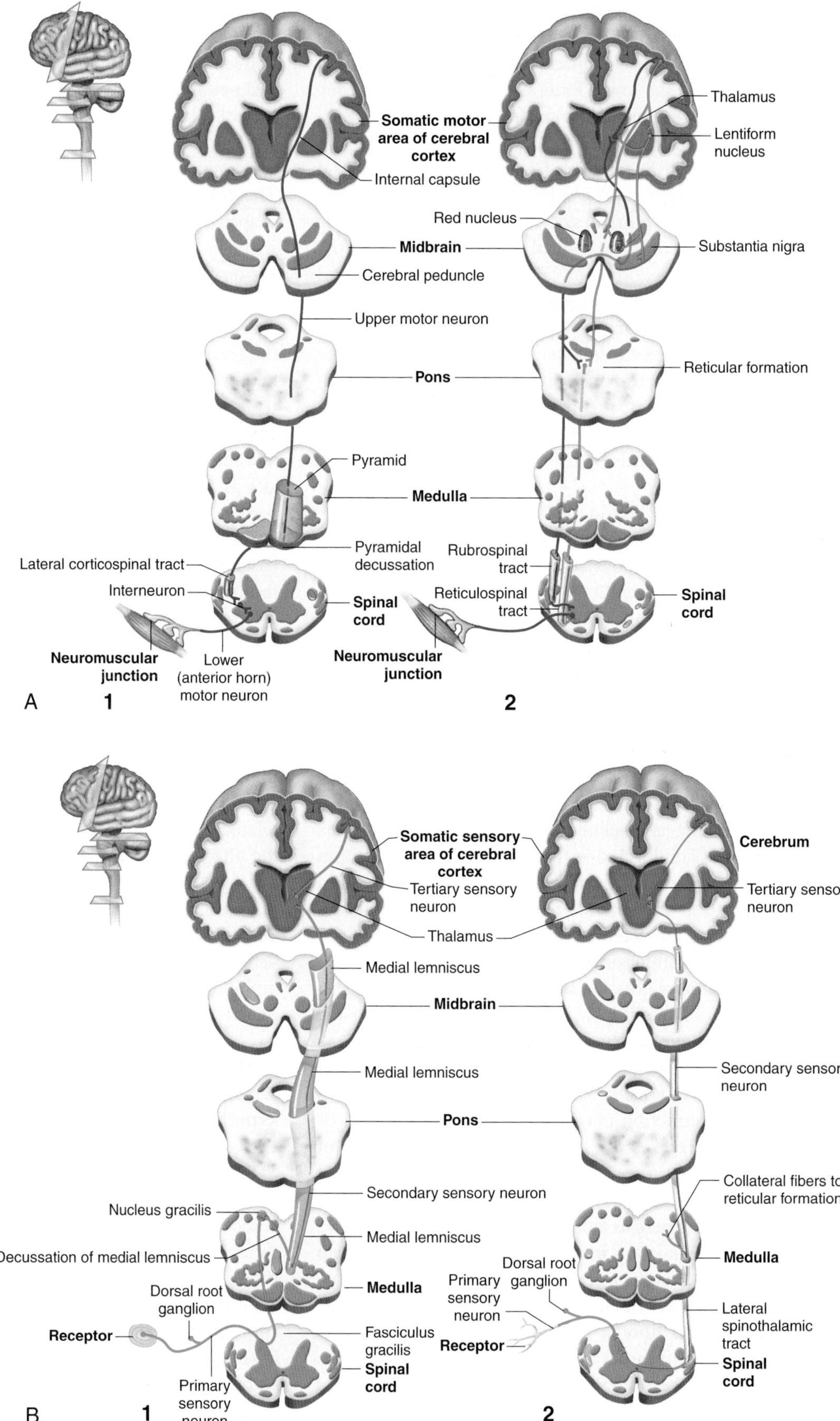

FIGURE 15-9 Examples of Somatic Motor and Sensory Pathways. **A,** Motor: **1,** the pyramidal pathway through the lateral corticospinal tract and **2,** the extrapyramidal pathways through the rubrospinal and reticulospinal tracts. Note that the pyramidal tracts decussate (cross over) to control the opposite side of the body. **B,** Sensory: **1,** pathways of the medial lemniscal system that conducts information about discriminating touch and kinesthesis and **2,** the spinothalamic pathway that conducts information about pain and temperature. (From Patton KT, Thibodeau GA: *Anatomy & physiology,* ed 8, St Louis, 2013, Mosby.)

BOX 15-2 INVASIVE TREATMENTS FOR PARKINSON DISEASE

Surgical treatment can provide gratifying relief from the disabling symptoms of Parkinson disease (PD) when pharmaceutical therapies are no longer effective or as an adjunct to pharmacotherapy. The forms of surgical intervention include deep brain stimulation (globus pallidus internus to improve motor symptoms and nucleus ventralis intermedius to improve tremor), ablation (thalamotomy, unilateral pallidotomy, and subthalamotomy), stem cell and fetal dopamine neuron replacement therapy, and gene therapy (mainly of the striatum to restore dopaminergic function). Deep brain stimulation with placement of brain electrodes is currently the surgical gold standard for treatment of PD because it results in symptom control with minimal tissue destruction. However, an ablation technique can be the preferable option for other individuals. Functional imaging during the procedures is contributing to the understanding of how these treatments affect neuronal activity. Stem cell grafts of dopamine neurons are being studied, but a number of problems still remain to be resolved, including poor cell survival of the grafted neurons and reinnervation into the host striatum. Gene therapy strategies include activation of dopamine-synthesizing enzyme genes in the subthalamic nucleus. Controlled trials are in progress and are showing some promise.

Data from Fasano A, Daniele A, Albanese A: *Lancet Neurol* 11(5):429–442, 2012; Freed CR, Zhou W, Breeze RE: *Neurotherapeutics* 8(4):549–561, 2011; Kahn E et al: *J Neurol Neurosurg Psychiatry* 83(2):164–170, 2012; Lindvall O, Björklund A: *Neurotherapeutics* 8(4):539–548, 2011; Obeso I et al: *Int Rev Psychiatry* 23(5):467–475, 2011; Politis M, Lindvall O: *BMC Med* 10:1, 2012; Schuepbach WM et al: *N Engl J Med* 368(7):610–616. 2013.

and cerebellum to appropriate cortical motor areas. Cerebral cortical information also projects to the thalamus, creating reverberating circuits.

The hypothalamus forms the base of the diencephalon. Hypothalamic function falls into two major areas: (1) maintenance of a constant internal environment and (2) implementation of behavioral patterns. Integrative centers control function of the ANS, regulation of body temperature, function of the endocrine system, and regulation of emotional expression. (Temperature regulation is discussed in Chapter 16.) The hypothalamus exerts its influence through the endocrine system, as well as through neural pathways (Box 15-3). (For endocrine functions of the hypothalamus and pituitary, see Chapter 21.)

The subthalamus flanks the hypothalamus laterally. The subthalamus contains the **subthalamic nucleus,** which is part of the basal ganglia system (p. 456).

BOX 15-3 FUNCTIONS OF THE HYPOTHALAMUS

Visceral and somatic responses
Affectual responses
Hormone synthesis
Sympathetic and parasympathetic activity
Temperature regulation
Feeding responses
Physical expression of emotions
Sexual behavior
Pleasure-punishment centers
Level of arousal or wakefulness

Midbrain

The **midbrain (mesencephalon)** (see Table 15-3) is composed of three structures: the **corpora quadrigemina,** or **tectum** (composed of the superior and inferior colliculi); the **tegmentum** (containing the red nucleus and substantia nigra); and the basis pedunculi. (The tegmentum and basis pedunculi are collectively termed the cerebral peduncles—see Figure 15-9, *A*.)

The **superior colliculi** are involved with voluntary and involuntary visual motor movements (e.g., the ability of the eyes to *track* moving objects in the visual field). The **inferior colliculi** accomplish similar motor activities but involve movements affecting the auditory system (e.g., positioning the head to improve hearing). The inferior colliculus is also a major relay center along the auditory pathway. The **red nucleus** is a major motor output center that is influenced by the cerebellum. The inferior-most portion of the basal ganglia is the **substantia nigra,** which synthesizes **dopamine,** a neurotransmitter and precursor of norepinephrine. Its dysfunction is associated with Parkinson disease (see Chapter 17) and drug addiction (see What's New? Nucleus Accumbens, Dopamine, and Drug Addiction). The **basis pedunculi** are made up of efferent fibers of the corticospinal, corticobulbar, and corticopontocerebellar tracts.

Other notable structures of this region are the nuclei and tracts of the third and fourth cranial nerves. The **cerebral aqueduct (aqueduct of Sylvius),** which carries cerebrospinal fluid (CSF), also traverses this structure. The obstruction of this aqueduct is often the cause of hydrocephalus.

Hindbrain

Metencephalon. The major structures of the **metencephalon** are the cerebellum and the pons. The **cerebellum** (see Figure 15-7, *A* and *B*) is composed of two cerebellar hemispheres covered with small convolutions called *folia.* Each hemisphere is divided by the primary fissure into two lobes (anterior and posterior) that are connected by a midline structure called the **vermis,** meaning worm.

The cerebellum is responsible for conscious and unconscious muscle synergy and for maintaining balance and posture. This is accomplished through extensive neural connections from the spinal cord and medulla oblongata through the inferior cerebellar peduncle and with the midbrain and higher structures through the superior cerebellar peduncle. The two cerebellar hemispheres receive massive cerebral cortical input through the middle cerebellar pedunculi. These connections allow extensive sampling of visual, vestibular, and proprioceptive data from other regions of the CNS and periphery. Damage to the cerebellum is characterized by ipsilateral (same side) loss of equilibrium, balance, and motor coordination. The cerebellum has ipsilateral control of the body, in contrast to the cerebral cortex, which has contralateral (opposite side) control of the body.

The **pons** (bridge) is easily recognized by its bulging appearance below the midbrain and above the medulla oblongata. Primarily, it transmits information from the cerebellum to the brainstem nuclei and relays motor information from the

WHAT'S NEW?

Nucleus Accumbens, Dopamine, and Drug Addiction

A small nucleus (see accompanying figure) in the septal area of the frontal lobe has become a center of intense research. The nucleus accumbens is considered to be the principal site of action for addictive drugs and the anatomic basis of positive reinforcement and reward. The nucleus accumbens has input from the mesencephalon (ventral tegmental area) and many other neural areas. Mesencephalon neurons project dopamine to the nucleus accumbens and can affect its activity. Other neurotransmitters involved in this positive feedback system are gamma-aminobutyric acid (GABA), serotonin, and glutamate. Opiates can interfere with this system by allowing excessive amounts of dopamine to travel to the nucleus accumbens, contributing to drug craving and addiction. Research is in progress to discover pharmaceutical agents that target specific neurotransmitter receptors for the treatment of drug addiction.

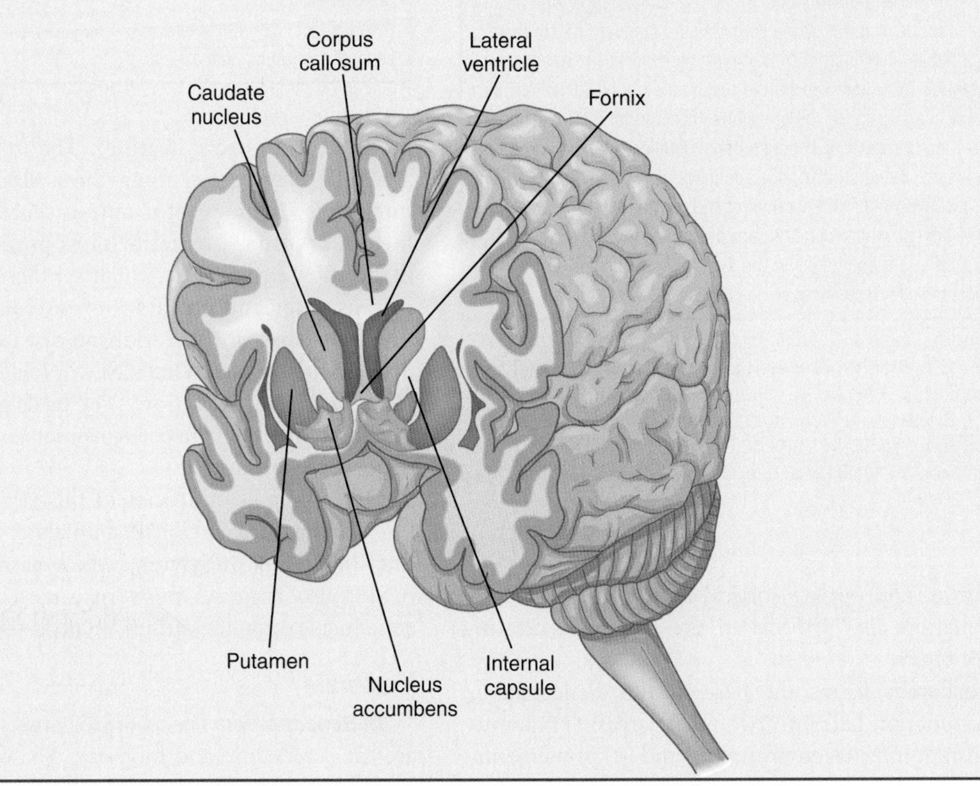

Data from Gardner EL: *Adv Psychosom Med* 30:22–60, 2011; Lee BR, Dong Y: *Neuropharmacology* 61(7):1060–1069, 2011; Morales M, Pickel VM: *Ann N Y Acad Sci* 1248:71–88, 2012; Hikida T et al: *Proc Natl Acad Sci U S A* 110(1):342–347, 2013.

cerebral cortex to the contralateral cerebellar hemisphere. The pons is an important center for the control of respiration (i.e., rate and relationship of inspiration to expiration). The nuclei of cranial nerves V through VIII are located in this structure.

Myelencephalon. The **medulla oblongata** comprises the **myelencephalon** and is the lowest portion of the brainstem. Reflex activities, such as heart rate, respiration, blood pressure, coughing, sneezing, swallowing, and vomiting, are controlled in this area. The nuclei of cranial nerves IX through XII (see Table 15-6 for discussion) are located in this region. The lowest portion of the reticular formation is found here as well.

A major portion of the descending motor pathways (i.e., corticospinal tracts) crosses to the contralateral side, or decussates, at the inferior medulla oblongata (see Figure 15-9, *A*). These pathways, together with other areas of decussation in the CNS, are the basis for the phenomenon of contralateral control.

Spinal Cord

The **spinal cord** is the portion of the CNS that lies within the vertebral canal and is surrounded and protected by the vertebral column. The spinal cord has many functions, which include being a long nerve tract that connects the brain and body, conducting somatic and autonomic reflexes, providing motor pattern control centers, and serving as a sensory and motor modulation center. It continues from the medulla oblongata and ends inferiorly at the level of the first or second lumbar vertebra in adults (Figure 15-10). The end of the spinal cord, the **conus medullaris,** is cone shaped (Figure 15-11). Spinal nerves continue from the end of the spinal cord and form a nerve bundle called the **cauda equina.** The thin filament anchor from the conus medullaris to the coccyx is the **filum terminale** (see Figure 15-10).

Grossly, the spinal cord is divided into sections (8 cervical, 12 thoracic, 5 lumbar, 5 sacral, and 1 coccygeal) that

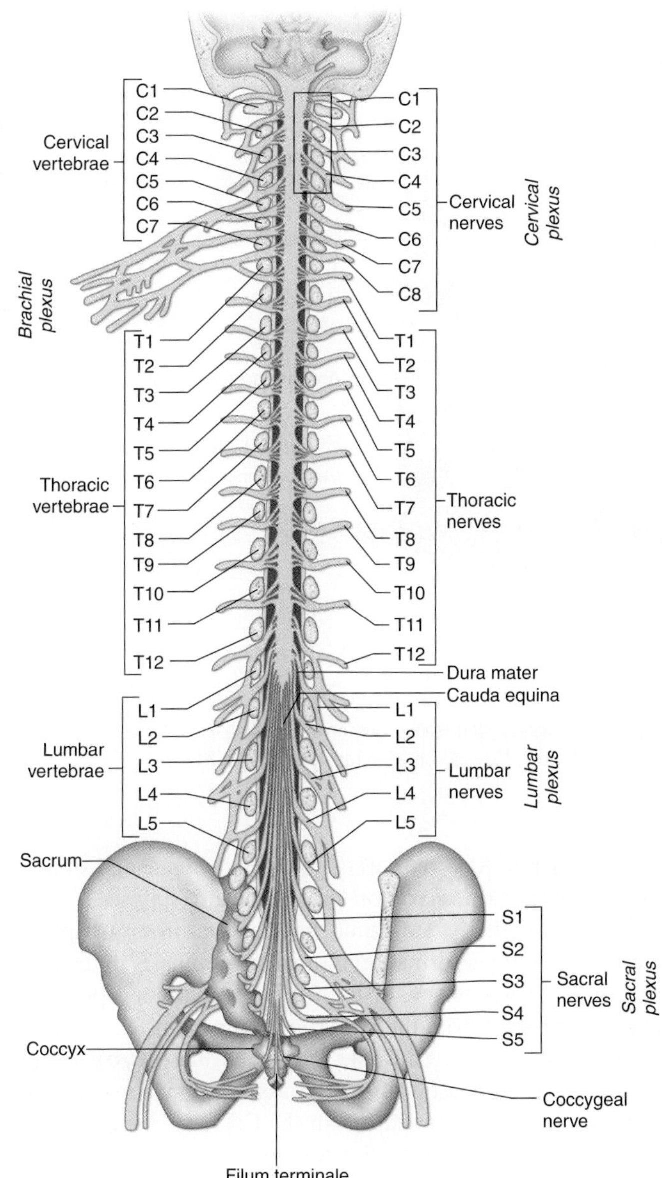

FIGURE 15-10 Spinal Cord Within Vertebral Canal and Exiting Spinal Nerves. Posterior view of brainstem and spinal cord in situ with spinal nerves and plexus. (From Patton KT, Thibodeau GA: *Anatomy & physiology,* ed 8, St Louis, 2013, Mosby.)

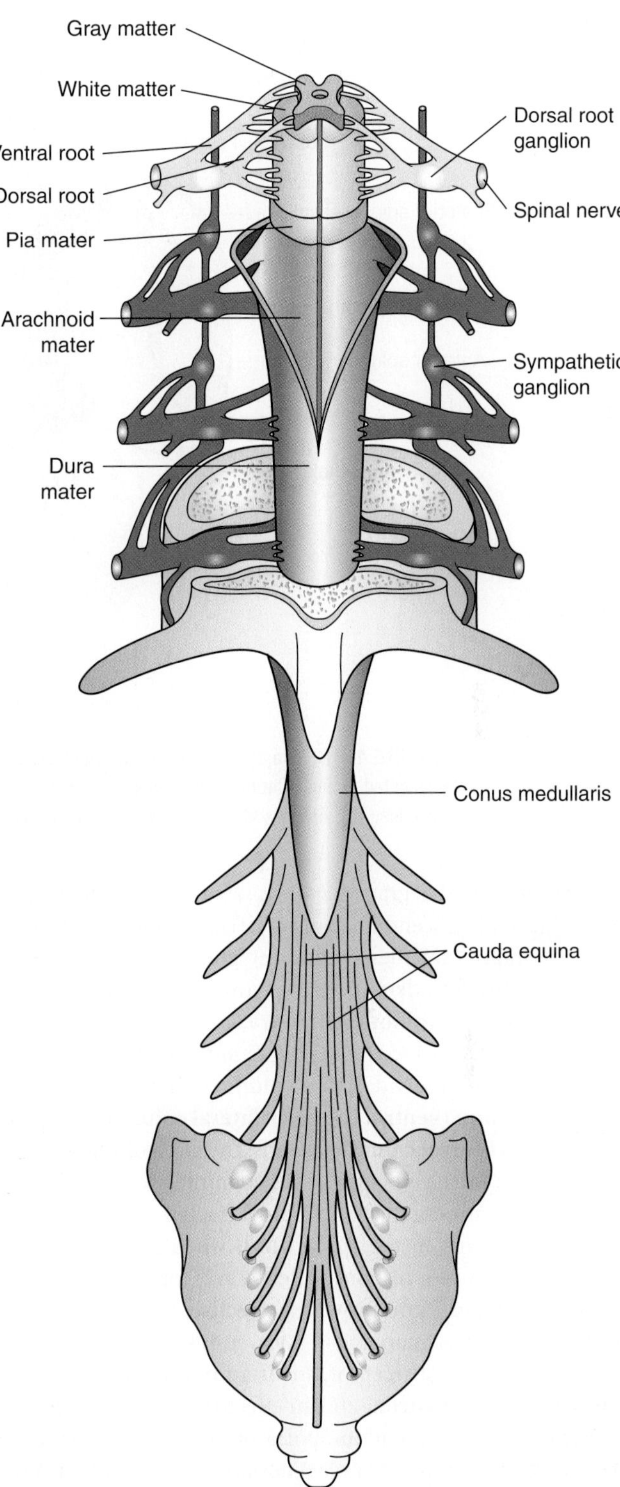

FIGURE 15-11 Spinal Nerves and Coverings of the Spinal Cord. Note how the dura mater extends to cover the spinal nerve roots and nerves. (Modified from Thibodeau GA, Patton KT: *Structure and function of the body,* ed 14, St Louis, 2012, Mosby.)

correspond to paired nerves (see Figure 15-10). A cross section of the spinal cord (see Figures 15-11 and 15-12) is characterized by a butterfly-shaped inner core of gray matter (containing nerve cell bodies). The **central canal** lies in the center of this region and extends through the spinal cord from its origin in the fourth ventricle. The gray matter of the spinal cord is divided into three regions with specific functional characteristics. These regions include the **posterior horn (dorsal horn),** which is composed primarily of interneurons and axons from sensory neurons whose cell bodies lie in the **sensory ganglion (dorsal root ganglion).** At the tip of the posterior horn is the **substantia gelatinosa,** a structure involved in pain transmission (see Chapter 16). The **intermediolateral gray horn (lateral horn)** contains cell bodies involved with the ANS. The **anterior horn (ventral horn)** contains the nerve cell bodies for efferent pathways leaving the spinal cord by way of spinal nerves. The terms *anterior* and *posterior* are preferred by many authors for describing human spinal cord anatomy, whereas *dorsal* and *ventral* are the common zoologic (veterinary) terms.

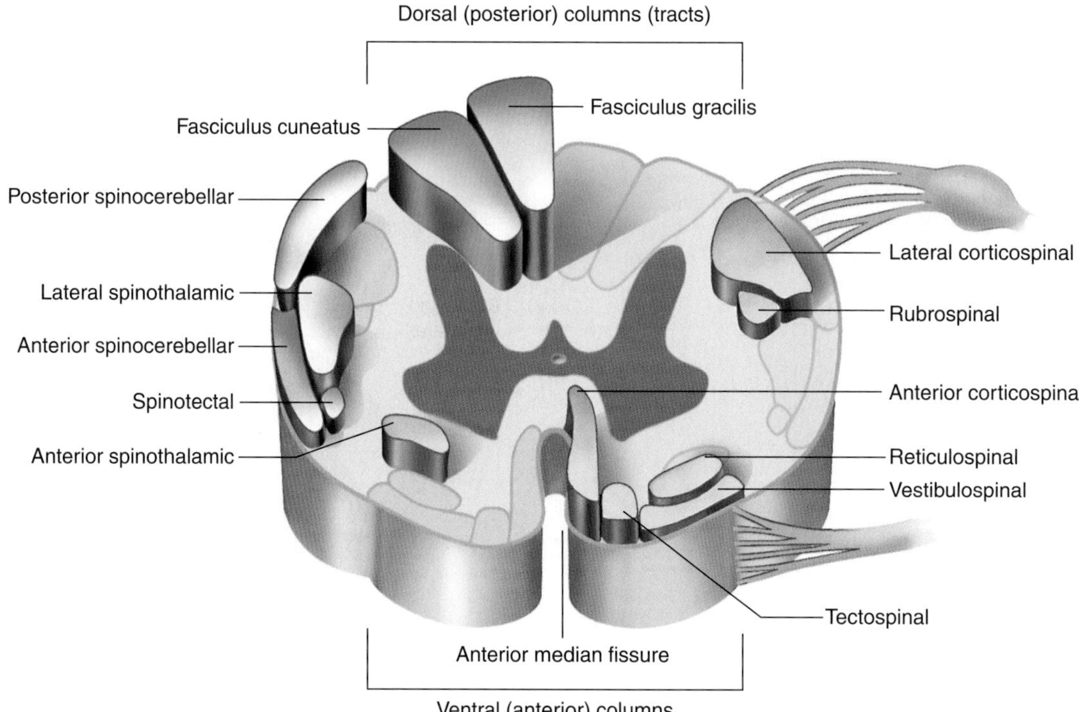

FIGURE 15-12 Major Tracts of the Spinal Cord. The major ascending (sensory) tracts, shown only on the left here, are highlighted in blue. The major descending (motor) tracts, shown only on the right, are highlighted in red. (From Patton KT, Thibodeau GA: *Anatomy & physiology,* ed 8, St Louis, 2013, Mosby.)

Surrounding the gray matter is white matter that forms ascending and descending pathways called **spinal tracts** and short ascending and descending integrative pathways. Spinal tracts are named to denote their beginning and ending points. For example, the **spinothalamic tract** carries nerve impulses from the spinal cord to the thalamus in the diencephalon. The white matter is subdivided into columns. These consist of the **anterior column (ventral column), lateral column,** and **posterior column (dorsal column),** that is, the fasciculus gracilis and fasciculus cuneatus. (Figure 15-12 identifies the location and principal activities of the major spinal tracts.)

Neural circuits in the spinal cord, when activated, display specific sets of motor responses. **Reflex arcs** form basic units that respond to stimuli and provide protective circuitry for motor output. Structures mandatory for a simple reflex arc (monosynaptic reflex) are a receptor, an **afferent (sensory) neuron,** an **efferent (motor) neuron,** and an effector muscle or gland. The afferent neuron is a pseudounipolar neuron, with its cell body in the sensory ganglion. A simple reflex arc contains only two neurons (e.g., knee jerk reflex). Most reflex arcs include one or more interneurons or association neurons between the afferent and efferent neurons (polysynaptic reflex). (Figure 15-13 illustrates a reflex arc.) The transmission time for polysynaptic reflexes is slower than that for monosynaptic reflexes because there are two or more synaptic delays. The afferent neuron of the reflex arc simultaneously sends sensory information to the effector organ and to higher CNS centers (see Figure 15-8, *B*; also see Figure 16-3). The motor effects from reflex arcs generally occur before perception of the event in the higher centers of the brain. Much of the regulation of the internal environment is mediated by polysynaptic ANS reflexes (e.g., cardiac muscle and smooth muscle contraction/relaxation and glandular responses).

Afferent pathways transmit information from peripheral receptors and the information ultimately terminates in the cerebral or cerebellar cortex, or both. Efferent pathways primarily relay information from the cerebrum to the brainstem or spinal cord (see Figure 15-9, *A*). **Upper motor neurons** (i.e., corticospinal and corticobulbar tracts) are the classification of motor pathways completely contained within the CNS (see Figure 17-31). Their primary roles include directing, influencing, and modifying reflex arcs, lower-level control centers, and motor (and some sensory) neurons. Generally, upper motor neurons form synapses with interneurons, which then form synapses with lower motor neurons before projecting into the periphery. **Lower motor neurons** (i.e., cranial and spinal efferent neurons) are responsible for direct influence on muscles. Their cell bodies lie in the gray matter of the spinal cord, but their processes extend into the PNS (see Figure 15-9, *A* and Figure 17-32). Destruction of upper motor neurons usually results in initial paralysis followed within days or weeks by partial recovery, whereas destruction of the lower motor neurons often leads to permanent paralysis, unless peripheral nerve damage is followed by nerve regeneration. (Injury to motor neurons is discussed in Chapter 18.)

Muscle activity (i.e., stimulation and contraction) is regulated by nerve impulses. Motor neurons innervate one or more muscle cells, forming **motor units** consisting of a neuron and the skeletal muscles it stimulates. The junction between the axon of the motor neuron and the plasma membrane of the muscle cell is called the **neuromuscular (myoneural) junction** (Figure 15-14). The skeletal muscle neuromuscular junction is

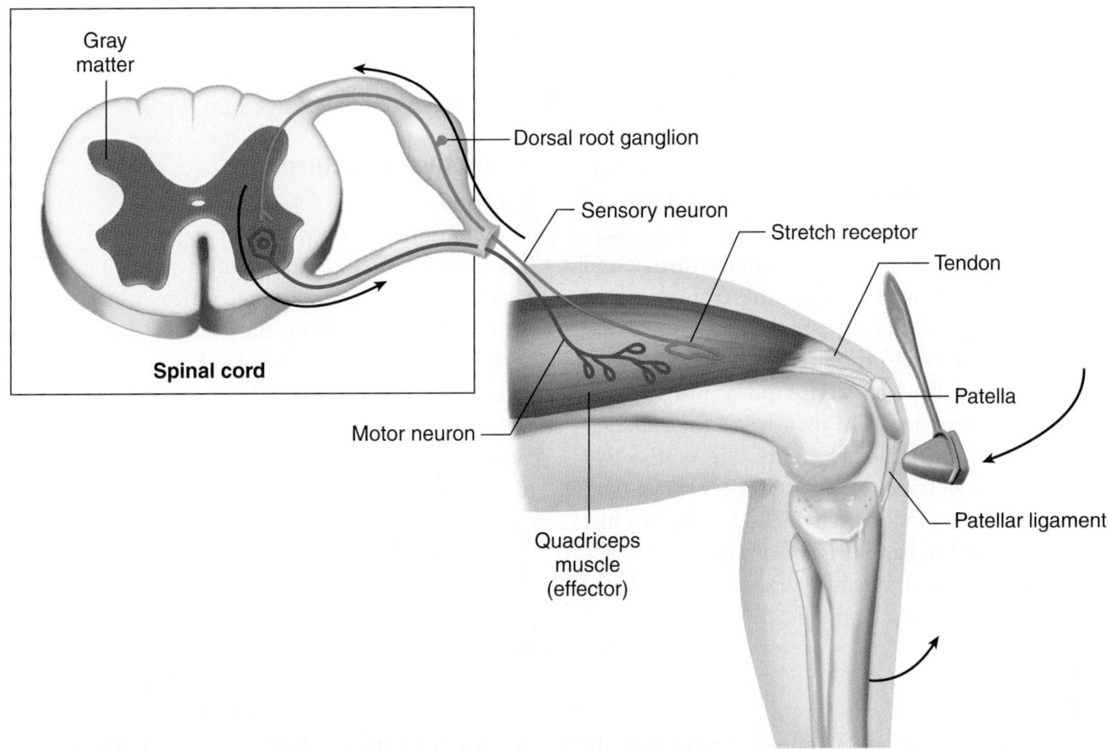

FIGURE 15-13 **Cross Section of Spinal Cord Showing Simple Reflex Arc.** (From Patton KT, Thibodeau GA: *Anatomy & physiology,* ed 8, St Louis, 2013, Mosby.)

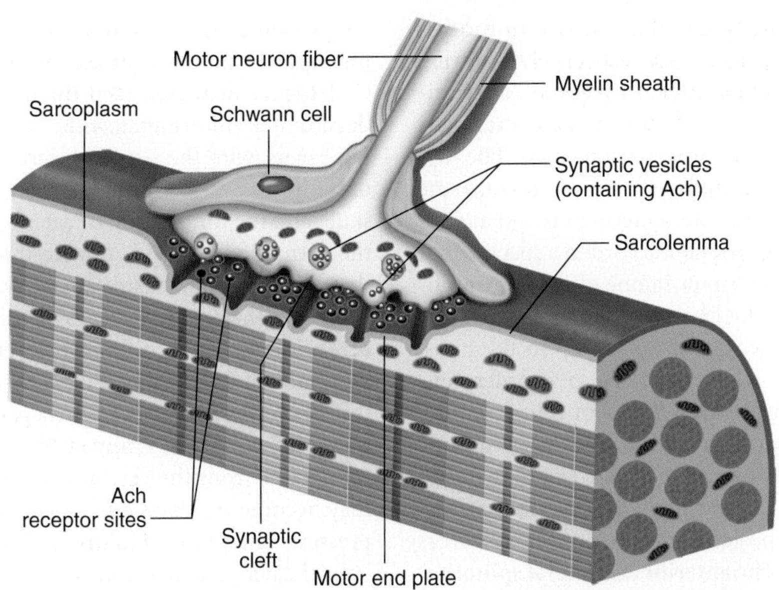

FIGURE 15-14 **Neuromuscular Junction.** This figure shows how the distal end of a motor neuron fiber forms a synapse, or "chemical junction," with an adjacent muscle fiber. Neurotransmitters (specifically, acetylcholine *[Ach]*) are released from the neuron's synaptic vesicles and diffuse across the synaptic cleft where they stimulate receptors in the motor end-plate region of the sarcolemma. (From Patton KT, Thibodeau GA: *Anatomy & physiology,* ed 8, St Louis, 2013, Mosby.)

more elaborate than the simpler smooth muscle neuromuscular junction.

Motor Pathways (Tracts)

The four clinically relevant motor pathways (tracts) are the **lateral corticospinal, corticobulbar** (upper motor neurons of cranial nerves), basal ganglia, and **vestibulospinal pathways.** The corticospinal (see Figure 15-9, *A*) and corticobulbar (see Figure 17-31) are essentially the same tract and consist of a two-neuron chain. The cell bodies originate in and around the precentral gyrus; pass through the corona radiata of the cerebrum, the internal capsule, and the middle three fifths of the basis pedunculus, pons, and pyramid; decussate (cross contralaterally) in the medulla oblongata; and form the lateral corticospinal tract of the spinal cord (see Figure 15-12). The lateral corticospinal tract axons (upper motor neurons) leave the tract to go to specific interneurons or motor neurons in the anterior horn. The lateral corticospinal tract has the same somatotopic organization as the body. These spinal motor neurons project to specific motor units and are lower motor neurons. The corticobulbar (bulbar refers to brainstem) tract can be thought of as the part of the corticospinal tract that innervates the cranial motor nuclei for eye, face, tongue, throat, and neck movement. This tract innervates all the cranial motor nuclei bilaterally except for the facial (spinal), accessory, and hypoglossal nuclei, which receive primarily contralateral innervation. These tracts are involved in precise motor movements. The basal ganglia are part of a system that drives the reticular descending tracts. (Figure 15-12 shows only one of the two reticulospinal tracts.) These tracts modulate motor movement by inhibiting and exciting spinal activity. The vestibulospinal tract is an extrapyramidal tract and arises from the lateral vestibular nucleus in the pons and causes the extensor muscles of the body to rapidly contract, most dramatically witnessed when a person starts to fall backward.

Sensory Pathways

The three clinically important spinal afferent pathways are the posterior (dorsal) column, anterior spinothalamic, and lateral spinothalamic (see Figure 15-12; also see Figures 16-2 and 16-3). The **posterior (dorsal) column pathway** has a somatotopic organization (looks like your body) with the fasciculus gracilis and fasciculus cuneatus, respectively, carrying lower body and upper body fine touch, two-point discrimination, and proprioceptive information (i.e., **epicritic**). The posterior column is formed by a three-neuron chain. The first neuron of the chain is the primary afferent neuron. It is also the sensory neuron of the reflex arc. After entering the spinal cord it sends its axon ipsilaterally up the spinal cord in a specific part of the posterior column and synapses in one of three posterior column nuclei in the hindbrain. A basketball center has primary afferent neurons that run from the great toe up to the pons, which could be more than 6 feet long. The second-order neuron has its cell body in one of the three posterior column nuclei and sends its axon contralaterally and ascends to a specific nucleus of the thalamus and synapses. The third-order neuron, originating in the thalamus, continues the tract into the internal capsule, corona radiata, and postcentral gyrus (Brodmann areas 3, 1, 2) (see Figure 15-7, *C*). The **anterior** and **lateral spinothalamic tracts** are responsible for vague touch and for pain and temperature, respectively (see Figure 15-9, *B*). These modalities are referred to as **protopathic.**

Today the anterior and lateral spinothalamic tracts are combined by many neuroanatomists into the anterolateral system because these modalities are difficult to localize into finite tracts in the spinal cord. These tracts also form a three-neuron chain. However, the primary afferent neurons synapse in the posterior horn of the spinal cord, not just at the level they enter the intervertebral foramen but in a number of spinal segments above and below their point of entry. This is an example of divergence. The axons of the second-order neurons in the posterior horn cross to the contralateral side in the spinal cord in the lateral column, and ascend to the same thalamic nucleus as the posterior column pathway and continue on with the posterior column pathway to the postcentral gyrus.

Protective Structures

Cranium

The cranium is composed of eight bones. The cranial vault functions to enclose and protect the brain and its associated structures. The **galea aponeurotica,** which is a thick, fibrous band of tissue overlying the cranium between the frontal and occipital muscles, affords added protection to the bony structure of the skull. The subgaleal space has venous connections with the dural sinuses, and with increased intracranial pressure, blood can be shunted to this space, thus reducing pressure in the intracranial cavity. The subgaleal space is also a common site for placement of wound drains after intracranial surgery.

The floor of the cranial vault is irregular and contains many foramina (openings) that act as exit sites for cranial nerves, blood vessels, and the spinal cord. The cranial floor is divided into three fossae (depressions). The frontal lobes lie in the **anterior fossa;** the temporal lobes and base of the diencephalon lie in the **middle fossa (temporal fossa);** and the cerebellum lies in the **posterior fossa.** These terms are commonly used anatomic landmarks to describe the location of intracranial lesions.

Meninges

Surrounding the brain and spinal cord are three protective membranes: the dura mater, the arachnoid, and the pia mater. Collectively they are called the **meninges** (Figure 15-15). The **dura mater** (meaning literally "hard mother") is composed of two layers, with the venous sinuses formed between them. The outermost layer forms the **periosteum (endosteal layer)** of the skull, and the **inner dura,** or **meningeal layer,** is responsible for the formation of rigid, double-thickness membranous plates that serve to support and separate various brain structures.

One of these membranous plates (see Figure 15-15), the **falx cerebri,** dips between the two cerebral hemispheres along the longitudinal fissure. The falx cerebri is anchored anteriorly to the base of the brain at the crista galli of the ethmoid bone. The **tentorium cerebelli** is a membrane that separates the cerebellum below from the cerebral structures above. The tentorium may become involved during periods of increased intracranial pressure caused by an injury to the brain. An injury within the cranial cavity tends to shift intracranial contents, and as structures shift, they tend to be compressed against these rigid membranes, resulting in damage or destruction. A common example is tentorial herniation.

Below the dura mater lies the **arachnoid membrane,** characterized by its filmy, weblike structure. It loosely follows the contours of the cerebral structures but lies over the sulci.

The **subdural space** lies between the dura and arachnoid. Many small bridging veins that have little support traverse the subdural space. Their disruption results in a subdural hematoma (see Chapter 18 and Figures 18-5 and 18-6). The **subarachnoid space,** which contains CSF, lies between the arachnoid and the pia mater (see Figure 15-15). Damage to

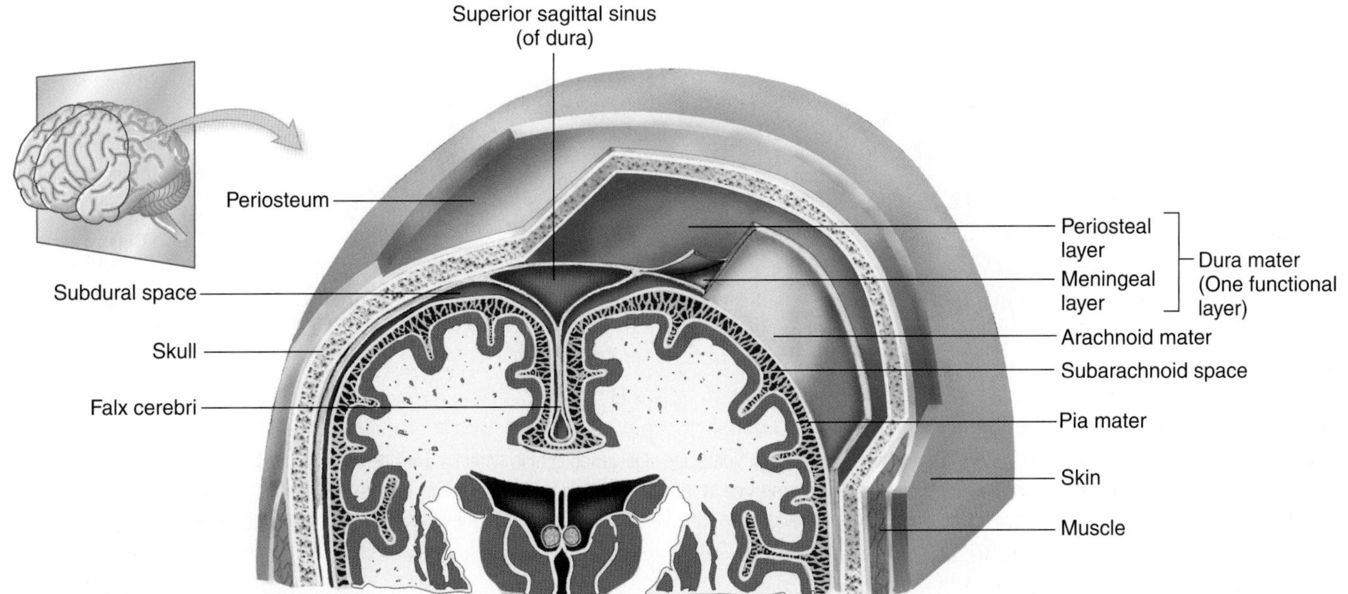

FIGURE 15-15 **Coverings of the Brain.** Frontal section of the superior portion of the head, as viewed from the front. The bony and the membranous coverings of the brain can be seen. (From Patton KT, Thibodeau GA: *Anatomy & physiology,* ed 8, St Louis, 2013, Mosby.)

intracranial vessels can lead to a condition called *subarachnoid hemorrhage,* which frequently results in signs of meningeal irritation, such as neck stiffness, positive Kernig sign, and low back pain.

Unlike the dura mater and arachnoid, the delicate **pia mater** (see Figure 15-15) closely adheres to the surface of the brain and spinal cord and even follows the sulci and fissures. It provides support for blood vessels serving brain tissue. The **choroid plexuses,** structures that produce cerebrospinal fluid (CSF), arise from the pia mater. The spinal cord is anchored to the vertebrae by extensions of the meninges called **denticulate ligaments.** The meninges continue beyond the end of the spinal cord to the lower portion of the sacrum. CSF, contained within the subarachnoid space, also circulates down to the large **lumbar cistern,** which extends from the second lumbar vertebra to the second sacral vertebra. Cisterns are expanded areas of the subarachnoid space. The **cerebellomedullary cistern (cisterna magna)** and the pontine cistern are two other important cisterns.

The meninges form potential and real spaces important to understanding functional and pathologic mechanisms. For example, between the dura mater and skull lies a potential space termed the **epidural space** (see Figure 15-15). In the spinal canal is a real epidural space filled with fatty tissue and a venous plexus. The arterial supply to the meninges consists of blood vessels that lie within grooves in the skull. As a result of trauma, the skull can be fractured and the blood vessels disrupted. The ruptured vessels can lead to an accumulation of blood within the epidural space, called an *epidural hematoma* (see Chapter 18 and Figure 18-4). Persons with alcoholism often fall and injure their head, resulting in an epidural hematoma. An inflammation of the meninges (meningitis) also can have life-threatening implications because of the relative proximity to the brain. (See Chapter 18.)

TABLE 15-4 COMPOSITION OF CEREBROSPINAL FLUID

CONSTITUENT	NORMAL VALUE
Na^+	148 mM
K^+	2.9 mM
Cl^-	125 mM
HCO_3^-	22.9 mM
Glucose (fasting)	50-75 mg/dl (60% of serum glucose)
pH	7.3
Protein	15-45 mg/dl
Albumin	80%
Gamma globulin	6-10%
Cells	
White (lymphocytes)	0-6/mm^3
Red (red blood cell [RBC])	0/mm^3

Cl^-, Chloride; *HCO_3^-*, bicarbonate; *K^+*, potassium; *Na^+*, sodium.

Cerebrospinal Fluid and the Ventricular System

Cerebrospinal fluid (CSF) is a clear, colorless fluid similar to blood plasma and interstitial fluid. The intracranial and spinal cord structures float in CSF and are thereby partially protected from jolts and blows. The buoyant properties of the CSF also prevent the brain from tugging on meninges, nerve roots, and blood vessels. (Constituents of CSF are listed in Table 15-4.) Between 125 and 150 ml of CSF, approximately the quantity of a small cup of coffee, is circulating within the **ventricles** (small cavities) and subarachnoid space at any given time. Approximately 600 ml of CSF is produced daily.

The choroid plexuses in the lateral, third, and fourth ventricles produce the major portion of CSF. (Ventricles are illustrated in Figures 15-15 and 15-16.) These plexuses are characterized by a rich network of blood vessels, supplied by the pia

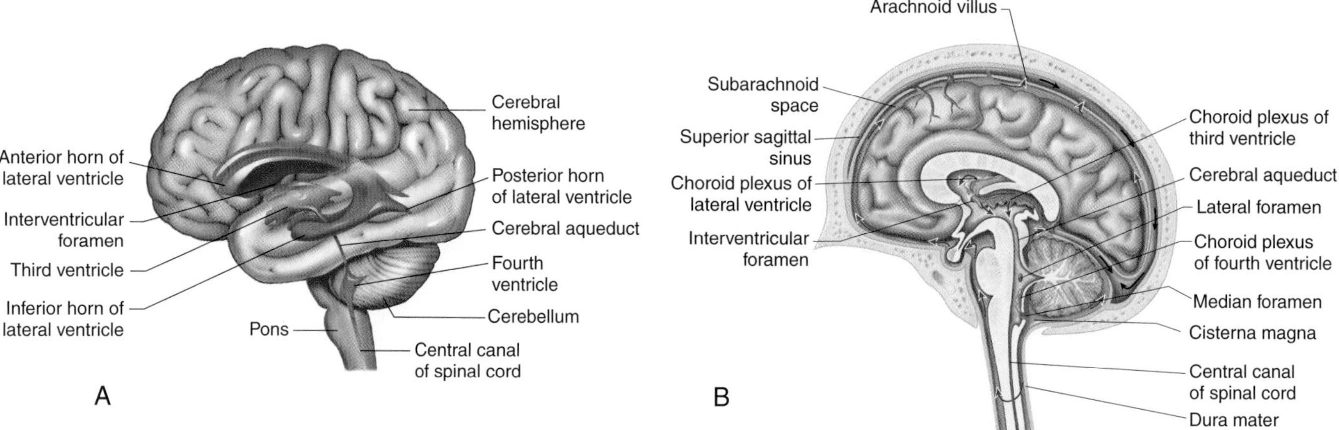

FIGURE 15-16 Flow of Cerebrospinal Fluid. **A,** Ventricles highlighted in blue within a translucent brain in a left lateral view. **B,** Flow of cerebrospinal fluid. The fluid is produced by filtration of blood by the choroid plexus of each ventricle, and from the ventricles flows to the subarachnoid space and then to the blood. (From Patton KT, Thibodeau GA: *Anatomy & physiology,* ed 8, St Louis, 2013, Mosby.)

mater, that lie in close contact with ventricular ependymal cells that secrete and absorb CSF.

The CSF exerts pressure within the brain and spinal cord. When a person is lying down, CSF pressure is approximately 120 to 180 mm of water pressure, or approximately 9 to 14 mmHg pressure. CSF flow is a result of a pressure gradient between the arterial system and the CSF-filled cavities. Beginning in the lateral ventricles, the CSF flows through the **interventricular foramen (foramen of Monro)** into the third ventricle and then passes through the cerebral aqueduct (aqueduct of Sylvius) into the fourth ventricle. From the fourth ventricle, the CSF may pass through either the paired **lateral apertures (foramina of Luschka)** into the pontine cisterns, located along the basal pons, or the midline **median aperture (foramen of Magendie)** into the cerebellomedullary cistern before communicating with the subarachnoid spaces of the brain and spinal cord. The CSF does not, however, accumulate. Instead, it is reabsorbed into the venous circulation through the arachnoid villi, primarily located superior to the falx cerebri in the **superior sagittal sinus.** The **arachnoid villi** protrude from the arachnoid space, through the dura mater, and lie within the blood flow of the venous sinuses. CSF is reabsorbed by means of a pressure gradient between the arachnoid villi and the cerebral venous sinuses. The villi function as one-way valves directing CSF outflow into the blood but preventing blood flow into the subarachnoid space. Thus CSF is derived from the blood, and after circulating throughout the CNS, it returns to the blood.

Samples of CSF are withdrawn for diagnostic purposes either (1) by inserting a needle between the third and fourth lumbar vertebrae into the lumbar cistern (subarachnoid space)—a procedure called **lumbar puncture**—or (2) by placing an intraventricular catheter. Spinal anesthesias (blocks) are administered in a manner similar to the lumbar puncture.

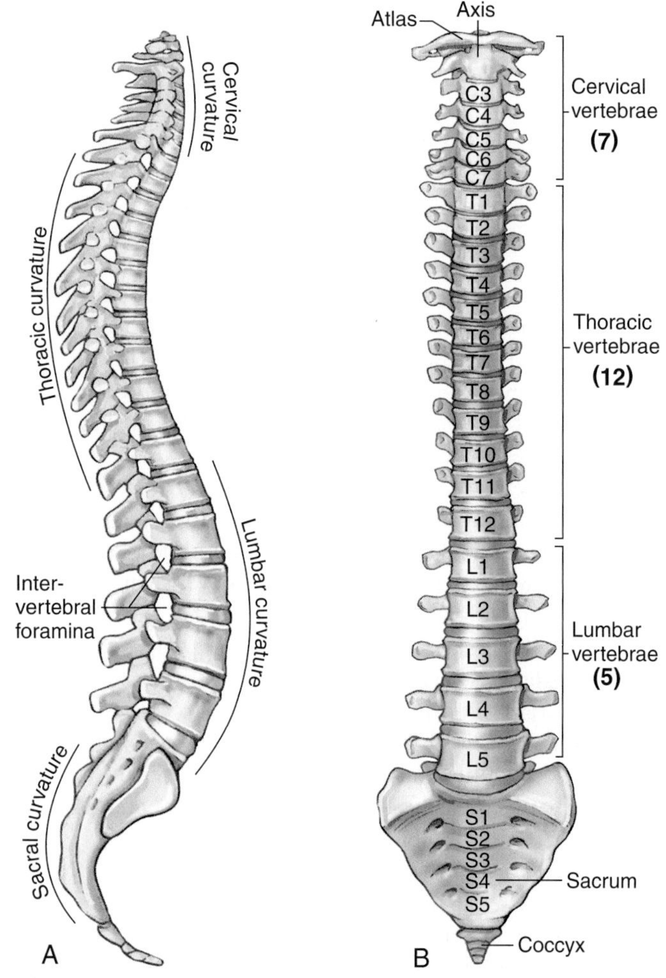

FIGURE 15-17 Vertebral Column. **A,** Right lateral view. **B,** Anterior view. (From Patton KT, Thibodeau GA: *Anatomy & physiology,* ed 8, St Louis, 2013, Mosby.)

Vertebral Column

The **vertebral column** (Figure 15-17) is composed of 33 vertebrae: 7 cervical, 12 thoracic, 5 lumbar, 5 fused sacral, and 4 fused coccygeal. Between each interspace (except the fused sacral and

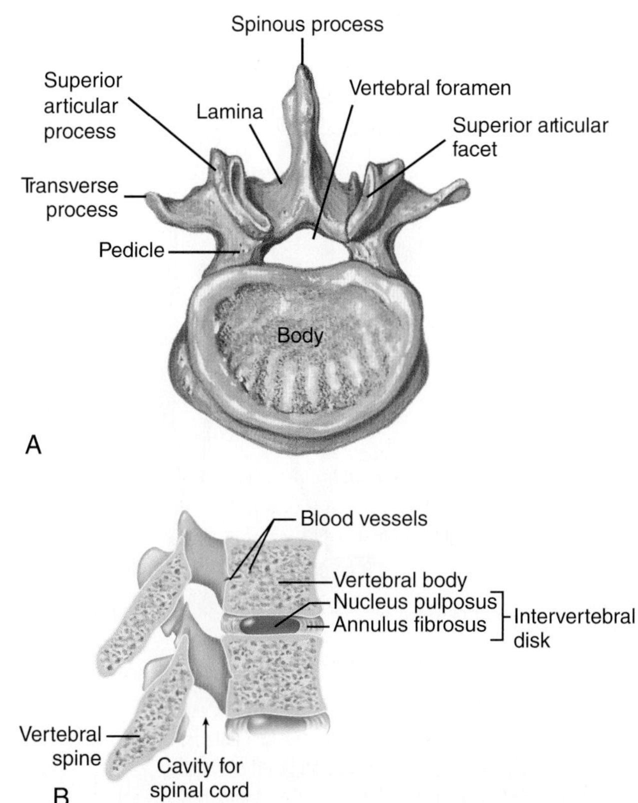

FIGURE 15-18 **A,** Lumbar Vertebra, Superior View. **B,** Intervertebral Disk. (**A** from Patton KT, Thibodeau GA: *Anatomy & physiology,* ed 6, St Louis, 2007, Mosby; **B** from Patton KT, Thibodeau GA: *Anatomy & physiology,* ed 8, St Louis, 2013, Mosby.)

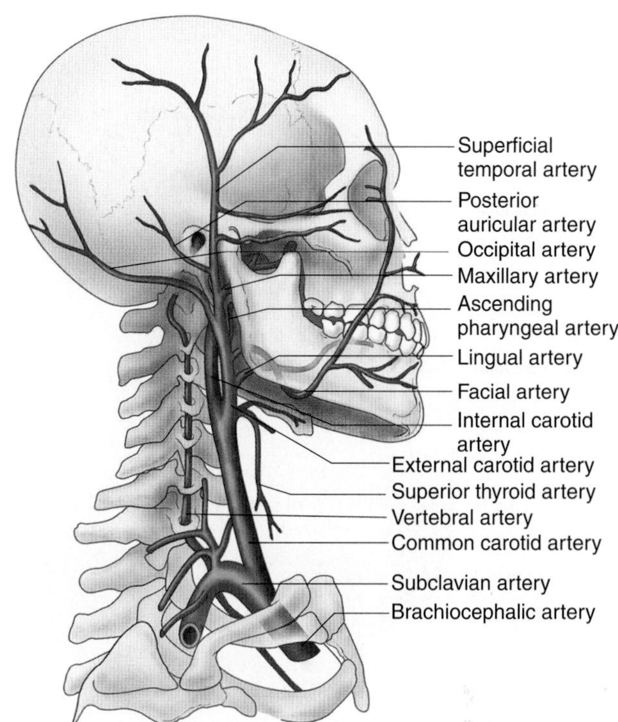

FIGURE 15-19 Major Arteries of the Head and Neck. (From Patton KT, Thibodeau GA: *Anatomy & physiology,* ed 8, St Louis, 2013, Mosby.)

coccygeal vertebrae) is an **intervertebral disk** (Figure 15-18). At the center of the intervertebral disk is the **nucleus pulposus,** a pulpy mass of elastic fibers. The intervertebral disk functions to absorb shocks, preventing damage to the vertebrae. The intervertebral disk is also a common source of back problems. If too much stress is applied to the vertebral column, the disk contents may rupture and protrude into the spinal canal, causing compression of the spinal cord or nerve roots. The disks also can degenerate.

Blood Supply

Blood Supply to the Brain

The brain receives approximately 20% of the cardiac output, or 800 to 1000 ml of blood flow per minute. Carbon dioxide serves as a primary regulator for blood flow within the CNS. It is a potent vasodilator in the CNS, and its effects ensure an adequate blood supply.

The brain derives its arterial supply from two systems: the **internal carotid arteries** and the **vertebral arteries** (Figure 15-19). The internal carotid arteries, anteriorly, supply a proportionately greater amount of blood flow. They originate from the common carotid arteries, enter the cranium through the base of the skull, and pass through the **cavernous sinus.** After giving off some small branches, they divide into the **anterior** and **middle cerebral arteries** (Figure 15-20). The vertebral arteries, posteriorly, originate as branches off the subclavian arteries, pass through the transverse foramina of the cervical vertebrae, and enter the cranium through the foramen magnum. They join at the junction of the pons and medulla oblongata to form the **basilar artery.** The basilar artery divides at the level of the midbrain to form paired **posterior cerebral arteries.** Three major paired arteries perfuse the cerebellum and brainstem and originate from the posterior arterial supply: the posterior inferior cerebellar artery, off the vertebral artery; and the anterior inferior cerebellar and superior cerebellar arteries, off the basilar artery. The basilar artery also gives rise to small pontine arteries. The large arteries on the surface of the brain and their branches are called **superficial arteries (conducting arteries).** The small branches that project into the brain are termed **projecting arteries (nutrient arteries).** Occluding any of these vessels can cause neurologic signs and symptoms that are often diagnostically unique.

The **arterial circle (circle of Willis)** (see Figure 15-20) is a structure credited with the ability to compensate for reduced blood flow from any one of the major contributors (collateral blood flow). The arterial circle is formed by the posterior cerebral arteries, posterior communicating arteries, internal carotid arteries, anterior cerebral arteries, and anterior communicating artery. The anterior cerebral, middle cerebral, and posterior cerebral arteries leave the arterial circle and extend to various brain structures. (Table 15-5 and Figure 15-21 illustrate structures served, functional relationships, and pathologic considerations related to occlusion of cerebral arteries.)

Cerebral venous drainage does not parallel (lie side by side) its arterial supply, whereas the venous drainage of the brainstem and cerebellum does parallel the arterial supply of the structures. The cerebral veins are classified as superficial veins and deep cerebral veins. The veins drain into venous plexuses and dural sinuses

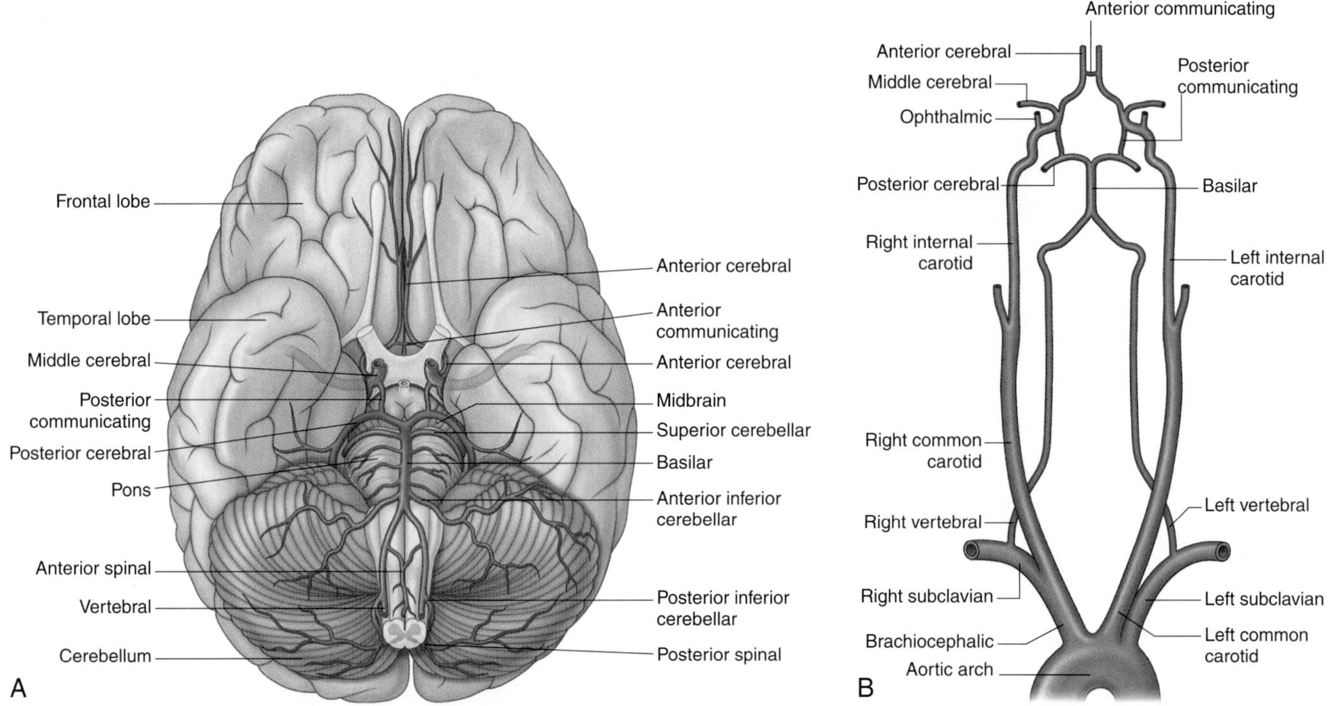

FIGURE 15-20 Arteries at the Base of the Brain. The arteries that compose the circle of Willis are the two anterior cerebral arteries, joined to each other by the anterior communicating two short segments of the internal carotids, off of which the posterior communicating arteries connect to the posterior cerebral arteries. (From Patton KT, Thibodeau GA: *Anatomy & physiology*, ed 8, St Louis, 2013, Mosby.)

TABLE 15-5 ARTERIAL SYSTEMS SUPPLYING THE BRAIN

ARTERIAL ORIGIN	STRUCTURES SERVED	CONDITIONS CAUSED BY OCCLUSION
Anterior cerebral artery	Basal ganglia; corpus callosum; medial surface of cerebral hemispheres; superior surface of frontal and parietal lobes	Hemiplegia on contralateral side of body, greater in lower than in upper extremities
Middle cerebral artery	Frontal lobe; parietal lobe; temporal lobe (primarily cortical surfaces)	Aphasia in dominant hemisphere and contralateral hemiplegia (see Chapter 17)
Posterior cerebral artery	Part of diencephalon and temporal lobe; occipital lobe	Visual loss; sensory loss; contralateral hemiplegia if cerebral peduncle affected

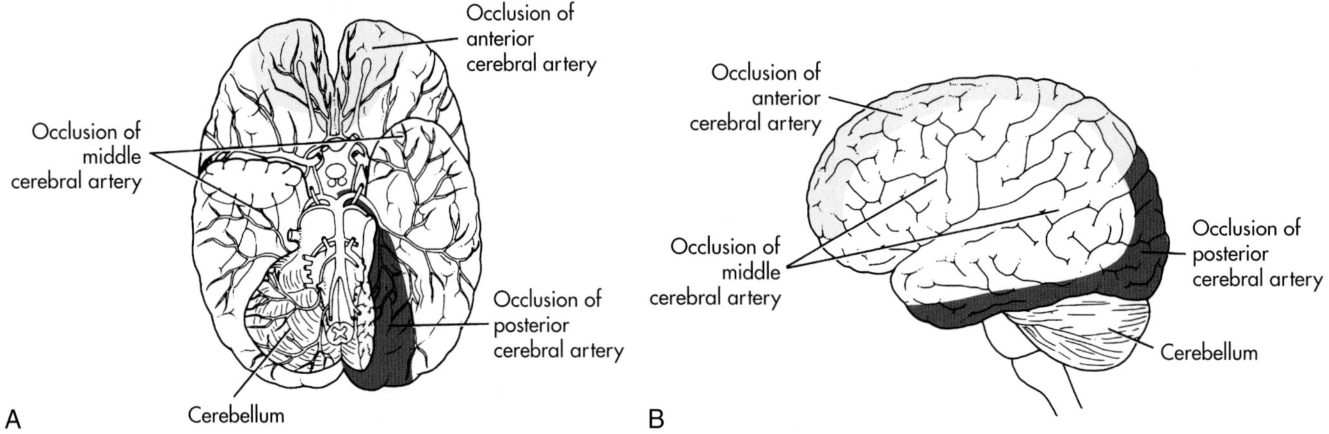

FIGURE 15-21 Areas of the Brain Affected by Occlusion of the Anterior, Middle, and Posterior Cerebral Artery Branches. **A,** Inferior view. **B,** Lateral view.

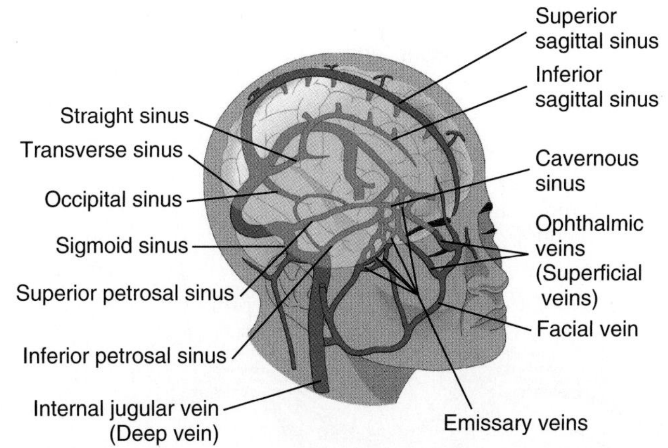

FIGURE 15-22 **Large Veins of the Head.** Deep veins and dural sinuses are projected on the skull. Note connections (emissary veins) between the superficial and deep veins. (From Patton KT, Thibodeau GA: *Anatomy & physiology,* ed 8, St Louis, 2013, Mosby.)

BOX 15-4 THE BLOOD-BRAIN BARRIER

The **blood-brain barrier (BBB)** is a term used to describe cellular structures that selectively inhibit certain substances in the blood from entering the interstitial spaces of the brain or cerebrospinal fluid (CSF). This term emphasizes the impermeability of the nervous system to large and potentially harmful molecules. Astrocytes wrap their foot processes around the epithelial cells of brain capillaries, contributing to the formation of the BBB. Tight junctions between capillary endothelial cells form a barrier that regulates the passage of ions (e.g., sodium and potassium) that could interfere with nerve transmission, prevent toxins from entering the brain, and promote transport of nutrients and removal of metabolites. Compromise of the BBB contributes to passage of molecules and immune cells into the brain causing disease. The BBB has substantial implications for drug therapy because certain types of antibiotics and chemotherapeutic drugs show a greater propensity than others for crossing the barrier. BBB permeability can be affected by hormones, neurotransmitters, and inflammatory mediators. Inhibiting these endogenous chemicals with drug therapy may reduce brain edema and slow the onset of degenerative brain diseases.

Data from Caraglia M et al: *Curr Cancer Drug Targets* 12(3):188–196, 2012; Cristante E et al: *Proc Natl Acad Sci U S A* 110(3):832–941, 2013; De Rosa G et al: *Curr Drug Metab* 13(1):61–69, 2012; Muldoon LL et al: *J Cereb Blood Flow Metab* 33(1):13–21, 2013; Rosenberg GA: *J Cereb Bood Flow Metab,* 2012 [Epub]; Van Sorge NM, Doran KS: *Future Microbiol* 7(3):383–394, 2012.

(formed between the dural layers) and eventually join the internal jugular veins at the base of the skull (Figure 15-22). Adequacy of venous outflow can have a significant effect on intracranial pressure. For example, in individuals with head injury, turning or letting the head fall to the side partially occludes venous return and can increase intracranial pressure because of decreased flow through the jugular veins.

The blood-brain barrier is discussed in Box 15-4.

Blood Supply to the Spinal Cord

The spinal cord derives its blood supply from branches off the vertebral arteries and from branches from various regions of the aorta (Figure 15-23). The **anterior spinal arteries** and the paired **posterior spinal arteries** branch off the vertebral artery at the base of the cranium and descend alongside the spinal cord. Arterial branches from vessels exterior to the spinal cord follow the spinal nerve through the intervertebral foramina, pass through the dura, and divide into the anterior and posterior radicular arteries.

The radicular arteries eventually reconnect to the spinal arteries. Branches from the radicular and spinal arteries form plexuses whose branches penetrate the spinal cord, supplying the deeper tissues. Venous drainage parallels the arterial supply closely and drains into venous sinuses located between the dura and periosteum of the vertebrae.

PERIPHERAL NERVOUS SYSTEM

The cranial and spinal nerves, including their branches and ganglia, constitute the PNS. A peripheral nerve (cranial or spinal) is composed of individual axons/dendrites, with most wrapped in a myelin sheath. These individual fibers are arranged in bundles called fascicles (see Figure 15-1 and Figure 15-24, *B*). The coverings provide structural support, a blood supply, and interstitial compartments necessary for the delivery of essential electrolytes to support nerve impulse conduction.

The 31 pairs of spinal nerves derive their names from the vertebral level from which they exit. There are eight cervical spinal nerves. The first cervical nerve exits above the first cervical vertebra, and the rest of the spinal nerves exit below their corresponding vertebrae. From the thoracic region (and inferiorly) nerves correspond to the vertebral level above their exit (see Figure 15-10).

Spinal nerves contain both sensory and motor neurons and are called **mixed nerves.** They arise as rootlets from the anterior and posterior horn cells of the spinal cord. These two spinal nerve roots converge in the region of the intervertebral foramen to form the spinal nerve (see Figure 15-11). Shortly after converging, the spinal nerve divides into anterior and posterior rami (branches). The anterior rami (except the thoracic) initially form plexuses (networks of nerve fibers), which then branch into the peripheral nerves. Instead of forming plexuses, the thoracic nerves pass through the intercostal spaces and innervate regions of the thorax.

The main spinal nerve plexuses innervate the skin and the underlying muscles of the limbs. The **brachial plexus,** for example, is formed by the last four cervical nerves (C5-C8) and the first thoracic nerve (T1). The brachial plexus innervates the nerves of the arm, wrist, and hand. The **lumbar plexus** (L2-L4) and **sacral plexus** (L5-S5) contain nerves that innervate the anterior and posterior portions of the lower body, respectively (see Figure 15-10).

The posterior rami of each spinal nerve, with their many processes, are distributed to a specific area in the body. Sensory signals thus arise from specific sites associated with a specific spinal cord segment. Specific areas of cutaneous (skin) innervation at these spinal cord segments are called **dermatomes.** The dermatomes of various spinal nerves are distributed in a fairly regular pattern, although adjacent regions between dermatomes can be innervated by more than one spinal nerve Figure 15-24, *D*.

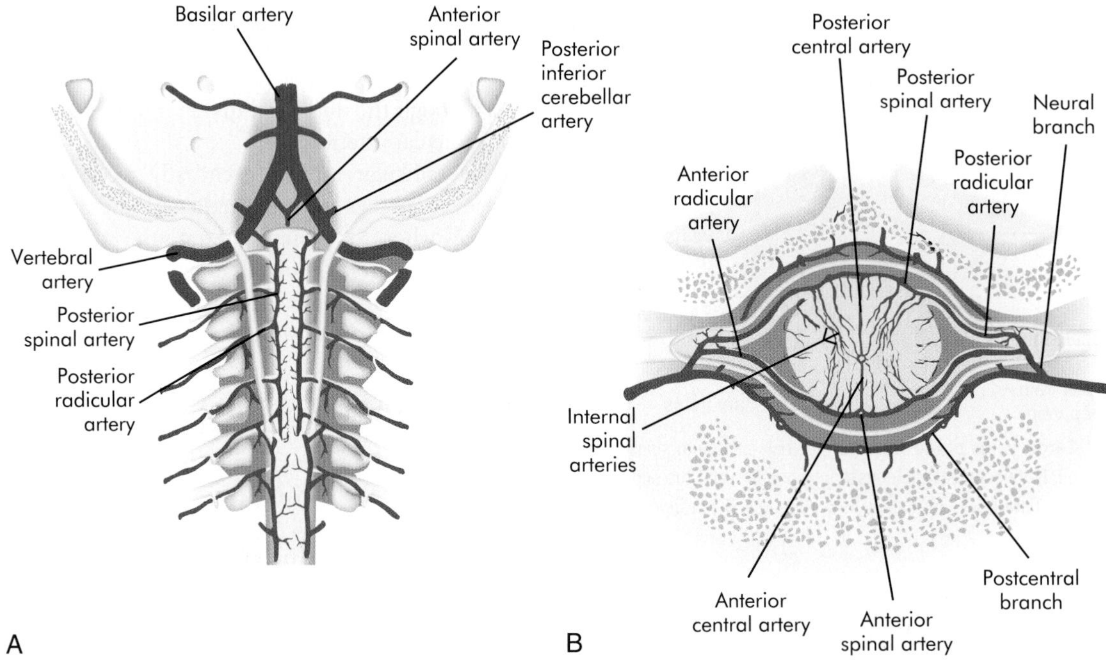

FIGURE 15-23 **Arteries of the Spinal Cord. A,** Arteries of cervical cord exposed *(posterior view).* **B,** Arteries of spinal cord diagrammatically shown in horizontal section. (From Rudy EB, editor: *Advanced neurological and neurosurgical nursing,* St Louis, 1984, Mosby.)

Like spinal nerves, cranial nerves are categorized as peripheral nerves. Most of these are mixed nerves (like the spinal nerves), although some are purely sensory or motor. Cranial nerves arise from nuclei in the brain and brainstem. (Figure 15-24, *A,* illustrates their location, and Table 15-6 describes structural and functional characteristics.)

AUTONOMIC NERVOUS SYSTEM

Components of the ANS are located in both the CNS and the PNS; however, the ANS is considered part of the efferent division of the PNS, even though visceral afferent neurons are an important part of this system. Many neurons of the ANS travel in spinal nerves and in certain cranial nerves. The widespread activity of this system indicates that its components are distributed over the entire body. The peripheral autonomic nerves carry mainly efferent fibers. The motor component of the ANS is a two-neuron system consisting of **preganglionic neurons** (myelinated) and **postganglionic neurons** (unmyelinated). This arrangement contrasts with the somatic nervous system, in which a single motor neuron travels from the CNS to the innervated structure. Visceral afferent neurons have their cell bodies in some sensory and cranial ganglia and their fiber processes traveling in peripheral nerves. The CNS has autonomic areas in the intermediolateral horns of the spinal cord, cardiovascular and respiratory centers in the reticular formation, and both sympathetic and parasympathetic areas in the hypothalamus. CNS pathways interconnect all these areas.

The ANS coordinates and maintains a steady-state among visceral (internal) organs, such as regulation of cardiac muscle, smooth muscle, and the glands of the body. This system is considered an involuntary system because one generally cannot *will* these functions to happen. The ANS is separated structurally and functionally into two divisions: (1) the **sympathetic nervous system** (Figure 15-25) and (2) the **parasympathetic nervous system** (Figure 15-26).

Anatomy of the Sympathetic Nervous System

The sympathetic nervous system functions to mobilize energy stores in times of need (e.g., in the fight-or-flight response) (see Chapter 11 and Figure 11-2). The sympathetic division receives its innervation from cell bodies located from the first thoracic (T1) through the second lumbar (L2) regions of the spinal cord and is therefore called the **thoracolumbar division.** The preganglionic axons of the sympathetic division form synapses shortly after leaving the spinal cord in the **sympathetic ganglia.** These preganglionic axons travel several different ways: (1) directly synapsing with postganglionic neurons in the sympathetic chain ganglion at their level, (2) traveling up or down the sympathetic chain ganglion before forming synapses with a higher or lower postganglionic neuron (divergence), or (3) passing through the sympathetic chain ganglion postganglionic neurons within collateral ganglia (see Figure 15-25). Some preganglionic axons form pathways called **splanchnic nerves,** which lead to **collateral ganglia** surrounding the abdominal aorta. The collateral ganglia are named according to the branches of the aorta nearest them, namely, the **celiac, superior mesenteric,** and **inferior mesenteric.** These postganglionic neurons leave the collateral ganglia and innervate the viscera below the diaphragm.

Preganglionic sympathetic neurons that innervate the adrenal medulla also travel in the splanchnic nerves and do not synapse before reaching the gland. The secretory cells in the adrenal medulla are considered modified postganglionic neurons.

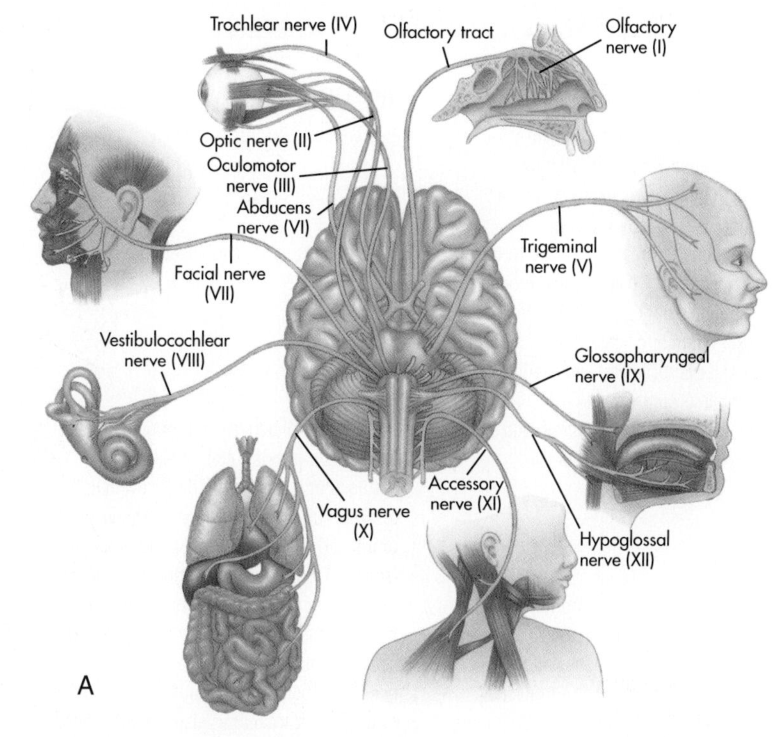

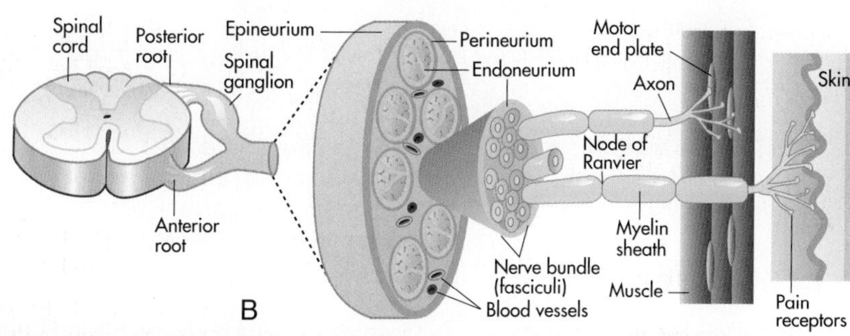

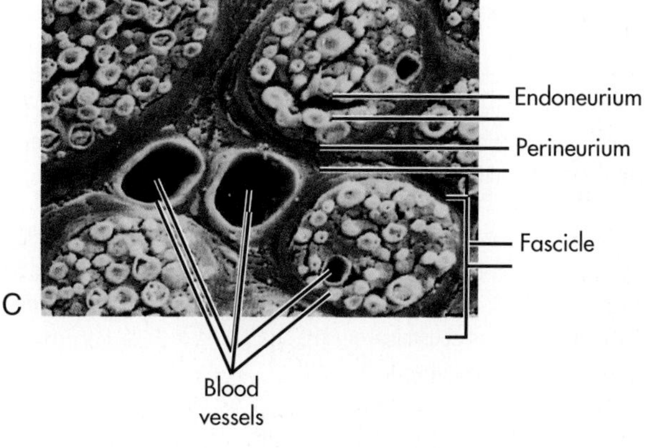

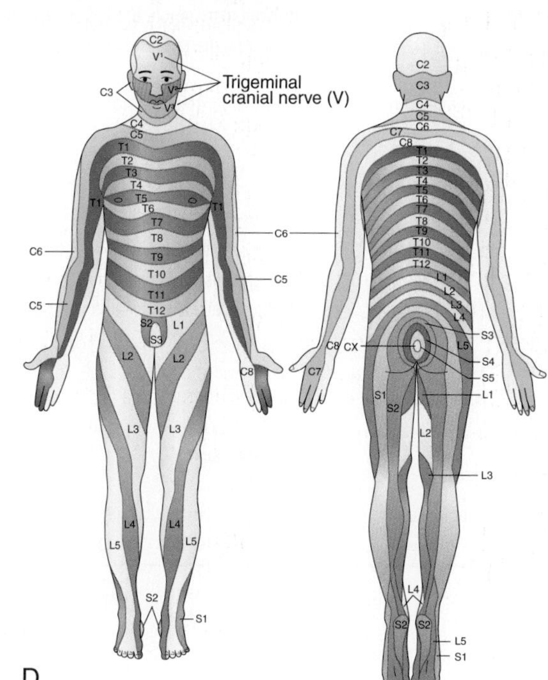

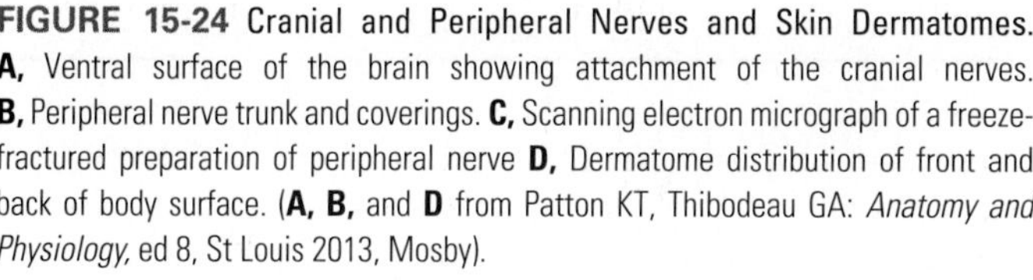
FIGURE 15-24 Cranial and Peripheral Nerves and Skin Dermatomes. **A,** Ventral surface of the brain showing attachment of the cranial nerves. **B,** Peripheral nerve trunk and coverings. **C,** Scanning electron micrograph of a freeze-fractured preparation of peripheral nerve **D,** Dermatome distribution of front and back of body surface. (**A, B,** and **D** from Patton KT, Thibodeau GA: *Anatomy and Physiology,* ed 8, St Louis 2013, Mosby).

TABLE 15-6 THE CRANIAL NERVES

NUMBER AND NAME	ORIGIN AND COURSE	FUNCTION	HOW TESTED
I. Olfactory	Fibers arise from nasal olfactory epithelium and form synapses with olfactory bulbs that transmit impulses to temporal lobe	Purely sensory; carries impulses for sense of smell	Person is asked to sniff aromatic substances, such as oil of cloves and vanilla, and to identify them
II. Optic	Fibers arise from retina of eye to form optic nerve, which passes through sphenoid bone; two optic nerves then form optic chiasma (with partial crossover of fibers) and eventually end in occipital cortex	Purely sensory; carries impulses for vision	Vision and visual field tested with an eye chart and by testing point at which person first sees an object (finger) moving into visual field; inside of eye is viewed with ophthalmoscope to observe blood vessels of eye interior
III. Oculomotor	Fibers emerge from midbrain and exit from skull and extend to eye	Contains motor fibers to inferior oblique and to superior, inferior, and medial rectus extraocular muscles that direct eyeball; levator muscles of eyelid; smooth muscles of iris and ciliary body; and proprioception (sensory) to brain from extraocular muscles	Pupils examined for size, shape, and equality; pupillary reflex tested with a penlight (pupils should constrict when illuminated); ability to follow moving objects
IV. Trochlear	Fibers emerge from posterior midbrain and exit from skull to run to eye	Proprioceptor and motor fibers for superior oblique muscle of eye (extraocular muscle)	Tested in common with cranial nerve III relative to ability to follow moving objects
V. Trigeminal	Fibers emerge from pons and form three divisions that exit from skull and run to face and cranial dura mater	Both motor and sensory for face; conducts sensory impulses from mouth, nose, surface of eye, and dura mater; also contains motor fibers that stimulate chewing muscles	Sensations of pain, touch, and temperature tested with safety pin and hot and cold objects; corneal reflex tested with a wisp of cotton; motor branch tested by asking subject to clench teeth, open mouth against resistance, and move jaw from side to side
VI. Abducens	Fibers leave inferior pons and exit from skull and extend to eye	Contains motor fibers to lateral rectus muscle and proprioceptor fibers from same muscle to brain	Tested in common with cranial nerve III relative to ability to move each eye laterally
VII. Facial	Fibers leave pons and travel through temporal bone and extend to face	Mixed: (1) supplies motor fibers to muscles of facial expression and to lacrimal and salivary glands, and (2) carries sensory fibers from taste buds of anterior part of tongue	Anterior two thirds of tongue tested for ability to taste sweet (sugar), salty, sour (vinegar), and bitter (quinine) substances; symmetry of face checked; subject asked to close eyes, smile, whistle, and so on; tearing tested with ammonia fumes
VIII. Vestibulocochlear (acoustic)	Fibers run from inner ear (hearing and equilibrium receptors in temporal bone) to enter brainstem just below pons	Purely sensory; vestibular branch transmits impulses for sense of equilibrium; cochlear branch transmits impulses for sense of hearing	Hearing checked by air and bone conduction by use of a tuning fork; vestibular tests: Bárány and caloric tests
IX. Glossopharyngeal	Fibers emerge from midbrain and leave skull and extend to pharynx, salivary glands, and tongue	Mixed: (1) motor fibers serve pharynx (throat) and salivary glands, and (2) sensory fibers carry impulses from pharynx, posterior tongue (taste buds), and pressure receptors of carotid artery	Gag and swallow reflexes checked; subject asked to speak and cough; posterior one third of tongue may be tested for taste
X. Vagus	Fibers emerge from medulla, pass through skull, and descend through neck region into thorax and abdominal region	Fibers carry sensory and motor impulses for pharynx; a large part of this nerve is parasympathetic motor fibers, which supply smooth muscles of abdominal organs; receives sensory impulses from viscera	Same as for cranial nerve IX (IX and X are tested in common) because they both serve muscles of the throat
XI. Spinal accessory	Fibers arise from medulla and superior spinal cord and extend to muscles of neck and back	Provides sensory and motor fibers for sternocleidomastoid and trapezius muscles and muscles of soft palate, pharynx, and larynx	Sternocleidomastoid and trapezius muscles checked for strength by asking subject to rotate head and shrug shoulders against resistance
XII. Hypoglossal	Fibers arise from medulla and exit from skull and extend to tongue	Carries motor fibers to muscles of tongue and sensory impulses from tongue to brain	Subject asked to stick out tongue, and any position abnormalities are noted

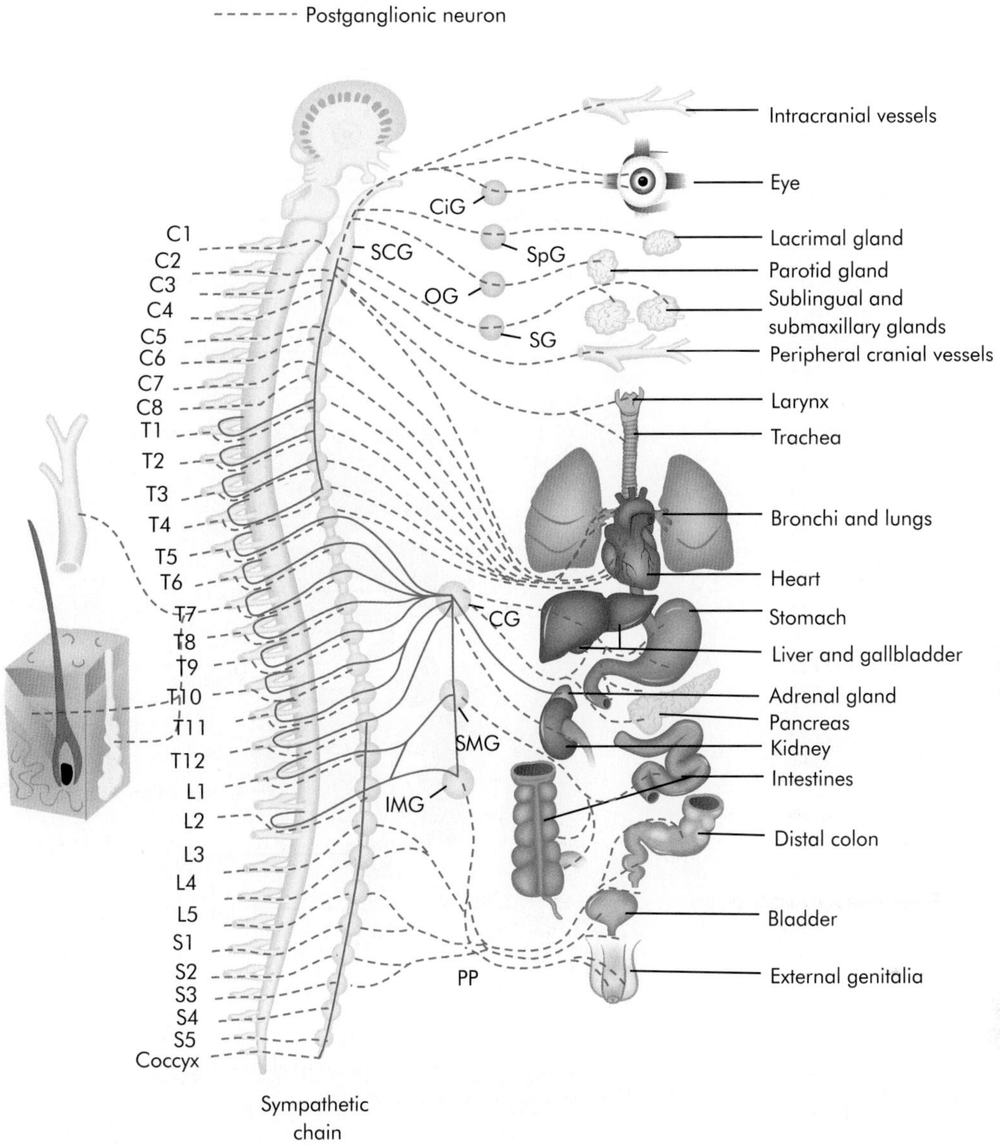

FIGURE 15-25 Sympathetic Division of the Autonomic Nervous System. *CG,* Celiac ganglion; *CiG,* ciliary ganglion; *IMG,* inferior mesenteric ganglion; *OG,* otic ganglion; *PP,* pelvic plexus; *SCG,* superior cervical ganglion; *SG,* submandibular ganglion; *SMG,* superior mesenteric ganglion; *SpG,* sphenopalatine ganglion. (Redrawn from Rudy EB, editor: *Advanced neurological and neurosurgical nursing,* St Louis, 1984, Mosby.)

Because preganglionic sympathetic fibers are all myelinated, nerve conduction to the adrenal medulla is quick, and innervation causes the rapid release of epinephrine and norepinephrine. Epinephrine and norepinephrine are mediators of the fight-or-flight response (see Chapter 11).

Anatomy of the Parasympathetic Nervous System

The parasympathetic nervous system functions to conserve and restore energy. The nerve cell bodies of this division are located in the cranial nerve nuclei and in the sacral region of the spinal cord, and therefore constitute the **craniosacral division.** Unlike the sympathetic division, the preganglionic fibers in the parasympathetic division travel to ganglia close to the organs they innervate before forming synapses with the relatively short postganglionic neurons (see Figure 15-26). Parasympathetic nerves arising from nuclei in the brainstem travel to the viscera of the head, thorax, and abdomen within cranial nerves—including the oculomotor (III), facial (VII), glossopharyngeal (IX), and vagus (X) nerves.

Preganglionic parasympathetic nerves that originate from the sacral region of the spinal cord run either separately or together with some spinal nerves. The preganglionic axons join to form the **pelvic nerve,** which innervates the viscera of the pelvic cavity. These preganglionic axons synapse with postganglionic neurons in terminal ganglia located close to the organs they innervate.

Neurotransmitters and Neuroreceptors

Sympathetic preganglionic fibers and parasympathetic preganglionic and postganglionic fibers release **acetylcholine**—the

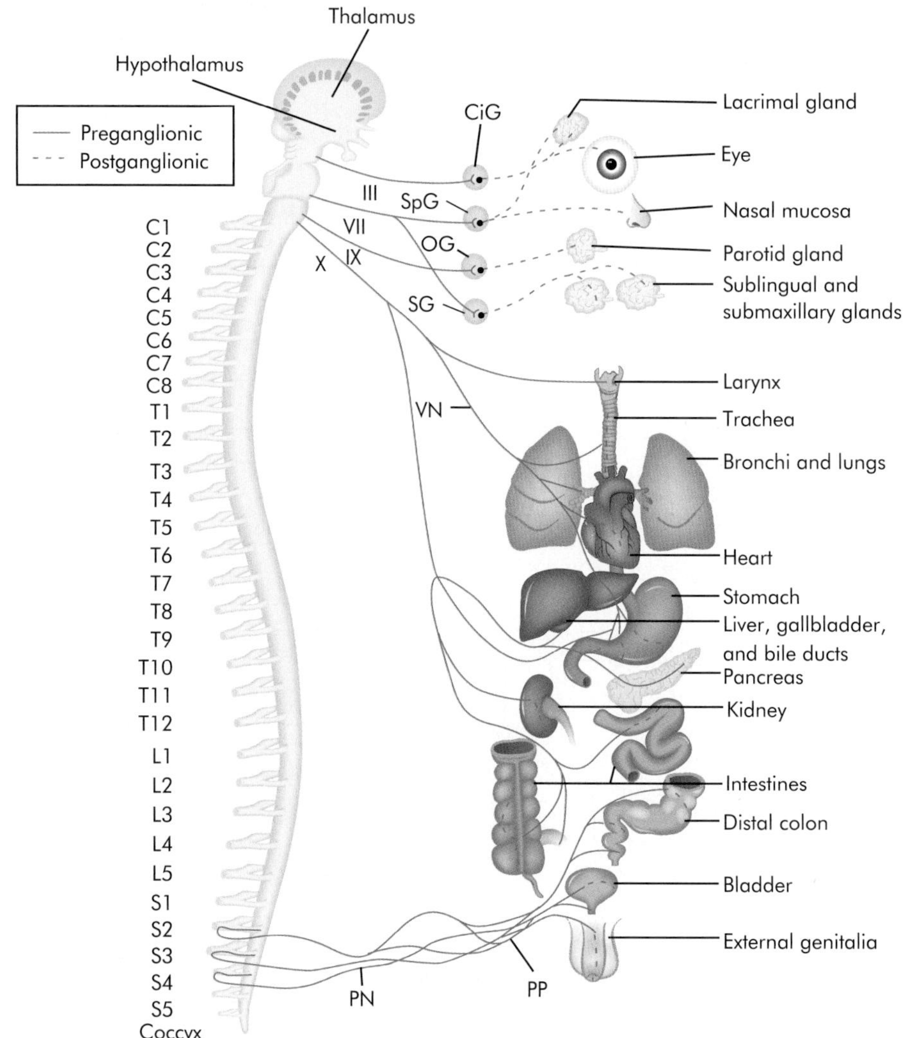

FIGURE 15-26 Parasympathetic Division of the Autonomic Nervous System. *CiG,* Ciliary ganglion; *OG,* otic ganglion; *PN,* pelvic nerve; *PP,* pelvic plexus; *SG,* submandibular ganglion; *SpG,* sphenopalatine ganglion; *VN,* vagus nerve. (From Rudy EB, editor: *Advanced neurological and neurosurgical nursing,* St Louis, 1984, Mosby.)

same neurotransmitter released by somatic efferent neurons (Figure 15-27). These fibers are characterized by **cholinergic transmission.** Most postganglionic sympathetic fibers release **norepinephrine** (adrenaline) and thus are considered to function by **adrenergic transmission.** A few postganglionic sympathetic fibers, such as those that innervate the sweat glands, release acetylcholine.

The action of catecholamines (epinephrine, norepinephrine, dopamine) varies with the type of neuroreceptor stimulated. It should be remembered that catecholamines also are released by the adrenal medulla gland that physiologically and biochemically resembles the sympathetic nervous system. Mainly two types of adrenergic receptors exist: α- and β-adrenergic receptors. Cells of the effector organs may have only one or both types of adrenergic receptors. The **α-adrenergic receptors** have been further subdivided according to the action produced: α_1-adrenergic activity is associated mostly with excitation or stimulation; α_2-adrenergic activity is associated with relaxation or inhibition. Most of the α-adrenergic receptors on effector organs belong to the α_1-adrenergic class. The **β-adrenergic receptors** are classified as β_1-adrenergic receptors (which facilitate increased heart rate and contractility and cause the release of renin from the kidney), β_2-adrenergic receptors (which facilitate all of the remaining effects attributed to β-adrenergic receptors), and β_3-adrenergic receptors (mediate lypolysis and thermogenesis and are up-regulated in cardiovascular disease).[6]

Norepinephrine stimulates all α-adrenergic and β_1-adrenergic receptors and β_3-adrenergic receptors, and only certain β_2-adrenergic receptors. The primary response from norepinephrine, however, is stimulation of the α_1-adrenergic receptors that cause vasoconstriction. Epinephrine strongly stimulates all four types of receptors and induces general vasodilation because of the predominance of β-adrenergic receptors in muscle vasculatures. (Table 15-7 summarizes the effects of neuroreceptors on their effector organs.)

Dopamine is a precursor of norepinephrine and epinephrine and is a brain neurotransmitter synthesized in the substantia

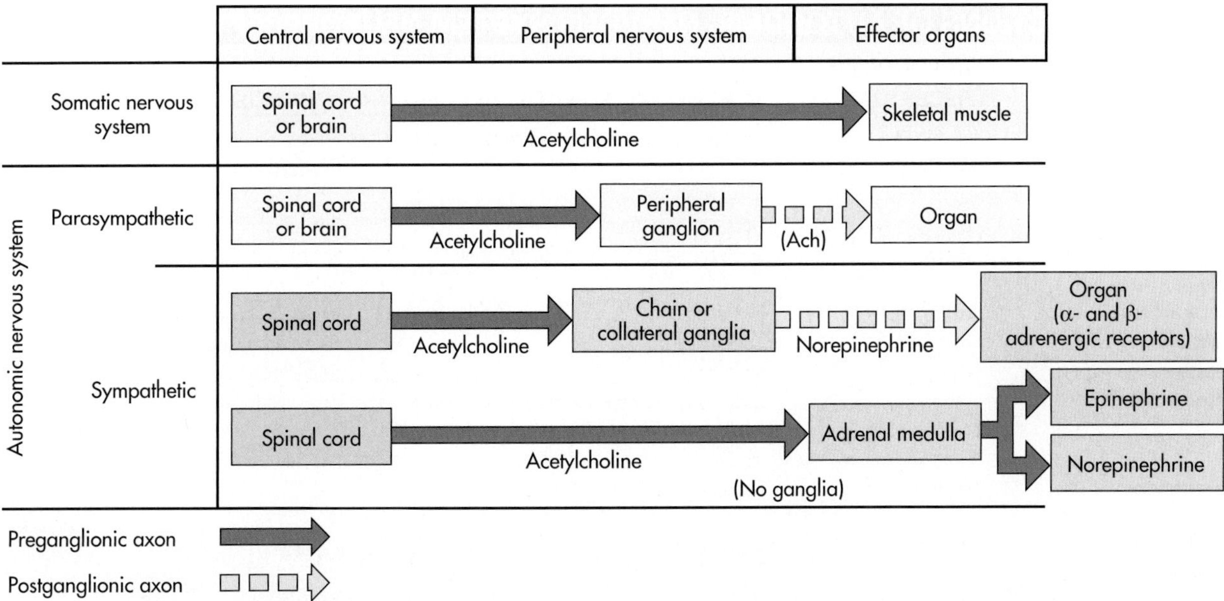

FIGURE 15-27 Autonomic Nervous System and Type of Neurotransmitters Secreted by Preganglionic and Postganglionic Fibers. Note that all preganglionic fibers are cholinergic (Ach). A somatic nerve is used for comparison.

TABLE 15-7 ACTIONS OF AUTONOMIC NERVOUS SYSTEM NEURORECEPTORS

EFFECTOR ORGAN OR TISSUE	ADRENERGIC RECEPTORS	ADRENERGIC EFFECTS	CHOLINERGIC EFFECTS (NICOTINE AND MUSCARINIC* RECEPTORS)
Eye			
Iris			
Radial muscle	α_1	Dilation	—
Sphincter muscle	—	—	Constriction
Ciliary muscle	β_2	Relaxation for far vision	Contraction for near vision
Lacrimal glands	α_1	Secretion	Secretion
Nasopharyngeal glands	—	—	Secretion
Salivary glands	α_1	Secretion of potassium and water	Secretion of potassium and water
	β	Secretion of amylase	—
Heart			
SA node	β_1, β_2	Increase heart rate	Decrease heart rate; vagus arrest
Atrial	β_1, β_2	Increase contractility and conduction velocity	Decrease contractility; shorten action potential duration
AV junction	β_1, β_2	Increase automaticity and propagation velocity	Decrease automaticity and propagation velocity
Purkinje system	β_1, β_2	Increase automaticity and propagation velocity	—
Ventricles	β_1, β_2	Increase contractility	Slight decrease in contraction
Arterioles			
Coronary	$\alpha_1, \alpha_2, \beta_2$	Constriction, dilation	Dilation
Skin and mucosa	α_1, α_2	Constriction	Dilation
Skeletal muscle	α, β_2	Dilation, constriction	Dilation
Cerebral	α_1	Constriction (slight)	Dilation
Pulmonary	α_1, β_2	Constriction, dilation	Dilation
Mesenteric	α_1	Constriction	Dilation
Renal	$\alpha_1, \beta_1, \beta_2$	Constriction, dilation	Dilation
Salivary glands	α_1, α_2	Constriction	Dilation
Veins, systemic	$\alpha_1, \alpha_2, \beta_2$	Constriction, dilation	—
Lung			
Bronchial muscle	α_2	Relaxation	Contraction
Bronchial glands	α_1, β_2	Decrease secretion; increase secretion	Stimulation
Stomach			
Motility	$\alpha_1, \alpha_2, \beta_1, \beta_2$	Decrease (usually)	Increase
Sphincters	α_1	Contraction (usually)	Relaxation (usually)
Secretion	α_2	Inhibition	Stimulation

Continued

TABLE 15-7 ACTIONS OF AUTONOMIC NERVOUS SYSTEM NEURORECEPTORS—cont'd

EFFECTOR ORGAN OR TISSUE	ADRENERGIC RECEPTORS	ADRENERGIC EFFECTS	CHOLINERGIC EFFECTS (NICOTINE AND MUSCARINIC* RECEPTORS)
Liver	α_1, β_2	Glycogenolysis and gluconeogenesis	—
Gallbladder and ducts	β_2	Relaxation	Contraction
Pancreas			
Acini	α	Decrease secretion	Secretion
Islet cells	α_2, β_2	Decrease secretion; increase secretion	—
Intestine			
Motility and tone	α_1, α_2, β_1, β_2	Decrease	Increase
Sphincters	α_1	Contraction	Relaxation (usually)
Secretion	α_2	Inhibition	Stimulation
Adrenal medulla	—	Secretion of epinephrine and norepinephrine (nicotinic effect)	
Kidney			
Renin secretion	α_1, β_1	Decrease; increase	—
Ureter			
Motility and tone	β_1	Increase	Increase (?)
Urinary bladder			
Detrusor	β_2	Relaxation	Contraction
Trigone and sphincter	α_1	Contraction	Relaxation
Sex organs, male	α_1	Ejaculation	Erection
Skin			
Pilomotor muscles	α_1	Contraction	—
Sweat glands	α_1	Localized secretion	—
Fat cells	α_2, β_1, β_2, β_3	Inhibition of lipolysis; stimulation of lipolysis	—
Pineal gland	β	Melatonin synthesis	—

Modified from Brunton LL et al, editors: *Goodman & Gilman's the pharmacological basis of therapeutics*, ed 12, New York, 2010, McGraw-Hill; Yagiela JA et al: *Pharmacology and therapeutics for dentistry*, ed 6, St Louis, 2011, Mosby.
*Muscarinic receptors respond to circulating muscarinic antagonists.

nigra and the ventral tegmental areas of the brain There are five types of dopamine receptors distributed throughout the brain, D_1, D_2, D_3, D_4, and D_5. They have varying functions including pleasure, motivation, cognition, memory, learning, and fine motor control (see What's New? Nucleus Accumbens, Dopamine, and Drug Addiction, p. 460).

Many body organs are innervated by the sympathetic and parasympathetic nervous systems. The two divisions frequently cause opposite responses; for example, sympathetic stimulation of the gastrointestinal (GI) tract causes decreased peristalsis, whereas parasympathetic stimulation of the GI tract increases peristalsis. In general, sympathetic stimulation promotes responses that are concerned with the protection of the individual. For example, sympathetic activity increases blood glucose levels and temperature and raises blood pressure. In emergency situations a generalized and widespread discharge of the sympathetic system occurs. This is accomplished by an increased firing frequency of sympathetic fibers and by activation of sympathetic fibers normally silent and at rest (fibers to the sweat glands, pilomotor muscles, and the adrenal medulla, as well as vasodilator fibers to muscle). Regulation of vasomotor tone is considered the single most important function of the sympathetic nervous system. (Figure 15-28 illustrates some of the most important functions of the sympathetic nervous system; also see Figure 11-2.)

Increased parasympathetic activity promotes rest and tranquility and is characterized by reduced heart rate and enhanced visceral functions leading to digestion. Stimulation of the vagus nerve in the GI tract increases peristalsis and secretion, as well as relaxation of sphincters. Activation of parasympathetic fibers in the head, provided by cranial nerves III, VII, and IX, causes pupillary constriction, tear secretion, and increased salivary secretion. Stimulation of the sacral division of the parasympathetic system contracts the urinary bladder and facilitates the process of genital erection.

The parasympathetic system lacks the generalized and widespread response of the sympathetic system. Specific parasympathetic fibers are activated to regulate particular functions. Although the actions of the parasympathetic and sympathetic systems usually are antagonistic, there are exceptions. Changes in the shape of the lens (for near vision) require only oculomotor parasympathetic activity. Most of the blood vessels involved in the control of blood pressure are innervated by sympathetic nerves. Peripheral vascular resistance is increased and decreased by the relative activity of the sympathetic division without a counteracting parasympathetic component. To decrease blood pressure, therefore, it is more important to block or paralyze the continuous (tonic) discharge of the sympathetic system than to promote parasympathetic activity.

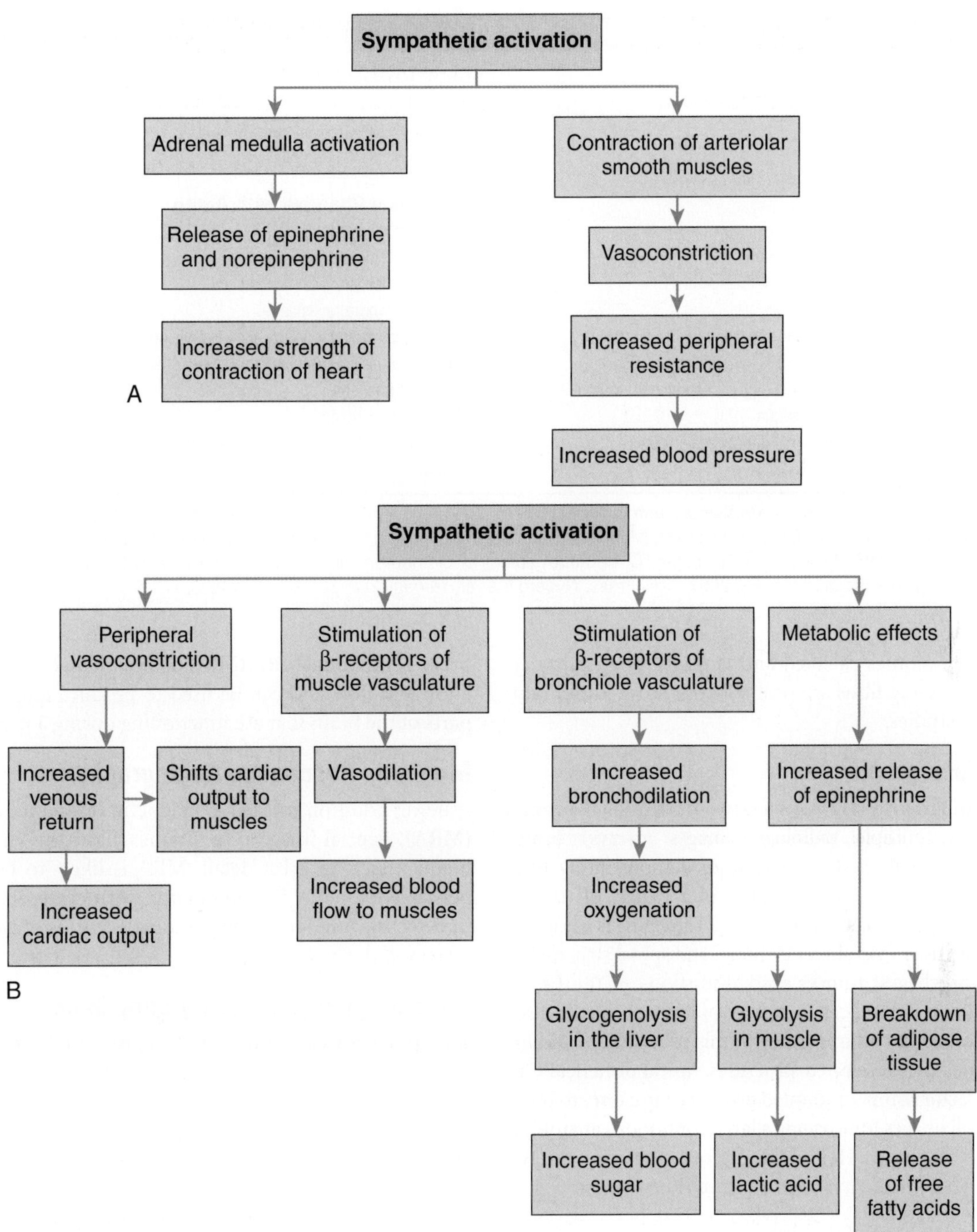

FIGURE 15-28 Some Important Functions of the Sympathetic Nervous System. **A,** Regulation of vasomotor tone. **B,** Regulation of strenuous muscular exercise (fight-or-flight response). (See also Chapter 11 and Figure 11-2 for more detail of the stress response.)

AGING AND THE NERVOUS SYSTEM

The CNS mechanisms involved in the aging process are extremely complex, and many questions concerning the neurologic effects of aging have yet to be answered. Some of the identified mechanisms associated with aging are pathologic, but the distinction between these mechanisms and those that are a part of the normal aging process remains somewhat ambiguous. Box 15-5 contains information on the structural, cellular, cerebrovascular, and functional changes that occur in the nervous system with aging.

TESTS OF NERVOUS SYSTEM FUNCTION

Skull and Spine Roentgenograms

Roentgenograms (x-ray films) of the skull or spine from multiple angles (views) are used primarily to localize bony defects, bone density, erosion, or calcified structures. The pineal gland

BOX 15-5 AGING AND THE NERVOUS SYSTEM

Structural Changes with Aging

Decreased brain weight and size, particularly frontal regions
Fibrosis and thickening of the meninges
Narrowing of gyri and widening of sulci
Increase in size of ventricles

Cellular Changes with Aging

Decrease in the number of neurons, not consistently related to changes in mental function
Decreased amount of myelin
Lipofuscin deposition (a pigment resulting from cellular autodigestion)
Decreased number of dendritic processes and synaptic connections
Formation of intracellular neurofibrillary tangles; significant accumulation in cortex associated with Alzheimer dementia
Imbalance in the amount and distribution of neurotransmitters

Cerebrovascular Changes with Aging

Arterial atherosclerosis (may cause infarcts and scars)
Increased permeability of the blood-brain barrier
Decreased vascular density

Functional Changes with Aging

Decreased tendon reflexes
Skeletal muscle atrophy
Progressive deficit in taste and smell
Decreased vibratory sense
Decrease in accommodation and color vision
Decrease in neuromuscular control with change in gait and posture
Sleep disturbances
Memory impairments
Cognitive alterations associated with chronic disease
Functional changes and nervous system aging have significant individual variation

Data from Brown WR, Thore CT: *Neuropathol Appl Neurobiol* 37(1):56–74, 2011; Crowley K: *Neuropsychol Rev* 21(1):41–53, 2011; Glorioso C, Sibille E: *Prog Neurobiol* 93(2):165–181, 2011; Hof PR, Mobbs C: *Neuroscience of aging,* Oxford, 2009, Academic Press; Jang YC, Van Remmen H: *Exp Gerontol* 46(2-3):193–198, 2011; Kumar A, Foster TC: Neurophysiology of old neurons and synapses. In Riddle DR, editor: *Brain aging: models, methods, and mechanisms,* Boca Raton, FL, 2007, CRC Press; Nyberg L et al: *Trends Cogn Sci* 16(5):292–305, 2012.

in older people becomes calcified and is useful as an internal brain landmark. X-ray films are probably the most commonly used radiologic studies.

Computed Tomography

Computed tomography (CT) creates two-dimensional reconstructions from multiple radiologic images (x-rays) using computer-assisted analysis. It is capable of demonstrating fine distinctions in shape, size, and densities of a variety of tissues based on differential absorption of x-rays. CT imaging is a noninvasive procedure used in evaluating cranial and spinal structures, as well as hemorrhages, tumors, and distortions in the brain caused by pressure differences. A variety of contrast media also are commonly used in conjunction with this procedure to aid in enhanced delineation of selected structures. **Spiral or helical CT** uses a multidetector scanner mounted on a rotating gantry to provide several axial images for imaging a large continuous anatomic area in a matter of seconds. **Helical CT angiography** uses contrast media for detection of aneurysms or ruptured aneurysms.

Magnetic Resonance Imaging

Magnetic resonance imaging (MRI) is a commonly used testing modality. It uses a static magnetic field, instead of x-rays, to orient physiologic atomic particles. Disruption of this orientation by excitation of the particles using serial radiofrequency pulsations provides the image data. The specific tissue reaction is computer-analyzed to give an image of exquisite detail, similar to that provided by CT. The MRI also provides reconstruction of images in three views at right angles (i.e., axial, sagittal, coronal). MRI is reported to have none of the adverse effects associated with radiation examinations. **Magnetic resonance spectroscopy** can be completed at the same time as a standard MRI by analyzing the chemical composition of proton (hydrogen) or phosphorus-based molecules and is useful for evaluating the chemical composition and function of various regions of the brain. **Functional MRI (fMRI)** detects changes in blood oxygenation and flow and can be used to produce maps showing the parts of the brain that are functioning during a mental process.

Magnetic Resonance Angiography

A newer addition to MRI is **magnetic resonance angiography (MRA).** Special imaging techniques allow the visualization of blood vessels in great detail. MRA is likely to become indispensable, alone or in conjunction with cerebral angiography, in detecting and localizing pathologic lesions of the circulatory system of the brain.

Positron-Emission Tomography Scan

The **positron-emission tomography (PET) scan** uses CT imaging to detect the emission of positive electrons from trace amounts of radioactive substances injected into the bloodstream or administered as inhaled gases. With radioactive decay, radioactive substances emit a positron. As they are distributed in tissues, they display characteristic patterns that indicate physiologic and metabolic processes, for example, glucose and oxygen uptake, cerebral blood flow, neural and neurotransmitter function, and the effects of drugs. As a research tool, PET is being used to visualize the specific brain sites that are involved in the processing of information in the brain.

Brain Scan

The **brain scan** images radionuclide substances (technetium [^{99m}Tc]) that have been introduced into the bloodstream. For example, visualization of tissue uptake of the radioactive agent provides an indication of blood-brain barrier integrity (increased uptake of the agent indicates disruption). This scanning technique also can identify abnormalities in blood flow dynamics and cellular metabolic function. The brain scan is particularly helpful in detecting abnormal vascularity resulting from neoplasms, abscesses, and vascular lesions.

TABLE 15-8 **CEREBROSPINAL FLUID ANALYSIS**

PARAMETERS	NORMAL	ABNORMAL	POSSIBLE CAUSE
Pressure (initial readings)	120-180 mm H_2O (9-14 mmHg)	<60 mm H_2O	Faulty needle placement Dehydration Spinal block along subarachnoid space Block of foramen magnum
		>200 mm H_2O	Muscle tension Abdominal compression Brain tumor Subdural hematoma Brain abscess Brain cyst Cerebral edema (any cause) Hydrocephalus
Color (turbidity)	Clear, colorless	Cloudy	Increased cell count Increased microorganisms
		Yellow	Xanthochromic (caused by red blood cell [RBC] pigments) High protein content
		Smoky	Presence of RBCs
Red blood cells	None	Blood-tinged	Traumatic tap
		Grossly bloody	Traumatic tap Subarachnoid hemorrhage
White blood cells	0-6/mm³	>10/mm³ (cell counts range from <100/mm³ to many thousands depending on causative factor; all are abnormal findings)	Occurs in many conditions: Bacterial infections of meninges Viral infections of meninges Neurosyphilis Tuberculous meningitis Metastatic neoplastic lesions Parasitic infections Acute demyelinating diseases Following introduction of air or blood into subarachnoid space
Protein*	15-45 mg/dl (1% of serum protein)	<10 mg/dl	Little clinical significance
		>60 mg/dl	Occurs in many conditions: Complete spinal block Guillain-Barré syndrome Carcinomatosis of meninges Tumors close to pial or ependymal surfaces or in cerebellopontine angle Acute and chronic meningitis Meningeal hemorrhage Demyelinating disorders Degenerative diseases
Glucose (CSF: Serum Ratio)	0.6: approximately 60% of blood glucose level - 50-55 mg/dl)	<0,4: <40 mg/dl >0,6: >60mg/dl	Acute bacterial meningitis Tuberculous meningitis Meningeal carcinomatosis Acute viral meningitis
		>100 mg/dl	Diabetes
Chloride	700-750 mg/dl	<625 mg/dl	Hypochloremia
	116-130 mEq/L	<110 mEq/L	Tuberculous meningitis
		>800 mg/dl	Not of neurologic significance; correlates with blood levels of chloride

Data from Rudy EB, editor: *Advanced neurological and neurosurgical nursing,* St Louis, 1984, Mosby; Marx JA editor in chief: *Rosen's emergency medicine,* Philadelphia, 2010, Saunders.
***Note:** If CSF contains blood, this will raise the protein level.

Isotope cisternography is another radionuclide imaging technique that uses brain scan imaging to detect CSF flow, CSF resorption, and integrity of CSF pathways. The radionuclide agent in this case is injected directly into the subarachnoid space. Under normal conditions the agent passes over the cortical surface and is resorbed through the arachnoid villi. Demonstration of the agent in the ventricular system after a specific period of time indicates CSF obstruction; that is, the CSF backflows from the subarachnoid space into the ventricles.

Cerebral Angiography

Angiography is a radiologic technique that demonstrates cerebrovascular blood flow. This technique commonly is performed by the introduction of a small catheter into the femoral artery. The catheter is then passed to the level of the cerebral circulation and through the aorta, and a contrast dye is injected. Serial x-ray films are then taken. These films demonstrate flow of the dye through the cerebral vasculature and provide information on patency, location, size, and flow pattern of the vessels. Another technique used in cerebral angiography is the retrograde (reverse flow) injection of the dye through catheterization of a brachial, axillary, subclavian, or femoral vein.

Myelography

A **myelogram** demonstrates intraspinal anatomy by the introduction of a radiographic dye into the lumbar subarachnoid space or the cerebellomedullary cistern (cisterna magna). The dye is allowed to flow in a cephalic direction, as in the case of a lumbar injection, or inferiorly in a cerebellomedullary cistern puncture. X-ray films are then obtained. The distribution of the dye delineates spinal cord and nerve root structure and integrity.

Echoencephalography (Ultrasound)

Echoencephalography, or **ultrasound,** is a safe, noninvasive procedure using sound waves that are deflected at differing rates, depending on the density of the tissue. Information is processed and displayed on an oscilloscope screen. It is useful primarily in the detection of structural characteristics of intracranial space–occupying mass lesions and the determination of ventricular dimensions, especially in newborns.

Electroencephalography

The **electroencephalograph (EEG)** is a recording of electrical impulses, arising from the cortical surface of the brain, which is detected by scalp electrodes. The recording of brain wave patterns is analyzed for alterations or localization (or both) of specific electrical activity. This test is especially useful in detecting and localizing foci that initiate seizure activity. It is also an important technique in determining, from a person's brain activity, whether the person is legally "brain dead."

Evoked Potentials

Evoked potentials (EPs) are a method of detecting electrical brain activity that results from a stimulus—primarily auditory, visual, or peripheral sensory. Electrical activity is computer formatted to display changes in trends. The primary uses of EPs include perioperative detection of sensory pathway integrity and disease- or drug-related sensory dysfunction.

Cerebrospinal Fluid Analysis

CSF generally is obtained from the lumbar or cisternal subarachnoid space by means of a hollow needle that allows passive flow. The lumbar puncture is performed most often at the L3-L4 interspace (below the level of the spinal cord at L1-L2). Cisternal puncture is performed by the insertion of a needle into the cerebellomedullary cistern using an approach from the back of the neck in the region of the foramen magnum. CSF pressure is commonly measured during these procedures. The CSF can be analyzed also for gross characteristics and constituents (color, blood cells, electrolytes, and protein) and cultured for microorganisms (Table 15-8).

SUMMARY REVIEW

Overview and Organization of the Nervous System

1. The divisions of the nervous system have been categorized as either structural (CNS and PNS) or functional (somatic nervous system and ANS).
2. The CNS is contained within the brain and spinal cord.
3. The PNS is composed of cranial and spinal nerves that carry impulses toward the CNS (afferent) and away from the CNS (efferent) to target organs or skeletal muscle.

Cells of the Nervous System

1. The neuron and neuroglial cells make up nervous tissue. The neuron is specialized to transmit and receive electrical and chemical impulses, and the neuroglial cell provides supportive functions. The neuron is further divided into unipolar, pseudounipolar, bipolar, and multipolar categories, according to structure and particular mechanics of impulse transmission.
2. The neuron is composed of a cell body, one or more dendrites, and an axon. A myelin sheath around selected axons forms an insulation that allows quicker nerve impulse conduction, referred to as *saltatory conduction.*
3. Neurons have four basic types of cell configuration: (a) unipolar, (b) pseudounipolar, (c) bipolar, and (d) multipolar. The three function types of neurons are sensory, associational, and motor.
4. Neuroglial cells ("nerve glue") support the CNS and comprise approximately half of the total brain and spinal cord volume.
5. Nerve injury triggers a sequence of events known as *wallerian degeneration.* The degree of nerve regeneration that occurs depends on many factors.

Nerve Impulse

1. The region between adjacent neurons is the synapse, and the region between the neuron and muscle is the myoneural junction.

SUMMARY REVIEW—cont'd

2. Neurotransmitters are responsible for chemical conduction across the synapse and myoneural junction. The nerve impulse is predominantly regulated by a balance of IPSPs and EPSPs, temporal and spatial summation, and convergence and divergence.

Central Nervous System

1. The brain is contained within the cranial vault and is divided into three distinct regions: (a) forebrain, (b) midbrain, and (c) hindbrain.
2. The forebrain comprises the two cerebral hemispheres and allows conscious perception of internal and external stimuli, thought and memory processes, and voluntary control of skeletal muscles. The deep portion of the forebrain is termed the *diencephalon* and processes incoming sensory data. The center for voluntary control of skeletal muscle movements is located along the precentral gyrus in the frontal lobe, whereas the center for perception is along the postcentral gyrus in the parietal lobe. The Broca area (rostral to the postcentral gyrus) and the Wernicke area (superoposterior temporal lobe) are major speech centers.
3. The midbrain is primarily a relay center for some motor and sensory tracts, as well as a center for auditory and visual reflexes.
4. The hindbrain allows sampling and comparison of sensory data from the periphery and motor impulses from the cerebral hemispheres for the purpose of coordination and refinement of skeletal muscle movement.
5. The spinal cord contains the majority of nerve fibers connecting the brain with the periphery. Reflex arcs are completed in the spinal cord and influenced by the higher centers in the brain.
6. The four clinically relevant motor pathways are the lateral corticospinal, corticobulbar, basal ganglia, and vestibulospinal.
7. The three clinically important afferent pathways are the posterior column, anterior spinothalamic, and lateral spinothalamic.
8. The CNS is protected by the scalp, bony cranium, meninges, vertebral column, and CSF. The CSF is formed from blood components in the choroid plexuses of the ventricles and is reabsorbed in the arachnoid villi (located in the dural venous sinuses) after circulating through the brain and spinal cord.
9. The paired carotid and vertebral arteries supply blood to the brain and connect to form the circle of Willis. The major branches projecting from the circle of Willis are the anterior, middle, and posterior cerebral arteries. Drainage of blood from the brain is accomplished through the venous sinuses and jugular veins.
10. Blood supply to the spinal cord originates from the vertebral arteries and branches arising from the aorta.

Peripheral Nervous System

1. The PNS functions to relay information from the CNS to muscle and effector organs through cranial and spinal nerve tracts arranged in fascicles (multiple fascicles bound together form the peripheral nerve).
2. The 31 pairs of spinal nerves contain sensory and motor neurons.

Autonomic Nervous System

1. The ANS is responsible for the maintenance of a steady-state in the internal environment. Two opposing systems constitute the ANS: (a) the sympathetic nervous system responds to stress by mobilizing energy stores and prepares the body to defend itself, and (b) the parasympathetic nervous system conserves energy and the body's resources.

Aging and the Nervous System

1. Major structural changes with aging include a decrease in number of neurons and a decrease in brain weight and size.
2. Decreased amounts of myelin, deposition of lipofuscin, and the presence of senile plaques, multiple neurofibrillary tangles, and Lewy bodies are common cellular changes with aging.
3. Cerebral atherosclerosis, decreased vascular density, and increased permeability of the blood-brain barrier occur with aging.
4. Functional changes with aging include diminished sensory functions, sleep disturbances, and memory impairments.

Tests of Nervous System Function

1. Tests of nervous system function include x-ray films, CT, MRI and MRA, PET, brain scan, cerebral angiography, myelography, echoencephalography, electroencephalography, EPs, and analysis of CSF.

KEY TERMS

Acetylcholine, 473
α-Adrenergic receptor, 474
β-Adrenergic receptor, 474
Adrenergic transmission, 474
Afferent pathway (ascending pathway), 448
Afferent (sensory) neuron, 462
Amygdala, 457
Angiography, 480
Anterior cerebral artery, 467
Anterior column (ventral column), 462
Anterior fossa, 464
Anterior horn (ventral horn), 461
Anterior spinal artery, 469
Anterior spinothalamic tract, 464
Arachnoid membrane, 464
Arachnoid villi, 466
Arterial circle (circle of Willis), 467
Association fiber, 457
Association neuron (interneuron), 449
Astrocyte, 449
Autonomic nervous system (ANS), 448
Axon, 448
Axon hillock, 448
Basal ganglia, 456
Basal ganglia system, 456
Basilar artery, 467
Basis pedunculi, 459
Bipolar neuron, 449
Brachial plexus, 469
Brain scan, 478

KEY TERMS—cont'd

Brainstem, 454
Broca speech area, 457
Cauda equina, 460
Cavernous sinus, 467
Celiac branch of aorta, 470
Central canal, 461
Central nervous system (CNS), 448
Central sulcus (fissure of Rolando), 456
Cerebellomedullary cistern (cisterna magna), 465
Cerebellum, 459
Cerebral aqueduct (aqueduct of Sylvius), 459
Cerebral cortex, 456
Cerebral nuclei, 457
Cerebrospinal fluid (CSF), 465
Cerebrum, 456
Cholinergic transmission, 474
Choroid plexus, 465
Collateral ganglia, 470
Computed tomography (CT), 478
Contralateral control, 457
Conus medullaris, 460
Convergence, 448
Corpora quadrigemina (tectum), 459
Corpus callosum (commissural fiber), 457
Corpus striatum, 457
Corticobulbar pathway, 463
Corticospinal tract, 457
Cranial nerves, 448
Craniosacral division, 473
Dendrite, 448
Dendritic zone, 448
Denticulate ligament, 465
Dermatome, 469
Diencephalon, 457
Divergence, 448
Dopamine, 459
Dura mater, 464
Echoencephalography (ultrasound), 480
Effector organ, 448
Efferent (motor) neuron, 462
Efferent pathway (descending pathway), 448
Electroencephalograph (EEG), 480
Endoneurium, 448
Ependymal cells, 449
Epicritic, 464
Epidural space, 465
Epithalamus, 457
Evoked potential (EP), 480
Excitatory postsynaptic potential (EPSP), 453
Facilitation, 453
Falx cerebri, 464
Fascicle, 448
Filum terminale, 460
Fissure, 456
Frontal lobe, 456
Functional MRI (fMRI), 478
Galea aponeurotica, 464
Ganglia, 448
Gray matter, 456
Helical CT angiography, 478
Hippocampus, 457
Hypothalamus, 457
Inferior colliculi, 459
Inferior mesenteric branch of aorta, 470
Inhibitory postsynaptic potential (IPSP), 453
Inner dura (meningeal layer), 464
Insula, 457
Intermediolateral gray horn (lateral horn), 461
Internal capsule, 457
Internal carotid artery, 467
Interventricular foramen (foramen of Monro), 466
Intervertebral disk, 467
Lateral aperture (foramen [*pl.*, foramina] of Luschka), 466
Lateral column, 462
Lateral corticospinal tract, 463
Lateral spinothalamic tract, 464
Lateral sulcus (sylvian fissure, lateral fissure), 456
Lentiform nucleus, 457
Limbic system, 457
Longitudinal fissure, 457
Lower motor neuron, 462
Lumbar cistern, 465
Lumbar plexus, 469
Lumbar puncture, 466
Magnetic resonance angiography (MRA), 478
Magnetic resonance imaging (MRI), 478
Magnetic resonance spectroscopy, 478
Median aperture (foramen of Magendie), 466
Medulla oblongata, 460
Meninges, 464
Metencephalon, 459
Microglia, 449
Microtubule, 448
Midbrain (mesencephalon), 459
Middle cerebral artery, 467
Middle fossa (temporal fossa), 464
Mixed nerve, 469
Motor neuron, 449
Motor unit, 462
Multipolar neuron, 449
Myelencephalon, 460
Myelin, 448
Myelin sheath, 448
Myelogram, 480
Neurilemma (Schwann sheath), 448
Neurofibril, 448
Neurofilament, 448
Neuroglia, 449
Neuroglial cell, 448
Neuromuscular (myoneural) junction, 462
Neuron, 448
Neurotransmitter, 451
Nissl substance, 448
Nodes of Ranvier, 448
Norepinephrine, 474
Nucleus (*pl.*, nuclei), 448
Nucleus pulposus, 467
Occipital lobe, 457
Oligodendrocyte, 449
Papez circuit, 457
Parasympathetic nervous system, 470
Parietal lobe, 457
Pelvic nerve, 473
Periosteum (endosteal layer), 464
Peripheral nervous system (PNS), 448
Pia mater, 465
Plasticity, 456
Plexus (*pl.*, plexuses), 448
Pons, 459
Positron-emission tomography (PET) scan, 478
Postcentral gyrus, 457
Posterior cerebral artery, 467
Posterior column (dorsal column), 462
Posterior (dorsal) column pathway, 464
Posterior fossa, 464
Posterior horn (dorsal horn), 461
Posterior spinal artery, 469
Postganglionic neuron, 470
Postsynaptic neuron, 451
Precentral gyrus, 456
Prefrontal area, 456
Preganglionic neuron, 470
Premotor area, 456
Presynaptic neuron, 451
Primary motor area, 456
Primary voluntary motor area, 456
Projecting artery (nutrient artery), 467
Protopathic, 464
Pseudounipolar neuron, 449
Red nucleus, 459
Reflex arc, 462
Reticular activating system, 454
Reticular formation, 454
Roentgenogram (x-ray film), 477
Sacral plexus, 469
Saltatory conduction, 448
Schwann cell (neurolemmocyte), 450
Sensory ganglion (dorsal root ganglion), 461
Sensory neuron, 449
Somatic nervous system, 448
Spatial summation, 453
Spinal cord, 460
Spinal nerve, 448
Spinal tract, 462
Spinothalamic tract, 462
Spiral (helical) CT, 478
Splanchnic nerve, 470
Subarachnoid space, 464
Subdural space, 464
Substantia gelatinosa, 461
Substantia nigra, 459
Subthalamic nucleus, 459
Subthalamus, 457
Sulci, 456
Summation, 453
Superficial artery (conducting artery), 467
Superior colliculi, 459
Superior mesenteric branch of aorta, 470
Superior sagittal sinus, 466
Sympathetic ganglia, 470
Sympathetic nervous system, 470
Synapse, 451
Synaptic cleft, 451
Synaptic knob (bouton), 451
Tegmentum, 459
Telencephalon, 456
Temporal lobe, 457
Temporal summation, 453
Tentorium cerebelli, 464
Thalamus, 457
Thoracolumbar division, 470
Unipolar neuron, 448
Upper motor neuron, 462
Ventricle, 465
Vermis, 459
Vertebral artery, 467
Vertebral column, 466
Vestibulospinal pathway, 463
Wallerian degeneration, 450
Wernicke area, 457
White matter, 456

REFERENCES

1. Haines DE: *Fundamental neuroscience for basic and clinical applications*, ed 3, Philadelphia, 2012, Churchill Livingstone.
2. Kandel ER et al: *Principles of neural science*, ed 5, New York, 2012, McGraw-Hill.
3. Purves D et al: *Neuroscience*, ed 4, Sunderland, 2008, Sinauer Associates.
4. Kolb B, Whishaw IQ: *An introduction to brain and behavior*, ed 3, New York, 2011, Worth.
5. Kovacs FE et al: Exogenous and endogenous cannabinoids suppress inhibitory neurotransmission in the human neocortex, *Neuropsychopharmacology* 37(5):1104–1114, 2012.
6. Dessy C, Balligand JL: Beta3-adrenergic receptors in cardiac and vascular tissues emerging concepts and therapeutic perspectives, *Adv Pharmacol* 59:135–163, 2010.

CHAPTER

16

Pain, Temperature Regulation, Sleep, and Sensory Function

Sue E. Huether, George Rodway, and Curtis DeFriez

evolve WEBSITE

http://evolve.elsevier.com/McCance/

- Review Questions and Answers
- Animations

CHAPTER OUTLINE

Alterations in sensory function may involve dysfunctions of the general or the special senses. Dysfunctions of the general senses include chronic pain and altered temperature regulation. Somatosensory alterations include tactile, proprioceptive, and vestibular dysfunction. Dysfunctions of the special senses include visual, auditory, olfactory, and gustatory (taste) dysfunction.

Pain is a unique sensory experience that, although universally described as unpleasant, is nonetheless essential to our survival. Pain provides protection by signaling the presence of disease or injury. Unlike pain, which need not be a part of everyday life, temperature is carefully monitored and regulated within clearly defined normal limits. Like pain, however, variations in temperature can signal disease. Fever is a common manifestation of dysfunction and is often the first symptom observed in an infectious or inflammatory condition.

Sleep is a normal, cyclic process that restores the body's energy and maintains normal functioning. Sleep is so essential to physiologic and psychologic function that sleep deprivation causes a wide range of clinical manifestations. Prolonged deprivation or disruption of sleep ultimately leads to serious dysfunction.

The special senses of vision, hearing, touch, smell, and taste are the means by which individuals perceive stimuli that are essential for interacting with the environment. Special sensory receptors are connected to specific areas of the brain through the afferent pathways of the peripheral and central nervous system (CNS). Each of the special senses thus involves a connected system of organs and tissues that receives stimuli and sends sensory messages to areas of the CNS, where they are processed and guide behavior.

PAIN

Pain is one of the body's most important adaptive and protective mechanisms and all definitions suggest it is a complex phenomenon and cannot be characterized as only a response to injury. A widely accepted definition of pain is that drafted by the International Association for the Study of Pain (IASP) and accepted by the American Pain Society and the World Health Organization: "Pain is an unpleasant sensory and emotional experience associated with actual or potential tissue damage or described in terms of such damage."[1] Waddell defines pain as "…a symptom, not a clinical sign, diagnosis or disease.…"[2] A clear understanding of the complexities of the pain experience—specifically one that encompasses an individual's emotions, cognition, motivation, prior history, and even issues of secondary gain—is needed to manage pain and to further understand the pain processes. "The inability to communicate verbally does not negate the possibility that an individual is experiencing pain and is in need of appropriate pain-relieving treatment. Pain is always subjective."[2]

Theories of Pain

The theories of pain include the specificity theory, pattern theory, gate control theory, and neuromatrix theory.

Specificity theory proposes that injury activates specific pain receptors and fibers that project to the brain. *Intensity of pain* is directly related to the amount of associated tissue injury (i.e., pricking one's finger with a needle would cause minimal pain, whereas cutting one's hand with a knife would produce more pain). The theory is useful when applied to specific injuries and the acute pain associated with them. It does not account for chronic pain or cognitive and emotional elements that contribute to more complex types of pain.[3]

Pattern theory describes the role of impulse intensity and the repatterning of the central nervous system (CNS). The pattern theory is limited because it does not account for all types of pain experiences.[4,5]

Gate control theory (GCT) integrates and builds upon features of the other theories to explain the complex multidimensional aspects of pain perception and pain modulation.[4] Pain transmission is modulated by a balance of impulses conducted to the spinal cord where cells in the substantia gelatinosa function as a "gate." The spinal gate regulates pain transmission to higher centers in the CNS. Large myelinated A-delta fibers and small unmyelinated C fibers respond to a broad range of painful stimuli (mechanical, thermal, and chemical). These fibers terminate on interneurons in the substantia gelatinosa (laminae in the dorsal horn of the spinal cord). **Nociceptive transmissions** on these fibers "open" the spinal gate and increase the perception of pain. Closure or partial closure of the spinal gates can occur from **non-nociceptive stimulation** (i.e., from touch sensors in the skin). These signals are carried on non-nociceptive larger A-beta fibers and decrease pain perception. This is why rubbing a painful area may alleviate some of the discomfort. Other efferent CNS pathways descend to the spinal cord and may close, partially close, or open the gate modulating the pain experience. The gate control theory, bolstered by progress in understanding neuronal pathways in the peripheral and central nervous systems, has greatly advanced our understanding of pain. As good as the GCT has been, however, there are observations about pain in paraplegics that "do not fit the theory."

Neuromatrix theory proposes that the brain produces patterns of nerve impulses drawn from various inputs, including genetic, psychologic, and cognitive experiences.[6] The qualities we normally feel from the body, including pain, also can be felt in the absence of inputs from the body (as noted with phantom limb pain). In other words, stimuli may trigger the patterns but do not produce them. Neuromatrix patterns are normally activated by sensory inputs from the periphery, but may originate independently in the brain with no external input.[7] The neuromatrix theory illustrates the plasticity (adaptable change in structure and function) of the brain. It does not supplant our understanding of the gate theory, and what we have learned about peripheral inflammation, spinal modulation, and midbrain descending control of pain. The neuromatrix theory expounds upon the gate control theory by explicating a body-self that provides a holistic, integrated, dynamic consideration of pain. However, there are many different kinds of pain and no single theory is adequate to explain the complex dynamics of the pain experience. Continuing research is advancing our understanding of the neural mechanisms of pain.[8,9]

Neuroanatomy of Pain

The integrated function of three portions of the nervous system is responsible for the sensation and perception of pain:

1. The afferent pathways, which begin in the peripheral nervous system (PNS), travel to the spinal gate in the dorsal horn and then ascend to higher centers in the central nervous system (CNS).
2. The interpretive centers located in the brainstem, midbrain, diencephalon, and cerebral cortex.
3. The efferent pathways that descend from the CNS to the dorsal horn of the spinal cord modulate pain.

The processing of potentially harmful (noxious) stimuli through a normally functioning nervous system is called **nociception.** Nociception involves four phases: transduction, transmission, perception and modulation.

Pain transduction begins when tissue is damaged by exposure to chemical, mechanical, or thermal noxious stimuli and is converted to electrophysiological activity. This causes activation of nociceptors,

Nociceptors

Nociceptors are free nerve endings in the afferent peripheral nervous system that selectively respond to different chemical, mechanical, and thermal stimuli. Nociceptors are located throughout the body (Table 16-1) but are not evenly distributed so the relative sensitivity to pain differs according to their location. The variable nature and distribution of nociceptors affects relative sensitivity to pain in different areas of the body. For example, fingertips have more nociceptors than the skin of the back, and all skin has many more nociceptors than the internal organs. Unlike sensory neurons of the special senses of vision, gustation, and olfaction (discussed later), which are required to detect only one type of sensory stimulus (e.g., light for the sense of vision), primary nociceptive afferents have the remarkable ability to detect a wide range of stimuli. To do this, nociceptors are equipped with an array of transduction channels that can sense different forms of noxious stimulation and at different intensities. In addition to the previously well studied voltage-gated potassium, sodium, and calcium channels, there are multiple types of transmembrane receptors (called *transient receptor potential* [*TRP*] *channels*), which reside on "naked nerve endings" and respond to a variety of physical, chemical, and thermal stimuli.[10]

TABLE 16-1 STIMULI THAT ACTIVATE NOCICEPTORS (PAIN RECEPTORS)

LOCATION OF RECEPTOR	PROVOKING STIMULI
Skin	Pricking, cutting, crushing, burning, freezing
Gastrointestinal tract	Engorged or inflamed mucosa, distention or spasm of smooth muscle, traction on mesenteric attachment
Skeletal muscle	Ischemia, injuries of connective tissue sheaths, necrosis, hemorrhage, prolonged contraction, injection of irritating solutions
Bone	Periosteal injury, inflammation, fractures, tumors
Joints	Synovial membrane inflammation
Arteries	Piercing, inflammation
Head	Traction, inflammation, or displacement of arteries, meningeal structures, and sinuses; prolonged muscle contraction
Heart	Ischemia and inflammation

Nociceptors *(primary order neurons)* are categorized according to the stimulus to which they respond and by the properties of the axons associated with them. **A-delta (Aδ) fibers** are lightly myelinated, medium-sized fibers that are stimulated by severe mechanical deformation *(mechanonociceptors)* or by mechanical deformation and/or extremes of temperature *(mechanothermal nociceptors)*. Aδ fibers rapidly transmit sharp, well-localized "fast" pain sensations. These fibers are responsible for causing reflex withdrawal of the affected body part from the stimulus before a pain sensation is perceived. The smaller **unmyelinated C fibers** are polymodal and are stimulated by mechanical, thermal, and chemical nociceptors. The unmyelinated C fibers slowly transmit dull, aching, or burning sensations that are poorly localized and longer lasting. **A-beta (Aβ) fibers** are large myelinated fibers that transmit touch and vibration sensations. They do not normally transmit pain but play a role in pain modulation.[11]

Pain transmission is the conduction of pain impulses along the Aδ and C fibers into the dorsal horn of the spinal cord and to the brainstem, thalamus, and cortex (Figure 16-1).

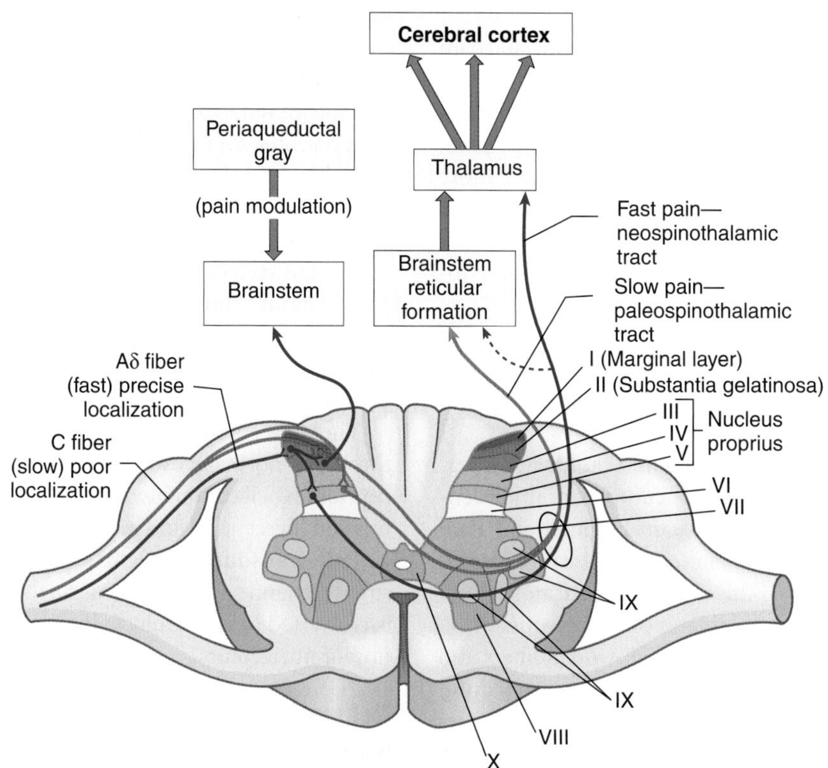

FIGURE 16-1 **Pain Fibers That Terminate Primarily in Laminae II and V of the Dorsal Horn.** The myelinated Aδ fibers (fast localized pain) synapse on a second set of neurons that carry the signal to the thalamus via the neospinothalamic tracts. The C fibers (slow pain) synapse on laminae II and V interneurons that connect with neurons in laminae II, IV, and V and carry the pain signal to the reticular formation and midbrain via the paleospinothalamic tract. The axons of the spinothalamic tracts cross over the spinal cord to ascend in the anterior and lateral spinal cord white matter.

Pathways of Nociception

The cell bodies of *primary-order neurons* or pain-transmitting neurons reside in the dorsal root ganglia just lateral to the spine along the sensory pathways that penetrate the posterior part of the cord. Once the axons of the Aδ and C fibers enter the cord they synapse with interneurons *(second-order neurons)* that may branch into ascending or descending collaterals for one or two cord segments in neuronal projections called the *dorsolateral tract*. Eventually all of the primary afferents terminate on interneurons in the *marginal layer* (laminae I) or *substantia gelatinosa* (laminae II) of the spinal cord (Figure 16-2).

Two classes of interneurons or second-order neurons are found in the dorsal horn: (1) *excitatory interneurons*, which relay nociceptive transmissions to projection cells, to other interneurons, or to motor cells concerned with local reflexes such as the pain withdrawal reflex; and (2) *inhibitory interneurons*, which modulate nociceptive transmission. The synaptic connections between cells of primary and second-order neurons located in the substantia gelatinosa and other spinal laminae function as a "pain gate." The "gate" in the spinal cord regulates the transmission of pain impulses that ascend to the brain for further processing and interpretation (see gate control theory, p. 485).

From the dorsal horn, nociception continues on the axons of projection neurons as they cross the midline of the cord and ascend to various areas of the brain. These ascending fibers are organized into tracts or funiculi that are found in the white matter of the spinal cord, and are named according to their location in the cord and to where they project—either to the higher cord and brainstem or to the diencephalon (thalamus and hypothalamus) and limbic structures. Most nociceptive information travels by means of ascending columns in the lateral spinothalamic tract (also called the anterolateral funiculus) (Figure 16-3).

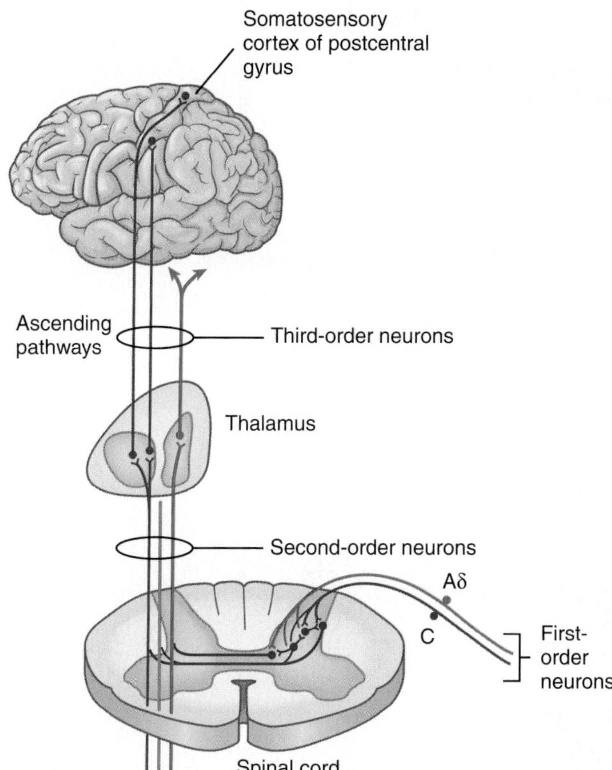

FIGURE 16-2 Nociception Pathways. Aδ and C fibers comprise the primary, first-order sensory afferents coming into the gate at the dorsal horn of the spinal cord. Second-order neurons cross the cord ("decussate") and ascend to the thalamus as part of the spinothalamic tract. Third-order afferents project to higher brain centers of the limbic system, the frontal cortex, and the primary sensory cortex of the postcentral gyrus of the parietal lobe.

Although the organization of all of the ascending tracts is complex, the principal target for nociceptive afferents is the thalamus (the major relay station of sensory information in general). Several other spinal cord projection systems convey nociceptive information directly or indirectly to the reticular formation of the brainstem and the periaqueductal gray (PAG) matter of the midbrain.

From the thalamus, brainstem, and midbrain, *third-order neurons* project to portions of the CNS and cortex involved in the processing and interpretation of pain and neuroendocrine responses (e.g., the response to fright or to surgical stress).[12] The extensive cortical networks that detect and react to pain are referred to as the "pain matrix."[13,14]

Pain perception is the conscious awareness of pain. Interpretation of pain is influenced by many factors including cultural preferences, male and female roles, and life experience, including past pain experiences and current expectations. Three systems interact to produce the perception of pain and individual responses to pain. The **sensory-discriminative system** is mediated by the somatosensory cortex and is responsible for identifying the presence, character, location, and intensity of pain. The **affective-motivational system** determines an individual's conditioned avoidance behaviors and emotional responses to pain. It is mediated through the reticular formation, limbic system, and brainstem with projections to the prefrontal cortex. The **cognitive-evaluative system** overlies the individual's learned behavior concerning the experience of pain and can modulate perception of pain. It is mediated through the cerebral cortex.

Pain Modulation

Pain modulation is the physiologic process of suppressing or facilitating pain. Pain modulation involves many different mechanisms that increase or decrease the transmission of pain signals throughout the nervous system. Depending on the mechanism, modulation can occur before, during, or after pain is perceived.[15]

Pathways of Modulation

Several mechanisms modulate pain both at the level of the spinal cord and in the brain (Figure 16-4). **Segmental inhibition of pain** occurs when Aβ fibers (which synapse in the dorsal horn along with their nociceptive Aδ and C fiber counterparts) close the pain gates through an inhibitory interneuron. These afferent Aβ fibers carry non-noxious low-threshold mechanical information gained by touch, vibration, and pressure. For example, hitting your thumb with a hammer and holding the thumb or putting it into your mouth provides distractive input that lessens the pain.

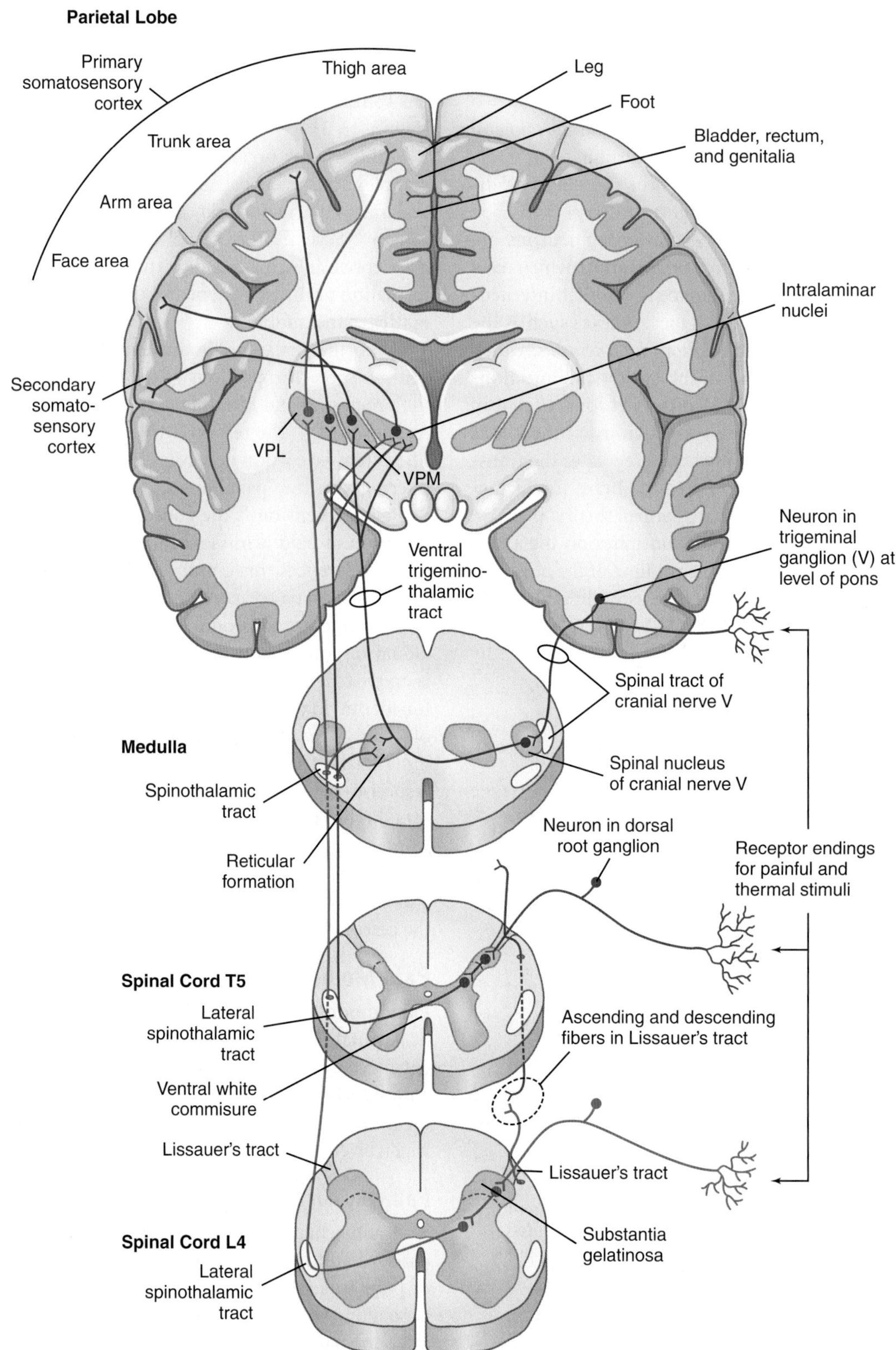

FIGURE 16-3 Central Nervous System Pathways That Mediate the Sensations of Pain and Temperature. *VPL,* Ventral posterior lateral thalamic nuclei; *VPM,* ventral posterior medial thalamic nuclei.

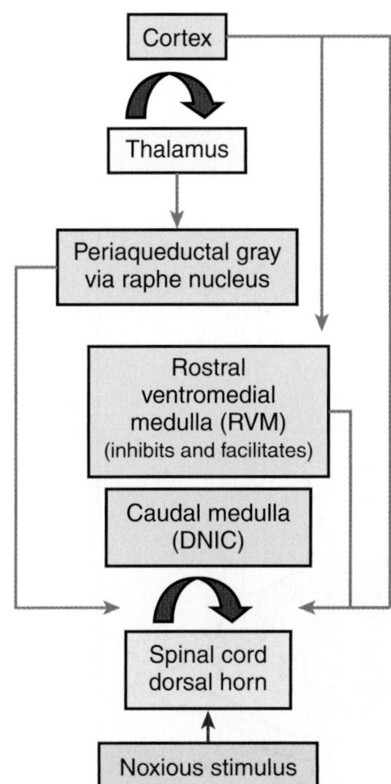

FIGURE 16-4 Diagram Representing the Central Mechanisms of Pain Modulation. A noxious peripheral stimulus activates both segmental and top-down (corticofugal and bulbospinal heterosegmental) modulatory mechanisms, which either accentuate or inhibit afferent pain transmission to the brain. The most important and widespread source of top-down (corticofugal) modulation arises from the cortex. Both thalamic and prethalamic nociceptive relays are under the influence of this top-down control. The dorsal horn of the spine is also under the influence of the caudal medulla through diffuse noxious inhibitory control (DNIC). (Modified from Villanueva L, Fields HL: *The pain system in normal and pathological states: a primer for clinicians*, Seattle, 2004, IASP Press.)

Descending modulation of pain arises from many brain areas. Powerful *heterosegmental control of nociception* probably originates from the cortex because almost all nociceptive relays within the CNS are under so-called top-down (corticofugal) modulation that often occurs even in the absence of painful stimuli.[16]

Diffuse noxious inhibitory controls (DNICs) are spinal-medullary-spinal pathways that are activated when peripheral pain stimulation remote from the pain site relieves pain (counter-irritation). It may be the basis for pain relief with acupuncture or deep massage. Several ascending and descending bulbospinal pathways (between the medulla and spinal cord) respond simultaneously to the noxious stimulus and participate in DNICs.[17]

Expectancy-related cortical activation can exert control over analgesic systems of the brainstem to attenuate or intensify pain. In other words, cognitive expectations (also known as the *placebo effect* or *nocebo [adverse] effect*) can cause real, measurable, often powerful physiologic effects that share some of the same descending corticofugal pathways as the pain modulation systems.[18,19]

The entire complex of modulatory pathways represents an integration of peripheral sensory axon terminals, spinal interneurons, and top-down control pathways that converge on the spinal dorsal horns. The result is to modify, dampen, or augment nociceptive transmission, depending on the many factors existing both within and without the organism.[20]

BOX 16-1 STIMULI THAT ACTIVATE NOCICEPTORS

Inflammatory Mediators (Excitatory)
Bradykinin
Leukotrienes
Prostaglandins
Serotonin
Substance P
Interleukins
Tumor necrosis factor-alpha
Nitric oxide
ATP
Neurokinins
Calcitonin gene–related peptide

Excitatory Transmitters
Glutamate (fast pain)
NMDA
AMPA
Tachykinins
Neurokinin A
Neurokinin B
Substance P
Other receptors
Calcitonin gene–related peptides
Somatostatins
Bombesins
Cholecystokinins

Inhibitory Transmitters
Gamma-aminobutyric acid (GABA)
Glycine
Descending pain modulators
Norepinephrine–α_2-receptors
Serotonin (5-hydroxytryptamine)
Opioids (μ, δ, κ receptors)
Endorphins, Enkephalins, Dynorphins — Released from PAG and NRM and other areas of the brain

AMPA, α-Amino-3-hydroxy-5-methyl-4-isoxazole-propionate; *ATP*, adenosine triphosphate; *NMDA*, *N*-methyl-D-aspartate; *NRM*, nucleus raphes magnus; *PAG*, periaqueductal gray.

Neurotransmitters of Pain Modulation

A wide variety of biogenic amines and other neurotransmitters act to modulate control over the transmission of pain impulses in the periphery, spinal cord, and brain. Pain neurotransmitters can be classified as inflammatory, pain excitatory, or pain inhibitory (Box 16-1). In the periphery, local injury and inflammation can result in direct or indirect excitation or inhibition of nociceptors.

Direct excitation occurs when nociceptors respond with a threshold depolarization initiated by the application of heat, radiation, toxic chemicals, or tissue trauma. *Indirect excitation* occurs when tissue injury results in inflammation and the release of inflammatory mediators including prostaglandins (PGE_2 and PGI_2), tumor necrosis factor-alpha (TNF-α), nitric oxide, bradykinins, histamine, and other cytokines (see Chapter 7). Activity within the nociceptors or damage to them causes them to release peptides and neurotransmitters, such as tachykinins (e.g., substance P and neurokinins), calcitonin gene–related peptide (CGRP), and adenosine triphosphate (ATP), which promote the spread of pain locally and further contribute to vasodilation, increased vascular permeability, and degranulation of even more mast cell cytokines. The resultant "inflammatory soup" serves to lower the threshold for nociceptive depolarization and increases the magnitude of the response to noxious stimulation, known as **hyperalgesia.** The consequence of some or all of these mechanisms is known as **peripheral sensitization.** Normally peripheral sensitization phenomena extinguish themselves as the tissue heals and inflammation subsides. However, when primary afferent function is altered in an enduring way by injury or disease, hyperalgesia may persist and cause chronic pain.

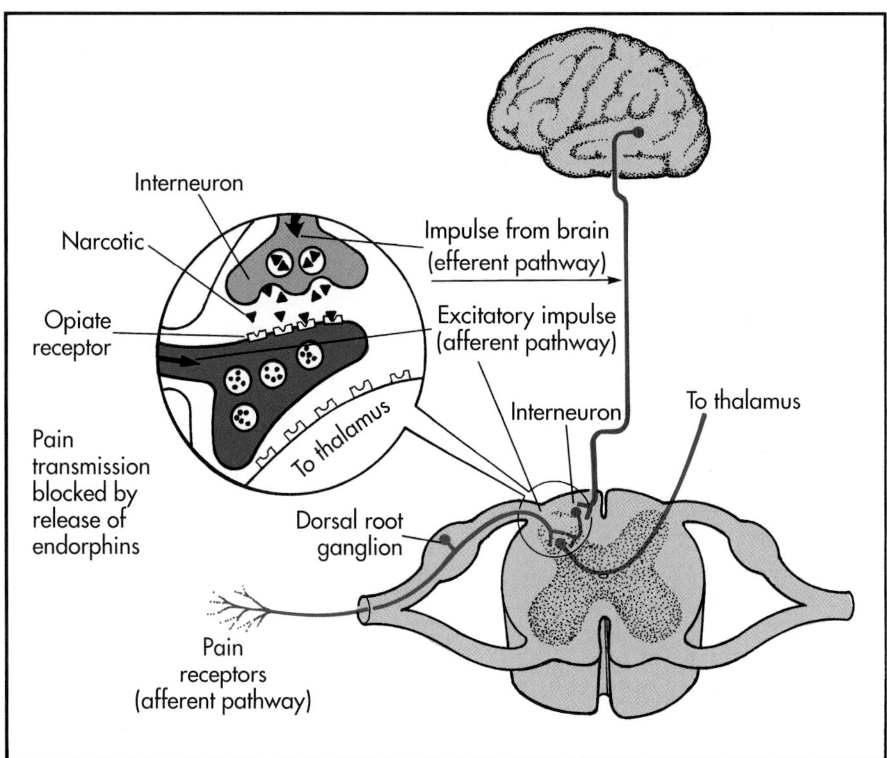

FIGURE 16-5 Descending Pathway and Endorphin Response. The biologic receptors of the enkephalins and endorphins are located close to known pain receptors in the periphery and ascending and descending pain pathways.

Excitatory Neurotransmitters. **Glutamate** is the most common excitatory neurotransmitter in the brain and spinal cord. Glutamate activates two different kinds of receptors: AMPA (α-amino-3-hydroxy-5-methyl-4-isoxazole propionate) receptors, which are very fast, and NMDA (*N*-methyl-D-aspartate) receptors, which are implicated in memory and long-term potentiation of synapses. Both of these receptors lead to nerve membrane excitation and depolarization of the cell. Glutamate receptors mediate many spinal and central responses to painful stimulation.[21] High levels of glutamate and aspartate have been found in the periaqueductal gray (PAG) as well as at the synapses of first-order nociceptors with ascending spinothalamic tract neurons. Repeated stimulation of nociceptive afferents results in an activity-dependent increase in the excitability of neurons in the dorsal horn of the cord. Glutamate, which accumulates in the dorsal horn, results in the displacement of a magnesium ion that serves to inhibit the NMDA receptor. With the loss of the blocking magnesium ion, receptor "*wind-up*" or sensitization in the CNS to further nociception becomes evident. This is known as **central sensitization** (increased excitability of neurons). Although central sensitization is triggered in dorsal horn neurons by activity in peripheral nociceptors, innocuous activation of fibers carrying low-threshold mechanoreception (light touch) will activate second-order nociceptive neurons, giving rise to **allodynia** (the induction of pain by normally nonpainful stimuli) and hypersensitivity. Changes in microglia, astrocytes, gap junctions, membrane excitability, and gene transcription also contribute to central sensitization.[22] Thus both peripheral and central sensitization can lead to chronic pain syndromes.

Inhibitory Neurotransmitters. **Gamma-aminobutyric acid (GABA)** and **glycine** have major inhibitory effects in the spinal cord and brain.[23] For example, dorsal horn laminae interneurons are rich in GABA (GABA-A, GABA-B, etc.) and function to inhibit release of pain neurotransmitters. Loss of GABAnergic interneurons in the dorsal horn after nerve injury may cause loss of pain inhibition, resulting in chronic pain.[24] Glycine receptors inhibit pain and also have anti-inflammatory, cytoprotective, and immune modulating effects. Norepinephrine and 5-hydroxytryptamine (serotonin) contribute to pain modulation (inhibition) in the medulla and pons.

Endogenous opioids are a family of morphine-like neuropeptides that inhibit transmission of pain impulses in the spinal cord, brain, and periphery. Their receptors also play a role in various central nervous system, gastrointestinal system, immune system, and other organ system disorders.[25] There are four types of opioid neuropeptides: (1) *enkephalins,* (2) *endorphins,* (3) *dynorphins,* and (4) *endomorphins.* These substances are neurohormones that act as neurotransmitters by binding to one or more G-protein–coupled opioid receptors. Three distinct types of **opioid receptors** are found in the body: mu (μ) meaning morphine (with subtypes μ_1 and μ_2), kappa (κ) (with subtypes κ_1 and κ_2), and delta (δ). A fourth receptor is nociceptin-opioid peptide (NOP) receptor. Its ligand is **nociceptin** and it is homologous to dynorphin.

Each receptor type binds differently with the various types of opioids. Agonist activity at the opioid receptors by endogenous opioids inhibits the release of excitatory neurotransmitters such as substance P in the dorsal horn (blocking the transmission of the painful stimulus) or in other areas of the brain such as the PAG or the rostral ventromedial nuclei in the brainstem (Figure 16-5).

Opioids from the midbrain release adrenergic and serotonergic descending pathways from GABAnergic inhibition and decrease pain. Leukocytes release opioids and participate in peripheral pain control. Because leukocyte opioids do not cross the blood-brain barrier, they do not have central nervous system side effects such as respiratory depression, somnolence, or addiction.[26]

Perhaps the best known and the most prevalent of these natural opioids are the **enkephalins.** There are two types of enkephalins: *methionine-enkephalin* (Met-enkephalin) and *leucine-enkephalin* (Leu-enkephalin), and their ratio is 4:1, respectively. They were the first endogenous opioids extracted in research. Enkephalins, like the other endogenous opioids, can be identified immunohistochemically. They are found concentrated in the hypothalamus, the PAG matter, the nucleus raphe magnus of the medulla, and the dorsal horns of the spinal cord.

Endorphins were first discovered in the human PAG with β-endorphin being the best studied of the group. The synthesis and activity of β-endorphin are concentrated in the hypothalamus and the pituitary gland. β-Endorphin is purported to produce a greater sense of exhilaration, or "high," than all of the other endorphin types. It is a strong μ-receptor agonist and is generally believed to provide substantial natural pain relief.

Dynorphins (the most potent of these endogenous neurohormones) are found in the hypothalamus, the brainstem, the PAG–rostral ventromedial medulla (PAG-RVM) system, and the spinal cord. Dynorphins and nociceptin, which bind strongly to κ-receptors located in the dorsal horn of the spinal cord and in areas of the brain, generally serve to impede pain signals but can, in certain circumstances, incite pain through mechanisms of up-regulation.[27]

Endomorphins have potent analgesic, gastrointestinal (GI), and anti-inflammatory effects. Endomorphin-1 and endomorphin-2 are peptides isolated from the brain and the spinal cord and show the highest affinity and selectivity for the μ-opiate receptor.[28,29]

In addition to analgesic effects, endogenous opioids are involved in a variety of other functions throughout the body including modulation of stress and anxiety, feeding behavior, cough suppression, immune and inflammatory responses, and alcohol intake.[30] Endogenous opioids of one type or another are found to bind to almost all tissues in the body and thus affect numerous biologic functions.[25]

Pain Threshold and Pain Tolerance

Pain threshold is the point at which a stimulus is perceived as pain and it does not vary significantly among people or in the same person over time. Intense pain at one location, however, may cause an increase in the threshold in another location. For example, a person with severe pain in one knee is less likely to experience chronic back pain that is less intense. This phenomenon is called **perceptual dominance.** Because of perceptual dominance, pain at one site may mask other painful areas.[3,31]

Pain tolerance is the duration of time or the intensity of pain that an individual will endure before initiating overt pain responses and is generally decreased with repeated exposure to pain. Pain tolerance is influenced by the person's cultural perceptions, expectations, role behaviors, physical and mental health, gender, fatigue, anger, boredom, apprehension, and sleep deprivation. Tolerance may be increased by alcohol consumption, persistent use of pain medication, hypnosis, warmth, distracting activities, and strong beliefs or faith.[32]

BOX 16-2 CATEGORIES OF PAIN

- **I. Neurophysiologic pain**
  - A. Nociceptive pain
    - 1. Somatic
    - 2. Visceral
    - 3. Referred
  - B. Neuropathic (non-nociceptive)
    - 1. Central pain (lesion/dysfunction in brain or spinal cord)
    - 2. Peripheral pain (lesion/dysfunction in peripheral nervous system [PNS])
- **II. Neurogenic pain**
  - A. Neuralgia (pain in the distribution of a nerve)
  - B. Constant
    - 1. Sympathetically independent
    - 2. Sympathetically dependent
- **III. Temporal pain (time related)**
  - A. Acute pain
  - B. Chronic
- **IV. Regional pain**
  - A. Abdominal pain
  - B. Chest pain
  - C. Headache
  - D. Low back pain
  - E. Orofacial pain
  - F. Pelvic pain
  - G. Joint pain
- **V. Etiologic pain**
  - A. Cancer pain
  - B. Dental pain
  - C. Inflammatory pain
  - D. Ischemic pain
  - E. Vascular pain
  - F. Postoperative pain

Adapted from Derasari MD: Taxonomy of pain syndromes: classification of chronic pain syndromes. In Raj PP, editor: *Practical management of pain,* ed 3, St Louis, 2000, Mosby.

Clinical Descriptions of Pain

Pain can be described in a variety of ways, including duration (acute vs. chronic), inferred neurophysiologic mechanisms (nociceptive vs. non-nociceptive [i.e., neuropathic]), etiology, and region affected. Because of the complex nature of pain, however, many terms overlap and more than one approach is often used. The broad categories of pain are summarized in Box 16-2. Some of the most common clinical pain presentations are summarized in the following sections.

Acute Pain

Acute pain is a protective mechanism that alerts the individual to a condition or experience that is immediately harmful to the body and mobilizes the individual to take prompt action to relieve it. Acute pain is transient, usually lasting seconds to days, and sometimes up to 3 months.[33] It begins suddenly and is

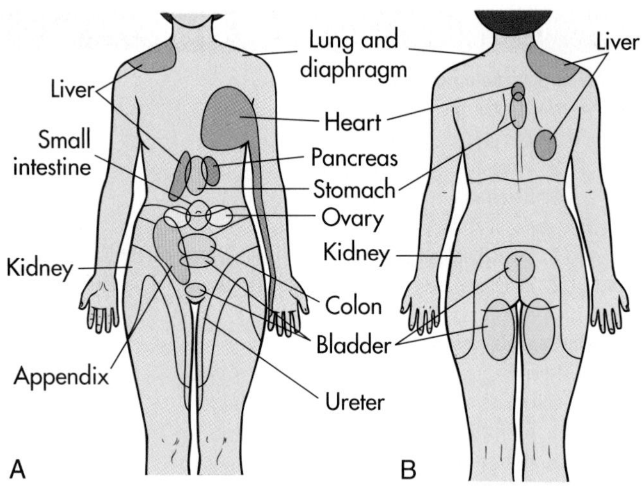

FIGURE 16-6 Sites of Referred Pain. **A,** Front. **B,** Back.

relieved after the chemical mediators that stimulate pain receptors are removed. Stimulation of the autonomic nervous system results in physical manifestations including increased heart rate, hypertension, diaphoresis, and dilated pupils. Anxiety related to the pain experience, including its cause, treatment, and prognosis, is common and there is expectation of limited duration.

Acute pain arises from cutaneous and deep somatic tissue, or from visceral organs and can be classified as (1) acute somatic, (2) acute visceral, and (3) referred.

Somatic pain is superficial, arising from connective tissue, muscle or bone, and skin. It is either sharp and well localized (especially fast pain carried by Aδ fibers) or dull, aching, throbbing, and poorly localized as seen in polymodal C fiber transmissions.

Visceral pain refers to pain in internal organs and the lining of body cavities with an aching, gnawing, throbbing, or intermittent cramping quality. It is transmitted by sympathetic afferents and is poorly localized because of the lesser number of nociceptors in the visceral structures. Visceral pain is associated with nausea and vomiting, hypotension, restlessness, and, in some cases, shock. It often radiates (spreads away from the actual site of the pain) or is referred.

Referred pain is pain that is felt in an area removed or distant from its point of origin—the area of referred pain is supplied by the same spinal segment as the actual site of pain. Impulses from many cutaneous and visceral neurons converge on the same ascending neuron, and the brain cannot distinguish between the two. Because the skin has more receptors, the painful sensation is experienced at the referred site instead of the site of origin. Referred pain can be acute or chronic. Figure 16-6 illustrates common areas of referred pain and their associated sites of origin.

Chronic Pain

Chronic pain is usually defined as lasting at least 3 months and lasting well beyond the expected healing time following the initial onset of tissue damage or injury. Chronic or persistent pain serves no purpose and is poorly understood. It often appears to be out of proportion to any observable tissue injury. It may be ongoing (e.g., low back pain) or intermittent (e.g., migraine headaches). Changes in the peripheral and central nervous systems that cause dysregulation of nociception and pain modulation processes (peripheral and central sensitization) are thought to lead to chronic pain.

The following mechanisms have been implicated in the initiation and entrenchment of chronic pain states[34,35]:

- Changes in sensitivity of neurons—lower threshold with peripheral and central sensitization
- Spontaneous impulses from regenerating peripheral nerves
- Alterations in the dorsal root ganglion in response to peripheral nerve injury and neurotransmitters—reorganization of nociceptive neurons (deafferentation pain)
- Loss of pain inhibition in the spinal cord
- Up-regulation of nociceptive chemokines and their receptors
- Structural and functional alterations in brain processing neural networks

Neuroimaging studies have demonstrated brain changes in individuals with chronic pain that may lead to cognitive deficits and decreased ability to cope with pain.[36,37] It is thought to be due, in part, to the stress of coping with continuous pain and may be reversible when pain is controlled.[38,39] Chronic pain often does not respond to usual therapy. Because it is not yet possible to predict when acute pain will develop into chronic pain, early and individualized prevention and treatment of acute pain is encouraged.[40,41]

Physiologic responses to intermittent chronic pain are similar to those associated with acute pain, whereas persistent pain allows for physiologic adaptation, producing normal heart rate and blood pressure. This leads many to mistakenly conclude that people with chronic pain are malingering because they do not appear to be in pain. As chronic pain progresses, certain behavioral and psychologic changes often emerge, including depression, difficulty eating and sleeping, preoccupation with the pain, and avoidance of pain-provoking stimuli.[42] The desire to relieve pain and the need to hide it become conflicting drives for those with chronic pain, who fear being labeled complainers.[43,44] Comparison of acute and chronic pain is summarized in Table16-2. Common chronic pain conditions are listed in Table 16-3.

Chronic Pain Syndromes. **Specific** (i.e., intervertebral disk degeneration) and **non–specific low back pain** (not attributable to a specific pathologic source) are global, common, chronic, and disabling pain conditions. The prevalence of non–specific low back pain is about 23% with 11% to 12% of those affected being disabled.[45,46] Prevalence estimates and definition of risk factors vary among studies depending on the definition of low back pain used. Acute back pain is relatively rare and many individuals of all ages have chronic recurrent back pain. Both cortical and spinal alterations in pain processing are associated with low back pain. Treatment is often ineffective and the personal and societal burden is great.[45,47,48]

Myofascial pain syndrome (MPS) is associated with injury to muscle, fascia, and tendons and includes myositis, fibrositis, myofibrositis, myalgia (see Chapter 44 for fibromyalgia),

TABLE 16-2 COMPARISON OF ACUTE AND CHRONIC PAIN

CHARACTERISTIC	ACUTE PAIN	CHRONIC PAIN
Experience	An event	A situation; state of existence
Source	External agent or internal disease usually known	Unknown; if known, treatment is prolonged or ineffective
Onset	Usually sudden	May be sudden or develop insidiously
Duration	Transient (up to 6 months)	Prolonged and persistent (months to years)
Pain identification	Painful and nonpainful areas generally well identified	Painful and nonpainful areas less easily differentiated: change in sensations becomes more difficult to evaluate
Clinical signs	Increased pulse rate, elevated blood pressure, increased respiratory rate, diaphoresis, dilated pupils	Response patterns vary; fewer overt signs (adaptation)
Significance	Significant (informs person something is wrong)	Person looks for significance
Pattern	Self-limiting or readily corrected	Continuous or intermittent; intensity may vary or remain constant
Course	Suffering usually decreases over time	Suffering usually increases over time
Actions	Leads to actions to relieve pain	Leads to actions to modify pain experience
Prognosis	Likelihood of eventual complete relief	Complete relief usually not possible

Data from Black RG: *Surg Clin North Am* 55(4):999, 1975.

TABLE 16-3 COMMON CHRONIC PAIN CONDITIONS

CONDITION	DESCRIPTION
Persistent low back pain	Most common chronic pain condition Results from poor muscle tone, inactivity, muscle strain, or sudden, vigorous exercise
Myofascial pain syndromes	Second most common chronic pain condition Pain results from muscle spasm, tenderness, and stiffness Examples include myositis, fibrositis, myofibrositis, myalgia, and muscle strain—conditions that involve injury to the muscle and fascia As disorder progresses, pain becomes increasingly generalized
Chronic postoperative pain	Chronic pain that can occur with disruption or cutting of sensory nerves
Cancer pain	Can be pain attributed to advance of disease, associated with treatment, or attributed to coexisting disease entities
Deafferentation pain	Painful condition resulting from damage to a peripheral nerve Common types include severe burning pain triggered by various stimuli, such as cold, light touch, or sound, and reflex sympathetic dystrophies (occur after peripheral nerve injury and are characterized by continuous, severe, burning pain associated with vasomotor changes and muscle wasting)
Hyperesthesias	Increased sensitivity and decreased pain threshold to tactile and painful stimuli Pain is diffuse, modified by fatigue and emotion, and mixed with other sensations May result from chronic irritations of central nervous system areas
Hemiagnosia	Loss of ability to identify source of pain on one side of the body Painful stimuli on that side produce discomfort, anxiety, moaning, agitation, and distress but no attempt to withdraw from the stimulus Associated with stroke
Phantom limb pain	Pain experienced in amputated limb after stump has completely healed; may be immediate or occur months later Influenced by emotions or sympathetic stimulation Trigger points—small hypersensitive regions in muscle or connective tissues that, when stimulated, produce pain in a specific area

and muscle strain. These conditions involve myofascial trigger points within a taut band of skeletal muscle. The pain may be the result of low-threshold mechanosensitive afferents projecting to sensitized dorsal horn neurons and the development of peripheral and central sensitization.[49] Neuroaxonal degeneration with alterations in neuromuscular transmission may occur. Compression of the trigger point causes referred pain, motor dysfunction, and autonomic responses. During the early stages of the disorder the pain is localized, but as the disorder progresses it becomes deep, aching, and more generalized. These, like many other chronic conditions, begin as a result of poor muscle tone, inactivity, muscle or tendon strain, or sudden vigorous exercise and can evolve into a chronic pain state.

Chronic postoperative pain occurs in some individuals and includes complex regional pain syndrome, phantom limb pain, chronic donor site pain, post-thoracotomy pain syndrome, postmastectomy pain syndrome, and joint arthroplasty pain. Plastic changes in the peripheral nervous system (PNS) and CNS contribute to allodynia and hypersensitivity. Multimodal approaches to analgesia are needed for pain management including adequate management of preoperative pain and postoperative management of acute pain.[41,50]

Cancer pain is often chronic and associated with neuropathies. The categories include[51]: (1) pain attributed to tumor growth and advance of the disease, (2) pain associated with treatment of the disease, and (3) pain attributed to coexisting entities (e.g., osteoarthritis) that are unrelated to the disease. Cancer and immune cells can release mediators that sensitize primary afferent nociceptors in the area of the tumor. Infection and inflammation, increasing pressure of a growing tumor on nerve endings, tissue destruction, distention of visceral surfaces, and obstruction of ducts and intestine also cause pain.[52] Alterations in the dorsal horn and other central pain processing pathways lead to central sensitization and chronic pain.[52] Therapeutic approaches to the management of cancer pain have advanced significantly in recent years, particularly in palliative care and hospice programs. Frequent assessment of pain, management of breakthrough pain, and implementation of individualized interdisciplinary therapeutic strategies (including pharmacotherapeutic, anesthetic, neurosurgical, psychologic, and rehabilitative techniques along with frequent evaluations) are essential to optimal cancer pain management.[53]

Neuropathic Pain

Neuropathic pain results from primary injury to the peripheral or central nervous system and is not the result of pain signaling from peripheral tissues or organs. Chronic neuropathic pain leads to long-term plastic changes along somatosensory pathways from the periphery to the cortex and abnormal processing of sensory information by the PNS and CNS. The pathogenesis of neuropathic pain syndromes includes both peripheral and central mechanisms of pain sensitization.[54]

Peripheral neuropathic pain is caused by peripheral nerve trauma, diabetic or alcohol abuse–induced neuropathy, carcinoma, nutritional deficiencies, and human immunodeficiency virus (HIV). When injured nerves become hyperexcitable, they generate ectopic discharges, resulting in spontaneous firing of some neurons with low thresholds for mechanical, chemical, or thermal stimuli. Pain sensation can occur in the absence of a stimulus and may be evoked by movement *(incident pain)*, and hypersensitivity and/or allodynia may be present in the involved body part.

Central neuropathic pain is caused by a lesion or dysfunction in the CNS (brain or spinal cord). Alterations of the sensory pathways and impairment of descending inhibitory mechanisms contribute to the pain. Examples of central causes of neuropathic pain include brain or spinal cord trauma, tumors, vascular lesions, multiple sclerosis, Parkinson disease, postherpetic neuralgia (PHN), phantom limb pain, and reflex sympathetic dystrophy.

Neuropathic pain is often paroxysmal with hyperesthesia and paresthesias (tingling sensations of pins and needles), burning, shooting, or stabbing sensations. Neuropathic pain is often described as "gnawing" and miserable. No single diagnostic test for neuropathic pain (or for pain in general) is available, and differentiating some neuropathies from other chronic somatic pain syndromes can be difficult.[55,56]

Lesions resulting in loss of sensory input to the dorsal column of the spinal cord from a part of the body are called *deafferentation*. **Deafferentation pain syndromes** are neuropathies that result from lesions in the peripheral nervous system (i.e., complex regional pain syndrome type II, postherpetic neuralgia, phantom limb pain, tumor infiltration of nerve tissue; damage from radiation, chemotherapy, brachial plexus avulsion, or surgical sectioning of a nerve) or lesions in the central nervous system that interrupt the spinothalamic pathways at any level of the nervous system (i.e., thalamic lesions or stroke). Deafferentation pain syndromes are associated with hyperexcitability of the somatosensory thalamus and cortex.[57] Deafferentation pain, which is poorly controlled by many analgesics, is usually described as a constant, dull, viselike ache, accompanied by paroxysms of burning or electric shock–like sensations. There may be loss of temperature sensation. The pain may manifest over a large and diffuse area or be well-defined and circumscribed. It is usually irritating and constant, can be difficult to treat, and can cause considerable suffering.[58,59]

Hemiagnosia pain is a form of central pain associated with stroke that produces paralysis and hypersensitivity/allodynia on one half of the body. In this painful condition, often a concomitant loss of ability to identify the source of pain through normal sensory pathways occurs. The result is a confusing presentation in which even mild stimulation of the affected side of the body produces discomfort, anxiety, moaning, agitation, and distress, with a diminished ability to withdraw from the offending stimulus.

Phantom limb pain is pain that an individual feels in an amputated limb after the stump has completely healed. Nonpainful phantom limb sensations occur in almost all amputees, but the sensations usually fade with time. This is distinguished from the syndrome of phantom limb pain, a chronic pain occurring in 80% to 100% of amputees.[60,61] It is more likely to appear in individuals who experienced pain in the limb before amputation. Theories about the cause of phantom limb pain include regeneration or hyperactivity of injured or cut peripheral nerves, scar tissue or neuroma formation in the cut peripheral nerves, spinal cord deafferentation, and alterations in the thalamus and cortex. It has been proposed that CNS integration, including reorganization and plastic changes of the somatosensory cortex, results in the perception of pain from receptors associated with the amputated limb even though the limb itself is no longer present.[62] The absence of inhibitory effects of sensory input from the missing peripheral body part may cause increased autonomous activity of dorsal horn neurons with pain transmission. The cause is likely multifactorial, contributing to the difficulty of prevention or effective treatment.[63]

Sympathetically mediated pain (SMP) is another type of neuropathic pain that can occur after peripheral nerve or extremity injury. The diseases formerly called *reflex sympathetic dystrophy* and *causalgia*, both thought to arise from sympathetic nervous system imbalance, are now called **complex regional pain syndromes (CRPSs)** type I (associated with injury but no apparent nerve injury) and type II (evidence of nerve injury). CRPS develops 1 to 2 weeks after an extremity injury (e.g., a fracture without identifiable nerve injury) (type I) or an injury to the brachial plexus or the median, sciatic, or other peripheral nerves (type II). The exact pathophysiologic mechanism is unclear. A combination of injury and the presence of inflammatory cytokines and neuropeptides may lead to peripheral nociceptive sensitization and physiologic change in pain transmission and autonomic and motor systems.[64] The severe, diffuse, burning, and persistent pain occurs in the extremity or area supplied by the injured nerve. Hypersensitivity and allodynia are common. Discoloration and changes in the texture of the skin may appear in the affected area. Vasomotor changes usually begin with vasodilation and are followed by vasoconstriction and cool, cyanotic, and edematous extremities. Swelling and stiffness of proximate joints may occur. Hair loss is usually noted and there are changes in skin color and temperature.[65]

In the evaluation and management of neuropathic pain, as well as all other chronic pain states, psychologic components (e.g., depression or anxiety), sleep disturbances, work-related issues of impairment and disability, treatment expectations, the availability of social support from family and friends (or lack thereof), and legal compensation should not be overlooked.[66]

PEDIATRICS AND PERCEPTION OF PAIN

Infants and children have the anatomic and functional ability to perceive pain. Pain pathways and cortical and subcortical centers for pain perception, as well as neurochemicals associated with pain transmission and modulation, are functional in preterm and newborn infants. The nociceptor system is functional in fetuses by 20 to 24 weeks of gestation although the cortical experience may be minimal.[67,68] Repetitive, painful experiences and prolonged exposure to analgesic drugs in infants, in children, and during the neonatal period may permanently alter synaptic and neuronal organization[69] and fetal pain may have an enduring effect on behavior and pain perception.[70,71]

Facial expression, crying, body movements, and lack of consolability are the most consistent expressions of pain in infants. The painful facial expression includes lowered brows drawn together; presence of a vertical bulge and furrows in the forehead between the brows; broadened nasal root; tightly closed, scourged eye fissures; and angular, tongue cupping, squarish mouth and chin quiver (Figure 16-7). Physiologic responses include increases in heart rate, blood pressure, and respiratory rate although these measures lack sensitivity and specificity. There may be flushing or pallor, sweating, and decreased oxygen saturation.[72] Toddlers also express pain with crying, facial expression, and body language (tensed body, guarding, and hands holding body). Older children, between ages 5 and 18 years, tend to have a lower pain threshold than do adults. Children, like adults, have highly individual responses to pain. Any behavioral and physiologic indicators of pain must be carefully and accurately assessed[73] and adequately treated for children of all ages.[74,75]

AGING AND PERCEPTION OF PAIN

Studies on pain perception in the older adult population have yielded conflicting evidence. Some studies show an increase in pain threshold with aging; others show no change.[76-78] The varied results are probably a function of independent variation in

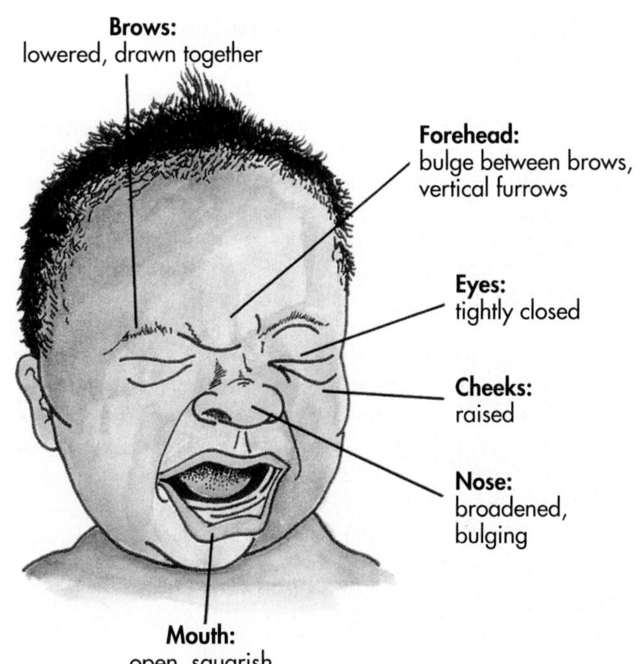

FIGURE 16-7 Painful Facial Expression of Infants. (From Hockenberry MJ: *Wong's nursing care of infants and children,* ed 7, St Louis, 2003, Mosby.)

the sensory-discriminative, motivational-affective, and cognitive-evaluative components of the pain experience. In general, studies confirm that an increase in the pain threshold occurs in some older adults. This change may be caused by peripheral neuropathies and changes in the thickness of the skin or cognitive impairment. (Neuropathies are discussed in Chapter 18.) A decrease in pain tolerance is also evident in some older adults, and women appear to be more sensitive to pain than are men[79,80] (see What's New? Pain and Gender). Pain in the older adult is also influenced by liver and renal function, including alterations in metabolism of drugs and metabolites and age-associated brain changes. Pain must be accurately assessed in relation to its effect on cognitive function, coexisting disease, drug interactions, other reactions to treatment, and an individual's ability to express pain and safety.[43] Poorly managed pain can result in depression, inactivity, and failure to maintain activities of daily living.[81]

TEMPERATURE REGULATION

In all homeothermic animals, temperature regulation is achieved through precise balancing of heat production, heat conservation, and heat loss. In humans, body temperature is maintained around 37° C (98.6° F) and rarely exceeds 41° C (105.8° F). The normal range is 36.2° to 37.7° C (97.2° to 99.9° F), but all parts of the body do not have the same temperature. The extremities, for example, are generally cooler than the trunk. The temperature at the core of the body (as measured by rectal temperature) is generally 0.5° C higher than the surface temperature (as measured by oral temperature) and has minimal fluctuations. The internal temperature varies normally in response to activity, environmental temperature, and daily

WHAT'S NEW?

Pain and Gender

Gender differences in the experience of pain and the response to analgesics have been studied in both animal and human research. Women report higher pain levels or have less tolerance for pain stimuli, such as heat, cold, pressure, and electrical stimulation. The differences may be related to mechanisms of excitatory and inhibitory control. Gender differences exist also in the prevalence of painful chronic diseases; for example, women are more affected by intestinal cystitis, fibromyalgia, and rheumatoid arthritis, and men are more affected by cluster headache. Pain symptoms differ for men and women for diseases such as coronary artery disease, irritable bowel syndrome, appendicitis, and cancer. Sex hormones are known to have an effect on the mechanisms and outcomes of opiate analgesia, and in rodents, morphine analgesia is more effective in males than in females. Pain sensitivities in women also vary across the phases of the menstrual cycle. Recent human and animal studies suggests that κ-opioid receptor analgesia is greater in women than in men and may reflect a difference in endogenous pain circuits mediated by different opiate receptor subtypes and influenced by effects of estrogen and progesterone. Gender differences with respect to pain also are influenced by role socialization, cognitive factors, and culture. Continuing research is needed to further understand gender differences in the operation of pain mechanisms and the development of more specific pain management strategies.

Data from Leresche L: *Clin Orthop Relat Res* 469(7):1871–1877, 2011; Mogil JS, Bailey AL: *Prog Brain Res* 186:141–157, 2010; Palmeira CC, Ashmawi HA, Posso Ide P: *Rev Bras Anestesiol* 61(6):814–828, 2011; Popescu A et al: *Pain* 150(2):309–318, 2010; Racine M et al: *Pain* 153(3):602–618, 2012; Racine M et al: *Pain* 153(3):619–635, 2012; Rasakham K, Liu-Chen LY: *Life Sci* 88(1-2):2–16, 2011.

fluctuation of **circadian rhythm** (the pattern of each 24-hour day). Oral temperatures generally fluctuate within 0.2° to 0.5° C during a 24-hour period. Women tend to have wider fluctuations that follow the menstrual cycle, with a sharp rise in temperature just before ovulation. In both genders the daily fluctuating temperature peaks around 6 PM and is at its lowest during sleep.[82] Maintenance of body temperature within the normal range is necessary for life.

Hypothalamic Control of Temperature

Temperature regulation (**thermoregulation**) is mediated by the hypothalamus. Peripheral thermoreceptors in the skin and abdominal organs (unmyelinated C fibers and thinly myelinated Aδ fibers) and central thermoreceptors in the spinal cord and other central locations provide the hypothalamus with information about skin and core temperatures. If these temperatures are low or high, the hypothalamus responds by triggering heat production, heat conservation, or heat loss mechanisms. The endocrine system also operates to control body temperature.[83]

Increased **heat production** is initiated by a series of hormonal mechanisms involving the hypothalamus and its connections with the endocrine system. The heat-producing mechanism begins with a hypothalamic hormone, thyroid-stimulating hormone–releasing hormone (TSH-RH). In turn, TSH-RH stimulates the anterior pituitary to release TSH, which acts on the thyroid gland, stimulating release of thyroxine (T_4), one of the thyroid hormones. This hormone then acts on the adrenal medulla, causing the release of epinephrine (a catecholamine and vasopressive hormone) into the bloodstream (see Chapter 21). Epinephrine causes vasoconstriction (improves thermal insulation), stimulates glycolysis, and increases metabolic rates, thus increasing heat production. Heat is distributed by the circulatory system.

The hypothalamus also triggers heat conservation. The mechanisms of heat conservation involve stimulating the sympathetic nervous system, which is responsible for stimulating the adrenal cortex, increasing skeletal muscle tone, initiating the shivering response, and producing vasoconstriction. The hypothalamus also functions in raising body temperatures by relaying information to the cerebral cortex. Awareness of cold provokes voluntary responses such as increasing body movement and wearing protective clothing.

The hypothalamus responds to warmer core and peripheral temperatures by reversing the same mechanisms. The TSH-RH pathway is shut down. The sympathetic pathway is prompted to produce cutaneous vasodilation, decreased muscle tone, and increased sweat production. Hypothalamic stimulation of the cerebral cortex provokes voluntary behavior to reduce heat production and promote heat loss.[84]

Mechanisms of heat production, heat loss, and heat conservation maintain body temperature within a narrow range of 98° F (36.6° C) and 100° F (37.7° C) when the ambient temperature is between 68° F (20° C) and 130° F (54.4° C).

Mechanisms of Heat Production

Chemical Reactions of Metabolism. The *chemical reactions* that occur during the ingestion and metabolism of food and those required to maintain the body at rest (basal metabolism) require energy and produce heat. These processes occur in the body core (primarily the liver) and are in part responsible for the maintenance of core temperature.

Skeletal Muscle Contraction. Skeletal muscles produce heat through two mechanisms: (1) gradual increase in muscle tone and (2) production of rapid muscle oscillations (*shivering*—which does not occur in neonates). Both increasing muscle tone and shivering are controlled by the posterior hypothalamus and occur in response to cold. As peripheral temperature drops, muscle tone increases and shivering begins. Shivering is a fairly effective method for increasing heat production because no work is performed and all the energy produced is retained as heat.[85]

Chemical Thermogenesis. Chemical thermogenesis, also called *nonshivering thermogenesis* or *adrenergic thermogenesis*, results from the release of epinephrine and norepinephrine. Epinephrine and norepinephrine produce a rapid, transient increase in heat production by raising the body's basal metabolic rate. Chemical thermogenesis seems to be different from hormone-triggered increases in the basal metabolic rate. Chemical thermogenesis produces a quick, brief rise in basal metabolic rate, whereas the hormone thyroxine triggers a slow, prolonged rise. Chemical thermogenesis occurs in brown adipose tissue. Brown adipose tissue is rich with mitochondria and blood vessels and is essential for nonshivering thermogenesis. White and brown adipocytes are found together in visceral and subcutaneous tissue. White adipocytes store energy and brown adipocytes produce heat. Adipocytes demonstrate transdifferentiation and such plasticity allows direct conversion of one cell type into the other. With chronic cold exposure white-to-brown conversion increases thermogenesis, whereas excessive food consumption induces brown-to-white conversion to meet the need for energy storage.[86]

Mechanisms of Heat Loss

Heat loss is achieved through many mechanisms: (1) radiation, (2) conduction, (3) convection, (4) vasodilation, (5) decreased muscle tone, (6) evaporation, (7) increased pulmonary ventilation, (8) voluntary measures, and (9) adaptation to warmer climates.

Radiation. **Radiation** refers to heat loss through electromagnetic waves. These waves emanate from surfaces with temperatures higher than the surrounding air temperature. Thus if the temperature of the skin is higher than that of the air, the skin and therefore the body lose heat to the air.

Conduction. **Conduction** refers to heat loss by direct molecule-to-molecule transfer from one surface to another. Through conduction, the warmer surface loses heat to the cooler surface. Thus the skin loses heat through direct contact with cooler air, water, or another surface. In the same manner, the core of the body loses heat to the cooler body surface.

Convection. **Convection** is the transfer of heat through currents of gases or liquids. It greatly aids heat loss through conduction by exchanging warmer air at the surface of the body with cooler air in the surrounding space. Convection occurs passively as warmer air at the surface of the body rises away from the body and is replaced by cooler air, but the process may be aided by fans or wind. (The combined effect of conduction and convection by wind is conventionally measured as the *windchill factor*.)

Vasodilation. Peripheral vasodilation increases heat loss by diverting core-warmed blood to the surface of the body. As the core-warmed blood passes through the periphery, heat is transferred by conduction to the skin surface and from the skin to the surrounding environment. Because heat loss through conduction depends on the surrounding temperature, it is minimal to nonexistent if the surrounding air or water is warmer than the body surface.

Vasodilation occurs in response to autonomic stimulation under the control of the hypothalamus. It is useful in instances of moderate temperature elevation. As core temperature increases, vasodilation increases until maximal dilation is achieved. At that point the body must use additional heat loss mechanisms.

Decreased Muscle Tone. To decrease heat production, muscle tone may be moderately reduced and voluntary muscle activity curtailed. These mechanisms explain in part the "washed-out" feeling associated with high temperatures and warm weather. Decreased muscle tone and reduced activity have a limited effect on decreasing heat production, however, because muscle tone and heat production cannot be reduced below basal body requirements.

Evaporation. Evaporation of body water from the surface of the skin and the linings of the mucous membranes is a major source of heat reduction. Insensible water loss (in the absence of perceptible sweating) accounts for a loss of about 600 ml of water per day. Heat is lost as surface fluid is converted to gas, so that heat loss by evaporation is increased if more fluids are available at the body surface. To speed this process, fluids are actively secreted through the sweat glands. As much as 2.2 L of fluid per hour may be lost by sweating. Electrolytes are lost with the water. Therefore, loss of large volumes through sweating may result in decreased plasma volume, decreased blood pressure, weakness, and fainting. (Alterations in fluid balance are discussed in Chapter 3.)

Like other heat reduction mechanisms, stimulation of sweating occurs in response to sympathetic neural activity and depends on a favorable temperature difference between the body and the environment. In addition, heat loss through evaporation is affected by the relative humidity of the air. If the humidity is low, sweat evaporates quickly, but if the humidity is high, sweat does not evaporate and instead remains on the skin or drips off.

Increased Pulmonary Ventilation. Exchanging air with the environment through the normal pulmonary ventilation provides some heat loss, although it is minimal in humans. As air is inhaled, the air draws heat from the upper respiratory tract. The air is further warmed in the alveoli by blood in the microcirculation. This warmed air then is exhaled into the environment. This normal process occurs faster at higher body temperatures through an increase in ventilatory rates. Thus hyperventilation is associated with hyperthermia. (Normal pulmonary function is discussed in Chapter 34.)

Voluntary Mechanisms. In response to high body temperatures, people physically "stretch out," thereby increasing the body surface area available for heat loss. They also "slow down" or "take it easy," thereby decreasing skeletal muscle work, and they "dress for warm weather" with light-colored, loose-fitting garments to reflect heat and promote convection, conduction, and evaporation.

Adaptation to Warmer Climates. The body of an individual who moves from a cooler to a much warmer climate undergoes a period of adjustment, a process that takes several days to weeks. At first the individual experiences feelings of lassitude, weakness, and faintness with even moderate activity. Body temperatures rise with any work. Within several days, however, the individual experiences an earlier onset of sweating, the volume of sweat is increased, and the sodium content is lowered. Heart rate is decreased and stroke volume increased so that cardiac output remains unchanged. Extracellular fluid volume increases, as does plasma volume. These physiologic adaptations result in improved warm weather functioning and decreased symptoms of heat intolerance. People's work output, endurance, and coordination increase, and their subjective feelings of discomfort decrease.[87]

Mechanisms of Heat Conservation

The body conserves heat and protects core temperature through two important mechanisms: (1) involuntary vasoconstriction mediated by the sympathetic nervous system and (2) voluntary mechanisms.[88] To preserve core temperature, the skin and periphery are used as an insulating cover.[87]

Vasoconstriction. By constricting peripheral blood vessels, centrally warmed blood is shunted away from the periphery (where radiation, conduction, and convection would allow heat loss) to the core of the body, where heat can be retained. This mechanism takes advantage of the insulating layers of the skin and subcutaneous fat to protect core temperature.

Voluntary Mechanisms. In response to lower body temperatures, individuals typically "bundle up," "keep moving," or "curl up in a ball." Bundling up involves dressing with several layers of clothes that allow air to be trapped between the skin and the clothing, thus providing an additional layer of insulation. Keeping moving, stamping feet, clapping hands, jogging, and other types of physical activity increase skeletal muscle activity and thus promote heat production. Curling up in a ball decreases the amount of skin surface available for heat loss through radiation, convection, and conduction.

PEDIATRICS AND TEMPERATURE REGULATION

Infants and older adults require special attention to maintenance of body temperature. Term infants produce sufficient body heat, primarily through the metabolism of brown fat, but they are unable to efficiently conserve heat because of the infant's small body size, greater ratio of body surface area to body weight with heat loss through conduction and convection, and inability to shiver. Infants have a thin layer of subcutaneous fat and thus are not as well insulated as adults.[89] Therefore, it is important to keep infants warm with hats, clothing, and blankets. Children also have a greater ratio of body surface area to body weight, lower sweating rate, higher peripheral blood flow in the heat, and a greater extent of vasoconstriction in the cold than adults. They can acclimatize to changes in environmental temperatures, but do so at a lower rate than that seen in adults.[90]

AGING AND TEMPERATURE REGULATION

Older adults have poor responses to environmental temperature extremes as a result of slowed blood circulation, structural and functional changes in the skin, an overall decrease in heat-producing activities, and the presence of disease (i.e., congestive heart failure, chronic lung disease, diabetes mellitus, or peripheral vascular disease). Cold stress in older adults also decreases coronary perfusion.[91] Other factors affecting thermal regulation in the older adult population include decreased shivering response (delayed onset and decreased effectiveness), slowed metabolic rate, sedentary lifestyle, decreased vasoconstrictor and vasodilator responses, diminished or absent sweating, desynchronization of circadian rhythm, undernutrition, and decreased perception of heat and cold.[92-94]

Pathogenesis of Fever

Fever (febrile response or pyrexia) is a temporary resetting of the hypothalamic thermostat to a higher level in response to endogenous or exogenous pyrogens.[95] The pathophysiologic mechanism of fever begins with the introduction of **exogenous pyrogens** or endotoxins produced by pathogens (Figure 16-8). The most frequently encountered exogenous pyrogens are the lipopolysaccharide complex in the cell wall of gram-positive bacteria and viruses. **Endogenous pyrogens,** including prostaglandin E_2 (PGE_2), interleukin-1 (IL-1), IL-6, tumor necrosis factor-alpha (TNF-α), and interferon-γ, are produced by phagocytic cells as they destroy microorganisms within the host. The endogenous pyrogens act on the preoptic nucleus of the hypothalamus. An integrated behavioral, endocrine, and autonomic nervous system response is then initiated. Centers in the hypothalamus and brainstem signal an increase in heat production and heat conservation to raise body temperature to the new set point. Peripheral vasoconstriction occurs with shunting of blood from the skin to the body core. Epinephrine release increases metabolic rate, and muscle tone increases. Decreased release of vasopressin reduces the volume of body fluid to be heated. Shivering also may occur. The individual dresses more warmly, decreases body surface area by curling up, and may go to bed in an effort to get warm. Body temperature is maintained at the new level until the fever "breaks."

During fever, arginine vasopressin (AVP), α-melanocyte-stimulating hormone (α-MSH), and corticotropin-releasing factor are released from the brain, and systemic anti-inflammatory cytokines (i.e., IL-1 receptor agonist and IL-10) can act as **endogenous cryogens** or **antipyretics** to help diminish and control the febrile response.[95] This antipyretic effect constitutes a negative-feedback loop (see Figure 16-8). The antipyretic effect may help explain fluctuations in the febrile response. When the fever breaks, the set point is returned to normal. The hypothalamus responds by signaling a decrease in heat production and an increase in heat reduction mechanisms. The result is decreased muscle tone, peripheral vasodilation, flushed skin, and sweating. The individual feels very warm, replaces warm clothing with cooler clothes, throws off the covers, and stretches out. Once the body has returned to a normal temperature, the individual feels more comfortable and the hypothalamus adjusts thermoregulatory mechanisms to maintain the new temperature.

Benefits of Fever

Moderate fever aids responses to infectious processes through several mechanisms.[96] A raised body temperature kills many microorganisms and has adverse effects on the growth and replication of others. Higher body temperatures decrease serum levels of iron, zinc, and copper, all of which are needed for bacterial replication. The body switches from burning glucose to a metabolism based on lipolysis and proteolysis, thereby depriving bacteria of a food source. Anorexia and somnolence reduce the demand for muscle glucose.[97,98] Increased temperature also causes lysosomal breakdown and autodestruction of cells, thus preventing viral replication in infected cells. Acute-phase proteins produced by the liver during inflammation bind cations necessary for bacterial reproduction. Heat increases lymphocytic transformation and motility of polymorphonuclear neutrophils, thus facilitating the immune response. Phagocytosis is enhanced, and production of antiviral interferon may be augmented.[99]

Because fever is a beneficial response to infection, suppressing fever with antipyrogenic medications should be reviewed

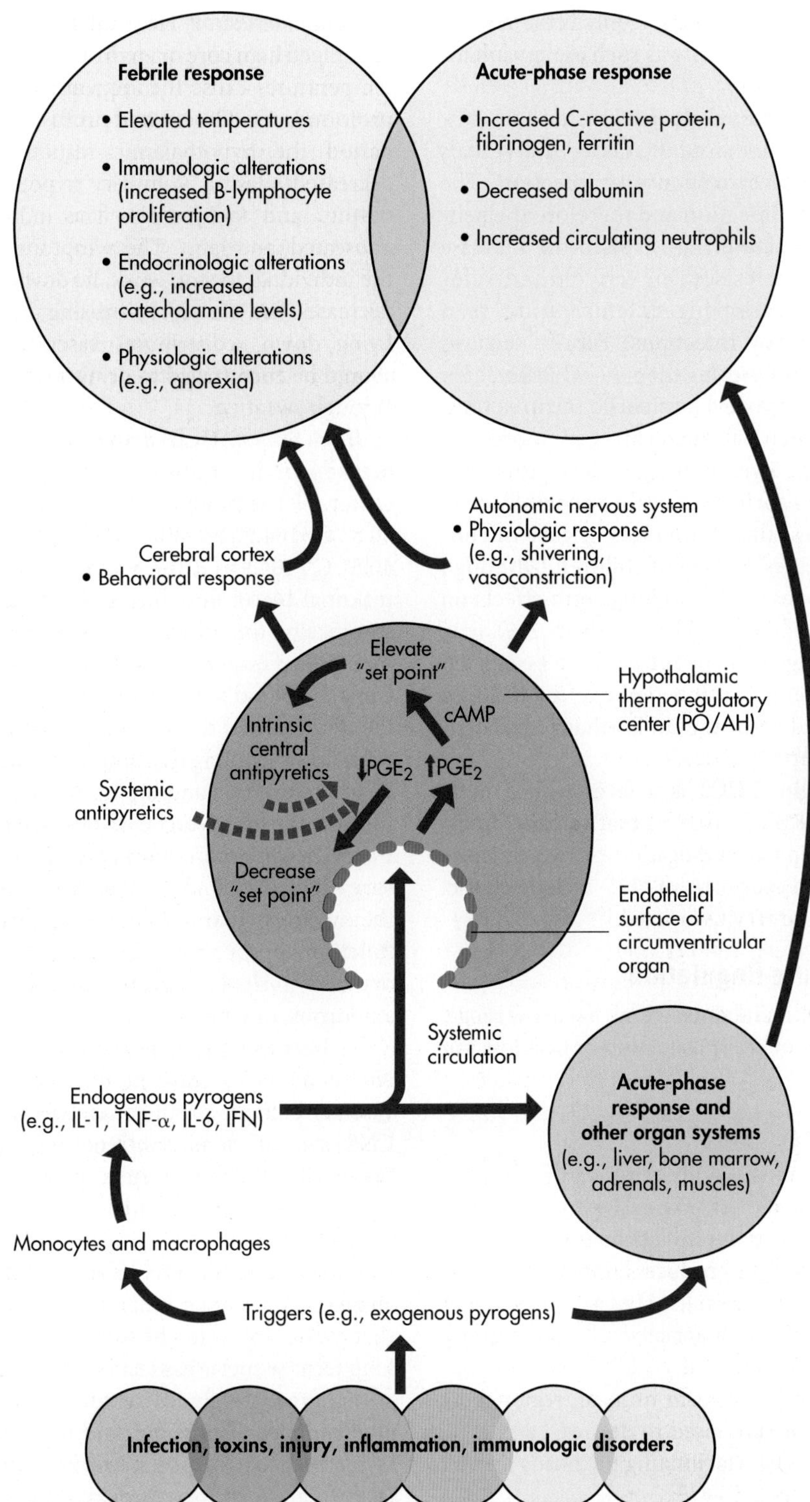

FIGURE 16-8 **Pathogenesis of Fever and Acute-Phase Response.** Certain disease states, through the elaboration of exogenous pyrogens, stimulate monocytes and macrophages to produce endogenous pyrogens such as IL-1, IL-6, TNF-α, and interferon-γ. These pyrogenic cytokines act at the endothelial surface of the circumventricular organ of the preoptic area of the anterior hypothalamus *(PO/AH)* to induce the production of PGE_2, which elevates the body's thermal set point. Physiologic and behavioral responses may be invoked to raise body temperature to a new set point. This febrile response must be considered in the context of an overlapping acute-phase response as a global nonspecific response to the original insult. Intrinsic central antipyretics and systemic antipyretics exert their effects by decreasing levels of PGE_2, thus decreasing the "set point" and lowering body temperature. The red dotted line represents a negative feedback response. *cAMP,* Cyclic adenosine monophosphate; *IFN,* interferon; *IL-1, IL-6,* interleukin-1, interleukin-6; *PGE_2,* prostaglandin E_2; *TNF-α,* tumor necrosis factor-alpha. (Modified from Armstrong D, Cohen J: *Infectious diseases,* ed 2, St Louis, 2004, Mosby.)

carefully.[100] Such treatment should be used only if the fever is high enough to produce serious side effects such as nerve damage or convulsion.

Infection and fever responses in older adults and in children may vary from those in the adult. Older individuals may have decreased or no fever response to infection. The absence of fever responses to infection and therefore the beneficial aspects of fever production may explain the increase in morbidity and mortality rates seen in very old individuals.[101] In contrast, children develop higher temperatures than do adults for relatively minor infections. Febrile seizures may occur with temperatures greater than 39° C (102.2° F), although most children do not develop febrile seizures until temperatures are much higher. Febrile seizures are more predominant in boys before age 5 years, and genetic factors contribute to susceptibility.[102] Febrile seizures are generally brief and self-limiting, lasting less than 5 minutes in 40% of children and less than 20 minutes in 75% of children. Although in most instances there appear to be no long-term effects on the child, a small percentage of children (1% to 2%) may develop epilepsy.[103] Prolonged febrile seizures are associated with the development of temporal lobe epilepsy in children and are probably associated with functional changes in neurons and neural networks.[104,105]

Fever of unknown origin (FUO) is a fever with a body temperature greater than 38.3° C (101° F) that remains undiagnosed after 3 days of hospital investigation or two or more outpatient visits. The clinical categories of FUO include classic, nosocomial, neutropenic, and HIV associated.[106]

Disorders of Temperature Regulation

Internal body temperature is maintained within a narrow range. Alterations in the regulation of heat production or heat loss can be life-threatening.

Hyperthermia

Hyperthermia is elevation of the body temperature without an increase in the hypothalamic set point. Hyperthermia can produce nerve damage, coagulation of cell proteins, and death. At 41° C (105.8° F), nerve damage produces convulsions in the adult. At 43° C (109.4° F), death results. Hyperthermia is not mediated by pyrogens, and may be associated with brain injury or applied therapeutically.

Therapeutic hyperthermia is a form of local, regional, or whole-body induced hyperthermia used to destroy pathologic microorganisms or tumor cells by facilitating the host's natural immune process or tumor blood flow.[107]

Accidental hyperthermia includes: (1) heat cramps, (2) heat exhaustion, (3) heat stroke, and (4) malignant hyperthermia.[108]

Heat Cramps. **Heat cramps** are severe spasmodic cramps in the abdomen and extremities that follow prolonged sweating and associated sodium loss. Heat cramps usually appear in individuals who are not accustomed to heat or in those who are performing strenuous work in very warm climates. Fever, rapid pulse rate, and increased blood pressure often accompany the cramps. Treatment involves administration of dilute salt solutions through oral or parenteral routes.

Heat Exhaustion. **Heat exhaustion,** or collapse, is a result of prolonged high core or environmental temperatures. These high temperatures cause the appropriate hypothalamic response of profound vasodilation and profuse sweating. Over a prolonged period the hypothalamic responses produce dehydration, decreased plasma volumes, hypotension, decreased cardiac output, and tachycardia. The individual feels weak, dizzy, nauseated, and faint. The symptoms of heat exhaustion cause the individual to stop work, lie down, and rest. Ceasing activity decreases muscle work, causing decreased heat production. Lying down redistributes vascular volume. The individual should be encouraged to drink warm fluids to replace fluid lost through sweating.

Heat Stroke. **Heat stroke** is a potentially lethal result of a breakdown in control of an overstressed thermoregulatory center.[109] The brain cannot tolerate temperatures greater than 40.5° C (104.9° F). When core temperature reaches or exceeds 40.5° C (104.9° F), the brain may be preferentially cooled by maximal blood flow through the veins of the head and face, specifically the forehead. Sweat production on the face is maintained even during dehydration. Evaporation of the sweat cools the blood in the veins of the face and forehead; the blood then is returned to the endocranial venous network and sinus cavernosus, cooling the blood in the cerebral arterial vessels that lie in proximity. Fanning the face enhances this mechanism. In this way the brain can be maintained temporarily at 40° C (104° F), even when core temperatures are higher. In instances of very high core temperatures (40° to 43° C [104° to 109.4° F]), the cardiovascular and thermoregulatory centers may cease to function appropriately. Sweating ceases, and the skin becomes dry and flushed. The individual may be irritable, confused, stuporous, or comatose. Visual disturbances may occur.

As heat loss through the evaporation of sweat ceases, core temperatures increase rapidly. High core temperatures and vascular collapse produce cerebral edema, degeneration of the CNS, swollen dendrites, renal tubular necrosis, and multiple organ failure. Death results unless immediate, effective treatment is initiated. Individuals who recover from heat stroke may have permanent damage to the thermoregulatory center and thus may have difficulty tolerating environmental temperature changes. A systemic inflammatory response syndrome (SIRS) that ensues following heat-induced tissue injury may cause the long term sequelae associated with heat-injured tissue.[110]

Treatment includes removing the person from the warm environment, if possible, and using a cooling blanket or cool water bath or ice packs on the head, neck, groin, and axillae.[108] Care must be taken to prevent too rapid cooling of the surface, which causes peripheral vasoconstriction and prevents core cooling. Children are more susceptible to heat stroke than adults because (1) they produce more metabolic heat when exercising, (2) they have a greater surface area to body mass ratio, and (3) their sweating capacity is less than that of adults.

Malignant Hyperthermia. **Malignant hyperthermia** is a potentially lethal hypermetabolic complication of a rare inherited muscle disorder. The condition is precipitated by the administration of volatile anesthetics and neuromuscular-blocking agents. There is wide variability in incidence ranging from 1:5000 to 1:50,000. Malignant hyperthermia is caused by either increased myoplasmic calcium release or decreased calcium uptake with muscle contraction. This allows intracellular calcium levels to rise, producing sustained, uncoordinated muscle contractions, which in turn increase muscle work, oxygen consumption, and lactic acid production. As a result of these contractions, acidosis develops and temperature rises (body temperature may rise 1° C [1.8° F] every 5 minutes); approximately 5% of those who develop malignant hyperthermia do not survive.[111] Malignant hyperthermia occurs most often in children and young adults immediately after the induction of anesthesia. Sympathetic responses and acidosis produce tachycardia and cardiac dysrhythmias, followed by hypotension, decreased cardiac output, and, eventually, cardiac arrest. Increasing temperature, acidosis, hyperkalemia, and hypoxia produce coma-like symptoms in the CNS (including unconsciousness, absent reflexes, fixed pupils, apnea, and sometimes a flat electroencephalogram [EEG]). Oliguria and anuria are common, probably resulting from shock, ischemia, and low cardiac output.[112]

Treatment includes withdrawal of the provoking agents and administration of dantrolene sodium (a skeletal relaxant that inhibits calcium release during muscle contraction). Procainamide (Pronestyl) is used to treat cardiac dysrhythmias. Sodium bicarbonate is used for acidosis. Hyperkalemia can be treated with insulin and glucose. Body temperature can be decreased through use of ice bags, a cooling blanket, and iced saline lavage.

Hypothermia

Hypothermia (core body temperature less than 35° C [95° F]) is caused by prolonged exposure to cold. Hypothermia produces vasoconstriction, shivering, alterations in microcirculation, coagulation, and ischemic tissue damage. In a controlled situation, such as a surgical procedure, most tissues can tolerate temperatures as low as 33° C (91.4° F). In severe hypothermia (less than 28° C [82.4° F]), ice crystals forming on the inside of the cell cause cells to rupture and die. Tissue hypothermia slows the rate of chemical reactions (tissue metabolism), increases the viscosity of the blood, slows blood flow through the microcirculation, facilitates blood coagulation, and stimulates profound vasoconstriction. Hypothermia may be accidental or therapeutic. In accidental hypothermia, high-energy phosphates (e.g., ATP) are depleted, and in therapeutic hypothermia, ATP storage is preserved.[113,114]

Accidental Hypothermia. Accidental hypothermia is generally the result of sudden immersion in cold water or prolonged exposure to cold environments.[114] At particular risk for accidental hypothermia are young persons and older adults, because thermoregulatory mechanisms are altered in these two groups. Also at risk are individuals with conditions that diminish the ability to generate heat. Such conditions include hypothyroidism, hypopituitarism, decreased liver function, malnutrition, Parkinson disease, and rheumatoid arthritis. Other risk factors include chronic increased vasodilation and decreased thermoregulatory control caused by cerebral injuries, ketoacidosis, uremia, and drug overdoses. In acute hypothermia, peripheral vasoconstriction shunts blood away from the cooler skin to the core in an effort to decrease heat loss, which produces peripheral tissue ischemia. Intermittent reperfusion of the extremities (the Lewis phenomenon) helps preserve peripheral oxygenation. Intermittent peripheral perfusion continues until core temperatures drop dramatically.

The hypothalamic center stimulates **shivering** in an effort to increase heat production. Severe shivering occurs at core temperatures of 35° C (95° F) and continues until core temperature drops to about 30° to 32° C (86° to 89.6° F). Prolonged shivering can lead to exhaustion of liver glycogen stores. Thinking becomes sluggish and coordination is decreased at 34° C (93.2° F). As hypothermia deepens, paradoxical undressing may occur as hypothalamic control of vasoconstriction is lost and vasodilation occurs with loss of core heat to the periphery. The hypothermic individual therefore feels suddenly warm and begins to remove clothing.[115]

At 30° C (86° F), the individual becomes stuporous, heart rate and respiratory rate decline, and cardiac output is diminished. Cerebral blood flow is decreased. Metabolic rate declines, further decreasing core temperature. Sinus node depression occurs with slowing of conduction through the atrioventricular node. In severe hypothermia (core temperature of 26° to 28° C [78.8° to 82.4° F]), pulse and respirations may be undetectable. Acidosis is moderate to severe. Coagulopathy, ventricular fibrillation, and asystole are common.[116] Surface cooling may cause frostbite and fat necrosis.

If hypothermia is mild, passive rewarming may be sufficient. If core temperature is greater than 30° C (86° F), active rewarming also may be required. Active rewarming uses warm-water baths, warm blankets, heating pads, and warm oral fluids when the individual is fully alert. Core rewarming may be accomplished through administration of warm intravenous (IV) solutions, warm gastric lavage, warm peritoneal lavage, inhalation of warmed gases, and, in extreme cases, exchange transfusions, warming blood in a pump oxygenator circuit, and mediastinal lavage.[113]

Rewarming generally should proceed no faster than a few degrees per hour. Short-term complications of rewarming include acidosis, rewarming shock, and dysrhythmias. Long-term complications include congestive heart failure, hepatic and renal failure, abnormal erythropoiesis, myocardial infarction, pancreatitis, and neurologic dysfunctions.

Therapeutic Hypothermia. Therapeutic hypothermia is used to slow metabolism and preserve ischemic tissue after brain trauma or during brain surgery, after cardiac arrest, and in neonatal hypoxic encephalopathy.[117] Hypothermia protects the brain by reduction in metabolic rate, ATP consumption, oxidative stress, and the critical threshold for oxygen delivery; modulation of excitotoxic neurotransmitters and calcium antagonism; preservation of protein synthesis and the blood-brain barrier; decreased edema formation; and modulation of the inflammatory response.[118,119]

Trauma

Major body trauma has varying effects on temperature regulation, depending on the body systems involved. Five types of traumatic injury that usually affect temperature regulation are: (1) CNS trauma (discussed in Chapter 18), (2) accidental injury, (3) hemorrhagic shock, (4) major surgery, and (5) thermal burns.

Central Nervous System Trauma. CNS trauma that causes CNS damage, inflammation, increased intracranial pressures, or intracranial bleeding typically produces a temperature greater than 39° C (102.2° F). This temperature, often referred to as *neurogenic or central fever,* appears with or without relative bradycardia and is not caused by infection. The temperature is sustained, does not induce sweating, and is highly resistant to antipyretic therapy.[120]

Accidental Injuries. Mild accidental injuries may produce a slight elevation in core temperature. Moderate to severe injuries result in peripheral vasoconstriction with decreased surface and core temperatures. Core temperature is thought to be inversely related to the severity of the injury and may be a result of decreased oxygen transport to the tissues. In severe injuries, shivering is absent and some alteration in thermoregulation is evident.[121]

Hemorrhagic Shock. Loss of blood volume in hemorrhage triggers peripheral vasoconstriction and hypoxia, contributing to hypothermia. Risk for subsequent decreases in core temperature occurs when hemorrhagic shock is treated with unwarmed, volume-expanding solutions and surgery. Volume expansion with warmed solutions is recommended to prevent the deleterious effects of hypothermia on cardiac output, cardiac rhythm, and the immune system.

Major Surgery. Major surgery often induces significant hypothermia through exposure of body cavities to the relatively cool operating room environment, irrigation of body cavities with room temperature solutions, infusion of room temperature intravenous solutions, use of drugs that impair thermoregulatory mechanisms, and inhalation of unwarmed anesthetic agents. Anesthesia induces hypothermia, reduces platelet function, and impairs the coagulation cascade, contributing to transfusion requirements and postoperative complications. Use of warmed irrigating and intravenous solutions and perioperative forced air and skin warming procedures reduces intraoperative hypothermia and postoperative complications.[122]

Thermal Burns. Large burn injuries produce significant hypothermia because of the loss of the skin barrier to fluid evaporation and the loss of control of the microcirculation in the skin. Severe burns also compromise the normal insulation of the skin and subcutaneous tissues. (Burns are discussed in Chapter 48.)

SLEEP

Sleep is an active, multiphase, complex brain process that provides restorative functions and promotes memory consolidation. Several areas of the brain are associated with sleep and sleep-wake cycles. A small group of hypothalamic nerve cells, the **suprachiasmatic nucleus (SCN),** controls the timing of the sleep-wake cycle and coordinates this cycle with circadian rhythms (24-hour rhythm cycles) in other areas of the brain and body tissues using electrical, endocrine, and metabolic signaling pathways.[123] Normal sleep has two phases that can be documented by electroencephalography (EEG): rapid eye movement (REM) sleep and non-REM (NREM), or slow-wave, sleep. REM and NREM sleep succeed each other in 90- to 110-minute intervals in a predictable pattern.[124] Four to six cycles occur during a normal sleep period in an adult. NREM sleep is divided into three stages based on changes in the EEG pattern (Figure 16-9) followed by REM sleep[125]:

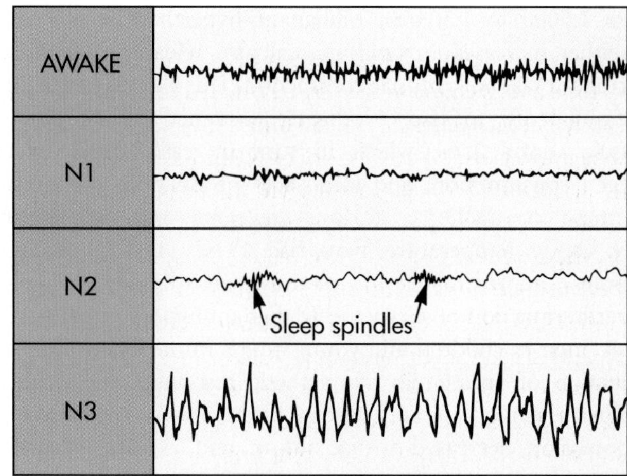

FIGURE 16-9 Electroencephalogram (EEG) Stages of Wakefulness and NREM Sleep. *Awake,* Low-voltage fast activity; *stage N1,* falling asleep; *stage N2,* light sleep with sleep spindles; *stage N3,* slow delta waves. Rapid eye movement (REM) sleep looks similar to awake and stage N1 sleep. Sleep spindles are bursts of brain activity associated with onset of sleep.

Awake—Wakefulness with eyes closed and predominated by alpha waves (8 to 25 Hz)

N1—Light sleep, with alpha waves (6 to 8 Hz) interspersed with low-frequency theta waves; slow eye movements (3% to 8% of sleep time)

N2—Further slowing of the EEG (4 to 7 Hz) with the presence of sleep spindles and slow eye movements (45% to 55% of sleep time)

N3—Low-frequency (1 to 3 Hz) high-amplitude delta waves with occasional sleep spindles—also known as *slow-wave sleep;* no slow eye movements (15% to 20% of sleep time)

REM sleep—time of most dreaming (20% to 25% of sleep time)

Non–Rapid Eye Movement (NREM) Sleep

NREM (slow-wave) sleep accounts for 75% to 80% of sleep time and is initiated by the withdrawal of neurotransmitters from the reticular formation and by the inhibition of arousal mechanisms in the cerebral cortex. During NREM sleep, respiration is controlled by metabolic processes.[126] The basal metabolic rate is decreased by 10% to 15%. Temperature is decreased 0.5° to 1° C (0.9° to 1.8° F). Heart rate decreases by 10 to 30 beats per minute. Respiration, blood pressure, and muscle tone all decrease. Knee-jerk reflexes are absent. Pupils are constricted. During stages N1 and N2, cerebral blood flow to the brainstem and cerebellum is decreased. During stage N3, cerebral blood flow to the cortex is decreased.[127] Growth hormone is released during stage N3, and levels of corticosteroids and catecholamines are depressed.

Rapid Eye Movement Sleep

Rapid eye movement (REM) sleep accounts for 20% to 25% of sleep time and is characterized by desynchronized, low-voltage, fast activity that occurs for 5 to 60 minutes about every 90 minutes beginning after 1 to 2 hours of NREM sleep. The brain is quite active in REM sleep with vivid dreaming. REM sleep is also known as *paradoxic sleep* because the EEG pattern is similar to the normal awake pattern. Alternating periods of REM and NREM sleep occur throughout the night, with lengthening intervals of REM sleep and fewer intervals of deeper stages of NREM sleep toward morning. REM sleep is characterized by bursts of conjugate rapid eye movement in all directions; atonia of antigravity muscles; suppressed temperature regulation; alteration in heart rate, blood pressure,[127,128] and respiration; penile erection in men and clitoral engorgement in women; and a high rate of memorable dreams. Steroids are released in short bursts. During REM sleep, respiratory control is thought to be largely independent of metabolic requirements and oxygen variation. Loss of normal voluntary muscle control in the tongue and upper pharynx may produce some respiratory obstruction. Cerebral blood flow to both hemispheres is increased. REM sleep is controlled by the pontine reticular formation.

An individual progresses through REM and NREM sleep in a predictable cycle while asleep. The first cycle of the night begins with stage N1. The individual then progresses through stages N2, N3, and REM sleep. A new cycle, beginning with stage N2, follows each REM sleep. With each successive cycle, the amount of time spent in stage N3 sleep decreases and the amount of time spent in REM sleep increases (Figure 16-10). The individual who is awakened begins the next cycle with stage N1.

The hypothalamus as a major sleep center secretes hypocretins (orexins), neuropeptides that promote wakefulness and REM sleep as well as appetite, energy consumption, and pleasure or reward. In addition to the hypocretins, acetylcholine and glutamate are important waking factors. The preoptic area of the hypothalamus promotes sleep through inhibitory modulation of multiple arousal systems with involvement of the inhibitory neurotransmitter GABA.[129] The reticular formation is primarily responsible for generating REM sleep and projections from the reticular formation and other areas of the mesencephalon and brainstem produce NREM sleep.[127]

Many neurotransmitters are associated with excitatory and inhibitory sleep mechanisms. Sleep-promoting neurotransmitters include prostaglandin D_2, L-tryptophan, serotonin, adenosine, melatonin, GABA, and growth hormones. Awake-promoting neurotransmitters include hypocretin (orexin), acetylcholine, and glutamate.[130] Their mechanism of action is complex and not clearly understood. Growth hormone is associated with initiation of sleep, and cortisol levels rise in the morning just before waking.[131] Acetylcholine and somatostatin play a role in stages of sleep transition. Forced awakenings in the middle of the night may result in increased difficulty returning to sleep or may alter the normal progression of sleep, or both.[130,132] The purpose of sleep is unknown, although restorative processes, particularly neuronal repair and generation of new neural pathways, have been proposed.[133] Loss of REM sleep impairs learning and memory. Sleep is important enough that people spend about one third of their life sleeping.

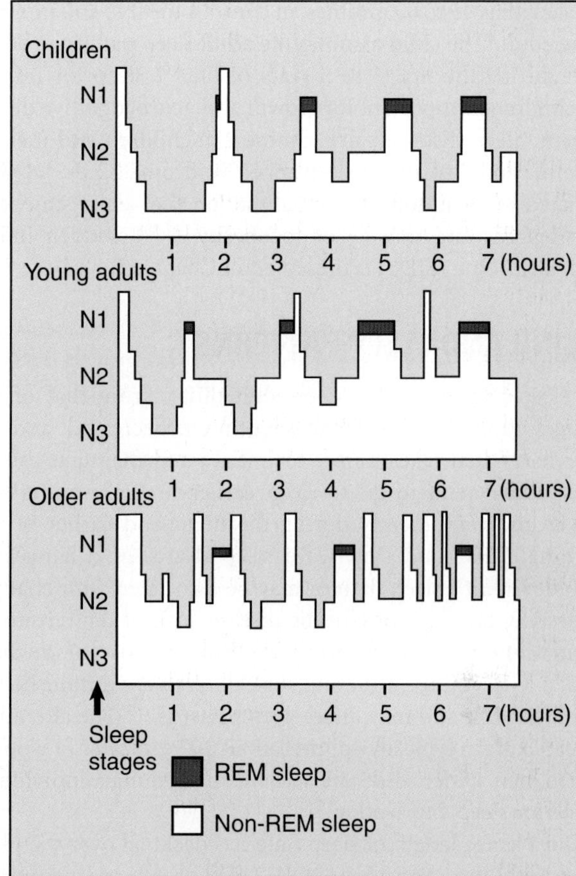

FIGURE 16-10 Normal Sleep Cycles. Rapid eye movement *(REM)* sleep occurs cyclically throughout the night at intervals of approximately 90 minutes in all age groups. REM sleep shows little variation in the different age groups, whereas stage N3 sleep decreases with age. In addition, older adults awaken frequently and show a marked increase in total time awake.

PEDIATRICS AND SLEEP PATTERNS

The sleep patterns of the newborn and young child vary from those of the adult in total sleep time, cycle length, and percentage of time spent in each sleep cycle.[134] Newborns sleep about 16 to 17 hours per day. About 53% of that time is spent in active sleep (REM sleep), 23% in quiet sleep (NREM sleep), and the remainder in an indeterminate phase. The infant sleep cycle is approximately 50 to 60 minutes long, with 20 minutes of NREM sleep and 10 to 45 minutes of REM sleep, in contrast to the adult sleep cycle. Newborns enter REM sleep immediately on falling asleep.[135] At about 1 year of age, an infant spends approximately 45% of total sleep time in quiet sleep and 41% in REM sleep. Total sleep time decreases slightly from birth to 1 year. Bottle-fed infants that do not share sleeping space with the mother increase maximum sleep time from 4 to 5 hours to 8 to 10 hours by 4 months of age. They begin to "sleep through the night." Infants who are breast-fed for up to 2 years and share sleeping space with the mother continue to sleep in short bouts and wake frequently to nurse.[135] In the young child, the sleep cycle length is 45 to 60 minutes, in contrast to 90 to 100 minutes in the adult. The child assumes the adult sleep pattern at some point during the first 2 to 5 years of life.[136] Sleep for infants and children is important for growth and neurocognitive development. Sleep disorders are common in children and include insomnia and obstructive sleep apnea syndrome (OSAS). OSAS is related to adenotonsillar inflammation (i.e., enlargement of the adenoids and tonsils) or to obesity.[137,138] Sudden infant death syndrome (SIDS) is presented in Chapter 36.

AGING AND SLEEP PATTERNS

The sleep pattern of the older adult differs from that of the younger adult or child. Total sleep time is decreased, and the older individual takes longer to initiate and maintain asleep. Older adults tend to go to sleep earlier in the evening and awaken more frequently during the night and earlier in the morning. REM and slow-wave sleep decreases. Changes in the older adult's sleep pattern may be associated with changes in lifestyle, presence of chronic disease, lack of daily routine, desynchronization of circadian rhythm, and use of medications.[139] Growth hormone and cortisol levels are diminished in the older adult and may affect sleep patterns.[132] The alteration in sleep pattern typically appears about 10 years later in women than in men. Older adults are less able than younger individuals to tolerate sleep deprivation.[140]

The average length of sleep time has declined over the years for both children and adults.[141,142] Daily sleep loss accumulates as a sleep debt that becomes evident in reduced neurobehavioral capability that, in turn, results in decline of executive function and lapses in vigilance.[143,144] Individuals responsible for public health and safety, including but not limited to healthcare workers, often work night shifts and long hours that make them prone to sleep-related errors.[145,146]

Sleep Disorders

Sleep disorders can be primary or secondary and can occur as a result of many medical and psychiatric conditions. The focus of this section is on primary sleep disorders. The classification of primary sleep disorders is complex and a system has been produced by the American Academy of Sleep Medicine[147] that includes four general classifications: (1) dyssomnias (intrinsic and extrinsic sleep disorders and circadian rhythm sleep disorders); (2) parasomnias (arousal and sleep-wake transition disorders and REM sleep disorders); (3) sleep disorders associated with mental, neurologic, or other medical disorder; and (4) proposed sleep disorders. The most common dyssomnias and parasomnias are presented here.

Common Dyssomnias

The **dyssomnias** are sleep disorders related to difficulty in initiating or maintaining sleep or the presence of excessive sleepiness. The most common dyssomnias include insomnia, obstructive sleep apnea syndrome, restless leg syndrome, circadian rhythm disorder, and hypersomnia.

Insomnia is the inability to fall or stay asleep and is more common in women.[148] Primary insomnia may be transient, lasting a few days, and related to travel across time zones, disrupted sleep schedules, or acute stress. Secondary insomnia is associated with drug or alcohol abuse, chronic pain disorders, or chronic depression, obesity, and aging.[149] Drugs known to produce insomnia include amphetamines, steroids, central adrenergic blockers, bronchodilating agents, and caffeine.[150]

Obstructive sleep apnea syndrome (OSAS) is a disorder of breathing during sleep related to upper airway obstruction that is associated with reduced blood oxygen saturation and hypercapnia. The typical classification of the severity of this disease uses the Apnea Hypopnea Index (AHI). This index represents how many apnea (total airway closure) or hypopnea (partial airway closure) episodes occur per night—the number of which is then divided by the night's total sleep time to give an average number of apnea or hypopnea episodes per hour. The AHI severity scale is as follows:

- *Normal:* fewer than 5 episodes of abnormal sleep episodes per hour
- *Mild:* between 5 and 15 episodes of abnormal sleep episodes per hour
- *Moderate:* between 15 and 30 episodes of abnormal sleep episodes per hour
- *Severe:* more than 30 episodes of abnormal sleep episodes per hour

The prevalence of OSAS associated with accompanying daytime sleepiness is common with an occurrence of approximately 3% to 7% for adult men and 2% to 5% for adult women,[151] or approximately 10 million adults in the United States. Some estimates suggest between 12 and 20 million people in the United States have diagnosable OSAS.[152] Risk factors include obesity, male gender, menopause, and age.[153]

OSAS is increasingly prevalent in our rapidly expanding older adult population.[154,155] Premenstrual women may be protected from sleep-disordered breathing because the female hormone progesterone is a respiratory stimulant.[156] The longer pharyngeal airway in males also may contribute to increased risk for OSAS. Obese individuals often have a short, thick neck; pharyngeal airway collapse; impaired respiratory mechanics; and depressed respiratory control, particularly during sleep.[157] **Obesity hypoventilation syndrome** (obesity, daytime hypoventilation, and sleep-disordered breathing not related to other causes) may be related to leptin resistance because leptin is also a respiratory stimulant.[158]

OSAS is, as reflected in the preceding discussion of AHI, characterized by repetitive increases in resistance to airflow within the upper airway with loud snoring, gasping, intervals of apnea lasting from 10 to 30 seconds, fragmented sleep, and chronic daytime sleepiness. The obstruction is caused by the soft palate or base of the tongue, or both, collapsing against the pharyngeal walls because of decreased muscle tone especially during REM sleep. In the supine position, the tongue may fall farther back, obstructing the airway. The level of negative intrathoracic pressure is the most likely stimulus for arousal, possibly mediated by mechanoreceptors in the upper airway. Potentially fatal cardiac and vascular illnesses associated with OSAS include hypertension, pulmonary hypertension, heart failure, nocturnal cardiac dysrhythmias, myocardial infarction, and ischemic stroke.[159]

The pathophysiologic consequences of mechanical and neurochemical responses present during apneic episodes may be causal factors in the cardiovascular disease commonly seen in OSAS. Such hypoxia-induced vascular dysfunction impairs blood flow regulation and compromises tissue perfusion and oxygen delivery during episodes of OSAS. The combination of intermittent hypoxia and hypercapnia, increased number of arousals, increased sympathetic tone, altered baroreflex control during sleep, oxidative stress, hormonal changes, and cardiovascular changes induced by increased negative intrathoracic pressure contribute to these complications.[160] OSAS also contributes to the development of metabolic syndrome, which is associated with cardiovascular disease mortality[161] (see Chapter 22). Many individuals are not aware of their heavy snoring and nocturnal arousals and may remain undiagnosed. Fatigue, decline in cognitive function, car accidents, and poor work performance are common.

Diagnosis of OSAS is confirmed with polysomnography. Treatments include continuous positive airway pressure (CPAP), dental devices that modify the position of the tongue or jaw, upper airway surgical reconstruction, and weight reduction.[162] Treatment with CPAP utilizes positive air pressure to maintain an open airway and has been shown to result in a reversal of abnormalities associated with OSAS, including systemic and pulmonary hypertension and decreased cardiovascular disease mortality.[163,164]

Restless leg syndrome (RLS) is a common sensorimotor disorder associated with unpleasant sensations (prickling, tingling, crawling) that occurs at rest and is worse in the evening or at night. There is a compelling urge to move the legs for relief, with a significant effect on sleep and quality of life. The disorder is more common in women, older adults, and individuals with iron deficiency. RLS has a familial tendency and is associated with a circadian fluctuation of dopamine in the substantia nigra. Iron is a cofactor in dopamine production, and some individuals respond to iron administration as well as dopamine agonists.[165,166]

Hypersomnia is excessive daytime sleepiness and is commonly associated with voluntary sleep deprivation. There may also be an underlying sleep disorder such as OSAS or narcolepsy. Individuals may fall asleep while driving, working, or even conversing, resulting in significant concerns for safety. Treatment is symptomatic with reinforcement of good sleeping habits.

Narcolepsy is characterized by hypersomnia, cataplexy (brief spells of muscle weakness), hallucinations, and sleep paralysis. The disorder is associated with hypothalamic hypocretin (orexin) deficiency and may be related to immune-mediated destruction of hypocretin-secreting cells. There is a genetic component to the disorder in animals.[167]

Circadian rhythm sleep disorders are common disorders of the sleep-wake schedule and include rapid time-zone changes (jet-lag syndrome), alterations in sleep schedule with an advance or a delay of 3 hours or more in sleep time, or changes in total sleep time from day to day. These changes in the timing of established sleep schedules have been shown to desynchronize circadian rhythm.[168] Degree of vigilance, performance of psychomotor tasks, and subjective reports of levels of arousal are markedly depressed after alterations in the sleep-wake schedule. Individuals may experience short sleep episodes called *microsleeps* without being aware of decreased vigilance.[169,170]

It is well established that industrial shift workers exhibit a decrease in accuracy, an increase in accident proneness, and an increase in likelihood of poor work performance.[168] For similar reasons, people suffering from jet-lag syndrome require several days to adapt to a new time zone. Travel across time zones requires 2 days to adjust the sleep-wake schedule, 5 days to adjust the body temperature cycle, and 8 days to adjust cortisol level secretion. Transmeridian travel requires up to 10 days to adjust the body clock when traveling from east to west. Timed bright light exposure and administration of exogenous melatonin provide some success in retiming or resetting the body clock before or after time-zone shifts.[171,172]

Sleep deprivation can result in significant neurocognitive decline, particularly in the domains of executive control, working memory, and attention.[173] Neuropsychologic effects of sleep loss include[174]:

1. A marked impact on performance through decreases in cognitive functions and specific effects on brain regions that support cognitive function
2. Decreased speed of mental processing
3. Declines in attention and vigilance with distinct intraindividual variability
4. Abnormal activation in the prefrontal cortex, parietal lobes, thalamus, and temporal lobes as shown by functional neuroimaging
5. Task performance decreases as sleep debt accumulates in a manner that is "dose dependent"

Common Parasomnias

Parasomnias are complex behaviors related to awakening from REM sleep or partial arousal from NREM sleep and disorders of sleep stage transitions. Three types of parasomnias include *arousal disorders* such as confusional arousals, sleepwalking (somnambulism), night terrors (dream anxiety attacks), rearranging furniture, eating food, violent behavior, bruxism (teeth grinding), and sleep enuresis; *sleep-wake transition disorders* such as rhythmic movements (head banging), sleep talking, and nocturnal leg cramps; and *disorders associated with REM sleep* such as sleep paralysis and nightmares, sleep apnea, and SIDS. SIDS affects children primarily in the first 2 years of life and may be related to central sleep apnea (a disorder of thalamic breathing control) episodes (see Chapter 36). Parasomnias are more common in children and may be familial.[175-177]

Sleep Disorders Associated with Mental, Neurologic, or Medical Disorders

Many mental and physical disorders are associated with alterations in sleep (secondary sleep disorders). Many disorders produce alterations in the quantity and quality of sleep or affect sleep stages, including mental disorders (e.g., depression and anxiety), disorders of neurocognitive function (e.g., dementia or Parkinson disease), and physical disorders (e.g., alterations in thyroid hormone levels, pain, and many acute and chronic diseases). In other instances, sleep stages may contribute to disease (sleep-provoked disorders) such as chronic obstructive pulmonary disease (COPD), asthma, cardiac ischemia, diabetes mellitus, and gastroesophageal reflux.

REM sleep behavior disorder is loss of normal skeletal muscle atonia during REM sleep and may cause injury from acting-out of dreams. It is more common in older adult men and is associated with Parkinson disease and other neurodegenerative diseases.[178]

Individuals who are depressed have difficulty falling asleep and exhibit less slow-wave sleep, less time spent in REM sleep, early awakening, and less total sleep time. In addition, depressed individuals move through the sleep stages more quickly than do individuals who are not depressed. The same neurotransmitters that may be disturbed in depression also regulate sleep.[175,179]

Coronary artery disease is most affected during REM sleep. During REM, dreams may provoke nocturnal angina, increased heart rate, and electrocardiogram (ECG) changes. In adults, attacks of bronchial asthma may occur at any time during the night. The attacks cause the individual to spend more of the sleep period awake and thus result in a decrease in stage N3 sleep time. In children, bronchial asthma attacks are uncommon during the first one third of the night, when stage N3 sleep predominates, and occur more frequently during the final two thirds of the night. Stage N3 sleep time is decreased overall in the child with bronchial asthma. In addition to these changes, asthmatic individuals may experience bronchial spasm during REM sleep.[180-182]

People with COPD experience significantly lowered oxygen tension and increases in carbon dioxide retention during sleep. The lowered oxygen tension is most significant in the tonic phase of REM sleep when voluntary neuromuscular control, including intercostal muscle function, is depressed. Pulmonary spasm and transient pulmonary hypertension result. These changes are particularly evident in the "blue bloater" individual and may contribute to early pulmonary hypertension and cor pulmonale in these people.[183,184]

Because blood glucose levels vary during sleep, individuals with uncontrolled diabetes may need to pay careful attention to blood glucose levels. Studies show that people with duodenal ulcers secrete 3 to 20 times more gastric acid during REM sleep than do people without duodenal ulcers. This increased gastric acid secretion often produces nocturnal epigastric pain.

SOMATOSENSORY FUNCTION AND THE SPECIAL SENSES

The somatosensory system includes the peripheral receptors and central nervous system pathways that detect internal and external information, which is then processed and interpreted by the brain. This system includes touch, proprioception and vestibular function, and the special senses—sight, hearing, smell, and taste.

Touch

Touch is not a uniform sensory experience. The sensation of touch involves the fusion of several qualities, including modality, intensity, location, and duration of the sensory stimulus. Receptors sensitive to touch are present in the skin. Meissner and pacinian corpuscles are rapidly adapting receptors, whereas Merkel disks and Ruffini endings are slowly adapting touch receptors. Touch receptors are most numerous in the skin of the fingers and lips and are more scarce in the skin of the trunk. Specific sensory input is carried to the higher levels of the CNS by the dorsal column of the spinal cord and the anterior spinothalamic tract.

Much of the development of the cutaneous senses takes place before birth, but structural growth of the cutaneous senses continues into early adulthood at a reduced rate. Then a gradual decline occurs.[185] Studies have documented loss in tactile sensitivity with advancing age.[186,187] This occurs simultaneously with an increase in the size of pacinian corpuscles and a decrease in the number of corpuscles.

Abnormal tactile perception may be caused by alterations at any level of the nervous system, from the receptor to the cerebral cortex. Any factor that interrupts or impairs reception, transmission, perception, or interpretation of touch also alters tactile sensation. Trauma, tumor, infection, metabolic changes, vascular changes, and degenerative diseases thus may cause tactile dysfunction, which may involve heightened or diminished tactile perceptions.

In addition, most tactile sensations evoke affective responses that determine whether the sensation is unpleasant, pleasant, or neutral. Cerebral and hypothalamic centers influence this response. Sedative drugs and prefrontal injury, which interrupt connections between the prefrontal cortex and subcortical centers, diminish the interpretation of tactile sensations.

Proprioception

Perception and awareness of the position of the body and its parts depend on impulses from the inner ear and from receptors in joints and ligaments. The role of muscle, tendon, and cutaneous receptors is indefinite. Sensory data are transmitted to higher centers, primarily through the dorsal columns and the spinocerebellar tracts, with some data passing through the medial lemnisci and thalamic radiations to the cortex. These stimuli are necessary for the coordination of movements, the grading of muscular contraction, and the maintenance of equilibrium.

A progressive loss of proprioception has been reported in older adults with increased risk for falls and injury.[188] Proprioceptive dysfunction may be caused by alterations at any level of the nervous system. As with tactile dysfunction, any factor that interrupts or impairs the reception, transmission, perception, or interpretation of proprioceptive stimuli also alters proprioception. Two common causes of proprioceptive dysfunction are vestibular dysfunction and neuropathy.

Specific vestibular dysfunctions are vestibular nystagmus and vertigo. **Vestibular nystagmus** is the constant, involuntary movement of the eyeball caused by ear disturbances. This condition occurs when the semicircular canal system is overstimulated. **Vertigo** (dizziness) is the sensation of spinning that occurs with inflammation of the semicircular canals in the ear. The individual may feel either that he or she is moving in space or that the world is revolving. Vertigo often causes loss of balance. Vertigo and nystagmus may occur in a variety of conditions, including labyrinthitis, vestibular neuritis, acute toxic labyrinthitis, benign paroxysmal positional vertigo, migrainous vertigo, and Ménière disease.[189]

Ménière disease (endolymphatic hydrops) is an idiopathic episodic vestibular disorder resulting from abnormalities in the quantity, composition, and pressure of the endolymph in the middle ear.[190] The individual with Ménière disease experiences vertigo, hearing loss, tinnitus, and aural fullness and may have proprioceptive dysfunction. Standing or walking may be impossible because of loss of balance. **Ménière syndrome,** or secondary endolymphatic hydrops, is secondary to other conditions that alter the production or absorption of endolymph.

Peripheral neuropathies also can cause proprioceptive dysfunctions. Neuropathies may be caused by a variety of conditions and commonly are associated with renal disease and diabetes mellitus. Although the exact sequence of events is unknown, neuropathies are thought to be caused by a metabolic disturbance of the neuron itself. The result is a diminished or absent sense of body position or position of body parts. Gait changes often occur. (Neuropathies are further discussed in Chapter 18.)

Vision

The eyes are complex sense organs responsible for vision. Within a protective casing, each eye has receptors, a lens system for focusing light on the receptors, and a system of nerves for conducting impulses from the receptors to the brain. Visual dysfunction may be caused by abnormal ocular movements or alterations in visual acuity, refraction, color vision, or accommodation. Visual dysfunction also may be the secondary effect of another neurologic disorder.

The External Eye

Protective external eye structures include the eyelids (palpebrae), conjunctivae, and lacrimal apparatus (Figure 16-11). The eyelids are used to control the amount of light reaching the eyes, and the conjunctivae line the eyelids. Tears released from the lacrimal apparatus bathe the surface of the eye and prevent friction, maintain hydration, and wash out foreign bodies and other irritants.

Infection and inflammatory responses are the most common conditions affecting the supporting structures of the eyes. **Blepharitis** is an inflammation of the eyelids caused by *Staphylococcus* or seborrheic dermatitis. Redness, edema, tearing, and itching are common symptoms.[191]

An external **hordeolum (stye)** is an infection of the sebaceous glands of the eyelids, and an internal hordeolum is an infection of the eyelid margin. A **chalazion** is a noninfectious lipogranuloma of the meibomian (oil-secreting) gland and may be associated with an internal hordeolum. These conditions present with redness, swelling, and tenderness and are treated symptomatically.[192] **Entropion** is a common eyelid malposition in which the lid margin turns inward against the eyeball. There are both surgical and nonsurgical treatments to reposition the lid margin.

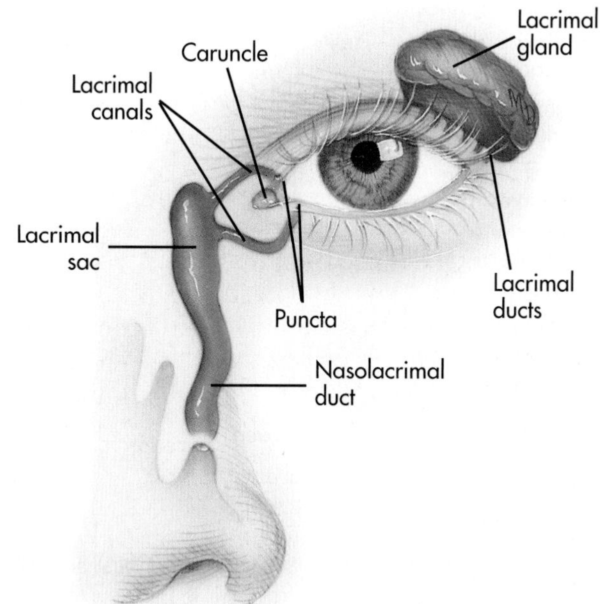

FIGURE 16-11 Lacrimal Apparatus. Fluid produced by lacrimal glands (tears) streams across the eye surface, enters the canals, and then passes through the nasolacrimal duct to enter the nose. (From Patton KT, Thibodeau GA: *Anatomy & physiology,* ed 8, St Louis, 2013, Mosby.)

Conjunctivitis

Conjunctivitis is an inflammation of the conjunctiva (mucous membrane covering the front part of the eyeball). Conjunctivitis may be caused by bacteria, viruses, allergies, or chemical irritations. The inflammatory response produces redness, edema, pain, and lacrimation. Treatment is related to cause.[193]

Acute bacterial conjunctivitis (pinkeye) is highly contagious and often is caused by gram-positive organisms *(Staphylococcus, Haemophilus, Proteus),* although other bacteria may be involved. The onset is acute, characterized by mucopurulent drainage from one or both eyes. In children younger than 6 years, *Haemophilus* infection often leads to otitis media (conjunctivitis-otitis syndrome). Preventing spread of the organism with meticulous handwashing and use of separate towels is important. The disease often is self-limiting and resolves spontaneously in 10 to 14 days. Antibiotic eyedrops usually are effective.

Viral conjunctivitis is caused by an adenovirus. Symptoms vary from mild to severe. Some strains of virus cause conjunctivitis and pharyngitis (pharyngoconjunctival fever), and others cause keratoconjunctivitis. Both diseases are contagious, with watering, redness, and photophobia. Treatment is symptomatic.

Allergic conjunctivitis is associated with a variety of antigens, including pollens. Ocular itching is associated with photophobia, burning, and gritty sensations in the eye. Treatment is symptomatic and may include antihistamines, low-dose corticosteroids, mast cell stabilizers, and vasoconstrictors.

Chronic conjunctivitis is the result of any persistent conjunctivitis. The cause requires identification for effective treatment.

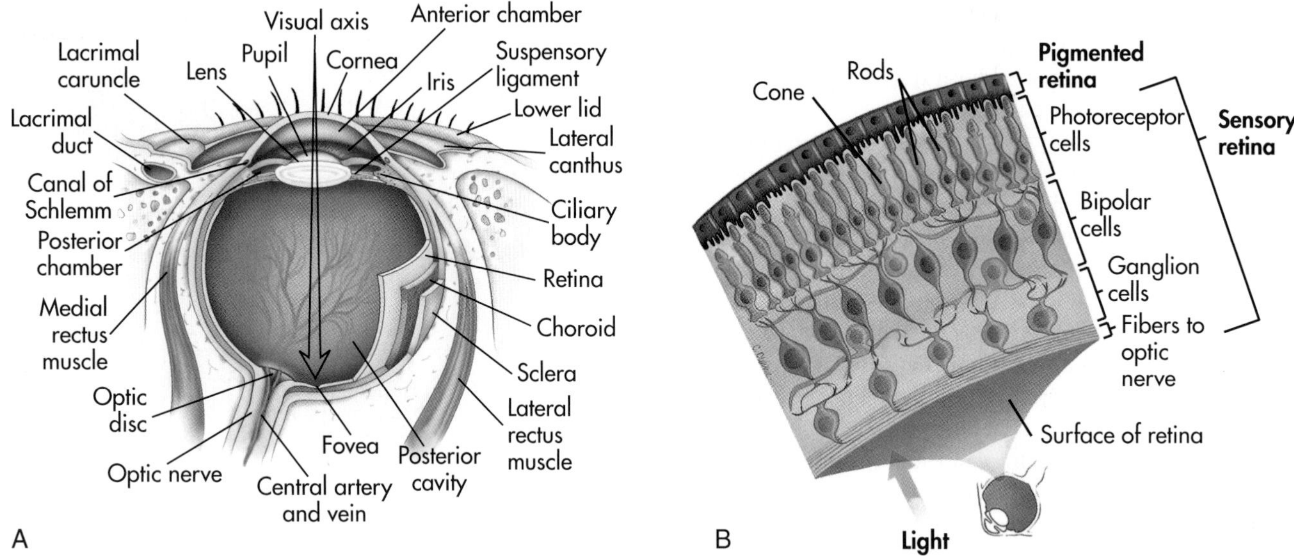

FIGURE 16-12 Structure of the Eyeball and Cell Layers of the Retina. **A,** Horizontal section through the left eyeball. The eye is viewed from above. **B,** Pigmented and sensory layers of the retina. (From Patton KT, Thibodeau GA: *Anatomy & physiology,* ed 8, St Louis, 2013, Mosby.)

Trachoma (chlamydial conjunctivitis) is caused by *Chlamydia trachomatis.* It often is associated with poor hygiene and is the leading cause of preventable blindness in the world. The severity of the disease varies, but it can involve inflammation with scarring of the conjunctiva and eyelids causing distorted lashes to abrade the cornea, leading to corneal scarring and blindness. Chlamydial organisms are sensitive to local or systemic antibiotics. The World Health Organization aims to eliminate trachoma as a public health problem by 2020 using the SAFE Strategy: Surgery for inturned lashes, Antibiotics, Facial cleanliness, and Environmental improvement.[194]

Keratitis. **Keratitis** is an inflammation of the cornea that can be noninfectious or caused by bacteria, viruses, or fungus. Bacterial infections often cause corneal ulceration and require intensive antibiotic treatment. *Staphylococcus aureus* is the most common bacterial infection. Type 1 herpes simplex virus can involve the cornea and conjunctiva. Predisposing factors include contact lens use, trauma, and penetrating keratoplasty (corneal grafting). Common symptoms include photophobia, pain, and lacrimation. Severe ulcerations with residual scarring require corneal transplantation.[195]

The Eye

The wall of the eye is formed of three layers: sclera, choroid, and retina (Figure 16-12). The **sclera** is the thick, white, outermost layer. It becomes transparent at the **cornea,** the portion of the sclera in the central anterior region that allows light to enter the eye. The **choroid** is the deeply pigmented middle layer that prevents light from scattering inside the eye. The **iris,** part of the choroid, has a round opening, the **pupil,** through which light passes. Smooth muscle fibers control the size of the pupil so that in close vision and bright light the pupil constricts and in distant vision and dim light the pupil dilates.

The **retina** is the innermost layer of the eye, and contains millions of rods and cones, special photoreceptors that convert light energy into nerve impulses. **Rods** mediate peripheral and dim light vision and are densest at the periphery. **Cones,** densest in the center of the retina, are color and detail receptors. The photoreceptive rods and cones are distributed over the entire retina, except where the optic nerve leaves the eyeball. Lack of rods and cones in this area results in the **optic disc,** or blind spot. Lateral to each optic disc is the **fovea centralis,** a tiny area that contains only cones and provides the greatest visual acuity (see Figure 16-12).

The **optic nerve** (second cranial nerve) is composed of retinal cell axons. As shown in Figure 16-13, nerve impulses pass through the optic nerves after leaving the retinas. At the optic chiasm the fibers from the inner (nasal) halves of the retinas cross to the opposite side, where they join fibers from the outer (temporal) halves of the retinas to form the optic tracts. The fibers of the optic tracts synapse in the dorsal lateral geniculate nucleus, and from there the geniculocalcarine fibers pass by way of the optic radiation (or geniculocalcarine tract) to the primary visual cortex in the occipital lobe of the brain. Some fibers terminate in the suprachiasmatic nucleus (located above the optic chiasm) and are involved in regulating the sleep-wake cycle.

Light entering the eye is focused on the retina by the **lens**—a flexible, biconvex, crystal-like structure. In youth the lens is transparent and has the consistency of hardened jelly. The flexibility of the lens allows a change in curvature with contraction of the ciliary muscles. This is called **accommodation** and it allows the eye to focus on objects at different distances. Anterior to the lens are the iris and the aqueous chamber, which is filled with **aqueous humor**. The aqueous humor helps to maintain the pressure inside the eye and provides nutrients to the lens and cornea. Aqueous humor is free-flowing fluid, secreted by the ciliary processes and reabsorbed into the canal of Schlemm. If drainage is blocked, pressure within the eye increases (as it does with glaucoma). Posterior to the lens is the vitreous chamber and it is filled with a gel-like substance called **vitreous humor**. Vitreous humor helps prevent the eyeball from collapsing inward.

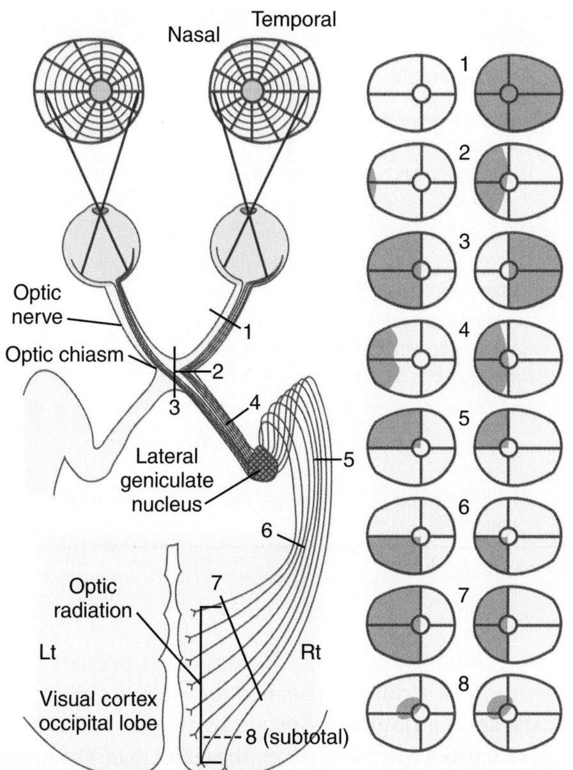

FIGURE 16-13 Visual Fields and Defects That Accompany Damage to the Right Visual Pathways. **1,** Optic nerve: blindness. **2,** Lateral optic chiasm: grossly incongruous, incomplete (contralateral) homonymous hemianopsia. **3,** Central optic chiasm: bitemporal hemianopsia. **4,** Optic tract: incongruous, incomplete homonymous hemianopsia. **5,** Temporal loop of the optic radiation: congruous partial or complete (contralateral) homonymous superior quadrantanopia. **6,** Parietal *(superior)* projection of the optic radiation: congruous partial or complete homonymous inferior quadrantanopia. **7,** Complete parieto-occipital interruption of the optic radiation: complete congruous homonymous hemianopsia with psychophysical shift of the foveal point, often sparing central vision and resulting in "macular sparing." **8,** Incomplete (subtotal) damage to the visual cortex: congruous homonymous scotomas, usually encroaching at least acutely on central vision. (From Goldman C, editor: *Goldman's Cecil medicine,* ed 24, vol 2, Philadelphia, 2012, Saunders.)

The central retinal artery provides blood to the inner retinal surface. Nutrients and oxygen are supplied to the outer surface of the retina by the choroid, a vascular layer that lies between the retina and sclera. Six extrinsic eye muscles, attached to the outer surface of each eye, allow gross eye movements and permit the eyes to follow a moving object (Figure 16-14).

AGING AND VISION

Changes in the visual and motor components of the eye caused by aging begin at an early age, particularly in the lens of the eye. Changes caused by aging are summarized in Table 16-4. Structural changes combined with chronic diseases, including dementias and diabetes mellitus, result in a decline in visual acuity and extraocular motor muscle function.[196,197]

Visual Dysfunction

Alterations in Ocular Movements. Abnormal ocular movements occur as a result of oculomotor, trochlear, or abducens cranial nerve dysfunction (see Table 15-6). The three types of eye movement disorders are (1) strabismus, (2) nystagmus, and (3) paralysis of individual extraocular muscles.

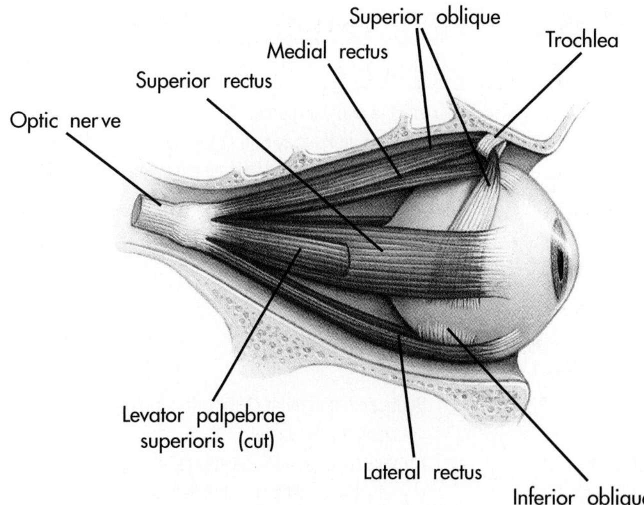

FIGURE 16-14 Extrinsic Muscles of the Right Eye, Superior View. (From Patton KT, Thibodeau GA: *Anatomy & physiology,* ed 8, St Louis, 2013, Mosby.)

Strabismus is the deviation of one eye from the other when a person is looking at an object; it results in failure of the two eyes to simultaneously focus on the same image and therefore loss of binocular vision. The deviation may be upward, downward, inward, or outward, resulting from a weak or hypertonic muscle in one of the eyes. Strabismus may be caused by a neuromuscular disorder of the eye muscle, diseases involving the cerebral hemispheres, or thyroid disease.[198] The primary symptom of strabismus is **diplopia** (double vision). Strabismus in children requires early intervention to prevent the development of amblyopia (reduced vision in the affected eye without ocular pathology and with full optical correction). Surgery may be helpful to both children and adults with strabismus.[199]

Nystagmus is an involuntary unilateral or bilateral rhythmic movement of the eyes and can occur in infants (congenital) or adults (acquired). It may be present at rest, or it may occur with eye movement. The two major forms of nystagmus are pendular nystagmus and jerk nystagmus. **Pendular nystagmus** is characterized by a regular alternating forward and backward movement of the eyes in which both phases of the movement are equal in length. In **jerk nystagmus** one phase of the eye movement is faster than the other. Nystagmus may be caused by an imbalance in the normally coordinated reflex activity of the inner ear, vestibular nuclei (connecting the vestibular nerve with vestibulospinal tracts), cerebellum, medial longitudinal fascicle (connecting the mesencephalon with the upper portion of the spinal cord), or nuclei of the oculomotor, trochlear, and abducens cranial nerves (see Table 15-6). Drugs, retinal disease, and diseases involving the cervical cord also may produce nystagmus. Acquired untreated nystagmus can lead to loss of visual acuity.[200]

Paralysis of specific extraocular muscles may cause a variety of abnormalities, including limited abduction, abnormal closure of the eyelid, ptosis (drooping of the eyelid), and diplopia.

TABLE 16-4 CHANGES IN THE EYE CAUSED BY AGING

STRUCTURE	CHANGE	CONSEQUENCE
Cornea	Thicker and less curved	Increase in astigmatism
	Formation of a gray ring at the edge of cornea (arcus senilis)	Not detrimental to vision
Anterior chamber	Decrease in size and volume caused by thickening of lens	Occasionally exerts pressure on Schlemm canal and may lead to increased intraocular pressure and glaucoma
Lens	Increase in opacity	Decrease in refraction with increased light scattering and decreased color vision (green and blue); decreased dark adaptation; cataracts
	Loss of elasticity	Loss of accommodation (presbyopia: loss of focus for near objects)
Ciliary muscles	Reduction in pupil diameter, atrophy of radial dilation muscles	Persistent constriction (senile miosis); decrease in critical flicker frequency*
Retina	Reduction in number of rods at periphery, loss of rods and associated nerve cells	Increase in the minimum amount of light necessary to see an object
Macula	Atrophy (age-related macular degeneration)	Loss of vision
Vitreous	Liquefaction of vitreous and decrease in gel volume	Posterior vitreous detachment causing "floaters;" risk for retinal detachment

*The rate at which consecutive visual stimuli can be presented and still be perceived as separate.

The abnormalities occur as a result of unopposed muscle activity. Trauma or pressure in the area of the cranial nerves may cause paralysis of specific extraocular muscles. Diseases such as diabetes mellitus and myasthenia gravis also may affect specific extraocular muscles.

Alterations in Visual Acuity. Visual acuity is the ability to see objects in sharp detail. With advancing age the eye's lens becomes less flexible and less adjustable. In addition, the sclera changes shape, causing light to fall on the **macula** (an opaque portion of the cornea). Thus visual acuity declines with age. Visual acuity also may change or diminish for many other reasons. Specific causes of visual acuity changes include: (1) amblyopia, (2) scotoma, (3) cataracts, (4) papilledema, (5) dark adaptation, (6) glaucoma, (7) retinal detachment, and (8) macular degeneration.

Amblyopia (lazy eye) is a reduction or dimness of vision for unknown reasons. It does not result from a change in refraction (i.e., deviation of light rays) or from any visible changes in the eye. Amblyopia is associated with strabismus and anisometropia (refractive error in one eye differs from that of the other eye); with diseases such as diabetes mellitus, renal failure, and malaria; and with toxic substances such as alcohol and tobacco. Amblyopia is the most common cause of vision loss in children and is usually treated either by patching the unaffected eye for extended times to ensure a period of use of the affected eye or by administering atropine eyedrops.[201] Refractive errors are treated with corrective lenses.

A **scotoma** is a circumscribed defect of the central field of vision. It can be a sequel to demyelinating optic neuritis, an inflammatory lesion of the optic nerve frequently associated with optico-spinal multiple sclerosis (see Chapter 18). Age-related macular degeneration is associated with scotoma. Less common causes include the compression of one optic nerve by a retroorbital tumor, neuromyelitis optica (autoantibody-related inflammation of the optic nerve and spinal cord), pernicious anemia, and toxic or metabolic causes such as methyl alcohol poisoning and use of tobacco. The precise mechanisms for these conditions causing a scotoma are uncertain, but the result is always a serious impairment in visual acuity.[202]

A **cataract** is a cloudy or opaque area in the ocular lens and leads to visual loss when located on the visual axis. The incidence of cataracts increases with age as the lens enlarges. Cataracts develop because of alterations of metabolism and transport of nutrients within the lens. Although the most common form of cataract is degenerative, cataracts also may occur congenitally or as a result of infection, radiation, trauma, drugs, or diabetes mellitus. Cataracts cause decreased visual acuity, blurred vision, glare, and decreased color perception. Cataracts are treated by removal of the entire lens and replacement with an intraocular artificial lens.[203]

Dark adaptation also affects visual acuity. Low illumination causes impaired visual acuity, particularly in older adults. The average 80-year-old person needs more than twice as much light as a 20-year-old person to see equally well. Changes in the quantity and quality of rhodopsin, a substance found in the rods and responsible for low-light vision, are thought to be responsible for reduced dark adaptation in older adults.[204] Vitamin A deficiencies can cause the same phenomenon in individuals of any age.

Glaucoma is a leading cause of visual impairment and blindness. It is characterized by intraocular pressures greater than the normal pressures of 12 to 20 mmHg maintained by the aqueous fluid. Family history is a risk factor, and glaucoma can be inherited.[205] The types of glaucoma are summarized in Table 16-5 and Figure 16-15. Open-angle glaucoma is the most common. Chronic increased intraocular pressure causes death of retinal ganglions and optic nerve degeneration with loss of peripheral vision, followed by central vision impairment and blindness. Extremely high pressures can cause blindness within days or hours. Loss of visual acuity results from pressure on the optic nerve, which is believed to block the flow of cytoplasm from neuronal bodies in the retina to peripheral optic nerve fibers entering the brain. Lack of nutrients, ischemia, cytotoxic factors, and altered immune mechanisms may lead to death of the

TABLE 16-5 TYPES OF GLAUCOMA

TYPE	MECHANISM OF INCREASED PRESSURE
Open-angle	Obstruction of outflow of aqueous humor at trabecular meshwork or Schlemm canal; myopia may be a risk factor
Normal or low-tension	Form of open-angle glaucoma with symptomless damage to the optic nerve and gradual vision loss when intraocular pressure is within normal range (12-20 mmHg)
Narrow-angle (angle-closure)	Forward displacement of iris toward cornea with narrowing of iridocorneal angle and obstruction to outflow of aqueous humor from anterior chamber
Acute angle-closure	Acute closure of iridocorneal angle with a sudden rise in intraocular pressure, producing pain, redness, and visual disturbances
Chronic angle-closure	Progressive, permanent closure of anterior chamber angle
Secondary	Open- or closed-angle obstruction caused by, for example, uveitis, hemorrhage, rupture of lens or tumors
Congenital glaucoma	Malformation of trabecular meshwork and excess extracellular matrix in outer meshwork

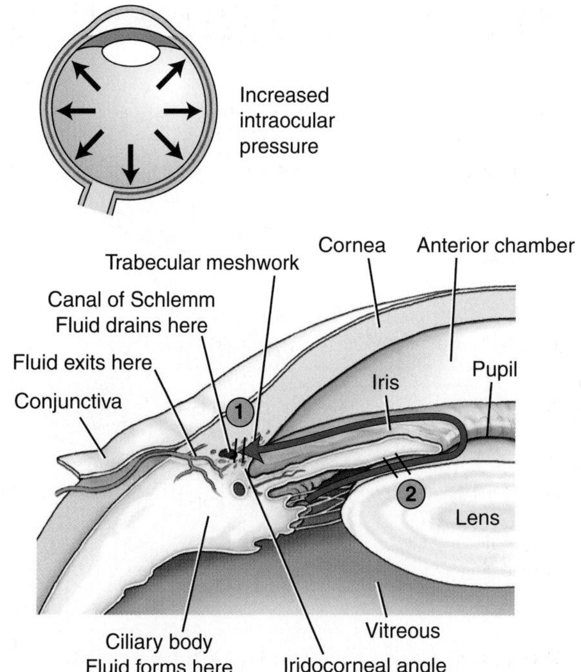

FIGURE 16-15 Glaucoma. **1,** Open-angle glaucoma. The obstruction to aqueous flow lies in the trabecular meshwork. **2,** Closed-angle glaucoma. The iris presses against the lens, blocking aqueous flow into the anterior chamber and raising intraocular pressure.

involved neurons.[206] Acute pain may result and there is loss of peripheral vision and progression to blindness. Early detection and treatment prevent optic neuropathy and visual impairment. Glaucoma often is treated with pharmaceutical eyedrops to reduce secretion or increase absorption of aqueous humor. Surgery may be needed to open the spaces of the trabeculae and reduce intraocular pressure. Neuroprotective therapies are being evaluated.[207]

Retinal detachment is a common cause of visual impairment and blindness. Risk factors include retinal holes and vitreoretinal traction. Fluid (exudate, hemorrhage, or liquid vitreous) separates the photoreceptors from the retinal pigment epithelium. The separation deprives the outer retina of oxygen and nutrients because the diffusion distance is increased. Communication is also disrupted between the pigment epithelium and photoreceptors. **Rhegmatogenous retinal detachment** (retinal breaks caused by vitreoretinal traction) is the most common form of retinal detachment. Causes include intracapsular cataract extraction, severe myopia, lattice degeneration, vitreoretinal traction, and trauma. Contraction of fibrous membranes can cause tractional separation of the retinal layers as occurs in proliferative diabetic retinopathy. Treatment involves surgical retinal reattachment.[208]

Age-related macular degeneration (AMD) is a process in which "drusen" or retinal waste products accumulate within the deep retinal layers. There are two forms of AMD: wet and dry. The *dry* or *atropic form* of AMD is most prevalent and involves loss of retinal pigment epithelium and photoreceptors with overall atrophy of cells. The *wet exudative form* (neovascular AMD) is the more severe form and involves proliferation of abnormal choroidal vessels, which leak and bleed, causing retinal detachment. Hypertension, cigarette smoking, cataract surgery, diabetes mellitus, higher plasma fibrinogen levels, and genetic predisposition are risk factors for AMD.[209] Symptoms include blurred vision, loss of central vision, difficulty reading, and poor night vision. AMD is the major cause of blindness in individuals older than 50 years. Progress is being made in antiangiogenic and vascular endothelial growth factor treatments. Understanding genetic factors contributing to AMD will assist with identifying a biomarker for the disease.[210]

Alterations in Accommodation. Accommodation is the process whereby the thickness of the lens changes with contraction of the ciliary muscles. Accommodation is needed for clear vision and is mediated through the oculomotor nerve (cranial nerve III). Pressure, inflammation, and disease of the oculomotor nerve may alter accommodation. Symptoms include diplopia, blurred vision, and headache. Loss of accommodation in older adults is termed **presbyopia,** a condition in which the ocular lens becomes larger, firmer, and less elastic. The major symptom is reduced near vision, causing the individual to hold reading material at arm's length. Correction of presbyopia is accomplished through reading glasses or bifocal lenses, accommodative intraocular lenses, or surgical treatment.[211]

Alterations in Refraction. Alterations in refraction are the most common visual problem. Errors in refraction are caused by irregularities of the corneal curvature, the focusing power of the lens, and the length of the eye. The major symptoms of refraction alterations are blurred vision and headache. Three types of refraction alterations are myopia, hyperopia, and astigmatism (Figure 16-16).

In **myopia** (nearsightedness), light rays are focused in front of the retina when a person is looking at a distant object, resulting in blurred vision. A concave lens is needed for correction.

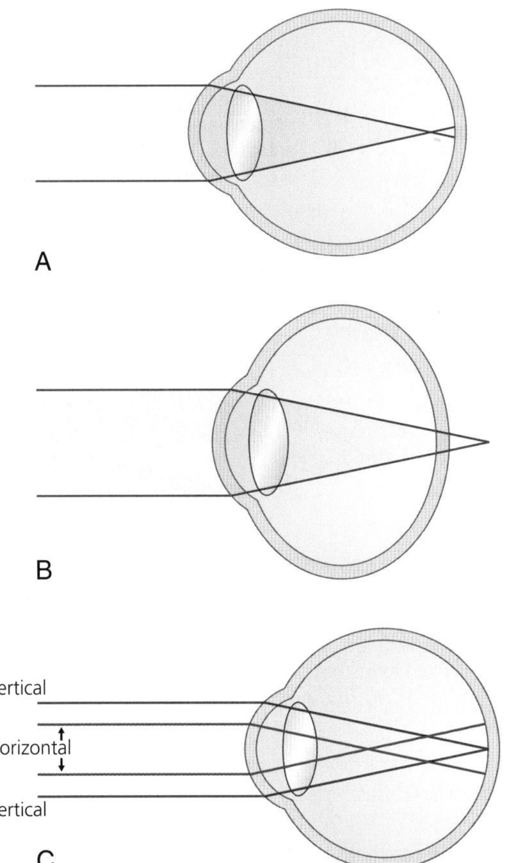

FIGURE 16-16 Alterations in Refraction. **A,** Myopic eye. Parallel rays of light are brought to a focus in front of the retina. **B,** Hyperopic eye. Parallel rays of light come to a focus behind the retina in the nonaccommodative eye. **C,** Simple myopic astigmatism. The vertical bundle of rays is focused on the retina; the horizontal rays are focused in front of the retina and the image is blurred. (From Stein HA, Stein RM, Freeman MI: *The ophthalmic assistant: a text for allied and associated ophthalmic personnel,* ed 9, Philadelphia, 2013, Saunders.)

Myopia requires frequent changes of eyeglasses while the eyeball is lengthening in childhood. Myopia is a risk factor for retinal detachment and cataract formation.

In **hyperopia** (farsightedness), light rays are focused behind the retina when a person is looking at a near object. Hyperopia is corrected with a convex lens. **Astigmatism** is caused by an unequal curvature of the cornea. In astigmatism, light rays are bent unevenly and do not come to a single focus on the retina. Astigmatism may coexist with myopia, hyperopia, or presbyopia. Correction is accomplished with a cylinder lens.

Alterations in Color Vision. Normal sensitivity to color diminishes with age because of the progressive yellowing of the lens that occurs with aging. All colors become less intense, although color discrimination for blue and green is most greatly affected. Color vision deteriorates more rapidly for individuals with diabetes mellitus than for the general population. The deterioration is thought to be an accelerated version of senile color vision deterioration.

Abnormal color vision also may be caused by **color blindness,** an inherited trait. Color blindness is generally an X-linked recessive characteristic affecting 8% of the male population and 0.5% of the female population. Although many forms of color blindness exist, most commonly the affected individual cannot distinguish red from green.[212,213]

Neurologic Disorders Causing Visual Dysfunction. Various neurologic disorders may cause visual dysfunction. Vision may be disrupted at many points along the visual pathway, causing a variety of defects in fields of vision. Visual changes do not always cause defects or blindness in the entire visual field; **hemianopia** is the term that describes defective vision in half of a visual field. (Figure 16-13 illustrates the many areas along the visual pathway that may be damaged and the associated visual changes.) Because of the anatomy of the optic nerves, injury to the optic nerve causes ipsilateral (same side) blindness but a normal contralateral (opposite side) visual field. Injury to the **optic chiasm** (the X-shaped crossing of the optic nerves), often caused by atherosclerotic ischemia or external compression from trauma or aneurysm, can cause a variety of defects, depending on the location of injury. These defects vary because at the optic chiasm, nerve fibers from the medial half of each retina separate from the lateral half and enter the opposite optic tract.

Because of the normal structure of the visual pathways, destruction of one optic tract causes **homonymous hemianopsia** (complete loss of vision in the inner half of one eye and the outer half of the other). Thus, if an injury to the left optic tract occurs, the individual is blind in the right eye's medial (inner) field and the left eye's lateral (outer) field. If the compression of the optic tract is asymmetric, an incongruous (or uneven) homonymous defect results. Injury to one optic radiation (an ocular pathway in the internal capsule, temporal lobe, or occipital lobe) also causes a homonymous (same field) defect. A major injury in the optic radiation causes homonymous hemianopsia. A lesser injury may cause an upper quadrant homonymous defect. Generally the defects are the same size in both eyes. When the homonymous hemianopsia is caused by an occipital lobe lesion, the area of hemianopsia is split. Although visual acuity may remain unimpaired, reading is difficult because of the inability to group words.

Papilledema is edema of the optic nerve at its point of entrance into the eyeball. Papilledema is caused by increased intracranial pressure (e.g., brain tumors, intracranial hemorrhage, hydrocephalus). The subarachnoid space of the brain is continuous with the optic nerve sheath. As cerebrospinal fluid (CSF) pressure increases, the pressure is transmitted to the optic nerve and the optic nerve sheath compresses the nerve and impedes axoplasmic transport. This leads to accumulation of axoplasmic substances at the level of the lamina cribrosa (a meshlike structure in the sclera where the retinal nerves exit the eye and form the optic nerve), resulting in the characteristic swelling of the optic disc. Obliteration of the physiologic cup (a bright area normally located in the center of the optic disc) follows. Later the optic disc becomes raised above the level of the surrounding retina, and the margins become blurred and indistinct. With severe swelling, hemorrhage and patches of white exudate (caused by nerve infarcts) surround the disc margins. The edematous nerves compress the small retinal veins, causing venous stasis and engorgement. Headache is common and

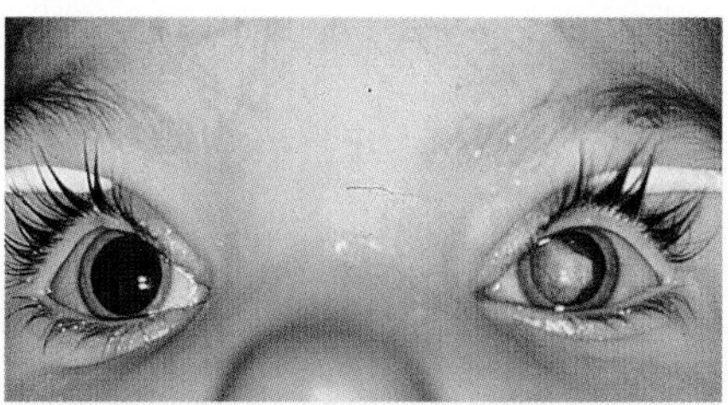

FIGURE 16-17 **Retinoblastoma.** The tumor occupies a large portion of the inside of the eye globe. (From Damjanov I: *Pathology for the health professions,* ed 3, St Louis, 2006, Saunders. Courtesy Dr. Walter Richardson and Dr. Jamsheed Khan, Kansas City, Kansas.)

there may be no visual changes, blurred vision, or constriction of visual fields.

Retinoblastoma. **Retinoblastoma** is a rare congenital eye tumor of young children that originates in the retina of one or both eyes (Figure 16-17). Retinoblastoma demonstrates both an inherited and an acquired form. Retinoblastoma rarely is diagnosed after the child is 5 years of age. The inherited form of the disease generally is diagnosed during the first year of life and often involves multiple tumors and sometimes both eyes (40%).[214] The acquired disease is commonly diagnosed in children 2 to 3 years of age and involves unilateral disease. Although retinoblastoma is the most common pediatric intraocular tumor, only about 300 cases are diagnosed in the United States each year and 1 in 4 cases involves both eyes.[215]

PATHOPHYSIOLOGY. Approximately 40% of retinoblastomas are inherited as an autosomal dominant disorder caused by mutations in the *RB1* tumor-suppressor gene. The remaining 60% are acquired. In the early 1970s Knudson proposed the "two-hit" hypothesis to explain the occurrence of hereditary and acquired forms of the disease. This hypothesis predicts that two separate transforming events or "hits" must occur in a normal retinoblast cell to cause the cancer. Further, it proposes that in the inherited form the first hit or mutation occurs in the germ cell (inherited from either parent), and the mutation is contained in every cell of the child's body. Only a second, random mutation in a retinoblast cell is necessary to transform that cell into cancer. Multiple tumors are observed in the inherited form because these second mutations are likely to occur in several of the approximately 1 to 2 million retinoblast cells. In contrast, the acquired form of retinoblastoma requires that two independent hits or mutations occur in the same somatic cell (after the egg is fertilized) for transformation to cancer. This is much less likely to happen.[216] Figure 16-18 illustrates the two-mutation model for these two patterns of mutation.

The gene location in which the initial retinoblastoma mutation occurs is on the long arm of chromosome 13, band q14.[216] The gene responsible for retinoblastoma, a tumor-suppressor gene, is called the *RB* gene. The first hit inactivates one allele of the *RB* gene, and the second hit inactivates the other allele of the gene. Without the normal functioning of the *RB* gene, production of protein growth regulators that control retinal cell growth is lacking. Because the gene is inactivated, lack of cell growth control results in unregulated proliferation and tumor development. Epigenic effects are under investigation.[216a]

Retinoblastoma grows as one or more tumors in the retina and extends into the vitreous humor. Free-floating, small tumors in the vitreous humor may attach to the surface of the retina in multiple areas and proliferate (Figure 16-19). The tumor also can invade the optic nerve by infiltrating the cribriform plate of the ethmoid bone or can spread through the sheath around the nerve. In either case the tumor can gain access to the subarachnoid space and the CNS. The tumor spreads into the choroid in 25% of children with retinoblastoma. Because the choroid is highly vascular, metastasis by means of hematogenous spread is possible. When hematogenous spread occurs, metastatic sites include the bone marrow, long bones, lymph nodes, and liver. If the tumor invades the orbit, lymphatic spread is possible. Spontaneous regression occurs, although infrequently, and may be caused by the tumor outgrowing its blood supply.

CLINICAL MANIFESTATIONS. The two most frequent symptoms of retinoblastoma are leukokoria, a white pupillary reflex also called **cat's-eye reflex** caused by the mass behind the lens (see Figure 16-17), and strabismus. At that point, the tumor is large enough that a light shone into the eye is reflected back by the tumor, making the pupil appear white. Note that an ophthalmologic examination is not necessary to detect this tumor but only a simple examination of the pupils with a flashlight. If leukokoria is noted, the child should be referred for a complete dilated ophthalmologic exam. Other signs and symptoms include a red, painful eye and limited vision. Any of these signs and symptoms in a child younger than 4 years of age warrants careful ophthalmologic examination of both eyes. Similarly, any newborn with a known genetic risk for retinoblastoma should have routine ophthalmologic examinations.

EVALUATION AND TREATMENT. Diagnostic evaluation for retinoblastoma includes documentation of family history; complete ophthalmologic examination; and metastatic studies that include bone marrow aspiration, lumbar puncture for spinal fluid examination, bone scan, and additional ultrasound, radiologic, and CT studies of the orbit and brain. Because of the potential hereditary risk to a child's siblings, all siblings younger than 4 years also should receive ophthalmologic evaluations.

Retinoblastoma is a treatable tumor, and dual priorities are saving the child's life and restoring useful vision. Early diagnosis and new chemotherapeutic agents have led to a more conservative approach to treatment. Chemoreduction of the tumor occurs with intravenous chemotherapy to reduce tumor volume. Focal treatments using hyperthermia, laser photocoagulation, or cryotherapy then destroy residual tumor. Large or multiple tumors, indicating more advanced disease, require external beam or plaque radiotherapy and in some cases enucleation (removal) of the eye. Every attempt is made to preserve vision in at least one eye without jeopardizing the child's survival.[217]

The prognosis for most children with retinoblastoma is excellent, with a greater than 90% long-term survival, although children with bilateral or metastatic disease at diagnosis have a poor prognosis. Approximately 75% of children have useful vision in the treated eye.

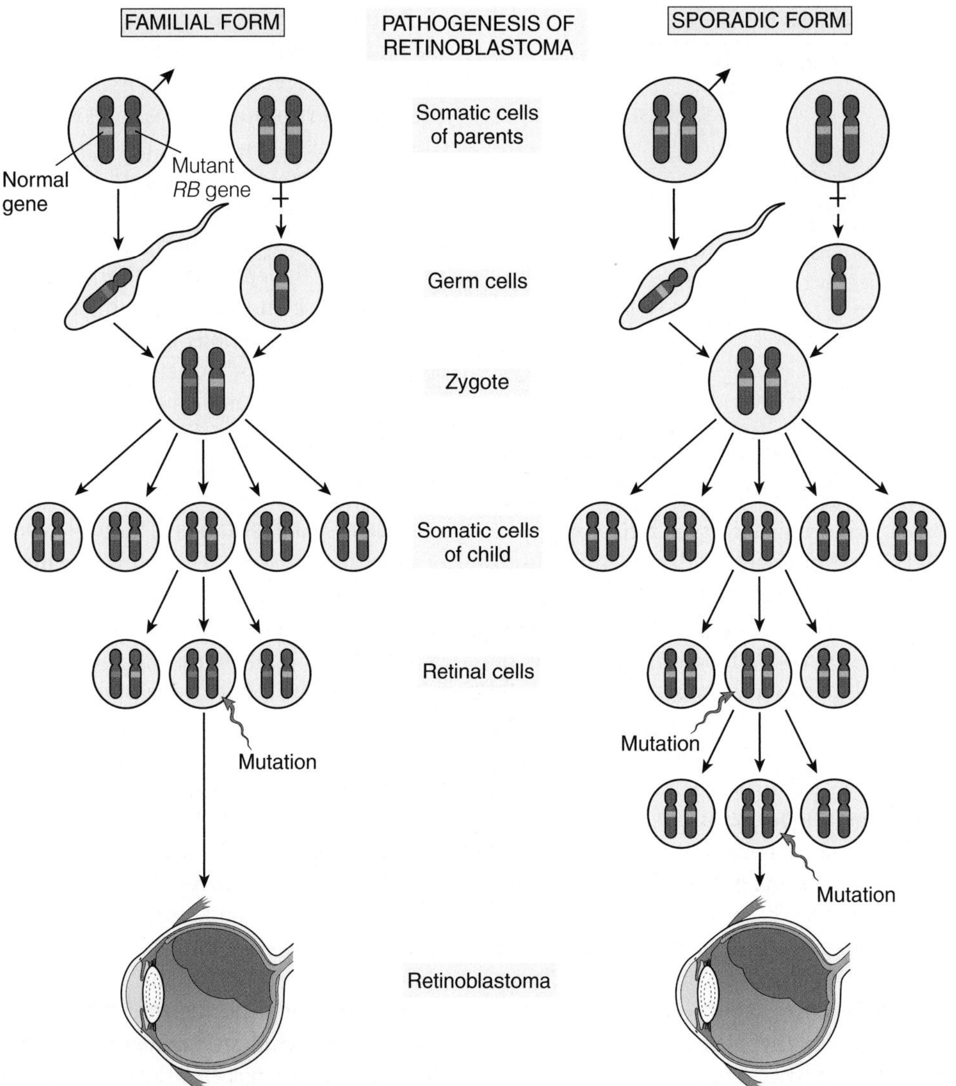

FIGURE 16-18 The Two-Mutation Model of Retinoblastoma Development. In inherited (familial) retinoblastoma, mutations of the *RB* locus on chromosome 13q14 lead to neoplastic proliferation of retinal cells. The first mutation is transmitted through the germline of an affected parent. The second mutation occurs somatically in a retinal cell, leading to development of the tumor. In sporadic retinoblastoma, development of a tumor requires two somatic mutations. (From Kumar V, Cotran RS, Robbins SL: *Robbins basic pathology,* ed 8, Philadelphia, 2010, Saunders.)

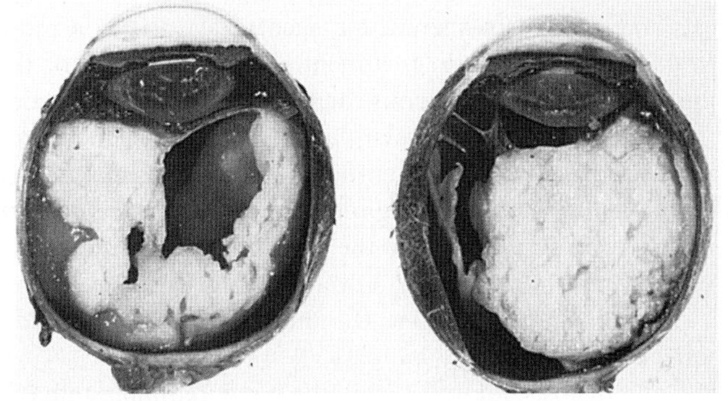

FIGURE 16-19 Bilateral Retinoblastoma. Presence of white mass consisting of detached retina and neoplastic tissue immediately behind lens in each eye. (From Kissane JM, editor: *Anderson's pathology,* ed 8, St Louis, 1985, Mosby.)

Hearing

The **external auditory canal** is surrounded by the bones of the cranium. Its opening (meatus) is just above the **mastoid process** (Figure 16-20), which contains air-filled sinuses called **mastoid air cells.** These promote conductivity between the external and the middle ear.

The Ear

The ear is divided into three areas: (1) the external ear, involved only with hearing; (2) the middle ear, involved only with hearing; and (3) the inner ear, involved with both hearing and equilibrium. The external ear is composed of the **pinna** (auricle), which is the visible portion of the ear, and the external auditory canal, a tube that leads to the middle ear (see Figure 16-20). Sound waves entering the external auditory canal hit

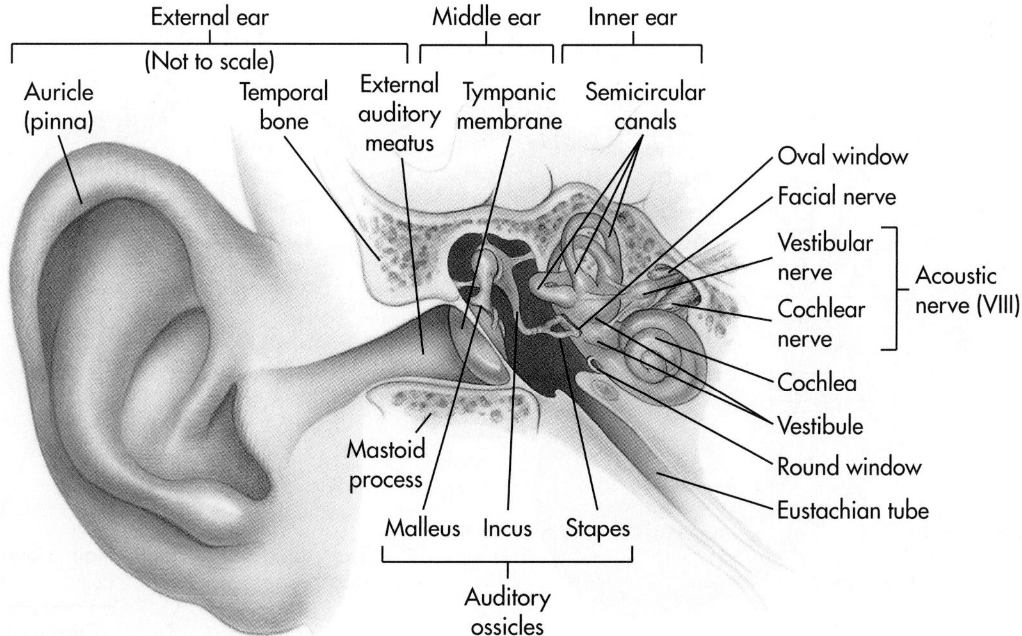

FIGURE 16-20 The Ear. External, middle, and inner ear structures. (Anatomic structures are not drawn to scale. Middle and inner ears enlarged for better visualization here.) (From Patton KT, Thibodeau GA: *Anatomy & physiology,* ed 8, St Louis, 2013, Mosby.)

the **tympanic membrane** (eardrum) and cause it to vibrate. The tympanic membrane separates the external ear from the middle ear.

The middle ear is composed of the **tympanic cavity,** a small chamber in the temporal bone. Three ossicles (small bones) transmit the vibration of the tympanic membrane to the inner ear. The three ossicles are termed the **malleus (hammer), incus (anvil),** and **stapes (stirrup)**. When the tympanic membrane moves, the malleus moves with it and transfers the vibration to the incus, which passes it on to the stapes. The stapes presses against the **oval window,** a small membrane of the inner ear. The movement of the oval window sets the fluids of the inner ear in motion (Figure 16-21).

The **eustachian (pharyngotympanic) tube** connects the middle ear with the thorax. Normally flat and closed, the eustachian tube opens briefly when a person swallows or yawns, and it equalizes the pressure in the middle ear with atmospheric pressure. Equalized pressure permits the tympanic membrane to vibrate freely. Through the eustachian tube the mucosa of the middle ear is contiguous with the mucosal lining of the throat.

The inner ear is a system of osseous labyrinths (bony, mazelike chambers) filled with a fluid called **perilymph.** The bony labyrinth is divided into the **cochlea,** the **vestibule,** and the **semicircular canals** (see Figure 16-21). Suspended in the perilymph is a membranous labyrinth that basically follows the shape of the bony labyrinth. The membranous labyrinth is filled with a thicker fluid called **endolymph.**

Within the cochlea is the **organ of Corti,** which contains **hair cells** (hearing receptors). Sound waves that reach the cochlea through vibrations of the tympanic membrane, ossicles, and oval window set the cochlear fluids into motion. Receptor cells on the basilar membrane are stimulated when their hairs are bent or pulled by the movement. Once stimulated, hair cells transmit impulses along the cochlear nerve (a division of the vestibulocochlear nerve) to the auditory cortex of the temporal lobe in the brain (see Figure 16-21), where interpretation of the sound occurs. Directional hearing is controlled by the angle of the sound source to both ears and by the axonal delay in conduction in groups of neurons.

The semicircular canals and vestibule of the inner ear contain **equilibrium receptors.** In the semicircular canals the dynamic equilibrium receptors respond to changes in direction of movement. Within each semicircular canal is the **crista ampullaris,** a receptor region composed of a tuft of hair cells covered by a gelatinous cupula. When the head is rotated, the endolymph in the canal lags behind and moves in the direction opposite to the head's movement. The hair cells are stimulated, and impulses are transmitted through the vestibular nerve (a division of the vestibulocochlear nerve) to the cerebellum.

The vestibule in the inner ear contains maculae, receptors essential to the body's sense of static equilibrium. As the head moves, **otoliths** (small pieces of calcium salts) move in a gel-like material in response to changes in the pull of gravity. The otoliths pull on the gel, which in turn pulls on the hair cells in the maculae. Nerve impulses in the hair cells are triggered and transmitted to the brain (see Figure 16-21). Thus the ear not only permits the hearing of a large range of sounds but also assists with maintaining balance through the sensitive equilibrium receptors.

AGING AND HEARING

Auditory changes caused by aging are common and incremental. Changes in hearing with aging are summarized in Table 16-6. Approximately one third of people older than 65 years have hearing loss caused by genetic and environmental

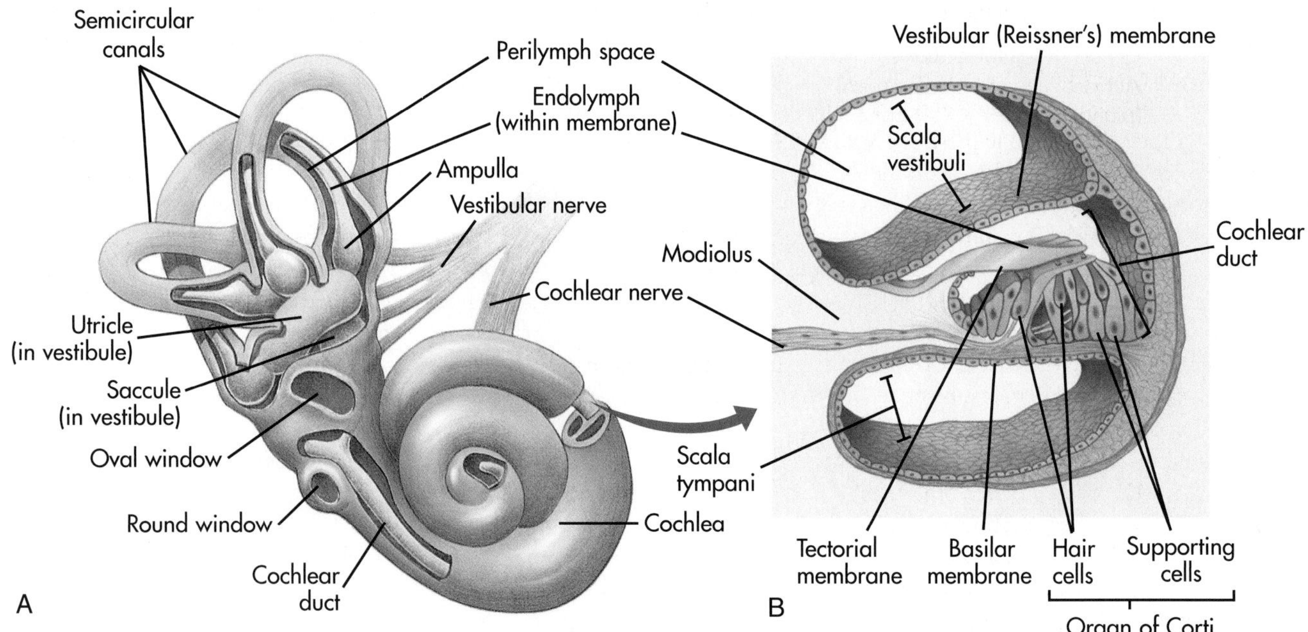

FIGURE 16-21 The Inner Ear. **A,** The bony labyrinth *(orange)* is the hard outer wall of the entire inner ear and includes semicircular canals, vestibule, and cochlea. Within the bony labyrinth is the membranous labyrinth *(purple),* which is surrounded by perilymph and filled with endolymph. Each ampulla in the vestibule contains a crista ampullaris that detects changes in head position and sends sensory impulses through the vestibular nerve to the brain. **B,** The inset shows a section of the membranous cochlea. Hair cells in the organ of Corti detect sound and send the information through the cochlear nerve. The vestibular and cochlear nerves join to form the eighth cranial nerve. (From Patton KT, Thibodeau GA: *Anatomy & physiology,* ed 8, St Louis, 2013, Mosby.)

TABLE 16-6 CHANGES IN HEARING CAUSED BY AGING

CHANGES IN STRUCTURE	CHANGES IN FUNCTION
Cochlear hair cell degeneration	Inability to hear high-frequency sounds (presbycusis, sensorineural loss); interferes with understanding speech; hearing may be lost in both ears at different times
Loss of auditory neurons in spiral ganglia of organ of Corti	Inability to hear high-frequency sounds (presbycusis, sensorineural loss); interferes with understanding speech; hearing may be lost in both ears at different times
Degeneration of basilar (cochlear) conductive membrane of cochlea	Inability to hear at all frequencies, but more pronounced at higher frequencies (cochlear conductive loss)
Decreased vascularity of cochlea	Equal loss of hearing at all frequencies (strial loss); inability to disseminate localization of sound
Loss of cortical auditory neurons	Equal loss of hearing at all frequencies (strial loss); inability to disseminate localization of sound

factors.[218] Changes may occur in the structural and functional components of the peripheral or central auditory system. Loss of hearing for sounds in the high-frequency range (**presbycusis**) is most common and interferes with understanding speech, particularly high-frequency consonant sounds (e.g., *s, sh, f*). Hearing may be lost in both ears but not at the same time. Older adults from rural areas have less hearing loss than those in noisy cities. The ability to discriminate localization of sound varies with high and low frequencies and diminishes with age.[219] In the low-frequency range, sound localization is a function of the timing of sound arrival between the two ears; localization of high-frequency sounds is a function of sound intensity. Because older adults tend to lose high-frequency hearing first, they may have difficulty localizing high-frequency sounds.

Ear Infections

Otitis Externa. Ear infections can occur in the ear canal (otitis externa) or in the middle ear (otitis media). Otitis media is the leading cause of healthcare visits and drug prescriptions throughout the world with 50% occurring in the under 5-year age group.[220]

Otitis externa is the most common infection of the outer ear usually caused by bacteria and less commonly a fungus.[221] The most frequently found microorganisms are *Pseudomonas, Escherichia coli,* and *Staphylococcus aureus.* Infection usually follows prolonged exposure to moisture (swimmer's ear). The earliest symptoms are inflammation with swelling and clear drainage progressing to purulent drainage with obstruction of the canal. Tenderness and pain with earlobe retraction accompany inflammation.

Otitis Media. **Otitis media** is an infection of the middle ear and is the most common infection of infants and children. Most children have one episode by 3 years of age. The most common pathogens are *Streptococcus pneumoniae, Haemophilus influenzae,* and *Moraxella catarrhalis.* Respiratory viruses also may have an etiologic role.[222] Predisposing factors include allergy, sinusitis, submucous cleft palate, adenoidal hypertrophy, and immune deficiency. Breast-feeding is a protective factor.

Acute otitis media (AOM) is associated with ear pain, fever, irritability, inflamed tympanic membrane, and fluid in the middle ear. The tympanic membrane progresses from erythema to opaqueness with bulging as fluid accumulates. An increasing prevalence of AOM is caused by methicillin-resistant microorganisms. Otitis media with effusion (OME) is the presence of fluid in the middle ear without symptoms of acute infection. Treatment includes antimicrobial therapy for AOM, particularly in children 2 years and younger.

Chronic otitis media is persistent or recurring infection of the middle ear. Placement of tympanostomy tubes is considered when bilateral effusion persists for 3 months and for significant hearing loss.[223] Mastoidectomy combined with tympanostomy tubes may be required when there is cholesteatoma (skin growth into the middle ear associated with perforation of the eardrum).[224] Complications include mastoiditis, brain abscess, meningitis, and chronic otitis media with hearing loss. Speech, language, and cognitive disabilities may be affected by persistent middle ear effusions.

Auditory Dysfunction

Between 5% and 10% of the general population have a hearing impairment. The major categories of auditory dysfunction are conductive hearing loss, sensorineural hearing loss, mixed hearing loss, and functional hearing loss.

Conductive Hearing Loss. **Conductive hearing loss** occurs when a change in the outer or middle ear impairs sound from being conducted from the outer to the inner ear. Conductive hearing loss occurs when there is interference in air conduction. Conditions that commonly cause a conductive hearing loss include impacted cerumen, foreign bodies lodged in the ear canal, benign tumors of the middle ear, carcinoma of the external auditory canal or middle ear, eustachian tube dysfunction, otitis media, acute viral otitis media, chronic suppurative otitis media, cholesteatoma, and otosclerosis (impaired mobility of the stapes footplate in the presence of dense sclerotic bone).

Symptoms of conductive hearing loss include diminished hearing and soft speaking voice. The voice is soft because often the individual hears his or her voice, conducted by bone, as loud. In addition, although the cause is unknown, the individual often hears better in a noisy environment than in a quiet one (a condition called *paracusia willisiana*). Treatment of the underlying cause generally improves hearing and a hearing aid can improve quality of life.[225]

Sensorineural Hearing Loss. A **sensorineural hearing loss** is caused by impairment of the organ of Corti or its central connections. The hearing loss may be gradual or sudden. Conditions that commonly cause sensorineural hearing loss include congenital and hereditary factors, noise exposure, aging, Ménière disease, ototoxicity, and systemic disease (syphilis, Paget disease, collagen diseases, diabetes mellitus). Congenital and neonatal sensorineural hearing loss may be caused by maternal rubella, ototoxic drugs, prematurity, traumatic delivery, erythroblastosis fetalis, and congenital hereditary malfunction. Diagnosis often is made when delayed speech development is noted.

Presbycusis is age-related hearing loss usually in the high frequencies. It is the most common form of sensorineural hearing loss and is especially common in older adutls.[218] Presbycusis may occur because of atrophy of the basal end of the organ of Corti, a loss in the number of auditory receptors, changes in vasculature, or stiffening of the basilar membranes. Because of the slow progression of hearing loss, onset of symptoms is gradual. In addition, drug ototoxicities (drugs that cause destruction of auditory function) have been observed after exposure to a variety of chemicals, for example, antibiotics such as streptomycin, neomycin, gentamicin, and vancomycin; diuretics such as ethacrynic acid and furosemide; and chemicals such as salicylate, quinine, carbon monoxide, nitrogen mustard, arsenic, mercury, gold, tobacco, and alcohol. Because of increased concentrations of antibiotics in the endolymph, these drugs generally cause damage to the cells of the cristae and maculae (located in the inner ear) or the cells of the organ of Corti. The increased concentration of drugs in the endolymph is preferentially toxic to the cells.

Diuretics affect hearing primarily by altering the sodium-potassium balance, causing extracellular fluid accumulation and changes in the microstructure of secretory cells. Quinine, mercury, and lead affect the neural pathways of hearing, including the spinal ganglia, the eighth cranial nerve, and the cochlear nucleus. The site of action for the other chemicals, including alcohol and tobacco, has not yet been determined. In most instances the drugs and chemicals listed previously initially cause **tinnitus** (ringing in the ear), followed by a progressive high-tone sensorineural hearing loss. Care is aimed at prevention of further hearing loss because the loss is usually permanent.

Mixed Hearing Loss. A **mixed hearing loss** is caused by a combination of conductive and sensorineural losses.

Functional Hearing Loss. A **functional hearing loss** occurs for no organic reason. The individual does not respond to voice and appears not to hear. Functional hearing loss is thought to be caused by emotional or psychologic factors. It occurs only rarely.

Olfaction and Taste

Olfaction (smell) dysfunction and taste (gustation) dysfunction may occur separately or jointly. The strong relationship between smell and taste creates the sensation of flavor. If either sensation is impaired, the perception of flavor is altered. (Olfactory structures are illustrated in Figure 16-22.)

Olfaction is a function of cranial nerve I (olfactory) and part of cranial nerve V (trigeminal). The receptor cells for smell are located in the olfactory epithelium. Seven primary classes of olfactory stimulants have been identified: (1) camphoraceous, (2) musky, (3) floral, (4) peppermint, (5) ethereal, (6) pungent, and (7) putrid.

Olfactory dysfunctions include hyposmia, anosmia, hallucinations, and parosmia. **Hyposmia** is the impaired sense of smell, and **anosmia** is the complete loss of smell. Both conditions are associated with aging, neurodegenerative and nasal/sinus disorders, and head trauma.[226] When hyposmia or anosmia occurs bilaterally, it is usually the result of rhinitis

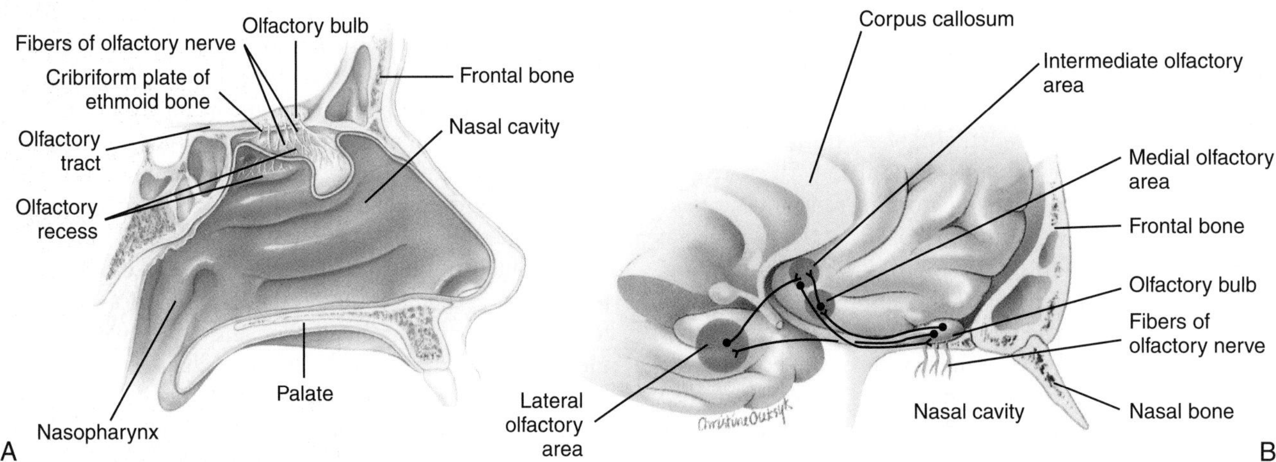

FIGURE 16-22 **Olfaction.** Location of olfactory epithelium, olfactory bulb, and neuronal pathways involved in olfaction. **A,** Midsagittal section of the nasal area shows the locations of major olfactory sensory structures. **B,** Major olfactory integration centers of the brain. (Modified from Patton KT, Thibodeau GA: *Anatomy & physiology,* ed 8, St Louis, 2013, Mosby.)

(inflammation of nasal mucosa), sinusitis, nasal polyps, or excessive smoking. Unilateral hyposmia or anosmia may indicate compression of one olfactory bulb (a bulblike portion of the olfactory nerves) or nerve tract (olfactory nerve pathway), possibly by tumor or head trauma. **Olfactory hallucinations** arise from hyperactivity in cortical neurons and involve smelling odors that are not really present. They are associated with temporal lobe seizures and rarely with schizophrenia. **Parosmia,** an abnormal or perverted sense of smell, may occur with severe depression.[227]

Taste is a function of multiple nerves in the tongue, soft palate, uvula, pharynx, and upper esophagus, including cranial nerves VII (facial) and IX (glossopharyngeal). The primary sensations of taste are sour, salty, sweet, bitter, and umami (savoriness). Taste buds sensitive to each of the primary sensations are located on the circumvallate, fungiform, and foliate papillae in specific areas of the tongue. Taste receptors also are found on airway smooth muscle (bitter) and in the gastrointestinal tract (bitter and sweet). Their function is not for taste. In the lung they stimulate bronchodilation and in the gastrointestinal tract they may participate in metabolic and digestive regulation.[228,229]

Alterations in taste can be caused by injury, medications, oral infections, or aging. A change in taste also may be attributable to impairment of smell associated with injury near the hippocampus.

Hypogeusia is a decrease in taste sensation, and **ageusia** is the absence of taste. Ageusia affecting the entire tongue may follow head injury. Damage to the glossopharyngeal nerve (cranial nerve IX, which innervates the posterior one third of the tongue) causes the loss of the ability to detect bitterness. This loss occurs because the receptors for bitter are located on the base of the tongue. Damage to the facial nerve (cranial nerve VII, which innervates the anterior two thirds of the tongue) causes loss of the ability to detect sour, sweet, and salty tastes. Only bitter tastes can be detected. These losses occur because sour, sweet, and salt receptors are located on the anterior portion of the tongue. **Parageusia** is a perversion of taste in which substances possess an unpleasant flavor. Parageusia occasionally develops for no apparent reason in older adults and is common in individuals receiving chemotherapy for cancer. In both cases, parageusia often leads to anorexia and malnutrition.

AGING AND OLFACTION AND TASTE

Sensitivity to odors declines steadily with aging.[230,231a] A study of odor identification indicates an increasing ability from childhood to adolescence and then a decline after 60 years of age. The sense of smell begins to degenerate with loss of olfactory sensory neurons and loss of cells from the olfactory bulbs. Loss of olfactory sensitivity and odor identification may diminish appetite and food selection and thus may lead to malnutrition. Safety also may be compromised by an inability to smell spoiled food or hazardous gases.[226]

The decline in taste sensation is more gradual than that of smell and is associated with loss of olfaction. Higher concentrations of flavors are required, and older adults have difficulty differentiating combinations of flavors. Taste changes with aging are associated with decline in the number of fungiform papillae on the tongue, and changes in taste receptor function.[231] Taste also may be affected by decreased salivary gland secretion. Amylase, contained in saliva, facilitates perception of sweet flavors.

SUMMARY REVIEW

Pain

1. Pain is a protective and a complex phenomenon composed of sensory experiences (time, space, intensity) and emotion, cognition, and motivation.
2. The gate control theory of pain describes the modulation of pain in the dorsal horn of the spinal cord by sensory afferent stimulation and central descending impulses that influence the "pain gate" within the substantia gelatinosa of the spinal cord.
3. The neuromatrix theory proposes that sensory inputs to the brain produce patterns of pain but the stimuli may originate independently in the brain with no external input.
4. The portions of the nervous system responsible for the sensation and perception of pain may be divided into three areas: (a) the afferent fibers, (b) the afferent pathways, and (c) the CNS.
5. The afferent system is composed of nociceptors, Aδ and C fibers (first-order neurons); the dorsal horn of the spinal column (second-order neurons); and afferent neurons in the spinothalamic tract (third-order neurons).
6. Nociceptors detect a wide range of stimuli and respond to chemical, mechanical, and thermal stimulation.
7. Myelinated Aδ receptor transmission is fast and conveys mechanical and thermal, sharp, localized pain. Unmyelinated polymodal C fiber transmission is slower and conveys diffuse burning and aching sensations. These primary-order neurons terminate on second-order neurons.
8. Three classes of second-order neurons modulate pain transmission: projection cells, excitatory interneurons, and inhibitory interneurons. The second-order neurons are located in the spinal cord laminae and function as a pain gate to regulate pain transmission.
9. Second-order neurons cross over the cord and ascend primarily in the lateral spinothalamic tract to projection centers including the thalamus, reticular formation, and PAG matter.
10. Third-order neurons carry information to the sensory cortex and reticular and limbic systems for pain processing and interpretation.
11. Efferent pathways from the PAG are responsible for modulation or inhibition of afferent pain signals. The thalamus, cortex, and postcentral gyrus perceive, describe, and localize pain. The reticular formation and limbic system control the emotional and affective response to pain.
12. Pain can be modulated by segmental inhibition, which is the peripheral stimulation of nociceptors by touch, vibration, or pressure resulting in closure of the spinal cord pain gate. The higher brain center also can influence painful stimuli (heterosegmental control of nociception) as well as inhibition from the caudal medulla (diffuse noxious inhibitory controls). Thus pain can be modulated with stimulation from the periphery or by descending impulses from the brain.
13. Pain neurotransmitters can be classified as inflammatory, excitatory, and inhibitory modulators of pain. Inflammatory neurotransmitters are usually excitatory.
14. Pain threshold is the point at which pain is perceived. Pain threshold does not vary significantly among people or within the same person over time.
15. Pain tolerance is the duration of time or the intensity of pain that an individual will endure before initiating overt pain response. Tolerance varies widely among individuals and in the same individual over time.
16. Classifications of pain include nociceptive pain (with a known physiologic cause), non-nociceptive pain (neuropathic pain), acute pain (signal to the person of a harmful stimulus), and chronic pain (persistence of pain of unknown cause or unusual response to therapy).
17. Acute pain may be (a) somatic (superficial), (b) visceral (internal), or (c) referred (present in an area distant from its origin).
18. Somatic pain arises from connective tissue, muscle, bone, and skin and is sharp and localized.
19. Visceral pain is from internal organs and is transmitted by sympathetic afferents and is poorly localized.
20. Referred pain usually arises from the viscera and terminates in an area of the spinal cord that is conjoined with fibers originating in the skin and other areas and thereby produces the perception of pain at the referred site.
21. Physiologic responses to acute pain include increased heart rate, respiratory rate, and blood pressure; pallor or flushing; dilated pupils; and diaphoresis. Blood glucose level is elevated; gastric secretion and motility are decreased; and blood flow to the viscera and skin is decreased.
22. Chronic pain generally lasts at least 3 months and may be persistent, for example, low back pain or intermittent migraine headache pain, myofascial pain syndromes, chronic postoperative pain, and chronic pain associated with cancer.
23. Neuropathic pain is usually chronic, results from nerve trauma or disease, and leads to abnormal peripheral and central pain processing. Types of neuropathic pain include deafferentation pain, sympathetically maintained pain, central pain, and phantom pain.
24. Newborns and young children have the anatomic and functional ability to perceive pain. Pain experienced by infants may have prolonged effects on brain organization and responses to pain.
25. Older individuals may or may not have an increased pain threshold. In all age groups, women appear to be more sensitive to pain than are men.
26. Pain in older adults is influenced by liver and renal function, including alterations in the metabolism of drugs and metabolites.

Temperature Regulation

1. Temperature regulation (thermoregulation) is achieved through precise balancing of heat production, heat conservation, and heat loss. Body temperature is maintained around 37° C (98.6° F).
2. Temperature regulation is mediated by the hypothalamus. Peripheral thermoreceptors in the skin and central

SUMMARY REVIEW—cont'd

thermoreceptors in the hypothalamus, spinal cord, and abdominal organs provide the hypothalamus with information about skin and core temperatures.

3. Heat is produced through chemical reactions of metabolism, skeletal muscle contraction (shivering), and chemical thermogenesis.
4. Heat is lost through radiation, conduction, convection, vasodilation, decreased muscle tone, evaporation of sweat, increased ventilation, and voluntary mechanisms.
5. Heat conservation is accomplished through vasoconstriction and voluntary mechanisms.
6. Fever is triggered by the release of pyrogens from leukocytes and other cells involved in the immune response (endogenous pyrogens) and bacteria (exogenous pyrogens). Fever is both a symptom of a disease and a normal immunologic mechanism.
7. Fever involves resetting the hypothalamic thermostat to a higher level. When a fever breaks, the set point is returned to normal.
8. Fever production aids responses to infectious processes. Higher temperatures kill many microorganisms and decrease serum levels of iron, zinc, and copper that are needed for bacterial replication.
9. Infants and older adults require special attention to maintenance of body temperature. Because of their greater body surface area to mass ratio and decreased subcutaneous fat, infants do not conserve heat well. Older individuals have poor responses to environmental temperature extremes as a result of slowed blood circulation, structural and functional changes in skin, and an overall decrease in heat-producing activities.
10. Hyperthermia (marked warming of core temperature) can produce nerve damage, coagulation of cell proteins, and death. Forms of accidental hyperthermia include heat cramps, heat exhaustion, heat stroke, and malignant hyperthermia. Heat stroke and malignant hyperthermia are potentially lethal developments.
11. Hypothermia (marked cooling of core temperature) slows the rate of chemical reaction (tissue metabolism), increases the viscosity of the blood, slows blood flow through the microcirculation, facilitates blood coagulation, and stimulates profound vasoconstriction. Hypothermia may be accidental or therapeutic.

Sleep

1. Sleep may be divided into REM and NREM stages, each of which has its own series of stages. While asleep, an individual progresses through the three stages of NREM (slow-wave) sleep and REM sleep in a predictable cycle.
2. NREM sleep is initiated by the withdrawal of neurotransmitters from the afferent formation and by the inhibition of arousal mechanisms in the cerebral cortex. REM sleep is controlled by mechanisms in the hypothalamus and pontine reticular formation.
3. During sleep the body is actively engaged in restoring and repairing itself. Sleep deprivation can cause profound changes in personality and functioning.
4. The restorative, reparative, and growth processes occur during slow-wave sleep.
5. The sleep patterns of the newborn and young child vary from those of the adult in total sleep time, cycle length, and percentage of time spent in each sleep cycle. Older adults experience a total decrease in sleep time.
6. Sleep disorders include: (a) dyssomnias, (b) parasomnias, (c) sleep disorders associated with mental, neurologic, or other medical disorder, and (d) proposed sleep disorders.
7. Common dyssomnias include insomnia, OSAS, RLS, circadian rhythm disorder, and hypersomnia.
8. Common parasomnias include arousal disorders, sleep-wake transition disorder, and disorders associated with REM sleep.
9. Sleep and disease are interrelated. Some diseases may produce alterations in the quantity and quality of sleep or affect sleep stages. These are referred to as *secondary sleep disorders*. In some instances sleep stages produce alterations in certain disease states. These are referred to as *sleep-provoked disorders*.

Somatosensory Function and the Special Senses

Somatosensory Function

1. The sensation of touch involves the fusion of several qualities, including modality, intensity, location, and duration of the sensory stimulus.
2. Receptors sensitive to touch are present in the skin; these include Meissner and pacinian corpuscles and Merkel disks and Ruffini endings. The sensory response is conducted to the brain through the dorsal column and anterior spinothalamic tract.
3. Abnormal tactile perception may be caused by alterations at any level of the nervous system, from the receptor to the cerebral cortex.
4. Proprioception is the perception of the position and location of the body and its parts. Proprioceptors are located in the inner ear, joints, and ligaments. Proprioceptive stimuli are necessary for balance, coordinated movement, and grading of muscular contraction.
5. Disorders of proprioception can be caused by alterations at any level of the nervous system. Two common causes of proprioceptive dysfunction are vestibular dysfunction and neuropathy.

Vision

1. The eyelids, conjunctivae, and lacrimal apparatus protect the eye. Infections are the most common disorders; they include blepharitis, conjunctivitis, chalazion, and hordeolum.
2. Conjunctivitis can be acute or chronic, bacterial, viral, or allergic. Redness, edema, pain, and lacrimation are common symptoms. Trachoma (chlamydial conjunctivitis) is

SUMMARY REVIEW—cont'd

the leading cause of blindness in the world and is associated with poor sanitary conditions.
3. Keratitis is a bacterial or viral infection of the cornea that can lead to corneal ulceration. Photophobia, pain, and tearing are common symptoms.
4. The wall of the eye has three layers: sclera, choroid, and retina. The retina contains millions of photoreceptors known as rods and cones that receive light through the lens and then convey signals to the optic nerve and subsequently to the visual cortex of the brain.
5. The eye is filled with vitreous and aqueous humor, which prevent it from collapsing.
6. Structural eye changes caused by aging or chronic disease result in decreased visual acuity.
7. The major alterations in ocular movement include strabismus, nystagmus, and paralysis of the extraocular muscles.
8. Alterations in visual acuity can be caused by amblyopia, scotoma, cataracts, papilledema, macular degeneration, retinal detachment, and glaucoma.
9. Alterations in accommodation develop with increased intraocular pressure, inflammation, and disease of the oculomotor nerve. Presbyopia is loss of accommodation caused by loss of lens elasticity with aging.
10. Alterations in refraction, including myopia, hyperopia, and astigmatism, are the most common visual disorders.
11. Alterations in color vision occur with disorders of the cornea and the inherited trait of color blindness.
12. Trauma or disease of the optic nerve pathways, or optic radiations, can cause blindness in the visual fields. Homonymous hemianopsia is caused by damage of one optic tract.
13. Retinoblastoma is a congenital eye tumor that has a hereditary and a nonhereditary form.

Hearing

1. The ear is composed of external, middle, and inner structures. The external structures are the pinna, auditory canal, and tympanic membrane. The tympanic cavity (containing three bones: malleus, incus, and stapes), oval window, eustachian tube, and fluid comprise the middle ear and transmit sound vibrations to the inner ear.
2. The inner ear includes the bony and membranous labyrinths that transmit sound waves through the cochlea to the division of the eighth cranial nerve (i.e., vestibulocochlear). The semicircular canals and vestibule help maintain balance through the equilibrium receptors.
3. Approximately one third of all people older than 65 years have hearing loss.
4. Otitis externa is an infection of the outer ear. Otitis media, an infection of the middle ear, is common in children and can be acute or chronic.
5. Acute otitis media is an infection of the middle ear associated with ear pain, fever, an inflamed tympanic membrane, and fluid in the middle ear.
6. Chronic otitis media is persistent or recurrent middle ear infection.
7. Hearing loss can be classified as conductive, sensorineural, mixed, or functional.
8. Conductive hearing loss occurs when sound waves cannot be conducted through the middle ear.
9. Sensorineural hearing loss develops with impairment of the organ of Corti or its central connections. Presbycusis is age-related hearing loss and is the most common form of sensorineural hearing loss.
10. A combination of conductive and sensorineural loss is a mixed hearing loss.
11. Loss of hearing with no known organic cause is a functional hearing loss.

Olfaction and Taste

1. The perception of flavor is altered if olfaction or taste dysfunctions occur. Sensitivity to odor and taste decreases with aging.
2. Hyposmia is a decrease in the sense of smell, and anosmia is the complete loss of smell. Inflammation of the nasal mucosa and trauma or tumors of the olfactory nerve lead to a diminished sense of smell.
3. Hypogeusia is a decrease in taste sensation, and ageusia is the absence of taste. Loss of taste buds or trauma to the facial or glossopharyngeal nerves decreases taste sensation.

KEY TERMS

A-beta (Aβ) fiber, 486
Accidental hyperthermia, 500
Accommodation, 508
Acute bacterial conjunctivitis (pinkeye), 507
Acute otitis media (AOM), 517
Acute pain, 491
A-delta (Aδ) fiber, 486
Affective-motivational system, 487
Age-related macular degeneration (AMD), 511
Ageusia, 518
Allergic conjunctivitis, 507
Allodynia, 490
Amblyopia, 510
Anosmia, 517
Antipyretic, 498
Aqueous humor, 508
Astigmatism, 512
Blepharitis, 507
Cancer pain, 494
Cataract, 510
Cat's-eye reflex, 513
Central neuropathic pain, 494
Central sensitization, 490
Chalazion, 507
Choroid, 508
Chronic conjunctivitis, 507
Chronic otitis media, 517
Chronic pain, 492
Chronic postoperative pain, 493
Circadian rhythm, 496
Circadian rhythm sleep disorder, 505
Cochlea, 515
Cognitive-evaluative system, 487
Color blindness, 512
Complex regional pain syndrome (CRPS), 494
Conduction, 497
Conductive hearing loss, 517
Cone, 508
Conjunctivitis, 507
Convection, 497
Cornea, 508
Crista ampullaris, 515
Dark adaptation, 510
Deafferentation pain syndrome, 494
Descending modulation of pain, 489

KEY TERMS—cont'd

REFERENCES

1. International Association for the Study of Pain: *IASP taxonomy*. Available at www.iasp-pain.org/AM/Template.cfm?Section=Pain_Definitions&;Template=/CM/HTMLDisplay.cfm&ContentID=1728. Accessed March 20, 2013.
2. Waddell G: *The back pain revolution*, ed 2, London, 2004, Churchill Livingstone.
3. Melzack R, Wall PD: Pain mechanisms: a new theory, *Science* 150:971, 1965.
4. Arnstein P: *Clinical coach for effective pain management*, Philadelphia, 2010, FA Davis.
5. Helms JE, Barone CP: Physiology and treatment of pain, *Crit Care Nurs* 28:38–49, 2008.
6. Melzak R: Toward a new concept of pain for the new millenium. In Waldman SD, editor: *Interventional pain management*, ed 2, Philadelphia, 2001, Saunders.
7. Melzack R: Evolution of the neuromatrix theory of pain, *Pain Practice* 5(2):85–94, 2005.
8. Chen J: History of pain theories, *Neurosci Bull* 27(5):343–350, 2011.
9. Perl ER: Pain mechanisms: a commentary on concepts and issues, *Prog Neurobiol* 94(1):20–38, 2011.
10. Chung MK, Jung SJ, Oh SB: Role of TRP channels in pain sensation, *Adv Exp Med Biol* 704:615–636, 2011.
11. Todd AJ: Neuronal circuitry for pain processing in the dorsal horn, *Nat Rev Neurosci* 11(12):823–836, 2010.
12. Moffat R, Colin RP: Anatomy physiology and pharmacology of pain, *Anaesth Intensive Care Med* 12(1):12–15, 2011.
13. Lamm C, Decety J, Singer T: Meta-analytic evidence for common and distinct neural networks associated with directly experienced pain and empathy for pain, *Neuroimage* 54(3):2492–2502, 2011.
14. Legrain V et al: The pain matrix reloaded: a salience detection system for the body, *Prog Neurobiol* 93(1):111–124, 2011.
15. Marchand S: The physiology of pain mechanisms: from the periphery to the brain, *Rheum Dis Clin North Am* 34:285–309, 2008.
16. Xie YF, Huo FQ, Tang JS: Cerebral cortex modulation of pain, *Acta Pharmacol Sin* 30(1):31–41, 2009.
17. van Wijk G, Veldhuijzen DS: Perspective on diffuse noxious inhibitory controls as a model of endogenous pain modulation in clinical pain syndromes, *J Pain* 11(5):408–419, 2010.
18. Benedetti F, Carlino E, Pollo A: How placebos change the patient's brain, *Neuropsychopharmacology* 36(1):339–354, 2011.
19. Dobrila-Dintinjana R, Nacinović-Duletić A: Placebo in the treatment of pain, *Coll Anthropol* 35(Suppl 2):319–323, 2011.

20. Ossipov MH, Dussor GO, Porreca F: Central modulation of pain, *J Clin Invest* 120(11):3779–3787, 2010.
21. Larsson M, Broman J: Synaptic plasticity and pain: role of ionotropic glutamate receptors, *Neuroscientist* 17(3):256–273, 2011.
22. Woolf CJ: Central sensitization: implications for the diagnosis and treatment of pain, *Pain* 152(Suppl 3):S2–S15, 2011.
23. Zeilhofer HU, Wildner H, Yévenes GE: Fast synaptic inhibition in spinal sensory processing and pain control, *Physiol Rev* 92(1):193–235, 2012.
24. Kuner R: Central mechanisms of pathological pain, *Nat Med* 16(11):1258–1266, 2010.
25. Sauriyal DS, Jaggi AS, Singh N: Extending pharmacological spectrum of opioids beyond analgesia: multifunctional aspects in different pathophysiological states, *Neuropeptides* 45(3):175–188, 2011.
26. Guillot X et al: Pain and immunity, *Joint Bone Spine* 79(3):228–236, 2012.
27. Mika J, Obara I, Przewlocka B: The role of nociceptin and dynorphin in chronic pain: implications of neuro-glial interaction, *Neuropeptides* 45(4):247–261, 2011.
28. Jessop DS et al: Endomorphins in rheumatoid arthritis, osteoarthritis, and experimental arthritis, *Ann N Y Acad Sci* 1193:117–122, 2010.
29. Fichna J et al: The endomorphin system and its evolving neurophysiological role, *Pharmacol Rev* 59(1):88–123, 2007.
30. Bodnar RJ: Endogenous opiates and behavior, *Peptides* 31(12): 2325–2359, 2009.
31. Sterzer P, Kleinschmidt A: A neural basis for inference in perceptual ambiguity, *Proc Natl Acad Sci U S A* 104(1):323–328, 2007.
32. Defrin R, Eli I, Pud D: Interactions among sex, ethnicity, religion, and gender role expectations of pain, *Gend Med* 8(3):172–183, 2011.
33. American Pain Society: *Principles of analgesic use in the treatment of acute pain and cancer pain*, ed 6, Glenview, IL, 2008, Author.
34. Gao YJ, Ji RR: Chemokines, neuronal-glial interactions, and central processing of neuropathic pain, *Pharmacol Ther* 126(1):56–68, 2010.
35. White FA, Jung H, Miller RJ: Chemokines and the pathophysiology of neuropathic pain, *Proc Natl Acad Sci U S A* 104(51):20151–20158, 2007.
36. Lee MC, Tracey I: Unravelling the mystery of pain, suffering, and relief with brain imaging, *Curr Pain Headache Rep* 14(2):124–131, 2010.
37. Seifert F, Maihöfner C: Functional and structural imaging of pain-induced neuroplasticity, *Curr Opin Anaesthesiol* 24(5):515–523, 2011.
38. Davis KD: Neuroimaging of pain: what does it tell us? *Curr Opin Support Palliat Care* 5(2):116–121, 2011.
39. Siemionow M, Mendiola A: Methods of assessment of cortical plasticity in patients following amputation, replantation, and composite tissue allograft transplantation, *Ann Plast Surg* 65(3):344–348, 2010.
40. Lavand'homme P: The progression from acute to chronic pain, *Curr Opin Anaesthesiol* 24(5):545–550, 2011.
41. Voscopoulos C, Lema M: When does acute pain become chronic? *Br J Anaesth* 105(Suppl 1):i69–i85, 2010.
42. Turk DC, Wilson HD: Fear of pain as a prognostic factor in chronic pain: conceptual models, assessment, and treatment implications, *Curr Pain Headache Rep* 14(2):88–95, 2010.
43. Catananti C, Gambassi G: Pain assessment in the elderly, *Surg Oncol* 19(3):140–148, 2010.
44. Cornally N, McCarthy G: Help-seeking behaviour for the treatment of chronic pain, *Br J Commun Nurs* 16(2):90–98, 2011.
45. Balagué F et al: Non-specific low back pain, *Lancet* 379(9814):482–491, 2012.
46. Hoy D et al: The epidemiology of low back pain, *Best Pract Res Clin Rheumatol* 24(6):769–781, 2010.
47. Pransky G, Buchbinder R, Hayden J: Contemporary low back pain research—and implications for practice, *Best Pract Res Clin Rheumatol* 24(2):291–298, 2010.
48. Wand BM et al: Cortical changes in chronic low back pain: current state of the art and implications for clinical practice, *Man Ther* 16(1):15–20, 2011.
49. Shah JP, Gilliams EA: Uncovering the biochemical milieu of myofascial trigger points using in vivo microdialysis: an application of muscle pain concepts to myofascial pain syndrome, *J Body Mov Ther* 12(4):371–384, 2008.
50. Nett MP: Postoperative pain management, *Orthopedics* 33(Suppl 9):23–26, 2010.
51. Goudas LC et al: The epidemiology of cancer pain, *Cancer Invest* 23(2):182–190, 2005.
52. Schmidt BL et al: Mechanism of cancer pain, *Mol Interv* 10(3):164–178, 2010.
53. Portenoy RK: Treatment of cancer pain, *Lancet* 377(9784):2236–2247, 2011.
54. Baron R, Binder A, Wasner G: Neuropathic pain: diagnosis, pathophysiological mechanisms, and treatment, *Lancet Neurol* 9(8):807–819, 2010.
55. Vranken JH: Elucidation of pathophysiology and treatment of neuropathic pain, *Cent Nerv Syst Agents Med Chem* 12(4):304–314, 2012.
56. Vinik A: The approach to the management of the patient with neuropathic pain, *J Clin Endocrinol Metab* 95(11):4802–4811, 2010.
57. De Ridder D et al: Somatosensory cortex stimulation for deafferentation pain, *Acta Neurochir Suppl* 297(Pt 2):67–74, 2007.
58. Giummarra MJ, Moseley GL: Phantom limb pain and bodily awareness: current concepts and future directions, *Curr Opin Anaesthesiol* 24(5):524–531, 2011.
59. Raslan AM et al: Motor cortex stimulation for trigeminal neuropathic or deafferentation pain: an institutional case series experience, *Stereotact Funct Neurosurg* 89(2):83–88, 2011.
60. Giummarra MJ, Moseley GL: Phantom limb pain and bodily awareness: current concepts and future directions, *Curr Opin Anaesthesiol* 24(5):524–531, 2011.
61. Mercier C, Léonard G: Interactions between pain and the motor cortex: insights from research on phantom limb pain and complex regional pain syndrome, *Physiother Can* 63(3):305–314, 2011.
62. Flor H: Maladaptive plasticity, memory for pain and phantom limb pain: review and suggestions for new therapies, *Exp Rev Neurother* 8(5):809–818, 2008.
63. Giummarra MJ et al: The menacing phantom: what pulls the trigger? *Eur J Pain* 15(7):691, 2011.
64. Marinus J et al: Clinical features and pathophysiology of complex regional pain syndrome, *Lancet Neurol* 10(7):637–648, 2011.
65. Lee J, Nandi P: Early aggressive treatment improves prognosis in complex regional pain syndrome, *Practitioner* 255(1736):3, 23–26, 2011.
66. Tunks ER, Crook J, Weir R: Epidemiology of chronic pain with psychological comorbidity: prevalence, risk, course, and prognosis, *Can J Psychiatry* 53(4):224–234, 2008.
67. Derbyshire SW: Fetal pain: do we know enough to do the right thing? *Reprod Health Matters* 16(Suppl 31):117–126, 2008.
68. Lowery CL et al: Neurodevelopmental changes of fetal pain, *Semin Perinatol* 31(5):275–282, 2007.
69. Hays SR, Deshpande JK: Newly postulated neurodevelopmental risks of pediatric anesthesia, *Curr Neurol Neurosci Rep* 11(2):205–210, 2011.
70. Bellieni CV, Bounocore G: Is fetal pain a real evidence? *J Matern Fetal Neonatal Med* 25(8):1203–1208, 2012.
71. Van de Velde M et al: Fetal pain perception and pain management, *Semin Fetal Neonatal Med* 11(4):232–236, 2006.
72. Raeside L: Physiological measures of assessing infant pain: a literature review, *Br J Nurs* 20(21):1370–1376, 2011.
73. Drendel AL, Kelly BT, Ali S: Pain assessment for children: overcoming challenges and optimizing care, *Pediatr Emerg Care* 27(8):773–781, 2011.
74. Bellieni CV: Pain assessment in human fetus and infants, *AAPS J* 14(3):456–461, 2012.
75. Pillai Riddell R et al: Nonpharmacological management of procedural pain in infants and young children: an abridged Cochrane review, *Pain Res Manag* 16(5):321–330, 2011.
76. Yezierski RP: The effects of age on pain sensitivity: preclinical studies, *Pain Med* 13(Suppl 2):S27–S36, 2012.
77. Gagliese L et al: Age-related patterns in adaptation to cancer pain: a mixed-method study, *Pain Med* 10(6):1050–1061, 2009.
78. Gibson SJ, Farrell M: A review of age differences in the neurophysiology of nociception and the perceptual experience of pain, *Clin J Pain* 20(4):227–239, 2004.
79. Defrin R, Eli I, Pud D: Interactions among sex, ethnicity, religion, and gender role expectations of pain, *Gend Med* 8(3):172–183, 2011.
80. Palmeira CC, Ashmawi HA, Posso Ide P: Sex and pain perception and analgesia, *Rev Bras Anesesiol* 61(6):814–828, 2011.
81. Chai E, Horton JR: Managing pain in the elderly population: pearls and pitfalls, *Curr Pain Headache Rep* 14(6):409–417, 2010.
82. Dinarello CA, Wolff SM: Pathogenesis of fever in man, *N Engl J Med* 298(11):607–612, 1978.
83. Nakamura K: Central circuitries for body temperature regulation and fever, *Am J Physiol Regul Integr Comp Physiol* 301(5):R1207–R1228, 2011.
84. Morrison SF, Nakamura K: Central neural pathways for thermoregulation, *Front Biosci* 16:74–104, 2011.

85. Pitoni S, Sinclair HL, Andrews PJ: Aspects of thermoregulation physiology, *Curr Opin Crit Care* 17(2):115–121, 2011.
86. Cinti S: Between brown and white: novel aspects of adipocyte differentiation, *Ann Med* 43(2):104–115, 2011.
87. Yousef MK: Effects of climatic stresses on thermoregulatory processes in man, *Experientia* 43(1):14–19, 1987.
88. Rintamaki H: Human responses to cold, *Alaska Med* 49(Suppl 2):29–31, 2007.
89. Lyon AJ, Freer Y: Goals and options in keeping preterm babies warm, *Arch Dis Child Fetal Neonatal Ed* 96(1):F71–F74, 2011.
90. Falk B, Dotan R: Temperature regulation and elite young athletes, *Med Sport Sci* 56:126–149, 2011.
91. Gao Z et al: Altered coronary vascular control during cold stress in healthy older adults, *Am J Physiol Heart Circ Physiol* 302(1):H312–H318, 2012.
92. Hansen A et al: Older persons and heat-susceptibility: the role of health promotion in a changing climate, *Health Promot J Austr* 22:S17–S20, 2011.
93. Blatteis CM: Age-dependent changes in temperature regulation—a mini review, *Gerontology* 58(4):289–295, 2012.
94. Kingma BR et al: Increased systolic blood pressure after mild cold and rewarming: relation to cold-induced thermogenesis and age, *Acta Physiol (Oxford)* 203(4):419–427, 2011.
95. Ogoina D: Fever, fever patterns and diseases called 'fever'—a review, *J Infect Public Health* 4(3):108–124, 2011.
96. Launey Y et al: Clinical review: fever in septic ICU patients—friend or foe? *Crit Care* 15(3):222, 2011.
97. Hopkins SJ: Central nervous system recognition of peripheral inflammation: a neural, hormonal collaboration, *Acta Biomed* 78(Suppl 1): 231–247, 2007.
98. Luheshi G, Rothwell N: Cytokines and fever, *Int Arch Allergy Immunol* 109(4):301–307, 1996.
99. Bartfai T, Conti B: Fever, *Scientific World Journal* 10:490–503, 2010.
100. Carey JV: Literature review: should antipyretic therapies routinely be administered to patients with [corrected] fever? *J Clin Nurs* 19: 2377–2393, 2010.
101. Matheï C et al: Infections in residents of nursing homes, *Infect Dis Clin North Am* 21(3):761–772, 2007.
102. Nakayama J, Arinami T: Molecular genetics of febrile seizures, *Epilepsy Res* 70(Suppl 1):S190–S198, 2006.
103. Gordon KE et al: Is temperature regulation different in children susceptible to febrile seizures? *Can J Neurol Sci* 36(2):192–195, 2009.
104. Cross JH: Fever and fever-related epilepsies, *Epilepsia* 53(Suppl 4):3–8, 2012.
105. Graves RC, Oehler K, Tingle LE: Febrile seizures: risks, evaluation, and prognosis, *Am Fam Physician* 85(2):149–153, 2012.
106. Hayakawa K, Ramasamy B, Chandrasekar PH: Fever of unknown origin: an evidence-based review, *Am J Med Sci* 344(4):307–316, 2012.
107. Habash RW et al: Principles, applications, risks and benefits of therapeutic hyperthermia, *Front Biosci (Elite Ed)* 3:1169–1181, 2011.
108. Becker JA, Stewart LK: Heat-related illness, *Am Fam Physician* 83(11):1325–1330, 2011.
109. Hashim IA: Clinical biochemistry of hyperthermia, *Ann Clin Biochem* 47(Pt 6):516–523, 2010.
110. Leon LR, Helwig BG: Heat stroke: role of the systemic inflammatory response, *J Appl Physiol* 109(6):1980–1988, 2010.
111. Lehmann-Horn F, Klingler W, Jurkat-Rott K: Nonanesthetic malignant hyperthermia, *Anesthesiology* 115(5):915–917, 2011.
112. Bandschapp O, Girard T: Malignant hyperthermia, *Swiss Med Wkly* 142:w13652, 2012.
113. Lantry J, Dezman Z, Hirshon JM: Pathophysiology, management and complications of hypothermia, *Br J Hosp Med (Lond)* 73(1):31–37, 2012.
114. Polderman KH: Mechanisms of action, physiological effects, and complications of hypothermia, *Crit Care Med* 37(Suppl 7):S186–S202, 2009.
115. Jurkovich GJ: Environmental cold-induced injury, *Surg Clin North Am* 87(1):247–267, 2007.
116. Ireland S et al: The incidence and significance of accidental hypothermia in major trauma—a prospective observational study, *Resuscitation* 82(3):300–306, 2011.
117. Lampe JW, Becker LB: State of the art in therapeutic hypothermia, *Annu Rev Med* 62:79–93, 2011.
118. Delhaye C, Mahmoudi M, Waksman R: Hypothermia therapy: neurological and cardiac benefits, *J Am Coll Cardiol* 59(3):197–210, 2012.
119. Gancia P, Pomero G: Brain cooling and eligible newborns: should we extend the indications? *J Matern Fetal Neonatal Med* 24(Suppl 1):53–55, 2011.
120. Agrawal A, Timothy J, Thapa A: Neurogenic fever, *Singapore Med J* 48(6):492–494, 2007.
121. Block J et al: Evidence-based thermoregulation for adult trauma patients, *Crit Care Nurs Q* 35(1):50–63, 2012.
122. Moola S, Lockwood C: Effectiveness of strategies for the management and/or prevention of hypothermia within the adult perioperative environment, *Int J Evid Based Healthc* 9(4):337–345, 2011.
123. Albrecht U: Timing to perfection: the biology of central and peripheral circadian clocks, *Neuron* 74(2):246–260, 2012.
124. Chokroverty S: Overview of sleep & sleep disorders, *Indian J Med Res* 131:126–140, 2010.
125. Iber C et al: *The AASM manual for the scoring of sleep and associated events*, Westchester, IL, 2007, American Academy of Sleep Medicine.
126. Schäffer T: Respiratory physiology in sleep and wakefulness, *Handb Clin Neurol* 98:371–381, 2011.
127. Brown RE et al: Control of sleep and wakefulness, *Physiol Rev* 92(3):1087–1187, 2012.
128. Monti JM: The role of dorsal raphe nucleus serotonergic and non-serotonergic neurons, and of their receptors, in regulating waking and rapid eye movement (REM) sleep, *Sleep Med Rev* 14(5):319–327, 2010.
129. Tsujino N, Sakurai T: Orexin/hypocretin: a neuropeptide at the interface of sleep, energy homeostasis, and reward system, *Pharmacol Rev* 61(2):162–176, 2009.
130. Murillo-Rodriguez E et al: Basic sleep mechanisms: an integrative review, *Cent Nerv Syst Agents Med Chem* 12(1):38–54, 2012.
131. Steiger A: Neurochemical regulation of sleep, *J Psychiatr Res* 41(7): 537–552, 2007.
132. Pace-Schott EF, Spencer RM: Age-related changes in the cognitive function of sleep, *Prog Brain Res* 191:75–89, 2011.
133. Rial RV et al: Evolution of wakefulness, sleep and hibernation: from reptiles to mammals, *Neurosci Biobehav Res* 34(8):1144–1160, 2010.
134. Meltzer LJ, Mindell JA: Sleep and sleep disorders in children and adolescents, *Psychiatr Clin North Am* 29(4):1059–1076, 2006.
135. Danker-Hopfe H: Growth and development of children with a special focus on sleep, *Prog Biophys Mol Biol* 107(3):333–338, 2011.
136. Leo G: Parasomnias, *World Med J* 102(1):32–35, 2003.
137. Byars KC et al: Prevalence, patterns, and persistence of sleep problems in the first 3 years of life, *Pediatrics* 129(2):e276–e284, 2012.
138. Lazaratou H, Soldatou A, Dikeos D: Medical comorbidity of sleep disorders in children and adolescents, *Curr Opin Psychiatry* 25(5):391–397, 2012.
139. Neikrug AB, Ancoli-Israel S: Sleep disorders in the older adult—a minireview, *Gerontology* 56(2):181–189, 2010.
140. Roepke SK, Ancoli-Israel S: Sleep disorders in the elderly, *Indian J Med Res* 131:302–310, 2010.
141. Wolfson AR, Carskadon MA: Sleep schedules and daytime functioning in adolescents, *Child Dev* 69(4):875–887, 1998.
142. Wolfson AR, Carskadon MA: Understanding adolescents' sleep patterns and school performance: a critical appraisal, *Sleep Med Rev* 7(6): 491–506, 2003.
143. Belenky G et al: Patterns of performance degradation and restoration during sleep restriction and subsequent recovery: a sleep dose-response study, *J Sleep Res* 12(1):1–12, 2003.
144. Czeisler CA: Impact of sleepiness and sleep deficiency on public health—utility of biomarkers, *J Clin Sleep Med* 7(Suppl 5):S6–S8, 2011.
145. Howard SK et al: Simulation study of rested versus sleep-deprived anesthesiologists, *Anesthesiology* 98(6):1345–1355, 2003.
146. Sallinen M et al: The effects of sleep debt and monotonous work on sleepiness and performance during a 12-h dayshift, *J Sleep Res* 13(4):285–294, 2004.
147. American Academy of Sleep Medicine: *Diagnostic Classification Steering Committee: International classification of sleep disorders, revised: diagnostic and coding manual*, Westchester, IL, 2005, Author.
148. Mong JA et al: Sleep, rhythms, and the endocrine brain: influence of sex and gonadal hormones, *J Neurosci* 31(45):16107–16116, 2011.
149. Buysse DJ: Insomnia, *JAMA* 309(7):706–716, 2013.
150. Neubauer DN, Flaherty KN: Chronic insomnia, *Semin Neurol* 29(4):340–353, 2009.
151. Punjabi NM: The epidemiology of adult obstructive sleep apnea, *Proc Am Thorac Soc* 5:136–143, 2008.
152. Sieck GC: Highlighted topics series: physiological and genomic consequences of intermittent hypoxia, *J Appl Physiol* 90:1187–1188, 2001.
153. Lurie A: Obstructive sleep apnea in adults: epidemiology, clinical presentation, and treatment options, *Adv Cardiol* 46:1–42, 2011.

154. Cherniack EP, Cherniack NS: Obstructive sleep apnea, metabolic syndrome, and age: will geriatricians be caught asleep on the job? *Aging Clin Exp Res* 22(1):1–7, 2010.
155. Edwards BA et al: Aging and sleep: physiology and pathophysiology, *Semin Respir Crit Care Med* 31(5):618–633, 2010.
156. Caufriez A et al: Progesterone prevents sleep disturbances and modulates GH, TSH, and melatonin secretion in postmenopausal women, *J Clin Endocrinol Metab* 96(4):E614–E623, 2011.
157. Isono S: Obesity and obstructive sleep apnoea: mechanisms for increased collapsibility of the passive pharyngeal airway, *Respirology* 17(1):32–42, 2012.
158. Carpagnano GE et al: The role of obstructive sleep apnea syndrome and obesity in determining leptin in the exhaled breath condensate, *J Breath Res* 4(3):036003, 2010.
159. Lurie A: Cardiovascular disorders associated with obstructive sleep apnea, *Adv Cardiol* 46:197–266, 2011.
160. Fava C et al: Obstructive sleep apnea syndrome and cardiovascular diseases, *Semin Thromb Hemost* 37(3):280–297, 2011.
161. Baguet JP et al: Mechanisms of cardiac dysfunction in obstructive sleep apnea, *Nat Rev Cardiol* 9(12):679–688, 2012.
162. Park JG, Ramar K, Olson EJ: Updates on definition, consequences, and management of obstructive sleep apnea, *Mayo Clin Proc* 86(6):549–554, 2011.
163. Butt M et al: Obstructive sleep apnea and cardiovascular disease, *Int J Cardiol* 139(1):7–16, 2010.
164. Marrone O et al: Blood pressure changes after automatic and fixed CPAP in obstructive sleep apnea: relationship with nocturnal sympathetic activity, *Clin Exp Hypertens* 33(6):373–380, 2011.
165. Natarajan R: Review of periodic limb movement and restless leg syndrome, *J Postgrad Med* 56(2):157–162, 2010.
166. Rye DB, Trotti LM: Restless legs syndrome and periodic leg movements of sleep, *Neurol Clin* 30(4):1137–1166, 2012.
167. Akintomide GS, Rickards H: Narcolepsy: a review, *Neuropsychiatr Dis Treat* 7:507–518, 2011.
168. Arendt J: Shift work: coping with the biological clock, *Occup Med (Lond)* 60(1):10–20, 2010.
169. Chou YH et al: An fMRI study of abrupt-awake episodes during behavioral microsleeps, *Conf Proc IEEE Eng Med Biol Soc* 2011:5060–5063, 2011.
170. Poudel GR et al: The relationship between behavioural microsleeps, visuomotor performance and EEG theta, *Conf Proc IEEE Eng Med Biol Soc* 2010:4452–4455, 2010.
171. Bittencourt LR et al: Chronobiological disorders: current and prevalent conditions, *J Occup Rehabil* 20(1):21–32, 2010.
172. Forbes-Robertson S et al: Circadian disruption and remedial interventions: effects and interventions for jet lag for athletic peak performance, *Sports Med* 42(3):185–208, 2012.
173. Killgore WD: Effects of sleep deprivation on cognition, *Prog Brain Res* 185:105–129, 2010.
174. Waters F, Bucks RS: Neuropsychological effects of sleep loss: implication for neuropsychologists, *Int Neuropsychol Soc* 17:571–586, 2011.
175. España RA, Scammell TE: Sleep neurobiology from a clinical perspective, *Sleep* 34(7):845–858, 2011.
176. Provini F et al: Arousal disorders, *Sleep Med* 12(Suppl 2):S22–S26, 2011.
177. Vetrugno R, Montagna P: Sleep-to-wake transition movement disorders, *Sleep Med* 12(Suppl 2):S11–S16, 2011.
178. Boeve BF: REM sleep behavior disorder: Updated review of the core features, the REM sleep behavior disorder-neurodegenerative disease association, evolving concepts, controversies, and future directions, *Ann N Y Acad Sci* 1184:15–54, 2010.
179. Edge LC: The role of emotional brain processing during sleep in depression, *J Psychiatr Ment Health Nurs* 17(10):857–861, 2010.
180. Greenberg H, Cohen RI: Nocturnal asthma, *Curr Opin Pulm Med* 18(1):57–62, 2012.
181. Schiza SE et al: Sleep patterns in patients with acute coronary syndromes, *Sleep Med* 11(2):149–153, 2010.
182. Schiza SE et al: Sleep disordered breathing in patients with acute coronary syndromes, *J Clin Sleep Med* 8(1):21–26, 2012.
183. Kent BD, Mitchell PD, McNicholas WT: Hypoxemia in patients with COPD: cause, effects, and disease progression, *Int J Chron Obstruct Pulmon Dis* 6:199–208, 2011.
184. Owens RL, Malhotra A: Sleep-disordered breathing and COPD: the overlap syndrome, *Respir Care* 55(10):1333–1344, 2010.
185. Besne I, Descombes C, Breton L: Effect of age and anatomical site on density of sensory innervation in human epidermis, *Arch Dermatol* 138(11):1445–1450, 2002.
186. Kalisch T, Tegenthoff M, Dinse HR: Repetitive electric stimulation elicits enduring improvement of sensorimotor performance in seniors, *Neural Plast* 2010:690531, 2010.
187. Shaffer SW, Harrison AL: Aging of the somatosensory system: a translational perspective, *Phys Ther* 87(2):193–207, 2007.
188. Barin K, Dodson EE: Dizziness in the elderly, *Otolaryngol Clin North Am* 44(2):437–454, x, 2011.
189. Post RE, Dickerson LM: Dizziness: a diagnostic approach, *Am Fam Physician* 82(4):361–369, 2010.
190. Semaan MT, Megerian CA: Ménière's disease: a challenging and relentless disorder, *Otolaryngol Clin North Am* 44(2):383–403, ix, 2011.
191. Bernardes TF, Bonfioli AA: Blepharitis, *Semin Ophthalmol* 25(3):79–83, 2010.
192. Lindsley K, Nichols JJ, Dickersin K: Interventions for acute internal hordeolum, *Cochrane Database Syst Rev*(9):CD007742, 2010.
193. Cronau H, Kankanala RR, Mauger T: Diagnosis and management of red eye in primary care, *Am Fam Physician* 81(2):137–144, 2010.
194. Baneke A: Review: Targeting trachoma: Strategies to reduce the leading infectious cause of blindness, *Travel Med Infect Dis* 10(2):92–96, 2012.
195. Dargin JM: The painful eye, *Emerg Med Clin North Am* 26(1):199–216, viii, 2008.
196. Owsley C: Aging and vision, *Vision Res* 51(13):1610–1622, 2011.
197. Pelak VS: Ocular motility of aging and dementia, *Curr Neurol Neurosci Rep* 10(6):440–447, 2010.
198. Doshi NR, Rodriquez ML: Amblyopia, *Am Fam Physician* 74(3):361–367, 2007.
199. Kushner BJ: The efficacy of strabismus surgery in adults: a review for primary care physicians, *Postgrad Med J* 87(1026):269–273, 2011.
200. Thurtell MJ, Leigh RJ: Nystagmus and saccadic intrusions, *Handb Clin Neurol* 102:333–378, 2011.
201. Stewart CE, Moseley MJ, Fielder AR: Amblyopia therapy: an update, *Strabismus* 19(3):91–98, 2011.
202. Brass SD, Zivadinov R, Bakshi R: Acute demyelinating optic neuritis: a review, *Front Biosci* 13:2376–2390, 2008.
203. Pershing S, Kumar A: Phacoemulsification versus extracapsular cataract extraction: where do we stand? *Curr Opin Ophthalmol* 22(1):37–42, 2011.
204. Jackson RG, Owsley C, McGwin G Jr: Aging and dark adaptation, *Vision Res* 39(23):3975–3982, 1999.
205. Rao KN, Nagireddy S, Chakrabarti S: Complex genetic mechanisms in glaucoma: an overview, *Indian J Ophthalmol* 59(Suppl):S31–S42, 2011.
206. Pan Y, Varma R: Natural history of glaucoma, *Indian J Ophthalmol* 59(Suppl):S19–S23, 2011.
207. Bagnis A et al: Current and emerging medical therapies in the treatment of glaucoma, *Expert Opin Emerg Drugs* 16(2):293–307, 2011.
208. Schaal S et al: Primary retinal detachment repair: comparison of 1-year outcomes of four surgical techniques, *Retina* 31(8):1500–1504, 2011.
209. Chakravarthy U et al: Clinical risk factors for age-related macular degeneration: a systematic review and meta-analysis, *BMC Ophthalmol* 10:31, 2010.
210. Deangelis MM et al: Genetics of age-related macular degeneration: current concepts, future directions, *Semin Ophthalmol* 26(3):77–93, 2011.
211. Lichtinger A, Rootman DS: Intraocular lenses for presbyopia correction: past, present, and future, *Curr Opin Ophthalmol* 23(1):40–46, 2012.
212. Neitz J, Neitz M: The genetics of normal and defective color vision, *Vision Res* 51(7):633–651, 2011.
213. Simunovic MP: Colour vision deficiency, *Eye (Lond)* 24(5):747–755, 2010.
214. Aerts I et al: Retinoblastoma, *Orphanet J Rare Dis* 1:31, 2006.
215. American Cancer Society: *What are the key statistics about retinoblastoma?* Last revised August 16, 2012. Available at www.cancer.org/Cancer/Retinoblastoma/DetailedGuide/retinoblastoma-key-statistics.
216. Saxena P, Kaur J: Differential expression of genes in retinoblastoma, *Clin Chim Acta* 412(23-24):2015–2021, 2011.
261a. Reis AH, Vargas FR, Lemos B: More epigenetic hits than meets the eye: microRNAs and genes associated with the tumorigenesis of retinoblastoma, *Front Genet* 3:284, 2012.
217. Ali MJ et al: Orbital retinoblastoma: where do we go from here? *J Cancer Res Ther* 7(1):11–14, 2011.
218. Huang Q, Tang J: Age-related hearing loss or presbycusis, *Eur Arch Otorhinolaryngol* 267(8):1179–1191, 2010.
219. Humes LE et al: Measures of hearing threshold and temporal processing across the adult lifespan, *Hear Res* 264(1-2):30–40, 2010.
220. Monasta L et al: Burden of disease caused by otitis media: systematic review and global estimates, *PLoS One* 7(4):e36226, 2012.
221. Narayan S, Swift A: Otitis externa: a clinical review, *Br J Hosp Med (Lond)* 72(10):554–558, 2011.

222. Pettigrew MM et al: Viral-bacterial interactions and risk of acute otitis media complicating upper respiratory tract infection, *J Clin Microbiol* 49(11):3750–3755, 2011.
223. Lous J, Ryborg CT, Thomsen JL: A systematic review of the effect of tympanostomy tubes in children with recurrent acute otitis media, *Int J Pediatr Otorhinolaryngol* 75(9):1058–1061, 2011.
224. Yoon TH et al: Tympanoplasty, with or without mastoidectomy, is highly effective for treatment of chronic otitis media in children, *Acta Otolaryngol Suppl*(558):44–48, 2007.
225. Banga R et al: Bone-anchored hearing aids versus conventional hearing aids, *Adv Otorhinolaryngol* 71:132–139, 2011.
226. Gaines AD: Anosmia and hyposmia, *Allergy Asthma Proc* 31(3):185–189, 2010.
227. Nguyen AD, Shenton ME, Levitt JJ: Olfactory dysfunction in schizophrenia: a review of neuroanatomy and psychophysiological measurements, *Harv Rev Psychiatry* 18(5):279–292, 2010.
228. Behrens M, Meyerhof W: Gustatory and extragustatory functions of mammalian taste receptors, *Physiol Behav* 105(1):4–13, 2011.
229. Robinett KS et al: Agonist-promoted homologous desensitization of human airway smooth muscle bitter taste receptors, *Am J Respir Cell Mol Biol* 45(5):1069–1074, 2011.
230. Pinto JM: Olfaction, *Proc Am Thorac Soc* 8(1):46–52, 2011.
231. Boyce JM, Shone GR: Effects of ageing on smell and taste, *Postgrad Med J* 82(966):239–241, 2006.
231a. Methven L et al: Ageing and taste, *Proc Nutr Soc* 71(4):556–565, 2012.

CHAPTER

17

Alterations in Cognitive Systems, Cerebral Hemodynamics, and Motor Function

Barbara J. Boss and Sue E. Huether

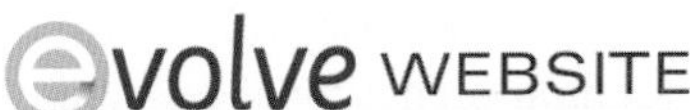

WEBSITE

http://evolve.elsevier.com/McCance/

- Review Questions and Answers
- Animations

CHAPTER OUTLINE

A person achieves functional adequacy (competence) through complex integrated processes. Three major neural systems account for this functional adequacy: cognitive systems, sensory systems, and motor systems. Alterations in any or all of these affect functional adequacy. Alterations in cognitive and sensory systems and motor function are associated with many central and peripheral nervous system injuries and pathologies. The purpose of this chapter is to present the concepts and processes of these alterations as an approach to understanding the manifestation of neurologic dysfunction. Some specific diseases are also presented (i.e., Parkinson disease, Huntington disease, and amyotrophic lateral sclerosis) because they fit best here. The manifestations of these concepts and processes are integrated with specific central and peripheral nervous system disorders and are presented in Chapter 18. Alterations in sensory function are presented in Chapter 16.

The neural systems essential to cognitive function are: (1) attentional systems that provide arousal and maintenance of attention over time; (2) memory and language systems by which information is communicated; and (3) affective or emotive systems that mediate mood, emotion, and intention. These core systems are fundamental to the processes of abstract thinking and reasoning. The products of abstraction and reasoning are organized and made operational through the executive attentional networks. The normal functioning of these systems manifests through the motor system in a behavioral array viewed by others as being appropriate to human activity and successful living. Nervous system disorders can be acquired (i.e., from trauma, infection, or related to systemic disease) or have a genetic basis.

ALTERATIONS IN COGNITIVE SYSTEMS

Full **consciousness** is a state of awareness both of oneself and of the environment and appropriate responses to that environment. The fully conscious individual responds to external stimuli with a wide array of responses. Any decrease in this state of awareness and varied responses is thus a decrease in consciousness.

Consciousness has two distinct components: arousal (state of awakeness) and awareness (content of thought). **Arousal** is mediated by the reticular activating system, which regulates aspects of attention and information processing and maintains consciousness (see Figure 15-6). Cognitive cerebral functions require a functioning reticular activating system. **Awareness** encompasses all cognitive functions and is mediated by attentional systems, memory systems, language systems, and executive systems.

Alterations in Arousal

Alterations in level of arousal may be caused by structural, metabolic, or psychogenic (functional) disorders.

PATHOPHYSIOLOGY. **Structural alterations in arousal** are divided according to original location of the pathologic condition or lesion: supratentorial (above the tentorium cerebelli); infratentorial (subtentorial, below the tentorium cerebelli); subdural (below the dura mater [see Figure 17-17]); extracerebral (outside the brain tissue); and intracerebral (within the brain tissue). Structural alterations can be caused by infectious, vascular, neoplastic, traumatic, congenital (developmental), degenerative, genetic, and metabolic disorders.

Supratentorial disorders produce changes in arousal by either diffuse or localized dysfunction. Diffuse dysfunction may be caused by disease processes affecting the cerebral cortex or the underlying subcortical white matter (e.g., encephalitis). Disorders outside the brain but within the cranial vault (extracerebral) also can produce diffuse dysfunction, including neoplasms, closed-head trauma with subsequent bleeding, and subdural empyema (accumulation of pus). Localized dysfunction is generally caused by masses that directly impinge on diencephalic structures (i.e., thalamus and hypothalamus) or that secondarily compress these structures in the process of herniation. Disorders within the brain substance (intracerebral)—bleeding, infarcts, emboli, and tumors—function primarily as masses. Such localized destructive processes directly impair function of the thalamic or hypothalamic activating systems.

Infratentorial disorders produce a decline in arousal in one of two ways: (1) there may be a direct destruction of the reticular activating system (RAS) and its pathways, or (2) the brainstem may be destroyed either by direct invasion or by indirect impairment of its blood supply. The most common cause of direct destruction is cerebrovascular disease. Demyelinating diseases, neoplasms, granulomas, abscesses, and head injury also may cause brainstem destruction by tissue compression. This compression may occur because of (1) direct pressure on the pons and midbrain, producing ischemia and edema of the neurons of the RAS; (2) upward herniation of the cerebellum through the tentorial notch, thus compressing the upper midbrain and diencephalon; or (3) downward herniation of the cerebellum through the foramen magnum, compressing and displacing the medulla oblongata.

Metabolic alterations in arousal are caused by alterations in delivery of energy substrates (e.g., hypoxia, electrolyte disturbances, or hypoglycemia) or alterations in neuronal excitability caused by drugs and toxins (both exogenous and endogenous [e.g., liver or renal failure]). All the systemic diseases that eventually produce nervous system dysfunction are part of this metabolic category.

Psychogenic alterations in arousal (unresponsiveness), although uncommon, may signal general psychiatric disorders (see Chapter 19). Despite apparent unconsciousness, the person actually is physiologically awake and the neurologic examination reflects a normal response.

CLINICAL MANIFESTATIONS AND EVALUATION. Patterns of clinical manifestations assist in determining the extent of brain dysfunction and serve as indexes for identifying increasing or decreasing central nervous system (CNS) function. Distinctions are made between metabolic and structurally induced manifestations (Table 17-1). The types of manifestations suggest the

TABLE 17-1 CLINICAL MANIFESTATIONS OF METABOLIC AND STRUCTURAL CAUSES OF ALTERED AROUSAL

MANIFESTATION	METABOLICALLY INDUCED	STRUCTURALLY INDUCED
Blink to threat (cranial nerves II, VII)	Equal	Asymmetric
Discs (cranial nerve II)	Flat, good pulsation	Papilledema
Extraocular movement (cranial nerves III, IV, VI)	Roving eye movements; normal doll's eyes and calorics	Gaze paresis, nerve III palsy, medial longitudinal fasciculus (MLF) syndrome (internuclear ophthalmoplegia)
Pupils (cranial nerves II, III)	Equal and reactive; may be large (e.g., atropine), pinpoint (e.g., opiates), or midposition and fixed (e.g., glutethimide [Doriden])	Asymmetric and/or nonreactive; may be midposition (midbrain injury), pinpoint (pons injury), large (tectal injury)
Corneal reflex (cranial nerves V, VII)	Symmetric response	Asymmetric response
Grimace to pain (cranial nerve VII)	Symmetric response	Asymmetric response
Motor function movement	Symmetric	Asymmetric
Tone	Symmetric	Paratonic, spastic, flaccid, especially if asymmetric
Posture	Symmetric	Decorticate, especially if symmetric; decerebrate, especially if asymmetric
Deep tendon reflexes	Symmetric	Asymmetric
Babinski sign	Absent or symmetric response	Present
Sensation	Symmetric	Asymmetric

cause of the altered arousal state (Table 17-2). Five categories of neurologic function are critical to the evaluation process: (1) level of consciousness, (2) pattern of breathing, (3) pupillary changes, (4) oculomotor responses, and (5) motor responses.

Level of Consciousness

Level of consciousness is the most critical clinical index of nervous system function or dysfunction. Changes can indicate either improvement or deterioration of the individual's condition and state of awakeness. A person who is alert and oriented to self, others, place, and time is considered to be functioning at the highest level of consciousness, which implies full use of all the person's cognitive capacities. From this normal alert state, levels of consciousness diminish in stages from confusion to coma, each of which is clinically defined (Table 17-3).

Pattern of Breathing

Respiratory patterns help to evaluate level of brain dysfunction and level of coma. Rate, rhythm, and pattern of breathing should be assessed. The breathing patterns can be categorized as hemispheric or brainstem breathing patterns (Table 17-4 and Figure 17-1).

With normal breathing, a neural center in the forebrain (cerebrum) produces a rhythmic breathing pattern. When consciousness decreases, lower brainstem centers regulate the breathing pattern by responding only to changes in $Paco_2$ levels. This irregular breathing pattern is called **posthyperventilation apnea (PHVA).**

Cheyne-Stokes respiration is an abnormal rhythm of breathing (periodic breathing) with alternating periods of hyperventilation and apnea (crescendo-decrescendo pattern).

TABLE 17-2 DIFFERENTIAL CHARACTERISTICS OF DISORDERS CAUSING ALTERED AROUSAL

MECHANISM	MANIFESTATIONS
Supratentorial mass lesions compressing or displacing diencephalons or brainstem	Initiating signs usually of focal cerebral dysfunction Signs of dysfunction progress rostral to caudal Neurologic signs at any given time point to one anatomic area (e.g., diencephalon, mesencephalon, medulla) Motor signs often asymmetric
Infratentorial mass of destruction, causing coma	History of preceding brainstem dysfunction or sudden onset of coma Localizing brainstem signs precede or accompany onset of coma and always include oculovestibular abnormality Cranial nerve palsies; usually manifest "bizarre" respiratory patterns that appear at onset
Metabolic coma Exogenous toxins (drugs) Endogenous toxins (organ system failure)	Confusion and stupor commonly precede motor signs Motor signs usually are symmetric Pupillary reactions usually are preserved Asterixis, myoclonus, tremor, and seizures are common Acid-base imbalance with hyperventilation or hypoventilation is common
Psychiatric unresponsiveness	Lids close actively Pupils reactive or dilated (cycloplegics) Oculocephalic reflexes are unpredictable; oculovestibular reflexes are physiologic (nystagmus is present) Motor tone is inconsistent or normal Eupnea or hyperventilation is usual No pathologic reflexes are present Electroencephalogram (EEG) is normal

TABLE 17-3 LEVELS OF ALTERED CONSCIOUSNESS

STATE	DEFINITION
Confusion	Loss of ability to think rapidly and clearly; impaired judgment and decision making
Disorientation	Beginning loss of consciousness; disorientation to time followed by disorientation to place and impaired memory; lost last is recognition of self
Lethargy	Limited spontaneous movement or speech; easy arousal with normal speech or touch; may not be oriented to time, place, or person
Obtundation	Mild to moderate reduction in arousal (awakeness) with limited response to the environment; falls asleep unless stimulated verbally or tactilely; answers questions with minimum response
Stupor	A condition of deep sleep or unresponsiveness from which the person may be aroused or caused to open eyes only by vigorous and repeated stimulation; response is often withdrawal or grabbing at stimulus
Coma	No verbal response to the external environment or to any stimuli; noxious stimuli such as deep pain or suctioning yields motor movement
Light coma	Associated with purposeful movement on stimulation
Coma	Associated with nonpurposeful movement only on stimulation
Deep coma	Associated with unresponsiveness or no response to any stimulus

TABLE 17-4 PATTERNS OF BREATHING

BREATHING PATTERN	DESCRIPTION	LOCATION OF INJURY
Hemispheric Breathing Patterns		
Normal	After a period of hyperventilation that lowers the arterial carbon dioxide pressure ($Paco_2$), the individual continues to breathe regularly but with a reduced depth.	Response of the nervous system to an external stressor—not associated with injury to the CNS
Posthyperventilation apnea	Respirations stop after hyperventilation has lowered the Pco_2 level below normal. Rhythmic breathing returns when the Pco_2 level returns to normal. (Usually an intact cerebral cortex will trigger breathing within 10 seconds regardless of Pco_2.)	Associated with diffuse bilateral metabolic or structural disease of the cerebrum
Cheyne-Stokes respirations	Breathing pattern has a smooth increase (crescendo) in the rate and depth of breathing (hyperpnea), which peaks and is followed by a gradual smooth decrease (decrescendo) in the rate and depth of breathing to the point of apnea when the cycle repeats itself. The hyperpneic phase lasts longer than the apneic phase (represents an amplitude change).	Bilateral dysfunction of the deep cerebral or diencephalic structures; seen with supratentorial injury and metabolically induced coma states unrelated to neurologic dysfunction; may see also in CHF
Brainstem Breathing Patterns		
Central reflex hyperpnea (central neurogenic hyperventilation)	A sustained deep rapid but regular pattern (hyperpnea) occurs, with a decreased $Paco_2$ and a corresponding increase in pH and increased Po_2.	May result from CNS damage or disease that involves the lower midbrain and upper pons; seen after increased intracranial pressure and blunt head trauma
Apneusis	A prolonged inspiratory cramp (a pause at full inspiration) occurs. A common variant of this is a brief end-inspiratory pause of 2 or 3 seconds, often alternating with an end-expiratory pause.	Indicates damage to the respiratory control mechanism located at the pontine level; most commonly associated with pontine infarction but documented with hypoglycemia, anoxia, and meningitis
Cluster breathing	A cluster of breaths has a disordered sequence with irregular pauses between breaths.	Dysfunction in the lower pontine and high medullary areas
Ataxic breathing	Completely irregular breathing occurs, with random shallow and deep breaths and irregular pauses. Often the rate is slow.	Originates from a primary dysfunction of the lower pons or upper medulla
Gasping breathing pattern (agonal gasps)	A pattern of deep "all-or-none" breaths is accompanied by a slow respiratory rate.	Indicative of a failing medullary respiratory center

CHF, Congestive heart failure; *CNS,* central nervous system.

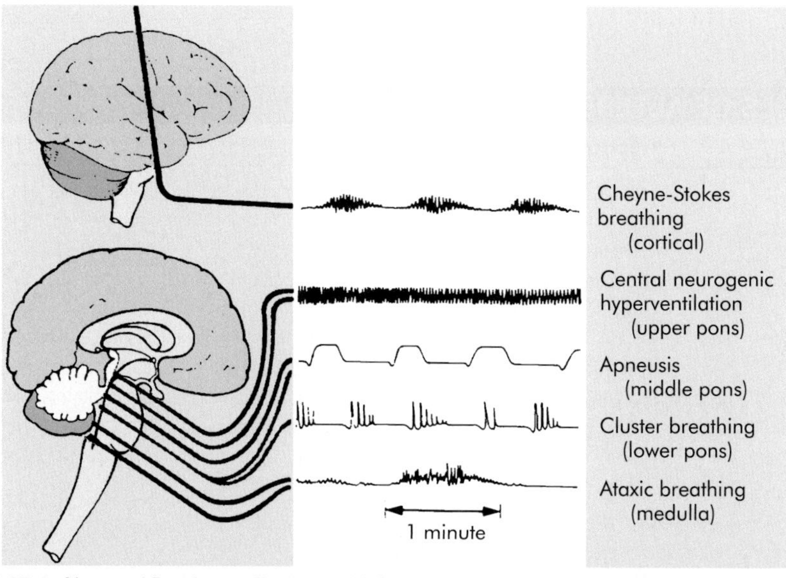

FIGURE 17-1 Abnormal Respiratory Patterns with Corresponding Level of Central Nervous System Activity.

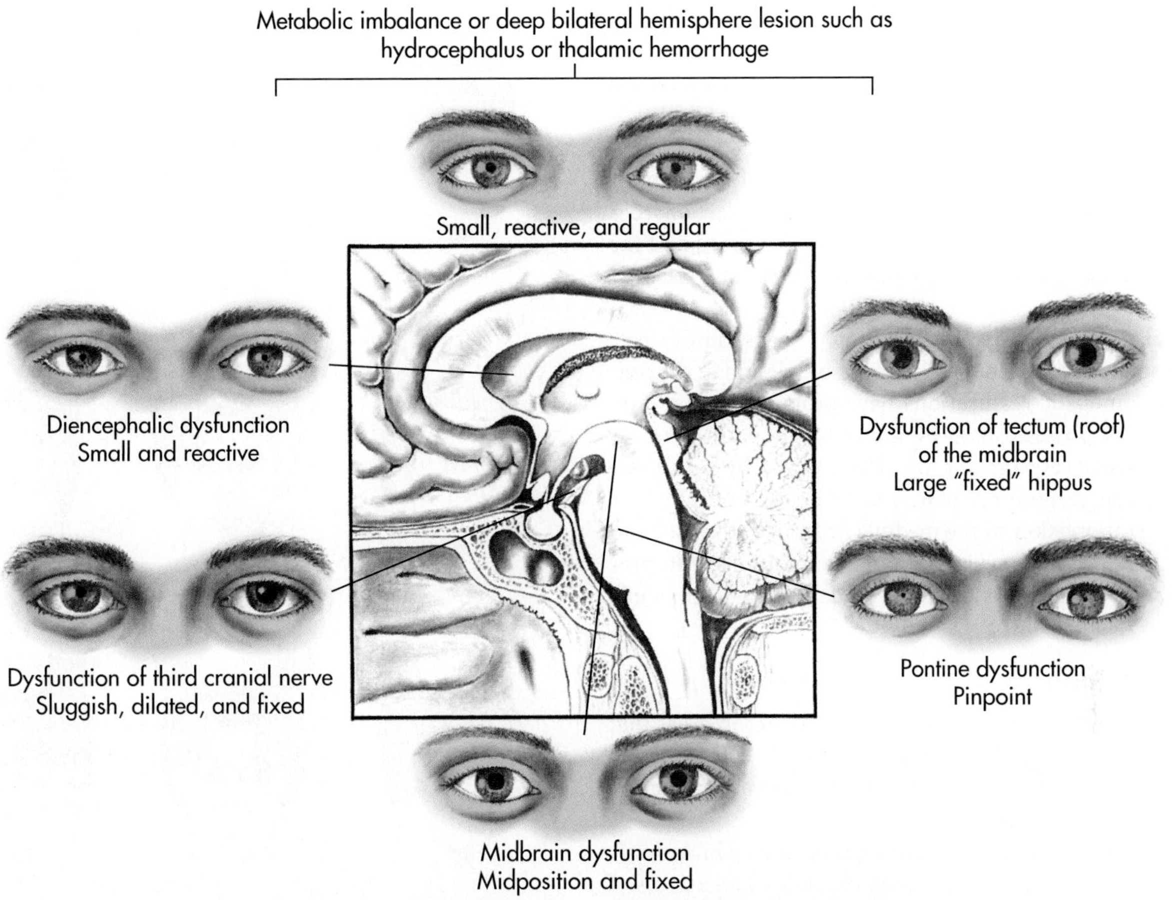

FIGURE 17-2 Appearance of Pupils at Different Levels of Consciousness.

TABLE 17-5 CHANGES IN OCULOMOTOR RESPONSES

STATE	RESTING AND SPONTANEOUS EYE MOVEMENTS	REFLEXIVE EYE MOVEMENTS
Full consciousness	Eyes at rest, still (cortical gaze centers inhibit spontaneous roving eye movements)	Eyes move as the head turns Oculocephalic responses not elicited or inconsistently elicited (frontal gaze centers inhibit brainstem reflexes that fix gaze straight ahead) Oculovestibular (caloric) stimulation produces nystagmus
Cortical dysfunction or disruption of efferent pathways	Conjugate, horizontal, roving eye movements may well be present (cortical gaze centers no longer inhibit these brainstem-generated roving eye movements)	Gaze fixed straight ahead regardless of head position—positive doll's eyes reaction (normal oculocephalic reflexes are no longer inhibited by frontal gaze centers)
Diffuse anoxic damage to cortex	"Ocular dipping"—slow, dysrhythmic downward movement followed by faster, upward movement	Nystagmus is no longer induced by caloric stimulation (normally a cold-water stimulus produces deviation of the eyes opposite the irrigated ear; a warm-water stimulus deviates the eyes to the same [ipsilateral] side) With an injury that depresses cortical gaze center function, the eyes (and often the entire head) deviate or appear to look toward the side of the injured hemisphere With an injury that irritates (stimulates) the neurons of the cortical gaze center, the eyes (and often the entire head) deviate away from the injured hemisphere (all fibers from the frontal gaze centers decussate and therefore control the function of the contralateral pontine gaze center, which moves the eyes in the ipsilateral direction)
Mesencephalon dysfunction	Roving eye movements cease and the eyes become immobile and directed ahead (roving eye movements require an intact brainstem) Eyes may turn down and inward	Oculovestibular reflexes become inconsistent and abnormal Loss of Bell phenomenon (upward deviation of eyes on stimulation) (requires intact eye movement pathways from the mesencephalon to pons)
Pontine dysfunction	Loss of spontaneous blinking (requires an intact pons) "Ocular bobbing"—brisk, conjugate, downward movement of eyes with loss of horizontal eye movements	

The pathophysiology of Cheyne-Stokes respiration involves a hyperventilatory response to carbon dioxide stimulation. In the damaged brain, higher levels of $Paco_2$ (hypercapnia) are required to stimulate ventilation, and the response is hyperventilation. As a result, the $Paco_2$ level decreases to below normal and breathing stops (PHVA) until carbon dioxide reaccumulates and stimulates hyperventilation. In cases of opiate or sedative drug overdose, the respiratory center is depressed and the rate of breathing gradually decreases until respiratory failure occurs.

Central neurogenic hyperventilation is a respiratory pattern of sustained hyperventilation caused by a lesion in the central pons. **Apneustic respirations** have prolonged inspiratory and expiratory phases caused by injury to the pons or upper medulla. **Cluster respirations** are characterized by periods or clusters of rapid respirations of near equal depth resulting from trauma or compression to the medulla or from chronic opioid abuse. **Ataxic respirations** are irregular respirations with prolonged periods of apnea associated with damage to the medulla (see Figure 17-1).

Pupillary Changes

Brainstem areas that control arousal are adjacent to areas that control the pupils. Pupillary changes thus are a valuable guide to evaluating the presence and level of brainstem dysfunction (Figure 17-2).

Some drugs affect pupils and must be considered in the evaluation of pupillary responses in comatose states. Large doses of atropine, scopolamine, amphetamines, mydriatics, and cycloplegics can fully dilate and fix pupils. Sedatives (e.g., glutethimide) in sufficient amounts to produce a coma cause the pupils to become midposition or moderately dilated (4 to 5 mm in diameter), unequal, and frequently fixed to light. Opiates (heroin and morphine) and barbiturates, as well as extensive pontine damage, cause pinhole pupils (1 mm). Severe barbiturate intoxication may produce fixed pupils.

Severe ischemia and hypoxia produce bilaterally wide (5 mm) and fixed pupils usually caused by severe midbrain damage. Occasionally the pupils remain small (1 to 2.5 mm) or midposition even in the presence of profound hypoxia. Hypothermia also may cause fixed pupils.

Oculomotor Responses

Resting, spontaneous, and reflexive eye movements and oculovestibular (caloric) reflexes change at various levels of brain dysfunction (Table 17-5). Persons with metabolically induced coma, except in cases of barbiturate-hypnotic and phenytoin (Dilantin) poisoning, generally retain ocular reflexes, however, even when other signs of brainstem damage, such as central neurogenic hyperventilation, are present.

The presence of brisk oculocephalic reflexes and roving eye movements, as well as the failure to elicit nystagmus with instillation of cold or warm water into the external ear canal, indicates a decrease in consciousness (loss of cortical influence) but an intact brainstem (Figures 17-3 and 17-4).

Destructive or compressive injury to the brainstem causes specific abnormalities of the oculocephalic and oculovestibular reflexes. For example, a skewed deviation, in which one eye diverges downward and the other looks upward, indicates brainstem dysfunction. Destructive or compressive disease processes that involve an oculomotor nucleus or nerve cause the involved eye to deviate outward, producing a resting dysconjugate lateral position of the eyes (each eye diverges laterally). Unilateral abducens paralysis (paralysis of cranial nerve VI) results in an upward deviation of the ipsilateral eye. With bilateral abducens paralysis, the eyes come together (converge). Reflexive eye movements may be suppressed by drugs, most commonly phenytoin, tricyclics, and barbiturates. Occasionally alcohol, phenothiazines, and diazepam may alter reflex eye movements.

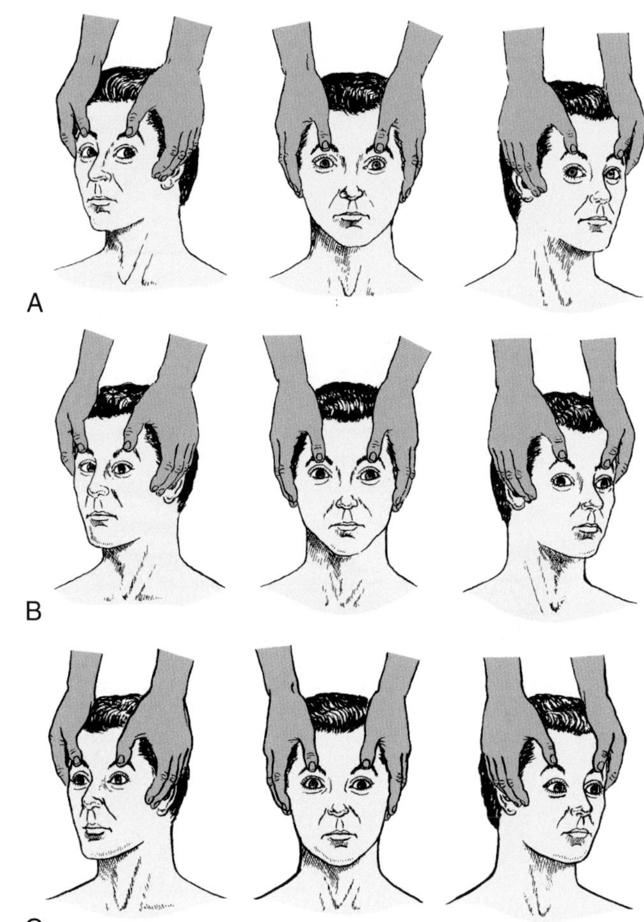

FIGURE 17-3 Test for Oculocephalic Reflex Response (Doll's Eyes Phenomenon). **A,** Normal response—eyes turn together to side opposite from turn of head. **B,** Abnormal response—eyes do not turn in conjugate manner. **C,** Absent response—eyes do not turn as head position changes. (**A** and **C** from Rudy EB: *Advanced neurological and neurosurgical nursing,* St Louis, 1984, Mosby.)

Motor Responses

Assessment of motor responses helps to evaluate the level of brain dysfunction and determine the side of the brain that is maximally damaged. The pattern of response noted may be (1) purposeful (a defensive or withdrawal movement of limbs to noxious stimuli); (2) inappropriate, or not purposeful (generalized motor movement, posturing, grimacing, or groaning); or (3) not present (unresponsive, no motor response).

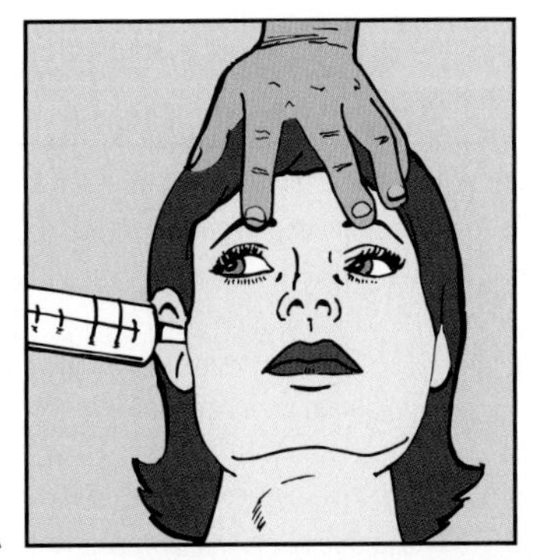

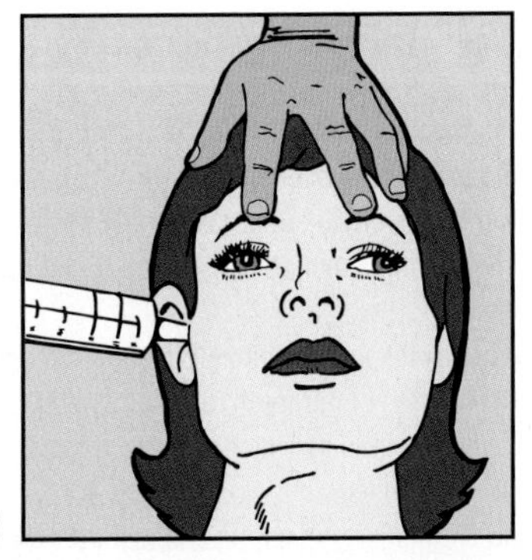

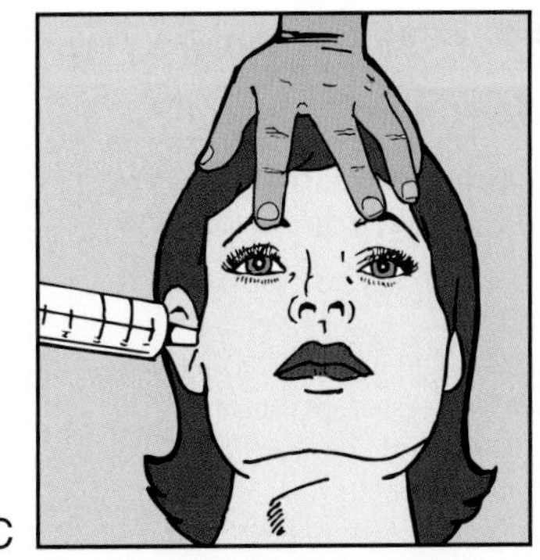

FIGURE 17-4 Test for Oculovestibular Reflex (Caloric Ice-Water Test). **A,** Normal response—conjugate eye movements. **B,** Abnormal response—dysconjugate or asymmetric eye movements. **C,** Absent response—no eye movements.

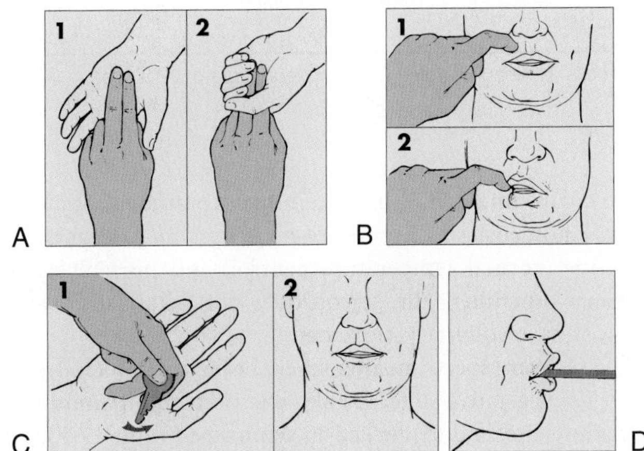

FIGURE 17-5 Pathologic Reflexes. **A,** Grasp reflex. **B,** Snout reflex. **C,** Palmomental reflex. **D,** Suck reflex.

Purposeful movement requires an intact corticospinal system. Nonpurposeful movement is evidence of severe dysfunction of the corticospinal system.

Motor signs indicating loss of cortical inhibition are commonly associated with decreased consciousness. These signs include contralateral or bilateral (depending on whether the process is localized or diffuse) reflex grasping, reflex sucking, snout reflex, palmomental reflex, and rigidity (paratonia) (Figure 17-5). Abnormal flexor and extensor responses, particularly in the upper extremities, are defined in Table 17-6 and illustrated in Figure 17-6.

Vomiting, yawning, and **hiccups** are complex reflex-like motor responses that are integrated by neural mechanisms in the lower brainstem. These responses may be produced by compression or diseases involving tissues of the medulla oblongata (e.g., infection, neoplasm, infarct, or other more benign stimuli to the vagal nerve). Most CNS disorders produce nausea and vomiting. Vomiting without nausea indicates direct involvement of the central neural mechanism (or pyloric obstruction). Vomiting often accompanies CNS injuries that (1) involve the vestibular nuclei or its immediate projections, particularly when double vision (diplopia) also is present; (2) impinge directly on the floor of the fourth ventricle; or (3) produce brainstem compression secondary to increased intracranial pressure.

Outcomes of Alterations in Arousal

Outcomes of alterations in arousal fall into two categories: *extent of disability (morbidity)* and *mortality*. Outcomes depend on the cause and extent of brain damage and the duration of coma. Some individuals may recover consciousness and an original level of function, some may have permanent disability, and some may never regain consciousness and experience neurologic death. Two forms of neurologic death—brain death and cerebral death—result from severe pathologic conditions and are associated with irreversible coma. Other possible outcomes include a vegetative state, a minimally conscious state, akinetic mutism, or locked-in syndrome. Extent of disability has four subcategories: recovery of consciousness, recovery of residual cognitive function, recovery of psychologic function, and recovery of vocational function.

Brain death (total brain death) occurs when irreversible brain damage is so extensive that the brain has no potential for recovery and no longer can maintain the body's internal homeostasis. State laws define brain death as irreversible cessation of function of the entire brain, including the brainstem and cerebellum. The brain is autolyzing (self-digesting) or already autolyzed on postmortem examination.

Clinical criteria for brain death include the absence of discernible evidence of cerebral hemisphere function or function of the brainstem's vital centers for an extended period. There is no detectable function above the level of the foramen magnum so there is whole brain death. In addition, the abnormality of brain function must result from structural or known metabolic disease and *not* be caused by a depressant drug, alcohol poisoning, neuromuscular blockage, or hypothermia. An isoelectric, or flat, electroencephalogram (EEG) (electrocerebral silence) for a period of 6 to 12 hours in a person who is not hypothermic and has not ingested depressant drugs indicates that no mental recovery is possible. This usually means that the brain is already dead. A task force to determine brain death in children recommended the same criteria as those used for adults[1] but with a longer observation period.

The following summary of medical criteria determines brain death[2-5]:

1. Completion of all appropriate and therapeutic procedures with no possibility of brain function recovery
2. Unresponsive coma (absence of motor and reflex movements)

TABLE 17-6 ABNORMAL MOTOR RESPONSES WITH DECREASED RESPONSIVENESS

MOTOR RESPONSE	DESCRIPTION OF MOTOR RESPONSES	LOCATION OF INJURY
Decorticate posturing/rigidity: upper extremity flexion, lower extremity extension (Figure 17-6)	Slowly developing flexion of the arm, wrist, and fingers with abduction in the upper extremity and extension, internal rotation, and plantar flexion of the lower extremity	Hemispheric damage above midbrain releasing medullary and pontine reticulospinal systems
Decerebrate posturing/rigidity: upper and lower extremity extensor responses (Figure 17-6)	Opisthotonos (hyperextension of the vertebral column) with clenching of the teeth; extension, abduction, and hyperpronation of the arms; and extension of the lower extremities	Associated with severe damage involving midbrain or upper pons
	In acute brain injury, shivering and hyperpnea may accompany unelicited recurrent decerebrate spasms	Acute brain injury may cause limb extension regardless of location
Extensor responses in the upper extremities accompanied by flexion in the lower extremities		Pons
Flaccid state with little or no motor response to stimuli		Lower pons and upper medulla

Data from Goetz CG: *Textbook of clinical neurology,* ed 3, Philadelphia, 2007, Saunders; Nadeau SE et al: *Medical neuroscience,* Philadelphia, 2004, Saunders.

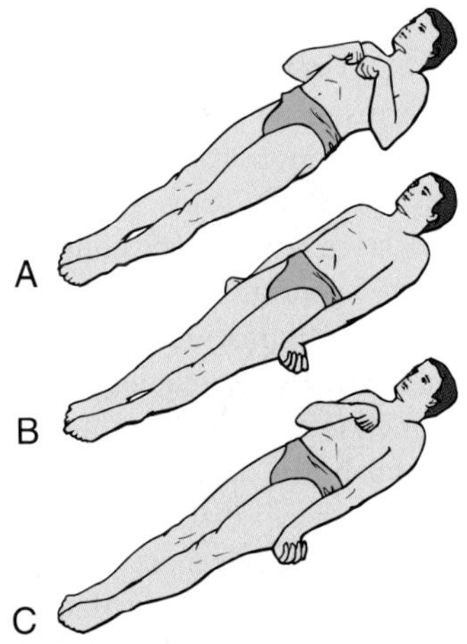

FIGURE 17-6 Decorticate and Decerebrate Responses. **A,** *Decorticate response (flexor posturing):* bilateral flexion of elbows and wrists with shoulder adduction in upper extremities. Extension, internal rotation of lower extremities. **B,** *Decerebrate response (extensor posturing):* all four extremities in rigid extension, internal rotation of shoulders with hyperpronation of forearms. **C,** *Decorticate response on right side of body and decerebrate response on left side of body:* the most pronounced response differences are in the upper body. (From Rudy EB: *Advanced neurological and neurosurgical nursing,* St Louis, 1984, Mosby.)

3. No spontaneous respiration (apnea)—a $Paco_2$ that rises above 60 mmHg without breathing efforts, providing evidence of a nonfunctioning respiratory center (apnea challenge)
4. No brainstem function (ocular responses to head turning or caloric stimulation; dilated, fixed pupils; no gag or corneal reflex)
5. Isoelectric (flat) EEG (electrocerebral silence)
6. Persistence of these signs for an appropriate observation period

Cerebral death or **irreversible coma** is death of the cerebral hemispheres exclusive of the brainstem and cerebellum. Brain damage is permanent and sufficiently severe that the individual is unable to ever respond behaviorally in any significant way to the environment. The brainstem may continue to maintain internal homeostasis (normal respiratory and cardiovascular functions, normal temperature control, and normal gastrointestinal function). The person does not follow commands, speak, or have voluntary movement.

The recovery spectrum after severe brain injury includes: (1) coma, (2) vegetative state, (3) akinetic mutism, (4) minimally conscious state, and (5) locked-in syndrome (Table 17-7). The survivor of cerebral death may remain in a coma or emerge into a vegetative state. In coma (a state of unarousable neurobehavioral unresponsiveness) the eyes are usually closed with no evidence of eye opening either spontaneously or in response to external stimuli. The person does not follow commands, does not verbalize or mouth words, and has no goal-directed or volitional behavior. There are no sustained visual pursuit movements beyond a 45-degree arc.

A **persistent vegetative state (VS)** is complete unawareness of the self or surrounding environment and complete loss of cognitive function. The Multi-Society Task Force on Persistent Vegetative States (MSTF) identified the diagnostic criteria for VS as: (1) periods of eye opening (spontaneous or following stimulation); (2) the potential for subcortical responses to external stimuli, including generalized physiologic responses to pain, such as posturing, tachycardia, and diaphoresis, and subcortical motor responses, such as grasp reflex; (3) return of so-called vegetative (autonomic) functions, including sleep-wake cycles and normalization of respiratory and digestive system functions; and (4) occasional roving eye movements without concomitant visual tracking ability.[6] The person's eyes open spontaneously or following stimulation, or both. There may be random hand, extremity, or head movements. The individual maintains blood pressure and breathing without support. Brainstem reflexes (pupillary, oculocephalic, chewing, swallowing) are intact. No discrete localizing motor responses are present, and the individual does not speak any comprehensible words or follow commands.[7]

TABLE 17-7 COMPARATIVE CLINICAL FEATURES OF ALTERATIONS IN LEVELS OF AROUSAL

DIAGNOSIS	AROUSAL	AWARENESS	COMMUNICATION
Coma	Eyes do not open spontaneously or in response to stimulation	No evidence of perception, communication ability, only reflexes and postural responses	None
Persistent vegetative state	Eyes open spontaneously; no visual tracking; sleep-wake cycle resumes or state of chronic wakefulness; arousal often sluggish	No evidence of cognitive function or purposeful motor activity	None
Akinetic mutism	Eyes open spontaneously; normal sleep-wake cycle; arousal level is normal	Visual tracking present; little or no following of commands	Little or no volitional speech or movement
Minimally conscious state	Eyes open spontaneously; normal to abnormal sleep-wake cycle; arousal level ranges from obtunded to normal	Inconsistent evidence of perception, communication ability, or purposeful motor activity; visual tracking often intact	Inconsistent verbalization, and gesturing
Locked-in syndrome	Full arousal; sleep-wake cycle present; quadriplegic	Perceptions and emotions intact	Cannot speak or move muscles except vertical eye movement and blinking

Data from Giacino JT et al: *Neurology* 58(3):349-353, 2002; Owen AM: *Ann N Y Acad Sci* 1125:225–238, 2008.

In a **minimally conscious state (MCS),** an individual demonstrates minimal but defined behavioral evidence of self or environmental awareness.[6,8] The clinical features include: (1) following simple commands, (2) manipulating objects, (3) responding with gestural or verbal "yes/no" responses, (4) demonstrating intelligible verbalization, and (5) blinking and smiling that occur in a meaningful relationship to the eliciting stimulus and are not attributable to reflexive activity.

Akinetic mutism (AM) is a neurobehavioral state characterized by a severe disturbance in behavioral drive (motivation). Generally, these individuals evidence eye opening with visual tracking and have little or no spontaneous speech or following of commands. Little movement is present. This is not attributable to decreased wakefulness or motor weakness or impairment. The pathology involves damage to the frontal lobe or cingulate gyrus (a component of the limbic system) (also see p. 538).[9]

With **locked-in syndrome** there is complete paralysis of voluntary muscles with the exception of eye movement. Content of thought and level of arousal are intact but the efferent pathways are disrupted (injury at the base of the pons with the reticular formation intact, often caused by basilar artery occlusion).[10] Thus the individual cannot communicate either through speech or through body movement but is fully conscious, with intact cognitive function. The upper cranial nerves (I through IV) often are preserved, so that the person possesses vertical eye movement and blinking as a means of communication.

Alterations in Awareness

Awareness (content of thought) encompasses all cognitive functions, including awareness of self, environment, and affective states (i.e., moods). Awareness is mediated by the core networks (selective attention and memory) under the guidance of executive attention networks (i.e., the networks that involve abstract reasoning, planning, decision making, judgment, error correction, and self-control). Each attentional function is not localized in a single brain area but is a network of interconnected brain circuits.

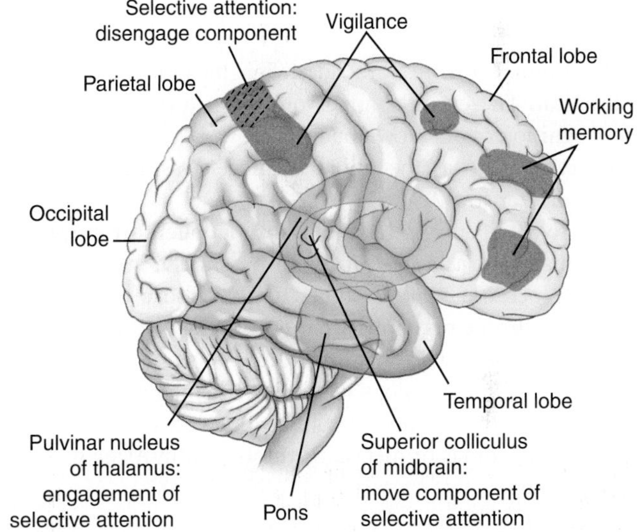

FIGURE 17-7 Right Cortical, Subcortical, and Brainstem Areas of the Brain-Mediating Cognitive Functions. (From Boss BJ, Wilkerson R: Communication: language and pragmatics. In Hoeman SP, editor: *Rehabilitation nursing: prevention, intervention, & outcomes,* ed 4, p 508, St Louis, 2008, Mosby.)

Selective attention (orienting) refers to the ability to select specific information to be processed from available, competing environmental and internal stimuli and to focus on those stimuli.[11] Frontal and parietal regions of the right hemisphere contribute to selective attention. The engage component is mediated by the pulvinar nucleus of the thalamus (Figure 17-7). The disengagement mechanism is mediated by the right parietal lobe. The move component is mediated by the superior colliculi for visual orienting. A weak orienting network results in a neglect syndrome.

Sensory inattentiveness is a form of neglect and may be visual, auditory, or tactile. The person with sensory inattentiveness is able to recognize individual sensory input from the dysfunctional side when asked to do so but ignores (i.e., neglects, extinguishes) the sensory input from the dysfunctional side

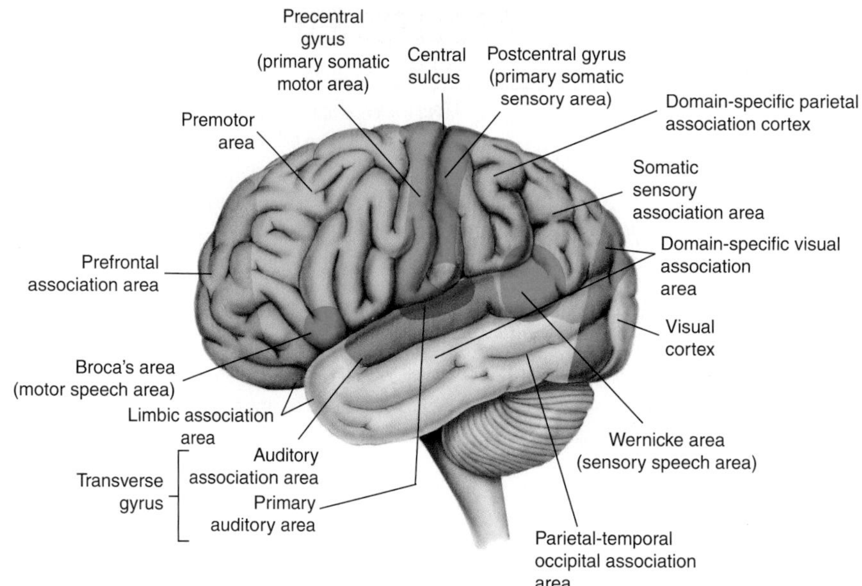

FIGURE 17-8 Cortical Areas of the Left (Dominant) Hemisphere. (From Patton KT, Thibodeau GA: *Anatomy & physiology,* ed 8, St Louis, 2013, Mosby.)

when stimulated from both sides. This phenomenon is called **extinction.** The entire complex of denial of dysfunction, loss of recognition of one's own body parts, and extinction is sometimes referred to as the **unilateral neglect syndrome** and is common after stroke.

An isolated (pure) **selective attention deficit (orientation),** which manifests as a neglect syndrome, rarely, if ever, occurs clinically because typically other deficits also are present. A neglect syndrome may appear temporarily as a result of seizure activity or a postictal state. Temporary or permanent deficits may occur with contusions or subdural hematomas, encephalitis, and ischemic stroke. Progressive neglect deficits may be found with gliomas or metastatic tumor and in Alzheimer and Pick diseases.

Memory is the recording, retention, and retrieval of knowledge. Two types of memory exist: declarative and nondeclarative (Figure 17-10). **Declarative memory** involves the learning and remembrance of *episodic memories* (personal history, events, and experiences) and *semantic memories* (facts and information). Declarative memory is mediated by domain-specific cortical areas of the association areas. This includes: (1) areas of the temporal, parietal, and occipital lobes (Figure 17-8), where long-term memories are thought to be stored; and (2) domain-independent areas of the medial temporal lobe (i.e., hippocampus), the diencephalon (thalamic structures and hypothalamus), and the basal forebrain (located ventral to the striatum and produces acetylcholine) (Figure 17-9), where it is thought distinct domain-specific features of an experience are related or bound.[12]

Nondeclarative memory (nonconscious), also called *reflexive, procedural,* or *implicit memory,* is the memory for actions, behaviors (habits), skills, and outcomes.[13] It is not a language memory but a motor memory. Nondeclarative memory involves the construction of the motor pattern for the motor performance so that the action, behavior, or skill becomes increasingly more automatic. The striatum of the basal ganglia supports this learning across trials (stimulus-response learning), as well as probabilistic classification learning, which supports outcome prediction.[14] All skills and habits are stored in this memory network. *Cerebellar memory* was originally thought to be related to only motor learning but it is now believed to involve nonmotor functions of cognition, emotion, and memory.[15] *Emotional memory* is mediated by the amygdala (located on the inner surface of the temporal lobe) (see Figure 17-9). The amygdala attaches positive (e.g., pleasure) or negative (e.g., fear) dispositions to stimuli in the absence of conscious recollection of the circumstances of the emotional experience. Additionally, the amygdala modulates the event memory during and after the event (memory-enhancing effect).[16] The reflex pathways mediate nonassociative learning (e.g., habituation [decreased response to a stimulus] and sensitization [increased response to a stimulus]) (see Figure 17-10).

Dysmnesia is a disorder of the domain-independent declarative memory network. Dysmnesia is defined as the loss of past memories (retrograde amnesia) coupled with an inability to form new memories (anterograde amnesia) despite intact attentional networks. The hippocampus and other temporal lobe structures are often involved. *Isolated (pure) domain-independent dysmnesia* is caused by only a limited number of conditions, such as transient global dysmnesia (episodic global dysmnesia), amnestic stroke, and Korsakoff psychosis (amnestic or dysmnesic syndrome), as well as after temporal lobectomy. Many disorders may temporarily or permanently produce domain-independent dysmnesia that accompanies other deficits of the cognitive systems.[16a] A *temporary domain-independent dysmnesia* is found during complex partial seizures that persist for a time in the postictal state, in postconcussive states, and in mild posttraumatic brain injury states. A *permanent domain-independent dysmnesia* may be seen in several

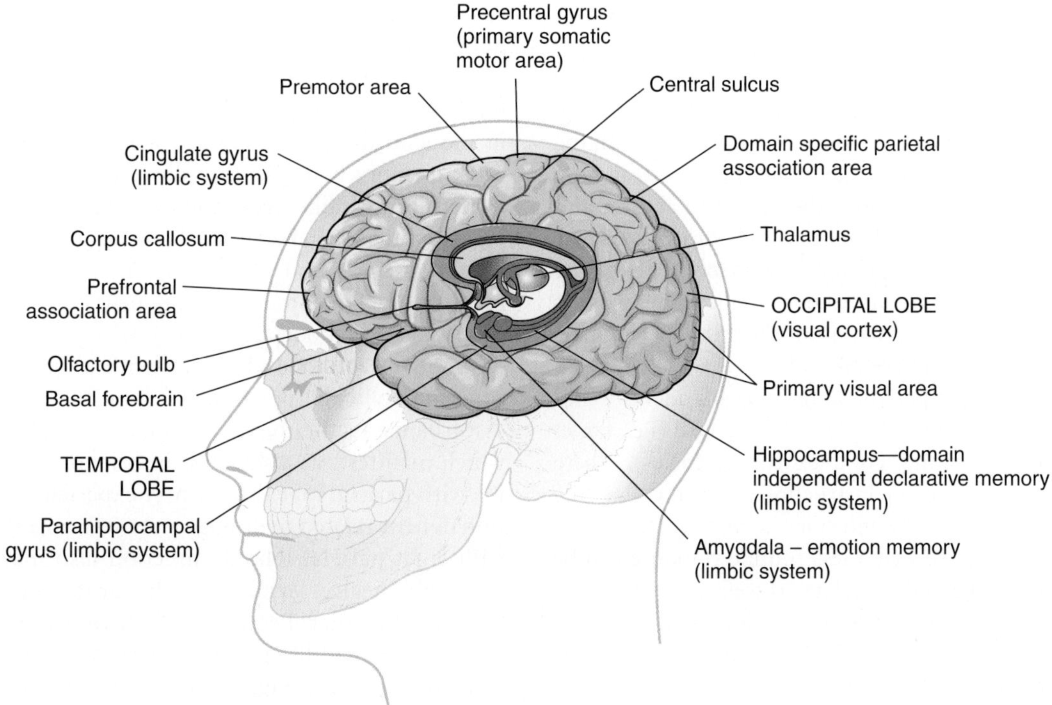

FIGURE 17-9 Midline Cortical and Deep Areas of the Cerebral Hemisphere.

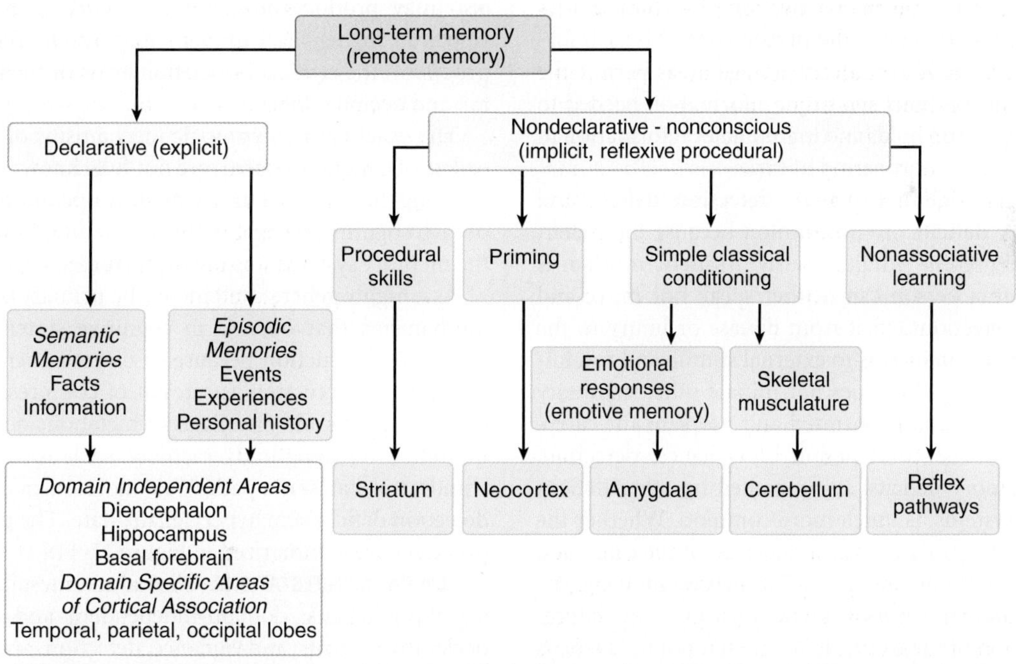

FIGURE 17-10 Types of Memory and Associated Brain Systems. (From Miller RD et al: *Miller's anesthesia,* ed 7, Philadelphia, 2010, Churchill Livingstone.)

disorders including subarachnoid hemorrhage or moderate or severe posttraumatic brain injury states; carbon dioxide poisoning and other hypoxic or anoxic states; Wernicke encephalopathy, viral encephalitis, and granulomatous meningitides; tumors; and Alzheimer and Pick diseases.

A pure *auditory* or *visual domain–specific declarative memory deficit* manifests as an isolated agnosia (see Table 17-9). An isolated (pure) domain-specific declarative memory deficit of tactile sensations rarely occurs clinically because selective attention would likely be affected as well. A temporary auditory, visual, or tactile pattern recognition (remote memory) deficit may appear as a result of seizure activity or a postictal state. A temporary or permanent deficit can occur with temporal, occipital, or parietal lobe contusion; with subdural hematoma or ischemic stroke; and in encephalitis. A *progressive domain-specific declarative memory deficit* may occur in temporal, occipital, or parietal gliomas; in metastatic tumors; and in Alzheimer and Pick diseases.

The prefrontal areas mediate several cognitive functions, called *executive attention functions* (planning, problem solving, goal setting). The *vigilance system* provides the person with the ability to maintain a sustained state of alertness for searching and scanning activities and involves the right frontal areas and the locus ceruleus (LC) (located in the rostral pons) (see Figure 17-7). Through the neurotransmitter norepinephrine from the LC, the speed of the orienting (selective attention) network is increased and the detection function of the anterior cingulate gyrus (see Figure 17-9) is decreased.

Detection is the recognition of the object's identity and the realization that the object fulfills a desired goal (i.e., target selection among competing, complex contingencies). There is conscious execution of an instruction, ensuring that the instructions are followed. The anterior cingulate cortex inhibits automatic responses so that a less routine response can be given. The basal ganglia and cingulate, as well as other frontal areas, function in color, motion, and form detection.

The anterior cingulate plus the ventrolateral and dorsolateral prefrontal cortex (see Figure 17-7) are involved in the representations of information in the absence of a stimulus, such as spatial position of visual events in memory when the event is removed from view (i.e., *working memory* [short-term representation memory]). Control of activation of such memories is also in these areas. This gives the person control over information processing. These temporary storage areas permit the brain to retrieve instructions and other information needed to guide behavior. A person holds and manipulates information in working memory for a short period of time.

Isolated (pure) vigilance deficit, detection deficit and **working memory deficits** are uncommon because these deficits generally are present simultaneously. **Akinetic mutism** is a condition where a person can neither speak nor move and it exemplifies a detection deficit from disease or injury to the frontal lobe. The person orients to external stimuli and can follow with his or her eyes but does not initiate other voluntary activity. There are no goals generated and no plans for carrying out the goals. The combination of vigilance, detection, and working memory deficits, accompanied by other deficits of the cognitive systems, is much more common. Whether the deficits are temporary or permanent depends on the cause and severity of injury. Deficits caused by CNS-depressant drugs, by seizure activity, and (it is hoped) by neurosurgical procedures involving retraction of the frontal lobes are temporary. Deficits in postconcussive and mild traumatic brain injury states may prove to be temporary and resolve over time. Permanent deficits are more likely to be found with frontal lobe contusions, moderate or severe posttraumatic brain injury states, ischemic frontal lobe stroke, and neurosurgery that required frontal lobe resection. Progressive deficits in vigilance, detection, and working memory functions are caused by frontal lobe gliomas, frontal lobe infarcts associated with hypertensive vascular disease, and late stages of Alzheimer and Pick diseases. People with schizophrenia have difficulty in clearing working memory of information that is irrelevant to the task. Additionally, recently encountered visual material that is no longer in plain view cannot be preserved in working memory.

Higher-level thought involves the same neural areas used for sensory-specific computations, but when used voluntarily in thought, these areas are activated from the detection and work memory networks (top-down processing from the prefrontal cortex) rather than from bottom-up automatic processing (from the medial temporal lobe) beginning in sensory areas with a specific sensory stimulus. There is a voluntary search for a feature. By reordering component computation, a person produces novel thoughts.

PATHOPHYSIOLOGY. Individuals with a disease affecting the superior colliculi (positioned below the thalamus) have a disturbance in the move component of selective attention, which manifests as a slowness in orienting attention.[17] People with parietal lobe disease may experience selective attention deficits related to disengagement from a stimulus. Those with right parietal lobe dysfunction also may experience a unilateral neglect syndrome, the prototype of a selective attention disorder. People with a disease affecting the pulvinar of the thalamus (posterior part of the thalamus) have a disturbance in the engage component of selective attention (see Figure 17-9).

A disorder in vigilance may be produced by disease in the right frontal areas. A pathologic condition in the frontal areas also may produce detection and working memory deficits. Impaired higher-level thought may result from a pathologic process in the cortical association areas of the parietal, temporal, and occipital lobes.

The exact pathophysiologic mechanisms of the various disorders of cognitive systems are not fully known. Researchers are studying the defects in the elementary operations (components) of each cognitive system. In the past, pathophysiology related to the memory systems was the most studied component.

As a highly general statement, the primary pathophysiologic mechanisms that operate in cognitive system disorders are: (1) direct destruction because of direct ischemia and hypoxia or indirect destruction as a result of compression and (2) the effects of toxins and chemicals or metabolic derangement. Disinhibition resulting in overactivity, such as seen in some drug withdrawal states, is a pathologic mechanism that can produce detection deficits or a hypervigilant state. The pathophysiologic processes are summarized in Figure 17-11.

CLINICAL MANIFESTATIONS. Clinical manifestations of selective attention deficits; domain-independent and domain-specific declarative deficits; and vigilance, detection, and working memory deficits are presented in Table 17-8.

EVALUATION AND TREATMENT. Immediate medical management is directed at diagnosing the cause and treating reversible factors. Rehabilitative measures for cognitive system deficits generally are either compensatory or restorative in nature and have been greatly facilitated by computer technology and other electronic-assisted devices. Approaches based on behavioral techniques tend to be compensatory, whereas process-oriented approaches, it is hoped, are restorative.

Selective attention and executive attention deficits masquerade as other cognitive deficits. Differential diagnosis of other cognitive deficits is blocked, and learning potential is largely obscured, by the presence of an attention deficit. Therefore, diagnosis and treatment of attention deficits are fundamental.

Data Processing Deficits

Data processing deficits include specific disorders of awareness (content of thought): agnosias, dysphasias, acute confusional states, and dementias including Alzheimer disease.

Agnosia

Agnosia is a defect of pattern recognition—a failure to recognize the form and nature of objects. The disorder involves the loss of recognition through one sense, although the object or person may still be recognized by other senses. Agnosia can be tactile, visual, or auditory. For example, an individual may be unable to identify a safety pin by touching it with a hand but able to name it when looking at it. Agnosia may be as minimal as a finger agnosia (failure to identify by name the fingers of one's hand) or more extensive, such as a color agnosia.

Agnosia is produced by dysfunction in the primary sensory area or in the interpretive areas of the cerebral cortex (temporo-occipital area) (see Figure 17-8). The types of agnosia and the associated area that is most commonly involved with each are presented in Table 17-9. Although agnosia most commonly is associated with cerebrovascular accidents, it may arise from any pathologic process that injures these specific areas of the brain.

Dysphasia

Dysphasia is impairment of comprehension or production of language (semantic processing). With dysphasia, comprehension or use of symbols, in either written or verbal language, is disturbed or lost. **Aphasia** is loss of comprehension or production of language.

Dysphasias usually are associated with cerebrovascular accidents involving the middle cerebral artery or one of its many

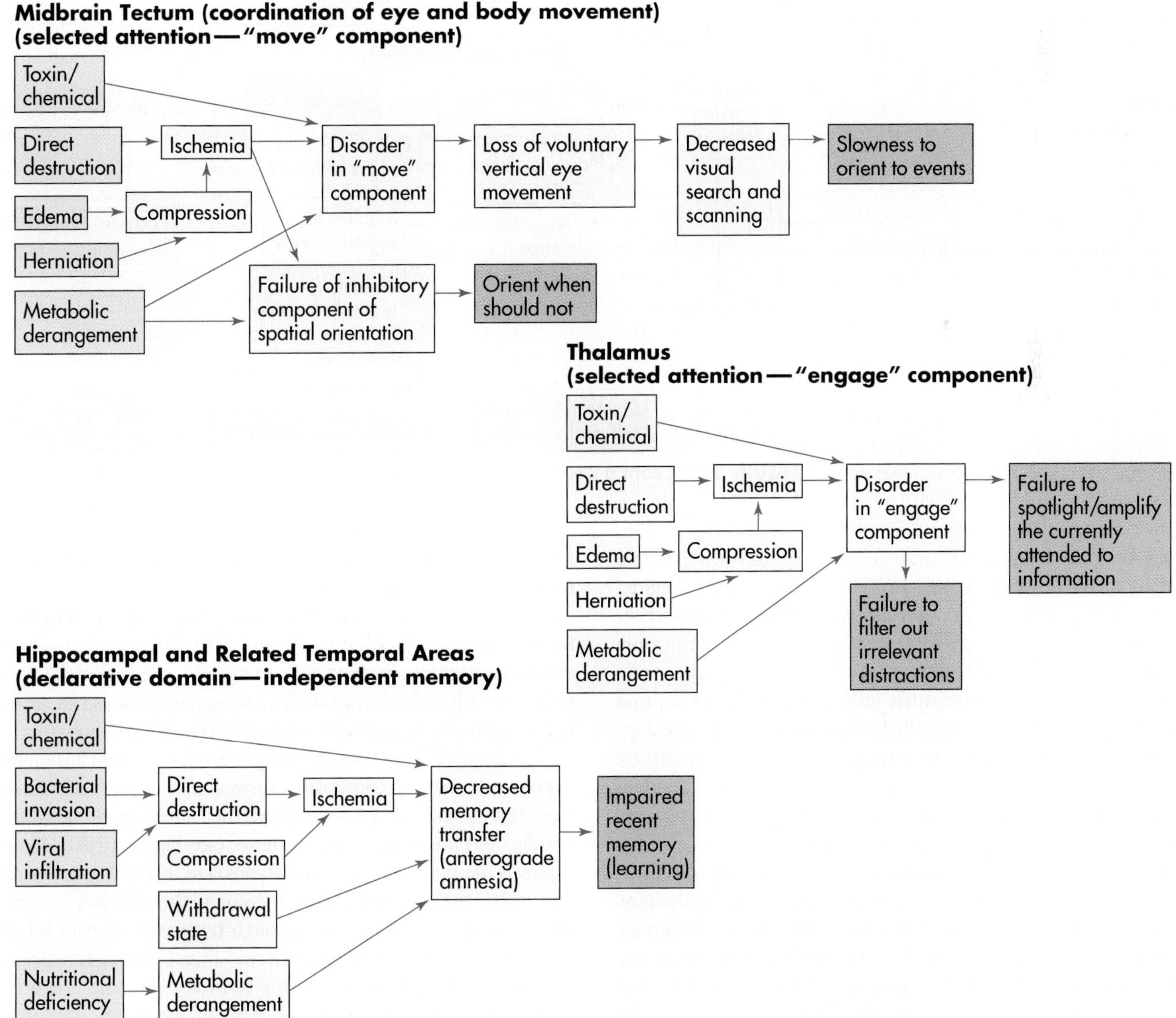

FIGURE 17-11 Cognitive Network Deficits. General pathophysiologic mechanisms underlying cognitive network deficits.

Continued

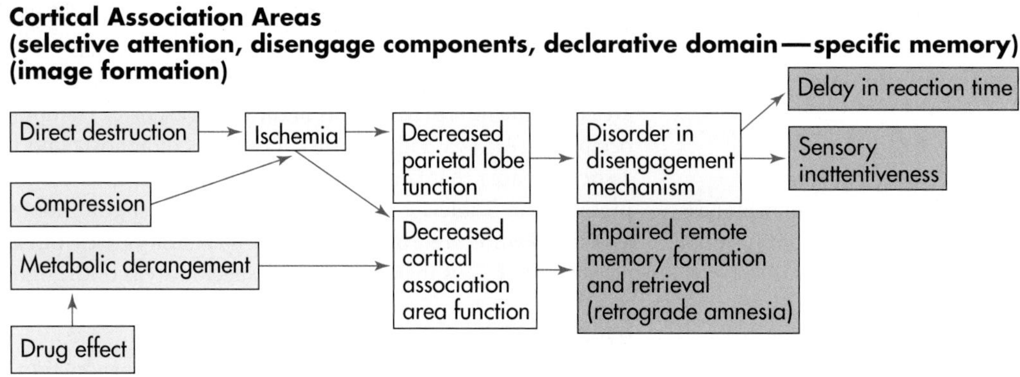

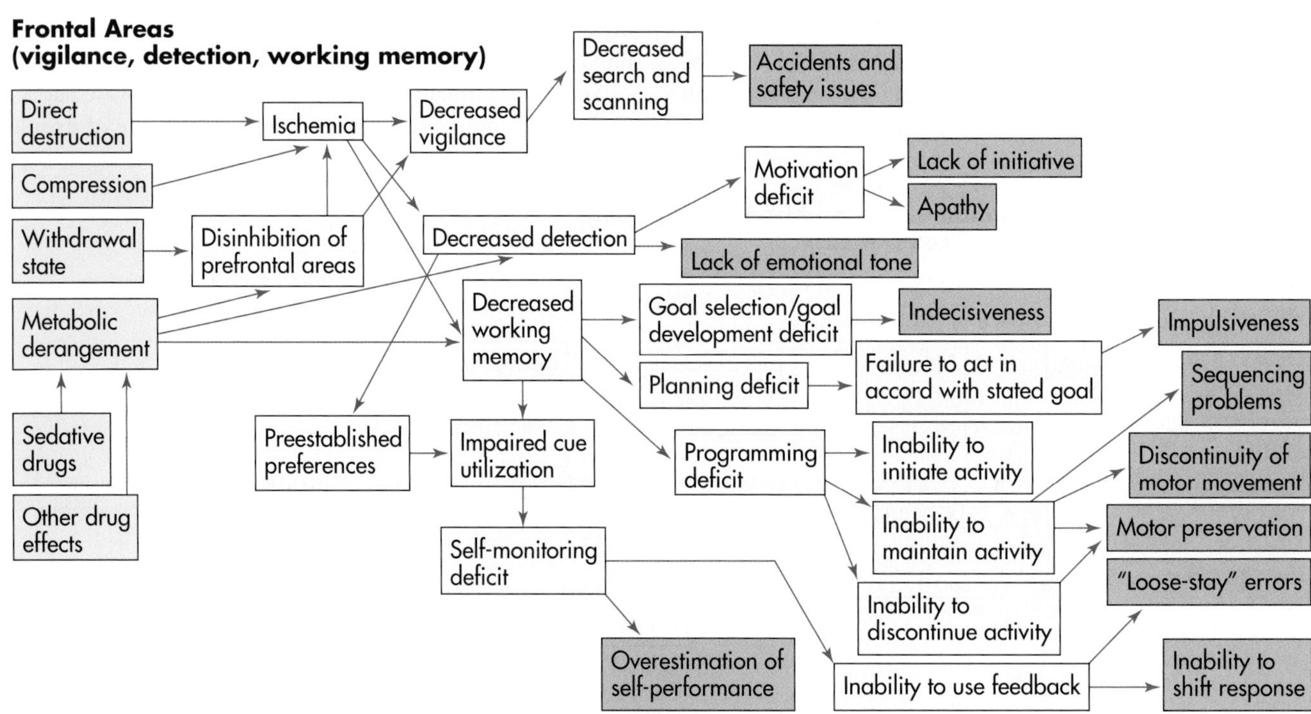

FIGURE 17-11, cont'd Cognitive Network Deficits.

branches. The language disorders, however, may arise from a variety of injuries and diseases—vascular, neoplastic, traumatic, degenerative, metabolic, or infectious. Dysphasia results from dysfunction in the left cerebral hemisphere, most commonly in the frontotemporal region, particularly around the insula (insular cortex) deep within the lateral sulcus. Genes located on several chromosomes have been linked to language development and disorders.[18] Most language disorders are caused by acute processes that either resolve or cause a chronic residual deficit. Some language disorders are caused by degenerative disorders that make the dysfunction progressive.

Dysphasias have been classified anatomically and functionally. Other classifications are linguistic and describe fluency, volume, or quantity of speech. Pure forms of any language dysfunction, however, are rare. Expressive dysphasias are characterized primarily by expressive deficits, but a verbal comprehension (auditory-receptive element) deficit may be present. Receptive dysphasias may have expressive deficits. (Table 17-10 compares types of dysphasias; Table 17-11 illustrates some of the language disturbances.)

Dysphasias referred to as **transcortical dysphasias (transcortical sensory dysphasia, mixed transcortical dysphasia, isolated speech center)** involve the ability to repeat (called **echolalia**) and recite. Speech is fluent but with striking paraphrases. The individual cannot read and write, and comprehension is impaired.

Transcortical dysphasias are caused by hypoxia from prolonged hypotension, carbon monoxide poisoning, or other mechanisms that destroy the border zone (watershed area) of the anterior, middle, and posterior cerebral arteries (see Figure 15-20). Blood supply is marginal in this region. Hypoxia in this area occasionally may isolate the posterior speech areas or all the speech areas from the remainder of the cortex, although both areas remain intact. The sensory and motor speech areas therefore are functional, but connections with other sensory or motor areas are impaired. Information from the remaining areas of the cortex cannot be transmitted to the Wernicke area to be transformed into language.

TABLE 17-8 **CLINICAL MANIFESTATIONS OF COGNITIVE NETWORK DEFICITS**

DEFICIT	CLINICAL SIGNS	SYMPTOMS
Attention		
Selective attention (orienting)	Inability to focus attention; decreased eye, head, and body movements associated with focusing on the stimuli; decreased search and scanning; faulty orientation to stimuli causing safety problems	Person reports inability to focus attention, failure to perceive objects and other stimuli (history of injuries, falls, and safety problems)
Memory (Long Term, Remote)		
Domain-independent declarative	*Left hemisphere:* disorientation to time, situation, place, name, person (verbal identification); impaired language memory (e.g., names of objects); impaired semantic memory *Right hemisphere:* disorientation to self, person (visual), place (visual); impaired episodic memory (personal history); impaired emotional memory *Either or both hemispheres:* confusion; behavioral change	Person reports disorientation, confusion, "not listening," "not remembering"; reports by others of person being disoriented, not able to remember, not able to learn new information
Domain-specific declarative	*Left hemisphere:* inability to retrieve personal history, past medical history; unaware of recent current events *Right hemisphere:* inability to recognize persons, places, objects, music, etc. from the past	Person reports remote memory problems; others report that person cannot recall formerly known information
Image processing (semantic processing)	Inability to categorize (identify similarities and differences), sort; inability to form concepts; inability to analyze relationships; misinterpretation; inability to interpret proverbs	Reports by others of frequent misinterpretation of data; failure to conceptualize or generalize information
	Inability to perform deductive reasoning (convergent reasoning); inability to perform inductive reasoning (divergent reasoning); inability to abstract; concrete reasoning demonstrated; delusions	Reports by others of predominantly concrete thinking; lack of understanding of everyday situations, healthcare regimens, delusional thinking
Executive Attentional Network		
Vigilance	Failure to search and scan environment	Person reports accidents, safety issues
Detection	Lack of initiative (anergy); lack of ambition; lack of motivation; flat affect; no awareness of feelings; appears depressed, apathetic, and emotionless; fails to appreciate deficit; disinterested in appearance; lacks concern about childish or crude behavior	Reports by others of laziness or apathy, flat affect or lack of emotional expression, failing to exhibit or be aware of feelings
Mild	Responds to immediate environment but no new ideas; grooming and social graces are lacking	Reports by others of lack of ambition, motivation, or initiative, failure to carry out adult tasks, lack of social graces and new ideas
Severe	Motionless, lack of responding to even internal cues; does not respond to physical needs; does not interact with surroundings	Reports by others of failure to groom or toilet self, unawareness of surroundings and own physical needs
	Inability to use feedback regarding behavior; failure to recognize omissions and errors in self-care, speech, writing, and arithmetic; impaired cue utilization; overestimation of performance	Reports by others of not changing behavior when requested; unawareness of limitations; does not recognize and correct errors in dressing, grooming, toileting, eating; fails to recognize speech and arithmetic errors; careless speech
	Failure to shift response set; failure to change behavior when conditions change; cue utilization may be impaired	Reports by others of failure to use feedback; inability to incorporate feedback (does not correct when feedback is given)
Working memory (recent memory, short-term memory)	Inability to set goals or form goals; indecisiveness	Reports by others of failure to set goals, indecisiveness
	Failure to make plans; inability to produce a complete line of reasoning; inability to make up a story; appears impulsive	Reports by others of failure to plan, impulsiveness, "does not think things through"
	Failure to initiate behavior; failure to maintain behavior; failure to discontinue behavior; slowness to alternate response for the next step; motor perseveration	Reports by others of not knowing where to begin, inability to carry out sequential acts (maintain a behavior), inability to cease a behavior

TABLE 17-9 TYPES OF AGNOSIA (CONCEPT DISORDERS)

TYPE OF AGNOSIA	DEFINITION	LOCATION OF INJURY
Tactile agnosia (astereognosis)	Inability to recognize objects by touch	Parietal lobe
Spatial agnosia	Incapacity to find one's way around familiar places; disturbance of perception of space (disorders of [1] topographic [extrapersonal] orientation or [2] topographic and geographic memory [construction])	Parietal lobe
Gerstmann syndrome	Loss of spatial orientation of fingers, body, sides, and numbers	Left angular gyrus (parietal lobe)
Finger agnosia (digital agnosia)	Inability to identify the names of one's fingers	
Right-left confusion	Inability to distinguish right from left	
Agraphia	Inability to write	
Acalculia	Inability to perform mathematic calculations	
Visual agnosia		
Object agnosia	Inability to recognize objects and pictures	Temporo-occipital area
Prosopagnosia	Inability to recognize faces	Temporo-occipital ventromesial region
Color agnosia	Inability to understand colors as qualities of objects; faulty color concepts and inability to evoke color images in the absence of color blindness; specific types: (1) "hue" problem, (2) color anomia (cannot name color)	Inferior occipital cortex in left hemisphere
Body image agnosias (may be spatial)		
Anosognosia	Ignorance or denial of existence of the disease	Right parietal lobe
Autotopagnosia	Loss of ability to identify the body, in whole or in part, or to recognize relationships among various parts	Right parietal lobe
Word blindness (alexia/dyslexia)	Inability to recognize written symbols	Left parietotemporal region
Auditory agnosia (pure word deafness)	Inability to recognize speech sounds	Superior temporal area
Amusia (music deafness)	Loss of capacity to recognize tones and melodies	Right superior temporal area

Acute Confusional States

Acute confusional states (ACSs) (also may be known as acute organic brain syndromes) are transient disorders of awareness. They are associated with cerebral dysfunction secondary to drug intoxication, alcohol or drug withdrawal, metabolic disorders (hypoglycemia, thyroid storm), nervous system disease, trauma or surgery (following anesthesia), febrile illnesses or heat stroke, and electrolyte imbalance; in addition, ACSs may be associated with systemic diseases (such as heart, kidney, or liver failure), head injury, anesthesia administration, or the presence of certain focal cerebral lesions.[19] The complex of symptoms is characterized by deficits in attention and coherence of thoughts and actions. Often the symptoms are associated with an altered level of arousal, global cognitive dysfunction, perceptual disturbances, sleep-wake cycle disruption, affective disturbance, and emotional liability. Hospitalized older individuals are at greatest risk for ACS.[20]

PATHOPHYSIOLOGY. Acute confusional states arise from disruption of a widely distributed neural network involving the reticular activating system of the upper brainstem and its projections to the thalamus, basal ganglion, and specific association areas of the cortex and limbic areas. **Delirium** (hyperkinetic confusional state) is an acute state of brain dysfunction associated with right middle temporal gyrus or left temporo-occipital junction disruption.[21] These areas receive extensive input from the limbic areas and modulate motivational and affective aspects of attention. Several neurotransmitters are involved, including increased levels of acetylcholine, dopamine, and serotonin, and increased or decreased levels of gamma-aminobutyric acid (GABA). Inflammatory cytokines, including interleukins, interferon, and tumor necrosis factor-alpha (TNF-α), may contribute to delirium by altering the blood-brain barrier permeability and further affecting the neurotransmission and subsequent neurobehavioral and cognitive symptoms.[22]

Excited delirium syndrome (ExDS), also known as agitated delirium, is a type of hyperkinetic delirium that can lead to sudden death. The exact signs and symptoms are difficult to precisely define. There is altered mental status, combativeness, aggressiveness, tolerance to significant pain, rapid breathing, sweating, severe agitation, elevated temperature, noncompliance or poor awareness to direction from police or medical personnel, lack of fatiguing, unusual or superhuman strength, and inappropriate clothing for the current environment. Hypoglycemia, thyroid storm, certain kinds of seizures, cocaine or methamphetamine intoxication, and/or catecholamine-induced fatal arrhythmias are associated with ExDS. Individuals with ExDS are at high risk for sudden death and represent a true medical emergency.[23]

Hypokinetic confusional states (hypokinetic delirium) are more likely associated with right-sided frontal–basal ganglion disruption.[21] These areas modulate motor exploratory aspects of attention. Most metabolic disturbances that produce a confusional state interfere with neuronal metabolism or synaptic transmission. Many drugs and toxins also interfere with neurotransmission function at the synapse. Cholinergic pathways critical for attention and arousal are often disrupted.

CLINICAL MANIFESTATIONS. The predominant feature of an acute confusional state is impaired or lost detection. Symptoms can fluctuate and include confusion, inability to focus or maintain attention, delusions, and hallucinations. Because of dysfunction of the anterior cingulate gyrus (see Figure 17-9 and Figure 15-7, *B*), the ability to focus, sustain, or shift attention is seriously impaired or completely lost. The person is highly distractible and unable to concentrate on incoming sensory information or on any particular mental or motor task, and loses coherence of thought and actions. The person may persist in thoughts or actions that are no longer appropriate (perseveration) and be unable to monitor the

TABLE 17-10 MAJOR TYPES OF DYSPHASIA

TYPE	EXPRESSION	VERBAL COMPREHENSION	REPETITION	NAME	READING COMPREHENSION	WRITING	LOCATION OF LESION	CAUSE OF LESION
Expressive (Broca Dysphasia, Motor)								
	Nonfluent; impairment of ability to find words, difficulty in writing	Relatively intact	Impaired	Impaired	Variable	Impaired	Left posteroinferior frontal lobe (Broca area)	Occlusion of one or several branches of middle cerebral artery, trauma, tumor, infection, abscess
Receptive								
Wernicke dysphasia, sensory	Fluent: able to produce verbal language but language is meaningless; words are often inappropriate; words with similar sounds or words with similar meaning are substituted for the correct words; words that are not part of the language may be present; these neologisms may be so extensive as to make the speech entirely incomprehensible; because the person has no means to monitor the language for correctness, errors are not recognized; intonation, accent, cadence, rhythm, and articulation are normal	Impaired (disturbance in understanding all language)	Impaired	Impaired	Impaired	Impaired	Left posterosuperior temporal lobe (Wernicke area)	Occlusion of inferior division of left middle cerebral artery, temporal abscess
Global (sensorimotor receptive-expressive)	Nonfluent, produces little speech; at best speaks a few words or phrases	Impaired or completely lost; person understands only the simplest things said	Impaired; not able to repeat	Impaired	Reading out loud—impaired or completely lost Reading silently intact	Impaired; produces little written language	Frontotemporal lobe (left sylvian region); anterior and posterior speech areas extensively impaired	Occlusion of the left middle cerebral artery of left internal carotid artery; trauma, infection, tumors, other mass lesions, and hemorrhage may be the cause

Continued

TABLE 17-10 MAJOR TYPES OF DYSPHASIA—cont'd

TYPE	EXPRESSION	VERBAL COMPREHENSION	REPETITION	NAME	READING COMPREHENSION	WRITING	LOCATION OF LESION	CAUSE OF LESION
Conduction	Fluent but with paraphrasia in self-initiated speech and writing or reading aloud	Relatively intact	Impaired; unable to repeat	Impaired	Variable	Impaired	Arcuate fasciculus, deep in supramarginal gyrus, disruption of the large bundle of fibers that arise from the temporal lobe and pass posteriorly around the sylvian fissure and then project anteriorly to the premotor area	Typical cause is embolic occlusion of the ascending parietal or posterior temporal branch of the middle cerebral artery, angular branch of middle cerebral artery
Anomic, nominal, amnesic (anomia)	Fluent but impaired ability to name objects, persons, qualities, or characteristics; knows what he or she wants to say but cannot find words; may even use desired word in another context but still cannot isolate word when needed	Relatively intact; able to recognize word when it is given	Intact	Impaired	Variable	Variable	Angular gyrus—posterosuperior temporal lobe	Residual of other aphasias, degenerative disorders
Transcortical motor	Nonfluent	Relatively intact	Intact	Impaired	Variable	Impaired	Left dorsolateral frontal cortex (anterior presylvian fissure)	Occlusion of left anterior cerebral artery or anterior border zone vascular infarct
Transcortical sensory	Fluent	Impaired	Intact	Impaired	Impaired	Impaired	Left temporo-parietooccipital junction (posterior presylvian fissure)	Occlusion of left internal carotid with posterior border zone infarct, tumor, trauma, intracerebral hemorrhage, and degenerative disease

TABLE 17-11 EXAMPLES OF LANGUAGE DISTURBANCES

DISORDER		EXAMPLE
Verbal paraphrasia	Question:	What did the car do?
	Response:	The car would spit sweetly down the road. (The car sped swiftly down the road.)
Literal paraphrasia	Request:	Say "persistence is essential to success."
	Response:	Mesastence is instans to success.
Neologism	Question:	What do you call this? (Pointing to a plant.)
	Response:	It's a logper.
Circumlocution	Question:	What do you call this? (Pointing to a plant.)
	Response:	Something that grows.
Anomia	Question:	What do you call this? (Pointing to a plant.)
	Response:	It's...
		Or
	Question:	What did you do this morning?
	Response:	Reading.
	Question:	Were you reading a book or a newspaper?
	Response:	One of those.
Telegraphic style	Question:	Where is your daughter?
	Response:	New Orleans...home...Monday.

From Boss BJ: *J Neurosurg Nurs* 16(3):151–160, 1984.

TABLE 17-12 COMPARISON OF DELIRIUM AND DEMENTIA

FEATURE	DELIRIUM	DEMENTIA
Age	Usually older	Usually older
Onset	Acute—common during hospitalization	Usually insidious; acute in some cases of strokes/trauma
Associated conditions	Urinary tract infection, thyroid disorders, hypoxia, hypoglycemia, toxicity, fluid-electrolyte imbalance, renal insufficiency, trauma, multiple medications	May have no other conditions Brain trauma
Course	Fluctuating; remits with treatment	Chronic slow decline
Duration	Hours to weeks	Months to years
Attention	Impaired	Intact early; often impaired late
Sleep-wake cycle	Disrupted	Usually normal or fragmented
Alertness	Impaired	Normal
Orientation	Impaired	Intact early; impaired late
Behavior	Agitated, withdrawn/depressed	Intact early
Speech	Incoherent, rapid/slowed	Word-finding problems
Thoughts	Disorganized, delusions	Impoverished
Perceptions	Hallucinations/illusions	Usually intact early

Adapted from Caplan JP, Rabinowitz T: *Med Clin North Am* 94(6):1103–1116, ix, 2010.

environment for events of importance (impaired vigilance). The person demonstrates irrelevant or inappropriate responses.

The onset of an acute confusional state usually is abrupt rather than insidious. Later there are top-down processing problems, including misperceptions, delusions, and hallucinations. Obsessions, compulsive behavior, and rituals may be evident.

Delirium is associated with autonomic nervous system overactivity and typically develops over 2 to 3 days, most commonly in critical care units, after surgery, or during withdrawal from central nervous system depressants (e.g., alcohol or narcotic agents). Delirium initially manifests as difficulty in concentrating, restlessness, irritability, insomnia, tremulousness, and poor appetite. Some persons experience seizures. Unpleasant, even terrifying, dreams or hallucinations may occur. In a fully developed delirium state, the individual is completely inattentive and perceptions are grossly altered with delusions or hallucinations. The person appears distressed and often perplexed; conversation is incoherent. Frank tremor and high levels of restless movement are common. Violent behavior may be present. The individual cannot sleep, is flushed, and has dilated pupils, a rapid pulse rate (tachycardia), temperature elevation, and profuse sweating (diaphoresis). Delirium typically abates suddenly or gradually in 2 to 3 days, although delirium states occasionally persist for weeks.

In hypokinetic acute confusional states (hypokinetic/hypoactive delirium), the individual exhibits decreases in mental function. Alertness is decreased, as are attention span, accurate perception, and interpretation of the environment. Forgetfulness is prominent. Reactions to the environment are slowed and indecisive. The individual dozes frequently. Hypoactive ACS can be mistaken for depression or dementia although individuals may have underlying depression or dementia with an incident of ACS.

EVALUATION AND TREATMENT. An ACS is an acute medical problem. The initial goal is to establish that the individual is confused, and to identify the cause and contributing factors. Hypokinetic delirium will need to be differentiated from depression. An underlying dementia may be present (Table 17-12). A complete history and physical examination, as well as laboratory tests, is needed including an electrocardiogram and blood, urine, cerebral spinal fluid (CSF), and radiologic studies. Several assessment scales are available to guide evaluation.[24]

Once the cause is established, treatment is directed at controlling the primary disorder. In an acute confusional state, all drugs that may be contributing to or causing the condition are discontinued unless the problem is the result of drug withdrawal. Supportive measures are designed to enhance coping skills and to minimize the individual's need for altered cortical functions. Supportive and protective management also involves maintaining the person's intact cortical functions by promoting use of these functions. Delirium is preventable in some individuals.[25,26]

Dementia

Dementia is the progressive failure (an acquired deterioration) of many cerebral functions that includes impairment of intellectual function with a decrease in orienting, memory,

BOX 17-1 CAUSES OF DEMENTIA

Potentially Reversible Causes of Dementia
- Infection
  - Encephalitis
  - Meningitis
  - Neurosyphilis
- Normal Pressure Hydrocephalus
- Chronic Subdural Hematoma
- Nutritional Deficiencies
  - Vitamin B_1 (thiamine) deficiency
  - Vitamin B_{12} (cobalamin) deficiency
  - Nicotinic acid (pellagra) deficiency
- Chronic Drug Intoxication
  - Alcohol*
  - Sedatives
- Metabolic Disorders
  - Thyroid abnormalities
  - Chronic hepatic encephalopathy
  - Cerebral vasculitis
  - Sarcoidosis
- Some Types of Tumors
  - Frontal and temporal lobe
  - Pseudodementia of depression
- Medical Side Effects
  - Anticholinergics
  - Antihypertensives
  - Antihistamines

Irreversible Causes of Dementia
- Neurodegenerative Disorders
  - Alzheimer disease*
  - Dementia with Lewy bodies
  - Frontotemporal dementia
  - Pick disease
  - Huntington disease
  - Parkinson disease
- Vascular Disease
  - Vascular dementia*
  - Multi-infarct
  - Strategic single infarct
  - Binswanger disease* (diffuse white matter disease)
  - Amyloid angiopathy
- Infection
  - Creutzfeldt-Jakob disease (CJD)
  - Postencephalitic dementia
  - Dementia associated with HIV

*Most common; *HIV*, human immunodeficiency virus.

language, executive attentional functions, and alterations in behavior. The greatest risk factor is age.[27] More than 26 million people in the world have Alzheimer disease and by 2050 the number is expected to triple with nearly 50% requiring a high level of care.[28]

Dementias can be classified according to etiologic factors (e.g., trauma, tumors, vascular disorders, infections) and to associated clinical and laboratory signs. Dementing processes have been grouped as cortical, subcortical, or both. Box 17-1 lists the potentially reversible and irreversible causes of dementia. Alzheimer disease (AD) is the most common cause followed by vascular disease, then dementia associated with Lewy bodies (i.e., Parkinson disease).[27] In people younger than 60 years, frontotemporal dementia (FTD) rivals AD in terms of frequency.[29] Disruption in cerebral neural circuits is present. The culmination of a progressive dementing process is nerve cell degeneration and brain atrophy involving the cerebral cortex, diencephalon, and basal ganglia.

PATHOPHYSIOLOGY. Mechanisms leading to dementia include: (1) neurodegeneration, possibly caused by genetics, inflammation, or biochemical alterations; (2) atherosclerosis, multiple foci of infarction throughout the thalami, basal ganglia, cerebral projection pathways, and associated areas; (3) trauma, lesions in the cerebral convolutions (mainly frontal and temporal), corpus callosum, and mesencephalon; and (4) compression, increased intracranial pressure, and chronic hydrocephalus. Genetic predisposition associated with neurodegenerative diseases is summarized in Table 17-13. CNS infections, including the human immunodeficiency virus (HIV) and Creutzfeldt-Jakob disease (human prion disease or transmissible spongiform encephalopathies), are associated with dementia in addition to changes in motor function (i.e., ataxia, rigidity, and shuffling gait). Progressive dementias produce nerve cell degeneration and brain atrophy.

CLINICAL MANIFESTATIONS. A summary of the clinical manifestations of the degenerative dementias is presented in Table 17-14.

EVALUATION AND TREATMENT. Establishing the cause for a dementing process may be complicated, but anyone evidencing the clinical manifestations of dementia should be evaluated with laboratory and neuropsychologic testing and brain imaging.

If a specific treatable cause is identified, the appropriate treatment is initiated. For example, an infectious process requires the appropriate antibiotic, and a potentially resectable mass may require neurosurgery. Nutritional deficiencies are corrected. If the cause is metabolic, the imbalance is corrected or the metabolic disorder is treated, or both.

Unfortunately no specific treatment or cure exists for most progressive dementias. The goal is to discover the pathogenetic mechanisms underlying dementia and to delay the conversion of cognitive decline and mild cognitive impairment to full dementia. Therapy is directed at maintaining and maximizing the remaining capacities, restoring functions if possible, accommodating to lost abilities, and controlling behavioral changes.[30] Delusions, paranoia, and hallucinations often respond to neuroleptic medications. If coexisting depression is suspected, a trial of antidepressants is appropriate. Assisting the family to understand the dementing process and to learn ways to assist the demented individual is an essential component of supportive management.

Alzheimer Disease

Alzheimer disease (dementia of Alzheimer type [DAT], senile disease complex) is the leading cause of dementia and one of the most common causes of severe cognitive dysfunction in older adults. Nonhereditary, or sporadic, late-onset AD (70% of cases) is the most prevalent form. It is estimated that 5.4 million Americans have AD and by 2050 the numbers are expected to range from 11 to 16 million.[31] The greatest risk factors are age and family history. Other proposed risk factors include diabetes, midlife hypertension, hyperlipidemia, midlife obesity, smoking, depression, cognitive inactivity or low educational attainment, female gender, estrogen deficit at the time of menopause, physical inactivity, head trauma, elevated serum homocysteine and cholesterol levels, oxidative stress, and neuroinflammation (Figure 17-12). Proposed protective factors include lifelong activity, the presence of *apoE2* and antioxidant substances, estrogen replacement at the time of menopause, low-calorie diet, and use of nonsteroidal anti-inflammatory agents. Statins are being investigated for their role in preventing AD.[32-34]

PATHOPHYSIOLOGY. The exact cause of AD is unknown and there is no clear understanding of this complex disease process. Early-onset familial Alzheimer disease (FAD) is autosomal dominant and has been linked to three gene defects: amyloid precursor protein *(APP)* gene on chromosome 21, presenilin 1 *(PSEN1)* on chromosome 14, and *PSEN2* on chromosome 1.[35,36] Late-onset AD may be associated with chromosome 19 involved with

TABLE 17-13 THE MOLECULAR BASIS FOR DEGENERATIVE DEMENTIA

DEMENTIA	MOLEULAR MECHANISM	CAUSAL GENES (CHROMOSOME)	SUSCEPTIBILITY GENES (CHROMOSOME)	PATHOLOGY
Alzheimer disease (familial)	Amyloid beta protein (AB)	*Early onset: autosomal dominant:* <2% carry these mutations *APP* (21), *PSEN1* (14), *PSEN2* (1) (most mutations are in *PSEN1*)	*Late onset: risk gene apoE4* (19) *CUGBP2* (10p)	Amyloid plaques, neurofibrillary tangles; neuronal and synaptic loss in the brain
Creutzfeldt-Jakob disease (hereditary form)	PrP^SC proteins type 1 and 2	Prion (20) (up to 15% of cases carry these dominant mutations)	*PRNP* codon 129 homozygosity for methionine or valine	Tau inclusions, spongiform changes, gliosis
Dementia with Lewy bodies	Alpha-synuclein	Very rare alpha-synuclein (4) (dominant)	Unknown	Alpha-synuclein inclusions (Lewy bodies)
Behavioral variant frontotemporal dementia	Microtubule-associated protein tau (MAPT)	Tau exon and intron mutation (17) (about 10% of familial cases)	Tau haplotypes *(H1* and *H2)*	Tau inclusions, Pick bodies, neurofibrillary tangles
	Progranulin (PGRN)	*PGRN* (17) (10% of familial cases)		
Huntington disease (autosomal dominant)	Huntingtin protein (polyglutamine)	*Autosomal dominant: HD-IT15* (4) (trinucleotide repeat expansion)	None known	Neuronal degeneration, astrogliosis
Parkinson disease dementia	*Autosomal dominant:* Alpha-synuclein Leucine-rich repeat kinase 2 *Autosomal recessive:* Parkin (juvenile onset) DJ-1 protein PTEN-induced putative kinase 1	*Autosomal dominant:* *SNCA-PARK1* (4) *LRRK2-PARK8* (12) *Autosomal recessive:* *PARK2* (4) oncogene DJ-1 *(PARK7)* *PINK1 (PARK6)*	*GBA* (glucosidase beta acid) *SNCAIP* (alpha-synuclein interacting protein) *NR4A2* (orphan nuclear receptor) *UCH-L1 (PARK5)* ubiquitin C-terminal hydrolase Other low-risk genes	Neuronal degeneration, alpha-synuclein inclusions (Lewy bodies), gliosis; neuronal degeneration

Data from Premi E, Padovani A, Borroni B: *Adv Exp Med Biol* 724:114–127, 2012; Sikorska B et al: *Adv Exp Med Biol* 724:76–90, 2012; Wijsman EM et al: *PLoS Genet* 7(2):e1001308, 2011; Zimprich A: *Curr Opin Neurol* 24(4):318–323, 2011.
APP, Amyloid precursor protein; *PRNP,* prion protein; *PrP^SC,* prion protein scrapie form; *PSEN,* presenilin.

TABLE 17-14 CLINICAL DIFFERENTIATION OF THE MAJOR DEGENERATIVE DEMENTIAS

DISEASE	MENTAL STATUS	NEUROBEHAVIOR	NEUROLOGIC EXAMINATION
Alzheimer disease	Memory loss, disorientation to place and time, loss of facial recognition	Initially normal; progressive cognitive, language, abstraction, and judgment impairment	Initially normal
Creutzfeldt-Jakob disease	Variable, frontal/executive, focal cortical, memory	Depression, anxiety, decreased cognitive function and memory loss	Myoclonus, rigidity, parkinsonism
Dementia with Lewy body (Lewy body dementia)	Initially affects concentration and attention, then memory or cognition loss but unpredictable levels of ability, attention, or alertness; delirium prone	Visual hallucinations, depression, sleep disorder, delusions, transient loss of consciousness	Parkinsonism Changes in walking or movement may present first
Frontotemporal disorders/ degeneration/ dementia	PPA variant Language loss with talking less and speech becoming hesitant or loss of understanding of language, may precede memory loss; spares drawing	Behavioral variant FTD Loss of empathy (emotional blunting), apathy, increased inappropriate or decline in personal or social conduct, loss of judgment and reasoning, hyperorality, euphoria, depression	Caused by CBD and PSP variants
Huntington disease		Apathy, loss of interest early; impaired cognition, judgment, and memory occur later	Chorea, bradykinesia, dystonia
Vascular dementia	Frontal/executive, cognitive slowing; memory can be intact	Often but not always sudden, usually within 3 months of a stroke; variable; apathy, falls, focal weakness, delusions, anxiety	Usually motor slowing, spasticity; can be normal or may have symptom improvement with stroke recovery

CBD, Cortical basal degeneration; *FTP,* frontotemporal dementia; *PPA,* primary progressive aphasia; *PSP,* progressive supranuclear palsy.

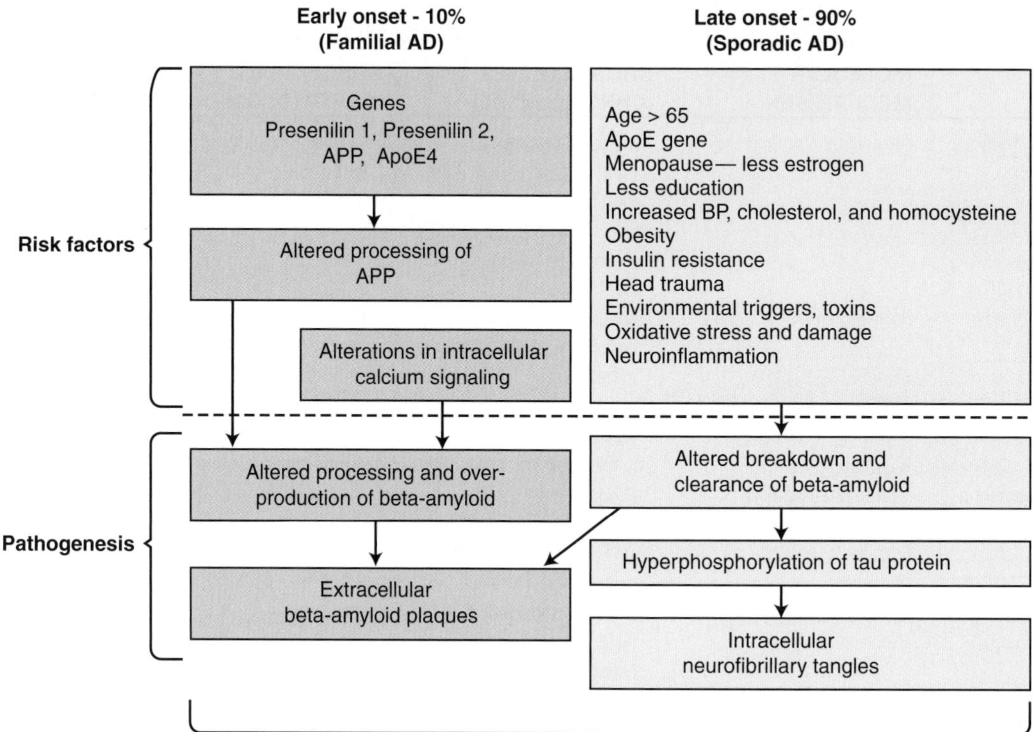

FIGURE 17-12 Proposed Risk Factors and Pathogenesis of Alzheimer Disease. *ApoE,* Apolipoprotein E; *APP,* amyloid precursor protein; *BP,* blood pressure. (Data from Barnes DE, Yaffe K: The projected effect of risk factor reduction on Alzheimer's disease prevalence, *Lancet Neurol* 10[9]:819–828, 2011; de la Monte SM: Contributions of brain insulin resistance and deficiency in amyloid-related neurodegeneration in Alzheimer's disease, *Drugs* 72[1]:49–66, 2012; Daviglus ML et al: Risk factors and preventive interventions for Alzheimer disease: state of the science, *Arch Neurol* 68[9]:1185–1190, 2011; Hasan MK, Mooney RP: The predisposing factors, biological markers, neuroimaging techniques and medical complications associated with Alzheimer's disease, *W V Med J* 107[3]:26–29, 2011.)

the apolipoprotein E gene-allele 4 *(apoE4)*.[37] Sporadic AD is the most common and does not have a specific genetic association; however, the cellular pathologic mechanisms are the same as those seen in early- and late-onset AD. Pathologic alterations in the brain include the formation of **neuritic plaques** containing a core of amyloid beta protein, the formation of neurofibrillary tangles, and the degeneration of basal forebrain cholinergic neurons with loss of acetylcholine. Failure to process and clear amyloid precursor protein results in the accumulation of toxic fragments of amyloid beta protein that leads to formation of diffuse neuritic plaques, disruption of nerve impulse transmission, and death of neurons. Amyloid also is deposited in cerebral arteries, causing an amyloid angiopathy and disturbance in blood flow (Figure 17-13). The tau protein, a microtubule-binding protein, in neurons detaches and forms an insoluble filament called a **neurofibrillary tangle,** which contributes to neuronal death. Tangles are flame shaped (Figure 17-14). Senile plaques and neurofibrillary tangles are more concentrated in the cerebral cortex and hippocampus (important for memory). The loss of neurons results in brain atrophy with decreases in

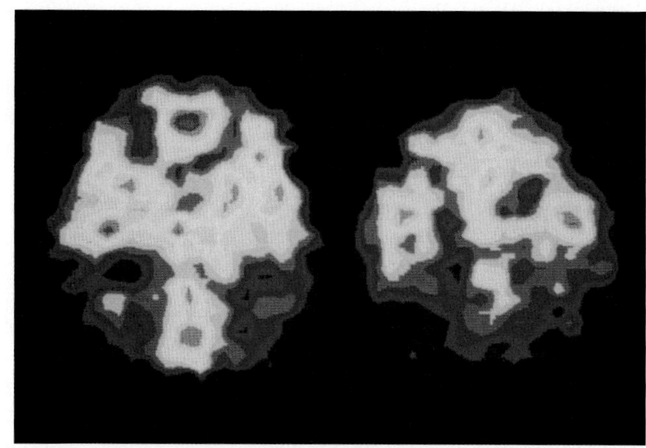

FIGURE 17-13 Altered Cerebral Blood Flow in Alzheimer Disease. Single photon emission computerized tomography scan showing reduction of temporoparietal blood flow *(right)* compared with normal blood flow *(left).* (From Perkin GD et al: *Atlas of clinical neurology,* ed 3, Philadelphia, 2011, Saunders.)

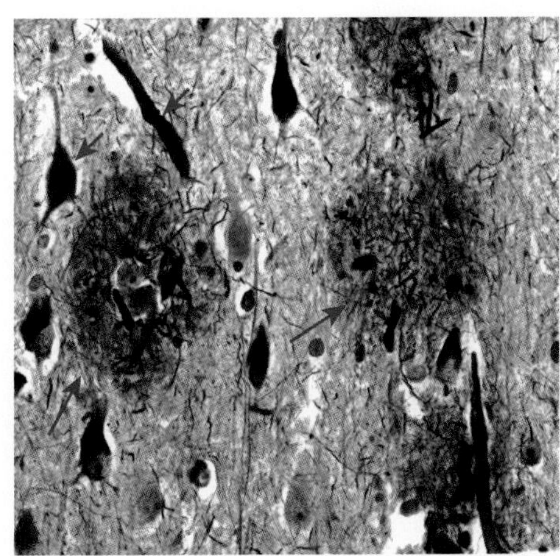

FIGURE 17-14 Major Histopathologic Changes in Alzheimer Disease. Beta-amyloid protein deposits (plaques) in the neutrophil *(long arrows)* and neurofibrillary tangles *(short arrows)*. (From Kumar V, Abbas AK, Aster J: *Robbins basic pathology*, ed 9, Philadelphia, 2013, Saunders.)

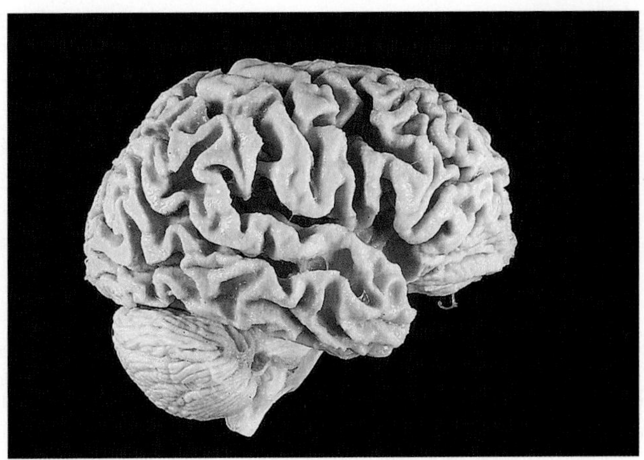

FIGURE 17-15 Alzheimer Disease. The brain decreases in volume and weight, the sulci widen, and the gyri thin, especially in the temporal and frontal lobes. The ventricles enlarge to fill the space. (From Kumar V, Cotran RS, Robbins SL: *Robbins basic pathology*, ed 7, p 843, Philadelphia, 2007, Saunders.)

weight and volume. The sulci widen and the gyri thin, especially in the frontal and temporal lobes, and the ventricles enlarge to fill the space (Figure 17-15). Loss of acetylcholine and other neurotransmitters contributes to the decline of memory and attention and the decline of other cognitive functions associated with AD. Neuroinflammation is evident in the pathophysiology of AD but the exact mechanisms are still being determined.[38] Alterations in intracellular calcium levels are functionally linked to presenilin mutations, *apoE4* expression, amyloid plaques, tau tangles, and synaptic dysfunction. Aging and injury may result in changes that contribute to the development and progression of this disease. Such changes include oxidative stress and neuroinflammation, decreased oxygen and glucose transport, molecular changes in vascular smooth muscle and in the blood-brain barrier, and mitochondrial defects that alter cell metabolism and processing of proteins, including amyloid *(apoE4)*.[39-41]

CLINICAL MANIFESTATIONS. AD has a long preclinical and prodromal course while pathophysiologic changes can occur decades before the appearance of the clinical dementia syndrome. The disease progresses from mild short-term memory deficits and culminates in total loss of cognition and executive functions. Initial clinical manifestations are subtle and nonspecific and often attributed to forgetfulness, emotional causes, or other illness. The individual becomes progressively more forgetful over time, particularly in relation to recent events. Memory loss increases as the disorder advances, and the person becomes disoriented and confused. The ability to concentrate declines. Abstraction, problem solving, and judgment gradually deteriorate. A failure in mathematic calculation ability, language, and visuospatial orientation occurs. Dyspraxia may appear. The mental status changes induce behavioral changes, including irritability, agitation, and restlessness. Mood changes also result from the deterioration in cognition. The person may become anxious, depressed, hostile, emotionally labile, and prone to mood swings. Motor changes may occur if the posterior frontal lobes are involved. The individual exhibits rigidity (paratonia, gegenhalten), with flexion posturing, propulsion, and retropulsion. Weight loss can be significant (see Nutrition & Disease: Diet and Alzheimer Disease). Great variability in age of onset, intensity and sequence of symptoms, and location and extent of brain abnormalities occurs among individuals with AD. Table 17-15 presents the clinical findings in each stage of AD.

NUTRITION & DISEASE

Diet and Alzheimer Disease

Weight loss is a major concern for older adults with Alzheimer disease and it may precede onset of the classic motor symptoms. Weight loss may be a result of (1) increased incidence of infection, (2) increased energy output because of constant pacing, (3) olfactory and taste changes making food less appealing, (4) inadequate food intake, and (5) decreased independence and difficulty in self-feeding. Dementia may lead to memory loss, social isolation, depression, and poor food intake with resultant weight loss. Individuals may forget or refuse to eat, fail to communicate the need to eat, throw or hide food, eat spoiled food or nonfood substances, eat favorite foods to the exclusion of other foods, take a long time to eat, have difficulty in preparing foods, and be unable to feed themselves. Reduced lean body mass has been associated with brain atrophy and declining cognitive performance. Oral nutritional supplementation can improve nutritional status.

Data from Burns JM et al: *Arch Neurol* 67(4):428–433, 2010; Pivi GA et al: *Nutr J* 26(10):98, 2011; Soto ME et al: *J Alzheimers Dis* 28(3):647–654, 2012.

EVALUATION AND TREATMENT. The specific diagnosis of AD is made by postmortem examination.[42] The clinical history, cognitive testing, course of the illness, laboratory tests, and brain imaging are used for diagnostic evaluation. The course of the disorder is highly variable, usually developing over 5 years or more. Genetic susceptibility tests for *PSEN1*, *PSEN2*, and *APP* are used to screen for early-onset AD.[43]

There are no disease-arresting therapies available for AD. Cholinesterase inhibitors (ChE-Is) are used in mild to moderate AD to enhance cholinergic transmission. Drugs for moderate to severe AD block the activity of glutamate (an excitatory neurotransmitter and modulator of neuroplasticity) and work as an noncompetitive *N*-methyl-D-aspartate (NMDA) receptor (a glutamate receptor) antagonist.[44]

TABLE 17-15 PROGRESSION OF ALZHEIMER DISEASE

STAGE	MILD COGNITIVE IMPAIRMENT	EARLY STAGE	MIDDLE STAGE	LATE STAGE	END STAGE
Cognitive	Mild memory loss, particularly for recent event (episodic memory) and new information (semantic memory)	Measurable short-term memory loss; difficulty planning; disorientation to location	Significant forgetfulness; easy to get lost; may dress inappropriately; may have hallucinations	Little cognitive ability; language not clear; personality change; does not recognize family members; wandering; repetitive behavior	No significant cognitive function; loss of word speech
Functional	Possibly depression (vs. apathy); mild anxiety	Mild IADL problems	IADL-dependent; some ADL problems	ADL-dependent; incontinent; difficulty eating	Nonambulatory/bedbound; unable to eat

Adapted from National Conference of Gerontological Nurse Practitioners and the National Gerontological Nursing Association, *Counseling Points* 1(1):6, 2008.
ADL, Activities of daily living; *IADL,* instrumental activities of daily living.

Treatment of AD also is directed at decreasing impaired cognitive function by implementing compensation techniques (such as memory aids), maintaining cognitive functions that are not impaired, and retaining or improving the general state of hygiene, nutrition, and health. Environmental management, counseling, education, pharmacotherapy, and health promotion measures provide the foundation on which a comprehensive individualized treatment program is built.[45]

Frontotemporal Dementia

Frontotemporal dementia (FTD), previously known as **Pick disease,** is a rare, severe degenerative disease of the frontal and anterior frontal lobes that produces death of tissue and dementia. Age of onset is less than 60 years. Three different clinical presentations have been described: behavioral variant frontotemporal dementia (bvFTD), semantic dementia (SD), and progressive nonfluent aphasia (PNFA) (see What's New? The Frontotemporal Disorders). Each clinical presentation is associated with a distinct region of brain atrophy and patterns of cellular atrophy. There is an autosomal dominant pattern of inheritance in 30% to 50% of cases. The majority of cases involve mutations of genes encoding tau protein or progranulin (may be important for nerve repair). The disease is difficult to distinguish clinically and pathologically from Alzheimer disease.[46]

WHAT'S NEW?

The Frontotemporal Disorders

Although marked by progressive damage to the anterior temporal or frontal lobes of the brain, or both, specific subtypes of frontotemporal degeneration (FTD) have been identified with distinct clinical presentations associated with the brain area most affected. Behavioral variant FLTD (bvFTD, Pick disease, or frontal variant FTD) has a predominant behavioral presentation characterized by loss of empathy and increasingly inappropriate social behavior. The right frontal lobe is most affected by bvFTD. A predominant language presentation known as primary progressive aphasia (PPA) can manifest as a nonfluent/agrammatic PPA with the person talking less and the speech becoming hesitant or with a progressive deterioration in understanding language and recognizing objects. The left language areas are most affected in this subtype. A third variant is marked by deteriorating ability to retrieve (recall) words and is associated with left temporal areas. A predominant movement presentation occurs in corticobasal syndrome (CBS) characterized by decreased movement unilaterally and rigidity accompanied by a tremor initially and in progressive supranuclear palsy (PSP) characterized by gait and balance problems and inability to coordinate eye movements.

Data from Gorno-Tempini ML et al: *Neurology* 15:76(11):1006–1014, 2011; Sieben A et al: *Acta Neuropathol* 124(3):353–372, 2012.

Seizure Disorders

Seizure disorders represent a manifestation of disease and not a specific disease entity. A **seizure** is a sudden, transient disruption in brain electrical function caused by abnormal excessive hypersynchronous discharges of cortical neurons.[47] **Epilepsy** is the recurrence of seizures and a type of seizure disorder for which no underlying correctable cause for the seizure can be found. The term **convulsion** is sometimes applied to seizures and refers to the tonic-clonic (jerky, contract-relax) movement associated with some seizures. Seizures in children are presented in Chapter 20.

Diseases and Conditions Associated with Seizure Disorders

Any condition that changes the neuronal environment may produce seizure activity; therefore, in theory, anyone can have a seizure. The seizure threshold of some individuals, however, is genetically lower.

Diseases or other processes that involve the nervous system may cause a seizure disorder. The onset of seizures may point to the presence of an ongoing primary neurologic disease. Etiologic factors in seizures include: (1) cerebral lesions, (2) biochemical disorders, (3) cerebral trauma, and (4) epilepsy. Conditions that may produce a seizure are metabolic defects, congenital malformations, genetic predisposition, perinatal injury, postnatal trauma, myoclonic syndromes, infection, brain tumor, and vascular disease.

Seizures also may be precipitated by hypoglycemia; fatigue or lack of sleep; emotional or physical stress; fever; large amounts of water ingestion (hyponatremia); constipation; use of stimulant drugs; withdrawal from depressant drugs or alcohol; hyperventilation (respiratory alkalosis); and some environmental stimuli, such as blinking lights, a poorly adjusted television screen, loud noises, certain odors, or merely being startled. Immediately before or during menses women may have increased seizure activity.[48]

Types of Seizure

Seizures are classified in different ways—by clinical manifestations, site of origin, EEG correlates, or response to therapy.[49,50] Types of seizures are presented in Table 17-16. **Generalized seizures,** 30% of seizures, involve neurons bilaterally, often do not have a local (focal) onset, and usually originate from a subcortical or deeper brain focus. Generalized seizures result from cellular, biochemical, or structural abnormalities of a widespread nature.[47] With a generalized seizure, consciousness always is impaired or lost. **Focal seizures (partial seizures)**

TABLE 17-16 TYPES OF SEIZURES AND CLINICAL MANIFESTATIONS

TYPE	CLINICAL MANIFESTATIONS	SITE
I. Focal (partial) seizures	Seizures originating in one hemisphere	
A. Simple		
1. With motor symptoms		
a. Without jacksonian march (focal motor seizure—the motor movements do not extend into adjacent areas)	Motor activity is usually clonic Motor movement elicited by the seizure activity depends on the anatomic-physiologic portion of the irritated cortex, but motor seizures most often begin in the face and hands Focal seizures begin with slow, repetitive jerking of the body part, which increases in strength and rate over 5 to 15 seconds The seizure can cease spontaneously, with a gradual decrease in clonic movement	Primary motor area
b. With jacksonian march (jacksonian seizure—the seizure activity spreads in an orderly fashion to adjacent areas)	Seizure activity spreads to adjacent areas after the initial clonic movement increases; motor movements, for example, begin in the fingers of one side and spread to the hand, wrist, forearm, arm, face, and finally the lower extremity on the same side of the body After spreading, the jerking movements in all areas spontaneously stop	Primary motor area
c. Adversive seizure	Turning movement of hand and eyes to the side opposite the irritative focus occurs Often it is associated with contractions of the trunk and extremities It may remain local or develop into a generalized seizure	Frontal lobe anterior to the primary motor area
2. With special sensory or somatosensory symptoms (focal sensory seizure); less common than focal motor seizures; any age may be affected	Sensory experience is subjective and confined to the primary sensory modalities (somesthetic, visual, auditory-vestibular, or olfactory) If sensory seizure begins on the hand area of the sensory cortex, the person experiences numbness, tingling, or "pins and needles" phenomena. Other sensory experiences include burning, a crawling sensation, or a feeling of movement of the body part Areas most often affected include lips, fingers, and toes May remain local or develop into a generalized seizure	Sensory cortex Postcentral gyrus (parietal lobe) with involvement of the primary sensory area
B. Complex (temporal lobe or psychomotor seizure)		
1. Simple partial onset followed by impairment of consciousness—common seizures found in children and adults but in most persons occurs before 20 years of age	The person is able to interact with the environment with purposeful, although inappropriate, movements; although the body muscles stiffen, the person does not fall and may even continue the complex activity in which he or she was involved, such as driving (perseverative automatisms); the person may appear "wide eyed" A wide variety of sensory experiences precede the automatism and include illusions; formed hallucinations; primitive visceral, olfactory, and gustatory sensations; and affective and cognitive symptoms Most characteristic event of a temporal lobe seizure is the automatism; common examples of automatisms are lip smacking, chewing, facial grimacing, swallowing movements, and patting, picking, or rubbing oneself or one's clothing Temporal lobe seizures generally last 11 seconds to 8 minutes (average 2 minutes) and are followed by several minutes of postictal confusion	Temporal lobe and its connections Frontal lobes Other areas
2. Impaired consciousness at onset—with or without automatisms	See B1 above	
C. Secondarily generalized	Unconsciousness appears General symptoms are produced	
II. Generalized seizures	Seizures involve both hemispheres and without local onset	
A. Absence (petit mal seizures) 1. Typical 2. Atypical	Characterized by lapses in consciousness that rarely last longer than 10 seconds. Often associated with additional subtle signs and symptoms such as clonic movements, changes in postural tone, automatisms, and autonomic changes Immediate return to normal consciousness without a postictal period Hyperventilation will induce a typical absence seizure Lapses in consciousness occur almost always accompanied by motor signs, especially changes in tone and lasts from 10 to 25 seconds Often occurs on awakening and with drowsiness A postictal period of confusion may follow Hyperventilation does *not* induce an atypical absence seizure	Multifocal

Continued

TABLE 17-16 TYPES OF SEIZURES AND CLINICAL MANIFESTATIONS—cont'd

TYPE	CLINICAL MANIFESTATIONS	SITE
B. Myoclonus and myoclonic seizures	Characterized by sudden uncontrollable jerking movements of one or more extremities or the entire body Seizures usually occur in the morning Consciousness is thought to be preserved Person often is flung violently to the ground; injury is a real possibility Myoclonic seizures can occur in clusters	Multifocal
C. Clonic	Characterized by repetitive clonic jerks of constant amplitude and diminishing frequency	
D. Tonic (affects infants and children)	Loss of postural tone without evidence of clonicity, with flexion of the upper limbs and extension of the lower limbs	
E. Tonic-clonic (grand mal seizure) (affects children and adults)	Assumes an abnormal posture for seconds or minutes without losing consciousness A prodromal period of irritability and tension may precede a tonic-clonic seizure by several hours or days; however, usually seizures begin without warning Characteristically tonic-clonic seizures begin with a sudden loss of consciousness and brief flexion; the person falls to the ground and the body stiffens in an opisthotonos position with legs and, usually, arms extended; the jaw snaps shut; a shrill cry may be heard as a result of forceful exhalation of air through the closed vocal cords as the thoracic muscles initially contract; the bladder and, less often, the bowel may evacuate; during the tonic phase, the person is apneic with subsequent cyanosis; pupils are dilated and unresponsive to light The tonic phase lasts less than 1 minute (average 10-15 seconds) The clonic phase is characterized by flexion spasms of the whole body interrupted by muscular relaxation; muscular contractions are accompanied by strenuous hyperventilation; the face is contorted; the eyes roll, and there is excessive salivation with frothing from the mouth; profuse sweating and a rapid pulse rate are evident. The tongue is often bitten. The clonic jerking subsides in frequency and amplitude over a period of about 30 seconds The tonic-clonic seizure lasts 2-5 minutes After the clonic phase, the person is in a stupor or coma for about 5 minutes; the extremities are limp; breathing is quiet; and the pupils begin to respond to light When the person awakens, he or she may be confused and disoriented with complaints of headache, muscle aching, and fatigue There is no recollection of the attack Tonic-clonic seizures may occur at any time of day or night, whether the person is awake or asleep The frequency of recurrence may vary from hours to weeks, months, or years	Multifocal
F. Atonic (drop attack)	Characterized by sudden loss of postural muscle tone; the tone loss may be mild, resulting in a head nod, or more dramatic, including falls	Multifocal
III. Unclassified epileptic seizures		
A. Neonatal seizures	Occurs within first 28 days of life Myoclonic or tonic Presents as blinking, chewing, bicycling, or apnea	
B. Epileptic (infantile) spasms	Neck and trunk flexion and arm abduction with a jackknife pattern Extension may occur Epileptic spasms occur in clusters recurring every 5 to 40 seconds	

involve neurons only unilaterally, often have a local (focal) onset, and originate from discrete areas usually associated with structural abnormalities localized to the cortical brain tissue, thereby having a superficial focus. Consciousness may be maintained as long as the seizure activity is limited to one hemisphere in simple partial seizures, but partial seizures may become generalized to involve neurons of the other hemisphere and the deeper brain nuclei. This process is called **secondary generalization.** Consciousness is lost at the point of generalization. In complex partial seizures, consciousness is impaired; that is, the person is unable to respond normally to exogenous stimuli. Sixty percent of seizures are either complex partial seizures or seizures with secondary generalization.

PATHOPHYSIOLOGY. Seizures occur when there is disruption in the balance of excitation and inhibition of electrical impulses.[51] The primary abnormality may be a membrane defect leading to instability in resting potential, abnormalities of potassium conductance or calcium channels, defects of the gamma-aminobutyric acid (GABA) inhibitory system, or an abnormality in excitatory transmission enhancement, particularly of the *N*-methyl-D-aspartate type (NMDA). In animal models, a defect in the GABA inhibitory system is the mechanism causing generalized seizures. Three groups of physiologic mechanisms are involved in seizures and epilepsies: (1) mechanisms of seizure initiation and propagation (excitation and inhibition), (2) mechanisms of epileptogenesis, and (3) genetics.[52]

Seizure initiation is characterized by two simultaneous events in a group of neurons: (1) high-frequency bursts of action potentials and (2) hypersynchronization. The burst activity is produced by a relatively long-lasting depolarization of the neuron caused by an influx of extracellular calcium that opens the voltage-dependent sodium channel. The influx of sodium generates repetitive action potentials.[47] The firing of involved neurons becomes increasingly greater in frequency and amplitude. With sufficient neuronal activation, recruitment of surrounding neurons occurs through a variety of mechanisms. The discharge spreads or propagates to adjacent normal neurons through corticocortical synapses. If uninhibited at this point, the cortical excitation spreads through interhemispheric tracts to the contralateral cortex and through projection pathways to the subcortical areas of the basal ganglia, thalamus, and brainstem. The excitation spread to the subcortical, thalamic, and brainstem areas corresponds to the **tonic phase** (phase of muscle contraction associated with increased muscle tone) and is associated with *loss of consciousness.* Autonomic clinical manifestations also may emerge at this point, and *apnea* may be present for a few seconds. The excitation is further projected downward to the spinal cord neurons through the corticospinal and reticulospinal pathways.

The **clonic phase** (phase of alternating contraction and relaxation of muscles) begins as inhibitory neurons in the cortex, anterior thalamus, and basal ganglia begin to inhibit the cortical excitation. This inhibition causes an interruption in the seizure discharge, producing an intermittent contract-relax pattern of muscle contractions. The intermittent clonic bursts gradually become more and more infrequent until they finally cease. At this point the epileptogenic neurons are exhausted and the neuronal membranes probably are hyperpolarized.

The maintenance of seizure activity demands a 250% increase in the concentration of adenosine triphosphate (ATP). Cerebral oxygen consumption is increased by 60%. Although cerebral blood flow also increases approximately 250% during seizure activity, available glucose and oxygen are readily depleted. With a severe seizure the brain tissue may require more ATP than can be produced by the tissues from the available oxygen and glucose. A deficiency of ATP, phosphocreatine, and glucose then occurs, and lactate accumulates in the brain tissues. Severe seizures thus may produce secondary hypoxia, acidosis, and lactate accumulation, all of which are imbalances that may result in progressive brain tissue injury and destruction. Cellular exhaustion and destruction are consequences of these events.

Epileptogenesis refers to the transformation of a normal neuronal network into one that is chronically hyperexcitable **(epileptogenic focus)**.[53] A delay of months to years often occurs between the initiating injury and the first seizure. Some forms of epileptogenesis involve structural changes in the neuronal network. Reorganization or "sprouting" of surviving neurons (plasticity) also has been found to affect the excitability of the network.

If a seizure focus is active for a prolonged period, a secondary focus, called a **mirror focus,** may develop in normal tissue. This process apparently is caused by the interhemispheric communication, inasmuch as the mirror focus is located in the contralateral cortical area. Seizure threshold in some individuals is genetically lower. Research is in progress to identify alterations in gene transcription that affect seizure threshold.[54,55]

Status epilepticus in adults is a state of continuous seizures lasting more than 5 minutes, or rapidly recurring seizures before the person has fully regained consciousness from the preceding seizure, or a single seizure lasting more than 30 minutes. Status epilepticus can arise from abnormal persistence of excessive excitation or ineffective recruitment of inhibition.[56] The person is still in a **postictal state** (a state that follows an epileptic seizure and returns to baseline) when the next seizure begins. Status epilepticus most often results from abrupt discontinuation of antiseizure medications but also may occur in untreated or inadequately treated persons with seizure disorders. The situation is a medical emergency because of the resulting cerebral hypoxia. Mental retardation, dementia, other brain damage, and even death are serious threats. Aspiration also is a great risk.

The term **epilepsy,** meaning "to be seized by a force from without," generally is applied to conditions in which there is no underlying correctable cause for the seizures. The seizure activity recurs without treatment because of a primary underlying brain abnormality. Epilepsy therefore is a general term for the primary condition that causes the symptoms of seizures.[57] It is now considered to be the result of the interaction of complex genetic mutations with environmental effects that cause abnormalities in brain wiring, an imbalance in the brain's neurotransmitters, or the development of abnormal nerve connections after injury.[58] Epilepsy is estimated to affect about 2.7 million people in the United States with 150,000 new cases of epilepsy reported in 2010.[59] Incidence is highest in early childhood and declines to plateau in adulthood. However, incidence rises again in older people to early childhood levels.

Epileptic syndromes are epileptic disorders characterized by specific clusters of signs and symptoms.[60] Two categories are based on clinical history, EEG manifestations, and etiology and include: (1) localization (focal) related (e.g., temporal lobe epilepsy) and (2) generalized. Localization-related epilepsies and syndromes are typified by seizures that originate from a localized cortical region and are characterized by seizures that have a focal or partial onset. Generalized epilepsies are characterized by seizures with initial activation of neurons within both cerebral hemispheres.

Epilepsy syndromes are further subdivided into idiopathic, symptomatic, or cryptogenic. **Idiopathic epilepsy** refers to syndromes that arise spontaneously without a known cause, presumably having a genetic basis. The genetic basis may be through a specific inherited trait in which the seizures are the principal expression of the genetic defect (e.g., childhood absence epilepsy). In two thirds of cases, the etiology of the epilepsy is not identified. **Symptomatic epilepsy** denotes epilepsies with an identified cause. One third of seizures can be classified as symptomatic (provoked or secondary). Some symptomatic epilepsies also have a genetic basis in which the inherited trait is expressed in a neurologic or systemic disorder that is associated with seizures (e.g., neurofibromatosis). The term **cryptogenic epilepsy** describes syndromes that are presumed to be symptomatic but have no known etiology, and occur in persons with or without abnormalities on neurologic examination. Box 17-2 presents the international classification of epilepsies, and Table 17-17 groups the etiology of recurrent seizures by age group.

CLINICAL MANIFESTATIONS. The clinical manifestations associated with seizure depend on the type of seizure (see Table 17-16). Two types of symptoms often signal an impending generalized tonic-clonic seizure: an **aura,** a partial seizure that immediately precedes the onset of a generalized tonic-clonic

BOX 17-2 INTERNATIONAL CLASSIFICATION OF THE EPILEPSIES

I. Localization related (focal, partial)
  A. Idiopathic
    1. Benign childhood epilepsy with centrotemporal spikes
    2. Childhood epilepsy with occipital paroxysms
    3. Primary reading epilepsy
  B. Symptomatic
    1. Temporal lobe epilepsy
    2. Frontal lobe epilepsy
    3. Parietal lobe epilepsy
    4. Occipital lobe epilepsy
    5. Chronic progressive epilepsia partialis continua of childhood
  C. Cryptogenic defined by:
    1. Seizure type
    2. Clinical features
    3. Etiology
    4. Anatomic localization
II. Generalized
  A. Idiopathic
    1. Benign neonatal familial convulsions
    2. Benign neonatal convulsions
    3. Benign myoclonic epilepsy in infancy
    4. Childhood absence epilepsy
    5. Juvenile absence epilepsy
    6. Juvenile myoclonic epilepsy
    7. Epilepsies with grand mal seizures on awakening
    8. Other generalized idiopathic epilepsies
  B. Cryptogenic or symptomatic
    1. West syndrome
    2. Lennox-Gastaut syndrome
    3. Epilepsy with myoclonic-astatic seizures
    4. Epilepsy with myoclonic absences
    5. Other symptomatic generalized epilepsies
  C. Symptomatic
    1. Nonspecific etiology
    2. Early myoclonic encephalopathy
    3. Early infantile epileptic encephalopathy with suppression bursts
III. Undetermined epilepsies
  A. Generalized and focal features
    1. Neonatal seizures
    2. Severe myoclonic epilepsy in infancy
    3. Epilepsy with continuous spike wave during slow-wave sleep
    4. Acquired epileptic aphasia
IV. Special syndromes
  A. Situation-related seizures
    1. Febrile convulsions
    2. Isolated seizures or isolated status epilepticus
    3. Seizures occurring only when there is an acute or toxic event attributable to factors such as alcohol, drugs, eclampsia, nonketotic hyperglycemia

TABLE 17-17 CAUSES OF RECURRENT SEIZURES IN DIFFERENT AGE GROUPS

AGE AT ONSET	PROBABLE CAUSE
Neonates (<1 month)	Acute CNS infection (e.g., sepsis, meningitis, encephalitis) Cortical malformation Drug withdrawal or toxicity Genetic disorders Intracranial hemorrhage and trauma Kernicterus Metabolic disturbances (e.g., hypoglycemia, hypocalcemia, hypomagnesemia, pyridoxine deficiency) Perinatal hypoxic and ischemic encephalopathy
Infants and children (1 month to 12 yr)	Degenerative disorders (e.g., tuberous sclerosis, neurofibromatosis, Tay-Sachs disease) Febrile seizures Genetic disorders (e.g., metabolic, degenerative, primary epilepsy syndromes) Idiopathic Infantile spasms Trauma
Children (5-11 yr)	Early onset and childhood absence seizures Meningoencephalitis
Adolescents (12-18 yr)	Acute CNS infection (e.g., sepsis, meningitis, encephalitis) Brain tumor Genetic disorders Idiopathic Illicit drug use (e.g., cocaine, amphetamines) Trauma
Young adults (18-35 yr)	Alcohol or drug withdrawal (e.g., barbiturates, benzodiazepines) Brain tumor Idiopathic Illicit drug use (e.g., cocaine, amphetamines) Trauma
Older adults (>35 yr)	Alcohol or drug withdrawal (e.g., barbiturates, benzodiazepines) Brain tumor Cerebrovascular disease (e.g., stroke, aneurysm, arteriovenous malformations) CNS degenerative diseases (e.g., Alzheimer disease, multiple sclerosis) Idiopathic Metabolic disorders (e.g., uremia, hepatic failure, electrolyte abnormalities, hypoglycemia)

Data from Goetz CG, editor: *Textbook of clinical neurology,* ed 3, Philadelphia, 2007, Saunders; Nabbout R, Dulac O: *Curr Opin Neurol* 21(2):16106, 2008; Neubauer BA, Gross S, Hahn A: *Dtsch Arztebl Int* 105(17):319–327, 2008; Waterhouse E, Towne A: *Cleve Clin J Med* 72(Suppl 3):S26–S37, 2005.
CNS, Central nervous system; *yr,* year(s).

TABLE 17-18 TERMINOLOGY USED TO DESCRIBE A SEIZURE

TERM	DEFINITION
Aura	A partial seizure experienced as a peculiar sensation preceding the onset of a generalized seizure or complex partial seizure that may take the form of gustatory, visual, or auditory experience; a feeling of dizziness or numbness; or just "a funny feeling"
Prodroma	Early clinical manifestations, such as malaise, headache, or a sense of depression, that may occur hours to a few days before the onset of a seizure
Tonic phase	A state of muscle contraction in which there is excessive muscle tone
Clonic phase	A state of alternating contraction and relaxation of muscles
Postictal state	The period immediately following the cessation of seizure activity

seizure; and a **prodroma,** an early manifestation that may occur hours to days before a seizure (Table 17-18). Both manifestations may become familiar to the person experiencing recurrent generalized seizures and so may help in preventing injuries during the seizure.

EVALUATION AND TREATMENT. Health history is the most critical aspect in diagnosing a seizure disorder and establishing the cause and onset. The health history is supplemented by the physical examination and laboratory tests of blood and urine (blood glucose, serum calcium, blood urea nitrogen, urine sodium, and creatinine clearance measurements) to identify any systemic diseases known to have seizures as a clinical manifestation. Brain imaging and cerebrospinal fluid (CSF) examination are useful for identifying any neurologic diseases associated with seizures. The EEG is useful in assessing the type of seizure and may help determine its focus. Combined EEG and functional magnetic resonance imaging (MRI) are useful in identifying neural networks involved in epileptic activity.[61]

Treatment for a seizure disorder is first to correct or control its cause, if possible. If this is not possible, the major means of management is the judicious administration of antiseizure medications. The therapeutic goal is complete suppression of seizure activity without intolerable side effects of the drug or drug resistance. Dietary treatments (e.g., ketogenic diet) are effective for some individuals with epilepsy.[62] Surgical interventions can improve seizure control and quality of life in people with drug-resistant epilepsy.[63] Vagus nerve stimulation can reduce seizure frequency in persons with drug-resistant partial seizures.[64] Educational programs may reduce seizure frequency and improve psychologic functioning but it is not known if behavioral and psychologic treatments are beneficial.[65]

ALTERATIONS IN CEREBRAL HEMODYNAMICS

An injured brain reacts with structural, chemical, and pathophysiologic changes called secondary brain injuries (see Chapter 18). The primary injury is the original trauma and the secondary injury is a consequence of ischemia often related to cerebral hemorrhage and edema. Critical features of these injuries include alterations in cerebral blood flow, intracranial pressure, and oxygen delivery. Several relevant features of cerebral hemodynamics relate to cerebral oxygenation (Box 17-3).

BOX 17-3 CEREBRAL HEMODYNAMICS

Cerebral blood volume (CBV) is the amount of blood in the intracranial vault at a given time (normally about 10%). Most of this CBV is in the low-pressure venous system. CBV is determined by autoregulatory mechanisms that control **cerebral blood flow** (CBF). CBF is the flow of blood through the brain and is normally maintained at a rate that matches local oxygen need and removal of metabolic wastes. CBF is sensitive to concentrations of carbon dioxide, hydrogen ion, and oxygen. CBF decreases 3% for every 1-mmHg decrease in CO_2 pressure attributable to vasoconstriction. CBF increases at a Pao_2 of less than 50 mmHg; CBF is stable (maintained) at a Pao_2 of greater than 80 mmHg.

CBF to the brain is maintained at a rate that matches local metabolic needs of the brain, about 750 to 900 ml/minute (15% to 20% of the cardiac output). Blood flow to neuronal cell bodies of gray matter is about three to four times greater than that to white matter because of the increased metabolic activity. CBF is calculated as follows: CBF + CPP **(cerebral perfusion pressure)**/CVR (cardiovascular resistance). CPP is the net pressure gradient required to perfuse the cells of the brain. CPP is calculated as follows: CPP = mean arterial pressure (MAP) – intracranial pressure (ICP). Normal CPP is 60 to 100 mmHg. The CPP determines the CBF. As the CPP decreases to 70 to 80 mmHg in the injured brain, vasodilation occurs, which increases the CBV, also increasing the ICP. An increased ICP will decrease CPP.

Cerebral oxygen saturation is measured in the internal jugular vein (Sjo_2) at the jugular bulb and reflects the amount of oxygen still bound as the blood leaves the cranial vault. Cerebral extraction of oxygen (CEo_2) is calculated using the formula $Sao_2 - Sjo_2/Sao_2 \times 100$. Normal CEo_2 is 20% to 24%; normal Sjo_2 is 55% to 70%. When oxygen demand exceeds oxygen supply, extraction increases, increasing the Sjo_2. A CEo_2 less than 24% or an Sjo_2 greater than 75% indicates cerebral hyperemia. Acid-base balance and temperature influence oxyhemoglobin dissociation (see Figure 34-16).

Data from Arshi B, Mack WJ, Emanuel B: *Neural Res Int* 2013:987934, 2013; Brady KM et al: *Anesth Analg* 108(4):1278–1283, 2009; Verweij BH, Amelink GJ, Muizelaar JP: *Prog Brain Res* 161:111–124, 2007.
CO_2, Carbon dioxide; *PaO_2*, arterial oxygen pressure; *SaO_2*, oxygen saturation in arterial blood; *SjO_2*, oxygen saturation in the jugular vein.

Alterations in cerebral blood flow may be related to three injury states: (1) cerebral oligemia (inadequate cerebral perfusion), (2) cerebral perfusion pressure (CPP) in the normal range (60 to 100 mmHg) but with an elevated intracranial pressure (ICP), and (3) cerebral hyperemia (excessive cerebral blood volume). In the treatment algorithms, oxygen saturation measured in the internal jugular vein (Sjo_2) is categorized as less than 55%, greater than 55% but less than 70%, or greater than 75%. After Sjo_2 is categorized, the ICP must be added to the equation as less than 20 mmHg or greater than 20 mmHg. Depending on the Sjo_2 and ICP values, treatment algorithms are implemented that address not only ICP but also CPP. The therapeutic goal is to balance ICP and Sjo_2. Target values for relevant clinical parameters are presented in Table 17-19.

Increased Intracranial Pressure

Intracranial pressure normally is 5 to 15 mmHg, or 60 to 180 mm H_2O. **Increased intracranial pressure (IICP)** may result from an increase in intracranial content (as occurs with tumor growth), edema, excess CSF, or hemorrhage. It necessitates an equal reduction in volume of the other cranial contents. The most readily displaced content is CSF. If intracranial pressure remains high after CSF displacement out of the cranial vault, cerebral blood volume and blood flow are altered.

In *stage 1 of intracranial hypertension,* vasoconstriction and external compression of the venous system occur in an attempt to further decrease the intracranial pressure. Thus, during the first stage of intracranial hypertension, ICP may not change because of the effective compensatory mechanisms and there may be few symptoms (Figure 17-16). Small increases in volume, however, cause an increase in pressure, and the pressure may take longer to return to baseline. This can be detected with ICP monitoring.

In *stage 2 of intracranial hypertension,* there is continued expansion of intracranial contents. The resulting increase in ICP may exceed the brain's compensatory capacity to adjust. The pressure begins to compromise neuronal oxygenation, and systemic arterial vasoconstriction occurs in an attempt to elevate the systemic blood pressure sufficiently to overcome the IICP. Clinical manifestations at this stage are usually subtle and transient, including episodes of confusion, restlessness, drowsiness, and slight pupillary and breathing changes (see Figure 17-16).

In *stage 3 of intracranial hypertension,* the ICP begins to approach arterial pressure, the brain tissues begin to experience hypoxia and hypercapnia, and the individual's condition rapidly deteriorates. Clinical manifestations include decreasing levels of arousal or central neurogenic hyperventilation, widened pulse pressure, bradycardia, and pupils that become small and sluggish (see Figure 17-16).

Dramatic sustained rises in ICP are not seen until all compensatory mechanisms have been exhausted. Then dramatic rises in ICP occur over a very short period. **Autoregulation,** the compensatory alteration in the diameter of the intracranial blood vessels designed to maintain a constant blood flow during changes in cerebral perfusion pressure, is lost with progressively increased ICP. Accumulating carbon dioxide may still cause vasodilation locally, but without autoregulation this vasodilation causes the hydrostatic (blood) pressure in the vessels to drop and blood volume to increase. The brain volume is thus further enhanced, and ICP continues to rise. Small increases in volume cause dramatic increases in ICP, and the pressure takes much longer to return to baseline. As the ICP begins to approach systemic blood pressure, cerebral perfusion pressure falls and cerebral perfusion slows dramatically. The brain tissues experience severe hypoxia, hypercapnea, and acidosis.

TABLE 17-19 THERAPEUTIC MANAGEMENT GOALS FOR INDIVIDUALS WITH ALTERED CEREBRAL HEMODYNAMICS

CLINICAL PARAMETER	TARGET VALUE
Central perfusion pressure	>70 mmHg
Intracranial pressure	<20 mmHg
Arterial CO_2 pressure ($Paco_2$)	35 mmHg
Mean arterial pressure	90 mmHg
Temperature	34-36° C (93.2-96.8° F)
Pulmonary capillary wedge pressure	10-15 mmHg

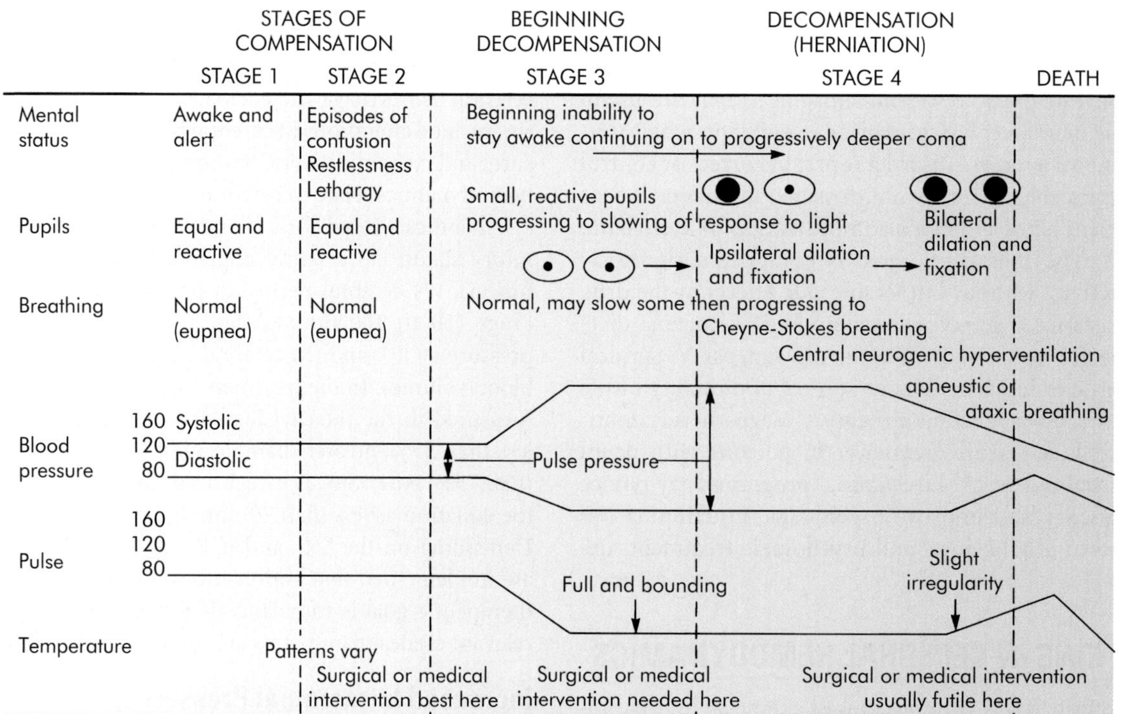

FIGURE 17-16 Clinical Correlates of Compensated and Uncompensated Phases of Intracranial Hypertension. (From Beare PG, Myers JL: *Principles and practice of adult health nursing,* ed 3, St Louis, 1998, Mosby.)

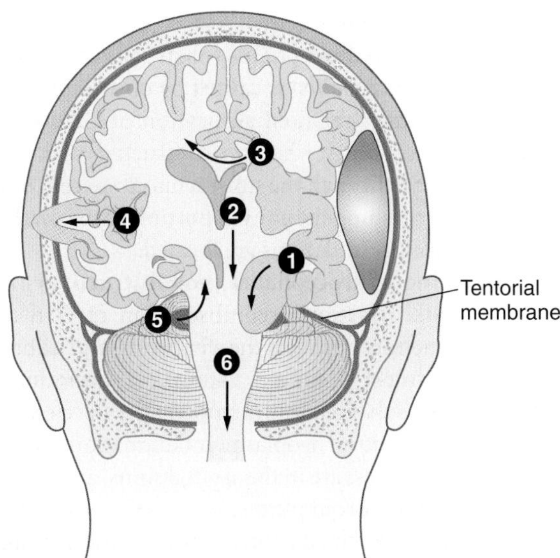

FIGURE 17-17 **Brain Herniation.** Herniations can occur both above and below the tentorial membrane. *Supratentorial:* **1,** uncal (transtentorial); **2,** central; **3,** cingulate; **4,** transcalvarial (external herniation through an opening in the skull). *Infratentorial:* **5,** upward herniation of cerebellum; **6,** cerebellar tonsillar moves down through foramen magnum.

In *stage 4 of intracranial hypertension,* brain tissue shifts (herniates) from the compartment of greater pressure to a compartment of lesser pressure and IICP in one compartment of the cranial vault is not evenly distributed throughout the other vault compartments (see Figures 17-16 and 17-17). With this shift in brain tissue, the herniating brain tissue's blood supply is compromised, causing further ischemia and hypoxia in the herniating tissues. The volume of content within the lower pressure compartment increases, exerting pressure on the brain tissue that normally occupies that compartment, and impairing its blood supply. Small hemorrhages often develop in the involved brain tissue. Obstructive hydrocephalus may develop. The herniation process markedly and rapidly increases intracranial pressure. Mean systolic arterial pressure soon equals ICP and cerebral blood flow ceases at this point. The types of **herniation syndromes** are outlined in Box 17-4.

Cerebral Edema

Cerebral edema is an increase in the fluid content of brain tissue, a net accumulation of water within the brain (Figures 17-18 and 17-19). Cerebral edema causes an increase in extracellular or intracellular tissue volume after brain insult from trauma, infection, hemorrhage, tumor, ischemia, infarct, or hypoxia. The harmful effects of cerebral edema are caused by the distortion of blood vessels, the displacement of brain tissues, and the eventual herniation of brain tissue from one brain compartment to another.

Three types of cerebral edema are (1) vasogenic edema, (2) cytotoxic (metabolic) edema, and (3) interstitial edema. **Vasogenic edema** is clinically the most important type. It is caused by the increased permeability of the capillary endothelium of the brain after injury to the vascular structure. The result

BOX 17-4 BRAIN HERNIATION SYNDROMES

Supratentorial Herniation

1. *Uncal herniation.* This occurs when the uncus or hippocampal gyrus, or both, shifts from the middle fossa through the tentorial notch into the posterior fossa, compressing the ipsilateral third cranial nerve, the contralateral third cranial nerve, and the mesencephalon. Uncal herniation generally is caused by an expanding mass in the lateral region of the middle fossa. The classic manifestations of uncal herniation are a decreasing level of consciousness, pupils that become sluggish before fixing and dilating (first the ipsilateral, then the contralateral pupil), Cheyne-Stokes respirations (which later shift to central neurogenic hyperventilation), and the appearance of decorticate and then decerebrate posturing.
2. *Central herniation.* This is the straight downward shift of the diencephalon through the tentorial notch. It may be caused by injuries or masses located around the outer perimeter of the frontal, parietal, or occipital lobes; extracerebral injuries around the central apex (top) of the cranium; bilaterally positioned injuries or masses; and unilateral cingulate gyrus herniation. The individual rapidly becomes unconscious; moves from Cheyne-Stokes respirations to apnea; develops small, reactive pupils and then dilated, fixed pupils; and passes from decortication to decerebration.
3. *Cingulate gyrus herniation.* This occurs when the cingulate gyrus shifts under the falx cerebri. Little is known about its clinical manifestations.
4. *Transcalvarial herniation.* The brain shifts through a skull fracture or a surgical opening in the skull. This type of external herniation may occur during a craniectomy—surgery in which a flap of skull is removed, preventing the piece of skull from being replaced.

Infratentorial Herniation

The most common syndrome is *cerebellar tonsillar.* The cerebellar tonsil shifts through the foramen magnum because of increased pressure within the posterior fossa. The clinical manifestations are an arched stiff neck, paresthesias in the shoulder area, decreased consciousness, respiratory abnormalities, and pulse rate variations. Occasionally the force produces an *upward transtentorial* herniation of a cerebellar tonsil or the lower brainstem. There is increased ICP but no specific set of clinical manifestations associated with infratentorial herniation (see Figure 17-17).

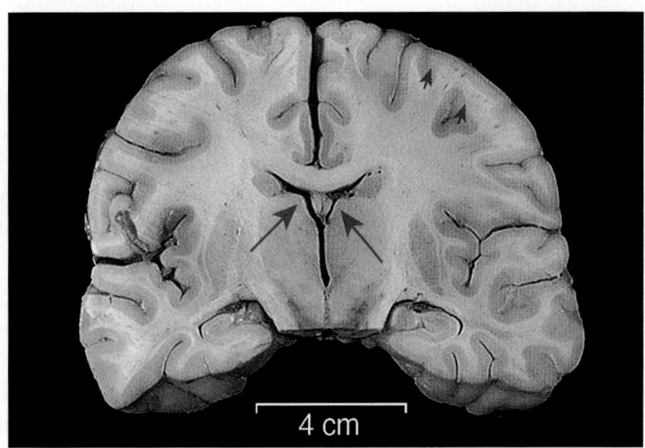

FIGURE 17-18 **Cerebral Edema.** This coronal section of cerebrum demonstrates marked compression in the lateral ventricles *(long arrows)* and flattening of gyri *(short arrows)* from extensive bilateral cerebral edema. Edema increases intracranial pressure, leading to herniation. (From Klatt EC: *Robbins and Cotran atlas of pathology,* ed 2, Philadelphia, 2010, Saunders.)

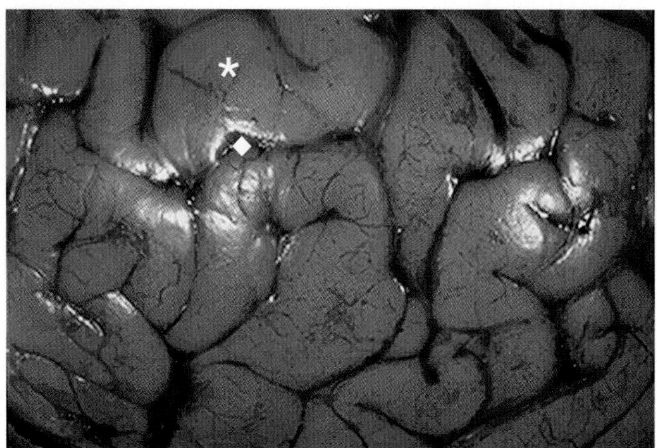

FIGURE 17-19 Cerebral Edema, Gross. The surface of the meninges of the brain with cerebral edema shows widened, flattened gyri (*) with narrowed sulci (◇). (From Klatt EC: *Robbins and Cotran atlas of pathology,* ed 2, Philadelphia, 2010, Saunders.)

is a disruption in the blood-brain barrier (selective permeability of brain capillaries). Plasma proteins leak into the extracellular spaces, drawing water to them, and the water content of the brain parenchyma increases. Vasogenic edema begins in the area of injury and spreads with preferential accumulation in the white matter of the ipsilateral side because the parallel myelinated fibers separate more easily. Edema then promotes more edema because of ischemia from increasing pressure.

Clinical manifestations of vasogenic edema include focal neurologic deficits, disturbances of consciousness, and a severe increase in intracranial pressure. Vasogenic edema resolves by slow diffusion.

In **cytotoxic (metabolic) edema,** toxic factors directly affect the cellular elements of the brain parenchyma (neuronal, glial, and endothelial cells), causing failure of the active transport systems. The blood-brain barrier is not disrupted. The cells lose their potassium and gain larger amounts of sodium. Water follows by osmosis into the cell so that the cells swell. Cytotoxic edema occurs principally in the gray matter and may increase vasogenic edema.

Interstitial edema is seen most often with noncommunicating hydrocephalus (see following section and Chapter 20). The edema is caused by transependymal movement of CSF from the ventricles into the extracellular spaces of the brain tissues. The brain fluid volume thus is increased predominantly around the ventricles. The hydrostatic pressure within the white matter increases, and the size of the white matter is reduced because of the rapid disappearance of myelin lipids.

Hydrocephalus

The term **hydrocephalus** refers to various conditions characterized by an excess of fluid within the cerebral ventricles, subarachnoid space, or both (see Figures 15-15 and 15-16). Hydrocephalus occurs because of interference with CSF flow caused by increased fluid production, obstruction within the ventricular system, or defective reabsorption of the fluid. A papilloma (i.e., epithelial tumor) may, in rare instances, cause overproduction of CSF (Figure 17-20).

Types of Hydrocephalus

Noncommunicating hydrocephalus (obstructive) *(internal or intraventricular hydrocephalus)* is caused by obstruction within the ventricular system. Impaired absorption of CSF from the subarachnoid space occurs when an obstructive process disrupts the flow of CSF through the subarachnoid space. The fluid is prevented from reaching the convex portion of the cerebrum, where the arachnoid granulations are located.

Communicating hydrocephalus (nonobstructive) *(extraventricular)* results from impaired absorption of CSF in the absence of obstruction between the ventricles and subarachnoid space. The most common causes of communicating hydrocephalus are subarachnoid hemorrhage, developmental malformation, head injury, neoplasm, inflammation (i.e., meningitis), high venous pressure in the sagittal sinus, and increased CSF secretion by the choroid plexus.

Hydrocephalus ex vacuo is a form of communicating hydrocephalus that arises from cerebral atrophy. CSF fills the unoccupied space. The amount of CSF is increased, but the fluid is not under pressure.

Normal-pressure hydrocephalus (low-pressure, adult, or **occult hydrocephalus)** is a form of communicating hydrocephalus that occurs mostly in late middle age. The ventricles are enlarged and the cerebrospinal fluid pressure is minimally elevated. This form of hydrocephalus is idiopathic or occurs secondarily as a complication of head injury or subarachnoid hemorrhage.

Acute hydrocephalus may develop in several hours in persons who have sustained head injuries. Acute hydrocephalus contributes significantly to increased ICP.

PATHOPHYSIOLOGY. The obstruction of CSF flow associated with hydrocephalus produces dilation of the ventricles proximal to the obstruction. Obstructed CSF is under pressure, causing atrophy of the cerebral cortex and degeneration of the white matter tracts. There is selective preservation of gray matter. When excess CSF fills a defect caused by atrophy, a degenerative disorder, or a surgical excision, this fluid is not under pressure; therefore, atrophy and degenerative changes are not induced.

CLINICAL MANIFESTATIONS. Most cases of hydrocephalus develop gradually and insidiously over time. Acute hydrocephalus presents with signs of rapidly developing increased intracranial pressure. The person deteriorates rapidly into a deep coma if not promptly treated. Normal-pressure hydrocephalus has a long-term presentation and develops slowly over time. A triad of symptoms, including declining memory with loss of cognitive function (frontal lobe and subcortical dementia); unsteady, broad-based gait; and urinary urgency and incontinence from detrusor overactivity, are common and make diagnosis difficult to differentiate from other causes of dementia. Additional clinical manifestations are apathy, inattentiveness, and indifference to self, family, and the environment.[66,67]

EVALUATION AND TREATMENT. The diagnosis is made on the basis of clinical history and physical examination, evaluation of CSF pressure and volume, and results of brain imaging. Hydrocephalus can be treated by surgery to resect cysts, neoplasms, or hematomas or by ventricular bypass into the normal intracranial channel or into an extracranial compartment using a shunt.

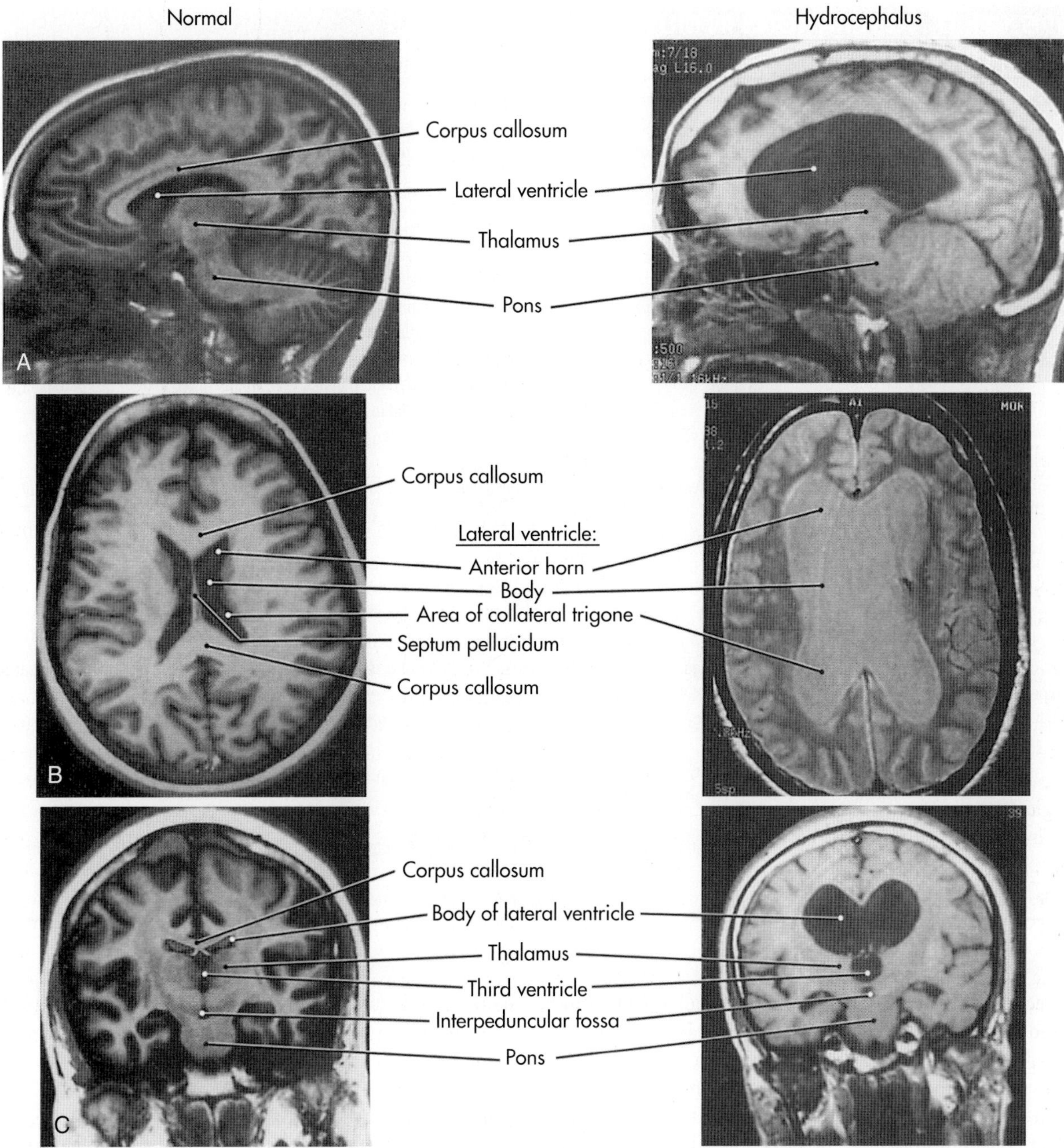

FIGURE 17-20 Comparison of Normal and Hydrocephalic Brains. **A,** Sagittal; **B,** axial; and **C,** coronal planes as seen in magnetic resonance imaging (MRI). (From Haines DE, editor: *Fundamental neuroscience for basic and clinical applications,* ed 4, Philadelphia, 2013, Saunders.)

Excision or coagulation of the choroid plexus is needed occasionally when a papilloma is present.

ALTERATIONS IN NEUROMOTOR FUNCTION

Movements are complex patterns of activity controlled by the cerebral cortex, the pyramidal system, the extrapyramidal system, and the muscle motor units. Dysfunction in any of these areas can cause motor dysfunction. General motor dysfunctions are associated with changes in muscle tone, movement, and complex motor performance.[68,69]

Alterations in Muscle Tone

Normal muscle tone involves a slight resistance to passive movement. The resistance is smooth, constant, and even throughout the range of motion. Abnormalities of muscle tone are presented in Table 17-20.

Hypotonia

In **hypotonia (decreased muscle tone),** passive movement of a muscle occurs with little or no resistance to stretching. Hypotonia is a symptom of alterations in nervous control of muscles. It is thought to be caused by decreased muscle spindle

TABLE 17-20 ALTERATIONS IN MUSCLE TONE

ALTERATIONS	CAUSE	CHARACTERISTICS
Hypotonia	Thought to be caused by decreased muscle spindle activity as a result of decreased excitability of neurons Occurs typically when nerve impulses necessary for muscle tone are lost	Passive movement of a muscle mass with little or no resistance Difficult to detect; extremity is floppy and allows excessive movement when displaced Muscles may be rapidly moved without resistance
Flaccidity		Associated with limp, atrophied muscles and paralysis
Hypertonia	Results when the lower motor unit reflex arc continues to function but is not mediated or regulated by higher centers	Increased muscle resistance to passive movement May be associated with paralysis May be accompanied by muscle hypertrophy (see Figure 17-24)
Spasticity	Exact mechanism unclear; appears to arise from an increased excitability of the alpha motor neurons to any input because of absence of the descending inhibition of the pyramidal systems	A gradual increase in tone causing increased resistance until tone suddenly is reduced, which results in clasp-knife phenomenon Velocity dependent (may be absent with slow speed of displacement) Selective distribution (predominates in flexors of upper extremities and extensors of lower extremities and in pronators compared with supinators)
Gegenhalten (paratonia)	Exact mechanism unclear: associated with frontal lobe injury	Resistance to passive movement, which varies in direct proportion to force applied
Dystonia	Loss of CNS inhibitory function with sustained muscular contraction	Sustained involuntary twisting and repetitive movements or abnormal posture
Rigidity	Occurs as a result of constant, involuntary contraction of muscle	Muscle resistance to passive movement of a rigid limb that is uniform in both flexion and extension throughout the motion Not velocity dependent Activated by contraction of muscles in contralateral extremities Uniform through range in displacement
Plastic or lead-pipe	Associated with basal ganglion damage	Increased muscular tone relatively independent of degree of force used in passive movement; does not vary throughout the passive movement
Cogwheel	Associated with basal ganglion damage	The uniform resistance may be interrupted by a series of brief jerks resulting in movements much like a ratchet, "cogwheel" phenomenon
Gamma	Loss of excitation of extensor inhibitory areas by the cerebral cortex, decreasing the inhibition of alpha and gamma motor neurons	Characterized by extensor posturing (decerebrate rigidity)
Alpha	Loss of cerebellum input to lateral vestibular nuclei	Impaired relaxation characterized by extensor rigidity of skeletal muscle after the contraction
Myotonia		Impaired relaxation of skeletal muscle after the contraction

activity secondary to decreased excitability of neurons. Hypotonia caused by pure pyramidal tract damage (a rare occurrence) produces hypotonia and weakness. Hypotonia contributes to the ataxia and intention tremor in cerebellar damage and manifests with minimal weakness and normal or slightly exaggerated reflexes. Hypotonia, often described as flaccidity (a state in which the muscle may be moved rapidly without resistance), occurs when nerve impulses necessary for muscle tone are lost, such as in spinal cord injury or cerebrovascular accident.

Individuals with hypotonia report that they tire easily (asthenia) or are weak, signs that can be observed during their activity attempts. They may have difficulty rising from a sitting position, sitting down without using arm support, or walking up and down stairs, as well as an inability to stand on their toes. Because of their weakness, accident proneness during locomotion and self-care activities is common. Inasmuch as the joints become hyperflexible in hypotonic states, people with hypotonia may be able to assume positions that require extreme joint mobility. The joints may appear loose, and the knee jerks are pendulous.

The muscle mass atrophies because of decreased input entering the motor unit. Muscle cells gradually are replaced by connective tissue and fat. The muscles are flabby on palpation and are flat in appearance. Fasciculations may be present in some cases.

Hypertonia

In **hypertonia (increased muscle tone),** passive movement of a muscle occurs with resistance to stretch and is caused by upper motor neuron damage. Four types of hypertonia are described: spasticity, gegenhalten (paratonia), dystonia, and rigidity.

Spasticity results from hyperexcitability of the stretch reflexes (overactivation of the alpha motor neurons) and is associated with damage to the motor, premotor, and supplementary motor areas, as well as lateral corticospinal tract damage (Figure 17-21). Spasticity is accompanied by increased deep tendon reflexes (hyperreflexia) and the spread of reflexes (clonus).

Gegenhalten (paratonia) is resistance to passive movement that increases with velocity of movement. **Dystonia** is increased involuntary muscle contraction, manifested as sustained, involuntary twisting movements. It is caused by slow muscle contraction and may be caused by a failure in appropriate reciprocal inhibition of the muscles (Figures 17-22 and 17-23).

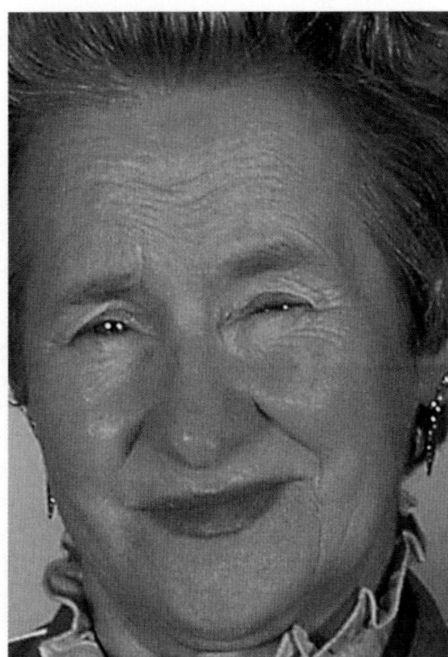

FIGURE 17-21 Left-Sided Hemifacial Spasm. (From Perkin GD: *Mosby's color atlas and text of neurology,* London, 1998, Mosby-Wolfe.)

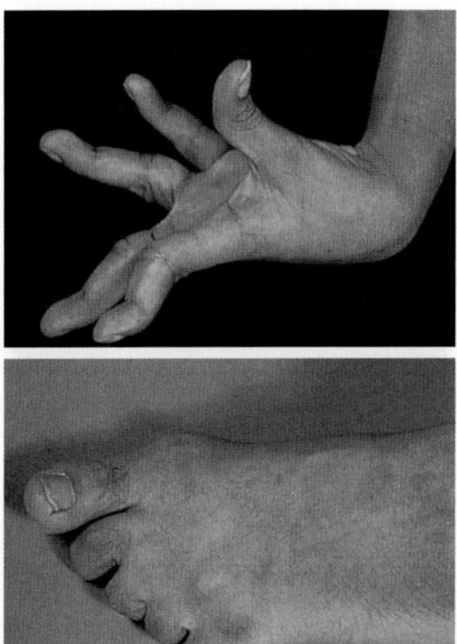

FIGURE 17-22 Dystonic Posturing of the Hand and Foot. (From Perkin GD: *Mosby's color atlas and text of neurology,* London, 1998, Mosby-Wolfe.)

Injury to the putamen or its outflow tracts also is associated with hemidystonia.

Rigidity produced by tonic reflex activity mediated by gamma motor neurons may be continuous or intermittent. The involved muscles are firm and tense; the increase in muscle movement is even and uniform throughout the range of passive movement. Four types of rigidity are described: plastic, or lead-pipe; cogwheel; gamma; and alpha (see Table 17-20).

Individuals with hypertonia may tire easily (asthenia) or be weak. Passive movement and active movement are equally affected, except in gegenhalten, in which more active than passive movement is possible. As a result of hypertonia and weakness, accident proneness during locomotion and self-care activities is common.

The muscles may atrophy because of decreased use. However, hypertrophy occasionally may occur in some diseases. Hypertrophy results from overstimulation of muscle fibers. Overstimulation occurs when the motor unit reflex arc remains intact and functioning but is not inhibited by higher centers. The loss of inhibition and the constant state of excitation cause continual muscle contraction, resulting in enlargement of the muscle mass. The muscles are firm on palpation (Figure 17-24).

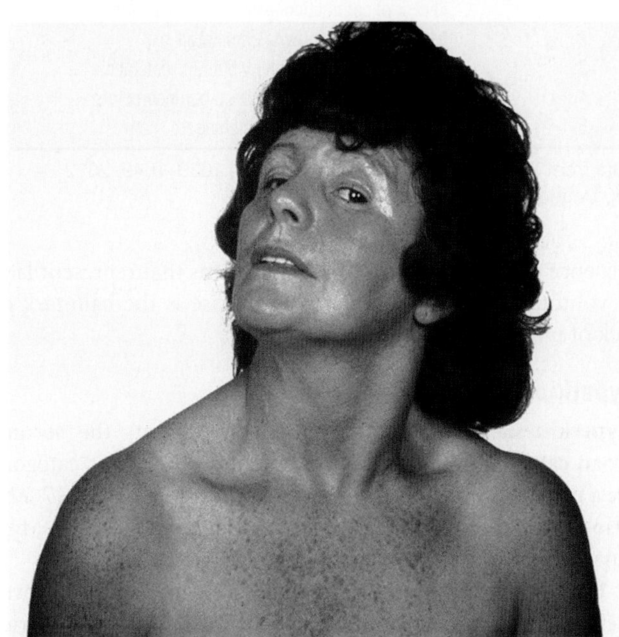

FIGURE 17-23 Spasmodic Torticollis. A characteristic head posture. (From Perkin GD et al: *Atlas of clinical neurology,* ed 3, Philadelphia, 2011, Saunders.)

Alterations in Movement

Movement requires a change in the contractile state of muscles. Abnormal movements may occur when a variety of CNS dysfunctions alter muscular innervation. The neurotransmitter *dopamine* has a role in motor function. Some movement disorders (e.g., the akinesias) result from too little dopaminergic activity, whereas others (e.g., chorea, ballism, tardive dyskinesia) result from too much dopaminergic activity. Still others are not related primarily to dopamine function. Movement disorders are not associated necessarily with mass, strength, or tone but are neurologic dysfunctions with either an excess of movement or a lack of voluntary movement. Muscle strength is quantitatively evaluated on a scale of 0 to 4+ or 0 to 5, in which 4+ or 5 is normal and 0 indicates an inability to move against gravity (Table 17-21).

Hyperkinesia (excessive movements), *dyskinesias* (unnatural movements), and *abnormal involuntary movements* represent excess movement. Huntington disease is the hallmark of excess movement. *Hypokinesia* (decreased amplitude of movement), *bradykinesia* (decreased speed of movement), and *akinesia*

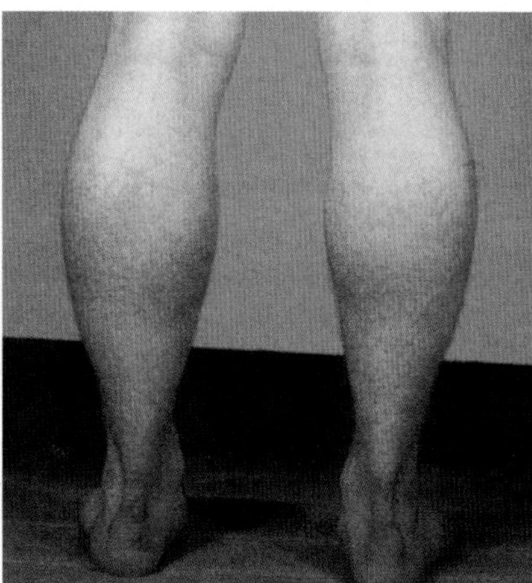

FIGURE 17-24 Pseudohypertrophy of the Calf Muscles. (From Perkin GD et al: *Atlas of clinical neurology,* ed 3, Philadelphia, 2011, Saunders)

TABLE 17-21 UK MEDICAL RESEARCH COUNCIL CLASSIFICATION OF MUSCLE POWER

GRADE	DEFINITION
0	Total paralysis—no muscle contraction
1	Flicker of contraction—no joint movement
2	Movement with gravity eliminated
3	Movement against gravity but not resistance
4	Movement against resistance but incomplete
5	Normal power against resistance

Data from Vanhoutte EK et al: *Brain* 135(Pt 5):1639–1649, 2012.
UK, United Kingdom.

(absence of voluntary movement) are terms that represent lack of voluntary movement. Parkinson disease is the hallmark of lack of movement.

Hyperkinesia

Hyperkinesia (excessive movement) represents the second broad category of abnormal movements. Within this category are a number of specific hyperkinesia syndromes (Table 17-22). Also included in the general category of hyperkinesias are dyskinesias, that is, abnormal involuntary movements.

Paroxysmal dyskinesias are abnormal, involuntary movements that occur as spasms. The type of dyskinesia varies depending on the specific disorder.

Tardive (slow onset) **dyskinesia** is the involuntary movement of the face, trunk, and extremities. Although the condition occurs occasionally in individuals with Parkinson disease, it usually occurs as a side effect of prolonged use of first- or second-generation antipsychotic drugs.[70] The antipsychotic drugs cause denervation hypersensitivity, thereby mimicking the effect of excessive dopamine. The most common symptom of tardive dyskinesia is rapid, repetitive, stereotypic movements. The most characteristic movements of tardive dyskinesia include continual chewing with intermittent protrusions of the tongue, lip smacking, and facial grimacing. Stereotypic movements are believed to be a form of excessive dopaminergic activity.

WHAT'S NEW?

Tourette Syndrome

There is growing evidence that Tourette syndrome (TS) occurs worldwide and, has common features across all races and cultures. No specific genetic mutations have been found. The hallmark of TS is the presence of multiple motor and vocal tics. The tics may be simple, involving only an individual muscle group (for example, eye blinking or a grunt), or complex, requiring coordinated movement of muscle groups (for example, head banging or repeating of another person's words). Sensory tics involve unpleasant sensations in the face, head, and neck areas. Onset of TS is typically between the ages of 2 and 15 years, is more common in males, and is probably underdiagnosed. The tics lessen in adulthood. The syndrome has a complex, multifactorial etiology with as yet to be determined genetic, environmental, immune, and hormonal factors. The pathophysiology of TS is unclear and currently under study. There is evidence of basal ganglia dysfunction and, in some cases, altered dopaminergic neurotransmission. TS is often diagnosed in association with anxiety, depression, attention-deficit/hyperactivity disorder (ADHD), and obsessive-compulsive disorder.

Data from Bloch M, State M, Pittenger C: *Curr Opin Neurol* 24(2):119–125, 2011; Deng H, Gao K, Jankovic J: *Nat Rev Neurol* 8(4):203–213, 2012; Jankovic J, Kurlan R: *Mov Disord* 26(6):1149–1156, 2011; State MW: *Curr Opin Genet Dev* 21(3):302–309, 2011.

Other movement disorders under this category are (1) complex repetitive movements, including automatism, stereotype, complex tics (e.g., Tourette syndrome [see What's New? Tourette Syndrome]), compulsions, perseverations, and mannerisms; (2) positivism (excessive reactions to certain stimuli); and (3) paroxysmal excessive activity, including cataplexy and excessive startle reaction.

Huntington Disease

Huntington disease (HD), also known as *chorea,* is a relatively rare, autosomal dominant disease with high penetrance. The onset of HD is usually between 25 and 45 years of age, when the trait may already have been passed to the person's children. The disorder has a prevalence rate of approximately 2 to 8 per 100,000 persons and occurs in all races.[71]

PATHOPHYSIOLOGY. The genetic defect of HD is on the short arm of chromosome 4. There is an abnormally long polyglutamine tract in the huntingtin (htt) protein that is toxic to neurons and is caused by a cytosine-adenine-guanine (CAG) trinucleotide repeat expansion (40 to 70 repeats instead of 9 to 34). Age of symptom onset is related to the length of the repeat sequences and mechanisms of toxicity. Repeat lengths greater than 60 cause the juvenile form of the disease.[72]

The principal pathologic feature of HD is severe degeneration of the basal ganglia, particularly the caudate and putamen nuclei and the frontal cerebral cortex. The degeneration of the basal ganglia leaves enlarged lateral ventricles (Figure 17-25). Expression of the *huntingtin* gene produces tangles of protein that collect in brain cells and chains of glutamine on the abnormal molecules that adhere to each other.[73] The mechanism of neuronal death is unknown. The excitotoxic theory of striatal and cortical degeneration proposes that the mutated huntingtin protein produces excitotoxic pathways meditated by glutamate function that also induce concomitant dysregulation of

TABLE 17-22 TYPES OF HYPERKINESIA SYNDROMES

TYPE	CHARACTERISTICS	CAUSES
Chorea*	Nonrepetitive muscular contractions, usually of the extremities of the face; random pattern of irregular, involuntary rapid contractions of groups of muscles; disappears with sleep, decreases with resting; increases with emotional stress and attempted voluntary movement	Associated with excess concentration of or a supersensitivity to dopamine within basal ganglia
Athetosis*	Disorder of distal-muscle postural fixation; slow, twisting, sinuous, irregular movements most obvious in the distal extremities, more rhythmic than choreiform movements and always much slower; movements accompany characteristic hand posture; slowly fluctuating grimaces	Occurs most commonly as a result of injury to the putamen of the basal ganglion; exact pathophysiologic mechanism is not known
Ballism	Disorder of proximal-muscle postural fixation with wild flinging movement of the limbs; movement is severe and stereotyped, usually lateral; does not lessen with sleep; ballism is most common on one side of the body, a condition termed hemiballism	Results from injury (vascular disease) to the subthalamic nucleus (one of the nuclei that comprise the basal ganglia); thought to be caused by reduced inhibitory influence in the nucleus, a release phenomenon; hemiballism results from injury to the contralateral subthalamic nucleus
Hyperactivity	State of prolonged, generalized, increased activity that is largely involuntary but may be subject to some voluntary control; not highly stereotyped but rather manifests as continual changes in total body posture or in excessive performance of some simple activity, such as pacing under inappropriate circumstances	May be caused by frontal and reticular activating system injury
Wandering	Tendency to wander without regard for environment	"Release" phenomenon; associated with bilateral injury to globus pallidus or putamen
Akathisia	Special type of hyperactivity; mild compulsion to move (usually more localized to legs); severe frenzied motion possible; movements are partly voluntary and may be transiently suppressed; carrying out the movement brings a sense of relief; a frequent complication of antipsychotic drugs	Dopaminergic transmission may be involved
Tremor at Rest	Rhythmic, oscillating movement affecting one or more body parts	Caused by regular contraction of opposing groups of muscles
Parkinsonian tremor	Regular, rhythmic, slow flexion-extension contraction; involves principally the metacarpophalangeal and wrist joints; alternating movements between thumb and index finger described as "pill rolling"; disappears during voluntary movement	Loss of inhibitory influence of dopamine in the basal ganglia, causing instability of basal ganglia feedback circuit within the cerebral cortex
Postural Tremor		
Asterixis (tremor of hepatic encephalopathy)	Irregular flapping movement of the hands accentuated by outstretching arms	Caused by transient inhibition of muscles that maintain posture; thought to be related to accumulation of products normally detoxified by the liver
Metabolic	Rapid, rhythmic tremor affecting fingers, lips, and tongue; accentuated by extending the body part; enhanced physiologic tremor	Occurs in conditions associated with disturbed metabolism or toxicity, as in thyrotoxicosis (hyperthyroidism), alcoholism, and chronic use of barbiturates, amphetamines, lithium, amitriptyline (Elavil); exact mechanism responsible unknown
Essential (familial)	Tremor of fingers, hands, and feet; absent at rest but accentuated by extension of body part, prolonged muscular activity, and stress	Not associated with any other neurologic abnormalities; cause unknown
Intentional Tremor		
Cerebellar	Tremor initiated by movement, maximal toward end of movement	Occurs in disease of the dentate nucleus (one of the deep cerebellar nuclei responsible for efferent output) and the superior cerebellar peduncle (a stalklike structure connected to the pons); caused by errors in feedback from the periphery and errors in preprogramming goal-directed movement
Rubral	Rhythmic tremor of limbs that originates proximally by movement	Results from lesions involving the dentatorubrothalamic tract (a spinothalamic tract connecting the red nucleus in the reticular formation and the dentate nucleus in the cerebellum)
Myoclonus	Series of shocklike, nonpatterned contractions of a portion of a muscle, entire muscle, or group of muscles that cause throwing movements of a limb; usually appear at random but frequently triggered by sudden startle; do not disappear during sleep	Associated with an irritable nervous system and spontaneous discharge of neurons; structures associated with myoclonus include the cerebral cortex, cerebellum, reticular formation, and spinal cord

*Choreoathetosis involves chorea and athetosis; precise pathophysiology unknown.

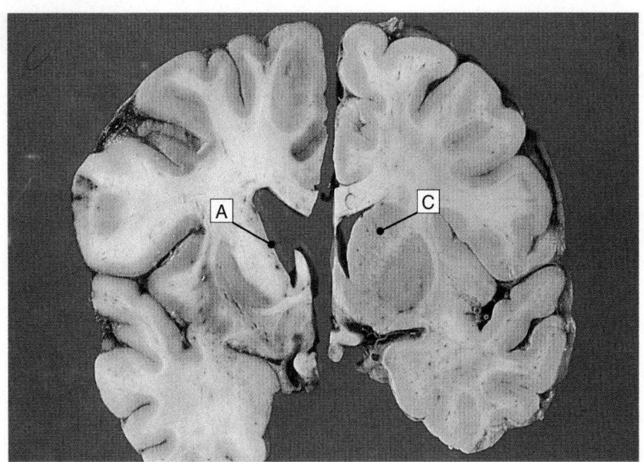

FIGURE 17-25 Huntington Disease. On the right is a normal brain with a normal caudate *(C)*; on the left is a brain from an individual with Huntington disease showing severe atrophy of the caudate *(A)* and an enlarged lateral ventricle. (From Stevens A, Lowe J, Scott I: *Core pathology*, ed 3, London, 2009, Mosby.)

dopaminergic function. The huntingtin protein also may alter mitochondrial function, which in turn activates apoptotic pathways and causes neuronal death. Neurotrophic factors also may be depleted, leading to loss of neurons.[73-75]

Early in the disease, selective loss of the striatal GABA/dopamine-enkephalin pathway to the lateral aspect of the pallidum occurs. The striatum of the basal ganglia normally contains a preponderance of GABAergic (GABA-secreting) neurons, including the pathway between the basal ganglia and substantia nigra (pallidonigral pathway–express dopamine D_1-receptors, dynorphin, and substance P). Basal ganglia and nigral depletion of GABA, an inhibitory neurotransmitter, is the principal biochemical alteration in HD. Degeneration of the GABAergic pallidonigral pathway causes GABA depletion in the substantia nigra with decreased inhibitory GABA activity on dopaminergic neurons in the substantia nigra and a relative excess of dopaminergic activity in the basal ganglia feedback circuit within the cerebral cortex. A relative excess of dopaminergic activity in this circuit, as in HD, is manifested by hypotonia and hyperkinesia (involuntary, fragmentary movements such as chorea). Loss of excitatory glutamate may liberate the pathway from the thalamus to the premotor cortex, impairing modulation of movement later in the course of the disease. Producing energy for brain activity is difficult and there is resultant buildup of lactic acid.

CLINICAL MANIFESTATIONS. The classic manifestations of HD are abnormal movements that occur without conscious effort, emotional lability, and progressive dysfunction of cognitive processes (dementia). Any one of these features may mark the onset of the disease. Cognitive impairment may precede motor symptoms by up to 15 years.[76] Chorea is the most common type of abnormal movement and begins in the face and arms, eventually affecting the entire body. It can be combined with athetosis (twisting and writhing). Symptoms of frontal lobe dysfunction include executive attention deficits and short-term memory loss (working memory); reduced capacity to plan, organize, and sequence, as well as bradyphrenia (slow thinking); and apathy. Restlessness, disinhibition, and irritability are common. Affectively, euphoria or depression or both may be present. Progression of the disease is fatal.

EVALUATION AND TREATMENT. The diagnosis of HD is based on family history, clinical presentation of the disorder, and genetic testing. No known treatment is effective in halting the degeneration or progression of symptoms. Chorea is treated with dopamine receptor–blocking or dopamine receptor–depleting agents. Medication and nonmedical care for depression and aggressive behavior may be required. Efforts are in progress to identify biomarkers for early diagnosis and to monitor disease progression.[77,78]

Hypokinesia

Hypokinesia (decreased movement) is loss of voluntary movement despite preserved consciousness and normal peripheral nerve and muscle function. Types of hypokinesia include akinesia, bradykinesia, and loss of associated movement.

Akinesia. **Akinesia** is an absence, poverty, or lack of control of associated and voluntary muscle movements. There is a disturbance in the time it takes to perform a movement. Akinesia is related to dysfunction of the extrapyramidal system, as in parkinsonism. Pathogenesis is related to either a deficiency of dopamine or a defect of the postsynaptic dopamine receptors, which occurs in parkinsonism (see Parkinson disease below).

Bradykinesia. **Bradykinesia** is slowness of voluntary movements. There is a disturbance in the time it takes to perform a movement. In bradykinesia all voluntary movements become slow, labored, and deliberate. Bradykinesia consists of: (1) difficulty in initiating movements, (2) difficulty in continuing movements smoothly, and (3) difficulty in performing synchronous (at the same time) and consecutive tasks. Difficulty in initiating movements ranges from slight hesitancy to severe **freezing** (transient, helpless immobility). Each intended movement requires effort. Difficulty in continuing motions smoothly causes jerky, irregular, rapid movements, which then decrease in rate and amplitude until they stop. The individual is scarcely aware of the cessation. Difficulty in performing synchronous and consecutive tasks means that each motor act is performed separately. The individual is unable to integrate two acts or to change from one motor pattern to the next with a single smooth motion.

Loss of Associated Movement. In hypokinesia the normal, habitually associated movements that provide skill, grace, and balance to voluntary movements are lost. Decreased associated movements accompanying emotional expression cause an expressionless face, a statue-like posture, absence of speech inflection, and absence of spontaneous gestures. Decreased associated movements accompanying locomotion cause reduction in arm and shoulder movements, in hip swinging, and in rotary motion of the cervical spine.

Parkinson Disease

Parkinson disease (PD) is a complex motor disorder accompanied by systemic nonmotor and neurologic symptoms. The main disease feature is degeneration of the basal ganglia (corpus striatum, globus pallidus, subthalamic nucleus, and substantia nigra) involving the dopaminergic (dopamine-secreting) nigrostriatal pathway. Nigrostriatal disorders produce a

BOX 17-5 PRIMARY AND SECONDARY CAUSES OF PARKINSONISM

Primary Parkinsonism

Sporadic (idiopathic); most common form

Genetic: autosomal dominant; autosomal recessive

Phenotype may be influenced by gene-environment interactions

Secondary Parkinsonism

Neurodegenerative disorders (sporadic or genetic)

- Disorders associated with alpha-synuclein pathology
  - Multiple system atrophies (glial and neuronal inclusions)
    - Nigrostriatal degeneration
    - Olivopontocerebellar atrophy
    - Shy-Drager syndrome
    - Motor neuron disease with PD features
  - Dementia with Lewy bodies (cortical and brainstem neuronal inclusions)
- Disorders associated with primary tau pathology ("tauopathies")
  - Progressive supranuclear palsy
  - Corticobasal degeneration
  - Frontotemporal dementia
- Disorders associated with primary amyloid pathology ("amyloidopathies")
  - Alzheimer disease with parkinsonism

Genetically mediated disorders with occasional parkinsonian features

- Wilson disease
- Hallervorden-Spatz disease
- Chédiak-Higashi syndrome
- SCA-3 spinocerebellar ataxia
- X-linked dystonia-parkinsonism *(DYT3)*
- Fragile X permutation associated with ataxia-tremor-parkinsonism syndrome
- Huntington disease (Westphal variant)
- Prion disease

Miscellaneous acquired conditions

- Vascular parkinsonism: atherosclerosis, amyloid angiopathy
- Normal pressure hydrocephalus
- Catatonia
- Cerebral palsy

Repeated head trauma ("dementia pugilistica" with parkinsonian features)

Infectious and postinfectious diseases

- Postencephalitic PD
- Creutzfeldt-Jakob disease
- Neurosyphilis

Metabolic conditions

- Hypoparathyroidism or pseudohypoparathyroidism with basal ganglia calcifications
- Non-wilsonian hepatolenticular degeneration

Multiple sclerosis

Neoplastic disease

Drugs

- Neuroleptics (typical antipsychotics)
- Selected atypical antipsychotics
- Antiemetics (e.g., compazine, metoclopramide)
- Dopamine-depleting agents (reserpine, tetrabenazine)
- α-Methyldopa
- Lithium carbonate
- Valproic acid
- Fluoxetine

Toxins

- 1-Methyl-1,2,4,6-tetrahydropyridine (MPTP)
- Manganese
- Cyanide
- Methanol
- Carbon monoxide
- Carbon disulfide
- Hexane

Data from Delong MR, Juncos IL: Parkinson's disease and other extrapyramidal movement disorders. In Fauci AS et al, editors: *Harrison's principles of internal medicine,* ed 17, p 2553, New York, 2008, McGraw-Hill; Lang A: Parkinsonism. In Goldman L, Ausiello D, editors: *Cecil medicine,* ed 23, p 2726, Philadelphia, 2008, Saunders.

syndrome of abnormal movement called **parkinsonism (Parkinson syndrome, parkinsonian syndrome).**

Etiologic classification of parkinsonism includes primary parkinsonism and secondary parkinsonism (Box 17-5). The onset of PD occurs after 40 years of age, with mean onset of 60 years of age.[79] PD is one of the most prevalent of the primary CNS disorders and a leading cause of neurologic disability in individuals older than 60 years. Approximately 60,000 people in the United States are diagnosed each year and an estimated 10 million people worldwide are living with PD. Men are 150% more likely to have PD than women.[80] The familial form represents about 10% of PD; however, the majority of cases are sporadic or idiopathic.

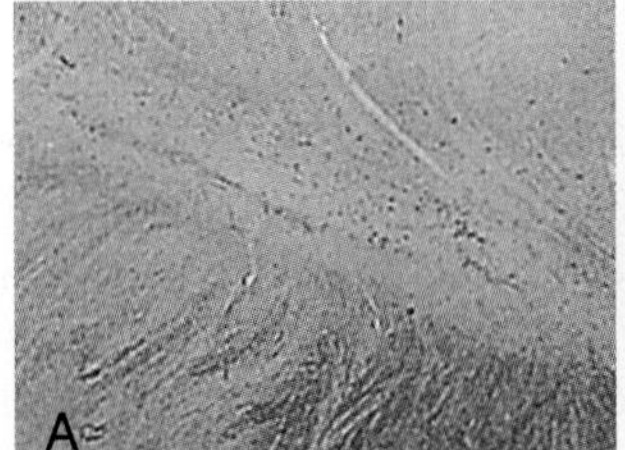

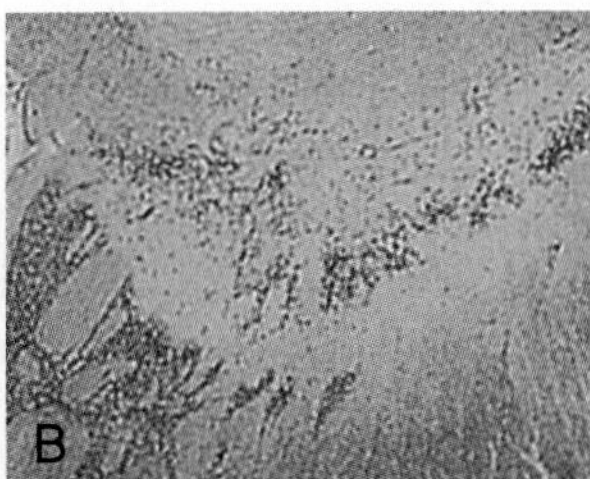

FIGURE 17-26 Atrophic Substantia Nigra (A) Compared with Normal Control (B). (From Perkin GD et al: *Atlas of clinical neurology,* ed 3, Philadelphia, 2011, Saunders.)

PATHOPHYSIOLOGY. The pathogenesis of primary PD is unknown. Several PD genes have been identified, the most significant of which are listed in Table 17-13 (p. 547). The hallmark pathologic features of PD are loss of dopaminergic pigmented neurons in the substantia nigra (SN) pars compacta with dopaminergic deficiency in the putamen portion of the striatum (the striatum includes the putamen and caudate nucleus) (Figure 17-26). Dopamine loss in other brain areas including the brainstem, thalamus, and cortex also occurs.[81] Degeneration of the dopaminergic nigrostriatal pathway to the basal ganglia results in underactivity of the direct motor pathway (normally facilitates movement) (Figure 17-27) and overactivity of the indirect motor loop (normally inhibits movement). This results in inhibition of the motor cortex manifested with *bradykinesia* and *rigidity*. The subthalamic nucleus (STN) overactivity also influences the limbic system,[79] accounting for emotional signs and symptoms. Neuronal loss within the cerebral cortex is found in half of individuals with PD. Mechanisms of cell dysfunction and death

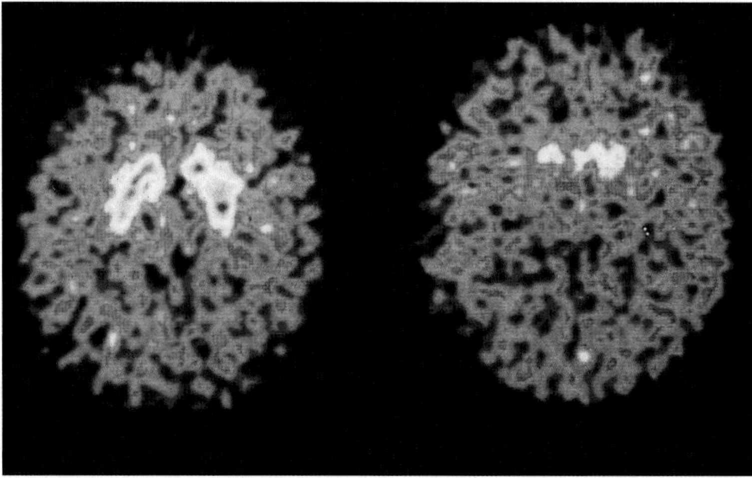

FIGURE 17-27 Reduced Fluorodopa in Parkinson Disease. Positron-emission tomography scan showing reduced fluorodopa uptake in the basal ganglia consistent with neurodegeneration *(right)* compared with a normal control *(left).* (From Perkin GD et al: *Atlas of clinical neurology,* ed 3, Philadelphia, 2011, Saunders.)

include mitochondrial dysfunction, oxidative stress, altered protein handling, and inflammatory changes with autophagy and apoptosis.[82]

Lewy bodies, fibrillar intracellular eosinophilic inclusions, and high concentrations of alpha-synuclein, ubiquitin, tau protein, tuberculin, and other proteins are found in the substantia nigra (SN), locus ceruleus (LC), and other areas of the brain. They are a marker for neuronal degeneration.[83] Degeneration of the LC, which contains noradrenergic neurons, also occurs in PD. Norepinephrine is thought to be neuroprotective and loss of LC neurons may be associated with a worsening of disease progression and the behavioral symptoms of PD.[84] Molecular events thought to be associated with the neurodegeneration of PD include mitochondrial dysfunction, oxidative stress, abnormal folding and accumulation of alpha-synuclein, abnormal phosphorylation, and dysfunction of the ubiquitin proteasome system (regulates intracellular protein processing)[85,86] (Figure 17-28).

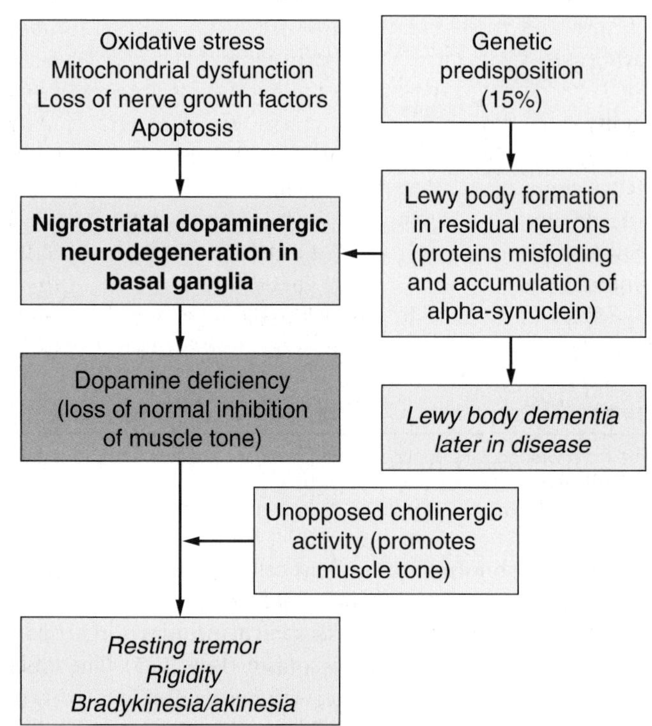

FIGURE 17-28 Pathophysiology of Parkinson Disease.

CLINICAL MANIFESTATIONS. Onset of symptoms is insidious and symptoms appear after a 70% to 80% loss of pigmented nigral neurons and a 60% to 90% loss of striatal dopamine.[87] The classic motor manifestations of PD are resting tremor, bradykinesia/akinesia (poverty of movement), rigidity (muscle stiffness), and postural abnormalities. These manifestations may develop alone or in combination; however, as the disease progresses, all four are usually present to at least some degree. There is no true paralysis. A modified Hoehn and Yahr scale[88] can be used to assess progression of symptoms:

0 No visible disease
1 Unilateral involvement, may have tremor of one limb
2 Bilateral involvement, balance intact
3 Bilateral involvement, slowing of body movement, mild to moderate postural instability, and gait difficulty
4 Bilateral involvement with severe postural instability, rigidity, and bradykinesia present
5 Bilateral involvement with inability to walk, confinement to wheelchair, cachexia present

In early stages of the disease, reflex, sensory, and mental status are usually normal. Nonmotor symptoms associated with PD include hyposmia, fatigue, pain, autonomic dysfunction, sleep fragmentation, depression, and dementia with or without psychosis.[89]

Parkinsonian tremor, the most conspicuous and most variable symptom, is usually the first motor symptom to appear. It is a tremor at rest, disappearing briefly during the course of a voluntary movement and reappearing when the limb is held in a stationary position. Intensity and amplitude of the tremor vary. The arm is more affected than the leg. Most individuals with PD have this tremor and tremors are increased by stress and anxiety.

Parkinsonian tremor appears to result from instability of feedback from the basal ganglia to the cerebral cortex caused by loss of the inhibitory influence of dopamine in the basal ganglia. Increased oscillation in the normal feedback cycles of the motor outflow feedback circuit when the muscles are at rest produces the tremor. When the individual performs voluntary movements, the tremor becomes temporarily blocked, presumably because other motor control signals arriving in the thalamus override the abnormal basal ganglia signals. As the disorder worsens, tremor may lessen as rigidity supervenes. The postural tremor is associated with damage to the cerebellofugal pathway to the red nucleus, a pathway that subserves communication from muscle spindles to the thalamus and motor cortex.

Parkinsonian rigidity is an increased resistance to the passive movement of a joint that impedes active and passive movement. The first symptoms of rigidity may be painful muscle cramps in the toes or hands. More commonly the limb feels stiff, heavy, tired, or aching. **Plastic rigidity** is constant throughout the entire range of motion and is felt as lead-pipe resistance during passive movement. **Cogwheel rigidity,** brief palpable jerks, is accompanied by tremor. The mechanism underlying rigidity is unclear, but there is increased resting muscle activity of antagonistic muscle groups with enhancement of the long-latency component of the stretch reflex.[79]

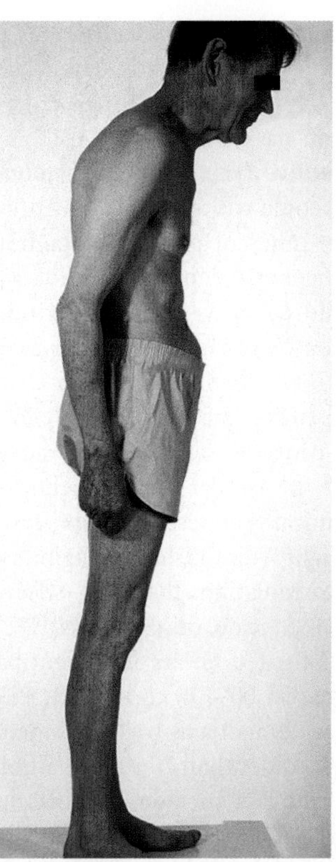

FIGURE 17-29 Stooped Posture of Parkinson Disease. (From Perkin GD et al: *Atlas of clinical neurology,* ed 3, Philadelphia, 2011, Saunders.)

Parkinsonian bradykinesia is poverty of associated and voluntary movements. It is the most prevalent and crippling symptom and often is overlooked in the early stages. The pathophysiology underlying the bradykinesia is an overactive subthalamic nucleus (STN) that inhibits the motor thalamus and motor cortex.[79] It is associated with dopamine deficiency and failure of the mechanism programming movement patterns manifested as a defect in the voluntary production of smooth motions at different speeds.[90]

All striated muscles—extremity, trunk, ocular, facial—are affected eventually, including muscles of mastication (chewing), deglutition (swallowing), and articulation. Micrographia (small handwriting) is present. Extreme underactivity in the individual with PD makes the person appear stiff, even when resistance to passive movement cannot be felt. Bradykinesia is a separate phenomenon from rigidity and may be severe even in the presence of rigidity. Individuals state that they feel "wooden" (as though moving against resistance) and complain of rapid, severe fatigue.

Hypokinesia, or decreased frequency or absence of associated movements, is one of the earliest symptoms. Individuals with PD sit and lie motionless for long periods without the little shifts an unaffected person makes to prevent discomfort and stiffness. Bradykinesia, or slowness of voluntary movements, is characterized by difficulty initiating, continuing, or synchronizing movements. Both associated and voluntary movements are interspersed by freezing (an inability to continue movement). Freezing may be precipitated by (1) increasing the effort to move, (2) turning, and (3) initiating certain types of tactile and visual contact.

Postural Abnormalities. Three types of postural abnormalities occur in individuals with PD: (1) disorders of postural fixation, (2) disorders of equilibrium, and (3) disorders of righting. The disorder of postural fixation associated with PD is involuntary flexion of the head and neck. The individual is unable to maintain an upright position of the trunk while standing or walking. Postural abnormalities of the hands and feet also occur. Postural abnormalities are caused by a loss of normal postural reflexes, muscular rigidity, axial dystonia, weakness caused by myopathy, and impaired proprioception.[91]

Disorders of equilibrium result from loss of postural stability. The person with PD is unable to make the appropriate postural adjustment to tilting or falling and falls like a post when starting to tilt. The festinating gait (short, accelerating steps) of the person with PD is an attempt to maintain an upright position while walking (Figure 17-29). Individuals also are unable to right themselves when changing from a reclining or crouching position to a standing position and when rolling over from a supine to a lateral or prone position.

Autonomic and Neuroendocrine Symptoms. Autonomic and neuroendocrine dysfunctions in PD produce nonmotor symptoms that are distressing but not incapacitating. The basal ganglia influence hypothalamic function (autonomic and neuroendocrine) through pathways connecting the hypothalamus with the basal ganglia and cerebral cortex. Common autonomic symptoms in PD include inappropriate diaphoresis, gastric retention, constipation, and urinary retention. Cardiac sympathetic denervation is common and causes neurogenic orthostatic hypotension. A symptom attributed to neuroendocrine dysfunction is seborrhea. Hypothalamic hypersecretion of hormone-releasing factors acting on the anterior pituitary causes hypersecretion of androgenotropic hormones, producing sebum hypersecretion by sebaceous glands. The resulting seborrhea is characterized by oily skin with seborrheic dermatitis along the hairline and in chin-nasal creases.[92]

Cognitive-Affective Symptoms and Dementia. Approximately 30% to 40% of people with PD have a depression that is now believed to be an inherent part of the pathologic state of the disease (an endogenous depression), not a response to the situation.[93,94] Mild cognitive impairment not associated with either dementia or depression is associated with dopaminergic dysmodulation. *Bradyphrenia* (slowness of thinking) also is present. These disorders may appear early in the course of the disease and may progress to dementia. Bradyphrenia is caused by disruption of the caudal basal ganglion connections and outflows. The clinical manifestations are slowness of thinking, poverty of thought (diminished imagination and insight), and difficulty formulating thoughts (decreased ability to conceptualize, plan, decide, or improvise).[95]

Of individuals treated on an outpatient basis for PD, 30% have a dementia, and 80% of those with PD requiring institutional care have dementia as well.[96] Dementia is more common in individuals older than 70 years. Pathologically, in those with dementia, findings include loss of cholinergic cells in the basal nucleus of Meynert (nucleus basalis); neuronal loss, senile plaques, and neurofibrillary tangles in the neocortex; and amyloid changes in small blood vessels. Lewy bodies (alpha-synuclein inclusions) are distributed diffusely in many neurons, making this a Lewy body dementia.[97] The individual evidences disorientation; confusion; memory loss; distractibility; and difficulty with concept formation, abstraction, calculations, thinking, and judgment. Although the symptoms fluctuate, they progressively worsen. Anxiety disorders, impulse-control disorders, and punding (a disorder of stereotypical motor behavior in which there is intense fascination with repetitive handling and examining of mechanical objects) are recognized features of PD.

Other nonmotor symptoms are common in PD including sensory dysfunction with anosmia, ageusia, pain, paresthesias, fatigue and weight loss, sweating, urinary and gastrointestinal dysfunction, and eye tremor.[98,99] Sleep disorders are common including disturbances in the sleep-wake cycle, excessive daytime sleepiness, obstructive sleep apnea, and restless leg syndrome.[100]

Influence of Symptoms. Early in the disease, people often experience a sleep benefit; that is, symptoms decrease with sleep. Symptoms also fluctuate in an on-off pattern. Stress influences symptoms adversely, but the underlying mechanism is unclear. The person's mental status may be further compromised by the side effects of the medication taken to control symptoms.

The combination of all the parkinsonian symptoms gives the individual a characteristic appearance: a wide-eyed, unblinking, staring expression with the facial muscles smoothed out and almost immobile. Saliva frequently drools from the corners of the slightly open mouth. The skin of the face is frequently greasy. The gait is pathognomonic: the individual walks with slow, short, shuffling steps; the arms are flexed, abducted, and held stiffly at the side; and the trunk is bent slightly forward. The person may break into a run spontaneously or when pushed forward or backward. Because of the disorder of postural fixation, the tendency is to fall to the side. Postural instability, sleep disorders, and difficulty concentrating are some of the most depressing symptoms for people with PD.[101]

EVALUATION AND TREATMENT. The diagnosis of primary PD is made on the basis of the four cardinal symptoms: (1) resting tremor, (2) cogwheel rigidity, (3) akinesia, and (4) postural instability. This group of symptoms has the acronym TRAP.[102] The exclusion of other causes of parkinsonism and a combination of imaging techniques, clinical evaluations, biochemical markers, and genetic tests support the diagnosis of PD.[103,104] Early nonmotor symptoms of PD can precede motor symptoms and their identification may assist early diagnosis and guide disease-modifying strategies.[103,105] Median time between diagnosis and death is between 7 and 15 years. Disease progression varies with age of disease onset, comorbidities, quality of care, and among different populations.[106,107]

The aim of drug therapy is to restore striatal dopamine levels using oral drugs such as levodopa (L-dopa), a precursor of dopamine (dopamine does not cross the blood-brain barrier), dopamine agonists that directly stimulate dopamine receptors, anticholinergic drugs, antihistamines, and amantadine; L-dopa is effective in reducing symptoms in early PD but can cause motor fluctuations, "off" periods, and dyskinesia in the long term. Monoamine oxidase B inhibitors, which inhibit the breakdown of endogenous dopamine, may improve symptoms, reduce motor fluctuations, and delay the need for L-dopa but can cause adverse effects. Adding catechol-*O*-methyltransferase (COMT) inhibitor prolongs the half-life of dopamine (COMT metabolizes dopamine in the synapse). Dopamine agonists to L-dopa or a dopamine agonist alone may reduce "off" time or improve symptoms but can also increase disability.[108] Surgery may be considered in later stages of PD. Thalamotomy and pallidotomy are surgical options. Deep brain stimulation is an approach to controlling medically resistant motor symptoms and L-dopa–related peak dose dyskinesia.[109] Gene- and cell-based therapies hold promise for future treatment.[110] Dysphagia and general immobility are special problems of the individual with PD requiring preventive, symptomatic, supportive, and rehabilitative management, such as physiotherapy and speech therapy.[99] Nursing interventions, occupational therapy (OT), physical therapy (PT), and speech, language, and swallowing therapy are effective and safe for improving functional status.

Upper and Lower Motor Neuron Syndromes

Paresis and paralysis are symptoms of upper and lower motor neuron syndromes (Table 17-23).

Paresis (weakness) is impairment of motor function, that is, partial paralysis with incomplete loss of muscle power. **Paralysis** is loss of motor function, that is, inability of a muscle group to overcome gravity. The characteristics of paresis or paralysis are related to involvement of either the upper or the lower motor neurons.

Upper Motor Neuron Syndromes. **Upper motor neuron paresis/paralysis** is known also as *spastic paresis/paralysis* and different terms are used to describe the specific disorders. **Hemiparesis** or **hemiplegia** is paresis or paralysis, respectively,

TABLE 17-23 UPPER AND LOWER MOTOR NEURON SIGNS AND SYMPTOMS

UPPER MOTOR NEURON (PYRAMIDAL CELLS [MOTOR CORTEX])	LOWER MOTOR NEURON (VENTRAL HORN [SPINAL CORD], MOTOR NUCLEI [BRAINSTEM])
Muscle groups are affected	Individual muscles may be affected
Mild weakness	Mild weakness
Minimal disuse muscle atrophy	Marked muscle atrophy
No fasciculations	Fasciculations
Increased muscle stretch reflexes (clasp-knife spasticity; resistance to passive flexion that releases abruptly to allow easy flexion)	Decreased muscle stretch reflexes
	Clonus not present
Clonus may be present	Hypotonia, flaccidity
Hypertonia, spasticity	Hyporeflexia
Pathologic reflexes (Babinski and Hoffmann signs, loss of abdominal reflexes)	No Babinski sign
Often initial impairment of only skilled movements	Asymmetric and may involve one limb only in beginning to become generalized as disease progresses

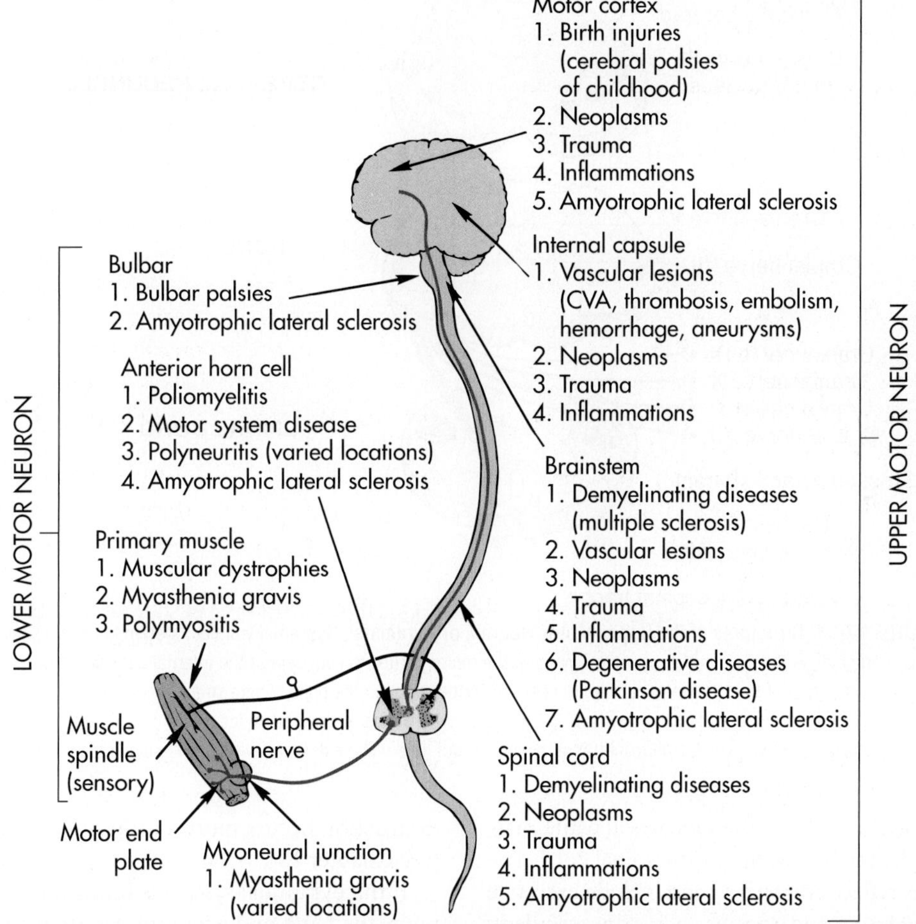

FIGURE 17-30 Disturbances in Motor Function. Disturbances in motor function are classified pathologically along upper and lower motor neuron structures. It should be noted that neoplasms occur at more than one site in an upper motor neuron *(above right)*. A few pathologic conditions, such as amyotrophic lateral sclerosis, involve upper and lower motor neuron structures. Other lesion sites include myoneural junctions and primary muscles, making it possible to classify conditions as neuromuscular and muscular, respectively. *CVA,* Cerebrovascular accident.

of the upper and lower extremities on one side. **Diplegia** is the paralysis of both upper and lower extremities as a result of cerebral hemisphere injuries. **Paraparesis** or **paraplegia** refers to weakness or paralysis, respectively, of the lower extremities. **Quadriparesis** or **quadriplegia** refers to paresis or paralysis of all four extremities. Paraparesis or paraplegia and quadriparesis or quadriplegia may be caused by dysfunction of the spinal cord. Upper cord damage results in quadriparesis or quadriplegia, and lower cord damage preserves upper extremity function and causes paraparesis or paraplegia (spinal cord injury is discussed in Chapter 18).

Upper motor neuron paresis/paralysis is associated with a pyramidal motor syndrome. The **pyramidal motor syndrome** is a series of motor dysfunctions that result from interruption of the pyramidal system (Figures 17-30 and 17-31). The

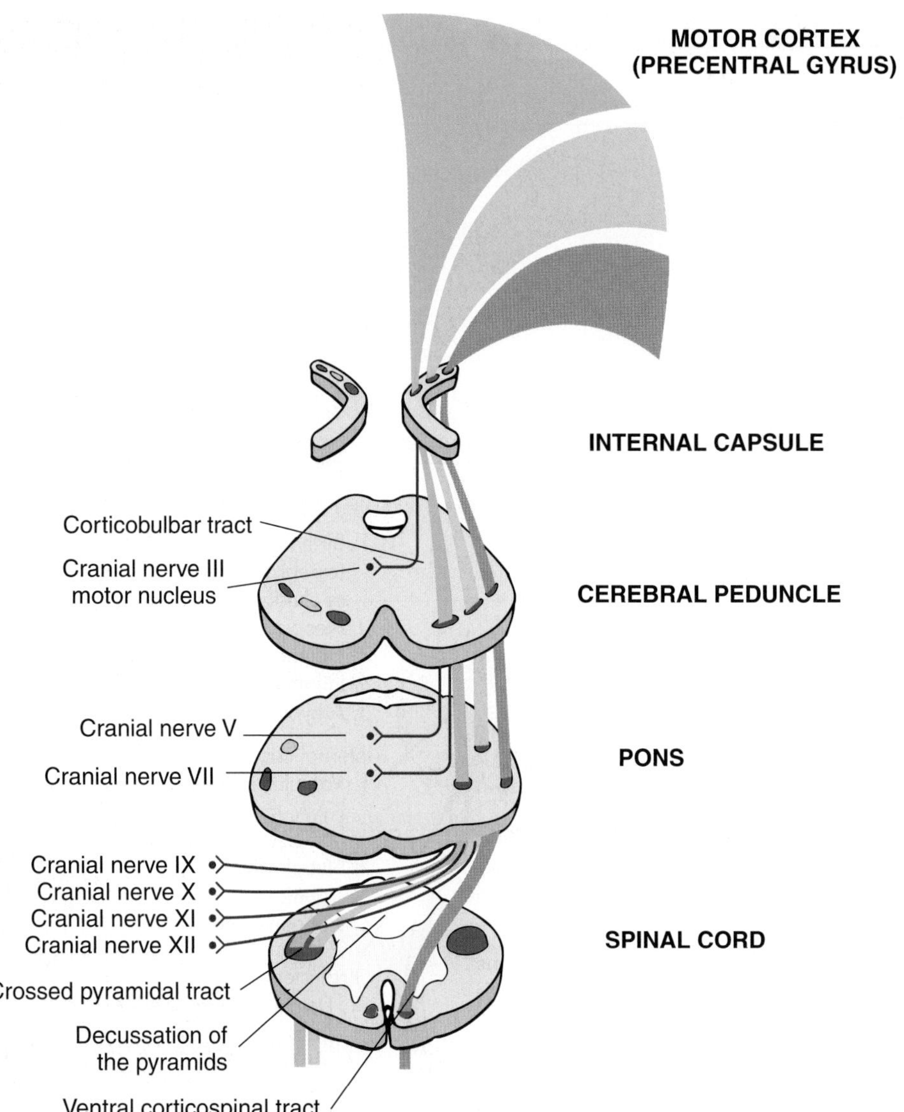

FIGURE 17-31 **Structures of the Upper Motor Neuron, or Pyramidal, System.** Pyramidal system fibers are shown to originate primarily in the cells in the precentral gyrus of the motor cortex; to converge at the internal capsule; to descend to form the central third of the cerebral peduncle; to descend farther through the pons, where small fibers supply cranial nerve motor nuclei along the way; to form pyramids at the medulla, where most of the fibers decussate; and then to continue to descend in the lateral column of the white matter of the spinal cord. A few fibers descend without crossing at the medulla level.

injury may be in the cerebral cortex, the subcortical white matter, the internal capsule, the brainstem, or the spinal cord. The clinical manifestations reflect overactivity and include excessive movements, such as clonus and spasms, occurring regularly as a result of loss of higher motor control. The distribution of clinical manifestations varies, depending on the location of the lesion, although certain features are constant. There is great variation depending on the suddenness of onset and the age of the individual.

Spinal shock is the complete cessation of spinal cord function below the lesion. When the pyramidal system is destroyed below the level of the pons, spinal shock occurs. It is characterized by complete flaccid paralysis, absence of reflexes, and marked disturbances of bowel and bladder function. The reasons for spinal shock are not fully understood, but a major factor is the sudden destruction of the efferent pathways. If destruction occurs more slowly, spinal shock may not develop (see Chapter 18).

If the pyramidal system is interrupted above the level of the pons, the hand and arm muscles are greatly affected. Paralysis rarely involves all the muscles on one side of the body, however, even when the hemiplegia results from complete damage to the internal capsule. Bilateral movements, such as those of the eye, jaw, and larynx, are affected only slightly, if at all. Predominantly the limbs are affected. Because of their bilateral control, trunk muscles are much less influenced.

Paralysis associated with a pyramidal motor syndrome rarely remains flaccid for a prolonged time. After a few days or weeks, a gradual return of spinal reflexes marks the end of spinal shock. Reflexes then become hyperactive, and muscle tone is increased significantly, particularly in antigravity muscles. Spasticity is common, although rigidity occasionally occurs. Most often,

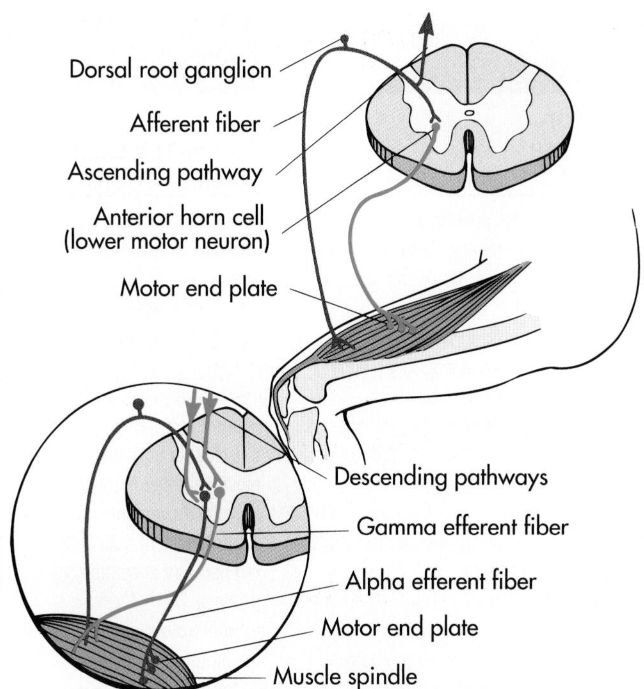

FIGURE 17-32 Component Structure of a Lower Motor Neuron, Including Motor (Efferent) and Sensory (Afferent) Elements. *Top,* Anterior horn cell (in anterior gray column of spinal cord and its axon), terminating in motor end plate as it innervates extrafusal muscle fibers in the quadriceps muscle. *Detailed enlargement:* Sensory and motor elements of the gamma loop system. The gamma efferent fiber is shown innervating the polar, or end, region of the muscle spindle (sensory receptor of skeletal muscle). Contraction of muscle spindle fibers stretches the central portion of the spindle and causes the afferent spindle fiber to transmit the impulse centrally to the cord. Muscle spindle afferent fibers in turn synapse on the anterior horn cell and are transmitted by way of gamma efferent fibers to skeletal (extrafusal) muscle, causing it to contract. Muscle spindle discharge is interrupted by active contraction of extrafusal muscle fibers.

passive range of motion causes the "clasp-knife" phenomenon, probably because of the activation of the two varieties of stretch receptors: (1) the muscle spindles and (2) the Golgi tendon organ. (Muscle function is discussed in Chapter 43.) With pyramidal motor syndrome, predominantly the flexors of the arms and the extensors of the legs are affected.

Lower Motor Neuron Syndromes. Lower (primary, alpha) motor neurons are the large motor neurons in the anterior (ventral) horn of the spinal cord and the motor nuclei of the brainstem. The axons from these nerve cell bodies bring nerve impulses from upper motor neurons to the skeletal muscles through the anterior spinal roots or cranial nerves (Figure 17-32). **Lower motor neuron syndromes** impair voluntary and involuntary movement. The degree of paralysis or paresis is proportional to the number of lower motor neurons affected. If only a portion of the motor units that supply a muscle is affected, only partial paralysis or paresis results. If all the motor units are affected, a complete paralysis results. Other clinical manifestations also are proportional to the degree of dysfunction, but the precise manifestations depend on the location of the dysfunction in the motor unit and in the CNS.

Small motor (gamma) neurons, which function to maintain muscle tone and protect the muscle from injury, also are necessary for normal motor movement. These neurons depend on input from the muscle spindle (arriving through an afferent limb rising to the cord). Dysfunction in this motor system impairs tone and reduces the tendon reflexes, causing hyporeflexia. The muscle is lax and soft, with a decrease in normal tone, or hypotonia, which impairs voluntary and involuntary motor movements. The muscles become susceptible to damage from hyperextensibility because the normal protective mechanisms that prevent muscle fiber injury are impaired. The degree of tone loss and the loss of tendon reflexes are proportional to the dysfunction in these reflex motor units.

Generally in a pathologic process the large and small motor neuron systems are equally affected. Therefore, the paresis and paralysis caused by a disorder of the lower motor neurons are called **flaccid paresis/flaccid paralysis** because the muscle has reduced or absent tone and is accompanied by hyporeflexia or **areflexia** (loss of tendon reflexes).

A few **gamma neuropathies** (small motor neuron disorders) affect only the gamma motor system of the spinal cord. A manifestation of these disorders is a marked reduction in the deep tendon reflexes, which are strikingly out of proportion to the degree of muscle weakness present.

Denervated muscles (i.e., muscles that have lost their nervous system input) undergo atrophy over weeks to months, mostly from disuse. Denervated muscles also demonstrate fasciculations, which are seen as muscle rippling or quivering under the skin. Occasionally denervated muscles cramp. Fibrillation (isolated contraction of a single muscle fiber) also may occur, although this manifestation is not visible clinically.

Motor Neuron Diseases

Motor neuron diseases result from progressive degeneration of upper or lower motor neurons in the spinal cord, brainstem, or cortex. Amyotrophic lateral sclerosis and paralytic poliomyelitis (now almost nonexistent because of the polio vaccine) are examples of these diseases.

Several pathologic processes may generate motor neuron diseases, which can be sporadic or inherited. A virally induced or postinfectious or postvaccination inflammatory process may injure or destroy anterior horn cells or cranial nerve cell bodies. Most of these inflammatory processes are mild and are followed by rapid cellular recovery (see What's New? Bell Palsy).

In motor neuron disease, muscle strength, muscle tone, and muscle bulk are affected in the muscles innervated by the involved motor neurons. The paresis and paralysis associated with anterior horn cell injury are segmental, but because each muscle is supplied by two or more roots, the segmental character of the weakness may be difficult to recognize. When cranial nerve motor nuclei are affected (these lack nerve roots and have only small rootlets near the point of exit from the brainstem), the distribution of the motor weakness follows that of the peripheral nerve. The weakness may involve distal muscles, proximal muscles, and the muscles of midline structures. Hypotonia and hyporeflexia or areflexia are present.

The atrophy associated with motor neuron disease is segmental when the anterior horn cells of the spinal cord are involved and follows the distribution of the peripheral nerve

WHAT'S NEW?

Bell Palsy

The etiology of Bell palsy (facial nerve palsy) remains unknown. There is usually an inflammatory reaction compressing the facial nerve in the fallopian canal, particularly in the narrowest labyrinthine segment, followed by demyelinating neural change. The most distressing symptoms are unilateral facial weakness and inability to smile or whistle. Bell palsy may be caused by reactivation of herpesviruses in cranial nerve VII (facial) geniculate ganglia. Herpes simplex type 1 has been detected in up to 78% of cases and herpes zoster in 30% of cases. Severe pain with facial palsy and a vesicular rash in the ear or mouth suggest herpes zoster infection. Ramsay Hunt syndrome (herpes zoster oticus) is rare but complete recovery is less than 50%. Recovery from Bell palsy is usually complete. Both disorders may be treated with antivirals, corticosteroids, or both. Treatment should be individualized according to severity of symptoms.

Data from Arbusow V et al: *J Med Virol* 82(11):1917–1920, 2010; Gronseth GS, Paduga R: *Neurology* 79(22):2209–2213, 2012; Linder TE, Abdelkafy W, Cavero-Vanek S: *Otol Neurotol* 31(2):319–327, 2010; Santos Rde F, Brasileiro BF: *Gen Dent* 59(4):266–271, 2011.

when the motor nuclei of the cranial nerves are affected. The atrophy may be in distal, proximal, or midline muscles. Fasciculations are particularly associated with primary motor neuron injury, and muscle cramps are common. Mild fatigue is a common complaint. If the pathologic process is limited to the primary motor neuron, no sensory changes are evident.

Because degenerative disorders can cause loss of nerve cells in the anterior horn or motor nuclei, the surviving cells are small and shrunken and filled with lipofuscin. Lost neurons are replaced by astrocytes. The roots or rootlets are thin, and the muscles show denervation and atrophy.

Several brainstem syndromes involve damage to one or more of the cranial nerve nuclei. These are called cranial nerve palsy (Table 17-24) and may be caused by vascular occlusion, tumor, aneurysm, tuberculosis, or hemorrhage.

The anterior horn cells and the motor nuclei of the cranial nerves may be affected secondarily in many severe pathologic processes that primarily involve the peripheral nerves. The condition may extend proximally to affect the nerve roots or rootlets and the motor neurons themselves, a process commonly seen, for example, in Guillain-Barré syndrome (see Chapter 18). If sufficient numbers of motor neurons are destroyed, permanent loss of motor function results because regeneration of the damaged axons requires a living neuronal cell body.

A group of degenerative disorders principally cause progressive motor cell atrophy. One of these is **progressive spinal muscular atrophy,** in which the degenerated anterior horn cells of the spinal cord are the affected motor neurons. This disorder occurs in adults and closely resembles the familial progressive muscular atrophies that occur in infants and children and that are considered inherited metabolic disorders (see Chapter 45). If the motor nuclei of the cranial nerves are affected instead of the anterior horn cells, the disorder is labeled **progressive bulbar palsy,** so named because the myelencephalon (medulla and upper cranial nerves) originally was called the *bulb* and a degenerative process causes a progressively more serious condition. When any lower motor neuron syndrome involves the cranial

TABLE 17-24 EXAMPLES OF CRANIAL NERVE PALSIES

TYPE OF NUCLEAR PALSY	CAUSES	ASSOCIATED CLINICAL MANIFESTATIONS
Ocular	Upper brainstem tumor Cerebrovascular disease in the vertebrobasilar system Aneurysm Intramedullary bleeding	Other cranial nerve signs Contralateral spastic hemiparesis/hemiplegia Contralateral hyperreflexia Contralateral extensor plantar reflex
Facial	Pontine tumor Cerebrovascular disease in the vertebrobasilar system	Paresis/paralysis of both upper and lower facial muscles for both voluntary movement and emotionally induced movement
Vagal	Intramedullary tumor	Ipsilateral loss of pain and temperature sensations of the face
	Cerebrovascular disease in the vertebrobasilar system	Contralateral spastic arm and leg paresis/hemiplegia Ipsilateral cerebellar signs
Hypoglossal	Intramedullary tumor	Contralateral loss of position sense and vibration in the arm and leg
	Cerebrovascular disease in the vertebrobasilar system	Contralateral spastic hemiparesis/hemiplegia

nerves that arise from the bulb (i.e., cranial nerves IX, X, and XII), the dysfunction is called a **bulbar palsy.**

The clinical manifestations of bulbar palsy include paresis or paralysis of the jaw, face, pharynx, and tongue musculature. Articulation is affected, especially articulation of the lingual *(r, n, l),* labial *(b, m, p, f),* dental *(d, t),* and palatal *(k, g)* consonants. Modulation is impaired, making the voice rasping or nasal. Pharyngeal reflexes are diminished or lost. Palate and vocal cord movement during phonation is impaired, and chewing and swallowing are affected. The facial muscles are weak, and the face appears to droop. The jaw jerk reflex is decreased. Atrophy eventually becomes apparent, as do fasciculations. All these manifestations become progressively worse, leading to aspiration, malnutrition, possible dehydration, and an inability to communicate verbally.

Amyotrophic Lateral Sclerosis

Amyotrophic lateral sclerosis (ALS) (sporadic motor system disease, sporadic motor neuron disease, motor neuron disease, Lou Gehrig disease) is a worldwide degenerative disorder diffusely involving lower and upper motor neurons. Progressive muscle weakness leads to respiratory failure and death, usually 2 to 5 years from symptom onset. There are no racial, ethnic, or socioeconomic boundaries. The prevalence rate is about 6 to 8 cases per 100,000. ALS may begin at any time from the fourth decade of life; its peak occurrence is in the early fifties. Male/female ratio is 1:4 to 2:5, equalizing at about age 70 years.[111]

The term *amyotrophic* (without muscle nutrition or progressive muscle wasting) refers to the predominant lower motor neuron component of the syndrome. Lateral sclerosis, or scarring of the corticospinal tract in the lateral column of the spinal cord, refers to the upper motor neuron component of the syndrome. ALS differs from other motor neuron disorders in that upper and lower motor neurons are both involved.

Most cases of ALS are sporadic. In familial ALS (5% to 10% of cases), mutations have been found in 12 different genes with the superoxide dismutase *(SOD1)* gene on chromosome 21 the most common.[112] The defective *SOD1* gene leads to an autosomal dominant pattern with age-dependent penetrance and accounts for 15% to 20% of the cases of familial ALS. Mutated TAR DNA-binding protein 43 *(TDP-43)* is a major constituent of the ubiquitinated protein inclusions in ALS, and provides a possible link between the genetic mutation and cellular pathology of motor neuron injury.[113]

PATHOPHYSIOLOGY. The pathogenesis of ALS is not clear. Apoptotic factors, abnormal synthesis of filament units, defects in axonal transport, glutamate excitotoxicity, oxidative stress, growth factors, mitochondrial dysfunction, and neuroinflammation are under study for a possible contribution to the pathogenesis.[114] The principal pathologic feature of ALS is lower and upper motor neuron degeneration. The number of large motor neurons in the spinal cord, brainstem, and cerebral cortex (premotor and motor areas) is reduced, with ongoing degeneration in the remaining motor neurons. The nuclei of cranial nerves III, IV, and VI usually are not involved. Death of the motor neuron results in axonal degeneration and secondary demyelination with glial proliferation and sclerosis (scarring) along the corticospinal tract. Inclusion bodies containing the protein *ubiquitin* are found in surviving neurons. However, there also is widespread neural degeneration of nonmotor neurons in the spinal cord and motor cortices, as well as in the premotor, sensory, and temporal cortices.[115] Altered astrocytes and microglial functions are suspected to exist. Lower motor neuron degeneration denervates motor units. Adjacent, still-viable lower motor neurons attempt to compensate by a process of distal intramuscular sprouting, reinnervation, and enlargement of motor units.

CLINICAL MANIFESTATIONS. The initial onset of ALS can be subtle with cramping or weakness that affects a limb, incoordination, slurring of speech, and difficulty swallowing. Muscle weakness in ALS exhibits the following characteristics:

1. Paresis usually begins in a single muscle group.
2. Corresponding muscle groups are asymmetrically affected in a mottled distribution.
3. Gradual involvement occurs in all striated muscles, except extraocular and heart muscles, and progresses to paralysis with no remissions.
4. Flaccid and spastic paresis may coexist in a single muscle group; flaccid paresis may mask spasticity, which is usually mild.
5. Urethral and anal sphincter weakness is uncommon.

The lower motor neuron syndrome of flaccid paresis consists of weakness of individual muscles, progressing to paralysis, associated with hypotonia and primary muscle atrophy (i.e., atrophy caused by denervation). Hypotonia is manifested by (1) decreased resistance to passive movement, (2) hypoactive or absent deep tendon reflexes, (3) absent abdominal and cremasteric reflexes, and (4) absent Babinski sign. Primary atrophy is manifested by (1) severe, irreversible muscular wasting; (2) fasciculations; (3) metabolically related changes in the skin and appendages; and (4) specific electromyographic (EMG) findings. Fasciculations, along with fibrillations, are prominent features of ALS. Metabolic changes include: (1) thinning of the skin, (2) thickening of the nails, (3) loss of body hair, and (4) decreased perspiration.

The upper motor neuron syndrome of spastic paresis consists of weakness of movement patterns, progressing to paralysis, associated with spasticity and, in some cases, atrophy secondary to disuse. Spasticity is manifested by (1) clasp-knife phenomenon, evident with passive movement; (2) hyperactive deep tendon reflexes and clonus with severe spasticity; (3) absent abdominal and cremasteric reflexes; and (4) presence of Babinski sign. The coexistence of a dementia has been demonstrated to be higher than previously thought.

EVALUATION AND TREATMENT. The diagnosis of ALS is based predominantly on medical history and physical examination.[116] Nerve conduction studies are important to exclude other diagnoses. There must be upper and lower motor neuron symptoms not attributable to other causes. Riluzole (Rilutek), an antiglutamate, is the standard treatment for ALS and prolongs life for months. Treatment also is directed at relief of symptoms, prevention of complications, maintenance of maximal function, and maintenance of optimal quality of life. Special problems requiring preventive and symptomatic management are communication difficulties caused by dysmasesis and dysphonia, salivation problems with either thick saliva or excessively thin saliva (sialorrhea), and dyspnea caused by diaphragmatic and intercostal weakness. Ventilatory issues become prominent. Supportive and rehabilitation management is directed toward preventing complications of immobility. Psychologic support of the affected individual and the family is extremely important in this disorder. ALS is fatal from respiratory failure usually within 3 years of diagnosis. A small percentage of individuals live 5 to 10 years or longer.[117]

Extrapyramidal Motor Syndromes

Because the extrapyramidal system encompasses all the motor pathways except the pyramidal system, two types of motor dysfunction comprise the **extrapyramidal motor syndromes:** (1) the basal ganglia motor syndromes and (2) the cerebellar motor syndromes. Unlike pyramidal motor syndromes, both extrapyramidal motor syndromes result in movement or posture disturbance without significant paralysis, along with other distinctive symptoms (Table 17-25).

Basal ganglia motor syndromes are movement disorders that involve either a paucity or an excess of movements. Stress and nervous tension typically worsen the symptoms, whereas relaxation improves motor performance. Akinesia may occur despite normal strength. Involuntary movements, such as tremor, chorea, ballism, athetosis, and dystonia, also may occur and probably are caused by the loss of the normal modulating effects of the corpus striatum and other parts of the basal ganglia.

Basal ganglia motor syndromes also are characterized by alterations in muscle tone and posture. Rigidity, together with the cogwheel phenomenon, is present in all muscle groups but is most prominent in those that maintain flexed position. Postural

TABLE 17-25 PYRAMIDAL VS. EXTRAPYRAMIDAL MOTOR SYNDROMES

MANIFESTATIONS	PYRAMIDAL MOTOR SYNDROME	EXTRAPYRAMIDAL MOTOR SYNDROME
Unilateral movement	Paralysis of voluntary movement	Little or no paralysis of voluntary movement
Tendon reflexes	Increased tendon reflexes	Normal or slightly increased tendon reflexes
Babinski sign	Present	Absent
Involuntary movements	Absence of involuntary movements	Presence of tremor, chorea, athetosis, or dystonia
Muscle tone	Spasticity in muscles (e.g., clasp-knife phenomenon)	Plastic (equal throughout movement) rigidity or intermittent (generalized but predominantly in flexors of limbs and trunk) rigidity (cogwheel rigidity)
	Hypertonia present in flexors of arms and extensors of legs	Hypotonia, weakness and gait disturbance in cerebellar disease

abnormalities result from the loss of normal postural reflexes. Dysfunctional equilibrium results from the loss of postural stability.

Cerebellar motor syndromes involve the cerebellum and may result in (1) acute loss of muscle tone; (2) difficulty with coordination of voluntary movements (ataxia); (3) minor degrees of muscle weakness, tendency toward fatigue, and impairment of associated movements; and (4) disorders of equilibrium, posture, and gait. Cerebellar effects are chiefly ipsilateral (primarily affecting the same side of the body), so damage to the right cerebellum generally causes symptoms on the right side of the body. Predominant symptoms depend on the area of damage within the cerebellum. The four cerebellar syndromes are the rostral vermis, caudal vermis, cerebellar hemisphere, and pancerebellum[118] (Table 17-26).

Diagnosis of a cerebellar motor syndrome is based on the symptoms, but these may vary because of the individual's attempts at compensation. Further, the nervous system often can operate well despite destruction of parts of the cerebellum, although the mechanisms responsible for this retained function are not fully understood.

TABLE 17-26 CEREBELLAR MOTOR SYNDROMES

ANATOMIC LOCATION OF DYSFUNCTION	CHARACTERISTICS
Rostral vermis (so-called *anterior lobe*)	Ataxia of stance and gait with varying degrees of instability of the trunk and ataxia of legs; anteroposterior body sway; presence of Romberg sign
Caudal vermis (including flocculonodular lobe)	Truncal, postural, and gait ataxia; omnidirectional body sway; Romberg negative; tendency to fall; saccadic slow pursuit, nystagmus; inability to suppress vestibulo-ocular reflex (doll's eyes)
Cerebellar hemisphere (neocerebellar syndrome)	Severe disturbance in ipsilateral limb movements; hypotonia in acute situation; dysmetria (extremity overshooting its target); decomposition of movement; kinetic tremor, past-pointing; deviation of gait; dysarthria
Pancerebellum	Ataxia of trunk and bilateral limbs; ataxia of gait and stance; dysarthria; oculomotor disturbance

Data from Timmann D, Diener HC: Coordination and ataxia. In Goetz GC, editor: *Textbook of clinical neurology,* St Louis, 2007, Saunders.

Alterations in Complex Motor Performance

The alterations in complex motor performance include disorders of posture (stance), disorders of gait, and disorders of expression.

Disorders of Posture (Stance)

An inequality of tone in muscle groups because of a loss of normal postural reflexes results in a posturing of limbs. Many reflex systems govern tone and posture, but the most important factor in posture control is the stretch reflex, in which stretching of extensor (antigravity) muscles causes increased extensor tone and inhibited flexor tone. Four types of disorders of posture are described: (1) dystonic posture, (2) decerebrate posture, (3) basal ganglion posture, and (4) senile posture. Equilibrium and balance are disrupted when postural disorders are present.

Dystonia is the maintenance of an abnormal posture through muscular contractions. When muscular contractions are sustained for several seconds, they are called **dystonic movements,** such as in choreoathetoid movements associated with high levels of L-dopa. When contractions last for longer periods, they are called **dystonic postures,** such as in torticollis. Dystonic postures may last for weeks, causing permanent fixed contractures. Dystonia has been associated with basal ganglia abnormality, but the exact pathophysiologic mechanisms are unknown (Box 17-6). One particularly relevant dystonic posture already discussed in this chapter is decorticate posture (striatal posture or upper motor neuron dysfunction posture), which may be unilateral or bilateral in occurrence. **Decorticate posture** (also referred to as **antigravity posture** or **hemiplegic posture**) is characterized by upper extremities that are flexed

BOX 17-6 BOTULINUM TOXIN THERAPEUTIC EFFECTIVENESS IN DYSTONIA

Botulinum toxin, both A and B, is effective in relieving cervical dystonia (spasmodic torticollis) symptoms in adults and is the mainstay of modern treatment for focal dystonia. The effectiveness of other drugs (benodiazepines, gamma-aminobutyric acid [GABA] inhibitors, atypical anticonvulsants, dopaminergic agonists and antagonists), as well as the effect of surgical interventions or physical therapies, is not empirically known.

Data from Nijmeijer SW et al: *Parkinsonism Relat Disord* 18(6):731–736, 2012; Truong D: *Neurol Sc* 316(1-2):9–14, 2012; Colosimo C, Tiple D, Berardelli A: *Neurotox Res* 22(4):265–273, 2012.

at the elbows and held close to the body and by lower extremities that are externally rotated and extended (see Figure 17-6). Decorticate posture is believed to occur when the brainstem, which facilitates the antigravity position, is not inhibited by the motor function of the cerebral cortex. Upper motor neuron posture is more commonly described as the arm flexed at the elbow, with a wristdrop; the leg inadequately bent at the knee, with the hip excessively circumabducted; and the presence of a footdrop.

Decerebrate posture refers to increased tone in extensor muscles and trunk muscles, with active tonic neck reflexes. When the head is in a neutral position, all four limbs are rigidly extended (see Figure 17-6). The decerebrate posture is caused by severe injury to the brain and brainstem, resulting in overstimulation of the postural righting and vestibular reflexes.

Basal ganglion posture refers to a stooped, hyperflexed posture with a narrow-based, short-stepped gait. This posture abnormality results from the loss of normal postural reflexes and not from defects in proprioceptive, labyrinthine, or visual function. Dysfunctional equilibrium results from the loss of postural stability, and thus the individual is unable to make the appropriate postural adjustment to tilting or loss of balance and consequently falls. Dysfunctional righting is the inability to right oneself when changing from a lying or crouching to a standing position or when rolling from the supine to the lateral or prone position. Dysfunctional postural fixation is the involuntary flexion of the head and neck, causing the person difficulty in maintaining an upright trunk position while standing or walking. Basal ganglion dysfunction accounts for this posture.

Senile posture is characterized by an increasingly flexed posture similar to that caused by basal ganglion dysfunction. The posture is associated with frontal lobe dysfunction, but the primary pathophysiology is not well described.

Disorders of Gait

Four predominant types of gait disorder are: (1) upper motor neuron dysfunction gait, (2) cerebellar (ataxic) gait, (3) basal ganglion gait, and (4) senile (frontal lobe, pseudoparkinsonian) gait. As with posture, equilibrium and balance are affected with gait disturbances.

Several upper motor neuron gaits exist. In the presence of mild upper motor neuron dysfunction, a footdrop may appear only with fatigue. The individual may complain of hip and leg pain. A **spastic gait,** which is associated with unilateral injury, is manifested by a shuffling gait with the leg extended and held stiff, causing a scraping over the floor surface. An impaired leg swing around the body rather than an appropriate lifting and placing of the leg is noted. The foot may drag on the ground, and the person tends to fall to the affected side. A **scissors gait** is associated with bilateral injury and spasticity. The legs are abducted, causing them to touch each other. As the person walks, the legs are still swung around the body but then cross in front of each other because of adduction. Injury to the pyramidal system accounts for these gaits.

A **cerebellar gait** manifests as a wide-based gait with the feet apart and often turned outward or inward for greater stability. The pelvis is held stiff, and it seems to be independent of the trunk. The individual staggers when walking. Cerebellar dysfunction accounts for this particular gait.

A **basal ganglion gait** and a **senile gait** are both broad-based gaits. The person walks with small steps and a decreased arm swing. The head and body are flexed and the arms are semiflexed and abducted, whereas the legs are flexed and rigid in more advanced states. Basal ganglion and frontal lobe dysfunction, respectively, account for these two gaits.

Disorders of Expression

Disorders of expression involve the motor aspects of communication and include (1) hypermimesis, (2) hypomimesis, and (3) dyspraxias and apraxias. **Hypermimesis** is a disinhibition phenomenon that most commonly manifests as pathologic laughter or crying. Pathologic laughter is associated with right hemisphere injury, and pathologic crying is associated with left hemisphere injury. The exact pathophysiology is not known. **Hypomimesis** manifests as aprosody, or the loss of voice modulation (pitch, speed, emphasis, emotion). Receptive aprosody involves an inability to *understand* emotion in speech and facial expression, whereas expressive aprosody involves the inability to *express* emotion in speech and facial expression. Aprosody is associated with right hemisphere damage.

Dyspraxia is the partial inability and **apraxia** is the complete inability to perform purposeful or skilled motor acts in the absence of paralysis, sensory loss, abnormal posture and tone, abnormal involuntary movement, incoordination, or inattentiveness. These are disorders of learned skilled movements.[119] Dyspraxia and apraxia are associated with left hemisphere vascular disorders, trauma, tumor, degenerative disorders, infections, and metabolic disorders. The medial premotor cortex, including the supplementary motor area (SMA), appears to play a role in skilled movements as does the convexity premotor areas[119] (Table 17-27).

True dyspraxias occur when the connecting pathways between the left and right cortical areas are interrupted, causing language-motor and motor representation disconnections between the hemispheres. Dyspraxias may result from any pathologic process that disrupts the cortical areas necessary for the conceptualization and execution of a complex motor act or the communication pathways within the left hemisphere or between the hemispheres.

TABLE 17-27 DYSPRAXIAS AND APRAXIAS

TYPES	DESCRIPTION	LOCATION
Ideomotor apraxia	Impairment in selecting, sequencing, and spatial orientation of movements involved in gestures (spatial and temporal production errors)	Left parietal cortex (angular gyrus) or supramarginal gyrus
Posterior form	Difficulty performing in response to command and imitation; cannot discriminate well between poorly performed and well-performed acts	Left parietal cortex (angular gyrus or supramarginal gyrus) lesion
Anterior form	Performs poorly to command and imitation but comprehends and discriminates pantomime	Lesions anterior to the supramarginal gyrus, which disconnects visual kinesthetic motor engrams from premotor and motor areas
Conduction apraxia	Greater impairment in performance when imitating movements than when pantomiming to command; comprehends pantomime and gesture but cannot perform the movements	Location unknown at this time
Disassociation apraxia	Inability to gesture normally to command and required verbal mediation; has good performance with imitation and actual tools and objects	Callosal abnormalities but not all locations known
Ideational apraxia	Inability to carry out an ideational plan or a series of acts in the proper sequence	Location unclear at this time
Conceptual apraxia	Cannot recall type of action associated with specific tools, utensils, or objects (content and tool selection errors; may be unable to recall which tool is associated with a specific object or may have impaired mechanical knowledge)	Bilateral frontal and parietal dysfunction

SUMMARY REVIEW

Alterations in Cognitive Systems

1. Full consciousness is an awareness of oneself and the environment and includes an ability to respond to external stimuli with a wide variety of responses.
2. Consciousness has two components: arousal (state of awakeness) and awareness (content of thought).
3. Alterations in level of arousal may be caused by structural, metabolic, or psychogenic disorders.
4. Levels of consciousness can diminish in stages from alert and oriented to confusion and coma.
5. An alteration in breathing pattern and level of coma reflects the level of hemispheric and brainstem dysfunction.
6. Pupillary changes reflect changes in level of brainstem function, drug action, and response to hypoxia and ischemia.
7. Abnormal eye movements, including nystagmus and divergent gaze, reflect alterations in brainstem function.
8. Level of brain function manifests by changes in generalized motor responses or the presence of no responses.
9. Loss of cortical inhibition associated with decreased consciousness includes abnormal flexor and extensor movements.
10. Brain death represents irreversible total brain damage including an inability to maintain cardiac, respiratory, and other vital functions.
11. Arousal returns in the vegetative state and minimally conscious state, but content of thought is absent or markedly reduced, respectively.
12. Alterations in awareness encompass all cognitive functions including awareness, selective attention, and memory.
13. With a deficit in selective attention, mediated by the brainstem, the parietal lobe structures, and the pulvinar nucleus of the thalamus, the individual cannot focus on selective stimuli and thus neglects those stimuli, causing a neglect syndrome.
14. In dysmnesia and amnesia, some memories are not retrieved and new memories cannot be stored.
15. Frontal areas mediate vigilance, detection, and working memory. With a vigilance deficit, the person cannot maintain search and scanning activities. With a detection deficit, the person is unmotivated and unable to use feedback.
16. Some specific disorders of awareness (content of thought) are data processing deficits: agnosias, dysphasias, acute confusional states, and dementias, including AD.
17. Agnosias are a defect of recognition and may be tactile, visual, or auditory. They are caused by dysfunction in the primary sensory area or the interpretive areas of the cerebral cortex.
18. Dysphasia is an impairment of comprehension or production of language. Dysphasia may be expressive or sensory.
19. Aphasia is loss of language comprehension or production.
20. Wernicke dysphasia is a disturbance in understanding all language—verbal and reading comprehension.
21. Conductive dysphasias result from disruption of temporal lobe fibers, with a failure to repeat words but an ability to initiate speech, writing, and reading aloud.
22. Anomic dysphasia is an inability to name objects, people, or qualities.
23. Transcortical dysphasias involve an ability to repeat and recite.
24. Broca aphasia is an expressive dysphasia of speech and writing but with retention of comprehension.
25. Global aphasia involves anterior and posterior speech areas, with expressive and receptive aphasia.
26. Acute confusional states are characterized chiefly by defects in attention and coherence of thoughts and actions and, in the case of delirium, an intense autonomic nervous system hyperactivity.
27. Dementia is impairment of intellectual function, memory, and language with alteration in behavior and can be caused by trauma, vascular disease, infection, and progressive neurodegeneration.

SUMMARY REVIEW—cont'd

28. AD is the most common chronic, irreversible dementia.
29. Seizures represent abnormal, excessive hypersynchronous discharges of cerebral neurons with transient alterations in brain function. Seizures may be generalized or focal. There are three categories of epileptic syndrome: location-related, generalized, and cryptogenic (undetermined).

Alterations in Cerebral Hemodynamics

1. Cerebral oxygenation is a critical management issue.
2. Cerebral perfusion pressure determines cerebral blood flow.
3. An injured brain may experience cerebral oligemia, normal cerebral blood flow but with increased intracranial pressure, or cerebral hyperemia.
4. Increased intracranial pressure may result from edema, excess CSF, hemorrhage, or tumor growth. When intracranial pressure approaches arterial pressure, hypoxia and hypercapnia produce brain damage.
5. Cerebral edema is an increase in the fluid content of the brain resulting from infection, hemorrhage, tumor, ischemia, infarct, or hypoxia.
6. The shifting or herniation of brain tissue from one compartment to another disrupts the blood flow of both compartments and damages brain tissue.
7. Supratentorial herniation involves temporal lobe and hippocampal gyrus shifting from the middle fossa to the posterior fossa; transtentorial herniation with a downward shift of the diencephalon through the tentorial notch; and shifting of the cingulate gyrus herniation under the falx.
8. The most common infratentorial herniation is a shift of the cerebellar tonsils through the foramen magnum.
9. Hydrocephalus comprises a variety of disorders characterized by an excess of fluid within the cranial vault, subarachnoid space, or both. Hydrocephalus occurs because of interference with CSF flow caused by increased fluid production or obstruction within the ventricular system or by defective reabsorption of the fluid.

Alterations in Neuromotor Function

1. Motor dysfunction may be characterized as alterations of motor tone, movement, and complex motor performance.
2. Hypotonia and hypertonia are the main categories of altered muscle tone.
3. Four types of hypertonia exist: spasticity, gegenhalten, dystonia, and rigidity.
4. Alteration in muscle movement includes hyperkinesia (excessive movement), hypokinesia (slow movement), and dyskinesias (abnormal voluntary movement).
5. Included in the category of hyperkinesia are chorea, athetosis, ballism, akathisia, tremor, and myoclonus.
6. HD (chorea) is a rare hereditary irreversible disease involving the basal ganglia and frontal cerebral cortex with a depletion of neurons that secrete GABA (an inhibitory neurotransmitter) that causes involuntary, fragmentary movements accompanied by emotional lability and progressive dementia.
7. Types of hypokinesia include akinesia, bradykinesia, and loss of associated movements.
8. PD is a common degenerative disorder of the basal ganglia (corpus striatum) involving degeneration of the dopamine-secreting nigrostriatal pathway resulting in overactivity by the subthalamic nucleus, causing tremor, rigidity, and bradykinesia. Involvement of the limbic system causes emotional lability. Progressive dementia may be associated with an advanced stage of the disease.
9. Two subtypes of paresis and paralysis are described: upper motor neuron and lower motor neuron.
10. An upper motor neuron syndrome is characterized by spastic paresis or paralysis, hypertonia, and hyperreflexia.
11. Interruption of the pyramidal tract below the pons results in spinal shock.
12. Lower motor neuron syndromes manifest with impaired voluntary and involuntary movements and flaccid paralysis.
13. Partial paralysis occurs with only partial loss of alpha motor neurons, and total paralysis is complete loss of alpha motor neurons. Loss of gamma motor neurons impairs muscle tone and decreases deep tendon reflexes.
14. Motor neuron diseases result from progressive degeneration of upper or lower motor neurons in the spinal cord, brainstem, or cortex.
15. Nuclear palsies involve damage to the cranial nerve nuclei.
16. Bulbar palsies involve cranial nerves IX, X, and XII.
17. ALS is a motor neuron disease. The pathogenesis of ALS is not fully known; however, lower and upper motor neuron degeneration occurs as well as degeneration of the nonmotor neurons in the cortices and spinal cord. Clinical manifestations of ALS may include weakness in all muscles that may begin in a single muscle group, slurring of speech, and difficulty swallowing. Flaccid paresis progressing to paralysis is characteristic of the lower motor neuron syndrome.
18. Extrapyramidal motor syndromes include basal ganglia and cerebellar motor syndromes.
19. Basal ganglia disorders manifest with alterations in muscle tone and posture, including rigidity, involuntary movements, and loss of postural reflexes.
20. Cerebellar motor syndromes result in loss of muscle tone, difficulty with coordination, and disorders of equilibrium and gait.
21. Alterations in complex motor performance include disorders of posture (stance), disorders of gait, and disorders of expression.
22. Disorders of posture include dystonic posture, decerebrate posture, basal ganglion posture, and senile posture.
23. Disorders of gait include upper motor neuron gaits, cerebellar gait, basal ganglion gait, and senile gait.
24. Disorders of expression include hypermimesis, hypomimesis, and dyspraxia or apraxia.
25. Dyspraxia is the partial inability and apraxia is the complete inability to perform purposeful or skilled motor acts.

KEY TERMS

Acute confusional state (ACS), 542
Acute hydrocephalus, 558
Agnosia, 539
Akinesia, 564
Akinetic mutism (AM), 535, 538
Alzheimer disease (dementia of Alzheimer type [DAT], senile disease complex), 546
Amyotrophic lateral sclerosis (ALS) (sporadic motor system disease, sporadic motor neuron disease, motor neuron disease, Lou Gehrig disease), 572
Aphasia, 539
Apneustic respiration, 532
Apraxia, 575
Areflexia, 571
Arousal, 528
Ataxic respiration, 532
Aura, 553
Autoregulation, 556
Awareness (content of thought), 528, 535
Basal ganglia motor syndrome, 573
Basal ganglion gait, 575
Basal ganglion posture, 575
Bradykinesia, 564
Brain death (total brain death), 533
Bulbar palsy, 572
Central neurogenic hyperventilation, 532
Cerebellar gait, 575
Cerebellar motor syndrome, 574
Cerebral blood flow, 555
Cerebral blood volume, 555
Cerebral death (irreversible coma), 534
Cerebral edema, 557
Cerebral oxygen saturation, 555
Cerebral perfusion pressure, 555
Cheyne-Stokes respiration, 529
Clonic phase, 553
Cluster respiration, 532
Cogwheel rigidity, 567
Communicating hydrocephalus (nonobstructive), 558
Consciousness, 527
Convulsion, 550
Cryptogenic epilepsy, 553
Cytotoxic (metabolic) edema, 558
Decerebrate posture, 575
Declarative memory, 536
Decorticate posture (antigravity posture, hemiplegic posture), 574
Delirium, 542
Dementia, 545
Detection, 538
Detection deficit, 538
Diplegia, 569
Dysmnesia, 536
Dysphasia, 539
Dyspraxia, 575
Dystonia, 560, 574
Dystonic movement, 574
Dystonic posture, 574
Echolalia, 540
Epilepsy, 550, 553
Epileptic syndrome, 553
Epileptogenesis, 553
Epileptogenic focus, 553
Excited delirium syndrome (ExDS), 542
Extinction, 536
Extrapyramidal motor syndrome, 573
Flaccid paresis/paralysis, 571
Focal seizure (partial seizure), 551
Freezing, 564
Frontotemporal dementia (FTD) (Pick disease), 550
Gamma neuropathy, 571
Gegenhalten (paratonia), 560
Generalized seizure, 551
Hemiparesis, 568
Hemiplegia, 568
Herniation syndrome, 557
Hiccups, 533
Huntington disease (HD), 562
Hydrocephalus, 558
Hydrocephalus ex vacuo, 558
Hyperkinesia (excessive movement), 564
Hypermimesis, 575
Hypertonia (increased muscle tone), 560
Hypokinesia (decreased movement), 564
Hypokinetic confusional state, 542
Hypomimesis, 575
Hypotonia (decreased muscle tone), 559
Idiopathic epilepsy, 553
Increased intracranial pressure (IICP), 555
Interstitial edema, 558
Irreversible coma, 534
Isolated (pure) vigilance deficit, 538
Locked-in syndrome, 535
Lower motor neuron syndrome, 571
Memory, 536
Metabolic alterations in arousal, 528
Minimally conscious state (MCS), 535
Mirror focus, 553
Neuritic plaque, 548
Neurofibrillary tangle, 548
Noncommunicating hydrocephalus (obstructive), 558
Nondeclarative memory (nonconscious), 536
Normal-pressure hydrocephalus (low-pressure, adult, occult hydrocephalus), 558
Paradoxysmal dyskinesias, 562
Paralysis, 568
Paraparesis, 569
Paraplegia, 569
Paresis (weakness), 568
Parkinson disease (PD), 564
Parkinsonian bradykinesia, 567
Parkinsonian rigidity, 567
Parkinsonian tremor, 566
Parkinsonism (Parkinson syndrome, parkinsonian syndrome), 565
Paroxysmal dyskinesia, 562
Persistent vegetative state (VS), 534
Pick disease, 550
Plastic rigidity, 567
Posthyperventilation apnea (PHVA), 529
Postictal state, 553
Prodroma, 555
Progressive bulbar palsy, 572
Progressive spinal muscular atrophy, 572
Psychogenic alterations in arousal (unresponsiveness), 528
Pyramidal motor syndrome, 569
Quadriparesis, 569
Quadriplegia, 569
Rigidity, 561
Scissors gait, 575
Secondary generalization, 552
Seizure, 550
Seizure disorder, 550
Seizure initiation, 552
Selective attention, 535
Selective attention deficit (orientation), 536
Senile gait, 575
Senile posture, 575
Sensory inattentiveness, 535
Spastic gait, 575
Spasticity, 560
Spinal shock, 570
Status epilepticus, 553
Structural alterations in arousal, 528
Symptomatic epilepsy, 553
Tardive dyskinesia, 562
Tonic phase, 553
Transcortical dysphasia (transcortical sensory dysphasia, mixed transcortical dysphasia, isolated speech center), 540
Unilateral neglect syndrome, 536
Upper motor neuron paresis/paralysis, 568
Vasogenic edema, 557
Vomiting, 533
Working memory deficit, 538
Yawning, 533

REFERENCES

1. Nakagawa TA et al: Guidelines for the determination of brain death in infants and children: an update of the 1987 task force recommendations, *Crit Care Med* 39(9):2139–2155, 2011.
2. Gardiner D et al: International perspective on the diagnosis of death, *Br J Anaesth* 108((Suppl 1):i14–i28, 2012.
3. Scripko PD, Greer DM: An update on brain death criteria: a simple algorithm with complex questions, *Neurologist* 17(5):237–240, 2011.
4. Teitelbaum J, Shemi SD: Neurologic determination of death, *Neurol Clin* 29(4):787–799, 2011.
5. Wijdicks EF et al: Evidence-based guideline update: determining brain death in adults: report of the Quality Standards Subcommittee of the American Academy of Neurology, *Neurology* 74(23):1911–1918, 2010.
6. Boss BJ, Fletcher A: Severe brain injury rehabilitation: what's going to happen after critical care? *Crit Care Nurs Clin* 13(3):421–431, 2001.
7. Owen AM et al: Detecting awareness in the vegetative state, *Science* 313(5792):1402, 2006.
8. Owen AM: Disorders of consciousness, *Ann N Y Acad Sci* 1124:225–238, 2008.
9. Shetty AC, Morris J, O'Mahony P: Akinetic mutism—not coma, *Age Ageing* 38(3):350–351, 2009.
10. Lacroix G et al: Transient locked-in syndrome and basilar artery vasospasm, *Neurocrit Care* 16(1):145–147, 2012.
11. Carrasco M: Visual attention: the past 25 years, *Vision Res* 51(13):1484–1525, 2011.
12. Deiana S, Platt B, Riedel G: The cholinergic system and spatial learning, *Behav Brain Res* 221(2):389–411, 2011.
13. LaVoie DJ, Cobia DJ: Recollecting, recognizing and other acts of remembering: an overview of human memory, *J Neurol Phys Ther* 31(3):135–144, 2007.
14. Shohamy D: Learning and motivation in the human striatum, *Curr Opin Neurobiol* 21(3):408–414, 2011.
15. Schmahmann JD: The role of the cerebellum in cognition and emotion: personal reflections since 1982 on the dysmetria of thought hypothesis, and its historical evolution from theory to therapy, *Neuropsychol Rev* 20(3):236–260, 2010.

16. Markowitsch HJ, Staniloiu A: Amygdala in action: relaying biological and social significance to autobiographical memory, *Neuropsychologia* 49(4):718–733, 2011.
16a Markowitsch HJ, Staniloiu A: Amnesic disorders, *Lancet* 380(9851):1429–1440, 2012.
17. Krauzlis R, Zenon A: Superior colliculus inactivation impairs covert selective attention to motion but does not alter gain modulation of motion signals in areas MT and MST, *J Vis* 11(1):495, 2011.
18. Li N, Bartlett CW: Defining the genetic architecture of human developmental language impairment, *Life Sci* 90(13-14):469–475, 2012.
19. Hughes CG, Patel MB, Pandharipande PP: Pathophysiology of acute brain dysfunction: what's the cause of all this confusion? *Curr Opin Crit Care* 18(5):518–526, 2012.
20. Mittal V et al: Review: delirium in the elderly: a comprehensive review, *Am J Alzheimers Dis Other Demen* 26(2):97–109, 2011.
21. Josephson SA, Miller BL: Confusion and delirium. In Fauci AS et al: *Harrison's principles of internal medicine*, ed 15, New York, 2008, McGraw-Hill.
22. Cerejeira J et al: The neuroinflammatory hypothesis of delirium, *Acta Neuropathol* 119(6):737–754, 2010.
23. Vilke GM et al: Excited delirium syndrome (ExDS): treatment options and considerations, *J Forensic Leg Med* 19(3):117–121, 2012.
24. Adamis D et al: Delirium scales: a review of current evidence, *Aging Ment Health* 14(5):543–555, 2010.
25. Popeo DM: Delirium in older adults, *Mt Sinai J Med* 78(4):571–582, 2011.
26. Brummel NE, Girard TD: Preventing delirium in the intensive care unit, *Crit Care Clin* 29(1):51–65, 2013.
27. Bird TD, Miller BL: Dementia. In Fauci AS et al: *Harrison's principles of internal medicine*, ed 15, New York, 2008, McGraw-Hill.
28. Rocca WA et al: Trends in the incidence and prevalence of Alzheimer's disease, dementia, and cognitive impairment in the United States, *Alzheimers Dement* 7(1):80–93, 2011.
29. Rabinovici GD, Miller BL: Frontotemporal lobar degeneration: epidemiology, pathophysiology, diagnosis and management, *CNS Drugs* 24(5):375–398, 2010.
30. Simmons BB, Hartmann B, Dejoseph D: Evaluation of suspected dementia, *Am Fam Physician* 84(8):895–902, 2011.
31. Alzheimer's Association: 2012 Alzheimer's disease facts and figures, *Alzheimers Dement* 8(2):131–168, 2010.
32. Barnes DE, Yaffe K: The projected effect of risk factor reduction on Alzheimer's disease prevalence, *Lancet Neurol* 10(9):819–828, 2011.
33. Daviglus ML et al: Risk factors and preventive interventions for Alzheimer disease: state of the science, *Arch Neurol* 68(9):1185–1190, 2011.
34. Grimm A et al: Alzheimer's disease, oestrogen and mitochondria: an ambiguous relationship, *Mol Neurobiol* 46(1):151–160, 2012.
35. Bettens K, Sleegers K, Van Broeckhoven C: Genetic insights in Alzheimer's disease, *Lancet Neurol* 12(1):92–104, 2013.
36. Guerreiro RJ, Gustafson DR, Hardy J: The genetic architecture of Alzheimer's disease: beyond APP, PSENs and APOE, *Neurobiol Aging* 33(3):437–456, 2012.
37. Bekris LM et al: Genetics of Alzheimer disease, *J Geriatr Psychiatry Neurol* 23(4):213–227, 2010.
38. Johnston H, Boutin H, Allan SM: Assessing the contribution of inflammation in models of Alzheimer's disease, *Biochem Soc Trans* 39(4): 886–890, 2011.
39. Harrington CR: The molecular pathology of Alzheimer's disease, *Neuroimaging Clin North Am* 22(1):11–22, 2012.
40. Nicolakakis N, Hamel E: Neurovascular function in Alzheimer's disease patients and experimental models, *J Cereb Blood Flow Metab* 31(6):1354–1370, 2011.
41. Selfridge JE et al: Role of mitochondrial homeostasis and dynamics in Alzheimer's disease, *Neurobiol Dis*, 2012 Jan 10. [Epub ahead of print.].
42. Montine TJ et al: National Institute on Aging—Alzheimer's Association guidelines for the neuropathologic assessment of Alzheimer's disease: a practical approach, *Acta Neuropathol* 123(1):1–11, 2012.
43. Goldman JS et al: Genetic counseling and testing for Alzheimer disease: joint practice guideline of the American College of Medical Genetics and the National Society of Genetic Counselors, *Genet Med* 13(6):597–605, 2011.
44. Herrmann N et al: Current and emerging drug treatment options for Alzheimer's disease: a systematic review, *Drugs* 71(15):2031–2065, 2011.
45. Hampel H et al: The future of Alzheimer's disease: the next 10 years, *Prog Neurobiol* 95(4):718–728, 2011.
46. Premi E, Padovani A, Borroni B: Frontotemporal lobar degeneration, *Adv Exp Med Biol* 724:114–127, 2012.
47. Lowenstein DH: Seizures and epilepsy. In Fauci AS et al: *Harrison's principles of internal medicine*, ed 15, New York, 2008, McGraw-Hill.
48. Berg AT et al: Revised terminology and concepts for organization of seizures and epilepsies: report of the ILAE Commission on Classification and Terminology, 2005-2009, *Epilepsia* 51(4):676–685, 2010.
49. Berg AT, Scheffer IE: New concepts in classification of the epilepsies: entering the 21st century, *Epilepsia* 52(6):1058–1062, 2011.
50. Panayiotopoulos CP: The new ILAE report on terminology and concepts for the organization of epilepsies: critical review and contribution, *Epilepsia* 53(3):399–404, 2012.
51. Huff JS, Fountain NB: Pathophysiology and definitions of seizures and status epilepticus, *Emerg Med Clin North Am* 29(1):1–13, 2011.
52. Scharfman HE: The neurogiology of epilepsy, *Curr Neurol Neurosci Rep* 7(4):348–354, 2007.
53. Pitkänen A, Lukasiuk K: Mechanisms of epileptogenesis and potential treatment targets, *Lancet Neurol* 10(2):173–186, 2011.
54. DiFrancesco JC et al: Recessive loss-of-function mutation in the pacemaker HCN2 channel causing increased neuronal excitability in a patient with idiopathic generalized epilepsy, *J Neurosci* 31(48):17327–17337, 2011.
55. Maroso M et al: Interleukin-1 type 1 receptor/toll-like receptor signaling in epilepsy: the importance of IL-1beta and high-mobility group box 1, *J Intern Med* 270(4):319–326, 2011.
56. Nair PP, Kalita J, Misra UK: Status epilepticus: why, what, and how, *J Postgrad Med* 57(3):242–252, 2011.
57. Jefferys JG: Advances in understanding basic mechanisms of epilepsy and seizures, *Seizure* 19(10):638–646, 2010.
58. Baulac S, Baulac M: Advances on the genetics of mendelian idiopathic epilepsies, *Neurol Clin* 27(4):1041–1061, 2009.
59. Centers for Disease Control and Prevention (CDC): *Epilepsy: epilepsy fast facts*. Available at www.cdc.gov/epilepsy/basics/fast_facts.htm. Last updated January 16, 2013.
60. Berg AT, Blackstone NW: Concepts in classification and their relevance to epilepsy, *Epilepsy Res* 70(Suppl 1):S11–S19, 2006.
61. Laufs H: Functional imaging of seizures and epilepsy: evolution from zones to networks, *Curr Opin Neurol* 25(2):194–200, 2012.
62. Lee PR, Kossoff EH: Dietary treatments for epilepsy: management guidelines for the general practitioner, *Epilepsy Behav* 21(2):115–121, 2011.
63. Privitera M: Current challenges in the management of epilepsy, *Am J Manag Care* 17(Suppl 7):S195–S203, 2011.
64. Englot DJ, Chang EF, Auguste KI: Vagus nerve stimulation for epilepsy: a meta-analysis of efficacy and predictors of response, *J Neurosurg* 115(6):1248–1255, 2011.
65. Elliott J, Shneker B: Patient, caregiver, and health care practitioner knowledge of, beliefs about, and attitudes toward epilepsy, *Epilepsy Behav* 12(4):547–556, 2008.
66. Paidakakos N, Borgarello S, Naddeo M: Indications for endoscopic third ventriculostomy in normal pressure hydrocephalus, *Acta Neurochir Suppl* 113:123–127, 2012.
67. Shprecher D, Schwalb J, Kurlan R: Normal pressure hydrocephalus: diagnosis and treatment, *Curr Neurol Neurosci Rep* 8(5):371–376, 2008.
68. Fahn S: Classification of movement disorders, *Mov Disord* 26(6):947–957, 2011.
69. Moore AP: Classification of movement disorders, *Neuroimaging Clin North Am* 20(1):1–6, 2010.
70. Lerner V, Miodownik C: Motor symptoms of schizophrenia: is tardive dyskinesia a symptom or side effect? A modern treatment, *Curr Psychiatry Rep* 13(4):295–304, 2011.
71. Olanow CW: Hyperkinetic movement disorders. In Fauci AS et al: *Harrison's principles of internal medicine*, ed 15, New York, 2008, McGraw-Hill.
72. Benraiss A, Goldman SA: Cellular therapy and induced neuronal replacement for Huntington's disease, *Neurotherapeutics* 8(4):577–590, 2011.
73. Jones L, Hughes A: Pathogenic mechanisms in Huntington's disease, *Int Rev Neurobiol* 98:373–418, 2011.
74. Giacomello M, Hudec R, Lopreiato R: Huntington's disease, calcium, and mitochondria, *Biofactors* 37(3):206–218, 2011.
75. Vonsattel JP, Keller C, Cortes Ramirez EP: Huntington's disease—neuropathology, *Handb Clin Neurol* 100:83–100, 2011.
76. Paulsen JS: Cognitive impairment in Huntington disease: diagnosis and treatment, *Curr Neurol Neurosci Rep* 11(5):474–483, 2011.

77. Roos RA: Huntington's disease: a clinical review, *Orphanet J Rare Dis* 5(1):40, 2010.
78. Ross CA, Tabrizi SJ: Huntington's disease: from molecular pathogenesis to clinical treatment, *Lancet Neurol* 10(1):83–98, 2011.
79. Galvez-Jiminez H: Parkinson's disease. In Gilman S, editor: *Neurobiology of disease*, ed 1, Burlington, MA, 2007, Academic Press.
80. Parkinson Disease Foundation: *Statistics on Parkinsons's*. Available at www.pdf.org/en/parkinson_statistics. Accessed May 13, 2013.
81. Galvan A, Wichmann T: Pathophysiology of parkinsonism, *Clin Neurophysiol* 119(7):1459–1474, 2008.
82. Schapira AH, Jenner P: Etiology and pathogenesis of Parkinson's disease, *Mov Disord* 26(6):1049–1055, 2011.
83. Wakabayashi K et al: The Lewy body in Parkinson's disease: molecules implicated in the formation and degradation of alpha-synuclein aggregates, *Neuropathology* 27(5):494–506, 2007.
84. Rommelfanger KS, Weinshenker D: Norepinephrine: the redheaded stepchild of Parkinson's disease, *Biochem Pharmacol* 74(2):177–190, 2007.
85. Fasano M, Lopiano L: Alpha-synuclein and Parkinson's disease: a proteomic view, *Exp Rev Proteomics* 5(2):239–248, 2008.
86. Thomas B, Beal MF: Parkinson's disease, *Hum Mol Genet* 16(Spec No 2):R183–R194, 2007.
87. Probst A, Block A, Tolnay M: New insights into the pathology of Parkinson's disease: does the peripheral autonomic nervous system become central? *Eur J Neurol* 15(Suppl 1):1–4, 2008.
88. Hoehn M, Yahr M: Parkinsonism: onset, progression and mortality, *Neurology* 17(5):427–442, 1967.
89. Wolters E: Variablility in the clinical expression of Parkinson's disease, *J Neurol Sci* 266(1-2):197–203, 2008.
90. Jankovic J: Parkinson's disease: clinical features and diagnosis, *J Neurol Neurosurg Psychiatry* 79(4):368–376, 2008.
91. Doherty KM et al: Postural deformities in Parkinson's disease, *Lancet Neurol* 10(6):538–549, 2011.
92. Jain S: Multi-organ autonomic dysfunction in Parkinson disease, *Parkinsonism Relat Disord* 17(2):77–83, 2011.
93. Blonder LX, Slevin JT: Emotional dysfunction in Parkinson's disease, *Behav Neurol* 24(3):201–217, 2011.
94. Schwarz J et al: Depression in Parkinson's disease, *J Neurol* 258(Suppl 2):S336–S338, 2011.
95. Kehagia AA, Barker RA, Robbins TW: Neuropsychological and clinical heterogeneity of cognitive impairment and dementia in patients with Parkinson's disease, *Lancet Neurol* 9(12):1200–1213, 2010.
96. Aarsland D, Kurz MW: The epidemiology of dementia associated with Parkinson disease, *J Neurol Sci* 289(1-2):18–22, 2010.
97. Steiner JA, Angot E, Brundin P: A deadly spread: cellular mechanisms of α-synuclein transfer, *Cell Death Differ* 18(9):1425–1433, 2011.
98. Gitchel GT et al: Pervasive ocular tremor in patients with Parkinson disease, *Arch Neurol*, April 9, 2012. Published online.
99. Seppi K et al: The Movement Disorder Society evidence-based medicine review update: treatments for the non-motor symptoms of Parkinson's disease, *Mov Disord* 26(Suppl 3):S42–S80, 2011.
100. Schulte EC, Winkelmann J: When Parkinson's disease patients go to sleep: specific sleep disturbances related to Parkinson's disease, *J Neurol* 258(Suppl 2):S328–S335, 2011.
101. Baker JH: The symptom experience of patients with Parkinson disease, *J Neurosci Nurs* 38(1):51–57, 2006.
102. Defer GL et al: Core assessment program for surgical interventional therapies in Parkinson's disease (CAPSIT-PD), *Mov Disord* 14(4):572–584, 1999.
103. Chahine LM, Stern MB: Diagnostic markers for Parkinson's disease, *Curr Opin Neurol* 24(4):309–317, 2011.
104. Janikivic J: Parkinson's disease: clinical features and diagnosis, *J Neurol Neurosurg Psychiatry* 79:368–376, 2008.
105. Winkler J et al: Parkinson's disease risk score: moving to a premotor diagnosis, *J Neurol* 258(Suppl 2):S311–S315, 2011.
106. Forsaa EB et al: What predicts mortality in Parkinson disease: a prospective population-based long-term study, *Neurology* 75(14):1270–1276, 2010.
107. Posada IJ et al: Mortality from Parkinson's disease: a population-based prospective study (NEDICES), *Mov Disord* 26(14):2522–2529, 2011.
108. Jann MW: Advanced strategies for treatment of Parkinson's disease: the role of early treatment, *Am J Manag Care* 17(Suppl 12):S315–S321, 2011.
109. Fox SH et al: The Movement Disorder Society evidence-based medicine review update: treatments for the motor symptoms of Parkinson's disease, *Mov Disord* 26(Suppl 3):S2–S41, 2011.
110. Hickey P, Stacy M: Available and emerging treatments for Parkinson's disease: a review, *Drug Des Devel Ther* 5:241–254, 2011.
111. Amyotrophoic Lateral Sclerosis Association: *Epidemiology of ALS and suspected clusters*. Available at www.alsa.org/als-care/resources/publications-videos/factsheets/epidemiology.html. Accessed May 13, 2013.
112. Andersen PM, Al-Chalabi A: Clinical genetics of amyotrophic lateral sclerosis: what do we really know? *Nat Rev Neurol* 7(11):603–615, 2011.
113. Redler RL, Dokholyan NV: The complex molecular biology of amyotrophic lateral sclerosis (ALS), *Prog Mol Biol Transl Sci* 107:215–262, 2012.
114. Liscic RM, Breljak D: Molecular basis of amyotrophic lateral sclerosis, *Prog Neuropsychopharmacol Biol Psychiatry* 35(2):370–372, 2011.
115. Wijesekera LC, Leigh PN: Amyotrophic lateral sclerosis, *Orphanet J Rare Dis* 4:3, 2009.
116. Hardiman O, van den Berg LH, Kiernan MC: Clinical diagnosis and management of amyotrophic lateral sclerosis, *Nat Rev Neurol* 7(11):639–649, 2011.
117. Mateen FJ, Carone M, Sorenson EJ: Patients who survive 5 years or more with ALS in Olmsted County, 1925-2004, *J Neurol Neurosurg Psychiatry* 81(10):1144–1146, 2010.
118. McGee S: *Evidence-based physical diagnosis*, ed 3, Philadelphia, 2012, Saunders.
119. Heilman KM, Watson RT, Gonzalez-Rothi LJ: Praxis. In Goetz CG, editor: *Textbook of clinical neurology*, Philadelphia, 2003, Saunders.

CHAPTER 18

Disorders of the Central and Peripheral Nervous Systems and the Neuromuscular Junction

Barbara J. Boss and Sue E. Huether

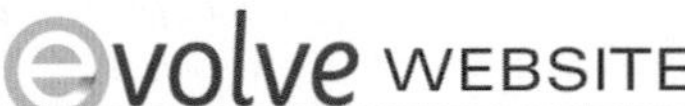

http://evolve.elsevier.com/McCance/

- Review Questions and Answers
- Animations
- Online Course: Module 9

CHAPTER OUTLINE

Alterations in central nervous system (CNS) structure and function are caused by traumatic injury, vascular disorders, tumor growth, infectious and inflammatory processes, metabolic derangements (including those arising from nutritional deficiencies and drugs/chemicals), and degenerative processes. Alterations in peripheral nervous system function involve the nerve roots (radiculopathies), a nerve plexus, the nerves themselves (neuropathies), or the neuromuscular junction.

CENTRAL NERVOUS SYSTEM DISORDERS

Traumatic Brain and Spinal Cord Injury

Traumatic Brain Injury

Traumatic brain injury (TBI) is an alteration in brain function or other evidence of brain pathology caused by an external force.[1] An estimated 1.7 million people sustain TBI in the United States each year with approximately 53,000 deaths. Those at highest risk for TBI are children 4 years and younger, adolescents 15 to 19 years, and adults 65 years and older. Males have the highest incidence in every age group.[2] TBI is highest among American Indian/Alaska Natives and blacks and in lower- and median-income families. TBIs are caused by falls (35%), motor vehicle–related injuries (17%), and a strike or blow to the head from or against an object (e.g., workplace or sports-related injuries [16.5%], assaults [10%], and other and unknown causes [21%]).[3]

TBI survival is improving because of advancements in safety measures (e.g., passive seat restraints, air bags, protective head gear), reduced transport time to hospitals or trauma centers, and improved on-scene and follow-up medical management. Prevention and management of secondary and tertiary brain injuries also have improved outcomes. TBI is capable of producing physical, intellectual, emotional, social, and vocational changes.

TABLE 18-1 **SEVERITY OF BLUNT TRAUMA, TRAUMA STATE INDUCED, AND ONSET AND PERSISTENCE OF CLINICAL MANIFESTATIONS**

SEVERITY OF TRAUMA	TRAUMA STATE INDUCED: FOCAL INJURY	TRAUMA STATE INDUCED: DIFFUSE AXONAL INJURY (DAI)	ONSET OF CLINICAL MANIFESTATIONS	PERSISTENCE OF DAI CLINICAL MANIFESTATIONS
Mild blunt trauma		Mild concussion	Immediate	Hours to days
Moderate blunt trauma		Classic cerebral concussion	Immediate	Up to 6 months or longer
	Paraplegia (associated with injury to top of head)		Immediate	
	Blindness (associated with occipital injury)		Immediate	
	Delayed development of unresponsiveness (vasomotor or vasovagal syncopal episode)		Delayed	
Severe blunt trauma		Mild DAI	Immediate	Recovery in days to weeks
		Moderate DAI	Immediate	Residual manifestation
		Severe DAI	Immediate	Permanent severe disability
	Acute epidural hemorrhage		Immediate to delayed (2-3 hours)	
	Acute contusional swelling		Delayed onset (few hours after injury)	
	Acute subdural hematoma		Delayed onset (few hours to 1 week after injury)	
	*Subacute subdural hematoma**		Delayed onset (1 to few weeks)	
	Subdural hygroma (fluid accumulation)		Delayed onset	
	*Traumatic cerebral hemorrhage**		Delayed onset (as late as 1 week after injury)	

*May be seen after moderate head injury, especially in elderly people.

Traumatic brain injury can be caused by closed (blunt) trauma and open (penetrating) trauma. **Closed (blunt) trauma** is more common and involves either the head striking a hard surface or a rapidly moving object striking the head. The dura mater remains intact, and brain tissues are not exposed to the environment. Most closed (blunt) trauma is mild (75% to 90%) and causes mild concussion and classic cerebral concussion (see pp. 587-588 and Table 18-1). **Open (penetrating) trauma** occurs when a break in (penetration of) the dura mater results in exposure of the cranial contents to the environment.

The Glasgow Coma Scale (GCS) is used to assess severity of injury.[4] The hallmark of a severe TBI is loss of consciousness for 6 hours or more. TBI classifications using the GCS are: (1) mild TBI with GCS score of 13 to 15, associated with mild concussion; (2) moderate TBI with GCS score of 9 to 12, associated with structural injury such as hemorrhage or contusion; and (3) severe TBI with GCS score of 3 to 8, associated with cognitive and/or physical disability or death. Age and admission GCS score are important diagnostic factors in TBI.[5] Mild TBI is characterized by five features: a GCS score between 13 and 15, a brief period of unconsciousness or dazed consciousness, posttraumatic amnesia, negative neuroimaging studies, and recovery within weeks to months without sequelae or the need for specific medical intervention.

Three mechanisms produce brain damage: primary, secondary, and tertiary injury. Primary injury is caused by the impact and involves neural injury, primary glial injury, vascular responses, and shearing and rotational forces. Secondary injury is an indirect consequence of the primary injury and includes a cascade of cellular and molecular brain events (Figure 18-1). Tertiary injury can develop days or months later as a consequence of systemic complications, such as pneumonia, fever, infections, and immobility, which contribute to further brain injury or delays in repair.

Primary Brain Injury. Primary brain injuries can be classified as focal, affecting one area of the brain, or diffuse (diffuse axonal injury [DAI]), involving more than one area of the brain (see Table 18-1). Both types of injury can be associated with the same initiating event and can occur with brain trauma or stroke syndromes (see Figure 18-1). Focal brain injury accounts for more than two thirds of head injury deaths; DAI accounts for less than one third. However, more severely disabled survivors, including those in an unresponsive state or reduced level of consciousness, have DAI.

Focal Brain Injury. Focal brain injuries are specific, grossly observable brain lesions that occur in a precise location (e.g., cortical contusions, epidural hemorrhage, subdural hematoma, intracerebral hematoma). Focal brain injuries can occur

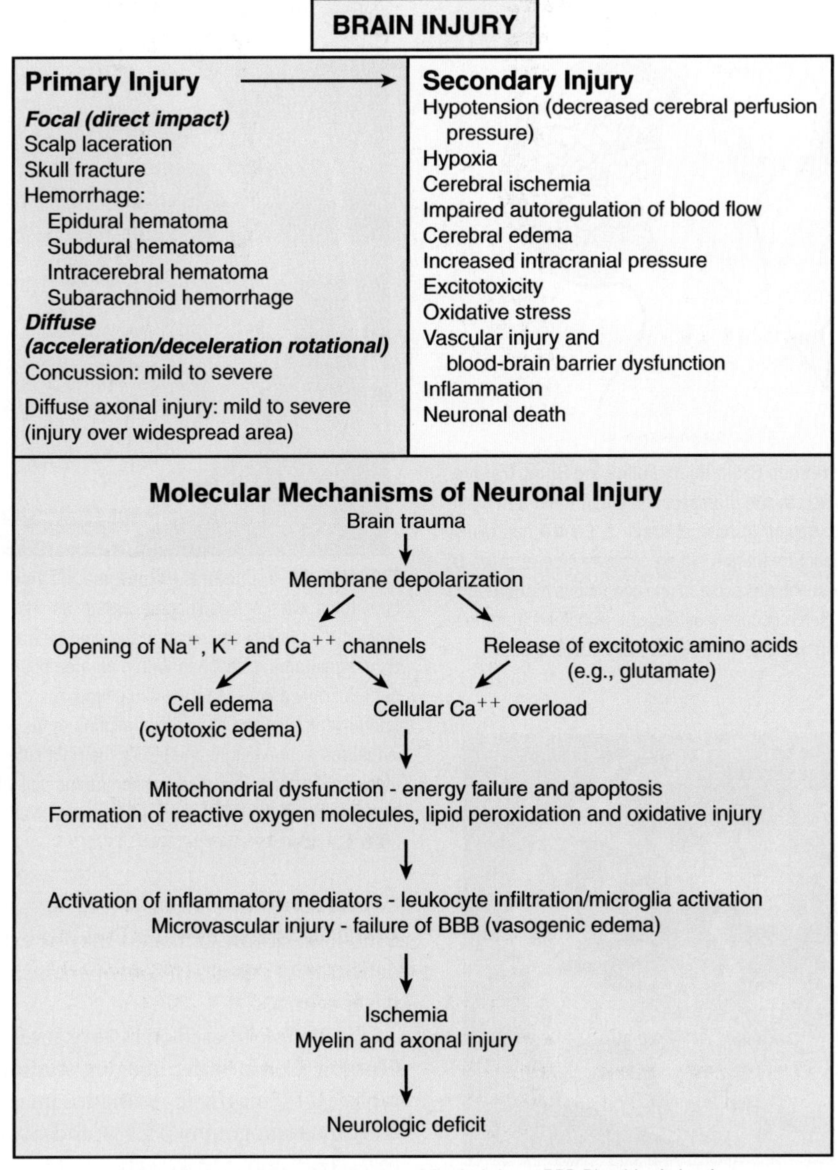

FIGURE 18-1 Pathophysiology of Brain Injury. *BBB,* Blood-brain barrier.

with both blunt and open brain trauma and can be associated with skull fractures.

Focal brain injury results from compression of the skull at the point of impact and rebound effects. The focal injury may be a **coup injury** (directly below the point of impact) or **contrecoup** (on the pole opposite the site of impact) (Figure 18-2). Objects (e.g., baseball bat, weapon) striking the front of the head usually produce only coup injuries (contusions and fractures) because the inner skull in the occipital area is smooth. Objects striking the back of the head usually result in both coup and contrecoup injuries because of the irregularity of the inner surface of the frontal bones. Objects striking the side of the head may produce coup or contrecoup injuries. The force of impact (translational acceleration) typically produces localized brain contusions. Injury to the vault, other vessels, and supporting structures can produce epidural hemorrhage and subdural and intracerebral hematomas.

Contusions (blood leaking from an injured vessel) (Figure 18-3) are found most commonly in the frontal lobes, particularly at the poles and along the inferior orbital surfaces; in the temporal lobes, especially at the anterior poles and along the inferior surface; and at the frontotemporal junction. Contusion severity varies with the amount of impact energy transmitted by the skull to underlying brain tissue. The smaller the area of impact, the greater the severity of injury because the force is concentrated into a smaller area. Brain edema forms around and in damaged neural tissues, contributing to increasing intracranial pressure (ICP). Within the contused areas are infarction and necrosis, multiple hemorrhages, and edema. The tissue has a pulpy quality. The maximum effects of injury related to contusion, bleeding, and edema peak 18 to 36 hours after severe head injury.

Contusions cause changes in attention, memory, executive attentional function (motivation, goal selection or formation, planning, self-monitoring, and use of feedback), affect, emotion, and behavior. Less commonly, contusions occur in the parietal and occipital lobes. Focal cerebral contusions are

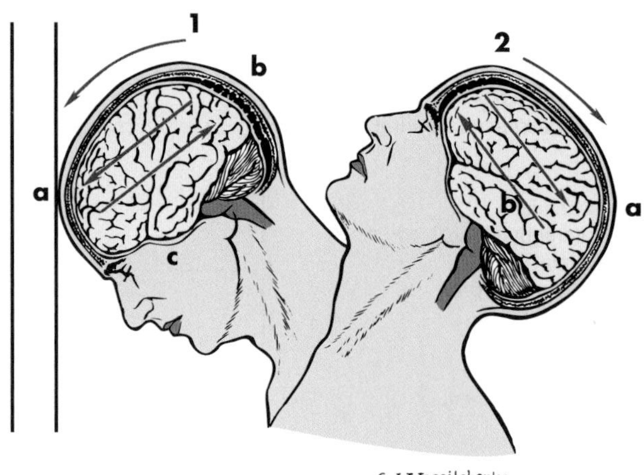

FIGURE 18-2 **Coup and Contrecoup Brain Injury Following Blunt Trauma.** **1,** Coup injury: impact against object; ***a,*** site of impact and direct trauma to brain; ***b,*** shearing of subdural veins; ***c,*** trauma to base of brain. **2,** Contrecoup injury: impact within skull; ***a,*** site of impact from brain hitting opposite side of skull; ***b,*** shearing forces through brain. These injuries occur in one continuous motion—the head strikes the wall (coup) and then rebounds (contrecoup). (Modified from Rudy EB: *Advanced neurological and neurosurgical nursing,* St Louis, 1984, Mosby.)

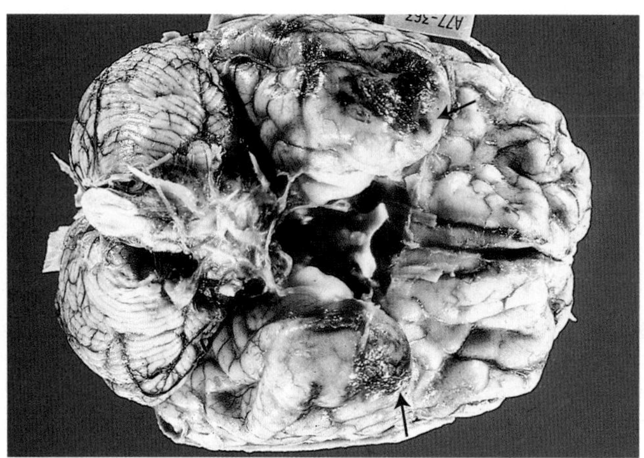

FIGURE 18-3 **Cerebral Contusions.** The temporal poles are discolored by areas of hemorrhage *(arrows).* Such lesions represent "bruises" on the surface of the brain caused by violent contact between the delicate brain parenchyma and the hard inner surface of the skull. (From Kumar V, Cotran RS, Robbins SL: *Robbins basic pathology,* ed 7, Philadelphia, 2003, Saunders.)

superficial, involving just the gyri. Hemorrhagic contusions may coalesce into a large, confluent intracranial hematoma.

The clinical manifestations of a *contusion* may include immediate loss of consciousness (generally accepted to last no longer than 5 minutes); loss of reflexes, which results in the individual falling to the ground; transient cessation of respiration; brief period of bradycardia; and decrease in blood pressure (lasting 30 seconds to a few minutes). A momentary increase in cerebrospinal fluid (CSF) pressure and changes on electrocardiogram (ECG) and electroencephalogram (EEG) recordings have been demonstrated to occur on impact. Vital signs may stabilize to normal values in a few seconds. Reflexes return next and the person begins to regain consciousness. Returning to being fully awake and alert can vary from minutes to days. Regaining

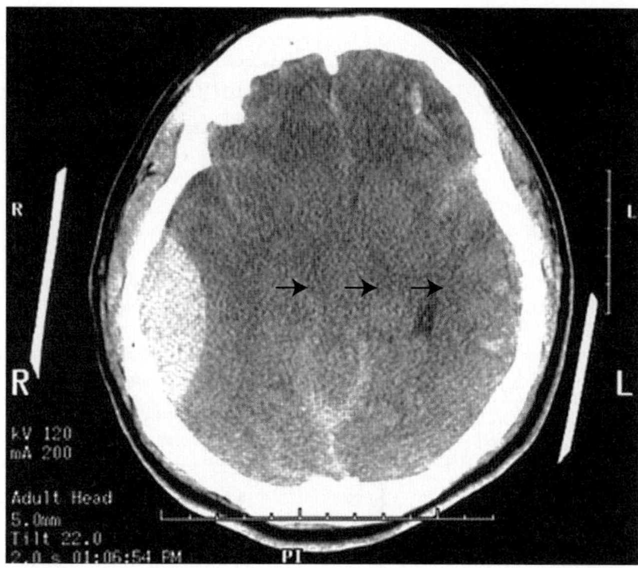

FIGURE 18-4 **Epidural Hematoma, CT Image.** Note the large right epidural hematoma with a lens-shaped outline as the smooth dura becomes indented against the underlying cortex on the right lateral aspect of the cerebrum. The epidural hematoma is confined within an area bounded by cranial sutures where the dura is firmly adherent to the skull. Note the mass effect with effacement of the lateral ventricles and the shift of midline to the left *(arrows).* In this case the individual fell from a height and struck the right side of his head, severing the middle meningeal artery. This epidural hematoma collected within hours. *CT,* Computed tomography. (From Klatt EC: *Robbins and Cotran atlas of pathology,* Philadelphia, 2006, Saunders.)

a full level of consciousness may be extremely slow and residual deficits may persist. In some persons, full level of consciousness never returns.

Evaluation is based on history, level of consciousness using the Glasgow Coma Scale, imaging studies (e.g., computed tomography [CT], magnetic resonance imaging [MRI], and positron-emission tomography [PET]), and assessment of vital parameters (e.g., ICP and EEG). Large contusions and lacerations with hemorrhage may be excised surgically.[6] Otherwise, treatment is directed at controlling ICP and managing symptoms.

Extradural hematomas (bleeding between the dura mater and the skull [i.e., epidural hematomas or epidural hemorrhages]) represent 1% to 2% of major head injuries and occur in all age groups, but most commonly in those 20 to 40 years of age. Extradural hematomas are caused most commonly by motor vehicle accidents (MVAs) and occasionally by falls and sporting accidents. A temporal fracture causes 90% of temporal lobe extradural hematomas. Direct frontal lobe trauma is associated with frontal extradural hematomas. Posterior extradural hematomas are associated with a fracture across the transverse sinus from an occipital blow.

An artery is the source of bleeding in 85% of extradural hematomas (Figure 18-4); 15% result from injury to the meningeal vein or dural sinus. Ninety percent of individuals also have a skull fracture. The temporal fossa is the most common site of extradural hematoma caused by injury to the middle meningeal artery or vein. The resulting shift of the temporal lobe medially precipitates uncal and hippocampal gyrus herniation

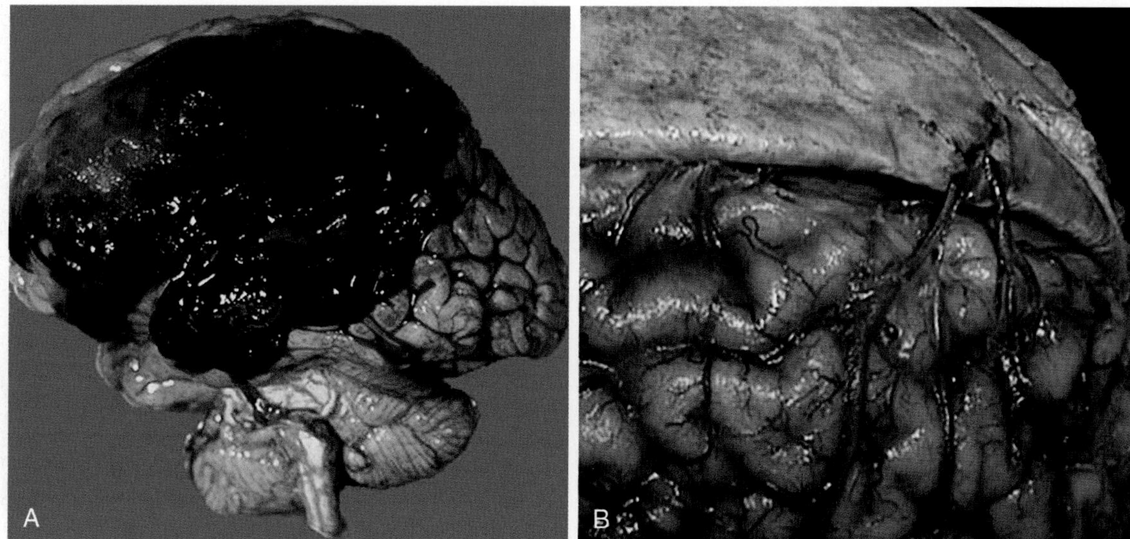

FIGURE 18-5 Subdural Hematoma, Gross, and Bridging Veins, Gross. A large subdural hematoma **(A)** is seen in the frontoparietal region. A subdural hematoma forms after head trauma that severs the bridging veins from dura to brain, shown in the right panel **(B)**, where the dura has been reflected to reveal the normal appearance of the bridging veins that extend across to the superior aspect of the cerebral hemispheres. Older adults and the very young are at greater risk because their cerebral veins are more vulnerable to injury. Because the bleeding is venous, blood collects over hours to weeks, with variable onset of symptoms. Because the blood collects beneath the dura, a subdural hematoma can be seen to cross the region of cranial sutures. (From Klatt EC: *Robbins and Cotran atlas of pathology,* Philadelphia, 2006, Saunders.)

through the tentorial notch. Extradural hemorrhages are found occasionally in the subfrontal area (especially in the young and older adult populations), caused by injury to the anterior meningeal artery or a venous sinus, and in the occipital-suboccipital area, which results in herniation of the posterior fossa contents through the foramen magnum. CT and MRI show a lens-shaped mass over the surface of the cortex.

Individuals with classic *temporal extradural hematomas* (i.e., over the temporal lobe) experience loss of consciousness at the time of injury, followed by a lucid period that lasts from a few hours to a few days in one third of individuals (if bleeding from a vein). As the hematoma accumulates, a headache of increasing severity, vomiting, drowsiness, confusion, seizure, and hemiparesis may develop. Level of consciousness may dwindle rapidly as temporal lobe herniation begins. Clinical manifestations of temporal lobe herniation also include ipsilateral pupillary dilation and contralateral hemiparesis.

The diagnosis of an extradural hematoma is usually made by CT or MRI. In some instances, diagnosis is made by history and clinical findings, because time for a CT or MRI is not available. The prognosis is usually good if intervention is initiated before bilateral dilation of the pupils. Surgical therapy is evacuation of the hematoma through burr holes, followed by ligation of the bleeding vessel or vessels. Extradural hematomas are almost always medical emergencies.

Subdural hematomas arise in 10% to 20% of TBIs. MVAs are the most common cause of subdural hematomas; 50% of subdural hematomas are associated with skull fractures. Falls, especially in older adults or in those with long-term alcohol abuse, are associated with chronic subdural hematomas.

Acute subdural hematomas rapidly develop (within 48 hours) and usually are located at the top of the skull (the cerebral convexities). On CT they appear as a high-density mass. *Bilateral hematomas* occur in 15% to 20% of persons. *Subacute subdural hematomas* develop more slowly, often over 48 hours to 2 weeks. On CT they appear as a mixed-density mass. Chronic subdural hematomas (commonly found in older adults and those who abuse alcohol and have some degree of brain atrophy with a subsequent increase in the extradural space) develop over weeks to months. Tearing of the bridging veins is the major cause of rapidly developing and subacutely developing subdural hematomas, although torn cortical veins or venous sinuses and contused tissue may be the source. These subdural hematomas act as expanding masses, giving rise to increased ICP that eventually compresses the bleeding vessels (Figures 18-5 and 18-6). The displacement of brain tissue can result in a herniation syndrome.

In *acute, rapidly developing subdural hematomas* the expanding clots directly compress the brain, giving rise to the clinical manifestations. As the ICP rises the bleeding veins are compressed and thus bleeding is self-limiting, although cerebral compression and displacement of brain tissue can cause temporal lobe herniation.

An *acute subdural hematoma* classically begins with headache, drowsiness, restlessness or agitation, slowed cognition, and confusion. These symptoms worsen over time and progress to loss of consciousness, respiratory pattern changes, and pupillary dilation (the symptoms of temporal lobe herniation). These manifestations are more pronounced than focal manifestations such as dysphasia, dyspraxia, or hemiparesis. Other clinical manifestations may include homonymous hemianopsia (defective vision in either the right or the left field), dysconjugate gaze, and gaze palsies.

The pathogenesis of a *chronic subdural hematoma* is different. The existing subdural space gradually fills with blood.

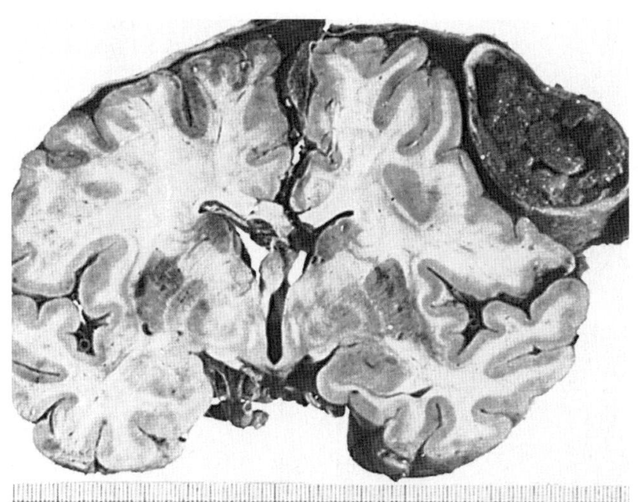

FIGURE 18-6 Chronic Subdural Hematoma. Compression of underlying brain and lateral ventricle. (From Kissane JM, editor: *Anderson's pathology,* ed 9, St Louis, 1993, Mosby.)

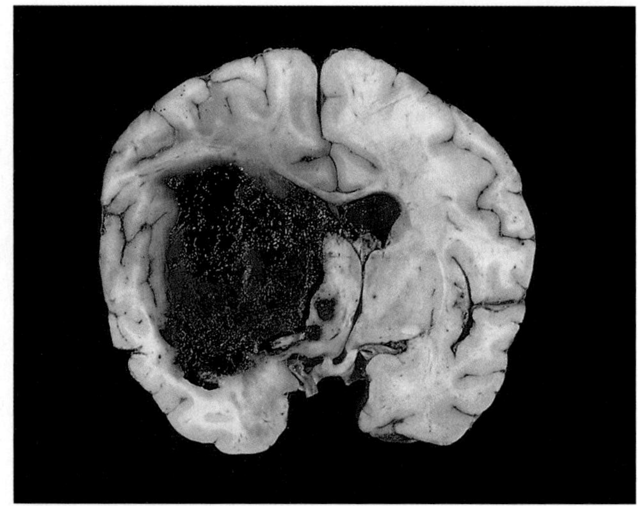

FIGURE 18-7 Acute Intracerebral Hemorrhage. A fresh hematoma has disrupted and expanded the left cerebral hemisphere, causing the midline structures to shift to the right. Uncontrolled hypertension is an important cause of this catastrophic lesion. (From Kumar V, Cotran RS, Robbins SL: *Robbins basic pathology,* ed 7, Philadelphia, 2003, Saunders.)

A vascular membrane forms around the hematoma in approximately 2 weeks. Further enlargement takes place in some persons, but the mechanism of this enlargement is unclear.

Presenting manifestations of *chronic subdural hematomas* vary. Of those affected, 80% have chronic headaches and tenderness over the hematoma on percussion. Most appear to have a progressive dementia accompanied by generalized rigidity (paratonia).

Whereas most acute and subacute subdural hematomas are treated with clot evacuation through a burr hole, chronic subdural hematomas (and some that are subacute) require a craniotomy to evacuate the gelatinous blood. The membrane around a chronic subdural hematoma is then dissected away from the dura mater and arachnoid membranes. A technique for percutaneous drainage for chronic subdural hematomas has proved successful.

Intracerebral hematomas occur in 2% to 3% of head injuries and are usually associated with MVAs and falls from some distance. Intracerebral hematomas may be single or multiple, and they are associated with contusions. Although most commonly located in the frontal and temporal lobes, intracerebral hematomas may occur in the hemispheric deep white matter. Small blood vessels are traumatized by penetrating injury or shearing forces. The intracerebral hematoma then acts as an expanding mass, resulting in increased ICP and compression of brain tissues with resultant edema and ischemia (Figure 18-7). Delayed intracerebral hematomas may appear 3 to 10 days after the head injury.

A decreasing level of consciousness is associated with an *intracerebral hematoma.* Coma or a confusional state from other injuries, however, can make the cause of this increasing unresponsiveness difficult to detect. Contralateral hemiplegia also may occur. As the ICP rises, clinical manifestations of temporal lobe herniation may appear. In delayed intracerebral hematoma, the presentation is similar to that of hypertensive brain hemorrhage: sudden, rapidly progressive decreased level of consciousness with pupillary dilation; breathing pattern changes; hemiplegia; and bilateral positive Babinski reflexes.

Evacuation of a singular intracerebral hematoma has only occasionally been helpful, mostly for subcortical white matter hematomas. Otherwise, treatment is directed at reducing the ICP to maintain cerebral perfusion pressure and allowing the hematoma to reabsorb slowly. Secondary brain injury is common (see p. 588).

Open brain trauma produces both focal and diffuse injuries and includes compound skull fractures and missile injuries (e.g., bullets, rocks, shell fragments, knives, and blunt instruments). A compound fracture opens a communication between the cranial contents and the environment and should be investigated whenever there are lacerations of the scalp, tympanic membrane, a sinus, an eye, or mucous membranes. Such fractures may involve the cranial vault or the base of the skull (basilar skull fracture). A basilar skull fracture can involve the temporal, sphenoid, and occipital bones. The cranial nerves may be damaged and the meninges torn, causing leakage of cerebrospinal fluid from the ear and nose, or both. Severity of brain damage is related to the severity of skull fracture. Infection is a significant complication. Injury incurred from bone fragments is mainly a tangential injury (injury caused by direct contact) and occasionally a penetrating injury. Bone fragments may lacerate or contuse brain tissues or blood vessels.

The mechanisms of open brain trauma are crush injury (laceration and crushing of tissue touched by the missile) and stretch injury (damage of blood vessels and nerves not directly contacted, occurring as a result of stretching). *Crush injury* is the laceration and crushing of whatever tissue the missile touches, with the amount of crush related to the degree of fragmentation, deformity, size, and shape. The tangential injury is injury to the coverings of the brain (scalp and brain lacerations) and also may include skull fractures and meningeal and cerebral lacerations. When driven into the brain substance, projectiles and debris from scalp and skull injury produce a penetrating brain injury. Occasionally projectiles are so forceful that they exit the cranial vault in addition to entering it, producing a through-and-through injury (e.g., high-velocity bullets). Primary damage is localized along the path of the penetrating object, and direct tissue disruption along the projectile tract results.

Stretch injury involves blood vessels and nerves that are damaged without direct contact as a result of the amount of tissue stretched secondary to shape, deformation, and striking velocity. Air compressed in front of a bullet exerts an explosive effect on entry, producing extreme distant tissue damage and an immediate primary increase in ICP; a cavity many times greater than the size of the bullet is produced because the brain tissue is propelled away from the tract. The cavity and pressure produce contrecoup injuries. The intracranial volume is increased directly by the projectile and the debris. The temporary cavity collapses back onto itself, leaving a smaller, permanent cavity. Intracranial bleeding occurs into the permanent cavity and may cause the cavity to expand. Edema in and around the injured brain tissue rapidly develops; edema and bleeding contribute markedly to increased ICP. This second rise in ICP to 60 to 100 mmHg may last 2 to 5 minutes. Because of acute ischemic damage to the tract, necrosis of tissue begins. Within hours after bullet-induced injury, tissue within 1 cm adjacent to the tract disintegrates. Demyelination of white matter affected by hemorrhage and edema occurs by the second day. Clinical manifestations such as unconsciousness, flaccidity, or decerebrate posture (see Chapter 17) are associated with high mortality.

Most victims lose consciousness with open-head injury. The depth of the coma and the length of the unresponsive state are related to the location of injury, extent of damage, and amount of bleeding. The diagnosis of a compound fracture is made through physical examination, skull radiographs, or both. The diagnosis of a basilar skull fracture is made on the basis of clinical findings. Skull radiographs often do not demonstrate the fracture, although intracranial air or air in the sinuses on radiograph, CT, or MRI is indirect evidence of a basilar skull fracture.

A compound linear fracture is débrided nonsurgically in cooperative adults and surgically in children and uncooperative adults. Cranioplasty with insertion of bone or an artificial graft may be necessary but often is delayed until antibiotics have been given. Antibiotics are administered after surgery. Open-head injury often requires surgery to débride the traumatized tissues to prevent infection and to remove blood clots to help reduce the ICP. ICP also is managed with dehydrating agents, osmotic diuretics, or a combination of these drugs. Broad-spectrum antibiotics are administered to prevent infection. Use of prophylactic antibiotics is controversial because studies have failed to demonstrate that they reduce the rate of infection.[7] Bed rest and close observation for meningitis and other complications are prescribed for a basilar skull fracture.

Diffuse Brain Injury. Diffuse brain injury (diffuse axonal injury [DAI]) involves widespread areas of the brain. Damage to delicate axonal fibers and white matter tracts that project to the cerebral cortex causes concussion. Mechanical effects from high levels of acceleration and deceleration (whiplash) and rotational and twisting movements are the primary mechanisms of injury, producing strains and distortions within the brain (see Figure 18-2). As a result of the skull's motion caused

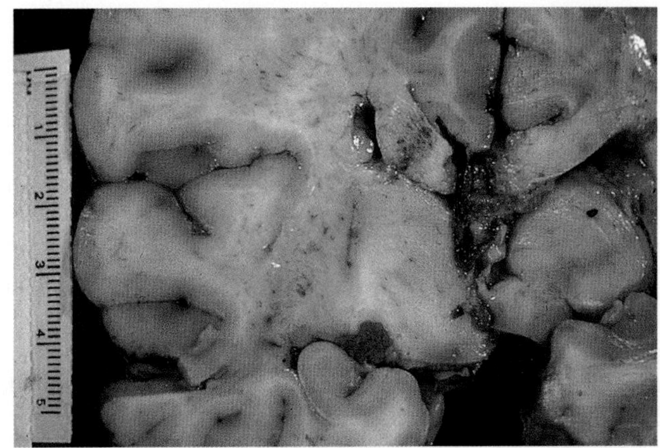

FIGURE 18-8 Diffuse Axonal Injury. Gross photograph demonstrating characteristic hemorrhage lesions within the corpus callosum. (Courtesy Walter Kemp, MD, Department of Pathology, University of Texas Southwestern Medical School, Dallas. From Kumar V, Cotran RS, Robbins SL: *Robbins basic pathology,* ed 7, Philadelphia, 2003, Saunders.)

by its attachment to the neck, striking the head causes rotational forces that can trigger shearing forces on brain tissues. Stretching and tearing of nerve fibers result in axonal damage. The most severe axonal injuries are located more peripheral to the brainstem, causing extensive cognitive and affective impairments, as seen in survivors of traumatic brain injury from vehicular crashes. Axonal damage reduces the speed of information processing and response and disrupts the individual's attention span.

Pathophysiologically, axonal damage can be seen only with an electron microscope and involves numerous axons alone or axonal injury in conjunction with actual tissue tears (Figure 18-8). Areas where axons and small blood vessels are torn appear as small hemorrhages, located particularly in the corpus callosum and dorsolateral quadrant of the rostral brainstem at the superior cerebellar peduncle. Increasingly more damaged axons are visible 12 hours to several days after the injury and secondary brain injury also is occurring (see p. 588). The severity of diffuse injury correlates with how much shearing force was applied to the brain. DAI is not associated with intracranial hypertension immediately after injury; however, secondary brain injury causes acute brain swelling from increased intravascular blood flow within the brain, vasodilation, and increased cerebral blood volume.

Several categories of diffuse brain injury exist: mild concussion, classic concussion, mild DAI, moderate DAI, and severe DAI (see Table 18-1 and Figure 18-1).

Mild concussion (mild traumatic brain injury) is characterized by immediate but transitory clinical manifestations. CSF pressure rises, and ECG and EEG changes occur without loss of consciousness. The Glasgow Coma Scale score is 13 to 15.[8] The initial confusional state lasts from 1 to several minutes, possibly with amnesia for events preceding the trauma (retrograde amnesia). Anterograde amnesia also may exist transiently. Persons may experience head pain and complain of nervousness and "not being themselves" for up to a few days. Three grades have been described:

Grade I: Transient confusion and disorientation accompanied by amnesia (momentary); no loss of consciousness; symptoms resolve within 15 minutes

Grade II: Transient confusion and retrograde amnesia that develops after 5 to 10 minutes (memory loss involves only events occurring several minutes before injury); symptoms last more than 15 minutes

Grade III: Any loss of consciousness (seconds or minutes); confusion and retrograde and anterograde amnesia remain present from impact and persist for several minutes

Classic cerebral concussion (Grade IV) is any loss of consciousness (can last up to 6 hours) accompanied by retrograde and anterograde amnesia. Transient cessation of respiration can occur with brief periods of bradycardia, and a decrease in blood pressure lasting 30 seconds or less occurs. Vital signs stabilize within a few seconds to within normal limits. This is a phenomenon of physiologic, neurologic dysfunction without substantial anatomic disruption. A confusional state persists for hours to days. The individual experiences head pain, nausea, and fatigue. Attentional and memory system impairments may persist for weeks to months and may include inability to concentrate and forgetfulness. Mood and affect changes may persist for weeks to months and may include nervousness, anxiety reactions, depression, irritability, fatigability, and insomnia. There are two forms of Grade IV classic cerebral concussion: uncomplicated classic cerebral concussion (without focal injury) and complicated classic cerebral concussion (accompanied by focal injury [e.g., a cerebral contusion that yields focal signs]).

Some of the effects of a concussion may persist for weeks or months, depending on the severity of the injury. Approximately 15% to 30% of persons have a **postconcussive syndrome** that includes headache, nervousness or anxiety, irritability, insomnia, depression, inability to concentrate, forgetfulness, and fatigability.[9] Treatment entails reassurance, symptomatic relief, and close observation for 24 hours with follow-up care for persistent symptoms.

DAI produces prolonged traumatic coma lasting more than 6 hours because of axonal disruption. Three forms of DAI exist: mild, moderate, and severe. In **mild diffuse axonal injury,** posttraumatic coma lasts 6 to 24 hours. Death is uncommon but residual cognitive, psychologic, and sensorimotor deficits may persist. Mild DAI is a relatively uncommon lesion, occurring in 8% of all severe head injuries and 19% of all cases of DAI. In mild DAI 30% of persons display decerebrate or decorticate posturing (see Figure 17-6); they may experience prolonged periods of stupor or restlessness.

In **moderate diffuse axonal injury,** widespread physiologic impairment exists throughout the cerebral cortex and diencephalon. Actual tearing of some axons in both hemispheres occurs. Basal skull fracture, a focal injury, is commonly associated with moderate DAI. Prolonged coma lasting more than 24 hours is present but prominent brainstem signs do not exist with moderate DAI. Recovery often is incomplete in 93% of those individuals who survive. Moderate DAI is the most common type of DAI and is found in 20% of severe head injuries and 45% of all cases of DAI.

In moderate DAI, the GCS score is 4 to 8 initially and 6 to 8 by 24 hours following the injury. Thirty-five percent of victims have transitory decerebration or decortication. The person often remains unconscious for days or weeks and on awakening is confused. He or she experiences a long period of posttraumatic anterograde and retrograde amnesia and often has permanent deficits in memory, selective attention, vigilance, detection, working memory, data processing, vision or perception, and language, as well as mood and affect changes ranging from mild to severe.

Severe diffuse axonal injury involves severe mechanical disruption of many axons in both cerebral hemispheres and those extending to the diencephalon and brainstem. Severe DAI represents 16% of all severe head injuries and 36% of all cases of DAI. With an initial GCS score of 3, the mortality is 78%;[5] with an initial score between 3 and 8, the mortality is 36%; 16% of persons have either a moderate or a severe disability and 5% survive in a coma (unresponsive) state.[5]

Severe DAI is associated with brainstem signs that disappear in a few weeks. The person experiences immediate autonomic dysfunction that resolves in a few weeks. Increased ICP appears 4 to 6 days after injury. Pulmonary complications occur frequently, with profound sensorimotor and cognitive system deficits. Severely compromised coordinated movements and verbal and written communication, inability to learn and reason, and inability to modulate behavior also are evident.

High-resolution CT scans and MRIs assist in the diagnosis of focal and diffuse brain injuries.[5,10] The goal of treatment is to maintain cerebral perfusion and oxygenation and promote neuroprotection. Implementation of traumatic brain injury guidelines decreases deaths and improves neurologic outcome.[11,12] Specifically, the evidence is inconclusive about the effectiveness of hyperventilation and mild hypothermia. Hypertonic saline or mannitol is used selectively to manage increased intracranial pressure (IICP).[13] Barbiturates have not been shown to be effective in reducing intracranial pressure or preventing adverse outcomes after TBI. The Corticosteroid Randomisation After Significant Head Injury (CRASH) trial showed corticosteroids increase mortality with acute TBI, so these drugs are no longer used. Antiepileptic drugs may be recommended to reduce the onset of early and late seizures. Prophylactic antibiotics have not been shown to reduce the risk of meningitis or death with a skull fracture. Progesterone is under investigation and may improve neurologic outcome.[14] Extensive research is underway to discover effective therapeutic interventions. Fluid and nutrition management has emerged as critically important in the care of individuals with severe brain injuries.[15]

Secondary Brain Injury. **Secondary neuronal injury** occurs when there is brain or spinal cord trauma and in stroke syndromes. It occurs within hours to days of the primary injury. **Secondary brain injury** is the result of both systemic and intracranial processes and is an indirect result of primary brain injury. Systemic hypotension, hypoxia, anemia, hypoglycemia, hyperglycemia, and hypercapnia contribute to secondary brain insults. Mechanisms of secondary injury include altered cerebral blood flow, ischemia, inflammation, cerebral edema, decreased cerebral perfusion pressure (CPP), IICP, and brain herniation. Molecular alterations occur with stretching and tearing of axonal membranes and ischemia (see Figure 18-1). The complex pathophysiology of secondary brain injury underlies the functional, cognitive, and behavioral changes associated with brain injury and the motor and sensory losses associated with spinal cord injury.

Cerebrovascular autoregulation (constriction or dilation in response to increases or decreases in CPP) is impaired after brain injury and may be transient or persistent with alterations in CO_2 reactivity (i.e., CO_2 vasodilation). Vasospasm commonly occurs, contributing to brain hypoperfusion, and is caused by chronic depolarization of vascular smooth muscle, release of endothelin (vasoconstrictor), and decreased availability of nitric oxide (vasodilator).

Widespread release of excitatory neurotransmitters (e.g., glutamate and aspartate) causes calcium and sodium influx that is neurotoxic (excitotoxicity). Mitochondrial loading with calcium leads to mitochondrial failure, anaerobic metabolism, lactic acid production, and increased levels of reactive oxygen species (ROS), phospholipases, and other enzymes. ROS and phospholipase damage proteins and the phospholipid components of cell and organelle membranes, causing cell swelling, vacuolization, and, ultimately, necrotic or programmed cell death (apoptosis). Energy metabolism is depressed with alteration of gene expression. These events lead to failure of the capillary blood-brain barrier and *vasogenic edema*. The influx of sodium attracts water and results in intracellular cytotoxic edema in neurons, astrocytes, and microglia irrespective of the integrity of the vascular endothelial wall. Edema increases intracranial pressure, contributing to tissue hypoxia and cerebral ischemia.[16,17]

Both primary and secondary injuries cause inflammation (see Chapter 7), which occurs immediately and persists for weeks. Inflammation is critical for wound healing; immune cells, including neutrophils, macrophages, and T-cell lymphocytes, need to infiltrate injured tissue and clear debris, thus promoting formation of scar tissue. However, an overactive response leads to occlusion of the microvasculature with leukocytes and platelets. The release of inflammatory cytokines (e.g., tumor necrosis factor-alpha [TNF-α], interleukins, and interferons), proteases, free radicals, prostaglandins, and complement alters the blood-brain barrier and causes vasoconstriction, brain edema, increased intracranial pressure, reduced cerebral perfusion, and ischemia, aggravating secondary brain injury.[17,18]

Intracranial hemorrhage, whether traumatic or related to a stroke syndrome, may contribute to secondary brain injury. The bleeding is often accompanied by increased ICP, ischemia, oxidative damage, and vasogenic and cytotoxic edema as previously described. In addition, the vascular injury can cause activation of platelets, which contribute to vasoconstriction in large arteries and vasodilation in small arteries. Activated platelets also trigger the release of free radicals from granulocytes, enhancing oxidative stress. Vascular injury causes coagulation disorders from release of increased amounts of tissue factor from endothelial cells, which initiates the coagulation cascade and overwhelms the normal factors that control coagulation. Free heme and free iron are released from red blood cells and both cause the induction of free radicals, lipid peroxidation, and nerve damage.[19]

WHAT'S NEW?

Progesterone for Treatment of Traumatic Brain Injury (TBI)

There currently are no pharmacologic agents approved for the treatment of TBI. Animal studies and phase II clinical trials, using intravenous progesterone for treatment of moderate to severe brain trauma, have shown preliminary benefits for improved outcome and decreased mortality. Progesterone is lipid soluble; readily crosses the blood-brain barrier; is safe for administration in both men and women; is inexpensive; and is known for its multiple anti-inflammatory, anti-apoptotic, trophic growth–promoting, and neuroprotective properties. Unlike other steroid hormones, progesterone is synthesized directly in the brain by oligodendrocytes and in excitatory neurons, so it can be considered a "neurosteroid" beyond its role as a sex hormone. A phase III clinical trial is now evaluating progesterone for moderate-to-severe TBI in 1140 individuals with final results to be reported in 2015. Additionally, the SyNAPSe trial is evaluating intravenous progesterone in 1200 individuals with severe closed-head trauma in 100 to 120 medical centers throughout the world. These long-term, multicenter studies will contribute evidence to confirm the safety, efficacy, and generalizability of using progesterone for treatment of TBI.

Data from BHR Pharma, LLC: *SyNAPSe: the global Phase 3 study of progesterone in severe traumatic brain injury,* © 2012, BHR Pharma, LLC, a Besins Healthcare Co. Available at www.synapse-trial.com/; Feeser VR, Loria RM: *J Neuroimmunol* 237(1-2):4–12, 2011; National Institutes of Health: *Clinical trials Gov: progesterone for the treatment of traumatic brain injury (ProTECT III)*. Available at http://clinicaltrials.gov/ct2/show/record/NCT00822900; Stein DG: *Neuroscience* 191: 101–106, 2011.

The management of secondary brain trauma is related to prevention and includes removal of hematomas and management of hypotension, hypoxemia, anemia, intracranial pressure, body temperature, ventilation, fluid replacement, and nutrition. Research is in progress to find specific pharmacologic interventions and neuroprotective agents that limit the progression of secondary injury and to identify biomarkers to guide prevention, prognosis, and treatment[20,21] (see What's New? Progesterone for Treatment of Traumatic Brain Injury [TBI]).

Genetics of Head Injury. Certain genes are up-regulated and others are down-regulated after head trauma. The attention of researchers has been focused predominantly on the *apolipoprotein E (apoE)* gene and its various alleles. Certain alleles have been correlated with increased susceptibility to and severity of head injury. Other alleles have been associated with improved or diminished recovery after head injury. The clinical significance of these findings is not clearly known.[22,23]

Spinal Cord Trauma

The number of spinal cord injuries (SCIs) in the United States is approximately 273,000, with 12,000 new cases annually; of these, 80.7% are males, mostly young adults. The average age is 40.7 years. Since 2010 the causes include vehicular (36.5%), falls (28%), violence (14%), and sports (9%). The extent of injury has been 41% incomplete quadriplegia, 16% complete quadriplegia, 18.7% incomplete paraplegia, and 18% complete paraplegia.[24]

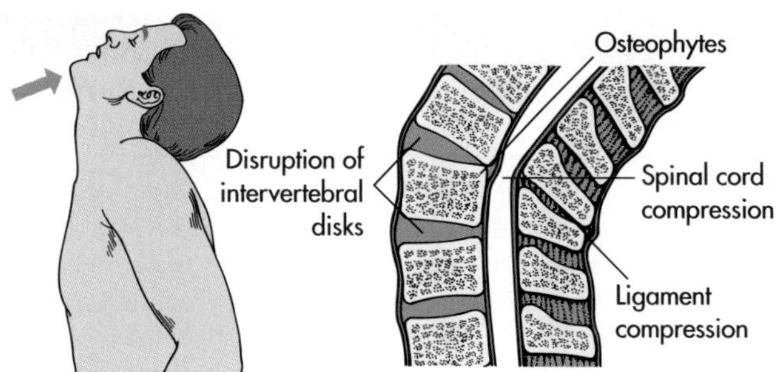

FIGURE 18-9 Hyperextension Injuries of the Spine. Hyperextension can result in fracture or nonfracture injuries with spinal cord damage.

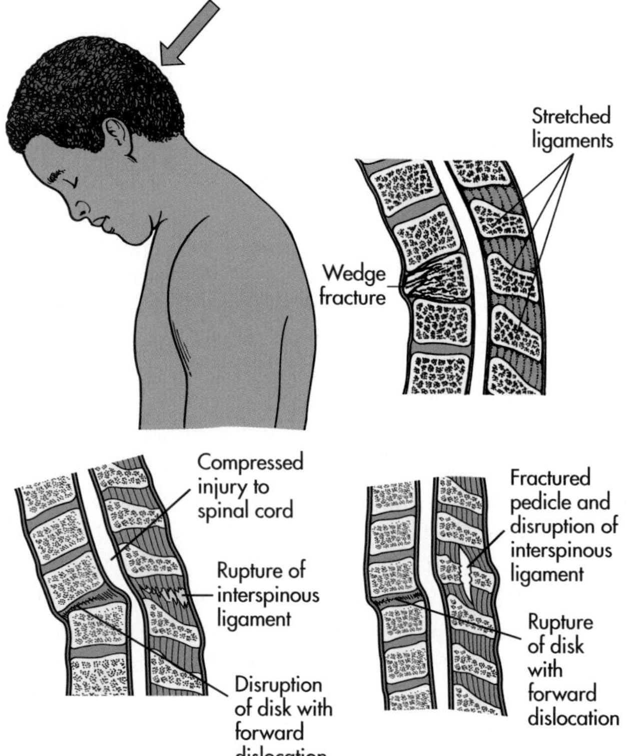

FIGURE 18-10 Hyperflexion Injury of the Spine. Hyperflexion produces translation (subluxation) of vertebrae, which compromises the central canal and compresses spinal cord parenchyma or vascular structures.

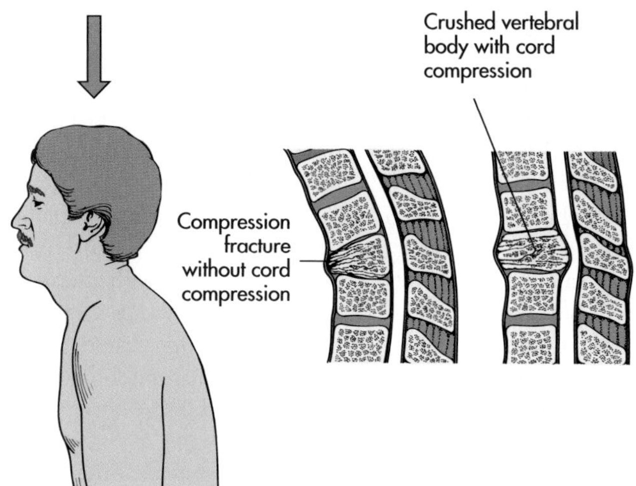

FIGURE 18-11 Axial Compression Injuries of the Spine. In axial compression the spinal cord is contused directly by retropulsion of bone or disk material into the spinal canal.

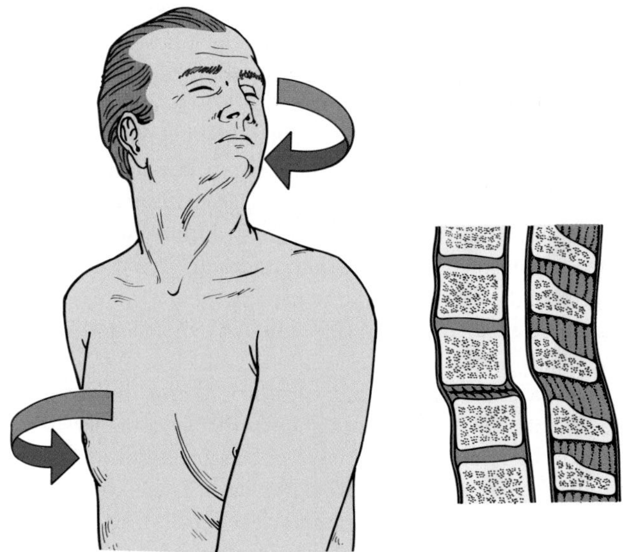

FIGURE 18-12 Flexion-Rotation Injuries of the Spine.

PATHOPHYSIOLOGY. Primary spinal cord injury occurs with the initial mechanical trauma and immediate tissue destruction. Vertebral fractures or dislocations can cause bone fragments or connective tissues to compress and damage nerve fibers. Vertebral injuries result from acceleration, deceleration, or deformation forces at impact. These forces cause compression, traction, or shearing of tissues. The bones, ligaments, joints, and neural tissue of the vertebral column may be damaged by hyperextension, hyperflexion, vertical compression, or rotation (Figures 18-9 through 18-12). Vertebral fracture and often compression of one or more elements, dislocation of its elements, or both fracture and dislocation can occur (see Figure 15-17 for the structure of the vertebral column). Vertebral injuries can be classified as (1) simple fracture, a single break usually affecting transverse or spinous processes; (2) compressed (wedged) vertebral fracture, in which a vertebral body is compressed anteriorly; (3) comminuted (burst) fracture, in which a vertebral body is shattered into several fragments; and (4) dislocation.

Vertebrae fracture readily with direct and indirect trauma. When the supporting ligaments are torn, the vertebrae move out of alignment, and dislocations occur. A horizontal force moves the vertebrae straight forward; if the individual is in a flexed position at the time of injury, the vertebrae are then in an angulated position. Flexion and extension injuries may result in dislocations. (Mechanisms of vertebral injury are presented in Table 18-2.) Vertebral injuries occur mostly at vertebrae C1-C2 (cervical), C4-C7, and T1-L2 (thoracic-lumbar) (see Figure 15-17). These are the most mobile portions of the vertebral column. The cord occupies most of the vertebral canal in the cervical and lumbar regions. The size makes the cord in these areas more easily injured. The *primary spinal cord injuries* are summarized in Table 18-3. Noncontiguous vertebral injuries are common. Further, primary injury occurs if an injured

TABLE 18-2 MECHANISMS OF VERTEBRAL INJURY

MECHANISMS OF INJURY	VERTEBRAL INJURY	FORCES OF INJURY	LOCATION OF INJURY
Hyperextension	Fracture and dislocation of posterior elements such as spinous processes, transverse processes, laminae, pedicles, or posterior ligaments	Results from forces of acceleration-deceleration and the sudden reduction in the anteroposterior diameter of the spinal cord	Cervical area
Hyperflexion	Fracture or dislocation of the vertebral bodies, disks, or ligaments	Results from sudden and excessive force that propels the neck forward or causes an exaggerated lateral movement of the neck to one side	Cervical area
Vertical compression (axonal loading)	Shattering fractures	Results from a force applied along an axis from the top of the cranium through the vertebral bodies	T12-L2
Rotational forces (flexion-rotation)	Ruptures support ligaments in addition to producing fractures	Adds shearing force to acceleration-deceleration forces	Cervical area

TABLE 18-3 SPINAL CORD INJURIES

INJURY	DESCRIPTION
Cord concussion	Results in a temporary disruption of cord-mediated functions
Cord contusion	Bruising of the neural tissue causing swelling and temporary loss of cord-mediated functions
Cord compression	Pressure on the cord causing ischemia to tissues; must be relieved (decompressed) to prevent permanent damage to the spinal cord
Laceration	Tearing of the neural tissues of the spinal cord; may be reversible if only slight damage is sustained by the neural tissues; may result in permanent loss of cord-mediated functions if spinal tracts are disrupted
Transection	Severing of the spinal cord, causing permanent loss of function
Complete	All tracts in the spinal cord are completely disrupted; all cord-mediated functions below the transection are completely and permanently lost
Incomplete	Some tracts in the spinal cord remain intact, together with functions mediated by these tracts; has the potential for recovery although function is temporarily lost
Preserved sensation only	Some demonstrable sensation below the level of injury
Preserved motor nonfunctional	Preserved motor function without useful purpose; sensory function may or may not be preserved
Preserved motor functional	Preserved voluntary motor function that is functionally useful
Hemorrhage	Bleeding into the neural tissue because of blood vessel damage; usually no major loss of function
Damage or obstruction of spinal blood supply	Causes local ischemia

spine is not adequately immobilized. Primary spinal cord injury may occur in the absence of vertebral fracture or dislocation from longitudinal stretching of the cord with or without flexion and/or extension of the vertebral column. The stretching causes altered axon transport, edema, myelin degeneration, and retrograde or wallerian degeneration.

Secondary spinal cord injury is a pathophysiologic cascade of vascular, cellular, and biochemical events that begins within a few minutes after injury and continues for weeks. The edema, ischemia, excitotoxicity, inflammation, oxidative damage, and activation of necrotic and apoptotic cell death signaling events are similar to those previously described for secondary brain injury.[25] By 5 minutes after injury, venules of the gray matter are congested and distended by erythrocytes. In 15 to 30 minutes, small hemorrhages occur with extravasation of erythrocytes into perivascular spaces of postcapillary and muscular venules. *Microscopic hemorrhages* appear in the central gray matter and pia arachnoid that increase in size within 2 hours. *Edema* in the white matter impairs the microcirculation of the cord. Within 4 hours, numerous swollen axis cylinders develop. Localized hemorrhaging and edema are followed by loss of autoregulation, vasospasm, impaired venous drainage, and reduced vascular perfusion with *development of ischemic areas*. There is myelin disruption, axonal degeneration, and necrosis. The microscopic hemorrhages and edema are maximal at the level of injury and for two cord segments above and below it. Impaired perfusion is aggravated by systemic responses including neurogenic or hemorrhagic shock, and arrhythmias.[26]

Cord swelling increases an individual's degree of dysfunction; therefore distinguishing the functions to be lost permanently from those that are impaired just temporarily becomes difficult. In the cervical region, cord swelling may be life threatening because of the possibility of resulting impairment of diaphragm function (phrenic nerves exit C3-C5) and vegetative functions mediated by the medulla oblongata. Within the first few days of injury, progressive axonal changes occur and necrotic zones develop. Progressive cavitation and coagulation necrosis at the site of injury are termed *posttraumatic infarction*.

Circulation in the white matter tracts of the spinal cord returns to normal in about 24 hours, but gray matter circulation remains altered. Phagocytes appear 36 to 48 hours after injury. Proliferation of microglia and changes in astrocytes occur. Red cells then begin to disintegrate, and resorption of hemorrhages begins. Degenerating axons are engulfed by macrophages in the first 10 days after injury. A cyst with fluid forms. The traumatized cord is replaced by acellular collagenous tissue (a scar), usually in 3 to 4 weeks. Meninges thicken as part of the scarring process.

CLINICAL MANIFESTATIONS. Immediately after cord injury, normal activity of spinal cord cells at and below the level of injury ceases because of loss of the continuous tonic discharge from the brain or brainstem and inhibition of suprasegmental impulses, thus causing spinal shock. **Spinal shock** is characterized by a complete loss of reflex function, flaccid paralysis, sensory deficit, and loss of bladder and rectal control in all segments below the level of the lesion. Disruption of central communication with sympathetic spinal nerves causes a transient drop in blood pressure, poor venous circulation, and disturbed thermal regulation. This damage causes faulty control of diaphoresis (sweating) and heat radiation through capillary dilation. The hypothalamus cannot regulate body heat through vasoconstriction and increased metabolism; therefore, the individual's body temperature assumes the temperature of the air. Spinal shock may persist for as short a time as a few days or as long as 3 months. Indications that spinal shock is terminating include the reappearance of reflex activity, hyperreflexia, spasticity, and reflex emptying of the bladder.

Neurogenic shock occurs with cervical or upper thoracic cord injury and may be seen in addition to spinal shock. Neurogenic shock is caused by the absence of sympathetic activity through loss of supraspinal control and unopposed parasympathetic tone mediated by the intact vagus nerve. Symptoms include vasodilation, hypotension, bradycardia, and hypothermia.

Continued loss of motor and sensory function depends on the extent and level of injury. All motor, sensory, reflex, and autonomic functions cease below any transected area and may cease below concussive, contused, compressed, or ischemic areas (Table 18-4). Paralysis of the lower half of the body with both legs involved is termed *paraplegia.* Paralysis involving all four extremities is termed *quadriplegia* (tetraplegia). In complete quadriplegia the level of injury is above C6, and all upper extremity function is lost. In incomplete quadriplegia, function at or above C6 is preserved, leaving the shoulder, upper arm, and some forearm muscle control intact. With acceleration injuries the greatest stress point is C4-C5. With a deceleration force the greatest stress point is at C5-C6.

TABLE 18-4 CLINICAL MANIFESTATIONS OF SPINAL CORD INJURY

STAGE	MANIFESTATIONS
Spinal Shock Stage	
Complete spinal cord transection	Loss of motor function
	1. Quadriplegia with injuries of cervical spinal cord
	2. Paraplegia with injuries of thoracic spinal cord
	Muscle flaccidity
	Loss of all reflexes below level of injury
	Loss of pain, temperature, touch, pressure, and proprioception below level of injury
	Pain at site of injury caused by a zone of hyperesthesia above the injury
	Atonic bladder and bowel
	Paralytic ileus with distention
	Loss of vasomotor tone in lower body parts; low and unstable blood pressure
	Loss of perspiration below level of injury
	Loss or extreme depression of genital reflexes such as penile erection and bulbocavernous reflex
	Dry and pale skin, possible ulceration over bony prominences
	Respiratory impairment
Partial spinal cord transection	Asymmetric flaccid motor paralysis below level of injury
	Asymmetric reflex loss
	Preservation of some sensation below level of injury
	Vasomotor instability less severe than with complete cord transection
	Bowel and bladder impairment less severe than that seen with complete cord transection
	Preservation of ability to perspire in some portions of the body below level of injury
	Brown-Séquard syndrome (associated with penetrating injuries, hyperextension and flexion, locked facets, and compression fractures)
	1. Ipsilateral paralysis or paresis below level of injury
	2. Ipsilateral loss of touch, pressure, vibration, and position senses below level of injury
	3. Contralateral loss of pain and temperature sensations below level of injury
	Central cervical cord syndrome (acute cord compression between bony bars or spurs anteriorly and thickened ligamentum flavum posteriorly associated with hyperextension)
	1. Motor deficits in upper extremities, especially hands; more dense than in lower extremities
	2. Varying degrees of bladder dysfunction
	Burning hand syndrome (variant of central cord syndrome; half of cases have an underlying spine fracture/dislocation present)
	1. Severe burning paresthesias and dysesthesias in the hands and/or feet
	Anterior cord syndrome (compromise of anterior spinal artery by occlusion or pressure effect of disk)
	1. Loss of motor function below level of injury
	2. Loss of pain and temperature sensations below level of injury
	3. Touch, pressure, position, and vibration senses intact

TABLE 18-4 CLINICAL MANIFESTATIONS OF SPINAL CORD INJURY—cont'd

STAGE	MANIFESTATIONS
	Posterior cord syndrome (associated with hyperextension injuries with fractures of vertebral arch) 1. Impaired light touch and proprioception *Conus medullaris syndrome* (compression injury at T12 from disk herniation or burst fracture of body of T12) 1. Flaccid paralysis of legs 2. Flaccid paralysis of anal sphincter 3. Variable sensory deficits *Cauda equina syndrome* (compression of nerve roots below L1 caused by fracture and dislocation of spine or large posterocentral intervertebral disk herniation) 1. Lower extremity motor deficits 2. Variable sensorimotor dysfunction 3. Variable reflex dysfunction 4. Variable bladder, bowel, and sexual dysfunction *Syndrome of neuropraxia* (seen as post–athletic injury, associated with congenital spinal stenosis) 1. Dramatic but transient neurologic deficits including quadriplegia *Horner syndrome* (injury to preganglionic sympathetic trunk or postganglionic sympathetic neurons of superior cervical ganglion) 1. Ipsilateral pupil smaller than contralateral pupil 2. Sunken ipsilateral eyeball 3. Ptosis of affected eyeball 4. Lack of perspiration on ipsilateral side of face
Heightened Reflex Activity Stage	
	Emergence of Babinski reflexes, possibly progressing to a triple reflex; possible development of still later flexor spasms Reappearance of ankle and knee reflexes, which become hyperactive Contraction of reflex detrusor muscle, leading to urinary incontinence Appearance of reflex defecation Mass reflex with flexion spasms, profuse sweating, piloerection, and bladder and occasional bowel emptying may be evoked by an autonomic stimulation of skin or from a full bladder Episodes of hypertension Defective heat-induced sweating Eventual development of extensor reflexes, first in muscles of hip and thigh, later in leg Possible paresthesias below level of transaction: dull, burning pain in lower back, abdomen, buttocks, and perineum

Return of spinal neuron excitability occurs slowly. Depending on the degree of damage, either of the following can occur: (1) motor, sensory, reflex, and autonomic functions return to normal; or (2) autonomic neural activity in the isolated segment develops. The sequence of hyperactivity phases, which vary in length, may include: (1) minimal reflex activity, (2) flexor spasms, (3) alternation between flexor and extensor spasms, and (4) predominant extensor spasms.

The initial clinical manifestations associated with acute spinal cord injury are: (1) rapid loss of voluntary movements in body parts below the level of injury, (2) sensations in the lower extremities and possibly lower trunk (depending on the level of injury), and (3) spinal and autonomic reflexes below the level of injury. The duration of this areflexic state is highly variable. In most persons, reflex activity returns in 1 to 2 weeks.

Gradually reflexes return and become increasingly easier to elicit. A pattern of flexion reflexes emerges first, involving the toes and later the feet and legs. Reflex voiding and bowel elimination appear. Flexor spasms accompanied by profuse sweating, piloerection, and automatic bladder emptying (together called a **mass reflex**) may develop. The ability to sweat when overheated may be disrupted, and extensor spasms may develop, usually after full development of flexor spasms. Sometimes after several months, episodes of autonomic hyperreflexia occur.

Autonomic hyperreflexia (dysreflexia) is a syndrome of sudden, massive reflex sympathetic discharge associated with spinal cord injury at level T5-T6 or above. Supraspinal control of the sympathetic nervous system is disrupted, causing an imbalance between the sympathetic and the parasympathetic nervous systems. The pathophysiology of hyperreflexia involves the stimulation of sensory receptors below the level of the cord lesion. The sensory input ascends the spinal cord and activates the thoracolumbar sympathetic nerves. The intact sympathetic nervous system reflexively responds with vasoconstriction of the muscular, splanchnic, and cutaneous vascular beds. The paroxysmal increase in blood pressure causes baroreceptors in the cerebral vessels, the carotid sinus, and the aorta to stimulate parasympathetic vasodilation above the level of the cord lesion. The heart rate decreases but not enough to overcome the hypertension. The visceral and peripheral vessels do not dilate because efferent impulses cannot pass through the injured cord (Figure 18-13).

Autonomic hyperreflexia is characterized by debilitating symptoms: paroxysmal hypertension (up to 300 mmHg systolic), bradycardia (30 to 40 beats/minute), a pounding headache, blurred vision, sweating above the level of the lesion with flushing of the skin, nasal congestion, nausea, and piloerection caused by pilomotor spasm. The symptoms may develop singly

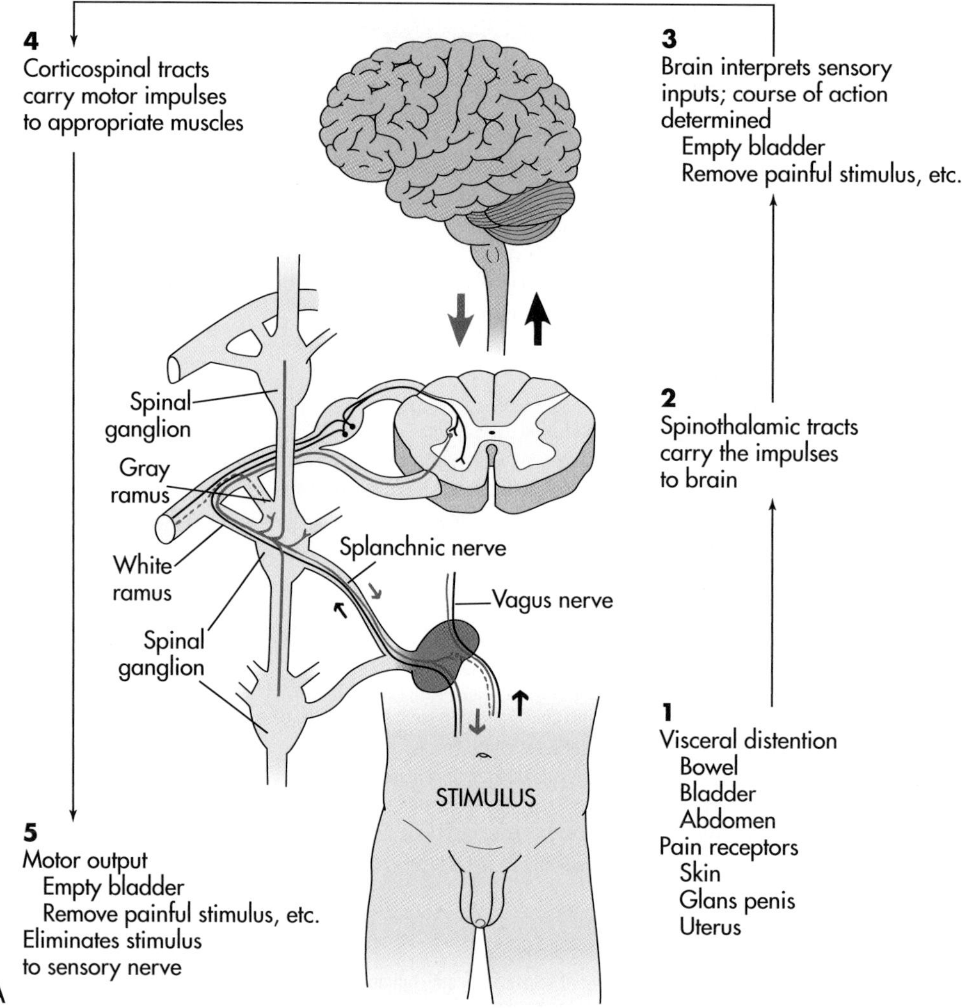

FIGURE 18-13 Autonomic Hyperreflexia. **A,** Normal response pathway.

or in combination (syndrome) and often are associated with somatic (distended bladder or rectum) or sensory stimulation. The condition is life threatening and requires immediate treatment because cerebrovascular accident (CVA) is possible. The head of the bed should be elevated and the stimulus should be determined and removed. Emptying of the bladder or bowel usually relieves the syndrome. Medical treatment may include topical nitroglycerin paste above the level of the lesion, calcium channel blockers (e.g., nefedipine), or α-adrenergic receptor blocking agents.[27] Prevention of autonomic hyperreflexia with bowel and bladder management programs is an effective approach.

EVALUATION AND TREATMENT. Diagnosis of spinal cord injury is made on the basis of physical examination and imaging (e.g., MRI). For a suspected or confirmed vertebral fracture or dislocation, regardless of the presence or absence of spinal cord injury, the immediate intervention is immobilization of the spine to prevent further injury. Decompression and surgical fixation may be necessary and performed early. Corticosteroids may be given at the time of injury to decrease secondary cord injury and continued for 24 to 48 hours, depending on time of initiation following injury. Therapeutic hypothermia has shown some encouraging evidence for improved outcomes, particularly for cervical cord injuries, but more research is needed.[28] Several clinical trials are in progress that address treatment of acute spinal cord injury, including cell-based therapies, immune modulators, vasculature selective treatments, and functional electrical stimulation.[29] Nutrition, lung function, skin integrity, and bladder and bowel management must be addressed. Plans for rehabilitation require early consideration. Impairments are permanent because endogenous repair events fail to restore the damaged axonal circuits.[30,31]

Degenerative Disorders of the Spine

Degenerative Disk Disease

Degenerative disk disease (DDD) is a common finding in individuals 30 years of age and older. It is, in part, a process of normal aging and includes a genetic component and environmental interactions that may increase susceptibility to lumbar disk disease by disrupting normal building and maintenance of cartilage.[32] Causes include biochemical (e.g., inflammatory mediators) and biomechanical alterations (e.g., mechanical loading and compression) of the intervertebral disk tissue. Diminished blood supply and loss of disk proteoglycans cause

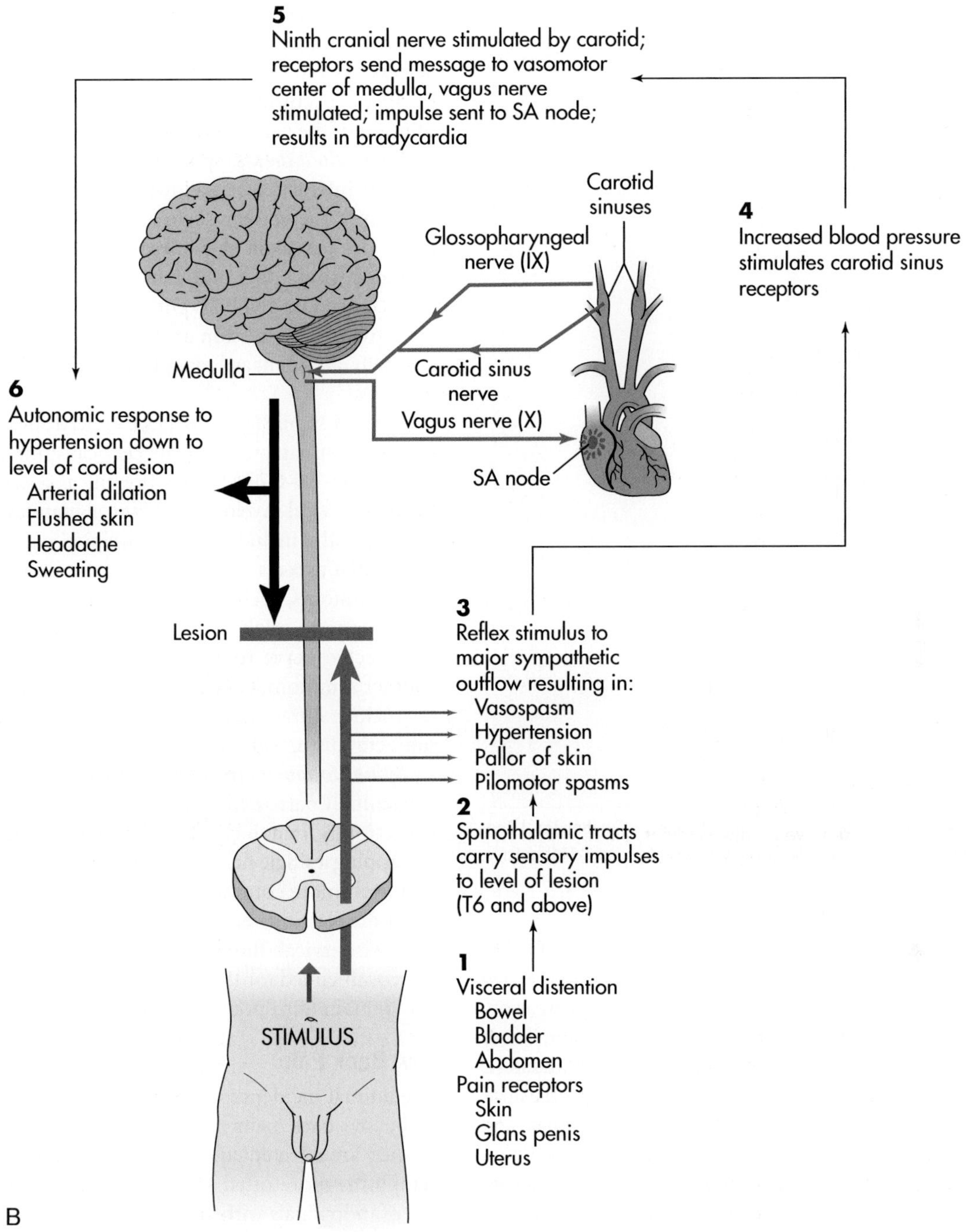

FIGURE 18-13, cont'd B, Autonomic dysreflexia pathway. *SA,* Sinoatrial. (Modified from Rudy EB: *Advanced neurological and neurosurgical nursing,* St Louis, 1984, Mosby.)

subsequent disk dehydration and alterations in disk structure and function. Splits in the annulus fibrosis can permit herniation of the nucleus pulposus, compressing nerves or placing strain on the spine. Fibrocartilage replaces the gelatinous mucoid material of the nucleus pulposus as the disk changes with age. There may be shrinkage of the nucleus pulposus that produces prolapse or folding of the annulus with secondary osteophyte formation at the margins of the adjacent vertebral body. The pathologic findings in DDD include disk protrusion, spondylolysis or subluxation (or both), degeneration of vertebrae (spondylolisthesis), and spinal stenosis.[33]

Symptoms result from either (1) protrusion of the disk or annulus or (2) narrowing of the spinal canal or intervertebral foramen by osteophytes. A congenital narrow canal or congenitally short pedicles may be present. Posterior disk protrusion in the cervical, thoracic, and lumbar regions leads to spinal cord compression causing *myelopathy* (pathology in the spinal cord). Posterolateral disk protrusions, with or without a contribution from the vertebral body or apophyseal joint osteophytes, lead to nerve root compression causing *radiculopathy* (nerve root damage).

Thoracic disk disease is rarely symptomatic. Lumbosacral disk disease *(lumbar spondylosis)* involves degeneration of the

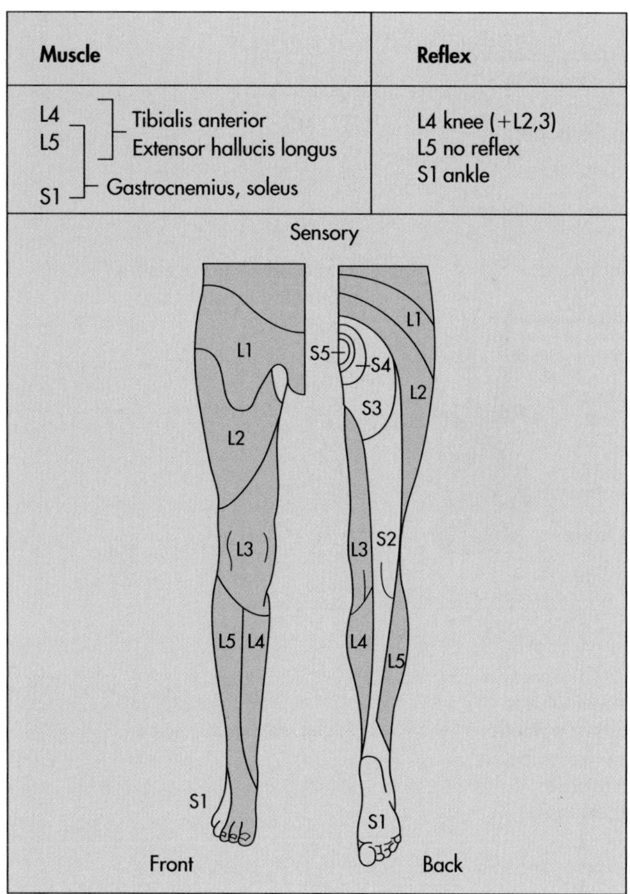

FIGURE 18-14 Motor, Sensory, and Reflex Changes in Lumbosacral Root Disorders. (From Perkin DG et al: *Atlas of clinical neurology,* ed 3, Philadelphia, 2011, Saunders.)

lower two lumbar disks in 90% of persons. There may be (1) lateral disk protrusion (10% of cases), manifesting as pain referred to the anterior thigh and leg; (2) posterolateral disk protrusion; or (3) central disk protrusion, manifesting with pain, lower extremity weakness, impaired sphincter function, and saddle anesthesia. Clinical manifestations of posterolateral protrusions (Figure 18-14) include pain in the back, the sacroiliac joint, and the medial aspect of the buttock and upper thigh; radicular pain exacerbated by movement and straining (medial calf suggests L5, lateral calf suggests S1 root compression); sensory symptoms that are common and segmental in distribution; focal tenderness on palpation of the back; limited range of motion in the back and scoliosis secondary to paravertebral spasms; restricted straight-leg raising (root at or below L5); positive femoral stretch test (roots of L2, L3, or L4); and focal signs that are determined by the root affected.

Spondylolysis. **Spondylolysis** is a degenerative process of the vertebral column and associated soft tissue. It is characterized by a structural defect of the spine involving the lamina or neural arch of the vertebra. The most common site affected is the lumbar spine. This defect occurs in the portion of the lamina between the superior and inferior articular facets called the *pars interarticularis.* Mechanical pressure may cause a forward displacement of the deficient vertebra called *spondylolisthesis.*

Heredity plays a significant role, and spondylolysis is associated with an increased incidence of other congenital spinal defects. As a result of torsional and rotational stress, "microfractures" occur at the affected site and eventually cause dissolution of the pars interarticularis.

Spondylolisthesis. **Spondylolisthesis** is an osseous defect of the pars interarticularis allowing a vertebra to slide forward in relation to the vertebra below, commonly occurring at L5-S1. It is more prevalent in adolescent athletes.[34] Spondylolisthesis is graded from 1 to 4 on the basis of the percentage of slip that has occurred. Individuals with grade 3 or 4 are considered for operative decompression or stabilization, or both. Grades 1 and 2 usually are managed symptomatically and with nonsurgical methods.

Cervical spondylolysis is facet hypertrophy and disk degeneration with narrowing in the cervical spine predominantly at C5-C6 and C6-C7.[35] It may present as a cervical radiculopathy or a cervical myelopathy. Clinical manifestations of cervical radiculopathy include neck or occipital pain as well as pain in the medial aspects of the scapula, the shoulder, or arm. Sensory symptoms, such as tingling or numbness, follow a dermatomal pattern; weakness follows the pattern of innervation of the affected nerve root. Occipital or suboccipital headache is another symptom. Clinical manifestations of cervical myelopathy include difficulty walking, altered sensation in the feet, and sphincter disturbances (occurs late).

Spinal Stenosis. In **spinal stenosis** the spinal canal may be congenitally narrowed or narrowed by a bulging annulus, a facet hypertrophy, or a thick/ossified posterior longitudinal ligament entrapping a single nerve involving many roots. It is classified as acquired (more common) or developmental (such as occurs in achondroplastic dwarfism). It is categorized by area of the spine affected: cervical, thoracic, or lumbar. Surgical decompression is recommended for those with long-term symptoms and those who remain unresponsive to medical management.

Low Back Pain

The annual incidence of, or percentage of population affected with, low back pain ranges from 6.3% to 15.4%. Men and women are affected equally; however, women report low back symptoms more often after the age of 60 years. About 1% to 2% of individuals with acute low back pain are disabled.[36] Several risk factors have been identified in the pathogenesis of low back pain. They include involvement caused by occupations that require repetitious lifting in the forward bent-and-twisted position, exposure to vibrations caused by vehicles or industrial machinery, psychosocial workplace factors, and obesity. Osteoporosis increases the risk of spinal compression fractures and may be the reason older adult women report more symptoms than men. Genetic predispositions for low back pain include isthmic spondylolisthesis (vertebra slides forward or slips in relation to a vertebra below), spinal osteochondrosis, and spinal stenosis associated with achondroplasia.[37]

PATHOGENESIS. Most cases of low back pain are idiopathic or nonspecific, and clinicians are unable to provide a precise diagnosis for most individuals with this disorder.[38] Local processes may be involved in low back pain, including tension caused by tumors or disk prolapse, bursitis, synovitis, rising venous and tissue pressures (found in degenerative joint disease), abnormal bone pressures, problems with spinal mobility, inflammation caused by infection (as in osteomyelitis), bony fractures, ligamentous sprains, and inflammation of the lumbar facet joints. Pain can be referred from viscera or the posterior peritoneum. Other causes of low back pain include bone diseases, such as osteoporosis or osteomalacia, and hyperparathyroidism.[39]

Anatomically, low back pain must come from innervated structures, but deep pain is widely referred and varies from person to person. The nucleus pulposus has no intrinsic innervation; however, when extruded or herniated through a prolapsed disk, it irritates the dural membranes and is responsible for pain referred to the associated segmental area (see Figure 18-14). The interspinous bursae can be a source of low back pain between L3, L4, L5, and S1, but also may affect L1, L2, and L3 spinous processes, depending on the closeness of the adjacent pair of spines. The anterior and posterior longitudinal ligaments of the spine and the interspinous and supraspinous ligaments are abundantly supplied with pain receptors, as is the ligamentum flavum. All of these ligaments are vulnerable to traumatic tears (sprains) and fracture. The role of muscle injury in the production of low back pain remains uncertain, even though sprains and strains are the most common diagnoses. The muscle spasms that often are produced during sieges of low back pain are thought to be produced by as yet unknown sensory or motor-reflex pathways. The most commonly encountered causes of low back pain include lumbar disk herniation, degenerative disk disease, spondylolysis, spondylolisthesis, and spinal stenosis. (For a discussion of disk herniation and rupture, see following text.) Chronic low back pain can cause central sensitization (see Chapter 16) and abnormal endogenous pain modulation.

CLINICAL MANIFESTATIONS. Low back pain affects the area between the lower rib cage and gluteal muscles and often radiates into the thighs. About 1% of individuals with acute low back pain have sciatica or pain in the distribution of the sciatic nerve or lumbar and sacral nerve roots. Sciatica often is accompanied by neurosensory and motor deficits, such as weakness. Major or progressive motor or sensory deficit, cauda equina syndrome (new-onset bowel or bladder incontinence or urinary retention, loss of anal sphincter tone, saddle anesthesia), history of cancer metastatic to bone, and suspected spinal infection can be associated with chronic low back pain.

EVALUATION AND TREATMENT. Diagnosis of low back pain is made by personal history; physical examination; electromyography (EMG), epidurography, diskography, and imaging (MRI and CT) for specific clinical conditions; and nerve conduction studies. Most individuals with acute low back pain benefit from a nonspecific short-term treatment regimen including nonsteroidal anti-inflammatory medications, exercises, physical therapy, and education. Individuals with chronic low back pain (pain for more than 3 months) can be treated with anti-inflammatory and muscle relaxant medications, exercise programs, massage, topical heat, spinal manipulation, cognitive-behavioral therapy, and interdisciplinary care.[39] Surgical treatments for identified pathologic conditions include diskectomy and spinal fusions. Radiotherapy is used for treatment of facet-related pain after diagnostic nerve block. Evaluation of treatment outcomes should include pain, function, and quality of life.[40]

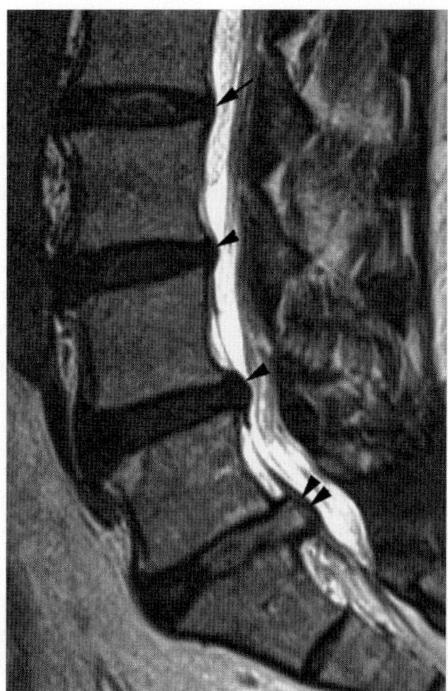

FIGURE 18-15 **Disk Bulge, Protrusion, and Herniation.** Sagittal T2-weighted image demonstrates examples for all stages of disk pathology. Viewing from rostral to caudal, a disk bulge *(arrow)*, a small and more prominent protrusion *(arrowheads)*, and a herniation *(double arrowhead)* are seen. (From Daroff RB et al: *Bradley's neurology in clinical practice*, Philadelphia, 2012, Saunders.)

Herniated Intervertebral Disk

Herniation of an intervertebral disk is a displacement of the disk material (nucleus pulposus or annulus fibrosis) beyond the intervertebral disk space (Figure 18-15). Men are more affected than women, with the highest incidence in the 30- to 50-year age group. The lumbosacral disks (L4-L5, L5-S1) are most commonly affected. Disk herniation occasionally occurs in the cervical area, usually at C5-C6 and C6-C7. Herniations at the thoracic level are extremely rare. Risk factors for herniation include weightlifting sports and certain work activities, such as repeated lifting. Rupture of an intervertebral disk usually is caused by trauma or degenerative disk disease, or both. The injury may occur immediately, within a few hours, or months to years after injury.

PATHOPHYSIOLOGY. In a herniated disk the ligament and posterior capsule of the disk usually are torn, allowing the gelatinous material (the nucleus pulposus) to extrude. This extrusion compresses the nerve root, compromising the vascular supply and causing inflammatory-like changes. Occasionally the injury tears the entire disk loose, and it protrudes onto the nerve root or compresses the spinal cord. One or more nerve roots may be compressed. This multiple nerve root compression is found especially at the L5-S1 level, where the cauda equina may be compressed. Large amounts of extruded nucleus pulposus or complete disk herniation (i.e., of both the capsule and the nucleus pulposus) may compress the spinal cord.

CLINICAL MANIFESTATIONS. The location and size of the herniation into the spinal canal, together with the amount of space that exists inside the spinal canal, determine the clinical manifestations associated with the injury. A herniated disk in the lumbosacral area is associated with pain that radiates along the sciatic nerve course over the buttock and into the calf or ankle. The pain occurs with straining, including coughing and sneezing, and usually on straight-leg raising. Other clinical manifestations include limited range of motion of the lumbar spine; tenderness on palpation in the sciatic notch and along the sciatic nerve; impaired pain, temperature, and touch sensation in the L5-S1 or L4-L5 dermatomes of the leg and foot; decreased or absent ankle jerk reflex; and mild weakness of the foot.

With the herniation of a lower cervical disk, paresthesias and pain are present in the upper arm, forearm, and hand in the affected nerve root distribution. Neck and nerve root pain may be increased by neck motion and straining, including coughing and sneezing. Neck range of motion is diminished. Slight weakness and atrophy of biceps or triceps may occur; the biceps or triceps reflex may decrease. Occasionally signs of corticospinal and sensory tract impairments appear. These include motor weakness of the lower extremities, sensory disturbances in the lower extremities, and presence of a Babinski reflex.

EVALUATION AND TREATMENT. Diagnosis of a herniated intervertebral disk is made on the basis of the history and physical examination, EMG results, imaging procedures when there are signs of systemic disease, and nerve conduction studies. Radiologic evidence of disk herniation does not reliably correlate with symptoms or predict low back pain. Many individuals with disk herniation on imaging have no symptoms.[41] Clinical improvement occurs in most people over weeks to months. The herniated disk portion on serial imaging tends to regress over time.[42] There is little evidence to support drug treatments, including the use of analgesics, antidepressants, or muscle relaxants.[43] Randomized controlled trials are needed to evaluate conservative therapy (e.g., nonsteroidal anti-inflammatory drugs [NSAIDs], bed rest, epidural injections of nonsteroidals, activity, acupuncture, massage, exercise, heat, or ice).[44,45] A surgical approach is indicated if there is evidence of progressive neurologic deficit (e.g., weakness, decreased deep tendon reflexes, and bladder/bowel reflexes) or cauda equina syndrome (saddle anesthesia, decreased or absent reflexes in the lower extremities, and neurogenic bowel or bladder dysfunction).[46]

Cerebrovascular Disorders

Cerebrovascular disease is the most frequently occurring neurologic disorder. More than 50% of persons admitted to general hospitals with neurologic problems have cerebrovascular disease. Any abnormality of the brain caused by a pathologic process in the blood vessels is referred to as a *cerebrovascular disease*. Included in this category are lesions of the vessel wall (e.g., aneurysm or malformations) and strokes or cerebrovascular accidents.

Cerebrovascular Accidents (Stroke Syndromes)

The incidence of new and recurrent stroke is 795,000, and approximately 185,000 of these are recurrent. Strokes are the third leading cause of death in the United States, resulting in about 134,148 deaths. The incidence of stroke is about two times higher in blacks than whites. Stroke tends to run in families. Of all strokes, 87% are ischemic (thrombotic or embolic), 10% are intracerebral hemorrhagic, and 3% are subarachnoid hemorrhagic.[47] No identifiable cause can be established by conventional diagnostic tests in many ischemic strokes and they are classified as "undetermined" or "cryptogenic." Strokes in children are presented in Chapter 20.

The mildest outcome of a cerebrovascular accident (CVA) is so minimal as to be almost unnoticed. The most severe outcomes are hemiplegia, coma, and death. Strokes are classified according to pathophysiology: ischemic (thrombotic or embolic) is the most common, global hypoperfusion (as in shock), or intracerebral hemorrhage.[47] Hypertension is the single greatest risk factor for stroke.[48] Risk factors for stroke include the following[49]:

1. Arterial hypertension
2. Intracranial atherosclerosis
3. Insulin resistance and diabetes mellitus
4. High total cholesterol or low high-density lipoprotein (HDL) cholesterol level, elevated lipoprotein-A level
5. Hyperhomocysteinemia
6. Congestive heart disease and peripheral vascular disease
7. Asymptomatic carotid stenosis
8. Polycythemia and thrombocythemia
9. Atrial fibrillation and patent ductus arteriosus
10. *Chlamydia pneumoniae* infection promotes atherosclerosis[50]
11. Sickle cell disease
12. Postmenopausal hormone therapy
13. High sodium intake, >2300 mg; low potassium intake, <4700 mg
14. Smoking
15. Physical inactivity
16. Obesity
17. Chronic sleep deprivation
18. Depression

Ischemic Stroke

PATHOPHYSIOLOGY. Thrombotic strokes (cerebral thrombosis) arise from arterial occlusions caused by thrombi formed in the arteries supplying the brain or in the intracranial vessels. The development of a cerebral thrombosis most frequently is attributed to atherosclerosis and inflammatory disease processes (arteritis) that damage arterial walls. Increased coagulation can lead to thrombus formation. Conditions causing inadequate cerebral perfusion (e.g., dehydration, hypotension, prolonged vasoconstriction from malignant hypertension) increase the risk of thrombosis. Over 20 to 30 years, atheromatous plaques (stenotic lesions) tend to form at branchings and curves in the cerebral circulation. The smooth stenotic area can degenerate, forming an ulcerated area of vessel wall. Platelets and fibrin adhere to the damaged wall, and clots form, gradually occluding the artery. The thrombus may enlarge both distally and proximally in the vessel. Portions of the clot detach and travel up the vessel to distant sites where occlusion occurs, producing a stroke syndrome.

Transient ischemic attacks (TIAs) are transient episodes of neurologic dysfunction (weakness, numbness, sudden confusion, loss of balance, loss of vision, sudden severe headache) resulting from focal cerebral ischemia. However, use of brain imaging techniques (e.g., diffusion-weighted imaging) in persons with symptoms lasting less than 24 hours often reveals a brain infarction that requires treatment intervention to prevent stroke. About 30% of individuals experiencing a TIA will have a stroke within 1 year. Risk stratification for early stroke is enhanced when imaging is combined with a risk stratification score (e.g., the ABCD2 score, which considers age, neurologic symptoms, symptom duration, and diabetes).[51]

Embolic stroke involves fragments that break from a thrombus formed outside the brain or in the heart, aorta, or common carotid artery. Other sources of embolism include fat, air, tumor, bacterial clumps, and foreign bodies. The embolus usually involves small vessels and obstructs at a bifurcation or other point of stenosis, thus causing ischemia. An embolus may obstruct the lumen entirely and remain in place or shatter into fragments and become part of the vessel's blood flow. Risk factors for an embolic stroke are atrial fibrillation (15% to 25% of strokes), left ventricular aneurysm or thrombus, left atrial thrombus, recent myocardial infarction, rheumatic valvular disease, mechanical prosthetic valve, nonbacterial thrombotic endocarditis, bacterial endocarditis, patent foramen ovale, and primary intracardiac tumors.[52] In persons who experience an embolic stroke, a second stroke usually follows at some point because the source of emboli continues to exist. Embolization is usually in the distribution of the middle cerebral artery (the largest cerebral artery).

Cerebral Infarction. Cerebral infarction results when an area of the brain loses blood supply and becomes ischemic because of vascular occlusion (embolic or thrombotic). The pathologic manifestation is either (1) a global process that affects neurons most susceptible to ischemia (pyramidal and striatal neurons), Purkinje cells of the cerebral hemispheres, and the border zones at the very end of the circulation of the artery; or (2) a focal process with a central zone of infarction surrounded by a zone of reversible ischemia, the ischemic penumbra, which if perfused in 1 hour will survive. Proposed pathogenesis may include: (1) abrupt vascular occlusion (e.g., embolus), (2) gradual vessel occlusion (e.g., atheroma), and (3) vessels that are stenosed but not completely occluded. Cerebral thrombi and cerebral emboli are the most common causes of occlusion, but atherosclerosis and hypotension are the dominant underlying processes.

Cerebral infarctions are ischemic. In ischemic infarcts (pale infarcts, "white stroke"), cytotoxic ischemic events and interaction between blood elements and blood vessels combine to produce brain injury. The affected area becomes slightly discolored and softens about 6 to 12 hours after the occlusion. Necrosis, swelling around the insult, and mushy disintegration have appeared by 48 to 72 hours after infarction. At a microscopic level, neuronal cell bodies change, myelin sheaths and axis cylinders are interrupted and disintegrate, and loss of oligodendrites and astrocytes occurs. Secondary cellular and biochemical events contribute to neuronal injury and death (see Secondary Brain Injury, p. 588).

A syndrome of luxury perfusion (increased blood flow to the brain but decreased O_2 uptake by cerebral tissue) in areas adjacent to the infarct develops first from the loss of autoregulation. The vascular bed in this area dilates. Later, capillary sprouting (neovascularization) supports this luxury perfusion syndrome.

In hemorrhagic infarcts ("red strokes"), bleeding occurs into the infarcted area as a result of restoration of blood flow. Reperfusion occurs when the embolus fragments, or lysis or compressive forces lessen, allowing blood flow to be reestablished into the infarcted area. Most hemorrhagic infarcts are located in the cerebral cortex. Unfortunately, reperfusion can compromise recovery by accelerating the sequence of metabolically damaging events including oxidative stress (reperfusion injury).

Lacunar Stroke. A **lacunar stroke (lacunar infarct)** is a microinfarct smaller than 1 cm in diameter and involves occlusion of the small perforating arteries, predominantly in the basal ganglia, internal capsules, and pons. Lacunar infarcts are caused by lipohyalinosis, subintimal lipid-loading foam cells, and fibrinoid materials that thicken the arterial walls. The small arterioles lengthen, become tortuous, and develop subintimal dissections and microaneurysms. They are associated with hyperlipidemia, smoking,[53] hypertension, and diabetes mellitus. Because of the subcortical location and small area of infarction, these strokes may have pure motor and sensory deficits.

CLINICAL MANIFESTATIONS. Because neurons surrounding the ischemic or infarcted areas undergo changes that disrupt plasma membranes, cellular edema results, causing compression of capillaries. Most persons survive an initial hemispheric ischemic stroke unless massive cerebral edema develops. Massive brainstem infarcts, caused by basilar thrombosis or embolism, are almost always fatal.

Clinical manifestations of thrombotic or ischemic stroke vary, depending on the artery obstructed. Different sites of obstruction create different occlusion syndromes (Table 18-5).

EVALUATION AND TREATMENT. Treatment of ischemic stroke is focused on (1) restoring brain perfusion in a timeframe that does not contribute to reperfusion injury, (2) counteracting the ischemic cascade pathways, (3) lowering cerebral metabolic demand so that the susceptible brain tissue is protected against impaired perfusion, (4) preventing recurrent ischemic events, and (5) promoting tissue restoration. Thrombolysis (i.e., tissue-type plasminogen activator [tPA]) given within 3 and up to 4.5 hours of onset of symptoms reduces dependency at 6 months when the diagnosis of ischemic stroke has been confirmed and contraindications are eliminated. Endovascular intra-arterial thrombolysis can be used to treat those who cannot receive tPA.[54] Because of the short time window of efficacy, some individuals are not eligible for tPA therapy and antiplatelet agents are administered. Aspirin, clopidogrel, or aspirin plus extended-release dipyridamole have been shown to effectively reduce death and dependency at 6 months when initiated within 48 hours. Systemic anticoagulants (unfractionated heparin, low-molecular-weight heparin, or fondaparinux) are used to prevent venous thromboembolism, particularly in immobilized individuals.[55] Acute ischemic stroke frequently presents with hypertension, but the systemic blood pressure should not be treated unless the systolic pressure exceeds 220 mmHg or the

TABLE 18-5 STROKE SYNDROMES SECONDARY TO OCCLUSION OR STENOSIS

LOCATION/VESSEL	AREA OF BRAIN INFARCTED	SIGNS AND SYMPTOMS NOTED
Anterior and Central Circulation		
Note: The internal carotid artery enters the circle of Willis and supplies the lateral anterior and central portions of the cerebral hemispheres through the middle cerebral artery and the paramedial frontal lobe superior to the corpus callosum through the anterior cerebral artery; penetrating branches serve the deeper layers of the hemispheres.		
Internal carotid	If collateral circulation is intact, commonly no infarction has occurred; if infarcted, location is same as in the middle cerebral artery	• Arterial pressure may be low in the retina • Bruit over the internal carotid artery • Possible retinal emboli • History of transient ischemic attacks (TIAs) • Positive noninvasive studies
Middle cerebral artery (MCA) (most common area); either stem or branches of MCA	Cortical motor area (face, arm, leg) and/or posterior limb, internal capsule, corona radiata	• **Motor:** contralateral hemiparesis or hemiplegia, greater in face and arm than leg
	Cortical sensory area (face, arm, leg) and/or posterior limb of internal capsule	• **Sensation:** contralateral loss in same distribution as motor loss
	Broca area and deep fibers in the dominant hemisphere	• **Speech:** expressive (motor) disorder with anomia (left hemisphere most commonly affected) with nonfluent aphasia and some comprehension defects
	Broca area and deep fibers in the nondominant hemisphere	• **Speech:** dysarthria
	Optic radiations deep in the temporal lobe	• **Vision:** contralateral homonymous hemianopsia or quadranopsia • **Motor:** mirror movement
	Location not known	• **Respirations**: Cheyne-Stokes respirations, contralateral hyperhidrosis, occasional mydriasis
	Posterior limb or internal capsule and adjacent corona radiate	• **Motor:** pure motor hemiplegia
	Penetrating branches of MCA (lenticulostriate branches) into the basal nuclei	• **Motor:** varying degrees of contralateral weakness of face, arm, or leg • **Sensory:** little or no loss; if present, contralateral following the motor distribution • **Speech:** transcortical sensory aphasia (communicating pathways are interrupted) • **Perception:** transient visual and sensory neglect on the left if a right lesion
Anterior cerebral artery (ACA) (least common)	Proximal segment: corona radiata (rarely) Main stem (complete occlusion is uncommon, thus areas affected differ and collateral circulation may alleviate signs or symptoms); medial aspect of frontal lobes, caudate nucleus, and corpus callosum are supplied by the ACA	• **Motor:** when present, a mild contralateral hemiparesis, greater in leg; with bilateral occlusion of ACA, cerebral paraplegia in both legs can occur • **Motor:** contralateral paralysis or paresis (greater in foot and thigh); mild upper extremity weakness • **Sensory:** mild contralateral lower extremity deficiency with loss of vibratory and/or position sense, loss of two-point discrimination • **Speech:** may have transcortical motor and sensory aphasia if left hemisphere • Frontal lobe releasing signs • Apraxia
Posterior Circulation		
Note: The posterior circulation includes the posterior cerebral artery, the vertebral arteries, and the basilar artery; the anatomic territory covered includes the posterior aspects of the hemispheres, the central areas of the thalamus and midbrain, and the brainstem; occlusion of the vessels is most commonly by emboli; effects of infarct in these vessels and their penetrating vessels can be specific or devastatingly global; many complex syndromes have been identified.		
Vertebral arteries	Medulla and spinal cord tracts, anterior spinal artery and penetrating branches (medial medullary syndrome)	• **Motor:** contralateral hemiparesis (face spared) and/or impaired contralateral proprioception; flaccid weakness or paralysis of the tongue and/or dysarthria

TABLE 18-5 STROKE SYNDROMES SECONDARY TO OCCLUSION OR STENOSIS—cont'd

LOCATION/VESSEL	AREA OF BRAIN INFARCTED	SIGNS AND SYMPTOMS NOTED
Basilar artery (three sets of branches)	Midline structures of pons (paramedian branches); three general areas of infarction are common: (1) medial inferior pontine syndrome, (2) medial midpontine syndrome, and (3) medial superior pontine syndrome Corticospinal and corticobulbar tracts in pons, sensory tracts of medial and lateral lemnisci, vestibular nuclei, inferior and middle cerebellar peduncles, cranial nerve nuclei and/or fibers, cerebellar connections in tectum, descending sympathetic pathways, central brainstem, pontine tegmentum (vertebrobasilar syndrome)	• **Motor:** contralateral hemiparesis or hemiplegia, ipsilateral lower motor neuron facial palsy, "locked-in syndrome" • **Sensory:** contralateral loss of vibratory sense, sense of position with dysmetria, loss of two-point discrimination, impaired rapid alternating movements • **Visual:** inferior pontine: diplopia; impaired abduction of ipsilateral eye: internuclear ophthalmoplegia; medial superior: diplopia, internuclear ophthalmoplegia, skewed deviation • **Motor:** upper motor neuron type of weakness: paralysis in combinations involving face, tongue, throat, and extremities; dysphagia, facial weakness, dysmetria, ataxia (either trunk or extremities), weak mastication muscles • **Sensation:** combinations of impaired sensation (vibratory, two-point, position sense, pain, temperature), facial hypesthesia, anesthesia of cranial nerve V
Posterior cerebral artery (PCA)	Central territory (thalamic area, dentothalamic tract, cerebral peduncle, red nucleus, subthalamic nucleus, and cranial nerve III)	• **Motor:** contralateral hemiplegia with possible dysmetria, dyskinesia, hemiballism or choreoathetosis, dystaxia, cerebellar ataxia, and tremor; contralateral upper motor neuron palsy; several syndromes are associated: (1) Weber: cranial nerve III palsy and contralateral hemiplegia; (2) thalamoperforate syndrome: superior crossed cerebellar ataxia or inferior crossed cerebellar ataxia with cranial nerve III palsy (Claude syndrome); (3) decerebrate attacks • **Sensory:** contralateral sensory loss of all modalities without agraphia • **Function:** prosopagnosia (inability to recognize familiar faces), topographic disorientation, memory deficits, alexia, inability to read, color anomia • **Level of consciousness:** in bilateral PCA syndromes, coma with absent doll's eyes reflex or loss of alertness may occur; if tegmentum of midbrain near hypothalamus and third ventricle is damaged, akinetic mutism may occur
Small Vessel Disease		
Note: Small penetrating vessels in brain parenchyma that supply areas near the basal ganglia are most vulnerable to infarction although any small vessels can occlude deep in the brain and cause injury, producing neurologic signs or symptoms; such infarcts are commonly called *lacunes* (small pit or hollow), a term that is changing in meaning; they can be caused by emboli but are most commonly associated with microatheromas; although they can be found in otherwise healthy people, those with concurrent atherosclerosis, arterial hypertension, and/or diabetes have a higher incidence of this type of infarct.		
	Internal capsule, most commonly	• **Motor:** contralateral hemiparesis on a single side, with equal deficit in face, arm, and leg; often unaccompanied by detectable signs of sensory, visual, and speech loss, depending on location; old term is "pure motor stroke" although evidence suggests that other neurologic signs are present but overlooked because of low intensity
	Thalamus, most commonly	• **Sensory:** complete or partial loss in face, arm, trunk, and leg that appears exactly midline; may be accompanied by pain, hyperesthesias, and uncomfortable sensations (hemisensory stroke)
	Pons	• Dysarthria, clumsy hand
	Pons, midbrain, capsule or parietal white matter	• Hemiparesis, ataxia on same side

diastolic pressure exceeds 120 mmHg. Overly aggressive treatment of hypertension can compromise collateral perfusion of the ischemic penumbra.[56] When the pathophysiology of stroke is stabilized, all individuals should receive BP-lowering therapy to maintain BP lower than 140/90 mmHg.[57-59] Hypothermia has been used for neuroprotection in ischemic stroke with some promising results, but additional studies are needed to determine clinical practice guidelines.

Neuroprotective agents (calcium channel antagonists, citicoline, gamma-aminobutyric acid [GABA] agonists, glycine antagonists, magnesium, *N*-methyl-D-aspartate antagonists, tirilazad) have not been shown to significantly reduce the risk

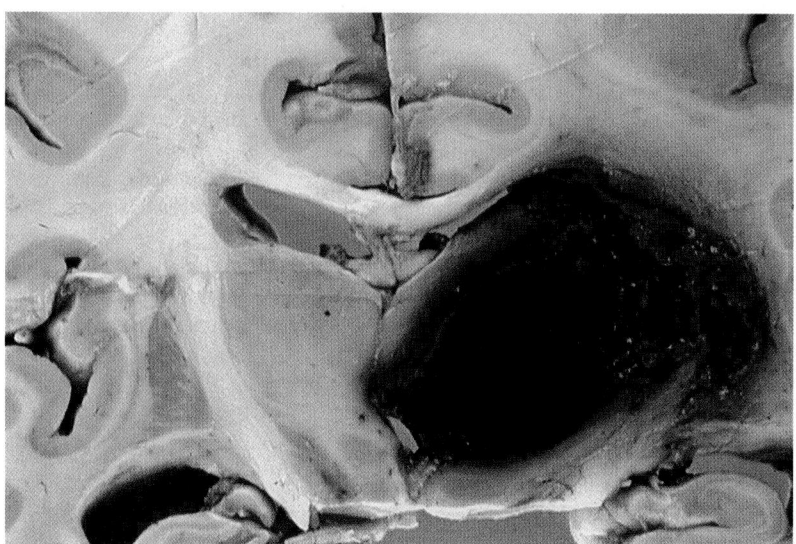

FIGURE 18-16 Hypertensive Hemorrhage. Cross section of the pons showing a hypertensive hemorrhage. (From Damjanov I: *Pathology for the health professions*, Philadelphia, 2012, Saunders.)

of poor outcome including death or improve outcomes with ischemic stroke. New neuroprotective agents are being evaluated.[60] For acute ischemic stroke, cholesterol reduction using statins appears to provide neuroprotection and improve both incidence and survival.[61]

Hemorrhagic Stroke. **Hemorrhagic stroke (spontaneous intracranial hemorrhage [ICH])** is spontaneous bleeding into the brain. It is the third most common cause of CVA and accounts for 8% to 18% of CVAs in whites but 30% in blacks and Asians.[53] There are about 40,000 ICHs in the United States per year.[62] Risk factors for hemorrhagic stroke include hypertension, previous cerebral infarct, coronary artery disease, and diabetes mellitus. The most common causes of spontaneous primary hemorrhagic strokes are hypertension (56% to 81%), ruptured aneurysms, arteriovenous malformation and fistula, amyloid angiopathy, and cavernous angioma.[62] ICH can occur secondary to traumatic brain injury, bleeding into ischemic brain infarction or tumor, or bleeding disorder or anticoagulation therapy.

PATHOPHYSIOLOGY. A hypertensive hemorrhage is associated with a significant increase in systolic and diastolic pressure over several years and usually occurs within the brain tissue. The pathogenesis of hypertensive cerebral hemorrhage is not fully understood. Hypertension involves primarily smaller arteries and arterioles, resulting in thickening of the vessel walls and increased cellularity of the vessels and hyalinization. Necrosis may be present. Microaneurysms in these smaller vessels or arteriolar necrosis precipitates the bleeding.

Hemorrhages are described as massive, small, slit, or petechial. A massive hemorrhage is several centimeters in diameter; a small hemorrhage is 1 to 2 cm in diameter; a slit hemorrhage lies in the subcortical area; and a petechial hemorrhage is the size of a pinhead bleed. The most common sites for hypertensive hemorrhages are in the putamen of the basal ganglia (a portion of the lentiform nucleus) (40%), the thalamus (15%), the cortex and subcortex (22%), the pons (8%) (Figure 18-16), caudate (7%), and cerebellar hemispheres (8%).

With bleeding, a mass of blood is formed and its volume increases. In massive intracerebral hemorrhage (volume greater than 150 ml), cerebral perfusion falls to zero and cerebral blood flow stops, resulting in death. In strokes with less than massive hemorrhage, adjacent brain tissue is displaced and compressed. Necrosis around the hematoma is present within 6 hours. Edema forms and the blood-brain barrier is disrupted. An inflammatory reaction in surrounding brain tissue appears rapidly and peaks in several days.[62] Figure 18-17 illustrates additional detail. Rupture or seepage of blood into the ventricular system occurs in many cases.[62] The cerebral hemorrhage resolves through reabsorption. Macrophages and astrocytes appear to dissipate the blood. A cavity forms, which is surrounded by a dense gliosis after removal of the blood.

CLINICAL MANIFESTATIONS. With hemorrhagic stroke, clinical manifestations vary according to the location and size of the bleed. Focal neurologic deficits are found in 80% of individuals experiencing hemorrhagic strokes; altered consciousness occurs in 50%. Once a deep unresponsive state occurs the immediate prognosis is grave, and the individual rarely survives. If the person survives, however, recovery of function frequently is possible.

Individuals experiencing intracranial hemorrhage from a ruptured or leaking aneurysm have one of three sets of symptoms: (1) onset of an excruciating generalized headache with an almost immediate lapse into an unresponsive state; (2) headache, but with consciousness maintained; and (3) sudden lapse into unconsciousness. If the hemorrhage is confined to the subarachnoid space, there may be no local signs. If bleeding spreads into the brain tissue, hemiparesis/paralysis, dysphasia, or homonymous hemianopsia may be present. Warning signs of an impending aneurysm rupture may include headache, transient unilateral weakness, transient numbness and tingling, and transient speech disturbance. Warning signs, however, often are not present.

EVALUATION AND TREATMENT. Clinical guidelines for the management of spontaneous intracerebral hemorrhage have been published by the American Heart Association/American Stroke

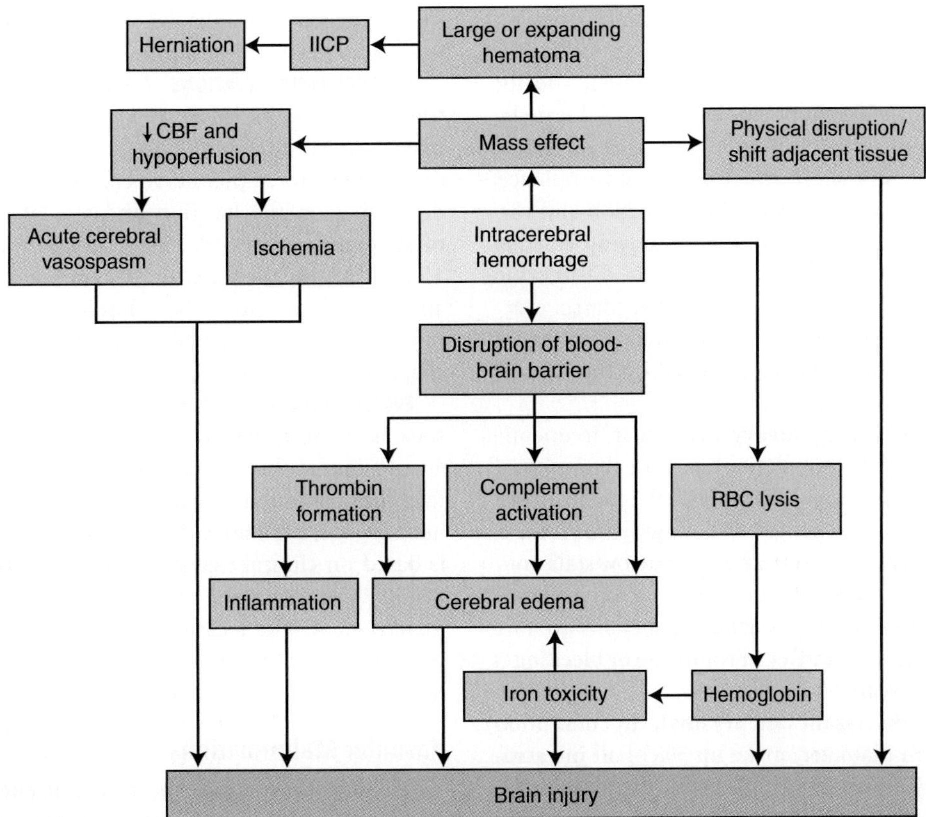

FIGURE 18-17 Injury Mechanisms Promoted by Intracerebral Hemorrhage. Hemorrhages can induce neuronal injury through mass effect, particularly in large hematomas that can *cause* increased intracranial pressure and herniation. Hemorrhages may also cause tissue damage through cerebral edema and secondary "neurotoxic" mechanisms caused by activation of the coagulation cascade and inflammation. Not all potential interactions are shown (e.g., thrombin may potentiate iron-induced injury; the complement and inflammatory systems overlap and several factors contribute to cerebral edema). *CBF,* Cerebral blood flow; *IICP,* increased intracranial pressure; *RBC,* red blood cell. (Data from Mocco J et al: *Neurosurg Focus* 15:22[5]:E7, 2007; Schubert GA, Thome C: *Front Biosci* 13:1594–1603, 2008; Xi G, Keep RF, Hoff JT: *Lancet Neurol* 5[1]:53–63, 2006.)

Association.[63] Diagnosis of hemorrhagic stroke considers the health history, clinical presentation, laboratory tests, and neuroimaging procedures (CT and MRI). Treatment needs to be initiated within 3 to 4 hours of symptom onset for reversibility of brain ischemia. Care in multidisciplinary stroke rehabilitation units appears to be most effective at reducing disability, dependency and length of hospital stay for all stroke syndromes.[64]

Treatment of a hemorrhagic stroke, regardless of cause, is focused on: (1) stopping or reducing the bleeding, (2) controlling increased ICP, (3) preventing a rebleed, (4) preventing vasospasm, and (5) promoting tissue restoration. Treatment for hemorrhagic stroke includes limiting hematoma enlargement and preventing or controlling seizures and cerebral edema. Known coagulopathies should be corrected and oral anticoagulation reversed. Hematoma enlargement is limited when recombinant activated factor VII is given within 4 hours of onset but it does not improve outcome and is associated with thromboembolic complications.[65] Surgical evacuation does not appear to be an effective treatment for supratentorial ICHs but may be indicated for a large posterior fossa hematoma.[66] Hypertension management is individualized. Elevated blood pressure can expand the hematoma and low blood pressure can contribute to ischemia.[58,67]

Prophylactic treatment of seizures is controversial and when used it is on a short-term basis (e.g., 3 days).[68] Osmotic therapies (e.g., mannitol) are used for the treatment of increased intracranial pressure and cerebral edema in hemorrhagic stroke.[69] Supportive care is provided for airway management; respiratory function; blood pressure control; avoidance of fever; and maintenance of fluids, glucose, electrolytes, and nutrition.

Intracranial Aneurysm. Intracranial aneurysms (weak bulging areas of an arterial vessel wall) may result from arteriosclerosis, congenital abnormality, trauma, inflammation, or infection. Cocaine use has been linked to aneurysm formation. The size of the aneurysm may vary from 2 mm to 3 cm. Most aneurysms are located at bifurcations in or near the circle of Willis, in the vertebrobasilar arteries, or within the carotid system—85% to 95% are in the anterior portion of the circle of Willis (see Figure 15-20 and p. 420). Aneurysms may be single, but in 20% to 25% of cases, more than one is present. In these instances the aneurysms may be unilateral or bilateral. The incidence of rupture is 11 in 100,000 per year. Peak incidence of rupture is from 50 to 60 years of age. Women have a slightly greater incidence of aneurysms.

PATHOPHYSIOLOGY. No single pathologic mechanism exists.[69a] A combination of genetic, congenital, and acquired factors (hypertension) is present.[70] Abnormalities in multiple layers of the blood vessel are found. The endothelial layer is thin, the internal elastic lamina is not present or fragmented, and the muscularis layer of the media ends at the aneurysm. Atherosclerotic changes are found. Aneurysm development is attributed to hemodynamic and wall shear stress and flow turbulence, particularly at bifurcations, and sites of inflammation and vascular remodeling. They are a symptom of underlying vascular disease. Hypertension and certain connective tissue disorders in which there are abnormalities in the extracellular matrix exacerbate aneurysm formation.[70] The aneurysm wall is composed of fibrous tissue. Aneurysms may be classified on the basis of shape and form (Figure 18-18).[71]

Saccular aneurysms (berry aneurysms) occur frequently (in approximately 2% of the population) and are the result of a combination of a congenital abnormality in the media of the arterial wall and degenerative changes. The sac grows over time. A saccular aneurysm may be (1) round with a narrow stalk connecting it to the parent artery (Figure 18-19), (2) broad based without a stalk, or (3) cylindrical. Saccular aneurysms are rare in childhood; their highest incidence of rupturing or bleeding is among people 20 to 50 years of age.

Fusiform aneurysms (giant aneurysms), by definition greater than 25 mm in diameter, make up 5% of all intracranial aneurysms. They occur as a result of diffuse arteriosclerotic changes and are found most commonly in the basilar arteries or terminal portions of the internal carotid arteries. They act as space-occupying lesions. **Mycotic aneurysms** result from arteritis caused by bacterial emboli (e.g. associated with bacterial endocarditis); these aneurysms are uncommon. **Traumatic (dissecting) aneurysms** are caused by a weakening of the arterial wall by a fracture line, by a penetrating missile, or after neurosurgical or imaging (e.g., angiographic) procedures.

What causes an aneurysm to rupture is not known.[70] Rupture causes hemorrhage into the subarachnoid space (subarachnoid hemorrhage) (see p. 605) with rapid spread, producing localized changes in the cerebral cortex and focal irritation of nerves and arteries. Because of compression, bleeding ceases with the formation of a fibrin-platelet plug at the point of rupture. Blood undergoes reabsorption through arachnoid villi within 3 weeks.

CLINICAL MANIFESTATIONS. Aneurysms are frequently asymptomatic. In routine autopsy, 5% of persons are found to have one or more intracranial aneurysms. Clinical manifestations may arise from cranial nerve compression, but the signs vary, depending on the location and size of the aneurysm. Most often, cranial nerves III, IV, V, and VI are affected (see Table 15-6). Unfortunately the most common first indication of an aneurysm is an acute subarachnoid hemorrhage, intracerebral hemorrhage, or combined subarachnoid-intracerebral hemorrhage (see pp. 602 and 605).

EVALUATION AND TREATMENT. Diagnosis before a bleeding episode is made using arteriographic examination. Intracranial aneurysms may be found incidently during CT or MRI imaging for other conditions. After a subarachnoid or an intracerebral hemorrhage, a tentative diagnosis of an aneurysm that has bled is based on clinical manifestations, history, and CT and MRI results. The treatment of choice for an aneurysm is surgical management. The location and size of the aneurysm and the person's clinical status determine whether invasive therapy is feasible.[72,73]

Vascular Malformations

Vascular malformations are rare congenital vascular lesions. They are about one-tenth as common as aneurysms and can cause hemorrhagic stroke, epilepsy, chronic headache, or focal neurologic deficits.[74] Four types of vascular malformation exist: arteriovenous malformation, cavernous angioma, capillary telangiectasis, and venous angioma. Most are sporadic, although multiple lesions are observed in families.[75] In an **arteriovenous malformation (AVM),** arteries feed directly into veins through a vascular tangle of malformed vessels without a true capillary bed. AVMs occur as frequently in males as in females, and occasionally are found in families. Although usually present at birth, AVMs exhibit a delayed age of onset and symptoms most commonly occur before 30 years of age. They usually rupture in the

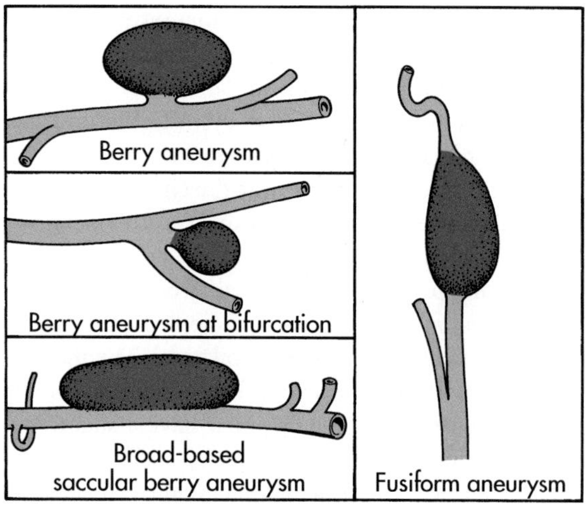

Berry aneurysm
Berry aneurysm at bifurcation
Broad-based saccular berry aneurysm
Fusiform aneurysm

FIGURE 18-18 Types of Aneurysms.

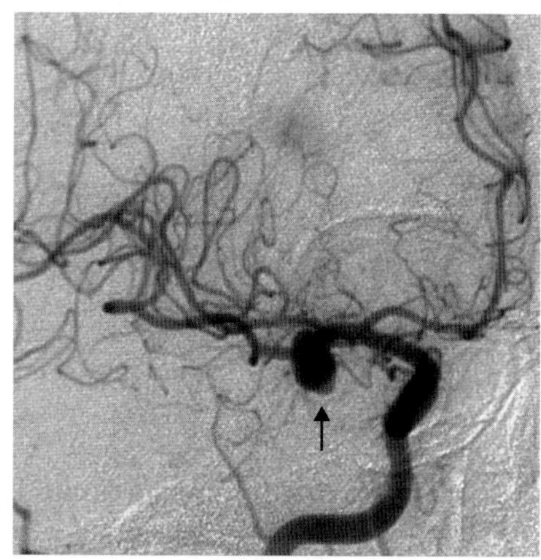

FIGURE 18-19 Berry Aneurysm, Angiogram. In this lateral view with contrast filling a portion of the cerebral arterial circulation can be seen a berry aneurysm *(arrow)* involving the middle cerebral artery of the circle of Willis at the base of the brain. (From Klatt EC: *Robbins and Cotran atlas of pathology,* Philadelphia, 2006, Saunders.)

second and third decades of life. **Cavernous angiomas (malformations)** are sinusoidal collections of blood vessels without interspersed normal brain tissue. They rarely hemorrhage and comprise 2% to 4% of hemorrhagic strokes. A **capillary telangiectasis** is dilated capillaries with interspersed normal brain tissue found deep in the brain, particularly in the brainstem; hemorrhage is rare. These vascular malformations are associated with Rendu-Osler-Weber disease (AVM in various areas of the body). **Venous angioma,** the most common vascular malformation found at autopsy (3% of cases), is considered a subset of developmental venous anomalies that occur secondary to arrested development. The result is primitive embryologic veins in a radial pattern feeding a central vein. These rarely hemorrhage.[76]

PATHOPHYSIOLOGY. AVMs are developmental abnormalities that represent persistence of embryonic patterns of blood vessels, do not have a normal blood vessel structure, and are abnormally thin (Figure 18-20). The involved vessels are considered by some researchers to enlarge over time. Their size is highly variable, from malformations of a few millimeters to large ones that extend from the cortex to the ventricle. The large AVMs also may involve the dura mater, including the falx cerebri and the tentorium cerebelli. The AVM may be fed by one or several arteries. There is usually high flow through the feeding arteries and draining veins. These feeder vessels become tortuous over time and often are dilated. With moderate to large AVMs, sufficient blood is shunted into the malformation to deprive surrounding tissue of adequate blood perfusion. There also are theories that propose sporadic AVMs develop as a postnatal consequence of an active angiogenic and inflammatory response to some inciting vascular event, such as trauma or infection.[77]

CLINICAL MANIFESTATIONS. Clinical manifestations vary: about 20% of persons with an AVM have a characteristic chronic nondescript headache, although some experience migraine; about 20% to 25% experience seizure disorders caused by compression. Initially, the seizures tend to be focal or jacksonian; generalization often occurs over time. (Seizures are discussed in Chapter 17.) About 40% to 70% suffer an intracerebral, a subarachnoid, or a subdural hemorrhage.[74] Bleeding from an AVM into the subarachnoid space causes clinical manifestations identical to those associated with a ruptured aneurysm. If bleeding is into the brain tissue, focal signs that develop resemble a stroke-in-evolution. Ten percent of persons experience hemiparesis or other focal signs. Hemiparesis usually is caused by compression or rupture. At times, noncommunicating hydrocephalus (see Chapters 17 and 20) develops with a large AVM that extends into the ventricle lining. AVMs account for up to 1% of all sudden deaths.[78]

EVALUATION AND TREATMENT. A systolic bruit over the carotid in the neck, the mastoid process, or (in a young person) the eyeball is almost diagnostic of an AVM. CT, magnetic resonance angiography (MRA), transcranial Doppler (TCD), and MRI are used in initial diagnosis, followed by an arteriogram to identify feeding vessels. Treatment options are microsurgery, embolization, stereotactic radiosurgery (SRS), or combinations of treatment. Observation only depends on age, overall health, lesion-specific factors (size, location, and angiographic anatomy), and individual-specific factors. The risk of bleeding is about 6% in the first year and 2% to 4% each year thereafter with no intervention.[79]

Subarachnoid Hemorrhage

With a **subarachnoid hemorrhage (SAH),** blood escapes from a defective or injured vasculature into the subarachnoid space (Figure 18-21). Previous family history of SAH is one of the strongest predictors of aneurysmal SAH. Heavy alcohol use, hypertension, smoking, anticoagulation use, and oral contraceptive use are associated with SAH. Individuals at risk for a SAH are those with a saccular intracranial aneurysm (80% of cases), intracranial AVM, or hypertension and those who have sustained head injuries. The mortality is approximately 50%,

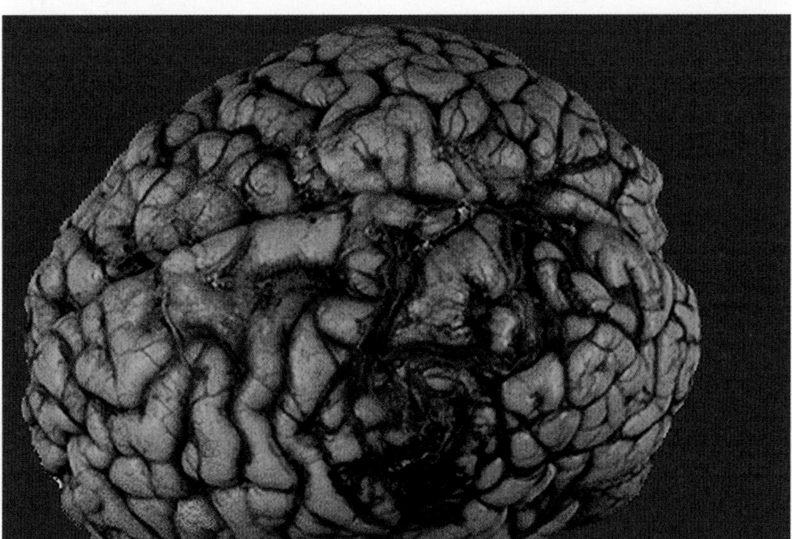

FIGURE 18-20 Vascular Malformation, Gross. A vascular malformation represented by a mass of irregular tortuous vessels over the left posterior parietal region of the brain. (From Klatt EC: *Robbins and Cotran atlas of pathology*, Philadelphia, 2006, Saunders.)

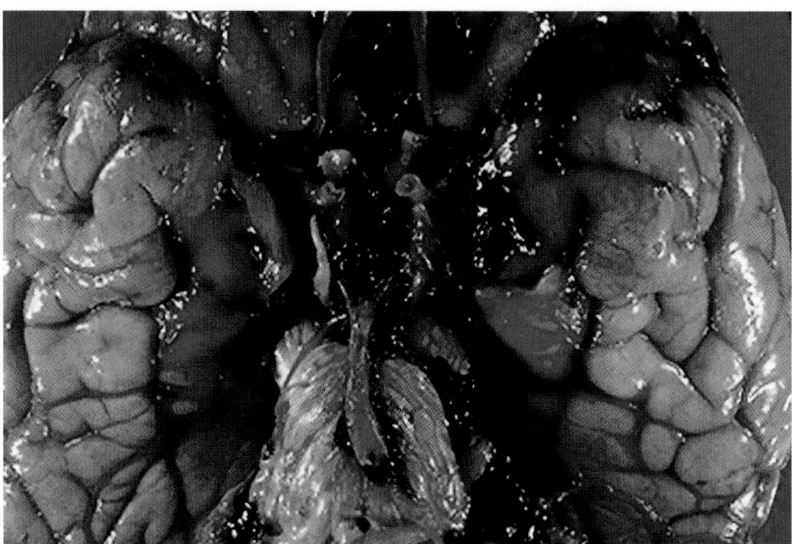

FIGURE 18-21 Subarachnoid Hemorrhage, Gross. Subarachnoid hemorrhage resulting from rupture of a berry aneurysm. (From Klatt EC: *Robbins and Cotran atlas of pathology,* Philadelphia, 2006, Saunders.)

and about one third of survivors are dependent. SAHs often recur, especially from a ruptured intracranial aneurysm.[80]

PATHOPHYSIOLOGY. When a vessel is leaking, blood oozes into the subarachnoid space. When a vessel tears, blood under pressure is pumped into the subarachnoid space. The blood is extremely irritating to the meningeal and other neural tissues and so produces an inflammatory reaction in these tissues. Additionally, the blood coats nerve roots, clogs arachnoid granulations (impairing CSF reabsorption), and clogs foramina within the ventricular system (impairing CSF circulation). ICP immediately increases to almost diastolic levels. ICP returns to near baseline in about 10 minutes. Cerebral blood flow and cerebral perfusion pressure (CPP) decrease. The expanding hematoma acts like a space-occupying lesion, compressing and displacing brain tissue. Granulation tissue is formed and scarring of the meninges, with resulting impairment of CSF reabsorption and secondary hydrocephalus, often results.

Subarachnoid hemorrhage has a unique pathophysiologic cascade triggered by the sudden appearance of blood in the subarachnoid space. Eighty percent of persons with SAH have infarction on MRI, which is the major cause of death and disability, and 33% of persons have asymptomatic vasospasm in the first 2 weeks following an SAH.[81]

The cause for **cerebral vasospasm (CVS)** and **delayed cerebral ischemia (DCI)** is unclear. DCI is related to but not explained by the CVS. Development of CVS requires the presence of blood and its breakdown products as a consequence of the SAH. It also appears that oxyhemoglobin is a powerful precipitator of CVS. It scavenges nitric oxide (a vasodilator), and its breakdown triggers a free radical cascade that disrupts multiple blood vessel layers and initiates release of inflammatory factors. It appears that CVS, disruption of cerebral autoregulation, microthrombi, and spreading cortical depression contribute to DCI. Autoregulation may be impaired in SAH and the combination of narrowed blood vessels, because of spasm and disrupted autoregulation, impairs perfusion, resulting in ischemia and infarction.[82]

CLINICAL MANIFESTATIONS. Early manifestations associated with leaking vessels are episodic headache, transient changes in mental status or level of consciousness, nausea or vomiting, focal neurologic defects including visual or speech disturbances, cranial nerve palsies, or stiff neck. A ruptured vessel often is accompanied by a sudden throbbing, "explosive" headache that is associated with nausea and vomiting, visual disturbances, motor deficits, and loss of consciousness. These signs can be related to a dramatic rise in ICP as blood is released directly into the CSF. Meningeal irritation and inflammation often occur, causing neck stiffness (nuchal rigidity), photophobia, blurred vision, irritability, restlessness, and low-grade fever. A positive Kernig sign (in which straightening the knee with the hip and knee in a flexed position produces pain in the back and neck regions) and a positive Brudzinski sign (in which passive flexion of the neck produces neck pain and increased rigidity) may appear. No localizing signs are present if the bleed is confined completely to the subarachnoid space.

The Hunt and Hess SAH grading system is based on description of the clinical manifestations (Table 18-6). Rebleeding is a significant risk with a high mortality (up to 70%). The period of greatest risk is the first month, with the peak incidence of rebleeding during the first 2 weeks after the initial bleed. Rebleeding is manifested by a sudden increase in blood pressure and ICP, along with a deteriorating neurologic status.

EVALUATION AND TREATMENT. The diagnosis of a subarachnoid hemorrhage is based on the clinical presentation, imaging results, and cerebrospinal fluid evaluation.[83,84] Treatment is directed at control of intracranial pressure, prevention of ischemia and hypoxia of neural tissues, and prevention of rebleeding episodes. Antifibrinolytic drugs may be used to stop rebleeding in selected cases. Blood pressure is allowed to remain in the high normal range or is elevated to that level. Calcium channel blockers, such as nimodipine, are used to prevent or reverse vasospasm. Volume expansion or hemodilution through continuous or bolus administration of hetastarch and administration of plasma protein factors to maintain a hematocrit of 33%

are used to expand blood volume and augment cerebral perfusion in selected cases. Surgical clipping of the aneurysm may be done. Endovascular placement of platinum coils and balloon embolization to occlude the aneurysm are used. Cerebral angioplasty can be tried for vasospasm. Evaluation of new treatments is in progress.[85-87]

Headache Syndromes

Headache is a common neurologic disorder and is usually a benign symptom. However, it can be associated with serious disease, such as brain tumor, meningitis, giant cell arteritis, and cerebrovascular disease. The primary headache syndromes discussed here are the chronic, recurring type not associated with structural abnormalities or systemic disease and include migraine, cluster, paroxysmal hemicrania, and tension headaches. Characteristics of the major types of headache syndromes are summarized in Table 18-7.

Migraine

Migraine is an episodic neurologic disorder whose marker is headache lasting 4 to 72 hours. Migraine is more common in those 25 to 55 years of age, and can occur in young children. The incidence of migraine by age 85 years is about 18% in males and 44% in females. Onset after 55 years of age is rare.[88] Hormonal factors account for most of the gender differences. A positive family history is common as is a genetic predisposition.

Migraine is diagnosed when it is not attributable to any other disorder and when any two of the following features occur: unilateral head pain, pulsating pain, pain worsening with activity, moderate or severe pain intensity, and at least one of the following: nausea or vomiting, or both, or photophobia and phonophobia.[89]

Migraine is a multifactorial disorder caused by a combination of multiple genetic and environmental factors. Specific gene associated migraine includes familial hemiplegic migraine, sporadic hemiplegic migraine, and cerebral autosomal dominant arteriopathy with subcortical infarcts and leukoencephalopathy. Migraine sufferers have an increased risk for epilepsy, depression, anxiety disorders, and stroke.[90] Migraine may be precipitated by triggers. Individuals with migraine are likely to have a genetically determined reduced threshold for triggers with further reduced threshold caused by endogenous factors (e.g., altered sleep patterns [becoming tired or too much sleep], missed meals, overexertion, weather change, stress or relaxation from stress, hormonal changes [such as menstrual periods], excess afferent stimulation [bright lights, strong smells], and chemicals [alcohol or nitrates]).[88]

The International Headache Society has broadly classified episodic migraine into two major subtypes: migraine with aura and migraine without aura.[91] In migraine with aura, at least some of the attacks are temporarily associated with distinct aura symptoms suggestive of focal brain dysfunction (flashing lights, visual loss). There are no associated focal neurologic symptoms in migraine without aura. Two thirds of those with migraines have migraine without aura. **Chronic migraine** is a progression of episodic migraine with a prevalence of about 2%. Criteria for these headaches include the following: it occurs on more than 15 days per month for at least 3 months; no excessive use of opiate or barbiturate medications is involved; and on more than 8 days per month there is migraine without aura or treatment provides relief before symptoms develop.[91]

The pathophysiologic basis for migraine is complex and not clearly established. It includes neurologic, vascular, hormonal, and neurotransmitter components. Migraine pain appears to be related to activation of the peripheral and central arms of the

TABLE 18-6 SUBARACHNOID HEMORRHAGE CLASSIFICATION SCALE

CATEGORY	DESCRIPTION
Grade I	Neurologic status intact; mild headache, slight nuchal rigidity
Grade II	Neurologic deficit evidenced by cranial nerve involvement; moderate to severe headache with more pronounced meningeal signs (e.g., photophobia, nuchal rigidity)
Grade III	Drowsiness and confusion with or without focal neurologic deficits; pronounced meningeal signs
Grade IV	Stuporous with pronounced neurologic deficits (e.g., hemiparesis, dysphasia); nuchal rigidity
Grade V	Deep coma state with decerebrate posturing and other brainstem dysfunction

From Cook HA: Aneurysmal subarachnoid hemorrhage: neurosurgical frontiers and nursing challenges. In Winkleman C, editor: *AACN clinical issues in critical care nursing,* Philadelphia, 1991, Lippincott; Hunt WE, Hess RM: *J Neurosurg* 28(1):14–20, 1968.

TABLE 18-7 CHARACTERISTICS OF COMMON HEADACHES

	MIGRAINE WITH OR WITHOUT AURA	CLUSTER HEADACHE/PROXIMAL HEMICRANIA	TENSION TYPE OF HEADACHE
Age of onset	Childhood, adolescence, or young adulthood	Young adulthood, middle age	Young adulthood, middle age
Gender	Female	Male	Not gender specific
Family history of headaches	Yes	No	Yes
Onset and evolution	Slow to rapid	Rapid	Slow to rapid
Time course	Episodic	Clusters in time	Episodic, may become constant
Quality	Usually throbbing	Steady	Steady
Location	Variable, often unilateral	Orbit, temple, cheek	Variable
Associated features	Prodrome, vomiting	Lacrimation, rhinorrhea, Horner syndrome	None

trigeminal system, cortical spreading depression, and distinct activity of brainstem nuclei.

The clinical phase of a migraine attack and associated pathophysiology are as follows[92-95]:

1. *Premonitory phase:* Up to one third of migraine patients have premonitory symptoms at least some of the time for several hours before aura or headache onset (e.g., neck pain, depression, yawning, food cravings); the pathogenesis is unknown but evidence suggests dopaminergic/hypothalamic involvement.[96]
2. *Migraine aura:* Up to one third of migraine patients have aura symptoms at least some of the time that may last 1 hour or sometimes much longer; migraine aura is defined as a spreading, focal, neurologic disturbance manifested as visual, sensory, or motor symptoms; the pathophysiologic mechanism appears to be a cortical spreading depression (CSD) (focal hyperemia [vasodilation] followed by spreading oligemia [vasoconstriction]), a reduction in electrical activity, and a decrease in blood flow that slowly spreads across the cerebral cortex from the occipital region.[97]
3. *Headache phase:* This phase includes associated symptoms and may last from 4 to 72 hours (usually about 1 day). The genesis of migraine pain is unknown and there is debate about whether the initiating mechanisms are central or peripheral, vascular or nonvascular.[98] Proposed pain mechanisms include: (1) activation of trigeminal cervical afferent neurons (arise from the ophthalmic division of the trigeminal ganglion and in the upper cervical dorsal roots in the posterior fossa) that innervate cerebral vessel nociceptors—activation of trigeminal sensory nerves releases vasoactive peptides that cause a sterile, inflammatory response around vessels in the meninges; (2) abnormal processing of trigeminal pain from the dural vessels and upper cervical muscles by the diencephalon (thalamus and hypothalamus), brainstem, or high cervical spinal cord; (3) central sensitization from an increased response of thalamic neurons to stimulation—allodynia; (4) dilation of the terminal branches of the external carotid artery.[99-101]
4. *Recovery phase*: This phase may take several hours to days.

Migraine without aura is often located on one side of the head. In migraine with aura, the most common prodromal symptoms are visual (scotomas with luminous angles and scintillating edges, and hemianopsia). Sensory deficits and aphasia also may be present. The aura develops within 5 to 20 minutes and remits within 60 minutes, followed by headache and other symptoms, including nausea, vomiting, photophobia, and scalp tenderness; 10% experience diarrhea.

In susceptible women, migraine occurs most frequently before and during menstruation and is decreased during pregnancy and menopause. Excessive levels of estrogen during menstruation stimulate receptors in the trigeminal ganglia and periaqueductal gray that manifest as menstrual migraine.[102] Estrogens also may act directly on vascular smooth muscle, modulate activity of vasoactive substances at the neurovascular junction, and activate vasoregulatory responses in the hypothalamus. However, no direct evidence has been found to link circulating female sex hormones with the frequency and severity of migraine.

The diagnosis of migraine is made from health history and physical examination. Clinicians must be skilled in their understanding of different types of headaches, risk factors, family history, and clinical features. Differential diagnosis is confirmed with CT, MRI, and EEG. A significant number of individuals with migraine have depression as a comorbidity.

The management of migraine includes education that migraine is a chronic physiologic, not psychosomatic, disorder. Avoidance of triggers, adequate sleep, regular eating habits, and daily relaxation and meditation can create a headache-protective environment. With the onset of acute migraine, a dark room, ice, and sleep can provide relief. The pharmacologic management of migraine varies with each individual and is related to the severity of the attack. Drug considerations should include antiemetics, NSAIDs, ergotamine and dihydroergotamine, and serotonin receptor agonists (e.g., sumatriptan). Triptans, transcutaneous estrogen, and magnesium administration may help some women with menstrual migraine. Gastric absorption may be decreased during an attack, and routes of administration other than oral (e.g., nasal sprays, intravenous, and rectal) may be used. There are several emerging drugs that may target the molecular pathophysiology of migraine pain.[103] The prophylaxis of migraine is considered when attacks cannot be treated effectively. Several drugs may be considered and should *not* be used in combination. Examples include beta-blockers, a calcium antagonist (flunarizine), serotonin antagonists (lisuride, methysergide), NSAIDs, dihydroergotamine (DHE), valproic acid, and amitriptyline. There are many new drugs under evaluation.[104]

Cluster Headache

Cluster headaches are one of a group of disorders referred to as trigeminal autonomic cephalagia[105] and occur primarily in men between 20 and 50 years of age. Cluster headache has been known also as *histamine cephalalgia, Horton syndrome,* and *erythromelalgia.* These uncommon headaches occur in clusters for a period of days followed by a long period of spontaneous remission. Cluster headache has an episodic and a chronic form with extreme pain intensity and short duration. If the cluster of attacks occurs more frequently without sustained spontaneous remission, they are classified as *chronic cluster headaches* (20% of cases) (see Table 18-7). Triggers are similar to those that cause migraine headache.

Trigeminal activation occurs but the mechanism is unclear. There is unilateral trigeminal distribution of severe pain with ipsilateral autonomic manifestations, including tearing on the affected side, ptosis of the ipsilateral eye, and congestion of the nasal mucosa. The pathogenic mechanism for pain is related to the release of vasoactive peptides, the formation of neurogenic inflammation, and the activation of the pain matrix. Autonomic dysfunction is characterized by sympathetic underactivity and parasympathetic activation. The rhythmicity of attacks is associated with changes in the inferior posterior hypothalamus. There may be altered serotonergic nerve transmission, but at different loci than in migraine headache.[106]

The headache attack usually begins without warning and is characterized by severe, unilateral tearing; and burning, periorbital, and retrobulbar or temporal pain lasting 30 minutes to 2 hours. One or several attacks may occur in a day, usually at the same time of day or night. The same side is affected in subsequent episodes, and the attack activates the trigeminal-autonomic reflex. Associated symptoms include lacrimation, reddening of the eye, nasal stuffiness, eyelid ptosis, and nausea. Pain often is referred to the midface and teeth. Alcohol can stimulate an attack during a cluster headache in about 50% to 70% of cases, but it is not a triggering factor during remission.

Prophylactic drugs are used to treat cluster headache, as well as avoidance of triggers. The most effective are calcium channel antagonists (verapamil), lithium carbonate, topiramate, valproic acid, gabapentin, and baclofen. Acute attacks are managed with oxygen inhalation and intravenous sumatriptan, or inhaled ergotamine administration and nerve stimulation.[107]

Chronic paroxysmal hemicrania (CPH) is a cluster-type headache with unilateral head pain that occurs with more daily frequency (4 to 12 times per day) but with shorter duration (20 to 120 minutes). The remission phases are often shorter. The attacks are more common in women, usually after pregnancy. The symptoms are similar to cluster headache. As with cluster headache, there is an episodic and a chronic form. The pathophysiology involves a disorder of sympathetic hyperactivity, but the mechanism is different from that of cluster headache because there is effective relief of symptoms with indomethacin.[108]

Tension-Type Headache

Tension-type headache (TTH) is the most prevalent type of primary headache. It is not a vascular or migrainous headache. The average age of onset is during the second decade of life. It is a mild to moderate bilateral headache with a sensation of a tight band or pressure around the head. The onset of pain is usually gradual. *Episodic tension-type headache* may last for several hours or several days. It is not aggravated by physical activity. *Chronic tension-type headache* evolves from episodic tension-type headache and represents headache that occurs at least 15 days per month for at least 3 months.[91] Many individuals have both tension-type and migraine headaches.

The pathogenesis of TTH is not clear; however, there is a probable genetic predisposition. Both a central mechanism and a peripheral mechanism operate in causing tension headache. The central mechanism probably involves hypersensitivity of pain fibers from the trigeminal nerve that leads to central sensitization. The peripheral sensitization of myofacial sensory afferents may contribute to muscular hypersensitivity and the development of chronic TTH.[109] Headache sufferers have more localized pain and tenderness of pericranial muscles.

Mild headaches are treated with ice, and more severe forms are treated with aspirin or NSAIDs. Chronic tension-type headaches are best managed with a tricyclic antidepressant, such as amitriptyline. Cognitive-behavioral therapy and relaxation training reduce symptoms of chronic tension-type headache. Long-term use of analgesics or other drugs, such as muscle relaxants, antihistamines, tranquilizers, caffeine, and ergot alkaloids, should be avoided.[110]

Infection and Inflammation of the Central Nervous System

The CNS may be infected by bacteria, viruses, fungi, parasites, and mycobacteria. Viruses causing acute and chronic CNS infections are listed in Table 18-8. The infecting microorganisms gain entry to the nervous system by (1) hematogenous spread through arterial blood or (2) direct extension from another site of infection.[111] Neurologic infections produce disease by several mechanisms: direct neuronal or glial infection; mass lesion formation; inflammation with subsequent edema; interruption of cerebrospinal fluid pathways; neuronal damage, or vasculopathy; and secretion of neurotoxins (Figures 18-22 through 18-24). Syndromes are acute and subacute bacterial meningitis, epidural and brain abscess, encephalitis, peripheral neuropathy, or neurosyphilis depending on the infecting microorganism. Signs and symptoms are produced because of (1) interference with the function of the nervous system tissue being invaded or compressed or (2) the inflammatory response produced by the body in response to infection. The cardinal signs of CNS infection are fever, head or spine pain, and generalized or focal neurologic dysfunction.[112]

Meningitis

Meningitis is inflammation of the brain or spinal cord. Infectious meningitis may be caused by bacteria, viruses, fungi, parasites, or toxins. (The pathophysiology of infection is discussed in Chapter 10.) The infection may be acute, subacute, or chronic with the pathophysiology, clinical manifestations, and treatment differing for each type of microorganism. In **aseptic meningitis** no specific pathogen can be identified and the disease is treated symptomatically.

Bacterial meningitis is primarily an infection of the pia mater and arachnoid villi, the subarachnoid space, the ventricular system, and the CSF. About 1 in 100,000 persons are affected annually.[113] Meningococcus *(Neisseria meningitidis)* and pneumococcus *(Streptococcus pneumoniae)* are the most common causes of bacterial meningitis. Meningococcus has been identified worldwide. Meningococcal meningitis occurs predominantly in men and boys and in the fall, winter, and spring of the year. Epidemics of meningococcal meningitis occur in approximately 10-year cycles, predominantly affecting children and adolescents. With pneumococcal meningitis, young persons and those more than 40 years of age are mostly affected. Predisposing conditions are otitis or sinusitis (25%), immunocompromised status (16%), and pneumonia (12%).[113,114]

Meningitis (viral meningitis, nonpurulent meningitis, lymphocytic meningitis) is believed to be limited to the meninges. An identifiable bacteria cannot be found in the cerebrospinal fluid. The most at-risk populations and the time of year when occurrences are seen depend on the virus and on the immune status of the individual. Viral meningitis produces a variety of symptoms and is caused by a variety of viruses. The most common are enteroviral viruses (echovirus, coxsackievirus, and nonparalytic poliomyelitis), arboviruses, and herpes simplex type 2.[115] Treatment is primarily supportive and the disease usually resolves within 7 to 10 days.

TABLE 18-8 VIRUSES CAUSING ACUTE AND CHRONIC CNS DISEASES

VIRUS	FAMILY	NUCLEIC ACID	CNS DISEASE	CELL TROPISM	NONHUMAN HOST	ROUTE OF ENTRY TO CNS	TREATMENT
Viruses Causing Acute CNS Diseases							
Herpes simplex viruses 1 and 2	Herpesviridae	DNA	Meningoencephalitis	Neuron	ND	Intraneuronal	Acyclovir
Rabies virus	Rhabdoviridae	RNA	Encephalomyelitis	Neuron	Carnivores	Intraneuronal	Postexposure prophylaxis; RIG and vaccine
West Nile virus	Flaviviridae	RNA	Meningoencephalomyelitis	Neuron	Birds, horses	Hematogenous	IVIG, interferon-alpha
Nipah virus	Paramyxoviridae	RNA	Encephalitis	Neuron, endothelia	Pigs, fruit bats	Hematogenous	Ribavirin
Equine encephalitis viruses	Togaviridae	RNA	Meningitis, encephalitis	Neuron, astrocytes	Horses	Hematogenous	Supportive care
Mumps virus	Paramyxoviridae	RNA	Meningitis, encephalitis, myelitis	Neuron, ependymal cell	ND	Hematogenous	IVIG
Rubella virus	Togaviridae	RNA	Meningitis, encephalitis	Not specified	ND	Hematogenous	Plasmapheresis
Coxsackievirus, echovirus	Picornaviridae	RNA	Meningitis, meningoencephalitis, myelitis	Neuron	ND	Hematogenous	Pleconaril
Poliovirus	Picornaviridae	RNA	Meningitis, myelitis	Neuron	ND	Hematogenous	Pleconaril
California encephalitis virus	Bunyaviridae	RNA	Meningitis, encephalitis	Neuron	Small mammals	Hematogenous	Ribavirin
Viruses Causing Chronic CNS Disease							
Human immunodeficiency virus	Retroviridae	RNA	Encephalitis, meningitis, myelitis	Microglia, macrophage, astrocytes	ND	Hematogenous	HAART and neuroprotective agents
Human T-cell leukemia viruses 1 and 2	Retroviridae	RNA	Myelitis	Astrocyte, leukocyte	ND	Hematogenous	Zidovudine, lamivudine, glucocorticoids
JC virus	Polyomaviridae	DNA	Progressive multifocal leukoencephalopathy	Oligodendrocyte, astrocyte	ND	Hematogenous	Interferon-alpha, cidofovir
Varicella-zoster virus	Herpesviridae	DNA	Leukoencephalitis, cerebellitis, meningitis, myelitis	Neurons, satellite cell	ND	Hematogenous	Acyclovir, valacyclovir
Measles virus	Paramyxoviridae	RNA	Encephalitis; SSPE	Neuron	ND	Hematogenous	Ribavirin, interferon-alpha, isoprinosine
Cytomegalovirus	Herpesviridae	DNA	Encephalitis	Neuron, ependymal cell, oligodendrocyte, monocytoid cell, endothelia	ND	Hematogenous	Foscarnet, ganciclovir, cidofovir, fomivirsen, valganciclovir
Epstein-Barr virus	Herpesviridae	DNA	Encephalitis, meningitis, myelitis	Infiltrating mononuclear cells	ND	Hematogenous	Acyclovir, ganciclovir (?)

From Lindquist L, Vapalahti O: *Lancet* 371(9627):1861–1871, 2008; Power C, Noorbakhsh F: Central nervous system viral infections: clinical aspects and pathogenic mechanism. In Gilman S, editor: *Neurobiology of disease,* pp 487-488, Burlington, MA, 2007, Elsevier.

CNS, Central nervous system; *DNA,* deoxyribonucleic acid; *HAART,* highly active antiretroviral therapy; *IVIG,* intravenous immunoglobulin; *JC,* John Cunningham; *ND,* not determined; *RIG,* rabies immune globulin; *RNA,* ribonucleic acid; *SSPE,* subacute sclerosing panencephalitis.

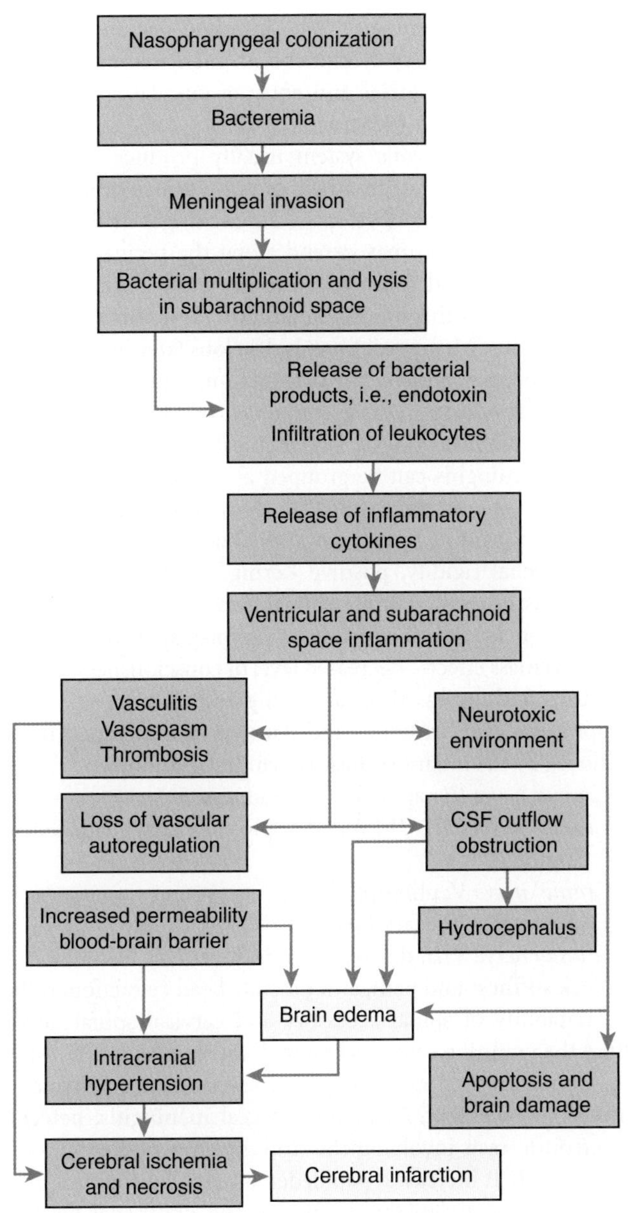

FIGURE 18-22 Pathogenesis of Meningitis. (Adapted from Cohen J, Powderly WG: *Infectious diseases,* ed 2, Mosby, 2004, Edinburgh.)

Fungal meningitis is a chronic, much less common condition than bacterial or viral meningitis. The most common fungal infections of the nervous system are histoplasmosis, cryptococcosis, coccidioidomycosis, mucormycosis, candidiasis, and aspergillosis. The infection occurs most often in persons with impaired immune responses or alterations in normal body flora. It develops insidiously, usually over days or weeks.

Tubercular meningitis is a common and serious form of CNS tuberculosis especially in persons with acquired immunodeficiency syndrome (AIDS). Miliary tubercles form in the brain and meninges. At some point the tuberculomas erode the pia mater, and the mycobacteria enter the CSF, producing a hypersensitivity reaction that results in a purulent exudate involving the basal meninges, cerebrum, and spinal nerves. Cerebral ischemia and infarction occur from vasculitis. Symptoms include headache, low-grade fever, nausea and vomiting,

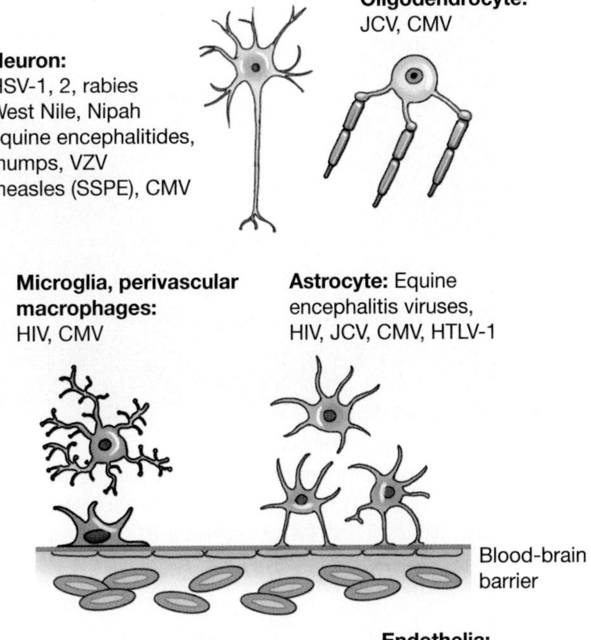

FIGURE 18-23 Viral Infection in the Central Nervous System (CNS). Viruses infect specific cell types within the CNS depending on the specific properties of the virus together with individual cell membrane proteins expressed on permissive cell types. Normally the brain is protected from circulating pathogens and toxins by the blood-brain barrier. *CMV,* Cytomegalovirus; *HIV,* human immunodeficiency virus; *HSV,* herpes simplex virus; *HTLV-1,* human T-cell lymphotropic virus type 1 (causes T-cell leukemia); *JCV,* John Cunningham virus (a polyomavirus causing progressive multifocal leukoencephalopathy); *SSPE,* subacute sclerosing panencephalitis; *VZV,* varicella-zoster virus. (Adapted from Power C, Noorbakhsh G: Central nervous system viral infections: clinical aspects and pathogenic mechanisms. In Gilman S, editor: *Neurobiology of disease,* p 488, Burlington, MA, 2007, Elsevier.)

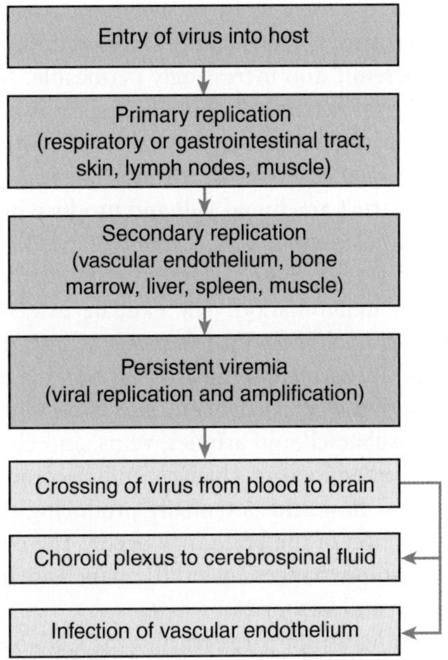

FIGURE 18-24 Hematogenous Spread of Viral Pathogens to the Central Nervous System. (Adapted from Cohen J, Powderly WG: *Infectious diseases,* Mosby, 2007, Edinburgh.)

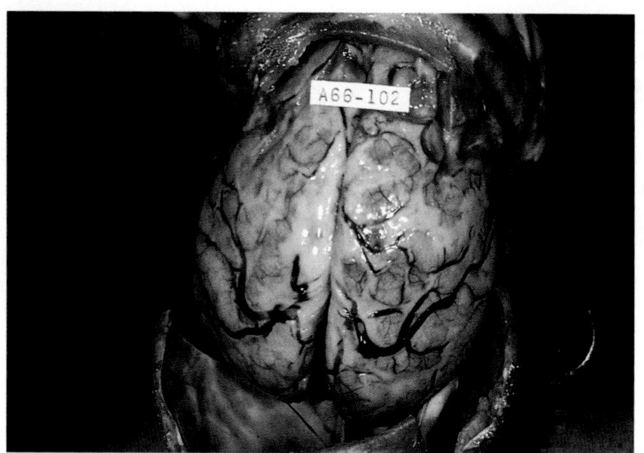

FIGURE 18-25 Acute Leptomeningitis. The leptomeninges contain abundant creamy, purulent exudate, most prominently over the superior surface of the cerebrum. The underlying brain is swollen, and the vessels are congested. (From Kumar V, Cotran RS, Robbins SL: *Robbins basic pathology,* ed 7, Philadelphia, 2003, Saunders.)

irritability, difficulty sleeping, and fatigue. These signs and symptoms increase to confusion, stiff neck, significant behavioral changes, and seizures. Hydrocephalus and cranial nerve palsies or cerebral infarcts may occur. Recovery rate is 90% with early diagnosis and treatment with appropriate antituberculosis therapy.[116]

PATHOPHYSIOLOGY. In bacterial meningitis, a systemic or bloodstream infection or a direct extension from an infected area (e.g., from a respiratory tract, ear, or paraspinal infection; as a result of dental work) is the access route to the subarachnoid space. The method of CNS entry is through the choroid plexuses or areas of altered blood-brain barrier or by hematogenous spread. Bacteria multiply in the subarachnoid space. The bacteria or their toxins function as irritants and induce an inflammatory reaction by the meninges (pia mater and arachnoid), the CSF, and the ventricles. The meningeal vessels undergo change, becoming hyperemic and increasingly permeable. Neutrophils migrate into the subarachnoid space, producing an exudate that thickens the CSF and interferes with normal CSF flow around the brain and spinal cord (Figure 18-25). The exudate has the potential to obstruct arachnoid villi and produce hydrocephalus and interstitial edema. The amount of purulent exudate increases rapidly (especially around the base of the brain), causing further inflammation. The exudate extends into the sheaths of the cranial and spinal nerves and into the perivascular spaces of the cortex. Meningeal cells become edematous. The exudate and vasogenic edema increase ICP. The small and medium-sized subarachnoid arteries, veins, and choroid plexuses undergo inflammatory changes and become engorged, disrupting blood flow and potentially producing thrombosis. Secondary infection of the brain may occur. The cortical neurons also show some changes, including an increase in the number of microglia and astrocytes.

In viral meningitis, the virus reaches the CNS by hematogenous spread. The virus enters the brain either directly or indirectly, through infected migrating leukocytes, and then infects vascular endothelial cells. The virus then enters the subarachnoid space, leading to meningitis. The immune response leads to release of inflammatory cytokines with increased permeability of the blood-brain barrier and entry of circulating immunoglobulins that combat the virus.

Fungi in the nervous system usually produce a granulomatous reaction with formations of granulomas or gelatinous masses. These usually develop in the meninges at the base of the brain. Fungi also may extend along the perivascular sites in the subarachnoid space and into the brain tissue, producing arteritis with thrombosis, infarction, and communicating hydrocephalus. Meningeal fibrosis develops later in the inflammatory process. Cranial nerve dysfunction, caused by compression, often results from the granulomas and fibrosis.

CLINICAL MANIFESTATIONS. The clinical manifestations of a bacterial meningitis can be grouped as: (1) inflammation and irritation—generalized meningeal signs, throbbing headache that becomes more severe, photophobia that becomes more severe, nuchal rigidity, positive Kernig and Brudzinski signs; (2) local tissue dysfunction—cranial nerve palsies, focal neurologic deficits (such as hemiparesis/hemiplegia, ataxia), and seizures; (3) mass effect—decreased level of consciousness, nausea, vomiting, and increased intracranial pressure; and (4) vascular compromise. The irritation and damage to the cranial nerves produced by the inflamed sheaths manifest as follows:

Cranial nerve II: papilledema, blindness
Cranial nerves III, IV, and VI: ptosis, visual field deficits, diplopia
Cranial nerve V: photophobia
Cranial nerve VII: facial paresis
Cranial nerve VIII: deafness, tinnitus, vertigo

Neck stiffness and pain, and possibly head retraction, reflect the irritability of spinal accessory and cervical spinal nerves. Often the vomiting center is irritated, causing projectile vomiting. Confusion and decreasing responsiveness are evidence of cortical involvement. In meningococcal meningitis, petechial or purpuric rash involving the skin and mucous membranes occurs. As ICP increases, papilledema may develop and delirium may progress to the point that the individual becomes unconscious.

The clinical manifestations of viral meningitis are mild compared with those associated with bacterial meningitis. Mild generalized throbbing headache, mild photophobia, mild neck pain, stiffness, fever, and malaise are manifestations of viral meningitis. Symptoms of aseptic meningitis are similar to those of viral meningitis.

Fungal meningitis develops slowly and insidiously. The first manifestations are often those of dementia or communicating hydrocephalus (see Chapter 17). The individual is characteristically afebrile.

EVALUATION AND TREATMENT. Diagnosis of bacterial meningitis is based on physical examination and the results of nasopharyngeal smear and antigen tests. CSF cultures are required to diagnose fungal meningitis. Bacterial meningitis and fungal meningitis are treated with appropriate antibiotic therapy, but resistant strains are an increasing problem. Other supportive measures may be needed. Viral meningitis is managed pharmacologically with antiviral drugs and corticosteroids in

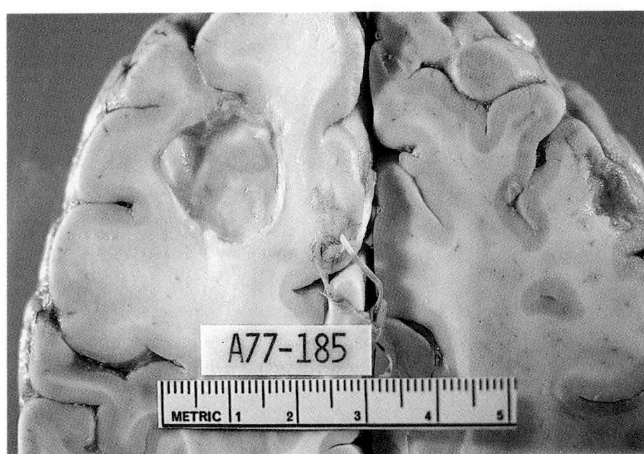

FIGURE 18-26 Brain Abscess. The abscess is sharply demarcated, indicating that it has been present for some time. Purulent exudate is visible in the center of the abscess. Because antibiotics penetrate very poorly into abscesses, surgical drainage is often necessary to treat such lesions. (From Kumar V, Cotran RS, Robbins SL: *Robbins basic pathology,* ed 7, Philadelphia, 2003, Saunders.)

addition to supportive care. There are vaccinations to prevent meningococcal, pneumococcal, and *Haemophilus influenzae* meningitis.[117]

Brain or Spinal Cord Abscess

Abscesses are localized collections of pus within the parenchyma of the brain or spinal cord and include subdural and extradural empyemas. They are rare and develop in about 1 per 100,000 hospital admissions and are more common in males. Abscesses occur (1) after open trauma and during neurosurgery; (2) from contiguous spread of infection, such as the middle ear, mastoid cells, nasal cavity, and nasal sinuses; (3) through metastatic or hematogenous distribution from distant foci, such as the heart, lungs, pelvic organs, skin, tonsils, abscessed teeth, osteomyelitis (with the exception of cranial bones), and dirty needles (especially in compromised hosts); and (4) from cryptogenic (unknown) factors arising without other associated areas of infections. *Streptococci, Staphylococci,* and *Bacteroides,* often in combination with anaerobes, are the most common bacteria that cause abscesses; however, yeast and fungi also have been found in CNS abscesses. *Toxoplasma gondii* is producing an ever-increasing number of CNS abscesses in persons with acquired immunodeficiency syndrome (AIDS). Most CNS abscesses are located in the frontal and temporal lobes (Figure 18-26). Immunosuppressed persons are particularly at risk.

Brain abscesses are classified as extradural, subdural, or intracerebral. **Extradural brain abscesses (empyemas)** are associated with osteomyelitis in a cranial bone. **Subdural brain abscesses (empyemas)** arise from a sinus infection or a vascular source. **Intracerebral brain abscesses** arise from a vascular source. **Spinal cord abscesses** are classified as epidural or intramedullary. Epidural spinal abscesses usually originate as osteomyelitis in a vertebra; the infection then spreads into the epidural space. (Osteomyelitis is discussed in Chapter 44.)

PATHOPHYSIOLOGY. Microorganisms gain entrance to the CNS from adjacent sites by direct extension from osteomyelitis or spread along the wall of a vein. Infective emboli carry the microorganisms from distant sites. The virulence of the pathogen and the immune response of the host are important determinants of outcome.[118] Brain abscess evolves through four stages regardless of infecting microorganism except in the immunosuppressed host, where the process may be incomplete. The stages are as follows:

1. *Early cerebritis* (days 1 to 3): A localized inflammatory process develops in which perivascular infiltration or inflammatory cells, composed of neutrophils, plasma cells, and mononuclear cells, surround a central core of coagulative necrosis; marked cerebral edema surrounds the area.
2. *Late cerebritis* (days 4 to 9): The necrotic center is surrounded by an inflammatory infiltrate of macrophages and fibroblasts; rapid new blood vessel formation occurs around the abscess; a thin capsule of fibroblasts and reticular fibers gradually develops; the area is still surrounded by cerebral edema.
3. *Early capsule formation* (days 10 to 13): The necrotic center decreases in size; the inflammatory infiltrate changes in character and contains an increasing number of fibroblasts and macrophages; mature collagen evolves, forming a capsule.
4. *Late capsule formation* (days 14 and longer): A well-formed necrotic center surrounded by a dense collagenous capsule develops.[119]

A free (nonencapsulated) abscess is associated with a higher mortality. Existing abscesses also tend to spread and form daughter abscesses.

Abscesses arising from the ear frequently are located in the middle or inferior temporal lobe or in the anterolateral cerebellar hemispheres. Abscesses originating from the oral, nasal, or sinus areas most commonly are located in the frontal and temporal lobes. Abscesses from distant foci often occur in multiple numbers in the distal portion of the middle cerebral arteries. In extradural abscesses, pus and granulation tissue accumulate in the extradural space.

CLINICAL MANIFESTATIONS. Clinical manifestations of brain abscesses are associated with (1) intracranial infection, such as fever and increased sedimentation rate; or (2) an expanding intracranial mass, such as headache, nausea, vomiting, decreasing cognitive abilities, paresis, and seizures. Early clinical manifestations of brain abscesses are low-grade fever, headache, neck pain and stiffness with mild nuchal rigidity, confusion, drowsiness, sensory deficits, and communication deficits. Headache is the most common early symptom. Later clinical manifestations may include inattentiveness (distractibility), memory deficits, decreased visual acuity and narrowed visual fields, papilledema, ocular palsy, ataxia, and dementia. Symptoms depend on the location of the abscess. The development of symptoms may be very insidious, often making an abscess difficult to diagnose. Extradural brain abscesses are associated with localized pain, purulent drainage from the nasal passages or auditory canal, fever, localized tenderness, and neck stiffness; occasionally the individual experiences a focal seizure. Clinical manifestations of spinal cord abscesses have four stages: (1) spinal aching; (2) root pain, which is usually severe, accompanied by spasms of the back

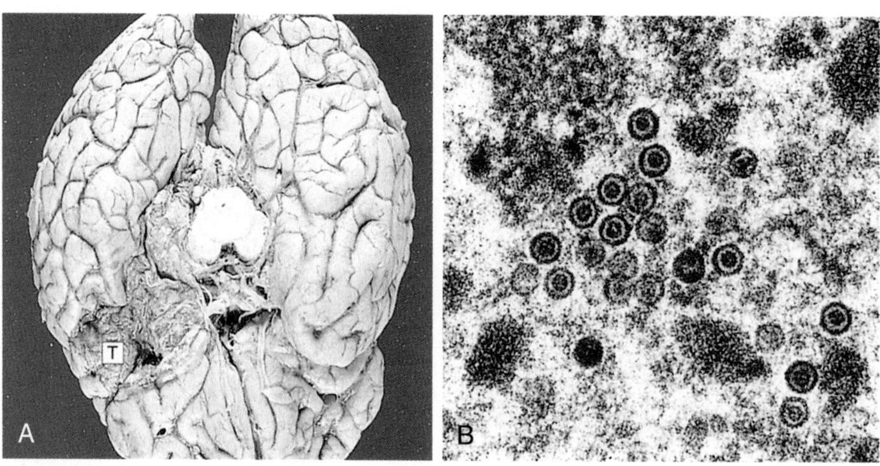

FIGURE 18-27 Herpes Simplex Encephalitis. In herpes simplex encephalitis **(A)** necrosis of the temporal lobes *(T)* is a typical development. Brain biopsy is useful in diagnosis when the virus can be seen by electron microscopy **(B)** as rounded particles with a dense core. Virus also can be identified by immunostaining or culture. In early cases, polymerase chain reaction (PCR) can be used to identify viral deoxyribonucleic acid (DNA) in cerebrospinal fluid samples. (From Stevens A, Lowe JS, Scott I: *Core pathology,* ed 3, London, 2009, Mosby.)

muscles and limited vertebral movement because of pain and spasm; (3) weakness caused by progressive cord compression; and (4) paralysis.[120]

EVALUATION AND TREATMENT. The diagnosis is suggested on the basis of clinical features and confirmed with MRI or contrast-enhanced CT. Surgical aspiration or excision is usually indicated.[121] Multiple or surgically inaccessible abscesses are treated with antibiotics, often in conjunction with corticosteroid therapy to treat the cerebral edema. In addition, ICP may require management.[122] Because decompression is necessary, spinal cord abscesses are treated with surgical excision or aspiration. Antibiotic administration and supportive therapy also are instituted.

Encephalitis

Encephalitis is an acute febrile illness, usually of viral origin, with nervous system involvement. The most common encephalitides are caused by arthropod-borne (mosquito-borne) viruses and herpes simplex viruses, almost exclusively herpes simplex type 1 in adults (Figure 18-27). Etiologic agents for viral encephalitis are presented in Table 18-8. Referred to as *infectious viral encephalitides,* encephalitis also may occur as a complication of systemic viral diseases such as poliomyelitis, rabies, mononucleosis, rubella, or rubeola. Encephalitis also may follow vaccination with a live attenuated virus vaccine if the vaccine has an encephalitis component. Such vaccines include measles, mumps, rubella; varicella; rotavirus; and yellow fever. Typhus, trichinosis, malaria, and schistosomiasis also are associated with encephalitis. Toxoplasmosis may acutely reactivate in immunosuppressed hosts when the once-dormant parasite in cyst form disseminates in brain tissues.

With the exception of the California viral encephalitis, which is endemic, the arthropod-borne encephalitides occur in epidemics, varying in geographic and seasonal incidence (Table 18-9). Eastern equine encephalitis is the most serious but least common of the encephalitides.[123] West Nile virus is presented in Box 18-1.

PATHOPHYSIOLOGY. Viruses gain access to the CNS through the bloodstream, olfactory bulb, or choroid plexus, or through an intraneuronal route from peripheral nerves.[124] Evidence of meningeal involvement appears in all encephalitides. The arthropod-borne viral encephalitides cause widespread nerve cell degeneration. Edema and areas of necrosis with or without hemorrhage develop. Increased ICP develops and may progress to herniation. Large degenerative injuries are found in eastern equine encephalitis, whereas the other arthropod-borne viral encephalitides have microscopic areas of injury and degeneration. Infectious encephalitis may result from a postinfectious autoimmune response to the virus or from direct invasion of the CNS by the virus. Herpes simplex type 1 has a tendency to infect the inferomedial surfaces of the temporal and frontal lobes and causes hemorrhagic necrosis.

CLINICAL MANIFESTATIONS. Encephalitis may range from a mild infectious disease to a life-threatening disorder. The dramatic clinical manifestations of encephalitis are fever, delirium, or confusion progressing to unconsciousness, seizure activity, cranial nerve palsies, paresis and paralysis, involuntary movement, and abnormal reflexes. Signs of marked ICP may be present.

EVALUATION AND TREATMENT. Diagnosis is based on health history and clinical presentation aided by CSF examination and culture, serologic examination, white blood cell (WBC) count, CT scan, or MRI. (Treatment available for the viral encephalitides is listed in Table 18-8.) Supportive therapy is initiated, and measures to control ICP are paramount.

Neurologic Complications of Acquired Immunodeficiency Syndrome

Approximately 40% to 60% of all persons with AIDS have neurologic complications (see Chapter 10 for the pathophysiology of AIDS). On postmortem examination, 75% have nervous system pathologic findings. The CNS pathologic findings result from (1) the primary human immunodeficiency virus (HIV) infection; (2) the immune dysregulation of early HIV infection and progressive immunosuppression in late HIV infections

TABLE 18-9 CLASSIFICATION AND CHARACTERISTICS OF ARTHROPOD VIRUSES CAUSING ENCEPHALITIS

VIRUSES	INCUBATION PERIOD (DAYS)	VIRUS	LOCATION	VECTOR	SEASON	AFFECTED POPULATION
Eastern equine encephalitis	5-10	Togaviridae *Alphavirus* (formerly group A arbovirus)	Swampy areas of eastern United States and Michigan	Mosquito	June to October	Infants, children, and adults >50 years
Western equine encephalitis	5-10	Same as above	All parts of United States: eastern, central, and western	Mosquito	July to October	All ages
Venezuelan equine encephalitis	2-5	Same as above	Texas, Florida, Mexico; Central and South America	Mosquito	All year	Infants and young children
St. Louis encephalitis	4-21	Flaviviridae *Flavivirus*	All parts of United States: eastern, central, and western	Mosquito	June to October	Adults >40 years; older adults more often affected than younger ages
La Cross encephalitis including California	5-15	Bunyaviridae *Bunyavirus* (California virus serogroup)	Midwestern United States, eastern seaboard, and Canada	Woodland mosquito	July to September	Children <15 years
West Nile encephalitis	3-14	Flaviviridae *Flavivirus*	Lower 48 states of United States	Mosquito	Summer and fall	Older adults most seriously

BOX 18-1 EMERGENCE OF WEST NILE VIRUS

West Nile (WN) virus, a *Flavivirus* transmitted predominantly by the *Culex* mosquito, emerged in New York state in 1999. By the end of 2004, human cases had been found in the 48 contiguous states. Humans and horses, as well as other mammals, are incidental hosts. Birds and mosquitoes are life cycle hosts. Summer and fall are peak times of infection incidence. The highest amount of virus carried by mosquitoes is in early fall. Besides mosquito transmission, WN virus can be transmitted through blood transfusions and organ transplants. Health experts believe transmission from mother to unborn child and through breast milk is possible. Novel strains are emerging increasing the risk for epidemics.

Three clinical forms of West Nile virus have emerged: WN fever, WN encephalitis; and WN meningitis, although some individuals have other clinical manifestations. Some persons develop WN fever. The febrile illness of acute onset may be clinically unrecognizable as WN. About 20% of those infected have mild symptoms that last 4 to 6 days; symptoms generally include fever and may include weakness, nausea, vomiting, headache, mental status changes, diarrhea, rash, and lymphadenopathy. WN encephalitis is marked by disorientation, stupor, coma, seizures, and movement disorders including tremor, ataxia, extrapyramidal signs, and paralysis. WN meningitis is characterized by meningeal signs of severe headache, high fever, and nuchal rigidity. Myelitis and polyradiculitis also may be present. Myocarditis, pancreatitis, and fulminant hepatitis are rare. Abnormalities in the brain stem, thalamus, basal ganglia, and cerebellum are often seen on MRI in people with severe infection—about 1 in 150 develop nervous system involvement. Identifiable risk factors for this are very young or advanced age, immunocompromised status, and pregnancy.

A preliminary diagnosis is made if IgM for the virus is found in serum or CSF. A rapid test became available in 2007. Plaque reduction neutralization assay (PRNA) is the confirmatory test. Interferon-alpha is used during treatment along with supportive care for those with severe infection. Several vaccines are under development.

Data from National Institute of Allergy and Infectious Diseases, Department of Health and Human Services, National Institutes of Health: *NIAID Research on West Nile Virus, January 2010.* Available at www.niaid.nih.gov; Cho H, Diamond MS: *Viruses* 4(12):3812–3830, 2012; Leis AA, Stokic DS: *Front Neurol* 3:37, 2012.

CSF, cerebrospinal fluid; *IgM,* immunoglobulin M; *MRI,* magnetic resonance imaging.

resulting in opportunistic infections, neoplasms, and systemic illness; and (3) the complications of therapy.[125] A variety of CNS complications of HIV exist (Box 18-2). Multiple CNS pathologic conditions may be experienced by one person. The most common neurologic disorder is HIV-associated dementia; others are peripheral neuropathies, vacuolar (spongy softening) myelopathy, opportunistic infections of the CNS, neoplasms, and, less commonly, stroke syndromes.[126]

HIV-infected macrophages/monocytes in blood are attracted to the brain by up-regulation of proinflammatory mediators such as monocyte chemoattractant protein-1 (MCP-1), tumor necrosis factor-alpha (TNF-α), and adhesion molecules on endothelial cells. Up-regulation enables transendothelial migration of activated macrophages/monocytes and causes neuroinflammation. Brain HIV-infected macrophages and microglia may be a sanctuary site for HIV because drugs have more difficulty crossing the blood-brain barrier, and there may be drug-resistant viral mutations and reinfection of the vascular system.[127]

Human Immunodeficiency Virus–Associated Neurocognitive Disorders (HANDs). A variety of names have been used for **human immunodeficiency virus–associated neurocognitive disorders (HANDs),** including HIV-associated dementia (HAD), HIV-associated cognitive dysfunction, HIV encephalopathy,

BOX 18-2 NERVOUS SYSTEM COMPLICATIONS OF HIV-1 INFECTIONS

CNS Complications of HIV-1 Infection

- Diffuse cerebral disorders
  - Minor cognitive and motor deficits (MCMDs)
  - HIV-associated dementia neurocognitive disorder (HAND)
- Meningitis
  - Atypical aseptic meningitis
    - Acute: typical meningitis signs
    - Chronic: headache syndrome
  - Nonviral infection
    - *Cryptococcus neoformans*
  - Other fungal infections
    - Mycobacterial infections
- Myelopathy
  - Spinal vacuolar myelopathy
- Focal brain disorders
  - Opportunistic viral infections
    - Progressive multifocal leukoencephalopathy
  - Herpesviruses
  - Nonviral infections
    - *Toxoplasma gondii*
  - Bacterial infections
  - Neoplasms
    - Primary CNS neoplasms
    - Metastatic neoplasms
  - Cerebrovascular complications
  - Complications resulting from systemic HIV therapy

Peripheral Nervous System Complications of HIV-1 Infections

- Distal symmetric peripheral neuropathy (polyneuropathy)
- Inflammatory demyelinating polyradiculoneuropathy
- Mononeuropathy multiplex
- Progressive polyradiculopathy
- Other causes of peripheral nervous system dysfunction
- Herpes zoster radiculitis
- Cranial neuropathies

CNS, Central nervous system; *HIV,* human immunodeficiency virus.

subacute encephalitis, HIV-associated dementia complex, HIV cognitive motor complex, AIDS encephalopathy, AIDS dementia complex, or AIDS-related dementia. Both adults and children may be affected with progressive cognitive dysfunction in conjunction with motor and behavioral alterations. The syndrome typically develops later in the disease but may be an early or a singular manifestation. The syndrome is more prevalent in drug users with HIV.[128]

The neurologic syndromes develop from properties of the virus, genetic characteristics of the host, and interactions with the environment (including treatment). At the time of primary HIV infection, HIV infects the perivascular macrophages, microglial cells, and astrocytes, particularly in the basal ganglia and deep white matter. Affected macrophages, macrophage-derived multinucleated cells, and microglia cause an immune-mediated demyelination process in white matter. Focal and diffuse demyelination of white matter and spongy changes of the spinal cord are present.

HIV-associated neurocognitive disorder is insidious in onset and unpredictable in its course. Most individuals experience a steady progression of mental decline characterized by abrupt accelerations of signs over several months to more than 1 year, although some experience an abrupt onset or an accelerated course. The triad of clinical manifestations are neurocognitive impairment, behavioral disturbance, and motor abnormalities. Clinical manifestations are summarized in Table 18-10.

Diagnosis is difficult, especially in early stages. The individual's health history, along with physical examination findings and supporting CSF, CT, and MRI data, helps establish the diagnosis although the brain may appear normal until there is advanced disease. Specific screening tools have been developed to assist in diagnosis. Highly active antiretroviral therapy (HAART) with more efficient CNS drug penetration has reduced the prevalence and improved survival for severe HAND, but milder forms of the disease may persist because of

TABLE 18-10 CLINICAL MANIFESTATIONS OF HIV-RELATED DEMENTIA

Early Stages

- *Cognitive impairments*
  - Short-term memory deficit
  - Decreased concentration/attention
  - Confusion and disorientation
  - Visuospatial perception deficits
- *Changes in personality or behavior*
  - Apathy, depression
  - Impaired judgment, erratic behavior
  - Social withdrawal
  - Rigidity of thought
  - Speech impairment
- *Psychotic symptoms*
  - Hallucinations and delusions
  - Suspiciousness and delusions
  - Agitation and inappropriate behavior
- *Motor symptoms*
  - Ataxia, loss of coordination, weakness
  - Tremors
- *Generalized systemic symptoms*
  - Fatigue, sleep changes (hypersomnia)
  - Anorexia, weight loss
  - Enuresis
  - Hypersensitivity to drugs and alcohol

Advanced Stages

- *Cognitive symptoms*
  - Global cognitive impairment
  - Impaired social relationship
  - Disorientation
  - Psychomotor retardation, decreased spontaneity
  - Agitation (e.g., nighttime delusions)
  - Coma, vegetative state
- *Motor symptoms*
  - Ataxia
  - Spastic weakness
  - Paraplegia, quadriparesis
  - Hyperreflexia, myoclonus, seizures
  - Bladder and bowel incontinence

Data from Clark C: Psychiatric aspects of AIDS, Chapter 71. In Jacobson JL, Jacobson AM, editors: *Psychiatric secrets,* ed 2, Philadelphia, 2001, Hanley & Belfus; Stern TA et al: *Massachusetts General Hospital comprehensive clinical psychiatry,* ed 1, St Louis, 2008, Mosby.

longer life. Research is continuing to evaluate the best treatment protocols and the possible neurotoxicity of HAART.[129]

HIV Myelopathy. **HIV myelopathy** involving diffuse degeneration of the spinal cord may occur with HIV. **Vacuolar myelopathy** is believed to be a direct consequence of HIV. The lateral and posterior columns of the lumbar spinal cord are affected. A progressive spastic paraparesis with ataxia is the predominant clinical manifestation. Leg weakness, upper motor neuron signs, incontinence, and posterior column sensory loss may be present. Diagnosis is made on the basis of history, physical findings, and supporting data from diagnostic procedures. Vacuolar myelopathy is treated supportively and does not respond to antiretrovirals.[125]

HIV-Associated Peripheral Neuropathy. Some **HIV-associated peripheral neuropathies** occur early, may coincide with seroconversion, are immune-mediated, and respond to standard immunotherapies. Other peripheral neuropathies primarily develop with advanced HIV infection and immunocompromised states and are facilitated by HIV replication, neurotoxicity from antiretroviral therapies, and coinfection with opportunistic pathogens.

HIV neuropathy may have one or a combination of several presentations: a predominantly sensory neuropathy, an autonomic neuropathy, a mononeuritis multiplex, an inflammatory demyelinating polyneuropathy (e.g., a Guillain-Barré–like syndrome), and a myopathy. The peripheral nervous system may sustain injury in HIV, manifesting as a peripheral neuropathy or radiculopathy. A progressive radiculopathy of predominantly the dorsal roots of the lumbar and sacral nerves may occur, involving severe myelin and axonal loss.

HIV-associated distal symmetric polyneuropathy, a sensory neuropathy occurring late in the disease, is the most commonly occurring neuropathy with slowly progressive numbness and paresthesias and burning sensations in the extremities and feet. Weakness and decreased or absent distal reflexes may be present.

The most common myopathy is polymyositis; it may be present initially or develop later. Inflammation leads to muscle cell degeneration and necrosis resulting in weakness of extremities with myalgia and fatigue.

Viral Meningitis and HIV. Some people develop an acute viral meningitis at approximately the time of seroconversion. This may well represent the initial infection of the nervous system by the HIV. Symptoms include headache, fever, and meningismus.

Opportunistic Infections and HIV. Opportunistic infections may be bacterial, fungal, protozoal, or viral in origin and produce nervous system disease. Typically bacterial infections are caused by unusual microorganisms. Cryptococcal infection is the most common fungal disorder and the third leading cause of neurologic disease with HIV. In *Cryptococcus neoformans,* small granulomas and cysts are found in the cerebral cortex and later may be present in deep cerebral tissues. The symptoms are vague, such as fever, headache, malaise, and meningismus. Herpes encephalitis and herpes varicella-zoster radiculitis may develop. Papovavirus (especially JC virus) in the immunocompromised person with HIV may produce a demyelinating disorder called *progressive multifocal leukoencephalopathy (PML).* This virus is found in 90% of healthy persons but is dormant. The virus reactivates to cause PML in 15% of persons with HIV. Sensory and motor deficits, aphasia, and apraxia are common clinical manifestations. The condition is progressive and there is no effective treatment.[130]

Cytomegalovirus Infection. Cytomegalovirus encephalitis is common with AIDS but often not diagnosed while a person is alive. The encephalitis may be present as an acute illness with encephalitis features accompanied by nystagmus and cranial nerve signs. Retinitis is found in 50% of those affected.

Parasitic Infection. Toxoplasmosis is the most common opportunistic infection and occurs in one third of persons with HIV. CNS toxoplasmosis typically manifests as focal encephalitis. *Toxoplasma gondii,* a protozoan, is thought to reactivate from latent lesions to produce a well-demarcated necrotizing process. Lesions may be multiple and exist throughout the cerebral hemispheres.

Clinical manifestations of CNS toxoplasmosis are focal but highly variable and include clumsiness to hemiplegia, aphasia, seizures, ataxia, cognitive changes, and constitutional symptoms. Fever and headache are common. Toxoplasmosis is difficult to diagnose but is treated effectively with pyrimethamine and sulfadiazine.

HIV-Associated Central Nervous System Neoplasms. HIV-associated CNS neoplasms have declined significantly with HAART, particularly primary CNS lymphoma. Other neoplasms associated with HIV include systemic non-Hodgkin lymphoma and metastatic Kaposi sarcoma. Metastasis of a Kaposi sarcoma to the CNS is uncommon.[131]

Lyme Disease

Lyme disease, a tick-borne spirochete bacterial infection, is a common arthropod-borne infection in the United States. It affects all age groups and involves the peripheral and central nervous systems. Transmission is most likely in the late summer or early fall in areas where there are deer, mice, and other animals that are primary reservoirs for infected ticks. Infected ticks are endemic in the Midwest, Western wooded and coastal areas, the mid- to northeast Atlantic, Europe, and eastern Asia. Lyme disease is caused by *Borrelia burgdorferi (B.b.)* introduced by tick bite, requiring about 36 to 72 hours of attachment and feeding. During feeding the microorganism is transferred from the gut of the tick to the salivary glands and then into the skin of the host. *B.b.* larvae evade immune surveillance by inhibiting complement killing, producing surface proteins that block phagocytic recognition (antigenic variation), and hiding in the extracellular matrix. *B.b.* incubates for 3 to 32 days and then migrates to the skin, lymph nodes, and other body systems. The pathologic process progresses through three stages[132]:

Stage I (acute localized): Within 1 month after the bite, the disease is characterized by a bull's-eye–like (5 cm in diameter) burning and centrifugally expanding erythema migrans rash followed by acute disseminated disease with general malaise, flulike symptoms (fever, muscle pain), stiff neck, and headache (seen in 50% to 90% of cases).

Stage II (systemic infection): Skin manifestations continue with or without acute widespread dissemination of antibodies and immune complexes and cardiac and neurologic involvement (within a week up to a month). About 10% of cases show cardiac signs and symptoms (palpitations, dizziness, shortness of breath, arrhythmias, and first-degree heart block). Neurologic signs occur in 10% to 15% of those affected and include headache, chronic aseptic (lymphocytic) meningitis, Bell palsy, encephalitis, and radiculitis. Pathologically, there is meningeal inflammation, perivascular inflammatory cell formation, and focal demyelination.

Stage III (chronic stage): The third stage may occur up to 2 years after the bite and involves arthritis and involvement of brain parenchyma with encephalitis, chronic neuropathy (paresthesias, radiculopathy), and encephalopathy (cognitive deficits, memory loss).

B.b. infection can be difficult to diagnoses. Treatment of choice is antibiotic therapy. Minor recurring symptoms are common in 50% of individuals. Some individuals experience post–Lyme disease syndrome after antibiotic treatment, with fatigue, musculoskeletal pain, and short-term memory difficulty.[133]

Demyelinating Disorders

Demyelinating disorders are the result of damage to the myelin nerve sheath. They can occur in either the central (e.g., multiple sclerosis) or the peripheral (e.g., Guillain-Barré syndrome, which also involves a polyneuropathy [see p. 622]) nervous system. Causes of the disorders include genetics, infections, autoimmune reactions, environmental toxins, and unknown factors. Multiple sclerosis is the most common and is presented in the next section.

Multiple Sclerosis

Multiple sclerosis (MS) is a chronic inflammatory disease involving degeneration of CNS myelin, scarring or formation of plaque, and loss of axons. MS is caused by an autoimmune response to self-antigens in genetically susceptible individuals. About 0.1% of the population is affected (400,000 persons in the United States and 2.1 million worldwide).[134] Prevalence rates vary with geographic location (higher in temperate regions far above the equator) and racial groups (highest in whites, although it occurs in all races).

The onset of MS is usually between 20 and 40 years of age with a peak of age 30. Male to female ratio is about 1:2. MS is the most prevalent CNS demyelinating disorder and a leading cause of neurologic disability in early adulthood. Life expectancy is not greatly altered by MS and the disease course often extends over 30 years. The etiology of MS is unknown. Genetic and environmental factors and interactions are implicated in disease onset. Although the disorder does not exhibit a defined inheritance pattern, 15% of those with MS have an affected relative. Multiple genes affect risk of development of MS. A genetic link exists in the human leukocyte antigen (HLA) complex, a large cluster of genes responsible for many immune functions. Several genetic polymorphisms are probably involved.[135] Vitamin D deficiency, cigarette smoking, and Epstein-Barr virus infection are environmental risk factors.[136]

The first demyelinating event, or "clinically isolated syndrome" (CIS), is a single episode of neurologic dysfunction lasting greater than 24 hours that can be a prelude to MS. Characteristic episodes include optic neuritis, solitary brainstem lesions, and transverse myelitis.[137]

PATHOPHYSIOLOGY. MS is a diffuse and progressive CNS disease that affects white and gray matter. Autoreactive T and B cells recognize myelin autoantigens and trigger inflammation in the CNS, leading to the loss of myelin sheaths and nerve conductivity and subsequently to the death of neurons (Figure 18-28). MS is described as occurring when a previous infectious insult to the nervous system has occurred in a genetically susceptible individual with a subsequent abnormal CNS immune response. Various mechanisms cause irreversible tissue damage (inflammation,

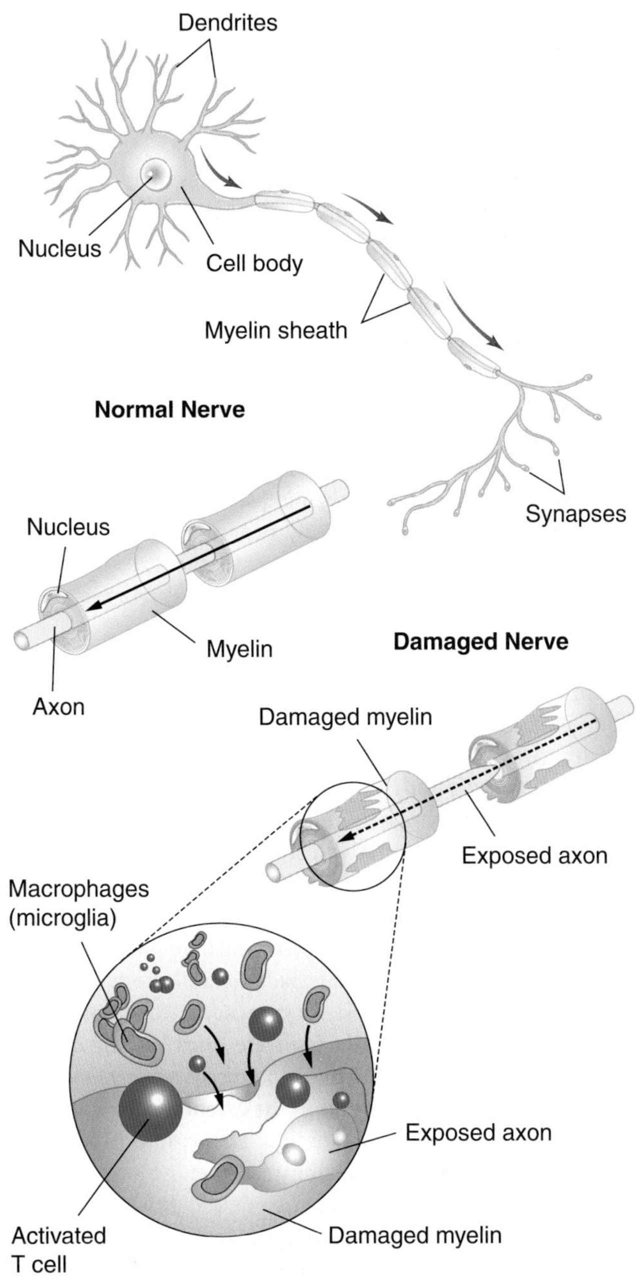

FIGURE 18-28 Pathogenesis of Multiple Sclerosis.

oligodendrocyte injury, demyelination, scarring or plaque formation, and axonal degeneration) that characterizes MS. These degenerative processes begin early in the course of the disease and continue to progress throughout a person's life. Demyelinated axons are more fragile and susceptible to further damage and, when degeneration exceeds self-repair ability (remyelination), permanent disability results. Myelin destruction and axonal damage begin before symptom onset (early inflammatory demyelination).

The innate and adaptive immune systems are activated in the pathology of MS. The immunopathology of MS involves[138] the following events:

1. Activation of CD4+ and CD8+ T cells; cells cross the blood-brain barrier and enter the CNS and attack myelin
2. Production of interleukin-12 (IL-12) and IL-23 (proinflammatory cytokines)
3. Lack of IL-10 (an anti-inflammatory cytokine)
4. Production of IL-17 (proinflammatory cytokine) by Th17 cells
5. Expression of integrins to facilitate adherence and passage of immune cells into the CNS
6. Promotion of chemokine migration of immune cells into the CNS that is up-regulated in MS
7. Contribution of B lymphocytes and plasma cells to the inflammatory response and direct damage to myelin and axons; B cells are more active in chronic or progressive forms of MS (B cells produce autoantibodies, secrete inflammatory cytokines, and activate T cells by presenting antigen)[139,140]
8. Activation of complement (promotes inflammation) during the acute phase; may be neuroprotective during relapse[141]
9. Presence of cells of inflammation including eosinophils, neutrophils, and macrophages

As the disease progresses, inflammatory changes in the CNS increase, and loss of brain volume progresses more rapidly.[142,143] The demyelination disrupts sodium, calcium, and potassium ion channels and calcium influx is proinflammatory and neurotoxic. Activated microglia and macrophages release nitric oxide and oxygen free radicals. Activated immune cells also produce glutamate, a neurotoxin.[144]

MS is characterized not only by focal inflammatory changes but also by diffuse injury throughout the CNS (MS lesions) (Figure 18-29). MS lesions may occur anywhere in white or gray matter. In addition, other neurodegenerative processes that involve the entire CNS are taking place, including: (1) changes in gray matter in the cortex, basal ganglia, brainstem, and spinal cord with substantial loss over time; (2) brain atrophy that begins early in the disease and is highly correlated with disability and progressive MS; and (3) direct dysfunction of or damage to oligodendrocytes that manufacture myelin.[145,146] Normal-appearing white matter also is highly abnormal microscopically with the presence of wallerian degeneration, diffuse inflammation, extensive microglial activation, neurotoxic substances, and gene activation that disrupt cellular processes.[145] Iron deposits in both gray and white matter have been found in MS, and the pathologic significance may be associated with mitochondrial and oxidative injury.[147] Research is in progress to determine if chronic cerebrospinal venous insufficiency is a pathogenic factor in MS.[148] In established disease the multifocal, multistaged feature of MS lesions gives rise to the aphorism that the lesions are "scattered in space and time." Symptoms therefore are multiple and variable among individuals with the disease.

CLINICAL MANIFESTATIONS. A variety of events (e.g., infection, trauma, or pregnancy) occurring immediately before the onset or exacerbation of symptoms are regarded as precipitating factors related to MS. Most of the pregnancy-related exacerbations

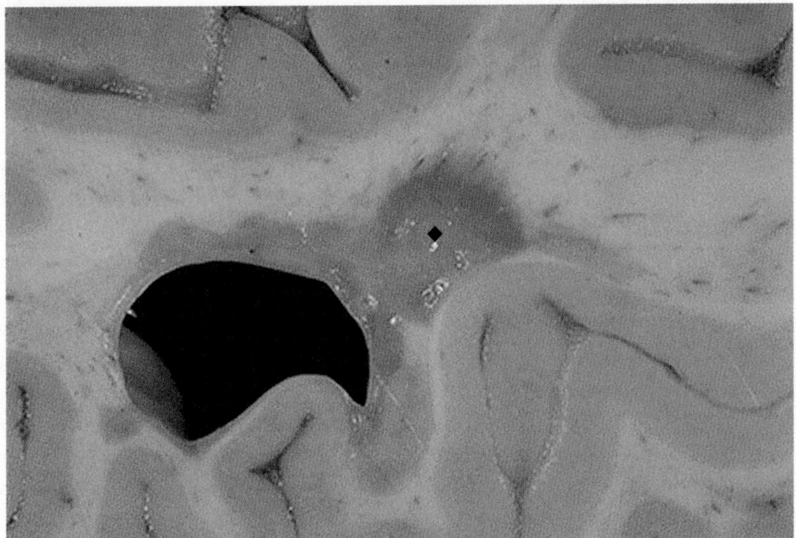

FIGURE 18-29 Multiple Sclerosis, Gross. Seen here in periventricular white matter is a large "plaque" (◆) of demyelination that has a sharp border with adjacent normal white matter. Such plaques have a gray-tan appearance and are typically associated with the clinical appearance of transient or progressive loss of neurologic function in multiple sclerosis (MS). Because MS is often multifocal, and the lesions appear in various white matter locations in the central nervous system over time, the clinical course and findings can be quite varied. (From Klatt EC: *Robbins and Cotran atlas of pathology,* Philadelphia, 2006, Saunders.)

BOX 18-3 ESTABLISHED SYNDROMES OF MULTIPLE SCLEROSIS

Mixed or Generalized Type (50% of Persons)
Optic signs—optic neuritis
- Brainstem signs—internuclear ophthalmoplegia, diplopia, vertigo (vomiting), nystagmus, dysarthria
- Cerebellar signs—see below

Spinal Type (30% to 40% of Persons)
Spastic ataxia
- Deep sensory changes in the extremities
- Bladder and bowel symptoms

Cerebellar or Pontobulbar-Cerebral Type (5% of Persons)
Motor ataxia
- Hypotonia
- Asthenia

Amaurotic Form (5% of Persons)
Blindness

occur 3 months postpartum, suggesting a relation to the stresses of labor and the increased fatigue during the postpartum period rather than to the pregnancy itself.[149] The major classifications of MS are relapsing-remitting, primary progressive, secondary progressive, and progressive-relapsing. Initially 90% of persons present with a relapsing, remitting course; 10% present with a primary progressive course; and 90% develop a progressive course in 10 to 20 years after onset of the disease. However, once walking problems develop, disease progression occurs quickly regardless of disease type. Usually persons with late MS have one of the established syndromes—mixed, spinal, or cerebellar (Box 18-3). The initial syndrome depends on the portion of the CNS that is most involved. After years of disease, 50% of individuals appear to have established syndromes of mixed involvement.

Optico-Spinal Multiple Sclerosis. **Optico-spinal multiple sclerosis (OSMS)** has the manifestations of optic nerve and spinal cord axonal loss. The condition usually evolves rapidly over hours to days and is highly suggestive of MS. Involvement may be unilateral or bilateral. Subjective symptoms are impaired central vision (blurring, fogginess, haziness) and impaired color perception. Signs are decreased central visual acuity; central or paracentral scotoma (area of diminished vision); acquired color vision deficit, especially to red and green; and defective pupillary reaction to light. A variety of field defects may occur. In the acute phase these symptoms may reflect optic papillitis (inflammation and swelling of the optic disc) or retrobulbar neuritis with a normal disc. Immune injury damages the optic nerve and inflammatory edema compresses the blood supply in the tight optic canal. One third of persons recover completely, and most others improve significantly.[150]

The brainstem lesions involve cranial nerves III through XII at the root, nuclear, or corticobulbar (upper motor neuron) level. Internuclear ophthalmoplegia, nystagmus, and dysarthria are the most common brainstem symptoms, followed by deafness, vertigo and vomiting, tinnitus, facial weakness, and facial sensory deficit. Internuclear ophthalmoplegia is lateral gaze paralysis caused by involvement of the medial longitudinal fasciculus, the brainstem pathway that coordinates eye movement. Diplopia and eyeball pain are common complaints. Bilateral internuclear ophthalmoplegia in a young adult is virtually diagnostic of MS.

Cognitive dysfunction has been demonstrated to occur early in the disease course. The person experiences decreased short-term memory, recent memory impairment, decreased concentration, word-finding problems, and planning difficulties. Mood alterations are common in MS. Depression is far more common than euphoria.

Neuromyelitis optica (NO; Devic disease) is a demyelinating disease that also selectively affects the optic nerve and spinal cord (usually grouped within three to four vertebrae). It was previously considered to be a severe variant of MS because of the similar pathologic features and its resemblance to optico-spinal MS that occurs in the Asian population. However, aquaporin-4 (AQP4) IgG autoantibodies play a pathogenic role in NO and it may be a distinct disorder or overlap with OSMS.[151]

Spinal Multiple Sclerosis. The spinal type of MS is the second most common type, chiefly involving the spinal tracts and dorsal column. Weakness, numbness, or both in one or more limbs are initial symptoms in 50% of cases of MS. Subjective corticospinal (upper motor neuron) symptoms (stiffness, slowness, weakness) are often unilateral and are a component of fatigability. Spinal signs are usually bilateral (symmetric), with lower limbs more often and more severely affected than upper limbs; spastic paraparesis is probably the most common single neurologic finding in MS.

Bladder and bowel symptoms occur with major spinal cord involvement. Urgency and hesitancy generally precede incontinence. Bladder dysfunction most often involves a small, spastic bladder, although occasionally a large, flaccid bladder may develop with retention problems. Neurogenic impotence often occurs when sphincter symptoms are present. Bowel incontinence is rare, but constipation is common with severe disease. Subjective dorsal column symptoms are symmetric paresthesias (tingling and numbness) in an unpredictable pattern but with a predilection for lower extremities over upper extremities. Dorsal column signs are vibration, position, and two-point discrimination deficits. Sensory complaints often are not substantiated by objective physical findings but by further diagnostic tests.

Cerebellar Multiple Sclerosis. Nystagmus and ataxia can present initially and reflect cerebellar and corticospinal involvement. Cerebellar deficits are usually symmetric, with all four limbs involved. With combined corticospinal and cerebellar involvement, the individual has a spastic ataxic gait and ataxia of the arms. Pure cerebellar symptoms are those of motor ataxia, hypotonia, and asthenia (weakness). Manifestations of motor ataxia are decomposition of movement, inability to perform rapid alternating movements (dysdiadochokinesia), and dysmetria. Charcot triad describes a combination of dysarthria, intention tremor, and nystagmus associated with cerebellar multiple sclerosis. Hypotonia is manifested by decreased resistance to passive movement, hypoactive deep tendon reflexes, and pendular knee jerk reflex.

TABLE 18-11 DIAGNOSTIC EVALUATION FOR MULTIPLE SCLEROSIS

	FINDINGS IN MULTIPLE SCLEROSIS
Clinical Signs and Symptoms	Signs and symptoms indicating disease of the brain or spinal cord not attributable to another diagnosis with two or more episodes lasting at least 24 hours and occurring at least 1 month apart
Tests	
Magnetic resonance imaging	
T2 weighted	Demyelinated plaques, both active and inactive
Gadolinium enhanced	Active demyelinating plaques
Cerebrospinal fluid analysis	Oligoclonal bands of immunoglobulin G Elevated immunoglobulin G index
Evoked potentials	Slowed nerve impulse conduction

Short-lived attacks of neurologic deficits are the temporary appearance or worsening of symptoms. The mechanism of these attacks is complete reversible conduction block in partially demyelinated axons. Conditions that cause short-lived attacks include: (1) minor increases in body temperature or serum Ca^{++} concentration and (2) functional demands exceeding conduction capacity. An increase in body temperature or serum Ca^{++} level increases current leakage through demyelinated neurons. Individuals with MS may become dramatically worse when body temperature is raised. Hypercalcemia induced by decreased serum pH may aggravate symptoms of MS. Physical and emotional stress imposes functional demands that may exceed conduction capacity of affected neurons.

Paroxysmal attacks are sensory or motor symptoms of abrupt onset and short duration (a few seconds or minutes). These symptoms include paresthesias, dysarthria and ataxia, and tonic head turning. The mechanism of paroxysmal attacks is nonsynaptic transmission in which nerve impulses are directly transmitted between adjacent demyelinated axons. These impulses arise focally and spuriously in the cervical portion of the spinal cord or in the brainstem. A common paroxysmal symptom, called *Lhermitte sign,* is the momentary paresthesia (shock-like or tingling sensation) that shoots down the trunk or limbs during active or passive flexion of the neck. Bending the neck evokes nonsynaptic impulses in demyelinated axons of the dorsal column in the spinal cord. A person with MS may have many paroxysmal attacks each day. Inciting events include sensory stimulation, voluntary movement, hyperventilation, and emotional stress. Paroxysmal attacks tend to persist for weeks or months and may be followed by progressive symptoms of MS.

EVALUATION AND TREATMENT. The diagnostic criteria for MS were revised in 2010 and are known as the McDonald criteria.[152] Clinical examination in combination with MRI, to demonstrate MS lesions in time and space, and CSF findings are used to make an early diagnosis (Table 18-11) so that treatment may begin sooner. Persistently elevated CSF immunoglobulin G (IgG) index is found in about two thirds of individuals with MS, and oligoclonal bands of IgG on electrophoresis are found in more than 90% of persons. Evoked response (ER) studies aid diagnosis by detecting decreased conduction velocity in visual, auditory, and somatosensory pathways. MRI is used to assist diagnosis and assess prognosis although there are limitations to detecting the full extent of the lesions.[153]

The treatment goal in MS is prevention of permanent neurologic damage. Acute relapses are treated with corticosteroids to speed recovery. Both oral and injectable disease-modifying drugs are used to decrease the number of relapses, promote remyelination and repair, prevent demyelination, suppress selective B-cell and T-cell function, and prevent disability.[154] Vitamin D supplementation may reduce the risk of MS and promote a more favorable progression.[155]

Symptom management for fatigue, weakness, vertigo, ataxia, tremor, heat intolerance, spasticity, bladder dysfunction, bowel dysfunction, sexual dysfunction, sensory sensations, pain, cognitive difficulties, depression, and psychosocial issues is essential. Many treatments are only partially effective, particularly for fatigue and spasticity. Supportive and rehabilitative management is directed toward preventing the complications of immobility, especially pressure sores and infections of the pulmonary and genitourinary systems. Interdisciplinary inpatient rehabilitation may improve function in the short term.[156]

PERIPHERAL NERVOUS SYSTEM AND NEUROMUSCULAR JUNCTION DISORDERS

Peripheral Nervous System Disorders

Neuropathies

The axons traveling to and from the brainstem and spinal cord neuronal cell bodies may be injured by a multitude of disease processes. Distinct anatomic areas of the axon may be injured or the spinal nerves may be affected at the spinal roots, at the plexus before peripheral nerve formation, or at the peripheral nerves themselves. Cranial nerves do not have roots or plexuses so are affected only within the nerves. Autonomic nerve fibers may be injured as they travel within certain cranial nerves or emerge through the ventral root and plexuses to travel in the peripheral nerves of the body.

Neuropathies can be classified as (1) generalized symmetric polyneuropathies, (2) generalized neuropathies, and (3) focal or multifocal neuropathies. **Generalized symmetric polyneuropathies** are characterized by symmetric involvement of sensory, motor, or autonomic fibers although, with clinical signs, one type of fiber may predominate. Generalized symmetric polyneuropathies further subdivide into **distal axonal polyneuropathy** and **demyelinating polyneuropathy.** Distal axonal polyneuropathy affects peripheral axons and is the generalized peripheral neuropathy commonly seen. The clinical feature of distal axonal polyneuropathy is involvement of the longest nerves of the body, those going to the feet, first. Sensory impairment is greater than motor impairment. Symptoms are burning pain, tingling, and numbness of the feet. Small nerve fiber damage produces decreased pain and temperature sensation, as well as burning, numbness, and tingling. Large nerve fiber injury causes decreased light touch, vibration, and position sense.

The two most common causes are diabetes mellitus and alcohol abuse; occasionally, neurotoxic therapeutic agents also are the cause. Within the classification of distal axonal neuropathies is another group of neuropathies called *autonomic neuropathy*. This neuropathy can involve virtually any sympathetic or parasympathetic nerve fiber with impairment of cardiovascular, gastrointestinal, urogenital, thermoregulatory, sudomotor, and pupillomotor autonomic function. Autonomic neuropathies have a progressive course and are usually reversible. The myelin or Schwann cells are affected in demyelinating polyneuropathy, which occurs far less frequently. Weakness is the predominant sign with far less sensory impairment. Acute and chronic inflammatory demyelinating neuropathies comprise this group, of which Guillain-Barré syndrome is the most widely recognized disorder (see below).

Generalized neuropathies affect the cell body of only one type of peripheral neuron. The dorsal root ganglion cell is affected in sensory neuropathies, producing numbness that may begin in a focal or asymmetric distribution or in a distal symmetric pattern. **Sensory neuropathies** are seen in leprosy, some industrial solvent poisonings, some hereditary disorders, and chloramphenicol toxicity. **Motor neuropathies** are caused by anterior horn cell disease, such as amyotrophic lateral sclerosis or paralytic poliomyelitis. There is weakness or paralysis that may be symmetric or asymmetric.

Focal neuropathy or **multifocal neuropathies** affect sensory and motor fibers in one or more nerves, as is seen in common compression neuropathies such as carpal tunnel syndrome (median nerve compression), ulnar nerve compression (at the elbow), peroneal nerve compression, or sciatic nerve compression. Focal neuropathies can involve one or more cranial nerves. Plexus injuries and radiculopathies also fall into this category.

PATHOPHYSIOLOGY. Although distinct pathophysiologic processes are recognized in a neuropathy, these are not disease specific and may exist simultaneously in any one neuropathy. Wallerian degeneration, in which the axon and myelin distal to the site of axonal interruption degenerate, may be present (see Chapter 15). This type of degeneration is characteristic of a traumatic nerve injury in which the nerve is severed. In demyelinating neuropathies the axon may be spared and only the myelin degenerates. In axonal degeneration distal degeneration of the axon occurs first and is followed by degeneration of the myelin and the axis cylinder. Many pathologic processes may give rise to neuropathy, and one or more nerves may be involved.

CLINICAL MANIFESTATIONS. When the axons are affected, muscle strength, muscle tone, and muscle bulk also are affected. Whole muscles or groups of muscles are paretic or paralyzed, and the muscles of the feet and legs often are affected first and more severely. These long, large axons are thought to (1) be more vulnerable to injury because of their size and length, (2) have more Schwann cells available to be injured, and (3) exhibit a "dying back" phenomenon caused by difficulty of the nerve cell body in maintaining the terminal portion of the axon. If unchecked, the pathologic process tends to involve the hands and arms because these have the next longest and largest axons.

Tone and the deep tendon reflexes in the affected muscles generally are decreased in a neuropathy. Atrophy is distributed according to the peripheral nerves involved. The degree and distribution of the atrophy probably depend on the extent of the injury. Fasciculation may be present, especially with associated ventral root or motor neuron changes, or both, as in Guillain-Barré syndrome, diabetic neuropathy, and porphyric neuropathy. Mild fatigue may be experienced. A few disorders, notably Guillain-Barré syndrome, produce a pattern of paresis and paralysis that involves all limbs, the trunk, and the neck. Peripheral bifacial and other cranial nerve palsies may be seen with a variety of disorders. Tenderness of the nerve trunks and associated sensory alterations help to distinguish neuropathy from amyotrophy. These include paresthesias and dysesthesias as well as decreased or absent primary sensations (e.g., of temperature, touch, light pain, position, or vibration). Ataxia of gait or limb may arise from the loss of position and vibratory sensations (i.e., proprioceptive sensory loss) and may be enhanced by motor weakness.

Reflexes may be altered. Reflex-mediated autonomic nervous system functions, such as sweating and pupillary size, may be affected. Neuropathies associated with autonomic disturbances include diabetes mellitus, alcoholism and related nutritional neuropathies, amyloidosis, porphyria, Guillain-Barré syndrome, Riley-Day syndrome, and familial sensory neuropathy. In many chronic polyneuropathies, the feet, hands, and spine become deformed. Metabolic changes may arise secondary to nerve dysfunction.

EVALUATION AND TREATMENT. The diagnostic workup to determine the cause of a neuropathy is often extensive. Early diagnosis and treatment before irreversible neuronal cell damage ensues are of paramount importance. Although axonal regrowth and recovery of function may take months, many neuropathies can be reversed. The therapeutic management is directed first at elimination of the cause, if possible. At least the primary disorder, such as diabetes mellitus, should be controlled. Further damage to the axon must be prevented by avoiding (1) trauma from premature demand for reuse of the nerve, (2) accidents that cause tissue damage, and (3) hypoxia and ischemia or other deprivation of essential substrates.

Guillain-Barré Syndrome. **Guillain-Barré syndrome (GBS) (Landry-Guillain-Barré syndrome, idiopathic polyneuritis, acute inflammatory demyelinating polyradiculopathy, acute autoimmune neuropathy)** is an acquired acute inflammatory demyelinating or axonal polyneuropathy with four subtypes. The subtypes and their clinical features are presented in Table 18-12. These subtypes occur throughout the world, affect children and adults of both genders and all age groups equally, and occur in all seasons of the year. The annual incidence rate is 1 to 2 per 100,000 with a 4% to 6% mortality, and a 5% to 10% morbidity rate (permanent disabling weakness, imbalance, or sensory loss).[157]

PATHOPHYSIOLOGY. GBS is considered to be an autoimmune disease triggered by a preceding bacterial or viral infection. Molecular mimicry (cross-activation of self-epitopes and pathogen-derived peptides by autoreactive T and B cells) is associated with the immune injury.[158] It has been recognized that glycolipids, particularly gangliosides, are immune targets in the subtypes of GBS. Different gangliosides predominate in different locations in peripheral nerves and in different nerve fiber types. Table 18-12 presents the pathology and pathogenesis of the four axonal subtypes of GBS. The muscle innervated by the damaged peripheral nerves undergoes denervation and atrophy. If the cell body survives, regeneration of the peripheral nerve takes place and recovery of function is likely. If the cell body dies from intense root involvement in the inflammatory-degenerative process, no regeneration is possible. Collateral reinnervation from surviving axons and regenerating axons may take place. In this case, motor recovery is less complete and residual deficits persist.

CLINICAL MANIFESTATIONS. Clinical manifestations may vary depending on subtype. Typical first manifestations are numbness, pain, paresthesias, or weakness in the limbs. Motor signs manifest as an acute or subacute progressive paralysis. Proximal muscles may be involved earlier and more significantly than distal muscles. The paresis/paralysis may be present in an ascending pattern involving limbs, respiratory muscles, and bulbar muscles. Only bulbar muscles may be involved, resulting in dysphagia and dysarthria. Weakness usually plateaus or improves by the fourth week in 90% of cases. After weakness plateaus, strength improves over a period of days to months, with the majority of individuals reaching activity levels similar to their predisease state. If sensory symptoms are present in the subtype they may include paresthesias/dysthesias (tingling, burning, shocklike sensations, particularly in the limbs), pain (throbbing and aching, particularly in the lower back, buttocks, and legs), and numbness. Position and vibratory sensations are more affected than superficial sensation. Respiratory muscle weakness leads to the need for ventilatory support in 10% to 30% of individuals. Cranial nerve weakness manifests as facial weakness and bulbar weakness involving chewing, swallowing, and coughing. Autonomic dysfunction may manifest as tachycardia or, less frequently, bradycardia; hypotension or

TABLE 18-12 EXPANDED CLASSIFICATION OF GUILLAIN-BARRÉ SYNDROME (GBS)

SUBTYPES	CLINICAL FEATURES	PATHOLOGY	PATHOGENESIS
Acute inflammatory demyelinating polyneuropathy (AIDP accounts for most cases of GBS)	Ascending paralysis with typically distant start	Macrophages invade myelin sheaths and denude axons Lymphocytic inflammation Demyelination	T-cell–mediated lymphocytic infiltration into nerves is common
	Early sensory symptoms Loss of DTRs	Endoneurial edema Some degree of axon loss (all findings most prominent in the spinal roots and nerve terminals) CD4 and CD8 lymphocytes and macrophages are present Complement is deposited on the outermost Schwann cell plasmalemma	Antibody-mediated pathogenesis not yet demonstrated
Acute motor axonal neuropathy (AMAN)	Acute progressive weakness with no sensory impairment	Macrophages invade nodes of Ranvier, leaving the myelin sheath intact (absence of demyelination) Axonal degeneration in ventral root in severe cases	Selective antibody-mediated attack on axon (presence of IgG and complement deposits on axolemma along with macrophage recruitment) Associated with *Campylobacter jejuni* enteritis
		Lymphocyte infiltration sparse	GM1 autoantibodies play a direct pathogenic role through molecular mimicry
Acute motor and sensory axonal neuropathy (AMSAN)	Ascending paralysis Early sensory symptoms	Similar to AMAN Absence of demyelination Evidence of axonal loss in dorsal and ventral roots Lymphocytic infiltration sparse Extensive sensory nerve fiber degeneration	Undetermined
Fisher syndrome (FS) (5% of cases of GBS)	In purist form have ophthalmoparesis, areflexia, and ataxia	Pathologic features similar to those in AIDP, but are atypical FS	Antibodies to ganglioside GQ1b measured in serum in 90% of cases
	In atypical FS also have features of AIDP	Deposition of antiganglioside antibodies initially causes reversible conduction block followed by axonal degeneration	Anti-GQ1b antibodies cross-react with other gangliosides (typically GT1a, but in many cases with GD3, GD1b, and GT1b)
	Infections are common triggers for FS (*Campylobacter jejuni* enteritis)		

Data from Hardy TA et al: *Curr Allergy Asthma Rep* 11(3):197–204, 2011; Shahrizaila N, Yuki N: *Exp Rev Neurother* 11(9):1305–1313, 2011.

hypertension; and loss of or significant increase in sweating in those more severely affected. Persons may undergo a respiratory arrest or cardiovascular collapse, a cause of death. Hyponatremia caused by the syndrome of inappropriate antidiuretic hormone (SIADH) is common, especially in individuals whose lungs have been ventilated.

EVALUATION AND TREATMENT. Clinical history helps diagnose GBS and its subtypes. The major diagnostic tests are the examination of the CSF, nerve conduction studies, and EMG. The CSF findings include an unusually high protein level (500 mg/dl) without cellular abnormality. Nerve conduction studies help identify the subtype. Ventilatory support and management of the autonomic nervous system dysfunction are two dominant aspects of the therapeutic management. Intravenous immunoglobulin, plasmapheresis, or plasma exchanges or combination therapy within the first 2 weeks of onset of clinical manifestations may be indicated. After the disorder begins to remit, aggressive rehabilitation should be instituted.[159]

Radiculopathies. **Radiculopathies** are disorders of spinal nerve roots. As the spinal roots emerge from or enter the vertebral canal, they may be injured or damaged by compression, infection, inflammation, ischemia, or direct trauma whereby the roots are stretched or torn. **Radiculitis (radiculoneuritis)** refers to an inflammatory disorder of the spinal nerve roots. One or more roots may be affected.

PATHOPHYSIOLOGY. Many different pathologic conditions may cause tearing, compression, or inflammation of nerve roots.[160] Roots may be traumatized by a forceful tearing of a nerve, termed *avulsion,* often associated with injuries to the head and shoulders. An acute intervertebral disk prolapse (herniated disk), degenerative spondyloarthropathies, or a benign tumor may compress nerve roots. Metastatic tumors of the lung, breast, and gastrointestinal tract may produce a carcinomatous meningitis, causing compression and inflammatory changes in nerve roots. Other causes of inflammatory changes in nerve roots are chronic meningitis, neurosyphilis, sarcoidosis, and inflammatory arachnoiditis produced by myelography and lumbar punctures.

CLINICAL MANIFESTATIONS. The strength, tone, and bulk of the muscles innervated by the involved roots are affected. The pattern and distribution of weakness and atrophy are similar to those of the amyotrophies. Tone and deep tendon reflexes are decreased, but rarely absent, because the involved muscles are usually innervated by two or more spinal roots. Fasciculations often are present, and mild fatigue may be experienced. Because pathologic processes usually affect the ventral as well as the dorsal roots, sensory alterations are common.

Diseases that involve spinal roots typically produce local pain; pain on local percussion; pain and paresthesias in the sensory root distribution (called **radicular pain** and **radicular paresthesia**); increased pain with movement, stretching of the root, and maneuvers that transiently increase CSF pressure; sensory loss in a radicular pattern; and spasms of the muscles surrounding the vertebral column (i.e., paravertebral muscle spasms).

EVALUATION AND TREATMENT. Diagnostic measures may include physical examination, spinal films, nerve conduction studies, EMG, lumbar puncture with CSF examination, myelography, and biopsy of tumor masses.[161]

Treatment is directed at the cause of the injury and may take the form of surgical intervention, antibiotic administration, removal of the injurious agent, corticosteroid use, and radiation therapy and chemotherapy. Supportive management may include control of the discomfort, protection from further injury, prevention of complications, and rehabilitation when appropriate.

Plexus Injuries. **Plexus injuries** involve the nerve plexus distal to the spinal roots but proximal to the formation of the peripheral nerves. Such injuries may be caused by trauma, compression (entrapment), or infiltration, or they may be iatrogenic, caused by positioning during surgery or by an intramuscular injection. Clinical manifestations include motor weakness, muscle atrophy, and sensory loss in affected areas. Paralysis can occur with complete plexus lesions.[162]

The diagnosis is made on the basis of history and clinical manifestations. Therapeutic treatment is directed at removal of the cause, repair and approximation of nervous tissue, prevention of further injury, control of discomfort, prevention of complications, and rehabilitation when appropriate. Acetyl-L-carnitine (ALCAR) or *N*-acetylcysteine (NAC) can provide neuroprotection.[163]

Neuromuscular Junction Disorders

Transmission of the nerve impulse at the neuromuscular junction requires the release of adequate amounts of neurotransmitter from the presynaptic terminals of the axon and effective binding of the released transmitter to the receptors on the membranes of muscle cells (see Figure 15-14). Four neuromuscular junction disorders (NMJDs), whose pathogenesis is thought to be autoantibodies, are described: myasthenia gravis, muscle-specific kinase (MuSK) protein antibody–associated myasthenia gravis, Lambert-Eaton myasthenic syndrome, and acquired neuromyotonia. In addition, there are rare **inherited (congenital) myasthenic syndromes** that result from mutations in different key proteins for the acetylcholine receptor, ion channels, and motor end plates at the neuromuscular junction.[164] Nutritional deficits; certain drugs (e.g., reserpine or methyldopa [Aldomet]); certain toxins (e.g., botulism); some snake, scorpion, or spider venoms; certain plant extracts; and some insecticides also affect the neuromuscular junction. The most common autoimmune neuromuscular junction disorder (NMJD) is myasthenia gravis caused by the binding of autoantibodies to the acetylcholine receptor on the postsynaptic membrane. MuSK antibody–associated myasthenia gravis is also postsynaptic and is a severe form of the disease.[165] Presynaptic autoimmune diseases include **neurotonia** with autoantibodies to the potassium channels and the rare **Lambert-Eaton myasthenic syndrome** with autoantibodies to calcium channels on presynaptic nerve terminals, which presents with muscle weakness and is commonly associated with small-cell lung carcinoma.[166]

Myasthenia Gravis

Myasthenia gravis is a chronic autoimmune disease mediated by acetylcholine receptor (AchR) antibodies that act at the neuromuscular junction (Figure 18-30 and Table 18-13). About 20,000 to 70,000 people in the United States have the disease.

Myasthenia gravis is associated with an increased incidence of other autoimmune diseases, including systemic lupus erythematosus, rheumatoid arthritis, polymyositis, and thyrotoxicosis. (Autoimmune mechanisms are discussed in Chapter 9.) The etiology of myasthenia gravis is unknown. Some persons have genetic susceptibility related to variants in AchR genes, as well as the major histocompatibility genes, and they can present with varying clinical phenotypes.[167]

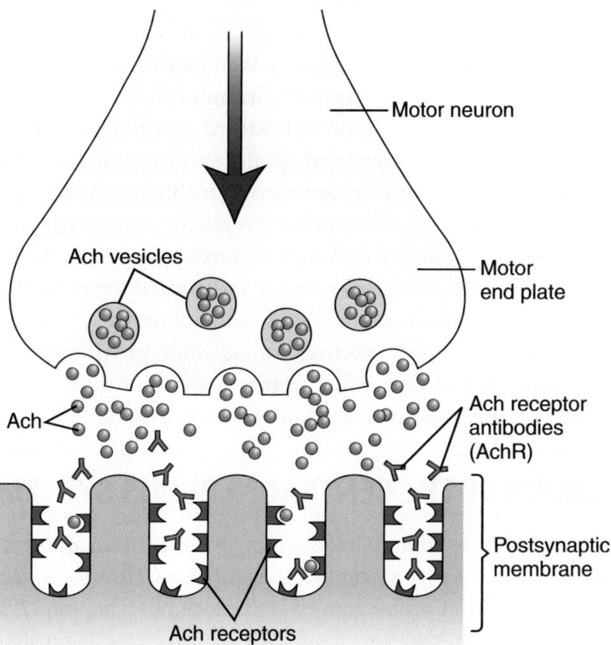

FIGURE 18-30 Antibodies and Myasthenia Gravis. Acetylcholine receptor antibodies block the acetylcholine receptor and inhibit the stimulating effect of acetylcholine on the postsynaptic membrane. *AchR,* Acetylcholine receptor. (Data from Juel VC, Massey JM: *Orphanet J Rare Dis* 2:44, 2007; Mahadeva B, Phillips LH 2nd, Juel VC: *Semin Neurol* 28[2]:212–227, 2008; Shigemoto K: *Acta Mycol* 26[3]:185–191, 2007.)

The subtypes of autoimmune myasthenia gravis are generalized AchR, ocular, and neonatal. Generalized AchR myasthenia gravis is further subdivided based on age and thymic pathology into the following categories:

1. Young persons, mostly female, with thymic hyperplasia
2. Older adults, both genders, with normal or involuted thymus glands
3. Persons of both genders with thymomas

Generalized AchR myasthenia involves the proximal musculature throughout the body and has several courses: (1) a course with periodic remissions, (2) a slowly progressive course, (3) a rapidly progressive course, or (4) a fulminating course. Classification by disease severity is as follows:

Grade I: ocular disease
Grade II: generalized mild weakness
Grade IIa: mild weakness
Grade IIb: moderate weakness
Grade III: severe generalized weakness
Grade IV: myasthenic "crisis" with respiratory failure[168]

About 10% to 15% of those with signs and symptoms of myasthenia gravis often involving severe swallowing and breathing (bulbar) problems do not have AchR antibodies on testing. Some of these have MuSK antibodies (an IgG4). This is now subtyped as MuSK antibody–associated myasthenia gravis.

In **neonatal myasthenia,** transitory signs of myasthenia gravis are present in 10% to 15% of infants born to mothers with myasthenia gravis. The signs appear 1 to 3 days after birth and persist for a few days to a few weeks. Myasthenia immunoglobulin is transferred from the mother to the neonate through the placenta. **Ocular myasthenia,** which is more common in males, involves weakness of the eye muscles and eyelids and may include swallowing difficulties and slurred speech as well.

PATHOPHYSIOLOGY. Myasthenia gravis results from a defect in nerve impulse transmission at the neuromuscular junction. The main defect is T-cell–dependent formation of autoantibodies (an IgG antibody) against receptors at the Ach-binding site on the postsynaptic membrane. The autoantibodies block the AchR or cause complement-mediated loss of AchRs from

TABLE 18-13 ANTIBODIES AND MECHANISMS OF ACTION AT NEUROMUSCULAR JUNCTION

FEATURES	MYASTHENIA GRAVIS (MG)	MUSCLE-SPECIFIC KINASE MG	LAMBERT-EATON MYASTHENIC SYNDROME	NEUROMYOTONIA
Target	AchR	MuSK	α1A VGCC	VGKC
Principal subclass of antibody	IgG1, IgG3 (autoantibodies against AchR)	IgG4 (autoantibody against MuSK)	Autoantibodies not known (possibly IgG4)	IgG4 (autoantibody against voltage-gated K^+ channels)
Principal mechanisms of action at NMJ	Complement-mediated destruction of folds (includes loss of AchR and sodium channels), increased turnover, direct block of function	Not clear yet; complement not activated; may involve mutations in end-plate protein Dok-7	Increased turnover	Increased turnover
Compensatory mechanisms identified	Increased presynaptic Ach release, increased postsynaptic AchR synthesis	Not clear yet	Involvement of other VGCCs in release process	Probable up-regulation of other VGKCs

Data from Farrugia ME, Vincent A: *Curr Opin Neurol* 23(5):489–495, 2010; Pal J et al: *J Neuroimmunol* 231(1-2):43–54, 2011.
AchR, Acetylcholine receptor; *Ig,* immunoglobulin; *MuSK,* muscle-specific kinase; *NMJ,* neuromuscular junction; *VGCC,* voltage-gated calcium channel; *VGKC,* voltage-gated potassium channel.

the neuromuscular junction (see Figure 18-30).[169] The cause of this autosensitization is unknown. Destruction of receptor sites occurs, decreasing the number of receptors on the plasma membrane and causing diminished transmission of nerve impulses across the neuromuscular junction. Muscle depolarization is incomplete or unsuccessful.

CLINICAL MANIFESTATIONS. Myasthenia gravis typically has an insidious onset. Clinical manifestations may first appear during pregnancy, during the postpartum period, or in conjunction with the administration of certain anesthetic agents. Hallmark symptoms are exertional fatigue and weakness that worsens with activity, improves with rest, and recurs with resumption of activity. The individual often complains of fatigue after exercise and has a recent history of recurring upper respiratory tract infections. The muscles of the eyes, face, mouth, throat, and neck usually are affected first. The extraocular (eye) muscles and the levator muscles are most affected. Manifestations include diplopia, ptosis, and ocular palsies.

The muscles of facial expression, mastication, swallowing, and speech are the next most involved. The results are facial droop and an expressionless face; difficulty chewing and swallowing associated with dietary changes and weight loss; drooling; episodes of choking and aspiration; and a nasal, low-volume but high-pitched monotonous speech pattern.

The muscles of the neck, shoulder girdle, and hip flexors are affected less frequently. When these muscles do become involved, however, the person experiences fatigue requiring periods of rest, weakness of the arms and legs that improves with rest, and difficulty in maintaining head position. The respiratory muscles of the diaphragm and chest wall become weak, and ventilation is impaired. Impairment in deep breathing and coughing predisposes the individual to atelectasis and congestion. In the advanced stage of the disease, all the muscles are weak.

Myasthenic crisis occurs when severe muscle weakness causes extreme quadriparesis or quadriplegia, respiratory insufficiency with shortness of breath and a markedly decreased tidal volume and vital capacity, and extreme difficulty in swallowing. The individual in myasthenic crisis is in danger of respiratory arrest. Myasthenic crisis usually occurs 3 to 4 hours after the person takes medication.

Cholinergic crisis may develop secondary to drug overdose (anticholinesterase drug toxicity). The clinical picture resembles that of myasthenic crisis but the weakness occurs 30 to 60 minutes after taking anticholinergic medication. Other symptoms are also present. Intestinal motility increases and is associated with episodes of diarrhea and complaints of cramping; fasciculation, bradycardia, pupillary constriction, increased salivation, and increased sweating are present. These clinical manifestations are caused by the smooth muscle hyperactivity secondary to excessive accumulation of acetylcholine at the neuromuscular junctions and excessive parasympathetic-like activity. As in myasthenic crisis, the individual is in danger of respiratory arrest.

EVALUATION AND TREATMENT. The diagnosis of myasthenia gravis is made on the basis of a response to edrophonium chloride (Tensilon), results of repetitive single-fiber EMG, and detection of AchR and MuSK antibodies. The antibodies are found in 80% of generalized autoimmune myasthenia and 70% of individuals with ocular myasthenia. With intravenous administration of Tensilon, immediate improvement in muscle strength usually persists for 5 to 10 minutes. The EMG is diagnostic in that the muscle fiber weakens readily. Mediastinal CT and MRI are used to determine whether a thymoma is present. The progression of myasthenia gravis is highly variable. In some individuals it is mild and spontaneously remits. There is usually a series of relapses, with symptom-free intervals ranging from weeks to months. Over time the disease can progress, leading to death; however, current treatments have improved prognosis, including ocular myasthenia.

Treatment of myasthenia gravis is individualized. Anticholinesterase drugs, corticosteroids, immunosuppressant drugs (e.g., Rituximab, a chimeric monoclonal antibody against the protein CD20, primarily found on the surface of B cells), azathioprine, and cyclosporine are used to treat myasthenia gravis and myasthenic crisis. Plasmapheresis may be lifesaving during myasthenic crisis, before and after thymectomy, and at the start of immunosuppressant therapy. For individuals with cholinergic crisis, treatment is to withhold anticholinergic drugs until blood levels fall out of the toxic range while providing ventilatory support and preventing respiratory complications. Thymectomy is the treatment of choice for a thymoma.[170]

TUMORS OF THE CENTRAL NERVOUS SYSTEM

Central nervous system (CNS) tumors include brain and spinal cord tumors. No proven causative agents for CNS tumors have been established. Carcinogenesis is discussed in Chapter 12.

Cranial Tumors

Tumors within the cranium can be either primary or metastatic as follows:

- *Primary:* Intracerebral tumors originate from brain substance, including neuroglia, neurons, cells of blood vessels, and connective tissue (Table 18-14). Extracerebral tumors originate outside substances of the brain and include meningiomas, acoustic nerve tumors, and tumors of pituitary and pineal glands.
- *Metastatic (secondary):* These tumors arise in organ systems outside the brain and spread to the brain.

Sites of intracranial tumors are illustrated in Figure 18-31.

Primary brain tumors (both malignant and nonmalignant) had an estimated incidence rate of 23,130 with 14,080 deaths in the United States in 2013.[171] The incidence of CNS tumors increases to age 70 years and then decreases. CNS tumors are the second most common group of tumors occurring in children. Approximately 70% of all intracranial tumors in children are located infratentorially (see Chapter 20), and in adults 70% to 75% are located supratentorially. Peripheral nerve tumors are rare in children and common in adults.

Cranial tumors cause local and generalized clinical manifestations. The local effects are caused by the destructive action of the tumor itself on a particular site in the brain and compression causing decreased cerebral blood flow. The effects are

TABLE 18-14 BRAIN AND SPINAL CORD TUMORS

NEOPLASM	LOCATION	CHARACTERISTICS	CELL OF ORIGIN
Gliomas			
Pilocytic astrocytoma	Anywhere in brain or spinal cord	Slow growing, well circumscribed	Astrocytes
Diffuse astrocytoma	Anywhere in brain	Slow growing; marked cellular differentiation; infiltrative; undergoing malignant progression over time	Astrocytes
Oligodendroglioma	Most commonly in frontal lobes deep in white matter; may arise in brainstem, cerebellum, and spinal cord	Well differentiated; diffusely infiltrative; well-demarcated borders	Oligodendrocytes
Oligoastrocytoma	Same as with diffuse astrocytoma and oligodendroglioma	Most common mixed glioma	At least two distinct populations of neoplastic cell types—astrocytes and oligodendrocytes
Anaplastic astrocytoma	Anywhere in brain or spinal cord, but predominantly in cerebral hemispheres	Anaplastic features demonstrated	Astrocytes
Anaplastic oligoastrocytoma	Same as with anaplastic astrocytoma	Same as anaplastic astrocytoma or anaplastic oligodendroglioma	Astrocytes and oligodendrocytes
Glioblastoma multiforme	Predominantly in cerebral hemispheres	Poorly differentiated neoplastic cells; extensive cellular heterogeneity; well-developed microvascular proliferation; necrosis	Astrocytes
Ependymoma	Intramedullary: wall of ventricles, may arise in caudal tail of spinal cord	More common in children, variable growth rates; more malignant, invasive form is called *ependymoblastoma;* may extend into ventricle or invade brain tissue	Ependymal cells
Neuronal Cell			
Medulloblastoma	Posterior cerebellar vermis, roof of fourth ventricle	Well demarcated, rapid growing, fills fourth ventricle	Embryonic cells
Mesodermal Tissue			
Meningioma	Intradural, extramedullary: sylvian fissure region, superior parasagittal surface of frontal and parietal lobes, olfactory groove, wing of sphenoid bone, superior surface of cerebellum, cerebellopontine angle, spinal cord	Slow growing, circumscribed, encapsulated, sharply demarcated from normal tissues, compressive in nature	Arachnoid cells, may be from fibroblast
Choroid Plexus			
Papillomas	Choroid plexus of ventricular system, lateral ventricle in children, fourth ventricle in adults	Usually benign, slow expansion inducing hemorrhage and hydrocephalus; malignant tumor is rare	Epithelial cells
Cranial Nerves and Spinal Nerve Roots			
Schwannoma (neuroma, neurolemma)	Cranial nerves (most commonly vestibular division of cranial nerve VIII)	Slow growing	Sheath of Schwann cells
Neurofibroma (NF1 and NF2)	NF1 primarily PNS, occasionally CNS NF2 primarily CNS	Both types slow growing	Nerve sheath
Pituitary Tumors	Pituitary gland; may extend to or invade floor of third ventricle	Age linked, several types, slow growing, macroadenomas and microadenomas	Pituitary cells, pituitary chromophobes, basophils, eosinophils
Germ Cell Tumors	Neurohypophysis, hypothalamus, pineal region	Rare, 0.5% of all primary brain tumors; primarily in adolescents; male more common than female; variable prognosis	Several types: germinoma, embryonal carcinoma, yolk sac tumor, choriocarcinoma, teratoma, mixed germ cell tumor, with different cell origins
Blood Vessel Tumors			
Angioma	Predominantly in posterior cerebral hemispheres	Slow growing	Arising from congenitally malformed arteriovenous connections
Hemangioblastomas	Predominantly in cerebellum	Slow growing	Embryonic vascular tissue

CNS, Central nervous system; *PNS,* Peripheral nervous system.

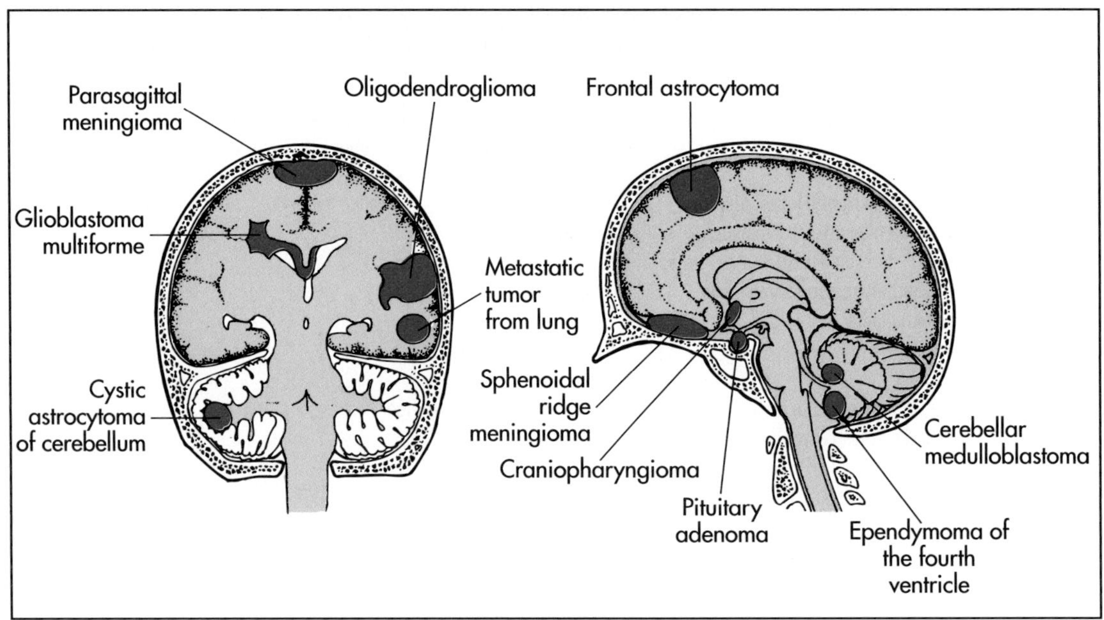

FIGURE 18-31 Common Sites of Intracranial Tumors.

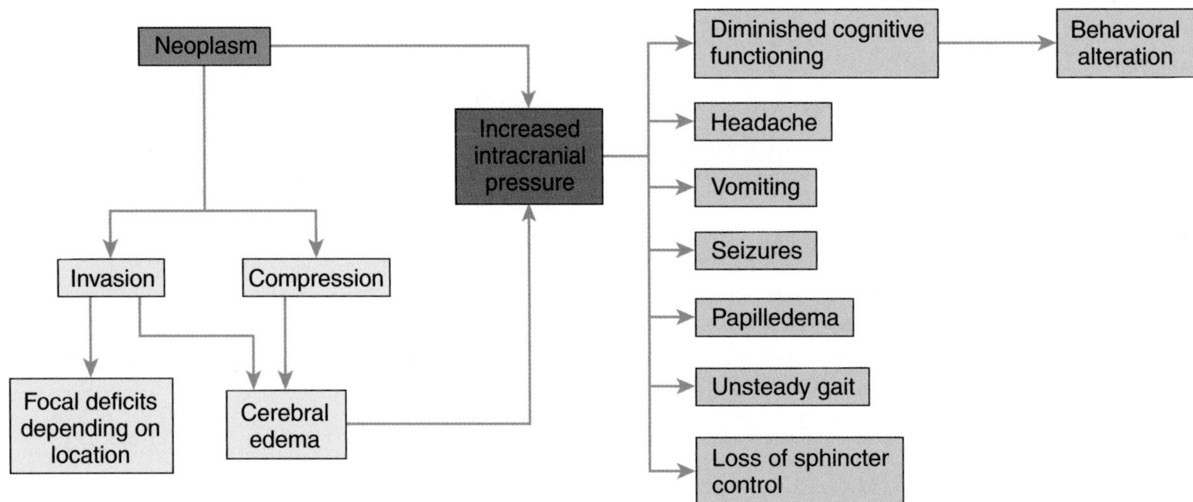

FIGURE 18-32 Origin of Clinical Manifestations Associated with an Intracranial Neoplasm.

varied and include seizures, visual disturbances, unstable gait, and cranial nerve dysfunction. The generalized effects result from increased ICP (Figure 18-32). Increased ICP may occur because of obstruction of the ventricular system, hemorrhages occurring in and around the tumor, cerebral edema caused by tumors or expansion of the tumor mass.

Intracranial brain tumors do not metastasize as readily as tumors in other organs because there are no lymphatic channels within the brain substance. If metastasis does occur, it is usually through seeding of cerebral blood, through CSF, during cranial surgery, or through artificial shunts.

Primary Brain (Intracerebral) Tumors

Primary brain tumors constitute about 2% of all cancers in the United States. **Gliomas** comprise 50% to 60% of all adult primary brain tumors and include astrocytomas, oligodendrogliomas, mixed oligoastrocytomas, and glioblastoma multiforme. Gliomas are divided into four grades based on histopathologic features, cellular density, atypia, mitotic activity, microvascular proliferation, and necrosis (Table 18-15). Other CNS tumors include meningiomas, ependymomas, nerve sheath tumors (schwannomas), and neurofibromas.

Pilocytic astrocytomas are more common in children and most often present with a median age of 12 years.[172] All other gliomas generally present after age 30 with secondary glioblastomas occurring more frequently in younger adults and primary glioblastomas usually presenting in older adults.[173]

Etiology for primary brain tumors is unclear and ionizing radiation is the only known environmental risk factor. Exposure to radiofrequency electromagnetic fields (cell phones) is under investigation.[174]

Mutation of the isocitrate dehydrogenase 1 *(IDH1)* gene, or less commonly mutation of the related *IDH2* gene, has been identified in the vast majority of World Health Organization

TABLE 18-15 CLASSIFICATION OF GLIOMAS

GRADE*	TYPE	DESCRIPTION	CHARACTERISTICS
I	Pilocytic astrocytoma	Common in children and young adults and people with neurofibromatosis type 1; common in cerebellum	Least malignant, well differentiated; grows slowly; near-normal microscopic appearance, noninfiltrating
II	Diffuse, low-grade astrocytoma (fibrillary, gemistocytic, protoplasmic) Oligodendroglioma	Common in young adults; more common in cerebrum but can occur in any part of brain	Abnormal microscopic appearance; grows slowly; infiltrates to adjacent tissue; may recur at higher grade
III	Anaplastic (malignant) astrocytoma Anaplastic oligodendroglioma	Common in young adults	Malignant; many cells undergoing mitosis; infiltrates adjacent tissue; frequently recurs at higher grade
IV	Glioblastoma (glioblastoma multiforme)	Common in older adults, particularly men Predominant in cerebral hemispheres	Poorly differentiated; increased number of cells undergoing mitosis; bizarre microscopic appearance; widely infiltrates; neovascularization; central necrosis

Data from American Brain Tumor Association: *Brain tumor primer,* ed 9, Chicago, IL, 2010, Author. Available at http://neurosurgery.mgh.harvard.edu/abta/; Louis DN et al: *Acta Neuropathol* 114(2):97–109, 2007.
*World Health Organization Grading of Central Nervous System Tumors.

(WHO) grades II and III astrocytic, oligodendroglial, and oligoastrocytic gliomas. Silencing of the *MGMT* gene (methylated-DNA-protein-cysteine methyltransferase) is found in astrocytomas. Chromosome 1p and 19q deletions are associated with oligodendrogliomas. Alterations in tumor-suppressor genes (e.g., mutations, *TP53*) are common. Alterations also occur in growth factor signaling[175] and gliomas may arise from cancer-initiating resident stem cells.[176]

The principal treatment for cerebral tumors is surgical or radiosurgical excision or surgical decompression if total excision is not possible. Chemotherapy, radiation therapy, or their combination may be used. The blood-brain barrier is an obstacle to the delivery of chemotherapeutic agents. New methods are in progress for penetration of this barrier.[177] Specificity of treatment is advancing with the development of immunotherapy techniques.[178] (Cancer treatment is discussed in Chapter 12.)

Astrocytoma. Astrocytomas are a type of glioma and the most common primary CNS tumor (50% of all brain and spinal cord tumors). Astrocytomas develop from astrocytes and grow by expansion and infiltration into the normal surrounding brain tissues. These tumor cells are believed to have lost normal growth restraint, and thus they proliferate uncontrollably.

One third of astrocytomas are classified at diagnosis as grade I or grade II. These slow-growing but infiltrative gliomas tend to form cavities (pseudocysts); however, some are firm, noncavitating, avascular, gray-white masses that are difficult to distinguish from normal white matter of the brain. Although these tumors may occur anywhere in the brain or spinal cord, they are located most commonly in the cerebrum, hypothalamus, or pons. Low-grade astrocytomas in adults tend to have a lateral or supratentorial location, and they tend to be midline or near midline in position in children, often in the posterior fossa.

Headache and subtle neurobehavioral changes may be an early symptom. Approximately half of persons with low-grade astrocytomas experience a focal or generalized seizure. Onset of a focal seizure disorder between the second and sixth decades of life is suggestive of an astrocytoma. Other general or focal neurologic manifestations develop gradually. Increased ICP is usually a late clinical manifestation.

Grade I astrocytomas are treated with surgery and follow-up CT scans. Grade II astrocytomas are treated surgically if they are accessible or by conventional external radiation, local radiation, or stereotactic radiosurgery. Following surgery alone, the 5-year survival rate is 25%; with surgery followed by radiotherapy, the 5-year survival rate is 50%.

Grades III and IV astrocytomas are found predominantly in the frontal lobes and cerebral hemispheres (Figures 18-33 and 18-34). These tumors also may be located in the brainstem. They are found twice as frequently in men as in women. Grades III and IV astrocytomas are the third most common cancer in the 15- to 34-year-old age group and the fourth most common in the 35- to 54-year-old age group.[179] Grades III and IV astrocytomas are often large and well circumscribed with a variegated pattern. The peripheral rim is pinkish gray and solid with a soft, yellow necrotic center and points of hemorrhage. Microscopically, there is increased cellularity, vascular proliferation, cellular pleomorphism, and necrosis. Necrosis is the main histologic difference between an anaplastic grade III tumor and a grade IV glioblastoma multiforme.

Grade IV astrocytomas (glioblastoma multiforme) account for about 55% of all gliomas. They are highly vascular and extensively infiltrative with heterogeneity in their molecular pathology. They may become large enough to extend from the meningeal surface through the ventricular wall. Fifty percent of glioblastomas are bilateral or at least occupy more than one lobe at the time of death. There are reports of grade IV astrocytomas found outside the central nervous system.[180,181]

The typical clinical presentation for a glioblastoma multiforme is that of diffuse, nonspecific clinical manifestations, such as headache, irritability, and personality changes, that progress to more clear-cut manifestations of increased ICP, such as headache on position change; papilledema; or vomiting. Of those affected, 30% to 40% experience seizure activity. Symptoms may progress to definite focal signs, such as hemiparesis, dysphasia, dyspraxia, cranial nerve palsies, and visual field deficits, in addition to the generalized signs from increased ICP.

Diagnosis of high-grade astrocytomas most commonly takes 3 to 6 months from onset of the first clinical manifestations

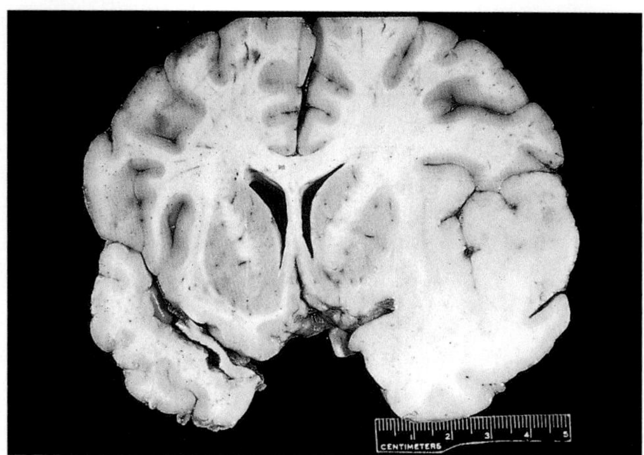

FIGURE 18-33 Well-Differentiated Infiltrating Astrocytoma. The right temporal lobe contains an infiltrative, homogeneous lesion that has expanded the lobe and obscured the normal boundaries between gray and white matter (compare to left temporal lobe). Because of the ill-defined borders, surgical resection rarely removes all of the tumor in such cases. (From Kumar V, Cotran RS, Robbins SL: *Robbins basic pathology,* ed 7, Philadelphia, 2003, Saunders.)

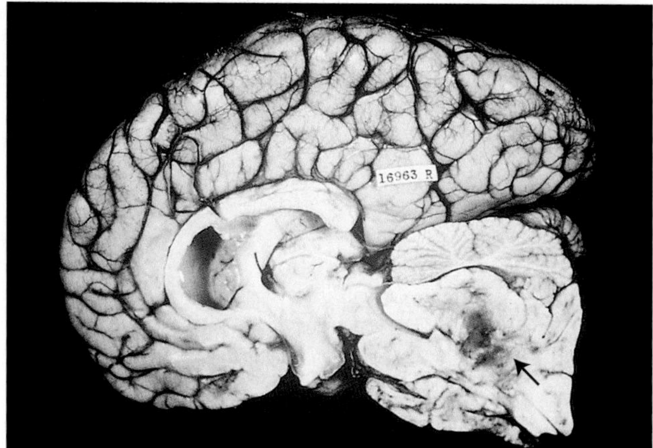

FIGURE 18-35 Ependymoma. These tumors may arise in both the intracranial compartment and the spine. Intracranial tumors typically originate from a ventricular surface, as in the case of this large lesion arising in the fourth ventricle *(arrow).* (From Kumar V, Cotran RS, Robbins SL: *Robbins basic pathology,* ed 7, Philadelphia, 2003, Saunders)

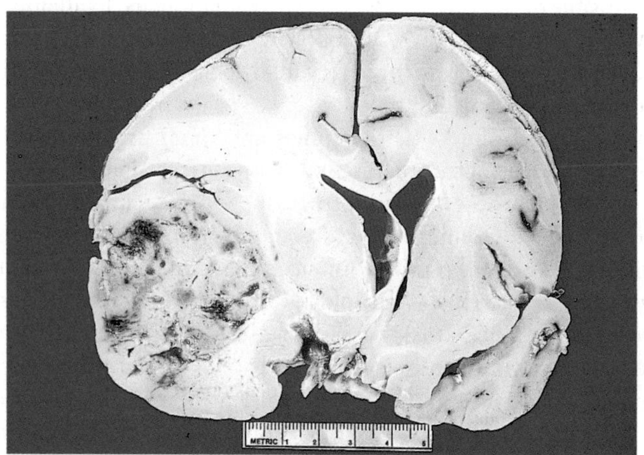

FIGURE 18-34 Glioblastoma Multiforme. In contrast to the well-differentiated infiltrating astrocytoma in Figure 18-33, this glioblastoma contains irregular areas of discoloration and cystic change, reflecting the presence of necrosis and hemorrhage. These lesions are widely infiltrative and associated with considerable mass effect. Note the shift of midline structures to the right. (From Kumar V, Cotran RS, Robbins SL: *Robbins basic pathology,* ed 7, Philadelphia, 2003, Saunders.)

because the person does not recognize the need to consult a healthcare provider. Survival at 5 years for grades III and IV astrocytomas is about 5% to 10%.

Oligodendroglioma. A far less commonly occurring glioma is **oligodendroglioma,** comprising 2% of all brain tumors and 10% to 15% of all gliomas. Oligodendrogliomas are typically slow-growing well-differentiated tumors, often with cysts and calcification present. Most are macroscopically indistinguishable from other gliomas. They occur most often from 30 to 50 years of age and are more common in males than females. Their etiology is unknown. Most oligodendrogliomas are in the frontal and temporal lobes, often in deep white matter; 20% are in both hemispheres. They may be found also in other parts of the cerebrum, third ventricle, brainstem, cerebellum, and spinal cord. A high incidence of this tumor occurs in young adults with a history of temporal lobe epilepsy. Approximately half of these tumors generally classified as oligodendrogliomas (a grade II tumor) are actually oligoastrocytomas (a grade III tumor).[182] Malignant degeneration occurs in approximately one third of persons with oligodendrogliomas. If there is extension to the pia mater (see Figure 15-15) or ependymal wall (epithelial layer surrounding choroid plexus and separating brain tissue from cerebrospinal fluid), oligodendrogliomas may metastasize to distant CNS sites through the ventriculoarachnoid spaces.

More than 50% of individuals experience a focal or generalized seizure as the first clinical manifestation; approximately half have experienced increased ICP at the time of diagnosis and surgery, and only one third develop any focal manifestations. The time from first clinical manifestation to surgical intervention often ranges from 2 to 6 years. Median survival, when surgery and radiotherapy are both used, is 5 to 10 years and prognosis is better than for other astrocytomas.[179]

Ependymoma. **Ependymomas** are rare gliomas that arise from ependymal cells that form the walls of the ventricles or the spinal canal. They are not encapsulated (Figure 18-35 and see Table 18-14). They comprise 6% of all primary brain tumors in adults and 10% in children and adolescents. Intracranial locations are more common among children and spinal cord location is more common among adults. The clinical presentation of spinal ependymoma is neurologic deficit (e.g., pain and dysthesias) corresponding to the level of the lesion. Lateral and third ventricle ependymomas that involve the cerebral hemispheres present with seizures, visual changes, and contralateral weakness of a body part on one side of the body. Etiology for these tumors is unknown.[183]

Clinical manifestations and progression of dysfunction associated with ependymomas may follow a short or long course. The interval between first manifestations and surgery may be as short as 4 weeks with some ependymoblastomas to as long as 7 to 8 years with others.

Ependymomas are treated surgically and with radiotherapy of the tumor region and operative site (possibly of the entire brain and spine). The 5-year survival rate is between 20% and

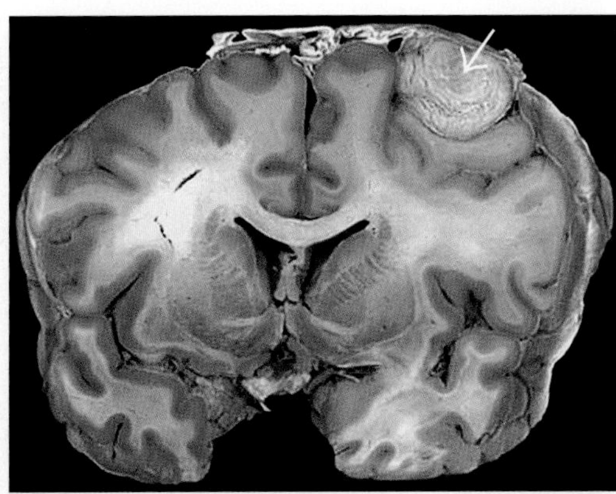

FIGURE 18-36 Meningioma, Gross. Meningioma beneath the dura with compression of underlying cerebral hemisphere. (From Klatt EC: *Robbins and Cotran atlas of pathology,* Philadelphia, 2006, Saunders.)

50%. Some persons benefit from a shunting procedure when the ependymoma has caused a noncommunicating hydrocephalus (see Chapter 17 and Chapter 20).

Primary Extracerebral Tumors

Meningioma. **Meningioma** constitutes about 30% of all intracranial tumors. The annual incidence is 6 cases per 100,000, with a peak incidence in the sixth and seventh decades, and this tumor is more common in women.[184] Predisposing factors to developing a meningioma are having neurofibromatosis (NF) type 2 (NF2, see Nerve Sheath Tumors at right) and undergoing ionizing radiation after a several-decade latency period. Genetically, formation of benign meningiomas has been linked to *NF2* gene mutation and chromosome 22q loss along with *DAL-1* loss on chromosome 18. Atypical and anaplastic meningiomas have been linked to additional gene alterations involving other multiple chromosomes.[185]

A meningioma is a sharply circumscribed mass that derives its shape from the space it occupies; the cause is unknown. These slow-growing, often encapsulated tumors arise from arachnoidal (meningeal) cap cells in the dural coverings of the brain. Rarely do meningiomas arise from arachnoid cells of the choroid plexus of the ventricles. Most are attached to the dura mater and arise within the intracranial cavity, the spinal cavity, or, rarely, the orbit (Figure 18-36). A meningioma may extend to the dural surface and erode the cranial bones or produce an osteoblastic reaction. Small meningiomas (less than 2 cm in diameter) are often found on postmortem examination in middle-aged and older adults who had experienced no clinical manifestations and died of totally unrelated causes. A few meningiomas exhibit malignant, invasive qualities.

Only when meningiomas reach a certain size—at which time they begin to indent the brain parenchyma—do they begin to produce clinical manifestations. Focal seizures are frequently the first manifestation. Other clinical manifestations depend on the tumor's location. Clinical features based on site of origin are as follows:

1. *Sphenoidal wing:* ophthalmoplegia, mild proptosis, and involvement of the ophthalmic division of the trigeminal nerve
2. *Olfactory groove:* anosmia, personality change, and visual failure
3. *Parasagittal:* focal seizures of a focal motor or sensory deficit
4. *Parasellar:* evidence of chiasmatic compression; urinary incontinence; dementia; gradual paraparesis, hormonal failure; optic atrophy; bitemporal hemianopia
5. *Lateral convexity:* variable depending on structures compressed, including slow hemiparesis, speech abnormalities[179]

Because of the extremely slow-growing nature of most meningiomas, increased ICP is less common than with gliomas. The most common symptom is seizures (40%). Diagnosis is made using contrast-enhanced CT, MRI, or both. The primary treatment is surgical resection. Stereotactic radiotherapy is used with incomplete resection or recurrence (20% rate). Conventional radiotherapy also is used. Hydroxyurea and somatostatin are used in cases of tumor recurrence.[186]

Nerve Sheath Tumors. Nerve sheath tumors are either neurofibromas or schwannomas (neuroma, neurolemma). Neurofibromatosis (NF) is an inherited autosomal dominant disorder accounting for 5% of all neuromas and is divided into two types: NF1 and NF2, which are clinically and genetically distinct disorders. The gene products are neurofibromin and merlin (schwannomin), both of which are thought to be tumor suppressors.[187]

Alterations in chromosomes 17 (17q11.2 for NF1) and 22 (NF2) are associated with both neurofibromas and schwannomas. NF1 is associated with cutaneous manifestations, iris hamartomas, and tumors primarily involving the peripheral nervous system and, occasionally, the CNS.[188] NF2 is associated with cataracts, hearing loss, and tumors primarily in the CNS, most commonly vestibular schwannoma and meningioma.[189] Criteria for the diagnosis of neurofibromatosis types 1 and 2 are presented in Box 18-4. The remaining neuromas are benign tumors that arise from the sheath of Schwann cells surrounding the axons of the cranial nerves. The tumors most commonly affect people older than 50 years, women more often than men. The vestibular division of cranial nerve VIII is most commonly affected, although neuromas of the acoustic division of cranial nerves V, VII, VIII, and IX are found (Figure 18-37).

The tumor originates most commonly just distal to the junction between the nerve root and the brainstem. As the tumor grows, it extends into the posterior fossa to occupy the cerebropontine angle and compress adjacent nerves. Eventually the brainstem is displaced, and the CSF flow is obstructed.

Initial clinical manifestations may include headache, tinnitus, hearing loss, impaired balance, unsteady gait, facial pain, and loss of facial sensations. Later, vertigo with nausea and vomiting, a sense of pressure in the ear, and moderate to severe unsteadiness with rapid position changes may appear. CT or MRI can establish the diagnosis. Posterior fossa dye studies may be required. Treatment is by surgical excision and radiotherapy of the neuroma. Pituitary tumors are discussed in Chapter 22, and cerebral tumors in children are discussed in Chapter 20.

Brain Metastases. Brain metastases are approximately 10 times more common than primary brain tumors and the incidence is increasing with improved local control of systemic

BOX 18-4 NIH DIAGNOSTIC CRITERIA FOR NEUROFIBROMATOSIS

Criteria for the Diagnosis of NF1

Two of the following eight criteria:

- Six or more café-au-lait macules greater than 5 mm in greatest diameter in prepubertal individuals and greater than 15 mm in greatest diameter in postpubertal individuals (adults)
- Multiple axillary or inguinal freckles
- One plexiform neurofibroma or two or more neurofibromas of any types
- Optic glioma
- Two or more Lisch nodules (iris hamartomas)
- A distinctive osseous lesion such as sphenoid dysplasia or thinning of the cortex of long bones with or without pseudoarthrosis
- A first-degree relative with NF1 by the above criteria

Criteria for the Diagnosis of NF2

Either one of the following criteria:

- Bilateral masses of the eighth cranial nerve seen with appropriate imaging techniques (e.g., CT or MRI)
- A first-degree relative with NF2 and either:
  a. Unilateral mass of the eighth cranial nerve or
  b. Two of the following:
    1. Neurofibroma
    2. Meningioma
    3. Glioma
    4. Schwannoma
    5. Juvenile posterior subcapsular lenticular opacity

From *NIH diagnostic criteria for neurofibromatosis*. Available at www.medicalcriteria.com/criteria.neuro_nf.htm. Last modified October 23, 2010. Accessed April 1, 2013.

CT, Computed tomography; *MRI*, magnetic resonance imaging; *NF*, neurofibromatosis.

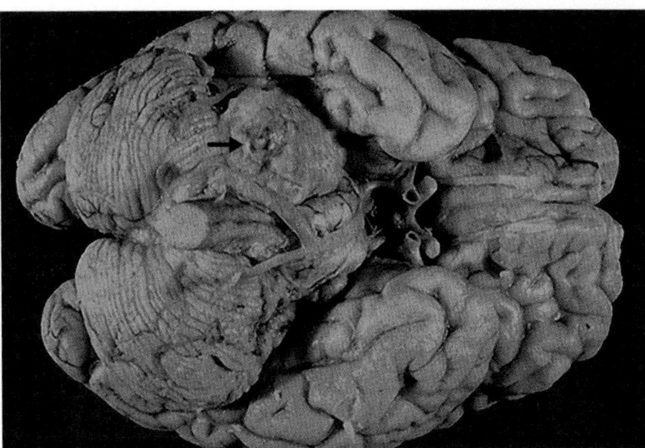

FIGURE 18-37 Acoustic Neuroma (Schwannoma), Gross. A mass lesion arising in the right vestibular branch of the eighth cranial nerve at the cerebellopontine angle *(arrow)*. (From Klatt EC: *Robbins and Cotran atlas of pathology*, Philadelphia, 2006, Saunders.)

tumors. The incidence is estimated at up to 250,000 new cases per year. At autopsy, about 25% of persons with metastases have brain metastases. Lung and breast cancer are the most common tumors to have brain metastases within 1 to 3 years, followed by renal cell carcinoma, gastrointestinal cancer, and malignant melanomas. Carcinoma of the gallbladder, liver, thyroid, testes, uterus, ovary, and pancreas also may metastasize to the brain. Other tumors, besides carcinomas, that metastasize only occasionally are rhabdomyosarcomas, Ewing tumors, chorioepithelioma, and lymphoma.[190]

Metastasis of a cancer to the brain parenchyma or the meninges is a late occurrence in the disease process and is believed to be hematogenous in origin. Two thirds of metastatic tumors are located within the brain and one third are located in extradural spaces. The cerebral hemispheres are the site of 75% of metastases, most predominantly in the frontal lobes followed by the parietal, occipital, and temporal lobes in order of frequency of location. Tumors of the pelvis or retroperitoneal space have a predilection to metastasize to the cerebellum, pons, or their coverings.[191] In more than three fourths of persons with metastasis, the metastases are multiple and found in both the cerebrum and the cerebellum in a scattered distribution. The metastatic tumors often are located in the meninges and near the brain surface in the gray matter and subcortical white matter. These tumors produce little glial cell reaction in the brain tissue but do cause vasogenic, peritumoral edema in the surrounding brain tissue attributable to blood-brain barrier incompetence.[192]

The brain metastatic process requires a series of sequential events, called the "metastatic cascade," as follows:

1. Invasion of primary tumor border
2. Extravasation of the circulatory system
3. Survival and persistence/quiescence in the circulation
4. Extravasation at the distant CNS site
5. Formation of micrometastasis
6. Progressive colonization and growth

Hematogenous metastasis to the CNS is an inherently inefficient process depending on an interaction between tumor cells with host defenses and the microenvironment. To produce brain metastasis, tumor cells must reach the brain vasculature by attaching themselves to the endothelial cells of the brain microvessels in the blood-brain barrier, extravasate into the brain parenchyma, induce blood vessel development (angiogenesis), and proliferate in response to growth factors. Local brain invasion, in itself, is a process requiring mechanisms for cell motility, cell adhesion, enzymatic remodeling of the extracellular components, tumor cell survival, and proliferation. Cytokines, chemokines, and growth factors have been demonstrated to participate in the process.[193]

The clinical manifestations of parenchymal brain metastasis are headache, seizures, or alteration in cognition, mental status, and behavior,[192] although several unusual syndromes do exist. Carcinomatous encephalopathy causes headache, nervousness, depressed mood, trembling, confusion, and forgetfulness. In carcinomatosis of the cerebellum, headache, dizziness, and ataxia are found. Carcinomatosis of the craniospinal meninges (carcinomatous meningitis) manifests with headache, confusion, and manifestations of cranial or spinal nerve root dysfunction.

Contrast-enhanced imaging is the most sensitive imaging procedure for metastatic brain tumors. Prognosis is poor. If one to three tumors are found, surgical excision is indicated. Radiotherapy is commonly used to treat solitary as well as multiple tumors and may be combined with whole brain radiation.[194]

BOX 18-5 MOST COMMON PRIMARY SPINE TUMORS

Benign Tumors	Malignant Tumors
Osteoid osteoma/osteoblastoma	Chondrosarcoma
Giant cell tumors	Chordoma
Hemangiomas	Ewing sarcoma
Aneurysmal bone cyst	Osteosarcoma

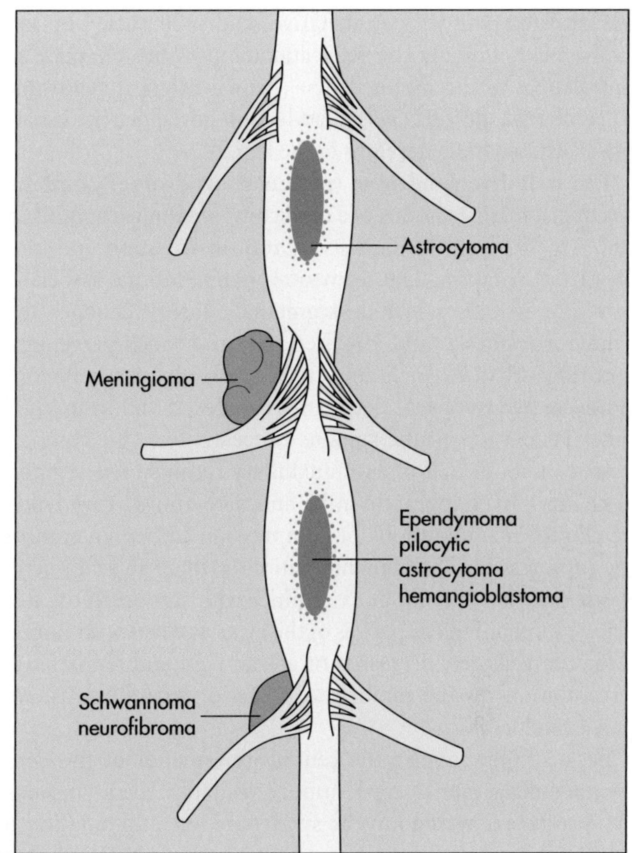

FIGURE 18-38 Distribution of Some Spinal Tumors. (From Perkin DG: *Mosby's color atlas and text of neurology,* London, 1998, Mosby-Wolfe.)

Spinal Cord Tumors

Primary spinal cord tumors are relatively rare, about 2% to 4% of CNS neoplasms. The most common primary spinal cord tumors are listed in Box 18-5 and shown in Figure 18-38. Spinal cord tumors are named to reflect their cell type, growth rate, and structure of origin. They are classified as **intramedullary tumors** (originating within the neural tissues) or **extramedullary tumors** (originating from tissues outside the spinal cord). Extramedullary tumors arise from the meninges or roots (forming **intradural tumors**) or from epidural tissue or vertebral structures (forming **extradural tumors**). About 5% of spinal cord tumors seen in general hospital settings are intramedullary, 40% are intradural-extramedullary, and 55% are extradural.

Metastatic spinal cord tumors are three to four times more common than primary spinal cord tumors. They are usually carcinomas from breast, lung, and prostate; lymphomas; or myelomas; 25% to 70% involve the vertebral body and are asymptomatic. Metastatic spinal cord tumors are extradural in location. Of extradural tumors, 50% are metastatic and have spread to the spine through direct extension from tumors of the vertebral structures or from extraspinal sources extending through the interventricular foramen or through the bloodstream.

The most common primary extramedullary spinal cord tumors are neurofibromas and meningiomas. These tumors are intradural more often than extradural. Neurofibromas are found most commonly in the thoracic and lumbar regions. Meningiomas are more evenly distributed throughout the spine. Other extramedullary tumors in order of frequency of occurrence are sarcomas, vascular tumors, chordomas, and epidermoid and similar tumors. Of intradural-extramedullary tumors, 70% are meningiomas, neurofibromas, or sarcomas.

Intramedullary tumors have the same cellular origins as brain tumors. Ependymomas are the most common intramedullary tumors. Astrocytomas, glioblastomas, oligodendrogliomas, ganglioneuromas, medulloblastomas, hemangiomas, and hemangioblastomas are more or less equally distributed in frequency of occurrence.[195]

PATHOPHYSIOLOGY. Extramedullary spinal cord tumors produce dysfunction by compression of adjacent tissue, not by direct invasion. The spinal cord is compressed by the tumor from without, and destruction of the white matter tracts occurs. The spinal canal around the cord becomes filled by tumor.

Intramedullary spinal cord tumors produce dysfunction by invasion and compression. The cord enlarges as a result of the tumor that is enlarging inside the cord. In addition, distortion of adjacent white matter tracts occurs. Metastases from spinal cord tumors occur from seeding through the CSF; medulloblastomas and ependymomas establish distant implants in this manner.

CLINICAL MANIFESTATIONS. The acute onset of clinical manifestations suggests a vascular insult caused by thrombosis of vessels supplying the spinal cord. Clinical manifestations that are gradual and progressive suggest compression. The clinical manifestations associated with spinal cord tumors fall into three major categories: (1) a compressive syndrome (sensorimotor syndrome), (2) an irritative syndrome (radicular syndrome), and rarely (3) a syringomyelic syndrome.

The **compressive syndrome (sensorimotor syndrome)** is associated with compression and is caused less frequently by invasion and destruction of the spinal cord tracts. Symptoms are usually gradual and progressive, and initial manifestations may be asymmetric. With tumors located in the cervical area, the motor dysfunction usually has the following pattern: ipsilateral arm involvement, followed by ipsilateral and contralateral leg involvement, and finally involvement of the opposite arm. With thoracic tumors the pattern of motor involvement is paresis and spasticity of one leg, followed by involvement of the opposite leg. The sensory clinical manifestations of tingling paresthesias have a pattern similar to that of the motor signs. Pain and temperature dysfunctions are found more commonly than touch, vibration, and proprioceptive changes, although posterior column signs also are found frequently. Pain is less well localized than with an irritative syndrome caused by root involvement. Initially the pain and temperature changes are contralateral to the motor deficit (Brown-Séquard syndrome, see Table 18-4, pp. 592-593). Bladder and bowel deficits usually appear when paresis develops in the legs.

The **irritative syndrome (radicular syndrome)** combines the clinical manifestations of a cord compression with radicular pain, which is pain in the sensory root distribution and indicates root irritation. The segmental manifestations associated with root irritation include segmental sensory changes that include paresthesias and impaired pain and touch perception; motor disturbances, including cramps, atrophy, fasciculations, and decreased or absent deep tendon reflexes; and ache in the spine. Tenderness of the spinous processes over the tumor is present in about half of extramedullary tumors. The segmental changes may appear months and sometimes years before the clinical manifestations of compression in benign tumors. The compressive clinical manifestations include an asymmetric spastic paresis of the lower extremities with tumors in the thoracic or lumbar region, paresis of the arms and legs with tumors in the cervical area, decreased or absent pain and temperature perception below the tumor site, posterior column signs, and spastic bladder.

Because they involve the central gray matter of the cord, intramedullary spinal cord tumors (notably ependymomas) may produce a **syringomyelic syndrome,** or inflammation of the spinal cord. Inflammation results in the development of tubular (syrinx) cavities in the spinal cord. Occasionally an extramedullary tumor may produce the same effect, although the mechanisms are unknown.

EVALUATION AND TREATMENT. The diagnosis of a spinal cord tumor is made through bone scan, needle biopsy guided by CT and positron-emission tomography (PET), or open biopsy. Involvement of specific cord segments is established. Spinal tumors are not staged but can be classified as slow growing (low-grade) or rapidly growing (high-grade).

Treatment varies, depending on the nature of the tumor and the person's clinical status. Indications for surgery include establishment of a tissue diagnosis, neurologic palliation, spinal stabilization, pain relief, and cancer therapy. Surgical resection may involve curettage (piecemeal removal of the tumor) or may be performed en bloc (removal of tumor in one piece). Surgical approaches to the spine include the posterior approach (decompression laminectomy), lateral approach, anterior approach (most favored), and combined approaches. Posterior and anterior reconstructive surgery may be necessary. Oncologic surgical procedures are classified as intralesional, marginal, wide excision, or radical excision. Indications for external radiation vs. surgery are a radiosensitive tumor (e.g., lymphoma), soft tissue compression without instability, a person who is a poor surgical candidate, paraplegia or advanced paraparesis of greater than 24 hours' duration, and an expected survival of less than 3 to 4 months. Chemotherapy, hormonal therapy, and pain management protocols may be appropriate.

SUMMARY REVIEW

Central Nervous System Disorders

1. Traumatic brain injury (TBI) is an alteration in brain function or other evidence of brain pathology caused by an external force.
2. MVAs are the major cause of traumatic CNS injury. Traumatic injuries are classified as closed-head trauma (blunt) or open-head trauma (penetrating). Closed-head trauma is the more common type of trauma.
3. Primary brain injury is caused by an impact and can be classified as focal or diffuse.
4. Focal brain injury includes coup and contrecoup, contusion (bruising of the brain), laceration (tearing of brain tissue), extradural hematoma (accumulation of blood above the dura mater), subdural hematoma (blood between the dura mater and arachnoid membrane), intracerebral hematoma (bleeding into the brain), and open-head trauma.
5. Open-head trauma involves a skull fracture with exposure of the cranial vault to the environment. The types of open-head trauma (compound fracture, perforated fracture) are linear, comminuted, compound, and basilar skull fracture (in the cranial vault or at the base of the skull).
6. Diffuse axonal injury (DAI) results from the effects of head rotation. The brain experiences shearing stresses resulting in axonal damage ranging from concussion to a severe DAI state. Categories of diffuse brain injury include mild concussion; classic cerebral concussion; and mild, moderate, and severe DAI.
7. Secondary neuronal injury occurs as an indirect result of primary brain injury and is the result of both systemic and intracranial processes. Secondary injury results from ischemia, excitotoxicity, inflammation, cerebral edema, increased intracranial pressure, and brain herniation.
8. Spinal cord injuries occur most often in young men who sustain various kinds of injuries (recreational or travel related) and older adults because of preexisting degenerative vertebral disorders.
9. Primary spinal cord injury involves damage to vertebral or neural tissues from compression, traction, or shearing forces.
10. Secondary spinal cord injury is related to ischemia, excitotoxicity, inflammation, edema, oxidative damage, and activation of necrotic and apoptotic cell death, and begins within minutes after injury and continues for weeks.
11. Spinal cord injury often causes spinal shock with cessation of all motor, sensory, reflex, and autonomic functions below any transected area. Loss of motor and sensory function depends on the level of injury.
12. Paralysis of the lower half of the body with both legs involved is called paraplegia. Paralysis involving all four extremities is called quadriplegia.
13. Return of spinal neuron excitability occurs slowly. Reflex activity can return in 1 to 2 weeks in most people with acute spinal cord injury. A pattern of flexion reflexes emerges, involving first the toes and then the feet and legs. Eventually

SUMMARY REVIEW—cont'd

reflex voiding and bowel elimination appear, and mass reflex (flexor spasms accompanied by profuse sweating, piloerection, and automatic bladder emptying) may develop.

14. Autonomic hyperreflexia (dysreflexia) is a syndrome of sudden massive reflex sympathetic discharge associated with spinal cord injury at level T5-T6 or above and can cause life-threatening hypertension.
15. Immobilization of the spine is the immediate intervention for a suggested or confirmed vertebral fracture.
16. The pathologic findings in degenerative disk disease (DDD) include disk protrusion, spondylosis and/or subluxation, degeneration of the vertebrae (spondylolisthesis), and spinal stenosis.
17. Low back pain is pain between the lower rib cage and gluteal muscles and often radiates into the thigh.
18. Low back pain has a high prevalence, affecting 75% to 90% of the population at some time. Sciatica affects about 1% of those with low back pain.
19. Most causes of low back pain are unknown; however, some secondary causes are disk prolapse, tumor, bursitis, synovitis, DDD, osteoporosis, fracture, inflammation, and sprain.
20. Diagnosis of injury to the lower back is made on the basis of physical examination, EMG results, and imaging procedures.
21. Treatment for low back pain includes use of analgesics and NSAIDs, exercise, physical therapy, education, and surgery.
22. Herniation of an intervertebral disk is a protrusion of part of the nucleus pulposus. Herniation most commonly affects the lumbosacral disks (L5-S1 and L4-L5). The extruded pulposus compresses the nerve root, causing pain that radiates along the sciatic nerve.
23. Clinical improvement occurs in most cases; only 10% have sufficient pain after 6 weeks to consider surgery. There is little evidence that drug treatments are effective.
24. Cerebrovascular disease is the most frequently occurring neurologic disorder. Any abnormality of the blood vessels of the brain is referred to as a cerebrovascular disease.
25. Cerebrovascular disease is associated with two types of brain abnormalities: (a) ischemia with or without infarction and (b) hemorrhage.
26. The most common clinical manifestation of cerebrovascular disease is a CVA (stroke syndrome), and the most common risk factor is hypertension.
27. CVAs are classified according to pathophysiology and include ischemic (thrombotic, embolic, and global hypoperfusion), lacunar, and hemorrhagic strokes.
28. A transient ischemic attack is a transient episode of neurologic dysfunction resulting from focal cerebral ischemia.
29. Aspirin, systemic anticoagulation, and thrombolysis improve outcomes with ischemic stroke. Antiplatelet therapy and statins decrease recurrence. Endarterectomy is effective if carotid stenosis is greater than 50%.
30. Treatment of hemorrhagic stroke includes control of bleeding, prevention of increased intracranial pressure, and prevention of cerebral edema and seizures.
31. Intracranial aneurysms result from defects in the vascular wall and are classified on the basis of form and shape. They are commonly asymptomatic, but the signs vary according to the location and size of the aneurysm.
32. Surgical intervention is the treatment of choice before a cerebral aneurysm ruptures.
33. An AVM is a tangled mass of dilated blood vessels. Although sometimes present at birth, AVM exhibits a delayed age of onset with symptoms ranging from headache and dementia to seizures and ICH or SAH. Vasospasm and delayed cerebral ischemia are serious complications.
34. Migraine is an episodic disorder whose marker is headache. Migraine is classified as a headache with and without aura and is precipitated by a triggering event.
35. The clinical phases of a migraine attack are the premonitory phase, the migraine aura, the headache phase, and the recovery phase.
36. Migraine is associated with activation of the peripheral and central arms of the trigeminal system, cortical spreading depression, and distinct activity of brainstem nuclei.
37. Cluster headaches occur in episodes several times during a day for a period of days at different times of the year. The pain is unilateral, intense, tearing, and burning. Associated symptoms include ptosis, lacrimation, reddening of the eye, and nausea. The cause of trigeminal activation is unknown. There is sympathetic nervous system underactivity and parasympathetic overactivity. The two forms are acute and chronic.
38. Chronic paroxysmal hemicrania is a cluster headache with more frequent daily attacks; it occurs primarily in women. It responds to treatment with indomethacin.
39. Tension-type headache is the most common type of headache. Both a central mechanism and a peripheral mechanism are associated with the etiology. The headache is bilateral, with the sensation of a tight band around the head. The pain may last for hours or days. There are acute and chronic forms.
40. Infection and inflammation of the CNS can occur by bacteria, viruses, fungi, parasites, and mycobacteria. The resulting infection by bacteria is pus producing, or pyogenic.
41. Meningitis is inflammation of the brain or spinal cord. Bacterial meningitis is primarily an infection of the pia mater and arachnoid villi and of the fluid of the subarachnoid space. Viral meningitis is believed to be limited to the meninges. Fungal and tubercular meningitis are less common and occur in immunosuppressed individuals in particular.
42. The meningeal vessels become hyperemic, and neutrophils migrate into the subarachnoid space with bacterial meningitis. An inflammatory reaction occurs, and exudation ensues and increases rapidly.
43. The variety of clinical manifestations depends on the type of meningitis and ranges from throbbing headache to neck stiffness and rigidity and decreasing responsiveness. Specific cranial nerve dysfunction is a common occurrence.
44. Bacterial meningitis and fungal meningitis are treated with appropriate antibiotic therapy; viral meningitis is treated with antiviral drugs or corticosteroids and supportive care.
45. Brain abscesses often originate from infections outside the CNS. Microorganisms gain access to the CNS from adjacent sites or spread along the wall of a vein. A localized

SUMMARY REVIEW—cont'd

inflammatory process develops with exudate formation, vessel thrombosis, and leukocyte degeneration. After a few days the infection becomes delimited, with a center of pus and a wall of granular tissue.

46. Clinical manifestations of brain abscesses include headache, nuchal rigidity, confusion, drowsiness, and sensory and communication deficits. Treatment includes antibiotic therapy and surgical excision or aspiration.
47. Encephalitis is an acute febrile illness of viral origin with nervous system involvement. The most common encephalitides are caused by arthropod-borne viruses and herpes simplex virus. Meningeal involvement appears in all encephalitides.
48. Clinical manifestations of encephalitis include fever, delirium, confusion, seizures, abnormal and involuntary movement, and increased intracranial pressure.
49. Most encephalitides are treated by administration of an antiviral agent or an immune globulin and by control of intracranial pressure.
50. The common neurologic complications of AIDS are HIV-associated neurocognitive disorder (HAND), HIV neuropathy, HIV myelopathy, opportunistic infections, cytomegalovirus infection, parasitic infection, and neoplasms. Pathologically, there may be diffuse CNS involvement, focal pathologic findings, and obstructive hydrocephalus. Neurologic involvement associated with HIV has declined with HAART.
51. Lyme disease is a tick-borne spirochete bacterial infection involving the peripheral and central nervous systems that progresses through three stages of symptoms with acute and chronic manifestations.
52. MS is a chronic inflammatory disease involving degeneration of CNS myelin. The cause is unknown and an immune system dysfunction produces the pathology. The demyelination is thought to result from a previous viral insult to the nervous system in a genetically susceptible individual with a subsequent abnormal immune response in the CNS.
53. The clinical manifestations of MS involve different types: relapsing-remitting, primary progressive, secondary progressive, and progressive-relapsing. Optico-spinal MS involves the optic nerve and cranial nerves III through XII. Spinal MS primarily involves the spinal tracts and dorsal column with spastic paresis and bowel and bladder dysfunction. Cerebellar MS manifests with motor ataxia and weakness.
54. There is no cure for MS. Corticosteroid and immune therapy is used to acutely manage relapses or reduce frequency of relapses.

Peripheral Nervous System and Neuromuscular Junction Disorders

1. Neuropathies are the syndromes that result when the peripheral nerves are affected. Axon and myelin degeneration may be present. Neuropathies are classified as generalized symmetric polyneuropathies, generalized neuropathy, and focal or multifocal neuropathies.
2. Therapy for the neuropathies is directed at the primary cause, such as diabetes mellitus. Axonal regrowth and recovery of function may take months, but many neuropathies can be reversed.
3. Guillain-Barré syndrome is an acquired, acute inflammatory demyelinating or axonal disorder caused by a humoral or cell-mediated immunologic response, or both, directed at peripheral nerves. Four subtypes have been identified and clinical manifestations depend on the subtype.
4. Radiculopathies are disorders of the roots of spinal cord nerves. The roots may be compressed, inflamed, or torn. Clinical manifestations include local pain or paresthesias in the sensory root distribution. Treatment may involve surgery, antibiotics, corticosteroids, radiation therapy, and chemotherapy.
5. Myasthenia gravis results from a defect in nerve impulse transmission at the neuromuscular junction. Autoantibodies, complement deposits, and membrane attack complex destroy the acetylcholine receptor (AchR) sites, causing decreased transmission of the nerve impulse.
6. Clinical manifestations of myasthenia gravis include weakness of voluntary muscles, including muscles of the face and throat, and may involve muscles of the diaphragm and chest wall.
7. Treatment of myasthenia gravis involves symptom relief and immunotherapy. The progression of the disease is highly variable; in some individuals it is mild and spontaneously remits.

Tumors of the Central Nervous System

1. Tumors that occur within the cranium are either primary or metastatic (secondary). Primary tumors arise from brain tissue and are classified as intracerebral or extracerebral. Metastatic tumors to the brain arise in organs outside the brain and are much more common than primary brain tumors.
2. CNS tumors cause local and generalized manifestations. Gliomas are the most common primary tumor in adults. The effects are varied; local manifestations include seizures, visual disturbances, loss of equilibrium, and cranial nerve dysfunction.
3. The principal treatment for brain tumors is surgical or radiosurgical excision or decompression if total excision is not possible. Chemotherapy and radiation therapy also are used.
4. Spinal cord tumors are classified as intramedullary (within the neural tissues) or extramedullary (outside the spinal cord). Metastatic spinal cord tumors are usually carcinomas, lymphomas, or myelomas.
5. Extramedullary spinal cord tumors produce dysfunction by compression of adjacent tissue, not by direct invasion. Intramedullary spinal cord tumors produce dysfunction by invasion and compression.
6. The onset of clinical manifestations of spinal cord tumors is gradual and progressive, suggesting compression. Specific manifestations depend on the location of the tumor; for example, there may be paresis and spasticity of one leg with thoracic tumors, followed by involvement of the opposite leg.
7. Spinal cord tumors are treated by surgery, radiation therapy, chemotherapy, and hormonal therapy.

KEY TERMS

Arteriovenous malformation (AVM), 604
Aseptic meningitis, 609
Autonomic hyperreflexia (dysreflexia), 593
Bacterial meningitis, 609
Brain abscess, 613
Capillary telangiectasis, 605
Cavernous angioma (malformation), 605
Cerebral vasospasm (CVS), 606
Cholinergic crisis, 626
Chronic migraine, 607
Chronic paroxysmal hemicrania (CPH), 609
Classic cerebral concussion (Grade IV), 588
Closed (blunt) trauma, 582
Cluster headache, 608
Compressive syndrome (sensorimotor syndrome), 633
Contrecoup injury, 583
Contusion, 583
Coup injury, 583
Degenerative disk disease (DDD), 594
Delayed cerebral ischemia (DCI), 606
Demyelinating polyneuropathy, 621
Diffuse brain injury (diffuse axonal injury [DAI]), 587
Distal axonal polyneuropathy, 621
Embolic stroke, 599
Encephalitis, 614
Ependymoma, 630
Extradural brain abscess (empyema), 613
Extradural hematoma, 584
Extradural tumor, 633
Extramedullary tumor, 633
Focal brain injury, 582
Focal neuropathy, 622
Fungal meningitis, 611
Fusiform aneurysm (giant aneurysm), 604
Generalized AchR myasthenia, 625
Generalized neuropathy, 622
Generalized symmetric polyneuropathy, 621
Glioma, 628
Guillain-Barré syndrome (GBS) (Landry-Guillain-Barré syndrome, idiopathic polyneuritis, acute inflammatory polyradiculopathy, acute autoimmune neuropathy), 622
Hemorrhagic stroke (spontaneous intracranial hemorrhage [ICH]), 602
HIV-associated peripheral neuropathy, 617
HIV myelopathy, 617
HIV neuropathy, 617
Human immunodeficiency virus–associated neurocognitive disorder (HAND), 615
Inherited (congenital) myasthenic syndrome, 624
Intracerebral brain abscess, 613
Intracerebral hematoma, 586
Intradural tumor, 633
Intramedullary tumor, 633
Irritative syndrome (radicular syndrome), 634
Lacunar stroke (lacunar infarct), 599
Lambert-Eaton myasthenic syndrome, 624
Lyme disease, 617
Mass reflex, 593
Meningioma, 631
Meningitis (viral meningitis, nonpurulent meningitis, lymphocytic meningitis), 609
Migraine, 607
Mild concussion (mild traumatic brain injury), 587
Mild diffuse axonal injury, 588
Moderate diffuse axonal injury, 588
Motor neuropathy, 622
Multifocal neuropathy, 622
Multiple sclerosis (MS), 618
Myasthenia gravis, 624
Myasthenic crisis, 626
Mycotic aneurysm, 604
Neonatal myasthenia, 625
Neurogenic shock, 592
Neuromyelitis optica (NO; Devic disease), 620
Neurotonia, 624
Ocular myasthenia, 625
Oligodendroglioma, 630
Open brain trauma, 586
Open (penetrating) trauma, 582
Optical-spinal multiple sclerosis (OSMS), 620
Plexus injury, 624
Postconcussive syndrome, 588
Primary spinal cord injury, 590
Radicular pain, 624
Radicular paresthesia, 624
Radiculitis (radiculoneuritis), 624
Radiculopathy, 624
Saccular aneurysm (berry aneurysm), 604
Seconary brain injury, 588
Secondary neuronal injury, 588
Secondary spinal cord injury, 591
Sensory neuropathy, 622
Severe diffuse axonal injury, 588
Spinal cord abscess, 613
Spinal shock, 592
Spinal stenosis, 596
Spondylolisthesis, 596
Spondylolysis, 596
Subarachnoid hemorrhage (SAH), 605
Subdural brain abscess (empyema), 613
Subdural hematoma, 585
Syringomyelic syndrome, 634
Thrombotic stroke (cerebral thrombosis), 598
Toxoplasmosis, 617
Transient ischemic attack (TIA), 599
Traumatic (dissecting) aneurysm, 604
Traumatic brain injury (TBI), 581
Tubercular meningitis, 611
Vacuolar myelopathy, 617
Venous angioma, 605

REFERENCES

1. Menon DK et al: Demographics and Clinical Assessment Working Group of the International and Interagency Initiative toward Common Data: elements for research on traumatic brain injury and psychological health: position statement: definition of traumatic brain injury, *Arch Phys Med Rehabil* 91(11):1637–1640, 2010.
2. Centers for Disease Control and Prevention: *Injury prevention and control: traumatic brain injury*. Available at www.cdc.gov/traumatic braininjury/statistics.html. Updated March 18, 2013.
3. Faul M et al: *Traumatic brain injury in the United States: emergency department visits, hospitalizations, and deaths, 2002-2006*, Atlanta, GA, 2010, Centers for Disease Control and Prevention, National Center for Injury Prevention and Control.
4. Symptoms of traumatic brain injury: *Glasgow Coma Scale*. Available at www.traumaticbraininjury.com/content/symptoms/glasgowcomascale.html. Accessed April 1, 2013 .
5. *BJM clinical evidence handbook*, London, 2007, BJM Publishing Group Ltd.
6. Alahmadi H, Vachhrajani S, Cusimano MD: The natural history of brain contusion: an analysis of radiological and clinical progression, *J Neurosurg* 112(5):1139–1145, 2010.
7. Ratilal BO et al: Antibiotic prophylaxis for preventing meningitis in patients with basilar skull fractures, *Cochrane Database Syst Rev* (8):CD004884, 2011.
8. Jagoda AS: Mild traumatic brain injury: key decisions in acute management, *Psychiatr Clin North Am* 33(4):797–806, 2010.
9. Hou R et al: When a minor head injury results in enduring symptoms: a prospective investigation of risk factors for postconcussional syndrome after mild traumatic brain injury, *J Neurol Neurosurg Psychiatry* 83(2):217–223, 2012.
10. Gallagher CN, Hutchinson PJ, Pickard JD: Neuroimaging in trauma, *Curr Opin Neurol* 20(4):402–409, 2007.
11. Hesdorffer DC, Ghajar J: Marked improvement in adherence to traumatic brain injury guidelines in United States trauma centers, *J Trauma* 63(4):841–847, 2007.
12. Protheroe RT, Gwinnutt CL: Early hospital care of severe traumatic brain injury, *Anaesthesia* 66(11):1035–1047, 2011.
13. Sakellaridis N et al: Comparison of mannitol and hypertonic saline in the treatment of severe brain injuries, *J Neurosurg* 114(2):545–548, 2011.
14. Ma J et al: Progesterone for acute traumatic brain injury, *Cochrane Database Syst Rev* 10:CD008409, 2012.
15. Chiang YH et al: Early enteral nutrition and clinical outcomes of severe traumatic brain injury patients in acute stage: a multi-center cohort study, *J Neurotrauma* 29(1):75–80, 2012.
16. Park E, Bell JD, Baker AJ: Traumatic brain injury: can the consequences be stopped? *CMAJ* 178(9):1163–1170, 2008.
17. Signoretti S et al: The pathophysiology of concussion, *PM R* 3(10 Suppl 2):S359–S368, 2011.
18. Zink BJ, Szmydynger-Chodobska J, Chodobski A: Emerging concepts in the pathophysiology of traumatic brain injury, *Psychiatr Clin North Am* 33(4):741–756, 2010.
19. Lok J et al: Intracranial hemorrhage: mechanisms of secondary brain injury, *Acta Neurochir Suppl* 111:63–69, 2011.
20. Finnoff JT, Jelsing EJ, Smith J: Biomarkers, genetics, and risk factors for concussion, *PM R* 3(10 Suppl 2):S452–S459, 2011.
21. Topolovec-Vranic J et al: The value of serum biomarkers in prediction models of outcome after mild traumatic brain injury, *J Trauma* 71 (5 Suppl 1):S478–S486, 2011.
22. McAllister TW: Genetic factors modulating outcome after neurotrauma, *PM R* 2(12 Suppl 2):S241–S252, 2010.

23. Ponsford J et al: The association between apolipoprotein E and traumatic brain injury severity and functional outcome in a rehabilitation sample, *J Neurotrauma* 28(9):1683–1692, 2011.
24. National Spinal Cord Injury Statistical Center: *Spinal cord injury facts and figures at a glance*, February, 2013. Available at www.nscisc.uab.edu/.
25. Oyinbo CA: Secondary injury mechanisms in traumatic spinal cord injury: a nugget of this multiply cascade, *Acta Neurobiol Exp (Wars)* 71(2):281–299, 2011.
26. Sinescu C et al: Molecular basis of vascular events following spinal cord injury, *J Med Life* 3(3):254–261, 2010.
27. Rabchevsky AG, Kitzman PH: Latest approaches for the treatment of spasticity and autonomic dysreflexia in chronic spinal cord injury, *Neurotherapeutics* 8(2):274–282, 2011.
27a. Milligan J et al: Autonomic dysreflexia: recognizing a common serious condition in patients with spinal cord injury, *Can Fam Physician* 58(8):831–835, 2012.
28. Dietrich WD et al: Hypothermic treatment for acute spinal cord injury, *Neurotherapeutics* 8(2):229–239, 2011.
29. Rabchevsky AG, Patel SP, Springer JE: Pharmacological interventions for spinal cord injury: where do we stand? How might we step forward? *Pharmacol Ther* 132(1):15–29, 2011.
30. Fehlings MG, Cadotte DW, Fehlings LN: A series of systematic reviews on the treatment of acute spinal cord injury: a foundation for best medical practice, *J Neurotrauma* 28(8):1329–1333, 2011.
31. Thibault-Halman G et al: Acute management of nutritional demands after spinal cord injury, *J Neurotrauma* 28(8):1497–1507, 2011.
32. Kao PY et al: Genetics of lumbar disk degeneration: technology, study designs, and risk factors, *Orthop Clin North Am* 42(4):479–486, vii, 2011.
33. Chan WC et al: Structure and biology of the intervertebral disk in health and disease, *Orthop Clin North Am* 42(4):447–464, vii, 2011.
34. Leone A et al: Lumbar spondylolysis: a review, *Skeletal Radiol* 40(6): 683–700, 2011.
35. Jiang SD, Jiang LS, Dai LY: Degenerative cervical spondylolisthesis: a systematic review, *Int Orthop* 35(6):869–875, 2011.
36. Friedly J, Standaert C, Chan L: Epidemiology of spine care: the back pain dilemma, *Phys Med Rehabil Clin North Am* 21(4):659–677, 2010.
37. Hoy D et al: The epidemiology of low back pain, *Best Pract Res Clin Rheumatol* 24(6):769–781, 2010.
38. Balagué F et al: Non-specific low back pain, *Lancet* 379(9814):482–491, 2012.
39. Casazza BA: Diagnosis and treatment of acute low back pain, *Am Fam Physician* 85(4):343–350, 2012.
40. Chapman JR: Evaluating common outcomes for measuring treatment success for chronic low back pain, *Spine* (Phila Pa 1976) 36(Suppl 21): S54–S68, 2011.
41. Maus T: Imaging the back pain patient, *Phys Med Rehabil Clin North Am* 21(4):725–766, 2010.
42. Casey E: Natural history of radiculopathy, *Phys Med Rehabil Clin North Am* 22(1):1–5, 2011.
43. Legrand E et al: Sciatica from disk herniation: medical treatment or surgery? *Joint Bone Spine* 74(6):530–535, 2007.
44. Jacobs WC et al: Surgery versus conservative management of sciatica due to a lumbar herniated disc: a systematic review, *Eur Spine J* 20(4):513–522, 2011.
45. Jegede KA, Ndu A, Grauer JN: Contemporary management of symptomatic lumbar disc herniations, *Orthop Clin North Am* 41(2):217–224, 2010.
46. Bruggeman AJ, Decker RC: Surgical treatment and outcomes of lumbar radiculopathy, *Phys Med Rehabil Clin North Am* 22(1):161–177, 2011.
47. Roger VL et al: Heart disease and stroke statistics—2013 update: a report from the American Heart Association, *Circulation* 127:e6–e245, 2013.
48. Dubow J, Fink ME: Impact of hypertension on stroke, *Curr Atheroscler Rep* 13(4):298–305, 2011.
49. Aoki J, Uchino K: Treatment of risk factors to prevent stroke, *Neurotherapeutics* 8(3):463–474, 2011.
50. Bandaru VC et al: Outcome of *Chlamydia pneumoniae* associated acute ischemic stroke in elderly patients: a case-control study, *Clin Neurol Neurosurg* 114(2):120–123, 2012.
51. Sorensen AG, Ay H: Transient ischemic attack: definition, diagnosis, and risk stratification, *Neuroimaging Clin North Am* 21(2):303–313, x, 2011.
52. Freeman WD, Aguilar MI: Prevention of cardioembolic stroke, *Neurotherapeutics* 8(3):488–502, 2011.
53. Ihle-Hansen H et al: Risk factors for and incidence of subtypes of ischemic stroke, *Funct Neurol* 27(1):35–40, 2012.
54. Kelley RE, Martin-Schild S: Ischemic stroke: emergencies and management, *Neurol Clin* 30(1):187–210, ix, 2012.
55. Broussalis E et al: Current therapies in ischemic stroke. Part A. Recent developments in acute stroke treatment and in stroke prevention, *Drug Discov Today* 17(7-8):296–309, 2012.
56. Ntaios G, Bath P, Michel P: Blood pressure treatment in acute ischemic stroke: a review of studies and recommendations, *Curr Opin Neurol* 23(1):46–52, 2010.
57. Arima H, Chalmers J: PROGRESS: prevention of recurrent stroke, *J Clin Hypertens (Greenwich)* 13(9):693–702, 2011.
58. Dubow J, Fink ME: Impact of hypertension on stroke, *Curr Atheroscler Rep* 13(4):298–305, 2011.
59. Owens WB: Blood pressure control in acute cerebrovascular disease, *J Clin Hypertens (Greenwich)* 13(3):205–211, 2011.
60. Pandya RS et al: Central nervous system agents for ischemic stroke: neuroprotection mechanisms, *Cent Nerv Syst Agents Med Chem* 11(2): 81–97, 2011.
61. Montecucco F et al: Statins in the treatment of acute ischemic stroke, *Curr Pharm Biotechnol* 13(1):68–76, 2012.
62. RF Xi G, Hoff JT: Intracerebral hemorrhage and intraventricular hemorrhage-induced brain injury. In Gilman S, editor: *Neurobiology of disease*, Burlington, MA, 2007, Elsevier.
63. Jauch EC et al: American Heart Association Stroke Council; Council on Cardiovascular Nursing; Council on Peripheral Vascular Disease; Council on Clinical Cardiology: Guidelines for the early management of patients with acute ischemic stroke: a guideline for healthcare professionals from the American Heart Association/American Stroke Association, *Stroke* 44(3):870–947, 2013.
64. Langhorne P, Bernhardt J, Kwakkel G: Stroke rehabilitation, *Lancet* 377(9778):1693–1702, 2011.
65. Flower O, Smith M: The acute management of intracerebral hemorrhage, *Curr Opin Crit Care* 17(2):106–114, 2011.
66. Elliott J, Smith M: The acute management of intracerebral hemorrhage: a clinical review, *Anesth Analg* 110(5):1419–1427, 2010.
67. Arima H et al: Lower treatment blood pressure is associated with greatest reduction in hematoma growth after acute intracerebral hemorrhage, *Hypertension* 56(5):852–858, 2010.
68. Gilmore E et al: Seizures and CNS hemorrhage: spontaneous intracerebral and aneurysmal subarachnoid hemorrhage, *Neurologist* 16(3): 165–175, 2010.
69. Helbok R et al: Effect of mannitol on brain metabolism and tissue oxygenation in severe haemorrhagic stroke, *J Neurol Neurosurg Psychiatry* 82(4):378–383, 2011.
69a. Sehba FA et al: The importance of early brain injury after subarachnoid hemorrhage, *Prog Neurobiol* 97(1):14–37, 2012.
70. Penn DL, Komotar RJ, Sander Connolly E: Hemodynamic mechanisms underlying cerebral aneurysm pathogenesis, *J Clin Neurosci* 18(11):1435–1438, 2011.
71. Pritz MB: Cerebral aneurysm classification based on angioarchitecture, *J Stroke Cerebrovasc Dis* 20(2):162–167, 2011.
72. Krings T et al: Intracranial aneurysms: from vessel wall pathology to therapeutic approach, *Nat Rev Neurol* 7(10):547–559, 2011.
73. Washington CW et al: The current surgical management of intracranial aneurysms, *J Neurosurg Sci* 55(3):211–231, 2011.
74. Laakso A, Hernesniemi J: Arteriovenous malformations: epidemiology and clinical presentation, *Neurosurg Clin North Am* 23(1):1–6, 2012.
75. Brouillard P, Vikkula M: Genetic causes of vascular malformations, *Hum Mol Genet* 16(Spec No. 2):R140–R149, 2007.
76. San Millán Ruíz D, Gailloud P: Cerebral developmental venous anomalies, *Childs Nerv Syst* 26(10):1395–1406, 2010.
77. Kim H et al: Brain arteriovenous malformation pathogenesis: a response-to-injury paradigm, *Acta Neurochir Suppl* 111:83–92, 2011.
78. Matschke J, Lockemann U, Schulz F: Intracranial arteriovenous malformations presenting as sudden unexpected death: a report of 3 cases and review of literature, *Am J Forensic Med Pathol* 28(2):173–176, 2007.
79. Barr JC, Ogilvy CS: Selection of treatment modalities or observation of arteriovenous malformations, *Neurosurg Clin North Am* 23(1):63–75, 2012.
80. Zacharia BE et al: Epidemiology of aneurysmal subarachnoid hemorrhage, *Neurosurg Clin North Am* 21(2):221–233, 2010.
81. Wang HC et al: Time course of cerebral hemodynamics in aneurysmal subarachnoid hemorrhage, *J Clin Ultrasound* 40(2):91–98, 2012.
82. Dorsch N: A clinical review of cerebral vasospasm and delayed ischaemia following aneurysm rupture, *Acta Neurochir Suppl* 110(Pt 1):5–6, 2011.
83. Smith SD, Eskey CJ: Hemorrhagic stroke, *Radiol Clin North Am* 49(1):27–45, 2011.

84. Mehrotra P et al: Investigation of subarachnoid haemorrhage: does the buck stop with CT? *J Med Life* 3(3):338–342, 2010.
85. Coppadoro A, Citerio G: Subarachnoid hemorrhage: an update for the intensivist, *Minerva Anestesiol* 77(1):74–84, 2011.
86. Currie S, Mankad K, Goddard A: Endovascular treatment of intracranial aneurysms: review of current practice, *Postgrad Med J* 87(1023):41–50, 2011.
87. Kimball MM et al: Critical care guidelines on the endovascular management of cerebral vasospasm, *Neurocrit Care* 15(2):336–341, 2011.
88. Bigal ME, Lipton RB: The epidemiology, burden, and comorbidities of migraine, *Neurol Clin* 27(2):321–334, 2009.
89. International Headache Society: *HIS classification ICHD-II: 1. Migraine.* Available at http://ihs-classification.org/en/02_klassifikation/02_teil1/01.00.00_migraine.html. Accessed April 1, 2013.
90. Ferrari MD, Goadsby PJ: Migraine as a cerebral ionopathy with abnormal central sensory processing. In Gilman S, editor: *Neurobiology of disease*, Burlington, MA, 2007, Elsevier.
91. Mathew NT: Pathophysiology of chronic migraine and mode of action of preventive medications, *Headache* 51(Suppl 2):84–92, 2011.
92. Akerman S, Holland PR, Goadsby PJ: Diencephalic and brainstem mechanisms in migraine, *Nat Rev Neurosci* 12(10):570–584, 2011.
93. Davies P: What has imaging taught us about migraine? *Maturitas* 70(1):34–36, 2011.
94. Kelman L: The biological basis of headache, *Expert Rev Neurother* 11(3):363–378, 2011.
95. Shevel E: The extracranial vascular theory of migraine: an artificial controversy, *J Neural Transm* 118(4):525–530, 2011.
96. Akerman S, Goadsby PJ: Dopamine and migraine: biology and clinical implications, *Cephalagia* 27(11):1208–1214, 2007.
97. Cutrer FM, Huerter K: Migraine aura, *Neurologist* 13(3):118–125, 2007.
98. Chakravarty A, Sen A: Migraine, neuropathic pain and nociceptive pain: towards a unifying concept, *Med Hypotheses* 74(2):225–231, 2010.
99. Aurora SK, Kulthia A, Barrodale PM: Mechanism of chronic migraine, *Curr Pain Headache Rep* 15(1):57–63, 2011.
100. Burstein R et al: Thalamic sensitization transforms localized pain into widespread allodynia, *Ann Neurol* 68(1):81–91, 2010.
101. Mathew NT: Pathophysiology of chronic migraine and mode of action of preventive medications, *Headache* 51(Suppl 2):84–92, 2011.
102. Dhillon KS, Singh J, Lyall JS: A new horizon into the pathobiology, etiology and treatment of migraine, *Med Hypotheses* 77(1):147–151, 2011.
103. Olesen J, Ashina M: Emerging migraine treatments and drug targets, *Trends Pharmacol Sci* 32(6):352–359, 2011.
104. Barbanti P et al: Migraine prophylaxis: what is new and what we need? *Neurol Sci* 32(Suppl 1):S111–S115, 2011.
105. O'Neilck: Pain management. In Chisholm-Burns MS et al: *Pharmacotherapy principles and practices*, New York, 2008, McGraw-Hill.
106. Iacovelli E et al: Neuroimaging in cluster headache and other trigeminal autonomic cephalalgias, *J Headache Pain* 13(1):11–20, 2012.
107. Ashkenazi A, Schwedt T: Cluster headache—acute and prophylactic therapy, *Headache* 51(2):272–286, 2011.
108. Sjaastad O, Vincent M: Indomethacin responsive headache syndromes: chronic paroxysmal hemicrania and hemicrania continua. How they were discovered and what we have learned since, *Funct Neurol* 25(1): 49–55, 2010.
109. Rossi P et al: The contribution of clinical neurophysiology to the comprehension of the tension-type headache mechanisms, *Clin Neurophysiol* 122(6):1075–1085, 2011.
110. Bendtsen L, Jensen R: Treating tension-type headache—an expert opinion, *Expert Opin Pharmacother* 12(7):1099–1109, 2011.
111. Bleck TP: Bacterial and fungal infections of the nervous system. In Gilman S, editor: *Neurobiology of disease*, Burlington, MA, 2007, Elsevier.
112. Roos KL: Nonviral infections. In Goetz CG, editor: *Textbook of clinical neurology*, ed 2, Philadelphia, 2003, Saunders.
113. Thigpen MC et al: Emerging Infections Programs Network. Bacterial meningitis in the United States, 1998-2007, *N Engl J Med* 364(21): 2016–2025, 2011.
114. van de Beek D et al: Clinical features and prognostic factors in adults with bacterial meningitis, *N Engl J Med* 351(18):1849–1859, 2004.
115. Irani DN: Aseptic meningitis and viral myelitis, *Neurol Clin* 26(3): 635–655, vii-viii, 2008.
116. van der Harst JJ, Luijckx GJ: Treatment of central nervous system tuberculosis infections and neurological complications of tuberculosis treatment, *Curr Pharm Des* 17(27):2940–2947, 2011.
117. Centers for Disease Control and Prevention (CDC): Updated recommendations for use of meningococcal conjugate vaccines—Advisory Committee on Immunization Practices (ACIP), 2010, *MMWR Morb Mortal Wkly Rep* 60(3):72–76, 2011.
118. Muzumdar D, Jhawar S, Goel A: Brain abscess: an overview, *Int J Surg* 9(2):136–144, 2011.
119. Roos KL: Nonviral infections. In Goetz CG, editor: *Textbook of clinical neurology*, ed 2, Philadelphia, 2003, Saunders.
120. Honda H, Warren DK: Central nervous system infections: meningitis and brain abscess, *Infect Dis Clin North Am* 23(3):609–623, 2009.
121. Ratnaike TE et al: A review of brain abscess surgical treatment—78 years: aspiration versus excision, *World Neurosurg* 76(5):431–436, 2011.
122. Hakan T: Management of bacterial brain abscesses, *Neurosurg Focus* 24(6):E4, 2008.
123. Centers for Disease Control and Prevention: *Eastern equine encephalitis*, June 2011. Available at www.cdc.gov/EasternEquineEncephalitis/tech/epi.html.
124. Hollidge BS, González-Scarano F, Soldan SS: Arboviral encephalitides: transmission, emergence, and pathogenesis, *J Neuroimmune Pharmacol* 5(3):428–442, 2010.
125. Singer EJ et al: Neurologic presentations of AIDS, *Neurol Clin* 28(1): 253–275, 2010.
126. Connor M: Human immunodeficiency virus (HIV) and stroke: targets for intervention, *Infect Disord Drug Targets* 10(2):76–83, 2010.
127. Gras G, Kaul M: Molecular mechanisms of neuroinvasion by monocytes-macrophages in HIV-1 infection, *Retrovirology* 7:30, 2010.
128. Gannon P, Khan MZ, Kolson DL: Current understanding of HIV-associated neurocognitive disorders pathogenesis, *Curr Opin Neurol* 24(3):275–283, 2011.
129. Mothobi NZ, Brew BJ: Neurocognitive dysfunction in the highly active antiretroviral therapy era, *Curr Opin Infect Dis* 25(1):4–9, 2012.
130. White MK, Khalili K: Pathogenesis of progressive multifocal leukoencephalopathy—revisited, *J Infect Dis* 203(5):578–586, 2011.
131. Malfitano A et al: Human immunodeficiency virus-associated malignancies: a therapeutic update, *Curr HIV Res* 10(2):123–132, 2012.
132. Bhate C, Schwartz RA: Lyme disease: part I. Advances and perspectives, *J Am Acad Dermatol* 64(4):619–636, 2011.
133. Lantos PM: Chronic Lyme disease: the controversies and the science, *Exp Rev Anti Infect Ther* 9(7):787–797, 2011.
134. National Multiple Sclerosis Society: *Multiple sclerosis: just the facts, 2012.* Available at www.nationalmssociety.org/about-multiple-sclerosis/index.aspx. Accessed April 1, 2013.
135. Kallaur AP et al: Genetic polymorphisms associated with the development and clinical course of multiple sclerosis (review), *Int J Mol Med* 28(4):467–479, 2011.
136. Mowry EM: Natural history of multiple sclerosis: early prognostic factors, *Neurol Clin* 29(2):279–292, 2011.
137. Miller E: Multiple sclerosis, *Adv Exp Med Biol* 724:222–238, 2012.
138. Wu GF, Alvarez E: The immunopathophysiology of multiple sclerosis, *Neurol Clin* 29(2):257–278, 2011.
139. Disanto G et al: The evidence for a role of B cells in multiple sclerosis, *Neurology* 78(11):823–832, 2012.
140. Nylander A, Hafler DA: Multiple sclerosis, *J Clin Invest* 122(4):1180–1188, 2012.
141. Gonsette RE: Endogenous neuroprotection in multiple sclerosis, *Acta Neurol Belg* 110(1):26–35, 2010.
142. Nylander A, Hafler DA: Multiple sclerosis, *J Clin Invest* 122(4): 1180–1188, 2012.
143. Owens GP et al: Viruses and multiple sclerosis, *Neuroscientist* 17(6): 659–676, 2011.
144. Cambron M et al: White-matter astrocytes, axonal energy metabolism, and axonal degeneration in multiple sclerosis, *J Cereb Blood Flow Metab* 32(3):413–424, 2012.
145. Costello K: *New insights into MS immunotherapy: implications for treatment and long-term outcomes*, New York, 2008, Bioscience Communications.
146. Zeis T, Schaeren-Wiemers N: Lame ducks or fierce creatures? The role of oligodendrocytes in multiple sclerosis, *J Mol Neurosci* 35(1):91–100, 2008.
147. Williams R et al: Pathogenic implications of iron accumulation in multiple sclerosis, *J Neurochem* 120(1):7–25, 2012.
148. Flynn LC, Moster ML: Current thoughts on chronic cerebrospinal venous insufficiency in multiple sclerosis, *Curr Opin Ophthalmol* 22(6):463–467, 2011.
149. Tsui A, Lee MA: Multiple sclerosis and pregnancy, *Curr Opin Obstet Gynecol* 23(6):435–439, 2011.
150. Kira J: Neuromyelitis optica and opticospinal multiple sclerosis: mechanisms and pathogenesis, *Pathophysiology* 18(1):69–79, 2011.

151. Kira J: Autoimmunity in neuromyelitis optica and opticospinal multiple sclerosis: astrocytopathy as a common denominator in demyelinating disorders, *J Neurol Sci* 311(1-2):69–77, 2011.
152. Polman CH et al: Diagnostic criteria for multiple sclerosis: 2010 revisions to the McDonald criteria, *Ann Neurol* 69(2):292–302, 2011.
153. Giesser BS: Diagnosis of multiple sclerosis, *Neurol Clin* 29(2):381–388, 2011.
154. Derwenskus J: Current disease-modifying treatment of multiple sclerosis, *Mt Sinai J Med* 78(2):161–175, 2011.
155. Munger KL, Ascherio A: Prevention and treatment of MS: studying the effects of vitamin D, *Mult Scler* 17(12):1405–1411, 2011.
156. Zwibel HL, Smrtka J: Improving quality of life in multiple sclerosis: an unmet need, *Am J Manag Care* 17(Suppl 5 Improving):S139–S145, 2011.
157. Sejvar JJ et al: Population incidence of Guillain-Barré syndrome: a systematic review and meta-analysis, *Neuroepidemiology* 36(2):123–133, 2011.
158. Shahrizaila N, Yuki N: Guillain-Barré syndrome animal model: the first proof of molecular mimicry in human autoimmune disorder, *J Biomed Biotechnol* 829129:2011, 2011.
159. Bowyer HR, Glover M: Guillain-Barré syndrome: management and treatment options for patients with moderate to severe progression, *J Neurosci Nurs* 42(5):288–293, 2010.
160. Tsao B: The electrodiagnosis of cervical and lumbosacral radiculopathy, *Neurol Clin* 25(2):473–494, 2007.
161. De Luigi AJ, Fitzpatrick KF: Physical examination in radiculopathy, *Phys Med Rehabil Clin North Am* 22(1):7–40, 2011.
162. Fox IK, Mackinnon SE: Adult peripheral nerve disorders: nerve entrapment, repair, transfer, and brachial plexus disorders, *Plast Reconstr Surg* 127(5):105e–118e, 2011.
163. Terenghi G, Hart A, Wiberg M: The nerve injury and the dying neurons: diagnosis and prevention, *J Hand Surg Eur* 36(9):730–734, 2011.
164. Farrugia ME: Myasthenic syndromes, *J R Coll Physic Edinb* 41(1):43–47, 2011.
165. Gomez AM et al: Antibody effector mechanisms in myasthenia gravis—pathogenesis at the neuromuscular junction, *Autoimmunity* 43(5-6): 353–370, 2010.
166. Titulaer MJ, Lang B, Verschuuren JJ: Lambert-Eaton myasthenic syndrome: from clinical characteristics to therapeutic strategies, *Lancet Neurol* 10(12):1098–1107, 2011.
167. Verschuuren JJ, Palace J, Gilhus NE: Clinical aspects of myasthenia explained, *Autoimmunity* 43(5-6):344–352, 2010.
168. Bartt R, Shannon KM: Autoimmune and inflammatory disorders. In Goetz CG, editor: *Textbook of clinical neurology*, ed 2, Philadelphia, 2003, Saunders.
169. Tüzün E, Huda R, Christadoss P: Complement and cytokine based therapeutic strategies in myasthenia gravis, *J Autoimmun* 37(2):136–143, 2011.
170. Kumar V, Kaminski HJ: Treatment of myasthenia gravis, *Curr Neurol Neurosci Rep* 11(1):89–96, 2011.
171. American Cancer Society: *Cancer facts and figures*, 2013. Available at http://www.cancer.org/acs/groups/content/@epidemiologysurveilance/documents/document/acspc-036845.pdf. Accessed April 1, 2013.
172. Fisher JL et al: Epidemiology of brain tumors, *Neurol Clin* 25(4): 867–890, vii, 2007.
173. Persson AI et al: Glioma. In Gilman S, editor: *Neurobiology of disease*, Burlington, MA, 2007, Elsevier.
174. Little MP et al: Mobile phone use and glioma risk: comparison of epidemiological study results with incidence trends in the United States, *BMJ* 344:e1147, 2012.
175. Riemenschneider MJ et al: Molecular diagnostics of gliomas: state of the art, *Acta Neuropathol* 120(5):567–584, 2010.
176. Siebzehnrubl FA et al: The origins of glioma: E Pluribus Unum? *Glia* 59(8):1135–1147, 2011.
177. Etame AB et al: Focused ultrasound disruption of the blood-brain barrier: a new frontier for therapeutic delivery in molecular neurooncology, *Neurosurg Focus* 32(1):E3, 2012.
178. Jackson C et al: Challenges in immunotherapy presented by the glioblastoma multiforme microenvironment, *Clin Dev Immunol* 732413:2011, 2011.
179. Janus TJ, Yung KA: Primary neurological tumors. In Goetz CG, editor: *Textbook of clinical neurology*, ed 2, Philadelphia, 2003, Saunders.
180. Nicholas MK et al: Molecular heterogeneity in glioblastoma: therapeutic opportunities and challenges, *Semin Oncol* 38(2):243–253, 2011.
181. Templeton A et al: Extraneural spread of glioblastoma—report of two cases, *Onkologie* 31(4):192–194, 2008.
182. Belda-Iniesta C et al: Molecular biology of malignant gliomas, *Clin Transl Oncol* 8(9):635–641, 2006.
183. Gilbert MR, Ruda R, Soffietti R: Ependymomas in adults, *Curr Neurol Neurosci Rep* 10(3):240–247, 2010.
184. Wiemels J, Wrensch M, Claus EB: Epidemiology and etiology of meningioma, *J Neurooncol* 99(3):307–314, 2010.
185. Mawrin C, Perry A: Pathological classification and molecular genetics of meningiomas, *J Neurooncol* 99(3):379–391, 2010.
186. Chamberlain MC, Barnholtz-Sloan JS: Medical treatment of recurrent meningiomas, *Expert Rev Neurother* 11(10):1425–1432, 2011.
187. Uhlmann EJ, Plotkin SR: Neurofibromatoses, *Adv Exp Med Biol* 724:266–277, 2012.
188. Jouhilahti EM et al: The pathoetiology of neurofibromatosis 1, *Am J Pathol* 178(5):1932–1939, 2011.
189. Evans GR, Lloyd SK, Ramsden RT: Neurofibromatosis type 2, *Adv Otorhinolaryngol* 70:91–98, 2011.
190. Fox BD et al: Epidemiology of metastatic brain tumors, *Neurosurg Clin North Am* 22(1):1–6, v, 2011.
191. Benjamin RK, Das A, Hochberg FH: Metastatic neoplasms and paraneoplastic syndrome. In Goetz CG, editor: *Textbook of clinical neurology*, ed 2, Philadelphia, 2003, Saunders.
192. Well JR: Central nervous system metastasis. In Gilman S, editor: *Neurobiology of disease*, Burlington, MA, 2007, Elsevier.
193. Beasley KD, Toms SA: The molecular pathobiology of metastasis to the brain: a review, *Neurosurg Clin North Am* 22(1):7–14, v, 2011.
194. Lo SS et al: Advances in radiation therapy of brain metastasis, *Prog Neurol Surg* 25:96–109, 2012.
195. Chamberlain MC, Tredway TL: Adult primary intradural spinal cord tumors: a review, *Curr Neurol Neurosci Rep* 11(3):320–328, 2011.

CHAPTER

19

Neurobiology of Schizophrenia, Mood Disorders, and Anxiety Disorders*

Lorey K. Takahashi

***Treatment and prevention of mental disorders are currently being debated.**

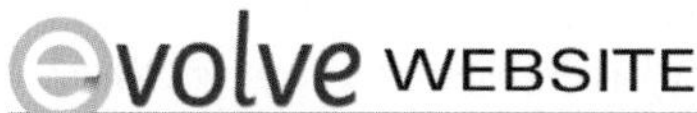

http://evolve.elsevier.com/McCance/

- Review Questions and Answers

CHAPTER OUTLINE

Mental illnesses are common and found in different cultures and across the socioeconomic spectrum. When left untreated, the consequences can be devastating. This chapter provides an introduction to the neurobiology of schizophrenia, mood disorders, and some anxiety disorders. The etiology and pathophysiology of mental illnesses are diverse and complex. Diagnostic criteria are constantly being updated to more precisely diagnose and effectively treat the disorders. Every mental disorder manifests a range of symptoms that vary in intensity. Symptom variations likely reflect individual differences in neural pathologic brain structures or functions, or both, which affect treatment. Risk factors, such as exposure to uncontrollable psychosocial stress, may precipitate the onset of mental disorders and point to the challenge in understanding how diseased genes and environmental factors interact.

The development of visual and quantitative structural and functional neuroimaging techniques provides insight into the pathophysiologic basis of mental disorders. In schizophrenia, neuroanatomic, functional, and neurochemical alterations associated with this debilitating illness have uncovered abnormal brain regions along with a host of candidate genes that confer risk. Similarly, in mood and anxiety disorders, brain scans are revealing structural and functional abnormalities. Notably, many brain regions implicated in normal cognitive and emotional processing are found in schizophrenia, mood, and anxiety disorders. The future lies in unraveling how the highly interconnected brain structures modulated by neurotransmitters, neuropeptides, and hormones operate in normal to abnormal mental states.

Knowledge of the pathophysiology associated with a specific mental illness has guided the development of pharmacologic medications. Although second- and third-generation drugs with fewer side effects are now available, many individuals continue to suffer; and to complicate diagnosis and treatment, psychiatric disorders, such as depression and anxiety, often coexist. Identifying and characterizing diseased genes and environmental triggers in mental illness will offer hope in developing effective therapies that alleviate symptoms and lessen or reverse the pathophysiologic alterations.

SCHIZOPHRENIA

Schizophrenia is a serious psychiatric illness that strikes 1% of the world's population. The illness is equally prevalent in males and females and emerges in young adults during the late teens and early twenties, with a slightly earlier onset in males than in females. **Schizophrenia** is the term coined originally by Eugen Bleuler in 1911 to describe a collection of illnesses characterized by **thought disorders,** which reflect a break in reality or splitting of the cognitive from the emotional side of one's personality. A schizophrenic individual may exhibit a feeling of happiness when recollecting a terrible event or emotional indifference when describing a joyful occasion. Today, disorganized thought in schizophrenia is characterized by positive and negative symptoms including auditory hallucinations, paranoid delusions, and cognitive deficits that have devastating effects on the individual and the individual's family.

Etiology and Pathophysiology

Genetic Predisposition

Schizophrenia is a heritable disorder. In monozygotic twins, the concordance rate varies from 30% to 50%. This variability may stem from different diagnostic criteria and methodologic or sampling differences across studies. In dizygotic twins and siblings the concordance rate decreases to 12%, which is still considerably higher than the 1% figure found in the general population.

Nonetheless, schizophrenia is not a simple genetic disorder in which inherited disease alleles will always lead to illness. Schizophrenia likely involves several genes located on different chromosomes and differs from mendelian disorders, in which genes are fully penetrant and recognized as the primary cause of disease (e.g., genes for Huntington disease). As indicated by the 50% concordance rate in monozygotic twins, the genes for schizophrenia show reduced penetrance, resulting in individuals who carry the disease genes without manifesting the illness. Further complicating the search for the specific genes that confer risk of schizophrenia is the variability in biologic and phenotypic traits among individuals who manifest the illness (see What's New? Copy Number Variations Increase in Schizophrenia and in Offspring of Older Fathers).

Prenatal and Perinatal Vulnerability Factors. Because the concordance rate of schizophrenia in monozygotic twins is never 100% as in mendelian disorders, environmental factors likely play an important role in increasing the risk of developing the disorder. A leading hypothesis suggests that early environmental factors interfere with genetically programmed neural developmental alterations that eventually compromise normal brain structures and functions.[1] An early brain defect may remain silent and not dramatically affect the individual until subsequent development requires adaptive use of brain structures.[2] Several hypothesized early environmental factors that may alter brain development and increase the risk of developing schizophrenia include exposure to prenatal infection, prenatal nutritional deficiencies, perinatal complications (such as birth defects and neonatal hypoxia), and upbringing in an urban environment.[3]

WHAT'S NEW?

Copy Number Variations Increase in Schizophrenia and in Offspring of Older Fathers

Copy number variations (CNVs) involving deletions or duplications of several million base pairs of DNA sequence of the genome are increasingly recognized to elevate the risk of serious neurodevelopmental disorders including schizophrenia, autism, epilepsy, and mental retardation. Concerning schizophrenia, large CNV deletions involving multiple genes show increased penetrance accompanied with severe phenotypic symptoms of the disease. For example, CNV deletion at 22q11.2, which consists of 1.5 to 3.0 megabases of DNA, is reported to increase the risk of schizophrenia by 20- to 30-fold in comparison to the general population. Research linking 22q11.2 deletion to schizophrenia as well as other recently identified CNV deletions occurring at distinct loci will accelerate our genetic understanding of the pathogenesis of the disease and have implications for genetic counseling and clinical management.

Of further potential clinical relevance of the role of CNVs in schizophrenia, offspring of fathers who are age 50 or more have a twofold to threefold increased risk of the disease when compared to fathers who are in their twenties. Although the causal mechanisms remain unclear, a recent study using a mouse model reported that offspring sired by older male mice exhibited an increase in spontaneously occurring (de novo) CNVs. Six de novo CNVs were found in the offspring of aged male mice and none from the younger control group. When the CNVs in the mouse brain were then mapped to the human genome, three de novo CNVs were found to have genes on human chromosomes linked to brain development and schizophrenia. These results suggest that paternal-age–related mutations in the germline contribute to offspring de novo CNVs that may underlie schizophrenia.

Data from Bassett AS et al: *Am J Psychiatry* 167:899–914, 2010; Flatscher-Bader T et al: *Transl Psychiatry* 1:e34, 2011; Moreno-DeLuca D, Cubells JF: *Curr Psychiatry Rep* 13:129–137, 2011.

Neuroanatomic and Functional Abnormalities

Neuroanatomic Alterations. Advanced neuroimaging techniques have revealed evidence of structural brain abnormalities in schizophrenia.[4,5] A consistent finding is the enlargement of the lateral and third ventricles and the widening of frontocortical fissures and sulci (Figure 19-1). Schizophrenics with cerebral ventricular enlargement often exhibit cognitive impairments and negative symptoms, and respond poorly to treatment. Other studies reported a reduction in the thalamus and temporal lobe areas (e.g., amygdala, hippocampus, and parahippocampal gyrus).[6] A reduction in thalamus size may disrupt neurotransmission between the cortex and primary sensory and motor areas. Temporal lobe alterations may contribute to the production of positive schizophrenic symptoms, such as hallucinations, delusions, and thought disorder.

Brain imaging studies in adolescents with early onset schizophrenia reveal progressive loss of cortical gray matter in temporal lobes, somatosensory and motor cortices, and the dorsolateral cortex (Figure 19-2). Of clinical concern is the loss of cortical tissue, which is evident by the time the individual seeks treatment and continues throughout the course of the illness despite the use of antipsychotic medication.[7] The progressive loss in frontal lobe volume is accompanied by increased severity of negative symptoms and further reductions in cognitive functioning. These results highlight the ineffectiveness of

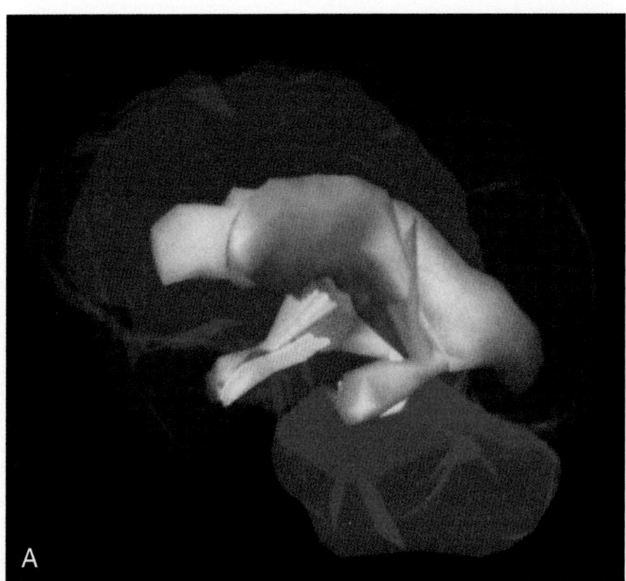

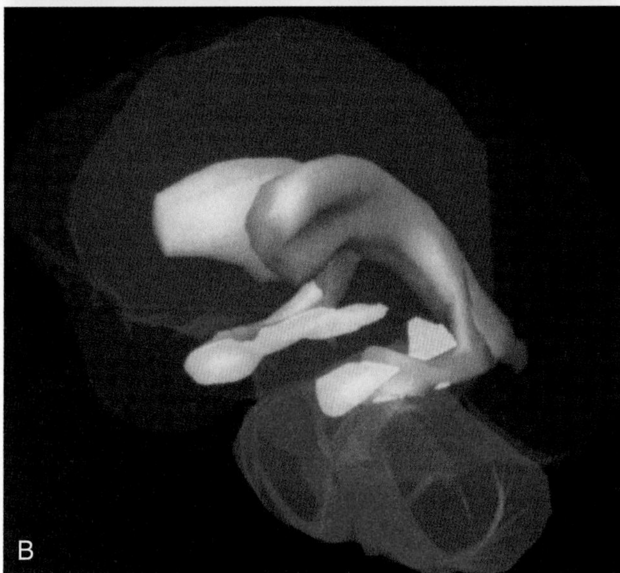

FIGURE 19-1 Magnetic Resonance Imaging (MRI) Comparison of Normal Brain and Brain with Schizophrenia. Three-dimensional MRI reconstructions showing **A,** the cerebroventricles *(gray regions)* and hippocampus *(yellow regions)* of a schizophrenic patient, and **B,** those of a healthy individual. Note the enlarged cerebroventricles and reduced hippocampal volume of the brain of the schizophrenic individual. (From Gershon ES, Rieder RO: *Sci Am* 267:128, 1992. Original illustrations by Nancy C. Andreason, University of Iowa.)

current medications for schizophrenia to attenuate or reverse the loss of frontal brain tissue.

Brain abnormalities in schizophrenia are believed to originate in the prenatal period of cell proliferation and migration. Reelin, an extracellular matrix protein involved in neuronal migration during development and in synaptic function during adulthood, is reduced in the prefrontal cortex and hippocampus of schizophrenic individuals.[8,9] Reelin is concentrated in interneurons that contain **gamma-aminobutyric acid (GABA),** the most widespread inhibitory neurotransmitter. Furthermore, in the dorsal prefrontal cortex of schizophrenic brains, the level of glutamic acid decarboxylase, the major enzyme in

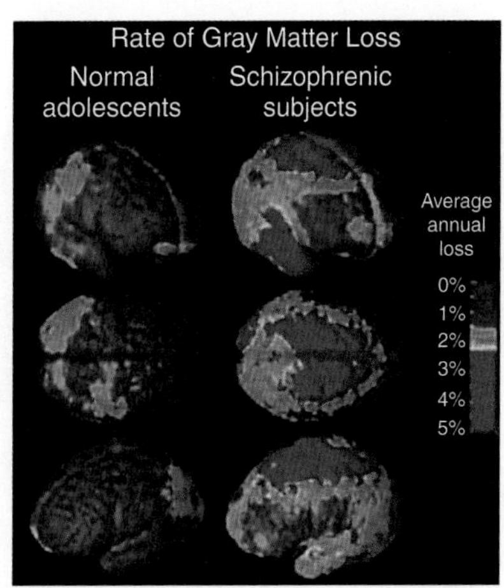

FIGURE 19-2 Accelerated Gray Matter Loss in Brains of Early Onset Schizophrenic Adolescents. Annual gray matter loss ranging from 2% to 5% was found in 13- to 18-year-old schizophrenics—compared with age-matched healthy adolescents. (From Thompson PM et al: *Proc Natl Acad Sci U S A* 98:11650, 2001.)

GABA biosynthesis, is reduced, which likely impairs normal cognitive/emotional functions.

Pathophysiologic changes in the dorsal prefrontal cortex are believed to contribute to the production of negative symptoms in schizophrenia (Figure 19-3). In particular, the **dorsolateral prefrontal cortex (DLPFC)** (Brodmann areas 9, 10, 46, 47) is intricately involved in the initiation and maintenance of goal-directed activities and in solving cognitive problems related to working memory. **Working memory** involves the brief storage and use of information to complete cognitive tasks such as language comprehension, learning, and reasoning. Blood flow and metabolism normally increase in the DLPFC during working memory processing but not in schizophrenics, who also perform poorly in tests of working memory. Thus the dorsolateral prefrontal cortex appears to be hypoactive in schizophrenia.

Neurotransmitter Alterations. The onset of schizophrenia was initially hypothesized to stem from abnormally high concentrations of the brain neurotransmitter dopamine. This **dopamine hypothesis** of schizophrenia was proposed on the basis of pharmacologic studies showing that antipsychotic drugs were potent blockers of brain dopamine receptors. A strong positive correlation was found between the clinical potencies of first-generation antipsychotic drugs (e.g., chlorpromazine, fluphenazine, and haloperidol) and their affinity for the dopamine D_2 receptor. In addition, drugs at high doses that dramatically increased dopaminergic transmission—such as levodopa (L-dopa), cocaine, and amphetamine—produced schizophrenic-like psychosis, which was reversed by dopamine blockers.

A current view of the dopamine hypothesis of schizophrenia is that brain dopamine pathways are altered in different ways (Figure 19-4). For example, the negative symptoms and cognitive alterations in schizophrenia are proposed to result from reduced dopaminergic neurotransmission in the mesocortical dopamine pathway.[10] This hypodopaminergic transmission in the prefrontal cortex contrasts with the hypothesized hyperdopaminergic secretion, in mesolimbic brain regions, which may

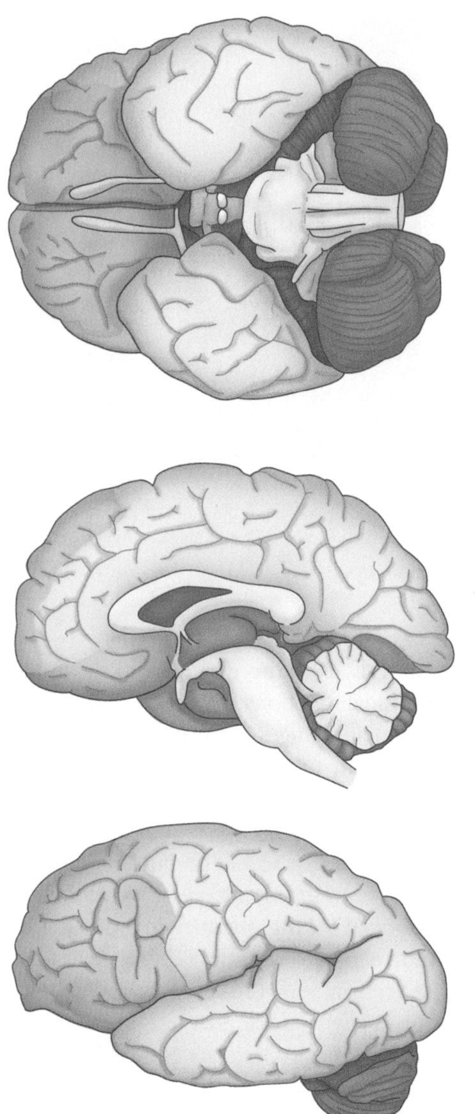

FIGURE 19-3 **The Prefrontal Cortex.** The prefrontal cortex consists of a dorsolateral *(blue)* and an orbitofrontal *(green)* region.

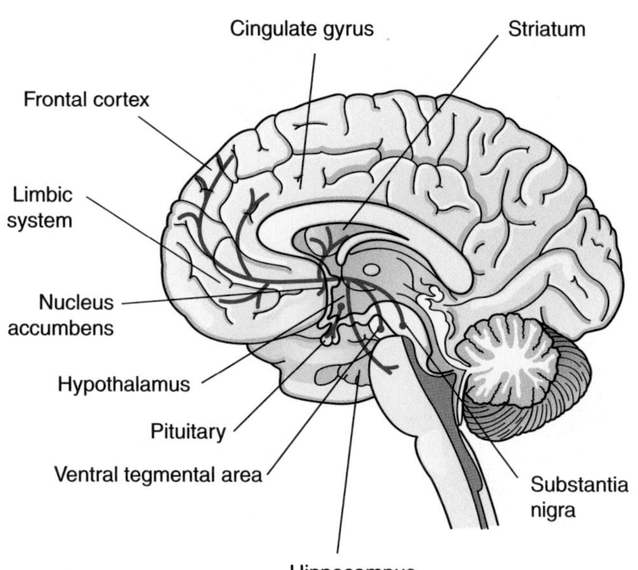

FIGURE 19-4 **The Dopamine System.** Dopamine cell bodies are located in the substantia nigra, where they project to the stratum (nigrostriatal pathway); and in the ventral tegmental area, where they project to the frontal and cingulate cortex (mesocortical pathway), the striatum, the hippocampus, and other limbic structures (mesolimbic pathway). Dopamine nuclei are also located in the hypothalamus and project to the pituitary.

contribute to the production of positive schizophrenic symptoms. The mesolimbic dopamine pathway innervates temporal lobe structures including the hippocampal formation and amygdala, as well as the nucleus accumbens and anterior cingulate cortex.

Another neurotransmitter system that may underlie the pathogenesis of schizophrenia is the excitatory neurotransmitter glutamate and its actions on the *N*-methyl-D-aspartate (NMDA) receptor subtype. The **glutamate hypothesis** of schizophrenia proposes that underactivation of glutamate receptors contributes to schizophrenia.[11] In schizophrenia, glutamate concentrations in the cerebrospinal fluid (CSF) are reduced along with a decrease in cortical glutamate synthesis. Furthermore, in unaffected individuals, blocking the glutamate NMDA receptor with antagonists, such as phencyclidine (PCP) and ketamine, facilitates the positive and negative symptoms of schizophrenia. PCP users report auditory hallucinations and disorientation, and may become violent from their delusions. In monkeys, chronic PCP treatment impairs cognitive performance in a test associated with prefrontal cortical damage.[12]

Clinical Manifestations

The symptoms of schizophrenia are currently divided into three broad categories of positive, negative, and cognitive symptoms (Box 19-1). *Positive symptoms* frequently occur during a **psychotic episode,** when an individual loses touch with reality and experiences something that should be absent (e.g., hallucinations). *Negative symptoms* are characterized by disruptions in normal emotional states and expressions. Cognitive symptoms are fairly common and involve problems with thought processes that severely impair the ability to perform routine daily tasks that involve attention, planning, and social skills. According to the *Diagnostic and Statistical Manual of Mental Disorders (DSM-IV-TR),*[13] schizophrenia is diagnosed when an individual exhibits delusions, hallucinations, negative symptoms, or social/occupational dysfunctions for at least 6 months and at least two of the common symptoms of the disorder—delusions, hallucinations, disorganized speech, disorganized or catatonic behavior, or presence of negative symptoms—must occur for 1 month (or less if successfully treated).

Psychotic Dimension

Psychotic dimension refers to hallucinations and delusions and reflects a person's confusion or loss of touch with the external world. Hallucinations and delusions are classified as positive symptoms and are the most common in schizophrenia.

Hallucinations. A **hallucination** is a perception experienced without external stimulation of the sense organs. Sensory hallucinations can be auditory, tactile, visual, gustatory, and olfactory. For example, the schizophrenic individual may hear

BOX 19-1 MAJOR SYMPTOMS OF SCHIZOPHRENIA

Positive Symptoms

Hallucinations
Auditory
Olfactory
Somatic-tactile
Visual
Voices commenting
Voices conversing

Delusions
Delusions of being controlled
Delusions of mind reading
Delusions of reference
Grandiosity
Guilt
Persecutory
Religious
Somatic
Thought broadcasting
Thought insertion
Thought withdrawal

Positive Formal Thought Disorder
Circumstantiality
Derailment
Distractible speech
Illogicality
Incoherence
Pressure of speech
Tangentiality

Bizarre Behavior
Aggressive, agitated
Clothing, appearance
Repetitive, stereotyped
Social, sexual behavior

Negative Symptoms

Affective Flattening
Affective nonresponsivity
Decreased spontaneous movements
Inappropriate affect
Lack of vocal inflections
Paucity of expressive gestures
Poor eye contact
Unchanging facial expression

Alogia
Blocking
Increase in response latency
Poverty of speech
Poverty of speech content

Anhedonia-Asociality
Few recreational interests
Few social relationships
Impaired intimacy
Little sexual interest

Attention
Social inattentiveness
Inattentiveness during testing

Avolition-Apathy
Impaired personal hygiene
Lack of persistence
Physical anergia

Cognitive Symptoms
Inability to understand information and make proper decision to complete a task
Difficulty paying attention
Problems with working memory or the inability to use recently learned information
Lack of insight

WHAT'S NEW?

Controversies in Mental Health Research

The *Diagnostic and Statistical Manual of Mental Disorders*—or *"DSM"* —is published by the American Psychiatric Association, and has been considered the authoritative guide to diagnosing mental disorders. First published in 1952, the *DSM* has undergone several revisions, and not until the 1980 publication of the *DSM-III* did the manual dramatically impact mental health professionals, including psychiatrists, clinical psychologists, social workers, and nurses. The *DSM-III* became known as the "bible of psychiatry" because it introduced a new set of criteria to standardize the diagnoses of mental disorders by categorizing symptoms presumably unique to each mental illness, such as schizophrenia and bipolar disorder. This categorical symptom approach stimulated research on the etiology and pathophysiology of diverse mental disorders and began to impact public health policy, education, and reimbursement decisions made by insurance companies. Modest categorical changes were subsequently made in the 1994 edition of *DSM-IV* and a text revision of *DSM-IV*, called *DSM-IV-TR*, was published in 2000.

The highly anticipated *DSM-5* published in 2013 and represents the culmination of more than 10 years of revision work involving more than 1500 experts in the psychiatric, psychologic, psychiatric nursing, pediatric, neurologic, social work, and related disciplines from 39 countries. Users familiar with earlier *DSM* versions will encounter two major changes in *DMS-5*. One major change includes reordering the chapters based on the relatedness of disorders in terms of similar underlying vulnerabilities and symptoms. This change in each chapter is intended to align the *DMS-5* with the *World Health Organization's International Classification of Diseases*, ed 11, in order to further facilitate communication and diagnosis of disorders.

The second major change is to replace the multiaxial system of diagnosis with a nonaxial documentation by combining the former Axes I, II, and III with separate notations for psychosocial and contextual factors (formerly Axis IV) and disability (formerly Axis V). Notably, the *DSM-5* will not increase the number of mental disorders; instead, fewer disorders will be found in *DSM-5* than in *DSM-IV*. However, any change by *DSM* in the diagnosis of mental health that defines "normal" behavior will be of concern, especially by advocacy groups and insurance companies. For example, one controversial change in the *DSM-5* will be to potentially diagnose any child over the age of 6 who displays irritability or frequent angry outbursts with "disruptive mood dysregulation disorder." This new diagnosis was included to provide parents or caregivers the opportunity to plan interventions for children who exhibit problems controlling their emotions. However, advocacy groups questioned whether such a diagnosis would stigmatize children and may lead to unnecessary drug prescriptions. Another change is a grief and depression diagnosis. Whereas previous *DSM* versions prevented a diagnosis of depression in a person grieving the death of a loved one, the *DMS-5* will allow depression diagnoses in the bereaved. The rationale was to provide those with chronic grief to be diagnosed with, and obtain treatment for, depression. However, some healthcare professionals questioned whether diagnosing normal grieving as depression is necessary at all, as in the previous *DSM*.

Although the new *DSM-5* is expected to be used by many clinicians for diagnosing and treating mental disorders, some prominent researchers and clinicians have begun to question the way mental illnesses are currently viewed by categorizing and diagnosing symptoms. In particular, the current categorical symptom diagnoses guide to mental disorders does not guarantee effective treatment. A patient may exhibit multiple symptoms that overlap with a diagnosis for different disorders and that may explain why specific clinical treatment will not always relieve or temper mental illness. What appears to be missing in our present understanding of mental disorders are the causes and underlying brain mechanisms that trigger the onset of the illness.

To address this issue, Dr. Thomas Insel, Director of the National Institute of Mental Health, and other prominent scientists are hoping to steer psychiatric research away from classifying symptoms to a fundamental approach of identifying the genes, molecules, and pathophysiologic brain circuits that cause mental disorders. To do so, Dr. Insel started a federal project called Research Domain Criteria to fund research that investigates the biologic basis, and not the symptom categories, of mental disorders. Research projects are beginning to unravel brain functions that broadly implicate neural systems linked to memory, fear, anhedonia, and stress, which affect many people with mental illness. Future treatments that target pathophysiologic neural systems with new drugs or with cognitive-behavioral methods may be more beneficial to psychiatric patients than currently available treatments for psychiatric symptoms.

Data from Adam D: *Nature* 496:416–418, 2013; American Psychiatric Association: www.dsm5.org; Halter MJ et al: *J Psychosoc Nurs* 51:30–39, 2013; Insel TR et al: *Neurosci Biobehav Rev* (in press); Stringaris A: *J Child Psychol Psychiatr* 54:501, 2013.

voices, experience touch or electrical sensations, report images of animate and inanimate objects, or complain of unpleasant tastes and odors. These hallucinations may occur alone or together.

Delusions. A **delusion** is a persistent belief contrary to the educational and cultural background of the individual. Delusions may involve grandiose, nihilistic, persecutory, somatic, sexual, and religious themes. Paranoid beliefs are common and may involve spying, conspiracy, persecution, and ridicule. Delusions also may be referential in that particular stimuli or events become highly personalized, such as believing a television talk show host is directing information specifically at them.

Disorganized Behavior

Disorganized behavior includes disorganized speech and disorganized or bizarre behavior. Incongruity of affect is another dimension of disorganized behavior.

Disorganized Speech. A common form of disorganized speech is **formal thought disorder,** which involves fluent speech that is difficult to comprehend. The speech often moves from one topic to another unexpectedly (loose associations) and illogically and the person becomes easily distracted when talking.

Another form of disorganized speech is called **poverty of content.** Here, the use of vocabularies to convey information is severely retarded despite a fair amount of spoken words. For instance, the same phrases are used repeatedly throughout a conversation.

Disorganized Behavior. Disorganized (or bizarre) behavior is the conceptual equivalent of disorganized speech. The individual has difficulty engaging in goal-directed activities. Repetitive (e.g., stereotyped rocking) or aimless behavior and poor personal hygiene are exhibited. Another feature is the incongruity of affect or the manifestation of inappropriate situational affect as exemplified by hostility without provocation or childlike silliness in sober situations.

Negative Dimensions

Negative dimensions reflect a deficit in normal functioning and are characterized by affective flattening, anhedonia, alogia (poverty of speech), and avolition. **Affective flattening** is the near absence of emotional or facial expressions throughout a conversation or in different situations. In **anhedonia,** individuals are unable to experience emotions such as pleasure or pain and report a sense of detachment from the environment. **Alogia** is the absence of spontaneous speech production for the purpose of answering questions or expressing oneself. **Avolition** is a deficit in spontaneous or goal-directed behavior, such as completing simple daily tasks.

Treatment

The use of chlorpromazine in the mid-1950s dramatically altered the treatment of schizophrenia, which previously required extensive institutional hospitalization. The drug was especially effective in reducing positive symptoms such as hallucinations and delusions as well as thought disorders and hyperactivity. The beneficial effects of chlorpromazine and similar first-generation antipsychotic drugs like haloperidol on positive symptoms were believed to stem from their ability to block the dopamine D_2-receptor subtype, especially in the overly active mesolimbic dopamine pathways.

BOX 19-2 MEDICATIONS USED IN THE TREATMENT OF SCHIZOPHRENIA

GENERIC NAME	BRAND NAME
Conventional Antipsychotics	
Chlorpromazine	Thorazine
Fluphenazine	Prolixin
Haloperidol	Haldol
Perphenazine	Trilafon
Pimozide	Orap
Prochlorperazine	Compazine
Thioridazine	Mellaril
Thiothixene	Navane
Trifluoperazine	Stelazine
Second-Generation Atypical Antipsychotics	
Aripiprazole	Abilify
Clozapine	Clozaril
Loxapine	Loxitane
Molindone	Moban
Olanzapine	Zyprexa
Paliperidone	Invega
Quetiapine	Seroquel
Risperidone	Risperdal
Ziprasidone	Geodon

However, D_2-receptor blockade, such as in the striatum, produces a notable neurologic side effect resembling Parkinson disease—a disorder associated with degeneration of dopamine cell bodies in the substantia nigra that project to the striatum. A related side effect of conventional antipsychotics that develops in 15% to 20% of schizophrenics after several years of treatment is a condition called **tardive dyskinesia.** This condition is characterized by tic-like jerky movements, such as smacking the lips or flicking the tongue, unsteady gait, or rocking back and forth when seated. Other side effects may include sedation, hypotension, akathisia (motor restlessness), constipation, weight gain, amenorrhea, and, less frequently, hepatotoxicity and electrocardiographic changes.

Although the majority of schizophrenic individuals obtained some positive symptom relief from the first-generation or conventional antipsychotics, approximately 20% failed to respond to D_2-blocking drugs (Box 19-2), especially those with pronounced symptoms of apathy, disorientation, and social withdrawal. However, some of these treatment-resistant individuals responded to a second generation of drugs that became known as atypical antipsychotic drugs.[14] Atypical antipsychotics also were shown to have superior efficacy in reducing not only the positive but also the negative symptoms in comparison with conventional antipsychotics. For example, clozapine improve some cognitive functions (such as verbal fluency, verbal learning, and memory) and some physical functions (such as psychomotor speed). In addition, the notable neurologic side effects that accompany the use of the conventional antipsychotics were diminished.

Unlike conventional antipsychotics, atypical drugs appear to work by blocking a range of neurotransmitter receptors. For example, clozapine blocks not only D_2 receptors but also D_1, D_3, D_4, and D_5 receptors and serotonin (5-hydroxytryptamine, i.e., HT_2, 5-HT_6, 5-HT_7); norepinephrine; and cholinergic and histamine receptors. Risperidone and ziprasidone have higher affinity for blocking 5-HT_2 than D_2 receptors. The higher 5-HT_2/D_2-receptor–binding ratio of atypical antipsychotics in comparison with conventional drugs may reflect a normalization of serotonin-dopamine interactions leading to clinical efficacy not observed with D_2-receptor blockade alone.

Atypical antipsychotics are not without adverse effects, most notably metabolic abnormalities including regulation of glucose and lipid levels and weight gain. For example, long-term clozapine or olazapine treatment increases body weight gain, which becomes a risk factor for diabetes and cardiovascular disease. Schizophrenics treated with clozapine also are at risk of developing **agranulocytosis,** a potentially lethal blood disorder involving the loss of white blood cells and a compromised immune system.

In conjunction with antipsychotic medication, psychosocial therapy can facilitate the management of schizophrenia. Psychosocial relationships assist the individual in developing coping strategies and in identifying stressors and relapse symptoms. Cognitive-behavioral therapy (CBT), a talking therapy that initiates cognitive and behavioral change based on an individualized reappraisal of the person's faulty beliefs, is effective in treating schizophrenics with stabilized antipsychotic medications.[15] An important benefit of psychosocial and family support is the encouragement of compliance with antipsychotic medication that requires a period before the emergence of clinical efficacy.

MOOD DISORDERS: DEPRESSION AND BIPOLAR DISORDER

Mood refers to a sustained emotional state as opposed to brief emotional feelings, which are termed *affective states.* Healthy individuals are normally capable of experiencing a variety of affective states including euphoria, joy, surprise, fear, sadness, anxiety, and depression. When emotional states, such as sadness, become chronic and uncontrollable, individuals may be diagnosed with a mood disorder called *depression.* The two major classifications of mood disorder are: (1) unipolar or major depressive disorder, also known as *major depression* or *clinical depression,* which consists of episodes of depression; and (2) **bipolar disorder,** which is further classified into bipolar I and bipolar II disorders. Bipolar I disorder features manic episodes and at least one major depressive episode and bipolar II disorder is characterized by recurrent major depressive episodes with one or more hypomanic (milder than manic) episodes. Box 19-3 presents the major criteria of depression and bipolar disorder according to the American Psychiatric Association's *DSM-IV-TR.*[13]

Major (unipolar) depression is the most common mood disorder and the leading cause of disability in the United States and throughout the world. Unipolar depression appears in all age groups including young children. In the United States, the lifetime prevalence rate of depression is 16.2% of the population with a twofold greater risk in women than men after adolescence. In children and adolescents, 2% to 6% suffer from depression. The prevalence of bipolar disorder ranges from 3% to 5% in the general population. Bipolar I disorder occurs equally in men and women in comparison with bipolar II disorder, which afflicts more women than men. When left untreated, a number of depressed and bipolar individuals are at risk of developing a host of medical illnesses, including cardiovascular disease, obesity, diabetes, and thyroid disease.

BOX 19-3 MAJOR SYMPTOMS OF DEPRESSION AND MANIA

Symptoms of Depression*

- Depressed or irritable mood
- Loss of interests and pleasure
- Significant (>5%) weight gain or loss in a month
- Insomnia or hypersomnia
- Psychomotor agitation or retardation
- Fatigue or loss of energy
- Feelings of worthlessness or excessive guilt
- Poor concentration or indecisiveness
- Recent thoughts of death or suicide

Symptoms of Manic Episode†

- Elevated mood
- Irritable mood
- Inflated self-esteem
- Decreased need for sleep
- Excessive talking
- Racing/crowded thoughts
- Distractibility
- Increase in goal-directed activity
- Excessive risky activities

*Five or more of the symptoms are present in a 2-week period and at least one of the symptoms is either depressed mood or loss of interests or pleasure.

†Three or more symptoms (four if the mood is only irritable) during a distinct period of abnormally and persistently elevated, expansive, or irritable mood occurring for at least 1 week.

Etiology and Pathophysiology

Genetic Predisposition and Environmental Influences

Family and twin studies indicate a strong basis for mood disorders. Using *DSM-III* or *DSM-III-R* criteria, concordance rates for bipolar disorder ranged up to 62% and 42% for monozygotic and dizygotic twins, respectively.[16] For unipolar disorder, concordance rates of 62% and 28% were reported in monozygotic and dizygotic twins, respectively. Even among adoptees with a biologic family history of mood disorders, the incidence of developing major depression or manic-depressive illness is higher than among control adoptees. The strong tendency for mood disorders to run in families has encouraged a search for the abnormal gene or genes. Interestingly, loci on chromosomes 18 and 22 have been linked to both bipolar disorder and schizophrenia. Bipolar individuals, who may exhibit psychotic behavior, have deficits in reelin expression linked to genetic loci, located on chromosome 22, which confers susceptibility to schizophrenia (see preceding section on schizophrenia, p. 642). However, the large variation in clinical symptoms suggests that developmental and environmental factors are as important as genetic factors in contributing to the etiology of mood disorders.

A current view of mood disorders is that the illness stems from a complex interplay between susceptible genes and environmental influences. For example, the interplay between life stressors and a potentially dysfunctional serotonin (5-HT) system appears to elevate the risk of depression.[17] Researchers have identified a polymorphic variant of the serotonin transporter (5-HT-T) that exists either as a short *(s)* allele or as a long *(l)* allele. The serotonin transporter serves in the reuptake of serotonin at the synapse and may moderate the serotonergic response to stress. However, individuals with two copies of the *s* allele were more likely to develop major depression and have suicidal thoughts in response to stressful events than individuals homozygous for the *l* allele. In addition, among individuals who carry two *s* alleles, the risk of a major depressive episode increased twofold after experiencing four or more stressful events. This work[17] suggests that exposure to both adverse life events and a genetic alteration in 5-HT function increases the risk of developing major depression.

Neurochemical Dysregulation

Modern theories of mood disorders began with the important observations that drugs such as imipramine that elevated norepinephrine levels within the synapse reduced depression whereas drugs that depleted monoamine levels (e.g., reserpine) increased depression. These studies led to the dominant **monoamine hypothesis of depression,** in which a deficit in the concentration of brain norepinephrine, dopamine, and/or serotonin is the underlying cause of depression, in contrast to mania, which results from elevated concentrations of monoamines. Three major classes of antidepressant drugs were initially developed and included monoamine oxidase inhibitors (MAOIs), tricyclic antidepressants (TCAs), and selective serotonin reuptake inhibitors (SSRIs). These antidepressants shared the common property, albeit through different mechanisms, that increasing monoamine neurotransmitter levels within the synapse is the basis for their antidepressant effects (Figure 19-5).

Additional support for the monoamine hypothesis of depression came from studies showing a reduction of monoamine metabolites in the cerebral spinal fluid (CSF) of depressed people. Other work demonstrated that dietary depletion of tryptophan, the precursor of serotonin synthesis, or alpha-methylparatyrosine (AMPT), a drug that inhibits dopamine and norepinephrine synthesis, produced a rapid return to depression in individuals successfully treated with antidepressants.[18]

Neuroendocrine Dysregulation

Stress and Hypothalamic-Pituitary-Adrenal System Dysregulation. The hypothalamic-pituitary-adrenal (HPA) system plays an essential role in an individual's ability to cope with stress (see Chapter 11). However, chronic activation of the HPA system and elevated glucocorticoid secretion are found in a large percentage (30% to 70%) of people with major depression, suggesting that mechanisms responsible for increased HPA hormone secretion contribute to the pathophysiology of depression.[19] Notably, antidepressant drugs effective in normalizing the HPA system are associated with a good clinical response, whereas persistent dysregulation of the HPA system is related to continued depression or relapse.

Uncontrollable stress activates not only the HPA system but also the immune system, which may further contribute to the development of depression. Psychosocial stress-induced activation of the immune system increases secretion of proinflammatory cytokines, such as interleukin-1α (IL-1α) and IL-β, tumor necrosis factor-alpha (TNF-α), and IL-6, which modulates signaling pathways throughout the periphery and brain and augments further secretion of HPA hormones and monoamine metabolism. A potential consequence of prolonged cytokine-induced activation is dysregulation in feedback and feed-forward control mechanisms of the HPA system, leading to chronic elevations in cortisol level, as observed in major depression. Persistent elevations in cortisol level also may induce immunosuppression that compromises the body's immune systems to control inflammation and infectious diseases. Increasing evidence suggests that inflammation is another risk factor that triggers the onset of depression. For example, inflammation is a significant contributor to coronary heart disease and the prevalence of comorbid depression in people with heart disease is threefold higher than that in the general population.[20]

Increasing evidence from animal models of stress-induced depression shows that depression-like behavior is accompanied by atrophy of neurons in the hippocampus, a reduction in the development of new hippocampal neurons (i.e., **neurogenesis**), and a deficit in hippocampal **brain-derived neurotrophic factor (BDNF)** levels.[21,22] Consistent with animal studies, human postmortem work indicates low hippocampal BDNF levels in depression. Because the growth factor BDNF supports the survival of neurons and facilitates neurogenesis from hippocampal stem cells, a neurotrophic hypothesis of depression has been proposed as an extension of the monoamine hypothesis of depression to broadly account for the pathophysiologic basis of depression. That is, stress-induced depression and the accompanying reduction in levels of monoamines are caused by deficits in neurogenesis and BDNF levels. Of clinical relevance, administration of antidepressants to animals reverses the depression-like state and increases the development of neurogenesis and BDNF levels (see What's New? Hippocampal Neurogenesis and the Glucocorticoid Receptor Play Essential Roles in Deterring Depression).

Hypothalamic-Pituitary-Thyroid System Dysregulation. Approximately 20% to 30% of persons with major depression have an altered hypothalamic-pituitary-thyroid (HPT) system. These individuals exhibit increased CSF levels of thyrotropin-releasing hormone (TRH), blunted thyroid-stimulating hormone (TSH) response to TRH challenge, and decreased nocturnal rise in TSH level that normally occurs between midnight and the early morning hours.[23] Persistent blunting of the TSH response to TRH is associated with an increased

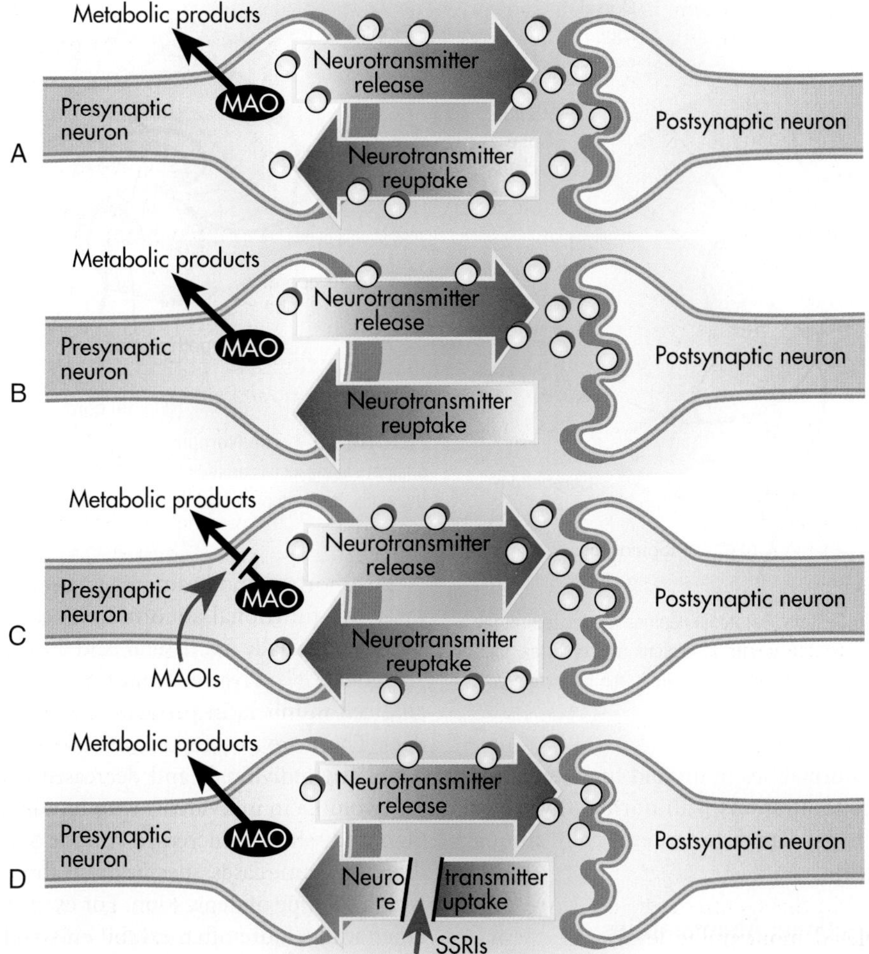

FIGURE 19-5 Schematic Diagrams Showing the Sites of Actions of Antidepressants and Their Effects on Neurotransmitter Levels. **A,** In healthy individuals an action potential generated in the presynaptic neuron results in neurotransmitter release into the synapse. Some neurotransmitters bind to receptors on the postsynaptic neuron that leads to activation of second messenger systems (not shown). Neurotransmitters are also removed from the synapse by reuptake into the presynaptic neuron and deaminated by monoamine oxidase *(MAO)*. **B,** In depressed individuals, neurotransmitter levels are hypothesized to be reduced. The mechanisms responsible for this reduction are not understood. **C,** MAO inhibitors act by preventing the degradation of neurotransmitters, such as norepinephrine and serotonin. As a result, neurotransmitter levels are elevated. **D,** The tricyclic antidepressants (TCAs) and selective serotonin reuptake inhibitors *(SSRIs)* act by reducing the uptake of neurotransmitters from the synapse, leading to increased neurotransmitter levels. TCAs, such as nortriptyline and desipramine, tend to block norepinephrine reuptake, whereas amitriptyline and imipramine also have effects on serotonin reuptake. SSRIs are highly effective in blocking serotonin reuptake.

WHAT'S NEW?

Hippocampal Neurogenesis and the Glucocorticoid Receptor Play Essential Roles in Deterring Depression

The hippocampus contains glucocorticoid receptors that play a negative feedback role in modulating the inhibition of the HPA hormone system. Chronic stress induces a persistent elevation in secretion of the glucocorticoid cortisol and may precipitate depression as well as a reduction in hippocampal neurogenesis. However, the specific effects of hippocampal neurogenesis on depression are not well understood. Two recent studies examined the role of hippocampal neurogenesis in depression. One study reported that hippocampal neurogenesis–deficient mice were more likely to exhibit increases in depression-like behavior and deficits in glucocorticoid negative feedback in comparison to control mice. The results suggest an essential role of hippocampal neurogenesis in dampening stress-induced HPA hormone secretion and buffering the effects of stress on depression. The other study examined whether hippocampal glucocorticoid receptors are involved in antidepressant-induced stimulation of neurogenesis. Using human hippocampal progenitor cells, the antidepressant sertraline was found to increase neuronal differentiation via a glucocorticoid receptor–dependent mechanism. Furthermore, drugs that block the actions of the glucocorticoid receptor reduced the effects of sertraline on progenitor cell proliferation. The results of this study highlight a role of the glucocorticoid receptor in the antidepressant-induced facilitation of hippocampal neurogenesis in humans.

Data from Anacker et al: *Mol Psychiatry* 16:738–750, 2011; Snyder JS et al: *Nature* 476:458–461, 2011.

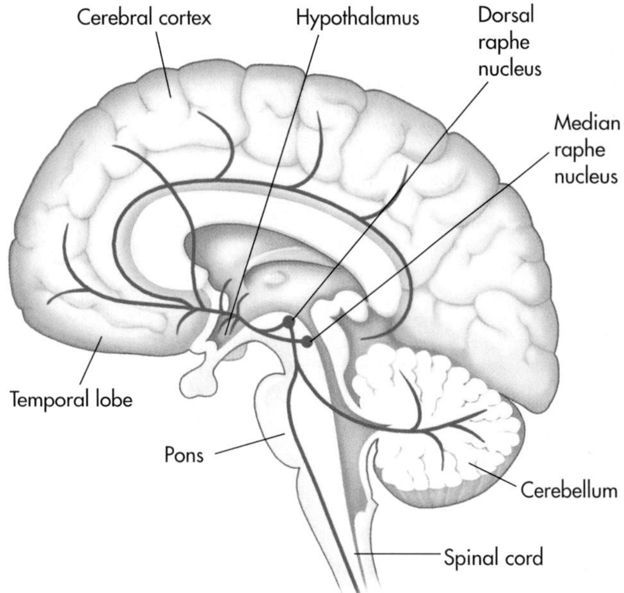

FIGURE 19-6 The Serotonin System. Serotonin neurons are located in the brainstem raphe nuclei. They project diffusely to all regions of the cortex, temporolimbic regions, hypothalamus, basal ganglia, cerebellum, the brainstem, and spinal cord.

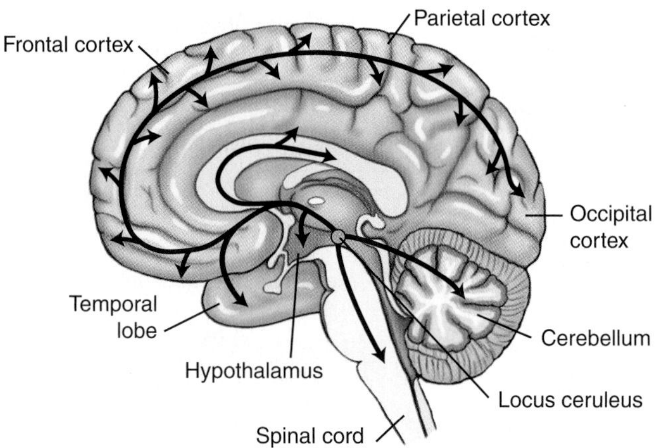

FIGURE 19-7 The Norepinephrine System. The norepinephrine cell bodies originate in the locus ceruleus and project throughout the brain, including the hypothalamus, the temporal lobe, the entire cortex, the cerebellum, and spinal cord.

probability of relapse. Abnormalities in thyroid function, such as increased basal TSH concentrations with normal thyroxine levels, also are observed in bipolar disorder, especially among individuals with rapid cycling.

Neuroanatomic and Functional Abnormalities

The dorsal and median raphe nuclei, located in the central gray of the caudal mesencephalon and rostral pons, contain a large group of serotonin-synthesizing neurons that project extensively to all regions of the cortex, basal ganglia, limbic system, hypothalamus, cerebellum, and brainstem (Figure 19-6). Postmortem and/or brain imaging studies of depressed individuals revealed a widespread decrease in serotonin 5-HT_{1A} receptor subtype binding in the frontal, temporal, and limbic cortex as well as serotonin transporter binding in the cerebral cortex and hippocampus. Mood disorders in some people may reflect a dysfunctional raphe-serotonin system, which normally modulates homeostasis, emotionality, and tolerance to aversive experiences.

A group of norepinephrine-containing cells located in the locus ceruleus of the rostral pons project to vast areas of the forebrain, brainstem, and spinal cord (Figure 19-7). The locus ceruleus–norepinephrine system is implicated in global psychologic processes including attention, vigilance, and orientation to novel, aversive, or threatening stimuli. Activation of the locus ceruleus–norepinephrine system is also capable of inhibiting the raphe-serotonin system, suggesting an indirect role in modulating serotonin functions. Norepinephrine receptor alterations (e.g., α- and β-adrenergic receptor subtypes) are found in the frontal cortex of some suicide victims with major depression. Alterations in norepinephrine systems may be linked to attention or concentration difficulties as well as sleep and arousal disturbances in depression.

Postmortem and brain imaging studies further reveal structural and functional abnormalities associated with mood disorders, especially in frontal and limbic regions such as the amygdala.[24,25] Postmortem studies report a reduction in glial cell numbers in people with unipolar and bipolar disorders. There are also reports of reduced frontal lobe volume in depressed individuals and decreased or asymmetric temporal lobe volume in individuals with bipolar illness and depression. One study showed increased volume of the amygdala in bipolar illness. In some cases, specific brain abnormalities are associated with a subtype of depression. For example, late onset depressed older adults more often exhibit enlarged lateral ventricles than midlife depressed individuals, depressed older adults with an early age of illness, or bipolar individuals.

Functional neuroimaging studies indicate decreased cerebral blood flow and glucose metabolism in the dorsolateral and dorsomedial prefrontal cortex of individuals affected by major depression or bipolar disorder. Dorsolateral prefrontal abnormalities in depression may be responsible for the retardation in cognitive processing and speech deficits similar to those found in schizophrenia. Dorsomedial frontal dysfunction may be associated with mnemonic and attentional impairments that accompany mood disorders. Other frontocortical regions, including the ventrolateral, ventromedial, and orbital areas, exhibit increased blood flow and metabolism in unipolar depression (Figure 19-8). These frontal brain areas have extensive interconnections with the amygdala, and increased blood flow and metabolism, especially in the right amygdala, is positively related to negative affect in depressed individuals. These functional changes in brain activity begin to normalize with successful antidepressant treatments, suggesting they are state rather than trait related.

Clinical Manifestations

Depression

Major **depression** is characterized by unremitting feelings of sadness and despair (see Box 19-3). The **dysphoric mood** or intensely painful mood is accompanied frequently by insomnia, loss of appetite and body weight, and reduced interest in

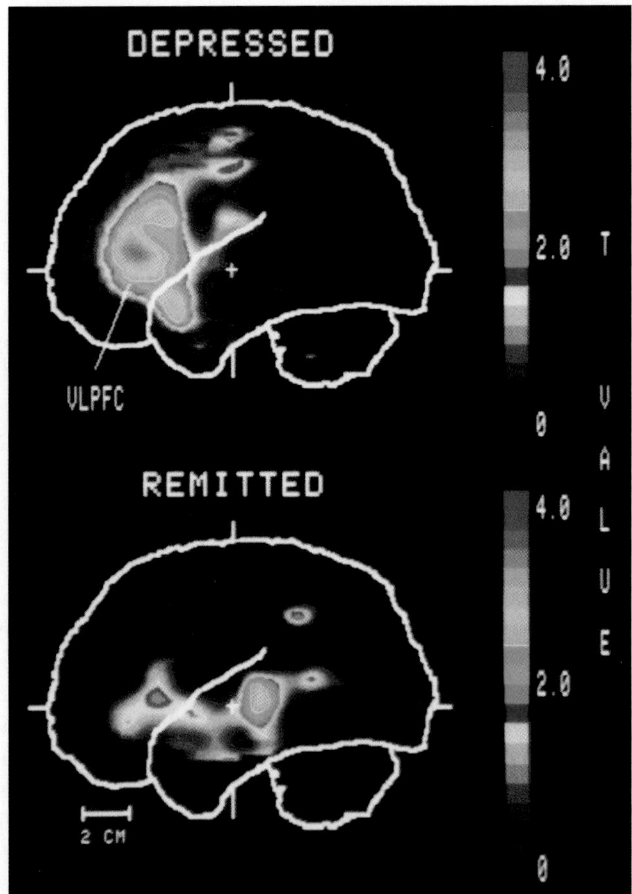

FIGURE 19-8 **Positron-Emission Tomography (PET) Comparison of Brain Activity in Depression and in Remittance.** PET scan showing increased activity in the left prefrontal cortex in a depressed person but not in the remitted person. *VLPFC,* Ventrolateral prefrontal cortex. (From Drevets WC et al: *J Neurosci* 12:3628, 1992. Copyright ©1992 by the Society for Neuroscience.)

pleasurable activities and interpersonal relationships. Sleep disturbances may include difficulty in initially falling asleep and awakening in the middle of the night, lying awake for several hours with an inability to subsequently fall asleep. Individuals may have reduced motor activity and suffer marked fatigue. Others complain of restlessness and agitation. Feelings of worthlessness and guilt are common, and pessimistic or negative outcomes are often perceived even in routine situations. The ability to function (e.g., work) and concentrate is greatly diminished. Depressive episodes may occur or recur suddenly or gradually and continue from a few weeks to months, and 20% may exhibit a chronic form of depression.

Suicidal risk increases in depression. Factors such as living alone or being divorced, having a prior history of drug abuse or suicide attempt, or having depression at midlife or older ages contribute to suicide in 10% to 15% of depressed individuals.

Bipolar Disorder: Mania

Manic individuals experience elevated levels of euphoria and self-esteem and feelings of grandiosity. Energy levels are greatly enhanced even after only a few hours of sleep each night. The increased energy, however, does not lead to organized plans and thoughts. The individual may show poor judgment in spending money, may become hypersexual, or may make poor business commitments. Other hallmarks of mania are excessive, rapid, loud, and pressured speech. The manic person frequently skips from one topic of conversation to another and is easily distracted both when speaking and when performing tasks. Approximately 50% of manic individuals develop psychotic symptoms, such as delusions or hallucinations, which require hospitalization. The onset and termination of manic symptoms (see Box 19-3) are usually abrupt and may last for a few days or months followed by depression. The risk of recurrence of bipolar disorder is high, especially without immediate treatment.

Treatment

Depression

Approximately 80% of depressed persons will respond to antidepressant drugs such as MAOIs, TCAs, and SSRIs (Box 19-4); psychotherapy; or a combination of both treatment modalities. Although SSRIs have become the standard first-line treatment for major depression, initial selection of an antidepressant often includes an assessment of the person's symptoms and age as well as the side effects, safety, cost, and convenience of the prescribed medication. For example, medications that produce sedation may be helpful for the treatment of sleep disturbances. Approximately 50% of depressed individuals may not show a favorable response during initial treatment to an antidepressant drug, and 10% to 20% may continue to exhibit symptoms after 2 years. Individuals who are nonresponsive to a specific antidepressant during a 2-month period may be given another antidepressant medication. Atypical antidepressants, such as nefazodone, trazodone, and mirtazapine, presumably produce their clinical effects by blocking specific receptors (e.g., 5-HT_{2A}). A new generation of antidepressants that selectively block serotonin and norepinephrine reuptake is available in the United States (e.g., venlafaxine) and Europe (i.e., milnacipran, reboxetine). At present, there are no criteria to determine whether selection of the next antidepressant will be efficacious. Among children and adolescents, only fluoxetine is currently approved for use in children by the U.S. Food and Drug Administration (FDA)[26] (see What's New? Comprehensive Treatment of Risk Factors May Promote Resilience and Rapid Recovery from Depression).

In bipolar depression, antidepressant medications may lead to cycle acceleration or induction of mania. However, SSRIs and bupropion may be less likely to induce these effects than MAOIs or TCAs.

A number of side effects are reported with MAOIs, TCAs, and SSRIs. Commonly reported side effects of MAOIs include sedation or agitation, insomnia, dry mouth, impotence, and weight gain. MAOIs also may induce acute and heightened elevations in blood pressure (e.g., hypertensive crisis) after intake of tyramine-rich foods, such as aged cheeses, sour cream, pods of broad beans, pickled herring, liver, canned figs, raisins, and avocados. In addition, MAOI interactions with TCAs, SSRIs, stimulants, and over-the-counter flu medications are dangerous and should be avoided. Because of these adverse side effect issues, MAOIs are used less often than other antidepressants.

BOX 19-4 FDA-APPROVED MEDICATIONS USED IN THE TREATMENT OF DEPRESSION AND ANXIETY DISORDERS

GENERIC NAME	BRAND NAME
Monoamine Oxidase Inhibitors	
Isocarboxazid	Marplan
Phenelzine	Nardil
Tranylcypromine	Parnate
Selegiline	Emsam
Tricyclics	
Amitriptyline	Elavil
Amoxapine	Asendin
Clomipramine	Anafranil
Desipramine	Norpramin, Pertofrane
Doxepin	Adapin, Sinequan
Imipramine	Tofranil
Maprotiline	Ludiomil
Nortriptyline	Aventyl, Pamelor
Protriptyline	Vivactil
Trimipramine	Surmontil
Selective Serotonin Reuptake Inhibitors	
Citalopram	Celexa
Escitalopram	Lexapro
Fluoxetine	Prozac
Fluvoxamine	Luvox
Paroxetine	Paxil
Sertraline	Zoloft
Serotonin and Norepinephrine Reuptake Inhibitors	
Desvenlafaxine	Pristiq
Duloxetine	Cymbalta
Venlafaxine	Effexor
Serotonin Reuptake Inhibitor and 5-HT$_{1A}$ Receptor Partial Agonist	
Vilazodone	Viibryd
Norepinephrine and Specific Serotonergic Modulator	
Mirtazapine	Remeron
Norepinephrine–Dopamine Reuptake Inhibitor	
Bupropion	Wellbutrin
Serotonin Modulator	
Nefazodone	Serzone
Trazodone	Desyrel

TCAs may produce sedation, insomnia, orthostatic hypotension, seizures, and weight gain. Some TCAs have moderate anticholinergic side effects, including constipation, urinary hesitancy or retention, dry mouth, blurred vision, and memory impairment. These side effects may be an issue when considering TCA treatment of older adults, in which case the TCAs desipramine and nortriptyline may be preferred because of their reduced anticholinergic, cardiovascular, and sedating effects.

Common side effects of SSRIs include sleep disturbances (e.g., insomnia) and nausea. However, agitation, allergic skin reactions, dry mouth, anxiety, altered appetite, and sexual dysfunction have been reported. Unlike MAOIs and TCAs, SSRIs do not have pronounced effects on the cardiovascular or cholinergic systems. SSRIs are potent inhibitors of cytochrome P-450 isoenzymes, which are involved in drug metabolism. Therefore, SSRIs may lead to dangerous elevations in blood concentrations of other psychiatric medications when taken together. SSRIs should not be taken with MAOIs or immediately after discontinuing MAOI treatment. A serotonin syndrome characterized by excitement or autonomic hyperactivity, abdominal pain, rigidity, and hyperthermia may develop, leading to coma or death.

Side effects of atypical antidepressants may include sedation, dry mouth, weight gain, and constipation. Nefazodone and trazodone have been associated with hepatic toxicity. Venlafaxine and reboxetine lack many of the serious side effects associated with TCAs; however, sweating, dry mouth, and some sedation may occur.

Electroconvulsive therapy (ECT) is used when individuals fail to respond to antidepressants or when they are severely depressed, pregnant, suicidal, or psychotic. ECT effectively alleviates depressive symptoms in about 50% to 80% of people, who may then begin to respond to antidepressant medications. Although the mechanism of action of ECT is not clear, the procedure is known to produce alterations in monoamine systems. Deep brain stimulation (DBS) is another treatment showing promise to alleviate major depression in people resistant to current antidepressant medications, ECT, and psychotherapy.[27,28] The treatment involves implanting electrodes during neurosurgery into the subcallosal cingulate gyrus (SCG [Brodmann area 25 and parts of 24 and 32]) and attaching them to an implanted pulse generator through subcutaneous extension wires. This SCG region is targeted because abnormal SCG brain activity, a suggested pathophysiologic cause of major depression, is reversed by effective antidepressant treatment. A 3- to 6-year follow-up study of 20 treatment-resistant depressed individuals who received DBS in the SCG found that more than half eventually returned to work and improved their quality of life.[29]

Bipolar Disorder

FDA-approved treatments are available for bipolar disorders.[30] Individuals with bipolar I disorder are usually treated with lithium, the first choice of treatment to control mania and rapid cycling and to reduce the risk of suicide. In some cases, lithium in combination with SSRIs is used to treat bipolar disorder. In addition to lithium, several medications are used including anticonvulsants (e.g., carbamazepine, valproate, gabapentin, lamotrigine, topiramate) or atypical antipsychotics (e.g., clozapine, risperidone, ziprasidone, quetiapine, and a combination of olanzapine with the SSRI fluoxetine). Some bipolar individuals benefit from thyroid augmentation (levothyroxine). As in depression, ECT is administered when manic individuals fail to respond to medication, are pregnant, or have cardiovascular disease.

Frequently reported side effects of lithium treatment include increased thirst, tremors, diarrhea, and weight gain, which diminish over time. A potentially serious side effect is lithium

WHAT'S NEW?

Comprehensive Treatment of Risk Factors May Promote Resilience and Rapid Recovery from Depression

Environmental stressors and genetic predisposition

	Depression risk factors	Therapeutic intervention	Resilience protective factors
Cognitive/behavioral	Weak executive function: weak coping self-efficiency; negative attention bias; cognitive inflexibility	Cognitive behavioral therapy with cognitive reappraisal; positive emotion exercises, coping skill development, and training; well-being therapy	Strong executive function; high coping self-efficacy; positive emotions; realistic optimism; cognitive flexibility
Emotion regulation	Weak regulation (e.g., anhedonia; slow stress recovery)	Mindfulness; training; antidepressant medications	Strong regulation (e.g., delay gratification; rapid stress recovery)
Social	Weak social skills; minimal social network; no resilient role models	Social emotional training; network support treatment	Strong social skills; diverse social network; resilient role models
Physical health	Sleep deprivation; poor cardiovascular fitness; poor nutrition; obesity	Teach sleep hygiene; exercise regimen; improve diet	Strong sleep habits; physically fit; good nutrition
Neurobiology	Dysregulated HPA axis and SNS in response to stress; attenuated prefrontal cortical executive function and stress-induced limbic system hyperactivity	Neural circuit training; novel medications (corticotropin-releasing factor, NPY, GABA, glutamate)	Effective regulation of HPA axis and SNS in response to stress; robust prefrontal cortical executive function and capacity to regulate limbic reactivity to stress

Genetic and environmental factors, such as uncontrollable stress, interact to increase the risk of developing major depression. These factors interact in complex ways that are not fully understood to dysregulate neurobiologic systems that compromise adaptive cognitive, emotional, social, and physiologic/health functions. For example, exaggerated stress-induced arousal of sympathetic and neuroendocrine systems may be due, in part, to genetic polymorphisms in serotonin, endocrine, and neuropeptide systems. However, the extent to which a genetic predisposition contributes to severe depression also may arise from the individual's inability to cope with stressors, inexperience in exhibiting flexible psychosocial and emotional skills, and lack of physical health, among others. Identifying and addressing these varied genetic and cognitive/behavioral/socioemotional/health risk factors of depression may open new doors to effective treatment. In particular, combined treatments or behavioral programs that promote resilience, the ability to recover from adversity—such as cognitive-behavioral therapy; social support; and improved diet, sleep, and exercise used in conjunction with current or novel drug medications that lessen or reverse the neuropathophysiology associated with heightened activation of stress systems—may quickly lead to remission. Although, at its early stages, the development of comprehensive resilience programs holds promise not only for treating depressed individuals but also for proactively serving to diminish or prevent the risk of acquiring stress-related disorders.

Data from Karatsoreos IN, McEwen BS: *Trends Cogn Neurosci* 15(12):576–584, 2011; Southwick SM, Charney DS: *Science* 338(6103):79–82, 2012. Figure from Southwick SM, Charney DS: *Science* 338(6103):79–82, 2012.

toxicity. Lithium is normally removed from the kidneys; however, when the body is sodium depleted, the kidneys will reabsorb sodium along with lithium. Individuals receiving lithium treatment are advised to avoid physically demanding activities that may dehydrate the body and to seek medical attention during fever or other conditions that may increase sweating. Anticonvulsant treatment may produce unsteadiness, dizziness, tremors, nausea, and blurry vision.

In addition to pharmacotherapy, psychotherapy can be beneficial for those who have difficulty with psychosocial stressors, such as low self-esteem, legal problems, fear of recurrence, and interpersonal conflicts. Treatment is effective when the individual becomes aware of the bipolar disorder, copes with psychosocial stressors, engages in drug compliance, and monitors symptom recurrences.

Unlike treatment of mania in bipolar I disorder, a major focus in the treatment of bipolar II disorder, the less severe form of mania, is on the recurrent depressive symptoms. Here, antidepressants alone (e.g., escitalopram, fluoxetine, venlafaxine) are reported to be effective in treating bipolar II disorder.

The treatment of bipolar II in children has raised concerns because of complications with its diagnosis. For example, bipolar II and attention-deficit/hyperactivity disorder (ADHD) share the common features of elevated behavioral activity levels, excessive talking, restlessness, and distractibility. Misdiagnosing bipolar II for ADHD has negative consequences for treatment because the stimulant drugs Ritalin and Adderall, which are frequently used to treat ADHD, will potentially exacerbate the symptoms of a child with bipolar II disorder. On the other hand, when ADHD is misdiagnosed with bipolar disorder, the child may begin an ineffective treatment regimen. To reduce misdiagnosis of children with bipolar and other similar symptomatic characteristics, such as ADHD as well as conduct disorder and oppositional defiant disorder, the upcoming *DSM-5*[31] includes a new category called *disruptive mood dysregulation disorder*. This new disorder diagnosis will be used to describe a young child (6 to 10 years of age) who exhibits only some of the symptoms of bipolar II, such as frequent temper outbursts, irritability, and bad moods. This category is hoped to exclude children from being diagnosed with bipolar disorder and reduce possible unwarranted treatment with strong medications.[32]

ANXIETY DISORDERS

Fear and anxiety are normal feelings expressed in threatening or harmful situations. The symptoms may include arousal, tenseness, and increased autonomic activity such as heart rate, blood pressure, and respiration. In addition, individuals often engage in protective behavioral responses such as flight or avoidance. These physiologic and behavioral responses allowed humans to adapt and cope under a variety of situational challenges. However, when fear and anxiety become too intense and undermine the ability to function on a daily basis, the individual may develop an anxiety disorder. **Anxiety disorders** are the most prevalent psychiatric illness, occurring in approximately 10% to 30% of the general population. Notably, many individuals with anxiety disorders develop major depression, and the high comorbidity of anxiety disorders and depression suggests a common neural pathophysiologic basis linking these two mental illnesses.

The *DMS-IV-TR* lists eight recognized anxiety disorders: panic disorder, agoraphobia, generalized anxiety disorder, social phobia, specific phobia, obsessive-compulsive disorder, posttraumatic stress disorder, and acute stress disorder. This section presents an overview of panic disorder, generalized anxiety disorder, posttraumatic stress disorder, and obsessive-compulsive disorder.

Panic Disorder

Panic disorder consists of multiple disabling panic attacks and is characterized by intense autonomic arousal involving a wide variety of symptoms, including lightheadedness, a rapid heart rate (tachycardia), difficulty breathing, chest discomfort, generalized sweating, general weakness, trembling, abdominal distress, and chills or hot flashes. Between panic attacks the individual often worries about future panic attacks and fear of losing control and dying. Symptoms originally occur spontaneously and vary in length from several minutes to an hour.

A notable complication of panic disorder is the development of **agoraphobia** or phobic avoidance of places or situations where escape or help is not readily available. The agoraphobic individual will avoid being away from home, standing in line or in a crowd, or traveling in a train, plane, or automobile. Severe agoraphobic individuals become housebound.

ETIOLOGY AND PATHOPHYSIOLOGY. Genetic factors play a major role in panic disorder. The risk is nearly 20% among first-degree relatives and the prevalence of panic disorder is about 1.5% in men and up to 3.0% in women with no family history of the illness. Some studies suggest that the cholecystokinin (CCK) receptor gene on chromosome 11p may be linked to panic disorder.[33]

The etiology of panic disorder is not known but the ability to elicit physical symptoms of panic attacks by chemicals, called panicogens, provides insight into its pathophysiology. Panic-prone individuals respond to panicogens that include carbon dioxide, caffeine, cholecystokinin, sodium lactate, and adrenergic receptor agonists, such as yohimbine. Carbon dioxide and sodium lactate, two well-studied panicogens, alter brain pH balance that panic-prone people are sensitive in detecting. Brain pH chemosensors are located in the brainstem medulla and pons, the midbrain serotonergic raphe neurons, the hypothalamus, and the amygdala. Heightened pH sensitivity in the amygdala may play a key role in generating fearful perceptions and activating the cerebral cortex and neural circuits in the temporal lobe and brainstem, which further facilitate the production of panic symptoms (see Figures 19-7 and 19-9).[34] Exaggerated activation of physiologic and behavioral arousal stemming from the noradrenergic locus ceruleus neurons also may enhance the symptoms of panic. Thus, panic-prone people appear especially sensitive in detecting pH alterations in brain sites that modulate fear and arousal.

Panic disorder also may involve the GABA-benzodiazepine (BZ) receptor system. BZ increases the $GABA_A$ ion channel response to GABA, thereby elevating chloride ion influx and producing a neuronal inhibitory effect. Brain imaging work reveals a reduction in BZ receptor binding in brain regions including the hippocampus, insular, and prefrontal cortex.[35] Drugs that block the benzodiazepine receptor are reported to increase panic attacks and feelings of anxiety, suggesting an alteration in inhibitory neuromodulation contributes to panic disorder.

TREATMENT. Up to 80% of individuals affected by panic disorder respond to CBT and antidepressant drugs, either separately or in combination. In CBT, the individual learns that the physical symptoms are not fatal and attempts to exert control over the anxiety and panic. For example, breathing exercises to

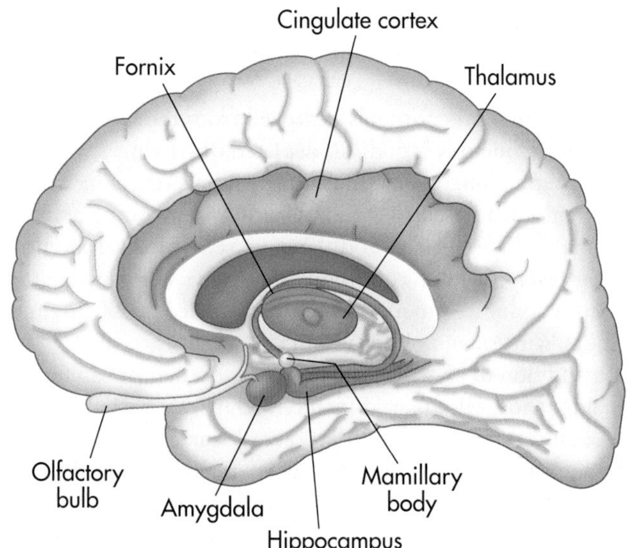

FIGURE 19-9 The Limbic System. Structures of the limbic system play important roles in emotion, learning, and memory. Pathophysiology in limbic structures is frequently found in mental disorders.

control hyperventilation serve to lessen the intense physiologic symptoms of panic, such as elevated heart and respiration rates. Another benefit of CBT is awareness of compliance with drug medications. However, for individuals with mild agoraphobia, CBT alone may be effective.

Antidepressants such as SSRIs are considered first-line medications for panic disorder. Among the SSRIs, paroxetine and sertraline have received FDA approval specifically for panic disorder. Venlafaxine, a serotonin-norepinephrine reuptake blocker, also is effective.

BZs, such as alprazolam and clonazepam, are other medications for treating panic disorder. These drugs also serve as an adjunct or augmentation therapy for individuals who do not fully respond to SSRIs. Short-term effects of BZs include sedation, ataxia, and cognitive impairments. Long-term BZ treatment may lead to physiologic and psychologic dependence. Abrupt BZ withdrawal induces a withdrawal syndrome of heightened reemergence of anxiety, insomnia, photophobia, and diarrhea. A gradual reduction in BZ medication or adjunct CBT may reduce the reliance and withdrawal symptoms of BZs.

Generalized Anxiety Disorder

Excessive and persistent worries are the hallmarks of **generalized anxiety disorder (GAD).** The individual worries about life events such as marital relationships, job performance, health, money, or social status. The lifetime prevalence rates of GAD range from 4.1% to 6.6%, with somewhat higher rates in women than in men. GAD usually emerges in the early twenties, but can occur in childhood. Six major symptoms of GAD have been identified and include restlessness, muscle tension, irritability, being easily fatigued, difficulty concentrating, and difficulty sleeping. The individual startles easily and frequently suffers from depression and panic attacks. The severity of symptoms fluctuates over time and may be linked to the changing nature of stress. Although GAD tends to be chronic, the symptoms may lessen with age. A frequent complication of GAD is substance abuse, which may result from self-medication with alcohol or drugs to relieve anxiety symptoms.

ETIOLOGY AND PATHOPHYSIOLOGY. Female twin studies suggest a concordance rate of 30%, but disease genes linked to specific chromosomes have yet to be identified. Abnormalities in the norepinephrine and serotonin systems were reported in GAD.[36] For example, there is a reduction in α_2-adrenergic receptor binding, a decrease in serotonin levels in CSF, and reduced platelet binding of paroxetine, an SSRI. Another reported alteration in GAD is a reduction of BZ binding in the left temporal hemisphere.[37]

Two functional magnetic resonance imaging (fMRI) studies have revealed alterations in specific brain regions in adults and adolescents with GAD. One study in GAD adults showed increased anticipatory anxiety was associated with elevated cingulate cortex activity and both the heightened anxiety and cingulate cortex activation were reduced after 8 weeks of treatment with venlafaxine, a serotonin and norepinephrine reuptake inhibitor.[38] This study suggests that a decrease in pathophysiologic cingulate cortex activity is a predictor of GAD treatment efficacy. In children and adolescents with GAD, brief exposure to masked angry faces induced heightened right amygdala activation, which correlated positively with severity of anxiety.[39] This study underscores the role of abnormal amygdala activity in attentional bias or vigilance to threats in GAD.

TREATMENT. GAD is diagnosed when a person spends at least 6 months worrying excessively and engages in at least three of the six major symptoms.[12] 5-HT/norepinephrine (NE) reuptake inhibitors, such as venlafaxine or the SSRIs paroxetine and escitalopram, have become first-line therapeutics for managing GAD. These medications may produce relief of GAD symptoms within 1 week and are effective in treating comorbid symptoms of depression. Buspirone, which has an affinity for serotonin receptors (5-HT_{1A}), is another treatment option, although the onset of clinical efficacy may take 2 weeks. The primary side effects of buspirone, which lessen over time, include dizziness, headaches, nausea, and mild nervousness. GAD nonresponders to 5-HT/NE reuptake inhibitors or buspirone may be treated with BZs. However, because GAD tends to be chronic, and comorbid with depression or other anxiety disorders,[40] BZs are usually limited to uncomplicated cases of GAD. In addition to drug therapy, behavioral therapy is used to acquire relaxation techniques that control anxiety.

Posttraumatic Stress Disorder

Exposure to a terrifying or life-threatening event may produce **posttraumatic stress disorder (PTSD).**[41, 42] Although the disorder was initially described in combat situations and called "shell shock," "war neurosis," or "traumatic neurosis," PTSD does not develop only from exposure to traumatic experiences in the battlefield. Any horrific experience involving intense fear, threat of death, or helplessness, including serious accidents, natural disasters (such as earthquakes), child abuse, kidnapping, and violent attacks (such as rape or assault), may induce PTSD. The disorder may develop within hours of the traumatic experience or after several months or years. In PTSD, the individual reexperiences the traumatic event with intrusive flashbacks and persistent nightmares. During a flashback, images, odors, sounds, and negative emotions are recalled and lead to marked distress. The duration of the flashback varies from seconds to hours or, in rare cases, several days. Nightmares of the traumatic experiences often prevent further sleep. Exposure to cues associated with the life-threatening event triggers psychologic distress, intense autonomic arousal, and avoidance behavior. The individual shows emotional numbing or detachment from others and often avoids activities that may lead to a recollection of thoughts, feelings, or contact to places or people involved in the trauma. Additional characteristics of PTSD include irritability, lack of concentration, hypervigilance, and exaggerated startle response.

The lifetime prevalence rate of PTSD is 7% to 8%. In men, PTSD is usually found among combat veterans, whereas PTSD in women is often related to rape or assault. Abused children also may develop PTSD. Individuals with a history of psychiatric illness (major depression, panic disorder) or those lacking strong social support appear more sensitive to the effects of traumatic stress.

ETIOLOGY AND PATHOPHYSIOLOGY. The primary etiology of PTSD is exposure to a terrifying life-threatening event and likely involves stress-induced alterations in several neural structures and neurotransmitter systems. The amygdala and prefrontal cortex are highly involved in the pathophysiology of PTSD because these brain structures normally play important roles in how fearful memories are stored, retrieved, and extinguished. Individuals with PTSD who are exposed to trauma-related stimuli generally exhibit increased activity in the amygdala and diminished activity in prefrontal cortical areas. Persistent dysregulation of this fear-based memory system may underlie chronic PTSD—that is, the failure of prefrontal cortical inhibition to control amygdala-induced activation of fear compromises the extinction of fear memory.[43] Structural brain imaging studies show that combat-exposed PTSD victims also have a smaller hippocampus, a brain structure involved in endocrine functions and memory formation. Pediatric PTSD studies reveal a more generalized effect of trauma on reducing total brain volume. Other brain sites exhibiting increased activity in PTSD are the dorsal anterior cingulate cortex and insula, albeit similar findings were reported in other anxiety disorders (e.g., GAD, obsessive-compulsive disorder [OCD]).[44]

As in panic disorder, BZ binding is altered in PTSD as indicated by a reduced distribution of BZ receptor binding in the prefrontal cortex compared with healthy controls.[45] This reduction in prefrontal BZ receptor distribution was not found in other brain regions.

TREATMENT. PTSD is diagnosed according to the duration and timing of symptoms *(DSM-IV-TR)*. When the duration of symptoms is less than 3 months, PTSD is diagnosed as acute whereas a chronic diagnosis is made when symptoms persist for 3 months or longer or when the delay of onset is longer than 6 months after the trauma. As in GAD, the severity of symptoms fluctuates over time. Among war veterans, financial coverage for group or family therapy is supported by the Veterans Administration. CBT is another therapy used for the individual to learn to control their anxiety symptoms and the emotionally distressing memories of the traumatic event.

Chronic PTSD lasting for years may occur in 30% of diagnosed individuals. Paroxetine and sertraline are considered first-line SSRI medications for chronic PTSD because of their tendency to lessen the recurrent nightmares and flashbacks and to treat the high accompanied prevalence of depression and substance abuse. Other antidepressants, such as the TCAs (amitriptyline and imipramine), have moderate effects and are second-line drugs; drugs such as nefazodone and bupropion may provide benefits. BZs may be used in the aftermath of a traumatic event to control hyperarousal symptoms such as irritability, insomnia, and muscle tension. However, there is no clear evidence that BZs have clinical efficacy or provide prophylaxis against the development of chronic PTSD, and BZs should be carefully monitored among individuals with a history of drug abuse.

Obsessive-Compulsive Disorder

Repetitive, intrusive thoughts and/or compulsions are the hallmarks of **obsessive-compulsive disorder (OCD).** These thoughts and acts impair normal functioning and cause marked distress. Obsessions may involve a preoccupation with contamination, doubting, religious or sexual themes, or the belief that a negative outcome will occur if a specific act is not performed. Compulsions are physical and mental ritualized acts such as washing, cleaning, checking, counting, organizing, hoarding, and repeating specific thoughts or prayers. The lifetime prevalence rates of OCD range from 1.2% to 3.3% with an age of onset between 20 and 25 years. OCD occurs equally in adult men and women; however, many begin to experience symptoms during childhood or adolescence.

OCD is diagnosed when obsessions or compulsions cause severe distress, consume time, or interfere with normal daily activities.[13] In many cases the OCD individual also is diagnosed with major depression, panic disorder, or GAD.[46] Among children, tic disorders, attention-deficit/hyperactivity disorder, and depression coexist with OCD.

ETIOLOGY AND PATHOPHYSIOLOGY. The risk of developing OCD is about 10% to 12% among first-degree relatives. These first-degree relatives are also at increased risk (4.6%) of Tourette syndrome and tics in comparison with control relatives (1%). Thus OCD and Tourette syndrome may share common genes and pathophysiology.

Abnormalities of the basal ganglia–frontocortical circuitry are found in OCD.[47] Some studies have shown increased orbitofrontal and thalamic volumes in OCD but not in the caudate nucleus of the basal ganglia (Figure 19-10). More consistent data report an increase in orbitofrontal and anterior cingulate cortical activity, which may be responsible for intrusive thoughts, obsessions, and anxiety, which drive the basal ganglia to engage in compulsive ritualized acts as a means to alleviate the anxious obsessions. Furthermore, when provoked, OCD individuals consistently show increased activity in the orbitofrontal, anterior cingulate, and caudate nucleus areas of the brain. Of relevance to prognosis, OCD individuals with very high frontocortical activity are likely to respond poorly to treatment.

Abnormalities in serotonin and dopamine functions may further contribute to the pathophysiology of OCD. Serotonin

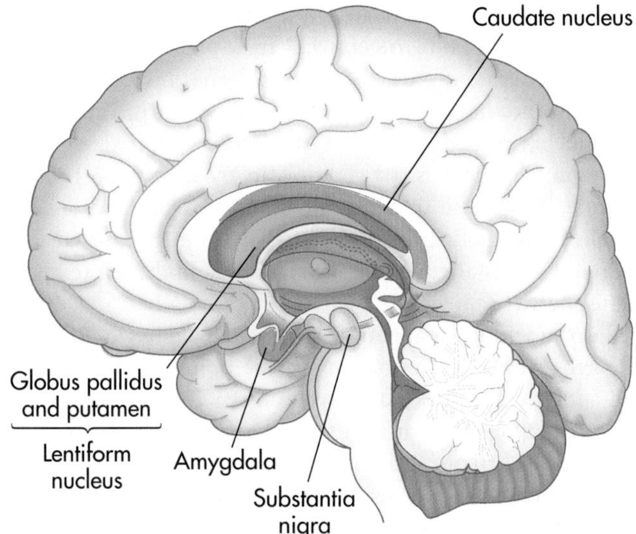

FIGURE 19-10 **Basal Ganglion.** Structures of the basal ganglion, which include the caudate nucleus, putamen, globus pallidus, and substantia nigra, are important in movement.

agonists exacerbate the symptoms of OCD, and serotonin synthesis is decreased in the prefrontal cortex and caudate nucleus. Stimulation of the dopamine system also increases repetitive acts, which may be blocked by dopamine antagonists. However, the dopamine stimulant–induced compulsions are not accompanied by anxiety and, therefore, suggest that lack of serotonin control over the dopamine system may be a primary defect in OCD.

TREATMENT. Because of the chronic nature of OCD, long-term treatment often involves a combination of pharmacotherapy and CBT. SSRIs, including citalopram, fluvoxamine, paroxetine, and sertraline, are the first drugs of choice for OCD.[48] Approximately 70% to 80% of OCD individuals show a partial positive response that may be further improved by other medications. For example, clonazepam, a BZ, is found to improve the effects of fluoxetine and clomipramine therapy. Antipsychotic drugs (e.g., haloperidol and risperidone) in combination with SSRIs are also effective especially in comorbid OCD and tic disorders. Normalization of dysfunctional serotonin and dopamine systems in OCD may be the basis for the therapeutic effects of SSRIs and dopamine receptor–related drugs.

CBT and response prevention therapy involve exposure to cues that elicit distress followed by preventing the individual from engaging in compulsive rituals for at least an hour or until the anxiety subsides. Both therapies can produce long-term symptom remission in adults and children who are able to tolerate the exposure-induced anxiety component.

For individuals with severe treatment-resistant OCD, neurosurgery is used to disconnect the basal ganglia from the frontal cortex.[49] This lesioning procedure results in significant relief of obsessions and compulsions in nearly 50% of individuals and provides further evidence of pathophysiology in the basal ganglia–frontocortical circuitry in OCD. An alternative treatment to ablative neurosurgery is deep brain stimulation, which also is used for intractable depression.[27] Deep brain stimulation in the anterior limb of internal capsule, striatum/ventral capsule, nucleus accumbens, subthalamic nucleus, and inferior thalamic peduncle is effective in alleviating some OCD symptoms.[50,51] Stimulating these brain regions may be reducing abnormal neuronal firing in the neuroanatomic circuitry linked to OCD.

SUMMARY REVIEW

Schizophrenia

1. Schizophrenia is characterized by thought disorders that reflect a break between the cognitive and the emotional sides of one's personality.
2. Schizophrenic symptoms are classified into positive, negative, and cognitive categories. Positive symptoms include hallucinations, delusions, formal thought disorder, and bizarre behavior. Negative symptoms include flattened affect, alogia, anhedonia, attention deficits, and apathy. Cognitive symptoms are the inability to perform daily tasks requiring attention and planning.
3. Schizophrenia has a strong genetic predisposition and environmental factors (e.g., viral infection, nutritional deficiencies, prenatal birth complications, urban upbringing) may interfere with genetically programmed neural development to alter brain structure and function.
4. Brain imaging studies reveal structural brain abnormalities including an enlargement of the cerebroventricles and widening of the fissures and sulci in the frontal cortex. In addition, there is a reduction in the volumes of both the thalamus, which may disrupt communication among cortical brain regions, and the temporal lobe, which may be responsible for the manifestations of positive symptoms.
5. In schizophrenia the frontal lobe shows a progressive loss in volume and a worsening of negative symptoms despite the use of antipsychotic medications. Blood flow and metabolism are reduced in the dorsolateral prefrontal cortex, which compromise the ability to engage in goal-directed and cognitive problem-solving behavior.
6. Neurochemical abnormalities in dopamine and glutamate systems are found in schizophrenia.
7. The first generation of antipsychotic drugs block the dopamine D_2 receptor. The second generation, called atypical antipsychotics, block not only D_2 receptors but also dopamine, serotonin, and other neurotransmitter receptors. Antipsychotic medications, however, are not always effective in treating schizophrenic individuals with severe negative symptoms. Talk therapies are used to increase drug compliance and to encourage coping strategies.

Mood Disorders: Depression and Bipolar Disorder

1. Major depression and bipolar disorder are two common mood disorders. Major depression is characterized by an intense and sustained unpleasant state of sadness and hopelessness. In bipolar disorder, individuals show recurrent patterns of depression and mania, the latter characterized by extreme levels of energy and euphoria.
2. Environmental triggers such as psychosocial stress appear to facilitate the onset of depression in individuals with a genetic vulnerability.
3. A reduction in brain monoamine neurotransmission is linked to depression, whereas an elevated monoamine level is associated with mania.
4. Exposure to uncontrollable stress elevates secretion of the stress hormone cortisol, which increases both the secretion of proinflammatory cytokines and the risk of developing depression. Abnormalities involving thyroid hormones also are found in depression.
5. Stress-induced depression is accompanied by deficits in brain-derived neurotrophic factor (BDNF) and neurogenesis in the hippocampus. In animal models, stress-induced depression-like behavior and the accompanying deficits in hippocampal BDNF and neurogenesis are reversed by antidepressant treatment.
6. The frontal lobe and limbic system volumes are reduced in major depression and bipolar illness. In addition, blood flow is altered in prefrontal and limbic brain regions that include the amygdala, a structure implicated in emotional behavior.

SUMMARY REVIEW—cont'd

7. Pharmacotherapy involves the use of MAOIs, TCAs, SSRIs, and atypical antidepressants. Manic and bipolar individuals are treated with lithium or mood stabilizers. Severely depressed and manic people may be administered ECT. Deep brain stimulation is another promising treatment for intractable depression.

Anxiety Disorders

1. When normal fear and anxiety mental states persist and become uncontrollable, an individual may develop an anxiety disorder. PD, GAD, PTSD, and OCD are examples of uncontrollable fear and anxiety states that require medical attention.
2. Panic disorder consists of panic attacks characterized by intense autonomic arousal that occurs spontaneously and is accompanied by symptoms including lightheadedness, tachycardia, and difficulty breathing. In addition, the intense occurrence of autonomic responses is accompanied by heightened fear and anxiety that often continue between panic attacks.
3. Panic-prone people are sensitive in detecting pH alterations in the amygdala, a brain structure that modulates fear. An activated amygdala recruits the cerebral cortex and neural circuits in the temporal lobe and brainstem, which may further exacerbate symptoms of panic.
4. A reduction in BZ receptor binding in brain regions, including the hippocampus, insular, and prefrontal cortex, also may contribute to the pathophysiology of panic disorder.
5. Panic disorder is generally treatable with CBT and antidepressants such as TCAs and SSRIs. BZs are used as an adjunct or augmentation therapy for individuals who are nonresponsive to SSRIs or TCAs.
6. GAD is characterized by excessive and persistent worries about life events. Individuals exhibit varying levels of motor disturbances, irritability, and fatigue that may be linked to fluctuations in psychosocial stress. Many GAD individuals manifest symptoms of depression.
7. Pathophysiologic changes in the cingulate cortex and amygdala may have prominent roles in stimulating anticipatory anxiety and attentional bias to threats in people with GAD.
8. Treatment of GAD usually involves a combination of behavioral therapy and drug medications, especially serotonin/norepinephrine reuptake inhibitors.
9. PTSD develops after exposure to a life-threatening or traumatic experience. Individuals experience recurring thoughts and flashbacks and nightmares of the terrifying event.
10. In PTSD structural and/or functional alterations exist in the amygdala, prefrontal cortex, and hippocampus, which likely contribute to dysfunction in an emotional fear memory system.
11. Treatment of chronic PTSD is difficult and involves psychotherapy and SSRI pharmacotherapy.
12. OCD is a chronic illness characterized by irrational obsessions and ritualized acts that impair normal functioning and cause severe distress.
13. Pathophysiologic alterations in the basal ganglia–frontocortical circuitry and serotonin and dopamine functions are linked to OCD.
14. OCD requires long-term treatment consisting of CBT and drug medication, such as SSRIs and talk therapies. Severe OCD may require neurosurgery to disconnect the basal ganglia from the frontal cortex. Deep brain stimulation may be another option for uncontrollable OCD.

KEY TERMS

REFERENCES

1. Lewis DA, Levitt P: Schizophrenia as a disorder of neurodevelopment, *Annu Rev Neurosci* 25:409–432, 2002.
2. Marenco S, Weinberger DR: The neurodevelopmental hypothesis of schizophrenia: following a trail of evidence from cradle to grave, *Dev Psychopathol* 12(3):501–527, 2000.
3. van Os J, Kenis G, Rutten BPF: The environment and schizophrenia, *Nature* 468:203–212, 2010.
4. Berman KF, Meyer-Lindenberg A: Functional brain imaging studies in schizophrenia. In Charney DS, Nestler EJ, editors: *Neurobiology of mental illness*, ed 2, New York, 2004, Oxford.
5. Shenton LD et al: A review of MRI findings in schizophrenia, *Schizophr Res* 49(1-2):1–52, 2001.
6. Ross CA et al: Neurobiology of schizophrenia, *Neuron* 52(1):139–153, 2006.
7. Ho BC et al: Progressive structural brain abnormalities and their relationship to clinical outcome, *Arch Gen Psychiatry* 60:585–594, 2003.
8. Costa E et al: Dendritic spine hypoplasticity and downregulation of reelin and GABAergic tone in schizophrenia vulnerability, *Neurobiol Dis* 8(5):723–742, 2001.
9. Fatemi SH, Earle JA, McMenomy T: Reduction in reelin immunoreactivity in hippocampus of subjects with schizophrenia, bipolar disorder and major depression, *Mol Psychiatry* 5(6):654–663, 2000.

10. Duncan GE, Sheitman BB, Lieberman JA: An integrated view of pathophysiological models of schizophrenia, *Brain Res Brain Res Rev* 29(2-3): 250–264, 1999.
11. Coyle JT, Tsai G, Goff D: Converging evidence of NMDA receptor hypofunction in the pathophysiology of schizophrenia, *Ann N Y Acad Sci* 1003:318–327, 2003.
12. Jentsch JD et al: Enduring cognitive deficits and cortical dopamine dysfunction in monkeys after long-term administration of phencyclidine, *Science* 277:953–955, 1997.
13. American Psychiatric Association: *Diagnostic and statistical manual of mental disorders.* Text Revision (DSM-IV-TR), ed 4, Washington, DC, 2000, Author.
14. Tamminga CA: Principles of the pharmacotherapy of schizophrenia. In Charney DS, Nestler EJ, editors: *Neurobiology of mental illness*, ed 2, New York, 2004, Oxford.
15. Tai S, Turkington D: The evolution of cognitive behavior therapy for schizophrenia: current practice and recent developments, *Schizophr Bull* 35(5):865–873, 2009.
16. Shih RA, Belmonte PL, Zandi PP: A review of the evidence from family, twin and adoption studies for a genetic contribution to adult psychiatric disorders, *Internat Rev Psychiatry* 16:260–283, 2004.
17. Caspi A et al: Influence of life stress on depression: moderation by a polymorphism in the 5-HTT gene, *Science* 301(5631):386, 2003.
18. Heninger GR et al: The revised monoamine theory of depression: a modulatory role for monoamines, based on new findings from monoamine depletion experiments in humans, *Pharmacopsychiatry* 29(1):2–11, 1996.
19. Holsboer F: The corticosteroid receptor hypothesis of depression, *Neuropsychopharmacology* 23:477, 2000.
20. Krishnadas R, Cavanagh J: Depression: an inflammatory illness? *J Neurol Neurosurg Psychiatry* 83:495–502, 2012.
21. Masi G, Brovedani P: The hippocampus, neurotrophic factors and depression. Possible implications for the pharmacotherapy of depression, *CNS Drugs* 25(11):913–931, 2012.
22. Pittenger C, Duman RS: Stress, depression, and neuroplasticity: a convergence of mechanisms, *Neuropsychopharmacol Rev* 33:88–109, 2008.
23. Bartalena L et al: Nocturnal serum thyrotropin (TSH) surge and the TSH response to TSH-releasing hormone: disassociative behavior in untreated depression, *J Clin Endocrinol Metab* 71(3):650–655, 1990.
24. Drevets WC: Prefrontal cortical-amygdalar metabolism in major depression, *Ann N Y Acad Sci* 877:614–637, 1999.
25. Rajkowska G: Depression: what we can learn from postmortem studies, *Neuroscientist* 9(4):273–284, 2003.
26. Whittington CJ et al: Selective serotonin reuptake inhibitors in childhood depression: systematic review of published versus unpublished data, *Lancet* 363(9418):1341–1345, 2004.
27. Goodman WK, Alterman RL: Deep brain stimulation for intractable psychiatric disorders, *Annu Rev Med* 63:511–524, 2012.
28. Hamani C et al: The subcallosal cingulate gyrus in the context of major depression, *Biol Psychiatry* 69:301–308, 2011.
29. Kennedy SH et al: Deep brain stimulation for treatment-resistant depression: follow-up after 3 to 6 years, *Am J Psychiatry* 168:502–510, 2011.
30. Goldberg JF: What psychotherapists should know about pharmacotherapies for bipolar disorder, *J Clin Psychol* 63(5):475–490, 2007.
31. American Psychiatric Association: *Diagnostic and statistical manual of mental disorders. (DSM-5)*, ed 5, 2013, Washington, DC.
32. Parens E, Johnston J: Controversies concerning the diagnosis and treatment of bipolar disorder in children, *Child Adolesc Psychiatry Mental Health* 4:9, 2010.
33. Kennedy JL et al: Investigation of cholecystokinin system genes in panic disorder, *Mol Psychiatry* 4(3):284, 1999.
34. Wemmie JA: Neurobiology of panic and pH chemosensation in the brain, *Dialogues Clin Neurosci* 13:475–483, 2011.
35. Malizia AL et al: Decreased brain $GABA_A$-benzodiazepine receptor binding in panic disorder, *Arch Gen Psychiatry* 55(8):715–720, 1998.
36. Jetty PV et al: Neurobiology of generalized anxiety disorder, *Psychiatr Clin North Am* 24(1):75, 2001.
37. Tiihonen J et al: Cerebral benzodiazepine receptor binding and distribution in generalized anxiety disorder, *Mol Psychiatry* 2(6):463–471, 1997.
38. Nitschke JB et al: Anticipatory activation in the amygdala and anterior cingulate in generalized anxiety disorder and prediction of treatment response, *Am J Psychiatry* 166:302–310, 2009.
39. Monk CS et al: Ventrolateral prefrontal cortex activation and attentional bias in response to angry faces in adolescents with generalized anxiety disorder, *Am J Psychiatry* 163:1091–1097, 2006.
40. Bruce SE: Infrequency of "pure" GAD: impact of psychiatric comorbidity on clinical course, *Depress Anxiety* 14(4):219–225, 2001.
41. Charney DS et al: Psychobiologic mechanisms of posttraumatic stress disorder, *Arch Gen Psychiatry* 50(4):294–305, 1993.
42. Southwick SM et al: Neurotransmitter alterations in PTSD: catecholamines and serotonin, *Semin Clin Neuropsychiatry* 4(4):242–248, 1999.
43. Bremner JD et al: Structural and functional plasticity of the human brain in posttraumatic stress disorder, *Prog Brain Res* 167:171–186, 2008.
44. Shin LM, Liberzon I: The neurocircuitry of fear, stress, and anxiety disorders, *Neuropsychopharmacology* 35(1):169–191, 2010.
45. Bremner JD et al: Decreased benzodiazepine receptor binding in prefrontal cortex in combat-related posttraumatic stress disorder, *Am J Psychiatry* 157(7):1120–1126, 2000.
46. Fireman B et al: The prevalence of clinically recognized obsessive-compulsive disorder in a large health maintenance organization, *Am J Psychiatry* 158(11):1904–1910, 2001.
47. Saxena S, Rauch SL: Functional neuroimaging and the neuroanatomy of obsessive-compulsive disorder, *Psychiatr Clin North Am* 23(3):563–586, 2000.
48. Swedo SE, Snider LA: The neurobiology and treatment of obsessive-compulsive disorder. In Charney DS, Nestler EJ, editors: *Neurobiology of mental illness*, ed 2, New York, 2004, Oxford.
49. Greenberg BD, Murphy DL, Rasmussen SA: Neuroanatomically based approaches to obsessive-compulsive disorder, *Psychiatr Clin North Am* 23(3):671–686, 2000.
50. de Koning PP et al: Current status of deep brain stimulation for obsessive-compulsive disorder: a clinical review of different targets, *Curr Psychiatry Rep* 13:274–282, 2011.
51. Holtzheimer PE, Mayberg HS: Deep brain stimulation for psychiatric disorders, *Annu Rev Neurosci* 34:289–307, 2011.

CHAPTER

20

Alterations of Neurologic Function in Children

Lynne M. Kerr and Sue E. Huether

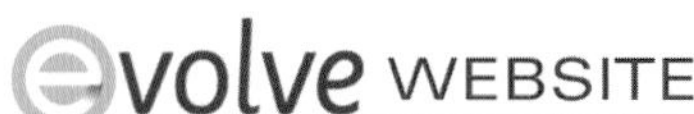

http://evolve.elsevier.com/McCance/
- Review Questions and Answers

CHAPTER OUTLINE

Neurologic disorders in children can occur before birth through adolescence and include congenital malformations, genetic defects in metabolism, brain injuries, infection, tumors, and other disorders that affect neurologic structure and function. The symptoms, diagnosis, and management of neurologic disorders in children are often different than those of adults. It is important to note that with better proactive care and advances in treatment, many of the children with these disorders will live into adulthood and physicians who care for adults will be seeing these disorders in adults in increasing numbers.

STRUCTURE AND FUNCTION OF THE NERVOUS SYSTEM IN CHILDREN

Embryology is a highly complex and often difficult science to understand fully. A basic knowledge of this science is essential because it is the process of embryonic development that explains many of the malformations that occur in children.

Both genetics and environment shape nervous system development. The proper proportions of essential nutrients are necessary for growth and proliferation of the nervous system tissue (see Nutrition & Disease: Iron and Cognitive Function). Maternal lifestyle, nutrition, exposure to potential toxins, and state of health also have a crucial effect on nervous system development at critical periods of fetal maturation.

The central nervous system (CNS) develops from a dorsal thickening of the ectoderm known as the **neural plate.** This plate appears around the middle of the third gestational week and unfolds to form a **neural groove** and **neural folds.** During the fourth gestational week the neural groove deepens, its folds develop laterally, and it closes dorsally to form the **neural tube,** epithelial tissue that ultimately becomes the CNS. The neural tube closes first in the cervical region and then "zippers" in two directions—cranially and caudally (Figure 20-1).

In the developmental process, some neuroectodermal cells separate from the neural tube but remain between the tube and the surface ectoderm, creating the **neural crest.** This cellular band develops into the cranial and spinal ganglia, more commonly referred to as the *peripheral nervous system.* Other structures associated with the nervous system arise from mesoderm (**somite**) and include blood vessels, microglial cells, dural and arachnoid layers of the meninges, the capsule of

NUTRITION & DISEASE

Iron and Cognitive Function

Iron deficiency (ID) is the single most significant nutrient deficiency, affecting 15% of the world population and causing anemia in 40% to 50% of children. Iron is essential for neurologic activity, including synthesis of dopamine, serotonin, and catecholamine and, possibly, formation of myelin. Children with ID have decreased attentiveness, short attention span, and perceptual restrictions. ID also may contribute to attention-deficit/hyperactivity disorder. In some studies, cognitive deficits in iron can be reversed with iron supplements. In one randomized study, supplementation with iron or zinc, or both, during infancy did not lead to long-term cognitive improvement in 9-year-old children. Research is in progress to determine the effects of acute vs. chronic ID and the relationships between severity of deficiency and cognitive functioning. Alterations in the hippocampus and the brain striatal dopaminergic-opiate system function have been found in ID.

Data from Congdon EL et al: *J Pediatr* 160(6):1027–1033, 2012; Khor GL, Misra S: *Asia Pac J Clin Nutr* 21(4): 476–486, 2012; Lozoff B: *J Nutr* 141(4):740S–746S, 2011; Madan N et al: *Indian J Pediatr* 78(1):58–64, 2011; Pongcharoen T et al: *Am J Clin Nutr* 93(3):636–643, 2011; Yadav D, Chandra J: *Indian J Pediatr* 78(1):65–72, 2011.

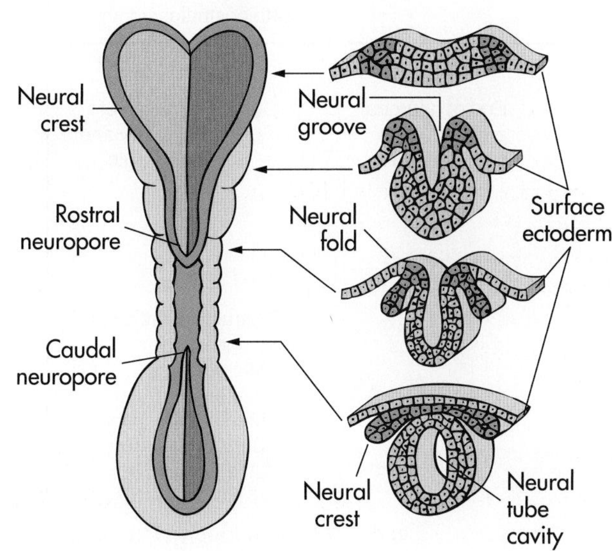

FIGURE 20-1 Neural Tube at 3 Weeks of Gestation. Neural folds have begun to fuse at the cervical level of the future spinal cord. *Right,* Cross sections of the neural tube at four different levels; at any given level the embryonic central nervous system (CNS) goes through a series of stages resembling these four cross sections. Total length of neural tube at this time is about 2.5 mm.

some peripheral sensory nerve endings, and peripheral nerve coverings.

The cranial end of the neural tube forms the brain, and the remainder develops into the spinal cord. The lumen of the neural tube becomes the ventricles of the brain and the central canal of the spinal cord (Figure 20-2). On either side of the neural tube's inner surface is a longitudinal groove (**sulcus limitans**). Anterior to this region (**basal plate**) the gray matter differentiates into the nuclei of the lower motor neurons. The region posterior to the sulcus (**alar plate**) differentiates into the sensory nuclei of the spinal cord.

Embryonic development of the nervous system occurs in six stages: (1) dorsal (posterior) induction, (2) ventral (anterior)

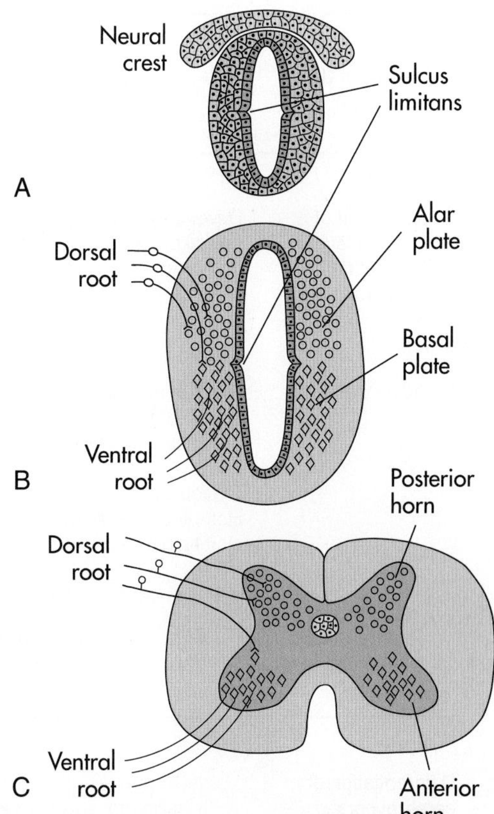

FIGURE 20-2 Sulcus Limitans and Alar and Basal Plates. A, Neural tube during the fourth week of gestation. **B,** Embryonic spinal cord during the sixth week of gestation; dorsal root ganglion cells, derived from the neural crest, send their central processes into the spinal cord to terminate mainly in alar plate cells; basal plate cells become motor neurons, whose axons exit in the ventral roots. **C,** Adult spinal cord.

induction, (3) proliferation, (4) migration, (5) organization, and (6) myelination. Figure 20-3 summarizes the embryonic development of the nervous system and identifies disorders associated with interference in any of these stages. Many different events happen simultaneously, and critical periods must pass uninterrupted if the vulnerable fetus is to develop normally.

Brain Development

When an infant is born, the bones of the skull are separated at the suture lines, thus forming two fontanels or "soft spots": one diamond-shaped anterior fontanel and one triangular-shaped posterior fontanel. The posterior fontanel may be open until 2 to 3 months of age; the anterior fontanel normally closes by 18 months (Figure 20-4). The fact that the sutures are not closed allows for increases in head circumference as part of normal growth for 5 to 8 years after birth; in fact, the head is the fastest growing body part during infancy. Although basically all of the neurons that an individual will ever have are present at birth, the development of skills, such as walking, talking, and thinking, depends on these cells making correct connections with other cells and on myelination of the axons making those connections. This leads to brain and then to skull growth. Increased intracranial pressure may result in an increased head circumference in excess of that expected with normal growth.

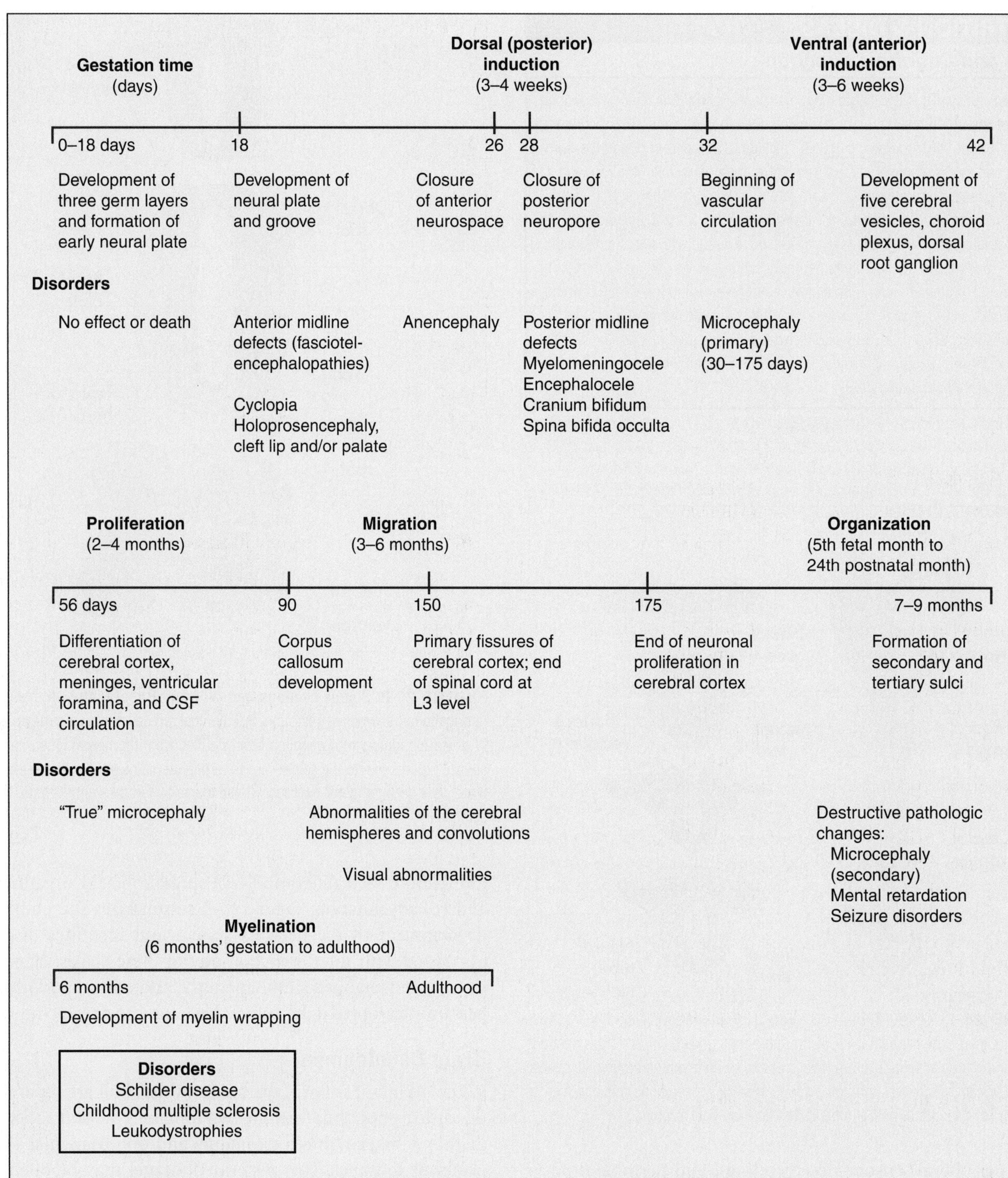

FIGURE 20-3 Disorders Associated with Specific Stages of Embryonic Development. *CSF,* Cerebrospinal fluid.

Healthcare providers carefully monitor head growth during the first 5 years of life by measuring head circumference and comparing the results with a standardized growth chart. In contrast, the adult cranium is a closed cavity with sutures firmly holding the cranial bones together. An adult's head size will not expand regardless of intracranial events, e.g., tumor growth, bleeding, or increased production of cerebrospinal fluid (CSF).

Most neurons are formed during fetal life but the connections between brain circuits, myelination of those connections, and dendritic development are most significant after birth. Human neurologic functioning is primarily at a subcortical level at birth with many reflex patterns mediated by brainstem and spinal cord mechanisms that disappear at predictable times during infancy while brain axons are myelinated and connecting pathways develop. Myelination is a process by which lipid-protein material made by specialized connective tissue cells (Schwann cells in the peripheral nervous system and oligodendrocytes in the central nervous system) covers the axons of neurons, allowing electrical signals to travel more quickly (see Chapter 16). The development of myelin in the brain follows

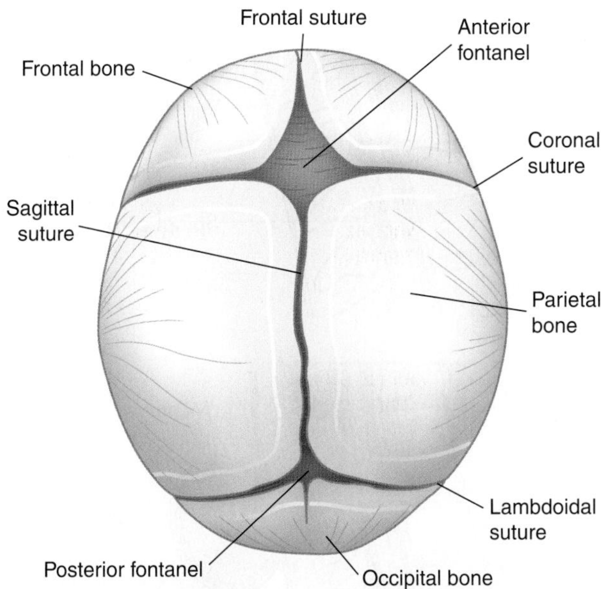

FIGURE 20-4 Cranial Sutures and Fontanels in Infancy. Fibrous union of suture lines and interlocking of serrated edges (occurs by 6 months; solid union requires approximately 12 years).

predictable patterns over time and is most extensive after birth and throughout childhood. The primitive reflex pathways require myelination and by 6 months of age they are integrated and inhibited for progression to voluntary movement. Table 20-1 summarizes the ages at which primitive reflexes appear and disappear. Testing for the presence or absence of these reflexes at various times enables the examiner to evaluate the function and development of the nervous system.

Absence of expected reflex responses at the appropriate age indicates general depression of central or peripheral motor function. Asymmetric responses may indicate lesions in the motor cortex on the opposite side or may occur with fractures of bones after traumatic delivery or postnatal injury. While the infant matures, the primitive reflexes disappear in a predictable order as voluntary motor functions supersede them. Abnormal persistence of these reflexes is seen in infants with developmental delays or with central nervous system lesions.

TABLE 20-1 **REFLEXES OF INFANCY**

REFLEX	AGE AT APPEARANCE OF REFLEX	AGE AT WHICH REFLEX SHOULD NO LONGER BE OBTAINABLE
Stepping	Birth	6 weeks
Moro	Birth	3 months
Sucking	Birth	4 months awake 7 months asleep
Rooting	Birth	4 months awake 7 months asleep
Palmar grasp	Birth	6 months
Plantar grasp	Birth	10 months
Tonic neck	2 months	5 months
Neck righting	4-6 months	24 months
Landau	3 months	24 months
Parachute reaction	9 months	Persists for life

WHAT'S NEW?

Reduction of Risks for Neural Tube Defects (NTDs)

Studies indicate that ingestion of multivitamins with folic acid before conception or early in pregnancy may offer protection against neural tube defects and reduction of stillbirths caused by NTDs. Folate is a coenzyme essential for DNA and RNA synthesis and cellular methylation. Recent repeated studies demonstrate a 60% to 86% reduction of risks for neural tube defects with periconceptional ingestion of vitamins containing the U.S. recommended daily allowance of 400 mcg of folic acid. There may also be an increased risk associated with maternal obesity.

Data from Branum AM, Bailey R, Singer BJ: *J Nutr* 143(4):486–492, 2013; Centers for Disease Control and Prevention: *MMWR Morb Mortal Wkly Rep* 53(36):847–850, 2004; Imdad A, Yakoob MY, Bhutta ZA: *BMC Public Health* 11(Suppl 3):S4, 2011; Mastroiacovo P, Leoncini E: *Biofactors* 37(4):272–279, 2011; Wolff T et al: *Ann Intern Med* 150(9): 632–639, 2009.

STRUCTURAL MALFORMATIONS

Defects of Neural Tube Closure

Neural tube defects (NTDs) are caused by an arrest of the normal development of the brain and spinal cord during the first month of embryonic development and occur in about 3000 pregnancies in the United States each year.[1] There is a strong association of fetal death with NTDs, reducing the actual prevalence of neural defects at birth. Maternal folate deficiency is associated with NTDs. The specific mechanism that relates to how folate supplements prevent these anomalies is unknown but genes involving folate metabolism and environmental factors are involved.[2] In 1996 the United States mandated folate fortification in many foods and since that time neural tube defects have decreased by 20% to 30%[3] (see What's New? Reduction of Risks for Neural Tube Defects [NTDs]).

Defects of neural tube closure are divided into two categories: posterior defects and anterior midline defects. Posterior defects are more common and will be discussed further below. These include anencephaly (*an,* "without"; *enkephalos,* "brain"), encephalocele, and a group of disorders collectively referred to as the *myelodysplasias* (*dys,* "bad"; *plassein,* "to form"). Although **myelodysplasia** is defined as a defect in formation of the spinal cord, the term is used to refer to anomalies of both the vertebral column and the spinal cord. Birth defects in which there is failure of closure of the vertebrae are known as spina bifida (split spine). Myelomeningocele is a form of spina bifida with incomplete development of the spine and protrusion of both the spinal cord and meninges through the skin. Meningocele is a form of spina bifida in which there is protrusion of the meninges but the spinal cord remains in the spinal canal. There is a broad spectrum of abnormalities within each of these categories depending on the location of the defect, the tissue involved, and other factors.

Anencephaly

Anencephaly is an anomaly in which the soft, bony component of the skull and much of the brain are missing. This is a

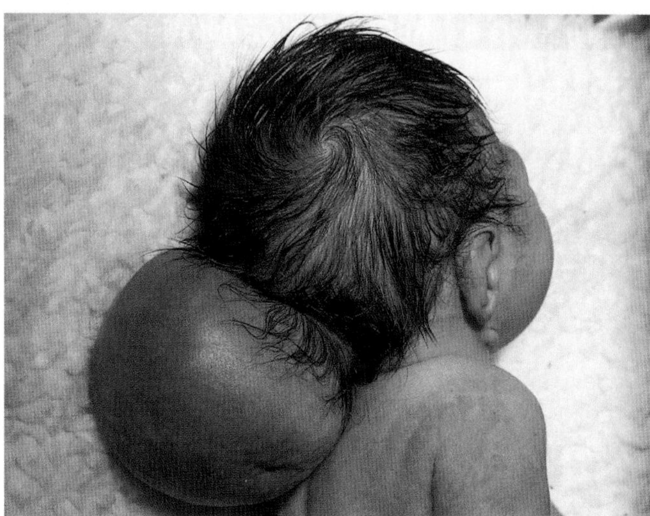

FIGURE 20-5 **Meningoencephalocele of the Occipital Region.** (From Gilbert-Barness: *Potter's pathology of the fetus, infant and child,* ed 2, Philadelphia, 2007, Mosby.)

relatively common disorder, with an incidence rate of approximately 1 per 4859 live births in the United States each year.[4] These infants are stillborn or die within a few days after birth. The pathologic mechanism is unknown. Diagnosis is often made prenatally using ultrasound or evaluating maternal serum alpha fetoprotein (AFP).[5]

Encephalocele

Encephalocele refers to a herniation or protrusion of various amounts of brain and meninges through a defect in the skull, resulting in a saclike structure. The incidence rate is approximately 1 in 10,000 live births in the United States each year.[6]

PATHOPHYSIOLOGY. Encephalocele occurs during the first weeks of pregnancy. When the defect contains only meninges, it is referred to as a **cranial meningocele.** Most encephaloceles, which contain neural tissue as well as meninges, occur in the occipital area, with the remainder found in the frontal, parietal, or nasopharyngeal regions.

CLINICAL MANIFESTATIONS. Encephalocele usually is seen at birth as a midline skull defect through which a large mass protrudes (Figure 20-5). If the defect is located in the nasopharynx, no external anomaly is visible, but the child may experience nasal airway obstruction. On examination with a nasal speculum, a smooth, round mass will be visible in the nasal passages. A frontal encephalocele may extend into the orbit of the eye and produce proptosis on the affected side.

EVALUATION AND TREATMENT. Diagnosis is based on clinical manifestations and examination of the meningeal sac. With cranial meningocele, surgical repair of the cranial defect affords a good prognosis for most affected infants whose intellectual and motor functioning is normal. An occipital encephalocele may be associated with other findings, such as blindness and cognitive impairment. The size, location, and involvement of the encephalocele help determine a child's development and intellectual outcome.

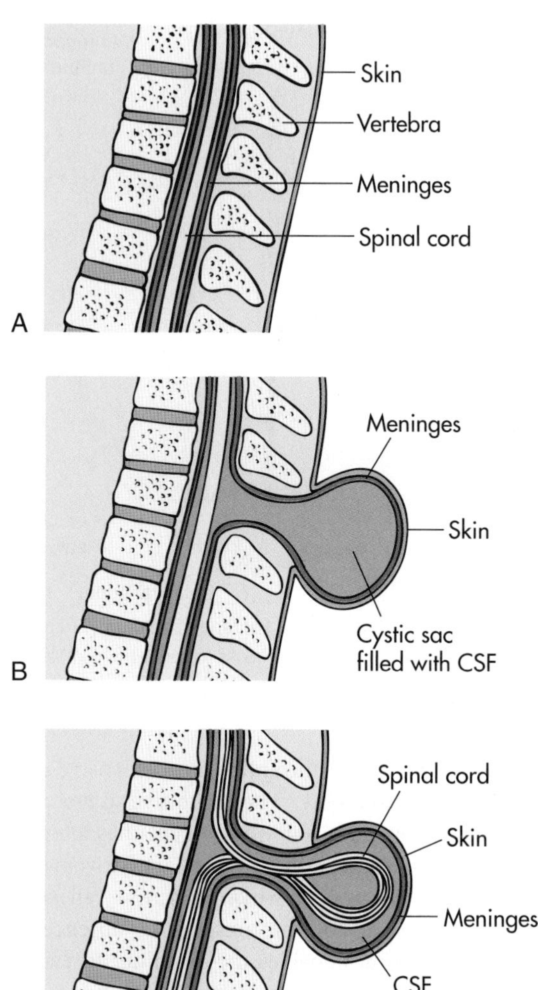

FIGURE 20-6 **Comparison of Normal Spine and Spine with Meningocele and Myelomeningocele Neural Tube Defects.** Diagram depicts section through normal spine **(A)**, spine with meningocele **(B)**, and spine with myelomeningocele **(C)**.

Meningocele and Myelomeningocele

Meningocele and myelomeningocele are different types of spina bifida that occur because of an incompletely formed or absent posterior vertebral arch in the spinal column, allowing protrusion of either a saclike cyst of meninges filled with spinal fluid (a meningocele) or a similar saclike cyst that also has neural tissue, spinal cord, or nerves in it, in which case it is a myelomeningocele. Both develop during the first 4 weeks of pregnancy when the neural tube fails to close completely (Figure 20-6). Meningoceles occur with equal frequency in the cervical, thoracic, and lumbar spine areas, whereas 80% of myelomeningoceles are located in the lumbar and lumbosacral regions, the last regions of the neural tube to close. Myelomeningocele is much more common than meningocele and has an incidence rate ranging from 0.5 to 1 per 1000 pregnancies in the United States.[7] It is thus is one of the most common developmental anomalies of the nervous system.

PATHOPHYSIOLOGY. **Meningocele** is a cystlike dilation of meninges protruding through a defect in the posterior arch of the vertebra. The dura mater may be missing and the arachnoid layer of the meninges bulges beneath the skin. This defect does not involve the spinal cord. A **myelomeningocele** results in a cystic dilation of meninges and protuberance of various amounts of the spinal cord through the vertebral defect and is associated with more severe complications than those associated with a meningocele. Both defects occur during the first 4 weeks of the gestational period; at the end of this time the neural tube is normally closed anteriorly and posteriorly.

Because of changes in cerebrospinal fluid (CSF) flow, myelomeningoceles also are likely to be associated with a Chiari II malformation, which is a downward displacement of the cerebellum, brainstem, and fourth ventricle (Figure 20-7). The Chiari II malformation compresses and essentially stretches the posterior region of the cerebellum and brainstem downward through the foramen magnum. The brainstem houses cranial nerve nuclei and pressure on this region may result in altered function of these nerves or actual palsies. The Chiari II malformation is associated with hydrocephalus, an increase in intracranial pressure attributable to obstruction of the flow of CSF; syringomyelia, an abnormality causing cysts at multiple levels within the spinal cord; and cognitive and motor deficits.[8]

Other forms of Chiari malformation include type I, which is usually asymptomatic; type III, in which the brainstem or cerebellum extends into a high cervical myelomeningocele; and type IV, which is characterized by lack of cerebellar development.[9]

Seizures are present in about 30% of children with myelomeningocele,[10] and visual problems (perceptual and astigmatism) and intellectual deficits (ranging from learning problems to intellectual disability) also are common.[11]

CLINICAL MANIFESTATIONS. Myeloceles and myelomeningoceles are evident at birth as a pronounced skin defect on the infant's back (see Figure 20-6). The severity of the clinical presentation will depend on the amount of tissue involved (generally the more neural tissue that is included in the sac, the worse the clinical presentation; some children with meningocele will not have any functional problems) and the level of the defect (thoracic vs. sacral; a sacral defect will cause fewer problems than a defect higher in the neural axis). The bony prominences of the unfused neural arches can be palpated at the lateral border of the defect. The defect is usually covered by a transparent membrane that may have neural tissue attached to its inner surface. This membrane may be intact at birth or may leak CSF, thereby increasing the risks of infection and neuronal damage. Until the defect is closed surgically, CSF may accumulate and cause increased dilation and enlargement of the sac, which may further endanger the nervous system.

Motor and sensory functions below the level of the lesions are altered. Dysfunction may include degrees of weakness, paralysis, spasticity, and bowel and bladder dysfunction. These problems often worsen as the child grows. As the cord ascends within the vertebral canal, primary scar tissue can tether the cord. Several musculoskeletal deformities are related to myelomeningocele, including clubfoot, dislocation of hip or hips, and poor spinal alignment. Spinal deformities, such as scoliosis and kyphosis, are common.

Tethered cord syndrome may develop in children with myelomeningocele.[12] The cord becomes abnormally attached or tethered as a result of scar tissue that develops as the cord transcends the vertebral canal with growth. Traction decreases blood flow and impairs oxidative metabolism. Symptoms are related to excessive tension on the lumbosacral cord and can include scoliosis, altered gait pattern, changes in muscle strength at or below the lesion, disturbance in urinary and bowel patterns, and back pain. The cord can be untethered surgically.[12]

It is possible for a defect to occur without any visible exposure of meninges or neural tissue. There is a cleft in the spine

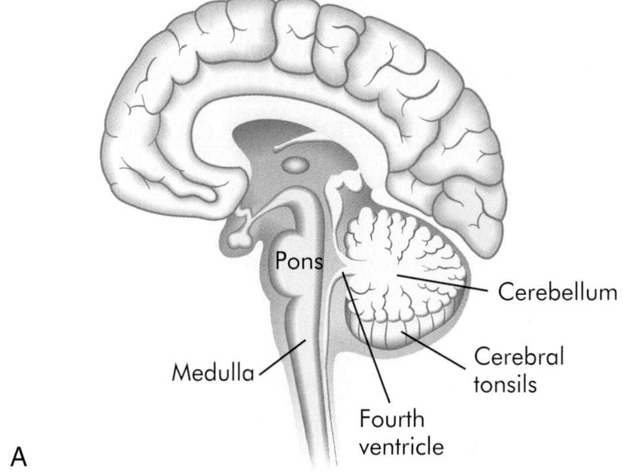

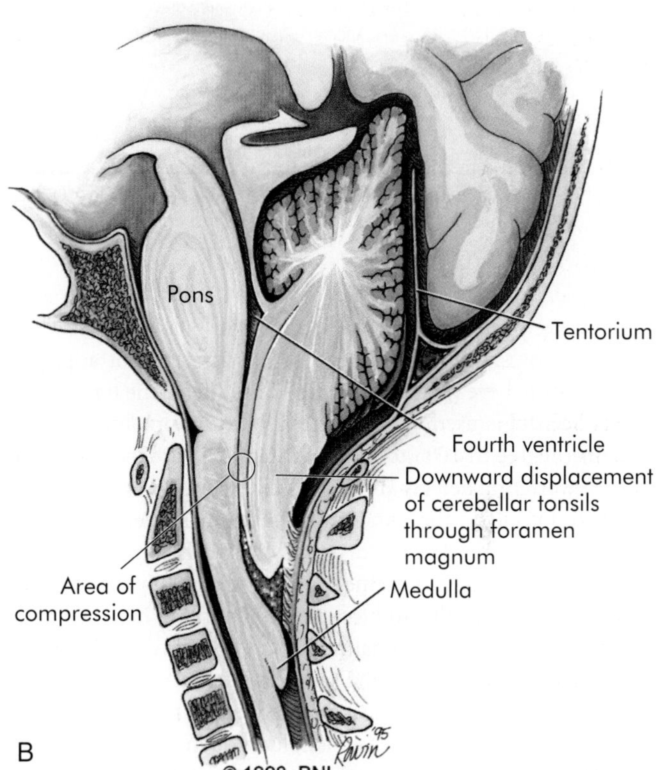

FIGURE 20-7 Normal Brain and Chiari Type II Malformation. **A,** Diagram of normal brain. **B,** Diagram of Chiari II malformation with downward displacement of cerebellar tonsils and medulla through foramen magnum causing compression and obstruction to flow of CSF. (**B** modified from Barrow Neurological Institute of St. Joseph's Hospital and Medical Center, Phoenix, Arizona. Reprinted with permission.)

TABLE 20-2 FUNCTIONAL ALTERATIONS IN MYELODYSPLASIA RELATED TO LEVEL OF LESION

LEVEL OF LESION	FUNCTIONAL IMPLICATIONS
Thoracic	Flaccid paralysis of lower extremities; variable weakness in abdominal trunk musculature; high thoracic level may mean respiratory compromise; absence of bowel and bladder control
High lumbar	Voluntary hip flexion and adduction; flaccid paralysis of knees, ankles, and feet; may walk with extensive braces and crutches; absence of bowel and bladder control
Midlumbar	Strong hip flexion and adduction; fair knee extension; flaccid paralysis of ankles and feet; absence of bowel and bladder control
Low lumbar	Strong hip flexion, extension, and adduction and knee extension; weak ankle and toe mobility; may have limited bowel and bladder function
Sacral	Normal function of lower extremities; normal bowel and bladder function

Data from Farley JA, Dunleavy MJ: Myelodysplasia. In Allen PJ, Vessey JA, editors: *Primary care of the child with a chronic condition,* ed 4, St Louis, 2004, Mosby.

because the posterior vertebral laminae have failed to fuse and the overlying skin is intact. Because the defect is not apparent to the unaided eye (i.e., it is "occult" or hidden), the term **spina bifida occulta** is used.[13] This extremely common defect occurs to some degree in 10% to 25% of infants. Approximately 80% of these vertebral defects are located in the lumbosacral regions, most commonly in the fifth lumbar vertebra and the first sacral vertebra. Spina bifida occulta usually causes no serious neurologic dysfunctions because the spinal cord and spinal nerves are generally anatomically and functionally normal, but the spinal defect can cause hydrocephalus.[14]

EVALUATION AND TREATMENT. Diagnosis is based on clinical manifestations and examination of the meningeal sac. Prenatal diagnosis of myelomeningocele is possible through ultrasonography. In the United States, most pregnant women receive triple or quad screening between 15 and 20 weeks of a pregnancy. The presence of a neural tube defect may result in an elevated amniotic fluid AFP level and subsequent maternal serum AFP levels. Additional testing is then performed if screening tests are positive, including a detailed ultrasound, which may allow for prenatal diagnosis of spina bifida. Prenatal diagnosis offers the parents the option to terminate the pregnancy or become a candidate for fetal intrauterine repair.[15] Cesarean delivery may be recommended to minimize trauma to the open myelomeningocele.[16]

In an effort to preserve neuronal function and minimize damage that may occur from infection and manipulation of the fragile sac, surgical closure is optimal prenatally or during the first 72 hours of life, as recommended by the management of Myelomeningocele Study (MOMS).[17] Functional implications depend on the level and severity of the defect (Table 20-2) and the presence of associated conditions, such as abnormal renal structure or function, or both, and the presence of a Chiari II malformation (see p. 665). These conditions are screened at birth in any child born with myelomeningocele or meningocele.

Because myelodysplasia affects several other body systems (e.g., renal, gastrointestinal, musculoskeletal), these infants require a comprehensive, multidisciplinary approach to treatment. The prognosis depends on the extent of the involvement at birth and the success of prophylactic and acute treatment for potential and actual complications that affect the many body systems. Symptomatic Chiari II malformations require surgical decompression and/or placement of cerebrospinal fluid shunts.

Craniosynostosis

Craniosynostosis (craniostenosis) is the premature closure of one or more of the cranial sutures during the first 18 to 20 months of an infant's life. The incidence of craniosynostosis is 1 in 1800 to 2200 live births.[18] Males are affected twice as often as females. Craniosynostosis can occur as part of a syndrome or, more commonly, as an isolated defect.[19] **Nonsyndromic craniosynostosis** is classified as *simple craniosynostosis* when only one suture is involved and *compound* or *complex craniosynostosis* when two or more sutures are involved. Craniosynostosis prevents normal skull expansion and causes asymmetric skull growth. Premature closure of a suture causes failure of the growth of the bone located at a right angle to the involved suture. Compensatory growth occurs in regions where the sutures are patent, and this causes the various cosmetic deformities of head shape. Where sutures are fused, cerebral growth may exceed the space present. Brain growth may be restricted, and compression may cause neurologic symptoms (Figure 20-8). Clinically, however, most children who present with small heads and developmental delay have microcephaly (see below) caused by defects in brain growth, not compression by prematurely closed sutures.

PATHOPHYSIOLOGY. The exact causes of craniosynostosis are unknown, but are associated with defects in multiple genes that control the fibroblast growth factor receptor family.[20]

Syndromic craniosynostosis refers to synostosis that occurs as part of a genetic syndrome. It is associated with various dysmorphisms involving the face, skeleton, and nervous system and is usually accompanied by developmental delay.

CLINICAL MANIFESTATIONS. Craniosynostosis is classified according to head contour or suture involvement. Final skull contour is determined by the sutures that close, the duration and order of closure, and the ability of other sutures to compensate by expansion (see Figures 20-8 and 20-9).

Premature closure of the sagittal suture, the most common form of craniosynostosis, causes elongation of the skull in the anteroposterior direction. Other anomalies are seen in 25% of these children. When the coronal suture fuses prematurely, the brain expands in a lateral direction. This type of craniosynostosis is associated with a 33% to 66% incidence of associated anomalies.

EVALUATION AND TREATMENT. Craniosynostosis must be differentiated from the more benign skull deformity known as positional plagiocephaly (flattening of one side of the head), which is quite common and may be related to the amount of time an infant spends on his or her back. When the American Academy

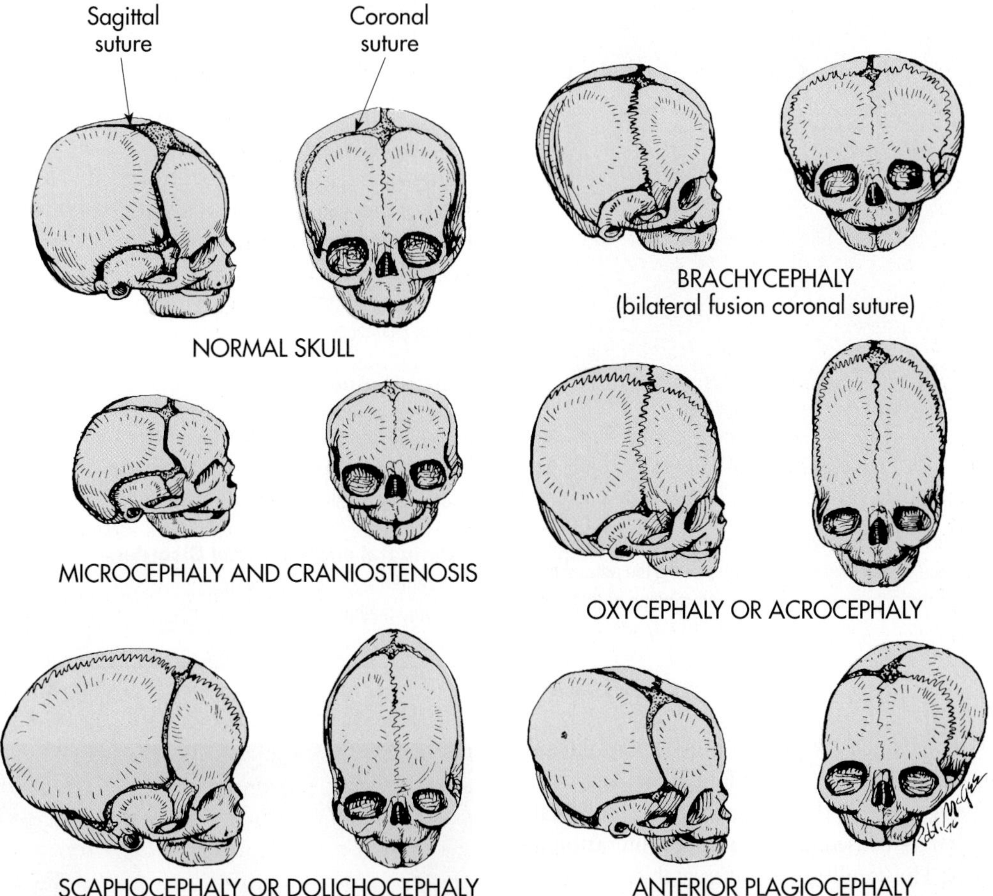

FIGURE 20-8 Types and Frequency of Craniosynostosis. Abnormal head configuration resulting from premature closing of cranial sutures. *Normal skull:* Bones separated by membranous seams until sutures gradually close. *Microcephaly and craniostenosis:* Microcephaly is head circumference more than 2 standard deviations below the mean for age, gender, race, and gestation and reflects a small brain; craniosynostosis is premature closure of sutures. *Scaphocephaly or dolichocephaly* (frequency 56%): Premature closure of sagittal suture, resulting in restricted lateral growth. *Brachycephaly:* Premature closure of coronal suture, resulting in excessive lateral growth. *Oxycephaly or acrocephaly* (frequency 5.8% to 12%): Premature closure of all coronal and sagittal sutures, resulting in accelerated upward growth and small head circumference. *Anterior plagiocephaly* (frequency 13%): Unilateral premature closure of coronal suture, resulting in asymmetric growth. (From Hockenberry JH et al: *Wong's nursing care of infants and children,* ed 9, St Louis, 2011, Mosby.)

of Pediatrics recommended that babies should sleep on their backs instead of their stomachs, the incidence of positional plagiocephaly increased (whereas the incidence of sudden infant death syndrome decreased). A custom-molded helmet or headband applied at about 4 months of age can correct plagiocephaly before closure of fontanels and sutures.

Diagnosis of craniosynostosis is made on the basis of physical examination, head circumference measurements, and radiologic examination. Surgical treatment is often indicated for craniosynostosis and is performed when closure of multiple sutures causes chronic increased intracranial pressure. Surgery then limits the extent of brain damage. In children with craniosynostosis of one suture, surgery often is performed for cosmetic purposes.[21]

Malformations of Cortical Development

Structural malformations of cortical development are a diverse, heterogeneous group of disorders caused by abnormal neuronal cell migration, abnormal neuronal and glial proliferation, and malformations secondary to abnormal postmigrational neuronal development. The processes of malformation can occur at any time during fetal development and after birth. There is a specific genetic defect for some of these disorders; others are multifactorial or acquired (i.e., intrauterine trauma or infection). Most increase the risk for seizures that are difficult to control, developmental delay, and motor dysfunction. Diagnosis is made by magnetic resonance imaging (MRI), family history, and clinical information. Genetic testing is done to assess risk in other family members and to guide prospective therapy.[22-25]

Microcephaly

Reduced proliferation or accelerated apoptosis causes congenital microcephaly (microencephaly—small brain), whereas increased proliferation causes megalencephaly (abnormally large brain). **Microcephaly** is a rare defect in brain growth as a whole (see Figure 20-8). The word *microcephaly* is derived

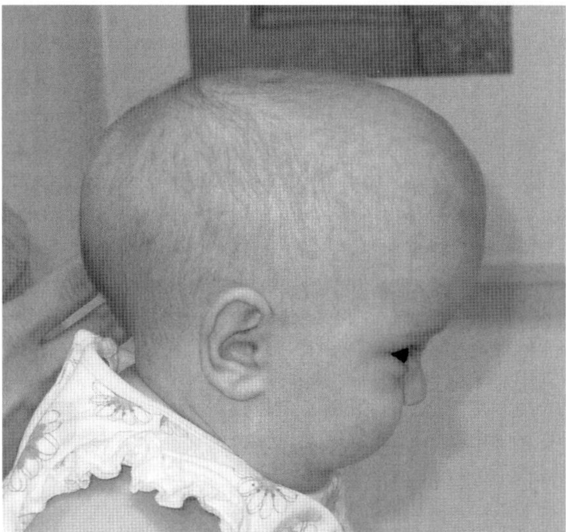

FIGURE 20-9 Lateral View of a Child with Scaphocephaly Resulting from Sagittal Synostosis. Note the frontal bossing, elongation along the anteroposterior (AP) axis, and prominent occiput, all of which are characteristic of this condition. (From Coran A et al: *Pediatric surgery,* ed 7, St Louis, 2012, Mosby.)

BOX 20-1 CAUSES OF MICROENCEPHALY

Defects in Brain Development
Hereditary (recessive) microcephaly
Down syndrome and other trisomy syndromes
Fetal ionizing radiation exposure
Maternal phenylketonuria
Seckel syndrome
Cornelia de Lange syndrome
Rubinstein-Taybi syndrome
Smith-Lemli-Opitz syndrome
Fetal alcohol syndrome

Intrauterine Infections
Congenital rubella
Cytomegalovirus infection
Congenital toxoplasmosis
Congenital syphilis

Perinatal and Postnatal Disorders
Intrauterine or neonatal anoxia
Severe malnutrition in early infancy
Neonatal herpesvirus infection

from the Greek (*mikro,* "small"; *kephale,* "head"). Cranial size is significantly below average for the infant's age, sex, race, and gestation. The small size of the skull reflects a small brain (microencephaly) that is caused by reduced proliferation or accelerated apoptosis. The condition is not treatable.

True (primary) microcephaly is present at birth and can be caused by genetic alterations, including autosomal dominant, autosomal recessive, or X-linked genetic abnormalities, or various chromosomal abnormalities. Environmental causes include toxin or radiation exposure or intrauterine infection during the period of induction and neural cell migration (Box 20-1). *Secondary microcephaly* develops postnatally (the baby's head size is normal at birth but then fails to grow as expected) and is associated with a variety of causes including infection, trauma, metabolic disorders, maternal anorexia experienced during the third trimester of pregnancy, and the presence of some genetic syndromes (e.g., Rett syndrome).[26]

Microcephalic brain weight may be as low as 25% of normal, and the number and size of the cortical gyri may be diminished. Growth of the frontal lobes is severely stunted, and the cerebellum often is disproportionately large. In microcephaly caused by perinatal or postnatal disorders, neuronal loss and gliosis may be present in the cerebral cortex. Children with microcephaly are usually developmentally delayed.

Cortical Dysplasias

Cortical dysplasias are a heterogeneous group of disorders caused by defects in neuronal cell migration and subsequent abnormalities in connections between cells. These disorders may range from a small area of abnormal tissue (e.g., heterotopia, which are pieces of gray matter that did not migrate to their normal position in the cortex of the brain; or focal cortical dysplasias, where brain organization in one small area is abnormal) to an entire brain that is smooth without the normal configuration of gyri and sulci of a developed brain (lissencephaly) (Figure 20-10).

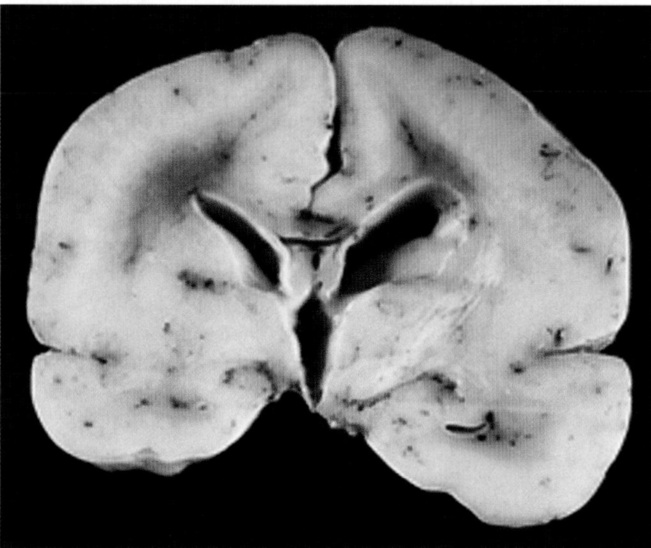

FIGURE 20-10 Lissencephaly. The absence of cortical gyri defines this abnormality, seen here in the brain from a full-term infant. (From Kumar V et al: *Robbins & Cotran pathologic basis of disease,* ed 8, Saunders, 2010, Philadelphia.)

Congenital Hydrocephalus

Congenital hydrocephalus is present at birth and characterized by increased intracranial pressure (ICP). This increase may be caused by a blockage within the ventricular system in which the CSF flows, an imbalance in the production of CSF, or a reduced reabsorption of CSF that results in ventricular enlargement and increased ICP. The pressure within the ventricular system dilates the ventricles and pushes and compresses the brain tissue against the skull. When hydrocephalus develops before fusion

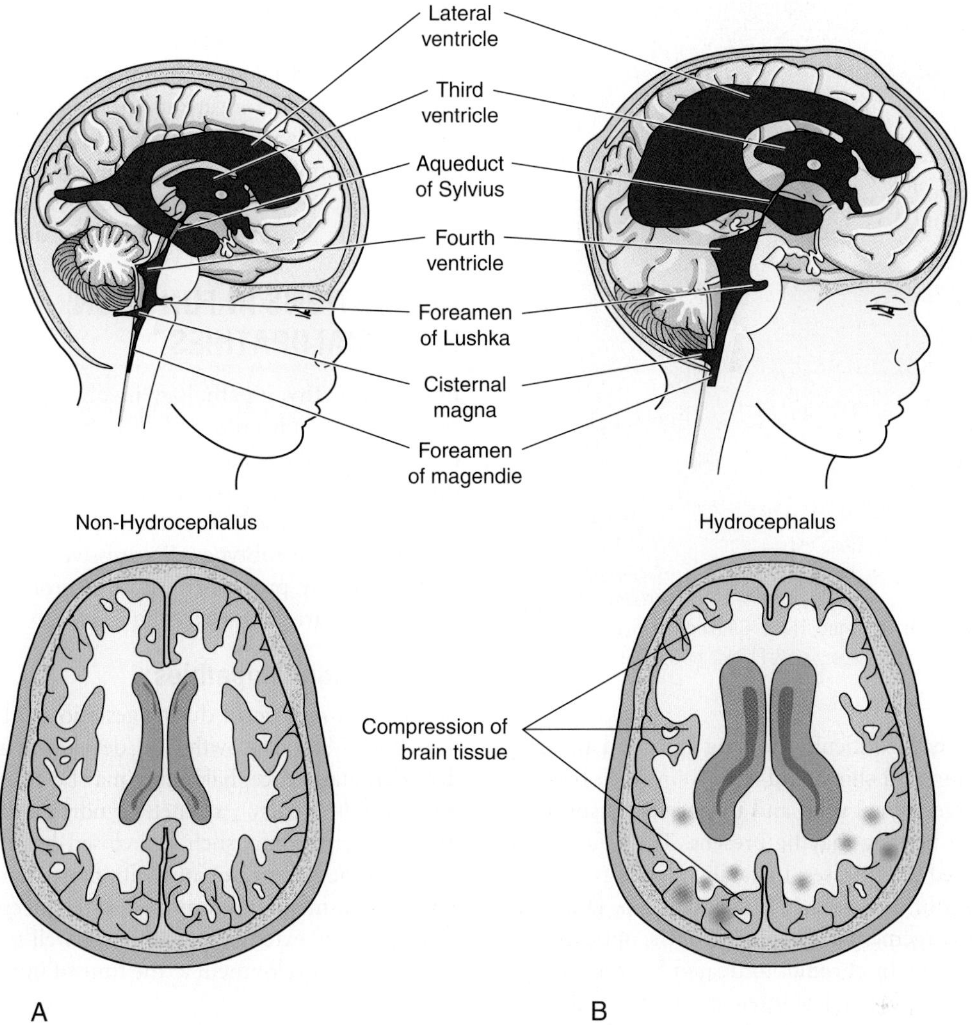

FIGURE 20-11 Hydrocephalus. A block in the flow of cerebrospinal fluid (CSF). **A,** Patent cerebrospinal fluid circulation. **B,** Enlarged lateral and third ventricles caused by obstruction of circulation—stenosis of aqueduct of Sylvius.

of the cranial sutures, the skull has the capacity to increase its size to accommodate this additional space-occupying volume and to preserve neuronal function. The overall incidence of hydrocephalus is approximately 1 to 3 per 1000 live births.[27] The incidence of hydrocephalus, excluding the hydrocephalus associated with myelomeningocele, is approximately 0.5 to 1 per 1000 live births, with aqueductal stenosis as the cause for approximately one third of these cases.[28] (Types of hydrocephalus are discussed in Chapter 17.)

PATHOPHYSIOLOGY. *Obstructive hydrocephalus* is caused most commonly by congenital aqueductal stenosis. The cerebral aqueduct, which connects the third ventricle to the fourth ventricle, is narrowed or replaced by multiple channels that end blindly. In a small number of children the stenosis is transmitted as an X-linked recessive trait. The **Dandy-Walker malformation** is a congenital defect of midline cerebellar structures and the fourth ventricle in which hydrocephalus is caused by atresia of the foramina of Luschka or Magendie, which normally allow the fourth ventricle to empty into the areas surrounding the brain, leading the ventricular flow of CSF into a "blind pouch." Other causes of obstructions within the ventricular system that can result in hydrocephalus include brain tumors, cysts, trauma, arteriovenous malformations, blood clots, infection, and spina bifida.

CSF travels throughout the ventricular system, surrounds the brain, and is reabsorbed into the venous system by the arachnoid villi. Blockage of the arachnoid villi may occur in conditions such as bacterial or viral meningitis, intraventricular hemorrhage, and subarachnoid hemorrhage, or may result from congenital malformations within this area. In this instance CSF flows or communicates effectively but is unable to be reabsorbed, resulting in hydrocephalus.

CLINICAL MANIFESTATIONS. Congenital hydrocephalus is present at birth, whereas acquired hydrocephalus usually becomes apparent in the first weeks to months of life. Symptoms of this condition depend directly on the cause and rate of hydrocephalus development. Typically, the fontanels enlarge and become full and bulging (Figures 20-11 and 20-12). The eyes may assume a staring expression, with sclera visible above the iris, a finding called *sunsetting eyes.*

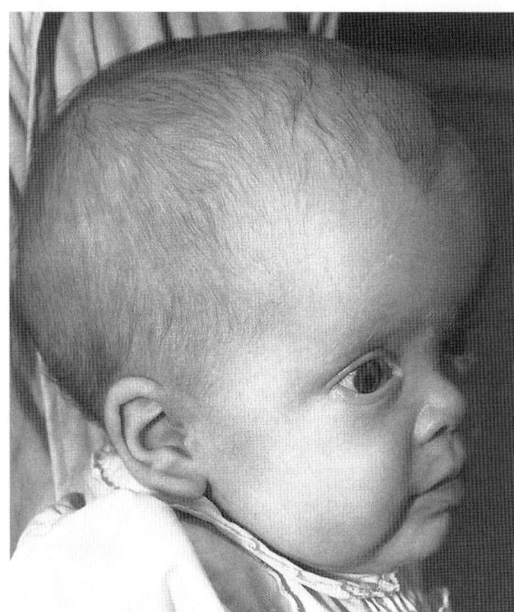

FIGURE 20-12 Child with Enlarged Head Caused by Hydrocephalus. (From McLaurin DC: *Pediatric neurosurgery,* ed 2, Philadelphia, 1989, Saunders.)

The infant may have difficulty holding the head upright. The scalp skin is thin and shiny, and scalp veins may become prominent. The large cranial vault and the face are disproportionate, and frontal bossing may be present. The infant's cry becomes high pitched as ICP rises; irritability, lethargy, vomiting, and other signs of increased ICP may develop. Dramatic head growth and enlargement, compression of the optic nerves, and optic chiasm occur in chronic, untreated hydrocephalus. However, because of early surgical intervention, these signs of hydrocephalus rarely are seen in developed countries. When hydrocephalus develops late in childhood, the head may not have the capacity to enlarge, and symptoms of increased ICP occur quickly (see Chapter 17).

The relationship between hydrocephalus and intellectual disability has been heavily debated. Correlation between the degree of hydrocephalus and impaired cognitive function often is a result of additional complications, such as severe congenital malformations, acute or chronic infections, or progressive brain tumors. Approximately two thirds of children with uncomplicated congenital hydrocephalus treated successfully with shunting may have normal to borderline intelligence.[29]

EVALUATION AND TREATMENT. Both cranial ultrasound and computed tomography (CT) are used to evaluate hydrocephalus. Magnetic resonance imaging (MRI) may add information about the specific cause of the hydrocephalus. In infancy, head circumference measurements are obtained and monitored, and if the head is enlarging too quickly the child is referred for imaging first and then, if needed, to neurosurgery for further evaluation. The treatment is surgical placement of a shunt to divert the excess CSF from the ventricular cavity to other areas of the body. Several types of shunts are available. The main objective of any shunt system is to decrease ICP and preserve neuronal function. With neurosurgical intervention and follow-up, the 5-year survival usually is greater than 80%. Most deaths that occur within this category result from severe congenital malformations and/or progressive disorders such as brain tumors. Children with hydrocephalus depend on the internal shunt system to maintain safe ICPs and therefore are at risk for sudden failure of this system, which leads to acute increased ICP and death. Endoscopic ventriculostomy with choroid plexus cauterization are two newer procedures performed together and offer hope to replace shunts, and avoiding shunt blocks, malfunction, and infection.[29a]

ALTERATIONS IN FUNCTION: ENCEPHALOPATHIES

Encephalopathy, a pathology involving the brain, is a general category of syndromes and diseases that include infections, ischemia, metabolic and toxic causes, and others. Encephalopathies in children are associated with a great variety of known and suspected causes. They can be divided into non-progressive and progressive subtypes. Progressive subtypes can be either acute or slowly progressive. Rare neurologic disorders with a genetic basis are summarized in Table 20-3.

Static Encephalopathies

Brain injury may occur during gestation or birth or at any time during childhood growth and development, causing a static disorder. Static encephalopathy may be a result of trauma near birth (cerebral palsy); a genetic syndrome (intellectual disability); or later trauma, such as a closed-head injury, which may cause a static encephalopathy with motor and cognitive deficits. The clinical manifestations of a static encephalopathy depend on the site and extent of the injury, as well as the age of the child and stage of development at the time of injury.

Cerebral Palsy

Cerebral palsy (CP) is a disorder of movement, muscle tone, or posture that is caused by injury or abnormal development in the immature brain, before, during, or after birth up to 1 year of age. CP is one of the most common crippling disorders of childhood, affecting nearly 500,000 children in the United States alone. Although the exact incidence is unknown, studies suggest that the prevalence is approximately 3.3 per 1000 live births in the United States.[30] Although the term cerebral palsy refers specifically to the motor deficits, associated intellectual disability, seizures, and other problems also are common in children with this disorder.

PATHOPHYSIOLOGY. Several factors, alone or in combination, can produce brain damage that leads to CP (Table 20-4). Prenatal factors that affect the developing nervous system may be endogenous or exogenous. The fetus may be affected by impaired embryo implantation, chromosomal abnormalities, infection, trauma, radiation exposure, and toxic substances. Maternal toxemia, diabetes mellitus, and maternal nutritional deficiencies can produce neurologic damage in the fetus. Anoxia, trauma, and infections are the most common factors that cause injury to the nervous system in the perinatal period. Low birth weight and birth asphyxia are commonly identified risk factors for cerebral palsy. Vascular abnormalities, arterial or venous stasis, and thrombosis can occur as a result of tissue

TABLE 20-3 SELECTED NEUROLOGIC DISORDERS WITH A GENETIC BASIS

SYNDROME/ DISORDERS	CURRENTLY KNOWN GENETIC COMPONENTS	PATHOPHYSIOLOGY	MAJOR NEUROLOGIC FEATURES
Angelman syndrome	Loss of function mutation of the *UBE3A* gene (ubiquitin protein ligase) can be acquired from mother (chromosome 15)	Protein, important in degradation of proteins in the brain	Little to no verbal language, mental retardation, seizure disorder, sleep disorder, movement/ balance disorder
Batten disease	Autosomal recessive; mutation of the *CLN3* gene (ceroid-lipofuscinosis, neuronal 3) (chromosome 16)	Lysosomal storage defect resulting in abnormal storage of cerebral lipofuscins	Develops normally until 6 months to 2 years of age when progressive brain disease becomes apparent; seizures, mental retardation, blindness, and death
Branched-chain ketoaciduria (maple syrup urine disease)	Autosomal recessive; most common type is classic caused by mutation of the *BCKDHA* gene (2-oxoisovalerate dehydrogenase subunit alpha, a mitochondrial enzyme) (chromosome 19)	All types result in inability to metabolize three amino acids; these acids accumulate and are toxic at high levels	Without early diagnosis and treatment, mental retardation, seizures, and death
Cri du chat syndrome	Autosomal dominant; deletion on the short arm of chromosome 5 (also called 5p minus syndrome)	Deletion of multiple genes responsible for phenotype; evidence that deletion of telomerase reverse transcriptase gene contributes to phenotype	High-pitched cry; mental retardation, microcephaly, low birth weight, failure to thrive; widely spaced eyes (ocular hypertelorism), unusually small jaw (micrognathia)
Lesch-Nyhan syndrome	X-linked recessive; mutation of the *HPRT* gene (hypoxanthine phosphoribosyltransferase 1)	Metabolism disturbance of purines; excessive production of uric acid	Mental retardation, progressive neurologic disorder, compulsively bitten lips and fingers; self-mutilating
Neurofibromatosis (NF)	Autosomal dominant	Variable expressivity	Multiple café-au-lait spots, neurofibromas, learning disability, seizure disorder
NF1 (von Recklinghausen disease)	Mutation of the *NF1* gene (neurofibromin) (chromosome 17)	A large, complex protein; this protein may act as a switch to regulate cell growth; mutation may lessen or inhibit the normal output of this protein and allow irregular cell growth that may lead to tumor development	Increased risk for nerve sheath tumors and brain tumors
NF2 (bilateral acoustic NF)	Autosomal dominant: mutation of either the *merlin* (moesin-ezrin-radixin-like protein or schwannomin) or the *NF2* gene (chromosome 22)	A tumor-suppressor protein (*merlin* or *schwannomin*)	Multiple tumors (schwannomas) on cranial and spinal nerves, acoustic neuromas, hearing loss
Progressive myoclonus epilepsy			
Unverricht-Lundborg disease	Autosomal recessive; mutation *CSTB* gene (cystatin B, a cysteine protease inhibitor) (chromosome 21)	This protein regulates enzymes that break down other proteins	Onset at age 6-15 years, severe incapacitating stimulus-sensitive progressive myoclonus, tonic-clonic epileptic seizures, and characteristic abnormalities on electroencephalogram; also may develop other neurologic symptoms. such as ataxia, incoordination, dysarthria
Lafora disease	Autosomal recessive; mutation of the *EMP2A* gene (epilepsy, progressive myoclonus type 2A or laforin) and *EMP2B* gene (malin) (chromosome 6)	Concentric amyloid (Lafora) bodies found in neurons, liver, skin, bone, and muscle; defects in protein degradation and clearance	Grand mal seizures and/or myoclonus at about age 15; rapid and severe motor and coordination impairments, rapid mental deterioration, often with psychotic features; survival is short, less than 10 years after onset
Rett syndrome	X-linked dominant; appears to occur only in girls; defective *MeCP2* gene (methyl CpG binding protein 2) (X-chromosome)	Protein involved in regulation of gene expression; defects in this gene allow other genes to be expressed at inappropriate times in development	Progressive neurologic disorder; develops normally in first year of life, then loss of mental capacity and motor skills begins; loss of purposeful hand movements; stereotypical hand wringing and flapping
Tay-Sachs disease	Autosomal recessive; mutation of the *HEXA* gene (chromosome 15)	Caused by a deficiency of hexosaminidase, an enzyme, which results in accumulation of a material that damages the brain	Failure to thrive, blindness, seizures, progressive paralysis; usually death by age 4
Tuberous sclerosis	Autosomal dominant; mutation of either the *TSC1* gene (hamartin) (chromosome 9) or the *TSC2* gene (tuberin) (chromosome 16)	These proteins act as tumor growth suppressors	Develops in early childhood; seizures, mental retardation, skin and eye lesions; multiple benign tumors in brain and other vital organs

TABLE 20-4 CEREBRAL PALSY: PREDISPOSING FACTORS AND KNOWN CAUSES

RISK FACTORS	ASSOCIATED CAUSES
Prenatal	
Maternal	Metabolic diseases
	Nutritional deficiencies (e.g., anemia)
	Twin or multiple births
	Bleeding
	Toxemia
	Blood incompatibilities
	Exposure to radiation
	Infection (e.g., rubella, toxoplasmosis, cytomegalic inclusion disease)
	Premature labor
Prematurity	Asphyxia leading to cerebral hemorrhage
Genetic factors	Absence of corpus callosum, aqueductal stenosis, cerebellar hypoplasia
Congenital anomalies of the brain	Unknown causes not evident on clinical examination
Perinatal	Anesthesia or analgesia during labor and delivery
	Mechanical trauma during delivery
	Immaturity at birth
	Metabolic disorders (e.g., hyperbilirubinemia, hypoglycemia, amino acid disorders, hyperosmolality)
	Electrolyte disturbances (e.g., hypernatremia, hypoglycemia)
Postnatal	Head trauma
	Infections (e.g., meningitis, encephalitis)
	Cerebrovascular accidents
	Toxicosis
	Environmental toxins (e.g., lead ingestion, methyl mercury ingestion from contaminated fish)

hypoxia or as unrelated structural alterations. These anomalies may result in direct brain trauma that leads to infarction, intraventricular hemorrhage, and subarachnoid hemorrhage. Physical trauma to the central nervous system can occur during the birthing process. Genetic, teratogenic, and early pregnancy influences on the development of cerebral palsy are multifactorial and not yet fully understood.[31,32] The severity of the damage depends on the gestational age at the time of the injury and the type and degree of injury sustained. Magnesium sulfate in preterm newborns and head cooling during or after resuscitation at birth may reduce brain damage and risk of CP.[33,34]

CLINICAL MANIFESTATIONS. Although CP is by definition nonprogressive, its clinical manifestations change with growth and maturation of the child. Associated problems are common and may involve vision and hearing impairment, intellectual disability, seizures, swallowing problems, and more.[35,36]

The syndromes associated with CP can be classified according to the areas of the brain that are damaged and the part of the body that is affected. Brain damage may affect the pyramidal system, causing spasticity, or the extrapyramidal system, leading to dyskinetic, ataxic, or hypotonic CP. **Pyramidal/spastic cerebral palsy** results from damage or defects in the brain's corticospinal pathways (upper motor neuron) in either one or both hemispheres and accounts for approximately 70% to 80% of cerebral palsy cases. It is associated with increased muscle tone, prolonged primitive reflexes, exaggerated deep tendon reflexes, clonus, rigidity of the extremities, scoliosis, and contractures. Cognitive impairment occurs in about 30% of children.[37] If spasticity occurs throughout the body, the child has *spastic quadriparesis;* if it occurs in primarily one half of the body, the child has *hemiparetic cerebral palsy*. The latter type can occur after a stroke in the middle cerebral artery territory before or at the time of birth.

Extrapyramidal/nonspastic cerebral palsy is caused by damage to cells in the basal ganglia, thalamus, or cerebellum and includes two subtypes: dyskinetic and ataxic. **Dyskinetic cerebral palsy** is associated with extreme difficulty in fine motor coordination and purposeful movements. Movements are jerky, uncontrolled, and abrupt, resulting from injury to the basal ganglia or thalamus. This form of CP accounts for approximately 20% to 25% of cases. **Ataxic cerebral palsy** is associated with damage to the cerebellum and manifests with gait disturbances and instability. The infant with this form of CP may have hypotonia at birth, but develops stiffness of the trunk muscles later in infancy. This lack of flexibility exaggerates the infant's inability to balance body position without support. This form of CP accounts for approximately 5% of cases. A child may have symptoms of each of these CP types, which leads to a mixed-variety disorder seen in approximately 13% of children with this disorder.

A few decades ago, a large percentage of children were identified as having CP for unknown reasons. Many had no history of trauma or other cause for their CP. As imaging techniques and other testing methods have improved, there is an increased chance that the underlying cause of a child's CP will be delineated. A small percentage of these children may actually have a treatable and slowly progressive condition; therefore, every attempt to find an underlying cause for a child's CP should be made. One example of such an underlying cause is glucose transporter deficiency, a condition where the concentration of glucose in the cerebral spinal fluid is very low. Children with this condition have ataxic movements that may be misidentified as CP and also have intractable seizures. If this defect is identified, the child is treated with the ketogenic diet (see Epilepsy section) with amelioration of some of the symptoms. Because of examples like this, the American Academy of Neurology has made specific recommendations regarding the evaluation of a child with CP of an unknown cause as it may actually be a slowly progressive encephalopathy.[38]

EVALUATION AND TREATMENT. Although the brain injury is static, the clinical picture of CP may change with growth and development. The use of intrathecal baclofen pumps, botulinum toxin, and selective dorsal rhizotomy for spasticity has led to improvement in selected children with CP.[39,40]

The management of children with CP varies with age, type and severity of involvement, and associated disorders. Thus the scope of care required by the child and family includes ongoing medical, social, and educational intervention, and a family-focused multidisciplinary team approach.[41]

TABLE 20-5 INHERITED METABOLIC DISORDERS OF THE CENTRAL NERVOUS SYSTEM PRESENTING AT DIFFERENT AGES

AGE OF ONSET	DISORDER
Neonatal period	Pyridoxine dependency, galactosemia, maple syrup urine disease and its variant, phenylketonuria (PKU)
Early infancy	Tay-Sachs disease and its variants, infantile Gaucher disease, infantile Niemann-Pick disease, Krabbe disease (leukodystrophy), Farber lipogranulomatosis, Pelizaeus-Merzbacher disease and other sudanophilic leukodystrophies, spongy degeneration, Alexander disease, Alpers disease, Leigh disease (subacute necrotizing encephalomyelopathy), congenital lactic acidosis, Zellweger encephalopathy, Lowe disease (oculocerebrorenal disease)
Late infancy and early childhood	Disorders of amino acid metabolism, metachromatic leukodystrophy, late infantile GM1 gangliosidosis, late infantile Gaucher and Niemann-Pick diseases, neuroaxonal dystrophy, mucopolysaccharidosis, mucolipidosis, fucosidosis, mannosidosis, aspartylglycosaminuria, amaurotic idiocy (Jansky-Bielschowsky disease, Batten disease, Vogt-Spielmeyer disease, neuronal ceroid lipofuscinosis), Cockayne syndrome
Later childhood and adolescence	Progressive cerebellar ataxias of childhood and adolescence, hepatolenticular degeneration (Wilson disease), Hallervorden-Spatz disease, Lesch-Nyhan syndrome and other uremic states, familial calcification of vessels in basal ganglia and cerebellum, familial polymyoclonus, chronic familial leukodystrophy, homocystinuria, Fabry disease

For more information regarding screening and parent education see Medical Home Portal at www.medicalhomeportal.org/.

Inherited Metabolic Disorders of the Central Nervous System

A large number of inherited metabolic disorders have been identified. The advent of newborn metabolic screening for 28 metabolic conditions (in some states as many as 50) has led to many of these children being identified before symptoms develop. In these disorders, there is either a deficiency of an essential product or an accumulation of a substrate with damage induced either by overaccumulation or toxicity or by a combination of both. Inborn errors of metabolism are present at birth, although they may not manifest until childhood or even adulthood, and most cause disturbances of the nervous system. Restrictive diets can prevent symptoms from developing for many children and those with these disorders can lead relatively normal lives. The following website contains a list of the newborn metabolic screening tests: www.marchofdimes.com/professionals/bringinghome_screening.html. Table 20-5 lists some of these inherited metabolic disorders. Defects in amino acid and lipid metabolism are more common than rarely occurring defects in carbohydrate metabolism.

Defects in Amino Acid Metabolism. Biochemical defects in amino acid metabolism are examples of defects in inherited metabolic disorders. They may be classified as (1) those in which the transport of an amino acid is impaired; (2) those involving an enzyme or cofactor deficiency; and (3) those grouped around certain chemical components, such as sulfur-containing amino acids.[42] Most of the disorders in the literature described to date suggest that the absence of enzymatic activity most often is caused by the genetically determined absence of the enzyme protein. Diseases caused by an enzymatic deficiency are associated with increased blood concentrations of the amino acid whose degradation pathway is impaired and with the appearance of the amino acid in the urine. With the exception of phenylketonuria, the estimated incidence of each of these defects is about 1 in 100,000 to 200,000 live births, although this number may increase with newborn screening.

Phenylketonuria. Phenylketonuria (PKU) is an example of an inborn error in the metabolism of amino acids. PKU is an autosomal recessive inborn error of metabolism characterized by mutations of the phenylalanine hydroxylase *(PAH)* gene. PKU has a prevalence rate of about 1 per 15,000 live births in the United States.[43] Because of its genetic component and distribution, this statistical prevalence varies widely on the basis of geographic and ethnic differences.[44] Most natural food proteins contain about 15% phenylalanine. The body uses tyrosine in the biosynthesis of protein, melanin, thyroxine, and the catecholamines in the brain and adrenal medulla. Loss of *PAH* activity results in phenylalanine hydroxylase deficiency and the inability of the body to convert the essential amino acid phenylalanine to tyrosine, leading to the accumulation of phenylalanine in the serum. It is the accumulation of phenylalanine and associated metabolites that causes damage to the central nervous system (Figure 20-13). One of these phenyl acids, phenylpyruvic acid, gives the urine a characteristic musty odor and is responsible for the name given to the disorder. High blood levels of phenylalanine prevent sufficient neutral amino acid entry into the brain, which contributes to the neuropathologic process of PKU. A baby with the genetic defect of PKU born to a mother without PKU or to a mother with PKU who is well controlled on a phenylalanine-restricted diet will not have any problems because he or she is receiving nutrients from the mother. When a baby is born with PKU and begins a regular diet high in phenylalanine without treatment, buildup of phenylalanine occurs, brain growth slows, and the child exhibits developmental delay or intellectual disability, concomitant with jerking movements, seizures, skin rashes, and attention problems. Because of the lack of tyrosine and its relationship to the biosynthesis of melanin, children with PKU have a characteristic phenotype that includes blond hair, blue eyes, and fair skin. Children with genetically darker complexions may be red haired or brunette.

Less severe variants of this disorder are caused by defects in the phenylalanine hydroxylase system rather than the phenylalanine hydroxylase enzyme itself. This related disorder, known as **hyperphenylalaninemia (HPA),** occurs when plasma phenylalanine levels rise above normal but do not rise as high as in PKU.[45] Individuals with PKU also need to be screened for response to BH4 (6-*R*-L-erythro-5,6,7,8-tetrahydrobiopterin), which significantly decreases blood phenylalanine levels when given as an oral supplement (sapropterin dihydrochloride).[46]

When infants are treated appropriately, growth and development are normal. Treatment for PKU involves restriction of phenylalanine in the diet to maintain a nontoxic level and supplementation with other essential amino acids. Treatment must be continued for life and strict adherence to the diet is especially important for pregnant women with PKU so that damage does not occur prenatally to the fetus. The diet also must be supplemented with adequate sources of energy, protein, and nutrients to allow for optimal growth and brain development. Supplementation of tyrosine also may be required if plasma levels are low. Enzyme replacement and gene and cell therapies are under investigation.[47]

Storage Diseases. Some metabolic disorders are caused by abnormal accumulation of metabolites. These disorders are generally not included in newborn screening. Lysosomal storage diseases and Tay-Sachs disease will be discussed as examples of storage diseases.

Lysosomal Storage Disease. Lipids are fat-like substances that are important parts of the membranes found within and between each cell and in the myelin sheath that coats and protects the nerves. Lipids include oils, fatty acids, waxes, steroids (such as cholesterol and estrogen), and other related compounds. Although these compounds accumulate to some extent in cells, excess amounts are broken down in lysosomes (vesicles within the cell whose primary function is to degrade the breakdown products of cellular metabolism as discussed

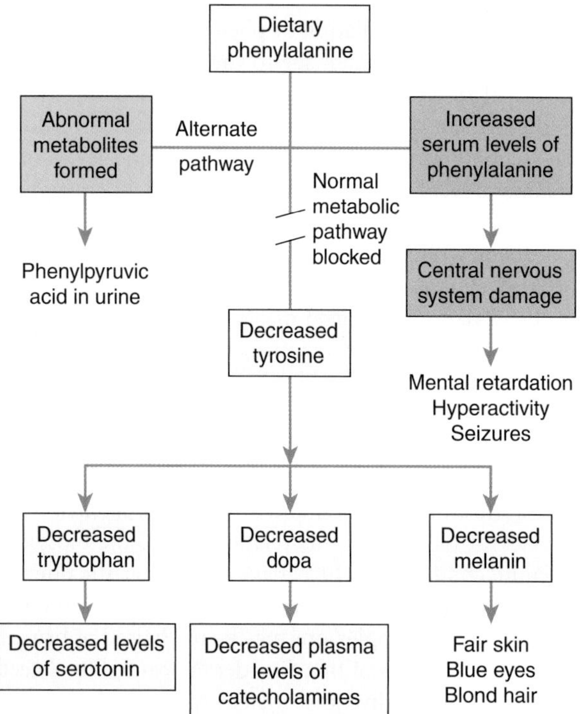

FIGURE 20-13 Metabolic Errors and Consequences in Phenylketonuria. (Redrawn from Hockenberry MJ et al: *Wong's nursing care of infants and children,* ed 9, St Louis, 2011, Mosby.)

in Chapter 1). An estimated 25 to 30 enzymes within lysosomes participate in the breakdown of excess compounds. A genetic defect resulting in a missing or defective enzyme, such as lysosomal hydrolase, causes an excessive accumulation of the enzyme's substrate, which alters cell function. The enzyme defect may occur in the brain, liver, spleen, bone, or lung, thus involving several organ systems. Prenatal diagnosis is available. Enzyme replacement therapy and stem cell therapy have been successful in some cases.[48]

Tay-Sachs Disease. Tay-Sachs disease (GM2 gangliosidosis) is an example of a lysosomal storage disease. It is a fatal autosomal recessive disorder (*HexA* gene on chromosome 15) caused by deficiency of the lysosomal enzyme hexosaminidase A (HexA), an enzyme that degrades GM2 gangliosides (fatty acids) within nerve cell lysosomes. Consequently, there is accumulation of gangliosides (**gangliosidosis**), which causes toxicity to nerve cells.[49] French Canadians, Louisiana Cajuns, and Ashkenazi Jews are all considered high-risk with a carrier rate of 1 per 27.[50] Prenatal screening is available.

In Tay-Sachs disease, GM2 ganglioside accumulates in neurons throughout the body, although the pathologic progressive changes prevail in the CNS. With time, neurons become distorted and balloon, and microglial cells, which also are swollen and filled with large granules, proliferate. Cystic degeneration of the cerebral white matter and atrophy of the cerebellar hemispheres often occur. The number of neurons is diminished. Changes in the spinal cord, particularly in the motor cells of the anterior horn of the cord, also are characteristic. Involvement of this region of the spinal cord results in hypotonia, hyporeflexia, and overall weakness.

Onset of symptoms usually occurs when the infant is 3 to 6 months old. A loss of milestones is associated with an excessive startle response. Seizures, muscular rigidity, and blindness become prominent after the first year of life, and head size may increase. Death usually occurs by 2 to 5 years of age. No beneficial therapy has been developed. Genetic counseling programs are available, and some states require screening techniques for couples and those at risk who may be carriers.[51]

Acute Encephalopathies

Intoxications of the Central Nervous System

Drug-induced encephalopathies always must be considered in the child with unexplained neurologic changes. Such encephalopathies may result from accidental ingestion, therapeutic overdose, intentional overdose, or ingestion of environmental toxins (the most commonly ingested poisons are listed in Box 20-2). Approximately 1.6 million children were exposed to poisons and approximately 263 children died in the United States in 2010 as a result of poisoning.[52]

Lead Poisoning. High blood levels of lead occur in lead poisoning. If lead poisoning is not treated, lead encephalopathy will result and cause serious and irreversible neurologic damage[53,54] (Figure 20-14). Those at greatest risk are children 2 to 3 years of age and those with pica or living in lead-contaminated environments. **Pica** is the habitual, purposeful, and compulsive ingestion of nonfood substances such as clay, dirt, or paint chips. Lead intoxication also may occur from long-term exposure to smelters, sniffing of gasoline, exposure to lead-based paint, and ingestion of airborne lead.[55]

An estimated 203,000 U.S. children have excessive amounts of lead in their blood, which leads to varying amounts of intellectual disability depending on level and length of exposure time.[56] Young children are more likely to be exposed to lead-containing materials than older children and also absorb lead more easily than older children. Levels continue to be highest among non-Hispanic black children, Mexican American, and non-Hispanic white children, with the greatest risk being in the non-Hispanic black population.[57] The American Academy of Pediatrics has published recommendations for the treatment of lead poisoning depending on blood lead level.[58]

BOX 20-2 COMMON POISONS

PHARMACOLOGIC AGENTS	HEAVY METALS	MISCELLANEOUS AGENTS
Acetaminophen	Lead	Botulinum toxin
Amphetamines	Acute	Alcohols
Anticonvulsants	Chronic	Ethyl, isopropyl, methyl
Antidepressants	Mercury	Pesticides
Antihistamines	Thallium	Organophosphates
Atropine	Arsenic	Chlorinated hydrocarbons
Barbiturates		Mushrooms
Methadone		Venoms
Phencyclidine		Snake bite
Salicylates		Tick paralysis
Tranquilizers		Ethylene glycol

Data from Swaiman KF et al: *Swaiman's pediatric neurology: principles and practice,* vol 2, ed 5, St Louis, 2012, Mosby.

Infections of the Central Nervous System

Meningitis is inflammation of the meninges and subarachnoid space surrounding the brain and spinal cord, whereas the word **encephalitis** reflects inflammation within the brain. In many infections of the meninges, encephalitis also is present and the term *meningo-encephalitis* is used. The origin of such inflammation and acute encephalopathy can be caused by bacteria, viruses, or other microorganisms. **Aseptic meningitis** has no evidence of bacterial infection but may be associated with viral infection, systemic disease, or drugs.

Bacterial Meningitis. **Acute bacterial meningitis** is one of the most serious infections to which infants and children are susceptible. In the United States approximately 4100 cases of bacterial meningitis occurred each year between 2003 and 2007,

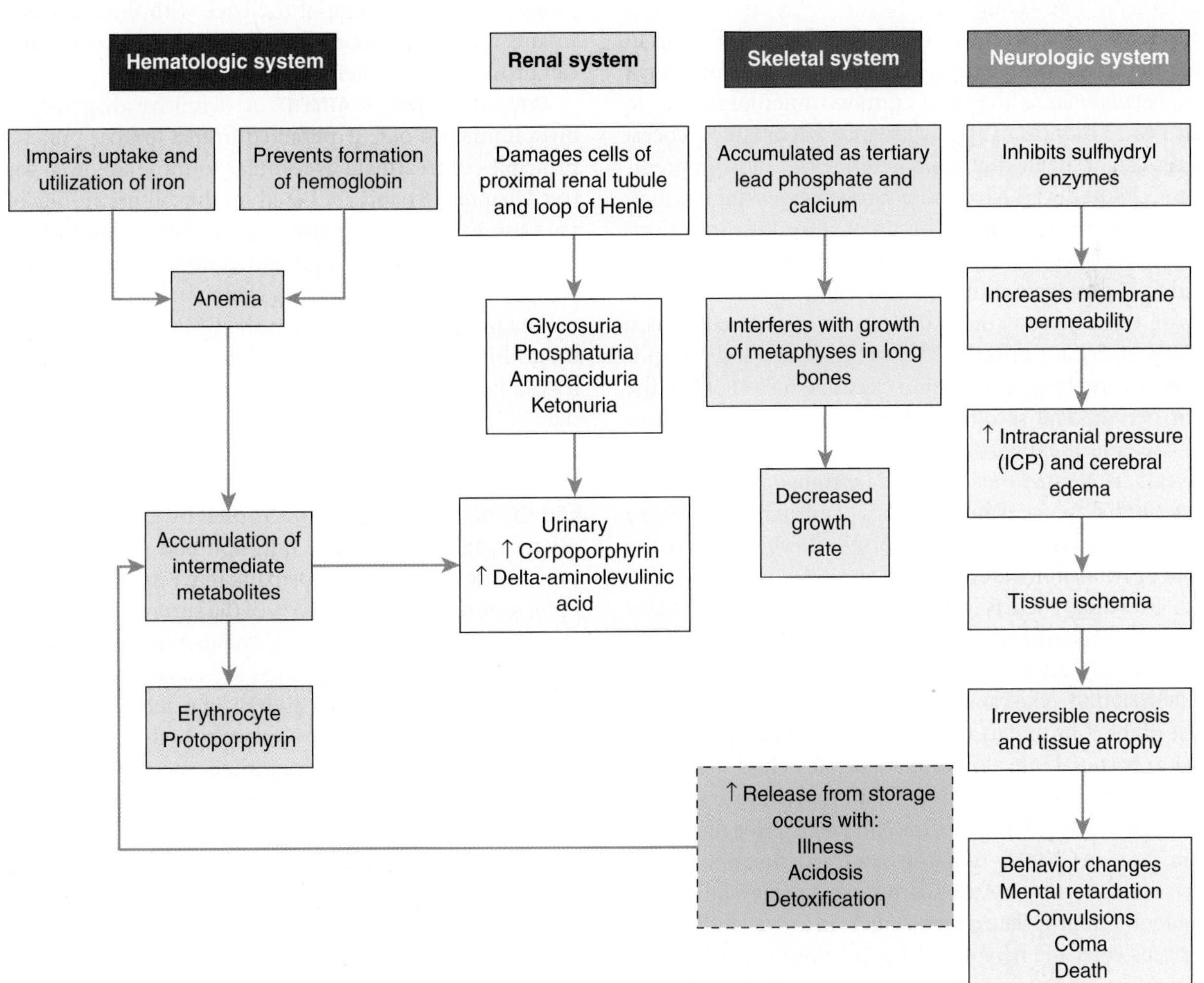

FIGURE 20-14 Systemic Effects of Increased Lead Absorption in Children.

TABLE 20-6 CAUSES OF BACTERIAL MENINGITIS

AGE GROUP	COMMON BACTERIAL PATHOGENS
Newborns	Group B *Streptococcus, Escherichia coli, Listeria monocytogenes*
Infants and children	*Streptococcus pneumoniae, Neisseria meningitidis, Haemophilus influenzae* type b
Adolescents and young adults	*Neisseria meningitidis, Streptococcus pneumoniae*

including 500 deaths.[59] About half of these cases occurred in children younger than 18 years of age. The microorganisms accountable for this illness are summarized in Table 20-6.

The introduction of conjugate vaccines against *Haemophilus influenzae* type B, *Streptococcus pneumoniae,* and *Neisseria meningitidis* (meningococcus) has decreased the incidence of bacterial meningitis.[60] Vaccines for serogroup B *N. meningitidis* are not yet available but clinical trials are in progress.[61] Meningitis is still prevalent in countries without access to the vaccine.[59] (Note that although many families are worried about giving their infants vaccines, the change in incidence of many illnesses has been drastically reduced with their introduction; bacterial meningitis is just one example.)

Group B *Streptococcus* causes lethal meningitis and sepsis in neonates and is transmitted to the child from the mother's birth canal. *S. pneumoniae* is the most common microorganism in children 1 to 23 months of age. Staphylococcal or streptococcal meningitis can occur in children of any age but shows a predilection for children who have had neurosurgery, skull fracture, or a complication of systemic bacterial infection. Infections that originate in the middle ear, sinuses, or mastoid cells also may lead to *S. pneumoniae* infection in children. Children who have sickle cell disease or have undergone a splenectomy are particularly at risk for infection.[62] *Escherichia coli* and group B streptococcus are the most common causes of meningitis in the newborn period. The second most common microorganism causing bacterial meningitis, particularly in children younger than 4 years, is *Neisseria meningitidis* (meningococcus) and it has the potential to occur in epidemics. Approximately 2% to 5% of healthy children are carriers of *N. meningitidis.* As the incidence of *N. meningitidis* infection increases in adolescence and with crowding, such as in dormitories and among military personnel, it is recommended that all individuals 11 to 18 years of age receive two immunizations against this pathogen.[63]

PATHOPHYSIOLOGY. The cause of bacterial meningitis is related to the age of the child and to a number of factors that predispose the child to bacterial infection or that alter the child's response to an invading microorganism. *Staphylococcus aureus* or *Pseudomonas aeruginosa* may develop in the child with cystic fibrosis or severe burns. (See Chapter 10 for further discussion of bacterial virulence and infection.) Any microorganism may be pathogenic under the appropriate circumstances in a given individual.

Pathogens enter the nervous system by direct extension (i.e., paranasal sinuses or mastoid cells) or, more commonly, by hematogenous spread (see Figure 18-32). Infection may travel through the blood to the meninges in children with infective endocarditis, pneumonia, or thrombophlebitis, or to those who have undergone recent procedures or been severely burned. Many bacteria are very successful at evading normal defenses (see Chapter 10). Pathogens cross the blood-brain barrier, enter the cerebrospinal fluid, and multiply. Bacterial toxins increase cerebrovascular permeability, causing alterations in blood flow and edema. Thrombosis and increased ICP can cause neurologic damage. As a result of meningitis, thickened meninges and fibrous exudate in the subarachnoid space at the base of the brain can obstruct CSF resorption, resulting in nonobstructing hydrocephalus. Untreated, this can cause brainstem herniation and death.

CLINICAL MANIFESTATIONS. Acute bacterial meningitis often is preceded by an upper respiratory tract or a gastrointestinal tract infection. Inflammation leads to the general symptoms of fever, headache, vomiting, and irritability and the CNS symptoms of photophobia, nuchal and spinal rigidity, decreased level of consciousness, and seizures. Irritation of the meninges and spinal roots causes pain and resistance to neck flexion (nuchal rigidity), a positive Kernig sign (resistance to knee extension in the supine position with the hips and knees flexed against the body), and a positive Brudzinski sign (flexion of the knees and hips when the neck is flexed forward rapidly). With severe meningeal irritation the child may demonstrate opisthotonic posturing (rigid arching of the back with the head extended). Infants may have bulging fontanels. Meningococcal meningitis can produce a characteristic petechial rash.

EVALUATION AND TREATMENT. A definitive diagnosis is made by examination of CSF obtained from a lumbar puncture. The principles of treatment are similar to those followed for adults (see Chapter 18) and are based on the culture results in which the causative microorganism is identified. Empirical antibiotic therapy should be initiated and continued until CSF cultures are negative[64] or changed if the empirical therapy is not correct for the bacteria cultured from the CSF. Bacterial lysis induced by antibiotics can cause subarachnoid inflammation; the severity can be reduced with corticosteroid treatment.[65] The factors that influence outcomes are the age of the child (mortality is highest in infants younger than 1 year), the infective microorganisms (the lowest mortality is in meningococcal meningitis and the highest in meningitis caused by gram-negative enteric microorganisms), and the duration and extent of inflammation before treatment. Approximately 8% of children with *H. influenzae* meningitis die; 35% of the survivors have serious and permanent sensory or motor dysfunction caused by pressure on the peripheral nerves during the early phases of the illness. Approximately 5% of the children who survive meningitis have hearing deficits; 10% to 15% have cerebral damage, hydrocephalus, motor deficits, or sensory impairments.[66,67]

Viral Meningitis. The hallmark of **viral meningitis** is a mononuclear response in the CSF and the presence of normal blood glucose level, although the findings with aseptic meningitis are similar to those seen in bacterial meningitis in some cases.

The clinical manifestations are similar to those in bacterial meningitis, although usually milder. Isolation of the specific virus is difficult. An exception is when the virus responsible is the herpes simplex virus, which can occur in infants after exposure to the herpes virus type 2 in the birth canal, or sporadic cases caused by herpes virus type 1, which is the type that causes cold sores. It is possible to test for the herpes virus and, unlike most of the other viruses, there is a specific antiviral medication.[68] When a child has symptoms of bacterial or viral meningoencephalitis, antibiotic and antiviral treatments are administered until the cause is determined.

Human Immunodeficiency Virus Encephalopathy. Human immunodeficiency virus type 1 (HIV-1) causes a syndrome called HIV-1 encephalopathy (see Chapter 10 for details of HIV infection which results in developmental delays and impaired brain growth in children not directly related to opportunistic infections in the brain).

PATHOPHYSIOLOGY. The CNS is a distinct reservoir for HIV-1 but the pathogenesis of HIV encephalopathy in children is not clearly understood. HIV-1 invades the CNS early in infection, primarily through infected monocytes/macrophages and CD4+ T lymphocytes. The presence of viral products and inflammatory mediators and overstimulation of the *N*-methyl-D-aspartate–type receptor system lead to neuronal injury and death, particularly in the immature brain, and this is thought to cause the HIV-1 encephalopathy.[69]

CLINICAL MANIFESTATIONS. The 1994 classification from the Centers for Disease Control and Prevention (CDC) requires one of the following progressing findings to be present for at least 2 months,[70] in the absence of a concurrent illness other than HIV that could explain the findings:

1. Failure to attain or loss of developmental milestones, or loss of intellectual ability, verified by standard developmental scale or neuropsychologic tests
2. Impaired brain growth or acquired microcephaly demonstrated by head circumference measurements or brain atrophy established by CT or MRI, with serial imaging required in children younger than 2 years
3. Acquired symmetric motor deficits manifested by affecting a child 1 month of age or older

The onset of progressive encephalopathy may be a prognostic indicator of a poor outcome and it may be difficult to completely differentiate the effects of HIV infection on the CNS from the effects of prenatal and perinatal exposure. In addition, other insults may accompany HIV in a young child and affect growth and development, such as drug exposure, prematurity, and chronic illness.

EVALUATION AND TREATMENT. A definite diagnosis of HIV is made by patient history, viral culture, and clinical manifestations. Monitoring CD8+ T lymphocytes and monocytes, in addition to CD4+ T lymphocytes, has been suggested for predicting risk for progressive encephalopathy. Decreases in CD8+ T lymphocytes diminish defenses against viral infection and facilitate infected monocytes to cross the blood-brain barrier. In general, treatment is focused on preservation and maintenance of the immune system, aggressive response to opportunistic infections, and support and relief of symptomatic occurrences by administration of highly active antiretroviral therapy (HAART). (HIV treatment is discussed in Chapter 10.) Progressive HIV encephalopathy is an infrequent and reversible complication of HIV infection because the disease responds to HAART.[71,72]

BOX 20-3 STROKE IN CHILDREN

- Risk factors different than those for adult (i.e., hypertension, atherosclerosis, diabetes, smoking, obesity)
- Important risk factors (causes) include:
  Ischemic stroke—heart disease or cardiac disorders (most common), blood disorders, clotting or coagulation disorders, sickle cell anemia, infections (chickenpox, meningitis, encephalitis, moyamoya disease), and arterial dissection
  Hemorrhagic stroke—vascular malformations, including arteriovenous malformations (AVMs) and aneurysms; blood disorders, including thrombocytopenia and leukemia; and malignancy, including intracranial tumors
- Vascular occlusion occurs more often in intracranial vessels, including internal carotid, middle cerebral, and basilar arteries; infarcts more often limited to deep regions of the cerebral hemispheres, mostly basal ganglion and internal capsule areas
- Intracerebral hemorrhage and subarachnoid hemorrhage account for a much higher percentage of strokes in children

From *Causes and outcome in childhood stroke.* Available at www.pediatricstroke.org/child_stroke.htm. Accessed April 4, 2013.

CEREBROVASCULAR DISEASE IN CHILDREN

Perinatal Stroke

Perinatal arterial ischemic stroke is estimated to occur in 1 in 4000 live births and is a leading cause of perinatal brain injury, cerebral palsy, and lifelong disability.[73] Children with perinatal stroke may not be diagnosed until later in infancy or childhood when it becomes apparent that the child is not moving one side of the body as much as the other. Early signs may consist of the family noticing that one hand is preferred over the other at an early age—typical "handedness" does not usually occur until 16 to 18 months of age—or one foot is dragging. An MRI is often performed at this point and is most likely to show evidence of a previous middle cerebral artery stroke. The clinical pattern that usually results from this type of stroke is contralateral hemiplegia with the arm more affected than the leg. Children with hemiplegia caused by perinatal stroke (hemiplegic CP) are prone to seizures although generally do well cognitively. Testing for abnormalities in blood-clotting mechanisms, such as antithrombin enzyme activity, protein C and protein S deficiencies, or abnormal factor V Leiden, is often performed in children with prenatal stroke. Although often normal, abnormalities in these clotting mechanisms should be assessed because they may make the child prone to further vascular events.

Childhood Stroke

Childhood stroke occurs in about 1 to 13 per 100,000 live births (Box 20-3).[74]

Ischemic Stroke

PATHOPHYSIOLOGY. Ischemic stroke is rare in children and may result from embolism, arteriopathy, or, rarely, sinovenous thrombosis leading to a decreased flow of blood and oxygen to areas of the brain. Children with arterial ischemic stroke do not have the typical adult risk factors of atherosclerosis and hypertension. Approximately 40% of children with ischemic stroke have no identifiable underlying risk factors. Sickle cell disease, cerebral arteriopathies, and cardiac anomalies are the most common disorders that lead to **arterial ischemic stroke.**[75,76] Treatment options for children with stroke are investigational.[77,78]

Hemorrhagic Stroke

PATHOPHYSIOLOGY. Congenital cerebral arteriovenous malformations are the most common cause of intracranial bleeding and hemorrhagic stroke in children.[79] Hemorrhagic stroke may result from vascular anomalies that lead to rupture, such as aneurysm, or from congenital arteriovenous malformation; the cause of hemorrhagic stroke is more likely to be found than the cause of ischemic stroke. The rupture of a cerebral aneurysm is rare in children younger than 19 years. Intraventricular hemorrhage associated with premature birth is related to immature blood vessels and unstable blood pressure. There is a high risk of developing posthemorrhagic hydrocephalus.[80,81]

Moyamoya disease is a rare, chronic, progressive stenosis of the anterior circulation, such as the internal carotid arteries and middle cerebral arteries. Obstruction of arterial flow to the brain occurs slowly, allowing time for new blood vessels to form and increase collateral blood flow to ischemic areas. *Moyamoya* is a Japanese term that means "puff of smoke," which describes the vascular appearance on cerebral angiogram. Moyamoya vasculopathy may be idiopathic or may be associated with certain genetic or metabolic syndromes, or it can develop as a result of cranial radiation therapy. Complications are developmental delay/intellectual disability, and cerebral hemorrhage.[82] Treatment is surgical bypass of the ischemic region.

CLINICAL MANIFESTATIONS. Symptoms of ischemic or hemorrhagic stroke may include degrees of hemiplegia (flaccid, spastic), weakness, seizures, headache, high fever, nuchal rigidity, hemianopia, sensory changes, facial palsy, and temporary aphasia.

EVALUATION AND TREATMENT. Diagnosis of cerebrovascular disease is made through a series of tests, including imaging studies.[83] History of evolving symptoms and medical history are of vital importance in attaining an accurate diagnosis of stroke etiology, although causative factors often cannot be determined. Prophylactic medications may be prescribed in those children who have suffered an ischemic stroke (e.g., from aspirin). Arteriovenous malformations that may leak and cause hemorrhagic stroke vary in size, location, and symptoms and these factors determine treatment. If a malformation is present, treatment options include surgery, radiation therapy, and embolic occlusion of the malformation[84] (see Chapter 18).

Excellent collateral circulation in the child's brain allows for more rapid recovery of motor function, as compared to adults. The developing brain, however, may suffer more global, long-term effects leading to intellectual disability, behavior disorders, and seizures.[85]

EPILEPSY

Epilepsy is the occurrence of seizures. The incidence of epilepsy varies greatly with age, geographic location, and study design. The incidence is estimated to be 40 to 95 cases per 100,000, with highest onset during the first 12 months of life. Incidence then decreases with age. Approximately 181,000 persons in the United States are newly diagnosed each year.[86,87]

PATHOPHYSIOLOGY. Seizures are caused by abnormal discharge of electrical activity within the brain. When a sufficient number of neurons become overexcited, they discharge abnormally, which sometimes results in clinical manifestations (seizures). Dysregulation of inhibitory $GABA_A$ neurotransmission with imbalance of excitatory and inhibitory mechanisms is speculated to be a cause of early childhood seizures. Dysregulation of other types of voltage- and ligand-gated ion channels (i.e., sodium, calcium, potassium, and chloride) is associated with genetically determined epileptic syndromes.[88,89] If seizures develop, the specific physical activity that occurs depends on the origin of the electrical activity and its extent within the brain. If a child has more than one unprovoked seizure, that child is said to have **epilepsy,** although there are a few exceptions—one example being febrile seizures. Either seizures can be symptoms of an underlying disorder (e.g., meningitis or a brain tumor) or seizures may, themselves, be diseases; the latter may have a genetic or a familial predisposition (for instance, childhood absence epilepsy and juvenile myoclonic epilepsy) (see Tables 17-16 and 17-17). Nearly half of childhood epilepsy is of unknown etiology.[90,91]

Seizures and seizure patterns may change as a child grows and develops. The differences between the immature and mature nervous systems may help explain the changing patterns of clinical seizures with age. For example, febrile seizures manifest in children 6 months to 3 years of age and juvenile myoclonic epilepsy is first noted in adolescence. The immature nervous system has a reduced capacity for sustaining well-organized seizures and, therefore, infants are prone to have seizures that occur only in small parts of the body compared to generalized tonic-clonic seizures in older children. This is because intracortical connections are poorly developed in children and the sending of impulses throughout the cortex is limited. At the cellular level, neurons are less capable of firing in repetitive high-frequency bursts. The excitatory output of a seizure focus is further diminished because the affected neurons do not act synchronously. In addition, changing neurotransmitters, immaturity of cells, and ongoing postnatal factors affect seizure expression in children.

During the newborn period, asphyxia, intracranial hemorrhage, CNS infections, injury, electrolyte imbalances, and inborn errors of metabolism may cause seizures, although often, despite an extensive search for a cause, the etiology remains unknown. Infants and children may have seizures based on earlier brain damage (e.g., cerebral palsy) or may manifest specific epilepsy syndromes (childhood absence epilepsy, Lennox-Gastaut syndrome). Adolescents may have seizures caused by juvenile myoclonic epilepsy or because of other underlying conditions. There is a peak new seizure occurrence in adolescents with autism for unknown reasons.

CLINICAL MANIFESTATIONS. The clinical manifestations at the time of the seizures vary depending on the primary cause and the extent and involvement of abnormal electrical discharges within the neuronal tissue. Because of the diversity and complexity that seizure activity invariably displays, an international classification system was adopted. This classification system groups seizures with similar clinical manifestations (see Table 17-16). Its general purpose is to assist the clinician with the type of evaluation needed, the identification of the most appropriate treatment, and the evaluation of the individual's response to treatment.

The international classification system of epilepsy contains three major groupings: (1) partial seizures, (2) generalized seizures, and (3) unclassified epileptic seizures. Each major grouping is then divided into subsets on the basis of clinical manifestations and electroencephalogram (EEG) findings.

Partial seizures are characterized by seizure activity that begins in and usually is limited to one part of either the left or the right hemisphere. A *simple partial seizure* refers to seizure activity that occurs without loss of consciousness. A *complex partial seizure* refers to seizure activity that occurs with impairment of consciousness. The clinical activity displayed by the individual is contingent on the particular part of the cortex from which the seizure is generated. For example, partial seizures may result in abnormal motor activity, such as twitching or loss of tone, or sensory changes, such as tingling or numbness.

Both simple and complex partial seizures may evolve into a generalized tonic-clonic, tonic, or clonic convulsion. Partial seizures are more likely to be caused by an abnormality in a specific part of the brain, and thus brain imaging is usually performed in children whose seizures have started in a localized manner, even if they generalize later. Possibilities include brain tumors, small areas of localized brain damage, and other causes.

Generalized seizures are those in which the first clinical manifestations indicate that the seizure activity starts in or involves both cerebral hemispheres. Because both hemispheres are involved, the clinical manifestations are almost always bilateral. Consciousness may be impaired in this grouping of seizures. The clinical manifestations may include convulsive activity (tonic-tonic, tonic, or clonic activity) or nonconvulsive activity (absence seizures). Generalized seizures are more likely than partial seizures to have a genetic component; although the genetics of some of the epilepsy syndromes have been identified, many appear to have a multifactorial genetic etiology.[92-94]

Childhood absence epilepsy (also called petit mal seizures or nonconvulsive epilepsy) is a type of generalized epilepsy. The age of onset is 4 to 10 years. The genetic causes are unknown and probably multifactorial; it also can be sporadic. Mutations in inhibitory $GABA_A$ receptor subunit genes are associated with absence seizures. The seizures are initiated at a cortical site and spread to other cortical areas and to the thalamus. The EEG shows a characteristic 3- to 4-Hz spike-wave discharge.[95] The characteristic absence seizure is of sudden onset and sudden termination with impairment of consciousness and unresponsiveness usually lasting less than 10 seconds with no residual deficits. There is interruption of ongoing voluntary activity accompanied by staring, mild eyelid fluttering, or myoclonic jerks. There is no aura. Seizures may be provoked by about 3 minutes of hyperventilation. Hundreds of seizures can occur per day, disrupting school work and socialization. Antiepileptic drugs provide beneficial treatment.[96,97]

Unclassified epileptic seizures are seizure disorders that do not fit neatly into a classified grouping. These seizures characteristically have a wide variety of abnormal clinical activity. Examples of this activity include rhythmic eye movements, chewing, and swimming movements. These activities are commonly seen in neonatal seizures.[98]

Epilepsy Syndromes

In addition to the seizures classified by the international system, there are several types of epileptic syndromes. These are seizure disorders that display a group of signs and symptoms that occur collectively and that characterize or indicate a particular condition. Several syndromes associated with epilepsy occur in infants and children. The four syndromes that occur most often are febrile seizures, infantile spasms, Lennox-Gastaut syndrome, and juvenile myoclonic epilepsy.

Febrile seizures are defined as seizures associated with fever in the absence of central nervous system infection. They are divided into two types: simple febrile seizures and complex febrile seizures. **Simple febrile seizures** occur in 2% to 5% of children. They are benign and the most common childhood seizure.

The pathogenesis of simple febrile seizures is unknown. A familial incidence of simple febrile seizures indicates a genetic predisposition to the problem. Factors that contribute to susceptibility include age, degree and rate of temperature elevation, and nature of the particular fever-inducing illness. Any disorder producing a high fever may provoke benign febrile seizures in susceptible children.

The following characteristic features distinguish simple febrile seizures from complex seizures precipitated by fever:

1. Simple febrile seizures are rare before 9 months of age or after 5 years of age.
2. The convulsion occurs with a rise in temperature greater than 39° C (102.2° F).
3. An acute respiratory tract or ear infection usually is present, with no evidence of CNS infection or inflammation.
4. Most seizures occur during the first 24 hours of the illness.
5. The convulsion is short (15 minutes or less), generalized, and predominantly tonic.
6. Interictal (period between seizures) EEG is normal.
7. The seizure usually does not recur during the same infection.
8. No acute systemic metabolic disorder is present.

Complex febrile seizures have characteristic features similar to those of simple febrile seizure except that (1) they have a longer duration than do benign febrile seizures, usually longer than 15 minutes; (2) they have focal characteristics; and (3) they usually occur more than once in a 24-hour period. Complex febrile seizures are considered a risk factor for the development of epilepsy.[99]

Infantile spasms (also known as West syndrome) are a severe form of epilepsy characterized by a variety of clinical manifestations.[100] The infant may have episodes of sudden flexion or extension movements involving the neck, trunk, and extremities. Infantile spasms in some children are caused by underlying brain abnormalities such as intrauterine stroke or tuberous sclerosis, whereas others may be caused by mutations in several genes.[101] Clinical manifestations of the resulting spasms may range from subtle head nods to violent body contractions, commonly referred to as *jackknife seizures*. Onset of infantile spasms usually is between 4 and 8 months of age and may be idiopathic or may occur in response to a CNS insult.[102] An EEG will display the classic hypsarrhythmic chaotic pattern of epileptic discharges on a slow, disorganized background. After infantile spasms begin, there is usually a typical clinical course. The "spasms" usually occur in clusters and transpire 5 to 150 times per day. They are usually worse when the infant is waking up or falling asleep. Once begun, the seizure activity increases in intensity and severity over time. Invariably, a loss of developmental milestones and disability is associated with this syndrome. A short-term course of high-dose oral corticosteroids (usually prednisolone) is effective in many cases of infantile spasms.[103]

Infantile spasms are present in about 30% of children with **tuberous sclerosis complex (TSC).**[104] TSC develops from mutations in hamartin *(TSC1)* or tuberin *(TSC2)* genes. *Tubers* are cortical developmental malformations in the brain; they also form in other organs. Epilepsy associated with TSC is often difficult to treat. Vigabatrin, which may cause vision defects, is the medication of choice for children with infantile spasms attributable to tuberous sclerosis because it seems to be particularly effective in these children.[105]

Lennox-Gastaut syndrome is an epileptic syndrome characterized by an onset of seizures early in childhood; it occurs in males more often than females and begins between 1 and 8 years of age. This syndrome includes a variety of generalized seizures—predominantly tonic-clonic, atonic (drop attacks), akinetic, absence, and myoclonic activity and a specific pattern on EEG (slow spike and wave). Seizures associated with this syndrome are usually very difficult to treat; children may be prescribed multiple medications and alternate therapies, such as a ketogenic diet or a vagal nerve stimulator. Epilepsy surgery may be necessary. Although children may be developmentally on track when manifestations of this syndrome begin, development is usually affected and the future manifestation of intellectual disability is common.[106]

Juvenile myoclonic epilepsy is a primary, generalized epilepsy that usually affects adolescents and young adults. Although not fully understood, the genetics are in the process of being elucidated. It is a relatively benign form of epilepsy involving myoclonic jerks of the neck, shoulders, and arms as well as generalized tonic-clonic seizures. The seizures may occur singularly or repetitively. This form of epilepsy is commonly associated with a normal neurologic examination, normal intelligence, and a family history of seizures. It is often underdiagnosed.[107] Children with this syndrome will usually need to take medications for life.

EVALUATION AND TREATMENT OF EPILEPSY. Diagnoses of epilepsy and seizure classification are based on history, clinical presentation, physical and developmental examination, and the record of milestone achievements. The first step in the evaluation is to rule out other entities that may appear to be seizures; examples include breath-holding spells and syncope. If the diagnosis of seizure is confirmed, evaluation and testing include an EEG to isolate the focus or origin and involvement of seizure activity and an MRI brain scan to investigate the presence of a lesion or abnormal tissue if the seizure semiology (the appearance of the seizure to the observer) or the EEG shows a focal onset of abnormal electrical activity. Depending on associated symptoms, a complete metabolic workup or genetic testing, or both, may be performed to explore the possibility of deficiency or malabsorption.[108]

Specific treatment for epilepsy is directed at the particular clinical manifestations or syndrome of seizure activity and its underlying causes. Treatment usually begins with the use of anticonvulsant medications. Although seizures in most children are controlled by one medication, the epileptic pattern and clinical course may require more than one drug to control the seizures.[109] A ketogenic diet may be effective as a supplement treatment for epilepsy that is difficult to control with drugs (see Nutrition & Disease: Ketogenic Diet in Children with Epilepsy).

Surgery provides treatment for some forms of epilepsy that cannot be controlled with drugs. As with medical interventions, surgical therapy focuses on the particular clinical manifestations of seizure activity. Surgical interventions include resection of the epileptogenic zone of brain tissue (i.e., the temporal lobe for partial seizures or partial or complete severing of the corpus callosum for intractable generalized epilepsy). Children with intractable epilepsy have shown some benefit from using a vagal nerve stimulator.[110]

NUTRITION & DISEASE

Ketogenic Diet in Children with Epilepsy

The goal of the ketogenic diet is to maintain a state of ketosis, which appears to facilitate reduced seizure frequency and severity for difficult-to-control seizures in children. The diet may be helpful to children who do not respond to conventional therapy or have intolerable side effects. Seizure reduction can occur within 5 to 14 days of initiating the diet and usually within 6 months. Two basic approaches to the ketogenic diet are: (1) a traditional approach with four parts fat to one part carbohydrate/protein in the diet, and (2) the medium-chain triglyceride (MCT) approach, in which MCTs make up about 50% to 70% of the diet. Either diet may be unpalatable and difficult to follow, particularly if the child has free access to food. Carbohydrates can be added by 5-g increments after 3 to 6 months if there has been no seizure activity, provided ketosis is maintained. Both dietary approaches include adequate protein for growth. A medium-chain triglyceride diet, modified Atkins diet, and low glycemic index treatment can also induce ketosis and does not restrict protein, fluid, or calories. The mechanisms are not clearly understood, but enhanced mitochondrial respiration, adenosine triphosphate (ATP) production, and reduced reactive oxygen species formation may influence the dynamics of excitatory and inhibitory neurotransmitter systems in the brain and may be neuroprotective. Side effects can include acidosis, kidney stones, hypoglycemia, gastrointestinal distress, dehydration, lethargy, and poor growth. Most side effects are treatable.

Data from Groomes LB et al: *J Child Neurol* 26(2):160–165, 2011; Jóźwiak S, Kossoff EH, Kotulska-Jóźwiak K: *Neurol Neurochir Pol* 45(4):370–378, 2011; Kessler SK et al: *Epilepsy Behav* 22(1):17–22, 2011; Lee PR, Kossoff EH: *Epilepsy Behav* 21(2):115–121, 2011; Wang HS, Lin KL: *Biomed J* 36(1):16–17, 2013.

For febrile seizures, the cause of the child's fever should be determined and meningitis should be considered in the differential diagnosis. Phenobarbital may be an effective medication for preventing recurrence of simple febrile seizures in selected children who have frequent, prolonged febrile seizures but it is rarely used because it needs to be given daily to be effective.[111]

Status epilepticus is defined as the state of continuing or recurring seizure activity in which the recovery from seizure activity is incomplete. Seizure activity is unrelenting and usually lasts for 30 minutes or more. Any one of the seizure activities discussed can evolve into status epilepticus. Status epilepticus is a medical emergency that requires immediate intervention. Most emergency departments have a structured algorithm of how to respond to a child in status epilepticus.[112]

The prognosis for epilepsy greatly depends on the type and severity of the disorder; the age of onset; coexisting factors; and the type and success of medical, surgical, and nutritional therapy. Many children will become seizure free or have sustained seizure remission after initiation of treatment.[113]

CHILDHOOD TUMORS

Brain Tumors

Brain tumors are the most common solid tumor and the second most common primary neoplasm in children, second only to leukemia. Approximately 45% of primary brain tumors in children are nonmalignant.[114] Overall, primary brain tumors account for nearly 20% of all childhood cancers, with an annual incidence of 3.82 per 100,000 for malignant tumors and 3.44 per 100,000 for nonmalignant tumors in the United States; approximately 4300 new cases will be diagnosed in 2013.[115] Brain tumors remain the leading cause of death from disease in children ages 1 to 15 years.[116]

Primary brain tumors arise from brain tissue and do not metastasize outside the brain. The cause of brain tumors is largely unknown.

PATHOPHYSIOLOGY. Most childhood brain tumors arise from glial tissue, the supportive tissue of the brain. Tumors also may originate in other tissue such as nerve cells, cranial nerves, the pineal and pituitary glands, blood vessels, or neuroepithelium. Brain tumors are classified by the tissue and location from which they arise. Because a uniform pathologic nomenclature has yet to be established, inconsistencies occur when statistical data are compared.

Two thirds of all pediatric brain tumors are found in the posterior fossa region of the brain. This area also may be referred to as infratentorial because it is located below the tentorium. The tentorium is the layer of dura mater that separates the cerebellum from the hemispheres or cerebrum. Thus the area above the tentorium is referred to as the *supratentorial region*. Approximately one third of childhood brain tumors are located in the supratentorial space, whereas in the adult population two thirds of brain tumors are located in the supratentorial region and only one third in the infratentorial region. The types and characteristics of childhood brain tumors are summarized in Table 20-7.

TABLE 20-7 BRAIN TUMORS IN CHILDREN

TYPE	CHARACTERISTICS	TREATMENT	PROGNOSIS
Astrocytoma	Arises from astrocytes, often in cerebellum or lateral cerebral hemisphere Slow growing, solid or cystic Often very large before diagnosed Varies in degree of malignancy	*Cerebellar astrocytoma* Surgery; possibly curative Radiation and chemotherapy not proved successful but may delay recurrence *Cerebral astrocytoma* Surgery used if resection is possible Radiation useful for all grades of astrocytoma Chemotherapy beneficial in higher grade tumors but further study required	*Cerebellar astrocytoma* 90-100% 5-year survival rate if pilocytic type (most common); if tumor recurs, it does so very slowly *Cerebral astrocytoma* 75% 5-year survival rate with lower grade tumors 20% 5-year survival rate if high-grade tumor
Optic pathway glioma	Arises from optic chiasm or optic nerve (association with neurofibromatosis type 1) Slow-growing, low-grade astrocytoma	In setting of visual impairment or progression (increase in size), chemotherapy is usual initial treatment Radiation therapy for tumors that progress or recur in spite of chemotherapy Surgery for large tumors, or hydrocephalus, or other complications; rarely for diagnosis	100% 5-year survival when confined to optic nerve 70% 5-year survival for tumor progression beyond optic chiasm
Medulloblastoma (infiltrating glioma)	Often located in cerebellum, extending into fourth ventricle and spinal fluid pathway Can extend outside CNS Rapidly growing malignant tumor	Type of treatment is age and tumor type dependent Surgery, primarily as partial resection to relieve increased intracranial pressure and "debulk" tumor Radiation as primary treatment; may include spinal radiation Chemotherapy showing some promise in conjunction with craniospinal radiation	65-85% 5-year survival rate depending on stage/type
Brainstem glioma	Arises from pons Numerous cell types Compresses cranial nerves V through X	Surgery, resection occasionally possible Radiation, primarily palliative treatment Chemotherapy not yet proven beneficial, but new protocols being studied	20-40% 5-year survival rate

Continued

TABLE 20-7 BRAIN TUMORS IN CHILDREN—cont'd

TYPE	CHARACTERISTICS	TREATMENT	PROGNOSIS
Ependymoma	Arises from ependymal cells lining ventricles Circumscribed, solid, nodular tumors	Tumor possibly indolent for many years Surgery rarely curative; risk of resecting an infratentorial tumor too great Radiation for palliation (current controversy over whether local or craniospinal radiation is best) Chemotherapy used for recurrent disease but with disappointing results	20-80% 5-year survival rate dependent on total resection
Craniopharyngioma	Arises near pituitary gland, optic chiasm, and hypothalamus Cystic and solid tumors that affect vision, pituitary, and hypothalamic functions	Surgery possibly successful when complete resection is performed (partial resection usually requires further treatment) Radiation after partial surgical resection Chemotherapy not commonly used	80-95% 5-year survival rate

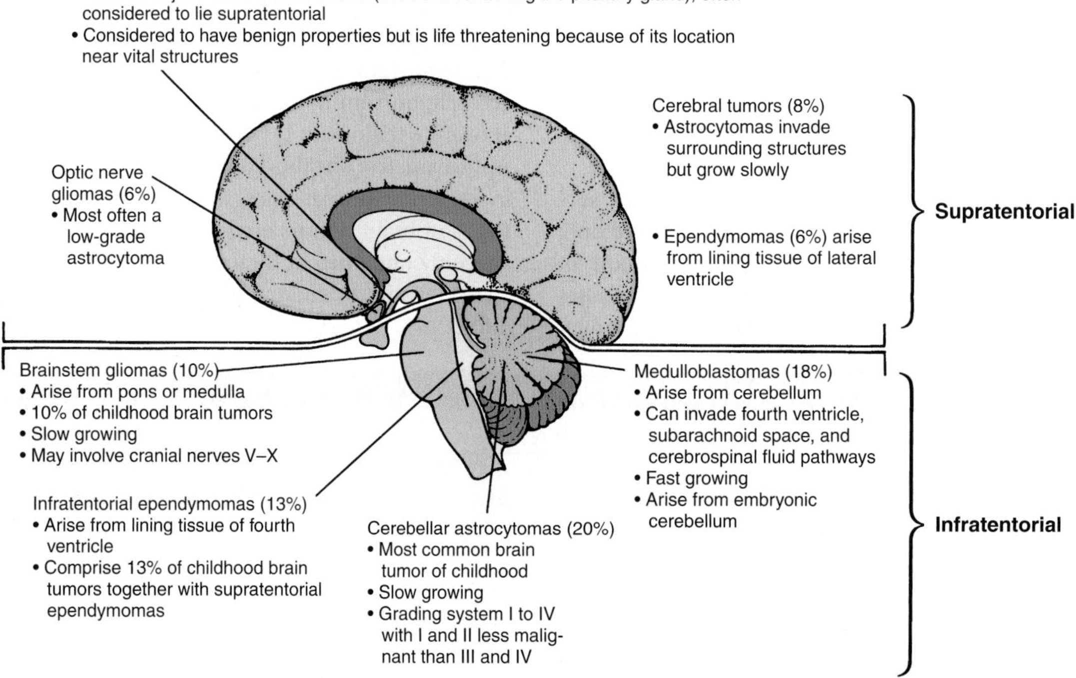

FIGURE 20-15 Location of Brain Tumors in Children.

Brain tumors, by virtue of their location, have unique characteristics that distinguish them from tumors found elsewhere in the body. A number of brain tumors in children may be considered histologically benign yet clinically malignant and life threatening because of their location. For example, a tumor located in the brainstem region may appear benign under the microscope, but the clinical presentation threatens and all too often overrides the vital functions of the brainstem.

Types

Medulloblastoma, ependymoma, gliomas (astrocytoma, brainstem glioma, and optic nerve glioma), and craniopharyngioma comprise approximately 75% to 80% of all pediatric brain tumors.[115] The location of brain tumors in children is illustrated in Figure 20-15; specific characteristics, treatment strategies, and prognoses are listed in Table 20-7.

CLINICAL MANIFESTATIONS. The location of the brain tumor, cell type, and rate of growth dictate the presenting signs and symptoms (discussed in greater detail with each particular brain tumor type). The ability of the brain and intracranial cavity to compensate for tumor growth is directly related to the rate of its growth. This compensatory mechanism allows the components of the intracranial space (blood, brain, and CSF) to adapt temporarily to slow changes in increased intracranial pressure. Therefore slow-growing tumors can grow to enormous size before signs and symptoms are apparent. Conversely, fast-growing tumors allow little time for compensation of the space-occupying lesion, and clinical symptoms occur quickly. Clinical symptoms may range from changes in personality to paralysis, depending on the location of the tumor.

Signs and symptoms of brain tumors in children vary from generalized and vague to those that are localized and related specifically to the anatomic area. If the tumor is located in the posterior fossa region, the fourth ventricle may become blocked, which leads to hydrocephalus and signs of increased ICP. Increased ICP also may occur because of the additional mass volume within the fixed container of the skull vault. The symptoms of increased ICP include headache, vomiting, lethargy, and irritability. If a young child complains of a headache, a thorough investigation should take place because headache is an uncommon complaint in young children. Headache caused by increased ICP usually is worse in the morning and gradually improves during the day when the child is upright and venous drainage is enhanced. Frequency of headache and other symptoms worsens as the tumor grows. A headache related to increased ICP generally occurs because of expansion of the lateral ventricle and cerebral hemisphere, which causes a stretching of the pain-sensitive dura mater. Irritability or possible apathy and increased somnolence also may result from increased ICP. Like headache, vomiting occurs more commonly in the morning. It frequently is not preceded by nausea and may become projectile, differing from a gastrointestinal disturbance in that the child may be ready to eat immediately after vomiting. Other signs and symptoms that can accompany increased ICP include increased head circumference with bulging fontanel in children younger than 2 years, cranial nerve palsies, and papilledema.

Localized findings relate to the degree of disturbance in physiologic functioning in the area where the tumor is located (see Table 18-14). Infratentorial tumors exhibit localized signs of impaired coordination and balance, including ataxia, gait difficulties, truncal ataxia, and loss of balance. A **medulloblastoma** is an embryonal tumor and the most common childhood malignant tumor. It occurs as a fast-growing, invasive tumor that develops in the vermis of the cerebellum and may extend into the fourth ventricle.[117] Angiogenesis is the hallmark of progressive medulloblastomas. The **ependymoma** develops in the fourth ventricle and arises from the ependymal cells that line the ventricular system. The histologic appearance of the ependymoma varies, which makes the treatment course and prognosis difficult to establish. They may contain cysts and areas of calcification. Because both tumors are located in the posterior fossa region along the midline, presenting signs and symptoms are similar. In addition to those already described, they may obstruct the fourth ventricle, resulting in hydrocephalus and generalized increased ICP, headache, nausea and vomiting, and nystagmus (involuntary eye movement).

In contrast, **cerebellar astrocytomas** are located on the surface of the right or left cerebellar hemisphere. Most cerebellar astrocytomas are low-grade, localized cystic tumors. They cause unilateral symptoms (occurring on the same side of the tumor), such as head tilt, limb ataxia, and nystagmus when the eyes are turned toward the tumor.

Brainstem gliomas often cause a combination of cranial nerve involvement, cerebellar signs of ataxia, and corticospinal tract dysfunction. A common clinical pattern includes unilateral paralysis of cranial nerves with contralateral paralysis of the arm and leg, hyperreflexia, and extensor plantar responses. Increased ICP generally does not occur. Children with diffuse tumors usually die within 1 to 2 years.[118]

The area of the sella turcica, the structure containing the pituitary gland, is the site of several childhood brain tumors, including **craniopharyngioma** (the most common and is benign) and pituitary adenoma (see Chapter 22). These tumors may originate from the pituitary gland or the hypothalamus. They are usually slow growing and may be quite large by the time of diagnosis. Obstruction of the interventricular foramen can increase ICP. Symptoms include headache, seizures, diabetes insipidus, early onset of puberty, and growth delay. Other tumors located in this region of the brain include **optic gliomas.** Tumors that involve the optic tract may cause complete unilateral blindness and hemianopia of the other eye. Optic atrophy is another common finding. Optic gliomas are common in children with neurofibromatosis, a relatively common genetic condition.

Supratentorial tumors of the cerebral hemispheres in children are not very common. **Pilocytic astrocytomas** are the most common supratentorial tumors. These are localized (grade I) slow-growing, cyst-filled tumors that are often completely removed surgically. Tumors located in the cortex may cause focal cerebral dysfunction, weakness, hemiparesis, seizures, and visual changes. Involvement of particular lobes may result in more specific localized symptoms. For example, a tumor located in the frontal lobe may cause changes in affect and behavior, and a tumor in the occipital lobe may cause cortical blindness or blindness in half of the visual field.

EVALUATION AND TREATMENT. A child with signs and symptoms of a brain tumor requires a complete workup, including a neurologic, developmental, and ophthalmic examination. CT with contrast enhancement allows direct visualization of the tumor mass. MRI provides advanced, dramatic examination of the brain and neoplasms. Small low-grade tumors not seen on CT may be detected by MRI. Although less commonly used, magnetic resonance angiography (MRA) is very helpful in assessing the vascularity of the tumor and its relationship to major blood vessels. Spine MRI examination may be used to evaluate tumor dissemination along the spinal column. Lumbar puncture to examine CSF for tumor cells also may be performed. Tumors more likely to spread throughout the neuraxis include medulloblastomas and ependymomas.

The most useful treatment for brain tumors is surgical resection. Surgery to establish the diagnosis by biopsy or to excise the tumor is part of the initial treatment for most brain tumors. Some brain tumors may be cured with complete resection alone, such as low-grade cerebellar astrocytomas. Contraindications to such interventions are tumors in which surgical resection and biopsy carry a high risk of mortality or serious morbidity (brainstem gliomas). In these instances, diagnosis is made on the basis of radiologic evidence and clinical manifestations.

Most brain tumors require additional radiation and chemotherapy. Although these treatments are essential for potential eradication of the brain tumor, radiation to the child's brain is associated with significant morbidity, including acute- and long-term sequelae. Prognosis varies according to the type and location of the brain tumor (see Table 20-7). Historically, survival rates have been low; however, advances have been made with the combination of surgery, radiation therapy, and chemotherapy. Comprehensive care and management of these children and their families are vital. Multidisciplinary teams composed of neurosurgeons, neurologists, radiation therapists, oncologists, nurses, social workers, physical therapists, and other providers are necessary to provide the continuity and consistency needed to care for these children.

Embryonal Tumors

Neuroblastoma

Neuroblastoma is an embryonal aggressive tumor that originates outside the CNS in the developing sympathetic nervous system (sympathetic ganglia and the adrenal medulla). The primitive neural crest cells (also called *sympathogonia*) are pluripotential (i.e., they develop into several cell types) and mature into sympathetic ganglion cells, pheochromocytes (which are found in the sympathetic nervous system), or neurofibrous tissue. Thus tumors that develop from neural crest cells reflect the varying degrees of differentiation of the cells. **Ganglioneuroblastomas** are tumors of an intermediate level of cellular differentiation. The most differentiated tumor is a **ganglioneuroma,** which is considered benign and does not metastasize.

Because neuroblastoma involves a defect of embryonal tissue, it is most commonly diagnosed in infants and young children. Although it accounts for 8% to 10% of pediatric malignancies, neuroblastoma causes approximately 50% of all solid tumors in children in the first year, and about 15% of cancer deaths in children of all ages.[119] Although familial tendency has been noted in individual cases, a nonfamilial or sporadic pattern is found in most children with neuroblastoma. Familial cases of neuroblastoma are considered to have an autosomal dominant pattern of inheritance (mechanisms of inheritance are discussed in Chapter 4).

PATHOPHYSIOLOGY. Neuroblastoma is the most primitive, or immature, form of the sympathetic nervous system tumors. Areas of necrosis and calcification often are present in the tumor. Neuroblastomas also are known to regress or mature into benign lesions.[120]

The cause of neuroblastoma is elusive. The tumor has been associated with a number of conditions, including neurofibromatosis and Hirschsprung disease, but most children with neuroblastoma have neither of these conditions.

CLINICAL MANIFESTATIONS. The most common location of neuroblastoma is in the retroperitoneal region (65% of cases), most often the adrenal medulla. The tumor is evident as an abdominal mass and may cause anorexia, bowel and bladder alteration, and sometimes spinal cord compression. The second most common location of neuroblastoma is the mediastinum (15% of cases), where the tumor may cause dyspnea or infection related to airway obstruction. Less commonly, neuroblastoma may arise from the cervical sympathetic ganglion (3% to 4% of cases). Cervical neuroblastoma often causes Horner syndrome, which consists of miosis (pupil contraction), ptosis (drooping eyelid), enophthalmos (backward displacement of the eyeball), and anhidrosis (sweat deficiency). Neuroblastoma can present with a neurologic syndrome called opsoclonus-myoclonus syndrome (jerky movements of the limbs, ataxia, and chaotic eye movements in all directions).[121]

A number of systemic signs and symptoms are characteristic of neuroblastoma, including weight loss, irritability, fatigue, and fever. Intractable diarrhea occurs in 7% to 9% of children and is caused by tumor secretion of a hormone called *vasoactive intestinal polypeptide (VIP).*

More than 90% of children with neuroblastoma have increased amounts of catecholamines and associated metabolites in their urine. High levels of urinary catecholamines and serum ferritin are associated with a poor prognosis.

EVALUATION AND TREATMENT. Initial diagnostic studies are dictated by the location of the primary tumor. Diagnosis begins with a complete physical and neurologic examination. Imaging studies provide further information. Laboratory analyses include measurement of levels of urinary catecholamines; plasma ferritin; serum neuron-specific enolase (NSE), an enzyme produced by neuronal tissues; and gangliosides, lipid molecules that may be shed from the surface of tumor cells.[122] The diagnosis of neuroblastoma is confirmed by surgical biopsy and histopathologic results. Antenatal ultrasound may detect the tumor in the antenatal period.

Treatment is based on the extent of the disease and prognostic markers, such as age, *MYCN* copy numbers (a proto-oncogene), chromosome 11q status and DNA ploidy, and high serum ferritin or NSE levels.[123] Low-risk disease is treated surgically. Chemotherapy is used if there is recurrence. Intermediate-risk tumors are treated with surgery and chemotherapy. High-risk neuroblastomas are being treated with high-dose chemotherapy and radiotherapy followed by transplantation of purged autologous bone marrow. Monoclonal antibody–based immunotherapy has been shown to be effective for high-risk tumors.[124] Approximately 60% of children with high-risk disease will die despite intensive therapy, although this percentage is improving over time.

SUMMARY REVIEW

Structure and Function of the Nervous System in Children

1. The central nervous system develops from the neural tube, which is ectodermal in origin. The cranial end of the tube forms the brain, and the spinal cord is formed from the remainder of the tube.
2. The cranial and spinal ganglia (peripheral nervous system) develop from the neural crest.
3. The nervous system develops in six stages, and disruption of any of the stages can lead to malfunction of the nervous system.
4. The bones of the skull are joined by sutures; the wide, membranous junctions of the sutures, known as *fontanels,* close by 20 months of age.
5. Myelin is a sheath that develops around axons to facilitate speed of nerve impulse conduction. Progressive development of reflexes corresponds to normal maturation of nerve tissue and development of voluntary movement.
6. Neurologic functioning at birth is at the subcortical level with reflex patterns mediated by the brainstem and spinal

SUMMARY REVIEW—cont'd

cord. With maturation, neonatal reflexes disappear and voluntary motor functions develop.
7. The fontanels allow for cranial expansion because the head is the fastest growing body part during infancy. Sutures close by 5 to 8 years after birth.

Structural Malformations

1. Defects of neural tube closure include anencephaly (absence of part of the brain and soft, bony part of skull), encephalocele (protrusion of brain and meninges through a skull defect), and myelodysplasias: meningocele (cystlike defect with protrusion of spinal fluid–filled meninges through a vertebral defect), myelomeningocele (a defect like meningocele only also containing the spinal cord), and spina bifida (failure of the vertebrae to close with protrusion of neural tube contents with intact skin).
2. Craniosynostosis (craniostenosis) is premature closure of one or more of the cranial sutures and prevents normal skull expansion, causing compression of growing brain tissue.
3. Microcephaly is lack of brain growth and retarded mental and motor development.
4. Cortical dysplasias are a heterogeneous group of disorders caused by defects in neuronal cell migration and subsequent abnormalities in connections between cells.
5. Congenital hydrocephalus results from an imbalance between the production and reabsorption of cerebrospinal fluid.

Encephalopathies

1. Static encephalopathies (i.e., cerebral palsy and epilepsy) are nonprogressive disorders of the brain that can occur during gestation, birth, or childhood and can be caused by trauma or genetic factors.
2. Cerebral palsy (CP) is a group of nonprogressive syndromes that can be caused by prenatal cerebral hypoxia or perinatal or postnatal trauma with symptoms of mental retardation, seizure disorders, or developmental disabilities. CP can be **extrapyramidal/nonspastic or pyramidal/spastic.**
3. Inherited disorders that damage the nervous system include metabolic defects in amino acid metabolism (phenylketonuria) and storage diseases.
4. Storage diseases include lysosomal storage disease, such as Tay-Sachs disease (GM2 gangliosidosis). Both inherited disorders and storage diseases result in abnormal behavior, seizures, and deficient psychomotor development.
5. Accidental poisonings from a variety of toxins can cause serious neurologic damage.
6. Bacterial meningitis is commonly caused by *H. influenzae* type B, *S. pneumoniae,* or *N. meningitidis* and may result from respiratory tract or gastrointestinal tract infections with symptoms of fever, headache, photophobia, seizure, rigidity, and stupor.
7. Viral meningitis presents similar to bacterial meningitis, and the specific virus is often unknown.
8. HIV-1 encephalopathy is a CNS infection that can occur in infants and children.

Cerebrovascular Disease in Children

1. Ischemic stroke is rare in children and may result from embolism, arteriopathy, or, rarely, sinovenous thrombosis.
2. Hemorrhagic stroke results from congenital arteriovenous malformations that rupture and cause intracranial bleeding.

Seizure Disorders in Children

1. Epilepsy is the occurrence of seizures. Seizures are the abnormal discharge of electrical activity within the brain. Seizure disorders are associated with numerous nervous system disorders and more often are a generalized rather than a partial type of seizure.
2. Generalized forms of seizures involve both brain hemispheres and include tonic-clonic, myoclonic, atonic, akinetic, and infantile spasms.
3. Partial seizures suggest more localized brain dysfunction.
4. Childhood absence epilepsy (petit mal seizures or nonconvulsive epilepsy) is a type of generalized epilepsy.
5. Epilepsy syndromes include febrile seizures, infantile spasms, Lennox-Gastaut syndrome, and juvenile myoclonic epilepsy.

Childhood Tumors

1. Brain tumors are the most common primary neoplasm in children and the second most common type of childhood cancer. The most common tumors include medulloblastoma, ependymoma, gliomas (astrocytoma, brainstem glioma, and optic nerve glioma), and craniopharyngioma.
2. Tumors in children are most often located below the tentorial membrane in the posterior fossa.
3. Fast-growing tumors produce symptoms early in the disease, whereas slow-growing tumors may become very large before symptoms appear.
4. Symptoms of brain tumors may be generalized or localized. The most common general symptom is increased ICP (headache, irritability, vomiting, somnolence, and bulging of fontanels).
5. Localized signs of infratentorial tumors in the cerebellum include impaired coordination and balance. Cranial nerve signs occur with tumors near the brainstem.
6. Supratentorial tumors may be located near the cortex or deep in the brain. Symptoms depend on the specific location of the tumor.
7. Neuroblastoma is an embryonal tumor of the sympathetic nervous system and can be located anywhere there is sympathetic nervous tissue. It is the most common type of solid tumor occurring in the first year.
8. Symptoms are related to tumor location and size of metastasis.

KEY TERMS

Acute bacterial meningitis, 675
Alar plate, 661
Anencephaly, 663
Arterial ischemic stroke, 678
Aseptic meningitis, 675
Ataxic cerebral palsy, 672
Basal plate, 661
Brainstem glioma, 683
Cerebellar astrocytoma, 683
Cerebral palsy (CP), 670
Childhood absence epilepsy, 679
Complex febrile seizure, 679
Congenital hydrocephalus, 668
Cortical dysplasia, 668
Cranial meningocele, 664
Craniopharyngioma, 683
Craniosynostosis (craniostenosis), 666
Dandy-Walker malformation, 669
Dyskinetic cerebral palsy, 672
Encephalitis, 675
Encephalocele, 664
Encephalopathy, 670
Ependymoma, 683
Epilepsy, 678
Extrapyramidal/nonspecific cerebral palsy, 672
Febrile seizure, 679
Ganglioneuroblastoma, 684
Ganglioneuroma, 684
Gangliosidosis, 674
Generalized seizure, 679
Hyperphenylalaninemia (HPA), 673
Infantile spasm, 679
Juvenile myoclonic epilepsy, 680
Lennox-Gastaut syndrome, 680
Medulloblastoma, 683
Meningitis, 675
Meningocele, 664
Microcephaly, 667
Moyamoya disease, 678
Myelodysplasia, 663
Myelomeningocele, 665
Neural crest, 660
Neural fold, 660
Neural groove, 660
Neural plate, 660
Neural tube, 660
Neural tube defect (NTD), 663
Neuroblastoma, 684
Nonsyndromic craniosynostosis, 666
Optic glioma, 683
Partial seizure, 679
Phenylketonuria (PKU), 673
Pica, 674
Pilocytic astrocytoma, 683
Pyramidal/spastic cerebral palsy, 672
Simple febrile seizure, 679
Somite, 660
Spina bifida occulta, 666
Status epilepticus, 681
Sulcus limitans, 661
Syndromic craniosynostosis, 666
Tay-Sachs disease (GM2 gangliosidosis), 674
Tethered cord syndrome, 665
Tuberous sclerosis complex (TSC), 680
Unclassified epileptic seizure, 679
Viral meningitis, 676

REFERENCES

1. National Center on Birth Defects and Developmental Disabilities: *Folic acid: reducing folic acid-preventable neural tube defects.* Updated April 2, 2012. Available at www.cdc.gov/ncbddd/aboutus/birthdefects-folicacid.html.
2. De Marco P et al: Human neural tube defects: genetic causes and prevention, *Biofactors* 37(4):261–268, 2011.
3. Centers for Disease Control and Prevention: *Spina bifida: data and statistics in the United States.* Updated March 18, 2011. Available at www.cdc.gov/ncbddd/spinabifida/data.html.
4. Centers for Disease Control and Prevention: *Facts about anencephaly.* Updated March 26, 2013. Available at www.cdc.gov/ncbddd/birthdefects/anencephaly.html.
5. Krantz DA, Hallahan TW, Sherwin JE: Screening for open neural tube defects, *Clin Lab Med* 30(3):721–725, 2010.
6. Centers for Disease Control and Prevention: *Facts about encephalocele.* Updated February 25, 2011. Available at www.cdc.gov/ncbddd/birthdefects/encephalocele.html.
7. Shaer CM, Chescheir N, Schulkin J: Myelomeningocele: a review of the epidemiology, genetics, risk factors for conception, prenatal diagnosis, and prognosis for affected individuals, *Obstet Gynecol Surv* 62(7):471–479, 2007.
8. Salman MS: Posterior fossa decompression and the cerebellum in Chiari type II malformation: a preliminary MRI study, *Childs Nerv Syst* 27(3):457–462, 2011.
9. Vidmer S et al: The neurophysiological balance in Chiari type 1 malformation (CM1), tethered cord and related syndromes, *Neurol Sci* 32(Suppl 3):S311–S316, 2011.
10. Reigel DH: Infancy through the school years. In Rowley-Kelly F, Reigel DH, editors: *Teaching the student with spina bifida,* Baltimore, 1993, Brookes.
11. Salman MS et al: Smooth ocular pursuit in Chiari type II malformation, *Dev Med Child Neurol* 49(4):289–293, 2007.
12. Mehta VA et al: Spinal cord tethering following myelomeningocele repair, *J Neurosurg Pediatr* 6(5):498–505, 2010.
13. Sandler AD: Children with spina bifida: key clinical issues, *Pediatr Clin North Am* 57(4):879–892, 2010.
14. Behrman RE, Kleigman RM, Jenson HB: *Nelson's textbook of pediatrics,* ed 17, Philadelphia, 2004, Saunders.
15. Danzer E, Johnson MP, Adzick NS: Fetal surgery for myelomeningocele: progress and perspectives, *Dev Med Child Neurol* 54(1):8–14, 2012.
16. Hamrick SE: Cesarean delivery and its impact on the anomalous infant, *Clin Perinatol* 35(2):395-406 (review), 2008. *Erratum in Clin Perinatol* 36(1):xvii, 2009.
17. Adzick NS et al: MOMS Investigators. A randomized trial of prenatal versus postnatal repair of myelomeningocele, *N Engl J Med* 364(11):993–1004, 2011.
18. Hukki J, Saarinen P, Kangasniemi M: Single suture craniosynostosis: diagnosis and imaging, *Front Oral Biol* 12:79–90, 2008.
19. Kimonis V et al: Genetics of craniosynostosis, *Semin Pediatr Neurol* 14(3):150–161, 2007.
20. Melville H et al: Genetic basis of potential therapeutic strategies for craniosynostosis, *Am J Med Genet A* 152A(12):3007–3015, 2010.
21. Ursitti F et al: Evaluation and management of nonsyndromic craniosynostosis, *Acta Paediatr* 100(9):1185–1194, 2011.
22. Barkovich AJ, et al: A developmental and genetic classification for malformations of cortical development: update 2012, *Brain* 135(Pt 5):1348–1369, 2012.
23. Kanekar S, Gent M: Malformations of cortical development, *Semin Ultrasound CT MR* 32(3):211–227, 2011.
24. Manzini MC, Walsh CA: What disorders of cortical development tell us about the cortex: one plus one does not always make two, *Curr Opin Genet Dev* 21(3):333–339, 2011.
25. Raybaud C, Widjaja E: Development and dysgenesis of the cerebral cortex: malformations of cortical development, *Neuroimaging Clin N Am* 21(3):483–543, vii, 2011.
26. Ashwal S et al: Practice parameter: evaluation of the child with microcephaly (an evidence-based review): report of the Quality Standards Subcommittee of the American Academy of Neurology and the Practice Committee of the Child Neurology Society, *Neurology* 73(11):887–897, 2009.
27. Garton HJ, Platt JH Jr: Hydrocephalus, *Pediatr Clin North Am* 51(2):305–325, 2004.
28. Jackson PL: Hydrocephalus. In Jackson PL, Vessey JA, editors: *Primary care of the child with a chronic condition,* ed 4, St Louis, 2003, Mosby.
29. Lindquist B et al: Very long-term follow-up of cognitive function in adults treated in infancy for hydrocephalus, *Childs Nerv Syst* 27(4):597–601, 2011.

29a Warf BC et al: Long-term outcome for endoscopic third ventriculostomy alone or in combination with choroid plexus cauterization for congenital aqueductal stenosis in African infants, *J Neurosurg Pediatr* 10(2):108–111, 2012.

30. Centers for Disease Control and Prevention: *Cerebral palsy, what should you know about cerebral palsy,* Updated September 7, 2012. Available at www.cdc.gov/ncbddd/cp/index.html.
31. Himmelmann K et al: Risk factors for cerebral palsy in children born at term, *Acta Obstet Gynecol Scand* 90(10):1070–1081, 2011.
32. Longo M, Hankins GD: Defining cerebral palsy: pathogenesis, pathophysiology and new intervention, *Minerva Ginecol* 61(5):421–429, 2009.
33. Cahill AG et al: Magnesium sulfate therapy for the prevention of cerebral palsy in preterm infants: a decision-analytic and economic analysis, *Am J Obstet Gynecol* 205(6):542.e1–542.e7, 2011.

34. Chalak LF, Rouse DJ: Neuroprotective approaches: before and after delivery, *Clin Perinatol* 38(3):455–470, 2011.
35. Aisen ML et al: Cerebral palsy: clinical care and neurological rehabilitation, *Lancet Neurol* 10(9):844–852, 2011.
36. Novak I et al: Clinical prognostic messages from a systematic review on cerebral palsy, *Pediatrics* 130(5):e1285–e1312, 2012.
37. Jones MW et al: Cerebral palsy: introduction and diagnosis (part I), *J Pediatr Health Care* 21(3):146–152, 2007.
38. Ashwal S et al: Practice parameter: diagnostic assessment of the child with cerebral palsy: report of the Quality Standards Subcommittee of the American Academy of Neurology and the Practice Committee of the Child Neurology Society, *Neurology* 62(6):851–863, 2004.
39. Chung CY, Chen CL, Wong AM: Pharmacotherapy of spasticity in children with cerebral palsy, *J Formos Med Assoc* 110(4):215–222, 2011.
40. van Schie PE et al: Short- and long-term effects of selective dorsal rhizotomy on gross motor function in ambulatory children with spastic diplegia, *J Neurosurg Pediatr* 7(5):557–562, 2011.
41. Liptak GS, Murphy NA: Council on Children with Disabilities: Providing a primary care medical home for children and youth with cerebral palsy, *Pediatrics* 128(5):e1321–e1329, 2011.
42. Gleason CA, Devaskar S: *Avery's diseases of the newborn*, ed 9, Philadelphia, 2012, Saunders.
43. National Institutes of Health Consensus Development Panel: National Institutes of Health Consensus Development Conference Statement: phenylketonuria: screening and management, *Pediatrics* 108(4):972–982, 2001.
44. Blau N, van Spronsen FJ, Levy HL: Phenylketonuria, *Lancet* 376(9750):1417–1427, 2010.
45. Mitchell JJ, Trakadis YJ, Scriver CR: Phenylalanine hydroxylase deficiency, *Genet Med* 13(8):697–707, 2011.
46. Burton BK et al: Safety of extended treatment with sapropterin dihydrochloride in patients with phenylketonuria: results of a phase 3b study, *Mol Genet Metab* 103(4):315–322, 2011.
47. Bélanger-Quintana A et al: Up to date knowledge on different treatment strategies for phenylketonuria, *Mol Genet Metab* 104(Suppl):S19–S25, 2011.
48. Urbanelli L et al: Developments in therapeutic approaches for lysosomal storage diseases, *Recent Pat CNS Drug Discov* 6(1):1–19, 2011.
49. Bley AE et al: Natural history of infantile G(M2) gangliosidosis, *Pediatrics* 128(5):e1233–e1241, 2011.
50. National Tay-Sachs & Allied Diseases: *Tay-Sachs disease.* Available at www.ntsad.org/index.php/tay-sachs. Accessed March 1, 2012.
51. Schneider A et al: Population-based Tay-Sachs screening among Ashkenazi Jewish young adults in the 21st century: hexosaminidase A enzyme assay is essential for accurate testing, *Am J Med Genet A* 149A(11):2444–2447, 2009.
52. Bronstein AC et al: 2010 annual report of the American Association of Poison Control Centers' National Poison Data System (NPDS): 28th annual report, *Clin Toxicol (Phil)* 49(10):910–941, 2011.
53. Abelsohn AR, Sanborn M: Lead and children: clinical management for family physicians, *Can Fam Physician* 56(6):531–535, 2010.
54. Bellinger DC: Very low lead exposures and children's neurodevelopment, *Curr Opin Pediatr* 20(2):172–177, 2008.
55. Woolf AD, Goldman R, Bellinger DC: Update on the clinical management of childhood lead poisoning, *Pediatr Clin North Am* 54(2):271–294, 2007.
56. Centers for Disease Control and Prevention: *Lead.* Available at www.cdc.gov/nceh/lead/. Updated January 27, 2012.
57. Jones RL et al: Trends in blood lead levels and blood lead testing among U.S. children aged 1 to 5 years, 1988-2004, *Pediatrics* 123(3):e376–e385, 2009.
58. American Academy of Pediatrics: Lead exposure in children: prevention, detection, and management, *Pediatrics* 116(4):1036–1046, 2005.
59. Thigpen MC et al: Bacterial meningitis in the United States, 1998-2007, *N Engl J Med* 364(21):2016–2025, 2011.
60. Kim KS: Acute bacterial meningitis in infants and children, *Lancet Infect Dis* 10(1):32–42, 2010.
61. Gossger N et al: Immunogenicity and tolerability of recombinant serogroup B meningococcal vaccine administered with or without routine infant vaccinations according to different immunization schedules: a randomized controlled trial, *J Am Med Assoc* 307(6):573–582, 2012.
62. Ramakrishnan M et al: Increased risk of invasive bacterial infections in African people with sickle-cell disease: a systematic review and meta-analysis, *Lancet Infect Dis* 10(5):329–337, 2010.
63. Centers for Disease Control and Prevention: *Vaccines and preventable diseases: meningococcal: who needs to be vaccinated?* Available at www.cdc.gov/vaccines/vpd-vac/mening/who-vaccinate.htm. Accessed May 20, 2013.
64. Brouwer MC, Tunkel AR, van de Beek D: Epidemiology, diagnosis, and antimicrobial treatment of acute bacterial meningitis, *Clin Microbiol Rev* 23(3):467–492, 2010.
65. Borchorst S, Møller K: The role of dexamethasone in the treatment of bacterial meningitis: a systematic review, *Acta Anaesthesiol Scand* 56(10):1210–1221, 2012.
66. Ahmed MN, Steele RW: Meningitis in a young infant, *Clin Pediatr* 43(5):495–497, 2004.
67. Chandran A et al: Long-term sequelae of childhood bacterial meningitis: an underappreciated problem, *Pediatr Infect Dis J* 30(1):3–6, 2011.
68. Stahl JP et al: Epidemiology of viral encephalitis in 2011, *Med Mal Infect* 41(9):453–464, 2011.
69. Govender R et al: Neurologic and neurobehavioral sequelae in children with human immunodeficiency virus (HIV-1) infection, *J Child Neurol* 26(11):1355–1364, 2011.
70. Centers for Disease Control and Prevention: 1994 revised classification system for human immunodeficiency virus infection in children less than 13 years of age, *MMWR Morb Mortal Wkly Rep* 43(12):1, 1994. Available at www.cdc.gov/mmwr/preview/mmwrhtml/00032890.htm.
71. AIDS Info: Guidelines for the use of antirefroviral agents in pediatric HIV infection. Available at http://aidsinfo.nih.gov/guidelines/html/2/pediatric-arv-guidelines/62/treatment-recommendations. Updated November 1, 2012.
72. Wright E: Neurocognitive impairment and neuroCART, *Curr Opin HIV AIDS* 6(4):303–308, 2011.
73. Kirton A et al: Symptomatic neonatal arterial ischemic stroke: the International Pediatric Stroke Study, *Pediatrics* 128(6):e1402–e1410, 2011.
74. Mallick AA, O'Callaghan FJ: The epidemiology of childhood stroke, *Eur J Paediatr Neurol* 14(3):197–205, 2010.
75. Chabrier S et al: New insights (and new interrogations) in perinatal arterial ischemic stroke, *Thromb Res* 127(1):13–22, 2011.
76. Munot P, Crow YJ, Ganesan VL: Paediatric stroke: genetic insights into disease mechanisms and treatment targets, *Lancet Neurol* 10(3):264–274, 2011.
77. Freundlich CL, Cervantes-Arslanian AM, Dorfman DH: Pediatric stroke, *Emerg Med Clin North Am* 30(3):805–828, 2012.
78. Roach ES et al: Management of stroke in infants and children: a scientific statement from a Special Writing Group of the American Heart Association Stroke Council and the Council on Cardiovascular Disease in the Young, *Stroke* 39(9):2644–2691, 2008.
79. Beslow LA, Jordan LC: Pediatric stroke: the importance of cerebral arteriopathy and vascular malformations, *Childs Nerv Syst* 26(10):1263–1273, 2010.
80. Cárdenas JF, Rho JM, Kirton A: Pediatric stroke, *Childs Nerv Syst* 27(9):1375–1390, 2011.
81. Tsitouras V, Sgouros S: Infantile posthemorrhagic hydrocephalus, *Childs Nerv Syst* 27(10):1595–1608, 2011.
82. Smith ER, Scott RM: Moyamoya: epidemiology, presentation, and diagnosis, *Neurosurg Clin N Am* 21(3):543–551, 2010.
83. Yock-Corrales A, Barnett P: The role of imaging studies for evaluation of stroke in children, *Pediatr Emerg Care* 27(10):966–974, 2011.
84. Hartmann A et al: Treatment of arteriovenous malformations of the brain, *Curr Neurol Neurosci Rep* 7(1):28–34, 2007.
85. Galvin J et al: Functional outcome following paediatric stroke, *Dev Neurorehabil* 14(2):67–71, 2011.
86. Durá-Travé T et al: Incidence of epilepsies and epileptic syndromes among children in Navarre, Spain: 2002 through 2005, *J Child Neurol* 23(8):878–882, 2008.
87. Wirrell EC et al: Incidence and classification of new-onset epilepsy and epilepsy syndromes in children in Olmsted County, Minnesota from 1980 to 2004: a population-based study, *Epilepsy Res* 95(1-2):110–118, 2011.
88. Briggs SW, Galanopoulou AS: Altered GABA signaling in early life epilepsies, *Neural Plast* 527–605, 2011.
89. Mantegazza M et al: Epileptogenic ion channel mutations: from bedside to bench and, hopefully, back again, *Epilepsy Res* 92(1):1–29, 2011.
90. Berg AT et al: Revised terminology and concepts for organization of seizures and epilepsies: report of the ILAE Commission on Classification and Terminology, 2005-2009, *Epilepsia* 51(4):676–685, 2010.
91. Panayiotopoulos CP: The new ILAE report on terminology and concepts for the organization of epilepsies: critical review and contribution, *Epilepsia* 53(3):399–404, 2012.
92. Baulac S, Baulac M: Advances on the genetics of Mendelian idiopathic epilepsies, *Clin Lab Med* 30(4):911–929, 2010.
93. Brooks-Kayal A: Molecular mechanisms of cognitive and behavioral comorbidities of epilepsy in children, *Epilepsia* 52(Suppl 1):13–20, 2011.
94. Van Hove JL, Lohr NJ: Metabolic and monogenic causes of seizures in neonates and young infants, *Mol Genet Metab* 104(3):214–230, 2011.

95. Crunelli V, Cope DW, Terry JR: Transition to absence seizures and the role of GABA(A) receptors, *Epilepsy Res* 97(3):283–289, 2011.
96. Groomes LB et al: Do patients with absence epilepsy respond to ketogenic diets? *J Child Neurol* 26(2):160–165, 2011.
97. Verrotti A et al: Early-onset pure absence epilepsy: a distinct epileptic syndrome, *Acta Paediatr* 100(5):647–650, 2011.
98. Siverstein FS, Jensen FE: Neonatal seizures, *Ann Neurol* 62(2):112–120, 2007.
99. Hampers LC, Spina LA: Evaluation and management of pediatric febrile seizures in the emergency department, *Emerg Med Clin North Am* 29(1):83–93, 2011.
100. Frost JD Jr, Hrachovy RA: Pathogenesis of infantile spasms: a model based on developmental desynchronization, *J Clin Neurophysiol* 22(1):25–36, 2005.
101. Paciorkowski AR, Thio LL, Dobyns WB: Genetic and biologic classification of infantile spasms, *Pediatr Neurol* 45(6):355–367, 2011.
102. Guggenheim MA, Frost JD Jr, Hrachovy RA: Time interval from a brain insult to the onset of infantile spasms, *Pediatr Neurol* 38(1):34–37, 2008.
103. Mytinger JR et al: Outcomes in treatment of infantile spasms with pulse methylprednisolone, *J Child Neurol* 25(8):948–953, 2010.
104. Petrova LD: Tuberous sclerosis and epilepsy, *Am J Electroneurodiagnostic Technol* 51(1):5–15, 2011.
105. Gaily E: Vigabatrin monotherapy for infantile spasms, *Expert Rev Neurother* 12(3):275–286, 2012.
106. Crumrine PK: Management of seizures in Lennox-Gastaut syndrome, *Paediatr Drugs* 13(2):107–118, 2011.
107. Mantoan L, Walker M: Treatment options in juvenile myoclonic epilepsy, *Curr Treat Options Neurol* 13(4):355–370, 2011.
108. Skjei KL, Dlugos DJ: The evaluation of treatment-resistant epilepsy, *Semin Pediatr Neurol* 18(3):150–170, 2011.
109. Desai J, Mitchell WG: Does one more medication help? Effect of adding another anticonvulsant in childhood epilepsy, *J Child Neurol* 26(3):329–333, 2011.
110. Elliott RE et al: Vagus nerve stimulation for children with treatment-resistant epilepsy: a consecutive series of 141 cases, *J Neurosurg Pediatr* 7(5):491–500, 2011.
111. Subcommittee on Febrile Seizures, American Academy of Pediatrics: Neurodiagnostic evaluation of the child with a simple febrile seizure, *Pediatrics* 127(2):389–394, 2011.
112. Shearer P, Riviello J: Generalized convulsive status epilepticus in adults and children: treatment guidelines and protocols, *Emerg Med Clin North Am* 29(1):51–64, 2011.
113. Sillanpää M, Schmidt D: Predicting antiepileptic drug response in children with epilepsy, *Expert Rev Neurother* 11(6):877–885, 2011.
114. Kohler BA et al: Annual report to the nation on the status of cancer, 1975-2007, featuring tumors of the brain and other nervous system, *J Natl Cancer Inst* 103(9):714–736, 2011.
115. Central Brain Tumor Registry of the United States: Fact sheet. Available at http://www.cbtrus.org/factsheet/factsheet.html. Accessed May 20, 2013.
116. Kaatsch P: Epidemiology of childhood cancer, *Cancer Treat Rev* 36(4):277–285, 2010.
117. Taylor MD et al: Molecular subgroups of medulloblastoma: the current consensus, *Acta Neuropathol* 123(4):465–472, 2012.
118. Khatua S et al: Diffuse intrinsic pontine glioma—current status and future strategies, *Childs Nerv Syst* 27(9):1391–1397, 2011.
119. Janoueix-Lerosey I, Schleiermacher G, Delattre O: Molecular pathogenesis of peripheral neuroblastic tumors, *Oncogene* 29(11):1566–1579, 2010.
120. Owens C, Irwin M: Neuroblastoma: the impact of biology and cooperation leading to personalized treatments, *Crit Rev Clin Lab Sci* 49(3):85–115, 2012.
121. Brunklaus A et al: Outcome and prognostic features in opsoclonus-myoclonus syndrome from infancy to adult life, *Pediatrics* 128(2):e388–e394, 2011.
122. Maris JM: Neuroblastoma, *Lancet* 369(9579):2106–2120, 2007.
123. Jeison M, Yaniv I, Ash S: Genetic stratification of neuroblastoma for treatment tailoring, *Future Oncol* 7(9):1087–1099, 2011.
124. Seeger RC: Immunology and immunotherapy of neuroblastoma, *Semin Cancer Biol* 21(4):229–237, 2011.

CHAPTER

21

Mechanisms of Hormonal Regulation

Valentina L. Brashers, Robert E. Jones, and Sue E. Huether

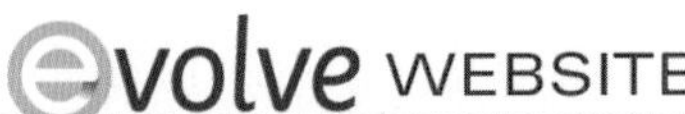

http://evolve.elsevier.com/McCance/

- Review Questions and Answers

CHAPTER OUTLINE

The endocrine system is composed of various glands located throughout the body (Figure 21-1). These glands are capable of synthesizing and releasing special chemical messengers called **hormones.** The endocrine system has five general functions:

1. Differentiation of the reproductive and central nervous systems in the developing fetus
2. Stimulation of sequential growth and development during childhood and adolescence
3. Coordination of the male and female reproductive systems, which makes sexual reproduction possible
4. Maintenance of an optimal internal environment throughout the life span
5. Initiation of corrective and adaptive responses when emergency demands occur

Hormones convey specific regulatory information among cells and organs and are integrated with the nervous system to maintain communication and control. The mechanisms of communication include autocrine (within cell), paracrine (between local cells), and endocrine (between remote cells).

MECHANISMS OF HORMONAL REGULATION

The endocrine glands respond to specific signals by synthesizing and releasing hormones into the circulation. Although a wide variety of hormones function within the body, they share certain general characteristics:

1. Hormones have specific rates and rhythms of secretion. Three basic secretion patterns are: (1) circadian or diurnal patterns, (2) pulsatile and cyclic patterns, and (3) patterns that depend on levels of circulating substrates (e.g., calcium, sodium, potassium, or the hormones themselves).
2. Hormones operate within feedback systems, either positive or negative, to maintain an optimal internal environment.
3. Hormones affect only cells with appropriate receptors and then act on those cells to initiate specific cell functions or activities.
4. Steroid hormones are either excreted directly by the kidneys or metabolized (conjugated) by the liver, which

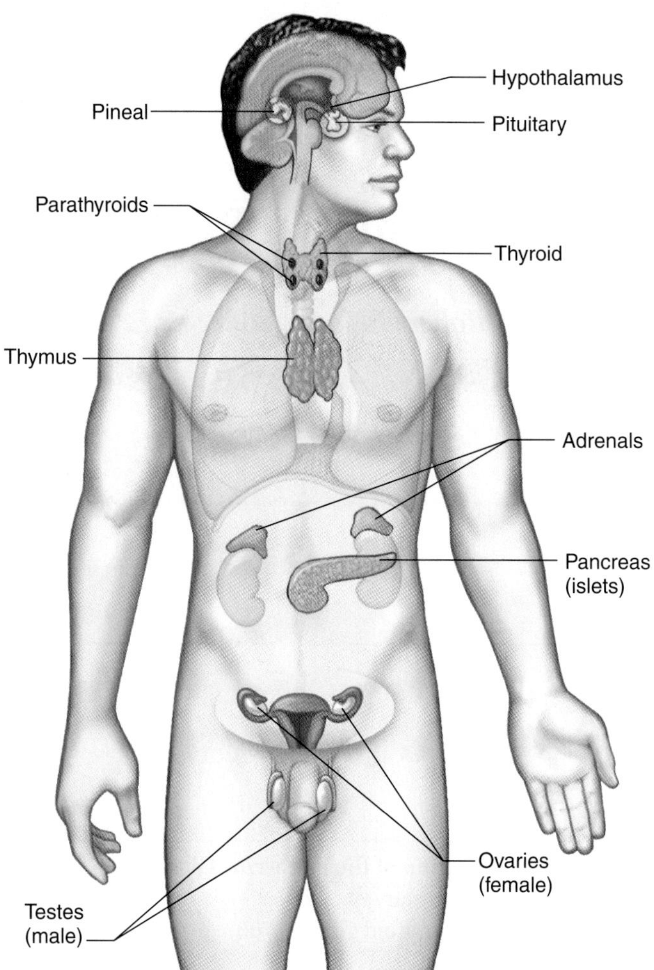

FIGURE 21-1 Principal Endocrine Glands. (From Patton KT, Thibodeau GA: *Anatomy & physiology*, ed 8, St Louis, 2013, Mosby.)

TABLE 21-1 STRUCTURAL CATEGORIES OF HORMONES

STRUCTURAL CATEGORY	EXAMPLES
Water Soluble	
Peptides	Growth hormone
	Insulin
	Leptin
	Parathyroid hormone
	Prolactin
Glycoproteins	Follicle-stimulating hormone
	Luteinizing hormone
	Thyroid-stimulating hormone
Polypeptides	Adrenocorticotropic hormone
	Antidiuretic hormone
	Calcitonin
	Endorphins
	Glucagon
	Hypothalamic hormones
	Lipotropins
	Melanocyte-stimulating hormone
	Oxytocin
	Somatostatin
	Thymosin
	Thyrotropin-releasing hormone
Amines	Epinephrine
	Norepinephrine
Lipid Soluble	
Thyroxine (an amine but lipid soluble)	Thyroxine (both thyroxine [T_4] and triiodothyronine [T_3])
Steroids (cholesterol is a precursor for all steroids)	Estrogens
	Glucocorticoids (cortisol)
	Mineralocorticoids (aldosterone)
	Progestins (progesterone)
	Testosterone
Derivatives of arachidonic acid (autocrine or paracrine action)	Leukotrienes
	Prostacyclins
	Prostaglandins
	Thromboxanes

inactivates them and renders the hormone more water soluble for renal excretion. Peptide hormones are catabolized by circulating enzymes and eliminated in the feces or urine.

Hormones may be classified according to their structure, gland of origin, effects, or chemical composition. (Table 21-1 categorizes hormones based on structure.) The secretion and mechanisms of action of hormones represent an extremely complex system of integrated responses. Although much has been learned about these complex systems, many of the specific mechanisms of action are not yet understood. The endocrine and nervous systems work together to regulate responses to the internal and external environments.

Regulation of Hormone Release

The release of hormones occurs either in response to an alteration in the cellular environment or in the process of maintaining a regulated level of certain hormones or certain substances. Hormone release is regulated by one or more of the following mechanisms: (1) chemical factors (such as blood glucose or calcium levels); (2) endocrine factors (a hormone from one endocrine gland controlling another endocrine gland); and (3) neural control (such as stress-induced release of catecholamines from the adrenal medulla).

Feedback systems provide precise monitoring and control of the cellular environment. The most common feedback system, **negative feedback,** occurs because the changing chemical, neural, or endocrine response to a stimulus negates the initiating change that triggered the release of the hormone. An example of hormone negative feedback is shown in Figure 21-2, *A*. Thyroid-stimulating hormone (TSH) secretion from the anterior pituitary is stimulated by **thyrotropin-releasing hormone (TRH)** from the hypothalamus. Secretion of TSH stimulates the synthesis and secretion of thyroid hormones. Increasing levels of T_4 (thyroxine) and T_3 (triiodothyronine) then generate negative feedback on the pituitary and hypothalamus to inhibit TRH and TSH synthesis.

Negative-feedback systems are important in maintaining hormone concentrations within physiologic ranges. The lack of negative-feedback inhibition on hormonal release often results in pathologic conditions. As discussed in Chapter 22, various

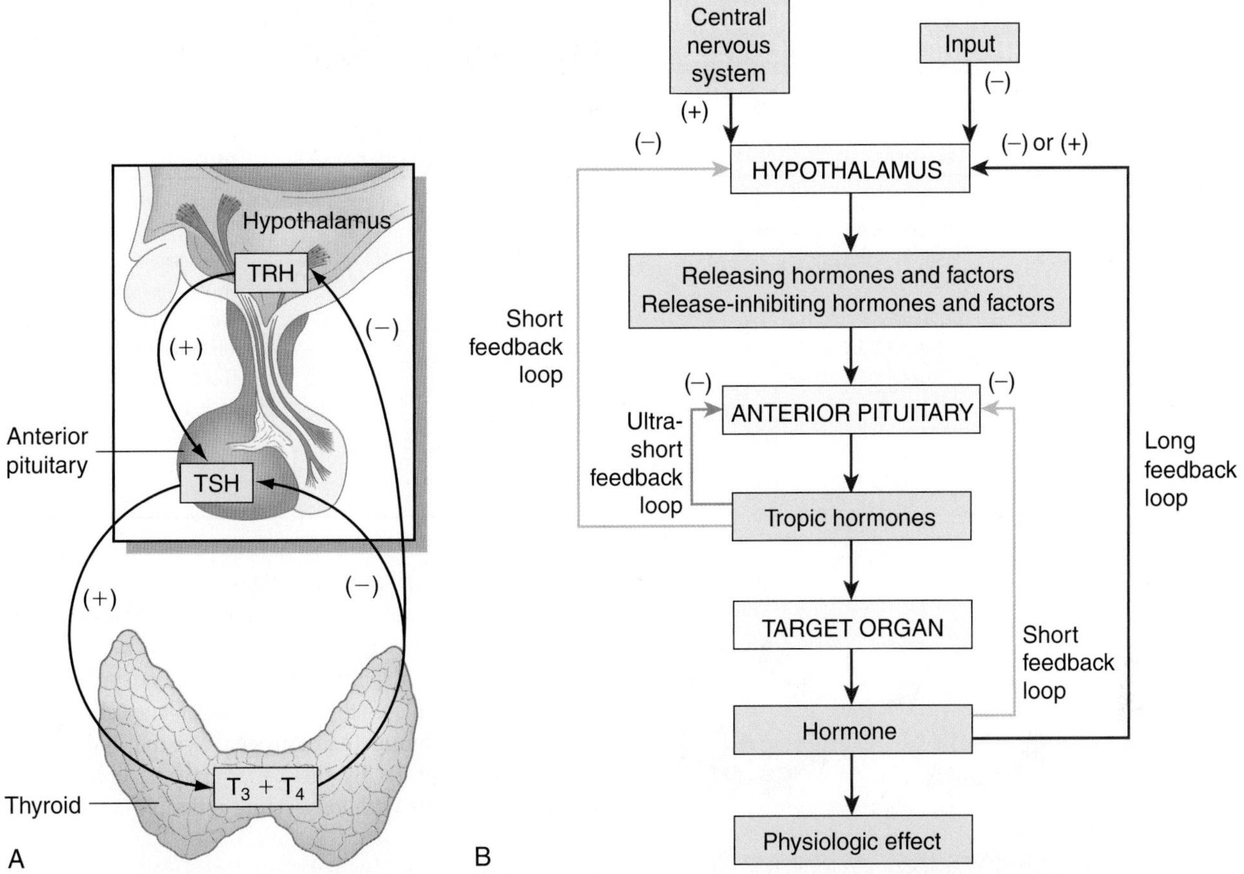

FIGURE 21-2 **Feedback Loops. A,** Endocrine feedback loops involving the hypothalamus-pituitary gland and end organs; in this example, the feedback loops for the thyroid gland (endocrine regulation). **B,** General model for control and negative feedback to hypothalamic-pituitary target organ systems. Negative-feedback regulation is possible at three levels: target organ (ultrashort feedback), anterior pituitary (short feedback), and hypothalamus (long feedback). *TRH,* Thyrotropin-releasing hormone; *TSH,* thyroid-stimulating hormone; T_3, triiodothyronine; T_4, tetraiodothyronine (thyroxine).

hormonal imbalances and related conditions are caused by excessive hormone production, which is the result of failure to "turn off" the system. These negative-feedback regulatory systems are diagrammed in Figure 21-2, *B*.

Hormone Transport

Once hormones are released into the circulatory system, they are distributed throughout the body. Peptide or protein hormones (pituitary, hypothalamic, and parathyroid hormones; and insulin) are water soluble and circulate in free (unbound) forms. Water-soluble hormones generally have a short half-life because they are catabolized by circulating enzymes. For example, insulin has a half-life of 3 to 5 minutes and is catabolized by insulinases. Lipid-soluble hormones, such as cortisol and adrenal androgens, are transported bound to a carrier or transport protein (Table 21-2) and can remain in the blood for hours to days. Only free hormones (those not bound to the carrier protein) can signal a target cell. Because an equilibrium exists between the concentrations of free hormones and hormones bound to plasma proteins, a significant change in the concentration of binding proteins can affect the concentration of free hormones in the plasma (see Table 21-2). (Mechanisms of hormone binding are discussed in Chapter 1.)

Hormone Receptors

When a hormone is released into the circulatory system, it is distributed throughout the body, but only those cells with appropriate **hormone receptors** for that hormone are affected. The target cell hormone receptors have two main functions: (1) to recognize and bind with high affinity to their particular hormones and (2) to initiate a signal to appropriate intracellular effectors. See Chapter 1 for cell signaling pathways, particularly Figures 1-19 and 1-20 on pp. 21-22.

The sensitivity of the target cell to a particular hormone is related to the total number of receptors per cell: the more receptors, the more sensitive the cell. Low concentrations of hormone increase the number of receptors per cell, called **up-regulation** (Figure 21-3, *A*). High concentrations of hormone decrease the number of receptors, called **down-regulation** (Figure 21-3, *B*). Thus the cell can adjust its sensitivity to the concentration of the signaling hormone. The receptors on the plasma membrane are continuously synthesized and degraded, so that changes in receptor concentration may occur within hours. Various physiochemical conditions also can affect both the receptor number and the affinity of the hormone for its receptor. Some of these physiochemical conditions are the fluidity and structure of the plasma membrane, pH, temperature, ion concentration, diet, and the presence of other

TABLE 21-2 BINDING PROTEINS, THEIR HORMONES, AND VARIABLES THAT AFFECT THEIR CIRCULATING LEVELS

BINDING PROTEIN	HORMONE	FACTORS THAT INCREASE BINDING PROTEIN LEVELS	FACTORS THAT DECREASE BINDING PROTEIN LEVELS
Corticosteroid-binding globulin	Cortisol Progesterone	Estrogen	Liver disease
Sex hormone–binding globulin	Dihydrotestosterone Testosterone Estradiol	—	Androgens Hypothyroidism Liver disease
Thyroid-binding globulin	Thyroxine (T_4) Triiodothyronine (T_3)	Estrogen Hyperthyroidism	Testosterone Glucocorticoids Liver disease
Albumin	All lipid-soluble hormones	Estrogen	Liver disease Malnutrition Renal disease

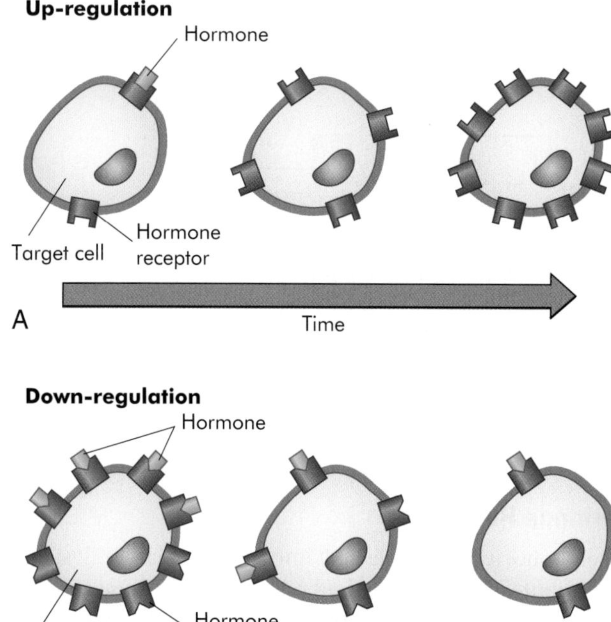

FIGURE 21-3 Regulation of Target Cell Sensitivity. **A,** Low hormone level and up-regulation, or an increase in the number of receptors. **B,** High hormone level and down-regulation, or a decrease in the number of receptors. (From Patton KT, Thibodeau GA: *Anatomy & physiology,* ed 8, St Louis, 2013, Mosby.)

chemicals (e.g., drugs). Finally, mutations in receptor structure can affect target cell activation such that normal cellular responses are increased or decreased. For example, mutations in thyroid hormone receptors can lead to resistance to thyroid hormone and can contribute to the development of tumors.[1,2]

Hormone receptors may be located in or on the plasma membrane or in the intracellular compartment of the target cell (Figure 21-4). Water-soluble hormones (see Table 21-1) have a high molecular weight and cannot diffuse across the cell membrane. They interact or bind with receptors in or on the cell membrane and mediate short-acting responses.[3] Lipid-soluble steroids, vitamin D, retinoic acid, and thyroid hormones diffuse freely across the plasma and nuclear membranes and bind with cytosolic or nuclear receptors (see Figure 21-4). The hormone-receptor complex binds to a specific region in the deoxyribonucleic acid (DNA) and stimulates the expression of a specific gene. Some lipid-soluble hormones (e.g., estrogen) also may bind with plasma membrane receptors. By these mechanisms, lipid-soluble hormones can mediate both long-acting and rapid-acting responses.[4]

Plasma Membrane Receptors and Signal Transduction

First Messenger

A hormone is the **first messenger,** is secreted into the bloodstream, and carries a message to a target cell. **Signal transduction** is the process by which this message is communicated into a cell. In general, signal transduction involves a series of steps that includes receptor activation or binding of a hormone to its receptor, activation of a G protein (transducer) and membrane-associated enzyme (effector enzyme), and production of a second messenger (see Figure 1-22, p. 24, and Figure 21-5). The final event is activation of an intracellular enzyme, such as protein kinase A or C, which causes alterations in gene transcription and the resulting target cell response to the hormone.

Cell surface receptors are usually classified according to how they initiate signal transduction: (1) G-protein–linked receptors, (2) ion-channel receptors, and (3) enzyme-linked receptors (including tyrosine kinase, serine kinase, and the cytokine-receptor superfamily with intrinsic enzyme activity—such as the Janus family of tyrosine kinases [JAK] and signal transducers and activators of transcription [STAT] molecules). With the exception of insulin, growth hormone, and prolactin, most water-soluble hormones—such as adrenocorticotropic hormone (ACTH), glucagon, norepinephrine, and epinephrine—activate G-protein–linked receptors. Other hormones, such as angiotensin II, activate G-protein–linked and ion-channel receptors. Insulin activates a tyrosine kinase receptor. Growth hormones, prolactin, and cytokines—such as interleukins—activate the JAK/STAT receptors.

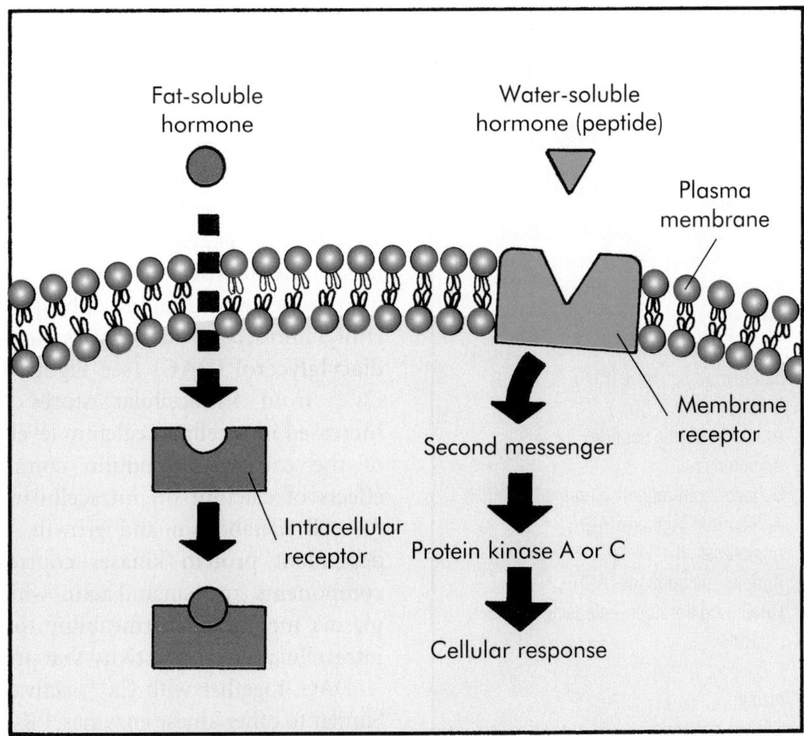

FIGURE 21-4 Hormone Binding at Target Cell.

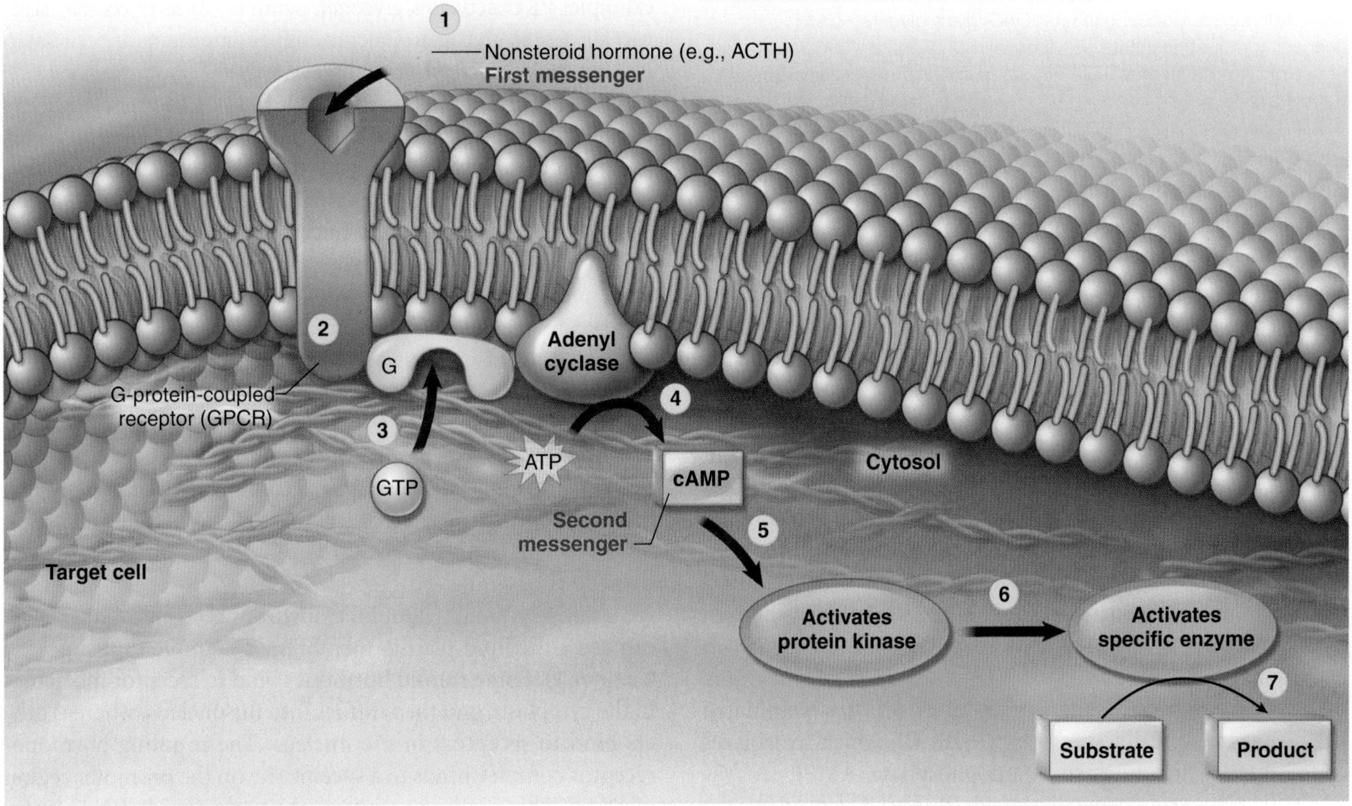

1 Nonsteroid hormone (e.g., ACTH)
First messenger
2
G-protein-coupled receptor (GPCR)
G
Adenyl cyclase
3
GTP
ATP
4
cAMP
Cytosol
Second messenger
5
Target cell
Activates protein kinase
6
Activates specific enzyme
7
Substrate
Product

FIGURE 21-5 Examples of First- and Second-Messenger Signaling. A nonsteroid hormone (first messenger) binds to a fixed receptor of the target cell **(1).** The hormone-receptor complex activates the G protein **(2).** The activated G protein *(G)* reacts with guanosine triphosphate *(GTP),* which in turn activates the membrane-bound enzyme adenylyl cyclase **(3).** Adenylyl cyclase catalyzes the conversion of adenosine triphosphate *(ATP)* to cyclic adenosine monophosphate (*cAMP;* second messenger) **(4).** cAMP activates protein kinase **(5).** Protein kinases activate specific intracellular enzymes **(6).** These activated enzymes then influence specific cellular reactions and metabolic pathways, thus producing the target cell's response to the hormone **(7).** (From Patton KT, Thibodeau GA: *Anatomy & physiology,* ed 8, St Louis, 2013, Mosby). *ACTH,* Adrenocorticotropic hormone.

TABLE 21-3 SECOND MESSENGERS IDENTIFIED FOR SPECIFIC HORMONES

SECOND MESSENGER	ASSOCIATED HORMONES
Cyclic AMP	Adrenocorticotropic hormone (ACTH) Luteinizing hormone (LH) Human chorionic gonadotropin (hCG) Follicle-stimulating hormone (FSH) Thyroid-stimulating hormone (TSH) Antidiuretic hormone (ADH) Thyrotropin-releasing hormone (TRH) Parathyroid hormone (PTH) Glucagon
Cyclic GMP	Atrial natriuretic peptide
Calcium	Angiotensin II Gonadotropin-releasing hormone (GnRH) Antidiuretic hormone (ADH)
IP_3 and DAG	Angiotensin II Antidiuretic hormone (ADH) Luteinizing hormone–releasing hormone (LHRH)
Tyrosine phosphorylation	
Tyrosine kinase	Insulin
JAK-STAT	Growth hormone Leptin Prolactin

AMP, Adenosine monophosphate; *DAG,* diacylglycerol; *GMP,* guanosine monophosphate; *IP_3,* inositol triphosphate; *JAK,* Janus family of tyrosine kinases; *STAT,* signal transducers and activators of transcription.

Second-Messenger Molecules: cAMP, cGMP, and Ca^{++}

Cyclic Adenosine Monophosphate (cAMP). **Second-messenger** molecules are the initial link between the first signal (hormone) and the inside of the cell (Table 21-3). For example, binding of epinephrine to a β-adrenergic receptor subtype activates (through a stimulatory G protein [G_s]) the enzyme adenylyl cyclase. Adenylyl cyclase catalyzes the conversion of adenosine triphosphate (ATP) to the second messenger 3′,5′-cAMP. Elevation of cAMP activates the enzyme cAMP-dependent *protein kinase A (PKA).* PKA phosphorylates and activates nuclear transcription factors (cAMP response element–binding [CREB] proteins) that influence numerous cellular functions.[5] For example, CREB proteins associated with the L-type channel in cardiac muscle increase the influx of calcium into the cell, which increases myocardial contractility. Alterations in CREB activity have been implicated in many disease states including diabetes and cancer.[6,7] The actions of cAMP are terminated by the enzyme phosphodiesterase (PDE) III, which hydrolyzes cAMP into inactive adenosine monophosphate (AMP).

Cyclic Guanosine Monophosphate (cGMP). Guanylyl cyclase is an enzyme that converts guanosine triphosphate (GTP) to the second-messenger 3′,5′-cGMP. cGMP activates cGMP-dependent kinase (protein kinase G), which in turn activates a number of physiologic processes. The effects of various ligands, such as atrial natriuretic hormone (vascular smooth muscle relaxation) and nitric oxide (e.g., vascular smooth muscle relaxation and platelet inhibition), are mediated by the second-messenger cGMP. Drugs that target the actions of cGMP are being explored for the treatment of vascular and pulmonary disorders.[8]

Calcium (Ca^{++}). In addition to being an important ion that participates in a multitude of cellular actions, Ca^{++} is considered an important second messenger. The binding of a hormone (such as norepinephrine or angiotensin II) to a surface receptor activates the enzyme *phospholipase C* through a G protein inside the plasma membrane. This enzyme breaks down membrane phospholipid phosphatidylinositol biphosphate (PIP_2) into second-messengers **inositol triphosphate (IP_3)** and **diacylglycerol (DAG)** (see Figure 1-22, p. 24) IP_3 mobilizes Ca^{++} from intracellular stores (endoplasmic reticulum). Increased intracellular calcium levels can lead to the formation of the calcium-calmodulin complex, which mediates the effects of calcium on intracellular activities that are crucial for cell metabolism and growth. For example, calmodulin-dependent protein kinases control intracellular contractile components (myosin and actin, which cause contraction), alter plasma membrane permeability to calcium, and regulate the intracellular enzyme activity that promotes hormone secretion.

DAG, together with Ca^{++}, activates *protein kinase C (PKC).* Similar to other kinase enzymes, PKC activates (by phosphorylation) other proteins or enzymes. PKC initiates a variety of cellular responses that are linked to cell metabolism and growth. For example, PKC activates glycogen synthase in liver cells to convert glucose to glycogen. Calcium signaling systems are crucial to healthy functioning of virtually every tissue system in the body including heart, brain, bone, smooth muscle, and many others.[9]

Some hormones, such as insulin, growth hormone, and prolactin, bind to surface receptors that directly activate tyrosine kinases. These tyrosine kinases include the Janus family of tyrosine kinases (JAK) and signal transducers and activators of transcription (STAT). They regulate a wide range of intracellular processes that contribute to cellular metabolism and growth, and are being targeted in emerging treatments for diabetes.[10] An example of first- and second-messenger systems is presented in Figure 21-5.

Steroid (Lipid-Soluble) Hormone Receptors

The lipid-soluble hormones are steroid hormones and are synthesized from cholesterol. They include androgens, estrogens, progestins, glucocorticoids, mineralocorticoids, vitamin D, and retinoid. Thyroid hormones are lipid soluble but are not synthesized from cholesterol (see p. 701). Because these hormones are relatively small, lipophilic, hydrophobic molecules, they can cross the lipid plasma membrane by simple diffusion (see Chapter 1). Some steroid hormones bind to receptor molecules in the cytoplasm and then diffuse into the nucleus, whereas others bind to receptors in the nucleus. The resulting hormone-receptor complex binds to a specific site on the promoter region of DNA. This binding activates ribonucleic acid (RNA) polymerase, which stimulates DNA transcription and increased synthesis of specific proteins (increased gene expression) (Figure 21-6). Modulation of gene expression can take hours to days.

Steroid hormone receptors also may be found in the plasma membrane and are associated with rapid responses (seconds or minutes) that have nongenomic and genomic effects. Crosstalk

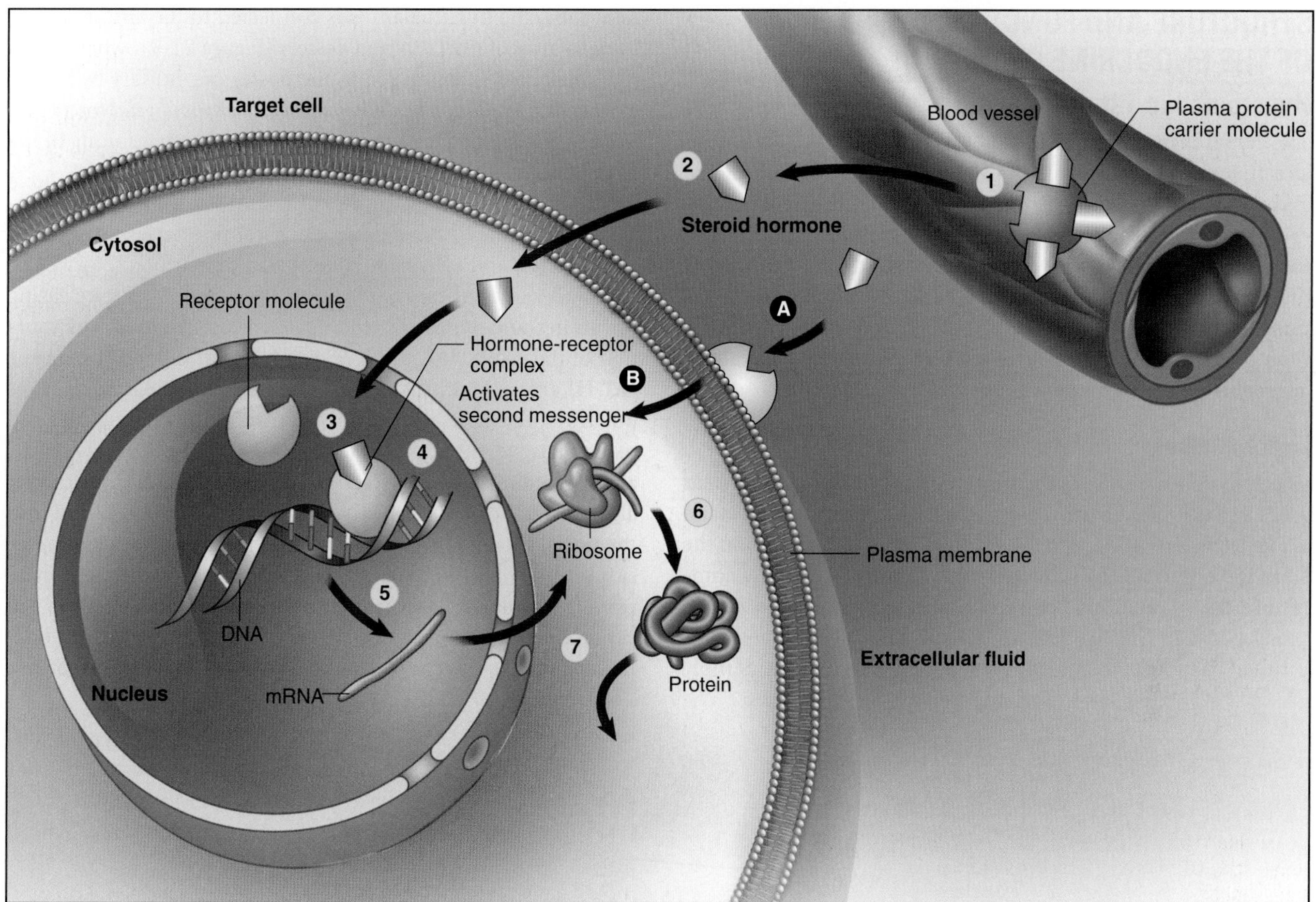

FIGURE 21-6 Steroid Hormone Mechanism. Lipid-soluble steroid hormone molecules detach from the carrier protein **(1)** and pass through the plasma membrane **(2).** Hormone molecules then diffuse into the nucleus, where they bind to a receptor to form a hormone-receptor complex **(3).** This complex then binds to a specific site on a DNA molecule **(4),** triggering transcription of the genetic information encoded there **(5).** The resulting messenger ribonucleic acid *(mRNA)* molecule moves to the cytosol, where it associates with a ribosome, initiating synthesis of a new protein **(6).** This new protein—usually an enzyme or channel protein—produces specific effects on the target cell **(7).** The classic genomic action is typically slow *(red arrows).* Steroids also may exact rapid effects by binding to receptors on the plasma membrane **(A)** and activating an intercellular second messenger **(B).** (Modified from Patton KT, Thibodeau GA: *Anatomy & physiology,* ed 8, St Louis, 2013, Mosby.)

between gene transcription and nongenomic responses modulate each other, allowing cells to adapt rapidly to environmental changes. Thyroid hormone, a nonsteroid lipid-soluble hormone, also has been found to use a cell surface receptor for its nongenomic actions. It first binds to an integrin receptor on the plasma membrane, and then uses a specific transport mechanism to gain access to its nuclear receptors where it can influence cell division and metabolic function.[11]

Hormone Effects

The binding of hormones with their receptors stimulates three general types of effects by:

1. Acting on pre-existing channel-forming proteins to alter membrane channel permeability
2. Activating pre-existing proteins through a second-messenger system
3. Activating genes to cause protein synthesis

Hormones have two general types of effects on target cells: direct and permissive. **Direct effects** are the obvious changes in cell function that specifically result from stimulation by a particular hormone. **Permissive effects** are less obvious hormone-induced changes that facilitate the maximal response or functioning of a cell. For example, insulin has a direct effect on skeletal muscle cells with insulin receptors, causing increased glucose transport into these cells. Insulin also has a permissive effect on mammary cells, facilitating the response of these cells to the direct effects of prolactin.

Some hormones have biphasic pharmacologic effects that are dependent on the concentration of the hormone. For example, low or physiologic levels of antidiuretic hormone (ADH, or arginine-vasopressin) stimulate renal tubular reabsorption of sodium and water. However, at supraphysiologic levels (i.e., those that can be achieved by exogenous administration), ADH acts as a vasoconstrictor.

STRUCTURE AND FUNCTION OF THE ENDOCRINE GLANDS

Hypothalamic-Pituitary Axis

The hypothalamic-pituitary axis (HPA) forms the structural and functional basis for central integration of the neurologic and endocrine systems, creating what is called the **neuroendocrine system.** The HPA produces a number of releasing/inhibitory hormones and tropic hormones that affect a number of diverse body functions (Figure 21-7). For example, the functions of the thyroid gland, adrenal gland, and male and female reproductive glands, as well as somatic growth and lactation, are regulated by hormones originating from the HPA.

Hypothalamus

The hypothalamus is divided into several nuclei and nuclear areas and is located at the base of the brain. The pituitary gland is located at the sella turcica, a saddle-shaped depression on the superior surface of the sphenoid bone (Figure 21-8). The communication or anatomic connection (blood vessels and neural tract) between the hypothalamus and anterior and posterior pituitary is quite elaborate and well described. However, simply described, the hypothalamus is connected to the anterior pituitary by way of portal blood vessels (Figure 21-9), whereas the hypothalamus is connected to the posterior pituitary by way of a nerve tract referred to as the *supraopticohypophysial tract* (Figure 21-10). These connections are vital to the functioning of the hypothalamus-pituitary system.[12]

The special cells of the hypothalamus are like other neurons in that they have similar electrical properties, organelles, membranes, and synapses. Hypothalamic neurosecretory cells, however, can synthesize and secrete the hypothalamic-releasing hormones and synthesize the hormones of the posterior portion of the pituitary gland. For example, **antidiuretic hormone (ADH)** and **oxytocin** are synthesized in hypothalamic neurons but are stored and secreted by the posterior pituitary. ADH and oxytocin travel to the posterior pituitary by way of the hypothalamohypophysial nerve tract. Releasing/inhibitory hormones also are synthesized in the hypothalamus and are secreted into the portal blood vessels, through which they travel to the anterior pituitary and control the release of tropic hormones. These releasing/inhibitory hormones from the hypothalamus include **prolactin-inhibiting factor (PIF), thyrotropin-releasing hormone (TRH), gonadotropin-releasing hormone (GnRH),**

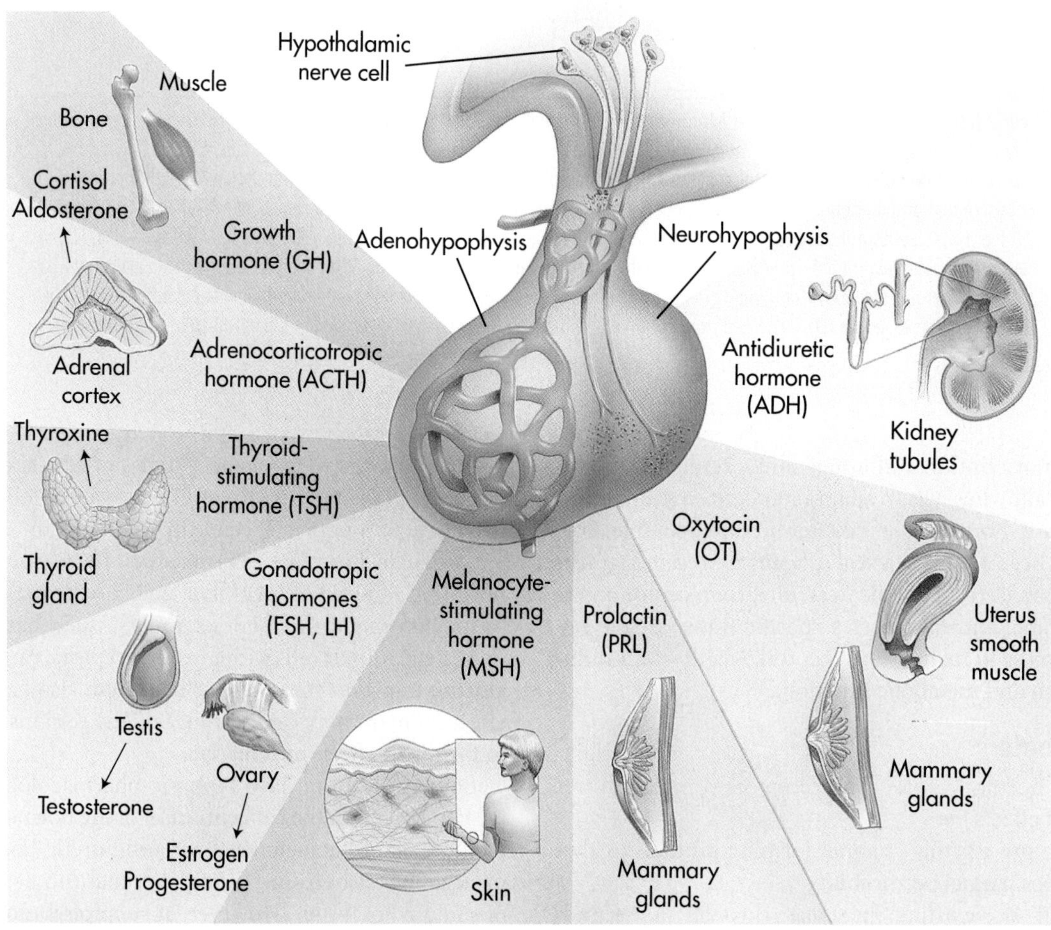

FIGURE 21-7 **Pituitary Hormones and Their Target Organs.** *FSH,* Follicle-stimulating hormone; *LH,* luteinizing hormone. (Modified from Patton KT, Thibodeau GA: *Anatomy & physiology,* ed 8, St Louis, 2013, Mosby.)

somatostatin, growth hormone–releasing factor (GRF), corticotropin-releasing hormone (CRH), and **substance P.** These hormones are summarized in Table 21-4.

Pituitary Gland

The **anterior pituitary** (adenohypophysis) accounts for 75% of the total weight of the pituitary gland. It is composed of three regions: (1) the pars distalis, (2) the pars tuberalis, and (3) the pars intermedia. The **pars distalis** is the major component of the anterior pituitary and the source of the anterior pituitary hormones. The **pars tuberalis** is a thin layer of cells on the anterior and lateral portions of the pituitary stalk. The **pars intermedia** lies between the two. In the adult the distinct intermediate lobe disappears, and the individual cells are distributed diffusely throughout the pars distalis and **pars nervosa (neural lobe),** which are part of the posterior pituitary.

The **posterior pituitary** (neurohypophysis) arises embryologically from an outpouching of the floor of the third ventricle within the brain. The posterior pituitary consists of three parts: (1) the median eminence located at the base of the hypothalamus, (2) the pituitary stalk, and (3) the infundibular process, also known as the *pars nervosa* or *neural lobe*. The **median eminence** is composed largely of the nerve endings of axons that arise primarily in the ventral hypothalamus. The median eminence often is designated as part of the posterior pituitary but contains at least 10 biologically active hypothalamic-releasing hormones, as well as the neurotransmitters dopamine, norepinephrine, serotonin, acetylcholine, and histamine. The median eminence therefore might be more appropriately considered part of the hypothalamus. The **pituitary stalk** contains the axons of neurons that originate in the supraoptic and paraventricular nuclei of the hypothalamus. Axons originating in the hypothalamus terminate in the pars nervosa, which secretes the hormones of the posterior pituitary.

Because of the anatomic location and connection of the pituitary gland to the brain, several neurotransmitters as well as physical and emotional stressors influence the release of specific hypothalamic releasing–inhibitory hormones and their respective tropic hormones. This allows for the integrated and coordinated function of the hypothalamic-pituitary axis. Interestingly, hypothalamic hormones also are synthesized outside the HPA. For example, CRH is synthesized in cells of the immune system, female and male reproductive organs, and the placenta. These peripherally synthesized neuropeptides are thought to play a role in the reproductive and immune responses to stress.[13,14]

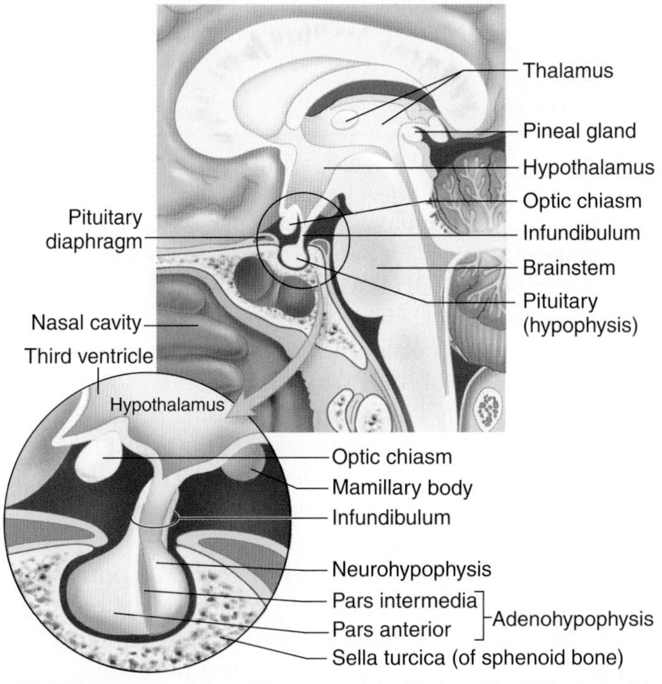

FIGURE 21-8 Location and Structure of the Pituitary Gland (Hypophysis). The pituitary gland is located within the sella turcica of the skull's sphenoid bone and is connected to the hypothalamus by a stalklike infundibulum. The infundibulum passes through a gap in the portion of the dura mater that covers the pituitary (the pituitary diaphragm). The inset shows that the pituitary is divided into an anterior portion, the adenohypophysis, and a posterior portion, the neurohypophysis. The adenohypophysis is further subdivided into the pars anterior and pars intermedia. The pars intermedia is almost absent in the adult pituitary. (Modified from Patton KT, Thibodeau GA: *Anatomy & physiology,* ed 8, St Louis, 2013, Mosby.)

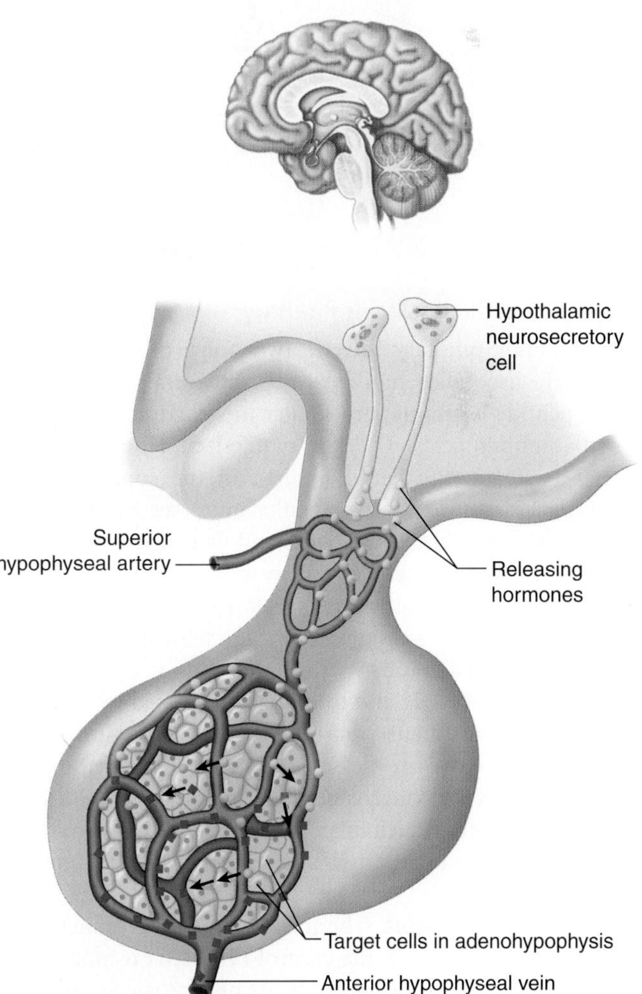

FIGURE 21-9 Hypophyseal Portal System. Neurons in the hypothalamus secrete releasing hormones into veins that carry the releasing hormones directly to the vessels of the adenohypophysis, thus bypassing the normal circulatory route. (From Patton KT, Thibodeau GA: *Anatomy & physiology,* ed 8, St Louis, 2013, Mosby.)

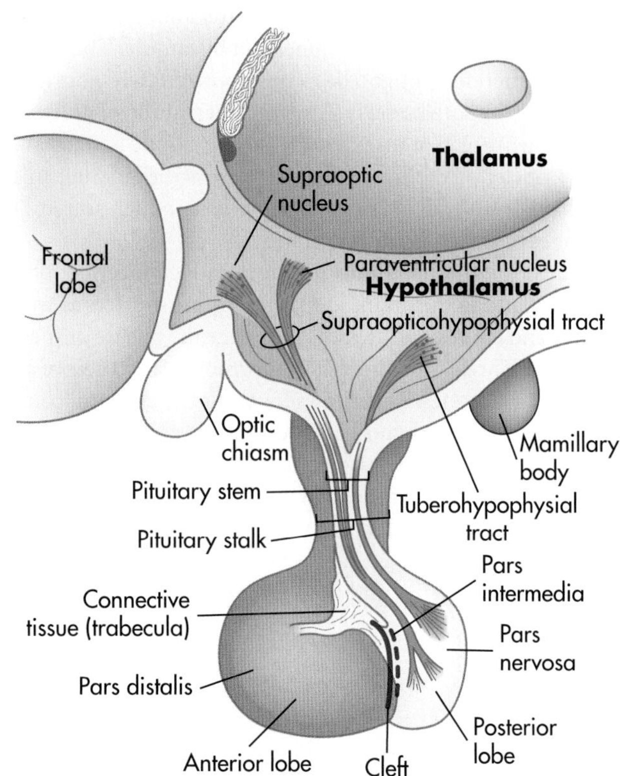

FIGURE 21-10 Nerve Tracts from Hypothalamus to Posterior Lobe of Pituitary Gland.

TABLE 21-4 HYPOTHALAMIC HORMONES (HYPOPHYSIOTROPIC HORMONES)

HORMONE	TARGET TISSUE	ACTION
Thyrotropin-releasing hormone (TRH)	Anterior pituitary	Stimulates release of thyroid-stimulating hormone (TSH) Modulates prolactin secretion
Gonadotropin-releasing hormone (GnRH)	Anterior pituitary	Stimulates release of follicle-stimulating hormone (FSH) and luteinizing hormone (LH)
Somatostatin	Anterior pituitary	Inhibits release of growth hormone (GH) and TSH
Growth hormone–releasing hormone (GHRH)	Anterior pituitary	Stimulates release of GH
Corticotropin-releasing hormone (CRH)	Anterior pituitary	Stimulates release of adrenocorticotropic hormone (ACTH) and β-endorphin
Substance P	Anterior pituitary	Inhibits synthesis and release of ACTH Stimulates secretion of GH, FSH, LH, and prolactin
Dopamine	Anterior pituitary	Inhibits synthesis and secretion of prolactin
Prolactin-releasing factor (PRF)	Anterior pituitary	Stimulates secretion of prolactin

Hormones of the Posterior Pituitary

The posterior pituitary secretes two polypeptide hormones: (1) ADH, also called *arginine-vasopressin;* and (2) oxytocin. These peptide hormones are similar in structure, differing by only two amino acids. They are synthesized, along with their carrier proteins (the neurophysins), in the supraoptic and paraventricular nuclei of the hypothalamus (see Figure 21-10). Once synthesized, these hormones and their neurophysins are packaged in secretory vesicles and are moved down the axons of the pituitary stalk to the pars nervosa for storage. The posterior pituitary thus can be seen as a storage and releasing site for hormones synthesized in the hypothalamus.

The release of ADH and oxytocin is mediated by cholinergic and adrenergic neurotransmitters. The major stimulus to both ADH and oxytocin release is glutamate, whereas the major inhibitory input is through gamma-aminobutyric acid (GABA). Before release into the circulatory system, ADH and oxytocin are split from the neurophysins and are secreted in unbound form.[15]

Antidiuretic Hormone. The major homeostatic function of the posterior pituitary is the control of plasma osmolality, as regulated by ADH (see Chapter 3). At physiologic levels, ADH acts on the vasopressin 2 (V2) receptors of the renal tubular cells to increase their permeability (see Chapter 37). This increased permeability leads to an increase in water reabsorption into the blood and the production of more concentrated urine. These effects may be inhibited by hypercalcemia, prostaglandin E, and hypokalemia. At pathophysiologically high serum levels, ADH acts on vasopressin 1 (V1) receptors and causes vasoconstriction.

The secretion of ADH is regulated primarily by the osmoreceptors of the hypothalamus, located near or in the supraoptic nuclei. As plasma osmolality increases, these osmoreceptors are stimulated, the rate of ADH secretion increases, more water is reabsorbed from the kidney, and the plasma is diluted to its set-point osmolality (approximately 280 mOsm/kg).[15] ADH has no direct effect on electrolyte levels, but by increasing water reabsorption, serum electrolyte concentrations may decrease because of a dilutional effect.

ADH secretion also is increased by changes in intravascular volume, which are monitored by mechanoreceptors in the left atrium and in the carotid and aortic arches. A volume loss of 7% to 25% acts through these receptors to stimulate ADH secretion. Stress, trauma, pain, exercise, nausea, nicotine, exposure to heat, and drugs such as morphine also increase ADH secretion. ADH secretion decreases with a decrease in plasma osmolality; an increase in intravascular volume; hypertension; an increase in estrogen, progesterone, and angiotensin II levels; and alcohol ingestion.

As mentioned previously, ADH at high serum levels acts on the V1 receptors and causes vasoconstriction and a resulting

TABLE 21-5 TROPIC HORMONES OF THE ANTERIOR PITUITARY AND THEIR FUNCTIONS

HORMONE	SECRETORY CELL TYPE	TARGET ORGANS	FUNCTIONS
Adrenocorticotropic hormone (ACTH)	Corticotropic	Adrenal gland (cortex)	Increased steroidogenesis (cortisol and androgenic hormones) Synthesis of adrenal proteins contributing to maintenance of the adrenal gland
Melanocyte-stimulating hormone (MSH)	Melanotropic	Anterior pituitary	Promotes secretion of melanin and lipotropin by anterior pituitary; makes skin darker
Somatotropic hormones			
Growth hormone (GH)	Somatotropic	Muscle, bone, liver	Regulates metabolic processes related to growth and adaptation to physical and emotional stressors, muscle growth, increased protein synthesis, increased liver glycogenolysis, increased fat mobilization
		Liver	Induces formation of somatomedins, or insulin-like growth factors (IGFs) that have actions similar to insulin
Prolactin	Lactotropic	Breast	Milk production
Glycoprotein hormones			
Thyroid-stimulating hormone (TSH)	Thyrotropic	Thyroid gland	Increased production and secretion of thyroid hormone Increased iodide uptake Promotes hypertrophy and hyperplasia of thymocytes
Luteinizing hormone (LH)	Gonadotropic	In women: granulosa cells In men: Leydig cells	Ovulation, progesterone production Testicular growth, testosterone production
Follicle-stimulating hormone (FSH)	Gonadotropic	In women: granulosa cells In men: Sertoli cells	Follicle maturation, estrogen production Spermatogenesis
β-Lipotropin	Corticotropic	Adipose cells	Fat breakdown and release of fatty acids
β-Endorphins	Corticotropic	Adipose cells Brain opioid receptors	Analgesia; may regulate body temperature, food and water intake

increase in arterial blood pressure. This baroreceptor-mediated response is much less sensitive than the ADH response to changes in osmolarity. Therefore, physiologic levels of ADH do not significantly affect vessel tone. However, significant vasoconstriction may be achieved pharmacologically. For example, high doses of ADH (given as the drug vasopressin) may be administered to achieve hemostasis during hemorrhage and to raise blood pressure in shock states.[16]

Oxytocin. Oxytocin is responsible for contraction of the uterus and milk ejection in lactating women and may affect sperm motility in men. In a woman, oxytocin is secreted in response to suckling and mechanical distention of the female reproductive tract. Stimulated by sucking, oxytocin binds to its receptors on myoepithelial cells in the mammary tissues and causes contraction of those cells. This results in increased intramammary pressure and milk expression ("let down" reflex). In response to distention of the uterus, oxytocin stimulates contractions. Oxytocin functions near the end of labor to enhance the effectiveness of contractions, promote delivery of the placenta, and stimulate postpartum uterine contractions, thereby preventing excessive bleeding. The function of this hormone is discussed in more detail in Chapter 23.

Oxytocin has been implicated in behavior responses, especially in women. It has been suggested that oxytocin and its receptor play a role in the brain's responsiveness to stressful stimuli, especially in the pregnant and postpartum states. Its potential role in the treatment of maternal child neglect and a variety of anxiety disorders is being explored.[17,18]

Hormones of the Anterior Pituitary

The anterior pituitary is composed of two main cell types: (1) the **chromophobes,** which appear to be nonsecretory; and (2) the **chromophils,** which are considered the secretory cells of the adenohypophysis. The chromophils are subdivided into seven secretory cell types, each type secreting one or more specific hormones (Table 21-5). In general, the regulation of the anterior pituitary hormones is achieved by (1) feedback of hypothalamic releasing–inhibitory hormones and factors, (2) feedback from target gland hormones (i.e., cortisol, estrogen), and (3) direct effects of neurotransmitters.

The major tropic hormones secreted by the anterior pituitary include ACTH, melanocyte-stimulating hormone (MSH), luteinizing hormone (LH), growth hormone (GH), prolactin, follicle-stimulating hormone (FSH), and TSH. The actions of these anterior pituitary tropic hormones are summarized in Table 21-5. These major hormones can be grouped into three categories: corticotropin-related hormones (ACTH and MSH), glycoproteins (LH, FSH, and TSH), and somatomammotropins (GH and prolactin). The corticotropin-related hormones are all derived from the precursor pro-opiomelanocortin (POMC). The role of ACTH is discussed later in this chapter. MSH promotes the secretion of melanin, which makes the skin darker. β-Lipotropin and β-endorphins are minor corticotropic hormones also released from the anterior pituitary. β-Lipotropin plays a role in fat catabolism and β-endorphins impact pain perception, body temperature, and food and water intake. The glycoprotein gonadotropins FSH and LH control reproductive processes in men and women and are discussed in Chapter 23. TSH and its effects on the thyroid gland are discussed later in this chapter. Growth hormone and prolactin have diverse and important effects on body tissues and are discussed next.

Growth Hormone (GH). GH secretion is controlled by two hormones from the hypothalamus: growth hormone–releasing hormone (GHRH), which increases GH secretion; and somatostatin, which inhibits it. GH is released from the pituitary in a pulsatile fashion, and overall secretion peaks during adolescence. This hormone is essential to normal tissue growth and maturation, and affects aging, sleep, nutritional status, stress, and reproductive hormones. In the bone, GH stimulates epiphyseal growth and increases osteoclast and osteoblast activity, resulting in increased bone mass. GH also increases amino acid transport in muscles. Other functions of GH include lipolysis and enhancement of hepatic protein synthesis.

Many of the anabolic functions of GH are mediated, at least in part, by the insulin-like growth factors (IGFs), also known as the somatomedins. There are two primary forms of IGF: IGF-1 and IGF-2, of which IGF-1 is the most biologically active. They both circulate bound to a group of binding proteins (IGFBP). IGF-1 binds to both insulin receptors, providing an insulin-like effect on skeletal muscle, and with the IGF-1 receptor, which mediates the anabolic effects of GH. IGF-2 causes a negative effect on tissue growth, thus balancing the activity of the IGF-1. Because of the anabolic effects of GH and IGF, they can be used to treat growth disorders and increase muscle mass but their use also has been linked to increased rates of cancer.[19] Interestingly, deficiencies in the growth hormone receptor have been linked to decreased risk of cancer and diabetes.[20]

Prolactin. Prolactin functions to induce milk production during pregnancy and lactation. It also has effects on reproduction and immune function. Its synthesis is stimulated by vasoactive intestinal polypeptide, serotonin, and growth factors. Its release is inhibited by dopamine. Hyperprolactinemia is a complication of tumors of the pituitary gland and some medications and is discussed in Chapter 22.

Pineal Gland

The pineal gland is located within the brain itself (see Figure 21-1) and is composed of photoreceptive cells that secrete melatonin. It is innervated by noradrenergic sympathetic nerve terminals controlled by pathways within the hypothalamus. **Melatonin** release is stimulated by exposure to dark and inhibited by light exposure. It is synthesized from tryptophan, which is first converted to serotonin and then to melatonin. Melatonin regulates circadian rhythms and reproductive systems, including the secretion of GnRH and the onset of puberty. It also plays an important role in immune regulation and is postulated to affect the aging process. Further effects of melatonin include increasing nitric oxide release from blood vessels, removing toxic oxygen free radicals, and decreasing insulin secretion. Melatonin has been used therapeutically in humans to help with sleep disturbances, jet lag, and psychologic disorders. Its utility for numerous other disorders is being explored.[21,22]

Thyroid and Parathyroid Glands

The thyroid gland, located in the neck just below the larynx, produces hormones that control the rates of metabolic processes throughout the body. The four parathyroid glands are located near the posterior side of the thyroid and function to control serum calcium levels.

Thyroid Gland

The **thyroid gland** is composed of two lobes that lie on either side of the trachea, inferior to the thyroid cartilage (Figure 21-11). The lobes are joined by a small band of tissue, the **isthmus,** which crosses the anterior surface of the trachea and larynx at the cricoid cartilage. The normal thyroid gland is not visible on inspection, but it may be palpated on swallowing, which causes upward displacement of the gland.

The thyroid gland is composed of **follicles** (Figure 21-12). The follicles are composed of follicular cells that surround a viscous substance called *colloid.* The follicular cells synthesize and secrete some of the thyroid hormones. Neurons of the autonomic nervous system terminate on blood vessels within the thyroid gland and on the follicular cells themselves. Acetylcholine, catecholamines, and other peptides directly affect secretory activity of the follicular cells and thyroid blood flow.

Regulation of Thyroid Hormone Secretion. **Thyroid hormone (TH)** is regulated through a negative-feedback loop involving the hypothalamus, the anterior pituitary, and the thyroid gland (see Figure 21-2). Thyrotropin-releasing hormone (TRH), which is synthesized and stored within the hypothalamus, initiates this loop. TRH is released into the hypothalamic-pituitary portal system and circulates to the anterior pituitary, where it stimulates the release of TSH. TRH levels increase with exposure to cold or stress and from decreased levels of T_4.

Thyroid-stimulating hormone (TSH) is a glycoprotein hormone synthesized and stored within the anterior pituitary. Once TSH is secreted by the anterior pituitary, it circulates to

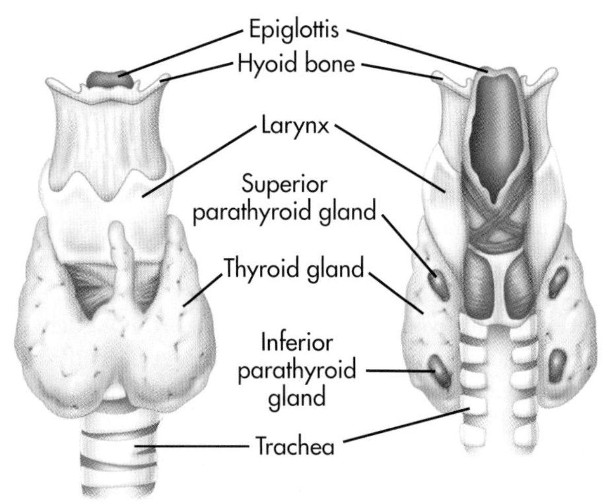

FIGURE 21-11 Thyroid and Parathyroid Glands. Note the relationship of the thyroid and parathyroid glands to each other, to the larynx (voice box), and to the trachea. (From Thibodeau GA, Patton KT: *Structure & function of the body,* ed 14, St Louis, 2012, Mosby.)

bind with TSH receptor sites located on the plasma membrane of the thyroid follicular cells. The effects of TSH on the thyroid include: (1) an immediate increase in the release of stored thyroid hormones, (2) an increase in iodide uptake and oxidation, (3) an increase in thyroid hormone synthesis, and (4) an increase in the synthesis and secretion of prostaglandins by the thyroid. TSH is also important in stimulating the growth and maintenance of the thyroid gland by stimulating thyrocyte hypertrophy and hyperplasia and decreasing apoptosis.[23] Thyroid gland hormones and their regulation and function are summarized in Table 21-6.

Thyroid hormones have a negative-feedback effect and inhibit TRH and TSH, which decreases TH synthesis and secretion. Thyroid hormone synthesis is also controlled by circulating enzymes called deiodinases that inactivate the precursor molecule thyroxine.

Synthesis of Thyroid Hormone. Thyroid hormone synthesis is summarized in the following steps:

1. Uniodinated thyroglobulin (a large glycoprotein) is produced by the endoplasmic reticulum of the follicular cells.
2. Tyrosine is incorporated into the thyroglobulin as it is synthesized.

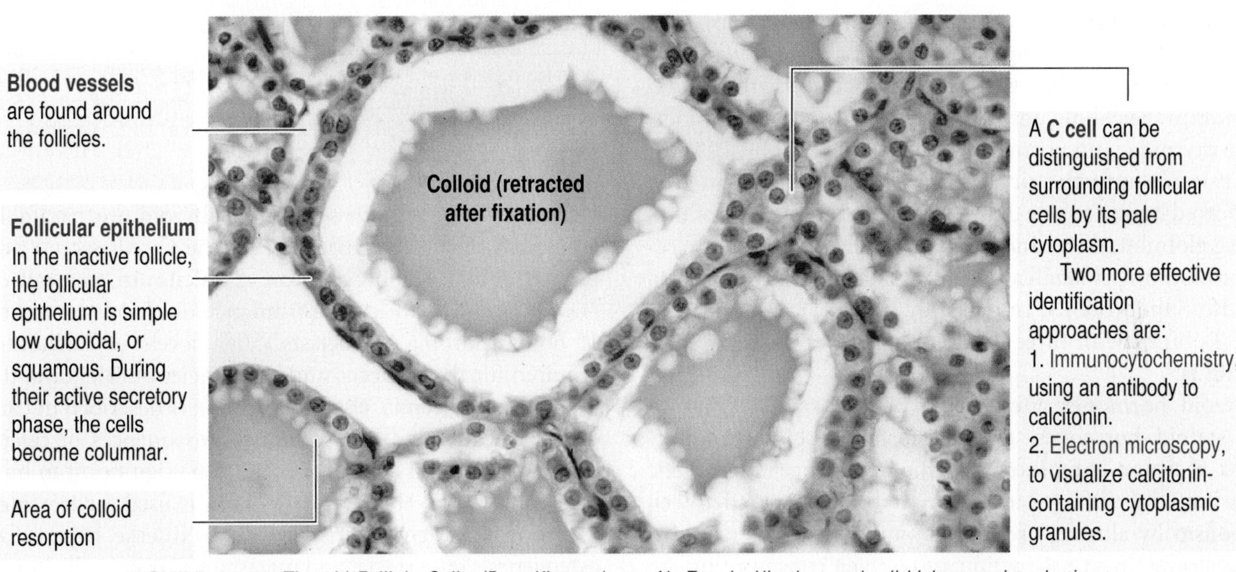

FIGURE 21-12 Thyroid Follicle Cells. (From Kierszenbaum AL, Tres L: *Histology and cell biology: an introduction to pathology*, ed 3, Philadelphia, 2012, Mosby.)

TABLE 21-6 THYROID GLAND HORMONES AND THEIR REGULATION AND FUNCTIONS

HORMONE	REGULATION	FUNCTIONS
Thyroxine (T_4) and triiodothyronine (T_3)	T_4 and T_3 levels are controlled by TSH Released in response to metabolic demand Influences on amount secreted: Gender Pregnancy Gonadal and adrenocortical-increased steroids = ↑ levels Exposure to extreme cold = ↑ levels Nutritional state Chemicals GHIH = ↓ levels Dopamine = ↓ levels Catecholamines = ↑ levels	Regulates protein, fat, and carbohydrate catabolism in all cells Regulates metabolic rate of all cells Regulates body heat production Insulin antagonist Maintains growth hormone secretion, skeletal maturation Affects CNS development Necessary for muscle tone and vigor Maintains cardiac rate, force, and output Maintains secretion of GI tract Affects respiratory rate and oxygen utilization Maintains calcium mobilization Affects RBC production Stimulates lipid turnover, free fatty acid release, and cholesterol synthesis
Calcitonin	Elevated serum calcium—major stimulant for calcitonin Other stimulants Gastrin Calcium-rich foods (regardless of serum Ca^{++} levels) Pregnancy Lowered serum calcium—suppresses calcitonin release	Lowers serum calcium by opposing bone-resorbing effects of PTH, prostaglandins, and calciferols by inhibiting osteoclastic activity Lowers serum phosphate levels May also decrease calcium and phosphorus absorption in GI tract

From Monahan FD et al: *Phipps' medical-surgical nursing: health and illness perspectives*, ed 8, St Louis, 2007, Mosby.
CNS, Central nervous system; *GHIH*, growth hormone–inhibiting hormone; *GI*, gastrointestinal; *PTH*, parathyroid hormone; *RBC*, red blood cell; *TSH*, thyroid-stimulating hormone.

3. Iodide (the inorganic form of iodine) is actively transferred (pumped) from the blood into the colloid by carrier proteins located in the outer membrane of the follicular cells. This active transport system is called the *iodide trap* and is very efficient at accumulating the trace amounts of iodide from the blood.
4. Iodide is oxidized and quickly attaches to tyrosine within the thyroglobulin molecule.
5. Coupling of iodinated tyrosine forms thyroid hormones. Triiodothyronine (T_3) is formed from coupling of monoiodotyrosine (one iodine atom and tyrosine) and diiodotyrosine (two iodine atoms and tyrosine). Tetraiodothyronine (T_4), commonly known as thyroxine, is formed from coupling of two diiodotyrosines.
6. Thyroid hormones are stored attached to thyroglobulin within the colloid until it is released into the circulation.

The thyroid gland normally produces 90% T_4 and 10% T_3. Once released into the circulation, T_3 and T_4 are primarily transported bound to one of three carrier proteins: thyroxine-binding globulin, thyroxine-binding prealbumin (transthyretin), or albumin. A small amount of thyroid hormone is also carried by lipoproteins. In the body tissues, T_4 is converted to T_3. T_3 binds with three different receptors (TRα1, TRβ1, and TRβ2).

Thyroid hormones affect many body tissues. Similar to some steroid hormones, thyroid hormones bind to intracellular receptor complexes and then influence the genetic expression of specific proteins. Thyroid hormones affect cell metabolism by altering protein, fat, and glucose metabolism and, as a result, heat production and oxygen consumption are increased. Thus these hormones are essential for maintaining healthy metabolic processes and normal growth and maturation. Their use is being explored for the therapy of many metabolic disorders.[24,25]

It is important to note that thyroid hormones exert a number of permissive effects on many organs, which are rather modest at physiologic thyroid hormone levels. However, these effects can become very pronounced when there are either high or low levels of circulating thyroid hormones. For example, in the heart, T_3 stimulates the synthesis of specific contractile proteins (e.g., α-myosin heavy chain), sarcolemmal ion pumps (Na^+-K^+-ATPase pump, Ca^{++}-ATPase pump), and membrane receptors (β-adrenergic receptors). Therefore, in hyperthyroidism, which is associated with elevated levels of thyroid hormones, cardiac effects include increased heart rate and cardiac output, as well as the development of cardiomyopathy. Thyroid hormones also affect the respiratory center, contributing to the normal hypoxic and hypercapnic drives. In severe hypothyroidism, ventilation can become very depressed. Thyroid hormone also stimulates bone resorption, and hyperthyroidism is associated with osteopenia, hypercalcemia, and hypercalciuria. Thyroid hormone is essential for normal neurologic development in the fetus and infant and affects neurologic functioning in adults. Other manifestations of thyroid hormone alteration are explained in Chapter 22. A newly described group of hormones called thyronamines have effects that oppose those of thyroid hormone (see What's New? Thyronamines).[26]

WHAT'S NEW?

Thyronamines

Thyronamines (TAMs) are a newly identified class of endogenous signaling compounds. Their structure is nearly identical to that of thyroid hormone but they have very different effects on tissues. Two TAMs, 3-iodothyronamine (T1AM) and thyronamine (TAM), have been identified in humans. Among the physiologic effects of TAMs found in experimental models are hypothermia, decreased metabolic rate, decreased cardiac contractility, hyperglycemia, and changes in adipose tissue metabolism. T1AM has been implicated in heart failure and insulin resistance. TAMs may have future therapeutic uses because they can induce hypothermia as a potential neuroprotective treatment for stroke, and affect metabolism in many kinds of cells including cancer cells.

Data from Galli E et al: *J Clin Endocrinol Metab* 97:E69–E74, 2012; Piehl S et al: *Endocr Rev* 32(1):64–80, 2011; Roy G, Placzek E, Scanlan T: *J Biol Chem* 287:1790–1800, 2012; Saba A et al: *Endocrinology* 151:5063–5073, 2010.

Also found in the tissue of the thyroid are parafollicular cells, or **C cells** (see Figure 21-12). The C cells secrete various polypeptides, including calcitonin. **Calcitonin,** also called *thyrocalcitonin,* acts to lower serum calcium levels by inhibition of bone-resorbing osteoclasts. High levels of calcitonin are required for these effects, and deficiencies of calcitonin do not lead to hypocalcemia. (Bone resorption is described in Chapter 43.) Consequently, the metabolic consequences of calcitonin deficiency or excess do not appear to be significant in humans (see Table 21-6). However, calcitonin is used for treatment of osteoporosis, osteoarthritis, Paget bone disease, hypercalcemia, osteogenesis imperfecta, and metastatic cancer of the bone. The precursor molecule to calcitonin, called procalcitonin, is a stress hormone that is elevated in infectious and inflammatory disorders and its measurement can aid in the diagnosis of these serious diseases.[27,28]

Parathyroid Glands

Two pairs of parathyroid glands normally are present, but the number may range from two to six. They are small and located behind the upper pole and lower pole of the thyroid gland (see Figure 21-11). The parathyroid glands produce **parathyroid hormone (PTH),** which works in concert with vitamin D to increase serum calcium concentration (Figure 21-13).[29] The overall effect of PTH secretion is to increase serum calcium concentration and decrease serum phosphate level. Magnesium and phosphate levels also affect PTH secretion. Hypomagnesemia in persons with normal calcium levels acts as a mild stimulant to PTH secretion, whereas in hypocalcemic individuals, hypomagnesemia decreases PTH secretion. Hyperphosphatemia leads to hypocalcemia because of calcium phosphate precipitation in soft tissue and bone. Alterations in serum phosphate levels therefore may indirectly influence PTH secretion by affecting serum calcium levels.

Once the parathyroid gland is stimulated, PTH is secreted. On release, PTH enters the circulation in unbound form. The hormone attaches to plasma membrane receptors in target tissues, where the biologic effects of PTH are mediated primarily by activation of the adenylyl cyclase system (see Chapter 1).

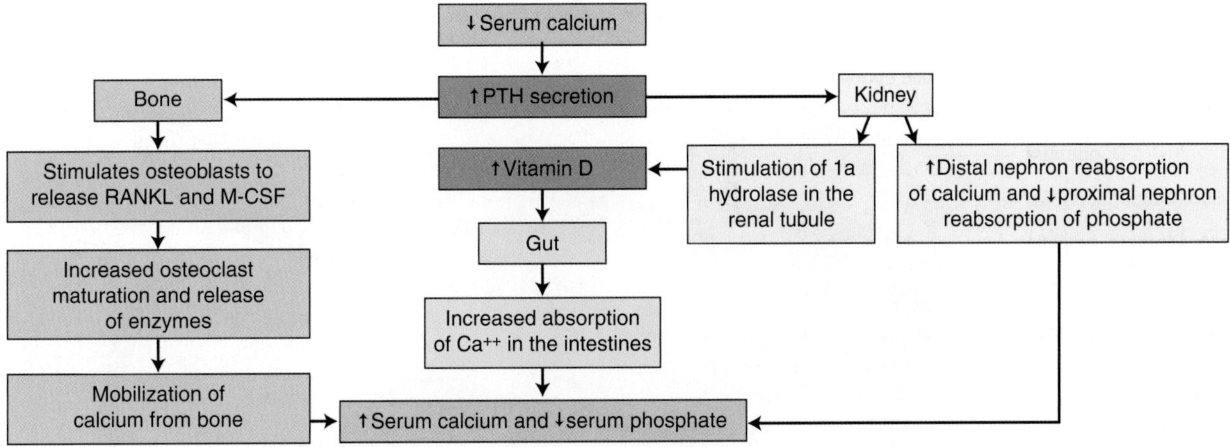

FIGURE 21-13 Normal Calcium Metabolism Regulated by PTH and Vitamin D. *M-CSF,* Macrophage-colony stimulating factor; *PTH,* parathyroid hormone; *RANKL,* receptor activator of NF-κβ ligand.

To achieve regulation of serum calcium concentration, PTH acts directly on bone and the kidneys. In bone, PTH has at least two effects. In acute hypocalcemia, PTH secretion stimulates osteoblasts to release receptor activator for nuclear factor–kappa beta (NF-κβ) ligand (RANKL) and macrophage-colony stimulating factor (M-CSF), which results in osteoclast proliferation, maturation, and release of acidic enzymes, such as cathepsin.[30] These enzymes mobilize calcium release from bone, which increases the serum calcium level. Chronic stimulation by PTH results in bone remodeling, a process in which bone is broken down and re-formed. Chronic stimulation can occur because of parathyroid tumors (primary hyperparathyroidism) or because of chronic hypocalcemia, such as that seen in end-stage renal disease (secondary hyperparathyroidism).[29] This process can weaken the bone, leading to an increased risk for fracture (e.g., renal osteodystrophy).[31] Paradoxically, intermittent therapeutic bursts of PTH can actually strengthen bone and this treatment modality is used in individuals with osteoporotic fractures.[32,33]

In the kidneys, PTH acts on its plasma membrane receptor in the distal tubules of the nephron to increase reabsorption of calcium. It acts on the proximal tubules to decrease reabsorption of phosphorus and bicarbonate. In renal cells, PTH stimulates the activity of 1α-hydroxylase, which mediates a step in the formation of the biologically active form of vitamin D (1,25-dihydroxy-vitamin D_3). The primary role of vitamin D_3 is to serve as a cofactor with PTH to increase gastrointestinal absorption of calcium. Vitamin D also increases PTH-mediated osteoclast stimulation. Vitamin D deficiency is associated with poor bone health and has been implicated in many other disorders (see What's New? Vitamin D).

Another hormone that plays an important role in calcium and bone physiology is parathyroid hormone–related peptide (PTHrP). This hormone is synthesized in many adult and fetal tissues and affects tissues around it in a paracrine fashion. It has similar biologic properties to PTH and utilizes the same receptors; however, it also plays a role in placental calcium transport, lactation, and tooth development in the fetus. It was discovered as the primary hormone involved in malignancy-related hypercalcemia (paraneoplastic disorders).[30]

WHAT'S NEW?

Vitamin D

Vitamin D is essential for bone health and is widely used for the prevention and treatment of postmenopausal osteoporosis and renal osteodystrophy. More recently, vitamin D deficiency has been associated with an increased risk for infections, cancer, asthma, heart disease, dementia, diabetes, chronic pain syndromes, and autoimmune disorders. Controversies continue as to whether these associations indicate a direct cause and effect between low levels of vitamin D and the pathophysiology of these diseases, and whether vitamin D supplementation reduces risk or improves outcomes. However, many health organizations recommend increased intake of vitamin D–containing foods (seafood, vitamin D–fortified juices, and milk products), increased exposure to sunlight, and supplementation with vitamin D. The Institute of Medicine currently recommends 400 to 600 IUs of vitamin D per day for adults.

Data from De-Regil LM et al: *Cochrane Database Syst Rev* 2:CD008873, 2012; Fleet JC et al: *Biochem J* 441(1):61–76, 2012; Holick MF et al: *J Clin Endocrinol Metab* 96(7):1911–1930, 2011; Hollis BW: *Curr Opin Clin Nutr Metab Care* 14(6):598–604, 2011; Institute of Medicine: *Dietary reference intakes for calcium and vitamin D,* Washington, DC, 2010, National Academies Press; Karakas M et al: *J Clin Endocrinol Metab* 98(1):272–280, 2013; Paul G et al: *Am J Respir Crit Care Med* 185(2):124–132, 2012.

Endocrine Pancreas

The **pancreas** is both an endocrine gland that produces hormones and an exocrine gland that produces digestive enzymes. (The exocrine pancreas is discussed in Chapter 40.) A major disorder of the endocrine pancreas is diabetes mellitus.

The pancreas is located behind the stomach, between the spleen and the duodenum. It houses the **islets of Langerhans.** The islets of Langerhans have four types of hormone-secreting cells: **alpha cells,** which secrete glucagon; **beta cells,** which secrete insulin and amylin; **delta cells,** which secrete gastrin and somatostatin; and **F (or PP) cells,** which secrete pancreatic polypeptide that stimulates gastric secretion and antagonizes cholecystokinin. These hormones regulate carbohydrate, fat,

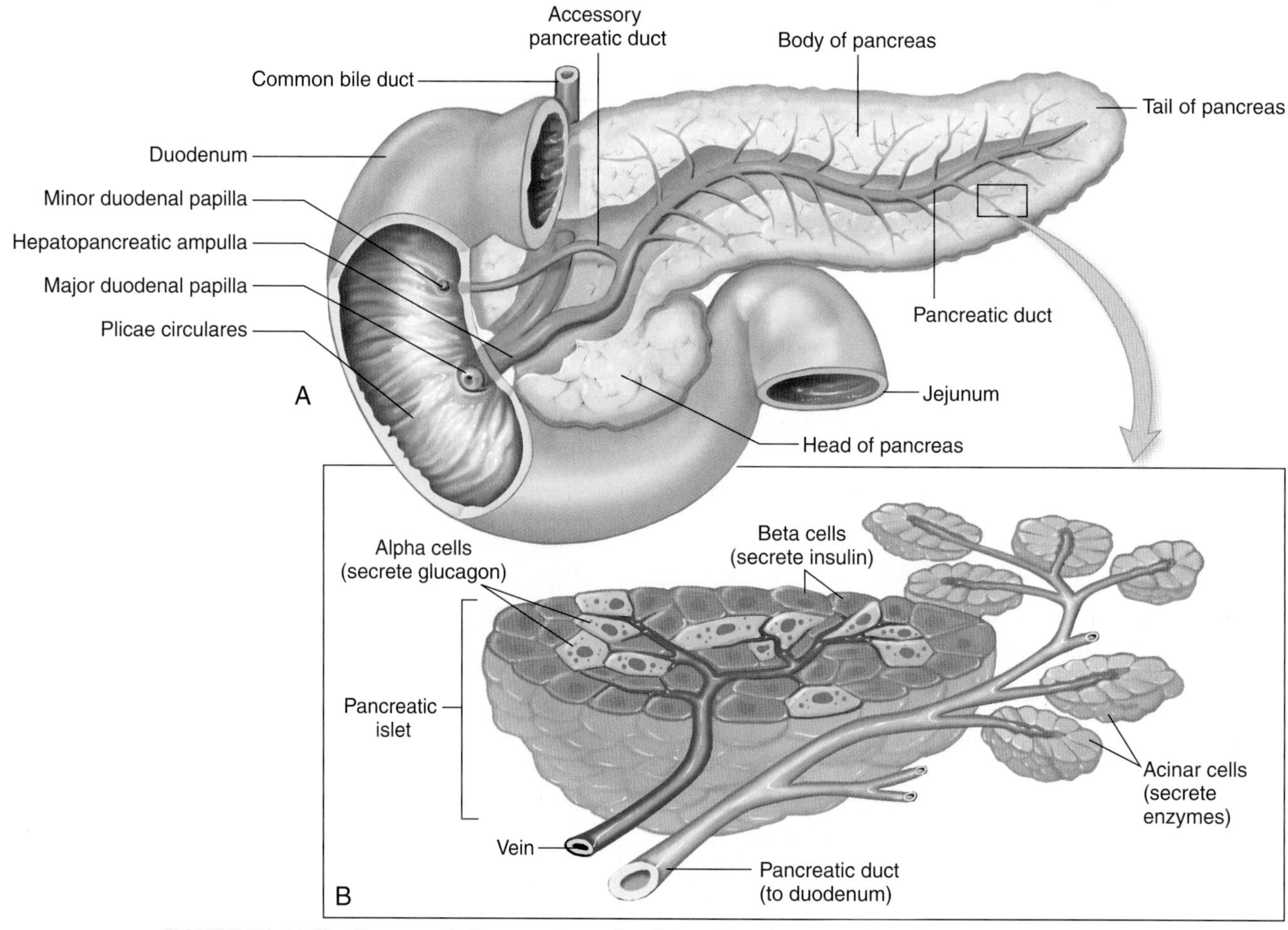

FIGURE 21-14 The Pancreas. **A,** Pancreas dissected to show main and accessory ducts. The main duct may join the common bile duct, as shown here, to enter the duodenum by a single opening at the major duodenal papilla, or the two ducts may have separate openings. The accessory pancreatic duct is usually present and has a separate opening into the duodenum. **B,** Exocrine glandular cells (around small pancreatic ducts) and endocrine glandular cells of the pancreatic islets (adjacent to blood capillaries). Exocrine pancreatic cells secrete pancreatic juice, alpha endocrine cells secrete glucagon, and beta cells secrete insulin. (From Patton KT, Thibodeau GA: *Anatomy & physiology,* ed 8, St Louis, 2013, Mosby.)

and protein metabolism. (The pancreas is illustrated in Figure 21-14.) Nerves from both the sympathetic and the parasympathetic divisions of the autonomic nervous system innervate the pancreatic islets.

The perfusion of the anterior lobe of the pancreas, where alpha, beta, and delta cells are most numerous, comes from branches of the superior mesenteric artery. The posterior lobe is perfused by branches of the celiac artery. The pancreatic islets receive 10% of the pancreatic blood flow but represent only 1% of pancreatic mass. This is necessary for oxygenation and delivery of islet hormones to target cells.

Insulin

The beta cells of the pancreas synthesize **insulin** from the precursor proinsulin. Proinsulin is formed from a larger and earlier precursor molecule, preproinsulin. Proinsulin is composed of an A peptide and a B peptide connected by a C peptide and two disulfide bonds. C peptide is cleaved by proteolytic enzymes, leaving the bonded A and B peptide chains that become insulin. Insulin circulates freely in the plasma and is not bound to a carrier. C peptide can be measured in the blood as an indirect measure of serum insulin synthesis. Recent studies have shown that C peptide has biologic activity and binds to cells through a G-protein receptor, resulting in increased intracellular calcium levels. Its role in diabetic complications is being explored.[34]

Secretion of insulin is regulated by chemical, hormonal, and neural control. Insulin secretion is promoted when blood levels of glucose, amino acids (arginine and lysine), and gastrointestinal hormones (glucagon, gastrin, cholecystokinin, secretin) increase, and when the beta cells are stimulated parasympathetically. Insulin secretion diminishes in response to low blood levels of glucose (hypoglycemia), high levels of insulin (through negative feedback to the beta cells), and sympathetic stimulation of the alpha cells in the islets. Prostaglandin (PGE_2) also inhibits insulin secretion.

Insulin facilitates the rate of glucose uptake into many cells within the body. At the target cell, insulin binds with an enzyme-linked plasma membrane receptor that contains tyrosine kinase on the cytosolic surface. Insulin receptor binding sends a cascade of signals to activate glucose transporters

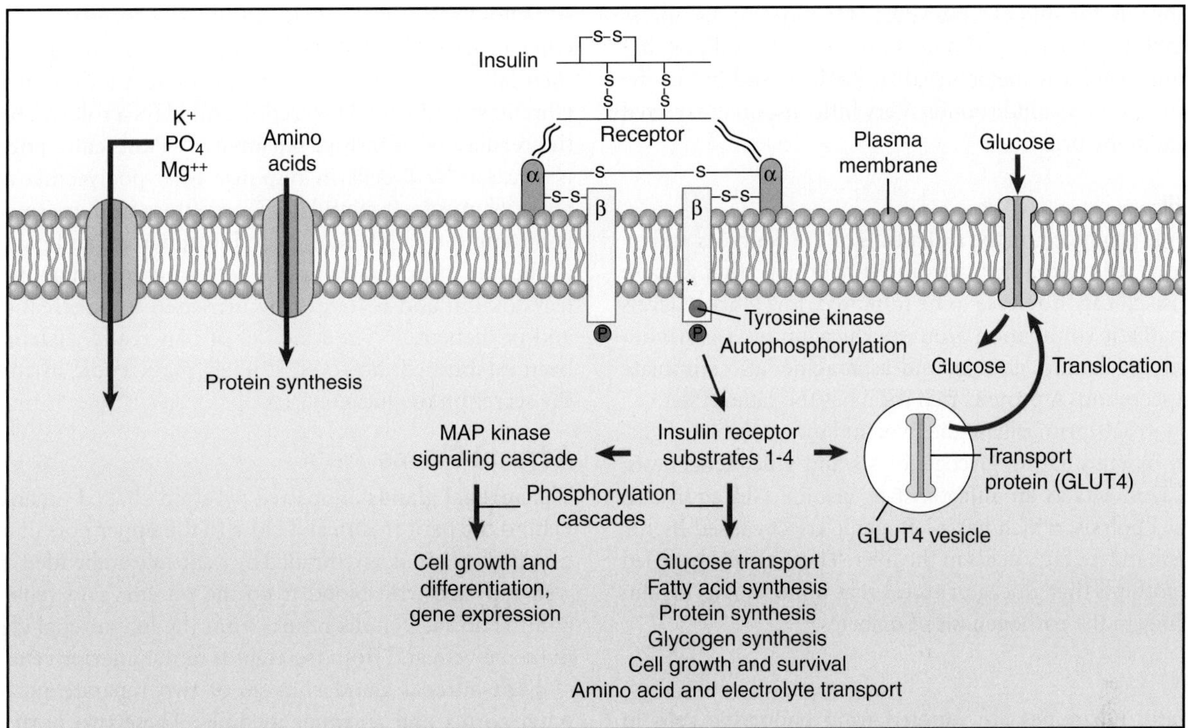

FIGURE 21-15 Insulin Action on Cells. Binding of insulin to its receptor causes autophosphorylation of the receptor, which then itself acts as a tyrosine kinase that phosphorylates insulin receptor substrate 1. Numerous target enzymes, such as protein kinase B and MAP kinase, are activated, and these enzymes have a multitude of effects on cell function. The glucose transporter, GLUT4, is recruited to the plasma membrane, where it facilitates glucose entry into the cell. The transport of amino acids, potassium, magnesium, and phosphate into the cell is also facilitated. The synthesis of various enzymes is induced or suppressed, and cell growth is regulated by signal molecules that modulate gene expression. *MAP,* Mitogen-activated protein. (Redrawn from Levy MN, Koeppen BM, Stanton BA: *Principles of physiology,* ed 4, St Louis, 2006, Mosby.)

TABLE 21-7 INSULIN ACTIONS

	SITES OF INSULIN-PROMOTED SYNTHESIS		
ACTIONS	**LIVER CELLS**	**MUSCLE CELLS**	**ADIPOSE CELLS**
Glucose uptake	Increased	Increased	Increased
Glucose use	—	—	Increased glycerol phosphate
Glycogenesis	Increased	Increased	—
Glycogenolysis	Decreased	Decreased	—
Glycolysis	Increased	Increased	Increased
Gluconeogenesis	Increased	—	—
Other	Increased fatty acid synthesis Decreased ketogenesis Decreased urea cycle activity	Increased amino acid uptake Increased protein synthesis Decreased proteolysis	Increased fat esterification Decreased lipolysis Increased fat storage

(GLUT) for entry of glucose into the cell.[35] The primary GLUT is called GLUT4. It is stored in cellular vesicles until activated by the insulin receptor and is then translocated to the cell surface where it facilitates the diffusion of glucose into the cell. Translocation of GLUT4 to the cell surface is associated with a 10- to 21-fold increase in glucose diffusion into the cell, particularly in skeletal and cardiac muscle, liver, and adipose cells (Figure 21-15). The sensitivity of the insulin receptor is a key component in maintaining normal cellular function, and insulin resistance has been implicated in numerous cardiovascular diseases, including hypertension and diabetes. Adipocytes release a number of hormones that are altered in obesity and have an important effect on insulin sensitivity.

Insulin is an anabolic hormone that promotes not only the uptake of glucose but also the synthesis of proteins, carbohydrates, lipids, and nucleic acids. It functions mainly in the liver, muscle, and adipose tissue. Table 21-7 summarizes the actions of insulin. The net effect of insulin in these tissues is to stimulate protein and fat synthesis and decrease blood glucose level. The brain, red blood cells, kidney, and lens of the eye do not require insulin for glucose transport. Insulin also facilitates the intracellular transport of potassium (K^+), phosphate, and magnesium. Insulin is metabolized in the liver and kidney by enzymes that split disulfide bonds. Very little insulin is excreted unchanged in the urine.

Glucagon

Glucagon is produced by the alpha cells of the pancreas and by a number of cells lining the gastrointestinal tract. High glucose levels cause glucagon release to be inhibited; low glucose levels and sympathetic stimulation promote glucagon release. Amino acids, such as alanine, glycine, and asparagine, also stimulate glucagon secretion. A protein-rich meal has the same effect.

Glucagon acts primarily in the liver and increases blood glucose level by stimulating glycogenolysis and gluconeogenesis; thus glucagon acts as an antagonist to insulin. Glucagon also stimulates lipolysis, which has a ketogenic effect caused by the metabolism of free fatty acids in the liver. These effects have led to the hypothesis that glucagon excess is as important as insulin insufficiency in the pathogenesis of diabetes.[36]

Incretins

The incretin hormones are secreted from endocrine cells in the gastrointestinal tract in the presence of carbohydrates, proteins, and fats. The major incretin hormones are glucagon-like peptide-1 (GLP-1) and glucose-dependent insulinotropic polypeptide (GIP). They control postprandial glucose levels by promoting glucose-dependent insulin secretion, inhibiting glucagon synthesis, and delaying gastric emptying.[37] Incretins also enhance beta-cell mass and replenish intracellular stores of insulin. Incretins are broken down by an enzyme called dipeptidyl peptidase 4 (DPP IV) and drugs that inhibit this enzyme (called 'gliptins') increase incretin levels. The gliptins and other drugs are incretin agonists used for the treatment of type 2 diabetes.[38,39]

Amylin

Amylin (islet amyloid polypeptide) is a peptide hormone co-secreted with insulin by beta cells in response to nutrient stimuli. It regulates blood glucose level by delaying nutrient uptake and suppressing glucagon secretion after meals. Amylin also has a satiety effect. Through these mechanisms, amylin has an antihyperglycemic effect. Aggregated amylin has cytotoxic properties and contributes to the loss of beta cells in type 2 diabetes and in islet cell transplants.[40,41] New drugs that serve as amylomimetics are used for treatment of both type 1 and type 2 diabetes.[42]

Somatostatin

Pancreatic **somatostatin** is produced by delta cells of the pancreas and is a hormone essential in carbohydrate, fat, and protein metabolism (i.e., homeostasis of ingested nutrients). It differs from hypothalamic somatostatin, which inhibits release of growth hormone and TSH. Pancreatic somatostatin is involved in regulating alpha-cell and beta-cell function within the islets by inhibiting secretion of insulin, glucagon, and pancreatic polypeptide.

Ghrelin, Pancreatic Polypeptide, and Gastrin

Ghrelin levels increase before a meal and stimulate appetite, then fall soon after a meal and promote a feeling of satiety.[43] Ghrelin stimulates GH secretion and plays a role in obesity and the regulation of insulin sensitivity.[44] **Pancreatic polypeptide** is released by F cells in response to hypoglycemia and protein-rich meals. It stimulates Y receptors in numerous tissues, including the gallbladder, exocrine pancreas, and parietal cells in the gut. It promotes gastric secretion and antagonizes cholecystokinin and is frequently increased in pancreatic tumors and in diabetes.[45] The function of pancreatic **gastrin** has not been established; however, it likely plays a role in controlling the secretion of glucagon.

Adrenal Glands

The **adrenal glands** are paired pyramid-shaped organs located behind the peritoneum and close to the upper pole of each kidney. Each gland is surrounded by a capsule embedded in fat and well supplied with blood from the phrenic and renal arteries and the aorta. Venous return from the left adrenal gland is to the renal vein and from the right is to the inferior vena cava.

Each adrenal gland consists of two separate portions: an outer cortex and an inner medulla. These two portions have different embryonic origins, different structures, and different hormonal functions. In effect, each adrenal gland functions like two separate glands, although there are interrelationships between functions of each portion (Figure 21-16).

Adrenal Cortex

The **adrenal cortex,** or outer region of the gland, accounts for 80% of the weight of the adult gland. The cortex is histologically subdivided into the following three zones:

1. The **zona glomerulosa,** the outer layer, constitutes about 15% of the cortex and primarily produces the mineralocorticoid aldosterone.
2. The **zona fasciculata,** the middle layer, constitutes 78% of the cortex and secretes the glucocorticoids cortisol, cortisone, and corticosterone.
3. The **zona reticularis,** the inner layer, constitutes 7% of the cortex and secretes mineralocorticoids (aldosterone), adrenal androgens and estrogens, and glucocorticoids.

The cells of the adrenal cortex are stimulated by the anterior pituitary hormone ACTH. The adrenal cortex secretes several steroid hormones, including the glucocorticoids (mainly cortisol), the mineralocorticoids (mainly aldosterone), and the adrenal androgens and estrogens. These hormones are all synthesized from cholesterol. The best-known pathway of steroidogenesis involves the conversion of cholesterol to pregnenolone, which is then converted to the major corticosteroids.[46]

Glucocorticoids. The **glucocorticoids** have metabolic, neurologic, anti-inflammatory, and growth-suppressing effects. They act through nuclear and nongenomic pathways in the cell. The term glucocorticoid refers to those steroid hormones that have direct effects on carbohydrate metabolism. These hormones increase blood glucose concentration by promoting gluconeogenesis in the liver and by decreasing uptake of glucose into muscle cells, adipose cells, and lymphatic

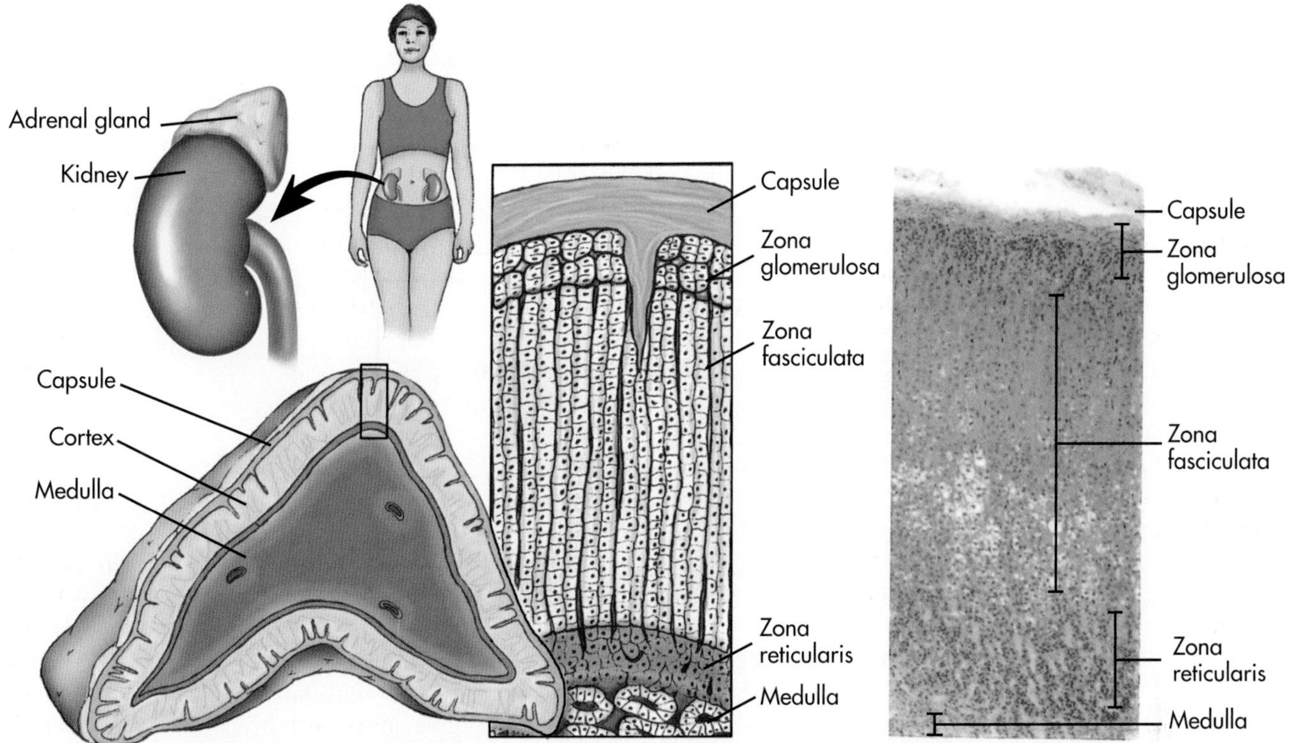

FIGURE 21-16 Structure of the Adrenal Gland Showing Cell Layers (Zones) of the Cortex. Zona glomerulosa secretes aldosterone. Zona fasciculata secretes abundant amounts of glucocorticoids, chiefly cortisol. Zona reticularis secretes minute amounts of sex hormones and glucocorticoids. A portion of the medulla is visible at lower right in the photomicrograph (×35) and at the bottom of the drawing. (From Patton KT, Thibodeau GA: *Anatomy & physiology,* ed 6, St Louis, 2007, Mosby.)

cells.[47] In extrahepatic tissues, the glucocorticoids stimulate protein catabolism and inhibit amino acid uptake and protein synthesis. The ultimate effect on the body is protein breakdown (catabolism).

The glucocorticoids act at several sites to influence immune and inflammatory reactions (described in Chapters 7 and 11).[48] They affect innate immunity through several pathways, including decreasing the activity of pattern receptors on the surface of macrophages (see Chapter 7). Another major immune suppressant effect is a glucocorticoid-mediated decrease in the proliferation of T lymphocytes, primarily T-helper lymphocytes.[48] There is a greater effect on T-helper 1 cytokine production (including antiviral interferons) than there is T-helper 2 cytokine production and therefore greater depression of cellular immunity than humoral immunity (see Chapter 8). Glucocorticoids also decrease immune and inflammatory responses by decreasing natural killer cell activity and suppressing the synthesis, secretion, and actions of chemical mediators involved in inflammatory and immune responses. Glucocorticoids suppress the inflammatory response by blocking phospholipase A and the synthesis of prostaglandins, thromboxanes, and leukotrienes; and by inhibiting inflammatory gene expression.[48] In addition, glucocorticoids stimulate anti-inflammatory cytokines (e.g., interleukin-10 [IL-10] and transforming growth factor-beta). Lysosomal membranes are also stabilized, decreasing the release of proteolytic enzymes. This suppression of innate and adaptive immunity by glucocorticoids means that infection and poor wound healing are some of the most problematic complications of the use of glucocorticoids in the treatment of disease. Similarly, psychologic and physiologic stress increases glucocorticoid production, which provides a pathway for the well-described decrease in immunity seen in both acute and chronic stress conditions (see Chapter 11).

Other effects of glucocorticoids include inhibition of bone formation, inhibition of ADH secretion, and stimulation of gastric acid secretion. Glucocorticoids appear to potentiate the effects of catecholamines, including sensitizing the arterioles to the vasoconstrictive effects of norepinephrine. Thyroid hormone and growth hormone effects on adipose tissue also are potentiated by glucocorticoids. A metabolite of cortisol may act like a barbiturate and depress nerve cell function in the brain, accounting for the noted effects on mood associated with steroid level fluctuation in disease or stress.

Pathologically high levels of glucocorticoids increase the number of circulating erythrocytes (leading to polycythemia), increase the appetite, promote fat deposition in the face and cervical areas, increase uric acid excretion, decrease serum calcium levels (possibly by inhibiting gastrointestinal absorption of calcium), suppress the secretion and synthesis of ACTH, and interfere with the action of growth hormone so that somatic growth is inhibited.[49]

The most potent of the naturally occurring glucocorticoids is **cortisol.** It is the main secretory product of the adrenal cortex and is necessary for the maintenance of life and for protection from stress (see Chapter 11, particularly Figure 11-2). Cortisol

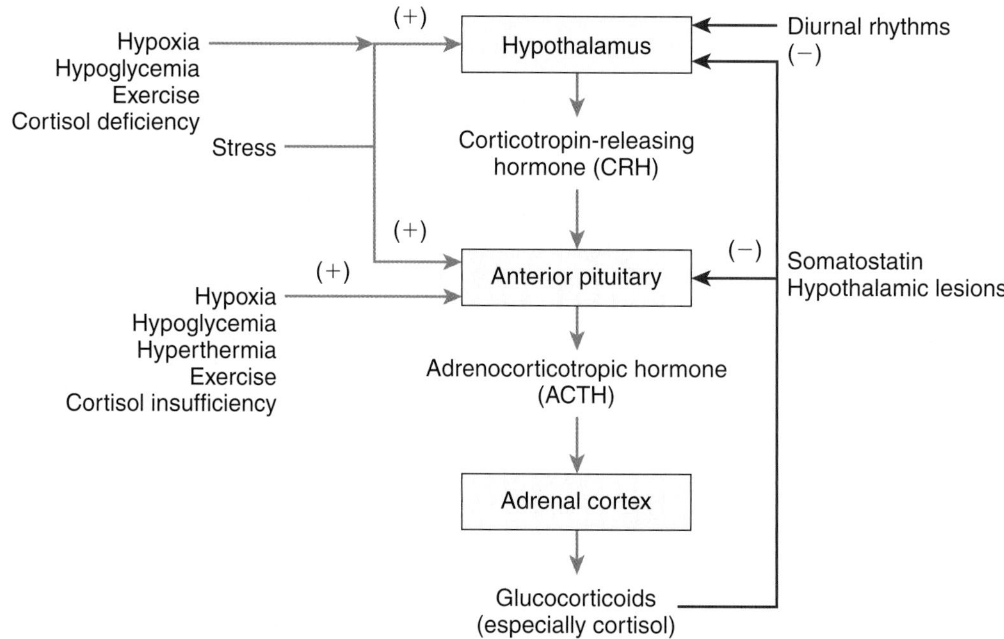

FIGURE 21-17 Feedback Control of Glucocorticoid Synthesis and Secretion.

has a biologic half-life of approximately 90 minutes, with the liver primarily responsible for its deactivation.

The secretion of cortisol is regulated primarily by the hypothalamus and the anterior pituitary gland (Figure 21-17). In the hypothalamus, CRH is produced in several nuclei and stored in the median eminence. Once released, CRH travels through the portal vessels to stimulate the production of ACTH from POMC, β-lipotropin, γ-lipotropin, endorphins, and enkephalins by the anterior pituitary. ACTH is the main regulator of cortisol secretion and adrenocortical growth.

Three factors appear to be primarily involved in regulating the secretion of ACTH: (1) high circulating levels of cortisol and synthetic glucocorticoids suppress CRH and ACTH, whereas low cortisol levels stimulate their secretion; (2) diurnal rhythms affect ACTH and cortisol levels (in persons with regular sleep-wake patterns, ACTH peaks 3 to 5 hours after sleep begins and declines throughout the day; and cortisol levels follow a similar pattern, peaking just before awakening); and (3) psychologic and physiologic (e.g., hypoxia, hypoglycemia, hyperthermia, exercise) stress increases ACTH secretion, leading to increased cortisol levels.[50,51] (Neurologic mechanisms regulating sleep are discussed in Chapter 16.) A form of immunoreactive ACTH (ir ACTH) is produced by the cells of the immune system and may account, in part, for integration of the immune and endocrine systems.

Once ACTH is secreted, it binds to specific plasma membrane receptors on the cells of the adrenal cortex and on other extra-adrenal tissues. Because both adrenal and extra-adrenal tissues have ACTH receptors, a number of effects result from stimulation by ACTH (these effects are summarized in Box 21-1). In addition to increasing adrenocortical secretion of cortisol, ACTH maintains the size and synthetic functions of the adrenal cortex through activation of crucial enzymes and storage of cholesterol for metabolism into steroid hormones.

BOX 21-1 EFFECTS OF ADRENOCORTICOTROPIC HORMONE

Adrenal
Maintenance of gland size
Depletion of ascorbic acid
Activation of adenylyl cyclase
Conversion of cholesterol to pregnenolone
Maintenance of enzymes active in converting pregnenolone to other steroids
Accumulation of cholesterol
Secretion of cortisol and adrenal androgens

Extra-Adrenal
Activation of tissue lipase

Extra-adrenal effects of ACTH include stimulation of melanocytes and activation of tissue lipase.

Once ACTH stimulates the cells of the adrenal cortex, cortisol synthesis and secretion immediately occur. In the healthy person, the secretory patterns of ACTH and cortisol are nearly identical. After secretion, most cortisol circulates in bound form: 15% to 30% is bound to albumin, 55% to 75% is tightly but reversibly bound to a plasma glycoprotein called *transcortin,* and 10% to 15% is unbound. The levels of transcortin play a role in the HPA feedback system controlling cortisol secretion. Transcortin levels are significantly elevated by increased estrogen levels that occur with pregnancy and hormone therapy. The unbound portion is free to diffuse into cells, but only those cells with specific intracellular glucocorticoid receptors respond to cortisol stimulation. ACTH is rapidly inactivated in the circulation, and the liver and kidneys remove the deactivated hormone.

Mineralocorticoids: Aldosterone. **Mineralocorticoid** steroids directly affect ion transport by epithelial cells, causing sodium retention and potassium and hydrogen loss.

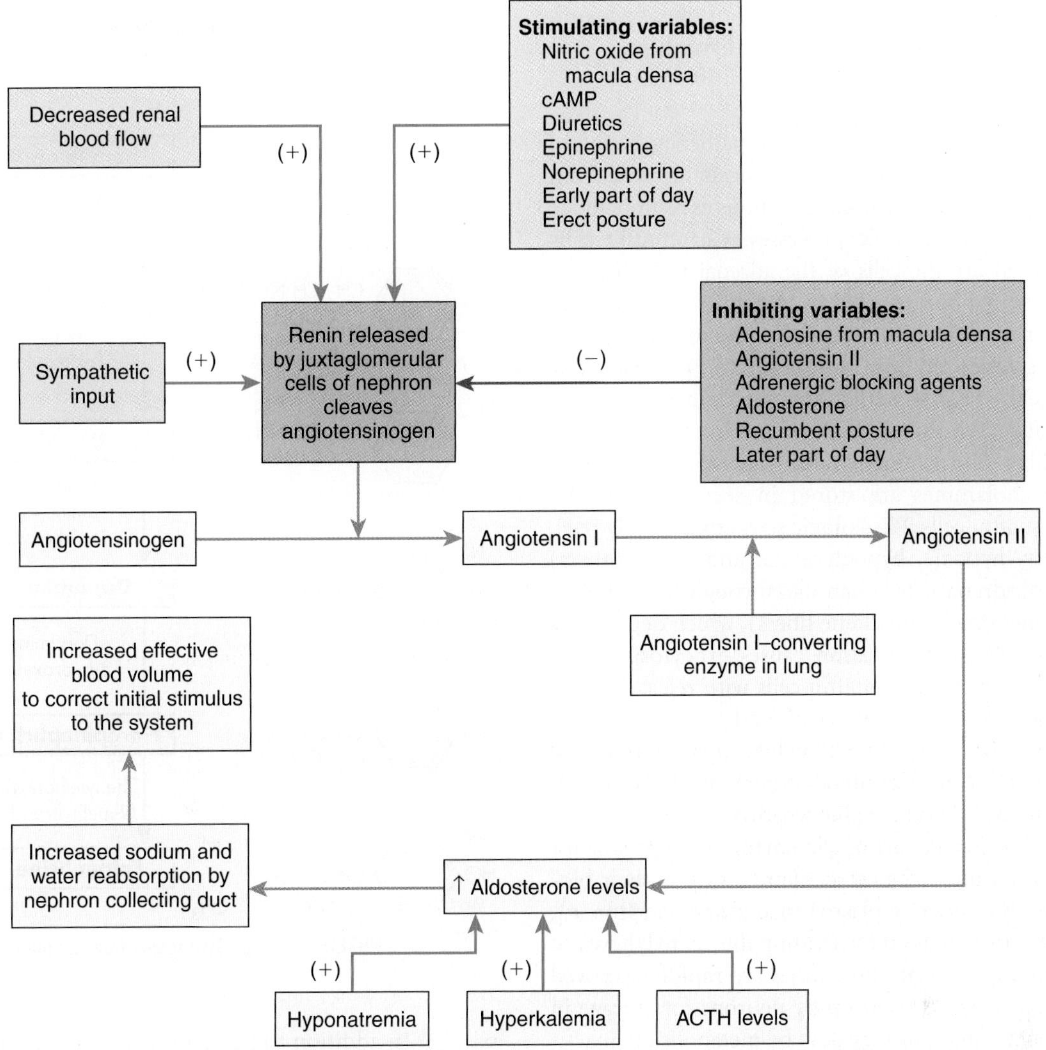

FIGURE 21-18 Feedback Mechanisms Regulating Aldosterone Secretion. *ACTH,* Adrenocorticotropic hormone; *cAMP,* cyclic adenosine monophosphate.

Aldosterone is the most potent of the naturally occurring mineralocorticoids and acts to conserve sodium by increasing the activity of the sodium pump of the epithelial cells in the nephron. (The sodium pump is described in Chapter 1.)

The initial stages of aldosterone synthesis occur in the zona fasciculata and zona reticularis. The final conversion of corticosterone occurs in the zona glomerulosa. Aldosterone synthesis and secretion are regulated primarily by the renin-angiotensin-aldosterone system (described in Chapter 3 and Chapter 37; see Figures 3-4 and 37-10), although other factors also may be involved. The renin-angiotensin system is activated by sodium and water depletion, increased potassium levels, and a diminished effective blood volume (Figure 21-18). Angiotensin II is the primary stimulant of aldosterone synthesis and secretion; however, sodium and potassium levels also may directly affect aldosterone secretion.

When sodium and potassium levels are within normal limits, approximately 50 to 250 mg of aldosterone is secreted daily. Of the secreted aldosterone, 50% to 75% binds to plasma proteins. Aldosterone is degraded in the liver and is excreted by the kidney.

Aldosterone maintains extracellular volume by acting on distal nephron epithelial cells to increase sodium reabsorption and potassium and hydrogen excretion.[52] This renal effect takes 90 minutes to 6 hours. Other effects of aldosterone include enhancement of cardiac muscle contraction, stimulation of ectopic ventricular activity through secondary cardiac pacemakers in the ventricles, stiffening of blood vessels with increased vascular resistance, and decreased fibrinolysis. Pathologically elevated levels of aldosterone have been implicated in the myocardial changes associated with heart failure.[53,54]

Adrenal Estrogens and Androgens. The healthy adrenal cortex secretes small amounts of estrogen and androgens. ACTH appears to be the major regulator. The biologic effects and metabolism of the adrenal sex steroids do not vary from those produced by the gonads (see Chapter 23).

Some of the weak androgenic substances secreted by the cortex (dehydroepiandrosterone [DHEA], androstenedione) are converted by peripheral tissues to stronger androgens, such as testosterone, thus accounting for some androgenic effects initiated by the adrenal cortex. Peripheral conversion of adrenal androgens to estrogens is enhanced in aging or obese persons, as well as in those with liver disease or hyperthyroidism.

Adrenal Medulla

The **adrenal medulla,** together with the sympathetic division of the autonomic nervous system, is embryonically derived from neural crest cells. The adrenal medulla functions as a sympathetic ganglion without postganglionic processes. **Chromaffin cells (pheochromocytes)** are the cells of the adrenal medulla. The major products stored and secreted by the chromaffin cells are the catecholamines epinephrine (adrenaline) and norepinephrine, which are synthesized from the amino acid phenylalanine (Figure 21-19). Only 30% of circulating epinephrine comes from the adrenal medulla; the other 70% is released from nerve terminals. The medulla is only a minor source of norepinephrine.[55]

Adrenal catecholamines are stored in secretory granules within the chromaffin cells. Physiologic stress to the body (e.g., traumatic injury, hypoxia, hypoglycemia, and many others) triggers release of adrenal catecholamines through acetylcholine (from the preganglionic sympathetic fibers), which depolarizes the chromaffin cells. Depolarization causes exocytosis of the storage granules from the chromaffin cells with release of epinephrine and norepinephrine into the bloodstream; therefore, the catecholamines from the adrenal medulla are hormones and not neurotransmitters.[55] Secretion of adrenal catecholamines is also increased by ACTH and the glucocorticoids.

Once released, the catecholamines remain in the plasma for only seconds to minutes. The catecholamines exert their biologic effects after binding to a plasma membrane receptor (α_1, α_2, β_1, β_2, β_3) in target cells and activating the adenylyl cyclase system (see Table 15-7). Catecholamines are rapidly removed from the plasma by being taken up by neurons for storage in new cytoplasmic granules, or they may be metabolically inactivated and excreted in the urine.

Catecholamines have diverse effects on the entire body. Their release and the body's response have been characterized as the "fight or flight" response (see Chapter 11).

In general, the metabolic effects of catecholamines promote hyperglycemia through a variety of mechanisms and through interference with usual glucose regulatory feedback mechanisms.

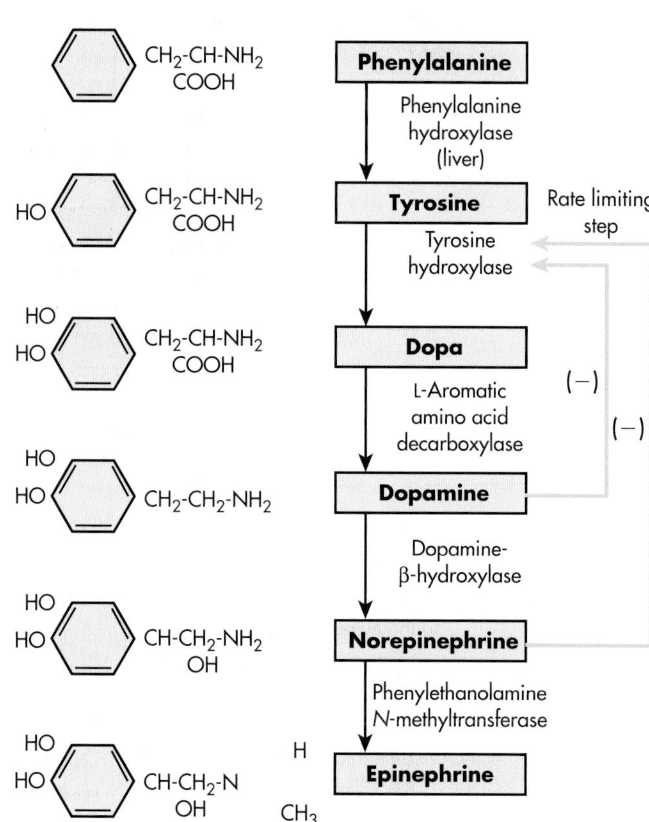

FIGURE 21-19 Synthesis of Catecholamines.

Neuroendocrine Response to Stressors

The endocrine system acts together with the nervous system to respond to stressors. The integrated response to stressors also includes the immune system. Hormones of the neuroendocrine system affect components of the immune system, and mediators produced by immune components regulate the neuroendocrine response.

Perception that an event is stressful may be essential to the emotional arousal and initiation of the stress response. Some events, such as bacterial invasion, can activate the stress response without emotional arousal. The hypothalamus receives input from a variety of areas within the brain and ultimately directs the neuroendocrine response to stress through the actions of CRH, the locus ceruleus–norepinephrine autonomic (sympathetic) nervous system, and the pituitary-adrenal axis.[50,56] In addition to the neuroendocrine components of the stress response, the gamma motor neuron system is activated to increase skeletal motor tone. Enhanced availability of vital substrates occurs, and growth and reproduction are inhibited to preserve energy for protective responses. Details of the stress response are presented in Chapter 11.

Tests of Endocrine Function

Evaluation of the endocrine system is challenging because of: (1) the complexity of the clinical presentation because of multiple organ system involvement, (2) the nonspecific nature of complaints frequently associated with endocrine dysfunction, and (3) the inappropriate use of laboratory test interpretations.

Tests of the endocrine system involve several general types of clinical evaluation. Measurement of hormone level is accomplished by radioimmunoassay, by enzyme-linked immunosorbent assay, and less commonly by bioassay. **Radioimmunoassay (RIA)** is a technique for measuring the minute quantities of hormones in the blood that uses antibodies and radiolabeled hormones to determine the quantity of hormone in the plasma. **Enzyme-linked immunosorbent assay (ELISA)** also is used to determine circulating hormone levels. This method is similar to that of RIA but is less expensive and easier to conduct. Instead of radiolabeled hormones, an enzyme-labeled hormone is used. A **bioassay** involves the use of graded doses of hormone in a reference preparation and then comparison of the results with an unknown sample. Bioassays are used more commonly in investigative endocrinology than in clinical laboratories. If the serum level is greater or less than the reference values, more definitive tests are required to determine the source of the problem.

Measurement of individual hormones does not always permit differentiation between normal and abnormal values when hormone levels are changing over time. For an accurate interpretation, the broad normal range of some hormones requires a knowledge of previous hormonal levels and timed sampling. Stimulation and suppression tests that determine the response to exogenous stimulants or inhibitors can help to decipher some of these complexities.

Indirect assessment of hormonal function often includes measurement of concentrations of serum glucose and electrolytes that are affected by the endocrine process. Evaluation of hormonal function also may include radiographic imaging of specific glands.

AGING AND THE ENDOCRINE SYSTEM

The precise relationship between aging and the endocrine system is not clear. Perhaps most important, the question of whether changes in endocrine function are a consequence or a cause of aging has yet to be resolved. These relationships have been difficult to identify, in part because of a number of age-related variables that may coexist, such as acute and chronic non–endocrine disease; use of medications; alterations in diet, body composition, and weight; and changes in sleep-wake cycles. However, the endocrine system is so integral to health that changes in endocrine function have been used as "biomarkers" for unhealthy aging.

Effects of Aging on the Endocrine System

Investigation into the role of the endocrine glands and their interactions in the aging process has generated much data, although the evidence is contradictory. There are complex changes within the HPA; and altered biologic activity of hormones, altered circulating levels of hormones, altered secretory response of the endocrine glands, altered metabolism of hormones, and loss of circadian control of hormone secretion are among the findings. Changes in secretion of hypothalamic regulatory factors and hormones or changes in hypothalamic feedback sensitivity may contribute to alterations in control of an optimal internal environment.[57] The dynamic equilibrium of the endocrine system also may be affected by altered secretion of neurotransmitters within certain areas of the brain, affecting hypothalamic and pituitary function. Such alterations may include an excess or deficit in secretion of pituitary hormones and loss of appropriate secretory pattern of those hormones. Loss of endocrine steady states may be associated with or contribute to aging.

The most studied changes in hormone function with aging affect the levels of reproductive hormones and gonadotropins (menopause and andropause) (discussed in Chapter 23). Two of the most important endocrine changes associated with aging affect the thyroid gland and the pancreas. Other important hormone changes associated with aging include a decline in serum levels of growth hormone and IGF-1, parathyroid hormone, dehydroepiandrosterone, and ADH.

Thyroid Gland. Changes in thyroid structure and function occur with aging.[58] Structurally, some glandular atrophy and fibrosis occur with nodularity and increasing inflammatory infiltrates. These infiltrative changes may reflect age-related autoimmune damage. Clinical signs of thyroid disease are more difficult to detect in older adults. Overall, it is estimated that there is some evidence of thyroid dysfunction in 5% to 10% of older adult women. The presence of thyroid nodules increases after the age of 70 years. Changes relative to thyroid hormone and its function are more difficult to assess and much of the available data are contradictory. Most evidence, however, supports the following age-related changes:

1. Overall TSH secretion is diminished, although centenarians have elevated TSH.[58a]
2. Responsiveness of plasma TSH concentration to TRH administration is reduced, especially in men.
   a. T_4 secretion and degradation are decreased.
   b. Plasma levels of T_3 decline, especially in men, but are generally in the normal range.
   c. Hypothyroidism is seen with increasing frequency as age advances.

Treatment for thyroid deficiency is also affected by aging. The appropriate dose for thyroid hormone (TH) replacement is often lower in older adults because the peripheral metabolism of TH decreases with age. In addition, TH must be replaced slowly in elderly individuals with coronary artery disease to prevent angina and myocardial infarction.[58]

Pancreas. It is estimated that 40% to 50% of individuals older than age 65 have impaired glucose tolerance or diabetes. With aging, the pancreatic cells are increasingly replaced with fat tissue.[59] Dysfunction of the pancreas with decreased insulin secretion of beta cells and insulin receptors and increased insulin resistance have all been documented and may be related to changes in adipokine physiology.[60-62]

These changes have significant implications for many target organs, particularly the cardiovascular system, which is increasingly at risk for both vascular (hypertension, atherosclerosis, glomerulosclerosis) and cardiac (infarction, failure) disorders. Exciting research is exploring the relationship between insulin and activation of genes for the "sirtuins," which are a group of proteins that have been linked with the aging process.[63]

Growth Hormone and Insulin-like Growth Factors. The amounts of GH and IGF decline with aging, a process that has been called the "somatopause."[64] This decline in anabolic stimuli is linked to decreases in muscle size and function, decreased amounts of fat and bone mass, and changes in reproductive and cognitive function[65] (see What's New? Growth Hormone [GH] and Insulin-like Growth Factor [IGF] in Aging).

Parathyroid Glands. An age-related alteration in PTH secretion has been proposed to explain alterations in calcium homeostasis that have been noted in older adults.[66] Calcium intake, especially in women, tends to decrease with aging and may contribute to osteoporosis (see Chapter 44). The average daily intake of 450 to 500 mg/day causes a negative calcium

WHAT'S NEW?

Growth Hormone (GH) and Insulin-like Growth Factor (IGF) in Aging

Aging is a multifactorial process that is influenced by genetic and environmental factors. The aging process is associated with many hormonal and metabolic changes. The amounts of GH and IGF decline with aging, a process that has been called the "somatopause." Clinical findings related to somatotropic hormone changes with aging include increased visceral fat, decreased lean body mass, decreased bone density, and changes in reproductive and cognitive function. The underlying mechanisms of aging and its relationship to GH and IGF are complex. For example, not only do these hormones promote bone and muscle growth, but also a recent study suggests that the brain IGF-1 receptor may be a significant factor in determining overall life span and ability to respond to physiologic stress. GH and IGF effects on inflammation and immunity also are important in the aging process. Unfortunately, there remains much confusion and controversy over the role of these hormones. Although most studies suggest that it is a deficiency of these hormones that leads to an acceleration of the aging process, there are several studies suggesting that lower lifetime levels of these hormones may confer longevity by providing protection from cancer and other age-related diseases. As these hormones are used to treat a wider range of disorders and for different age groups, more information about their safety is emerging. Despite the initial enthusiasm for the use of therapeutic doses of recombinant human growth hormone (rhGH) as a way to slow the aging process, studies have not been consistently positive and the risk for GH- and IGF-mediated oncogenesis is being explored.

Data from Allen DB: *J Clin Endocrinol Metab* 96(10):3042–3047, 2011; Bartke A: *Exp Gerontol* 46(2-3):108–111, 2011; Bartke A: *Trends Endocrinol Metab* 22(11):437–442, 2011; Birzniece V, Nelson AE, Ho KK: *Trends Endocrinol Metab* 22(5):171–178, 2011; Di Somma C et al: *Minerva Endocrinol* 36(3):243–255, 2011; Holzenberger M: *Nestle Nutr Workshop Ser Pediatr Program* 68:237–245, 2011; Kokshoorn NE et al: *Eur J Endocrinol* 164(5):657–665, 2011; Rosenfeld RG et al: *J Clin Endocrinol Metab* 97(1):68–72, 2012.

balance greater than 40 mg/day and may be related to the absolute bone loss of approximately 1.5% per year. Older adults show decreased intestinal adaptation to variations in calcium intake. Hyperparathyroidism may occur secondary to calcium malabsorption and hypocalcemia with increased bone remodeling that results in cortical bone thinning and porosity. Elevated levels of parathyroid hormone have been linked with an increase in mortality in older adults, many of whom also have a mild, persistent hypercalciuria, which indicates a defective renal mechanism for responding to decreased calcium intake. Decreased circulating levels of vitamin D are common in older adults, especially those in long-term care institutions. Vitamin D deficiency has been linked to not only osteoporosis but also cancer, autoimmune diseases, diabetes, cardiovascular disease, and mental health disorders.

Adrenal Glands. The adrenal cortex loses some weight and has more fibrous tissue after the age of 50 years. Age does not appear to affect the feedback mechanisms involved in maintaining glucocorticoid levels, but the decrease in the metabolic clearance rate of the glucocorticoids is age related.

The metabolic clearance of cortisol decreases with an age-related decline in liver and kidney function. Further, less cortisol appears to be used by the body when aging is accompanied by a loss of lean body mass. Decreased clearance and reduced use of cortisol contribute to higher circulating cortisol levels, but diurnal variation is maintained. Because feedback mechanisms are intact, the higher cortisol levels cause a decrease in cortisol secretion. Circadian patterns of ACTH and cortisol secretion may change with aging.

Plasma levels of the adrenal androgens, as well as urinary excretion of the metabolic end products, decrease gradually but dramatically with age, to as much as 50% to 70% of the young adult level. This change in adrenal function has been called the "adrenopause" and is correlated with decreased synthesis activity of dehydroepiandrosterone (DHEA).[67] This change appears to reflect a decline in the function of the zona reticularis. In postmenopausal women, this decline in adrenal androgen secretion is especially important because nearly all sex steroids after menopause come from adrenal and ovarian production of androgen precursors converted to estrogens in the periphery. In older adult men, adrenal androgen production accounts for more than half of circulating testosterone levels.

Antidiuretic Hormone. Although hyponatremia is a common finding in older adults, it appears related to changes in renal function rather than to ADH-related mechanisms. Morphologic studies have not shown significant age-related degenerative changes in the neuroendocrine pathways that regulate the synthesis and secretion of ADH. It appears that ADH secretion is augmented when stimulated by changes in osmotic concentration, whereas baroreceptor-mediated ADH secretion is reduced.

SUMMARY REVIEW

Mechanisms of Hormonal Regulation

1. The endocrine system has diverse functions, including sexual differentiation, growth and development, continuous maintenance of the body's internal environment, and adaptive responses to stress.
2. Hormones are chemical messengers synthesized by endocrine glands and released into the circulation; they work with the nervous system to maintain communication and control.
3. Hormones have specific negative- and positive-feedback mechanisms. Most hormone levels are regulated by negative feedback, in which tropic hormone secretion raises the level of a specific hormone. The elevated level of the specific hormone then causes negative feedback, decreasing secretion of the tropic hormone.
4. Endocrine feedback is described in terms of short and long feedback loops.

SUMMARY REVIEW—cont'd

5. Water-soluble hormones circulate throughout the body in unbound form, whereas lipid-soluble hormones (i.e., steroid and thyroid hormones) circulate throughout the body bound to carrier proteins.
6. Hormones serve as first messengers and affect only target cells with appropriate receptors and then act on those cells to initiate specific cell functions or activities.
7. Hormones have two general types of effects on cells: direct effects, or obvious changes in cell function; and permissive effects, or less obvious changes that facilitate cell function.
8. Receptors for hormones are proteins and may be located on or in the plasma membrane or in the cytosol or nucleus of the target cell. Receptors may be G protein linked, ion channels, or enzyme linked.
9. Water-soluble hormones act as first messengers, binding to receptors on the cell's plasma membrane. The signals initiated by hormone-receptor binding are then transmitted into the cell by the action of second messengers.
10. Second messengers that have been identified include cAMP, cGMP, and calcium, which associates with IP_3 and DAG to produce physiologic effects.
11. For cells that have cAMP as their second messenger, a series of interactions within the plasma membrane must activate adenylyl cyclase.
12. Cells that have cGMP as their second messenger are activated by the enzyme guanylyl cyclase.
13. For cells that have calcium as their second messenger, an increase in intracellular calcium concentration causes calcium to bind with calmodulin, a regulatory protein. This step then initiates other intracellular processes.
14. Lipid-soluble hormones (including steroid and thyroid hormones) may have rapid effects by binding to a plasma membrane or receptor or crossing the plasma membrane through diffusion. These hormones then either bind to cytoplasmic proteins or diffuse directly into the cell nucleus and bind to nuclear receptors.
15. Hormones have direct effects (specific changes in cell function) or permissive effects (facilitate the effects of other hormones).

Structure and Function of the Endocrine Glands

1. The pituitary gland, consisting of anterior and posterior portions, is connected to the central nervous system through the hypothalamus.
2. The hypothalamus regulates anterior pituitary function by secreting releasing hormones into the portal circulation.
3. Hypothalamic hormones include dopamine, which inhibits prolactin secretion; TRH, which affects release of thyroid hormones; CRH, which facilitates release of ACTH and endorphins; and substance P, which inhibits ACTH release and stimulates release of a variety of other hormones. ADH and oxytocin are synthesized in the hypothalamus and stored and secreted by the posterior pituitary.
4. The posterior pituitary stores and secretes ADH, also called arginine-vasopressin, and oxytocin.
5. ADH controls serum osmolality, increases the permeability of the renal tubules to water, and causes vasoconstriction when administered pharmacologically in high doses. ADH also may regulate some central nervous system functions.
6. Oxytocin causes uterine contraction and lactation in women and may have a role in sperm motility in men. In men and women, oxytocin has an antidiuretic effect similar to that of ADH.
7. Hormones of the anterior pituitary are regulated by (a) secretion of hypothalamic-releasing hormones or factors, (b) negative feedback from hormones secreted by target organs, and (c) mediating effects of neurotransmitters.
8. Hormones of the anterior pituitary include ACTH, MSH, somatotropic hormones (GH and prolactin), and glycoprotein hormones (FSH, LH, and TSH).
9. Growth hormone stimulates bone growth, increased protein metabolism in muscles, and lipolysis. Its effects are mediated in part by IGFs.
10. Prolactin functions to produce milk during pregnancy and lactation.
11. The pineal gland produces melatonin, which affects sleep, immune function, and aging.
12. The two-lobed thyroid gland contains follicles, which secrete some of the thyroid hormones, and C cells, which secrete calcitonin and somatostatin.
13. Regulation of TH levels is complex and involves the hypothalamus (TRH), anterior pituitary (TSH), thyroid gland, and numerous biochemical variables.
14. TH secretion is regulated by TRH through a negative-feedback loop that involves the anterior pituitary and hypothalamus.
15. TSH, which is synthesized and stored in the anterior pituitary, stimulates secretion of TH by activating intracellular processes, including uptake of iodine necessary for the synthesis of TH.
16. Synthesis of TH depends on the glycoprotein thyroglobulin, which contains a precursor of TH, tyrosine. Tyrosine then combines with iodide to form precursor molecules of the thyroid hormones T_4 and T_3.
17. When released into the circulation, T_3 and T_4 are bound by carrier proteins in the plasma that store these hormones and provide a buffer for rapid changes in hormone levels.
18. Thyroid hormones alter protein synthesis and have a wide range of metabolic effects on proteins, carbohydrates, lipids, and vitamins. TH also affects heat production and cardiac function.
19. Parafollicular cells or C cells secrete calcitonin and lower serum calcium concentration by inhibiting bone-resorbing osteoclasts.
20. The paired parathyroid glands normally are located behind the upper and lower poles of the thyroid gland. These glands secrete PTH, an important regulator of serum calcium and phosphate levels.

SUMMARY REVIEW—cont'd

21. PTH secretion is regulated by levels of ionized calcium in the plasma and by cAMP within the cell. Some other substances—hormones, neurotransmitters, and ions—affect PTH secretion by inhibiting cAMP or by changing calcium levels.
22. In bone, PTH causes bone breakdown and resorption. In the kidney PTH increases reabsorption of calcium, decreases reabsorption of phosphorus and bicarbonate, and stimulates synthesis of vitamin D.
23. Parathyroid hormone–related peptide (PTHrP) has properties similar to those of PTH and plays a role in placental calcium transport, lactation, and fetal tooth development.
24. The endocrine pancreas contains the islets of Langerhans, which secrete hormones responsible for much of the carbohydrate metabolism in the body.
25. The islets of Langerhans consist of alpha cells, beta cells, delta cells, and F cells.
26. Beta cells synthesize insulin, a hormone that regulates blood glucose concentrations and overall body metabolism of fat, protein, carbohydrates, and amylin.
27. Alpha cells produce glucagon, which is secreted inversely to blood glucose concentrations and stimulates glycogenolysis, gluconeogenesis, and lipolysis.
28. Incretin hormones are produced by endocrine cells of the gastrointestinal tract that promote glucose-dependent insulin secretion, inhibit glucagon synthesis, and delay gastric emptying.
29. Amylin promotes glucose-dependent insulin secretion, inhibits glucagon synthesis, and delays gastric emptying, producing an antihyperglycemic effect.
30. Delta cells secrete somatostatin, which inhibits glucagon, insulin, and polypeptide secretion.
31. F cells secrete pancreatic polypeptide, which stimulates Y receptors, promotes gastric secretion, and antagonizes cholecystokinin.
32. The paired adrenal glands are situated on the kidneys. Each gland consists of an adrenal medulla, which secretes catecholamines, and an adrenal cortex, which secretes steroid hormones.
33. The steroid hormones secreted by the adrenal cortex are all synthesized from cholesterol. These hormones include glucocorticoids, mineralocorticoids, and adrenal androgens and estrogens.
34. Glucocorticoids directly affect carbohydrate metabolism by increasing blood glucose concentration through gluconeogenesis in the liver and by decreasing use of glucose. Glucocorticoids also inhibit immune and inflammatory responses, inhibit bone formation and ADH secretion, and stimulate gastric secretion.
35. Cortisol secretion is related to secretion of ACTH, which is stimulated by CRH. ACTH binds with receptors of the adrenal cortex, which activates intracellular mechanisms (specifically cAMP) and leads to cortisol release.
36. Mineralocorticoids, especially aldosterone, are steroid hormones that directly affect ion transport by epithelial cells, causing sodium retention and potassium and hydrogen loss.
37. Aldosterone secretion is controlled by the renin-angiotensin-aldosterone system and acts by binding to a site on the cell nucleus and altering protein production within the cell. Its principal site of action is the kidney, where it causes sodium reabsorption and potassium and hydrogen excretion.
38. Androgens and estrogens secreted by the adrenal cortex act in the same way as those secreted by the gonads.
39. The adrenal medulla secretes the catecholamines epinephrine and norepinephrine. Catecholamines are synthesized from the amino acid phenylalanine. Their release is stimulated by sympathetic nervous system stimulation, ACTH, and glucocorticoids.
40. Catecholamines bind with various target cells and are taken up by neurons or excreted in the urine. They cause a range of metabolic effects that generally are characterized as the "flight or fight" response.
41. The endocrine system acts together with the nervous and immune systems to respond to stressors, providing an integrated and protective response.
42. Several assay methods are used to measure levels of hormones in the plasma. RIA compares the proportion of radiolabeled and nonradiolabeled hormone against standard reference curves.
43. ELISA is a method similar to RIA, but uses a radiolabeled enzyme rather than a radiolabeled hormone.
44. Bioassays use graded doses of hormone in a reference preparation and then compare the results with an unknown sample to determine the hormone level.

Aging and the Endocrine System

1. Endocrine changes that may be associated with aging include altered biologic activity of hormones, altered circulating levels of hormones, altered secretory responses of endocrine glands, altered metabolism of hormones, loss of circadian control of hormone release, and changes in secretion of hypothalamic regulatory hormones.
2. Cellular damage associated with aging, genetically programmed cell change, and chronic wear and tear may contribute to endocrine gland dysfunction or alterations in the responsiveness of target organs.
3. Aging apparently causes atrophy of the thyroid gland and is associated with infiltrative glandular changes. Secretion of thyroid hormones may diminish with age.
4. Aging causes pancreatic fat deposition and is associated with a decrease both in insulin secretion and in insulin sensitivity.
5. Growth hormone levels decrease with aging, leading to decreased bone and muscle mass.
6. Aging is associated with alterations in calcium steady states, which may be related to alterations in PTH secretion from the parathyroid glands.
7. Age-related changes in adrenal function include decreased clearance of glucocorticoids and a decrease in levels of adrenal androgens. The effects of these changes, however, are offset by feedback mechanisms that maintain glucocorticoid levels and by gonadal secretion of androgens.

KEY TERMS

Adrenal cortex, 706
Adrenal gland, 706
Adrenal medulla, 710
Aldosterone, 709
Alpha cell, 703
Amylin, 706
Anterior pituitary, 697
Antidiuretic hormone (ADH), 696
Beta cell, 703
Bioassay, 710
C cell, 702
Calcitonin, 702
Chromaffin cell (pheochromocyte), 710
Chromophil, 699
Chromophobe, 699
Corticotropin-releasing hormone (CRH), 697
Cortisol, 707
Delta cell, 703
Diacylglycerol (DAG), 694
Direct effect, 695
Down-regulation, 691
Enzyme-linked immunosorbent assay (ELISA), 710
F (or PP) cell, 703
First messenger, 692
Follicle, 700
Gastrin, 706
Glucagon, 706
Glucocorticoid, 706
Gonadotropin-releasing hormone (GnRH), 696
Ghrelin, 706
Growth hormone–releasing factor (GRF), 697
Hormone, 689
Hormone receptor, 691
Inositol triphosphate (IP_3), 694
Insulin, 704
Islets of Langerhans, 703
Isthmus, 700
Median eminence, 697
Melatonin, 700
Mineralocorticoid, 708
Negative feedback, 690
Neuroendocrine system, 696
Oxytocin, 696
Pancreas, 703
Pancreatic polypeptide, 706
Parathyroid hormone (PTH), 702
Pars distalis, 697
Pars intermedia, 697
Pars nervosa (neural lobe), 698
Pars tuberalis, 697
Permissive effect, 695
Pituitary stalk, 697
Posterior pituitary, 697
Prolactin-inhibiting factor (PIF), 696
Radioimmunoassay (RIA), 710
Second messenger, 694
Signal transduction, 692
Somatostatin, 697, 706
Substance P, 697
Thyroid gland, 700
Thyroid hormone (TH), 700
Thyroid-stimulating hormone (TSH), 700
Thyrotropin-releasing hormone (TRH), 690, 696
Up-regulation, 691
Zona fasciculata, 707
Zona glomerulosa, 706
Zona reticularis, 706

REFERENCES

1. Bochukova E et al: A mutation in the thyroid hormone receptor alpha gene, *N Engl J Med* 366(3):243–249, 2012.
2. Lu C, Cheng SY: Extranuclear signaling of mutated thyroid hormone receptors in promoting metastatic spread in thyroid carcinogenesis, *Steroids* 76(9):885–891, 2011.
3. Gonzalez-Maseo J, Selafon SC: Hormone signaling via G protein-coupled receptors. In Jamerson JL, Degroot LJ, editors: *Endocrinology*, ed 6, Philadelphia, 2010, Saunders.
4. McKenna NJ, Moore DD: Nuclear receptors: structure, functions and coregulators. In Jamerson JL, Degroot LJ, editors: *Endocrinology*, ed 6, Philadelphia, 2010, Saunders.
5. Lefrancois-Martinez AM et al: Transcriptional control of adrenal steroidogenesis: novel connection between Janus kinase (JAK) 2 protein and protein kinase A (PKA) through stabilization of cAMP response element-binding protein (CREB) transcription factor, *J Biol Chem* 286(38): 3276–3285, 2011.
6. Cho EC, Mitton B, Sakamoto KM: CREB and leukemogenesis, *Crit Rev Oncog* 16(1-2):37–46, 2011.
7. Favre D et al: Impaired expression of the inducible cAMP early repressor accounts for sustained adipose CREB activity in obesity, *Diabetes* 60(12):3169–3174, 2011.
8. Schlossmann J, Schinner E: cGMP becomes a drug target, *Naunyn Schmiedebergs Arch Pharmacol* 385(3):243–252, 2012.
9. Martin TFJ: Control of hormone secretion. In Jamerson JL, Degroot LJ, editors: *Endocrinology*, ed 6, Philadelphia, 2010, Saunders.
10. Agostino NM et al: Effect of the tyrosine kinase inhibitors (sunitinib, sorafenib, dasatinib, and imatinib) on blood glucose levels in diabetic and nondiabetic patients in general clinical practice, *J Oncol Pharm Pract* 17(3):197–202, 2011.
11. Lin HY et al: Identification and functions of the plasma membrane receptor for thyroid hormone analogues, *Discov Med* 11(59):337–347, 2011.
12. Molina PE: The hypothalamus and posterior pituitary gland, *Endocrine physiology*, ed 3, New York, 2010, McGraw-Hill.
13. Bonfiglio JJ et al: The corticotropin-releasing hormone network and the hypothalamic-pituitary-adrenal axis: molecular and cellular mechanisms involved, *Neuroendocrinology* 94(1):12–20, 2011.
14. Vrachnis N et al: Immune aspects and myometrial actions of progesterone and CRH in labor, *Clin Dev Immunol* 937618:2012, 2012.
15. Carmody D, Hannon MJ, Thompson C: Vasopressin, diabetes insipidus and the syndrome of inappropriate antidiuretic hormone secretion. In Jamerson JL, Degroot LJ, editors: *Endocrinology*, ed 6, Philadelphia, 2010, Saunders.
16. Anand T, Skinner R: Arginine vasopressin: the future of pressure-support resuscitation in hemorrhagic shock, *J Surg Res* 178(1):321–329, 2012.
17. Strathearn L: Maternal neglect: oxytocin, dopamine and the neurobiology of attachment, *J Neuroendocrinol* 23(11):1054–1065, 2011.
18. Matsuzaki M et al: Oxytocin: a therapeutic target for mental disorders, *J Physiol Sci* 62(6):441–444, 2012.
19. Rosenfeld RG et al: Long-term surveillance of growth hormone therapy, *J Clin Endocrinol Metab* 97(1):68–72, 2012.
20. Guevara-Aguirre J et al: Growth hormone receptor deficiency is associated with a major reduction in pro-aging signaling, cancer, and diabetes in humans, *Sci Transl Med* 70(3):ra13–ra16, 2011.
21. Hickie I, Rogers N: Novel melatonin-based therapies: potential advances in the treatment of major depression, *Lancet* 378:621–631, 2011.
22. Kostoglou-Athanassiou I: Therapeutic applications of melatonin, *Ther Adv Endocrinol Metab* 4(1):13–24, 2013.
23. Gordon DF et al: Thyroid-stimulating hormone: physiology and secretion. In Jamerson JL, Degroot LJ, editors: *Endocrinology*, ed 6, Philadelphia, 2010, Saunders.
24. Arsanjani R et al: Translational potential of thyroid hormone and its analogs, *J Mol Cell Cardiol* 51(4):506–511, 2011.
25. Tancevski I, Rudling M, Eller P: Thyromimetics: a journey from bench to bed-side, *Pharmacol Ther* 131(1):33–39, 2011.
26. Piehl S et al: Thyronamines—past, present, and future, *Endocr Rev* 32(1):64–80, 2011.
27. Bohnhorst B et al: Procalcitonin and valuable clinical symptoms in the early detection of neonatal late-onset bacterial infection, *Acta Paediatr* 101(1):19–25, 2012.
28. Horie M et al: Diagnostic and prognostic value of procalcitonin in community-acquired pneumonia, *Am J Med Sci* 343(1):30–35, 2012.
29. Kumar R, Thompson JR: The regulation of parathyroid hormone secretion and synthesis, *J Am Soc Nephrol* 22(2):216–224, 2011.
30. Lippuner K: The future of osteoporosis treatment—a research update, *Swiss Med Wkly* 142:w13624, 2012.
31. Qunibi W, Kalantar-Zadeh K: Target levels for serum phosphorus and parathyroid hormone, *Semin Dial* 24(1):29–33, 2011.
32. Lecart MP, Reginster JY: Current options for the management of postmenopausal osteoporosis, *Exp Opin Pharmacother* 12(16):2533–2552, 2011.
33. Silverman SL, Nasser K: Teriparitide update, *Rheum Dis Clin North Am* 37(3):471–477, vii, 2011.
34. Luppi P, Cifarelli V, Wahren J: C-peptide and long-term complications of diabetes, *Pediatr Diabetes* 12(3 Pt 2):276–292, 2011.
35. Siddle K: Signalling by insulin and IGF receptors: supporting acts and new players, *J Mol Endocrinol* 47(1):R1–R10, 2011.
36. Unger RH, Cherrington AD: Glucagonocentric restructuring of diabetes: a pathophysiologic and therapeutic makeover, *J Clin Invest* 122(1):4–12, 2012.

37. Wu T et al: Effects of different sweet preloads on incretin hormone secretion, gastric emptying, and postprandial glycemia in healthy humans, *Am J Clin Nutr* 95(1):78–83, 2012.
38. Campbell RK: Clarifying the role of incretin-based therapies in the treatment of type 2 diabetes mellitus, *Clin Ther* 33(5):511–527, 2011.
39. Cefalu WT: Evolving treatment strategies for the management of type 2 diabetes, *Am J Med Sci* 343(1):21–26, 2012.
40. Pillay K, Govender P: Amylin uncovered: a review on the polypeptide responsible for type II diabetes, *Biomed Res Int* 2013:826706, 2013.
41. Westermark GT et al: Further evidence for amyloid deposition in clinical pancreatic islet grafts, *Transplant* 93(2):219–223, 2012.
42. Younk LM, Mikeladze M, Davis SN: Pramlintide and the treatment of diabetes: a review of the data since its introduction, *Exp Opin Pharmacother* 12(9):1439–1451, 2011.
43. Stengel A, Tache Y: Interaction between gastric and upper small intestinal hormones in the regulation of hunger and satiety: ghrelin and cholecystokinin take the central stage, *Curr Protein Pept Sci* 12(4):293–304, 2011.
44. Park CW, Torquati A: Physiology of weight loss surgery, *Surg Clin North Am* 91(6):1149–1161, 2011, vii.
45. Walther C, Morl K, Beck-Sickinger AG: Neuropeptide Y receptors: ligand binding and trafficking suggest novel approaches in drug development, *J Pept Sci* 17(4):233–246, 2011.
46. Auchus RJ, Miller WL: The principles, enzymes and pathways of human steroidogenesis. In Jamerson JL, Degroot LJ, editors: *Endocrinology*, ed 6, Philadelphia, 2010, Saunders.
47. Munck AU, Náray-Fejes-Tóth A: Glucocorticoid action: physiology. In Jameson JL, De Groot LJ, editors: *Endocrinology*, ed 6, Philadelphia, 2010, Saunders.
48. Flammer JR, Rogatsky I: Minireview: glucocorticoids in autoimmunity: unexpected targets and mechanisms, *Mol Endocrinol* 25(7):1075–1086, 2011.
49. Cavagnini F, Pecori Giraldi F: Adrenal causes of hypercortisolism. In Jamerson JL, Degroot LJ, editors: *Endocrinology*, ed 6, Philadelphia, 2010, Saunders.
50. Cutolo M, Buttgereit F, Straub RH: Regulation of glucocorticoids by the central nervous system, *Clin Exp Rheumatol* 29(5 Suppl 68):S19–S22, 2011.
51. Kageyama K, Tamasawa N, Suda T: Signal transduction in the hypothalamic corticotropin-releasing factor system and its clinical implications, *Stress* 14(4):357–367, 2011.
52. Toney GM, Vallon V, Stockand JD: Intrinsic control of sodium excretion in the distal nephron by inhibitory purinergic regulation of the epithelial Na(+) channel, *Curr Opin Nephrol Hypertens* 21(1):52–60, 2012.
53. Gandhi MS et al: Cellular and molecular pathways to myocardial necrosis and replacement fibrosis, *Heart Fail Rev* 16(1):23–34, 2011.
54. Nappi JM, Sieg A: Aldosterone and aldosterone receptor antagonists in patients with chronic heart failure, *Vasc Health Risk Manag* 7:353–363, 2011.
55. Pacak K, Timmers HJLM, Eisenhofer G: Pheochromocytoma. In Jamerson JL, Degroot LJ, editors: *Endocrinology*, ed 6, Philadelphia, 2010, Saunders.
56. Groeneweg FL et al: Rapid non-genomic effects of corticosteroids and their role in the central stress response, *J Endocrinol* 209(2):153–167, 2011.
57. Aguilera G: HPA axis responsiveness to stress: implications for healthy aging, *Exp Gerontol* 46(2-3):90–95, 2011.
58. Mitrou P, Raptis SA, Dimitriadis G: Thyroid disease in older people, *Maturitas* 70(1):5–9, 2011.
58a. Gesing A, Lewiński A, Karbownik-Lewińska M: The thyroid gland and the process of aging; what is new? *Thyroid Res* 5(1):16, 2012.
59. Li J et al: Noninvasive quantification of pancreatic fat in healthy male population using chemical shift magnetic resonance imaging: effect of aging on pancreatic fat content, *Pancreas* 40(2):295–299, 2011.
60. Carrascosa JM et al: Development of insulin resistance during aging: involvement of central processes and role of adipokines, *Curr Protein Pept Sci* 12(4):305–315, 2011.
61. Hupfield CJ, Courtney CH, Olefsky JM: Type 2 diabetes mellitus: etiology, pathogenesis and natural history. In Jamerson JL, Degroot LJ, editors: *Endocrinology*, ed 6, Philadelphia, 2010, Saunders.
62. Phielix E, Szendroedi J, Roden M: Mitochondrial function and insulin resistance during aging: a mini-review, *Gerontology* 57(5):387–396, 2011.
63. Mahlknecht U, Zschoernig B: Involvement of sirtuins in life-span and aging related diseases, *Adv Exp Med Biol* 739:252–261, 2012.
64. Di Somma C et al: Somatopause: state of the art, *Minerva Endocrinol* 36(3):243–255, 2011.
65. Bartke A: Pleiotropic effects of growth hormone signaling in aging, *Trends Endocrinol Metab* 22(11):437–442, 2011.
66. Chapurlat RD, Delmas PD, Genant HK: Bone density and imaging of osteoporosis. In Jamerson JL, Degroot LJ, editors: *Endocrinology*, ed 6, Philadelphia, 2010, Saunders.
67. Allan CA, McLachlan RI: Androgen deficiency disorders. In Jamerson JL, Degroot LJ, editors: *Endocrinology*, ed 6, Philadelphia, 2010, Saunders.

CHAPTER

22

Alterations of Hormonal Regulation

Valentina L. Brashers, Robert E. Jones, and Sue E. Huether

evolve WEBSITE

http://evolve.elsevier.com/McCance/

- Review Questions and Answers
- Animations
- Online Course: Module 10

CHAPTER OUTLINE

The function of the endocrine system involves complex interrelationships and interactions that maintain dynamic steady-states, provide growth and reproductive capabilities, and allow for adaptive changes in times of stress. Alterations in function were thought only to be caused by either hypersecretion or hyposecretion of the various hormones, leading to abnormal hormone concentrations in the blood. Techniques for studying the various components of the endocrine system have improved, and evidence has shown that dysfunction may also result from abnormal receptor function or from altered intracellular response to the hormone-receptor complex.

MECHANISMS OF HORMONAL ALTERATIONS

Significantly elevated or depressed hormone levels may result from a variety of causes (Table 22-1). Dysfunction of an endocrine gland may involve the gland's failure to produce adequate amounts of biologically free or active hormone forms. This failure may occur when the secretory cells are unable to produce or obtain an adequate quantity of required hormone precursors or when they are unable to convert the precursors to the active hormone. A gland also may synthesize or release excessive amounts of hormone. For example, feedback systems that recognize the need for a particular hormone may fail to function properly or may respond to inappropriate signals. Once hormones are released into the circulation, they may be degraded at an altered rate or they may be inactivated by antibodies before reaching the target cell. Ectopic sources of hormones (hormones produced by nonendocrine tissues) may result also in abnormally elevated hormone levels without benefit of the normal feedback system for hormone control. In these cases the ectopic hormone production is said to be *autonomous.*

Target cells may fail to respond to its hormone *(hormone insensitivity)* (see Table 22-1). The general types of abnormal

TABLE 22-1 MECHANISMS OF HORMONE ALTERATIONS

INAPPROPRIATE AMOUNTS OF HORMONE DELIVERED TO TARGET CELL	INAPPROPRIATE RESPONSE BY TARGET CELL
Inadequate hormone synthesis	**Cell surface receptor–associated disorders**
Inadequate quantity of hormone precursors	Decrease in the number of receptors
Secretory cell unable to convert precursors to active hormone	Impaired receptor function (altered affinity for hormones)
Failure of feedback systems	Presence of antibodies against specific receptors
Do not recognize positive feedback leading to inadequate hormone synthesis	Unusual expression of receptor function
Do not recognize negative feedback leading to excessive hormone synthesis	**Intracellular disorders**
Hormones inactive	Acquired defects in postreceptor signaling cascades
Inadequate biologically free hormone	Inadequate synthesis of a second messenger
Hormone degraded at an altered rate	Intracellular enzymes or proteins are altered
Circulating inhibitors	Alterations in nuclear co-regulators
Dysfunctional delivery system	Altered protein synthesis
Inadequate blood supply	
Inadequate carrier proteins	
Ectopic production of hormones	

target cell responses currently recognized are receptor-associated disorders and intracellular disorders. Receptor-associated disorders have been identified primarily in water-soluble hormones, such as insulin. These types of disorders usually involve one of the following: (1) a decrease in the number of receptors, leading to decreased or defective hormone-receptor binding; (2) impaired receptor function, resulting in insensitivity to the hormone; (3) presence of antibodies against specific receptors that either reduce available binding sites or mimic hormone action; or (4) unusual expression of receptor function, as occurs in some tumor cells.

Intracellular disorders may involve acquired defects in postreceptor signaling cascades or inadequate synthesis of a second messenger, such as cyclic adenosine monophosphate (cAMP), needed to transduce the hormonal signal into intracellular events. The target cell for water-soluble hormones may have a faulty response to hormone-receptor binding and thus fail to generate the required second messenger, or the cell also may have an abnormal response to the second messenger if levels of intracellular enzymes or proteins are altered. (Second messengers for various hormones are listed in Table 21-3.) Both of these pathogenic mechanisms result in failure of the target cell to express the usual hormonal effect. Pathogenic mechanisms affecting target cell response for lipid-soluble hormones, such as thyroid hormone or glucocorticoids, are recognized less often than those affecting the water-soluble hormones. These hormone-resistant states have been generally linked to mutations in the nuclear receptor for the hormone. The number of receptors may be decreased, or those receptors may have an altered affinity or selectivity for hormones.[1] In other cases, hormone responsiveness may be linked to alterations in nuclear co-regulators, which are proteins (such as cAMP response element–binding protein [CREB], see Chapter 21 p. 694) that facilitate or inhibit the transcription of the target gene.[2] Alterations in generation of new messenger ribonucleic acid (mRNA) or absence of substrates for new protein synthesis also may occur, resulting in altered target cell response.

ALTERATIONS OF THE HYPOTHALAMIC-PITUITARY SYSTEM

Perhaps the most common cause of apparent hypothalamic dysfunction is interruption of the pituitary stalk, which can be caused by destructive lesions, rupture after head injury, surgical transection, or tumor. The absence of hypothalamic releasing or inhibiting hormones (Figure 22-1) causes a variety of manifestations that present clinically as pituitary disease. For example, if there is an absence of gonadotropin-releasing hormone (GnRH) from the hypothalamus, then there is a lack of stimulation of gonadotropin follicle-stimulating hormone (FSH) and luteinizing hormone (LH) from the pituitary; thus, menses cease in women and spermatogenesis is impaired in men.

Diseases of the Posterior Pituitary

Diseases of the posterior pituitary usually cause abnormal secretion of antidiuretic hormone (ADH, arginine vasopressin). An excess amount of this hormone results in water retention and a hypoosmolar state, whereas deficiency in the amount or response to ADH results in serum hyperosmolarity. These complex pathophysiologic states not only have significant clinical effects on the modulation of body fluids and electrolytes, but also affect cognitive and emotional responses to stress.

Syndrome of Inappropriate Antidiuretic Hormone Secretion

Syndrome of inappropriate antidiuretic hormone (SIADH) secretion is characterized by high levels of ADH in the absence of normal physiologic stimuli for its release. SIADH can complicate malignancies, pulmonary disorders, central nervous system disorders, surgical procedures, and the use of certain medications.[3] SIADH is associated with ectopic secretion of ADH by several types of tumor cells. Tumors that have been reported in association with SIADH include small cell carcinoma of the lung, duodenum, stomach, and pancreas; cancers of the bladder, prostate, and endometrium; lymphomas; and sarcomas. Pulmonary disorders associated with SIADH include pneumonia (e.g., tuberculosis), asthma, cystic fibrosis, and respiratory failure requiring mechanical ventilation. Central nervous system disorders that may cause SIADH include encephalitis, meningitis, intracranial hemorrhage, tumors, and trauma. A nephrogenic form of SIADH has recently been described. In these individuals, mutations in arginine vasopressin (AVP) genes lead to chronic activation of tubular V2 receptor and resulting excessive free water reabsorption.[4] Any surgery can result in postoperative fluid volume shifts and transient SIADH for as long as 5 to 7 days after surgery. The precise

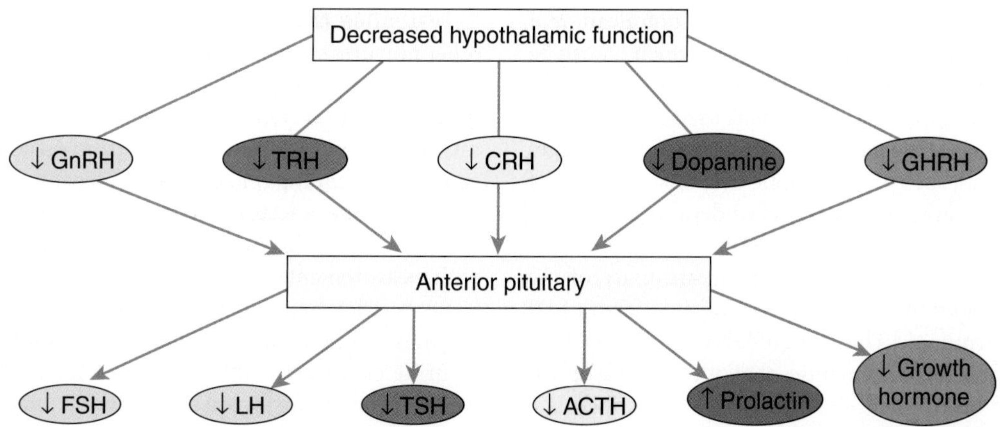

FIGURE 22-1 Loss of Hypothalamic Hormones. *ACTH,* Adrenocorticotropic hormone; *CRH,* corticotropin-releasing hormone; *FSH,* follicle-stimulating hormone; *GHRH,* growth hormone–releasing hormone; *GnRH,* gonadotropin-releasing hormone; *LH,* luteinizing hormone; *TRH,* thyrotropin-releasing hormone; *TSH,* thyroid-stimulating hormone.

mechanism is uncertain but is likely related to fluid and volume changes following surgery, the amount and type of intravenous fluids given, and the use of narcotic analgesics. Transient SIADH is especially common after pituitary surgery because stored ADH is released in an unregulated fashion. Medications are an important cause of SIADH, especially in older adults. These include antidepressants, antipsychotics, narcotics, general anesthetics, chemotherapeutic agents, nonsteroidal anti-inflammatory drugs, quinolone antibiotics, and synthetic ADH analogs.[3] These drugs serve either to simulate ADH release, to enhance the physiologic effects of ADH, or to have a biologic action similar to that of ADH.

PATHOPHYSIOLOGY. The pathophysiologic features of SIADH are the result of enhanced renal water retention. Water retention results from the action of ADH on renal collecting ducts, where it increases their permeability to water, thus increasing water reabsorption by the kidneys. (Renal function is discussed in Chapter 37.) This results in an expansion of extracellular fluid volume that leads to dilutional hyponatremia (low serum sodium concentration), hypoosmolarity, and urine that is inappropriately concentrated with respect to serum osmolarity.

CLINICAL MANIFESTATIONS. The symptoms of SIADH result from hypotonic (dilutional) hyponatremia and are associated with hypervolemia and weight gain. The severity and rapidity of onset of the hyponatremia determine the extent of the symptoms. Thirst, impaired taste, anorexia, dyspnea on exertion, fatigue, and dulled sensorium occur when the serum sodium level decreases rapidly from 140 to 130 mEq/L. Peripheral edema is usually absent. Severe gastrointestinal symptoms, including vomiting and abdominal cramps, occur with a drop in sodium concentration from 130 to 120 mEq/L. With a serum sodium level below 115 mEq/L, confusion, lethargy, muscle twitching, and seizures may occur. Even if hyponatremia develops slowly, serum sodium levels below 110 to 115 mEq/L are likely to cause severe and sometimes irreversible neurologic damage. Symptoms resolve with correction of hyponatremia.

EVALUATION AND TREATMENT. A diagnosis of SIADH requires documentation of the following manifestations: (1) serum hypoosmolality (<280 mOsm/kg) and hyponatremia (serum sodium level <135 mEq/L); (2) urine hyperosmolarity (i.e., the osmolality of the urine is always higher than the concurrent serum osmolality); (3) urine sodium excretion that matches sodium intake; (4) normal renal, adrenal, and thyroid function; and (5) absence of conditions that can alter volume status (e.g., recent diuretic use, heart failure, hypervolemia from any cause, or renal insufficiency).[3] Individuals with neurologic injury also may develop hyponatremia caused by cerebral salt wasting syndrome. This can be differentiated from SIADH because cerebral salt wasting is characterized by hypovolemia and weight loss. In addition, urine sodium levels are elevated.[5]

The treatment of SIADH involves the correction of the underlying causal problems; emergency correction of severe hyponatremia by administration of hypertonic saline; and, most importantly, fluid restriction to 800 to 1000 ml/day. Careful monitoring is important. Resolution usually occurs within 3 days, with a 2- to 3-kg weight loss resulting from enhanced free water clearance. If hyponatremia is corrected too rapidly, a severe neurologic syndrome called central pontine myelinolysis can ensue. No drug therapy is available to suppress ectopically produced ADH; however, demeclocycline, which causes the renal tubules to develop resistance to ADH, may be used to treat resistant or chronic SIADH. An ADH receptor agonist, conivaptan, has been approved for the treatment of hospitalized individuals with hyponatremia caused by ADH excess.[6] An oral form of ADH receptor antagonists has been developed.[7]

Diabetes Insipidus

Diabetes insipidus (DI) is an insufficiency of ADH, leading to polyuria (frequent urination) and polydipsia (frequent drinking). There are three forms: neurogenic (hypothalamic), nephrogenic (renal), and polydipsic (polydipsia-polyuria syndrome).

Neurogenic DI is the form encountered most often in clinical practice and is caused by insufficient amounts of ADH. It occurs when any organic lesion of the hypothalamus, pituitary stalk, or posterior pituitary interferes with ADH synthesis, transport, or release.[3] Causative lesions include primary or secondary brain tumors, aneurysms, thrombosis, infections, and immunologic disorders. DI is a well-recognized complication of closed-head trauma and of pituitary surgery in which DI can be transient or permanent.[8] Neurogenic DI can be a complication of pregnancy. In rare cases, it also can be caused by hereditary disorders that affect ADH genes or result in structural changes in the pituitary gland, such as septo-optic dysplasia (absence of the septum pellucidum in the brain and underdevelopment of the optic nerve).[9]

Nephrogenic DI is associated with an insensitivity of the renal collecting tubules to ADH. The nephrogenic form of DI can be genetic or acquired.[3] This form of DI is often idiopathic, although several genetic abnormalities that affect the vasopressin receptor have been noted. One of the best described is a mutation in the gene that codes for aquaporin-2, which is one of the four water transport channels in the renal tubule.[9]

Acquired nephrogenic DI is generally related to disorders and drugs that damage the renal tubules or inhibit the generation of cAMP in the tubules. These disorders include pyelonephritis, amyloidosis, destructive uropathies, polycystic disease, and intrinsic renal disease, all of which lead to irreversible DI. Drugs that may induce a reversible form of nephrogenic DI include lithium carbonate, colchicine, amphotericin B, loop diuretics, general anesthetics such as methoxyflurane, and demeclocycline.

Dipsogenic DI occurs when excessive fluid intake lowers the plasma osmolarity to the point that it falls below the threshold for ADH secretion.[3] This condition may be associated with psychiatric disorders but also has been found in individuals who have a low osmotic threshold for inducing thirst. Chronic ingestion of extremely large quantities of fluid dilute the renal medullary concentration gradient, which results in a partial resistance to ADH. This condition resolves with effective management of water ingestion.

PATHOPHYSIOLOGY. Neurogenic, nephrogenic, and dipsogenic DI are all characterized by the inability of the kidney to increase permeability to water. This causes excretion of large volumes of dilute urine and an increase in plasma osmolality. In conscious individuals, the thirst mechanism is stimulated and induces polydipsia. For unknown reasons the person usually craves cold drinks. The urine output is varied but can increase from the normal output of 1 to 2 L/day to as much as 8 to 12 L/day. The urine specific gravity is low, from 1.00 to 1.005, which is consistent with the failure to reabsorb water. Dehydration develops rapidly without ongoing fluid replacement. If the individual with DI cannot maintain balance with the urinary loss of water, serum hypernatremia and hyperosmolality occur. Other serum electrolytes generally are not affected.

CLINICAL MANIFESTATIONS. The signs and symptoms of DI include polyuria, nocturia, continuous thirst, and polydipsia. Untreated individuals with long-standing DI may develop a large bladder capacity and hydronephrosis (see Chapter 38). Idiopathic neurogenic DI usually has an abrupt onset, and many individuals can specifically recall the date of onset of their symptoms. Those with posttraumatic or postneurosurgical DI may develop a classic three-phase syndrome: (1) diuresis, (2) antidiuresis, and (3) polyuria/polydipsia.[8] Nephrogenic DI usually has a more gradual onset.

EVALUATION AND TREATMENT. DI must be distinguished from other polyuric states, including diabetes mellitus. The basic criteria for the diagnosis of DI include polyuria, polydipsia, low urine specific gravity (<1.010), low urine osmolality (<200 mOsm/kg), hypernatremia, high serum osmolality (300 mOsm or more depending on adequate water intake), and continued diuresis despite a serum sodium level of 145 mEq/L or greater.

The first step in the diagnosis of DI uses water deprivation with measurement of serum osmolarity and plasma ADH levels. Water restriction is a useful test because individuals without DI respond with a rapid decrease in urine volume and an increase in urine osmolality, whereas those with DI have no decrease in urine volume or increase in urine osmolality. In individuals with severe DI, water deprivation testing can be hazardous. If the individual loses more than 3% of the pretest body weight, circulatory collapse and shock can ensue. Neurogenic DI can be differentiated from nephrogenic DI by measuring the response to administered desmopressin. Neurogenic DI will respond with an increased ability to concentrate the urine, whereas nephrogenic DI will not respond.[3] The diagnosis of dipsogenic DI can be extremely difficult, and differentiation from nephrogenic DI is based on plasma ADH levels. Copeptin, a stable fragment of the ADH precursor molecule, is a reliable surrogate measurement for ADH secretion and can be used for the diagnosis of dipsogenic DI.[10]

Treatment for neurogenic DI is based on the extent of the ADH deficiency and on individual variables such as age, endocrine and cardiovascular status, and lifestyle. Replacement therapy for symptomatic neurogenic DI includes administration of the synthetic vasopressin analog desmopressin acetate (DDAVP) given intranasally or orally.[11]

Treatment for nephrogenic DI requires treatment of any reversible underlying disorders, discontinuation of etiologic medications, and correction of associated electrolyte disorders. Although the use of thiazide diuretics has been implicated as a cause for DI, they improve salt and water absorption at the proximal tubule and may be helpful in moderate DI.[3] New treatments for genetic abnormalities involving the V2 receptor are being evaluated.[9,12]

Diseases of the Anterior Pituitary

Disorders of the anterior pituitary may involve either hypofunction or hyperfunction of the gland.

Hypopituitarism

Hypopituitarism can be characterized by the absence of selective pituitary hormones or the complete failure of all pituitary hormone functions. Hypopituitarism results from either an inadequate supply of hypothalamic-releasing hormones, damage to the pituitary stalk, or an inability of the gland to produce hormones. The most common causes of hypopituitarism lie within the pituitary gland itself. An important cause is pituitary infarction resulting from severe shock, pituitary apoplexy, aneurysms, sickle cell disease, or pregnancy.[13,14] Space-occupying lesions, such as pituitary adenomas or aneurysms, also can compress the gland. Head trauma is another important cause of panhypopituitarism and may be transient or permanent.[15,16] Other causes of hypopituitarism include surgical removal or destruction of the gland, infections (e.g., meningitis, syphilis, tuberculosis), sarcoidosis, autoimmune hypophysitis, or certain drugs (e.g., bexarotene, carbamazepine).[14] A rare form of hypopituitarism is characterized by combined hormonal deficiencies and is related to mutations of the prophet of pituitary transcription factor *(PROP-1)* gene involved in early embryonic pituitary development.[17,18]

PATHOPHYSIOLOGY. The pituitary gland is highly vascular and is therefore extremely vulnerable to ischemia and infarction. It relies heavily on portal blood flow from the hypothalamus. In traumatic brain injury, disruption of blood flow can cause infarction with subsequent necrosis and fibrosis of pituitary tissue.[14] After tissue necrosis, edema with swelling of the gland occurs. Expansion of the pituitary within the fixed compartment of the sella turcica further impedes blood supply to the pituitary. Over time the pituitary undergoes shrinkage, and symptoms of hypopituitarism develop.

CLINICAL MANIFESTATIONS. The signs and symptoms of hypofunction of the anterior pituitary are variable and depend on which hormones are affected. In **panhypopituitarism,** all hormones are deficient and the individual suffers from multiple complications including cortisol deficiency from lack of adrenocorticotrophic hormone (ACTH), thyroid deficiency from lack of thyroid-stimulating hormone (TSH), and loss of secondary sex characteristics from lack of FSH and LH. Low levels of growth hormone (GH) and insulin-like growth factor 1 (IGF-1) affect growth in children and can cause physiologic and psychologic symptoms in adults. In addition, postpartum women cannot lactate because of decreased or absent prolactin.

ACTH deficiency is a potentially life-threatening disorder because cortisol is required for many aspects of cellular metabolism. ACTH deficiency is usually encountered with generalized pituitary hypofunction and rarely occurs as an isolated event.[19] Within 2 weeks of the complete absence of ACTH, symptoms of cortisol insufficiency develop, including nausea, vomiting, anorexia, fatigue, and weakness. Hypoglycemia is caused by increased insulin sensitivity, decreased glycogen reserves, and decreased gluconeogenesis associated with hypocortisolism. In women, loss of body hair and decreased libido may be caused by decreased adrenal androgen production. ACTH deficiency also limits maximum aldosterone secretion, although the renin-angiotensin system can stimulate some aldosterone secretion with resultant hypotension and decreased urine output.

TSH deficiency also is rarely seen in isolation but most often occurs in conjunction with other pituitary hormone deficiencies. The symptoms of decreased TSH levels may become apparent in 4 to 8 weeks and may include cold intolerance, dryness of skin, mild myxedema, lethargy, and decreased metabolic rate. The symptoms are usually less severe than those associated with primary hypothyroidism, in which lack of thyroxine is related to disease in the thyroid gland (see p. 728).

The onset of **FSH** and **LH deficiencies** in women of reproductive age is associated with amenorrhea and with atrophic changes in the vagina, uterus, and breasts. In postpubertal males, atrophy of the testes and decreased beard growth occur. Men as well as women experience a decrease in body hair and diminished libido.

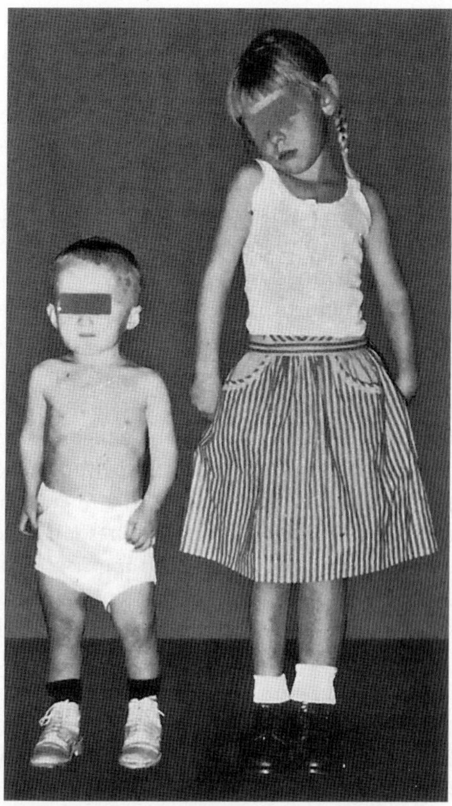

FIGURE 22-2 **Hypopituitary Dwarfism.** A 4-year-old boy whose height is 25 inches. The girl is also 4 years old and has a normal height of 39 inches. Dwarf has a normal face, as well as head, trunk, and limbs of approximately normal proportions. (From Brashear HR, Raney RB: *Shands' handbook of orthopaedic surgery,* ed 10, St Louis, 1986, Mosby.)

GH deficiency occurs in children and adults. As described previously, GH deficiency may result from any of the causes of hypopituitarism. In children it may be genetic or it may be the result of tumors such as craniopharyngiomas. Several genetic defects have been identified in the GH axis that account for impaired GH action. These include a recessive mutation in the *GHRH* gene, resulting in a failure of GH secretion, and mutations that cause GH insensitivity by affecting the GH receptor, insulin-like growth factor 1 (IGF-1) biosynthesis, IGF-1 receptors, or defects in GH signal transduction.[20,21] GH deficiency in children is manifested by growth failure (Figure 22-2). Another feature of GH deficiency in children is fasting hypoglycemia, likely attributable to impaired substrate mobilization for gluconeogenesis and enhanced insulin sensitivity.

In both children and adults, acute GH and IGF-1 deficiency has been implicated in significant metabolic perturbations seen with critical illness.[22] Symptoms of chronic adult GH deficiency syndrome include increased body fat, decreased muscle bulk and strength, reduced sweating, dry skin, and psychologic problems, including depression, social withdrawal, fatigue, loss of motivation, and a diminished feeling of well-being.[14] Several studies also have documented increased mortality in adults who are GH deficient. Osteoporosis and alterations in body composition (i.e., reduced lean body mass) are common concomitants of adult GH deficiency. A decline in GH production is an inevitable consequence of aging.[23]

EVALUATION AND TREATMENT. The diagnostic evaluation of suspected pituitary disease is often challenging and must be carefully interpreted together with the individual's signs and symptoms. Simultaneous measurements of the tropic hormones from the pituitary and target endocrine glands are crucial and, in some cases, dynamic testing of the various axes is indicated.[14] Radiographic assessment of the pituitary (magnetic resonance imaging [MRI] or computed tomography [CT] scans) may demonstrate enlargement of the pituitary, abnormal areas of enhancement suggestive of an adenoma, deviation of the pituitary stalk, or evidence of a locally aggressive tumor.

In general, treatment of hypopituitarism involves replacing target gland hormone(s) that are deficient. In cases of circulatory collapse, immediate therapy with glucocorticoids and intravenous fluids is critical. Thyroid and cortisol replacement therapy must be maintained. Gender-specific sex steroid replacement therapy is also initiated to improve general well-being and to prevent osteoporosis. Recombinant human GH (rhGH) is used for treatment of GH deficiency in children and results in both improved stature and metabolism.[24] Treatment of adult GH deficiency improves quality of life, metabolism, body composition, and physical performance in some individuals.[14,25] The use of GH to treat otherwise healthy aging is more controversial.[23]

Hyperpituitarism: Primary Adenoma

Pituitary adenomas are usually benign slow-growing tumors that arise from cells of the anterior pituitary, most commonly those that secrete GH and prolactin. They are very common in the population with prevalence rates estimated to be around 17%. However, most are microadenomas found incidentally on high-resolution MRI scanning and are hormonally silent and do not pose significant hazards to the individual.[26,27] More significant adenomas are associated with morbidity and mortality attributable to alterations in hormone secretion or to invasion or impingement of surrounding structures. The pathogenesis of pituitary adenomas includes hypothalamic and intrapituitary factors, including altered expression of pituitary cell cycle genes, activation of pituitary selective oncoproteins, or loss of pituitary suppressor factors.[28] Several associated gene mutations have been identified, including those associated with multiple endocrine neoplasia (MEN) syndromes.[29] Primary pituitary carcinomas are rare, representing about 0.2% of all pituitary tumors.

PATHOPHYSIOLOGY. Local expansion of pituitary adenomas may cause both neurologic and secretory defects. Neurologically, the tumor may impinge on the optic chiasm if it extends upward from the sella turcica. This causes a variety of visual disturbances, depending on the area of the optic chiasm that is compressed. If the tumor is locally aggressive, it may invade the cavernous sinus and cause cavernous sinus thrombosis with impairment of the function of the oculomotor, trigeminal, trochlear, and abducens cranial nerves, evoking symptoms relative to their function. Extension also may involve the hypothalamus, disturbing hypothalamic control of wakefulness, thirst, appetite, and temperature.

Hormonal effects of adenomas include hypersecretion from the adenoma itself, and hyposecretion from surrounding pituitary cells. The adenomatous tissue secretes the hormone of the cell type from which it arose, without regard to physiologic needs and without benefit of regulatory feedback mechanisms.

CLINICAL MANIFESTATIONS. The clinical manifestations of pituitary adenomas are related to tumor growth and hormone hypersecretion or hyposecretion. Effects from an increase in tumor size include such nonspecific complaints as headache and fatigue. Visual changes produced by pressure on the optic chiasm include visual field impairments (occasionally beginning in one eye and progressing to the other) and temporary blindness. If the tumor infiltrates other cranial nerves, neurologic function is affected.

Pituitary adenomas arise from hormone-producing cells of the pituitary, and most often are associated with increased secretion of GH and prolactin. Paradoxically, the pressure produced by a pituitary adenoma is also associated with decreased function of neighboring anterior pituitary cells, which results in hyposecretion of other anterior pituitary hormones. For example, gonadotropic hyposecretion often results in menstrual irregularity in women, decreased libido, and receding secondary sex characteristics in men and women. If the tumor exerts sufficient pressure, thyroid and adrenal hypofunction may occur because of lack of TSH and ACTH, respectively. These result in the respective symptoms of hypothyroidism and hypocortisolism.

EVALUATION AND TREATMENT. Diagnosis of pituitary adenoma involves physical and laboratory evaluations, including pertinent hormone assays and radiographic examination of the skull (MRI [preferred] or contrast-enhanced CT). The goal of treatment is to protect the individual from the effects of tumor growth, to control hormone hypersecretion (if present), and to replace deficient hormones while minimizing damage to appropriately secreting portions of the pituitary. Depending on the tumor size and type, individuals may be treated with specific medications to suppress tumor growth, transsphenoidal tumor resection, or radiation therapy. Simple observation and close follow-up is commonly employed for individuals who have no evidence of hormonal hypersecretion and no suggestion of anatomic aggressiveness.[27,30]

Hypersecretion of Growth Hormone: Acromegaly

Acromegaly occurs in adults who are exposed to continuously excessive levels of GH and concomitant elevation of IGF-1. In children and adolescents whose epiphyseal plates have not yet closed, the effect of increased GH levels on long bone growth is termed **giantism** (Figure 22-3).

Approximately 15% of all pituitary tumors release excessive GH. The most common cause of acromegaly is a primary autonomous GH-secreting pituitary adenoma. Acromegaly occurs more often in women than men and is diagnosed most often in adults in their forties and fifties, although the disease is usually present for years preceding the diagnosis.

Acromegaly is a slowly progressive disease that, if untreated, is associated with a decreased life expectancy. The increased number of deaths associated with acromegaly are caused by

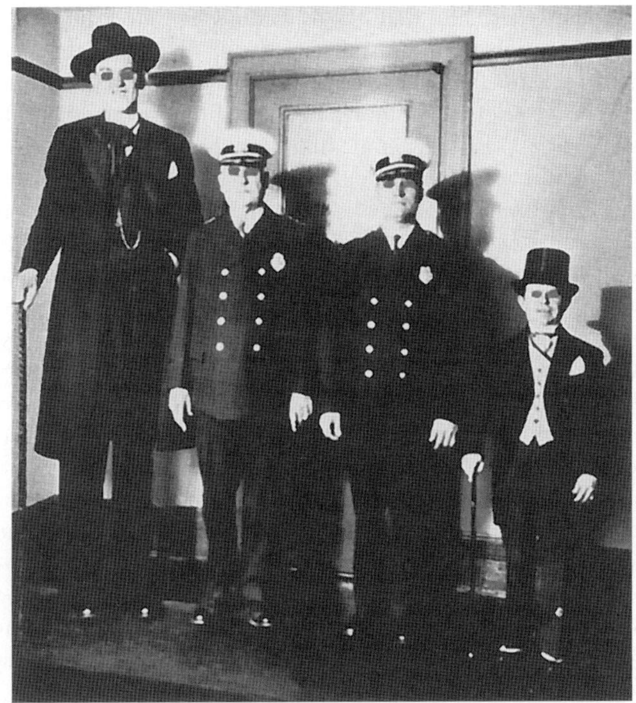

FIGURE 22-3 Giantism. A pituitary giant and dwarf contrasted with normal-size men. Excessive secretion of growth hormone by the anterior lobe of the pituitary gland during the early years of life produces giants of this type, whereas deficient secretion of this hormone produces well-formed dwarfs. (From Patton K, Thibodeau GA: *Anatomy & physiology*, ed 8, St Louis, 2013, Mosby.)

cardiac hypertrophy, hypertension, atherosclerosis, and type 2 diabetes mellitus that lead to coronary artery disease. Malignancies, including colon, breast, and lung cancer, are also more common in individuals with acromegaly.

PATHOPHYSIOLOGY. With a GH-secreting adenoma, the usual GH baseline secretion pattern and sleep-related GH peaks are lost, and an unpredictable secretory pattern ensues. With only slight elevations of GH, IGF-1 levels increase, stimulating growth. In children and adolescents whose epiphyseal plates have not yet closed, the effect of increased GH levels causes excessive skeletal growth, with some individuals becoming 8 or 9 feet tall. In the adult, epiphyseal closure has occurred and increased amounts of GH and IGF-1 cause connective tissue proliferation and increased cytoplasmic matrix, as well as bony proliferation that results in the characteristic appearance of acromegaly (Figures 22-4 and 22-5).

GH also has significant effects on glucose, lipid, and protein metabolism.[31] Hyperglycemia results from GH's inhibition of peripheral glucose uptake and increased hepatic glucose production, followed by compensatory hyperinsulinism and, finally, insulin resistance.[32] Excessive levels of GH and IGF-1 also affect the cardiovascular system. Although the associated pathophysiology is not clearly understood, hypertension and left heart failure are seen in one third to one half of individuals with acromegaly. Cardiomyopathy associated with progressive and unrestrained myocardial growth is a significant factor.[33,34]

GH also acts on the renal tubules to increase phosphate reabsorption, leading to mild hyperphosphatemia. The adenoma increasingly becomes a space-occupying lesion and

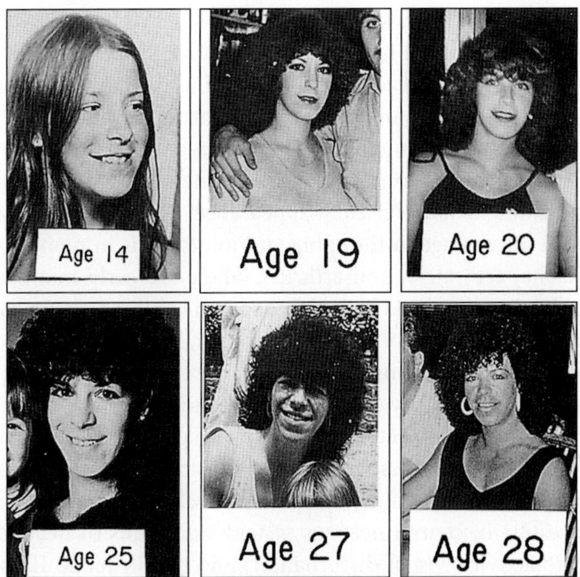

FIGURE 22-4 Acromegaly in a female. Chronologic sequence of photographs showing slow development of acromegaly. (From Belchetz P, Hammond P: *Mosby's color atlas and text of diabetes and endocrinology*, Edinburgh, 2003, Mosby.)

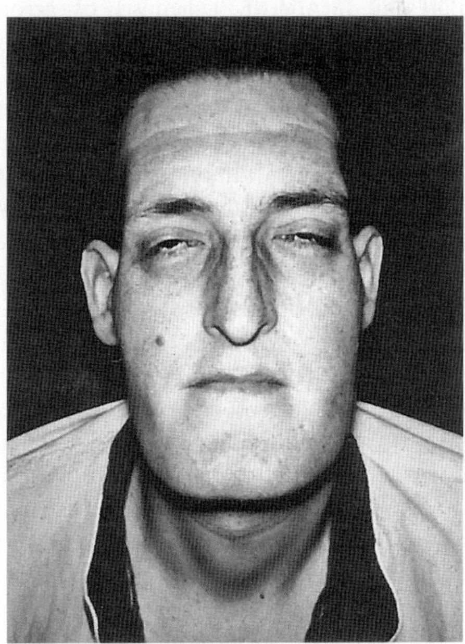

FIGURE 22-5 Acromegaly in a male. Note large head, forward projection of jaw, and protrusion of frontal bone. (Thibodeau GA, Patton K: *The human body in health & disease*, ed 5, St Louis, 2010, Mosby.)

hypopituitarism may occur because of compression of surrounding hormone-secreting cells.

CLINICAL MANIFESTATIONS. As a result of connective tissue proliferation, individuals with acromegaly have enlarged tongues, interstitial edema, increase in the size and function of sebaceous and sweat glands (leading to increased body odor), and coarse skin and body hair. The coarse skin condition becomes very apparent when procedures such as inserting an intravenous needle are performed; the skin is very thick and difficult to penetrate. Bony proliferation results in large joint arthropathy with swelling and decreased range of motion and periosteal vertebral growth, which causes kyphosis. Enlargement of the facial bones and the bones of the hands and feet result in protrusion of the lower jaw and forehead and a need for increasingly larger sizes of shoes, hats, rings, and gloves (see Figures 22-4 and 22-5).

Because IGF-1 stimulates cartilaginous growth, the increased IGF-1 levels cause elongation of ribs at the bone-cartilage junction, leading to a barrel-chest appearance, and increased proliferation of cartilage in the spine and joints. This in turn causes backache, arthralgia, and arthritis. These are early manifestations of acromegaly. With continued bony and soft tissue overgrowth, entrapment of nerves may occur, leading to peripheral nerve damage as manifested by weakness, muscular atrophy, footdrop, and sensory changes in the hands.

Symptoms of diabetes, such as polyuria and polydipsia, may occur. Acromegaly-associated hypertension is usually asymptomatic until heart failure symptoms develop. Increased tumor size results in central nervous system symptoms of headache, seizure activity, visual disturbances, and papilledema. If compression hypopituitarism occurs, gonadotropin secretion may be affected, causing amenorrhea in women and sexual dysfunction in men. Approximately 20% of growth hormone–secreting tumors also secrete prolactin, resulting in hypogonadism.

EVALUATION AND TREATMENT. Diagnosis of acromegaly is accomplished by documenting elevated IGF-1 levels and GH suppression during oral glucose tolerance testing. The goals of treatment are to normalize GH and IGF-1 serum levels, restoring normal pituitary function and relieving or preventing complications related to tumor expansion. The treatment of choice for acromegaly is transsphenoidal surgery or endonasal endoscopic surgery for removal of the GH-secreting adenoma.[35] Treatment by radiation therapy may be effective when rapid control of GH levels is not essential, when the individual is not a good surgical candidate, or when hyperfunction persists after subtotal resection. Octreotide, octreotide long-acting, and lanreotide are somatostatin analogs that have been shown to be effective in lowering elevated GH levels, reversing many of the clinical manifestations of the disease, and causing tumor shrinkage.[36] Dopaminergic agonists, such as cabergoline, also may be helpful, especially if the tumor also secretes prolactin. Pegvisomant is an effective drug that induces tissue insensitivity to GH by blocking the GH receptor.[37]

Hypersecretion of Prolactin: Prolactinoma

Pituitary tumors that secrete prolactin are called **prolactinomas** and are the most common of the hormonally active pituitary tumors encountered in clinical medicine. These tumors can be classified as microprolactinomas (<1 cm in size) or macroprolactinomas (>1 cm in size). Microprolactinomas are usually encapsulated and noninvasive, whereas macroprolactinomas commonly expand into the optic chasm and invade local structures.[38] The physiologic actions of prolactin include breast development during pregnancy, postpartum milk production, and suppression of ovarian function in nursing women.

In addition to pituitary tumors, many conditions or medications can elevate prolactin level in the absence of pituitary pathologic condition. For example, renal failure, hepatic cirrhosis, polycystic ovarian disease (see Chapter 24), breast stimulation, or chest wall lesions can increase prolactin levels. Because thyrotropin-releasing hormone (TRH) stimulates prolactin secretion, in addition to enhancing TSH release, prolactin level may be elevated in individuals with primary hypothyroidism. Prolactin is under tonic inhibitory hypothalamic control through the secretion of dopamine (prolactin inhibitor factor [PIF]). Thus medications that block the effects of dopamine at the pituitary can increase prolactin production and stimulate proliferation of prolactin-secreting cells (lactotropes). These include antipsychotics (risperidone, chlorpromazine), metoclopramide, tricyclic antidepressants, methyldopa, and estrogens. Any process that interferes with the delivery of dopamine from the hypothalamus to the lactotropes (pituitary stalk tumor, pituitary stalk transection, or compressive pituitary tumor) also results in hyperprolactinemia.

PATHOPHYSIOLOGY. The hallmark of a prolactinoma is sustained increases in serum prolactin concentration. Because the adenoma becomes increasingly a space-occupying lesion, hypopituitarism may occur because of compression of surrounding hormone secreting cells. Central nervous system symptoms may develop because of growth and pressure of the adenoma within the sella turcica.

CLINICAL MANIFESTATIONS. Women with hyperprolactinemia generally present with galactorrhea (nonpuerperal milk production) and menstrual disturbances, including amenorrhea. In susceptible women, hirsutism develops because of estrogen deficiency. If not detected until after many years, this estrogen deficiency also may result in osteoporosis. Men often develop hypogonadism and erectile dysfunction but may not seek care until symptoms related to the increasing size of the adenoma (i.e., headache or visual impairment) develop.[39]

EVALUATION AND TREATMENT. The diagnostic evaluation of hyperprolactinemia starts with a careful history to exclude medications that may cause elevations in prolactin level. A careful search for a nonpituitary cause should be pursued if prolactin concentration is less than 50 ng/ml. Symptoms of hypothyroidism should be elicited, and screening with a serum TSH measurement is indicated. Prolactin levels more than 200 ng/ml are usually associated with a prolactinoma and are an indication for MRI scanning of the pituitary.

Dopaminergic agonists (bromocriptine, cabergoline, and pergolide) are the treatment of choice for prolactinomas, and their use is often associated with both a rapid reduction in the size of the tumor and a reversal of the gonadal effects of hyperprolactinemia.[40] Restoration of fertility in previously anovulatory women is common. Although there is an association between valvular heart disease and cabergoline used in the treatment of parkinsonism, a similar association has not been found when cabergoline is used to treat prolactinoma.[41,42] In individuals resistant or intolerant to these medications, transsphenoidal surgery, endonasal endoscopic surgery, and radiotherapy are options.[38]

ALTERATIONS OF THYROID FUNCTION

Disorders of thyroid function develop as a result of primary dysfunction or disease of the thyroid gland or, secondarily, as a

WHAT'S NEW?

Thyroid Disease and Iodinated Contrast Media (ICM)

Large amounts of circulating iodide can be associated with either hyperthyroidism or hypothyroidism. Iodinated contrast medium is commonly used for both CT and radiographic imaging. A recent case controlled study of 178 and 213 incident hyperthyroid and hypothyroid cases, respectively, was matched to 655 and 779 euthyroid controls, respectively. The cases exposed to ICM did not have preexisting hyperthyroidism or hypothyroidism. Large amounts of iodide inhibit the oxidation of iodide within the thyroid follicle and decrease the release of thyroid hormones into the bloodstream, an autoregulatory process (known as the Wolff-Chaikoff effect), with return of normal thyroid function over weeks to months. This mechanism may explain the incident hypothyroidism found in this study. However, there was no incident hypothyroidism overall.

Normally, uptake of iodide and the subsequent synthesis and release of triiodothyronine and thyroxine are tightly controlled. However, supraphysiologic levels of iodide administered as ICM may overwhelm regulatory capacity and precipitate hyperthyroidism. In this study there was a significant association between ICM exposure and incident hyperthyroidism, and incident overt hyperthyroidism.

Further research is needed to confirm the findings of this study, to establish causality, and to provide guidance for clinical practice. However, individuals unable to tolerate thyroid dysfunction (e.g., unstable cardiovascular disease) should be monitored for thyroid disease after iodide exposure.

Data from Pearce EN: *Arch Intern Med* 172(2):159–161, 2012; Rhee CM et al: *Arch Intern Med* 172(2):153–159, 2012.

result of pituitary or hypothalamic alterations. **Primary thyroid disorders** result in alterations of thyroid hormone (TH) levels with secondary feedback effects on pituitary TSH levels. For example, when there are primary elevations in TH level, TSH level will secondarily decrease because of negative feedback. When TH level is decreased because of a condition affecting the thyroid gland, TSH level will be elevated. Thyroid disease also can present with no or minimal symptoms but with abnormal laboratory values. This is known as **subclinical thyroid disease.** **Central (secondary) thyroid disorders** are related to disorders of pituitary gland TSH production. When there is excessive TSH production, TH level is elevated secondary to the primary elevation of TSH level. The reverse is true with inadequate TSH production. Exposure to iodinated contrast media has been shown to be associated with development of both hyperthyroidism and hypothyroidism (see What's New? Thyroid Disease and Iodinated Contrast Media [ICM]).

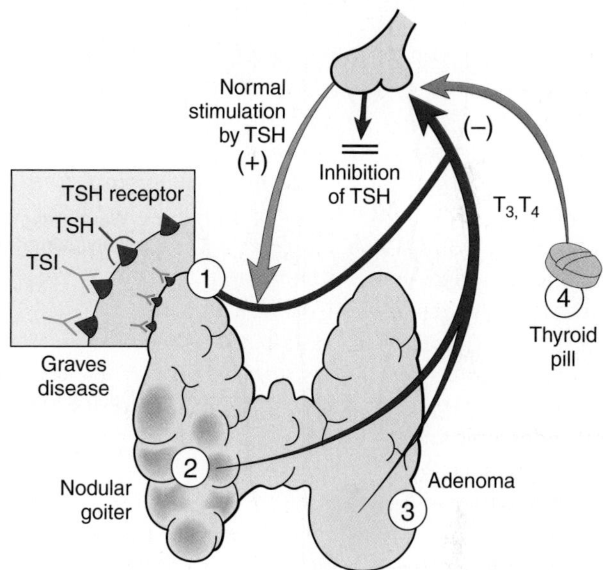

FIGURE 22-6 Causes of Hyperthyroidism. Hyperthyroidism may have several causes, among them: **1,** Graves disease; **2,** toxic multinodular goiter; **3,** follicular adenoma; **4,** thyroid medication. *TSH,* Thyroid-stimulating hormone; *TSI,* thyroid-stimulating immunoglobulin. (From Damjanov I: *Pathology for the health professions,* ed 4, St Louis, 2012, Saunders.)

Hyperthyroidism

Thyrotoxicosis

PATHOPHYSIOLOGY. **Thyrotoxicosis** is a condition that results from any cause of increased amounts of TH. Hyperthyroidism is a form of thyrotoxicosis in which excess amounts of TH are secreted from the thyroid gland. The terms *thyrotoxicosis* and *hyperthyroidism* are often used interchangeably. The prevalence of hyperthyroidism is estimated to be 0.7% to 2.1% in the United States, of which 0.7% is subclinical and is more prevalent in women and in iodine-deficient geographical areas.[43] Common diseases that cause **primary hyperthyroidism** include Graves disease, toxic multinodular goiter, a solitary toxic adenoma (Figure 22-6), and, very rarely, follicular thyroid carcinoma. **Central (secondary) hyperthyroidism** is less common and is caused by TSH-secreting pituitary adenomas. Thyrotoxicosis not associated with hyperthyroidism includes subacute thyroiditis, ectopic thyroid tissue, and ingestion of excessive TH. TSH progressively decreases in **subclinical hyperthyroidism** and can be caused by thyroid hormone therapy or iatrogenic exogenous disease. It is more prevalent in iodine-deficient populations.[44] Identifying the cause is important because the treatment and expected outcome vary accordingly. Each condition is associated with specific pathophysiology and manifestations; however, all forms of thyrotoxicosis share some common characteristics.

CLINICAL MANIFESTATIONS. The clinical features of thyrotoxicosis are attributable to the metabolic effects of increased circulating levels of TH (Figure 22-7). This usually results in an increased metabolic rate with heat intolerance and increased tissue sensitivity to stimulation by the sympathetic division of the autonomic nervous system. The major manifestations are summarized in Table 22-2. Enlargement of the thyroid gland (goiter) is common in hyperthyroid conditions caused by stimulation of TSH receptors.

EVALUATION AND TREATMENT. The diagnosis of thyrotoxicosis is based on symptoms of TH excess and documentation of increased circulating thyroid hormone levels. Elevated serum thyroxine (T_4) and triiodothyronine (T_3) levels and decreased serum TSH levels are diagnostic for primary hyperthyroidism. By contrast, central (secondary) hyperthyroidism caused by

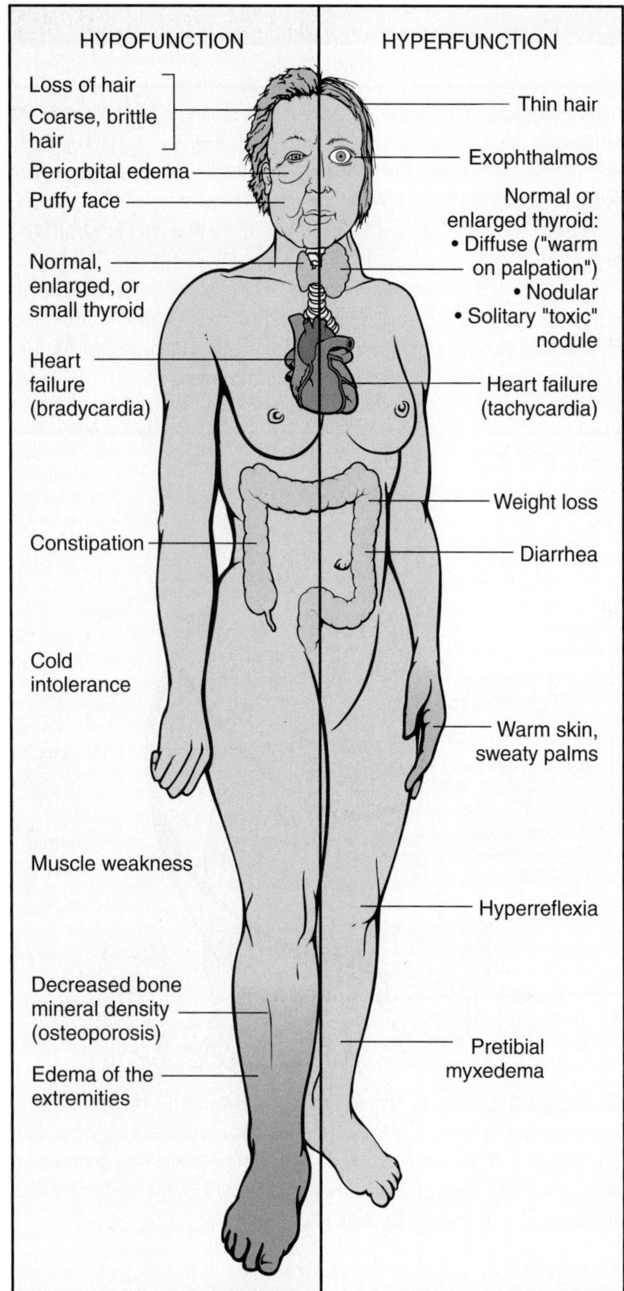

FIGURE 22-7 Clinical Manifestations of Hyperthyroidism and Hypothyroidism. (From Damjanov I: *Pathology for the health professions,* ed 4, St Louis, 2012, Saunders.)

TSH-secreting pituitary tumors is characterized by normal to increased TSH levels in the face of elevated thyroid hormone concentrations. Radioactive iodine is used to test for increased uptake in primary hyperthyroidism (Figure 22-8).

Treatment is directed at controlling excessive TH production, secretion, or action. The major types of therapy currently used to achieve these goals include antithyroid drug therapy (methimazole or propylthiouracil), radioactive iodine therapy, and surgery. Guidelines for the treatment of hyperthyroidism and thyrotoxicosis have been published.[45] Treatment of subclinical hyperthyroidism is based on levels of TSH and clinical symptoms.[44] A major complication of all forms of treatment for hyperthyroidism is hypothyroidism.[46]

Hyperthyroid Conditions

Graves Disease. **Graves disease** is the underlying cause of 50% to 80% of cases of hyperthyroidism and has a prevalence of approximately 0.5% in the U.S. population.[47] It occurs more commonly in women. Although the cause of Graves disease is not known, genetic factors interacting with environmental triggers play an important role in the pathogenesis of this autoimmune thyroid disease. Graves disease results from a form of type II hypersensitivity (see Chapter 9) in which there is stimulation of the thyroid by autoantibodies directed against the TSH receptor. These autoantibodies, called thyroid-stimulating immunoglobulins (TSIs; also called thyroid-stimulating antibodies [TSAbs] or thyroid receptor antibodies [TRAbs]), override normal regulatory mechanisms. The TSI stimulation of TSH receptors in the gland results in hyperplasia of the gland (goiter) and increased synthesis of TH, especially of triiodothyronine (T_3). Increased levels of TH affect every physiologic system and result in the classic signs and symptoms of hyperthyroidism illustrated in Figure 22-8. TSH production by the pituitary is inhibited through the usual negative feedback loop.

TSIs also contribute to two major distinguishing clinical manifestations of Graves disease: ophthalmopathy and pretibial myxedema (Graves dermopathy). Graves ophthalmopathy affects more than half of individuals with Graves disease. There are two categories of ocular manifestations: (1) functional abnormalities resulting from hyperactivity of the sympathetic division of the autonomic nervous system (lag of the globe on upward gaze or a lag of the upper lid on downward gaze) and (2) infiltrative changes involving the orbital contents with enlargement of the ocular muscles. The infiltrative changes result from TSH receptor autoantibodies reacting with receptors on orbital fibroblasts (Figure 22-9). Increased secretion of hyaluronic acid, orbital fat accumulation, inflammation, and edema of the orbital contents result in **exophthalmos** (protrusion of the eyeball). Periorbital edema and extraocular muscle weakness lead to diplopia (double vision). The individual may experience irritation, pain, lacrimation, photophobia, blurred vision, decreased visual acuity, papilledema, visual field impairment, exposure keratosis, and corneal ulceration.[48]

A small number of individuals with Graves disease and very high levels of TSI experience **pretibial myxedema (Graves dermopathy),** characterized by subcutaneous swelling on the anterior portions of the legs and by indurated and erythematous skin (Figure 22-10). Graves dermopathy is associated with thyrotropin receptor antigens on fibroblasts and recruited T lymphocytes that stimulate excess amounts of hyaluronic acid production in the dermis and subcutis. The manifestations occasionally appear on the hands giving the appearance of clubbing of the fingers (thyroid acropachy).[49]

Therapy for Graves disease includes antithyroid drugs, radioactive iodine (used with caution in Graves ophthalmopathy because it may worsen the condition), or surgery. Unfortunately, current treatment for Graves disease does not reverse the infiltrative ophthalmopathy or the pretibial myxedema. Surgical orbital decompression and glucocorticoids can help many individuals with progressive ophthalmopathy.[50] Skin lesions

TABLE 22-2 SYSTEMIC MANIFESTATIONS OF HYPERTHYROIDISM

SYSTEM	CLINICAL MANIFESTATIONS	MECHANISMS UNDERLYING CLINICAL MANIFESTATIONS
Endocrine	Enlarged thyroid gland (goiter) (97-99% of cases); systolic or continuous bruit over thyroid; increased cortisol degradation; hypercalcemia and decreased PTH secretion; diminished sensitivity to exogenous insulin	Hyperactivity of the thyroid gland; excess bone resorption leading to hypercalcemia and a disruption of PTH-regulating mechanisms; increased insulin degradation
Reproductive	Oligomenorrhea or amenorrhea; erectile dysfunction and decreased libido; increased serum estradiol and estrone levels but lower than normal levels of free estradiol and estrone	Menstrual cycle alterations that may be related to hypothalamic or pituitary disturbances; increase in sex hormone–binding globulin
Gastrointestinal	Weight loss; increased peristalsis leading to less formed and more frequent stools; nausea, vomiting, anorexia, abdominal pain; increased use of hepatic glycogen stores and of adipose and protein stores; decrease in serum lipid levels (including triglycerides, phospholipids, and cholesterol); changes in vitamin metabolism leading to decrease in tissue stores of vitamins	Increased catabolism leading to the body's inability to meet its metabolic needs; increased glucose absorption; increase in cholesterol excretion in feces and cholesterol conversion to bile salts; impaired conversion of B vitamins to their coenzymes, causing increased need for water-soluble and fat-soluble vitamins
Integumentary	Excessive sweating, flushing, and warm skin; heat intolerance; hair fine, soft, and straight; temporary hair loss; nails that grow away from nail beds, palmar erythema	Hyperdynamic circulatory state
Sensory (eyes)	Ocular manifestations including elevated upper eyelid leading to decreased blinking and a staring quality; fine tremor of lid; infiltrative ocular changes associated with Graves disease	Overactivity of Müller muscle; inflammation of retroorbital contents
Cardiovascular	Increased cardiac output and decreased peripheral resistance; tachycardia at rest; loud heart sounds; supraventricular dysrhythmias, left ventricular dilation and hypertrophy	Hypermetabolism and need to dissipate heat
Nervous	Restlessness; short attention span; compulsive movement; fatigue; tremor; insomnia; increased appetite; emotional lability	Not clearly defined; alterations in cerebral metabolism resulting from excess thyroid hormone
Pulmonary	Dyspnea; reduced vital capacity	Weakness of respiratory muscles

PTH, Parathyroid hormone.

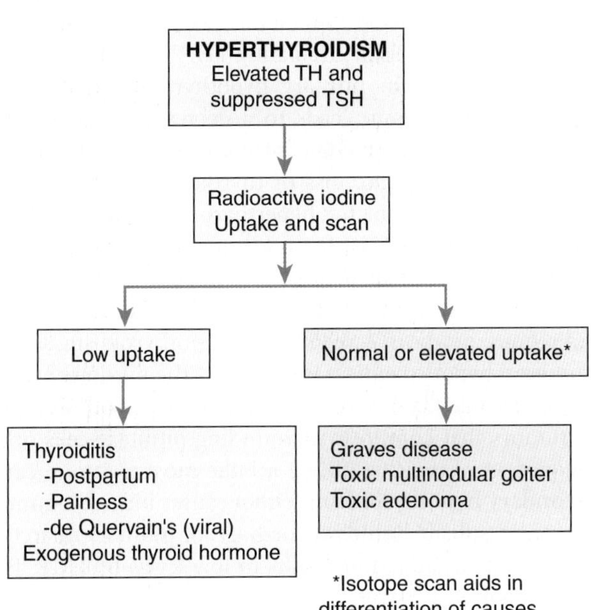

FIGURE 22-8 Evaluation of Hyperthyroidism. Radioactive iodine is used in the differential diagnosis of hyperthyroidism. *TH,* Thyroid hormone; *TSH,* thyroid-stimulating hormone.

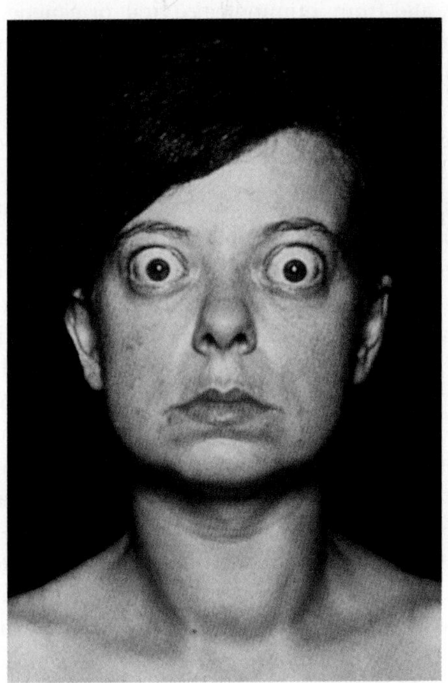

FIGURE 22-9 Thyrotoxicosis (Graves Disease). Note large and protruding eyeballs in association with a large goiter. (From Stein HA, Slatt BJ, Stein RM: *The ophthalamic assistant: fundamentals and clinical practice,* ed 7, Philadelphia, 2000, Mosby.)

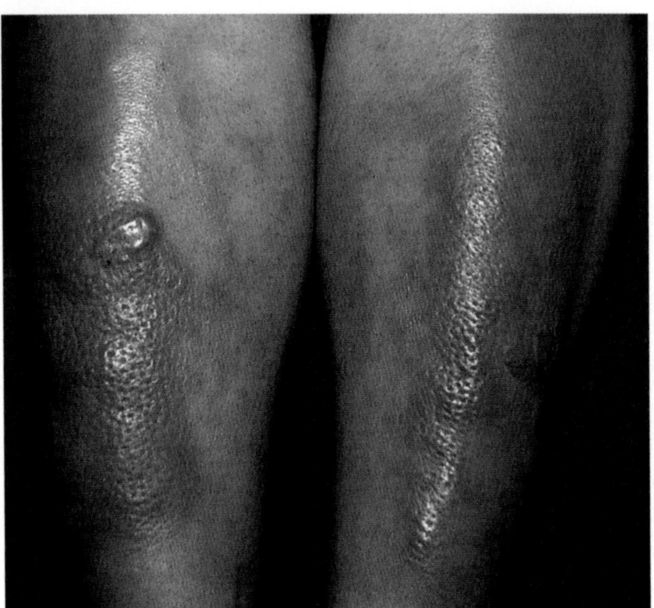

FIGURE 22-10 Pretibial Myxedema. Purple-brown edematous plaques on shins of individual with Graves disease. Note orange peel appearance. (From Bolognia JL, Jorizzo JL, Schaffer JV: *Dermatology,* ed 3, New York, 2013, Saunders.)

rarely require treatment, but if they are symptomatic they may respond to topical glucocorticoids.[51]

Hyperthyroidism Resulting from Nodular Thyroid Disease. The thyroid gland normally enlarges in response to an increased secretion of TSH that occurs in puberty, pregnancy, or iodine deficiency, and from immunologic, viral, or genetic disorders. The increased number of follicles is a compensatory mechanism in response to increased TSH levels. When the condition requiring increased TH resolves, TSH secretion normally subsides and the thyroid gland returns to its original size.

Irreversible changes may occur in some follicular cells and these cells function autonomously and produce excessive amounts of TH. On the other hand, some follicular cells may cease to function. The balance between the amount of TH produced by hyperfunctioning nodules and that produced by the remainder of the gland determines whether an individual becomes euthyroid or hyperthyroid. **Toxic multinodular goiter** occurs when there are several hyperfunctioning nodules leading to hyperthyroidism. If only one nodule becomes hyperfunctioning it is termed **solitary toxic adenoma.** This condition is more common in iodine-deficient regions. The classic clinical manifestations of hyperthyroidism (see Figure 22-7) usually develop slowly and exophthalmos and pretibial myxedema do not occur. Nodules may be palpable on physical examination. The incidence of malignancy in toxic multinodular goiter is estimated to be as high as 9% and 10.5%, so most individuals should undergo a fine needle aspiration biopsy of suspicious nodules before treatment.[52] Treatment consists of a combination of radioactive iodine, surgery, or antithyroid drugs. Mutations of the TSH receptor have been found in most solitary toxic adenomas.[53,54]

Thyrotoxic Crisis (Thyroid Storm). **Thyrotoxic crisis (thyroid storm)** is a rare but dangerous worsening of the thyrotoxic state, in which death can occur within 48 hours without treatment. The condition may develop spontaneously, but it occurs in individuals who have undiagnosed or partially treated severe hyperthyroidism and who are subjected to excessive stress from other causes. These causes may include infection, pulmonary or cardiovascular disorders, trauma, burns, seizures, surgery (especially thyroid surgery), obstetric complications, emotional distress, or dialysis. The symptoms of thyroid crisis are caused by the increased action of thyroxine (T_4) and triiodothyronine (T_3) exceeding metabolic demands.[55]

The systemic symptoms of thyrotoxic crisis include hyperthermia; tachycardia, especially atrial tachydysrhythmias; high-output heart failure; agitation or delirium; and nausea, vomiting, or diarrhea, contributing to fluid volume depletion. Treatment includes: (1) the use of drugs that block TH synthesis (i.e., propylthiouracil or methimazole), (2) the use of beta-blockers for control of cardiovascular symptoms, (3) administration of corticosteroids or (4) iodine (e.g., saturated solution of potassium iodide [SSKI]), and (5) supportive care.

Hypothyroidism

Hypothyroidism is caused by a deficient production of TH by the thyroid gland. Hypothyroidism is the most common disorder of thyroid function; it affects between 0.1% and 2% of individuals in the United States and is more common in women and the elderly. It may be primary or secondary. **Primary hypothyroidism** is the most prevalent. **Central (secondary) hypothyroidism,** which is much less common, includes conditions that cause either pituitary or hypothalamic failure with failure to stimulate normal thyroid function. **Subclinical hypothyroidism** is mild thyroid failure and is estimated to occur in 4% to 8% of U.S. adults. It is defined as an elevation in TSH level with normal levels of circulating TH.[44]

PATHOPHYSIOLOGY. In primary hypothyroidism the loss of functional thyroid tissue leads to a decreased production of TH. Causes in adults include autoimmune thyroiditis (Hashimoto disease), iatrogenic loss of thyroid tissue after surgical or radioactive treatment for hyperthyroidism, head and neck radiation therapy, medications, and endemic iodine deficiency. Infants and children may present with hypothyroidism because of congenital defects in the pituitary or thyroid glands.[56] Most states require newborn screening for hypothyroidism. Central (secondary) hypothyroidism is caused by the pituitary's failure to synthesize adequate amounts of TSH or a lack of TRH. Pituitary tumors that compress surrounding pituitary cells or the consequences of their treatment are the most common causes of **secondary hypothyroidism.** Other causes include traumatic brain injury, subarachnoid hemorrhage, or pituitary infarction. Hypothalamic dysfunction results in low levels of TRH, TSH, and TH (Figure 22-11).

CLINICAL MANIFESTATIONS. Hypothyroidism generally affects all body systems and occurs insidiously over months or years. The extent of the symptoms is closely related to the degree of TH deficiency (see Figure 22-7). The lowered levels of TH result in decreased energy metabolism and decreased heat production. The individual develops a low basal metabolic rate, cold intolerance, lethargy, tiredness, and slightly lowered basal body

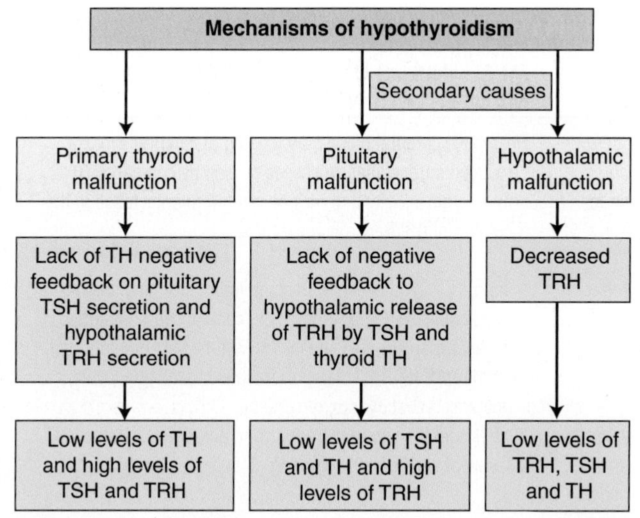

FIGURE 22-11 Mechanisms of Primary and Central (Secondary) Hypothyroidism. *TH,* Thyroid hormone; *TRH,* Thyroid-releasing hormone; *TSH,* Thyroid-stimulating hormone.

temperature and also may have diastolic hypertension. Many organ systems are affected (Table 22-3). The decrease in the level of TH leads to increases in TSH production and may cause goiter.

The characteristic sign of severe or long-standing hypothyroidism is **myxedema,** which is histologically similar to the pretibial myxedema deposits that often occur with Graves disease. Myxedema is a result of an alteration in the composition of the dermis and other tissues. The connective fibers are separated by an increased amount of protein and mucopolysaccharides. This protein-mucopolysaccharide complex binds water, producing nonpitting, boggy edema, especially around the eyes, hands, and feet and in the supraclavicular fossae. Myxedema is also responsible for thickening of the tongue and the laryngeal and pharyngeal mucous membranes. This results in thick, slurred speech and hoarseness, both of which are common in hypothyroidism.

Myxedema coma, a medical emergency, is a diminished level of consciousness associated with severe hypothyroidism. Precipitating events include infections and discontinuation of thyroid supplements, overuse of narcotics or sedatives, or a consequence of an acute illness in individuals who have hypothyroidism. Older individuals with severe vascular disease and with moderate or untreated hypothyroidism are particularly at risk for developing myxedema coma. Signs and symptoms include hypothermia without shivering, hypoventilation, hypotension, hypoglycemia, lactic acidosis, and coma.[57] Symptoms of hypothyroidism in older adults should not be attributed to normal aging changes.

EVALUATION AND TREATMENT. The diagnosis of primary hypothyroidism is made by documentation of the clinical symptoms of hypothyroidism, and by measurement of increased levels of TSH and decreased levels of TH (total T_3 and both total and free T_4). When hypothyroidism is caused by pituitary deficiencies, serum TSH levels are decreased or are inappropriately normal in the face of low levels of TH. Hormone replacement therapy is the treatment of choice for hypothyroidism. Levothyroxine (a synthetic hormone) is preferred over desiccated thyroid (the crude extract from animal thyroid glands). Treatment of myxedema coma with TH, combined with circulatory and ventilatory support and management of hyponatremia and hypothermia, is usually effective. Mortality can be as high as 25%.[55] Treatment of subclinical hypothyroidism is related to elevated levels of TSH and clinical symptoms.[58] The goal of treatment is maximal metabolic restoration consistent with the individual's overall well-being and normalization of TSH levels in primary hypothyroidism or normalization of TH levels in central hypothyroidism.

Hypothyroid Conditions

Primary Hypothyroidism. **Primary hypothyroidism** has several causes. **Iodine deficiency (endemic goiter)** is the most common cause worldwide, but is relatively rare in the United States because of the use of iodized table salt and fortified foods. The most common cause of hypothyroidism in the United States is **autoimmune thyroiditis (Hashimoto disease,** chronic **lymphocytic thyroiditis),** which results in gradual inflammatory destruction of thyroid tissue by infiltration of lymphocytes and circulating thyroid autoantibodies (antithyroid peroxidase and antithyroglobulin antibodies). Autoreactive T lymphocytes, antibody activation of natural killer cells (antibody-dependent cell-mediated cytotoxicity), cytokines, and induction of apoptosis also are involved in the tissue destruction seen in Hashimoto thyroiditis.[59] Variants in major histocompatibility complex (MHC) antigens have been associated with autoimmune thyroiditis that are different from those found in Graves disease. Hashimoto disease occurs in genetically predisposed individuals and is associated with high iodine intake, selenium deficiency, smoking, chronic hepatitis C, and interferon-alpha (IFN-α).[60] Epigenetic mechanisms are probably involved.[61] Goiter formation is commonly observed.

Spontaneous recovery of thyroid function is seen in three conditions: subacute thyroiditis, painless thyroiditis, and postpartum thyroiditis.[62] **Subacute thyroiditis (subacute granulomatous thyroiditis,** or **de Quervain thyroiditis)** is an uncommon nonbacterial inflammation of the thyroid often preceded by a viral infection. It is accompanied by fever, tenderness, and enlargement of the thyroid. The inflammatory process initially results in elevated levels of TH caused by release of stored thyroglobulin, and then is associated with transient hypothyroidism before the gland recovers normal activity. Symptoms may last 2 to 4 months and nonsteroidal anti-inflammatory agents, corticosteroids, beta-blockers, and, possibly, TH supplementation may be required during the course of the illness. **Painless thyroiditis (silent** or **subacute lymphocytic thyroiditis)** has a course similar to that of subacute thyroiditis but is pathologically identical to Hashimoto disease. **Iatrogenic hypothyroidism** results from radioiodine thyroid ablation, thyroidectomy, and medications (lithium and amiodarone). **Postpartum thyroiditis** generally occurs within 6 to 12 months of delivery, develops in up to 5.4% of all women, and has a course similar to that of painless thyroiditis. Pathologic specimens suggest it is related to Hashimoto disease. Spontaneous recovery is seen in most women affected with this form of thyroiditis; however, persistent hypothyroidism does occur.[63,64]

TABLE 22-3 **SYSTEMIC MANIFESTATIONS OF HYPOTHYROIDISM**

SYSTEM	CLINICAL MANIFESTATIONS	MECHANISMS UNDERLYING CLINICAL MANIFESTATIONS
Neurologic	Confusion, syncope, slowed speech and thinking, memory loss; lethargy, headaches, hearing loss, night blindness; slow, clumsy movements; cerebellar ataxia; slow alpha-wave activity and loss of amplitude in EEG; reduced cAMP response to epinephrine, glucagons, and PTH stimulation; decreased appetite	Decreased cerebral blood flow leading to cerebral hypoxia; reduced intracellular processes caused by decreased β-adrenergic activity that may be related to a decrease in the number of β-adrenergic receptor sites
Endocrine	Increased TSH production in primary hypothyroidism; enlarged pituitary thyrotropes, increase in serum prolactin levels with galactorrhea; decreased rate of cortisol turnover but with normal serum cortisol levels	Impaired TH synthesis or defects in iodide trapping leading to compensatory TSH production; chronic overstimulation of thyrotropes of TRH and by TSH synthesis; stimulation of lactotropes by TRH related to increased prolactin levels; decreased deactivation of cortisol
Reproductive	Decreased androgen secretion in men, increased estriol formation in women; low total hormone values but with increased amounts of unbound hormone; anovulation, decreased libido, menorrhagia, and a high incidence of spontaneous abortion in women; erectile dysfunction, decreased libido, and oligospermia in men	Altered metabolism of estrogens and androgens; decreased levels of sex hormone–binding globulin
Hematologic	Decrease in red cell mass leading to normocytic, normochromic anemia; macrocytic anemia associated with vitamin B_{12} deficiency and inadequate folate or iron absorption in the gastrointestinal tract	Decreased basal metabolic rate and reduced oxygen requirements; decreased production of erythropoietin; possible relationship between TH and optimal hematologic response to vitamin B_{12}
Cardiovascular	Reduction in stroke volume and heart rate causing lowered cardiac output; increased peripheral vascular resistance to maintain systolic blood pressure can cause hypertension; normal response to exercise but with alterations in circulatory system at rest (prolonged circulation time and decreased blood flow to tissues); cool skin and cold tolerance; enlarged heart; decreased intensity of heart sounds and variety of ECG changes (sinus bradycardia, prolonged PR interval, depressed P waves, flattened or inverted T waves, and low-amplitude QRS complexes); cardiac tamponade (although rare) (see Chapter 32)	Decreased metabolic demands and loss of regulatory and rate-setting effects of TH; protein-mucopolysaccharide–rich fluid in the pericardial sac associated with enlarged heart; pericardial effusions associated with heart sounds and ECG changes Increases in peripheral vascular resistance and increased blood volume can cause hypertension
Pulmonary	Dyspnea; myxedematous changes in respiratory muscles leading to hypoventilation and carbon dioxide retention, which contribute to myxedema coma	Pleural effusions associated with dyspnea, although effusions may be asymptomatic
Renal	Reduced renal blood flow and glomerular filtration rate leading to decreased renal excretion of water; increase in total body water and dilutional hyponatremia; reduced production of erythropoietin	Hemodynamic alterations associated with reduced blood flow and filtration; increased total body water related to decreased excretion and mucinous deposits in tissue
Gastrointestinal	Constipation, weight gain, and fluid retention; decreased absorption of most nutrients; decreased protein metabolism leading to retarded skeletal and soft tissue growth and slightly positive nitrogen balance; edema; decreased glucose absorption and delayed glucose uptake; elevated serum lipid values	Reduced intake and reduced peristaltic activity that may progress to fecal impaction; water absorption related to prolonged transit time; fluid retention associated with myxedematous changes; edema associated with high concentrations of exchangeable albumin in the extravascular space caused by increased capillary permeability to proteins; depressed insulin degradation; depressed lipid synthesis and degradation
Musculoskeletal	Muscle aching and stiffness; slow movement and slow tendon jerk reflexes; decreased bone formation and resorption, increased bone density; aching and stiffness in joints	Decreased rate of muscle contraction and relaxation contributing to slow movement and reflexes
Integumentary	Dry, flaky skin; dry, brittle head and body hair; reduced growth of nails and hair; slow wound healing	Reduced sweat and sebaceous gland secretion
	Myxedema	Accumulation of hyaluronic acid, which binds water and causes a puffy appearance
	Cool skin	Decreased circulation to skin

cAMP, Cyclic adenosine monophosphate; *ECG,* electrocardiogram; *EEG,* electroencephalogram; *PTH,* parathyroid hormone; *TH,* thyroid hormone; *TRH,* thyrotropin-releasing hormone; *TSH,* thyroid-stimulating hormone.

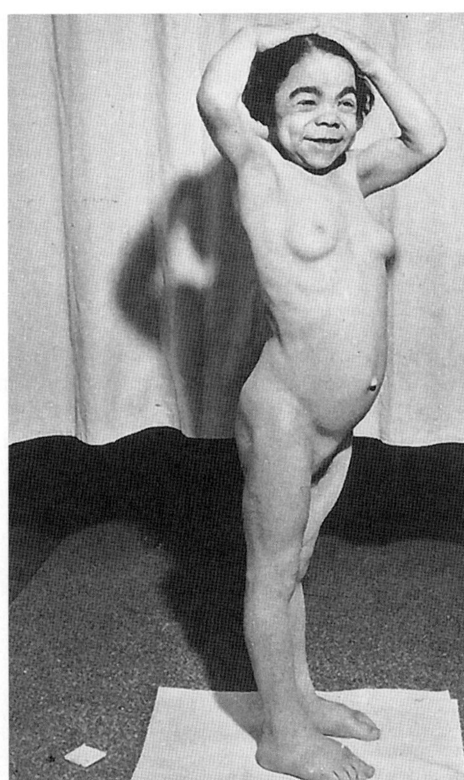

FIGURE 22-12 Adult Cretin. Note characteristic facial features, dwarfism (44 inches), absent axillary and scant pubic hair, poorly developed breasts, potbelly, and small umbilical hernia. (From Schneeberg NG: *Essentials of clinical endocrinology,* St Louis, 1970, Mosby.)

Congenital Hypothyroidism. **Congenital hypothyroidism (CH)** is thyroid hormone deficiency present at birth. It occurs as a result of absent thyroid tissue (thyroid agenesis) or with hereditary defects in TH synthesis. Thyroid agenesis occurs more often in female infants, with permanent abnormalities in 1 of every 3000 to 4000 live births.[65] Because TH is essential for embryonic growth, particularly of brain tissue, the infant will be mentally retarded if there is no T_4 available during fetal life.

Clinical manifestations at birth are not the typical signs of hypothyroidism and this is most likely caused by transplacental passage of some maternal thyroid hormone in addition to some residual neonatal thyroid function. Without treatment, symptoms may not be evident until after 4 months of age. Hypothyroidism is difficult to identify at birth, but high birth weight, hypothermia, delay in passing meconium, and neonatal jaundice are suggestive signs. Without treatment, symptoms include difficulty eating, hoarse cry, and protruding tongue caused by myxedema of oral tissues and vocal cords; hypotonic muscles of the abdomen with constipation, abdominal protrusion, and umbilical herniation; subnormal temperature; lethargy; excessive sleeping; slow pulse rate; and cold, mottled skin. Skeletal growth is stunted because of impaired protein synthesis, poor absorption of nutrients, and lack of bone mineralization. The individual will become dwarfed, with short limbs, if not treated (cretinism) (Figure 22-12). Dentition is often delayed. Mental retardation is a function of the severity of hypothyroidism and the delay before initiation of treatment.

Cord blood can be screened in the first days of life for T_4 and TSH levels. Neonatal screening has resulted in eradication of mental retardation related to CH where screening is available. Treatment is administration of T_4. The probability of normal growth and intellectual function is high if treatment is started within 2 weeks and before the child is 3 or 4 months old. The earlier TH replacement is initiated, the better the child's outcome. Permanent congenital hypothyroidism will require treatment for life.[66]

Thyroid Carcinoma. **Thyroid carcinoma** is the most common endocrine malignancy, accounting for 60,220 estimated new cases and 1850 estimated cancer deaths in 2013 in the United States, less than 4% of all neoplasms.[67] Exposure to ionizing radiation, especially during childhood, is the most consistent causal factor. Papillary and follicular thyroid carcinomas are the most frequent, and medullary and anaplastic thyroid carcinomas are less common. Most tumors are well differentiated.[68]

Most individuals with thyroid carcinoma have normal T_3 and T_4 levels and are therefore euthyroid. Thyroid cancer typically is discovered as a small thyroid nodule or as a metastatic tumor most commonly occurring in the regional lymph nodes, lungs, brain, or bone. Changes in voice and swallowing and difficulty in breathing are related to tumor growth impinging on the trachea or esophagus. The diagnosis of thyroid carcinoma is generally made by fine-needle aspiration of a thyroid nodule. Ultrasonographic characteristics may be suggestive of malignancy, and staging requires appropriate imaging.[69]

Treatment for well-differentiated thyroid carcinoma remains somewhat controversial mainly because of its protracted nature and the relatively low mortality regardless of the method of treatment. Treatment of well-differentiated tumors includes surgical dissection (e.g., a near-total or total thyroidectomy), postoperative radioactive iodine therapy to treat any microscopic residual tumor, and suppression of TSH with levothyroxine to replace TH and suppress TSH on any tumor cells.[68] Anaplastic thyroid carcinoma carries a grave prognosis, and palliation with surgical debulking, external beam radiotherapy, and chemotherapy may be offered.[70]

ALTERATIONS OF PARATHYROID FUNCTION

Hyperparathyroidism

Hyperparathyroidism is characterized by greater than normal secretion of parathyroid hormone (PTH) and hypercalcemia. Hyperparathyroidism is classified as primary, secondary, or tertiary. Calcium levels are either low or normal in secondary hyperparathyroidism. Normocalcemic hyperparathyroidism is characterized by increased levels of intact PTH, normal total and ionized serum calcium concentrations, and no underlying etiology. Increased PTH screening for osteoporosis has led to the development of this diagnosis. There may be tissue resistance to PTH or the elevated level of PTH may represent an early phase of primary hyperparathyroidism.[71]

PATHOPHYSIOLOGY. Primary hyperparathyroidism is usually a sporadic disease characterized by inappropriate excess secretion of PTH by one or more of the parathyroid glands. PTH secretion

TABLE 22-4 MANIFESTATIONS OF PRIMARY HYPERPARATHYROIDISM

SYMPTOMS	RESPONSIBLE DERANGEMENTS	MECHANISMS
Renal colic, nephrolithiasis, recurrent urinary tract infections, renal failure	Hypercalciuria, hyperphosphaturia, proximal renal tubular bicarbonate leak, urine pH >6	Calcium phosphate salts precipitate in alkaline urine, renal pelvis, and collecting ducts; calcium oxalate stones also formed
Abdominal pain, peptic ulcer disease	Hypercalcemia-stimulated hypergastrinemia	Elevated hydrochloric acid secretion
Pancreatitis	Hypercalcemia	Etiology of relationship unknown
Bone disease, osteitis fibrosa and osteitis cystica, osteoporosis	PTH-stimulated bone resorption, metabolic acidosis	Osteoporosis now more commonly encountered, but other disorders are more specific for hyperparathyroidism
Muscle weakness, myalgia	PTH excess, possible direct effect on striated muscle and on nerves	Characteristic myopathic changes in muscle histology (neuropathy of type I and type II muscle fibers)
Neurologic and psychiatric problems (impaired memory, confusion, depression, anxiety, psychosis)	Hypercalcemia	Neuropathy; electroencephalographic changes present
Polyuria, polydipsia	Hypercalcemia	Direct effect on renal tubule to decrease responsiveness to antidiuretic hormone
Constipation	Hypercalcemia	Decreased peristalsis of gastrointestinal tract
Anorexia, nausea, and vomiting	Hypercalcemia	Central stimulation of vomiting center
Hypertension	Renal disease, direct effect of calcium on arterial smooth muscle, pheochromocytoma	Plasma rennin activity elevated or normal
Arthralgia and arthritis	Gout, pseudogout, periarticular classification	Hyperuricemia, chronic renal failure with high calcium- phosphate product

Data from Flint PW et al: *Cummings otolaryngology: head & neck surgery,* ed 5, St Louis, 2010, Mosby.
PTH, Parathyroid hormone.

is increased and is not under the usual feedback control mechanisms. The calcium level in the blood increases because of increased bone resorption and gastrointestinal absorption of calcium, but fails to inhibit PTH secretion.

Primary hyperparathyroidism is one of the most common endocrine disorders: 80% to 85% of cases are caused by parathyroid adenomas, another 10% to 15% result from parathyroid hyperplasia, and approximately 1% are caused by parathyroid carcinoma.[72] Normal feedback mechanisms, such as elevated serum levels of ionized calcium, fail to normally inhibit PTH secretion by the parathyroid gland.

The cause of primary hyperparathyroidism is unknown; however, recent data suggest that there are two mechanisms for the development of this condition. The first is a monoclonal proliferation of parathyroid cells with a higher threshold for calcium feedback, and the second is generalized growth of parathyroid tissue. The former is most likely the cause of adenomas, and the latter is probably the cause for hyperplasia. There is also a familial form of the disease that includes a wide range of inherited endocrine disorders including multiple endocrine neoplasia syndromes (MEN-1 and MEN-2a).[73] Hypercalcemia and hypophosphatemia are the hallmarks of primary hyperparathyroidism. The effects of excessive PTH secretion and primary hyperparathyroidism on various organ systems are summarized in Table 22-4.

Secondary hyperparathyroidism is caused by an increase in PTH secondary to a chronic disease state, such as chronic kidney disease or intestinal malabsorption, which causes a decrease in serum ionized calcium levels (hypocalcemia) or chronic vitamin D deficiency. Hypercalcemia does not occur in secondary hyperparathyroidism because the parathyroid tissue is not autonomous and is only responding to a physiologic stimulus of hypocalcemia.

The most common cause of secondary hyperparathyroidism is chronic kidney disease (with failure of glomerular filtration), which results in hyperphosphatemia, reduced levels of activated vitamin D, and hypocalcemia, which stimulates PTH secretion. Disturbances in calcium and vitamin D metabolism that arise in chronic renal disease diminish activation of the parathyroid calcium-sensing receptor leading to increases in PTH secretion. Because vitamin D metabolism is impaired in kidney failure, eucalcemia cannot be restored unless vitamin D supplements are administered.[74] Other causes of secondary hyperparathyroidism include chronic vitamin D or calcium deficiency; decreased intestinal absorption of vitamin D or calcium; and ingestion of drugs, such as phenytoin, phenobarbital, and laxatives, which either accelerates the metabolism of vitamin D or decreases intestinal absorption of calcium.

Tertiary hyperparathyroidism is excessive secretion of PTH and hypercalcemia that occurs after long-standing secondary hyperparathyroidism. The etiology is unknown but represents autonomous secretion of PTH from persistent parathyroid stimulation even after withdrawal of calcium and calcitriol therapy. It develops in individuals with chronic secondary hyperparathyroidism and after renal transplantation.

Two other conditions must be differentiated from primary and secondary hyperparathyroidism. **Pseudohypoparathyroidism** is an inherited condition that presents with increased PTH levels, hypocalcemia, and hyperphosphatemia. These individuals are resistant to PTH and cannot produce cAMP in response to PTH (a postreceptor defect in PTH action).[75] **Familial hypocalciuric hypercalcemia (FHH)** is a benign autosomal dominant condition that can mimic hyperparathyroidism and is characterized by a high serum calcium level, low serum phosphate level, and low urine calcium excretion. It is caused by a mutation in the calcium-sensing receptor in the parathyroid gland. It can be differentiated from primary hyperparathyroidism by measurement of 24-hour urine calcium excretion.[76]

CLINICAL MANIFESTATIONS. Most individuals with primary hyperparathyroidism are asymptomatic. Hypercalcemia and hypophosphatemia commonly occur in primary hyperparathyroidism. Hypercalcemia may be asymptomatic or affected individuals may present with symptoms related to the muscular, nervous, and gastrointestinal systems, including fatigue, headache, depression, anorexia, and nausea and vomiting. There also is an increased risk for cardiovascular disease including hypertension.[77] Excessive osteoclastic and osteocytic activity resulting in bone resorption may cause pathologic fractures, kyphosis of the dorsal spine, and compression fractures of the vertebral bodies. (Bone resorption is discussed in Chapter 43.)

In primary hyperparathyroidism, hypercalcemia affects proximal renal tubular function, causing hypercalciuria, metabolic acidosis, and production of abnormally alkaline urine. PTH also enhances the renal excretion of phosphate, which results in hypophosphatemia (low serum phosphate concentration) and hyperphosphaturia (increased urine phosphate level). The combination of these three variables—hypercalciuria, alkaline urine, and hyperphosphaturia—predisposes the individual to the formation of calcium stones. Kidney stones are often formed in the renal pelvis or in the renal collecting ducts and may be associated with infections. Kidney stones and renal infection may lead to impaired renal function.[78] Hypercalcemia also impairs the concentrating ability of the renal tubule by decreasing its response to ADH. Chronic hypercalcemia of hyperparathyroidism is associated with mild insulin resistance, necessitating increased insulin secretion to maintain normal glucose levels. Hypercalcemia also affects the muscular, nervous, and gastrointestinal systems. Elevated levels of PTH increase the risk for cardiovascular disease.[79]

Secondary hyperparathyroidism caused by renal disease presents clinically not only with bone resorption but also with the symptoms of hypocalcemia and hyperphosphatemia. Hypocalcemia can cause many significant clinical problems (see Chapter 3). Hyperphosphatemia can cause deleterious effects on the cardiovascular system.[80]

EVALUATION AND TREATMENT. The concurrent findings of increased ionized calcium concentration in the face of elevated intact PTH level (which documents an abnormal feedback mechanism) are suggestive of primary hyperparathyroidism. Sestamibi (a radioisotope) scanning, CT, or ultrasound is used to localize adenomas before surgery.[81] Definitive treatment of severe primary hyperparathyroidism involves surgical removal of the solitary adenoma or, in the case of hyperplasia, complete removal of three and partial removal of the fourth hyperplastic parathyroid glands. In those individuals who fail surgery, other treatments such as bisphosphonates, corticosteroids, and calcimimetics (e.g., cinacalcet) may be considered. Calcimimetics increase the parathyroid calcium receptor sensitivity, thus lowering PTH levels.[82]

If hypercalcemia is documented but PTH levels are low, the differential diagnosis shifts to hypercalcemia of malignancy, granulomatous diseases (sarcoidosis), excessive calcium ingestion, or to hypervitaminosis A or D. Treatment of these conditions depends on the underlying cause.

If serum calcium level is low but PTH level is elevated, secondary hyperparathyroidism is likely. Evaluation for renal function frequently documents chronic renal disease. Treatment for secondary hyperparathyroidism in chronic kidney disease requires calcium replacement, dietary phosphate restriction and phosphate binders, and vitamin D replacement. Treatment also may include calcimimetics.[83]

Hypoparathyroidism

Hypoparathyroidism (abnormally low PTH levels) most commonly is caused by damage to the parathyroid glands during thyroid surgery and occurs because of the anatomic proximity of the parathyroid glands to the thyroid. Hypoparathyroidism also is associated with genetic syndromes, including familial hypoparathyroidism and DiGeorge syndrome (velocardiofacial syndrome) and an idiopathic or autoimmune form of the disease.[84] Hypomagnesemia also can cause a decrease in PTH secretion and function.[85]

PATHOPHYSIOLOGY. A lack of circulating PTH causes depressed serum calcium levels and increased serum phosphate levels. In the absence of PTH, resorption of calcium from bone and regulation of calcium reabsorption from the renal tubules are impaired. The phosphaturic effects of PTH are lost, resulting in hyperphosphatemia.

The effects of hypomagnesemia on the peripheral metabolism and clearance of PTH are not clearly understood. Once serum magnesium levels return to normal, however, PTH secretion returns to normal, as does the responsiveness of peripheral tissues to PTH. Hypomagnesemia may be related to chronic alcoholism, malnutrition, malabsorption, increased renal clearance of magnesium caused by the use of aminoglycoside antibiotics or certain chemotherapeutic agents, or prolonged magnesium-deficient parenteral nutritional therapy.

CLINICAL MANIFESTATIONS. Symptoms associated with hypoparathyroidism are related to hypocalcemia. Hypocalcemia causes a lowering of the threshold for nerve and muscle excitation so that a nerve impulse may be initiated by a slight stimulus anywhere along the length of a nerve or muscle fiber. This creates tetany manifested as muscle spasms, hyperreflexia, tonic-clonic convulsions, laryngeal spasms, and, in severe cases, death from asphyxiation. Chvostek and Trousseau signs may be used to evaluate for neuromuscular irritability. Chvostek sign is elicited by tapping the cheek, resulting in twitching of the upper lip. Trousseau sign is elicited by sustained inflation of a sphygmomanometer placed on the upper arm to a level above the systolic blood pressure with resultant painful carpal spasm.[85] Other symptoms of hypocalcemia are caused by mechanisms that are not yet understood. These symptoms include dry skin, loss of body and scalp hair, hypoplasia of developing teeth, horizontal ridges on the nails, cataracts, basal ganglia calcifications (which may be associated with a parkinsonian syndrome), and bone deformities, including brachydactyly and bowing of the long bones.

Phosphate retention caused by increased renal reabsorption of phosphate is associated also with hypoparathyroidism. Hyperphosphatemia is associated with inhibition of the renal enzyme necessary for the conversion of vitamin D to its most active form. This enzyme, 25-hydroxy-vitamin D 1α-hydroxylase, also is required by PTH. This tends to depress serum calcium levels further by reducing gastrointestinal absorption of calcium.

EVALUATION AND TREATMENT. A low serum calcium level and a high phosphorous level in the absence of renal failure, intestinal disorders, or nutritional deficiencies suggest hypoparathyroidism. Intact PTH levels are low in hypoparathyroidism, and measurement of serum magnesium and urinary calcium excretion can help in diagnosis.[85]

The treatment of hypoparathyroidism is directed toward the alleviation of hypocalcemia. In acute states this involves parenteral administration of calcium, which allows correction of serum calcium deficit within minutes. Maintenance of serum calcium level is achieved with pharmacologic doses of an active form of vitamin D and oral calcium. PTH hormone replacement therapy is being evaluated and results are encouraging.[86] Hypoplastic dentition, cataracts, bone deformities, and basal ganglia calcifications do not respond to the correction of hypocalcemia; however, the other symptoms of hypocalcemia are reversible.

As serum calcium levels return to normal, phosphaturia usually is stimulated. This leads to a return to normal serum phosphate levels. In some individuals, however, the absence of the phosphaturic effect of PTH causes a persistent hyperphosphatemia. Significant elevations of phosphorous concentration should be treated with drugs that inhibit gastrointestinal absorption of phosphate (phosphate binders).[85]

DYSFUNCTION OF THE ENDOCRINE PANCREAS: DIABETES MELLITUS

Diabetes mellitus (DM) is a group of metabolic diseases characterized by hyperglycemia resulting from defects in insulin secretion, insulin action, or both. It affects 8.3% of the U.S. population and 27% of Americans older than age 65.[87] The American Diabetes Association (ADA) classifies four categories of diabetes mellitus[88] (Table 22-5):

1. Type 1 (beta-cell destruction, usually leading to absolute insulin deficiency)
2. Type 2 (ranging from predominantly insulin resistance with relative insulin deficiency to predominantly an insulin secretory defect with insulin resistance)
3. Other specific types
4. Gestational diabetes

The diagnosis of diabetes mellitus is based on glycosylated hemoglobin (HbA_{1c}) levels, fasting plasma glucose (FPG) levels, 2-hour plasma glucose level during oral glucose tolerance testing (OGTT) using a 75-g oral glucose load, or random glucose

TABLE 22-5 CLASSIFICATION AND CHARACTERISTICS OF DIABETES MELLITUS

NAME	CHARACTERISTICS
Type 1	Cellular-mediated autoimmune destruction of pancreatic beta cells
Beta-cell destruction leading to absolute insulin deficiency; immune-mediated diabetes is most common form (≈90%)	Individual prone to ketoacidosis Little or no insulin secretion Insulin dependent 75% of individuals develop before 30 years of age; can occur up to the tenth decade Usually not obese
Idiopathic (≈10%)	No defined etiologies; absolute requirement for insulin replacement therapy in affected individuals may be sporadic
Type 2	Usually not insulin dependent but may be insulin requiring
May range from predominantly insulin resistant with relative insulin deficiency to predominantly secretory defect with insulin resistance	Individual not ketosis prone (but may form ketones under stress) Obesity common in the abdominal region Generally occurs in those older than 40 years, but the frequency is rapidly increasing in children Strong genetic predisposition Often associated with hypertension and dyslipidemia
Other Specific Types	
Genetic defects of beta-cell function	Genetic abnormalities that decrease the ability of the beta cell to secrete insulin: 1. Maturity-onset diabetes of youth (MODY) includes 6 specific autosomal dominant mutations including genes for hepatocyte nuclear factor-1α (HNF-1α; MODY 3), glucokinase (MODY 2), HNF-4α (MODY 1), insulin-promoter factor-1(IPF-1; MODY 4), HNF-1β (MODY 5), and NeuroD1 (MODY 6) 2. Defects in mitochondrial deoxyribonucleic acid (DNA) 3. Other (including an inability to convert proinsulin to insulin)
Genetic defects in insulin action	Mutations in the insulin receptor with hyperinsulinism or hyperglycemia or severe diabetes
Diseases of the exocrine pancreas	Any process that diffusely injures the pancreas, including pancreatitis, neoplasia, and cystic fibrosis
Endocrinopathies	Endocrine disorders including acromegaly, Cushing syndrome, glucagonoma, pheochromocytoma, hyperthyroidism, somatostatinoma, and aldosteronoma
Drug- or chemical-induced beta-cell dysfunction	Commonly associated drugs include glucocorticoids and thiazide diuretics, although many others may be implicated

TABLE 22-5 CLASSIFICATION AND CHARACTERISTICS OF DIABETES MELLITUS—cont'd

NAME	CHARACTERISTICS
Infections	Beta-cell destruction by viruses including cytomegalovirus, congenital rubella
Uncommon forms of immune-mediated diabetes mellitus	Anti–insulin receptor antibodies Reported with "stiff man syndrome" and individuals receiving interferon-α
Other genetic syndromes sometimes associated with diabetes mellitus	Down, Klinefelter, Turner, and Wolfram syndromes
Gestational Diabetes Mellitus (GDM)	
Any degree of glucose intolerance with onset or first recognition during pregnancy	Insulin resistance combined with inadequate insulin secretion in relation to hyperglycemia Women who are obese, older than 25 years of age, have a family history of diabetes, have a history of previous GDM, or are of certain ethnic groups (Hispanic, Native American, Asian, or African American) are at increased risk of developing GDM The metabolic stress of pregnancy may uncover a genetic tendency for type 2 diabetes mellitus

Data from Agency for Healthcare Research & Quality, U.S. Preventive Services Task Force (USPSTF): *Screening for gestational diabetes mellitus recommendation statement,* May 2008. Available at www.ahrq.gov/clinic/uspstf08/gestdiab/gdrs.htm; American Diabetes Association (Committee Report): *Diabetic Care* 26(Suppl 1):S5–S20, 2003.

BOX 22-1 DIAGNOSTIC CRITERIA FOR DIABETES MELLITUS

1. HbA_{1c} (as measured in a DCCT-referenced assay) ≥6.5%*

OR

2. FPG ≥126 mg/dl (7.0 mmol/L); fasting is defined as no caloric intake for at least 8 hr*

OR

3. 2-hr plasma glucose ≥200 mg/dl (11.1 mmol/L) during an OGTT*

OR

4. In a patient with classic symptoms of hyperglycemia or hyperglycemic crisis, a random plasma glucose ≥200 mg/dl (11.1 mmol/L)

Categories of Increased Risk for Diabetes

1. FPG 100 to 125 mg/dl
2. 2-hr PG in the range of 75 to 199 mg/dl during an OGTT
3. HbA_{1c} 5.7% to 6.4%

From American Diabetes Association: *Diabetes Care* 33:S62–S69, 2010.

*In the absence of unequivocal hyperglycemia, criteria 1 through 3 should be confirmed by repeat testing.

DCCT, Diabetes Control and Complications Trial; *FPG,* fasting plasma glucose; *HbA_{1c},* hemoglobin A_{1c}; *hr,* hour(s); *OGTT,* oral glucose tolerance test; *PG,* plasma glucose.

levels in an individual with symptoms (Box 22-1). Glycosylated hemoglobin refers to the permanent attachment of glucose to hemoglobin molecules and reflects the average plasma glucose exposure over the life of a red blood cell (approximately 120 days).

The ADA classification "...categories at increased risk for diabetes..."[88] describes nondiabetic elevations of HbA_{1c}, FPG, or the 2-hour plasma glucose value during OGTT (see Box 22-1). This classification includes impaired glucose tolerance (IGT), which results from diminished insulin secretion, and impaired fasting glucose (IFG), which is caused by enhanced hepatic glucose output. Individuals with IGT and IFG are at increased risk of cardiovascular disease and premature death and carry a 3% to 7% yearly risk of developing diabetes.[88]

Types of Diabetes Mellitus

Type 1 Diabetes Mellitus

Although type 2 diabetes affects a larger percentage of children and adolescents each year, **type 1 diabetes mellitus** remains the most common form of diabetes in those under age 12, affecting 1 in 300 individuals in the United States. Diagnosis is rare during the first 9 months of life and peaks at 12 years of age. It is the result of a loss of beta cells in the pancreatic islets. Table 22-6 summarizes the epidemiology of diabetes mellitus (DM).

PATHOPHYSIOLOGY. Two distinct types of type 1 diabetes have been identified: autoimmune and nonimmune. In autoimmune-mediated diabetes mellitus, environmental-genetic factors are thought to trigger cell-mediated destruction of pancreatic beta cells. Autoimmune type 1 diabetes is called *type 1A.* Nonimmune type 1 diabetes is far less common than autoimmune. It occurs secondary to other diseases, such as pancreatitis, or to a more fulminant disorder termed *idiopathic (type 1B) diabetes.* Type 1B diabetes occurs mostly in people of Asian or African descent and affected individuals have varying degrees of insulin deficiency.

Genetic Susceptibility. Between 10% and 13% of individuals with newly diagnosed type 1 diabetes have a first-degree relative (parent or sibling) with type 1 diabetes. There is a 50% concordance rate in twins.[89] The exact nature of genetic susceptibility to type 1A diabetes is not clearly understood. The strongest association is with major histocompatibility complex, or MHC (histocompatibility leukocyte antigen [HLA] class II alleles HLA-DQ and HLA-DR). Numerous other mutations involving single genes both within and outside of the MHC complex have been associated with an increased risk of type 1 DM.[90]

Environmental Factors. Environmental factors are thought to have a significant contribution to the development of type 1 diabetes mellitus. Several types of viral infections have been implicated with autoimmune damage to beta cells, especially enteroviruses, although a cause-and-effect relationship has not yet been proven[91,92] (see What's New? The Role of Viruses in the Etiology of Type 1 Diabetes). Exposure to other infectious

TABLE 22-6 EPIDEMIOLOGY AND ETIOLOGY OF DIABETES MELLITUS IN THE UNITED STATES

	TYPE 1 DIABETES: PRIMARY BETA-CELL DEFECT OR FAILURE	TYPE 2 DIABETES: INSULIN RESISTANCE WITH INADEQUATE INSULIN SECRETION
Incidence		
Frequency	One of the most common childhood diseases (5-10% of all cases of diabetes mellitus) Prevalence rate is 0.17%	Accounts for most cases (≈90-95%) Prevalence rate for ages 45-64 yr is 10.5%, for ages 65-74 yr is 18.4%
Change in incidences	No documented increase in incidence in the United States	Incidence in all age groups has doubled since 1980
Characteristics		
Age at onset	Peak onset at age 11-13 yr (slightly earlier for girls than for boys) Rare in children younger than 1 yr and adults older than 30 yr	Risk of developing diabetes increases after age 40 yr; in general, incidence increases with age into the 70s; among Pima Indians, incidence peaks between ages 40 and 50 yr, then falls
Gender	Similar in males and females	Similar in males and females overall, although black females have the highest incidence and prevalence of all groups
Racial distribution	Rates for whites 1.5-2 times higher than those for nonwhites Higher rates for those of Scandinavian descent than for those of central or southern European descent	Risk is highest for blacks and Native Americans
Obesity	Generally normal or underweight	Frequent contributing factor to precipitate type 2 diabetes among those susceptible; a major factor in populations recently exposed to westernized environment Increased risk related to duration, degree, and distribution of obesity
Etiology		
Common theory	*Autoimmune:* Genetic and environmental factors, resulting in gradual process of autoimmune destruction in genetically susceptible individuals *Nonautoimmune:* Unknown Strong association with *HLA-DQA* and *HLA-DQB* genes	Disease results from genetic susceptibility (polygenic) combined with environmental determinants and other risk factors; inherited defects in beta-cell mass and function combined with peripheral tissue insulin resistance Associated with long-duration obesity
Heredity	Risk to sibling: 5-10% Risk to offspring: 2-5%	Risk to first-degree relative (child or sibling): 10-15%
Presence of antibody	Islet cell autoantibodies (ICAs) and/or autoantibodies to insulin, and autoantibodies to glutamic acid decarboxylase (GAD_{65}) and tyrosine phosphatases IA-2 and IA-2β are present in 85-90% of individuals when fasting; hyperglycemia is initially detected	Islet cell antibodies not prevalent
Insulin resistance	Insulin resistance at diagnosis is unusual, but insulin resistance may occur as the individual ages and gains weight	Insulin resistance is generally caused by altered cellular metabolism and an intracellular postreceptor defect
Insulin secretion	Severe insulin deficiency or no insulin secretion at all	Typically increased at time of diagnosis, but progressively declines over the course of the illness

Data from American Diabetes Association: *Diabetic Care* 30(Suppl 1):S42–S47, 2007.

WHAT'S NEW?

The Role of Viruses in the Etiology of Type 1 Diabetes

The etiology of type 1 diabetes is believed to be the result of genetic and environmental interactions. The role of viral infection in the etiology of type 1 diabetes continues to be debated. The most recent studies focus on the association between type 1 diabetes and enteroviruses, especially coxsackieviruses B (CV-B). Enteroviruses have been implicated both epidemiologically and immunologically. In one recent study, type 1 diabetes incidence was found to have increased after epidemics because of enteroviruses; in addition, enteroviral RNA can be detected in the blood of more than half of individuals with type 1 diabetes at the time of diagnosis. Enteroviruses can infect pancreatic beta cells and establish persistent infection. This is postulated to initiate both innate and adaptive immune responses with consequent effects ranging from functional damage to cell death. T-cytotoxic T cells play an important role in the autoimmune destruction of beta cells, and enteroviruses are potent stimulators of T-cytotoxic cell activation. Another postulated mechanism by which enteroviral infection might induce beta-cell autoimmunity is by infecting thymic epithelial cells, resulting in an increase in autoreactive thymocytes. Further investigation into the relationship between viral infection and type 1 diabetes may lead to prevention or treatment through vaccination or immune modulation.

Data from Coppieters KT, von Herrath MG: *Clin Rev Allergy Immunol* 41(2):169–178, 2011; Galleri L et al: *Adv Exp Med Biol* 771:252–271, 2012; Grieco FA et al: *Clin Exp Immunol* 168(1):24–29, 2012; Hober D et al: *Clin Exp Immunol* 168(1):47–51, 2012; Lind K, Huhn MH, Flodstrom-Tullberg M: *Clin Exp Immunol* 168(1):30–38, 2012; Stene LC, Rewers M: *Clin Exp Immunol* 168(1):12–23, 2012.

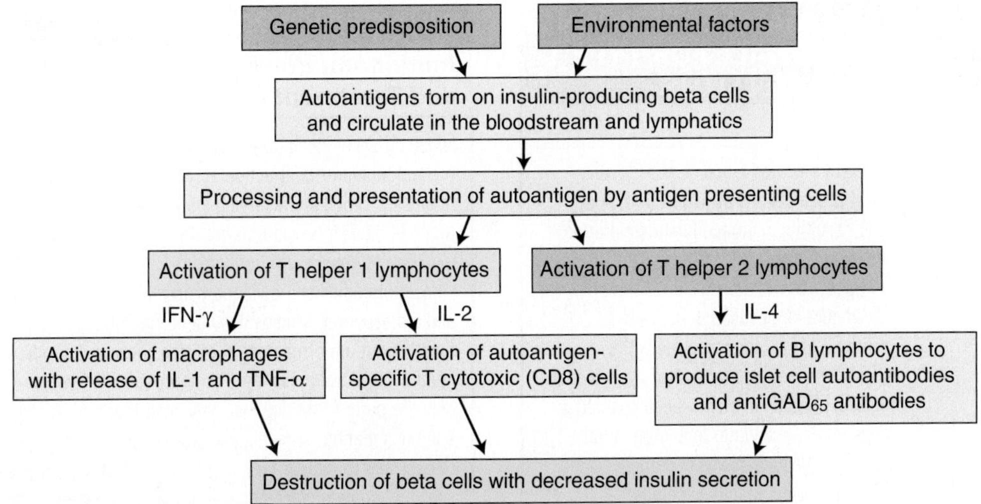

FIGURE 22-13 **Pathophysiology of Type 1 Diabetes Mellitus.** *GAD_{65},* Glutamic acid decarboxylase; *IFN-γ,* interferon-gamma; *IL,* interleukin; *TNF-α,* tumor necrosis factor-alpha.

microorganisms (such as *Helicobacter pylori*), exposure to cow's milk proteins, and a relative lack of vitamin D also have been implicated.[93,94] Despite intensive research, the number of identified possible environmental factors remains small.

Immunologically Mediated Destruction of Beta Cells. Type 1 diabetes mellitus is a slowly progressive autoimmune T cell–mediated disease that occurs in genetically susceptible individuals (Figure 22-13 and see Chapter 9). The destruction of beta cells progresses through the following stages:

1. *Lymphocyte and macrophage infiltration of the islets resulting in inflammation (insulinitis) and islet beta-cell death.* Autoantigens are expressed on the surface of pancreatic islet cells and circulate in the bloodstream and lymphatics (see Figure 22-13). Circulating autoantigens are ingested by antigen-presenting cells that activate CD4+ T helper 1 (Th1) lymphocytes.[95] The activated T helper lymphocytes secrete interleukin-2 (IL-2) that activates beta-cell autoantigen-specific T cytotoxic lymphocytes, causing them to proliferate and attack islet cells through secretion of toxic perforins and granzymes.[96] T helper lymphocytes also secrete interferon that activates macrophages and stimulates the release of inflammatory cytokines (including IL-1 and tumor necrosis factor [TNF]), which cause further beta-cell destruction and apoptosis.[97]
2. *Production of autoantibodies against islet cells, insulin, glutamic acid decarboxylase (GAD), and other cytoplasmic proteins.* Activated T helper 2 (Th2) lymphocytes produce IL-4, which stimulates B lymphocytes to proliferate and produce antibodies (see Figure 22-13). Islet cell autoantibodies (ICAs) precede evidence of beta-cell deficiency and can be found in the serum years before symptoms occur.[98] Anti–glutamic acid decarboxylase (antiGAD$_{65}$) antibodies (an enzyme in beta cells that is involved in coordinating insulin release) are more persistent, which makes them clinically useful in differentiating the etiology of diabetes in a given individual. Autoantibodies against insulin (insulin autoantibodies [IAAs]) also have been noted. It is likely that IAAs may form during the process of active islet cell and beta-cell destruction.[99] Finally, another islet antigen against which antibodies are produced in type 1 diabetes can now be measured in the serum. It is called the zinc transporter 8 (Znt8) protein and is associated with variation in disease progression.[100,101]

An additional autommune mechanism being explored in the pathogenesis of type 1 diabetes is a relative inactivity of T regulatory cells. These T lymphocytes normally serve to inhibit the immune response and maintain self tolerance.[102] Over time these immune mechanisms lead to a decrease in beta-cell mass and insulin production.

Hyperglycemia, Glucagon, and Hyperketonemia. Before hyperglycemia occurs, 80% to 90% of the function of the insulin-secreting beta cells in the islet of Langerhans must be lost. Beta-cell abnormalities are present long before the acute clinical onset of type 1 diabetes.

A disequilibrium of hormones produced by the islets of Langerhans occurs in diabetes mellitus. Alpha-cell and beta-cell functions are abnormal. Lack of insulin and amylin (produced by beta cells) and a relative excess of glucagon (produced by alpha cells) exist in type 1 diabetes. The ratio of insulin to glucagon in the portal vein controls hepatic glucose and fat metabolism. The paracrine action of insulin and amylin normally suppresses secretion of glucagon. Considerable data have documented that high levels of glucagon relative to insulin levels contribute to the generation of hyperglycemia and hyperketonemia. Thus, both alpha-cell and beta-cell functions are abnormal and both a lack of insulin and amylin and a relative excess of glucagon contribute to hyperglycemia in type 1 diabetes. Relative hyperglucagonemia occurs in every form of diabetes mellitus, leading some researchers to suggest that it is important in propagating the metabolic abnormalities in diabetes.[103-105]

CLINICAL MANIFESTATIONS. Historically, type 1 diabetes mellitus has been thought to have an abrupt onset. It is now known, however, that the natural history involves a long preclinical

TABLE 22-7 CLINICAL MANIFESTATIONS AND RATIONALE FOR TYPE 1 DIABETES MELLITUS

MANIFESTATIONS	RATIONALE
Polydipsia	Because of elevated blood glucose levels, water is osmotically attracted from body cells, resulting in intracellular dehydration and hypothalamic stimulation of thirst
Polyuria	Hyperglycemia acts as an osmotic diuretic; the amount of glucose filtered by the glomeruli of the kidneys exceeds the amount that can be reabsorbed by the renal tubules; glycosuria results, accompanied by large amounts of water lost in the urine
Polyphagia	Depletion of cellular stores of carbohydrates, fats, and protein results in cellular starvation and a corresponding increase in hunger
Weight loss	Weight loss occurs because of fluid loss in osmotic diuresis and the loss of body tissue as fat and proteins are used for energy as a result of the effects of insulin deficiency
Fatigue	Metabolic changes result in poor use of food products, contributing to lethargy and fatigue; sleep loss from severe nocturia also contributes to fatigue

WHAT'S NEW?

Immunomodulation in the Prevention and Treatment of Type 1 Diabetes

Many different kinds of immunologic approaches are being tested to prevent the autoimmune destruction of beta cells in type 1 diabetes. These treatments are aimed at preserving insulin synthesis early in the course of disease. Some of these interventions create generalized immunosuppression, including mycophenolate mofetil, monoclonal antibodies to B cells (rituximab), monoclonal antibodies to T cells (otelixizumab, teplizumab), interleukin-1 blockade, and cyclosporine. Studies document their effectiveness in stabilizing beta-cell function but, unfortunately, they also cause many side effects. More focused immunologic therapies are "antigen specific," which means they suppress only the parts of the immune response that are attacking the beta cells. One approach that has shown some promising (but mixed) results has been the use of vaccines to induce T-regulatory cells that suppress the immune attack on specific antigens. Vaccines that have been tested so far include insulin, glutamic acid decarboxylase 65 (GAD-Alum), and heatshock proteins (DiaPep277). Another ambitious new approach to preserving beta-cell function is through the introduction of stem cells, which decrease autoimmune responses and may engraft and become insulin-producing beta cells.

Data from Chen W, Xie A, Chan L: *Transl Res* 161(4):217–229, 2013; Godfrey KJ et al: *Diabetic Med* 29(1):14–23, 2012; Li CR, Baaten BJ, Bradley LM: *J Mol Cell Biol* 4(1):38–47, 2012; Ludvigsson J et al: *N Engl J Med* 366(5):433–442, 2012; Miller SA, St Onge E: *Exp Opin Biol Ther* 11(11):1525–1532, 2011; Pozzilli P et al: *Curr Pharm Design* 17(29):3224–3228, 2011; Sherry N et al: *Lancet* 378:487–497, 2011; Tooley JE, Waldron-Lynch F, Herold KC: *Trends Mol Med* 18(3):173–181, 2012; Zhao Y et al: *BMC Med* 10:3, 2012.

period with gradual destruction of beta cells, eventually leading to insulin deficiency and hyperglycemia. Generally, this latent period is longer in older individuals with type 1 diabetes and often results in misclassification of those affected as having type 2 diabetes.

Type 1 diabetes mellitus affects the metabolism of fat, protein, and carbohydrates. Glucose accumulates in the blood and appears in the urine as the renal threshold for glucose is exceeded, producing an osmotic diuresis and symptoms of polyuria and polydipsia. Wide fluctuations in blood glucose levels occur. In addition, protein and fat breakdown occur because of the lack of insulin, resulting in weight loss (Table 22-7).

Insulin normally stimulates lipogenesis and inhibits lipolysis, thus preventing fat catabolism. With insulin deficiency, lipolysis is enhanced and there is an increase in the amount of nonesterified fatty acids delivered to the liver. The consequence is increased glyconeogenesis contributing to hyperglycemia. In the absence of insulin, the release of free fatty acids from adipocytes increases production of ketone bodies (acetoacetate, hydroxybutyrate, and acetone) by the mitochondria of the liver at a rate that exceeds peripheral use. Accumulation of ketone bodies causes a drop in pH and triggers the buffering system associated with metabolic acidosis. Diabetic ketoacidosis (DKA), caused by increased levels of circulating ketones in the absence of the antilipolytic effect of insulin, may occur (p. 744).

EVALUATION AND TREATMENT. The criteria for diagnosis of type 1 diabetes are the same as those for type 2 diabetes (see Box 22-1). The diagnosis of diabetes is not difficult when the symptoms of polydipsia, polyuria, polyphagia, weight loss, and hyperglycemia are present in fasting and postprandial states. C-peptide, a component of proinsulin released during insulin production, can be measured in the serum as a surrogate for insulin levels and is indicative of residual beta-cell mass and function. Other important aspects of evaluation include assessing for evidence of the chronic complications of type 1 diabetes, including renal, nervous system, cardiac, peripheral vascular, retinal, and bony tissue damage.

Nearly half of children aged 4 years and younger and nearly one fourth of those between the ages of 5 and 15 with type 1 diabetes are first diagnosed when they present with the signs and symptoms of DKA.[106] In DKA, acetone (a volatile form of ketones) is exhaled by hyperventilation and gives the breath a sweet or "fruity" odor. Occasionally, diabetic coma is the initial symptom of the disease.

Many different kinds of approaches are being tested to prevent the autoimmune destruction of beta cells that is characteristic of type 1 diabetes. Avoidance of cow's milk, utilization of a gluten-free diet, and increased intake of omega-3 fatty acids and vitamin D are all being explored.[107] Pharmacologic prevention trials include immunosuppression with antirejection drugs (e.g., mycophenolate mofetil, rituximab, monoclonal antibodies to CD3, and cyclosporine), immunomodulation therapies, and oral or intranasal insulin[108] (see What's New? Immunomodulation in the Prevention and Treatment of Type 1 Diabetes).

Treatment regimens are designed to achieve optimal glucose control (as measured by the HbA_{1c} value) without causing episodes of significant hypoglycemia. Successful management

BOX 22-2 CRITERIA FOR THE DIAGNOSIS OF METABOLIC SYNDROME

Three of the following five traits:

- Increased waist circumference (>40 inches in men; >35 inches in women)
- Plasma triglycerides ≥150 mg/dl
- Plasma high-density lipoprotein (HDL) cholesterol <40 mg/dl (men) or <50 mg/dl (women)
- Blood pressure ≥130/85 mmHg
- Fasting plasma glucose ≥100 mg/dl

Data from Grundy SM et al: *Circulation* 109:433–438, 2004.

requires individual planning according to type of disease, age, and activity level. All individuals with type 1 diabetes require some combination of insulin supplementation, meal planning, exercise program, and self-monitoring of blood glucose level. Several different types of insulin preparations are available, as well as new technologies for more physiologic insulin delivery systems, such as modern insulin pumps.[109] The use of pramlintide, a synthetic analog of amylin, can replace this hormone in individuals with type 1 and type 2 diabetes.[110] Blood glucose monitoring is an essential part of management and there are numerous types of monitoring devices for both self and "real-time" blood glucose monitoring.[111] Individuals also should be screened at least yearly for complications of diabetes. Finally, islet cell and whole pancreas transplantation has been successful in selected individuals.

Type 2 Diabetes Mellitus

Type 2 diabetes mellitus is much more common than type 1 and has been rising in incidence since 1940. In the United States, type 2 diabetes affects 10.5% of those aged 45 to 64 years and 18.4% of those aged 65 to 74 years, and has doubled in all adult age groups in the past two decades.[112] Prevalence varies by ethnic group and gender and is highest in African American women with an overall prevalence of 34% in those aged 65 to 74. There also is a greatly increased prevalence of type 2 diabetes in children, especially in Native American and obese children (see Table 22-6).

An environmental-genetic interaction appears to be responsible for type 2 diabetes.[113] The most well-recognized risk factors are age, obesity, hypertension, physical inactivity, and family history. The *metabolic syndrome* is a constellation of disorders (central obesity, dyslipidemia, prehypertension, and an elevated fasting blood glucose level) that together confer a high risk of developing type 2 diabetes and associated cardiovascular complications (Box 22-2). The metabolic syndrome develops during childhood and is highly prevalent among overweight children and adolescents and affects approximately 55 million Americans. These individuals should be screened on a regular basis for diabetes mellitus. Early recognition and treatment, including vigorous lifestyle changes, are critical to reducing cardiovascular events and improving clinical outcomes.[114] Polycystic ovary syndrome (PCOS) also is associated with insulin resistance and risk of diabetes seven times the average risk for women without PCOS.[115]

PATHOPHYSIOLOGY. Many organs contribute to the insulin resistance and chronic hyperglycemia associated with type 2 diabetes mellitus (Figure 22-14). Additionally, genes have been identified that are associated with type 2 diabetes, including those that code for beta-cell mass, beta-cell function (ability to sense blood glucose levels, insulin synthesis, and insulin secretion), proinsulin and insulin molecular structure, insulin receptors, hepatic synthesis of glucose, glucagon synthesis, and cellular responsiveness to insulin stimulation. Genetic abnormalities also are the result of epigenetic changes that occur in response to environmental influences that span generations.[116,117] The combination of genetic, epigenetic, and environmental influences results in the basic pathophysiologic mechanisms of type 2 diabetes: insulin resistance and decreased insulin secretion by beta cells (Figure 22-15). All of these mechanisms are essential to the development of type 2 diabetes. Although many individuals with risk factors for type 2 diabetes (including obesity, metabolic syndrome, and hypertension) are insulin resistant, only those individuals who are genetically predisposed to beta-cell dysfunction (and therefore a relative deficiency in insulin) will develop type 2 diabetes.[118]

Insulin resistance is defined as a suboptimal response of insulin-sensitive tissues (especially liver, muscle, and adipose tissue) to insulin. Several mechanisms are involved in abnormalities of the insulin signaling pathway and contribute to insulin resistance. These include an abnormality of the insulin molecule, high amounts of insulin antagonists, down-regulation of the insulin receptor, decreased or abnormal activation of post-receptor kinases, and alteration of glucose transporter (GLUT) proteins. Obesity is present in 60% to 80% of those with type 2 diabetes and is a major contributor to insulin resistance through several important mechanisms:

1. Adipokines are hormones produced in adipose tissue. A nuclear receptor, called peroxisome proliferator–activated receptor gamma (PPARγ), is highly expressed in adipose cells and is responsible for modulating changes in adipokines in obese individuals, including increased serum levels of leptin (leptin resistance) and resistin and decreased levels of adiponectin. Changes in adipokines have effects not only on tissues but also on hypothalamic and pancreatic function.[119,120] A group of insulin-sensitizing drugs, called the thiazolidinediones that modulate PPARγ activity, have been used in the treatment of type 2 diabetes for many years.
2. Elevated levels of serum free fatty acids (FFAs) and intracellular deposits of triglycerides and cholesterol are found in obese individuals who have what has been termed "metabolic overload" (high caloric and lipid intake). FFAs bind to G-protein–coupled receptors, which modulate several responses. These changes interfere with intracellular insulin signaling, decrease tissue responses to insulin, cause alterations in insulin incretin and glucagon secretion, and promote inflammation.[121]
3. Obesity causes release of inflammatory cytokines (TNF-α, IL-6) from intra-abdominal adipocytes or adipocyte-associated mononuclear cells and from activated macrophages in other tissues. These cytokines

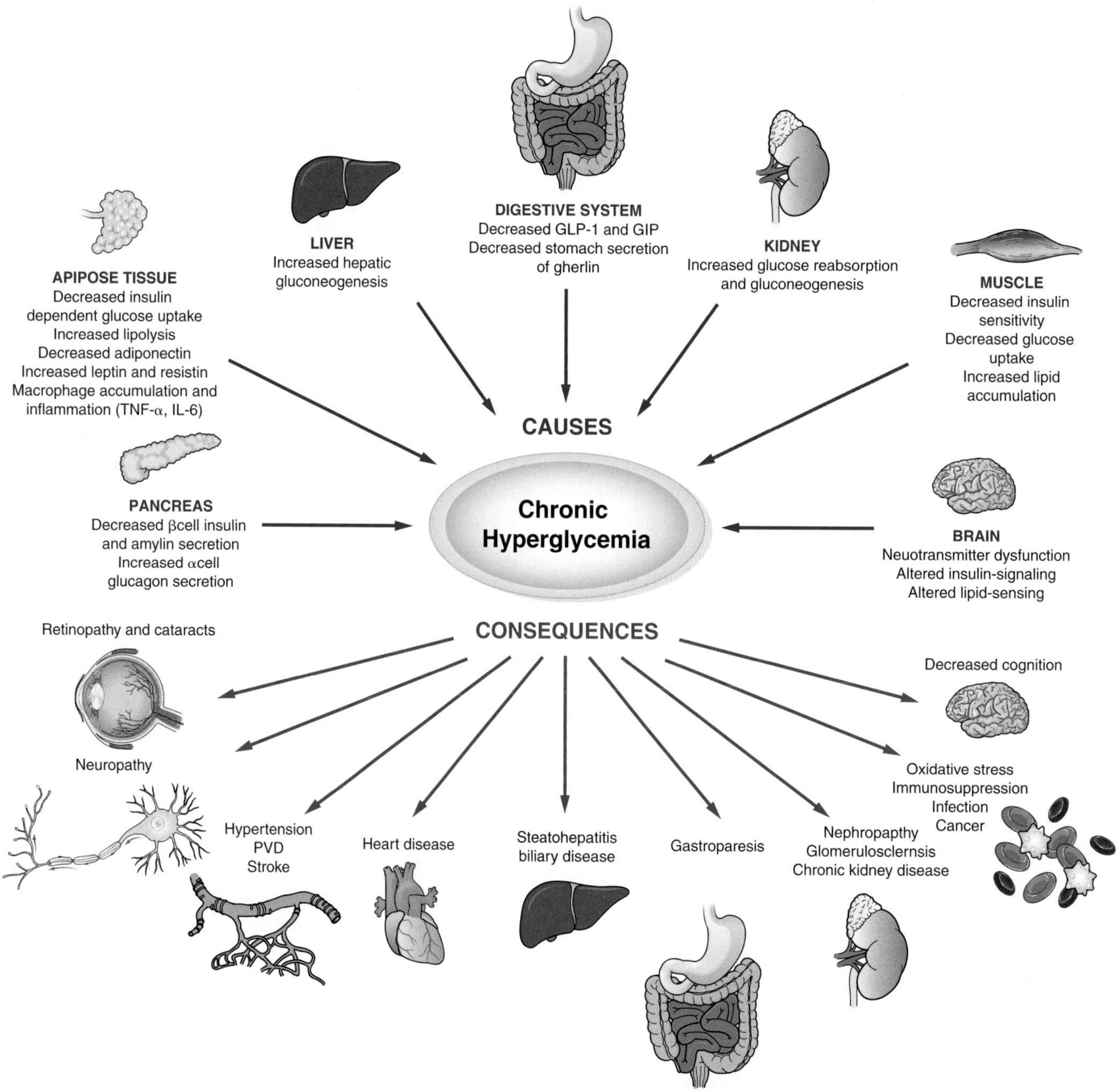

APIPOSE TISSUE
Decreased insulin dependent glucose uptake
Increased lipolysis
Decreased adiponectin
Increased leptin and resistin
Macrophage accumulation and inflammation (TNF-α, IL-6)
LIVER
Increased hepatic gluconeogenesis
DIGESTIVE SYSTEM
Decreased GLP-1 and GIP
Decreased stomach secretion of gherlin
KIDNEY
Increased glucose reabsorption and gluconeogenesis
MUSCLE
Decreased insulin sensitivity
Decreased glucose uptake
Increased lipid accumulation
CAUSES
PANCREAS
Decreased βcell insulin and amylin secretion
Increased αcell glucagon secretion
Chronic Hyperglycemia
BRAIN
Neuotransmitter dysfunction
Altered insulin-signaling
Altered lipid-sensing
CONSEQUENCES
Retinopathy and cataracts
Neuropathy
Hypertension
PVD
Stroke
Heart disease
Steatohepatitis
biliary disease
Gastroparesis
Nephropapthy
Glomerulosclernsis
Chronic kidney disease
Decreased cognition
Oxidative stress
Immunosuppression
Infection
Cancer

FIGURE 22-14 Multiorgan Causes and Common Consequences of Chronic Hyperglycemia in Type 2 Diabetes Mellitus. *IL*, Interleukin; *PVD*, Peripheral vascular disease; *TNF*, Tumor necrosis factor.

Genetic predisposition
Obesity
Diet, inactivity
Adipokines, ↑free fatty acids inflammatory cytokines
↓Activity of ghrelin
↓Beta cell mass and function
Insulin resistance
↓Activity of incretins
↑Demand for insulin synthesis
↓Amylin
Hypoinsulinemia
Hyperinsulinemia
↑Glucagon
Tissue effects and hyperglycemia (type 2 diabetes)
Tissue effects without hyperglycemia (insulin resistance without diabetes)

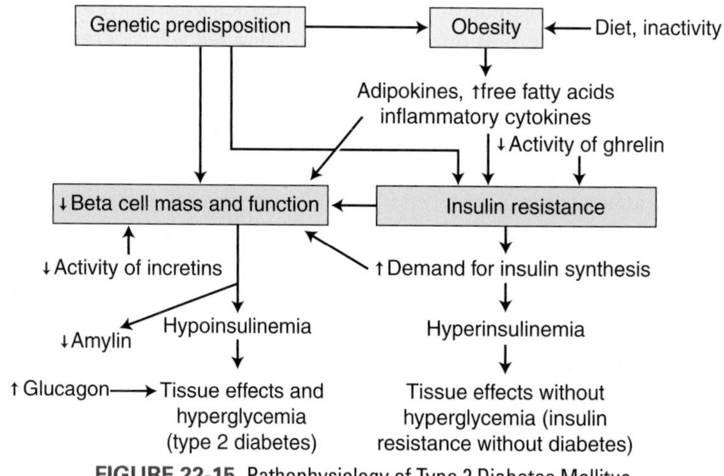

FIGURE 22-15 Pathophysiology of Type 2 Diabetes Mellitus.

induce insulin resistance through a postreceptor mechanism and play an important role in the genesis of fatty liver, atherosclerosis and dyslipidemia.[122,123]

4. Alterations in oxidative phosphorylation in cellular mitochondria have been documented, resulting in reduced insulin-stimulated mitochondrial activity and insulin resistance, especially in skeletal muscle and hepatocytes.[124,125]
5. Obesity is correlated with hyperinsulinemia and decreased insulin receptor density.

In most individuals with type 2 diabetes, compensatory hyperinsulinemia prevents the clinical appearance of diabetes for many years. Eventually, however, islet cell dysfunction develops and leads to a relative deficiency of insulin activity. **Beta-cell dysfunction** is caused, in part, by a decrease in beta-cell mass. A progressive decrease in the weight and number of beta cells occurs in type 2 diabetes, and several different mechanisms have been implicated. Beta cells are extremely sensitive to high levels of glucose and free fatty acids and, under these so-called glucolipotoxic conditions, beta-cell endoplasmic reticulum function is interrupted and beta cells undergo apoptotic cell death.[126] Beta-cell dysfunction also is caused by inflammation and changes in adipokines. A variety of inflammatory cytokines, including TNF-α, IL-1β, and IL6, also have been shown to be toxic to beta cells, and autoimmune beta-cell destruction has been described in type 2 diabetes.[127] The adipokine leptin decreases insulin synthesis in the beta cell. Thus many of the obesity-related causes of insulin resistance (elevated free fatty acid [FFA] hyperglycemia, adipokines, and inflammatory cytokines) also promote programmed cell death in beta cells.

Glucagon is a hormone produced by the alpha cells of the pancreas and acts primarily in the liver to increase blood glucose level by stimulating glycogenolysis and gluconeogenesis. Glucagon acts as an antagonist to insulin. In healthy individuals, high glucose levels cause glucagon release to be inhibited. As in type 1 diabetes, pancreatic alpha cells in type 2 diabetes are less responsive to glucose inhibition, resulting in increased glucagon secretion. These abnormally high levels of glucagon have long been known to play a role in the increased hepatic production of glucose and resultant hyperglycemia seen in type 2 diabetes.[103,128]

Amylin (islet amyloid polypeptide) is another beta-cell hormone that is decreased in both type 1 and type 2 diabetes. Amylin increases satiety and suppresses glucagon release from the alpha cells. It also contributes to islet cell destruction through the deposition of abnormal (misfolded) amyloid polypeptide in the pancreas.[129,130] Pramlintide, a synthetic analog of amylin, is used for treatment in both type 1 and type 2 diabetes.[104,131]

The **incretins, glucagon-like peptide-1 (GLP-1)** and **glucose-dependent insulinotropic polypeptide (GIP),** are a class of peptides released from the gastrointestinal tract in response to food intake. They increase the sensitivity of beta cells to circulating glucose levels, thus improving insulin responsiveness to meals. They are then inactivated by the enzyme **dipeptidyl peptidase IV (DPP-IV)**. These peptides are important in maintaining glycemic control, and currently two GLP-1 agonists and four DPP-IV inhibitors are approved for use in the United States[131,132] (see What's New? Incretin-Based Therapies for Diabetes Mellitus).

WHAT'S NEW?

Incretin-Based Therapies for Diabetes Mellitus

The incretin hormone system is being explored as a possible therapeutic target in diabetes. Incretin hormones are secreted by enteroendocrine cells of the large and small intestines. The major component of this system, glucagon-like peptide-1 (GLP-1), has many positive effects on glucose metabolism. GLP-1 augments glucose-dependent insulin secretion without causing hypoglycemia, stimulates insulin gene expression, inhibits glucagon secretion, delays gastric emptying, and induces a feeling of satiety through an effect on the central nervous system. GLP-1 also has been shown to induce new beta-cell differentiation (neogenesis) from pancreatic ductal cells and to protect beta cells from apoptosis (programmed cell death). There are two classes of incretin-related therapies: GLP-1 receptor agonists (GLP-1 RAs) and dipeptidyl peptidase IV (DPP-IV) inhibitors. Two incretin GLP-1 RAs (exenatide and liraglutide) are approved for use in the United States and three are in development. They lower postprandial plasma glucose level with little risk of hypoglycemia, assist individuals with weight loss, and augment endogenous insulin secretion. A recent study documented that nearly two thirds of persons treated with GLP-1 RAs alone achieved target HbA_{1c} levels after 12 weeks of therapy. The available DPP-IV inhibitors (sitagliptin, saxagliptin, vildagliptin, and linagliptin) also improve metabolic control but to a lesser degree than the GLP-1 RAs; however, they have been shown to improve levels of serum lipids. Both classes are well tolerated: GLP-1 RAs are associated with nausea and DPP-IV inhibitors are associated with headaches and certain infections. Pancreatitis has been reported in both but appears to be a rare complication.

Data from Blonde L, Montanya E: *Diabetes Obes Metab* 14(Suppl 2):20–32, 2012; Esposito K et al: *Diabetes Obes Metab* 14(3):228–233, 2012; Israili ZH: *Am J Ther* 18(2):117–152, 2011; Karagiannis T et al: *BMJ* 344:e1369, 2012; Monami M et al: *Adv Therapy* 29(1):14–25, 2012; Scheen AJ: *Exp Opin Pharmacol* 13(1):81–99, 2012.

Ghrelin is a peptide produced in the stomach and pancreatic islets. Hyperinsulinemia and hyperleptinemia are associated with decreased levels of ghrelin in type 2 diabetes.[133] Decreased levels of circulating ghrelin have been associated with alterations in insulin secretion, insulin resistance, and obesity. Its use as a potential treatment for type 2 diabetes is being investigated.[134,135]

CLINICAL MANIFESTATIONS. Clinical manifestations of type 2 diabetes are nonspecific. The affected individual often is overweight, dyslipidemic, hyperinsulinemic, and hypertensive. Classic symptoms of polyuria and polydipsia may present, but more often individuals will complain of nonspecific symptoms such as fatigue, pruritus, recurrent infections, visual changes, or symptoms of neuropathy (paresthesias or weakness). In those whose diabetes has progressed without treatment, symptoms related to coronary artery, peripheral artery, and cerebrovascular disease may develop (Table 22-8).

EVALUATION AND TREATMENT. The diagnostic criteria for type 2 diabetes are the same as those for type 1 (see Box 22-1). Prevention of type 2 diabetes hinges on diet and exercise to reduce weight. Pharmacologic therapy may be considered for those at highest risk for diabetes, especially if HbA_{1c} levels continue to rise despite lifestyle modifications. Annual monitoring for diabetes is indicated in those with prediabetes.[136]

TABLE 22-8 CLINICAL MANIFESTATIONS AND RATIONALE FOR TYPE 2 DIABETES MELLITUS

MANIFESTATION	RATIONALE
Recurrent infections (e.g., boils and carbuncles; skin infections) and prolonged wound healing	Growth of microorganisms is stimulated by increased glucose levels; impaired blood supply hinders healing
Genital pruritus	Hyperglycemia and glycosuria favor fungal growth; candidal infections, resulting in pruritus, are a common presenting symptom in women
Visual changes	Blurred vision occurs as water balance in the eye fluctuates because of elevated blood glucose levels; diabetic retinopathy is another cause of visual loss
Paresthesias	Paresthesias are common manifestations of diabetic neuropathies
Fatigue	Metabolic changes result in poor use of food products, contributing to lethargy and fatigue

WHAT'S NEW?

Bariatric Surgery in the Treatment of Diabetes

The American Diabetes Association has endorsed bariatric surgery for the treatment of type 2 diabetes in individuals with body mass indexes (BMIs) ≥35 kg/m^2. Gastric bypass surgery is now the procedure of choice, although gastric banding procedures also have beneficial results. There is current powerful evidence that bariatric surgery improves glycemic control in up to 80% of individuals with type 2 diabetes, even before there is any significant weight loss. The proposed mechanisms for these effects continue to be researched. Current hypotheses relate to changes in neuroendocrine control involving the hypothalamus, pancreas, liver, and gut. Hormones that have been implicated include changes in the concentrations of ghrelin, leptin, and the incretins. Long-term studies are now confirming the safety and efficacy of bariatric surgery in achieving persistent glycemic control and reduced risk for diabetes-associated cardiovascular complications. Further study is needed to determine the mechanisms by which bariatric surgery has such profound effects on type 2 diabetes, and whether similar outcomes might be achieved with less-invasive techniques.

Data from Dixon JB et al: *Obes Rev* 13(1):57–67, 2012; Ismail-Beigi F: *N Engl J Med* 366(14):1319–1327, 2012; Li Q et al: *Diabetes Obes Metab* 14(3):262–270, 2012; McKenney RL, Short DK: *Surg Clin North Am* 91(6):1139–1148, vii, 2011; Noria SF, Grantcharov T: *Can J Surg* 56(1):47–57, 2013; Park CW, Torquati A: *Surg Clin North Am* 91(6):1149–1161, vii, 2011; Sala PC et al: *Obes Surg* 22(1): 167–176, 2012.

The first step in management is to establish an appropriate glycemic goal. Although treatment regimens that reduce HbA_{1c} to around 7% have been shown to reduce long-term complications, intensive lowering of glucose concentration to near-normal levels through the use of multiple agents is not correlated with better outcomes and is associated with a greater risk for hypoglycemic episodes and weight gain.[136-140]

Dietary measures, including restriction of the total caloric intake, are of primary importance in both the prevention and the treatment of type 2 diabetes.[136] As the obese individual loses weight, the body's resistance to insulin often diminishes. Nonobese individuals with type 2 diabetes should consume calories consistent with their ideal weight and pattern of activity. The emphasis of medical nutrition therapy (MNT) in type 2 diabetes mellitus should be focused on achieving glucose, lipid, and blood pressure goals.[141]

Exercise is an important aspect of prevention and treatment of type 2 diabetes.[136] Exercise reduces postprandial blood glucose levels, diminishes insulin requirements, lowers triglyceride and cholesterol levels, and increases the level of high-density lipoprotein (HDL) cholesterol. In addition, exercise is a valuable adjunct to weight loss for the overweight individual. Hypoglycemia may result, however, when the exercising individual receives sulfonylurea or insulin therapy.

In those individuals with morbid obesity unresponsive to diet and exercise interventions, bariatric surgery may be indicated. Studies suggest that gastric bypass surgery is associated with marked improvements in glycemic control in those with established diabetes[138] (see What's New? Bariatric Surgery in the Treatment of Diabetes).

For most individuals with type 2 diabetes, medications are needed for optimal management. Although many older individuals continue to use insulin injections, oral hypoglycemic agents are the treatment of choice for most people.[142] There are currently nine classes of oral agents available[139] (Table 22-9). Insulin therapy may be needed in the later stages of type 2 diabetes because of loss of beta-cell function; however, the risks of treatment-related hypoglycemia must be considered.[143]

Other Specific Types of Diabetes Mellitus and Gestational Diabetes Mellitus

As described in Table 22-5 (p. 734), the American Diabetes Association (ADA) classification of diabetes mellitus encompasses not only the most common forms of diabetes (type 1 and type 2) but also "other specific types of diabetes mellitus" and "gestational diabetes mellitus." Other specific types of diabetes include genetic defects in beta-cell function, genetic defects in insulin action, diseases of the exocrine pancreas, endocrinopathies, drug- or chemical-induced beta-cell dysfunction, infections, and other uncommon autoimmune and inherited disorders that are associated with diabetes.

The most well described of these other specific types of diabetes is termed **maturity-onset diabetes of youth (MODY).** MODY accounts for 1% to 2% of diabetes and should be considered in children who lack beta-cell antibodies. It also may account for up to 5% of individuals diagnosed with gestational diabetes.[144] MODY includes six specific autosomal dominant mutations including genes for hepatocyte nuclear factor-1α (HNF-1α; MODY 3), glucokinase (MODY 2), HNF-4α (MODY 1), insulin promoter factor-1 (IPF-1; MODY 4), HNF-1β (MODY 5), and NeuroD1 (MODY 6).[145] Interestingly, the gene mutations found in MODY are not commonly found in type 2 diabetes. The clinical diagnosis of MODY is based on the following criteria: family history of diabetes with an autosomal

TABLE 22-9 TYPES OF ORAL HYPOGLYCEMIC DRUGS

DRUG TYPE	MECHANISMS OF METABOLIC CONTROL
α-Glycosidase inhibitor (miglitol and voglibose)	Delays carbohydrate absorption in gut by inhibiting disaccharidases
Biguanide (metformin)	Decreases hepatic glucose production and increases insulin sensitivity and peripheral glucose uptake
Meglitinides (glinides) (repaglinide and nateglinide)	Stimulate insulin release from pancreatic beta cells
Sulfonylureas (glyburide, glipizide, gliclazide, glimepiride)	Stimulate insulin release from pancreatic beta cells
Peroxisome proliferator-activated-receptor-gamma agonists (thiazolidinediones, pioglitazone, and rosiglitazone)	Increase insulin sensitivity, particularly in adipose tissue
Bile acid sequestrant (colesevelam)	Unknown; theories include decreased hepatic glucose production, increased insulin secretion, and increased incretin release
GLP-1 receptor agonists (exenatide and liraglutide)	Increase insulin secretion, decrease glucagon secretion, decrease rate of gastric emptying, decrease appetite, weight loss
DPP-IV inhibitors (sitagliptin, saxagliptin, vildagliptin, and linagliptin)	Increase insulin secretion, decrease glucagon secretion, decrease rate of gastric emptying, decrease appetite
Amylin mimetics (pramlintide)	Decrease glucagon secretion, decrease rate of gastric emptying, and decrease appetite
SGLT2 inhibitor (sodium-glucose co-transporter 2) In clinical trials: canagliflozin, dapagliflozin, empagliflozin	Inhibits proximal tubular renal transport of glucose, decreasing glucose reabsorption and increasing renal excretion of glucose independent of insulin

Data from Ismail-Beigi F: *N Engl J Med* 366(14):1319–1327, 2012; Misra M: *J Pharm Pharmacol*, published online August 9, 2012.

dominant mode of inheritance, insulin independence (nonketotic diabetes mellitus), and age at onset younger than 25 years. Genetic testing confirms the diagnosis. It is important to identify those with MODY because many can be effectively treated with an oral hypoglycemic agent (sulfonylureas) rather than with injections of insulin.[145,146]

Gestational diabetes mellitus (GDM) has long been defined as any degree of glucose intolerance with onset or first recognition during pregnancy. However, the recent dramatic increase in type 2 diabetes prevalence has led to the recommendation that high-risk women found to have diabetes at their initial prenatal visit receive a diagnosis of overt diabetes.[88] GDM complicates approximately 7% of all pregnancies. The exact mechanism of GDM is unknown, but insulin resistance and inadequate insulin secretion are contributing factors. The American Diabetes Association recommends that pregnant women with risk factors be screened for type 2 diabetes at their first prenatal visit. Those without a history of DM also should be screened with an oral glucose tolerance test at 24 to 28 weeks' gestation. Women with GDM should be monitored after delivery.[136] Often there are no symptoms and careful glucose level control prenatally, during pregnancy, and after delivery is essential to both the short-term and the long-term health of mother and baby.[147] There is an increased risk for type 2 diabetes and associated complications later in life in women who develop gestational diabetes.[148]

Acute Complications of Diabetes Mellitus

Hypoglycemia

Hypoglycemia is a lowered plasma glucose level. In general, hypoglycemia occurs when blood glucose levels are less than 35 mg/dl in newborns for the first 48 hours of life and less than 45 to 60 mg/dl in children and adults. Its causes may be exogenous (medications, alcohol, or exercise), endogenous (tumors of the pancreas or inherited disorders), or functional (hyperalimentation, spontaneous, or liver disease). Hypoglycemia in diabetes is sometimes called *insulin shock* or *insulin reaction.* Individuals with type 2 diabetes are at less risk for hypoglycemia than those with type 1 diabetes because they retain relatively intact glucose counterregulatory mechanisms. However, hypoglycemia does occur in type 2 diabetes when treatment involves insulin secretogogues (e.g., sulfonylureas) or exogenous insulin (Table 22-10).

Symptoms of hypoglycemia result either from activation of the sympathetic nervous system (neurogenic adrenergic symptoms) or from an abrupt cessation of glucose delivery to the brain (neuroglycopenic symptoms), or both.[149,150]

Neurogenic reactions occur when the decrease in blood glucose level is rapid and present with tachycardia, palpitations, diaphoresis, tremors, pallor, and arousal anxiety. Neuroglycopenia causes further symptoms including headache, dizziness, irritability, fatigue, poor judgment, confusion, visual changes, hunger, seizures, and coma. Hypoglycemia unawareness is a phenomenon that occurs in individuals without appropriate autonomic warning symptoms. Autonomic symptoms are blunted, symptoms are reduced, and recovery from hypoglycemia may be delayed because of impaired glycogenolysis and hampered delivery of gluconeogenic substrates to the liver.

The American Diabetes Association recommends that glucose (15 to 20 g) be given to the conscious individual with hypoglycemia. Doses of glucagon should be prescribed for emergency use for all individuals at significant risk of severe hypoglycemia, and caregivers should be instructed in their use. Individuals with hypoglycemia unawareness or who have had episodes of severe hypoglycemia should raise their glycemic treatment targets to reduce risk of future episodes.[136]

TABLE 22-10 COMMON ACUTE COMPLICATIONS OF DIABETES MELLITUS (DM)

HYPOGLYCEMIA IN PERSONS WITH DM	DIABETIC KETOACIDOSIS	HYPERGLYCEMIC NONKETOTIC SYNDROMES
Synonyms		
Insulin shock, insulin reaction	Diabetic coma syndrome	Hyperosmolar hyperglycemia nonketotic coma
Persons at Risk		
Individuals taking insulin Individuals with rapidly fluctuating blood glucose levels Individuals with type 2 diabetes taking sulfonylurea agents	Individuals with type 1 diabetes Individuals with nondiagnosed diabetes	Older adults or very young individuals with type 2 diabetes, nondiabetic individuals with predisposing factors, such as pancreatitis; individuals with undiagnosed diabetes
Predisposing Factors		
Excessive insulin or sulfonylurea agent intake, lack of sufficient food intake, excessive physical exercise, abrupt decline in insulin needs (e.g., renal failure, immediately postpartum), simultaneous use of insulin-potentiating agents or beta-blocking agents that mask symptoms	Stressful situation such as infection, accident, trauma, emotional stress; omission of insulin; medications that antagonize insulin	Infection, medications that antagonize insulin, comorbid condition
Typical Onset		
Rapid	Slow	Slowest
Presenting Symptoms		
Adrenergic reaction: pallor, sweating, tachycardia, palpitations, hunger, restlessness, anxiety, tremors Neurogenic reaction: fatigue, irritability, headache, loss of concentration, visual disturbances, dizziness, hunger, confusion, transient sensory or motor defects, convulsions, coma, death	Malaise, dry mouth, headache, polyuria, polydipsia, weight loss, nausea, vomiting, pruritus, abdominal pain, lethargy, shortness of breath, Kussmaul respirations, fruity or acetone odor to breath	Polyuria, polydipsia, hypovolemia, dehydration (parched lips, poor skin turgor), hypotension, tachycardia, hypoperfusion, weight loss, weakness, nausea, vomiting, abdominal pain, hypothermia, stupor, coma, seizures
Laboratory Analysis		
Serum glucose <30 mg/dl in newborn (first 2-3 days) and <55-60 mg/dl in adults	Glucose levels >250 mg/dl, reduction in bicarbonate concentration; increased anion gap; increased plasma levels of β-hydroxybutyrate, acetoacetate, and acetone	Glucose levels >600 mg/dl, lack of ketosis, serum osmolarity >320 mOsm/L, elevated blood urea nitrogen and creatinine

Diabetic Ketoacidosis

Ketoacidosis, a serious complication of diabetes mellitus, is a common cause for hospital admissions. **Diabetic ketoacidosis (DKA)** develops when there is an absolute or relative deficiency of insulin and an increase in the levels of insulin counterregulatory hormones.[151] This is most common in individuals with type 1 diabetes but can occur in those with type 2 diabetes as well. In addition, a syndrome called *ketosis-prone diabetes (KPD)* has been described and occurs most frequently in obese, middle-aged men with a strong family history of type 2 diabetes. These individuals do not fit the criteria for diagnosis of type 1 or type 2 diabetes but exhibit significantly impaired insulin secretion spontaneously or in response to physiologic stress such as infection.[152] The most common precipitating factor for DKA is intercurrent illness, such as infection, trauma, surgery, or myocardial infarction. Interruption of insulin administration also may result in DKA. Factors associated with increased risk are younger or older age, diagnostic error, ethnic minority, lack of health insurance in the United States, lower body mass index, preceding infection, and delayed treatment.[153]

PATHOPHYSIOLOGY. In a state of relative insulin deficiency there is an increase in the concentrations of insulin counterregulatory hormones including catecholamines, cortisol, glucagon, and GH. These counterregulatory hormones antagonize insulin by increasing glucose production and decreasing tissue use of glucose. Profound insulin deficiency results in decreased glucose uptake, increased fat mobilization with release of fatty acids, and accelerated gluconeogenesis and ketogenesis (Figure 22-16).[151] Relatively increased glucagon levels also contribute to activation of the gluconeogenic (glucose-forming) and ketogenic (ketone-forming) pathways in the liver. Because of the insulin deficiency, hepatic overproduction of β-hydroxybutyrate and acetoacetic acids causes increased ketone concentrations. Ordinarily ketones are used by tissues as an energy source to regenerate bicarbonate. This balances the loss of bicarbonate, which occurs when the ketone is formed. Hyperketonemia (increased blood ketone levels) may be a result of impairment in the use of ketones by peripheral tissue, which permits strong organic acids to circulate freely. Bicarbonate buffering then does not occur, and the individual develops a metabolic acidosis.

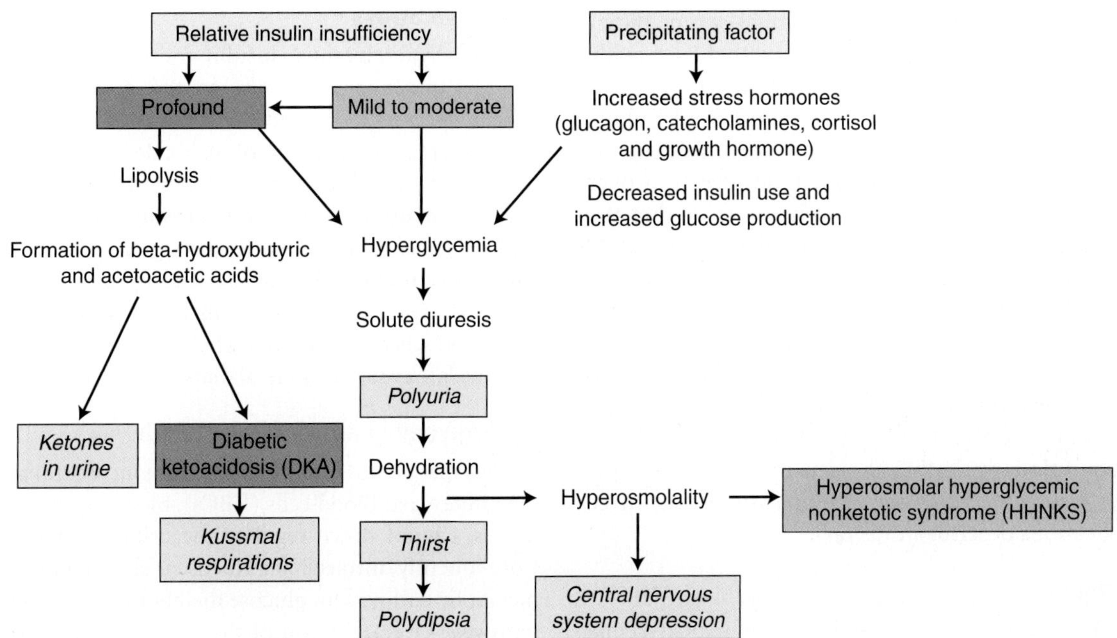

FIGURE 22-16 Pathophysiology of DKA and HHNKS in Diabetes Mellitus.

CLINICAL MANIFESTATIONS. The signs and symptoms of DKA are nonspecific. Polyuria and dehydration result from the osmotic diuresis associated with hyperglycemia. In this case, the plasma glucose level is higher than the individual's renal threshold, allowing significant amounts of glucose to be lost in the urine. Deficits of sodium, phosphorus, and magnesium are common. The most important electrolyte disturbance, however, is a marked deficiency in the level of total body potassium. Although the serum potassium concentration may appear normal or elevated because of volume contraction and a shift of potassium out of the cell and into the blood caused by metabolic acidosis, the total body deficiency of potassium may reach 3 to 5 mEq/kg. Symptoms of diabetic ketoacidosis include Kussmaul respirations (hyperventilation in an attempt to compensate for the acidosis), postural dizziness, central nervous system depression, ketonuria, anorexia, nausea, abdominal pain, thirst, and polyuria (see Table 22-10).

EVALUATION AND TREATMENT. The diagnosis of ketoacidosis is suggested when individuals have symptoms of vomiting, abdominal pain, dehydration, an acetone odor on the breath, and change in sensorium. The American Diabetes Association criteria for the diagnosis of DKA are: (1) a serum glucose level >250 mg/dl, (2) a serum bicarbonate level <18 mg/dl, (3) a serum pH <7.30, (4) the presence of an anion gap, and (5) the presence of urine and serum ketones.[154]

Treatment of DKA involves administration of insulin to decrease glucose levels. Fluids are administered to replace lost fluid volume. Electrolyte deficits become apparent as fluid volume is replaced, and intravenous sodium, potassium, and phosphorus are administered as needed. Fluids and electrolytes should be monitored closely.[155] After the administration of insulin, the concentration of β-hydroxybutyrate promptly begins to decrease, and after a slight increase, acetoacetate concentration also begins to decrease. A persistent ketonuria may be observed for several days after treatment. Continuous monitoring of the individual is essential to ensure an uncomplicated recovery from DKA. Health teaching emphasizes predisposing factors and strategies for avoiding DKA.

Hyperosmolar Hyperglycemic Nonketotic Syndrome

Hyperosmolar hyperglycemic nonketotic syndrome (HHNKS), or **hyperglycemic hyperosmolar state (HHS),** is a life-threatening emergency most often precipitated by infections, medications, nonadherence to diabetes treatment, or coexisting disease.[151] HHNKS is more commonly seen with type 2 diabetes. It can also occur in individuals with pancreatic destruction from other causes such as chronic pancreatitis.

PATHOPHYSIOLOGY. HHNKS differs from DKA in the degree of insulin deficiency (which is more profound in DKA) and the degree of fluid deficiency (which is more marked in HHNKS) (see Figure 22-16). HHNKS is characterized by a lack of ketosis. Because the amount of insulin required to inhibit fat breakdown is less than that needed for effective glucose transport, insulin levels are sufficient to prevent excessive lipolysis but not to use glucose properly.[151] Glucose levels are considerably higher in HHNKS than in DKA because of volume depletion.

CLINICAL MANIFESTATIONS. Glycosuria and polyuria in HHNKS result from the extreme serum glucose level elevation. As much as 19 g of glucose per hour may be lost in diuresis, which also causes severe volume depletion, increased serum osmolarity, intracellular dehydration, and loss of electrolytes including potassium. Neurologic changes, such as stupor, correlate with the degree of hyperosmolarity and are common in HHNKS; thus, this syndrome is sometimes called *hyperosmolar hyperglycemic coma.*

EVALUATION AND TREATMENT. The diagnostic features of HHNKS include a very high serum glucose concentration (often more than 600 mg/dl), a near-normal serum bicarbonate level and pH, a serum osmolarity that is usually greater than 320 mOsm/L, and either absent or low levels of ketones in the urine and serum.[151] DKA and HHNKS show considerable overlap in symptoms and treatment. Insulin infusion should be combined with fluid repletion over 24 hours.[156] An important distinction, however, is that the dehydration in HHNKS is far more severe than that in DKA. Thus fluid replacement, with both crystalloids and colloids, is more rapid. Potassium deficits may be extreme and require several days of treatment. Phosphorus and sodium also may be needed. HHNKS is a significant risk factor for infection, sepsis, and venous thrombosis.[151] Mortality also is high in HHNKS, and is related to the age of the individual and comorbid conditions including the severity of the precipitating illness (see Table 22-10 for a comparison of the three acute complications described thus far).

Somogyi Effect

The **Somogyi effect** is a unique combination of hypoglycemia followed by rebound hyperglycemia. The rise in blood glucose concentration occurs because counterregulatory hormones (epinephrine, GH, corticosteroids), which are stimulated by hypoglycemia, cause gluconeogenesis. Excessive carbohydrate intake may contribute to the rebound hyperglycemia. The clinical occurrence of Somogyi effect is controversial.

Dawn Phenomenon

The **dawn phenomenon** is an early morning rise in blood glucose concentration with no hypoglycemia during the night. It is related to nocturnal elevations of GH, which decrease metabolism of glucose by muscle and fat. Increased clearance of plasma insulin also may be involved. Altering the time and dose of insulin administration manages the problem.

Chronic Complications of Diabetes Mellitus

A number of serious complications are associated with any type of DM, including microvascular (e.g., retinopathy, nephropathy, and neuropathy) and macrovascular disease (e.g., coronary artery disease, stroke, and peripheral vascular disease), and infection. Most complications are associated with chronic hyperglycemia (see Figure 22-14). Strict control of blood glucose level significantly reduces some complications, particularly microvascular events. Oxidative stress (overproduction of reactive oxygen species) and activation of several complex metabolic pathways have been associated with persistent hyperglycemia and the chronic complications of DM. They include shunting of glucose into the polyol pathway, activation of protein kinase C isoforms, increased formation of advanced glycation end products (AGEs), increased expression of the receptor for AGEs (RAGE), and increased activation of the hexosamine pathway.[157] It has been proposed that hyperglycemia induces mitochondrial overproduction of oxygen free radicals and this is a key pathologic mechanism for the activation of the metabolic pathways associated with the chronic complications of DM.[158,159] Genetic and epigenetic factors contribute to the etiology of diabetic complications.[160,161]

Oxidative Stress

Chronic hyperglycemia, insulin resistance, hyperinsulinemia, and dyslipidemia contribute to the production of reactive oxygen species (ROS) and the detrimental effects of oxidative stress. Increased formation of AGEs, defects in the polyol pathway, and uncoupling of nitric oxide synthase, xanthine oxidase, and nicotinamide adenine dinucleotide phosphate (NADPH) oxidase generate ROS, which damage large and small vessels and contribute to atherogenesis and to micro- and macrovascular disease. Direct cellular injury, as well as the formation of gene products that cause endothelial cellular injury, contributes to these late complications of diabetes mellitus.[157]

Hyperglycemia and the Polyol Pathway

Tissues that do not require insulin for glucose transport, such as the kidney, red blood cells (RBCs), blood vessels, eye lens, and nerves, cannot down-regulate the cellular uptake of glucose. Consequently, intracellular glucose is shunted into an alternate metabolic pathway for glucose metabolism known as the **polyol pathway**. Overactivation of the polyol pathway results in two processes that may contribute to the complications of diabetes. One is the excessive accumulation of sorbitol (a polyol-sugar alcohol) through the action of the enzyme **aldose reductase.** The accumulated sorbitol increases intracellular osmotic pressure and attracts water in tissue. Swelling occurs along with visual changes and predisposition to cataracts in the lens of the eye. Sorbitol interferes with ion pumps in the nerves, damages Schwann cells, and disrupts nerve conduction. RBCs become swollen and stiff and interfere with perfusion. Second, activation of the polyol pathway reduces glutathione, an important antioxidant, contributing to oxidative injury in cells and tissues, particularly blood vessels. Aldose reductase inhibitors are being evaluated for treatment of these complications.[162]

Hyperglycemia and Protein Kinase C

Protein kinase C (PKC) is a family of intracellular signaling proteins that can become inappropriately activated in different tissues by hyperglycemia. Intracellular hyperglycemia increases the second-messenger diacylglycerol (DAG)-PKC pathway, which in turn activates protein kinase C. Various consequences have been observed, including insulin resistance, extracellular matrix and cytokine production, vascular cell proliferation, enhanced contractility, angiogenesis, and increased permeability. These effects may contribute to the microvascular complications of diabetes. Specific PKC inhibitors are under investigation and have shown some promise in stabilizing or preventing retinopathy, nephropathy, and neuropathy.[163]

Hyperglycemia and Glycation

Glycation is a normal non-enzymatic process that involves the *reversible* attachment of glucose to proteins, lipids, and nucleic acids without the action of enzymes. With recurrent or persistent hyperglycemia, glucose becomes *irreversibly* bound to collagen and other proteins in red blood cells (e.g., glycated hemoglobin), blood vessel walls, interstitial tissue, and within cells. The products of this binding are known as **advanced glycation end products (AGEs),** and their receptor (RAGE). They have a number of properties that may cause tissue injury or pathologic conditions associated with diabetes[164,165]:

1. Cross-linking and trapping of proteins, including albumin, low-density lipoprotein (LDL), immunoglobulin, and complement, with thickening of the basement membrane or increased permeability in small blood vessels and nerves
2. Binding to cell receptors, such as macrophages and glomerular mesangial cells, and inducing release of inflammatory cytokines and growth factors that stimulate cellular proliferation in the glomeruli, smooth muscle of blood vessels, and collagen synthesis with fibrosis
3. Induction of lipid oxidation, oxidative stress, and inflammation
4. Inactivation of nitric oxide with loss of vasodilation and diminished endothelial function
5. Procoagulant changes on endothelial cells with promotion of platelet adhesion and reduced fibrinolysis

Pharmacologic agents that inhibit AGE formation or block their receptor (RAGE) are being evaluated.[166]

Hyperglycemia and the Hexosamine Pathway

Chronic intracellular hyperglycemia causes shunting of excess intracellular glucose into the hexosamine pathway and leads to O-linked glycosylation (an enzymatic process) of several proteins with alteration in signal transduction pathways and oxidative stress. The O-linked attachment of *N*-acetylglucosamine (O-GlcNAc) on serine and threonine residues of nuclear and cytoplasmic proteins is associated with insulin resistance and cardiovascular complications of diabetes mellitus.[167]

Microvascular Disease

Diabetic microvascular complications (disease in capillaries) are a leading cause of blindness, end-stage renal failure, and various neuropathies. Thickening of the capillary basement membrane, endothelial cell hyperplasia, thrombosis, and pericyte degeneration are characteristic of diabetic microangiopathy and emerge over a period of 1 to 2 years. The thickening eventually results in decreased tissue perfusion. Hyperglycemia is a prerequisite for these microvascular changes and may be related to glycation of structural proteins, which results in the accumulation of AGEs. The frequency and severity of the lesions appear to be proportional to the duration of the disease and blood glucose control. In the Diabetes Control and Complications Trial—the Epidemiology of Diabetes Intervention and Complications Study (DCCT-EDIC), the intensively treated cohort continued to have significantly fewer complications (metabolic memory) even though their HbA_{1c} values were essentially equivalent to those of the conventional therapy group.[168,169] Hypoxia and ischemia accompany microangiopathy, particularly in the retina, the kidney, and nerves. Many individuals with type 2 diabetes present with microvascular complications because of the long duration of asymptomatic hyperglycemia that generally precedes diagnosis. This underscores the need for diabetes screening.

Diabetic Retinopathy. The retina is the most metabolically active structure per weight of tissue in the body. Thus the retina is a vulnerable target for microvascular disease in diabetes mellitus. **Diabetic retinopathy** is a leading cause of blindness worldwide and in U.S. adults younger than age 60.[170] In comparison to type 1 diabetes, retinopathy seems to develop more rapidly in individuals with type 2 diabetes because of the likelihood of long-standing hyperglycemia before diagnosis. Most individuals with diabetes will eventually develop retinopathy and they also are more likely to develop cataracts and glaucoma (see Chapter 16). Diabetic retinopathy is associated with increased risk of life-threatening systemic vascular complications, including stroke, coronary heart disease, and heart failure.[171] The prevalence and severity of the retinopathy are strongly related to the age of the individual, the duration of diabetes, and the extent of glycemic control.

Diabetic retinopathy results from relative hypoxemia, damage to retinal blood vessels and vasoconstriction, red blood cell (RBC) and platelet aggregation, influence of vascular endothelial growth factors and growth hormone, and angiogenesis. The following three stages of retinopathy lead to loss of vision: stage I: *nonproliferative*—characterized by thickening of the retinal capillary basement membrane and an increase in retinal capillary permeability, vein dilation, microaneurysm formation, and superficial (flame-shaped) and deep (blot) hemorrhages; stage II: *preproliferative*—progression of retinal ischemia with areas of poor perfusion that culminate in infarcts; and stage III *proliferative*—neovascularization (angiogenesis) and fibrous tissue formation within the retina or optic disc (see Figures 22-17 and 22-18, and Table 22-11 for details). Traction of the new vessels on the vitreous humor may cause retinal detachment or hemorrhage into the vitreous humor. **Maculopathy** is a progressive process that may accompany the increased retinal capillary permeability, vessel occlusion, and ischemia. If formation of exudates, edema, or ischemia occurs near the fovea, serious loss of vision may result. **Macular edema** (fluid accumulation and retinal thickening near the center of the macula) is the leading cause of vision loss among persons with diabetes. Blurring of vision also can be a consequence of hyperglycemia and sorbitol accumulation in the lens. Dehydration of the lens, aqueous humor, and vitreous humor also reduces visual acuity.[172] Cataracts, optic neuropathy, and defects in eye muscle function also are associated with the chronic complications of hyperglycemia and diabetes mellitus.

Laser treatments are used to reduce the rate of vision loss from diabetic macular edema and neovascularization. Vitrectomy is a surgical procedure used to treat an intravitreal hemorrhage secondary to rupture of a neovascular capillary tuft. Intravitreal delivery of steroids, antivascular endothelial growth factor preparations, and renin-angiotensin system (RAS) inhibitors is being evaluated.[173]

Diabetic Nephropathy. Diabetes is the most common cause of end-stage kidney disease in the Western world. Without appropriate management, approximately 30% of individuals with type 1 and 40% of those with type 2 diabetes develop nephropathy.[174] The early phases of nephropathy are asymptomatic and begin to develop after 10 years with type 1 diabetes or after 5 to 8 years with type 2 diabetes. There are some differences in renal lesions in type 1 and type 2 diabetes,

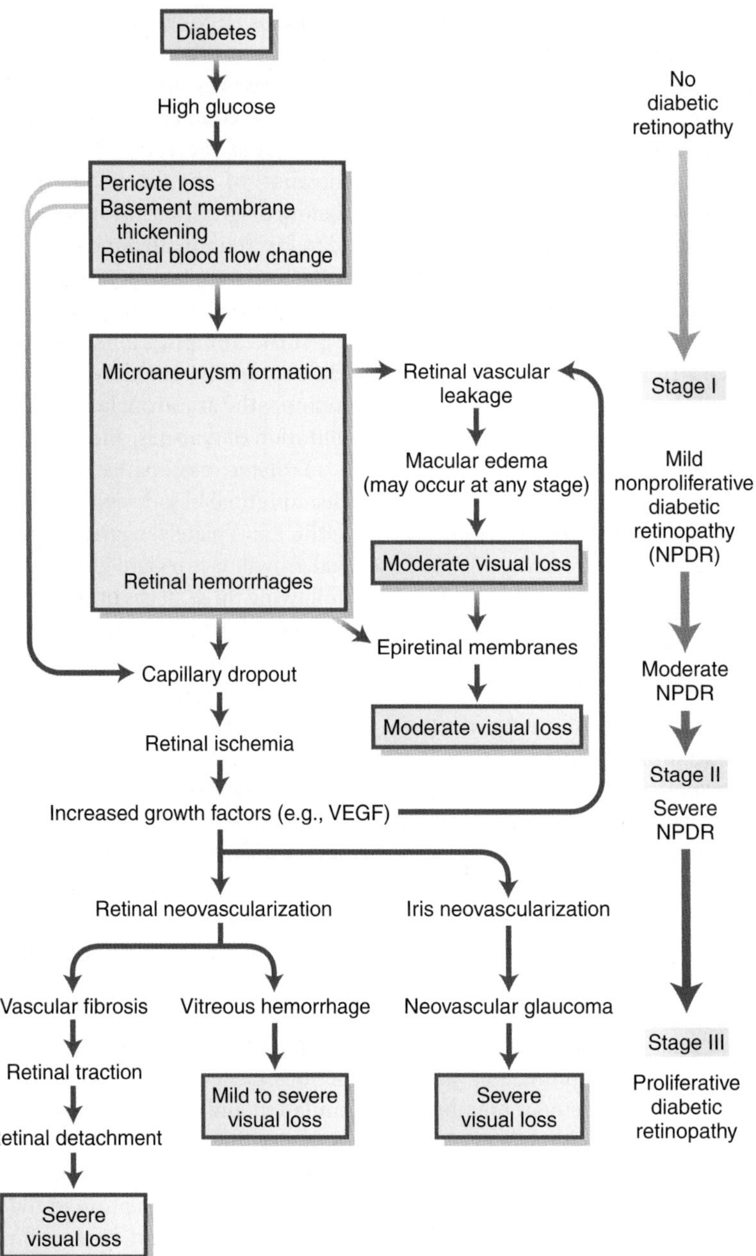

FIGURE 22-17 **Pathophysiology of Diabetic Retinopathy.** *VEGF,* Vascular endothelial growth factor. (From Mehlmed S et al: *Williams textbook of endocrinology,* ed 12, Philadelphia, 2012, Saunders.)

with glomerular changes and earlier microalbuminuria in type 1 being most prominent; however, hyperglycemia is the major initiating factor in both types.

The exact process responsible for destruction of the kidneys in diabetes is unknown. Multiple mechanisms contribute to nephropathy, including chronic hyperglycemia, systemic hypertension, hyperperfusion, hyperfiltration, increased blood viscosity, increased glomerular pressure, albuminuria, protein kinase C, growth factors, advanced glycation end products, the polyol pathway, inflammatory cytokines, oxidative stress, the renin-angiotensin-aldosterone system, and hypercholesterolemia.[175-178]

The glomeruli are injured by protein denaturation, hyperglycemia with high renal blood flow (hyperfiltration), and intraglomerular hypertension exacerbated by systemic hypertension. Renal glomerular changes can occur early in diabetes mellitus and occasionally may precede the overt manifestations of the disease (Figure 22-19). Progressive changes include glomerular enlargement, glomerular basement membrane thickening with proliferation of mesangial cells, and proliferation of the mesangial matrix. This results in diffuse and nodular glomerulosclerosis (Kimmelstiel-Wilson nodule), loss of podocytes, resistance to glomerular capillary blood flow, and decreased glomerular filtration rates (GFRs). Alterations in glomerular membrane permeability occur with loss of negative charge and albuminuria. Tubular and interstitial fibrosis contributes to loss of function.[179]

Microalbuminuria is usually the first manifestation of kidney dysfunction (30 to 300 mg/day). Continuous untreated proteinuria generally heralds a life expectancy less than 10 years.

Microalbuminuria is an independent risk factor for cardiovascular disease and progressive renal impairment.[180] The determinants of proteinuria in diabetic nephropathy are not completely understood.[181] Glycated albumin generates ROS and directly damages glomerular membrane epithelial cells, vascular smooth muscle, and mesangial cells. Glomerular endothelial dysfunction also promotes albuminuria.[182] As renal failure progresses, extensive vascular and extravascular changes occur.

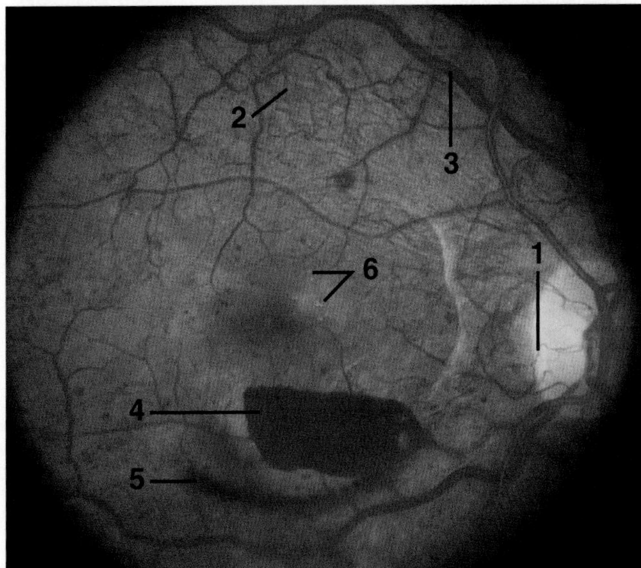

FIGURE 22-18 Proliferative Diabetic Retinopathy. Neovascularization is present at the optic nerve **(1)** and along the vascular arcades **(2).** Retinal veins are engorged **(3),** and a preretinal hemorrhage **(4)** is present inferior to the fovea. This boat-shaped hemorrhage blocks the view of the retinal vessels. A more diffuse hemorrhage **(5)** is present in an arcuate pattern just inferior to the preretinal hemorrhage that represents a mild vitreous hemorrhage. A few small, hard exudates are visible in the fovea **(6).** (From Palay D, Krachmer J: *Ophthalmology,* ed 2, St Louis 2005, Mosby.)

Before the development of clinical proteinuria (more than 300 mg/day), no clinical signs or symptoms of progressive glomerulosclerosis are likely to be evident. Later, hypoproteinemia, reduction in plasma oncotic pressure, fluid overload, anasarca (generalized body edema), and hypertension may occur. In type 1 DM, about 24% of individuals have a decline in GFR without albuminuria.[183] As renal function continues to deteriorate, individuals with type 1 diabetes may experience hypoglycemia, which necessitates a decrease in insulin therapy. The hypoglycemia occurs because the kidney's ability to metabolize insulin is lost along with other renal functions. As the glomerular filtration rate drops below 10 ml/minute, uremic signs such as nausea, lethargy, acidosis, anemia, and uncontrolled hypertension occur (see Chapter 38 for a discussion of renal failure). Impaired kidney function accelerates retinopathy and cardiovascular disease. Control of hypertension and hyperglycemia delays the onset of end-stage kidney disease.

The development of more sensitive tests has permitted the detection of small amounts of urinary albumin (i.e., microalbuminuria). Earlier intervention with tight glucose control and angiotensin-converting enzyme (ACE) inhibitors or angiotensin II receptor blockers has reduced proteinuria and slowed the progression of nephropathy. Aggressive treatment of hypertension is another therapeutic intervention definitively shown to slow the progression of established renal disease.[184]

Diabetic Neuropathies. Diabetic neuropathy is the most common cause of neuropathy in the Western world and is probably the most common complication of diabetes. Nerves do not require insulin for glucose transport and are particularly vulnerable to the pathologic effects of chronic hyperglycemia. Peripheral neuropathy affects up to 50% of individuals with diabetes.[185]

The underlying pathologic mechanism includes both metabolic and vascular factors related to chronic hyperglycemia. Inflammation, ischemia, oxidative stress, advanced glycation

TABLE 22-11 FINDINGS IN DIABETIC RETINOPATHY

STAGES OF RETINOPATHY	PATHOLOGIC FINDINGS
Nonproliferative Retinopathy (Stage I)	
Venous abnormalities	Increased tortuosity, dilation with irregular constriction; frequency increases with increased severity of retinopathy
Microaneurysms	Mostly thin walled; 15-50 mcg in diameter; pathogenesis controversial
Interretinal hemorrhage	Circular and small; may take several months to resorb
Macular edema	Caused by serum leakage through incompetent vessel walls; may resorb in several weeks
Hard exudates	Characteristically "hard" exudates with pattern of exudation irregular in shape and sharply defined may appear and disappear over months to years; common with hypertension; "soft" exudates may appear and disappear more often; related to increased retinal capillary permeability
Preproliferative Diabetic Retinopathy (Stage II)	
Cotton-wool patches	Infarcts of the nerve fiber layer caused by retinal ischemia
Intraretinal microvascular shunts	Tortuous shunts between patent and occluded retinal vessels
Proliferative Diabetic Retinopathy (Stage III)	
Neovascularization	New vessels surrounded by connective tissue; five distinct groups representing different hazards to the eye
Glial proliferation	Often produced to reinforce neovascularization; may occur on optic disc and along vascular arcades
Vitreoretinal traction hemorrhage; retinal detachment	Traction occurring from the vitreous jelly; eventually causes small blood vessels to hemorrhage and retinal detachment to occur

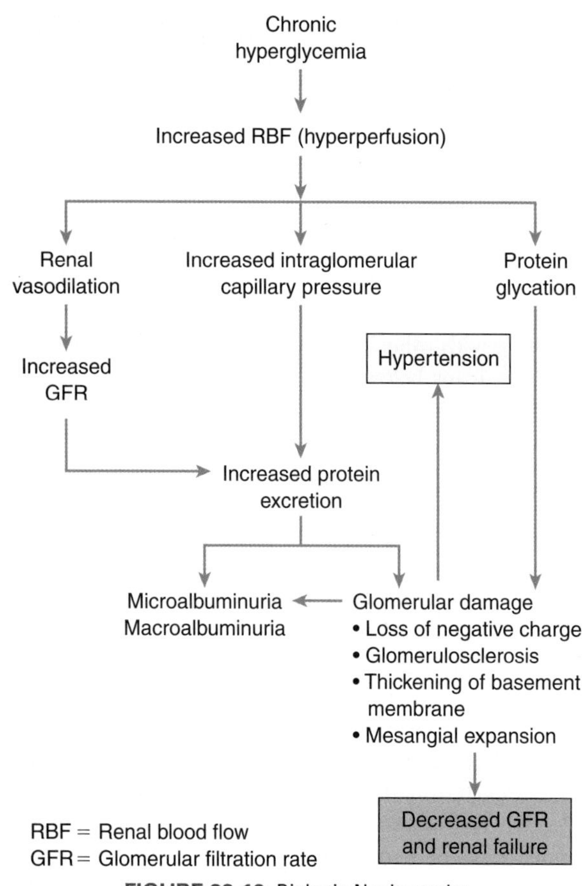

FIGURE 22-19 Diabetic Nephropathy.

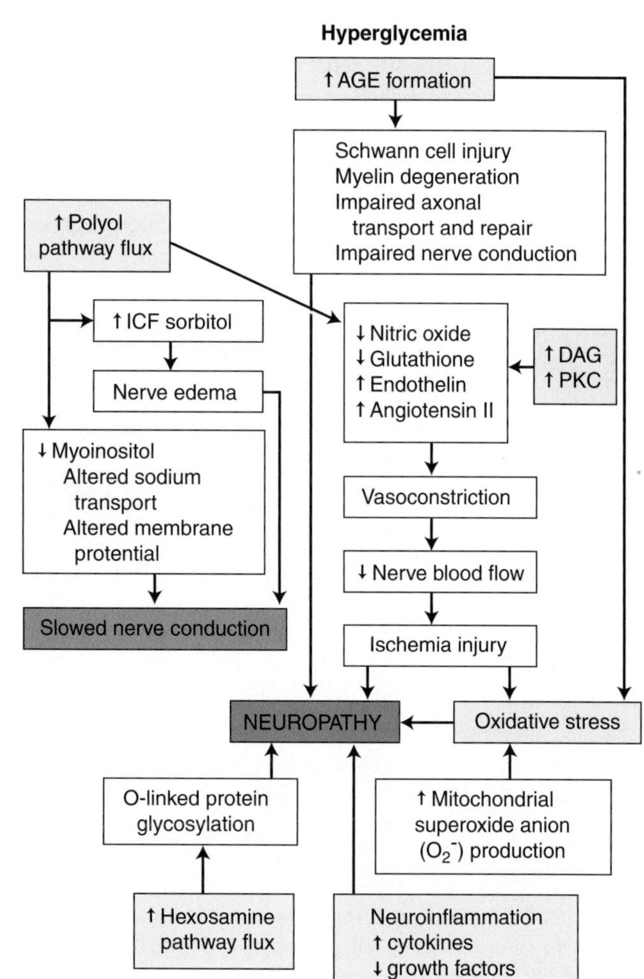

FIGURE 22-20 Multifactorial Pathogenesis of Diabetic Neuropathy. The yellow boxes represent the consequences of chronic hyperglycemia in the development of neuropathy. *AGE,* Advanced glycation end product; *DAG,* diacylglycerol; *ICF,* intracellular fluid; *PKC,* protein kinase C.

end products and increased formation of polyols contribute to demyelination, nerve degeneration, and delayed conduction (Figure 22-20).[186] Both somatic and peripheral nerve cells show diffuse or focal damage resulting in polyneuropathy. Sensory deficits generally precede motor involvement. The extremities are involved first in a "stocking and glove" pattern.

Diabetic neuropathy is a form of "dying back" neuropathy, in which the distal portions of the neurons are initially and eventually more severely affected. The earliest morphologic change is axonal degeneration that preferentially involves sensory nerve fibers, particularly the smaller polymodal unmyelinated peripheral C fibers and the larger myelinated Aδ fibers. Metabolic activity of Schwann cells is disturbed, causing segmental loss of myelin and a characteristic pattern of demyelination and remyelination observed in long-term diabetic neuropathy. The location of the pathologic condition can include the spinal cord, the posterior root ganglia, or the peripheral nerves. These changes may occur alone or in combination. Nerve degeneration begins in the periphery.

Distal symmetric polyneuropathy (sensory, autonomic, and motor nerve involvement) is the most common neuropathy with involvement of both large and small nerve fibers. Loss of small nerve fiber function includes neuropathic pain and loss of sensation, and carries high risk for development of foot ulceration with subsequent gangrene and amputation. Large nerve fiber involvement results in sensory loss of proprioception and vibration with ataxia, loss of coordination, and risk for falls and fractures. Motor involvement results in weakness and muscle atrophy, particularly in the lower legs and feet.[187]

Involvement of the autonomic nervous system can occur early. Multiple alterations can develop affecting gastrointestinal enteric nerves (nausea, bloating, gastroparesis, diarrhea, or constipation), bladder and sexual function (loss of bladder sensation, urine retention, recurrent infection, erectile dysfunction), sweating, and body temperature regulation. Cardiovascular autonomic neuropathy is a serious complication with heart rate variability, changes in baroreceptor reflexes, postural hypotension, dysrhythmias, exercise intolerance, painless myocardial infarction, and sudden death.[188] Alterations in cognitive function and increased risk for dementia may accompany long-term complications in the brain, particularly in persons with type 2 diabetes. The neurodegenerative mechanisms are not clear.[189]

There are varying manifestations of diabetic neuropathies involving both the somatic and the autonomic nerves (Table 22-12). Some of the neuropathic syndromes are progressive, but many—such as painful peripheral neuropathy, mononeuropathy (wristdrop, footdrop), diabetic amyotrophy, diabetic

TABLE 22-12 CLASSIFICATION OF DIABETIC NEUROPATHIES

TYPE OF NEUROPATHY	CHARACTERISTICS
Hyperglycemic neuropathy	Hyperesthesia, tingling and pain associated with hyperglycemia that resolves with glycemic control
Distal symmetric polyneuropathy (sensorimotor neuropathy)	Loss of large and small myelinated and unmyelinated nerve fibers Longest nerves affected first with numbness, tingling, and pain (sharp, burning, aching) in toes and feet and then ascending to hands (stocking and glove pattern); loss of vibration and proprioception (large nerve fiber); loss of sensory light touch and temperature and pain (small nerve fiber) Motor nerves affected later with weakness, depressed reflexes, and gait disturbances
Autonomic neuropathy	Cardiovascular: postural hypotension; exercise intolerance; silent myocardial infarction Gastrointestinal: decreased esophageal motility, gastroparesis and delayed gastric emptying, diabetic constipation or diarrhea Genitourinary tract: neurogenic bladder, urine retention, erectile dysfunction and retrograde ejaculation in men Sudomotor: anhidrosis, gustatory sweating Cranial nerve III: pain and ptosis and may spare the pupil
Mononeuropathies (focal neuropathies)	Compression and entrapment syndromes: carpel tunnel syndrome, radial nerve (wristdrop), peroneal nerve (footdrop), femoral nerve Cranial neuropathies: cranial nerve III, pain and ptosis and may spare the pupil Truncal mononeuropathy: abdominal or lower chest pain or hyperesthesia, abdominal muscle weakness Asymmetric lower limb neuropathy (diabetic amyotrophy; diabetic polyradiculopathy): involvement of lower thoracic and lumbar nerve roots (upper leg weakness, upper leg muscle atrophy, diminished knee and ankle tendon reflexes); may have paresthesia, hyperesthesia, pain

neuropathic cachexia, and visceral manifestations associated with autonomic neuropathy (e.g., diabetic diarrhea and orthostatic hypotension)—may spontaneously improve. *Charcot neuroarthropathy* (Charcot joint) is the progressive degeneration and structural disorganization of a joint, particularly in the feet of individuals affected by long-term diabetes. The pathogenesis is not clear but may be related to loss of sensation or neurally mediated vascular alterations with osteoclastic bone resorption, or both.[190]

Macrovascular Disease

Macrovascular disease (lesions in large and medium sized arteries) increases morbidity and mortality and increases risk for accelerated atherosclerosis and myocardial infarction, stroke, and peripheral vascular disease, particularly among individuals with type 2 diabetes mellitus. Children with poorly controlled diabetes have high risk for macrovascular disease within one or two decades.[191] Unlike microangiopathy, atherosclerotic disease is unrelated to the severity of diabetes and is often present in those with insulin resistance and impaired glucose tolerance.[192] The premature atherosclerosis of diabetes has many contributing factors, including hyperinsulinemia (insulin resistance), hyperglycemia, hypertriglyceridemia, low levels of high-density lipoprotein (HDL), high levels of low-density lipoprotein (LDL), lipoprotein oxidation, and platelet abnormalities. Advanced glycosylated end products attach to their receptor (RAGE) in the walls of blood vessels, promoting oxidative stress, inflammation, and endothelial and vascular smooth muscle dysfunction (Figure 22-21). The process tends to be more severe and accelerated with the presence of other risk factors, including hyperlipidemia, hypertension, and smoking.[193]

Coronary Artery Disease. Coronary artery disease (CAD) is the most common cause of morbidity and mortality (up to 75%) in both men and women with diabetes mellitus. In general, the prevalence of CAD increases with the duration but not the severity of diabetes. Risk factors contributing to disease include hyperglycemia and insulin resistance, high levels of LDLs and triglycerides (lipotoxicity), low levels of HDLs, increased levels of apolipoprotein B, platelet abnormalities, and endothelial cell dysfunction.[194]

Myocardial infarction (death of heart muscle as a result of coronary artery occlusion) is the cause of death in up to 75% of those with diabetes. Individuals with diabetes mellitus have a higher mortality during the acute phase of myocardial infarctions than do nondiabetic individuals because they are often asymptomatic as a result of sensory and autonomic neuropathy. Atherosclerotic CAD is accelerated in diabetes because of hyperglycemia-induced endothelial dysfunction, impaired fibrinolysis, increased platelet aggregation, plaque instability, dysfunctional arterial remodeling, and fibrotic and calcified coronary arteries.[195] In addition, the incidence of cardiomyopathy (heart failure or myocardial dysfunction in the absence of CAD and hypertension) is higher in individuals with diabetes. The reason is unclear but may be related to metabolic remodeling of the myocardium with the presence of increased amounts of collagen in the ventricular wall, which reduces the mechanical compliance of the heart during filling, inflammation, and changes in calcium management.[195a] Diastolic dysfunction is the earliest symptom.[196] Guidelines have been developed to reduce the risk and improve prevention, screening, and treatment of cardiovascular and coronary artery disease in individuals with diabetes.[136]

Stroke. Stroke is twice as common in those with diabetes (particularly type 2 diabetes) as in the nondiabetic population. Ischemic stroke is more common than hemorrhagic stroke. The survival rate for an individual with diabetes after a massive stroke is typically shorter than that for a person without

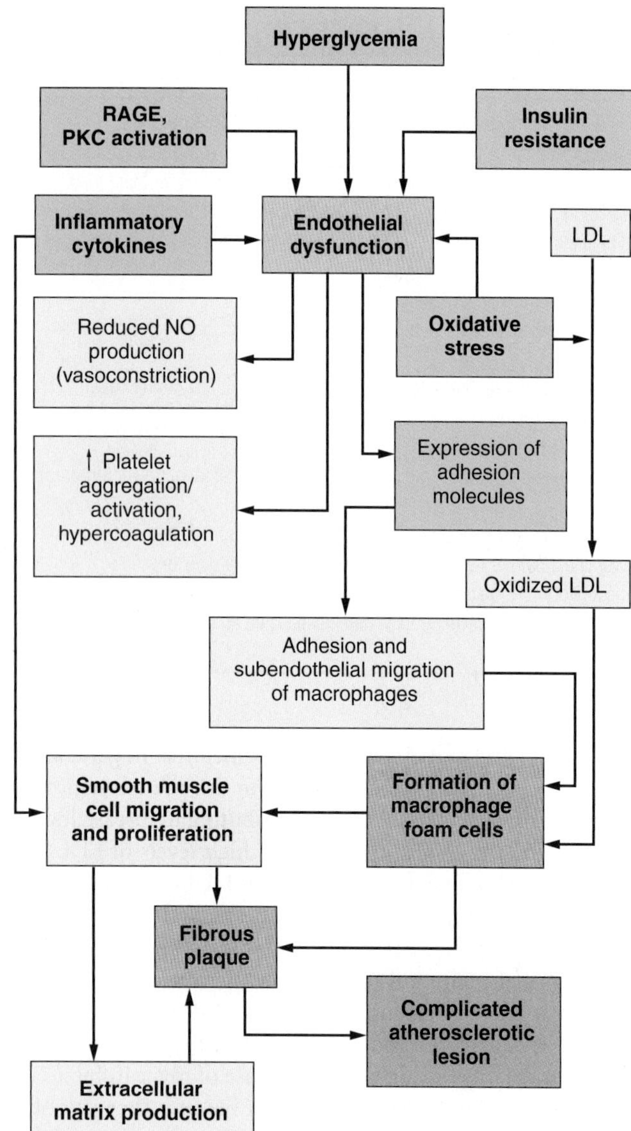

FIGURE 22-21 Diabetes Mellitus and Atherosclerosis. Diabetes with its associated hyperglycemia, relative hypoinsulinemia, oxidative stress, and proinflammatory state contributes to atherogenesis by causing arterial endothelial dysfunction (impaired vasodilation and adhesion of inflammatory cells), dyslipidemia, and smooth muscle proliferation. *LDL,* Low-density lipoprotein; *NO,* nitric oxide; *PKC,* protein kinase; *RAGE,* receptor for advanced glycation end product; *TG,* triglyceride. (Data from D'Souza A et al: *Mol Cell Biochem* 331[1-2]:89–116, 2009; Stratmann B, Tschoepe D: *Best Pract Res Clin Endocrinol Metab* 23[3]:291–303, 2009.)

diabetes. Hypertension, hyperglycemia, hyperlipidemia, and thrombosis are definite risk factors (see Chapters 17 and 32), and aggressive management of blood pressure, hyperglycemia, and lipidemia in individuals with diabetes has been shown to reduce the incidence of stroke.[197]

Peripheral Arterial Disease. There is an increased incidence of peripheral arterial disease (PAD), neuropathy, gangrene, and amputation in diabetic persons, particularly in individuals with type 2 diabetes.[198,199] The atherosclerotic process in diabetic persons is more common, appears at a younger age, and advances more rapidly than vascular changes in nondiabetic persons.[200] The prevalence of PAD is nearly equal in males and females with diabetes. Age, duration of diabetes, glycemic control, genetics, and additional risk factors influence the development of PAD.[201]

Atherosclerosis combined with peripheral neuropathy causes the occlusions, ulcers, and gangrenous changes of the lower extremities. They tend to occur in patchy areas of the feet and toes.[202] Smaller vessels often have more occlusion than larger vessels in the same individuals. Figure 22-22 illustrates how foot lesions of diabetes can lead to amputation. More than 60% of nontraumatic amputations in the United States are performed on individuals with diabetes. Referral to specialists can reduce amputation rates by 45% to 85%.[203]

Infection

Increased morbidity and mortality from infectious agents have been documented in those with diabetes.[204] The individual with diabetes is at increased risk for infection for several reasons[205,206]:

1. *The senses.* Impaired vision caused by retinal changes and impaired touch caused by sensory neuropathy lead to loss of protection with injury. Repeated trauma increases risk for infection in open wounds, soft tissue, or bones (osteomyelitis).
2. *Hypoxia.* Once skin integrity is compromised, tissues' susceptibility to infection increases as a result of vascular disease and hypoxia. In addition, the glycosylated hemoglobin in the RBCs impedes the release of oxygen to tissues.
3. *Pathogens.* Some pathogens proliferate rapidly because of increased glucose in body fluids, which provides an excellent source of energy.
4. *Blood supply.* Decreased blood supply results from vascular changes and autonomic dysfunction, which decreases the supply of white blood cells to the affected area.
5. *Suppressed immune response.* Chronic hyperglycemia impairs both the innate and the adaptive immune responses, including abnormal vasoactive responses and defective chemotaxis and phagocytosis. Clinical signs of infection may be absent.
6. *Delayed wound healing.* Slower collagen synthesis and decreased angiogenesis increase the opportunity for infection.

The risk of infection is especially high for individuals undergoing surgery and for those taking immunosuppressant medications.[207]

ALTERATIONS OF ADRENAL FUNCTION

Disorders of the Adrenal Cortex

Disorders of the adrenal cortex are related to either hyperfunction or hypofunction. Hyperfunction that causes increased levels of circulating cortisol leads to Cushing disease, or Cushing syndrome; hyperfunction that causes increased secretion of adrenal androgens and estrogens leads to virilization or feminization; and hyperfunction that causes increased levels of aldosterone leads to hyperaldosteronism, which may be primary or

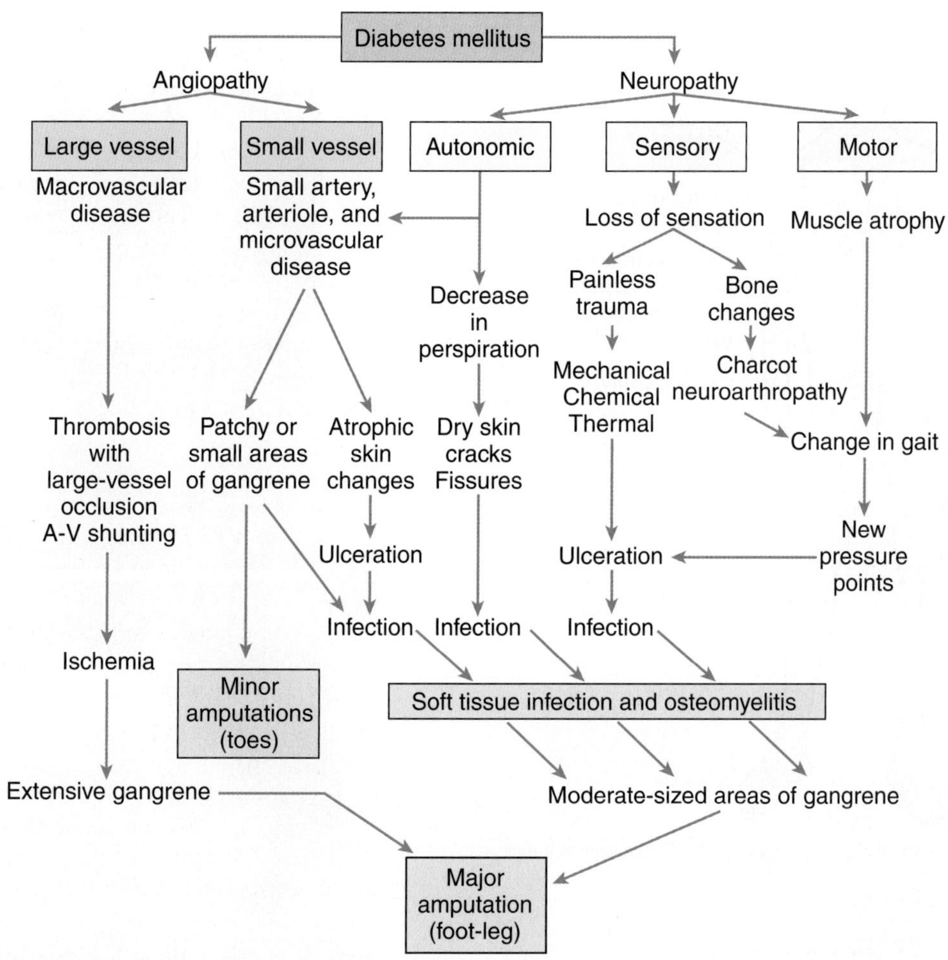

FIGURE 22-22 How Foot Lesions of Diabetes Can Lead to Amputation. (From Levin ME, O'Neal LW, Bowker JH: *The diabetic foot,* ed 5, St Louis, 1993, Mosby.)

secondary. Hypofunction of the adrenal cortex leads to Addison disease.

Adrenocortical Hyperfunction: Cushing Disease, Cushing Syndrome

Cushing syndrome refers to the complex of clinical manifestations resulting from chronic exposure to excess cortisol. **Cushing disease** is overproduction of pituitary ACTH by a pituitary adenoma (can occur at any age). Ectopic secretion of ACTH by an ectopic-secreting non–pituitary tumor (e.g., a small cell carcinoma of the lung; more common in older adults) also can cause hypercortisolism. Rarely, *ACTH-independent hypercortisolism* is caused by cortisol secretion from a benign or malignant tumor of one or both adrenal glands (more common in children). All are rare. A **Cushing-like syndrome** may develop as a result of the exogenous administration of glucocorticoids.[208]

PATHOPHYSIOLOGY. With ACTH-dependent hypercortisolism, the excess ACTH stimulates excess production of cortisol and there is loss of feedback control of ACTH secretion. Whatever the cause, two observations consistently apply to individuals with Cushing syndrome: (1) they do not have diurnal or circadian secretion patterns of ACTH and cortisol, and (2) they do not increase ACTH and cortisol secretion in response to a stressor.[209] In individuals with ACTH-dependent hypercortisolism, secretion of both cortisol and adrenal androgens is increased, and corticotropin-releasing hormone (CRH) secretion is inhibited. ACTH-independent secreting tumors of the adrenal cortex, however, generally secrete only cortisol. Elevated cortisol levels suppress CRH and ACTH secretion from the hypothalamus and anterior pituitary, respectively, which leads to low levels of ACTH. Low levels of ACTH cause atrophy of the remaining normal portions of the adrenal cortex, which over time will alter the cortisol-secreting activity of normal cells. When the secretion of cortisol by the tumor exceeds normal cortisol levels, symptoms of hypercortisolism develop.

CLINICAL MANIFESTATIONS. Weight gain is the most common feature and results from the accumulation of adipose tissue in the trunk, facial, and cervical areas. These characteristic patterns of fat deposition have been described as "truncal [central] obesity," "moon face," and "buffalo hump" (Figures 22-23 and 22-24). Transient weight gain from sodium and water retention may be present because of the mineralocorticoid effects of cortisol, exhibited when cortisol is present in high levels.

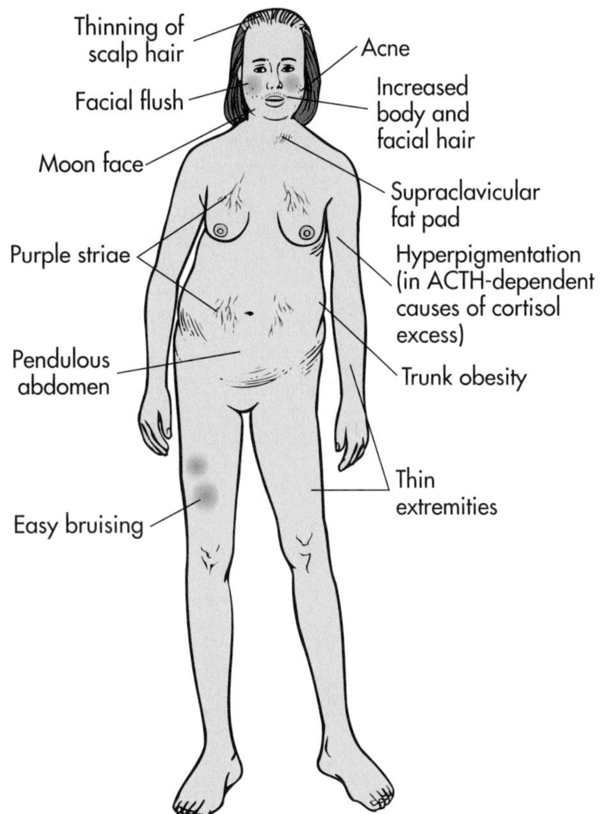

FIGURE 22-23 Symptoms of Cushing Disease. *ACTH,* Adrenocorticotropic hormone.

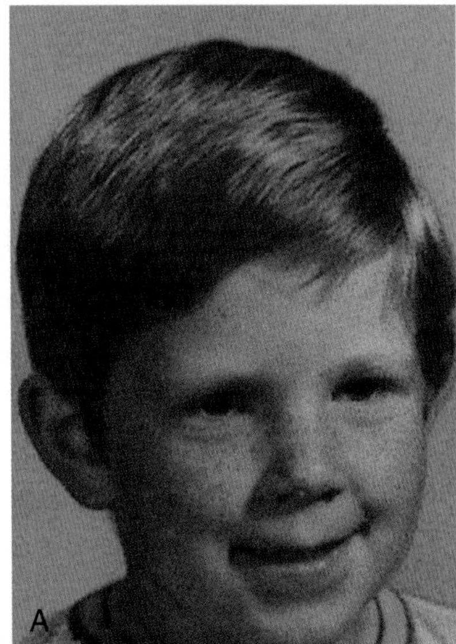

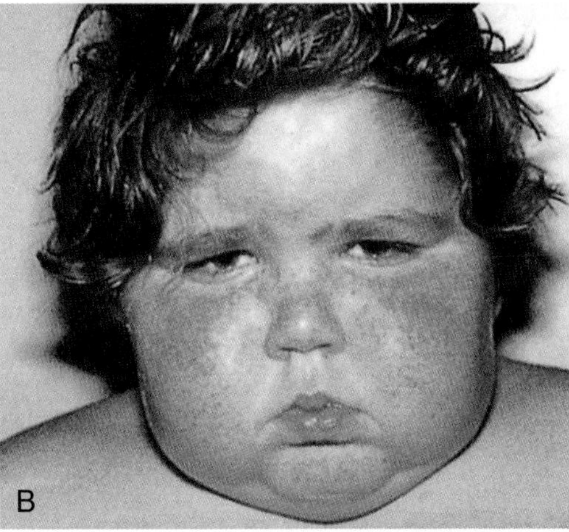

FIGURE 22-24 Cushing Syndrome. **A,** Patient before onset of Cushing syndrome. **B,** Patient 4 months later. Moon facies is clearly demonstrated. (From Zitelli BJ, McIntire SC, Nowalk AJ: *Zitelli and Davis' atlas of pediatric physical diagnosis,* ed 6, London, 2012, Saunders.)

Glucose intolerance occurs because of cortisol-induced insulin resistance and increased gluconeogenesis and glycogen storage by the liver. Overt diabetes mellitus develops in approximately 20% of individuals with hypercortisolism. Polyuria is a manifestation of hyperglycemia and resultant glycosuria.

Protein wasting is caused by the catabolic effects of cortisol on peripheral tissues. Muscle wasting leads to muscle weakness and is especially obvious in the muscles of the extremities with thinning of the limbs. In bone, loss of the protein matrix and increases in bone resorption lead to osteoporosis and can result in pathologic fractures, vertebral compression fractures, bone and back pain, kyphosis, and reduced height. Hypercalciuria may result in renal stones, which are experienced by approximately 20% of individuals with this disease. Loss of collagen also leads to thin, weakened integumentary tissues through which capillaries are more visible; the tissues are easily stretched by adipose deposits. Together these changes account for the characteristic purple striae most often observed in the truncal area. Loss of collagenous support around small vessels makes them susceptible to rupture, leading to easy bruising, even with minor trauma. Thin, atrophied skin is also easily damaged, leading to skin breaks and ulcerations. Bronze or brownish hyperpigmentation of the skin, mucous membranes, and hair occurs when there are very high levels of ACTH. This is caused by increased levels of melanocyte-stimulating hormones resulting from excess conversion of pro-opiomelanocortin when ACTH concentration is elevated.[210]

With elevated cortisol levels, vascular sensitivity to catecholamines is increased significantly, leading to vasoconstriction and hypertension. Metabolic syndrome with abdominal obesity, hypertension, glucose intolerance, and dyslipidemias is a common complication (see Box 22-2, p. 739). Individuals with Cushing syndrome are at increased risk for cardiovascular complications (CAD, heart failure, and stroke).[211] Chronically elevated cortisol levels also cause suppression of the immune system, increased susceptibility to infections, and poor wound healing.

Approximately 50% of individuals with Cushing syndrome experience alterations in their mental status, caused by the effects of cortisol on hippocampal neurons and the subsequent implications on learning, memory, and other neurologic functions when cortisol levels are elevated. These may range from irritability and depression to severe psychiatric disturbances such as schizophrenia.[212]

Females may experience symptoms of increased adrenal androgen levels, increased hair growth (especially facial hair), acne, and oligomenorrhea. Rarely do androgen levels become high enough to cause changes of the voice, recession of the hairline, and clitoral hypertrophy unless an adrenal carcinoma is involved. Infertility is more common among women.[213]

EVALUATION AND TREATMENT. A variety of laboratory tests must be used to diagnose hypercortisolism and to determine the underlying disorder.[214] These include urinary free cortisol concentration higher than 50 mcg per 24 hours, abnormal dexamethasone suppressibility of either urinary or serum cortisol, and simultaneous measurement of ACTH and cortisol levels. Late evening salivary cortisol levels are used as a screening test and to document alterations in the diurnal variation of cortisol level. Routine laboratory examinations may reveal hyperglycemia, glycosuria, hypokalemia, and metabolic alkalosis. Tumors are diagnosed using imaging procedures. Guidelines are available for the diagnosis of Cushing syndrome.[215]

Treatment is specific for the cause of hypercorticoadrenalism and includes medication, radiation, and surgery. Differentiation among pituitary, ectopic, and adrenal causes is essential for effective treatment. Without treatment, approximately 50% of individuals with Cushing syndrome die within 5 years of onset as a result of overwhelming infection, suicide, complications from generalized arteriosclerosis, and hypertensive disease.[216]

Congenital Adrenal Hyperplasia

Congenital adrenal hyperplasia is an autosomal recessive disorder that causes the deficiency of an enzyme that is critical in cortisol biosynthesis. Because cortisol production is low, ACTH concentration increases and causes adrenal hyperplasia, which results in the overproduction of either mineralocorticoids or androgens. The most common form is a 21-hydroxylase deficiency that involves both mineralocorticoid and cortisol synthesis. Affected female infants are virilized and infants of both genders exhibit salt wasting.[217]

Hyperaldosteronism

Hyperaldosteronism is characterized by excessive aldosterone secretion by the adrenal cortex. There are both primary and secondary forms of hyperaldosteronism.

Primary hyperaldosteronism (Conn disease, primary aldosteronism) is caused by excessive secretion of aldosterone from an abnormality of the adrenal cortex, usually a single benign aldosterone-producing adrenal adenoma. Bilateral adrenal nodular hyperplasia and adrenal carcinomas account for the remainder of cases. The incidence is estimated to be between 1% and 2% of all hypertensive individuals and is the most common cause of secondary hypertension.[218]

Secondary hyperaldosteronism (secondary aldosteronism) involves excessive aldosterone secretion from an extra-adrenal stimulus, most often angiotensin II through a renin-dependent mechanism. (Factors that affect renin and aldosterone secretion are summarized in Table 22-13). This occurs in various situations, including decreased circulating blood volume (e.g., in dehydration, shock, or hypoalbuminemia) and decreased delivery of blood to the kidneys (e.g., renal artery stenosis, heart failure, or hepatic cirrhosis). Here the activation of the renin-angiotensin system and subsequent aldosterone secretion may be seen as compensatory, although in some instances (e.g., congestive heart failure) the increased circulating volume further worsens the condition. Other causes of secondary hyperaldosteronism include renin-secreting tumors of the kidney and Bartter syndrome, an inherited renal tubular defect in tubular reabsorption of sodium and resulting elevated aldosterone levels and hypokalemia. Diuretic use is perhaps the most common cause of secondary hyperaldosteronism. (Renal disorders are discussed in Chapter 38.) Apparent mineralocorticoid excess can be seen in individuals who consume excess licorice (glycyrrhizic acid) or chewing tobacco.

TABLE 22-13 PHYSIOLOGIC FACTORS AFFECTING RENIN AND ALDOSTERONE SECRETION

FACTORS	RENIN SECRETION
Age	Highest in infants; lowest in older adults
Menstrual cycle	Highest in luteal phase (see Chapter 23)
Sodium intake	Increased by salt restriction Decreased by salt loading
Potassium status	Increased by K^+ excess
Posture	Increased with erect posture
Sympathetic nervous system	Renin increased by catecholamine stimulation
Time of sampling	Highest before noon; lowest in evening

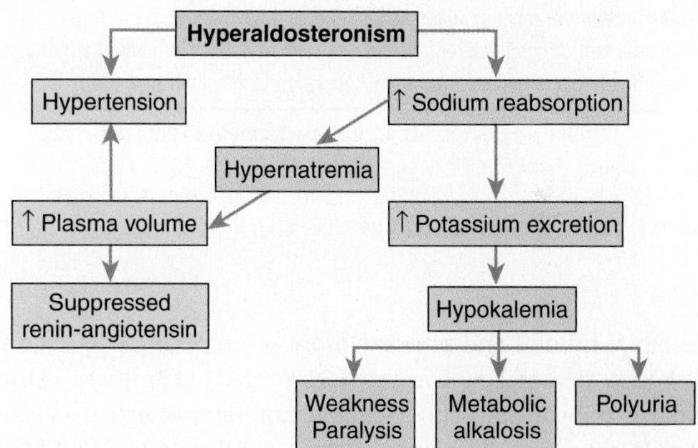

FIGURE 22-25 Pathophysiology of Primary Hyperaldosteronism. (From Bonow RO et al: *Braunwald's heart disease: a textbook of cardiovascular medicine*, ed 9, Philadelphia, 2012, Saunders.)

PATHOPHYSIOLOGY. In *primary hyperaldosteronism,* pathophysiologic alterations are caused by excessive aldosterone secretion and the fluid and electrolyte imbalances that ensue (Figure 22-25). Hyperaldosteronism promotes (1) increased renal sodium and water reabsorption with corresponding hypervolemia (see Chapter 3) and hypertension and (2) renal excretion of potassium. The extracellular fluid volume overload and suppression of normal feedback mechanisms of renin secretion are characteristic of primary disorders.

Edema usually does not occur with primary aldosteronism. Sodium loss and water loss are maintained by hypervolemia-induced atrial natriuretic factor release, pressure natriuresis, and aldosterone escape (spontaneous diuresis). The escape phenomenon changes or resets the rate of sodium excretion in the

WHAT'S NEW?

Aldosteronism and Metabolic Syndrome

Increased aldosterone production and mineralocorticoid receptor (MR) activation are associated with genomic and nongenomic actions that contribute to pancreatic fibrosis, impaired beta-cell function, and components of metabolic syndrome, including insulin resistance, hypertriglyceridemia, low levels of high-density lipoprotein, resistant hypertension, and obesity. Insulin resistance may be related to increased levels of aldosterone and decreased insulin responsiveness of GLUT4 in skeletal muscle and GLUT2 in the liver, as has been found in animal studies, or be a result of direct effects on insulin signaling and hepatic gluconeogenesis. Aldosterone increases oxidative stress and the number of proinflammatory cytokines; combined with insulin resistance, it contributes to reduced endothelial-mediated vasorelaxation, vascular injury, and atherosclerosis, causing hypertension, cardiac disease, and renal disease. High levels of aldosterone are associated with left ventricular hypertrophy, cardiac fibrosis, and diastolic dysfunction, and promote both glomerular and tubulointerstitial renal disease. MR antagonists have a significant role in the management of complications associated with metabolic syndrome although the side effects of gynecomastia and hypokalemia may limit their use.

Data from Briet M, Schiffrin EL: *Curr Hypertens Rep* 13(2):163–172, 2011; Briet M, Schiffrin EL: *J Vasc Res* 50(2):89–99, 2013; Ronconi V et al: *Curr Vasc Pharmacol* 10(2):238–246, 2012; Tirosh A, Garg R, Adler GK: *Curr Hypertens Rep* 12(4):252–257, 2010.

proximal tubules and prevents more severe sodium retention. Although this mechanism provides protection from excessive sodium reabsorption and edema, it can increase urinary losses of potassium and cause hypokalemia (see Figure 22-24). Metabolic syndrome (hypertension, obesity, dyslipidemia, insulin resistance, and hyperglycemia) is associated with primary aldosteronism (see What's New? Aldosteronism and Metabolic Syndrome). Activation of the aldosterone receptor induces insulin resistance; promotes inflammation, endothelial dysfunction, and cardiovascular remodeling; and affects adipose tissue differentiation and function.[219,220]

In *secondary hyperaldosteronism* the effect of increased extracellular volume on renin secretion may vary. If renin secretion is being stimulated by variables other than pressure-initiated cellular changes at the juxtaglomerular apparatus (see Chapter 37), increased circulating blood volume may not decrease renin secretion through feedback mechanisms. This physiologic process is normal in pregnancy and related to increased levels of plasma estrogen.

Potassium secretion also is promoted by aldosterone, so that with excessive circulating levels of aldosterone, hypokalemia occurs (see Chapter 3). In hyperaldosteronism, hypokalemic alkalosis, myocardial conduction changes, and skeletal muscle alterations may be seen, particularly with severe potassium depletion (i.e., the renal tubules may become insensitive to ADH, thus promoting excessive loss of free water). Rarely, this may result in mild hypernatremia because water is not able to follow the sodium that is reabsorbed.

CLINICAL MANIFESTATIONS. Hypertension, hypokalemia, renal potassium wasting, and neuromuscular manifestations are the hallmarks of hyperaldosteronism.[221] Hypertension is resistant to treatment and may result from increased intravascular volume or from a state of aldosterone-mediated vasoconstriction, although the latter mechanism requires very high levels of aldosterone. If hypertension is sustained, the long-term effects of elevated arterial pressure become evident, which include the development of left ventricular dilation and hypertrophy, vascular disease, and renal disease. Because of the increased arterial pressure, renin secretion is typically suppressed, although it is elevated in secondary hyperaldosteronism, which provides a means to clearly differentiate between these conditions.

Aldosterone-stimulated potassium loss can be variable. Serum potassium levels below 3.0 mEq/L result in the typical manifestations of hypokalemia. Hypokalemic alkalosis is caused by the movement of potassium from the intercellular to extracellular space in exchange for hydrogen ions as well as renal loss of hydrogen ions to facilitate sodium reabsorption (see Chapter 3).

EVALUATION AND TREATMENT. Various clinical and laboratory measurements are useful in the assessment of hyperaldosteronism and include the following[222]:

1. Blood pressure: elevated
2. Serum and urinary electrolyte levels: serum sodium level is normal or elevated; serum potassium level is normal or depressed, but urinary potassium level is elevated
3. Serum and urinary levels of aldosterone increase
4. Aldosterone suppression testing: fludrocortisone acetate (Florinef) is used
5. Plasma renin activity: suppressed
6. Plasma aldosterone concentration/plasma renin activity ratio can be high

Serum aldosterone and plasma renin activity both must be measured under controlled situations and after careful dietary regulation of sodium and potassium intake (see Table 22-13).

Imaging techniques, such as CT and nuclear magnetic resonance (NMR), may be used to localize an aldosterone-secreting adenoma. Sampling from both adrenal veins is also useful.

Treatment includes management of hypertension and hypokalemia, as well as correction of any underlying causal abnormalities. If an aldosterone-secreting adenoma is present, it is generally approached surgically. Medical management with aldosterone receptor antagonists, such as spironolactone or eplerenone (a drug without the side effects of spironolactone), is a viable option in selected cases.[222]

Hypersecretion of Adrenal Androgens and Estrogens

Hypersecretion of adrenal androgens and estrogens may be caused by adrenal tumors (either adenomas or carcinomas), Cushing syndrome, or defects in steroid synthesis. The clinical syndrome that results depends on the hormone secreted, the gender of the individual, and the ages at which the hypersecretion was initiated. Hypersecretion of estrogens causes **feminization,** the development of female sex characteristics. Hypersecretion of androgens causes **virilization,** the development of male sex characteristics (Figure 22-26).

The effects of an estrogen-secreting tumor are most evident in men and result in gynecomastia (breast enlargement) (98% of cases), testicular atrophy, and decreased libido. In female children such tumors may lead to early development of secondary

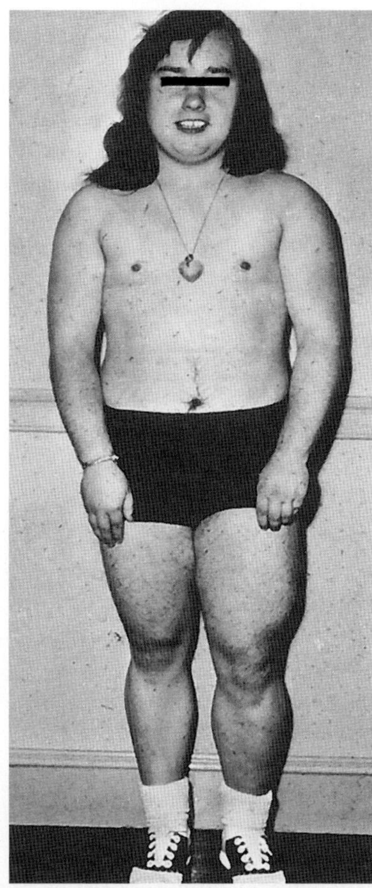

FIGURE 22-26 Virilization. Virilization of a young girl by an androgen-secreting tumor of the adrenal cortex. Masculine features include lack of breast development, increased muscle bulk, and hirsutism. (From Thibodeau GA, Patton KT: *The human body in health & disease,* ed 4, St Louis, 2010, Mosby.)

sex characteristics. An androgen-secreting tumor indicates changes more easily observed in women, including hirsutism, clitoral enlargement, deepening of the voice, amenorrhea, acne, and breast atrophy. In children, virilizing tumors promote precocious sexual development and bone aging. Treatment of androgen-secreting tumors usually involves surgical excision.

Adrenocortical Hypofunction

Hypocortisolism (low levels of cortisol secretion) develops because of either inadequate stimulation of the adrenal glands by ACTH or a primary inability of the adrenals to produce and secrete the adrenocortical hormones. In some syndromes, however, there is partial dysfunction of the adrenal cortex so that only synthesis of cortisol and aldosterone or the adrenal androgens is affected. Hypofunction of the adrenal cortex may affect glucocorticoid or mineralocorticoid secretion or a combination of both.

Addison Disease. **Primary adrenal insufficiency** is termed **Addison disease.** Addison disease is relatively rare, occurring most often in adults 30 to 60 years of age, although it may appear at any time. Addison disease, caused by autoimmune mechanisms, is more common in women.

The most common cause of Addison disease in the United States is autoimmune destruction of the adrenal cortex and it is more common in women. Other causes include infections (tuberculosis, fungal infections, human immunodeficiency virus [HIV]), infiltrative diseases (amyloidosis, metastatic carcinoma), or bilateral adrenal hemorrhage. Adrenoleukodystrophy and adrenomyeloneuropathy are two rare types of X-linked adrenal deficiency that lead to symptoms of hypocortisolism and progressive neurologic symptoms.

PATHOPHYSIOLOGY. Addison disease is characterized by inadequate corticosteroid and mineralocorticoid synthesis and elevated serum ACTH levels. Before clinical manifestations of hypocortisolism are evident, more than 90% of total adrenocortical tissue must be destroyed. Thus the adrenal glands are smaller and may be misshapen.

Idiopathic Addison disease (organ-specific autoimmune adrenalitis), which causes adrenal atrophy and hypofunction, generally is recognized as an organ-specific autoimmune disease. (Autoimmunity is discussed in Chapter 9.) 21-Hydroxylase autoantibodies and autoreactive T cells specific to adrenal cortical cells are present in 50% to 70% of individuals with idiopathic Addison disease; this percentage increases in younger persons and in those with other autoimmune diseases. Apparently, a genetic defect in immune surveillance mechanisms causes a deficiency of immune-suppressor cells. This deficiency allows the proliferation of immunocytes directed against specific antigens within the adrenocortical cells. The adrenal glands in idiopathic Addison disease are smaller than normal and may be misshapen.[223,224] Several genes have been identified.[225]

Idiopathic Addison disease often is associated with other autoimmune diseases and in such cases is known as *autoimmune polyendocrine syndrome (APS).* APSI (APS type I) is inherited as autosomal recessive with childhood onset and includes Addison disease, hypoparathyroidism, mucocutaneous candidiasis, and other less common symptoms. APSII (APS type II) is more common and involves Addison disease, immune thyroid disease, diabetes mellitus, celiac disease, and hypogonadism.[226] (Mechanisms of inheritance are described in Chapter 4.)

CLINICAL MANIFESTATIONS. The symptoms of Addison disease are primarily a result of hypocortisolism and hypoaldosteronism. With mild to moderate hypocortisolism, symptoms usually begin with weakness and easy fatigability. Skin changes, including hyperpigmentation and vitiligo, may occur. As the condition progresses, anorexia, nausea, vomiting, and diarrhea may develop. Of greatest concern is the development of hypotension that can progress to complete vascular collapse and shock.

Decreased adrenal androgen secretion is usually not clinically obvious in men because the adrenals are not a major source of male androgens. Women may experience a loss of some secondary sexual characteristics, such as pubic and axillary hair, normally maintained by the adrenal androgens.[227] Disturbances in mood and motivation are common. The symptoms of Addison disease are summarized in Table 22-14.

EVALUATION AND TREATMENT. Serum and urine levels of cortisol are depressed with primary hypocortisolism and ACTH levels are increased. Because of dehydration, blood urea nitrogen levels may increase. Serum glucose concentration is low. Eosinophil and lymphocyte counts are often elevated. Hyperkalemia is seen in Addison disease and may cause mild alkalosis (see

TABLE 22-14 CLINICAL MANIFESTATIONS AND PATHOPHYSIOLOGIC MECHANISMS OF ADDISON DISEASE

CLINICAL MANIFESTATIONS	PATHOPHYSIOLOGIC MECHANISM
Weakness and easy fatigability that worsen as the day progresses, seen especially after exposure to stressors	Not known, may be related to hypoglycemia, hypotension, decreased metabolism of proteins
Gastrointestinal disturbances: anorexia, nausea, vomiting, diarrhea, abdominal pain, weight loss	May be associated with celiac disease or electrolyte abnormalities
Hypoglycemia, manifested by fatigue, mental confusion, apathy, psychosis	Absence of cortisol leads to decreased gluconeogenesis, decreased glycogen storage by liver, decreased metabolism of proteins, increased insulin sensitivity
Hyperpigmentation	Elevations of ACTH that lead to stimulation of melanocytes
Vitiligo (white patchy areas of depigmented skin)	Autoimmune destruction of melanocytes
Addisonian crisis: severe hypotension and vascular collapse	Combined effects of hypocortisolism, hypoaldosteronism, extracellular volume depletion, and some precipitating stressor (e.g., infection, vomiting, diarrhea); decreased vasomotor tone caused by cortisol deficiency

ACTH, Adrenocorticotropic hormone.

Chapter 3). The ACTH stimulation test may be used to evaluate serum cortisol levels.

The treatment of Addison disease involves lifetime glucocorticoid and mineralocorticoid replacement therapy, together with dietary modifications and correction of any underlying disorders. In the event of acute stressors, additional cortisol must be administered to approximate the amount of cortisol that might be expected to be secreted if normal adrenal function were present (approximately 100 to 300 mg/day).[228] The individual's diet should include at least 150 mEq of sodium per day, with sodium intake increased in the event of excessive sweating or diarrhea.

Secondary Hypocortisolism. **Secondary hypocortisolism** commonly results from prolonged administration of exogenous glucocorticoids, which suppress ACTH secretion. This causes adrenal atrophy and results in inadequate corticosteroidogenesis once the exogenous glucocorticoids are withdrawn. Decreased ACTH secretion also can result from pituitary infarction, pituitary tumors that compress ACTH-secreting cells, or hypophysectomy. In all instances of low ACTH levels, adrenal atrophy occurs and endogenous adrenal steroidogenesis is depressed. Clinical manifestations of secondary hypocortisolism are similar to those of Addison disease, although hyperpigmentation usually does not occur. The renin-angiotensin system usually is normal, so aldosterone and potassium levels also tend to be normal.

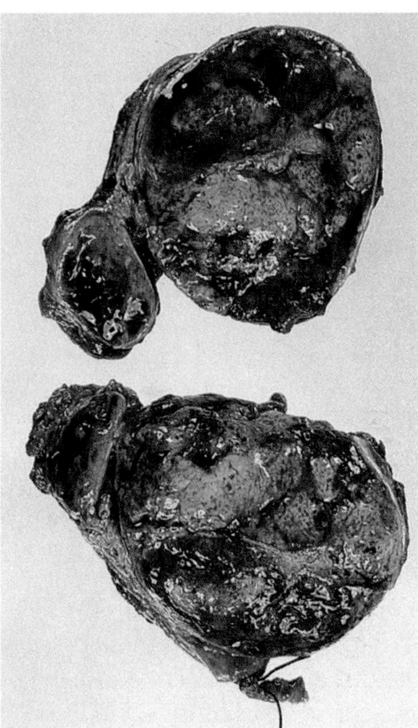

FIGURE 22-27 **Pheochromocytoma.** Gross appearance of adrenal pheochromocytoma. (From Rosai J: *Rosai and Ackerman's surgical pathology,* ed 10, Philadelphia, 2011, Mosby.)

Disorders of the Adrenal Medulla

Tumor of the Adrenal Medulla

Adrenomedullary hyperfunction is caused by **pheochromocytomas** (chromaffin cell tumors) of the adrenal medulla, which secrete catecholamines (Figure 22-27). They are rare and less than 10% of cases are malignant. Most pheochromocytomas produce norepinephrine, although large tumors secrete epinephrine and norepinephrine.

The true incidence of pheochromocytoma in the general population is not known. About one tenth of 1% of the adult hypertensive population has a pheochromocytoma. The tumors are most common in people 40 to 60 years of age, with men and women equally affected. Familial forms of the disease are associated with mutations in the *RET* proto-oncogene, the von Hippel-Lindau *(VHL)* gene, and the neurofibromatosis type 1 gene *(NF1)*. Any of the succinate dehydrogenase complex subunit genes can lead to pheochromocytoma (and paragangliomas).[229]

PATHOPHYSIOLOGY. Pheochromocytomas cause excessive production of norepinephrine, although large tumors secrete epinephrine and norepinephrine because of autonomous functioning of the tumor. Approximately 5% of people with pheochromocytomas have no symptoms because the tumor appears to be nonfunctioning; however, these tumors can release catecholamines in response to stressors, such as abdominal surgery.

CLINICAL MANIFESTATIONS. The clinical manifestations of a pheochromocytoma are related to the chronic effects of catecholamine secretion. Hypertension is the most common sign and it may be sustained or paroxysmal. Other symptoms include diaphoresis, tachycardia, palpitations, and severe headache.[230] Hypertension is a result of increased peripheral vascular resistance. Headaches appear because of sudden changes in catecholamine levels in the blood, affecting cerebral blood flow. Hypermetabolism and sweating are related to chronic activation of sympathetic receptors in adipocytes, hepatocytes, and other tissues. Glucose intolerance may occur because of catecholamine-induced inhibition of insulin release by the pancreas. Complaints of warmth, heat intolerance, weight loss, and constipation are common despite a normal or an increased appetite.

An acute episode of hypertension related to hypersecretion of catecholamines may follow specific events. Exercise, excessive ingestion of tyrosine-containing foods (e.g., aged cheese, red wine, beer, yogurt), ingestion of caffeine-containing foods, external pressure on the tumor, and induction of anesthesia all can increase secretion of catecholamines by the tumor.

These tumors tend to be extremely vascular and can rupture. Such an event can cause massive and potentially fatal hemorrhage. Rupture of a pheochromocytoma is characterized by a sudden, unexplained decrease in blood pressure; sudden, severe abdominal pain; and a rigid abdomen.

EVALUATION AND TREATMENT. A diagnosis of pheochromocytoma is made when increased catecholamine production is demonstrated in the blood or urine. Individuals with this disorder can have total urine catecholamine levels greater than 250 mg/day. After elevation of urinary or plasma catecholamine levels is documented, the site of the tumor is determined using MRI. Because of the possibility of metastasis, whole-body scanning may be done.

Management of catecholamine excess is essential to prevent hypertensive emergencies and requires the use of α- and β-adrenergic blockers. The usual treatment of pheochromocytoma is laparoscopic surgical excision of the tumor with adjunctive radiopharmaceuticals or chemotherapy. Medical therapy is continued to stabilize blood pressure before surgery. Drugs used include α-adrenergic blocking agents and, possibly later, β-adrenergic blocking agents. Open resection is completed for large tumors or when metastasis is suspected. Malignant pheochromocytoma is rarely curable and is usually managed by a combination of surgical debulking of the tumor combined with chemotherapy.[231]

SUMMARY REVIEW

Mechanisms of Hormonal Alterations

1. Abnormalities in endocrine function may be caused by hypersecretion or hyposecretion of hormones, causing alterations in normal hormone levels.
2. Endocrine abnormalities also may be caused by alterations in receptor function through a variety of mechanisms: (a) a decrease in the number of receptors, (b) receptor insensitivity to the hormone, (c) antibodies against specific receptors, and (d) defects in second-messenger generation or postreceptor defects.
3. Abnormally high levels of circulating hormones sometimes are caused by hormone release from tissues outside the endocrine system (ectopic foci) that may not respond to normal feedback mechanisms, in which case they are said to function autonomously.

Alterations of the Hypothalamic-Pituitary System

1. Dysfunction in the release of hypothalamic hormones probably is related to interruption of the connection between the hypothalamus and pituitary—namely, the pituitary stalk.
2. Disorders of the posterior pituitary include SIADH secretion and DI. SIADH secretion is characterized by abnormally high ADH secretion; DI is characterized by abnormally low ADH secretion.
3. In SIADH, high ADH levels interfere with renal free water clearance, leading to hyponatremia and hypoosmolality. SIADH secretion is associated with certain forms of cancer, apparently because of ectopic secretion of ADH by tumor cells.
4. DI may be neurogenic, caused by insufficient amounts of ADH, or nephrogenic, caused by an inadequate response to ADH. Its principal clinical features are failure to concentrate urine with polyuria and polydipsia. Dipsogenic DI occurs when excessive fluid intake lowers the plasma osmolarity to the point that it falls below the threshold for ADH secretion.
5. Hypopituitarism is dysfunction of the anterior pituitary that causes failure of hormonal functions. Symptoms may be mild to severe.
6. Causes of hypopituitarism include pituitary infarction, space-occupying lesions such as tumor or aneurysm, surgical removal, or infections. Symptoms are variable depending on which hormones are deficient (e.g., TSH, ACTH, or GH).
7. Hyperpituitarism is caused by pituitary adenomas. These are usually benign slow-growing tumors that arise from cells of the anterior pituitary.
8. Expansion of a pituitary adenoma causes neurologic and secretory effects. Pressure from the expanding tumor causes hyposecretion of cells, dysfunction of the optic chiasm (leading to visual disturbances), and dysfunction of the hypothalamus and some cranial nerves.
9. Hypersecretion of GH causes acromegaly in adults and giantism in children. Pituitary adenoma is the most common cause of acromegaly.
10. Prolonged, abnormally high levels of GH lead to proliferation of body and connective tissues. Renal, thyroid, cardiovascular, and reproductive dysfunctions develop slowly, together with a change in bony proportions and insulin resistance.
11. GH deficiency in children results in growth failure and fasting hypoglycemia. Adult GH deficiency results in fatigue, osteoporosis, and increased mortality.
12. Pituitary prolactinomas, renal failure, and medications can result in increased levels of prolactin and affect reproductive organs and function in both men and women.

SUMMARY REVIEW—cont'd

Alterations of Thyroid Function

1. Thyrotoxicosis is a general condition in which TH levels are elevated and produce an exaggerated physiologic response in tissues. The condition can be primary, secondary, or subclinical.
2. In general, hyperthyroidism has a range of endocrine, reproductive, gastrointestinal, integumentary, and ocular manifestations. These are caused by increased circulating levels of TH and by stimulation of the sympathetic division of the autonomic nervous system.
3. Graves disease, the most common form of hyperthyroidism, is caused by thyroid-stimulating immunoglobulins that stimulate thyroid TSH receptors, resulting in thyroid hyperplasia and increased synthesis of TH.
4. Manifestations of Graves disease can include symptoms of hyperthyroidism, diffuse thyroid enlargement, disorders of the skin, and enlargement of extraocular muscles.
5. The cutaneous manifestation of Graves disease is pretibial myxedema, a condition characterized by subcutaneous swelling of the legs and, occasionally, the hands.
6. Ocular manifestations of Graves disease are caused by hyperactivity of the sympathetic division of the autonomic nervous system and by immune-induced infiltration of extraocular muscles, orbital fat accumulation, and edema (exophthalmos).
7. Toxic multinodular goiter and solitary toxic adenoma occur when some hyperplastic, hyperfunctioning thyroid nodules autonomously secrete TH, causing hyperthyroidism and producing symptoms similar to those of Graves disease.
8. Toxic multinodular goiters result from multiple functioning adenomas.
9. Thyrotoxic crisis (thyroid storm) is a severe form of hyperthyroidism that often is associated with physiologic stress. Without treatment, death occurs quickly.
10. Hypothyroidism is caused by deficient production of TH by the thyroid gland. The condition may be primary, secondary, or subclinical.
11. Causes of primary hypothyroidism include iodine deficiency, autoimmune thyroiditis, subacute or painless thyroiditis, silent or subacute lymphocytic thyroiditis, iatrogenic hypothyroidism, and postpartum thyroiditis.
12. Autoimmune thyroiditis (Hashimoto disease) is associated with lymphocyte infiltration, antibody activation of natural killer cells, induction of apoptosis with gradual loss of thyroid function, and hypothyroidism.
13. Subacute thyroiditis, a form of hypothyroidism, is a self-limited nonbacterial inflammation of the thyroid gland. The inflammatory process damages follicular cells, causing leakage of triiodothyronine (T_3) and thyroxine (T_4). Hyperthyroidism then is followed by transient hypothyroidism, which is corrected by cellular repair and a return to normal levels in the thyroid.
14. Secondary hypothyroidism is caused by hypothalamic-pituitary dysfunction in which TRH and TSH are not produced in sufficient amounts.
15. Thyroid carcinoma is a relatively rare cancer. The most consistent causal risk factor associated with thyroid carcinoma is exposure to ionizing radiation, especially in childhood.
16. Hypothyroidism affects all body systems. Symptoms depend on the degree of TH deficiency. Common manifestations include decreased energy metabolism and loss of heat production.
17. Myxedema is the characteristic sign of hypothyroidism. Myxedema is caused by alterations in connective tissue with water-binding proteins. The excess water leads to thickened mucous membranes and edema, particularly around the eyes and in the hands and feet.
18. Myxedema coma is a severe form of hypothyroidism, which may be life threatening without emergency medical treatment.
19. Congenital hypothyroidism is TH deficiency at birth; it occurs with thyroid agenesis and results in hypothyroidism, growth failure, and mental retardation from absence of thyroxine.
20. Papillary and follicular thyroid carcinomas are the most common thyroid malignancies probably caused by exposure to ionizing radiation, particularly during childhood. Thyroid nodules are present with normal thyroxine levels.

Alterations of Parathyroid Function

1. Hyperparathyroidism may be primary, secondary, or tertiary and is characterized by greater than normal secretion of PTH.
2. Primary hyperparathyroidism is usually caused by a parathyroid adenoma with interruption of the normal mechanisms that regulate calcium and PTH levels. Manifestations include chronic hypercalcemia, increased bone resorption, and hypercalciuria.
3. Secondary hyperparathyroidism is a compensatory response to hypocalcemia and often occurs with chronic renal failure or chronic vitamin D deficiency.
4. Tertiary hyperparathyroidism is excessive secretion of PTH and hypercalcemia that occurs after long-standing secondary hyperparathyroidism.
5. Pseudohypoparathyroidism and familial hypocalciuric hypercalcemia are inherited conditions. In pseudohypoparathyroidism there is resistance to PTH action and familial hypocalciuric hypercalcemia mimics hyperparathyroidism with failure of calcium sensing by the parathyroid gland.
6. Hypoparathyroidism, defined by abnormally low PTH levels, is caused by thyroid surgery, autoimmunity, or genetic mechanisms.
7. The lack of circulating PTH in hypoparathyroidism causes depressed serum calcium levels, increased serum phosphate levels, decreased bone resorption, and eventual hypocalciuria.

SUMMARY REVIEW—cont'd

Dysfunction of the Endocrine Pancreas: Diabetes Mellitus

1. Diabetes mellitus is a group of diseases characterized by hyperglycemia resulting from defects in insulin secretion or insulin action, or both. The two most common types of diabetes mellitus are type 1 and type 2.
2. A diagnosis of diabetes mellitus is based on glycosylated hemoglobin (HbA_{1c}) levels, fasting plasma glucose (FPG) levels, and 2-hour plasma glucose levels during oral glucose tolerance testing (OGTT).
3. Type 1 diabetes mellitus includes an autoimmune (most common) and a nonimmune type. The immune type (type 1A) is associated with genetic susceptibility, environmental factors, and autoantibody, T-cell, and macrophage destruction of pancreatic beta cells with loss of insulin production and a relative excess of glucagon. Antibodies also can be formed against glutamic acid decarboxylase and insulin. Nonimmune type diabetes (type 1B) occurs secondary to other disease.
4. A diagnosis of diabetes mellitus is based on elevated plasma glucose concentrations and classic signs and symptoms.
5. Type 2 diabetes mellitus is caused by genetic susceptibility that is triggered by environmental factors. The most compelling environmental risk factor is obesity. Insulin production continues but the weight and number of beta cells decrease.
6. Several mechanisms of insulin resistance (hyperinsulinemia) cause reduced glucose uptake and metabolism in type 2 diabetes. These mechanisms include alteration in the production of adipokines by adipose tissue (i.e., leptin resistance), elevated levels of serum free fatty acids and intracellular lipid deposits, release of inflammatory cytokines from adipose tissue, reduced insulin-stimulated mitochondrial activity, and obesity-associated insulin resistance.
7. In type 2 diabetes amylin deficiency results in increased glucagon secretion and hyperglycemia. Deposition of amyloid in the pancreas contributes to beta-cell loss.
8. Decreased ghrelin levels have been associated with insulin resistance and hyperleptinemia in type 2 diabetes.
9. Other specific types of diabetes mellitus include MODY associated with autosomal dominant gene mutations and gestational diabetes associated with onset of glucose intolerance during pregnancy.
10. Acute complications of diabetes mellitus include hypoglycemia, DKA, HHNKS, the Somogyi effect, and the dawn phenomenon.
11. Hypoglycemia is a lowered blood glucose level that may be related to exogenous (i.e., insulin shock or insulin reaction), endogenous, or functional causes.
12. Symptoms of hypoglycemia are divided into adrenergic, caused by activation of the sympathetic nervous system; and neuroglycopenic, reflecting defective central nervous system metabolism resulting from impaired energy generation.
13. DKA develops when there is an absolute or relative deficiency of insulin and an increase in the amounts of insulin counterregulatory hormones of catecholamines, cortisol, glucagon, and GH; increased lipolysis; and accelerated gluconeogenesis and ketogenesis. It is most common in type 1 diabetes, but also occurs in type 2.
14. HHNKS is pathophysiologically similar to DKA, although levels of FFAs are lower in HHNKS and lack of ketosis indicates that some level of insulin is present. The hyperosmolar state can cause osmotic diuresis and profound dehydration, causing coma.
15. The Somogyi effect is a combination of hypoglycemia with rebound hyperglycemia caused by effects of counterregulatory hormones. It is most common in persons with type 1 diabetes mellitus and in children.
16. The dawn phenomenon is an early morning rise in glucose levels caused by nocturnal elevations of GH concentration.
17. Chronic complications of diabetes mellitus are related to chronic hyperglycemia and include microvascular disease (e.g., retinopathy, nephropathy, and neuropathy), macrovascular disease (e.g., CAD, stroke, and peripheral vascular disease), and infection. Metabolic changes contributing to complications include oxidative stress, shunting of glucose to the polyol pathway, activation of protein kinase C, formation of AGEs, and accumulation of hexosamines.
18. Microvascular complications are associated with vascular alterations in the endothelium and the basement membrane as well as thrombosis.
19. Diabetic retinopathy is caused by several mechanisms including microvascular changes and thrombosis that lead to microvascular occlusion, retinal ischemia, increased vascular permeability, microaneurysm formation, hemorrhages, and neovascularization with loss of vision.
20. Diabetic nephropathy is related to hyperglycemia, hyperperfusion, oxidative stress, and inflammation with glomerular enlargement and glomerular basement membrane thickening, diffuse intercapillary glomerulosclerosis, expansion of the mesangial matrix, and progressive renal failure.
21. Diabetic neuropathies may be caused by vascular and metabolic mechanisms, or by a combination of both, with axonal and Schwann cell degeneration and abnormalities in sensory and motor nerve conduction velocity, and involvement of the autonomic nervous system.
22. Macrovascular disease associated with diabetes mellitus is associated with hyperglycemia, hyperlipidemia, inflammation, and altered endothelial function.
23. The incidence of coronary heart disease, peripheral vascular disease, and stroke is greater in persons with diabetes than in nondiabetic individuals.
24. CAD and stroke in diabetes are a consequence of accelerated atherosclerosis, hypertension, and increased risk for thrombus formation.
25. Peripheral vascular disease is a consequence of neuropathy and occlusion of large and small arteries with an increased risk of ischemia, necrosis, and amputation.

SUMMARY REVIEW—cont'd

26. Individuals with diabetes are at risk for a variety of infections related to sensory impairment, vascular complications, impaired white blood cells and suppressed immunity, rapid proliferation of pathogens, and delayed wound healing.

Alterations of Adrenal Function

1. Disorders of the adrenal cortex are related to hyperfunction or hypofunction. No known disorders are associated with hypofunction of the adrenal medulla, but medullary hyperfunction causes clinically defined syndromes.
2. Hypercortisolism is divided into ACTH-dependent (Cushing disease or ectopic ACTH syndrome) and ACTH-independent (adrenal adenoma or adenocarcinoma) mechanisms.
3. Cushing disease is excessive anterior pituitary ACTH production most commonly by an ACTH-secreting pituitary microadenoma.
4. Cushing syndrome occurs whenever there is an excessive level of cortisol regardless of cause. Exogenous forms result from exogenous administration of glucocorticoids. Endogenous forms are either corticotropin dependent (most common and caused by an ACTH-secreting pituitary tumor) or corticotropin independent (usually caused by an adrenal cortical tumor).
5. Individuals with Cushing disease lose diurnal and circadian patterns of ACTH and cortisol secretion, and they lack the ability to increase secretion of these hormones in response to a stressor. Individuals experience weight gain, glucose intolerance, protein wasting, bone disease, hyperpigmentation, and immunosuppression.
6. Congenital adrenal hyperplasia is an autosomal recessive disorder with inadequate synthesis of cortisol and increased levels of ACTH that cause adrenal hyperplasia and overproduction of mineralocorticoids or androgens.
7. Primary hyperaldosteronism is a disorder of excessive aldosterone secretion usually caused by an adrenal cortical adenoma or bilateral nodular hyperplasia. The condition is characterized by hypertension, hypokalemia, renal potassium wasting, and neuromuscular manifestations.
8. Secondary hyperaldosterone secretion is related to a variety of conditions associated with elevated renin release and activation of angiotensin II. These include decreased circulating blood volume, decreased renal blood supply, elevated estrogen levels, Bartter syndrome, and renin-secreting tumors.
9. Adrenal tumors, either adenomas or carcinomas, can autonomously secrete androgens or estrogens.
10. Hypofunction of the adrenal cortex can affect glucocorticoid or mineralocorticoid secretion or both. Hypofunction can be caused by a deficiency of ACTH or by a primary deficiency in the gland itself.
11. Hypocortisolism (low levels of cortisol) is caused by inadequate adrenal stimulation by ACTH or by primary cortisol hyposecretion. Primary adrenal insufficiency is termed Addison disease.
12. Addison disease is characterized by elevated ACTH levels with inadequate corticosteroid synthesis and output. Causes include idiopathic autoimmune disease, tuberculosis of the adrenal gland, familial adrenal insufficiency, amyloidosis, metastatic destruction of the adrenal glands, and adrenal hemorrhage.
13. Manifestations of Addison disease are related to hypocortisolism and hypoaldosteronism. Symptoms include weakness, fatigability, hypoglycemia and related metabolic problems, lowered response to stressors, vitiligo, hyperpigmentation, and manifestations of hypovolemia and hyperkalemia.
14. Secondary hypercortisolism is characterized by low to absent ACTH levels, leading to inadequate adrenal stimulation, adrenal atrophy, and decreased corticosteroidogenesis. The most common cause is withdrawal of exogenous administration of glucocorticoids. Manifestations are similar to those of Addison disease only without hyperpigmentation.
15. Hyperfunction of the adrenal medulla is caused by a pheochromocytoma, which is a catecholamine-producing tumor. Symptoms of catecholamine excess are related to their sympathetic nervous system effects and include hypertension, palpitations, tachycardia, glucose intolerance, excessive sweating, and constipation.

KEY TERMS

KEY TERMS—cont'd

REFERENCES

1. McKenna NJ, Moore DD: Nuclear receptors: structure, functions and coregulators. In Jameson JL, Degroot LJ, editors: *Endocrinology*, ed 6, Philadelphia, 2010, Saunders.
2. Schoenmakers N et al: A mutation in the thyroid hormone receptor alpha gene, *N Engl J Med* 366(3):243–249, 2012.
3. Carmody D et al: Vasopressin, diabetes insipidus and the syndrome of inappropriate antidiuretic hormone secretion. In Jameson JL, Degroot LJ, editors: *Endocrinology*, ed 6, Philadelphia, 2010, Saunders.
4. Vandergheynst F et al: Lack of responsiveness to 1-desamino-D arginine vasopressin (desmopressin) in male patients with nephrogenic syndrome of inappropriate antidiuresis: from bench to bedside, *Eur J Clin Invest* 42(3):254–259, 2012.
5. Rabinstein AA, Bruder N: Management of hyponatremia and volume contraction, *Neurocrit Care* 15(2):354–360, 2011.
6. Gross P: Clinical management of SIADH, *Ther Adv Endocrinol Metab* 3(2):61–73, 2012.
7. Dasta JF et al: Update on tolvaptan for the treatment of hyponatremia, *Expert Rev Pharmacoecon Outcomes Res* 12(4):399–410, 2012.
8. Merenkov VV, Kovalev AN, Gorbunov VV: Water-electrolyte disturbances after pituitary surgery, *J Neurosurg Anesthesiol* 24(1):79–80, 2012.
9. Babey M, Kopp P, Robertson GL: Familial forms of diabetes insipidus: clinical and molecular characteristics, *Nat Rev Endocrinol* 7(12): 701–714, 2011.
10. Fenske W, Allolio B: Clinical review: current state and future perspectives in the diagnosis of diabetes insipidus: a clinical review, *J Clin Endocrinol Metab* 97(10):3426–3437, 2012.
11. Chanson P, Salenave S: Treatment of neurogenic diabetes insipidus, *Ann Endocrinol (Paris)* 72(6):496–499, 2011.
12. Los EL, Deen PM, Robben JH: Potential of nonpeptide (ant)agonists to rescue vasopressin V2 receptor mutants for the treatment of X-linked nephrogenic diabetes insipidus, *J Neuroendocrinol* 22(5):393–399, 2010.
13. Karaca Z, Kelestimur F: Pregnancy and other pituitary disorders (including GH deficiency), *Best Pract Res Clin Endocrinol Metab* 25(6):897–910, 2011.
14. Lee P, Ho K: Hypopituitarism and growth hormone deficiency. In Jameson JL, Degroot LJ, editors: *Endocrinology*, ed 6, Philadelphia, 2010, Saunders.
15. Heather NL et al: Permanent hypopituitarism is rare after structural traumatic brain injury in early childhood, *J Clin Endocrinol Metab* 97(2):599–604, 2012.
16. Gasco V et al: Hypopituitarism following brain injury: when does it occur and how best to test? *Pituitary* 15(1):20–24, 2012.
17. Castinetti F et al: Pituitary stem cell update and potential implications for treating hypopituitarism, *Endocr Rev* 32(4):453–471, 2011.
18. Romero CJ, Pine-Twaddell E, Radovick S: Novel mutations associated with combined pituitary hormone deficiency, *J Mol Endocrinol* 46(3):R93–R102, 2011.
19. Hannon MJ, O'Halloran DJ: Isolated acquired ACTH deficiency and primary hypothyroidism: a short series and review, *Pituitary* 14(4): 358–361, 2011.
20. Alatzoglou KS, Dattani MT: Genetic causes and treatment of isolated growth hormone deficiency—an update, *Nat Rev Endocrinol* 6(10): 562–576, 2010.
21. Mullis PE: Genetics of GHRH, GHRH-receptor, GH and GH-receptor: its impact on pharmacogenetics, *Best Pract Res Clin Endocrinol Metab* 25(1):25–41, 2011.
22. Elijah IE et al: The GH/IGF-1 system in critical illness, *Best Pract Res Clin Endocrinol Metab* 25(5):759–767, 2011.
23. Antonopoulou M et al: Hypopituitarism in the elderly, *Maturitas* 72(4):277–285, 2012.
24. Miller BS: rhGH safety and efficacy update, *Adv Pediatr* 58(1):207–241, 2011.
25. Molitch ME et al: Evaluation and treatment of adult growth hormone deficiency: an Endocrine Society clinical practice guideline, *J Clin Endocrinol Metab* 96(6):1587–1609, 2011.
26. Fernandez-Balsells MM et al: Natural history of nonfunctioning pituitary adenomas and incidentalomas: a systematic review and metaanalysis, *J Clin Endocrinol Metab* 96(4):905–912, 2011.
27. Lleva RR, Inzucchi SE: Diagnosis and management of pituitary adenomas, *Curr Opin Oncol* 23(1):53–60, 2011.
28. Rostad S: Pituitary adenoma pathogenesis: an update, *Curr Opin Endocrinol Diabetes Obes* 19(4):322–327, 2012.
29. Vasilev V et al: Familial pituitary tumor syndromes, *Endocrine Pract* 17(Suppl 3):41–46, 2011.
30. Mehta GU, Jane JA Jr: Pituitary tumors, *Curr Opin Neurol* 25(6):751–755, 2012.
31. Golkowski F et al: Goiter, cardiovascular and metabolic disorders in patients with acromegaly, *Endocr Regul* 45(4):191–197, 2011.

32. Espinosa-de-los-Monteros AL et al: Clinical and biochemical characteristics of acromegalic patients with different abnormalities in glucose metabolism, *Pituitary* 14(3):231–235, 2011.
33. Colao A et al: Determinants of cardiac disease in newly diagnosed patients with acromegaly: results of a 10 year survey study, *Eur J Endocrinol* 165(5):713–721, 2011.
34. Jayasena CN et al: The effects of long-term growth hormone and insulin-like growth factor-1 exposure on the development of cardiovascular, cerebrovascular and metabolic co-morbidities in treated patients with acromegaly, *Clin Endocrinol* 75(2):220–225, 2011.
35. Katznelson L et al: American Association of Clinical Endocrinologists medical guidelines for clinical practice for the diagnosis and treatment of acromegaly—2011 update: executive summary, *Endocr Pract* 17(4):636–646, 2011.
36. Sherlock M, Woods C, Sheppard MC: Medical therapy in acromegaly, *Nat Rev Endocrinol* 7(5):291–300, 2011.
37. Higham CE et al: Effective combination treatment with cabergoline and low-dose pegvisomant in active acromegaly: a prospective clinical trial, *J Clin Endocrinol Metab* 97(4):1187–1193, 2012.
38. Oh MC et al: Medical versus surgical management of prolactinomas, *Neurosurg Clin N Am* 23(4):669–678, 2012.
39. Klibanski A: Clinical practice. Prolactinomas, *N Engl J Med* 362(13):1219–1226, 2010.
40. Melmed S et al: Diagnosis and treatment of hyperprolactinemia: an Endocrine Society clinical practice guideline, *J Clin Endocrinol Metab* 96(2):273–288, 2011.
41. Maiter D, Primeau V: 2012 Update in the treatment of prolactinomas, *Ann Endocrinol (Paris)* 73(2):90–98, 2012.
42. Steffensen C et al: Heart valve disease among patients with hyperprolactinemia: a nationwide population-based cohort study, *J Clin Endocrinol Metab* 97(5):1629–1634, 2012.
43. Seigel SC, Hodak SP: Thyrotoxicosis, *Med Clin North Am* 96(2):175–201, 2012.
44. Cooper DS, Biondi B: Subclinical thyroid disease, *Lancet* 379(9821):1142–1154, 2012.
45. Bahn Chair RS et al: Hyperthyroidism and other causes of thyrotoxicosis: management guidelines of the American Thyroid Association and American Association of Clinical Endocrinologists, *Thyroid* 21(6):593–646, 2011.
46. Franklyn JA, Boelaert K: Thyrotoxicosis, *Lancet* 379(9821):1155–1166, 2012.
47. Brent GA: Clinical practice. Graves' disease, *N Engl J Med* 358(24):2594–2605, 2008.
48. Stan MN, Garrity JA, Bahn RS: The evaluation and treatment of Graves ophthalmopathy, *Med Clin North Am* 96(2):311–328, 2012.
49. Reddy SV, Gupta SK, Jain M: Dermopathy of Graves' disease: clinico-pathological correlation, *Indian J Endocrinol Metab* 16(3):460–462, 2012.
50. Boboridis KG, Bunce C: Surgical orbital decompression for thyroid eye disease, *Cochrane Database Syst Rev* 7(12):CD007630, 2011.
51. Fatourechi V: Pretibial myxedema: pathophysiology and treatment options, *Am J Clin Dermatol* 6(5):295–309, 2005.
52. Cerci C et al: Thyroid cancer in toxic and non-toxic multinodular goiter, *J Postgrad Med* 53(4):157–160, 2007.
53. Krohn K et al: Molecular pathogenesis of euthyroid and toxic multinodular goiter, *Endocr Rev* 26(4):504–524, 2005.
54. Paschke R: Molecular pathogenesis of nodular goiter, *Langenbecks Arch Surg* 396(8):1127–1136, 2011.
55. Klubo-Gwiezdzinska J, Wartofsky L: Thyroid emergencies, *Med Clin North Am* 96(2):385–403, 2012.
56. Almandoz JP, Gharib H: Hypothyroidism: etiology, diagnosis, and management, *Med Clin North Am* 96(2):203–221, 2012.
57. Mathew V et al: Myxedema coma: a new look into an old crisis, *J Thyroid Res* 493462:2011, 2011.
58. Khandelwal D, Tandon N: Overt and subclinical hypothyroidism: who to treat and how, *Drugs* 72(1):17–33, 2012.
59. Stuart A: The changing scene in Hashimoto's disease: a review, *Med Hypotheses* 77(3):424–426, 2011.
60. Saranac L et al: Why is the thyroid so prone to autoimmune disease? *Horm Res Paediatr* 75(3):157–165, 2011.
61. Eschler DC, Hasham A, Tomer Y: Cutting edge: the etiology of autoimmune thyroid diseases, *Clin Rev Allergy Immunol* 41(2):190–197, 2011.
62. Samuels MH: Subacute, silent, and postpartum thyroiditis, *Med Clin North Am* 96(2):223–233, 2012.
63. Samuels MH: Subacute, silent, and postpartum thyroiditis, *Med Clin North Am* 96(2):223–233, 2012.
64. Stagnaro-Green A et al: American Thyroid Association Taskforce on Thyroid Disease During Pregnancy and Postpartum. Guidelines of the American Thyroid Association for the diagnosis and management of thyroid disease during pregnancy and postpartum, *Thyroid* 21(10):1081–1125, 2011.
65. Abduljabbar MA, Afifi AM: Congenital hypothyroidism, *J Pediatr Endocrinol Metab* 25(1-2):13–29, 2012.
66. LaFranchi SH: Approach to the diagnosis and treatment of neonatal hypothyroidism, *J Clin Endocrinol Metab* 96(10):2959–2967, 2011.
67. American Cancer Society: *Cancer facts & figures 2013*, Atlanta, 2013, Author.
68. Pauci F, Castagna MG: Approach to and treatment of differentiated thyroid carcinoma, *Med Clin North Am* 96(2):369–383, 2012.
69. Saindane AM: Pitfalls in the staging of cancer of thyroid, *Neuroimaging Clin N Am*(1)123–145, 2013.
70. Wein RO, Weber RS: Anaplastic thyroid carcinoma: palliation or treatment? *Curr Opin Otolaryngol Head Neck Surg* 19(2):113–118, 2011.
71. Carneiro-Pla D, Solorzano C: A summary of the new phenomenon of normocalcemic hyperparathyroidism and appropriate management, *Curr Opin Oncol* 24(1):42–45, 2012.
72. Pepe J et al: Sporadic and hereditary primary hyperparathyroidism, *J Endocrinol Invest* 34(Suppl 7):40–44, 2011.
73. Cetani F et al: Molecular pathogenesis of primary hyperparathyroidism, *J Endocrinol Invest* 34(Suppl 7):35–39, 2011.
74. Nuti R, Merlotti D, Gennari L: Vitamin D deficiency and primary hyperparathyroidism, *J Endocrinol Invest* 34(Suppl 7):45–49, 2011.
75. Mantovani G: Clinical review: pseudohypoparathyroidism: diagnosis and treatment, *J Clin Endocrinol Metab* 96(10):3020–3030, 2011.
76. Varghese J, Rich T, Jimenez C: Benign familial hypocalciuric hypercalcemia, *Endocr Pract* 17(Suppl 1):13–17, 2011.
77. Broulik PD et al: Improvement of hypertension after parathyroidectomy of patients suffering from primary hyperparathyroidism, *Int J Endocrinol* 309068:2011, 2011.
78. Rejnmark L, Vestergaard P, Mosekilde L: Nephrolithiasis and renal calcifications in primary hyperparathyroidism, *J Clin Endocrinol Metab* 96(8):2377–2385, 2011.
79. Anderson JL et al: Parathyroid hormone, vitamin D, renal dysfunction, and cardiovascular disease: dependent or independent risk factors? *Am Heart J* 162(2):331–339, e2, 2011.
80. Ellam TJ, Chico TJ: Phosphate: the new cholesterol? The role of the phosphate axis in non-uremic vascular disease, *Atherosclerosis* 220(2):310–318, 2012.
81. Johnson NA, Carty SE, Tublin ME: Parathyroid imaging, *Radiol Clin North Am* 49(3):489–509, vi, 2011.
82. Khan AA: Medical management of primary hyperparathyroidism, *J Clin Densitom* 16(1):60–63, 2013.
83. Vestergaard P, Thomsen SS: Medical treatment of primary, secondary, and tertiary hyperparathyroidism, *Curr Drug Saf* 6(2):108–113, 2011.
84. Bilezikian JP et al: Hypoparathyroidism in the adult: epidemiology, diagnosis, pathophysiology, target-organ involvement, treatment, and challenges for future research, *J Bone Miner Res* 26(10):2317–2337, 2011.
85. Al-Azem H, Khan AA: Hypoparathyroidism, *Best Pract Res Clin Endocrinol Metab* 26(4):517–522, 2012.
86. Cusano NE et al: Mini-review: new therapeutic options in hypoparathyroidism, *Endocrine* 41(3):410–414, 2012.
87. Centers for Disease Control and Prevention: *2011 National diabetes fact sheet*. Available at www.cdc.gov/diabetes/pubs/estimates11.htm#1.
88. American Diabetes Association: Diagnosis and classification of diabetes mellitus, *Diabetes Care* 35:S64–S71, 2012.
89. Ferrannini E et al: Progression to diabetes in relatives of type 1 diabetic patients: mechanisms and mode of onset, *Diabetes* 59(3):679–685, 2010.
90. Baker PR Jr, Steck AK: The past, present, and future of genetic associations in type 1 diabetes, *Curr Diabetes Rep* 11(5):445–453, 2011.
91. Grieco FA et al: Immunology in the clinic review series; focus on type 1 diabetes and viruses: how viral infections modulate beta cell function, *Clin Exp Immunol* 168(1):24–29, 2012.
92. Stene LC, Rewers M: Immunology in the clinic review series; focus on type 1 diabetes and viruses: the enterovirus link to type 1 diabetes: critical review of human studies, *Clin Exp Immunol* 168(1):12–23, 2012.
93. Vehik K, Dabelea D: The changing epidemiology of type 1 diabetes: why is it going through the roof? *Diabetes Metab Res Rev* 27(1):3–13, 2011.
94. Wherrett DK, Daneman D: Prevention of type 1 diabetes, *Pediatr Clin North Am* 58(5):1257–1270, xi, 2011.
95. Calderon B, Unanue ER: Antigen presentation events in autoimmune diabetes, *Curr Opin Immunol* 24(1):119–128, 2012.

96. Roep BO, Peakman M: Diabetogenic T lymphocytes in human type 1 diabetes, *Curr Opin Immunol* 23(6):746–753, 2011.
97. Haskins K, Cooke A: CD4 T cells and their antigens in the pathogenesis of autoimmune diabetes, *Curr Opin Immunol* 23(6):739–745, 2011.
98. Zhang L, Eisenbarth GS: Prediction and prevention of type 1 diabetes mellitus, *J Diabetes* 3(1):48–57, 2011.
99. Culina S, Brezar V, Mallone R: Insulin and type 1 diabetes: immune connections, *Eur J Endocrinol* 168(2):R19–R31, 2013.
100. Long AE et al: Rising incidence of type 1 diabetes is associated with altered immunophenotype at diagnosis, *Diabetes* 61(3):683–686, 2012.
101. Nielsen LB et al: Relationship between *ZnT8Ab*, the *SLC30A8* gene and disease progression in children with newly diagnosed type 1 diabetes, *Autoimmunity* 44(8):616–623, 2011.
102. Cabrera SM, Rigby MR, Mirmira RG: Targeting regulatory T cells in the treatment of type 1 diabetes mellitus, *Curr Mol Med* 12(10):1261–1272, 2012.
103. Unger RH, Cherrington AD: Glucagonocentric restructuring of diabetes: a pathophysiologic and therapeutic makeover, *J Clin Invest* 122(1):4–12, 2012.
104. Lebovitz HE: Adjunct therapy for type 1 diabetes mellitus, *Nat Rev Endocrinol* 6(6):326–334, 2010.
105. Tomita T: Islet amyloid polypeptide in pancreatic islets from type 1 diabetic subjects, *Islets* 3(4):166–174, 2011.
106. Bui H et al: Is diabetic ketoacidosis at disease onset a result of missed diagnosis? *J Pediatr* 156(3):472–477, 2010.
107. Wherrett DK, Daneman D: Prevention of type 1 diabetes, *Pediatr Clin North Am* 58(5):1257–1270, xi, 2011.
108. Gallagher MP, Goland RS, Greenbaum CJ: Making progress: preserving beta cells in type 1 diabetes, *Ann N Y Acad Sci* 1243:119–134, 2011.
109. Pickup JC: Insulin-pump therapy for type 1 diabetes mellitus, *N Engl J Med* 366(17):1616–1624, 2012.
110. Traina AN, Kane MP: Primer on pramlintide, an amylin analog, *Diabetes Educ* 37(3):426–431, 2011.
111. Szypowska A et al: Beneficial effect of real-time continuous glucose monitoring system on glycemic control in type 1 diabetic patients: systematic review and meta-analysis of randomized trials, *Eur J Endocrinol* 166(4):567–574, 2012.
112. Centers for Disease Control and Prevention: *Diabetes data and trends.* Available at http://apps.nccd.cdc.gov/DDTSTRS/default.aspx. Accessed May 20, 2013.
113. Temelkova-Kurktschiev T, Stefanov T: Lifestyle and genetics in obesity and type 2 diabetes, *Exp Clin Endocrinol Diabetes* 120(1):1–6, 2012.
114. Prasad H et al: Metabolic syndrome: definition and therapeutic implications, *Postgrad Med* 124(1):21–30, 2012.
115. Barber TM, Franks S: The link between polycystic ovary syndrome and both type 1 and type 2 diabetes mellitus: what do we know today? *Women's Health (Lond Engl)* 8(2):147–154, 2012.
116. Gluckman PD: Epigenetics and metabolism in 2011: epigenetics, the life-course and metabolic disease, *Nat Rev Endocrinol* 8(2):74–76, 2012.
117. Pinney SE, Simmons RA: Metabolic programming, epigenetics, and gestational diabetes mellitus, *Curr Diabetes Rep* 12(1):67–74, 2012.
118. Ashcroft FM, Rorsman P: Diabetes mellitus and the beta cell: the last ten years, *Cell* 148(6):1160–1171, 2012.
119. Marino JS, Xu Y, Hill JW: Central insulin and leptin-mediated autonomic control of glucose homeostasis, *Trends Endocrinol Metab* 22(7):275–285, 2011.
120. Wolfson N et al: Relation of adiponectin to glucose tolerance status, adiposity, and cardiovascular risk factor load, *Exp Diabetes Res* 250621:2012, 2012.
121. Vinolo MA, Hirabara SM, Curi R: G-protein-coupled receptors as fat sensors, *Curr Opin Clin Nutr Metab Care* 15(2):112–116, 2012.
122. Bhargava P, Lee CH: Role and function of macrophages in the metabolic syndrome, *Biochem J* 442(2):253–262, 2012.
123. Stienstra R et al: The inflammasome puts obesity in the danger zone, *Cell Metab* 15(1):10–18, 2012.
124. Ma ZA, Zhao Z, Turk J: Mitochondrial dysfunction and beta-cell failure in type 2 diabetes mellitus, *Exp Diabetes Res* 2012:703538, 2012.
125. Szendroedi J, Phielix E, Roden M: The role of mitochondria in insulin resistance and type 2 diabetes mellitus, *Nat Rev Endocrinol* 8(2):92–103, 2012.
126. Karunakaran U et al: Guards and culprits in the endoplasmic reticulum: glucolipotoxicity and beta-cell failure in type II diabetes, *Exp Diabetes Res* 639762:2012, 2012.
127. Brooks-Worrell B, Palmer JP: Immunology in the Clinic Review Series; focus on metabolic diseases: development of islet autoimmune disease in type 2 diabetes patients: potential sequelae of chronic inflammation, *Clin Exp Immunol* 167(1):40–46, 2012.
128. Cryer PE: Minireview: glucagon in the pathogenesis of hypoglycemia and hyperglycemia in diabetes, *Endocrinology* 153(3):1039–1048, 2012.
129. Cheng B et al: Silibinin inhibits the toxic aggregation of human islet amyloid polypeptide, *Biochem Biophys Res Commun* 419(3):495–499, 2012.
130. Loomes KM: Survival of an islet beta-cell in type-2 diabetes: curbing the effects of amyloid cytotoxicity, *Islets* 3(1):38–39, 2011.
131. Israili ZH: Advances in the treatment of type 2 diabetes mellitus, *Am J Ther* 18(2):117–152, 2011.
132. Garber AJ: Novel GLP-1 receptor agonists for diabetes, *Expert Opin Investig Drugs* 21(1):45–57, 2012.
133. Hamed EA et al: Circulating leptin and insulin in obese patients with and without type 2 diabetes mellitus: relation to ghrelin and oxidative stress, *Diabetes Res Clin Pract* 94(3):434–441, 2011.
134. Delhanty PJ, van der Lely AJ: Ghrelin and glucose homeostasis, *Peptides* 32(11):2309–2318, 2011.
135. Ukkola O: Ghrelin in type 2 diabetes mellitus and metabolic syndrome, *Mol Cell Endocrinol* 340(1):26–28, 2011.
136. American Diabetes Association: Standards of medical care in diabetes 2012, *Diabetes Care* 35(Suppl 1):S11–S63, 2012.
137. Boussageon R et al: Effect of intensive glucose lowering treatment on all cause mortality, cardiovascular death, and microvascular events in type 2 diabetes: meta-analysis of randomised controlled trials, *BMJ* 343:d4169, 2011.
138. Colagiuri S: Optimal management of type 2 diabetes: the evidence, *Diabetes Obes Metab* 14(Suppl 1):3–8, 2012.
139. Ismail-Beigi F: Clinical practice. Glycemic management of type 2 diabetes mellitus, *N Engl J Med* 366(14):1319–1327, 2012.
140. Kansagara D et al: Intensive insulin therapy in hospitalized patients: a systematic review, *Ann Intern Med* 154(4):268–282, 2011.
141. Igel LI et al: Advances in medical therapy for weight loss and the weight-centric management of type 2 diabetes mellitus, *Curr Atheroscler Rep* 14(1):60–69, 2012.
142. Qaseem A et al: Oral pharmacologic treatment of type 2 diabetes mellitus: a clinical practice guideline from the American College of Physicians, *Ann Intern Med* 156(3):218–231, 2012.
143. Currie CJ, Johnson JA: The safety profile of exogenous insulin in people with type 2 diabetes: justification for concern, *Diabetes Obes Metab* 14(1):1–4, 2012.
144. Konig M, Shuldiner AR: The genetic interface between gestational diabetes and type 2 diabetes, *J Matern Fetal Neonatal Med* 25(1):36–40, 2012.
145. Steck AK, Winter WE: Review on monogenic diabetes, *Curr Opin Endocrinol Diabetes Obes* 18(4):252–258, 2011.
146. Thanabalasingham G, Owen KR: Diagnosis and management of maturity onset diabetes of the young (MODY), *BMJ* 343:d6044, 2011.
147. Ballas J, Moore TR, Ramos GA: Management of diabetes in pregnancy, *Curr Diabetes Rep* 12(1):33–42, 2012.
148. Sullivan SD, Umans JG, Ratner R: Gestational diabetes: implications for cardiovascular health, *Curr Diabetes Rep* 12(1):43–52, 2012.
149. Beall C, Ashford ML, McCrimmon RJ: The physiology and pathophysiology of the neural control of the counterregulatory response, *Am J Physiol Regul Integr Comp Physiol* 302(2):R215–R223, 2012.
150. McCrimmon RJ: Update in the CNS response to hypoglycemia, *J Clin Endocrinol Metab* 97(1):1–8, 2012.
151. Foster DW, Esser V: Ketoacidosis and hyperosmolar coma. In Jamerson JL, Degroot LJ, editors: *Endocrinology*, ed 6, Philadelphia, 2010, Saunders.
152. Tan H, Wang C, Yu Y: H1N1 influenza: the trigger of diabetic ketoacidosis in a young woman with ketosis-prone diabetes, *Am J Med Sci* 343(2):180–183, 2012.
153. Usher-Smith JA et al: Factors associated with the presence of diabetic ketoacidosis at diagnosis of diabetes in children and young adults: a systematic review, *BMJ* 343:d4092, 2011.
154. Kitabchi AE, Nyenwe EA: Hyperglycemic crises in diabetes mellitus: diabetic ketoacidosis and hyperglycemic hyperosmolar state, *Endocrinol Metab Clin North Am* 35(4):725–751, viii, 2006.
155. Savage MW: Management of diabetic ketoacidosis, *Clin Med* 11(2): 154–156, 2011.
156. Nyenwe EA, Kitabchi AE: Evidence-based management of hyperglycemic emergencies in diabetes mellitus, *Diabetes Res Clin Pract* 94(3): 340–351, 2011.
157. Folli F et al: The role of oxidative stress in the pathogenesis of type 2 diabetes mellitus micro- and macrovascular complications: avenues for a mechanistic-based therapeutic approach, *Curr Diabetes Rev* 7(5): 313–324, 2011.

158. Pangare M, Makino A: Mitochondrial function in vascular endothelial cell in diabetes, *J Smooth Muscle Res* 48(1):1–26, 2012.
159. Naudi A et al: Cellular dysfunction in diabetes as maladaptive response to mitochondrial oxidative stress, *Exp Diabetes Res* 696215:2012, 2012.
160. Doria A: Genetics of diabetes complications, *Curr Diabetes Rep* 10(6):467–475, 2010.
161. Reddy MA, Natarajan R: Epigenetic mechanisms in diabetic vascular complications, *Cardiovasc Res* 90(3):421–429, 2011.
162. Tang WH, Martin KA, Hwa J: Aldose reductase, oxidative stress, and diabetic mellitus, *Front Pharmacol* 3:87, 2012.
163. Geraldes P, King GL: Activation of protein kinase C isoforms and its impact on diabetic complications, *Circ Res* 106(8):1319–1331, 2010.
164. Win MT et al: Regulation of RAGE for attenuating progression of diabetic vascular complications, *Exp Diabetes Res* 894605:2012, 2012.
165. Yamagishi S: Role of advanced glycation end products (AGEs) and receptor for AGEs (RAGE) in vascular damage in diabetes, *Exp Gerontol* 46(4):217–224, 2011.
166. Ramasamy R, Yan SF, Schmidt A: The diverse ligand repertoire of the receptor for advanced glycation endproducts and pathways to the complications of diabetes, *Vascul Pharmacol* 57(5-6):160–167, 2012.
167. Teo CF, Wollaston-Hayden EE, Wells L: Hexosamine flux, the O-GlcNAc modification, and the development of insulin resistance in adipocytes, *Mol Cell Endocrinol* 318(1-2):44–53, 2010.
168. Pop-Busui R et al: DCCT and EDIC studies in type 1 diabetes: lessons for diabetic neuropathy regarding metabolic memory and natural history, *Curr Diabetes Rep* 10(4):276–282, 2010.
169. White NH et al: Effect of prior intensive therapy in type 1 diabetes on 10-year progression of retinopathy in the DCCT/EDIC: comparison of adults and adolescents, *Diabetes* 59(5):1244–1253, 2010.
170. Fante RJ, Jurairaj VD, Oliver SC: Diabetic retinopathy: an update on treatment, *Am J Med* 123(3):213–216, 2010.
171. Cheung N, Mitchell P, Wong TY: Diabetic retinopathy, *Lancet* 376(9735):124–136, 2010.
172. Romero-Aroca P: Managing diabetic macular edema: the leading cause of diabetes blindness, *World J Diabetes* 2(6):98–104, 2011.
173. Abbate M et al: Prevention and treatment of diabetic retinopathy: evidence from clinical trials and perspectives, *Curr Diabetes Rev* 7(3): 190–200, 2011.
174. Dronavalli S, Duka I, Bakris GL: The pathogenesis of diabetic nephropathy, *Nat Clin Pract Endocrinol Metab* 4(8):444–452, 2008.
175. Kanwar YS et al: A glimpse of various pathogenetic mechanisms of diabetic nephropathy, *Annu Rev Pathol* 6:395–423, 2011.
176. Najafian B, Alpers CE, Fogo AB: Pathology of human diabetic nephropathy, *Contrib Nephrol* 170:36–47, 2011.
177. Ritz E: Clinical manifestations and natural history of diabetic kidney disease, *Med Clin North Am* 97(1):19–29, 2013.
178. Van Buren PN, Toto R: Hypertension in diabetic nephropathy: epidemiology, mechanisms, and management, *Adv Chronic Kidney Dis* 18(1):28–41, 2011.
179. Tang SC, Leung JC, Lai KN: Diabetic tubulopathy: an emerging entity, *Contrib Nephrol* 170:124–134, 2011.
180. Williams ME: The goal of blood pressure control for prevention of early diabetic microvascular complications, *Curr Diabetes Rep* 11(4):323–329, 2011.
181. Thomas MC: Pathogenesis and progression of proteinuria, *Contrib Nephrol* 170:48–56, 2011.
182. Gorriz JL, Martinez-Castelao A: Proteinuria: detection and role in native renal disease progression, *Transplant Rev (Orlando)* 26(1):3–13, 2012.
183. Macisaac RJ, Jerums G: Diabetic kidney disease with and without albuminuria, *Curr Opin Nephrol Hypertens* 20(3):246–257, 2011.
184. Van Buren PN, Toto RD: The pathogenesis and management of hypertension in diabetic kidney disease, *Med Clin North Am* 97(1):31–51, 2013.
185. Tesfaye S, Selvarajah D: Advances in the epidemiology, pathogenesis and management of diabetic peripheral neuropathy, *Diabetes Metab Res Rev* 28(Suppl 1):8–14, 2012.
186. Tomlinson DR, Gardiner NJ: Diabetic neuropathies: components of etiology, *J Peripher Nerv Syst* 13(2):112–121, 2008.
187. Andersen H: Motor dysfunction in diabetes, *Diabetes Metab Res Rev* 28(Suppl 1):89–92, 2012.
188. Vinik AI, Erbas T, Casellini CM: Diabetic cardiac autonomic neuropathy, inflammation, and cardiovascular disease, *J Diabetes Investig* 4(1):4–18, 2013.
189. Umegaki H: Neurodegeneration in diabetes mellitus, *Adv Exp Med Biol* 724:258–265, 2012.
190. Pappalardo J, Fitzgerald R: Utilization of advanced modalities in the management of diabetic Charcot neuroarthropathy, *J Diabetes Sci Technol* 4(5):1114–1120, 2010.
191. Giannini C et al: Macrovascular angiopathy in children and adolescents with type 1 diabetes, *Diabetes Metab Res Rev* 27(5):436–460, 2011.
192. Ford ES, Zhao G, Li C: Pre-diabetes and the risk for cardiovascular disease: a systematic review of the evidence, *J Am Coll Cardiol* 55(13): 1310–1317, 2010.
193. Yamagishi S et al: Role of advanced glycation end products (AGEs) and oxidative stress in vascular complications in diabetes, *Biochim Biophys Acta* 1820(5):663–671, 2012.
194. Chopra S, Peter S: Screening for coronary artery disease in patients with type 2 diabetes mellitus: an evidence-based review, *Indian J Endocrinol Metab* 16(1):94–101, 2012.
195. Nandish S et al: Implementing cardiovascular risk reduction in patients with cardiovascular disease and diabetes mellitus, *Am J Cardiol* 108(Suppl 3):42B–51B, 2011.
195a. Battiprolu PK et al: Diabetic cardiomyopathy and metabolic remodeling of the heart, *Life Sci* 92(11):609–615, 2013.
196. Tarquini R et al: The diabetic cardiomyopathy, *Acta Diabetol* 48(3): 173–181, 2011.
197. Luitse MJ et al: Diabetes, hyperglycaemia, and acute ischaemic stroke, *Lancet Neurol* 11(3):261–271, 2012.
198. Gazis A et al: Mortality in patients with diabetic neuropathic osteoarthropathy (Charcot foot), *Diabetes Med* 21(11):1243–1246, 2004.
199. Al-Delaimy WK et al: Effect of type 2 diabetes and its duration on the risk of peripheral arterial disease among men, *Am J Med* 116(4): 236–240, 2004.
200. Mohler ER: III: Therapy insight: peripheral arterial disease and diabetes—from pathogenesis to treatment guidelines, *Nat Clin Pract Cardiovasc Med* 4(3):151–162, 2007.
201. Faglia E: Characteristics of peripheral arterial disease and its relevance to the diabetic population, *Int J Low Extrem Wounds* 10(3):152–166, 2011.
202. Kalish J, Hamdan A: Management of diabetic foot problems, *J Vasc Surg* 51(2):476–486, 2010.
203. Centers for Disease Control and Prevention: *National diabetes fact sheet: national estimates and general information on diabetes and prediabetes in the United States, 2011*, Atlanta, GA, 2011, Author.
204. Jude EB, Unsworth PF: Optimal treatment of infected diabetic foot ulcers, *Drugs Aging* 21(13):833–850, 2004.
205. Gupta S et al: Infections in diabetes mellitus and hyperglycemia, *Infect Dis Clin North Am* 21(3):617–638, 2007.
206. Hobizal KB, Wukich DK: Diabetic foot infections: current concept review, *Diabetic Foot Ankle* 3, 2012.
207. Shilling AM, Raphael J: Diabetes, hyperglycemia, and infections, *Best Pract Res Clin Anaesthesiol* 22(3):519–535, 2008.
208. De Martin M et al: Cushing's disease, *Best Pract Res Clin Endocrinol Metab* 23(5):607–623, 2009.
209. Castinetti F et al: Cushing's disease, *Orphanet J Rare Dis* 7:41, 2012.
210. Newell-Price J: Proopiomelanocortin gene expression and DNA methylation: implications for Cushing's syndrome and beyond, *Endocrinology* 177(3):365–372, 2003.
211. De Leo M et al: Cardiovascular disease in Cushing's syndrome: heart versus vasculature, *Neuroendocrinology* 92(Suppl 1):50–54, 2010.
212. Pereira AM, Tiemensma J, Romijn JA: Neuropsychiatric disorders in Cushing's syndrome, *Neuroendocrinology* 92(Suppl 1):65–70, 2010.
213. Unuane D et al: Endocrine disorders & female infertility, *Best Pract Res Clin Endocrinol Metab* 25(6):861–873, 2011.
214. Alexandraki KI, Grossman AB: Novel insights in the diagnosis of Cushing's syndrome, *Neuroendocrinology* 92(Suppl 1):35–43, 2010.
215. Nieman LK et al: The diagnosis of Cushing's syndrome: an Endocrine Society clinical practice guideline, *J Clin Endocrinol Metab* 93(5): 1526–1540, 2008.
216. Tritos NA et al: Management of Cushing disease, *Nat Rev Endocrinol* 7(5):279–289, 2011.
217. Witchel SF, Azziz R: Congenital adrenal hyperplasia, *J Pediatr Adolesc Gynecol* 24(3):116–126, 2011.
218. Mulatero P, Monticone S, Veglio F: Diagnosis and treatment of primary aldosteronism, *Rev Endocr Metab Disord* 12(1):3–9, 2011.
219. Briet M, Schiffrin EL: The role of aldosterone in the metabolic syndrome, *Curr Hypertens Rep* 13(2):163–172, 2011.
220. Fallo F, Pilon C, Urbanet R: Primary aldosteronism and metabolic syndrome, *Horm Metab Res* 44(3):208–214, 2012.

221. Mattsson C, Young WF Jr: Primary aldosteronism: diagnostic and treatment strategies, *Nat Clin Pract Nephrol* 2(4):198–208, 2006.
222. Rossi GP: Diagnosis and treatment of primary aldosteronism, *Endocrinol Metab Clin North Am* 40(2):313–332, vii-viii, 2011.
223. Napier C, Pearce SH: Autoimmune Addison's disease, *Presse Med* 41(12 P2):e626–e635, 2012.
224. Harris KB, Pass KA: Increase in congenital hypothyroidism in New York state and in the United States, *Mol Genet Metab* 91(3): 268–277, 2007.
225. Bratland E, Husebye ES: Cellular immunity and immunopathology in autoimmune Addison's disease, *Mol Cell Endocrinol* 336(1-2):180–190, 2011.
226. Larsen RP et al: *Williams textbook of endocrinology*, ed 10, Philadelphia, 2003, Saunders.
227. Nieman LK, Chanco Turner ML: Addison's disease, *Clin Dermatol* 24(4):276–280, 2006.
228. Betterle C, Morlin L: Autoimmune Addison's disease, *Endocr Dev* 20:161–172, 2011.
229. Fishbein L, Nathanson KL: Pheochromocytoma and paraganglioma: understanding the complexities of the genetic background, *Cancer Genet* 205(1-2):1–11, 2012.
230. Zuber SM, Kantorovich V, Pacak K: Hypertension in pheochromocytoma: characteristics and treatment, *Endocrinol Metab Clin North Am* 40(2):295–311, vii, 2011.
231. Gimm O et al: Malignant pheochromocytomas and paragangliomas: a diagnostic challenge, *Langenbecks Arch Surg* 397(2):155–177, 2012.

CHAPTER

23

Structure and Function of the Reproductive Systems

*Gillian Tufts, George Rodway, Sue E. Huether, and Angela Deneris**

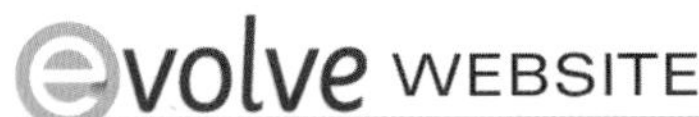

http://evolve.elsevier.com/McCance/

- Review Questions and Answers

CHAPTER OUTLINE

The male and female reproductive systems have several anatomic and physiologic features in common. Most obvious is their major function, reproduction, through which a 23-chromosome female gamete, the **ovum,** and a 23-chromosome male gamete, the **spermatozoon (sperm cell),** unite to form a 46-chromosome zygote that is capable of developing into a new individual. The male reproductive system produces sperm and delivers them to the female reproductive tract. The female reproductive system produces the ovum and, if it is fertilized, can nurture and protect it (at that point called the **embryo** and **developing fetus**) and expel it at birth. These functions are determined not only by anatomic structures but also by complex hormonal, neurologic, and psychogenic factors.[1]

*Angela Deneris contributed to the previous edition.

DEVELOPMENT OF THE REPRODUCTIVE SYSTEMS

The structure and function of male and female reproductive systems depend on steroid hormones called **sex hormones** and their precursors. Hormonal effects on the reproductive systems begin well before birth and continue for life.

Sexual Differentiation and Hormone Production In Utero

Initially in embryonic development, the reproductive structures of male and female embryos are homologous (the same) and consist of one pair of primary sex organs, or **gonads,** and two pairs of ducts, the mesonephric ducts (wolffian ducts) and the paramesonephric ducts (müllerian ducts) (Figure 23-1). Both pairs of ducts empty into an opening called the *urogenital sinus.*

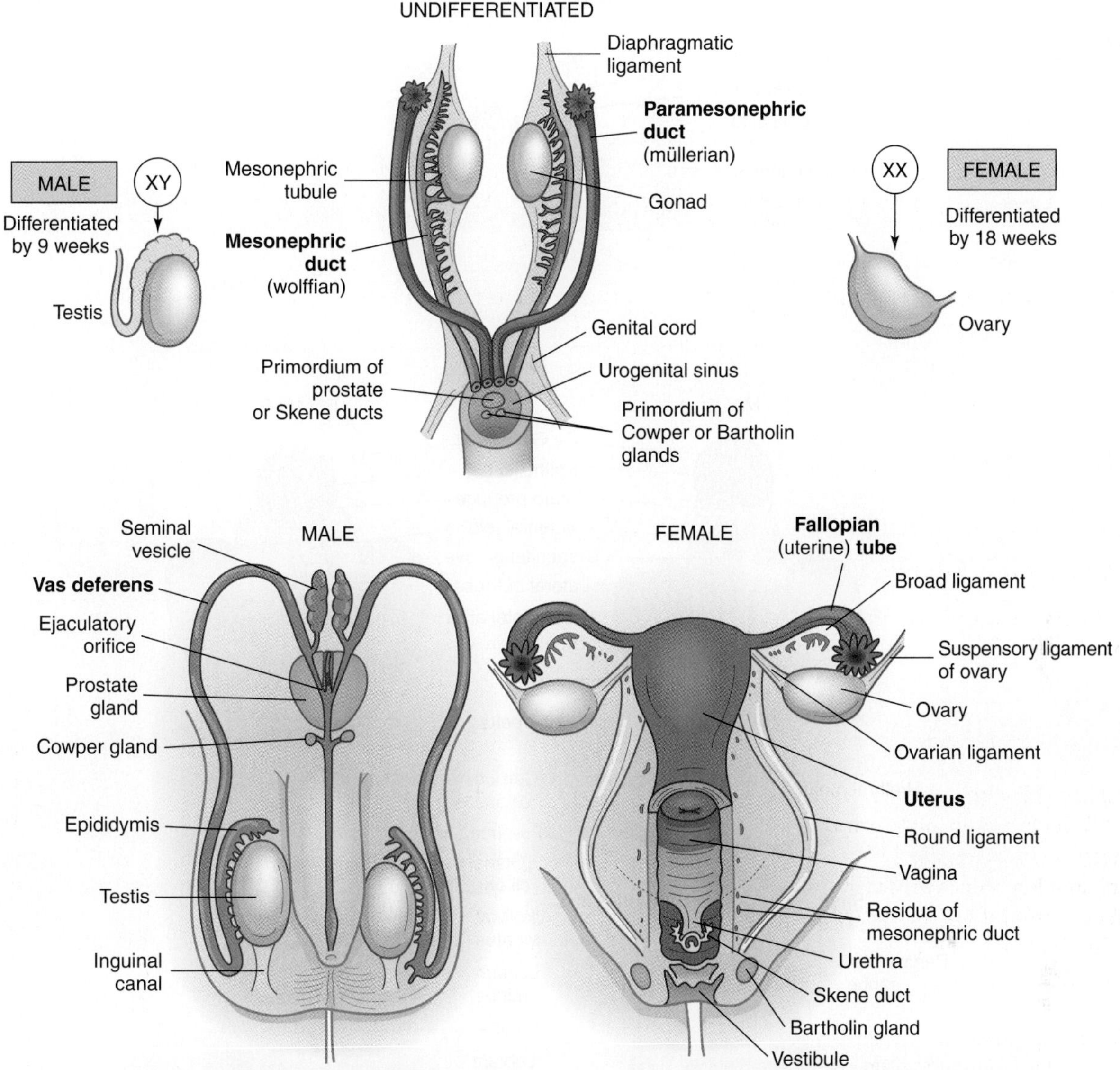

FIGURE 23-1 **Internal Genitalia Development.** Embryonic and fetal development of the internal genitalia.

Between 6 and 7 weeks of gestation, the male embryo will differentiate under the influence of testes-determining factor (TDF), a protein expressed by a gene in the sex-determining region on the Y chromosome (SRY). When the *SRY* gene is expressed, male gonadal development prevails. TDF stimulates the male gonads to develop into the two testes and by 8 weeks of gestation testosterone secretion begins. By 9 months' gestation, the male gonads (testes) have descended into the scrotum. The testes produce sperm after puberty.

Female gonadal development occurs in the absence of *SRY* expression and with the expression of other genes.[2] The presence of *estrogen* and the absence of *testosterone* cause regression of the wolffian system and, at 6 to 8 weeks' gestation, the two female gonads develop into ovaries, which will produce ova. By the tenth week, the loss of wolffian ducts allows the müllerian ducts to join and become the uterus, fallopian tubes, cervix, and upper two thirds of the vagina. The fallopian tubes carry ova from the ovaries to the uterus during a woman's reproductive years.

Like the internal reproductive structures, the external structures develop from homologous embryonic tissues. During the first 7 to 8 weeks of gestation, both male and female embryos develop an elevated structure called the *genital tubercle* (Figure 23-2). **Testosterone** is necessary for the genital tubercle to differentiate into male genitalia; otherwise, female genitalia develop, which may occur even in the absence of ovaries possibly because of the presence of placental estrogens.

Anterior pituitary gland development starts between the 4th and 6th weeks of fetal life, and the vascular connection between the hypothalamus and the pituitary is established by the 12th week. **Gonadotropin-releasing hormone (GnRH)** is produced in the hypothalamus by 10 weeks' gestation and controls the production of two gonadotropins by the anterior pituitary gland, **luteinizing hormone (LH)** and **follicle-stimulating hormone (FSH).** In the female fetus, high levels of FSH and LH are excreted. FSH and LH stimulate the production of estrogen and progesterone by the ovary. The production of FSH and LH rises until about 28 weeks' gestation, until the production of

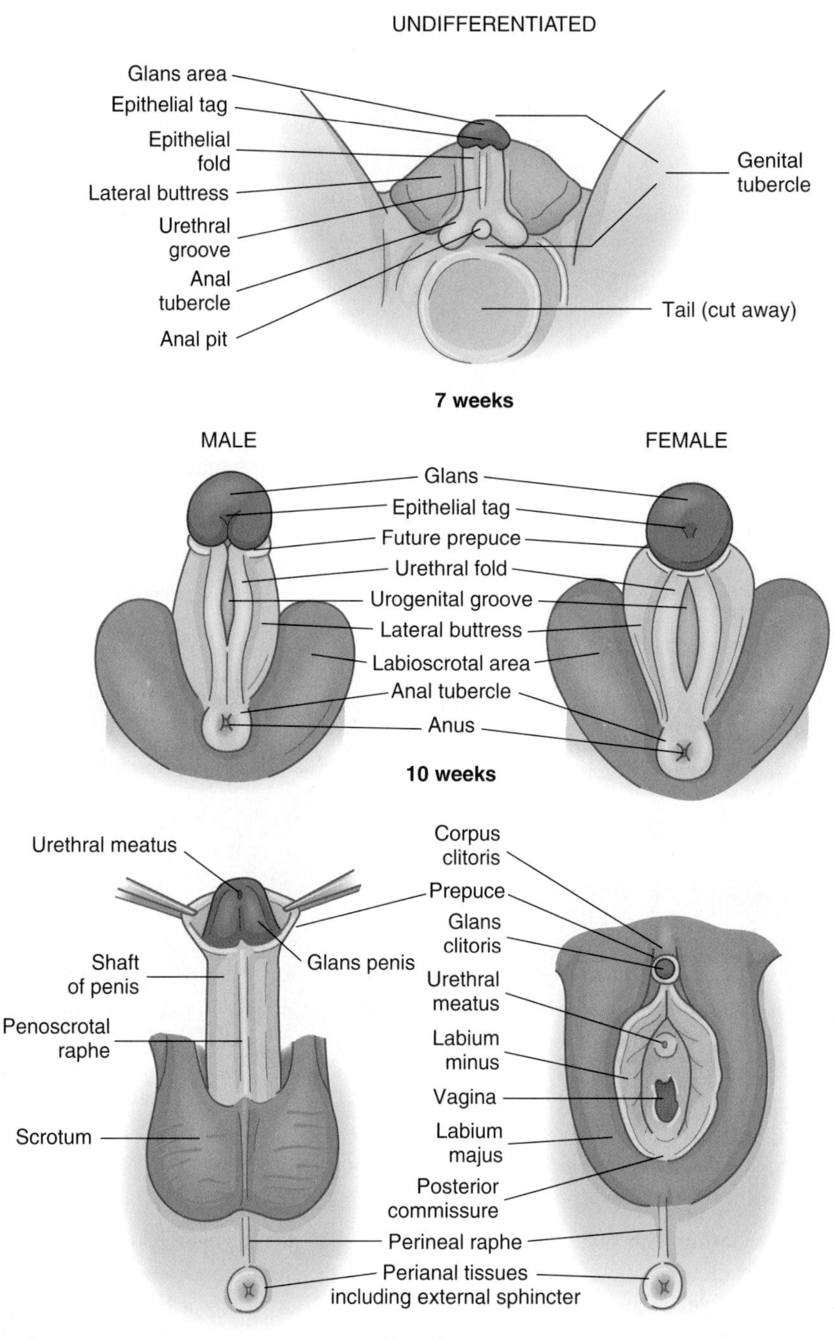

FIGURE 23-2 **External Genitalia Development.** Embryonic and fetal development of the external genitalia.

estrogen and progesterone by the ovaries and placenta is high enough to result in the decline of gonadotropin production.[1] Production of primitive female gametes (ova) occurs solely during fetal life. From puberty to menopause, one female gamete matures per menstrual cycle. Production of the male gametes (sperm) begins at puberty; after that millions are produced daily, usually for life.

By the end of pregnancy a sensitive negative-feedback system, which includes the **gonadostat** (also known as the **gonadotropin-releasing hormone pulse generator**), is operative in the human fetus. The gonadostat responds to high placental estrogens by releasing low levels of GnRH. Soon after birth steroid hormones levels drop because of withdrawal of maternal placental hormones. Hypothalamic pulsatile GnRH is secreted and gonadotropins LH and FSH are released and peak at 3 to 6 months for boys and 12 to 18 months for girls, and then fall steadily. The gonadotropins will be suppressed until the onset of puberty.

Puberty and Reproductive Maturation

Puberty is the onset of sexual maturation and differs from adolescence. Adolescence is the stage of human development

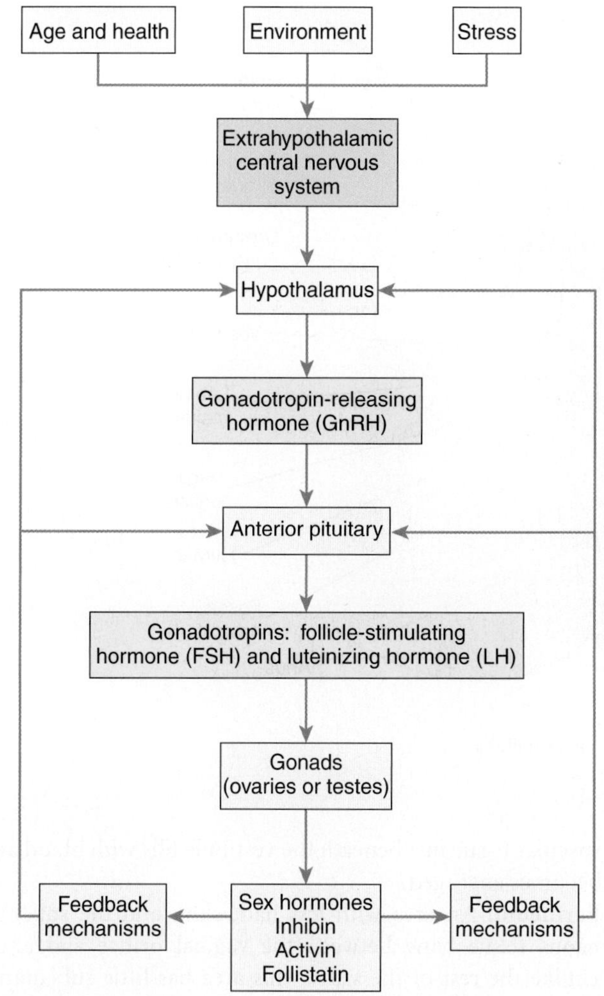

FIGURE 23-3 Hormonal Stimulation of the Gonads. The hypothalamic-pituitary-gonadal axis.

between childhood and adulthood and includes social, psychologic, and biologic changes. In girls, puberty begins at about ages 8 to 9 years with thelarche (breast development). In boys, it begins later—at about age 11 years. Genetics, environment, ethnicity, general health, and nutrition can influence the timing of puberty. Girls who are obese mature earlier, perhaps from higher estrogen levels related to leptin and gonadotropin secretion,[3] and girls who have low body fat, reduced body weight, and intense exercise may experience delayed maturation.[4] Although leptin is not the trigger for puberty onset, it plays an important permissive role.

Reproductive maturation involves the hypothalamic-pituitary-gonadal (HPG) axis, the central nervous system, and the endocrine system (Figure 23-3). A sequential series of hormonal events promotes sexual maturation as puberty approaches. About 1 year before puberty in girls, there is an increase in frequency and amplitude of nocturnal pulses of gonadotropin secretion, LH, and FSH and an increased response in the pituitary to GnRH. This, in turn, stimulates gonadal maturation (**gonadarche**) with estradiol secretion in girls and testosterone secretion in boys. Estradiol causes breast development (**thelarche**), maturation of the reproductive organs (vagina, uterus, ovaries), and fat deposit in hips in girls. Estrogen and increased production of growth factors cause rapid skeletal growth in both boys and girls. Testosterone causes growth of the testes, scrotum, and penis. A positive feedback loop is created with gonadotropins stimulating the gonads to produce more sex hormones. The most important hormonal effects occur in the gonads. In males the testes begin to produce mature sperm that are capable of fertilizing an ovum. Male puberty is complete with the first ejaculation that contains mature sperm. In females, the ovaries begin to release mature ova. Female puberty is complete with the first ovulatory menstrual period; however, this can take up to 1 to 2 years after menarche. **Adrenarche** is the increased production of adrenal androgens (dehydroepiandrosterone and androstenedione, which is converted to testosterone and estrogen) prior to puberty, which occurs in both sexes, and is exhibited by axillary and pubic hair growth and body odor. Puberty is complete when an individual is capable of reproduction.

THE FEMALE REPRODUCTIVE SYSTEM

The function of the reproductive system is to produce mature ova and, when they are fertilized, protect and nourish them through embryonic and fetal life and expel them at birth. In females the most important internal reproductive organs in females are the ovaries, fallopian tubes, uterus, and vagina. The external genitalia protect body openings and play an important role in sexual functioning.[1,5,6]

External Genitalia

Figure 23-4 shows the external female genitalia, which are known collectively as the **vulva,** or pudendum. The major structures are as follows:

- **Mons pubis** (*mons veneris*). A fatty layer of tissue over the pubic symphysis (joint of the pubic bones). During puberty the mons pubis becomes covered with pubic hair, and sebaceous and sweat glands become more active. Estrogen causes fat to be deposited under the skin, giving the mons pubis a moundlike shape. This cushion of tissue protects the pubic symphysis during sexual intercourse.
- **Labia majora** (*singular,* **labium majus**). Two folds of skin that arise at the mons pubis and extend back to the fourchette, forming a cleft. Like the mons pubis, the labia majora undergo changes at puberty: the amount of fatty tissue increases, pubic hair grows on the lateral surfaces, and sebaceous glands on the hairless medial surfaces begin to secrete lubricants. Because of an extensive network of nerve endings, the labia majora are highly sensitive to temperature, touch, pressure, and pain and are homologous to the male scrotum (see Figures 23-2 and 23-15). The principal function of the labia majora is to protect the inner structures of the vulva.
- **Labia minora** (*singular,* **labium minus**). Two smaller, thinner folds of skin lie within the labia majora. Anteriorly they form the clitoral hood, or prepuce, and frenulum then split to enclose the vestibule and converge near the anus, forming the fourchette. The labia minora are hairless, pink, and

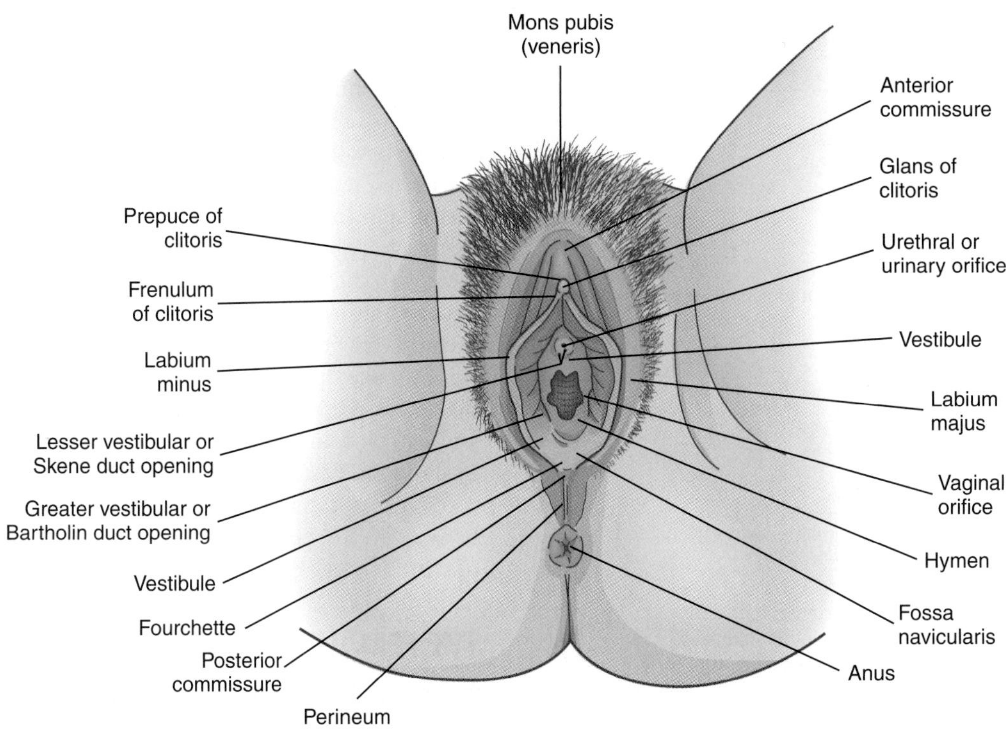

FIGURE 23-4 External Female Genitalia.

moist and are well supplied with nerves, blood vessels, and sebaceous glands. These glands secrete a bactericidal fluid that has a distinctive odor and lubricates and waterproofs the vulvar skin. During sexual arousal the labia minora become swollen with blood.

- **Clitoris.** A richly innervated, erectile organ that lies anterior between the labia minora. It is a small, cylindric structure having a glans that is visible and a shaft that lies beneath the skin (see Figure 23-4). The clitoris is homologous to the male penis. Like the penis the clitoris is a major site of sexual stimulation and orgasm. With sexual arousal erectile tissues in the clitoris fill with blood, causing it to enlarge somewhat. Similar to other vulvar glands, the clitoris secretes a fluid, called *smegma,* which has a unique odor and may be erotically stimulating to the male.
- **Vestibule.** An area protected by the labia minora and contains the external opening of the vagina, called the **introitus,** or vaginal orifice. A thin, perforated membrane called the **hymen** may cover the introitus. The vestibule also contains the opening of the urethra, or **urinary meatus** (orifice). These structures are lubricated by two pairs of glands: Skene glands and Bartholin glands. The ducts of **Skene glands** (also called the **lesser vestibular** or **paraurethral glands**) open on both sides of the urinary meatus. The ducts of **Bartholin glands (greater vestibular** or **vulvovaginal glands)** open on either side of the introitus. In response to sexual stimulation, Bartholin glands secrete mucus that lubricates the inner labial surfaces, as well as enhances the viability and motility of sperm. Skene glands help lubricate the urinary meatus and the vestibule. Secretions from both sets of glands facilitate coitus. Also, in response to sexual excitement, the highly vascular tissue just beneath the vestibule fills with blood and becomes engorged.
- **Perineum.** An area with less hair, skin, and the subcutaneous tissue lying between the vaginal orifice and anus. Unlike the rest of the vulva, this area has little subcutaneous fat so that the skin is close to the underlying muscles. The perineum covers the muscular **perineal body,** a fibrous structure that comprises elastic fiber, connective tissue, and the common attachment of the **bulbocavernosus,** the external anal sphincter, and the levator ani muscles (see Figure 23-4). The perineum varies in length from 2 to 5 cm or more and stretches remarkably. The length of the perineum and the elasticity of the perineal body influence tissue resistance and injury during childbirth.

Internal Genitalia

Vagina

The **vagina** is an elastic fibromuscular canal, 9 to 10 cm long in a reproductive-aged female, which extends up and back from the introitus to the lower portion of the uterus. As Figure 23-5 shows, it lies between the urethra (and part of the bladder) and the rectum. Mucosal secretions from the upper genital organs, menstrual fluids, and products of conception leave the body through the vagina, which also receives the penis during coitus. During sexual excitement the vagina lengthens and widens and the lower third becomes congested with blood.

The vaginal wall is composed of four layers:

1. Its lining is a mucous membrane of squamous epithelial cells. (Types of epithelium are described and illustrated in Chapter 1, Table 1-7.) This layer thickens and thins in response to hormones, particularly estrogen. The

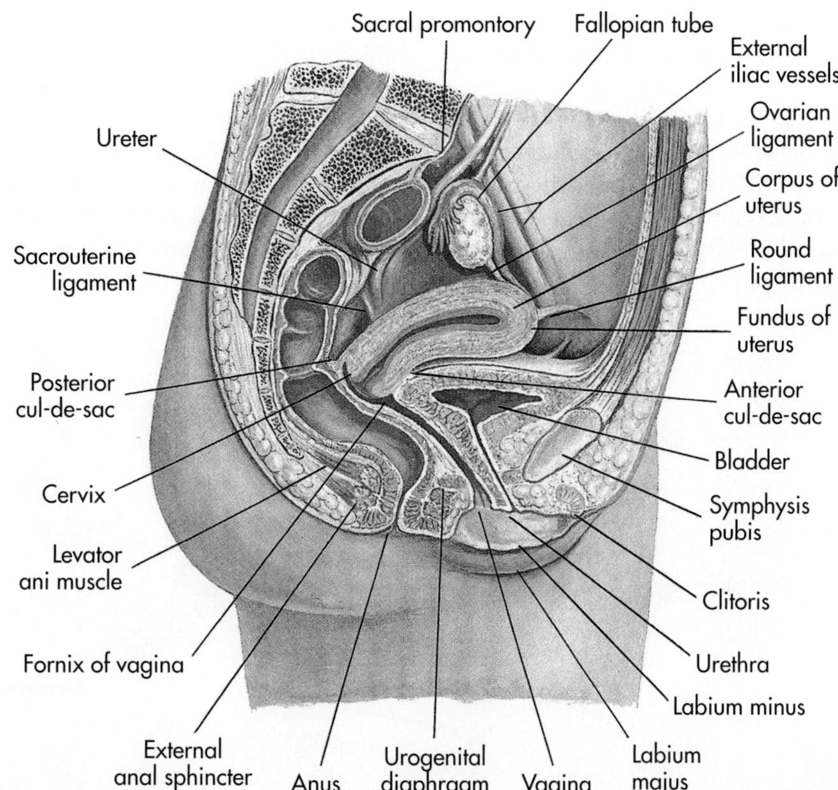

FIGURE 23-5 Internal Female Genitalia and Other Pelvic Organs. Midsagittal view. (Modified from Seidel HM et al: *Mosby's guide to physical examination,* ed 7, St Louis, 2011, Mosby.)

squamous epithelial membrane is continuous with the membrane that covers the lower part of the uterus. In women of reproductive age, the mucosal layer is arranged in transverse wrinkles, or folds, called **rugae** (*singular,* **ruga**) that permit stretching during coitus and childbirth.

2. Fibrous connective tissue containing numerous blood and lymphatic vessels
3. Smooth muscle
4. Connective tissue and a rich network of blood vessels.

The upper part of the vagina surrounds the cervix, the lower end of the uterus (see Figure 23-5). The recessed space around the cervix is called the **fornix** of the vagina. The posterior fornix is "deeper" than the anterior fornix because of the angle at which the cervix meets the vaginal canal. In most women this angle is about 90 degrees. A pouch called the **cul-de-sac** separates the posterior fornix and the rectum.

Its elasticity and relatively sparse nerve supply enhance the vagina's function as the birth canal. During sexual arousal the vaginal wall becomes engorged with blood, like the labia minora and clitoris. Engorgement pushes some fluid to the surface of the mucosa, enhancing lubrication. The vaginal wall does not contain mucus-secreting glands; rather, secretions drain into the vagina from the endocervical glands or enter from the vestibule, from the Bartholin and Skene glands.

Two factors help maintain the self-cleansing action of the vagina and defend it from infection, particularly during the reproductive years: (1) an acid-base balance that discourages the proliferation of most pathogenic bacteria and (2) the thickness of the vaginal epithelium. Before puberty, vaginal pH is about 7 (neutral) and the vaginal epithelium is thin. At puberty the pH becomes more acidic (4 to 5) and the squamous epithelial lining thickens. These changes are maintained until menopause (cessation of menstruation), at which time the pH rises again to more alkaline levels and the epithelium thins out. Therefore, protection from infection is greatest during the years when a woman is most likely to be sexually active. Between puberty and menopause, vulnerability to infection varies somewhat with cyclic changes in pH and epithelial thickness. Both defenses are greatest when estrogen levels are high and the vagina contains a normal population of *Lactobacillus acidophilus,* a harmless resident bacterium that helps maintain pH at acidic levels. Any condition that causes vaginal pH to rise, such as douching or use of vaginal sprays or deodorants, low estrogen levels, or destruction of *L. acidophilus* by antibiotics, lowers vaginal defenses against infection.

Uterus

The **uterus** is a hollow pear-shaped organ whose lower end opens into the vagina. The functions of the uterus are to anchor and protect a fertilized ovum, provide an optimal environment while it develops, and push the fetus out at birth. In addition, the uterus plays an important role in sexual response and conception. During sexual excitement the opening of the uterus (the cervix) dilates slightly. At the same time, the uterus increases in size and moves upward and backward, creating a tenting effect in the midvagina that results in the cervix "sitting" in a pool of semen. During orgasm, rhythmic contractions facilitate movement of sperm through the cervical os while also enhancing physical pleasure.

At puberty the uterus attains its adult size and proportions and descends from the abdomen to the lower pelvis, between the bladder and the rectum (see Figure 23-5). The uterus of a mature, nonpregnant female is approximately 7 to 9 cm long and 6.5 cm wide, with muscular walls 3.5 cm thick. It is held loosely in position by ligaments, peritoneal tissue folds, and pressure of adjacent organs, especially the urinary bladder, sigmoid colon, and rectum. In most women the uterus is anteverted; that is, it is tipped forward so that it rests on the urinary bladder. However, it may be retroverted, or tipped backward. Various degrees of flexion are normal (Figure 23-6).

Figure 23-7 shows a cross section of the uterus. The uterus has two major parts: the body, or **corpus,** and the cervix. The top of the corpus, above the insertion of the fallopian tubes, is called the **fundus.** The diameter of the uterine cavity is widest at

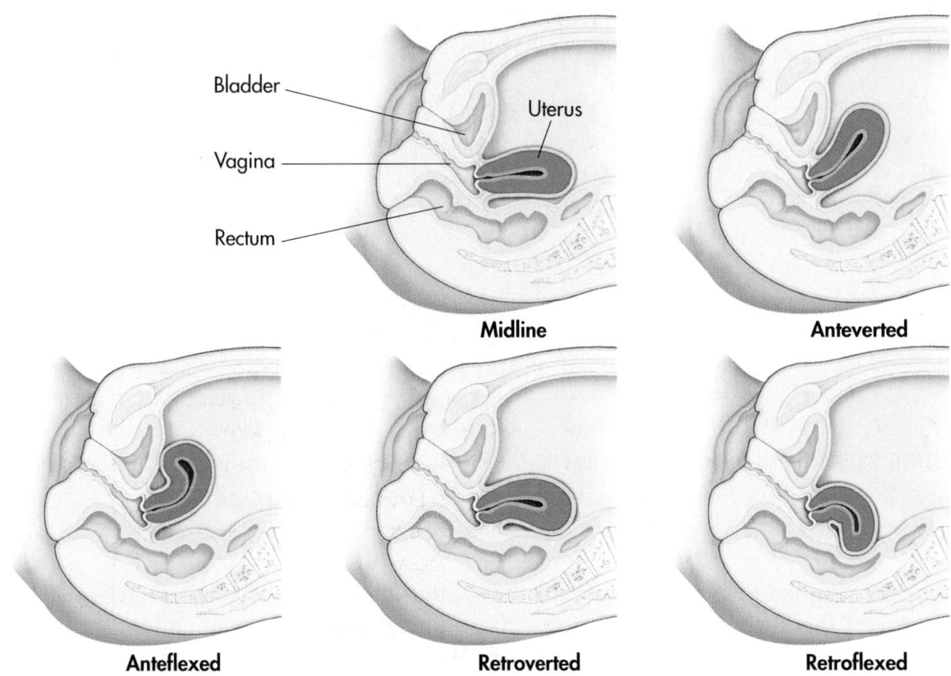

FIGURE 23-6 Variations in Uterine Position.

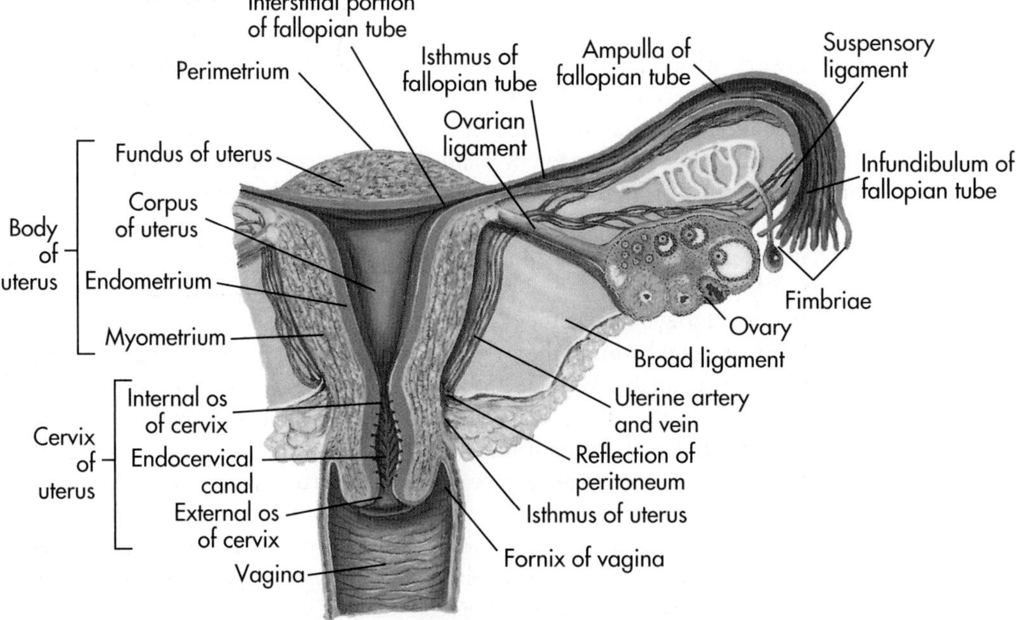

FIGURE 23-7 Cross Section of Uterus, Fallopian Tube, and Ovary. (From Seidel HM et al: *Mosby's guide to physical examination,* ed 7, St Louis, 2011, Mosby.)

the fundus and narrowest at the **isthmus,** which is the narrowed part of the corpus just above the cervix. The **cervix,** or neck of the uterus, extends from the isthmus to the vagina. The passageway between the cervix's upper opening (the internal os) and its lower opening (the external os) is called the **endocervical canal.** The entire uterus, like the upper vagina, is innervated exclusively by motor and sensory fibers of the autonomic nervous system.

The uterine wall is composed of three layers: the perimetrium, the myometrium, and the endometrium (see Figure 23-7). The **perimetrium (parietal peritoneum)** is the outer serous membrane that covers the uterus. The **myometrium** is the thick muscular middle layer. The myometrium is thickest at the fundus, apparently to facilitate birth. The **endometrium,** or uterine lining, is composed of a functional layer (superficial compact layer and spongy middle layer) and a basal layer. The functional layer of the endometrium is responsive to sex hormones. Between puberty and menopause this layer proliferates and sloughs off monthly. The basal layer, which is attached to the myometrium, regenerates the functional layer after it sloughs (menstruation).

The endocervical canal does not have an endometrial layer. Rather, it is lined with columnar epithelial cells (see Table 1-7). The endocervical lining is continuous with that of the outer cervix and vagina, but it is not made up of the same type of epithelial cells. The point at which the columnar epithelium of the cervix meets the squamous epithelium of the vagina is called the *transformation zone,* or the **squamous-columnar junction.** The transformation zone is especially susceptible to the oncogenic human papillomavirus (HPV), especially HPV types 16 and 18, which can lead to cervical dysplasia and, ultimately, cervical cancer (see What's New? Human Papillomavirus (HPV) Vaccine and Cancer Prevention in Women and Men); these are the cells sampled during the Papanicolaou test (Pap test).[7]

The cervix acts as a mechanical barrier to infectious microorganisms that may be present in the vagina. The external cervical os is a very small opening that contains thick, sticky mucus (the *mucous plug*) during the luteal phase of the menstrual cycle and all of pregnancy. During ovulation the mucus changes under the influence of estrogen and forms watery strands, or spinnbarkeit mucus, to facilitate the transport of sperm into the uterus. In addition, the downward flow of cervical secretions moves microorganisms away from the cervix and uterus. In women of reproductive age, the pH of these secretions is inhospitable to most bacteria. Furthermore, mucosal secretions contain enzymes and antibodies (mostly immunoglobulin A) of the secretory (humoral) immune system (see Chapter 8). These defenses do not always prevent infection, even if they are intact. Besides infection, uterine pathophysiology includes displacement of the uterus within the pelvis, benign growths (fibroids) of the uterine wall, hyperplasia of the endometrium, endometriosis, and cancer.

Fallopian Tubes

The two **fallopian tubes (oviducts, uterine tubes)** enter the uterus bilaterally just beneath the fundus (see Figure 23-7). Their function is to conduct the ova from the spaces around the ovaries to the uterus. From the uterus the fallopian tubes curve up and over the two ovaries. Each tube is 8 to 12 cm long and about 1 cm in diameter, except at its ovarian end, which flares out like the bell of a trumpet. This widened end, called the **infundibulum,** is fringed or fimbriated. The **fimbriae** (*singular,* **fimbria**) (fringes) move, creating a current that draws the ovum into the infundibulum. Once the ovum has entered the fallopian tube, cilia and peristalsis (muscle contractions) keep it moving toward the uterus.

The ampulla, or distal third, of the fallopian tube is the usual site of fertilization (see Figure 23-7). Sperm released into the vagina travel upward through the endocervical canal and uterine cavity and enter the fallopian tubes. If an ovum is present in either tube, fertilization can occur. Whether or not the ovum encounters sperm, it continues to travel through the fallopian tube to the uterus. If fertilized, the ovum (then called a *blastocyst*) implants itself in the endometrial layer of the uterine wall. If not fertilized, the ovum breaks down within 12 to 24 hours.

WHAT'S NEW?

Human Papillomavirus (HPV) Vaccine and Cancer Prevention in Women and Men

Two HPV vaccines are approved in the United States: the quadrivalent HPV recombinant vaccine in males and females (HPV 6, 11, 16, and 18); and the bivalent HPV recombinant vaccine (HPV 16 and 18) in females. HPV types 16 and 18 are oncogenic and can cause cervical dysplasia, cervical cancer, anal cancer, penile cancer, and cancer of the head and neck. Types 6 and 11 cause genital warts. HPV is responsible for 99.7% of cervical cancer cases, 40% of penile cancers, and an estimated 5% of all cancers worldwide. Symptoms of infection are often silent, and approximately 50% of women are estimated to be infected, usually during adolescence. Men who have sex with men are at high risk. The incidence of genital warts and cancer is reduced in those receiving the vaccine. The vaccine is administered by intramuscular injection and the recommended schedule is a three-dose series with the second and third doses administered 2 and 6 months after the first dose. The recommended age for vaccination of females is 11 to 12 years. The vaccine can be administered as young as age 9 years. Catch-up vaccination is recommended for females ages 13 to 26 years who have not been previously vaccinated. The vaccine is not disease treatment, and disease may develop related to non–vaccine-related HPV infection. Pap smear screening for cervical cancer should be continued. Efforts are in progress to make the vaccine affordable in less-developed countries, with the hope of eradicating cervical cancer.

Vaccination programs target women to prevent cervical cancer. The quadrivalent vaccine has been approved for males 9 to 26 years of age to prevent genital warts. Rates of vaccination among men and low income minority women are low, and education and financing efforts need to be expanded for these groups. Cost effectiveness of vaccinating men is controversial. There are no antiviral therapies for this disease.

Data from Alexander KA, Giuliano AR: *Am J Med* 125(7):S1, 2012; Fontenot HB, Morelock N: *Nurs Womens Health* 16(1):57–65, 2012; Laz TH, Rahman M, Berenson AB: *Cancer* 119(7):1386–1392, 2013; Low GM et al: *Viral Immunol* 25(3):174–186, 2012; Stanley MA: *J Gen Virol* 93(Pt 4): 681–691, 2012; Stupiansky NW, Alexander AB, Zimet GD: *Curr Opin Infect Dis* 25(1):86–91, 2012.

Disorders that affect the fallopian tubes (e.g., congenital malformations, infection, and inflammation) can block the path of sperm and ovum and cause infertility or ectopic (tubal) pregnancy.

Ovaries

The **ovaries,** the female gonads, are the primary female reproductive organs. Their two main functions are secretion of female sex hormones and development and release of female gametes, or ova.

The almond-shaped ovaries are located on both sides of the uterus and are suspended and supported by the mesovarian portions of the broad ligament, ovarian ligaments, and suspensory ligaments (see Figure 23-7). The ovaries are smaller than their male homologs, the testes. In women of reproductive age, each ovary is 3 to 5 cm long, 2.5 cm wide, and 2 cm thick and weighs 4 to 8 g. Size and weight vary somewhat from phase to phase of the menstrual cycle (see p. 778).

Figure 23-8, *A* shows a cross section of an ovary. The central part, or medulla, is composed of connective tissue and contains many small arteries, veins, and lymphatics that enter at the hilum. Surrounding the medulla is the cortex. At birth the cortex of each ovary contains approximately 2 million ova within primordial (immature) **ovarian follicles.** Follicles grow and undergo atresia continuously and irrevocably throughout a woman's life. By puberty the number ranges between 300,000 and 500,000 ova. Between puberty and menopause the ovarian cortex always contains follicles and ova in various stages of development, including the primary and secondary follicles (see Figure 23-8, *A*). Once every menstrual cycle (about every 28 days), usually only one of the follicles reaches maturation (see Figure 23-8, *B* and *C*) and discharges its ovum through the ovary's outer covering, the germinal epithelium. During the reproductive years, 400 to 500 ovarian follicles mature completely and release an ovum **(ovulation).** The rest either fail to develop at all or degenerate without maturing completely and are known as atretic follicles[1] (see Figure 23-8).

After release of the mature ovum (ovulation), the follicle develops into another structure, the **corpus luteum** (see Figure 23-8). The immediate fate of the corpus luteum depends on whether the ejected ovum is fertilized. If fertilization occurs, the corpus luteum enlarges and begins to secrete hormones that maintain and support pregnancy. If fertilization does not occur, the corpus luteum secretes these hormones for approximately 14 days and then degenerates, which triggers the maturation of another follicle. The **ovarian cycle**—the process of follicular maturation, ovulation, corpus luteum development, and corpus luteum degeneration—is continuous from puberty to menopause, except during pregnancy or hormonal contraceptive use. At menopause this process ceases and the ovaries atrophy to the point that they cannot be felt during pelvic examination.

Sex hormones are secreted by cells within the ovarian cortex including two types of cells in the ovarian follicle **(theca cells** and **granulosa cells)** and cells of the corpus luteum (see Figure 23-8). These cells all contain receptors for the gonadotropins (LH, FSH) or for the sex hormones, which are discussed in the next section.

Female Sex Hormones

The sex hormones are all steroid hormones and are synthesized from cholesterol (see Chapter 21). Male and female sex hormones are present in all adults. However, the female body contains low levels of testosterone and other androgens, and the male body contains low levels of estrogen. Individual effects of sex hormones depend on their amount and concentration in the blood.

The dominant female sex hormones, estrogen and progesterone, are produced primarily by the ovaries. During fetal development, infancy, and childhood, sex hormone production is low. At puberty hormone production surges, triggering sexual maturation and development of secondary sex characteristics. From puberty to menopause, the sex hormones control the menstrual cycle and are produced cyclically, that is, production surges and diminishes monthly, creating the ovarian and uterine changes associated with the menstrual cycle. These hormones also are produced in higher levels during pregnancy by the placenta, inhibiting ovulation. Androgens are produced in small amounts by the ovaries and the adrenals and have important functions in women.

Estrogens and Androgens

Estrogen is a generic term for three similar hormones: estradiol, estrone, and estriol. **Estradiol (E_2)** is the most potent and plentiful of the three and is principally produced (95%) by the ovaries (ovarian follicle and corpus luteum). Androgens are converted to estrone in the ovary and peripheral adipose tissue. Estriol is the peripheral metabolite of estrone and estradiol.

Estrogen has numerous biologic effects, many of which involve interactions with other hormones, and is needed for maturation of reproductive organs, development of secondary sex characteristics (differentiating male and female physical characteristics that are not directly related to reproduction), closure of long bones after the pubertal growth spurt, regulation of the menstrual cycle, and endometrial regeneration after menstruation. Estrogen also has metabolic effects on the bones, liver, blood vessels, brain and central nervous system, kidneys, and skin. After menopause ovarian production of estradiol and estrone is markedly diminished (see Menopause, p. 791). At this time the majority of estrogen is derived from extraovarian and extraglandular production of estrones.[1]

Like other steroid hormones, estrogens are derived from cholesterol in a complex, enzyme-mediated series of reactions. (Mechanisms of hormone synthesis and action are described in Chapter 21.) The hypothalamus secretes GnRH in a pulsatile manner that stimulates gonadotropin (LH and FSH) release from the anterior pituitary. Gonadotropins trigger ovarian production of estrogen. The primary function of LH is to stimulate theca cells of the ovarian follicle to produce androgens, mainly androstenedione. (Androgens are discussed further on p. 789 and in the section on male reproductive function.) Some of these androgens are converted to estrogen by the theca cells themselves, and others diffuse into the granulosa cells. Within the granulosa layer, FSH induces conversion (aromatization) of androgens to estrogens. Estrogens are then released into the bloodstream. Estrogen and FSH together increase FSH

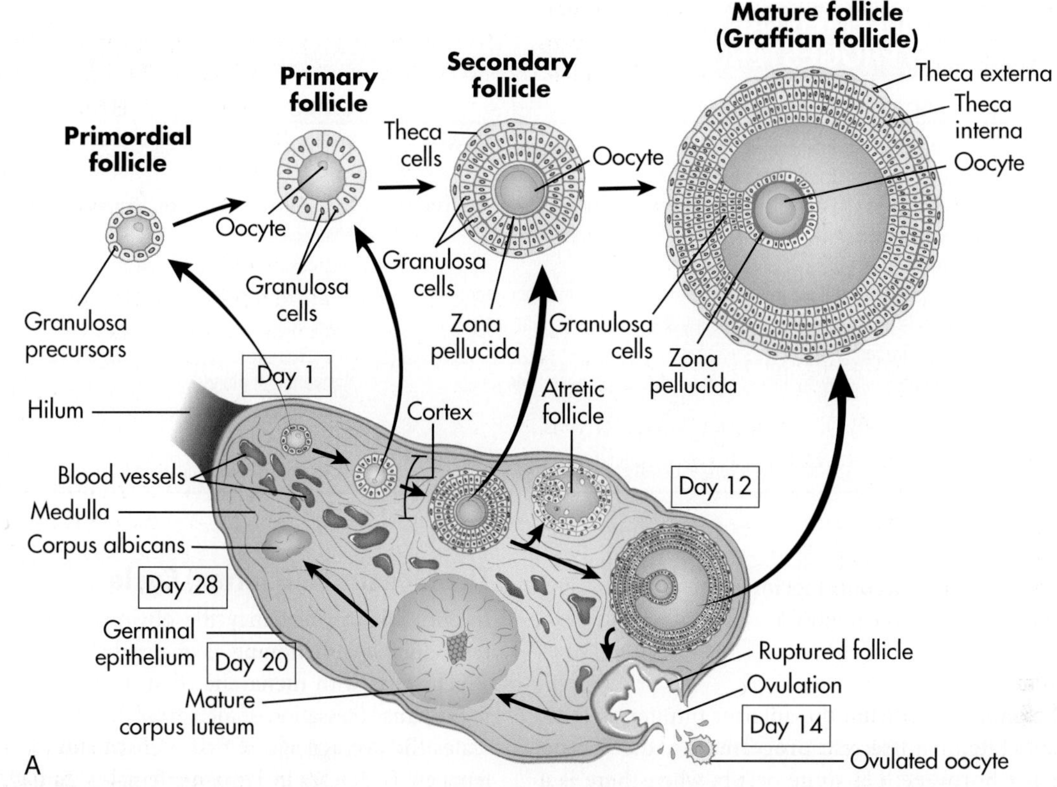

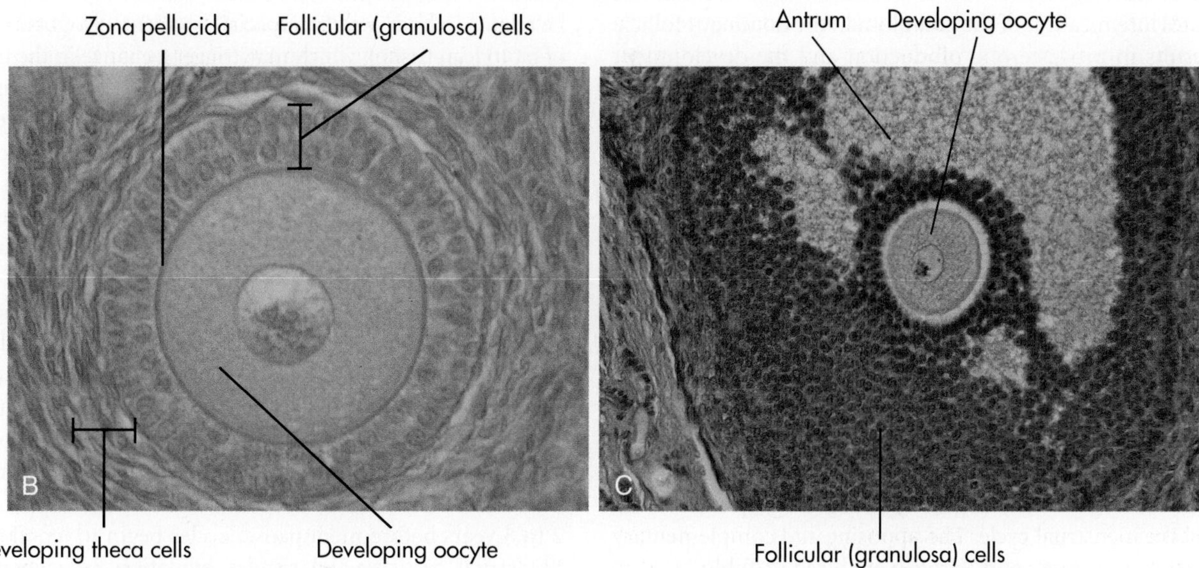

FIGURE 23-8 Cross Section of Ovary and Development of an Ovarian Follicle. **A,** Schematic representation (not to scale) of the structure of the ovary, showing the various stages in the development of the follicle and its successor structure, the corpus luteum. **B,** A developing oocyte surrounded by hormone-secreting follicular (granulosa) cells. **C,** A more mature ovarian follicle has a fluid-filled cavity called the *antrum.* (**A** adapted from Berne RM, Levy MN, editors: *Physiology,* ed 5, St Louis, 2003, Mosby. **B** and **C** from Patton KT, Thibodeau GA: *Anatomy & physiology,* ed 8, St Louis, 2013, Mosby.)

receptors in the follicle, stimulating additional granulosa cells until a dominant follicle is determined.

Disturbances of estrogen production can be caused by abnormalities that affect (1) secretion of GnRH by the hypothalamus, (2) secretion of LH or FSH by the anterior pituitary, (3) hormonal feedback mechanisms, or (4) structural integrity of the ovaries. Estrogen's role in the menstrual cycle is described on page 781.

Although **androgens** are primarily male sex hormones produced by the testes, small amounts are produced in the adrenal cortex in both men and women and in the ovaries. Some androgens (dehydroepiandrosterone and its metabolite androstenedione) are precursors of estrogens (estrone, estradiol). At puberty, androgens contribute to the skeletal growth spurt and cause growth of pubic and axillary hair. The androgens also

TABLE 23-1 COMPLEMENTARY AND OPPOSING EFFECTS OF ESTROGEN AND PROGESTERONE

STRUCTURE	EFFECT OF ESTROGEN	EFFECT OF PROGESTERONE
Vaginal mucosa	Proliferation of squamous epithelium; increase in glycogen content of cells; layering (cornification) of cells	Thinning of squamous epithelium; decornification
Cervical mucosa	Production of abundant fluid secretions that favor survival and enhance motility of sperm	Production of thick, sticky secretions that tend to "plug" the cervical os
Fallopian tube	Increase of motility and ciliary action	Decrease of motility and ciliary action
Uterine muscle	Increase of blood flow; increase of contractile proteins and uterine muscle and myometrial excitability and action potential; increase of sensitization to oxytocin	Relaxation of myometrium; decrease of sensitization to oxytocin
Endometrium	Stimulation of growth; increase in number of progesterone receptors	Activation of glands and blood vessels; accumulation of glycogen and enzymes; decrease in number of estrogen receptors
Breasts	Growth of ducts; promotion of prolactin effects	Growth of lobules and alveoli; inhibition of prolactin effects

activate sebaceous glands, accounting for some cases of acne during puberty, and play a role in libido.

Progesterone

Luteinizing hormone (LH) from the anterior pituitary stimulates the corpus luteum to secrete **progesterone,** the second major female sex hormone. LH surge occurs when there is a peak level of estrogen, about 24 to 36 hours before ovulation. LH promotes luteinization of the granulosa in the dominant follicle and results in progesterone production and the development of blood vessels and connective tissue. A rising level of progesterone can be detected from the preovulatory follicle as early as day 10 of the menstrual cycle. Small amounts of progesterone also are secreted steadily by the adrenal cortex. Before ovulation the ovary and the adrenal glands each contribute approximately 50% of total progesterone production. Conversely, large amounts are secreted from the ovary while the corpus luteum is active for about 9 to 13 days after ovulation. Progesterone secreted by the corpus luteum stimulates the thickened endometrium to become more complex in preparation for implantation of a blastocyst. If conception and implantation do occur, the corpus luteum persists and secretes progesterone (and estrogen) until the placenta is well established at approximately 8 to 10 weeks' gestation. Together, estrogen and progesterone control the menstrual cycle. The opposing and complementary effects of progesterone and estrogen are listed in Table 23-1.

Progesterone is sometimes called the *hormone of pregnancy.* Progesterone's effects in pregnancy include: (1) maintaining the thickened endometrium; (2) relaxing smooth muscle in the myometrium, which prevents premature contractions and helps the uterus expand; (3) thickening (hypertrophy) of the myometrium, which prepares it for the muscular work of labor; (4) promoting growth of lobules and alveoli in the breast in preparation for lactation but prevents lactation until the fetus is born; (5) preventing additional maturation of ova by way of suppressing FSH and LH, thereby stopping the menstrual cycle; (6) providing immune modulation allowing tolerance against fetal antigens (the mother's immune system does not attack the fetus); and preventing preterm birth.[8-10]

The Menstrual (Ovarian) Cycle

In addition to pregnancy the obvious manifestation of female reproductive functioning is menstrual bleeding (the menses), which starts with **menarche** (first menstruation) and ends with **menopause** (cessation of menstrual flow for 1 year). In the United States the average age of first menstruation is 12 years in black females, 12.5 years in Hispanic females, and 12.6 years in white females, with a range from 9 to 17 years.[11] Menarche appears to be related to body weight, especially percentage of body fat (ratio of fat to lean tissue), which may trigger a change in the metabolic rate and lead to hormonal changes associated with early menarche.[12] There is an increased sensitivity to **leptin** (a regulatory hormone of appetite and energy metabolism) during puberty and, in theory, the adolescent consumes more calories to meet caloric needs of the pubertal growth spurt.[13] The percent of body fat and leptin levels in girls continue to increase, whereas muscle mass increases in boys.[14]

At first, cycles are anovulatory and may vary in length from 10 to 60 days or more. As adolescence proceeds into adulthood, regular patterns of menstruation and ovulation are established at intervals ranging from 25 to 35 days. The length of the menstrual cycle varies considerably among women. The commonly accepted cycle average is 28 (27 to 30) days, with rhythmic intervals of 21 to 35 days considered normal. Approximately 2 to 8 years before menopause, cycles begin to lengthen again. Menstrual cyclicity and regular ovulation are dependent on (1) the activity of the gonadostat (GnRH pulse generator); (2) the initial pituitary secretion of the gonadotropin FSH; and (3) estrogen (estradiol) positive feedback for the preovulatory FSH and LH surge, oocyte maturation, and corpus luteum formation and production of progesterone.[15]

Phases of the Menstrual Cycle

The menstrual (ovarian) cycle (Figure 23-9) consists of ovulation, which occurs in two phases: the follicular/proliferative and the luteal/secretory phase and each lasts about 14 days. Ovulation occurs between the follicular and luteal phases. If implantation of the blastocyst does not occur in the late luteal phase, **menstruation (menses)** occurs, also known as the ischemic/menstrual phase.[16]

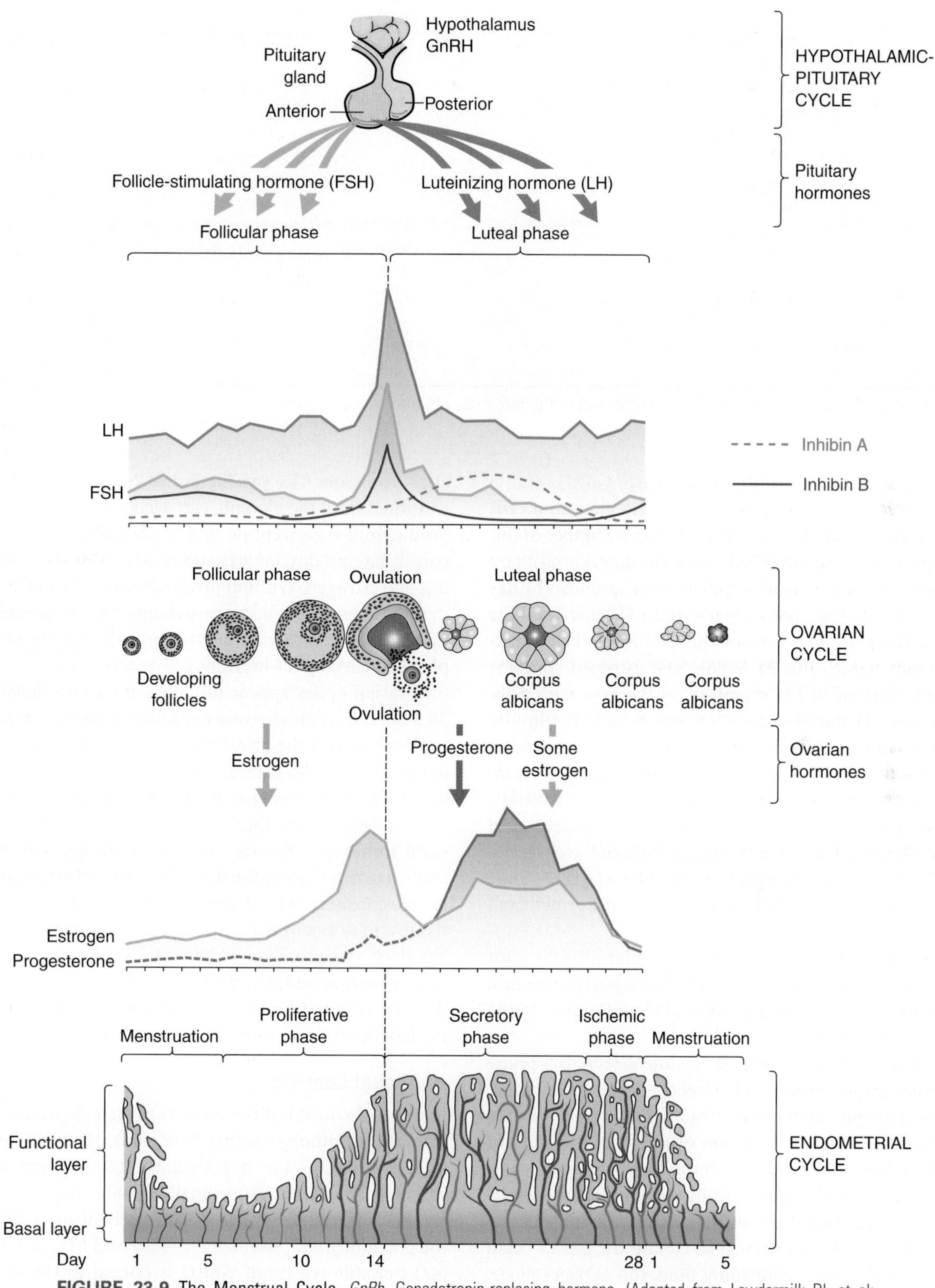

FIGURE 23-9 The Menstrual Cycle. *GnRh,* Gonadotropin-replacing hormone. (Adapted from Lowdermilk DL et al: *Maternity and women's health care,* ed 10, St Louis, 2012, Mosby.)

TABLE 23-2 **HORMONAL FEEDBACK MECHANISM IN THE MENSTRUAL CYCLE**

PHASE OF CYCLE AND OVARIAN HORMONE LEVELS	FEEDBACK TO HYPOTHALAMUS AND ANTERIOR PITUITARY	RESULTANT GnRH, FSH, AND LH LEVELS	OVARIAN AND MENSTRUAL EVENTS
Early follicular phase: estrogen levels low; minute amount of progesterone secreted	Negative and inhibitory	All low	Ovarian follicle develops; endometrium proliferates
Late follicular (preovulatory) phase: estrogen levels high; progesterone increases with small surge before ovulation	Positive and stimulatory	All surge; LH dominates	Process of ovulation begins; endometrial proliferation complete
Ovulatory phase: estrogen levels dip; progesterone levels begin to rise	Negative and inhibitory	All fall sharply	Corpus luteum begins to develop; endometrium enters secretory phase
Early luteal phase: estrogen and progesterone levels high; progesterone dominates	Negative and inhibitory	All continue to decline, but gradually	Corpus luteum fully developed; endometrium ready for implantation
Late luteal phase: estrogen and progesterone levels fall sharply	Negative and inhibitory; feedback lessens slightly	All rise slightly	Corpus luteum regresses; endometrium breaks down; menstruation begins
Menstrual phase: estrogens levels low; minute amount of progesterone secreted	Negative and inhibitory	All low	More ovarian follicles begin to develop; functional layer of endometrium is shed

FSH, Follicle-stimulating hormone; *GnRH,* gonadotropin-releasing hormone; *LH,* luteinizing hormone.

During the **follicular/proliferative phase** GnRH and a balance between activin and inhibin from the granulosa cells contribute to the rise of FSH, which stimulates a number of follicles. The pulsatile secretion of FSH from the anterior pituitary gland rescues a dominant ovarian follicle from apoptosis by day 5 to 7 of the cycle. Together estrogen and FSH increase FSH receptors in the granulosa cells of the primary follicle, making them more sensitive to FSH. FSH and estrogen combine to induce production of LH receptors on the granulosa cells, thus promoting LH stimulation to combine with FSH stimulation, causing a more rapid secretion of follicular estrogen. As estrogen increases, FSH levels drop because of an increase in inhibin-B secreted by the granulosa cells in the dominant follicle. This drop in FSH decreases the growth of less-developed follicles (see Figure 23-9). Estrogen causes cells of the endometrium to proliferate and stimulates production of LH. A surge in both FSH and LH are required for final follicular growth and ovulation.

Increase in stromal tissue in the late follicular phase is associated with a rise in androgen levels. Androgen production enhances the process of follicle atresia and may stimulate libido at the point of ovulation.[1]

Ovulation marks the beginning of the **luteal/secretory phase** of the menstrual cycle. The ovarian follicle begins its transformation into a corpus luteum (see Figure 23-8, *A*), hence the name *luteal phase.* Pulsatile secretion of LH from the anterior pituitary stimulates the corpus luteum to secrete progesterone, which in turn initiates the secretory phase of endometrial development. Glands and blood vessels in the endometrium branch and curl throughout the functional layer, and the glands begin to secrete a thin glycogen-containing fluid, the *secretory phase.* If conception occurs, the nutrient-laden endometrium is ready for implantation. Human chorionic gonadotropin (HCG) is secreted 3 days after fertilization by the blastocytes and maintains the corpus luteum once implantation occurs at about day 6 or 7. HCG can be detected in maternal blood and urine 8 to 10 days after ovulation. The production of estrogen and progesterone continues until the placenta can adequately maintain hormonal production. If conception and implantation do not occur, the corpus luteum degenerates and ceases production of progesterone and estrogen. Without progesterone or estrogen to maintain it, the endometrium becomes ischemic (blood-starved) and disintegrates. Menstruation then occurs—the **ischemic/menstrual phase**—marking the beginning of another cycle.

Ovarian cycles appear to have a minimum length of 24 to 26.5 days: the primary ovarian follicle requires 10 to 12.5 days to develop, and the luteal phase appears relatively fixed at 14 days (±3 days). Menstrual blood flow usually lasts 3 to 7 days, but it may last as long as 8 days or stop after 1 to 2 days and still be considered within normal limits. Bleeding is consistently scant to heavy and varies from 30 to 80 ml, with most blood loss occurring during the first 3 days of menses. Menstrual discharge consists of blood, mucus, and desquamated endometrial tissue and does not clot under normal circumstances. It is usually dark and produces a characteristic musty odor on oxidation. Environmental factors such as severe emotional stress, illness, malnutrition, obesity, and seasonal variation may affect the length of the menstrual cycle.[1,17-19]

Hormonal Controls

Hormonal control of the menstrual cycle depends on complex interactions among the hypothalamus, the anterior pituitary, and the ovaries (or hypothalamic-pituitary-ovarian [HPO] axis)[20] (Table 23-2). Hormonal control is dependent on negative and positive ovarian feedback mechanisms. GnRH controls the gonadotropin production of FSH and LH, and the constant and pulsatile release of GnRH is critical to the timing of the menstrual cycle. GnRH is secreted by the hypothalamus into the hypophyseal portal system and travels to the anterior pituitary, where it stimulates the secretion of LH and FSH. FSH and LH are released from the anterior pituitary in pulses that correspond to the pulsatile secretion of GnRH.

During the early follicular phase, estrogen levels rise steadily and, through negative feedback, suppress FSH and positively increase the production of LH. During the late follicular phase, the preovulatory rise in progesterone facilitates the positive feedback of estrogen; estrogen levels begin to increase, stimulating a surge of LH secretion from the anterior pituitary. The midcycle surge of LH and FSH induces ovulation. A nonsteroidal ovarian factor, gonadotropin surge-attenuating factor (GnSAF), may antagonize the effect of estrogen on the pituitary and regulate the surge of LH at midcycle.[21] Rising estrogen and progesterone levels during the luteal phase may inhibit the anterior pituitary, and thus reduce LH and FSH secretion. Just before the onset of menstruation, FSH and LH levels begin to increase slightly, probably because of declining estrogen and progesterone levels (see Figure 23-9).

A variety of growth factors and autocrine/paracrine peptides influence hormonal control and follicular response.[1] During the early follicular stage, FSH stimulates FSH and LH receptors, insulin-like growth factor 1, and production of inhibin and activin in the ovary. **Activin** from granulosa cells stimulates the secretion of FSH and increases the pituitary response to GnRH, and increases FSH-binding in the granulosa cells in the dominant follicle. FSH stimulates **inhibin** secretion from granulosa cells and it in turn suppresses FSH synthesis. Inhibin B is primarily secreted in the follicular phase of the cycle but sharply spikes when ovulation occurs. Inhibin A is secreted in the luteal phase and further suppresses FSH. Inhibin also restrains prolactin and growth hormone release, interferes with GnRH receptors, and promotes breakdown of intracellular gonadotropins. In summary, the balance between activin and inhibin regulates FSH secretion, and **follistatin** inhibits activin and boosts inhibin activity. Inhibin and activin also regulate LH stimulation of androgen synthesis in theca cells.[22,23] Figure 23-9 depicts fluctuating estrogen, progesterone, gonadotropin, and inhibin levels. Research continues to advance understanding of the function and structural complexity of these polypeptides and their interaction with GnRH, gonadotropins, and sex hormones.[24]

Ovarian Cycle

By stimulating follicles, gonadotropins initiate their growth and maturation. The most important hormonal event is a rise in FSH. The decline in the late luteal phase of estrogen, progesterone, and inhibin secretion allows FSH to rise; concurrently there is a slight increase in LH levels (see Figure 23-9). FSH stimulates granulosa cell growth and initiates estrogen production in these cells in the next cycle. At this time a group of ovarian follicles is recruited and begins to mature; the exact number depends on the remaining pool of inactive follicles. As the follicles mature, granulosa cells multiply, increasing estradiol secretion. Within a few days of the cycle, one follicle becomes dominant and the others atrophy. The mechanism for follicular recruitment or dominance is unknown.[25] The dominant follicle begins to secrete progressively larger amounts of estrogen (estradiol), which exerts an increase in GnRH receptor concentration and an increase in pituitary sensitivity to GnRH, creating a positive-feedback effect causing an FSH and LH surge. Ovulation generally occurs 1 to 2 hours before the final progesterone surge, or about 12 to 36 hours after the onset of the FSH and LH surge. Progesterone, proteolytic enzymes, and prostaglandins (E and F series) trigger mechanisms controlling follicular rupture and release of the ovum.[1] Possible mechanisms include thinning, stretching, degradation, and digestion of the follicular wall and contraction of smooth muscle cells of the follicle. The role of prostaglandins is essential to ovulation, and infertility patients should be advised to avoid the use of drugs that inhibit prostaglandin synthesis.[26]

The FSH and LH surge also transforms the granulosa cells of the ovulatory follicle into the corpus luteum. The corpus luteum secretes estrogen and progesterone in amounts that depend in part on adequate development of the follicle before ovulation. Progesterone acts centrally and locally within the ovary to suppress new follicular growth during the early and midluteal phases. If pregnancy does not occur, the corpus luteum persists for 11 to 14 days, then regresses and eventually disappears. An increase in pulse frequency of GnRH from a low level of estrogen and progesterone reactivates hormonal control of the menstrual cycle and FSH secretion increases.

Uterine Phases

Uterine phases of the menstrual cycle—proliferative, secretory, and ischemic/menstrual phases—involve cyclic endometrial changes controlled by estrogen and progesterone. Hormonal effects are influenced by the presence of receptors and numerous growth factors, peptides, and enzymes that act as intermediaries between the sex steroids and the endometrium.[27] During the midfollicular phase, increasing levels of estrogen contribute to endometrial repair and proliferation, increasing endometrial thickness. Once ovulation occurs and serum progesterone levels increase, the endometrial tissue develops secretory characteristics. If implantation of a fertilized ovum does not take place, endometrial tissue begins to break down approximately 11 days after ovulation. The period of breakdown is sometimes called the *ischemic phase* (see Figure 23-9). Sloughing of tissue (menstrual bleeding) begins about 14 days after ovulation.

Cervical mucus also undergoes cyclic changes. During the proliferative phase the cervical mucus is thin and watery. Peak estrogen levels occur just before ovulation and maximally stimulate the cervical glands to produce mucus. Cervical mucus becomes abundant and more elastic (spinnbarkeit). In the presence of estrogen, tiny channels develop in the mucus, which allows sperm access to the interior of the uterus. Changes in the consistency of cervical mucus can be used to identify fertile intervals.

Vaginal Response

Vaginal endothelium also responds to cyclic hormonal changes. Under the influence of estrogen, epithelial cells of the vagina grow maximally during the follicular/proliferative phase. After ovulation, layers of keratinized cells overgrow the basal epithelium, a process known as **cornification.** Near the end of the luteal phase, leukocytes invade vaginal epithelium, removing the outer layers in a process termed **decornification.**

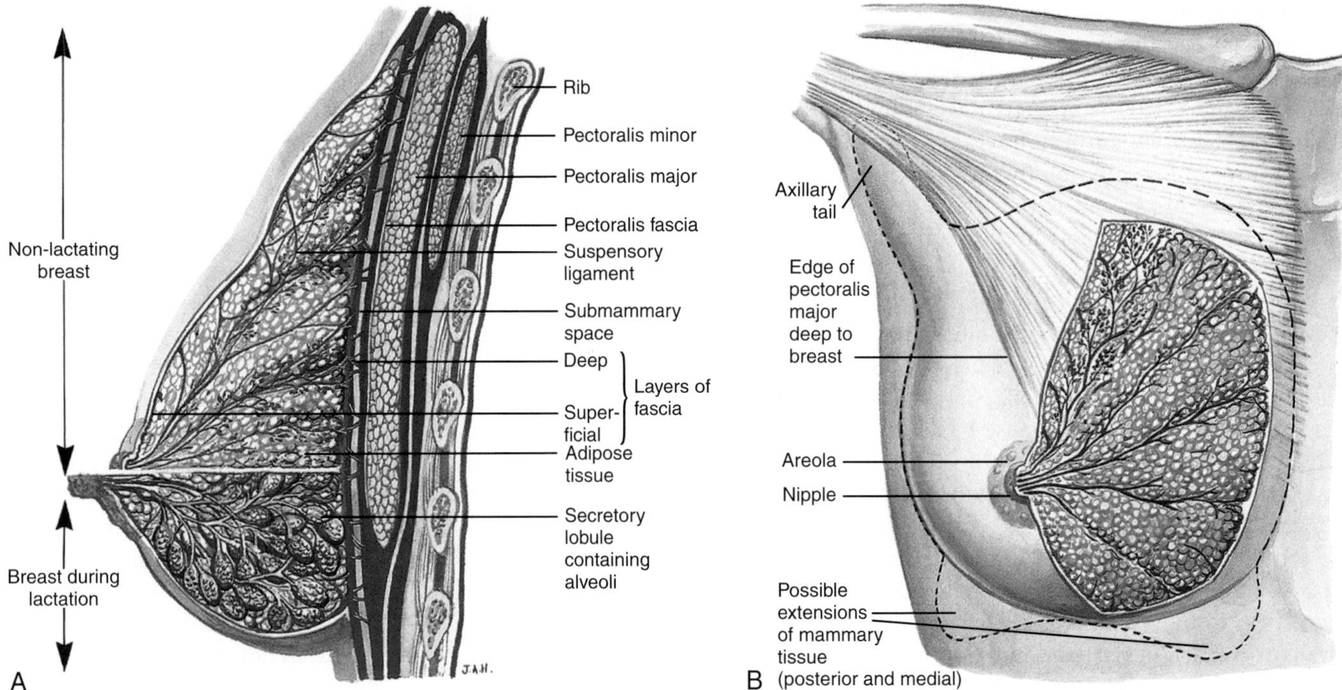

FIGURE 23-10 Schematic Diagram of Breast. A, Lactating breast. **B,** Structures of the breast. (From Shah P: Breast. In Standring S, editor: *Gray's anatomy*, ed 39, London, 2005, Elsevier Churchill Livingstone.)

Body Temperature

Basal body temperature (BBT) undergoes characteristic biphasic changes during menstrual cycles in which ovulation occurs. During the follicular phase the BBT fluctuates around 37° C (98° F). After the LH surge, the average temperature increases by 0.2° to 0.5° C (0.4° to 1° F). At the end of the luteal phase, 1 to 3 days before the onset of menstruation, BBT declines to follicular-phase levels. The shift in temperature is related to ovulation, corpus luteum formation, and increased serum progesterone levels. Progesterone probably acts on the thermoregulatory center of the hypothalamus to increase body temperature. Changes in BBT are used to document ovulatory cycles but when used alone are not the best method to predict the exact timing of ovulation.

STRUCTURE AND FUNCTION OF THE BREAST

The adult **breast** lies on the ventral surface of the thorax, within the superficial fascia of the chest wall, extending vertically from the second rib to the sixth or seventh intercostal space and laterally from the side of the sternum to the midaxillary line. Breast tissue also may extend into the axilla; this tissue is known as the *tail of Spence.*

The Female Breast

The female breast is composed of 15 to 20 pyramid-shaped lobes that are separated and supported by suspensory (Cooper) ligaments (Figure 23-10). Each lobe contains 20 to 40 lobules that are subdivided into glandular alveoli. The lobes and lobules are surrounded and separated by muscle strands and fatty connective tissue. The amount of fatty connective tissue varies from individual to individual, depending on weight and genetic and endocrine factors, and contributes to the diversity of breast size and shape and function of the mammary epithelium. During pregnancy the alveoli further develop, becoming composed of secretory acini that synthesize milk (lactation) (see Figure 23-10). Given this function, it is only during a pregnancy/lactation cycle and subsequent hormonal changes that the gland remodels into a milk-secreting organ and reaches its ultimate mature development stage.[28] The breast has the capacity to regress to a resting state after cessation of lactation and then undergo the same cycle of expansion and regression in subsequent pregnancies, a process possibly maintained by stem cells.[28,29] This remarkable plasticity of the breast suggests tight hormonal control and dramatic tissue-stromal restructuring. Investigators are focusing on the anatomy as a tool to advance knowledge on normal and aberrant breast development and to understand the origin of breast cancer.[30-32] After pregnancy, the milk is continuously secreted into the alveolar lumen and is stored there until the myoepithelial cells are stimulated by oxytocin to contract, which triggers the let-down reflex.[33] The alveoli empty into a network of lactiferous ducts. These ducts reach the skin through 9 or 10 openings (pores) in the nipple. The lobes and lobules are surrounded and separated by muscle strands and fatty connective tissue.

An extensive capillary network surrounds the alveoli and is supplied by perforating branches of the internal mammary, the thoracoacromial, the internal and lateral thoracic, and the intercostal arteries. Venous return follows arterial supply, with relatively rapid emptying into the superior vena cava. The breasts receive sensory innervation from branches of the second through sixth intercostal nerves and the cervical plexus. This accounts for the fact that breast pain may be referred to the

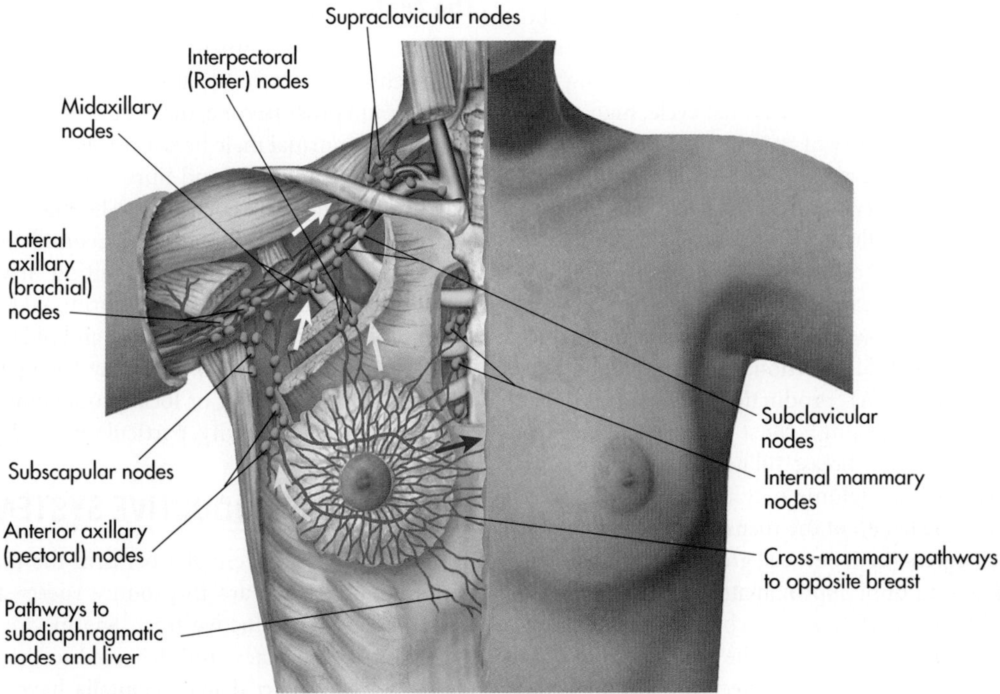

FIGURE 23-11 **Lymphatic Drainage of the Female Breast.** Arrows indicate the direction of lymphatic drainage. (From Seidel HM et al: *Mosby's guide to physical examination,* ed 7, St Louis, 2011, Mosby.)

chest, back, scapula, medial arm, and neck. Lymphatic drainage of the breast occurs largely through axillary nodes with minor drainage through the superficial mammary routes (Figure 23-11). There may be asymmetry between the breasts.[34,35]

The **nipple** is a pigmented, cylindric structure that is located within the central area of the areola. It measures 0.5 to 1.3 cm in diameter and is approximately 10 to 12 mm in height when erect. On its surface lie multiple openings, one from each lobe. The **areola** is the pigmented circular area in the center of the breast surrounding the nipple. It may be 15 to 60 mm in diameter. A number of sebaceous glands, the **glands of Montgomery,** are located within the areola and aid in lubrication of the nipple during lactation. The nipple and areola contain smooth muscles that receive motor innervation from the sympathetic nervous system. Breast-feeding, sexual stimulation, and exposure to cold cause the nipple to become erect.

Fetal and early postnatal breast tissue development occurs independently from the sex hormones, but the fetal breast tissue becomes progressively responsive to hormonal stimulation at birth. The neonatal breasts are rudimentary, containing 10 to 12 branching ducts. During childhood, breast, nipple, and areola growth is slow, keeping pace with other body tissues. (Male breast development normally does not progress any further.) At the onset of puberty in the female, estrogen secretion stimulates mammary growth. Breast development, or **thelarche,** is usually the first sign of puberty in the female. Full differentiation and maturation of breast tissue occur over approximately 4 years and are mediated by a variety of hormones, including estrogen, progesterone, prolactin, growth hormone, thyroxine, insulin, and cortisol. Estrogen promotes the increase in size of the breast by the formation of a mass of tissue under the areola, increases the size and pigmentation of the areola, and promotes development of the lobular ducts. The breast cells of parous women are different than those of women who never become pregnant. During menopause the lobules of the parous breast regress to prepregnancy composition and become identical to the nulliparous breast. Variations in breast development are listed in Box 23-1.

BOX 23-1 VARIATIONS IN BREAST DEVELOPMENT

- Ectopic breast development may occur in males and females with tissue in the axilla, abdomen, labia in females, or back and buttocks (less common). The breast tissue develops from the milk line, an embryonic mammary ridge of ectoderm.
- Accessory nipples (polythelia) or mammary glands (polymastia) are caused by cellular migration along the milk line; polythelia occurs in approximately 1% of the population and is slightly more common in men.
- Inverted nipples usually revert to normal during the first month; persistence into adulthood may cause concerns with lactation.
- Failed development of the nipple (athelia) or entire mammary gland (amastia) is rare and may include a complete lack of development, unilateral failure, or extreme asymmetry. This is caused by complete involution of the mammary ridge in the milk lines.
- Symmetric or asymmetric hyperplasia occurs in approximately 1% to 4% of all females.

Data from DeSilva NK, Merritt DF: Chapter 545, Breast concerns. In Kliegman RM et al, editors: *Nelson textbook of pediatrics,* ed 19, p 834, Philadelphia, 2011, Saunders; Greydanus DE, Matytsina L, Gains M: *Prim Care* 33(2):455–502, 2006.

During the reproductive years the breast undergoes cyclic changes in response to changes in the levels of estrogen and progesterone associated with the menstrual cycle. During the follicular/proliferative phase of the menstrual cycle, high estradiol levels increase the vascularity of breast tissue and stimulate proliferation of ductal and alveolar tissue. This effect is sustained into the luteal/secretory phase of the cycle. During this phase progesterone levels influence the growth of the alveoli and increase and contribute to the breast changes induced by estradiol. Specific effects of estrogen and progesterone include dilation of the ducts and conversion of the alveolar cells into secretory cells, as well as fluid secretion, mitotic activity, and deoxyribonucleic acid (DNA) production of nonglandular tissue and glandular epithelium.[1] Most women experience some degree of premenstrual breast fullness, tenderness, and increased nodularity. Breast volume may increase as much as 10 to 30 ml. Because the length of the menstrual cycle does not allow for complete regression of new cell growth, breast growth continues at a slow rate until approximately 35 years of age. Because of the cyclic changes that occur in breast tissue, clinical breast examination is recommended at the conclusion of or a few days after menses, when hormonal effects are minimal and breasts are at their smallest and least tender.

During pregnancy the breast reaches its maximum development. With increased levels of estrogen the lobules further differentiate. Progesterone stimulates development of cells lining the alveoli to produce milk. Lactation (milk production) occurs after childbirth in response to increased levels of prolactin. Prolactin secretion, in turn, increases by continued breast-feeding. Oxytocin, another hormone released during and after delivery, controls milk ejection from alveolar cells. Milk is continuously secreted into the alveolar lumen and is stored there until the myoepithelial cells are stimulated by suckling stimulation of oxytocin, which triggers the let-down reflex.[33] The alveoli empty into a network of lactiferous ducts. These ducts reach the skin through 9 or 10 openings (pores) in the nipple.

The function of the female breast is primarily to provide a source of nourishment for the newborn. Physiologically, breast milk is the most appropriate nourishment for newborns. Not only does its composition change over time to meet the changing digestive capabilities and nutritional requirements of the infant but it also contains immune cells, specific immunoglobulins, especially immunoglobulin A (IgA), and nonspecific antimicrobial factors, such as lysozymes and lactoferrin, that protect the infant against infection, allergies, and asthma. Evidence suggests breast-feeding decreases future incidence in the infant of adult obesity, lowers atherosclerotic disease, and lowers the incidence of types 1 and 2 diabetes.[36] During lactation high prolactin levels interfere with hypothalamic-pituitary hormones that stimulate ovulation. Lactation usually suppresses the menstrual cycle (lactational amenorrhea) and prevents ovulation for the first 6 months postpartum.[37] In many parts of the world breast-feeding is the major means of contraception. Breasts are also a source of pleasurable sexual sensation and in Western cultures have become a sexual symbol.

The Male Breast

Until puberty, development of the male breast is similar to that of the female breast. In the absence of sufficiently high levels of estrogen and progesterone, the male breast does not develop any further. The normal male breast consists of a small underdeveloped nipple, some fatty and fibrous tissue, and a few ductlike structures in the subareolar area. The male breast may appear enlarged in obese men because of accumulation of fatty tissue. Physiologic gynecomastia is a condition in which the breasts temporarily enlarge as a result of hormonal fluctuations and is common in newborns, adolescents, and older men. Of men 50 to 80 years of age, 30% to 60% may have palpable breast tissue related to circulating or local production of estrogen from elevated aromatase activity, particularly in adipose tissue.[38,39]

THE MALE REPRODUCTIVE SYSTEM

In men the external genitalia perform the major functions of reproduction, which are to produce sperm and deliver them to the female reproductive tract. Sperm, are produced in the male gonads, the testes, and delivered to the female vagina by the penis. The internal male genitalia have a more accessory function. They consist of conducting tubes and fluid-producing glands, all of which aid in the transport of sperm from the testes to the urethral opening of the penis. The male reproductive and urinary structures are shown in Figure 23-12.

External Genitalia

Testes

In men the **testes** (*singular,* testis) are the essential organs of reproduction. Like the ovaries, the testes have two functions: (1) production of gametes (in this case, sperm), and (2) production of sex hormones (in this case, androgens and testosterone). The testes are suspended outside the pelvic cavity because sperm production requires an environment that is 1° or 2° C (1.6° to 3.6° F) cooler than body temperature.

During embryonic and fetal life, the testes develop within the abdomen (see Figure 23-1). About 3 months before birth, the testes start to descend toward the developing scrotum. About 1 month before birth they enter twin passageways called **inguinal canals.** The inguinal canals are vaginal processes created by outpouchings of the peritoneum (lining of the abdominal cavity). The descent of a testis is shown in Figure 23-13. Each testis moves down outside the peritoneum until it is suspended in the scrotal sac by its supply lines: the ducts, blood vessels, lymphatic vessels, and nerves of the **spermatic cord.** When descent is complete, the abdominal end of each vaginal process closes up and the inguinal canal disappears. If peritoneal closure at the site of the inguinal canal is incomplete or weak, an inguinal hernia may occur later in life. The scrotal end of each vaginal process becomes the outer covering of the testis, the **tunica vaginalis.**

Figure 23-14 shows a sagittal section of a mature testis. The adult testis is ovoid and varies considerably in length (3 to 6 cm), width (2 to 3.5 cm), depth (3 to 4 cm), and weight (10 to 40 g). The testis is almost entirely surrounded by an outer covering, the tunica vaginalis, which separates the testis from the scrotal wall, and an inner covering, the **tunica albuginea.** Inward extensions

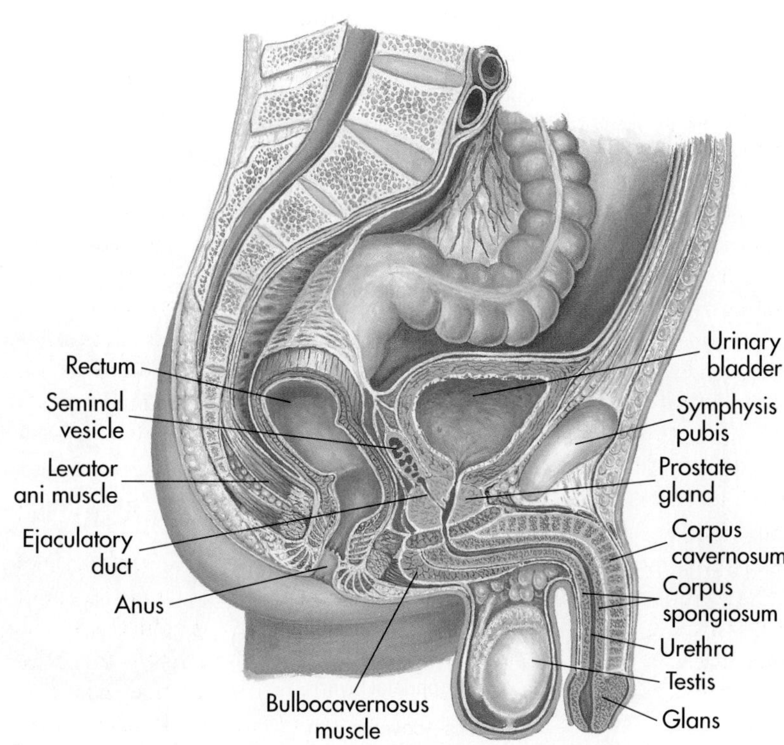

FIGURE 23-12 Structure of the Male Reproductive Organs. (From Seidel HM et al: *Mosby's guide to physical examination,* ed 7, St Louis, 2011, Mosby.)

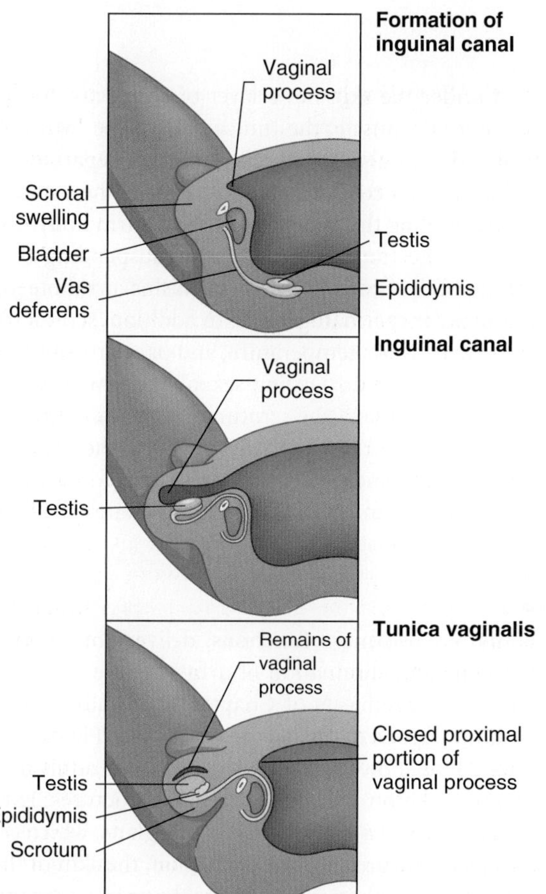

FIGURE 23-13 Descent of a Testis. The testes descend from the abdominal cavity to the scrotum during the last 3 months of fetal development.

of the tunica albuginea form septa that separate the testis into about 250 compartments, or lobules, each of which contains several tortuously coiled ducts called **seminiferous tubules.** The seminiferous tubules constitute the bulk (80%) of testicular volume and are the site of sperm production. (Sperm production, termed **spermatogenesis,** is described on p. 789.) Tissue surrounding these ducts contains blood and lymphatic vessels, fibroblastic support cells, macrophages, mast cells, and Leydig cells. **Leydig cells,** which occur in clusters and account for about 1% to 5% of testicular volume, produce androgens, chiefly testosterone.

The two ends of each seminiferous tubule join and leave the lobule through a short, straight section called the **tubulus rectus.** Sperm travel from the seminiferous tubules into these straight sections, which lead to the central portion of the testis, the **rete testis.** From the rete testis, sperm move through the **efferent tubules,** or vasa efferentia, to the epididymis, where they mature.

The testes are innervated by adrenergic fibers, whose sole function apparently is to regulate blood flow to the Leydig cells. The testes receive arterial blood from the internal spermatic and differential arteries. Arterial blood flows over the surface of the testes before entering the parenchyma (functional tissues). Surface flow cools the blood to temperatures that promote spermatogenesis, approximately 1° to 2° C (34° to 36° F) below body core temperature.[40] Additionally, the testes are suspended outside the pelvic cavity to facilitate cooling.

Epididymis

The **epididymis** (*plural,* epididymides) is a comma-shaped structure that curves over the posterior portion of each testis

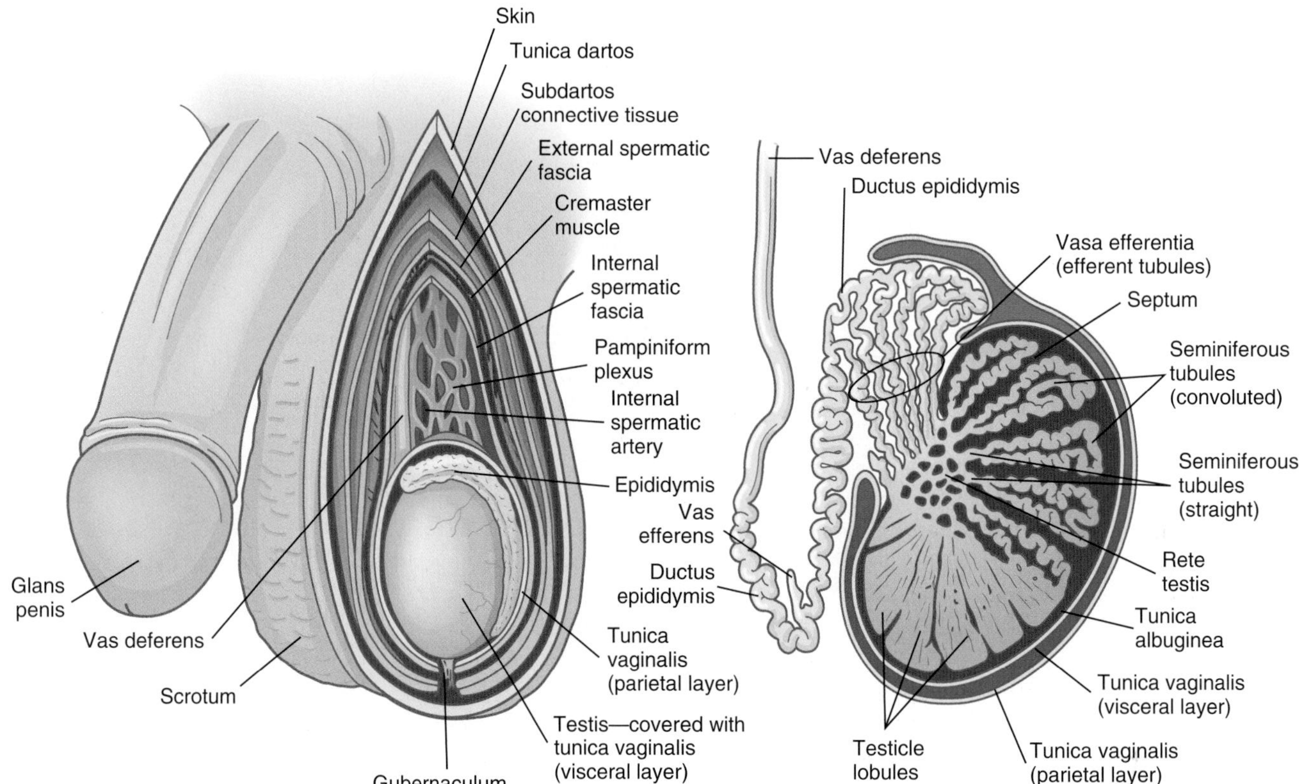

FIGURE 23-14 The Testes. External and sagittal views showing interior anatomy. (From Seidel HM et al: *Mosby's guide to physical examination,* ed 6, St Louis, 2006, Mosby.)

(see Figure 23-14). It consists of a single highly packed and markedly coiled (about 6 meters when uncoiled) duct measuring 5 cm long, whose structural function is to conduct sperm from the efferent tubules to the vas deferens. The duct can become inflamed from infection by microorganisms that ascend the urethra or from the prostate, causing epididymitis. The epididymis has physiologic functions as well. When sperm enter the head of the epididymis, they are not fully mature or motile, nor are they capable of fertilizing an ovum. During the 12 days (or more) sperm take to travel the length of the epididymis, they receive nutrients and testosterone from the epididymal epithelium, and some biochemical or physiologic mechanism enhances their capacity for fertilization.[41]

The tail of the epididymis is continuous with the **vas deferens (ductus deferens),** a duct with muscular layers capable of powerful peristalsis that transports sperm toward the urethra. After traveling the length of the epididymis, sperm are stored in the epididymal tail and vas deferens. The vas deferens enters the pelvic cavity through the spermatic cord.

Scrotum

The testes, epididymides, and spermatic cord are enclosed and protected by the scrotum. The **scrotum** is a skin-covered fibromuscular sac that is homologous to the female labia majora (see Figure 23-2). The skin of the scrotum is thin and has rugae (wrinkles or folds) that enable it to enlarge or relax away from the body. At puberty the scrotal skin darkens, develops active sebaceous glands, and becomes sparsely covered with hair. Just under the skin lies a layer of connective tissue (fascia) and smooth muscle, the tunica dartos (see Figure 23-14). The **tunica dartos** also forms a septum that separates the two testes. Exposure to cold temperatures causes the tunica dartos to contract, pulling the testes close to the warm body. In warm temperatures the tunica dartos relaxes, suspending the testes away from body heat. These mechanisms promote optimal temperatures for spermatogenesis. In addition, scrotal sensitivity to touch, pressure, temperature, and pain protects the testes against potential harm. During sexual excitement the scrotal skin and tunica thicken, the scrotum tightens and lifts, and the spermatic cords shorten, partially elevating the testes toward the body. As excitement plateaus, the engorged testes increase 50% in size, rotate anteriorly, and flatten against the body, signaling impending ejaculation.

Penis

The **penis** has two main functions: delivery of sperm to the female vagina and elimination of urine. (Urine formation and excretion are the subjects of Chapter 37.) Embryonically, the penis is homologous to the female clitoris (see Figure 23-2).

Figure 23-12 shows a sagittal section of the adult penis and its anatomic relation to other urogenital structures. Externally the penis consists of a shaft with a tip, the **glans,** which contains the opening of the urethra. For protection, the skin of the glans folds over the tip of the penis, forming the prepuce, or **foreskin.** At birth, the foreskin is adhered to the glans. Penile erections, which commonly occur, cause the adhesions to break so that

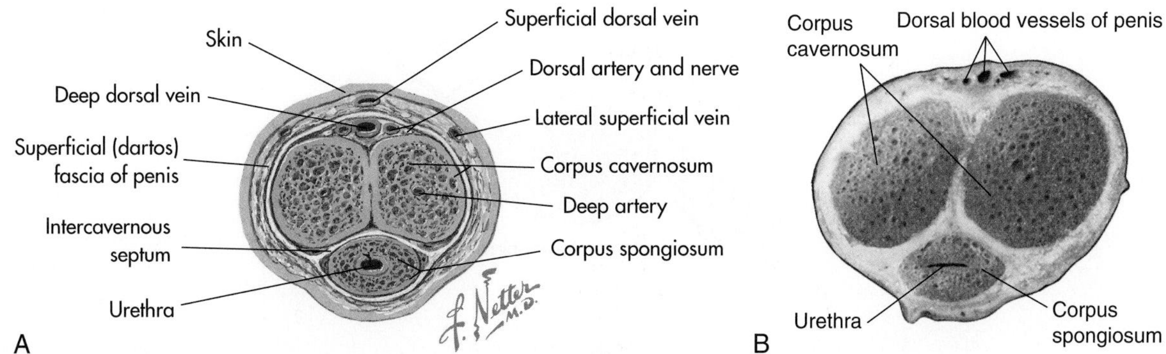

FIGURE 23-15 **The Penis.** **A,** Cross section of the penis. **B,** Cross section of the shaft of the penis showing three columns of erectile, or cavernous, tissue. (**A** Netter illustration from www.netterimages.com. Copyright © Elsevier Inc. All rights reserved. **B** from Vidic B, Suarez RF: *Photographic atlas of the human body*, St. Louis, 1984, Mosby.)

by age 3 years the foreskin becomes completely retractable. The skin of the penis is continuous with that of the groin, scrotum, and inner thighs. It is hairless, movable, and darker than surrounding skin.

Internally the penis consists of the urethra and three compartments: two **corpora cavernosa** (*singular,* corpus cavernosum) and the **corpus spongiosum** (Figure 23-15). The three compartments are separated by Buck fascia and, like the testes, are enclosed by a tunica albuginea. The **urethra** passes through the corpus spongiosum and ends at a sagittal slit in the glans. If the urethra is not completely surrounded by the corpus spongiosum, the meatus may open on the ventral surface of the penile shaft (hypospadias) or on the dorsal surface (epispadias).

Penetration of the female vagina is made possible by the **erectile reflex,** a process in which erectile tissues within the corpora cavernosa and corpus spongiosum become engorged with blood, generally 20 to 50 ml. The erectile tissues consist of vascular spaces, or chambers, that are supplied with blood by arterioles (small arteries). Most of the time the arterioles are constricted through tonic noradrenaline release from sympathetic nerves so that not much blood flows through the erectile tissues. Sexual stimulation, however, causes the arterioles to dilate through release of nitric oxide and fill with blood.[42] Their rapid expansion fills the erectile tissues, causing an erection. Erection apparently is maintained by compression or constriction of veins that drain the corpora cavernosa and corpus spongiosum. When sexual stimulation ceases or orgasm and ejaculation occur, these veins open up, blood flows out of the arterioles, and the penis becomes flaccid (soft and pendulous).

Erection is under the control of the autonomic nervous system but can be stimulated or inhibited by central nervous system input. Stimulation of mechanoreceptors of the penis, particularly of the glans, causes parasympathetic nerves of the autonomic nervous system to relax smooth muscle in the walls of penile arterioles. At the same time, the effects of sympathetic nerves, which normally cause arteriolar smooth muscle to constrict, are inhibited.

Erections begin in utero and continue throughout life, but ejaculation does not occur until sperm production begins at puberty. Growth of the penis and scrotal contents continues well past puberty, however, and may not be complete until the late teens or early 20s. Penis size, when flaccid, varies considerably; with an erection, differences in penis size diminish. Sexual excitement causes the corpora cavernosa to increase in length and width and become rigid; the penis becomes erect. Stimulation of the glans, which is endowed with copious sensitive nerve endings, provides maximum erotic sensation. With sexual arousal, skin color deepens, the glans doubles in size, and the urethral meatus dilates. Ejaculation occurs with frequent, strong contractions of the vas deferens, epididymis, seminal vesicles, prostate, urethra, and penis. Erection and ejaculation can occur independently of each other.[43]

Internal Genitalia

Figure 23-13 shows the anatomy of the internal genitalia and their relation to other pelvic organs. The internal genitalia consist of ducts and glands. The ducts—the two vasa deferentia, the ejaculatory duct, and the urethra—conduct sperm and glandular secretions from the testes to the urethral opening of the penis. The glands—the prostate gland, two seminal vesicles, and two Cowper (or bulbourethral) glands—secrete fluids that serve as a vehicle for sperm transport and create an alkaline, nutritious medium that promotes sperm motility and survival. Together the sperm and the glandular fluids comprise **semen.**

Sperm leave the epididymides and travel rapidly through the internal ducts in a process called **emission.** Emission occurs just seconds before ejaculation, at the moment when sexual arousal peaks. Emission always leads to ejaculation.

Emission occurs as smooth muscle in the walls of the epididymides and vasa deferentia begins to contract rhythmically, pushing sperm and epididymal secretions through the vasa deferentia. Each vas deferens is a firm, elastic fibromuscular tube that begins at the tail of the epididymis, enters the pelvic cavity within the spermatic cord, loops up and over the bladder, and ends in the prostate gland (Figure 23-16; see also Figure 23-12). Sperm are moved along by peristaltic contractions of smooth muscle in the walls of the vas deferens.

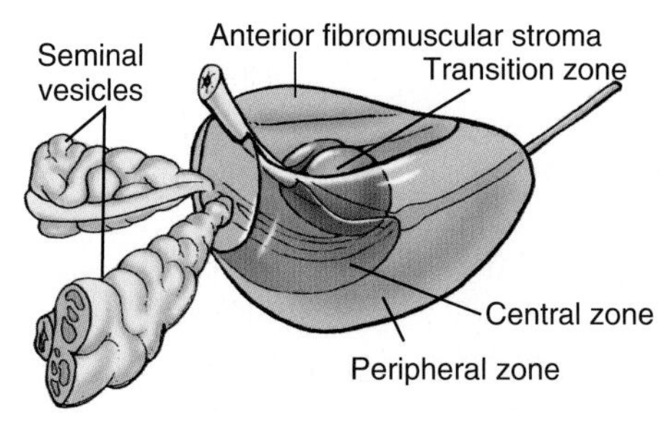

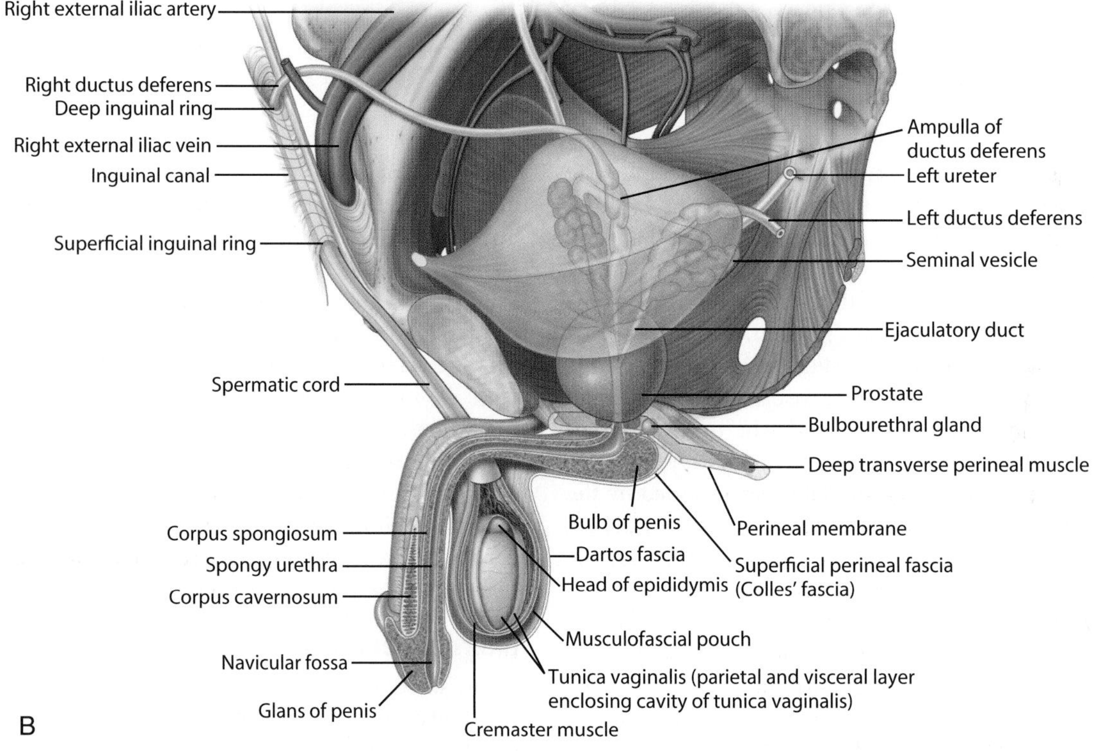

FIGURE 23-16 **Zones of the Prostate Gland and Seminal Vesicles. A,** Zones of the prostate. The peripheral zone, accounting for 70% of the prostate gland, is the site of origin of ≤70% of prostate cancers; the central zone, approximately 25% of the prostate gland, gives rise to only 1% to 5% of prostate cancers; and the transition zone, ≈5% to 10% of the prostate gland, gives rise to 20% of prostate cancers and is the site of origin of benign prostatic hyperplasia (BPH). **B,** Prostate gland within the male reproductive system. (**A** copyright Baylor College of Medicine, Houston, TX. **B** from Drake et al: *Gray's atlas of anatomy*, Philadelphia, 2008, Churchill Livingstone.)

As sperm leave the ampulla (wide portion) of the vas deferens, the seminal vesicles secrete a nutritive glucose-rich fluid into the ejaculate (semen). The **seminal vesicles** are a pair of glands, each about 4 to 6 cm long, that lie behind the urinary bladder and in front of the rectum. The seminal vesicles provide fructose as a source of energy for ejaculated sperm, and secrete prostaglandins that promote smooth muscle contraction assisting with sperm transport. The ducts of the seminal vesicles join the ampulla of the vas deferens to become the **ejaculatory duct,** which contracts rhythmically during emission and ejaculation. As can be seen in Figures 23-12 and 23-16, the ejaculatory duct joins the urethra, where both pass through the prostate gland. During emission and ejaculation a sphincter (muscle surrounding a duct) closes, preventing urine from entering the prostatic urethra.[44]

The **prostate gland** is about the size of a walnut, has three zones, and surrounds the urethra (see Figure 23-16). It is composed of glandular alveoli and ducts embedded in fibromuscular tissue. Prostate growth, development, and function are regulated by androgens and the androgen receptor. Without them the prostate is at risk for hyperplastic and malignant growth[45] (see Chapter 25). Nerves required for penile erection travel along the posterolateral surface of the prostate. Included in prostate epithelial secretions are prostate-specific antigen (PSA), cytokeratins, prostate-specific membrane antigen (PSMA), and prostate-specific acid phosphatase. Prostate secretions contribute to the ejaculate. While semen moves through the prostatic portion of the urethra, the prostate gland contracts rhythmically and secretes prostatic fluid into the mixture. Prostatic fluid is a thin, milky substance with an alkaline pH that helps sperm survive in the acid environment of the female reproductive tract. In addition, clotting enzymes and fibrinolysin in prostatic fluids help mobilize sperm after ejaculation.

Cowper glands (bulbourethral glands), whose ducts secrete mucus into the urethra near the base of the penis, are the last pair of glands to add fluid to the ejaculate. Ejaculation occurs as semen reaches the base of the penis and muscles there begin the rhythmic contractions that push semen out. Normally a man ejaculates between 2 and 6 ml of semen, containing 75 million to 400 million sperm. About 98% of the ejaculate consists of glandular fluids; 60% to 70% of volume comes from the seminal vesicles and 20% from the prostate. Therefore, the ejaculate of a man who has undergone vasectomy (a surgical procedure that prevents sperm from entering the vas deferens) is not reduced by much: about 2%. During vasectomy, the vas deferens are severed and then tied in order to prevent sperm from entering the ejaculate; this procedure is used for permanent male birth control.

Spermatogenesis

Spermatogenesis begins at puberty and continues for life. In this respect, spermatogenesis differs markedly from oogenesis (production of primordial ova), which occurs during fetal life only.

Spermatogenesis takes place within the seminiferous tubules of the testes (see Figure 23-14). The basement membrane of each seminiferous tubule is lined with diploid (46-chromosome) germ cells called **spermatogonia** (*singular,* spermatogonium). These cells undergo continuous mitotic division. (Mitotic division, in which a cell divides into two identical cells, is described in Chapter 1.) Some of the spermatogonia move away from the basement membrane and mature, becoming **primary spermatocytes** (Figure 23-17). The primary spermatocytes undergo meiosis, a type of cell division that results in two haploid (23-chromosome) cells called **secondary spermatocytes.** (Meiosis is described and illustrated in Chapter 4.) The two secondary spermatocytes then undergo meiosis, resulting in four **spermatids.** It is the spermatids that differentiate into spermatozoa, or sperm, each of which contains 23 chromosomes (Figure 23-18).

The development of spermatids into sperm depends on the presence of **Sertoli cells (nondividing support cells)** within the seminiferous tubules. The spermatids attach themselves to Sertoli cells, from which they receive the nutrients and the hormonal signals (i.e., testosterone) they need to develop into sperm.[46] The process of spermatogenesis, from mitotic division of a spermatogonium to maturation of the spermatids, takes about 70 to 80 days. Mature sperm migrate from the seminiferous tubules to the epididymis, where their capacity for fertilization continues to develop. Although they are completely mature by the time they are ejaculated, the sperm do not become motile (capable of movement) until they are activated by biochemicals in semen and in the female reproductive tract.

Male Sex Hormones

The male sex hormones are androgens and **testosterone** is the primary male sex hormone. Leydig cells of the testes and, to a lesser degree, the adrenal glands produce testosterone and other androgens. In men, sex hormone production is relatively constant with some diurnal variation.

The androgens have a number of physiologic actions related to growth and development of male tissues and organs. They are responsible for fetal differentiation and development of the male urogenital system and have some effects on the fetal brain. After birth, the Leydig cells become quiescent until activated by the gonadotropins during puberty. At puberty, androgens cause the sex organs to grow and secondary sex characteristics to develop.

Testosterone affects nervous and skeletal tissues, bone marrow, skin and hair, and sex organs. It has an anabolic effect on skeletal muscle tissue, thereby contributing to the difference in body weight and composition between men and women. Testosterone also stimulates growth of the musculature and cartilage of the larynx, causing a permanent deepening of the voice. Testosterone directly stimulates the bone marrow and indirectly stimulates renal erythropoietin production to achieve increased hemoglobin and hematocrit levels. Because sebaceous gland activity is stimulated by testosterone, acne may develop. In the presence of testosterone, hair becomes coarser in texture, and facial hair, axillary hair, and pubic hair grow in male patterns. Later in life, testosterone causes baldness in genetically susceptible individuals. Testosterone is required for spermatogenesis and for secretion of fluid by the prostate gland, seminal vesicles, and Cowper glands. Testosterone is also associated with an increase in **libido** (sex drive). Other, less-understood, effects of testosterone include alterations in fatty acid and cholesterol metabolism.

The regulation of androgen production and spermatogenesis is achieved by a complex feedback system involving the extrahypothalamic central nervous system, the hypothalamus, the anterior pituitary, the testes, and the androgen-sensitive end organs. These relationships, which are essentially the same in women, are summarized in Figure 23-3. Extrahypothalamic influences include such variables as physiologic and psychologic stress, which may inhibit or augment hypothalamic activity. In the hypothalamus, neurotransmitters regulate GnRH synthesis and pulsatile release (about every 3 hours) into the hypophyseal portal veins. Norepinephrine stimulates GnRH secretion, and serotonin and dopamine inhibit GnRH secretion. GnRH is transported by portal flow to the median eminence of the pituitary gland, where it binds to receptors and stimulates the synthesis and secretion of gonadotropins, LH, and FSH. LH and FSH, which are named for their effects in the female reproductive system, have important effects on the male system as well. LH acts on the Leydig cells to regulate testosterone secretion. FSH acts on the seminiferous tubule Sertoli cells to promote spermatogenesis. FSH secretion is inhibited by inhibin secreted by the Sertoli cells. Similar to their action in the female gonad, inhibin functions as an autocrine/paracrine regulator in the male gonad. Inhibin inhibits proliferation of spermatogonia by

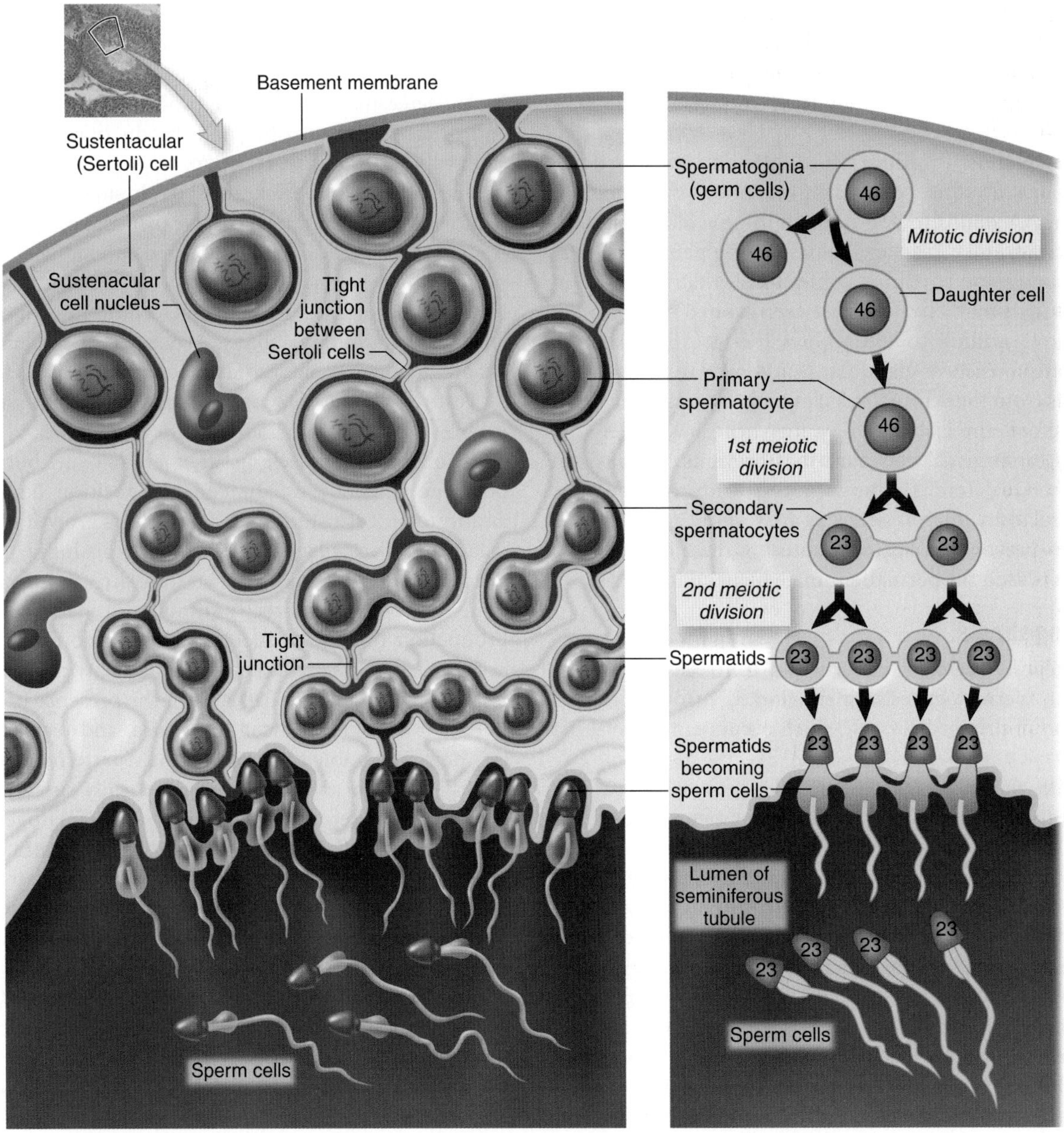

FIGURE 23-17 **Seminiferous Tubule.** Section shows process of meiosis and sperm cell formation. (From Patton KT, Thibodeau GA: *Anatomy & physiology*, ed 8, St Louis, 2013, Mosby.)

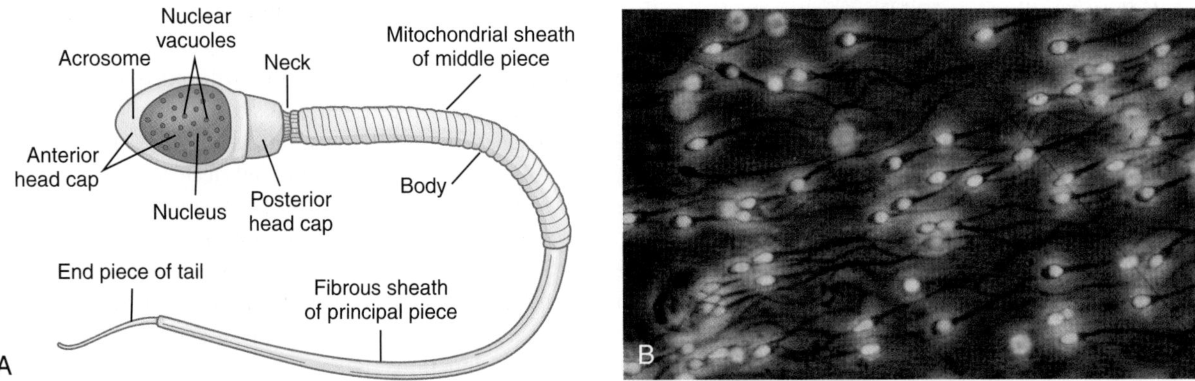

FIGURE 23-18 **Mature Sperm Cell (Spermatozoon). A,** Anatomy of mature sperm cell. **B,** Human sperm with nuclear material glowing with a fluorescent dye. (**B** from Lennart Nilsson.)

regulating pituitary FSH levels. In addition, inhibin facilitates LH stimulation of androgen biosynthesis in Leydig cells.

Ninety-eight percent of testosterone, the major steroid hormone produced by the testes, binds to either **sex hormone–binding globulin (SHBG)** (40%) or albumin (48%). The remaining 2% remains unbound in the plasma and is free to enter cells and wield its metabolic effects. Changes in the amount of available SHBG affect the amount of testosterone within tissues. The testes secrete only 25% of circulating estrogen (estradiol). The majority is produced by peripheral conversion of testosterone and androstenedione. Estrogens help regulate GnRH and LH secretion. Peripheral conversion of testosterone by 5-alpha-reductase also produces **dihydrotestosterone (DHT),** another potent androgen. DHT is necessary for external virilization during embryogenesis and androgen activity beginning at puberty and continuing throughout adulthood. **Prolactin,** a polypeptide synthesized and secreted from the pituitary, helps maintain biosynthesis of testosterone. However, elevated prolactin levels may suppress biosynthesis.[47]

In summary, hormones secreted at each level of the hypothalamic-pituitary-testicular (HPT) axis control and coordinate testicular function (Figure 23-19). This control is exerted through positive and negative feedback signals by (1) sex steroids that inhibit hypothalamic GnRH secretion and pituitary LH responsiveness to GnRH; and (2) testicular inhibin that inhibits pituitary FSH and, possibly, circulating estrogens (E_2). Any disruption along the HPT axis may lead to hypogonadism or infertility.

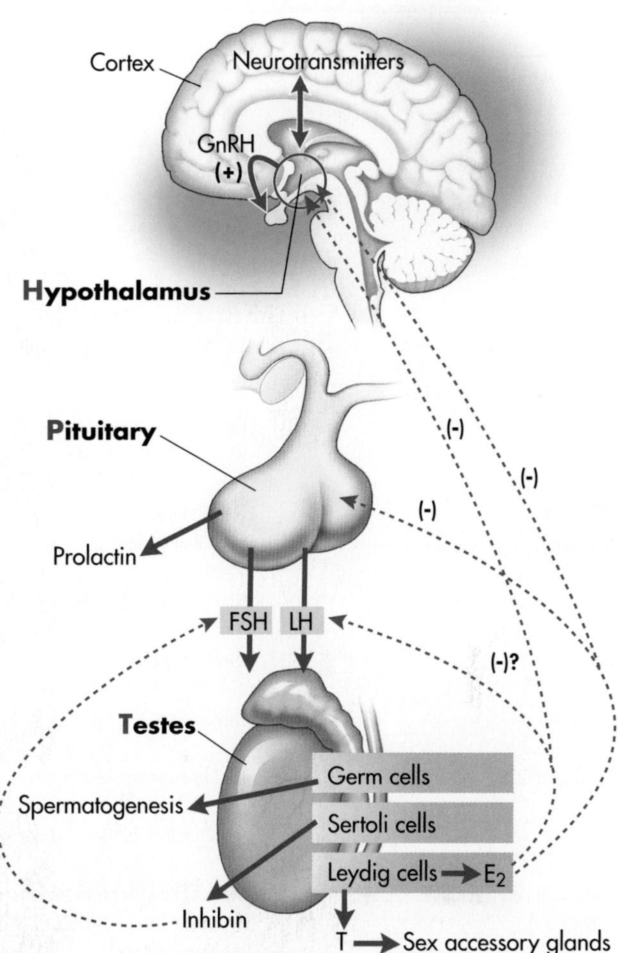

FIGURE 23-19 Schematic Representation of Activity Along the Hypothalamus-Pituitary-Testicular (HPT) Axis. *E_2,* Estrogen; *FSH,* follicle-stimulating hormone; *GnRH,* gonadotropin-releasing hormone; *LH,* luteinizing hormone; *T,* testosterone.

TESTS OF REPRODUCTIVE FUNCTION

Diagnostic tests of the male and female reproductive systems are performed to determine the cause of infertility, to detect the presence of cancerous lesions, or to identify the presence of sexually transmitted infections. (Alterations of the female reproductive system including carcinoma are discussed in Chapter 24. Alterations of the male reproductive system including carcinoma are discussed in Chapter 25. Sexually transmitted infections are discussed in Chapter 26.)

Tests of reproductive function are performed most commonly when infertility exists. Both partners are examined, and several diagnostic evaluations may be completed. The types of tests and their normal values are summarized in Tables 23-3 and 23-4. The man is evaluated for number, amount, structure, and motility of sperm and obstruction along the reproductive tract. Tests for women determine whether (1) the reproductive tract (cervix, uterus, fallopian tubes) is adequately patent to allow for passage of ovum and sperm, (2) ovulation occurs normally, (3) the endometrium is responding normally to hormones, and (4) reproductive tissues are free of tumors or infections. Hormonal assays evaluate the adequacy of pituitary function and target organ response. The position and size of organs or the presence of tumors can be detected by direct observation procedures using a laparoscope or by radiographic studies, such as plain films, computerized scans, or tomography.[48]

AGING AND REPRODUCTIVE FUNCTION

Aging and the Female Reproductive System

Natural **menopause** is a normal developmental event marking the end of reproduction. It is universally experienced by midlife women at the average age of 50.5 to 51.4 years in North America with variability between 40 and 60 years.[49,50] A number of factors are thought to influence the age of menopause, including genetics, socioeconomic status, race, parity, oral contraceptive use, and lifestyle, such as smoking or weight.[51] It can occur 2 years sooner on average for smokers; thinner women also tend to experience menopause at a slightly younger age. However, it is genetically predetermined and has been documented by family history. Menopause is the cessation of ovulation due to loss of ovarian follicles resulting in reduced ovarian production of estradiol, increased FSH and LH, and decreased inhibin (inhibits release of FSH). The primary changes of menopause are as follows:[52]

- *Perimenopause:* This is the transitional period between reproductive and nonreproductive years, a transition lasting

TABLE 23-3 TESTS AND NORMAL VALUES OF REPRODUCTIVE FUNCTION/FERTILITY

TEST	DESCRIPTION	NORMAL VALUE
Basic Assessment		
Semen analysis (two samples at least 2 weeks apart)	Determines number, motility, and structure of sperm cells	Volume = 2-6 ml Number = >20 million/ml Motility = >50% with forward progression
White blood cells	Determines presence of bacteria/leukocytes	Morphology = >50% normal shape
Immunologic tests	Detects antibody to sperm	Immunobead test = <20% with adherent particles Sperm MAR test (mixed antiglobulin reaction) = <10% with adherent particles $<10^6$ WBC/ml No sperm agglutinins present
Other Assessments		
Basal body temperature	Determines whether ovulation has occurred	Decrease in basal body temperature before ovulation followed by a rise in temperature at the time of ovulation
FSH level	Day 3 of cycle	Lab specific results
Estradiol	Days 3 of cycle	Low FSH in conjunction with low estradiol—lab specific results
Progesterone	Midluteal phase – one week before menses	Lab specific results—low level associated with decreased or absent ovulation.
Prolactin	Day 3 of cycle	Lab specific results—high levels can interfere with ovulation
TSH level	Day 3 of cycle	Lab specific results—elevated value associated with hypothyroidism
Cervical mucus	Evaluates presence of ovulation from estrogenic effects at ovulation; mucus also may be examined for pH, glucose, or proteins or cultured for presence of infection	Fern pattern appears when cervical mucus dries on a clean slide; mucus is clear, watery, and elastic (spinnbarkeit ≥8-10 cm) with no inflammatory cells
Postcoital cervical mucus (Sims-Huhner test)	Tests ability of sperm to penetrate and maintain motility in cervical mucus 2-4 hours after coitus approximately 1 day before ovulation	≥10 motile sperm in each high-power field; motility in one direction; previous sperm analysis normal
Zona binding test or hamster penetration test	Nonliving oocytes are surgically removed and bisected; sperm added to the hemi-oocyte to test fertilizing capability	Bonding <30% predicted failed fertilization 70% of the time Bonding >30% predicted successful fertilization 85% of the time Results may vary with lab
Ultrasound vaginal scanning	Provides superior quality resolution of the uterine, fallopian, and ovarian structures; also can be used to study folliculogenesis, ovulation, and luteogenesis to detect abnormalities	Normal structures visualized
More Specialized Tests		
Endometrial biopsy	Determines whether ovulation has occurred by obtaining endometrial tissue on day 26 of 28-day menstrual cycle (or postovulatory day 12)	Finding is "secretory-type" endometrium if ovulation has occurred; read in conjunction with day of cycle and serum progesterone levels
Hysterosalpingogram	Assessment of uterus and fallopian tubes for obstructions using transuterine injection of contrast material and radiography; performed 1-2 days after cessation of menses	No obstruction evident
Laparoscopy (pelvic endoscopy)	Visualization of reproductive organs using a laparoscope inserted within the pelvic cavity through the abdomen to assess structure or determine presence of adhesions, endometriosis, tumors, or infection	Normal structure and position of organs
Hysteroscopy	Visualization of uterine cavity using modified cystoscope inserted through cervical os; best done during first 14 days of cycle	Absence of intrauterine lesions

FSH, Follicle-stimulating hormone; *TSH,* thyroid-stimulating hormone; *WBC,* white blood cell.

TABLE 23-4 SERUM HORMONE VALUES

HORMONE	VALUE
Serum progesterone	Normal = >10 ng/dl, presumptive evidence of ovulation; draw level between days 20-25 of 28-day cycle or 6-10 days postovulation <10 ng/ml = inadequate luteal function <3 ng/ml suggests anovulation
Serum testosterone	Normal = 300-1200 ng/dl; must be interpreted with serum LH and FSH levels
Resulting from diurnal and pulsatile pattern, need serial blood draws	Low values in male hypogonadism
Serum FSH and LH	FSH = <22 international units/L
Resulting from diurnal and pulsatile pattern, need serial blood draws	LH = 4-24 international units/L High levels in males indicate primary testicular disease; low levels in males indicate hypogonadism caused by hypothalamic-pituitary dysfunction

FSH, Follicle-stimulating hormone; *LH,* luteinizing hormone.

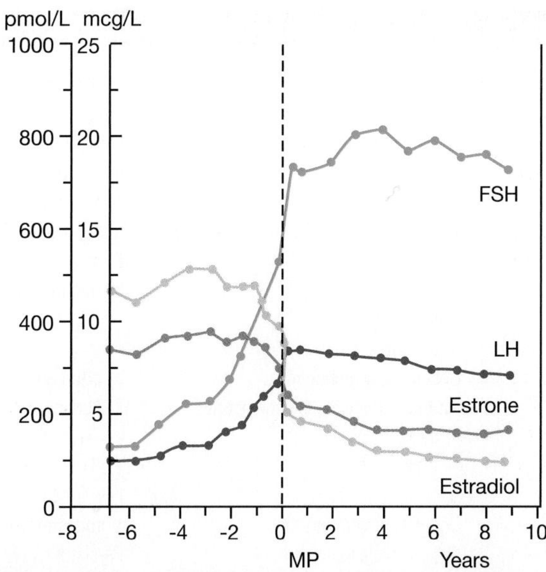

FIGURE 23-20 The Perimenopausal Hormone Transition. Mean circulating hormone levels. *FSH,* Follicle-stimulating hormone; *LH,* luteinizing hormone.

2 to 8 years.[1,52] Five to 10 years before menopause, approximately 90% of women note mild to extreme variability in frequency and quality of menstrual flow. Changes in hormones occur during this time including erratically higher estradiol levels, decreased progesterone levels (in normal ovulatory, short luteal phase, or anovulatory cycles), and a disturbed ovarian-pituitary-hypothalamic feedback relationship with higher LH levels. A decrease in the sensitivity of the target tissue receptors and the development of perimenopausal symptoms commonly are experienced. Symptoms usually begin with a lengthening of the menstrual cycle, which correlates with anovulatory cycles. Unpredictable or irregular ovulation uniformly precedes menopause.[53] The perimenopause experience varies among women and from cycle to cycle in the same woman. Estradiol levels remain in the normal to slightly elevated range until about 1 year before menopause.[1]

- *Ovarian changes:* Beginning in utero, the number of follicles steadily decreases through activation, maturation, and atresia. Starting in the late 30s, 10 to 15 years before menstruation ceases, this process accelerates until the supply of follicles is depleted.[54] This accelerated loss correlates with increased FSH stimulation, delayed and attenuated LH surges, and a decrease in inhibin. Increased FSH stimulation seems to accelerate follicular loss, declining inhibin production, slightly elevated estradiol levels, and decreasing anti-müllerian hormone. Attenuated LH surges are associated with impaired hypothalamic responses to estradiol positive feedback[55] (Figure 23-20 and Box 23-2). The ovarian response to high FSH recruits increasing numbers of follicles; these follicles only partially develop, with a net effect of irregular ovulation, lower progesterone levels, depleted follicle reserve, and infertility. The ovaries begin to decrease in size around age 30; this decrease accelerates after age 60.[1,55] Of the 500,000 follicles present at the onset of puberty, the number dwindles to approximately 1000 with menopause. Table 23-5 summarizes endocrine events occurring during

BOX 23-2 CHANGES IN OVARIAN FOLLICULOGENESIS DURING THE PERIMENOPAUSE LEADING TO ENDOGENOUS OVERSTIMULATION

- ↑ FSH → ovarian hyperstimulation → ↑ number of follicles recruited (net effect of follicular depletion) → ↑ estradiol
- ↓ Follicular reserve → ↓ inhibin and ↑ activin in FP and LP → ↑ FSH → ↑ number of follicles recruited, partial development, infrequent ovulation → ↑ estrogen (E_2) and ↓ progesterone

FP, Follicular phase; *FSH,* follicle-stimulating hormone; *LP,* luteal phase.

TABLE 23-5 ENDOCRINE EVENTS ASSOCIATED WITH PERIMENOPAUSE

HORMONE CHANGES	EFFECTS
Estradiol (E_2) levels	Erratic and intermittent increase
Mean FP level 1 greater than mean FP level in younger women	First in FP (inverse relationship between length of FP and estradiol level)
FP level may be greater than midcycle peak level in fertile women	Later during premenstrual phase
Ovulatory cycles	Short or insufficient LP (decreased fertility)
Progesterone levels	Decreased in ovulatory cycle; minimal during anovulatory cycles
Anovulatory cycles	Increased to about 50%; perhaps more in later perimenopause
FSH levels	Variable, then increased
LH levels	Normal initially, then increased
Inhibin levels	Correlate with progesterone levels

FP, Follicular phase; *FSH,* follicle-stimulating hormone; *LH,* luteinizing hormone; *LP,* luteal phase.

TABLE 23-6 POSTULATED PERIMENOPAUSAL TRANSITION TIMELINE

PHASE	MENSTRUAL PHYSIOLOGY	HORMONAL CHANGES	SYMPTOMATOLOGY
A	Regular, ovulatory cycles Short cycles, short FP	Intermittent ↑ E_2 FSH usually normal Intermittent ↑ FP FSH Low inhibin	Increased breast tenderness, mood swings, fluid retention, premenstrual symptoms Early morning night sweats (vasomotor symptoms) Weight gain, migraine headaches, heavy flow
B	Regular cycles with disturbances in ovulation Short LP Insufficient LP Anovulatory cycles	Intermittent ↑ FP FSH E_2 often ↑ Inhibin inappropriately low	Heavy flow ↑ Premenstrual symptoms ↑ Dysmenorrhea Predictable or ↑ vasomotor symptoms before flow
C	Onset of perimenopause Alternating short, long, or skipped cycles	E_2 often quite ↑ E_2 normal or low ↑ FSH (slight) ↑ LH Low inhibin	Vasomotor symptoms during waking hours Vasomotor symptoms more persistent, remain cyclic before flow
D	Onset of oligomenorrhea 50% of cycles anovulatory Heavy flow may predict onset of oligomenorrhea	↑ Progesterone with ovulation Persistent ↓ FSH ↑ LH ↑ E_2 Low inhibin	↑ Vasomotor symptoms ↑ Signs/symptoms of high estrogen after long periods without flow Flow light but unpredictable
E	Final menstrual period plus 1 year	↑ FSH and LH ↓ or normal E_2 Consistent low inhibin ↓ Progesterone	↑ Intensity and frequency of vasomotor symptoms (although vasomotor symptoms may disappear) ↓ Cramps and premenstrual-type symptoms without subsequent flow ↓ Breast, mood, and fluid symptoms

E_2, Estradiol; *FP*, follicular phase; *FSH*, follicle-stimulating hormone; *LP*, luteal phase.

the perimenopause. Table 23-6 provides a template to visualize the complex physiology of the perimenopause and the dynamic changes that occur during this time.

- *Uterine changes:* Uterine changes occur primarily in the endometrium. The increase in anovulatory cycles allows for proliferative growth of the endometrium. The longer exposure to estrogen alone results in greater thickness of the endometrium, and 50% of perimenopausal women will experience dysfunctional uterine bleeding that is heavy and unpredictable. Increased endometrial bleeding is correlated with a change from ovulatory to anovulatory cycles and is associated with unopposed high estrogen levels the week before menses. Estrogen causes endometrial tissue to thicken. However, without corresponding stromal support from progesterone, estrogen production leads to heavier periods, menorrhagia (heavy bleeding), or metrorrhagia (midcycle bleeding)[6] (Table 23-7). In the past this has put women at high risk for hysterectomy. Newer treatment includes progesterone administration or endometrial ablation by laser or electrocautery. New methods of decreasing the function of the endometrial tissue are being developed.
- *Systemic changes:* **Vasomotor flushes** are characterized by a rise in skin temperature, dilation of peripheral blood vessels, increased blood flow in the hands, increased skin conductance, and a transient increase in heart rate followed by a temperature drop and profuse perspiration over the area of flush distribution. This usually occurs in the face and neck and may radiate into the chest and other parts of the body. Night sweats, dizziness, nausea, headaches, or palpitations

TABLE 23-7 IMPACT OF HIGH ESTROGEN LEVELS ON MENSTRUAL CYCLE AND SYMPTOMATOLOGY

ASSOCIATED PHYSIOLOGIC CHANGE	SIGNS/SYMPTOMS
Short follicular phase (FP)	Short cycles
Long FP	Long cycles
Thickened endometrium*	Heavy, long, or unpredictable flow (including clotting and flooding)*
Increase in glandular cells without stromal support produced by progesterone → unstable endometrium	Midcycle spotting Menorrhagia
Possible increased production of prostaglandins within endometrial tissue	Metrorrhagia Dysmenorrhea Breast tenderness, modularity, enlargement Water retention Emotional stress; new or unpredictable mood swings Weight gain Vasomotor symptoms New onset of migraine headaches; exacerbation of headaches Increased premenstrual symptoms

*Symptoms aggravated by anovulatory cycles; leads to dysfunctional uterine bleeding (see Chapter 24).

may accompany the flush. These flushes can vary in frequency, intensity, and duration and are experienced by up to 85% of perimenopausal to postmenopausal women from 1 to 15 years (mean 1 to 5 years). The physiology of vasomotor flushes is poorly understood. One theory proposes that rapid changes in estrogen may result in loss of negative feedback over hypothalamic noradrenaline synthesis, the primary neurotransmitter involved in thermoregulation.[56] Estrogen modulates adrenergic receptors. The decrease in estrogen in menopause is thought to decrease the number of receptors leading to increased noradrenaline levels and hot flushes. Interestingly, emerging evidence shows that the intensity of vasomotor flushes may be associated with increased risk for cardiovascular disease.[57]

- *Menopause:* Menopause is defined by the point that marks 12 consecutive months of amenorrhea. This means that it is determined retrospectively after a woman has not had a menstrual period for 1 year. It is characterized by loss of ovarian function, low estrodiol and progesterone levels, high FSH and LH levels, and decreased follicular inhibin secretion[49,58] (see Figure 23-20). Less androgens are produced but sensitivity to them is increased because of the lost opposition of estrogen.
- *Breast tissue changes:* Glandular breast tissue becomes involuted; fat deposits and connective tissue increase; and breasts are reduced in size and firmness.
- *Urogenital tract changes:* The ovaries shrink; the uterus atrophies; and the vagina shortens, narrows, and loses some elasticity. Lubrication of the vagina diminishes and vaginal pH increases, creating higher incidence of vaginitis. The cervix atrophies, cervical os shrinks; vaginal epithelium atrophies; labia majora and minora become less prominent; some pubic hair is lost; urethral tone declines along with muscle tone throughout the pelvic area; urinary frequency or urgency, urinary tract infections, and incontinence are associated with estrogen deficiency. Regular sexual activity and orgasm may diminish some of these changes. Sexually active women have less vaginal atrophy.
- *Skeletal changes:* Postmenopausal bone mass is reduced, leading to increased brittleness and porosity and increases the risk osteoporosis and fracture. Healthy bone is maintained through a balance of breakdown and reformation. Estrogen promotes positive bone mass during the childbearing years; however, once menopause occurs with the resultant low estrogen levels, the balance tips toward reabsorption and reduced bone mass.[59]
- *Cardiac change:* The risk of coronary heart disease (CHD) increases significantly after menopause. Estrogen is known to foster favorable lipid profiles and to have beneficial effects on vessel endothelium through production of nitric oxide. Once postmenopausal, blood pressure and LDL levels rise, central adiposity and weight increases, and HDL levels lower, together increasing the risk of CHD.[60,61]
- *Other changes:* Emotional stress with unpredictable mood swings, weight gain, migraine headaches, and insomnia often accompany the change in estrogen levels.[62,63] Lower estrogen levels decrease skin thickness and diminish skin elasticity, thereby causing increased skin dryness and wrinkling.[64]

Aging and the Male Reproductive System

Men maintain reproductive capacity longer than women. There is no known discrete event, comparable to menopause, that characterizes aging of the male reproductive system, although the term *andropause* is sometimes used to describe the changes associated with male aging. Gradual changes do occur, and aging in the male reproductive system is characterized by hypogonadism, testosterone deficiency, erectile dysfunction, and proliferative disorders of the prostate gland[65] (see Chapter 25). Aging changes are also influenced by chronic diseases and use of medications.

Components of male sexual behavior include both sexual drive and erectile and ejaculatory capacity. Libido, or sexual drive, is a complex phenomenon that requires a baseline hormonal milieu but is influenced significantly by health status and environmental, social, and psychologic factors. In men older than 40 years, organic factors and chronic disease (e.g., vascular, endocrine, and neurologic disorders) are involved in more than half of the cases of male sexual dysfunction. Aging causes specific physical changes that may influence erectile and ejaculatory capabilities. Alterations in sexual response include the need for longer stimulation to achieve full erection; slower and less forceful ejaculation, with less pelvic muscle involvement; decreased vasocongestive response; and longer refractory period (time during which erection and ejaculation are not possible), up to 24 hours in some men.

The testes undergo several age-related structural changes, including decreased weight, atrophy, and softening. Degenerative changes in the seminiferous tubules may include thickening of the basement membrane; increase in lumen size; germ cell (spermatogonium) arrest and a decrease in spermatogenic activity; and collapse of tubules, followed by complete obstruction caused by sclerosis and fibrosis. Areas of mild to severe degenerative change may be interspersed with areas having intact tubules. These morphologic changes may result from atherosclerosis (arterial clogging) in the testicular vascular bed.[66] Alterations of the seminiferous tubules do not appear to diminish sperm counts (20 million sperm per milliliter of semen is estimated as the minimum concentration for fertility),[67] but they do reduce fertility because a greater percentage of the sperm lack motility or have structural abnormalities.

Aging probably causes changes in the production of male sex hormones, levels of SHBG, and responsiveness of target tissues. Hormone synthesis by the testes and testicular responsiveness to the gonadotropins (FSH and LH) are diminished, and pituitary secretion of these gonadotropins is elevated.[68] The reduced levels of testosterone may be related to alterations in the Leydig cells, the testosterone producers of the testes. The number of Leydig cells and their function decreases as age increases, perhaps because of decreased arterial perfusion of the testes and decreased responsiveness to LH.[69] Even if testosterone levels are not decreased, older men may have less unbound testosterone in their blood, decreasing the amount of unbound hormone available to stimulate target tissues. Decreased testosterone levels have several effects, including functional deterioration of the accessory sex organs (the prostate gland, seminal vesicles, epididymis, and ductus deferens); loss of muscle mass, strength, and endurance; increased visceral fat, osteopenia, and cognitive decline; and, in many men, decrease in libido. This last effect also may be caused by alterations in other variables that affect libido.[70] Modifiable risk factors for low testosterone and symptoms of androgen deficiency include health status and waist circumference.[71]

SUMMARY REVIEW

Development of the Reproductive Systems

1. Differentiation of female and male genitalia begins around weeks 7 to 8 of embryonic development, when the gonads of genetically male embryos begin to secrete male sex hormones, primarily testosterone. Until that time the primitive reproductive organs of males and females are homologous (the same).
2. The structure and function of male and female reproductive systems are controlled by the hypothalamic-pituitary-gonadal (HPG) axis, a set of complex neurologic and hormonal interactions that accelerate at puberty and lead to sexual maturation and reproductive capability.
3. Extrahypothalamic factors cause the hypothalamus to secrete GnRH, which stimulates the anterior pituitary to secrete gonadotropins—FSH and LH—that stimulate the gonads (ovaries or testes) to secrete female or male sex hormones. Paracrine hormones (inhibin, activin, and follistatin) influence the positive and negative feedback loops that occur along the HPG axis.
4. Production of primitive female gametes (ova) occurs solely during fetal life. From puberty to menopause, one female gamete matures per menstrual cycle. Production of the male gametes (sperm) begins at puberty; after that, millions are produced daily, usually for life. Females release a mature ova at the time of puberty.

The Female Reproductive System

1. The function of the reproductive system is to produce mature ova and, when fertilized, to protect and nourish them through embryonic and fetal life, and expel them at birth.
2. The external female genitalia are the mons pubis, labia majora, labia minora, clitoris, vestibule (urinary and vaginal openings), Bartholin glands, and Skene glands.
3. The internal female genitalia are the vagina, uterus, fallopian tubes, and ovaries.
4. The vagina is a fibromuscular canal that receives the penis during sexual intercourse and is the exit route for menstrual fluids and products of conception. The vagina leads from the introitus (its external opening) to the cervical portion of the uterus.
5. The uterus is the hollow, muscular organ in which a fertilized ovum develops. The uterine walls have three layers: the endometrium (lining), myometrium (muscular layer), and perimetrium (outer covering, which is continuous with the pelvic peritoneum). The endometrium proliferates (thickens) and sloughs off in response to cyclic hormonal changes. The cervix is the narrow, lower portion of the uterus that opens into the vagina.
6. The two fallopian tubes extend from the uterus to the ovaries. Their function is to conduct ova from the spaces around the ovaries to the uterus. Fertilization normally occurs in the distal third of the fallopian tubes.
7. From puberty to menopause, the ovaries are the site of (1) ovum maturation and release and (2) production of female sex (estrogen and progesterone) and male (androgens) hormones. Female sex hormones predominate and are involved in sexual differentiation and development, the menstrual cycle, pregnancy, and lactation. Androgens in women contribute to prepubertal growth spurt, pubic and axillary hair growth, and activation of sebaceous glands.
8. Developing ovarian follicles (structures that enclose the ovum) produce estrogen (primarily estradiol). The corpus luteum, the structure that develops from the ruptured ovarian follicle after ovulation or ovum release, produces progesterone. Androgens are produced within the ovarian follicle, adrenal glands, and adipose tissue.
9. The average menstrual cycle lasts 27 to 30 days and consists of three phases, which are named for ovarian and endometrial changes: the follicular/proliferative phase, the luteal/secretory phase, and the ischemic/menstrual phase.
10. Ovarian events of the menstrual cycle are controlled by gonadotropins. High FSH levels stimulate follicle and ovum maturation (follicular phase), then a surge of LH causes ovulation, which is followed by development of the corpus luteum (luteal phase).
11. Ovarian hormones control the uterine (endometrial) events of the menstrual cycle. During the follicular/proliferative phase of the ovarian cycle, estrogen produced by the follicle causes the endometrium to proliferate (proliferative phase) and induces the LH surge and progesterone production in the granulosa layer. During the luteal/secretory phase, estrogen maintains the thickened endometrium, and progesterone causes it to develop blood vessels and secretory glands (secretory phase). As the corpus luteum degenerates, production of both hormones drops sharply, and the "starved" endometrium degenerates and sloughs off, causing menstruation, the ischemic/menstrual phase.
12. Cyclic changes in hormone levels also cause thinning and thickening of the vaginal epithelium, thinning and thickening of cervical secretions, and changes in basal body temperature.

Structure and Function of the Breast

1. Until puberty the female and male breasts are similar, consisting of a small underdeveloped nipple, some fatty and fibrous tissue, and a few ductlike structures under the areola.

SUMMARY REVIEW—cont'd

At puberty, however, a variety of hormones (estrogen, progesterone, prolactin, growth hormone, insulin, cortisol) cause the female breast to develop into a system of glands and ducts that is capable of producing and ejecting milk.

2. The basic functional unit of the female breast is the lobe, a system of ducts that branches from the nipple to milk-producing units called lobules. The lobules contain alveolar cells, which are convoluted spaces lined with epithelial cells that secrete milk and subepithelial cells that contract, moving the milk into the system of ducts that leads to the nipple.
3. Each breast contains 15 to 20 lobes, which are separated and supported by Cooper ligaments.
4. Milk production occurs in response to prolactin, a hormone that is secreted by alveolar epithelial cells in larger amounts after childbirth. Milk ejection is under the control of oxytocin which causes contraction of myoepithelial cells.
5. During the reproductive years breast tissue undergoes cyclic changes in response to hormonal changes of the menstrual cycle.
6. Prior to puberty the male breast development is similar to female development. Lack of high levels of estrogen and progesterone prevents further development of the male breast.

The Male Reproductive System

1. The function of the male reproductive system is to produce male gametes (sperm) and deliver them to the female reproductive tract.
2. The external male genitalia are the testes, epididymides, scrotum, and penis. The internal genitalia are the vas deferens, ejaculatory duct, prostatic and membranous sections of the urethra, seminal vesicles, prostate gland, and Cowper glands.
3. The testes (male gonads) are paired glands suspended within the scrotum. The testes have two functions: spermatogenesis (sperm production) and production of male sex hormones (androgens, chiefly testosterone).
4. The epididymis is a long coiled tube arranged in a comma-shaped compartment that curves over the top and rear of the testis. The epididymis receives sperm from the testis and stores them while they develop further. Sperm travel the length of the epididymis and then are ejaculated into the vas deferens.
5. The scrotum is a skin-covered fibromuscular sac that encloses the testes and epididymides, which are suspended within the scrotum by the spermatic cord. The scrotum keeps these organs at optimal temperatures for sperm survival (about 1° to 2° C lower than body temperature) by contracting in cold environments and relaxing in warm environments.
6. The penis is a cylindric organ consisting of three longitudinal compartments (two corpora cavernosa and one corpus spongiosum) and the urethra. The urethra runs through the corpus spongiosum. The corpora cavernosa and corpus spongiosum consist of erectile tissue. Externally the penis consists of a shaft and a tip, which is called the glans. The glans contains sebaceous glands and the opening of the urethra and is covered by a flap of skin (the foreskin).
7. The penis has two functions: delivery of sperm to the female vagina and elimination of urine. These two fluids are never in the urethra at the same time.
8. Sexual intercourse is made possible by the erectile reflex, in which tactile or psychogenic stimulation of the parasympathetic nerves causes arterioles in the corpora cavernosa and corpus spongiosum to dilate and fill with blood, causing the penis to enlarge and become firm.
9. Emission, which occurs at the peak of sexual arousal, is the movement of semen from the epididymides to the penis. Ejaculation, which is a continuation of emission, is the pulsatile ejection of semen from the penis. Both emission and ejaculation involve rhythmic contractions of smooth muscle within the internal glands and ducts.
10. The prostate gland is about the size of a walnut and surrounds the urethra. Prostatic secretions are alkaline and contribute to the ejaculate.
11. Cowper glands (bulbourethral glands) secrete mucus in the urethra and add fluid to the ejaculate.
12. Spermatogenesis is a continuous process because spermatogonia, the primitive male gametes, undergo continuous mitosis within the seminiferous tubules of the testes. Some of the spermatogonia develop into primary spermatocytes, which divide meiotically into secondary spermatocytes and then spermatids. The spermatids develop into sperm with the help of nutrients and hormonal signals from Sertoli cells.
13. Production of the male sex hormones is controlled (like production of the female sex hormones) by the HPG axis and by complex feedback mechanisms. The male hormones are produced steadily, with diurnal variations.

Tests of Reproductive Function

1. Diagnostic tests are performed to evaluate fertility.
2. Evaluation of fertility includes reproductive hormone assays and assessment of structural alteration or infections and the determination of normal ovulation or adequate sperm motility and count.

Aging and Reproductive Function

1. In women the transition from fertility to menopause (perimenopause) starts about 2 to 8 years before the last menstrual period and ends the following year. During this transition period the ovaries produce erratic and high levels of estrogen that contribute to such symptoms as hot flashes, breast tenderness and nodularity, and migraine headaches. Menstrual cycles shorten and then become irregular as anovulation occurs. Menstruation ceases, and women move into menopause.
2. Men maintain reproductive capacity into their later years. In some men there are gradual changes with testosterone deficiency, hypogonadism, proliferative disorders of the prostate, and erectile dysfunction.

KEY TERMS

Activin, 781
Adrenarche, 771
Androgen, 777
Areola, 783
Bartholin gland (greater vestibular or vulvovaginal gland), 772
Breast, 782
Bulbocavernosus, 772
Cervix (neck of the uterus), 775
Clitoris, 772
Cornification, 781
Corpora cavernosa (*singular*, corpus cavernosum), 787
Corpus luteum, 776
Corpus spongiosum, 787
Corpus of the uterus (body of uterus), 774
Cowper gland (bulbourethral gland), 789
Cul-de-sac, 773
Decornification, 781
Developing fetus, 768
Dihydrotestosterone (DHT), 791
Efferent tubule, 785
Ejaculatory duct, 788
Embryo, 768
Emission, 787
Endocervical canal, 775
Endometrium, 775
Epididymis (*plural,* epididymides), 785
Erectile reflex, 787
Estradiol (E_2), 776
Estrogen, 776
Fallopian tube (oviduct, uterine tube), 775
Fimbriae (*singular,* fimbria), 775
Follicle-stimulating hormone (FSH), 769
Follicular/proliferative phase, 780
Follistatin, 781
Foreskin (prepuce), 786
Fornix, 773
Fundus of the uterus, 774
Glands of Montgomery, 783
Glans, 786
Gonad, 768
Gonadarche, 771
Gonadostat, 770
Gonadotropin-releasing hormone (GnRH), 769
Gonadotropin-releasing hormone pulse generator, 770
Granulosa cell, 776
Hymen, 772
Infundibulum, 775
Inguinal canal, 784
Inhibin, 781
Introitus, 772
Ischemic/menstrual phase, 780
Isthmus of the uterus, 775
Labia majora (*singular,* labium majus), 771
Labia minora (*singular,* labium minus), 771
Leptin, 778
Leydig cell, 785
Libido, 789
Luteal/secretory phase, 780
Luteinizing hormone (LH), 769, 778
Menarche, 778
Menopause, 778, 791
Menstruation (menses), 778
Mons pubis, 771
Myometrium, 775
Nipple, 783
Ovarian cycle, 776
Ovarian follicle, 776
Ovaries, 776
Ovulation, 776
Ovum, 768
Penis, 786
Perimetrium (parietal peritoneum), 775
Perineal body, 772
Perineum, 772
Primary spermatocyte, 789
Progesterone, 778
Prolactin, 791
Prostate gland, 788
Puberty, 770
Rete testis, 785
Rugae (*singular,* ruga; pertains to vagina and testes), 773
Scrotum, 786
Secondary spermatocyte, 789
Semen, 787
Seminal vesicle, 788
Seminiferous tubule, 785
Sertoli cell (nondividing support cell), 789
Sex hormone, 768
Sex hormone–binding globulin (SHBG), 791
Skene gland (lesser vestibular or paraurethral gland), 772
Spermatic cord, 784
Spermatid, 789
Spermatogenesis, 785
Spermatogonia (*singular,* spermatogonium), 789
Spermatozoon (sperm cell), 768
Squamous-columnar junction, 775
Testes (*singular,* testis), 784
Testosterone, 769, 789
Theca cell, 776
Thelarche, 771, 783
Tubulus rectus, 785
Tunica albuginea, 784
Tunica dartos, 786
Tunica vaginalis, 784
Urethra, 787
Urinary meatus, 772
Uterus, 773
Vagina, 772
Vas deferens (ductus deferens), 786
Vasomotor flush, 794
Vestibule, 772
Vulva, 771

REFERENCES

1. Fritz MA, Speroff L: *Clinical gynecologic endocrinology and infertility*, ed 8, Philadelphia, 2011, Lippincott Williams & Wilkins.
2. Di Vall SA, Radovick S: Pubertal development and menarche, *Ann N Y Acad Sci* 1135:19–28, 2008.
3. Biro FM, Greenspan LC, Galvez MP: Puberty in girls of the 21st century, *J Pediatr Adolesc Gynecol* 25(5):289–294, 2012.
4. Kaplowitz PB: Link between body fat and the timing of puberty, *Pediatrics* 121(Suppl 3):S208–S217, 2008.
5. Koeppen BM, Stanton BA, editors: *Berne and Levy physiology*, ed 6, St Louis, 2010, Mosby.
6. Lowdermilk DL, Perry SE: *Maternity and women's health care*, ed 10, St Louis, 2012, Mosby.
7. Guo M et al: The role of human papillomavirus type 16/18 genotyping in predicting high-grade cervical/vaginal intraepithelial neoplasm in women with mildly abnormal Papanicolaou results, *Cancer Cytopathol* 121(2):79–85, 2013.
8. Pang WW, Hartmann PE: Initiation of human lactation: secretory differentiation and secretory activation, *J Mammary Gland Biol Neoplasia* 12(4):211–221, 2007.
9. Society for Maternal-Fetal Medicine Publications Committee, with assistance of Vincenzo Berghella: Progesterone and preterm birth prevention: translating clinical trials data into clinical practice, *Am J Obstet Gynecol* 206(5):376–386, 2012.
10. Wetendorf M, DeMayo FJ: The progesterone receptor regulates implantation, decidualization, and glandular development via a complex paracrine signaling network, *Mol Cell Endocrinol* 357(1–2):108–118, 2012.
11. Vital and Health Statistics: *Fertility, family planning, and reproductive health of U.S. women: data from the 2002 National Survey of Family Growth* (Series 23, Number 25, p. 69), Hyattsville, MD, 2005, U.S. Department of Health and Human Services, Centers for Disease Control and Prevention, National Center for Health Statistics.
12. Karapanou O, Papadimitriou A: Determinants of menarche, *Reprod Biol Endocrinol* 8:115, 2010.
13. Euling SY et al: Examination of U.S. puberty-timing data from 1940 to 1994 for secular trends; panel findings, *Pediatrics* 121(Suppl 3): S172–S191, 2008.
14. Rogol AD: Sex steroids, growth hormone, leptin and the pubertal growth spurt, *Endocr Dev* 17:77–85, 2010.
15. Maybin JA, Critchley HO: Progesterone: a pivotal hormone at menstruation, *Ann N Y Acad Sci* 1221:88–97, 2011.
16. Mihm M, Gangooly S, Muttukrishna S: The normal menstrual cycle in women, *Anim Reprod Sci* 124(3-4):229–236, 2011.
17. Trealor AE et al: Variation of the human menstrual cycle through reproductive life, *Int J Fertil* 12:77–126, 1970.
18. Peacock A, Alvi NS, Mushtaq T: Period problems: disorders of menstruation in adolescents, *Arch Dis Child* 97(6):554–560, 2012.
19. Scheid JL, De Souza MJ: Menstrual irregularities and energy deficiency in physically active women: the role of ghrelin, PYY and adipocytokines, *Med Sport Sci* 55:82–102, 2010.
20. Richards JS, Pangas SA: The ovary: basic biology and clinical implications, *J Clin Invest* 120(4):963–972, 2010.
21. Karligiotou E et al: FSH modulatory effect on human granulosa cells: a gene-protein candidate for gonadotrophin surge-attenuating factor, *Reprod Biomed Online* 23(4):440–448, 2011.
22. Makanji Y, Harrison CA, Robertson DM: Feedback regulation by inhibins A and B of the pituitary secretion of follicle-stimulating hormone, *Vitam Horm* 85:299–321, 2011.
23. Sirotkin AV: Cytokines: signalling molecules controlling ovarian functions, *Int J Biochem Cell Biol* 43(6):857–861, 2011.
24. Knight PG, Satchell L, Glister C: Intra-ovarian roles of activins and inhibins, *Mol Cell Endocrinol* 359(1-2):53–65, 2012.
25. Son WY et al: Mechanisms of follicle selection and development, *Minerva Ginecol* 63(2):89–102, 2011.

26. Singh M, Chaudhry P, Asselin E: Bridging endometrial receptivity and implantation: network of hormones, cytokines, and growth factors, *J Endocrinol* 210(1):5–14, 2011.
27. Ferin M, Lobo RA: Chapter 4. Reproductive endocrinology: neuroendocrinology, gonadotropins, sex steroids, prostaglandins, ovulation, menstruation, hormone assay. In Lenz GM et al: *Comprehensive gynecology*, ed 8, St Louis, 2013, Mosby.
28. Hassiotou F, Geddes D: Anatomy of the human mammary gland: current status of knowledge, *Clin Anat* 26(1):29–48, 2013.
29. Gusterson BA, Stein T: Human breast development, *Semin Cell Dev Biol* 23(5):567–573, 2012.
30. O'Brien J et al: Macrophages are crucial for epithelial death and adipocyte repopulation during mammary gland involution, *Development* 139:269–275, 2012.
31. Ahmad A: Pathways to breast cancer recurrence, *ISRN Oncol* 290568:2013, 2013.
32. Schedin P et al: Mammary ECM composition and function are altered by reproductive state, *Mol Carcinog* 41:207–220, 2004.
33. Riordan J: *Breastfeeding and human lactation*, ed 3, Sudbury, MA, 2005, Jones & Bartlett.
34. Coad J, Dunstall M: *Anatomy and physiology for midwives*, ed 2, London, 2006, Churchill Livingstone.
35. Shuiling KD, Likis FE: *Women's gynecologic health*, Sudbury, MA, 2006, Jones & Bartlett.
36. Owen CG, Whincup PH, Cook DG: Breast-feeding and cardiovascular risk factors and outcomes in later life: evidence from epidemiological studies, *Proc Nutr Soc* 70(4):478–484, 2011.
37. King J: Contraception and lactation, *J Midwifery Womens Health* 52(6):614–620, 2007.
38. Dickson G, Gynecomastia: *Am Fam Physician* 85(7):716–722, 2012.
39. Iuanow E, Kettler M, Slanetz PJ: Spectrum of disease in the male breast, *AJR Am J Roentgenol* 196(3):W247–W259, 2011.
40. Jung A, Schuppe HC: Influence of genital heat stress on semen quality in humans, *Andrologia* 39(6):203–215, 2007.
41. Hinton BT et al: How do you get six meters of epididymis inside a human scrotum? *J Androl* 32(6):558–564, 2011.
42. Andersson KE: Mechanisms of penile erection and basis for pharmacological treatment of erectile dysfunction, *Pharmacol Rev* 63(4):811–859, 2011.
43. Giuliano F: Neurophysiology of erection and ejaculation, *J Sex Med* 8(Suppl 4):310–315, 2011.
44. Ohi DA et al: Anejaculation and retrograde ejaculation, *Urol Clin North Am* 35(2):211–220, viii, 2008.
45. Meeks JJ, Schaeffer EM: Genetic regulation of prostate development, *J Androl* 32(3):210–217, 2011.
46. Walker WH: Molecular mechanisms of testosterone action in spermatogenesis, *Steroids* 74(7):602–607, 2009.
47. Walia R et al: Recovery pattern of hypothalamo-pituitary-testicular axis in patients with macroprolactinomas after treatment with cabergoline, *Indian J Med Res* 134:314–319, 2011.
48. Lenz GM et al: *Comprehensive gynecology*, ed 8, St Louis, 2013, Mosby.
49. Gold EB: The timing of the age at which natural menopause occurs, *Obstet Gynecol Clin North Am* 38(3):425–440, 2011.
50. Palacios S et al: Age of menopause and impact of climacteric symptoms by geographical region, *Climacteric* 13(5):419–428, 2010.
51. Voorhuis M et al: Human studies on genetics of the age at natural menopause: a systematic review, *Hum Reprod Update* 16(4):364–377, 2010.
52. Hacker NF, Gambone JC, Hobel CJ, editors: *Hacker and Moore's essentials of obstetrics and gynecology*, ed 5, Phildelphia, 2010, Saunders.
53. Prior JC, Hitchcock CL: The endocrinology of perimenopause: need for a paradigm shift, *Front Biosci (Schol Ed)* 3:474–486, 2011.
54. Broekmans FJ, Soules MR, Fauser BC: Ovarian aging: mechanisms and clinical consequences, *Endocr Rev* 30(5):465–493, 2009.
55. Devoto L et al: Neuroendocrinology and ovarian aging, *Gynecol Endocrinol* 28(Suppl 1):14–17, 2012.
56. Vilar-González S, Pérez-Rozos A, Cabanillas-Farpón R: Mechanism of hot flashes, *Clin Transl Oncol* 13(3):143–147, 2011.
57. Thurston RC, Joffe H: Vasomotor symptoms and menopause: findings from the Study of Women's Health Across the Nation, *Obstet Gynecol Clin North Am* 38(3):489–501, 2011.
58. Lobo RA: Chapter 14. Menopause and care of the mature woman: endocrinology, consequences of estrogen deficiency, effects of hormone replacement therapy, and treatment regimens. In Lenz GM et al: *Comprehensive gynecology*, ed 8, St Louis, 2013, Mosby.
59. Lo JC, Burnett-Bowie SA, Finkelstein JS: Bone and the perimenopause, *Obstet Gynecol Clin North Am* 38(3):503–517, 2011.
60. Hutter R et al: Coronary artery disease in aging women: a menopause of endothelial progenitor cells? *Med Clin North Am* 96(1):93–102, 2012.
61. Wellons M et al: Early menopause predicts future coronary heart disease and stroke: the multi-ethnic study of atherosclerosis, *Menopause*, 2012, Jun 11. [Epub ahead of print.].
62. Bromberger JT, Kravitz HM: Mood and menopause: findings from the Study of Women's Health Across the Nation (SWAN) over 10 years, *Obstet Gynecol Clin North Am* 38(3):609–625, 2011.
63. MacGregor EA: Perimenopausal migraine in women with vasomotor symptoms, *Maturitas* 71(1):79–82, 2012.
64. Emmerson E, Hardman MJ: The role of estrogen deficiency in skin ageing and wound healing, *Biogerontology* 13(1):3–20, 2012.
65. Pines A: Male menopause: is it a real clinical syndrome? *Climacteric* 14(1):15–17, 2011.
66. Hafez ESE, Hafez B, Hafez SD: *An atlas of reproductive physiology in men*, London, 2003, Taylor & Francis Group.
67. Walsh TJ, Smith JF: Male infertility. In McAninch JW, Lue TF, editors: *Smith and Tanagho's general urology*, ed 18, Norwalk CT, 2012, McGraw-Hill Lange.
68. Araujo AB, Wittert GA: Endocrinology of the aging male, *Best Pract Res Clin Endocrinol Metab* 25(2):303–319, 2011.
69. Perheentupa A, Huhtaniemi I: Aging of the human ovary and testis, *Mol Cell Endocrinol* 299(1):2–13, 2009.
70. Corona G et al: Update in testosterone therapy for men, *J Sex Med* 8(3):639–654, 2011.
71. Hall SA et al: Correlates of low testosterone and symptomatic androgen deficiency in a population-based sample, *J Clin Endocrinol Metab* 93(10):3870–3877, 2008.

CHAPTER

24

Alterations of the Female Reproductive System

Julia C. Phillippi, Gwen A. Latendresse, and Kathryn L. McCance

evolve WEBSITE

http://evolve.elsevier.com/McCance/

- Review Questions and Answers
- Animations
- Online Course: Module 11

CHAPTER OUTLINE

Alterations of the reproductive system span a wide range of concerns, from delayed sexual development and suboptimal sexual performance to structural and functional abnormalities. Many common reproductive disorders carry potentially serious physiologic or psychologic consequences. Sexual or reproductive dysfunction, such as impotence or infertility, can dramatically affect self-concept, relationships, and overall quality of life. Conversely, organic and psychosocial problems, such as alcoholism, depression, situational stressors, chronic illness, and medications, can affect ovulation and menstruation, sexual performance, and fertility and may be risk factors for the development of some types of reproductive tract cancers.[1] Breast cancer is the second leading cause of cancer death in women. Diagnosis and treatment of reproductive system disorders are complicated because of the stigma and symbolism associated with the reproductive organs and the emotion-laden beliefs and behaviors related to reproductive health.[2] Treatment and diagnosis for related problems may be delayed because of embarrassment, guilt, fear, or denial.

ABNORMALITIES OF REPRODUCTIVE TRACT DEVELOPMENT

As discussed in Chapter 23, normal development of the female reproductive tract requires absence of testosterone during embryonic/fetal life. The resulting fusion of the two paramesonephric (müllerian) ducts produces the normal cervix and the uterus with an internal cavity. The distal portions of the paramesonephric ducts remain independent and form the two fallopian/uterine tubes. Alterations in the normal process include errors in cellular sensitivity to testosterone (androgen insensitivity) or failures of cell line migration, resulting in changes in structure of the reproductive organs.

Androgen insensitivity occurs in its most extreme form in about 1 in 20,000 people[3] and it is discussed briefly in this chapter because of the often-resulting female phenotype, despite a male genotype. Children with complete androgen insensitivity may have testes palpable within the labia majora but are often not diagnosed until puberty.[4] Breast development may be

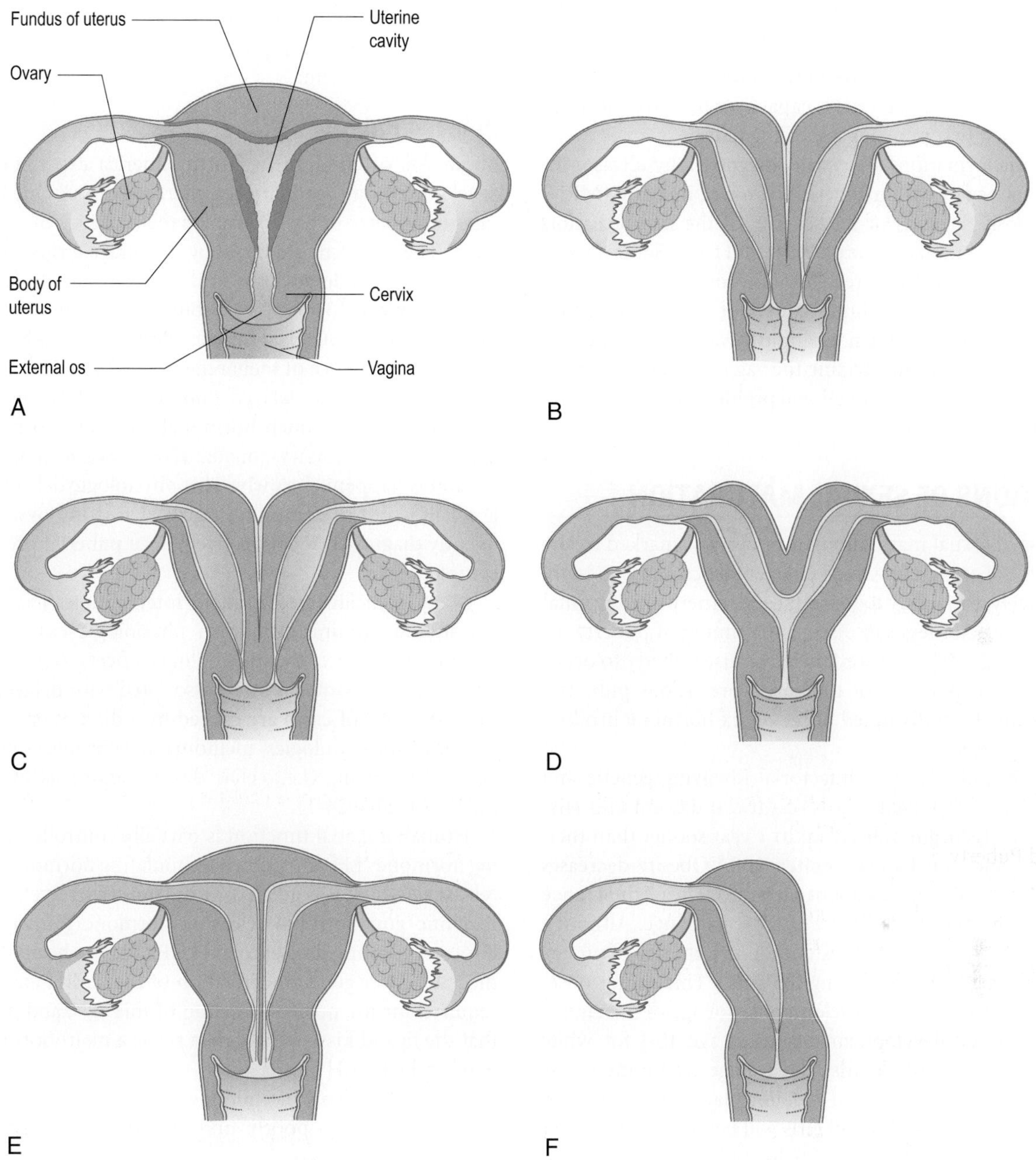

FIGURE 24-1 Uterine Malformations. Congenital uterine abnormalities. **A,** The normal configuration of the uterus and the ovaries. **B,** Double uterus with a double vagina and **C,** a single vagina. **D,** Bicornuate uterus. **E,** A uterus with a midline septum. **F,** Unicornuate uterus. (From de Bruyn R: *Pediatric ultrasound,* ed 2, London, 2010, Churchill Livingstone.)

normal, but pubic and axillary hair is often sparse and menarche does not occur because of the absence of a cervix, uterus, and ovaries.[4] A short vagina that ends blindly also may be present. Milder forms of androgen insensitivity (also a common cause of male infertility)[3] are much more common and have less dramatic phenotypic manifestations with many affected having normal male genitalia. A genetic karyotype reveals a male, genotype (XY).[4]

Other abnormalities of the uterus, cervix, and fallopian/uterine tubes have multi-factorial origins, often the result of an interaction between genetic predisposition and environmental factors. Such interactions result in müllerian duct abnormalities.[5] Some medications, chemicals, and toxins have been implicated as a direct cause of uterine abnormalities. For instance, diethylstilbestrol (DES) was prescribed from 1938 until 1971 as a drug to prevent miscarriages.[6] Although it was not effective at preventing miscarriage, DES did affect cell development and cause abnormal internal reproductive anatomy in exposed fetuses,[6] causing uterine malformations and a predisposition to cancer.

Most uterine abnormalities stem from abnormal cell migration in the müllerian ducts during key moments in fetal development (Figure 24-1). About 5% of the general female population has some sort of uterine abnormality but the rate is much higher in populations of women who have experienced infertility or miscarriage.[7] Uterine abnormalities are rarely diagnosed until the woman has trouble becoming pregnant or carrying a baby to term because the uterus is capable of menstruation but may have difficulty supporting a growing fetus.[5]

Uterine malformations are usually diagnosed by ultrasound during pregnancy or with magnetic resonance imaging (MRI). Their prognosis depends of the severity of the malformation and the location and size of the placenta and fetus. Some abnormalities can be surgically corrected to improve the outcome of subsequent pregnancies.[5] Abnormalities of the lower genital tract also can result in women having two vaginas or a vaginal septum (a thin membrane dividing the vaginal vault). For most women this does not create functional problems but can be surgically corrected if needed.

ALTERATIONS OF SEXUAL MATURATION

The process of sexual maturation, or puberty, is marked by the development of secondary sexual characteristics, rapid growth, and, ultimately, the ability to reproduce. A variety of congenital and endocrine disorders can disrupt the timing of puberty, or sexual maturation. These disorders may cause puberty to occur too late (delayed puberty) or too early (precocious puberty). Both types involve a disrupted onset of sex hormone production by the gonads.

The age of puberty is multifactorial involving genetic and environmental components. Girls of African descent and Hispanic/Latina girls begin puberty up to 1 year sooner than their non-African and non-Latina counterparts.[8] Obesity decreases the age at onset of puberty by about 6 months. The normal range for the onset of puberty is now 8 to 13 years of age. Although there are conflicting and inconsistent reports, the age of pubertal onset appears to be decreasing for girls.[8] This earlier onset appears primarily in breast development, not age of menarche. On average breast development begins at age 10.4 for white girls and 9.5 years for black girls. The average age for menarche is 12.6 years for white girls and 12.1 for black girls. However, 5% of white girls and 15% of all girls will begin puberty before age 8.[8] Both early puberty, known as precocious puberty, and delayed puberty have implications for the child's social interactions and self-esteem.

Delayed Puberty

About 3% of children in North America experience delayed development of secondary sex characteristics.[9] One of the first signs of puberty in girls is usually thelarche, or breast development. Thelarche should begin by the time a girl is 13 years old. Puberty is considered delayed if there are no clinical signs of puberty by age 13 in girls (2 standard deviation [SDs] above the mean age of pubertal onset). Clinical diagnosis also can be made in the absence of menarche by age 15 or 16.

In 95% of cases, delayed puberty is a physiologic (constitutional) delay in which hormonal levels are normal and the hypothalamic-pituitary-gonadal (HPG) axis is intact, but maturation is happening slowly. This physiologic delay tends to be familial, is not as common in girls as it is in boys, and is frequently diagnosed retrospectively once pubertal progression is complete.[10]

Many clinicians recommend intervention (i.e., exogenous sex steroid administration) in physiologic cases of delayed puberty to reduce the psychologic effects (e.g., self-esteem issues, embarrassment) often associated with delayed puberty. The other 5% of cases are caused by a disruption of the HPG axis of various etiologies, including any chronic condition that delays bone aging (i.e., celiac disease, anorexia, hypothyroidism)[10,11] (Table 24-1).

Human gonadal function is partially controlled by luteinizing hormone (LH) and follicle-stimulating hormone (FSH), the release of which is regulated by the pulsatile secretion of hypothalamic gonadotropin-releasing hormone (GnRH).[12,13] The G-protein–coupled receptor 54 (GPR54) has been identified as the gatekeeper gene for activation of the GnRH axis. GPR54 is required for the normal function of this axis, and data suggest that the ligand kisspeptin-1 may act as a neurohormonal regulator of the GnRH axis.[14]

The mechanisms of childhood inhibition of GnRH release and activation are poorly understood but appear to involve

TABLE 24-1 FREQUENCY AND COMMON CAUSES OF DELAYED PUBERTY OTHER THAN CONSTITUTIONAL DELAY OF GROWTH AND PUBERTY

DELAYED PUBERTY	HYPERGONADOTROPIC HYPOGONADISM	PERMANENT HYPOGONADOTROPIC HYPOGONADISM	FUNCTIONAL HYPOGONADOTROPIC HYPOGONADISM
Frequency (%)			
Boys	5-10	10	20
Girls	25	20	20
Common causes	Turner syndrome, gonadal dysgenesis, chemotherapy, or radiation therapy	Tumors or infiltrative diseases of the central nervous system, GnRH deficiency (isolated hypogonadotropic hypogonadism, Kallmann syndrome), combined pituitary-hormone deficiency, chemotherapy, or radiation therapy	Systemic illness (inflammatory bowel disease, celiac disease, anorexia nervosa, or bulimia), hypothyroidism, excessive exercise

From Palmert MR, Dunkel L: *N Engl J Med* 366(5):443–453, 2012.
GnRH, Gonadotropin-releasing hormone.

feedback inhibition by sex steroids and presumably other central nervous system (CNS) pathways.[14] Given the numerous etiologies contributing to the occurrence of delayed puberty, a thorough evaluation should be conducted that includes physical examination and medical and family history that specifically targets known contributors to delayed puberty. Laboratory workup may consist of x-ray studies for bone age, measurement of thyroid function, serum levels of prolactin and adrenal and gonadal steroids, radioimmunoassay of plasma gonadotropins, and screening for systemic disorders. Adolescents with high gonadotropin levels require a karyotype to rule out genetic causes, and those with low levels need skull imaging (lateral skull film, computed tomography [CT], or MRI) to rule out pituitary or other CNS infiltrate or tumor. Treatment of delayed puberty depends on the cause; the goal of treatment is the development of secondary sex characteristics and fertility, when possible. Insufficient sex hormone secretion can be corrected by hormone replacement therapy, such as estrogen. Idiopathic hypogonadotropic hypogonadism is treated with synthetic GnRH or sex hormone administration, or both, and may be lifelong.[11]

Precocious Puberty

Precocious puberty is a rare event, affecting about 1 in 10,000 girls and fewer than 1 in 50,000 boys. Precocious puberty has been redefined as sexual maturation before age 6 in black girls or age 7 in white girls, and before age 9 in boys.[15] This reflects a trend toward earlier puberty, primarily for breast development in girls (see What's New? Precocious Puberty). There have been many postulated causes of precious puberty (Box 24-1), including increased obesity, an increase in protein consumption,[16,17] and the growing prevalence of molecular compounds known as endocrine disruptors in common household products.[18] However, because precocious puberty can be a sign of pathology, all cases of precocious puberty require thorough evaluation.

Precocious puberty may be partial, complete, or mixed types (Box 24-2) and can be further categorized into central (GnRH dependent) and peripheral (GnRH independent)

WHAT'S NEW?

Precocious Puberty

Studies implicate obesity, leptin, ghrelin, and environmental endocrine disruptor chemicals (EDCs) as possible contributors to precocious puberty in girls. Obesity may affect the production and secretion of leptin and ghrelin, powerful communicators of satiety, hunger, metabolic rate, and in timing of puberty. EDCs may mimic, block, or alter the normal signaling systems involved in sex hormone secretion, uptake, and use. EDCs include agrochemicals, widespread industrial compounds, and persistent pollutants.

Data from Bluher S, Mantzoros CS: *Curr Opin Endocrinol Diabetes Obes* 14(6):458–464, 2007; Buck Louis GM et al: *Pediatrics* 121(Suppl 3):S192–S207, 2008; Caserta DL et al: *Hum Reprod Update* 14(1): 59–72, 2008; Euling SY et al: *Pediatrics* 121(Suppl 3):S167–S171, 2008; Kaplowitz PB: *Pediatrics* 121(Suppl 3):S208–S217, 2008; Rasier G et al: *Mol Cell Endocrinol* 254–255:187-201, 2006; Tena-Sempere M: *Vitam Horm* 77:285–300, 2008.

BOX 24-1 CAUSES OF PRECOCIOUS PUBERTY

Central (Gonadotropin-Releasing Hormone [GnRH] Dependent)
Idiopathic
Central nervous system (CNS) disorders
- Congenital anomalies (hydrocephalus)
- Hypothalamic hamartoma
- Postinflammatory/infectious condition
- Trauma
- Tumors (hypothalamic, pineal, other)

Hypothyroidism (severe)
Imprinted gene (MKRN3)

Peripheral Puberty (GnRH Independent)
Adrenal hyperplasia or tumor
Environmental endocrine disruptors
Exogenous sex steroid exposure
Exogenous anabolic steroids
Familial Leydig cell hyperplasia
Gonadal tumors or cysts
Human chorionic gonadotropin (hCG)–secreting tumors (hepatoblastomas, intracranial lesions)
McCune-Albright syndrome
Testotoxicosis

From Abreu AP et al: *NEJM*, 2013 [Epub ahead of print.]; Bhagavath B, Layman LC: *Semin Reprod Med* 25(4):272–286, 2007; Burchett MLR et al: Endocrine and metabolic diseases. In Burns CE et al, editors: *Pediatric primary care*, St Louis, 2009, Saunders; Caserta DL et al: *Hum Reprod Update* 14(1):59–72, 2008; Cesario SK, Hughes LA: *J Obstet Gynecol Neonatal Nurs* 36(3):263–274, 2007; Jospe N: Disorders of pubertal development. In Osborn LM et al, editors: *Pediatrics*, Philadelphia, 2005, Mosby.

BOX 24-2 PRIMARY FORMS OF PRECOCIOUS PUBERTY

Complete Precocious Puberty
Premature development of appropriate characteristics for the child's sex
Hypothalamic-pituitary-ovarian axis working normally but prematurely
In about 10% of cases, lethal central nervous system tumor may be the cause

Partial Precocious Puberty
Partial development of appropriate secondary sex characteristics
Premature thelarche (breast budding) seen in girls between 6 months and 2 years of age
Does not progress to complete puberty (ovulation and menstruation)
Premature adrenarche (growth of axillary and pubic hair) tends to occur between 5 and 8 years of age
Can progress to complete precocious puberty; may be caused by estrogen-secreting neoplasms or may be a variant of normal pubertal development

Mixed Precocious Puberty
Causes the child to develop some secondary sex characteristics of the opposite sex
Common causes: adrenal hyperplasia or androgen-secreting tumors

Data from Burchett MLR et al: Endocrine and metabolic diseases. In Burns CE et al, editors: *Pediatric primary care*, St Louis, 2009, Saunders; Jospe N: Disorders of pubertal development. In Osborn LM et al, editors: *Pediatrics*, Philadelphia, 2005, Mosby.

(see Box 24-1). **Central precocious puberty** is GnRH dependent and occurs when the HPG axis is working normally but prematurely. Besides the premature development of secondary sex characteristics, precocity causes premature closure of the epiphysis of long bones, which results in lifelong short stature.[10] Central precocious puberty results from failure of central inhibition of the GnRH pulse generator (the gonadostat). The diagnosis of central precocious puberty is one of exclusion.[10] Because a CNS lesion may be missed, children with presumed central precocious puberty require long-term surveillance. Peripheral puberty is GnRH independent and develops when sex hormones are produced by some mechanism other than stimulation by the gonadotropins. Sex steroid–producing tumors (i.e., gonadal tumors), testotoxicosis, and exposure to exogenous sex steroids (i.e., hormonal contraceptives and environmental endocrine disruptors) are some of the causes (see Box 24-1). Mutations in the imprinted gene MKRN3 was recently reported as a cause of central precocious puberty.[18a]

Partial precocious puberty is the partial development of appropriate secondary sex characteristics alone or in combination. A girl with incomplete precocious puberty might undergo thelarche or pubarche and, rarely, premature menarche. Premature thelarche is seen in girls between 6 months and 2 years of age. Premature pubarche tends to occur between ages 5 and 8 years. Premature pubarche is usually the consequence of an early increase in the adrenal androgens that leads to early growth of pubic hair and possibly a transient acceleration in growth and bone maturation that has no significant effect on timing of puberty or final height. Sparse hair growth on the genitalia, in the absence of thelarche or menarche, does not represent precocious puberty.

The diagnosis and cause of premature development are often straightforward.[8] A thorough history and physical examination are done to determine the velocity of the process and to rule out life-threatening CNS, ovarian, or adrenal neoplasms. Family occurrence helps exclude tumors. Children with precocious puberty also have a tendency toward obesity.[8]

Treatment for all forms of precocious puberty includes identifying and removing the underlying cause or administering appropriate hormones (see Boxes 24-1 and 24-2). If needed, precocious puberty can be reversed. Management goals include diagnosing and treating intracranial disease; arresting maturation until developmentally appropriate; maximizing eventual adult height; reducing emotional problems. The most common form, central precocious puberty, is usually treated with potent GnRH agonist analogs, which induce reversible, selective suppression of the HPG axis. Because many of these children are obese and childhood obesity is predictive of morbidity in adolescence and adulthood, it is important for clinicians to include assessment and management of obesity as part of the treatment for central precocious puberty.

Complete precocious puberty refers to the onset and progression of all pubertal features (i.e., thelarche, pubarche, and menarche). **Mixed precocious puberty** (virilization of a girl or feminization of a boy) causes the child to develop some secondary sex characteristics of the opposite sex. This condition is usually evident at birth and is rare in older children (Box 24-3).

BOX 24-3 CAUSES OF MIXED PRECOCIOUS PUBERTY

Female (Virilization)

- Congenital adrenal hyperplasia
- Androgen-secreting tumors
  - Adrenal
  - Ovarian
  - Teratoma
  - Exogenous androgens

Male (Feminization)

- Estrogen-producing tumors
  - Adrenal
  - Teratoma
  - Hepatoma
  - Testicular
- Exogenous estrogens
- Increased peripheral conversion of androgens to estrogens

From Jospe N: Disorders of pubertal development. In Osborn LM et al, editors: *Pediatrics,* Philadelphia, 2005, Mosby.

DISORDERS OF THE FEMALE REPRODUCTIVE SYSTEM

Hormonal and Menstrual Alterations

Primary Dysmenorrhea

Primary dysmenorrhea is painful menstruation associated with the release of prostaglandins in ovulatory cycles, but not with pelvic disease. Approximately 50% of all women experience dysmenorrhea, 10% of whom are incapacitated for 1 to 3 days because of pain severity. Primary dysmenorrhea usually begins with the onset of ovulatory cycles, around age 15 or 16 years with prevalence highest during adolescence.[19] In contrast, **secondary dysmenorrhea** is related to pelvic pathology (i.e., ovarian cysts, endometriosis) which manifests in later reproductive years and may occur any time in the menstrual cycle.[20]

PATHOPHYSIOLOGY. Primary dysmenorrhea is attributed to excessive endometrial prostaglandin production.[20,21] Women with painful periods produce 10 times as much prostaglandin F ($PGF_2\alpha$), a potent myometrial stimulant and vasoconstrictor, as asymptomatic women. Elevated levels of prostaglandins (especially $PGF_2\alpha$ and $PGE_2\alpha$) cause uterine hypercontractility, decreased blood flow to the uterus, and increased nerve hypersensitivity, thus resulting in pain.[20] Women with dysmenorrhea may have up-regulated cyclo-oxygenase (COX) enzyme activity, which contributes to increased synthesis of prostaglandins. Furthermore, leukotriene production is elevated further contributing to increased levels of pain.[20] Prostaglandins are primarily released during the first 48 hours of menstruation, when symptoms are the most intense. Women who are anovulatory because they use oral contraceptives rarely have primary dysmenorrhea. Secondary dysmenorrhea results from disorders such as endometriosis (the most common cause), endometritis (infection), pelvic inflammatory disease, obstructive uterine or vaginal anomalies, uterine fibroids, polyps, tumors, ovarian cysts, pelvic congestion syndrome, or nonhormonal intrauterine devices (IUDs).[20]

CLINICAL MANIFESTATIONS. The chief symptom of dysmenorrhea is pelvic pain associated with the onset of menses. The pain often radiates into the groin and may be accompanied by backache, anorexia, vomiting, diarrhea, syncope, and headache. The latter symptoms are caused by entry of prostaglandins and prostaglandin metabolites into the systemic circulation. Usually the discomfort associated with primary dysmenorrhea begins shortly before the onset of menstruation and persists for the first 1 to 3 days of menstrual flow.[20]

EVALUATION AND TREATMENT. Primary dysmenorrhea can be differentiated from secondary dysmenorrhea by a thorough history and pelvic examination. Nonsteroidal anti-inflammatory medication (NSAIDs, e.g., ibuprofen) is the treatment of choice as these reduce COX enzyme activity, thus prostaglandin production. NSAIDs work in the majority of women with primary dysmenorrhea and are most effective if started at the first sign of bleeding or cramping.[22] In women who desire contraception, dysmenorrhea may be relieved with hormonal contraceptives.[23] Hormonal contraception stops ovulation and creates an atrophic endometrium, thereby decreasing prostaglandin synthesis and myometrial contractility. Regular exercise and stress reduction are thought to prevent or reduce symptoms.[24] Other nonpharmacologic approaches with some evidence of effectiveness in pain relief include local application of heat; acupuncture;[25] high-frequency transcutaneous electrical nerve stimulation (TENS); supplements, such as thiamine and vitamin E; and Chinese herbal treatment.[26]

Amenorrhea

Amenorrhea means lack of menstruation, and the most common causes (aside from pregnancy) are caused by hypothalamic dysfunction, polycystic ovarian syndrome, hyperprolactinemia, and ovarian failure.27 **Primary amenorrhea** is the failure of menarche and the absence of menstruation by age 13 years without the development of secondary sex characteristics or by age 15 regardless of the presence of secondary sex characteristics (see p. 802 for discussion of delayed puberty).[28] Primary amenorrhea differs from delayed puberty in that most cases of delayed puberty require only reassurance, but when the diagnosis of primary amenorrhea is reached, a thorough evaluation is needed. **Secondary amenorrhea** is the absence of menstruation for a time equivalent to three or more cycles in women who have previously menstruated. Pregnancy is the most common condition to rule out prior to further evaluation.

PATHOPHYSIOLOGY. There are numerous classifications of the etiologies of primary amenorrhea. One approach to understanding the pathophysiology is through compartmentalization. *Compartment IV disorders* include CNS disorders, in particular hypothalamic disorders. In some of the congenital syndromes that cause primary amenorrhea, the hypothalamic-pituitary-ovarian (HPO) axis is dysfunctional. The hypothalamus is unable to synthesize GnRH, so the pituitary fails to secrete LH and FSH. Therefore, the ovary does not receive the hormonal signals required to stimulate estrogen production, and ovulation and menstruation do not occur. Because the ovarian hormones are absent, estrogen-dependent sex characteristics do not develop.

Compartment III disorders are disorders of the anterior pituitary, including tumors. Some anatomic defects of the CNS, whether congenital or acquired, impinge on the hypothalamic-pituitary unit so as to interfere with or interrupt the secretion of GnRH or FSH and LH. Examples of such defects include hydrocephalus, craniopharyngiomas, and other space-occupying lesions of the CNS. Again the target organ, the ovary, does not receive the necessary signals, and ovulation and menstruation do not occur. In some cases these lesions develop between the onset and conclusion of puberty. Therefore, skeletal growth may occur and secondary sex characteristics may develop, but sexual maturation is interrupted before menarche.

Compartment II disorders involve the ovary and are often linked with genetic abnormalities. These include gonadal dysgenesis (Turner syndrome), androgen insensitivity syndrome (AIS), formerly known as *testicular feminizing syndrome* or *male pseudohermaphroditism.* Turner syndrome involves the lack of two functional and complete X chromosomes in at least some body tissues (45,X/46,XX; structural X or Y abnormalities; mosaicism),[29] which results in the ovaries lacking gametes and ovarian failure. Without primitive gametes and follicles, follicular development and estrogen secretion cannot occur. Lack of estrogen accounts for failure of secondary sex characteristic development and amenorrhea, although there are high levels of circulating FSH and LH.[29]

In AIS, the individual is male genetically but female morphologically. The individual does not develop male genitalia because even though testosterone is produced in the fetus as a result of the presence of the Y chromosome, the cells are not sensitive to testosterone because androgen receptors are absent in target cells forming the reproductive tract.[30] In individuals with AIS, the gonads are found either in the abdomen or in the inguinal canal, and they may produce both androgens and estrogens. Because target tissues lack androgen receptors but have estrogen receptors, most individuals with AIS have female external genitalia and female secondary sex characteristics. With the exception of a small vagina, internal female genitalia are absent, accounting for amenorrhea and infertility.[30]

Compartment I disorders are anatomic defects of the outflow tract associated with primary amenorrhea. They include congenital absence of the vagina and uterus and congenital uterine hypoplasia (infantile uterus). Genetically normal females without a uterus or vagina usually have normal ovarian function. Therefore, skeletal growth occurs and secondary sex characteristics develop in the proper sequence, but menstruation does not occur because the uterus is too small or malformed to produce substantial endometrium.

CLINICAL MANIFESTATIONS. The major clinical manifestation of primary amenorrhea is the absence of the first menstrual period. The cause of the amenorrhea determines whether secondary sex characteristics and height are affected.

EVALUATION AND TREATMENT. Diagnosis of primary amenorrhea is based on history and physical examination and whether secondary sexual characteristics are present or absent. Absence of these sexual characteristics indicates that a girl or woman has never been exposed to estrogen. If ovarian steroid hormone levels are low, the individual has the appearance of an immature female. Physical examination may show structural or physiologic alterations of the reproductive tract as outlined at the beginning of the chapter. Laboratory studies may be required to document karyotype, abnormal levels of gonadotropins, and ovarian hormones. Diagnostic imaging is used to document structural abnormalities (see Figure 24-1).

Treatment involves correction of any underlying disorders and hormone replacement therapy to induce the development of secondary sex characteristics as necessary (see p. 802 for a discussion of delayed puberty). Although surgical alteration of the genitalia may be undertaken to correct structural abnormalities, surgery should be delayed until the affected individual can make a truly informed decision. Hormonal manipulation or embryo transplantation may make pregnancy possible for women with primary amenorrhea who have a normal uterus.

Secondary Amenorrhea

A wide variety of disorders and physiologic conditions are associated with secondary amenorrhea. Besides disease, secondary amenorrhea can be triggered by dramatic weight loss, whether the loss results from malnutrition or excessive exercise. Secondary amenorrhea is common during early adolescence and the perimenopausal period, pregnancy, and lactation. The most common causes (after pregnancy) are thyroid disorders (e.g., hypothyroidism), hyperprolactinemia, HPO interruption

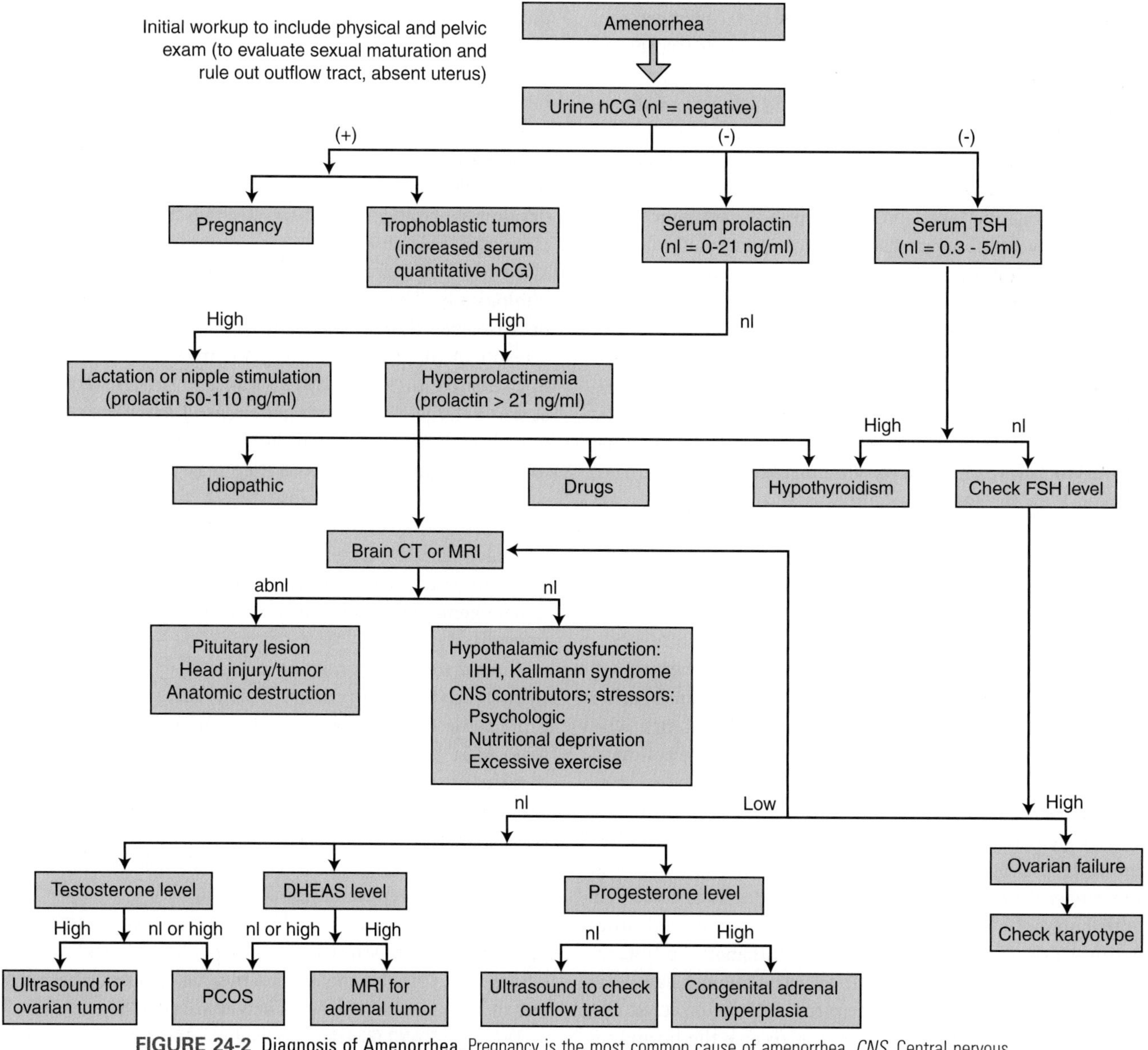

FIGURE 24-2 Diagnosis of Amenorrhea. Pregnancy is the most common cause of amenorrhea. *CNS,* Central nervous system; *CT,* computed tomography; *DHEAS,* dehydroepiandrosterone sulfate; *FSH,* follicle-stimulating hormone; *hCG,* human chorionic gonadotropin; *IHH,* idiopathic hypogonadotropic hypogonadism; *MRI,* magnetic resonance imaging; *nl,* normal; *PCOS,* polycystic ovary syndrome; *TSH,* thyroid-stimulating hormone. (Adapted from Schorge JO et al, editors: *Williams gynecology,* New York, 2008, McGraw-Hill.)

secondary to excessive exercise, stress, weight loss, and polycystic ovary syndrome (PCOS).

PATHOPHYSIOLOGY. The causes of secondary amenorrhea are summarized in Figure 24-2. In women with normal ovarian steroid hormone levels, secondary amenorrhea may be caused by structural abnormalities (müllerian anomalies), Asherman syndrome (removal of the endometrial decidua basalis), or removal of the uterus. In women with elevated ovarian steroid hormone levels, inhibited ovulation leads to amenorrhea. An excess of ovarian hormones disrupts feedback relationships within the HPO axis, preventing ovulation. Depressed ovarian hormone levels, which are associated with a variety of clinical disorders, also cause amenorrhea by preventing ovulation. Lack of ovulation, termed **anovulation,** may result from increased levels of prolactin, decreased levels of gonadotropins, irregular secretion of gonadotropins, or abnormally low levels of CNS neurotransmitters (i.e., dopamine and GnRH). Any of these variables alters the feedback effects that the ovarian hormones have on the hypothalamus and pituitary.

High levels of prolactin are physiologic during lactation because it increases milk production and suppresses ovulation, preventing closely spaced pregnancies. However, high levels of prolactin not related to lactation are abnormal and will disrupt the menstrual cycle. **Hyperprolactinemia** (overproduction of prolactin by the pituitary) may have indirect effects that lead to decreased secretion of GnRH by the hypothalamus. The result is a reduction in FSH and LH secretion followed by anovulation and secondary amenorrhea. Hyperprolactinemia should be diagnosed through blood testing that specifically tests for both normal-size and large molecular prolactin (macroprolactin). Hyperprolactinemia can have many causes including medication side effects, hypothyroidism, excessive nipple stimulation, and pituitary tumors[31] (see pp. 724 and 837 for additional information).

CLINICAL MANIFESTATIONS. The major manifestation of secondary amenorrhea is the absence of menses after previous menstrual periods. Infertility, vasomotor flushes, vaginal atrophy, acne, osteopenia, and **hirsutism** (abnormal hairiness) also may be present, depending on the underlying cause of the amenorrhea.

EVALUATION AND TREATMENT. Pregnancy is the most common cause of amenorrhea and must be ruled out prior to other evaluations. The menstrual cycle also may stop or become irregular in response to stress, extreme exercise, large dietary changes, eating disorders, or sleep abnormalities. A thorough history of the woman's life and stressors is important in assessing amenorrhea. Diagnosis of the organic cause of secondary amenorrhea involves the identification of underlying hormonal or anatomic alterations. A woman with secondary amenorrhea and normal secondary sex characteristics should have a complete history and physical examination. After ruling out pregnancy and performing an in-depth history, initial laboratory evaluation includes measurement of thyroid-stimulating hormone (TSH) and prolactin levels (Figure 24-3). Elevated prolactin levels warrant further investigation, including a complete medication history, TSH, and brain CT or MRI if warranted.[31] If these initial tests are normal, further testing would include measurement of gonadotropins (FSH), estrogen and testosterone, ultrasonography of the outflow tract and ovaries or adrenal MRI, or both.

Treatment of amenorrhea depends on the cause and the woman's psychologic need for cycle stability. Treatments may include replacing deficient hormones (e.g., estrogens, thyroid

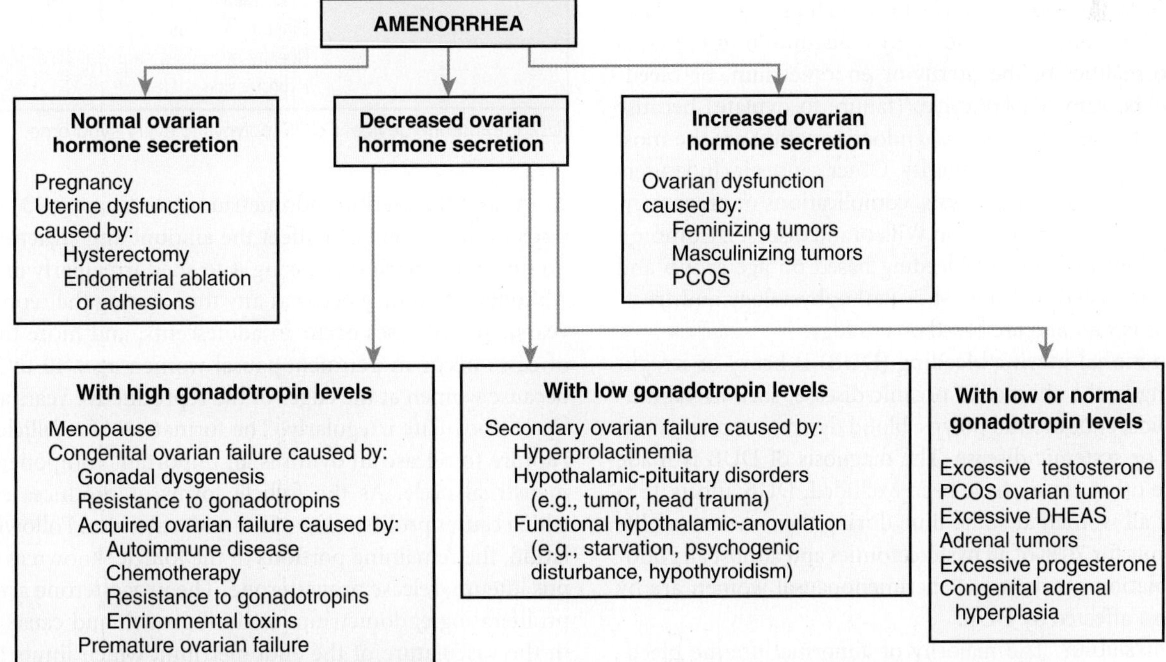

FIGURE 24-3 Causes of Secondary Amenorrhea. Of note, hypothyroidism is a relatively common condition and should be ruled out as the cause of hyperprolactinemia before more extensive evaluation (i.e., computed tomography or magnetic resonance imaging) occurs. *DHEAS*, Dehydroepiandrosterone sulfate; *PCOS*, polycystic ovary syndrome.

TABLE 24-2 ABNORMAL MENSTRUAL BLEEDING

TERM	DEFINITION
Polymenorrhea	Cycles shorter than 3 wk; may indicate disturbance in endocrine control of ovulation
Oligomenorrhea	Cycles longer than 6-7 wk; may indicate disturbance in endocrine control of ovulation
Metrorrhagia	Intermenstrual bleeding or bleeding of light character occurring irregularly between cycles; may be a sign of organic disease
Hypermenorrhea	Excessive flow; may be a sign of organic disease
Menorrhea	Prolonged duration of flow
Menorrhagia	Increased amount and duration of flow
Menometrorrhagia	Prolonged flow associated with irregular and intermittent spotting between bleeding episodes

hormone, glucocorticoids, gonadotropins) or correcting underlying pathology (e.g., tumor removal).[32,33] A diagnosis of PCOS might be treated with an insulin-sensitizing agent, such as metformin, as well as ovulation-inducing drugs if fertility is desired (a discussion of PCOS is on p. 810).

Some treatments for amenorrhea prevent pregnancy, whereas others may restore fertility; the choice of treatment may be influenced by the woman's childbearing plans. After pathologies have been corrected and the menstrual cycle stabilized, fertility may return. Occasionally, women with secondary amenorrhea may need additional ovulation-inducing drugs to assist conception, whereas others are able to conceive naturally.[33]

Abnormal Uterine Bleeding

Menstrual irregularity or abnormal bleeding patterns (Table 24-2) account for approximately 33% of all gynecologic visits. Abnormal bleeding can be caused by a disruption in the HPG axis, abnormalities of the uterus or endometrium, or bleeding disorders. Anovulatory cycles (failure to ovulate) because of various etiologies (age, stress, endocrinopathy) are the most common cause of cycle irregularity. Other causes include uterine tumors, polyps, ovarian cysts, complications of pregnancy, and bleeding disorders (e.g., von Willebrand disease). Common causes of abnormal uterine bleeding based on age group and frequency are listed in Table 24-3. Pathophysiology and treatment options vary and are based on etiology.[34]

Dysfunctional uterine bleeding (DUB) is heavy or irregular bleeding in the absence of organic disease, such as submucous fibroids, endometrial polyps, blood dyscrasias, pregnancy, infection, or systemic disease. The diagnosis of DUB is made once these other causes have been excluded. DUB affects 15% to 20% of all women at some time during their menstrual life and accounts for 70% of all hysterectomies and almost all endometrial ablation procedures.[35] Perimenopausal women are by far the most affected by DUB.

PATHOPHYSIOLOGY. The majority of abnormal uterine bleeding, commonly known as dysfunctional bleeding, is due to lack of ovulation.[34] Normal, regular periods are the result of a complex interplay between the hypothalamus, the pituitary, the

TABLE 24-3 COMMON CAUSES OF ABNORMAL (VAGINAL/GENITAL) BLEEDING IN DESCENDING ORDER OF FREQUENCY

AGE GROUP	CAUSE
Prepubescence	Sexual assault
	Trauma
	Foreign bodies
	Precocious puberty
Adolescence	Anovulation (immature hypothalamic-pituitary-ovarian axis)
	Trauma and sexual abuse
Reproductive years	Pregnancy
	Pelvic inflammatory disease
	Coagulation disorder
	Hormonal contraceptives
	Endometriosis
	Anovulation
	IUDs
	Ovarian cysts
	Uterine polyps/tumors
	PCOS
	Bleeding disorders (e.g., von Willebrand)
	Trauma/rape
Perimenopause	Anovulation
	Malignancy
	Pregnancy
	Endometriosis
	Benign neoplasms (myomas, adenomyosis)
Postmenopause	Malignancy
Other: Non–age specific	Chronic conditions
	Adrenal conditions
	Thyroid disorders
	Liver disease
	Diabetes mellitus
	Obesity
	Hypertension

IUD, Intrauterine device; *PCOS,* polycystic ovary syndrome.

ovary, and the uterine endometrium (see Chapter 23). Disruptions in this system can affect the amount and structure of the uterine endometrium, causing it to shed irregularly or heavily. Although DUB may occur at any time during the reproductive years, 20% of cases occur in adolescents, and more than 50% of cases occur in perimenopausal women ages 40 to 50 years because women at the edges of the reproductive years are more likely to ovulate irregularly. The formation of a follicle and its rupture to release an ovum is an important component of the menstrual cycle. As the follicle forms, it produces estrogen, which causes proliferation of the endometrium. Following ovulation, the remaining portions of the follicle, known as the corpus luteum, release progesterone. The progesterone acts on the proliferating endometrium to limit growth and cause changes in the vasculature of the endometrium, which limits bleeding during endometrial shedding.

If a follicle forms but never releases the ovum, the follicle may continue to produce estrogen (estradiol [E_2]) encouraging endometrial proliferation beyond the normal 14-day time window. In addition, the lack of progesterone causes the thickened endometrium to be unable to shed in a predictable fashion without excessive blood loss. Women who fail to ovulate experience irregularities in their menstrual bleeding related to the lack of progesterone and, in some cases, an excess of estrogen.

Many conditions are associated with irregular ovulation. Women at the edges of their reproductive life span, both young and old, are more likely to experience anovulatory cycles. In older women this is a result of having fewer viable follicles for ovulation (see Chapter 23 for a description of the many hormonal changes associated with the time before and just after menopause). Other conditions associated with chronic anovulation include PCOS, in which follicles begin to form but never reach maturation and rupture; obesity because adipose tissue excretes estrogen, which can suppress the HPG axis; hyperthyroidism and hypothyroidism; and estrogen-secreting ovarian neoplasms.

Without ovulation, menstrual flow may become irregular (metrorrhagia) and excessive (menorrhagia) or both (menometrorrhagia), resulting from the large quantity of tissue available for bleeding and the random breakdown of tissue that results in exposure of vascular channels. In the absence of adequate progesterone levels, usual endometrial control mechanisms are missing, such as vasoconstrictive rhythmicity, tight coiling of spiral vessels, and orderly collapse, and stasis does not occur. Unopposed estrogen induces a progression of endometrial responses beginning with proliferation, hyperplasia, and adenomatous hyperplasia; over a course of many years, unopposed estrogen may end with atypia and carcinoma.

Abnormal menstrual bleeding also can result from defects of the corpus luteum, resulting in progesterone deficiencies or from abnormalities of the uterus or cervix, such as endometrial polyps, uterine fibroids, or even uterine or cervical cancers. (These conditions are covered in more detail later in the chapter.) Coagulation defects also can cause heavy and abnormal uterine bleeding and should be suspected in younger women with a history of extensive bruising.

CLINICAL MANIFESTATIONS. Abnormal uterine bleeding is characterized by unpredictable and variable bleeding. Especially during perimenopause, abnormal bleeding also may involve greatly increased menstrual flow and the passage of large clots, leading to excessive blood loss. Excessive bleeding can lead to iron deficiency anemia and associated symptoms (fatigue, shortness of breath).

EVALUATION AND TREATMENT. The first step in assessing abnormal bleeding is to determine the cause of bleeding. If an organic cause can be found, the focus is on eliminating the pathology or mitigating its effects. To determine the cause of the bleeding, a complete and thorough history and physical examination is needed. The woman's age and risk factors for other abnormal conditions are important in assessing the likely cause of the bleeding. If no cause can be found, it is usually assumed that the bleeding is caused by lack of regular ovulation because this is the cause of the majority of abnormal bleeding. Irregular menstrual bleeding because of anovulation is often referred to as DUB. Treatment goals include preventing or controlling abnormal bleeding, identifying underlying disease, and inducing regular menstrual cycles. Treatment varies greatly by the age of the woman and her desire for current and future fertility.

NSAIDs, such as ibuprofen and naproxen, are often first-line treatments for excessive menstrual bleeding because they reduce prostaglandin synthesis within the endometrial tissues, which causes vasoconstriction and decreased menstrual blood loss. NSAIDs can reduce menstrual bleeding significantly with minimal side effects.[36] For best effect they should be taken in the few days preceding the beginning of the menstrual period and be continued through the days of heaviest bleeding. NSAIDs are not as effective in controlling menstrual blood loss as hormonal therapies but they are readily available without a prescription.[36]

Young women and those of childbearing age with abnormal bleeding are often treated with hormonal therapies to override the HPG axis and mimic normal menstrual bleeding or suppress it entirely. Common treatments include oral contraceptive pills that contain both estrogen and progesterone, long-term treatment with medroxyprogesterone (Depo-Provera) (though the U.S. Food and Drug Administration [FDA] black box warning about potential bone loss has drastically curtailed the use of this therapy), and the levonorgestrel intrauterine device (LNG-IUD). The LNG-IUD has a dual indication from the FDA for both birth control and suppression of abnormal menstrual bleeding. The device releases a steady amount of progesterone directly into the uterus to stabilize and suppress the uterine lining. In addition, the progesterone works to suppress the HPG axis and prevent ovulation. There is no strong evidence to differentiate whether estrogen and progesterone or progesterone alone is superior in the treatment of abnormal uterine bleeding; the woman should be allowed to select a treatment regimen that is compatible with her life and needs.[37]

Women who are greater than 35 years old and smoke cigarettes may not be candidates for oral contraceptive pills as the estrogen increases their risk of cardiovascular incidents, such as myocardial infarction. However, the LNG-IUD can still be used because it contains only progesterone. The LNG-IUD is widely used as a first step in controlling perimenopausal bleeding because it can be inserted in a clinic office and is easily removed if the treatment is ineffective. The LNG-IUD decreases blood loss by 86% to 97% by decreasing endometrial proliferation and has similar success rates as more invasive procedures.[38] Women who do not wish to have future pregnancies also can opt for treatments that permanently suppress their uterine lining. These treatments include ablation, where the lining is burned to prevent future proliferation of the endometrial cells, and complete removal of the uterus in hysterectomy.[38] If a woman is menopausal, and has not had a menstrual period for greater than 1 year, all vaginal bleeding should be investigated to rule out uterine and other cancers. Appropriate initial evaluation includes ultrasound and endometrial biopsy to rule out uterine cancer.[39]

Women with coagulation disorders may have excessive menstrual bleeding because they have a genetic predisposition to bleeding or because they are taking anticoagulant medications to overcome a genetic predisposition to excessive clotting.[40] To control their menstrual bleeding, these women can opt for cycle suppression. Provision of birth control for these women is important because pregnancy may be risk to their health.[41]

Polycystic Ovary Syndrome

Polycystic ovary syndrome (PCOS) has at least two of the following conditions: oligo-ovulation or anovulation, elevated levels of androgens, or clinical signs of hyperandrogenism and polycystic ovaries. Polycystic ovaries do not have to be present to diagnose PCOS, and conversely their presence alone does not establish the diagnosis. PCOS remains one of the most common endocrine disturbances affecting women, especially young women, and is a leading cause of infertility in the United States, where prevalence rates are estimated at between 4% and 12%, afflicting between 3.2 and 5.4 million young women.[42] PCOS appears to be familial, and various features of the syndrome may be differentially inherited.[43,44] Confusing the issue is the frequency, expression, and timing of PCOS symptoms and diagnosis. From 22% to 30% of women have polycystic ovaries on ultrasound, with 80% having one or more symptoms of the syndrome; 80% of women with normal ovaries also experience one or more PCOS symptoms. Signs and symptoms of women with PCOS may change over time, with metabolic syndrome becoming more prominent with age. In addition, polycystic ovaries may be associated with Cushing syndrome, acromegaly, premature ovarian failure, simple obesity, congenital adrenal hyperplasia, thyroid disease, androgen-producing adrenal tumors or ovarian tumors (Figure 24-4), and syndromes with hyperprolactinemia. Thus diagnosing PCOS can be difficult. In addition, several diagnostic criteria are proposed by different agencies, resulting in nonstandard application of the diagnosis.[45]

PATHOPHYSIOLOGY. Although the underlying cause of PCOS is unknown, a genetic basis is suspected. Initial identification of genes involved in steroid biosynthesis, androgen biosynthesis, and insulin receptors within the ovary indicate genetic involvement. No single factor fully accounts for the abnormalities of PCOS.[44,46-48] A hyperandrogenic state is a cardinal feature in the pathogenesis of PCOS. However, glucose intolerance/insulin resistance (IR) and hyperinsulinemia often run parallel and markedly aggravate the hyperandrogenic state, thus contributing to the severity of signs and symptoms of PCOS.[44,49] Obesity adds to and worsens IR. Although 50% of normal weight women with PCOS have IR, all obese women with PCOS do. Insulin stimulates androgen secretion by the ovarian stroma and reduces serum sex hormone–binding globulin (SHBG) directly and independently. The net effect is an increase in free testosterone levels. Excessive androgens affect follicular growth, and insulin affects follicular decline by suppressing apoptosis and enabling follicles, which would normally disintegrate, to survive[50] (Figure 24-5). Further, there appears to be a genetic ovarian defect in PCOS, which makes the ovary either more susceptible to or sensitive to insulin's stimulation of androgen production. Recent research suggests that decreased intraovarian receptors for estrogen receptor-α or insulin-like growth factor 1 (IGF-1), increased leptin levels, or direct IR within selective ovarian cells (fibroblasts) may contribute to this phenomenon.[50] Intrauterine and early childhood environments may also contribute to the development of PCOS (see What's New? Early Programming for PCOS?).

Weight gain tends to aggravate symptoms, whereas weight loss may ameliorate some of the endocrine and metabolic

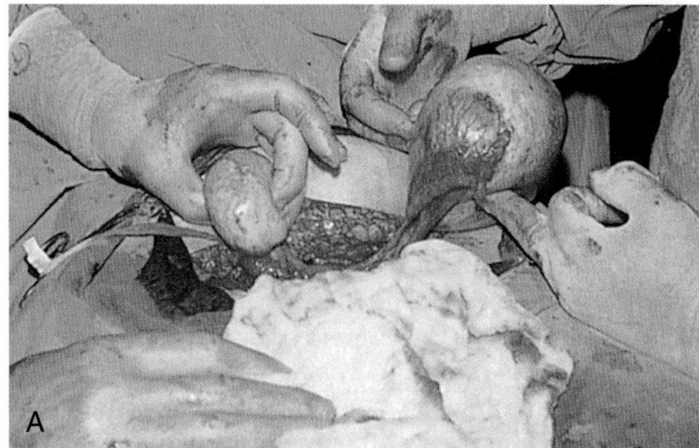

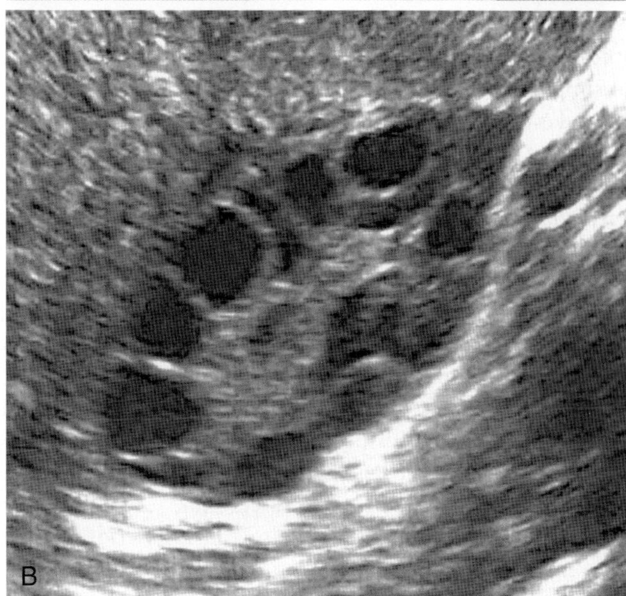

FIGURE 24-4 Polycystic Ovary. **A,** Surgical view of polycystic ovaries. **B,** Ultrasound of polycystic ovary. (**A** from Symonds EM, Macpherson MBA: *Diagnosis in color: obstetrics and gynecology,* London, 1997, Mosby-Wolfe. **B** from King J: *J Midwifery Womens Health* 51[6]:415–422, 2006. Reprinted with permission.)

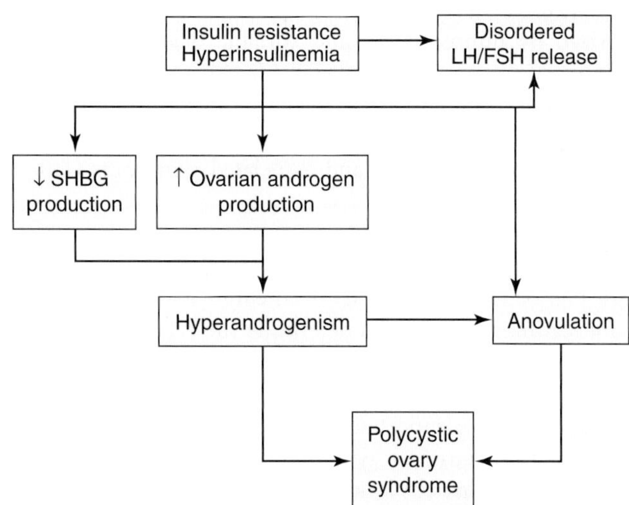

FIGURE 24-5 Insulin Resistance and Hyperinsulinemia in Polycystic Ovary Syndrome (PCOS). See text. *FSH,* Follicle-stimulating hormone; *LH,* luteinizing hormone; *SHBG,* sex hormone–binding globulin. (From Franks S, Berga SL: *Fertil Steril* 97[1]:2–6, 2012.)

WHAT'S NEW?

Early Programming for PCOS?

A fetal environment containing abnormal levels of pollutants, hormones, and other factors yet undefined can induce epigenetic modifications of the DNA and increased risk for adult disease. Female fetuses exposed to testosterone at levels normally found with male fetuses appear programmed to develop altered TGF-β signaling and increased risk of hyperinsulinemia and hyperandrogenism related to PCOS.

Kosova G, Urbanek M, *Mol Cell Endocrinol* 373(1-2):29–38, 2013; Witchel SF et al: *Endocrine* 42(3):526–534, 2012; Xita N, Tsatsoulis A: *Ann NY Acad Sci* 1205:148–155, 2010.

events and thus decrease symptoms. Women with PCOS tend to have increased leptin levels (leptin levels are increased in thin as well as overweight women with PCOS).[51] Leptin influences the hypothalamic pulsatility of GnRH and consequent interaction along the entire HPO axis. Feedback from the polycystic ovary is disturbed because of changes in ovarian steroid and nonsteroidal (inhibins and related proteins) hormones.

In PCOS there is dysfunction in follicle development.[50] Inappropriate gonadotropin secretion triggers the beginning of a vicious cycle that perpetuates anovulation. Typically, levels of FSH are low or below normal and LH levels and LH bioactivity are elevated. An increased frequency of GnRH pulses appears to cause increased frequency of LH pulses.[52,53] Persistent LH elevation causes an increase in androgens (dehydroepiandrosterone sulfate [DHEAS] from the adrenal glands and testosterone, androstenedione, and DHEAS from the ovary). Androgens are converted to estrogen in peripheral tissues, and increased testosterone levels cause a significant reduction (approximately 50%) in SHBG, which in turn causes increased levels of free estradiol. Elevated estrogen levels trigger a positive-feedback response in LH and a negative-feedback response in FSH. Because FSH levels are not totally depressed, new follicular growth is continuously stimulated, but not to full maturation and ovulation. The accumulation of follicular tissue in various stages of development allows an increased and relatively constant production of steroids in response to gonadotropin stimulation. Thus PCOS is characterized by excessive production of both androgen and estrogen.

Increased androgen secretion by the ovaries contributes to premature follicular failure (atresia) and persistent anovulation. In turn, persistent anovulation causes enlarged polycystic ovaries characterized by a smooth, pearly white capsule. This characteristic appearance is caused by an increase of surface area and increased volume of up to 2.8 times, doubling of growing and atretic follicles, thickening of the tunica (outermost area) by 50%, increasing cortical stromal thickening by one third and a fivefold increase in subcortical stroma, and escalating hyperplasia. With advancing age, menstrual irregularities may improve while metabolic syndrome and type 2 diabetes mellitus increases. Women with PCOS have a three times greater incidence of uterine cancer in later life than normally cycling women related to the anovulatory lack of progesterone in PCOS. Without treatment for anovulation, women with PCOS have a 9% lifetime risk for endometrial cancers related to the effects of unopposed estrogen.[54]

CLINICAL MANIFESTATIONS. Clinical manifestations of PCOS usually appear within 2 years of puberty but may appear after a variable period of normal menstrual function and, possibly, pregnancy. The symptoms are related to anovulation and hyperandrogenism and include dysfunctional bleeding or amenorrhea, hirsutism, acne, and infertility. Approximately 41% of women with PCOS are obese.[46] Box 24-4 contains a list of signs and symptoms, summary of hormonal disturbances, and complications of PCOS. In addition, women with PCOS are more likely to experience sleep apnea than unaffected women, which results in impaired sleep and may reduce their overall quality of life.[45]

BOX 24-4 CLINICAL MANIFESTATIONS OF POLYCYSTIC OVARY SYNDROME

Presenting Signs and Symptoms (% of Women Affected)

Obesity (41%)
Menstrual disturbance (70% [i.e., dysfunctional uterine bleeding])
Oligomenorrhea (47%)
Amenorrhea (19%)
Regular menstruation (48%)
Hyperandrogenism (69% to 74%)
Infertility (73% of anovulatory infertility)
Asymptomatic (20% of those with PCOS)

Hormonal Disturbances

Increased insulin (independent of obesity)
Decreased SHBG
Increased androgens (testosterone, androstenedione)
Increased DHEA (occurs in 50% of women)
Increased LH (genetic variant LH-β subunit)
Increased prolactin
Increased leptin, especially in obesity (independent of insulin)
Suggested decreased insulin-like growth factor (IGF-1) receptors on theca cells
Possible decreased estrogen receptors (intraovarian and along hypothalamic-pituitary axis)

Possible Late Sequelae

Dyslipidemia: increased low-density lipoproteins, decreased high-density lipoproteins, increased triglycerides
Diabetes mellitus (30% of women with or without obesity develop type 2 diabetes mellitus by age 30)
Cardiovascular disease; hypertension
Endometrial hyperplasia and carcinoma (anovulatory women are hyperestrogenic)

Other

Women with PCOS are at increased risk of gestational diabetes mellitus, pregnancy-induced hypertension, preterm birth, and perinatal mortality

Adapted from Azziz R et al: *Fertil Steril*, October 22, 2008 [Epub ahead of print]; Boomsma CM et al: *Semin Reprod Med* 26(1):72–84, 2008; Diamanti-Kandarakis E: *Expert Rev Mol Med* 10(2):e3, 2008; Simoni M et al: *Hum Reprod Update* 14(5):459–484, 2008.
DHEA, Dehydroepiandrosterone; *LH,* luteinizing hormone; *PCOS,* polycystic ovary syndrome; *SHBG,* sex hormone–binding globulin.

EVALUATION AND TREATMENT. Diagnosis of PCOS is based on evidence of androgen excess, chronic anovulation, and inappropriate gonadotropin secretion. Tests for impaired glucose tolerance are recommended. As stated, polycystic ovaries do not have to be present and, conversely, their presence alone does not establish the diagnosis. Goals of treatment include reversing signs and symptoms of androgen excess, instituting cyclic menstruation, restoring fertility, and ameliorating any associated metabolic or endocrine, or both, disturbances.[55,56] Traditionally, treatment of PCOS focused on correcting anovulation and the effects of hyperandrogenism with combined oral contraceptives (COCs), antiandrogens, and fertility agents. With a greater understanding of the role that IR and hyperinsulinemia play in this disease, insulin sensitizers, such as metformin,[50,57] may be used to decrease insulin, prevent diabetes and heart disease (by reducing microvascular events), and restore fertility if desired. Progesterone therapy is recommended to oppose estrogen's effects on the endometrium and as a means to initiate monthly withdrawal bleeding (at the expense of continued hirsutism). For infertile women desiring pregnancy, clomiphene citrate, an antiestrogen, can be used to facilitate ovulation, although better effects are achieved (75% ovulation rates and 30% to 40% pregnancy rates) if therapy is combined with an insulin sensitizer.[58-60]

Women who are primed with human chorionic gonadotropin (hCG) before in vitro fertilization have greater success in achieving and maintaining pregnancy (58% to 82%).[58] Only a small reduction of weight has shown a restoration of ovulation and increased insulin sensitivity by 71% in obese women with PCOS. Lifestyle changes are therefore encouraged, particularly weight loss and exercise. Reduction of IR by loss of abdominal fat appears crucial in restoring ovulation.[61] However, lifestyle changes alone have not been shown to reverse the hyperlipidemia and hyperinsulinemia of PCOS, and pharmacologic treatment is often needed to prevent later health complications.[62] Management of PCOS is a near lifelong process because the effects of the syndrome persist past childbearing years. Appropriate primary care is needed to control the systemic features of PCOS so that it has minimal impact on a woman's life.

Premenstrual Disorders

Premenstrual syndrome (PMS) and **premenstrual dysphoric disorder (PMDD)** are the cyclic recurrence (in the luteal phase of the menstrual cycle) of distressing physical, psychologic, or behavioral changes that impair interpersonal relationships or interfere with usual activities.[52] The prevalence of PMS and PMDD is difficult to determine, in part because of the wide-ranging nature of accepted symptoms. Symptoms of PMS and PMDD begin after ovulation during the luteal phase and persist up to 4 days into the menstrual cycle.[63]

It has been estimated that 91% of women experience some form of distress around their menstrual period but a much smaller number, as low as 3.1%, meet the criteria for PMDD.[64] Sources vary but suggest that around 30% of women experience enough distress to interrupt their daily life and routine.[65]

The psychologic and physiologic changes of PMS/PMDD occur in the luteal phase of ovulatory cycles and are linked with the complex hormonal changes of the menstrual cycle. There are many theories on the cause(s) of the disorder, including that the fall in estrogen following ovulation and the immediate rise in progesterone interacts with hormones and neurotransmitters to cause symptoms.[66] However, the mechanisms involved are not known and may involve an individual sensitivity to the hormones more than hormonal levels. Furthermore, the neurotransmitters serotonin, gamma-aminobutyric acid (GABA), and noradrenaline may have mediating or moderating roles on symptom manifestation. These neurotransmitters have demonstrated interactions with estrogen and progesterone and *all* of these are neuroactive with known mood and behavior effects, including negative mood, irritability, aggression, and impulse control.[66] Sex steroids also interact with the renin-angiotensin-aldosterone system (RAAS), which could explain some PMS/PMDD signs and symptoms (e.g., water retention, bloating, weight gain). A predisposition to PMS runs in families, perhaps because of genetics or shared environment. Although research is limited, evidence supports a relationship between the severity and frequency of premenstrual symptoms and reports of low general well-being, history of major affective disorder, and personality characteristics, such as perfectionism, increased stress, poor nutrition, lack of exercise, low self-esteem, history of sexual abuse, and family conflict.[64] In turn, when premenstrual symptoms are perceived as distressing, the quality of interpersonal relationships and self-image are negatively affected.

CLINICAL MANIFESTATIONS. The pattern of symptom frequency and severity is more important than specific complaints. Nearly 300 physical, emotional, and behavioral symptoms have been attributed to PMS/PMDD. Emotional symptoms, particularly depression, anger, irritability, and fatigue, have been reported as the most prominent and the most distressing, whereas physical symptoms seem to be the least prevalent and problematic. Underlying physical or psychologic disease may be aggravated premenstrually and must be diagnosed and treated independently from PMS/PMDD.

EVALUATION AND TREATMENT. Diagnosis of PMS/PMDD is based on prospective health history and symptoms. Diagnostic criteria for PMDD are presented in Box 24-5. Because the cause of PMS is not known and cannot be reduced to a single biologic

BOX 24-5 AMERICAN COLLEGE OF OBSTETRICIANS AND GYNECOLOGISTS (ACOG) CRITERIA: PMDD

A problem with premenstrual dysphoric disorder (PMDD) diagnosis is that many women with clinically relevant premenstrual syndrome/premenstrual dysphoric disorder (PMS/PMDD) symptoms do not meet the full criteria of the *Diagnostic and Statistical Manual of Mental Disorders-IV* (DSM-IV). The ACOG attempts to rectify this problem by using the following definitions: "Presence of at least one psychological or physical symptom that causes significant impairment and is confirmed by means of prospective ratings (i.e., 2 cycles of a symptom diary)."

Data from American College of Obstetricians and Gynecologists: *ACOG Pract Bull* 15, 2000; Yonkers KA et al: *Lancet* 371(9619): 1200–1210, 2008.

NUTRITION & DISEASE

Premenstrual Syndrome

Women who are affected by premenstrual syndrome (PMS) often look for ways to decrease their symptoms. Dietary interventions that can help are multiple: eating six small meals each day; increasing intake of complex carbohydrates, fiber, and water; and decreasing caffeine, alcohol, refined sugar, and animal fat consumption. A low-fat vegetarian diet has been associated with decreased symptoms, possibly because of an increase in serum sex hormone–binding globulin concentration that lowers serum estrogen levels. It also may be helpful to limit sodium intake, and some limited evidence suggests that moderate doses (50 mg/day) of vitamin B_6 may reduce emotional symptoms of depression, irritability, and tiredness. This finding needs to be confirmed.

Some researchers have suggested links between serotonin, endorphins, and high sugar intake and PMS risk. One interesting craving is chocolate. Some researchers suggest that a craving for chocolate is an unconscious desire for a compound called phenylethylamine (PEA) in chocolate that stimulates the release of the neurotransmitter dopamine, which regulates mood.

Data from Barnard ND et al: *Obstet Gynecol* 95(2):245, 2000; Mahan LK, Escott-Stump S: *Krause's food, nutrition, and diet therapy,* ed 10, Philadelphia, 2000, Saunders; Mura Kami K et al: *Nutrition* 24(6):554–561, 2008.

explanation, and because the occurrence and severity of PMS are mediated by lifestyle and social and psychologic factors, treatment for PMS is symptomatic. Nonpharmacologic therapies, with or without medication, tend to be more effective in controlling symptoms than medication alone (see Nutrition & Disease: Premenstrual Syndrome). Initial treatment focuses on validation of the premenstrual experience, education on PMS and self-help techniques, and elimination of contributing factors or treatment of coexisting or underlying disorders.

After a trial of nonpharmacologic therapies or if criteria for PMDD are met, medications may be beneficial. Two major forms of treatment that have been well substantiated through research include the use of hormonal cycle regulation and use of selective serotonin reuptake inhibitor (SSRI) antidepressants.

If a woman does not desire immediate fertility, hormonal cycle regulation may be beneficial in regulating her menstrual cycle and decreasing the amount of circuiting steroidal hormones. The oral contraceptive pill containing estrogen and progesterone has shown benefits in decreasing PMS/PMDD.[67] Pills containing drospirenone have been shown to be particularly helpful in decreasing bloating and other PMS/PMDD signs[68] but have an increased risk of blood clots when compared with pills using another form of progestin.[69] Oral contraceptive pills also can be used continuously for up to 3 months to decrease the frequency of menstrual periods and PMS/PMDD.[67] SSRIs have been well studied for use in prevention and treatment of PMS/PMDD.[70] They relieve symptoms in about 60% to 90% of women and may be given continually or only during the premenstrual period but may have undesired side effects such as sexual problems.

In severe cases, menses can be abolished using GnRH agonists. However, if GnRH analogs are prescribed, continuous estrogen replacement therapy should be used to avoid side effects of "medical menopause."[71]

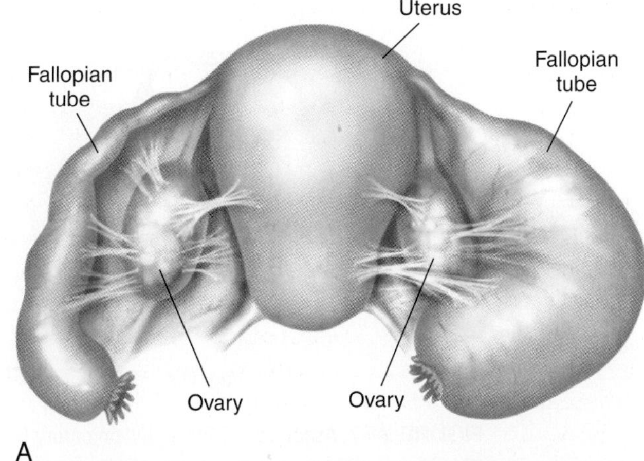

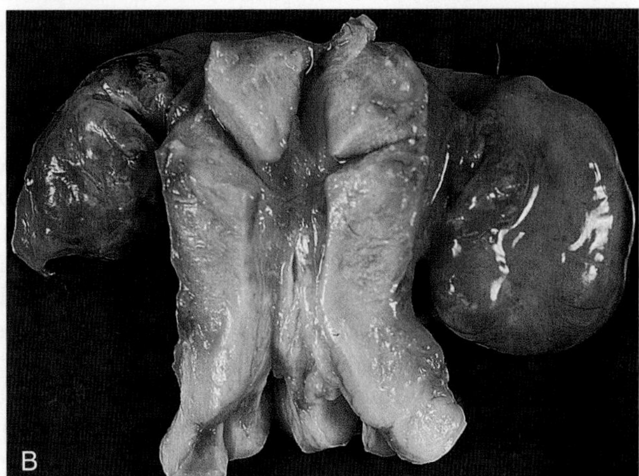

FIGURE 24-6 Salpingitis. **A,** Advanced pyosalpinx. Note the swollen fallopian tubes. **B,** Bilateral, retort-shaped, swollen, sealed tubes and adhesions of ovaries are typical of salpingitis. (**A** from Seidel HM et al: *Mosby's guide to physical examination,* ed 7, St Louis, 2011, Mosby. **B** from Damjanov I, Linder J, editors: *Anderson's pathology,* ed 10, St Louis, 1996, Mosby.)

Infection and Inflammation

Infections of the genital tract may result from exogenous or endogenous microorganisms. Exogenous pathogens are most often sexually transmitted (see Chapter 26). Endogenous causes of infection include microorganisms that are normally present in the vagina, bowel, or vulva. Infection occurs if these microorganisms migrate to a new location or overproliferate or if the immune system and other defense mechanisms are impaired.

A number of skin disorders can affect the vulva. They include reactive dermatitis, contact dermatitis, psoriasis, and impetigo. (See Chapter 46 for a discussion of skin disorders.) Many infectious disorders that affect the vulva and vagina are sexually transmitted; these disorders are described in Chapter 26.

Pelvic Inflammatory Disease

Pelvic inflammatory disease (PID) is an acute inflammatory process caused by infection. PID may involve any organ, or combination of organs, of the upper genital tract—the uterus, fallopian tubes, or ovaries—and, in its most severe form, the entire peritoneal cavity. Inflammation of the fallopian tubes is termed **salpingitis** (Figure 24-6); inflammation of the ovaries is

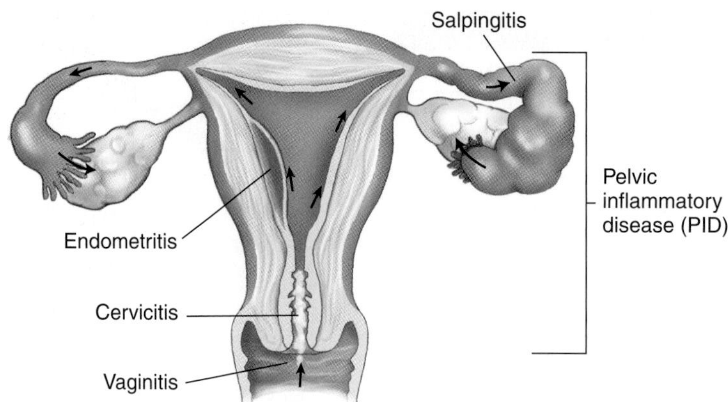

FIGURE 24-7 Ascension of Pelvic Inflammatory Disease (PID). Microorganisms from the lower genital tract ascend into the endometrium, fallopian tubes, and peritoneum to cause endometritis-salpingitis-peritonitis (pelvic inflammatory disease). The *arrows* indicate the "flow" of microorganisms from the lower genital tract to the upper genital tract. This is noted as an ascending infection in the text. (Adapted from Brooks ML: *Exploring medical language,* ed 8, St Louis, 2012, Mosby.)

called **oophoritis.** Sexually transmitted microorganisms, such as chlamydia and gonorrhea, that migrate from the vagina to the uterus, fallopian tubes, and ovaries cause most cases of PID. The ascension of these microorganisms into the upper genital tract may be facilitated by disruptions in the normal vaginal flora.[72] Some cases of PID occur after invasive procedures, such as IUD placement, when microorganisms are pushed up into the upper genital tract.[73]

Pelvic inflammatory disease is very common in the United States and around the world and has both immediate and long-term health implications for women. Infections of the upper reproductive tract cause changes to the delicate cells of the fallopian/uterine tubes, which can affect fertility and increase the risk of ectopic pregnancy.[74]

PATHOPHYSIOLOGY. The development of upper genital tract infections is mediated by the failure of a number of defense mechanisms that usually are effective in preventing PID. Virulence of the organism, size of the inoculum, and defense status of the individual determine whether an infectious process results. Gonorrhea and chlamydia are the main infectious causes of PID.[75,76] These microorganisms can infect the vagina and cervix but do not ascend into the upper genital tract and cause PID (Figure 24-7). However, when the normal vaginal microbial flora is disrupted the pathogens can more easily ascend through the cervix. Many anaerobic bacteria have been implicated in increasing the risk of PID because they alter the pH of the vaginal environment and may decrease the integrity of the mucus blocking the cervical canal. Bacterial vaginosis (BV) is present in up to 66% of women with PID and other anaerobes, such as *Bacteroides,* and *Gardnerella vaginalis, Haemophilus influenzae,* and genital tract mycoplasmas *(Mycoplasma hominis, Mycoplasma genitalis* and *Ureaplasma urealyticum)* are frequently isolated from women with PID (see Chapter 26 for further discussion of BV). *Escherichia coli* may contribute to pelvic infections in older women. Therefore, although gonorrhea and chlamydia are the main pathogens in PID, the disease is really polymicrobial in origin and is treated with a broad spectrum of antibiotics to ensure that all the causative agents are eliminated.[75,76]

Once the infection is established within the uterus and fallopian/uterine tubes, gonorrhea or chlamydia, or both, may induce changes in the columnar epithelium that lines the upper reproductive tract, causing permanent damage and facilitating invasion by other microorganisms. The resultant inflammatory response causes localized edema and occasionally necrosis of the area. Gonorrhea gonococci attach to the fallopian tubes and excrete a substance toxic to the tubal mucosa, causing further inflammation and damage. Chlamydia enters the tubal cells and replicates, bursting the cell membrane as it reproduces, causing permanent scarring. Gonorrhea and chlamydia can spread to the abdominal cavity through the openings of the fallopian/uterine tubes. Other mechanisms that may contribute to PID include lymphatic drainage with parametrial spread of the infection.

Luckily, the rate of mortality from PID in the United States is fairly low. However, PID infection results in permanent changes to the ciliated epithelium of the fallopian or uterine tubes. A recent study found that one episode of mild, subclinical PID resulted in a 40% decrease in later pregnancy rates, and multiple episodes of PID further increase the risk of infertility.[72] Scarring caused by PID greatly increases the risk of later ectopic pregnancy by up to 10-fold.[77] Scarring and adhesions also can result in chronic pelvic pain[77] and, potentially, an increased risk of later uterine cancer.[78]

CLINICAL MANIFESTATIONS. The clinical manifestations of PID vary from sudden, severe abdominal pain with fever to no symptoms at all. An asymptomatic cervicitis may be present for some time before PID develops. Of women with salpingitis, 67% to 75% may have a subclinical infection. The first sign of the ascending infection may be the onset of low bilateral abdominal pain, most often characterized as dull and steady with a gradual onset. Symptoms are more likely to develop during or immediately after menstruation. The pain of PID may worsen with walking, intercourse, or other activities involving movement. Other manifestations of PID include dysuria (difficult or painful urination) and irregular bleeding.

BOX 24-6 DIAGNOSTIC CRITERIA FOR PELVIC INFLAMMATORY DISEASE

Minimum Criteria (One or More Needed for Diagnosis)

Cervical motion tenderness, *or*
Uterine tenderness, *or*
Adnexal tenderness

Additional Criteria That Increase Specificity of Diagnosis

Fever >38.3° C (101° F)
Mucopurulent cervical or vaginal discharge
Numerous white blood cells on saline wet prep
Elevated C-reactive protein
Elevated erythrocyte sedimentation rate
Documented infection with *Chlamydia trachomatis* or *Neisseria gonorrhoeae*

Definitive Criteria (*Not* Needed for Treatment)

Transvaginal ultrasound, magnetic resonance imaging, *or*
Doppler studies showing thickened and fluid-filled tubes
Laparoscopic visualization of PID-related abnormalities

Data from: Centers for Disease Control and Prevention: *MMWR* 59(RR-12), 2010; Yudin MH, Ross JDC: Pelvic Inflammatory disease. In Zenilman JM, Shahmanesh M, editors: *Sexually transmitted diseases*, pp 67–76, Sudbury, MA, 2012, Jones & Bartlett Learning.
PID, Pelvic inflammatory disease.

EVALUATION AND TREATMENT. PID often has limited or vague clinical symptoms, leading to undertreatment and long-term health effects.[72] Because PID is a substantial health risk to a woman, the Centers for Disease Control and Prevention (CDC) encourage clinicians to consider PID as a likely diagnosis when a sexually active woman has abdominal or pelvic tenderness and *one* of the following: cervical motion tenderness, uterine tenderness, or adnexal tenderness.[75] Box 24-6 lists the diagnostic criteria for PID. No labs or studies are needed to begin treatment, however, additional information can improve the specificity of diagnosis.[75] Abdominal pain in women can have many causes, and it is important to rule out other diagnoses (Figure 24-8); however, further studies to rule out other diagnoses can be done while treating for PID.[75]

Because of the significance of the complications of PID, rapid treatment is recommended even before the causative pathogen can be identified. Because treatment is empiric, it needs to be effective against a broad range of pathogens, especially chlamydia, gonorrhea, and anaerobic bacteria.[75] Treatment is usually outpatient unless the woman has symptoms of advanced infection, cannot take oral medications, is pregnant, or other pathologies cannot be excluded. The CDC-recommended outpatient regimen is shown in Box 24-7.[79] Although alternative treatment regimens are available, the growing antibiotic

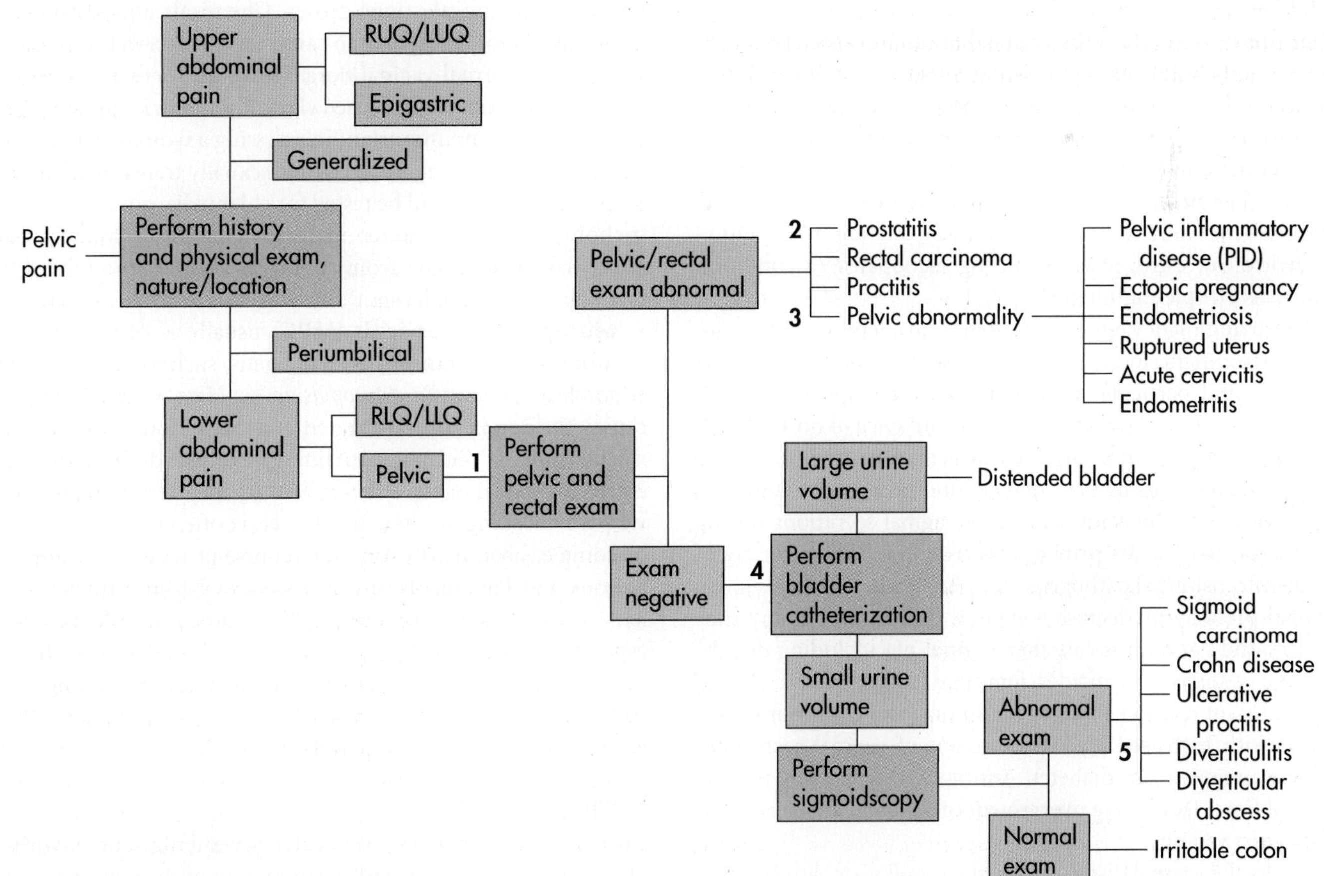

FIGURE 24-8 Diagnostic Algorithm for Pelvic Pain. *LLQ*, Left lower quadrant; *LUQ*, left upper quadrant; *RLQ*, right lower quadrant; *RUQ*, right upper quadrant.

BOX 24-7 CDC RECOMMENDED ORAL TREATMENT FOR PELVIC INFLAMMATORY DISEASE

Ceftriaxone: 250 mg IM in a single dose
Doxycycline: 100 mg orally twice a day for 14 days
WITH or WITHOUT
Metronidazole: 500 mg orally twice a day for 14 days

Data from Workowski KA, Berman S, Centers for Disease Control and Prevention (CDC): *MMWR Recom Rep* 59(RR-12):1–110, 2010; Centers for Disease Control and Prevention (CDC): *MMWR Morb Mortal Wkly Rep* 61(31):590–594, 2012.

resistance of gonorrhea limits antibiotic choices. The CDC is closely monitoring gonorrhea's antibiotic sensitivity and updates treatment guidelines periodically to reflect new information.[79] The most up-to-date treatment guidelines can be found on the CDC website.

Sexual partners of women with PID also should also receive treatment, even if they are asymptomatic. Women receiving treatment should be reevaluated by their care provider in 3 days to ensure antibiotic treatment is effective.[75] Because women with a history of PID are at increased risk for ectopic pregnancy, they should seek care as soon as they know they are pregnant because ectopic pregnancy is a major cause of maternal mortality.[74]

Vaginitis

Vaginitis is irritation of the vagina that can be caused by a variety of microorganisms, irritants, pathologies, or a disruption of the normal flora of the vagina. Vaginitis is characterized by an increase in white blood cells on saline wet prep examination. Vaginal irritation without white blood cells is known as **vaginosis.**[80] The major causes of vaginitis are overgrowth of normal flora, sexually transmitted diseases, and vaginal irritation related to low estrogen levels during menopause (a condition known as atropic vaginitis).[81]

The irritation of vaginitis is related to an alteration in the vaginal environment, including changes in skin integrity, immune reaction, and particularly vaginal pH. The pH of the vagina depends on cervical secretions and the presence of normal flora that help maintain an acidic environment. A neutral or alkaline pH normally occurs before puberty, after menopause, and during pregnancy. The acidic nature of vaginal secretions during the reproductive years provides protection against a variety of sexually transmitted pathogens (see Chapter 26). Changes in the vaginal pH may predispose a woman to infection. Many substances and conditions can alter vaginal pH including douching; use of soaps, spermicides, feminine hygiene sprays, semen, or deodorant menstrual pads or tampons; and conditions associated with increased glycogen content of vaginal secretions, such as pregnancy or diabetes. Antibiotics can destroy normal vaginal flora, facilitating overgrowth of *Candida albicans,* causing a yeast vaginitis.

Normally vaginal discharge is a clear, milky, or cloudy secretion with a slippery or clumpy texture. It is nonirritating, has a mild smell, and may yellow after drying. Throughout the menstrual cycle the amount and texture of a woman's discharge change in response to hormonal fluctuation. Vaginal secretions increase at the time of ovulation, during pregnancy (because of increased estrogen levels), and with sexual arousal; just before menstruation, vaginal discharge becomes thick and sticky. Unusual changes in the amount, color, or texture of vaginal discharge may signal an infection, especially if the discharge is copious, malodorous, or irritating. Irritation of the vaginal area may be the result of many factors.

Diagnosis of the cause of vaginitis is based on history, physical examination, and examination of the discharge by wet mount; treatment by physical symptoms alone is inadequate.[81] Treatment involves developing and maintaining an acidic environment, relieving symptoms (usually pruritus), and administering antimicrobial or antifungal medications to eradicate the infectious organism. If the infection can be sexually transmitted, a woman's partner also will be treated. Research suggests that probiotics, especially *Lactobacillus crispatus,* can encourage normal vaginal flora and decrease the incidence of vaginitis in women at risk for vaginitis.[82,83]

Cervicitis

Cervicitis is a nonspecific term used to describe inflammation of the cervix. The CDC defines cervicitis as having two diagnostic signs: a purulent or mucopurulent discharge from the cervical os or endocervical bleeding, or both, induced by gently introducing a cotton swab into the cervix.[75] Cervicitis can have infectious or noninfectious causes. Chemicals and substances introduced into the vagina can cause cervicitis as well as disruptions in the normal vaginal flora. However, there are conflicting definitions of cervicitis used clinically and in research.[84] Age and risk factors are important in assessing a woman with cervicitis. Younger women are at risk for sexually transmitted infections (STIs) and should be tested for chlamydia, gonorrhea, and trichomonas. Older women with cervicitis may have STIs but are at risk for irritation from abnormal vaginal flora related to low vaginal estrogen levels.

Mucopurulent cervicitis (MPC) usually is caused by one or more sexually transmitted pathogens, such as *Trichomonas,* gonorrhea, *Chlamydia, Mycoplasma,* or *Ureaplasma.* Infection causes the cervix to become red and edematous. A mucopurulent (mucus- and pus-containing) exudate drains from the external cervical os, and the individual may report vague pelvic pain, bleeding, or dysuria. The cervix often becomes friable, bleeding easily during sexual intercourse or with pelvic examinations and Papanicolaou (Pap) smears. Because mucopurulent cervicitis is a symptom of PID, women at risk for STIs, especially those less than 26 years old, should receive treatment for PID while awaiting results of microbial testing.[75] If the woman is not at risk for STIs, a thorough evaluation often reveals another cause for the inflammation.

Vulvodynia

Vulvodynia (also referred to as vulvitis, vestibulitis, or vulvovestibulitis) is chronic pain and inflammation of the vulva or vestibule, or both. In many cases it may represent several disorders without an identifiable cause. Vulvodynia is fairly common,

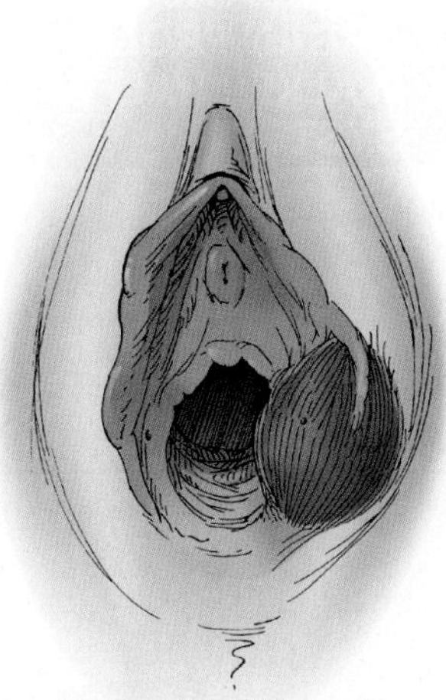

FIGURE 24-9 Inflammation of Bartholin Gland. (Modified from Gershenson DM et al: *Operative gynecology,* ed 2, Philadelphia, 2001, W.B. Saunders. In Fuller JK: *Surgical technology,* ed 6, Philadelphia, 2013, Saunders.)

affecting approximately 8% of women at some point in life.[85] Whereas the inflammation of vulvodynia may be caused by contact dermatitis (i.e., exposure to soaps, detergents, lotions, sprays, shaving, menstrual pads/tampons, perfumed toilet paper, tight-fitting clothes), the condition may be more complex and represent abnormalities in multiple systems, including vestibular mucosa, pelvic floor musculature, and CNS pain regulatory pathways.[86] The condition may also represent an autoimmune reaction, similar to fibromyalgia. Genetic and psychologic links have also been proposed and studied.[86] The mechanisms are poorly understood; thus vulvodynia is difficult to evaluate and treat. Vulvodynia can be classified as generalized or localized and provoked and unprovoked.[86] Assessment includes ruling out and treating conditions that may contribute to or cause vulvar inflammation (e.g., *Candida,* STI, seborrhea, psoriasis, lichen sclerosus, and contact dermatitis) and testing for vulvodynia with a cotton-tipped swab along the inner edge of the labia minora.

Women are advised to avoid potential irritants and to wear loose, cotton clothing. Vulvodynia may increase susceptibility to vaginal infection; likewise, it may be caused by vaginal infections (e.g., candidiasis, trichomoniasis) that spread to the labia, where they cause inflammation and edema. Studies on treatments are limited but suggest that women may benefit from behavioral treatment, topical lidocaine (Xylocaine), topical or systemic antidepressants, Botox injections into the affected nerve, or vestibulectomy.[86,87] Other skin diseases, such as tinea cruris, psoriasis, lichen sclerosus, and inflammation of the apocrine (sweat) glands, can involve the vulva (see Chapter 46).

Bartholinitis

Bartholinitis, or **Bartholin cyst,** is an inflammation of one or both of the ducts that lead from the introitus (vaginal opening) to the Bartholin/greater vestibular glands (Figure 24-9). The usual causes of bartholinitis are microorganisms that infect the lower female reproductive tract, such as streptococci, staphylococci, and sexually transmitted pathogens.

Infection or trauma causes inflammatory changes that narrow the distal portion of the duct, leading to obstruction and stasis of glandular secretions. The obstruction, or cyst, varies from 1 to 8 cm in diameter and is located in the posterolateral portion of the vulva. The cyst may be reddened and painful, and pus may be visible at the opening of the duct. Any exudate should be cultured and tested for gonorrhea and chlamydia. The individual may have symptoms of the initiating infection, fever, and malaise. Diagnosis of a Bartholin cyst is based on the clinical manifestations and the identification of infectious microorganisms.

Most Bartholin cysts are asymptomatic and require no treatment. However, if they are uncomfortable or show signs of infection, treatment is advised to prevent abscess formation. Treatment is controversial but involves broad-spectrum antibiotics for suspected infection. Some clinicians also attempt to drain the cyst using hot soaks, needle aspiration, insertion of a catheter, or marsupialization of the infected gland. No one treatment has proved to be superior in symptom relief and prevention of recurrence.[88]

Pelvic Organ Prolapse

The bladder, urethra, and rectum are supported by the endopelvic fascia and the perineal muscles, particularly the levator ani group. This muscular and fascial tissue loses tone and strength with aging and may fail to maintain the pelvic organs in the proper position. The pelvic area contains many organs and has the force of gravity and the abdominal contents pushing down on it. If the pelvic fascia and musculature is not firm, the pelvic organs to move to fill any space voids. With weak support, the bladder and rectum tend to push into the vagina and vaginal wall. The vagina is an opening in the pelvic musculature for intercourse and childbirth. (Chapter 23 contains a discussion of pelvic support structures.) However, as gravity acts on the pelvis, this opening becomes a weakness in the musculature support of the entire pelvic cavity and without proper support from the vaginal muscles and fascia, the uterus and bulging vaginal walls can begin to herniate through the vaginal opening.

Pelvic organ prolapse (POP) is the descent of one or more of the following: the vaginal wall, the uterus, or the apex of the vagina (after a hysterectomy).[89] Up to 61% of women have some version of POP on physical examination. However, most women have no symptoms. As the degree of prolapse increases, women feel more vaginal pressure. When prolapse becomes severe, the function of the surrounding organs can be altered. For instance, as the bladder is pulled posterior, incontinence and incomplete voiding become more common. As the bowel bulges into the vaginal space, defecation becomes more difficult. The severity of POP and its symptoms increase with age, and half of women older than age 50 have symptoms of POP. By 2050 it is estimated that 43.8 million women will have symptoms of POP.[90]

POP is thought to be caused by direct trauma, such as childbirth or pelvic surgery or damage to pelvic innervation, particularly the pudendal nerve. A strong familial tendency and possibly a multifactorial genetic component place some women at risk for the development of prolapse. Black and Asian women have the lowest risk of POP, and Hispanic women appear to

BOX 24-8 RISK FACTORS ASSOCIATED WITH PELVIC ORGAN PROLAPSE

Pregnancy
Menopause
- Aging*
- Hypoestrogenism

Chronically increased intra-abdominal pressure
- Coughing (lung disease)
- Constipation
- Obesity*

Pelvic floor trauma
- Vaginal childbirth
- Hysterectomy*

Genetic factors
- Race
- Connective tissue disorders

From Hughes D: Pelvic organ prolapse. In Schorge JO et al, editors: *Williams gynecology*, New York, 2008, McGraw-Hill.
*Most frequently cited factors.

BOX 24-9 PHYSICAL EXAMINATION TERMS FOR DESCRIPTION OF SUPPORT ABNORMALITIES

- Anterior vaginal wall prolapse
- Apical vaginal wall prolapse
- Posterior vaginal wall prolapse
- Cervical prolapse
- Perineal prolapse
- Rectal prolapse

Data from Hughes D: Pelvic organ prolapse. In Schorge JO et al, editors: *Williams gynecology*, pp 532–555, New York, 2008, McGraw-Hill; Jelovsek JE et al: *Lancet* 369(9566):1027–1038, 2007.

BOX 24-10 EVALUATION OF PELVIC ORGAN PROLAPSE (BADEN-WALKER HALFWAY SCORING SYSTEM)

Grade 0: Normal position, no prolapse
Grade 1: Descent halfway to the hymen
Grade 2: Descent reaches the hymen
Grade 3: Descent halfway past hymen
Note: Any type of prolapse (posterior, apical, anterior vaginal, uterine, etc.) can be graded using this system.

From Baden WF, Walker TA: *Clin Obstet Gynecol* 15:1070–1072, 1972.

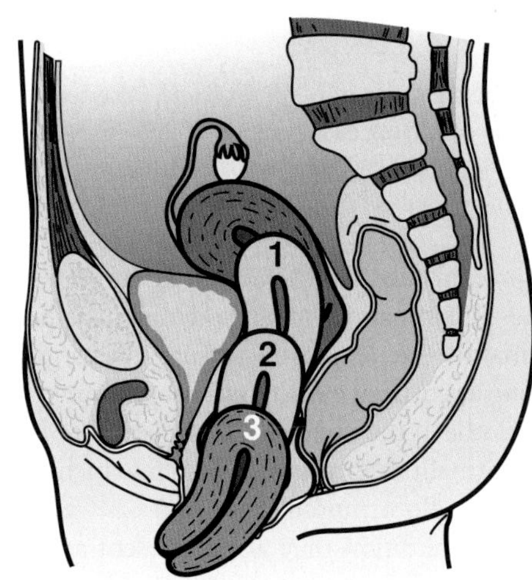

FIGURE 24-10 Degrees of Uterine Prolapse. **Grade 1** is minimal and rarely requires correction; **Grade 2** prolapse has moderate symptoms, and **Grade 3** prolapse is severe. The uterus is so low that the cervix protrudes from the vagina. (From Phillips N: *Berry & Kohn's operating room technique*, ed 12, Philadelphia, 2013, Mosby.)

have the highest risk.[91] Risk factors in nulliparous women are occupational activities that require heavy lifting or chronic medical conditions, such as chronic lung disease or refractory constipation. Some have neural abnormalities that interfere with the innervation of the levator ani. A list of risk factors is contained in Box 24-8.

The trend is to use terminology that describes physical examination findings, thus avoiding assumptions about structural involvement (Box 24-9). The terms *cystocele* and *rectocele* may be used when the structures involved (bladder, rectum) have been definitively identified (i.e., an anterior vaginal wall prolapse may or may not be a cystocele involving the urinary bladder) (see Figure 24-11, p. 819). Examining the woman in multiple positions and straining maximally provides the best information about the degree of pelvic organ relaxation.[89] Physical examination may be augmented with imaging by ultrasound, or magnetic resonance. Several systems are used to describe prolapse. One in widespread clinical use is based on physical examination findings (see Box 24-9) and uses a grading system to describe the extent of the prolapse (Box 24-10). Subjective reports regarding the symptoms and effects of POP can be assessed through direct questioning or questionnaires such as the Pelvic Floor Impact Questionnaire or the Pelvic Floor Distress Inventory.

Uterine prolapse is decent of the cervix or entire uterus into the vaginal canal (Figure 24-10). In severe cases the uterus falls completely through the vagina and protrudes from the introitus. Symptoms of other pelvic floor disorders also may be present. Treatment depends on the severity of symptoms and the physical condition of the woman. A common first-line treatment is a **pessary,** which is a removable mechanical device that holds the uterus in position. The pelvic fascia may be strengthened through Kegel exercises (repetitive isometric tightening and relaxing of the pubococcygeal muscles) or by estrogen therapy in menopausal women. Maintaining a healthy body mass index (BMI), preventing constipation, and treating chronic cough may help as well. Surgical repair with or without hysterectomy is the treatment of last resort. Women should be active participants in the decision-making surrounding treatment because they need to balance expectations for improvement with potential side effects.[92]

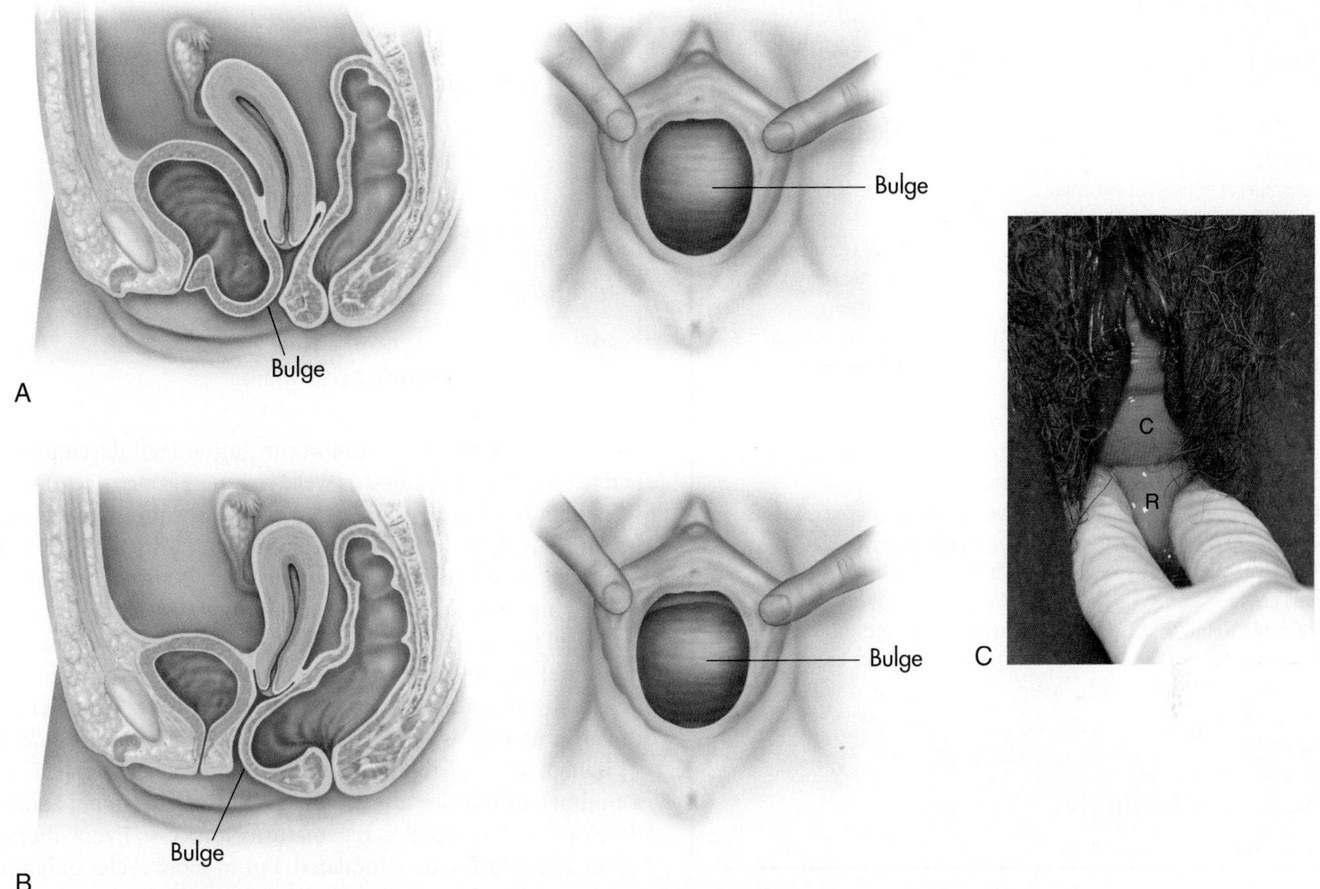

FIGURE 24-11 **Cystocele and Rectocele.** **A,** Grade 2: anterior vaginal wall prolapse. **B,** Grade 2: posterior wall prolapse. **C,** Photo showing cystocele *(C)* and rectocele *(R)*. (**A** and **B** from Seidel H et al: *Mosby's guide to physical examination,* ed 4, St Louis, 1999, Mosby. **C** from Seidel HM et al: *Mosby's guide to physical examination,* ed 7, St Louis, 2011, Mosby.)

Figure 24-11 shows vaginal prolapse caused by cystocele and rectocele. **Cystocele** is descent of a portion of the posterior bladder wall and trigone into the vaginal canal and usually is caused by the trauma of childbirth. In severe cases the bladder and anterior vaginal wall bulge outside the introitus. Usually symptoms are insignificant in mild to moderate cases. Increased bulging and descent of the anterior vaginal wall and urethra can be aggravated by vigorous activity, prolonged standing, sneezing, coughing, or straining and can be relieved by rest or assumption of a recumbent or prone position. If the prolapse is large, women may complain of vaginal pressure. Occasionally a cystocele causes significant residual urine and an increased rate of bladder infections.

Medical management can include vaginal pessary, Kegel exercises (prophylactic use produces the best outcome), and estrogen therapy for postmenopausal women. Surgical correction is used for severe anatomic injury unresponsive to medical treatment (see What's New? Vaginal Mesh).

A **rectocele** is the bulging of the rectum and posterior vaginal wall into the vaginal canal. During childbirth women may sustain damage that can lead to a rectocele, but symptoms usually do not occur until several years after menopause.[89] Familial and genetic predisposition and bowel habits contribute to rectocele development. Lifelong chronic constipation and straining may

WHAT'S NEW?

Vaginal Mesh

Because pelvic organ prolapse is often a result of weakened pelvic fascia and musculature, a surgical mesh was developed to improve pelvic support. This mesh was designed to be placed surgically along the area needing support. The goal was to have the woman's tissues grow through the mesh and provide consistent, long-term support. However, women who received the surgical mesh had a high rate of complications, including infection and persistent post-operative pain. In many cases the mesh eroded through the tissue, protruding into the vagina and perforating other organs. In addition, the mesh may shrink over time causing vaginal shortening, tightening, and pain.

Some large studies have shown a benefit from mesh use for some women. However, once implanted, the mesh is difficult to remove if not effective, resulting in long-term pain and the need for intensive surgeries and repairs. The U.S. Food and Drug Administration has issued several warnings about the mesh to caution women and practitioners and encourage fully informed consent about the risks and benefits of mesh placement.

Data from U.S. Food and Drug Administration: FDA safety communication: UPDATE on serious complications associated with transvaginal placement of surgical mesh for pelvic organ prolapse, 2010. Available at http://www.fda.gov/MedicalDevices/Safety/AlertsandNotices/ucm262435.htm. Accessed January 21, 2013; Maher C et al: *Cochrane Database Syst Rev* (4):CD004014, 2010.

BOX 24-11 PELVIC ORGAN PROLAPSE: SYMPTOMS AND TREATMENTS

SYMPTOMS	TREATMENT
Urinary Sensation of incomplete emptying of bladder Urinary incontinence Urinary frequency/urgency Bladder "splinting" to accomplish voiding **Bowel** Constipation or feeling of rectal fullness or blockage Difficult defecation Stool or flatus incontinence **Urgency** Manual "splinting" of posterior vaginal wall to accomplish defecation **Pain and Bulging** Vaginal, bladder, rectum Pelvic pressure, bulging, pain Lower back pain **Sexual** Dyspareunia Decreased sensation, lubrication, arousal	Depending on age of woman and cause and severity of the condition: Isometric exercise to strengthen the pubococcygeal muscle (Kegels) Estrogen to improve tone and vascularity of fascial support (postmenopausal) Pessary (a removable device) to hold pelvic organs in place **Surgical** Reconstructive: autologous grafts; synthetic mesh/sling Obliterative (most extreme) Weight loss Avoidance of constipation Treatment of cough/lung conditions

produce or aggravate a rectocele. Although most rectoceles are asymptomatic, larger ones cause vaginal pressure, rectal fullness, and incomplete bowel evacuation. If rectoceles are severe, defecation is difficult and can be facilitated by applying manual pressure to the posterior vaginal wall. Medical treatment focuses on the management and prevention of constipation and, if needed, the use of a pessary. Rectocele alone (without associated enterocele, uterine prolapse, and cystocele) seldom requires surgery.[92]

An **enterocele** is herniation of the rectouterine pouch into the rectovaginal septum (between the rectum and posterior vaginal wall). It can be congenital or acquired. Congenital enterocele rarely causes symptoms or progresses in size. Enteroceles also can result from a muscular weakness caused by previous surgery, especially surgeries through the vagina, or pelvic relaxation disorders, such as uterine prolapse, cystocele, and rectocele. Most large enteroceles are found in grossly obese and older adults and can be complicated by rupture or complete eversion of the vagina with trophic ulceration, edema, and fibrosis. Treatment is surgical. Box 24-11 summarizes the symptoms and treatments of POP.

Benign Growths and Proliferative Conditions

Benign Ovarian Cysts

Benign cysts of the ovary may occur at any time during the life span, but are most common during the reproductive years and, in particular, at the extremes of those years (Figure 24-12). An increase in benign ovarian cysts occurs when hormonal imbalances are more common, around puberty and menopause.[93]

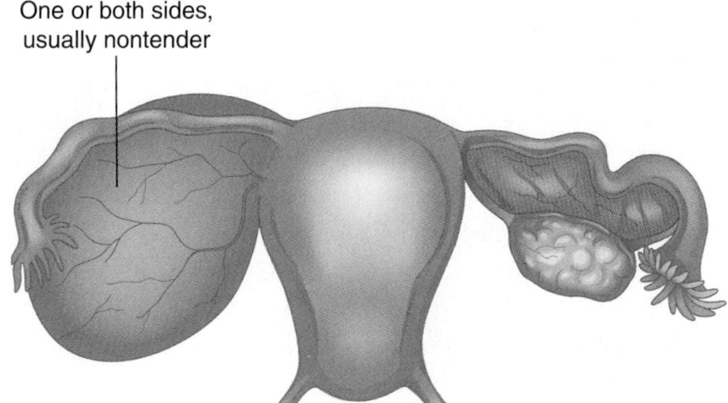

FIGURE 24-12 Ovarian Cyst.

However, ovarian masses can occur during fetal development and throughout childhood as well.[94]

Benign ovarian cysts are quite common and are the fourth leading diagnosis for gynecologic hospital admissions.[95] Two common causes of benign ovarian enlargement in ovulating women are follicular cysts and corpus luteum cysts. These cysts are called **functional cysts** because they are caused by variations of normal physiologic events. Follicular and corpus luteum cysts are usually unilateral. They are typically 5 to 6 cm in diameter but can grow as large as 8 to 10 cm. Most women are asymptomatic.

Benign cysts of the ovary are produced when a follicle or a number of follicles are stimulated but no dominant follicle develops and completes the maturity process. Every month about 120 follicles are stimulated, but in most cycles only one succeeds in ovulating a mature ova. Normally, during the early follicular phase of the menstrual cycle, follicles of the ovary respond to hormonal signals from the pituitary gland. The pituitary produces FSH to mature follicles in the ovary. As the follicles enlarge, granulosa cells in the follicle multiply and secrete estradiol (a form of estrogen). As a dominant follicle develops, it secretes higher levels of estradiol, which stimulates the LH surge that comes from the pituitary. A small cyst on the ovary during the follicular phase is normal. The LH surge stimulates the follicle to rupture, releasing the ova and transforming the granulosa cells of the dominant follicle into the corpus luteum. If the dominant follicle develops properly before ovulation, the corpus luteum becomes vascularized and secretes progesterone. Progesterone arrests development of other follicles in both ovaries in that cycle. LH, proteolytic enzymes, and prostaglandins trigger follicular rupture and release of the ovum.

Follicular cysts can be caused by a transient condition in which the dominant follicle fails to rupture or one or more of the nondominant follicles fail to regress. This disturbance is not well understood. It may be that the hypothalamus does not receive or send a message strong enough to increase FSH levels needed to develop or mature a dominant follicle. The hypothalamus monitors blood levels of estradiol and progesterone; when FSH is low, estradiol does not increase enough to stimulate LH. Evidence indicates that when progesterone is not being produced, the hypothalamus releases GnRH to increase the FSH level.[96] FSH continues to stimulate follicles to mature, and the granulosa cells grow and, presumably, estradiol increases. This abnormal cycle continues to stimulate follicular size and causes follicular cysts to develop. Clinical symptoms of follicular cysts or even a single cyst are bloating, swollen and tender breasts, and heavy or irregular menses. After several subsequent cycles in which hormone levels once again follow a regular cycle and progesterone levels are restored, cysts usually are absorbed or regress.

Follicular cysts can vary in size and symptoms from one episode to the next and often can recur. Most are fluid filled; the more solid an ovarian cyst, the greater the chance of malignancy. Follicular cysts can be treated with oral contraceptives because they block the HPG axis, effectively quieting the ovary.

A **corpus luteum cyst** is normally formed by the granulosa cells left behind after ovulation. This cyst is highly vascularized but limited in size and spontaneously regresses as part of the normal menstrual cycle. However, an abnormal or hemorrhagic cyst may develop because of a hormonal imbalance in low LH and progesterone levels causing an inadequate development of the corpus luteum. In some cases, however, large cysts can rupture, causing hemorrhage.[33]

Corpus luteum cysts are less common than follicular cysts, but luteal cysts typically cause more symptoms, particularly if they rupture. Manifestations include dull pelvic pain and amenorrhea or delayed menstruation, followed by irregular or heavier than usual bleeding. Rupture occasionally occurs and can cause massive bleeding with excruciating pain; immediate surgery may be required. Corpus luteum cysts usually regress spontaneously in nonpregnant women. A corpus luteum cyst is a normal finding within the first trimester of pregnancy as the corpus luteum produces progesterone to support the pregnancy until the placenta is established.[97] Following the development of a large, painful, or hemorrhagic cyst, oral contraceptives can be used to suppress ovarian function and prevent future cysts.

Dermoid cysts are ovarian teratomas that contain elements of all three germ layers; they are common ovarian neoplasms. These growths may contain mature tissue including skin, hair, sebaceous and sweat glands, muscle fibers, cartilage, and bone. Dermoid cysts are usually asymptomatic and are found incidentally on pelvic examination. However, cysts should be carefully evaluated for removal because they have malignant potential.[98]

Torsion of the ovary is a rare complication of ovarian cysts or tumors or enlargement of the ovary and can occur in girls or women. If a cyst is large enough it can cause the ovary to twist on its ligaments, pinching off blood supply to the ovary and causing extreme pain. Ovarian torsion is rare but is a gynecologic emergency. Individuals present with acute, severe unilateral abdominal or pelvic pain. Ovarian torsion is treated surgically.[99]

Endometrial Polyps

An **endometrial polyp** is a benign mass of endometrial tissue, covered by a surface epithelium, and contains a variable amount of glands, stroma, and blood vessels. Endometrial polyps can occur anywhere within the uterus. Polyps are morphologically diverse and usually classified as hyperplastic, atrophic (or inactive), or functional. In the last case, the surface epithelium may be "out of phase" with other endometrial tissue. Hyperplastic polyps are often pedunculated and may be mistaken for endometrial hyperplasia or, if large, adenosarcoma (Figure 24-13).

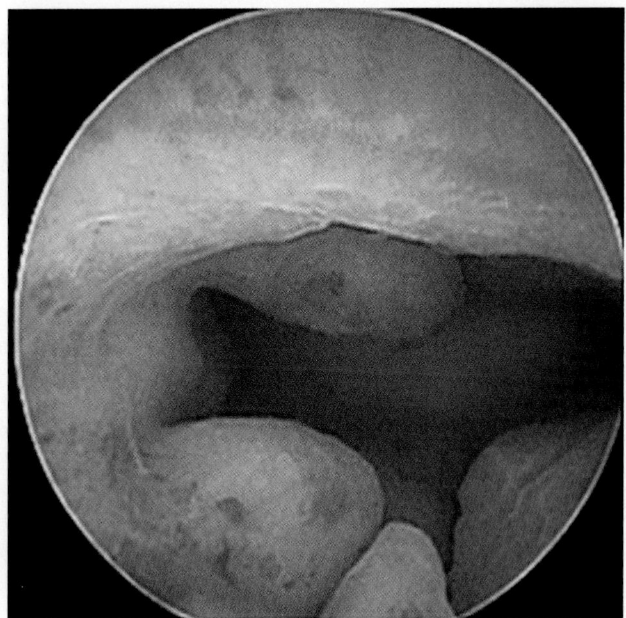

FIGURE 24-13 Uterine Polyps Visible Through Hysteroscopy. (From Cheng C et al: *J Minim Invasive Gynecol* 16[6]:739–742, 2009.)

Although polyps most often develop in women between ages 40 and 50, they can occur at all ages. These are often related to estrogen stimulation. As many as 35% of women with abnormal uterine bleeding are found to have polyps.[100]

Endometrial polyps are a common cause of intermenstrual or excessive menstrual bleeding. Diagnosis is made by transvaginal sonography or hysteroscopy. Risk factors include obesity, tamoxifen use, hypertension, and estrogenic states (i.e., anovulatory cycles and unopposed estrogen). Malignancy is rare (up to 4.7% of polyps have evidence of malignancy) and polyps that cause abnormal bleeding have twice the rate of malignancy of asymptomatic polyps.[101] Coexistence of a separate endometrial atypical hyperplasia or adenocarcinoma is common. Uterine polyps have a high rate of spontaneous resolution but have been associated with suboptimal fertility.[102] Polypectomy can be performed through hysteroscopy for symptomatic women, for those at risk for malignancy, or women who are struggling to conceive.

Leiomyomas

Leiomyomas, commonly called **myomas** or **uterine fibroids,** are benign smooth muscle tumors in the myometrium (Figure 24-14). Leiomyomas are the most common benign tumors of the uterus, affecting as many as 70% to 80% of all women, and most remain small, asymptomatic, and clinically insignificant.[103] Prevalence increases in women ages 30 to 50 but decreases with menopause. The incidence of leiomyomas in black and Asian women is two to five times higher than that in white women.[103] Complications related to leiomyomas are the number one reason for gynecologic hospitalizations.[95]

The cause of uterine leiomyomas is unknown, although their size appears to be related to estrogen, progesterone, growth factors, angiogenesis, and apoptosis. There is a genetic component to fibroids, and the leiomyomas exhibit chromosomal

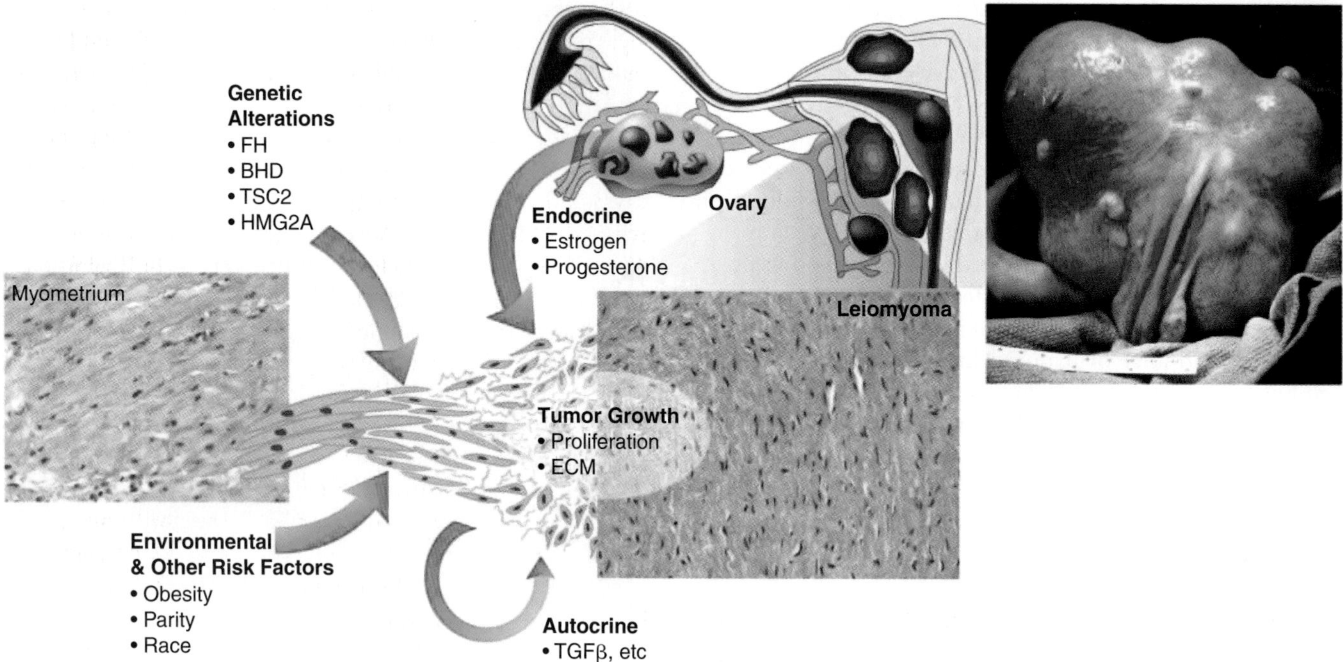

FIGURE 24-14 **Etiology of Uterine Leiomyomas.** Leiomyomas are heterogeneous in their natural history and etiology. Hereditary defects in *FH, BHD,* and *TSC2* genes and somatic alterations affecting *HMG2A* genes contribute to the development of leiomyomas, as do risk factors such as obesity, parity, and race. Tumor growth occurs by an increase in tumor cell number and extracellular matrix production and is promoted by both endocrine and autocrine growth factors. (From Walker CL, Stewart EA: *Science* 308:1589–1592, 2005.)

changes within their tissues.[103] Leiomyomas are estrogen- and progesterone-sensitive and are found to have increased numbers of estrogen receptors.[104] Uterine leiomyomas are not seen before menarche, and those that develop during the reproductive years generally decrease in size after menopause. Occurrence is multifactorial but often linked with estrogen exposure. Tumors in pregnant women may enlarge rapidly but often decrease in size after the end of the pregnancy. Risk factors for fibroids include nulliparity, obesity, PCOS, diabetes mellitus, black race, and hypertension.[104]

PATHOPHYSIOLOGY. Most leiomyomas occur in multiples in the fundus of the uterus, although they may occur singly and throughout the uterus. Leiomyomas are classified as subserous, submucous, or intramural according to their location within the various layers of the uterine wall (Figure 24-15). Uterine leiomyomas are usually firm and surrounded by a connective tissue layer. Unlike cancer, leiomyomas are unable to cause blood vessel proliferation to support their growth. Degeneration and necrosis may occur when a large leiomyoma outgrows its blood supply; the ensuing tissue necrosis causes pain.

CLINICAL MANIFESTATIONS. The major clinical manifestations of leiomyomas are abnormal uterine bleeding, pain, and symptoms related to pressure on nearby structures. Fibroids also may contribute to infertility and subfertility. The leiomyoma may distort the uterine cavity and increase the endometrial surface area. This increase may account for the increased menstrual bleeding that is associated with leiomyomas. Pain is not an early symptom but tends to occur with the devascularization of larger leiomyomas. It is also associated with blood vessel compression that limits blood supply to adjacent structures. Symptoms of abdominal pressure are slow to develop, apparently because the tumor is relatively slow growing, enabling adjacent structures to adapt to pressure. Pressure on the bladder may contribute to urinary frequency, urgency, and dysuria. Pressure on the ureter may cause it to become distended "upstream" from the pressure point; rectosigmoid pressure may lead to constipation. A sensation of abdominal or genital heaviness may be felt with larger tumors.

EVALUATION AND TREATMENT. Uterine leiomyomas are suspected when the bimanual examination discloses uterine enlargement and irregular, nontender nodularity of the uterus. Pelvic sonography or MRI confirms diagnosis.[104] Treatment depends on the symptoms, tumor size, age, reproductive status, overall health of the individual, and the woman's preference.[103] Most myomas are asymptomatic and can be managed by observation only. Medical treatment for symptomatic women not desiring pregnancy is aimed at shrinking the myoma, or reducing symptoms, or both. Some leiomyomas shrink in response to oral contraceptives, however, oral contraceptive pills (OCPs) may enhance growth, so should be monitored carefully. An LNG-IUD may be helpful for women who wish to reduce their bleeding and decrease the size of the tumors, if their uterine cavity is not completely blocked by large fibroids. GnRH agonists are usually a temporary management for those close to menopause or as a presurgical treatment. GnRH side effects related to decreased estrogen, including hot flashes and osteoporosis, limit its usefulness. Various selective estrogen receptor modulators have been studied in conjunction with GnRH agonists and appear effective.[103] Progesterone receptor agonists, such as mifepristone (RU486), also have shown some effectiveness in shrinking

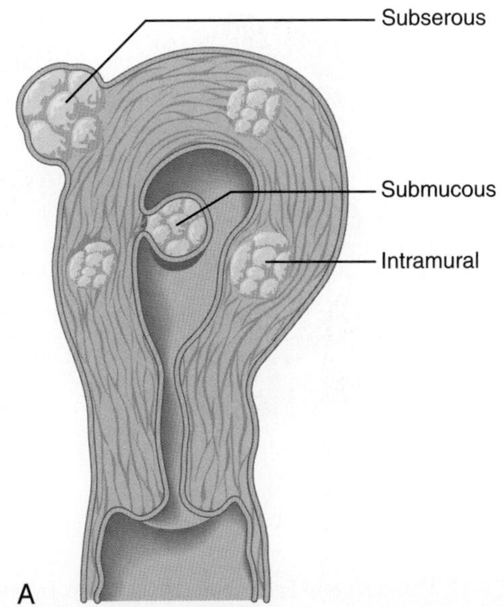

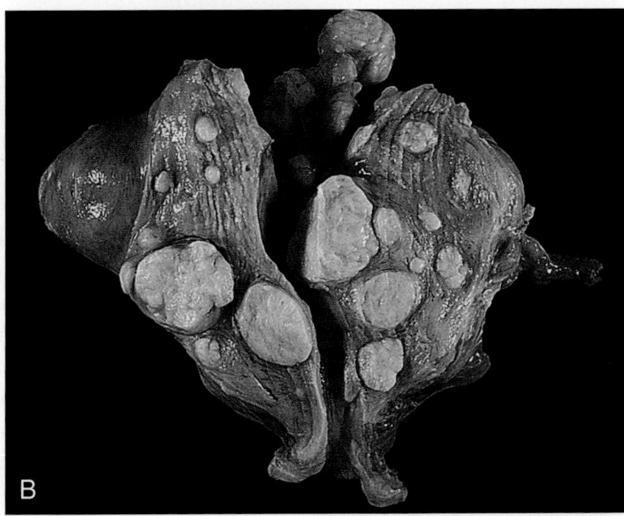

FIGURE 24-15 Leiomyomas. A, Uterine section showing whorl-like appearance and locations of leiomyomas, which are also called uterine fibroids. **B,** Multiple leiomyomas in sagittal section. Typical, well-circumscribed, solid, light gray nodules distort uterus. (**B** from Damjanov I, Linder J: *Pathology: a color atlas,* St Louis, 2000, Mosby.)

leiomyomas. Surgical treatments are commonly used but may be decreasing in frequency. Hysterectomy is commonly performed for bleeding and pain related to fibroids. Myomectomy, or removal of the fibroid from the muscle of the uterus, may be less invasive than a full hysterectomy and remains the standard of cure for women wishing to preserve their fertility. Newer less-invasive treatments that show promise include uterine artery embolization, mifepristone, and MRI-guided ultrasonography to coagulate areas of the fibroid, causing tissue destruction and involution. The benefits and risks of each therapy should be carefully explored with women who experience severe symptoms.[103]

Adenomyosis

Adenomyosis is the presence of islands of endometrial glands surrounded by benign endometrial stroma within the uterine myometrium. Endometrial cells migrate into the myometrial layer because of an unknown mechanism. Estrogen and progesterone likely play a role and, perhaps, metaplasia of müllerian tissue. Unlike endometriosis, this tissue does not respond to cyclic hormone changes. It is more commonly found during the late reproductive years; however, because adenomyosis is generally diagnosed after hysterectomy, time of diagnosis may not correspond with incidence. Adenomyosis has been found in up to 48% of hysterectomy specimens from otherwise normal women; rates are higher for women taking tamoxifen.[105] Parity also increases the risk for adenomyosis. Adenomyosis may be asymptomatic or may be associated with abnormal menstrual bleeding, dysmenorrhea, uterine enlargement, and uterine tenderness during menstruation. Secondary dysmenorrhea becomes increasingly severe as disease progresses. On bimanual examination the uterus is diffusely enlarged, globular, and most tender just before or after menstruation. Diagnosis is confirmed with ultrasound or MRI.[106] Treatment is symptomatic, similar to dysmenorrhea (i.e., NSAIDs, combined oral contraceptives [COCs], and perhaps LNG-IUDs). Surgical treatment includes resection of localized areas of adenomyosis (though this is difficult) or, if severe, hysterectomy. Uterine artery embolization and LNG-IUDs have shown good initial results but need further testing.[107,108]

Endometriosis

Endometriosis is the presence of functioning endometrial tissue or implants outside the uterus. Like normal endometrial tissue, the ectopic (out of place) endometrium responds to the hormonal fluctuations of the menstrual cycle.

The incidence of endometriosis is difficult to determine, particularly in asymptomatic adolescent and fertile women. It is estimated that 11% of reproductive-age women have endometriosis, though for most it is mild.[109] In addition, as many as 50% of women evaluated for pelvic pain, infertility, or a pelvic mass are diagnosed as having endometriosis. Moreover, the frequency and severity of symptoms do not correlate well with the extent or site of lesions.[109] A large study has found that women with endometriosis are at greater risk for cancers, especially ovarian cancer.[110]

The cause of endometriosis is not known, but several theories have been proposed. In 1927 Sampson[111] proposed that endometriosis is caused by the implantation of endometrial cells during **retrograde menstruation,** in which menstrual fluids move through the fallopian tubes and into the pelvic cavity (Figure 24-16). It is now known that retrograde menstruation occurs in almost all women; however, not all women develop endometriosis.

Another theory is that women with endometriosis have impaired cellular and humoral immunity. Alterations in cytokine and growth factor signaling have been identified. Cytotoxic T-cell and natural killer (NK) cell activity has been found to be depressed. At the same time, increased numbers of macrophages appear to be stimulating endometrial cell proliferation outside the uterus. An autoimmune response is also suspected.[112] Such alterations may cause the body to tolerate ectopic implantation of endometrial cells. Researchers also have proposed that endometrial cells spread through the lymphatic

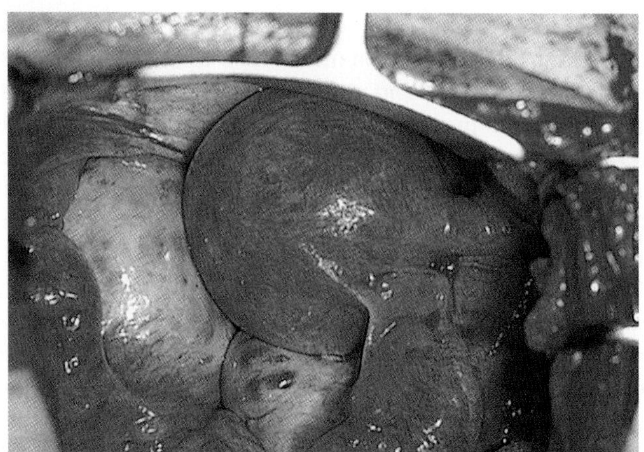

FIGURE 24-16 Endometriosis. The uterus is distended, and retrograde spill of menstrual loss has led to the development of endometriosis *(dark purple patches).* (From Symonds EM, Macpherson MBA: *Color atlas of obstetrics and gynecology,* London, 1994, Mosby-Wolfe.)

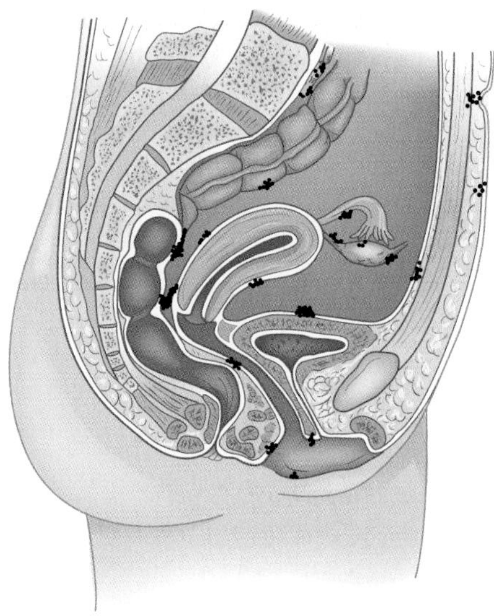

FIGURE 24-17 Pelvic Sites of Endometrial Implantation. Endometrial cells may enter the pelvic cavity during retrograde menstruation.

or vascular systems or that multipotential cells in the epithelial coverings of reproductive organs are somehow stimulated to develop into endometrial and metaplastic cells. A genetic predisposition to endometriosis has been documented. Some genetic polymorphisms have been identified.

PATHOPHYSIOLOGY. Endometrial implants can occur throughout the body but generally occur in the pelvic and abdominal cavities. The most common sites of implantation are the ovaries, uterine ligaments, rectovaginal septum, and pelvic peritoneum (Figure 24-17). Other sites of implantation are the sigmoid colon, small intestine, rectum, appendix, bladder, uterus, vulva, vagina, cervix, lymph nodes, extremities, pleural cavity, lungs, laparotomy scars, and hernial sacs.

Cyclic changes depend on the blood supply of the implants and the presence of glandular and stromal cells. Given that blood supply is sufficient, the ectopic endometrium proliferates, breaks down, and bleeds with the normal menstrual cycle. The bleeding causes inflammation, triggering a cascade of cellular inflammatory mediators, including cytokines, chemokines, growth factors, and protective factors such as secretory leukocyte protease inhibitor and superoxide dismutase.[112] The inflammation may lead to fibrosis, scarring, adhesions, and pain.

CLINICAL MANIFESTATIONS. The clinical manifestations of endometriosis can mimic other disease processes (i.e., PID, irritable bowel syndrome, ovarian cysts). Symptoms are variable in frequency and severity and include primarily infertility and pain,[112] dysmenorrhea, dyschezia (pain on defecation), dyspareunia (pain on intercourse), and, less commonly, constipation and abnormal vaginal bleeding. If implants are located within the pelvis they can cause an asymptomatic pelvic mass having irregular, movable nodules and a fixed, retroverted uterus. Most symptoms of endometriosis can be explained by the proliferation, breakdown, and bleeding of the ectopic endometrial tissue with subsequent formation of adhesions. In most instances, however, the degree of endometriosis is not related to the frequency or severity of symptoms.[109] Dysmenorrhea, for example, does not appear to be related to the degree of endometriosis. With involvement of the rectovaginal septum or the uterosacral ligaments, dyspareunia develops. Dyschezia occurs with bleeding of ectopic endometrium in the rectosigmoid musculature and subsequent fibrosis.

Twenty-five percent to 40% of women with infertility have endometriosis. The link between endometriosis and infertility is strong, yet the degree of disease and infertility is not as closely associated. That is, women with untreated minimal to mild disease may have high pregnancy rates or may experience infertility.[112] The exact mechanism for infertility in women with endometriosis is unknown. Infertility may result from mechanical interference with ovulation or ovum transport through the fallopian tube because of adhesions and the effects of inflammation and cytokine activity. However, the infertility also could be a result of the underlying autoimmune disorder that caused the endometriosis.[112] There are conflicting reports regarding the effect of endometriosis on sperm activity. An increased phagocytosis of spermatozoa by macrophages has been observed. The uterine endometrium in women with endometriosis appears to have an overactive response to estrogen and an underactive response to progesterone, impairing the endometrial receptivity to blastocyst implantation, decreasing the chance of successful pregnancy.[113]

EVALUATION AND TREATMENT. A presumptive diagnosis can be made based on clinical manifestations but laparoscopy is required for definitive diagnosis of endometriosis. A uniform classification system that includes both extent and severity has been developed (Table 24-4) but still does not correlate well with a woman's symptoms. Treatment is aimed at preventing or decreasing progression and spread, alleviating pain, and restoring fertility. Current therapies include suppression of ovulation with noncyclic estrogen-progestin COCs, depomedroxyprogesterone acetate (DMPA), danazol (which diminishes midcycle LH surge), GnRH agonists/analogs (to block the menstrual cycle), gestrinone (a 19-nortestosterone derivative and antiprogestational steroid), mifepristone (RU486) (an

TABLE 24-4 CLASSIFICATION SYSTEM FOR ENDOMETRIOSIS (REQUIRES LAPAROSCOPIC VISUALIZATION)

STAGE	DEGREE OF INVASIVENESS
I	Minimal
II	Mild
III	Moderate

Data from *Fertil Steril* 67(5):817–821, 1997.
Classification system also documents the location of lesions and presence of adhesions.

antiprogestational and antiglucocorticoid agent that can inhibit ovulation and disrupt endometrial integrity), and atrophy of endometrium with progestins, including DMPA, oral progestins, or an LNG-IUD.[112,114] A newer therapy is an injectable GnRH antagonist, which produces immediate inhibition of gonadotropin release but does not have substantially improved success rates when compared with other therapies.[115] Conservative surgical treatment includes laparoscopic removal of endometrial implants with conventional or laser techniques and presacral neurectomy for severe dysmenorrhea. Effectiveness may be increased when medical regimens are combined with surgical techniques. All treatments have risks or side effects, and recurrent symptoms develop in the majority of women within a few years, even with surgical treatments. Women should be fully informed about all options and carefully weigh the risk-to-benefit ratio of nonreversible treatments.[114]

Cancer

Malignant tumors of the female reproductive system are common. Cancers of the female reproductive tract can often grow large before causing pain because the pelvis and abdomen are poorly innervated and designed to accommodate a growing fetus. Reproductive tract cancers are more likely to be diagnosed early if there are symptoms. Uterine cancer is the fourth leading cancer diagnosis in women but is only the eighth leading cause of death in part because symptoms of vaginal bleeding prompt women to seek treatment. Ovarian cancer, on the other hand occurs less frequently, at 3% of total cancer diagnoses in women, but is the fifth leading cause of death from cancer related to its lack of symptoms and difficult detection.[1] Cervical cancer also has minimal symptoms until late in the process, but is easy to detect early with Pap smears. Three percent of cancers in women begin in the cervix but the death rate from cervical cancer has plummeted since the advent of screening techniques.[1]

Cervical Cancer

Cancer of the cervix is the leading cancer-related death in most of Africa, Central America, and South-Central Asia; however, it has a lower prevalence in the United States.[1,116] In the United States, the rates of invasive cancer have steadily decreased (a 75% reduction since the 1960s) and mortality rates caused by cervical cancer have declined (more than 45% since the early 1970s) largely because of the increased prevalence and frequency of cervical cancer screening with the Pap smear. In 2013, the American Cancer Society estimated 12,340 new cases of cervical invasive cancer and 4030 cervical cancer deaths.[1]

PATHOGENESIS. It is established that cervical cancer is almost exclusively caused by cervical human papillomavirus (HPV) infection. Infection with "high-risk" (oncogenic) types of HPV (predominantly 16 and 18) is a necessary precursor to development of the precancerous cell changes, known as dysplasia, of the cervix that leads to invasive cancer (also see Chapter 12). Precancerous dysplasia, also called *cervical intraepithelial carcinoma (CIN)* and *cervical carcinoma in situ (CIS),* is a more advanced form of the cell changes. Luckily, these cell changes can be detected noninvasively through examination of the cervical cells. The cells can be destroyed to prevent cancer development if dysplasia can be detected early.

Fifty percent of adolescents and young women acquire HPV (predominantly high-risk types) within 3 years of initiation of sexual intercourse, and it is estimated that 8.8% of all women ages 14 to 59 have persistent infection with high-risk HPV strains[117] (also see Chapter 26). Young women are especially vulnerable to HPV because of their cervical anatomy. There are two main cell types of the cervix: squamous epithelium cells and columnar epithelial cells. Squamous epithelial cells in older women cover the portions of the cervix that protrude into the vagina, and columnar epithelial cells line the inner portions of the cervical canal. The line where the two cells types meet, known as the transformation zone, is very vulnerable to the oncogenic effects of HPV. The location of the transformation zone changes as girls and women age and in response to estrogen and vaginal pH changes. In girls and young women a large portion of their cervix is covered with columnar epithelium, a condition known as squamous metaplasia.[118] As women age, the transformation zone moves as the squamous epithelium covers the surface of the cervix. Therefore, the younger a woman is when she contacts HPV, the more sensitive cervical cells are exposed. This is one reason vaccinations against HPV are aimed at women prior to the initiation of sexual activity.[118]

Most HPV infections are cleared by the immune system; the vast majority of infections do not cause cervical cancer. For this reason, screening for cervical cancer prior to age 21 is not recommended. Previous efforts at early screening resulted in many young women receiving treatments on their cervix. These treatments destroyed or removed cervical cells and in many cases altered the structural integrity of the cervix, resulting in an increase in preterm births in women treated without substantially decreasing the later rates of cervical cancer.[119]

It is unknown why some women are able to clear HPV infection and others cannot. Smoking has been shown to increase the risks of persistent infection and later development of cervical cancer.[120] In addition, certain gene polymorphisms on the genes that control epidermal growth factor increase the risk that HPV infection will lead to invasive cancer.[121] Anything that affects the integrity of the immune system may affect the later risk of cervical cancer including poor nutrition and chronic stress.[122] HIV infection greatly increases the risk that women infected with HPV will develop cervical cancer, and women with HIV should be screened for cervical cancer more

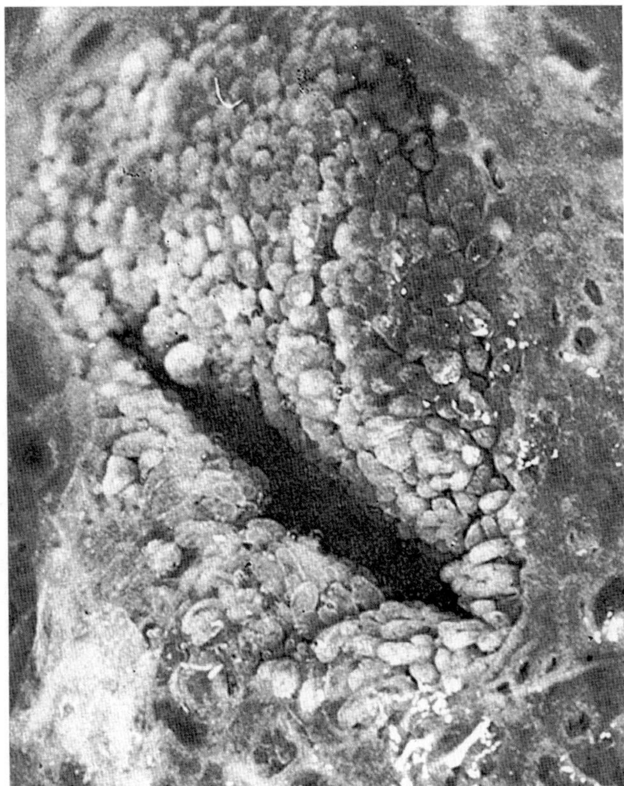

FIGURE 24-18 Cervical Carcinoma In Situ. Typical transformation zone, where the columnar (grapelike) epithelium is replaced by metaplastic epithelium. At its outer edge the metaplastic epithelium adjoins the squamous epithelium, which extends into the vagina. (From Coppleson M, Pixley E, Reid B: *Colposcopy: a scientific approach to the cervix in health and disease,* Springfield, IL, 1971, Charles C Thomas.)

frequently than women without HIV.[123] In addition, infection with *Chlamydia trachomatis* has been correlated with later risk for cancer.[120] It is hoped that the widespread use of the HPV vaccine in boys and girls will decrease rates of invasive cervical, genital, and anal cancers over the next several decades.[124]

Carcinoma in situ is most likely to develop in the squamous-columnar junction—the transformation zone—where the columnar epithelium of the cervical lining meets the squamous epithelium of the outer cervix and vagina (Figure 24-18). In this zone, columnar epithelium is constantly being replaced by squamous epithelium in a process known as *metaplasia.* Metaplasia is thought to be affected by hormonal levels; change in cervical epithelium is not understood as well as endometrial tissue change in response to fluctuating hormones. Because metaplastic cells are at increased risk of incorporating foreign or abnormal genetic material, neoplastic changes are most common in the transformation zone.

Many chromosomes may contain genes that relate to HPV-linked cervical cancer.[125] Like other cancers, cervical cancer requires the accumulation of genetic alterations for carcinogenesis to occur. However, the discrete tumor-suppressor gene locations have yet to be identified.[125] Several chromosome regions with recurrent loss of heterozygosity (LOH) have been identified (also see Chapter 12). In addition, other genes may influence a woman's receptivity to HPV.[121] For instance, HPV

WHAT'S NEW?

Cervical Cancer Screening in the Developing World

The problem with the use of the conventional Papanicolaou (Pap) smear in screening for cervical cancer is the low sensitivity of the test, which ranges between 44% and 77%. This means that a large number of cervical abnormalities (23% to 56%) can be missed with a single test! Thus the success of Pap smear screening in reducing cervical cancer in the United States lies in the frequency of screenings and that cervical cancer is a slowly progressive condition. However, a high frequency of Pap smear screenings is often not feasible, either economically, socially, culturally, or logistically, in many countries and in some regions leads to much higher rates of invasive cervical cancer for women in such populations or locales. Multiple, large, well-conducted studies have demonstrated that human papillomavirus (HPV) testing is considerably more sensitive (between 97% and 98%) than either conventional or liquid-based Pap testing. HPV infection is known to be the required precursor to cervical cancer. With sensitive HPV tests now widely available, requiring less frequent screening (every 3 to 5 years), the future of cervical cancer screening may rely on HPV screening, not on conventional cervical cytology testing.

In settings where there is not even adequate infrastructure for HPV testing, several studies have shown that simple visualization with acetic acid (VIA) can be used to diagnosis women with HPV infection and then immediately provide onsite cryotherapy to reduce rates of later cervical cancer. Although not ideal, this approach shows promise in low-resources settings, especially when the baseline rate of HIV infection is high, because it allows women to be screened and treated on the same visit.

Data from Hoppenot C, Stampler K, Dunton C: *Obstet Gynecol Surv* 67(10):658–667, 2012.

may up-regulate the E6 oncoprotein in certain gene sequences, causing a greater production of vascular epidermal growth factor, which allows the tumor to promote blood vessel growth toward the proliferating cells, fueling growth.[121,126]

CLINICAL MANIFESTATIONS. Cervical neoplasms are predominantly asymptomatic; therefore, regular Pap test or HPV screening is necessary for early detection (see Chapter 26 for screening frequency guidelines). About 90% of cervical cancer cases can be detected through early use of regular screening tests (see What's New? Cervical Cancer Screening in the Developing World). If symptoms exist, they may include vaginal bleeding or abnormal discharge. Bleeding is variable and may occur after intercourse or between menstrual periods. Vaginal discharge is a less common presenting symptom and may be serosanguineous or yellowish with a foul odor. Bleeding and discharge are subtle and are likely to be disregarded by premenopausal women. Postmenopausal women are more likely to seek medical attention if these signs appear. Advanced disease may cause urinary or rectal symptoms and pelvic or back pain along with anemia.

EVALUATION AND TREATMENT. Women should be screened for cervical cancer and risk for future cervical cancer through Pap smear and HPV testing.[127] HPV testing is now recommended at the same time as the Pap smear because it is noninvasive and identifies women at later risk for cellular abnormalities leading to cancer. HPV is often detectable for more than a decade prior to any noticed cellular changes.[127]

A Pap smear involves noninvasively taking a cell sample from the surface of the cervix during a pelvic examination using a

TABLE 24-5 CERVICAL EPITHELIAL CELL ABNORMALITIES (PRECANCEROUS CERVICAL NEOPLASIAS)

CYTOLOGY REPORT	TYPE OF INTRAEPITHELIAL LESION
Atypical squamous cells of undetermined significance (ASC-US)	Suggestive of but do not meet criteria for LSIL (mild dysplasia)
Atypical squamous cells—cannot exclude HSIL (ASC-H)	Do not meet criteria for HSIL but do not preclude HSIL (potentially CIN I/II; moderate to severe dysplasia)
LSIL	CIN 1 (mild dysplasia)
HSIL	CIN 2 and 3 (moderate to severe dysplasia and CIS)

CIN, Cervical intraepithelial neoplasia; *CIS,* carcinoma in situ; *HSIL,* high-grade squamous intraepithelial lesion; *LSIL,* low-grade squamous intraepithelial lesion.

speculum to allow for visualization of the cervix. Cervical cytology is most accurate if cells are obtained from both the endo- and ectocervix, which involves placing the collection device (a small brush or broom) into the cervical os. These cells are then sent to a laboratory for analysis. When dysplasia is detected, further testing is indicated for diagnosis. Colposcopy involves examining the cervix visually and taking needed biopsies. An acetic acid (vinegar) solution is applied to the cervix, making areas of HPV infection stand out in a white color, known as *aceto-white.* The cervix is then viewed under magnification for aceto-white areas, changes in the epithelium, and the presence of abnormal vascular patterns.[128] Abnormal areas of the cervix are biopsied. Because the vulnerable transformation zones move into the cervical canal as a woman ages, the endocervix is sampled using curettage for diagnosis (Table 24-5).

The progressive neoplastic changes of cervical cells are classified on a continuum from cervical intraepithelial neoplasia (dysplasia), to cervical carcinoma in situ (full epithelial thickness of the cervix is involved), to invasive carcinoma (see Tables 23-5 and 23-6). Various terms are used to describe the cellular changes in the cervix based on how the cells were obtained. Screening for cervical cancer is done with a Pap smear, and the cytology report describes Pap smear findings; these terms are outlined on the left side of Table 23-5. If a Pap smear has abnormal findings, a biopsy of the affected tissue is taken during a colposcopy. The biopsy reveals the actual extent of the lesion within the cervix. Terminology used in pathology reports is listed on the right side of Table 23-5. Pathology reports that involve cancer changes begin with the abbreviation CIN or CIS.

Cervical dysplasia is replacement of some epithelial cells by atypical neoplastic cells, and is "staged" depending on the depth of epithelial involvement (Figure 24-19). Risk of progression to invasive carcinoma rises steadily with the severity of dysplasia; however, women with intact immune systems are likely to resolve dysplasia on their own. More than half (57%) of HIV-infected women with CIN 1, 42% of women with CIN 2, and 32% of women with CIN 3 have a natural "regression" of lesions. At least a third or more of all cervical intraepithelial lesions persist without progression or regression. Women with CIN 1 (low-grade squamous intraepithelial lesion [LSIL] or mild dysplasia) have an 11% chance of progression to CIS and a 1% chance of progression to cervical invasion. Women with CIN 2 have a 22% chance of progression to CIS and a 5% chance of invasive lesions. In cervical CIN 3 or HSIL (high-grade squamous intraepithelial lesion), all or most of the cervical epithelium shows cellular features of carcinoma; however, underlying tissue is not affected. At least 12% of women with CIN 3 (CIS) progress to cervical invasion.

CIS is generally a precursor of invasive carcinoma of the cervix. A number of factors, including tumor type, contribute to the rate at which CIS becomes invasive. Because of the ease of Pap smear screening, invasive cervical cancer is rare within the United States, but much more common in the developing world, where screening is not available. **Invasive carcinoma of the cervix** consists of cancer invasion into adjacent tissues and metastasis. Adjacent tissues most often involved are the ureters and structures of the lateral pelvic wall, the vaginal stroma and epithelium, and the lower uterine segment and myometrium. The internal, external, and common iliac lymph nodes and the obturator nodes are common sites of lymphatic involvement. Invasive cervical cancer is most often discovered through Pap smears, tentatively diagnosed with a biopsy during a colposcopy, and then further diagnosed using surgery and lymphangiography, CT scan, MRI, ultrasonography, or radioimmunodetection methods. The staging system for carcinoma of the cervix is shown in Table 24-6.

Treatment depends on the degree of neoplastic change, the size and location of the lesion, and the extent of metastatic spread. For premalignant cellular changes and CIS, the goal is to kill or remove abnormal cells; these procedures can be done in a clinic with local anesthetic. Invasive carcinoma requires surgery, including removal of the cervix and other affected tissues.

Common treatments can be classified as ablative, when the cells are killed without being removed, or excisional in which the abnormal cells are physically removed from the cervix. Ablative therapies are appropriate for lower levels of cervical dysplasia because the treatment does not produce a sample for analysis. However, ablative therapies leave the cervix intact, which may be beneficial for later childbearing. Ablative surgeries include cryotherapy and cold coagulation in which extreme cold is applied to the surface of the cervix. Carbon dioxide laser and electrocoagulation also are used to kill abnormal cells and coagulate vessels supporting their growth. Excisional therapies are appropriate if a more advanced lesion is suspected because they produce tissue for analysis. Excisional therapies include conization, in which a cone-shaped portion of the cervix is removed, and the loop electrosurgical excision procedure (LEEP), in which a small looped wire with electric current generates heat and burns off cancer cells. Heat, cold, or lasers are used in excisional procedures to simultaneously excise the tissue and obliterate abnormal blood vessels.

For invasive cervical carcinoma, treatment depends on the stage of the tumor. Surgical intervention may include a hysterectomy, pelvic lymphadenectomy, or pelvic exenteration (radical

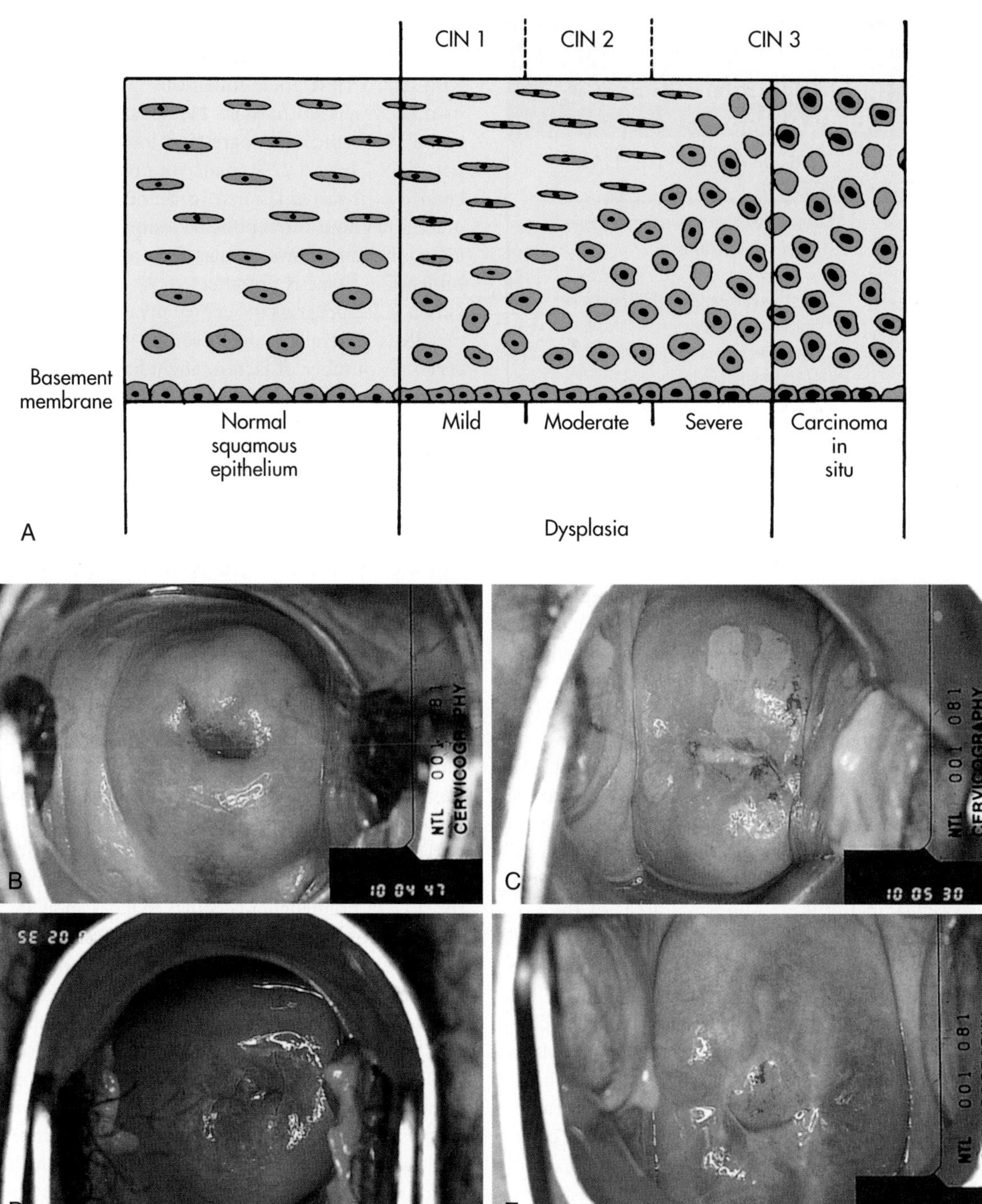

FIGURE 24-19 Cervical Intraepithelial Neoplasia (CIN). A, Diagram of cervical endothelium showing progressive degrees of CIN. **B,** Normal multiparous cervix. **C,** CIN stage 1. Note the white appearance of part of the anterior lip of the cervix associated with neoplastic changes. **D,** CIN stage 2. Lesions reflected in distant capillaries. **E,** CIN stage 3. Lesion predominantly around the external os. (**A** from Herbst AL et al: *Comprehensive gynecology,* ed 2, St Louis, 1992, Mosby. **B-E** from Symonds EM, Macpherson MBA: *Color atlas of obstetrics and gynecology,* London, 1994, Mosby-Wolfe.)

removal of contents of body cavity). Multidrug chemotherapy regimens also have been used alone or in combination with radiation.[129] Smokers tend to have a higher stage of disease at diagnosis, and their cancer is more resistant to radiation treatment.

With early detection and treatment, prognosis is excellent. Overall, the 5-year survival rate is 95% for stage IA or lower (e.g., early detection). A cure rate of 100% is possible for women with dysplasia or CIS.[1] The prevention of HPV infection may be the key to substantially reducing the risk of cervical cancer. FDA-approved vaccines for two of the high-risk types of HPV show excellent promise, and studies are underway to quantify their benefit; however, it may take 10 to 20 years to see the full effect of widespread vaccination due to the slow progression of cervical cancer.[124,130]

TABLE 24-6 CLINICAL STAGING FOR CANCER OF THE CERVIX

STAGE	CHARACTERISTICS
0	Cancer in situ, intraepithelial carcinoma; earliest stage of cancer; cancer confined to its original site
I	Carcinoma confined to cervix (extension to corpus disregarded)
IA	Earliest form of stage I; there is very small amount of cancer, which is visible only under a microscope
IA1	Area of invasion is <3 mm (about ⅛ inch) deep and <7 mm (about ⅓ inch) wide
IA2	Area of invasion is between 3 and 5 mm (about ⅕ inch) deep, and <7 mm (about ⅓ inch) wide
IB	Includes cancers that can be seen without a microscope; also includes cancers seen only with a microscope that have spread deeper than 5 mm (about ⅕ inch) into connective tissue of the cervix or are wider than 7 mm
IB1	IB cancer that is no larger than 4 cm (about 1⅓ inches)
IB2	IB cancer that is >4 cm
II	Cancer has spread beyond the cervix to the upper part of the vagina; cancer does not involve the lower third of the vagina
IIA	Cancer has spread beyond the cervix to the upper part of the vagina; cancer does not involve the lower third of the vagina
IIB	Cancer has spread to the tissue next to the cervix, called the *parametrial tissue*
III	Cancer has spread to the lower part of the vagina or the pelvic wall; cancer may be blocking the ureters (tubes that carry urine from the kidneys to the bladder)
IIIA	Cancer has spread to the lower third of the vagina but not to the pelvic wall
IIIB	Cancer extends to the pelvic wall, blocks urine flow to the bladder, or both
IV	Most advanced stage of cervical cancer; cancer has spread to other parts of the body
IVA	Cancer has spread to the bladder or rectum, which are organs close to the cervix
IVB	Cancer has spread to distant organs beyond the pelvic area, such as the lungs

Reprinted from the American Cancer Society's Cancer Information Database with permission.

Vaginal Cancer

Cancer of the vagina is the rarest of the female genital cancers and accounts for less than 2% of gynecologic cancers.[131] Vaginal and cervical cancers are thought to have similar epidemiology. Both start as intraepithelial lesions, occur in sexually active women, and are associated with HPV infection. Prior carcinoma of the cervix places a woman at higher risk for developing vaginal cancer.[132] In utero exposure to nonsteroidal estrogens is a risk factor. It has been estimated that 100,000 to 160,000 women were exposed in utero to such nonsteroidal estrogens as DES, dienestrol, or hexestrol from 1960 to 1971.[133] Exposure to such hormones during the first 3 months of gestation inhibits the normal replacement of columnar epithelium by squamous epithelium in the vagina of the fetus. The columnar epithelium, which is not normally found in the vagina, may then undergo malignant transformation. Not all women exposed to DES in utero develop neoplastic changes in the vagina, however.[133]

Vaginal cancer is usually diagnosed in women in their 60s and 70s but the cellular changes begin many years prior to clinically visible signs of the disease.[131] The most common type of vaginal cancer is squamous cell carcinoma. About 90% of tumors are squamous cell–type cancers; the remaining 10% are adenocarcinomas, sarcomas (rare), and melanomas (rare). Nonsquamous types of cancer are more common in younger women. Vaginal sarcomas can develop in children younger than 5 years and adenocarcinomas are the most common in women less than 30 years old.[131]

Vaginal cancer is generally asymptomatic until fairly late in the disease process. The major symptom of invasive cancer is vaginal bleeding or bloody discharge. Other symptoms can include vaginal discharge, vulvar pruritus, rectal or bladder symptoms, pain, or leg edema.

Several mechanisms can be used to diagnose vaginal cancer including Pap testing of abnormal vaginal skin, colposcopy, and biopsy. Once a diagnosis of cancer is established, size and extent of the lesion are determined using MRI, prior to surgery.[131] Like cervical neoplasms, vaginal cancers are classified as intraepithelial neoplasia (dysplasia), CIS, or invasive carcinoma and are staged based on extension into local tissues and metastasis to distant organs. Treatment depends on the type and extent of the cancer and the overall health and expectations of the woman.[131] Potential treatment modalities include removal of the affected tissues (vagina, uterus, bladder, and rectum), excision of lymph nodes, radiation, and chemotherapy. Many women with invasive vaginal cancer develop recurrent pelvic cancer and need intensive monitoring for recurrence. Recurrence and survival rates vary greatly by the type and extent of cancer and the aggressiveness of the treatment regimen.[131]

Vulvar Cancer

Cancer of the vulva is responsible for about 3% to 5% of all gynecologic cancers; however, there has been a steady increase in the incidence of vulvar cancers over the last 30 years. The majority (90%) are squamous cell carcinomas, although melanoma (5%), Bartholin gland carcinoma (2%), sarcoma (2%), and adenosquamous carcinoma (1%) may occur. A history of HPV infection is a risk factor with 40% of lesions related to infection with HPV subtype 16.[134] Previous squamous dysplasia of the vagina or cervix also is a major risk factor, as are smoking and HIV infections.[135] Although it usually affects postmenopausal women (median age of presentation is women in their 60s), vulvar cancer has been diagnosed in women between ages 30 and 90.[134,135] Usually women have a history of vulvar irritation and pruritus (70%); urinary symptoms and discharge are less common. In addition, there may be a hard ulcerated area of the vulva, large cauliflower lesions, or lesions similar to those of chronic dermatitis. Biopsy confirms the diagnosis. Treatment options include primarily ablative or excisional surgery,

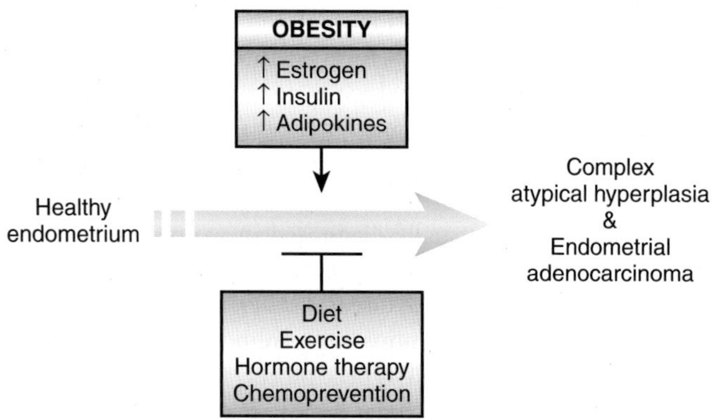

FIGURE 24-20 **Endometrial Cancer.** Overview of the contribution of obesity to endometrial cancer progression and preventive strategies. (From Schmandt RE et al: *Am J Obstet Gynecol* 205[6]:518–525, 2011.)

and sometimes radiation with or without chemotherapy. Less extensive removal of vulvar tissue is being studied to decrease postsurgical morbidity and maintain function.[136] Prognosis depends on lesion size and location, histology, and lymph involvement; risk of metastasis increases with tumor size. The 5-year survival rate depends on the extent of the lesion, the treatment, and the overall health of the woman. Cancer caught in the early stages has a greater than 90% 5-year survival rate with progressively poorer prognosis with advancing stages.[136]

Endometrial Cancer and Uterine Sarcoma

Endometrial carcinomas arise within the glandular epithelium of the uterine lining. Estimates include 49,560 new cases in 2013, with approximately 8190 deaths.[1] Most cases occur in postmenopausal women (Figure 24-20), with peak incidence occurring in the late 50s to early 60s.[137] Women have a 3% lifetime risk of developing uterine cancer. Although incidence rates are higher in white than in black women, mortality rates in black women are nearly twice as high. The primary risk factor is prolonged exposure to estrogen without the presence of progesterone. Estrogen causes endometrial proliferation, whereas progesterone changes the uterine lining to limit proliferation and encourage normal shedding. Estrogen without the presence of progesterone is known as *unopposed estrogen* because its proliferating effects are not restrained. Exposure to unopposed estrogen includes estrogen-only hormone replacement therapy, tamoxifen, early menarche, late menopause, never having children, and a failure to ovulate (i.e., PCOS and anovulatory cycles typical of the late reproductive years). Obesity also is a known source of endogenous estrogen and is a risk factor for endometrial cancer (see Figure 24-20).[138] Other risk factors not directly related to estrogen include diabetes, gallbladder disease, and hypertension, though obesity may be a mediating factor for these risks. A family history of colon, endometrial, or ovarian cancer could signal hereditary nonpolyposis colorectal cancer (HNPCC); women with this family history may wish to explore genetic testing and more aggressive screening.[139]

Although estrogen and obesity increase the risk of endometrial cancer, several interventions have been shown to decrease the risk of cancer. A review of modifiable risk factors and prevention for endometrial hyperplasia and cancer indicates that controlling obesity, hypertension, and diabetes may reduce an individual's risk of endometrial cancer.[140] Exposure to progesterone also decreases the risk of endometrial cancer both immediately and long term. Large amounts of progesterone are released during pregnancy. Smaller, but still effective, amounts of progesterone are in OCPs and the progestin-containing IUD. The use of birth control pills can decrease the risk of endometrial cancer by 80% even for more than a decade after use.[141] The progestin-containing IUD is used to prevent endometrial abnormalities in women who need to take tamoxifen as part of breast cancer prevention.[142]

About 75% of endometrial cancers are adenocarcinomas. Abnormal vaginal bleeding is the most common clinical manifestation of endometrial cancer. The bleeding is caused by disruption of the endometrial surface by neoplastic processes. Pain and weight loss are symptoms of late disease.

Screening methods for early detection of endometrial cancer are as effective as those for cervical cancer. Pap tests, which are highly effective in detecting cervical dysplasia, are ineffective in detecting early endometrial cancer. Transvaginal ultrasound (TVUS) may be used to measure endometrial thickness and screen postmenopausal and high-risk premenopausal women. If the endometrium is abnormally thick (defined as >5 mm), then further testing, such as endometrial biopsy, is warranted to rule out cancer, especially in high-risk women.[143] Endometrial biopsies can be performed in a normal clinic with minimal additional equipment. The biopsy involves placement of a small thin tube through the cervix to collect a specimen of the endometrium for analysis.[141] Once cancer is confirmed by biopsy, a laparoscopy and MRI may be performed to determine stage of disease.

Uterine cancers can be divided into two types by histology. Type I tumors are by far the most common and result from estrogen exposure leading to endometrial hyperplasia. Type II cancers make up 10% of endometrial cancers but are more likely to be invasive into the uterine muscle and metastasize beyond their original location resulting in a much greater risk for death.[144] Treatment is based on the cancer type and the extent of the disease. For women with simple hyperplasia, progestin therapy (orally or through LNG-IUD) may often suffice. However, treatment for atypical hyperplasia or invasive disease usually includes surgical intervention, such as curettage for carcinoma in situ, total abdominal hysterectomy with bilateral salpingo-oophorectomy, and lymphadenectomy.[141] Chemotherapy and radiation also may be used. The 1-year relative survival rate for endometrial cancer is 92%; the 5-year relative survival rate is 95% with early diagnosis and 16% if diagnosis occurred in the late stage. Survival rates for white women exceed those for black women by 8% at every stage.[1]

Uterine sarcomas are rare neoplasms that arise from mesenchymal tissues of and near the uterus, including myometrial smooth muscle, endometrial stroma, or adjacent connective tissues. Uterine sarcomas are rare, constituting up to 3% of all genital tract cancers and 3% to 5% of all uterine malignancies. The average age at diagnosis is the early 50s, though some sarcomas can form in childhood. Uterine sarcomas can be divided into endometrial stromal sarcoma, leiomyosarcoma, and adenosarcoma based on the involved tissue types. The

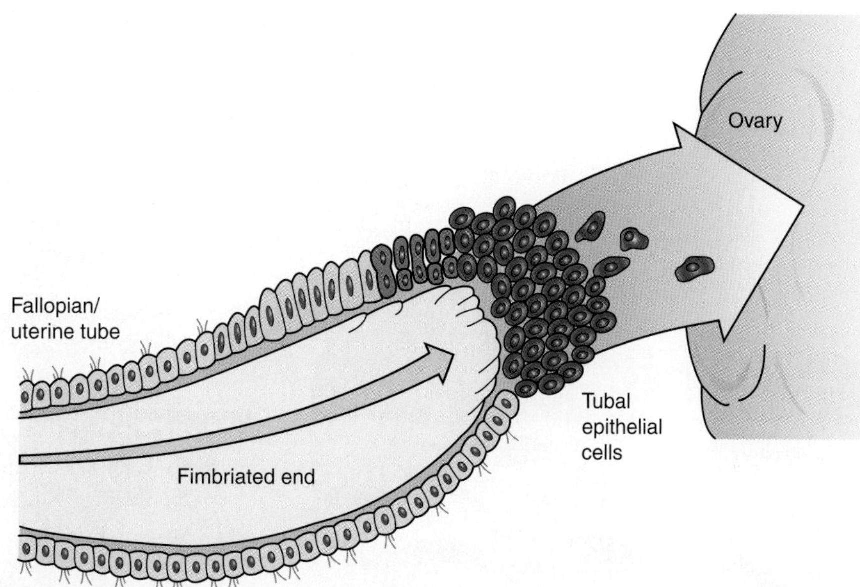

FIGURE 24-21 Migration of epithelial cells from the fallopian/uterine tubes to the ovary. (Adapted from Kurman RJ, Shih IM: *Am J Surg Pathol* 34[3]:433, 2010.)

very low occurrence and diversity of cellular composition of these tumors explains the lack of epidemiologic and treatment data.[145] Thus relatively few risk factors have been identified. However, chronic excess estrogen exposure, tamoxifen, and black race have been cited as risks. Symptoms include abnormal uterine bleeding, awareness of a mass, and pelvic pressure or pain. Vaginal discharge may be profuse and foul. Gastrointestinal and genitourinary complaints are common. Treatment consists of total hysterectomy, which may include bilateral salpingo-oophorectomy and selective lymphadenectomy followed by radiation therapy or chemotherapy, or both. Molecularly targeted therapies are also under investigation.[146] Five-year survival rates range from 50% in early disease to 5% in advanced disease. Like most cancers, stage and histopathology are the most important determinant of prognosis. The survival rate at 5 years for stage I disease is 50%. Few women survive advanced-stage disease.[145]

Ovarian Cancer

The incidence of ovarian cancer is estimated at 22,240 women in the United States in 2013. In 2013 ovarian cancer accounted for 3% of all cancers among women and caused more deaths (14,030) than any other female reproductive cancer in part because of the limited availability of early screening programs. From 2005 to 2009, the incidence declined at a rate of 0.9% per year.[1] Ovarian cancer in women older than 40 years is associated with conditions associated with increased ovulation over the lifetime, such as early menarche, late menopause, nulliparity, and the use of fertility drugs (especially in women who fail to carry a child after using fertility drugs).[146-148] Race and prior pelvic radiation also appear to increase risk.[147] Factors that suppress ovulation decrease the risk of ovarian cancer and include pregnancies, prolonged lactation, and the use of hormonal contraceptives that limit ovulation, including the birth control pill.[147,149]

PATHOGENESIS. There is controversy about the pathogenesis of ovarian cancer. The great majority (approximately 90%) of ovarian cancers are sporadic and not associated with a known pattern of inheritance.[150] Of the 5% to 10% that are familial, the majority are associated with the breast cancer susceptibility gene 1 *(BRCA1)* and a smaller number with mutations of *BRCA2* or mismatched repair genes (HNPCC syndrome). Various pathways have been proposed. Women and families who are more susceptible to cancer may have errors in the ability to repair cellular DNA, related to abnormalities in RAD51D, which is an enzyme crucial to DNA repair,[151] which allows aberrant cellular proliferation that occurs with repetitive ovulatory tissue repair in the ovary. In sporadic ovarian cancer, *BRCA1* and *BRCA2* are rarely mutated. A newer theory proposes that many spontaneous, nonhereditary ovarian tumors arise from the migration of cells from tissues of mesoderm origin to the surface of the ovary.[152,153] Cells from a variety of intra-abdominal locations, including endometrial tissue and epithelium of the fallopian/uterine tubes, can attach to the ovary (Figure 24-21). The local ovarian environment, including the ovarian stroma, may then interact with the transplanted cells to enhance cellular growth and encourage metastasis[154] (Figure 24-22).

The two major types of ovarian cancer are epithelial ovarian neoplasms and germ-cell neoplasms. Most ovarian malignancies are epithelial ovarian neoplasms that usually develop from the surface epithelium of the ovary or that which line cysts immediately beneath the ovarian surface, or may be cells that have migrated from the fallopian/uterine tubes.[153] Most epithelial cancers seem to arise from a single cell (i.e., clonal) because of a loss of tumor-suppressor genes and activation of oncogenes (see Chapter 12). Epithelial ovarian tumors may have cellular similarities to other tissues within the abdomen, including the lining of the fallopian/uterine tubes, or the endometrium, or be undifferentiated. Tumors are often classified as type I (low grade) and type II (high grade) based on their cellular type.

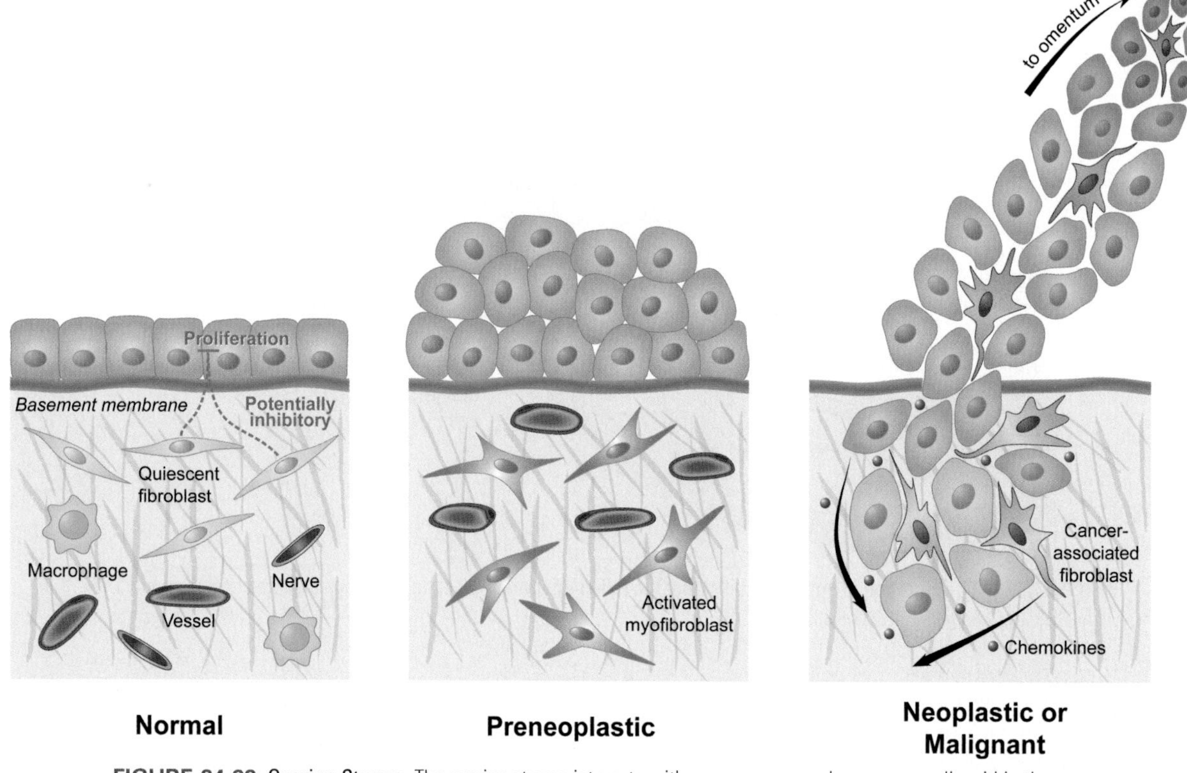

FIGURE 24-22 Ovarian Stroma. The ovarian stroma interacts with precancerous and cancerous cells within the ovary. (From Schauer IG et al: *Neoplasia* 13[5]:393, 2011)

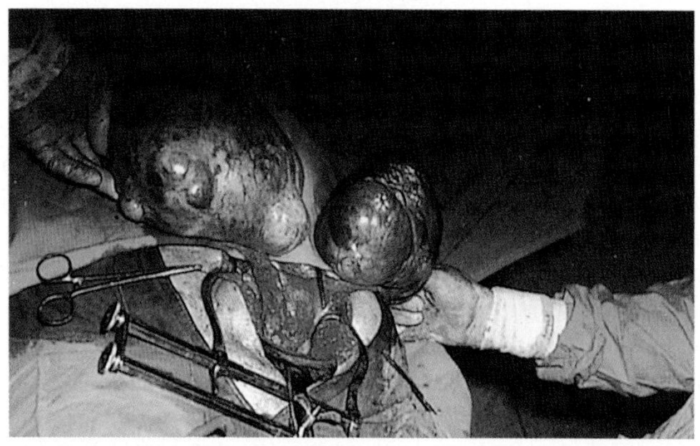

FIGURE 24-23 Ovarian Tumors. Bilateral multicystic ovarian tumors. (From Symonds EM, Macpherson MBA: *Color atlas of obstetrics and gynecology,* London, 1994, Mosby-Wolfe.)

Type I tumors grow more slowly but are more resistant to chemotherapy. Type II tumors often grow rapidly and aggressively but respond well to chemotherapy[153,155] (Figure 24-23). The 5-year survival rate is 92% if treated in stage I; however, only 15% of ovarian cancers are diagnosed this early. Five-year survival rates decline with stage of disease: women with regional spread of the cancer have a 5-year survival rate of 72%, whereas women with distant metastasis have only a 5-year survival rate of 27%.[1]

Germ-cell tumors are derived from the primitive germ cells (gametes) of the embryonic gonad and may be malignant or benign. The benign cystic teratoma accounts for approximately 10% of all ovarian tumors. These tumors represent an error in meiosis that results in the formation of ectoderm, endoderm, and mesoderm cell lines. Hair, teeth, and skin can be visualized within cystic teratomas. If the germ-cell tumor is malignant, it tends to be highly aggressive and rapidly growing with a poor prognosis. Cystic hygromas and other germ-cell tumors can occur on the ovaries of girls and women. Germ-cell tumors in children can be particularly aggressive.

CLINICAL MANIFESTATIONS. Ovarian cancer is commonly asymptomatic until the tumors have grown very large. Given the location of the ovaries, assessing abnormalities on routine gynecologic examination poses difficulty, especially in obese women. There is no sensitive and specific test for ovarian cancer for screening low-risk women, and routine screening of women without risk factors has not been shown to be beneficial and may cause harm because more women have unnecessary surgical procedures.[156]

Common first symptoms of ovarian cancer are vague and include persistent abdominal distention, loss of appetite due to early satiety, and pelvic pain. Screening is warranted if women have a new onset of these symptoms that persist for more than 12 days each month. However, many women fail to notice the very first signs of ovarian cancer because they are vague and fairly common in older women. The disease is most commonly diagnosed after metastasis has occurred. Consequently, ovarian cancer is often termed the *silent killer*. Symptoms of advanced disease include pain and abdominal swelling from the primary ovarian mass or ascites and abdominal distention (Figure 24-24). Gastrointestinal manifestations may include dyspepsia,

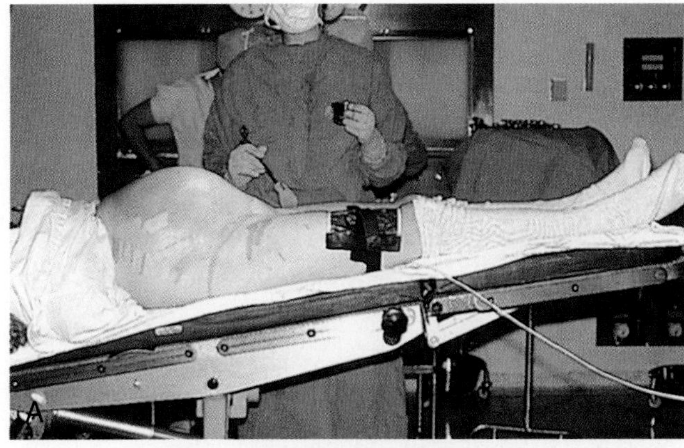

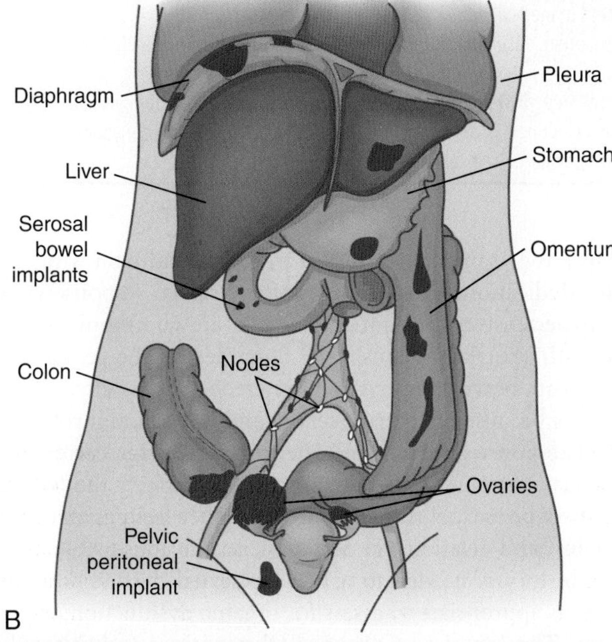

FIGURE 24-24 Large Malignant Ovarian Tumor and Metastasis of Ovarian Cancer. **A,** Tumor has caused massive abdominal distention. **B,** Pattern of spread for epithelial cancer of the ovary. (**A** from Symonds EM, Macpherson MBA: *Color atlas of obstetrics and gynecology,* London, 1994, Mosby-Wolfe.)

vomiting, and alterations in bowel habits caused by mechanical obstruction. Abnormal vaginal bleeding may occur if the postmenopausal endometrium is stimulated by a hormone-secreting tumor. The tumor also may cause ulcerations through the vaginal wall that result in bleeding. There also can be a feeling of pressure in the pelvis and leg pain.

Tumor obstruction of vascular channels can cause venous and, occasionally, arterial thrombosis. Alterations in coagulability also occur, contributing to clot formation. Metastasis often causes pleural effusion.

EVALUATION AND TREATMENT. Because ovarian cancer has no early symptoms and there is no cost-effective screening techniques for early detection, disease usually is advanced by the time treatment is sought. Women with symptoms of disease, as outlined earlier, should be assessed with minimally invasive tests first. Screening commonly begins with a CA-125 blood test looking for specific cancer markers and a transvaginal ultrasound.[157] Increased CA-125 levels are found in about 78% to 80% of nonmucinous ovarian cancers; however, elevated levels are produced in 29% of nongynecologic tumors and in a variety of noncancerous conditions, for example, endometriosis, PID, benign ovarian cysts, myomas, and pregnancy.

Women less than 40 years of age are more likely to have nonepithelial cells tumors and should be assessed with the blood tests to look for the CA-125 marker, alpha fetoprotein (AFP), and β-human chorionic growth hormone to screen for tumors of nonepithelial cell origin.[157] Some types of germ cells and, rarely, adenocarcinoma may be associated with increased levels of AFP, hCG, or CA-125.

If initial tests are suspicious for a cancerous mass, diagnosis is confirmed by biopsy and extent of the disease is determined by ultrasound, CT, MRI, or other imaging techniques. Women undergoing surgery for ovarian cancer staging receive a thorough assessment for metastasis. The International Federation of Gynecologists and Obstetricians (FIGO) staging system is described in Table 24-7. Other studies may be used to determine the extent of metastasis. These include an upper gastrointestinal series, barium enema, intravenous pyelogram (IVP), mammography, and lymphography.

TABLE 24-7 FIGO STAGING OF CARCINOMA OF THE OVARY

STAGE	CHARACTERISTICS
I	Growth limited to the ovaries
IA	Growth limited to one ovary; no ascites
IA1	No tumor on the external surface; capsule intact (90% 5-year survival with treatment)
IA2	Tumor present on the external surface, or capsule(s) ruptured, or both
IB	Growth limited to both ovaries; no ascites
IB1	No tumor on the external surface; capsule intact
IB2	Tumor present on the external surface, or capsule(s) ruptured, or both
IC	Tumor either stage IA or stage IB, with ascites present or with positive peritoneal washings
II	Growth involving one or both ovaries with pelvic extension
IIA	Extension and/or metastases to the uterus and/or tubes
IIB	Extension to other pelvic tissues
IIC	Tumor either stage IIA or stage IIB but with ascites present or with positive peritoneal washings
III	Growth involving one or both ovaries with intraperitoneal metastases outside the pelvis, or positive retroperitoneal nodes, or both; tumor limited to the true pelvis with histologically proven malignant extension to small bowel or omentum
IV	Growth involving one or both ovaries with distant metastases; if pleural effusion is present, there must be positive cytology to allot a case to stage IV; parenchymal liver metastases indicate stage IV
Special category	Unexplored cases that are thought to be ovarian carcinoma

FIGO, International Federation of Gynecologists and Obstetricians.

TABLE 24-8 **POSSIBLE EFFECTS OF CHRONIC DISEASE ON SEXUAL FUNCTIONING IN WOMEN**

DISEASE	SEXUAL FUNCTION
Cerebral palsy	Intact genital sensations, decreased lubrication; difficulty with sexual activity/positioning because of muscle spasticity, rigidity, and/or weakness; pain with positioning caused by contracture of knees and hips or because of increased spasms with arousal
Cerebrovascular accident (CVA)	Difficulties in sexual positioning and sensitivity because of impaired motor strength, coordination or paralysis; decreased sex drive with stroke on the dominant side of the brain
Diabetes	Diminished intensity of orgasm and gradual decline in ability to achieve orgasm; decreased lubrication and/or recurrent vaginal infections with resultant dyspareunia
Chronic renal failure	Decreased arousal; increasingly rare and less intense orgasms; decreased lubrication
Rheumatoid arthritis (RA)	Painful sexual activity/positions because of swollen, painful joints, muscular atrophy and joint contracture; decreased sex drive because of pain, fatigue, and/or medication; genital sensations remain intact
Systemic lupus erythematosus (SLE)	Similar to RA; decreased lubrication and vaginal lesions result in painful penetration
Myocardial infarction (MI)	Most literature male oriented; problems related to medications
Multiple sclerosis (MS)	Diminished genital sensitivity; decreased lubrication; declining orgasmic ability; difficulty with sexual activity because of muscle weakness, pain, or incontinence
Spinal cord injury	Reflex sexual response with injury above sacral area; disrupted response with lesion at or below sacrum; loss of sensation, decreased lubrication; spasticity, incontinence, or pain with arousal; continued orgasmic sensations or sensations diffused in general or to specific body parts, such as breast or lips

The initial approach to treatment is surgery, which is performed to determine the stage of disease and to remove as much of the tumor as possible. Future treatment is then customized based on the clinical stage of the cancer, the woman's desires, and the cell type and sensitivity of the cancer cells. Ideally treatment plans are developed and implemented by a multidisciplinary team from a variety of disciplines including surgeons, pathologists, and oncologists.[158]

Radiation therapy and chemotherapy with an agent containing platinum are common treatments.[159] Even after initially effective treatment, 55% to 75% of women relapse, and less than 20% survive long term with stage III or IV disease. New therapies under investigation include small-molecular-weight inhibitors, monoclonal antibodies, epidermal growth factor receptors, and gene therapy.[160]

Sexual Dysfunction

Sexual dysfunction is the lack of satisfaction with sexual function resulting from pain or a deficiency in sexual desire, arousal, or orgasm/climax.[161,162] Sexual function and dysfunction result from a complex interplay of the individual, culture, and physiology.[162] Sexual problems are multifaceted and often difficult to diagnose; adequate research is still needed. Sexual dysfunction can have organic or psychogenic causes or, more commonly, a combination of both.[162] Studies show that at any given time up to 45% of adult women have some form of sexual dysfunction.[163]

The sexual response cycle is complex, involving the brain/mind, sympathetic and parasympathetic nervous systems, the systemic and local vasculature, and local innervation. Any disruption in these systems can affect sexual response. Chronic medical conditions can greatly affect both sexual desire and sexual function (Table 24-8). Acute illness and infections also can affect the woman's desire and ability to engage in fulfilling sexual activity. Vaginal infections are especially problematic because they can lead to vaginal irritation and pain with friction. Medications also can disrupt the sexual response cycle. Antihypertensives and antidepressants are commonly associated with sexual problems.[161,163] Surgeries on the genital area can disrupt nerve pathways and hysterectomy may affect sexual function because the uterus, cervix, and vagina are involved in sexual response and orgasm. The mind is a large component of sexual response, and any stressor that affects the woman can affect her sexual response, including her feelings about her sexuality and relationship and past sexual abuse.[163] A thorough history is needed to assess for sexual dysfunction, and testing is appropriate to assess for organic dysfunction (Figure 24-25). The American College of Obstetricians and Gynecologists divide sexual dysfunction into four categories: disorders of desire, arousal, orgasm, and sexual pain.[161]

Disorders of desire (hypoactive sexual desire, decreased libido) is the most common sexual dysfunction in women.[163] The prevalence of hypoactive sexual desire increases with age and may be a biologic manifestation of depression, alcohol or other substance abuse, prolactin-secreting pituitary tumors, or testosterone deficiency. β-Adrenergic blockers used for heart disease also may inhibit sexual desire. Short-term treatment with testosterone has been shown to improve sexual desire and may be used to treat women who wish to improve their sexual interest.[161]

Anorgasmia, or **orgasmic dysfunction,** is the inability of the woman to reach or achieve orgasm. Dysfunction follows a continuum from difficulty in arousal to lack of orgasm. Any chronic illness may affect arousal. Diabetes, alcoholism, neurologic disturbances, hormonal deficiencies, and pelvic disorders, such as infections, trauma, and surgical scarring, may block orgasm. Narcotics, tranquilizers, antidepressants (especially SSRIs), and antihypertensive medications also can inhibit orgasm.[163]

Dyspareunia (painful intercourse) is common. Women may experience pain during arousal, at the time of orgasm, at

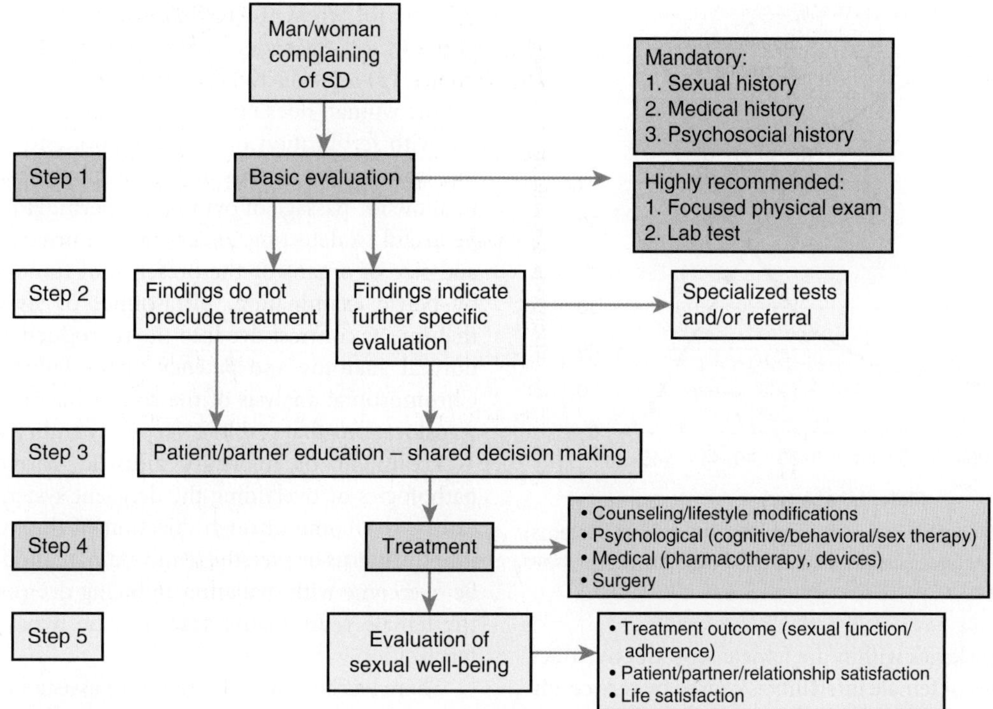

FIGURE 24-25 **Diagnostic and Treatment Algorithm for Sexual Dysfunction.** The International Consultation in Sexual Medicine (ICSM) stepwise diagnostic and treatment algorithm for sexual dysfunction in men and women. (From Hatzichristou D et al: *J Sex Med* 7[1pt2]:337–348, 2010.)

the initiation of intercourse, midway during intercourse, or after intercourse. The pain may have a burning, sharp, searing, or cramping quality and may be described as external, vaginal, deep abdominal, or pelvic. A variety of psychosocial and organic causes have been identified.

Inadequate lubrication may make penetration or intercourse difficult or painful. Low estrogen levels, as are common with menopause and lactation, can decrease vaginal lubrication. Drugs with a drying effect, such as antihistamines, certain tranquilizers, and marijuana, can decrease lubrication. Infections and skin problems of the vulva and vagina are a frequent cause of acute onset dyspareunia. The use of products such as spermicides and fragrances on the sensitive vaginal mucosa may increase the risk of irritation. Disorders of the vaginal opening, such as scarring from female genital mutilation, episiotomy, or an intact hymen, also can be problematic. Deep pelvic disorders such as infection, tumors, and cervical or uterine abnormalities can cause pain with intercourse.

Vaginismus is an involuntary muscle spasm in response to attempted penetration. Vaginismus is often a response to previous painful penetration. Common causes include prior sexual trauma or fear of sex; organic causes are less common and are similar to those that cause dyspareunia, including vulvovestibulitis. Even after the underlying organic problem is detected and successfully treated, vaginismus may persist.

Sexual dysfunction may develop as a coping mechanism. Women with a history of sexual trauma—rape, incest, or molestation—often have problems of desire, arousal, or orgasm or experience pain with sexual activity. In extreme cases total sexual aversion may develop.[163] At other times sexual dysfunction may be a symptom of marital or relationship problems. Because sexual dysfunction has many causes, assessment and treatment should be holistic and culturally sensitive.

Impaired Fertility

Infertility affects approximately 15% of all couples and is defined as the inability to conceive after 1 year of unprotected intercourse with the same, opposite-sex partner. However, many sources believe that medical intervention is indicated for women who are older than 35 years old if they fail to conceive after 6 months of unprotected intercourse.[164] The rate of infertility may be increasing because of an increase in sexually transmitted disease and a delay in the start of childbearing but the increase in incidence rates may also reflect the greater utilization of medical services for infertility.[165] Fertility can be impaired by factors in the man or the woman or both partners. The male is the sole cause of the infertility in 20% of cases, and a co-contributor to infertility in 30% to 40% of cases.[166] The majority of cases of infertility involve the female, caused in part by the complexity of the female reproductive cycle and tract. Ovulatory factors account for 40% of female infertility.[33] Regular ovulation occurs as a result of a functioning hypothalamic/pituitary axis. Ovulation can be disrupted by a wide variety of factors, including imbalances in a diversity of hormones (TSH, estrogen, progesterone, etc.), chronic conditions, and stress. Age is a major factor in female fertility because the regularity of ovulation and the quality of ova decrease with age (Figure 24-26). Abnormalities of the reproductive tract, including tubal pathologies, cause another 40% of cases of infertility.[33] Endometriosis and adhesions and scarring from PID are major

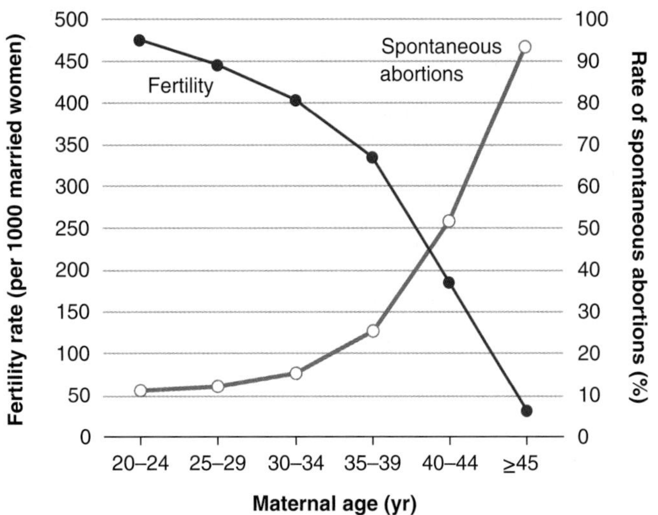

FIGURE 24-26 Relationship of Fertility and Miscarriage with Maternal Age. (From Heffner LJ: Advanced maternal age: how old is too old? *N Engl J Med* 351(19):1927–1929, 2004.)

contributors to blockages within the female reproductive tract. The remaining 20% of female infertility is caused by rare conditions or unknown etiology.[33]

Male infertility has a variety of causes, many of which can be corrected. Hormonal disorders, such as thyroid disturbances or low testosterone levels, can be diagnosed and corrected.[167] Throughout the 82 days of their creation and maturation, the sperm must be kept cooler than body temperature.[33] Elevations in temperature caused by illness, abnormal placement of the testes, varicoceles near the testes, or exposure to high temperatures in hot tubs or saunas may kill or disable sperm. Male infertility is also linked to abnormalities of the seminal tract and sexual dysfunction that disrupts ejaculation.[167] A number of diagnostic procedures are required in the routine investigation of the infertile couple (see Table 23-3). In many instances no cause may be identified.

Fertility Tests

Prior to the performance of even basic fertility tests, a complete history should be obtained that includes coital (sex) timing and frequency in relation to the menstrual cycle; an in-depth assessment and charting of the menstrual cycle; a reproductive history, including all previous pregnancies from both partners and their outcome; a medical history of systemic disease; current medications; past surgeries; a sexual history including any previous STIs; and any exposure to toxins.[168] The history allows the clinician to home in on the most useful tests. Testing starts with the least invasive test or procedure and increases in invasiveness and complexity as the duration of infertility increases. The types of tests and their normal values are summarized in Table 22-4.

The most common test for male infertility is the basic semen analysis, the man is evaluated for volume of semen and the concentration, morphology, and forward motility of sperm.[166,168] More advanced semen analysis also examines the function of the sperm including their ability to bind to and penetrate eggs. In-depth analysis may also analyze the sperm's DNA for number, fragmentation, and ability to merge with the egg's DNA.[168]

Tests for women determine whether: (1) ovulation occurs normally, (2) the endometrium is responding normally to hormones, (3) reproductive tissues are free of tumors or infections, (4) the woman does not have any chronic conditions interfering with fertilization or implantation, and (5) the reproductive tract (cervix, uterus, fallopian tubes) is adequately patent to allow for passage of ovum and sperm. Hormonal assays can be useful to detecting underlying abnormalities. The position and size of organs or the presence of tumors can be assessed by pelvic examination, ultrasound, or hysterosalpingogram that injects contrast dye into the reproductive tract to look for normal anatomy and patency of the fallopian/uterine tubes. Chromosomal analysis of the couple may reveal mutations or translocations that result in very early embryo loss.[33]

Treatment of infertility aims at correcting underlying pathologies or overriding the deficient system. Male infertility can be overcome through injection of the male DNA directly into the uterus or even the ovum. Anovulation in the female can be overcome with ovulation-inducing drugs. Blockages within the female reproductive tract can be bypassed with in vitro fertilization.

There has been a proliferation in assisted reproductive technologies (ART) that enable women and couples to conceive and bear children. ART results in more than 50,000 live births per year in the United States, and the rate is rising.[169] However, there are questions about the health and long-term safety of infants conceived with assisted reproduction; for instance, concerns about the high rate of twins and preterm birth in pregnancies conceived with ART. In addition, children born through ART have a higher rate of birth defects, even when other variables are controlled.[170] The many theories about the cause of this increase suggest that the birth defects may be the result of epigenetic changes when the expression of the embryo's DNA is affected by the very early environment of the blastocysts.[171] Research in this area and the field of epigenetics is ongoing.[171]

DISORDERS OF THE BREAST

Galactorrhea

Galactorrhea (inappropriate lactation) is the persistent and sometimes excessive secretion of a milky fluid from the breasts of a woman who is not pregnant or nursing an infant. It can occur in men, may involve one or both breasts, and is not associated with breast cancer.

Incidence is difficult to estimate because of differences among definitions of the condition, examination techniques, and populations of women who have been studied. Prevalence has been documented as 0.1% to 32% of all women.

PATHOPHYSIOLOGY. Galactorrhea is a manifestation of pathophysiologic processes in the body, rather than a breast disorder. These processes are chiefly hormone imbalances caused by hypothalamic/pituitary disturbances, pituitary tumors, or neurologic damage. Exogenous causes include drugs, estrogen, and manipulation of the nipples. When caused by hyperprolactinemia it is manifested by the spontaneous appearance of a milky secretion from multiple duct openings, usually from both breasts. Galactorrhea caused by oral contraceptives (OCs)

BOX 24-12 COMMON CAUSES OF HYPERPROLACTINEMIA

Physiologic Causes
Exercise
Idiopathic
Pregnancy and postpartum period
Sleep (rapid eye movement [REM] phase)
Stress (trauma, surgery)
Suckling

Drug Causes
Amoxapine
Amphetamines
Anesthetic agents
Butyrophenones
Cimetidine
Estrogens
Hydroxyzine
Methyldopa
Metoclopramide
Narcotics
Phenothiazines
Progestins
Reserpine
Tricyclic antidepressants
Verapamil

Pathophysiologic Causes
Acromegaly
Chronic chest wall stimulation (e.g., post-thoracotomy, postmastectomy, herpes zoster)
Cirrhosis
Hypothalamic disease
Hypothyroidism
Pressure on pituitary stalk
Prolactin-secreting tumors
Pseudocyesis (false pregnancy)
Renal failure (especially with zinc deficiency)
Spinal cord lesions

is more likely to occur with high-dose use; is characterized by clear, serous, or milky discharge from multiple ducts; and is noticeable during the drug-free interval between OC packets. In premenopausal women, unilateral or bilateral spontaneous multiple duct discharge that increases before menstruation often is caused by fibrocystic change. Unilateral, spontaneous, serous, or serosanguineous discharge from a single duct usually is caused by an intraductal papilloma; bloody discharge suggests cancer; bilateral, sticky, multicolored discharge from multiple ducts is often caused by duct ectasia; and purulent discharge indicates a subareolar abscess.[172]

The most common cause of galactorrhea is **nonpuerperal hyperprolactinemia,** or excessive amounts of prolactin (the pituitary hormone that stimulates milk production) in the blood not related to pregnancy or childbirth. Nonpuerperal hyperprolactinemia can be caused by any factor that (1) stimulates or overstimulates the prolactin-secreting units of the pituitary gland; (2) interferes with production of **prolactin-inhibiting factor (PIF),** a neurotransmitter (probably dopamine) that inhibits prolactin secretion; or (3) interferes with pituitary receptors for PIF. A variety of exogenous agents (such as drugs) and disorders can trigger one of these three mechanisms, thereby causing hyperprolactinemia (Box 24-12).

Hypothyroidism causes increased secretion of hypothalamic TSH that stimulates prolactin release from the pituitary. Hypothyroidism also is associated with reduced metabolic clearance of prolactin, which prolongs its effects.

Many types of pituitary tumors cause hyperprolactinemia. Prolactinomas cause hyperprolactinemia by secreting prolactin, decreasing production of PIF, or putting pressure on the pituitary stalk such that delivery of PIF to the anterior pituitary is prevented. Growth hormone–secreting pituitary tumors may cause galactorrhea through the intrinsic lactogenic effect that growth hormone appears to have on mammary tissue. Prolactin-secreting lung and kidney tumors also cause hyperprolactinemia.

Chronic stress may cause hyperprolactinemia by inhibiting PIF release. Cervical spinal injuries, head trauma, encephalitis, meningitis, herpes zoster, or thoracotomy scars may stimulate the afferent portion of the suckling reflex arc, which is carried in the second to sixth thoracic nerves. The suckling reflex increases prolactin secretion.

CLINICAL MANIFESTATIONS. A small amount of breast milk expressed from the nipples of parous women usually is not a concern, and normal breast milk color can be other than white. Inappropriate lactation is manifested by the appearance of a milky breast secretion in nonpregnant, nonlactating women from one or both breasts. Most women with galactorrhea experience menstrual abnormality. If a pituitary process is involved, the woman usually experiences hirsutism and infertility; if a hypothalamic lesion is present, she may report such CNS symptoms as intractable headache, visual field disturbances, sleep disturbances, and abnormal temperature, thirst, or appetite.

EVALUATION AND TREATMENT. Galactorrhea requires evaluation when it (1) occurs in nulliparous women or in parous women who have not been pregnant or have not breast-fed for 12 months, or (2) is associated with amenorrhea, headache, visual field abnormalities, or other symptoms implying systemic illness. Evaluation includes a variety of diagnostic tests. When amenorrhea accompanies galactorrhea, the assessment is the same as for amenorrhea. Breast secretions are examined for fat globules and neoplastic cells to verify their source. Serum prolactin levels are measured. Because such variables as eating, sleeping, stress, and breast examinations increase prolactin levels, at least two positive results are needed for a diagnosis of hyperprolactinemia. Prolactin levels greater than 25 to 30 ng/ml (by radioimmunoassay) are elevated. Those in the range of 75 to 100 ng/ml are considered to be caused by a pituitary tumor until proved otherwise. Serum thyroxine and TSH levels are measured to rule out hypothyroidism, and LH and FSH levels are obtained if the individual is amenorrheic. MRI may assist in locating adenomas.

Treatment is specific to the underlying cause and occurs after identification of the cause. Medical therapy is usual and surgery or radiation therapy is rarely required.

Benign Breast Disease

Benign breast disease (BBD) is a spectrum of noncancerous changes in the breast. Numerous benign alterations in ducts and lobules occur in the breast, including irregular lumps, cysts, sensitive nipples, and itching. The most common symptoms reported by women are pain, palpable mass, or nipple discharge; the majority of these prove to have a benign cause. After a diagnosis of BBD, however, major determinants of breast cancer risk include degree of family history; histologic or biologic features, or both; and previous biopsy.[173] This risk varies according to the histologic category of BBD (moderate in women with proliferative lesions without atypia [deviation from normal]) and substantial in women with atypical (atypia) hyperplasia (AH)[174] (see p. 841). Among premenopausal women, the risk appears to be greater for those with atypical lobular hyperplasia (ALH) than with atypical ductal hyperplasia (ADH) (see p. 841). For postmenopausal women, the risk of breast cancer was similar between those with ALH or ADH.[174] Family history is reported as an independent risk factor for breast cancer. Women with atypia and a family history had a breast cancer risk four times the expected risk.[175] Risk was lower among those with atypia and no family history.

The College of American Pathologists has classified biopsy tissue according to breast cancer risk. These classifications are listed in Box 24-13. Benign epithelial lesions can be broadly classified according to their risk of developing breast cancer as: (1) nonproliferative breast lesions, (2) proliferative breast disease, and (3) atypical (atypia) hyperplasia. Table 24-9 includes examples of benign breast tumors.

BOX 24-13 CLASSIFICATION OF BREAST BIOPSY TISSUE ACCORDING TO RISK FOR BREAST CANCER

No Increased Risk

- Adenosis (sclerosing or florid)
  - Apocrine metaplasia
  - Macrocysts or microcysts
  - Fibroadenoma
  - Fibrosis
- Mild hyperplasia
  - Mastitis or periductal mastitis
  - Squamous metaplasia

Slightly Increased Risk (1.5 to 2 Times)

- Moderate or florid hyperplasia
  - Papilloma

Moderately Increased Risk (4 to 5 Times)

- Atypical hyperplasia (ductal or lobular)

Data from Dupont WD, Page DL: *NEJM* 312(3):146–151, 1985.

Nonproliferative Breast Lesions

The term *nonproliferative* has been used to discriminate from the *proliferative* changes commonly associated with increased risk for development of breast cancer. Nonproliferative breast lesions are generally not associated with an increase risk in breast cancer.[173] Terms such as **fibrocystic changes (FCCs)** or physiologic nodularity and cysts, fibrocystic disease, chronic cystic mastitis, and mammary dysplasia refer to nonproliferative lesions and are not clinically definitive because they encompass a heterogeneous group of diagnoses.[173] **Cysts** (fluid-filled sacs) are a specific type of lump that commonly occurs in women in their 30s, 40s, and early 50s. Cysts feel "squishy" when they occur close to the surface of the breast but when deeply embedded they can feel hard (Figure 24-27). An

TABLE 24-9 BENIGN BREAST TUMORS

BENIGN BREAST TUMOR	RISK FACTORS	PATHOPHYSIOLOGY	CLINICAL MANIFESTATIONS	TREATMENT
Fibroadenoma	Puberty, early adulthood; occurs earlier and more frequently in young black women	Slow-growing lesion composed of variable proportions of epithelial and connective tissue; thought to be under influence of estrogen	Painless, firm, elastic, solitary, well-circumscribed mass ≈1-5 cm in diameter	Excision with person under local anesthesia; or careful observation
Phyllodes tumor	Middle age	Fibroepithelial tumor characterized by marked proliferation of connective tissue stroma and great size; initially slow growing; 10%-25% may be malignant	Spheric, firm, usually well-circumscribed multinodular tumor with a diameter of 2-20 cm; trophic cutaneous ulceration is a late manifestation	Local excision of benign or small tumor; simple mastectomy if voluminous or malignant tumor
Intraductal papilloma	Ages 30-50 yr; relatively uncommon	Subareolar tumor consists of epithelial vegetation with central connective tissue axis; found in lactiferous duct	Spontaneous or induced watery, serous, or bloody nipple discharge; small soft, friable, yellow or red, ≈5 mm, papillomatous growth attached to duct wall by short, thin stalk; rare nipple retraction	Excision of involved duct
Mammary duct ectasia	After menopause or during pregnancy and lactation	Principal lactiferous ducts become dilated and filled with cellular debris; secondary inflammatory reaction; possible rupture of ducts	Subareolar induration or nipple retraction; spontaneous, bloody, sticky, thick, multiple duct discharge; burning pain and swelling of areolar area; palpable mass after rupture	Antibiotic and anti-inflammatory therapy
Fat necrosis	Ages 14-80 yr; average age 50 yr; increased in women with fatty, voluminous breasts; trauma	50% are posttraumatic; necrosis secondary to inflammation is more rare	Poorly circumscribed indurated area with yellow or gray necrotic foci	Leave alone or local excision

estimated 50% to 80% of women normally experience some of these changes. The prevalence of fibrocystic lesions is probably related to hormonal changes, which in turn are affected by genetic background, age, parity, history of lactation, caffeine consumption, and use of exogenous hormones.[176] Based on experimental animal studies, it is assumed that breast cysts are the result of ovarian alterations, but the exact mechanism is unknown. Calcifications, found in cysts and adenosis or an increase in the number of acini per lobule, can form mammographically suspicious alterations.[177] Cysts also can be associated with unilateral nipple discharge. A variety of substances are secreted into cyst fluid, including polypeptide hormones and male and female sex steroid hormones. Cysts often rupture with release of secretory material into the adjacent tissue. The resulting chronic inflammation and scarring fibrosis contribute to the palpable firmness of the breast.[177] Fibrous tissue increases progressively until menopause and regresses thereafter. Papillary apocrine (glandular) change, epithelial-related calcifications, and mild hyperplasia of the usual type are all considered nonproliferative breast lesions.[173] Genetic aberrations are more common in proliferative than in nonproliferative lesions.[177]

Proliferative Breast Lesions Without Atypia

These disorders are characterized by proliferation of ductal epithelium and/or stroma without cellular signs of **atypia** or deviation from normal. Criteria for the diagnosis of intraductal proliferative lesions have been the subject of much research and controversy and include the following structurally diverse lesions:

1. **Usual ductal hyperplasia (UDH).** In the normal breast, only myoepithelial cells and a single layer of luminal cells are present above the basement membrane.[177] UDH is defined by the presence of *more* than two cell layers above the basement membrane within the ductal space. Cytologically they are benign cells, not monoclonal, and cells can vary in size and shape.[173,178] The additional or proliferating epithelial cells fills and distends the ducts and lobules by both luminal and myoepithelial cells. Moderate to **florid hyperplasia** is more than four cell layers above the basement membrane. Ductal hyperplasia is usually found as an incidental finding on biopsy of mammographic abnormalities.
2. **Intraductal papillomas.** Solitary papillomas are a monotonous (sameness) array of papillary cells that grow from the wall of a cyst into the lumen of the duct. Growth occurs within a dilated duct often near or beside the nipple causing benign nipple discharge (Figure 24-28). These papillomas *can* harbor areas of atypia or ductal carcinoma in situ (DCIS) (see p. 841). Solitary intraductal papillomas may present as a breast mass (mammogram), a nodule (ultrasound) or image from MRI, or ductography (galactogram).[178] Hyperplasia and metaplasia can be present within the ducts. Atypical hyperplasia may be present within or adjacent to papilloma, making the distinction from DCIS difficult (see p. 866). The presence of

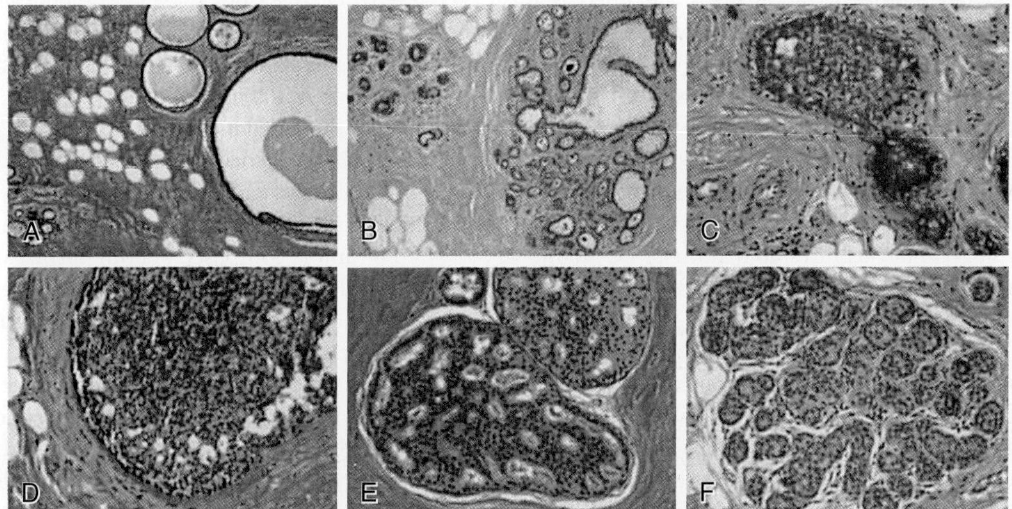

FIGURE 24-27 Benign Breast Disease. **A,** *Nonproliferative fibrocystic changes:* The architecture of the terminal-duct lobular unit is distorted by the formation of microcysts, associated with interlobular fibrosis. **B,** *Proliferative hyperplasia without atypia:* This is adenosis, a distinctive form of hyperplasia characterized by the proliferation of lobular acini, forming crowded glandlike structures. For comparison, a normal lobule is on the left side. **C,** *Proliferative hyperplasia without atypia:* There is moderate ductal hyperplasia, which is characterized by a duct that is partially distended by hyperplastic epithelium within the lumen. **D,** *Proliferative hyperplasia without atypia, which is florid ductal hyperplasia:* The involved duct is greatly expanded by a crowded, jumbled-appearing epithelial proliferation. **E,** *Atypical ductal hyperplasia:* These proliferations are complex and partially formed secondary lumens and mild nuclear hyperchromasia in the epithelial cell population. The peripheral spaces are irregular and slitlike. **F,** *Atypical lobular hyperplasia:* Monomorphic, small, rounded loosely cohesive cells fill the lumens of partially distended acini in this terminal-duct lobular unit (hematoxylin and eosin). (From Elmore JG, Gigerenzer G: *N Engl J Med* 353[3]:231, 2005.)

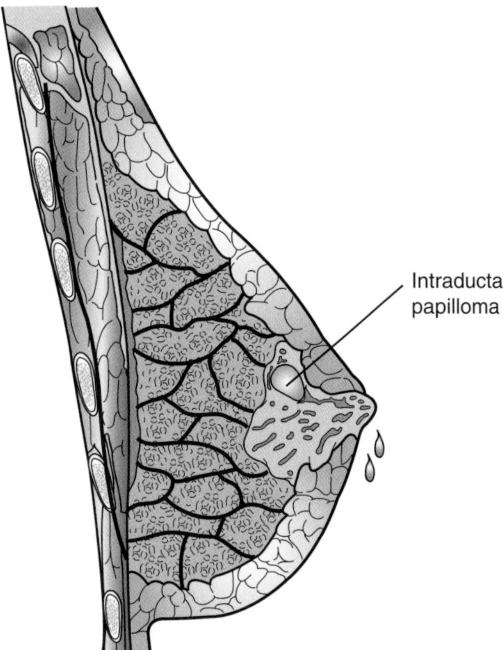

FIGURE 24-28 Intraductal Papilloma.

atypia (ductal or lobular) coexisting with a single papilloma (atypical papilloma) does not appreciably modify the breast cancer risk attributable to just atypia.[179] A solitary papilloma without atypia conveys a risk similar to proliferative fibrocystic lesions. Although the breast cancer risk is small, **multiple papillomas,** called **diffuse papillomatosis,** even without identified atypia, can increase breast cancer risk. Diffuse papillomatosis is defined as a minimum of five papillomas within a localized segment of breast tissue.[173]

3. **Sclerosing adenosis.** Sclerosing adenosis is a lobular lesion with increased fibrous tissue and scattered glandular cells.[173] Calcification is commonly present within the lumens; however, the normal lobular arrangement is maintained. It can present as a mass or suspicious finding from mammogram but requires no treatment. Occasionally, stromal fibrosis may mimic the appearance of invasive carcinoma.[177]
4. **Radial scar.** Radial scar (RS) refers to an irregular, radial proliferation of ductlike small tubules entrapped in a densely fibrotic stroma (Figure 24-29). The term *scar* refers to the structural appearance only because these lesions are not associated with scarring and fibrosis from a prior injury, biopsy, or surgery. RS also has been called *radial sclerosing lesions* and *sclerosing papillary proliferation.* RSs are usually discovered when a breast lesion or radiologic abnormality is biopsied or removed. Occasionally RSs are large enough to be detected by mammography, which, however, cannot reliably differentiate between these lesions and spiculated (spiky with pointed features) carcinoma. Controversy exists about the need for surgical excision when RSs are found. There is some evidence that RSs may be premalignant lesions, and the possibility of finding an unrecognized in situ or invasive component suggests that they be surgically excised.[173] Yet a retrospective study of 9556 women found that although RSs mildly elevate the risk of invasive breast cancer, the risk was largely attributed to the coexistent presence of proliferative disease.[180] Invasive breast cancer risk was further increased in women with AH.[180,181] No additional treatment is needed beyond excision and the risk of subsequent breast cancer is small.[173]

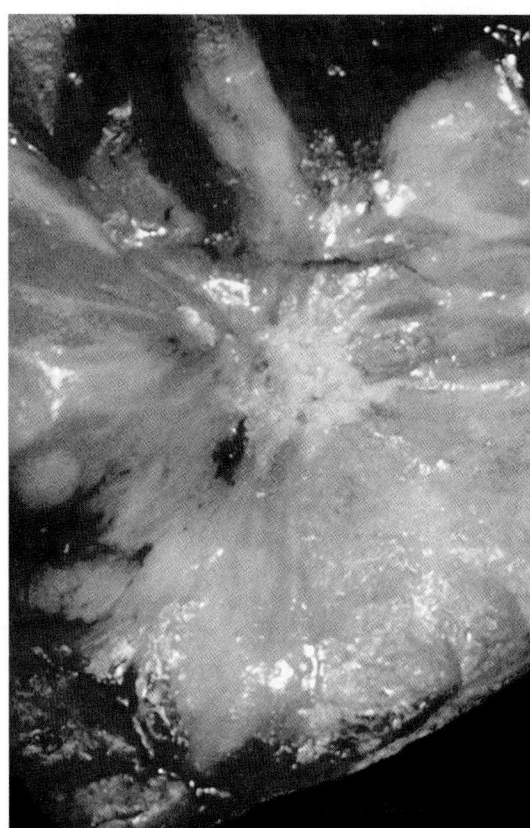

FIGURE 24-29 Radial Scar. Gross pathologic specimen of radial scar. (From the Armed Forces Institute of Pathology.)

5. **Simple fibroadenoma.** Simple fibroadenomas are benign solid tumors composed of both fibrous and glandular tissue.[178] Fibroadenomas are now considered proliferative lesions and the histologic features influence the risk of breast cancer.[178,182] If the fibroadenoma is complex with adjacent proliferative disease or if there is a family history of breast cancer the risk of breast cancer is slightly elevated. There is no increased risk of breast cancer in the majority of women with a simple fibroadenoma. Multiple fibroadenomas occur in the same breast or bilaterally in about 20% of cases.[178] Fibroadenomas are found most commonly in women between the ages of 15 and 35 years but they can occur at any age, especially in older women on hormone therapy.[183] The etiology is unknown, but a hormonal role is likely because they persist during the reproductive years, increase in size during pregnancy or with estrogen therapy, and usually regress after menopause. Fibroadenomas usually present as a well-defined mobile mass—smooth and hard like a marble—on physical examination or a well-defined solid mass on

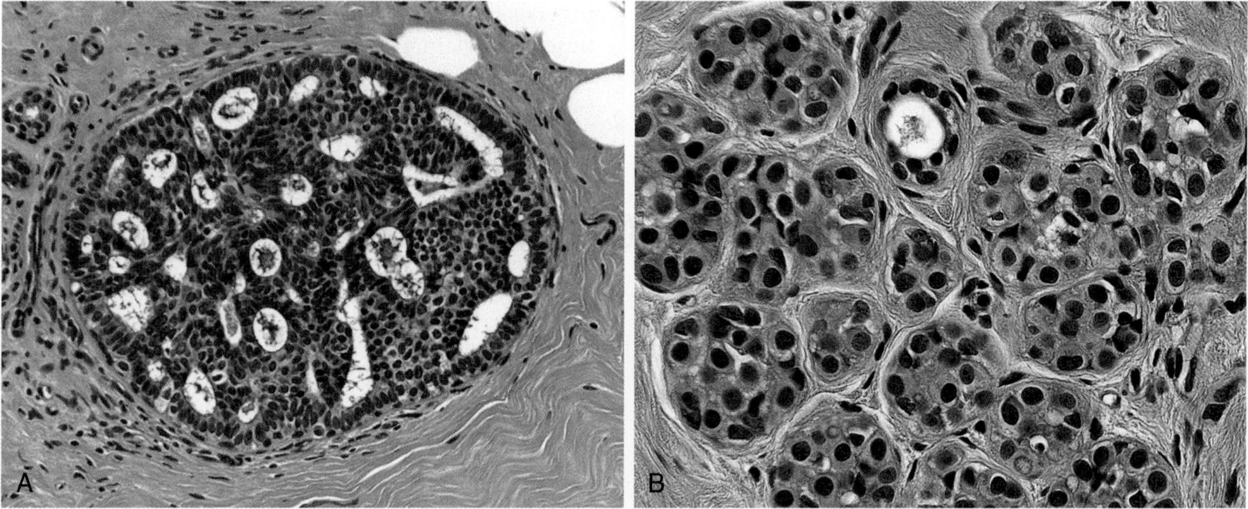

FIGURE 24-30 Atypical Ductal and Lobular Hyperplasias. A, Atypical ductal hyperplasia. A duct is filled with a mixed population of cells. Although some of the spaces are round and regular, the peripheral spaces are irregular and slitlike. These features are highly atypical but fall short of a diagnosis of ductal carcinoma in situ (DCIS). **B,** Atypical lobular hyperplasia. A population of monomorphic small, rounded, loosely cohesive cells partially fill a lobule. (From Kumar V: *Robbins & Cotran pathologic basis of disease,* ed 8, Philadelphia, 2008, Saunders.)

ultrasound. Not all biopsy-proven lesions require surgical excision. If a fibroadenoma increases in size or is symptomatic, surgical excision is mandated to know if the lesion is malignant.[178]

Proliferative Breast Lesions with Atypia

Proliferative breast lesions with some abnormal structure or *atypia* include **atypical ductal hyperplasia (ADH),** or abnormal proliferating cells in breast ducts, and **atypical lobular hyperplasia (ALH),** or abnormal proliferating cells in breast lobules.[177,178] ALH also can involve ducts.[178] **Atypical hyperplasia (AH)** is an increase in the number of cells with some variation in cellular structure but lacks sufficient qualitative or quantitative features of carcinoma. Studies continue to indicate that women with AH have an increased risk (about fourfold) of breast cancer compared with women who have nonproliferative lesions.[174] AH is associated with an increased risk of both ipsilateral (same side as lesion) and contralateral breast cancer indicating some evidence of underlying breast abnormalities that predispose to breast cancer.[178] Major determinants of breast cancer risk include histologic/biologic findings, degree of family history, and previous (age of) biopsy (see p. 843).[174] Recent findings from the Nurses' Health Study (NHS) found adolescent alcohol consumption is associated with increased risk of proliferative BBD.[184] Among premenopausal women at the time of their benign biopsy, the risk of breast cancer was substantially increased among women with AH (Odds ratio [OR], 7.3) than among women with ADH (OR, 2.72). The risks for women who were postmenopausal at the time of benign biopsy were similar for women with ALH and those with ADH.[174]

Ductal hyperplasia is an increased number of uniform epithelial cells within the lumen of the terminal ducts (Figure 24-30, *A*). Atypical ductal hyperplasia includes a continuum of changes—cell structure and placement—ranging from an increase in cellularity to features of DCIS (see p. 866). In ADH, the cells fail to completely fill ductal spaces as compared with DCIS.

Lobular hyperplasia refers to proliferation of small uniform cells in the lumen of lobular units. The abnormal cells of ALH and lobular carcinoma in situ (LCIS) share some of the cytologic and structural features, but the cells in ALH do not distend more than 50% of the acini within a lobule (see Figure 24-30, *B*). ALH can extend into ducts, and this is associated with an increased risk of invasive carcinomas.[177] Other benign conditions are summarized in Table 24-10.

EVALUATION AND TREATMENT. Breast problems should be diagnosed from a multimodal approach that combines physical examination, mammogram when applicable, sonogram, possibly MRI, and careful consideration of a biopsy. The principal mammographic signs of breast carcinoma are densities and calcifications. However, the dense breast tissue often seen in young women can make interpretation extremely difficult. Newer screening and diagnostic methods are being tested including those without compression and ionizing radiation such as different technologies using MRI. Ultrasonography (ultrasound) is used to differentiate a solid mass from a cystic (fluid-filled) mass, which is generally benign.

Treatment consists largely of relieving symptoms. Risk reduction for AH includes avoiding hormone therapy and oral contraceptives, careful diet choices, and exercise. Certain selective estrogen modulators, such as tamoxifen and raloxifene, or an aromatase inhibitor may be considered after a thorough discussion of risks and benefits.[178] Breast pain may be minimized by wearing a brassiere that provides good support. Reduction of caffeinated beverages, cola, root beer, and chocolate, which can cause overstimulation of breast tissue for some women, may reduce pain and nodularity. Given time the cysts may disappear without treatment. Although still controversial and possibly dose-dependent, isoflavone exposure has been associated with a decreased risk of proliferative benign fibrocystic changes, nonproliferative changes, and breast cancer.[185,186]

Iodine deficiency may increase fibrocystic breast change, thus may be useful for relieving pain.[187] Although unknown, increasing omega-3 fatty acids may decrease associated pain caused by inflammation as well as the application of castor oil packs to the breasts. The use of anti-inflammatories also may decrease inflammation. Drugs used to treat severe breast pain are listed in Table 24-11.

TABLE 24-10 OTHER BENIGN BREAST CONDITIONS

TYPE	COMMENT
Developmental	
Milk-line remnants	Increase in number of nipples or breasts results from persistent epidermal thickening along the milk line
Accessory axillary breast tissue	Ductal system may extend into subcutaneous tissue of the chest wall and axillary region; this tissue can undergo lactational changes and give rise to tumors
Congenital nipple inversion	Is common and may be unilateral; can spontaneously correct during pregnancy; can be confused with retraction of nipple, which is sometimes part of invasive cancer or inflammation
Macromastia	Juvenile hypertrophy may be caused by unusual tissue response to hormonal stimulus
Iatrogenic	
Reconstruction or augmentation	Breast tissue can be replaced or augmented by skin and muscle flaps for synthetic prostheses; silicone implants, the most common, are rubbery silicone filled with either silicone gel or saline; a common complication of implants is formation of a thick fibrous capsule (i.e., chronic inflammatory responses) that can cause cosmetic deformity; the capsule can limit the spread of a ruptured implant but if the capsule ruptures silicone gel can escape; long-term consequences of rupture are unknown
Inflammation	
Acute mastitis	Inflammatory diseases of the breast are rare; acute mastitis is confined to the lactating period of nursing; the nipples can become dry, cracked, and fissured, increasing risk of bacterial infection; infection may lead to abscess formation
Periductal mastitis	Women or men present with a painful subareolar mass thought to be infectious; not associated with lactation; 90% of individuals are smokers; vitamin A deficiency associated with smoking may alter the differentiation of the ductal epithelium; keratin is trapped within the ductal system causing dilation and rupture; antibiotic therapy and surgery are usually indicated
Mammary duct ectasia	Affects 50- and 60-year-olds, usually multiparous women, not associated with smoking; dilation of ducts with chronic granulomatous inflammatory reaction; fibrosis may eventually lead to skin and nipple retraction, thus mistaken for cancer; may have white nipple secretions
Fat necrosis	Painless, palpable mass, skin thickening or retraction; mammographic density or calcification; may have hemorrhage; most women will give a history of prior surgery or trauma; can be confused with breast carcinoma
Lymphocytic mastopathy	Single or multiple hard, palpable masses; can be so hard that interferes with biopsy; lesion includes collagenized stroma surrounding atrophic ducts and lobules; the breast membrane is frequently thickened; a prominent lymphocytic infiltrate surrounds epithelium and blood vessels; most common in women with type 1 diabetes or autoimmune thyroid disease

Data from Lester SC: The breast. In Kumar V, Abbas AK, Fausto N, editors: *Robbins & Cotran pathologic basis of disease*, ed 7, Philadelphia, 2005, Saunders.

TABLE 24-11 DRUGS USED TO TREAT SEVERE BREAST PAIN (MASTALGIA)

AGENTS	COMMENTS
Definitely Effective	
Danazol	Causes a decrease in cyclic pain and nodularity believed to reduce estrogen; also used for endometriosis; some side effects include changes in menstrual cycle regularity, weight gain, acne, and flushing
Bromocriptine	Decreases cyclic pain, nodularity, and tenderness; decreases prolactin levels and may alter dopamine receptors; is also used to suppress lactation after childbirth; can cause nausea, vomiting, hypotension, and dizziness
Tamoxifen	As an antiestrogen it can decrease cyclic pain; increase clot formation (phlebitis, emboli, strokes); cause hot flashes, amenorrhea, weight gain, and increased risk of uterine cancers
Evening primrose oil (linoleic acid)	Can decrease cyclic pain, nodularity, and tenderness; women with mastalgia believed to have low levels of breast linoleic acid; reduces PGE2 prostaglandins and inflammation; too much oil, however, has been associated with increasing inflammation (>1000 mg/day)
Possibly Effective	
Iodine	Can decrease cyclic pain and nodularity (see Nutrition & Disease: Premenstrual Syndrome, p. 813)
Vaginal progesterone	Decrease in cyclic pain and tenderness; not as effective for decreasing tenderness; antagonist to estrogen; can cause weight gain
Insufficiently Studied	
Progestins	May decrease estrogenic effects; however, related to endothelial vasospasms, weight gain, and increased risk of breast cancer

TABLE 24-12 CHANCE OF BEING DIAGNOSED WITH BREAST CANCER

BY AGE (Years)	BY RATIO
30-39	1 in 238
40-49	1 in 69
50-59	1 in 38
60-69	1 in 27
Ever*	1 in 8
Never	7 in 8

Data from Reis LAG et al: *Cancer statistics review,* 1975-2005, Bethesda, MD, 2008, National Cancer Institute. Available at http://seer.cancer.gov/csr/1975_2005. Based on November 2007 SEER data, posted SEER website, 2008.
NOTE: These calculations are averages. An individual's risk may be higher or lower depending on several factors (e.g., family history, reproductive history, race/ethnicity, and others).
*Absolute lifetime risk.

Cancer

Breast cancer, the most common cancer in American women, is the leading cause of death in women ages 40 to 44 years and the second most common killer after lung cancer of women of all ages. The incidence of breast cancer has risen steadily since the 1970s and started leveling off from 1998 to 1999; incidence for all races combined is about 125 cases per 100,000 women per year. It is estimated that 234,580 women and 2240 men will be diagnosed with breast cancer, and 40,030 women and 410 men will die from breast cancer in 2013.[1] Age and the chance of being diagnosed with breast cancer are presented in Table 24-12. The breast cancer death rate in the United States has been declining from 1989 to 1990, peaking at a rate of 33 deaths per 100,000 women.[188] The age-adjusted death rate from 2005 to 2009 in the United States is 23 per 100,000 women per year. Breast cancer comprises clinically distinct subtypes. The National Cancer Institute (NCI) reported subtypes by race including estrogen receptor (ER), progesterone receptor (PR), HER2/neu, and triple negative (ER negative, PR negative, and HER2 negative). The luminal breast cancer subtype predominates across racial/ethnic groups with lifetime risk lowest in Hispanic women and highest in white women. Triple negative breast cancer is highest in black women compared with Asians, followed by Hispanics and whites.[189] Overall, black women have lower incidence of breast cancer but a 41% higher mortality than white women.[190] Black women in all age groups experience the highest mortality rates for breast cancer although the reason for this disparity is not clearly understood but includes diagnoses at later stages, excess obesity, and triple negative breast cancer, which has a more aggressive phenotype.[190] More than two thirds of breast cancer cases occur in women older than 55 years. From 2005 to 2009, the median age for breast cancer diagnosis was 61 years of age. The median age at death for breast cancer was 68 years of age.[191] Because DCIS is almost exclusively detected by mammography, the large increase in incidence of DCIS over the past 20 years can be attributed to screening (see What's New? Screening Mammography: Why It Has Not Lived Up to Expectations, Chapter 12, p. 393).

Risk factors and possible causes of breast cancer can be classified as reproductive, hormonal, environmental and lifestyle, and familial (Table 24-13). However, two factors emerging as important are postpartum involution of the mammary gland and breast density, which are not as easily classified.

Reproductive Factors: Pregnancy

A clearer understanding of mammary gland structure (morphology) and function from fetal development, to puberty, pregnancy, and aging will help elucidate fundamental changes to breast development and disease. A key element is "branching morphogenesis," in which the mammary gland produces and delivers copious amounts of milk by forming a rootlike network of branched ducts from a rudimentary epithelial bud.[192] Branching morphogenesis begins in fetal development, pauses after birth, starts again in response to estrogens at puberty, and is modified by cyclic ovarian hormonal action. This systemic hormonal action elicits local paracrine interactions between the developing epithelial ducts and their adjacent mesenchyme (embryonic) or postnatal stroma. Then the local cellular crosstalk directs the tissue remodeling, ultimately producing a mature ductal tree.[192] The gland is unique because it undergoes most of its branching during adolescence and not fetal development. This allows experimental manipulation of the gland not possible with any other organ.[193]

A woman's age when her first child is born affects her risk for developing breast cancer—the younger she is, the lower the risk. Overall, lifetime risk of breast cancer is reduced in parous women compared to nulliparous women, but pregnancy must occur at a young age.[194] A complete pregnancy before age 25 reduces the risk of breast cancer by about 36%, this protective effect is weakened in multiparous women if their age at first birth is greater than 30.[195,196] The protective factor is especially observed in the years of peak incidence, the postmenopausal years.[197] The risk reduction is limited to hormone receptor–positive breast cancer.[195] The influence of pregnancy on the risk of breast cancer also depends on family history, lactation postpartum, and overall parity.[196] Paradoxically, women of all ages have a transient *increase* in breast cancer risk with a recent pregnancy and after each subsequent pregnancy.[196,198] **Pregnancy-associated breast cancer (PABC)** is defined as breast cancers diagnosed up to 5 years after a completed pregnancy; however, risk may persist for a decade.[196,199] Delayed childbearing observed in the United States and all developing countries is expected to show a rise in diagnosed breast cancers.[196] The transient increase in breast cancer risk for all parous women includes events associated with pregnancy, including pregnancy-related hormones, such as estrogen, progesterone, and growth hormone, that promote or initiate cancer cells, immune suppressive effects of pregnancy, and breast tissue involution.[196] Breast gland *involution* after pregnancy and lactation uses some of the same tissue remodeling pathways activated during wound healing (i.e., proinflammatory pathways). The proinflammatory environment, although physiologically normal, promotes tumor progression. One mechanism identified links fibrillar collagen deposition, noted during normal involution, to high levels of COX-2 expression in tumor cells

TABLE 24-13 FACTORS ASSOCIATED WITH INCREASED RISK OF BREAST CANCER*

CATEGORY	RISK FACTOR	RELATIVE RISK†
Race	Blacks have higher incidence up to age 40 yr; whites have higher incidence after age 40	1.1-1.9
Family history	Breast cancer in first-degree relative before age 60	2-3
	Premenopausal or bilateral breast cancer	>4
	Postmenopausal in first-degree relative	≤2
	Breast cancer in two first-degree relatives	4-6
	BRCA1 or *BRCA2*	≤4
	TP53 (Li-Fraumeni syndrome)	≤4
Previous medical history	Moderate or florid mammary hyperplasia	1.5-2
	Mammary papilloma	1.5-2
	Atypical mammary hyperplasia	4-5
	DCIS, LCIS‡	8-10
Estrogen exposure	Early menarche (before age 12 yr)	1.1-1.9
	Late menopause (after age 55)	1.1-1.9
	Postmenopausal hormone therapy	1.4
	Oral contraceptive use	1.5
Pregnancy	Nulliparous or late first pregnancy (after age 35)	1.1-1.9
Radiation	Atomic bomb	3
	Repeated fluoroscopy	1.5-2§
Obesity and stature	Postmenopausal	1.2
	Tallness	≤2
Dietary/alcohol	High alcohol consumption	1.4-2
	High energy intake	≤2
	Advanced age	2-4
	Xenobiotics	≤2
Social	Smoking	2-4
	Higher socioeconomic status	≤2
	Low physical activity	≤2
Environmental	Excess radiation to breasts	??‡
	Chemical carcinogens	≤2-??
	Infectious agents	≤2-??

*Normal lifetime risk in white non-Hispanic women: 1 in 8.
†Relative risk is defined and discussed in Chapter 5.
‡Data from Lester SC: The breast. In Kumar V, Abbas AK, Fausto N, editors: *Robbins & Cotran pathologic basis of disease,* ed 7, Philadelphia, 2005, Saunders.
§Currently debated.
DCIS, Ductal carcinoma in situ; *LCIS,* lobular carcinoma in situ.

and subsequent tumor cell metastasis.[194] This alteration provides support to the tissue change in stroma for driving carcinogenesis.[200] The presence of macrophages in the involuting mammary gland contributes to carcinogenesis.[198,201] Immature macrophages are capable of suppressing cytotoxic T-cell function causing an immunosuppressive stroma conducive to tumor cell promotion. Macrophage and T-cell abundance in breast cancer represent prognostic indicators for tumor recurrence and overall survival.[202] (Involution and pathophysiology are discussed on p. 845.)

The main mechanisms for the *protective* effect of pregnancy are controversial including: (1) induction of breast differentiation with lasting protective phenotypic (morphologic) changes; (2) altered cell fate with removal or modification of vulnerable cells, possibly stem cells; (3) enhancement of the ability for DNA repair or apoptosis, or both; (4) altered systemic hormonal regulation and possible persistent changes in intracellular pathways regulating proliferation; (5) decreased proliferation in the parous involuted gland; and (6) early-life hormonal and dietary exposures.[197] Longer duration of breast-feeding (at least 1 year) is associated with a decreased risk of both hormone receptor–positive and hormone receptor–negative breast cancer.[203] In older first-time mothers, there is theoretically a greater chance for precancerous breast lesions to continue to develop with pregnancy or with events related to pregnancy, for example, postpartum gland involution[196] (see p. 845).

Amphiregulin (AREG) was found to be a major paracrine mediator of ductal morphogenesis and plays an important role in mammary stem cell self-renewal and differentiation.[204] Recent studies show that AREG modulates WNT and NOTCH signaling and functions in regulating the invasive phenotype.[205] Investigators are focusing on the *TP53* tumor-suppressor gene, which has been demonstrated to be important in pregnancy-related hormone-induced protection. The function of *TP53* is required for hormone-mediated protection against the carcinogens dimethylbenz(*a*)anthracene (DMBA)-induced carcinogenesis in mice.[193] The functions of cadherins or adhesion molecules and p53 (protein) are closely linked. A pivotal role for p53 is the regulation of a balance between apoptosis and cell proliferation.[206] Russo and colleagues[207] have found that the postpregnancy involuted mammary gland exhibits elevated expression of genes involved in DNA repair and apoptosis. Pregnancy may induce a protective mechanism at the post-transcriptional level (epigenetically) that maintains the faithfulness of the transcriptional process.[208]

Lobular Involution and Age and Postlactational Involution

Part of the uniqueness of the mammary gland is its profound physiologic changes throughout the phases of a woman's life: puberty, pregnancy, lactation, postlactational involution, and aging. The human breast is organized to 15 to 20 major lobes, each with lobules containing milk-forming acini (see Figure 23-19). With aging, breast lobules regress or involute with a decrease in the number and size of acini per lobule and replacement of the intralobular stroma with the more dense collagen of connective tissue.[209] Over time the glandular elements and collagen are replaced with fatty tissue. This process is called **lobular involution** whereby, over many years, the parenchymal elements progressively atrophy and disappear. A first study of its kind found lobular involution was associated with reduced risk of breast cancer. Breast cancer risk decreased with increasing extent of involution in both high- and low-risk subgroups defined by family history of breast cancer, epithelial atypia, reproductive history, and age. Based on histologic and epidemiologic factors, these investigators propose that delayed involution (persistent glandular epithelium) is a major risk factor for breast cancer.[209] Widely appreciated is that as women age, their risk of breast cancer increases. But the *rate* of increase of breast cancer *slows* at about 50 years of age.[210] This slowing has been attributed to a reduction in ovarian hormone production. Milanese and colleagues[209] observed a definite increase in the process of involution at about 50 years of age with complete involution present in 5.8% of women ages 40 to 49 years and 21.6% of women ages 50 to 59 years. Investigators propose that involution may contribute to this slowing in the rate of increase of breast cancer among women older than 50 years. Importantly, investigators found an inverse association between lobular involution and parity.[209] Other investigators have reported that the more children a woman has, the more likely she is to have persistent lobular tissue,[211] which Milanese and colleagues[209] found was associated with increased risk of breast cancer. However, multiparity also has been found to reduce risk of breast cancer.[212,213] This apparent contradiction may be explained by studies documenting that full-term pregnancies after 35 years of age are correlated with an increased risk of breast cancer.[214] In the Milanese study, age of the mother at each child's birth was unknown.

Henson and colleagues[215] propose that late pregnancy with its concomitant increase in the proliferation of the ductal-alveolar epithelium is likely to interrupt the process of involution, which typically begins between 30 and 40 years of age. The activated stromal environment in the process of involution is similar to that in invasive breast cancer. The long-term protective effects of pregnancy with hormones released during pregnancy affect remodeling of the stromal microenvironment by causing apoptosis and involution. However, an increase in breast cancer risk following pregnancy may be caused by the *process* of mammary gland involution, which returns the tissue back to its prepregnant state and is co-opted by processes of wound healing resulting in a proinflammatory environment that although physiologically normal can promote carcinogenesis.[201] Postpartum involution uses the biologically coordinated programs of epithelial cell death and stromal remodeling to change the gland back to its original nonsecretory state before the next pregnancy.[194] In a mouse model, human breast cancer cells exposed to the involuting mammary microenvironment form large tumors with abundant fibrillar collagen, high COX-2 expression, and further evidence of an invasive phenotype.[194] Additionally, macrophages, specifically M2-polarized macrophages, are necessary for the epithelial cell death during normal postpartum mammary gland involution.[216] Therefore, the re-emerging stroma and activated immune cells seem key for understanding the pathogenesis of pregnancy-associated breast cancer. An important transcriptional regulator of genes, **Stat3,** is associated with inflammation, wound healing, mammary macrophages, and mast cells. Stat3 appears to have an important role in modulating cell death and involution.[217] In postlactational involution the mammary gland regresses and remodels to its prepregnant state whereby fibroblasts secrete proteases that degrade the extracellular matrix proteins. Consequently, the increased release of bioactive matrix fragments can promote tumor growth, motility, and invasion.[199] The extracellular matrix (ECM) is very different between nulliparous, lactating, and involuting glands as shown in Figure 24-31 (see What's New? Breastfeeding and a New Emerging Target—NSAIDs for the Prevention of Pregnancy-Associated Breast Cancer).

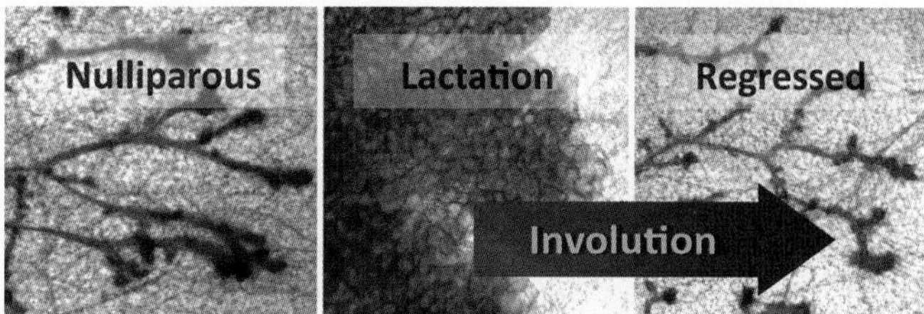

FIGURE 24-31 Extracellular Matrix (ECM) Is Different in Nulliparous, Lactating, and Involuting Glands. Several ECM differences between nulliparous, lactational, and involuting mammary glands are related to collagen-fiber organization, cell motility and attachment, and cytokine regulation in a rodent model. Many protumorigenic ECM proteins are mediators of breast cancer progression specific to the involutional window, and systemic ibuprofen experimental treatment during involution decreases its tumor promotional changes. (From O'Brien JH et al: *J Proteome Res* 11:4894–4905, 2012.)

Interestingly, oophorectomy, which is associated with a decrease in risk of breast cancer, leads to atrophy of breast parenchyma in young women as is noted in older women. Thus the risk reduction of oophorectomy may be caused by an accelerated involution.[215]

Hormonal Factors

The link between breast cancer and hormones is based on six factors that affect risk: (1) the protective effect of an early (i.e., in the 20s) first pregnancy; (2) the protective effect of removal of the ovaries and pituitary gland; (3) the increased risk associated

WHAT'S NEW?

Breastfeeding and a New Emerging Target—NSAIDs for the Prevention of Pregnancy-Associated Breast Cancer?

A longer duration of breast-feeding is correlated with a lower risk of breast cancer.[1] In reports of large sample sizes, the risk-reducing effect was observed for both pre-and postmenopausal women.[1,2] Longer duration of breast-feeding reduced the risk of triple-negative cancers but not for luminal cancers.[3] The longer the duration of breast-feeding per child was related to lowered risks of breast cancer.[4,5] Although it has not been adequately studied, one hypothesis for why longer duration of breast-feeding is protective against breast cancer is that a slow-paced weaning may decrease the stromal inflammatory reaction during the breast involution.[6] Pregnancy and postpartum involution both affect a woman's risk for breast cancer. The postpartum period is associated with a transient 5- to 10-year period of increased risk crossing over to a protective effect.[7-9] Recent pregnancy correlates with decreased survival for breast cancer patients compared with nonpregnancy-associated breast cancer.[10] Postpartum breast cancers are known as type II pregnancy-associated breast cancer (PABC). Mechanisms of postpartum mammary gland involution in which the physiologic programs similar to those involved in wound healing are activated to remodel the lactationally competent mammary gland back to a nonsecretory state likely account for the poorer prognosis of PABC.[11] Recently, having breast-fed and the total duration of breast-feeding conferred a substantial reduction in breast cancer risk among *BRCA1* but not *BRCA2* mutation carriers, of 32%.[12]

Investigators using the lactogenic microenvironment to discover new therapies that would promote breast differentiation (thus decrease the risk of cell transformation) developed a lactogenic mouse model. These investigators showed that the loss of a single gene, caveolin-3 (cav-3) expressed in myoepithelial cells within the mammary gland, conferred protection against mammary tumor formation.[13] These results support the fact that the lactogenic microenvironment is a critical factor in preventing mammary tumor onset, progression, and metastases.[13]

Investigators demonstrated that cyclo-oxygenase 2 (COX-2), an enzyme involved in initiating inflammatory responses, is up-regulated in the mammary gland during involution. COX-2 inhibition is considered an important target for prevention and treatment of several cancers.[14] NSAID treatment (ibuprofen) in animal models of PABC decreases tumor-promotional attributes of postpartum involution mammary extracellular matrix.[14] Treatment inhibited tumor progression, in part, by suppressing COX-2–dependent collagen deposition. Investigators assessed drug effects on the process of mammary gland involution. They demonstrated that COX-2 inhibition by NSAIDs can decrease COX-2 activity in the gland without interruption of involution.[14] NSAIDs suppress tenascin-C, a glycoprotein, expressed in mesenchymal tissues during development and re-expressed during carcinogenesis.[14] Studies investigating promotion of breast cancers that develop in the postpartum period have identified fibrillar collagen as an ECM mediator of progression that can be targeted by ibuprofen treatment.[15,16] Organization of collagen into radially aligned fibers, called tumor-associated collagen, predicts survival in women with breast cancer.[17] M2-polarized macrophages are necessary for epithelial cell death during normal postpartum mammary gland involution.[18] Macrophages and their monocytic precursors can change their functional state (e.g., exhibit plasticity) in response to cues from the microenvironment. For example, macrophages can be functionally polarized into M1 (proinflammatory) and M2 (alternatively activated),

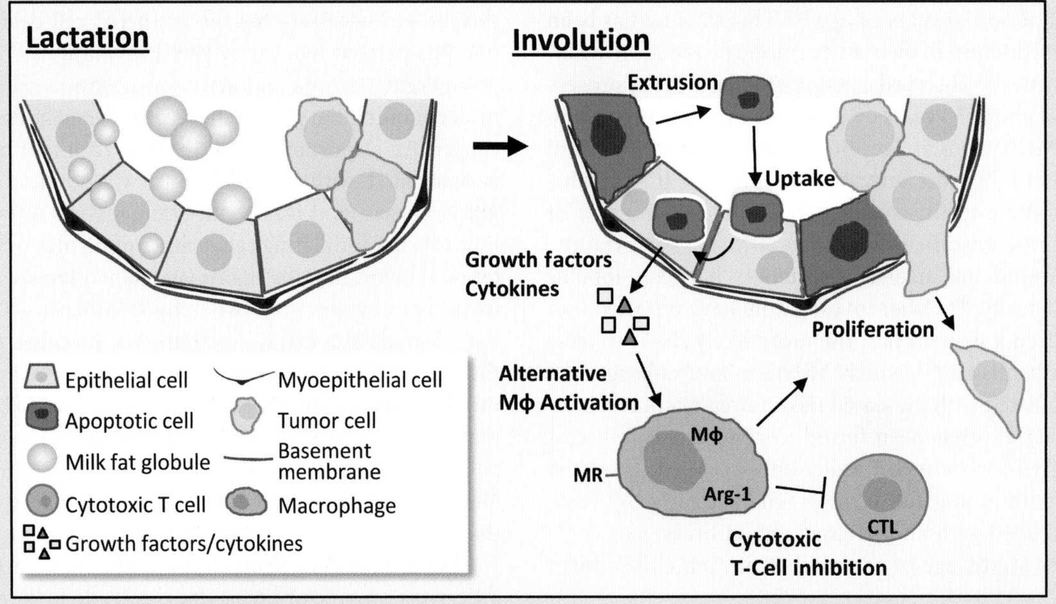

Mammary Epithelial Cells, Immune Modulation, Tumor Supportive. The switch from lactation *(left)* to involution *(right)* promotes milk-producing epithelial cells to undergo apoptosis *(dark blue cells)* and then the cells extrude into the alveolar lumen. Other milk-producing cells are activated to become phagocytic cells *(light blue cells)* and engulf the shed apoptotic (dead) cells. Clearance by the immune system of apoptotic cells is thought to result in release of Th2 cytokines and growth factors from the phagocytic mammary cells. This changed cytokine environment is anticipated to promote alternative activation of macrophages (see text) and inhibition of a protective immune response or cytotoxic T lymphocyte (CTL) cells, resulting in an immunosuppressive environment and promoting a tumor microenvironment *(green cells)*. (From Fornetti J et al: *Cell Cycle* 11[4]:639–640, 2012.)

WHAT'S NEW?—cont'd

Breastfeeding and a New Emerging Target—NSAIDs for the Prevention of Pregnancy-Associated Breast Cancer?

called M2-polarized macrophages.[19] Interleukin-4 (IL-4) and IL-13, cytokines of the Th2 response, are the major inducers of the "alternative activation" of macrophages that play an important role in the immune response to parasites, in allergy, wound healing, and tissue remodeling.[19] The figure on p. 846 represents a recent model of phagocytic mammary epithelial cells and a protumorigenic microenvironment.

NSAIDs potentially represent a promising treatment for type II PABC without interrupting postpartum remodeling. Elucidation on the mechanisms of lobular involution is very important for understanding breast carcinogenesis and factors that reduce breast cancer risk. Factors related to the risk of breast cancer are diverse and not just limited to reproductive factors. However, with later age of first full-term birth around the world, concern is for increasing the baseline risk of breast cancers.

References

1. Collaborative Group on Hormonal Factors in Breast Cancer: *Lancet* 360(9328):187–195, 2002.
2. Ursin G et al: *Br J Cancer* 93(3):364–371, 2005.
3. Gaudet MM et al: *Breast Cancer Res Treat* 130(2):587–597, 2011.
4. Chang-Claude J: *Cancer Causes Control* 11(8):687–695, 2000.
5. DeSilva M et al: *Cancer Epidemiol* 34(3):267–273, 2010.
6. Kobayashi S et al: *Breast Cancer* 19:302–308, 2012.
7. Albrektsen G et al: *Br J Cancer* 92(1):167–175, 2005.
8. Lambe M et al: *N Engl J Med* 331(1):5–9, 1994.
9. Lyons TR, Schedin PJ, Borges VF: *J Mammary Gland Biol Neoplasia* 14(2):87–98, 2009.
10. Schedin P: *Nat Rev Cancer* 6(4):281–291, 2006.
11. Fornetti J et al: *Cell Cycle* 11(4):639–640, 2012.
12. Kotsopoulos J et al: *Breast Cancer Res* 14(2):R42, 2012.
13. Sotgia F et al: *Am J Pathol* 174(2):613–629, 2009.
14. O'Brien O et al: *Int J Dev Biol* 55:745–755, 2011.
15. Lyons TR et al: *Nat Med* 17(9):1109–1115, 2011.
16. O'Brien J et al: *Am J Pathol* 176(3):1241–1255, 2010.
17. Conklin MW: *Am J Pathol* 178(3):1221–1232, 2011.
18. O'Brien J et al: *Development* 139:269–275, 2012.
19. Cassetta L, Cassol E, Poli G: *Sci World J* 11:2391–2402, 2011.

with early menarche, late menopause, and nulliparity; (4) the relationship between types of fat, free estrogen levels, and oxidative changes in estrogen metabolism; (5) the hormone-dependent development and differentiation of mammary gland structures; and (6) the efficacy of antihormone therapies for treatment and prevention of breast cancer. Throughout its existence, the mammary gland epithelium proceeds through critical "exposure periods" of rapid growth or cycles of proliferation, including neonatal growth, pubertal development, pregnancy, lactation, and involution (after pregnancy and postmenopause; see p. 845).[201,218]

Our understanding of the role of systemic hormones as powerful regulators of mammary gland development is shifting. Evidence is pointing to the wide-ranging effects of systemic hormones as possibly not due to their *direct* hormone action but rather their *induced* actions from multiple secondary paracrine effectors—thus the term *hierarchical*.[192] Unraveling is a complex model of hormone, paracrine, and adhesion molecule-signaling pathways affecting epithelial and stromal cell fate in development and cancer (Figure 24-32). Despite differences between the organized process of development and the less, even chaotic, environment of invasive cancer, both processes share many identical mechanisms and signaling pathways. Key is *tissue remodeling* that applies to pubertal growth, immediately after pregnancy and during involution (see previous section).[201,219,220]

The female reproductive hormones (estrogens, progesterone, and prolactin) have a major role and effect on mammary gland development and breast cancer (Figure 24-33).[219] A vast majority of breast cancers are *initially* hormone dependent (estrogen receptor positive [ER+] and/or progesterone receptor positive [PR+]), with estrogens playing a crucial role in their development.[221] Estrogens control processes critical for cellular functions by regulating activities and expression of key signaling molecules. These processes include regulation of receptor activity, its interaction with other intracellular proteins, and DNA.[221] Estrogens thus play prominent roles in cellular proliferation, differentiation, and apoptosis.[221-223] Estrogens affect microtubules that are essential for establishing cell shape and cell polarity, processes necessary for epithelial gland organization.[221]

Depending on the experimental model system used, progesterone in animal and in vitro studies show both an increase and decrease in breast cancer risk[224-226] (see following discussion). These data question the continuing view that PR is co-expressed in every ER+ luminal cell, highlighting the potential for ER and PR to *individually* contribute to the biology of normal breast development, function, and role in breast carcinogenesis[227] (Figure 24-34, and see p. 849). Additionally these data identify a novel cell population that may be very important in understanding the cancer-causing effects of synthetic progestins in hormone replacement therapy (HRT) (see p. 853).

Prolactin, produced by the pituitary gland, travels through the blood and exerts multiple metabolic and reproductive effects especially on the breast as the key regulator of lactation. Prolactin is also produced in other tissues, including the breast (known as extrapituitary prolactin).[228,229] Recently, investigators reported that autocrine prolactin is required for terminal mammary epithelial differentiation during pregnancy and production is regulated by the signaling pathway Pten-PI3K-Akt.[228] Although this finding is critical for normal breast development, differentiation, and lactation it may also be important in breast carcinogenesis because the PI3K-Akt signaling pathway is commonly activated in human cancers. This suggests the important possibility that autocrine prolactin may play a role in breast cancer.

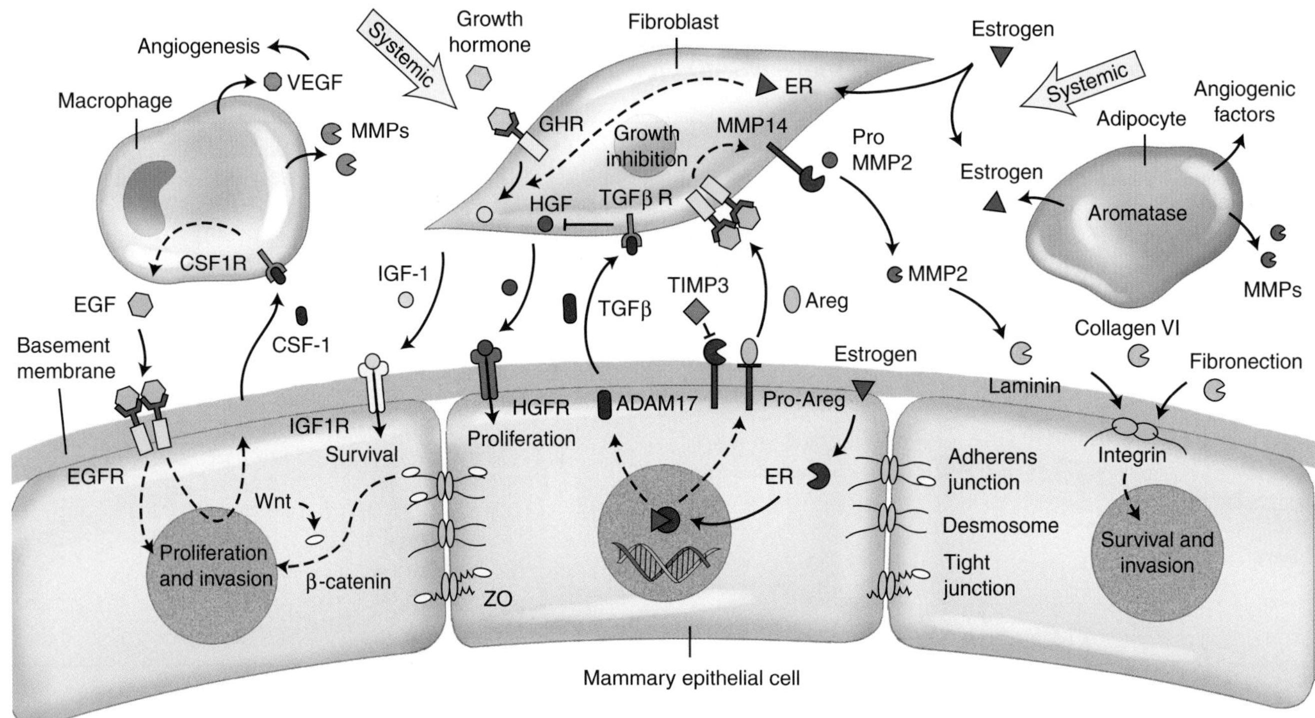

FIGURE 24-32 Figure of the Current Hypothesis of Mammary Gland During Development and Cancer. A tissue model of interacting endocrine, paracrine, and adhesion signaling pathways that modulate epithelial and stromal cell behavior. Some of the pathways depicted are not exclusive to one type of stromal cell. Dotted arrows indicate indirect interactions. (From Lanigan F et al: *Cell Mol Life Sci* 64:3165, 2007.)

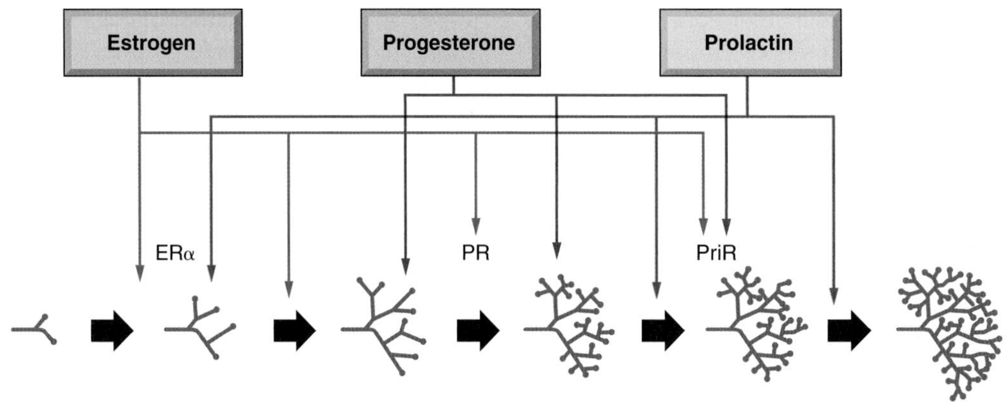

FIGURE 24-33 Factors Involved in Mammary Gland Development. Work of numerous laboratories led to the identification of many genes important in mammary gland development that are summarized in the scheme. (Adapted from Brisken C, O'Malley B: *Cold Spring Harb Perspect Biol* 2[12]:a003178. [Epub 2010 Aug 25.])

It is possible to consider four major hormonal hypotheses for breast cancer: (1) ovarian androgen excess (testosterone, for example), (2) estrogens and progesterone levels (ovarian and hormonal replacement), (3) estrogens alone (ovarian and hormone replacement), and, (4) local biosynthesis of estrogens in breast tissue. These hypotheses, however, may not be mutually exclusive. HRT is discussed later in a separate section; the present discussion is concerned with endogenous levels of hormones.

The first hypothesis that breast cancer risk is increased among women who have ovarian androgen excess also includes chronic anovulation and reduction of luteal-phase (menstrual cycle) progesterone production. Therefore, it is also called the "ovarian hyperandrogenism/luteal inadequacy hypothesis." This hypothesis, proposed by Grattarola in the 1960s, was based on the observation that women with breast cancer also reveal hyperplasia of the endometrium—a common symptom of ovarian, androgen excess chronic anovulation, and progesterone deficiency.[219] These findings have been confirmed and extended[230] in several studies including prospective studies. From a pooled analysis of nine prospective studies of postmenopausal women, all the androgens were positively (significantly) associated with breast cancer risk.[231] The majority of data from this pooled analysis were for testosterone. Similar findings were

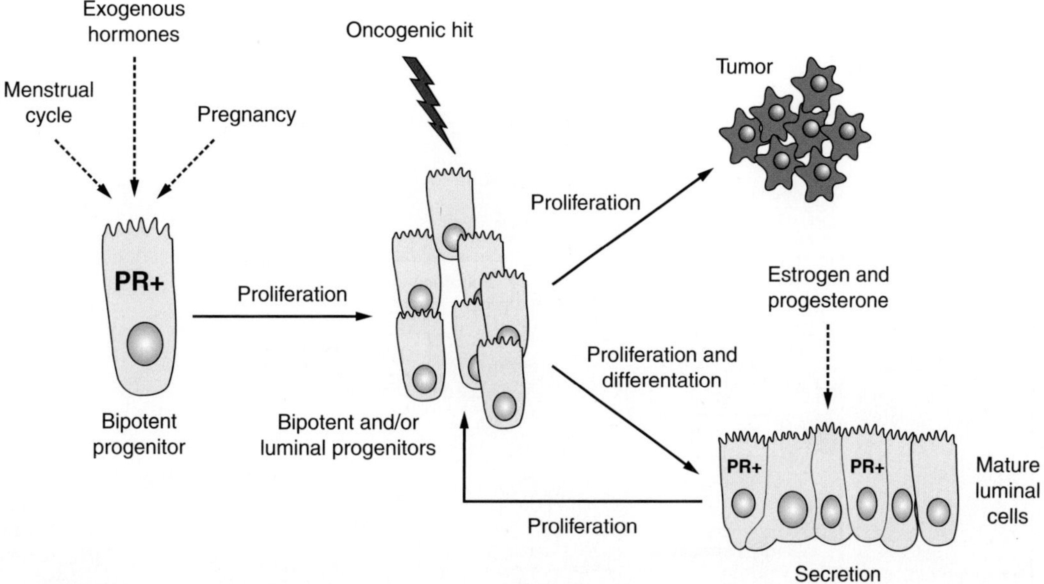

FIGURE 24-34 Progesterone Progenitor Cells, a Working Model. The fate of progesterone receptor–positive (PR+) progenitor cells is important to understand for normal breast development and breast carcinogenesis. When P levels peak during the second phase of the menstrual cycle and during pregnancy, a subset of PR+ bipotent (more than one type of cell) progenitor cells proliferate to expand the epithelial compartment providing a larger pool of cells susceptible to oncogenic mutation. These cells can then differentiate into mature luminal cells that can respond to the proliferative and secretory signals of both estrogen (E) and progesterone (P). This process is increased by the E induction of PR expression in this cell subtype. (Adapted from Hilton HN et al: *Mol Cell Endocrinol* 361:191–201, 2012.]

observed in the European Prospective Investigation into Cancer and Nutrition (EPIC) cohort study.[232] Four prospective studies have reported a positive association for premenopausal women between testosterone and risk of breast cancer.[233] A prospective Italian study showed a significant increase in breast cancer risk for premenopausal women who had elevated levels of testosterone and lower levels of progesterone.[234] In a recent case-control study serum androgens were associated with both ER+, PR+ and ER–, PR– cancers.[235] A case-control study nested with the New York University Women's Health Study showed premenopausal serum testosterone and free testosterone concentrations were positively associated with breast cancer risk.[236] Unclear from studies is whether the association with testosterone is direct or indirect (i.e., enzyme conversion by tissue aromatase of testosterone to estradiol) (Figure 24-35). Overall, the association between circulating testosterone in postmenopausal women and subsequent risk of breast cancer is now well established.[237] Indeed some investigators propose increased androgenic activity is the principal endocrine abnormality of women with hormone-dependent breast cancer called the androgen-excess theory.[238] These investigators suggest that androgen excess is the main growth stimulator of ER+ tumors through testosterone conversion into estrogens through the aromatase enzyme in stromal tissue (see the fourth hypothesis in the following text). Studies have demonstrated a correlation between the androgen receptor (AR) and ER/PR pathways, a potential role for AR in prognosis, carcinoma proliferative responses to androgen in several AR expressing cell lines, and expression of an androgen-dependent cascade of intracellular signaling in AR expressing breast tumors. AR is reported to be expressed in 50% to 100% of breast cancers; however, controversy exists about the percentages because of study methods used.[239] A subset of individuals with triple negative breast cancer (TNBC) has been reported to express AR in carcinoma cells leading to the treatment proposal of manipulation of androgen signaling or AR targeted therapies. Further study is needed because of the reported proliferative and antiproliferative effects of AR in TNBC.[239] For those women with high testosterone/AR-negative tumors, androgen excess does not stimulate tumor growth directly through conversions to estrogens but can by increasing the production of epidermal growth factor (EGF) and EGF inhibitors may be indicated.[238]

The second hypothesis is increased breast cancer risk among women with blood elevations of both estrogens and androgens. These observations revealed increased proliferation rates of breast epithelium during the luteal phase of the menstrual cycle when the ovaries produce both estradiol and progesterone. A recent reanalysis of 13 prospective studies showed that circulating concentrations of sex hormones are associated with several of the established or suspected risk factors for breast cancer. The hormones were all positively correlated with each other, implying they are all part of the same metabolic pathway.[240] The strongest associations were with BMI and all the hormones were higher in obese women with breast cancer than in women with a low BMI. Analyses related to increasing age found large decreases in circulating DHEAS and androstenedione, small changes in estrogens and testosterone, and increases in SHBG (consistent with other previous reports). The smaller decrease in estrogen blood concentrations may be caused by increased synthesis of estrogen in tissue by aromatization in older women

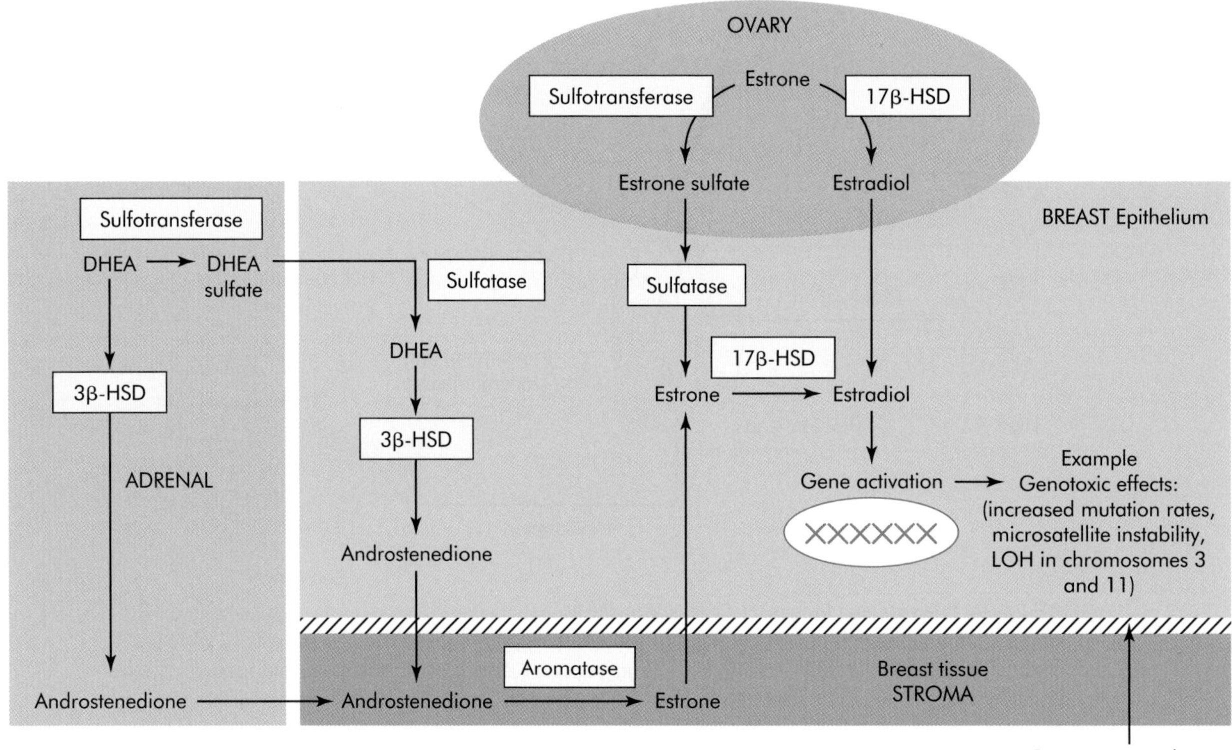

FIGURE 24-35 **Local Biosynthesis of Estrogens.** Three main enzyme complexes *(yellow)* involved in estrogen formation in breast tissue, including aromatase, sulfatase, and 17β-estradiol hydroxysteroid dehydrogenase (17β-HSD). Thus despite low levels of circulating estrogens in postmenopausal women with breast cancer, the tissue levels are several-fold higher than those in plasma, suggesting tumor accumulation of these estrogens. Data suggest that most abundant is sulfatase in both premenopausal and postmenopausal women with breast cancer. Numerous agents can block the aromatase action, exploration of progesterone, and various progestins to inhibit sulfatase and 17β-HSD or stimulate sulfotransferase (i.e., breast cancer cells cannot inactivate estrogens because they lack sulfotransferase) may provide new possibilities for treatment. *LOH,* Loss of heterozygosity (see Chapter 12). (Adapted from Russo J, Russo I: *Molecular basis of breast cancer: prevention and treatment,* Germany, 2004, Springer-Verlag, Berlin Heidelberg.)

or women with ovariectomy, or both.[240] Ovariectomy was associated with androgen levels about 30% lower than from women with natural menopause. Surprisingly, no significant differences in those women with ovariectomy were found for total estradiol or estrone (researchers excluded women using exogenous hormone therapies). Cigarette smoking and alcohol use were associated with moderate increases in all the hormones. Age at menarche, age at parity, age at first-term pregnancy, and family history of breast cancer were not strongly related to any of the hormones studies. From this study, type of hormone assay used affected some of the results and assays that used a purification step were more specific and sensitive.[240] Overall, older data are too few to draw any *firm* conclusions.[233] New data identify mammary stem cells (MaSCs) as critical targets for ovarian hormones, especially progesterone surges during the normal reproductive cycle and pregnancy increasing the proliferation of mammary stem cells.[241,242] Progesterone-expanded MaSC pools could accumulate mutations and acquire the properties of tumor-initiating cells. From these studies the progestin in HRT was proposed as a risk factor because of the presence of hidden or occult preinvasive breast cancer in postmenopausal women that contains ER–/PR–/CK5+ stem cells, which may be reactivated by progestins and function as tumor-initiating cells.[243] Overall, complex data indicate that progesterone as a proliferative hormone is a risk factor for breast cancer (promotes preneoplastic progression) and stimulates the normal breast epithelium through a complex paracrine mechanism (Figure 24-36, *A*). Paradoxically, however, in the more advanced stage of breast cancer, PR either independent of progesterone hormone or in response to progesterone is proposed to impede invasion and metastasis by maintaining epithelial cell differentiation and inhibiting epithelial-mesenchymal transition (EMT) a key developmental process often activated in cancer invasion and metastasis (see Figure 24-36, *B*, and Pathogenesis section). Dysregulation of the RANKL-RANK signaling pathway is implicated in both the initiation and progression of progesterone-dependent mammary carcinomas, and inhibitors of RANK or RANKL are suggested to have an effect on the development of breast cancer.[243]

The third hypothesis is often called the "estrogen-alone hypothesis." Substantial prospective data have accrued on circulating estrogens and breast cancer risk in postmenopausal women.[231,237,244] From the EPIC study,[232] increasing blood levels of estradiol also increased the risks for breast cancer (relative risks 1.4,1.2,1.8, 2). Updated analyses from two cohorts of the pooled analysis of nine prospective studies provide strong

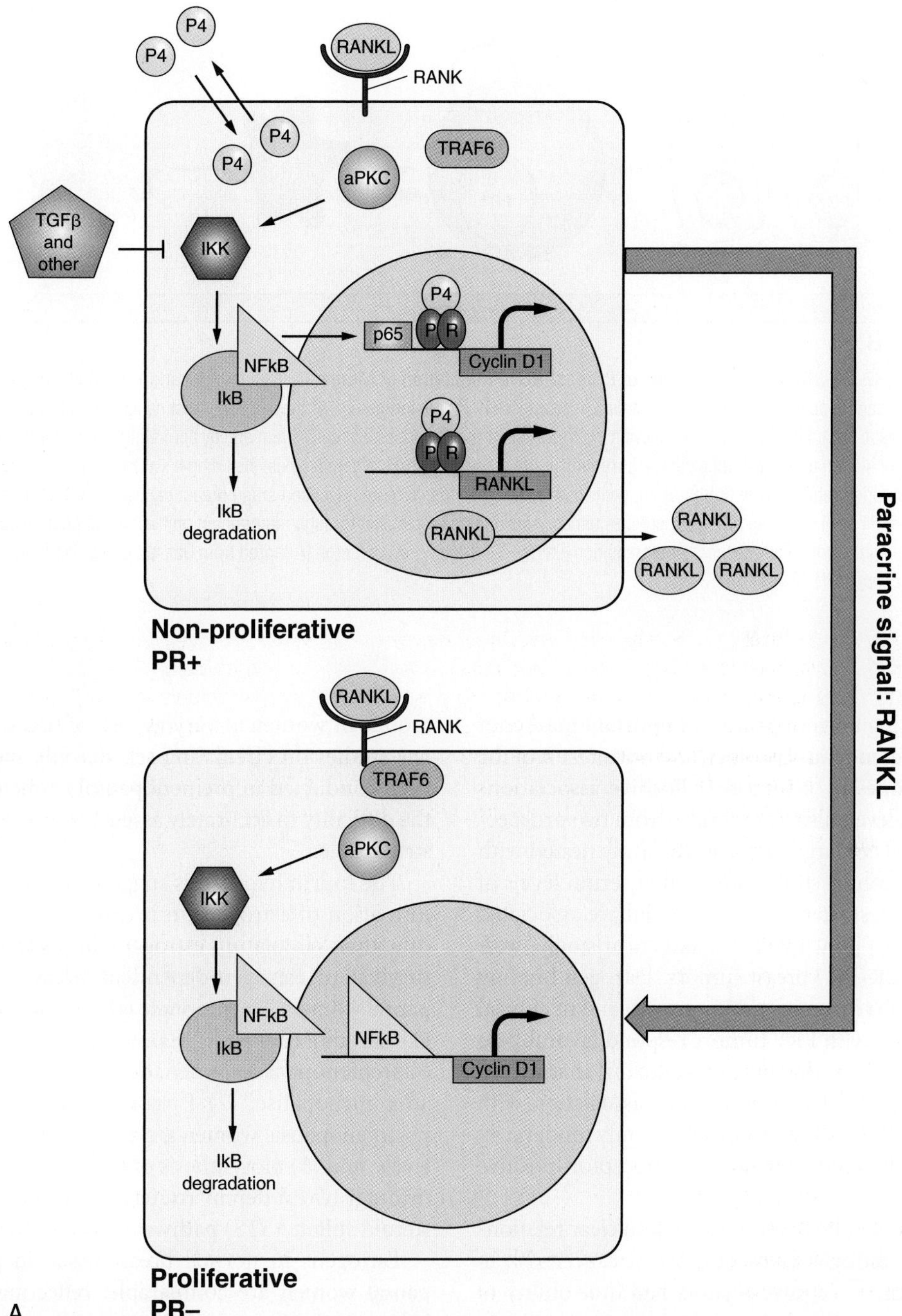

FIGURE 24-36 A Model of Progesterone Regulation of Mammary Cell Proliferation. A, Model for progesterone regulation of cell proliferation in the mammary epithelium mediated by the RANK-RANKL paracrine signaling pathway. This model is based on work with the mouse mammary gland; RANKL is a direct target of PR induced by progesterone (P4) and is then released to interact with the RANK receptor on either PR+ or PR– cells. In PR+ cells, RANKL activates the downstream IKK/IkB/NFkB/cyclin D1 signaling pathway to stimulate proliferation. RANKL does not generate a sustained activation of the NFkB/cyclin D1 proliferative pathway in PR+ cells because of the suppressive actions of TGF-β and/or other unknown mechanisms.

Continued

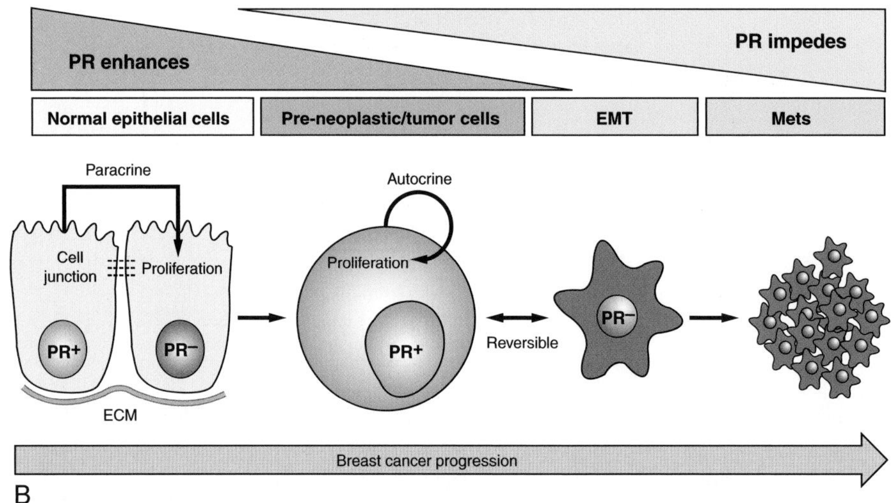

FIGURE 24-36, cont'd A Model of Progesterone Regulation of Mammary Cell Proliferation. **B,** Model for progesterone and PR action at stages of breast cancer progression. Progesterone is a risk factor for breast cancer and promotes preneoplastic progression by stimulating cyclic proliferation of the mature breast epithelium and by activating mammary stem cell pools or hidden tumor-initiating cells. Alterations in the progesterone/PR signaling axis, including a switch from a paracrine to an autocrine regulation of proliferation, contribute to progression. In more advanced stage breast cancer PR, either independent of P4 or in response to P4, suppresses tumor invasion and metastasis through maintaining epithelial cell phenotype and impeding the epithelial-mesenchymal transition (EMT). *TGF,* Tumor growth factor. (Adapted from Obr AE, Edwards DP: *Mol Cell Endocrinol* 357[1-2]:4–17, 2012.)

evidence that circulating hormones are an important marker of increased risk in postmenopausal women and not a result of the production of hormones by a tumor.[245] Positive associations with urinary estrogen levels also were similar from two prospective studies.[246,247] A recent large case-control study nested with the EPIC prospective cohort study showed that serum levels of total and bioavailable testosterone and estradiol are associated with risks of ER+, PR+, joint ER+PR+, and surprisingly, with ER–, PR–, and joint ER–PR– breast tumors. Estrogen binding to the receptor ER-alpha increases tumor growth and in clinical studies only individuals with ER+ tumors respond favorably to antiestrogenic therapy. It is, therefore, paradoxical that in this case-control study estrogens showed a direct association with ER–, PR–, and joint ER–PR– breast cancer and only moderately smaller (effect size) than seen for hormone receptor–positive disease.[235]

EPIC and other studies, however, observed no clear relationship between plasma estrogen levels and breast cancer risk in *premenopausal* women.[232] Yet investigators had little ability to evaluate hormonal levels with phases of the menstrual cycle. In premenopausal women, the NHS II found in the follicular phase of the menstrual cycle, but not the luteal phase, that circulating total and free estradiol was significantly associated with breast cancer risk.[248] Experimental studies have also provided strong and consistent evidence that estrogens can promote breast tumor development and growth[249] (see the Pathogenesis section).

Overall, the positive association between circulating estrogens in postmenopausal women and subsequent risk of breast cancer is well established. The association appears strongest for estrogen-positive tumors and is statistically robust across groups of women at varying risk of breast cancer.[237] Relatively few studies on circulating sex steroids and breast cancer have been conducted in premenopausal women, possibly because of the difficulty to accurately assess hormones levels over the menstrual cycle.

The fourth hypothesis suggests that *local* (in situ; paracrine) formation of estrogens in breast tumors may be more significant than circulating estrogens in *plasma* for the growth and survival of estrogen-dependent breast cancer in postmenopausal women. The rationale is based on the following evidence: (1) estradiol (E_2) levels in breast tumors are equivalent to those of premenopausal women, despite plasma E_2 levels being lower after menopause; (2) E_2 concentrations in breast tumors of postmenopausal women are at least 10 times higher than serum levels; and (3) biosynthesis of estrogens in breast tumors occurs through two different routes, the aromatase pathway and the steroid sulfate (STS) pathway[221] (see Figure 24-35).

Estrogens in normal breast tissue in pre- and postmenopausal women are comparable, reflecting other than ovarian biosynthesis of estrogens that occurs in several peripheral tissues including adipose, muscle, skin, bone, brain, aorta, and breast tissues.[250,251] A series of enzymes are involved in in situ production of estrogens in breast carcinoma tissues, but aromatase (member of the cytochrome P-450 family) is a key enzyme of estrogen production through conversion of adrenal androgens in estrogen-dependent postmenopausal breast cancer.[250] Breast tissue metabolism of estrogens through the aromatase-mediated pathway is correlated with the risk of breast carcinogenesis. Evidence suggests that the site of conversion of androgens to estrogens in breast cancer is the stroma and not the malignant

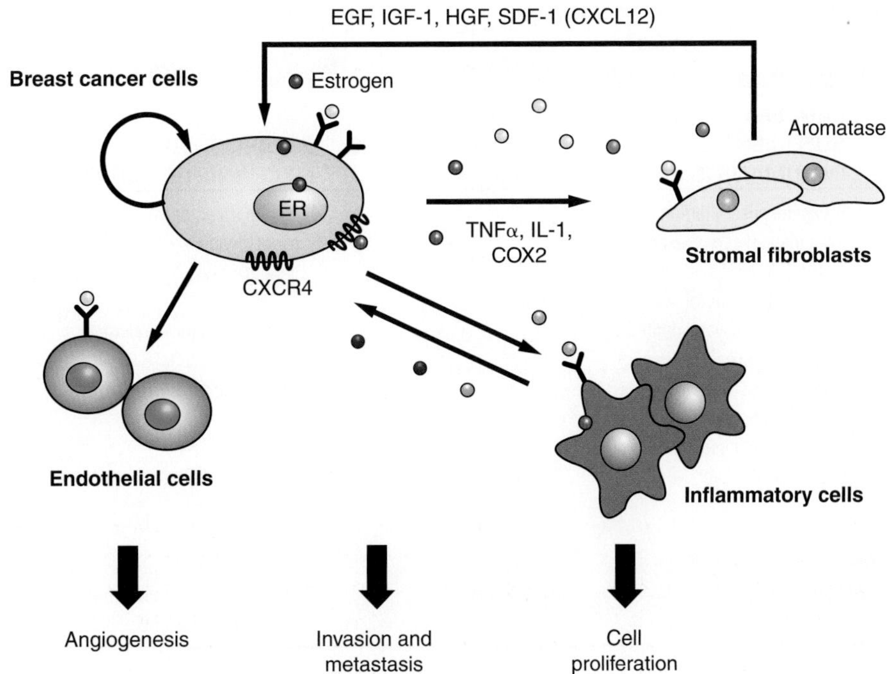

FIGURE 24-37 Breast Cancer Cells and Stromal Fibroblasts Produce Estrogen. In the microenvironment of breast carcinoma, breast cancer cells interact with different stromal cells through the secretion of growth factors and cytokines. Fibroblasts adjacent to cancer cells produce estrogen through the expression of the enzyme aromatase, which is induced by several factors including tumor necrosis factor alpha (TNF-α), interleukin 1 (IL-1), and cyclo-oxygenase 2 (COX-2). These interactions lead to cancer cell proliferation, angiogenesis, and metastasis. (Adapted from Yamaguchi Y, Hayashi S: *Endocr J* 56[1], 2009.)

epithelial cells.[252] Stromal fibroblasts adjacent to the tumor express aromatase and actively induce local estrogen production and signal crosstalk between estrogen and growth factors affecting the progression of breast carcinomas (Figure 24-37).

Investigators also have reported aromatase in adipocytes and carcinoma cells.[250] Stromal fibroblasts demonstrate multiple functions in the genesis and progression of breast cancers and carcinoma-associated fibroblast (CAFs) are potential therapeutic targets for many other cancers.

Breast tissue also contains high sulfatase activity and produces estrone through the hydrolysis of estrone sulfate[221] (see Figure 24-35). Thus quantitatively estrone sulfate may be the most important circulating estrogen in women; it increases the reservoir for the production of estrone and, ultimately, estradiol. It was found that E_2, itself, has antisulfatase action. This paradoxical effect of estradiol could be related to some studies that have found estrogen replacement therapy (ERT) to have either no effect or to decrease breast cancer mortality in postmenopausal women[253] (see p. 854). In summary, the blockage of estradiol through both the aromatase and sulfatase pathways, as well as the stimulation of sulfotransferase activity (i.e., sulfation is important to estrogens because the addition of the charged sulfonate group protects the hormones [estrogens] from binding to their receptors and, consequently, inhibiting cell growth) can provide new and potentially powerful applications in breast cancer.

Although experimental, clinical, and epidemiologic research have implicated endogenous estrogens in the etiology of breast and endometrial cancer and, possibly, ovarian cancer, the role of individual *patterns* of estrogen metabolism is a new focus, especially for epidemiology.[249] Estrogen metabolism from oxidation of the parent estrogens, estrone, and estradiol occurs at either the 2-, 4-, or 16-position of the carbon skeleton to yield 2-hydroxylated, 4-hydroxylated, or 16-hydroxylated estrogens, respectively. The 4- and 16-α-hydroxylated pathways are potentially tumor promoting; conversely, the 2-hydroxylated pathway has been demonstrated to be less tumor promoting and, possibly, inhibiting.[254] A recent prospective case-control study found nearly all estrogens, estrogen metabolites, and metabolic pathway groups were associated with an increased risk of breast cancer especially unconjugated estradiol. These investigators found more extensive 2-hydroxylation of estrogens is associated with lower risk and less methylation of potentially genotoxic 4-hydroxylation pathway with a higher risk of breast cancer in postmenopausal women.[255] Thus potential imbalances in estrogen metabolites in breast tissue correlate with the development of tumors and suggest possible biomarkers related to the risk of developing breast cancer.

Hormone Replacement Therapy (HRT) and Breast Cancer Risk: Estrogen Plus Progesterone and Estrogen Only (ERT). Most epidemiologic studies have found an increase in breast cancer risk related to HRT with combined estrogen and progestogens (HRT)[256,257] (Table 24-14). Evidence comes from observational studies and clinical trials and suggests an approximate 30% to 70% increase in breast cancer risk with HRT current use and

TABLE 24-14 HORMONAL TREATMENTS ASSESSED BY THE IARC MONOGRAPH WORKING GROUP

GROUP 1 AGENT	CANCER ON WHICH SUFFICIENT EVIDENCE IN HUMANS IS BASED	SITES WHERE CANCER RISK IS REDUCED	ESTABLISHED MECHANISTIC EVENTS	OTHER LIKELY MECHANISTIC EVENTS
Diethylstilbestrol	Breast (exposure during pregnancy), vagina and cervix (exposure in utero); limited evidence: testis (exposure in utero), endometrium	—	Estrogen receptor–mediated events (vagina, cervix), genotoxicity	Epigenetic programming
Estrogen-only menopausal therapy	Endometrium, ovary; limited evidence: breast	—	Estrogen receptor–mediated events	Genotoxicity
Combined estrogen-progestogen menopausal therapy	Endometrium (risk decreases with number days/month of progestogen use), breast	—	Receptor-mediated events	Estrogen genotoxicity
Combined estrogen-progestogen oral contraceptives	Breast, cervix, liver	Endometrium, ovary	Receptor-mediated events	Estrogen genotoxicity, hormone-stimulated expression of human papillomavirus genes
Tamoxifen	Endometrium	Breast	Estrogen receptor–mediated events, genotoxicity	—

From IARC Special Report: *Lancet* 10:13–14, 2009.

breast cancer risk disappearing a few years after treatment discontinuation.[258-260] Additional support for HRT to increase breast cancer risk was the *reduction* in risk reported by several countries with discontinuation of HRT use.[257,261]

Evidence on the route of administration of HRT, oral versus transdermal (gel or patch), and the risk of breast cancer has limited research. To date, epidemiologic data suggest the route has no effect on the risk of breast cancer and hip fracture.[262] Results on route of HRT on risk of coronary heart disease and colorectal cancer are inconsistent. Studies on the risks of diabetes and stroke are too few for clinical evidence. Additionally, there is a suggestion, that needs research confirmation, that oral route versus transdermal HRT may increase the risk of thromboembolism.[263]

HRT use has been associated with a greater breast cancer risk than ERT. Intense debate is whether ERT is associated with an increase in breast cancer risk compared with *never use* of hormone therapy. Use of ERT was associated with a *decreased* risk in the Women's Health Initiative (WHI) randomized trial even after cessation of treatment[264,265] but not in observational studies.[259,260,266,267] From the recent WHI report, women with a prior hysterectomy who were followed for 10.7 years and who used conjugated equine estrogen (CEE) for an average of 3.5 years (median of 5.9 years) were not associated with an increased or decreased risk of coronary heart disease (CHD), deep vein thrombosis, stroke, hip fracture, colorectal cancer, or total mortality, and the previous finding of a decrease in breast cancer risk persisted.[264] According to investigators, this decrease in risk is neither perplexing nor contradictory to other findings in which estrogen increases risk because of the underlying biology of breast cancer and estrogen. Laboratory data support a protective effect of estrogen under the right environment—that is, after a period of long-term natural (endogenous) estrogen deprivation. If this environment exists, then exogenous estrogen will induce apoptosis or cell death of the occult breast cancer cells.[225] The changing concepts in ERT are related to acquired resistance to long-term antihormonal therapy in breast cancer. This finding is the basis for the clinical use of estrogen to treat advanced antihormone-resistant breast cancer.[267,268] One hypothesis is long-term antiestrogen treatment or estrogen deprivation causes the development and progression of antihormone resistance (e.g., from tamoxifen).[267] Under these environments laboratory data support a mechanism of estrogen-induced apoptosis (estrogen E_2 suppressed ER alpha signaling) and produced stress responses, endoplasmic stress, and inflammatory stress responses, that led to apoptosis.[269] Other proposed causes of treatment resistance include the changes in the stroma with carcinomas (mesenchymal phenotype),[270] p53 status,[271] dysregulation of the estrogen receptor,[272] and low levels of nuclear Nu-Sta5a (signal transducer and activator of transcription-5a).[273] Nonetheless, careful debate has continued about ERT and breast cancer. Issues include: (1) a potential age effect (younger versus older women) on the risk-to-benefit profile of hormone therapy (HT), (2) overall duration and safety (short- and long-term) of HT use, (3) differential effects of HT in slender or overweight/obese women, and (4) estrogen decline or deprivation (menopause) for a specified time (length unknown) then followed by ERT replacement leads to apoptosis or cell killing of lingering breast cancer cells. Thus because the use of ERT in the WHI in 80% or greater (of study pills) was 3.5 years, longer use may still increase breast cancer risk. Longer use in animal studies has been linked with increasing cell proliferation, angiogenesis, and inhibiting apoptosis.[274] Longer use of ERT that may increase breast cancer risk was found in combined data of 16 studies and another analysis of 52,705 women with breast cancer.[267,268] In these studies and the Million Women Study, leaner women had an even higher risk of breast cancer.[275] Women in the WHI do not represent the typical woman who might be prescribed HT for menopausal symptoms.[276] For example, 68% of the women in the WHI were older than age 60 when enrolled in the study, thus an older population than the average woman entering menopause.

Insulin and Insulin-Like Growth Factors. IGFs regulate cellular functions involving cell proliferation, migratory, differentiation, and apoptosis. IGF-1 is a protein hormone with a structure similar to insulin. The growth hormone–IGF-1 axis can stimulate proliferation of both breast cancer and normal breast epithelial cells.[277] A pooled analysis of 17 studies showed a significant association of IGF-1 with breast cancer risk.[278] Interestingly, no significant difference was found according to menopausal status. Joint associations of IGF-1 and estradiol together showed they were related to risk and those women in the top thirds of estradiol and IGF-1 levels had the highest risk. Estradiol increases IGF-1 activity in the breast.[279] Insulin and IGF-1 receptor family are now known to have a role in macronutrient intake and cancer, diabetes and cancer, and obesity and cancer.[280]

Light at night (LAT) can accelerate tumor growth (in vivo), and one mechanism proposed is continuous activation of IGF-1 receptor (IGF-1R) signaling.[281] A recent case-control study of 1679 women exposed to LAT during sleep was significantly associated with breast cancer risk.[281] This study was the first to identify bedroom light intensity and breast cancer risk. Although inconclusive, shift-work and its disruptive effects on circadian rhythms and sleep deprivation at night have been suggested as a risk factor for breast cancer.[282]

Prolactin and Growth Hormone. Grown hormone (GH) injected in mice acts on mammary stroma.[283] GH induces the production of IGFs in the liver; IGF signaling is important for breast development and is implicated in breast carcinogenesis. Two studies, however, have reported a link with GH and breast cancer risk.[284,285] In the largest prospective analysis of circulating prolactin and breast cancer risk, those with the highest levels had the highest risk.[286] (For more on prolactin see p. 847.)

Human Chorionic Gonadotropin. hCG increases during the first trimester and then rapidly declines to a steady state throughout pregnancy. Data from rat studies indicate that hCG may be useful in developing new therapies because it has antiproliferative and anti-invasive effects.[287] However, insufficient data exist on the safety of hCG; its role in carcinogenesis is complex and much research needs to be done.[288]

Oral Contraceptives. The International Agency for Research on Cancer (IARC) group confirmed that combined estrogen-progestogen OCs increase the risk for breast, cervix, and liver cancers.[257] A recent meta-analysis of 66 studies showed current use of oral contraceptives, nulliparity, and 30 years or older at first birth were associated with a 1- to 1.5-fold increased risk of breast cancer.[289] Hormones are discussed further in the Pathogenesis section.

Mammographic Breast Density

Mammographic breast density (MBD) is the radiologic appearance of the breast (largely stromal and epithelial tissues) reflecting variations in breast tissue composition (Figure 24-38). Mammographic breast density appears white or dense on a mammogram, is expressed as a percentage of the mammogram (percent mammographic density), and is a strong and consistent risk factor for breast cancer.[290,291] **Percent mammographic density (PMD)** estimates the proportion of stromal and epithelial tissues in relation to fat tissue in the breast. Internationally, studies done in the United States, Canada, and Europe all found that a significant increase in risk associated with more extensive PMD; risk persisted for 8 to 10 years from the date of the mammogram, and increased with increasing PMD. Extensive PMD is associated with a markedly increased risk of invasive breast cancer.[290] Thus extensive breast density is one of the strongest risk factors for developing breast cancer and second only to age and carrying a *BRCA1* or *BRCA2* mutation.[290,292] Lifestyle factors, including age, parity, BMI, and exogenous hormone levels, explain about 20% to 30% of the variation in PMD among women. The estimate of 61% to 67% of the variation could be caused by genetic factors; however, linkage and candidate gene association studies have not reproducibly identified loci related to MBD.[293] A recent meta-analysis of five genome-wide studies of PMD discovered an association between common variants in ZNF365 and breast cancer. DNA methylation or other epigenetic studies of breast density are commencing.

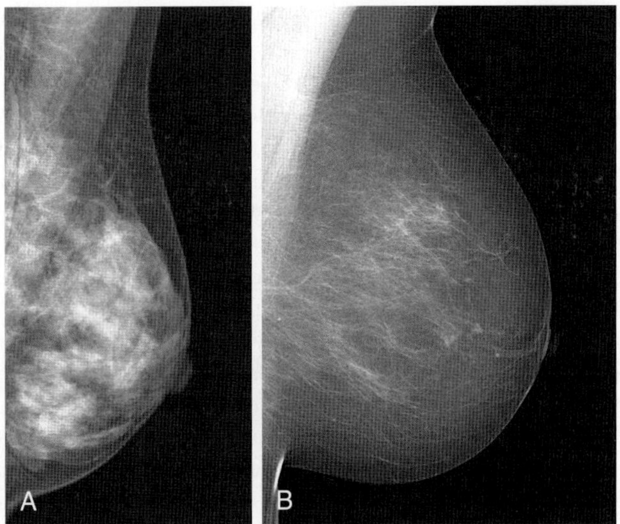

FIGURE 24-38 Breast Density Varies Among Women. The sensitivity of mammography for detecting malignancy is significantly reduced if the breast consists of a high proportion of fibroglandular (dense) breast tissue **(A)** compared to a breast that is fatty **(B)**. (From O'Malley FP, Pinder SE, Mulligan AM: *Breast pathology*, ed 2, Philadelphia, 2011, Saunders.)

Environmental Factors and Lifestyle

The environmental causes of breast cancer possibly affect the breast the most during critical phases or "windows" of development including early differential stages—that is, undifferentiated cells to alveolar buds and then lobules, puberty, pregnancy and lactation, involution, and menopause. During early phases, mitotic activity and cell division are greater than later in life.

Radiation. Ionizing radiation is a known mutagen and established carcinogen for breast cancer. To date, only accidentally or medically induced radiation has been demonstrated to exert a carcinogenic effect on the breast. The Institute of Medicine (IOM) reports that the two most strongly associated environmental factors are exposure to ionizing radiation and combined postmenopausal HT.[294] There are many sources of ionizing radiation, including x-rays, CT scans, fluoroscopy, and other medical radiologic procedures. CT imaging is frequently used in the absence of evidence[295,296] (see Chapter 13), and although only about 10% of diagnostic radiologic procedures in large U.S. hospitals are CTs, they contribute an estimated 65% of the effective radiation dose to the public from all medical x-ray examinations.[297] The IOM conclusion of a causal relationship between radiation exposure in the same range as CT and cancer is consistent from a large varied literature.[292] The IOM makes it clear that *avoidance* of medical imaging is an important and concrete step that women [girls] can take to reduce their risk of breast cancer.[295] Scientists and clinicians also have expressed concern about the increasing number of CT scans performed, including on children.[295,298]

The prevailing view has been that major predictors of risk from radiation are a young age at exposure and the radiation dose.[299] Yet, recent data in cell models and epidemiologic studies in older aged cells shows long-lasting and incomplete DSB repair.[299a,b,c] These data show increased carcinogenic risks of radiation exposure at older ages (see Chapters 2 and 13). Although protocols are continually updated, radiologic exposure of the upper spine, heart, ribs, lungs, shoulders and esophagus also can expose breast tissue to radiation. Breast tissue may be exposed from abdominal CT scans.[300] X-rays and fluoroscopy of infants may constitute whole-body irradiation. The duration of increased risks from radiation is unknown, but increased risk appears to have lasted at least 35 years in women treated for mastitis, those treated with fluoroscopy, and atomic-bomb survivors.

Cancer induction and exposure to low doses and low energy x-rays are controversial and the topic of much debate and research. Biologic understanding related to low doses of radiation is presented in Chapters 2 and 13. There is continuing debate and discussion of questionable radiation-induced cancers caused by mammographic screening,[302-304] especially among women with a positive family history of breast cancer.[305,306] Mammography is a low dose of low-energy x-rays usually of two views done within an interval of a few minutes. The computed average measure of the radiation absorbed by a fixed mass of biologic tissue (dose equivalent) used to account for the different biologic damage potential is about 2 mSv for low-energy x-rays, although this value has been suggested to be higher.[307,308] The mean glandular dose can increase with breast density,[309] volume of breast tissue, lack of breast compression,[310] breast augmentation prosthesis,[311] calling back individuals for more views, and technical variations in the setup of digital mammograms.[310] Radiosensitivity of individuals can vary and become a modifying factor of the radiation response[312-314] (see also Chapter 13).

Data from epidemiologic studies is challenging and controversial because they may lack sufficient statistical power to determine the health risks from low-dose radiation.[312] It is currently accepted that the benefits of screening mammography outweigh the possible risk of radiation-induced breast cancer in women 50 years and older. Still controversial and debated is screening mammography for women 40 to 49 years old and high-risk women especially those with genetic risk of breast cancer (Table 24-15 and Box 24-14). Women with genetic risk might be more susceptible to radiation-induced breast cancer because suppressor genes are implicated in the response to ionizing radiation.[312] Radiation-induced DNA double-strand breaks (DSBs) are considered the most critical lesions and their misrepair could lead to chromosomal instability.[312,315] Several studies have contributed to understanding the biologic responses of low-dose radiation but have not duplicated the protocols of mammographic screening (mGy doses, low-energy x-rays, and repeated exposures) or with an appropriate cellular model (i.e., nontumoral and untransformed breast epithelial cells).[307,315-324]

Investigators assessed in vitro mammographic radiation-induced DNA damage in mammary epithelial cells from 30 women with low (LR) or high (HR) family risk of breast cancer. From this study low and repeated doses simulating a two-view mammogram (2+2 mGy) created more damage than 2 mGy and, overall, more damage than 4 mGy.[312] The low and repeated dose effect was exacerbated in high-risk women, and these investigators even argue for avoidance of two view mammography. According to the National Cancer Institute, two-view examinations decrease the recall rate compared with single-view examinations.[299]

Continuing investigation is whether DSB repair is equally efficient after low and high doses. Using primary human fibroblasts in culture, investigators obtained the surprising finding that DSBs induced by low radiation doses (a few milligray) are repaired at a slower rate than DSBs produced by higher doses.[299c,325] Other investigators confirmed this finding and showed that pretreating cells with 10 μL of H_2O_2 generate single strand breaks and base damage, and improve the ability of cells to repair the DSBs induced by low radiation doses.[326] Overall, these data suggest that the cellular response to DSBs is very different for low versus high radiation doses. Confirmation with additional studies of DNA damage caused by mammographic exposures needs more subjects and analysis of DNA damage repair at more than 24 hours after mammography exposure.[312]

Women treated with chest radiation for a pediatric or young adult cancer have a substantially increased risk of breast cancer. Investigators from international studies have concluded that diagnostic chest irradiation or radiation therapy for benign or malignant diseases increases the risk of breast cancer for cumulative doses as low as 130 mGy. The breast cancer risk did not decrease when increasing the number of radiologic treatment fractions for delivering the same total dose but risk decreased greatly with increasing age of exposure to ionizing radiation.[327] International agencies are assessing the utility of screening MRI and mammography in these high-risk populations.

TABLE 24-15 BENEFITS AND HARMS OF SCREENING MAMMOGRAPHY: SUMMARY OF THE EVIDENCE FOR THE UNITED STATES

Benefit

Screening mammography in women ages 40 to 70 years decreases breast cancer mortality (see Magnitude of Effects below). The benefit is higher for older women, in part because their breast cancer risk is higher.

Evidence

- Study design: Meta-analysis of individual data from four randomized controlled trials (RCTs) and three additional RCTs.
- Internal validity: Validity of RCTs varies from poor to good; internal validity of meta-analysis is good.
- Overall consistency: Fair.
- Magnitude of effects on health outcomes: Relative breast cancer–specific mortality is decreased by 15% for follow-up analysis and 20% for evaluation analysis. Absolute mortality benefit for women screened annually starting at age 40 is 4 per 10,000 women screened over 10.7 years. The comparable number for women screened annually starting at age 50 years is approximately 50 per 10,000. Overall, the absolute benefit is approximately 1%, but depends on inherent breast cancer risk, which increases with age.

HARM	STUDY DESIGN	INTERNAL VALIDITY	CONSISTENCY	MAGNITUDE OF EFFECTS	EXTERNAL VALIDITY
Treatment of insignificant cancers (overdiagnosis, true positives) can result in breast deformity, lymphedema, thromboembolic events, or chemotherapy-induced toxicities	Descriptive population based, autopsy series, and series of mammary reduction specimens	Good	Good	Approximately 33% of breast cancers detected by screening mammograms represent overdiagnosis	Good
Additional testing (false-positives)	Descriptive population based	Good	Good	Estimated to occur in 50% of women screened annually for 10 years, 25% of whom will have biopsies	Good
False sense of security, delay in cancer diagnosis (false-negatives)	Descriptive population based	Good	Good	6% to 46% of women with invasive cancer will have negative mammograms, especially if young, with dense breasts or with mucinous, lobular, or fast-growing cancers	Good
Radiation-induced mutations can cause breast cancer, especially if exposed before age 30 years; latency is more than 10 years, and the increased risk persists lifelong	Descriptive population based	Good	Good	Between 9.9 and 32 breast cancers per 10,000 women exposed to a cumulative dose of 1 Sv; risk is higher for younger women	Good

Data from: National Cancer Institute: *Summary of evidence.* Available at www.cancer.gov/cancertopics/pdq/screening/breast/healthprofessional/page1update 03/30/2012; Nystrom L et al: *Lancet* 359(9310):909–919, 2002.

Currently an important topic is that radiation and other treatments can transform cancer cells into treatment-resistant breast cancer stem cells, even as the treatment kills half of all cells.[328] In some cases, cancer stem cells are generated by the therapy, and scientists are studying the mechanisms of how this occurs. DNA damage is a key factor for stem cell activation. DNA accumulates errors from environmental factors, including radiation, drugs (e.g., chemotherapy, hormones), chemicals, viruses, bacteria, or DNA replication errors.[329-330]

The risk of secondary lung malignancy (SLM) is an important concern for women treated with whole-breast radiation therapy after breast-conserving surgery for early-stage breast cancer.[331] Investigators studied SLM risk associated with several common methods of delivering whole-breast radiation therapy (RT). Compared with supine whole-breast irradiation (WBI), prone breast irradiation is associated with a significantly lower predicted risk of secondary lung malignancy.[331]

Accelerated partial breast irradiation with brachytherapy following lumpectomy versus traditional WBI has become a standard treatment. Use of brachytherapy can shorten treatment from 6 weeks to 5 days, theoretically with less risk for side effects to the heart and lungs (comparison studies are minimal and a randomized trial is ongoing). Concern is that brachytherapy increases the risk of acute skin and wound complications and may lead to increased rates of mastectomies. Retrospective data using Medicare claims data from older women indicate that brachytherapy is more likely than WBI to lead to certain complications, such as deep tissue and bone complications, and lung injury is higher with WBI; more data are needed on the severity of these complications.[332]

BOX 24-14 SUMMARY OF THE USPSTF RECOMMENDATIONS ON SCREENING FOR BREAST CANCER

- The USPSTF recommends against routine screening mammography in women in their 40s who are not at increased risk for breast cancer. The decision to start mammography before age 50 should be based on a woman's risk for breast cancer and personal preferences about the benefits and harms.
- The USPSTF recommends mammography every 2 years for women ages 50 to 74.
- Current evidence is not sufficient to assess the effectiveness of clinical breast examination in addition to screening mammography.
- The USPSTF recommends against clinicians teaching women breast self-examination.
- Current evidence is not sufficient to assess the additional effectiveness of digital mammography or breast magnetic resonance imaging instead of film mammography for breast cancer screening.

Data from U.S. Preventive Services Task Force (USPSTF): *Ann Intern Med* 716–726, 2009.

BOX 24-15 SUMMARY FOR UNDERSTANDING RADIATION EFFECTS FROM SCREENING MAMMOGRAPHY

The understanding of radiation-induced breast cancer from mammographic screening is not simple. The discussion is complex because of several issues: (1) ongoing debate about the significance of epidemiologic studies lacking sufficient statistical power to determine health risks from low-dose radiation; (2) these epidemiologic studies have determined the estimated mathematical extrapolations of low-dose health effects from high doses; (3) lacking are studies with exact protocols of mammographic procedures (mGy, low-energy x-rays, repeated exposures) or appropriate cell models (nontumoral, untransformed breast epithelial cells); (4) different reported mean glandular doses (MGDs) per screening view with changes in equipment over time and MGD can increase with breast density, volume (breast size), breast augmentation prosthesis, recall of women for additional views, and the variations in setup of digital mammographs; (5) differences in individual susceptibility to radiation (i.e., modifying factors such as genetic risk), and (6) carcinogenic effects at older ages.

Data from Colin C et al: *Int J Radiat Biol* 87(11):1103–1112, 2011; Hernandez L et al: *PLOS* 8(5):e63052, 2013.

The first study of its kind using surveillance, epidemiology, and end results (SEER) data examined trends from 1976 through 2008 of screening mammography on breast cancer incidence.[333] These investigators conclude that despite substantial increases in the number of cases of early-stage breast cancer detected, screening mammography has only marginally reduced the rate at which women present with advanced cancer. This imbalance suggests substantial overdiagnosis involving more than 1 million women in the last 30 years and, according to their estimate, more than 70,000 women in 2008 (31% of all breast cancers diagnosed in women 40 years and older) are overdiagnosed. In addition, these investigators report that because the absolute reduction in deaths (estimated at 20 deaths per 100,000 women) is larger than the number of cases of late-stage cancer (8 cases per 100,000 women), the contribution of early detection to decreasing numbers of death must be small.[333] This small reduction has been limited to regional (mostly node-positive) disease, a stage that is often treated successfully with an expected survival rate of 85% among women 40 years of age and older.[334,335] This study is important because overdiagnosis leads to overtreatment whereby women are treated for abnormalities that would not have caused illness and the harms of the treatment; surgery, radiation therapy, hormonal therapy for 5 years or more, chemotherapy, or a combination of the above can lead to significant future health concerns.

The estimated fatal radiation-induced cancer risk for breast-specific gamma imaging (BSGI), which involves a label-recommended dose of 740 to 1100 MBq (20-30 mCi) of technetium 99m-sestamibi is 20 to 30 times that of digital mammography in women age 40 years, and a single positron emission mammography (PEM) involving a labeled dose of 370 MBq (10 mCi) of fluorine 18 fluorodeoxyglucose is 23 times higher than that of digital mammography in women age 40 years.[336] The new 3D tomosynthesis uses a series of 15 low-dose mammographic images. This technology decreases the problem of overlapping breast tissue that occurs with mammography. The radiation is low dose and higher than regular mammography. No data are available on long-term effects and whether it saves lives.

Since the late 1990s, experimental evidence has shown that ionizing radiation can elicit secondary effects in nonirradiated cells.[337] These secondary or nontargeted effects include radiation-induced bystander effects (RIBEs) that are dependent on intercellular communication between the irradiated cells and the so-called innocent bystander cells. Included as a secondary effect is radiation-induced genomic instability (RIGI) in which the biologic effects include increased frequency of mutations and chromosomal aberrations that occur in descendants of irradiated cells. Several studies are ongoing and a comprehensive understanding of the RIBE response is emerging but is now incomplete. Box 24-15 includes a summary for understanding radiation effects from screening mammography.

Diet. Prospective epidemiologic studies on diet and breast cancer risk fail to show an association that is consistent, strong, and statistically significant except for alcohol intake, being overweight, and weight gain after menopause (see following discussion).[338] Diet has been postulated as important for breast cancer risk because of the international correlations of consumption of specific dietary factors (e.g., fats) and breast cancer incidence and mortality, and because migrant studies show greater incidence of breast cancer among descendants who relocated to another country compared with those in the country of origin. International variations also can occur because of differences in reproductive history, physical activity, obesity, and other factors.

Dietary Fat. Dietary fat and breast cancer risk is the subject of much study, controversy, and debate. Potential biologic mechanisms between fat intake and breast cancer risk include: (1) that fat may stimulate endogenous steroid hormone production (also affect weight gain, age of menarche), (2) fat interferes with immune or inflammatory function, and (3) fat influences gene expression. Evidence from large, prospective cohort studies has been mostly unsupportive, and clinical trials have not supported a strong association with total fat intake.[339] Cohort studies, however, suggest a modest positive association between fat intake and the risk of breast cancer,[340] but so far more than 70 studies of dietary fat during midlife on risk of breast cancer show the relationship is likely to be small. After 8.1 years of follow-up, the largest randomized controlled dietary trial conducted in the United States showed no significant difference in the number of newly diagnosed breast cancer cases in the women in the treatment group (intervention of a low-fat diet) compared with the control group (usual fat intake).[341] The World Cancer Research Fund/American Institute for Cancer Research (WCRF/AICR) report indicated that although the evidence is limited, there was an increase in breast cancer risk among postmenopausal women consuming higher-fat diets.[342] Concern also has been that any association with fat intake may be because of total energy intake. Moreover, there is limited evidence that modest reductions in fat intake (less than 20% of caloric intake) reduce breast cancer risk.

A meta-analysis of 57 international and national studies indicates that saturated fat intake is associated with an increased risk for postmenopausal disease, polyunsaturated fats were associated with increased risk regardless of menopausal status, and monounsaturated fats had no significant correlation with risk.[343]

Breast cancer risk may be determined earlier in life, before the period of investigations, and adult dietary exposures *may* have little influence on carcinogenesis. The hypothesis that exposures that occur between menarche and first pregnancy are especially important in determining subsequent risk of breast cancer is supported by several lines of evidence. Animal studies demonstrate increased susceptibility to mammary carcinogens before first pregnancy compared with administration at a later age,[344,345] and epidemiologic investigations of women who survived the atomic bomb in Hiroshima and Nagasaki show no increase in risk among women older than 35 at the time of the bombing but increased breast cancer risk among women younger than 20 years when exposed.[346] A recent and first prospective study of 39,268 premenopausal women observed a modest direct association between adolescent intake of fat and breast cancer.[347] This association persisted after adjusting for adult fat intake. Additionally, from this same study, milk, dairy, and total carbohydrate intake in adolescence, as well as the quality of carbohydrate as assessed by glycemic load, glycemic index, and dietary fiber, was not associated with breast cancer. Frequent consumption of fat, especially saturated fat, during adolescence was positively related to the incidence of hormone receptor–negative breast tumors.

Red Meat. Another area of study is how consumption of red meat could increase breast cancer risk. The hypotheses range from available iron content, growth-promoting hormones used in the cattle industry, and carcinogenic heterocyclic amines released from cooking the fatty acid content. Case-control and cohort studies have shown a modest association of red meat intake with breast cancer incidence but no association in a pooled analysis of prospective studies.[348] Research has reported an increased risk with red meat consumption.[349-351] However, a 2010 meta-analysis supported the WCRF/AICR report that suggested there was no conclusive evidence that red meat or processed meat acts as an independent risk factor for breast cancer.[342,352]

Fiber. Fiber intake could affect breast cancer risk by several mechanisms, including stimulation of the intestinal microflora and reduction of the enterohepatic estrogen circulation that could reduce overall body estrogen concentrations.[353,354] Dietary fiber has been shown to modify estrogen concentrations.[355] A recent meta-analysis of prospective cohort studies showed that every 10-g/day increment in dietary fiber was associated with a significant reduction in breast cancer risk.[356] A meta-analysis of prospective case-control studies also found an inverse association between dietary fiber intake and breast cancer risk.[357] Similar in structure to estrogens, lignans are biphenolic compounds in plant foods.[358] Primarily found in fiber-rich foods (seeds, grains, vegetables, and fruits), lignans are the major source of phytoestrogens in Western populations.[353,354] Plant lignans are converted in the human gut by intestinal bacteria to the enterolignans, enterolactone, and enterodiol, which are bioactive and are subsequently absorbed.[353] Enterolignans may protect against cancer and several mechanisms have been proposed and include: (1) they have weak estrogenic activity, therefore may bind to estrogen receptors (thus preventing other more powerful estrogens from binding to ERs); (2) inhibit tumor growth; (3) stimulate apoptosis; and (4) stimulate production of the carrier SHBG (which presumably lowers circulating free estrogen).[358] Two meta-analyses found lignans to be associated with a small risk reduction in postmenopausal breast cancer but not premenopausal,[359,360] and from a follow-up study those postmenopausal women with higher enterolignan levels may have better survival.[358]

Soy. Soy products are a hot topic because of their consumption in Asian countries that have low rates of cancer. These isoflavone compounds, including daidzein and genistein, can bind estrogen receptors but are far less potent than estradiol. Soy may act like other antiestrogens, such as tamoxifen, by blocking the action of endogenous estrogens to reduce breast cancer risk. Thus, depending on the estradiol concentration and the timing of administration, soy exhibits weak estrogenic or antiestrogenic activity. Isoflavones act through various mechanisms by which they may be cancer protective including antiproliferative effects, tyrosine kinase inhibition, induction of apoptosis, and inhibition of angiogenesis. They modulate enzyme activities, as well as signal transduction, and have antioxidant properties. In 2011 the North American Menopause Society held a symposium to review the latest evidence-based science on the role of soy and found that soy foods generally appear to be breast protective and recommended moderate lifelong soy consumption.[361] Specific recommendations for breast cancer survivors and soy or isoflavone consumption could not be reached, because animals studies indicate potential for risk and studies in humans imply a null or protective effect.[361,362] A recent large study of both American and Chinese women, however, suggested that moderate intake of soy (≥10 mg isoflavones/day) had a significant reduction in breast cancer recurrence as well as a nonsignificant trend toward reduced all-cause mortality.[363] In addition, soy may optimize extrarenal 1,25(OH)2 cholecalciferol or vitamin D_3 (a prodifferentiating vitamin D metabolite), which could result in growth control and, conceivably, inhibition of tumor progression.[364]

There is limited evidence on the role of dietary patterns and breast cancer risk modification. Some limited evidence supports the role of the Mediterranean diet.

Obesity. Obesity has been associated with a *reduced* risk of *premenopausal* breast cancer. One mechanism suggested is the direct relationship between irregular menstrual cycling, especially obesity and anovulatory cycling, which would result in a decrease in estrogens and progesterone and thus decrease the risk of breast cancer. It is possible that in obese women with hyperinsulinemia the higher insulin levels increase the enzymatic conversion of testosterone to dihydrotestosterone, rather than estradiol, lowering their estrogen levels.[365]

Obesity, however, is related to *increased* risk of breast cancer in *postmenopausal* women. Despite strong links with endogenous estrogen levels, body fat has been consistently but *weakly* related to increased postmenopausal risk.[366] This observation has been surprising because obese postmenopausal women have endogenous estrogen levels (estrone and estradiol) nearly double those of lean women.[366,367] This weak association is possibly related to two factors. First, the premenopausal reduction in breast cancer risk related to being overweight possibly persists, opposing the adverse effect of elevated estrogens after menopause. Thus *weight gain* should be more strongly related to postmenopausal breast cancer risk than attained weight. A meta-analysis of 11 studies suggests that adult weight gain is predictive of a twofold increase in the risk for ER+, as well as ER+/PR+, breast tumors with a greater risk in postmenopausal women.[368]

Premenopausal and postmenopausal weight gain also is associated with higher estradiol and estrone levels and lower SHBG as a transporter protein; low levels cause higher bioavailable estrogen.[369] This increase in estrogens, particularly estradiol, is from aromatization in the adipose tissue. Second, use of exogenous hormones postmenopausally obscures the variation in endogenous estrogens caused by adiposity and elevates breast cancer risk regardless of body weight.[366] Excess body fat and weight gain are stronger risk factors for women who do not use hormone therapy. However, a prospective study found weight gained at multiple time points throughout adulthood of 44 to 63 lbs was associated with a 56% higher risk of breast cancer, and weight gain of 88 to 108 lbs doubled the risk of breast cancer among hormone users.[370] A recent animal study showed obese animals deposited excess calories into the tumors themselves.[371] These tumors from obese animals had an increased expression of progesterone receptors.[371]

Weight loss after menopause reduces circulating estrogens and increases SHBG, making weight loss a potentially important prevention strategy especially for those women not on hormone therapy. Weight loss and postmenopausal cancer risk have been examined in prospective studies. In one of the largest studies, women who lost 22 lbs or more after menopause and maintained this weight loss halved their risk for breast cancer. This relationship was clearer in nonhormone users.[372]

The degree of obesity is an important indicator of risk as reported in the largest study to date, a prospective analysis of about 15,000 women with invasive breast cancer. Overweight (55 to 66 lbs) was not associated with any excess risk compared with normal weight. Similar associations were found for breast cancer death and non–breast cancer death but not recurrence of breast cancer. Women who were underweight and morbidly obese before breast cancer diagnosis were at the greatest risk of all-cause mortality. Morbidly obese women (BMI ≥ 88 lbs) were also at increased risk of death from breast cancer.[373]

Alcohol. Data on alcohol and risk of breast cancer continue to mount. From the analysis of the NHS, even low to moderate alcohol intake may increase breast cancer risk, particularly for postmenopausal women.[374] From this same study risk was increased regardless of source of alcohol, wine, beer, or spirits.[374] These investigators studied patterns of drinking and habits earlier in adulthood, as well as binge drinking and both may further increase risk. From the WHI an observational cohort of 87,724 postmenopausal women and 2944 cases of breast cancer over a 5-year follow-up, one drink daily was associated with an 82% greater risk for hormone receptor–positive lobular breast cancer.[375] A follow-up analysis from other investigators evaluated alcohol intake associated with ER+ disease and a lower risk for triple-negative disease.[376] Recently, a comprehensive study of lifetime alcohol intake and risk of breast cancer involved large numbers of Asian Americans.[377] Regular lifetime alcohol intake is a significant risk factor in U.S.-born Asian Americans but not in non–U.S.-born Asian Americans. Results by Asian ethnicity show that the prevalence of lifetime alcohol intake is significantly higher in Japanese than in Chinese and Filipino women and that lifetime alcohol intake is a significant risk factor in Japanese Americans (U.S. born and non-U.S. born) but not in Chinese- and Filipino-American women.[377]

The exact mechanism of how alcohol increases breast cancer risk is unknown. Suggested mechanisms include: (1) alcohol may hinder the liver's ability to rid the body of cancer-causing agents; (2) alcohol stimulates liver enzyme activity and greater sulfation of estrone, thus increasing the bioavailability of estrone and possibly breast exposure to higher levels of estrone/estradiol; (3) alcohol combined with hormone replacement therapy may synergistically enhance the risk; (4) alcohol can down-regulate the expression of *BRCA1* (i.e., the unmutated tumor-suppressor gene) thus increasing estrogen receptor-α responsiveness; (5) alcohol decreases folate levels causing changes in methyl donors for DNA stability and some studies show that folate intake may decrease this risk; and (6) alcohol decreases melatonin levels at night, which might increase circulating estrogen.

Iodine. Iodine deficiency is hypothesized as contributing to the development of breast pathology and cancer.[378-380] Iodine plays a significant role in breast health.[380-383] Although research is just beginning, some evidence reveals that iodine is an antioxidant and antiproliferative agent contributing to the integrity of normal mammary tissue. Seaweed, which is iodine-rich, is an important dietary item in Asian communities and has been associated with the *low* incidence of benign and breast cancer disease in Japanese women.[384] Other foods with iodine content include iodized salt (1 teaspoon = 400 mcg iodine), bread with iodate dough, haddock, shrimp, egg, cottage cheese, cheddar cheese, and ground beef.

Environmental Chemicals. Evidence for linking chemicals to the cause of breast cancer is difficult. It is challenging because it is a life history of exposure that is important, not just a single chemical but also complex mixtures of chemicals and their interaction with endogenous hormones and with radiation. The highest rates of breast cancer are found in superindustrialized countries—North America and Europe—and the lowest rates in central Africa and Asia. With industrial development, breast cancer rates increase. An estimated 85,000 synthetic chemicals are registered for use today in the United States, another 1000 or more are added each year, and toxicologic screening for these chemicals is minimal—only about 7%.[385] EPA researchers are going to change this serious challenge. They and their partners are teaming up and tapping modern technologies such as supercomputers and even robots to advance the scientific hazard identification and risk assessment. Chemicals persist in the environment, accumulate in adipose tissue, interact with local adipose tissue physiology in an endocrine-paracrine manner, and remain in breast tissue for decades. Some of these chemicals are known human carcinogens and many have been linked to mammary tumors in animals. Women who emigrate to the United States from Asian countries experience an enormous percent increase in risk within one generation. A generation later their daughters' risk approaches that of women born in the United States. This change in risk suggests that in utero exposures affect subsequent disease risk. However, it is difficult to know whether these changes in risk come from nutritional content, pollutants, cosmetics, food additives, or other factors.

Xenoestrogens are synthetic chemicals that mimic the actions of estrogens and are found in many pesticides, fuels, plastics, detergents, and drugs. Because many factors correlated with breast cancer (early menarche, delayed pregnancy and breastfeeding, late menopause, etc.) are associated with lifetime exposure to estrogens, investigators reasoned that environmental chemicals affect estrogen metabolism and contribute to breast cancer. The most significant chemicals may be polychlorinated biphenyls (PCBs), pesticides, BPA (pervasive in polycarbonate plastics), tobacco smoke (active and passive), dioxins (vehicle exhaust, incineration, contaminated food supply), alkylphenols (detergents and cleaning products), metals, phthalates (makes plastics flexible, some cosmetics), parabens (antimicrobials), food additives (recombinant bovine somatotropin [rBST] and zeranol to enhance growth in cattle and sheep), HRT, and others. Bisphenol A treatment of breast epithelial cells cultured from premalignant biopsied tissue elicited a genetic expression profile associated with large, high-histologic-grade breast tumors.[386] Some chemicals are fat soluble and the estrogenic effect would require that they either bind to the nuclear estrogen receptor and then cause cell division or gene transcription or they activate reactive oxygen species through oxidative catabolism of estrogens (see p. 853) (Table 24-16).

TABLE 24-16 SELECTED CHEMICALS AND RISK OF BREAST CANCER

CHEMICAL	COMMENTS
Bisphenol-A (BPA)	Studies have shown altered reproductive systems and breast tissue when exposed to BPA in utero[1]
	BPA is commonly found in plastics[2]
Polyvinyl chloride (PVC)	Used in food packaging, medical products, appliances, cars, toys, credit cards, rainwear[3]
	Has been found in the air near waste sites, landfills, and tobacco smoke
	Has been linked to increased mortality from breast and liver cancer among manufacturing workers[4,5]
Pesticides: aldrin and dieldrin (organochlorines)	Used in crops like corn and cotton from 1950s to 1970s
	Banned by the EPA in 1975 except for termite control; completely banned in 1987
	In vitro assays showed estrogenic activity and dieldrin found in 78% of women diagnosed with breast cancer[6]
	High incidence of breast cancer in Massachusetts study found associations with higher income and regular use of lawn services, termite treatments, and home pesticides[7]
Household products: methylene chloride	Spray paints and paint removers may contain methylene chloride, documented breast cancer in lab animals[8]
Diethylstilbestrol (DES)	Prescribed for women to avert miscarriages between 1941 and 1971
	Exposed daughters known to have higher rates of vaginal cancer, and in the mothers slight increased risk of breast cancer[9,10]
	Daughters now known to have slight increased risk of breast cancer[11]
Solvents (e.g., benzene, toluene, trichloroethylene, chlorinated organic solvents)	Used in manufacture of computers, also some in cosmetics
	In 2003 a Taiwanese study documented increased risk of breast cancer among electronic workers exposed to chlorinated organic solvents[12]
	A Danish study of women 22 to 55 years of age employed in industries (fabricated metal, lumber, furniture, printing, textiles) using solvents doubled the risk of breast cancer[13]
Styrene, carbon tetrachloride, formaldehyde	A 1995 study suggested increased risk with occupational exposure—validation in Finland, Sweden, and Italy[14–17]
Ethylene glycol methyl ether (EGME)	A Duke University study found it acts as hormone sensitizer in vivo and in vitro.[18,19] Compounds are found in semiconductor industry, varnishes, paints, dyes, and fuel additives
Valproic acid (anticonvulsant medication)	Found to be hormone sensitizing and prescribed for migraines and bipolar disorder[18,19]
1,3-butadiene	Air pollutant and synthetic rubber product and some fungicides and tobacco smoke. Causes mammary and ovarian tumors in female mice and rats[20,21]
Aromatic amines (heterocyclic, polycyclic, monocyclic)	Found in plastics, tobacco smoke, grilled meats and fish, combustion of wood chips and rubber. Exposure in adolescence before full-term pregnancy may increase risk[22]

Continued

TABLE 24-16 SELECTED CHEMICALS AND RISK OF BREAST CANCER—cont'd

CHEMICAL	COMMENTS
Dichlorodiphenyltrichloroethane (DDT) and polychlorinated biphenyls (PCBs)	PCB used in manufacture of electrical equipment[23] PCB and DDT are banned in the United States since 1970s but are still found in body fat, as well as breast milk[24] DDT was used as pesticide for insects on farms and swamps PCB deteriorates slowly in soil PCB is difficult to study because it is a diverse class of compounds A 1999 in vitro study showed PCBs proliferate in breast cancer cells[25] Conflicting results; several large studies failed to show relationship with PCBs
Polycystic aromatic hydrocarbons (PAHs, including tobacco)	Found in soot and fumes from fuels Increased DNA damage (DNA adducts) implicated from the Long Island Breast Cancer Study Project[26] Tobacco smoke also contains PAHs Smokers who began smoking as adolescents have an increased risk of breast cancer[27–29] In 2004 the California EPA concluded that environmental tobacco smoke (ETS) increases the risk of breast cancer, and the association appears stronger for premenopausal women[30] Tobacco smoke also contains the carcinogens polonium-210, vinyl chloride, benzene, and 1-3 butadiene[31]
Dioxin	Products containing PVC, PCBs, or other chlorinated compounds release dioxin from incineration Declared a known carcinogen by the EPA in 2000 It may be the most prevalent of all toxic chemicals Occurs in meat, poultry, dairy products, and human breast milk A United Kingdom study linked dioxin to the development of mammary tumors in mice[32] A study in Seveso, Italy, connected dioxin with breast cancer[33]
Ethylene oxide	Used to sterilize surgical instruments and in some cosmetics Linked to breast cancer in women exposed to ethylene oxide in commercial sterilization facilities[34]

References

1. Markey CM et al: *Biol Reprod* 65(4):1215–1223, 2001.
2. Infante PF, Pesak J: *J Occup Med* 36(8):826–831, 1994.
3. Chiazze L Jr., Ference LD: *Env Health Perspect* 41:137–143, 1981.
4. Hoyer AP et al: *Lancet* 352(9143):1816–1820, 1998.
5. Maxwell NI et al: *Newton Breast Cancer Study,* Newton, MA, 1999, Silent Spring Institute.
6. National Toxicology Program (NTP): *Chemicals associated with site-specific tumor induction in mammary glands,* 2003. Available at http://ntp-server.niehs.nih.gov/htdocs/sites/MAMM.html.
7. Colton T et al: *JAMA* 269(16):2096–2100, 1993.
8. Herbst AL, Scully RE: *Cancer* 25(4):745–757, 1970.
9. Palmer JR et al: *Cancer Causes Control* 13(8):753–758, 2002.
10. Chang YM et al: *Indust Health* 41(2):77–87, 2003.
11. Hansen J: *Am J Ind Med* 36(1):43–47, 1999.
12. Belli S et al: *Scand J Work Environ Health* 18(1):64–67, 1992.
13. Walrath J et al: *Am J Public Health* 75(8):883–885, 1985.
14. Weiderpass E et al: *Am J Ind Med* 36(1):48–53, 1999.
15. Wennborg H et al: *Am J Ind Med* 35(4):382–389, 1999.
16. Almekinder JL et al: *Fund Appl Toxicol* 38(2):191–194, 1997.
17. Jansen MS et al: *Proc Natl Acad Sci U S A* 101(18):7199–7204, 2004.
18. Melnick RL et al: *Carcinogenesis* 20(5):867–878, 1999.
19. National Toxicology Program (NTP), *U.S. Department of Health and Human Services: Toxicology and carcinogenesis studies of 1,3-butadiene (CAS No 106-99-0) in B6C3F1 mice (inhalation studies),* NTP TR 434, NIH Pub No 93-3165, Research Triangle Park, NC, 1993, National Institutes of Health.
20. DeBruin LS, Josephy PD: *Environ Health Perspect* 110(S1):119–128, 2002.
21. Evans N: *State of the evidence: what is the connection between the environment and breast cancer?* ed 3, San Francisco, 2004, Breast Cancer Fund.
22. Zheng T et al: *Am J Epidemiol* 150(5):453–458, 1999.
23. Hatakeyama M, Matsumura F: *J Biochem Molec Toxicol* 13(6):296–302, 1999.
24. Gammon MD et al: *Cancer Epidemiol Biomark Prev* 11(8):677–685, 2002.
25. Band PR et al: *Lancet* 360(9339):1044–1049, 2002.
26. Calle EE et al: *Am J Epidemiol* 139(10):1001–1007, 1994.
27. Johnson KC, Hu J, Mao Y: *Cancer Causes Control* 11(3):211–221, 2000.
28. California Environmental Protection Agency: *Draft Report Part B, chap* 7:147, 2004.
29. Kilthau GF: *Radiol Tech* 67(3):217–222, 1996.
30. Brown NM et al: *Carcinogenesis* 19(9):1623–1629, 1998.
31. Warner MB et al: *Environ Health Perspect* 110(7):625–628, 2002.
32. Steenland K et al: *Cancer Causes Control* 14(6):531–539, 2003.
33. Dorn J et al: *Med Sci Sports Exercise* 35(2):278–285, 2003.
34. Friedenreich CM, Orenstein MR: *J Nutr* 132(11 Suppl):3464S–3465S, 2002.

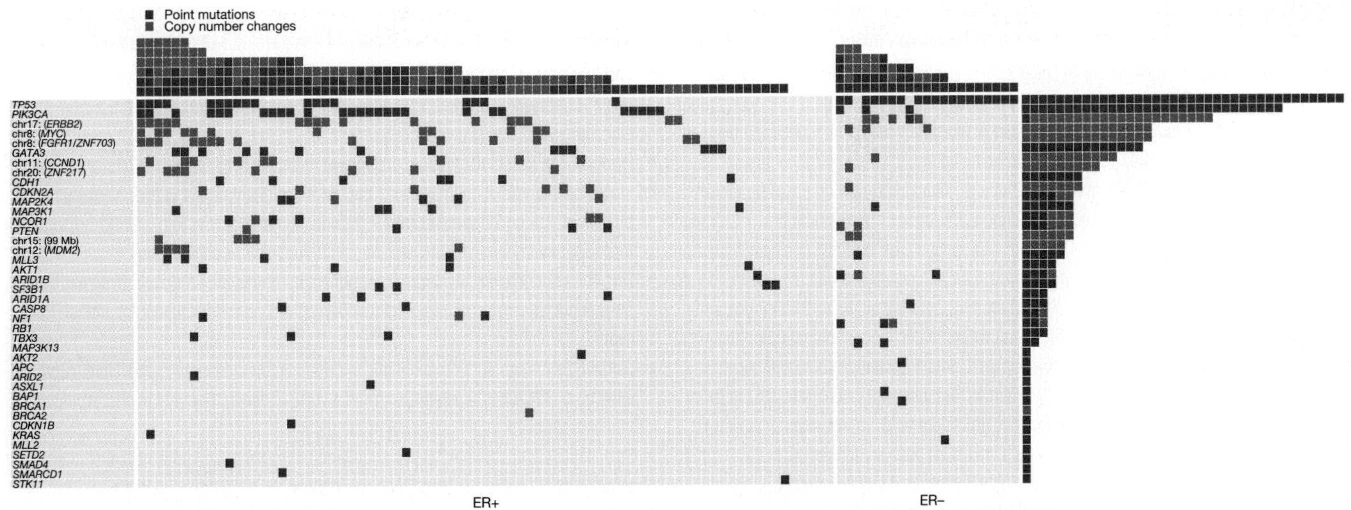

FIGURE 24-39 **Driver Mutations and Copy Number Changes in Breast Cancer.** The left side identifies each of the 40 cancer genes in which a driver mutation or copy number change has been identified. From investigation of 100 tumors, the number of mutations in each gene is shown (rows) as is the number of driver mutations in each breast cancer (columns). Point mutations are red and copy number changes are blue. (From: Stephens PJ et al: *Nature* 486:400–404, 2012.)

Physical Activity. Physically active individuals have lower rates of many cancers and improved cancer outcomes.[387,388] Activity also may reduce the invasiveness of breast cancer.[389] Consistent evidence from 27 observational studies showed physical activity is associated with all-cause, breast cancer–specific, and colon cancer–specific mortality.[387,390] A large prospective study found walking for 1 hour per day and additional weekly exercise seemed to be protective against breast cancer regardless of menopausal status.[391] Mechanisms for this protective effect are not known but include alterations in endogenous free radical formation and oxidative damage, effects on DNA repair capacity, changes in circulating insulin and insulin-related pathways, inflammation, alteration in carcinogen-metabolizing enzymes, increased intestinal transit times (i.e., reduced exposures to carcinogens), weight loss, changes in endogenous sex hormone, and possibly immunity levels.

Inherited Cancer Syndromes, Genes, Epigenetic Considerations

The causes of breast cancer have been difficult to define because each woman has a different genetic profile called **genetic heterogeneity.**[392] Genetic heterogeneity is common among individuals but also at the level of the tumor itself, involving both genetic and epigenetic processes. These facts are sobering and make the understanding of the genetic driving force behind tumor initiation, progression, and metastasis very complicated. Driver mutations are causally implicated in tumor development. Investigators examined the genomes of 100 tumors for somatic mutations and found they varied markedly between individual tumors.[392] Several new driver mutations were identified, including AKT2, ARIDIB, CASP8, CDKN1B, MAP3K1, MAP3K13, NCOR1, SMARCD1, and TBX3 (Figure 24-39).

A history of breast cancer in first-degree relatives (mother or sister) increases a woman's risk two to three times. Risk increases even more if two first-degree relatives are involved, especially if the disease occurred before menopause and was bilateral. In some families, breast cancer occurs at an earlier age and the frequency of bilateral tumors is greater. A small total proportion of breast cancers (incidence 5% to 10%, although the prevalence is significant) are the result of highly penetrant dominant genes (i.e., hereditary breast cancers). The most important of the dominant genes are the breast cancer susceptibility genes *(BRCA1, BRCA2). BRCA1* is located on chromosome 17 and *BRCA2* is located on chromosome 13. *BRCA1* and *BRCA2* (unmutated; normal) are tumor-suppressor genes. Box 24-16 summarizes key points about *BRCA1* and *BRCA2*.[393]

PATHOGENESIS. Most breast cancers arise from the ductal epithelium (Figure 24-40). Tumors of the infiltrating ductal type do not become large, but they metastasize early. Some types of breast carcinomas are summarized in Table 24-17.This type accounts for the majority of breast cancers. Breast cancer is a heterogeneous—not a single—disease with diverse molecular, biologic, phenotypic, and pathologic, changes.[394] Complex is that breast cancer also is heterogeneous *within* the same tumor (also see above). Despite heroic efforts, this diversity has greatly challenged the understanding of breast cancer evolution and the development of therapeutic strategies. Gene expression profiling studies have identified at least four major subtypes classified as luminal A, luminal B, HER2+, and basal-like.[395] Yet with mounting evidence it appears there are "subtypes within subtypes," and evidence is emerging suggesting that the biology of specific breast cancer subtypes reflects contributions from the tissue microenvironment.[396] In fact, in their updated article "Hallmarks of Cancer," Hanahan and Weinberg state, "In addition to cancer cells, tumors exhibit another dimension of complexity: they contain a repertoire of recruited, ostensibly normal cells that contribute to the acquisition of hallmark traits by creating the 'tumor microenvironment."[397, p. 646] Historically, many models of breast carcinogenesis have been suggested

BOX 24-16 KEY POINTS ABOUT *BRCA1* AND *BRCA2*

- A deleterious mutation in *BRCA1* or *BRCA2* increases a woman's risk of developing breast cancer or ovarian cancer, or both.
- Harmful *BRCA1* mutations may increase a woman's risk of developing cervical, uterine, pancreatic, and colon cancer.
- Men with harmful *BRCA1* mutations have an increased risk of breast cancer and possibly of pancreatic, testicular, and early-onset prostate cancer.
- Male breast cancer, however, and pancreatic and prostate cancer appear to be more strongly associated with harmful *BRCA2* mutations
- Harmful mutations in *BRCA1* or *BRCA2* are highest in families with a history of both breast and ovarian cancer, family members with tumors that develop from different sites in the body, or an Ashkenazi (Central European descent) Jewish background. However, not every woman in these families carries a harmful *BRCA1* or *BRCA2* mutation. Additionally, not every woman who has a harmful *BRCA1* or *BRCA2* mutation will develop breast or ovarian cancer, or both.
- A woman with a mutated *BRCA1* or *BRCA2* is about five times more likely to develop breast cancer than a woman without the mutation.
- Women with a harmful *BRCA1* or *BRCA2* have a probability of being diagnosed with ovarian cancer (150 to 400 out of 1000) compared with women without the mutation (14 out of 1000).
- The estimates of cancer risks are based on large families with multiple affected family members and may not accurately reflect other genetic and environmental risk factors.
- Options for those that have a positive test for a harmful *BRCA1* or *BRCA2* mutation include surveillance to find cancers early, prophylactic surgery (i.e., bilateral salpingo-oophorectomy), risk factor avoidance (e.g., avoid hormone replacement therapy [HRT], breast-feed), and chemoprevention.
- *BRCA1* and *BRCA2* function is a common pathway of genome protection. They work at different stages in the DNA damage response (DDR) and in DNA repair.
- *BRCA1* functions in both cell cycle check point activation and DNA repair, whereas *BRCA2* is a mediator of the DNA repair mechanism–homologous recombination.
- Both *BRCA1* and *BRCA2* work together to protect the genome from double-strand DNA damage during DNA replication.
- The prevalence and penetrance of both *BRCA1* and *BRCA2* vary with race; so far evidence indicates highest in whites compared to Asians and blacks.

Data from: National Cancer Institute: *BRCA1 and BRCA2: cancer risk & genetic testing.* Available at www.cancer.gov/cancertopics/factsheet/Risk/BRCA. Accessed February 2013.

including: (1) the multihits sequential acquisition model, (2) sporadic clonal evolution model, (3) telomere crisis, and (4) imprinted stem cell or cancer stem cell model.[398] In an effort to understand breast cancer biology three interrelated themes also have emerged and include: (1) gene addiction, (2) phenotypic plasticity, and (3) cancer stem cells.[399]

Cancer gene addiction includes oncogene addiction, whereby these genes play key roles in human breast cancer, and nononcogene addiction, whereby these genes may not initiate cancer but play major roles in cancer development and progression[399] (see p. 863). Phenotypic plasticity is exemplified by a distinctive phenotype called **epithelial to mesenchymal transition (EMT)** (see Chapter 12).[400] EMT is intimately involved in the generation of tissues and organs during embryogenesis, is essential for driving plasticity during development, and is an unintentional process during cancer progression. The EMT-associated reprogramming is involved not only in migration of cancer cells but also suppression of apoptosis and senescence, recapitulation during wound healing, weakening of cell-cycle progression, and resistance to radiotherapy and chemotherapy.[401] Much research is ongoing to define cancer stem cells in breast carcinogenesis including their origin and renewability properties. Numerous factors govern invasiveness and metastasis and include heterogeneity of cell subsets within the primary tumor, the interaction of tumor cells with the microenvironment, cell signaling factors, and the receptivity of metastatic colonization sites (the soil). EMT generates multiple epithelial cell subsets with different states of stemness relative to more differentiated cells.[402] In an effort to include all of these themes, it is striking that the same pathways and interactions observed in the normal mammary gland during development are exploited by tumors during their progression to metastatic disease (Figure 24-41).

The normal breast and breast tumors *share* molecular, cellular, systemic, and microenvironment components that are necessary for tumor progression.[396] The microenvironment is now recognized as a critical player in tumor progression and therapeutic responses.[403] Components of the microenvironment, including myoepithelial and endothelial cells, macrophages, and many ECM molecules, play a critical role in normal duct morphogenesis, and are increasingly recognized as major regulators of carcinogenesis[397] (see Figure 24-41).

Front and center for breast carcinogenesis is that cancer is a heterogeneous disease based on tumor anatomy, location, grade, lymph node metastasis, expression of growth factor receptors, and—emerging—several biomarkers assessed in the clinic.[396] Some breast tumors may be heterogeneous from their initial preinvasive stages,[398] but tumors are continuously evolving. Emerging is the understanding that the tumor microenvironment plays a major role in driving tumor heterogeneity.[396] Multiple microenvironment-related genes have been identified and include FGF, TGF-B, MMP, and collagen family members. Additionally, genetic signatures of genes involved in wound healing are thought to originate from fibroblasts of the tumor microenvironment. ECM-related gene expression modules are associated with tumor intrinsic subtypes and with clinical outcomes.[396] Gene expression prognostic signatures of motility and proliferation-related genes as well as stromal cells "reactive" phenotype during cancer progression show some commonality with normal branching morphogenesis and involution. Table 24-18 shows a comparison of similarities and differences between normal mammary gland branching and breast cancer invasion.[396]

The majority of studies evaluating gene expression stromal-derived signatures have focused on intratumoral stromal expression rather than the microenvironment surrounding normal breast or extratumoral expression.[404] Intratumoral stromal responses include: (1) elevated expression of immune mediators from stromal tissue,[405] (2) a signature of fibroblast

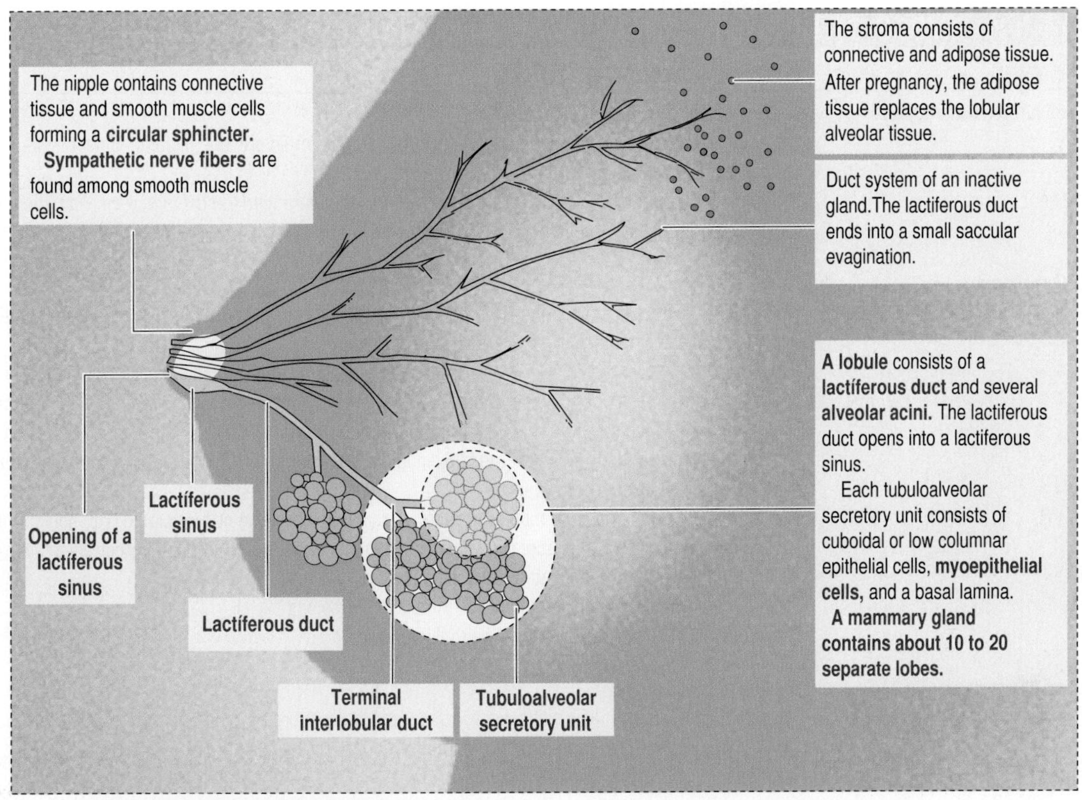

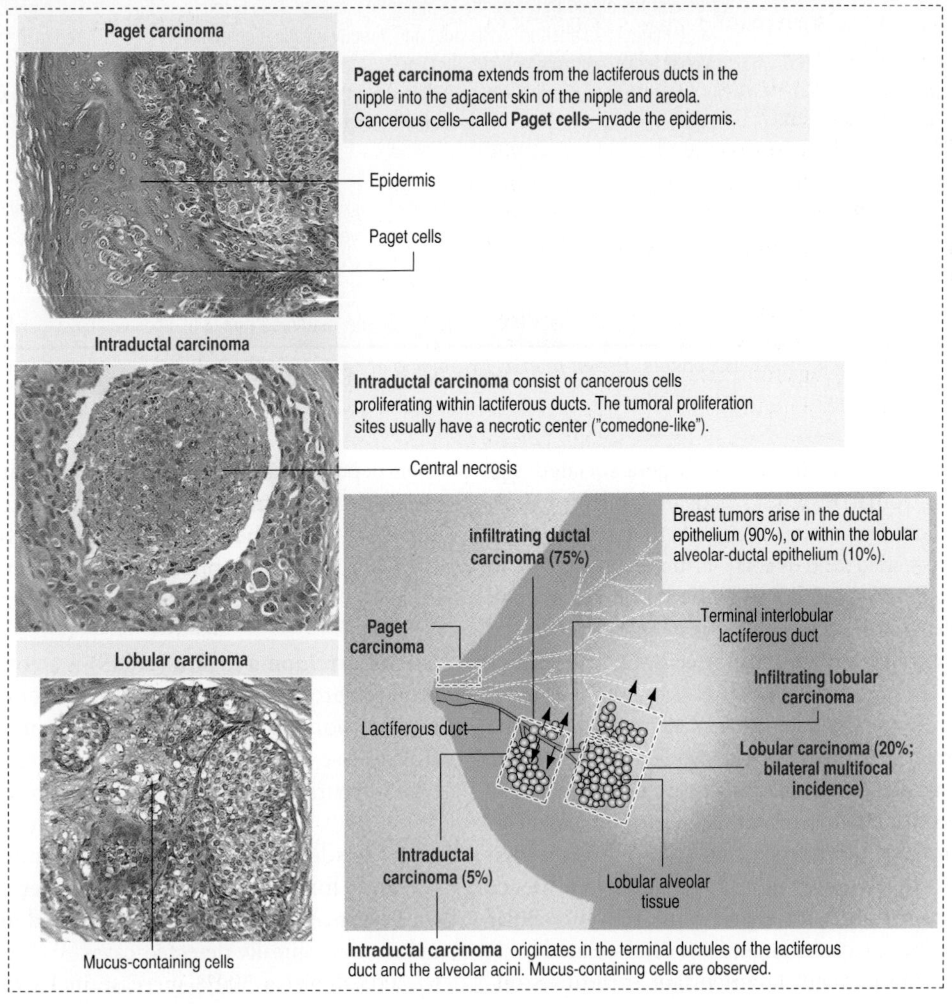

FIGURE 24-40 Normal Breast and Breast Cancer. **A,** Normal breast. **B,** Breast cancer. (From Kierszenbaum AL: *Histology and cell biology: an introduction to pathology,* ed 2, Philadelphia, 2007, Mosby.)

TABLE 24-17 TYPES OF BREAST CARCINOMAS AND MAJOR DISTINGUISHING FEATURES

HISTOLOGIC TYPE	DISTINGUISHING FEATURES
Carcinoma of Mammary Ducts	
Papillary	Well-delineated cystic masses in multiple areas; hemorrhage often present; majority appear in 40- to 60-year age group; often involves skin
Intraductal (comedo)	Often accompanied with evidence of inflammation; well-circumscribed tumors within the duct; well-differentiated tumor cells; rarely ulcerates the skin
Infiltrating Carcinoma	
Ductal (no specific type [NST])	Fibrous, firm, glistening, gray-tan mass with chalky streaks, mixture of patterns; may cause discharge from the nipple; represents about 79% of all breast cancer
Mucinous	Usually large (>3 cm in diameter), circumscribed, and encapsulated; glistening appearance, varies in color; two types: pure and mixed; pure tumor is surrounded by mucin; infrequent; found in the lateral half of the breast; tends to occur in women after age 70 years
Medullary	Encapsulated and grows to be very large (7-8 cm in diameter); commonly surrounded by lymphocytic inflammatory infiltrate; occurs after age 50 years
Tubular	Well differentiated with orderly tubules in center (stroma) of mass; can be associated with noninfiltrating ductal carcinoma; occurs in women about 50 years of age; nodal metastasis infrequent; occurrence rare
Adenoid cystic	Very rare; well-circumscribed, painless mass arising from the nipple and areola
Metaplastic	Involves cartilage or bone; mixed tumors or osteogenic sarcomas
Squamous cell	Frequent in blacks; originates in ductal epithelium
Carcinoma of Mammary Lobules	
Lobular carcinoma in situ	Found in individuals with fibrocystic disease; localized to upper breast quadrants; risk of 15%-35% becoming invasive; occurs frequently in mid-40s; infiltrating variety occurs in early 50s
Infiltrating lobular	Infiltrates from duct; firm mass with chalky streaks
Paget disease	Eczema of the nipple that extends to the areola; cancer usually found underneath the nipple; poorly circumscribed; large Paget cells arise from the duct and directly invade nipple; history of scaly, red rash spreading from the nipple; lesion palpable beneath the nipple, often bilateral; occurs in middle age
Inflammatory carcinoma	Not a histologic type; fairly diffuse within the breast tissue, diffuse edema of the overlying skin; extremely undifferentiated, very rare, most metastasize to axilla
Sarcoma of the Breast	
Cytosarcoma phyllodes	Usually large (>17 cm in diameter); mostly localized but can rupture through the skin; rarely metastasizes to lymph nodes; history of painless nodule present for years before it forms a large mass; ulceration and bleeding of skin often present; occurs in wide age range (ages 13-77 years)
Fibrosarcoma	Well circumscribed, firm, and usually does not involve the skin or nipple; well differentiated to extremely undifferentiated; arises from connective tissue; extremely rare (e.g., liposarcoma, angiosarcoma)

Data from Beahrs OH, Hutter RV, Kennedy BJ, editors: *Breast manual for staging of cancer,* ed 45, Philadelphia, 1992, Lippincott.

response,[406] (3) fibromatosis and macrophage-associated signature,[407] and (4) stromal responses activated early possibly before invasion.[408] Growing evidence suggests that extratumoral microenvironment—called field effects—also may play a role in tumor progression.[404] Normal homeostatic or developmental pathways and molecular processes, such as wound healing and TGF-β in the presence of initiated tumor cells, become tumor promoting.[404,409] The study of field effects has only just began in human cancer outcomes. Investigators demonstrated that wound responses may be divided into two types: active and inactive. Active cancer-adjacent tissue reveals characteristics of active EMT or cellular dedifferentiation (regression of specialized cellular features or simpler, more embryonic) and was associated with poor survival. Inactive extratumoral tissue has evidence of more differentiated tissue with higher expression of cellular adhesion genes and lower expression levels of EMT-related transcription factors.[404] Complicated and important are future studies to determine intra- and extratumoral changes to understand their dependence and independence on tumor characteristics. It seems clear that cancer heterogeneity and clinical outcome reflect signaling from a heterogeneous microenvironmental recurring theme that hopefully promises greater therapeutic outcomes.

Ductal Carcinoma In Situ

Ductal carcinoma in situ (DCIS) is a complex, heterogeneous group of proliferations limited to breast ducts and lobules without invasion of the basement membrane. About 84% of all in situ disease is DCIS; the remainder is mostly LCIS disease.[410] DCIS occurs predominantly in women but can occur in men. Since 1980, the widespread adoption of screening mammography has led to an epidemic of diagnoses of DCIS.[411] DCIS accounts for about 20% to 27% of newly diagnosed cases of breast cancer in the United States, and about 17% to 34% of mammographically detected cases.[411,412] SEER data from 1983 to 2003 depict a 500% increase in DCIS among women age 50 years and older and a decline of DCIS in 2003.[413] Among

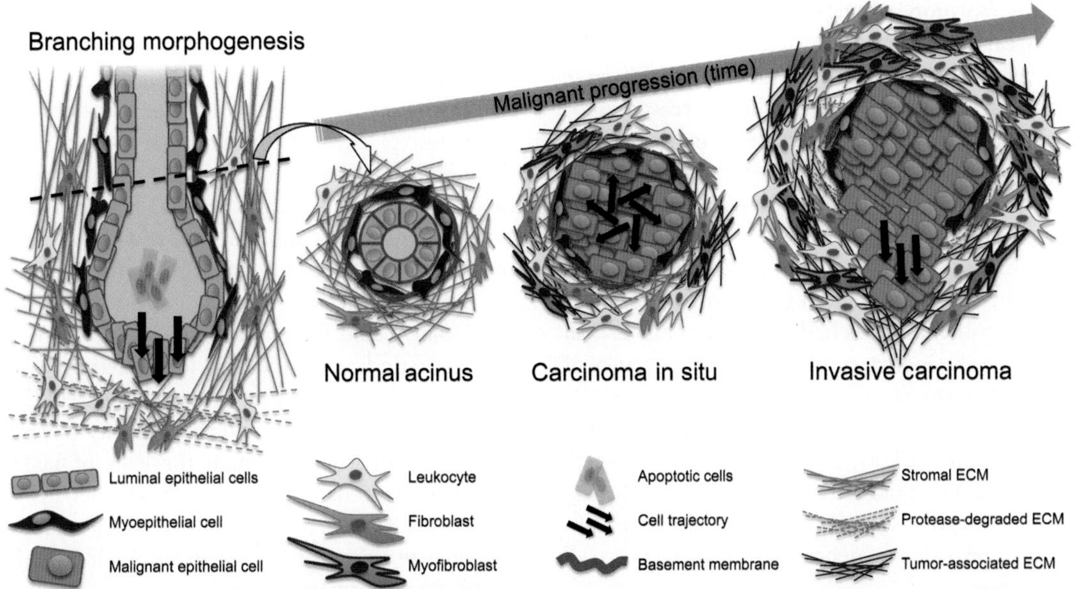

FIGURE 24-41 A Model of Breast Carcinogenesis: Dynamic Microenvironments Regulate Both Normal Breast Development and Breast Carcinogenesis. Anatomic changes during mammary gland development, called branching morphogenesis, require extensive dialogue between epithelial and stromal cells and their underlying extracellular matrix (ECM). These events are central and amplified during carcinogenesis and are often required for tumor progression. Loss of the myoepithelial cell layer and basement membrane is key for invasive progression. Potential crosstalk between cell–cell and cell–matrix interactions are abnormally regulated by autocrine and paracrine signaling networks of proteolytic enzymes and chemokines, and cytokines continue to attract leukocytes, modulate tumor remodeling, and increase tumor cell invasion eventually leading to metastasis. Tumors steal or "hack" the normal developmental program to manifest carcinogenesis. (From Boudreau A, van't Veer LJ, Bissell M: *Cell Adh Migr* 6[3]:236–248, 2012.)

TABLE 24-18 BREAST CANCER INVASION AND NORMAL MAMMARY GLAND BRANCHING SHARE MANY SIMILARITIES

	BRANCHING MORPHOGENESIS	BREAST TUMOR INVASION
Similarities	Requires heterotypic, paracrine interactions between epithelial cell proliferation and directional migration	
	Stromal cells secrete growth factors guiding epithelial cell proliferation and directional migration	
	Proliferative epithelial cells secrete growth factors to enrich their adjacent stroma	
	Conserved growth factors and receptors used, albeit at different amplitudes of signaling	
Differences	Regulated proliferation and migration	Aberrant mitogenic signaling and network substucture
	Transient stromal-epithelial interactions	Exaggerated stromal-epithelial interactions
	Migration confined by fat pad	Migration infiltrates adjacent tissues and beyond
	Epithelial cell apoptosis yields a lumen	Epithelial cell necrosis yields inflammation
	Deposition of basement membrane	Destruction of basement membrane
	Differentiation into polarized, bilayered ducts	Dedifferentiation; loss of polarity and myoepithelium
	End product is a functional tissue	End product is pathologic tissue

Data from Boudreau A, van't Veer LJ, Bissell M: *Cell Adh Migr* 6(3):236–248, 2012.

women younger than 50 years, there has been a 290% increase in DCIS since 1983 and the incidence is still increasing.[411] The American Cancer Society estimates about 64,640 new cases of carcinoma in situ in 2013.[414] The type of DCIS across all age groups not associated with subsequent DCIS or invasive cancer (i.e., noncomedo type) has mostly increased, and subsequent DCIS or invasive cancer has been constant or decreased. Importantly and despite 20 years of detecting DCIS by mammography, a decline in invasive cancer in the United States was not observed until the large decline in postmenopausal hormone therapy. Population data report screening rates of DCIS to be similar among white, black, and Asian/Pacific Islanders.[415] The majority of DCIS presents as linear or multiple clusters of calcifications on a mammogram.

Although risk factors for DCIS and invasive breast cancer are similar and therefore suggest a common etiology for both diseases, some characteristics are more strongly associated with invasive cancer. The risk factors that increase the risk of both DCIS and invasive cancers include family history of a first-degree relative, nulliparity or late age of first birth, history of biopsy, late age at menopause, long-term use of postmenopausal HRT, and increased BMI in postmenopausal women not taking hormone therapy.[415] A strong risk factor for invasive breast cancer and for DCIS is high mammographic breast density.[415,416] Conflicting studies for DCIS have been on smoking, lactation, early menarche, increased alcohol consumption, and oral contraceptive use. The prevalence of mutation carriers *BRCA1* and *BRCA2* is similar among women diagnosed with DCIS to that of women with invasive breast cancer.[415]

Recently it was shown that about 5900 genes are expressed in the epithelium during the transition from normal to DCIS and that only three epithelial genes had differential expression from DCIS to invasive carcinoma, suggesting the importance of the stroma in cancer progression.[396] Allinen and coworkers[417] performed the first systematic profiling of the various stromal cell types. They demonstrated gene expression alterations in all cell types within the tumor microenvironment accompanying progression from normal breast tissue to DCIS to invasive ductal carcinoma (IDC) provided evidence that these cell types all participate in tumorigenesis.[396]

Changes in the tumor microenvironment are observed early at the DCIS stage or even earlier.[396] With the secretion of chemokines causing accumulation of leukocytes and many other cells, stromal and epithelial cells participate in reciprocal and paracrine acting signaling loops (Figure 24-42). These communicating signaling links appear to stabilize the increased localization of macrophages, myofibroblasts, and fibroblasts at the DCIS stage, which ultimately remodel the ECM and promote tumor proliferation.[396] Depending on location, genetics, and other changes, the altered microenvironment may stiffen, increase blood vessel density, increase breast density, and result in calcifications. Although DCIS may remain stable and never progress (or may regress), for invasive DCIS the cells within the DCIS *breach* the myoepithelial layer and the basement membrane defining the moment when an invasive carcinoma is formed.[396] Importantly, the layer of myoepithelial cells is thought to be natural "tumor suppressors" and critical to maintaining tissue polarity (cell directional orientation) (see Figure 1-11), a role that is lost in invasive breast carcinomas. Investigators and clinicians are intensely studying this key step, or breach, in terms of cellular alterations because of tumor biology or iatrogenic stimuli, or both.

The natural history of DCIS is actually elusive and reflects the diversity of the condition. Preinvasive lesions do not invariably progress to invasive malignancy. DCIS is detected more often in younger women than in older women.

Although there is no universally accepted histopathologic classification, historically most pathologists divided DCIS into five subtypes (papillary, micropapillary, cribriform, solid, and comedo) and often compare the first four types, noncomedo, with comedo. In a single biopsy, however, several types may be mixed and some noncomedo types may express characteristics of the comedo type. Although the term *comedo type* is widely used it does not specify a grade or an architecture, so newer categories most often use nuclear grade (high, intermediate, or low) and record the architectural pattern separately.[418] When it comes to the architecture of DCIS, however, the literature is full of contradictory information.

Lobular Carcinoma In Situ

Lobular carcinoma in situ (LCIS) originates from the terminal duct–lobular unit (see Figure 24-40, *B*). Unlike DCIS, LCIS has a uniform appearance in which the cells occur in noncohesive (discohesive) clusters, primarily in lobules. Today, however, there is limited knowledge of the biology of LCIS.[419] Atypical lobular hyperplasia (ALH) and LCIS represent a spectrum of breast disease called **lobular neoplasia (LN).** Research suggests that some lobular and ductal carcinomas are closely related.[420] LCIS is not associated with calcifications or a stromal involvement that would form a density (lump). Thus it is usually an incidental finding from biopsy for something else. LCIS is fairly uncommon (up to 3.8% of all specimens).[421] LCIS is bilateral in 20% to 40% of women, and the majority (80% to 90%) occur before menopause. Although the cells of LCIS and invasive lobular carcinoma are identical,[177] whether LCIS is a true neoplasm or a marker of breast cancer risk remains controversial. Evidence to support LCIS as a precursor lesion of invasive carcinoma comes from molecular genetic data highlighting chromosomal alterations and that LOH on chromosome 16q is present in an invasive carcinoma.[47,422] Invasive carcinoma develops in 25% to 35% of women with LCIS, and the contralateral (opposite) breast also is at risk.[423] Chemoprevention is recommended for atypia types, including LCIS, to reduce breast cancer risk.[424]

Inflammatory Stroma in Breast Cancer

Dominating the cancer field is the idea that epithelial function depends on the *entire* tissue, including the stroma or microenvironment. The specific location where a tumor develops in the breast can have a major influence on its breast cancer outcome.[425] Variations in tumor development depend on the architecture and the microenvironment of the tumor in vivo and plays an important role in phenotypic outcome of genetic mutations.[426] Importantly, people can harbor potentially malignant tumors that remain dormant for many years.[425] The microenvironment surrounding a tumor may normally suppress tumor development by providing tumor-suppressive signals, and the loss of tissue homeostasis causes the development of an aberrant microenvironment and over time becomes a potent tumor promoter.[396,409,427-429] The stromal response (the "soil") is often associated with invasive breast cancer. Emerging are two views regarding the tissue stromal response to breast carcinogenesis—is the stromal response unique to the tumor or is the stromal response a host response, an individual's innate healing response to disrupted tissue? Embedded in these views is the stromal response, sometimes called an aberrant "wound" with an **inflammatory stromal (reactive stroma) component**[430] (see Chapter 12). This "wound response" is exemplified by expression of a set of genes associated with healing. Evidence of the link between wound healing and carcinogenesis is based on the fact that these two distinct pathologies share a common "footprint" or "signature," a common molecular gene expression signature.[201] Gene expression signatures derived from tumor stroma have been linked to clinical outcomes.[403] The genetic expression profile from a wound-healing model of fibroblasts actually predicted metastasis and death in several epithelial cancers. The "activated fibroblast gene signature" also

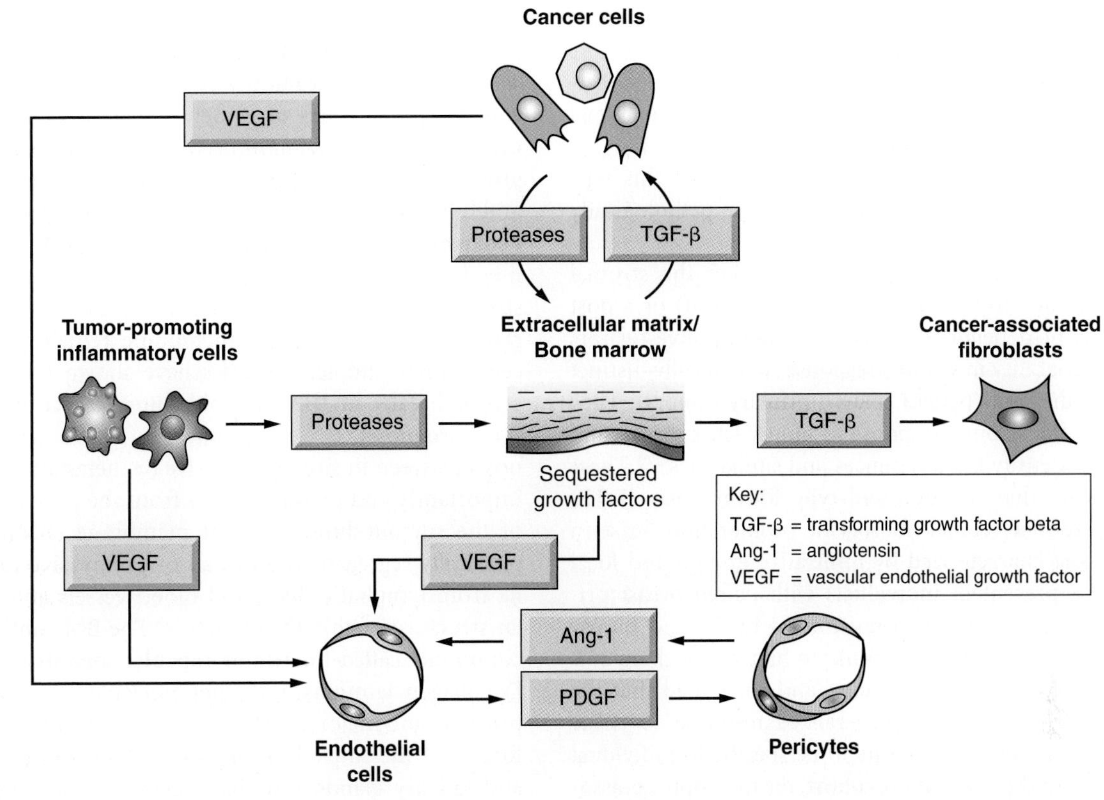

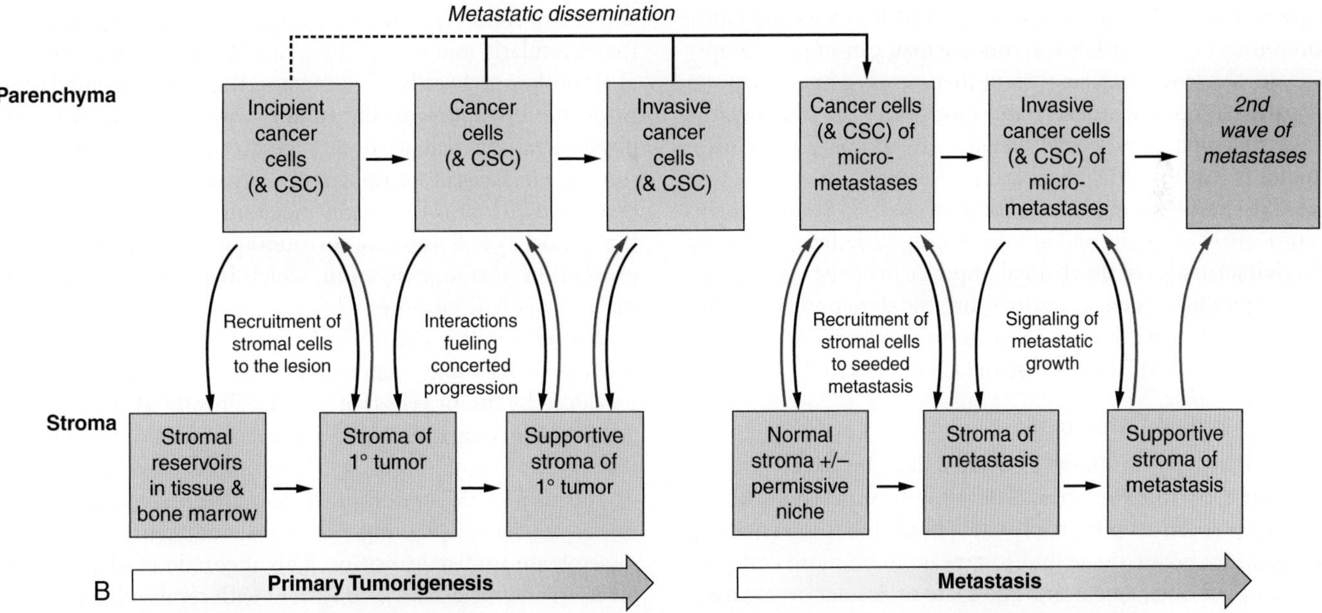

FIGURE 24-42 Signaling Interactions in the Tumor Microenvironment During Malignant Progression. **A,** Numerous cell types constitute the tumor microenvironment and are orchestrated and maintained by reciprocal interactions. **B,** The reciprocal interactions between the breast main tissue or parenchyma and the surrounding stroma are important for cancer progression and growth. Certain organ sites of "fertile soil" or "metastasis niches" facilitate metastatic seeding and colonization. Cancer stem cells are involved in some or all stages of tumor development and progression. (Adapted from Hanahan D, Weinberg R: *Cell* 144:646–674, 2011.) *CSC,* Cancer stem cells.

was shown to be an independent marker for local recurrence of breast cancer.[430,431]

Early alterations in the stroma that occur with wound healing and inflammation include activation of (1) mesenchymal cells (embryonic) fibroblasts; (2) endothelial cells; and (3) immune cells, including macrophages. Evidence of this type of activation is noted adjacent to tumors and is pathologically known as *desmoplastic stroma.*

To help answer the question as to whether the stromal response is unique to the tumor (tumor-provoked) or a host reaction (patient-dependent) to tissue alteration, investigators studied the variability in stromal responses in clinically distinct tumors from the same patient (paired primary tumors). They did studies of the stromal response to biopsy site changes and carcinoma to identify the differences and similarities.[279] These studies indicate that the **desmoid-type fibromatosis (DTF) fibroblast response** (clonal fibroblastic proliferations arise in deep soft tissue characterized by infiltrative growth and local recurrence) is present in individuals with paired breast primary tumors. Stroma taken from normal breast and biopsy site changes showed that the response to biopsy site changes is similar to the response to carcinoma and concluded that the DTF fibroblast response is a generalized response to tissue disruption and injury that appears to be specific to individual patients.[279] From the larger study cohort, the macrophage-associated pattern of gene overexpression called the **CSF1 response** showed no significant similarity or concordance in separate tumors within a given patient. The DTF fibroblast signature showed more concordance across normal, cancer, and biopsy site samples from within a patient than across a random group of patients' normal, cancer, and biopsy site samples but the CSF1 macrophage response did not. In summary from these studies is that the DTF fibroblast response is host-specific and the CSF1 response may be tumor-provoked.[279] Studies of this nature are challenging and are continuing to better understand the characteristics of the stromal response in breast carcinogenesis. Emerging evidence suggests that the development of this wound-reactive pattern and change in tumor tissue architecture creates an EMT (see p. 864 and Chapter 12).[400]

Invasive Breast Carcinoma

Invasive breast carcinoma is a malignant invasive epithelial lesion derived from the terminal duct lobular unit (Figure 24-40, *B*, p. 865). It can arise from anywhere in the breast parenchyma or accessory breast tissue, but it appears to be more common in the upper outer quadrant. The exact molecular events leading to invasion are complex and not completely understood. Because myoepithelial cells form a semi-continuous protective sheet separating the human breast epithelium and the surrounding stroma, it has been a major focus of understanding invasive carcinogenesis (Figure 24-43).

Two theories are proposed for the mechanism of tumor epithelial cells' progression from the in situ to invasive carcinogenesis stages.[432] The first theory of invasion is the result of proteolytic enzymes and their degradation capacities by myoepithelial cells and surrounding tumor cells. The second theory is that tumor invasion is a multistep process, involving dynamic interactions between damaged myoepithelial cells, and the immunoreactive cells initiate the release of basement membrane–degrading enzymes causing tumor progression.[432] Several lines of evidence suggest that myoepithelial cells block proliferation of breast carcinoma cells by inducing growth arrest and apoptosis. They also secrete many effector and inhibitor molecules that interfere or suppress the invasive behavior of tumor cells and block angiogenesis and basement membrane degradation.[433] Patterns of local dissemination are strongly constrained by the local ECM microenvironment and critically, if the basement membrane remains intact, cancer cells remain indolent. Studies have shown that even microscopic breaks in the myoepithelium are correlated with a poor prognosis.[434,435] The critical difference in clinical prognosis between in situ and invasive or metastatic cancer results importantly and predominantly from the presence or absence of the surrounding basement membrane (BM).[436] The BM physically segregates all normal or preinvasive tumor epithelia from lymphatic ducts and blood vessels and from vascular structures within the stroma.[436] The BM continuous sheet, commonly called the **tumor capsule,** consists of mainly type IV collagen, laminins, and other molecules[436] In human breast, prostate, and major salivary glands, the capsule is further reinforced by the single layer of myoepithelial cells in the breast and salivary glands and "basal cells" in the prostate.[436] The basal or myoepithelial cell layer lies between the epithelial cells and the BM. In the gastrointestinal tract, the normal mucosa and in situ cancer are further separated from the submucosa by the muscularis mucosa, a dense band composed of two layers of smooth muscle cells.[437] Because of these structural relationships, the disruption of the tumor capsule and its associated physical barriers is an absolute prerequisite for tumor cell invasion or metastasis.[436] Importantly, myoepithelial cells modulate the expression of matrix metalloproteinases (MMPs) in the tumor, as well as in the surrounding cells, and assist in the prevention of tumor invasion, which is possibly mediated by these proteolytic enzymes.[438]

A long-standing theory is that progression from in situ to invasive or metastatic cancer is caused by proteolytic enzymes produced by tumor cells that increase linearly with tumor progression, reaching their highest level at the in situ cancer stage. It has been hypothesized that these proteolytic enzymes cause degradation or disruption of the tumor capsule and allow the in situ cancer cells to migrate into the adjacent stroma or to disseminate to distant organs. This theoretic model of tumor invasion and metastasis is consistent with results obtained from tissue culture and animal model studies; however, it is debated because it appears inconsistent with a number of other well-established observations.[436] Therefore, other models exist for understanding tumor invasion and metastases and prominently include the role of the ECM, immune cells, and stem cells (Box 24-17). The intrinsic impact of focal myoepithelial cell degeneration, aberrant lymphocyte infiltration, and capsule disruptions is likely to be associated with tumor progression and invasion. Advanced breast cancer is associated with complete loss of the myoepithelial cell layer and basement membrane, invasion of epithelial cells, and angiogenesis (Figure 24-44).

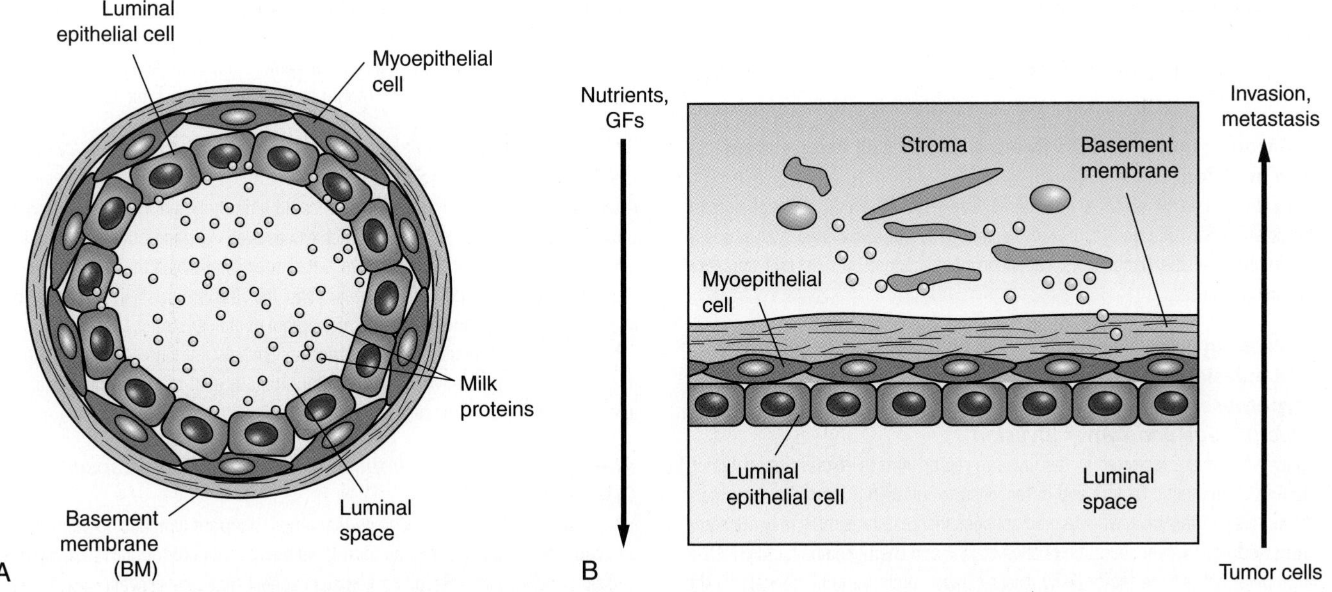

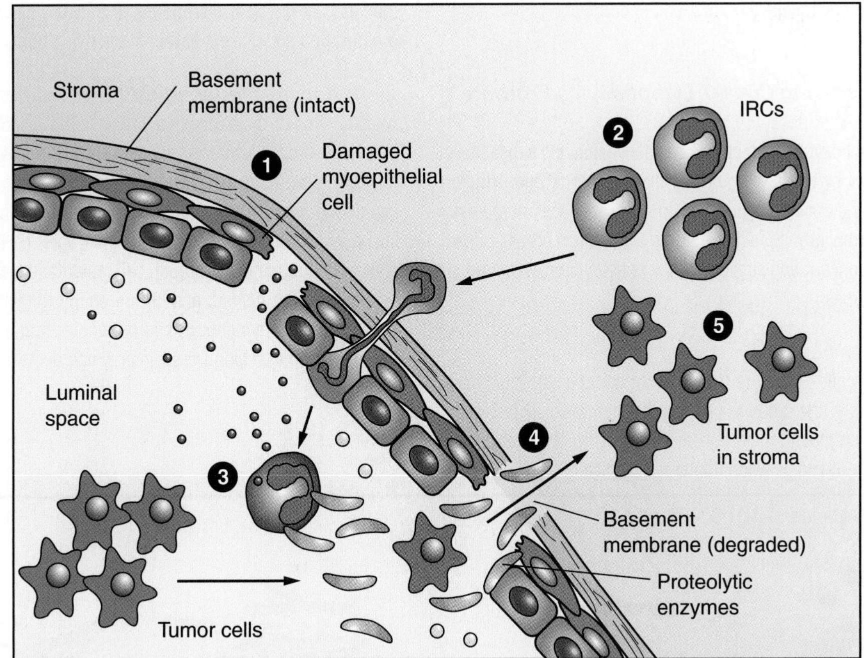

FIGURE 24-43 The Role of Myoepithelial Cells in Invasive Breast Cancer. A, Cross section of a normal mammary gland. **B,** Schematic of the anatomic relationship between mammary gland duct cells, basement membrane (BM), and stroma. **C,** With degradation of the normal "tumor suppressing" basement membrane tumor cells invade the stroma; **(1)** myoepithelial cells are damaged by various factors and release their inner contents (for example, diffusible molecules and chemoattractants); **(2)** immunoreactive cells (IRCs) are drawn to the luminal space by these chemoattractants; **(3)** IRCs become activated after contact with chemoattractants and secrete various proteolytic enzymes; **(4)** these enzymes then degrade the basement membrane resulting in gaps; and **(5)** tumor cells enter the stromal region through these gaps. (Data and adapted figures from Pandey PR, Saidou J, Watabe K: *Front Biosci* 15:226–236, 2011.) *GF,* Growth factor.

BOX 24-17 EXISTING THEORIES OF TUMOR INVASION AND METASTASES

Proteolytic Enzyme Theory

Proteolytic enzymes cause degradation or disruption of the tumor capsule and allow the in situ cancer cells to migrate into the adjacent stroma or to disseminate to distant organs.

Infiltrating Immune Cells Reduce Tumor Cell Progression and Invasion

Infiltration of immune cells into tumor tissues and direct physical contact between tumor cells and infiltrated immune cells are associated with physical destructions of the tumor cells, reduction of the tumor burden, and improved clinical prognosis.

Infiltrating Immune Cells Promote Tumor Cell Progression and Invasion

Hypotheses

Macrophage and Tumor Invasion

Macrophages are recruited to the invasive tumor front by expression of tumor-derived chemotactic factors and in response to the disruption of the basement membrane. At this invasive site macrophages increase tumor cell migration and invasion through their secretion of chemotactic and chemokinetic factors including epidermal growth factor (EGF). Macrophages promote angiogenesis by the synthesis of angiogenic factors including vascular endothelial growth factor (VEGF), and they remodel the extracellular matrix and in particular, regulate collagen fibrillogenesis.

Interleukin (IL)-4–Expressing CD4+ T Lymphocytes Promote Tumor Invasion

IL-4-expressing CD4+ T lymphocytes indirectly promote invasion and subsequent metastasis of breast cancer by directly regulating the phenotype and effector function of tumor-associated macrophages that in turn enhance metastasis through activation of epidermal growth factor receptor signaling in breast cancer epithelial cells. The same concept and similar pathways have been extended to lymphocytes and their subtypes.

Cancer Cell–Leukocyte Fusion

Macrophages ingest tumor cells leading to the fusion of genetic materials from the two cell types, resulting in the creation of a hybrid phenotype. This phenotype is associated with chemotactic migration in vitro toward fibronectin and shows high frequencies of metastasis when implanted in mice.

Regulatory T Cells (Treg) Induced Immunosuppression

Recruitment of Treg cells to the tumor supports disease progression through a dual mechanism: (1) the decrease of antitumor immunity, and (2) through the establishment of a proangiogenic reprogramming of the tumor microenvironment.

Monocyte-Mediated Protection Against Natural Killer (NK) Cell Lysis of Cancer Stem Cells

Alterations in NK cell effector function could ultimately aid in driving differentiation of a population of surviving healthy as well as transformed stem cells. Because the majority of NK cells have lost cytotoxic activity in those with cancer, they may eventually *contribute* rather than *halt* the progression of cancer by allowing the growth and expansion of the pool of cancer stem cells.

This hypothesis provides a general mechanism how immune cells may behave in inflammatory microenvironment for the ultimate goal of tissue regeneration and the resolution of inflammation.

Aberrant Lymphocyte Infiltration–Induced Focal Capsule Disruptions

Focal basal or myoepithelial cell degeneration, aberrant lymphocyte infiltration, and capsule disruptions may be correlated events that contribute to tumor progression and invasion. Research findings suggest that tumor invasion or metastasis is triggered by focal capsule degeneration–induced lymphocyte infiltration that causes physical disruptions within the capsule, which selectively favors proliferation and dissemination of overlying tumor stem cells.

Lymphocyte-Mediated Cell Dissemination and Metastasis

An extension of the above hypothesis is that aberrant tumor-infiltrating lymphocytes can trigger tumor metastasis through three correlated pathways: (1) the physical movement of infiltrated lymphocytes into the budding tumor cell nest can disrupt intercellular junctions and surface adhesion molecules, causing dissociation of some cells from the tumor core; (2) lymphocytes can conjoin with dissociated tumor cells through cell membrane fusion to form tumor-lymphocyte chimeras (TLCs; fusion); and (3) the ability to migrate and to cross intercellular barriers enables lymphocytes to physically drag tumor cells to remote sites and to intravasate into blood vessels or lymph ducts.

Data from Man YG et al: *J Cancer* 4:4(1):84–95, 2013.

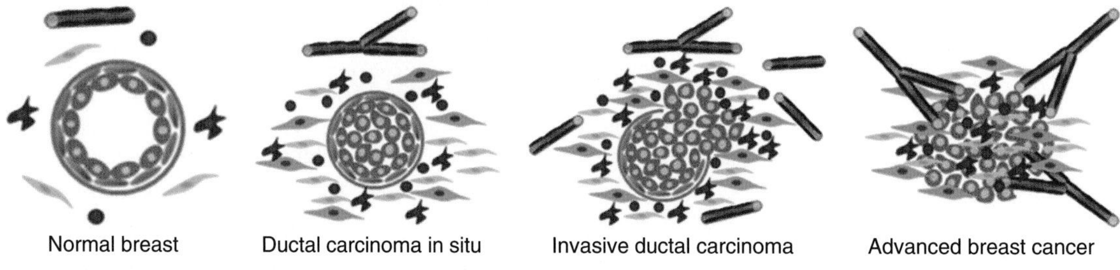

FIGURE 24-44 Breast Cancer Progression with Stromal Cells. The normal breast duct is composed of a layer of epithelial cells and a layer of myoepithelial cells, which is separated from the stroma by a basement membrane (BM). Examples of stromal cells include fibroblasts, bone marrow–derived cells (BMDCs), endothelial cells (important for angiogenesis), and other cells. Ductal carcinoma in situ (DCIS) is associated with luminal epithelial cell proliferation, and recruitment and expansion of stromal cells. In invasive ductal carcinoma, the myoepithelial cell layer is degraded with the underlying basement membrane and cancerous cells invade the surrounding microenvironment. Advanced breast cancer is associated with complete loss of myoepithelial cell layer and basement membrane, invasion of epithelial cells, proliferation of stromal cells, and angiogenesis. (From Khamis ZI, Sahab ZJ, Sang QX: *Int J Breast Cancer* 2012:574025, 2012.)

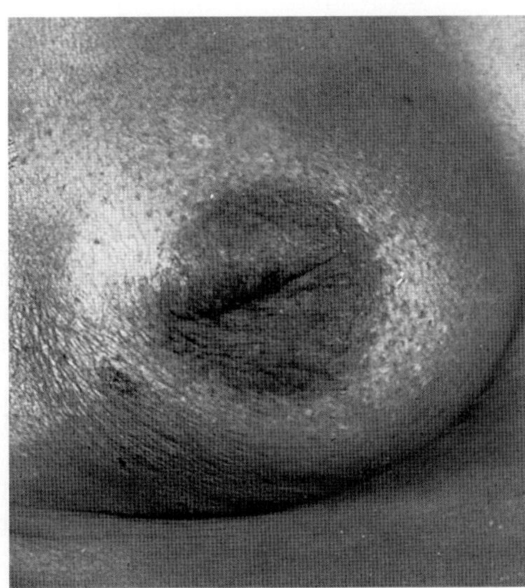

FIGURE 24-45 Retraction of Nipple Caused by Carcinoma. (From del Regato JA, Spjut HJ, Cox JD: *Ackerman and del Regato's cancer: diagnosis, treatment, and prognosis,* ed 6, St Louis, 1985, Mosby.)

CLINICAL MANIFESTATIONS. The first sign of breast cancer is usually a painless lump. Lumps caused by breast tumors do not have any classic characteristics. Other presenting signs include palpable nodes in the axilla, retraction of tissue (dimpling) (Figure 24-45), or bone pain caused by metastasis to the vertebrae. Table 24-19 summarizes the clinical manifestations of breast cancers. Manifestations vary according to the type of tumor and stage of disease.

EVALUATION AND TREATMENT. Clinical breast examination, mammography, ultrasound, thermography, MRI, biopsy or minimally invasive biopsy, hormone receptor assays, and gene expression profiling are used in evaluating breast alterations and cancer.

Treatment is based on the extent or stage of the cancer. The extent of the tumor at the primary site, the presence and extent of lymph node metastasis, and the presence of distant metastases are all evaluated to determine the stage of disease. Treatment includes surgery, radiation, chemotherapy, hormone therapy, and biologic therapy.

TABLE 24-19 CLINICAL MANIFESTATIONS OF BREAST CANCER

CLINICAL MANIFESTATION	PATHOPHYSIOLOGY
Chest pain	Metastasis to the lung
Dilated blood vessels	Obstruction of venous return by a fast-growing tumor; obstruction dilates superficial veins
Dimpling of the skin	Can occur with invasion of the dermal lymphatics because of retraction of Cooper ligament or involvement of the pectoralis fascia
Edema	Local inflammation or lymphatic obstruction
Edema of the arm	Obstruction of lymphatic drainage in the axilla
Hemorrhage	Erosion of blood vessels
Local pain	Local obstruction caused by the tumor
Nipple/areolar eczema	Paget disease
Nipple discharge in a nonlactating woman	Spontaneous and intermittent discharge caused by tumor obstruction
Nipple retraction	Shortening of the mammary ducts
Pitting of the skin (similar to the surface of an orange [peau d'orange])	Obstruction of the subcutaneous lymphatics, resulting in the accumulation of fluid
Reddened skin, local tenderness, and warmth	Inflammation
Skin retraction	Involvement of the suspensory ligaments
Ulceration	Tumor necrosis

Data from Griffiths MJ, Murray KH, Russo PC: *Oncology nursing: pathophysiology, assessment, and intervention,* New York, 1984, Macmillan.

SUMMARY REVIEW

Alterations of Sexual Maturation

1. Sexual maturation, or puberty, should begin in girls between ages 8 and 13 years. Delayed puberty is the onset of sexual maturation after these ages; precocious puberty is onset before these ages. The average age of puberty has been occurring earlier than in previous generations.
2. Alterations of sexual maturation can be idiopathic or caused by a disease or congenital anomaly. In most cases of delayed puberty, the hypothalamic pituitary gonadal (HPG) axis is intact but the surge of activity that stimulates puberty is delayed. Precocious puberty, more common in girls, also can be caused by mistiming of the stimulatory surge in a child whose HPG system is otherwise normal. Obesity is associated with younger pubertal age.
3. Precocious puberty can be complete (sex appropriate), mixed (not sex appropriate), or partial (development of one secondary sex characteristic only). Causes of delayed or incomplete puberty can be divided into categories based on gonadotropic secretion: hypergonadotropism (increased levels of FSH and LH), and hypogonadotropism (decreased LH and FSH levels).

Disorders of the Female Reproductive System

1. The female reproductive system can be altered by hormonal imbalances, infectious microorganisms, inflammation, structural abnormalities, and benign or malignant proliferative conditions.

SUMMARY REVIEW—cont'd

2. Menstrual disorders usually involve some disruption of the HPG axis and subsequent alteration of hormone production, reception by target organs, or feedback mechanisms.
3. Primary dysmenorrhea is painful menstruation not associated with pelvic disease. It often results from excessive synthesis of prostaglandins (or sensitivity to prostaglandins), which cause the myometrium to contract and constrict blood vessels, resulting in ischemic pain.
4. Primary amenorrhea is the continued absence of menarche and menstrual function by 14 years of age without the development of secondary sex characteristics or by age 16 years if these changes have occurred.
5. Secondary amenorrhea is the absence of menstruation for a time equivalent to more than three cycles or 6 months in women who have previously menstruated. Secondary amenorrhea is usually associated with anovulation.
6. Amenorrhea is divided into compartments that reflect the underlying disorder: compartment I, disorders of the outflow tract or uterine target organ; compartment II, disorders of the ovary; compartment III, disorders of the anterior pituitary; and compartment IV, disorders of the CNS or hypothalamic factors.
7. Dysfunctional uterine bleeding (DUB) is heavy or irregular bleeding caused by a disturbance of the menstrual cycle.
8. Polycystic ovary syndrome (PCOS) is a difficult syndrome to diagnose because several factors are involved. It is a syndrome in which at least two of the following are present: oligo-ovulation or anovulation, elevated levels of androgens, or clinical signs of hyperandrogenism and polycystic ovaries. Prolonged anovulation leads to infertility, menstrual bleeding disorders, hirsutism, acne, endometrial hyperplasia, cardiovascular disease, and diabetes mellitus in women with hyperinsulinemia.
9. PMS is the cyclic recurrence of physical, psychologic, or behavioral changes distressing enough to disrupt normal activities or interpersonal relationships. More than 200 emotional, physical, and behavioral symptoms have been attributed to PMS. Emotional symptoms, particularly depression, anger, irritability, and fatigue, are reported as the most distressing; physical symptoms tend to be less problematic. Treatment is symptomatic and includes self-help techniques, lifestyle changes, counseling, and selective serotonin reuptake inhibitors (SSRIs).
10. Infection and inflammation of the female genitalia can result from microorganisms from the environment or overproliferation of microorganisms that normally populate the genital tract.
11. Pelvic inflammatory disease (PID) is an acute ascending polymicrobial infection of the upper genital tract and is sexually transmitted.
12. Vaginitis, or vaginal infection, is usually caused by sexually transmitted pathogens or *C. albicans*, which causes candidiasis. Development is related to the overall health of a woman and local defense mechanisms, particularly vaginal pH. Variables such as antibiotics, douching, soaps, feminine hygiene sprays, and pregnancy alter vaginal pH or the bactericidal nature of secretions and predispose a woman to infection.
13. Cervicitis, which is inflammation of the cervix, can be acute (mucopurulent cervicitis) or chronic.
14. Vulvovestibulitis is an inflammation of the skin of the vulva. It can be caused by chemical and mechanical irritants, allergens, skin disorders, nerve problems, or vaginal infections, such as candidiasis.
15. Bartholinitis, also called Bartholin cyst, is an inflammation of the ducts that lead from the *Bartholin glands* to the surface of the vulva. Inflammation blocks the glands, preventing the outflow of glandular secretions, and is caused by trauma or infection.
16. Pelvic organ prolapse—uterine prolapse, cystocele, rectocele, and urethrocele—is caused by loss of support provided by the pelvic muscles and fascia. Age and pelvic trauma are associated. Women with a familial or genetic predisposition have a higher risk.
17. Benign growths and proliferative conditions of the female reproductive tract tend to affect the ovaries (benign ovarian cysts) or uterine tissues (endometrial polyps, leiomyomas, and endometriosis).
18. Benign ovarian cysts develop from mature ovarian follicles that do not release their ova (follicular cysts) or from a corpus luteum that persists abnormally instead of degenerating (corpus luteum cyst). Cysts usually regress spontaneously.
19. Endometrial polyps are overgrowths of endometrial tissue and often cause abnormal bleeding.
20. Leiomyomas, also called *uterine fibroids,* are tumors arising from the muscle layer of the uterus, the myometrium. Incidence increases in women between ages 30 and 50; most myomas remain small and asymptomatic. Adenomyosis is the presence of endometrial glands and stroma within the uterine myometrium.
21. Endometriosis is the presence of functional endometrial tissue (i.e., tissue that responds to hormonal stimulation) at sites outside the uterus. Endometriosis causes an inflammatory reaction at the site of implantation and is a cause of infertility.
22. Most cancers of the female genitalia involve the uterus (particularly the cervix) and the ovaries. Cancer of the vagina is rare.
23. Infection with high-risk HPV, a sexually transmitted infection, is a necessary precursor to developing CIN and cervical cancer. Smoking, immunosuppression, and poor nutrition are cofactors. HPV vaccination can substantially reduce the risk of cervical cancer.
24. Cervical cancer arises from the cervical epithelium. The progressively serious neoplastic alterations are: (1) cervical intraepithelial neoplasia (cervical dysplasia), (2) cervical carcinoma in situ, and (3) invasive cervical carcinoma.
25. Risk factors for vaginal cancer are in utero diethylstilbestrol (DES) exposure and prior or concurrent cervical cancer.

SUMMARY REVIEW—cont'd

Like cervical cancers, vaginal cancers arise from the epithelium and are identified as intraepithelial neoplasia (dysplasia), carcinoma in situ, or invasive carcinoma. Most are secondary in nature.

26. The major risk for vulvar cancer is a history of HPV infection or squamous dysplasia of the vagina or cervix. Symptoms include chronic vulvar irritation, pruritus, bloody discharge, and a hard, ulcerated area of the vulva or large cauliflower-like lesions. Peak incidence is in postmenopausal women, but younger women can be affected.
27. Endometrial cancer is the most common cancer of the pelvic region. Risk factors for endometrial cancer include unopposed estrogen exposure, obesity, infertility, failure to ovulate, early menarche or late menopause, and tamoxifen. Oral contraceptive use protects against endometrial and ovarian cancers. Peak incidence occurs at 58 to 60 years of age, approximately 10 years later than peak incidence of precursor lesions.
28. Risk factors for ovarian cancer include an increased number of total lifetime ovulations including early menarche, late menopause, nulliparity, use of fertility drugs. *BRCA1, BRCA2,* and HNPCC gene abnormalities also are linked with ovarian cancer. Ovarian cancer causes more deaths than any other genital cancer in women.
29. Awareness of sexual dysfunction is relatively new. Chronic illness, medications, infection, sexual trauma, and a variety of psychosocial concerns have been implicated as causes.
30. Infertility, or the inability to conceive after 1 year of unprotected intercourse, affects approximately 15% of all couples. Women's fertility decreases with age, and older women may opt for intervention sooner than younger women. Fertility can be impaired by factors in the male, female, or both partners. Treatment depends on the cause of the infertility; ovulation disorders and tubal blockages are the most common pathologies.

Disorders of the Female Breast

1. Most disorders of the breast are disorders of the mammary gland, that is, the female breast.
2. Galactorrhea, or inappropriate lactation, is the persistent secretion of a milky substance by one or both breasts in nonpregnant, nonlactating women. It can occur in men. Its most common cause is nonpuerperal hyperprolactinemia, a rise in serum prolactin levels that is not associated with pregnancy and childbirth. Hyperprolactinemia can be caused by medications, pituitary tumors, hypothyroidism, chronic stress, or persistent and repeated suckling.
3. Numerous benign conditions occur in ducts and lobules in the breast. Benign breast disease is a spectrum of noncancerous changes in the breast. Benign lesions are broadly classified as (1) nonproliferating breast lesions, (2) proliferative breast disease, and (3) atypical (atypia) hyperplasia.
4. The term *nonproliferative lesions* is used to discriminate such lesions from the "proliferative" changes associated with increased risk of breast cancer.
5. Fibrocystic changes or physiologic nodularity and cysts are not clinically definitive because they include a heterogeneous group of disorders and refer to nonproliferative lesions. Symptoms affect women ages 30 to 50 and include cyclic bilateral breast tenderness and transient breast lumps.
6. Proliferative breast lesions without atypia are characterized by proliferation of ductal epithelium and/or stroma. Criteria for the diagnosis of intraductal proliferative lesions have been the subject of much research and controversy and include the following structurally diverse lesions: (1) usual ductal hyperplasia, (2) intraductal papillomas, (3) sclerosing adenosis, and (4) simple fibroadenoma.
7. Proliferative breast lesions with atypia include ADH and ALH. ADH is an increased number of cells mostly within the lumen of the terminal ducts. It includes a continuum of changes—cell structure and placement—ranging from an increase in cellularity to features of DCIS. The cells in ALH do not distend more than 50% of the acini within a lobule.
8. Breast cancer is the most common form of cancer in American women and second only to lung cancer as the most frequent cause of cancer death. Most breast cancer occurs in women older than 50 years. The major risk factors for breast cancer are classified as reproductive, such as nulliparity; familial, such as inherited gene syndromes; and environmental and lifestyle, such as hormonal factors and radiation exposure. Important factors not easily classified are involution of the mammary gland and breast density.
9. Most breast cancers arise from the ductal epithelium and then may metastasize to the lymphatics, opposite breast, abdominal cavity, lungs, bones, kidneys, liver, adrenal glands, ovaries, and pituitary glands.
10. Breast cancer is a heterogeneous disease with diverse molecular, biologic, phenotypic, and pathologic changes. Breast cancer also is heterogeneous *within* the same tumor. With mounting evidence it appears there are "subtypes within subtypes" and that the biology of specific breast cancer subtypes reflect contributions from the tissue microenvironment.
11. Several models of pathogenesis exist for breast cancer. Evidence suggests multiple genetic and epigenetic pathways of complex crosstalking networks that progress toward malignancy. Components of the microenvironment, including myoepithelial and endothelial cells, macrophages, and many ECM molecules, play a critical role in normal duct morphogenesis and increasingly recognized as major regulators of carcinogenesis.
12. DCIS refers to a complex heterogeneous group of lesions limited to ducts and lobules without invasion to the basement membrane. Preinvasive lesions do not invariably progress to invasive malignancy. LCIS originates from the duct-lobular unit, and the biology of LCIS is limited.
13. Dominating the cancer field is the idea that epithelial function depends on the *entire* tissue including the stroma or microenvironment. Breast cancer and other types of cancer are getting known as tissue-based diseases with a possible

SUMMARY REVIEW—cont'd

abnormal aberrant wound healing and inflammatory stromal (reactive stroma) component. Early alterations in the stroma that occur with wound healing and inflammation include activation of (1) mesenchymal cells (embryonic) fibroblasts; (2) endothelial cells; and (3) immune cells, including macrophages

14. Epithelial-mesenchymal transition (EMT) is the distinctive phenotype created from the change in tumor tissue architecture (remodeled tissue).
15. The exact molecular events leading to invasion are complex and not completely understood. Because myoepithelial cells form a semi-continuous protective sheet separating the human breast epithelium and the surrounding stroma, it has been a major focus of understanding invasive carcinogenesis. The critical difference in clinical prognosis between in situ and invasive or metastatic cancer results importantly and predominantly from the presence or absence of the surrounding basement membrane (BM).
16. The first clinical manifestation of breast cancer is usually a small, painless lump in the breast. Other manifestations include palpable lymph nodes in the axilla, dimpling of the skin, nipple and skin retraction, nipple discharge, ulcerations, reddened skin, and bone pain associated with bony metastases.
17. Treatment is based on the extent or stage of the cancer and includes surgery, radiation, chemotherapy, hormone therapy, and biologic therapy.

KEY TERMS

REFERENCES

1. American Cancer Society: *Cancer facts & figures—2013*, Atlanta, 2013, American Cancer Society.
2. Greil AL et al: Variation in distress among women with infertility: evidence from a population-based sample, *Hum Reprod* 26(8): 2101–2112, 2011.
3. Geffner ME: Androgen insensitivity syndrome (AIS). In Shahram Yazdani MD et al: *Chronic complex diseases of childhood: a practical guide for clinicians*, Boca Raton, FL, 2011, Universal Publishers, pp 82–84.
4. Galani A et al: Androgen insensitivity syndrome: clinical features and molecular defects, *Hormones (Athens)* 7(3):217–229, 2008.
5. Reichman DE, Laufer MR: Congenital uterine anomalies affecting reproduction, *Best Pract Res Clin Obstet Gynaecol* 24(2):193–208, 2010.
6. Lauver D, Nelles KK, Hanson K: The health effects of diethylstilbestrol revisited, *J Obstet Gynecol Neonatal Nurs* 34(4):494–499, 2005.
7. Chan YY et al: The prevalence of congenital uterine anomalies in unselected and high-risk populations: a systematic review, *Hum Reprod Update* 17(6):761–771, 2011.
8. Bordini B, Rosenfield RL: Normal pubertal development: part II: clinical aspects of puberty, *Pediatr Rev* 32(7):281–292, 2011.
9. Jospe N: Disorders of pubertal development. In Osborn LM et al: *Pediatrics*, Philadelphia, 2005, Mosby.
10. Wales JKH: Disordered pubertal development, *Arch Dis Child Educ Pract Ed* 97:9–16, 2012.
11. Palmert MR, Dunkel L: Clinical practice. Delayed puberty, *N Engl J Med* 366(5):443–453, 2012.
12. Burchett MLR et al: Endocrine and metabolic diseases. In Burns CE et al: *Pediatric primary care*, St Louis, 2009, Saunders.
13. Foster DL et al: Programming of GnRH feedback controls timing puberty and adult reproductive activity, *Mol Cell Endocrinol* 254–255:109–119, 2006.

14. Dedes I: Kisspeptins and the control of gonadotrophin secretion, *Syst Biol Reprod Med* 58(3):121–128, 2012.
15. Euling SY et al: Examination of U.S. puberty-timing data from 1940 to 1994 for secular trends: panel findings, *Pediatrics* 121(Suppl 3): S172–S191, 2008.
16. Cheng G et al: Beyond overweight: nutrition as an important lifestyle factor influencing timing of puberty, *Nutr Rev* 70(3):133–152, 2012.
17. Gunther AL et al: Dietary protein intake throughout childhood is associated with the timing of puberty, *J Nutr* 140(3):565–571, 2010.
18. Toppari J, Juul A: Trends in puberty timing in humans and environmental modifiers, *Mol Cell Endocrinol* 324(1–2):39–44, 2010.
18a. Abreu AP: Central precocious puberty caused by mutations in the imprinted gene MKRN3, *NEJM* June 5, 2013. [Epub ahead of print].
19. Fedorowicz Z et al: Beta2-adrenoceptor agonists for dysmenorrhoea, *Cochrane Database Syst Rev* (5):CD008585, 2012.
20. Rapkin A, Nathan L: Pelvic pain and dysmenorrhea. In Berek J, editor: *Berek & Novak's gynecology*, Philadelphia, 2012, Lippincott Williams & Wilkins.
21. Morrow C, Naumburg EH: Dysmenorrhea, *Prim Care* 36(1):19–32, vii. 2009.
22. Marjoribanks J et al: Nonsteroidal anti-inflammatory drugs for dysmenorrhea, *Cochrane Database Syst Rev* (1):CD001751, 2010.
23. Zahradnik HP, Hanjalic-Beck A, Groth K: Nonsteroidal anti-inflammatory drugs and hormonal contraceptives for pain relief from dysmenorrhea: a review, *Contraception* 81(3):185–196, 2010.
24. Daley AJ: Exercise and primary dysmenorrhoea: a comprehensive and critical review of the literature, *Sports Med* 38(8):659–670, 2008.
25. Cho SH, Hwang EW: Acupuncture for primary dysmenorrhoea: a systematic review, *BJOG* 117(5):509–521, 2010.
26. Khan KS, Champaneria R, Latthe PM: How effective are non-drug, non-surgical treatments for primary dysmenorrhoea? *BMJ* 344:e3011, 2012.
27. Deligeoroglou E et al: Evaluation and management of adolescent amenorrhea, *Ann N Y Acad Sci* 1205:23–32, 2010.
28. Baker VL, Schillings WJ, McClamrock HD: Amenorrhea. In Berek J, editor: *Berek & Novak's gynecology*, Philadelphia, 2012, Lippincott Williams & Wilkins.
29. Zhong Q, Layman LC: Genetic considerations in the patient with Turner syndrome-45, X with or without mosaicism, *Fertil Steril* 98(4):775–779, 2012.
30. Hughes IA et al: Androgen insensitivity syndrome, *Lancet* 380(9851):1419–1428, 2012.
31. Melmed S et al: Diagnosis and treatment of hyperprolactinemia: an Endocrine Society clinical practice guideline, *J Clin Endocrinol Metab* 96(2):273–288, 2011.
32. Master-Hunter T, Heiman DL: Amenorrhea: evaluation & treatment, *Am Fam Physician* 73:1374–1382, 1387, 2006.
33. Speroff L, Fritz MA: *Clinical gynecologic endocrinology & infertility*, ed 8, Philadelphia, 2012, Lippincott Williams & Wilkins.
34. Munro MG: FIGO classification system (PALM-COEIN) for causes of abnormal uterine bleeding in nongravid women of reproductive age, *Int J Gynaecol Obstet* 113(1):3–13, 2011.
35. Pitkin J: Dysfunctional uterine bleeding, *BMJ* 334(7603):1110–1111, 2007.
36. Lethaby A et al: Nonsteroidal anti-inflammatory drugs for heavy menstrual bleeding, *Cochrane Database Syst Rev* (4):CD000400, 2007.
37. Hickey M, Higham JM, Fraser I: Progestogens with or without oestrogen for irregular uterine bleeding associated with anovulation, *Cochrane Database Syst Rev* (9):CD001895, 2012.
38. American College of Obstetricians and Gynecologists (ACOG): *Endometrial ablation*, Washington, DC, 2007, American College of Obstetricians and Gynecologists.
39. Bennett GL et al: *ACR appropriateness criteria abnormal vaginal bleeding*. [online publication], p 9, Reston, VA, 2010, American College of Radiology (ACR).
40. Munro MG, Critchley HOD, Fraser IS: The flexible FIGO classification concept for underlying causes of abnormal uterine bleeding, *Semin Reprod Med* 29(5):391–399, 2011.
41. Demers C et al: Gynaecological and obstetric management of women with inherited bleeding disorders, *Int J Gynaecol Obstet* 95(1):75, 2006.
42. Azziz R et al: The Androgen Excess and PCOS Society criteria for the polycystic ovary syndrome: the complete task force report, *Fertil Steril* 91(2):456–488, 2009.
43. Ehrmann DA: Genetic contributions to glucose intolerance in polycystic ovary syndrome, *Reprod Biomed Online* 9(1):28–34, 2004.
44. Franks S et al: Development of polycystic ovary syndrome: involvement of genetic and environmental factors, *Int J Androl* 29(1):278–285, 2006.
45. Shannon M, Wang Y: Polycystic ovary syndrome: a common but often unrecognized condition, *J Midwifery Womens Health* 57(3):221–230, 2012.
46. Ehrmann DA: Polycystic ovary syndrome, *N Engl J Med* 352(12): 1223–1236, 2005.
47. Milsom I: The levonorgestrel-releasing intrauterine system as an alternative to hysterectomy in peri-menopausal women, *Contraception* 75(Suppl 6):S152–S154, 2007.
48. Simoni M et al: Functional genetic polymorphisms and female reproductive disorders: part I: polycystic ovary syndrome and ovarian response, *Hum Reprod Update* 14(5):459–484, 2008.
49. Diamanti-Kandarakis E: Insulin resistance in PCOS, *Endocrine* 30(1):13–17, 2006.
50. Norman RJ et al: Polycystic ovary syndrome, *Lancet* 370(9588):685–697, 2007.
51. Mendonca HC et al: Positive correlation of serum leptin with estradiol levels in patients with polycystic ovary syndrome, *Braz J Med Biol Res* 37(5):729–736, 2004.
52. Schorge JO et al: *Williams gynecology*, New York, 2008, McGraw-Hill.
53. Diamanti-Kandarakis E: Polycystic ovarian syndrome: pathophysiology, molecular aspects and clinical implications, *Expert Rev Mol Med* 10(2):e3, 2008.
54. Haoula Z, Salman M, Atiomo W: Evaluating the association between endometrial cancer and polycystic ovary syndrome, *Hum Reprod* 27(5):1327–1331, 2012.
55. King J: Polycystic ovary syndrome, *J Midwifery Womens Health* 51(6):415–422, 2006.
56. Teede HJ et al: Insulin resistance, the metabolic syndrome, diabetes, and cardiovascular disease risk in women with PCOS, *Endocrine* 30(1): 45–53, 2006.
57. Palomba S et al: Outlook: metformin use in infertile patients with polycystic ovary syndrome: an evidence-based overview, *Reprod Biomed Online* 16(3):327–335, 2008.
58. Palomba S et al: Role of metformin in patients with polycystic ovary syndrome: the state of the art, *Minerva Ginecol* 60(1):77–82, 2008.
59. Nader S: Ovulation induction in polycystic ovary syndrome, *Minerva Ginecol* 60(1):53–61, 2008.
60. Sinawat S et al: Long versus short course treatment with metformin and clomiphene citrate for ovulation induction in women with PCOS, *Cochrane Database Syst Rev* (10):CD006226, 2012.
61. American College of Obstetricians and Gynecologists (ACOG): *Polycystic ovary syndrome*, Washington, DC, 2009, American College of Obstetricians and Gynecologists.
62. Moran LJ et al: Lifestyle changes in women with polycystic ovary syndrome, *Cochrane Database Syst Rev* (7):CD007506, 2011.
63. Hartlage S et al: Criteria for premenstrual dysphoric disorder: secondary analyses of relevant data sets, *Arch Gen Psychiatry* 69(3):300, 2012.
64. Tschudin S, Bertea PC, Zemp E: Prevalence and predictors of premenstrual syndrome and premenstrual dysphoric disorder in a population-based sample, *Arch Womens Ment Health* 13(6):485–494, 2010.
65. Steiner M et al: The Premenstrual Symptoms Screening Tool revised for adolescents (PSST-A): prevalence of severe PMS and premenstrual dysphoric disorder in adolescents, *Arch Womens Ment Health* 14(1): 77–81, 2011.
66. Cunningham J et al: Update on research and treatment of premenstrual dysphoric disorder, *Harv Rev Psychiatry* 17(2):120–137, 2009.
67. American College of Obstetricians and Gynecologists (ACOG): *Non-contraceptive uses of hormonal contraceptives*, Washington, DC, 2010, American College of Obstetricians and Gynecologists.
68. Lopez LM, Kaptein AA, Helmerhorst FM: Oral contraceptives containing drospirenone for premenstrual syndrome, *Cochrane Database Syst Rev* (2):CD006586, 2012.
69. U.S. Food and Drug Administration (FDA): *FDA drug safety communication: safety review update on the possible increased risk of blood clots with birth control pills containing drospirenone*, 2011. Available at www.fda.gov/drugs/drugsafety/ucm273021.htm. Accessed January 30, 2013.
70. Brown J et al: Selective serotonin reuptake inhibitors for premenstrual syndrome, *Cochrane Database Syst Rev* (2):CD001396, 2009.
71. Jungheim ES et al: Add-back regimens in patients using a GnRH agonist for premenstrual dysphoric disorder, *Am J Obstet Gynecol* 201(2): 221–222, 2009.
72. Wiesenfeld HC et al: Subclinical pelvic inflammatory disease and infertility, *Obstet Gynecol* 120(1):37–43, 2012.
73. Grimes DA, Lopez LM, Schulz KF: Antibiotic prophylaxis for intrauterine contraceptive device insertion, *Cochrane Database Syst Rev* (3): CD001327, 1999.
74. Bender N et al: Chlamydia infection, pelvic inflammatory disease, ectopic pregnancy and infertility: cross-national study, *Sex Transm Infect* 87(7):601–608, 2011.

75. Centers for Disease Control and Prevention (CDC): Sexually transmitted diseases treatment guidelines, *MMWR Morb Mortal Wkly Rep* 59(RR–12), 2010.
76. Soper DE: Pelvic inflammatory disease, *Obstet Gynecol* 116(2 Part 1): 419–428, 2010.
77. Yudin MH, Ross JDC: Pelvic inflammatory disease. In Zenilman JM, Shahmanesh M, editors: *Sexually transmitted diseases*, Sudbury, MA, 2012, Jones & Bartlett Learning, pp 67–76.
78. Lin HW et al: Risk of ovarian cancer in women with pelvic inflammatory disease: a population-based study, *Lancet Oncol* 12(9):900–904, 2011.
79. Centers for Disease Control and Prevention (CDC): Update to CDC's sexually transmitted diseases treatment guidelines, 2012: oral cephalosporins no longer recommended treatment for gonococcal infections, *MMWR Morb Mortal Wkly Rep* 61(31):590–594, 2012.
80. Fogel CI: Gynecologic infections. In Schuilling KD, Likis FE, editors: *Women's gynecologic health*, ed 2, Burlington, MA, 2013, Jones & Bartlett.
81. Singh RH et al: The role of physical examination in diagnosing common causes of vaginitis: a prospective study, *Sex Transm Infect*, 2012. Sep 27. [Epub ahead of print.].
82. Nyirjesy P et al: Alternative therapies in women with chronic vaginitis, *Obstet Gynecol* 117(4):856, 2011.
83. Ray A et al: Interventions for prevention and treatment of vulvovaginal candidiasis in women with HIV infection, *Cochrane Database Syst Rev* (8):CD008739, 2011.
84. Marrazzo J, Liss H: Cervicitis. In Zenilman JM, Shahmanesh M, editors: *Sexually transmitted infections*, Sudbury, MA, 2012, Jones & Bartlett Learning.
85. Reed BD et al: Prevalence and demographic characteristics of vulvodynia in a population-based sample, *Am J Obstet Gynecol* 206(2):170, 2011.
86. Cox KJ, Neville CE: Assessment and management options for women with vulvodynia, *J Midwifery Womens Health* 57(3):231–240, 2012.
87. Andrews JC: Vulvodynia interventions—systematic review and evidence grading, *Obstet Gynecol Surv* 66(5):299–315, 2011.
88. Wechter ME et al: Management of Bartholin duct cysts and abscesses: a systematic review, *Obstet Gynecol Surv* 64(6):395–404, 2009.
89. Haylen et al: An International Urogynecological Association (IUGA)/ International Continence Society (ICS) joint report on the terminology for female pelvic floor dysfunction, *Int Urogynecol J* 21(1):5–26, 2010.
90. Wu JM et al: Forecasting the prevalence of pelvic floor disorders in U.S. women: 2010 to 2050, *Obstet Gynecol* 114(6):1278, 2009.
91. Kim S et al: A review of the epidemiology and pathophysiology of pelvic floor dysfunction: do racial differences matter? *J Obstet Gynaecol Can* 27(3):251–259, 2005.
92. Abrams P et al: Fourth International Consultation on Incontinence Recommendations of the International Scientific Committee: Evaluation and treatment of urinary incontinence, pelvic organ prolapse, and fecal incontinence, *Neurourol Urodyn* 29(1):213–240, 2010.
93. Hoffman BL: Pelvic mass. In Schorge JO et al: *Williams gynecology*, New York, 2008, McGraw-Hill, pp 187–224.
94. de Silva KSH et al: Ovarian lesions in children and adolescents—an 11-year review, *J Pediatr Endocrinol Metab* 17(7):951–958, 2011.
95. Whiteman MK et al: Inpatient hospitalization for gynecologic disorders in the United States, *Am J Obstet Gynecol* 202(6):541, 2010.
96. McCartney CR et al: Hypothalamic regulation of cyclic ovulation: evidence that the increase in gonadotropin-releasing hormone pulse frequency during the follicular phase reflects the gradual loss of the restraining effects of progesterone, *J Clin Endocrinol Metab* 87(5): 2194–2200, 2002.
97. Blackburn ST: *Maternal, fetal, & neonatal physiology: a clinical perspective*, ed 4, Maryland Heights, MO, 2013, Elsevier.
98. Hoo WL et al: Expectant management of ultrasonically diagnosed ovarian dermoid cysts: is it possible to predict outcome? *Ultrasound Obstet Gynecol* 36(2):235–240, 2010.
99. Damigos E, Johns J, Ross J: An update on the diagnosis and management of ovarian torsion, *Obstetrician Gynaecol* 14(4):229–236, 2012.
100. Silberstein T et al: Endometrial polyps in reproductive-age fertile and infertile women, *Isr Med Assoc J* 8(3):192–195, 2006.
101. Lee SC: The oncogenic potential of endometrial polyps: a systematic review and meta-analysis, *Obstet Gynecol* 118(2, Part 1):361–362, 2011.
102. Lieng M, Istre O, Qvigstad E: Treatment of endometrial polyps: a systematic review, *Acta Obstet Gynecol Scand* 89(8):992–1002, 2010.
103. Laughlin SK, Stewart EA: Uterine leiomyomas: individualizing the approach to a heterogeneous condition, *Obstet Gynecol* 117(2, Part 1): 396, 2011.
104. Rice KE et al: Etiology, diagnosis, and management of uterine leiomyomas, *J Midwifery Womens Health* 57(3):241–247, 2012.
105. Weiss G et al: Adenomyosis a variant, not a disease? Evidence from hysterectomized menopausal women in the Study of Women's Health across the Nation (SWAN), *Fertil Steril* 91(1):201–206, 2009.
106. Champaneria R et al: Ultrasound scan and magnetic resonance imaging for the diagnosis of adenomyosis: systematic review comparing test accuracy, *Acta Obstet Gynecol Scand* 89(11):1374–1384, 2010.
107. Popovic M et al: Uterine artery embolization for the treatment of adenomyosis: a review, *J Vasc Interv Radiol* 22(7):901–909, 2011.
108. Sheng J et al: The LNG-IUS study on adenomyosis: a 3-year follow-up study on the efficacy and side effects of the use of levonorgestrel intrauterine system for the treatment of dysmenorrhea associated with adenomyosis, *Contraception* 79(3):189, 2009.
109. Buck Louis GM et al: Incidence of endometriosis by study population and diagnostic method: the ENDO study, *Fertil Steril* 96(2):360–365, 2011.
110. Vercellini P et al: Endometriosis and ovarian cancer, *Lancet Oncol* 13(5):e188–e189, 2012.
111. Sampson JA: Peritoneal endometriosis due to the menstrual dissemination of endometrial tissue into the peritoneal cavity, *Am J Obstet Gynecol* 14:422, 1927.
112. Giudice LC: Endometriosis, *N Engl J Med* 362(25):2389–2398, 2010.
113. Lessey BA, Young SL: Pathophysiology of infertility in endometriosis. In Giudice LC, Evers JLH, Healy DL, editors: *Endometriosis: science and practice*, Oxford, UK, 2012, Wiley-Blackwell.
114. American College of Obstetricians and Gynecologists (ACOG): *Management of endometriosis*, Washington DC, 2010, American College of Obstetricians and Gynecologists.
115. Brown J, Kives S, Akhtar M: Progestagens and anti-progestagens for pain associated with endometriosis, *Cochrane Database Syst Rev* (3): CD002122, 2012.
116. Arbyn M et al: Worldwide burden of cervical cancer in 2008, *Ann Oncol* 22(12):2675–2686, 2011.
117. Centers for Disease Control and Prevention (CDC): *Sexually transmitted disease surveillance*, Atlanta, 2011, Department of Health and Human Services.
118. Workowski KA, Berman S: Centers for Disease Control and Prevention: Sexually transmitted diseases treatment guidelines, 2010, *MMWR Recomm Rep* 59(RR–12):1–110, 2010.
119. Vesco KK et al: *Screening for cervical cancer: a systematic evidence review for the U.S. Preventive Services Task Force [Internet]*, Rockville, MD, 2011, Agency for Healthcare Research and Quality (U.S.).
120. Dahlström LA et al: Prospective seroepidemiologic study of human papillomavirus and other risk factors in cervical cancer, *Cancer Epidemiol Biomarkers Prev* 20(12):2541–2550, 2011.
121. Araújo AP et al: Epidermal growth factor genetic variation associated with advanced cervical cancer in younger women, *Am J Clin Oncol* 35(3):247, 2012.
122. González CA et al: Dietary factors and in situ and invasive cervical cancer risk in the European prospective investigation into cancer and nutrition study, *Int J Cancer* 129(2):449–459, 2011.
123. U.S. Preventive Services Task Force: Screening for cervical cancer: U.S. Preventive Services Task Force recommendation statement, *Ann Intern Med* 156(12):880–891, 2012.
124. Cuzick J, Castanon A, Sasieni P: Predicted impact of vaccination against human papillomavirus 16/18 on cancer incidence and cervical abnormalities in women aged 20–29 in the UK, *Br J Cancer* 102(5):933–939, 2010.
125. Narayan G, Murty VV: Integrative genomic approaches in cervical cancer: implications for molecular pathogenesis, *Future Oncol* 6(10): 1643–1652, 2010.
126. Delli Carpini J, Karam AK, Montgomery L: Vascular endothelial growth factor and its relationship to the prognosis and treatment of breast, ovarian, and cervical cancer, *Angiogenesis* 13(1):43–58, 2010.
127. Sankaranarayanan R et al: HPV screening for cervical cancer in rural India, *N Engl J Med* 360(14):1385–1394, 2009.
128. Carcio HA: Colposcopy. In Carcio HA, Secor MC, editors: *Advanced health assessment of women*, ed 2, New York, 2011, Springer.
129. Rosa DD et al: Adjuvant platinum-based chemotherapy for early stage cervical cancer, *Cochrane Database Syst Rev:* (6): CD005342, 2012.
130. Arbyn M et al: Prophylactic vaccination against human papillomaviruses to prevent cervical cancer and its precursors (protocol), *Cochrane Database Syst Rev* (4):CD009069, 2011.
131. Donato VD et al: Vaginal cancer, *Crit Rev Oncol Hematol* 81(3):286, 2012.

132. Brunner AH et al: The prognostic role of human papillomavirus in patients with vaginal cancer, *Int J Gynecol Cancer* 21(5):923–929, 2011.
133. Goodman A, Schorge J, Greene MF: The long-term effects of in utero exposures—the DES story, *N Engl J Med* 364(22):2083–2084, 2011.
134. Bodelon C et al: Is the incidence of invasive vulvar cancer increasing in the United States? *Cancer Causes Control* 20(9):1779–1782, 2009.
135. Lanneau GS et al: Vulvar cancer in young women: demographic features and outcome evaluation, *Am J Obstet Gynecol* 200:645, 2009.
136. Ansink AC et al: Surgical interventions for early squamous cell carcinoma of the vulva, *Cochrane Database Syst Rev* (4):CD002036, 1999.
137. Miller DS: Endometrial cancer. In Schorge JO et al: *Williams gynecology*, New York, 2008, McGraw-Hill, pp 687–705.
138. Dossus L et al: Reproductive risk factors and endometrial cancer: the European prospective investigation into cancer and nutrition, *Int J Cancer* 127(2):442–451, 2010.
139. Yurgelun MB et al: Impact of genetic testing on endometrial cancer risk-reducing practices in women at risk for Lynch syndrome, *Gynecol Oncol* 127(3):544–551, 2012.
140. Schmandt RE et al: Understanding obesity and endometrial cancer risk: opportunities for prevention, *Am J Obstet Gynecol* 205(6):518–525, 2011.
141. Modesitt SC: Missed opportunities for primary endometrial cancer prevention: how to optimize early identification and treatment of high-risk women, *Obstet Gynecol* 120(5):989–991, 2012.
142. Chin J, Konje JC, Hickey M: Levonorgestrel intrauterine system for endometrial protection in women with breast cancer on adjuvant tamoxifen, *Cochrane Database Syst Rev* (4):CD007245, 2009.
143. Jacobs I et al: Sensitivity of transvaginal ultrasound screening for endometrial cancer in postmenopausal women: a case-control study within the UKCTOCS cohort, *Lancet Oncol* 12(1):38–48, 2011.
144. Evans T et al: Differential trends in the rising incidence of endometrial cancer by type: data from a UK population-based registry from 1994 to 2006, *Br J Cancer* 104(9):1505–1510, 2011.
145. Altman AD et al: Uterine sarcoma and aromatase inhibitors: Tom Baker Cancer Centre Experience and review of the literature, *Int J Gynecol Cancer* 22(6):1006–1012, 2012.
146. Nam JH, Park JY: Update on treatment of uterine sarcoma, *Curr Opin Obstet Gynecol* 22(1):36, 2010.
147. Cramer DW: The epidemiology of endometrial and ovarian cancer, *Hematol Oncol Clin North Am* 26(1):1, 2012.
148. Kurta ML et al: Use of fertility drugs and risk of ovarian cancer: results from a U.S.-based case-control study, *Cancer Epidemiol Biomarkers Prev* 21(8):1282–1292, 2012.
149. Crane K: Oral contraceptives as ovarian cancer prevention in the news, *J Natl Cancer Inst* 103(17):1286–1288, 2011.
150. Jelovac D, Armstrong DK: Recent progress in the diagnosis and treatment of ovarian cancer, *CA Cancer J Clin* 61(3):183–203, 2011.
151. Loveday C et al: Germline mutations in RAD51D confer susceptibility to ovarian cancer, *Nat Genet* 43(9):879–882, 2011.
152. Kurman RJ, Shih IM: The origin and pathogenesis of epithelial ovarian cancer—a proposed unifying theory, *Am J Surg Pathol* 34(3):433, 2010.
153. Kurman RJ, Shih IM: Molecular pathogenesis and extraovarian origin of epithelial ovarian cancer—shifting the paradigm, *Hum Pathol* 42(7):918–931, 2011.
154. Schauer IG et al: Cancer-associated fibroblasts and their putative role in potentiating the initiation and development of epithelial ovarian cancer, *Neoplasia* 13(5):393, 2011.
155. Romero I, Bast RC: Minireview: human ovarian cancer: biology, current management, and paths to personalizing therapy, *Endocrinology* 153(4):1593–1602, 2012.
156. U.S. Preventive Services Task Force: Screening for ovarian cancer: U.S. Preventive Services Task Force reaffirmation recommendation statement, *Ann Intern Med* 157(12):900–904, 2012.
157. National Collaborating Centre for Cancer: Ovarian cancer. *The recognition and initial management of ovarian cancer*, London, 2011, National Institute for Health and Clinical Excellence (NICE).
158. Woo YL et al: Centralisation of services for gynaecological cancer, *Cochrane Database Syst Rev* (3):CD007945, 2012.
159. Winter-Roach BA, Kitchener HC, Lawrie TA: Adjuvant (post-surgery) chemotherapy for early stage epithelial ovarian cancer, *Cochrane Database Syst Rev* (3):CD004706, 2012.
160. Haldar K et al: Epidermal growth factor receptor blockers for the treatment of ovarian cancer, *Cochrane Database Syst Rev* (10):CD007927, 2011.
161. American College of Obstetricians and Gynecologists (ACOG): *Female sexual dysfunction*, Washington, DC, 2011, Author.
162. Hatzichristou D et al: Recommendations for the clinical evaluation of men and women with sexual dysfunction, *J Sex Med* 7(1pt2):337–348, 2010.
163. Lewis RW et al: Definitions/epidemiology/risk factors for sexual dysfunction, *J Sex Med* 7(4pt2):1598–1607, 2010.
164. Gurunath S et al: Defining infertility—a systematic review of prevalence studies, *Hum Reprod Update* 17(5):575–588, 2011.
165. Eisenberg ML et al: The frequency of the male infertility evaluation: data from the national survey of family growth, *J Urol* 189(3):1030–1034, 2013.
166. Practice Committee of the American Society for Reproductive Medicine: Diagnostic evaluation of the infertile male: a committee opinion, *Fertil Steril* 98(2):294–301, 2012.
167. Krausz C: Male infertility: pathogenesis and clinical diagnosis, *Best Pract Res Clin Endocrinol Metab* 25(2):271–285, 2011.
168. Natali A, Turek PJ: An assessment of new sperm tests for male infertility, *Urology* 77(5):1027–1034, 2011.
169. Sunderam S et al: Assisted reproductive technology surveillance—United States, 2009, *MMWR CDC Surveill Summ* 61:1–23, 2012.
170. Pinborg A et al: Congenital anomalies after assisted reproductive technology, *Fertil Steril* 99(2):327–332, 2013.
171. Pinborg A et al: Why do singletons conceived after assisted reproduction technology have adverse perinatal outcome? Systematic review and meta-analysis, *Hum Reprod Update*, 2012. Nov 14. [Epub ahead of print.].
172. Harney KA, Smith LF: The breast. In DeCherney AH, Pernoll ML, editors: *Current obstetric and gynecologic diagnosis and treatment*, ed 8, Norwalk, CT, 1994, Appleton & Lange.
173. Sabel MS: *Overview of benign breast disease*. Available at UpToDate Individual Web 2012, www.uptodate.com.
174. Collins LC et al: Magnitude and laterality of breast cancer risk according to histologic type of atypical hyperplasia: results from the Nurses' Health Study, *Cancer* 109(2):180–187, 2006.
175. Hartmann LC et al: Benign breast disease and the risk of breast cancer, *N Engl J Med* 353(3):229–237, 2005.
176. Friedenreich C et al: Risk factors for benign proliferative breast disease, *Int J Epidemiol* 29(4):634, 2000.
177. Lester SC: The breast. In Kumar V, Abbas AK, Fausto N, editors: *Robbins & Cotran pathologic basis of disease*, ed 7, Philadelphia, 2005, Saunders.
178. Costarelli L et al: Intraductal proliferative lesions of the breast—terminology and biology matter: premalignant lesions or preinvasive cancer? *Int J Surg Oncol* 2012:501905, 2012.
179. Lewis JT et al: An analysis of breast cancer risk in women with single, multiple, and atypical papilloma, *Am J Surg Pathol* 30(6):665–672, 2006.
180. Sanders ME et al: Interdependence of radial scar and proliferative disease with respect to invasive breast carcinoma risk to patients with benign breast biopsies, *Cancer* 106(7):1453–1461, 2006.
181. Berg JC et al: Breast cancer risk in women with radial scars in benign breast biopsies, *Breast Cancer Res Treat* 108(2):167–174, 2008.
182. Dupont WD et al: Long-term risk of breast cancer in women with fibroadenoma, *N Engl J Med* 331:10, 1994.
183. Love SM, Lindsey K: *Dr. Susan Love's breast book*, ed 5, Philadelphia, 2010, Merloyd Lawrence, Da Capo Press.
184. Liu Y et al: Intakes of alcohol and folate during adolescence and risk of proliferative benign breast disease, *Pediatrics* 129(5):e1192–e1198, 2012.
185. Lampe JW et al: Plasma isoflavones and fibrocystic breast conditions and breast cancer among women in Shanghai, China, *Cancer Epidemiol Biomarkers Prev* 16(12):2579–2586, 2007.
186. Guha N et al: Soy isoflavones and risk of cancer recurrence in a cohort of breast cancer survivors: the Life after Cancer Epidemiology Study, *Breast Cancer Res Treat* 118:395405, 2009.
187. Rohan TE et al: A randomized controlled trial of calcium plus vitamin D supplementation and risk of benign proliferative breast disease, *Breast Cancer Res Treat* 116(2):339–350, 2009.
188. National Cancer Institute: *Cancer advances in focus: breast cancer*, Bethesda, MD, 2010, National Cancer Institute.
189. Kuiren AW et al: Lifetime risks of specific breast cancer subtypes among women in four racial/ethnic groups, *Breast Cancer Res* 12(6):R99, 2010.
190. Centers for Disease Control and Prevention (CDC): Vital signs: racial disparities in breast cancer severity—United States, 2005–2009, *MMWR Morb Mortal Wkly Rep* 61:922, 2012.
191. Howlader N et al: *SEER cancer statistics review, 1975–2009 (vintage 2009 populations)*, Bethesda, MD, 2012, National Cancer Institute. Available at http://seer.cancer.gov/csr/1975_2009_pops09. Assessed January 2012.
192. Sternlicht MD et al: Hormonal and local control of mammary branching morphogenesis, *Differentiation* 74:365–381, 2006.

193. Medina D: Mammary developmental fate and breast cancer risk, *Endocr Relat Cancer* 12:483–495, 2005.
194. Lyons TR et al: Postpartum mammary gland involution drives progression of ductal carcinoma in situ through collagen and COX-2, *Nat Med* 17:1109–1115, 2011.
195. Lord SJ et al: Breast cancer risk and hormone receptor status in older women by parity, age of first birth, and breastfeeding: a case-control study, *Cancer Epidemiol Biomarkers Prev* 17(7):1723–1730, 2008.
196. Lyons TR, Schedin PJ, Borges VF: Pregnancy and breast cancer: when they collide, *J Mammary Gland Biol Neoplasia* 14:87–98, 2009.
197. Medina D: Breast cancer: the protective effect of pregnancy, *Clin Cancer Res* 10(1 Pt 2):380S–384S, 2004.
198. O'Brien J et al: Alternatively activated macrophages and collagen remodeling characterize the postpartum involuting mammary gland across species, *Am J Pathol* 176(3):1241–1255, 2010.
199. Schedin P: Pregnancy-associated breast cancer and metastasis, *Nat Rev Cancer* 6:281–291, 2006.
200. Fornetti J et al: Emerging targets for the prevention of pregnancy-associated breast cancer, *Cell Cycle* 11(4):639–640, 2012.
201. Schedin P et al: Microenvironment of the involuting mammary gland mediates mammary cancer progression, *J Mammary Gland Biol Neoplasia* 12:71–82, 2007.
202. DeNardo DG et al: Leukocyte complexity predicts breast cancer survival and functionally regulates response to chemotherapy, *Cancer Discov* 1:54–67, 2011.
203. Collaborative Group on Hormonal Factors in Breast Cancer: Breast cancer and breastfeeding: collaborative reanalysis of individual data from 47 epidemiological studies in 30 countries, including 50,302 women with breast cancer and 96,973 women without the disease, *Lancet* 360(9328):187–195, 2002.
204. LaMarca HL, Rosen JM: Hormones and mammary cell fate—what will I become when I grow up? *Endocrinology* 149(9):4317–4321, 2008.
205. Baillo A, Giroux C, Ethier SP: Knock-down of amphiregulin inhibits cellular invasion in inflammatory breast cancer, *J Cell Physiol* 226: 2691–2701, 2011.
206. Kotb AM et al: Replacement of E-cadherin by N-cadherin in the mammary gland leads to fibrocystic changes and tumor formation, *Breast Cancer Res* 13(5):R104, 2011.
207. Russo J et al: The protective role of pregnancy in breast cancer, *Breast Cancer Res* 8(3):131–142, 2005.
208. Peri S et al: Defining the genomic signature of the parous breast, *BMC Med Genomics* 5(1):46, 2012. [Epub ahead of print.].
209. Milanese TR et al: Age-related lobular involution and risk of breast cancer, *J Natl Cancer Inst* 98(2):1600–1607, 2006.
210. Cutler SY, Young JL: Third National Cancer Survey: incidence data, *Natl Cancer Inst Monog* 41, 1975.
211. Vorrherr H, editor: *The breast: morphology, physiology, and lactation*, New York, 1974, Academic Press.
212. Kelsey JL, Gammon MD, John EM: Reproductive factors and breast cancer, *Epidemiol Rev* 15:36–47, 1993.
213. Ursin G et al: Reproductive factors and subtypes of breast cancer defined by hormone receptor and histology, *Br J Cancer* 93:364–371, 2005.
214. Trichopoulos D et al: Age at any birth and breast cancer risk, *Int J Cancer* 31:701–704, 1983.
215. Henson DE, Tarone RE, Nsouli H: Lobular involution: the physiologic prevention of breast cancer, *J Natl Cancer Inst* 98(22):1589–1590, 2006.
216. O'Brien J et al: Macrophages are crucial for epithelial cell death and adipocyte repopulation during mammary gland involution, *Development* 139(2):269–275, 2012.
217. Hughes K et al: Conditional deletion of Stat3 in mammary epithelium impairs the acute phase response and modulates immune cell numbers during post-lactational regression, *J Pathol* 227(1):106–117, 2012.
218. Reis LAG et al: *Cancer statistics review, 1975–2005,* Bethesda, MD, 2008, National Cancer Institute. Available at http://seer.cancer.gov/csr/1975_2005.
219. Fenton SE: Endocrine-disrupting compounds and mammary gland development: early exposure and later life consequences, *Endocrinology* 147(Suppl 6):S18–S24, 2006.
220. Lanigan F et al: Molecular links between mammary gland development and breast cancer, *Cell Mol Life Sci* 64:3161–3184, 2007.
221. Cheskis BJ et al: Signaling by estrogens: mini review, *J Cell Physiol* 213(3):610–617, 2007.
222. Cheskis BJ et al: MNAR plays an important role in ERa activation of Src/MAPK and P13K/Akt signaling pathways, *Steroids* 73(9–10):901–905, 2008.
223. Kaaks R et al: Postmenopausal serum androgens, oestrogens, and breast cancer risk: the European prospective investigation into cancer and nutrition, *Endocr Relat Cancer* 12(4):1017–1082, 2005.
224. Lanaric C, Molinolo AA: Progesterone receptors—animal models and cell signaling in breast cancer. Diverse activation pathways for the progesterone receptor: possible implications for breast biology and cancer, *Breast Can Res* 4:240–243, 2002.
225. Rajkumar L et al: Long-term hormonal promotion overcomes genetic resistance to mammary cancer, *Steroids* 76(1–2):31–37, 2011.
226. Asselin-Labat M et al: Control of mammary stem cell function by steroid hormone signaling, *Nature* 465(7299):798–802, 2010.
227. Hilton HN et al: Progesterone and estrogen receptors segregate into different cell subpopulations in the normal human breast, *Mol Cell Endocrinol* 361:191–201, 2012.
228. Chen CC et al: Autocrine prolactin induced by the Pten-Akt pathway is required for lactation initiation and provides a direct link between the Akt and Stat5 pathways, *Genes Dev* 26(19):2154–2168, 2012.
229. McHale K et al: Altered expression of prolactin receptor-associated signaling proteins in human breast carcinoma, *Mod Pathol* 21(5):565–571, 2008.
230. Secreto G et al: Androgens and breast cancer. The hyperandrogenic theory of breast cancer: past, present, and future. In Ardis LI, editor: *Testosterone research trends*, New York, 2007, Nova Science publishers, pp 105–138.
231. Key TJ: Endogenous oestrogens and breast cancer risk in premenopausal and postmenopausal women, *Steroids* 76(8):812–815, 2011.
232. Key T et al: Endogenous sex hormones and breast cancer in postmenopausal women; reanalysis of nine prospective studies, *J Natl Cancer Inst* 94:606–616, 2002.
233. Micheli A et al: Endogenous sex hormones and subsequent breast cancer in premenopausal women, *Int J Cancer* 112:213–218, 2004.
234. Hankinson SE, Eliassen H: Endogenous estrogen, testosterone, and progesterone levels in relation to breast cancer risk, *J Steroid Biochem Mol Biol* 106(1–5):24–30, 2007.
235. James RE et al: Postmenopausal serum sex steroids and risk of hormone receptor positive and negative breast cancer: a nested case-control study, *Cancer Prev Res* 4(11):1626–1635, 2011.
236. Zeleniuch-Jacquotte A et al: Premenopausal serum androgens and breast cancer risk: a nested case-control study, *Breast Cancer Res* 14(1):R32, 2012.
237. Beral V et al: Breast cancer and hormone-replacement therapy in the Million Women Study, *Lancet* 362(9382):419–427, 2003.
238. Secreto G, Zumoff B: Role of androgen excess in the development of estrogen receptor-positive and estrogen receptor-negative breast cancer, *Anticancer Res* 32:3223–3228, 2012.
239. McNamara KM et al: Androgen receptor in triple negative breast cancer, *J Steroid Biochem Molec Biol* 133:66–76, 2013.
240. Endogenous Hormones and Breast Cancer Collaborative Group et al: Circulating sex hormones and breast cancer risk factors in postmenopausal women: reanalysis of 13 studies, *Br J Cancer* 105(5):709–722, 2011.
241. Joshi PA et al: Progesterone induces adult mammary stem cell expansion, *Nature* 465(7299):803–807, 2010.
242. Manjer J et al: Postmenopausal breast cancer risk in relation to sex steroid hormones, prolactin and SHBG (Sweden), *Cancer Causes Control* l4, 2003. 599–560, 2003.
243. Obr AE, Edwards DP: The biology of progesterone receptor in the normal mammary gland and in the breast, *Molec Cell Endocrinol* 35:4–17, 2012.
244. Zeleniuch-Jacquotte A et al: Premenopausal levels of oestrogen, androgen, and SHBG and breast cancer: long term results of a prospective study, *Br J Cancer* 90:153–159, 2004.
245. Key TJ et al: A prospective study of urinary oestrogen excretion and breast cancer risk, *Br J Cancer* 73:1615–1619, 1996.
246. Eliassen AH et al: Endogenous steroid hormone concentrations and risk of breast cancer among predominantly premenopausal women, *J Natl Cancer Inst* 98(19):1406–1415, 2006.
247. Onland-Moret NC et al: Urinary endogenous sex hormone levels and the risk of postmenopausal breast cancer, *Br J Cancer* 88:1394–1399, 2003.
248. Yager JD, Davidson NE: Estrogen carcinogenesis in breast cancer, *N Engl J Med* 354:270–282, 2006.
249. Foster PA: Steroid metabolism in breast cancer, *Minerva Endocrinol* 33:27–37, 2008.

250. Sasano H et al: *In situ* estrogen production and its regulation in human breast carcinoma: from endocrinology to intracrinology, *Pathol Int* 59:777–789, 2009.
251. Suzuki T et al: Sex steroid-producing enzymes in human breast cancer, *Endocrin Relat Cancer* 12:701–720, 2005.
252. Pasqualini JR, Chetrite GS: Recent insight on the control of enzymes involved in estrogen formation and transformation in human breast cancer, *J Steroid Biochem Mol Biol* 93(2–5):221–236, 2005.
253. Cavalieri E, Rogan E: Catechol quinines of estrogen in the initiation of breast, prostate, and other cancers: keynote lecture, *Ann N Y Acad Sci* 1089:286–301, 2006.
254. Cogliano V et al: Carcinogenicity of combined estrogen-progestogen contraceptives and menopausal treatment, *Lancet Oncol* 6:552–553, 2005.
255. Fuhrman BJ et al: Estrogen metabolism and risk of breast cancer in postmenopausal women, *J Natl Cancer Inst* 104(4):326–339, 2012.
256. IARC Special Report: Policy: a review of human carcinogens—part A: pharmaceuticals, *Lancet* 10:13–14, 2009.
257. Chlebowski RT et al: Breast cancer after use of estrogen plus progestin in postmenopausal women, *N Engl J Med* 360:573–587, 2009.
258. Collins JA, Blake JM, Crosinani PG: Breast cancer risk with postmenopausal hormone treatment, *Hum Reprod Update* 11:545–560, 2005.
259. Ringa V, Fournier A: Did the decrease in use of menopausal hormone therapy induce a decrease in the incidence of breast cancer in France (and elsewhere)? *Rev Epidemiol Sante Publique* 56:297–301, 2008.
260. Shah NR, Borenstein J, Dubois RW: Postmenopausal hormone therapy and breast cancer: a systematic review and meta-analysis, *Menopause* 12:668–678, 2005.
261. Fournier A: Should transdermal rather than oral estrogens be used in menopausal hormone therapy? A review, *Menopause Int* 16(1):23–32, 2010.
262. Canonico M et al: Postmenopausal hormone therapy and risk of idiopathic venous thromboembolism: results from the E3N cohort study, *Arterioscler Thromb Vasc Biol* 30:340–345, 2010.
263. Lacroix AZ et al: Health outcomes after stopping conjugated equine estrogens among postmenopausal women with prior hysterectomy: a randomized controlled trial, *J Am Med Assoc* 305(13):1305–1314, 2011.
264. Stefanick ML et al: Effects of conjugated equine estrogens on breast cancer and mammography screening in postmenopausal women with hysterectomy, *J Am Med Assoc* 295:1647–1657, 2006.
265. Collaborative Group on Hormonal Factors in Breast Cancer: Breast cancer and hormone replacement therapy: collaborative reanalysis of data from 51 epidemiological studies of 52,705 women with breast cancer and 108,411 women without breast cancer. Collaborative Group on Hormonal Factors in Breast Cancer, *Lancet* 350(9084):1047–1059, 1997.
266. Steinberg KK et al: A meta-analysis of the effect of estrogen replacement therapy on the risk of breast cancer, *J Am Med Assoc* 265(15):1985–1990, 1991.
267. Jordan VC, Ford LG: Paradoxical clinical effect of estrogen on breast cancer risk: a "new" biology of estrogen-induced apoptosis, *Cancer Prev Res (Phila)* 4(5):633–637, 2011.
268. Chlebowski RT, Anderson L: Changing concepts: menopausal hormone therapy and breast cancer, *J Natl Cancer Inst* 104(7):517–527, 2012.
269. Ariazi EA et al: Estrogen induces apoptosis in estrogen deprivation-resistant breast cancer through stress responses as identified by global gene expression across time, *Proc Natl Acad Sci U S A* 108(47): 18879–18886, 2011.
270. Marchini C et al: Mesenchymal/stromal gene expression signature relates to basel-like breast cancers, identifies bone metastasis and predicts resistance to therapies, *PLoS One* 5(11):e14131, 2010.
271. Fernandez-Cuesta L et al: p53 status influences response to tamoxifen but not to fulvestrant in breast cancer cell lines, *Int J Cancer* 128(8): 1831–1821, 2011.
272. Bailey ST et al: Estrogen receptor prevents p53-dependent apoptosis in breast cancer, *Proc Natl Acad Sci U S A* 109(44):18060–18065, 2012.
273. Peck A et al: Low levels of Stat5a protein in breast cancer are associated with tumor progression and unfavorable clinical outcomes, *Breast Cancer Res* 14:R130, 2012.
274. Beral V et al: Breast cancer risk in relation to the interval between menopause and starting hormone therapy, *J Natl Cancer Inst* 103(4):296–305, 2011.
275. Jungheim ES, Colditz GA: Short-term use of unopposed estrogen, *J Am Med Assoc* 305(13):1354–1355, 2011.
276. Pollack M: IGF-1 physiology and breast cancer, *Recent Results Cancer Res* 152:63–70, 1998.
277. Endogenous Hormones and Breast Cancer Collaborative Group et al: Insulin-like growth factor-1(IGF1), IGF binding protein 3 (IGFBP3), and breast cancer risk: pooled individual data analysis of 17 prospective studies, *Lancet Oncol* 11:530–542, 2010.
278. Kleinberg DL, Feldman M, Ruan W: IGF-1: an essential factor in terminal end bud formation and ductal morphogenesis, *J Mammary Gland Biol Neoplasia* 5(1):7–17, 2000, review.
279. Wu J et al: Light at night activates IGF-1R/PDK1 signaling and accelerates tumor growth in human breast cancer xenografts, *Cancer Res* 71(7):2622–2631, 2011.
280. Pollak M: The insulin and insulin-like growth factor receptor family in neoplasia: an update, *Nat Rev Cancer* 12(3):159–169, 2012.
281. Wang XS et al: Shift work and chronic disease: the epidemiological evidence, *Occup Med (Lond)* 61(2):78–89, 2011.
282. Wennbo H, Tornell J: The role of prolactin and growth hormone in breast cancer, *Oncogene* 19(8):1072–1076, 2000.
283. Renehen AG, Brennan BM: Acromegaly, growth hormone and cancer risk, *Best Pract Res Clin Endocrinol Metab* 22:639–657, 2008.
284. Schernhammer ES et al: Insulin-like growth factor-l, its binding protein (LGFBP-L and IBFBP-3), and growth hormone and breast cancer risk in The Nurses' Health Study II, *Endocr Relat Cancer* 13:583–592, 2006.
285. Tworoger SS et al: A prospective study of plasma prolactin concentrations and risk of premenopausal and postmenopausal breast cancer, *J Clin Oncol* 25:1482–1488, 2007.
286. Tanaka Y et al: Gonadotropins stimulate growth of MCF-7 human breast cancer cells by promoting intercellular conversion of adrenal androgens to estrogens, *Oncol* 59(Suppl 11):19–23, 2000.
287. Iles RK, Delves PJ, Butler SA: Does hCG or hCGβ play a role in cancer cell biology review? *Mol Cell Endocrinol* 329(1–2):62–70, 2010.
288. Boyd NF et al: Mammographic breast density as an intermediate phenotype for breast cancer, *Lancet Oncol* 6(10):798–808, 2005.
289. Nelson HP et al: Risk factors for breast cancer for women aged 40 to 49 years: a systematic review and meta-analysis, *Ann Int Med* 156(9): 635–648, 2012.
290. Boyd NF et al: Mammographic density and breast cancer risk: current understanding and future prospects, *Breast Cancer Res* 13(6):223, 2011.
291. McCormack VA, dos Santos Silva: Breast density and parenchymal patterns as markers of breast cancer risk: a meta-analysis, *Cancer Epidemiol Biomarkers Prev* 15:1159–1169, 2006.
292. Ginsburg ON et al: Mammographic density, lobular involution, and risk of breast cancer, *Br J Cancer* 4(99):1369–1374, 2008.
293. Lindstrom S et al: Common variants in ZNF365 are associated with both mammographic density and breast cancer risk, *Nat Genet* 43(3): 185–187, 2011.
294. Institute of Medicine of the National Academies: *Breast cancer and the environment: a life course approach*, Washington, DC, 2011, The National Academies Press.
295. Smith-Bindman R: Environmental causes of breast cancer and radiation from medical imaging, *Arch Intern Med* 172(13):1023–1027, 2012.
296. Baker LC, Atlas SW, Afendulis CC: Expanded use of imaging technology and the challenge of measuring value, *Health Aff (Millwood)* 2(6): 1467–1478, 2008.
297. National Cancer Institute: *Radiation risks and pediatric computed tomography (CT): a guide for health care providers*, 2002. Available at www.cancer.gov. Accessed December 2012.
298. Brenner DJ, Hall EJ: Computed tomography—an increasing source of radiation exposure, *N Engl J Med* 357(22):2277–2284, 2007.
299. National Cancer Institute: *Breast cancer screening concepts*, Bethesda, MD, modified, 2013, National Cancer Institute.
299a. Mullenders L et al: Assessing cancer risks of low-dose radiation, *Nat Rev Cancer* 9:596–604, 2009.
299b. Shuryah I et al: Cancer risks after radiation exposure in middle age, *J Natl Cancer Inst* 102:1628–1636, 2010.
299c. Hernandez L et al: Increased mammogram-induced DNA damage in mammary epithelial cells aged *in vitro*, *PLOS ONE* 8(5):e63052. doi:10.1371/journal.pone.0063052. Print 2013.
300. Hurwitz LM et al: Radiation dose to the female breast from 16-MDCT body protocols, *AJR Am J Roentgenol* 186(6):1718–1722, 2006.
301. Land CD: Radiation and breast cancer risk, *Prog Clin Biol Res* 396:115–124, 1997.
302. Berrington de Gonzalez A: Reeves G: Mammographic screening before age 50 years in the UK: comparison of the radiation risks with the mortality benefits, *Br J Cancer* 93(5):590–596, 2005.
303. Feig SA, Hendrick RE: Radiation risk from screening mammography of women aged 40–49 years, *J Natl Cancer Inst Monogr* 22:119–124, 1997.

304. Yaffe MJ, Mainprize JG: Risk of radiation-induced breast cancer from mammographic screening, *Radiology* 258:98–105, 2011.
305. Berrington de Gonzalez A et al: Estimated risk of radiation-induced breast cancer from mammographic screening for young BRCA mutation carriers, *J Natl Cancer Inst* 101:205–209, 2009.
306. Jansen-van der Weide MC et al: Exposure to low-dose radiation and the risk of breast cancer among women with a familial or genetic predisposition: a meta-analysis, *Eur Radiol* 20:2547–2556, 2010.
307. Heyes GJ, Mill AJ: The neoplastic transformation potential of mammography X rays and atomic bomb spectrum radiation, *Radiat Res* 162:120–127, 2004.
308. Heyes GJ, Mill AJ, Charles MW: Mammography-oncogenecity at low doses, *J Radiol Prot* 29:A123–A132, 2009.
309. Law J: Cancers detected and induced in mammographic screening: new screening schedules and younger women with family history, *Br J Radiol* 70:62–69, 1997.
310. Hendrick RE et al: Comparison of acquisition parameters and breast dose in digital mammography and screen-film mammography in the American College of Radiology Imaging Network Digital Mammographic Imaging Screening Trial, *Am J Roentgenol* 194:362–369, 2010.
311. Smathers RL et al: Radiation dose reduction for augmentation mammography, *Am J Roetgenol* 188:1414–1421, 2007.
312. Colin C et al: DNA double-strand breaks induced by mammographic screening procedures in human epithelial cells, *Int J Radiat Biol* 87(11):1103–1112, 2011.
313. Granzotto A et al: Individual susceptibility to radiosensitivity and to genomic instability; its impact on low doses phenomena, *Health Physics* 100:282, 2011a.
314. Granzotto A et al: Individual response to ionising radiation: what predictive assay(s) to choose? *Compte-rendus de l'Académie des Sciences, Biologies* 334:140–157, 2011b.
315. Jeggo PA, Lobrich M: Contribution of DNA repair and cell cycle checkpoint arrest to the maintenance of genomic stability, *DNA Repair (Amst)* 5:1192–1198, 2006.
316. Beyreuther E et al: DNA double-strand break signalling: X-ray energy dependence of residual co-localised foci of gamma-H2AX and 53BP1, *Int J Radiat Biol* 85:1042–1050, 2009a.
317. Beyreuther E et al: Relative biological effectiveness of 25 and 10 kV X-rays for the induction of chromosomal aberrations in two human mammary epithelial cell lines, *Radiat Environ Biophysics* 48:333–340, 2009b.
318. Ko SJ et al: Neoplastic transformation in vitro after exposure to low doses of mammographic-energy X rays: quantitative and mechanistic aspects, *Radiat Res* 162:646–654, 2004.
319. Lehnert A et al: RBE of 25 kV X-rays for the survival and induction of micronuclei in the human mammary epithelial cell line MCF-12A, *Radiat Environ Biophysics* 45:253–260, 2006.
320. Lehnert A et al: RBE of 10 kV X rays determined for the human mammary epithelial cell line MCF-12A, *Radiat Res* 169:330–336, 2008.
321. Panteleeva A et al: Clonogenic survival of human keratinocytes and rodent fibroblasts after irradiation with 25 kV x-rays, *Radiat Environ Biophysics* 42:95–100, 2003.
322. Redpath JL et al: Low doses of diagnostic energy X-rays protect against neoplastic transformation in vitro, *Int J Radiat Biol* 79:235–240, 2003.
323. Schmid E et al: The effect of 29 kV X rays on the dose response of chromosome aberrations in human lymphocytes, *Radiat Res* 158:771–777, 2002.
324. Slonina D et al: Induction of micronuclei in human fibroblasts and keratinocytes by 25 kV X-rays, *Radiat Environ Biophysics* 42:55–61, 2003.
325. Rothkamm K, Löbrich M: Evidence for a lack of DNA double-strand break repair in human cells exposed to very low x-ray doses, *Proc Natl Acad Sci U S A* 100:5057–5062, 2003.
326. Grudzenski S et al: Inducible response required for repair of low-dose radiation damage in human fibroblasts, *PNAS* 107(3):14205–14210, 2010.
327. Colin C et al: Update relevance of mammographic screening modalities in women previously treated with chest irradiation for Hodgkin disease, *Radiology* 265(3):669–676, 2012.
328. Lagadec et al: Radiation-induced reprogramming of breast cancer cells, *Stem Cells* 30:833–844, 2012.
329. Mathews LA, Cabarcas SM, Farrar WL: DNA repair: the culprit for tumor-initiating cell survival? *Cancer Metastasis Rev* 30(2):185–197, 2011.
330. O'Brien CA, Kreso A, Jamieson CH: Cancer stem cells and self-renewal, *Clin Cancer Res* 16(12):3113–3120, 2010.
331. Ng J et al: Predicting the risk of secondary lung malignancies associated with whole-breast radiation therapy, *Int J Radiat Oncol* 83(4): 1101–1106, 2012.
332. Presley CJ et al: Patterns of use and short-term complications of breast brachytherapy in the national Medicare population from 2008–2009, *J Clin Oncol* 30:4302, 2012.
333. Bleyer A, Welch HG: Effect of three decades of screening mammography on breast cancer incidence, *N Engl J Med* 367(21):1998–2005, 2012.
334. Early Breast Cancer Trialists' Collaborative Group (EBCTCG): Effects of chemotherapy and hormonal therapy for early breast cancer on recurrence and 15-year survival: an overview of the randomized trials, *Lancet* 365:1687–1717, 2005.
335. Surveillance, Epidemiology, and End Results (SEER) SEER Stat Database: Incidence-SEER 17 Regs Research Data+ Hurricane Katrina Impacted Louisiana Cases, Nov 2010 Sub (1973–2008 varying) Linked to County Attributes—Total U.S., 1969–2009 Counties, National Cancer Institute, DCCPS, Surveillance Research Program, Cancer Statistics Branch, released April 2011 (updated 10/28/2011).
336. Hendrick RE et al: Radiation doses and cancer risks from breast imaging studies, *Radiology* 257(1):246–253, 2010.
337. Nagasawa H, Little JB: Induction of sister chromatid exchanges by extremely low doses of alpha-particles, *Cancer Res* 52:6394–6396, 1992.
338. Michels KB et al: Diet and breast cancer: a review of the prospective observational studies, *Cancer* 109(Suppl 12):2712–2749, 2007.
339. Mahoney MC et al: Opportunities and strategies for breast cancer prevention through risk reduction, *CA Cancer J Clin* 58(6):347–371, 2008.
340. Smith-Warner SA, Stampfer MJ: Fat intake and breast cancer revisited, *J Natl Cancer Inst* 99(6):418–419, 2007.
341. Prentice RL et al: Low-fat dietary pattern and risk of invasive breast cancer: the Women's Health Initiative Randomized Controlled Dietary Modification Trial, *JAMA* 295(6):629–642, 2006.
342. World Cancer Research/American Institute for Cancer Research (WCR/AICR): *Food, nutrition, physical activity, and prevention of cancer: a global perspective*, Washington, DC, 2007, American Institute for Cancer Research.
343. Turner LB: Meta-analysis of fat intake, reproduction, and breast cancer risk: an evolutionary perspective, *Am J Hum Biol* 23:601–608, 2011.
344. Ariazi JL et al: Mammary glands of sexually immature rats are more susceptible than those of mature rats to the carcinogenic, lethal, and mutagenic effects of *N*-nitroso-*N*-methylurea, *Mol Carcinog* 43(3): 155–164, 2005.
345. Russo J, Russo IH: Cellular basis of breast cancer susceptibility, *Oncol Res* 11(4):169–178, 1999.
346. Land CE et al: Incidence of female breast cancer among atomic bomb survivors, Hiroshima and Nagasaki, 1950–1990, *Radiat Res* 160(6): 707–717, 2003.
347. Linos E et al: Adolescent diet and risk of breast cancer among premenopausal women, *Cancer Epidemiol Biomarkers Prev* 19(3):689–696, 2010.
348. Missner SA et al: Meat and dairy food consumption and breast cancer: a pooled analysis of cohort studies, *Int J Epidemiol* 31:78–85, 2002.
349. Cho E et al: Red meat intake and risk of breast cancer among premenopausal women, *Arch Intern Med* 166:2258–2259, 2006.
350. Taylor EF et al: Meat consumption and risk of breast cancer in the UK Women's Cohort Study, *Br J Cancer* 96:1139–1146, 2007.
351. Egeberg R et al: Meat consumption, N-acetyl transferase 1 and 2 polymorphism and risk of breast cancer in Danish postmenopausal women, *Eur J Cancer Prev* 17:39–47, 2008.
352. Alexander DD et al: A review and meta-analysis of red and processed meat consumption and breast cancer, *Nutr Res Rev* 23(2):349–365, 2010.
353. Aldercreutz H: Ligans and human health, *Rev Clin Lab Sci* 44(5–6): 483–525, 2007.
354. Sonestedt E, Wirfält E: Enterolactone and breast cancer: methodological issues may contribute to conflicting results in observational studies, *Nutr Res* 30:667–677, 2010.
355. Rock CL et al: Effects of a high-fiber, low-fat diet intervention on serum concentrations of reproductive steroid hormones in women with a history of breast cancer, *J Clin Oncol* 22(12):2379–2387, 2004.
356. Dong JY et al: Dietary fiber intake and risk of breast cancer: a meta-analysis of prospective cohort studies, *Am J Clin Nutr* 94(3):900–905, 2011.
357. Aune D et al: Dietary fiber and breast cancer risk: a systematic review and meta-analysis of prospective studies, *Ann Oncol* 23(6):1394–1402, 2012.
358. Buck K et al: Estimated enterolignans, lignan-rich foods, and fibre in relation to survival after postmenopausal breast cancer, *Br J Cancer* 105(8):1151–1157, 2011.

359. Buck K: Meta-analyses of lignans and enterolignans in relation to breast cancer risk, *Am J Clin Nutr* 92:141–153, 2010.
360. Velentzis LS et al: Lignans and breast cancer risk in pre-post-menopausal women: meta-analyses of observational studies, *Br J Cancer* 100:1492–1498, 2009.
361. North American Menopause Society (NAMS): The role of soy isoflavones in menopausal health: report of The North American Menopause Society/Wulf H. Utian Translational Science Symposium in Chicago, IL, *Menopause* 18(7):732–753, 2011.
362. Bedell S, Nachtigall M, Naftolin F: The pros and cons of plant estrogens for menopause, *J Steroid Biochem Mol Biol*, 2012 Dec 25. [Epub ahead of print.].
363. Nechuta SJ et al: Soy food intake after diagnosis of breast cancer and survival: an in-depth analysis of combined evidence from cohort studies of U.S. and Chinese women, *Am J Nutr* 96(1):123–132, 2012.
364. Cross HS et al: Phytoestrogens and vitamin D metabolism: a new concept for the prevention and therapy of colorectal, prostate, and mammary carcinomas, *J Nutr* 134(5):1207S–1212S, 2004.
365. Kuller LH: The etiology of breast cancer—from epidemiology to prevention, *Public Health Rev* 23(2):157–213, 1995.
366. Holmes MD, Willett WC: Does diet affect breast cancer risk? *Breast Cancer Res* 6(4):170–178, 2004.
367. Hankinson SE et al: Alcohol, height, and adiposity in relation to estrogen and prolactin levels in post-menopausal women, *J Natl Cancer Inst* 87(17):1297–1302, 1995.
368. Vrieling A et al: Adult weight gain in relation to breast cancer risk by estrogen and progesterone receptor status: a meta-analysis, *Breast Cancer Res Treat* 123:641–649, 2010.
369. Endogenous Hormones Breast Cancer Collaborative Group: Body mass index, serum sex hormones, and breast cancer risk in postmenopausal women, *J Natl Cancer Inst* 95(6):1218–1226, 2003.
370. Ahn J et al: Adiposity, adult weight gain, and postmenopausal breast cancer risk, *Arch Intern Med* 167:2091–2102, 2007.
371. Giles ED et al: Obesity and overfeeding affecting both tumor and systemic metabolism activates the progesterone receptor to contribute to postmenopausal breast cancer, *Cancer Res* 72(24):6490–6501, 2012.
372. Harvie M et al: Association of gain and loss of weight before and after menopause with risk of postmenopausal breast cancer in the Iowa Women's Health Study, *Cancer Epidemiol Biomarkers Prev* 14:656–661, 2005.
373. Kwan ML et al: Pre-diagnosis body mass index and survival after breast cancer in the After Breast Cancer Pooling Project, *Breast Cancer Res Treat* 132(2):729–739, 2012.
374. Chen WY et al: Moderate alcohol consumption during adult life, drinking patterns, and breast cancer risk, *JAMA* 306(17):1884–1890, 2011.
375. Li CI et al: Alcohol consumption and risk of postmenopausal breast cancer by subtype: the Women's Health Initiative observational study, *J Natl Cancer Inst* 102(18):1422–1431, 2010.
376. Kabat GC et al: Smoking and alcohol consumption in relation to risk of triple–negative breast cancer in a cohort of postmenopausal women, *Cancer Causes Control* 22(5):775–783, 2011.
377. Wu AH et al: Alcohol and breast cancer risk among Asian-American women in Los Angeles County, *Breast Cancer Res* 14:R151, 2012.
378. Iodine monograph, *Altern Med Rev* 15(3):273–278, 2010.
379. Venturi S: Is there a role for iodine in breast disease? *Breast* 10:379–382, 2001.
380. Aceves C, Anguiano B, Delgado G: Is iodine a gatekeeper of the integrity of the mammary gland? *J Mammary Gland Biol Neoplasia* 10(2): 189–196, 2005.
381. Cann SA, van Netten JP, van Netten C: Hypothesis: iodine, selenium and the development of breast cancer, *Cancer Causes Control* 11:121–127, 2000.
382. Eskin BA et al: Different tissue responses for iodine and iodide in rat thyroid and mammary glands, *Biol Trace Elem Res* 49:9–19, 1995.
383. Ghent WR et al: Iodine replacement in fibrocystic disease of the breast, *Can J Surg* 36:453–460, 1993.
384. Funahashi H et al: Seaweed prevents breast cancer, *Jpn J Cancer Res* 92(5):483–487, 2001.
385. *EPA Science Matters: The future of toxicity testing is here*, 2011. Available at www.EPA.Gov/Research. Accessed February 2012.
386. Dairkee SH et al: Bisphenol A induces a profile of tumor aggressiveness in high-risk cells from breast cancer patients, *Cancer Res* 68:2076–2080, 2008.
387. Loprinzi PD et al: Physical activity and the risk of breast cancer recurrence: a literature review, *Oncol Nurs Forum* 39(3):269–274, 2012.
388. Winzer BM et al: Physical activity and cancer prevention: a systematic review of clinical trials, *Cancer Causes Control* 22(6):811–826, 2011.
389. Sprague BL et al: Lifetime recreational and occupational physical activity and risk of in situ and invasive breast cancer, *Cancer Epidemiol Biomarkers Prev* 16(2):236–243, 2007.
390. Ballard-Barbash R et al: Physical activity, biomarkers, and disease outcomes in cancer survivors: a systematic review, *J Natl Cancer Inst* 104(11):815–840, 2012.
391. Suzuki S et al: Effect of physical activity on breast cancer risk: findings of the Japan Collaborative Cohort Study, *Cancer Epidemiol Biomarkers Prev* 17(12):3396–3401, 2008.
392. Stephens PJ et al: The landscape of cancer genes and mutational processes in breast cancer, *Nature* 486:400–404, 2012.
393. Yu-K Shao Z: Initiation, evolution, phenotype and outcome of BRCA1 and BRCA2 mutation-associated breast cancer, *Nat Rev Cancer* 12:372–373, 2012.
394. Polyak K: Heterogeneity in breast cancer, *J Clin Invest* 121:3786–3788, 2011.
395. Sorlie T et al: Gene expression patterns of breast carcinomas distinguish tumor subclasses with clinical implications, *Proc Natl Acad Sci U S A* 98:10869–10874, 2001.
396. Boudreau A, van't Veer LJ, Bissell M: An "elite hacker:" breast tumors exploit the normal microenvironment program to instruct their progression and biological diversity, *Cell Adh Migr* 6(3):236–248, 2012.
397. Hanahan D, Weinberg RA: Hallmarks of cancer: the next generation, *Cell* 144(5):646–674, 2011.
398. Damonte P et al: Mammary carcinoma behavior is programmed in the precancer stem cell, *Breast Cancer Res* 10(3):R50, 2008.
399. Cardiff RD, Couto S, Bolon B: Three interrelated themes in current breast cancer research: gene addiction, phenotypic plasticity, and cancer stem cells, *Breast Cancer Res* 13:216, 2011.
400. Acloque H, Thiery JP, Nieto MA: The physiology and pathology of the EMT, *EMBO Rep* 9(4):322–326, 2008.
401. Craene DB, Berx G: Regulatory networks defining EMT during cancer initiation and progression, *Nat Rev Cancer* 13(2):97–110, 2013.
402. Mani SA et al: The epithelial-mesenchymal transition generates cells with properties of stem cells, *Cell* 133:704–715, 2008.
403. Place AE, Jin Huh SJ: Polyak K: The microenvironment in breast cancer progression: biology and implications for treatment, *Breast Cancer Res* 13(6):227, 2011.
404. Román-Peréz E et al: Gene expression in extratumoral microenvironment predicts clinical outcome in breast cancer patients, *Breast Cancer Res* 14:R51, 2012.
405. Finak G et al: Stromal gene expression predicts clinical outcome in breast cancer, *Nat Med* 14:18–527, 2008.
406. Chang HY et al: Gene expression signature of fibroblast serum response predicts human cancer progression: similarities between tumors and wounds, *PLoS Biol* 2(2):E7, 2004.
407. Beck AH et al: The macrophage colony-stimulating factor 1 response signature in breast carcinoma, *Clin Cancer Res* 15:778–787, 2009.
408. Ma XJ et al: Gene expression profiling of the tumor microenvironment during breast cancer progression, *Breast Cancer Res* 11:R7, 2009.
409. Bissell MJ, Hines WC: Why don't we get more cancer? A proposed role of the microenvironment in restraining cancer progression, *Nat Med* 17(3):320–329, 2011.
410. Lee RJ et al: Ductal carcinoma in situ of the breast, *Int J Surg Oncol:* 2012:123549, 2012.
411. Kerlikowske K: Epidemiology of ductal carcinoma in situ, *J Natl Cancer Inst Monogr* 41:139–141, 2010.
412. DeSantis C, Breast cancer statistics, 2011 et al: *CA Cancer J Clin* 61(6):409–418, 2011.
413. Horner M et al: *SEER cancer statistics review, 1975–2006,* Bethesda, MD, 2009, National Cancer Institute. Available at http://seer.cancer.gov/csr/1975. Accessed February 24, 2012.
414. American Cancer Society (ACS): *Breast cancer*, 2013. Available at www.cancer.org/cancer/breastcancer/detailedguide/breast-cancer-key-statistics.
415. Kerlikowske K et al: Declines in invasive breast cancer and use of postmenopausal hormone therapy in a screening mammography population, *J Natl Cancer Inst* 99(17):1335–1339, 2007.
416. Reiner K, Vacek P, Geller B: Risk factors for breast carcinoma in situ versus invasive breast cancer in a prospective study of pre-and post-menopausal women, *Breast Cancer Res Treat* 103(3):343–348, 2007.
417. Allinen M et al: Molecular characterization of the tumor microenvironment in breast cancer, *Cancer Cell* 6:17–32, 2004.

418. Pinder SE, O'Malley FP: Morphology of ductal carcinoma in situ. In O'Malley FP, Pinder SE, editors: *Breast pathology*, Edinburgh, 2006, Churchill Livingstone.
419. Oppong BA, King TA: Recommendations for women with lobular carcinoma in situ (LCIS), *Oncology* 25(11):1051–1056, 2011.
420. Hanby AM, Hughes TA: In situ and invasive neoplasia of the breast, *Histopathology* 52(1):58–66, 2008.
421. Reis-Filho JS, Lakhani SR: Molecular genetics of ADH/DCIS and ALH/LCIS. In O'Malley FP, Pinder SE, editors: *Breast pathology*, New York, 2006, Churchill Livingstone/Elsevier.
422. Lakhani SR: Molecular genetics of solid tumors: translating research into clinical practice. What we could do now: breast cancer, *Mol Pathol* 54(5):281–284, 2001.
423. Page DL et al: Atypical lobular hyperplasia as a unilateral predictor of breast cancer risk: a retrospective cohort study, *Lancet* 361(9352): 125–129, 2003.
424. Coopey SB: The role of chemoprevention in modifying the risk of breast cancer in women with atypical breast lesions, *Breast Cancer Res Treat* 136(3):627–633, 2012.
425. Boghaert E et al: Host epithelial geometry regulates breast cancer cell invasiveness, *PNAS* 109(48):19632–19637, 2012.
426. Soto AM, Sonnenschein C: The tissue organization field theory of cancer: a testable replacement for the somatic mutation theory, *Bioessays* 33(5):332–340, 2011.
427. Kenny PA, Bissell MJ: Tumor reversion: correction of malignant behavior by microenvironment cues, *Int J Cancer* 107(5):688–695, 2003.
428. Sieweke MH et al: Mediation of wound-related Rous sarcoma virus tumorigenesis by TGF-beta, *Science* 248(4963):1656–1660, 1990.
429. Weaver VM et al: Reversion of the malignant phenotype of human breast cells in three dimensional culture and in vivo by integrin blocking antibodies, *J Cell Biol* 137(1):231–245, 1997.
430. Chang HY et al: Robustness, scalability, and integration of a wound-response gene expression signature in predicting breast cancer survival, *Proc Natl Acad Sci U S A* 102(10):3738–3743, 2004.
431. Nuyten DS et al: Predicting a local recurrence after breast-conserving therapy by gene expression profiling, *Breast Cancer Res* 8(5):R62, 2006.
432. Pandey PR, Saidou J, Watabe K: Role of the myoepithelial cells in breast tumor progression, *Front Biosci* 15:226–236, 2011.
433. Adriance MC et al: Myoepithelial cells: good fences make good neighbors, *Breast Cancer Res* 7(5):190–197, 2005.
434. Man YG, Sang QX: The significance of focal myoepithelial cell layer disruptions in human breast tumor invasion: a paradigm shift from the "protease-centered" hypothesis, *Exp Cell Res* 310:103–118, 2004.
435. Nguyen-Ngoc KV et al: ECM microenvironment regulates collective migration and local dissemination in normal and malignant mammary epithelium, *PNAS* 109(39):15543–15544, 2012.
436. Man YG et al: Tumor-infiltrating immune cells promoting tumor invasion and metastasis: existing theories, *J Cancer* 4(1):84–95, 2013.
437. Noffsinger A et al: *Gastrointestinal diseases*, Washington, DC, 2007, American Registry of Pathology and Armed Forces Institute of Pathology, pp 1–13.
438. Jones JL et al: Primary breast myoepithelial cells exert an invasion suppressor effect on breast cancer cells via paracrine down-regulation of MMP expression in fibroblasts and tumour cells, *J Pathol* 201(4):562–572, 2003.

CHAPTER

25

Alterations of the Male Reproductive System

George Rodway and Kathryn L. McCance

evolve WEBSITE

http://evolve.elsevier.com/McCance/

- Review Questions and Answers
- Animations
- Online Course: Module 11

CHAPTER OUTLINE

Alterations of the reproductive system span a wide range of concerns, from delayed sexual development and suboptimal sexual performance to structural and functional abnormalities. Many common male reproductive disorders carry potentially serious physiologic or psychologic consequences. Sexual or reproductive dysfunction, such as impotence or infertility, can dramatically affect self-concept, relationships, and overall quality of life. Conversely, organic and psychosocial problems, such as alcoholism, depression, situational stressors, chronic illness, and medications, can affect sexual performance and fertility and may be risk factors for the development of some types of reproductive tract cancers. Prostate cancer is the second leading cause of cancer death in men and is the most frequently diagnosed cancer in men aside from skin cancer. Incidence rates for prostate cancer changed substantially between the mid-1980s and mid-1990s and have since fluctuated widely from year to year, in large part reflecting changes in prostate cancer screening with the prostate specific antigen (PSA) blood test. Since 2004, incidence rates have act actually decreased by 2.7% per year among men 65 years of age and older and have remained stable among men younger than 65 years.[1] Diagnosis and treatment of male reproductive system disorders are, like female reproductive system disorders, complicated because of the stigma and symbolism associated with the reproductive organs and the emotion-laden beliefs and behaviors related to reproductive health. Treatment and diagnosis for related problems may be delayed because of embarrassment, guilt, fear, or denial.

ALTERATIONS OF SEXUAL MATURATION

The process of sexual maturation, or puberty, is marked by the development of secondary sexual characteristics, rapid growth, and, ultimately, the ability to reproduce. A variety of congenital and endocrine disorders can disrupt the timing of puberty, or sexual maturation. These disorders may cause puberty to occur too late (delayed puberty) or too early (precocious puberty). Both types involve a disrupted onset of sex hormone production by the gonads, although there is little change in the age of puberty for boys.

Delayed Puberty

About 3% of children in North America experience delayed development of secondary sex characteristics.[2] Normally, boys tend to mature later than girls, around 14 to 14.5 years of age. In boys the first sign is enlargement of the testes and thinning of the scrotal skin. Puberty is considered delayed if there are no clinical signs of puberty by age 14 in boys (2 standard deviations [SDs] above the mean age of pubertal onset). Boys especially tend to be embarrassed by sexual immaturity;[3] therefore, early diagnosis and treatment are recommended, as well as reassurance for boys as well as girls.

In 95% of cases delayed puberty is a physiologic delay, that is, hormonal levels are normal and the hypothalamic-pituitary-gonadal (HPG) axis is intact, but maturation is happening slowly.[4] This constitutional delay tends to be familial and is much more common in boys than in girls. Physiologic delay is difficult to distinguish from isolated gonadotropin deficiency and is usually diagnosed retrospectively once pubertal progression is complete.

Delayed puberty also may be related to consequences of any chronic condition that delays bone aging (i.e., lung disease, renal failure, cystic fibrosis) (Box 25-1).[2] Many clinicians recommend intervention (i.e., exogenous sex steroid administration) in physiologic cases of delayed puberty to reduce the psychologic effects (e.g., self-esteem issues, embarrassment) often associated with delayed puberty.[4]

The other 5% of cases are caused by a disruption of the HPG axis of various etiologies (see Box 25-1).[5] Human gonadal function is partially controlled by luteinizing hormone (LH) and follicle-stimulating hormone (FSH), the release of which is regulated by the pulsatile secretion of hypothalamic gonadotropin-releasing hormone (GnRH).[4,5] Most recently, the G-protein–coupled receptor 54 (GPR54) has been identified as the gatekeeper gene for activation of the GnRH axis based on loss of function studies in mice and humans. GPR54 is required for the normal function of this axis, and data suggest that the ligand kisspeptin-1 may act as a neurohormonal regulator of the GnRH axis.[6] The mechanisms of childhood inhibition of GnRH release and activation are poorly understood but appear to involve feedback inhibition by sex steroids and presumably other central nervous system (CNS) pathways.[7] Given the myriad etiologies contributing to the occurrence of delayed puberty, a thorough evaluation should be conducted that includes physical examination and medical and family history. Such evaluation should specifically target known contributors to delayed puberty.[4] Laboratory workup generally consists of x-ray studies for bone age, measurement of thyroid function, serum levels of prolactin and adrenal and gonadal steroids, radioimmunoassay of plasma gonadotropins, and screening for systemic disorders. Adolescents with high gonadotropin levels require a karyotype, to rule out genetic causes, and those with low levels need skull imaging (lateral skull film, computed tomography [CT], or magnetic resonance imaging [MRI]) to rule out pituitary or other CNS infiltrate or tumor.[2] Although several genes involved in the HPG maturation cascade have been characterized from familial or sporadic cases of primitive isolated hypogonadotropic hypogonadism, many genes regulating puberty onset remain undetermined. Treatment of delayed puberty depends on the cause; the goal of treatment is the development of secondary sex characteristics and fertility, when possible. Insufficient sex hormone secretion can be corrected by hormone replacement therapy, such as testosterone for boys.[8] Idiopathic hypogonadotropic hypogonadism is treated with synthetic GnRH or sex hormone administration, or both, and may be lifelong.[2,4,8]

BOX 25-1 CAUSES OF DELAYED OR ABSENT PUBERTY

Chronic or Systemic Conditions

- Chronic renal disease
- Cystic fibrosis
- Diabetes mellitus
- Excessive exercise
- Hematologic diseases
- Hypothyroidism
- Irritable bowel diseases
- Poor nutrition (eating disorders, GI diseases, poverty)
- Gonadal dysgenesis
  - Turner syndrome (genetic karyotype 45, XO)
- Bilateral gonadal failure
  - Autoimmune
  - Congenital anorchia
  - Postsurgical, postirradiation, postchemotherapy
  - Traumatic or infectious

Hypogonadotropic Hypogonadism (Deficient FSH/LH)

- Central nervous system defects (GnRH deficiency)
  - Craniopharyngioma
  - GPR54 mutations
  - Hemochromatosis
  - Hypopituitarism
  - Kallmann syndrome, Bardet-Biedl syndrome, Prader-Willi syndrome
  - Marijuana use
  - Pituitary adenoma/tumor
  - Prolactinomas

Disordered Puberty

Data from Burchett MLR, Hanna CE, Steiner RD: Endocrine and metabolic diseases. In Burns CE, Brady MA, Dunn AM, editors: *Pediatric primary care*, ed 4, St Louis 2009, Saunders; Jospe N: Disorders of pubertal development. In Osborn LM et al, editors: *Pediatrics*, Philadelphia, 2005, Mosby; Karagiannis A, Harsoulis F: *Eur J Endocrinol* 152(4):501–513, 2005.

FSH, Follicle-stimulating hormone; *GI,* gastrointestinal; *GnRH,* gonadotropin-releasing hormone; *LH,* luteinizing hormone.

Precocious Puberty

Precocious puberty is a rare event in boys, affecting less than 1 in 50,000. Precocious puberty in boys has been redefined as sexual maturation before age 9.[9] One study has noted observed mean ages of beginning male genital and pubic hair growth and early testicular volumes tending toward younger ages than earlier studies have suggested, although this seems to be dependent on race and ethnicity.[10] For instance, black boys are showing significantly earlier mean ages for stages 2 to 4 genital

BOX 25-2 PRIMARY FORMS OF PRECOCIOUS PUBERTY

Complete Precocious Puberty

Premature development of appropriate characteristics for the child's sex

Hypothalamic-pituitary-ovarian axis working normally but prematurely

In about 10% of cases, lethal central nervous system tumor may be the cause

Partial Precocious Puberty

Partial development of appropriate secondary sex characteristics

Premature thelarche (breast budding) seen in girls between 6 months and 2 years of age

Does not progress to complete puberty (ovulation and menstruation)

Premature adrenarche (growth of axillary and pubic hair) tends to occur between 5 and 8 years of age

Can progress to complete precocious puberty; may be caused by estrogen-secreting neoplasms or may be a variant of normal pubertal development

Mixed Precocious Puberty

Causes the child to develop some secondary sex characteristics of the opposite sex

Common causes: adrenal hyperplasia or androgen-secreting tumors

Data from Burchett MLR et al: Endocrine and metabolic diseases. In Burns CE et al, editors: *Pediatric primary care*, St Louis, 2009, Saunders; Jospe N: Disorders of pubertal development. In Osborn LM et al, editors: *Pediatrics,* Philadelphia, 2005, Mosby.

BOX 25-3 CAUSES OF PRECOCIOUS PUBERTY

Central (Gonadotropin-Releasing Hormone [GnRH] Dependent)

Idiopathic

Central nervous system (CNS) disorders

- Congenital anomalies (hydrocephalus)
- Hypothalamic hamartoma
- Postinflammatory/infectious condition
- Trauma
- Tumors (hypothalamic, pineal, other)

Hypothyroidism (severe)

Peripheral Puberty (GnRH Independent)

Adrenal hyperplasia or tumor

Environmental endocrine disruptors

Exogenous sex steroid exposure

Exogenous anabolic steroids

Familial Leydig cell hyperplasia

Gonadal tumors or cysts

Human chorionic gonadotropin (hCG)–secreting tumors (hepatoblastomas, intracranial lesions)

McCune-Albright syndrome

Testotoxicosis

From Bhagavath B, Layman LC: *Semin Reprod Med* 25(4):272–286, 2007; Burchett MLR et al: Endocrine and metabolic diseases. In Burns CE et al, editors: *Pediatric primary care*, St Louis, 2009, Saunders; Caserta DL et al: *Hum Reprod Update* 14(1):59–72, 2008; Cesario SK, Hughes LA: *J Obstet Gynecol Neonatal Nurs* 36(3):263–274, 2007; Jospe N: Disorders of pubertal development. In Osborn LM et al, editors: *Pediatrics,* Philadelphia, 2005, Mosby.

development and stages 2 to 4 pubic hair than white and Hispanic boys. All cases of precocious puberty require thorough evaluation.

Precocious puberty may be partial, complete, or mixed (heterosexual) types (Box 25-2) and can be further categorized into central (GnRH-dependent) and peripheral (GnRH-independent) (Box 25-3). **Central precocious puberty** is GnRH-dependent and occurs when the HPG axis is working normally but prematurely. Besides the premature development of secondary sex characteristics, precocity causes premature closure of the epiphysis of long bones, which results in shorter stature. Central precocious puberty results from failure of central inhibition of the GnRH pulse generator (the gonadostat). The diagnosis of central precocious puberty is one of exclusion. Because a CNS lesion may be missed, children with presumed central precocious puberty require long-term surveillance. Peripheral puberty is GnRH-independent and develops when sex hormones are produced by some mechanism other than stimulation by the gonadotropins. Sex steroid–producing tumors (i.e., gonadal tumors), testotoxicosis, and exposure to exogenous sex steroids (i.e., hormonal contraceptives and environmental endocrine disruptors) are some of the causes (see Box 25-3).

Complete precocious puberty refers to the onset and progression of all pubertal features. **Partial precocious puberty** is the partial development of appropriate secondary sex characteristics alone or in combination. Premature pubarche tends to occur between ages 5 and 8 years. Premature pubarche is usually the consequence of an early increase in the adrenal androgens that leads to early growth of pubic hair and possibly a transient acceleration in growth and bone maturation that has no significant effect on timing of puberty or final height.

The diagnosis and cause of premature development are often obvious. A thorough history and physical examination are done to determine the velocity of the process and to rule out life-threatening CNS or adrenal neoplasms. Family occurrence helps exclude tumors. Children with precocious puberty also have a tendency toward obesity.[7,11]

Treatment for all forms of precocious puberty includes identifying and removing the underlying cause (see Boxes 25-2 and 25-3) or administering appropriate hormones. In many cases precocious puberty can be reversed. Management goals include diagnosing and treating intracranial disease; arresting maturation until early teen years; maximizing eventual adult height; reducing emotional problems; and providing contraception, if necessary. The most common form, central precocious puberty, is usually treated with potent GnRH agonist analogs, which induce reversible, selective suppression of the HPG axis. Treatment does not seem to affect body composition or increase obesity in children with central precocious puberty. Because many of these children are obese and childhood obesity is predictive of morbidity in adolescence and adulthood, it is important for clinicians to include assessment and management of obesity as part of the treatment for central precocious puberty.

Mixed precocious puberty (e.g., feminization of a boy) causes the child to develop some secondary sex characteristics of the opposite sex. This condition is usually evident at birth and is rare in older children (Box 25-4).

BOX 25-4 CAUSES OF MIXED PRECOCIOUS PUBERTY

Female (Virilization)

Congenital adrenal hyperplasia
Androgen-secreting tumors
- Adrenal
- Ovarian
- Teratoma
- Exogenous androgens

Male (Feminization)

Estrogen-producing tumors
- Adrenal
- Teratoma
- Hepatoma
- Testicular

Exogenous estrogens
Increased peripheral conversion of androgens to estrogens

From Jospe N: Disorders of pubertal development. In Osborn LM et al, editors: *Pediatrics*, Philadelphia, 2005, Mosby.

DISORDERS OF THE MALE REPRODUCTIVE SYSTEM

Disorders of the Urethra

Urethritis and urethral strictures are common disorders of the male urethra. Urethral carcinoma occurs in men older than 60 years, but it is an extremely rare form of cancer.

Urethritis

Urethritis is an inflammatory process of the urethra without concurrent bladder infection that is usually, but not always, caused by a sexually transmitted microorganism. Biologic agents associated with infectious urethritis in males include *Neisseria gonorrhoeae* and *Chlamydia trachomatis, Ueaplasma urealyticum,* and other, less common, mycobacteria; parasites (e.g., *Trichomonas vaginalis*); and viruses (herpes simplex virus [HSV]).[12,13] Infectious urethritis caused by *N. gonorrhoeae* often is called *gonococcal urethritis (GU);* infection caused by other microorganisms is called *nongonococcal urethritis (NGU).*[14] (Sexually transmitted urethritis is described in Chapter 26.) Nonsexual origins of urethritis include inflammation or infection as a result of urologic procedures, insertion of foreign bodies into the urethra, anatomic abnormalities, or trauma.

Noninfectious urethritis is rare and is associated with the ingestion of wood alcohol, ethyl alcohol, or turpentine. It is seen also with Reiter syndrome, which involves a number of mucocutaneous lesions.

Symptoms of urethritis include urethral tingling, itching, or burning sensation on urination (dysuria), frequency, and urgency. The individual may note a purulent or clear mucus-like discharge from the urethra. Nucleic acid detection amplification tests allow easy detection of *N. gonorrhoeae* and *C. trachomatis* in first-void urine.[14] Treatment consists of appropriate antibiotic therapy for infectious urethritis and avoidance of future chemical or mechanical irritation.

Urethral Stricture

A **urethral stricture** is a fibrotic narrowing of the urethra caused by scarring. The scars may be congenital but are more likely to result from trauma or untreated or severe urethral infections, most often from long-term use of indwelling urinary catheters. It can present at any age and has a wide range of etiologic factors, including infection, trauma, and instrumentation. Large catheters and instruments cause internal trauma and ischemia, whereas external trauma, such as pelvic fracture, can partially or completely sever the urethra and cause severe and complex strictures.[15] In addition, a report has concluded that stricture may occur decades after initial hypospadias surgery.[16] Urethral carcinoma is a less common cause of urethral stricture. Prostatitis and infection secondary to urinary stasis are common complications. Severe and prolonged obstruction can result in hydronephrosis and renal failure. In addition, chronic, severe strictures may lead to urethral fistulas and periurethral abscesses.[15,17]

The clinical manifestations of urethral stricture are caused by bladder outlet obstruction. The primary symptom is diminished force and caliber of the urinary stream; other symptoms include urinary frequency and hesitancy, mild dysuria, double urine stream or spraying, and postvoiding dribbling. Symptoms of acute urinary retention may occur in the presence of infection or urinary obstruction. Induration at the stricture site may be palpable. Tender, enlarged masses along the urethra usually indicate periurethral abscesses. Urethral stricture often manifests itself as lower urinary tract symptoms or urinary tract infections with significant impairment in the quality of life.

Urethral stricture is diagnosed on the basis of history, physical examination, urinary flow rates, voiding cystourethrogram, and urethroscopy; biopsy confirms carcinoma. Treatment is usually surgical and may involve urethral dilation, urethrotomy, or a variety of open surgical techniques. The choice of surgical intervention depends on the age of the individual and the severity of the problem. Strictures may recur up to 1 year after treatment. Follow-up is necessary during this time; urinary flow measurements and urethrogram help determine extent of residual obstruction.

Disorders of the Penis

Phimosis and Paraphimosis

Phimosis and paraphimosis are disorders in which the foreskin (prepuce) is "too tight" to be moved easily over the glans penis. **Phimosis** is a condition in which the foreskin cannot be retracted back over the glans, whereas **paraphimosis** is the opposite: the foreskin is retracted and cannot be moved forward (reduced) to cover the glans (Figure 25-1). Both conditions can cause penile pathologic conditions.

The inability to retract the foreskin is normal in infancy and is caused by congenital adhesions. During the first 3 years of life these adhesions separate naturally with penile erections and are not an indication for circumcision. Although most cases occur in uncircumcised males, stenosis and resultant phimosis can occur in males with excessive skin remaining after circumcision.[17] Phimosis can occur at any age and is caused most commonly by poor hygiene and chronic infection. Chronic

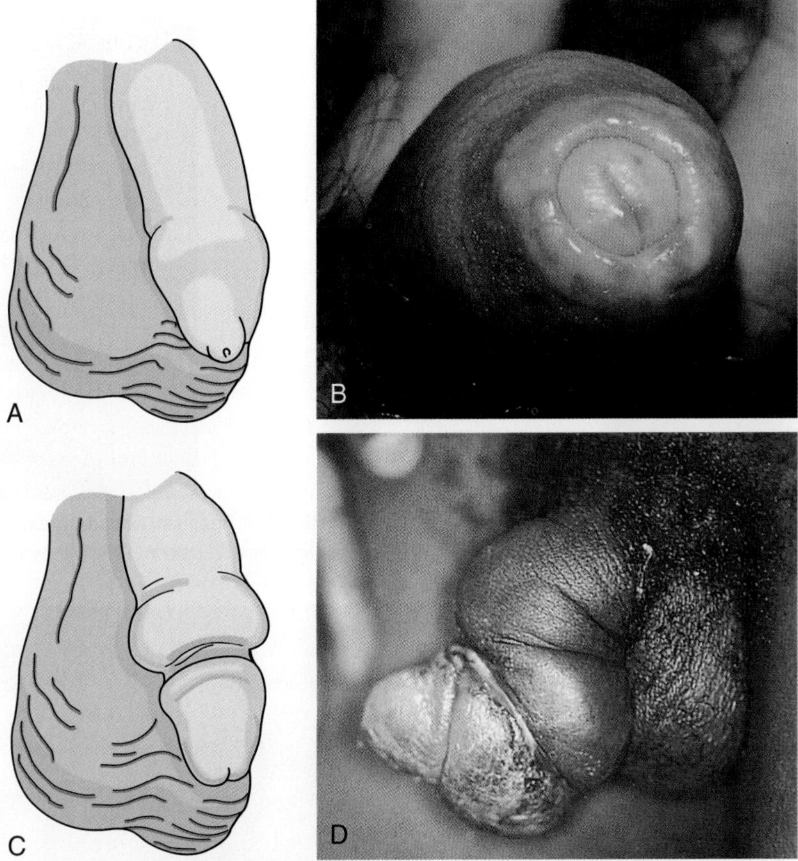

FIGURE 25-1 **Phimosis and Paraphimosis. A,** Phimosis: the foreskin has a narrow opening that is not large enough to permit retraction over the glans. **B,** Lesions on the prepuce secondary to infection cause swelling, and retraction of foreskin may be impossible. **C,** Paraphimosis: the foreskin is retracted over the glans but cannot be reduced to its normal position. Here it has formed a constricting band around the penis. **D,** Ulcer on the retracted prepuce with edema. (**A, C** from Monahan FD, et al: *Phipps' medical-surgical nursing,* ed 8, St Louis, 2007, Mosby; **B** from Taylor PK: *Diagnostic picture tests in sexually transmitted diseases,* London, 1995, Mosby-Wolfe; **D** from Morse SA, Holmes KK, Ballard RC: *Atlas of sexually transmitted diseases and AIDS,* ed 4, London, 2011, Saunders.)

balanoposthitis (inflammation of the glans and prepuce) predisposes older diabetic men to phimosis. It rarely occurs with normal foreskin.

Edema, erythema, and tenderness of the prepuce and purulent discharge are usually the reasons for seeking treatment; inability to retract the foreskin is a less common complaint. Circumcision, if needed, is performed after infection has been eradicated. Complications of phimosis include inflammation of the glans (balanitis) or prepuce (posthitis) and paraphimosis. There is a higher incidence of penile carcinoma in uncircumcised males, which is associated with morbidity and mortality, but chronic infection, most likely with HPV, is usually the underlying factor in such cases. Approximately 40% of invasive penile carcinomas are attributable to HPV.[17,18]

Paraphimosis, in which the foreskin is retracted, can constrict the penis, causing edema of the glans. If edema is such that the foreskin cannot be reduced manually, surgery must be performed to prevent necrosis of the glans caused by constricted blood vessels. Severe paraphimosis is a surgical emergency and phimosis may require immediate release if there is urinary obstruction.

Peyronie Disease

Peyronie disease (bent nail syndrome) is a fibrotic condition of the tunica albuginea of the penis resulting in varying degrees of curvature and sexual dysfunction[19] (Figure 25-2). Peyronie disease develops slowly and is characterized by tough, fibrous thickening of the fascia in the erectile tissue of the corpora cavernosa. A dense fibrous plaque is usually palpable on the dorsum of the penile shaft. The problem usually affects middle-age men and is associated with painful erection, painful intercourse (for both partners), and poor erection distal to the involved area. In some cases, impotence or unsatisfactory penetration occurs. There is no pain when the penis is flaccid.

Although the exact cause is unknown, a local vasculitis-like inflammatory reaction occurs and decreased tissue oxygenation results in fibrosis and calcification. Peyronie disease is associated with Dupuytren contracture (a flexion deformity of the fingers or toes caused by shortening or fibrosis of the palmar or plantar fascia), diabetes, tendency to develop keloids, and in rare cases, use of beta-blocker medications.

There is no definitive treatment for Peyronie disease. Spontaneous remissions occur in as many as 50% of cases. Treatment

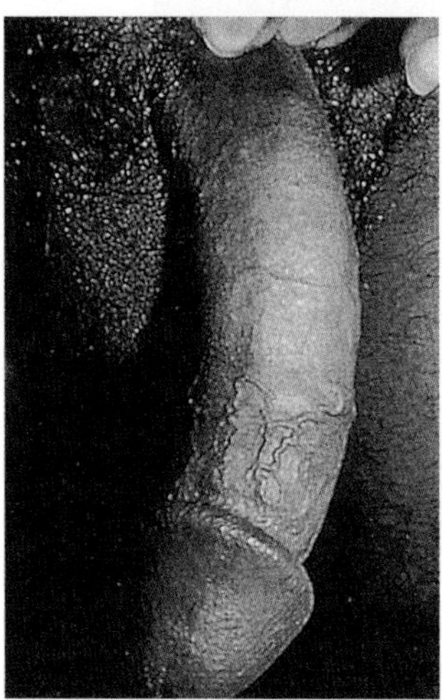

FIGURE 25-2 Peyronie Disease. (From Taylor PK: *Diagnostic picture tests in sexually transmitted diseases,* London, 1995, Mosby-Wolfe.)

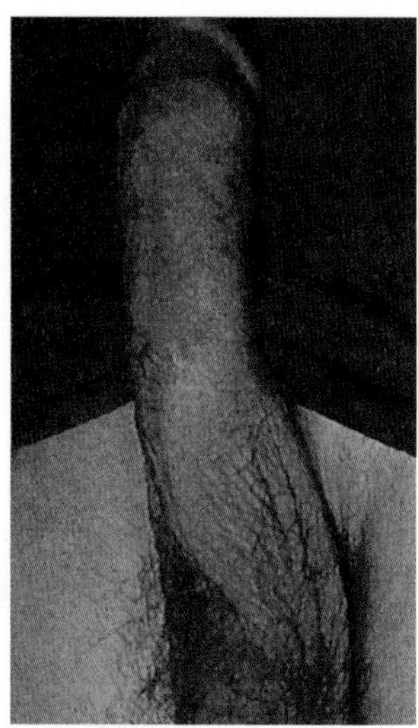

FIGURE 25-3 Priapism. (From Lloyd-Davies RW, Gow JG, Davies DR: *Color atlas of urology,* ed 2, London, 1994, Mosby-Wolfe.)

with pharmacologic therapies include colchicine, aminobenzoate potassium (Potaba), L-carnitine, and liposomal superoxide dismutase. Men suffering with Peyronie disease who have significant penile deformity precluding successful coitus can be appraised for surgical correction. Surgery is considered the gold standard and includes plication, incision and grafting, or penile-prosthesis-related procedures.[17,19]

Priapism

Priapism is an uncommon condition of prolonged penile erection. It is usually painful and is not associated with sexual arousal (Figure 25-3). Priapism is idiopathic in 60% of cases; the remaining 40% of cases are associated with spinal cord trauma, sickle cell disease, leukemia, pelvic tumors or infections, or penile trauma. Priapism also has been associated with cocaine use.[20,21] Intracavernous injection therapy for impotence seems to be the most common cause. Prolonged sexual stimulation often is associated with initial development of the idiopathic type.[17] The two corpora cavernosa within the erect penis are filled with blood and are tender to palpation; neither the corpus spongiosum nor the glans is engorged. The vascular congestion is thought to be associated with venous obstruction. If the erection remains over a period of days, edema and fibrosis develop, leading to erectile dysfunction (impotence).

Priapism is a urologic emergency. Treatment within hours is effective and prevents impotence. Conservative approaches include iced saline enemas, ketamine administration, and spinal anesthesia. Needle aspiration of blood from the corpus through the dorsal glans is often effective and is followed by catheterization and pressure dressings to maintain decompression. More aggressive surgical treatments include the creation of vascular shunts to maintain blood flow. Erectile dysfunction results in up to 50% of prolonged cases.

Balanitis

Balanitis is an inflammation of the glans penis (Figure 25-4) and usually occurs in conjunction with posthitis, an inflammation of the prepuce. It is associated with poor hygiene and

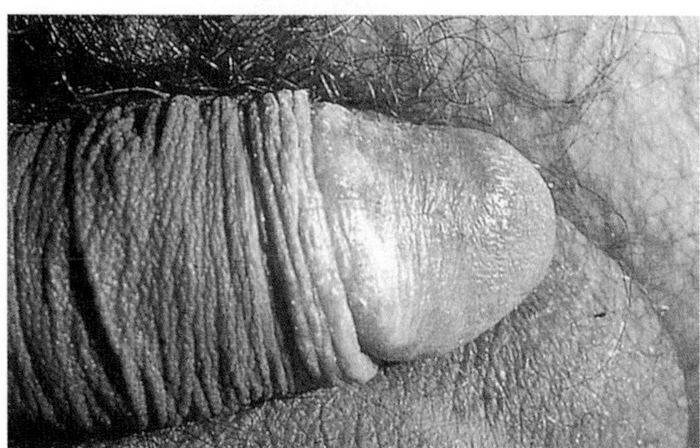

FIGURE 25-4 Balanitis. Itchy, red rash on glans of penis secondary to *Candida albicans.* (From Taylor PK: *Diagnostic picture tests in sexually transmitted diseases,* London, 1995, Mosby-Wolfe.)

phimosis. The accumulation under the foreskin of glandular secretions (smegma), sloughed epithelial cells, and *Mycobacterium smegmatis* can irritate the glans directly or lead to infection. Skin disorders (e.g., psoriasis, lichen planus, eczema) and candidiasis must be differentiated from inflammation resulting from poor hygienic practices. Balanitis is seen most commonly in men with poorly controlled diabetes mellitus and candidiasis. Antimicrobials are used to treat infection. Circumcision can prevent recurrences and can be considered after the inflammation has subsided.

Penile Cancer

In the United States, carcinoma of the penis is rare and affects about 1 in 100,000 men. Approximately 1570 cases and 310 deaths were estimated in the year 2012.[1] Although rare in North America and Europe, where it accounts for about 0.2% of cancers and 0.1% of cancer deaths in men, penile cancer may account for up to 10% of cancers in African and South American men.

In the United States, about four out of five cases of the disease are diagnosed in men older than age 55 years.[22] Major risk factors include infection with HPV (mainly serotypes 16 and

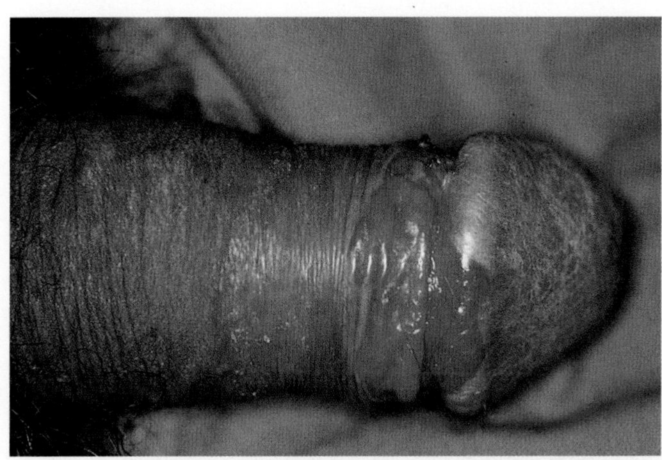

FIGURE 25-5 Squamous Cell Carcinoma Involving the Glans Penis. (From Callen JP et al: *Color atlas of dermatology,* Philadelphia, 1993, Saunders.)

18), smoking, and psoriasis treated with a combination involving the drug psoralen and ultraviolet (UV) light. Men circumcised at birth have less than half the chance of getting penile cancer than those who were not. Penile cancer is more common in men with phimosis and those with acquired immunodeficiency syndrome (AIDS).[22] About two thirds of men with penile cancer are diagnosed at more than 65 years of age.[1]

Before the development of penile cancer, signs of premalignant cancer or epidermal cancer in situ are present.[23] These include thick white plaque (leukoplakia) that typically involves the meatus; red, inflamed areas of Paget disease; red, velvety, ulcerative lesions of erythroplasia of Queyrat that usually involve the glans; large, invasive, scaly growths of Buschke-Löwenstein tumor; red plaque with encrustations of Bowen disease; and in situ carcinoma that generally affects the penile shaft. Men with leukoplakia or erythroplasia of Queyrat may have concurrent invasive penile carcinoma.[22,24] Pain and bleeding are late signs of penile cancer. Condylomata (genital warts) caused by HPV may be involved in the development of precancerous lesions (see Chapter 26 for a discussion of HPV). At times the penis might be the site of metastatic spread of solid tumors from the bladder, prostate, rectum, or kidney. Early squamous cell carcinoma and premalignant epidermal lesions are easily treated but are often ignored. Delays in seeking treatment are attributed to denial, embarrassment, failure to detect lesions under a phimotic foreskin, fear, guilt, and ignorance.

Penile cancer is mostly squamous cell carcinoma, which usually begins as a small, fat, ulcerative or papillary lesion on the glans or foreskin that grows to involve the entire penile shaft (Figure 25-5). Extensive lesions are associated with metastases and a poor prognosis.[23] These lesions are not as painful as the amount of tissue involvement would seem to indicate. The regional femoral and iliac nodes are common metastatic sites. Rarely the urethra and bladder are involved. Weight loss, fatigue, and malaise accompany chronic suppurative lesions. Untreated, progressive disease causes death within 2 years.

The specific diagnosis is made by biopsy after examination to document the location, size, and fixation of the lesion. After a positive biopsy the extent of cancer spread is determined by imaging tests such as ultrasound, CT, or MRI. Fine-needle aspiration of lymph tissue confirms absence or presence of regional adenopathy.[22] About 30% of penile cancers spread to lymph nodes before diagnosis. Distant metastases occur in less than 10% of cases and may involve lung, liver, bone, or brain.[24] The following stages are used for penile cancer: stage 0 (carcinoma in situ), stage I, stage II, stage III, and stage IV.[25]

Penile carcinoma is primarily managed with surgery. Newer, innovative surgical techniques can preserve as much penile tissue as possible without compromising cancer control. For invasive penile carcinoma, complete excision leaving adequate tumor-free margins is the goal. A simple circumcision may be sufficient for localized lesions of the prepuce. If the primary site is the glans and distal shaft, removal of the penis may be necessary. Although conventional radical surgery continues to be an effective approach, the emasculating nature of the treatment has serious psychologic and sexual consequences. Recent studies have challenged the conventional belief that a 2-cm margin was required for adequate cancer control.[23] Newer innovative surgical techniques can preserve as much penile tissue and functional integrity as possible without compromising cancer control. Inguinal lymph nodes also are removed if metastasis to these structures is known or suspected. Palliative treatment with radiation or chemotherapy may be used when the disease is inoperable and bulky inguinal metastases have occurred. Options for individuals with carcinoma in situ include local excision, radiation, laser surgery, cryosurgery, chemosurgery, or chemotherapy with topical (5%) 5-fluorouracil (5-FU). Differentiation, tumor stage, and age influence prognosis.[23,26] The 5-year survival rate for stage I disease is greater than 80%; average 5-year survival rate for all stages is 50%.[1,22]

Disorders of the Scrotum, Testis, and Epididymis

Disorders of the Scrotum

Men may seek treatment for painful or painless scrotal masses. Masses may be serious (cancer or torsion) or benign (hydrocele or cyst) and may require immediate surgical intervention or allow for careful observation.[27] Varicocele, hydrocele, and spermatocele are common intrascrotal disorders.[28-30] A **varicocele** is an abnormal dilation of a vein within the spermatic cord and is classically described as a "bag of worms" (Figure 25-6). Most (95%) occur on the left side and may be painful or tender. Varicocele occurs in 10% of males and is seen most often after puberty. Sudden development of a varicocele in an older man is a late sign of renal tumor.[31] Unilateral right-sided varicoceles are rare and result from compression or obstruction of the inferior vena cava by a tumor or thrombus. Color Doppler ultrasonography is used to confirm the diagnosis.[27]

The cause of varicocele is incompetent or congenitally absent valves in the spermatic veins. The valves that normally prevent backflow are absent or do not close adequately, permitting blood to pool in the veins rather than flow into the venous system. Varicocele decreases blood flow through the testis. This interferes with spermatogenesis and is a cause of infertility.[28,32] If infertility is a problem, treatment consists of ligation of the spermatic vein or occlusion of the vein by percutaneous methods, such as balloon catheter and sclerosing fluids.[32] If varicocele is mild and fertility is not an issue, a scrotal support

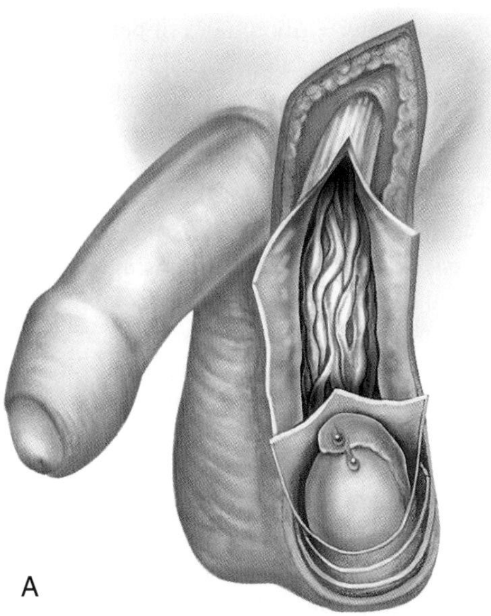

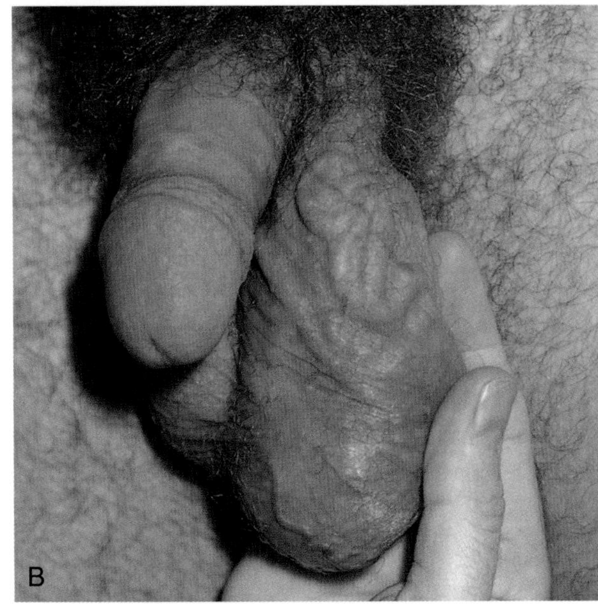

FIGURE 25-6 Varicocele. **A,** Dilation of veins within the spermatic cord. **B,** Varicocele on physical examination. (**A** from Seidel H et al: *Mosby's guide to physical examination,* ed 7, St Louis, 2011, Mosby. **B** from Swartz MH: *Textbook of physical diagnosis,* ed 6, Philadelphia, 2010, Saunders.)

usually is sufficient to relieve symptoms of scrotal heaviness or "dragging."

A **hydrocele** is a collection of fluid within the tunica vaginalis[28,33] (Figure 25-7). It is the most common cause of scrotal swelling. Hydroceles occur in 6% of male newborns and are congenital malformations (patent processus vaginalis) that often resolve spontaneously in the first year of life. Surgical ligation is recommended if hydrocele persists after age 1 year.[30] Hydroceles in adults may be caused by an imbalance between the secreting and absorptive capacities of scrotal tissues. Hydroceles range in size from slightly larger than the testes to the size of a grapefruit or larger and may be flaccid or tense. Compression of testicular blood supply may lead to atrophy.

The exact mechanism of idiopathic hydrocele is unknown. Secondary hydrocele may result from trauma or infection of the testis or epididymis or from a testicular tumor. Rapid accumulation of fluid occurs after local injury, radiotherapy, or infection (epididymitis or orchitis), or it may accompany testicular neoplasm. Chronic hydroceles are more common and occur in men older than 40 because of an imbalance between fluid secretion and reabsorption in the tunica vaginalis. A painless, extratesticular mass that easily transilluminates is found on physical examination. Ultrasonography of a large hydrocele, which may conceal a testicular tumor, is recommended. Treatment is usually not required unless a large, bulky hydrocele causes considerable physical discomfort or undesirable cosmetic appearance.[28] Treatment for uncomplicated hydrocele is aspiration of the fluid and injection of a sclerosing agent into the scrotal sac.[33-35] The goal of treatment is to remove the hydrocele and prevent recurrence by sclerosing or excising the tunica vaginalis.

Spermatoceles (epididymal cysts) are benign cystic collections of fluid of the epididymis located between the head of the epididymis and the testis. Efferent ducts of the epididymis have potential for cystic dilation to form a spermatocele [33,35] (Figure 25-8). Spermatoceles are filled with milky fluid that contains sperm. Spermatocele is differentiated from a hydrocele in that aspiration of the hydrocele recovers a clear, yellow fluid, and unlike a hydrocele, a spermatocele does not cover the entire anterior surface of the testis.

Spermatoceles manifest as discrete, firm, freely mobile masses distinct from the testis that may be transilluminated. Epididymal cysts do not require treatment.[33] A spermatic cord tumor may feel like a tense spermatocele but does not contain fluid and will not transilluminate.[27] Spermatoceles that cause pain or discomfort are excised. Usually, however, spermatoceles are asymptomatic or produce mild discomfort that is relieved by scrotal support.[35] Neither hydroceles nor spermatoceles are associated with infertility.

Cryptorchidism and Ectopy

Cryptorchidism is a condition of testicular maldescent, whereas an **ectopic testis** has strayed from the normal pathway of descent. Ectopy may be caused by an abnormal connection at the distal end of the gubernaculum testis that leads the gonad to an abnormal position, usually at the superficial inguinal site. In cryptorchidism the descent of one or both testes is arrested, with unilateral arrest occurring more often than bilateral arrest.[35] The testes may remain in the abdomen, or testicular descent may be arrested in the inguinal canal or the puboscrotal junction. Cryptorchidism is a common congenital anomaly, with an incidence of approximately 3% in full-term infants. However, this rate increases significantly with low birth weight infants; for instance, the rate of cryptorchidism at 3 months has been found to be 7.7% for infants with birth weights less than 2000 g, 2.5% for birth weights of 2000 to 2500 g, and 1.41% for birth weights of 2500 g or more.[35,36] The incidence of cryptorchidism in adults is 0.7% to 0.8%.[32] Cryptorchidism is commonly associated with vasal or epididymal abnormalities. These

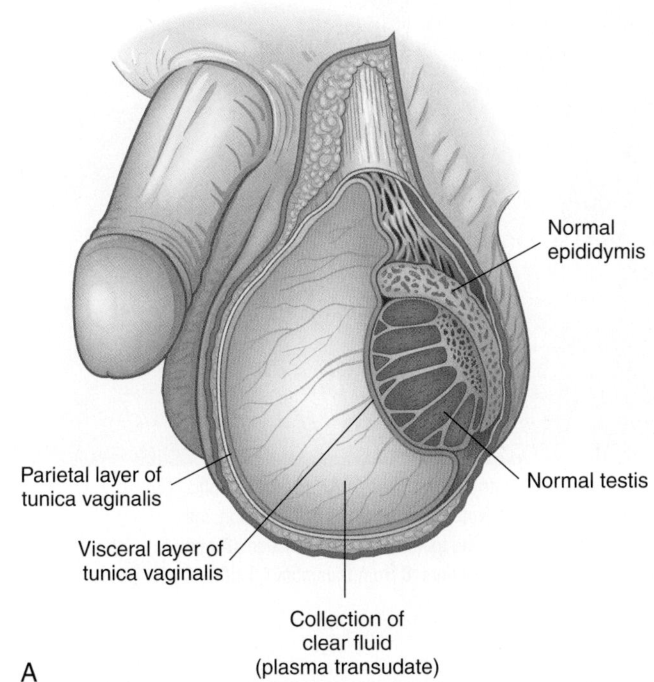

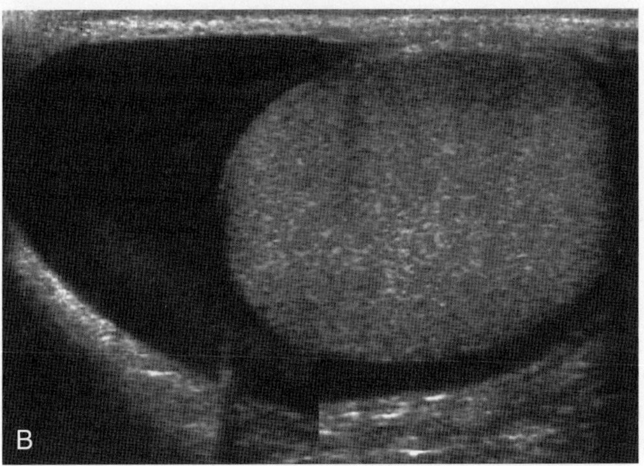

FIGURE 25-7 Depiction of a Hydrocele. A, Accumulation of clear fluid between the visceral (inner) and parietal (outer) layers of the tunica vaginalis. **B,** The appearance of a hydrocele on ultrasound examination. (**B** from Adam A, et al: *Grainger & Allison's diagnostic radiology,* ed 6, London, 2008, Churchill Livingstone.)

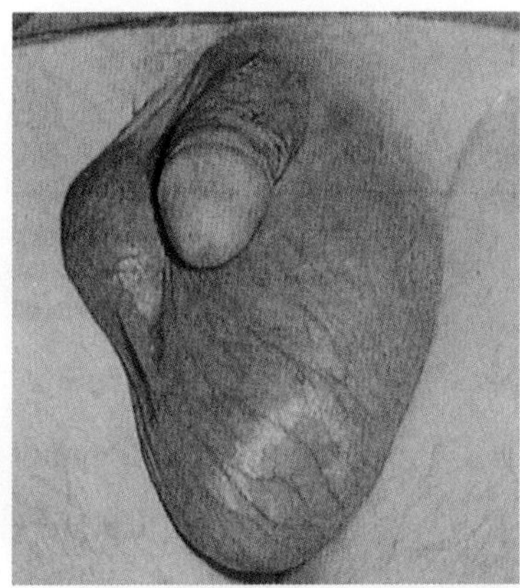

FIGURE 25-8 Spermatocele. Retention cyst of the head of the epididymis or of an aberrant tubule or tubules of the rete testis. The spermatocele lies outside the tunica vaginalis; therefore, on palpation it can be readily distinguished and separated from the testis. (From Lloyd-Davies RW, Gow JG, Davies DR: *Color atlas of urology,* ed 2, London, 1994, Mosby-Wolfe.)

congenital anomalies affect about one third to two thirds of newborns with cryptorchidism. Other structural anomalies include posterior urethral valves (less than 5%), upper tract abnormalities (less than 5%), and hypospadias. The presence of hypospadias as well as cryptorchidism raises the suspicion of mixed gonadal dysgenesis (intersex infant). It has been hypothesized that cryptorchidism may result from an absence or abnormality of the gubernaculum, a cordlike structure that extends from the lower pole of the testis to the scrotum; a congenital gonadal or dysgenetic defect that makes the testes insensitive to gonadotropins (a likely explanation for unilateral cryptorchidism); or lack of maternal gonadotropins (a likely explanation for bilateral cryptorchidism of prematurity).[32] Mechanical possibilities include a short spermatic cord, fibrous bands or adhesions in the normal path of the testes, or a narrowed inguinal canal. Chromosomal studies do not support a genetic component. Physiologic cryptorchidism, also called *retractile* or *migratory testis,* is an involuntary retraction of the testes out of the scrotum that occurs with excitement, physical activity, or exposure to cold and is caused by the small mass of prepubertal testis and the strength of the cremaster muscle. This is a common phenomenon that is self-limiting (descent occurs at puberty).

Physical examination discloses the absence of one or both testes in the scrotum and an atrophic scrotum on the affected side. If the undescended testis is in a vulnerable position, for example, over the pubic bone, an individual may complain of severe pain secondary to trauma. The adult male with bilateral cryptorchidism may be infertile. Ultrasonography, CT, or MRI can be used to locate an intra-abdominal or nonpalpable testis.

Testicular cancer is also a well-established complication of cryptorchidism. In men with a history of unilateral cryptorchidism, neoplasms also develop more commonly in the contralateral testis. This finding suggests cryptorchidism affects the testes and is a process more significant than simply the position of the testis in childhood.[35] The risk of testicular cancer is 35 to 50 times greater for men with cryptorchidism or a history of cryptorchidism than for the general male population. Because definite histologic change (decreased Leydig cells, loss of germ cells, and peritubular fibrosis) occurs in the cryptorchid testis by 1 year of age, surgical correction is recommended earlier.[37] Treatment often begins with administration of GnRH or human chorionic gonadotropin (hCG), hormones that may initiate descent, making surgery unnecessary. GnRH is given as a nasal spray in Europe and may enhance germ-cell counts even when the testis does not descend.[37] If hormonal therapy is not successful, the testis is located and moved surgically (orchiopexy) in young children or removed (orchiectomy) in adults and children older than 10 years.[37] The testis that is properly placed in the scrotum provides adequate hormonal function and gives the scrotum a normal appearance. A successful operation does not ensure fertility if the testis is congenitally defective. Approximately 20% of males with unilateral undescended testis remain infertile even

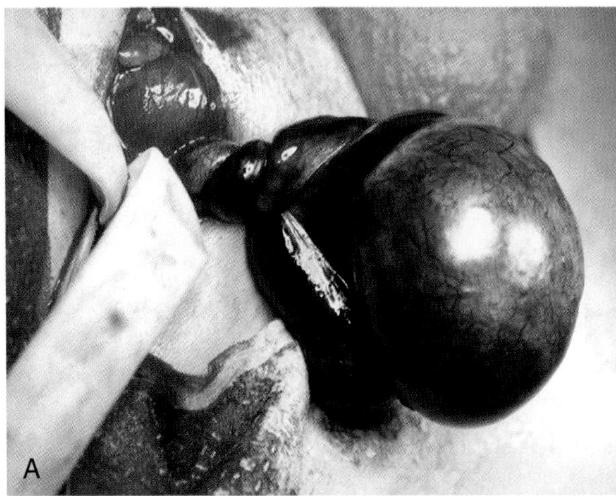

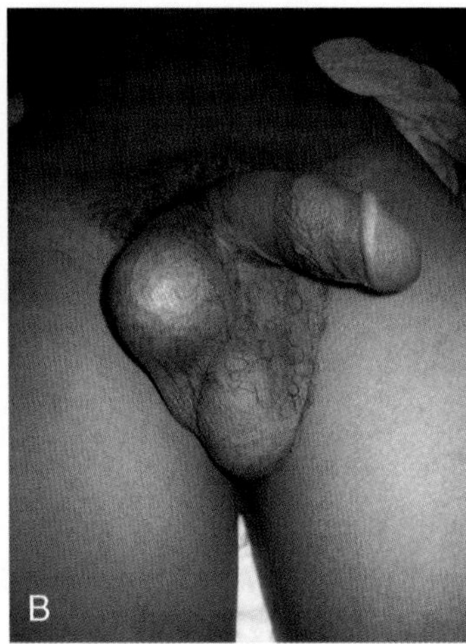

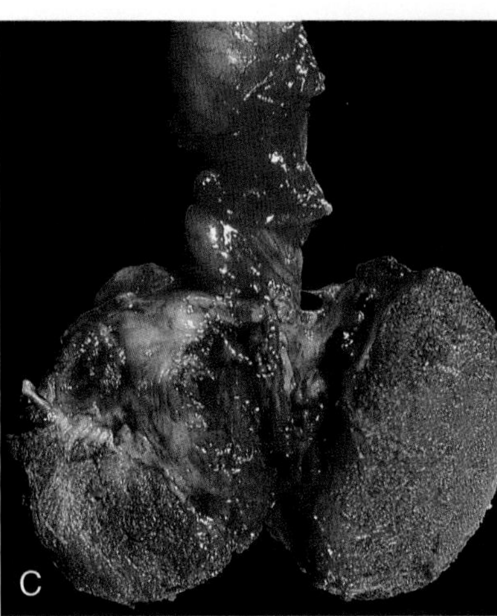

FIGURE 25-9 Torsion of the Testes. **A,** Left testicular torsion in an adolescent with acute scrotum; the testis is necrotic. **B,** Late phase torsion in an adolescent with severe testicular pain 1 month previously. Note the absence of inflammation and high position of testis in scrotum. **C,** The testes appear dark red and partially necrotic owing to hemorrhagic infarction. (**A** and **B** from Kliegman RM et al: *Nelson's textbook of pediatrics,* ed 19, Philadelphia, 2011, Saunders. **C** from Damjanov I, Linder J, editors: *Anderson's pathology,* ed 10, St Louis, 1996, Mosby.)

TABLE 25-1 DIAGNOSIS OF SELECTED CONDITIONS RESPONSIBLE FOR THE ACUTE SCROTUM

CONDITION	ONSET OF SYMPTOMS	AGE	TENDERNESS	URINALYSIS	CREMASTERIC REFLEX	TREATMENT
Testicular torsion	Acute	Early puberty	Diffuse	Negative	Negative	Surgical exploration
Appendiceal torsion	Subacute	Prepubertal	Localized to upper pole	Negative	Positive	Bed rest and scrotal elevation
Epididymis	Insidious	Adolescence	Epididymal	Positive or negative	Positive	Antibiotics

though orchiopexy is performed by age 1 year; most individuals with treated or untreated bilateral testicular maldescent have poor fertility. In addition, placement of the cryptorchid testis into the scrotal sac does not decrease the potential for malignancy; it does facilitate examination and tumor detection.

Torsion of the Testis

Torsion of the testis is rotation of a testis, which twists blood vessels in the spermatic cord. It causes an acute scrotum, which is testicular pain and swelling (Figure 25-9). Differentiation between testicular torsion and two other common causes of an acute scrotum is based on physical examination and history[35] (Table 25-1). This event is most common among neonates and pubertal adolescents, but it can occur in males at any age.[30] Onset may be spontaneous or follow physical exertion or trauma. Torsion twists the arteries and veins in the spermatic cord, reducing or stopping circulation to the testis. Vascular engorgement and ischemia develop, causing scrotal swelling and pain. These manifestations are not relieved by scrotal elevation (Prehn sign), rest, or scrotal support. On physical examination, men have a tender high-riding testis, a thickened spermatic cord, and an absent cremasteric reflex. Unlike epididymitis, the epididymis cannot be differentiated from the testis.[35] Diagnostic testing includes urinalysis (to rule out infection) and color Doppler ultrasonography.[32] Torsion of the testis is a surgical emergency. If the torsion cannot be reduced manually, surgery must be performed within 6 hours after the onset of symptoms to preserve normal testicular function. Surgery includes untwisting the spermatic cord and anchoring both testes in correct position within the scrotum to prevent recurrences. With successful manual detorsion, surgical fixation should be done within a few days.

Orchitis

Orchitis is an acute infection of the testes (Figure 25-10) and is uncommon except as a complication of systemic infection or as an extension of an associated epididymitis[38] (see p. 897). Infectious microorganisms may reach the testes through the blood or the lymphatics or, most commonly, by ascent through the urethra, vas deferens, and epididymis. Most cases of orchitis are actually cases of epididymo-orchitis. Occasionally, in middle-age men, a nonspecific, apparently noninfectious, inflammatory process (called *granulomatous orchitis*) occurs. It seems to be an autoimmune disease that triggers a granulomatous response to spermatozoa.

Mumps is the most common infectious cause of orchitis and usually affects postpubertal males. The onset is sudden, occurring 3 to 4 days after the onset of parotitis. Signs and symptoms include high fever, reaching 40° C (104° F), marked prostration, bilateral or unilateral erythema, edema and tenderness of the

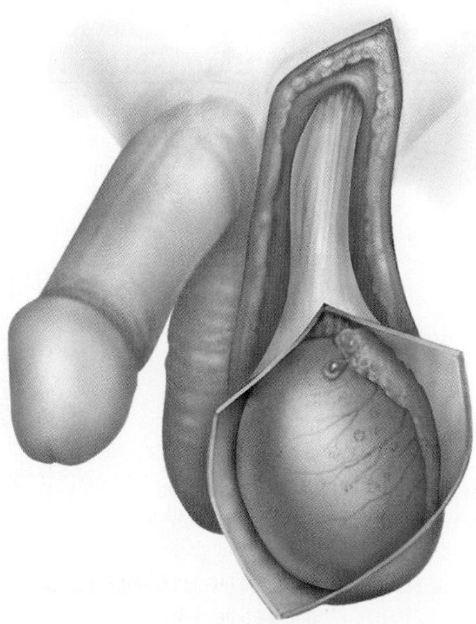

FIGURE 25-10 Orchitis. Inflammation of the testicle with enlargement or swelling. (From Seidel H et al: *Mosby's guide to physical examination,* ed 7, St Louis, 2011, Mosby.)

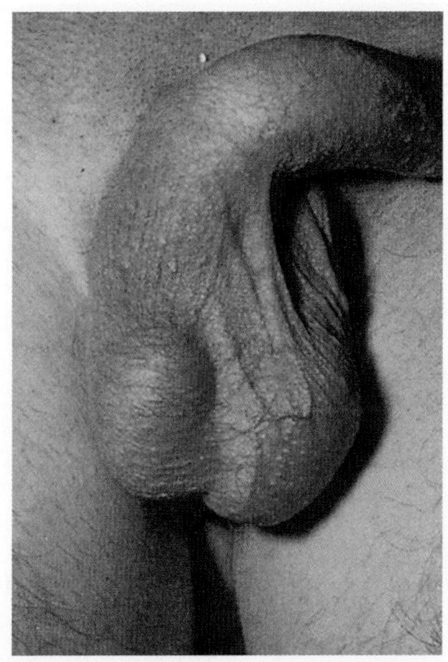

FIGURE 25-11 Testicular Tumor. (From Wolfe J: *400 Self assessment picture tests in clinical medicine,* London, 1984, Mosby.)

scrotum, and leukocytosis. An acute hydrocele may develop. Urinary signs and symptoms, which accompany epididymitis, are absent. Atrophy with irreversible damage to spermatogenesis may result in 30% of affected testes. Bilateral orchitis does not affect androgenic function but may cause permanent sterility.

Treatment is supportive and includes bed rest, scrotal support, elevation of the scrotum, hot or cold compresses, and analgesic agents for relief of pain. If an acute hydrocele develops, it is aspirated. Testicular abscess usually requires orchiectomy (removal of the testis). Appropriate antimicrobial drugs should be used for bacterial orchitis, and corticosteroids are indicated in proved cases of nonspecific granulomatous orchitis.

Cancer of the Testis

Testicular cancer is a highly treatable, usually curable, cancer that most often develops in young and middle-aged men. For men with seminoma (all stages combined), the cure rate exceeds 90%. For those with low-stage seminoma or nonseminoma, the cure rate approaches 100%.[39] Overall, testicular cancers are rare, yet they are the most common form of cancer in young men between ages 15 and 35. Approximately 8590 cases and 360 deaths were estimated for 2012.[1] In the United States, the lifetime probability of developing testicular cancer is 0.2% for white men, an incidence that is four times higher than for blacks. Testicular tumors are slightly more common on the right side than on the left, a pattern that parallels the occurrence of cryptorchidism; about 1% to 2% of primary testicular cancers are bilateral (Figure 25-11), and 50% of these tumors arise from treated or untreated cryptorchid testes.

PATHOGENESIS. Ninety percent of testicular cancers are germ-cell tumors arising from the male gametes. Germ-cell tumors constitute 90% of testicular cancers and can be broadly classified into two types: seminomas and nonseminomas. Seminomas are the most common, are the least aggressive, and make up about 30% to 35% of testicular cancers. Nonseminomas include embryonal carcinomas, teratomas, and choriocarcinomas, the most aggressive but rare (less than 1%) form of testicular cancer. Testicular cancers can include a mix of types.[40] In addition, testicular tumors can arise from specialized cells of the gonadal stroma. These tumors, which are named for their cellular origins, are Leydig cell, Sertoli cell, granulosa cell, and theca cell tumors and constitute less than 10% of all testicular cancers.[41]

The cause of testicular neoplasms is unknown. A genetic predisposition is suggested by the fact that the incidence is higher among brothers, identical twins, and other close male relatives. Genetic predisposition is supported further by statistics showing that the disease is relatively rare among black Africans, black Americans, Asians, and native New Zealanders. Familial testicular germ cell tumors may be associated with transgenerational inheritance of epigenetic events.[42] Risk factors include history of cryptorchidism, abnormal testicular development, human immunodeficiency virus (HIV) and AIDS, Klinefelter syndrome, and history of testicular cancer.[40]

CLINICAL MANIFESTATIONS. Painless testicular enlargement commonly is the first sign of testicular cancer. Enlargement is usually gradual and may be accompanied by a sensation of testicular heaviness or dull ache in the lower abdomen.[40] Occasionally, acute pain occurs because of rapid growth, resulting in hemorrhage and necrosis. Ten percent of affected men have epididymitis, 10% have hydroceles,[35] and 5% have gynecomastia or hydrocele. Incidence of gynecomastia increases considerably (30% to 45%) in men with Sertoli or Leydig tumors. Approximately 10% of individuals already have symptoms related to metastases at the time of initial diagnosis, which correlates with the typical delay of 3 to 6 months from initial recognition to definitive treatment. Lumbar pain may be present

TABLE 25-2 TESTICULAR TUMORS OF GERM CELL ORIGIN

CELL TYPES	OCCURRENCE	METASTATIC PATTERN	PROGNOSIS/REMISSION RATE
A. Seminoma (germinoma)	30%-35% of all testicular tumors	Rarely to retroperitoneal lymph nodes	Excellent; tumor usually remains localized and is responsive to radiation; cure rate stages I and II >95%; stages III and IV >80%
B. Nonseminomatous tumors	60% of all testicular tumors		
1. Single cell			
a. Embryonal carcinoma	20%-25% of all testicular tumors; most common testicular tumor in infants and children	Earlier to regional lymphatics, also lung, liver, bone	Good; complete remission rate stages I and II >95%; stages III and IV >70%-80%
b. Teratoma	5%-10% of all testicular tumors (occurs in children and adults)	Through lymphatics and bloodstream; affects same organ systems as embryonal type	Fair
c. Choriocarcinoma	<1% of all testicular tumors	Earliest and widest, initially through bloodstream	Poor; early metastasis
2. Mixed tumors	30%-40% of all testicular tumors		
a. Teratocarcinoma	20%-25% of all testicular tumors	Mixed pattern; depends on cell types	Variable; prognosis becomes that of the most malignant element
b. Other i. Teratocarcinoma with seminoma ii. Embryonal cancer with seminoma iii. Teratoma with seminoma iv. Any combination with choriocarcinoma	10%-15% of all testicular tumors	Mixed pattern; depends on cell types	Variable; prognosis becomes that of the most malignant element
3. Non–germ cell tumors (Leydig cell, Sertoli cell, granulosa cell, and thecal cell tumors)	<10%		

Data from American Cancer Society. In *Cancer response system document #10029,* New York, 1995, The Society; Cancer Net: *Cancer facts: questions and answers about testicular cancer,* National Cancer Institute, 2000. Available at www.cancernet.nci.nih.gov.

and usually is caused by retroperitoneal node metastasis. Signs of metastasis to the lungs include cough, dyspnea, and bloody sputum (hemoptysis). Supraclavicular node involvement may cause difficulty swallowing (dysphagia) and neck swelling. Alterations in vision or mental status, papilledema, and seizures may be experienced with metastasis to the CNS. Approximately 10% of affected individuals are asymptomatic; the tumor may be detected by the man's sexual partner or incidentally following trauma.

EVALUATION AND TREATMENT. An incorrect diagnosis at the initial examination occurs in as many as 25% of men with testicular cancer. Epididymitis and epididymo-orchitis are the most common misdiagnoses; others include hydrocele and spermatocele. Evaluation begins with careful physical examination, including palpation of the scrotal contents with the individual in the erect and supine positions. The abdomen and lymph nodes are palpated to rule out metastases. Signs of testicular cancer include abnormal consistency, induration, nodularity, or irregularity of the testis. A firm, nontender testicular mass or diffuse enlargement is found in the majority of cases. Primary testicular cancer can be assessed rapidly and accurately by scrotal ultrasonography. Tumor markers are higher than normal in the presence of a tumor and may help detect a tumor that is too small to be palpated during physical examination or seen on imaging.[35] Tumor type is identified after inguinal biopsy or orchiectomy. Scrotal incisions may cause dissemination of the tumor and increase the risk of local recurrence and therefore are avoided. Chest x-ray, lymphangiogram, intravenous pyelogram (IVP), abdominal ultrasound, and CT are used in clinical staging of disease. Treatment is based on type of tumor, stage of disease, general health, and age. Besides surgery, treatment involves radiation and chemotherapy singly or in combination. A number of factors influence the prognosis (Table 25-2). They include histology of the tumor, stage of the disease, and selection of appropriate treatment. Serum markers, such as alpha fetoprotein (AFP), β-hCG, and lactate dehydrogenase, are useful for detecting metastases and assessing responses to therapy. With appropriate treatment survival rates from testicular cancer are excellent, although some have persistent paresthesias, Raynaud phenomenon, or infertility. According to the National Cancer Institute, the overall 5-year survival rate from testicular cancer was 95.3% between 1999 and 2005. If the cancer was confined to the testis at the time of diagnosis, the survival rate was 99.2% and dropped only slightly to 95.9% with regional extension. For those with distant metastases, the survival rate was 71%.[35,40] Orchiectomy does not affect sexual function, but infertility can result from chemotherapy or surgical removal of affected abdominal lymph nodes if nerves

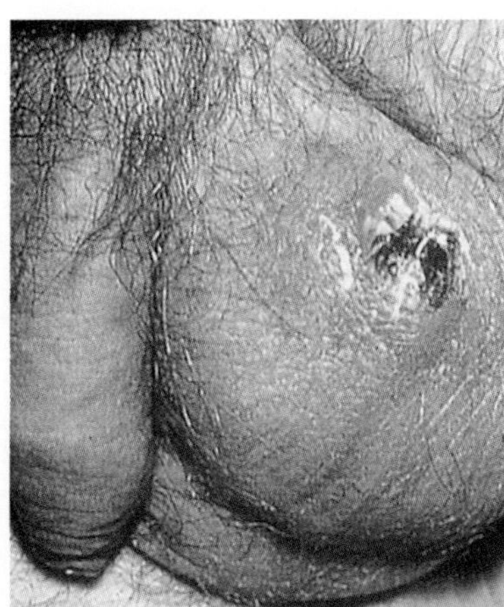

FIGURE 25-12 Epididymitis Secondary to Gonorrhea or Nongonococcal Urethritis. This infection spread to the testes, and rupture through the scrotal wall is threatened. (From Taylor PK: *Diagnostic picture tests in sexually transmitted diseases,* London, 1995, Mosby-Wolfe.)

necessary for ejaculation are severed. After orchiectomy, testicular silicone implants may be used to restore "normal" scrotal appearance.

Epididymitis

Epididymitis, or inflammation of the epididymis, generally occurs in sexually active young males (younger than 35 years) and is rare before puberty (Figure 25-12). In young men the usual cause is a sexually transmitted microorganism, such as *N. gonorrhoeae* or *C. trachomatis.* Men who practice unprotected anal intercourse may acquire sexually transmitted epididymitis because of *Escherichia coli, Haemophilus influenzae,* tuberculosis (especially in regions where incidence of pulmonary tuberculosis is high), *Cryptococcus,* or *Brucella.*[35] In men older than 35 years, enterobacteriaceae (intestinal bacteria) and *Pseudomonas aeruginosa* associated with urinary tract infections and prostatitis also may cause epididymitis. Besides an infectious etiology, epididymitis may result from a chemical inflammation caused by the reflux of sterile urine into the ejaculatory ducts.[43] It is associated with urethral strictures, congenital posterior valves, and excessive physical straining in which increased abdominal pressure is transmitted to the bladder. Chemical epididymitis is usually self-limiting and does not require evaluation or intervention unless it persists.

PATHOGENESIS. The pathogenic microorganism usually reaches the epididymis by ascending the vasa deferentia from an already infected urethra or bladder. The presence of bacteria initiates the inflammatory response, causing symptoms of bacterial epididymitis. Epididymitis caused by heavy lifting or straining results from reflux of urine from the bladder into the vas deferens and epididymis. Urine is extremely irritating to the epididymis and initiates an inflammatory response called *chemical epididymitis.*

CLINICAL MANIFESTATIONS. Pain is the main symptom of epididymitis. Scrotal or inguinal pain is caused by inflammation of the epididymis and surrounding tissues. The pain is usually acute and severe. Flank pain may occur if, as the urethra passes over the spermatic cord, edematous swelling of the cord obstructs the urethra. The individual may have pyuria and bacteriuria and a history of urinary symptoms, including urethral discharge. The scrotum on the involved side is red and edematous as a result of inflammatory changes. The tail of the epididymis near the lower pole of the testes usually swells first; then swelling ascends to the head of the epididymis. The spermatic cord also may be swollen and tender.

Complications of epididymitis include abscess formation, infarction of the testis, recurrent infection, and infertility. Infarction probably is caused by thrombosis (obstruction by blood clots) of the prostatic vessels secondary to severe inflammation. Recurrent epididymitis may result from inadequate initial treatment or failure to identify or treat predisposing factors. Chronic epididymitis can cause scarring of the epididymal endothelium. Once scarring has occurred, treatment with antibiotics is ineffective because adequate antibiotic levels cannot be achieved within the epididymis.[43]

EVALUATION AND TREATMENT. A history of recent urinary tract infection or urethral discharge suggests the diagnosis of epididymitis. The relief of pain when the inflamed testis and epididymis are elevated (Prehn sign) is also diagnostic. Definitive diagnosis is based on culture or Gram stain of a urethral swab. Epididymal aspiration may be necessary to obtain a specimen, especially if the individual has been taking antibiotics and has sterile urine.

Treatment includes antibiotic therapy for the infection itself (see Chapter 26). Analgesics, ice, and scrotal elevation can provide symptomatic relief. If the individual does not steadily improve, he should be reevaluated for possible complications, such as abscess formation, sepsis, or continued infection.[35] Bed rest and scrotal elevation are recommended until the scrotum is no longer tender. Scrotal elevation facilitates maximal lymphatic and venous drainage. Abscess formation is rare with antibiotic therapy. If an abscess occurs and persists, it is drained surgically and an orchiectomy may be indicated. Complete resolution of swelling and pain may take several weeks to months. The individual's sexual partner should be treated with antibiotics if the causative microorganism is a sexually transmitted pathogen.

Disorders of the Prostate Gland

Benign Prostatic Hyperplasia

Benign prostatic hyperplasia (BPH), also called **benign prostatic hypertrophy,** is the enlargement of the prostate gland (Figure 25-13). Because the major prostatic changes are caused by hyperplasia, not hypertrophy, benign prostatic hyperplasia is the preferred term. This condition becomes problematic as prostatic tissue compresses the urethra, where it passes through the prostate, resulting in frequency of lower urinary tract symptoms. The prevalence among U.S. men 60 years and older is about 50% and among men 70 years or older 90%.[44] BPH is common and involves a complex pathophysiology with several endocrine and local factors and remodeled microenvironment. Its relationship to aging is well documented. At birth the prostate is pea sized, and growth of the gland is gradual until puberty.

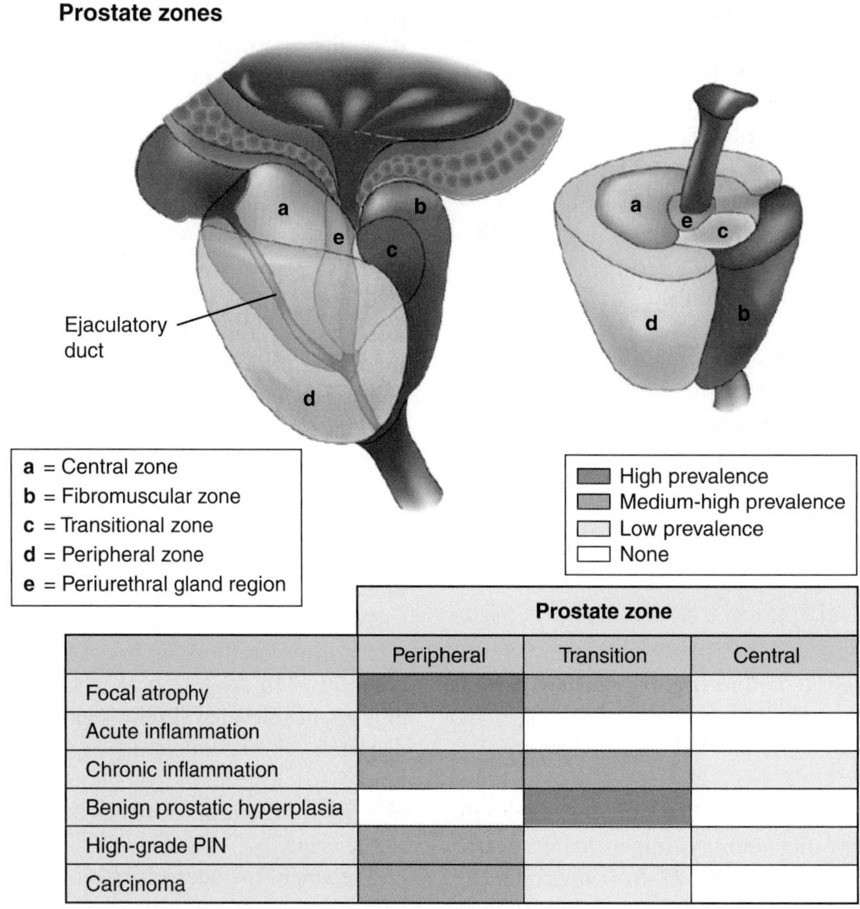

FIGURE 25-13 **Prostate Zones, Benign Prostatic Hyperplasia (BPH), and Prostate Cancer Locations.** BPH occurs in the peripheral zone of the prostate gland that can enlarge (not shown). BPH nodules and atrophy are associated with inflammation in the transition zone. Most cancer lesions occur in the peripheral zone. Carcinoma can involve the central zone but rarely occurs in isolation, suggesting that prostatic intraepithelial neoplasia (PIN) lesions do not easily progress to carcinoma in this region. (Adapted from De Marzo AM et al: *Nat Rev Cancer* 7:256–269, 2007.)

A period of rapid development continues until the third decade of life, when the prostate reaches adult size. Around 40 to 45 years of age, benign hyperplasia begins and continues slowly until death. Although dihydrotestosterone (DHT) is necessary for normal prostatic development, its role in BPH remains unclear. Among all androgen-metabolizing enzymes within the human prostate, 5α-reductase is the most powerful. This reductase corresponds to an age-dependent DHT level. Therefore, although 5α-reductase and DHT decrease with age in the epithelium, they remain relatively constant in the stroma of the prostate gland.

PATHOGENESIS. Current causative theories of BPH focus on levels and ratios of endocrine factors such as androgens, estrogens, gonadotropins, and prolactin and changes in the balance between autocrine/paracrine growth-stimulatory and growth-inhibitory factors. These factors include insulin-like growth factors (IGFs), epidermal growth factor, nerve growth factor, fibroblast factors, IGF binding proteins, and transforming growth factor-beta (TGF-β).[45]

Aging and circulating androgens are associated with BPH and enlargement. These factors are predisposed as disrupting the *balance* of growth factor signaling pathways and stromal/epithelial interactions creating a growth-promoting and tissue remodeling microenvironment. However, BPH is a multifactorial disease, and not all men respond well to available treatments, suggesting factors other than androgens are involved. Testosterone, the primary circulating androgen in men, also can be metabolized through CYP19/aromatase into the potent estrogen, estradiol-17β. The prostate is an estrogen target tissue and estrogens directly and indirectly affect growth and differentiation of prostate. The precise role of endogenous and exogenous estrogens in directly affecting prostate growth and differentiation in the context of BPH is an understudied area. Estrogens and selective estrogen receptor modulators have been shown to promote or inhibit prostate proliferation, signifying potential roles in BPH.[46] Taken together these interactions lead to an increase in prostate volume. The remodeled stroma promotes local inflammation with altered cytokine, reactive oxygen/nitrogen species, and chemoattractants.[47] The resultant increased oxygen demands of proliferating cells causes a local hypoxia that induces angiogenesis and changes to fibroblasts. Functional and phenotypic changes (transdifferentiation) of fibroblasts to the myofibroblasts is a hallmark of the remodeled microenviroment.[48]

BPH begins in the periurethral glands, which are the inner glands or layers of the prostate. The prostate enlarges as nodules form and grow (nodular hyperplasia) and glandular cells enlarge (hypertrophy). The development of BPH occurs over a prolonged period, and changes within the urinary tract are slow and insidious.

CLINICAL MANIFESTATIONS. As nodular hyperplasia and cellular hypertrophy progress, tissues that surround the prostatic urethra usually compress it but not always cause **bladder outflow obstruction.** These symptoms are sometimes called the spectrum of lower urinary tract symptoms (LUTS). Symptoms include the urge to urinate often, some delay in starting urination, and decreased force of the urinary stream. As the obstruction progresses, often over several years, the bladder cannot empty all the urine and the increasing volume leads to long-term urine retention. The volume of urine retained may be great enough to produce uncontrolled "overflow incontinence" with any increase in intra-abdominal pressure. At this stage the force of the urinary stream is significantly reduced, and much more time is required to initiate and complete voiding. Hematuria, bladder or kidney infection, bladder calculi, acute urinary retention hydroureter, hydronephrosis, and renal insufficiency are common complications.[49]

Some men initially have signs of uremia and renal failure. On digital rectal examination the hyperplastic prostate is a soft or firm enlargement with smooth mucosal surface and no discernible distinction between lobes; asymmetry is common. The palpated prostate does not always reflect the degree of BPH because a substantial portion of the enlargement is intravesicular.[50] Thirty percent of men with mild to moderate symptoms improve with watchful waiting.

EVALUATION AND TREATMENT. Diagnosis is made from a medical history, physical exam, and laboratory tests including urinalysis. Careful review of symptoms is necessary. Digital rectal examination (DRE) and PSA are conducted to determine hyperplasia. PSA alone, however, cannot determine whether symptoms are caused by BPH because PSA is elevated in both BPH and prostate cancer. Annual DREs are used to screen men older than 40 years of age for BPH, sooner in high-risk men.[51] If marked enlargement, moderate to severe symptoms, or complications are present, transrectal ultrasound (TRUS) is used to determine bladder and prostate volume and residual urine. Urinalysis, serum creatinine and blood urea nitrogen, uroflowmetry, postvoid residual (PVR) urine, pressure-flow study, cystometry, and cystourethroscopy are used to determine kidney and bladder function.[49] BPH has been treated successfully with drugs. α_1-Adrenergic blockers (prazosin and tamsulosin) are used to relax the smooth muscle of the bladder and prostate. Antiandrogen agents, such as finasteride (Proscar), selectively block androgens at the prostate cellular level and cause the prostate gland to shrink.[51] By shrinking the prostate, these drugs have been shown to improve BPH-related symptoms and reduce the risk of future urinary retention and BPH-related surgery. α_1-Adrenergic blockers do not affect PSA and have no effect on prostate cancer risk. However, antiandrogen agents lower PSA by 50% after 6 months of therapy.[51]

Newer minimally invasive procedures include interstitial laser therapy, transurethral radiofrequency procedure (TUNA), cooled Thermo Therapy and prostate artery embolization. When necessary, the hyperplastic tissue may be removed surgically to prevent the serious consequences of urethral obstruction. A permanent indwelling catheter is inserted if the individual cannot tolerate surgery.

BOX 25-5 NATIONAL INSTITUTES OF HEALTH CLASSIFICATION OF THE PROSTATITIS SYNDROMES

This system, developed for clinical research purposes, can be simplified for use in primary care practice.

Category I, or acute bacterial prostatitis (ABP), is an acute infection of the prostate and is manifested by systemic signs of infection and a positive urine culture.

Category II, or chronic bacterial prostatitis (CBP), is a chronic bacterial infection, in which bacteria are recovered in significant numbers from a purulent prostatic fluid. These bacteria are thought to be the most common cause of recurrent urinary tract infection in men.

Category III, or chronic pelvic pain syndrome (CPPS), is diagnosed when no pathogenic bacteria can be localized to the prostate (culture of expressed prostatic fluid or postprostatic massage urine specimen) and is further divided into IIIa and IIIb. Category IIIa refers to inflammatory CPPS in which a significant number of white blood cells (WBCs) are localized to the prostate, whereas, category IIIb is noninflammatory.

Category IV refers to asymptomatic inflammatory prostatitis, in which bacteria or WBCs are localized to the prostate, but individuals are asymptomatic.

Prostatitis

Prostatitis is an inflammation of the prostate. Some degree of prostatic inflammation is present in 4% to 36% of the male population, increasing to 50% in older men. Inflammation is usually limited to a few of the gland's excretory ducts.

Prostatitis syndromes have been classified by the National Institutes of Health as: (1) acute bacterial prostatitis (ABP), (2) chronic bacterial prostatitis (CBP), (3) chronic pelvic pain syndrome (CPPS), and (4) asymptomatic inflammatory prostatitis (Box 25-5). ABP and CBP are caused mostly by gram-negative enterobacteriaceae and enterococci species, which originate in the gastrointestinal flora. The most common microorganism is *E. coli,* which is identified in the majority of infections.[52] *Klebsiella* species, *P. aeruginosa,* and *Serratia* species are common gram-negative cultured microorganisms. Nonbacterial prostatitis (CP/CPPS) syndromes are caused by a cascade of inflammatory, immunologic, neuroendocrine, and neuropathic mechanisms in which the initiating cause is unknown.

Bacterial Prostatitis. **Acute bacterial prostatitis (ABP, category I)** is an ascending infection of the urinary tract that tends to occur in men between the ages of 30 and 50 years but also is associated with BPH in older men. Infection stimulates an inflammatory response in which the prostate becomes enlarged, tender, firm, or boggy. The onset of prostatitis may be acute and unrelated to previous illnesses or it may follow catheterization or cystoscopy.

Clinical manifestations of acute bacterial prostatitis are those of urinary tract infection or pyelonephritis. Sudden onset of malaise, low back and perineal pain, high fever (up to 40° C [104° F]) and chills is common, as are dysuria, inability to empty the bladder, nocturia, and urinary retention. The individual also may have symptoms of lower urinary tract obstruction, such as slow, small, "narrowed" urinary stream, which may be a medical emergency. Acute inflammatory prostatic edema can compress the urethra, causing urinary obstruction. Systemic signs of infection include sudden onset of a high fever, fatigue, arthralgia, and myalgia. Prostatic pain may occur, especially when the individual is in an upright position, because the pelvic floor muscles tighten with standing and the prostate gland is compressed. Some individuals experience low back pain, painful ejaculation, and rectal or perineal pain. Palpation discloses an enlarged, extremely tender and swollen prostate that is firm, indurated, and warm to the touch.

Because ABP is usually associated with a bladder infection caused by the same microorganism, urine cultures disclose its identity. Prostatic massage may express enough secretions from the urethra for direct bacterial examination, but massage may be painful and increases the risk that the infection will ascend to adjacent structures or enter the bloodstream and cause septicemia.

To resolve the infection and control its spread, individuals may require antibiotics. In severe cases, the individual is hospitalized and treated with intravenous antibiotics, followed by oral antibiotics. Analgesics, antipyretics, bed rest, and adequate hydration also are therapeutic. Complications include urinary retention that resolves with antibiotic therapy; prostatic abscess that may rupture into the urethra, rectum, or perineum; epididymitis; bacteremia; and septic shock. Urinary retention requiring drainage is best managed with a suprapubic catheter. Foley catheterization is contraindicated during acute infection.

Chronic bacterial prostatitis (CBP, category II) is characterized by recurrent urinary tract symptoms and persistence of pathogenic bacteria (usually gram negative) in urine or prostatic fluid. This form of prostatitis is the most common recurrent urinary tract infection in men. Symptoms may be similar to those of an acute bladder infection, such as frequency, urgency, dysuria, perineal discomfort, low back pain, myalgia, arthralgia, and sexual dysfunction. The prostate may only be slightly enlarged or boggy but it may be fibrotic because repeated infections can cause it to be firm and irregular in shape.

When the initial urine sample is bacteria-free, prostatic massage is used to express secretions. Subsequently, the first 10 ml of voided urine is collected and examined microscopically. Prostatic secretions showing more than 10 white blood cells (WBCs) per high-power field and macrophages containing fat are indicative of bacterial infection; diagnosis is confirmed by culture. A pelvic x-ray or TRUS may show prostatic calculi.

Treatment of chronic bacterial prostatitis is difficult because it is often caused by prostatic calculi. Calculi are silent and are found in up to 50% of men with prostatitis, and infected calculi can serve as a source of bacterial persistence and relapsing urinary tract infection.[53] Calculi harbor pathogens within the stone, and consequently pathogens cannot be eradicated from the urinary tract. Permanent cure is achieved by surgical intervention.

Chronic Prostatitis/Chronic Pelvic Pain Syndrome. **Chronic prostatitis/chronic pelvic pain syndrome (CPPS, category III)** is diagnosed when no pathogenic bacteria can be localized to the prostate and is further divided into categories IIIa and IIIb (see Box 25-5). Category IIIa refers to inflammatory chronic pelvic pain syndrome where WBCs are elevated and localized to the prostate. Symptoms tend to be milder but are persistent and annoying. Presumably, noninfectious prostatitis or pain is caused by reflux of sterile urine into the ejaculatory ducts because of high-pressure voiding.[53] Reflux may be triggered by spasms of the external or internal sphincters. Category IIIb is noninflammatory; in **category IV,** individuals are asymptomatic but have an increase in bacteria and WBCs localized to the prostate. Microorganisms suspected of causing CP/CPPS include *E. coli*, *Enterobacter*, *P. aeruginosa*, and *Helicobacter pylori*, a new suspect.[54]

Men with **nonbacterial prostatitis** may complain of pain or a dull ache that is continuous or spasmodic in the suprapubic, infrapubic, scrotal, penile, or inguinal area. Other symptoms are pain on ejaculation and urinary symptoms, such as frequency of urination. The prostate gland generally feels normal on palpation.

Nonbacterial prostatitis is a diagnosis by exclusion. Digital examination of the prostate, bacterial cultures of the urogenital tract, microscopic examination of expressed prostatic fluid, urethroscopy, and urodynamic studies are used to verify the diagnosis of nonbacterial prostatitis.

There is no generally accepted treatment for nonbacterial prostatitis. Hot sitz baths, bed rest, alpha-blockers, anticholinergics, and anti-inflammatory drugs can relieve symptoms.

Cancer of the Prostate

Prostate cancer is the most commonly diagnosed nonskin cancer in men in the United States, with a lifetime risk for diagnosis currently estimated at 15.9%.[55] The incidence varies greatly worldwide (Figure 25-14), but it is still considered to be the second most frequently diagnosed cancer and the sixth leading cause of death worldwide. Importantly, incidence rates vary by more than 25-fold worldwide, and the highest rates recorded mostly in developed countries include Oceania, Europe, and North America, largely because of the wide use or overuse of PSA testing.[56] Screening with PSA can amplify the incidence of prostate cancer by allowing detection of prostate lesions that although meeting the pathologic criteria for malignancy, may have low potential (e.g., latent, indolent, preclinical) for growth and metastasis. In countries with higher use of PSA testing, such as United States, Canada, Australia, and the Nordic countries, trends in incidence rates follow similar patterns.[56]

Different from Western countries, incidence and mortality rates are rising in several Asian (including Japan) and central and Eastern European countries.[56] Death rates have been decreasing in several countries including Australia, Canada, the United Kingdom, the United States, Italy, and Norway, in part from improved treatment. Males of African descent in the Caribbean have the highest mortality rates from prostate cancer in the world.[56] Most cases of prostate cancer have a good prognosis even without treatment but some cases are aggressive; the lifetime risk for dying of prostate cancer is 2.8%. Prostate cancer is rare before age 50 years and very few men die from it

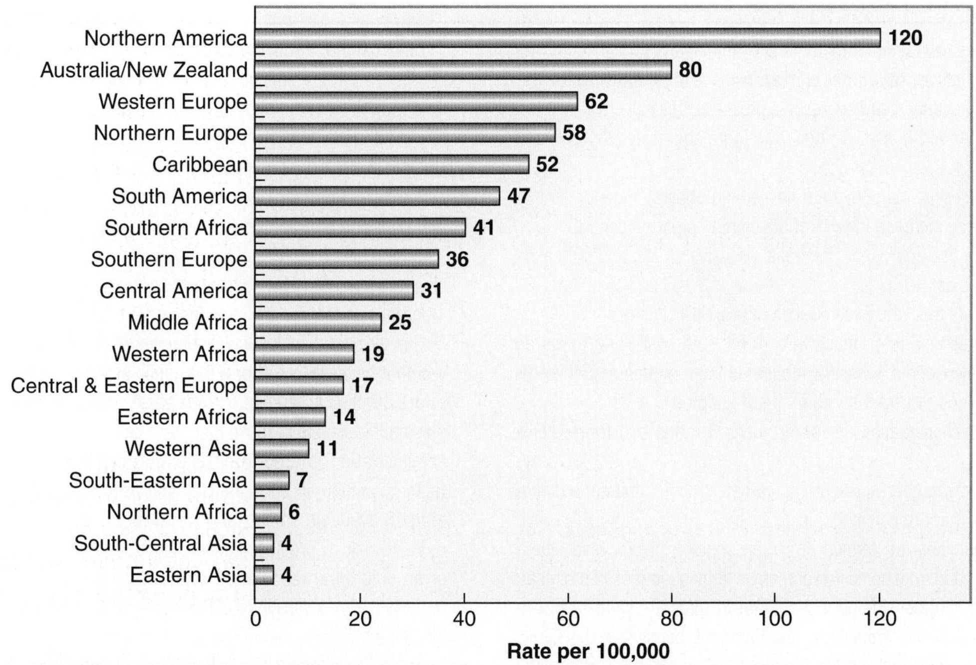

FIGURE 25-14 Selected World Population Age-Standardized (to the World Population) Incidence Rates of Prostate Cancer. (Modified from Jemal A et al: *Biomark Prev* 19:1893, 2010.)

before 60 years of age. Indeed, more than 75% of all prostate cancer is diagnosed in men older than 65.[55] With aging, most of the androgen-metabolizing enzymes undergo significant alteration and older age, race (black), and family history remain the well-established risk factors.[56]

Dietary Factors. Although evidence exists for a dietary role in prostate cancer, the epidemiologic evidence is inconsistent. The problem has been confounded by lack of biomarkers for certain nutrients, difficulties in measuring and quantifying diet, and a limitation of clinical trials to study diet over time. Important are the effects of diet on signaling pathways, hormones, oxidative stress, and reactive oxygen species (ROS). The nutrients in the epidemiology of prostate cancer that have received the most attention include carotenoids, fat, vitamin E, vitamin D/calcium, and selenium. Less studied are isoflavones, curcumin, lycopene, zinc, green tea, omega 3 polyunsaturated fats, and sulforaphane (see Nutrition & Disease: Summary of Diet for Prostate Cancer). Associations between obesity and prostate cancer are not clear, with some research inconsistencies, but obesity seems to be negatively associated with more indolent prostate cancer and positively associated with more aggressive disease and a worse outcome.[57] In process is a randomized clinical trial of diet and early-stage prostate cancer, Men's Eating and Living Study (MEAL). The hypothesis for MEAL is that a change in diet of higher intake of animal products to vegetables and fruits will slow the progression of the indolent to the aggressive form of prostate cancer.[57] As adipose tissue is increasingly being regarded as hormonally active tissue, high body fat and obesity need in-depth exploration to understand the associated risk of prostate problems. Adipose tissue is now known to affect circulating levels of several bioactive messengers and therefore could affect the risk of developing prostate problems in addition to several other well-recognized health problems.[58] High-energy intake (consumption of excess calories) indicates that this may indeed increase insulin levels and IGF-1, a powerful carcinogenic agent[59] (see Pathogenesis, p. 904). More robust, high-quality research trials are needed to guide understanding of the complex relationship between diet and prostate cancer.

Hormones. Prostate cancer develops in an androgen-dependent epithelium and is usually androgen sensitive. Androgens are synthesized not only in the testis, accounting for 50% to 60% of the total testosterone in the prostate, but also in the prostate gland itself. In a process called **intraprostatic conversion,** the hormone dehydroepiandrosterone (DHEA) produced by the adrenal glands[60,61] is converted to testosterone and then into DHT in the prostate (Figure 25-15). Additionally, prostate cancer cells have been reported to make androgens from cholesterol (i.e., de novo).[62] However, these overall relative contributions from intratumoral sources remain to be determined. Population studies have not, however, provided clear and convincing patterns involving associations between circulating hormone concentrations (e.g., not tissue concentrations) and prostate cancer risk.[63,64] Thus there is universal agreement that androgens are important for prostatic growth, development, and maintenance of tissue balance but their role in cancer is controversial.[65] Evidence for involvement of 5α-reductase activity, which is critical in androgen activity in the prostate, is contradictory and inconsistent[63,64] (see Figure 25-15). A prevention study has provided some of the strongest hormonal data with the drug finasteride, which inhibits 5α-reductase. The 7-year intervention study reduced prostate cancer risk in healthy men by about 25%.[66] Important, however, was that more high-grade tumors were found in those men who developed prostate cancer while on the drug. In men younger than 50 years, circulating levels of androgens

NUTRITION & DISEASE

Summary of Diet for Prostate Cancer

- Epidemiologic studies have found total fat intake, animal and saturated fat, red meat, and dairy products are associated with an increase in prostate cancer risk.
- Obesity is linked to advanced and aggressive prostate cancer.
- High body mass index (BMI) is associated with more aggressive disease and a worse outcome.
- Calorie-dense or excessive carbohydrate intake and obesity, independent of dietary fat intake, may increase the risk of developing prostate cancer.
- Dietary fat may increase androgens, increase oxidative stress, and increases reactive oxygen species (ROS).
- Monounsaturated fats may decrease the risk of prostate cancer.
- High levels of linoleic acid (e.g., found in corn oil; safflower) tend to act as a proinflammatory eicosanoid, which is implicated in promotion of cell proliferation and angiogenesis as well as inhibition of apoptosis.
- The Western diet has increased omega-6/omega-3 ratios and therefore is proinflammatory.
- Cooking meat at high temperatures produces heterocyclic amines and aromatic hydrocarbons that are carcinogenic.
- Carcinogenic nitrosamines are formed after consumption of processed meat that contains nitrites and from heme iron present in large quantities of red meat.
- Vitamin E has been long considered a candidate for prostate cancer prevention from in vitro and in vivo animal studies. Vitamin E belongs to the family of tocopherols and tocotrienols that exist as α, β, γ, and δ isoforms. Among these, δ-tocopherol is the major dietary isoform, whereas supplements contain α-tocopherol. Vitamin E is a fat-soluble vitamin obtained from vegetable oils, nuts, and egg yolk. It is a potent intracellular antioxidant known to inhibit peroxidation and DNA damage. The Alpha-Tocopherol, Beta-Carotene Cancer Prevention (ATBC) study showed supplementation with vitamin E could reduce the incidence of prostate cancer among men who smoked. In vitro studies demonstrate that γ- and δ-tocopherol induces cell cycle arrest in human prostate cancer cells (i.e., induces apoptosis) and inhibits the androgen receptor. Mouse studies show vitamin E can inhibit the growth-promoting effects of a high-fat diet; however, vitamin E in combination with selenium does not reduce the incidence of prostate cancer in lady mice models. In the prospective large clinical trial SELECT, the study found no apparent benefit of administering vitamin E.
- Selenium is a trace mineral and exists in food as selenomethionine and selenocysteine. It is essential for the functioning of many antioxidant enzymes and proteins in the body. Humans receive selenium in their diet through plant (dependent on soil concentrations) and animal products. Several large prospective studies reported 50% to 65% reductions in prostate cancer risk with high levels versus low levels of selenium as measured in toenails and plasma. The Nutritional Prevention of Cancer (NPC) trial reported a 50% reduction in risk of developing prostate cancer. No potential benefit was found in the SELECT trial, whereas a small insignificant increase was noted for type 2 diabetes. From these two trials two different forms of selenium were used—the NPC trial used selenized yeast and the SELECT trial used selenomethionine. A meta-analysis of 12 studies with 13,254 subjects and 5007 cases of prostate cancer showed that the risk of prostate cancer decreased with increasing plasma/serum selenium up to 170 ng/ml. Selenium has several modes of action depending on its form. Selenomethionine inhibits cell proliferation and induces cell cycle arrest of human prostate cells (i.e., apoptosis) and inhibits angiogenesis mediated in part by the androgen receptor. This also is true of methylselenic acid. Sodium selenite's anticancer effects are mediated through cellular antioxidants, leading to increased apoptosis and sensitizing cells to radiation-induced killing. Selenium and its derivatives can activate both intrinsic and extrinsic pathways of apoptosis. Selenium intervention may depend on individual genotype.
- Vitamin D may play an important role in prostate cancer prevention.
- Zinc may be important for prostate cancer; however, data are lacking.
- Soy contains isoflavones purported to have anticancer properties including inhibition of cell proliferation and angiogenesis and reduction in prostate specific antigen (PSA) and androgen receptor levels.
- Tomatoes or tomato products ingested daily seem to reduce prostate cancer risk. In vitro studies show lycopene inhibits DNA strand breaks. Unresolved is whether lycopene itself or a metabolic product is responsible for its biologic effect. In clinical studies tomato paste, which is high in lycopene, reduced plasma PSA levels in those men with benign prostatic hyperplasia. Lycopene administration is associated with cell cycle arrest (apoptosis) and growth factor signaling. In 2007 the U.S. Food and Drug Administration (FDA) evaluated 13 available studies and found the relationship between lycopene and reduced risk of prostate cancer inadequate. A Cochrane review found that given only three randomized controlled trials were included in the analysis and a high risk of bias in two, there is insufficient evidence to support or refute lycopene for the prevention of prostate cancer.
- Vegetables including broccoli, cabbage, cauliflower, Brussels sprouts, Chinese cabbage, and turnips (all crucifers) may be protective (several epidemiologic studies) against prostate cancer. In particular, a diet high in broccoli reduced cancer risk. By contrast, four studies revealed no cancer preventive effects. Cruciforms have anticancer properties mediated by the phytochemicals phenethyl isothiocyanate, sulforaphane, and indole-3-carbinol. Sulforaphane is a naturally occurring isothiocyanate that was first isolated in broccoli. It protects against carcinogen-induced cancer in many rodents. Mice given 240 mg of broccoli sprouts per day showed a significant reduction in growth of prostate cancer cells. Sulforaphane treatment lowered androgen receptor protein and gene expression.
- Green tea contains polyphenols, including epigallocatechin gallate (EGCG). Green tea consumption has been associated with a reduced incidence of several cancers including prostate cancer. Green tea consumed within a balanced controlled diet in humans improved overall antioxidant potential. The anticancer effect potential of green tea from in vitro and experimental studies shows these compounds bind directly to carcinogens and induce phase II enzymes that inhibit heterocyclic amines. EGCG administration decreased NF-$\kappa\beta$ activity. Green tea was shown to inhibit IGF-1 and increase IGFBP3, leading to inhibition of prostate cancer development and progression. Yet, in two small randomized studies in individuals with high-grade prostatic neoplasia, it showed no effects. In a population prospective large study ($n = 27{,}293$) green tea did not protect against prostate cancer and black tea showed a positive association with prostate cancer.
- Curcumin has anticarcinogenic potential with well-characterized anti-inflammatory, antiangiogenic, and antioxidant properties. Recent studies report curcumin modulates the Wingless signaling pathway (Wnt) that supports its antiproliferative potential.
- Overall, multiple signaling pathways are involved in prostate cancer development and progression, many of which are affected by dietary and lifestyle factors.

Data from: Astorg P: *Cancer Causes Control* 15:367–386, 2004; Beier R et al: *EMBO J* 19(21):5813–5823, 2000; Dagnelie PC et al: *BJ Int* 93(8):1139–1150, 2004; Demark-Wahnefried W, Moyad MA: *Curr Opin Urol* 17:168–174, 2007:737–743, 2001; Freedland SJ, Aronson WJ: *Urology* 65:433–439, 2005; Giovannucci E et al: *Int J Cancer* 121:1571–1578, 2007; Greenwald P: *J Nutr* 134(12 suppl):3507S–3512S, 2004; Hill P et al: *Cancer Res* 39:5101–5105, 1979; Hurst R et al: *Am J Clin Nutr* 96(1):111–122, 2012; Khan N, Mukhtar H: *Biochem Pharmacol*, 2012 [Epub ahead of print]; Kim DJ et al: *Cancer Causes Control* 11:65–77, 2000; Kobayashi N et al: *Clin Cancer Res* 12(15):4660–4670, 2006; Kolonel LN: *Epidemiol Rev* 23:72–81, 2001; Llic D, Forbes KM, Hassed C: *Cochrane Database Syst Rev* (11):CD008007, 2011; Lloyd JC et al: *J Urol* 183:1619–1624, 2010; Matsumara K et al: *Anticancer Res* 28:709–714, 2008; Montague JA et al: *Caner Causes Control* 23(10):1635–1641, 2012; Ngo TH et al: *Cancer Causes Control* 13:929–935, 2002; Ngo TH et al: *Clin Cancer Res* 9:2734–2743, 2003; Ni J, Yeh S: *Vitam Horm* 76:493–518, 2007; Rodriguez C et al: *Cancer Epidemiol Biomarkers Prev* 16:63–69, 2007; Sinha R et al: *Am J Epidemiol* 170:1165–1177, 2009; Teiten M et al: *Int J Oncol* 38:603–611, 2011; Yang CS, Suh N, Kong AN: *Cancer Prev Res (Phil)* 5(5):701–705, 2012.

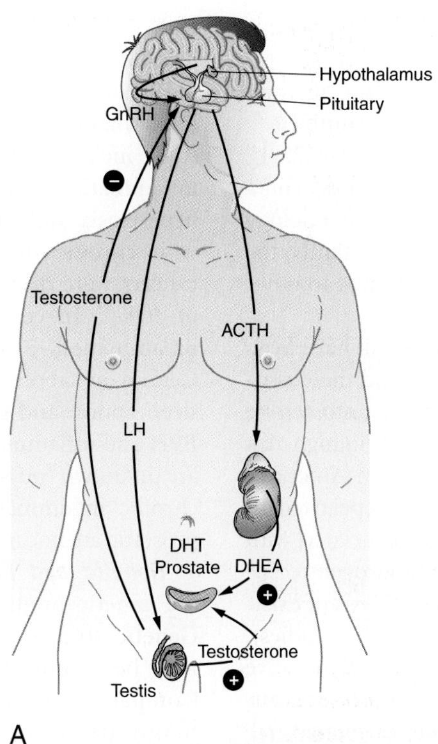

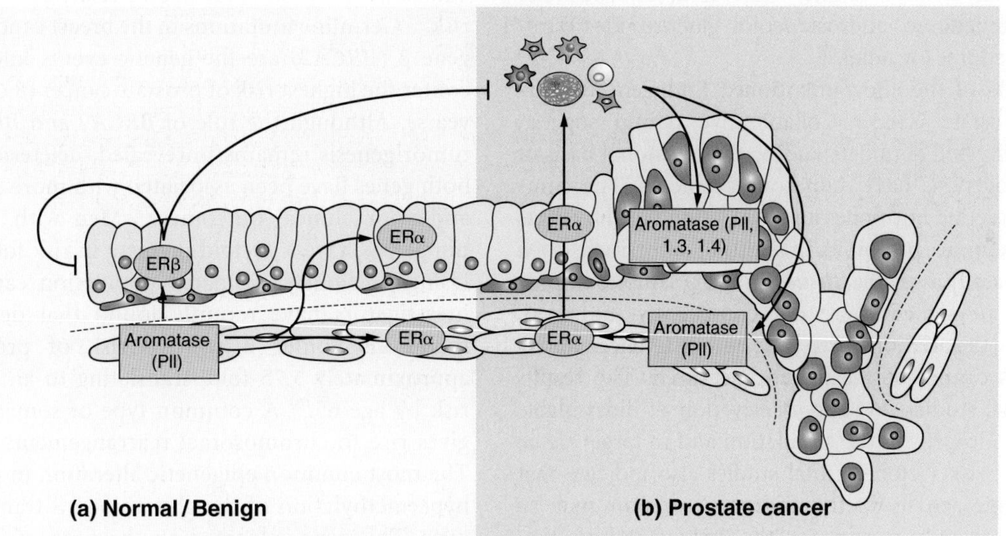

B

FIGURE 25-15 Sources of Androgens and Aromatase and Estrogen Signaling in the Prostate. **A,** Body sources of androgens in the prostate gland. Hypothalamic GnRH causes the release of LH from the anterior pituitary gland. LH stimulates the testes to produce testosterone, which then accumulates in the blood. Pituitary ACTH release stimulates the adrenal glands, which secrete the androgen precursor DHEA into the blood. DHEA is converted into testosterone and then into DHT in the prostate. **B,** Aromatase and estrogen signaling in the prostate. In normal and benign tissue, aromatase is expressed within the stroma and regulated by promoter PII. Estrogen then exerts its effects in an autocrine fashion through the stromal ER-α receptor and also in a paracrine fashion through both ER-α and ER-β receptors. With prostate cancer, aromatase is now expressed within the tumor cells and in stromal cells, and regulated by aromatase promoters 1.3, 1.4, and PII. Thus estrogen exerts its effects in an autocrine way through stromal and epithelial ER-α and ER-β. Consequently, the increased levels of estrogen and abnormal ER-α signaling promote inflammation, which increases aromatase expression and the development of a positive feedback cycle. Inflammation drives aromatase expression, thus increasing estrogen, which in turn promotes further inflammation. *ACTH,* Adrenocorticotropic hormone; *DHEA,* dehydroepiandrosterone; *DHT,* dihydrotestosterone; *GnRH,* gonadotropin-releasing hormone; *LH,* luteinizing hormone. (**A** adapted from Labrie F: *Nat Rev Urol* 8:73-80, 2011; **B** from Ellem SJ, Risbridger GP: *J Steroid Biochem Mol Biol* 118[4-5]:246–251, 2010.)

and estrogens appear to be higher in men of African descent than in European-American men.

Despite the well-documented importance of androgens, their pathophysiologic process in prostate diseases is incomplete.[65] Androgens also are metabolized to estrogens (see Figures 25-17 and 24-35) through the action of the enzyme aromatase, and a growing body of evidence implicates estrogens in the etiology of prostate disease (see Pathogenesis section). Importantly, the aberrant expression of aromatase has been implicated in other tissues, such as the breast and endometrium.[65]

Only a few associations with prostate cancer risk have been observed consistently (in at least three studies), and their associations are weak: (1) slightly higher circulating testosterone and estrogen levels and lower DHEA (sulfate) levels in high-risk black men as compared with lower-risk European-American men; and (2) a cytosine-adenine-guanine (CAG) repeat-length polymorphism in the androgen-receptor gene associated with increased risk and increased receptor activity (androgen receptor). Moreover, in a more recent collaborative analysis of existing worldwide epidemiologic data (18 prospective studies), the Endogenous Hormones and Prostate Cancer Collaborative Group found no associations between the risk of prostate cancer and serum concentrations of testosterone, calculated free testosterone, dihydrotestosterone, dehydroepiandrosterone sulfate, androstenedione, androstanediol glucuronide, estradiol, or calculated free estradiol.[67]

As the results of the above-mentioned Endogenous Hormones and Prostate Cancer Collaborative Group suggest, investigations directed at understanding the hormonal basis of prostate carcinogenesis have numerous problems. The complexities of interacting hormones and separating out the effects of a single hormone are profound. In addition, only single *blood* samples are generally available, *tissue* hormone samples important for paracrine signaling are not consistently measured, and within-subject variations over time and differences in circadian rhythms cannot be adequately measured. The results of several animal studies do support elevation of bioavailable and bioactive androgens in the circulation and in target tissue as an important risk factor. Animal studies also indicate that increased biologic activity of the androgen receptor may be associated with prostate cancer. See the Pathogenesis section for a more thorough discussion of the role of hormones in the pathogenesis of prostate cancer.

Vasectomy. Vasectomy has been identified as a possible risk factor for prostate cancer in case-controlled and cohort studies.[68-70] Three mechanisms by which vasectomy could increase risk are (1) elevation of circulating androgens; (2) immunologic mechanisms involving antisperm antibodies; and (3) reduction of seminal fluid levels of 5α-dihydrotestosterone, the active metabolite of testosterone in the prostate, in vasectomized men. These results suggest an elevation of circulating free testosterone following vasectomy. However, with these combined mechanisms it is unlikely that vasectomy plays a causal role.[71]

Chronic Inflammation. Data from the Medical Therapy of Prostatic Symptoms (MTOPS) study suggest the risk of BPH progression and acute urinary retention is greater in men with prostatic inflammation.[72,73] In certain mouse models prostatic hyperplasia is associated with inflammation.[74] The results of a 5-year longitudinal study of the influence of chronic inflammation and prostate cancer have been reported.[75] The study included 144 men, 33 of whom presented with chronic inflammation in their initial biopsy. Biopsies revealed prostatic hyperplasia and proliferative inflammatory atrophy in those with chronic inflammation. Upon repeat biopsy, 29 new cancers were diagnosed, representing a new cancer incidence of 20%.[75] In contrast, of the 33 men initially showing no inflammation, 2 (6%) were found to have adenocarcinoma. Certain metabolic comorbidities, including obesity, diabetes, sleep apnea, and erectile dysfunction may be linked to both BPH and inflammation.[76] The causes of chronic inflammation are unknown (possible causes are shown in Figure 25-16). Thus chronic inflammation may be an important risk factor for prostatic adenocarcinoma.

Genetic and Epigenetic Factors. Other possible causes are genetic predisposition (familial and hereditary forms). Genetic studies suggest that strong familial predisposition may be responsible for 5% to 10% of prostate cancers.[1] Compared with men with no family history, those with one first-degree relative with prostate cancer have twice the risk and those with two first-degree relatives have five times the risk.[77] Germline mutations in the breast cancer predisposition gene 2 *(BRCA2)* are the genetic events known to date that confer the highest risk of prostate cancer (8.6-fold in men ≤65 years). Although the role of *BRCA2* and *BRCA1* in prostate tumorigenesis remains unrevealed, deleterious mutations in both genes have been associated with more aggressive disease and poor clinical outcomes.[78] Men with *BRCA2* germline mutations have a 20-fold increase in risk for prostate cancer. Using previously estimated population carrier frequencies, investigators have recently found that deleterious *BRCA1* mutations confer a relative risk of prostate cancer of approximately 3.75-fold, translating to an 8.6% cumulative risk by age 65.[79] A common type of somatic mutation that gives rise to chromosomal rearrangements is the *ETS* gene. The most common epigenetic alteration in prostate cancer is hypermethylation of the glutathione S-transferase *(GST-P1)* gene. This gene is located on chromosome 11 and is part of the pathway that helps protect against carcinogen damage. More than 30 independent peer reviewed studies have reported a consistently high sensitivity and specificity of *GST-P1* hypermethylation in prostatectomy or biopsy tissue.[80] A number of other epigenetic modifications found on tumor suppressor genes include *PTEN, RB, p16/INK4a, MLH1, MSH21,* and *APC*.[81,82] There is no clear evidence of a causal link between BPH and prostate cancer even though they may often occur together. Variations in several other genes related to inflammatory pathways might affect the probability of developing prostate cancer.[83]

PATHOGENESIS. More than 95% of prostatic neoplasms are adenocarcinomas[84] and most occur in the periphery of the prostate. Prostatic adenocarcinoma is a heterogeneous group of tumors with a diverse spectrum of molecular and pathologic characteristics and therefore clinical behaviors and challenges.[85]

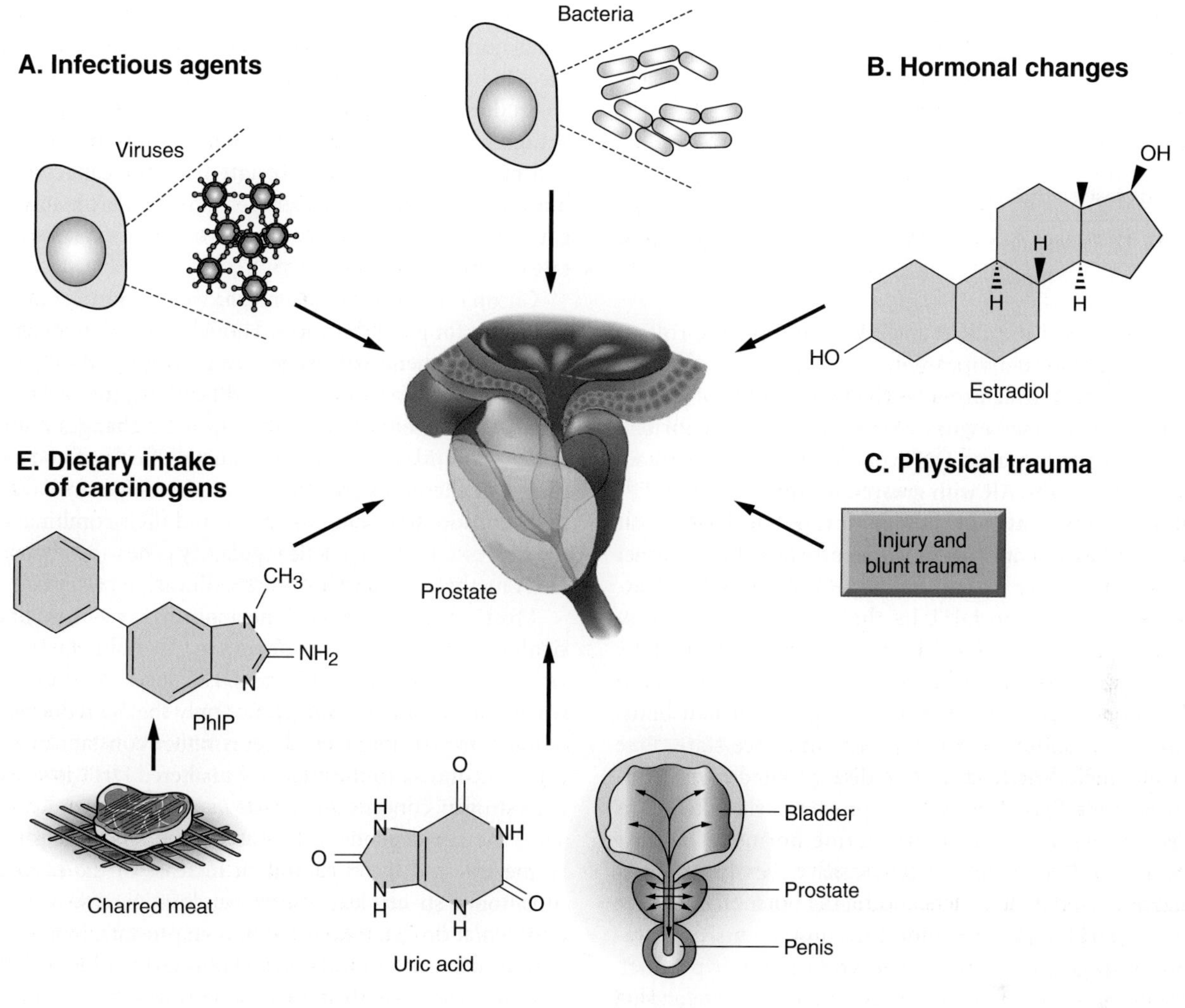

FIGURE 25-16 **Possible Causes of Prostate Inflammation. A,** Infection, including viruses, bacteria, fungi, and parasites. **B,** Hormones, for example, estrogen at key times during development. **C,** Physical trauma, any type of blunt physical injury. **D,** Urine reflex. **E,** Certain dietary factors (see text).

The biologic aggressiveness of the neoplasm appears to be related to the degree of differentiation rather than the size of the tumor (Box 25-6).

Hormonal. Just as the testicles are the male equivalent of the female ovaries, the prostate is the male equivalent of the female uterus; in both situations they originate from the same embryonic cells. This may be important in understanding the role of the associated hormones testosterone (T), DHT, and estrogens in prostate carcinogenesis. Testicular testosterone synthesis and serum testosterone levels fall as men age, remaining unchanged or increasing with age; however, the levels of estradiol do not decline.[86,87] The relationship between hormones and the pathophysiology of prostate carcinogenesis is incomplete and controversial. The main issues and controversies include: (1) sources of androgen production outside of the testes, or extratesticular sources (e.g., from adrenal DHEA and from prostate cholesterol [de novo], itself); (2) the role of prostatic androgen receptor (AR); (3) the role of estrogens, aromatase enzyme, and the

BOX 25-6 DETERMINING THE GRADE OF PROSTATE CANCER WITH THE GLEASON SCORE

Grade 1: The cancer cells closely resemble normal cells. They are small, uniformly shaped, evenly spaced, and well differentiated (i.e., they remain separate from one another).

Grade 2: The cancer cells are still well differentiated, but they are arranged more loosely and are irregular in shape and size. Some of the cancer cells have invaded the neighboring prostate tissue.

Grade 3: This is the most common grade. The cells are less well differentiated (some have fused into clumps) and are more variable in shape.

Grade 4: The cells are poorly differentiated and highly irregular in shape. Invasion of the neighboring prostate tissue has progressed further.

Grade 5: The cells are undifferentiated. They have merged into large masses that no longer resemble normal prostate cells. Invasion of the surrounding tissue is extensive.

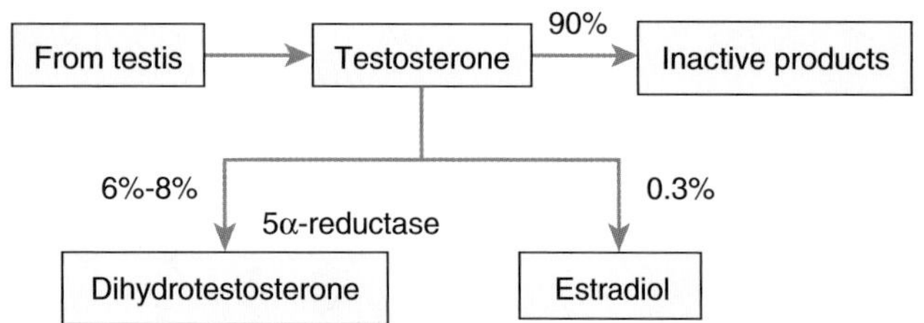

FIGURE 25-17 Testosterone and Conversion to Dihydrotestosterone (DHT).

estrogen receptors (ERs) ER-α and ER-β; and (4) the role of the surrounding microenvironment or stroma.

Testicular testosterone provides the main source of androgens in the prostate (see Figure 25-15) and is the major circulating androgen, whereas DHT predominates in prostate tissue and binds to the AR with greater affinity than does T.[88] The adrenal cortex contributes the far less potent DHEA that promotes synthesis of androgens in the prostate. In the target tissues and, to a lesser extent, in the testes themselves, testosterone is converted to DHT by the enzyme 5α-reductase (Figure 25-17). Thus DHT is the most potent intraprostatic androgen. About half of circulating testosterone is bound to sex hormone–binding globulin (SHBG), about half binds to albumin, and about 1% to 2% exists in a free state. Free testosterone, including testosterone disassociated from albumin and possibly SHBG, enters the prostate cell, where it is converted to DHT.[88] DHT is a paracrine hormone because it affects the local environment or stroma. Several intraprostatic enzymes encoded by genes, *HSD3A* and *HDS3B*, are activated by DHT and are important components of intraprostatic androgen regulation. The conjugated byproduct, 3α-androstenediol glucuronide (AAG), a terminal metabolite of DHT, can be measured in the circulation and used as an indicator of DHT levels.

Accumulating evidence shows that estrogens participate in the pathogenesis and development of BPH and prostate cancer by activating estrogen receptor-α. In contrast, estrogen receptor-β is involved in the differentiation and maturation of prostatic epithelial cells, and thus possesses antitumor effects in prostate cancer.[89] The effect of estrogen is determined by the two receptors ER-α and ER-β. ER-α leads to abnormal proliferation, inflammation, and the development of premalignant lesions. In contrast, ER-β leads to antiproliferative, anti-inflammatory, and potentially anticarcinogenic effects that act in concert or balance the actions of ER-α and androgens.[87] Increased expression of ER-α has been found to be associated with prostate cancer progression, metastasis, and the so-called castration-resistant (medical treatment that suppresses androgens) phenotype.[90] A specific oncogene is regulated by ERs, and those hormones that stimulate the ER-α receptor–like (i.e., agonists) endogenous estrogens can stimulate oncogene expression.[91]

Normally a small amount of estrogen is produced per day—estrone and estradiol—by the aromatization of androstenedione and testosterone, respectively. This reaction is catalyzed by the enzyme system aromatase. A small quantity of estradiol is released by the testes (see Figure 25-17); the rest of the estrogens in males are produced by adipose tissue, liver, skin, brain, and other nonendocrine tissue. Thus testosterone is a precursor of the two hormones, DHT and estradiol.

Studies show aromatase is expressed in stromal tissue in the benign human prostate gland.[92] Thus it appears that both normal prostate and benign prostate have the capacity to locally metabolize androgens to estrogens through aromatase. Investigators have demonstrated altered aromatase expression in prostate cancer[87,92] (see Figure 25-15, *B*).

Chronic exposure to arsenic, as well as estrogen, is a known risk factor for prostate cancer. Though the evidence suggests that exposure to arsenic or estrogens can disrupt normal DNA methylation patterns and histone modifications, the mechanisms by which these chemicals induce epigenetic changes are not fully understood. Moreover, the epigenetic effects of coexposure to these two chemicals are little known. Investigators have revealed that exposure to arsenic, estrogen, and their combination alters the expression of epigenetic regulatory genes and changes global DNA methylation and histone modification patterns.[93]

Most of the androgen-metabolizing enzymes undergo a significant age-dependent alteration. In epithelium, both the 5α-reductase activity and the DHT level decrease with age, whereas in stroma (prostate), not only the 5α-reductase activity but also the stromal DHT level is rather constant over the lifetime. In contrast to the relatively unaltered DHT level over time, the estrogen concentration follows an age-dependent increase. Thus the age-dependent decrease of the DHT accumulation in epithelium and the concomitant increase of the estrogen accumulation in stroma lead to a tremendous increase with age of the estrogen/androgen ratio in the human prostate. In animal studies chronic exposure to testosterone plus estradiol is strongly carcinogenic, whereas testosterone alone is weakly carcinogenic.[64] In mice studies elevated testosterone level in the absence of estrogen leads to the development of hypertrophy and hyperplasia but not malignancy. High estrogen and low testosterone levels have been shown to lead to inflammation with aging and the emergence of precancerous lesions.[87] The mechanism is not clearly understood and may involve estrogen-generated oxidative stress and DNA toxicity, and it requires androgen-mediated and estrogen receptor–mediated processes, such as changes in sex steroid metabolism and receptor status.[64] In addition, there are changes in the balance between autocrine/paracrine growth-stimulatory and growth-inhibitory factors, such as the IGFs.[94] When exogenous estradiol is added to testosterone treatment of rats, prostate cancer incidence is markedly increased, and even a short course of estrogen treatment results in a high incidence of prostate cancer.[64]

Androgen Receptor Signaling. The androgenic hormone responses in the normal prostate and prostate cancer are mediated by AR signaling. Exactly how AR drives the growth of prostate cancer cells is not fully known. Several mechanisms have been suggested,[95] and specific pathways of signaling are important because they can provide novel therapeutic targets. A study using animal models found that loss of androgen receptor function prevented prostatic carcinogenesis, malignant transformation, and metastasis. Tissue-specific evaluation of androgen hormone action demonstrated that epithelial androgen receptor was not necessary for prostate cancer progression, whereas stromal

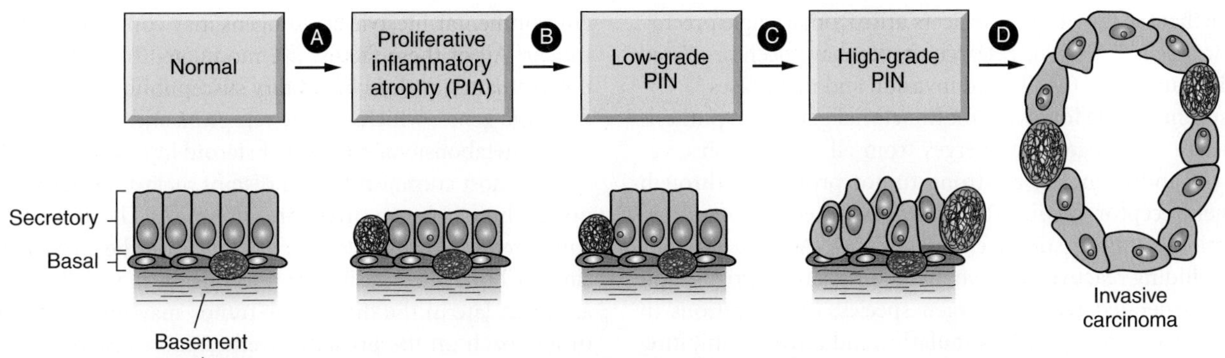

FIGURE 25-18 **Cellular and Molecular Model of Early Prostate Neoplasia Progression. A,** This stage includes infiltration of lymphocytes, macrophages, and neutrophils caused by repeated infections, dietary factors, urine reflux, injury, onset of autoimmunity (which triggers inflammation), and wound healing. **B,** Epigenetic alterations mediate telomere shortening. **C,** Genetic instability and accumulation of genetic alterations. **D,** Continued proliferation of genetically unstable cells leading to cancer progression. *PIN,* Prostatic intraepithelial neoplasia.

androgen receptor was essential for prostate cancer progression, malignant transformation, and metastasis.[96]

Prostate Epithelial Neoplasia. A precursor lesion, prostatic epithelial neoplasia (PIN), has been described. PIN may be more concentrated in prostates containing cancer and is noted in proximity to cancer.[81] However, the final fate of PIN is unknown, including the possibilities of latency, invasion, and even regression. The current working model of prostate carcinogenesis suggests that repeated cycles of injury and cell death occur to the prostate epithelium as a result of damage (i.e., from oxidative stress) from inflammatory responses.[97] The direct injury is hypothesized as a response to infections; autoimmune disease; circulating carcinogens or toxins, or both, from the diet; or urine that has refluxed into the prostate (see Figure 25-16). The resultant manifestation of this injury is focal atrophy or prostatic intraepithelial atrophy (PIA). Biologic responses cause an increase in proliferation and a massive increase in epithelial cells that possess a phenotype intermediate between basal cells and mature luminal cells (Figure 25-18).[97] In a small subset of cells, some may contain "stem cell" or tumor-initiating properties and telomere shortening (see Chapter 12). A subset of PIN cells may activate telomerase enzyme, causing the cells to become immortal.[98] Molecular, genetic, and epigenetic changes can increase genetic instability that might progress to high-grade PIN and early prostate cancer formation. This model of prostate carcinogenesis needs much more research.

Stromal Environment. The prostate gland is composed of secretory luminal epithelium, basal epithelium, neuroendocrine cells, and various cell types comprising supportive tissue or stroma. **Stroma,** or tissue microenvironment, produces autocrine/paracrine factors, as well as structural supporting molecules that help regulate normal cell behavior and organ homeostasis.[99] **Fibroblasts** are the most important cells during the reconstructive phase of wound healing (see Chapter 7). The collagen and connective tissue proteins produced by fibroblasts are deposited in wounded areas after fibroblasts have entered the lesion. Thus their presence is a signature of alterations in the stroma. Reactive tumor stroma is associated with an increased number of fibroblasts, increased capillary density, and collagen and fibrin deposition. These findings suggest that alteration in the prostate microenvironment, mediated by changes associated with aging or senescence, or both, promote epithelial responses that contribute to diseases. In animal studies, investigators have noted that the microenvironment has an increased number of cells that promote inflammation and a collapsed appearance of the smooth muscle cells within adjacent glandular stroma.[99] Fibroblast spreading has been proposed as indicative of decreased mechanical tension because of a lack of direct association of the fibroblasts with aged fragmented collagen fibrils.[100,101] These alterations in mechanical tension and cell shape are suggested as determinants in altering gene expression and cellular function. These alterations in aged prostate stroma for mice and men include significant enhancement for inflammation pathways (e.g., NF-κβ, collagens).[100,101] Inflammation can induce cell stress, and stressed mesenchymal cells can secrete inflammatory mediators (chemoattractants); however, it remains to be determined whether inflammatory infiltrates are a cause of or response to the alterations of aged stroma.[102] Evidence supports that inflammation has a role in the pathogenesis of prostate cancer.[97,103] Investigators have found that disruption of fibroblast growth factor signaling pathways leads to strongly activated and atypical stroma that preceded the development of mice PIN (mPIN).

Epithelial-mesenchymal transition (EMT) was first described in embryonic development, and is observed in a number of solid tumors[104] (also see Chapter 12). Cells that undergo EMT become more migratory and invasive and gain access to vascular vessels.[105] Numerous studies have shown that these transition states (EMT and mesenchymal-epithelial transition [MET]) are a consequence of tumor-stromal interactions.[105,106]

Investigators studying prostate cancer cells in vitro correlated EMT with increased growth, migration, and invasion. These investigators demonstrated that the microenvironment is a critical site for the transition of human prostate cancer cells from epithelial to mesenchymal structure, resulting in increased metastatic potential for bone and adrenal gland.[107]

Prostate cancer is known to be diverse and composed of multiple genetically distinct cancer cell clones. Studies, however, indicate that most metastatic cancers arise from a single precursor cancer cell.[108] Various research models have been proposed to understand EMT (MET) and invasion and metastases.[109]

In summary, the following multifactorial general hypothesis of prostate carcinogenesis emerges from all of these observations: (1) androgens act as strong tumor promoters through androgen receptor–mediated mechanisms to enhance the carcinogenic activity of strong endogenous DNA toxic carcinogens, including reactive estrogen metabolites and estrogen, and prostate-generated reactive oxygen species; (2) alterations in autocrine/paracrine growth-stimulating and growth-inhibiting factors between the prostate tumor cells and microenvironment influence cancer pathogenesis; and (3) possibly unknown environmental-lifestyle carcinogens may contribute to prostate cancer. All of these factors are modulated by diet and genetic determinants, such as hereditary susceptibility genes and polymorphic genes, which encode receptors and enzymes involved in the metabolism and action of steroid hormones.[64]

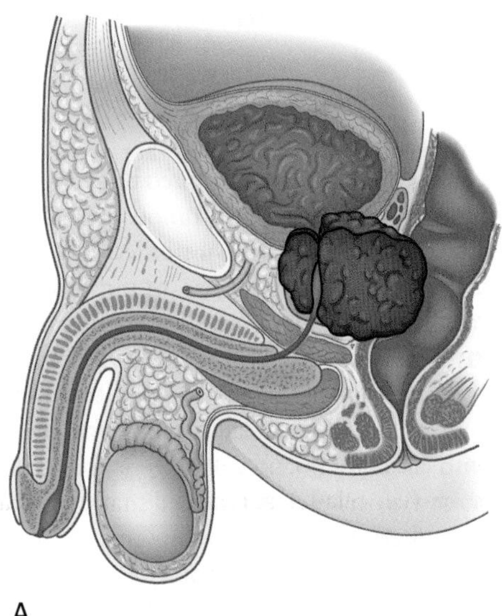

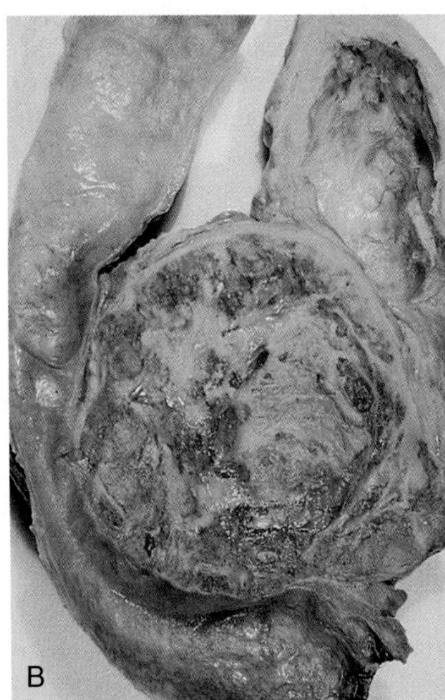

FIGURE 25-19 **Carcinoma of the Prostate. A,** Schematic of carcinoma of the prostate. **B,** Carcinoma of the prostate extending into the rectum and urinary bladder. (**B** from Damjanov I, Linder J, editors: *Pathology: a color atlas,* St Louis, 2000, Mosby.)

The most common sites of distant metastasis are the lymph nodes, bones, lungs, liver, and adrenals. The pelvis, lumbar spine, femur, thoracic spine, and ribs are the most common sites of bone metastasis. Local extension is usually posterior, although late in the disease the tumor may invade the rectum or encroach on the prostatic urethra and cause bladder outlet obstruction (Figure 25-19). The spread of cancer through blood vessels is illustrated in Figure 25-20.

CLINICAL MANIFESTATIONS. Prostatic cancer often causes no symptoms until it is far advanced. The first manifestations of disease are those of bladder outlet obstruction: slow urinary stream, hesitancy, incomplete emptying, frequency, nocturia, and dysuria. Unlike the symptoms of obstruction caused by BPH, the symptoms of obstruction caused by prostatic cancer are progressive and do not remit. Local extension of prostatic cancer can obstruct the upper urinary tract ureters as well. If rectal obstruction occurs, a man may experience a large bowel obstruction or difficulty in defecation. Symptoms of late disease include bone pain at sites of bone metastasis, edema of the lower extremities, enlargement of lymph nodes, liver enlargement, pathologic bone fractures, and mental confusion associated with brain metastases.

EVALUATION AND TREATMENT. Screening for prostatic cancer includes DRE, PSA blood tests, and TRUS. The most significant test used in the diagnosis and management of prostate cancer is **prostate-specific antigen (PSA).** DRE may detect early prostatic carcinomas but is has low sensitivity and specificity.[81] Cancer diagnosis is confirmed through tissue biopsy and microscopic examination of tissue. Lymphography, bone scans, MRI, and CT scans also may be used to determine metastasis to lymph, bone, or other adjacent tissue. Important for treatment is to accurately measure the size of the index (longest) tumor and its percentage Gleason grade of differentiation.[110]

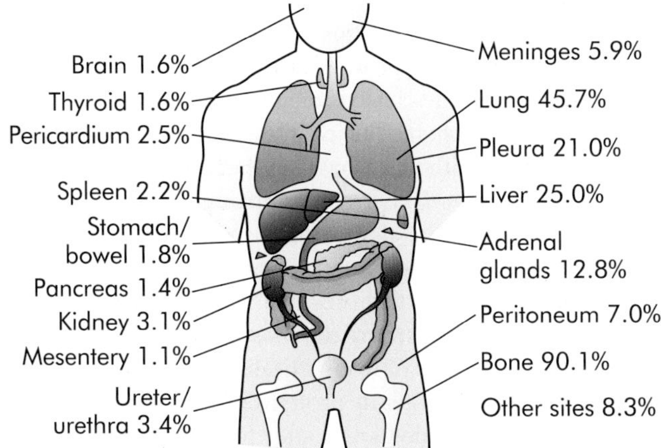

FIGURE 25-20 **Distribution of Hematogenous Metastases in Prostate Cancer.** Study of 556 individuals with metastatic prostate cancer. (Adapted from Budendorf L et al: *Hum Pathol* 31:578, 2000.)

PSA screening for prostate cancer has led to considerable controversy. A review of the evidence for the U.S. Preventive Services Task Force regarding screening for prostate cancer concluded that PSA-based screening results in small or no reduction in prostate cancer–specific mortality and is associated with harms related to subsequent evaluation and treatments, some of which may be unnecessary (See What's New? Summary of the American College of Physicians (ACP) Guidance Statement on Screening for Prostate Cancer).[111] Convincing evidence demonstrates that the PSA test unfortunately often produces false-positive results. Men who have a false-positive test are more likely to have additional testing, including one or more biopsies. Over a 10-year span, approximately 15% to 20% of men will have a PSA test result that triggers a biopsy, depending on the PSA threshold and testing interval used.[55] In addition, because PSA is organ specific and not cancer specific, it can increase and overlap with BPH, prostatitis, infarct, manipulation from instrumentation, and ejaculation.[81] The annual rate by which PSA rises is known as **PSA velocity** or doubling time (generally described as *PSA kinetics*). Its calculation has been judged to be far from straightforward. More than 20 different methods for calculation have been proposed, and many of these give divergent results. Evidence clearly shows that PSA kinetics are critical for understanding prognosis in advanced or relapsed prostate cancer. However, PSA kinetics have questionable value for men with an untreated prostate; neither PSA velocity nor doubling time has an established role in diagnosing prostate cancer or providing a prognosis for men before treatment.[112] In fact, investigators recently evaluated guidelines on the use of PSA velocity in prostate cancer detection and found that change in PSA levels over time is such a poor predictor of prostate cancer (in a previously untreated prostate) that it is highly likely many unnecessary biopsies have been performed.[113] It is thus somewhat doubtful at this juncture that PSA velocity adds any additional predictive accuracy to PSA alone or positive digital rectal examination, or both, for purposes of prostate cancer screening.

Older age is the strongest risk factor for the development of prostate cancer. However, neither screening nor treatment trials show benefit in men older than 70 years. Across age ranges, black men and men with a family history of prostate cancer have an increased risk of developing and dying of prostate cancer. Black men are approximately twice as likely to die of prostate cancer than other men in the United States and the reason for this disparity in unknown. Black men represent a very small minority of participants in randomized clinical trials of screening and, thus, no firm conclusions can be made about the balance of benefits and harms of PSA-based screening in this population. As such, it is a questionable practice to selectively recommend PSA-based screening for black men in the absence of data that support a more favorable balance of risks and benefits.[55] The ability to predict cancer rises significantly when TRUS is added to the annual DRE and PSA testing. Researchers are studying microRNAs as potential new biomarkers for prostate cancer.

Prostate cancer is now detected in greater numbers at lower stages of disease and is amenable to multiple forms of efficacious treatment. However, there is a lack of conclusive data demonstrating a definitive mortality benefit from this earlier diagnosis and treatment of prostate cancer. This is likely because of the treatment of a large proportion of indolent cancers that would have had little adverse effect on health or life span if left alone (Box 25-7).

Because of this "overtreatment" phenomenon, active surveillance with delayed intervention is gaining traction as a viable management approach in contemporary practice. The ability to distinguish clinically insignificant cancers from those with a high risk of progression or lethality, or both, is critical to the appropriate selection of surveillance protocols versus immediate intervention[114] (Box 25-8). The most important observation for pathologists to make to facilitate cure of any individual of prostate cancer is that of accurately measuring the size of the index (longest) tumor and Gleason score (degree of differentiation) (see Box 25-6).[115]

Treatment of prostatic cancer depends on the stage of the neoplasm (see Box 25-6); the anticipated effects of treatment; and the age, general health, and life expectancy of the individual. Options include no treatment; surgical treatments such as total prostatectomy, transurethral resection of the prostate (TURP), or cryotherapy; nonsurgical treatments such as radiation therapy, hormone therapy, or chemotherapy; watchful waiting; and any combination of these.[55] In addition, new approaches are using immunotherapy. Palliative treatment is aimed at relieving urinary, bladder outlet, or colon obstruction; spinal cord compression; and pain. Prognosis and survival rates have improved steadily since the early 1960s. According to the most recent data, 10- and 15-year relative survival rates are 98% and 91%, respectively.[1]

Treatment for prostate cancer may lead to loss of urinary control, which may or may not return to normal after several weeks or months. Stress incontinence can occur after surgery, and mild urge incontinence can occur after radiation therapy. Prostate cancer and its treatment can affect sexual functioning. Sensation of orgasm is not usually affected, but smaller amounts of ejaculate will be produced or men may experience a "dry" ejaculate because of retrograde ejaculation.

BOX 25-7 RETHINKING SCREENING FOR PROSTATE CANCER AND BREAST CANCER

In essence, it has become necessary to rethink screening for both prostate and breast cancer because since screening was introduced, the incidence of both prostate and breast cancer increased and never returned to prescreening levels, and the absolute number of advanced prostate and breast cancers diagnosed during this period has not decreased as predicted. Furthermore, whereas colon and cervical cancer screening detects precancerous treatable conditions, prostate and breast cancer screening detects so-called early cancers that may not be destined to grow or become lethal. Thus it is possible that prostate and breast cancer screening may be increasing the burden of low-risk cancers without any significant reduction of burden associated with aggressive lesions, thereby not resulting in the anticipated reduction in breast and prostate cancer mortality.

Data from Esserman L, Shieh Y, Thompson I: *J Am Med Assoc* 302(15):1685–1920, 2009.

WHAT'S NEW?

Summary of the American College of Physicians (ACP) Guidance Statement on Screening for Prostate Cancer

Disease or condition	Prostate cancer
Target audience	Internists, family physicians, other clinicians
Target patient population	All men
Screening tests	DRE and PSA
Interventions	Strategies to manage prostate cancer
Outcomes	Mortality and morbidity
Indications for discussing screening	• Men between the age of 50 and 69 years of age • Earlier age in men who are at increased risk for prostate cancer (African American race and first-degree relative (father or brother diagnosed with prostate cancer, especially before age 65 years)
Frequency of screening	• No clear evidence guides the periodically or frequency of screening • No clear evidence that PSA screening more frequently than every 4 years produces any additional benefit • PSA levels of 2.5 μg/L or greater may warrant yearly evaluation
Benefits of screening	Reduction in mortality
Harms of screening	• False alarms related to number of high false-positive results associated with DRE and especially PSA • High false-negative rates • Overdiagnosis (detection of cancer that is not destined to cause future morbidity and mortality) • Overtreatment and associated harms, including bleeding, pain, and hospitalization • Anxiety and discomfort • Positive screening results may lead to further testing, such as biopsies, which not only can be painful but also can lead to complications, such as infections
Recommendations	• *Guidance statement 1:* ACP recommends that clinicians inform men between the age of 50 and 60 years about the limited potential benefits and substantial harms of screening for prostate cancer. ACP recommends that clinicians base the decision to screen for prostate cancer using the prostate-specific antigen test on the risk for prostate cancer, a discussion of the benefits and harms of screening, the man's general health and life expectancy, and preferences. ACP recommends that clinicians should not screen for prostate cancer using the prostate-specific antigen test in men who do not express a clear preference for screening. • *Guidance statement 2:* ACP recommends that clinicians should not screen for prostate cancer using the prostate-specific antigen test in average-risk men under the age of 50 years, over the age of 69 years, or men with a life expectancy of less than 10 to 15 years. • Prostate cancer screening with the PSA test is controversial.
Talking points with patients	• PSA screening can detect prostate cancer, but for most men, the chances of harm from screening with the PSA test outweigh the chances of benefit. • A small number of prostate cancer cases are serious and can cause death; however, the vast majority of prostate cancer is slow-growing and does not cause death. • Most men who choose not to have PSA testing will not be diagnosed with prostate cancer and will die of something else. • Men who choose PSA testing are much more likely than those who decline PSA testing to be diagnosed with prostate cancer. • The PSA test often does not distinguish between cancer cases that are serious and those cases that are not serious; however, men with markedly elevated PSA levels (>10μg/L) may have a reduced chance of dying from prostate cancer by having surgical treatment. • The small potential benefit of prostate cancer screening corresponds to preventing, at most, 1 death caused by prostate cancer per 1000 men screened after 11 years of follow-up. • The potential harms of screening include: • Problems interpreting test results: the PSA test result may be high because of an enlarged prostate but not because of cancer, or it may be low even though cancer is present. • If a prostate biopsy is needed, it, too, is not free from risk—the biopsy involves multiple needles being inserted into the prostate under local anesthesia, and there is a risk for infection or significant bleeding as well as risk for hospitalization (1.4%). • If cancer is diagnosed, it will often be treated with surgery or radiation, which are associated with risks; there is a small risk for death with surgery, loss of sexual function (approximately 37% higher risk), and loss of control of urination (approximately 11% higher risk) compared with no surgery; these risks may vary depending on the man's and surgeon's characteristics and treatment method. • The PSA test is not "just a blood test;" it is a test that can open the door to more testing and treatment that a man may not actually want and that may actually harm him; a man's chances of being harmed are much greater than his chances of benefitting from the PSA test; thus, each man should have the opportunity to decide for himself whether to have the PSA screening test. • Studies are ongoing, so clinicians expect to learn more about the benefits and harms of screening, and recommendations may change over time; men also are welcome to change their minds at any time by asking for screening that they have previously declined or discontinue screening that they have previously requested.

DRE, digital rectal examination; *PSA*, prostate-specific antigen
Data from Qaseem A et al: *Ann Intern Med* 158(1):761, 2013.

BOX 25-8 PROSTATE SPECIFIC ANTIGEN–BASED SCREENING FOR PROSTATE CANCER

Why not screen for prostate cancer?

Screening may benefit a small number of men but will result in harm to many others. A person choosing to be screened should believe that the possibility of benefit is more important than the risk for harm. The U.S. Preventive Services Task Force assessment of the balance of benefits and harms in a screened population is that the benefits do not outweigh the harms.

What are the benefits and harms of screening 1000 men ages 55 to 69 years[1] with a prostate specific antigen (PSA) test every 1 to 4 years for 10 years?

Possible benefit of screening:	**Men, *n***
Reduced 10-year risk for dying of prostate cancer:	
Die of prostate cancer with no screening	5 in 1000
Die of prostate cancer with screening	4-5 in 1000
Do not die of prostate cancer because of screening	0-1 in 1000
Harms of screening:	
At least one false-positive screening PSA test result:	
Most positive test results lead to biopsy. Of men having biopsy, up to 33% will have moderate or major bothersome symptoms, including pain, fever, bleeding, infection, and temporary urinary difficulties; 1% will be hospitalized	100-120 in 1000
Prostate cancer diagnosis:	
Although a diagnosis of prostate cancer may not be considered a harm, currently 90% of diagnosed men are treated and thus are at risk for the harms of treatment. A large majority of the men who are being treated would do well without treatment. A substantial percentage of these men would have remained asymptomatic for life.	110 in 1000
Complications of treatment (among persons who are screened):[2]	
Develop serious cardiovascular events because of treatment	2 in 1000
Develop deep venous thrombosis or pulmonary embolus because of treatment	1 in 1000
Develop erectile dysfunction because of treatment	29 in 1000
Develop urinary incontinence because of treatment	18 in 1000
Die because of treatment	<1 in 1000

Data from Moyer VA, U.S. Preventive Services Task Force: *Ann Intern Med* 157(2):120–134, 2012. Also see Esserman L, Shieh Y, Thompson I: *J Am Med Assoc* 302(15):1685–1920, 2009 for further reading on this matter. A brief summary of the thinking of Esserman and colleagues is provided in the prostate cancer evaluation and treatment section (p. 908).

Calculations of the estimated benefits and harms rely on assumption and are, by nature, somewhat imprecise. Estimates should be considered in the full context of clinical decision making and used to stimulate shared decision making.

[1]The best evidence of possible benefit of PSA screening is in men ages 55 to 69 years.

[2]The rate of complications depends on the proportion of men having treatment and the method of treatment. The above reflects a distribution of 60% surgical treatment, 30% radiation treatment, and 10% observation. Other harms of radiation, such as bowel damage, are not shown.

Sexual Dysfunction

In men the normal sexual response involves three processes: erection, emission, and ejaculation. **Sexual dysfunction** is the impairment of any or all of these processes. Impairment can be caused by a number of physiologic and psychologic factors.

Until the late 1970s, most cases of male sexual dysfunction were thought to be psychogenic. Studies of this problem indicate that in men older than 40 years, organic factors are involved in more than 50% of cases. The causes of organic sexual dysfunction include: (1) vascular, endocrine, and neurologic disorders; (2) chronic disease, including renal failure and diabetes mellitus; (3) penile diseases and penile trauma; and (4) iatrogenic factors, such as surgery and pharmacologic therapies. Most of these disorders cause erectile dysfunction.

PATHOPHYSIOLOGY AND CLINICAL MANIFESTATIONS. Vascular disorders can prevent erection. Some arterial diseases diminish or interrupt circulation to the penis. This prevents engorgement of erectile tissues in the corpora cavernosa and corpus spongiosum. Rarely, excessive venous drainage of the corpora cavernosa prevents erection.

Endocrine disorders that reduce testosterone production affect sexual function and libido. The reduction may be caused by inadequate secretion of the gonadotropins caused by pituitary dysfunction or hyperprolactinemia. Feminizing tumors and estrogen therapy reduce relative levels of testosterone. Testicular atrophy from any cause also decreases testosterone levels and contributes to sexual dysfunction.

Neurologic disorders can interfere with the important sympathetic, parasympathetic, and CNS mechanisms required for erection, emission, and ejaculation. They include spinal cord injury or tumor, multiple sclerosis, and disorders that cause peripheral neuropathies, such as diabetes mellitus and chronic renal failure. Spinal cord injuries or tumors can alter one or more components of the sexual response, depending on the location of the lesion. For example, in most men with upper motor neuron lesions, reflexogenic erection is possible but emission and ejaculation (i.e., orgasm) are not possible. Lesions affecting the lower motor neurons usually prevent erection. In approximately 40% of such cases, emission and ejaculation are prevented.

Many chronic diseases are associated with sexual dysfunction. In some conditions the sexual dysfunction has a specific physiologic cause. Diabetes mellitus, for example, causes peripheral vascular and neurologic pathology that can lead to erectile dysfunction. Impotence occurs in about 50% of men undergoing dialysis due to decreased testosterone levels, autonomic neuropathy, accelerated vascular disease, multiple medications, worsening of primary disease, and psychologic stress. Potency may be restored by successful renal transplantation, except in bilateral transplantation if arterial flow is diminished or interrupted. Cirrhosis of the liver, scleroderma, chronic debilitation, and cachexia also are known to cause impotence. Emotional and psychologic response to chronic illness, such as anxiety, depression, and loss of self-esteem, can affect sexual functioning. In other chronic conditions, sexual dysfunction is associated with low energy levels and loss of libido. The pathophysiologic mechanisms responsible for such changes are not known.

Priapism causes fibrosis of trabeculae (erectile tissues) within the corpora cavernosa, making erection difficult. The penile curvature caused by Peyronie disease does not make erection impossible but may make it extremely painful and intercourse impossible. Penile trauma can damage the erectile tissue, disrupt the posterior urethra, and disrupt the pudendal arteries or nerves.

Iatrogenic factors, including drugs and surgery, have a significant effect on erectile function. The following surgical procedures carry the risk of erectile dysfunction: radical pelvic surgery; radical prostatectomy; transurethral, suprapubic, or simple retropubic prostatectomy; and aortoiliac surgery. Erectile dysfunction is caused by the severing of small nerve branches that are essential for erection. Aortoiliac surgery, retroperitoneal lymphadenectomy, and sympathectomy cause the loss of ejaculation capacity in some individuals.

A few pharmacologic agents enhance the sexual response, but most have the opposite effect. Men who are taking antihypertensives, antidepressants, antihistamines, antispasmodics, sedatives or tranquilizers, barbiturates, diuretics, sex hormone preparations, narcotics, or psychoactive drugs may experience some degree of sexual dysfunction. Drug-induced sexual dysfunction consists of decreased desire, decreased erectile ability, or decreased ejaculatory ability. Ethyl alcohol may induce alcoholic neuropathy or increased estrogens because of hepatic dysfunction; marijuana depresses testosterone levels; and cigarette smoking contributes to vasoconstriction and venous leakage. A number of pharmacologic agents also diminish the quality or quantity of sperm. A few may cause priapism. Drugs can assist in maintaining an erection.

EVALUATION AND TREATMENT. Evaluation of sexual dysfunction includes a physical examination, with particular attention to the genitalia, prostate, and nervous system, and basic laboratory tests to identify the presence of endocrinopathies or other underlying disorders that can cause the dysfunction. If no physiologic cause is found and the condition does not improve with psychotherapy, the man is referred for further investigation of organic causes. Psychologic evaluation is indicated for younger men with a sudden onset of sexual dysfunction or men of any age who are able to achieve but not maintain an erection.

Sophisticated diagnostic techniques can be used to assess penile blood flow, erectile tissue anatomy, nervous system function, and occurrence of erection or emission during sleep (nocturnal emission). Penile blood flow is measured by Doppler techniques and penile arteriography. Corpus cavernosography, in which contrast material is injected into the corpora cavernosa, provides anatomic information about the erectile tissue of the penis. Neuropathic causes of sexual dysfunction are evaluated by measuring the speed of the bulbocavernosus reflex. Nocturnal penile tumescence monitoring measures the frequency of nocturnal erections. Depending on the equipment used, this information may be correlated to rapid eye movement (REM) or non-REM sleep.

Treatments for organic sexual dysfunction include medical and surgical interventions. Nonsurgical interventions include correction of underlying disorders, particularly drug-induced dysfunction and endocrinopathy-related (e.g., reduced testosterone associated with chronic renal failure) dysfunction. Vasodilators and cessation of smoking can benefit individuals with vasculogenic erectile dysfunction. Surgical interventions include penile implants, penile revascularization, and correction of other anatomic defects contributing to sexual dysfunction.

Impairment of Sperm Production and Quality

Spermatogenesis requires adequate secretion of FSH and LH by the pituitary; sufficient secretion of testosterone by the Leydig cells; sufficient function of the Sertoli cells, including secretion of androgen-binding protein, growth factors, inhibin B, and a number of other important (but poorly understood) peptides; and adequate spermatogonia.[32,116] The Leydig cells are located in the testicular interstitium *between* the tubules, and the Sertoli cells and spermatogonia are located *within* the seminiferous tubules. The Sertoli cells extend from the basement membrane to the lumen, display tight junctions between adjacent cells, and form the blood-testis barrier. Inadequate secretion of gonadotropins may be caused by hypothyroidism, hyperadrenocortisolism, hyperprolactinemia, or hypogonadotropic hypogonadism. In these situations gonadotropin levels are low because of feedback inhibition or idiopathic hyposecretion. In the absence of adequate gonadotropin levels, the Leydig cells are not stimulated to secrete testosterone and sperm maturation is not promoted in the Sertoli cells. Spermatogenesis depends not only on appropriate stimulation by the gonadotropins but also an appropriate response by the testes. Defects in testicular response to the gonadotropins result in decreased secretion of testosterone and inhibin B and, as a result of normal feedback mechanisms, high levels of circulating gonadotropins. In the absence of adequate testosterone levels, spermatogenesis is impaired. Newer research demonstrates the significance of inhibin B as an important marker of the competence of Sertoli cells and spermatogenesis. Inhibin B is strongly correlated with severity of spermatogenic effects. A positive correlation exists between serum inhibin B levels and sperm concentration and testicular volume, and lower levels have been associated with azoospermia, testicular disorders, and infertility.[116]

Impaired spermatogenesis also can be caused by genetic disorders (such as Klinefelter syndrome), myotonic dystrophy, or testicular trauma. Other conditions associated with impaired spermatogenesis include systemic illness, such as renal failure, hepatic disease, or sickle cell disease; exposure to gonadotoxins, such as chemotherapy or radiation; varicocele; and cryptorchidism.

Fertility is adversely affected if spermatogenesis is normal but the sperm are chromosomally or morphologically abnormal or are produced in insufficient quantities. Chromosomal abnormalities are caused by genetic factors and by external variables, such as exposure to radiation or toxic substances. Ongoing research using small ribonucleic acids (RNAs) is elucidating the molecular mechanisms regulating spermatogenesis.[117] A sperm count of 20 million sperm per milliliter of semen has been suggested as the minimum concentration required for fertility. Average fertile men have 50 to 100 million sperm per milliliter.[32]

Sperm motility is another important variable affecting fertility. Motility appears to be affected by the sperm's chemical environment, that is, the characteristics of semen. Prostatic dysfunction, excessive semen viscosity, presence of drugs or toxins in the semen, and presence of antisperm antibodies are associated with impaired sperm motility. Approximately 3% to 7% of infertile males have antisperm antibodies in their semen. Antisperm antibodies may develop as a result of epididymitis or other inflammation of the genitourinary tract, testicular injury or torsion, a previous vasectomy or biopsy, and cryptorchidism. Antisperm antibodies may be (1) cytotoxic antibodies, which attack sperm and reduce their number in the semen; or (2) sperm-immobilizing antibodies, which impair sperm motility and reduce their ability to traverse the endocervical canal. Intrinsic, biologic factors leading to the production of antisperm antibodies seem to play a greater role than extrinsic factors. The exact mechanism remains unclear.[32]

A male factor contributes to the cause of up to 50% of cases of infertility. As understanding of the male factor in infertility increases, evaluation becomes more complex and essential to appropriate treatment (Box 25-9). Treatment for impaired spermatogenesis involves correction of any underlying disorders and avoidance of radiation or toxins. Androgens, human gonadotropins, and antiestrogens (e.g., clomiphene citrate, tamoxifen citrate) may enhance spermatogenesis. Semen can be modified to improve sperm motility. If conception is desired, the semen is obtained by masturbation (or mechanical device),[32] after which it can be diluted, concentrated, or washed to remove antisperm antibodies. These alterations are followed by artificial insemination.

BOX 25-9 EVALUATION OF MALE PARTNER OF INFERTILE COUPLES

- Thorough history and physical, including imaging for varicocele
- Two semen analyses and quantification of serum FSH, LH, testosterone levels, and prolactin if indicated
- Semen and urethral cultures
- Serum assays or monoclonal antibody testing for white blood cells
- Immunobead monoclonal antibody test
- Postcoital testing of semen activity and function
- Sperm penetration assay
- Inhibin B assays or testicular biopsy
- Vasogram, TRUS, or other imaging studies

FSH, Follicle-stimulating hormone; *LH,* luteinizing hormone; *TRUS,* transrectal ultrasonography.

DISORDERS OF THE MALE BREAST

Gynecomastia

Gynecomastia is the overdevelopment of breast tissue in a male. Gynecomastia accounts for approximately 85% of all masses that develop in the male breast and affects 32% to 40% of the male population. If only one breast is involved, it is typically the left. Incidence is greatest among adolescents and men older than 50 years.

Gynecomastia results from hormonal alterations, which may be idiopathic or caused by systemic disorders, drugs, or neoplasms. It usually involves an imbalance of the estrogen/testosterone ratio, which can be altered in one of two ways. First, estrogen levels may be excessively high, although testosterone levels are normal, as in drug-induced and tumor-induced cases of hyperestrogenism. Second, testosterone levels may be extremely low although estrogen levels are normal, as is the case in hypergonadism. Gynecomastia also can be caused by alterations in breast-tissue responsiveness to hormonal stimulation. Breast tissue may have increased responsiveness to estrogen or decreased responsiveness to androgen. Alterations of responsiveness may cause many cases of idiopathic gynecomastia.

Besides puberty and aging, estrogen-testosterone imbalances are associated with hypogonadism, Klinefelter syndrome, and testicular neoplasms. Hormone-induced gynecomastia is usually bilateral. Pubertal gynecomastia is a self-limiting phenomenon that usually disappears within 4 to 6 months. Senescent gynecomastia usually regresses spontaneously within 6 to 12 months.

Systemic disorders associated with gynecomastia include obesity, cirrhosis of the liver, infectious hepatitis, chronic renal failure, chronic obstructive lung disease, hyperthyroidism, tuberculosis, and chronic malnutrition. It may be that these disorders ultimately alter the estrogen/testosterone ratio, initiating gynecomastia.

Gynecomastia is often seen in men receiving estrogen therapy, either in preparation for a sex-change operation or for prostatic carcinoma. Other drugs that can cause gynecomastia include digitalis, cimetidine, spironolactone, reserpine, thiazide, isoniazid, ergotamine, tricyclic antidepressants, amphetamines, vincristine, and busulfan. Gynecomastia is usually unilateral in these instances.

Malignancies of the testes, adrenals, or liver can cause gynecomastia if they alter the estrogen/testosterone ratio. Pituitary adenomas and lung cancer also are associated with gynecomastia.

PATHOPHYSIOLOGY. The breast enlargement consists of hyperplastic stroma and ductal tissue. Hyperplasia results in a firm, palpable mass, at least 2 cm in diameter located beneath the areola.

EVALUATION AND TREATMENT. The diagnosis of gynecomastia is based on physical examination. Identification and treatment of the cause are likely to be followed by resolution of the gynecomastia. The man should be taught to perform breast self-examination and is examined at 6- and 12-month intervals if the gynecomastia persists. All unilateral breast enlargement in men warrants an evaluation for malignancy; workup includes fine-needle aspiration, cytology, mammography, ultrasound, and biopsy.

Cancer

Male breast cancer (MBC) accounts for 1% of all male cancers and less than 1% of all breast cancers. Global incidence rates were generally less than 1 per 100,000 man-years in contrast to much higher rates in females (see Chapter 24). The highest incidence rate for MBC is in Israel with 1.24 per 100,000, and the lowest incidence rates for males (0.16) and females (18.0) were observed in Thailand.[118] It occurs most commonly after age 60, with the peak incidence between 60 and 69 years (men tend to be diagnosed at an older age than women). It has, however, been reported in males as young as 6 years and in adolescents. Klinefelter syndrome is the strongest risk factor for developing male breast carcinoma. Other risk factors include germline mutation in *BRCA1* or *BRCA2*, but familial cases usually have *BRCA2* rather than *BRCA1* mutations.[119-121] Obesity increases the risk of MBC. Testicular disorders, including cryptorchidism, mumps, orchitis, and orchiectomy are related to risk.[122] The relationship between these factors and risk of disease is not clearly defined.

Recent data on most frequent molecular subtypes of male breast cancer appear to be different than female breast cancers with Luminal A and Luminal B the most common subtypes and basal-like, unclassifiable triple-negative, and HER2-driven male breast cancer subtypes are rare.[123-125] The majority of MBCs express estrogen and progesterone receptors.[126] The malignant male breast lesion is usually a unilateral solid mass located near the nipple. Because the nipple is commonly involved, crusting and nipple discharge are typical clinical manifestations. Other findings include skin retraction, ulceration of the skin over the tumor, and axillary node involvement. Patterns of metastasis are similar to those in females.

The diagnosis of cancer is confirmed by biopsy. Because of delays in seeking treatment, male breast cancer tends to be advanced at the time of diagnosis and therefore tends to have a poor prognosis. Treatment protocols are similar to those for female breast cancer, but endocrine therapy is used more often for males because a higher percentage of male tumors are hormone dependent. The mainstay of treatment is modified mastectomy with axillary node dissection to assess stage and prognosis. Because 90% of tumors are hormonal receptor positive, tamoxifen is standard adjuvant therapy. For metastatic disease, hormonal therapy is the main treatment but chemotherapy also can provide palliation.[119]

SUMMARY REVIEW

Alterations of Sexual Maturation

1. Sexual maturation, or puberty, should begin in boys between 9 and 14 years of age. Delayed puberty is the onset of sexual maturation after these ages; precocious puberty is onset before these ages.
2. Alterations of sexual maturation can be idiopathic or caused by a disease or congenital anomaly. In most cases of delayed puberty, the hypothalamic-pituitary-gonadal (HPG) axis is intact but the surge of activity that stimulates puberty is delayed. This situation is common in boys. Precocious puberty also can be caused by mistiming of the stimulatory surge in a child whose HPG system is otherwise normal.
3. Precocious puberty can be complete (sex appropriate), mixed (not sex appropriate), or partial (development of one secondary sex characteristic only). Causes of delayed or incomplete puberty can be divided into categories based on gonadotropic secretion: hypergonadotropism (increased levels of FSH and LH), and hypogonadotropism (decreased LH and FSH levels).

Disorders of the Male Reproductive System

1. Disorders of the urethra include urethritis (inflammation of the urethra) and urethral strictures (narrowing or obstruction of the urethral lumen caused by scarring).
2. Although noninfectious urethritis can occur, most cases of urethritis result from sexually transmitted pathogens. Symptoms of urethritis include dysuria, frequency, urgency, urethral tingling or itching, and clear or purulent discharge. Treatment consists of appropriate antibiotic therapy and avoidance of future chemical or mechanical irritation.
3. Acquired or congenital scarring that causes urethral stricture can be caused by trauma or by severe or untreated urethral infection. The primary symptom is diminished force and caliber of the urinary stream; other symptoms include urinary frequency and hesitancy, mild dysuria, double urine stream or spraying, and postvoiding dribbling. Treatment is usually surgical.
4. Phimosis and paraphimosis are penile disorders involving the foreskin (prepuce). In phimosis the foreskin cannot be retracted over the glans. In paraphimosis the foreskin is retracted and cannot be returned to its normal anatomic position over the glans. Phimosis is caused by poor hygiene and chronic infection and can lead to paraphimosis. Paraphimosis can constrict the penile blood vessels, preventing circulation to the glans.
5. Peyronie disease consists of fibrosis, affecting the corpora cavernosa, which causes penile curvature during erection. Fibrosis prevents engorgement on the affected side, causing a lateral curvature that can prevent intercourse.
6. Priapism, a prolonged painful erection not stimulated by sexual arousal, is a urologic emergency. The corpora cavernosa (but not the corpus spongiosum) fills with blood that does not drain out, probably because of venous obstruction. Priapism is associated with spinal cord trauma, sickle cell disease, leukemia, and pelvic tumors. It can also be idiopathic and can occur with cocaine use.
7. Balanitis is an inflammation of the glans penis and usually occurs in conjunction with posthitis. It is associated with phimosis, inadequate cleansing under the foreskin, skin disorders, and infections.
8. Cancer of the penis is rare; major risk factors include HPV, smoking, and consequences of treatment for psoriasis. Penile carcinoma in situ tends to involve the glans; invasive carcinoma of the penis involves the shaft as well.

SUMMARY REVIEW—cont'd

9. A varicocele is an abnormal dilation of the veins within the spermatic cord caused by either congenital absence of valves in the internal spermatic vein or acquired valvular incompetence.
10. A hydrocele is a collection of fluid between the testicular and scrotal layers of the tunica vaginalis. Hydroceles can be idiopathic or caused by trauma or infection of the testes.
11. A spermatocele is a cyst located between the testis and epididymis that is filled with fluid and sperm.
12. Cryptorchidism is a congenital condition in which one or both testes fail to descend into the scrotum. Uncorrected cryptorchidism is associated with infertility and a significantly increased risk of testicular cancer.
13. Testicular torsion is the rotation of a testis, which twists blood vessels in the spermatic cord. This interrupts blood supply to the testis, resulting in edema and, if not corrected within 4 to 6 hours, necrosis and atrophy of testicular tissues.
14. Orchitis is an acute infection of the testes. Pathogenic organisms may reach the testes through the blood or the lymphatics; most commonly, they reach the testes by ascending through the vas deferens and epididymis. Complications of orchitis include hydrocele and atrophy. Granulomatous orchitis, an autoimmune disease, is a nonspecific, noninfectious, inflammatory process that occurs in middle-aged men.
15. Testicular cancer is the most common malignancy in males ages 15 to 35 years. Although its cause is unknown, high androgen levels, genetic predisposition, and a history of cryptorchidism, trauma, or infection may contribute to tumorigenesis. Most testicular neoplasms are germ-cell tumors.
16. Epididymitis, an inflammation of the epididymis, is usually caused by a sexually transmitted pathogen that ascends through the vasa deferentia from an already infected urethra or bladder.
17. BPH is enlargement of the prostate gland. This condition becomes symptomatic as the enlarging prostate compresses the urethra, causing symptoms of bladder outlet syndrome and urine retention.
18. Prostatitis is inflammation of the prostate. Prostate syndromes have been classified by the National Institutes of Health as: (a) acute bacterial prostatitis (ABP), (b) chronic bacterial prostatitis (CBP), (c) chronic pelvic pain syndrome (CPPS), and (d) asymptomatic inflammatory prostatitis.
19. Prostate cancer is the most common cancer in American men, and the incidence varies greatly worldwide. Possible causes include genetic predisposition, environmental and dietary factors, inflammation, and alterations in levels of hormones (testosterone, dihydrotestosterone, and estradiol) and growth factors. Incidence is greatest among northwestern European and North American men (particularly blacks) older than 65 years of age.
20. Most cancers of the prostate are adenocarcinomas that develop at the periphery of the gland.
21. Sexual dysfunction in males can be caused by any physical or psychologic factor that impairs erection, emission, or ejaculation.
22. Spermatogenesis (sperm production by the testes) can be impaired by disruptions of the HPG axis that reduce testosterone secretion and by testicular trauma or atrophy from any cause. Sperm production is also impaired by neoplastic disease, cryptorchidism, or any factor that causes testicular temperature to rise.
23. Sperm quality is impaired by chromosomal abnormalities resulting from genetic factors, irradiation, or toxins. Sperm motility can be impaired by unfavorable constituents or characteristics of semen.

Disorders of the Male Breast

1. Gynecomastia is the overdevelopment (hyperplasia) of breast tissue in a male resulting from hormonal alterations, which may be idiopathic or caused by systemic disorders, drugs, or neoplasms. It usually involves an imbalance of the estrogen/testosterone ratio.
2. Gynecomastia affects 32% to 40% of the male population. The incidence is greatest among adolescents and men older than 50 years.
3. Gynecomastia is caused by hormonal or breast tissue alterations that cause estrogen to dominate. These alterations can result from systemic disorders, drugs, neoplasms, or idiopathic causes.
4. Breast cancer is relatively uncommon in males, but it has a poor prognosis because men tend to delay seeking treatment until the disease is advanced. The incidence is greatest in men in their 60s.
5. Most breast cancers in men are estrogen positive.

KEY TERMS

Acute bacterial prostatitis (ABP, category I), 899
Balanitis, 890
Benign prostatic hyperplasia (BPH) (benign prostatic hypertrophy), 897
Bladder outflow obstruction, 899
Central precocious puberty, 887
Chronic bacterial prostatitis (CBP, category II), 900
Chronic prostatitis/chronic pelvic pain syndrome (CPPS, category III), 900
Complete precocious puberty, 887
Cryptorchidism, 892
Ectopic testis, 892
Epididymitis, 897
Fibroblast, 907
Gynecomastia, 913
Hydrocele, 892
Intraprostatic conversion, 901
Mixed precocious puberty, 887
Nonbacterial prostatitis, 900
Orchitis, 894
Paraphimosis, 888
Partial precocious puberty, 887
Peyronie disease (bent nail syndrome), 889
Phimosis, 888
Precocious puberty, 886
Priapism, 890
Prostate-specific antigen (PSA), 908
Prostatitis, 899
PSA velocity, 909
Sexual dysfunction, 911
Spermatocele, 892
Stroma, 907
Torsion of the testis, 894
Urethral stricture, 888
Urethritis, 888
Varicocele, 891

REFERENCES

1. American Cancer Society: *Cancer facts & figures—2012*, Atlanta, 2012, American Cancer Society.
2. Jospe N: Disorders of pubertal development. In Osborn LM et al: *Pediatrics*, Philadelphia, 2005, Mosby.
3. Healtheon/WebMD: Hypothalamic disorders. *Scientific American Medicine*, 1999. Available at www.samed.com/sam/forms/index.htm.
4. Whittemore BJ et al: Endocrine and metabolic diseases. In Burns CE et al: *Pediatric primary care*, St Louis, 2012, Saunders.
5. Veldhuis JD, Keenan DM, Pincus SM: Regulation of complex pulsatile and rhythmic neuroendocrine systems: the male gonadal axis as a prototype, *Prog Brain Res* 181:79–110, 2010.
6. Pineda R et al: Physiological roles of the kisspeptin/GPR54 system in the neuroendocrine control of reproduction, *Prog Brain Res* 181:55–77, 2010.
7. Sørensen K et al: Recent secular trends in pubertal timing: implications for evaluation and diagnosis of precocious puberty, *Horm Res Paediatr* 77:137–145, 2012.
8. Fenichel P: Delayed puberty, *Endocr Dev* 22:138–159, 2012.
9. Euling SY et al: Examination of US puberty-timing data from 1940 to 1994 for secular trends: panel findings, *Pediatrics* 121(Suppl 3): S172–S191, 2008.
10. Herman-Giddens ME et al: Secondary sexual characteristics in boys: data from the pediatric research in office settings network, *Pediatrics* 130(5):e1058–e1068, 2012.
11. Burt Solorzano CM, McCartney CR: Obesity and the pubertal transition in girls and boys, *Reproduction* 140:399–410, 2010.
12. Howie SE et al: Immunity and vaccines against sexually transmitted *Chlamydia trachomatis* infection, *Curr Opin Infect Dis* 24(1):56–61, 2011.
13. Schollum JB, Walker RJ: Adult urinary tract infection, *Br J Hosp Med (Lond)* 73(4):218–223, 2012.
14. Brill JR: Diagnosis and treatment of urethritis in men, *Am Fam Physician* 81(7):873–878, 2010.
15. Hameed A et al: Management of bulbar urethral strictures: review of current practice, *Can J Urol* 18(3):5676–5682, 2011.
16. Tang SH et al: Adult urethral stricture disease after childhood hypospadias repair, *Adv Urol* 150315:2008, 2008.
17. McAninch JW: Disorders of the penis and male urethra. In McAninch JW, Lue TF, editors: *Smith and Tanagho's general urology*, ed 18, Norwalk, CT, 2012, McGraw-Hill Lange.
18. Anic GM, Giuliano AR: Genital HPV infection and related lesions in men, *Prev Med* 53(Suppl 1):S36–S41, 2011.
19. Gur S, Limin M, Hellstrom WJ: Current status and new developments in Peyronie's disease: medical, minimally invasive and surgical treatment options, *Exp Opin Pharmacother* 12(6):931–944, 2011.
20. Altman AL et al: Cocaine associated priapism, *J Urol* 161(6):1817–1818, 1999.
21. Minardi D et al: Persistent priapism and histological modifications of the erectile tissue. Two case reports, *Arch Ital Urol Androl* 76(2):97–99, 2004.
22. American Cancer Society: *Penile cancer resource center*, 2012. Available at www.cancer.org.
23. Letendre J, Saad F, Lattouf JB: Penile cancer: what's new? *Curr Opin Support Palliat Care* 5(3):185–191, 2011.
24. Presti JC: Genital tumors. In McAninch JW, Lue TF, editors: *Smith and Tanagho's general urology*, ed 18, Norwalk, CT, 2012, McGraw-Hill Lange.
25. National Cancer Institute: *Stages of penile cancer*, Bethesda, MD, 2011, National Cancer Institute, National Institutes of Health.
26. Lindegarrds JC et al: A retrospective analysis of 82 cases of cancer of the penis, *Br J Urol* 77(6):883, 1996.
27. Montgomery JS, Bloom DA: The diagnosis and management of scrotal masses, *Med Clin North Am* 95(1):235–244, 2011.
28. Benoff S, Marmar JL, Hurley IR: Molecular and other predictors for infertility in patients with varicoceles, *Front Biosci* 14:3641–3672, 2009.
29. Davis JE, Silverman M: Scrotal emergencies, *Emerg Med Clin North Am* 29(3):469–484, 2011.
30. Günther P, Rübben I: The acute scrotum in childhood and adolescence, *Dtsch Arztebl Int* 109(25):449–457, 2012.
31. Chen SS: Differences in the clinical characteristics between young and elderly men with varicocoele, *Int J Androl* 35(5):695–699, 2012.
32. Walsh TJ, Smith JF: Male infertility. In McAninch JW, Lue TF, editors: *Smith and Tanagho's general urology*, ed 18, Norwalk, CT, 2012, McGraw-Hill Lange.
33. Rioja J et al: Adult hydrocele and spermatocele, *BJU Int* 107(11): 1852–1864, 2011.
34. Rosenthal MS: *The fertility sourcebook*, Columbus, OH, 2002, McGraw-Hill.
35. Wampler SM, Llanes M: Common scrotal and testicular problems, *Prim Care* 37(3):613–626, 2010.
36. John Radcliffe Hospital Cryptorchidism Study Group: Cryptorchidism: a prospective study of 7500 consecutive male births, 1984–8, *Arch Dis Child* 67:892–899, 1992.
37. Walsh TJ et al: Prepubertal orchiopexy for cryptorchidism may be associated with lower risk of testicular cancer, *J Urol* 178(4 Pt 1):1440–1446, 2007.
38. Nguyen HT: Bacterial infections of the genitourinary tract. In McAninch JW, Lue TF, editors: *Smith and Tanagho's general urology*, ed 18, Norwalk, CT, 2012, McGraw-Hill Lange.
39. National Cancer Institute: *Testicular cancer incidence and mortality*, 2012. Available at www.cancer.gov/cancertopics/pdq/treatment/testicular.
40. National Cancer Institute: *Testicular cancer information*, 2012. Available at www.cancer.gov/cancertopics/pdq/treatment/testicular.
41. Shala C, Tripathi R, Mishra DP: Male germ cell apoptosis: regulation and biology, *Philos Trans R Soc Lond B Biol Sci* 365(1546):1501–1515, 2010.
42. Mirabello L et al: Promotor methylation of candidate genes associated with familial testicular cancer, *Int J Mol Epidemiol Genet* 3(3):213–227, 2012.
43. Trojian TH, Lishnak TS, Heiman D: Epididymitis and orchitis: an overview, *Am Fam Physician* 79:583–587, 2009.
44. Platz EA et al: Incidence and progression of lower urinary tract symptoms in a large prospective cohort of United States men, *J Urol* 188(2):496–501, 2012.
45. Timms BG, Hofkamp LE: Prostate development and growth in benign prostatic hyperplasia, *Differentiation* 82(4–5):173–183, 2011.
46. Nicholson TM, Ricke WA: Androgens and estrogens in benign prostatic hyperplasia: past, present and future, *Differentiation* 82(4–5):184–199, 2011.
47. Chughtai B et al: Inflammation and benign prostatic hyperplasia: clinical implications, *Curr Urol Rep* 12(4):274–277, 2011.
48. Sampson N, Madersbacher S, Berger P: [Pathophysiology and therapy of benign prostatic hyperplasia], *Wien Klin Wochenschr* 120(13–14): 390–401, 2008.
49. Bachmann A, de la Rosette J, editors: *Benign prostatic hyperplasia and lower urinary tract symptoms in men*, New York, 2012, Oxford University Press.
50. Cooperberg MR et al: Neoplasms of the prostate gland. In McAninch JW, Lue TF, editors: *Smith and Tanagho's general urology*, ed 18, Norwalk, CT, 2012, McGraw-Hill Lange.
51. Kapoor A: Benign prostatic hyperplasia (BPH) management in the primary care setting, *Can J Urol* 19(5 Suppl 1):10–17, 2012.
52. Touma NJ, Nickel JC: Prostatitis and chronic pelvic pain in men, *Med Clin North Am* 95:75–86, 2011.
53. Trottler H, Burchell AN: Epidemiology of mucosal human papillomavirus infection and associated diseases, *Public Health Genomics* 12(5-6):291–307, 2009.
54. Karatas OF et al: *Helicobacter pylori* seroprevalence in patients with chronic prostatitis: a pilot study, *Scand J Urol Nephrol* 44(2):91–94, 2010.
55. Moyer VA: U.S. Preventive Services Task Force: Screening for prostate cancer: U.S. Preventive Services Task Force recommendation statement, *Ann Intern Med* 157(2):120–134, 2012.
56. Jemal A et al: Global cancer statistics, *Ca Cancer J Clin* 61:69–90, 2011.
57. Marshall JR: Diet and prostate cancer prevention, *World J Urol* 30(2):157–165, 2012.
58. Tewari R et al: Diet, obesity, and prostate health: are we missing the link? *J Androl* 33(5):763–776, 2012.
59. Platz EA: Energy imbalance and prostate cancer, *J Nutr* 132(11 Suppl): 3471S–3481S, 2002.
60. Belanger B et al: Comparison of residual C-19 steroids in plasma and prostatic tissue of human, rat, guinea pig after castration: unique importance of extratesticular androgens in men, *J Scand Biochem* 32:695–698, 1989.
61. Labrie F: Blockage of testicular and adrenal androgens in prostate cancer treatment, *Nat Rev Urol* 8:73–80, 2011.
62. Montgomery RB: Maintenance of intratumoral androgens in metastatic prostate cancer: a mechanism for castration-resistant tumor growth, *Cancer Res* 68(11):4447–4454, 2008.
63. Bosland MC: The role of steroid hormones in prostate carcinogenesis, *J Natl Cancer Inst*(27)39–66, 2000.
64. Bosland MC: Sex steroids and prostate carcinogenesis: integrated, multifactorial working hypothesis, *Ann N Y Acad Sci* 1089:168–176, 2006.
65. Ellem SJ, Risbridger GP: The dual, opposing roles of estrogen in the prostate, *Ann N Y Acad Sci* 1155:174–186, 2009.
66. Thompson IM et al: The influence of finasteride on the development of prostate cancer, *N Engl J Med* 349:215–224, 2003.
67. Endogenous Hormones and Prostate Cancer Collaborative Group et al: Endogenous sex hormones and prostate cancer: a collaborative analysis of 18 prospective studies, *J Natl Cancer Inst* 100(3):170–183, 2008.

68. Ganesh B et al: Risk factors for prostate cancer: a hospital-based case-control study from Mumbai, India, *Indian J Urol* 27(3):345–350, 2011.
69. Lippman SM et al: Effect of selenium and vitamin E on risk of prostate cancer and other cancers: the Selenium and Vitamin E Cancer Prevention Trial (SELECT), *J Am Med Assoc* 301:39–51, 2009.
70. van Leeuwen PJ et al: Critical assessment of prebiopsy parameters for predicting prostate cancer metastasis and mortality, *Can J Urol*(6) 6018–6024, 2011.
71. Köhler TS, Fazili AA, Brannigan RE: Putative health risks associated with vasectomy, *Urol Clin North Am* 36(3):337–345, 2009.
72. McConnell JD et al: The long-term effect of doxazosin, finasteride, and combination therapy on the clinical progression of benign prostatic hyperplasia, *N Engl J Med* 349(25):2387–2398, 2003.
73. McVary KT: A review of combination therapy in patients with benign prostatic hyperplasia, *Clin Ther* 29(3):387–398, 2007.
74. Jiang M et al: Disruption of PPAR gamma signaling results in mouse prostatic intraepithelial neoplasia involving active autophagy, *Cell Death Differ* 17:469–481, 2010.
75. MacLennan GT et al: The influence of chronic inflammation in prostatic carcinogenesis: a 5-year follow-up study, *J Urol* 176(3):1012–1016, 2006.
76. Jiang M et al: PPARγ: a molecular link between systemic metabolic disease and benign prostate hyperplasia, *Differentiation* 82:220–236, 2011.
77. Albright F et al: Significant evidence for a heritable contribution to cancer predisposition: a review of cancer familiality by site, *BMC Cancer* 12:138, 2012.
78. Castro E, Eeles R: The role of BRCA1 and BRCA2 in prostate cancer, *Asian J Androl* 14(3):409–414, 2012.
79. Leongamornlert D et al: Germline BRCA1 mutations increase prostate cancer risk, *Br J Cancer* 106(10):1697–1701, 2012.
80. Van Neste L et al: The epigenetic promise for prostate cancer diagnosis, *Prostate* 72(11):1248–1261, 2012.
81. Epstein JI: The lower urinary tract and male genital system. In Kumar V, Abbas AK, Fausto N, editors: *Robbins & Cotran pathologic basis of disease*, ed 8, Philadelphia, 2009, Saunders.
82. Rubin MA: ETS rearrangements in prostate cancer, *Asian J Androl* 14(3):393–399, 2012.
83. Sciarra A et al: Inflammation and chronic prostatic diseases: evidence for a link? *Eur Urol* 52(4):964–972, 2007.
84. Lumen N et al: Screening and early diagnosis of prostate cancer: an update, *Acta Clin Belg* 67(4):270–275, 2012.
85. Mackinnon AC et al: Molecular biology underlying the clinical heterogeneity of prostate cancer: an update, *Arch Pathol Lab Med* 133(7):1033–1040, 2009.
86. Bonkoff H, Berges R: The evolving role of oestrogens and their receptors in the development and progression of prostate cancer, *Euro Urology* 55:533–542, 2009.
87. Ellem SJ, Risbridger GP: Aromatase and regulating the estrogen: androgen ration in the prostate gland, *J Steroid Biochem Mol Biol* 118(4-5):246–251, 2010.
88. Parnes HL, Thompson IM, Ford LG: Review article: prevention of hormone-related cancers: prostate cancer, *J Clin Oncol* 23(2):368–377, 2005.
89. Kawashima H, Nakatani T: Involvement of estrogen receptors in prostatic diseases, *Int J Urol* 19(6):512–522, 2012.
90. Bonkhoff H et al: Progesterone receptor expression in human prostate cancer: correlation with cancer progression, *Prostate* 48(4):285–291, 2001.
91. Setlur SR et al: Estrogen-dependent signaling in a molecular distinct subclass of aggressive prostate cancer, *J Natl Cancer Inst* 100:815–825, 2008.
92. Ellem SJ et al: Local aromatase expression in human prostate is altered in malignancy, *J Clin Endocrinol Metab* 89(5):2434–2551, 2004.
93. Treas JN, Tvagi T, Singh KP: Effects of chronic exposure to arsenic and estrogen on epigenetic regulatory genes expression and epigenetic code in human prostate epithelial cells, *PLoS One* 7(8):e43880, 2012.
94. Bosland MC, Mahmoud AM: Hormones and prostate carcinogenesis: androgens and estrogens, *J Carcinog* 10:33, 2011.
95. Vander Griend DJ et al: Cell autonomous intracellular androgen signaling drives the growth of human prostate cancer-initiating cells, *Prostate* 70(1):90–99, 2010.
96. Ricke EA et al: Androgen hormone action in prostatic carcinogenesis: stromal androgen receptors mediate prostate cancer progression, malignant transformation and metastasis, *Carcinogenesis* 33(7):1391–1398, 2012.
97. DeMarzo AM et al: Inflammation in prostate carcinogenesis, *Nat Rev Cancer* 7:256–269, 2007.
98. Marian CO, Shay JW: Prostate tumor initiating cells: a new target for telomerase inhibition therapy? *Biochim Biophys Acta* 1792:289–296, 2009.
99. Bianchi-Frias D et al: The effects of aging on the molecular and cellular composition of the prostate microenvironment, *PLoS* 5(9):e12501, 2010.
100. DeMagalhaes JP, Curado J, Church GM: Meta-analysis of age-related gene expression profiles identifies common signatures of aging, *Bioinformatics* 25:875–881, 2009.
101. Kim SK: Common aging pathways in worms, flies, mice and humans, *J Exp Biol* 210:1607–1612, 2007.
102. Kuilman T et al: Oncogene-induced senescence relayed by an interleukin-dependent inflammatory network, *Cell* 133:1019–1031, 2008.
103. Paapatto GS et al: Prostate carcinogenesis and inflammation: emerging insights, *Carcinogenesis* 26:1170–1181, 2005.
104. Thiery JP: Epithelial-mesenchymal transitions in tumor progression, *Nat Rev Cancer* 2(6):441–454, 2002.
105. Jossen S et al: Tumor-stromal interaction influence radiation sensitivity in epithelial versus mesenchymal-like prostate cancer cell, *J Oncol*, 2010. pii:232831.
106. Bhowmick NA, Moses HL: Tumor-stromal interactions, *Curr Opin Genet Develop* 15(1):97–101, 2005.
107. Xu J et al: Prostate cancer metastasis: role of the host microenvironment in promoting epithelial to mesenchymal transition and increase bone adrenal gland metastasis, *Prostate* 66:1664–1673, 2006.
108. Liu W et al: Copy number analysis indicates monoclonal origin of lethal metastatic prostate cancer, *Nat Med* 15(5):559–565, 2009.
109. Celia-Terrassa T et al: Epithelial-mesenchymal transition can suppress major attributes of human epithelial tumor-initiating cells, *J Clin Invest* 122(5):1849–1868, 2012.
110. Stamey TA: The era of serum prostate antigens as a marker for biopsy of the prostate and detecting prostate cancer is now over in the USA, *BJU Int* 94(7):963–964, 2004.
111. Chou R et al: Screening for prostate cancer: a review of the evidence for the U.S. Preventive Services Task Force, *Ann Intern Med* 155(11): 762–771, 2011.
112. Vickers AJ, Brewster SF: PSA velocity and doubling time in diagnosis and prognosis of prostate cancer, *Br J Med Surg Urol* 5(4):162–168, 2012.
113. Vickers AJ et al: An empirical evaluation of guidelines on prostate-specific antigen velocity in prostate cancer detection, *J Natl Cancer Inst* 103(6):462–469, 2011.
114. Nguyen CT, Kattan MW: Formalized prediction of clinically significant prostate cancer: is it possible? *Asian J Androl* 14(3):349–354, 2012.
115. Boorjian SA et al: The impact of discordance between biopsy and pathological Gleason scores on survival after radical prostatectomy, *J Urol* 181(1):95–104, 2009.
116. Toulis KA et al: Inhibin B and anti-Mullerian hormone as markers of persistent spermatogenesis in men with non-obstructive azoospermia: a meta-analysis of diagnostic accuracy studies, *Hum Reprod Update* 16(6):713–724, 2010.
117. He Z et al: Small RNA molecules in the regulation of spermatogenesis, *Reproduction* 137(6):901–911, 2009.
118. Ly D et al: An international comparison of male and female breast cancer incidence rates, *Int J Cancer*, 2012 Sept 14. [Epub ahead of print.].
119. Gómez-Raposo C et al: Male breast cancer, *Cancer Treat Rev* 36(6): 451–457, 2010.
120. Johansen Taber KA et al: Male breast cancer: risk factors, diagnosis, and management, *Oncol Rep* 24(5):1115–1120, 2010.
121. Ottini L et al: Male breast cancer, *Crit Rev Oncol Hematol* 73(2):141–155, 2010.
122. Zygogianni AG et al: Male breast carcinoma: epidemiology, risk factors and current therapeutic approaches, *Asian Pac J Cancer Prev* 13(1): 15–19, 2012.
123. Kornegoor R et al: Molecular subtyping of male breast cancer by immunochemistry, *Mod Pathol* 25(3):398–404, 2012.
124. Nilsson C et al: Molecular subtyping of male breast cancer using alternative definitions and its prognostic impact, *Acta Oncol*, 2012 Aug 29. [Epub ahead of print.].
125. Sanchez-Munoz A et al: Male breast cancer: immunohistochemical subtypes and clinical outcome characterization, *Oncology* 83(4):228–233, 2012.
126. Clark JL et al: Prognostic variables in male breast cancer, *Am Surg* 66(5):501, 2000.

CHAPTER

26

Sexually Transmitted Infections

Julia C. Phillippi and Gwen A. Latendresse

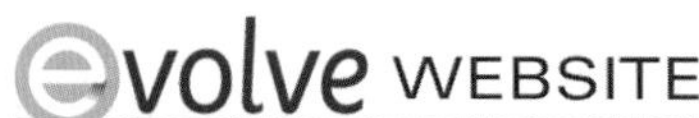

http://evolve.elsevier.com/McCance/

- Review Questions and Answers

CHAPTER OUTLINE

Throughout recorded history, infectious diseases have threatened humans. Even into the twentieth century, epidemics of diphtheria, typhoid, tuberculosis, cholera, and other catastrophic infections have decimated entire communities almost overnight (see Chapter 10). Despite medical advances, improved living standards, and better nutrition, epidemics still arise as major public health problems, and some pose lethal threats to individuals and communities. Some of these epidemics are caused by sexually transmitted infections (STIs). At this time, many people consider the number of individuals with acquired immunodeficiency syndrome (AIDS), human immunodeficiency virus (HIV), and human papillomavirus (HPV) infections to be at epidemic levels.

Sexually contracted infections affect more than 19 million Americans per year (see What's New? Sexually Transmitted Infection [STI] Statistical Summary from 2010 CDC Report), and half of those are younger than 25 years[1] and account for about one third of the reproductive mortality in the United States. They have been called the "hidden epidemic" by the Centers for Disease Control and Prevention (CDC)[2] because of their stigma and overall lack of knowledge of the prevalence and consequences of sexually transmitted infections. Complications of STIs include pelvic inflammatory disease, infertility, ectopic pregnancy, chronic pelvic pain, neonatal morbidity and mortality, and genital cancers. Long-term sequelae of untreated or undertreated STIs can affect a person's physical, emotional, and financial well-being.

In the past an infection transmitted through sexual intercourse was called a *venereal disease.* Because of its limited scope, the term venereal disease has been replaced with *sexually transmitted infection (STI).* STIs are contracted by intimate, as well as sexual, contact and include systemic infections, such as tuberculosis and hepatitis, that can be spread to a sexual partner. The etiology of an STI may be bacterial, viral, protozoal, parasitic, or fungal (Table 26-1). Although the majority of STIs can be treated, viral STIs cannot be cured, only treated naturally or pharmacologically. Many infected individuals do not seek treatment because symptoms are absent, minor, or transient or because health services are inaccessible, unaffordable, or culturally insensitive. High-risk sexual behaviors (e.g., multiple partners) and poor health habits (e.g., failure to use a condom in nonmonogamous or new relationships, drug use) increase an individual's risk of exposure or the severity of infection if exposed. Perhaps partly

WHAT'S NEW?

Sexually Transmitted Infection (STI) Statistical Summary from 2010 CDC Report

Each year in the United States:

- 19 million individuals contract a sexually transmitted infection; half of those infected are younger than 25 years
- 17 billion dollars are spent on STIs, not including long-term healthcare costs
- Only half of people who need STI screening receive needed services

Chlamydia cases:

- 1.3 million cases were reported and treated but an estimated 2.6 million additional cases remain untreated

Gonorrhea cases increased in 2010 and have become resistant to many previous treatments and may soon become resistant to remaining antibiotics

Syphilis cases have decreased for the first time in a decade:

- There was a 134% increase in the syphilis rate among young black men
- The syphilis rate is highest among men who have sex with men

Viral STIs affect more than 70 million people in the United States:

- 20 million currently infected with human papillomavirus; more than half of all sexually active people will get HPV in their lifetime
- 50 million with genital herpes
- 1 million with HIV

Data from Centers for Disease Control and Prevention: *Sexually transmitted disease surveillance, 2010,* Atlanta, 2011, U.S. Department of Health and Human Services. Available at www.cdc.gov/std/stats.

because of risk-taking behavior (unprotected intercourse or selection of high-risk partners), adolescents have the greatest risk for STI exposure and infection. In addition, adolescent women may have a physiologically increased susceptibility to infection because of cervical immaturity. Rates of gonorrhea, chlamydia, vaginitis, cervical condyloma, genital warts, and pelvic inflammatory disease (PID) are highest in adolescents and young women and decline exponentially with increasing age (Figure 26-1). The health consequences of STIs are both immediate and long-term. Women and infants bear the greatest health burden from STIs.

STIs are stereotyped as occurring only among urban poor and minority populations. Because the CDC does not require that all STIs be reported, private physicians may not report them. Thus reported STIs often are provided by public health clinics, giving the impression that a greater number of the urban poor and minority populations are infected with STIs. In fact, STIs are prevalent in all socioeconomic and racial/ethnic groups.

TABLE 26-1 CURRENTLY RECOGNIZED SEXUALLY TRANSMITTED INFECTIONS

CAUSAL MICROORGANISM	INFECTION
Bacteria	
Campylobacter	Campylobacter enteritis
Calymmatobacterium granulomatis	Granuloma inguinale
Chlamydia trachomatis	Urogenital infections; lymphogranuloma venereum
Polymicrobial	
Gardnerella vaginalis interaction with anaerobes (*Bacteroides* and *Mobiluncus spp.*) and genital mycoplasmas	Bacterial vaginosis
Haemophilus ducreyi	Chancroid
Mycoplasma	Mycoplasmosis
Neisseria gonorrhoeae	Gonorrhea
Shigella	Shigellosis
Treponema pallidum	Syphilis
Viruses	
Cytomegalovirus	Cytomegalic inclusion disease
Hepatitis B virus (HBV)	Hepatitis
Hepatitis C virus (HCV)	Hepatitis
Herpes simplex virus (HSV)	Genital herpes
Human immunodeficiency virus (HIV)	Acquired immunodeficiency syndrome (AIDS)
Human papillomavirus (HPV)	Condylomata acuminata, cervical dysplasia, and cervical cancer
Molluscum contagiosum virus	Molluscum contagiosum
Protozoa	
Entamoeba histolytica	Amebiasis; amebic dysentery
Giardia lamblia	Giardiasis
Trichomonas vaginalis	Trichomoniasis
Ectoparasites	
Phthirus pubis	Pediculosis pubis
Sarcoptes scabiei	Scabies
Fungus	
Candida albicans	Candidiasis

SEXUALLY TRANSMITTED UROGENITAL INFECTIONS

Bacterial Infections

Gonorrhea

Gonorrhea is caused by **gonococci** (singular, *gonococcus*), which are microorganisms of the species *Neisseria gonorrhoeae.* Neisser first identified gonococci in stained smears of vaginal, urethral, and conjunctival exudate in 1879. Until 1994 gonorrhea was the most commonly reported communicable infection in the United States. After reaching a record low in 2009, the rates for gonorrhea increased 2% between 2009 and 2010. Although the number of reported cases in 2010 was 309,341,[2] the actual number of cases is estimated to be twice as high.

Infection rates are highest in the southern region of the United States.[2] Other demographic and lifestyle risk factors may include transient or urban residence, early onset of sexual activity, multiple serial or consecutive sex partners, drug use, prostitution, and previous gonorrheal or concurrent STI.[2] The risk of developing gonorrhea from intercourse with an infected male partner is 50% to 80% for women, and with an infected female partner, it is 20% to 30% for men. The risk increases threefold to fourfold for men after four exposures to an infected partner. Men who have sex with infected men have a greater risk of contracting gonorrhea if they are the receptive partner in oral or anal intercourse.[2]

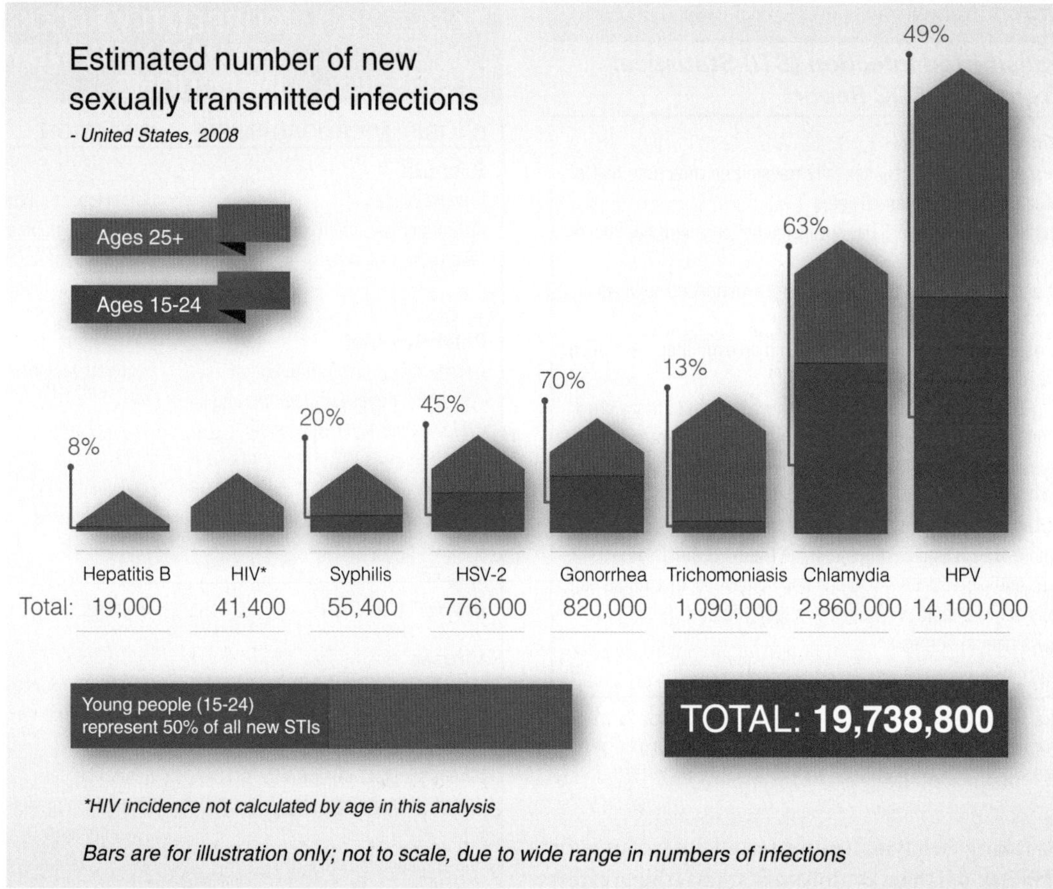

FIGURE 26-1 **Incidence and Prevalence of Sexually Transmitted Infections.** (From Centers for Disease Control and Prevention: *CDC fact sheet: incidence, prevalence, and cost of sexually-transmitted infections in the United States,* 2013. Available at www.cdc.gov/std/stats/STI-Estimates-Fact-Sheet-Feb-2013.pdf. Accessed February 24, 2013, using data from Satterwhite CL et al: *Sex Transm Dis* 40[3]:187–193, 2013.)

Transmission of gonococcal infection generally requires contact of epithelial (mucosal) surfaces, such as occurs during sexual, oral, or anal intercourse. A pregnant woman also can transmit gonorrhea to her fetus. The infection passes from mother to child predominantly through infected cervical and vaginal secretions. **Fomites** (contaminated objects) are rarely involved in the transmission of *N. gonorrhoeae,* primarily because the gonococcus requires a rich medium (e.g., body fluids) and an environment high in carbon dioxide (5% to 10%) for growth.

Treatment for gonorrhea is becoming more difficult because of rapidly developing resistance to available antibiotics. The CDC states that it is reasonable to expect that gonorrhea may become resistant to all known antibiotics in the near future.[3]

PATHOPHYSIOLOGY. Humans are the only natural hosts for *N. gonorrhoeae,* which is an aerobic, non–spore-forming, oxidase-positive gram-negative coccal (round) microorganism that usually appears in pairs (diplococci), with the adjacent sides slightly flattened. Hairlike filaments, called *pili,* appear to help the microorganisms attach themselves to host cells: the epithelial cells of mucous membranes (Figure 26-2). Columnar, transitional, and stratified squamous epithelial cells are infected most often. First the microorganisms become attached to the plasma membranes (cell walls) of these cells, and then they

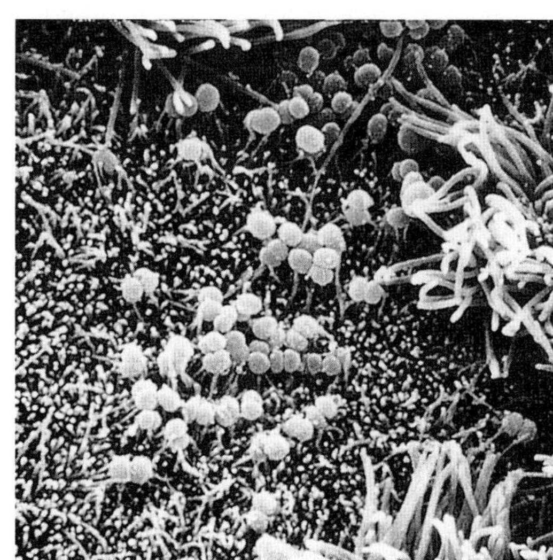

FIGURE 26-2 **Gonococci.** Scanning electron microscopy showing gonococci attaching to the nonciliated cells of human fallopian tube mucosa. (From Morse SA et al, editors: *Atlas of sexually transmitted diseases and AIDS,* ed 3, London, 2003, Mosby.)

invade the cells and begin to damage the mucosa. Generally a quick leukocytic (inflammatory) response and exudation at the site of infection occur.

In women the endocervical canal (inner portion of the cervix) is the usual site of initial gonococcal infection, although urethral colonization and infection of glands (paraurethral [Skene glands] and greater vestibular [Bartholin glands]) near the urethra and vagina also are common. Several factors can facilitate ascent of gonococci into the uterus and the fallopian tubes, where they cause PID. Among these factors are: (1) disintegration of the cervical mucous plug and an increase in vaginal pH to greater than 4.5 during menstruation, (2) uterine contraction that may cause retrograde menstruation into the fallopian/uterine tubes, and (3) various microbes that possess virulent potentiating factors for chlamydia or gonococcal PID. Bacteria *(N. gonorrhoeae, Chlamydia trachomatis)* also may adhere to sperm and be transported to the fallopian/uterine tubes. In the fallopian/uterine tubes, progressive mucosal and submucosal invasion and sloughing of normal, ciliated tubal epithelium are accompanied by a marked inflammatory response, causing the tubes to fill with exudate (see Chapter 25 for more on PID). In men the gonococci typically infect the urethra or rectum. Untreated urethral infection can cause epididymitis in men, and, if untreated, urethral stricture, fistula, and sterility.[4] Concurrent oropharyngeal and anorectal infection can be found in infected men and women.[2] Virulence is determined by variations in the bacterial properties and host response.

CLINICAL MANIFESTATIONS. The clinical manifestations of gonorrhea can be categorized as local or systemic and uncomplicated or complicated. Uncomplicated local infections are seen as urethral infections in men and urogenital infections in women. The majority of infected men will have sudden onset of painful urination or purulent penile discharge, or both, within a week of infection.[4] These severe symptoms encourage most men in developed countries to seek treatment.[2,4] However, some men have little discharge or urethral itching (i.e., pruritus) only, and 5% to 10% never have signs or symptoms. Most cases of untreated gonococcal urethritis resolve spontaneously after several weeks, and more than 95% of individuals are asymptomatic by 6 months after infection (although they may still be infectious). Some men develop urethritis even after being appropriately treated. If untreated, gonorrhea can cause penile abscesses, fistulae, and strictures.[4]

In women, the incubation period varies, but those who develop symptoms usually manifest within 10 days of exposure or within 1 to 2 days after the next menstrual period. More than half of gonorrhea infections in women are initially asymptomatic. Symptoms often do not appear until the infection has spread to the upper reproductive tract (uterus, fallopian/uterine tubes, and ovaries). Symptoms can include dysuria, increased vaginal discharge, abnormal menses (increased flow or dysmenorrhea), dyspareunia, lower abdominal/pelvic pain, and fever. Physical examination may disclose cervical friability and erythema (redness) and mucopurulent discharge from the cervical os (Figure 26-3). There may be a discharge from the paraurethral (Skene) or greater vestibular (Bartholin) glands if these sites are involved.

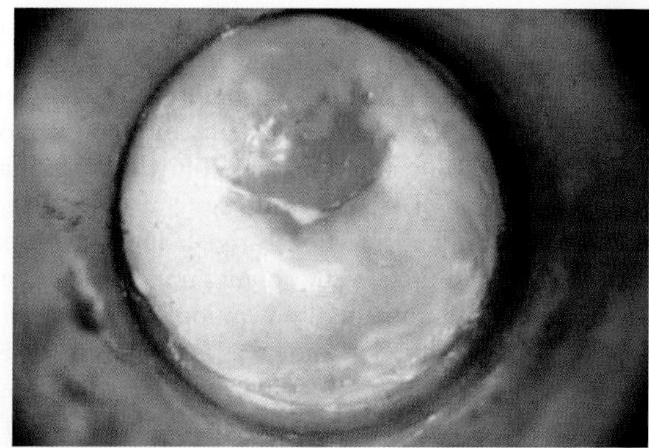

FIGURE 26-3 **Gonococcal Cervicitis.** The cervix is involved in 85% to 90% of cases in women, but the resultant discharge is profuse enough to be recognized in only 10%. (From Centers for Disease Control and Prevention: *STD clinical slides (website).* Available at www.cdc.gov/std/training/clinicalslides/slides-dl.htm. Accessed March 5, 2013.)

Anal and rectal gonococcal infection is found in 30% to 50% of women diagnosed with urogenital gonorrhea. In women, anorectal infection is usually asymptomatic and not necessarily related to anal intercourse. Symptomatic anorectal gonorrhea occurs more commonly in men who have sex with men.[2] Symptoms of anorectal gonorrhea range from mild anal pruritus (itching), mucopurulent rectal discharge, and slight rectal bleeding to severe rectal pain, tenesmus (painful and ineffectual straining at stool), and constipation. Physical examination findings include anal erythema and discharge and evidence of mucosal damage to the anus and rectum, such as friability, edema, and purulent exudate.

Gonococcal pharyngitis occurs after oral sexual contact with an infected partner. Symptomatic pharyngitis is indistinguishable from any other bacterial pharyngitis and can include fever, lymphadenopathy, and tonsillitis. Approximately 60% of these infections are asymptomatic.

Other sites of uncomplicated local infections include the eye, leading to conjunctivitis; however, this is rare in adults. Primary cutaneous infection also has been reported and is usually manifested as a localized ulcer of the genitalia, perineum, proximal lower extremities, or fingers. It is important to determine whether such infections are the result of *N. gonorrhoeae* or secondary colonization by a preexisting lesion.

Complicated gonococcal infections include prostatitis, epididymitis, lymphangitis, and urethral stricture in men and salpingitis, PID, and bartholinitis in women. Chronic salpingitis or perididymitis can cause scarring and adhesions that lead to sterility in men and women. Approximately 10%[2] of women with untreated cervical gonorrhea develop salpingitis or PID. Importantly, salpingitis has the potential for long-term sequelae, especially infertility and ectopic pregnancy.

The onset of symptoms for women may be rapid and usually occurs during menses. Women may experience chills, fever, nausea, vomiting, and lower abdominal/pelvic pain that worsen with movement, such as walking, coughing, sneezing, or intercourse. Abdominal palpation often discloses bilateral lower quadrant tenderness and rebound tenderness resulting from peritoneal irritation caused by tubal exudate. Marked tenderness of the internal genitalia is often noted during pelvic examination. Enlargement or masses may be palpable in the upper genital tract. Tubal infertility is found in 12% of women after one episode of PID. If a woman has three or more episodes of PID, she has a 50% risk of tubal infertility.[5] **Disseminated gonococcal infection (DGI)** is a rare systemic complication caused by the spread of infection through the bloodstream. Symptoms of this life-threatening condition include a generalized rash and severe joint pain. Proliferation of *N. gonorrhoeae* to the liver causes a condition known as **perihepatitis** or Fitz-Hugh–Curtis syndrome. *C. trachomatis* also has been identified as a causative agent of this condition. Inflammation of the capsule of the liver produces sudden and intense right upper quadrant pain.[6] This complication usually develops after acute salpingitis in women and is very rare in men.

If a mother has untreated gonorrhea at the time of birth, she can transmit the infection to her child, regardless of whether the baby is delivered vaginally or by cesarean section. Most states require all infants to receive prophylactic ophthalmic antibiotics to prevent gonococcal eye infection **(ophthalmia neonatorum)** (Figure 26-4) and risk for associated blindness. Newborns born to infected mothers also may develop gonorrheal rhinitis, anorectal infection, or an abscess at the site of electrode placement for fetal monitoring. Onset of symptoms generally occurs 1 to 12 days after birth, with a mean of 4 to 6 days. Affected newborns usually are born to mothers who have suffered from prolonged ruptured membranes. In these cases, immediate treatment with a topical antibiotic is not effective because the infection is already established. Established infection causes bilateral corneal ulceration, with a profuse yellow or gray purulent exudate, and is followed by necrosis, scarring, and permanent blindness.

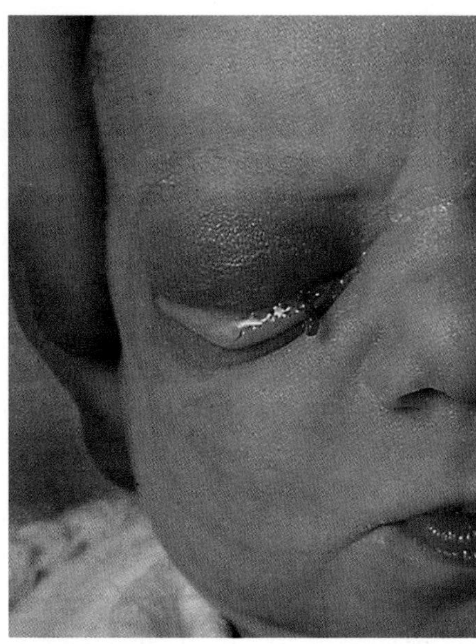

FIGURE 26-4 Gonococcal Ophthalmia Neonatorum. Examiner would be gloved. (From McMillan A, Scott GR: *Sexually transmitted infections,* ed 2, London, 2000, Churchill Livingstone.)

EVALUATION AND TREATMENT. Clinical signs and symptoms are not sufficient for the differential diagnosis of gonococcal infections. Microscopic evaluation of Gram-stained slides of clinical specimens is deemed positive for *N. gonorrhoeae* if gram-negative diplococci with typical "kidney bean" morphology are seen inside polymorphonuclear leukocytes. Such a finding is considered adequate for the diagnosis of gonococcal urethritis in a symptomatic man. For women, the Gram-stain technique is less accurate and reliable and is replaced with a single sample of endocervical secretions. Most clinic settings now use nucleic acid hybridization tests because these samples do not require an anaerobic incubation, are highly sensitive, and can be easily transported to a laboratory for testing. Because of the large percentage of infected women without symptoms, routine screening for at-risk women (i.e., those younger than age 25 or with a new sexual partner) is recommended. Samples can be obtained from the urine or the vagina, endocervix, urethra, rectum, or oropharynx. Although nucleic acid hybridization is acceptable for screening, the CDC prefers direct culture for testing because this will provide information about antibiotic susceptibility and help provide a cure.[3]

N. gonorrhoeae has developed resistance to many antibiotics and has the potential to become resistant to all current treatment drugs.[3] Several types of drug-resistant strains have been identified, including penicillinase-producing *N. gonorrhoeae* (PPNG), which is resistant to penicillin; tetracycline-resistant *N. gonorrhoeae* (TRNG), which is resistant to tetracycline; chromosomal control of mechanisms of resistance of *N. gonorrhoeae* (CMRNG), which is resistant to penicillin and tetracycline; and increasingly a fluoroquinolone-resistant *N. gonorrhoeae* (QRNG).[7,8] Until 2007 fluoroquinolones were the first-line treatment recommended by the CDC. In 2010 more than 27% of CDC-monitored samples were resistant to one or more antibiotics.[2] The only class of drugs still recommended for treatment of gonorrhea are the cephalosporins; however, there is increasing resistance to this type of medication in the United States, Canada, and around the world. There is currently only one CDC recommended drug, ceftriaxone, to treat gonorrhea although less-effective alternatives are available.[3] To prevent further drug resistance, the CDC recommends a multidrug treatment for gonorrhea that also is effective against chlamydia.[3]

The CDC is closely observing the drug resistance of gonorrhea through monitoring of samples obtained at sexually transmitted disease (STD) clinics around the country.[3] Treatment for gonorrhea is influenced by three factors: (1) the spread of infection caused by drug-resistant strains, (2) the high frequency of chlamydia infection accompanying gonorrhea, and (3) the recognition of the serious complications of chlamydia and gonorrhea infections. CDC treatment guidelines are updated regularly, and the most recent edition should be used. Current CDC treatment guidelines for uncomplicated gonorrheal infections are listed in Box 26-1; complicated infections require intravenous antibiotic therapy and possibly hospitalization.

Sexual partners also are assessed and treated according to these protocols, and sexual contact is avoided until treatment is completed. Condoms are strongly recommended to prevent future infection.

Syphilis

Syphilis, a disease with local and systemic manifestations, has been well-known throughout history. Many famous figures

BOX 26-1 OUTPATIENT TREATMENT FOR UNCOMPLICATED GONORRHEA INFECTION

- One of the following:
  Ceftriaxone, 125 mg IM in a single dose
- AND to prevent drug resistance and treat potential infection with chlamydia:
  Azithromycin, 1 g PO in a single dose
  or
  Doxycycline, 100 mg PO bid × 7 days

Data from Centers for Disease Control and Prevention: *MMWR Morb Mortal Wkly Rep* 61(31):590-594, 2012.
bid, Twice per day; *IM,* intramuscularly; *PO,* orally.

from the ancient world and from the royal families of Europe were thought or known to have had syphilis.[9] In the early half of the 1900s, an estimated 1 in 4 to 1 in 20 Americans were infected.[9] With the advent of antibiotics and intensive public health efforts during and after World War II, the prevalence of syphilis declined sharply. Rates of syphilis declined in the 1990s and reached a record low in 2000 (2.2 cases per 100,000). However, between 2000 and 2009, the syphilis rate in the United States increased. In 2010, the rate of syphilis infection was 7.9 cases per 100,000 population for men and 1.1 cases per 100,000 for women.[2] The rate of primary and secondary syphilis has risen dramatically among men. Data suggest this increase is driven by increased transmission of syphilis among men who have sex with men (MSM), and accounts for 67% of these cases. The rate of primary and secondary syphilis is now nearly six times greater in men than women, whereas rates were almost equivalent a decade ago. Syphilis remains a problem in certain geographic regions, particularly in the South. Syphilis facilitates the transmission of human immunodeficiency virus (HIV) infection and seems to contribute to HIV transmission in those parts of the United States where rates of both infections are high. From 2003 to 2009, the rates have increased for all groups; in 2010 the reported rate among non-Hispanic whites was 2.1 per 100,000, among Hispanics the rate was 4.6 per 100,000, among Asian/Pacific Islanders the rate was 1.3 per 100,000, among Native American/Alaskan Natives the rate was 2.5 per 100,000, and among blacks the rate was 16.8 per 100,000.

While rates in men have increased dramatically, rates in women have decreased slightly from a recent high in 2008.[2] There also has been a slight decline in the rate of congenital syphilis, currently reported as 8.7 cases of congenital syphilis per 100,000 live births.[2] During pregnancy, untreated early syphilis results in perinatal death in as many as 40% of cases and may lead to fetal infection in more than 70% of cases because the spirochete that causes syphilis can cross the placental membrane to infect the fetus.[10]

Race, ethnicity, and gender alone do not alter STI risk but rather act as risk markers that correlate with other more fundamental determinants of health status, such as poverty, access to quality care, and health-seeking behavior. Higher infection rates have been associated with urban areas, with the exchange of sex for drugs, and with prison populations.[2,11] A growing concern is the incidence of co-infection with HIV among MSM.[2] Since a syphilitic chancre is an open wound, it greatly increases the risk of acquiring other STIs such as HIV.

BOX 26-2 PROGRESSION OF UNTREATED SYPHILIS

Stage I, primary syphilis—local invasion: *Treponema pallidum* multiplies in epithelium, producing granulomatous tissue reaction (chancre); lymph-containing microorganisms drain into adjacent lymph nodes and stimulate immune responses

Stage II, secondary syphilis—systemic disease: blood-borne bacteria spread to all major organ systems; immune system suppresses infection and symptoms regress spontaneously

Stage III, latent syphilis—silent infection: transmission of infection possible even though there are no clinical signs of infection

Stage IV, tertiary syphilis—noninfectious disease: significant morbidity and mortality occur; destructive skin, bone, and soft tissue lesions, or gummas, result from severe hypersensitivity; cardiovascular complications (aneurysms, heart valve insufficiency, heart failure) and neurosyphilis develop

PATHOPHYSIOLOGY. *Treponema pallidum,* the cause of syphilis, is an anaerobic bacterium that cannot be cultured in vitro. The treponema (individual microorganism) resembles a corkscrew, with regular, tight spirals and a rotary motion; it can infect any organ or tissue. Because the bacterium is present in exudate from moist mucosal or cutaneous lesions, the spirochete is usually transmitted to others during the first few years of infection. Transmission generally occurs through minor abrasions during sexual intercourse but can occur extragenitally as well. Approximately 30% to 50% of partners who have sexual intercourse with an individual in early stage syphilis develop the disease.[2] Although condoms can decrease the likelihood of infection, syphilis can be easily transmitted by contact with areas not covered by the condom.

Syphilis becomes a systemic disease shortly after infection and can be transmitted from a pregnant woman to her fetus as early as the ninth week of gestation. The risk of transmission to the fetus gradually declines with each subsequent pregnancy; therefore, a mother who has given birth to several children with severe congenital syphilis may later have a healthy child.[12] The course of untreated syphilis consists of four stages: primary, secondary, latent, and tertiary (Box 26-2).

Primary syphilis begins at the site of bacterial invasion (Figure 26-5), where *T. pallidum* multiplies in the epithelium and produces a granulomatous tissue reaction called a **chancre.** Some microorganisms drain with lymph into adjacent lymph nodes. Within the nodes and at the site of the chancre, the cell-mediated and humoral immune responses are stimulated.

Secondary syphilis is systemic. During this stage, blood-borne bacteria spread to all major organ systems. The secondary stage is followed by a period during which the immune system is able to suppress the infection. Even without treatment, spontaneous resolution of the skin lesions occurs and the individual enters the latent stage of infection.

Latent syphilis may be subdivided into early and late stages; however, no specific criteria delineate one from the other.[11]

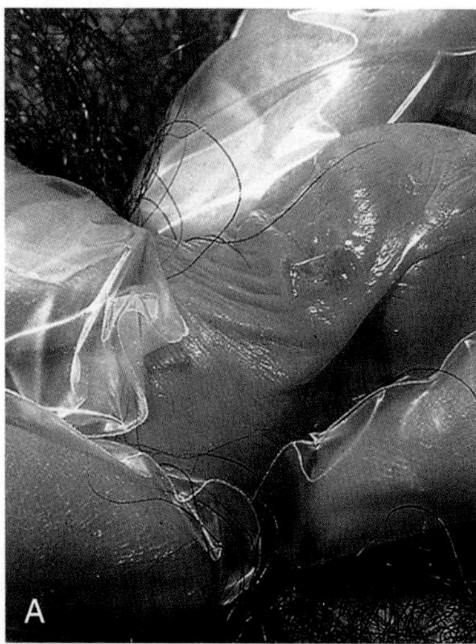

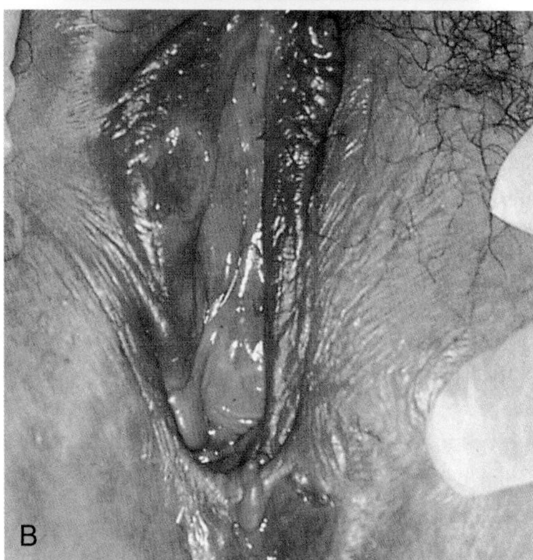

FIGURE 26-5 Primary Syphilis. **A,** Penile chancre. **B,** Vulval chancres; the labia and perineum show induration and edema of chancres. (**A** from McMillan A, Scott GR: *Sexually transmitted infections,* ed 2, London, 2000, Churchill Livingstone; **B** courtesy Barbara Romanowski, MD, from Morse SA et al, editors: *Atlas of sexually transmitted diseases and AIDS,* ed 4, London, 2013, Saunders.)

Medical history and serologic studies show that syphilis is present, but the individual has no clinical manifestations. Transmission is possible during the late and early latent stages.

Tertiary syphilis is the most severe stage, involving significant morbidity and mortality. The pathogenesis of syphilitic manifestations at this stage remains unclear. The destructive skin, bone, and soft tissue lesions (called **gummas**) of tertiary syphilis probably are caused by a severe hypersensitivity reaction to the microorganism. Within the cardiovascular system, infection with *T. pallidum* may cause aneurysms, heart valve insufficiencies, and heart failure. Within the central nervous system (CNS), the presence of *T. pallidum* in cerebrospinal fluid may cause the manifestations of neurosyphilis, which can occur within any stage of syphilis infection.[11]

Congenital syphilis is estimated to cause a half million fetal and neonatal deaths every year worldwide.[12] The risk of acquiring congenital syphilis (CS) is estimated at up to 80% in primary syphilis and declines with advancing stages of the disease. Intrauterine infection causes fetal or perinatal death in 40% of affected infants and many live-born infants have permanent lifelong morbidity.[12]

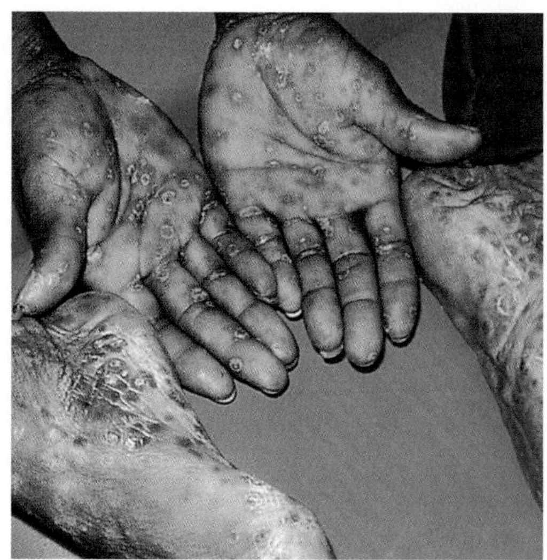

FIGURE 26-6 Secondary Syphilis. Secondary syphilis to the palms and plantar surfaces. (From Morse S et al, editors: *Atlas of sexually transmitted diseases and AIDS,* ed 4, London, 2013, Saunders.)

CLINICAL MANIFESTATIONS

Primary Stage. In adults, the incubation period of syphilis ranges from 12 days to 12 weeks after exposure and averages 3 weeks. A sore, or *hard chancre,* develops at the site of treponemal entry. Typically the chancre is an eroded, painless, firm, and indurated (hard) ulcer that may be a few millimeters to 2 cm in diameter. Firm, enlarged, and nontender regional lymph nodes accompany chancres. Figure 26-5 shows typical chancres of the penis and vulva. Syphilitic chancres are not always typical, however, and syphilis should be considered in the presence of any open lesion. Secondary infection can cause chancres to become necrotic and painful, and lesions on the fingers may be dry, scaly, and papular or moist and vegetative. If left untreated, the chancre of primary syphilis heals in 2 to 8 weeks and then spontaneously disappears, usually without leaving a scar.

Secondary Stage. Clinical manifestations of secondary syphilis usually develop 6 weeks after the first appearance of the chancre but may overlap with those of the primary stage. Typically this stage presents with variable systemic symptoms, including low-grade fever, malaise, sore throat, hoarseness, anorexia, generalized adenopathy, headache, joint pain, and skin or mucous membrane lesions or rashes. Cutaneous (skin) rashes are generally papulosquamous (raised and scaly), but any variation or combination of macular (flat), papular (raised), and pustular (pus-filled) lesions may be seen. Often lesions are widespread and bilateral and appear on the palms and soles (Figure 26-6). Some lesions become hypertrophied, flat, moist, and wartlike or vegetative (e.g., cauliflower-like). These lesions, called **condylomata lata,** are highly contagious and develop on the perineum, vulva, and groin of women (Figure 26-7) and around the inner thigh and the anal area in men and women. Besides skin sores, oral mucous membrane lesions (known as mucous patches), lymphadenopathy, pruritus, and alopecia are common. Some individuals develop anemia, leukocytosis, increased sedimentation rate, hepatitis, transitory proteinuria,

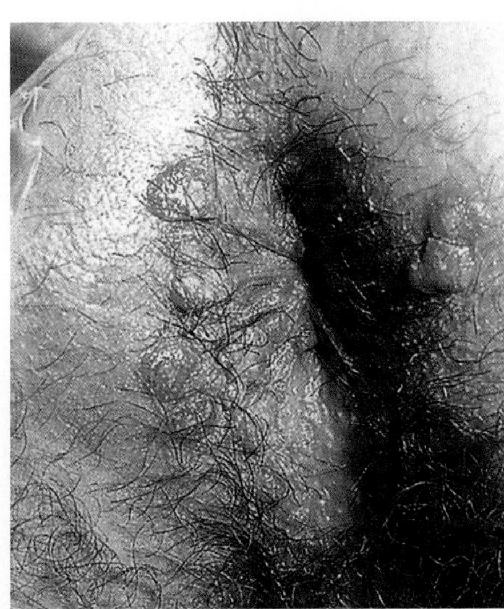

FIGURE 26-7 Condylomata Lata. Broad-based, moist, darkfield-positive condylomata lata of the perineum. (From McMillan A, Scott GR: *Sexually transmitted infections*, ed 2, London, 2000, Churchill Livingstone.)

arthritis, electrocardiographic abnormalities, and central nervous system (CNS) symptoms. Regardless of whether treatment is given, the cutaneous lesions generally heal in 2 to 10 weeks, but relapses may occur for several years.[11]

Latent and Tertiary Stages. The asymptomatic, latent stage of syphilis may be as short as 1 year or as long as a lifetime. After the latent stage, tertiary syphilis may present with gummas, cardiovascular lesions, and neurosyphilis. These manifestations of tertiary syphilis are quite rare because antibiotics can cure syphilis.

Congenital Syphilis. **Congenital syphilis (CS)** is characterized by vasculitis, necrosis, fibrosis, and distribution of *T. pallidum* throughout the tissues; it is divided into early and late stages. Signs and symptoms of early CS manifest in the first 2 years of life, and clinical manifestations of the late stage often occur near puberty. Affected newborns often are premature and have growth abnormalities, hepatosplenomegaly, bone marrow depression, destructive bone and skin lesions (see Figure 26-6), retinal inflammation, glaucoma, blood dyscrasia, nephrotic syndrome, and varying degrees of CNS involvement.[9] Late manifestations of classic congenital syphilis are rare and are similar to those of tertiary syphilis in the adult.

EVALUATION AND TREATMENT. Because *T. pallidum* cannot be cultured in vitro, early definitive diagnosis of primary or secondary syphilis depends on darkfield microscopy of a specimen taken from an infected site. If the initial result is negative, the darkfield examination is repeated on 2 successive days. In addition to darkfield microscopy, serologic testing is useful in diagnosis. An algorithmic approach to the diagnosis of genital ulcers is presented in Figure 26-8.

Two categories of serologic testing exist: nontreponemal antigen tests and treponemal antibody tests.[9] Nontreponemal antigen tests, which demonstrate the presence of *reagin* (a group of antibodies present in syphilis) in serum, provide indirect evidence of infection. Examples of nontreponemal analysis are the Venereal Disease Research Laboratory (VDRL) antigen and the rapid plasma reagin (RPR) tests (Box 26-3). These tests yield a positive result (presence of reagin) in more than 50% of individuals with primary syphilis and in 100% of individuals in the secondary phase of disease. Because the VDRL and RPR tests have high rates of false positives, a treponemal test is performed if the screening test is positive. Treponemal tests are serologic-specific tests that are used to assess antibody response to *T. pallidum* and include the fluorescent treponemal antibody absorption (FTA-ABS) test and the passive particle agglutination (TP-PA) assay.[9]

Numerous dermatologic disorders can mimic the skin lesions of secondary syphilis, making differential diagnosis difficult. Again, laboratory confirmation is important; darkfield microscopy of scrapings from condylomata lata or other skin lesions is diagnostic for the disease. Serologic blood tests are almost always strongly positive in this stage.

During the latent stage, individuals continue to have serologic evidence of untreated disease, but confirmation through darkfield microscopy is difficult. Examination of cerebrospinal fluid may confirm that the treponemata are present.

Preferred treatment for all stages of syphilis is parenteral injection of benzathine penicillin G. If the individual has manifested signs of the disease for less than 1 year, a single intramuscular dose is appropriate. If signs have been present for more than 1 year, the treatment is three weekly injections. This therapy is also appropriate for pregnant women.[9] There is no evidence to date that *T. pallidum* has developed resistance to penicillin. In fact, it is highly sensitive; but because of the slow replication time, serum levels must be maintained for 7 to 14 days. Nonpregnant women who are allergic to penicillin may receive oral doxycycline, 100 mg twice daily for 14 days. Pregnant women with a penicillin allergy should be desensitized and then treated with benzathine penicillin G as recommended by the CDC because tetracycline will cause permanent, lifelong discoloration of the forming teeth of the fetus.[9] Repeated assessment of VDRL or RPR titers is used to determine effectiveness of treatment. Titers should decrease fourfold if treatment has been successful. Sexual partners also are examined and treated, and the use of condoms is recommended until effective treatment is verified.

Newborns of mothers with documented syphilis need careful evaluation after birth. Definitive diagnosis of congenital syphilis is made by microscopic identification of *T. pallidum* in material from skin lesions, nasal discharge, or placental tissue. Nontreponemal tests are performed on the infant's blood and compared with maternal levels.[9] In all cases of maternal syphilis, the goal is to treat the mother to prevent congenital syphilis through early maternal treatment with penicillin. If the infant requires treatment, penicillin is the drug of choice. Such infants are then given serologic tests for syphilis every 2 to 3 months until the test becomes nonreactive or the titer has decreased fourfold.[9]

Chancroid

Chancroid, or soft chancre, is an acute infectious disease that was first differentiated from syphilis in 1852. It is caused by *Haemophilus ducreyi*, a gram-negative bacillus. The incidence of

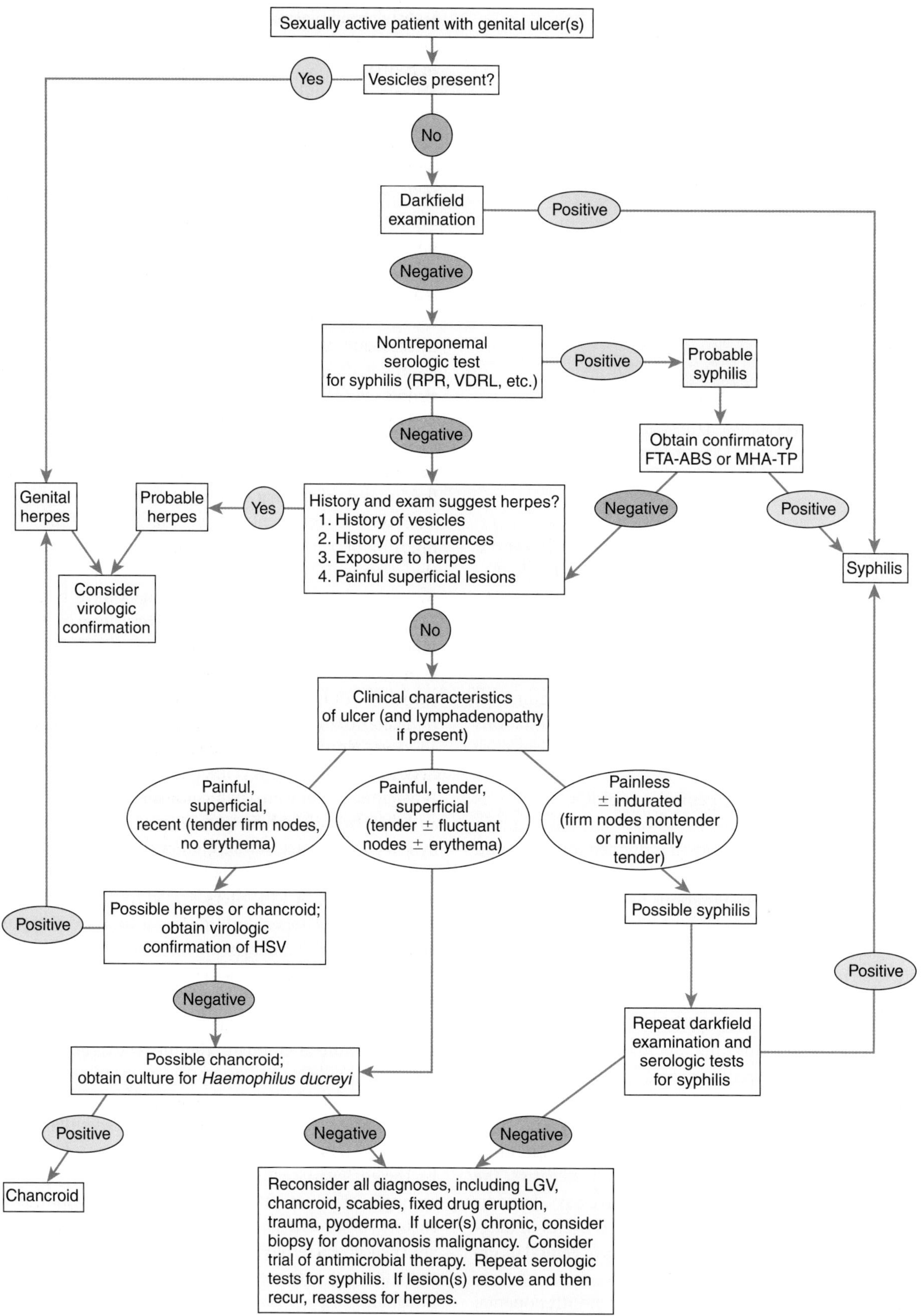

FIGURE 26-8 Genital Ulceration. Algorithm outlining an approach to the diagnosis of an individual who presents with a genital ulceration. *FTA-ABS,* Fluorescent treponemal antibody absorption; *HSV,* herpes simplex virus; *LGV,* lymphogranuloma venereum; *MHA-TP,* microhemagglutination assay–*Treponema pallidum; RPR,* rapid plasma reagin; *VDRL,* Venereal Disease Research Laboratory. (Redrawn from Pitot P, Plummer FA. In Holmes KK et al, editors: *Sexually transmitted diseases,* ed 2, New York, 1990, McGraw-Hill.)

BOX 26-3 FALSE-POSITIVE SEROLOGIC TESTS FOR SYPHILIS

Reasons for False-Positive, Nontreponemal Reactions (VDRL, RPR)

Transient Reactions (<6 Months)

Technical error (low titer)
Mycoplasma pneumonia
Enterovirus infections
Infectious mononucleosis
Pregnancy
Narcotic abuse
Advanced tuberculosis
Scarlet fever
Viral and atypical pneumonia
Brucellosis
Rat-bite fever
Leptospirosis
Measles
Mumps
Lymphogranuloma venereum
Malaria
Trypanosomiasis
Varicella

Chronic Reactions (>6 Months)

Malaria
Leprosy
Systemic lupus erythematosus
Narcotic abuse
Other connective tissue diseases
Elderly population
Hashimoto thyroiditis
Rheumatoid arthritis
Reticuloendothelial malignancy
Familial false-positive reaction
Idiopathic

Reasons for False-Positive, Treponemal-Specific Reactions (FTA-ABS)

Technical error
Inefficient sorbents
Healthy individuals without syphilis
Genital herpes simplex
Pregnancy
Lupus erythematosus (skin only or systemic)
Alcoholic cirrhosis
Scleroderma
Mixed connective tissue disease

FTA-ABS, Fluorescent treponemal antibody absorption; *RPR,* rapid plasma reagin; *VDRL,* Venereal Disease Research Laboratory.

chancroid is decreasing worldwide. The incidence in the United States is low; 24 cases were reported to the CDC in 2010.[2] Sporadic outbreaks occur throughout the world and tend to be associated with conditions such as poverty, prostitution, and illicit drug use, in which individuals continue to engage in intercourse in spite of the presence of a painful lesion.[2]

PATHOPHYSIOLOGY. *H. ducreyi* is a gram-negative bacillus with rounded ends. Under a microscope it is commonly observed in small chains or clusters along mucous strands. Transmission can occur through sexual contact and autoinoculation. There is no evidence of maternal-fetal transfer before or after delivery. Chancroid lesions usually are found throughout the genital region, most commonly on the internal surface of the foreskin or at its point of attachment to the penis (the frenulum) in men and on the labia, clitoris, or fourchette in women. Initially the papule enlarges; it then erodes into a soft, circumscribed ulcer containing a superficial exudate. Beneath the ulcer is a lesion characterized by edema, endothelial proliferation, and a base of granulation tissue that is full of lymphocytes and plasma cells. Adjacent lymph nodes are acutely inflamed and full of polymorphonuclear leukocytes and necrotic cells.[13]

CLINICAL MANIFESTATIONS. Chancroid has an incubation period of 3 to 10 days.[13] Generally, women are asymptomatic, but depending on the site of infection, can present with less obvious symptoms (dysuria, dyspareunia, vaginal discharge, pain on defecation, or rectal bleeding). Constitutional symptoms are unusual. At the site of inoculation, an initial vesicopustule lesion forms and erodes into a soft ulcer with a necrotic base, surrounding erythema, and a ragged, serpiginous (spreading) border (Figure 26-9). Unilateral, painful, local lymphadenopathy presents in about half of infected individuals—primarily men. (Women tend to have multiple lesions.) Inguinal **buboes** (unilocular abscess of the inguinal lymph nodes) develop 7 to 10 days after the initial chancre and fill with exudate. In 25% to 60% of cases, the buboes spontaneously rupture out onto the skin, spreading the infection through autoinoculation.

Ulcers on the prepuce may lead to phimosis or paraphimosis. Other complications of chancroid include balanitis, secondary infections, necrosis, and fistula formation. Recalcitrant, serpiginous lesions may take months or years to heal.

EVALUATION AND TREATMENT. Chancroid is easily confused with other types of genital ulcers, particularly those of syphilis, genital herpes, and granuloma inguinale (see Figure 26-9). Unlike the syphilitic ulcer, chancroidal ulcer is painful, tender, and nonindurated. Microscopic analysis of a Gram-stained smear from the chancroid helps to identify the microorganism. Definitive diagnosis depends on recovery of *H. ducreyi* from cultured specimens; however, the culture medium is not widely available.[9] Because 10% of infected individuals are coinfected with syphilis or herpes simplex virus (HSV), testing includes serologic examination for syphilis and viral culture for HSV. In addition, HIV testing is recommended: chancroid is a cofactor for transmission of HIV.

Resistance to recommended antibiotics has emerged in isolated instances worldwide. Recent treatment recommendations include a single intramuscular injection of ceftriaxone (250 mg) or a single dose of oral azithromycin (1 g). Effective oral multiple-dose regimens include ciprofloxacin, 500 mg orally twice daily for 3 days; or erythromycin, 500 mg three times daily for 7 days. Persons infected with HIV have higher rates of treatment failure with single-dose therapy and may require a longer treatment regimen. As a palliative measure, buboes can be aspirated through adjacent, healthy skin. In approximately 5% of cases, relapses at the site of original ulcer have occurred.[9] Simultaneous treatment of sexual partners and use of condoms are recommended to prevent reinfection.

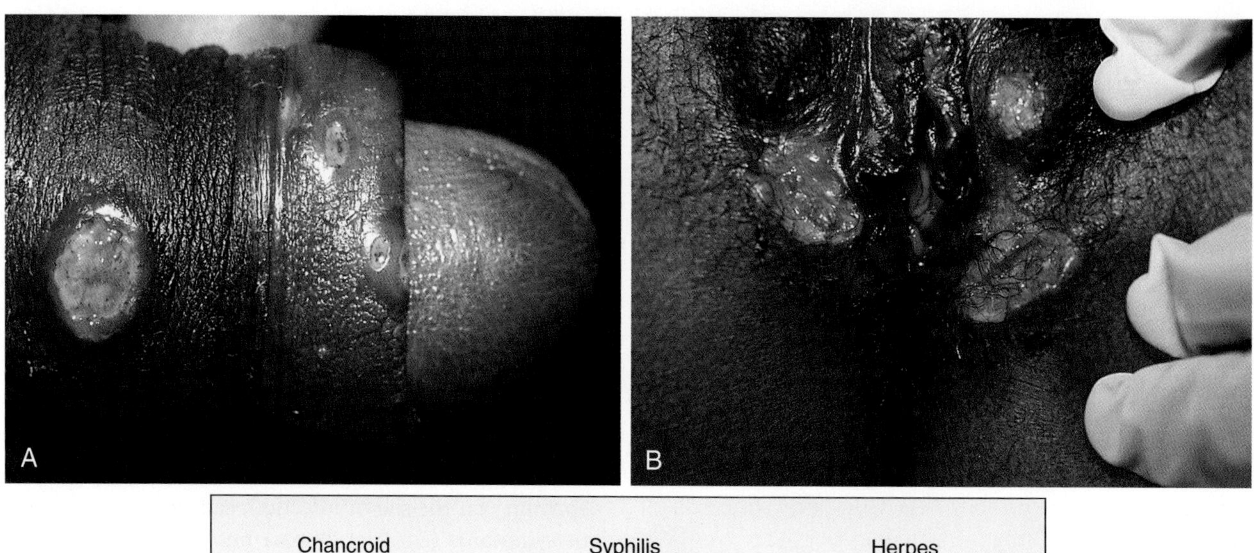

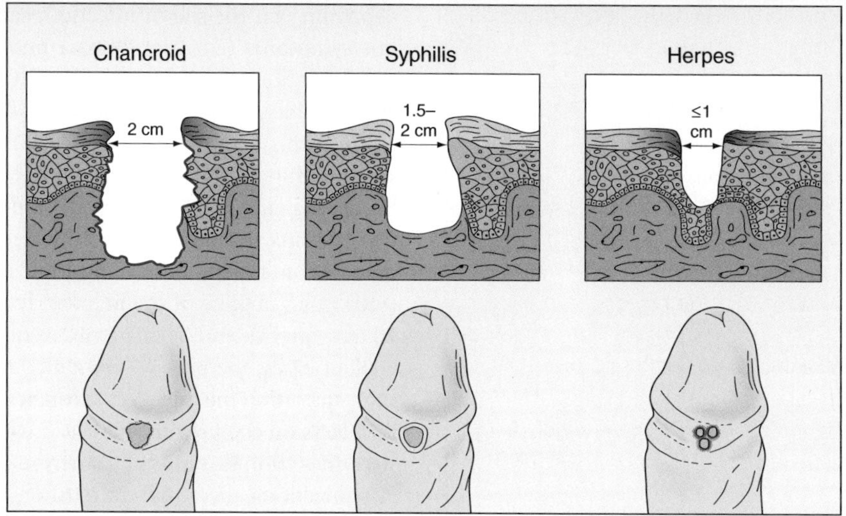

FIGURE 26-9 Chancroid. **A,** Ulcers on the penile shaft. **B,** Multiple vulvar lesions. **C,** Differences in clinical appearance among chancroid, syphilis, and genital herpes. (From Morse SA et al, editors: *Atlas of sexually transmitted diseases and AIDS,* ed 4, London, 2013, Saunders.)

Granuloma Inguinale

Granuloma inguinale (donovanosis) is a chronic, progressively destructive bacterial infection caused by *Calymmatobacterium granulomatis,* recently reclassified as *Klebsiella granulomatis.*[14] Although sexually transmissible, granuloma inguinale is only mildly contagious and repeated exposure is necessary to cause disease. Often, individuals are coinfected with syphilis.[15]

Granuloma inguinale very rarely occurs in the United States.[2] Yet it is more prevalent in some tropical and subtropical parts of the world (India, New Guinea, Africa, central Australia, and to a lesser extent the Caribbean and Brazil). Infection is usually acquired through sexual intercourse with an individual who has active disease or asymptomatic rectal infection. As with all genital ulcerative diseases, granuloma inguinale plays a role in HIV transmission.[2]

PATHOPHYSIOLOGY. *C. granulomatis* is a gram-negative, nonsporing, nonmotile, encapsulated rod that is not easily isolated in the laboratory. After exposure the bacteria survive and multiply within vacuoles of large histiocytic cells or polymorphonuclear leukocytes. The bacteria reproduce within these cells until a vacuole may contain 20 to 30 microorganisms. These bacteria-filled vacuoles were identified by Donovan in 1905 and are termed **Donovan bodies.** The presence of Donovan bodies in tissue smears of material from the lesions is considered the gold standard for diagnosis of lymphogranuloma inguinale, but this test is difficult even in well-equipped labs.[15,16]

The initial lesion is an indurated subcutaneous nodule that is often preceded and accompanied by itching. The primary sites for development of the lesions are the distal penis in men and the introitus in women. Single lesions often coalesce with nearby lesions or form new lesions by autoinoculation of nearby skin surfaces. Progression from the initial nodule to a large, granuloma-heaped ulcer occurs slowly. Secondary infection may occur, increasing tissue damage and residual scarring. The disease may spread to the bones, joints, and liver.

CLINICAL MANIFESTATIONS. The incubation period of granuloma inguinale is 8 to 80 days. The initial lesion is an indurated, sharply defined, painless, subcutaneous nodule that is often preceded and accompanied by itching. Nodules bleed easily and contain abundant red, beefy-looking granulation tissue.

Progression to a large granuloma-heaped ulcer occurs slowly; single lesions coalesce or form new lesions by autoinoculation of nearby skin surfaces. Secondary infection may occur, increasing tissue damage and residual scarring. Although systemic symptoms are rare, the disease may spread to the bones, joints, and liver. In some cases, infection spreads to the inguinal area and produces **pseudobuboes.** In these instances, the affected lymph nodes are not directly affected, but the surrounding area may be infected and abscessed.

EVALUATION AND TREATMENT. Although the clinical manifestations of this disease are important for diagnosis, confirmation in the developed world involves microscopic examination in which Donovan bodies are found in a smear or biopsy specimen. No FDA-cleared polymerase chain reaction (PCR) tests for the detection of *K. granulomatis* DNA exist.[13]

Many antibiotics have been used successfully against *K. granulomatis.* Because other STIs frequently coexist, individuals should be tested for chlamydia, gonorrhea, syphilis, hepatitis B, and HIV. Because of the persistent nature of the disease, duration of therapy tends to be relatively long. With effective antibiotic treatment, lesions begin to heal in 7 days, but treatment is continued for at least 3 weeks and until all lesions are completely healed. Oral therapy includes doxycycline, 100 mg twice a day; azithromycin, 1 g once a week for 3 weeks and until lesions are healed; ciprofloxacin, 750 mg twice a day for at least 3 weeks; erythromycin base, 500 mg four times a day for at least 3 weeks; or trimethoprim-sulfamethoxazole, 160 mg/800 mg, double-strength tablet twice a day for at least 3 weeks.[9] Relapses can occur 6 to 18 months later despite effective initial therapy, so prolonged follow-up is necessary, as is treatment of sexual partners.

Bacterial Vaginosis

Bacterial vaginosis (BV)—previously called nonspecific vaginitis; nonspecific vaginosis; or *Haemophilus, Corynebacterium,* or *Gardnerella* vaginitis—is a sexually associated condition, but is not necessarily considered an STI. The condition is associated with sexual contact including genital touching and digital penetration, oral sex, and penile penetration. Although BV occurs mostly in sexually active women of reproductive age, it can affect women, especially menopausal women, who are not sexually active. BV is diagnosed by the presence of characteristic symptoms and clinical findings. Prevalence rates vary from 17% among women in family planning clinics to 37% among some groups of pregnant women.[1] Fifty percent of women with signs of BV are asymptomatic.

PATHOPHYSIOLOGY. The exact etiology of BV is unknown but is thought to be a dysbiosis of normal vaginal flora that is associated with sexual contact. *Gardnerella vaginalis* and various anaerobes, including *Mycoplasma hominis, Bacteroides,* and *Mobiluncus,* interact and proliferate when lactobacilli (the normal predominant vaginal flora) are decreased or absent. Bacteria adhere to vaginal epithelium, and massive overgrowth occurs and causes a noninflammatory response. Catabolic enzymes degrade proteins into amines. In turn, amines elevate the vaginal pH and produce the characteristic fishy odor associated with BV. BV has been implicated in PID, chorioamnionitis, preterm labor, and postpartum endometritis. In addition, BV increases a woman's risk of contracting other STIs, such as HIV.

CLINICAL MANIFESTATIONS. BV is characterized by a thin, gray, homogeneous, and malodorous discharge that adheres to the vaginal walls but is often copious enough to drain into the vulva. Occasionally the discharge is bubbly or frothy. Usually the vaginal pH is 5 to 5.5, and women often complain of a strong, foul, fishy vaginal odor, particularly after intercourse and during menses. Odor is caused by contact with alkaline secretions, including semen and menstrual discharge. Male and female partners of infected women may harbor the microorganisms responsible for BV but have no signs or symptoms.

EVALUATION AND TREATMENT. Diagnosis of BV can be made on the basis of three of four of the following criteria, known as Amsel's criteria: (1) presence of adherent gray vaginal discharge, (2) vaginal pH greater than 4.5, (3) positive amine odor in the presence of an alkali such as potassium hydroxide, and (4) presence of clue cells on wet mount.[17] Clue cells are considered pathognomonic for BV. The saline wet mount also may show absence of lactobacilli and few or no leukocytes. Clue cells are vaginal epithelial cells that are covered with bacteria and look as if pepper has been sprinkled on them. A Gram stain is considered the "gold standard" for diagnosis but is difficult to perform quickly in a clinic laboratory.[18] Cultures for BV are not recommended; however, high-risk individuals should be screened for gonorrhea and chlamydia.

The most commonly used treatment for BV is a course of oral metronidazole (Flagyl), 500 mg twice daily for 7 days, or 0.75% vaginal gel once daily for 5 days.[9] Alternative regimens include tinidazole 2 g once daily for 2 days or 1 g orally for 5 days. Oral clindamycin, 300 mg twice daily for 7 days; or 2% vaginal cream, once daily for 7 days, is another choice for treatment.[9] Clindamycin vaginal suppositories are a 3-day treatment regimen in nonpregnant women. Clindamycin cream is oil based, and for up to 72 hours after completing therapy, it may weaken latex condoms and diaphragms. BV treatment in women infected with HIV is the same as that in individuals who are HIV-negative. In pregnancy, treatment decisions are more complex because even though the presence of BV is associated with preterm labor, the risk of preterm labor is actually increased with treatment. The CDC recommends that practitioners consider delaying treatment until 36 weeks and provide women with informed consent about the risk of preterm birth with treatment.[9] Treatment of sexual partners is not recommended.[9,19]

Chlamydial Infections

Urogenital Infections

Chlamydia is the common name for infections caused by *Chlamydia trachomatis* (CT). *C. trachomatis* is responsible for a variety of syndromes, including acute urethral syndrome, nongonococcal urethritis (NGU), mucopurulent cervicitis, and PID. Chlamydia, the most common reportable STI in the United States, affects about 3 million individuals annually and is a leading cause of preventable infertility and ectopic pregnancy.[2] In 2010, more than 1.3 million cases of chlamydial infections were reported, which was an increase of 5% from

2 years earlier.[2] Rates of chlamydia are increasing in all age groups, areas of the country, and racial/ethnic groups. This increase probably reflects the continued expansion of screening efforts and increased use of more sensitive diagnostic tests as well as an actual increase in incidence.[2] The majority of reported cases of chlamydia are in people less than 26 years old but the incidence in older adults is increasing.[2,20] Up to 90% of women with CT infection are asymptomatic, which can delay diagnosis and increase the risk of long-term health sequelae.[2]

Risk groups for chlamydia include age younger than 26 (with highest rates in people younger than 20 years old), recent new sexual partner, and drug use or other risky behaviors.[2] The incidence of CT infection in pregnancy has been estimated at between 2% and 21%.[2] Like gonorrhea, *Chlamydia* infection can be transmitted from mother to infant during birth and can cause eye infections and pneumonia in affected newborns.[9]

PATHOPHYSIOLOGY. *C. trachomatis* is an obligate, gram-negative intracellular bacterium that lacks the ability to reproduce independently. Like viruses, *Chlamydia* can reproduce only within host cells. It is differentiated from other bacteria by its unique two-part growth cycle. The first part consists of an elementary body that is small, resilient, metabolically inert, and able to survive extracellularly. Once this elementary body attaches itself to a receptor host cell, it is able to enter by endocytosis. Once inside the cell, the second part of the cycle begins and the microorganism becomes a metabolically active parasite, reproducing within the cell until the cell is destroyed and ruptures, disseminating up to 1000 new elementary bodies. Rarely does this cause a secondary infection. Infection with *C. trachomatis* produces a mononuclear inflammatory reaction rather than a polymorphonuclear inflammatory reaction. The mononuclear inflammatory reaction produces permanent scarring of tissues.[2]

Chlamydia microorganisms are always pathogens; they are not part of the normal flora of the urogenital tract, despite the fact that infection is often asymptomatic. Numerous serotypes, or strains, of *C. trachomatis* have been identified. Some cause urogenital infection; some, ocular trachoma; and others, lymphogranuloma venereum, which is discussed in the next section.

The strains of *C. trachomatis* that cause urogenital infection apparently require squamous-columnar and columnar-epithelial cells as hosts. *C. trachomatis* infects and disrupts epithelial tissues but does not seem to invade or destroy deeper tissues or organs.[21]

In newborns, several sites may be inoculated with *Chlamydia* during passage through the infected maternal cervix. These include the eye, nasopharynx, rectum, and vagina. The infant also may aspirate infected secretions with its first breaths, resulting in chlamydial pneumonitis and substantial newborn morbidity.

CLINICAL MANIFESTATIONS. Asymptomatic chlamydial infection in adults is common. Urogenital infections caused by *Chlamydia* closely parallel those caused by gonorrhea. Both microorganisms infect superficial genital tract tissues, such as mucosa of the urethra and cervix, and both can invade the epididymides, fallopian/uterine tubes, and (rarely) the hepatic capsule. Table 26-2 lists the pathophysiologic similarities of chlamydial and gonococcal infections.

TABLE 26-2 SIMILARITY OF CLINICAL SYNDROMES CAUSED BY *NEISSERIA GONORRHOEAE* AND *CHLAMYDIA TRACHOMATIS*

SITE OF INFECTION	CLINICAL SYNDROME: *N. GONORRHOEAE*	CLINICAL SYNDROME: *C. TRACHOMATIS*
Men		
Urethra	Urethritis	Nongonococcal urethritis; postgonococcal urethritis
Epididymis	Epididymitis	Epididymitis
Rectum	Proctitis	Proctitis
Conjunctiva	Conjunctivitis	Conjunctivitis
Systemic	Disseminated gonococcal infection	Reiter syndrome
Women		
Urethra	Acute urethral syndrome	Acute urethral syndrome
Bartholin gland	Bartholinitis	Bartholinitis
Cervix	Cervicitis	Cervicitis; cervical atypia
Fallopian tube	Salpingitis	Salpingitis
Conjunctiva	Conjunctivitis	Conjunctivitis
Liver capsule	Perihepatitis	Perihepatitis
Systemic	Disseminated gonococcal infection	Arthritis-dermatitis syndrome

Data from Stamm WE, Holmes KK: *Chlamydia trachomatis* infections in the adult. In Holmes KK et al, editors: *Sexually transmitted diseases*, ed 2, New York, 1990, McGraw-Hill.

Chlamydial infection accounts for 50% to 60% of cases of nongonococcal urethritis in men. Clinically, urethritis caused by gonorrhea and chlamydia cannot be differentiated: both have a 7- to 21-day incubation period and cause dysuria. Although urethral discharge in men may be similar in the two infections, chlamydial discharge tends to be more clear and gonococcal discharge more purulent. Men might note a clear, mucous discharge or mild burning with urination. Chlamydial urethritis is generally milder than gonorrheal urethritis and more likely to be asymptomatic. Gram-stained smears of the urethral discharge show numerous polymorphonuclear leukocytes, which indicate ongoing inflammation.

Chlamydial epididymitis can accompany chlamydial urethritis in men and is characterized by fever and a unilaterally painful, swollen scrotum. Chlamydial infection also causes proctitis (rectal inflammation) in people who have receptive anal intercourse. Chlamydial proctitis is generally mild, although it may, like gonorrheal proctitis, cause rectal bleeding, mucous discharge, and diarrhea. Reiter syndrome (urethritis, conjunctivitis, arthritis, and characteristic mucocutaneous lesions) is also associated with untreated chlamydial infections of the urogenital tract.

Chlamydia infection is the leading cause of tubal infertility in women. Risk factors for infertility include numbers of chlamydial infections and duration and severity of infection. Even

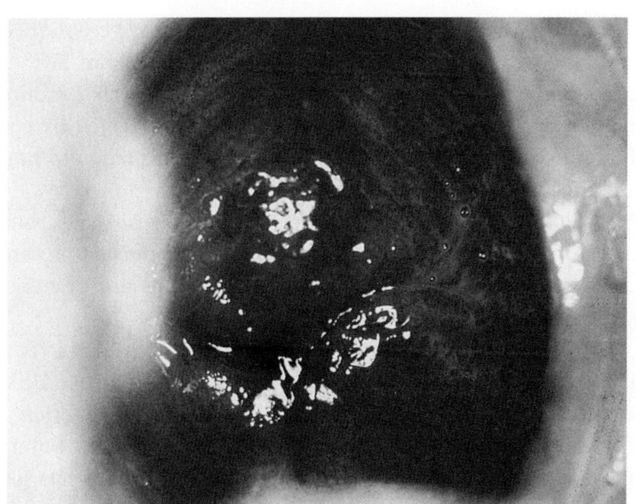

FIGURE 26-10 Chlamydial Cervicitis. Beefy red mucosa of columnar epithelium of cervix. (Courtesy Paul Weisner. From Morse SA et al, editors: *Atlas of sexually transmitted diseases and AIDS*, ed 4, London, 2013, Saunders.)

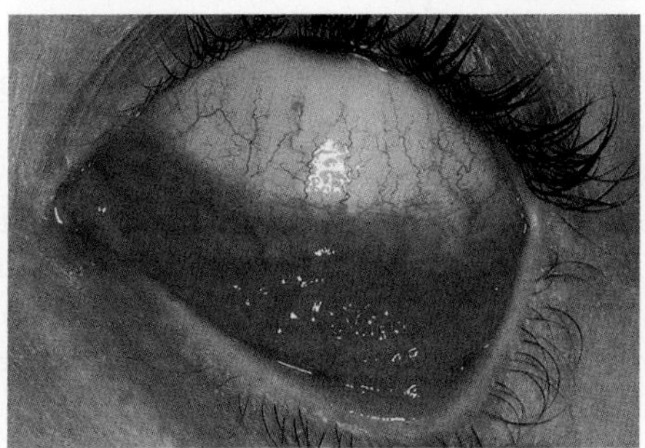

FIGURE 26-11 Chlamydial Ophthalmia. (From McMillan A, Scott GR: *Sexually transmitted infections*, ed 2, London, 2000, Churchill Livingstone.)

women with asymptomatic salpingitis have a risk of subsequent infertility. This may reflect an antigen-antibody response rather than inflammatory damage.[22]

In sexually active women, *C. trachomatis* can cause **acute urethral syndrome** (dysuria, urinary frequency, and presence of sterile pus in the urine). *C. trachomatis* also causes asymptomatic urethral infection in women. Chlamydial infection of Bartholin/greater vestibular glands can cause purulent discharge and formation of a Bartholin cyst. Women with chlamydial cervicitis may be asymptomatic or may have a yellow mucopurulent discharge from the cervical os and a hypertrophic, edematous, and friable area of cervical ectopy. The woman also may report intermenstrual or postcoital spotting. Although ectopy alone does not indicate a pathologic condition, an erythematous, raw, and friable cervix is suggestive of chlamydial cervicitis (Figure 26-10).

The most common clinical manifestations of chlamydial infections in the newborn are conjunctivitis and pneumonia. Prophylactic treatment with antibiotic eye ointment at birth does not provide complete protection against neonatal conjunctivitis and does not protect against neonatal pneumonia. Chlamydial conjunctivitis begins between 5 and 14 days after delivery, when the infant's eyes begin to water. This discharge may become purulent, and both eyes may become red and swollen (Figure 26-11).

Scarring of the conjunctivae may result, but this infection does not cause blindness, as does the ophthalmia neonatorum caused by *N. gonorrhoeae.* The pneumonia is mild or severe and may accompany the conjunctivitis. Infants with chlamydial pneumonia develop staccato coughing spells, nasal congestion, dyspnea, and minimal fever at 3 to 11 weeks of age. Affected infants may have persistently abnormal pulmonary function tests into childhood.[9]

EVALUATION AND TREATMENT. Methods for diagnosing chlamydial infections include tissue culture, direct chlamydial enzyme immunoassay, fluorescein-labeled monoclonal antibody tests, and nucleic acid amplification testing (NAAT). Currently, tests using chlamydia-specific nucleic acid sequences are the most sensitive and cost-effective tests available.[9] Concurrent testing for gonorrhea can be done using the same swab. NAAT can be performed on samples taken from the vagina, endocervix, urethra, or urine specimens. The ease of use means that screening can be performed without a clinician if needed.[9]

C. trachomatis is susceptible to inexpensive, readily accessible antibiotics. Treatment includes antibiotic therapy for infected individuals and all sexual contacts; abstinence or use of condoms during treatment and for 7 days after treatment is recommended. Azithromycin is given 1 g orally, as a single dose, or a 7-day course of oral doxycycline, 100 mg twice daily. Single-dose azithromycin is preferred if adherence to a multiple-dose, multiple-day regimen may not be feasible for the individual. Alternative regimens include a 7-day course of oral erythromycin, 500 mg four times a day; or erythromycin E, 800 mg four times daily for 7 days. Ofloxacin, 300 mg twice daily; and levofloxacin, 500 mg once daily for 7 days, are also effective alternatives.[9] Azithromycin is the drug of choice in pregnancy. Because of the asymptomatic nature of *Chlamydia* and the potential sequelae of untreated infection, the CDC recommends routine annual screening for chlamydia for all sexually active women who are less than 26 years old. In addition, the CDC recommends that all women, regardless of age, be screened if they have a new sexual partner or their partner is not monogamous.[9] Pregnant women should be routinely screened for *Chlamydia* at least once during pregnancy.[9]

Lymphogranuloma Venereum

C. trachomatis (invasive serovars of strains L1, L2, or L3) can cause a chronic STI known as **lymphogranuloma venereum (LGV),** which may be confused with syphilis, herpes, or chancroid. LGV was previously rare in the developed world but now is increasingly found in men who have sex with men and may spread to other populations. The infection is acquired during sexual intercourse or through contact with contaminated exudate from active lesions.[9]

PATHOPHYSIOLOGY. The strain of *C. trachomatis* that causes LGV probably penetrates skin and mucous membranes through tiny abrasions. LGV spreads to genital and rectal lymphatic tissue, where it causes marked inflammation, necrosis, buboes, abscesses of inguinal lymph nodes, and infection of surrounding tissues. Healing occurs by fibrosis after several weeks or months and results in scarring, damaging the lymph nodes and disrupting their function. LGV can cause permanent lymphatic disruption and genital disfigurement. Affected nodes become chronically swollen, hardened, and enlarged. *C. trachomatis* also spreads systematically through the bloodstream and can enter the CNS.[23]

CLINICAL MANIFESTATIONS. The primary lesion of LGV appears after an incubation period of 5 to 21 days. The lesion is most commonly a herpetiform (multivesicular) ulcer, but it can assume various forms. The ulcer generally is asymptomatic and inconspicuous and heals rapidly, leaving no scar. In men, the lesion is found most commonly on the penis or scrotum; in women, it is found on the vaginal wall, cervix, or labia. Other signs of primary LGV include a large, tender lymphatic nodule or bubo, urethritis, and cervicitis.

The secondary stage of untreated LGV in men is characterized by inflammation and swelling of the lymph nodes. At first the inguinal bubo is a firm, somewhat painful mass. As the bubo gradually enlarges, it becomes very painful, thereby restricting mobility, and is deep blue in color. This color change signals impending rupture of the bubo through the skin. Thick yellow pus may drain from the site for weeks or months. Healing is slow and results in scar formation. Systemic manifestations of secondary LGV include meningitis, pneumonitis, and other major infections. In some cases the bubo does not rupture but rather involutes and becomes firm. Bubo formation is most common in men and may result in a distinctive inguinal swelling, known as the "groove sign."[13] In women the path of pelvic lymph drainage is different and the inguinal lymph nodes are involved in less than one third of cases.

Anorectal LGV may be caused by direct inoculation during anal intercourse, or it may be a chronic or late manifestation of lymphatic spread from the inguinal area. Most individuals with anorectal LGV have had receptive anal intercourse with males. Clinical symptoms include multiple ulcerations of the rectal mucosa, chronic inflammation, mucopurulent rectal discharge, and rectovaginal fistulae in women. Individuals may have fever, rectal pain, and tenesmus. Rectal strictures, perirectal abscesses, and anal fissures may develop and are the cause of most of the severe morbidity associated with LGV.

EVALUATION AND TREATMENT. Clinical manifestations and laboratory tests are used to diagnose LGV. Tests include the LGV complement-fixation test, isolation of the microorganism in tissue culture, and monoclonal antibody tests. The diagnosis usually is made serologically and by excluding other causes of genital ulcers or inguinal lymphadenopathy. LGV is treated with oral doxycycline, 100 mg twice daily for 21 days. A 21-day course of erythromycin is also effective. Sexual partners also should be treated regardless of symptoms.[9]

Nongonococcal or Nonspecific Urethritis

Nongonococcal urethritis (NGU), also known as *nonspecific urethritis,* is a nonreportable STI. This terminology is slightly antiquated since it was originally developed to describe all forms of urethritis not associated with gonorrhea. At the time this term was first used, it was difficult to test for many microorganisms. However, with current lab tests clinicians are better able to diagnosis the exact cause of urethritis when test results are available. This diagnosis remains in use in part because it is clinically useful until definitive test results can be obtained. In student health centers and STI clinics, more than 50% of individuals with urethritis have NGU. Approximately 2 million men are affected each year. NGU may be complicated by epididymitis in men younger than 35 years or in men who have proctitis or Reiter syndrome, or both.

PATHOPHYSIOLOGY. Nongonococcal urethritis is a syndrome caused by a variety of microbes, including *C. trachomatis* and *Ureaplasma urealyticum.* Chlamydial infections are discussed earlier in this chapter (see p. 929).

C. trachomatis is the most common cause of NGU (15% to 55%). *Trichomonas vaginalis* and herpes simplex virus (HSV) sometimes cause NGU. However, *Mycoplasma genitalium* is implicated in as many as one third of the cases of NGU. Enteric bacteria also may cause NGU, especially if the man has had insertive anal intercourse.[9]

CLINICAL MANIFESTATIONS. Clinically, NGU infection caused by CT cannot be differentiated from NGU caused by another microbe. In both cases, men present after a 7- to 21-day incubation period with complaints of dysuria and mild to moderate white or clear urethral discharge. Discharge may be absent, and urethral itching may be the only symptom. Asymptomatic infection is common.

EVALUATION AND TREATMENT. NGU is a diagnosis of exclusion. Urethral exudate is Gram-stained, and an endourethral swab or a urine NAAT test may be taken for testing or culture. Urine sediment also may be examined. All individuals who have urethritis should be evaluated for the presence of gonococcal and chlamydial infection. A treatment of a single 1-g oral dose of azithromycin should be initiated as soon as possible after diagnosis. Doxycycline, 100 mg orally twice a day for 7 days, is also effective. Single-dose regimens have the advantage of improved compliance and of directly observed therapy.[9] These regimens have the advantage of providing coverage for a wide array of potential causes of urethritis, including *Trichomonas* and enteric bacteria. However, if improvement does not occur, the man should be evaluated again to rule out other pathologies.[9]

Viral Infections

Genital Herpes

Genital herpes, which causes blisters (cold sores), is the most common infectious cause of genital ulcerations in the United States. In fact, genital infection with HSV is an epidemic in the United States. Herpes simplex virus is not a reportable disease so national statistics are not available. However, HSV infections are estimated to affect 1 million new individuals each year. Recurrent infections are mostly asymptomatic (50% to 70%) and affect an estimated 50 million Americans annually.[2] Eighty percent of infected individuals do not know they have herpes.[2] Genital herpes can be caused by either of the two serotypes of HSV: HSV-1 or HSV-2. Although infections caused by the serotypes are clinically indistinguishable, serologic studies show that more than 80% of initial and 98% of recurrent genital HSV infections are caused by HSV-2.

The seroprevalence of HSV-2 is estimated to range from 16% to 20% of the total adult population to 50% for subgroups, for example, individuals treated at STI clinics and black women.

Genital herpes can be caused by either the HSV-1 or the HSV-2 subtype but HSV-2 has more virulent and frequent outbreaks.[9]

Herpes simplex virus infection is transmitted through genital skin or mucosal contact with a person who is shedding the virus. Persons without symptoms probably transmit most infections. Transmission rates are not well identified. However, women are more susceptible than men to contracting herpes related to prolonged semen contact with the vaginal or rectal mucosa. It is estimated that a woman has an 80% to 90% risk of developing genital herpes after being exposed to an infected man. In 1992 Mertz and colleagues[24] studied monogamous heterosexual couples in which one partner had HSV-2 infection. The noninfected partner seroconverted in 10% of couples over a 1-year period. As many as 70% of such infections seem to be acquired during periods of asymptomatic shedding. Uninfected female partners were at greater risk than men, especially if they were seronegative for HSV-1 antibodies as well. Both HSV-1 and HSV-2 can be transmitted through genital-genital contact or orogenital contact. The likelihood of nonsexual transmission of genital herpes, through aerosolized secretions of other fomites, is unlikely.[2,21]

Condoms do not fully protect against HSV infection because there is still contact between genital skin not covered by the latex. Female condoms offer a bit more protection from HSV since they cover and protect the vulva but they do not eliminate the risk of transmission.[25] HSV infection greatly increases the risk of HIV acquisition. People with HSV are four times more likely to contract HIV if exposed, potentially because of small skin splits that occur as a result of HSV infection.[2] Prevention of the spread of HIV and HSV through safer sex practices is essential for infected people.

Neonatal infections can begin in utero or, more commonly, during the intrapartum or postpartum period. The risk of transmission of HSV to the neonate varies from <3% among women with recurrence of known herpes at term who acquired HSV during the pregnancy to up to 30% to 60% in women who are exposed and acquire HSV near term.[26] Perinatal transmission can cause extensive morbidity and mortality.

Intrauterine transmission is rare but can occur through transplacental or ascending infection and can cause fetal malformations.[27] Eighty-five percent of infections are transmitted intrapartally. Infants are at greatest risk if the mother has a primary infection acquired near the time of delivery rather than a recurrent infection or an infection acquired during the first half of pregnancy. Ruptured membranes have a role in the development of HSV. Rupture of membranes for more than 4 hours increases the risk of the fetus for contracting HSV. Internal fetal monitoring devices also increase the risk of vertical transmission because they break the skin.[28] Infants also may be exposed after birth through mouth-to-mouth kissing by family members; there have been several cases of infants exposed during ritual circumcision involving direct orogenital suction.[29]

PATHOPHYSIOLOGY. After initial exposure and entry of the virus at mucocutaneous sites or abraded skin, the virus undergoes replication locally in the dermis and epidermis. This leads to cell destruction, transudation, and vesicle formation. The virus spreads to contiguous cells and eventually into sensory nerves. Eventually the virus is transported intra-axonally to the dorsal root, where it remains in a latent stage until it becomes reactivated. During the latent period the genome for the virus is maintained in the host cell nucleus without causing the death of the cell. After oral infection the latent virus resides in the trigeminal ganglion; after genital infection it resides in the dorsal sacral nerve roots.

Latent infections can become reactivated, often during times of physical or emotional stress, and cause a recurrent infection with similar manifestations. Reactivation of the HSV-2 infection is twice as common as HSV-1 infections, and the likelihood of HSV-2 recurrent infections is 8 to 10 times. Reactivation of HSV is not well understood but may be attributable to physical, hormonal, and immunologic stimuli. Other triggering events may be menstruation, stress, and sun exposure.[30] During reactivation the viral genomes are transported through the peripheral sensory nerves back to the dermal surface.

CLINICAL MANIFESTATIONS. Three distinct syndromes associated with HSV infection are first-episode primary genital infection, first-episode nonprimary HSV, and recurrent infections. The manifestations of each one depend on the individual's immune state. First-episode primary genital infection occurs when an individual has no antibodies to HSV-1 or HSV-2. Up to 60% of primary infections with HSV-2 and one third of primary infections with HSV-1 are asymptomatic.[31] If symptoms occur, the individual may have small (1 to 2 mm), multiple, vesicular lesions at the site of infection, usually on the labia minora, fourchette, penis, or mouth (Figure 26-12). They also may appear on the cervix, buttocks, and thighs and are often painful and pruritic. These lesions usually last about 10 to 20 days. The lesions of HSV-1 and HSV-2 are indistinguishable to the naked eye. These wet lesions actively shed virus for about 10 to 14 days, after which they heal by reepithelialization. Small lesions may coalesce into larger ulcers and become secondarily infected.

Systemic manifestations often accompany primary HSV infection, and an individual may experience fever, malaise, myalgias, lymphadenopathy, and urinary retention. Pharyngitis, aseptic meningitis, and hepatitis also may accompany primary HSV infection. Figure 26-13 illustrates the clinical course of primary genital HSV.

First-episode non-primary HSV occurs in individuals who have preexisting antibodies. In some individuals the primary infection may not have had any clinical manifestations, but the HSV virus has become latent in the nerve root and can reactivate later in life. Compared with primary infection, the first episode of nonprimary HSV is often milder with fewer lesions that are less painful and heal faster. Fewer systemic manifestations occur and viral shedding is of shorter duration.

Recurrent infections produce mild local symptoms. The number of lesions is greatly reduced, and the lesions are less painful. Lesions are often unilateral, with crusting within 4 to 5 days. Recovery and healing are usually complete within 10 days. Asymptomatic viral shedding can occur with both HSV-1 and HSV-2, but is more common with HSV-2.[9]

Individuals affected with HSV-2 are more likely to experience recurrent infections. Recurrent infections occur an average

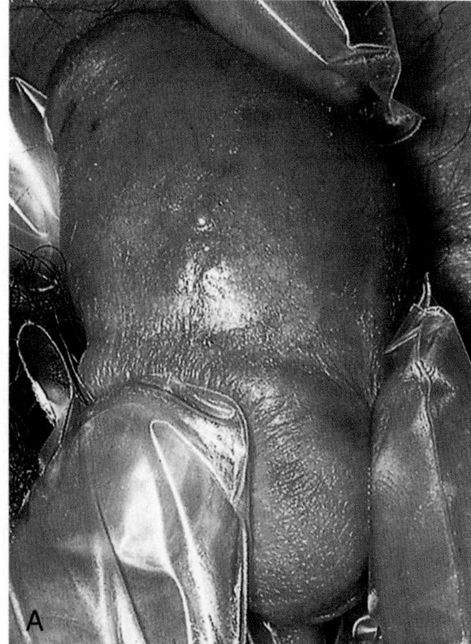

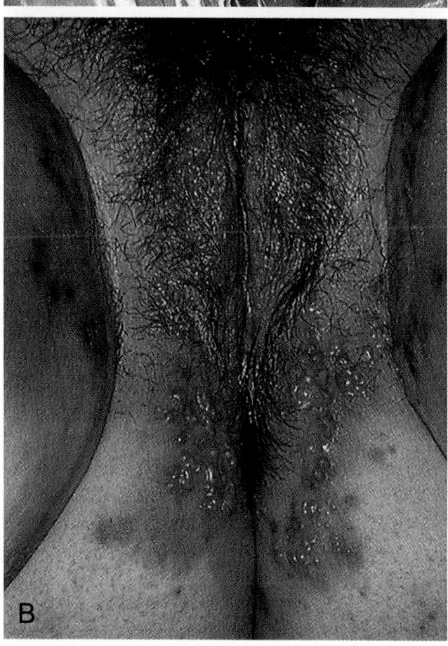

FIGURE 26-12 Herpes Lesions. A, Herpetic vesicles on the penis. **B,** Herpetic ulceration of the vulva. (From McMillan A, Scott GR: *Sexually transmitted infections,* ed 2, London, 2000, Churchill Livingstone.)

of five to eight times per year but may be as frequent as every month for many years. Individuals may experience prodromal symptoms (e.g., pruritus, tingling, dysesthesias) a few hours to 2 days before the eruption of lesions. Women may experience a vaginal discharge and dysuria, and 44% of men have dysuria.

Symptomatic HSV infection of the newborn may occur any time in the first month of life. Manifestations range from a local infection of the eyes, skin, or mucous membranes to a severe disseminated infection with CNS involvement. About 70% of affected infants present with skin lesions. CNS involvement includes seizures and is associated with a mortality of more than 50% and extensive neurologic sequelae in survivors. Eighty-five percent of untreated infants with disseminated disease will die.[27]

EVALUATION AND TREATMENT. Genital HSV infection is suggested if typical genital lesions are present. Diagnosis can be

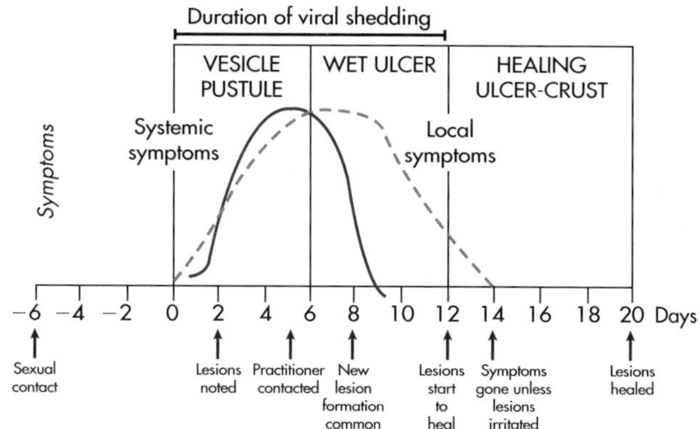

FIGURE 26-13 Clinical Course of Primary Genital Herpes. (From Corey L: Genital herpes. In Holmes KK et al, editors: *Sexually transmitted diseases,* ed 2, New York, 1990, McGraw-Hill.)

made after viral culture, but these cultures have a low sensitivity especially when lesions are healing. The CDC recommends serologic testing for diagnosis and to determine the virus subtype because the prognosis and the risk of transmission differ.[9]

There is no cure for HSV, only symptom management and viral suppression treatments. Oral acyclovir, valacyclovir, penciclovir, and famciclovir are used for primary and periodic outbreaks and to prevent recurrences. Acyclovir has a better safety profile for pregnant and nursing women, but there is ongoing research supporting the safety of valacyclovir as well.[26] Intravenous acyclovir is reserved for pregnant or severely immunocompromised individuals.[32] Suppressive treatment is recommended for individuals with more than six recurrences per year and pregnant women at term with a history of herpes. Suppressive treatment also may reduce asymptomatic viral shedding, decreasing transmission to sexual partners and vaginally-born infants. Although condoms offer some protection, individuals with HSV should refrain from all genital contact when prodromal or symptomatic and understand that an undetermined risk of transmission exists even during asymptomatic periods.

Human Papillomavirus Infection

Human papillomavirus (HPV) infection is the most common symptomatic viral STI in the United States. Although more than 5.5 million cases are diagnosed yearly, prevalence is considered underestimated because HPV infection is often subclinical. More sensitive measures of HPV indicate that 50% of all sexually active people are infected with the virus at some point in their lives.[9]

More than 120 different types of HPV have been identified. More than 40 serotypes are unique to the stratified squamous epitheliums of the genital area. These are divided into serotypes that have a high risk of causing cervical cancer and low-risk serotypes, which are associated with benign genital lesions or warts: *condylomata acuminata* of the vulva, vagina, penis, and perianal areas. High-risk types 16 and 18 are the most common, causing up to 70% of anogenital cancers.[9] Serotypes 6 and 11 are associated with 90% of genital warts. Low-risk subtypes can coexist with the high-risk types, but do not cause cancer. Although rare, these types also may cause oral lesions. It is now known that infection with persistent, high-risk serotypes of HPV is

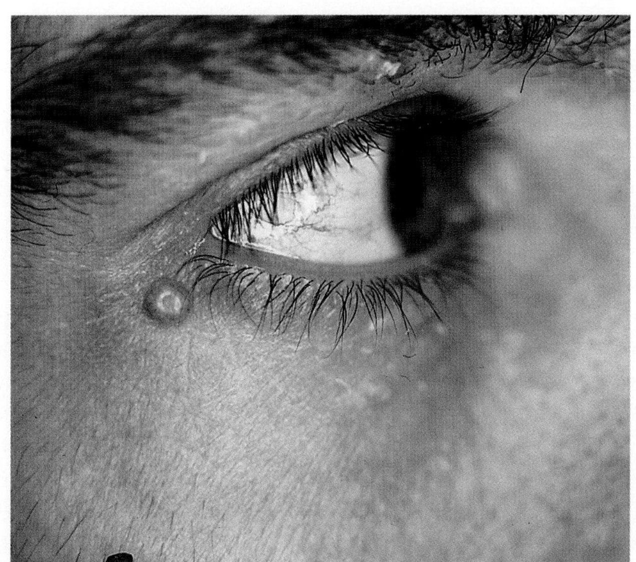

FIGURE 26-16 **Molluscum Contagiosum.** Flesh-colored papules of molluscum may be distinguished by their umbilicated centers. The papules contain a white cheesy substance that may be stained for the presence of viral inclusion bodies. (From Morse SA et al, editors: *Atlas of sexually transmitted diseases and AIDS,* ed 4, London, 2013, Saunders.)

Molluscum Contagiosum

Molluscum contagiosum is a benign viral infection of the skin in children and adults. Primarily the face, hands, lower abdomen, and genitalia are affected; papules found on other parts of the skin or widely distributed are not uncommon. Molluscum contagiosum also is a symptom of immunosuppression in HIV-positive individuals.[47]

Molluscum contagiosum occurs throughout the world and has been a common childhood disease in the developing world. It is much less common in the United States, where the incidence is highest among young adults. The childhood disease is transmitted by skin-to-skin contact and fomites (e.g., towels, wet surfaces and equipment) and affects the face, trunk, and limbs. Adult disease is more commonly sexually transmitted and affects the lower abdomen, genitalia, and perianal area.[47] Molluscum contagiosum in adults is most common in men 20 to 29 years of age and in those with multiple sexual partners. The molluscum contagiosum virus is taken into epithelial cells by phagocytosis and replicates within the cytoplasm, where it produces superficial cytoplasmic inclusions **(molluscum bodies)** and cellular hyperplasia. After an incubation period of 2 to 7 weeks, white or flesh-colored, round or oval dome-shaped papules appear. The lesions are relatively small (2 to 5 mm) but occasionally may coalesce to form larger lesions up to 15 mm. The surface has a characteristic central umbilication, from which a thick, creamy core material can be expressed (Figure 26-16). Generally the lesions are not painful or pruritic unless secondarily infected. The papules usually resolve in 6 to 12 months but may last several years and spread by autoinoculation.[47]

The appearance of the lesions is generally all that is needed to make the diagnosis, although direct microscopic examination of stained material from the core of the papule discloses molluscum bodies within the swollen and rounded epithelial cells. The lesions often heal spontaneously after several months but are contagious until completely healed. Other effective means of removing the lesions include curettage or application of liquid nitrogen (cryotherapy), silver nitrate, or topical creams; however, these treatments may cause scarring. Individuals tend to have lifetime immunity once lesions are healed.

Parasitic Infections

Trichomoniasis

Originally discovered in 1836, *T. vaginalis* was at first thought to be a harmless commensal microorganism. *T. vaginalis* is now known to be a common cause of sexually transmitted lower genital tract infection and urethritis.

Because **trichomoniasis** (infection by *T. vaginalis*) is not a reportable disease, its prevalence can only be estimated. The latest estimates suggest that as many as 3 million cases of trichomoniasis occur each year in the United States,[1,2] and that *T. vaginalis* accounts for one of four cases of infectious vaginitis. Although sexual transmission is clearly the most common means of disease spread, transmission through fomites is theoretically possible. To cause infection, the warm, moist fomite would have to introduce an inoculum of about 10,000 microorganisms directly into the vagina.[48]

PATHOPHYSIOLOGY. *T. vaginalis* is an anaerobic, unicellular, flagellated, parasitic protozoan that adheres to and damages squamous epithelial cells. Because this protozoan selectively affects squamous epithelia, vaginal and urethral tissue is often infected, as are periurethral (Skene) and greater vestibular (Bartholin) glands. The endocervical canal is not affected because it is lined with columnar epithelium. In men, the urethra is the most common site of infection, although the protozoa, called **trichomonads,** also can infect the epididymis and (rarely) the prostate.

Trichomoniasis is most common in men and women of reproductive age, and it is primarily an infection of the vagina. *T. vaginalis* can induce a marked inflammatory response in the vagina, causing a copious discharge that contains large numbers of polymorphonuclear neutrophils. Trichomonads adhere to but do not invade the squamous epithelial cells.

CLINICAL MANIFESTATIONS. Manifestations of vaginal trichomoniasis range from none to severe, with some women reporting an increase in distressing symptoms immediately after menses. Vaginal discharge and internal pruritus are the most common complaints. Dyspareunia and dysuria are also fairly common. Secretions are usually copious, frothy, malodorous, and yellow-green to gray-green. The vaginal walls may appear erythematous and sore. Small, punctate red marks, sometimes called *strawberry spots,* are sometimes visible on the vaginal walls and cervix. Vaginal pH is usually more than 4.5.[9] Most men with trichomoniasis are asymptomatic but may have scant intermittent discharge, slight pruritus, and mild dysuria.[9]

EVALUATION AND TREATMENT. History and symptoms are inadequate for diagnosis of trichomoniasis. Microscopic or laboratory confirmation of the presence of the trichomonads in vaginal secretions or urine provides a definitive diagnosis. In a fresh wet mount preparation that has been warmed slightly, the epithelial cells have relatively clean and sharp edges, the ratio of polymorphonuclear leukocytes to epithelial cells exceeds 1:1, and the trichomonads are visible. The ovoid microorganism is slightly larger than a polymorphonuclear leukocyte and has one rounded, flagellated end and one slightly pointed, flagellated end. The flagella give the trichomonads their characteristic twisting motility. Fresh secretions have a pH higher than 4.5 and a positive amine odor when mixed with 10% KOH (positive "whiff test"). In an acidic environment, such as urine, the trichomonads assume a "balled-up" or spherical shape and become less motile.

There are a variety of clinical tests for trichomoniasis, including microscopic examination of vaginal discharge and pH testing, as well as laboratory tests, such as an immunochromatographic dipstick (e.g., OSOM Trichomonas Rapid Test) and a nucleic acid probe (e.g., Affirm VPIII).[9] Many tests have a high false-negative rate that can delay adequate treatment of infected individuals.

The treatment of choice for trichomoniasis is a single 2-gram dose of metronidazole (Flagyl) or tinidazole. The single-dose therapy is effective, has fewer side effects than multiple-dose therapy, and eliminates the need for individual compliance with longer regimens. Sexual partners, even if asymptomatic, also should be treated for trichomoniasis. The 2-gram single dose of metronidazole can be used to treat pregnant women. However, lactating women should suspend breast-feeding for 12 to 24 hours after single-dose therapy.[9]

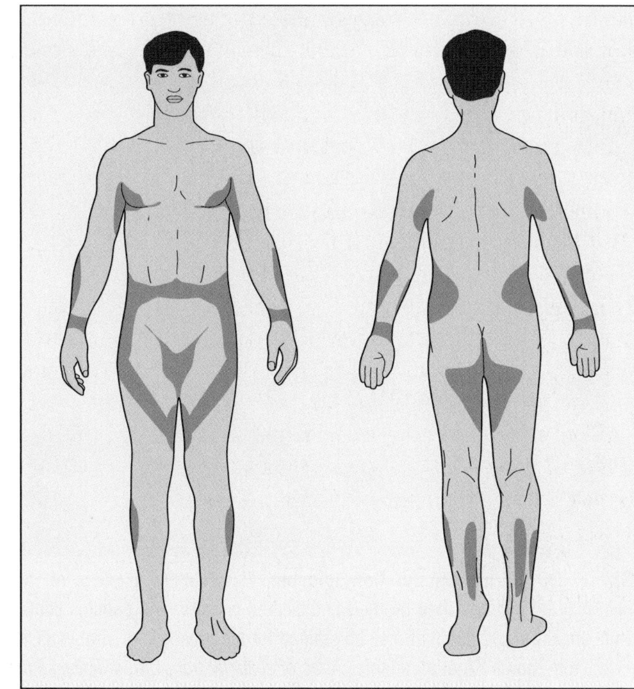

FIGURE 26-17 **Distribution of Skin Lesions of *Sarcoptes scabiei* Infestation.** Unshaded areas are rarely affected in healthy adults. (From Morse SA et al, editors: *Atlas of sexually transmitted diseases and AIDS,* ed 3, London, 2003, Mosby.)

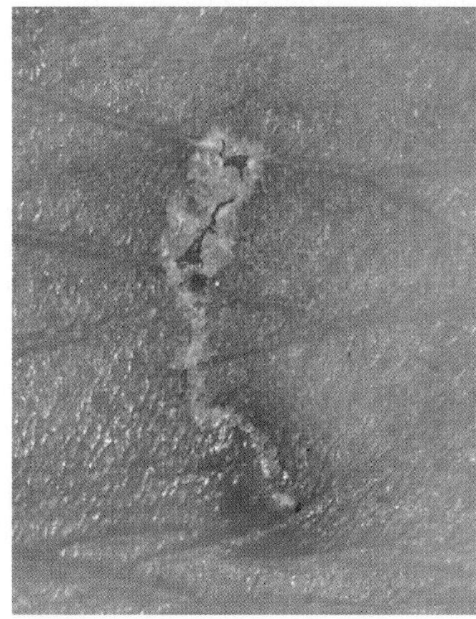

FIGURE 26-18 **Scabies Burrow.** An S-shaped burrow with a tiny vesicle at one end. (From Marks JG, Miller JJ: *Lookingbill and Marks' principles of dermatology,* ed 4, St Louis, 2006, Saunders.)

Scabies

Scabies is a common parasitic infection that can be spread by skin-to-skin and sexual contact. Discovered by Bonomo in 1687, it is considered to be the first human disease with a known cause.[49]

Scabies has a worldwide distribution, but actual prevalence is unknown.[14] Outbreaks are common in childcare centers, nursing homes, and prisons and are often spread to the larger community through familial contact. Transmission of scabies requires prolonged close skin-to-skin contact, which occurs within families or between sexual partners. Mites also can be transferred through infested bedding, clothes, and other fomites. Nonsexual transmission is common in residential institutions and hospitals, especially when crusted scabies, a highly contagious variant of scabies, is present.[50]

PATHOPHYSIOLOGY. Only 5 to 10 mites are needed to establish infection in a previously uninfected individual. The adult female itch mite, *Sarcoptes scabiei,* is 0.3 to 0.4 mm long and has a life span of about 30 days. Once deposited on human skin, it burrows through the horny layer of the stratum granulosum. Within hours of burrowing, the female begins laying two or three large eggs per day, each of which progresses through larval and nymphal stages to become an adult itch mite in about 10 days. The most common places for scabies to burrow are on the hands (between the fingers) and on the flexor surfaces of the wrists and the extensor surfaces of the elbows. The groin is a common location for sexually transmitted scabies. Lesions may occur on the penile shaft, glans, scrotum, and buttocks.[51,52] Figure 26-17 shows the typical sites of scabies burrows.

CLINICAL MANIFESTATIONS. The classic symptom of scabies is intense pruritus, which may increase at night. Pruritus is a result of a reaction to the presence of the *S. scabiei* mite. This reaction may take weeks to develop with initial infection, but only 24 hours if the person has been previously infected. The typical burrow of the *S. scabiei* is a short, linear, curved, or S-shaped line (Figure 26-18). There may be small, erythematous, excoriated larval papules near the burrows. Secondary infections are common and are caused by scratching. In some individuals a hypersensitivity reaction occurs a month or more after the infestation and causes multiple, reddish brown, pruritic nodules on the covered portions of the body—most commonly, the upper thighs, buttocks, male genitalia, and axillary regions. These nodules may persist for more than 1 year despite treatment with a scabicide. Even after successful treatment, some individuals will continue to experience pruritus for several weeks.[51]

EVALUATION AND TREATMENT. Although the diagnosis of scabies is often made clinically, microscopic identification of the mite or its eggs, larvae, or feces is recommended because the symptoms of scabies can imitate those of many other dermatologic conditions. Superficial scrapings from a recently developed unexcoriated papule or burrow can be observed easily under the microscope; the addition of KOH allows easier visualization of the mite.

Preferred treatment is topical application of 5% permethrin massaged into the skin and left for 8 to 14 hours, or ivermectin 1% dosed at 200 mcg/kg orally and repeated again in 2 weeks. Lindane (1%) lotion or cream also is effective if applied thinly to all areas of the body below the neck and washed thoroughly at 8 hours.[9] Close household and sexual contacts should be treated even if they are not yet symptomatic. Permethrin has been used safely in infants as young as 2 months and is the treatment of choice for children. Pregnant women should be treated with permethrin only if infestation with scabies can be documented. For population-based outbreaks, such as those in residential institutions, the CDC recommends treating the entire population; ivermectin has advantages in these settings because it is easy to administer and is not dependent on thorough topical treatment and bathing.[9] To prevent reinfestation, clothing and bed linens should be machine washed and dried at high temperatures, or kept away from body contact for 72 hours.[9]

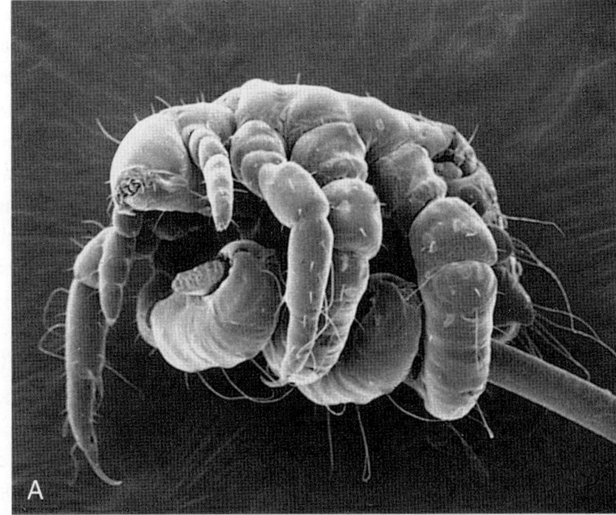

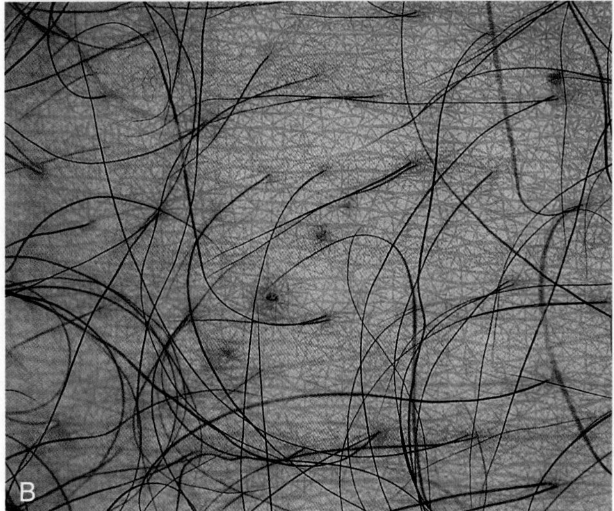

FIGURE 26-19 **Pubic Louse and Crab Louse. A,** Pubic louse *(Phthirus pubis)* encircling a pubic hair; the clawlike legs produce a firm grip. **B,** Crab louse bites *(P. pubis)*. (From Morse SA et al, editors: *Atlas of sexually transmitted diseases and AIDS*, ed 4, London, 2013, Saunders.)

Pediculosis Pubis

Phthirus pubis, the crab louse, is one of three species of lice that infest humans. *P. pubis* is commonly transmitted sexually and causes **pediculosis pubis,** or "crabs." Adolescents and young children are most commonly infected.

P. pubis is transmitted primarily by intimate sexual contact or contact with infected bed linens or clothing. It is highly contagious; there is a 95% chance of contracting the disease during a single sexual encounter. Fomites are another common method of infection because crabs can live away from the body for several days. The transfer of lice from pubic hair is probably mechanical, assisted by scratching, fingernails, towels, and other similar means rather than by self-propulsion. Pubic lice usually infect the perineal and axillary hair and occasionally the hair of the trunk, beard, scalp, and eyelashes.

PATHOPHYSIOLOGY. The crab louse has a 25- to 30-day life cycle from egg to egg that consists of five stages: an egg (or nit) stage, three nymphal stages, and an adult stage, all of which occur in the host. The nits of crab lice are found "glued" to hairs; they are oval, 0.8 by 0.3 mm, and whitish, and they hatch in 5 to 10 days (Figure 26-19). In the adult stage, pubic lice are grayish, are approximately 1 mm in length, and have a segmented body and claws particularly designed for clinging to pubic hairs. Because lice depend on blood for nutrition, they bite into the skin to obtain food.

CLINICAL MANIFESTATIONS. Symptoms range from mild pruritus to severe, intolerable itching, depending on the individual's sensitivity to louse bites. Allergic sensitization occurs in about 5 days, when itching, erythema, and inflammation may worsen. Excessive scratching may lead to secondary infection.

EVALUATION AND TREATMENT. The individual usually presents with a history of localized itching in the infected area. Because the lice and nits are visible to the naked eye, a thorough clinical examination permits definitive diagnosis. Pediculosis pubis is treated with 1% permethrin cream rinse or 1% lindane lotion, cream, or shampoo or with over-the-counter pyrethrin or piperonyl butoxide. Infection of the eyelashes should be treated with occlusive ophthalmic ointment for 10 days.[9] For nonocular infections, the pediculicide is applied to infested and adjacent hairy areas and removed after a specified length of time by thorough washing. Remaining nits can be removed with a fine-toothed comb. Permethrin is recommended for young children and pregnant women and has less potential toxicity with inappropriate use. On the other hand, lindane is the least expensive and nontoxic if used correctly. Lindane should not be used after a bath, or by persons with extensive dermatitis, by pregnant or lactating women, or by children less than 2 years of age.[53] Sexual contacts from the past month should be treated regardless of symptoms, and any other intimate household contacts also should be examined and treated if needed. Clothing and bed linens should be machine washed and dried at high temperatures or kept away from body contact for 72 hours. Treatment can be repeated in 7 days to eradicate any newly hatched lice.

Resistance to treatment is increasing and is widespread. If initial treatment fails, malathion 0.5% lotion is a second-line treatment but has an unpleasant odor and must be kept on the body for 8 to 12 hours.[9]

SEXUALLY TRANSMITTED INFECTIONS OF OTHER BODY SYSTEMS

There are a variety of infectious diseases, including some enteric bacterial and systemic viral diseases, in which the main mode of transmission is not through sexual contact. Some, however, are transmitted through sexual contact, more so among men who have sex with men. Although the major mode of transmission may be by ingestion (i.e., gastrointestinal system through hand-to-mouth or water or food consumption), respiratory exposure (i.e., hand to nose or eye, or inhalation), or direct contact with blood or body fluids (i.e., sharing of needles among drug users, blood transfusions, vertical transmission from mother to baby, health worker exposures), infection can be transmitted through intimate sexual contact as well. Among the most serious of these infections is acquired immunodeficiency syndrome (AIDS) caused by the human immunodeficiency virus (HIV) and hepatitis (all types). Worldwide, the main mode of transmission of HIV and hepatitis B is through sexual intercourse (primarily heterosexual), but nonsexual exposure to infected blood and body fluids contributes significantly to infection rates for both. The epidemiology, modes of transmission, pathophysiology, clinical manifestations, and evaluation and treatment of AIDS and hepatitis are discussed in detail in Chapters 10 and 41. Less serious, but often debilitating, are gastrointestinal infections, such as shigellosis and giardiasis, and systemic diseases, such as Epstein-Barr virus and cytomegalovirus infections. Table 26-3 provides a list of several gastrointestinal and systemic infections that are known to be transmitted by intimate sexual contact, but in which the mode of transmission is primarily through other routes.

TABLE 26-3 INFECTIONS WITH KNOWN SEXUAL TRANSMISSIBILITY: MAIN MODE OF TRANSMISSION BY OTHER MEANS

INFECTION/DISEASE	MAIN ROUTE OF TRANSMISSION
Gastrointestinal Infections	
Shigellosis caused by the *Shigella* bacteria	Contact with infected feces Hand-to-mouth
Campylobacter enteritis caused by the *Campylobacter jejuni* bacteria	Primarily an animal pathogen Hand-to-mouth
Giardiasis caused by the *Giardia lamblia* protozoa	Contaminated drinking water Hand-to-mouth
Amebiasis caused by the *Entamoeba histolytica* protozoa	Contaminated drinking water Hand-to-mouth
Hepatitis (liver infection and inflammation) A, C	Hepatitis A: contact with infected feces; hand-to-mouth Hepatitis C: blood-borne pathogen; direct exposure to contaminated blood; sexual transmission very uncommon
Systemic Diseases	
Epstein-Barr virus	Mucous membrane (oral) exposure
Cytomegalovirus	Body fluids; exposure via close interpersonal contact or direct transfer

Reported Cases of Acute Hepatitis C by Selected Risk Factors, United States, 1982–2001*

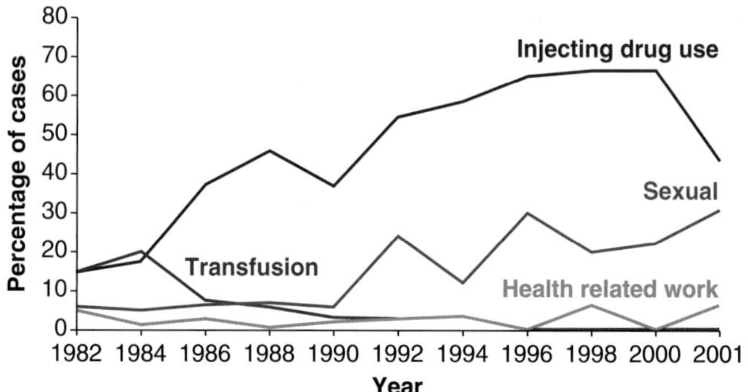

*1982–1990 based on non-A, non-B hepatitis

FIGURE 26-20 Risk for Hepatitis C Exposure. Comparison of injecting drug use *(blue)*, transfusions *(purple)*, health-related work *(green)*, and sexual exposure *(red)*. Note the rise in sexually transmitted incidences. (From Centers for Disease Control and Prevention: *Hepatitis C: What clinicians and other health professionals need to know, 2000.* Available at www.cdc.giv/ncid/diseases/hepatitis/c_training/edu/intro).

Hepatitis B Virus

Hepatitis is a liver infection that can be caused by six types of viruses: hepatitis A, hepatitis B, hepatitis C, hepatitis D, hepatitis E, and hepatitis G. Each virus causes a syndrome of acute, icteric (jaundice-producing) liver inflammation. Of the three types, the **hepatitis B virus (HBV)** is known to be sexually transmitted. (Hepatitis A, like most other predominantly enteric infections, may be considered an STI because of anal-oral transmission.) Although hepatitis C virus (HCV) is not recognized as an STI, the CDC has listed sexual exposure, particularly for individuals with multiple partners, as a potential HCV risk factor (Figure 26-20). Data indicate sexual transmission may occur in approximately 1% of HCV cases; however, the virus is inefficiently spread through this manner.[54] Additional information about hepatitis is found in Chapter 41.

The prevalence of HBV infection varies dramatically worldwide. Widespread screening of pregnant women and vaccination of all infants since 1991 has decreased the rate of infection in the United States by more than 80% and is expected to have lasting effects into future decades.[55] In the United States, approximately 5% to 20% of the general population has evidence of HBV infection, and more than 1.4 million are chronically infected.[2] Seropositivity generally increases with age. Serologic tests of STI clinic patients show evidence of past infection in 28% of individuals ages 25 years and older and 7% in those younger than 25 years.[53] Those at risk for HBV infection in the United States are infants born to hepatitis-infected mothers, healthcare workers, individuals who have sexual contact with HBV-infected persons, and immigrants from areas of high HBV prevalence. However, larger portions of the population are at risk in developing countries. For example, 60% to 80% of the population in Southeast Asia and Africa may harbor serologic evidence of past or current infection.

Transmission of HBV can occur through needle puncture, blood transfusion, cuts or abrasions in the skin, and absorption by mucosal surfaces. Direct contact with infected body fluids, such as tears, cerebrospinal fluid, synovial fluid, gastric juices, pleural fluid, semen, and urine, may pass the infection. The hepatitis B virus can survive dry and outside the body for up to 1 week, making it easily infectious on fomites, such as medical equipment. Only very high temperatures or bleach can kill the hepatitis virus.[9] Perinatal transmission of HBV is relatively common. Neonates whose mothers are infectious have a 90% chance of becoming chronically infected with HBV during labor or delivery if they do not receive treatment.[55] Infants of infected mothers should receive HBV vaccine and immunoglobulin against hepatitis within 12 hours of birth to reduce risk. The vaccine and immunoglobulin combination successfully prevents chronic carrier status 85% of the time.[55] Although HBV is in many maternal body fluids, it is not found in breast milk and breast-feeding is still encouraged for mothers with HBV.[56]

Hepatitis delta agent is a defective virus that is similar to HBV antigen but cannot cause hepatitis B by itself, requiring the presence of HBV to cause hepatitis. Hepatitis delta infection is rare in the United States, but cases have been documented in intravenous drug users and their sexual contacts and in recipients of contaminated blood. It is most commonly found in men who have sex with men, persons requiring kidney dialysis, and healthcare workers.

PATHOPHYSIOLOGY. After exposure, HBV passes through the bloodstream to the liver, where it infects liver cells and multiplies. The infection is usually self-limiting, with most patients mounting an effective immune response. Approximately 6% to 10% of infected adults cannot eradicate the virus and become chronic carriers of HBV. There is an inverse relationship between age and chronic carrier status, with younger individuals at greater risk for infection.[9]

CLINICAL MANIFESTATIONS. Most HBV infections are clinically asymptomatic and result in permanent immunity. Symptoms of hepatitis usually develop only after an HBV antigen has been circulating in the blood for 3 to 6 weeks. Approximately 15% to 20% of individuals develop a prodromal syndrome characterized by an erythematous rash, urticaria, polyarthralgias, and arthritis. Symptoms of infection also may include lassitude, anorexia, nausea, vomiting, headache, fever, dark urine, jaundice, and moderate liver enlargement with tenderness. Long-term sequelae include chronic persistent and chronic active hepatitis, cirrhosis, hepatocellular carcinoma, hepatic failure, and death. In neonates who contract HBV, the disease may be manifested in many ways from mild illness to a severe infection with liver damage.

EVALUATION AND TREATMENT. HBV infection is clinically indistinguishable from other types of hepatitis. Diagnosis can be made only through serologic testing. No specific therapy exists for HBV infection in adults. Treatment consists of supportive care and relief of symptoms. Since 1991, the CDC has promoted an aggressive vaccination campaign and recommends vaccination for all infants, children, and adolescents and a diversity of high-risk adults. The three-injection vaccine series is begun at birth for all infants.

Acquired Immunodeficiency Syndrome

Epidemiology, modes of transmission, pathophysiology, clinical manifestations, and evaluation and treatment of AIDS are discussed in detail in Chapter 10.

SUMMARY REVIEW

Sexually Transmitted Urogenital Infections

1. Gonorrhea is a sexually transmitted communicable disease that can be local or systemic. Complications include PID, sterility, and disseminated infection.
2. Gonorrhea passed to the fetus from the mother typically manifests as an eye infection and develops 1 to 12 days after birth. Usually ophthalmic antibiotic prophylaxis is not sufficient to prevent infection.
3. Gonorrhea is rapidly becoming resistant to available antibiotics. Multidrug therapy is now recommended to decrease drug resistance.
4. Syphilis is an STI that becomes systemic shortly after infection. The four stages of the disease are: (a) primary syphilis with a chancre at the site of infection; (b) secondary syphilis with systemic spread to all body systems; (c) latent syphilis with minimal symptoms or the development of skin lesions; and (d) tertiary syphilis, the most severe stage, with destruction of bone, skin, and soft and neurologic tissues.
5. Congenital syphilis contributes to prematurity of the newborn with bone marrow depression, CNS involvement, renal failure, and intrauterine growth retardation.
6. Syphilis is diagnosed by darkfield microscopy and serologic testing and is treated with injectable penicillin. Sexual partners also are treated.
7. With chancroid infection, women are generally asymptomatic and men may develop inflamed, painful genital ulcers

SUMMARY REVIEW—cont'd

and inguinal buboes. Incubation period is 1 to 14 days. Single-dose therapy with injectable ceftriaxone or oral azithromycin for both partners is recommended. Persons with HIV may require a longer treatment regimen.

8. Granuloma inguinale (donovanosis) is rare in the United States. The bacteria are gram negative and survive within macrophages. Localized nodules coalesce to form granulomas and ulcers on the penis in men and labia in women. Antibiotics provide effective treatment. Although rare and mildly infectious, granuloma inguinale is a chronic, progressively destructive bacterial infection.
9. Bacterial vaginosis (BV) is a sexually-associated condition caused by an overgrowth of anaerobic bacteria that produce aromatic amines and raise the pH of the vagina, promoting further bacterial growth (without an inflammatory response) and a fishy odor. "Clue cells" are found on the wet mount. Metronidazole (Flagyl) provides effective treatment. BV has been associated with PID, chorioamnionitis, preterm labor, and postpartum endometritis. Treatment of male sexual partners is not recommended.
10. Chlamydia is the most common bacterial STI in the United States and a leading preventable cause of infertility and ectopic pregnancy. The causative organism, *C. trachomatis,* localizes to epithelial tissue and can spread throughout the urogenital tract or pass from infected mother to the eyes and respiratory tract of newborn infants during birth. *C. trachomatis* is susceptible to inexpensive, readily accessible antibiotics. Single-dose azithromycin is the drug of choice. Antibiotic therapy for infected individuals and all sexual contacts is recommended. Because of the asymptomatic nature of chlamydia and the potential sequelae of untreated infection, extensive and widespread screening is recommended by the CDC.
11. Lymphogranuloma venereum is a chronic STI uncommon in the United States. The lesion begins as a skin infection and spreads to the lymph tissue, causing inflammation, necrosis, buboes, and abscesses of the inguinal lymph nodes. Primary lesions appear on the penis and scrotum in men and on the cervix, vaginal wall, and labia in women. Secondary lesions involve inflammation and swelling of the lymph nodes with formation of large blue buboes that rupture and form draining ulcerative lesions. A 21-day or longer course of oral doxycycline or erythromycin is needed for treatment. Treatment of sexual partners is recommended.
12. Genital herpes is the most common genital ulceration in the United States and is caused by either HSV-1 or HSV-2. Lesions initially appear as groups of vesicles that progress to ulceration with pain, lymphadenopathy, and fever. Herpes simplex virus passes from mother to fetus; thus, women with active lesions should give birth by cesarean section to avoid vertical transmission. Acyclovir reduces symptoms but does not cure the disease.
13. Herpes simplex virus (HSV) infection is lifelong and can result in an initial outbreak and subsequent outbreaks. Individuals are contagious during outbreaks and episodes of asymptomatic viral shedding. Recurrent infections are most often attributable to HSV-2 and are generally milder and of shorter duration.
14. Human papillomavirus (HPV) is associated with the development of cervical dysplasia and cancer as well as condylomata acuminata. The high-risk strains of HPV (HR-HPV) that are precursors to the development of cervical cancer do not cause genital warts. Testing is available to detect HR-HPV and a vaccine is now available for HPV types 16 and 18, which have the highest risk for cervical cancer.
15. Condylomata acuminata (genital warts) are sexually transmitted and highly contagious. The velvety cauliflower-like lesions occur in the genital and anal areas, vagina, and cervix and are painless. They can be transmitted to the infant at birth.
16. Molluscum contagiosum is a benign viral infection of the skin. It is transmitted by skin-to-skin contact in children and adults. In adults, it tends to occur on the genitalia and to be transmitted by sexual contact.
17. Trichomoniasis *(T. vaginalis)* causes vaginitis in women, and urethritis in men. Both partners usually are infected. Women usually have a copious, malodorous, gray-green discharge with pruritus. Men usually are asymptomatic. Metronidazole is the treatment for both partners.
18. Scabies is a common parasitic infection that can be spread by skin-to-skin contact and sexual contact. The scabies mite burrows through the skin, depositing two or three large eggs per day. Intense pruritus, especially at night, is the most pronounced clinical manifestation. Treatment consists of topical application of a pediculicide.
19. Pediculosis pubis (crabs) is commonly transmitted sexually and is caused by the crab louse, *P. pubis.* The lice bite into the skin for nutrition. Symptoms include mild and severe pruritus. Topical application of prescription or over-the-counter pediculicides is effective treatment.

Sexually Transmitted Infections of Other Body Systems

1. Systemic diseases known to be sexually transmitted include AIDS (see Chapter 9), cytomegalovirus infection, and Epstein-Barr virus.
2. Transmission of HBV can occur through needle puncture, blood transfusion, cuts in the skin, and contact with infected body fluids.
3. Hepatitis B infection poses significant health risks including chronic liver disease and hepatocellular cancer. Immunization against hepatitis B is the most effective means of preventing transmission. Universal vaccination of infants and children is recommended, as well as vaccination of high-risk adults.
4. The risk of perinatal transmission of HBV is high for infants of HBV-infected mothers unless they receive immunoglobulin and vaccination.
5. Hepatitis C is generally transmitted percutaneously but sexual transmission appears possible.

KEY TERMS

Acute urethral syndrome, 931
Bacterial vaginosis (BV), 929
Buboes, 927
Chancre, 923
Chancroid, 925
Chlamydia, 929
Condylomata acuminata, 935
Condylomata lata, 924
Congenital syphilis (CS), 925
Disseminated gonococcal infection (DGI), 922
Donovan body, 928
Fomite, 920
Genital herpes, 932
Gonococcus (*pl.*, gonococci), 919
Gonorrhea, 919
Granuloma inguinale (donovanosis), 928
Gummas, 924
Hepatitis B virus (HBV), 940
Hepatitis delta agent, 941
Human papillomavirus (HPV), 934
Latent syphilis, 923
Lymphogranuloma venereum (LGV), 931
Molluscum body, 937
Molluscum contagiosum, 937
Nongonococcal urethritis (NGU), 932
Ophthalmia neonatorum, 922
Pediculosis pubis, 939
Perihepatitis, 922
Primary syphilis, 923
Pseudobuboes, 929
Scabies, 938
Secondary syphilis, 923
Syphilis, 922
Tertiary syphilis, 924
Trichomonad, 937
Trichomoniasis, 937

REFERENCES

1. National Center for HIV/AIDS, Viral Hepatitis, STD, and TB Prevention: *Annual report 2008*, Atlanta, 2008, U.S. Department of Health and Human Services. Available at www.cdc.gov/std/stats.
2. Centers for Disease Control and Prevention: *Sexually transmitted disease surveillance, 2010*, Atlanta, 2011, U.S. Department of Health and Human Services. Available at www.cdc.gov/std/stats.
3. Centers for Disease Control and Prevention: Update to CDC's sexually transmitted diseases treatment guidelines, 2012: oral cephalosporins no longer recommended treatment for gonococcal infections, *MMWR Morb Mortal Wkly Rep* 61(31):590–594, 2012.
4. Zenilman JM: Gonorrhea and chlamydia. In Zenilman JM, Shahmanesh M, editors: *Sexually transmitted diseases*, Sudbury, MA, 2012, Jones & Bartlett Learning, pp 31–42.
5. Yudin MH, Ross JDC: Pelvic inflammatory disease. In Zenilman JM, Shahmanesh M, editors: *Sexually transmitted diseases*, Sudbury, MA, 2012, Jones & Bartlett Learning, pp 67–76.
6. Krieger JN: Sexually transmitted diseases in men. In Tanagho EA, McAninch JW, editors: *Smith's general urology*, ed 17, New York, 2007, McGraw-Hill.
7. Zenilman JM: Gonorrhea: clinical and public health issues, *Hosp Pract* 28(2a):29, 1993.
8. Sperling RS: Infection protocols: perihepatitis, *Contemp OB/GYN* 37(6):51, 1992.
9. Workowski KA, Berman S: Centers for Disease Control and Prevention: Sexually transmitted diseases treatment guidelines, 2010, *MMWR Recomm Rep* 59(RR-12):1–110, 2010.
10. World Health Organization (WHO): *The global elimination of congenital syphilis: rationale and strategy for action*, Geneva, 2007, Author.
11. Fenton KA, French P: Infectious syphilis. In Zenilman JM, Shahmanesh M, editors: *Sexually transmitted infections*, Sudbury, MA, 2012, Jones & Bartlett Learning.
12. World Health Organization: Division of Reproductive Health and Research: *Investment case for eliminating mother-to-child transmission of syphilis: promoting better maternal and child health and stronger health systems*, Geneva, 2012, Author.
13. Augenbraun M: Genital ulcer disease. In Zenilman JM, Shahmanesh M, editors: *Sexually transmitted infections*, Sudbury, MA, 2012, Jones & Bartlett Learning.
14. Wooldridge WE: Syphilis: a new visit from an old enemy, *Postgrad Med* 89(1):193–196, 199–202, 1991.
15. Para MF, Baird IM: Genital ulcer syndromes. In Spagna VA, Prior RB, editors: *Sexually transmitted diseases: a clinical syndrome approach*, New York, 1985, Marcel Dekker.
16. Committee on Infectious Disease: *Red Book 2000*, Elk Grove Village, IL, 2000, American Academy of Pediatrics.
17. Hart G: Donovanosis. In Holmes KK et al: *Sexually transmitted diseases*, ed 4, New York, 2008, McGraw-Hill.
18. Centers for Disease Control and Prevention: *Sexually transmitted disease surveillance, 2007*Atlanta, GA, December 2008, U.S. Department of Health and Human Services. Available at www.cdc.gov/std/stats.
19. Richens J: The diagnosis of treatment of donovanosis (granuloma inguinale), *Genitourin Med* 67(6):441–452, 1991.
20. Centers for Disease Control and Prevention (CDC): *NCHHSTP atlas* (online interactive database), 2012. Available at http://gis.cdc.gov/GRASP/NCHHSTPAtlas/main.html. Accessed August 31, 2012.
21. Amsel R et al: Nonspecific vaginitis. Diagnostic criteria and microbial and epidemiologic associations, *Am J Med* 74(1):14–22, 1983.
22. Kellogg ND et al: Comparison of nucleic acid amplification tests and culture techniques in the detection of *Neisseria gonorrhoeae* and *Chlamydia trachomatis* in victims of suspected child sexual abuse, *J Pediatr Adolesc Gynecol* 17(5):331–339, 2004.
23. Schachter J, Barnes R: Infections caused by *Chlamydia trachomatis*. In Morse SA, Moreland AA, Holmes KK, editors: *Atlas of sexually transmitted diseases and AIDS*, ed 2, London, 1996, Mosby-Wolfe.
24. Mertz GJ et al: Risk factors for the sexual transmission of genital herpes, *Ann Intern Med* 116(3):197, 1992.
25. Cates W, Harwood B: Vaginal barriers and spermicides. In Hatcher RA et al: *Contraceptive technology*, Atlanta, 2011, Ardent, pp 391–408.
26. American Academy of Obstetricians & Gynecologists: Management of herpes in pregnancy, *Obstet Gynecol* 109(6):1489–1498, 2007.
27. Knezevic A et al: Disseminated neonatal herpes caused by herpes simplex virus types 1 and 2, *Emerg Infect Dis* 13(2):302–304, 2007.
28. Chambers HF: Infectious diseases: bacterial and chlamydial. In McTierney LM, McPhee SJ, Papadakis MA, editors: *Current medical diagnosis and treatment*, ed 35, Norwalk, CT, 1996, Appleton & Lange.
29. Centers for Disease Control and Prevention (CDC): Neonatal herpes simplex virus infection following Jewish ritual circumcisions that included direct orogenital suction—New York City, 2000-2011, *MMWR Morb Mortal Wkly Rep* 61(22):405–409, 2012.
30. Hillier SL et al: Association between bacterial vaginosis and preterm delivery of a low-birth-weight infant, *N Engl J Med* 333(26):1737–1742, 1995.
31. Perine PI, Osoba AO: Lymphogranuloma venereum. In Holmes KK et al: *Sexually transmitted diseases*, ed 2, New York, 1990, McGraw-Hill.
32. Landenberg AG et al: A prospective study of new infections with herpes simplex virus type 1 and type 2. Chiron HSV Vaccine Study Group, *N Engl J Med* 341(19):1432–1438, 1999.
33. Stephenson J: Genital herpes vaccine shows limited promise, *JAMA* 284(15):1913–1914, 2000.
34. Centers for Disease Control and Prevention: *Sexually transmitted disease surveillance 2007 supplement, syphilis surveillance report*, Atlanta, GA, 2009, U.S. Department of Health and Human Services, Centers for Disease Control and Prevention, March 2009. Available at www.cdc.gov/std/stats.
35. Rose FB, Camp CJ: Genital herpes: how to relieve patients' physical and psychological symptoms, *Postgrad Med* 84(3):81–86, 1988.
36. Giuliano AR et al: Efficacy of quadrivalent HPV vaccine against HPV infection and disease in males, *N Engl J Med* 364(5):401–411, 2011.
37. Muñoz N et al: Safety, immunogenicity, and efficacy of quadrivalent human papillomavirus (types 6, 11, 16, 18) recombinant vaccine in women aged 24-45 years: a randomised, double-blind trial, *Lancet* 373(9679):1949–1957, 2009.
38. Wright TC et al: Interim guidance for the use of human papillomavirus DNA testing as an adjunct to cervical cytology for screening, *Obstet Gynecol* 103(2):304–309, 2004.
39. Derksen DJ: Children with condylomata acuminata, *J Fam Pract* 34(4):419–423, 1992.
40. Alary M et al: Strategy for screening pregnant women for chlamydial infection in a low-prevalence area, *Obstet Gynecol* 82(3):399, 1993.
41. Brandt AM: *No magic bullet: a social history of venereal disease in the United States since 1880, expanded edition*, New York, 1987, Oxford University Press.

42. Datta D et al: Human papillomavirus. In Zenilman JM, Shahmanesh M, editors: *Sexually transmitted infections*, Sudbury, MA, 2012, Jones & Bartlett Learning.
43. Vesco KK et al: *Screening for cervical cancer: a systematic evidence review for the U.S. Preventive Services Task Force [Internet]*, Rockville, MD, 2011, Agency for Healthcare Research & Quality.
44. U.S. Preventive Services Task Force: *Screening for cervical cancer: clinical summary of U.S. Preventive Task Force recommendation*, March 2012. Available at www.uspreventiveservicestaskforce.org/uspstf11/cervcancer/cervcancersum.htm. Accessed January 10, 2013.
45. Saslow D et al: American Cancer Society, American Society for Colposcopy and Cervical Pathology, and American Society for Clinical Pathology screening guidelines for the prevention and early detection of cervical cancer, *Am J Clin Pathol* 137(4):516–542, 2012.
46. Centers for Disease Control and Prevention: Human papillomavirus—associated cancers—United States, 2004-2008, *MMWR Morb Mortal Wkly Rep* 61(15):258–261, 2012.
47. Centers for Disease Control and Prevention, National Center for Emerging and Zoonotic Infectious Diseases, and Division of High-Consequence Pathogens and Pathology: *Clinical information: molluscum contagiosum*, 2011. Available at www.cdc.gov/ncidod/dvrd/molluscum/clinical_overview.htm. Accessed September 12, 2012.
48. Harper DM et al: Efficacy of a bivalent L1 virus-like particle vaccine in prevention of infection with human papillomavirus types 16 and 18 in young women: a randomised controlled trial, *Lancet* 364(9447):1757–1765, 2004.
49. Lambert DR, Yoder FW: Ectoparasites and molluscum contagiosum. In Spagna VA, Prior RB, editors: *Sexually transmitted diseases: a clinical syndrome approach*, New York, 1985, Marcel Dekker.
50. Bouvresse S, Chosidow O: Scabies in healthcare settings, *Curr Opin Infect Dis* 23(2):111–118, 2010.
51. Chosidow O: Clinical practice. Scabies, *N Engl J Med* 354(16):1718–1727, 2006.
52. Rein MR, Holmes KK: Nonspecific vaginitis, vulvovaginal candidiasis, and trichomoniasis: clinical features, diagnosis, and management. In Remington J, Schwartz MN, editors: *Current clinical topics in infectious diseases*, New York, 1983, McGraw-Hill.
53. Berger TG: Skin diseases of the external genitalia. In Tanagho EA, McAninch JW, editors: *Smith's general urology*, Norwalk, CT, 1995, Appleton & Lange.
54. Emmert DH, Kirchner JT: Sexually transmitted diseases in women: gonorrhea and syphilis, *Postgrad Med* 107(2):181–184, 189-190, 193–197, 2000.
55. Mast EE et al: A comprehensive immunization strategy to eliminate transmission of hepatitis B virus infection in the United States: recommendations of the Advisory Committee on Immunization Practices (ACIP) part 1: immunization of infants, children, and adolescents, *MMWR Recomm Rep* 54(RR-16):1–31, 2005.
56. Shi Z et al: Breastfeeding of newborns by mothers carrying hepatitis B virus: a meta-analysis and systematic review, *Arch Pediatr Adoles Med* 165(9):837–846, 2011.

CHAPTER

27

Structure and Function of the Hematologic System

Neal S. Rote and Kathryn L. McCance

evolve WEBSITE

http://evolve.elsevier.com/McCance/

- Review Questions and Answers
- Animations

CHAPTER OUTLINE

All the body's tissues and organs require oxygen and nutrients to survive. These essential needs are provided by the blood that flows through miles of vessels throughout the human body. The red blood cells provide the oxygen and remove carbon dioxide, and the fluid portion of the blood carries the nutrients and ions for proper acid-base balance. The blood also cleans discarded waste from the tissues; transports hormones; conveys cells (white blood cells), platelets, and other ingredients that are necessary for protecting the entire body from injury and infection and initiating healing; and provides thermal regulation to maintain organs and tissues within an acceptable range of temperatures.

COMPONENTS OF THE HEMATOLOGIC SYSTEM

Composition of the Blood

Blood consists of various cells that circulate in the cardiovascular system suspended in a solution of protein and inorganic materials (plasma), which is approximately 92% water and 8% dissolved substances (solutes) (Figure 27-1). The blood volume amounts to about 6 quarts (5.5 L) in adults. The continuous movement of blood guarantees that critical components are available to all parts of the body to carry out their chief functions: (1) delivery of substances needed for cellular metabolism in the tissues, (2) removal of the wastes of cellular metabolism, (3) defense against invading microorganisms and injury, and (4) maintenance of acid-base balance.

Plasma and Plasma Proteins

In adults, plasma accounts for 50% to 55% of blood volume. **Plasma** is a complex aqueous liquid containing a variety of organic and inorganic elements (Table 27-1). The concentration of these elements varies depending on diet, metabolic demand, hormones, and vitamins. Plasma differs from serum in that **serum** is plasma that has been allowed to clot in the laboratory in order to remove fibrinogen and other clotting factors that may interfere with some diagnostic tests.

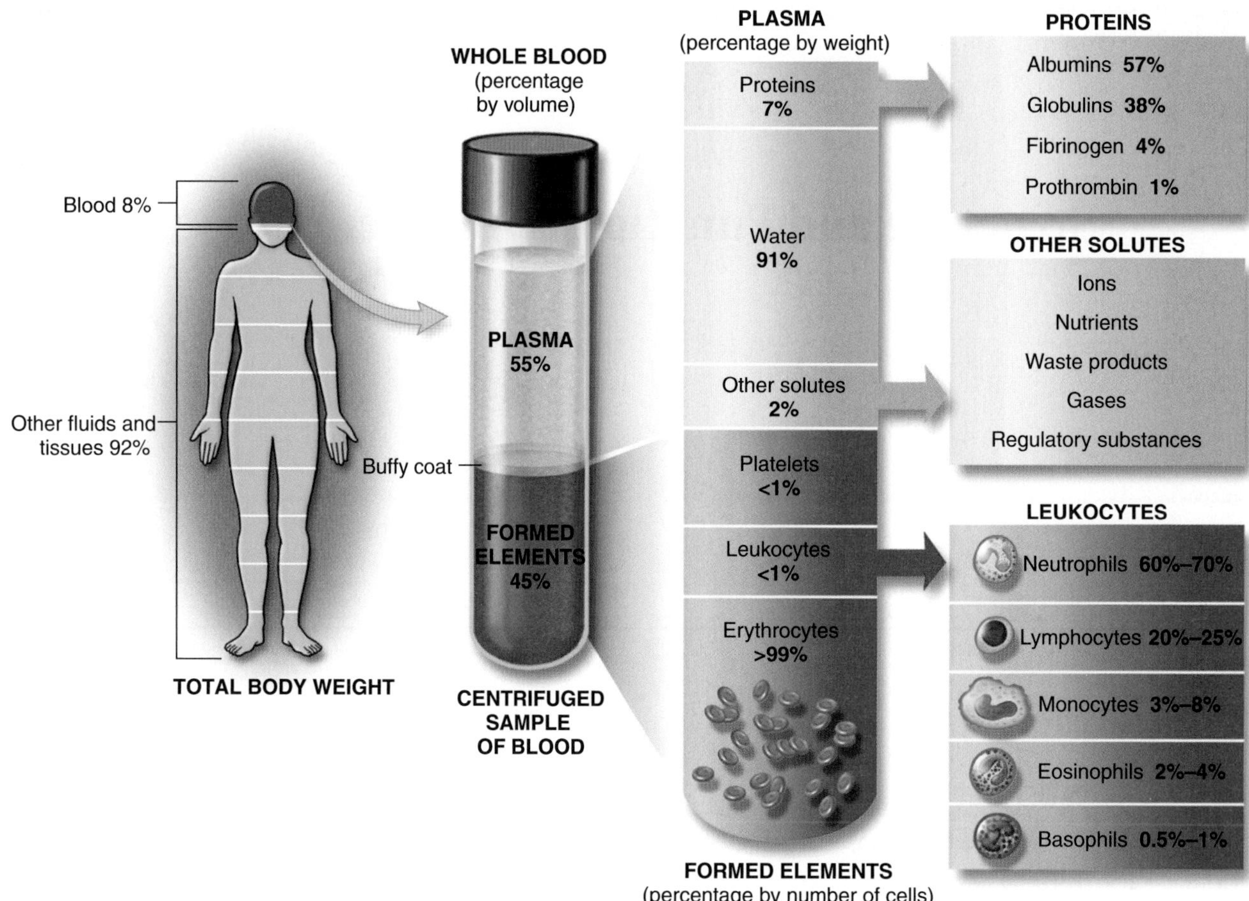

FIGURE 27-1 **Composition of Whole Blood.** Approximate values for the components of blood in a normal adult. (From Patton KT, Thibodeau GA: *Anatomy & physiology,* ed 8, St Louis, 2013, Mosby.)

The plasma contains a large number of proteins (**plasma proteins**) that constitute about 7% of the total plasma weight. These vary in structure and function and can be classified into two major groups, albumin and globulins. Most plasma proteins are produced by the liver. The major exception is antibodies (immunoglobulins), which are produced by plasma cells in the lymph nodes and other lymphoid tissues (see Chapter 8).

Albumin (about 60% of total plasma protein at a concentration of about 4 g/dl) serves as a carrier molecule for normal components of blood as well as drugs that have low solubility in water (e.g., free fatty acids, lipid-soluble hormones, thyroid hormones, bile salts). Its most essential role is regulation of the passage of water and solutes through the capillaries. Albumin molecules are large and do not diffuse freely through the vascular endothelium, and thus they maintain the critical colloidal osmotic pressure (or oncotic pressure) that regulates the passage of water and solutes into the surrounding tissues (see Chapters 1 and 3). Water and solute particles tend to diffuse out of the arterial portions of the capillaries because the blood pressure is greater in arterial than in venous blood vessels (see Chapter 3). Water and solutes move from tissue cells into the venous portions of the capillaries where the pressures are reversed, oncotic pressure being greater than intravascular pressure or hydrostatic pressure. In the case of decreased production (e.g., cirrhosis, other diffuse liver diseases, protein malnutrition) or excessive loss of albumin (e.g., certain kidney diseases, extensive burns), the reduced oncotic pressure leads to excessive movement of fluid and solutes into the tissue and decreased blood volume.

The remaining plasma proteins, or **globulins,** are often classified by their properties in an electric field (serum electrophoresis). Under the normal conditions used to perform serum electrophoresis, albumin is the most rapidly moving protein. The globulins are classified by their movement relative to albumin: alpha (α) globulins (those moving most closely to albumin), beta (β) globulins, and gamma (γ) globulins (those with the least movement). Depending on the electrophoretic procedure the alpha and beta globulins may be subdivided into subregions (α_1-, α_2-, β_1-, or β_2-globulins). Fibrinogen is a major plasma protein (about 4% of total plasma protein) that would move between the beta and gamma regions but is removed during the formation of serum. The gamma-globulin region consists primarily of immunoglobulin G (IgG) (see Chapter 8).

Plasma proteins can also be classified into groups by function: clotting, defense, transport, or regulation. The **clotting factors** promote coagulation and stop bleeding from damaged blood vessels. Fibrinogen is the most plentiful of the clotting factors and is the precursor of the fibrin clot. Proteins involved in defense, or protection, against infection include antibodies and complement proteins (see Chapters 7 and 8). Transport proteins

TABLE 27-1 ORGANIC AND INORGANIC COMPONENTS OF ARTERIAL PLASMA

CONSTITUENT	AMOUNT/CONCENTRATION	MAJOR FUNCTIONS
Water	93% of plasma weight	Medium for carrying all other constituents
Electrolytes	Total <1% of plasma weight	Maintain H_2O in extracellular compartment; act as buffers; function in membrane excitability
Na^+	142 mEq/L (142 mM)	
K^+	4 mEq/L (4 mM)	
Ca^{2+}	5 mEq/L (2.5 mM)	
Mg^{2+}	3 mEq/L (1.5 mM)	
Cl	103 mEq/L (103 mM)	
HCO_3^-	27 mEq/L (27 mM)	
Phosphate (mostly)	2 mEq/L (1 mM)	
Sulfate	1 mEq/L (0.5 mM)	
Proteins	7.3 g/dl (2.5 mM)	Provide colloid osmotic pressure of plasma; act as buffers; bind other plasma constituents (lipids, hormones, vitamins, minerals, etc.); clotting factors; enzymes; enzyme precursors; antibodies (immunoglobulins); hormones; transporters
Albumin	4.5 g/dl	
Globulins	2.5 g/dl	
Fibrinogen	0.3 g/dl	
Transferrin	250 mg/dl	
Ferritin	15-300 mcg/L	
Gases		
CO_2 content	22-32 mmol/L plasma	Byproduct of oxygenation, most CO_2 content is from HCO_3 and acts as a buffer
O_2	Pao_2 80 torr or greater (arterial); Pvo_2 30-40 torr (venous)	Oxygenation
N_2	0.9 ml/dl	Byproduct of protein catabolism
Nutrients		Provide nutrition and substances for tissue repair
Glucose and other carbohydrates	100 mg/dl (5.6 mM)	
Total amino acids	40 mg/dl (2 mM)	
Total lipids	500 mg/dl (7.5 mM)	
Cholesterol	150-250 mg/dl (4-7 mM)	
Individual vitamins	0.0001-2.5 mg/dl	
Individual trace elements	0.001-0.3 mg/dl	
Iron	50-150 mcg/dl	
Waste products		
Urea (blood urea nitrogen [BUN])	7-18 mg/dl (5.7 mM)	End product of protein catabolism
Creatinine (from creatine)	1 mg/dl (0.09 mM)	End product from energy metabolism
Uric acid (from nucleic acids)	5 mg/dl (0.3 mM)	End product from protein metabolism
Bilirubin (from heme)	0.2-1.2 mg/dl (0.003-0.018 mM)	End product of red blood cell destruction
Individual hormones	0.000001-0.05 mg/dl	Functions specific to target tissue

Data from Vander AJ, Sherman JH, Luciano DS: *Human physiology: the mechanisms of body function,* ed 8, New York, 2001, McGraw-Hill.

specifically bind and carry a variety of inorganic and organic molecules, including iron (transferrin), copper (ceruloplasmin), steroid hormones, and vitamins (e.g., retinol-binding protein). The plasma lipids, triglycerides, phospholipids, cholesterol, and fatty acids are carried through the blood as complexes with plasma proteins; they are known as *lipoproteins* (see Chapters 1 and 32). Regulatory proteins include a variety of enzymatic inhibitors (e.g., α_1-antitrypsin) that protect the tissues from damage, precursor molecules (e.g., kininogen) that are converted into active biologic molecules when needed, and protein hormones (e.g., cytokines) that communicate between cells.

Plasma also contains several charged inorganic ions (electrolytes) that regulate cell function, osmotic pressure, and blood pH. (Electrolytes are described in Chapters 1 and 3.)

Cellular Components of the Blood

The cellular elements of the blood are broadly classified as red blood cells (RBCs) (i.e., erythrocytes), white blood cells (WBCs) (i.e., leukocytes), and platelets (thrombocytes). The components of the blood are listed in Table 27-2.

Erythrocytes. In 1628 Robert Burton described blood as a "hot, temperate red humor whose office is to nourish the whole body, to give it strength and color being dispersed by the veins through every part of it."[1] A few years later, with the invention of the microscope, researchers learned that erythrocytes give blood its red color.

Erythrocytes (red blood cells [RBCs]) are the most abundant cells of the blood, occupying approximately 48% of the blood volume in men and about 42% in women. Erythrocytes are primarily responsible for tissue oxygenation. The erythrocyte contains hemoglobin, which carries the gases, and electrolytes, which regulate diffusion through a cell's plasma membrane. The mature erythrocyte lacks a nucleus and cytoplasmic organelles (e.g., mitochondria), so it cannot synthesize protein or carry out oxidative reactions. Because it cannot undergo mitotic division, the erythrocyte has a limited life span

TABLE 27-2 CELLULAR COMPONENTS OF THE BLOOD

CELL	STRUCTURAL CHARACTERISTICS*	NORMAL AMOUNTS OF CIRCULATING BLOOD	FUNCTION	LIFE SPAN
Erythrocyte (red blood cell)	Nonnucleated cytoplasmic disk containing hemoglobin	4.2-6.2 million/mm^3	Gas transport to and from tissue cells and lungs	80-120 days
Leukocyte (white blood cell)	Nucleated cell	5000-10,000/mm^3	Body defense mechanisms	See below
Lymphocyte	Mononuclear immunocyte	25-33% of leukocyte count (leukocyte differential)	Humoral and cell-mediated immunity (see Chapter 7)	Days or years depending on type
Monocyte and macrophage	Large kidney-shaped mononuclear phagocyte	3-7% of leukocyte differential	Phagocytosis; mononuclear phagocyte system	Months or years
Eosinophil	Segmented polymorphonuclear granulocyte with granules stainable by eosin dyes	1-4% of leukocyte differential	Phagocytosis; response to parasites, control of allergic reactions	8-12 days
Neutrophil	Segmented polymorphonuclear granulocyte with granules stainable by neutral staining	57-67% of leukocyte differential	Phagocytosis, particularly during early phase of inflammation, bacterial killing	4 days
Basophil	Lobate nuclear granulocyte with granules stainable by basic dyes	0-0.75% of leukocyte differential	Similar to mast cell, secretes inflammatory mediators (e.g., histamine, chemotactic factors for eosinophils and neutrophils), involved with allergic reactions	Few hours to days
Platelet	Irregularly shaped cytoplasmic fragment (not a cell)	140,000-340,000/mm^3	Hemostasis following vascular injury; normal coagulation and clot formation/retraction	8-11 days

*See bottom row of Figure 27-10 for illustrations of cells.

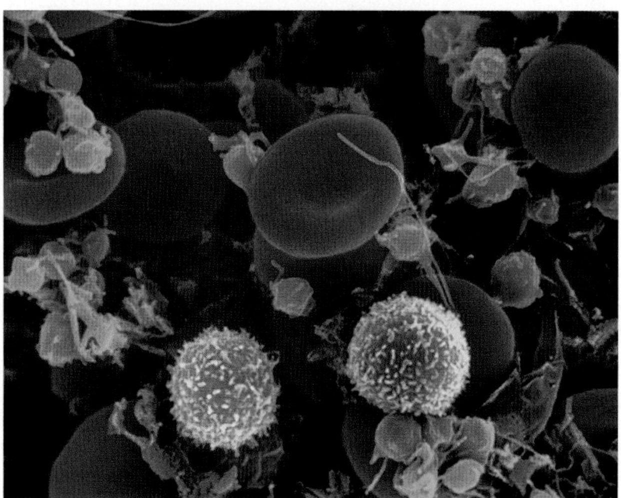

FIGURE 27-2 Blood Cells. Leukocytes are spherical and have irregular surfaces with numerous extending pili (appear as yellow). Erythrocytes are flattened spheres with a depressed center. Activated platelets are green. (Copyright Dennis Kunkel Microscopy, Inc.)

(approximately 100 to 120 days), ages, and is removed from the circulation to be replaced by new erythrocytes.

The erythrocyte's size and shape are ideally suited to its function as a gas carrier. An RBC is a small disk with two unique properties: (1) a *biconcave* shape and (2) the capacity to be *reversibly deformed* (Figure 27-2 and Figure 27-6). The flattened, biconcave shape provides a surface area/volume ratio that is optimal for gas diffusion into and out of the cell and for deformity.[2] During its life span, the erythrocyte, which is 6 to 8 μm in diameter, repeatedly circulates through sinusoids of the spleen and capillaries that are only 2 μm in diameter. Reversible deformity enables the erythrocyte to assume a more compact torpedo-like shape, squeeze through the microcirculation, and return to normal.

Leukocytes. **Leukocytes (white blood cells [WBCs])** defend the body against microorganisms that cause infection and remove debris, including dead or injured cells of all kinds (see Figure 27-2). The leukocytes act primarily in the tissues but are transported in the circulation. The average adult has approximately 5000 to 10,000 leukocytes/mm^3 of blood.

Leukocytes are classified according to structure as either **granulocytes** or **agranulocytes** and according to function as either **phagocytes** or **immunocytes.** The granulocytes, which include neutrophils, basophils, and eosinophils, are all phagocytes. (Phagocytic action is described in Chapter 7.) Of the agranulocytes, the monocytes and macrophages are phagocytes, whereas the lymphocytes are immunocytes (cells that create immunity; see Chapter 8).

Granulocytes. Granulocytes have many membrane-bound granules in their cytoplasm. These granules contain enzymes capable of killing microorganisms and catabolizing debris ingested during phagocytosis. The granules also contain powerful biochemical mediators with inflammatory and immune functions. These mediators, along with the digestive enzymes, are released from granulocytes in response to specific stimuli. The biochemical mediators have vascular and intercellular effects and the enzymes participate in the breakdown of debris from sites of infection or injury. Granulocytes are capable of amoeboid movement, by which they migrate through vessel walls (diapedesis) and then to sites where their action is needed (see Chapter 7).

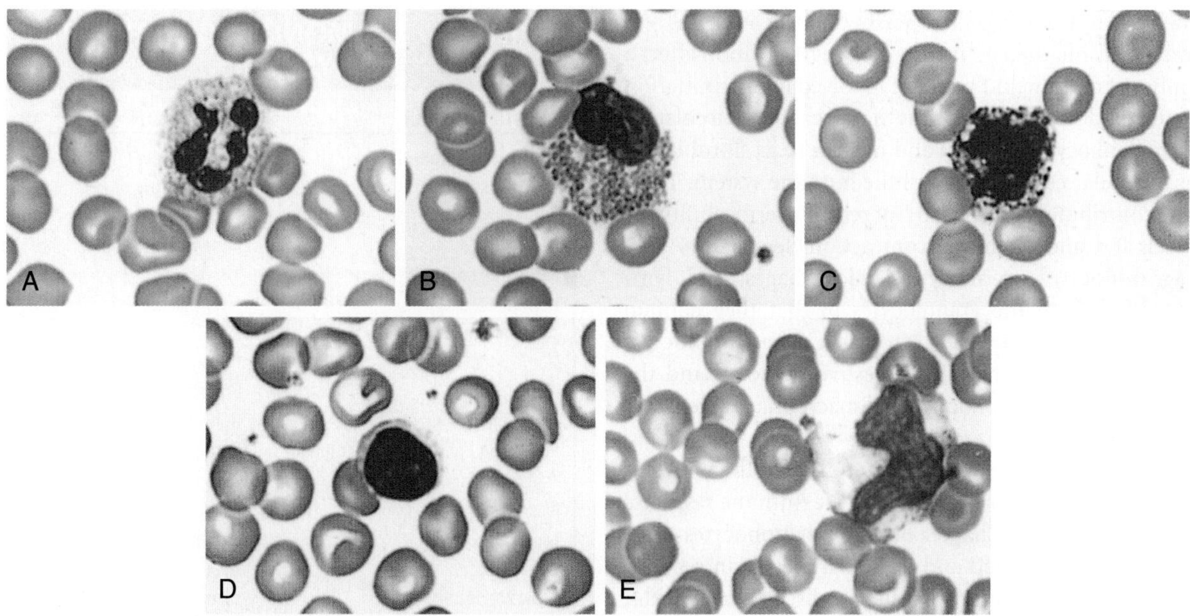

FIGURE 27-3 **Leukocytes.** An example of leukocytes in a human blood smear. **A,** Neutrophil. **B,** Eosinophil. **C,** Basophil. **D,** Lymphocyte. **E,** Monocyte. (From Erlandsen S, Magney J: *Color atlas of histology,* St Louis, 1992, Mosby.)

The **neutrophil (polymorphonuclear neutrophil [PMN])** is the most numerous and best understood of the granulocytes (Figure 27-3, *A*). Neutrophils constitute about 55% of the total leukocyte count in adults. The cytoplasm of neutrophils contains small lysosomal granules and a central nucleus with two to five distinct lobes. Immature neutrophils are called *bands* or *stabs.* Mature neutrophils are called *segmented neutrophils* because of the characteristic appearance of their nucleus. Neutrophils reach a fully mature state in the bone marrow, and these mature neutrophils are called the *marrow neutrophil reserve.* Normally it takes about 14 days for neutrophils to develop from early precursors, but this process is accelerated by infection and treatment with colony-stimulating factors.

Neutrophils are the chief phagocytes of early inflammation. Soon after bacterial invasion or tissue injury, neutrophils migrate out of the capillaries and into the inflamed site, where they ingest and destroy microorganisms and debris and then die in 1 or 2 days. The dissolution of dead neutrophils releases digestive enzymes from their cytoplasmic granules. These enzymes dissolve cellular debris and prepare the site for healing. (This final function, called *débridement,* is described in Chapter 7).

Eosinophils have large, coarse granules and constitute only 1% to 4% of the normal leukocyte count in adults (see Figure 27-3, *B*). Like neutrophils, eosinophils are capable of amoeboid movement and phagocytosis. Using a spectrum of pattern-recognition receptors, eosinophils ingest antigen-antibody complexes and viruses and are induced by mast cell chemotactic factors to attack parasites.[3] Eosinophil secondary granules contain toxic chemicals (e.g., major basic protein, eosinophil cationic protein, eosinophil peroxidase, eosinophil-derived neurotoxin) that are highly destructive to parasites and viruses. The eosinophil granules contain a variety of enzymes (e.g., histaminase) that help to control inflammatory processes. (Their function in inflammation and defense against parasites is described in Chapters 7 and 8.) Eosinophils also release leukotrienes, prostaglandins, platelet-activating factor (PAF), and a variety of cytokines (e.g., interleukin-1 [IL-1], IL-6, tumor necrosis factor-alpha [TNF-α], granulocyte-macrophage colony-stimulating factor [GM-CSF]) and chemokines (e.g., IL-8) that augment the inflammatory response.[4] Type I hypersensitivity allergic reactions and asthma are characterized by high numbers of circulating eosinophils, which may be involved in a dual role of regulation of inflammation and may contribute to the destructive inflammatory processes observed in the lungs of persons with asthma (see Chapter 9).

Basophils, which comprise less than 1% (0.01% to 0.3%) of the leukocytes, contain cytoplasmic granules that have an abundant mixture of biochemical mediators, including histamine, chemotactic factors, proteolytic enzymes (e.g., elastase, lysophospholipase), and an anticoagulant (heparin) (see Figure 27-3, *C*). Stimulation of basophils also induces synthesis of vasoactive lipid molecules (e.g., leukotrienes) and cytokines. Basophils produce IL-6 which induces IL-10 by Th1 cells and induction of Th2 cells that favor B-cell differentiation.[5] Basophils also are a particularly rich source of the cytokine IL-4, which preferentially guides B-cell differentiation toward plasma cells that secrete IgE (see Chapter 8).

The numbers of basophils are often increased at sites of allergic inflammatory reactions and parasitic infection, particularly exoparasites (e.g., ticks). IgE receptors on the basophil would induce degranulation at sites of IgE-mediated hypersensitivity reactions and contribute to the local inflammatory response.

Mast cells are highly similar to basophils, but are generated from a different set of precursor cells in the bone marrow, from which they migrate in an immature form into tissues.[6] They reside in vascularized connective tissues just beneath body epithelial surfaces, including the submucosal tissues of the gastrointestinal and respiratory tracts and the dermal layer that lies just below the surface of the skin. Mast cells play a central role in inflammation, and their activation and degranulation affect a great number of cells, including those involved in inflammation (e.g., vascular endothelial cells, smooth muscle cells, circulating platelets and leukocytes, nerves) and healing (e.g., fibroblasts), as well as glandular cells and cells of the immune system. Their activation contributes greatly to increased permeability of blood vessels and smooth muscle contraction (see Figure 7-11).

The **agranulocytes**—monocytes, macrophages, and lymphocytes—differ from the granulocytes in that they contain relatively fewer granules in their cytoplasm. The lymphocytes do not contain any enzyme-filled digestive vacuoles, and the digestive vacuoles of the monocytes and macrophages are larger and fewer than those of the granulocytes.

Lymphocytes constitute approximately 36% of the total leukocyte count and are the primary cells of the immune response (see Figure 27-3, *D,* and Chapter 8). Most lymphocytes transiently circulate in the blood and eventually reside in secondary lymphoid tissues as mature T cells, B cells, or plasma cells. The life span of the lymphocyte can be days, months, or years, depending on its type and subtype. (Lymphocyte function and dysfunction are described in detail in Unit III.)

Natural killer (NK) cells, which resemble large granular lymphocytes, kill some types of tumor cells (in vitro) and some virus-infected cells without being induced by previous exposure to these antigens (see Chapters 7 and 8). Hence they are named *natural killer cells* to differentiate them from T-cytotoxic cells, which are induced by antigen. NK cells also have the capacity to activate T cells and phagocytes and produce a variety of cytokines that can regulate immune responses. The predominant form of NK cells develops in the bone marrow and circulates in the blood, where it accounts for 5% to 10% of the circulating lymphoid pool, and is found mainly in the peripheral blood and spleen. NK cells develop independent of a thymus, although some NK precursors are found in the thymus and may develop into NKT cells that have markers of NK and T cells.

The monocytes and macrophages make up the **mononuclear phagocyte system (MPS),** formerly called the *reticuloendothelial system (RES)*.[7] Monocytes and macrophages are active phagocytes that participate in the immune and inflammatory responses. They also ingest dead or defective host cells, particularly blood cells.

Monocytes are the largest normal blood cell and have a horseshoe-shaped nucleus (see Figure 27-3, *E*). They are formed and released by the bone marrow into the bloodstream. Monocytes migrate into a variety of tissues and fully mature into tissue **macrophages** and myeloid **dendritic cells** (Table 27-3). Other monocytes may mature into macrophages in the circulation and migrate out of the vessels in response to infection or inflammation. Macrophages are generally larger and are more active as phagocytes than monocytes. Dendritic cells frequently extend projections *(dendrites)* into the tissue and take on a "neuron-like" appearance. The origin and turnover of many of the tissue macrophages are not precisely known. It seems clear that once monocytes leave the circulation, they do not return. They can survive many months or even years.

The normal role of macrophages is to remove old and damaged cells and large-molecular substances from the blood.

TABLE 27-3 MONONUCLEAR PHAGOCYTE SYSTEM*

NAME OF CELL	LOCATION
Committed Stem Cells†	Bone marrow
Monoblasts	Bone marrow
Promonoblasts	Bone marrow
Monocytes	Bone marrow and peripheral blood
Macrophages	Tissue
Kupffer cells	Liver macrophages
Alveolar macrophages	Lung
Histiocytes	Connective tissue
Macrophages	Bone marrow
Fixed and free macrophages	Spleen and lymph nodes
Pleural and peritoneal macrophages	Serous cavities
Adipose macrophages	Adipose (fat) tissue
Microglial cells	Nervous system
Mesangial cells	Kidney
Osteoclasts	Bone
Langerhans cells	Skin
Dendritic cells	Lymphoid tissue, lining of respiratory and gastrointestinal tracts

Modified from Kumar V et al: *Robbins & Cotran pathologic basis of disease,* ed 7, Philadelphia, 2005, Saunders.

*Formerly called the reticuloendothelial system.

†Development of blood cells from stem cells in the marrow is described on this page and illustrated in Figure 27-10.

Cellular targets of macrophage phagocytosis include circulating senescent or damaged erythrocytes and platelets (removed primarily in spleen), dead neutrophils (in the circulation and at sites of inflammation), and cells undergoing apoptosis. Noncellular targets include antigen-antibody complexes, cellular debris, products of coagulation, and macromolecules (such as lipids and carbohydrates synthesized by the body as the result of faulty metabolism, as in storage diseases). Macrophages remove and kill contaminating microorganisms in the blood (mostly in the liver and spleen) and at sites of infection. Macrophages and, particularly, dendritic cells are the major "antigen-processing" and "antigen-presenting" cells that initiate immune responses (see Chapter 8). Macrophages initiate wound healing and tissue remodeling and if activated by cytokines from T cells secrete a large array of biologically active chemicals that if uncontrolled result in chronic inflammation and tissue injury (see Chapter 7). Osteoclasts are multinucleated macrophage-like cells specialized for the function of lacunar bone resorptions and remodeling in addition to phagocytosis.[8]

Platelets. **Platelets (thrombocytes)** are not true cells but irregularly-shaped cytoplasmic fragments that are essential for blood coagulation and control of bleeding.[9] They are formed by fragmentation of very large (40 to 100 μm in diameter) cells known as **megakaryocytes** (Figure 27-4). They lack a nucleus and deoxyribonucleic acid (DNA), and are incapable of mitotic division. They do, however, contain cytoplasmic granules (i.e., dense granules, alpha granules) capable of releasing biochemical mediators when stimulated by injury to a blood vessel. The contents of the dense granules are generally proinflammatory (e.g., adenosine

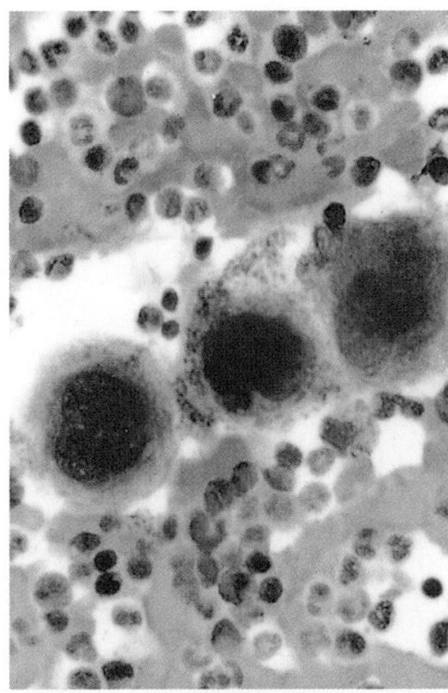

FIGURE 27-4 Megakaryocyte and Platelets. Note the large number of platelets *(purple)* surrounding the large megakaryocytes in the center. (From Miale JB: *Laboratory medicine: hematology,* ed 6, St Louis, 1982, Mosby.)

diphosphate [ADP], adenosine triphosphate [ATP], calcium, serotonin, and histamine).[10] The alpha granules contain a mixture of coagulation factors, growth and angiogenic factors (e.g., platelet-derived growth factor [PDGF], vascular endothelial growth factor [VEGF], and basic fibroblast growth factor), and angiogenesis inhibitors (e.g., platelet factor 4, thrombospondin, and inhibitors of metalloproteinases). Depending upon the particular stimulus, platelets may selectively release promoters or inhibitors of angiogenesis.[11] Activation also stimulates synthesis of arachidonic acid pathway products (e.g., thromboxane A_2) (see Chapter 7).

There are approximately 140,000 to 340,000 platelets/mm^3 of circulating blood. An additional one third of the body's available platelets are in a reserve pool in the spleen. A platelet circulates for approximately 10 days, ages, and is removed by macrophages of the MPS, mostly in the spleen.

Lymphoid Organs

The lymphoid system is closely integrated with the circulatory system. The lymphoid organs, some of which are merely aggregations of lymphoid tissue, are classified as primary or secondary. The primary lymphoid organs are the thymus and the bone marrow. The secondary lymphoid organs consist of the spleen, lymph nodes, tonsils, and Peyer patches of the small intestine (see Figure 8-3). All of the lymphoid organs link the hematologic and immune systems in that they are sites of residence, proliferation, differentiation, or function of lymphocytes and mononuclear phagocytes (monocytes and macrophages).[12] (The liver, which also has hematologic functions, is primarily a digestive organ and is described in Chapter 40.)

Spleen

The spleen is the largest of the secondary lymphoid organs. It is a site of fetal hematopoiesis; its mononuclear phagocytes filter and cleanse the blood; its lymphocytes mount an immune response to blood-borne microorganisms; and it serves as a blood reservoir (see Chapter 29).

The spleen is a concave, encapsulated organ that weighs approximately 150 g and is about the size of a fist. It is located in the left upper abdominal cavity, curved around a portion of the stomach (see Figure 8-3). Strands of connective tissue (trabeculae) extend from the capsule, dividing the spleen into compartments (Figure 27-5). The compartments contain masses of lymphoid tissue called *splenic pulp*. The spleen is interlaced with many blood vessels, some of which are capable of distending to store blood. Blood that circulates through the spleen comes from the splenic artery, which branches from the descending aorta and reenters the circulatory system through the splenic vein and into the portal vein.

The portion of arterial blood that enters the spleen first encounters the white splenic pulp, which consists of masses of lymphoid tissue containing macrophages and lymphocytes, primarily T lymphocytes in proximity to the arterioles (see Figure 27-5, *B* and *D*). Cellular clumps (lymphoid follicles) are formed in the white pulp around the splenic arterioles. The lymphoid follicles consist primarily of B lymphocytes. These are the chief sites of immune function within the spleen. Here blood-borne antigens encounter lymphocytes, initiating the immune response and the conversion of lymphoid follicles into germinal centers (see Chapter 8).[13]

Some of the blood that enters the terminal capillaries continues through the microcirculation and enters highly distensible storage areas called venous sinuses in the red pulp of the spleen. The venous sinuses are capable of storing more than 300 ml of blood. Passive dilation of the venous sinuses enables the spleen to increase its storage capacity as needed by the body. Sudden reductions in blood pressure cause the sympathetic nervous system to stimulate constriction of the sinuses, resulting in expulsion of as much as 200 ml of blood into the venous circulation, which helps restore blood volume and increases the hematocrit by as much as 4%.

The endothelial lining of the venous sinuses is discontinuous (having gaps between endothelial cells) and therefore extremely permeable so that blood cells are allowed to exit the circulation (Figure 27-6). The red pulp contains a system of loosely interconnected resident macrophages that provide the principal site of splenic filtration. Because of the slow circulation in the sinuses, the macrophages easily phagocytose old, damaged, or dead blood cells of all kinds (but chiefly erythrocytes), microorganisms, macromolecules, and particles of debris. Hemoglobin from phagocytosed erythrocytes is catabolized, and heme (iron) is stored in the cytoplasm of the macrophages or released back into the blood (see Figure 27-17). The macrophages also can remove particulate inclusions containing denatured hemoglobin (Heinz bodies) from erythrocytes without harming the cells themselves. Blood that filters through the red pulp also finds its way into the venous sinuses and hence into the portal circulation.

The spleen is not absolutely necessary for life or for adequate hematologic function. However, splenic absence from any cause (atrophy, traumatic injury, or removal because of disease) has several secondary effects on the body. For example, leukocytosis (high levels of circulating leukocytes) often occurs after

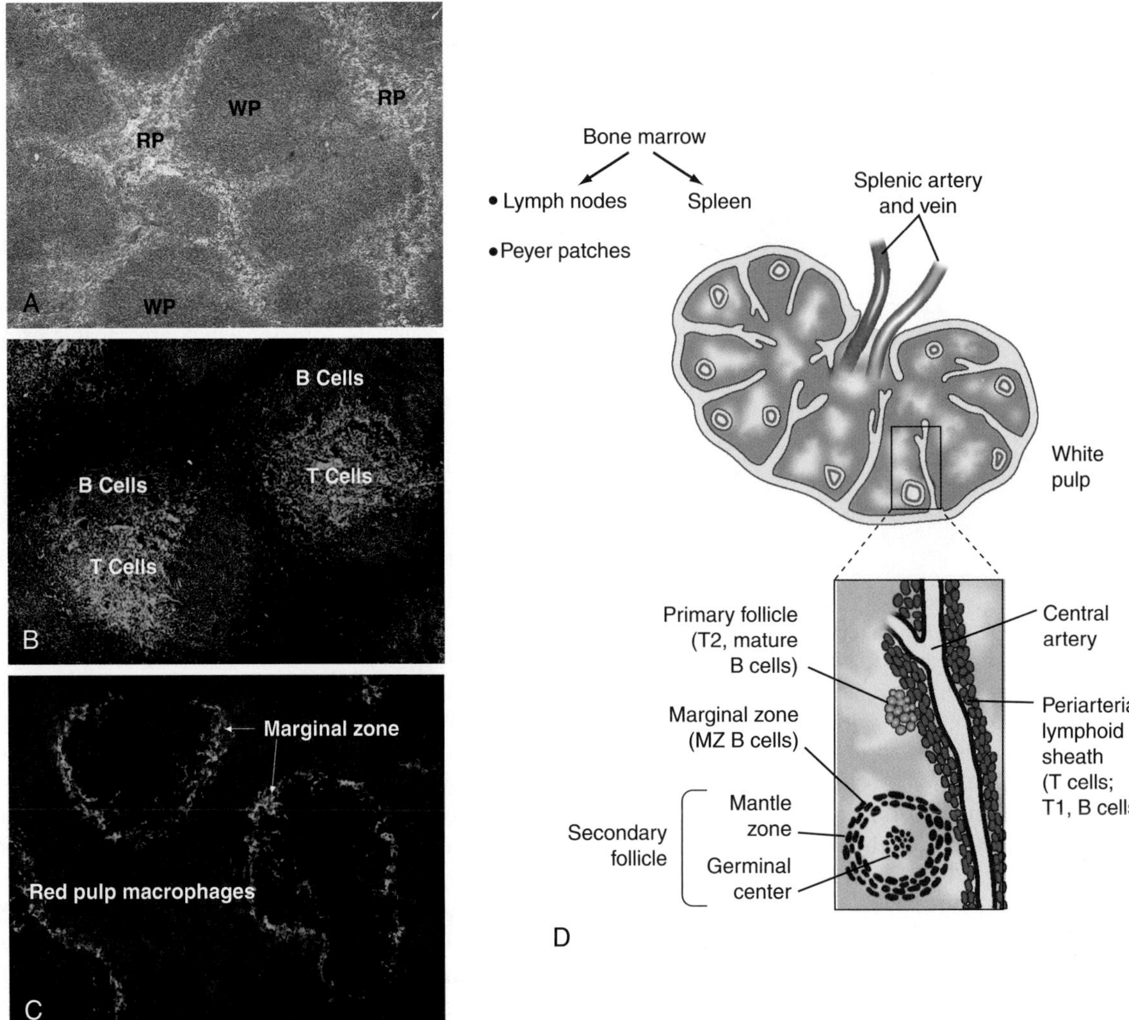

FIGURE 27-5 Spleen Architecture. **A,** Spleen section stained with hematoxylin and eosin shows areas of densely packed cells, referred to as the white pulp *(WP),* separated by areas with more dispersed cell populations, referred to as the red pulp *(RP).* **B,** Spleen section that has been stained with fluorescently labeled antibodies specific for B cells *(orange)* and T cells *(green)* shows the distinct localization of B cells and T cells within the white pulp. **C,** Staining for macrophages *(orange)* and the splenic marginal zone *(green)* shows the density of macrophages and phagocytic cells in the red pulp and marginal zone. **D,** The spleen is enclosed in a capsule with the interior pulp divided into compartments by strands of connective tissue. The splenic pulp contains regions that are rich in lymphocytes (white pulp) and those containing erythrocytes (red pulp). The central arteries are frequently surrounded by a periarterial lymphoid sheath, primarily containing T cells, B cells, and macrophages, with adjacent lymphoid follicles. The secondary lymphoid follicles contain B cells that are proliferating in response to antigen. (**A, B,** and **C** from Mandell G, Bennett J, Dolin R: *Mandell, Douglas, and Bennett's principles and practice of infectious diseases,* ed 7, Philadelphia, 2010, Churchill Livingstone; **D** from Hoffman R et al: *Hematology: basic principles and practice,* ed 6, Philadelphia, 2013, Churchill Livingstone.)

splenectomy, suggesting that the spleen exerts some control over the rate of proliferation of leukocyte stem cells in the bone marrow or their release into the bloodstream. Circulating levels of iron may also decrease, reflecting the spleen's role in the iron cycle. The immune response to encapsulated bacteria (e.g., *Streptococcus pneumoniae* [pneumococcus], *Neisseria meningitidis* [meningococcus], *Haemophilus influenzae*), which is primarily an IgM response, may be severely diminished, resulting in increased susceptibility to disseminated infections. Loss of the spleen results in an increase in morphologically defective blood cells in the circulation, confirming the spleen's role in removing old or damaged cells.

Lymph Nodes

Structurally, lymph nodes are part of the lymphatic system. Lymphatic vessels collect interstitial fluid from the tissues and transport it, as lymph, through vessels of increasing size to the thoracic duct, which drains into the superior vena cava returning the lymph to the circulation. Lymph nodes are distributed throughout the body and provide filtration of the lymph during its journey through the lymphatics. Each lymph node is enclosed in a fibrous capsule, branches of which (trabeculae) extend inward to partition the node into several compartments (Figure 27-7). Reticular fibers of connective tissue divide the compartments into a meshwork throughout the lymph node.

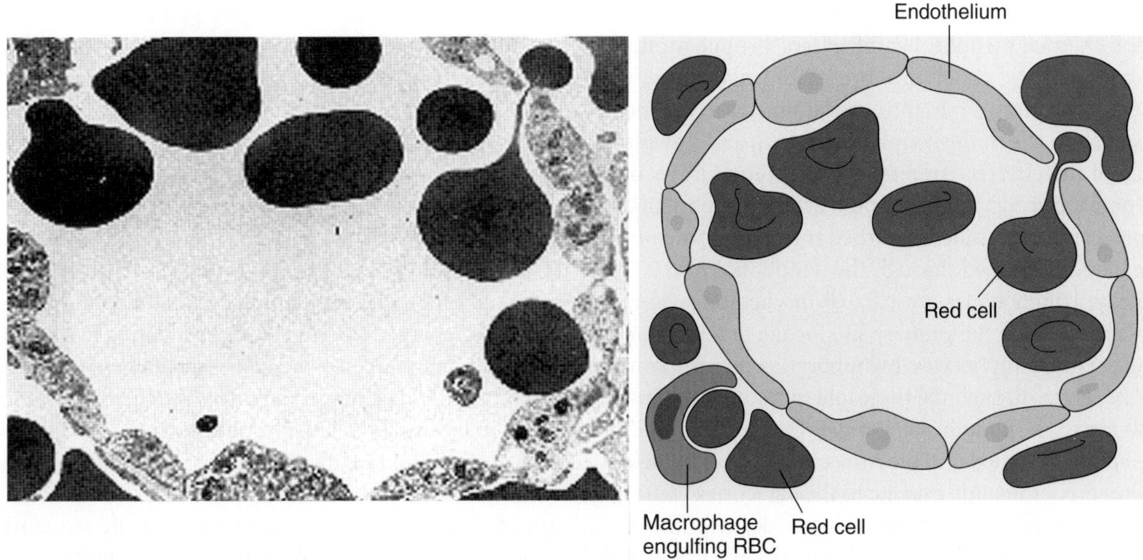

FIGURE 27-6 Splenic Sinus. Transmission electron micrograph and schematic of erythrocytes in the process of squeezing from the red pulp cords into the sinus lumen. Note the degree of deformability required for red cells to pass through the wall of the sinus. (From Damjanov I, Linder J, editors: *Anderson's pathology,* ed 10, St Louis, 1996, Mosby. Schematic from Kumar V, Fausto N, Abbas A: *Robbins & Cotran pathologic basis of disease,* ed 7, St Louis, 2005, Saunders.)

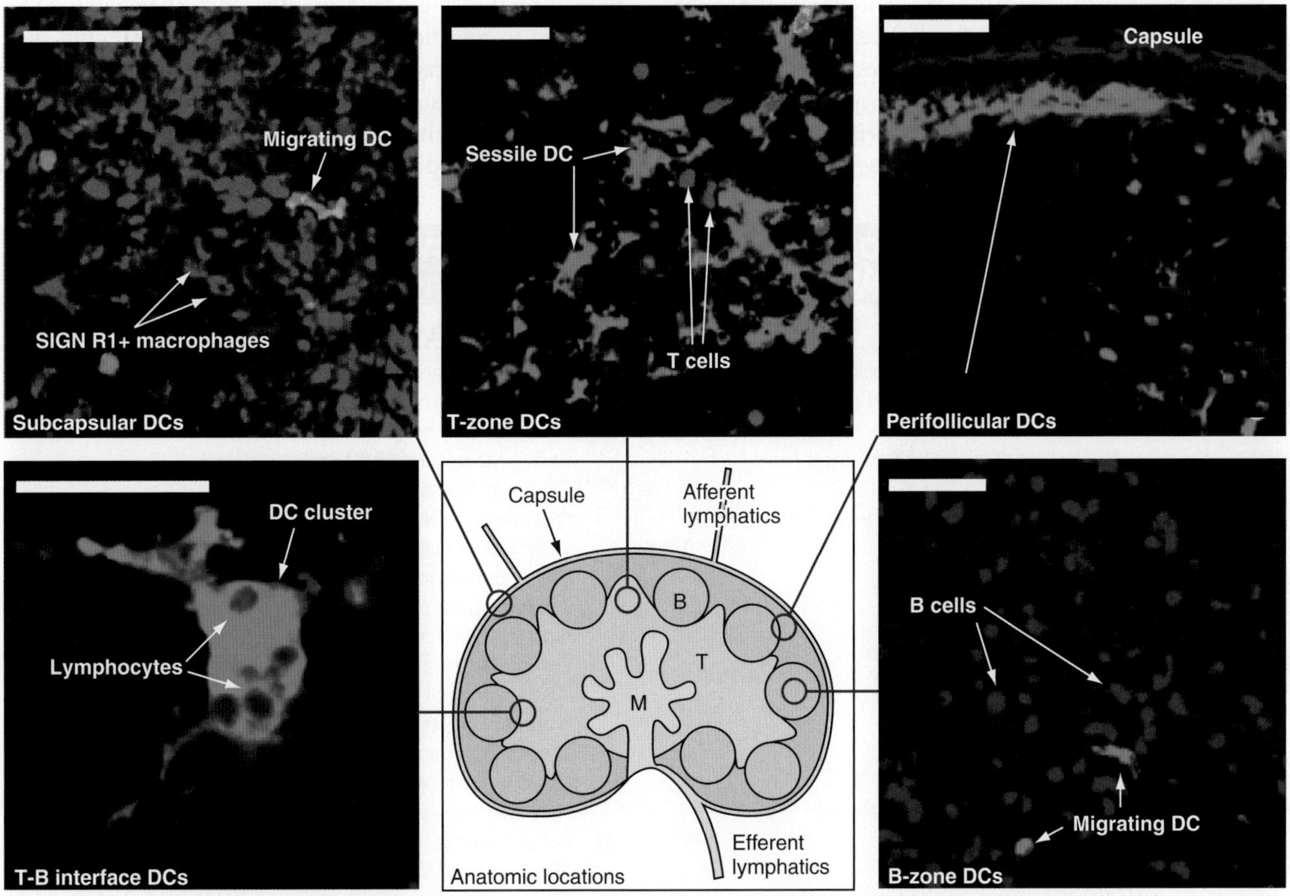

FIGURE 27-7 Lymph Node Architecture. *Drawing in lower center:* Lymph enters via the afferent lymphatics and exits via the efferent lymphatics. T cells enter the lymph nodes via the high endothelial venules and exit via the medulla to the efferent lymphatics. *B,* B-cell follicles; *M,* medullary cords; *T,* T-cell zone. Other structures are labeled. *Stained microscopic images:* All images are linked to the drawing of the lymph node. *DC,* Dendritic cell. (All scale bars 50 μm.) (From Lindquist RL et al: *Nat Immunol* 5:1243–1250, 2004, by permission from Macmillan Publishers Ltd.)

The node consists of outer (cortex) and inner (paracortex) cortical areas and an inner medulla. Lymph enters through multiple small afferent lymphatic vessels into the subcapsular sinus, just beneath the capsule; drains into the cortical sinuses to the medullary sinuses, from which the lymph is collected; and leaves the node by way of the efferent lymphatic vessel. Blood flows into the lymph nodes through the lymphatic artery, which ends in groups of postcapillary venules disturbed throughout the outer cortex. The blood is drained through the lymphatic vein.

Functionally, lymph nodes are part of the hematologic and immune systems and are the primary site for the first encounter between antigen and lymphocytes. Lymphocytes enter the lymph node from the blood through the postcapillary venules by means of diapedesis across the endothelial lining. B lymphocytes tend to migrate preferentially to nodes in the cortex and medulla, whereas T lymphocytes predominantly migrate to the paracortex (see Figure 27-7). Macrophages reside in the lymph node; help filter the lymph of debris, foreign substances, and microorganisms; and provide antigen-processing functions. The dendritic cells encounter and process antigens and microorganisms in other tissues, enter the lymph node through the afferent lymph vessels, and migrate throughout the nodes. The reticular network provides adhesive surfaces for trapping large numbers of phagocytes and lymphocytes and facilitating their organization into follicles or primary nodules. The presence of antigen, either removed from the lymph by macrophages or presented on the surface of dendritic cells, results in the production of secondary nodules containing germinal centers. In the germinal centers lymphocytes, particularly B cells, respond to antigenic stimulation by undergoing proliferation and further differentiation, including class-switch, into memory cells and plasma cells (see Chapter 8). Plasma cells migrate to the medullary cords. The B-lymphocyte proliferation in response to a great deal of antigen (e.g., during infection) may result in lymph node enlargement and tenderness (reactive lymph node).

DEVELOPMENT OF BLOOD CELLS

Hematopoiesis

The typical human requires about 100 billion new blood cells per day. Blood cell production, termed **hematopoiesis,** is constantly ongoing, occurring in the liver and spleen of the fetus and only in bone marrow *(medullary hematopoiesis)* after birth (see Chapter 30). This process involves the biochemical stimulation of populations of relatively undifferentiated cells to undergo mitotic division (i.e., proliferation) and maturation (i.e., differentiation) into mature hematologic cells (Table 27-4). Although proliferation and differentiation are usually sequential, certain blood cells proliferate and differentiate simultaneously. Erythrocytes and granulocytes generally differentiate fully before entering the blood, but monocytes and lymphocytes continue to mature in the blood and in secondary lymphatic organs.

Hematopoiesis continues throughout life, increasing in response to a need to replenish destroyed circulating cells (e.g., during hemorrhage, hemolytic anemia [peripheral destruction of erythrocytes], consumptive thrombocytopenia) or in response to infection. In general, long-term stimuli, such as chronic diseases, cause a greater increase in hematopoiesis than acute conditions, such as hemorrhage.

Various abnormalities in medullary hematopoiesis have been identified and are discussed in Chapter 28. Extramedullary

TABLE 27-4 HUMAN HEMATOPOIETIC GROWTH FACTORS (CYTOKINES, COLONY-STIMULATING FACTORS)

FACTOR	CELL ORIGIN	PRIMARY CELL STIMULATED
M-CSF	Macrophage, lymphocyte, fibroblast, endothelial cell, osteoblast	Monocyte progenitor to monocyte
GM-CSF	Macrophage, T cell, endothelial cell, fibroblast, mast cell	Common myeloid progenitor to granulocyte progenitor and monocyte progenitor
G-CSF	Macrophage, fibroblast, endothelial cell	Granulocyte progenitor to neutrophil
IL-2	Th cell	T-cell progenitor to T cell
IL-3	T cell, monocyte/macrophage, stromal cell	Common myeloid progenitor to progenitors for megakaryocyte, erythroid, granulocyte, and monocyte series
IL-4	Th cell	B-cell progenitor to B cell
IL-5	Th cell, mast cell	Common myeloid progenitor to eosinophil
IL-7	Stromal cell, intestinal epithelium	Hematopoietic stem cell to common lymphoid progenitor Common lymphoid progenitor to progenitor B cell, pro NK cell, and progenitor T cell Progenitor T cell to T cell and progenitor B cell to B cell
IL-11	Stromal cell	Megakaryocyte progenitor to megakaryocyte
IL-15	Monocyte/macrophage	NK progenitor to NK cell
Erythropoietin	Peritubular kidney cell and Kupffer cell	Common myeloid progenitor to erythrocyte progenitor Erythrocyte progenitor to erythrocyte
Thrombopoietin	Liver, kidney, skeletal muscle	All cells in megakaryocyte lineage from common myeloid progenitor to platelet
Stem cell factor (steel factor)	Stromal cell in bone marrow and many other cells	Hematopoietic progenitor to common myeloid progenitor Common myeloid progenitor to progenitors for megakaryocyte, erythroid, granulocyte, and monocyte series

G-CSF, Granulocyte colony-stimulating factor; *GM-CSF,* granulocyte-macrophage colony-stimulating factor; *IL,* interleukin; *M-CSF,* macrophage colony-stimulating factor; *NK,* natural killer; *pro,* progenitor; *Th,* T helper.

hematopoiesis—blood cell production in tissues other than bone marrow—of apparently normal blood cells has been reported in the spleen, liver, and, less frequently, lymph nodes, adrenal glands, cartilage, adipose tissue, intrathoracic areas, and kidneys. In adults, however, extramedullary hematopoiesis is usually a sign of disease, occurring in pernicious anemia, sickle cell anemia, thalassemia, hemolytic disease of the newborn (erythroblastosis fetalis), hereditary spherocytosis, and certain leukemias.

Bone Marrow

Bone marrow is confined to the cavities of bone and is the primary site of residence of hematopoietic stem cells (Figure 27-8). Adults have two kinds of bone marrow: red, or active (hematopoietic), marrow (also called **myeloid tissue**) and yellow, or inactive, marrow. The large quantity of fat in inactive marrow gives its characteristic yellow color. Not all bones contain active marrow. In adults, active marrow is found primarily in the flat bones of the pelvis (34%), vertebrae (28%), cranium and mandible (13%), sternum and ribs (10%), and in the extreme proximal portions of the humerus and femur (4% to 8%). Inactive marrow predominates in cavities of other bones. (Bones are discussed further in Chapter 43.)

Hematopoietic marrow is vascularized by the primary arteries of the bones, which terminate in a capillary network forming large venous sinuses. Hematopoietic marrow and fat fill the spaces surrounding the network of venous sinuses. Newly produced blood cells traverse narrow openings between endothelial cells in the venous sinus walls and thus enter the circulation. Normally, immature cells have not developed the appropriate surface receptors to interact with the endothelium and enter the circulation.

The hematologic compartment of the bone marrow consists of a variety of cellular microenvironments, called **niches,** that control differentiation of hematopoietic progenitor cells[14] (Figure 27-9). The cellular composition of niches includes osteoclasts, osteoblasts, sinusoidal endothelial cells, fibroblasts, megakaryocytes, macrophages, and nerve cells.[15] Osteoblasts are derived from fibroblasts and are responsible for construction of

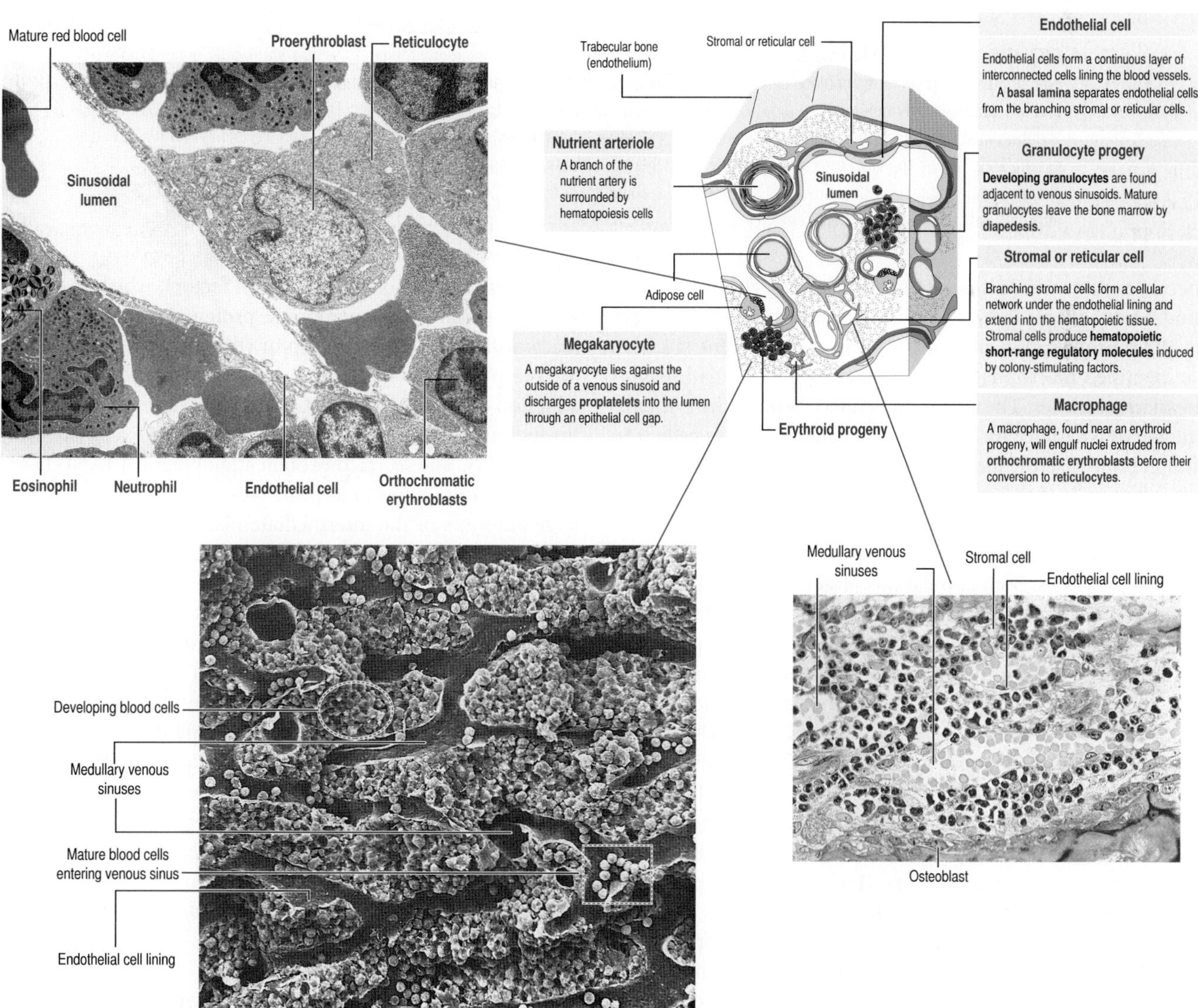

FIGURE 27-8 Bone Marrow: Structure and Vascularization. (From Kierszenbaum A, Tres L: *Histology and cell biology: an introduction to pathology,* ed 3, Philadelphia, 2012, Mosby. Scanning electron micrograph from Kessel RG, Kardon RH: *Tissues and organs,* New York, 1979, WH Freeman.)

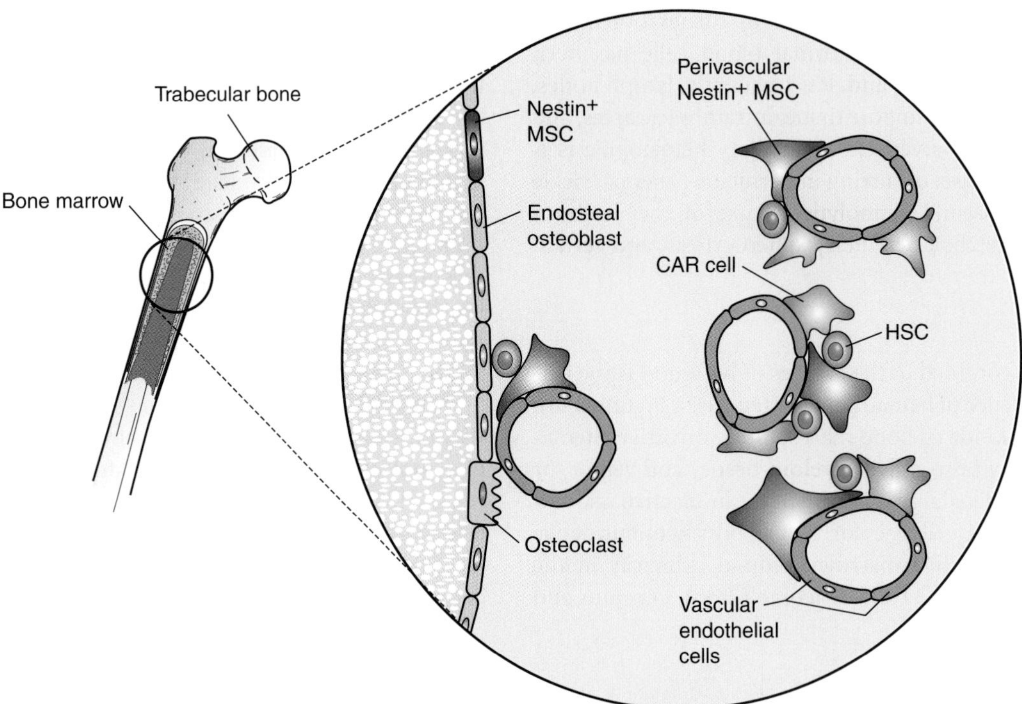

FIGURE 27-9 **Bone Marrow Stem Cell Niches.** Stem cell niches are microenvironments where stem cells undergo hematopoiesis into all forms of blood cells. Stem cell niches retain and maintain adult resting hematopoietic stem cells (HSCs) and are activated after cell injury to promote cell renewal or differentiation to form new tissues. The fate of individual HSCs is determined by interactions (intercellular adherence, cytokines, chemokines) with specialized cells within the niches. Within osteoblastic niches the HSC interacts primarily with the osteoblasts and specialized mesenchynal stem cells (MSCs) that include nestin-expressing (Nestin+) MSCs and CXCL12-abundant reticular (CAR) cells. Within the vascular niches, the HSC interacts with vascular endothelial cells, Nestin+ MSC, and a more abundant population of CAR cells.

bone. Osteoclasts are multinucleate cells of monocytic origin that remodel bone by resorption. Both cells can produce cytokines that affect proliferation of hematopoietic cells. Recent studies have identified macrophage and megakaryocyte populations in bone marrow niches. The area is innervated through the sympathetic nervous system. At least two populations of stem cells are found in bone marrow niches. **Mesenchymal stem cells (MSCs)** are stromal cells that can differentiate into a variety of cells, including osteoblasts, adipocytes, and chondrocytes (produce cartilage). **Hematopoietic stem cells (HSCs)** are progenitors of all hematologic cells. Both populations of stem cells also undergo self-renewal in the bone marrow so that additional MSCs and HSCs are produced to replace those undergoing differentiation.

Two distinct types of niches have been identified: the *osteoblastic* (also called endosteal) *niche* and the *vascular niche*. The **osteoblastic niche** is centralized around osteoblasts, which line the surface of bone, whereas the **vascular niche** is organized around sinusoidal endothelial cells. In both niches, HSCs are affected by direct cell-to-cell signaling and by soluble mediators produced by cells within each niche. Each niche also contains two specialized cells derived from MSCs: CXCL12-abundant reticular (CAR) cells and nestin-expressing cells.[16]

CAR cells resemble reticular cells with long cellular processes. CAR cells closely interact with HSCs and provide important intercellular signaling through several HSC regulatory molecules, including CXCL12, SCF, VCAM-1, and ANG1. Chemokine ligand 12 (CXCL12) is a chemokine that reacts with the C-X-C chemokine receptor type 4 (CXCR4) on HSCs. The cytokine stem cell factor (SCF; also known as steel factor), which is expressed as a cell surface transmembrane protein or a soluble protein, reacts with the HSC KIT receptor (named stem cell growth factor receptor, proto-oncogene c-Kit, or CD117). Vascular cell adhesion molecule 1 (VCAM-1) mediates intercellular adhesion through its receptor integrin $\alpha4\beta1$ (also called very late antigen 4, or VLA4). The secreted protein angiopoietin 1 (ANG1) reacts with a tyrosine kinase receptor. Nestin-expressing cells express large amounts of the intermediate filament protein nestin and, particularly, SCF and VCAM-1. Although both MSC-derived cells are present in the osteoblastic niche and vascular niche, the CAR cell is the predominant cell in the vascular niche.[17]

Each bone marrow niche affects HSCs differently. In the osteoblastic niche, HSCs are in direct contact with osteoblasts, CAR cells, and nestin-expressing cells. The effect is retention of HSCs in the bone marrow in a quiescent (dormant) state.[18] HSCs that traffic to the vascular niche directly contact endothelial cells, as well as nestin-expressing cells and larger numbers of perivascular CAR cells. The cumulative signaling events induce HSC activation, proceeding to increased cellular division and hematopoietic differentiation. Other cells in the bone marrow, including macrophages and adipocytes, contribute to regulation of hematopoiesis.

Cell Differentiation

Within the bone marrow niches, each type of blood cell originates from common hematopoietic stem cells that proliferate and differentiate under control of a variety of cytokines and growth factors (Figure 27-10 and see Table 27-4). During this

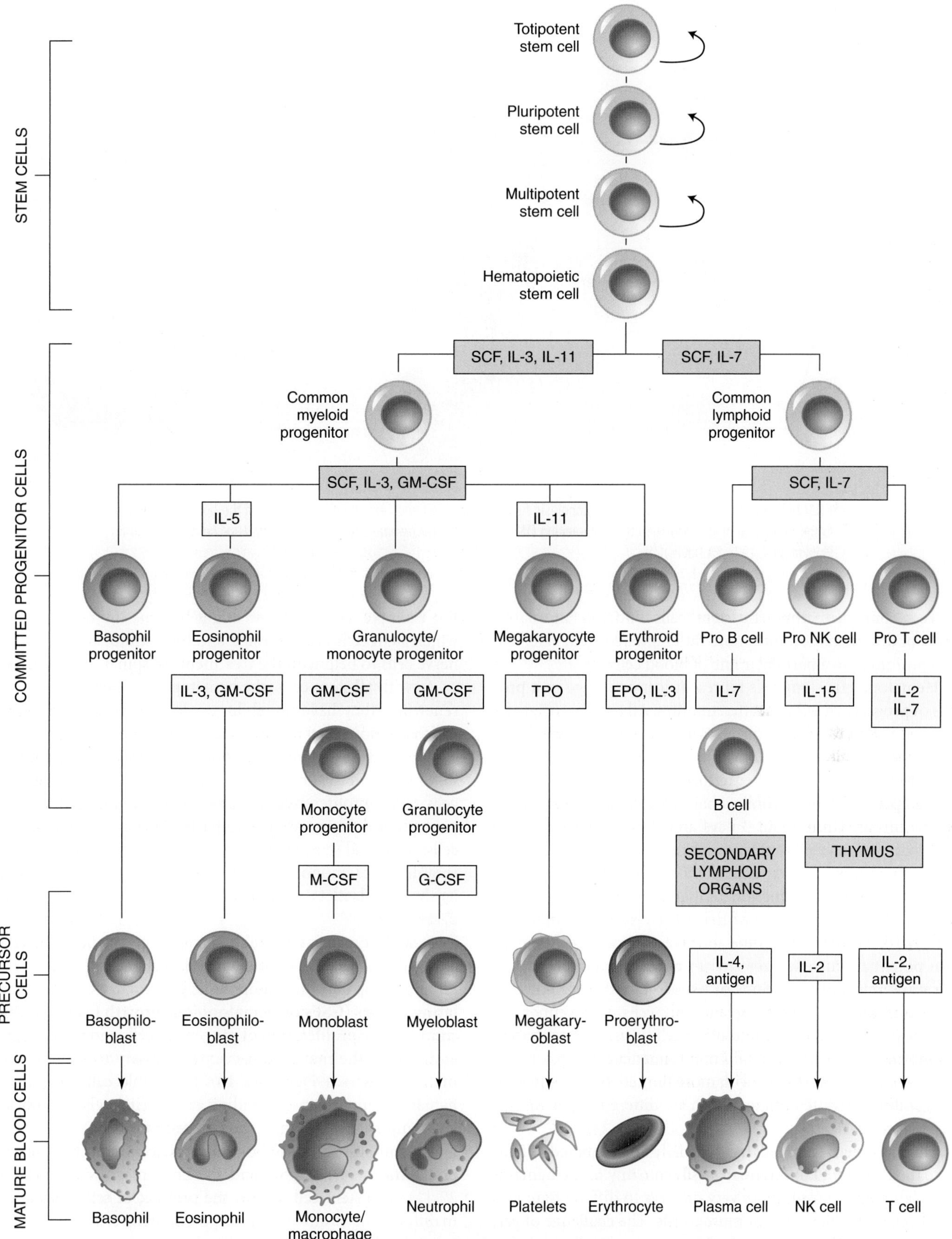

FIGURE 27-10 Differentiation of Hematopoietic Cells. Curved arrows indicate proliferation and expansion of prehematopoietic stem cell populations. *EPO,* Erythropoietin; *G-CSF,* granulocyte colony-stimulating factor; *GM-CSF,* granulocyte-macrophage colony-stimulating factor; *IL,* interleukin; *M-CSF,* macrophage colony-stimulating factor; *NK,* natural killer; *SCF,* stem cell factor; *TPO,* thrombopoietin.

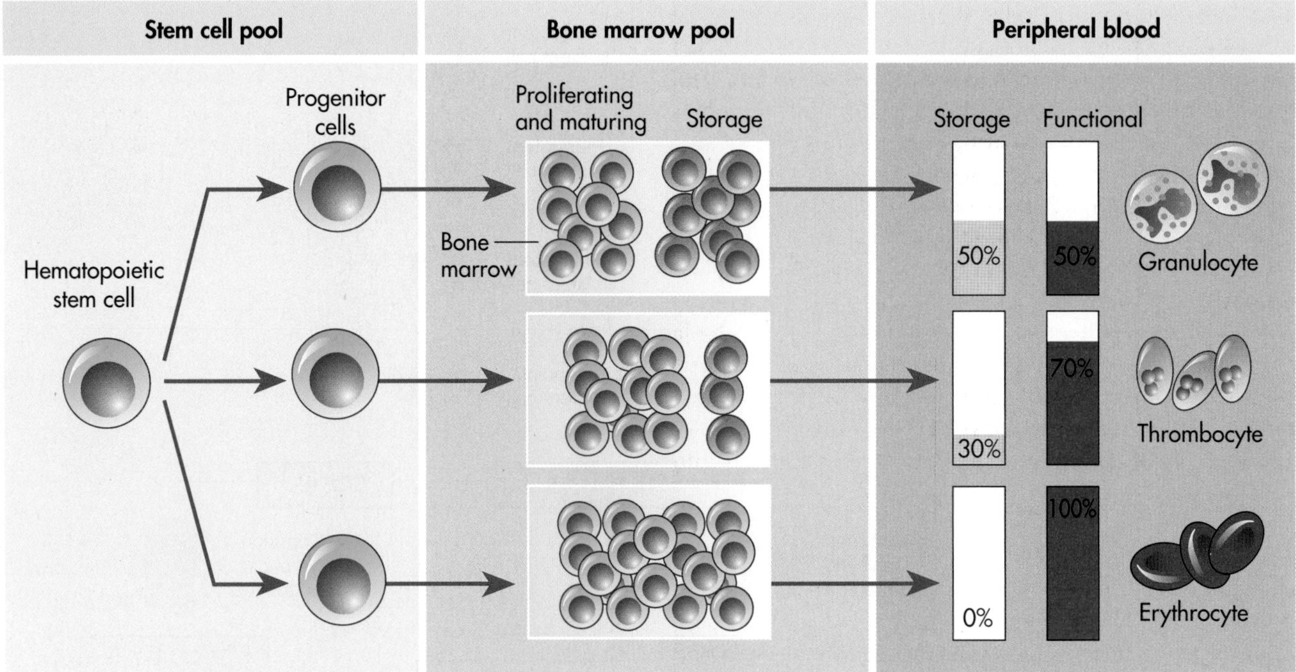

FIGURE 27-11 Hematopoiesis. Hematopoiesis from the stem cell pool; activity occurs mainly in the bone marrow and in the peripheral blood. (Modified from Harmening DM, editor: *Clinical hematology and fundamentals of hemostasis,* ed 3, Philadelphia, 1997, FA Davis.)

process some hematopoietic stem cells undergo alternative paths of differentiation into more differentiated stem cells that are committed to a particular line of blood cells.

Hematopoietic stem cells represent just one stage in a process of progressive cellular differentiation. All humans originate from a single cell (the fertilized egg) that has the capacity to proliferate and eventually differentiate into the huge diversity of cells of the human body. After fertilization, the egg divides over a 5-day period to form a hollow ball (blastocyst) that implants on the uterus. Until about 3 days after fertilization, each cell (blastomere) is undifferentiated and retains the capacity to differentiate into any cell type. In the 5-day blastocyst, the outer layer cells have undergone differentiation and commitment to become the placenta. Cells of the inner cell mass *(embryonic stem cells),* however, continue to have unlimited differentiation potential (currently referred to as being *pluripotent*) and can grow into different kinds of tissue—blood, nerves, heart, bone, and so forth. After implantation, cells of the inner cell mass begin differentiation into other cell types. Differentiation is a multistep process and results in intermediate groups of stem cells *(multipotent stem cells)* with more limited, but still impressive, abilities to differentiate into many different types of cells (see Figure 27-10).[19]

Hematopoietic stem cells have partially differentiated.[20] They have the capacity to differentiate easily into any of the hematologic cell populations but are very difficult to differentiate into other cell types, like nerve or muscle cells. The challenge of getting any partially committed multipotent stem cells to differentiate reliably involves coaxing them with identical chemical signals that the body uses naturally for differentiation. This is a daunting task with potentially astonishing clinical implications. For example, bone marrow might become the reservoir from which stem cells are harvested and then stimulated to produce nerve cells to help with the treatments of spinal cord injuries.

As with all stem cells, the hematopoietic stem cells are self-renewing (they have the ability to proliferate without further differentiation) so that a relatively constant population of stem cells is available. Some hematopoietic stem cells will continue differentiation into hematopoietic progenitor cells. Progenitor cells retain proliferative capacity but are committed to possible further differentiation into particular types of hematologic cells: lymphoid (lymphocytes, NK cells), granulocyte-monocyte (granulocytes, monocytes, macrophages), and megakaryocyte-erythroid (platelets, erythrocytes) progenitor cells (see Figure 27-10).

In addition to intercellular signaling events between HSCs and cells in the osteoblastic and vascular niches, several cytokines participate in hematopoiesis, particularly **colony-stimulating factors (CSFs** or **hematopoietic growth factors),** which stimulate the proliferation of progenitor cells and their progeny and initiate the maturation events necessary to produce fully mature cells (see Figure 27-10).[21] Multiple cell types in the hematopoietic organs, including endothelial cells, fibroblasts, and lymphocytes, produce the necessary CSFs.

Hematopoiesis in the bone marrow occurs in two separate pools: the stem cell pool and the bone marrow pool (Figure 27-11). The stem cell pool is the product of self-renewal that maintains the number of pluripotent stem cells and partially committed progenitor cells. The bone marrow pool contains cells that are proliferating and maturing in preparation for release into the circulation and mature cells that are stored for later release into the peripheral blood. The peripheral blood also contains two pools of cells: those in the circulation and those stored around the walls of the blood vessels (often called the **marginating storage pool**). The marginating storage pool primarily consists of neutrophils that adhere to the endothelium in vessels where the blood flow is relatively slow. These cells can rapidly move into tissues and mucous membranes when needed in an inflammatory response.

Under certain conditions of rapid depletion of the circulating pool, the circulating hematologic cells need to be rapidly replenished. Medullary hematopoiesis can be accelerated by any or all of three mechanisms: (1) conversion of yellow bone marrow, which does not produce blood cells, to hematopoietic red marrow by the actions of **erythropoietin** (a hormone that stimulates erythrocyte production); (2) faster differentiation of progenitor cells; and (3) faster proliferation of stem cells into progenitor cells (see Table 27-4).

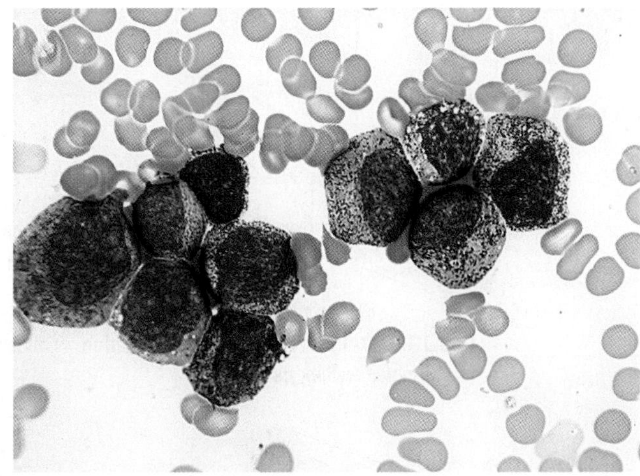

FIGURE 27-12 Colony-Stimulating Factor (CSF) Effects. Morphologic effects of growth factor. Marrow aspirate from a patient receiving granulocyte colony-stimulating factor (G-CSF) showing an early neutrophil response. There is a marked shift toward immaturity in the neutrophils with the majority at the promyelocyte and early myelocyte stages of maturation (Wright-Giemsa stain). (From Damjanov I, Linder J, editors: *Anderson's pathology,* ed 10, St Louis, 1996, Mosby.)

Clinical Uses of Colony-Stimulating Factors

Neutrophils are normally present in the blood in the range of 4000 to 6000 cells/μL, and in response to a bacterial infection, numbers usually increase to 10,000 to 20,000 cells/μL. Susceptibility to infection develops when levels drop below 1000 cells/μL, such as during congenital neutropenia or as a consequence of cytotoxic therapy for cancer. Similarly normal levels of other hematologic cells may be suppressed (e.g., congenital or acquired immune deficiencies and anemia; see Chapters 9 and 28).

The numbers of circulating hematologic cells are under the control of CSFs (see Table 27-4). Administration of CSFs can raise white cell numbers to extremely high levels in healthy individuals. These excessive levels of white blood cells may result in production of toxic products and tissue damage. Therapy with CSFs has been tested in individuals with subnormal levels of circulating blood cells, such as acquired immunodeficiency syndrome (AIDS), aplastic anemia, or congenital neutropenia or as a consequence of cytotoxic therapy lymphoma or leukemia (Figure 27-12). The results of CSF use in individuals with cancer have been disappointing. An analysis of 19 trials in which CSFs were administered postchemotherapy to those with acute myelogenous leukemia detected no effect on overall survival or infections.[22] Results of using CSF prophylactically to avoid neutropenia in individuals undergoing chemotherapy for metastatic solid tumors have been controversial.[23] An analysis of randomized trials of prophylactic use of granulocyte-macrophage CSF (GM-CSF) and granulocyte CSF (G-CSF) in individuals undergoing chemotherapy for metastatic breast cancer indicated a significant effect on prevention of febrile neutropenia and a decrease of general mortality and need for hospital care.[24] However, no effect was observed on the incidence of severe neutropenia, infections, or infection-related mortality. CSF therapy can stimulate increases in circulating granulocyte-monocyte populations, but the degree of response depends on the available numbers of stem and progenitor cells that have survived chemotherapy or the effects of disease. CSF treatment has corrected some cases of congenital neutropenia and resulted in reconstitution of hematopoiesis after bone marrow transplantation.[25] CSF treatment can result in shorter periods of intensive nursing and hospitalization. Recombinant CSFs (e.g., granulocyte colony-stimulating factor [G-CSF], GM-CSF, erythropoietin) are being mass-produced for therapeutic use.

Development of Erythrocytes

For almost 100 years it was believed that erythrocytes developed from lymphocytes that were transformed in the spleen. It was not until the 1850s that the bone marrow was identified as the site of **erythropoiesis,** or development of red blood cells.

Erythropoiesis

In the confines of the bone marrow erythroid progenitor cells proliferate and differentiate into large, nucleated **proerythroblasts,** which are committed into producing cells of the erythroid series (Figure 27-13). Erythroid development from the proerythroblast onward is contained in a compartment referred to as the *erythron.*[26] The proerythroblast, which has ribosomes and can produce protein, differentiates through several intermediate forms of **erythroblast** while synthesizing hemoglobin and progressively eliminating most intracellular structures, including the nucleus. Thus the maturing erythroblast becomes more compact and progressively assumes the shape and characteristics of an erythrocyte. Hemoglobin is readily apparent and increases in quantity as nuclear size shrinks throughout the basophilic and polychromatophilic stages. The orthochromatic erythroblast (**normoblast**) is the smallest of the nucleated erythrocyte precursors.

The last immature form of erythroblast is the **reticulocyte,** which is anucleate and contains a meshlike (reticular) network of ribosomal ribonucleic acid (rRNA) that is visible microscopically after staining with certain dyes. The reticulocyte contains polyribosomes (for globin synthesis) and mitochondria (for oxidative metabolism and heme synthesis). The

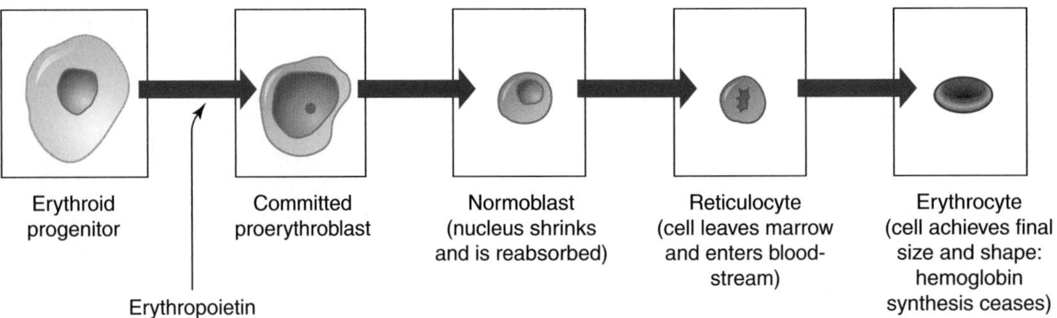

FIGURE 27-13 Erythrocyte Differentiation. Erythrocyte differentiation from large nucleated progenitor cells to small nonnucleated erythrocytes.

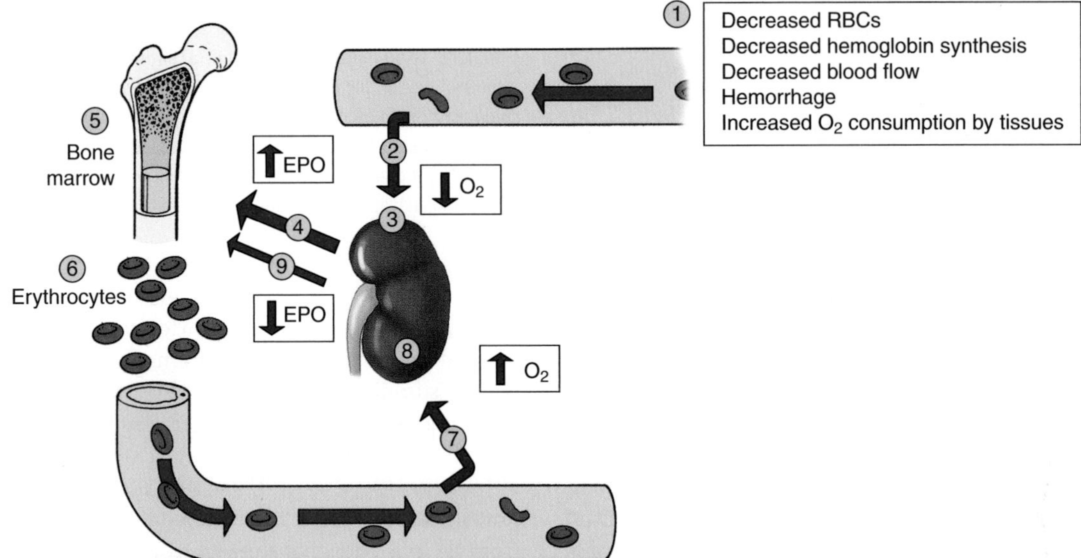

FIGURE 27-14 Role of Erythropoietin in Regulation of Erythropoiesis. (1) Decreased arterial oxygen levels result in **(2)** decreased tissue oxygen (hypoxia) that **(3)** stimulates the kidney to increase **(4)** production of erythropoietin. Erythropoietin is carried to the bone marrow **(5)** and binds to erythropoietin receptors on proerythroblasts, resulting in increased red cell production and maturation and expansion of the erythron **(6)**. The increased release of red cells into the circulation frequently corrects the hypoxia in the tissues **(7)**. **(8)** Perception of normal oxygen levels by the kidney causes **(9)** diminished production of erythropoietin (negative feedback) and return to normal levels of erythrocyte production. *EPO*, Erythropoietin; O_2, oxygen in the blood and tissue; *RBCs*, red blood cells.

reticulocyte matures into an erythrocyte within 24 to 48 hours. During this period, mitochondria and ribosomes disappear and the cell becomes smaller and more disk-like. With these final changes, the erythrocyte loses its capacity for hemoglobin synthesis and oxidative metabolism. Reticulocytes remain in the marrow approximately 1 day and are released into the venous sinuses. They continue to mature in the bloodstream and may travel to the spleen for several days of additional maturation. The normal reticulocyte count is 1% of the total red blood cell count. Approximately 1% of the body's circulating erythrocyte mass normally is generated every 24 hours. Therefore, the reticulocyte count is a useful clinical index of erythropoietic activity and indicates whether new red cells are being produced.

Regulation of Erythropoiesis

In healthy individuals, the total volume of circulating erythrocytes remains surprisingly constant. Most steps of erythropoiesis are primarily under the control of a feedback loop involving the glycoprotein erythropoietin (see Table 27-4). In conditions of tissue hypoxia, erythropoietin is secreted by the liver and, primarily, by the peritubular cells of the kidney (Figure 27-14).[27] Rising levels of circulating erythropoietin cause a compensatory increase in proliferation and differentiation of proerythroblasts in the bone marrow. The density of cellular erythropoietin receptor decreases progressively during erythroid maturation to almost undetectable levels on reticulocytes. The normal steady-state rate of production of approximately 2.5 million erythrocytes per second can increase to 17 million per second during anemia or under conditions of low oxygen concentration, such as high-altitude environments or pulmonary disease. Thus the body responds to reduced oxygenation of blood in two ways: (1) stimulation of chemoreceptors of the carotid body and aortic arch that signal the brain to increase respiration, and (2) stimulation of receptors on the kidney peritubular cells to increase erythropoietin synthesis and release.

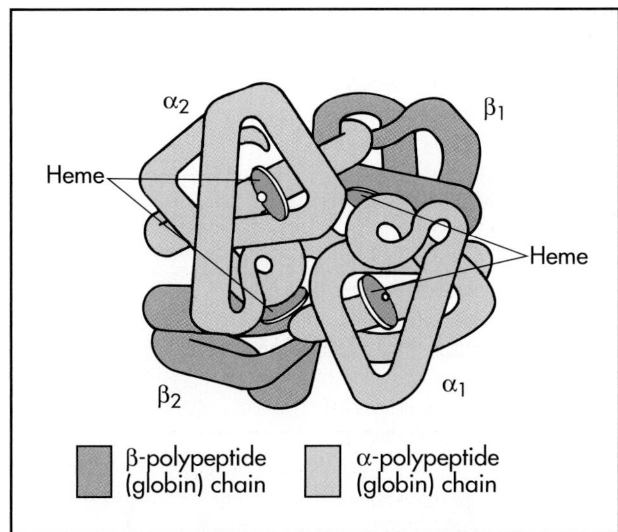

FIGURE 27-15 **Molecular Structure of Hemoglobin.** Molecule is a spherical tetramer weighing approximately 64,500 daltons. It contains a pair of α-polypeptide and a pair of β-polypeptide chains and several heme groups.

TABLE 27-5 STRUCTURE OF NORMAL HEMOGLOBIN MOLECULES

TYPE OF HEMOGLOBIN (Hb)	IDENTITY OF POLYPEPTIDE CHAIN	SIGNIFICANCE
HbA	$\alpha_2\beta_2$	92% of adult Hb
HbA_{1c}	α_2 (β-*NH*-glucose)	5% of adult Hb; increased in diabetes (see Chapter 22)
HbA_2	$\alpha_2\delta_2$	2% of adult Hb; increased in beta-thalassemia (see Chapter 30)
HbF	$\alpha_2\gamma_2$	Major fetal Hb from the third through ninth month of gestation; promotes oxygen transfer across platelets; increased in beta-thalassemia
Hb Gower I	ε_4 or $\zeta_2\beta_2$	Present in early embryo; function unknown
Hb Gower II	$\alpha_2\varepsilon_2$	Present in early embryo; function unknown
Hb Portland	$\zeta_2\gamma_2$	Present in early embryo; function unknown

NH, Amine.

One of the most significant advances in the study of hematopoietic growth factors has been the development of erythropoietin for use in individuals with chronic renal failure. In 1986 large amounts of recombinant human erythropoietin (r-HuEPO) became widely available for clinical research. Erythropoietin is administered intravenously or subcutaneously for the treatment of anemia caused by decreased production of erythropoietin. An immediate effect of increased endogenous or exogenous erythropoietin is an increase in the blood reticulocyte count, followed by increasing levels of erythrocytes. The most significant side effect associated with r-HuEPO is increased blood pressure.

Hemoglobin Synthesis

Hemoglobin (Hb), the oxygen-carrying protein of the erythrocyte, constitutes approximately 90% of the cell's dry weight. Hemoglobin-packed blood cells take up oxygen in the lungs and exchange it for carbon dioxide in the tissues. A single erythrocyte can contain as many as 300 hemoglobin molecules. Hemoglobin increases the oxygen-carrying capacity of blood by 100-fold. Each hemoglobin molecule is composed of two pairs of polypeptide chains (the **globins**) and four colorful complexes of iron plus protoporphyrin (the hemes) (Figure 27-15).[28] Hemoglobin is responsible for blood's ruby-red color.

Several variants of hemoglobin exist, but they differ only slightly in primary structure based on the use of different polypeptide chains; alpha, beta, gamma, delta, epsilon, or zeta (α, β, γ, δ, ε, or ζ) (Table 27-5). Each polypeptide chain contains approximately 150 amino acids and is arranged in the knotted-sausage configuration shown in Figure 27-15. The chains assemble to form a tetrahedron containing two pairs of identical chains. Hemoglobin A, the most common type in adults, is composed of two α- and two β-polypeptide chains ($\alpha 2\beta_2$). A normal variant, fetal hemoglobin (hemoglobin F), is a complex of two α- and two γ-polypeptide chains ($\alpha 2\gamma_2$) that binds oxygen with a much greater affinity than that found in adult hemoglobin.

Heme is a large, flat, iron-protoporphyrin disk that is synthesized in the mitochondria and can carry one molecule of oxygen (O_2). Thus an individual hemoglobin molecule with its four hemes can carry four oxygen molecules. If all four oxygen-binding sites are occupied by oxygen, the molecule is said to be saturated. Through a series of complex biochemical reactions, **protoporphyrin,** a complex four-ringed molecule, is produced and bound with ferrous iron. It is crucial that the iron be correctly charged; reduced ferrous iron (Fe^{2+}) can bind oxygen in the lungs and release it in the tissues, where oxygen concentration is less, whereas ferric iron (Fe^{3+}) cannot. Binding of oxygen to ferrous iron **(oxyhemoglobin)** temporally oxidizes Fe^{2+} to Fe^{3+}, but after the release of oxygen the body reduces the iron to Fe^{2+} (**deoxyhemoglobin** [reduced hemoglobin]) and reactivates the hemoglobin's capacity to bind oxygen. Without reactivation by methemoglobin reductase, the Fe^{3+}-containing hemoglobin **(methemoglobin)** cannot bind oxygen.

Several other molecules can competitively bind to deoxyhemoglobin. Carbon monoxide (CO) directly competes with oxygen for binding to ferrous ion with an affinity that is about 200-fold greater than that of oxygen. Thus even a small amount of CO can dramatically decrease the ability of hemoglobin to bind and transport oxygen. Hemoglobin also binds carbon dioxide (CO_2), but at a binding site separate from where oxygen binds. In the lungs, CO_2 is released, allowing hemoglobin to bind oxygen.

Erythrocytes may play a role in the maintenance of vascular relaxation. Nitric oxide (NO) produced by blood vessels is a major mediator of relaxation and dilation of the vessel walls. In the lungs, hemoglobin can concurrently bind oxygen to the ferrous ion and NO to cysteine residues in the globins. As

TABLE 27-6 NUTRITIONAL REQUIREMENTS FOR ERYTHROPOIESIS

NUTRIENT	ROLE IN ERYTHROPOIESIS	CONSEQUENCE OF DEFICIENCY
Protein (amino acids)	Structural component of plasma membrane	Decreased strength, elasticity, and flexibility of membrane; hemolytic anemia
	Synthesis of hemoglobin	Decreased erythropoiesis and life span of erythrocytes
Cobalamin (vitamin B_{12})	Synthesis of DNA, maturation of erythrocytes, facilitator of folate metabolism	Macrocytic (megaloblastic) anemia
Folate (folic acid)	Synthesis of DNA and RNA, maturation of erythrocytes	Macrocytic (megaloblastic) anemia
Vitamin B_6 (pyridoxine)	Heme synthesis	Microcytic-hypochromic anemia
Vitamin B_2 (riboflavin)	Oxidative reactions	Normocytic-normochromic anemia
Vitamin C (ascorbic acid)	Iron metabolism; acts as a reducing agent to maintain iron in its ferrous (Fe^{2+}) form	Normocytic-normochromic anemia
Pantothenic acid	Heme synthesis	Unknown in humans*
Niacin	None, but needed for respiration in mature erythrocytes	Unknown in humans
Vitamin E	Heme synthesis (?); protection against oxidative damage in mature erythrocytes	Hemolytic anemia with increased cell membrane fragility; shortens life span of erythrocytes in individuals with cystic fibrosis
Iron	Hemoglobin synthesis	Iron deficiency anemia
Copper	Required for optimal mobilization of iron from tissues to plasma	Microcytic-hypochromic anemia

Data from Ames BN, Atamna H, Killilea DW: Mineral and vitamin deficiencies can accelerate the mitochondrial decay of aging, *Mol Aspects of Med* 26(4-5), 367–378, 2005; Strine-Martin EA, Lotspeich-Steininger CA, Koepke JA: *Clinical hematology: principles, procedures, correlations,* ed 2, Philadelphia, 1998, Lippincott.

*Although pantothenic acid is important for optimal synthesis of heme, experimentally induced deficiency *failed* to produce anemia or other hematopoietic disturbances.

DNA, Deoxyribonucleic acid; *RNA,* ribonucleic acid.

hemoglobin transfers its oxygen to tissue, it may also shed small amounts of nitric oxide, contributing to dilation of the blood vessels and helping the oxygen gain access to tissues.

Nutritional Requirements for Erythropoiesis

Normal development of erythrocytes and synthesis of hemoglobin depends on an optimal biochemical milieu and adequate supplies of the necessary building blocks, including protein, vitamins, and minerals (Table 27-6). If these components are lacking for a prolonged time, erythrocyte production slows and anemia (insufficient numbers of functional erythrocytes) may result (see Chapter 28).

Erythropoiesis cannot proceed in the absence of vitamins, especially B_{12}, folate (folic acid), B_6, riboflavin, pantothenic acid, niacin, ascorbic acid, and vitamin E. Dietary vitamin B_{12} is a large molecule that requires a protein secreted by parietal cells into the stomach (intrinsic factor [IF]) for transport across the ileum. Once absorbed, vitamin B_{12} is stored in the liver and used as needed in erythropoiesis. Defects in IF production lead to decreased B_{12} absorption and pernicious anemia.

Folate is the second most important vitamin for erythrocyte production and maturation. Folate is necessary for DNA synthesis, being a component of three of the four DNA bases (thymine, adenine, and guanine), and RNA synthesis. Folate absorption occurs principally in the upper small intestine and is stored in the liver. Folate deficiency is more common than vitamin B_{12} deficiency and occurs more rapidly. Folate stores can be depleted within a few months, whereas vitamin B_{12} depletion can take years. Folate supplements are prescribed for pregnant women because pregnancy increases the demand for folate and may cause anemia.

Normal Destruction of Senescent Erythrocytes

After about 100 to 120 days in the circulation, old erythrocytes are removed by tissue macrophages, primarily in the spleen. Although mature erythrocytes lack nuclei, mitochondria, and endoplasmic reticulum, they do have cytoplasmic enzymes capable of glycolysis (anaerobic glucose metabolism) and production of small quantities of ATP, which provides the energy needed to maintain cell function and membrane pliability. Metabolic processes diminish as the erythrocyte ages, so less ATP is available to maintain plasma membrane function. Disruption of the anchorage between the cytoskeleton and the plasma membrane results in the senescent red cell becoming increasingly fragile and losing its reversible deformability, and thus becoming susceptible to rupture while passing through narrowed regions of the microcirculation.

Additionally, the plasma membrane of senescent red cells undergoes phospholipid rearrangement (movement of the phospholipid phosphatidylserine from the cytoplasmic surface of the membrane to the external surface) that is recognized by receptors for phosphatidylserine on macrophages (primarily in the spleen) that selectively remove and sequester the red cells.[29] If the spleen is dysfunctional or absent, macrophages in the liver (Kupffer cells) take over.

The erythrocytes are digested by proteolytic and lipolytic enzymes in the phagolysosomes (digestive vacuoles) of the macrophage. The heme and globin of methemoglobin dissociate easily, and the globin is broken down into its component amino acids. The iron in hemoglobin is oxidized, forming Fe^{3+} (methemoglobin), and recycled (see following section).

Porphyrin is reduced to bilirubin, which is transported to the liver, conjugated, and finally excreted in the bile as glucuronide (Figure 27-16). Approximately 6 g of hemoglobin is

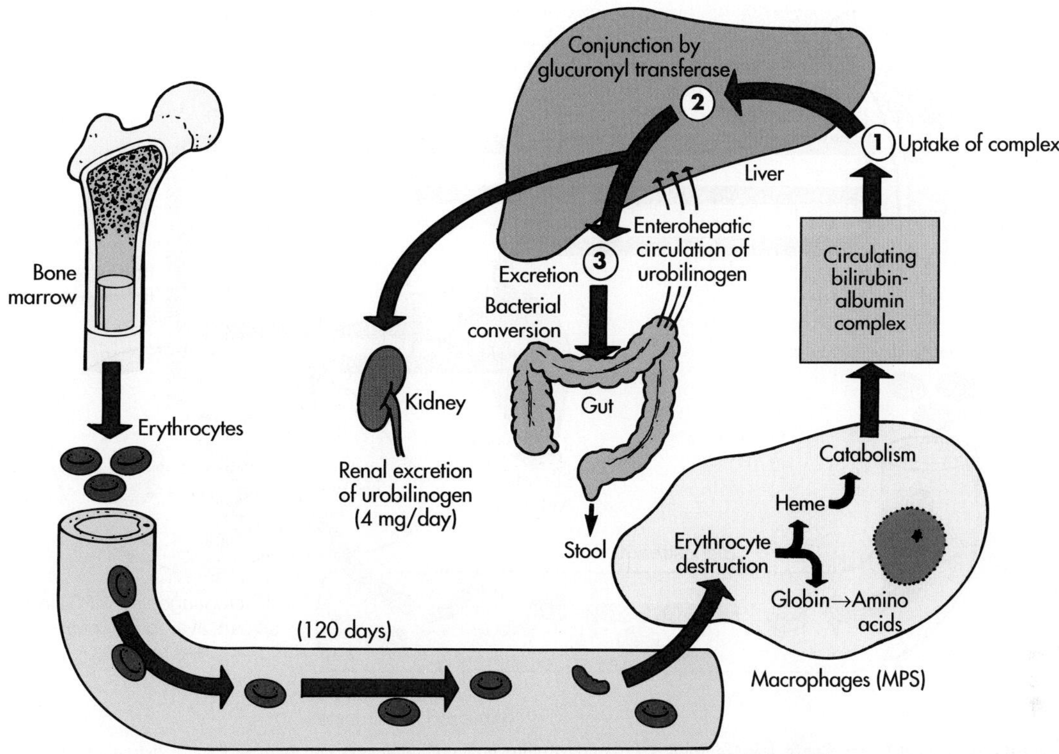

FIGURE 27-16 Metabolism of Bilirubin Released by Heme Breakdown.

catabolized daily, producing 200 mg of bilirubin. Bacteria in the intestinal lumen transform conjugated bilirubin into urobilinogen. Although a small portion is reabsorbed for further metabolism by the liver or excreted by the kidney into the urine, most urobilinogen is excreted in feces. Conditions causing accelerated erythrocyte destruction increase the load of bilirubin for hepatic clearance, leading to increased serum levels of unconjugated bilirubin and increased urinary excretion of urobilinogen. Gallstones (cholelithiasis) can result from a chronically elevated rate of bilirubin excretion.

Iron Cycle

Approximately 67% of total body iron is bound to heme in erythrocytes (hemoglobin) and muscle cells **(myoglobin),** and approximately 30% is stored in mononuclear phagocytes (i.e., macrophages) and hepatic parenchymal cells as either ferritin or hemosiderin. The remaining 3% (less than 1 mg) is lost daily in urine, sweat, bile, sloughing of epithelial cells from the skin and intestinal mucosa, and minor bleeding. Approximately 25 mg of iron is required daily for erythropoiesis; only 1 to 2 mg of iron is dietary and the remainder is obtained from iron recycling of erythrocytes.

Iron is continually recycled.[30] The methemoglobin released from the breakdown of senescent or damaged erythrocytes (see preceding section) is dissociated by the enzyme heme oxygenase, and the iron is released into the bloodstream, where it is free to bind again to transferrin or be stored in the macrophage's cytoplasm as ferritin or hemosiderin (Figure 27-17). A minute amount of iron is stored in muscle cells by the heme-containing protein myoglobin. Unavailable stores of iron are present in cytochromes, catalases, and peroxidase enzymes.

The protein ferritin is the major intracellular iron storage protein. **Apoferritin,** which is ferritin without attached iron, can store thousands of atoms of iron. Several apoferritin complexes combine to form the micelle ferritin. Large aggregates of micelles (if a large amount of iron is present) produce numerous ferritin micelles, known as **hemosiderin.** Hemosiderin is visible as an iron-based pigment under a light microscope as cell inclusions. The iron within deposits of hemosiderin is poorly available to supply iron when needed. The most common cause of hemosiderin deposition is simple bruising. Hemosiderin in small amounts within iron-rich tissues (i.e., spleen, liver, bone marrow) is considered normal. Large aggregates or its presence in tissue such as the lungs or subcutaneous tissue suggest a pathologic condition.

Iron from either dietary sources, release of iron stores, or erythrocyte catabolism is transported in the blood bound to **apotransferrin,** thus becoming **transferrin;** under normal conditions, only one third of the iron-binding sites on transferrin molecules are occupied.[31] Apotransferrin is a glycoprotein synthesized primarily by hepatocytes in the liver but also produced in small quantities by tissue macrophages, submaxillary and mammary glands, and ovaries or testes. Iron for hemoglobin production is carried by transferrin to the bone marrow, where it binds to transferrin receptors on erythroblasts. Transferrin receptors are on the plasma membrane of all nucleated cells, although at particularly high levels on erythroid precursors and rapidly proliferating cells (e.g., lymphocytes), and are thought to be the only route of cellular entry for transferrin-attached iron. Transferrin is recycled (transferrin cycle) in the following manner:

1. The transferrin-iron complex binds to a transferrin receptor on the erythroblast's plasma membrane.

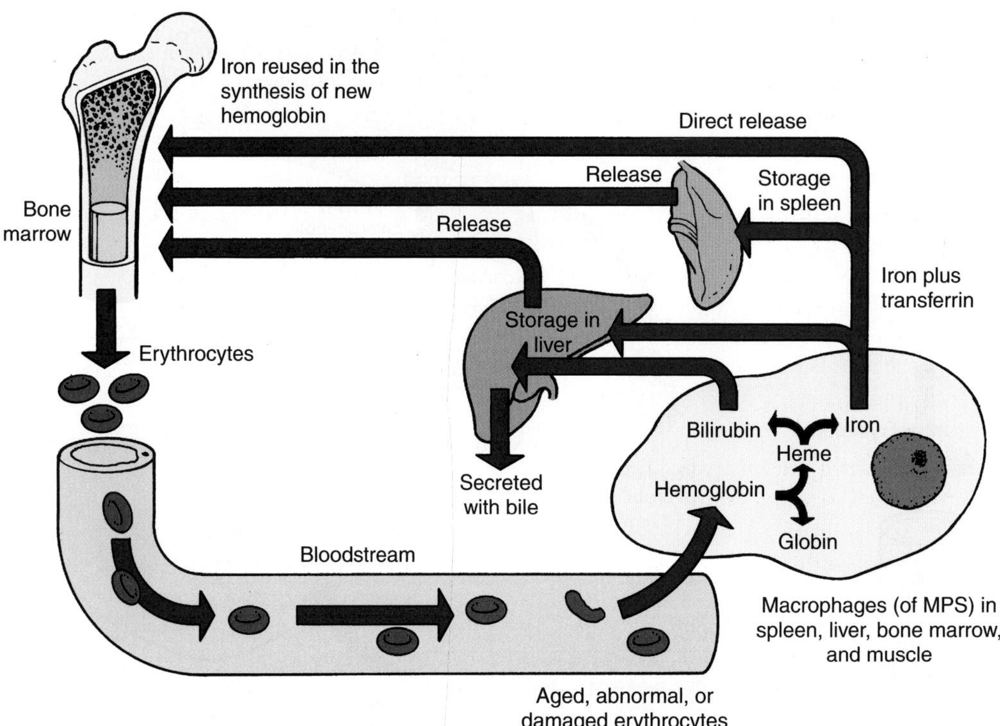

FIGURE 27-17 Iron Cycle. Iron (Fe) released from gastrointestinal epithelial cells circulates in the bloodstream associated with its plasma carrier, transferrin. It is delivered to erythroblasts in bone marrow, where most of it is incorporated into hemoglobin. Mature erythrocytes circulate for approximately 100 to 120 days, after which they become senescent and are removed by the mononuclear phagocyte system *(MPS)*. Tissue macrophages (mostly in spleen) break down ingested erythrocytes and return iron to the bloodstream directly or after storing it as a ferritin or hemosiderin.

2. The complex moves into the cell by receptor-mediated endocytosis.
3. Iron is released (dissociated) from transferrin.
4. The dissociated transferrin is returned to the bloodstream for reuse.

The iron is transported to the erythroblast's mitochondria (the site of hemoglobin production), where the enzyme heme synthetase inserts ferrous iron into protoporphyrin to form heme. Heme then is bound to globin to form hemoglobin. Iron not used in erythropoiesis is stored temporarily as ferritin or hemosiderin and later excreted.

The body's iron homeostasis is primarily controlled by the hormone hepcidin.[32] Hepcidin is synthesized in the liver and released as a 25 amino acid peptide, most of which is bound in the plasma with high affinity to α_2-macroglobulin and relatively lower affinity to albumin. Hepatocellular hepcidin production is regulated physiologically by the body's dietary absorption of iron, rate of erythropoiesis, and level of oxygen saturation.[33] Hepatocytes sense levels of circulating iron by means of receptors for transferrin, the major transporter of iron in the plasma. Excess iron is stored in hepatocytes and macrophages. Hepatocytes sense these levels by means of receptors for bone morphogenetic protein (BMP), most likely BMP-6, which is a growth factor produced to a large extent by bone marrow sinusoid endothelial cells. Hepcidin production also can be induced by inflammation by means of IL-6.

Hepcidin regulates iron levels through its binding capacity to ferroportin, which is a transmembrane iron exporter found in the plasma membrane of cells that transport or store iron, including macrophages, hepatocytes, and enterocytes. The body's total iron balance is maintained through controlled absorption rather than excretion.[34] Dietary iron (primarily as Fe^{2+}) is transported directly across the membranes of epithelial cells (enterocytes) in the duodenum and proximal jejunum.[35] (Transport mechanisms are described in Chapter 1.) Hepcidin induces internalization and degradation of ferroportin, thus leading to increased intracellular iron stores, decreased dietary iron absorption, and decreased levels of circulating iron.[36] Decreased production of hepcidin leads to release of stored iron and increased dietary absorption. Thus, if the body's iron stores are low or the demand for erythropoiesis increases, dietary iron is transported rapidly through the epithelial cell and into the plasma. If body stores are high and erythropoiesis is not increased, iron transport is stopped, although iron can cross the epithelial cells' plasma membrane passively and be stored as ferritin.

Development of Leukocytes

Leukocytes consist of lymphocytes, granulocytes, and monocytes. Most of the leukocytes arise from stem cells in the bone marrow (their pathways of differentiation are shown in Figure 27-10). Hematopoietic stem cells differentiate into two populations of progenitor cells: common lymphoid progenitors and common myeloid progenitors. Lymphoid progenitors that remain in the bone marrow undergo differentiation into the B-cell lineage, after which they are released into the circulation and undergo further maturation in the peripheral lymphoid organs (described in Chapter 8 [see Figure 8-3]). The common myeloid progenitors further differentiate into progenitors for basophils, mast cells, eosinophils, and megakaryocytes, and granulocyte/monocyte progenitors. The granulocyte/monocyte progenitors further differentiate into monocyte progenitors and granulocyte progenitors, which develop into monocytes/macrophages and neutrophils, respectively. Development from hematopoietic stem cells to common granulocyte-monocyte progenitors primarily is under the control of stem cell factor, IL-3, and GM-CSF, whereas further differentiation into granulocytic and monocytic progenitors is controlled by G-CSF and M-CSF, respectively (see Table 27-4).

Monocytic progenitors undergo development into monocytes within 24 hours and are released into the circulation. Monocytes mature into various forms of macrophages, a process that is usually completed within 1 or 2 days after their release (see Tables 27-3 and 27-4).[37]

Progenitor cells for granulocytes normally fully mature in the bone marrow into neutrophils, eosinophils, and basophils. The ultimate phenotype is determined by relative local bone marrow concentrations of early- and late-acting cytokines, including GM-CSF, G-CSF, IL-3, IL-5, stem cell factor, and others (see Table 27-4). Granulocytes are released into the blood within 14 days of development. The bone marrow selectively retains immature granulocytes as a reserve pool that can be rapidly mobilized in response to the body's needs.

Most leukocytes exist in the body from days to years, depending on type. Maintenance of optimal levels of granulocytes and monocytes in the blood depends on the availability of pluripotent stem cells in the marrow, induction of these into committed stem cells, timely release of new cells from the marrow, and mobilization of the granulocyte reserve pool. Leukocyte production increases in response to infection, to the presence of steroids, and to reduction or depletion of reserves in the marrow. It is also associated with strenuous exercise, convulsive seizures, heat, intense radiation, paroxysmal tachycardias, pain, nausea and vomiting, and anxiety.

Development of Platelets

Platelets (thrombocytes) are derived from stem cells and progenitor cells that differentiate into megakaryocytes.[38] During thrombopoiesis, the megakaryocyte progenitor is programmed to undergo an endomitotic cell cycle (**endomitosis**) during which DNA replication occurs, but anaphase and cytokinesis are blocked (see Chapter 1). Thus the megakaryocyte nucleus enlarges and becomes extremely polyploidy (up to 100-fold or more of the normal amount of DNA) without cellular division. Concurrently, the numbers of cytoplasmic organelles (e.g., internal membranes, granules) increase, and the cell develops cell surface proplatelet elongations into the sinusoidal blood vessels.[39] These branches progressively fragment into platelets. A single large (30 to 100 μm) megakaryocyte may produce thousands of smaller platelets (2 to 3 μm).[40] Like erythrocytes, platelets released from the bone marrow lack nuclei.

About two thirds of platelets enter the circulation; the remainder reside in the splenic pool. Platelets circulate in the bloodstream for about 8 to 10 days before losing their ability to carry out thrombogenic activity. Senescent platelets are sequestered and destroyed in the spleen by mononuclear cell phagocytosis.

An adequate level of committed platelet precursors (megakaryoblasts) in the bone marrow and differentiation into circulating platelets are controlled by specific interactions between megakaryocyte progenitors and stromal cells in the bone marrow as well as thrombopoietin (TPO, a hormonal growth factor primarily produced by the liver) and various cytokines and colony-stimulating factors and interleukins (see Table 27-4). Platelets express high-affinity receptors for TPO, and when circulating platelet levels are normal, TPO is adsorbed onto the platelet surface and prevented from accessing the bone marrow and initiating further platelet production.[41] TPO stimulates committed cells at further stages of differentiation to differentiate faster so that rates of megakaryocyte development, endomitosis, and platelet release are increased. During inflammation IL-6 induces increased production of TPO, which increases production of newly formed platelets, which are more thrombogenic.

MECHANISMS OF HEMOSTASIS

Hemostasis is defined as arrest of bleeding (Figure 27-18). As a result of hemostasis, damaged blood vessels maintain a relatively steady-state of blood volume, pressure, and flow. The importance of hemostasis clearly varies with vessel size. Damage to large vessels cannot easily be controlled by hemostasis but requires vascular contraction and dramatically decreased blood flow into the damaged vessels.

Three equally important components of hemostasis are the vasculature (endothelial cells and subendothelial matrix), platelets, and blood proteins (clotting factors). The following describes the general sequence of events in hemostasis: (1) vascular injury leads to a transient arteriolar vasoconstriction to limit blood flow to the affected site; (2) damage to the endothelial cell lining of the vessel exposes prothrombogenic subendothelial connective tissue matrix, leading to platelet adherence and activation and formation of a *hemostatic plug* to prevent further bleeding (primary hemostasis); (3) tissue factor, produced by the endothelium, collaborates with secreted platelet factors and activated platelets to activate the clotting (coagulation) system to form fibrin clots and further prevent bleeding (secondary hemostasis); and (4) the fibrin/platelet clot contracts to form a more permanent plug, and regulatory pathways are activated (fibrinolysis) to limit the size of the plug and begin the healing process.

Function of Blood Vessels

The vessel walls consist of a layer of endothelial cells that adhere to an underlying matrix of connective tissue. The matrix contains a variety of proteins, including collagen, fibronectin, and laminins. Endothelial cells adhere to the matrix and to each other through receptors (e.g., vascular endothelial cell–specific

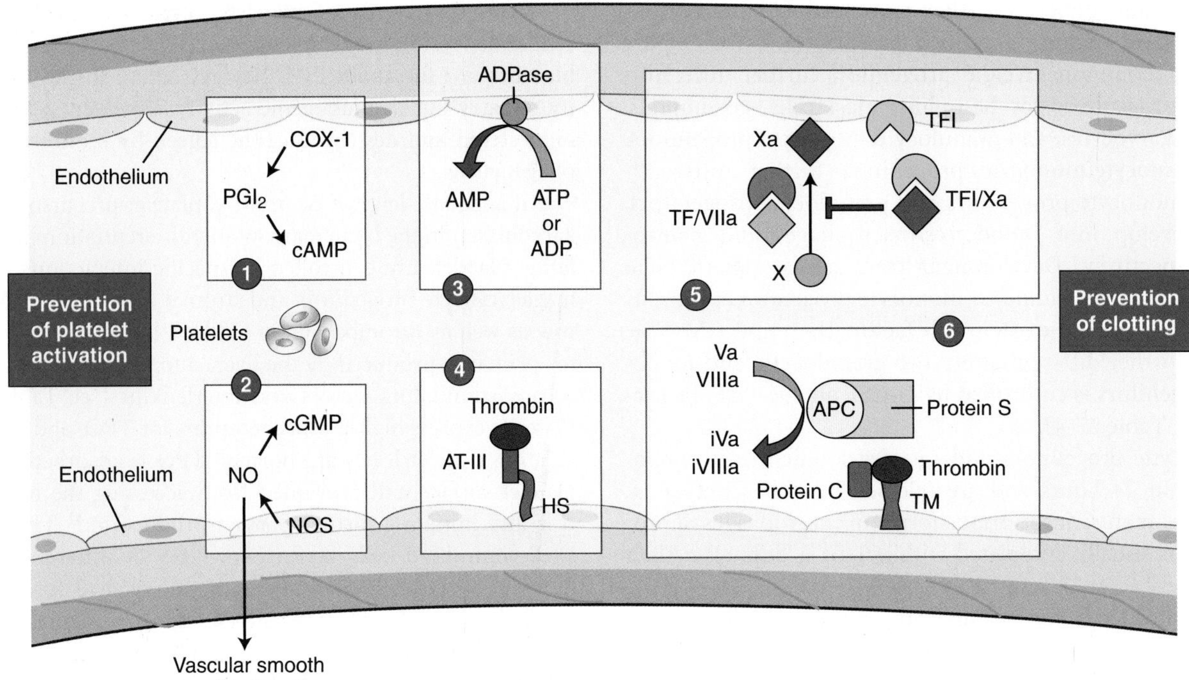

FIGURE 27-18 **Hemostasis.** Endothelium controls hemostasis by preventing platelet activation **(1-3)** and preventing activation of the clotting system **(4-6).** **(1)** *Prostacyclin production:* Injury activates inflammation (*COX-1,* arachidonic acid). Enzymes convert arachidonic acid into prostacylin I_2 *(PGI_2)* in endothelial cells. PGI_2 eventually increases intracellular cyclic adenosine monophosphate *(cAMP);* cAMP inhibits platelet aggregation and induces vasodilation. Nitric oxide *(NO)* formation is induced by NO synthases *(NOS)* and NO causes increased cyclic guanosine monophosphate *(cGMP).* **(2)** *Nitric oxide system:* Endothelial cell NOS produces nitric oxide, which controls platelet activation through cGMP-mediated signaling. **(3)** *ADPase:* Endothelial cells express a surface bound ADPase (CD39) that converts circulating ADP and ATP to AMP. **(4)** *Antithrombin III–heparan sulfate system:* Antithrombin III *(AT-III)* inhibits thrombin slowly when heparan sulfate *(HS)* is absent. When HS is present, it quickly activates thrombin because it binds to a specific site on AT-III that causes an instant conformational change in AT-III, allowing it to quickly activate thrombin. **(5)** *Tissue factor inhibitor (TFI) system:* Expression of TFI on the endothelial cells and secreted into the circulation complexes with factor IXa to form a competitive inhibitor of the tissue factor/factor VIIa complex *(TF/VIIa)* and prevent further activation of factor X to Xa. **(6)** *Protein C/protein S pathway (thrombomodulin):* Thrombin in the circulation binds to thrombomodulin on the endothelial cell, creating a complex that can bind and activate protein C to activated protein C *(APC)* that complexes in the blood or on the surface of active platelets with protein S. This complex degrades circulating clotting factors Va and VIIIa to inactive forms *(iVa, iVIIIa)* to prevent further activation of clotting.

cadherin [VE-cadherin], platelet-endothelial cell adhesion molecule 1 [PECAM-1], integrins [especially $\alpha 2\beta 1$ and $\alpha 5\beta 1$]) that are expressed only on the intercellular and basal surfaces.

Under normal conditions the endothelium actively regulates blood flow and prevents spontaneous activation of platelets and the clotting system (see Figure 27-18). Endothelial cells produce **nitric oxide (NO)** from L-arginine and synthesize **prostacyclin (PGI_2)** from arachidonic acid. Both NO, via cGMP, and PGI_2 are vasodilators that work in concert with endothelin (a vasoconstrictor) to maintain blood flow and pressure.[42] NO and PGI_2 also inhibit platelet adhesion and aggregation. Synergism between PGI_2 and NO is significant. PGI_2 production varies a great deal in response to stimuli, whereas NO is released continually to regulate vascular tone. NO has other biologic functions including cell signaling, free radical production, and possibly others. Endothelium also produces adenosine diphosphatase, which degrades ADP (a potent activator of platelets).

The endothelial cell surface contains antithrombotic molecules, such as glycosaminoglycans (e.g., heparan sulfate), thrombomodulin, and plasminogen activators. These limit platelet activation and fibrin deposition. Although thrombomodulin and plasminogen activators help control hemostasis in normal vessels, their effects are magnified during vascular damage and clot formation; therefore, further information is provided on these molecules in the following section on control of hemostatic mechanisms.

As a result of damage to the vessels, the endothelial cell barrier is frequently compromised, the remaining endothelial cells are activated by products of tissue damage, and the underlying matrix is exposed. Endothelial cells contain intracellular structures (Weibel-Palade bodies) that contain von Willebrand factor (vWF) that is released during damage. The matrix, in addition to collagen and other connective tissue, contains vWF and can bind additional vWF released by the endothelium.[43] The matrix itself and vWF are potent activators of platelets.

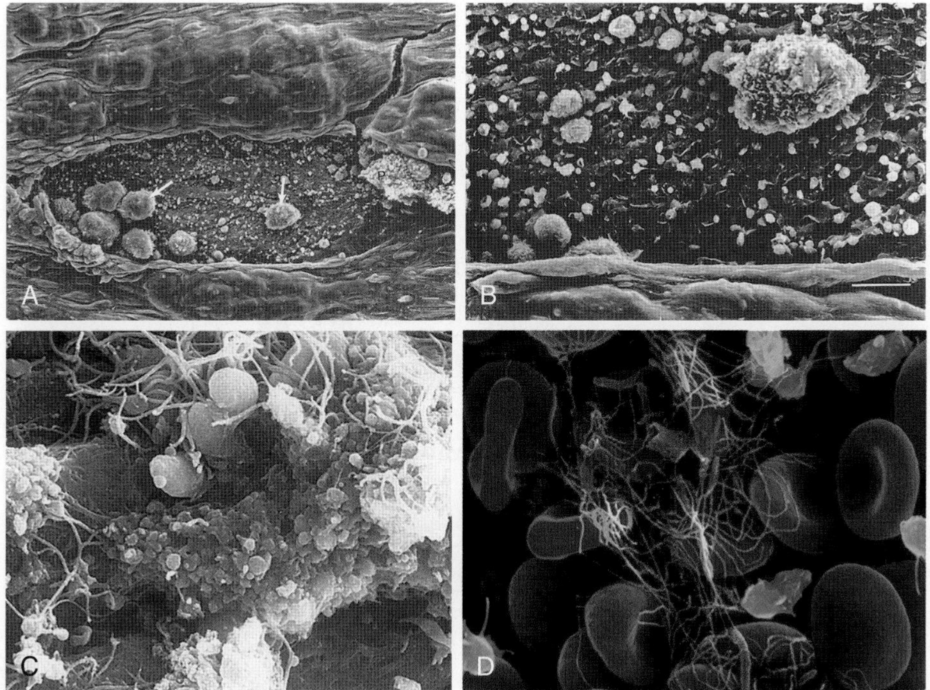

FIGURE 27-19 Platelet Activation. **A,** After endothelial denudation, platelets and leukocytes adhere to the subendothelium in a monolayer fashion. **B,** Higher-power view showing leukocytes and platelets adherent to the subendothelium. **C,** High magnification of a thrombus showing a mixture of red cells and platelets incorporated into the fibrin meshwork. **D,** An electron micrograph showing entrapped RBCs in a fibrin clot. (**A** and **B** from Libby P et al: *Braunwald's heart disease: a textbook of cardiovascular medicine,* ed 8, Philadelphia, 2007, Saunders, as reproduced from Faggiotto A, Ross R: *Arteriosclerosis* 341-356, 1984; **C** from Damjanov I, Linder J, editors: *Anderson's pathology,* ed 10, St Louis, 1996, Mosby; **D** copyright Dennis Kunkel Microscopy, Inc.)

Function of Platelets

Platelets normally circulate freely, suspended in plasma, in an unactivated state. The role of platelets is to (1) contribute to regulation of blood flow into a damaged site by induction of vasoconstriction (vasospasm), (2) initiate platelet-platelet interactions resulting in formation of a platelet plug to stop further bleeding, (3) activate the coagulation (or clotting) cascade to stabilize the platelet plug, and (4) initiate repair processes including clot retraction and clot dissolution **(fibrinolysis).** The normal platelet count ranges from 140,000 to 340,000/mm^3. If platelet counts drop below 100,000/mm^3 an individual is usually considered thrombocytopenic (abnormally low numbers of platelets) and may experience prolongation of normal clotting but is usually not at risk for spontaneous major bleeding episodes unless the platelet count falls below 20,000/mm^3. If platelet numbers are elevated (thrombocytosis) the risk for spontaneous blood clots (thrombosis), stroke, or heart attack is increased.

The state of platelet activation is primarily under the control of endothelial cells lining the vessels. Damage to the vessel initiates a process of platelet activation: (1) increased platelet *adhesion* to the damaged vascular wall; (2) *activation* leading to secretion of chemicals from platelet granules, which stimulate changes in platelet shape and biochemistry; and (3) *aggregation* as platelet–vascular wall and platelet-platelet adherence increases.[44] This process leads to activation of the clotting system and development of an immobilizing meshwork of platelets and fibrin (Figure 27-19).

Adhesion

Normally, platelets are generally observed "rolling" along the margins of vessels. At sites of vessel injury, however, platelets become adherent to the site of endothelial damage, where the subendothelial matrix is exposed and endothelial cells have released vWF and decreased their antithrombotic activities (Figure 27-20). **Platelet adhesion** is mostly mediated by the binding of platelet surface receptor glycoprotein-Ib (GPIb) (in a complex with clotting factors IX and V) to **von Willebrand factor (vWF).**[45] The vWF protein is found in the subendothelial matrix and is released by endothelial cells and platelets. Deficiencies in GPIb (Bernard-Soulier syndrome) or vWF (von Willebrand disease) lead to highly defective hemostasis and congenital bleeding disorders.[46] Platelet adhesion narrows the diameter of the blood vessel, resulting in increasing shear forces that could strip platelets off the vessel surface. However, those same forces induce conformational changes in the vWF molecule that result in increased affinity with GPIb, thus stabilizing the adherent platelet.[47]

Platelet adhesion is also facilitated by other interactions between platelet receptors and exposed molecules of the subendothelial matrix. For instance, adhesion is increased through binding of the platelet collagen receptors GPVI and integrin $\alpha 2\beta 1$ to exposed collagen in the matrix.

I. Subendothelial exposure

- Occurs after endothelial sloughing
- Platelets begin to fill endothelial gaps
- Promoted by thromboxane A_2 (TXA_2)
- Inhibited by prostacyclin I_2 (PGI_2)
- Platelet function depends on many factors, especially calcium

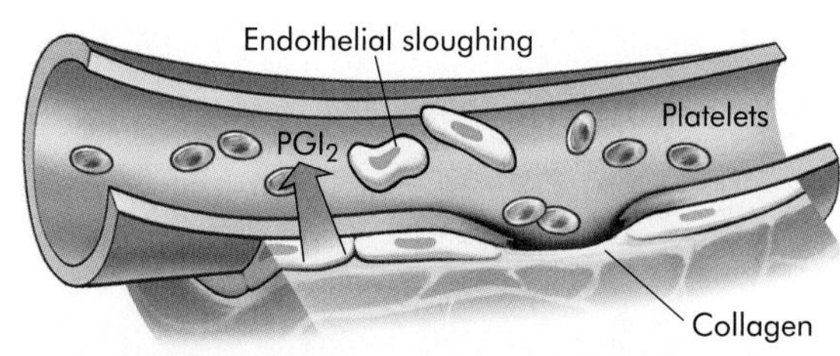

II. Adhesion

- Adhesion is initiated by loss of endothelial cells (or rupture or erosion of atherosclerotic plaque), which exposes adhesive glycoproteins such as collagen and von Willebrand factor (vWF) in the subendothelium. vWF and, perhaps, other adhesive glycoproteins in the plasma deposit on the damaged area. Platelets adhere to the subendothelium through receptors that bind to the adhesive glycoproteins (GPIb, GPIa/IIa, GPIIb/IIIa).

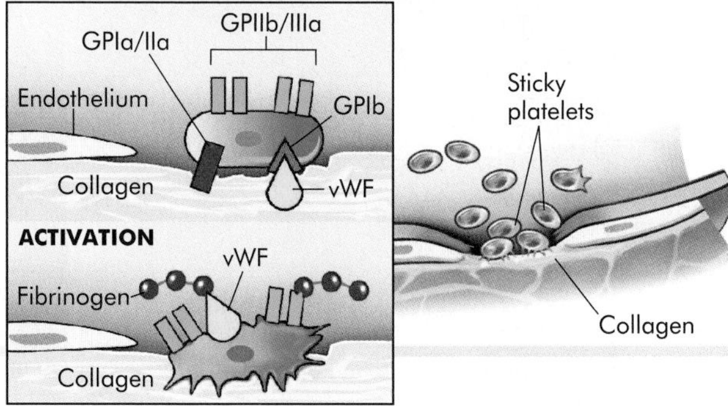

III. Activation

- After platelets adhere they undergo an activation process that leads to a conformational change in GPIIb/IIIa receptors, resulting in their ability to bind adhesive proteins, including fibrinogen and von Willebrand factor.
- Changes in platelet shape
- Formation of pseudopods
- Activation of arachidonic pathway

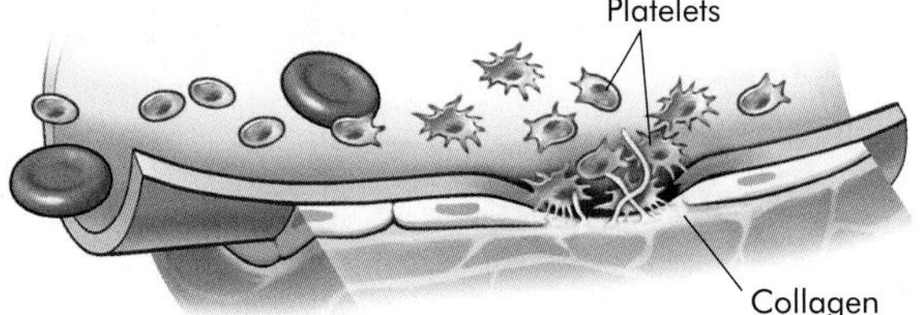

IV. Aggregation

- Induced by release of TXA_2
- Adhesive glycoproteins bind simultaneously to GPIIb/IIIa on two different platelets
- Stabilization of the platelet plug (blood clot) occurs by activation of coagulation factors, thrombin, and fibrin
- Heparin neutralizing factor enhances clot formation

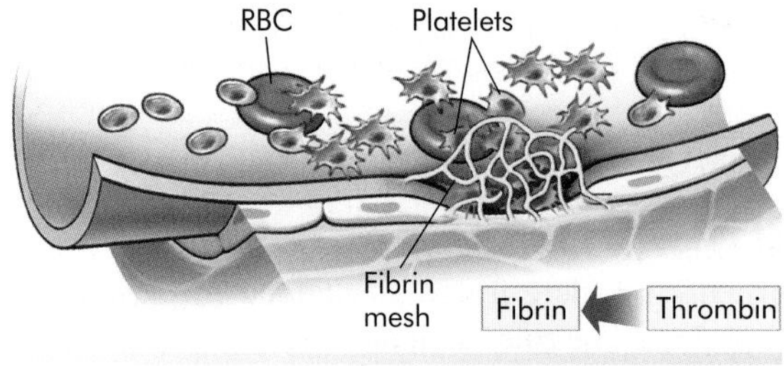

V. Platelet plug formation

- RBCs and platelets enmeshed in fibrin

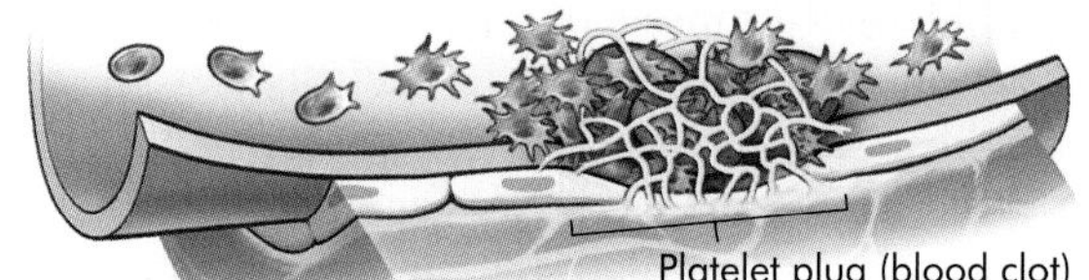

VI. Clot retraction and clot dissolution

- Clot retraction, using large number of platelets, joins the edges of the injured vessel.
- Clot dissolution is regulated by thrombin and plasminogen activators.

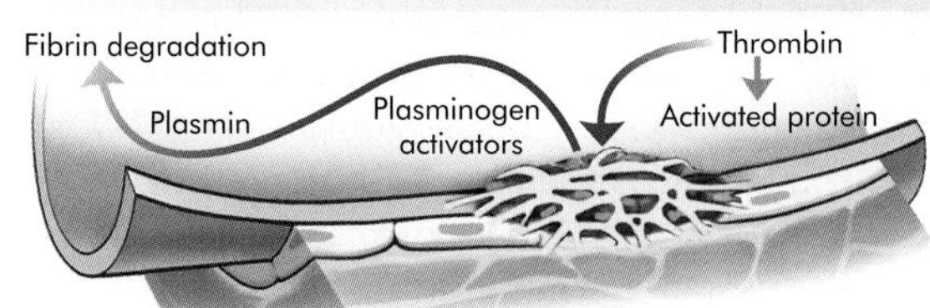

FIGURE 27-20 Blood Vessel Damage, Blood Clot, and Clot Dissolution.

Activation

As a result of interactions with the endothelium or the subendothelial matrix, as well as exposure to inflammatory mediators produced by the endothelium and other cells, the platelets are activated. Activation results in reorganization of the platelet cytoskeleton, leading to dynamic changes in platelet shape from smooth spheres to those with spiny projections and degranulation (also called the **platelet-release reaction**) and resulting in the release of various potent biochemicals (Figure 27-21).[48]

Platelets contain three types of granules: lysosomes, dense bodies, and alpha granules.[49] The contents of the dense bodies and alpha granules are particularly important in hemostasis. The dense bodies contain ADP, serotonin, and calcium. ADP recruits and activates other platelets through specific receptors. During activation the platelet plasma membrane undergoes several important changes, including becoming ruffled and sticky, undergoing cellular spreading to make tight contacts between neighboring platelets that cause the platelet plug to

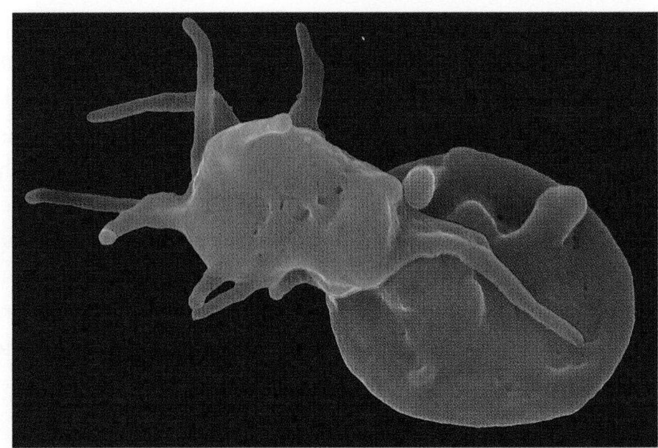

FIGURE 27-21 Micrograph of an Active and Moderately Active Platelet. (Copyright Dennis Kunkel Microscopy, Inc.)

seal the injured endothelium, and externalizing the phospholipid phosphatidylserine, which provides a matrix for activation of clotting factors (see Figure 27-20). Serotonin is a vasoactive amine that functions like histamine and increases vasodilation and vascular permeability. Calcium is necessary for many of the adhesive interactions as well as intracellular signaling mechanisms that control platelet activation.

Alpha granules contain a large number of clotting factors (e.g., fibrinogen, factor V), growth factors (e.g., PDGF), and heparin-binding proteins (e.g., platelet factor 4). Many of these mediators either promote or inhibit platelet activity and the eventual process of clot formation. PDGF stimulates smooth muscle cells and promotes tissue repair. Heparin-binding proteins enhance clot formation at the site of injury.

Platelets also initiate production of the prostaglandin derivative **thromboxane A_2 (TXA_2),** which counters the effects of PGI_2 that is produced by endothelial cells (see Figure 27-20). TXA_2 promotes the degranulation of platelets, increases expression of platelet fibrinogen receptors, and stimulates platelet aggregation. The balance between TXA_2 and PGI_2 affects platelet aggregation, which is favored by TXA_2 excess and inhibited by PGI_2 excess. An isoform of **cyclooxygenase (COX-1)** converts arachidonic acid to TXA_2 in platelets. Aspirin at low doses specifically and irreversibly inactivates COX-1, decreasing production of TXA_2 and decreasing platelet activation.[50] A few days of low doses of aspirin lead to more than 95% inhibition of TXA_2.

Other stimuli of platelet activation include epinephrine, thrombin, and collagen. Thrombin and collagen are particularly strong stimuli. Thrombin cleaves the extracellular domain of G-protein–coupled protease-activated receptors (PARs), thereby initiating transmembrane signaling.

Aggregation

Platelet aggregation is stimulated primarily by TXA_2 and ADP, which induce functional fibrinogen receptors on the platelet. The **GPIIb/IIIa complex** (also called integrin $\alpha IIb\beta 3$) undergoes a conformational change during activation to become a calcium-dependent receptor for fibrinogen (see Figure 27-20). It is a member of the integrin receptor family and binds other matrix proteins (e.g., fibronectin, fibrinogen, thrombospondin). Defects in expression of the GPIIb/IIIa complex (Glanzmann thrombasthenia) result in a failure to aggregate and diminished clotting times.[51] Although the GPIIb/IIIa complex is the most abundant aggregation receptor on the platelet, receptors for vWF (GPIb) and collagen (GPVI) also contribute to the process. Interplatelet aggregation and clot retraction that form the *primary hemostatic plug* are facilitated by fibrinogen bridges between receptors on the platelets. The GPIIb-IIIa–fibrinogen pathway is essential for the formation of a thrombus and as such is an important therapeutic target for blockage by antiplatelet drugs. In addition, fibrin strands within the clot shorten and become denser and stronger, helping the clot to approximate the edges of the injured vessel wall and sealing the site of injury. Contraction of myosin and actin filaments in the platelet cytoskeleton mediates *platelet contraction* and fusion of the platelet mass into a *secondary hemostatic plug.* Contraction expels serum from the fibrin meshwork, resulting in greater packing and increased strength. This process usually begins within a few minutes after a clot has formed, and most of the serum is expelled within 20 to 60 minutes.[52]

If blood vessel injury is minor, primary hemostasis is achieved by formation of the platelet plug within 3 to 5 minutes of injury. Platelet plugs seal the many minute ruptures that occur daily in the microcirculation, particularly in capillaries. With too few platelets, numerous small hemorrhagic areas called *purpuras* develop under the skin and throughout the tissues (see Chapter 29). If primary hemostasis is inadequate to prevent further bleeding, the process proceeds through secondary hemostasis to create a larger complex of more tightly interactive platelets within a matrix created by activation of the clotting system.

Function of Clotting Factors

A **blood clot** is a meshwork of protein strands that stabilizes the platelet plug and traps other cells, such as erythrocytes, phagocytes, and microorganisms. The strands are made of fibrin, which is produced by the **clotting (coagulation) system.** The clotting system was described in Chapter 7 and consists of a family of proteins that circulate in the blood in inactive forms (proenzymes). Initiation of the system results in sequential enzymatic activation (cascade) of multiple members of the system until a fibrin clot is created (Table 27-7).

The clotting system is usually presented as two pathways of initiation (intrinsic and extrinsic pathways) that join in a common pathway (Figure 27-22). The intrinsic pathway is activated when Hageman factor (factor XII) in plasma contacts negatively charged subendothelial substances exposed by vascular injury. Activated factor XII (XIIa) is an active enzyme with factor XI as a substrate. The extrinsic pathway is activated when **tissue factor (TF)** (also called **tissue thromboplastin**) reacts with a high affinity with circulating activated factor VII (TF/VIIa); approximately 1% of circulating factor VII has been spontaneously activated to VII.[53] TF is a transmembrane protein that exists in an inactive form on the endothelial membrane, but is activated into an active enzyme with factors IX and X as substrates.[54]

TABLE 27-7 COAGULATION FACTORS AND SYNONYMS

FACTOR	SYNONYM	PRIMARY FUNCTION
I	Fibrinogen	Source of fibrin to form clot
II	Prothrombin	Source of thrombin that activates fibrinogen, V, VII, VIII, XI, XIII, protein C, platelets
Tissue factor	Previously called factor III	Cofactor for factor VIIa
Calcium	Previously called factor IV	Cofactor for clotting factor binding to phosphatidylserine
V	Labile factor	Va is cofactor in the prothrombinase complex
VII	Stable factor, proconvertin	VIIa forms a complex with tissue factor and activates factors IX and X
VIII	Antihemophilic factor	VIIIa is a component of tenase complex
IX	Christmas factor	IXa is a component of tenase complex, activates factor X
X	Stuart-Prower factor	Xa is component of prothrombinase complex, activates prothrombin
XI	Plasma thromboplastin antecedent	XIa activates factor IX
XII	Hageman (contact) factor	XIIa activates factor XI
XIII	Fibrin-stabilizing factor	XIIIa cross-links fibrin

Activated platelets are important participants in clotting. The phosphatidylserine-rich surface produced during activation provides a matrix on which several important complexes of clotting factors are formed. These include the intrinsic pathway's *tenase complex* (factor X and activated factors VIII and IX) that activates factor X and the *prothrombinase complex* (prothrombin and activated factors X and V) that activates prothrombin into thrombin (see Figure 27-22). Thrombin then converts fibrinogen into fibrin, which polymerizes into a fibrin clot. Thrombin has broad reactivity in the inflammatory response.[55] In addition to producing fibrin, thrombin is an activator of other coagulation proteins (e.g., factors V, VIII, XI, XIII), platelets (e.g., aggregation, degranulation), endothelial cells (e.g., up-regulation of adhesion molecules for leukocytes, increased NO, PGI_2, PDGF), and monocytes (e.g., cytokine secretion, increased receptors for endothelial cells).

The extrinsic pathway is clearly predominant; individuals with deficiencies in intrinsic pathway components (i.e., factor XI, factor XII) do not have prolonged bleeding.[56] As with the complement cascade, the clotting system is complex with a large number of alternative activators and inhibitors, and the relative importance of particular factors may differ between in vivo hemostasis and in vitro testing of clotting or may depend on the particular mechanism by which the pathway is activated.[57] Also there is interaction between components of the intrinsic and extrinsic pathways so that an activated member of one pathway may activate a member of the other pathway (e.g., factor VIIa of the extrinsic pathway can directly activate factor IX of the intrinsic pathway).

Another similarity with the complement system is that some complexes may have biologic activities outside the predominantly described pathway. For instance, in vitro studies have showed that the TF/VIIa complex activates protease-activated receptors (PARs); thus TF may contribute to other biologic processes by facilitating signaling in vascular cells (Figure 27-23). Abnormal TF expression in the vessel wall and/or low circulating cells initiates life-threatening thrombosis in various diseases. TF also contributes to inflammation, tumor angiogenesis and metastasis, and cell migration (Figure 27-24).

Control of Hemostatic Mechanisms

The endothelium is the major site of hemostasis. Despite the continual presence of clotting factors and platelets in the circulation, blood normally remains fluid. Thus the major regulatory factors that control hemostasis reside where the greatest probability of clotting would occur: on the endothelial cell surface (see Figure 27-18). The primary anticoagulant mechanisms include thrombin inhibitors (e.g., antithrombin III), tissue factor inhibitors (e.g., tissue factor pathway inhibitor), and mechanisms for degrading activated clotting factors (e.g., protein C).[58] Antithrombotic mechanisms are listed in Table 27-8.

Antithrombin III (AT-III) is a circulating plasma serine protease inhibitor produced by the liver. Specifically, it inhibits thrombin and several activated clotting factors (e.g., VIIa, IXa, Xa, XIa, XIIa). Clinically administered heparin or heparan sulfate (on the surface of endothelial cells) binds to AT-III and induces a conformational change that greatly enhances its activity. Under normal conditions the presence of endothelial cell heparan sulfate and available AT-III in the circulation cooperate to protect the vessels from the effects of spontaneously activated thrombin (see Figure 27-18).

Acquired AT-III deficiencies can result from infection with bacteria that produce AT-III inhibitors, sepsis, liver disease, and nephrotic syndrome and lead to venous thrombosis and pulmonary embolism.

Tissue factor pathway inhibitor (TFPI) is produced by endothelial cells and platelets and complexes to, and reversibly inhibits, factor Xa.[59] The resultant TFPI/Xa complex inhibits TF/VIIa, which mediates feedback inhibition of tissue factor as well as factor VIIa (see Figure 27-18). Although the majority of TFPI remains associated with endothelial or platelet surfaces, about 20% circulates in plasma with lipoproteins. Heparin increases plasma levels of TFPI, which may contribute to heparin's antithrombotic effects.

Thrombomodulin is a membrane thrombin-binding protein on the surface of endothelial cells. **Protein C** in the circulation binds to thrombomodulin in a thrombin-dependent manner and is converted to activated protein C (see Figure 27-18).[60] Activated protein C, in association with a cofactor **(protein S),** degrades factors Va and VIIIa. Deficiencies of AT-III, protein C, or protein S are important causes of hypercoagulation (increased clotting).[61] Expression of thrombomodulin and the endothelial cell protein C receptor is down-regulated by cytokines and other products of inflammation (e.g., IL-1α, tumor necrosis factor-alpha [TNF-α], endotoxin). Decreased

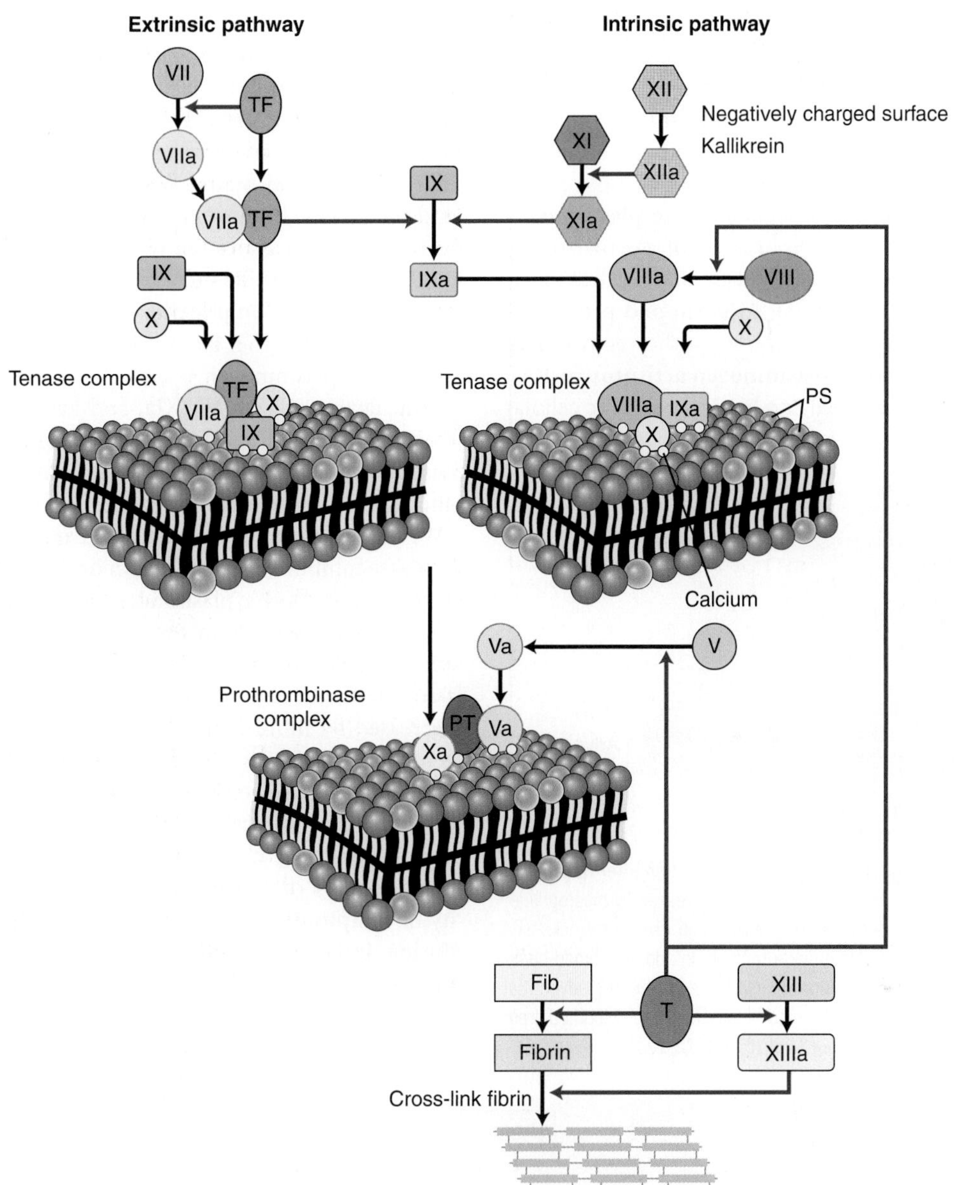

FIGURE 27-22 The Clotting System. The clotting system is frequently presented with two routes of initiation: the intrinsic and extrinsic pathways. The intrinsic pathway is initiated by activation of factor XII to XIIa by negatively charged molecules or surfaces or by the action of kallikrein, a member of the kinin system. Factor XIIa induces enzymatic activation of factor XI to XIa, which activates IX to IXa. A complex of factors IXa/VIIIa/X and calcium aggregate on the surface of activated platelets that have externalized the plasma membrane phospholipid phosphatidylserine *(PS)*. The IXa/VIIIa complex is an active enzyme ("tenase") that can activate factor X to Xa. The extrinsic pathway is the primary physiologic route of activation and is activated by exposure of tissue factor *(TF)* on endothelial cells or in the circulation. TF activates factor VII in the blood to factor VIIa. The TF/VIIa complex associates with circulating factors IX and X and calcium on the PS-rich surface of activated platelets. The TF/VIIa/IX complex is a tenase that produces Xa. The VIIa/TF complex also can activate factor IX to IXa and facilitate the formation of the VIIIa/IXa tenase. Factor Xa associates with activated factor V *(Va)* and prothrombin *(PT)* in a PS and calcium-dependent complex that is a "prothrombinase," which converts PT to thrombin *(T)*. Thrombin is an active enzyme that converts fibrinogen *(Fib)* to fibrin. Thrombin also activates factor XIII to XIIIa, which cross-links fibrin into a matrix that seals clots. Thrombin amplifies the clotting process by activating factor VIII to VIIIa and facilitating formation of the VIIIa/IXa tenase and by activating factor V to Va to create further prothrombinase complexes.

expression prevents protein C activation, thereby enhancing clot formation. Activated protein C inhibits the adhesion of neutrophils to the endothelium, but during inflammation the neutrophil enzyme elastase enzymatically removes thrombomodulin from the endothelial cell surface.[62]

Lysis of Blood Clots

Concurrent with activation of coagulation is the activation of pathways that limit the size of the clot and remove the clot after bleeding has ceased and repair has begun. The primary mechanism for lysis (breakdown) of blood clots is the

fibrinolytic system (plasminogen-plasmin system) that produces plasmin. **Plasmin** (also called *fibrinase* or *fibrinolysin*) is a serine protease that degrades fibrin polymers in clots.[63]

The inactive precursor of plasmin is **plasminogen,** which is produced in the liver (Figure 27-25). Plasminogen activation may occur by several means, although the most physiologically important is by the action of **tissue plasminogen activator (t-PA).**[64] Endothelial cells at a site of vascular injury express t-PA, which is also a serine protease that reaches maximal enzymatic activity after binding to fibrin and proteolytically activates plasminogen to plasmin. Another activator of plasminogen is **urokinase-like plasminogen activator (u-PA).** The u-PA is a serine protease that can bind to a specific cellular u-PA receptor (u-PAR), causing activation of plasminogen and resulting in plasmin generation. This urokinase is the major activator of fibrinolysis in the *extravascular* or tissue compartment, whereas t-PA is largely involved in *intravascular* fibrinolysis. Several cancers appear to use membrane-bound u-PA to digest intercellular matrix and greatly facilitate tumor invasion and metastasis. Both t-PA and u-PA have been used clinically to treat diseases associated with a blood clot (e.g., pulmonary embolism, myocardial infarction, stroke).

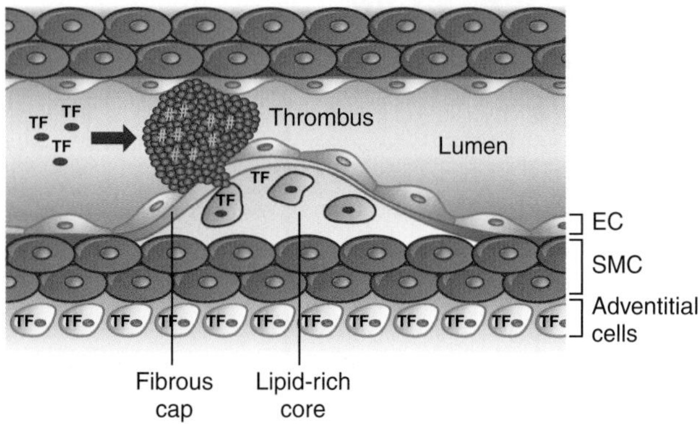

FIGURE 27-23 Tissue Factor (TF) in Thrombus Formation after Rupture of an Atherosclerotic Plaque. In atherosclerosis TF is expressed by macrophage-derived foam cells and within atherosclerotic plaque. High levels of TF exposed on rupture trigger thrombosis and myocardial infarction. In addition, blood-borne TF may contribute to thrombus propagation. TF is also expressed by adventitial cells *(blue)*. *EC,* Endothelial cells; *SMC,* smooth muscle cells. (Modified from Mackman N: *Arterioscler Thromb Vasc Biol* 24[6]:1015–1022, 2004.)

As with most components of inflammation, plasmin interacts greatly with other factors. In addition to activation by t-PA and u-PA, plasminogen is activated to plasmin by thrombin, fibrin, factor XIIa, factor XIa, and kallikrein. Plasmin is proteolytic to several substrates, including activation of collagenases, complement components C1 and C3, and factor XII, and cleaves fibronectin, fibrin, thrombospondin, laminin, and vWF. Plasmin activity is usually controlled directly by the serine protease inhibitor α_2-antiplasmin or by inhibiting plasminogen activation by specific plasminogen activator inhibitors (PAIs).

Congenital defects in the fibrinolytic system are very rare and variable in effects. Congenital plasminogen deficiency is associated with venous thrombosis if the plasminogen level is decreased by more than 50%. Apparent defects in plasminogen may result from dysfunctional plasminogen or an absence of fibrinogen. Congenital deficiencies of plasminogen activator or abnormal increases in plasminogen activator inhibitor also may increase the chance for spontaneous thrombosis. Alternative routes of fibrin degradation may mitigate the severity of symptoms in these deficiencies. Other enzymes released during inflammation (e.g., leukocyte elastase, cathepsin G, metalloproteinases [MMPs]) are fibrinolytic.

Cross-linked fibrin is deposited in tissues around wounds, inflammatory sites, and tumors. Fibrin removal is an

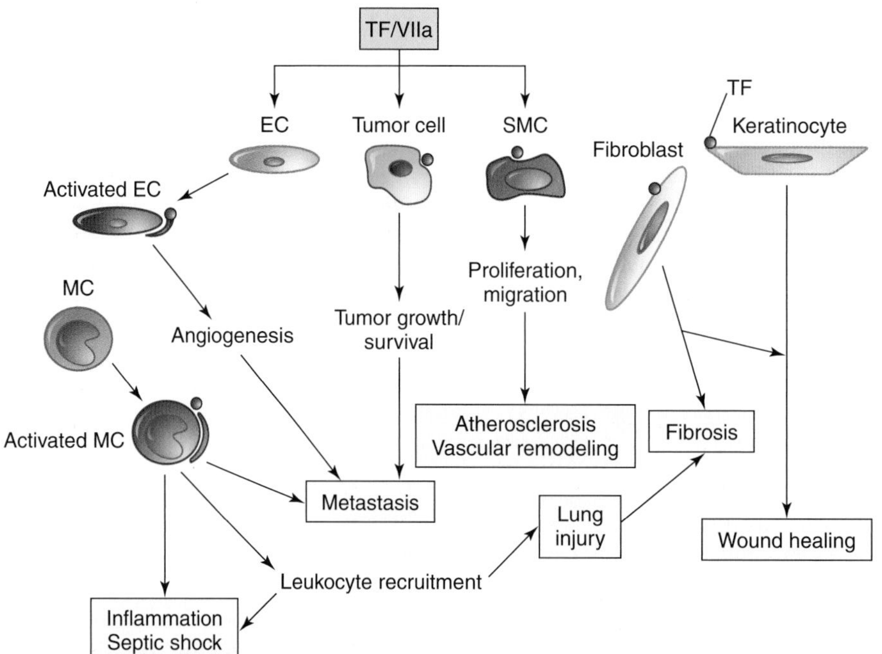

FIGURE 27-24 Factor VIIa Signaling Through Tissue Factor (TF) Expressed on the Surface of Cells Mediates Changes in Disease-Related Cellular Activities. *EC,* Endothelial cell; *MC,* monocyte/macrophage; *SMC,* smooth muscle cell. (Modified from Rao LV, Pendurthi UR: *Arterioscler Thromb Vasc Biol* 25[1]:47–56, 2005.)

TABLE 27-8 ANTITHROMBOTIC MECHANISMS OF ENDOTHELIAL CELLS

FUNCTION REGULATED	SUBSTANCES INVOLVED
Clotting cascade	Tissue factor pathway inhibitor Antithrombin III Heparan sulfate Thrombomodulin/protein C/protein S
Vessel and platelet activity	Covering of prothrombotic intercellular matrix molecules Prostacyclin (PGI_2) Nitric oxide (NO) Adenosine diphosphate
Eliminate fibrin clot	Plasminogen activators

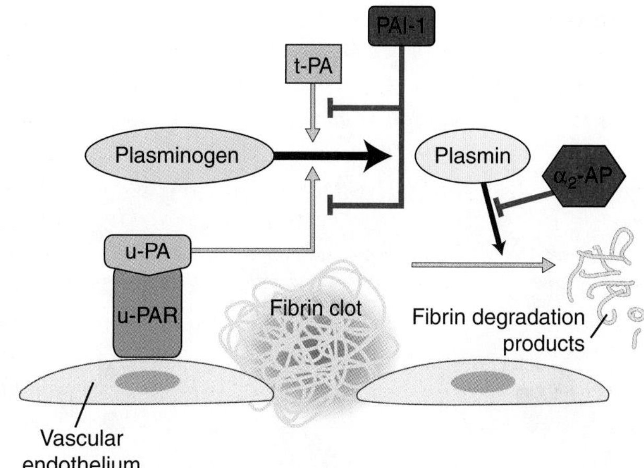

FIGURE 27-25 The Fibrinolytic System. Fibrinolysis is initiated by the binding of plasminogen to fibrin. Although tissue plasminogen activator *(t-PA)* initiates intravascular fibrinolysis, urokinase plasminogen activator *(u-PA)* is the major activator of fibrinolysis in tissue (extravascular). Inhibitors (indicated by red lines) of fibrinolysis include α_2-antiplasmin *(α_2-AP)* that inhibits plasmin and plasminogen activator inhibitor 1 *(PAI-1)* that inhibits t-PA. Plasmin digests the fibrin into smaller soluble pieces (fibrin degradation products). *u-PAR,* Urokinase-like plasminogen activator receptor.

important biologic process, for intravascular and extravascular spaces, with various controlling mechanisms that can lead to abnormalities of fibrin accumulation and thrombotic events and can be a structural barrier to tumor invasion (see Chapter 13).

Products of fibrinolysis include **fibrin degradation products (FDPs)** (see Figure 27-25). A major FDP is D-dimer. **D-dimer** is two D domains from adjacent fibrin monomers that are cross-linked by factor XIIIa and released as a result of enzymatic cleavage by plasmin. Measurement of levels of circulating D-dimer has been used for diagnosis of deep venous thrombosis (DVT) or pulmonary embolism (PE). Despite extensive literature, the diagnostic role of D-dimer is unclear because of the use of multiple D-dimer assays with different sensitivities and variabilities.[65]

CLINICAL EVALUATION OF THE HEMATOLOGIC SYSTEM

Tests of Bone Marrow Function

The bone marrow is the soft spongy tissue found within bones, especially the sternum, pelvis, and femur. Several abnormal conditions in the numbers or morphology of circulating blood cells or suspected infection of the marrow may justify further investigation of the bone marrow.

Usually bone marrow is aspirated from the sternum or pelvis using a needle. In children a bone marrow aspirate can be obtained from the vertebrae or the femur. The aspirate is examined microscopically and may be cultured if infection (e.g., fungi, mycobacteria, brucellosis, typhoid fever) is suspected. Microscopic evaluation may also include flow cytometry, chromosome analysis, or polymerase chain reaction (PCR) related to the presence of atypical cells, the presence of atypical numbers of normal cells, and the absence of particular cell types. A normal bone marrow aspirate contains stromal cells (fibroblasts, macrophages, osteoblasts, adipocytes), stem cells (hematopoietic, mesenchymal, and endothelial), and immature and mature forms of blood cells (erythrocytes, leukocytes, platelets) (Figure 27-26). The differential cell count of a bone marrow aspirate involves examining approximately 400 nucleated cells under oil-immersion magnification and counting populations of cells differentiated based on morphology. The relative number of each type of stem cell is expressed as a fraction of 400 (Table 27-9).

Bone marrow iron stores, primarily in macrophages, can be examined using special stains (e.g., Prussian blue) for iron-containing granules. A direct measure of iron stores also can be obtained only from liver biopsy specimens, although bone marrow is preferred as a safer procedure and because the bone marrow is the immediate source of iron destined for erythrocyte production.

Bone marrow aspiration is an important diagnostic test for severe central defects in hematopoiesis (e.g., aplastic anemia, metabolic anemias arising from insufficient iron or inadequate erythropoietin, thrombocytopenia, neutropenia; see Chapters 28 and 29). Examination of the bone marrow is also useful to diagnose B-lymphocyte immune deficiencies (see Chapter 9), nonmalignant myeloproliferative disorders (e.g., polycythemia vera), and lymphoid/monocytic malignancies (e.g., leukemias, myelomas, lymphomas; see Chapters 29 and 30). This test can also be used to monitor the effects of chemotherapy on malignancies that have invaded the bone marrow (see Figure 27-26). A marrow aspirate that is richly cellular implies normal or increased hematopoiesis but does not indicate whether marrow activity is effective.

Results from bone marrow aspiration are sometimes limited because this technique disturbs the architecture of the marrow and only provides an analysis of the general cellularity (numbers of constituent cells) of the marrow. On occasion, analysis of an aspirate may only suggest the presence of a malignancy or a central defect in hematopoiesis without being clearly confirmatory, or the sample may be inadequate for diagnosis of bone marrow fibrosis. In these cases the need for a bone marrow biopsy may be indicated.

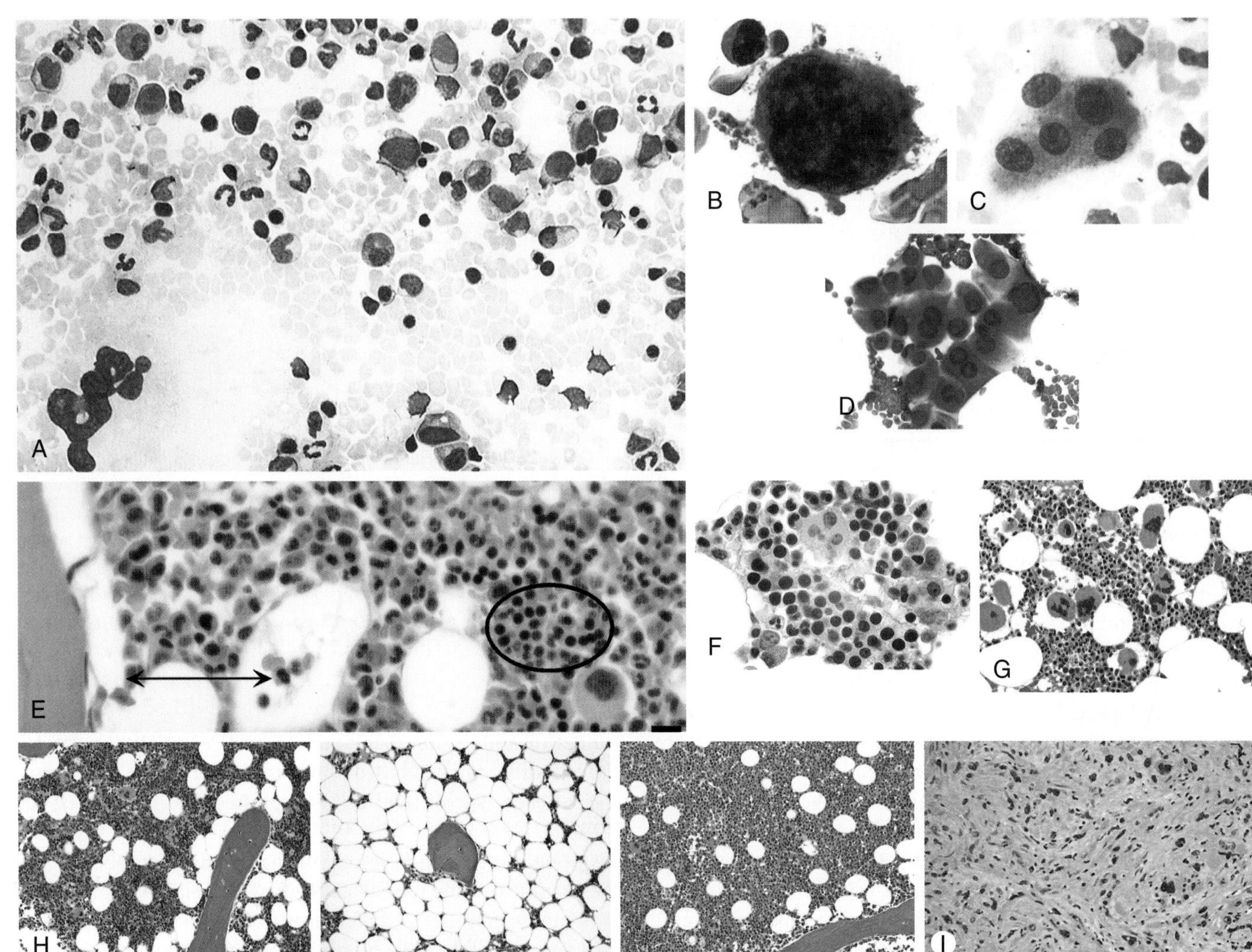

FIGURE 27-26 Bone marrow samples. Images **A** through **D** contain bone marrow aspirates; images **E** through **I** contain bone marrow biospy specimens. **A,** Normal bone marrow aspirate stained by the May-Grünwald/Giemsa technique. **B,** A normal megakaryocyte with budding platelets at the plasma membrane (Wright stain). **C,** Osteoclasts containing multiple nuclei that are separated by cytoplasm. These cells may be confused with megakaryocytes. **D,** Metastatic adenocarcinoma of the breast. **E,** Normal bone marrow biospy with paratrabecular space with immature myeloid cells (two-headed arrow) and circled erythron (site of erythrocyte production). **F,** A normal erythroid island in which several erythroid precursor clusters. **G,** Essential thrombocytopenia with normal cellularity, but increased numbers of large megakaryocytes. **H,** Bone marrow biopsies representing conditions of normal cellularity *(left),* hypocellularity *(middle)* as would be seen in conditions of bone marrow depletion such as aplastic anemia, and hypercellularity *(right)* as seen in malignant conditions. **I,** Advanced chronic idiopathic myelofibrosis marked by extensive replacement of the normal marrow stroma by fibrous tissue (stained pink; hematoxylin-eosin stain). (Sources for photographs: **A, C** from Hoffbrand V et al: *Color atlas of clinical hematology,* ed 4, Philadelphia, Mosby, 2013; **B** from Rodak BF et al: *Hematology,* ed 4, Philadelphia, Saunders, 2012; **D, F, G, H** from Jaffe E: *Hematology,* Philadelphia, Saunders, 2010; **E** from Young: *Clinical hematology,* ed 1, Mosby, 2005; **I** from Cleveland Clinic: *Current clinical medicine,* ed 2, Philadelphia, Saunders, 2010.)

TABLE 27-9 **DIFFERENTIAL CELL COUNTS IN BONE MARROW WITH AGE**

DEVELOPING CELLS IN MARROW	BIRTH	1 MONTH-1 YEAR	1-4 YEARS	4-12 YEARS	ADULT
Erythrocytic series	14	8	19	21	20
Lymphocytic series	14	47	22	18	17
Eosinophilic series	3	3	6	3	3
Neutrophilic series	60	33	50	52	57
Myeloid/erythroid ratio	4:3	4:0	1:3	2:5	1:3

NOTE: Values are percentages of cell types counted during examination of a marrow specimen containing approximately 400 nucleated cells.

During a biopsy, a special needle is used to obtain a "core" or cylindrical sample of bone and marrow in which the three-dimensional structure of the marrow is preserved. The biopsy specimens provide the most reliable and complete information about marrow cellularity (see Figure 27-26). Obtaining a bone marrow biopsy is, however, usually more painful and expensive than aspiration. Therefore, biopsy is not performed unless insufficient information is obtained from aspiration.

Blood Tests

Blood tests provide information about the absolute and relative numbers of blood cells in a specimen of blood, as well as various structural and functional characteristics of the cells, and usually provide the initial justification for performing a bone marrow aspiration. Deviations from the normal differential distribution and the presence of abnormal or immature cells can reflect disease, physiologic states (e.g., pregnancy, infancy, old age), injury, or dysfunction in almost any part of the body. Blood tests that reflect chiefly hematologic disorders are listed in Table 27-10.

PEDIATRICS AND THE HEMATOLOGIC SYSTEM

Blood cell counts tend to rise above adult levels at birth and then decline gradually throughout childhood. Table 27-11 lists normal ranges during infancy and childhood. The immediate rise in values is the result of accelerated hematopoiesis during fetal life, increased numbers of cells that result from the trauma of birth, and cutting of the umbilical cord.

Average blood volume in the full-term neonate is 85 ml/kg of body weight. The premature infant has a slightly larger blood volume of 90 ml/kg of body weight, with the mean increasing to 150 mg/kg during the first few days after birth. In both full-term and premature infants, blood volume decreases during the first few months. Thereafter the average blood volume is 75 to 77 ml/kg, which is similar to that of older children and adults.

The hypoxic intrauterine environment stimulates erythropoietin production in the fetus and accelerates fetal erythropoiesis, producing polycythemia (excessive proliferation of erythrocyte precursors) of the newborn. After birth the oxygen from the lungs saturates arterial blood, and more oxygen is delivered to the tissues. In response to the change from a placental to a pulmonary oxygen supply during the first few days of life, levels of erythropoietin and the rate of blood cell formation decrease.

The very active rate of fetal erythropoiesis results in a large number of immature erythrocytes (reticulocytes) in the peripheral blood of full-term neonates. After birth the number of reticulocytes decreases about 50% every 12 hours so that it is rare to find an elevated reticulocyte count after the first week of life. During this period of rapid growth, the rate of erythrocyte destruction is greater than that in later childhood and adulthood. In full-term infants, normal erythrocyte life span is 60 to 80 days; in premature infants, it may be as short as 20 to 30 days; and in children and adolescents, it is the same as that in adults—120 days.

The postnatal decrease in hemoglobin and hematocrit values is more marked in premature infants than in the full-term infant. In the preschool and school-age child, hemoglobin, hematocrit, and red blood cell counts gradually rise. Metabolic processes within the erythrocytes of neonates differ significantly from those of erythrocytes in the normal adult. Among other differences, the relatively young population of erythrocytes in the newborn consumes greater quantities of glucose than do erythrocytes in adults.

Children have quantitative and qualitative differences in clotting factors that result in decreased risk for thrombotic diseases and complications.[66] Levels of some clotting-related proteins are reduced in newborns (e.g., antithrombin III). Several clotting factors are initially produced in fetal forms (e.g., fibrinogen, antithrombin III) that are less active in thrombosis than adult forms.

At birth, the lymphocyte count is high and continues to rise during the first year of life, and then steadily declines until lower adult values are reached. The lymphocytes of children also tend to have more cytoplasm and less compact nuclear chromatin than do the lymphocytes of adults. A possible explanation is that children tend to have more frequent viral infections, some of which are subclinical, and are receiving vaccinations, both of which are associated with atypical lymphocytes.

The neutrophil count, like the lymphocyte count, is high at birth and rises during the first days of life. After 2 weeks the neutrophil count falls to within or below the normal adult range. By approximately 4 years of age, the neutrophil count is the same as that of an adult. The eosinophil count is high in the first year of life and higher in children than in teenagers or adults. Monocyte counts also are high in the first year of life but then decrease to adult levels. Platelet counts in full-term neonates are comparable with platelet counts in adults and remain so throughout infancy and childhood.

AGING AND THE HEMATOLOGIC SYSTEM

Blood composition changes little with age. Erythrocyte life span in older adults is normal, although erythrocytes are replenished more slowly after bleeding, probably because of iron depletion. Total serum iron, total iron-binding capacity, and intestinal iron absorption are all decreased in older adults. Iron deficiency is often responsible for the low hemoglobin levels noted in older adults. The plasma membranes of erythrocytes become increasingly fragile, presumably because of physical trauma inflicted during circulation.

Lymphocyte function decreases with age (see Chapters 8 and 9), causing changes in cellular immunity with some decline in T-cell function. The humoral immune system is less able to respond to antigenic challenge. No changes in platelet numbers or structure have been observed in elderly persons, yet platelet adhesiveness probably increases. Although fibrinogen levels and levels of factors V, VII, and IX tend to be increased in older adults, evidence concerning hypercoagulability is inconclusive.

TABLE 27-10 **BLOOD TESTS FOR HEMATOLOGIC DISORDERS**

CELL TYPE AND TEST	PROPERTY EVALUATED BY TEST	POSSIBLE HEMATOLOGIC CAUSE OF ABNORMAL FINDINGS
Erythrocyte		
Red cell count	Number (in millions) of erythrocytes/μL of blood	Altered erythropoiesis, anemias, hemorrhage, Hodgkin disease, leukemia
Mean corpuscular volume	Size of erythrocytes	Anemias, thalassemias
Mean corpuscular hemoglobin (MCH)	Amount of hemoglobin in each erythrocyte (by weight)	Anemias, hemoglobinopathy
Mean corpuscular hemoglobin concentration (MCHC)	Concentration of hemoglobin in each erythrocyte (percentage of erythrocyte occupied by hemoglobin)	Anemias, hereditary spherocytosis
Hemoglobin determination	Amount of hemoglobin (by weight)/dl of blood	Anemias
Hematocrit determination	Percentage of a given volume of blood that is occupied by erythrocytes	Hemorrhage, polycythemia, erythrocytosis, anemias, leukemia
Reticulocyte count	Number of reticulocytes/μL of blood (also expressed as percentage of reticulocytes in total red cell count)	Hyperactive or hypoactive bone marrow function
Erythrocyte osmotic fragility test	Cellular shape (biconcavity), structure of plasma membrane	Anemias, hemolytic disease caused by ABO or Rh incompatibility, Hodgkin disease, polycythemia vera, thalassemia major
Hemoglobin electrophoresis	Relative percentage of different types of hemoglobin in erythrocytes	Sickle cell disease, sickle cell trait, hemoglobin C disease, hemoglobin C trait, thalassemias
Sickle cell test	Presence of hemoglobin S in erythrocytes	Sickle cell trait, sickle cell anemia
Glucose-6-phospahte dehydrogenase (G6PD) deficiency test	Deficiency of G6PD in erythrocytes	Hemolytic anemia
Hemoglobin Metabolism		
Serum ferritin determination	Depletion of body iron (potential deficiency of heme synthesis)	Iron deficiency anemias
Total iron-binding capacity (TIBC)	Amount of iron in serum plus amount of transferrin available in serum (mcg/dl)	Hemorrhage, iron deficiency anemia, hemochromatosis, hemosiderosis, iron overload, anemias, thalassemias
Transferrin saturation	Percentage of transferrin that is saturated with iron	Acute hemorrhage, hemochromatosis, hemosiderosis, sideroblastic anemia, iron deficiency anemia, iron overload, thalassemias
Porphyrin analysis (protoporphyrin analysis)	Concentration of protoporphyrin in erythrocytes (mcg/dl); an indicator of iron-deficient erythropoiesis	Megaloblastic anemia, congenital erythropoietic porphyria
Direct antiglobulin test (DAT)	Antibody binding to erythrocytes	Hemolytic disease of the newborn, autoimmune hemolytic anemia, drug-induced hemolytic anemia, transfusion reaction
Antibody screen (indirect Coombs test)	Detection of antibodies to erythrocyte antigens (other than the ABO antigens)	Same as for DAT
Leukocytes		
Differential white cell count (absolute number of a type of leukocyte/μL of blood)	See below	See below
Neutrophil count	Neutrophils/μL	Myeloproliferative disorders, hematopoietic disorders, hemolysis, infection, immune deficiency
Lymphocyte count	Lymphocytes/μL	Infectious lymphocytosis, infectious mononucleosis, hematopoietic disorders, anemias, leukemia, lymphosarcoma, Hodgkin disease, primary immune deficiency
Plasma cell count	Plasma cells/μL	Infectious mononucleosis, lymphocytosis, plasma cell leukemia, primary immune deficiency
Monocyte count	Monocytes/μL	Hodgkin disease, infectious mononucleosis, monocytic leukemia, non-Hodgkin lymphoma, polycythemia vera, primary immune deficiency
Eosinophil count	Eosinophils/μL	Hematopoietic disorders
Basophil count	Basophils/μL	Chronic myelogenous leukemia, hemolytic anemias, Hodgkin disease, polycythemia vera

TABLE 27-10 BLOOD TESTS FOR HEMATOLOGIC DISORDERS—cont'd

CELL TYPE AND TEST	PROPERTY EVALUATED BY TEST	POSSIBLE HEMATOLOGIC CAUSE OF ABNORMAL FINDINGS
Platelets and Clotting Factors*		
Platelet count	Number of circulating platelets (in thousands)/μL of blood	Anemias, multiple myeloma, myelofibrosis, polycythemia vera, leukemia, disseminated intravascular coagulation (DIC), hemolytic disease of the newborn, idiopathic thrombocytopenic purpura, transfusion reaction, lymphoproliferative disorders
Bleeding time	Duration of bleeding following a standardized superficial puncture wound of the skin, integrity of the platelet plug, measured in minutes following puncture	Leukemia, anemias, DIC, fibrinolytic activity, purpuras, hemorrhagic disease of the newborn, infectious mononucleosis, multiple myeloma, clotting factor deficiencies, thrombasthenia, thrombocytopenia, von Willebrand disease
Clot retraction test	Platelet number and function, fibrinogen quantity and use, measured in hours required for expression of serum from a clot incubated in a test tube	Acute leukemia, aplastic anemia, factor XIII deficiency, increased fibrinolytic activity, Hodgkin disease, hyperfibrinogenemia or hypofibrinogenemia, idiopathic thrombocytopenic purpura, multiple myeloma, polycythemia vera, secondary thrombocytopenia, thrombasthenia
Platelet adhesion studies	Ability of platelets to adhere to foreign surfaces	Anemia, macroglobulinemia, Bernard-Soulier syndrome, multiple myeloma, myeloid metaplasia, plasma cell dyscrasias, thrombasthenia, thrombocytopathy, von Willebrand disease
Platelet aggregation tests	Ability of platelets to adhere to one another	Afibrinogenemia, Bernard-Soulier syndrome, thrombasthenia, hemorrhagic thrombocythemia, myeloid metaplasia, plasma cell dyscrasias, platelet release defects, polycythemia vera, preleukemia, sideroblastic anemia, von Willebrand disease, Waldenström macroglobulinemia, hypercoagulability
Whole blood clotting time (Lee-White coagulation time)	Overall ability of blood to clot, as measured in minutes in a test tube	Afibrinogenemia, clotting factor deficiencies, excessive fibrinolysis, hemorrhagic disease of the newborn, hypofibrinogenemia, hypoprothrombinemia, leukemia
Circulating anticoagulants (immunoglobulin G [IgG] or M [IgM] antibodies that inhibit coagulation)	Presence of antibodies that neutralize clotting factors and inhibit coagulation, as indicated by prolonged clotting time, prothrombin time, or partial thromboplastin time	Afibrinogenemia, presence of fibrin-fibrinogen degradation products, macroglobulinemia, multiple myeloma, DIC, plasma cell dyscrasias
Partial thromboplastin time (PTT)	Effectiveness of clotting factors (except factors VII and VIII), effectiveness of intrinsic pathway of coagulation cascade, as measured by a test tube (in seconds)	Presence of circulating anticoagulants, DIC, clotting factor deficiencies, excessive fibrinolysis, hemorrhagic disease of the newborn, hypofibrinogenemia and afibrinogenemia, prothrombin deficiency, von Willebrand disease, acute hemorrhage
Prothrombin time (PT)	Effectiveness of activity of prothrombin, fibrinogen, and factors V, VII, and X; effectiveness of vitamin K–dependent coagulation factors of the extrinsic and common pathways of the coagulation cascade as measured in a test tube (in seconds)	Hypofibrinogenemia, dysfibrinogenemia, and afibrinogenemia; presence of circulating anticoagulants; DIC; deficiency of factors V, VII, or X; presence of fibrin degradation products, increased fibrinolytic activity, hemolytic jaundice, hemorrhagic disease of the newborn; acute leukemia, polycythemia vera, prothrombin deficiency, multiple myeloma
Thrombin time	Quantity and activity of fibrinogen as measured in a test tube (in seconds)	Hypofibrinogenemia, dysfibrinogenemia, and afibrinogenemia; presence of circulating anticoagulants; hemorrhagic disease of the newborn, polycythemia vera; increase in fibrin-fibrinogen degradation products; increased fibrinolytic activity
Fibrinogen assay	Amount of fibrinogen available for fibrin formation	Acute leukemia, congenital hypofibrinogenemia or afibrinogenemia, DIC, increased fibrinolytic activity, severe hemorrhage
Fibrin-fibrinogen degradation products (fibrin-fibrinogen split products)	Fibrinogenic activity as measured by levels of fibrin-fibrinogen degradation products (in mcg/ml of blood)	Transfusion reactions, DIC, internal hemorrhage in the newborn, deep vein thrombosis, pulmonary embolism

Data from Byrne CJ et al: *Laboratory tests: implications for nursing care,* Menlo Park, CA, 1986, Addison-Wesley; Bick RL et al: *Hematology: clinical and laboratory practice,* St Louis, 1993, Mosby.

***Note:** See Figure 27-22 and Table 27-7 for information about clotting factors and their sequence of activation in the coagulation cascade.

TABLE 27-11 HEMATOLOGIC VALUES DURING INFANCY AND CHILDHOOD

					DIFFERENTIAL COUNTS				
AGE	**HEMOGLOBIN (g/dl):MEAN**	**HEMATOCRIT (%):MEAN**	**RETICULOCYTES (%):MEAN**	**LEUKOCYTES (WBC/mm^3):MEAN**	**NEUTROPHILS (%):MEAN**	**LYMPHOCYTES (%):MEAN**	**EOSINOPHILS (%):MEAN**	**MONOCYTES (%):MEAN**	**PLATELETS (10^3/mm^3)**
Cord blood	16.8	55	5.0	18,000	61	31	2	6	290
2 wk	16.5	50	1.0	12,000	40	48	3	9	252
3 mo	12.0	36	1.0	12,000	30	63	2	5	140-340
6 mo-6 yr	12.0	37	1.0	10,000	45	48	2	5	140-340
7-12 yr	13.0	38	1.0	8,000	55	38	2	5	140-340
Adult	13.0	40	1.0	8,000	55	35	2	5	140-340
Female	14	41	0.8-4.1	7,400	54-62	25-33	1-4	3-7	140-340
Male	16	47	0.8-2.5	7,400	54-62	25-33	1-4	3-7	140-340

WBC, White blood cell.

SUMMARY REVIEW

Components of the Hematologic System

1. Blood consists of cells suspended in a solution of about 90% water and 10% solutes. In adults the total blood volume is approximately 5.5 L.
2. Plasma, the liquid portion of the blood, contains two major groups of proteins: albumins and globulins.
3. The cellular elements of blood are the erythrocytes (red blood cells), leukocytes (white blood cells), and platelets (thrombocytes).
4. Erythrocytes are the most abundant cells of the blood, occupying approximately 48% of the blood volume in men and approximately 42% in women. Erythrocytes are responsible for tissue oxygenation.
5. Leukocytes are fewer in number than erythrocytes and constitute approximately 5000 to 10,000 cells/mm^3 of blood. Leukocytes defend the body against infection and remove dead or injured host cells.
6. Leukocytes are classified as either granulocytes (neutrophils, basophils, eosinophils) or agranulocytes (monocytes, macrophages, lymphocytes).
7. The neutrophil is the most abundant leukocyte (approximately 55% of the leukocytes) and is the primary granulocyte that defends against infections.
8. Lymphocytes are the primary cells of the immune response.
9. Platelets are not cells—they are disk-shaped cytoplasmic fragments. Platelets are essential for blood coagulation and control of bleeding.
10. The lymphoid organs are classified as primary (thymus and bone marrow) or secondary (spleen, lymph nodes, tonsils, and Peyer patches of the small intestine).
11. The lymphoid organs are sites of residence, proliferation, differentiation, and function of lymphocytes and mononuclear phagocytes.
12. The spleen is the largest of the secondary lymphoid organs and functions as the site of hematopoiesis in the fetus, filters and cleanses the blood, and is a reservoir for lymphocytes and other blood cells.
13. The lymph nodes are the site of development or activity of large numbers of lymphocytes, monocytes, and macrophages.
14. The MPS is composed of macrophages in tissue and lymphoid organs.
15. The MPS is the main line of defense against bacteria in the bloodstream and cleanses the blood by removing old, injured, or dead blood cells; antigen-antibody complexes; and macromolecules.

Development of Blood Cells

1. Hematopoiesis, or blood cell production, occurs in the liver and spleen of the fetus and in the bone marrow after birth.
2. Hematopoiesis involves two stages: (a) proliferation, and (b) maturation.
3. Hematopoiesis continues throughout life to replace blood cells that grow old and die, are killed by disease, or are lost through bleeding.
4. Bone marrow consists of red (hematopoietic) marrow (blood vessels, mononuclear phagocytes, stem cells, blood cells in various stages of differentiation, stromal cells) and yellow marrow (fatty tissue).
5. The bone marrow contains multiple populations of *stem cells;* mesenchymal stem cells develop into fibroblasts, osteoclasts, and adipocytes; and hematopoietic stem cells develop into blood cells.
6. Regulation of hematopoiesis occurs in specialized microenvironments (niches) in the bone marrow (an osteoblastic niche and a vascular niche) in which hematopoietic stem cells are signaled to undergo differentiation through the effects of multiple cytokines and chemokines and through direct contact with osteoblasts (osteoblastic niche) or vascular endothelial cells (vascular niche), as well as several other specialized cells, including CAR cells and nestin-expressing cells.
7. Specific hematopoietic growth factors (e.g., colony-stimulating factors) are necessary for the adequate production of myeloid, erythroid, lymphoid, and megakaryocytic lineages.
8. Erythropoiesis (production of erythrocytes) is regulated by erythropoietin. Erythropoietin is secreted by the kidneys in response to tissue hypoxia and causes a compensatory increase in erythrocyte production if the oxygen content of the blood decreases because of anemia, high altitude, or pulmonary disease.
9. Hemoglobin, the oxygen-carrying protein of the erythrocyte, enables the blood to transport 100 times more oxygen than could be transported dissolved in plasma alone.
10. The iron cycle reutilizes iron released from old or damaged erythrocytes. Iron binds to transferrin in the blood, is transported to macrophages of the MPS, and is stored in the cytoplasm as ferritin.
11. Iron homeostasis is controlled by hepcidin, a small hormone produced by hepatocytes, which regulates ferroportin, the principal transporter of iron from stores in hepatocytes and macrophages and from intestinal cells that take up dietary iron.
12. Granulocytes and monocytes in the blood develop from common myeloid progenitor cells in the bone marrow under the direction of several growth factors, including stem cell factor, IL-3, and GM-CSF.
13. Platelets develop from megakaryocytes by a process called *endomitosis,* which is controlled by thrombopoietin. During endomitosis the megakaryocytes undergo mitosis but not cell division and the cytoplasm and plasma membrane fragment into platelets.

Mechanisms of Hemostasis

1. Hemostasis, or arrest of bleeding in damaged vessels, involves: (a) vasoconstriction, (b) damage to the endothelium and exposure of connective tissue resulting in formation of a platelet plug, (c) activation of the clotting cascade, (d) formation of a blood clot, and (e) activation of fibrinolysis for clot retraction and clot dissolution.

SUMMARY REVIEW—cont'd

2. Platelet activation involves three linked processes: (a) adhesion, (b) activation, and (c) aggregation.
3. A blood clot is a meshwork of protein strands that stabilizes the platelet plug. The strands are made of fibrin. Fibrin is the end product of the coagulation cascade.
4. The coagulation cascade is composed of intrinsic and extrinsic pathways, with the extrinsic pathway being dominant. The intrinsic pathway is initiated by TF that forms a complex with the TF/VIIa complex.
5. The endothelium prevents the formation of spontaneous clots in normal vessels by several anticoagulant mechanisms, including by production of NO and PGI_2, thrombin inhibitors (antithrombin III), and tissue factor inhibitors (tissue factor pathway inhibitors) and by degradation of activated clotting factors (thrombomodulin–protein C).
6. Fibrinolysis (breakdown of blood clots) is the function of the plasminogen-plasmin system. Plasmin is a degrading enzyme of fibrin clots. It is produced from plasminogen by activation of plasminogen activators (t-PA, u-PA), thrombin, fibrin, factor XIIa, factor XIa, and kallikrein.
7. Products of fibrinolysis include fibrin degradation products, such as D-dimer.

Clinical Evaluation of the Hematologic System

1. Tests of bone marrow function include bone marrow aspiration and bone marrow biopsy.
2. Cells contained in the marrow specimen are assessed with respect to: (a) relative numbers of stem cells and their developing daughter cells, and (b) morphologic structure.

Pediatrics and the Hematologic System

1. Blood cell counts rise above adult levels at birth and then gradually decline throughout childhood.
2. The average blood volume of an infant is 75 to 77 ml/kg, which is similar to that of older children and adults.
3. In response to the change from a placental to a pulmonary oxygen supply during the first few days of life, levels of erythropoietin and the rate of blood cell formation decrease.
4. The normal erythrocyte life span is 60 to 80 days in full-term infants, 20 to 30 days in premature infants, and 120 days in children, adolescents, and adults.
5. The lymphocyte count is high at birth, rises further during the first year of life, and steadily declines until lower adult volumes are reached.
6. The neutrophil count is very high at birth, falls to adult ranges after 2 weeks, and is the same as that for adults by 4 years of age.
7. The eosinophil count is high in the first year of life and is higher in children than in adolescents and adults. Monocyte counts are high in the first year of life and decrease to adult levels.
8. Platelet counts in full-term infants are comparable with those in adults and remain so throughout childhood.

Aging and the Hematologic System

1. Blood composition changes little with age. A delay in erythrocyte replenishment may occur after bleeding, presumably because of iron deficiency.
2. Lymphocyte function appears to decrease with age. Particularly affected is a decrease in cellular immunity.
3. Platelet adhesiveness probably increases with age.

KEY TERMS

Agranulocyte, 948, 950
Albumin, 946
Antithrombin III (AT-III), 970
Apoferritin, 963
Apotransferrin, 963
Basophil, 949
Blood clot, 969
Bone marrow, 955
Clotting (coagulation) system, 969
Clotting factor, 946
Colony-stimulating factor (CSF, hematopoietic growth factor), 958
Cyclooxygenase (COX-1), 969
D-dimer, 973
Dendritic cell, 950
Deoxyhemoglobin, 961
Endomitosis, 965
Eosinophil, 949
Erythroblast, 959
Erythrocyte (red blood cell [RBC]), 947
Erythropoiesis, 959
Erythropoietin, 959
Fibrin degradation product (FDP), 973
Fibrinolysis, 967
Fibrinolytic system (plasminogen-plasmin system), 972
Globin, 961
Globulin, 946
GPIIb-IIIa complex, 969
Granulocyte, 948
Hematopoiesis, 954
Hematopoietic stem cell (HSC), 956
Heme, 961
Hemoglobin (Hb), 961
Hemosiderin, 963
Hemostasis, 965
Immunocyte, 948
Leukocyte (white blood cell [WBC]), 948
Lymphocyte, 950
Macrophage, 950
Marginating storage pool, 959
Mast cell, 949
Megakaryocyte, 950
Mesenchymal stem cell (MSC), 956
Methemoglobin, 961
Monocyte, 950
Mononuclear phagocyte system (MPS), 950
Myeloid tissue, 955
Myoglobin, 963
Natural killer (NK) cell, 950
Neutrophil (polymorphonuclear neutrophil [PMN]), 949
Niche, 955
Nitric oxide (NO), 966
Normoblast, 959
Osteoblastic niche, 956
Oxyhemoglobin, 961
Phagocyte, 948
Plasma, 945
Plasma protein, 946
Plasmin, 972
Plasminogen, 972
Platelet (thrombocyte), 950
Platelet adhesion, 967
Platelet aggregation, 969
Platelet-release reaction, 968
Proerythroblast, 959
Prostacyclin (PGI_2), 966
Protein C, 970
Protein S, 970
Protoporphyrin, 961
Reticulocyte, 959
Serum, 945
Thrombomodulin, 970
Thromboxane A_2 (TXA_2), 969
Tissue factor (TF, tissue thromboplastin), 969
Tissue factor pathway inhibitor (TFPI), 970
Tissue plasminogen activator (t-PA), 972
Transferrin, 963
Urokinase-like plasminogen activator (u-PA), 972
Vascular niche, 956
von Willebrand factor (vWF), 967

REFERENCES

1. Babior BM, Stossel TP: *Hematology: a pathophysiological approach*, New York, 1984, Churchill Livingstone.
2. Svetina S: Red blood cell shape and deformability in the context of the functional evolution of its membrane structure, *Cell Mol Biol Lett* 17(2):171–181, 2012.
3. Kvarnhammar AM, Cardell LO: Pattern–recognition receptors in human eosinophils, *Immunology* 136(1):11–20, 2012.
4. Valent P et al: Pathogenesis and classification of eosinophil disorders: a review of recent developments in the field, *Expert Rev Hematol* 5(2): 157–176, 2012.
5. Chirumbolo S: State-of-the-art review about basophil research in immunology and allergy: is the time right to treat these cells with the respect they deserve? *Blood Transfus* 10(2):148–164, 2012.
6. Gurish MF, Austen KF: Developmental origin and functional specialization of mast cell subsets, *Immunity* 37(1):25–33, 2012.
7. Sheel M, Engwerda CR: The diverse roles of monocytes in inflammation caused by protozoan parasitic diseases, *Trends Parasitol* 28(10):408–416, 2012.
8. Del Fattore A, Teti A, Rucci N: Bone cells and the mechanisms of bone remodelling, *Front Biosci* E4:2302–2321, 2012.
9. Projahn D, Koenen RR: Platelets: key players in vascular inflammation, *J Leukoc Biol* 92(6):1167–1175, 2012.
10. Flaumenhaft R: Monitoring granule traffic in megakaryocytes, *Blood* 120(19):3869–3870, 2012.
11. Italiano JE Jr: Unraveling mechanisms that control platelet production, *Semin Thromb Hemost* 39(1):15–24, 2013.
12. Boehm T, Hess I, Swann JB: Evolution of lymphoid tissues, *Trends Immunol* 33(6):315–321, 2012.
13. Junt T, Scandella E, Ludewig B: Form follows function: lymphoid tissue microarchitecture in antimicrobial immune defense, *Nat Rev Immunol* 8(10):764–775, 2008.
14. Shen Y, Nilsson SK: Bone, microenvironment and hematopoiesis, *Curr Opin Hematol* 19(4):250–255, 2012.
15. Ehninger A, Trumpp A: The bone marrow stem cell niche grows up: mesenchymal stem cells and macrophages move in, *J Exp Med* 208(3): 421–428, 2011.
16. Shi C: Recent progress toward understanding the physiological function of bone marrow mesenchymal stem cells, *Immunology* 136(2):133–138, 2012.
17. Sugiyama T, Nagasawa T: Bone marrow niches for hematopoietic stem cells and immune cells, *Inflammation Allergy Drug Targets* 11(3):201–206, 2012.
18. Lensch MW: An evolving model of hematopoietic stem cell functional identity, *Stem Cell Rev Rep* 8(2):551–560, 2012.
19. *Stem cell information*, Bethesda, MD, 2010, National Institutes of Health, U.S. Department of Health and Human Services. Available at http://stemcells.nih.gov/info. Accessed March 11, 2013.
20. Ratajczak MZ: Phenotypic and functional characterization of hematopoietic stem cells, *Curr Opin Hematol* 15(4):293–300, 2008.
21. Möhle R, Kanz L: Hematopoietic growth factors for hematopoietic stem cell mobilization and expansion, *Semin Hematol* 44(3):193–202, 2007.
22. Gurion R et al: Colony-stimulating factors for prevention and treatment of infectious complications in patients with myelogenous leukemia, *Cochrane Database Syst Rev* 6:CD008238, 2012.
23. Smith TJ, Hillner BE: A way forward on the medically appropriate use of white cell growth factors, *J Clin Oncol* 30(14):1584–1587, 2012.
24. Renner P et al: Primary prophylactic colony-stimulating factors for the prevention of chemotherapy-induced febrile neutropenia in breast cancer patients, *Cochrane Database Syst Rev* 10:CD007913, 2012.
25. Pusic I, DiPersio JF: The use of growth factors in hematopoietic stem cell transplantation, *Curr Pharm Des* 14(20):1950–1961, 2008.
26. Chasis JA, Mohandas N: Erythroblastic islands: niches for erythropoiesis, *Blood* 112(3):470–478, 2008.
27. Ingley E: Integrating novel signaling pathways involved in erythropoiesis, *IUBMB Life* 64(5):402–410, 2012.
28. Schechter AN: Hemoglobin research and the origins of molecular medicine, *Blood* 112(10):3927–3938, 2008.
29. De Oliveira S, Saldanha C: An overview about erythrocyte membrane, *Clin Hemorheol Microcirc* 44(1):63–74, 2010.
30. Edison ES, Bajel A, Chandy M: Iron homeostasis: new players, newer insights, *Eur J Haematol* 81(6):411–424, 2008.
31. Bartnikas TB: Known and potential roles of transferrin in iron biology, *Biometals* 25(4):677–686, 2012.
32. Kroot JJC et al: Hepcidin in human iron disorders: diagnostic implications, *Clin Chem* 57(12):1650–1669, 2011.
33. Goodnough LT: Iron deficiency syndromes and iron-restricted erythropoiesis, *Transfusion* 52(7):1584–1592, 2012.
34. Finberg KE: Unraveling mechanisms regulating systemic iron homeostasis, *Hematology Am Soc Hematol Educ Program* 2011(1):532–537, 2011.
35. West AR, Oates PS: Mechanisms of heme iron absorption: current questions and controversies, *World J Gastroenterol* 14(26):4101–4110, 2008.
36. Evstatiev R, Gasche C: Iron sensing and signalling, *Gut* 61(6):933–952, 2012.
37. Naito M: Macrophage differentiation and function in health and disease, *Pathol Int* 58(3):143–155, 2008.
38. Kaushansky K: Historical review: megakaryopoiesis and thrombopoiesis, *Blood* 111(3):981–986, 2008.
39. Thon JN, Italiano JE Jr: Does size matter in platelet production? *Blood* 120(8):1552–1561, 2012.
40. Thon JN, Italiano JE: Platelets: production, morphology and ultrastructure, *Handb Exp Pharmacol* 2012(210):3–22, 2012.
41. Marcucci R, Romano M: Thrombopoietin and its splicing variants: structure and functions in thrombopoiesis and beyond, *Biochim Biophys Acta* 1782(7-8):427–432, 2008.
42. Freestone B, Lip GY: The endothelium and atrial fibrillation. The prothrombotic state revisited, *Hämostaseologie* 28(4):207–212, 2008.
43. Reininger AJ: Function of von Willebrand factor in haemostasis and thrombosis, *Haemophilia* 14(Suppl 5):11–26, 2008.
44. Furie B, Furie BC: Mechanisms of thrombus formation, *N Engl J Med* 359(9):938–949, 2008.
45. Reininger AJ: VWF attributes—impact on thrombus formation, *Thromb Res* 122(Suppl 4):S9–S13, 2008.
46. Israels SJ, Rand ML: What we have learned from inherited platelet disorders, *Pediatr Blood Cancer* 60(Suppl 1):S2–S7, 2013.
47. Andrews RK, Berndt MC: Platelet adhesion: a game of catch and release, *J Clin Invest* 118(9):3009–3011, 2008.
48. Ren Q, Ye S, Whiteheart SW: The platelet release reaction: just when you thought platelet secretion was simple, *Curr Opin Hematol* 15(5):537–541, 2008.
49. Gleissner CA, von Hundelshausen P, Ley K: Platelet chemokines in vascular disease, *Arterioscler Thromb Vasc Biol* 28(11):1920–1927, 2008.
50. Krötz F, Sohn H-Y, Klauss V: Antiplatelet drugs in cardiological practice: established strategies and new developments, *Vasc Health Risk Manag* 4(3):637–645, 2008.
51. Nurden AT, Freson K, Selifsohn U: Inherited platelet disorders, *Haemophilia* 18(Suppl 4):154–160, 2012.
52. De Gaetano G, Crescente M, Cerletti C: Current concepts about inhibition of platelet aggregation, *Platelets* 19(8):565–570, 2008.
53. Mann KG, Krudysz-Ambio J, Butenas S: Tissue factor controversies, *Thromb Res* 129(Suppl 2):S5–S7, 2012.
54. Rao LVM, Kothari H, Pendurthi UR: Tissue factor encryption and decryption: facts and controversies, *Thromb Res* 129(Suppl 2):S13–S15, 2012.
55. Di Cera E: Thrombin, *Mol Aspects Med* 29(4):203–254, 2008.
56. Müller F, Renné T: Novel roles for factor XII-driven plasma contact activation system, *Curr Opin Hematol* 15(5):516–521, 2008.
57. Henry BL, Desai UR: Recent research developments in the direct inhibition of coagulation proteinases—inhibitors of the initiation phase, *Cardiovasc Hematol Agents Med Chem* 6(4):323–336, 2008.
58. Wang L, Bastarache JA, Ware LB: The coagulation cascade in sepsis, *Curr Pharm Des* 14(19):1860–1869, 2008.
59. Maroney SA, Mast AE: Platelet tissue factor pathway inhibitor modulates intravascular coagulation, *Thromb Res* 129(Suppl 2):S21–S22, 2012.
60. Morser J: Thrombomodulin links coagulation to inflammation and immunity, *Curr Drug Targets* 13(3):421–431, 2012.
61. Castoldi E, Hackeng TM: Regulation of coagulation by protein S, *Curr Opin Hematol* 15(5):529–536, 2008.
62. Jackson CJ, Xue M: Activated protein C—an anticoagulant that does more than stop clots, *Int J Biochem Cell Biol* 40(12):2692–2697, 2008.
63. Weisel JW, Litvinov RI: The biochemical and physical process of fibrinolysis and effects of clot structure and stability on the lysis rate, *Cardiovasc Hematol Agents Med Chem* 6(3):161–180, 2008.
64. Zorio E et al: Fibrinolysis: the key to new pathogenetic mechanisms, *Curr Med Chem* 15(9):923–929, 2008.
65. Bates SM: D-dimer assays in diagnosis and management of thrombotic and bleeding disorders, *Semin Thromb Hemost* 38(7):673–682, 2012.
66. Ignjatovic V, Mertyn E, Monagle P: The coagulation system in children: development and pathophysiological considerations, *Semin Thromb Hemost* 37(7):723–729, 2011.

CHAPTER

28

Alterations of Erythrocyte Function

Neal S. Rote and Kathryn L. McCance

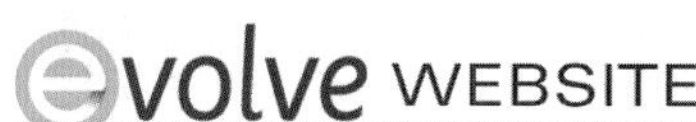

http://evolve.elsevier.com/McCance/

- Review Questions and Answers
- Animations
- Online Course: Module 12

CHAPTER OUTLINE

Alterations of erythrocyte function involve either insufficient or excessive numbers of erythrocytes in the circulation or normal numbers of cells with abnormal components. Anemias are conditions in which there are too few erythrocytes or an insufficient volume of erythrocytes in the blood. Polycythemias are conditions in which erythrocyte numbers or volume is excessive. Each of these conditions has many causes and is a pathophysiologic manifestation of a variety of disease states.

ANEMIA

Strictly speaking, **anemia** is a reduction in the total number of erythrocytes in the circulating blood or a decrease in the quality or quantity of hemoglobin. Anemias commonly result from (1) impaired erythrocyte production, (2) blood loss (acute or chronic), (3) increased erythrocyte destruction, or (4) a combination of these three factors.

Classification

Anemias are classified by their causes (e.g., anemia of chronic disease) or by changes that affect the size, shape, or hemoglobin content of the erythrocyte (Box 28-1). The most common classification is based on changes that affect the erythrocyte's size or hemoglobin content (Table 28-1). The terminology reflects these characteristics; terms that end in "-cytic" refer to cell size, whereas "-chromic" refers to hemoglobin content (Table 28-2). Additional descriptors of erythrocytes associated with some anemias include **anisocytosis** (assuming various sizes) or **poikilocytosis** (assuming various shapes) (Figure 28-1).

CLINICAL MANIFESTATIONS. The fundamental physiologic manifestation of anemia is a reduced oxygen-carrying capacity of the blood resulting in tissue hypoxia. Symptoms of anemia vary, depending on the body's ability to compensate for reduced oxygen-carrying capacity (Figure 28-2). Anemia that is mild and develops gradually is usually easier to compensate and may cause problems for the individual only during physical exertion. As the reduction in red blood cells (RBCs) continues, symptoms become more pronounced and alterations of specific organs and compensatory effects become more apparent. Compensation generally involves the cardiovascular, respiratory, and hematologic systems.

BOX 28-1 ETIOLOGIC (PATHOPHYSIOLOGIC) CLASSIFICATION OF ANEMIAS

Decreased or Defective Production of Erythrocytes

Altered hemoglobin synthesis
- Iron deficiency
- Thalassemia
- Anemia of chronic inflammation

Altered deoxyribonucleic acid (DNA) synthesis resulting from deficient nutrients

Pernicious anemia (decreased B_{12}, folate)

Stem cell dysfunction
- Aplastic anemia
- Myeloproliferative leukemia

Bone marrow infiltration
- Carcinoma
- Lymphoma

Pure red cell aplasia

Increased Erythrocyte Destruction

Blood loss
- Acute—hemorrhage, trauma
- Chronic—gastrointestinal bleeding, menorrhagia

Hemolysis (intracorpuscular defect)
- Membrane—hereditary spherocytosis
- Hemoglobin—sickle cell trait or disease
- Glycolysis—pyruvate kinase
- Oxidation—glucose-6-phosphate dehydrogenase (G6PD) deficiency

Hemolysis (extracorpuscular defect)
- Immune mechanisms—warm antibody/cold antibody
- Infection—clostridial, malarial
- Trauma to erythrocyte—hemolytic uremic syndrome
- Splenic sequestration—hypersplenism

TABLE 28-1 MORPHOLOGIC CLASSIFICATION OF ANEMIAS

MORPHOLOGY OF REMAINING ERYTHROCYTES	NAME AND MECHANISM OF ANEMIA	PRIMARY CAUSE
Macrocytic-normochromic anemia: large, abnormally shaped erythrocytes but normal hemoglobin concentrations	Pernicious anemia: lack of vitamin B_{12} (cobalamin) for erythropoiesis; abnormal deoxyribonucleic acid (DNA) and ribonucleic acid (RNA) synthesis in the erythroblast; premature cell death	Congenital or acquired deficiency of intrinsic factor (IF); genetic disorder of DNA synthesis
	Folate deficiency anemia: lack of folate for erythropoiesis; premature cell death	Dietary folate deficiency
Microcytic-hypochromic anemia: small, abnormally shaped erythrocytes and reduced hemoglobin concentration	Iron deficiency anemia: lack of iron for hemoglobin production; insufficient hemoglobin	Chronic blood loss; dietary iron deficiency; disruption of iron metabolism or iron cycle (see Chapter 27)
	Sideroblastic anemia: dysfunctional iron uptake by erythroblasts and defective porphyrin and heme synthesis	Congenital dysfunction of iron metabolism in erythroblasts; acquired dysfunction of iron metabolism as a result of drugs or toxins
	Thalassemia: impaired synthesis of α- or β-chain of hemoglobin A; phagocytosis of abnormal erythroblasts in the marrow	Congenital genetic defect of globin synthesis
Normocytic-normochromic anemia: normal size, normal hemoglobin concentration	Aplastic anemia: insufficient erythropoiesis	Depressed stem cell proliferation resulting in bone marrow aplasia
	Posthemorrhagic anemia: blood loss	Acute or chronic hemorrhage that stimulates increased erythropoiesis, which eventually depletes body iron
	Hemolytic anemia: premature destruction (lysis) of mature erythrocytes in the circulation	Increased fragility of erythrocytes
	Sickle cell anemia: abnormal hemoglobin synthesis, abnormal cell shape with susceptibility to damage, lysis, and phagocytosis	Congenital dysfunction of hemoglobin synthesis
	Anemia of chronic disease: abnormally increased demand for new erythrocytes	Chronic infection or inflammation; malignancy

TABLE 28-2 TERMS USED IN ASSESSMENT OF ERYTHROCYTES

	ERYTHROCYTE VOLUME	HEMOGLOBIN CONTENT
Normal	Normocytic	Normochromic
Increased	Macrocytic (higher mean corpuscular volume [MCV])	Hyperchromic (higher mean corpuscular hemoglobin concentration [MCHC])
Decreased	Microcytic (lower MCV)	Hypochromic (lower MCHC)

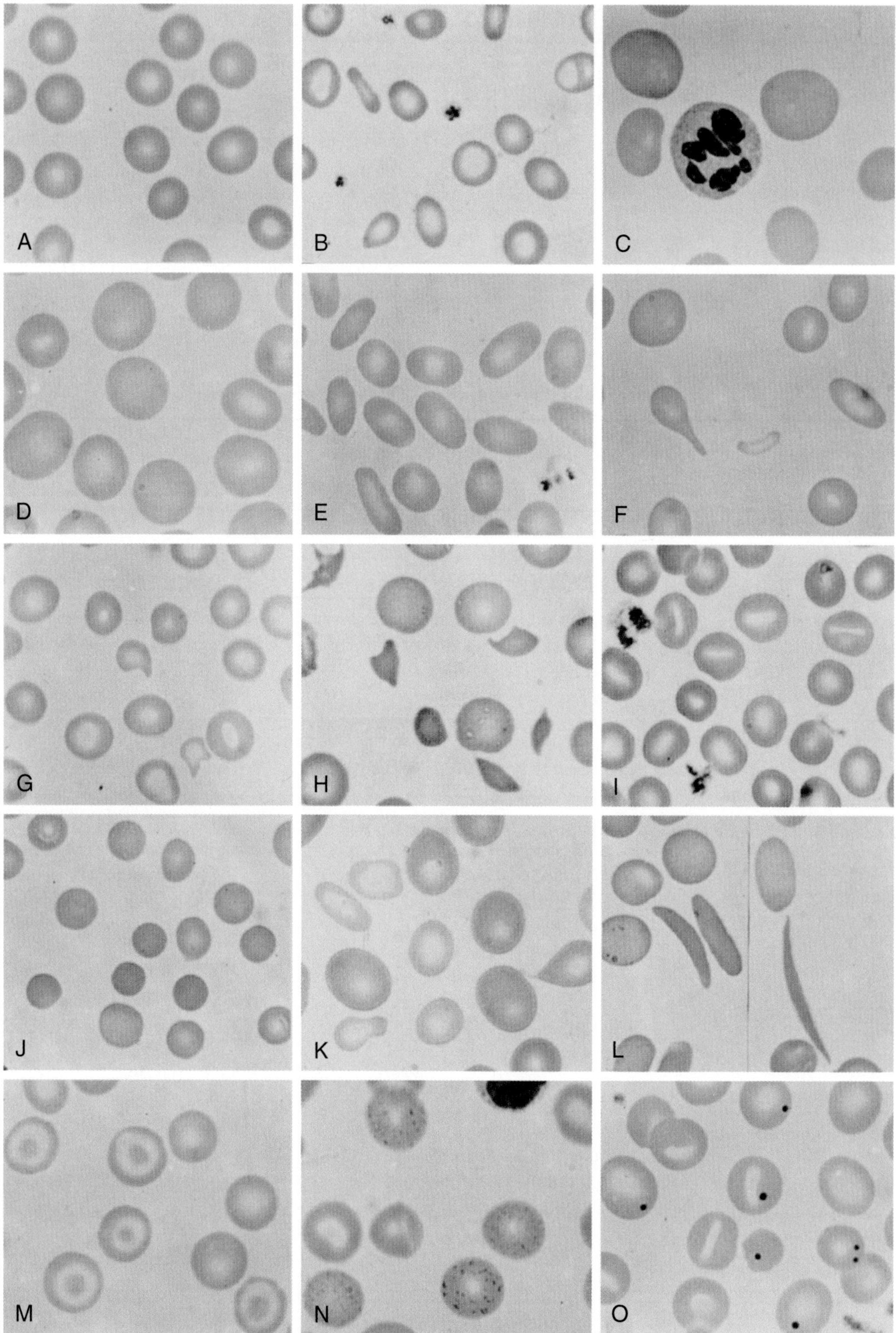

FIGURE 28-1 Appearance of Red Blood Cells in Various Disorders. **A,** Normal blood smear. **B,** Microcytic-hypochromic anemia (iron deficiency). **C,** Macrocytic anemia (pernicious anemia). **D,** Macrocytic anemia in pregnancy. **E,** Hereditary elliptocytosis. **F,** Myelofibrosis (teardrop). **G,** Hemolytic anemia associated with prosthetic heart valve. **H,** Microangiopathic anemia. **I,** Stomatocytes. **J,** Spherocytes (hereditary spherocytosis). **K,** Sideroblastic anemia; note the double population of red blood cells. **L,** Sickle cell anemia. **M,** Target cells (after splenectomy). **N,** Basophil stippling in case of unexplained anemia. **O,** Howell-Jolly bodies (after splenectomy). (From Wintrobe MM et al: *Clinical hematology,* ed 8, Philadelphia, 1981, Lea & Febiger.)

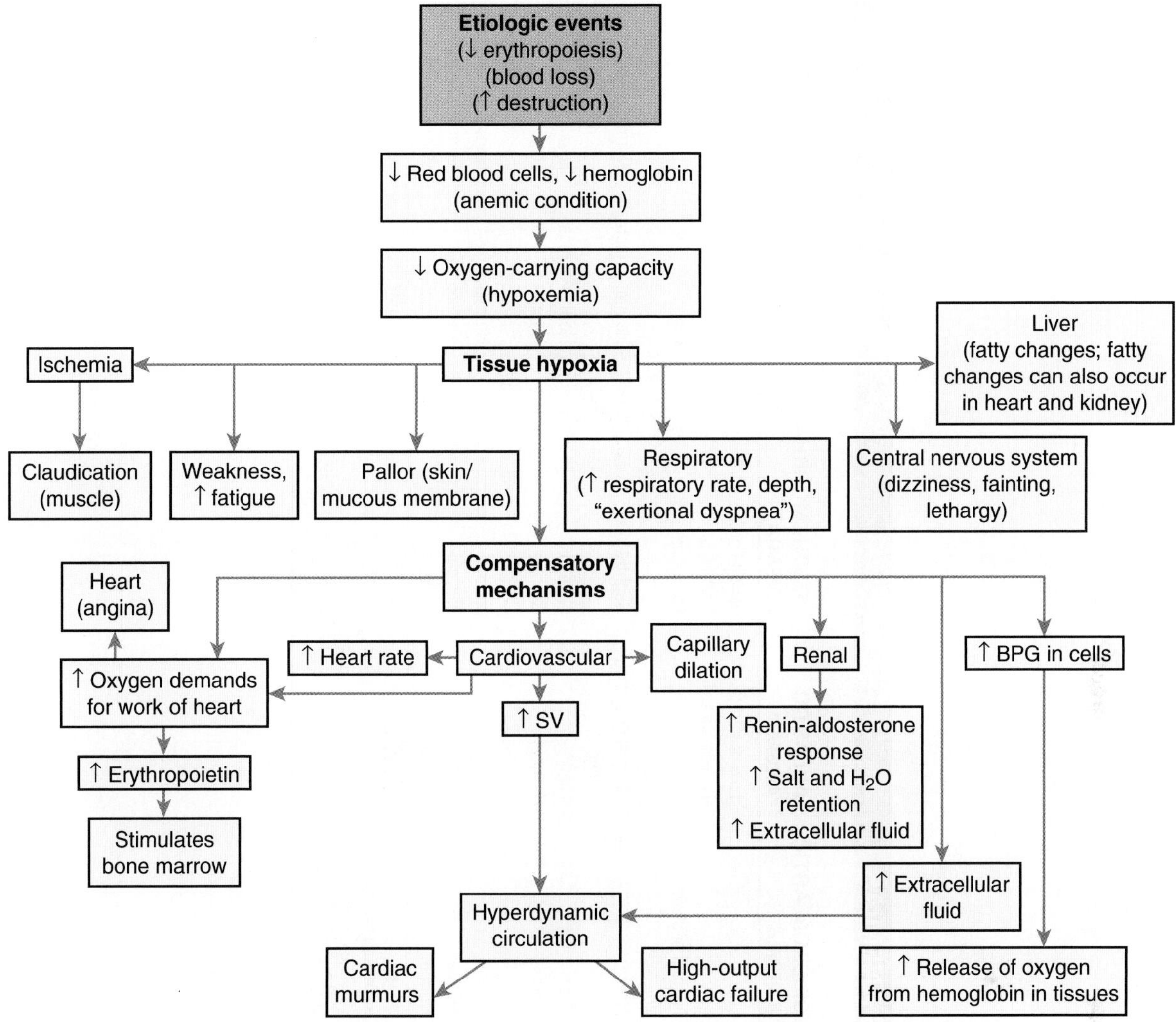

FIGURE 28-2 Progression and Manifestations of Anemia. *BPG,* Biphosphoglycerate; *SV,* stroke volume.

(Hematologic findings associated with various anemias are listed in Table 28-3 and progression and manifestations of anemias are shown in Figure 28-2.)

A reduction in the number of blood cells in the blood causes a reduction in the consistency and volume of blood. Compensation for a reduced blood volume causes interstitial fluid to move into the intravascular space, expanding plasma volume. This movement maintains adequate blood volume, but the viscosity (thickness) of the blood decreases. The diluted blood flows faster and more turbulently than normal blood, causing a hyperdynamic circulatory state. This hyperdynamic state creates cardiovascular changes—increased stroke volume and heart rate. These changes may lead to cardiac dilation and heart valve insufficiency if the underlying anemic condition is not corrected.

Hypoxemia, reduced oxygen levels in the blood, further contributes to cardiovascular dysfunction by causing dilation of arterioles, capillaries, and venules, thus leading to decreased vascular resistance and increased flow. Increased peripheral blood flow and venous return further contribute to an increase in heart rate and stroke volume in a continuing effort to meet normal oxygen demand and prevent cardiopulmonary congestion. These compensatory mechanisms may lead to heart failure.

Tissue hypoxia creates additional demands and compensatory actions on the pulmonary and hematologic systems. The rate and depth of breathing increase in an attempt to increase the availability of oxygen. These demands are accompanied by an increase in the release of oxygen from hemoglobin. (Mechanisms of oxygen transport and release by hemoglobin are described in Chapter 27.) All of these compensatory mechanisms may cause individuals to experience shortness of breath (dyspnea); a rapid, pounding heartbeat (palpitations); dizziness; and fatigue. In mild, chronic conditions, these symptoms might be present only when demand for oxygen is increased (e.g., during physical exertion), but in severe conditions they may be experienced at rest.

Manifestations of anemia may be observed in other parts of the body. The skin, mucous membranes, lips, nail beds, and

TABLE 28-3 LABORATORY FINDINGS FOR VARIOUS ANEMIAS

TEST	PERNICIOUS ANEMIA	FOLATE DEFICIENCY ANEMIA	IRON DEFICIENCY ANEMIA	SIDEROBLASTIC ANEMIA	APLASTIC ANEMIA	POSTHEMORRHAGIC ANEMIA	HEMOLYTIC ANEMIA	ANEMIA OF CHRONIC DISEASE
Hemoglobin	Low	Low	Low	Low	Low or normal	Normal or low	Low	Low
Hematocrit	Low	Low	Low	Low	Low or normal	Normal or low	Low	Low
Reticulocyte count	Low	Low	Normal or slightly high or low	Normal or slightly high	Low	Increased	High	Normal
Mean corpuscular volume	High	High	Low	Low	Normal or slightly high	Slightly low	Normal or high	Normal or low
Plasma iron	High	High	Low	High	High	Normal	Normal or high	Low
Total iron-binding capacity	Normal	Normal	High	Normal	Normal	Normal	Normal	Low
Ferritin	High	High	Low	High	Normal	Normal	Normal	Normal
Serum B_{12}	Low	Normal	Normal	Normal	Normal	Normal	Normal	Normal
Folate	Normal	Low	Normal	Normal	Normal	Normal	Normal	Normal
Bilirubin	Slightly high	Slightly high	Normal	High	Normal	Normal	Slightly high	Normal
Free erythrocyte protoporphyrin	Normal	Normal	High	Increased or normal	High	Normal	Normal	Normal or slightly high
Transferrin	Slightly high	Slightly high	Low	High	Normal	Normal	Normal	Slightly low

conjunctivae become pale as a result of reduced hemoglobin concentration. If anemia is caused by RBC destruction (hemolysis), the skin may become yellowish because of accumulation of the products of hemolysis. Tissue hypoxia of the skin results in impaired healing and loss of elasticity, as well as thinning and early graying of the hair. Nervous system manifestations can occur if the anemia is caused by a vitamin B_{12} deficiency. Myelin degeneration may occur, causing a loss of nerve fibers in the spinal cord and producing paresthesias (numbness), gait disturbances, extreme weakness, spasticity, and reflex abnormalities. Decreased oxygen supply to the gastrointestinal (GI) tract often produces abdominal pain, nausea, vomiting, and anorexia. A low-grade fever of less than 38.5° C (less than about 101° F) occurs in some anemic individuals and may result from the release of leukocyte pyrogens from ischemic tissues.

When the anemia is severe or acute in onset (e.g., hemorrhage), the initial compensatory mechanism is peripheral blood vessel constriction, diverting blood flow to vital organs. Decreased blood flow detected by the kidneys activates the renal renin-angiotensin response, causing salt and water retention in an attempt to increase blood volume. These situations are emergencies and require immediate intervention to correct the underlying problem that caused the acute loss of blood; therefore, long-term compensatory mechanisms do not develop.

Therapeutic interventions for slowly developing anemic conditions require treatment of the underlying disorder and palliation of associated symptoms. Therapies include transfusions, dietary correction, and administration of supplemental vitamins or iron.

Macrocytic-Normochromic Anemias

The **macrocytic (megaloblastic) anemias** are characterized by unusually large stem cells (megaloblasts) in the marrow that mature into erythrocytes that are unusually large in size (macrocytes), thickness, and volume.[1] The hemoglobin content is normal (normochromic). These anemias are the result of defective erythrocyte DNA synthesis, commonly caused by deficiencies of vitamin B_{12} (cobalamin) or folate (folic acid), coenzymes that are required for nuclear maturation and DNA synthesis. These defective erythrocytes die prematurely, which decreases their numbers in the circulation, causing anemia.

Premature death of damaged erythrocytes, **eryptosis,** is a common mechanism of cellular loss in individuals with anemias secondary to deficiencies of iron, infections (e.g., malaria, mycoplasma), chronic diseases (e.g., diabetes, renal disease), genetic diseases (e.g., beta-thalassemia, glucose-6-phosphate dehydrogenase [G6PD] deficiency, sickle-cell trait), and myelodysplastic syndrome.[2] The process is similar to the removal of old or senescent erythrocytes (see Chapter 27), but is triggered by erythrocyte damage before the cell's normal life span. Damaged erythrocytes undergo cell shrinkage, membrane changes (blebbing), and rearrangement of plasma membrane phospholipid distribution with efflux of phosphatidylserine (PS). Macrophages have receptors that recognize surface PS and remove the damaged erythrocytes from the circulation. The erythrocyte's life span may be decreased by as much as 50%.[3]

Defective DNA synthesis in megaloblastic anemias causes red cell growth and development to proceed at unequal rates. DNA synthesis and cell division are blocked or delayed. However, ribonucleic acid (RNA) replication and protein (hemoglobin) synthesis proceed normally. Asynchronous development leads to an overproduction of hemoglobin during prolonged cellular division, creating a larger-than-normal erythrocyte with a disproportionately small nucleus. With each cell division, the disproportion between RNA and DNA becomes more apparent.

Immature precursors of the megaloblastic erythrocytes have a greater chance of dying during maturation than do normoblastic precursors. Additionally, there is an increase in the amounts of lactic dehydrogenase, reflecting cellular destruction, and indirect bilirubin, from the breakdown of heme. Both of these substances may be measured in the blood, providing biochemical evidence of ineffective erythropoiesis.

Defective DNA synthesis also may result in significant enlargement of neutrophil precursors creating giant metamyelocytes with a tendency to have more nuclear lobes than normal. Other cells throughout the body also may demonstrate enlargement and nuclear abnormalities. Cells lining epithelium and those with high turnover rates are most affected.

Pernicious Anemia

Pernicious anemia (PA), the most common type of megaloblastic anemia, is caused by vitamin B_{12} deficiency, which is often associated with the end stage of type A chronic atrophic (congenital or autoimmune) gastritis (see Figure 28-1, *C*; Figure 28-3).[4] *Pernicious* means highly injurious or destructive and reflects the fact that this condition was once fatal. It most commonly affects individuals older than the age of 30 (60 being the median age of diagnosis) who are of Northern European descent, primarily those of Scandinavian, English, and Irish descent, and PA is less common in individuals of Greek or

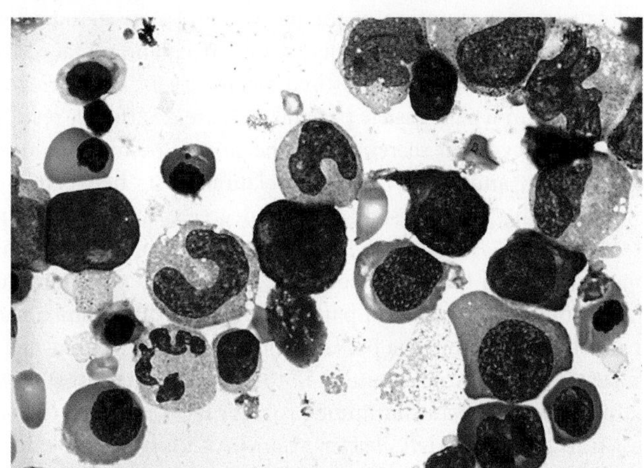

FIGURE 28-3 Bone Marrow Aspirate from Individual with Pernicious Anemia. Bone marrow aspirate smear from an individual with megaloblastic red blood cell precursors and giant metamyelocytes. The chromatin in the red blood cell nuclei is more dispersed than that in normal red blood cell precursors at comparable stages of maturation; the giant metamyelocytes have dispersed nuclear chromatin in contrast to a normal metamyelocyte, which has condensed chromatin (Wright-Giemsa stain). (From Damjanov I, Linder J, editors: *Anderson's pathology,* ed 10, St Louis, 1996, Mosby.)

Italian origin, Recently, PA has also been reported in blacks and Hispanics. Females are more prone to develop PA, with black females having an earlier onset.

PATHOPHYSIOLOGY. The principal disorder in PA is an absence of **intrinsic factor (IF),** a transporter required for absorption of dietary vitamin B_{12}, which is essential for nuclear maturation and DNA synthesis in erythrocytes. IF is secreted by gastric parietal cells and complexes with dietary vitamin B_{12} in the small intestine. The B_{12}-IF complex binds to cell surface receptors in the ileum and is transported across the intestinal mucosa.

Deficiency in IF secretion may be congenital or, more often, an autoimmune process directed against gastric parietal cells. Congenital IF deficiency is a genetic disorder that demonstrates an autosomal recessive inheritance pattern.[5] The autoimmune form of the disease also has a genetic component, as do most autoimmune diseases (see Chapter 9). Family clusters have been identified; 20% to 30% of individuals related to persons with PA also have PA. These relatives, particularly first-degree female relatives, also demonstrate a higher frequency of the presence of gastric autoantibodies. PA is also frequently a component of autoimmune polyendocrinopathy, which is a cluster of autoimmune diseases of endocrine organs (e.g., chronic autoimmune thyroiditis [Hashimoto thyroiditis], type 1 diabetes mellitus, Addison disease, primary hypoparathyroidism, Graves disease, and myasthenia gravis) that frequently present as comorbidities. Autoimmune thyroiditis and type 1 diabetes mellitus, in particular, are associated with PA.

Most cases of PA result from an autoimmune gastritis (type A chronic gastritis) in which gastric atrophy results from destruction of parietal and zymogenic cells. Individuals with PA commonly have autoantibodies against the gastric H^+-K^+ ATPase, which is the major protein constituent of parietal cell membranes. Early in the disease process the gastric submucosa becomes infiltrated with inflammatory cells, including CD4 lymphocytes, eventually extending into the lamina propria and causing degeneration of the parietal and zymogenic cells. The parietal and zymogenic cells are destroyed and replaced by mucous-containing cells (intestinal metaplasia). Gastric mucosal atrophy, in which gastric parietal cells are destroyed, results in a deficiency of all secretions of the stomach—hydrochloric acid, pepsin, and IF. A direct correlation exists between the severity of the gastric lesion and the degree of malabsorption of vitamin B_{12}.[6] Additionally, autoantibodies against IF prevent the formation of the B_{12}-IF complex. Thus, PA is secondary to autoimmune destruction of parietal cells, thus diminishing the production of IF, and the presence of autoantibodies that neutralize the capacity of remaining IF to transport vitamin B_{12}.

Initiation of the autoimmune process may be secondary to a past infection with *Helicobacter pylori*.[7] Although active infection with *H. pylori* is rare in individuals with PA, more than half of these individuals possess circulating antibodies against this microorganism, suggesting a history of infection. The current opinion is that in genetically prone individuals, antigens expressed by *H. pylori* mimic the parietal cell H^+-K^+ ATPase, resulting in production of an antibody that binds and damages the parietal cell (see Chapter 9 for a discussion of antigenic mimicry and autoimmune disease).

Environmental conditions also may contribute to chronic gastritis. These include excessive alcohol or hot tea ingestion and smoking. Complete or partial removal of the stomach (gastrectomy) causes IF deficiency. Drugs known as proton pump inhibitors (PPIs) are used to decrease gastric acidity, but also may decrease cobalamin absorption, although it is not thought that they actually cause PA. Although PA is a benign disorder, individuals with type A chronic gastritis also are at risk for developing gastric adenocarcinoma and gastric carcinoid type I. The incidence of carcinoma in these individuals is 2% to 3%.

CLINICAL MANIFESTATIONS. PA develops slowly (possibly over 20 to 30 years); 60 years of age is the median age at time of diagnosis. Because of the slow onset of symptoms, PA is usually severe by the time treatment is sought. Early symptoms are often ignored because they are nonspecific and vague and include infections, mood swings, and gastrointestinal, cardiac, or kidney ailments. When the hemoglobin level has decreased significantly (7 to 8 g/dl), the individual experiences the classic symptoms of anemia—weakness, fatigue, paresthesias of the feet and fingers, difficulty in walking, loss of appetite, abdominal pains, weight loss, and a sore tongue that is smooth and beefy red secondary to atrophic glossitis. The skin may become "lemon yellow" (sallow) as a result of a combination of pallor and icterus. Hepatomegaly, indicating right-sided heart failure, may be present in the elderly along with splenomegaly, which is nonpalpable.

Neurologic manifestations result from nerve demyelination that may produce neuronal death. The posterior and lateral columns of the spinal cord also may be affected, causing a loss of position and vibration sense, ataxia, and spasticity. These complications pose a serious threat because they are not reversible, even with appropriate treatment. The cerebrum also may be involved with manifestations of affective disorders, most commonly of the depressive types. An increased prevalence of serum vitamin B_{12} deficiency has been reported among individuals with Alzheimer disease.

EVALUATION AND TREATMENT. Diagnosis of PA is based on a variety of tests (see Table 28-3), which include blood tests, bone marrow aspiration, serologic studies, gastric biopsy, and clinical manifestations. A good test for PA was the Schilling test (no longer offered in most laboratories), which indirectly evaluated vitamin B_{12} absorption by administering radioactive B_{12} and measuring excretion in the urine. Low urinary excretion was significant for PA.

Serologic studies, however, have replaced the Schilling test for diagnosing PA. Measuring methylmalonic acid and homocysteine levels, which are elevated early in PA, is more sensitive. The presence of circulating antibodies against parietal cells and intrinsic factor is also useful in diagnosis.[8] Gastric biopsy reveals total achlorhydria (absence of hydrochloric acid), which is diagnostic for PA because it occurs only in the presence of this gastric lesion.

Replacement of vitamin B_{12} (cobalamin) is the treatment of choice. Initial injections of vitamin B_{12} are administered weekly until the deficiency is corrected, followed by monthly injections for the remainder of the individual's life. The effectiveness of cobalamin replacement therapy is determined by a rising reticulocyte count. Within 5 to 6 weeks, blood counts return to normal. PA cannot be cured so maintenance therapy is lifelong. Conventional wisdom and practice assumed that oral preparations were ineffective because there was no IF to facilitate absorption of vitamin B_{12}. However, recent experience has shown that higher doses of orally administered vitamin B_{12} will be absorbed across the small bowel and is beneficial.

Untreated PA is fatal, usually because of heart failure. Death occurs after a course of remissions and exacerbations lasting from 1 to 3 years. Since 1926, when replacement therapy began, mortality has been reduced significantly. Today, death from PA is rare, and any relapses that occur are usually the result of noncompliance with therapy.

Folate Deficiency Anemia

Folate (folic acid) is an essential vitamin for RNA and DNA synthesis within the maturing erythrocyte. Folates are coenzymes required for the synthesis of thymine and purines (adenine and guanine) and the conversion of homocysteine to methionine. Deficient production of thymine, in particular, affects cells undergoing rapid division (e.g., bone marrow cells undergoing erythropoiesis). Humans are totally dependent on dietary intake to meet the daily requirement of 50 to 200 mcg/day. Increased amounts are required for pregnant and lactating females. Absorption of folate occurs primarily in the upper small intestine and does not depend on the presence of any other facilitating factor, such as IF. After absorption, folate circulates through the liver, where it is stored. Folate deficiency is more common than B_{12} deficiency, particularly in alcoholics and individuals with chronic malnourishment. Alcohol interferes with folate metabolism in the liver, causing a profound depletion of folate stores. Fad diets and diets low in vegetables also may cause folate deficiency because of the absence of plant sources of folate. It is estimated that at least 10% of North Americans have a folate deficiency, although the incidence has been on the decrease in the United States since the fortification of foods with folate and the increased use of folate supplements.

PATHOPHYSIOLOGY. Impaired DNA synthesis secondary to a folate deficiency results in megaloblastic cells with clumped nuclear chromatin. Anemia may result from apoptosis of erythroblasts in the late stages of erythropoiesis. In addition to anemia, folate deficiency in pregnant women is associated with neural tube defects of the fetus. Folate is necessary for the reduction of circulating levels of homocysteine, a risk factor for the development of atherosclerosis (see Chapter 32); thus a folate deficiency increases the risk for developing coronary artery disease. A deficiency of folate also is implicated in the development of cancers, specifically colorectal cancers.

CLINICAL MANIFESTATIONS. Clinical manifestations are similar to the cachectic, malnourished appearance of individuals with PA. Specific symptoms include severe cheilosis (scales and fissures of the lips and corners of the mouth), stomatitis (inflammation of the mouth), and painful ulcerations of the buccal mucosa and tongue, characteristic of burning mouth syndrome. Burning mouth syndrome may be secondary to a large number of disorders (e.g., extremely dry mouth, infection, autoimmune disease, nutritional deficiencies, and other conditions). The mechanisms underlying folate deficiency as a cause remain unknown. Gastrointestinal symptoms may be present and include dysphagia (difficulty swallowing), flatulence, and watery diarrhea, as well as histologic and roentgenographic changes of the GI tract suggestive of sprue (a chronic malabsorption syndrome). Undiagnosed inflammatory bowel disease (e.g., Crohn disease, ulcerative colitis) may be the underlying cause of folate malabsorption in some individuals, and folate deficiency may suppress proliferation of the intestinal mucosa, leading to exacerbation of gastrointestinal damage. Neurologic manifestations, such as those that occur in PA, are generally not seen in folate deficiency anemia. Any neurologic symptoms are usually caused by a thiamine deficiency, which often accompanies folate deficiency.

EVALUATION AND TREATMENT. Evaluation of folate deficiency is based on measurement of serum folate levels and symptoms. Treatment requires daily oral administration of folate preparations until adequate blood levels are obtained and clinical symptoms are reduced or eliminated. One milligram per day is sufficient for most individuals, although persons with alcoholism may require 5 mg. Prophylactic dosages of 0.1 to 0.4 mg/day are sometimes given during pregnancy. Parenteral administration of folic acid (citrovorum factor or leucovorin) generally is not used except in situations in which an individual has been using drugs that inhibit dihydrofolate reductase. After administration of folate, the manifestations of anemia disappear within 1 to 2 weeks.

After the folate deficiency has been corrected, long-term treatment with folate is not necessary if the appropriate dietary adjustments are made to maintain adequate intake. An intake of folate (400 mcg/day) is recommended as a measure to prevent heart disease.

Microcytic-Hypochromic Anemias

The **microcytic-hypochromic anemias** are characterized by abnormally small erythrocytes that contain abnormally reduced amounts of hemoglobin (see Figure 28-1, *B*). Hypochromia occurs even in cells of normal size.

Microcytic-hypochromic anemia can result from (1) disorders of iron metabolism, (2) disorders of porphyrin and heme synthesis, or (3) disorders of globin synthesis. Specific disorders include iron deficiency anemia, sideroblastic anemia, and thalassemia (thalassemia is discussed in Chapter 30).

Iron Deficiency Anemia

Iron deficiency anemia (IDA) is the most common type of anemia worldwide, occurring in both developing and developed countries and affecting as many as one fifth of the world population. Certain populations are at high risk for developing hypoferremia and IDA and include individuals living in poverty, women of childbearing age, and children. Iron deficiency in children is associated with numerous adverse health-related manifestations, especially cognitive impairment, which may be irreversible. Teens with a history of iron deficiency as infants are likely to score lower on cognitive and motor tests, even if the iron deficiency was identified and treated in infancy.

Children in developing countries often are affected by chronic parasite infestations that result in intestinal blood and iron loss that outpaces dietary intake.[9] Treatment of helminth infections results in an improvement in the anemia as well as in appetite and growth. Iron deficiency also occurs in individuals with lead poisoning. Treatment of the iron deficiency is associated with a decrease in lead levels.

Females have a higher incidence of hypoferremia (13.9%) than do males (8.3%), as well as IDA— 4% to 6% in females and 4% in males. The incidence peaks in females during their reproductive years and decreases after menopause. Those at highest risk are black females living in urban poverty.[10] Males have a higher incidence during childhood and adolescence, a decrease occurring during young adulthood, and an upswing during late adulthood. In the United States, 720,000 children (9%) ages 1 to 2 years are estimated to be iron deficient, of whom 240,000 (3%) are anemic, which may be a result of increased iron requirements with growth. An increased prevalence of iron deficiency has been observed in overweight children.

PATHOPHYSIOLOGY. IDA can arise from one of two different etiologies or a combination of both—inadequate dietary intake or excessive blood loss. In both instances there is no intrinsic dysfunction in iron metabolism; however, both deplete iron stores and reduce hemoglobin synthesis. A second category is a metabolic or functional iron deficiency in which various metabolic disorders lead to either insufficient iron delivery to bone marrow or impaired iron use within the marrow. Paradoxically, iron stores may be sufficient but delivery is inadequate to maintain heme synthesis, thus producing a functional or relative iron deficiency.

The most common cause of IDA in developed countries is pregnancy and chronic blood loss.[11] Blood loss of 2 to 4 ml/day (1 to 2 mg of iron) is sufficient to cause iron deficiency and may result from erosive esophagitis, gastric and duodenal ulcers, colon adenomas, or cancers. *H. pylori* infections also have been found to cause IDA of unknown origin, although *H. pylori* impairs iron uptake. In females, menorrhagia (excessive bleeding during menstruation) is a common cause of primary IDA. Other causes of IDA for both genders are (1) use of medications that cause gastrointestinal bleeding (such as aspirin or nonsteroidal anti-inflammatory drugs [NSAIDs]); (2) surgical procedures that decrease stomach acidity, intestinal transit time, and absorption (e.g., gastric bypass); (3) insufficient dietary intake of iron; and (4) eating disorders, such as pica, which is the craving and eating of nonnutritional substances, such as dirt, chalk, and paper.

Iron in the form of hemoglobin is in constant demand by the body. Iron is recyclable; therefore, the body maintains a balance between iron that is contained in hemoglobin and iron that is in storage and available for future hemoglobin synthesis (see Chapter 27). Blood loss disrupts this balance by creating a need for more iron, thus depleting the iron stores more rapidly to replace the iron lost from bleeding.

Iron also contributes to immune function by regulating immune effector mechanisms (i.e., cytokine activities [interferon-gamma (IFN-γ)], nitric oxide formation, and T-cell proliferation). Acquired hypoferremia may be part of the body's response to infection. Anemia can be part of the nonspecific acute phase response to any type of inflammation of sufficient degree. Many pathogens require iron for survival; thus hypoferremia would hamper their growth. However, the precise benefits or detriments of iron deficiency and immunity are still controversial.

IDA occurs when the demand for iron exceeds the supply and develops slowly through three overlapping stages. In stage I, the body's iron stores are depleted. Erythropoiesis proceeds normally, with the hemoglobin content of erythrocytes remaining normal. In stage II, iron transportation to bone marrow is diminished, resulting in iron-deficient erythropoiesis. Stage III begins when the small hemoglobin-deficient cells enter the circulation to replace the normal aged erythrocytes that have been removed from the circulation. The manifestations of IDA appear in stage III when there is depletion of iron stores and diminished hemoglobin production.

CLINICAL MANIFESTATIONS. Symptoms of IDA begin gradually, and individuals usually do not seek medical attention until hemoglobin levels have decreased to about 7 to 8 g/dl. Early symptoms are nonspecific and include fatigue, weakness, shortness of breath, and pale earlobes, palms, and conjunctivae (Figure 28-4, *A*).

As the condition progresses and becomes more severe, structural and functional changes occur in epithelial tissue (see Figure 28-4). The fingernails become brittle, thin, coarsely ridged, and "spoon-shaped" or concave (koilonychia) as a result of impaired capillary circulation (Figure 28-4, *B*). IDA also is associated with unexplained burning mouth syndrome, as was

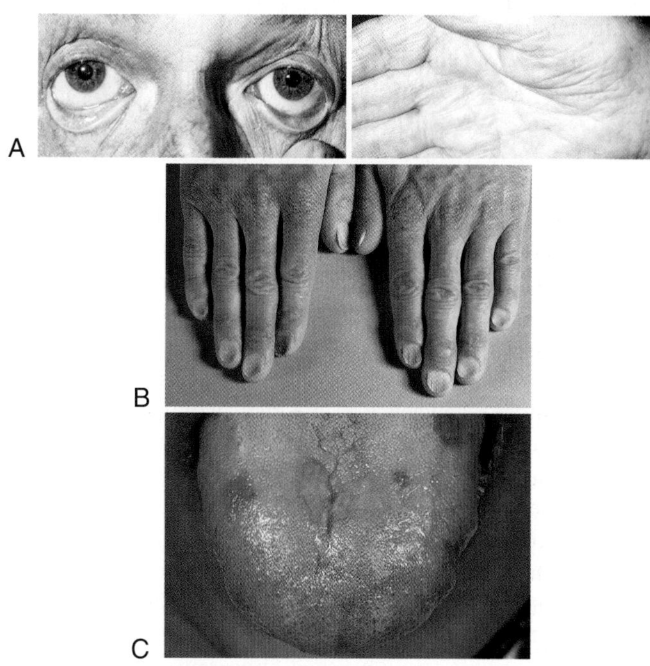

FIGURE 28-4 Manifestations of Iron Deficiency Anemia. **A**, Pallor and iron deficiency. Pallor of the skin, mucous membranes, and palmar creases in an individual with a hemoglobin level of 9 g/dl. Palmar creases become as pale as the surrounding skin when the hemoglobin level approaches 7 g/dl. **B,** Koilonychia. The nails are concave, ridged, and brittle. **C,** Glossitis. Tongue of individual with iron deficiency anemia has bald, fissured appearance caused by loss of papillae and flattening. (From Hoffbrand AV, Pettit JE, Vyas P: *Color atlas of clinical hematology,* ed 4, London, 2009, Mosby; **B** courtesy Dr. S.M. Knowles.)

discussed for folate deficiency. Tongue papillae atrophy and cause soreness along with redness and burning (glossitis) (Figure 28-4, *C*). The degree of pain experienced is directly associated with the amount of iron deficiency, and these changes can be reversed within 1 to 2 weeks of iron replacement therapy. Individuals also experience dryness and soreness in the epithelium at the corners of the mouth, known as *angular stomatitis.* Difficulty in swallowing is associated with an esophageal "web," a thin, concentric, smooth extension of normal esophageal tissue consisting of mucosa and submucosa at the juncture between the hypopharynx and esophagus. The duration of iron deficiency required for web formation is uncertain. Dysphagia also is exacerbated by hyposalivation. The pathophysiology associated with these epithelial lesions is not well understood, but the lesions have the potential to become cancerous.

Nonheme iron is a component of many enzymes in the body (e.g., cytochromes, myoglobin, catalases, peroxidases), particularly those involved in the metabolism of amine neurotransmitters, reduction of nucleotides, and biosynthesis of methionine. Abnormalities and deficiencies of iron-dependent enzymes may account for many of the clinical manifestations of IDA. Individuals with IDA also exhibit gastritis, neuromuscular changes, irritability, headache, numbness, tingling, and vasomotor disturbances. Gait disturbances are rare. The pathogenesis of neurologic symptoms is unknown but may be caused by hypoxia in already compromised cerebral vessels. In the elderly, mental confusion, memory loss, and disorientation are often associated with anemia and may be wrongly perceived as "normal" events related to aging.

EVALUATION AND TREATMENT. Initial evaluation is based on clinical symptoms and decreased levels of hemoglobin and hematocrit. Additional measurements, however, are needed to determine the cause of the anemia (see Table 28-3). Iron stores may be measured directly by bone marrow biopsy and iron staining or indirectly by laboratory tests for serum ferritin, transferrin saturation, or total iron-binding capacity. Serum ferritin is a widely accepted and available measurement of iron status that has been used for the past 25 years; 1 mcg/L serum ferritin corresponds to 8 to 10 mg or 120 mcg of storage iron/kg body weight. A limitation on interpretation of serum ferritin levels is that values may be elevated independently of iron status during acute or chronic inflammation, malignancy, liver disease, or alcoholism. A sensitive indicator of heme synthesis is the amount of free erythrocyte protoporphyrin (FEP) within erythrocytes. A test that determines the concentration of soluble fragment transferrin receptor differentiates primary IDA from IDA that is associated with chronic disease.

An indicator of iron levels is the level of serum transferrin receptor (sTfR). Transferrin receptors are membrane glycoproteins that bind circulating transferrin for transport into cells. Soluble forms of the receptor are found in serum. The ratio of serum levels of transferrin receptor to ferritin (R/F) estimates body iron stores and differentiates primary IDA from anemia secondary to chronic disease. A major drawback, however, is the lack of proper standardization for the sTfR assay.

The first step in treatment of IDA is to identify and eliminate sources of blood loss.[12] With ongoing bleeding, any replacement therapy is likely to be ineffective. Iron replacement therapy is required and very effective. Initial doses are 150 to 200 mg/day. Hematocrit levels should improve within 1 to 2 months of therapy; however, the serum ferritin level is a more precise measurement of improvement and total body stores of iron. Once the serum ferritin level reaches 50 mcg/L, adequate replacement of iron has occurred. A rapid decrease in fatigue, lethargy, and other associated symptoms is generally seen within the first month of therapy. Replacement therapy usually continues for 6 to 12 months after the bleeding has stopped but may continue for as long as 24 months. Menstruating females may need daily oral iron replacement therapy (325 mg/day) until menopause.

Parenteral iron replacement is used in instances of uncontrolled blood loss, intolerance to oral iron, intestinal malabsorption, or poor adherence to oral therapy. Iron dextran has been the only parenteral agent available in the United States. Intramuscular injection is the recommended method; however, intravenous (IV) administration is generally preferred because of the ability to administer larger doses. A significant concern in the use of IV dextran is the potential for severe anaphylactic reaction. Delayed allergic reactions are also major concerns.

Newer medications that have recently been approved for parenteral therapy in treating IDA are sodium ferric gluconate complex in sucrose (Ferrlecit) and iron sucrose injection (Venofer). Iron dextran is recommended as the first choice in spite of its higher rate of adverse reactions. For individuals who are intolerant of iron dextran, the two newer agents are safe and effective alternatives. Drawbacks to their use include higher cost and the need for multiple infusions.

Sideroblastic Anemia

Sideroblastic anemias (SAs) are a heterogeneous group of disorders characterized by anemia of varying severity caused by a defect in mitochondrial heme synthesis.[13] SA is characterized by the presence of ringed sideroblasts within the bone marrow. **Ringed sideroblasts** are erythroblasts that contain iron-laden mitochondria arranged in a perinuclear collar around one third or more of the nucleus (see Figure 28-1, *K*).[14] Individuals with SA also have increased levels of iron in their tissue. The blood contains hypochromic erythrocytes, either microcytic or macrocytic depending on the form of the disease.

PATHOPHYSIOLOGY. SAs have multiple etiologies but all share the commonality of altered heme synthesis in the erythroid cells in bone marrow. Mitochondrial aminolevulinic acid (ALA) synthase uses glycine to convert succinyl CoA into ALA.[15] ALA undergoes further enzymatic modification in the cytoplasm to the porphyrin structure, becoming coproporphyrinogen III, which reenters the mitochondria. Within the mitochondria the molecule is progressively converted to protophorphyrin IX, which has ferrous iron (Fe^{2+}) inserted by the enzyme ferrochelatase. Disruptions to this pathway lead to the accumulation of iron in the mitochondria and the characteristic sideroblasts.

SAs are either acquired or hereditary. **Acquired sideroblastic anemia,** which is the most common, occurs as a primary disorder with no known cause (idiopathic) or is associated with other myeloproliferative or myeloplastic disorders. Another form is described as reversible SAs; these are secondary to various conditions such as alcoholism, drug reactions, copper deficiency, and hypothermia. **Reversible sideroblastic anemia,** associated with alcoholism, results from nutritional deficiencies of folate. Alcohol impairs heme synthesis by reducing the activity of specific enzymes along the biosynthetic pathway and also by direct effects of alcohol or acetaldehyde, or both, on the heme biosynthetic steps or mitochondrial metabolism. Some specific drugs also cause reversible SA and include antituberculous agents (isoniazid [INH], pyrazinamide, cycloserine, and chloramphenicol) that interfere with B_{12} metabolism or directly injure the mitochondria. Copper deficiency also causes reversible SA by interfering with conversion of ferric iron to ferrous iron. This is extremely rare and is associated with gastrectomy and prolonged parenteral nutrition without copper supplements. Hypothermia causes decreased heme synthesis and incorporation into hemoglobin.

Hereditary sideroblastic anemia is rare and occurs almost exclusively in males, suggesting a predominant recessive X-linked transmission. Hereditary SA (X-linked sideroblastic anemia [XLSA]) has been linked to missense mutations in the erythroid-specific ALAS-E gene *Xp11.21*.[16] More than 25 missense mutations have been identified. ALAS is the first and rate-limiting enzyme in the heme biosynthesis pathway, and mutations lead to reduced synthesis of protoporphyrin IX and the characteristic accumulation of iron in the erythrocyte. An occasional autosomal recessive transmission affecting females occurs with mitochondrial mutations and deficiencies of ferrochelatase. Other genetic, chromosomal, or enzyme dysfunctions also have been associated with hereditary SA. The anemia of hereditary SA is usually present in infancy or childhood, but may remain undetected until midlife. In some instances, other symptoms (e.g., diabetes or cardiac failure resulting from tissue iron overload) may be the first manifestation of SA. Differentiation of SA from idiopathic hemochromatosis needs to be confirmed because both are characterized by tissue iron deposition.

The leading known cause of primary ASA, **myelodysplastic syndrome (MDS),** is a group of disorders of hematopoietic stem cells, with all three stem cell lines demonstrating dysplastic characteristics.[17] Initially, all ASAs associated with myelodysplastic syndrome were considered to be one and the same and identified as refractory anemia with ringed sideroblasts. This classification proved unsatisfactory because different outcomes were observed in individuals who had the same apparent disease. Further investigations discovered morphologic and chromosomal characteristics that predicted different clinical courses. Two subsets of myelodysplastic ringed sideroblasts were identified based on the cell lines that were affected. In one subset, dysplastic features were limited to the erythroid line and it was classified as pure SA. Individuals with pure SA require transfusions, which may produce iron overload.[18] With adequate chelation therapy, they are able to survive and thrive for many years. A significant outcome of this condition is the rare occurrence of conversion to leukemia.

The second subset of MDS was characterized by abnormalities of multiple cell lineages. In addition to SA, major alterations of neutrophil and platelet were observed. Infections, frequently fatal, are common secondary to neutropenia and neutrophil dysfunction. Bleeding from thrombocytopenia and platelet dysfunction also is prevalent. Of those who survive, 40% develop acute (myeloblastic) leukemia.

CLINICAL MANIFESTATIONS. The anemias of SA are generally moderate to severe, with hemoglobin levels varying from 4 to 10 g/dl. In addition to the cardiovascular and respiratory manifestations common to all anemias, individuals with SA may show signs of iron overload **(hemochromatosis).** Mild to moderate enlargement of the spleen (splenomegaly) and liver (hepatomegaly) occurs; however, liver function remains normal or only slightly impaired. Occasionally abnormal skin pigmentation (bronze-tinted) is seen. Neurologic and epithelial alterations commonly associated with other anemias are absent. Hemosiderosis of cardiac tissue resulting in heart rhythm disturbances and congestive heart failure are major life-threatening complications related to cardiac iron overload. These manifestations are fortunately rare and occur late in the progression of the disease. Young children and infants who are severely affected may demonstrate growth and developmental impairment.

EVALUATION AND TREATMENT. Initially, SA may be mistaken for deficiency of stem cells in the marrow **(hypoplastic anemia)** or iron deficiency anemia (laboratory findings are listed in Table 28-3). Bone marrow examination establishes the diagnosis. The marrow is packed with erythrocyte stem cells, and mononuclear phagocytes in the marrow are loaded with iron in the form of hemosiderin. The presence of sideroblasts confirms the diagnosis of SA. Platelet and leukocyte values are generally normal; however, they may be reduced if splenomegaly is evident.

The severity of the anemia is quite variable and qualitative alterations of the erythrocytes (e.g., decreased mean corpuscular volume [MCV] and increased erythrocyte volume distribution width) may be evident even when anemia is not present. **Dimorphism,** in which normocytic and normochromic cells are seen concomitantly with microcytic-hypochromic cells, may be present and is seen more commonly in individuals with mild anemia, in female carriers, or in those receiving treatment with pyridoxine. Anisocytosis and poikilocytosis also are seen on examination of the blood smear.

Initial treatment of SA is directed toward identification of a causative agent (i.e., drugs or toxins).[19] Treatment is supportive, with transfusions being the primary intervention. Following removal of the agent, oral pyridoxine (100 mg/day) may be administered on a trial basis. Acquired SA related to alcohol abuse and pyridoxine antagonists often demonstrates a complete response to pyridoxine. SA caused by other etiologies does not demonstrate the same improvement.

Individuals with hereditary SA are initially treated with pyridoxine therapy (50 to 200 mg/day), which is effective in approximately one third of individuals. An optimal response is reticulocytosis with blood hemoglobin levels and low free erythrocyte protoporphyrin levels also returning to normal within 1 to 2 months. Morphologic abnormalities of cells (microcytosis), however, do not disappear, even in the presence of normal ALA synthase activity and hemoglobin. Hemoglobin levels also may increase in response to therapy but stabilize at less than normal levels. When a response to pyridoxine therapy is observed, lifelong maintenance therapy at a lowered dosage is instituted. Discontinuing therapy initiates a relapse. Individuals not responding to pyridoxine require blood transfusions to relieve symptoms and permit growth and development.

Evidence of iron overload requires iron depletion therapy to prevent or minimize organ damage. Phlebotomy, or removal of blood from the circulation, is generally well tolerated and preferable for individuals who have a mild to moderate anemia without other complications (e.g., heart disease). Once all the stored iron is removed, maintenance phlebotomies are performed on a continuing basis. Individuals who have severe anemia and/or depend on transfusions become extremely overloaded with iron. When this occurs, therapy with deferoxamine (an iron chelating agent) is necessary to eliminate excess iron.

Individuals with acquired SA infrequently respond to pyridoxine. Fortunately, these individuals are rarely incapacitated by SA. In the absence of abnormalities of other blood cells and without iron overload, progression takes place over years. Transfusion and chelation therapy is the same as for hereditary SA when indicated.

Recent advances in treatment for SAs include prolonged administration of erythropoietin and stem cell transplant. Treatment with recombinant human erythropoietin improves anemia in 30% of those with myelodysplastic syndrome.[20] Individuals with the subset of MDS identified as refractory anemia have the overall best response rate. Congenital SA has been treated successfully with stem cell transplants; however, this treatment is in the early stages of use, and long-term efficacy has not yet been established. Death from SA is rare and often secondary to complications, such as infection, bone marrow failure, liver failure, or cardiac failure or arrhythmias, or both.

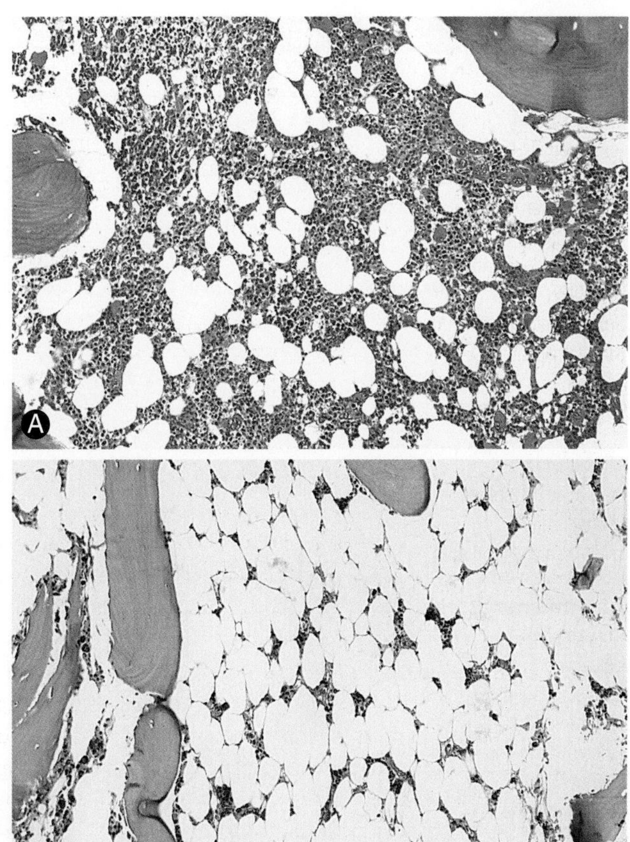

FIGURE 28-5 **Aplastic Anemia. A,** Normal bone marrow of an adult. Hematopoietic cells account for approximately 40% of marrow's cellularity. **B,** There is a marked reduction in hematopoietic cells with expansion of fat cells. (From Damjanov I, Linder J: *Pathology: a color atlas,* St Louis, 2000, Mosby.)

Normocytic-Normochromic Anemias

Normocytic-normochromic anemias (NNAs) are characterized by erythrocytes that are relatively normal in size and hemoglobin content but insufficient in number. These anemias have no common etiology, pathologic mechanisms, or morphologic characteristics. They are less frequent than macrocytic-normochromic and microcytic-hypochromic anemias. NNAs include five distinct groups: aplastic (damage to bone marrow erythropoiesis); posthemorrhagic (acute blood loss); acquired hemolytic (immune destruction of erythrocytes); hereditary hemolytic, such as sickle cell (destruction by eryptosis); and anemia of chronic inflammation (multiple causes). (Sickle cell anemia is discussed in Chapter 30.)

Aplastic Anemia

Aplastic anemia (AA) is a critical condition characterized by **pancytopenia,** a reduction or absence of all three blood cell types, resulting from failure or suppression of bone marrow to produce adequate amounts of blood cells (Figure 28-5). The rate or decline in the quantity of blood cells is related to their respective life span; thus erythrocytes (life span about 120 days) are last to demonstrate a reduction in numbers.

The incidence of AA is relatively rare (annual rate of 2 to 5 new cases per million per year). The incidence in developing countries is somewhat higher and may be related to greater exposure to certain chemicals known to cause AA. The incidence is bimodal, with one peak occurring between 15 and 25 years of age and a second peak occurring in individuals older than age 60. AA is equally distributed between genders.

AAs are the most common type, with idiopathic AA (primary acquired) accounting for approximately 75% of all confirmed cases and being an autoimmune disease. Secondary AA, which accounts for approximately 15% of cases, is caused by a variety of known chemical agents and ionizing radiation. Chemical agents include benzene, arsenic, and multiple drugs, including chloramphenicol and alkylating and antimetabolite chemotherapeutic drugs (6-mercaptopurine, vincristine, and busulfan).[21] Other drugs known to cause AA are identified in Table 28-4. The development of AA with use of these agents is generally dose related, and the effect can be controlled with diminished dosages. In other instances, AA might develop after the use of small amounts of these drugs (idiosyncratic), with the anemia following a severe, rapid, irreversible progression. Liver disease (seronegative hepatitis) is also recognized as a cause of AA.

AA is constitutional or familial in origin or is associated with one or more somatic abnormalities in approximately 5% to 10% of affected individuals. A subset of these is found to have defective telomerase RNA resulting in shortened telomeres. This abnormality also is found in some individuals with idiopathic AA.

TABLE 28-4 ANEMIAS SECONDARY TO DRUG EFFECTS*

DRUG	HEMOLYTIC	MEGALOBLASTIC	SIDEROBLASTIC	APLASTIC
Antibiotics				
Amphotericin B				X
Trimethoprim-sulfamethoxazole (Bactrim)		X		
Chloramphenicol (Chloromycetin)			XX	XXXX
Erythromycin	X			X
Sulfisoxazole (Gantrisin)				X
Penicillin	XXX			X
Sulfanilamide/sulfonamides	XX			X, X*
Streptomycin	X			X
Anticonvulsants				
Phenytoin (Dilantin)		XXX		XXX, X*
Mephenytoin		XXX		XXX
Primidone (Mysoline)		XX		
Phenobarbital		XX		
Trimethadione (Tridione)				XXX
Anti-inflammatories				
ASA (aspirin)				X*
Colchicine		X?		
Gold compounds				XX
Ibuprofen (Motrin)	X			X
Indomethacin (Indocin)				X
Phenacetin	XXX			X
Phenylbutazone				XX, X*
Antihypertensives/Diuretics				
Methyldopa (Aldomet)	XXX			
Acetazolamide (Diamox)				X
Thiazides	X			
Tranquilizers				
Chloridazepoxide (Librium)				X
Chlorpromazine (Thorazine)	XX			X
Meprobamate				X
Oral Hypoglycemics				
Chlorpropamide (Diabinese)	X			
Tolbutamide (Orinase)				X, X*
Immunosuppressants				
Azathioprine (Imuran)			X	X*
Cyclosporine	X			
Miscellaneous Agents				
Benzene	XX			XX
Cimetidine (Tagamet)				X
Heparin				X*
Antituberculous agents:				
INH (isoniazid)	XX			
PASA (*para*-aminosalicylic acid)	XX	X		
Pyridium (phenazopyridine HCl)				XX
Potassium perchlorate				XX
Quinine/quinidine	XX			
Acetaminophen (Tylenol)	X			X

X, Rare number of reported cases; *XXXX*, substantial number of reported cases; *XX, XXX*, intermediate number of reported cases; *X**, "pure red cell" aplasia; *X?*, uncertain.

Total body irradiation also causes AA and in certain instances may be used therapeutically for this effect. Infections are also known to cause AA, with viruses being the most common agent. These include infections with the human immunodeficiency virus (HIV), Epstein-Barr virus, and hepatitis (non-A, non-B, non-C, and non-G forms of the virus). Persistent parvovirus B19 infection also has been identified as producing bone marrow failure resulting in AA. Parvovirus B19 has been identified as the cause of aplastic crisis in children who have sickle cell hemoglobinopathies and hereditary spherocytosis.

Another condition associated with AA is **pure red cell aplasia (PRCA),** in which only the erythrocytes are affected. PRCA is a rare disorder and has been associated with autoimmune, viral, and neoplastic (leukemias) disorders; infiltrative disorders of the bone marrow (myelofibrosis); renal failure; hepatitis; mononucleosis; and systemic lupus erythematosus. It also is a well-recognized but infrequent complication of allogeneic bone marrow transplantation, particularly when there is donor-recipient ABO mismatch. A thymoma often is found in association with PRCA and is also present in Diamond-Blackfan syndrome, a congenital disorder.

A very small percentage of AA cases are linked to genetic alterations. **Fanconi anemia** is a rare genetic anemia characterized by pancytopenia resulting from defects in DNA repair.[22] This anemia develops early in life and is accompanied by multiple congenital anomalies.

PATHOPHYSIOLOGY. The characteristic lesion of AA is a hypocellular bone marrow that has been replaced with fat. Most cases of idiopathic AA result from an autoimmune disease directed against hematopoietic stem cells.[23] As with most autoimmune diseases, a genetic predisposition is apparent and has been attributed to polymorphisms in human leukocyte antigens (HLAs) and inhibitory cytokines (e.g., tumor necrosis factor-alpha [TNF-α], transforming growth factor-beta [TGF-β], and interferon-gamma [IFN-γ]).[24] The evidence supporting an autoimmune process includes the response of AA to immunosuppressive therapy including depletion of T cells by antithymocyte antibodies. Cytotoxic T cells (Tc cells) appear to be the main culprits, although the causative antigen has yet to be identified. Th1 cytokines (involved in the differentiation of Tc cells), such as IFN-γ and TNF-α, as well as cellular contact with Tc cells through FasL, induce apoptosis of CD34+ target cells, which includes most of the hematopoietic progenitors.

CLINICAL MANIFESTATIONS. The onset of symptoms is insidious and related to the rapidity with which the bone marrow is destroyed and replaced. Approximately 50% of AA cases progress rapidly, with a high risk of death from overwhelming infection or bleeding. In some cases the rate of decline is slow and the individual may adapt progressively to a new level of hematologic function. This condition is referred to as *hypoplastic anemia* rather than aplastic anemia.

Initial symptoms depend on which cell line is affected. Rapidly progressing disease is usually associated with hypoxemia, pallor (occasionally with a brownish pigmentation of the skin), and weakness along with fever and dyspnea with rapidly developing signs of hemorrhaging if platelets are affected (e.g., unexplained bruising, nosebleeds, bleeding gums, bleeding in the GI tract, prolonged bleeding at sites of minor injury). A slower onset over weeks or months is characterized by progressive weakness and fatigue with developing signs of hemorrhaging. Major hemorrhage may occur from any organ; however, it is generally observed in the late stages and is often secondary to other events. Menorrhagia and purpura also may be evident; however, purpura is not necessarily a classic indication of AA and may not be representative of the degree of thrombocytopenia. In both rapid and slow onset AA, diminished leukocyte production may result in a progressive frequency and prolongation of infections.

Late manifestations of the condition include ulcerations of the mouth and pharynx or a low-grade cellulitis in the neck. Splenomegaly is extremely rare, and if present, other conditions that may imitate AA should be ruled out. Neurologic changes are only evident when hemorrhages have occurred within the system; however, some individuals have complained of paresthesias.

EVALUATION AND TREATMENT. Diagnosis is made by blood tests and bone marrow biopsy. AA is suspected if levels of circulating erythrocytes, leukocytes, and platelets are diminished: a granulocyte count less than 500/μL, a platelet count less than 20,000/μL, and an absolute reticulocyte count less than or equal to 40×10^9/L. The diagnosis is confirmed by a bone marrow biopsy. The bone marrow usually has reduced cellularity (i.e., less than 25% normal cellularity). The morphology of the few remaining hematopoietic cells is usually normal. Occasionally the erythrocytes are macrocytic, with anisocytosis and poikilocytosis, and may appear immature.

Marrow biopsied from individuals with typical AA contains yellowish white material consisting mainly of fat, fibrous tissue, and lymphocytes. Pancytopenia is usually characterized by decreased stem cell and progenitor cell populations to approximately 1% or less of normal.

Up until 20 years ago, treatment involved determining the cause, removal of exposure to the potential causative agent, transfusion, and prevention and treatment of infection and hemorrhage. Stimulation of blood cell production also was used, and in some instances splenectomy was recommended. The prognosis with these forms of treatment was extremely poor. In acute cases, 25% of individuals succumbed within 4 months, and approximately 70% died within 5 years; only about 10% experienced complete recovery. Newer forms of treatment, such as bone marrow transplant (BMT), immunosuppression, and identification of high-risk individuals, have decreased mortality significantly.[25]

Bone marrow and, most recently, peripheral blood stem cell transplantation from a histocompatible sibling often cures the underlying bone marrow failure.[26] Survival rates of 75% to 80% have been reported, and death rates within the first 100 days have decreased. Before transplantation the recipient usually received radiation or chemotherapy to deplete the bone marrow of disease-causing lymphocytes. Thus an unsuccessful transplantation may leave the recipient with a depleted immune system and an increased vulnerability to infection. Graft-versus-host (GVH) disease remains a risk and is a major contributor to premature death.[27] Children demonstrate higher survival than adults.

For those individuals unable to undergo bone marrow transplantation or who lack a suitable sibling donor, immunosuppression remains the treatment of choice. Antithymocyte globulin (ATG) specifically suppresses lymphocytes, including those autoreactive lymphocytes destroying the bone marrow cells. Drugs like cyclosporine, which is often used in combination with ATG, broadly suppress the activity of immune cells. Response rates, that is, increased blood cell counts, of 40% to 50% may occur in individuals who receive ATG. The addition of cyclosporine has increased the response and survival rates to as much as 70% to 80%, with a 5-year survival rate between 80% and 90%. Cyclosporine as a single therapeutic agent is not as effective. Corticosteroids are often used concurrently with ATG and cyclosporine. Cyclophosphamide also has been used as an immunosuppressive agent and has produced the same effects as ATG; however, its use has been discontinued because of its toxicity. The addition of recombinant hematopoietic growth factors, such as granulocyte-macrophage colony-stimulating factor (GM-CSF), IL-6, and epoetin, to immunosuppressive therapy has produced significant additional benefit in both children and adults.

Immunosuppressive therapy is not without risk. Individuals receiving immunosuppressive therapy are at risk of experiencing treatment failure or late clonal/malignant conditions, or both. Late clonal/malignant conditions include paroxysmal nocturnal hemoglobinuria (PNH), MDS, acute leukemia, or solid tumor. Although quite rare (less than 3%), administration of ATG may cause an anaphylactic reaction in some individuals.

Posthemorrhagic Anemia (Acute Blood Loss)

Posthemorrhagic anemia is a normocytic-normochromic anemia caused by acute blood loss. Initial manifestations of this event depend on the severity of blood loss. If blood loss is severe, the significant manifestations are related to loss of blood volume rather than loss of hemoglobin.

A normal, healthy young adult can tolerate a blood loss of 500 to 1000 ml (10% to 20% of volume) without experiencing any symptoms. Additional losses up to 1500 ml do not cause obvious symptoms if the individual is recumbent—symptoms appear only when assuming an upright position. When blood loss exceeds 1500 ml, symptoms are apparent even in a recumbent position (Table 28-5).

Volume loss reduces mean systemic filling pressure, resulting in decreased venous return. The initial manifestations (increased sympathetic nerve activation and a reduction in blood pressure, cardiac output, and central venous pressure) are caused by cardiovascular adaptations to blood volume depletion. If blood loss exceeds 2000 ml, severe shock, lactic acidosis, and death occur. (Shock is discussed in Chapter 48.)

If the acute blood loss is not severe (does not cause the preceding manifestations), complete recovery is possible. Within 24 hours of blood loss, lost plasma is replaced by mobilizing water and electrolytes from tissues and interstitial spaces into the vascular system. The hemodilution that results lowers the hematocrit value; concurrently, there is often a rapid elevation of circulating neutrophils and platelets. Neutrophils can rise to levels between 10,000 and 30,000/μL within a few hours as a result of a shift of marginated leukocytes into the circulation and a release of leukocytes from the bone marrow. The platelet count can rise to levels of about 1 million/μL. In severe blood loss, more immature cells—metamyelocytes, myelocytes, and nucleated red blood cells—may enter the circulation. Reduction in tissue oxygenation stimulates production of erythropoietin and increasing production of erythrocytes (reticulocytes) in the bone marrow. Iron recovery from destroyed erythrocytes may occur if the acute blood loss is internal; however, if blood is lost externally, iron stores may be depleted and erythropoiesis may be impeded. Hemorrhage that is chronic (occult [i.e., bleeding ulcer or neoplasm]) produces adaptations that are less prominent, but the individual may experience an IDA when iron reserves become depleted.

TABLE 28-5 CLINICAL MANIFESTATIONS OF ACUTE BLOOD LOSS OF INCREASING SEVERITY*

VOLUME LOST		
% TBV	**ml**	**CLINICAL MANIFESTATIONS**
10	500	None; rarely notice vasovagal syncope in blood donors
20	1000	When person is at rest, it is difficult, if not impossible, to detect volume loss; tachycardia is common with exercise and a slight drop in blood pressure with postural change
30	1500	Neck veins are flat in supine position; exercise tachycardia and postural hypotension are usually present; resting supine blood pressure and pulse can still be normal
40	2000	Central venous pressure, cardiac output, and arterial blood pressure are below normal even at rest and supine position; person commonly has air hunger; a rapid, thready pulse; and cold, clammy skin
50	2500	Severe shock, lactic acidosis, death

Adapted from Hillman RS: Acute blood loss anemia. In Beutler E et al, editors: *Williams hematology*, ed 5, New York, 1995, McGraw-Hill.
*Data based on a 70-kg person with a total blood volume of 5000 ml.
TBV, Total blood volume.

Initial treatment for acute blood loss is restoration of blood volume by intravenous administration of saline, dextran, albumin, or plasma. Large volume losses may require transfusion of fresh whole blood.

Successful therapy is first indicated by a return of erythrocytes to their normal size and shape. As the bone marrow begins to produce more erythrocytes, an increase in the number of reticulocytes (10% to 15% after 7 days) is seen. Changes in the appearance of erythrocytes (polychromatophilia and macrocytosis) associated with reticulocytosis may give the impression that an underlying hemolytic process is occurring. A normal erythrocyte count is usually noted in 4 to 6 weeks, but hemoglobin restoration may take 6 to 8 weeks.

Hemolytic Anemia

The predominant event in **hemolytic anemias** is premature accelerated destruction of erythrocytes, either episodically or

TABLE 28-6 **CAUSES OF HEMOLYTIC ANEMIAS**

TYPE OF HEMOLYTIC DISORDER	PRIMARY CAUSE OR ASSOCIATED DISORDER	MECHANISMS OF ERYTHROCYTE DESTRUCTION
Acquired Forms		
Immune system–mediated hemolysis	Transfusion reaction Hemolytic disease of the newborn (see Chapter 30) Autoimmune hemolytic anemia (see text)	Antibody-mediated: intravascular hemolysis by activation of complement system; extravascular hemolysis by phagocytosis of antibody-coated erythrocytes in spleen (see Chapter 9)
Traumatic hemolysis	Presence of prosthetic heart valves Structural abnormalities of the heart Hemolytic uremic syndrome Disseminated intravascular coagulation Hemodialysis	Physical destruction of erythrocytes by "mechanical" means (trauma)
Infectious hemolysis	Bacterial infection Viral infection Protozoal infection Helminthic infection	Bacterial hemolysins (e.g., *Escherichia coli* 0157:H7 shiga toxin; *Clostridium perfringens* toxin) Initiate autoimmune hemolysis (e.g., *Mycoplasma pneumoniae:* cold agglutinin) Affects erythrocytes (e.g., parvovirus B19: infects erythroid progenitors) Infects erythrocytes (e.g., malaria) Intestinal bleeding (e.g., hookworm)
Drug or toxic (chemical) hemolysis	Exposure to toxic chemical agents Hemodialysis or uremia Venoms	Chemical injury of erythrocytes (see Chapter 2)
Physical hemolysis	Burns Radiation	Heat or radiation injury (see Chapter 2)
Hypophosphatemic hemolysis	Hypophosphatemia (phosphate deficiency in plasma; see Chapter 3)	Diminished cellular production of substances required for erythrocyte life and function
Hereditary Forms		
Structural defects	Plasma membrane defects	Fragility of the erythrocyte
Plasma membrane protein mutation	Deficient complement regulatory proteins (i.e., paroxysmal nocturnal hemoglobulinuria)	Complement activation on erythrocyte surface, intravascular lysis
Enzyme deficiencies	Deficiency of glycolytic enzymes Deficiency of metabolic enzymes (i.e., glucose-6-phosphate dehydrogenase deficiency)	Diminished cellular function
Defects of globin synthesis or structure	Sickle cell anemia	Increased membrane fragility and deformation during sickle crises
	Thalassemia	Defective hemoglobin structure and function
	Miscellaneous hemoglobin defects	Defective hemoglobin structure and function

From Lee GR et al: *Wintrobe's clinical hematology,* ed 9, Philadelphia, 1993, Lea & Febiger.

continuously. The consequences of the anemia are elevated levels of erythropoietin to induce accelerated production of erythrocytes and an increase in the products of hemoglobin catabolism.

Hemolytic anemias may be either congenital or acquired. Congenital hemolytic anemias result from intrinsic defects in erythrocytes, including the red cell membrane (e.g., hereditary spherocytosis, paroxysmal nocturnal hemoglobinuria), enzymatic pathways (e.g., glucose-6-phosphate dehydrogenase deficiency), and hemoglobin synthesis (e.g., the thalassemia syndromes, sickle cell anemia). (Glucose-6-phosphate dehydrogenase deficiency, thalassemia, and sickle cell disease are discussed in Chapter 30.) Acquired hemolytic anemias are usually immunologic (immune hemolytic anemias), such as erythrocyte destruction caused by autoantibodies against erythrocyte antigens (e.g., autoimmune hemolytic anemia), isohemagglutinins (e.g., mismatched erythrocyte transfusions), or allergic reactions against drug antigens adsorbed onto the erythrocyte surface (drug-induced hemolytic anemia). (Isohemagglutinins, erythrocyte antigens, autoantibodies, and allergic reactions are discussed in Chapter 9.) Acquired hemolytic anemia may also be secondary to erythrocyte damage caused by cardiac valve prostheses or by increased shear stresses in narrowed small vessels (e.g., during disseminated intravascular coagulation). Causes of acquired and hereditary hemolytic anemias are listed in Table 28-6.

PATHOPHYSIOLOGY. Hemolytic anemias can be classified by a variety of parameters, although no system is entirely satisfactory. Dividing these anemias into inherited or acquired is the preferred and most useful method. Pathophysiologic mechanisms also can be discussed in the context of where hemolysis occurs. Hemolysis occurs within blood vessels (intravascular) or lymphoid tissues (extravascular) that filter blood—that is, spleen and liver. Intravascular hemolysis is the least common and typically caused by physical destruction of erythrocytes in the circulation, frequently by antibody and complement. Extravascular hemolysis results from removal of damaged or opsonized erythrocytes by cells of the mononuclear phagocyte system (MPS). Erythrocytes continuously circulate through the spleen, passing through the thin-walled splenic cords into the splenic sinusoids, a spongelike labyrinth of macrophages with long dendritic processes. Normally, erythrocytes are able to alter their shape to allow passage through openings in the splenic cords. Macrophages will phagocytose erythrocytes with structure alterations of the membrane surface or that have become more rigid and are incapable of maneuvering through this network. In some cases, IgG antibodies or complement component C3b can coat erythrocytes without causing hemolysis, but can function as opsonins that are recognized by macrophages.

Paroxysmal nocturnal hemoglobinuria may be congenital or acquired secondarily to acquired aplastic anemia. The disease results from a mutation in the X-linked gene for phosphatidylinositol glycan—class A *(PIG-A),* which results in a defect in expression of glycosylphosphatidylinositol (GPI) in hematologic stem cells.[28] GPI is a lipid anchor that is necessary for attachment of a large number of proteins to the plasma membrane. Several GPI-anchored proteins on erythrocytes are complement regulatory proteins, including CD55 (decay-accelerating factor) and CD59 (membrane attack complex [MAC] inhibitory protein). Normally low levels of complement are activated on cell surfaces through the alternative pathway (see Chapter 7). Erythrocytes are protected from complement-mediated damage by CD55, which accelerates the degradation of any C3 convertase that forms on the cell surface, and by CD59, which prevents C9 aggregation and pore formation by the membrane attack complex. Thus erythrocytes deficient in CD55 and CD59 undergo complement-mediated intravascular lysis and release of hemoglobin.[29] In addition to anemia and hemoglobinuria, affected individuals also present with severe fatigue, abdominal pain, and thrombosis.[30] The cause of death is usually thrombosis of the abdominal or cerebral veins.[31] Thrombosis most likely results from a depletion of vascular nitric oxide (NO) by free hemoglobin, which has a high affinity for NO. The result is dysregulation of normal hemostasis and increased platelet vascular adherence and clot formation (see Chapter 27).

Autoimmune hemolytic anemias (AIHAs) are acquired disorders caused by autoantibodies against antigens normally on the surface of erythrocytes.[32] Three types of AIHAs have been described: (1) warm reactive antibody type, (2) cold agglutinin type, and (3) cold hemolysin type (paroxysmal cold hemoglobinuria). This classification is based on the optimal temperature at which the antibody binds to erythrocytes and the mechanism of erythrocyte destruction.

Warm autoimmune hemolytic anemia is uncommon (incidence of about 1 per 80,000 population annually), although it is the most common form of AIHA (80% to 90% of cases), and generally occurs in individuals older than the age of 40.[33] Approximately half of the cases are secondary to other diseases, especially lymphomas but also chronic lymphocytic leukemia, other neoplastic disorders, or systemic lupus erythematosus (SLE). The anemia is caused by IgG that binds optimally to erythrocytes at normal body temperature (37° C, 98.6° F). Most cases are related to antibody against Rh-related antigens other than the D epitope (Rh antigens are discussed in Chapter 9). The spectrum of antibody specificities includes antibodies against the e, E, or c antigens of the Rh complex. Other cases are caused by IgG antibodies against erythrocyte antigens outside the Rh complex and include antibodies against Wr^b, En^a, the Kell blood group, and many others. The warm reactive IgG antibodies usually do not activate complement because of the rather sparse distribution of antigens on the erythrocyte surface. (Activation of complement by antibody is discussed in Chapters 7, 8, and 9.) Erythrocyte destruction is caused by extravascular processes. The IgG-coated erythrocytes bind to the Fc receptors on monocytes and splenic macrophages and are removed by phagocytosis.

Cold agglutinin autoimmune hemolytic anemia is mediated by immunoglobulin M (IgM) antibodies and occurs less often than warm antibody hemolysis, affecting mostly middle-aged and older adults. Cold antibodies optimally bind to erythrocytes at colder temperatures (lower than 31° C [87.8° F]) with maximal binding capacity at 4° C (39.2° F). Cold agglutinin autoantibodies may appear acutely during recovery of certain infectious disorders, particularly infectious mononucleosis, mycoplasma pneumonia, and disseminated tuberculosis.[34] With these conditions, the individuals are usually younger than those with primary disease; the anemia may be severe but may be self-limiting. Chronic cold agglutinin AIHAs also can occur in association with lymphoid neoplasm and other unknown or idiopathic conditions.[35]

The IgM autoantibody is usually monoclonal and directed against erythrocyte carbohydrate antigens of the I system (i.e., i, I) or the P system (i.e., Pr).[36] In the colder areas of the body, particularly during cold weather (e.g., fingers, toes, nose, ears, exposed skin), the IgM autoantibodies bind to circulating erythrocytes. The IgM is rapidly released when the blood recirculates and warms. IgM is an extremely efficient activator of complement, resulting in the stable deposition of C3b on the cell surface. If an adequate amount of complement is deposited, the erythrocytes become vulnerable to recognition and rapid phagocytosis by mononuclear phagocytes in the liver and spleen (also see Chapter 9). The severity of hemolysis is variable and may result in a progressive chronic anemia. If the level of antibody is high or has particularly strong binding, hemagglutination may occur in the capillaries of exposed sites, such as fingers, toes, and ears, when temperatures are below 30° C (86° F). Obstruction of blood flow caused by erythrocyte agglutination may lead to a bluish discoloration of the skin (acrocyanosis) that resolves as the skin is warmed. Prolonged exposure to the cold may lead to gangrene.

Cold hemolysin autoimmune hemolytic anemia (paroxysmal cold hemoglobinuria) is a disorder in which exposure to cold initiates acute and severe intravascular hemolysis that, unlike cold agglutinin anemia, results in hemoglobulinuria. The chronic form of this anemia is extremely rare, but an acute form of paroxysmal cold hemoglobinuria is frequently observed

(30% to 40% of cases) in AIHA of childhood. The acute form occurs primarily in children younger than the age of 10 years and is usually preceded by an upper respiratory tract infection or flulike symptoms. Infections with measles, mumps, *Mycoplasma* (pneumonia), and *Varicella* have also been linked to an onset of paroxysmal cold hemoglobinuria. The anemia may be rapidly progressing and severe and associated with fever, reddish brown urine, hemoglobinuria, jaundice, abdominal pains, and pallor, with about 25% of individuals presenting with hepatomegaly and splenomegaly.

Paroxysmal cold hemoglobinuria is generally caused by IgG autoantibodies against the P blood group antigen. Antibody binding occurs in the colder portions of the body. As the erythrocyte recirculates, enzymes of the complement cascade are activated, and cells are destroyed in the vasculature by complement-mediated lysis. The involved antibody, also called *Donath-Landsteiner antibody,* was first recognized in individuals with anemia secondary to chronic syphilis infection. A transfusion reaction is an example of alloimmune hemolytic anemia (also see Chapter 9). Transfused blood that is mismatched for ABO antigens is destroyed by preexisting isohemagglutinins in the recipient. Isohemagglutinins, which are generally IgM antibodies, activate complement, resulting in a rapid intravascular hemolysis. The individual may immediately experience fever, chills, dyspnea, and hypotension and may progress to shock. In some cases the hemolytic reaction may be delayed and develop 3 to 10 days after transfusion. The delayed reaction is caused by a low titer of preexisting antibodies to minor erythrocyte antigens.

Drug-induced hemolytic anemia is a form of immune hemolytic anemia usually resulting from an allergic reaction against foreign antigens (e.g., antibiotics)[37] (also see Chapter 9). Usually the drug is low molecular weight, functions as a hapten, and binds to proteins on the surface of erythrocytes. This is sometimes called the *hapten model* and is based on anemia caused by penicillin, cephalosporins (more than 90% of cases), and, very recently, hydrocortisone (Figure 28-6, *A*).[38] IgG antibody against the drug or against the unique antigen formed by the interface of the drug and erythrocyte protein is formed and binds to the erythrocyte at normal body temperature. Hemolysis is usually extravascular because the opsonized erythrocytes are removed by phagocytes in the spleen and liver, although complement-dependent intravascular hemolysis may occur in some individuals. This form of drug-induced anemia usually follows a large intravenous infusion of an antibiotic and occurs 1 to 2 weeks after the initiation of therapy. Cessation of administration of the drug results in rapid resolution of the anemia.

The erythrocyte plasma membrane contains receptors of components of the complement system, such as C3b, and can bind circulating immune complexes that have activated the complement cascade (see Chapter 9 for a discussion of immune complexes). This forms the basis for the *immune complex model* of drug-induced hemolytic anemia and was first described for anemia resulting from administration of the drug quinidine (Figure 28-6, *B*). The drug or a metabolite of the drug, both of which are haptens, initially binds to plasma proteins and becomes immunogenic (see Chapter 8).

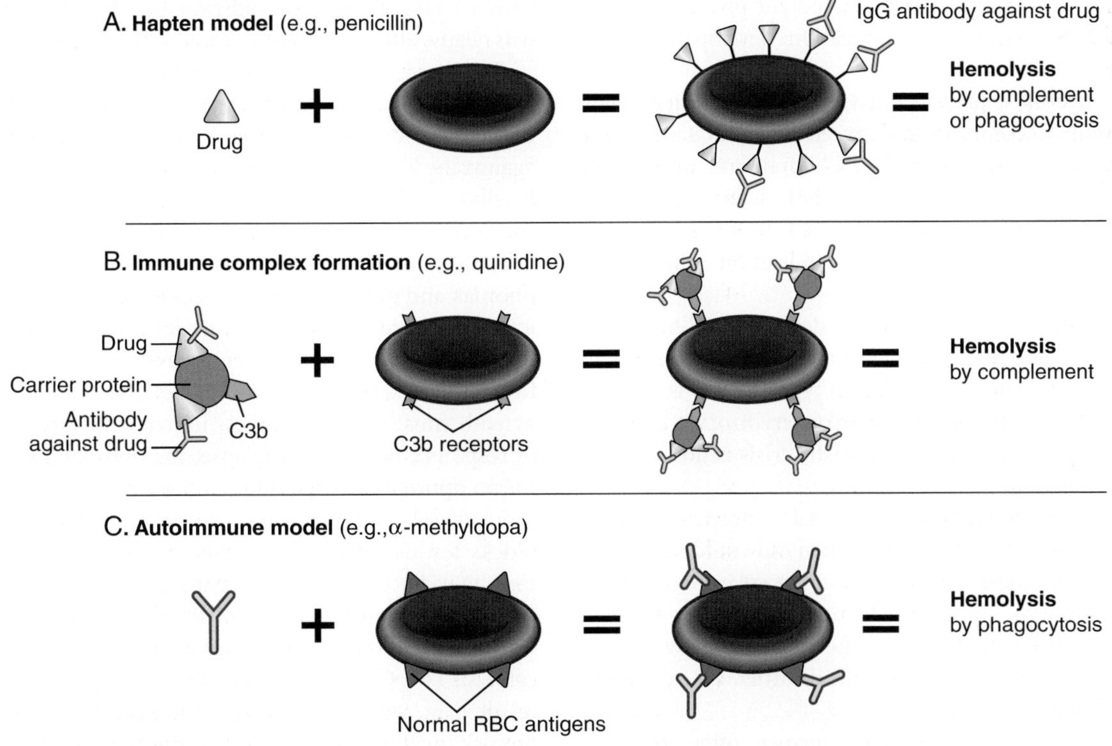

FIGURE 28-6 **Models of Drug-Induced Hemolytic Anemia.** See discussion in text. *IgG,* Immunoglobulin G; *RBC,* red blood cell.

The circulating drug/protein complex reacts with the resultant antibody (usually IgM, although IgG complexes have also been described) and activates the complement system, resulting in the deposition of C3b into the complex. Binding of the immune complexes to the erythrocyte surface results in further complement activation and intravascular hemolysis. This mechanism also may explain some of the anemia observed in other immune complex conditions, such as SLE.

In at least one instance, administration of the drug α-methyldopa induces an immune response against normal erythrocyte antigens and thus initiates a true AIHA *(autoimmune model)* (Figure 28-6, *C*). The autoantibody is usually against Rh blood group antigens. It is estimated that 20% of individuals taking α-methyldopa develop detectable antibodies, but only 1% actually develop clinically significant anemia. The mechanism by which α-methyldopa induces autoantibodies against the erythrocytes is unknown.

CLINICAL MANIFESTATIONS. The presence and severity of signs and symptoms of hemolytic anemia depend on the degree of anemia and hemolysis and the success of compensatory erythropoiesis. Adaptation to red cell destruction is facilitated by increased red cell production. Bone marrow is capable of increasing red cell production up to eight times its normal rate. Accelerated erythrocyte production that is incapable of keeping up with destruction develops into a true hemolytic anemia.

The severity of anemia varies widely from individual to individual, even in individuals who have the same illness. Severe disease is commonly diagnosed shortly after birth or within the first year of life. Mild to moderate anemia is more common because the shortened erythrocyte survival time is offset by increased erythropoiesis. Some individuals have no symptoms of anemia, and the underlying hemolytic process remains undetected unless some other complications develop during the course of the disease.

Jaundice (icterus) is present when heme destruction exceeds the liver's ability to conjugate and excrete bilirubin. Jaundice is first noticed in the neonatal period. Children and adults with congenital hemolytic anemia may not have icterus, or it may be mild enough that it remains unnoticed. In some individuals, faint scleral icterus may be the only indication of hemolytic disease.

Acute conditions that disrupt the delicate equilibrium of accelerated erythropoiesis and erythrocyte destruction may precipitate a crisis. The most common type of crisis is aplastic and results from failure of bone marrow erythrocyte production. The most common cause of aplastic crisis is human parvovirus B19 infection.

Commonly, individuals with congenital hemolytic disorders demonstrate splenomegaly, which is often only mild in nature. In some cases the spleen may become quite enlarged and may cause discovery of the underlying hemolytic disorder. Another underlying condition that may be the cause of inadvertently determining the presence of the anemic disorder is the development of gallstones.

Children who have hemolytic anemia often demonstrate skeletal abnormalities caused by expansion of erythroid bone marrow during the active phase of growth and development. These alterations are more pronounced in the bony structures of the face and skull and may result in pathologic fractures (see Chapter 30). Cardiovascular and respiratory manifestations vary with the degree of anemia. In spite of the disorder being characterized as hemolytic in nature, thromboembolism may occur. Pulmonary embolism is a common finding during autopsies of individuals with immune hemolytic anemia.

EVALUATION AND TREATMENT. Diagnosis is based on clinical manifestations, bone marrow studies, and blood tests (see Table 28-3). Abnormally increased numbers of erythrocyte stem cells are found in the marrow, a finding termed *erythroid hyperplasia.* Accelerated erythropoiesis causes large numbers of fragile and immature erythrocytes (stem cells and reticulocytes) to be released prematurely into the circulation. These cells are observed in blood smears. If the bone marrow is able to consistently maintain adequate compensation, the hemoglobin may remain stable. The mean corpuscular volume, however, may be decreased in the presence of reticulocytes. A blood smear is helpful in determining the presence of spherocytes or schistocytes, as well as examining white blood cells and platelets for coexisting hematologic or malignant conditions.

Acquired hemolytic anemias are treated by removing the cause or treating the underlying disorder. Corticosteroids are used for initial treatment. Approximately 75% of individuals initially respond to treatment with corticosteroids, but many of these relapse within a year. The most commonly used second-line treatments are splenectomy and administration of rituximab. Splenectomy is performed if the spleen is the major site of hemolysis and splenomegaly is significant. Analysis of multiple studies confirms that some response (complete or partial) is achieved in between 59% and 100% of individuals.[39] Although some individuals relapse after splenectomy, most achieve long-term remission.

The therapeutic use of monoclonal antibody has proven beneficial in individuals who relapse or are resistant to the effects of corticosteroids. Rituximab is a monoclonal antibody directed against the CD20 antigen and specifically depletes or suppresses B cells throughout the body. CD20 is expressed on most cells in the B-cell lineage, except hematopoietic stem cells and plasma cells. Rituximab is used to treat a variety of leukemias and lymphomas and autoimmune diseases (e.g., rheumatoid arthritis, idiopathic thrombocytopenia, multiple sclerosis, type 1 diabetes mellitus, systemic lupus erythematosus). It is used successfully in several types of immune hemolytic anemias, although, as with most other therapies, individuals vary in the degree of response, potential to relapse, the optimal dose and timing for an optimal response, and complications.[40] Eculizumab is a monoclonal antibody against complement protein C5, which blocks the enzymatic activation of C5 to C5a and C5b, and thus may be useful to treat paroxysmal nocturnal hemoglobinuria. Treatment with eculizumab prevents the formation of the membrane attack complex and complement-mediated cell lysis (see Chapter 7). In multiple trials, use of eculizumab resulted in reduced hemolysis, the need for transfusion, and the risk for thrombosis, as well as diminished other symptoms, including fatigue and abdominal pains.[41] Blockage of C5 activation mimics individuals who have congenital deficiencies in C5 (see Chapter 9). Lack of C5 increases the risk for disseminated infections with *Neisseria* sp., particularly *Neisseria meningitidis;* thus immunization with the meningococcal vaccine is recommended before treatment with eculizumab.[42]

Acute fulminating hemolytic anemia (hemolytic crisis) is treated with fluid and electrolyte replacement to prevent shock and renal damage, which may be caused by erythrocyte debris clogging the kidney tubules. Transfusions of blood products sometimes are given. Folate also is used in treating chronic hemolytic disease to prevent megaloblastic crisis because long-term erythrocyte turnover increases folate requirements.

Anemia of Chronic Disease

Anemia of chronic disease (ACD) is a mild to moderate anemia resulting from decreased erythropoiesis in individuals with conditions of chronic systemic disease or inflammation (e.g., infections, cancer, and chronic inflammatory or autoimmune diseases). These conditions include acquired immunodeficiency disease (AIDS), malaria (particularly that caused by *Plasmodium falciparum*), rheumatoid arthritis, systemic lupus erythematosus (SLE), acute and chronic hepatitis, and chronic renal failure (a condition in which almost all affected individuals are anemic).[43] This form of anemia also is commonly noted in the presence of congestive heart failure (CHF). The anemia develops after 1 to 2 months of disease activity. The initial severity is related to that of the underlying disorder but, although persistent, it usually does not progress. Individuals may be asymptomatic, or the anemia may be a coincidental clinical finding.

ACD is one of the most common conditions encountered in medicine and is probably only secondary to IDA in overall incidence. In individuals older than age 65, anemia is present in 10% of those who live in the community and more than 50% of those who reside in nursing homes, two thirds of which is ACD or unexplained anemia. The elderly may be predisposed to ACD related to age-associated hematopoietic restriction and generally have increased concentrations of inflammatory cytokines, which play a significant role in the development of ACD. The elderly who present with characteristics of ACD without an underlying malignancy or inflammatory condition are described as having primary defective iron-utilization syndrome.

PATHOPHYSIOLOGY. ACD results from a combination of (1) decreased erythrocyte life span, (2) suppressed production of erythropoietin, (3) ineffective bone marrow erythroid progenitor response to erythropoietin, and (4) altered iron metabolism and iron sequestration in macrophages.[44] During chronic inflammation a large variety of cytokines are released by lymphocytes, macrophages, and the affected tissue.[45] These include TNF-α, IFN-γ, interleukin-1β (IL-1β), IL-3, and IL-6 (also see Chapters 7 and 8).[46]

Impaired iron metabolism is partially the result of iron sequestration.[47] IL-6 in particular affects hepatocytes and increases the release of the peptide hepcidin, which regulates the activity of ferroportin. Ferroportin is the primary transporter for the export of iron from macrophages to the plasma, and increased levels of hepcidin result in decreased ferroportin activity and suppression of iron release (Figure 28-7).

Erythrocyte destruction is the result of eryptosis (described earlier in this chapter). Most of the diseases responsible for ACD damage erythrocytes, resulting in increased efflux of plasma membrane phosphatidylserine and susceptibility to removal by macrophages. Normal iron transport by transferrin also may be decreased as a result of competitive iron binding by inflammation-related increases in the levels of circulating lactoferrin and apoferritin. **Lactoferrin** is a member of the transferrin family of nonheme iron-binding glycoproteins, and under normal conditions is present in the blood in only small amounts. During inflammation neutrophils release lactoferrin to bind iron and reduce its availability for bacteria. However, the affinity of iron for lactoferrin is 260 times greater than that for transferrin. Lactoferrin-bound iron is removed by the mononuclear-phagocyte system and converted into ferritin, the storage form of iron. **Apoferritin** also has a higher affinity for iron and affects available iron in a similar manner.

The erythropoietic defect in ACD is failure to increase erythropoiesis in response to decreased numbers of erythrocytes. In part, decreased erythropoiesis results from diminished production of erythropoietin by the kidneys. The kidney is frequently affected by chronic inflammatory processes caused by circulating immune complexes and other factors that deposit in the kidney and activate secondary inflammatory mechanisms. In addition, the failure in erythropoiesis may reflect decreased responsiveness of erythroid progenitors to erythropoietin. Decreased availability of iron would diminish the rate of erythropoiesis. Proliferation of erythroid cells is also inhibited by proinflammatory cytokines, especially TNF-α, IFN-γ, and IL-1β. TNF-α also directly induces apoptosis of erythroid progenitors, thus diminishing the number of responsive cells. In individuals who had anemia secondary to rheumatoid arthritis, the bone marrow contained elevated levels of IL-3, which correlated with diminished expression of integrins on the surface of cells of the erythroid series.[48] Loss of integrins may prevent adequate interaction with stromal cells and matrix proteins and inhibit erythropoiesis.

Anemia associated with chronic renal failure may result from a variety of simultaneous mechanisms. Damage to the kidney affects the secretion of erythropoietin, a necessary hormone for production of erythrocytes in the bone marrow, thus resulting in diminished bone marrow erythropoiesis.[49] Uremic toxins (e.g., uric acid, sulfates, phosphates) that increase in the blood secondarily to renal failure may suppress bone marrow function and damage erythrocytes, which undergo eryptosis. Platelet function also may be defective in these individuals, which results in chronic bleeding and loss of erythrocytes.

Anemia may arise from the direct action of bacterial toxins. For example, *Clostridium perfringens* (gas gangrene and a cause of food poisoning) produces an alpha-toxin. This toxin has enzymatic activity (phospholipase C, sphingomyelinase) that disrupts the membrane of cells. If the cells are erythrocytes, hemolysis will result.

CLINICAL MANIFESTATIONS. The anemia of ACD is usually in the mild to moderate range, with few additional complications. If hemoglobin levels drop significantly, clinical manifestations of IDA appear.

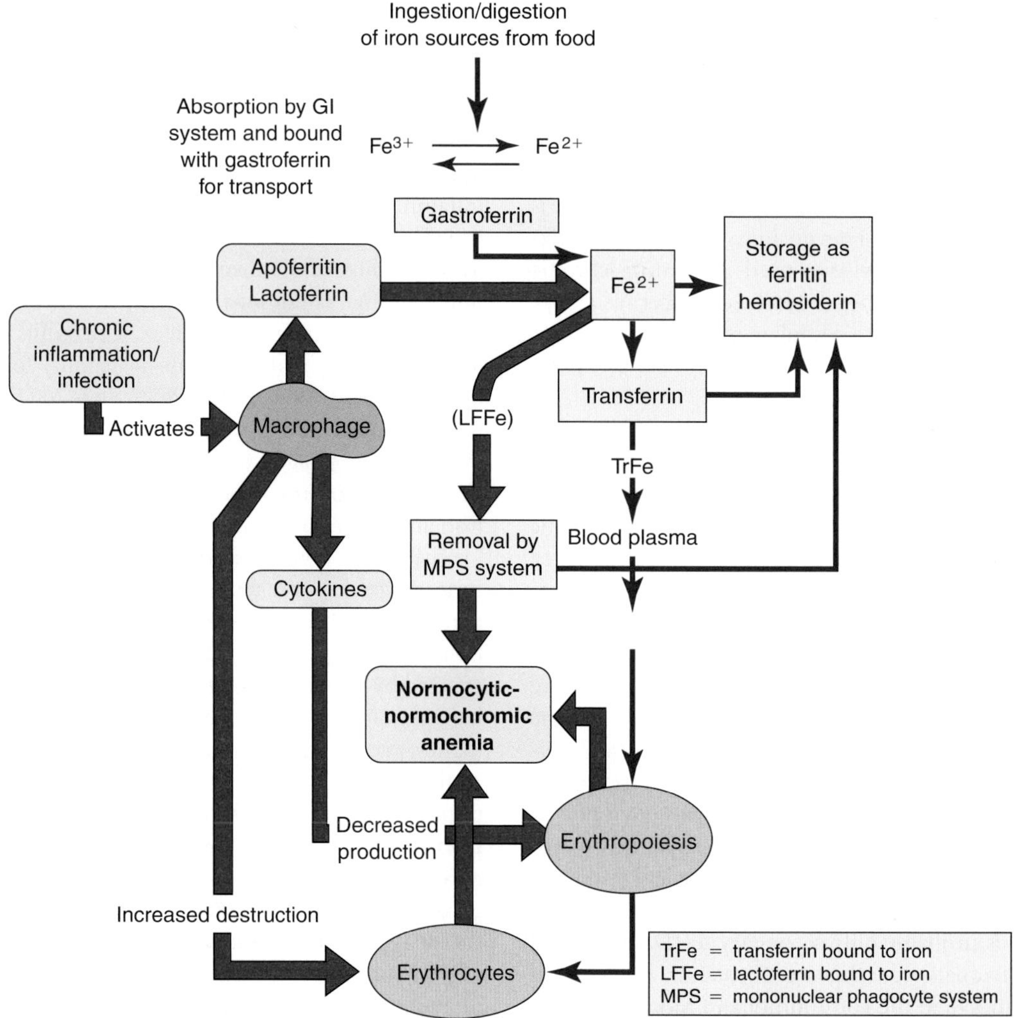

FIGURE 28-7 **Pathophysiology of Anemia of Chronic Disease.** Normal iron metabolism is indicated by the narrow arrows. Abnormal mechanisms that are instrumental in the development of anemia of chronic inflammation are indicated by thick arrows. (See discussion in text.) *GI,* Gastrointestinal.

EVALUATION AND TREATMENT. Morphologically, ACD is initially normocytic-normochromic, but as the condition persists it becomes hypochromic and microcytic. ACD is characterized by abnormal iron metabolism with low levels of circulating iron (less than 60 mcg/dl) and reduced levels of transferrin. The most significant finding of ACD is a very high total body iron storage, although inadequate iron is released from the bone marrow for erythropoiesis. Very often the first indication of ACD is a failure to respond to conventional iron replacement therapy. Levels of erythropoietin are generally lower than expected for the degree of anemia. The affected individuals also frequently present with low or normal total iron-binding capacity (TIBC), normal or high serum ferritin levels, and low concentrations of soluble transferrin receptor (blood test findings are listed in Table 28-3). Occasionally it may be difficult to differentiate ACD from IDA; however, measurement of sTfR may be useful. Levels of sTfR do not respond to iron supplementation in ACD but do so in IDA.

Use of erythropoietin in treatment of ACD associated with arthritis, malignancies, and AIDS has met with limited success. Individuals with severe anemia secondary to chronic kidney disease can be treated successfully with erythropoietin and treatments to increase iron stores.[43] However, the optimal degree of restoration of hemoglobin levels (a measure of anemia) has not been determined; achievement of normal levels increases the risk of hypertension, stroke, and death.[50] Transfusion of critically ill individuals may worsen the outcome and increase morbidity and mortality.[51] The principal treatment is alleviation of the underlying disorder. Individuals who have ACD but demonstrate no evidence of inflammatory or infectious conditions are screened for the presence of malignancies.

MYELOPROLIFERATIVE RED BLOOD CELL DISORDERS

Hematologic dysfunction results from an overproduction of cells as well as a deficiency. One or more hematopoietic lines may be overproduced in the marrow in response to exogenous (e.g., exposure to radiation, drugs) or endogenous (e.g., physiologic compensatory responses, immune disorders) signals. Excessive red blood cell production is classified as **polycythemia.** Polycythemia exists in two forms: relative and absolute. **Relative polycythemia** results from hemoconcentration of the blood associated with dehydration that may be caused by decreased water intake, diarrhea, excessive vomiting, or increased use of diuretics. Its development is usually of minor consequence and resolves with fluid administration or treatment of the underlying condition.

Absolute polycythemia consists of two forms: primary or secondary. *Secondary polycythemia,* the more common type, is a physiologic response resulting from increased erythropoietin secretion in response to chronic hypoxia. This hypoxia is noted in individuals who live at higher altitudes (i.e., above 10,000 feet), smokers with increased levels of carbon monoxide (CO), and individuals with chronic obstructive pulmonary disease or congestive heart failure, or both. Abnormal types of hemoglobin (e.g., $Hb_{San\ Diego}$ or $Hb_{Chesapeake}$), which have a greater affinity for oxygen, also can cause secondary polycythemia, as does secretion of erythropoietin by certain tumors (e.g., renal cell carcinoma, hepatoma, and cerebral hemiangioblastoma).

Polycythemia Vera

Polycythemia vera (PV) (also known as primary polycythemia) is one of several disorders collectively known as *chronic myeloproliferative disorders* (CMPDs).[52] Others in this group include essential thrombocytosis, chronic idiopathic myelofibrosis, chronic myeloid leukemia, chronic neutrophilic leukemia, and chronic eosinophilic leukemia. All result from abnormal regulation of the multipotent hematopoietic stem cells. The major characteristics shared by these disorders are: (1) involvement of a multipotent hematopoietic progenitor cell; (2) overproduction of one or more of the formed elements of the blood in the absence of a defined stimulus; (3) dominance of a transformed progenitor cell over the nontransformed progenitor cells; (4) marrow hypercellularity or fibrosis; (5) cytogenetic abnormalities; (6) predisposition to thrombus formation and hemorrhage; and (7) spontaneous transformation to acute leukemia. Determining a precise distinction between the CMPDs is difficult if not impossible because of overlapping clinical features and a lack of specific molecular markers. As a result, diagnosis is quite challenging.

PV is quite rare with an estimated incidence of 2.3 per 100,000 individuals; peak incidence is between the ages of 60 and 80 years, with a median incidence of 55 to 60. However, PV has been observed in individuals younger than the age of 40. Males are twice as likely as females to develop PV. PV is more common in whites, particularly those of Eastern European Jewish ancestry, than in blacks. PV is rarely found in children or in multiple members of a single family; however, an autosomal dominant form exists that is characterized by increased production of erythropoietin.

PATHOPHYSIOLOGY. **Polycythemia vera (PV)** is a chronic neoplastic, nonmalignant condition characterized by overproduction of red blood cells (frequently with increased levels of white blood cells [leukocytosis] and platelets [thrombocytosis]) and splenomegaly. Erythrocytosis is the essential component of PV. Clonal proliferation of erythroid progenitors occurs in the bone marrow independent of erythropoietin, although the cells express a normal erythropoietin receptor. However, more than 95% of individuals with PV possess an acquired mutation in Janus kinase 2 *(JAK2)*.[53] *JAK2* increases the activity of the erythropoietin receptor and is self-regulatory so that *JAK2* activity diminishes over time. The mutation associated with PV negates the self-regulatory activity of *JAK2* so that the erythropoietin receptor is constitutively active regardless of the level of erythropoietin.[54] These red blood cell precursors also demonstrate sensitivity to other growth factors, such as interleukin-3 (IL-3), granulocyte-macrophage colony-stimulating factor (GM-CSF), or insulin-like growth factor

CLINICAL MANIFESTATIONS. Almost every individual initially presents with an enlarged spleen, frequently with abdominal pain and discomfort. As the disease progresses many of the symptoms are related to the increased blood cellularity and viscosity. Increased viscosity, as well as thrombocythemia and increased platelet dysfunction, leads to a hypercoagulable state with formation of venous and arterial thrombosis and vessel occlusion.[55] Thrombi with occlusion of major and minor blood vessels lead to tissue and/or organ injury (ischemia) and death (infarction). Extreme thrombocythemia (greater than 1,500,000/mm^3 of blood) increases the risk for excessive bleeding, rather than thrombosis.

Increased blood viscosity results in a variety of circulatory alterations in PV, such as plethora (ruddy, red color of the face, hands, feet, ears, and mucous membranes) and engorgement of the retinal and cerebral veins. Individuals also may experience headache, drowsiness, delirium, mania, psychotic depression, chorea, and visual disturbances. Death from cerebral thrombosis is increased approximately fivefold in individuals with PV.

Cardiac workload and output remain essentially unchanged; however, increased blood volume may lead to elevated blood pressure. Coronary blood flow may be affected, precipitating angina, although cardiovascular infarctions are relatively rare. Other evidence of cardiovascular involvement is the development of Raynaud phenomenon and thromboangiitis obliterans.

Additionally, gastrointestinal gastric and duodenal thrombosis may occur with resultant hemorrhaging. The development of mesenteric thrombosis requires immediate medical intervention. Splenomegaly and hepatomegaly result from pooling of blood in these organs; consequently, individuals may develop portal hypertension. The respiratory system is generally not affected by PV, unless thrombosis and embolization occur.

A unique feature of PV, one helpful in diagnosis, is the development of intense, painful itching that is intensified by heat or exposure to water (aquagenic pruritus), particularly warm water when bathing or showering. The intensity of the itching is related to the concentration of mast cells in the skin and is generally not responsive to antihistamines or topical lotions.

EVALUATION AND TREATMENT. PV is frequently suspected on the basis of clinical features, such as a thrombotic event, splenomegaly, or aquagenic pruritus. Diagnosis of PV is made from blood and laboratory findings (Box 28-2). An absolute increase in the number of red blood cells and in total blood volume confirms the diagnosis. Hematocrit levels may range from 18 to 24 g/dl and red blood cell counts may range from 7×10^{12} to

BOX 28-2 DIAGNOSTIC CRITERIA FOR POLYCYTHEMIA VERA

Major Criteria (A)

Increased total red blood cell (RBC) volume (RBC mass):
- >25% above normal predicted value
- M ≥36 ml/kg (Hb >18.5 g/dl)
- F ≥32 ml/kg (Hb >16.5 g/dl)

O_2 saturation ≥92%

Splenectomy

Clonal genetic abnormality other than Philadelphia chromosome or *bcr/abl* fusion gene in marrow*

Endogenous erythroid formation in vitro*

Major Criteria (B)

Platelets ≥400,000/µL

WBC count ≥12,000/µL

LAP score >100

Serum B_{12} >900 pg/ml

$UB_{12}BC$ >2200 pg/ml

Panmyelosis (myeloid metaplasia with abnormal immature blood cells in spleen and/or liver) with prominent erythroid/megakaryocytic hyperplasia on marrow biopsy*

Decreased serum erythropoietin levels*

*World Health Organization (WHO) Criteria for Diagnosis: Elevated red cell mass (RCM) and any other major criteria or elevated RCM and any two minor criteria.

LAP, Leukocyte alkaline phosphatase; *$UB_{12}BC$,* unbound B_{12}-binding capacity; *WBC,* white blood cell.

$7 \times 10^{13}/mm^3$. Erythrocytes appear normal but anisocytosis may be present. A bone marrow examination may be done but is not very valuable unless performed in association with cytogenetic and molecular studies for relevant mutations in *JAK2*.[56] The presence of a *JAK2* mutation confirms the diagnosis.[57] Typically the marrow is hypercellular but not in such a manner as to differentiate it from other myeloproliferative disorders. Additional observations on abnormal megakaryocyte morphologies, formation of clusters of abnormal cells, and increased fibrosis add more specificity and usefulness to bone marrow analysis. Elevated serum levels of erythropoietin are not helpful because most individuals with PV have normal or low levels.

Treatment of PV is challenging and directed toward minimizing the risk of thrombosis and preventing progression to myelofibrosis and acute leukemia. In low-risk individuals (e.g., those younger than age 60 or with no history of thrombosis and without risk factors for cardiovascular disease), the recommended therapy is phlebotomy (300 to 500 ml at a time to reduce erythrocytosis and blood volume) and low-dose aspirin. Initial phlebotomies are done two or three times a week until the hematocrit drops sufficiently, and repeated every 3 to 4 months to maintain a safe hematocrit (less than 45%). Aspirin is used for its antithrombotic (decrease in thromboxane) properties.

Hydroxyurea, an antimetabolite that blocks DNA synthesis and reduces vascular cellularity, is the drug of choice for myelosuppression. Unlike other similar drugs, hydroxyurea reduces the risk of thrombotic complications, but does not increase the risk for developing leukemia.[53] Radioactive phosphorus (^{32}P) has been used to suppress erythropoiesis. Its effects may last up to 18 months. Side effects of ^{32}P treatment include suppression of hematopoiesis resulting in anemia, leukopenia, or thrombocytopenia. Acute leukemia also is a side effect, although most often it occurs after 7 or more years of treatment, making this therapy more useful in the elderly.

Interferon-alpha (IFN-α) has been used when other forms of treatment have failed. Interferon inhibits the growth of the abnormal progenitors and inhibits the actions of cytokines that may lead to the development of myelofibrosis. Therapy with IFN-α is complicated by its proinflammatory activities; thus fever, flulike symptoms, and more severe complications are common. IFN-α is not consistently effective in high-risk adult cases, but is considered in individuals who are intolerant to hydroxyurea, younger individuals, and individuals who are pregnant.

Treatment with inhibitors of the *JAK2* pathway has resulted in reduction of many associated disease symptoms (e.g., thrombosis) and a significant improvement in the quality of life.[58] However, the optimal target defining successful treatment (hematocrit) and the effects on life span have not yet been determined. Recent studies comparing the effects of phlebotomy or hydroxyurea, or both, concluded that a goal of maintaining a hematocrit of less than 45% was preferable to the goal of 45% to 50%.[59] The lower target goal resulted in a significantly lower rate of death from cardiovascular causes or major thrombotic events.

Survival for 10 to 15 years is common. However, without proper treatment, 50% of individuals with PV die within 18 months of the onset of initial symptoms. The primary cause of death is thrombosis, which is more prevalent in elderly individuals and those with prior vascular complications. Death because of hemorrhage is rare but more common in individuals with high platelet counts and those taking antiplatelet drugs. Conversion to acute myeloid leukemia (AML) occurs spontaneously in 10% of individuals within 15 years, increasing to 50% within 20 years. This leukemia is generally refractory to conventional treatment. Conversion to AML is most likely related to treatment with cytotoxic myelosuppressive agents, such as chlorambucil.[57] Those individuals treated only with IFN or hydroxyurea had the same incidence of conversion as those who received no treatment. Although PV is a chronic disorder, appropriate therapy results in remissions and prevention of significant morbidity.

Iron Overload

Iron overload can be primary, as in hereditary hemochromatosis, or secondary. The secondary causes of iron overload include anemias with inefficient erythropoiesis (e.g., sideroblastic anemia, aplastic anemia), dietary iron overload, or conditions that require repeated blood transfusions or iron dextran injections.

Hereditary hemochromatosis (HH) is a common inherited, autosomal recessive disorder of iron metabolism and is characterized by increased gastrointestinal iron absorption with subsequent tissue iron deposition. Excess iron is deposited in the liver, pancreas, heart, joints, and endocrine glands, causing tissue damage that can lead to diseases such as cirrhosis, diabetes, heart failure, arthropathies, and impotence.[60]

HH is caused by two genetic base-pair alterations, C282Y and H63D. These are mutations in the *HFE* gene on chromosome 6. Homozygosity of C282Y is the most common genotype and accounts for 82% to 90% of HH cases. The remaining cases appear to be caused by environmental factors or other genotypes. *HFE* mutations are common in the United States with 1 in 10 white individuals heterozygous for the *HFE* C282Y mutation and 4.4 in 1000 homozygous for the C282Y mutation. C282Y homozygosity is much lower among Hispanics (0.27 in 1000), Asian Americans (<0.001 per 1000), Pacific Islanders (0.12 per 1000), and blacks (0.14 per 1000).

PATHOPHYSIOLOGY. Studies in mice have confirmed that the *HFE* gene is responsible for HH. HFE protein, found in the crypt cells of the duodenum, facilitates transferrin receptor–dependent iron uptake into crypt cells. Mutant HFE protein loses its functional ability and causes a relative iron deficiency in duodenal crypt cells. The deficiency results in an increase in the expression of an iron transport protein, divalent metal ion transporter 1 (DMT-1), which is responsible for dietary iron absorption in the villus cells of the small intestine. This inappropriate intestinal iron absorption leads to iron overload and, eventually, end-organ damage that can result in cirrhosis, diabetes mellitus, hypothyroidism, cardiomyopathies, and arthritis.

Although the natural history of HH is not well understood, there appears to be a long latent period with individual variation in biochemical expression modified by environmental factors, such as blood loss from menstruation or donation, alcohol intake, and diet. Cirrhosis is a late-stage development of HH that can shorten life expectancy. Cirrhosis also is a risk factor for hepatocellular carcinoma that occurs between 40 and 60 years old. Cirrhosis prevention is a major goal of HH screening and treatment.

CLINICAL MANIFESTATIONS. Clinical manifestations of HH include symptoms such as fatigue, malaise, abdominal pain, arthralgias, and impotence, and clinical findings of hepatomegaly, abnormal levels of liver enzymes, bronzed skin, diabetes, and cardiomegaly. Many individuals are diagnosed as a result of serum iron studies as part of a health screening panel. Most (>75%) are asymptomatic and have a low frequency (<25%) of cirrhosis, diabetes, or skin pigmentation.

EVALUATION AND TREATMENT. Laboratory findings in individuals with HH show elevations in serum iron levels, transferrin saturation, and ferritin levels. Documentation of iron overload relies on quantitative phlebotomy with calculation of the amount of iron removed, or liver biopsy with determination of quantitative hepatic iron. With the advent of genetic testing, individuals who are C282Y homozygous or compound heterozygous, less than 40 years old, and have normal liver functions, no further workup is necessary.

Treatment of HH is simple and consists of phlebotomy of 550 ml of whole blood, which is equivalent to 200 to 250 mg of iron. Frequency of phlebotomy depends on ferritin levels and should continue until the ferritin level is between 20 and 50 ng/ml. Initially, phlebotomy may be needed weekly but once therapeutic ferritin levels are reached, phlebotomy may only be needed every 2 to 3 months. Blood banks now accept blood donations from persons with documented HH. Iron chelating agents are sometimes used in addition to phlebotomy, but this is not the mainstay of treatment. Individuals with HH should be instructed to refrain from taking iron and vitamin C supplements and consuming raw shellfish; in addition, alcohol should be used in moderation. Family screening is recommended and necessary for all first-degree relatives of a person with HH.

SUMMARY REVIEW

Anemia

1. Anemia is defined as a reduction in the number or volume of circulating erythrocytes or a decrease in hemoglobin level. Polycythemias are excessive levels of erythrocytes or volume.
2. Anemias can be classified according to (a) erythrocyte size or concentration of hemoglobin or (b) their cause.
3. Clinical manifestations of anemia may be demonstrated in all organs and tissues (tissue hypoxia) throughout the body. Decreased oxygen delivery to tissues causes fatigue, dyspnea, syncope, angina, compensatory tachycardia, and organ dysfunction.
4. Macrocytic-normochromic, or megaloblastic-normochromic, anemias are characterized by larger than normal erythrocytes with normal levels of hemoglobin. They most commonly are caused by deficiency of vitamin B_{12} (PA) or folate.
5. PA results from inadequate vitamin B_{12} absorption because of autoantibodies against the B_{12} transporter IF. Folate deficiency anemia is caused by inadequate dietary intake of folate. Both anemias respond to replacement therapy.
6. Microcytic-hypochromic anemias are characterized by abnormally small erythrocytes with insufficient hemoglobin content. This disorder results from disorders of (a) iron metabolism (IDA), (b) porphyrin and heme synthesis (SAs), or (c) globin synthesis (thalassemia).
7. IDA is the most common type of anemia worldwide. It usually develops slowly, with gradual insidious onset of symptoms. Fatigue, weakness, dyspnea, alteration of various epithelial tissues, and vague neuromuscular complaints result.
8. IDA is usually a result of blood loss or poor nutritional intake. Individuals at highest risk for developing IDA include older adults, women, infants, and those living in poverty. Anemia is also recognized as part of the nonspecific acute phase response to any type of inflammation. Once the source of blood loss is identified and corrected, oral iron replacement therapy can be initiated.
9. SA results from defects in mitochondrial metabolism leading to ineffective iron uptake and dysfunctional heme synthesis. The characteristic cell in the bone marrow, a ringed sideroblast, is an erythroblast containing iron granules arranged around the nucleus. SAs may be hereditary or acquired, and treatment varies depending on the cause.
10. Normocytic-normochromic anemias are characterized by insufficient numbers of normal erythrocytes. Included in this category are aplastic, posthemorrhagic, and hemolytic anemias and ACD.

SUMMARY REVIEW—cont'd

11. AA is a critical condition characterized by a reduction or absence of all three blood cell types (pancytopenia). Unless the cause is determined, bone marrow aplasia results in death.
12. Acute blood loss from hemorrhage results in posthemorrhagic anemia with the severity depending on the amount of hemorrhage. Restoration of blood volume by plasma expanders or transfusions may diminish subjective symptoms of anemia. Hemoglobin restoration may take 6 to 8 weeks.
13. Hemolytic anemia is a result of excessive destruction of erythrocytes and may be acquired or hereditary. Of the acquired forms, autoimmune reaction (immunohemolytic) and drug-induced hemolysis are the most common.
14. AIHAs include (a) warm reactive antibody type, (b) cold agglutinin type, and (c) cold hemolysin type (paroxysmal cold hemoglobinuria).
15. ACD results from decreased erythropoiesis secondary to chronic diseases. The anemia is mild to moderate and one of the most common conditions encountered in medicine.
16. Mechanisms associated with ACD include (a) decreased erythrocyte life span, (b) reduced production of erythropoietin, (c) ineffective bone marrow response to erythropoietin, and (d) iron sequestration in macrophages. In particular, the proinflammataory cytokine IL-6 increases hepatocyte release of hepcidin, which suppresses ferroportin transport of iron out of macrophages.

Myeloproliferative Erythrocyte Disorders (Polycythemia)

1. Polycythemia vera is a myeloproliferative disorder characterized by excessive proliferation of erythrocyte precursors in the bone marrow. Signs and symptoms result directly from increased blood volume and viscosity and a predisposition to thrombosis.
2. Therapeutic phlebotomy to remove excessive blood volume and the use of hydroxyurea have been helpful in decreasing the excessive erythrocyte population.

KEY TERMS

Absolute polycythemia, 1003
Acquired sideroblastic anemia, 991
Anemia, 982
Anemia of chronic disease (ACD), 1001
Anisocytosis, 982
Aplastic anemia (AA), 993
Apoferritin, 1001
Autoimmune hemolytic anemia (AIHA), 998
Cold agglutinin autoimmune hemolytic anemia, 998
Cold hemolysin autoimmune hemolytic anemia (paroxysmal cold hemoglobinuria), 998
Dimorphism, 992
Drug-induced hemolytic anemia, 999
Eryptosis, 987
Fanconi anemia, 995
Folate (folic acid), 989
Hemochromatosis, 992
Hemolytic anemia, 996
Hereditary hemochromatosis (HH), 1004
Hereditary sideroblastic anemia, 992
Hypoplastic anemia, 992
Hypoxemia, 985
Intrinsic factor (IF), 988
Iron deficiency anemia (IDA), 989
Lactoferrin, 1001
Macrocytic (megaloblastic) anemia, 987
Microcytic-hypochromic anemia, 989
Myelodysplastic syndrome (MDS), 992
Normocytic-normochromic anemia (NNA), 993
Pancytopenia, 993
Paroxysmal nocturnal hemoglobinuria, 998
Pernicious anemia (PA), 987
Poikilocytosis, 982
Polycythemia, 1003
Polycythemia vera (PV), 1003
Posthemorrhagic anemia, 996
Pure red cell aplasia (PRCA), 995
Relative polycythemia, 1003
Reversible sideroblastic anemia, 992
Ringed sideroblast, 991
Sideroblastic anemia (SA), 991
Warm autoimmune hemolytic anemia, 998

REFERENCES

1. Muñoz M, García-Erce JA, Remacha AF: Disorders of iron metabolism. Part II: iron deficiency and iron overload, *J Clin Pathol* 64(4):287–296, 2011.
2. Lang E, Qadri SM, Lang F: Killing me softly—suicidal erythrocyte death, *Int J Biochem Cell Biol* 44(8):1236–1243, 2012.
3. Handelman GJ, Levin NW: Red cell survival: relevance and mechanism involved, *J Renal Nutr* 20(5S):S84–S88, 2010.
4. Stabler SP: Vitamin B_{12} deficiency, *N Engl J Med* 368(2):149–160, 2013.
5. Banka S et al: Pernicious anemia—genetic insights, *Autoimmun Rev* 10(8):455–459, 2011.
6. Annibale B, Lahner E, Fave GD: Diagnosis and management of pernicious anemia, *Curr Gastroenterol Rep* 13(6):518–524, 2011.
7. Toh BH et al: Cutting edge issues in autoimmune gastritis, *Clin Rev Allerg Immunol* 42(3):269–278, 2012.
8. Vojdani A: Antibodies as predictors of complex autoimmune diseases, *Int J Immunopathol Pharmacol* 21(2):267–278, 2008.
9. West AR, Oates PS: Mechanisms of heme iron absorption: current questions and controversies, *World J Gastroenterol* 14(26):4101–4110, 2008.
10. Killip S, Bennett JM, Chambers MD: Iron deficiency anemia, *Am Fam Physician* 75(5):671–678, 2007.
11. Carmel R: Nutritional anemias and the elderly, *Semin Hematol* 45(4):225–234, 2008.
12. Alleyne M, Horne MK, Miller JL: Individualized treatment for iron-deficiency anemia in adults, *Am J Med* 121(11):943–948, 2008.
13. Finsterer J: Hematological manifestations of primary mitochondrial disorders, *Acta Haematol* 118(2):88–98, 2007.
14. Iolascon A, De Falco L, Beaumont C: Molecular basis of inherited microcytic anemia due to defects in iron acquisition or heme synthesis, *Haematologica* 94(3):395–406, 2009.
15. Edison ES, Bajel A, Chandy M: Iron homeostasis: new players, newer insights, *Eur J Haematol* 81(6):411–424, 2008.
16. Camaschella C: Recent advances in the understanding of inherited sideroblastic anaemia, *Br J Haematol* 143(1):27–38, 2008.
17. Garcia-Manero G: Myelodysplastic syndromes: 2012 update on diagnosis, risk-stratification, and management, *Am J Hematol* 87(7):693–701, 2012.
18. Dreyfus F: The deleterious effects of iron overload in patients with myelodysplastic syndromes, *Blood Rev* 22(Suppl 2):S29–S34, 2008.
19. Malcovati L, Nimer SD: Myelodysplastic syndromes: diagnosis and staging, *Cancer Contr* 15(Suppl):4–13, 2008.
20. Moyo V et al: Erythropoiesis-stimulating agents in the treatment of anemia in myelodysplastic syndromes: a meta-analysis, *Ann Hematol* 87(7):527–536, 2008.
21. Young NS, Calado RT, Scheinberg P: Current concepts in the pathophysiology and treatment of aplastic anemia, *Blood* 108(8):2509–2519, 2006.
22. Kee Y, D'Andrea AD: Molecular pathogenesis and clinical management of Fanconi anemia, *J Clin Invest* 122(11):3799–3806, 2012.
23. Bacigalupo A: Aplastic anemia: pathogenesis and treatment, *Hematology* 2007:23–28, 2007.
24. Mavroudi I, Papadaki HA: Genetic associations in acquired immune-mediated bone marrow failure syndromes: insights in aplastic anemia and chronic idiopathic neutropenia, *Clin Dev Immunol* 2012:1–7, 2012. (Article ID 123789).

25. Scheinberg P, Young NS: How I treat acquired aplastic anemia, *Blood* 120(6):1185–1196, 2012.
26. Armand P, Antin JH: Allogeneic stem cell transplantation for aplastic anemia, *Biol Blood Marrow Transplant* 13(5):505–516, 2007.
27. Davies JK, Guinan EC: An update on the management of severe idiopathic aplastic anaemia in children, *Br J Haematol* 136(4):549–564, 2007.
28. Brodsky RA: Narrative review: paroxysmal nocturnal hemoglobinuria: the physiology of complement-related hemolytic anemia, *Ann Intern Med* 148(8):587–595, 2008.
29. Risitano AM: Paroxysmal nocturnal hemoglobinuria and the complement system: recent insights and novel anticomplement strategies, *Adv Exp Med Biol* 735:155–172, 2013.
30. Ziakas PD, Poulou LS, Pomont A: Thrombosis in paroxysmal nocturnal hemoglobinuria at a glance: a clinical review, *Curr Vasc Pharmacol* 6(4):347–353, 2008.
31. Brodsky R: Advances in the diagnosis and therapy of paroxysmal nocturnal hemoglobinuria, *Blood Rev* 22(2):65–74, 2008.
32. Valent P, Lechner K: Diagnosis and treatment of autoimmune haemolytic anaemias in adults: a clinical review, *Wien Klin Wochenschr* 120(5–6), 2008.
33. Packman CH: Hemolytic anemia due to warm autoantibodies, *Blood Rev* 22(1):17–31, 2008.
34. Wu B, Rong R: Cold agglutinin syndrome with severe haemolytic anaemia in a patient diagnosed of disseminated tuberculosis and concomitant *Mycoplasma pneumonia* infection, *Transfus Med* 22(2):151–152, 2012.
35. Berentsen S, Belske K, Tjønnfjord GE: Primary chronic cold agglutinin disease: an update on pathogenesis, clinical features and therapy, *Hematology* 12(5):361–370, 2007.
36. Petz LD: Cold antibody autoimmune hemolytic anemias, *Blood Rev* 22(1):1–15, 2008.
37. Garratty G: Immune hemolytic anemia caused by drugs, *Expert Opin Drug Saf* 11(4):635–642, 2012.
38. Martinengo M et al: The first case of drug-induced immune hemolytic anemia due to hydrocortisone, *Transfusion* 48(9):1925–1929, 2008.
39. Crowther M et al: Evidence-based focused review of the treatment of idiopathic warm immune hemolytic anemia in adults, *Blood* 118(15):4036–4040, 2013.
40. Garvey B: Rituximab in the treatment of autoimmune haematological disorders, *Br J Haematol* 141(2):149–169, 2008.
41. Charneski L, Patel PN: Eculizumab in paroxysmal nocturnal haemoglobinuria, *Drugs* 68(10):1341–1346, 2008.
42. Hill A: Update on eculizumab for the treatment of paroxysmal nocturnal hemoglobinuria, *Clin Adv Hematol Oncol* 6(7):499–500, 2008.
43. Drüeke TB: Anemia treatment in patients with chronic kidney disease, *N Engl J Med* 368(4):387–389, 2013.
44. Handelman GJ, Levin NW: Iron and anemia in human biology: a review of mechanisms, *Heart Fail Rev* 13(4):393–404, 2008.
45. Kwaan HC: Infection and anemia, *Infect Disord Drug Targets* 11(1): 40–44, 2011.
46. Zarychanski R, Houston DS: Anemia of chronic disease: a harmful disorder or an adaptive, beneficial response? *Can Med Assoc J* 179(4):333–337, 2008.
47. Tussing-Humphreys L et al: Rethinking iron regulation and assessment in iron deficiency, anemia of chronic disease, and obesity: introducing hepcidin, *J Acad Nutr Diet* 112(3):391–400, 2012.
48. Jaworski J et al: Decreased expression of integrins by hematopoietic cells in patients with rheumatoid arthritis and anemia: relationship with bone marrow cytokine levels, *J Invest Allergy Clin Immunol* 18(1):17–21, 2008.
49. Portolés J et al: The development of anemia is associated to poor prognosis in NKF/KDOQI stage 3 chronic kidney disease, *BMC Nephrol* 14(1):2, 2013.
50. Jing Z et al: Hemoglobin targets for chronic kidney disease patients with anemia: a systematic review and meta-analysis, *PLoS One* 7(8):1–9, 2012.
51. Asare K: Anemia of critical illness, *Pharmacotherapy* 28(10):1267–1282, 2008.
52. Levine RL, Gilliland DG: Myeloproliferative disorders, *Blood* 112(6):2190–2198, 2008.
53. Finazzi G, Barbui T: Evidence and expertise in the management of polycythemia vera and essential thrombocythemia, *Leukemia* 22(8): 1494–1502, 2008.
54. Chen G, Prchal JT: Polycythemia vera and its molecular basis: an update, *Best Pract Res Clin Haemotol* 19(3):387–397, 2006.
55. Landolfi R, Cipriani MC, Novarese L: Thrombosis and bleeding in polycythemia vera and essential thrombocythemia: pathogenetic mechanisms and prevention, *Best Pract Res Clin Haematol* 19(3):617–633, 2006.
56. Tefferi A: The diagnosis of polycythemia vera: new tests and old dictums, *Best Pract Res Clin Haematol* 19(3):455–469, 2006.
57. Tefferi A: Polycythemia vera and essential thrombocytopenia: 2012 update on diagnosis, risk stratification, and management, *Am J Hematol* 87(3):285–293, 2012.
58. Tibes R, Bogenberger JM, Mesa RA: JAK inhibition: the key to treating myeloproliferative neoplasm? *Expert Rev Hematol* 5(6):583–585, 2012.
59. Marchioli R et al: Cardiovascular events and intensity of treatment in polycythemia vera, *N Engl J Med* 368(1):22–33, 2013.
60. Crownover BK, Covey CJ: Hereditary hemochromatosis, *Am Fam Physician* 87(3):183–190, 2013.

CHAPTER

29

Alterations of Leukocyte, Lymphoid, and Hemostatic Function

Anna Schwartz and Neal S. Rote

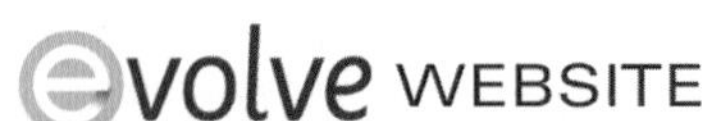

http://evolve.elsevier.com/McCance/
- Review Questions and Answers
- Animations
- Online Course: Module 13

CHAPTER OUTLINE

There are many disorders involving leukocytes, ranging from deficiencies in the quality and quantity of leukocytes (leukopenia) to increased numbers of leukocytes (leukocytosis) in response to infections or proliferative disorders, such as leukemia. Many hematologic disorders are malignancies, and many nonhematologic malignancies act like malignancies and can metastasize to bone marrow, affecting leukocyte production. Because of the complexity of hematologic disorders a large portion of this chapter is devoted to malignant disease.

The primary role of clotting (hemostasis) is to stop bleeding through an interaction among the vascular endothelium, platelets, and the clotting system. Many disease states are associated with clinically significant aberrations in any of these three necessary components of clotting. This chapter discusses various components of clotting and their control systems.

ALTERATIONS OF LEUKOCYTE FUNCTION

Leukocyte function is affected if too many or too few white cells are present in the blood or if the cells that are present are structurally or functionally defective. **Quantitative leukocyte disorders,** such as infections and leukemias, result from decreased production in the bone marrow or accelerated destruction of cells in the circulation. Other quantitative alterations, however, occur in response to infections.

Qualitative leukocyte disorders consist of disruptions of leukocyte function. Phagocytic cells (granulocytes, monocytes, macrophages) may lose their phagocytic capacity to function. Lymphocytes may lose their capacity to respond to antigens. (Qualitative disruptions of inflammatory and immune processes caused by leukocyte disorders are described in Chapter 9.) Other leukocyte alterations include infectious mononucleosis and cancers of the blood—leukemia and multiple myeloma.

Quantitative Alterations of Leukocytes

Leukocytosis is a leukocyte count that is higher than normal; conversely, **leukopenia** is a count that is lower than normal. Leukocytosis or leukopenia may affect all cell types or only a specific type of leukocyte and may result from a variety of physiologic conditions and alterations.

Leukocytosis occurs as a normal protective response to physiologic stressors, such as infection, strenuous exercise, emotional changes, temperature changes, anesthesia, surgery, pregnancy, and some drugs, hormones, and toxins. It is also caused by pathologic conditions, such as malignancies and hematologic disorders. Leukopenia is never normal and is defined as an absolute blood cell count less than 4000 cells/mm^3. Leukopenia is associated with a decrease in neutrophils, which increases risk for infection. The absolute neutrophil count (ANC) is calculated by multiplying the white blood cell count by the percent of band and segmented neutrophils. The ANC is classified as mild (1000 to 1500 cells/mm^3), moderate (500 to 1000 cells/mm^3), or severe (<500 cells/mm^3). When the ANC is less than 500/mm^3, the possibility for life-threatening infections is high. Leukopenia can be caused by radiation, anaphylactic shock, autoimmune disease (e.g., systemic lupus erythematosus), immune deficiencies (see Chapter 9), and exposure to certain drugs and chemotherapeutic agents.

Granulocytes and Monocytes

Increased numbers of circulating granulocytes (neutrophils, eosinophils, basophils) and monocytes are primarily a response to infection. Increased numbers also occur as a result of myeloproliferative disorders (i.e., polycythemia vera, chronic myelogenous leukemia, chronic neutrophilic leukemia, chronic eosinophilic leukemia) that increase stem cell proliferation in bone marrow.

Decreased numbers occur when infectious processes exhaust the supply of circulating granulocytes and monocytes by drawing them out of the circulation and into infected tissues faster than they can be replaced. Decreases also can be caused by disorders that suppress marrow function.

Granulocytosis—an increase in the number of granulocytes (neutrophils, eosinophils, basophils)—begins with the release of stored leukocytes from the venous sinuses of the marrow. **Neutrophilia** is another term that may be used to describe *granulocytosis* because neutrophils are the most numerous of the granulocytes (Table 29-1). Neutrophilia occurs in the early stages of infection or inflammation and is established when the absolute neutrophil count exceeds 7500/μL. Stored neutrophils are approximately 20 to 40 times greater in number than circulating neutrophils. On rare occasions when the neutrophil count increases greatly—more than 100,000/μL (usually seen only in those with myelocytic leukemia)—the blood viscosity may increase greatly so that thrombosis or occlusion of blood vessels occurs. Release and depletion of stored neutrophils from the venous sinuses stimulate granulopoiesis to replenish neutrophil reserves. Specific conditions associated with neutrophilia are identified in Table 29-1.

When the demand for circulating mature neutrophils exceeds the supply, the marrow begins to release immature neutrophils (and other leukocytes) into the blood. Premature release of the immature white cells is responsible for the phenomenon known as a **shift-to-the-left** or **leukemoid reaction.** This refers to the microscopic detection of disproportionate numbers of immature leukocytes in peripheral blood smears. Many diagrams present cellular differentiation and maturation progressing from left to right within the drawing, instead of vertically as shown in Figure 27-10. When immature leukocytes are released prematurely they cause a shift in the distribution of cells in the blood toward the left side, or immaturity side, of the diagram. This phenomenon is also seen in the blood smear of individuals with leukemia as well, hence the term *leukemoid reaction.* As infection or inflammation diminishes and as granulopoiesis replenishes circulating granulocytes, a shift back to normal occurs.

Neutropenia is a condition associated with a reduction in the number of circulating neutrophils. Clinically, neutropenia exists when the neutrophil count is less than 2000/μL.[1] The absolute neutrophil count reflects not only the degree of neutropenia but also the risk for infection (see preceding discussion of leukocytosis). A reduction in the number of neutrophils can occur in severe, prolonged infections when production of granulocytes cannot keep up with demand.

Other causes of neutropenia, in the absence of infection, may be (1) decreased neutrophil production or ineffective granulopoiesis, (2) reduced neutrophil survival, and (3) abnormal neutrophil distribution and sequestration. Neutropenia also is categorized as primary or secondary; primary disorders are further identified as congenital or acquired.

Congenital defects in neutrophil production include cyclic neutropenia and neutropenia with congenital immunodeficiency diseases, as well as multiple syndromes (e.g., Kostmann, Shwachman-Diamond, Diamond-Blackfan, Griscelli, Chédiak-Higashi, and Barth syndromes). Primary acquired neutropenia is associated with multiple conditions, for example, hypoplastic anemia or aplastic anemia, leukemia (acute myelogenous leukemia [AML]/chronic lymphocytic leukemia [CLL]), lymphomas (Hodgkin, non-Hodgkin), and myelodysplastic syndrome (MDS). The megaloblastic anemias (vitamin B_{12} and folate deficiency) as well as starvation and anorexia nervosa cause neutropenia because of an inadequate supply of vitamins and nutrients for protein production.

Reduced neutrophil survival and abnormal distribution and sequestration are usually secondary to other disorders. Neutropenia occurs in a variety of immunologic disorders, particularly systemic lupus erythematosus, rheumatoid arthritis, Felty and Sjögren syndromes, splenomegaly, and drug-related causes.

Severe neutropenia, **granulocytopenia** (less than 500/μL), or **agranulocytosis** (complete absence of granulocytes in the blood) is usually secondary to arrested hematopoiesis in the bone marrow or massive cell destruction in the circulation.

Chemotherapeutic agents used to treat hematologic and other malignancies cause generalized bone marrow suppression. Several other drugs and large doses of ionizing radiation cause agranulocytosis, which occurs rarely but carries a high mortality (10% to 50%). Clinical manifestations of agranulocytosis include recurrent and persistent life-threatening infection (particularly of the respiratory system) leading to septicemia, general malaise, fever, tachycardia, and ulcers in the mouth and colon. If untreated, sepsis caused by agranulocytosis results in death within 3 to 6 days.

Eosinophilia is an absolute increase (more than 450/μL) in the total numbers of circulating eosinophils. Allergic disorders (type I hypersensitivity) associated with asthma, hay fever, and drug reactions, as well as parasitic infections (particularly with metazoal parasites) are often cited as causes. Hypersensitivity

TABLE 29-1 OTHER CONDITIONS ASSOCIATED WITH NEUTROPHILS, EOSINOPHILS, BASOPHILS, MONOCYTES, AND LYMPHOCYTES

CONDITION	CAUSE	EXAMPLE
Neutrophil		
Neutrophilia (granulocytosis)	Inflammation or tissue necrosis	Surgery, burns, MI, pneumonitis, rheumatic fever, rheumatoid arthritis
	Infection	Bacterial: gram-positive (staphylococci, streptococci, pneumococci), gram-negative (*Escherichia coli, Pseudomonas* species)
	Physiologic	Exercise, extreme heat or cold, third-trimester pregnancy, emotional distress
	Hematologic	Acute hemorrhage, hemolysis, myeloproliferative disorder, chronic granulocytic leukemia
	Drugs or chemicals	Epinephrine, steroids, heparin, histamine, endotoxin
	Metabolic	Diabetes (acidosis), eclampsia, gout, thyroid storm
	Neoplasm	Liver, GI tract, bone marrow
Neutropenia	Decreased marrow production	Radiation, chemotherapy, leukemia, aplastic anemia, abnormal granulopoiesis
	Increased destruction	Splenomegaly, hemodialysis, autoimmune disease
	Infection	Gram-negative (typhoid), viral (influenza, hepatitis B, measles, mumps, rubella), severe infections, protozoal infections (malaria)
Eosinophil		
Eosinophilia	Allergy	Asthma, hay fever, drug sensitivity
	Infection	Parasites (trichinosis, hookworm), chronic (fungal, leprosy, TB)
	Malignancy	CML, lung, stomach, ovary, Hodgkin disease
	Dermatosis	Pemphigus, exfoliative dermatitis (drug-induced)
	Drugs	Digitalis, heparin, streptomycin, tryptophan (eosinophilia-myalgia syndrome), penicillins, propranolol
Eosinopenia	Stress response	Trauma, shock, burns, surgery, mental distress
	Drugs	Steroids (Cushing syndrome)
Basophil		
Basophilia	Inflammation	Infection (measles, chickenpox), hypersensitivity reaction (immediate)
	Hematologic	Myeloproliferative disorders (CML, polycythemia vera, Hodgkin lymphoma, hemolytic anemia)
	Endocrine	Myxedema, antithyroid therapy
Basopenia	Physiologic	Pregnancy, ovulation, stress
	Endocrine	Graves disease
Monocyte		
Monocytosis	Infection	Bacterial (subacute bacterial endocarditis, TB), recovery phase of infection
	Hematologic	Myeloproliferative disorders, Hodgkin disease, agranulocytosis
	Physiologic	Normal newborn
Monocytopenia	Rare	
Lymphocyte		
Lymphocytosis	Physiologic	4 months to 4 years
	Acute infection	Infectious mononucleosis, CMV infection, pertussis, hepatitis, mycoplasma pneumonia, typhoid
	Chronic infection	Congenital syphilis, tertiary syphilis
	Endocrine	Thyrotoxicosis, adrenal insufficiency
	Malignancy	ALL, CLL, lymphosarcoma cell leukemia
Lymphocytopenia	Immunodeficiency syndrome	AIDS, agammaglobulinemia
	Lymphocyte destruction	Steroids (Cushing syndrome), radiation, chemotherapy, Hodgkin lymphoma, CHF, renal failure, TB, SLE, aplastic anemia

AIDS, Acquired immunodeficiency syndrome; *ALL,* acute lymphocytic leukemia; *CHF,* congestive (left) heart failure; *CLL,* chronic lymphocytic leukemia; *CML,* chronic myelogenous leukemia; *CMV,* cytomegalovirus; *GI,* gastrointestinal; *MI,* myocardial infarction, *SLE,* systemic lupus erythematosus; *TB,* tuberculosis.

reactions and the normal defense against parasites trigger the release of eosinophil chemotactic factor of anaphylaxis (ECF-A) from mast cells, attracting eosinophils to the area. (These processes are described and illustrated in Chapters 8 and 9.) Tissues with abundant mast cells, such as the respiratory and gastrointestinal tracts, are particularly common sites for eosinophil invasion. Mast cells also release interleukin-5 (IL-5), which stimulates the bone marrow to produce and release more eosinophils into the blood. Eosinophilia may also be associated with dermatologic disorders, such as atopic dermatitis, eczema, and pemphigus. Various types of eosinophilic scleroderma-like diseases also have been reported to occur in association with hemato-oncogenic disorders (i.e., eosinophilic cellulitis [Wells syndrome] and eosinophilic fasciitis [Shulman syndrome]). Increased numbers of eosinophils have been observed in individuals with eosinophilia-myalgia syndrome (EMS), which is associated with ingestion of the supplement L-tryptophan. EMS may develop in individuals with fibromyalgia syndrome as an allergic reaction to L-tryptophan.[2]

Eosinopenia, a decrease in circulating numbers of eosinophils, generally is caused by migration of eosinophils into inflammatory sites. It also may be seen in Cushing syndrome and as a result of stress caused by surgery, shock, trauma, burns, or mental distress. Other conditions causing eosinopenia are detailed in Table 29-1.

Basophilia, an increase in circulating numbers of basophils, is rare and generally is a response to inflammation and immediate hypersensitivity reactions. Basophils contain histamine that is released during an allergic reaction. An increase in the levels of basophils is seen also in myeloproliferative disorders, such as chronic myeloid leukemia and myeloid metaplasia. Other conditions associated with basophilia are listed in Table 29-1.

Basopenia (also known as *basophilic leukopenia*), a decrease in circulating numbers of basophils, is seen in hyperthyroidism, acute infection, and long-term therapy with steroids. A decrease in the number of basophils may be seen during ovulation and pregnancy. Other conditions associated with basopenia are listed in Table 29-1.

Monocytosis is an increase (generally greater than 800/μL) in numbers of circulating monocytes. The condition is often transient and not related to a dysfunction of monocyte production. When present, it most commonly occurs with neutropenia associated with bacterial infections, particularly in the late stages or recovery stage, when monocytes are needed to phagocytize surviving microorganisms and debris. Monocytosis often is seen in chronic infections, usually with intracellular bacteria, such as tuberculosis (TB), brucellosis, listeriosis, and subacute bacterial endocarditis (SBE). Peripheral monocytosis has been found to correlate with the extent of myocardial damage following myocardial infarction. Increased numbers of monocytes also may indicate marrow recovery from agranulocytosis. Other conditions associated with monocytosis are identified in Table 29-1.

Monocytopenia, a decrease in numbers of circulating monocytes, is rare, and not much is known about this condition because of the small numbers of monocytes generally present in the blood. Monocytopenia, however, has been identified with hairy cell leukemia and prednisone therapy.

Lymphocytes

Quantitative alteration of lymphocytes occurs when lymphocytes are activated by antigenic stimuli, usually microorganisms (see Chapter 8). **Lymphocytosis** is rare in acute bacterial infections and occurs most commonly in acute viral infections, particularly those caused by the Epstein-Barr virus (EBV), a causative agent in infectious mononucleosis. Other specific disorders associated with lymphocytosis are listed in Table 29-1.

Lymphocytopenia may be attributable to (1) abnormalities of lymphocyte production associated with neoplasias and immune deficiencies, and (2) destruction by drugs, viruses, or radiation. It also can occur in individuals for no apparent reason. Other conditions associated with lymphocytopenia are identified in Table 29-1. The lymphocytopenia associated with heart failure and other acute illnesses may be caused by elevated levels of cortisol. Lymphocytopenia is a major problem in acquired immunodeficiency syndrome (AIDS) in which the human immunodeficiency virus (HIV) is cytopathic for T helper lymphocytes. (For a more detailed discussion of AIDS, see Chapter 10.)

Infectious Mononucleosis

Infectious mononucleosis (IM) is an acute, self-limiting, neoplastic lymphoproliferative clinical syndrome characterized by acute viral infection of B lymphocytes (B cells). The most common etiologic agent is EBV, a ubiquitous, lymphotrophic, gamma-group herpesvirus that was first recognized as the causative agent in IM in the late 1960s. EBV accounts for approximately 85% of all IM cases. Other etiologic agents that may cause symptoms resembling IM are viruses (cytomegalovirus [CMV], adenovirus, HIV, hepatitis A, influenza A and B, and rubella), as well as the bacteria *Toxoplasma gondii, Corynebacterium diphtheriae,* and *Coxiella burnetii.* IM caused by CMV is generally noted in older individuals, with fever and malaise the major complaints; the major manifestations of EBV-induced IM are the classic triad of symptoms of pharyngitis, lymphadenopathy, and fever.

Approximately 50% to 85% of children are infected with EBV by age 4, and more than 90% of adults have indications of subclinical EBV infections. These early infections are usually asymptomatic and provide immunity to EBV; thus early EBV infections rarely develop into IM. IM may arise when the initial infection occurs during adolescence or later, but still only results in IM in 35% to 50% of these individuals. Symptomatic IM usually affects young adults between ages 15 and 35 years, with the peak incidences occurring between 15 and 24 years; males have a later peak (18 to 24 years) than females. The overall incidence rate for this age group is 6 to 8 cases per 1000 persons per year. Children from low socioeconomic environments are particularly susceptible to infections with EBV. IM is uncommon in individuals older than age 40, but if it does occur, it is more commonly caused by CMV.

Transmission of EBV is usually by saliva through personal contact (e.g., kissing, hence the term "kissing disease"). The virus also may be present in other mucosal secretions of the genital, rectal, and respiratory tract, as well as blood. No evidence of aerosol transmission through sneezing or coughing has been documented. The disease begins with widespread infection of B lymphocytes, all of which possess receptors for EBV. The virus initially infects the oropharynx, nasopharynx, and salivary epithelial cells with later spread to the lymphoid tissue and B cells. Infection of B cells permits the virus to enter the bloodstream, which spreads the infection systemically.

PATHOPHYSIOLOGY. In the immunocompetent individual, unaffected B cells produce antibodies (IgG, IgM, IgA) against the virus. Concomitantly, there is a massive activation and proliferation of cytotoxic T cells (CD8) directed against EBV-infected cells; CD8 lymphocytes can account for greater than 50% of the total circulating lymphocytes. The immune response against EBV-infected cells (cellular infiltration, production of cytokines) is largely responsible for the cellular proliferation in the lymphoid tissues (lymph nodes, spleen, tonsils, occasionally liver). Sore throat and fever, two of the earliest manifestations, are caused by inflammation at the site of viral entry and initial infection (the mouth and throat).

CLINICAL MANIFESTATIONS. The incubation period of IM is approximately 30 to 50 days (4 to 8 weeks) followed by a 3- to 5-day prodrome of fever, malaise, and arthralgias that are often attributed to viral infection, although some individuals remain asymptomatic. These symptoms may vary in severity for the next 7 to 20 days. At the time of diagnosis the individual usually has the classic triad of symptoms: fever, pharyngitis, and lymphadenopathy of the cervical lymph nodes. The pharyngitis is usually diffuse and often accompanied by a whitish or grayish green, thick exudate. It also is quite painful and is the symptom that most often causes the individual to seek treatment. IM is usually self-limiting, and recovery occurs in a few weeks. Fatigue may last for 1 to 2 months after resolution of the infection.

Although severe clinical complications are rare, as the condition progresses generalized lymph node enlargement may develop and enlargement of the spleen and liver also may occur. Splenomegaly is clinically evident 50% of the time and is demonstrated radiologically 100% of the time. Difficulty in detecting splenomegaly with physical examination contributes to the underestimation of actual enlargement. Splenic rupture is rare (only 0.1% to 0.5% of all cases) and can occur spontaneously as a result of mild trauma, occurring primarily in men younger than 25 years of age and between days 4 and 21 after the onset of symptoms. It is the most common cause of death related to IM. Other causes of fatalities are hepatic failure, extensive bacterial infection, or viral myocarditis.

Other organ systems are rarely involved, but such involvement may result in additional symptoms, such as meningitis, encephalitis, Guillain-Barré syndrome, Bell palsy, optic neuritis, mental impairment, transverse myelitis, cerebellar ataxia, and demyelinating diseases. Ocular manifestations may include eyelid and periorbital edema, dry eyes, keratitis, uveitis, conjunctivitis, retinitis, oculoglandular syndrome, choroiditis, papillitis, and ophthalmoplegia. In children, Reye syndrome also has been associated with EBV infection.

Pulmonary involvement is rare, but when present may include hilar and mediastinal lymphadenopathy, interstitial pneumonitis, and pleural effusion. Pneumonia and respiratory failure have been documented; however, they are more likely to develop in immunocompromised individuals. Approximately 3% to 10% of adults older than 40 years of age have never been infected with EBV and are susceptible to IM later in life. In these individuals the classic symptoms are not generally present, making diagnosis more difficult. If an older individual has an elevated temperature that cannot be explained and persists for more than 2 weeks, EBV infection should be suspected, particularly in the presence of abnormal liver function tests with hepatomegaly and jaundice. Other neurologic manifestations that may be present include peripheral neuropathy and Guillain-Barré syndrome.

EVALUATION AND TREATMENT. The blood of affected individuals contains an increased number of atypical lymphocytes (Figure 29-1). Diagnosis of IM is commonly based on Hoagland's criteria of at least 50% lymphocytes and at least 10% atypical lymphocytes in the blood in the presence of fever,

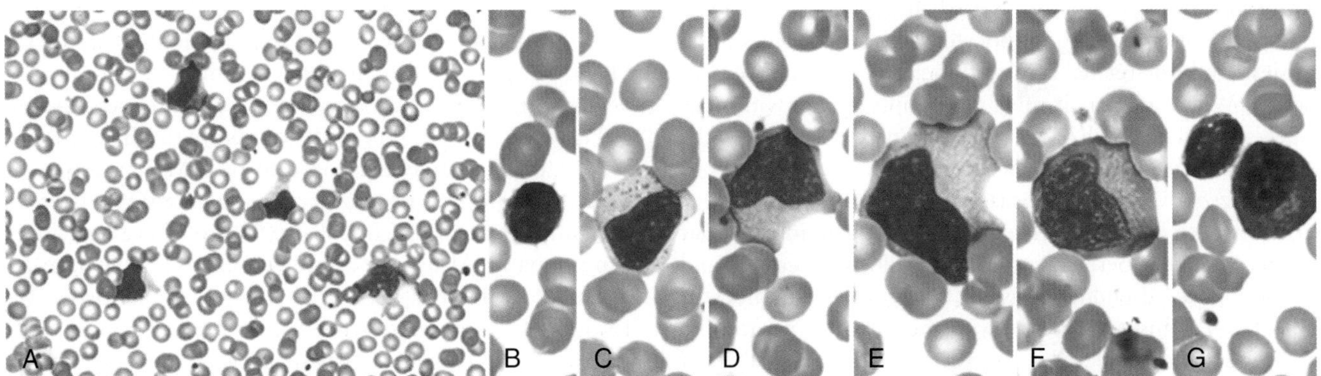

FIGURE 29-1 Peripheral Blood Smear in Infectious Mononucleosis. Low power **(A)** shows moderately high white blood cell count and high number of reactive, or "atypical," lymphocytes. Higher power **(B-G)** illustrates the spectrum of lymphoid morphology, including small resting lymphocyte **(B)** for comparison, large granular lymphocyte **(C)**, atypical forms **(D-F)**, also referred to as "reactive" lymphs, and circulating plasma cell **(G)**. (From Hoffman R et al: *Hematology: basic principles and practice,* ed 6, Philadelphia, 2013, Churchill Livingstone.)

pharyngitis, and adenopathy confirmed by a positive serologic test. Serologic tests are used to determine a heterophile antibody response.[3] **Heterophile antibodies** are a heterogeneous group of immunoglobulin M (IgM) antibodies that are agglutinins against nonhuman red blood cells (e.g., sheep, horse) and are detected by qualitative (Monospot) or quantitative methods (heterophile antibody test).

The Monospot test is limited because other infections (e.g., CMV, adenovirus) and toxoplasmosis also produce heterophilic antibodies. Thus 5% to 15% of Monospot tests yield false-positive results. Levels of heterophilic antibodies in the blood increase as the condition progresses, although some individuals and children younger than age 4 years do not produce them. These individuals give a false-negative result. Specificity for diagnosis of EBV infection may be increased with viral-specific serologic tests that identify EBV-specific antibodies (e.g., IgG or IgM against the viral capsid antigen [VCA], or IgG against the EBV nuclear antigen [EBNA]). These tests are more expensive and labor intensive; therefore they are reserved for instances in which the Monospot test is not appropriate.

Because IM is usually self-limiting, medical intervention is rarely required. Treatment of IM is supportive and includes rest and alleviation of symptoms with analgesics and antipyretics. Ibuprofen, *not aspirin,* is used with children and adolescents because of the reported incidence of Reye syndrome associated with EBV infection. Pharyngitis of streptococcal origin, which occurs in 20% to 30% of cases, is treated with penicillin or erythromycin. Ampicillin is contraindicated because it causes a rash in most individuals with IM.

Bed rest and avoidance of strenuous activity should be included in the therapy. Steroids may be used, but only in the presence of severe complications (e.g., impending airway obstruction) or other organ system involvement (e.g., nervous system manifestations, thrombocytopenic purpura, myocarditis, pericarditis). Acyclovir has been used with immunosuppressed individuals; however, clinical improvement has been minimal and therefore it is not recommended for standard treatment.

In the rare event of splenic rupture, the treatment has been removal of the spleen and continues to be the choice in hemodynamically unstable individuals. However, new research is suggesting that it may be better to repair the spleen to avoid overwhelming post-splenectomy infection (OPSI). Children are at greater risk of OPSI than adults. Post-splenectomy vaccinations for *Streptococcus pneumoniae, Haemophilus influenzae,* and *Meningococcus* are essential because these microorganisms are responsible for 92% of fatal infections. Treatment may also be necessary for airway obstruction from massive edema of the Waldeyer ring or for autoimmune hemolytic anemia, which occurs in approximately 3% to 5% of cases.

Fatal IM also is expressed with the inherited X-linked lymphoproliferative (XLP) syndrome (Duncan disease). Duncan disease is a rare disorder characterized by severe dysregulation of the immune system, often in response to EBV. The underlying cause leading to death is the absence of a functional SAP protein that allows for the unregulated proliferation of cytotoxic T cells and the concomitant production and release of cytokines.

Leukemias

Leukemia is a clonal malignant disorder of leukocytes in the blood and blood-forming organs. The common feature of all forms of leukemia is an uncontrolled proliferation of malignant leukocytes, causing an overcrowding of bone marrow and decreased production and function of normal hematopoietic cells. The first description of a "leukemic" individual was written by Velpeau in 1827.[4] Virchow, a pathologist, coined the term *white blood (Weissus blut)* and later originated the term *leukemia.* Since Virchow's initial discovery, the overall classification of leukemia has become increasingly complex and undergone several permutations.

The current classification of leukemia is based on (1) the predominant cell of origin (either myeloid or lymphoid) and (2) the rate of progression, which usually reflects the degree at which cell differentiation was arrested when the cell became malignant (acute or chronic) (Figure 29-2). **Acute leukemia** is characterized by undifferentiated or immature cells, usually a blast cell, and the onset of disease is abrupt and rapid with a short survival time. In **chronic leukemia** the predominant cell is more differentiated but does not function normally, with a relatively slow progression. There are four types of leukemia: acute lymphocytic (ALL), acute myelogenous (AML), chronic lymphocytic (CLL), and chronic myelogenous (CML). In 1976 the French-American-British Cooperative Group developed more extensive criteria for the classification of acute leukemias. This system is based on characteristics that may provide significant therapeutic prognostic information, such as structure, number of cells, genetics, identification of surface markers, and histochemical staining. Since this time, the World Health Organization has developed a classification that incorporates more recent research on the genetics and clinical features of AML that have prognostic and therapeutic relevance.[5]

Leukemia occurs with varying frequencies at different ages and is more common in adults than children (Figure 29-3). It is estimated that more than 44,600 cases of leukemia were newly diagnosed in 2011, with males having a slightly higher incidence than females (Table 29-2).[6] In all types of leukemia males have a higher incidence rate (56%) as do Americans of European descent. White children have higher rates of leukemia than children of other racial groups. ALL is the least common type overall, but is the most common in children (approximately 66% of ALL cases are diagnosed before the age of 20). Leukemia accounts for about 34% of all childhood cancers, and ALL accounts for almost 78% of all new cases of leukemia in children. CLL and AML are the most common types in adults. CML is found mostly in adults.

Over the past two decades the rates of induced remission and survival in most forms of leukemia have increased. Current survival rates range from 24% for AML to 81% for CLL, and as high as 91% for children and adolescents younger than 15 years of age with ALL.[7]

This progress is the result of more effective chemotherapeutic agents, improved blood product and antimicrobial support,

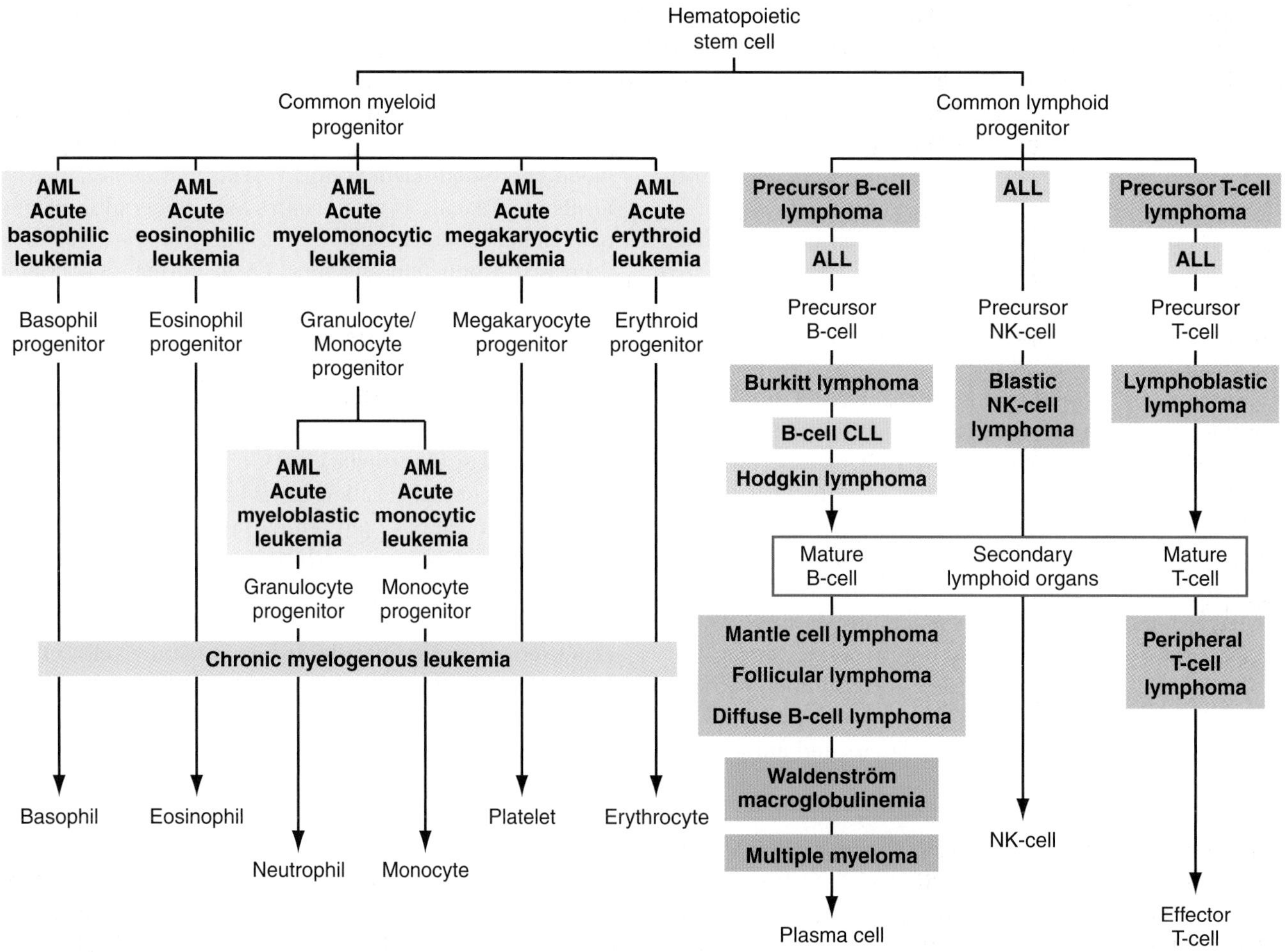

Hematopoietic stem cell
Common myeloid progenitor
Common lymphoid progenitor
AML Acute basophilic leukemia
AML Acute eosinophilic leukemia
AML Acute myelomonocytic leukemia
AML Acute megakaryocytic leukemia
AML Acute erythroid leukemia
Precursor B-cell lymphoma
ALL
Precursor T-cell lymphoma
ALL
ALL
Basophil progenitor
Eosinophil progenitor
Granulocyte/ Monocyte progenitor
Megakaryocyte progenitor
Erythroid progenitor
Precursor B-cell
Precursor NK-cell
Precursor T-cell
Burkitt lymphoma
Blastic NK-cell lymphoma
Lymphoblastic lymphoma
B-cell CLL
Hodgkin lymphoma
AML Acute myeloblastic leukemia
AML Acute monocytic leukemia
Mature B-cell
Secondary lymphoid organs
Mature T-cell
Granulocyte progenitor
Monocyte progenitor
Chronic myelogenous leukemia
Mantle cell lymphoma
Follicular lymphoma
Diffuse B-cell lymphoma
Peripheral T-cell lymphoma
Waldenström macroglobulinemia
Multiple myeloma
Basophil
Eosinophil
Platelet
Erythrocyte
Neutrophil
Monocyte
NK-cell
Plasma cell
Effector T-cell

FIGURE 29-2 Origins of Leukemias and Lymphomas. Differentiation pathways of blood-forming cells and reported sites from which specific leukemias and lymphomas originate. Tumors of similar types are given the same background coloring. *ALL,* Acute lymphocytic leukemia; *AML,* acute myelogenous leukemia; *CLL,* chronic lymphocytic leukemia; *NK,* natural killer.

Incidence (per 100,000)
35
30
25
20
15
10
5
0
ALL
AML
CLL
CML
<1
1–4
5–9
10–14
15–19
20–24
25–29
30–34
35–39
40–44
45–49
50–54
55–59
60–64
65–69
70–74
75–79
80–84
85+
Age at diagnosis

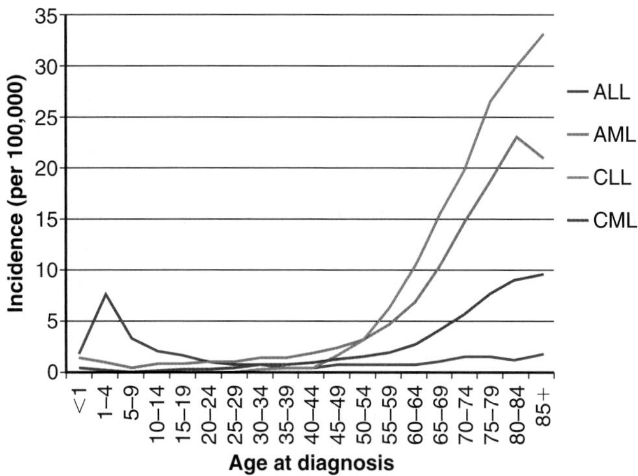

FIGURE 29-3 Age-Related Incidence at Diagnosis of Leukemias. The incidences of acute myelogenous leukemia (AML), chronic lymphocytic leukemia (CLL), and chronic myelogenous leukemia (CML) are relatively stable until middle age and then increase dramatically. The incidence of acute lymphocytic leukemia (ALL) peaks in childhood, and then diminishes until middle age when the incidence begins rising slowly with age. (Data obtained from Howlader N et.al, editors: *SEER cancer statistics review, 1975-2009 [vintage 2009 populations],* Bethesda, MD, 2012, National Cancer Institute. Available at http://seer.cancer.gov/csr/1975_2009_pops09/.)

and specialized nursing care. Chemotherapy and bone marrow transplants have significantly increased the survival time for individuals with acute leukemia.

PATHOPHYSIOLOGY. All leukemias have certain pathophysiologic features in common. Although the exact cause of leukemia is unknown, several risk factors and related genetic aberrations are associated with the onset of malignancy. There is a statistically significant tendency for leukemia to reappear in families. There is also an increased incidence of leukemia in association with other hereditary abnormalities such as Down syndrome, Fanconi aplastic anemia, Bloom syndrome, trisomy 13, Patau syndrome, and some immune deficiencies (i.e., ataxia-telangiectasia, Wiskott-Aldrich syndrome, and congenital X-linked agammaglobulinemia; see Chapter 9).

Genetic translocations (mitotic errors) are observed in leukemic cells. The most common genetic abnormality is the reciprocal translocation between chromosomes 9 and 22 t(9;22)(q34;q11), the **Philadelphia chromosome.**[8]

The Philadelphia chromosome was first observed in persons with CML, and is present in 95% of those with CML, 3% of individuals with AML, and 25% to 30% of adults with ALL and 2% to 10% of children with ALL.[9] This translocation results in the novel fusion of the *BCR1* gene region from

TABLE 29-2 ESTIMATED NEW CASES AND DEATHS: LEUKEMIA AND LYMPHOMA IN THE UNITED STATES IN 2013*

	ESTIMATED NUMBER AND PROPORTION (%) OF NEW CASES			ESTIMATED NUMBER OF DEATHS			5-YEAR SURVIVAL RATE (2005-2009)	
TYPE	TOTAL	MALE	FEMALE	TOTAL	MALE	FEMALE	OVERALL	<5 YEARS OF AGE
Leukemias	48,610	27,880	20,730	23,720	13,660	10,060	58%	
Acute lymphocytic leukemia	6050	3450	2600	1440	820	620	65.2%	90%*
Chronic lymphocytic leukemia	15,680	9720	5960	4580	2750	1830	78.8%	
Acute myelogenous leukemia	14,590	7820	6770	10,370	5930	4440	23.5%	55.2%
Chronic myelogenous leukemia	5920	3420	2500	610	340	270	59.1%	
Other leukemia	6350	3570	2780	6730	3820	2910		
Lymphomas	79,030	42,670	36,360	20,200	11,250	8950	70.6%	
Hodgkin lymphoma	69,740	5070	4220	1180	660	520	87%	
Non-Hodgkin lymphoma	19,020	37,600	32,140	19,020	10,590	8430	71%	
Multiple myeloma	22,350	12,440	9910	10,710	6070	4640	41.1%	

*Based on SEER Stat Fact Sheet, posted to the SEER website, NCI, 2013.

chromosome 22 and the proto-oncogene *ABL1* from chromosome 9 (Figure 29-4). The *BCR-ABL1* joining results in the expression of a unique fused oncoprotein, BCR-ABL1.[8] The ABL1 protein is a tyrosine kinase in the signaling pathway that promotes cell proliferation. The BCR-ABL1 variant possesses greater tyrosine kinase activity and has proven to be essential for transformation into leukemic cells. BCR-ABL1 appears to excessively activate intracellular pathways, leading to increased proliferation, decreased sensitivity to apoptosis, and premature release of immature cells into the circulation. In most leukemias and lymphomas a single major genetic abnormality, such as the t(9;22) translocation, does not lead to an aggressive malignancy. The initial event is usually followed by a series of secondary genetic changes.[10] Thus the original tumor becomes genetically unstable and diverse.

Risk factors for the onset of leukemia include environmental factors as well as other diseases. Increased risk in adults has been linked to exposure to cigarette smoke, benzene, and ionizing radiation. Large doses of ionizing radiation particularly result in an increased incidence of myelogenous leukemia. There is growing concern about the effect of low-dose radiation on subsequent risk of leukemia.[11] Infections with HIV or hepatitis C virus increase the risk for leukemia, and it is now widely accepted that some types of leukemia are caused by infection with the human T-cell leukemia/lymphoma virus type 1 (HTLV-1). Drugs that cause bone marrow depression (e.g., chloramphenicol, phenylbutazone, and certain alkylating agents, such as cytoxan) also can predispose an individual to leukemia. AML is the most frequently reported secondary cancer after high doses of chemotherapy for Hodgkin lymphoma, non-Hodgkin lymphoma, multiple myeloma, ovarian cancer, and breast cancer. Acute leukemia also may develop secondary to certain acquired disorders, including CML, CLL, polycythemia vera, myelofibrosis, Hodgkin lymphoma, multiple myeloma, ovarian cancer, and sideroblastic anemia.

Leukemias are considered clonal disorders in that a single progenitor cell undergoes malignant transformation. The leukemia blasts literally "crowd out" the marrow and cause cellular proliferation of the other cell lines to cease. Normal granulocytic-monocytic, lymphocytic, erythrocytic, and megakaryocytic progenitor cells cease to function, resulting in **pancytopenia** (a reduction in all cellular components of the blood). An interesting observation is that leukemic cells apparently divide more *slowly* and take longer to synthesize deoxyribonucleic acid (DNA) than other blood precursors. Leukemic cells accumulate relentlessly in the bone marrow causing overcrowding of the marrow, and they compete with cellular proliferation and function of normal hematopoietic cells. Thus leukemia has been termed an *accumulation* disorder, as well as a *proliferation* disorder. In the majority of cases, leukemic cells are ejected into the blood, where they accumulate. These cells also may infiltrate and accumulate in the liver, spleen, lymph nodes, and other organs throughout the body. The presentation of large numbers of leukemic cells in the blood may be one of the most dramatic indicators of leukemia; however, leukemia is still a primary disruption of the bone marrow.

Acute Leukemias

Acute leukemias consist of two types: **acute lymphocytic leukemia (ALL)** and **acute myelogenous leukemia (AML).** Acute leukemias are seen in both genders and in all ages, with the

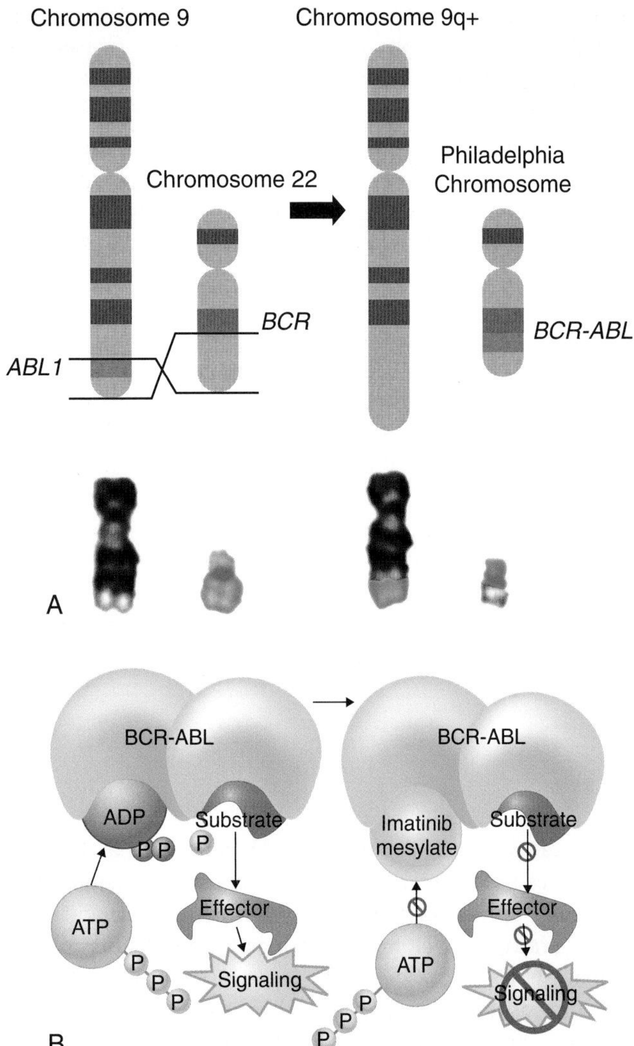

FIGURE 29-4 Philadelphia Chromosome. The Philadelphia chromosome is an example of a reciprocal chromosomal translocation that results in an abnormal gene product responsible for a clinical disorder. **A,** An exchange occurs between the long arm of chromosome 9 (black chromosome) and the long arm of chromosome 22 (blue chromosome); t(9;22)(q34;q11). **B,** Mechanism of action of imatinib. By occupying the ATP-binding pocket of the ABL kinase domain, imatinib prevents substrate phosphorylation and downstream activation of signals, thus inhibiting the leukemogenic effects of BCR-ABL on cells in chronic myelogenous leukemia. *ADP*, Adenosine diphosphate; *ATP*, adenosine triphosphate; *P*, phosphate group. (**A,** Top portion from Rakel R, Bope E: *Conn's current therapy 2008,* Philadelphia, 2008, Saunders. Lower portion from Yanoff M, Duker J: *Ophthalmology,* ed 3, Edinburgh, 2009, Mosby. **B** from Goldman L, Schafer AI: *Goldman's Cecil medicine,* ed 24, Philadelphia, 2012, Saunders.)

incidence increasing dramatically in individuals older than 50 years. Mortality for all acute leukemias in the United States is about 7 per 100,000. In children younger than 15 years, leukemia accounts for one third of all deaths from cancer. North American and Scandinavian countries have the highest mortality; Eastern European countries, Asia (except Japan), and Central America have the lowest mortality. Japan's higher mortality is the result of the atomic bombs dropped in World War II. Blacks have consistently shown a lower mortality than whites. More than 6070 new cases of ALL and 14,590 cases of AML are estimated in 2013, with more than 1430 deaths attributed to ALL and 10,370 to AML.[6,12,13]

PATHOPHYSIOLOGY. ALL is a progressive neoplasm defined by the presence of greater than 30% lymphoblasts in the bone marrow or blood. Most cases of ALL occur in children (80% of ALL), and it is the most common leukemia in children, most often occurring in the first decade. The median age of diagnosis of ALL is age 13. Although adults with ALL account for only 20% of all cases, their mortality is significantly higher (see Table 29-2). The 5-year survival rate for individuals 20 to 59 years old is about 30% to 40%, about 15% to 16% for persons older than 60 years, and 5% for persons older than 70 years. The survival rate in children is about 78%. The significant difference between the incidence of ALL in adults and children is thought to be determined by differences in the biology of the disease. Children with the highest survival rate (82% to 83%) have no radiographic manifestations, whereas children with five or more skeletal lesions have a survival rate of about 72% to 73%.[14]

Immunotyping of leukemic blast cells allows for the identification of subtypes of ALL. Approximately 75% of ALL cases in children originate from transformed precursor B cells, whereas adult ALL is a mixture of cancers of precursor B-cell or precursor T-cell origin (Table 29-3). A small percentage of ALL cases have neither B- nor T-cell origination and are called *null cell.* Precursor B-cell ALL can be subdivided into different phenotypes, depending on their progression through the B-cell maturation process before becoming malignant.[15,16] The general phenotype of precursor B-cell ALL expresses CD19, human leukocyte antigen DR (HLA-DR), and other B-cell–associated antigens in the cytoplasm. The most immature form (pro–B-cell ALL) occurs in about 5% of precursor B-cell ALL and is characterized by lack of expression of CD10. CD10 (common acute lymphocytic leukemia antigen [CALLA]) is a cell surface metalloprotease. Lack of CD10 is frequently associated with translocation of the myeloid/lymphoid leukemia *(MLL)* gene and a poor prognosis. The common precursor B-cell ALL comprises approximately 80% of precursor B-cell ALL cases; these express surface CD10, but have not yet undergone rearrangement of the immunoglobulin genes. The remaining individuals have a more mature form of precursor B-cell ALL (pre–B-cell ALL) in which the cells express immunoglobulin molecules in the cytoplasm. Less common variations include cells that are intermediate between the common precursor and pre–B-cell phenotypes and express immunoglobulin heavy chain, but no light chain, and cells that are more mature than the pre–B-cell ALL and express surface immunoglobulin and do not stain for the enzyme terminal deoxynucleotidyl transferase (TdT).

The T-cell lineage ALL (precursor T-cell ALL) is distinguished by T-cell–associated markers.[15,16] Cytoplasmic CD3 is the most common T-cell lineage specific marker, but CD7, CD2, and CD5 are frequently used. In addition to lymphoid markers, T-cell receptor (TCR) gene rearrangements are the most common genetic alteration in T-cell ALL. No specific cytogenetic abnormality, however, has been linked to the subtype of T-cell ALL. ALL blast cells also can express myeloid markers in 15% to 50% of adults and 5% to 35% of children.

Precursor B-cell ALL is strongly associated with aneuploidy of various types, ranging from hypodiploid to hyperdiploid with more than 50 chromosomes.[9,15,16] Individuals with hyperdiploid ALL usually have a better prognosis than those with fewer than 46 chromosomes. Individuals with precursor T-cell ALL generally have fewer cytogenetic abnormalities, and the majority of cases involve deletions. Genetic translocations between the *MYC* locus on chromosome 8 and one of the loci for the immunoglobulin (Ig) heavy- or light-chain genes (14q32, 2p12, and 22q11) are characteristic (also see Chapters 8 and 12). Several other translocations are commonly observed in ALL, including the Philadelphia chromosome and translocations involving the *ETV6 (formerly TEL)* and *MLL* genes (Figure 29-5).[9] Philadelphia chromosome–positive ALL carries the worst prognosis of all types of ALL and is found in 25% to 30% of adult ALL cases but less than 5% of childhood ALL cases. A translocation between chromosomes 12 and 21 (t[12;21]) results in fusion of the *ETV6* oncogene from chromosome 12 with the *AML1* (acute myeloid leukemia 1) gene on chromosome 21 to produce a fusion protein, ETV6-AML1. AML1 is a transcription factor for several genes important in hematopoiesis (e.g., IL-3, granulocyte-macrophage colony-stimulating factor [GM-CSF], CSF1 receptor).[9] The t(12;21) translocation occurs in 25% to 30% of childhood pre–B-cell ALL cases but in only 2% of adult ALL cases. This translocation significantly affects the prognosis of childhood ALL; children younger than 10 years with pre–B-cell ALL and the *ETV6-AML1* translocation have a 5-year cure rate of 90%, compared with 60% to 65% in those without the translocation.

Translocations of the *MLL* gene on chromosome 11 occur in about 10% of individuals with ALL and in 70% of infants with AML or ALL.[9] Infants and adults with this translocation develop a very aggressive form of leukemia with a very poor prognosis and frequent treatment failure, although children with this abnormality have better outcomes. The most common translocations involving *MLL* are t(4;11) and t(11;19). The t(4;11) translocation results in a fusion of *MLL* with the *AFF1* (ALL1 fused gene from chromosome 4) gene, and the t(11;19) translocation fuses *MLL* with the *MLLT1 (formerly ENL)* gene.

Specific causes of ALL are unknown, but multiple factors may contribute to its development.[15,16] Risk factors for childhood ALL include prenatal exposure to x-rays and postnatal exposure to high-dose radiation. Viral infections with HTLV-1 can cause a rare form of ALL and Epstein-Barr virus is linked to a form of ALL.[17]

Individuals with Down syndrome have an increased risk for developing ALL and AML. Increased risk for ALL is also seen in individuals with other genetic conditions, including neurofibromatosis, Shwachman syndrome, Bloom syndrome, and ataxia-telangiectasia (see Chapter 9). A unique characteristic of ALL, unlike other forms, is that ALL develops at different rates in different geographic locations, although the reason for this is unclear. Individuals in developed countries and in higher socioeconomic categories have an increased incidence of ALL. Prevention is almost impossible because there are no known causes.

AML is the most common adult leukemia; the mean age of diagnosis is 67 years of age. Approximately 60% to 70% of adults with AML can expect to attain complete remission status following appropriate induction therapy. Remission rates in adult AML are inversely related to age; remission rates for those younger than 60 years are more than 65%. AML[18] results from an abnormal proliferation of myeloid precursor cells, a decreased rate of apoptosis, and an arrest in cellular differentiation.[13] Therefore, the bone marrow and peripheral blood are characterized by leukocytosis and a predominance of blast cells. As the number of immature blasts increases, they replace normal myelocytic cells, megakaryocytes, and erythrocytes. This displacement eventually leads to complications of bleeding, anemia, and infection. AML increases with age, peaking in the sixth decade of life. Certain risk factors have been identified as possible causes, including exposure to radiation, benzene, and chemotherapy. Hereditary conditions, such as Down syndrome, Fanconi aplastic anemia, Bloom syndrome, ataxia-telangiectasia, trisomy 13 (Patau syndrome), Wiskott-Aldrich syndrome, and congenital X-linked agammaglobulinemia, are known to be associated with a higher risk for AML (see Table 29-2). AML subtypes are classified based on the stage of development the myeloblasts have reached at the time of diagnosis. These subtypes are included in Box 29-1.

More than 150 structural chromosomal abnormalities and several duplications or deletions within genes have been identified in AML.[9] The most common abnormalities are balanced translocations or inversions that disrupt genes critical to hematopoiesis of myeloid cells. The most common translocation is between chromosomes 8 and 21 in which the *RUNX1T1* (formerly *ETO*) (encodes a transcription factor) gene on chromosome 8 is fused with the *AML1* gene on chromosome 21, resulting in an *AML1-RUNX1T1* fusion gene and a fusion gene product, AML1-RUNX1T1. Production of AML1-RUNX1T1 disrupts the normal hematopoiesis process for myeloid cells and directly leads to the AML malignant phenotype.

Many kinds of mutations have been found in AML; however, a mutation in the receptor tyrosine kinase FLT3 occurs in about one third of persons affected by AML. FLT3 conveys a proliferation signal normally expressed early in the development of bone marrow stem cells, but mutated FLT3 remains active and promotes blast cell proliferation. Several FLT3 inhibitors are in various stages of clinical development. Another mutation in receptor tyrosine kinases is *KIT,* which also provides a proliferative and/or survival signal to progenitor cells. Together these mutations result in proliferation but not differentiation.

CLINICAL MANIFESTATIONS. The clinical manifestations of all the varieties of acute leukemia are generally similar. (Mechanisms associated with common manifestations are summarized in Table 29-4.) Signs and symptoms related to bone marrow depression include fatigue caused by anemia, bleeding resulting from thrombocytopenia (reduced numbers of circulating platelets), and fever caused by infection. Sites of infection include the oral cavity, throat, respiratory tract, lower colon, urinary tract, and skin. Common organisms include the gram-negative bacilli *Escherichia coli, Pseudomonas aeruginosa,* and *Klebsiella pneumoniae.* Fever is an early sign, often accompanied by chills. Bleeding can occur in skin, gums, mucous membranes, and gastrointestinal and genitourinary tracts. Visible signs of bleeding

TABLE 29-3 IMMUNOPHENOTYPE OF ADULT ACUTE LYMPHOCYTIC LEUKEMIA

LINEAGE	TDT	HLA-DR	CD34	CD19	CD22	CD79A	CD10	CYμ
Precursor B-cell ALL								
Pro-B ALL	+	+	+	+	+	+	−	−
CALL	+	+	−	+	+	−	+	−
Pre-B ALL	+	+	−	+	+	−	±	+
Transitional precursor B-cell ALL	±	+	−	+	+	−	−	−
Mature B-cell ALL	−	+	−	+	±	−	−	−
T-lineage ALL								
Pro-T ALL	+	±	±					
Pre-T ALL	+	±	±					
Cortical-T ALL	+	−	−					
Mature-T ALL	+	−	−					

From Faderl S et al: *Cancer* 98:1337-1354, 2003.
*Usually no surface light chain (L) expression.
ALL, Acute lymphoblastic leukemia; *cALL,* common acute lymphoblastic leukemia; *cy,* cytoplasmic; *TdT,* terminal deoxynucleotidyl transferase.

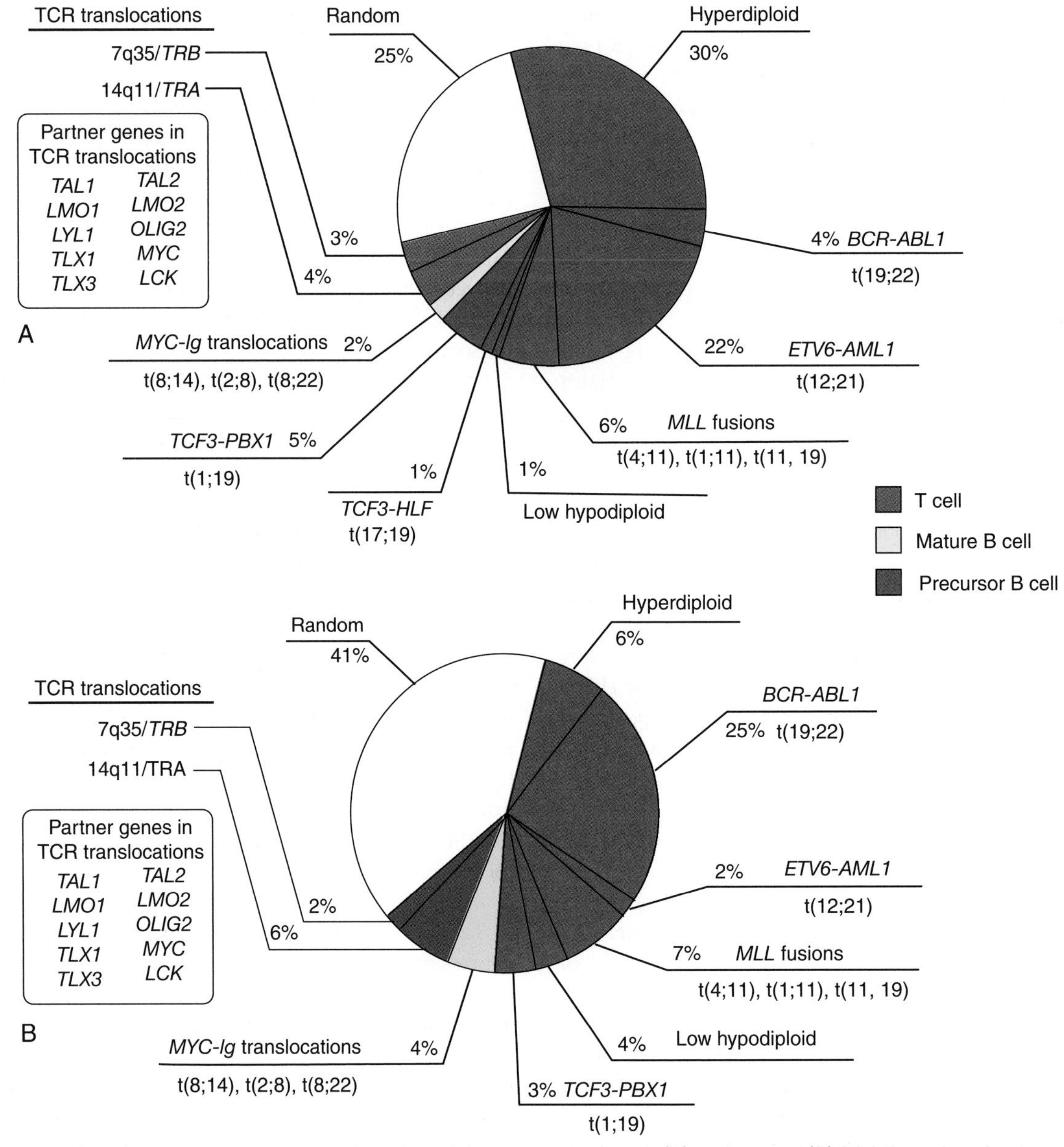

FIGURE 29-5 **Frequency of the Major Chromosomal Translocations in (A) Pediatric and (B) Adult Acute Lymphocytic Leukemia (ALL).** The genes affected by chromosomal translocation are shown. TCR translocations in T-ALL can activate a number of different proto-oncogenes as shown in the insert, including *TAL1, LMO1/2, TLX1, TLX3,* and *MYC.* (From Hoffman R et al: *Hematology: basic principles and practice,* ed 6, Philadelphia, 2013, Churchill Livingstone.)

CGκ/λ	SLGH/L	CYCD3	CD7	CD1A	CD2	CD5	SCD3	FREQUENCY (%)
								5-10
−	−							40-50
−	−							10
−	−							1
−	+*							1
+	+							5
		+	+	−	−	−	−	5
		+	+	−	+	+	−	
		+	+	+	+	+	−	10-15
		+	+	−	+	+	+	5-10

BOX 29-1 CLASSIFICATION OF ACUTE MYELOID LEUKEMIAS

Acute myeloblastic leukemia, minimally differentiated (AML-M0)
Acute myeloblastic leukemia without maturation (AML-M1)
Acute myeloblastic leukemia with maturation (AML-M2)
Acute promyelocytic leukemia (AML-M3)
  Hypergranular type
  Microgranular variant
Acute myelomonocytic leukemia (AML-M4)
  Increased marrow eosinophils (AML-M4-EO)
Acute monocytic leukemia (AML)
  Acute monoblastic leukemia (AML-M5A)
  Acute monocytic leukemia, differentiated (AML-M5B)
Erythroleukemia (AML-M6)
Acute megakaryoblastic leukemia (AML-M7)

From Damjanov I, Linder J: *Pathology: a color atlas,* St Louis, 2000, Mosby.

include petechiae and ecchymosis, as well as discoloration of the skin, gingival bleeding, hematuria, and midcycle or heavy menstrual bleeding.

Anorexia can occur in all varieties of acute leukemia and is associated with weight loss, diminished sensitivity to sour and sweet tastes, muscle atrophy, and difficulty in swallowing. Liver, spleen, and lymph node enlargement is more common in ALL than in AML (Figure 29-6). Splenomegaly and hepatomegaly usually occur together. The leukemic individual often experiences abdominal pain and tenderness and breast tenderness. Pain in the bones and joints is thought to result from leukemia infiltration with secondary stretching of the periosteum.

Central nervous system (CNS) involvement is common and may be caused by either leukemic infiltration or cerebral bleeding. Headache, vomiting, papilledema, facial palsy, blurred vision, auditory disturbances, and meningeal irritation can occur if leukemic cells infiltrate the cerebral or spinal meninges. CNS involvement at the time of diagnosis is rare, and less than 5% of children and less than 10% of adults are affected. Without CNS prophylaxis, approximately one third of individuals will develop CNS complications. Interventions associated with CNS prophylaxis include cranial irradiation, chemotherapy, and high doses of systemic chemotherapy. Specific treatment modalities or combinations of treatment vary and are determined by age and risk status.

EVALUATION AND TREATMENT. Leukemia is often confused with other conditions, making early detection difficult. Persistent symptoms need intensive medical investigation. The diagnosis is made through examination of blood cells and bone marrow. A stained peripheral blood smear will exhibit low red blood cell and platelet counts along with the presence of leukemic blast cells (Figure 29-7). Examination of bone marrow demonstrates hypercellularity with 60% to 100% blast cells, an occasional normal myeloid, erythroid precursors, and few to no megakaryocytes.

Chemotherapy, used in varying combinations, is the treatment of choice for leukemia.[15,16,19] Supportive measures include blood transfusions, antibiotics, antifungals, and antivirals. Allopurinol is used for preventing production of uric acid (which is elevated from cellular death because of treatment). Stem cell transplantation is now considered standard therapy for selected individuals with leukemia.

Bone marrow transplantation as a treatment has been increasing during the past two decades for both ALL and AML. Studies examining arsenic trioxide with *all-trans*-retinoic acid in combination with chemotherapy found that 80 of 85 subjects achieved remission. *all-trans*-Retinoic acid is made in the body from vitamin A and helps cells to grow and develop. In the leukemic individual, retinoic acid drives cells to develop into functional cells to alleviate the disease. It is a chemotherapeutic agent used to treat some forms of leukemia. In one study in which this chemical was utilized, although there were five deaths, the 5-year event-free survival rate was 89%, a remarkable improvement over historically bleak survival rates.[20]

The 5-year survival rate for those with leukemia is 38%, largely because of poor survival rates of individuals with certain types of leukemia (e.g., acute myelogenous). Since the 1970s, 5-year survival rates for those with ALL have increased from 38% to 65% for adults and from 53% to 85% for children. Factors influencing increased survival rate include the use of combined and multimodality treatment methods, improved supportive services such as blood banking and nutritional

TABLE 29-4 CLINICAL MANIFESTATIONS AND RELATED PATHOPHYSIOLOGY IN LEUKEMIA

CLINICAL MANIFESTATIONS	LABORATORY ABNORMALITIES	CAUSE	COMMENTS
Anemia	Key is the relative *proportion* of erythroblasts to total count (decreased in anemia)	Decreased stem cell input or ineffective erythropoiesis or both	In acute leukemia, anemia is usually present from the beginning, often the first symptom noticed, and severe; mild form without symptoms is common in CML and CLL; hemorrhage common in acute forms, occasional in CML, but rare in CLL
Bleeding (purpura, petechiae, ecchymosis, hemorrhage)	Decreased and possibly abnormal platelets	Reduction in megakaryocytes leading to thrombocytopenia	Bleeding more common in acute than in chronic leukemia
Infection	Increased multisegmented neutrophils	Opportunistic organisms; decreased protection resulting from granulocytopenia or immune deficiency secondary to chemotherapy, corticosteroids, and the disease process	Major sites of infection: oral cavity, throat, lower colon, urinary tract, lungs, and skin; prevention of infection focuses on restoration of host defenses, decreasing invasive procedures, and reducing colonization of organisms
Weight loss	Decreased 24-hr urinary creatinine excretion; hypoalbuminemia	Condition can be attributed to pain, depression, chemotherapy, radiation therapy, loss of appetite, and alterations in taste	Severe weight loss may be related to excess production of TNF-α
Bone pain	Often no radiographic evidence of bone problems	Result of bone infiltration by leukemic cells or intramedullary infection	If combination drug regimens are ineffective, radiation therapy is used
Liver, spleen, and lymph node enlargement	Biopsy abnormal for liver and spleen	Leukemic cell infiltration; lymph nodes also undergo leukemia proliferation in CLL	
Elevated uric acid	Normal excretion of uric acid is 300-500 mg/day; the leukemic individual can excrete 50 times more	Increased catabolism of protein and nucleic acid; urate precipitation increased from dehydration caused by anorexia or fever and drug therapy	Hyperuricemia is present in both acute leukemia and CML; increasing urine pH or decreasing acid production with the drug allopurinol

CLL, Chronic lymphocytic leukemia; *CML,* chronic myelogenous leukemia; *TNF,* tumor necrosis factor.

support, and the implementation of antimicrobial treatment. The presence of the Philadelphia chromosome (observed in about 5% of children with ALL, in 30% of adults with ALL, and occasionally in AML) is a poor prognostic indicator.

Myelosuppression is both a consequence of leukemia and its treatment. Hematologic support with blood products and granulocyte colony-stimulating factor (G-CSF) or granulocyte-macrophage colony-stimulating factor (GM-CSF) has effectively shortened the time of neutropenia and improved survival by reducing the risk for infection. A trial of individuals with CML demonstrated improved disease-free survival in the group receiving GM-CSF (23 months vs. 11 months; 2-year disease-free survival 48% vs. 21%).[21] The administration of colony-stimulating factors (CSFs) can increase white cell numbers and afford protection from infections.

Chronic Leukemias

The two main types of chronic leukemia are (1) **chronic myelogenous leukemia (CML)** and (2) **chronic lymphocytic leukemia (CLL)** (see Table 29-2). Several forms of CML can occur, depending on the lineage of the malignant cells (e.g., chronic neutrophilic leukemia [CNL], chronic eosinophilic leukemia [CEL]). Unlike cells in acute leukemia, chronic leukemic cells are well differentiated and can be readily identified. Individuals with chronic leukemia have a longer life expectancy, usually extending several years from the time of diagnosis.

The chronic leukemias account for the majority of cases in adults, comprising approximately 30% of leukemias in the Western world. It is estimated that in 2012 more than 15,680 cases of CLL and 5920 cases of CML were newly diagnosed in the United States.[22,23,23a] The incidences of CLL and CML increase significantly in individuals older than 40 years, with prevalence in the sixth through eighth decades. CML is a group of diseases called *myeloproliferative disorders,* which also include polycythemia vera, primary thrombocytosis, and idiopathic myelofibrosis (invasion of bone marrow by fibrous tissue).

PATHOPHYSIOLOGY. CLL involves malignant transformation and progressive accumulation of monoclonal B lymphocytes; rarely (less than 5%) are CLL malignancies of T-cell origin. The characteristic immunophenotype is expression of CD5, CD19, and CD23 molecules and low amounts of surface membrane Ig and CD20 molecules.[24] CD5 is a signal transduction molecule linked to the B-cell receptor (BCR); CD19 is a low-affinity antigen receptor expressed on maturing B cells, but is lost in plasma cells; and CD23 is a low-affinity receptor for the Fc portion of IgE. CLL is derived from a transformation of a partially mature B cell that has not yet encountered antigen. The gene for the variable region of the antibody heavy chain *(IGHV)* is frequently mutated (30% to 40% of persons). (See Chapter 8 concerning immunoglobulin heavy-chain structure.) Individuals with a mutated *IGHV* tend to have a more benign condition with a more slowly developing and less malignant disease.

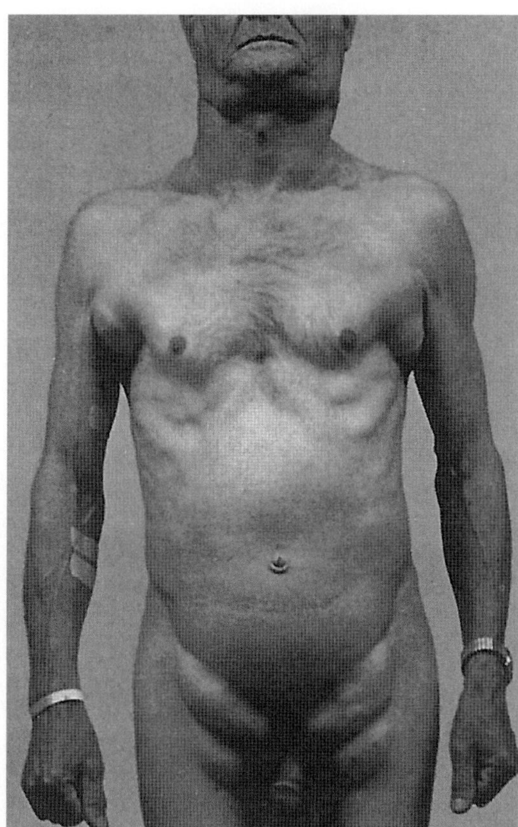

FIGURE 29-6 Lymphadenopathy. Individual with lymphocyte leukemia with extreme but symmetric lymphadenopathy. (Courtesy Dr. A.R. Kagan, Los Angeles. From Del Regato JA, Spjut HJ, Cox JD: *Ackerman and Del Regato's cancer,* ed 2, St Louis, 1985, Mosby.)

Significant numbers of this mutation are associated with a median survival in excess of 20 to 25 years, whereas the absence of mutations is associated with a poorer survival rate (median survival 8 to 10 years).[25]

The etiology of CLL is unknown. A familial tendency suggests a genetic linkage; first-degree relatives have a three times greater risk of developing the disease. It is rare in individuals younger than 45 years of age, and when diagnosed, 95% of individuals are older than age 50. Genetic anomalies occur in approximately 90% of cases, frequently as deletions, although none has been linked to the etiology of CLL.

CLL cells that accumulate in the marrow do not interfere with normal blood cell production to the extent found in acute leukemias. This is a significant feature explaining the reduced severity in the beginning stage of disease. Accumulation of malignant B cells is the result of cell cycle arrest in the G_0/G_1 phase. CLL cells tend to express increased levels of anti-apoptotic proteins (e.g., BCL2) and suppress pro-apoptotic proteins (e.g., BAX), which reduces their sensitivity to apoptosis. Because the major pathophysiologic deficit in CLL is the failure of B cells to mature into plasma cells that synthesize immunoglobulin, this often results in hypogammaglobulinemia (60% of clients).

CML is a member of the family of myeloproliferative disorders that also includes polycythemia vera (see Chapter 28), essential thrombocythemia, chronic idiopathic myelofibrosis (invasion of bone marrow by fibrous tissue), chronic neutrophilic leukemia, and chronic eosinophilic leukemia. CML is clonal and thought to arise from a hematopoietic stem cell. The cells observed in CML are heterogeneous in differentiation, depending on the stage of the disease.[26] During the chronic phase the predominant cell is a long-lasting hematopoietic stem cell. A leukemic granulocyte-monocyte progenitor cell is seen. The Philadelphia chromosome is present in more than 95% of CML, and the presence of the BCR-ABL1 protein is responsible for initiation of CML. In advanced disease, the accumulation of additional mutations leads to the more aggressive leukemic phenotype.

CLINICAL MANIFESTATIONS. Chronic leukemia advances slowly and insidiously. Approximately 70% of individuals with CLL are asymptomatic at the time of diagnosis. When symptoms do appear, the most common finding is lymphadenopathy. The most significant effect of CLL is suppression of humoral immunity and increased infection with encapsulated bacteria. Frequently the level of neutrophils is depressed, which adds to the risk of infection. Invasion of most organ cells is uncommon but infiltration does occur in lymph nodes, liver, spleen, and salivary glands. CNS involvement is rare. Approximately 10% of individuals develop a more aggressive malignancy, usually a diffuse large B-cell lymphoma. In these individuals, extreme fatigue, weight loss, night sweats, low-grade fever, elevated levels of the enzyme lactic dehydrogenase, hypercalcemia, anemia, and thrombocytopenia are common.

Individuals with CML may progress through three phases of the disease: a chronic phase lasting 2 to 5 years during which symptoms may not be apparent; an accelerated phase of 6 to 18 months during which the primary symptoms develop; and a terminal blast phase ("blast crisis") with a survival of only 3 to 6 months. The accelerated phase is characterized by excessive proliferation and accumulation of malignant cells. Splenomegaly is the most common finding, which may be prominent and painful, but lymphadenopathy generally is not present. Liver enlargement also occurs, but liver function is rarely altered. Hyperuricemia is common and produces gouty arthritis. Infections, fever, and weight loss also are frequent. The terminal blast phase is characterized by rapid and progressive leukocytosis with an increase in the number of basophils. In the later stages of the terminal phase, which then resembles AML, blast cells or promyelocytes predominate, and the individual experiences a blast crisis.

The acute effects of CML resemble those of acute leukemia but with more prominent and painful splenomegaly. Liver function rarely is altered despite enlargement, and lymphadenopathy generally is found only in the acute phase of the disease. Hyperuricemia invariably is present and produces gouty arthritis. Infections, fever, and weight loss are common findings in clients with CML.

EVALUATION AND TREATMENT. Diagnosis of chronic leukemia depends on laboratory analyses of peripheral blood and bone marrow samples. Diagnosis of CLL is based on detection of a monoclonal B-cell lymphocytosis in the blood. The cells must have the immunophenotype characteristic of CLL (CD5+, CD19+, CD20 [weak], CD23+), at levels in excess of 5000 cells/μL, over a sustained period of time (usually 4 weeks). Bone marrow may contain more than 30% lymphocytes and be normocellular or hypercellular.

Treatment is frequently based on prognostic indicators and ranges from observation with treatment of infection, hemorrhage, or immune complications to a variety of drug therapies. Because this disease typically occurs in older adults and the rate of progression is slow, it is often simply observed until the disease progresses. Meta-analysis of randomized trials shows no survival advantage for immediate vs. delayed treatment for those individuals with early stage disease.[27]

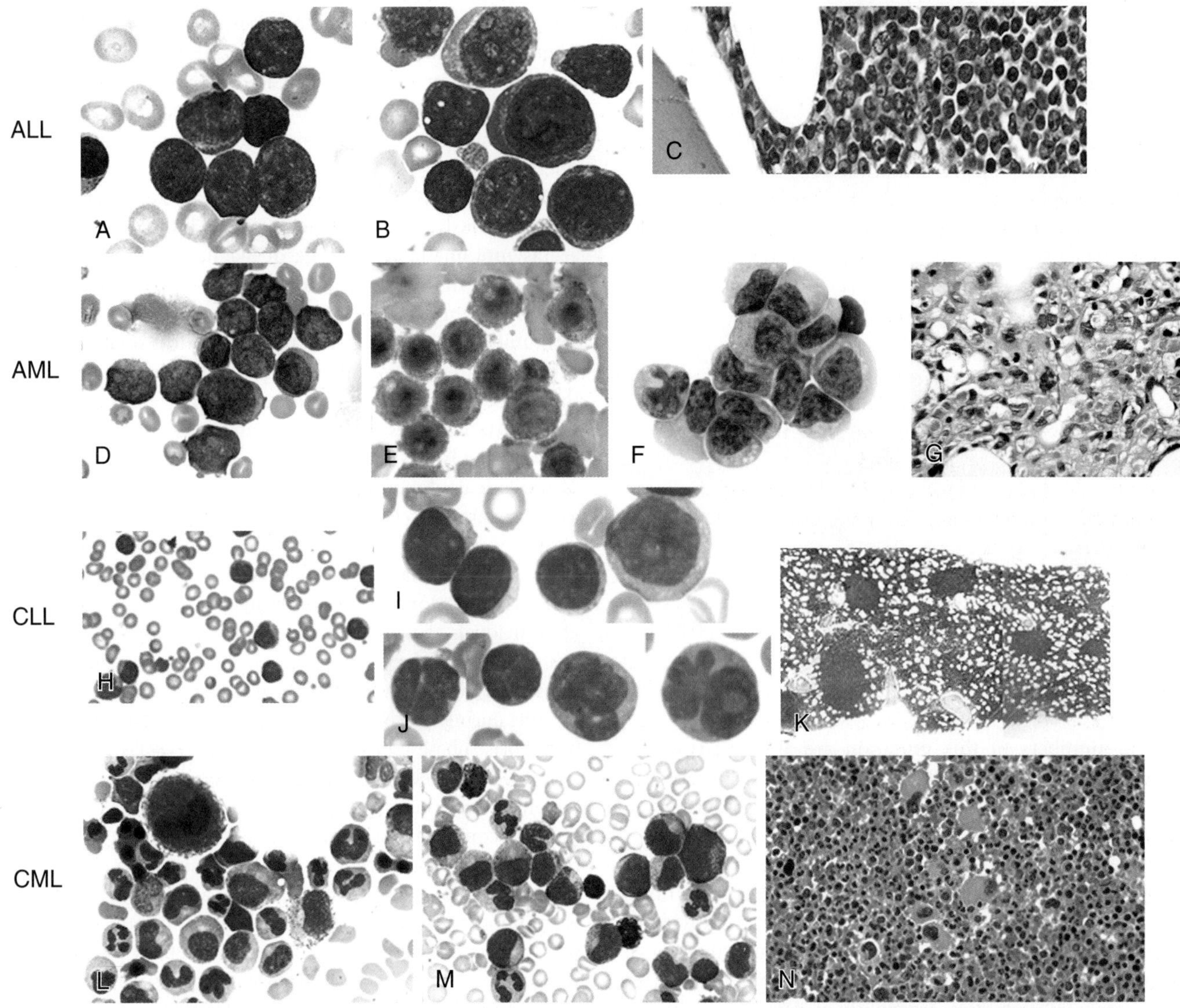

FIGURE 29-7 Morphologic Aspects of Leukemia Cells. *Acute lymphocytic leukemia (ALL)* **(A-C). A,** Typical uniform lymphoblasts with intermediate-sized nuclei, fine but "smudgy" chromatin, absence of nucleoli, and scant cytoplasm. **B,** Lymphoblasts with more cytologic variation, including variability in size, number of nucleoli, and amount of cytoplasm. **C,** Histologic features of ALL in bone core biopsy. *Acute myeloid leukemia (AML)* **(D-G). D,** Acute myeloblastic leukemia with minimal or no maturation. The cells are myeloblasts with dispersed chromatin and variable amounts of agranular cytoplasm. Some display medium-sized, poorly defined nucleoli. **E,** Acute monoblastic leukemia; characteristic monoblasts with round nuclei and delicate chromatin and prominent nucleoli. Cytoplasm is abundant. **F,** Acute monocytic leukemia with most of the cells in this field being promonocytes. Monoblasts and an abnormal monocyte also are present. **G,** Marrow biopsy of acute megakaryoblastic leukemia containing large and small blasts and atypical megakaryocytes. *Chronic lymphocytic leukemia (CLL)* **(H-K). H,** Peripheral blood smear typically shows lymphocytosis. Cytologic features of CLL cells differ. **I,** Classic cells have a small nucleus with a "soccer ball" chromatin pattern. **J,** Some cases have increased large cells, or prolymphocytes, with more open chromatin and prominent "punched-out" nucleoli (prolymphocyte, right side). **K,** The bone marrow can show nodular infiltrates of CLL cells. *Chronic myelogenous leukemia (CML)* **(L-N). L,** Peripheral smear shows marked leukocytosis attributable to a granulocytic proliferation of all stages with particularly increased myelocytes and absolute basophilia. **M,** Bone core biopsy illustrates markedly hypercellular marrow attributable to granulocytic proliferation and increased small hypolobated megakaryocytes. **N,** Bone marrow aspirate shows granulocytic proliferation and small, "dwarf" megakaryocyte. (**A-C, H-N** from Hoffman R et al: *Hematology: basic principles and practice,* ed 6, Philadelphia, 2013, Churchill Livingstone. **D-G** from Abeloff M et al: *Abeloff's clinical oncology,* ed 4, Philadelphia, 2008, Churchill Livingstone.)

Typically, individuals with CLL survive 10 years or more. However, those with certain risk markers have a more aggressive form of the disease that shortens survival to less than 3 years. Markers of high risk include anemia, thrombocytopenia, and the absence of mutations in the *IGHV* gene. Mutations in *IGHV* correlate very closely with levels of intracellular ZAP-70, detection of which may be substituted for tests of *IGHV* mutation. ZAP-70 is a tyrosine kinase that is linked to the T-cell receptor (see Chapter 8). ZAP-70 negativity is associated with improved mean survival.[28] It is not normally detected in CLL cells with mutated *IGHV*, but is easily detectable by immunohistologic analysis in cells with an unmutated *IGHV*.

Chlorambucil, administered with or without corticosteroids, on a daily or intermittent schedule is the most common treatment for individuals with the most aggressive disease. Relief of symptoms is often achieved, but there is no substantial effect on survival. Combination therapy (CHOP) that includes **c**yclophosphamide, **h**ydroxydaunomycin (Adriamycin), vincristine (**O**ncovin), and **p**rednisone has an improved response rate but still does not demonstrate improved survival. Fludarabine, a purine analog, has a higher response rate and disease-free intervals, although survival is not affected. Rituximab, a murine anti-CD20 monoclonal antibody, has shown limited promise in CLL (20% response rate). Ofatumumab is a human anti-CD20 monoclonal antibody that has shown overall response rates of 50% in persons with CLL.

Present treatment modalities for CML do not cure the disease, prevent blastic transformation, or prolong the average survival time. Standard treatment consists of combined chemotherapy, biologic response modifiers, and allogeneic stem cell transplant. Although transplantation is potentially curative, its use is limited by donor availability and high toxicity in older adults, thus limiting use to those older than 65 years. Allogeneic bone marrow transplantation has increased survival time significantly (20% to 30%) when used after high-dose radiation and chemotherapy and with concurrent treatment with interferon. Traditional chemotherapy agents used are hydroxyurea and busulfan. The development and introduction of the tyrosine kinase inhibitor imatinib mesylate (Gleevec) as a treatment modality have changed current management of CML. Imatinib mesylate is highly specific for CML and suppression of BCR-ABL kinase activity, and it produces a complete cytogenetic response in more than 80% of newly diagnosed persons. Suppression of hematologic symptoms occurs in 97% of treated individuals, and the use of imatinib mesylate has become the standard of care for CML. A small percentage of clients develop additional mutations in BCR-ABL that confer resistance to imatinib mesylate.[29] Several new tyrosine kinase inhibitors are under investigation as treatments for CML.

ALTERATIONS OF LYMPHOID FUNCTION

Lymphadenopathy

Lymphadenopathy is characterized by enlarged lymph nodes. Lymph node enlargement is caused by an increase in size and number of its germinal centers caused by proliferation of lymphocytes and monocytes or invasion by malignant cells. Normally, lymph nodes are not palpable or are barely palpable. Enlarged lymph nodes are characterized by being palpable and often also may be tender or painful to touch, although not in all situations (see Figure 29-6).

Localized lymphadenopathy usually indicates drainage of an area associated with an inflammatory process or infection (reactive lymph nodes). Generalized lymphadenopathy is generally a result of malignant or nonmalignant disease, particularly in adults. Palpable nodes, however, do not always indicate serious disease and may indicate only a reaction to minor trauma or infection of a specific structure. The location and size of the enlarged nodes are important factors in diagnosing the cause of the lymphadenopathy, as are the individual's age, gender, and geographic location. Generalized lymphadenopathy occurs with non-Hodgkin lymphomas, chronic lymphocytic leukemia, histiocytosis, and disorders that produce lymphocytosis. In general, lymphadenopathy results from one of four types of conditions: (1) neoplastic disease, (2) immunologic or inflammatory conditions, (3) endocrine disorders, or (4) lipid storage diseases. Diseases of unknown cause, including reactions to drugs, also may lead to generalized lymphadenopathy.

Malignant Lymphomas

Lymphomas consist of a diverse group of neoplasms that develop from the proliferation of malignant lymphocytes in the lymphoid system. The classification of lymphomas was published by the World Health Organization (WHO) and is derived from the Revised European-American Lymphoma (REAL) classification. This classification is based on the cell type from which the lymphoma probably originated (Box 29-2).[30] The groups include Hodgkin lymphoma and two that were previously classified as non-Hodgkin lymphoma (B-cell neoplasms, T-cell, and natural killer [NK] cell neoplasms). With the new classification, multiple myeloma, which was previously classified independently, is included as a B-cell lymphoma.

Incidence rates of lymphoma differ with respect to age, gender, geographic location, and socioeconomic class. The estimated number of new cases of lymphoma for 2013 is more than 79,030 individuals (see Table 29-2). It is estimated that more than 20,200 individuals will have died from lymphoma in 2013. Since the early 1970s, the incidence of non-Hodgkin lymphoma has nearly doubled. The exact reason for this increase remains a mystery; however, a modest portion of the increase had been attributed to lymphomas developing in association with immune deficiencies, including AIDS and organ transplants. Conversely, the incidence of Hodgkin lymphoma has declined over the same time period, especially among older adults.

In general, lymphomas are the result of genetic mutations or viral infection. Malignant transformation produces a cell with uncontrolled and excessive growth that accumulates in the lymph nodes and other sites, producing tumor masses. Lymphomas usually start in the lymph nodes or lymphoid tissues of the stomach or intestines.

Hodgkin Lymphoma

Hodgkin lymphoma (HL) is a malignant lymphoma first characterized by Thomas Hodgkin in 1832. It is estimated that more

BOX 29-2 WORLD HEALTH ORGANIZATION CLASSIFICATION OF LYMPHOID NEOPLASMS

B-Cell Neoplasms

Precursor B-Cell Neoplasms

- Precursor B-lymphoblastic leukemia/lymphoma
- Precursor B-cell acute lymphoblastic leukemia

Mature (Peripheral) B-Cell Neoplasms

- B-cell chronic lymphocytic leukemia/small lymphocytic lymphoma
- B-cell prolymphocytic leukemia
- Lymphoplasmacytoid lymphoma
- Splenic marginal zone B-cell lymphoma (with/without villous lymphocytes)
- Hairy cell leukemia
- Plasma cell myeloma/plasmacytoma
- Extranodal marginal zone B-cell lymphoma of mucosa-associated lymphoid tissue (MAL type)
- Nodal marginal zone B-cell lymphoma (with/without monocytoid B cells)
- Follicular lymphoma
- Mantle-cell lymphoma
- Diffuse large B-cell lymphoma
  - Mediastinal large B-cell lymphoma
  - Primary effusion lymphoma
- Burkitt lymphoma/Burkitt cell leukemia

T-Cell and NK-Cell Neoplasms

Precursor T-Cell Neoplasms

- Precursor T-lymphoblastic lymphoma/leukemia
- Precursor T-cell acute lymphoblastic leukemia

Mature (Peripheral) T-Cell Neoplasms

- T-cell prolymphocytic leukemia
- T-cell granular lymphocytic leukemia
- Aggressive NK-cell leukemia
- Adult T-cell lymphoma/leukemia (HTLV-1 positive)
- Extranodal NK/T-cell lymphoma, nasal type
- Enteropathy-type T-cell lymphoma
- Hepatosplenic gamma-delta T-cell lymphoma
- Subcutaneous panniculitis-like T-cell lymphoma
- Mycosis fungoides/Sézary syndrome
- Anaplastic large-cell lymphoma, T/null cell, primary cutaneous type
- Peripheral T-cell lymphoma, not otherwise characterized
- Angioimmunoblastic T-cell lymphoma
- Anaplastic large-cell lymphoma, T/null cell, primary systemic type

Hodgkin Lymphoma (Hodgkin Disease)

Nodular lymphocyte predominant Hodgkin lymphoma

Classic Hodgkin lymphoma

- Nodular sclerosis Hodgkin lymphoma (grades 1 and 2)
- Lymphocyte-rich classic Hodgkin lymphoma
- Mixed cellularity Hodgkin lymphoma
- Lymphocyte depletion Hodgkin lymphoma

From National Institutes of Health, National Cancer Institute: *Surveillance Epidemiology and End Results (SEER) program,* available at: http://training.seer.cancer.gov/module_coding_primary/table_who_class_hemo_2.html.
HTLV, Human T-cell leukemia virus; *NK,* natural killer.

than 9290 individuals will be newly diagnosed with HL in 2013 (see Table 29-2). The incidence of HL is approximately 26.6 per 100,000 men and 18.9 per 100,000 women.[31] The median age of diagnosis is 64. Incidence rates for HL have declined, especially among older adults. The decrease in incidence in older adults is attributed to improved diagnostic accuracy. The incidence is greater in whites than blacks. Denmark, the Netherlands, and the United States have the highest incidence of HL, and Japan and Australia have the lowest incidence. HL peaks at two different ages: early in life in the second and third decades and later in life during the sixth and seventh decades.

PATHOPHYSIOLOGY. HL is characterized by its progression from one group of lymph nodes to another, the development of systemic symptoms, and the presence of **Reed-Sternberg (RS) cells** (Figure 29-8). It is widely accepted that the RS cell represents the malignant transformed lymphocyte. The RS cells are often large and binucleate, with occasional mononuclear variants. RS cells are the hallmark of HL. RS cells are necessary for the diagnosis of HL; however, they are not specific to HL. In rare instances, cells resembling them can be found in benign illnesses, as well as in other forms of cancer, including non-Hodgkin lymphomas and solid tissue cancers and in infectious mononucleosis.

The triggering mechanism for the malignant transformation of cells remains unknown. Classic HL appears to be derived from a B cell in the germinal center that has not undergone successful immunoglobulin gene rearrangement (see Chapter 8) and would normally be induced to undergo apoptosis. Survival of this cell may be linked to infection with EBV. Laboratory and epidemiologic studies have linked HL with EBV infections and EBV DNA. RNA and proteins are frequently observed in HL cells. The RS cells secrete and release cytokines (e.g., IL-10, transforming growth factor-beta [TGF-β]) that result in the accumulation of inflammatory cells that produces the local and

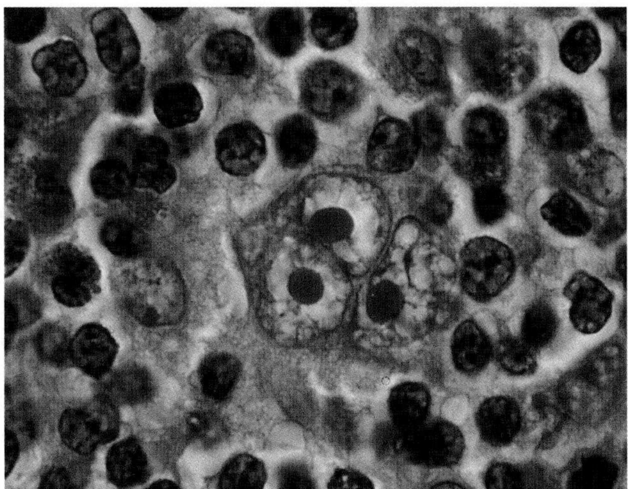

FIGURE 29-8 Reed-Sternberg Cell. A large multinucleated or multilobed cell *(center of photograph)* with inclusion body–like nucleoli surrounded by a halo of clear nucleoplasm. (From Damjanov I, Linder J, editors: *Anderson's pathology,* ed 10, St Louis, 1996, Mosby.)

TABLE 29-5 SUBTYPES OF HODGKIN LYMPHOMA

SUBTYPE	INCIDENCE	PRESENTATION
Nodular sclerosis Hodgkin lymphoma (HL)	Most common subtype in developing countries Found in all ages but most common in adolescents and young adults (median age of onset is about 28 years) Incidence in females exceeds that in males	Large tumor nodules with RS cells surrounded by collagen and fibrous bands
Mixed cellularity HL	Second most common subtype Incidence in males exceeds that in females	RS cells with mixed inflammatory cell (lymphocytes, monocytes/macrophages, eosinophils, plasma cells) infiltrates
Lymphocyte-rich classic HL	Uncommon subtype Found in all ages but most common in adults Incidence in males exceeds that in females	Few RS cells and predominantly lymphocytic infiltration Usually localized at diagnosis Survival is long with or without treatment
Lymphocyte depletion HL	Uncommon subtype Most common type in older adults, HIV-positive individuals, and persons in nonindustrialized countries Incidence in males exceeds that in females	Large number of RS cells with less additional cellular infiltrate Usually widespread disease: abdominal lymphadenopathy; spleen, liver, and bone marrow involvement, without peripheral lymphadenopathy Stage is usually more advanced at diagnosis

HIV, Human immunodeficiency virus; *RS,* Reed-Sternberg.

systemic effects. HL is subcategorized into two main types: classic Hodgkin and nodular lymphocyte–predominant Hodgkin. Classic HL is subclassified into four types (Table 29-5) based on the morphology of RS cells, and the characteristics of the inflammatory cell infiltrate in the tumor. Lymphocyte-predominant disease presents with earlier-stage disease, longer survival, and fewer treatment failures than classic HL.[32] However, despite a more favorable prognosis, lymphocyte-predominant HL has a tendency to histologically transform into diffuse large B-cell lymphoma by 10 years in approximately 10% of people.[33]

The molecular events causing malignant transformation remain controversial; although RS cells are apparently from B-cell lineage, they express very few B-cell markers and express markers normally not found on B cells. For instance, RS cells do not express immunoglobulin, but do express CD15 (a carbohydrate adhesion molecule found on neutrophils), TARC (a Th2-cell specific chemokine), and T-cell–associated antigens (e.g., β-chain of the T-cell receptor).[30] The precise genetic defects leading to development of HL are unknown, although several have been suggested. These generally include defects in immunoglobulin variable region gene rearrangement or defects in other B-cell–specific differentiation genes.

CLINICAL MANIFESTATIONS. Many of the characteristic clinical features (Box 29-3) of HL can be explained by the complex action of cytokines and other growth factors that are secreted by the malignant cells. These substances induce infiltration and proliferation of inflammatory cells, resulting in an enlarged, painless lymph node in the neck (often the first sign of HL) (Figure 29-9). The discovery of an asymptomatic mediastinal mass on routine chest x-ray is not uncommon and is often an initial sign of HL. The cervical, axillary, inguinal, and retroperitoneal lymph nodes are commonly affected in HL (Figure 29-10). Local symptoms caused by pressure and obstruction of the lymph nodes are the result of the lymphadenopathy.

About one third of individuals will have some degree of systemic symptoms.[34] Intermittent fever, without other symptoms

BOX 29-3 CLINICAL MANIFESTATIONS OF HODGKIN LYMPHOMA

Physical Findings
Adenopathy
Mediastinal mass
Splenomegaly
Abdominal mass

Symptoms
Fever, weight loss, night sweats
Pruritus

Laboratory Findings
Thrombocytosis
Leukocytosis
Eosinophilia
Elevated erythrocyte sedimentation rate (ESR)
Elevated alkaline phosphatase
Paraneoplastic syndromes

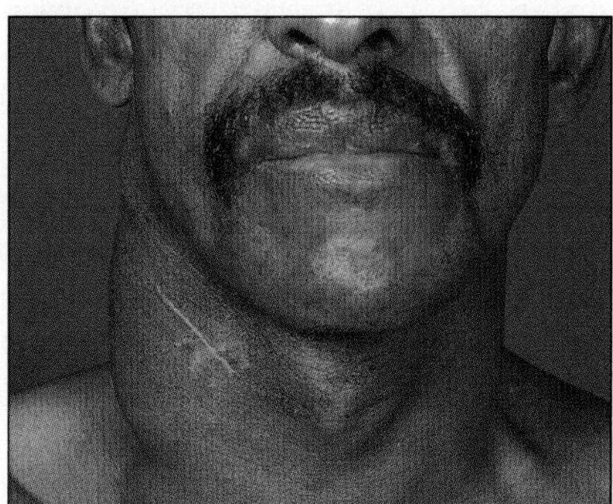

FIGURE 29-9 Hodgkin Lymphoma and Enlarged Cervical Lymph Node. Typical enlarged cervical lymph node in the neck of a man with Hodgkin lymphoma. The scar of previous biopsy incision is well healed. (From Hoffbrand AV, Pettit JE, Vyas P: *Color atlas of clinical hematology,* ed 4, Philadelphia, 2009, Mosby Elsevier.)

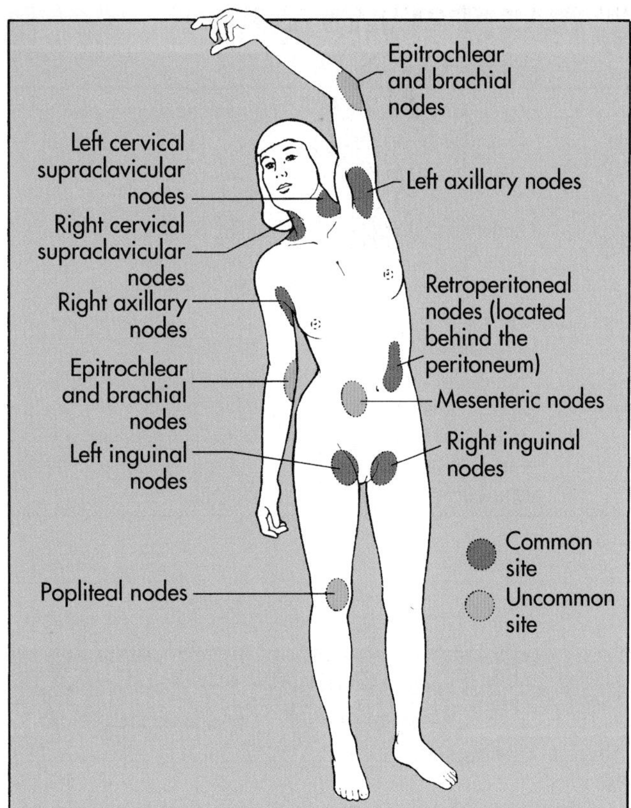

FIGURE 29-10 Common and Uncommon Involved Lymph Node Sites for Hodgkin Lymphoma.

of infection, drenching night sweats, itchy skin (pruritus), and fatigue are relatively common. These constitutional symptoms accompanied by weight loss are associated with a poor prognosis. The Cotswold staging classification system used for HL is able to establish a correlation between the anatomic extent of the disease and prognosis (Table 29-6). This classification system is based on the individual's medical history, examination (presence of symptoms and palpable lymph nodes), and other radiologic and hematologic results. Prognostic indicators include clinical stage, histologic type, tumor cell concentration and tumor burden, constitutional symptoms, and age.

Although HL rarely arises in the lung, mediastinal and hilar node adenopathy can cause secondary involvement of the trachea, bronchi, pleura, or lungs. Retroperitoneal nodes can involve vertebral bodies and nerves, causing displacement of ureters. Spinal cord involvement is more common in the dorsal and lumbar regions than in the cervical region. Although uncommon, skin manifestations include psoriasis and eczematoid lesions, causing itching and scratching.

As a result of direct invasion from mediastinal lymph nodes, pericardial involvement can cause pericardial friction rub, pericardial effusion, and engorgement of the neck veins. The gastrointestinal (GI) tract and urinary tract rarely are involved. Anemia often is found in individuals with HL, accompanied by a low serum iron level and decreased iron-binding capacity. Other laboratory findings include elevated sedimentation rate, leukocytosis, and eosinophilia. Leukopenia occurs in advanced states of HL.

TABLE 29-6 COTSWOLD STAGING CLASSIFICATION SYSTEM

STAGE	CRITERIA
I	Involvement of a single lymph node region or single extranodal organ or site
II	Involvement of two or more lymph node regions on the same side of the diaphragm or a single extranodal organ or site and its regional lymph nodes
III	Involvement of lymph node regions or structures on both sides of the diaphragm
IV	Disseminated involvement of one or more extralymphatic organs or an isolated extralymphatic organ with distant nodal involvement
	Modifying characteristics for all four stages:
	A: No B symptoms
	B: Unexplained fever of >38° C (100.4° F), drenching night sweats, unexplained loss of >10% of body weight in the 6 months preceding diagnosis
	E: Large mediastinal mass with direct extension into extranodal sites

Data from Lister TA, Crowther D: *Semin Oncol* 17:696, 1990.

Splenic involvement of HL depends on histopathologic type (see Table 29-5). The spleen is involved in 60% of cases of mixed cellularity and lymphocytic depletion types. With lymphocyte predominance and nodular sclerosis types, only 34% of cases reveal splenic involvement.

EVALUATION AND TREATMENT. Because of the variability in symptoms, early definitive detection may be difficult. Asymptomatic lymphadenopathy can progress undetected for several years. Careful evaluation, including chest x-rays, lymphangiography, and biopsy, should be carried out for individuals with fever of unknown origin and peripheral lymphadenopathy.[34] A lymph node biopsy with scattered RS cells and a cellular infiltrate is highly indicative of HL. The effectiveness of treatment is related to the age of the individual and the extent of the disease. Approximately 75% of individuals diagnosed with HL are cured, largely because of successful combined treatment with radiation therapy and chemotherapy (Figure 29-11). Over the past 50 years, the death rate has fallen more rapidly for HL than for any other malignancy. More recent treatments include high-dose chemotherapy with bone marrow or stem cell transplantation. Monoclonal antibodies also are being developed and nonmyeloablative allogeneic stem cell transplant has been found to help certain individuals even though this treatment is still under development.

The 5-year survival rate varies depending on the stage that is identified at diagnosis.[34] The 5-year survival rate for stages I and II is 90% to 95%, 80% to 85% for stage III, and 75% for stage IV. Those with stage I or II disease are candidates for chemotherapy, radiation therapy, or a combination of these treatment modalities. Individuals with stage III or IV disease, bulky disease (more than 10-cm mass or mediastinal disease with a transverse diameter exceeding 33% of the transthoracic diameter), or presence of B symptoms require combined chemotherapy with or without additional radiation treatment. Other factors, if

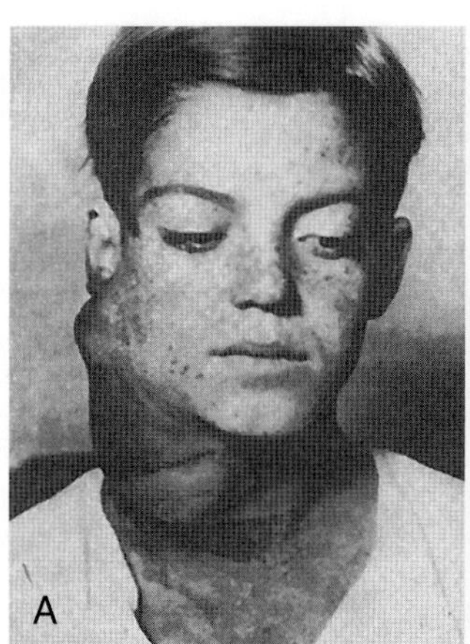

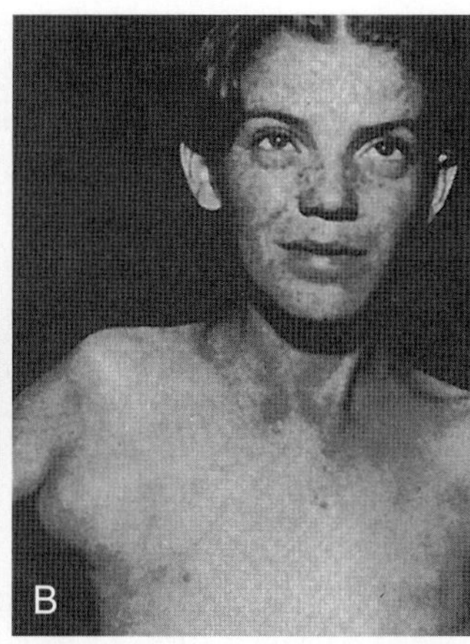

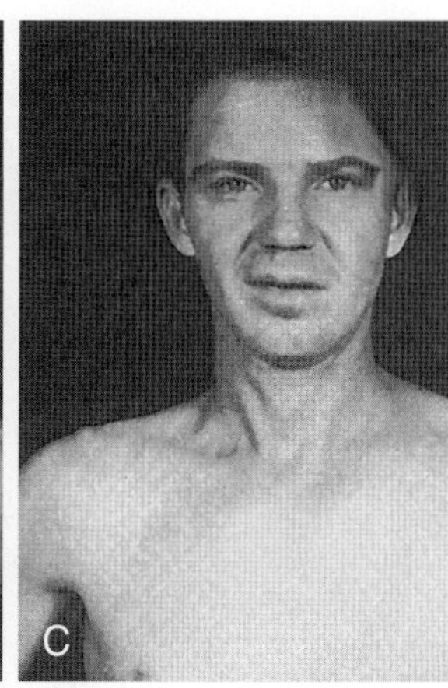

FIGURE 29-11 Cervical Hodgkin Lymphoma (Extreme Case). **A,** Young boy with extensive cervical Hodgkin lymphoma. **B,** Appearance several years later and after treatment, when axillary manifestations developed. **C,** Appearance 23 years after initial treatment with radiation. (From del Regato JA, Spjut HJ, Cox JD: *Ackerman and del Regato's cancer,* ed 2, St Louis, 1985, Mosby.)

present, have an influence on survival. Poorer survival is related to a high white blood cell count (greater than 15,000/μL) or low hemoglobin (Hb) level (less than 10.5 g/dl); low lymphocyte count (less than 600/μL); and male gender. Cure for HL can be achieved in 75% of cases with current therapies.

Non-Hodgkin Lymphoma

The previously used generic classification of **non-Hodgkin lymphoma (NHL)** has been reclassified in the WHO/REAL scheme into **B-cell neoplasms,** which include a variety of lymphomas including myelomas that originate from B cells at various stages of differentiation, and **T-cell** and **NK-cell neoplasms,** which include lymphomas that originate from either T or NK cells. These cancers are differentiated from HL by lack of RS cells and other cellular changes not characteristic of HL.

More than 69,740 cases of NHL and 19,020 deaths are predicted for 2013 (see Table 29-2).[35] The median age of diagnosis is 67 years of age. The incidence of NHL has increased from 8 persons per 100,000 in 1973 to 19.6 per 100,000 in 2009. Lymphomas from HIV and EBV have accounted for some of the increase but an actual cause has yet to be determined. Conversely, the mortality rate has risen at a slower rate. It is thought that newer treatment modalities are improving survival rates.

PATHOPHYSIOLOGY. NHL is best described as a progressive clonal expansion of B cells, T cells, or NK cells. The genetic lesions affecting proto-oncogenes or tumor-suppressor genes result in cell immortalization and the resultant increase in malignant cells. Oncogenes may be activated by chromosomal translocations or the tumor-suppressor loci may be inactivated by deletion or mutation of chromosomes. Oncogenic viruses also may alter the genome of certain subtypes. The various subtypes of NHL may be identified by specific diagnostic markers related to various cytogenic lesions.

Lymphomas most likely originate from mutations in cellular genes (many of which are environmentally induced) in a single cell that lead to loss of control of proliferation and other aspects of cell growth. The most common type of chromosomal alteration in NHL is translocation, which disrupts the genes encoded at the breakpoints. Risk factors include family history, exposure to a variety of mutagenic chemicals, irradiation, infection with certain cancer-related viruses (e.g., EBV, human herpesvirus-8, HIV, HTLV-1, hepatitis C), and immune suppression related to organ transplantation. Gastric infection with *Helicobacter pylori* increases the risk for gastric lymphomas. NHL is a disease of middle age, usually found in individuals more than 50 years old.

B cells account for 80% to 90% of NHLs, with T cells and NK cells accounting for the remaining percentage. A very small percent originates from macrophages. NHL tumors are categorized by the level of differentiation, cell of origin, and rate of cellular proliferation. Tumor aggressiveness of many B-cell NHLs may be predicted by the pattern of cell growth and size. Tumors with a characteristic nodular pattern, vaguely resembling lymphoid follicular structures, are generally less aggressive than lymphomas with a diffuse pattern of proliferation. Small lymphocyte lymphomas are less aggressive than large cell lymphomas, which are generally intermediate to high grade in aggressiveness. However, small cells are characteristic of some subtypes of high-grade lymphomas.

CLINICAL MANIFESTATIONS. Clinical manifestations of NHL usually begin as localized or generalized lymphadenopathy, similar to HL. The cervical, axillary, inguinal, and femoral chains are the most commonly affected sites. Generally, the swelling is painless and the nodes have enlarged and transformed over a period of months or years. Other sites of involvement are the nasopharynx, gastrointestinal (GI) tract, bone, thyroid, testes, and soft tissue. Some individuals have retroperitoneal and abdominal masses with symptoms of abdominal fullness, back pain, ascites (fluid in the peritoneal cavity), and leg swelling.

Lymphomas are classified as low, intermediate, or high grade. A low-grade lymphoma, which also may be termed *indolent,* has a slow progression. Individuals with low-grade lymphoma commonly present with a painless, peripheral adenopathy. Spontaneous regression of these nodes may occur, mimicking the presence of an infection. Night sweats with an elevated temperature (more than 38° C [100.4° F]) and weight loss, as well

TABLE 29-7 CLINICAL DIFFERENCES BETWEEN NON-HODGKIN LYMPHOMA AND HODGKIN LYMPHOMA

CHARACTERISTIC	NON-HODGKIN LYMPHOMA	HODGKIN LYMPHOMA
Nodal involvement	Multiple peripheral nodes Mesenteric nodes and Waldeyer ring commonly involved	Localized to single axial group of nodes (i.e., cervical, mediastinal, para-aortic) Mesenteric nodes and Waldeyer ring rarely involved
Spread	Noncontiguous	Orderly spread by contiguity
B symptoms*	Uncommon	Common
Extranodal involvement	Common	Rare
Extent of disease	Rarely localized	Often localized

*Fever, weight loss, night sweats.

TABLE 29-8 ANN ARBOR STAGING FOR HODGKIN LYMPHOMA

STAGE	CRITERIA
I	Involvement of single lymph node
II	Involvement of two or more lymph node regions
III	Involvement of lymph nodes on both sides of diaphragm
IV	Diffuse involvement of one or more extralymphatic organs with or without associated lymph node involvement
Subclassifications	
E	Involvement of adjacent extralymphatic site
S	Involvement of spleen
A	Asymptomatic
B	Fever, night sweats, weight loss

as extranodular involvement, are not commonly present in the early stages but are common in advanced or end stages of the disease. Cytopenia, reflective of bone marrow involvement, is often observed. Hepatomegaly is common; however, splenomegaly is present in approximately 40% of individuals. Fatigue and weakness are more prevalent with advanced stages.

Immediate and high-grade lymphomas, which are more aggressive, have a more varied clinical presentation. A high-grade lymphoma also may be termed *aggressive.* Adenopathy is common with more than one third of individuals having extranodal involvement. Common sites are the GI tract, skin, bone marrow, sinuses, genitourinary (GU) tract, thyroid, and CNS. Night sweats, with an increased temperature (more than 38° C [100.4° F]), as well as weight loss (more than 10% from baseline within 6 months) are present in approximately 30% to 40% of individuals. Some individuals have retroperitoneal and abdominal masses with symptoms of abdominal fullness, back pain, ascites (fluid in the peritoneal cavity), and leg swelling. Hepatomegaly and splenomegaly are often present. Differences in clinical features are noted in Table 29-7.

EVALUATION AND TREATMENT. Biopsy is considered the primary means for diagnosis of NHL. Staging of NHL is necessary to identify treatment and make a prognosis. In addition to biopsy, computed tomography (CT) scans of the neck, chest, abdomen, and pelvis, as well as bilateral bone marrow aspirate examination, are performed. Data from all three procedures are necessary for appropriate staging. A common finding in NHL is noncontiguous lymph node involvement, which is not common in HL. The Ann Arbor staging system is most commonly used to stage NHL (Table 29-8).

Treatment for NHL is quite diverse and depends on type (B or T cell), tumor stage, histologic status (low, intermediate, or high grade), symptoms, age, and any comorbidities. Depending on the type (B or T cell) of the tumor, the stage of the disease, and the aggressiveness of the tumor, treatment is usually initiated at the time of diagnosis. However, because treatment is not curative for some low-grade indolent lymphomas that are widely disseminated, observation without treatment may be the most appropriate choice. These indolent tumors are often not symptomatic for the individual and this approach improves quality of life. In some cases the disease may be so slow growing that treatment is not needed for an extended period of time.

Success of treatment is dependent on several parameters, including the type of lymphoma, stage of disease, cell type, involvement of organs outside the lymph nodes, age of the person, and the severity of the body's reaction to the disease (e.g., fever, night sweats, weight loss).[34,36] Treatment with chemotherapy alone may be adequate in many cases, although radiation therapy is frequently included. Low-dose chemotherapy has been followed by autologous stem cell transplantation in some NHLs or for recurrent disease. Treatment of B-cell lymphomas with rituximab has proven effective. Rituximab is a commercial monoclonal antibody against antigen CD20, which is expressed on the surface of all B cells, including those that are malignant. Administration of rituximab depletes most B cells and allows the replenishment of normal B cells from the lymphoid stem cell pool. It has also proven useful in a variety of autoimmune diseases, including immune thrombocytopenia purpura, autoimmune anemias, systemic lupus erythematosus, and rheumatoid arthritis.

Radioimmunotherapy, a newer treatment approach, combines radiation therapy with monoclonal antibody therapy and is used to improve rates of complete remission both in indolent forms of lymphoma (follicular and marginal zone) and in aggressive forms, including large B-cell and mantle cell lymphoma. Studies suggest improved complete remission rates and longer disease-free survival in persons with these types of lymphomas.

Individuals with NHL can survive for extended periods.[34,36] A partial remission may be achieved in some cases in which evidence of the disease remains but it does not progress. Survival with nodular lymphoma ranges up to 15 years, but those with diffuse disease generally do not survive as long. Overall,

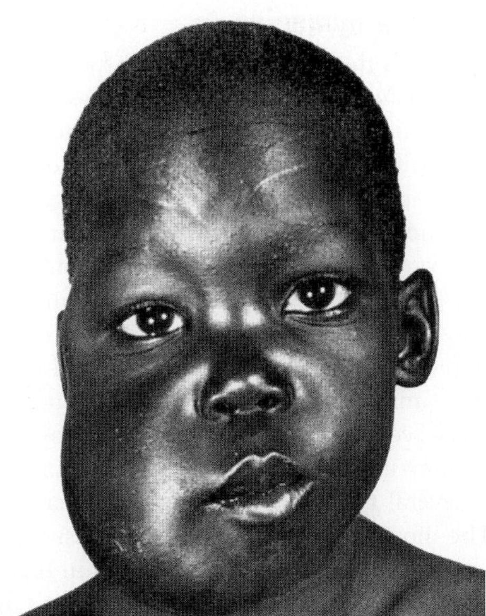

FIGURE 29-12 Burkitt Lymphoma. Burkitt lymphoma involving the jaw in a young African boy. (Courtesy I. Magrath, MD, Bethesda, MD. From Zitelli BJ, McIntire SC, Nowalk AJ: *Zitelli and Davis' atlas of pediatric physical diagnosis,* ed 6, Philadelphia, 2012, Saunders.)

the survival rates of NHL are less than those for Hodgkin lymphoma. For NHL, the survival rates are 1 year, 77%; 5 years, 59%; and 10 years, 42%. Many investigators believe that more aggressive treatment increases the cure rate. High-grade NHL is seen with increasing frequency in persons with AIDS and has an extremely poor prognosis.

Burkitt Lymphoma

Burkitt lymphoma is a B-cell tumor with unique clinical and epidemiologic features that accounts for 30% of childhood lymphomas worldwide. It is a highly aggressive B-cell non-Hodgkin lymphoma that is the fastest growing human tumor. It occurs in children from east-central Africa and New Guinea and is characterized by a rapidly growing tumor primarily in the jaw and facial bones (Figure 29-12). In the United States, Burkitt lymphoma is rare, usually involves the abdomen, and is characterized by extensive bone marrow invasion and replacement. EBV, found in nasopharyngeal secretions, is associated with Burkitt lymphoma in African children.

PATHOPHYSIOLOGY. EBV is associated with almost all cases (more than 90%) of Burkitt lymphoma. It is suspected that suppression of the immune system by other illnesses (e.g., HIV infection, chronic malaria) increases the individual's susceptibility to EBV. B cells are particularly sensitive because of specific surface receptors for EBV. As a result, the B cell undergoes chromosomal translocations that result in overexpression of the *C-MYC* proto-oncogene and loss of control of cell growth (Figure 29-13). The most common translocation (75% of individuals) is between chromosomes 8 (containing the *C-MYC* gene) and 14 (containing the immunoglobulin heavy-chain genes). Other translocations have been reported between chromosome 8 and chromosomes 2 or 22, which contain genes for immunoglobulin light chains.

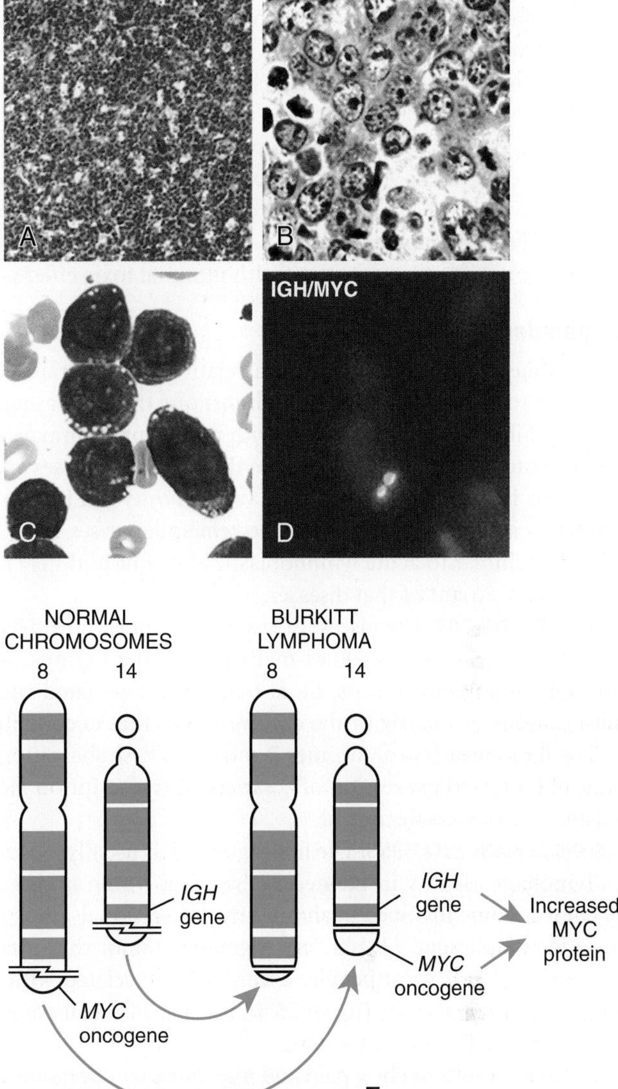

FIGURE 29-13 Burkitt Lymphoma Cells. A, A case of Burkitt lymphoma illustrated at low power showing the "starry sky" appearance. This is due to the dense proliferating cells producing the dark sky, and the scattered lighter-staining tingible body macrophages *(stars)* phagocytizing dying cells. **B,** Higher magnification illustrating the syncytia of intermediate-sized cells with coarse chromatin and multiple nucleoli. Note the tingible body macrophage with abundant light cytoplasm and ingested debris *(center bottom).* **C,** Burkitt cells as seen on a Wright-stained bone marrow aspirate in a person with Burkitt leukemia. Notice deep blue cytoplasm with numerous vacuoles. **D,** Fluorescence in situ hybridization (FISH) with probes to *MYC* and *IGH* illustrate the IGH/MYC fusion. **E,** The 8, 14 chromosomal translocation and associated oncogenes in Burkitt lymphoma. (**A-D** courtesy Dr. Y. Zhang, University of Chicago. From Hoffman R et al: *Hematology: basic principles and practice,* ed 6, Philadelphia, 2013, Churchill Livingstone. **E** from Kumar V et al: *Robbins & Cotran pathologic basis of disease,* ed 8, Philadelphia, 2010, Saunders.)

CLINICAL MANIFESTATIONS. In non-African Burkitt lymphoma the most common presentation is abdominal swelling. More advanced disease may involve other organs—eye, ovaries, kidneys, glandular tissue (breast, thyroid, tonsil)—and presents with type B symptoms (night sweats, fever, weight loss).

EVALUATION AND TREATMENT. The distribution of tumors and biopsies of enlarged lymph nodes or the bone marrow containing malignant B cells are usually indicative of Burkitt lymphoma. It is one of the most aggressive and quickly growing malignancies. However, the African variety in children has been successfully treated with radiotherapy and cyclophosphamide (60% survival overall; 90% survival with limited disease). The American type is more resistant to treatment. Adjuvant monoclonal antibody therapy with rituximab appears to be a promising agent for improving outcomes with minimal toxic effects.[37]

Lymphoblastic Lymphoma

Lymphoblastic lymphoma (LL) is a relatively rare variant of NHL (2% to 4%) but accounts for almost one third of cases of NHL in children and adolescents, with a male predominance. It is estimated that there will be more than 6000 new cases and more than 1400 deaths in 2012. The vast majority of LL (more than 85%) is of T-cell origin, and the remainder arises from B cells. LL is similar to acute lymphoblastic leukemia and may be considered a variant of that disease.

PATHOPHYSIOLOGY. The disease arises from a clone of relatively immature T cells that becomes malignant in the thymus. As with most lymphoid tumors, LL is frequently associated with translocations, primarily of the chromosomes that encode for the T-cell receptor (chromosomes 7 and 14). These aberrations result in increased expression of a variety of transcription factors and loss of growth control.

CLINICAL MANIFESTATIONS. The first sign of LL is usually a painless lymphadenopathy in the neck. Peripheral lymph nodes in the chest become involved in about 70% of individuals, mostly above the diaphragm. LL is a very aggressive tumor that presents as stage IV in most people. T-cell LL is associated with a unique mediastinal mass (up to 75%) because of the apparent origin of the tumor in the thymus.

The mass results in chest pain and may cause compression of bronchi or the superior vena cava. The tumor may infiltrate the bone marrow in about half of those affected, and suppression of bone marrow hematopoiesis leads to increased susceptibility to infections. Other organs, including the liver, kidney, spleen, and brain, may also be affected. Many individuals express type B symptoms: fever, night sweats, and significant weight loss.

EVALUATION AND TREATMENT. The most common therapeutic approach is combined chemotherapy with multiple drugs. In early disease, the response rate is high with increased survival; the 5-year survival in children is 80% to 90%, and 45% to 55% in adults. Although LL is easily treated, there is a high relapse rate: 40% to 60% of adults.

Conditions That Mimic Lymphomas

Certain other clinical conditions mimic the malignant lymphomas. These conditions include tuberculosis (TB), syphilis, systemic lupus erythematosus, lung cancer, and bone cancer. An important distinction between lymphomas and other conditions is that lymphomas usually involve localized lymphadenopathy. Infectious precursors of malignant lymphomas are characterized by more generalized lymphadenopathy with systemic signs and symptoms.

Plasma Cell Malignancies

The plasma cell is the end-stage cell of the humoral immune response (see Chapter 8). Immunocompetent B cells presented with antigen and stimulated with cytokines from T helper cells will undergo proliferation and differentiation into antibody-producing plasma cells. Antigen-reactive B cells have undergone rearrangement of immunoglobulin heavy-chain variable region genes *(V, D, J)* and express surface IgM or IgD, or both. After stimulation with antigen, the B cells may not undergo any further genetic rearrangement and develop into plasma cells that secrete IgM or selectively rearrange the immunoglobulin heavy-chain genes to irreversibly switch to secreting IgG, IgA, or IgE. During this process some cells may undergo malignant transformation, leading to one of several types of plasma cell malignancies (Figure 29-14). The most common and most aggressive plasma cell tumor is multiple myeloma. Other diseases in this classification include precursors to malignant myeloma (smoldering myeloma, monoclonal gammopathy of undetermined significance [MGUS]), solitary plasmacytoma of the bone, and Waldenström macroglobulinemia.[38] A common characteristic of these tumors is secretion of complete or partial immunoglobulin molecules.

Multiple Myeloma

Multiple myeloma (MM) is a clonal plasma cell cancer characterized by the slow proliferation of malignant cells as tumor cell masses in the bone marrow that usually results in destruction of the bone. Most MMs secrete large amounts of monoclonal proteins that resemble intact immunoglobulins. The reported incidence of myeloma has doubled in the past two decades, possibly as a result of more sensitive testing used for diagnosis. The annual incidence rate in the United States is 5.6 per 100,000, with more than 21,700 new cases and more than 10,700 deaths estimated for 2012.[39] Multiple myeloma occurs in all races, but the incidence in blacks is about twice that of whites. It rarely occurs before the age of 40 years—peak age of incidence is about 70 years. It is slightly more common in men than in women. Neoplastic cells of multiple myeloma reside in the bone marrow and are usually not found in the peripheral blood. Occasionally it may spread to other tissues, especially in very advanced disease.

PATHOPHYSIOLOGY. Many myelomas are aneuploidy, with chromosomal numbers ranging from 44 chromosomes to near tetraploid. Chromosomal translocations (breakpoints) are responsible for development of myeloma in most individuals. The primary translocation involves the immunoglobulin heavy chain on chromosome 14 that relocates to sites containing genes that cell cycle (cyclins) on chromosomes 11(q13), 12(p13), and 6(p21); oncogenes on chromosomes 16(q23), 8(q24), and 20; and fibroblast growth factor receptor on chromosome 4(p16).[9] A progression of further secondary genetic alterations causes development to an aggressive MM (Figure 29-15). The molecular pathogenesis of multiple myeloma also involves proto-oncogene mutations and, more rarely, inactivation of tumor-suppressor genes. The precise timing and reason for the genetic alteration and accumulation are unknown, but probably occur initially late in B-cell development after exposure to antigen. Investigators are studying various epigenetic alterations in multiple myeloma, for example, miRNAs and global changes in chromatin.[40]

Malignant plasma cells arise from one clone of B cells that produce abnormally large amounts of one class of immunoglobulin (usually IgG, occasionally IgA, and rarely IgD or IgE). The malignant transformation may begin early in B-cell development, possibly before encountering antigen in the secondary lymphoid organs. The myeloma cells return

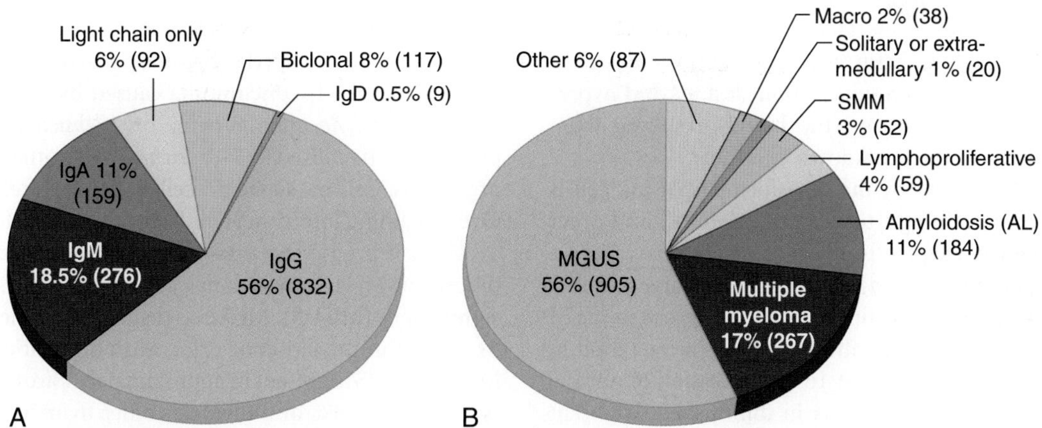

FIGURE 29-14 Distribution of Monoclonal Gammopathy Types. A, Distribution of serum monoclonal proteins in 1485 patients seen at the Mayo Clinic during 2008. **B,** Diagnoses in 1612 cases of monoclonal gammopathy seen at the Mayo Clinic during 2008. *Ig,* Immunoglobulin; *MGUS,* monoclonal gammopathy of undetermined significance; *PC,* plasmacytoma; *SMM,* smoldering multiple myeloma; *WM,* Waldenström macroglobulinemia. (From Goldman L, Schafer AI: *Goldman's Cecil medicine,* ed 24, Philadelphia, 2012, Saunders.)

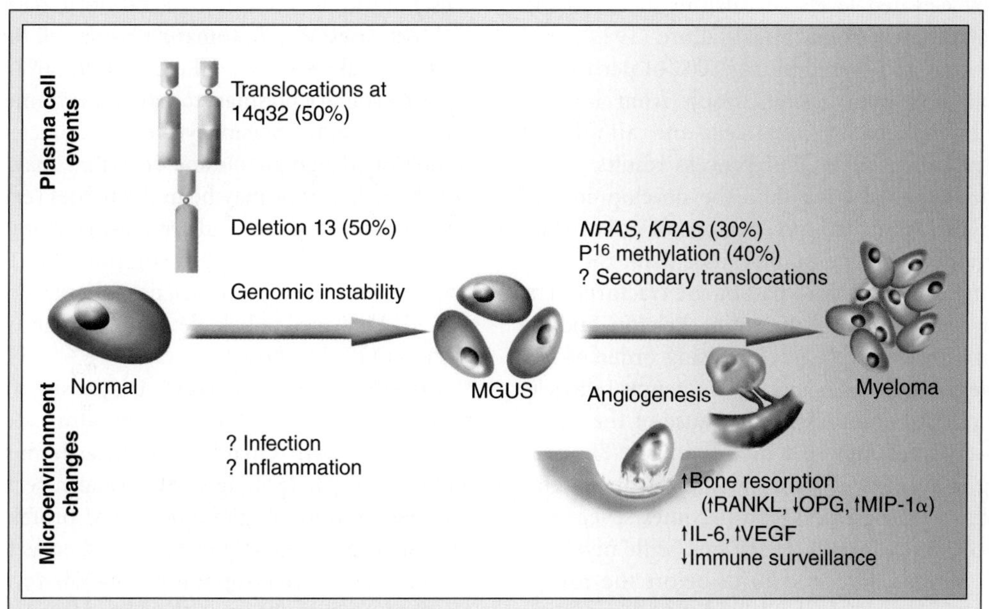

FIGURE 29-15 Myeloma Cell Proliferation and Disease Progression. Development of the malignant myeloma results from multiple genetic changes, initially a translocation involving the immunoglobulin heavy-chain genes on chromosome 14 or a deletion in chromosome 13. The intermediate phenotype is frequently genetically unstable, leading to further mutations that result in a myeloma. Interactions between myeloma cells and extracellular matrix proteins further increase adhesion molecule expression, anti-apoptotic pathways, angiogenesis, bone resorption, and cytokine secretion. *IL-6,* Interleukin-6; *KRAS,* V-Ki-ras Z Kirsten rat sarcoma viral oncogene homolog; *MGUS,* monoclonal gammopathy of undetermined significance; *MIP-1α,* macrophage inflammatory protein-1α; *NRAS,* neuroblastoma RAS viral (v-ras) oncogene homolog; *OPG,* osteoprotegerin; *RANKL,* receptor activator of nuclear factor-κB ligand; *VEGF,* vascular endothelial growth factor. (From Abeloff M et al: *Abeloff's clinical oncology,* ed 4, Philadelphia, 2008, Churchill Livingstone.)

either to the bone marrow or to other soft tissue sites. Their return is aided by cell adhesion molecules that help them target favorable sites that promote continued expansion and maturation.

Myeloma cells in the bone marrow directly secrete hepatocyte growth factor and parathyroid hormone–related peptide and adhere to stromal cells, inducing their production of several cytokines (e.g., IL-6, IL-1, TNF-α, TNF-β, IL-11, macrophage inflammatory protein). (Lymphocytes and cytokines are described in Chapter 8.) These factors, particularly IL-6, act as an osteoclast-activating factor and stimulate osteoclasts to reabsorb bone. This process results in bone lesions and hypercalcemia (high calcium levels in the blood) resulting from release of calcium from the breakdown of bone.

The antibody produced by the transformed plasma cell is usually defective, containing truncations, deletions, and other abnormalities, and is frequently referred to as a paraprotein (abnormal protein in the blood). Because of the large number of malignant plasma cells, the abnormal antibody, called the **M protein,** becomes the most prominent protein in the blood in 80% of myeloma clients (Figure 29-16). Suppression of normal plasma cells by the myeloma results in diminished or absent normal antibodies. The excessive amount of M protein also may contribute to many of the clinical manifestations of the disease. The myeloma may produce free immunoglobulin light chain **(Bence Jones protein)** that is present in the blood and urine in approximately 80% of clients and contributes to damage of renal tubular cells.

CLINICAL MANIFESTATIONS. The common presentation of MM is characterized by elevated levels of calcium in the blood (hypercalcemia) (13% of persons), renal failure (19%), anemia (72% of persons), and bone lesions (80% of persons).[41] The hypercalcemia and bone lesions result from infiltration of the bone by malignant plasma cells and stimulation of osteoclasts to reabsorb bone. This process results in the release of calcium (hypercalcemia) and the development of "lytic lesions" (round, "punched-out" regions of bone) (Figure 29-17). Destruction of bone tissue causes pain, the most common presenting symptom, and pathologic fractures. The pain may be felt in a single bone of the entire skeleton, and the bones most commonly involved, in decreasing order of frequency, are the vertebrae, ribs, skull, pelvis, femur, clavicle, and scapula. Spinal cord compression, because of the weakened vertebrae, occurs in about 10% of individuals. The pain is initially aching, intermittent, and aggravated by weight-bearing. As the disease progresses, pain becomes severe and prolonged. It is common for the individual with myeloma to be treated for a slipped disk or arthritis before the correct diagnosis of myeloma is established. The individual may complain of weakness, fatigue, weight loss, and anorexia in addition to pain.

Proteinuria is observed in 90% of individuals. Renal failure may be either acute or chronic and is usually secondary to the hypercalcemia. Bence Jones protein may lead to damage of the proximal tubules. Anemia is usually normocytic and normochromic and results from inhibited erythropoiesis caused by tumor cell infiltration of the bone marrow.

The high concentration of paraprotein in the blood may lead to hyperviscosity syndrome. The increased viscosity interferes with blood circulation to various sites (brain, kidneys, extremities). Hyperviscosity syndrome is observed in up to 20% of individuals with MM. Additional neurologic symptoms (e.g., confusion, headaches, blurred vision) may occur secondary to hypercalcemia or hyperviscosity.

Suppression of the humoral (antibody-mediated) immune response results in repeated infections, primarily pneumonias and pyelonephritis. The most commonly involved organisms are encapsulated bacteria that are particularly sensitive to the effects of antibody: pneumonia caused by *Streptococcus pneumoniae, Staphylococcus aureus,* or *Klebsiella pneumoniae* or pyelonephritis caused by *Escherichia coli* or other gram-negative organisms. Cell-mediated (T-cell) function is relatively normal. Overwhelming infection is the leading cause of death from MM.

MM is a progressive disorder and is often preceded by a condition known as **monoclonal gammopathy of undetermined significance (MGUS).** MGUS is diagnosed by the presence of an M protein in the blood or urine without additional evidence of MM.[41] MGUS is present in approximately 1% of the general population and in 3% of individuals older than 70 years. Although MGUS is considered nonpathologic and requires no treatment, about 2% of individuals with MGUS progress to malignant plasma cell disorders. Progression of MM following MGUS advances to asymptomatic MM and finally symptomatic MM. Asymptomatic MM also may be referred to as **smoldering myeloma** and indolent myeloma.[41] Smoldering myeloma is usually characterized by the presence of an M protein and clonal bone marrow plasma cells, but with no indication of end-organ damage.

Most cases of symptomatic plasma cell tumors are multiple myeloma (about 94%). The remaining 6% is divided equally between solitary plasmacytomas and extramedullary plasmacytomas.[38] **Solitary plasmacytoma** is characterized by a solitary tumor of malignant plasma cells that may result in a single lytic bone lesion or may be in the tissues (extramedullary plasmacytoma).[41] Extramedullary plasmacytoma can be found in a variety of soft tissues, but commonly in those of the upper respiratory tract (e.g., tonsils, nasopharynx, sinuses). Additionally, MM is staged to help determine prognosis and appropriate treatment (Table 29-9).

EVALUATION AND TREATMENT. Diagnosis of MM is made by symptoms, radiographic and laboratory studies, and a bone marrow biopsy. Quantitative measurements of immunoglobulins (IgG, IgM, IgA) are usually performed. Typically, one class of immunoglobulin (the M protein produced by the myeloma cell) is greatly increased, whereas the others are suppressed. Serum electrophoretic analysis reveals increased levels of M protein. Because the M protein is monoclonal, each molecule has the same electric change and migrates at about the same site on electrophoresis, resulting in a highly concentrated protein (M spike). Bence Jones protein is observed in the urine or serum by immunoelectrophoresis or in the serum using enzyme-linked immunosorbent assay (ELISA). Usually individuals with Bence Jones protein also have M protein in their blood. However, variants of MM include individuals in which free light chain only is produced and a rare variant that

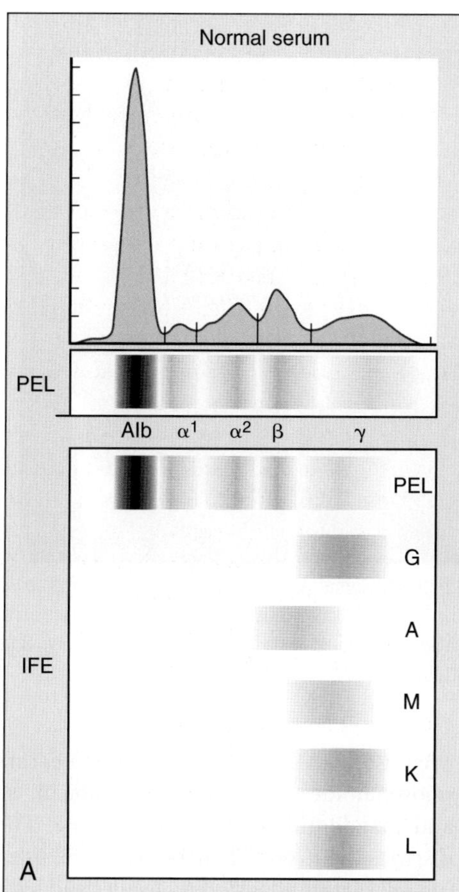

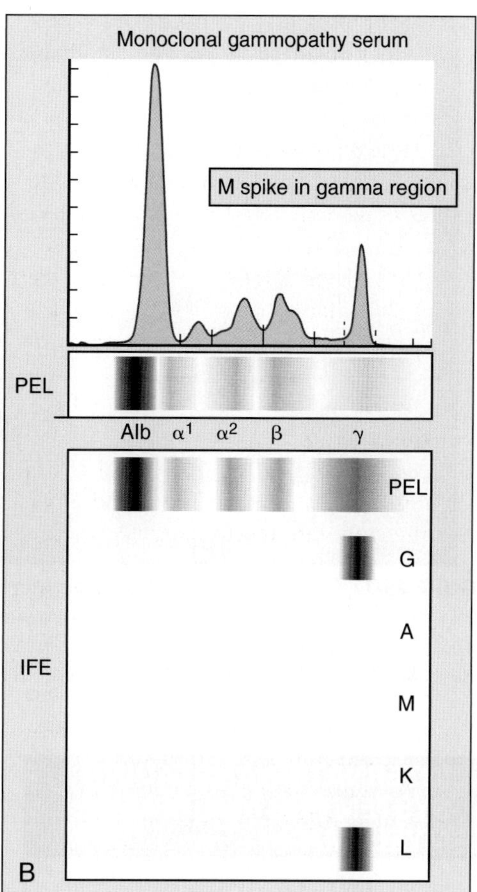

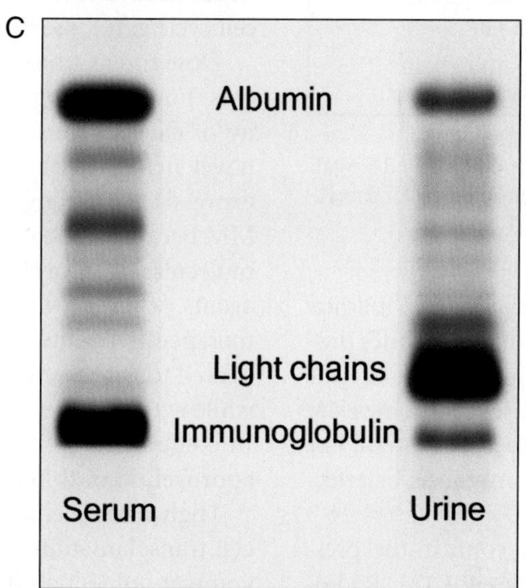

FIGURE 29-16 M Protein. Serum protein electrophoresis *(PEL)* is used to screen for M proteins in multiple myeloma. **A,** In normal serum the proteins separate into several regions between albumin *(Alb)* and a broad band in the gamma (γ) region, where most antibodies (gamma globulins) are found. Immunofixation *(IFE)* can identify the locations of IgG *(G),* IgA *(A),* IgM *(M),* and kappa *(K)* and lambda *(L)* light chains. **B,** Serum from an individual with multiple myeloma contains a sharp M protein *(M spike).* The M protein is monoclonal and contains only one heavy chain and one light chain. In this instance the IFE identifies the M protein as an IgG containing a lambda light chain. **C,** Serum and urine protein electrophoretic patterns in a client with multiple myeloma. Serum demonstrates an M protein *(immunoglobulin)* in the gamma region, and the urine has a large amount of the smaller-sized light chains with only a small amount of the intact immunoglobulin. (**A** and **B** from Abeloff M et al: *Abeloff's clinical oncology,* ed 4, Philadelphia, 2008, Churchill Livingstone. **C** from McPherson R, Pincus M: *Henry's clinical diagnosis and management by laboratory methods,* ed 22, Edinburgh, 2012, Saunders.)

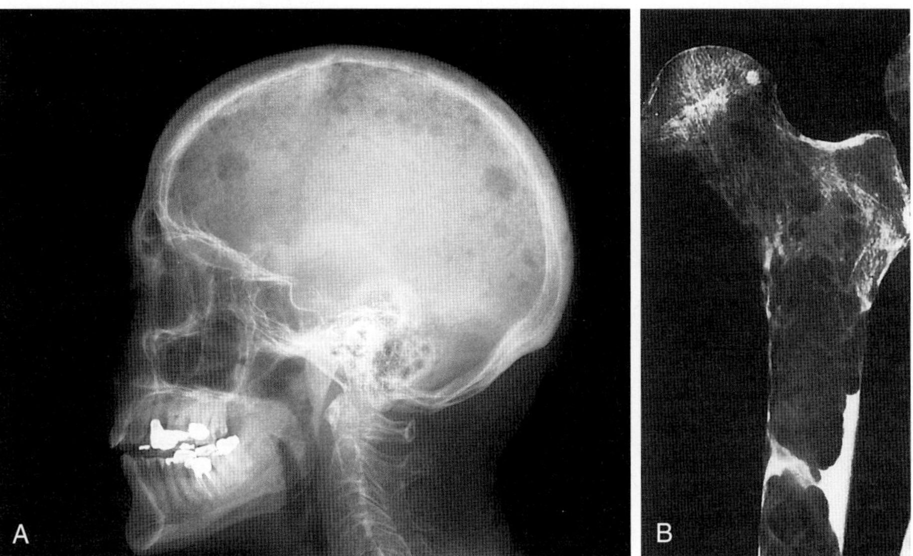

FIGURE 29-17 Osteolytic Lesions in Individuals with Multiple Myeloma. A, Lesions in the skull on radiograph in a client with myeloma. **B,** Roentgenogram of femur showing extensive bone destruction caused by tumor. Note absence of reactive bone formation. (**A** from Abeloff M et al: *Abeloff's clinical oncology,* ed 4, Philadelphia, 2008, Churchill Livingstone. **B** from Kissane JM, editor: *Anderson's pathology,* ed 9, St Louis, 1990, Mosby.)

TABLE 29-9 INTERNATIONAL STAGING SYSTEM FOR MULTIPLE MYELOMA

STAGE	CRITERIA
I	Serum β_2-microglobulin <3.5 mg/L Serum albumin ≥3.5 g/dl
II	Not stage I or III*
III	Serum β_2-microglobulin ≥5.5 mg/L

From Greipp PR et al: *J Clin Oncol* 23(15):3412–3420, 2005.
*There are two categories for stage II: serum β_2-microglobulin <3.5 mg/L but serum albumin <3.5 g/dl; or serum β_2-microglobulin 3.5 to <5.5 mg/L irrespective of the serum albumin level.

produces only free heavy chain, and approximately 1% are nonsecretory so that neither an M protein nor Bence Jones protein is produced. The amount of M protein in the blood may be used as a measure of the extent of the disease or as a measure of response to therapy. The serum level of another protein, free **β_2-microglobulin,** is a useful indicator of prognosis or effectiveness of therapy.

A bone marrow biopsy is performed to confirm the presence of myeloma cells in the marrow (Figure 29-18). Radiographic studies include x-ray, CT scans, and magnetic resonance imaging (MRI) to document the presence of bone lesions and areas of destruction. Diagnosis is based on findings and the degree of involvement. The individual must have all three major criteria (Box 29-4); however, new more sensitive and specific criteria have been proposed but not yet accepted into practice.[42]

Combinations of chemotherapy, radiation therapy, and plasmapheresis (exchange), and marrow transplantation have been the standards of treatment.[38] Conventional combinations of chemotherapeutic agents have included melphalan and prednisone (MP); MP with vincristine, carmustine, and cyclophosphamide; vincristine, doxorubicin, and dexamethasone; and thalidomide and dexamethasone. The drug thalidomide disrupts the stromal marrow–MM cell interaction by modulating cell surface adhesion molecules and inhibiting angiogenesis. In addition, it increases apoptosis and G_1 growth arrest (i.e., the cell cycle gap 1; see Chapter 1) of MM cells.

Dose intensification improves the outcomes in younger clients; however, long-term remissions are obtained in a minority of clients. Thus intensive research measuring the effect of novel new therapies is the objective of ongoing trials. Gene expression profiling (GEP) helps improve the treatment of MM because it identifies prognostic subgroups and defines the molecular pathways associated with these subgroups. Newer agents (e.g., bortezomib, lenalidomide) have broadened the therapeutic regimens for end-stage myeloma. Lenalidomide is related to thalidomide; however, it increases treatment efficacy while avoiding the adverse effects associated with thalidomide. In combination with dexamethasone, lenalidomide is now an approved second-line treatment for MM.

High-dose chemotherapy followed by blood-forming stem cell transplantation (SCT) has become standard treatment for younger individuals (up to 70 years old in some trials).[38,43] Survival is increased with SCT compared with chemotherapy alone. SCT uses the client's own blood-forming stem cells (autologous) or a donor's cells (allogeneic). Survival may be prolonged by performing a second autologous transplant, called *tandem transplant,* within 6 to 12 months from the first transplant.

Radiation with high-energy x-rays is used more for a localized effect rather than systemic. It is most often used to treat areas of the bone that have been damaged and are not responding to chemotherapy. In addition, it may be used to treat sites where tumor has led to collapse of vertebrae and spinal cord compression.

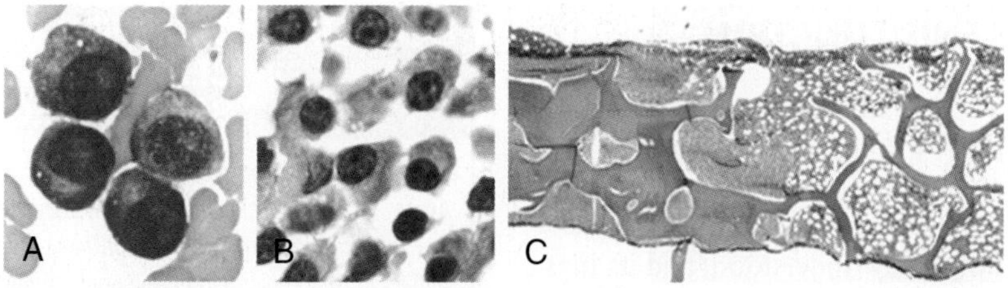

A B C

FIGURE 29-18 Myeloma Cells. The typical myeloma type has fairly mature-appearing plasma cells with eccentric nuclei on bone marrow aspirate **(A)** and biopsy **(B)**. **C,** Osteosclerotic myeloma in which the left side of the photograph shows bone sclerosis and the marrow cavity replaced by myeloma. (From Hoffman R et al: *Hematology: basic principles and practice,* ed 6, Philadelphia, 2013, Churchill Livingstone.)

BOX 29-4 DIAGNOSTIC CRITERIA FOR MULTIPLE MYELOMA

Major Criteria

Positive biopsy result
More than 30% plasma cells in bone marrow sample
Monoclonal antibody in blood/urine

Minor Criteria

10% to 30% plasma cells in bone marrow sample
Monoclonal antibody present but not enough to be a major criterion
Holes in bone from tumor seen on imaging studies
Normal antibody in blood abnormally low

Additional interventions are used to prevent and treat complications arising from progression of the disease. Drugs that inhibit bone resorption—bisphosphonates—reduce the incidence of skeletal damage, which also reduces hypercalcemia and decreases bone pain. Hydration and diuretics may be used to maintain a high urine output, and antibiotics to treat recurring infections.

The prognosis for persons with MM remains poor. The median survival for all states of MM is 3 years. Individuals with multiple bone lesions, if untreated, rarely survive more than 6 to 12 months. Individuals with inactive (indolent) myeloma, however, can survive for many years. With chemotherapy and aggressive management of complications, median survival may increase to 24 to 30 months, with a 10-year survival rate of 3%.

Waldenström Macroglobulinemia

Waldenström macroglobulinemia (WM), also called **lymphoplasmacytic lymphoma,** is a rare type of slow-growing plasma cell tumor that secretes a monoclonal IgM molecule. Approximately 1500 new cases are diagnosed yearly in the United States; the median age of diagnosis is 63 years of age.[44] WM shares a great deal of similarity with multiple myeloma regarding its plasma cell origin, diagnosis, and treatment. However, the overproduction of the macromolecule IgM leads to certain unique clinical characteristics.

PATHOPHYSIOLOGY. WM arises from plasma cells that have undergone genetic rearrangement of the variable region genes (*V, D, J*), but have not undergone class-switch. Therefore, the principal secretory product of the tumor is IgM. Although no definitive genetic defect has been identified, WM may originate from aberrant B-cell maturation and class-switch.

Most of the pathology is associated with the production of large amounts of IgM, a high-molecular-weight protein (about 900,000 daltons). Excessive production leads to thickening of the blood and abnormally high blood viscosity (hyperviscosity syndrome). The increased viscosity interferes with circulation to various sites (e.g., eyes, brain, kidneys, extremities). IgM paraprotein may also result in cryoglobulins (proteins that precipitate from the blood at lower than body temperature). Hyperviscosity syndrome is observed in up to 20% of individuals with WM.

CLINICAL MANIFESTATIONS. Many clients with WM are asymptomatic. The most common symptoms include weakness and fatigue, bleeding (from gums and nose), weight loss, and bruising. Bleeding may result secondary to formation of complexes among the macroglobulin, clotting factors, and platelets that diminish hemostatic capacity. If hyperviscosity syndrome occurs, the individual may develop neurologic problems (e.g., blurred vision, loss of vision, headaches, dizziness, vertigo). The macromolecules may also precipitate in colder regions of the body (cryoglobulins) leading to Raynaud phenomenon.

Although the malignant plasma cells invade the bone marrow, erosion of the bone is not commonly observed; less than 5% of individuals have lytic bone lesions. The tumor often disseminates to other organs, including the spleen, lymph nodes, and liver. Anemia occurs in about 10% of individuals, secondary to tumor infiltration of the bone marrow. Peripheral hemolysis can also result from production of cold agglutinins.

EVALUATION AND TREATMENT. Diagnosis is made on the basis of high levels of monoclonal IgM in the blood and the identification of malignant cells in bone marrow aspirates. Other hematologic abnormalities may be observed, especially anemia (80% of clients with symptomatic WM) but also thrombocytopenia and leukopenia. Bence Jones protein may be observed in almost half of individuals with WM.

Treatment is similar to that described for multiple myeloma.[45] First-line therapy includes combined chemotherapy with nucleoside analogs, alkylating agents, and monoclonal antibody (e.g., rituximab). Bone marrow stem cell transplantation has also proven effective in some individuals. The current recommendations include treatment with a combination of dexamethasone, rituximab, and cyclophosphamide, with the use of other drugs (e.g., doxorubicin, vincristine, and nucleoside analogs) in individuals with very high levels of M protein.

ALTERATIONS OF SPLENIC FUNCTION

The spleen has been an organ of mystery and perplexity in the study of medicine. Its relationship to other organs and disease processes, particularly the immune and hematologic systems, was not identified until the eighteenth century. The complexities of splenic function are not totally understood, and its mysteries are still being explored. The spleen is a useful organ, but its functions overlap those of other organs so that one is capable of living a normal, healthy life without the spleen. The relationship between asplenia and a higher risk for infection was not recognized until the early 1950s.

In the past, **splenomegaly** (enlargement of the spleen) was associated with various disease states. It is now recognized that splenomegaly is not necessarily pathologic; an enlarged spleen may be present in certain individuals without any evidence of disease. Splenomegaly may be, however, one of the first physical signs of underlying conditions, and its presence should not be ignored. In conditions in which splenomegaly is present, the normal functions of the spleen may become overactive, producing a condition known as **hypersplenism.**

Current criteria indicating the presence of hypersplenism include: (1) cytopenias (anemia, leukopenia, thrombocytopenia, or combinations of these); (2) cellular bone marrow; (3) splenomegaly; and (4) improvement after splenectomy. Some individuals may seek treatment for problems even though they have not met all these clinical criteria; therefore, the relevance and significance of hypersplenism are still uncertain. Primary hypersplenism is recognized when no etiologic factor has been identified; secondary hypersplenism occurs in the presence of another condition.

PATHOPHYSIOLOGY. Splenomegaly without a specific etiology is seen in 7% to 15% of individuals who are being evaluated for primary splenomegaly and is generally a diagnosis of exclusion. Specific conditions causing secondary splenomegaly and resulting hypersplenism are many and are related to all other categories of disease that affect individuals. Secondary splenomegaly may be classified according to the underlying cause. Specific conditions related to these various classifications of splenomegaly are detailed in Box 29-5. Different pathologic processes that produce splenomegaly are described briefly.

Acute inflammatory or infectious processes cause splenomegaly because of an increased demand for defensive activities. Acutely enlarged spleens secondary to infection may become so filled with erythrocytes that their natural rubbery resilience is lost and they become fragile and vulnerable to blunt trauma. Splenic rupture is a complication associated with infectious mononucleosis; rupture occurs mostly in males between the fourth and twenty-first day of acute illness.

Congestive splenomegaly is accompanied by ascites, portal hypertension, and esophageal varices and is most commonly seen in those with hepatic cirrhosis. Splenic hyperplasia develops in disorders that increase splenic workload and is associated most commonly with various types of anemia (hemolytic) and chronic myeloproliferative disorders (i.e., polycythemia vera).

BOX 29-5 DISEASES RELATED TO CLASSIFICATION OF SPLENOMEGALY

Inflammation or Infection

Acute: viral (hepatitis, infectious mononucleosis, cytomegalovirus), bacterial (*Salmonella*, gram negative), parasitic (typhoid)

Subacute or chronic: bacterial (subacute bacterial endocarditis, tuberculosis), parasitic (malaria), fungal (histoplasmosis), Felty syndrome, systemic lupus erythematosus, rheumatoid arthritis, thrombocytopenia

Congestive

Cirrhosis, heart failure, portal vein obstruction (portal hypertension), splenic vein obstruction

Infiltrative

Gaucher disease, amyloidosis, diabetic lipemia

Tumors or Cysts

Malignant: polycythemia vera, chronic or acute leukemias, Hodgkin lymphoma, metastatic solid tumors

Nonmalignant: hamartoma

Cysts: true cysts (lymphangiomas, hemangiomas, epithelial, endothelial); false cysts (hemorrhagic, serous, inflammatory)

Infiltrative splenomegaly is caused by engorgement by the macrophages with indigestible materials associated with various "storage diseases." Tumors and cysts cause actual growth of the spleen. Metastatic tumors in the spleen are rare and may result from primary tumors of the skin, lung, breast, and cervix.

CLINICAL MANIFESTATIONS. Overactivity of the spleen results in hematologic alterations that affect all blood components. Sequestering of red blood cells, granulocytes, and platelets results in a reduction of all circulating blood cells. The spleen may sequester up to 50% of the red blood cell population, thereby upsetting the normal physiologic concentration of red blood cells in the circulation. The rate of splenic pooling is directly related to spleen size and the degree of increased blood flow through it. Sequestering exposes the red blood cells to splenic conditions that accelerate destruction, further contributing to the decreased red blood cell concentration. Anemia is the result of these combined activities. Anemia may be further potentiated by an increase in blood volume, which produces a dilutional effect on the already reduced concentration of red blood cells. The dilutional effect, as well as the removal and destruction of red blood cells, depends primarily on the degree of splenomegaly.

White blood cells and platelets also are affected by sequestering, although not to the same degree as the red blood cell. Again, the size of the spleen is the determining factor in the number of cells sequestered.

EVALUATION AND TREATMENT. Treatment for hypersplenism is splenectomy; however, it is not always the treatment of choice. A splenectomy should be performed when its removal is considered necessary to alleviate the destructive effects on red blood cells. Clinical indicators should determine the need for splenectomy, not necessarily the specific condition. Splenectomy for splenic rupture no longer is considered mandatory in light of the possibility of overwhelming sepsis after removal. Repair and preservation of the ruptured spleen are now considered before the decision to remove the spleen. Splenectomy also may be performed as treatment for hairy cell leukemia, Felty syndrome, agnogenic myeloid metaplasia, thalassemia major, Gaucher disease, hemodialysis, splenomegaly, splenic venous thrombosis, and thrombotic thrombocytopenic purpura (TTP).

Individuals are able to lead normal lives after splenectomy, but hematologic abnormalities often exist after removal of the spleen. The red blood cells become thinner, broader, and wrinkled as a result of increases in surface area and membrane lipids. The white blood cell count increases dramatically 1 week after removal and then stabilizes to approximately 40% greater than normal. Platelet numbers also rise immediately after surgery and then equilibrate to above-normal levels for the duration of the individual's life. Increased platelet levels have been implicated in ischemic heart disease in males because of increased thrombocytosis and hypercoagulability.

A major postoperative complication following splenectomy is overwhelming post-splenectomy infection (OPSI). Unless treated in time, OPSI may rapidly progress to septic shock and possibly disseminated intravascular coagulation (DIC). Initial statistics indicate a death rate of 50% to 70%, with most deaths occurring within the first 48 hours after hospitalization. Prompt medical attention can reduce the death rate to 10%.

ALTERATIONS OF PLATELETS AND COAGULATION

Hemostasis is dependent on adequate numbers of platelets and levels of coagulation factors. Diminished or excessive levels may lead to defective hemostasis or spontaneous and unnecessary activation of clotting. (Hemostasis is described in Chapter 27.) Diminished hemostasis results in either internal or external hemorrhage. Diffuse hemorrhage into skin tissues that is visible through the skin causes a red-purple discoloration identified as a **purpura.** Purpuric disorders occur when there are not enough normal platelets to plug damaged vessels or prevent leakage from the many minute tears that occur daily in normal capillaries. Disorders of the clotting system tend to result in more serious internal bleeding than platelet defects and usually are caused by a deficiency of one or several clotting factors. Disorders that result in spontaneous clotting can result from genetic disorders of clotting system components or from acquired diseases that activate clotting. These disorders are known collectively as **thromboembolic disease.**

Disorders of Platelets

Quantitative or qualitative abnormalities of platelets can interrupt normal blood coagulation and prevent hemostasis.[46] The quantitative abnormalities are thrombocytopenia, a decrease in the number of circulating platelets, and thrombocythemia, an increase in the number of platelets. Qualitative disorders affect the structure or function of individual platelets and can coexist with the quantitative disorders. Qualitative disorders usually prevent platelet adherence and aggregation, preventing formation of a platelet plug.

Thrombocytopenia

Thrombocytopenia is defined as a platelet count less than 150,000 platelets/μL of blood, although most healthcare providers do not consider the decrease of significance unless the count falls to less than 100,000 platelets/μL of blood.[47] Hemorrhage resulting from minor trauma does not usually occur until the count falls below 50,000/μL. Spontaneous bleeding without apparent trauma can occur with counts between 10,000 and 15,000/μL, resulting in petechiae, ecchymoses, larger purpuric spots, or frank bleeding from mucous membranes. Severe spontaneous bleeding may result if the count is less than 10,000/μL and can be fatal if it occurs in the gastrointestinal tract, respiratory system, or CNS.

Before the diagnosis of thrombocytopenia is made, **pseudothrombocytopenia** must be ruled out. This phenomenon occurs in approximately 1 in 1000 to 1 in 10,000 laboratory samples and is an in vitro artifact that may occur when a blood sample is analyzed by an automated cell counter. Platelets in the sample may become nonspecifically agglutinated by immunoglobulins in the presence of ethylenediaminetetraacetic acid (EDTA), a preservative in banked blood. The agglutinated platelets are not counted, thus giving an apparent, but false, thrombocytopenia. Thrombocytopenia also may be falsely diagnosed because of a dilutional effect observed after massive transfusion of platelet-poor packed cells to treat a hemorrhage. This occurs when more than 10 units of blood have been transfused within a 24-hour period. The hemorrhage that necessitated the transfusion also accelerates the loss of platelets, which further contributes to the pseudothrombocytopenic state. Splenic sequestering of platelets secondary to hypersplenism (congestive) induces an apparent thrombocytopenia, as does hypothermia (less than 25° C [77° F]), which is reversed when temperatures return to normal, suggesting an increased platelet sequestration in response to chilling.

PATHOPHYSIOLOGY. Thrombocytopenia results from decreased platelet production, increased consumption, or both. The condition also may be congenital or acquired and primary or secondary to other acquired or congenital conditions. Thrombocytopenia secondary to congenital conditions occurs in a large number of different diseases, although each is relatively rare. These include thrombocytopenia with absence of radius (TAR) syndrome, Wiskott-Aldrich syndrome (see Chapter 9), various forms of *MYH9* gene mutation (e.g., May-Hegglin syndrome), X-linked thrombocytopenia, and many other examples.

Acquired thrombocytopenia is more common and may occur as a result of decreased platelet production secondary to viral infections (e.g., EBV, rubella, CMV, HIV), drugs (e.g., thiazides, estrogens, quinine-containing medications, chemotherapeutic agents, ethanol), nutritional deficiencies (vitamin B_{12} or folic acid in particular), chronic renal failure, bone marrow hypoplasia (e.g., aplastic anemia), radiation therapy, or bone marrow infiltration by cancer. Most common forms of thrombocytopenia are the result of increased platelet consumption. Examples include heparin-induced thrombocytopenia, idiopathic (immune) thrombocytopenic purpura, and thrombotic thrombocytopenic purpura.

Heparin-Induced Thrombocytopenia. Heparin is a common cause of drug-induced thrombocytopenia. Approximately 4% of individuals treated with unfractionated heparin develop **heparin-induced thrombocytopenia (HIT).** The incidence is lower (about 0.1%) with the use of low-molecular-weight heparin. HIT is an immune-mediated, adverse drug reaction caused by IgG antibodies against the heparin–platelet factor 4 complex leading to platelet activation through platelet FcγIIa receptors (Figure 29-19).[48] The release of additional platelet factor 4 from activated platelets and activation of thrombin lead to increased platelet consumption and a decrease in platelet counts beginning 5 to 10 days after administration of heparin.

CLINICAL MANIFESTATIONS. The hallmark of HIT is thrombocytopenia. A decrease of approximately 50% in the platelet count is seen in more than 95% of individuals. However, 30% or more of those with thrombocytopenia are also at risk for venous or arterial thrombosis.[48] Venous thrombosis is most common and results in deep venous thrombosis and pulmonary emboli. Arterial thromboses affect the large arteries of the lower extremities, causing acute limb ischemia. Arterial thrombosis also may lead to cerebrovascular accidents and myocardial infarctions. Other major arteries (renal, mesenteric, upper limb) also may be affected. Bleeding is uncommon in HIT, even with low platelet counts.

EVALUATION AND TREATMENT. Diagnosis is primarily based on clinical observations.[48] The individual presents with dropping platelet counts after 5 days or longer of heparin treatment. On average, platelet counts may reach 60,000/mm^3. Because most individuals develop this condition after surgery, and the onset of symptoms, including thrombosis, may be delayed until after release from the hospital, other possible causes of thrombocytopenia (e.g., infection, other drug reactions) must be considered.

Tests are available to measure antibodies against heparin–platelet factor 4.[49] The test sensitivity is extremely high (more than 90%), but the specificity is less because of false-positive reactions (e.g., persons receiving dialysis). HIT antibody titers may be measured, but the titers must be evaluated in the context of the clinical presentation. If HIT is not recognized and treated, intravascular aggregation of platelets causes rapid development of arterial and venous thrombosis. Although rare, heparin antibodies have caused anaphylactic shock.

Treatment is the withdrawal of heparin and use of alternative anticoagulants. A switch to low-molecular-weight heparin is not indicated, and warfarin should not be used until the symptoms of HIT have resolved because of an increased risk of initiating skin necrosis. The thrombocytopenia should progressively resolve. The chance of spontaneous blood clots can be diminished using thrombin inhibitors (e.g., lepirudin, argatroban).[48]

Immune Thrombocytopenic Purpura. The most common cause of thrombocytopenia secondary to increased platelet destruction is **immune thrombocytopenic purpura (ITP).** The incidence of ITP is estimated to be 5.8 to 6.6 per 100,000 in the general population. ITP was formerly known as *idiopathic thrombocytopenic purpura;* however, it is widely recognized

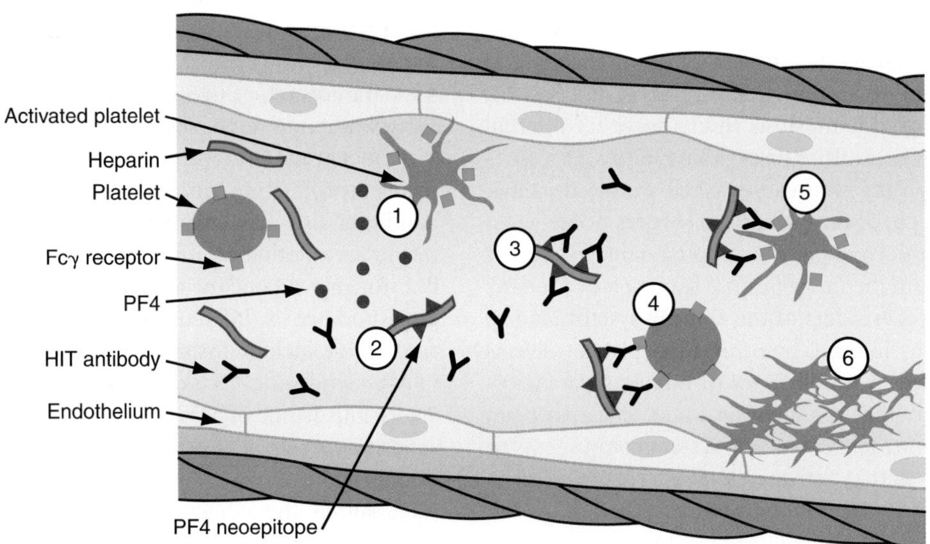

FIGURE 29-19 Pathogenesis of Heparin-Induced Thrombocytopenia (HIT). **(1)** Activated platelets release procoagulant proteins from α-granules, including platelet factor 4 *(PF4).* Administered heparin binds PF4 **(2),** which undergoes a conformational change and expresses a new antigen (neoepitope). Individuals with HIT produce an immunoglobulin G (IgG) antibody that specifically reacts **(3)** with multiple identical neoepitopes on the heparin-PF4 complex. The reaction forms heparin-PF4-IgG immune complexes. Platelets express FcγRIIa receptors (Fcγ receptor) that react **(4)** with the Fc portion of IgG in immune complexes. Cross-linking of Fc receptors **(5)** results in FcγRIIa-dependent platelet activation. The activated platelets mediate a series of events that lead to further activation of the coagulation cascade, resulting in thrombin generation. Further release of PF4 from newly activated platelets leads to a cycle of continuing platelet activation and **(6)** formation of a primary clot. The reaction can be enhanced by the release of platelet-derived microparticles that are rich in surface phosphatidylserine and increase activation of coagulation, and by the binding of heparin-PF4 complexes and HIT-IgG to the vascular endothelium (not shown.)

now as an immune process, hence the change from idiopathic to immune.[50] ITP may be acute or chronic. The acute form is frequently observed in children and typically lasts 1 to 2 months with a complete remission. In some instances it may last for up to 6 months, and some children (7% to 28%) may progress to the chronic condition. Acute ITP is usually secondary to infections (particularly viral) or other conditions that lead to large amounts of antigen in the blood, such as drug allergies or systemic lupus erythematosus (SLE) (see Chapter 9). Under these conditions the antigen usually forms immune complexes with circulating antibody, and it is thought that the immune complexes bind to Fc receptors on platelets, leading to their destruction in the spleen. The acute form of ITP usually resolves as the source of antigen is removed (e.g., the viral infection resolves).

Chronic ITP is associated with autoantibodies against platelet-specific antigens. This form is more commonly observed in adults, with highest prevalence in women between 20 and 40 years old, although it can develop at most any age. The chronic form tends to get progressively worse.

The autoantibodies are generally of the IgG class, although IgA and IgM antibodies also have been identified. They react against one or more of several platelet glycoproteins (e.g., GPIIb-IIIa, GPIb-IX, GPIa-IIa) (see Chapter 27).[51] The antibody-coated platelets are removed from the circulation by mononuclear phagocytes in the spleen through the Fc receptor.

CLINICAL MANIFESTATIONS. Initial manifestations are usually minor bleeding problems (development of petechiae and purpura) over the course of several days that progress to major hemorrhage from mucosal sites (epistaxis, hematuria, menorrhagia, bleeding gums). Rarely will an individual present with intracranial bleeding or internal bleeding at other sites.

During pregnancy, an individual with ITP may have a newborn that is also thrombocytopenic. In most individuals the antiplatelet antibody is an IgG that readily crosses the placenta (see Chapters 8 and 9). If the fetal platelets express the same antigen as the mother, the maternal antibody will coat the platelets, potentially resulting in thrombocytopenia in utero. A variant of neonatal thrombocytopenia (neonatal alloimmune thrombocytopenia) occurs when the mother does not have ITP, but makes IgG antibodies against an antigen inherited from the father and found on fetal platelets but not on maternal platelets.[52] Alloimmune neonatal thrombocytopenia occurs in 1 of 2000 pregnancies. The most common antibody in this condition is against the human platelet antigen-a (HPA-a) antigen on the GPIIIa protein. Neonatal thrombocytopenia, either secondary to maternal autoimmune thrombocytopenia or as alloimmune thrombocytopenia, may occur to various degrees. The most severe form results in fetal platelet counts below 20,000/mm^3 with a high associated risk of intracranial hemorrhage.

EVALUATION AND TREATMENT. Diagnosis of ITP is based on a history of bleeding and associated symptoms, such as weight loss, fever, and headache. Physical examination includes notations on the types of bleeding, location, and severity. Evidence of infections (bacterial, HIV, and other viral), medication history, family history, and evidence of thrombosis are also assessed. Other diagnostic tests include complete blood count (CBC) and peripheral blood smear. Unlike some other forms of thrombocytopenia, splenectomy is rarely observed. Testing for antiplatelet antibodies is usually not helpful. Although most cases of ITP are associated with elevated levels of IgG on platelets, other forms of thrombocytopenia also have a high incidence of platelet-associated antibodies; thus the specificity is low (50% to 65%).[53] In addition, some cases of ITP will not present with elevated platelet-associated antibodies; the sensitivity is 75% to 94%, so that a negative test does not completely rule out ITP.

The acute form of ITP usually resolves without major clinical consequences. As with most autoimmune diseases, the course of the chronic form is variable, with multiple remissions and exacerbations. For many individuals the platelet count may remain adequate enough to avoid clinically serious bleeding. However, the presence of spontaneous bleeding suggests more severe disease and requires immediate attention. Treatment is initiated when platelet counts are less than 30,000/μL or less than 50,000/μL with evidence of bleeding from mucous membranes or when the individual is at high risk to develop bleeding.

Treatment is palliative, not curative, focusing on prevention of platelet destruction. Initial therapy for ITP is infusion of glucocorticoids (e.g., prednisone), which suppresses the production of antiplatelet antibodies and prevents sequestering and further destruction of platelets. If platelet counts do not increase appropriately, other medications, such as prednisone, may be tried. Treatment with intravenous immunoglobulin (IVIG) is used to prevent major bleeding. The response rate is 80%, but the effects are transient, lasting only days or a few weeks. Anti-(Rh_o)D (RhoGAM), which is a preparation of antibody against the D antigen of the Rh blood group, has been used with limited success to treat individuals who are Rh-positive.

Newer treatments include romiplostim (trade name Nplate) and eltrombopag (trade name Promacta in the United States, Revolade in the European Union). Both drugs are thrombopoiesis–stimulating Fc-peptide fusion proteins (peptibody). Romiplostim is administered subcutaneously and eltrombopag is taken orally. These drugs increase platelet counts and decrease bleeding. Romiplostim is often used as a second-line treatment after IVIG or in individuals who experience relapse post-splenectomy.

If all other therapies are ineffective, splenectomy is considered to remove the primary site of platelet destruction.[54] The response rate (resolution of the thrombocytopenia) is 60% to 70%; however, the procedure is not without risk. Approximately 10% to 20% of individuals who undergo splenectomy suffer a relapse and require further treatment. It is thought that other reticuloendothelial organs, particularly the liver, can become major sites for platelet destruction. If splenectomy is unsuccessful and life-threatening thrombocytopenia persists, more aggressive immunosuppressive medications (e.g., azathioprine, cyclophosphamide) may be used. Because of potential major complications, these medications are reserved for individuals who are severely thrombocytopenic and refractive to other therapies.

Thrombotic Thrombocytopenic Purpura. **Thrombotic thrombocytopenic purpura (TTP)** is characterized by thrombotic microangiopathy in which platelets aggregate and cause occlusion of arterioles and capillaries within the microcirculation.[55] Aggregation may lead to increased platelet consumption and organ ischemia. TTP is relatively uncommon, occurring in about 5 per 1 million individuals per year. The incidence is increasing, which appears to be an actual increase in the number of affected individuals rather than a result of improved recognition. There are two forms of TTP: familial or acquired idiopathic. The familial form is the more rare and is usually chronic, relapsing, and seen in children. The child experiences predictable recurring episodes at approximately 3-week intervals and is responsive to treatment. Acquired TTP is more common, as well as more acute and severe. It occurs mostly in females in their thirties and is rarely observed in infants or older adults.

Platelet aggregation and microthrombi formation are found throughout the entire vascular system, causing damage to multiple organs. Organs most susceptible to damage are the kidney, brain, and heart. Other organs often affected are the pancreas, spleen, and adrenal glands. The thrombi are primarily composed of platelets with minimal fibrin and red cells, differentiating them from thrombi secondary to intravascular coagulation. Most cases of TTP are related to a dysfunction of the plasma metalloprotease ADAMTS13. This enzyme is responsible for digesting large precursor molecules of von Willebrand factor (vWF) produced by endothelial cells into smaller molecules. Defects in ADAMTS13 result in expression of large-molecular-weight vWF on the endothelial cell surface and the formation of large aggregates of platelets. The aggregates may break off and form occlusions in smaller vessels. Most individuals with TTP (about 80%) have less than 5% of normal plasma ADAMTS13 levels. TTP also is commonly associated with an IgG autoantibody against ADAMTS13 that is able to neutralize the enzyme's activity and accelerate its clearance from the plasma.

CLINICAL MANIFESTATIONS. The rare familial **chronic relapsing TTP** observed in children is usually recognized and successfully treated. The acquired **acute idiopathic TTP** is much more common and more severe.[55] Early diagnosis and treatment is important because the disease may be fatal within 90 days of onset. TTP is clinically related to and must be distinguished from other thrombotic microangiopathic conditions, including hemolytic uremic syndrome, malignant hypertension, preeclampsia, or the pregnancy-induced HELLP (**h**emolysis, **e**levated **l**iver enzymes, **l**ow **p**latelet count) syndrome. Hemolytic uremic syndrome (HUS) shares many of the clinical characteristics of TTP; however, HUS often follows a hemorrhagic, diarrheal illness.

EVALUATION AND TREATMENT. Acute idiopathic TTP is characterized by a "pathognomonic pentad" of symptoms. However, only 20% to 30% of people present with the classic pentad. These include extreme thrombocytopenia (less than 20,000 platelets/μL), intravascular hemolytic anemia, ischemic signs and symptoms most often involving the CNS (about 65% present with memory disturbances, behavioral irregularities, headaches, or coma), kidney failure (affecting about 65% of individuals), and fever (present in about 33%).[55] It is not mandatory that all five be present to begin treatment. A routine blood smear usually reveals fragmented red cells *(schizocytes)* produced by shear forces when red cells are in contact with the fibrin mesh in clots that form in the vessels. As a result of tissue injury, serum levels of lactate dehydrogenase (LDH) may be very high, and low-density lipoprotein (LDL) levels may be elevated. Tests for antibody on red cells are negative, excluding immune hemolytic anemia.

Untreated acute TTP has a death rate of 90%, which can be reduced to 10% to 20% with prompt treatment. Plasma exchange with fresh frozen plasma replenishes functional ADAMTS13 and is the treatment of choice, achieving a response rate of 70% to 85%. Additionally, steroids (glucocorticoids) are administered. In the absence of major organ damage, this approach may lead to complete recovery with no long-term complications. The anti-CD20 monocolonal antibody rituximab has shown some activity in people who are refractory to plasma exchange.[56] Relapses do occur at a rate of 13% to 36%, and recurrences have been reported, some as long as 9 years after the initial treatment. Individuals who do not respond to conventional treatment may be candidates for splenectomy; however, postoperative hemorrhage remains a dangerous complication. Immunosuppressive (azathioprine) therapy has been successful in some individuals.

Thrombocythemia

Thrombocythemia (also called **thrombocytosis**) is defined as a platelet count greater than 400,000/μL of blood.[57] Thrombocythemia may be primary or secondary (reactive) and is usually asymptomatic until the count exceeds 1 million/mm^3 of blood. Then intravascular clot formation (thrombosis), hemorrhage, or other abnormalities can occur.

PATHOPHYSIOLOGY. Secondary thrombocythemia may occur after splenectomy because platelets that normally would be stored in the spleen remain in circulating blood. The increase in the number of platelets may be gradual, with thrombocythemia not occurring for up to 3 weeks after splenectomy. Reactive thrombocythemia may occur during some inflammatory conditions, such as rheumatoid arthritis and cancers. In these conditions, excessive production of some cytokines (e.g., IL-6, IL-11) may induce increased production of thrombopoietin in the liver, resulting in increased megakaryocyte proliferation. Reactive thrombocythemia may also occur during a variety of physiologic conditions, such as after exercise. Because of the relatively self-resolving nature of secondary thrombocythemia, the remaining discussion will focus on the more severe primary form.

Essential (primary) thrombocythemia (ET) is a chronic myeloproliferative disorder characterized by excessive platelet production resulting from a defect in bone marrow megakaryocyte progenitor cells.[58] The overall incidence of ET is 0.8 per 100,000 in the United Kingdom, 2.53 in the United States, and 0.59 in Denmark. It is more common in middle-age individuals, with the majority of cases occurring between ages 50 and 60 years. There is no known gender preference. There also is a rare hereditary type of ET called *familial essential thrombocythemia (FET)* that is inherited in an autosomal dominant pattern.

The thrombocythemia is secondary to increased plasma thrombopoietin levels resulting from defects in the thrombopoietin receptor. The defective receptor cannot adequately bind and remove thrombopoietin from the blood, thus circulating levels remain high. Along with increased platelet levels, there may be a concomitant increase in red blood cells (RBCs), indicating a myeloproliferative disorder; however, the increase in red cells is not to the extent seen in polycythemia vera (see Chapter 28). The bone marrow of affected individuals with ET is characterized by hyperplasia of megakaryocytes. The platelets of affected individuals appear to have a normal survival time, compatible with a defect in production rather than an increase in platelet life span.

RBCs in ET tend to aggregate and contribute to the blockage of flow in the microvasculature and altered interactions between platelets and the vascular endothelium.[59] Increased adherence of erythrocytes to the endothelium appears to result from a mutation in an erythrocyte Janus kinase 2 (JAK2) that is responsible for phosphorylation of the erythrocyte receptor for endothelial laminin.[60,61] The frequency of JAK2 mutations in ET is about 30%. Increased platelet aggregation arises from several mutations that result in altered platelet membrane glycoproteins, particularly resulting in increased expression of GPIV, and increased secretion of thromboxane.

CLINICAL MANIFESTATIONS. Clinical manifestations vary significantly among individuals. Those with ET are at risk for large-vessel arterial or venous thrombosis, although the most common complication is **microvasculature thrombosis** leading to ischemia in the fingers, toes, or cerebrovascular regions.[59] The primary presenting symptoms of microvasculature thrombosis are erythromyalgia, headache, and paresthesias. **Erythromyalgia** is characterized by unilateral or bilateral warm, congested, red hands and feet with painful burning sensations, particularly in the forefoot sole and one or more toes. The lower extremities are affected more often, and only one side may be involved. The pain is initiated by standing, exercise, or warmth and relieved by elevation and cooling. In extreme situations, acrocyanosis and gangrene may result.

Arterial thrombosis is more common than venous thrombosis and may involve the coronary and renal arteries. The carotid, mesenteric, and subclavian arteries also may be affected. Myocardial ischemia and infarction have occurred without clear evidence of coronary artery disease. Deep venous thrombosis of the lower extremities and pulmonary embolism are the major sites for venous involvement. Intra-abdominal venous thrombosis of the portal and hepatic veins also is common. People older than 60 years of age or those with prior history of thrombotic events have as much as a 25% chance of developing a cerebral, cardiac, or peripheral arterial thrombus. Conversion to acute leukemia is found in less than 10%.[62]

Microvascular thrombosis in the CNS is usually associated with headache and dizziness, with paresthesias, transient ischemic attacks, strokes, visual disturbances, and seizures also being reported. Major thrombotic events, not directly related to the platelet count, occur in about 20% to 30% of individuals with ET. Prior history of thrombotic events, advanced age, and duration of thrombocytosis are predictors of future thrombotic complications. Individuals older than age 60 are at greatest risk.

Although thrombosis is the most common symptom, hemorrhage can also occur. Sites for bleeding include the gastrointestinal (GI) tract, skin, mucous membranes, urinary tract, gums, tooth sockets (after extraction), joints, eyes, and brain. GI bleeding may be mistaken for a duodenal ulcer. Hemorrhage is not severe, and generally occurs in the presence of very high platelet counts, and occasionally requires transfusion. Important is recognition that bleeding and clotting may exist simultaneously and individuals will not necessarily be "bleeders" or "clotters."

EVALUATION AND TREATMENT. Initial diagnosis is not difficult; as many as two thirds of affected individuals are diagnosed from a routine complete blood count (CBC). Secondary thrombocytosis may present as a moderate rise in the platelet count that resolves with treatment or resolution of the underlying condition. The World Health Organization (WHO) criteria for the diagnosis of ET require the following four conditions be met: (1) sustained platelet count of at least 450,000/μL; (2) bone marrow biopsy showing proliferation of enlarged mature megakaryocytes and no increase of granulocyte or erythocyte precursors; (3) failure to meet the criteria of polycythemia vera, myelofibrosis, CML, or other myelodysplastic syndrome; and (4) the presence of JAK2 617F or another clonal marker or evidence of reactive thrombocytosis.[63]

After diagnosis, these individuals may recall events related to thrombosis or hemorrhage. Manifestations of ET may be mistaken for CML; therefore, differentiation of the two is important because treatment varies significantly. Identification of the Philadelphia chromosome is recommended in all cases of ET.

Treatment of ET is directed toward preventing thrombosis or hemorrhage.[64] The importance of reducing the platelet count remains a significant treatment issue. Historically, treatment of ET relied on the use of alkylating agents (busulfan) or radiophosphorus (^{32}P) to suppress platelet production. Hydroxyurea, a nonalkylating myelosuppressive agent, has been the drug of choice to suppress platelet production: however, long-term use may cause progression to other myelodysplastic disorders, particularly AML or myelofibrosis.[64] Conversion to myelofibrosis occurs approximately 8% of the time and conversion to AML occurs approximately 3.5% of the time when treated with hydroxyurea as a single cytotoxic agent, but increases to 14% when more than one cytotoxic agent is used.

Interferon (IFN) also may be used and has a response rate of 80%. IFN may not be effective for everyone because it has many side effects and 20% of individuals may be intolerant. Anagrelide is now considered to be the drug of choice. Anagrelide specifically interferes with platelet maturation rather than production, thus not affecting erythropoiesis or leukopoiesis.

Aspirin also is used in the treatment of ET; however, its action is not to reduce the platelet count but to prevent adherence of platelets to each other and prevent thrombus formation. Early studies with aspirin found hemorrhage to be a major contraindication for its use; however, in lower doses (80 to 160 mg/daily) it effectively alleviates erythromyalgia and transient neurologic manifestations.

Prognosis and survival of individuals with ET have been somewhat difficult to establish. ET is not necessarily considered life threatening, but in those older than age 60 and who have a history of previous incidences of thrombosis, complications are more common and have a higher risk of mortality.

Alterations of Platelet Function

Qualitative alterations in platelet function occur with an increased bleeding time in the presence of a normal platelet count. Associated clinical manifestations include spontaneous petechiae and purpura, as well as bleeding from the GI tract, genitourinary tract, pulmonary mucosa, and gums. Congenital alterations in platelet function (thrombocytopathies) are quite rare and may be categorized into several types of disorders: (1) platelet–vessel wall adhesion, (2) platelet-platelet interactions, (3) platelet granules and secretion, (4) arachidonic acid pathways, and (5) membrane phospholipid regulation (coagulation protein–platelet interactions).[65]

Disorders of platelet–vascular wall adhesion result from aberrations of the platelet membrane glycoprotein GPIb-IX-V complex (Bernard-Soulier syndrome) or the collagen receptor GPVI, or deficiencies of vWF. The GPIb protein is the most commonly mutated in individuals with Bernard-Soulier syndrome. Lack of these proteins prevents platelets from adhering to collagen, resulting in impaired hemostasis and clinical hemorrhage.

Disorders of platelet-platelet interactions result in failure of platelets to aggregate in response to adenosine diphosphate (ADP), collagen, epinephrine, or thrombin because of a deficiency in the glycoprotein (αIIbβ3) that acts as a receptor for fibrinogen, vWF, and fibronectin (Glanzmann thrombasthenia). Lack of this protein results in a failure to build "fibrinogen bridges" between platelets (see Figure 27-20). Defects also can occur in platelet receptors for platelet activators. These include mutations in the receptors for thromboxane or ADP.

Disorders of platelet granules and secretion and arachidonic pathways are characterized by initial normal platelet aggregation with collagen or ADP; however, there is failure of subsequent processes, specifically secretion of prostaglandins and release of granules. Defective α-granule numbers or release (gray platelet syndrome) results from mutations in several aspects of granule function, including biosynthesis or loading of proteins normally found in these granules. Defects in dense granules include Hermansky-Pudlak syndrome, Chédiak-Higashi syndrome, and delta-storage pool disease. These usually result from mutations in proteins involved in formation of dense granules or their movement to the plasma membrane. Defects in the thromboxane pathway prevent the release of this mediator.

Externalization of plasma membrane phosphatidylserine (PS) is necessary for effective platelet function. In Scott syndrome, the enzyme responsible for PS efflux is defective; thus platelets are unable to support the activation of factor X and prothrombin. The reverse of Scott syndrome is Stormorken syndrome, in which platelets constitutively externalize PS.

Acquired disorders of platelet function are more common than the congenital disorders and may be categorized into three principal causes: (1) drug effects, (2) systemic inflammatory conditions, and (3) hematologic conditions.

Multiple drugs are known to affect platelet function in several ways: inhibition of platelet membrane receptors, inhibition of prostaglandin pathways, and inhibition of phosphodiesterase activity. Aspirin is the most commonly used drug that affects platelets and the only drug specifically used for its platelet effects. It irreversibly inhibits cyclooxygenase function for several days after administration. Nonsteroidal anti-inflammatory drugs also affect cyclooxygenase, although in a reversible fashion.

Systemic disorders that affect platelet function are chronic renal disease, liver disease, cardiopulmonary bypass surgery, severe deficiencies of iron or folate, and the presence of antiplatelet antibodies associated with autoimmune disorders. Hematologic disorders that cause platelet dysfunction are chronic myeloproliferative disorders, multiple myeloma, leukemias, myelodysplastic syndromes, and dysproteinemias.

Disorders of Coagulation

Disorders of coagulation usually are caused by defects or deficiencies of one or more of the clotting factors. (Normal function of the clotting factors is described in Chapter 27.) Qualitative or quantitative abnormalities of clotting factors interfere with or prevent the enzymatic reactions that transform circulating clotting proteins into a stable fibrin clot (see Figure 27-22).

Some clotting factor defects are inherited and usually involve a single factor, such as hemophilias and von Willebrand disease, caused by deficiencies of specific clotting factors (see Chapter 30). Other coagulation defects are acquired and tend to result from deficient synthesis of clotting factors by the liver. Causes include liver disease and dietary deficiency of vitamin K.

Other coagulation disorders are attributed to pathologic conditions that trigger coagulation inappropriately. For example, any cardiovascular abnormality that alters normal blood flow by acceleration, deceleration, or obstruction can result in spontaneous coagulation within the vessels. Coagulation is also stimulated by the presence of tissue factor, which is released by damaged or dead tissues. **Vasculitis,** or inflammation of the blood vessels, as well as vessel damage, activates platelets, which in turn activates the coagulation cascade. In extensive or prolonged vasculitis, blood clot formation can suppress mechanisms that normally control clot formation and breakdown, leading to clogging of the vessels. In each of these acquired conditions, normal hemostatic function proves detrimental to the body by consuming coagulation factors excessively or by overwhelming the normal control of clot formation and breakdown (fibrinolysis).

Impaired Hemostasis

Impaired hemostasis, or the inability to promote coagulation and the development of a stable fibrin clot, is commonly associated with liver disorders, either from the lack of vitamin K or from specific diseases of the liver.

Vitamin K Deficiency. Vitamin K, a fat-soluble vitamin, is necessary for synthesis and regulation of prothrombin, procoagulant factors (VII, IX, X), and anticoagulant regulators (proteins C and S) within the liver.[66] The primary dietary source of vitamin K is green, leafy vegetables. Vitamin K also is synthesized by intestinal flora, but its contribution to the overall supply of vitamin K is uncertain. The most common cause of vitamin K deficiency is the use of parenteral nutrition in combination with broad-spectrum antibiotics that destroy normal gut flora. Rarely is a deficiency caused by lack of dietary intake; however, bulimia can suppress vitamin K–dependent activity. Clinical manifestations of vitamin K deficiency are caused by a reduction of vitamin K–dependent proteins. The severity of manifestations is related to the degree of deficiency and ranges from laboratory abnormalities to significant hemorrhage.

Parenteral administration of vitamin K is the treatment of choice and usually results in correction of the deficiency. Improvement of clotting tests is usually noted within 8 to 12 hours. Fresh frozen plasma may be administered but usually is reserved for individuals with life-threatening hemorrhages or who require emergency surgery.

Liver Disease. Individuals who have liver disease (e.g., acute or chronic hepatocellular diseases, cirrhosis, vitamin K deficiency) or have undergone major liver surgery present with a broad range of hemostasis derangements that may be characterized by defects in the clotting or fibrinolytic systems or platelet function.[66] The hepatic parenchymal cells produce most of the factors involved in hemostasis. Thus damage to the liver frequently results in diminished production of factors involved in clotting, usually in proportion to the degree of hepatic parenchymal cell damage. For instance, factor VII is most sensitive to liver damage because of its rapid turnover. Factor IX levels are less affected and do not decline until liver destruction is well advanced. The liver is also a major site for production of plasminogen and α_2-antiplasmin of the fibrinolytic system, as well as thrombopoietin and the metalloprotease ADAMTS13. Diminished levels of thrombopoietin may lead to thrombocytopenia from decreased platelet production. Decreased production of ADAMTS13 results in increased levels of large precursor molecules of vWF, which leads to the formation of large aggregates of platelets.

In conditions of severe liver disease (e.g., cirrhosis) circulating levels of most clotting factors are significantly depressed. Concurrently, production of clotting system regulators (e.g., antithrombin, protein C, protein S) and of fibrinogen is diminished. The fibrinolytic system is commonly active because of decreased levels of plasmin inhibitor and unaffected levels of fibrinolytic activators (e.g., tissue plasminogen activator [tPA], urokinase-like plasminogen activator [uPA]). The affected individuals also are thrombocytopenic because of diminished thrombopoietin and ADAMTS13, as well as increased platelet sequestration in the spleen, which is frequently enlarged in cirrhosis and is associated with portal hypertension. Thus the individuals with cirrhosis may appear to have a condition similar to disseminated intravascular coagulation (DIC) (see next section).

Treatment of hemostatic alterations in liver disease must be comprehensive to cover all aspects related to platelet, clotting, and fibrinolytic dysfunctions. Fresh frozen plasma administration is the treatment of choice, but not all individuals tolerate the volume needed to adequately replace all deficient factors. Alternative modalities include the addition of exchange transfusions and platelet concentration to plasma administration.

Consumptive Thrombohemorrhagic Disorders

Consumptive thrombohemorrhagic disorders are a heterogeneous group of conditions that demonstrate the entire range of hemorrhagic and thrombotic pathologic conditions. Symptoms range from subtle to devastating and generally are considered to be intermediary disease processes that complicate many primary disease states. These disorders also are characterized by confusion and controversy regarding diagnosis, treatment, and management. No single definition can cover all possible varieties of these disorders; however, DIC is the most common term used in the clinical setting to describe a pathologic condition associated with hemorrhage and thrombosis.

Disseminated Intravascular Coagulation. **Disseminated intravascular coagulation** (DIC) is an acquired clinical syndrome characterized by widespread activation of coagulation, resulting in the formation of fibrin clots in medium and small vessels throughout the body. Disseminated clotting may lead to blockage of blood flow to organs, resulting in multiple organ failure. The magnitude of clotting may result in consumption of platelets and clotting factors, leading to severe bleeding. The Subcommittee on DIC of the International Society on Thrombosis and Hemostasis defined DIC as "an acquired syndrome characterized by the intravascular activation of coagulation with loss of localization arising from different causes. It can originate from and cause damage to the microvasculature, which if sufficiently severe, can produce organ dysfunction."[67,68]

The clinical course of DIC largely is determined by the intensity of the stimulus, host response, and comorbidities and ranges from an acute, severe, life-threatening process that is characterized by massive hemorrhage and thrombosis to a chronic low-grade condition. The chronic condition is characterized by subacute hemorrhage and diffuse microcirculatory thrombosis. DIC may be localized to one specific organ or generalized, involving multiple organs.

Because of the complexity and wide variations in manifestations of DIC, diagnosis has been confusing and difficult. Minimally acceptable diagnostic criteria have been established and include a systemic thrombohemorrhagic disorder with laboratory evidence of (1) clotting activation, (2) fibrinolytic activation, (3) coagulation inhibitor consumption, and (4) biochemical evidence of end-organ damage or failure.

DIC is secondary to a wide variety of well-defined clinical conditions, specifically those capable of activating the clotting cascade (Box 29-6). These include: (1) arterial hypotension, frequently accompanying shock; (2) hypoxemia; (3) acidemia; and (4) stasis of capillary blood flow.

Sepsis is the most common condition associated with DIC. Gram-negative microorganisms, as well as some gram-positive microorganisms, fungi, protozoa (malaria), and viruses (influenza, herpes), are capable of precipitating DIC by causing damage to the vascular endothelium. Gram-negative endotoxins are the primary cause of endothelial damage; DIC may occur in up

BOX 29-6 MAJOR ETIOLOGIES IDENTIFIED AS ANTECEDENTS TO THE INITIATION AND DEVELOPMENT OF DISSEMINATED INTRAVASCULAR COAGULATION (DIC)

- Malignancy: acute leukemias, metastatic solid malignancies
- Infections: bacterial (gram-negative endotoxin, gram-positive mucopolysaccharides), viral (hepatitis, varicella, cytomegalovirus), fungal, parasitic
- Pregnancy complications: eclampsia/preeclampsia, placental abruption, amniotic fluid embolism
- Severe trauma: head injury, burns, crush injuries, tissue necrosis
- Liver disease: obstructive jaundice, acute liver failure
- Intravascular hemolysis: transfusion reactions, drug-induced hemolysis
- Medical devices: aortic balloon, prosthetic devices
- Hypoxia and low blood flow states: arterial hypotension secondary to shock, cardiopulmonary arrest

Data from Bick RL et al: *Hematology: clinical and laboratory practice,* St Louis, 1993, Mosby.

to 50% of individuals with gram-negative sepsis. DIC occurs in approximately 10% to 20% of individuals with metastatic cancer or acute leukemia. Direct tissue damage (e.g., ischemia and necrosis, surgical manipulation, crushing injury) also results in release of tissue factor (TF) by the endothelium. Severe trauma, especially to the brain, can induce DIC. DIC occurs in about two thirds of individuals with a systemic inflammatory response to trauma. Some complications of pregnancy also are associated with DIC; incidences range from 50% for women with placental abruptions to less than 10% for women with severe preeclampsia. Other causes of DIC have been identified, most notably blood transfusion. Transfused blood dilutes the clotting factors, as well as circulating naturally occurring antithrombins. In hemolytic transfusion reactions, the endothelium is damaged by complement-mediated reactions.

PATHOPHYSIOLOGY. The coagulation system is designed to function at local areas of vascular damage, resulting in cessation of bleeding and activation of repair to the vessels. DIC results from abnormally widespread and ongoing activation of clotting (Figure 29-20). A variety of conditions are associated with DIC (see Box 29-6), primarily by activating the extrinsic clotting cascade. The common pathway for DIC appears to be excessive and widespread exposure of TF. This may occur by several mechanisms. Widespread damage to the vascular endothelium results in exposure of subendothelial TF. Several types of cells, either after stimulation by cytokines or constitutively, express TF on their surfaces. Endothelial cells and monocytes do not normally express surface TF unless stimulated by inflammatory cytokines (particularly IL-6 and TNF-α).[69] Many tumors express surface TF or produce cytokines that stimulate TF expression by endothelium or monocytes, or both.[70] These cytokines are abundantly produced during many of the conditions listed in Box 29-6. Endotoxin, in particular, triggers the release of multiple cytokines that play a significant role in the development and maintenance of DIC. Proinflammatory cytokines (TNF-α, interleukins [IL-1, IL-6, IL-8], and platelet activating factor [PAF]) are responsible for the clinical signs and symptoms associated with sepsis. They also contribute to the development of DIC by activating endothelial cells, causing release of TF and vWF, increasing plasminogen activator inhibitor-1 (PAI-1) synthesis and tissue factor activity, and decreasing thrombomodulin expression, thereby promoting development of thrombi. TF also may be released directly into the bloodstream from circulating white blood cells (monocyte/endotoxin interaction).

TF binds clotting factor VII, which leads to conversion of prothrombin to thrombin and formation of fibrin clots (see Figure 27-22). This pathway appears to be the primary route by which DIC is initiated; inhibition of TF or factor VIIa completely prevents the generation of thrombi by gram-negative bacterial endotoxin in animal models of DIC.

Not only is the clotting system extensively activated in DIC, but also the predominant natural anticoagulants (tissue factor inhibitor, antithrombin III [AT III], protein C) are greatly diminished (see Figure 27-18). During DIC the activation of clotting is prolonged by the increased rate of consumption because of persistent thrombin production, as well as decreased synthesis, of these inhibitors and protein S and by cytokine-mediated decreased expression of thrombomodulin on the endothelial cell surface. Hepatic dysfunction in sepsis results in decreased antithrombin synthesis and extravascular leakage of this protease inhibitor because of capillary leakage. Additionally, antithrombin is degraded by elastase released by activated neutrophils, and clotting is initiated concurrently with loss of regulation of the extent of thrombosis; thus the amount of thrombin produced during DIC exceeds the ability of the body's naturally occurring anticoagulants to regulate it.

The rate of fibrinolysis is also diminished in DIC. The primary component of fibrinolysis is plasmin, which exists in the circulation as an inactive precursor, plasminogen (see Figure 27-25). Plasminogen is activated to plasmin that digests fibrin clots, thus controlling the extent of fibrin deposition in the vessels. During DIC the activity of plasmin is diminished by increased production of its natural inhibitor, PAI-1. Although some fibrinolytic activity remains, the level is inadequate to control the systemic deposition of fibrin. The slow breakdown of fibrin by plasmin produces fibrin degradation products (FDPs) that are released into the blood. These are potent anticoagulants that are normally removed from blood by fibronectin and macrophages. FDPs, along with thrombin, induce further cytokine release from monocytes, contributing to endothelial damage and TF release. During DIC the presence of fibrin degradation products is prolonged, probably because of diminished production of fibronectin. Fibronectin is a glycoprotein with adhesive properties that mediate removal of particulate matter (e.g., fibrin clumps). Low levels of fibronectin suggest a poor prognosis.

Although thrombosis is generalized and widespread, individuals with DIC are paradoxically at risk for hemorrhage. Hemorrhage is secondary to the abnormally high consumption of clotting factors and platelets, as well as the anticoagulant properties of FDPs, which interfere with polymerization of fibrin monomers. Both thrombin and FDPs have a high affinity for platelets and cause platelet activation and aggregation—an event that occurs early in the development of DIC—which facilitates

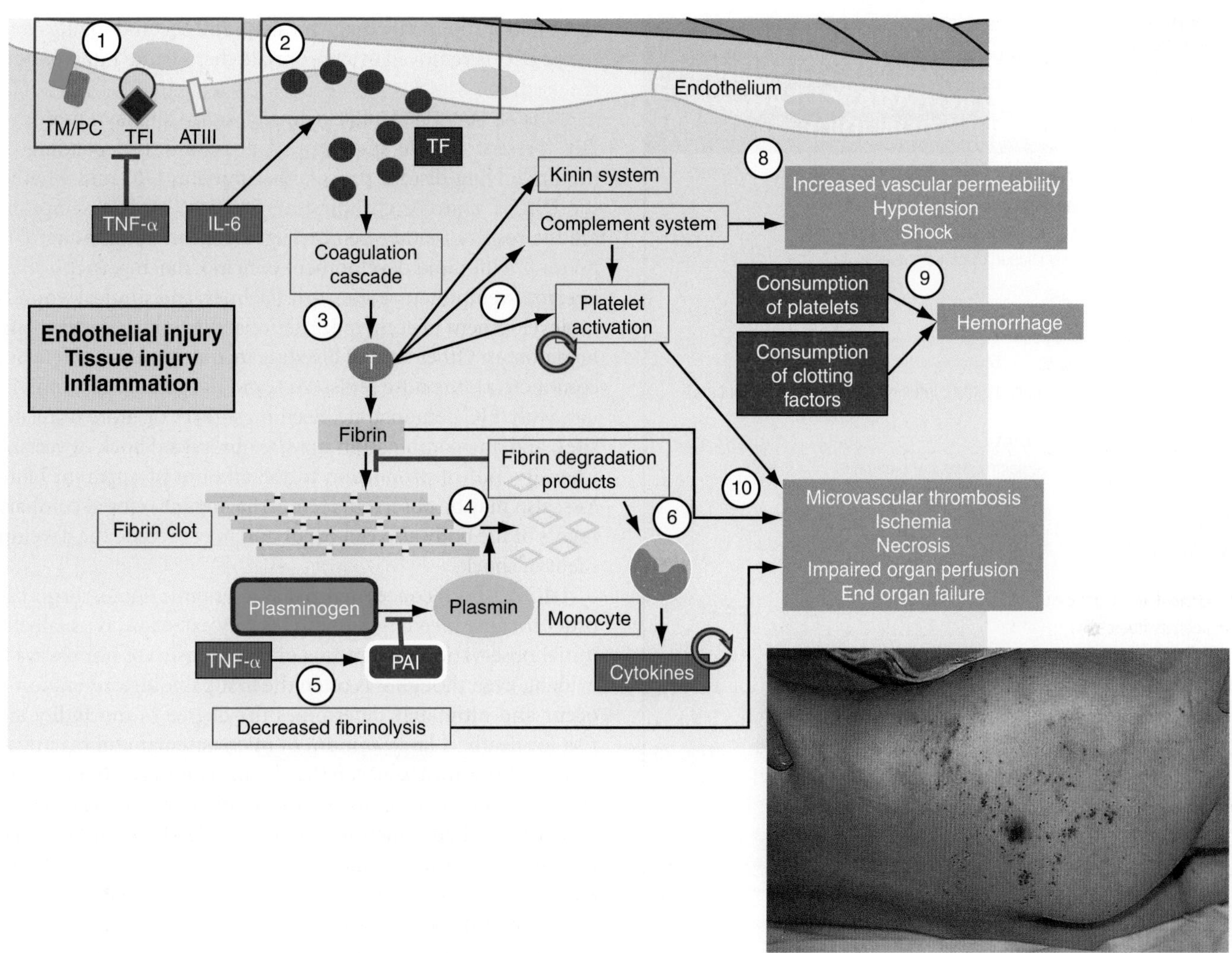

FIGURE 29-20 Pathophysiology of Disseminated Intravascular Coagulation (DIC). DIC is initiated by a variety of factors (endothelial injury, tissue injury, inflammation, and others), most of which either directly or indirectly result in release of large amounts of tissue factor. Many cytokines create a procoagulant environment by concurrently **(1)** suppressing normal control of homeostasis and **(2)** inducing tissue factor release by endothelium or monocytes. Tissue factor initiates the coagulation cascade **(3)** leading to the activation of thrombin, production of fibrin, and polymerization into a fibrin clot. Fibrinolysis normally digests clots **(4)** through the activity of plasmin, resulting in the production of various fibrin degradation products. However, during DIC, factors, such as TNF-α, induce **(5)** inhibitors of plasmin generation, thus leading to diminished fibrinolysis. Fibrin split products possess several biologic activities that affect DIC, including **(6)** the induction of further cytokine release by monocytes. Enzymatically active products of the coagulation cascade, including thrombin, activate **(7)** other inflammatory systems, including platelets and the kinin and complement systems. Activation of platelets and monocytes continues the procoagulant cycle (indicated by circular arrows) by inducing additional tissue factor and cytokines. Mediators produced from the kinin and complement system **(8)** affect vascular endothelium, leading to increased vascular permeability that contributes to hypotension and potential shock. The uncontrolled consumption of platelets and clotting factors **(9)** compromises the normal hemostatic mechanisms, resulting in potential systemic hemorrhages. Excess activation of the coagulation cascade and platelets, with decreased fibrinolysis, leads to systemic microvascular thrombosis **(10)** and blockage of the vessels with progressive ischemia. Uncontrolled DIC will eventually lead to multiple end-organ failure. For further details of these mechanisms see Chapters 7 and 27. *AT III,* Antithrombin III; *IL-6,* interleukin-6; *PAI,* plasminogen activator inhibitor; *T,* thrombin; *TF,* tissue factor; *TFI,* tissue factor inhibitor; *TM/PC,* thrombomodulin/protein C complex; *TNF-α,* tumor necrosis factor-alpha. The inset is an example of DIC resulting from staphylococcal septicemia. Note the characteristic skin hemorrhage ranging from small purpuric lesions to larger ecchymoses.

microcirculatory coagulation and obstruction in the initial phase. However, platelet consumption exceeds production, resulting in a thrombocytopenia that increases bleeding (Box 29-7).

Activation of clotting also leads to activation of other inflammatory pathways, including the kallikrein-kinin and complement systems (see Chapter 7). Factor XIIa, generated in DIC, converts prekallikrein to kallikrein, ultimately resulting in conversion to circulating kinins. Activation of these systems contributes to increased vascular permeability, hypotension, and shock. Activated complement components also induce platelet destruction, further contributing initially to the thrombosis and later to the thrombocytopenia.

BOX 29-7 CLINICAL MANIFESTATIONS ASSOCIATED WITH DISSEMINATED INTRAVASCULAR COAGULATION (DIC)

Integumentary System
Widespread hemorrhage and vascular lesions
Oozing from puncture sites, incisions, mucous membranes
Acrocyanosis (irregularly shaped cyanotic patches)
Gangrene

Central Nervous System
Subarachnoid hemorrhage
Altered state of consciousness (slight confusion to convulsions and coma)

Gastrointestinal System
Occult bleeding to massive gastrointestinal bleeding
Abdominal distention
Malaise
Weakness

Pulmonary System
Pulmonary infarctions
ARDS
Cyanosis
Tachypnea
Hypoxemia

Renal System
Hematuria
Oliguria
Renal failure

Modified from Bailes BK: *AORN J* 55(2):517–529, 1992.
ARDS, Acute respiratory distress syndrome.

The deposition of fibrin clots in the circulation interferes with blood flow, causing widespread organ hypoperfusion.

This condition may lead to ischemia, infarction, and necrosis, further potentiating and complicating the existing DIC process by causing further release of TF and eventually organ failure.

In addition to initiation of clotting by TF, DIC may be precipitated by direct proteolytic activation of factor X. This has been described as "thrombin mimicry" and is the result of activated factor X directly converting fibrinogen to fibrin. The proteases that activate factor X may come from snake venom, some tumor cells, or the pancreas and liver, where they are released during episodes of pancreatitis and various stages of liver disease. Direct proteolytic activity appears to be independent of any type of damage to the endothelium or tissue.

Vascular obstruction results from circulatory deposition of thrombin and clot formation that impedes blood flow, causing widespread organ hypoperfusion that can lead to tissue ischemia, infarction, and necrosis. The resulting tissue damage further potentiates and complicates the existing DIC process. Because organ perfusion is drastically impaired, manifestations of multisystem organ dysfunction and failure ultimately result. Multisystem organ dysfunction and failure are discussed in Chapter 48. Whatever initiates the process of DIC, the cycle of thrombosis and hemorrhage persists until the underlying cause of the DIC is removed or appropriate therapeutic interventions are used.

CLINICAL MANIFESTATIONS. Clinical signs and symptoms of DIC present a wide spectrum of possibilities, depending on the underlying disease process that initiates DIC and whether the DIC is acute or chronic (see Box 29-7). Most symptoms are the result of either hemorrhage or thrombosis. Acute DIC presents with rapid development of hemorrhaging, such as oozing from venipuncture sites, arterial lines, and surgical wounds, or development of ecchymotic lesions (purpura, petechiae) and hematomas. Other sites of bleeding include the eyes (sclera and conjunctiva), the nose (epistaxis), and the gums. Most individuals with DIC demonstrate bleeding at three or more unrelated sites, and any combination may be observed. Shock of variable intensity, out of proportion to the amount of apparent blood loss, also may be observed. Hemorrhaging into closed compartments of the body also can occur and may precede the development of shock.

DIC has been conceptualized as a systemic hemorrhagic disorder because bleeding, sometimes very extensive, is usually the initial observation. Symptoms of thrombosis are not always as evident, even though it is often the first pathologic alteration to occur and ultimately determines the degree of morbidity and risk for death. A large amount of microvascular and macrovascular occlusion may occur that is not clinically obvious. Several organ systems are susceptible to microvascular thrombosis that affects their function; these include the cardiovascular, pulmonary, central nervous, renal, and hepatic systems. Quick and accurate clinical diagnosis is critical to preventing further progression of DIC that may lead to multisystem organ dysfunction or failure. Indicators of multisystem failure include changes in level of consciousness, behavior, and mentation; confusion; seizure activity; oliguria; hematuria; hypoxia; hypotension; hemoptysis; chest pain; and tachycardia. Symmetric cyanosis of the fingers and toes ("blue finger/toe syndrome") and, in some instances, of the nose and breasts may be present. Symmetric parts are often affected and are indicative of microvascular thrombosis. This may progress to infarction and gangrene, requiring amputation. Jaundice also may be present and is believed to result from red blood cell destruction rather than hepatic dysfunction.

Individuals with chronic or low-grade DIC do not present with overt manifestations of hemorrhaging and thrombosis but instead have subacute bleeding and diffuse thrombosis and are described as having a **compensated DIC,** or non-overt DIC. The major characteristic of this state is an increased turnover and decreased survival time of the components of hemostasis: platelets and clotting factors. On occasion diffuse or localized thrombosis develops, but this is infrequent.

EVALUATION AND TREATMENT. No single laboratory test can be used to effectively diagnosis DIC. Diagnosis is based primarily on clinical symptoms and confirmed by a combination of laboratory tests. The individual must present with a clinical condition that is known to be associated with DIC. The most commonly used combination of laboratory tests usually confirms thrombocytopenia or a rapidly decreasing platelet count

BOX 29-8 LABORATORY DIAGNOSTIC CRITERIA FOR DISSEMINATED INTRAVASCULAR COAGULATION (DIC)*

Group I Tests (Indicators of Procoagulant Activation)

1. Elevated prothrombin fragment 1+2
2. Elevated fibrinopeptide A
3. Elevated fibrinopeptide B
4. Elevated thrombin-antithrombin (TAT) complex
5. Elevated D-dimer

Group II Tests (Indicators of Fibrinolytic Activity)

1. Elevated D-dimer
2. Elevated fibrin degradation products (FDPs)
3. Elevated plasmin
4. Elevated plasmin-antiplasmin (PAP) complex

Group III Tests (Indicators of Inhibitor Consumption)

1. Decreased antithrombin III
2. Decreased α_2-antiplasmin
3. Decreased heparin cofactor II
4. Decreased protein C or S
5. Elevated TAT complex
6. Elevated PAP complex

Group IV Tests (Indicators of End-Organ Damage/Failure)

1. Elevated lactic dehydrogenase (LDH)
2. Elevated creatinine
3. Decreased pH
4. Decreased Pa_{O_2}

Data from Bick RL: *Semin Thromb Hemost* 24(1):3, 1998.

*Satisfactory criteria for laboratory diagnosis of DIC require one abnormality in each of groups I through III and at least two abnormalities in group IV.

on repeated testing, prolongation of clotting times, the presence of fibrin degradation products, and decreased levels of coagulation inhibitors. The relationships among these criteria are summarized in Box 29-8. Platelet counts less than 100,000/mm^3 or a progressive decrease in platelet counts is very sensitive for DIC, although not greatly specific. These changes usually indicate consumption of platelets.

The standard coagulation tests (e.g., prothrombin time [PT], activated partial thromboplastin time [aPTT]) also have a high degree of sensitivity, but they are not highly specific for DIC. As a result of consumption of circulating clotting factors, these tests are usually abnormal, ranging from shortened to prolonged times. However, conditions other than DIC may prolong clotting times. Assays of specific clotting factors do not contribute meaningful diagnostic information.

Detection of various fibrin degradation products is more specific for DIC; of these tests the detection of D-dimers is the most widely used, reliable, and specific test.[71] A **D-dimer** is a molecule produced by plasmin degradation of cross-linked fibrin in clots. D-dimers in the blood can be quantified using enzyme-linked immunosorbent assay (ELISA) tests that include commercially available and highly specific monoclonal antibody against the D-dimer. Agglutination tests for other fibrin degradation products are available. Levels of fibrin degradation products, in general, are elevated in the plasma in 95% to 100% of cases; however, they are less specific and only document the presence of plasmin and its action of fibrin, whereas detection of D-dimers measures a specific DIC-related product.

ELISAs for markers of thrombin activity are sometimes used. Normal conversion of prothrombin to thrombin produces an inactive prothrombin fragment 1.2 (PF1+2).[71] This fragment is released from the prothrombin molecule, generating an intermediate factor, prethrombin 2. Once generated, prethrombin 2 can be split to produce thrombin that can then proteolyze fibrinogen, liberating fibrinopeptide A (FPA), or can combine with its major antagonist, antithrombin, and form a stable inactive enzyme-inhibitor complex, the thrombin-antithrombin (TAT) complex. Assays of these factors (PF1+2, FPA, TAT) are now generally available to quantify their blood levels, providing evidence of excessive factor Xa (PF1+2) and thrombin (FPA) generation.

Levels of coagulation inhibitors (e.g., AT III, protein C) can be measured by assays that rely on function or by ELISAs that quantify the amount of the specific inhibitor. AT III levels can provide key information for diagnosing and monitoring therapy of DIC. Initial levels of functional AT III are low in DIC because thrombin is irreversibly complexed with activated clotting factors and AT III.

Treatment of DIC is directed toward (1) eliminating the underlying pathology, (2) controlling ongoing thrombosis, and (3) maintaining organ function. Elimination of the underlying pathology is the initial intervention in the treatment phase in order to eliminate the trigger for activation of clotting. Once the stimulus is gone, production of coagulation factors in the liver leads to restoration of normal plasma levels within 24 to 48 hours.

Control of thrombosis is more difficult to attain. Heparin has been used for this; however, its use is controversial because its mechanism of action is binding to and activating AT III, which is deficient in many types of DIC. Currently heparin is indicated only in certain situations related to DIC. For instance, heparin seems to be effective in DIC caused by a retained dead fetus or associated with acute promyelocytic leukemia. Organ function is compromised by microthrombi, and there is a risk of losing an extremity because of vascular occlusion; thus heparin is also indicated in these conditions. Heparin's usefulness, however, for DIC that is precipitated by septic shock has not been established and so is contraindicated in that instance; heparin is also contraindicated when there is evidence of postoperative bleeding, peptic ulcer, or CNS bleeding.

Replacement therapy (interventions based on restoring the balance of coagulation factors, deficient coagulation factors, platelets, and other coagulation elements) is gaining recognition as an effective treatment modality. Components used in replacement therapy include platelets, fresh frozen plasma, and cryoprecipitate. Platelets are given for thrombocytopenia, plasma provides volume and replaces clotting factors, and cryoprecipitate replaces fibrinogen. Their use is not without controversy, however, because of the possible risk of adding components that will increase the rate of thrombosis. Clinical

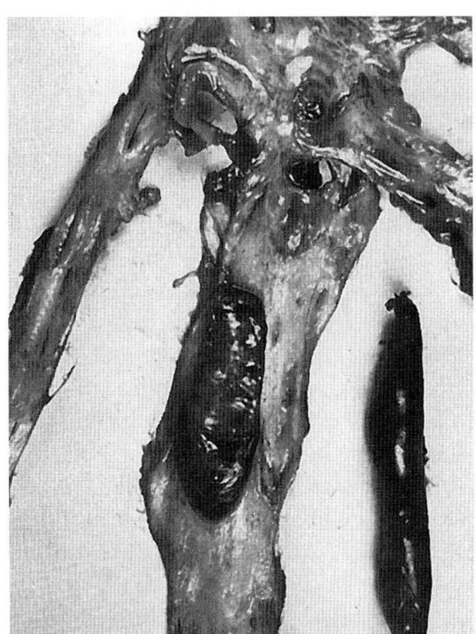

FIGURE 29-21 **Thrombus.** Thrombus arising in valve pocket at upper end of superficial femoral vein. Postmortem clot on the right is shown for comparison. (From McLachlin J, Paterson JC: *Surg Gynecol Obstet* 93:1, 1951.)

judgment is the key factor in determining whether replacement is to be used as a treatment modality.

Several clinical trials are evaluating replacement of anticoagulants (i.e., AT III, protein C). Replacement of AT III appears to be effective in DIC caused by sepsis. Low levels of AT III correlate with sepsis-initiated DIC, which makes a case for its use. AT III is an α_2-globulin that inactivates thrombin, factor Xa, factor IXa, and other activated components of the clotting system. Heparin augments AT III, but the increased benefit of a combination of heparin with AT III replacement has not been established. Antifibrinolytic drugs also are used in treatment but are limited to instances of life-threatening bleeding that have not been controlled by blood component replacement therapy.

Maintenance of organ function is achieved by fluid replacement to sustain adequate circulating blood volume and to maintain optimal tissue and organ perfusion. Fluids may be required to restore blood pressure, cardiac output, and urine output to normal parameters.

Thromboembolic Disease

Certain conditions within the blood vessels predispose an individual to develop clots spontaneously.[72] A stationary clot attached to the vessel wall is called a **thrombus** (Figure 29-21). A thrombus is composed of fibrin and blood cells and can develop in either the arterial or the venous system. **Arterial thrombi** form under conditions of high blood flow and are composed mostly of platelet aggregates held together by fibrin strands. **Venous thrombi** form in conditions of low flow and are composed mostly of red cells with larger amounts of fibrin and few platelets.

A thrombus may eventually grow large enough to reduce or obstruct blood flow to tissues or organs, such as the heart, brain, or lungs, depriving them of essential nutrients critical to survival. A thrombus also has the potential of detaching from the vessel wall and circulating within the bloodstream (referred to as an **embolus**). The embolus may become lodged in smaller blood vessels, blocking blood flow into the local tissue or organ and leading to ischemia. Whether episodes of thromboembolism are life threatening depends on the site of vessel occlusion.

Therapy consists of removal or lysis of the clot and supportive measures. Anticoagulant therapy is effective in treating or preventing venous thrombosis; it is not as useful in treating or preventing arterial thrombosis. Parenteral heparin is the major anticoagulant used to treat thromboembolism. Oral coumarin drugs also are widely used, particularly for individuals not hospitalized. More aggressive therapy may be indicated for such conditions as pulmonary embolism, coronary thrombosis, or thrombophlebitis. Streptokinase and urokinase activate the fibrinolytic system and are administered to accelerate the lysis of known thrombi. Thrombolytic therapy has limited uses and is prescribed with a high degree of caution because it can cause hemorrhagic complications.

The risk for developing spontaneous thrombi is related to several factors, referred to as the **Virchow triad:** (1) injury to the blood vessel endothelium, (2) abnormalities of blood flow, and (3) hypercoagulability of the blood.

Vascular endothelial injury can result from atherosclerosis (plaque deposits on arterial walls). Atherosclerosis initiates platelet adhesion and aggregation, promoting the development of atherosclerotic plaques that enlarge, causing further damage and occlusion. Other causes of vessel endothelial injury may be related to hemodynamic alterations associated with hypertension and turbulent blood flow. Injury also is caused by radiation injury, exogenous chemical agents (toxins from cigarette smoke), endogenous agents (cholesterol), bacterial toxins or endotoxins, or immunologic mechanisms. Whatever the precipitating cause of endothelial injury, it is a potent thrombogenic agent.

Sites of turbulent blood flow in the arteries and stasis of blood flow in the veins are at risk for thrombus formation. In areas of turbulence, platelets and endothelial cells may be activated, leading to thrombosis. In sites of stasis, platelets may remain in contact with the endothelium for prolonged times, and clotting factors that would normally be diluted with fresh-flowing blood are not diluted and may become activated. The most common clinical conditions that predispose to venous stasis and subsequent thromboembolic phenomena are major surgery (e.g., orthopedic surgery), acute myocardial infarction, congestive heart failure, limb paralysis, spinal injury, malignancy, advanced age, the postpartum period, and bed rest longer than 1 week. Turbulence and stasis occur with ulcerated atherosclerotic plaques (myocardial infarction), hyperviscosity (polycythemia), and conditions with deformed red cells (sickle cell anemia).

Hypercoagulability, or **thrombophilia,** is the condition in which an individual is at risk for thrombosis. Hypercoagulability is differentiated according to whether it results from primary (hereditary) or secondary (acquired) causes. Primary causes

BOX 29-9 CLINICAL CONDITIONS ASSOCIATED WITH HIGH RISK FOR THROMBOSIS OR THROMBOEMBOLISM

ARTERIAL	VENOUS
Atherosclerosis	General surgery
Cigarette smoking	Orthopedic surgery
Hypertension	Arthroscopy
Diabetes mellitus	Trauma
High LDL cholesterol	Malignancy
Hypertriglyceridemia	Immobility
Positive family history	Sepsis
Left ventricular failure	Congestive heart failure
Oral contraceptives	Nephrotic syndrome
Estrogens	Obesity
High lipoprotein A	Varicose veins
Polycythemia	Postphlebotic syndrome
Hyperviscosity syndrome	Oral contraceptives
Leukostasis syndrome	Estrogens
Thrombocythemia	Thrombocythemia

LDL, Low-density lipoprotein.

include defects in proteins involved in hemostasis. Secondary causes include a variety of clinical disorders or conditions (Box 29-9). It is unclear why the incidence of thrombosis formation in hypercoagulable states associated with various disease states and conditions is not more than anticipated.

Hereditary Thrombophilias. A large number of inherited conditions have been identified that increase the risk of developing thrombosis (Box 29-10).[73] Most are autosomal dominant; thus individuals who are homozygous for the mutation are at greatest risk for thrombosis. These include mutations in coagulation proteins, fibrinolytic proteins, platelet receptors, and other factors. The particular mutations that have been most strongly linked as risk factors for venous thrombosis or for arterial thrombosis leading to coronary artery disease or stroke include those that affect fibrinogen, prothrombin (G20210A variant), factor V (factor V Leiden) of the coagulation system, PAI-1 of the fibrinolytic system, the platelet receptor GPIIIa, and methylenetetrahydrofolate reductase (MTHFR), as well as mutations that result in excessive levels of homocysteine (hyperhomocysteinemia). Other inherited thrombophilias are risk factors primarily for venous thrombosis.[74,75] These include deficiencies in protein C, protein S, and AT III.[76]

Factor V Leiden results from a single nucleotide mutation of guanine to adenine at nucleotide 1691 (G1691A). Activated factor V (Va) is usually inactivated by protein C, but this single mutation results in a change in amino acid 506 from arginine to glutamine. The change alters the site where protein C would cleave factor Va and confers partial resistance, resulting in prolonged high levels of Va and prolongation of clot formation.[77] Although this mutation increases the risk for thrombosis, most individuals with factor V Leiden do not have clinically relevant thrombotic events. It is the most common hereditary thrombophilia and is found in about 30% of individuals presenting with deep venous thrombosis (DVT)

BOX 29-10 HEREDITARY AND ACQUIRED THROMBOPHILIC DISORDERS

Inherited Disorders (Primary)
- Activated protein C resistance
  - Factor V Leiden mutation
  - Factor V Cambridge mutation
  - Factor V Hong Kong
  - Factor V HR2 mutation
  - Prothrombin 20210A mutation
- Factor XII deficiency (Hageman trait)
- Dysfibrinogenemia
- Hyperhomocysteinemia
- Platelet defects
  - Wien-Penzing defect
  - Sticky platelet syndrome

Inherited and Acquired Disorders
- Antithrombin deficiency
- Heparin cofactor II deficiency
- Protein C deficiency
- Protein S deficiency
- Plasminogen deficiency
- Other fibrinolytic system defects

Acquired Disorders (Secondary)
- Antiphospholipid antibodies
  - Anticardiolipin antibodies
  - Lupus anticoagulant
  - Subgroup phospholipid antibodies
- Myeloproliferative syndromes
- Trousseau syndrome

From Bick RL: *Hematol Oncol Clin North Am* 17(1):115–147, 2003.

or pulmonary embolism. It is primarily observed in individuals of European ancestry and in about 5% of whites in the United States and Europe.

The second most common inherited thrombophilia is a mutation in the prothrombin gene, resulting in a replacement of guanine at nucleotide 20210 with an adenine (G20210A variant).[74] This mutation is observed in about 2% to 5% of individuals of European ancestry, but is found in 5% to 10% of individuals presenting with venous thrombosis. The G20210A variant leads to overproduction of prothrombin and prolongation of clot formation.

MTHFR mutation leads to alterations in the metabolism of the amino acid homocysteine into methionine and abnormally elevated levels of that amino acid in the blood (hyperhomocysteinemia).[78] Acquired hyperhomocysteinemia may result from deficiencies in vitamins B_6 or B_{12}, endocrine diseases (e.g., diabetes mellitus, hypothyroidism), pernicious anemia, inflammatory bowel disease, renal failure, and therapy with some drugs. Individuals with homocysteine levels above the 95th percentile are 2.5 times more likely to experience an episode of DVT.

More than 100 different known mutations lead to defects of proteins C, protein S, and AT III and increase the risk of venous thrombosis. Mutations may lead to either quantitative (low levels of protein) or qualitative (production of defective protein) changes.

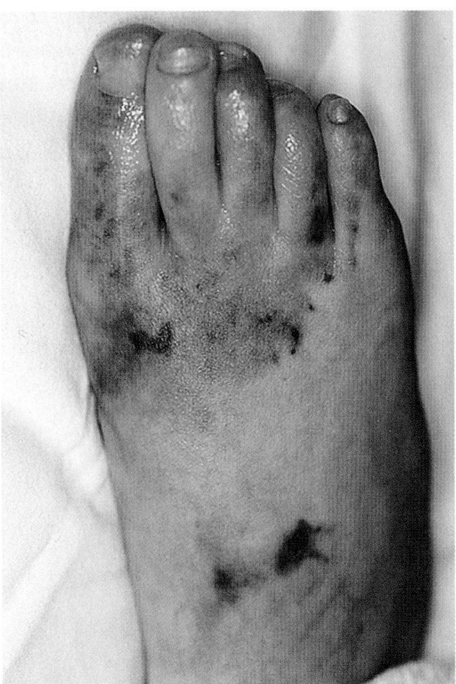

FIGURE 29-22 **Arterial Thrombosis Associated with Antiphospholipid Antibodies.** A 12-year-old girl with systemic lupus erythematosus and antiphospholipid antibodies with painful cutaneous vasculitis of the right foot. Arterial thrombosis documented by angiography resulted in cyanosis of the large toe. Symptoms resolved with treatment with heparin and corticosteroids. (From Kliegman R et al: *Nelson textbook of pediatrics,* ed 18, Philadelphia, 2007, Saunders.)

Tests to diagnose inherited thrombophilias include prothrombin time, partial thromboplastin time, and levels of protein C, protein S, and AT III. More elaborate tests to detect precise mutations in factor V, prothrombin, or MTHFR may be indicated.

Acquired Hypercoagulability. Deficiencies in proteins S and C and AT III may be acquired and contribute to a hypercoagulable state.[77] Conditions associated with an acquired protein deficiency include DIC, liver disease, infection, DVT, acute respiratory distress syndrome, l-asparaginase therapy, HUS, and TTP. The postoperative state also predisposes an individual to protein C or S deficiency; however, its role in contributing to DVT remains unclear.

Acquired hypercoagulable states include the antiphospholipid syndrome (APS), an autoimmune syndrome characterized by autoantibodies against plasma membrane phospholipids and phospholipid-binding proteins. As with most autoimmune diseases, the predominantly affected individual is female and of reproductive age. Those with APS are at risk for arterial and venous thrombosis and a variety of obstetric complications, including pregnancy loss and preeclampsia or eclampsia (Figure 29-22).[79] In severe cases the person may die from recurrent major thrombus formation.[80] The pathophysiology is related to autoantibodies directly reacting with platelets or endothelial cells (increasing the risk for thrombosis) or the placental surface (resulting in damage to the placenta). The predominant diagnostic tests measure prolongation of laboratory blood coagulation tests related to an antibody inhibitor (lupus anticoagulant) and specific ELISAs for antibodies against phospholipids (e.g., anticardiolipin antibody) or proteins that bind to phospholipids (e.g., β_2-glycoprotein I).[81,82] Highly effective therapy (i.e., unfractionated or low-molecular-weight heparin with low-dose aspirin) is available to prevent the obstetric complications.[83]

SUMMARY REVIEW

Alterations of Leukocyte Function

1. Quantitative alterations of leukocytes (too many or too few) can be caused by bone marrow dysfunction or premature destruction of cells in the circulation. Many quantitative changes in leukocytes occur in response to invasion by microorganisms.
2. Leukocytosis is a condition in which the leukocyte count is higher than normal and is usually a response to stress and invasion of microorganisms.
3. Leukopenia is a condition in which the leukocyte count is lower than normal and is caused by pathologic conditions such as malignancies and hematologic disorders.
4. Granulocytosis (particularly as a result of an increase in neutrophils) occurs in response to infection. The marrow releases immature cells, causing a shift-to-the-left, when responding to an infection that has created a demand for neutrophils that exceeds the supply in the circulation.
5. Eosinophilia results most commonly from parasitic invasion and ingestion or inhalation of toxic foreign particles.
6. Basophilia is seen in hypersensitivity reactions because of the high content of histamine and subsequent release.
7. Monocytosis occurs during the late or recuperative phase of infection when macrophages (mature monocytes) phagocytose surviving microorganisms and debris.
8. Granulocytopenia, a significant decrease in the number of neutrophils, can be a life-threatening condition if sepsis occurs; it is often caused by chemotherapeutic agents, severe infection, and radiation.
9. Infectious mononucleosis is an acute infection of B lymphocytes most commonly associated with EBV, a type of herpesvirus. Transmission of EBV is by personal contact, commonly through saliva, thus its nickname, the kissing disease.
10. Two of the earliest manifestations of mononucleosis are sore throat and fever caused by inflammation at the primary site of viral entry.
11. Most cases of EBV mononucleosis include fever lasting 7 to 10 days, sore throat, and enlargement and tenderness of the cervical lymph nodes. It is self-limiting, and treatment consists of rest and relief of symptoms.
12. The common pathologic feature of all forms of leukemia is an uncontrolled proliferation of leukocytes and overcrowding of the bone marrow, causing a decreased production and function of the other blood cell lines.

SUMMARY REVIEW—cont'd

13. All leukemias are classified by the cell type involved, lymphocytic or myelogenous, and are differentiated by onset, acute or chronic. Thus there are four major types of leukemia: ALL, CLL, AML, and CML.
14. Although the exact cause of leukemia is unknown, it is considered a clonal disorder. A higher incidence of acute leukemias and CLL is reported in certain families, suggesting a possible genetic predisposition.
15. The most common genetic abnormality in adult ALL is the Philadelphia chromosome.
16. In approximately one third of clients with AML, there is a mutation in the receptor tyrosine kinase FLT3.
17. In leukemia, blasts (precursor cells) "crowd out" the marrow and cause cellular proliferation of the other cell lines to cease.
18. The major clinical manifestations of leukemia include fatigue caused by anemia, bleeding caused by thrombocytopenia, fever secondary to infection, anorexia, and weight loss.
19. Chemotherapy is the treatment of choice for leukemia. Acute leukemias are associated with an increasing survival rate of 80% to 90%, with long-term survival of 30% to 40%. Chronic leukemias are associated with a longer life expectancy than are acute leukemias.
20. Chronic leukemias progress differently than acute leukemias, advancing slowly and without warning. The presence of the Philadelphia chromosome is a diagnostic marker for CML.

Alterations of Lymphoid Function

1. The number of lymphocytes is decreased (lymphocytopenia) in most acute infections and in some immunodeficiency syndromes.
2. Lymphocytosis occurs in viral infections (IM and infectious hepatitis, in particular), leukemia, lymphomas, and some chronic infections.
3. Lymphomas are tumors of primary lymphoid tissue (thymus, bone marrow) or secondary lymphoid tissue (lymph nodes, spleen, tonsils, intestinal lymphoid tissue). The two major types of malignant lymphomas are Hodgkin lymphoma (HL) and non-Hodgkin lymphoma (NHL).
4. Reed-Sternberg (RS) cells in lymph nodes are classically associated with HL. The RS cell is derived from a malignant B cell that usually becomes binucleate.
5. A virus might be involved in the pathogenesis of HL. Some familial clustering suggests an unknown genetic mechanism.
6. An enlarged painless mass or swelling, most commonly in the neck, is an initial sign of HL. Local symptoms are produced by lymphadenopathy, usually caused by pressure or obstruction.
7. Treatment of HL includes radiation therapy and chemotherapy. A cure is possible regardless of the stage of HL; however, individuals treated with chemotherapy who relapse in less than 2 years have a poor prognosis.
8. The cause of lymph node enlargement and cancerous transformation in NHL is unknown. Immunosuppressed persons have a higher incidence of NHL, suggesting an immune mechanism.
9. Generally, with NHL, the swelling of lymph nodes is painless, and the nodes enlarge and transform over months or years.
10. Individuals with NHL can survive for long periods. Treatment is chemotherapy.
11. Burkitt lymphoma involves the jaw and facial bones and occurs in children from east-central Africa and New Guinea.
12. Multiple myeloma (MM) is a neoplasm of B cells (immature plasma cells) and mature plasma cells. It is characterized by multiple malignant tumors of plasma cells scattered throughout the skeletal system and occasionally in soft tissue.
13. Myeloma cells usually secrete monoclonal protein (M protein) that is an abnormal antibody molecule. The myeloma cell may also secrete free antibody light chain that is excreted in the urine (Bence Jones protein).
14. The exact cause of MM is unknown, but genetic factors and chronic stimulation of the mononuclear phagocyte system by bacteria, viral agents, and chemicals have been suggested.
15. The major clinical manifestations for MM include recurrent infections caused by suppression of the humoral immune response and renal disease as a result of Bence Jones proteinuria.
16. Chemotherapy is the treatment of choice for MM. Treatment with tandem transplant or thalidomide, or both, is showing promise as an effective therapeutic agent in producing long-term remissions.
17. Waldenström macroglobulinemia is a rare type of slow-growing plasma cell tumor that secretes a monoclonal IgM molecule.

Alterations of Splenic Function

1. Splenomegaly (enlargement of the spleen) may be considered normal in certain individuals, but its presence should not be ignored.
2. Splenomegaly results from (a) acute inflammatory or infectious processes, (b) congestive disorders, (c) infiltrative processes, and (d) tumors or cysts.
3. Splenomegaly causes hypersplenism (overactivity of the spleen). Hypersplenism results in blood cell sequestration, causing destruction of red blood cells and the development of anemia.

Alterations of Platelets and Coagulation

1. Thrombocytopenia is characterized by a platelet count less than 100,000 platelets/μL of blood; a count less than 50,000/μL increases the potential for hemorrhage associated with minor trauma.

SUMMARY REVIEW—cont'd

2. Thrombocytopenia exists in primary or secondary forms and is commonly associated with autoimmune diseases and viral infections; bacterial sepsis with DIC also results in thrombocytopenia.
3. Heparin-induced thrombocytopenia develops in approximately 4% of individuals receiving unfractionated heparin.
4. Immune thrombocytopenic purpura (ITP) is a major cause of platelet destruction, often affecting females, and results in hemorrhaging that ranges from petechiae to bleeding from mucosal sites.
5. Thrombotic thrombycytopenic purpura (TTP) causes platelet aggregation leading to microcirculatory occlusion.
6. Thrombocythemia is characterized by a platelet count more than 400,000 platelets/μL of blood and is symptomatic when the count exceeds 1 million/μL, which increases the risk for intravascular clotting (thrombosis).
7. Thrombocythemia is caused by accelerated platelet production in the bone marrow.
8. Qualitative alterations in normal platelet adherence or aggregation prevent platelet plug formation and may result in prolonged bleeding times.
9. Prolonged bleeding can result from alterations in platelet function, including adhesion between platelets and the vessel wall, platelet-platelet adhesion, platelet granule secretion, arachidonic acid pathway activity, and membrane phospholipid regulation.
10. Disorders of coagulation are usually caused by defects or deficiencies of clotting factors.
11. Coagulation is impaired when there is a deficiency of vitamin K because of insufficient production of prothrombin and synthesis of clotting factors II, VII, IX, and X, often associated with liver diseases.
12. DIC is a complex syndrome that results from a variety of clinical conditions that release tissue factor, causing an increase in fibrin and thrombin activity in the blood and producing augmented clot formation and accelerated fibrinolysis. Sepsis is often associated with DIC.
13. DIC is characterized by a cycle of intravascular clotting followed by active bleeding caused by the initial consumption of coagulation factors and platelets and diffuse fibrinolysis.
14. Diagnosis of DIC is based on dysfunctional coagulation activity. Treatment is complex, nonstandardized, and focused on removing the primary cause, restoring hemostasis, and preventing further organ damage.
15. Thromboembolic disease results from a fixed (thrombus) or moving (embolus) clot that blocks flow within a vessel, denying nutrients to tissues distal to the occlusion; death can result when clots obstruct blood flow to the heart, brain, or lungs.
16. Hypercoagulability is the result of deficient anticoagulation proteins. Secondary causes are conditions that promote venous stasis.
17. The term Virchow triad refers to three factors that can cause thrombus formation: (a) vessel wall injury, (b) blood flow abnormalities, and (c) altered blood constituents leading to hypercoagulability.
18. Autoantibodies against phospholipids result in a state of acquired hypercoagulability, an increased risk for venous or arterial thrombosis, and a higher incidence of pregnancy complications.

KEY TERMS

Acute idiopathic TTP, 1040
Acute leukemia, 1013
Acute lymphocytic leukemia (ALL), 1015
Acute myelogenous leukemia (AML), 1015
Agranulocytosis, 1009
Arterial thrombus (*pl.*, thrombi), 1048
Basopenia, 1011
Basophilia, 1011
B-cell neoplasm, 1027
Bence Jones protein, 1032
β_2-microglobulin, 1034
Burkitt lymphoma, 1029
Chronic leukemia, 1013
Chronic lymphocytic leukemia (CLL), 1020
Chronic myelogenous leukemia (CML), 1020
Chronic relapsing TTP, 1040
Compensated DIC, 1046
Congestive splenomegaly, 1036
Consumptive thrombohemorrhagic disorders, 1043
D-dimer, 1047
Disseminated intravascular coagulation (DIC), 1043
Embolus, 1048
Eosinopenia, 1011
Eosinophilia, 1010
Erythromyalgia, 1041
Essential (primary) thrombocythemia (ET), 1040
Granulocytopenia, 1009
Granulocytosis, 1009
Heparin-induced thrombocytopenia (HIT), 1038
Heterophile antibody, 1013
Hodgkin lymphoma (HL), 1023
Hypercoagulability, 1048
Hypersplenism, 1036
Immune thrombocytopenic purpura (ITP), 1038
Impaired hemostasis, 1042
Infectious mononucleosis (IM), 1011
Infiltrative splenomegaly, 1036
Leukemia, 1013
Leukemoid reaction, 1009
Leukocytosis, 1009
Leukopenia, 1009
Lymphadenopathy, 1023
Lymphoblastic lymphoma (LL), 1030
Lymphocytopenia, 1011
Lymphocytosis, 1011
Lymphoplasmacytic lymphoma, 1035
Microvasculature thrombosis, 1041
Monoclonal gammopathy of undetermined significance (MGUS), 1032
Monocytopenia, 1011
Monocytosis, 1011
M protein, 1032
Multiple myeloma (MM), 1030
Neutropenia, 1009
Neutrophilia, 1009
NK-cell neoplasm, 1027
Non-Hodgkin lymphoma (NHL), 1027
Pancytopenia, 1015
Philadelphia chromosome, 1014
Pseudothrombocytopenia, 1037
Purpura, 1037
Qualitative leukocyte disorder, 1008
Quantitative leukocyte disorder, 1008
Reed-Sternberg (RS) cell, 1024
Shift-to-the-left, 1009
Smoldering myeloma, 1032
Solitary plasmacytoma, 1032
Splenomegaly, 1036
T-cell neoplasm, 1027
Thrombocythemia, 1040
Thrombocytopenia, 1037
Thrombocytosis, 1040
Thromboembolic disease, 1037
Thrombophilia, 1048
Thrombotic thrombocytopenic purpura (TTP), 1040
Thrombus, 1048
Vasculitis, 1042
Venous thrombus (*pl.*, thrombi), 1048
Virchow triad, 1048
Waldenström macroglobulinemia (WM), 1035

REFERENCES

1. Dubos F, Delebarre M, Martinot A: Predicting the risk of severe infection in children with chemotherapy-induced febrile neutropenia, *Curr Opin Hematol* 19(1):39–43, 2012.
2. Schwartz MJ et al: Evidence for an altered tryptophan metabolism in fibromyalgia, *Neurobiol Dis* 11(3):434–442, 2002.
3. Hanna B: Re: the diagnosis of infectious mononucleosis, *Clin Otolaryngol* 37(1):80–81, 2012.
4. Gunz FW: The dreaded leukemias and the lymphomas: their nature and their prospects. In Wintrobe MM, editor: *Blood, pure and eloquent: a story of discovery, of people, and of ideas*, New York, 1980, McGraw-Hill.
5. Brunning RD et al: Acute myeloid leukaemia: introduction. In Jaffe ES et al: *Pathology and genetics of tumours of haematopoietic and lymphoid tissues*, Lyon, France, 2001, IARC Press, World Health Organization Classification of Tumours, pp 77–80. Chapter 3.
6. *SEER stat fact sheets—leukemia,* Bethesda, MD, 2008, National Institutes of Health, U.S. Department of Health and Human Services. Available at http://seer.cancer.gov/statfacts/html/leuks.html. Accessed August 29, 2012.
7. *Seer cancer statistics review, 1975-2008*, Bethesda, MD, 2011, National Cancer Institute.
8. Druker BJ: Translation of the Philadelphia chromosome into therapy for CML, *Blood* 112(13):4808–4817, 2008.
9. Talpaz M et al: Dasatinib in imatinib-resistant Philadelphia chromosome-positive leukemias, *N Engl J Med* 354(24):2531–2541, 2006.
10. Dick JE: Stem cell concepts renew cancer research, *Blood* 112(13):4793–4807, 2008.
11. Wakeford R, Little MP, Kendall GM: Risk of childhood leukemia after low-level exposure to ionizing radiation, *Expert Rev Hematol* 3(3):251–254, 2010.
12. *SEER stat fact sheets—acute myeloid leukemia,* Bethesda, MD, 2008, National Institutes of Health, U.S. Department of Health and Human Services. Available at http://seer.cancer.gov/statfacts/html/amyl.html. Accessed August 29, 2012.
13. Appelbaum FM: The acute leukemias. In Goldman L, Schafer AI, editors: *Cecil medicine*, ed 24, Philadelphia, PA, 2001, Saunders Elsevier. Chapter 189.
14. Masera G et al: Prognostic significance of radiological bone involvement in childhood acute lymphoblastic leukaemia, *Arch Dis Child* 52:530–533, 1977.
15. *Childhood acute lymphoblastic leukemia treatment: health professional version*, Bethesda, MD, 2008, National Institutes of Health, U.S. Department of Health and Human Services. Available at www.cancer.gov/cancertopics/pdq/treatment/childALL/healthprofessional. Accessed August 30, 2012.
16. *Adult acute lymphoblastic leukemia treatment: health professional version* Available at Bethesda, MD, 2008, National Institutes of Health, U.S. Department of Health and Human Services. Accessed August 30, 2012 www.cancer.gov/cancertopics/pdq/treatment/adultALL/healthprofessional.
17. Levine AM: Lymphomas and leukemias due to infectious organisms, *Hematology* 17(Suppl 1):S87–S89, 2012.
18. Yanada M, Naoe T: Acute myeloid leukemia in older adults, *Int J Hematol* 96(2):186–193, 2012.
19. *Adult acute myeloid leukemia treatment: health professional version*. Available at Bethesda, MD, 2012, National Institutes of Health, U.S. Department of Health and Human Services. Accessed August 29, 2012. www.cancer.gov/cancertopics/pdq/treatment/adultAML/healthprofessional.
20. Hu J et al: Long-term efficacy and safety of all-trans retinoic acid/arsenic trioxide-based therapy in newly diagnosed acute promyelocytic leukemia, *Proc Natl Acad Sci U S A* 106(9):3342–3347, 2009.
21. Witz F et al: A placebo-controlled study of recombinant human granulocyte-macrophage colony-stimulating factor administered during and after induction treatment for de novo acute myelogenous leukemia in elderly patients, Groupe Ouest Est Leucémies Aiguës Myéloblastiques (GOELAM), *Blood* 91(8):2722–2730, 1998.
22. *SEER stat fact sheets—chronic lymphoblastic leukemia,* Bethesda, MD, 2008, National Institutes of Health, U.S. Department of Health and Human Services. Available at http://seer.cancer.gov/statfacts/html/clyl.html. Accessed August 30, 2012.
23. *SEER stat fact sheets—chronic myeloid leukemia,* Bethesda, MD, 2008, National Institutes of Health, U.S. Department of Health and Human Services. Available at http://seer.cancer.gov/statfacts/html/alyl.html. Accessed August 30, 2012.

23a. Howlader N et al, editors: *SEER Cancer Statistics Review, 1975-2010*, Bethesda, MD, 2013, National Cancer Institute. http://seer.cancer.gov/csr/1975_2010/, based on November 2012 SEER data submission, posted to the SEER web site.

24. Pinilla-Ibarz J, Flinn I: Expanding options for front-line treatment in patients with newly diagnosed CML, *Crit Rev Oncol Hematol*, April 7, 2012. [Epub ahead of print.].
25. Ouillette P et al: Acquired genomic copy number aberrations and survival in chronic lymphocytic leukemia, *Blood* 118(1):3051–3061, 2011.
26. Gora-Tybor J: Emerging therapy in chronic myeloid leukemia, *Curr Cancer Drug Targets* 12(5):458–470, 2012.
27. Friese CR et al: Timeliness and quality of diagnostic care for Medicare recipients with chronic lymphocytic leukemia, *Cancer* 117(7):1470–1477, 2011.
28. Orchard JA et al: ZAP-70 expression and prognosis in chronic lymphocytic leukaemia, *Lancet* 363(9403):105–111, 2004.
29. Rogers G et al: Dasatinib and nilotinib for imatinib-resistant or intolerant chronic myeloid leukaemia: a systematic review and economic evaluation, *Health Technol Assess* 16(22):1–410, 2012.
30. Bakshi N, Maghfoor I: The current lymphoma classification: new concepts and practical applications triumphs and woes, *Ann Saudi Med* 32(3), 2012. 296–205.
31. *SEER stat fact sheets—Hodgkin lymphoma,* Bethesda, MD, 2008, National Institutes of Health, U.S. Department of Health and Human Services. Available at http://seer.cancer.gov/statfacts/html/hodg.html. Accessed August 29, 2012.
32. Nogová L et al: Lymphocyte-predominant and classic Hodgkin's lymphoma: a comprehensive analysis from the German Hodgkin Study Group, *J Clin Oncol* 26(3):434–439, 2008.
33. Al-Mansour M et al: Transformation to aggressive lymphoma in nodular lymphocyte-predominant Hodgkin's lymphoma, *J Clin Oncol* 28(5):793–799, 2010.
34. *What you need to know about Hodgkin lymphoma,* Bethesda, MD, 2008, National Institutes of Health, U.S. Department of Health and Human Services. Available at http://cancer.gov/cancertopics/wyntk/hodgkin. Accessed August 30, 2012.
35. *SEER stat fact sheets—non-Hodgkin lymphoma,* Bethesda, MD, 2008, National Institutes of Health, U.S. Department of Health and Human Services. Available at http://seer.cancer.gov/statfacts/html/nhl.html. Accessed August 29, 2012.
36. *Adult non-Hodgkin lymphoma treatment: health professional version-* Bethesda, MD, 2008, National Institutes of Health, U.S. Department of Health and Human Services. Available at www.cancer.gov/cancertopics/pdq/treatment/myeloma/healthprofessional. Accessed August 30, 2012.
37. Molyneux EM et al: Burkitt's lymphoma, *Lancet* 379(9822):1234–1244, 2012.
38. *Multiple myeloma and other plasma cell neoplasms treatment: health professional version*, Bethesda, MD, 2008, National Institutes of Health, U.S. Department of Health and Human Services. Available at www.cancer.gov/cancertopics/pdq/treatment/adult-non-hodgkins/healthprofessional. Accessed August 30, 2012.
39. *SEER stat fact sheets—myeloma*, Bethesda, MD, 2008, National Institutes of Health, U.S. Department of Health and Human Services. Available at http://seer.cancer.gov/statfacts/html/mulmy.html. Accessed September 1, 2012.
40. Min DJ et al: MMSET stimulates myeloma cell growth through micro-RNA mediated modulation of c-MYC, *Leukemia*, 2012 Sep 1. [E-pub ahead of print.].
41. Rajkumar SV, Melini G: San Miguel JF: Haematological cancer: redefining myeloma, *Nat Rev Clin Oncol* 9(9):494–496, 2012.
42. Rajkumar SV: Treatment of multiple myeloma, *Nat Rev Clin Oncol* 8:479–491, 2011.
43. Eshaghian S, Berenson JR: Multiple myeloma: improved outcomes with new therapeutic approaches, *Curr Opin Support Palliat Care* 6(3):330–336, 2012.
44. *Waldenström macroglobulinemia: questions and answers: fact sheet,* Bethesda, MD, 2008, National Institutes of Health, U.S. Department of Health and Human Services. Available at http://cancer.gov/cancertopics/factsheet/Sites-Types/WM. Accessed September 1, 2012.
45. Gertz MA: Waldenström macroglobulinemia: 2012 update on diagnosis, risk stratification and management, *Am J Hematol* 87(5):503–510, 2012.
46. Ioannou A, Kannan L, Tsokos GC: *Platelets, complement and tissue inflammation*, August 28, 2012. [Epub ahead of print.].
47. *Thrombocytopenia*, Bethesda, MD, 2008, National Institutes of Health, U.S. Department of Health and Human Services. Available at www.nhlbi.nih.gov/health/dci/Diseases/thcp/thcp_all.html. Accessed September 1, 2012.
48. Selleng K, Selleng S, Greinacher A: Heparin-induced thrombocytopenia in intensive care patients, *Semin Thromb Hemost* 34(5):425–438, 2008.
49. Warkentin TE, Sheppard J-AI: Testing for heparin-induced thrombocytopenia antibodies, *Transfus Med Rev* 20(4):259–272, 2006.
50. Lakshmanan S, Cuker A: Contemporary management of primary immune thrombocytopenia (ITP) in adults, *J Thromb Haemost*, August 3, 2012. [Epub ahead of print.].

51. Curtis BR: Genotyping for human platelet alloantigen polymorphisms: applications in the diagnosis of alloimmune platelet disorders, *Semin Thromb Hemost* 34(6):539–548, 2008.
52. Kuhne T, Imback P: Management of children and adolescents with primary immune thrombocytopenia: controversies and solutions, *Vox Sang*, July 17, 2012. [Epub ahead of print.].
53. Bennett CM, de Jong JLO, Neufeld EJ: Targeted ITP strategies: do they elucidate the biology of ITP and related disorders? *Pediatr Blood Cancer* 47(Suppl 5):706–709, 2006.
54. Gomez-Almaguer D: Monocolonal antibodies in the treatment of immune thrombocytopenic purpura (ITP), *Hematology* 17(Suppl 1):S25–S27, 2012.
55. Zoller B et al: Autoimmune disease and venous thromboembolism: a review of the literature, *Am J Cardiovasc Dis* 2(3):171–183, 2012.
56. Scully M et al: A phase 2 study of the safety and efficacy of rituximab with plasma exchange in acute acquired thrombotic thrombocytopenic purpura, *Blood* 118(7):1746–1753, 2011.
57. *Thrombocytopenia & thrombocytosis,* Bethesda, MD, 2008, National Institutes of Health, U.S. Department of Health and Human Services. Available at www.nhlbi.nih.gov/health/dci/Diseases/thrm/thrm_all.html. Accessed September 1, 2012.
58. Cervantes F: Management of essential thrombocythemia, *Hematol Am Soc Hematol Educ Program*214–221, 2011. 2011.
59. Landolfi R: Fi Gennaro L: Thrombosis in myeloproliferative and myelodysplastic syndromes, *Hematology* 17(Suppl 1):S174–S176, 2012.
60. Santos FP, Verstovsek S: Breakthroughs in myeloproliferative neoplasms, *Hematology* 17(Suppl 1):S55–S58, 2012.
61. Tefferi A, Elliott M: Thrombosis in myeloproliferative disorders: prevalence, prognostic factors, and the role of leukocytes and *JAK2*V617F, *Semin Thromb Hemost* 33(4):313–320, 2007.
62. Wolanskyj AP et al: Essential thrombocythemia beyond the first decade: life expectancy, long-term complication rates, and prognostic factors, *Mayo Clin Proc* 81(2):159–166, 2006.
63. Tefferi A, Thiele J, Vardiman JW: The 2008 World Health Organization classification system for myeloproliferative neoplasms: order out of chaos, *Cancer* 115(17):3842–3847, 2009.
64. Barbui T, Finazzi MC, Finazzi G: Front-line therapy in polycythemia vera and essential thrombocythemia, *Blood Rec* 26(5):205–211, 2012.
65. Salles II et al: Inherited traits affecting platelet function, *Blood Rev* 22(3):155–172, 2008.
66. Lisman T et al: Hemostasis and thrombosis in patients with liver disease: the ups and downs, *J Hepatol* 53(2):362–371, 2010.
67. Levi M et al: Guidelines for the diagnosis and management of disseminated intravascular coagulation, British Committee for Standards in Haematology, *Br J Haematol* 145(1):24–33, 2009.
68. Hook KM, Abrams CS: The loss of homeostasis in hemostasis: new approaches in treating and understanding acute and disseminated intravascular coagulation in critically ill patients, *Clin Transl Sci* 5(1):85–92, 2012.
69. Kwaan HC, Vicuna B: Incidence and pathogenesis of thrombosis in hematologic malignancies, *Semin Thromb Hemost* 33(4):303–312, 2007.
70. Palumbo JS: Mechanisms linking tumor cell-associated procoagulant function to tumor dissemination, *Semin Thromb Hemost* 34(2):154–160, 2008.
71. Tripodi A: D-dimer testing in laboratory practice, *Clin Chem* 57(9): 1256–1262, 2011.
72. Sorensen B et al: Clinical review: prothrombin complex concentrates—evaluation of safety and thrombogenicity, *Crit Care* 15(1):201, 2011.
73. Chan MY, Andreotti F, Becker RC: Hypercoagulable states in cardiovascular disease, *Circulation* 118(22):2286–2297, 2008.
74. Lippi G, Franchini M: Pathogenesis of venous thromboembolism: when the cup runneth over, *Semin Thromb Hemost* 34(8):747–761, 2008.
75. Ho CH: Can very high level of D-dimer exclusively predict the presence of thromboembolic diseases, *J Chin Med Assoc* 74(4):151–154, 2011.
76. Bruce A, Massicotte MP: Thrombophilia screening: whom to test, *Blood* 120(7):1353–1355, 2012.
77. Baglin T: Inherited and acquired risk factors for venous thromoembolimsm, *Semin Respir Crit Care Med* 33(2):127–137, 2012.
78. Kearon C: Influence of hereditary or acquired thrombophilias on the treatment of venous thromboembolism, *Curr Opin Hematol* 19(5):363–370, 2012.
79. McNamee K, Dawood F, Farquharson R: Recurrent miscarriage and thrombophilia: an update, *Curr Opin Obstet Gynecol* 24(4):229–234, 2012.
80. Aksu K, Donmez A, Keser G: Inflammation-induced thrombosis: mechanisms, disease associations and management, *Curr Pharm Des* 18(11):1478–1493, 2012.
81. Wahl D et al: Definition and significance of high positivity aCL ELISA, *Lupus* 21(7):725–726, 2012.
82. Willis R, Harris EN, Pierangeli SS: Current international initiatives in antiphospholipid antibody testing, *Semin Thromb Hemost* 38(4):360–374, 2012.
83. Heilmann L et al: Pregnancy outcome in women with antiphospholipid antibodies: report on a retrospective study, *Semin Thromb Hemost* 34(8):794–802, 2008.

CHAPTER

30

Alterations of Hematologic Function in Children

Nancy E. Kline

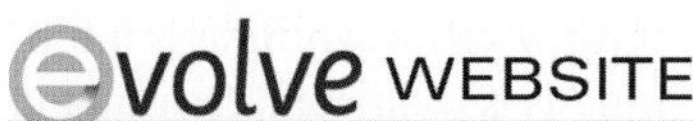

http://evolve.elsevier.com/McCance/

- Review Questions and Answers
- Animations

CHAPTER OUTLINE

This chapter briefly explains fetal and neonatal hematopoiesis and postnatal changes in blood as a foundation for understanding the pathophysiology of specific blood disorders in childhood. Among the diseases that affect erythrocytes are acquired disorders, such as iron deficiency anemia, hemolytic disease of the newborn, and anemia of infectious disease; and inherited disorders, such as glucose-6-phosphate dehydrogenase (G6PD) deficiency, hereditary spherocytosis, sickle cell disease, and the thalassemias. Disorders of coagulation and platelets include inherited hemorrhagic diseases, such as the hemophilias, and antibody-mediated hemorrhagic diseases, which include idiopathic thrombocytopenic purpura, autoimmune neonatal thrombocytopenias, and autoimmune vascular purpuras. Finally, leukocyte disorders, such as leukemia and the lymphomas (non-Hodgkin lymphoma as well as Hodgkin disease), are discussed.

FETAL AND NEONATAL HEMATOPOIESIS

As the developing embryo becomes too large for oxygenation of tissues by simple diffusion, the production of erythrocytes begins within the vessels of the yolk sac. Shortly after 2 weeks of gestation, circulating erythrocytes play a major role in delivering oxygen to the tissues. At approximately the eighth week of gestation, the site of erythrocyte production shifts from the vessels to the liver sinusoids, and the production of leukocytes and platelets begins in the liver and spleen. Erythropoiesis in the liver and, to a lesser extent, in the spleen and lymph nodes, reaches a peak at approximately 4 months. Hepatic blood formation declines steadily thereafter but does not disappear entirely during the remainder of gestation. By the fifth month of gestation, hematopoiesis begins to occur in the bone marrow and increases rapidly until hematopoietic (red) marrow fills the entire bone marrow space. By the time of delivery, the marrow is the only significant site of hematopoiesis.

In neonates and young infants, hematopoietic marrow progressively fills the bony cavities of the entire axial skeleton (skull, vertebrae, ribs, sternum), the long bones of the limbs, and many intramembranous bones. (These structures are described in Chapter 45.) Fatty (yellow) marrow gradually replaces hematopoietic marrow in some bones. During childhood, hematopoietic tissue retreats centrally to the vertebrae, ribs, sternum, pelvis, scapulae, skull, and proximal ends of the femur and humerus.

In diseases characterized by hemolysis, erythrocyte production can increase as much as eight times the normal because erythropoietin causes hematopoietic marrow to increase in volume. Initially, hematopoietic marrow expands from the ends of the long bones toward the middle of the shafts, replacing fatty marrow. Next, blood cell production begins to occur outside the marrow cavities, especially in the liver and spleen. Extramedullary hematopoiesis is more likely to occur in children than in adults because the bony cavities of children already are filled with red marrow (Figure 30-1). This is why hemolytic disease causes especially pronounced enlargement of the spleen and liver in children.

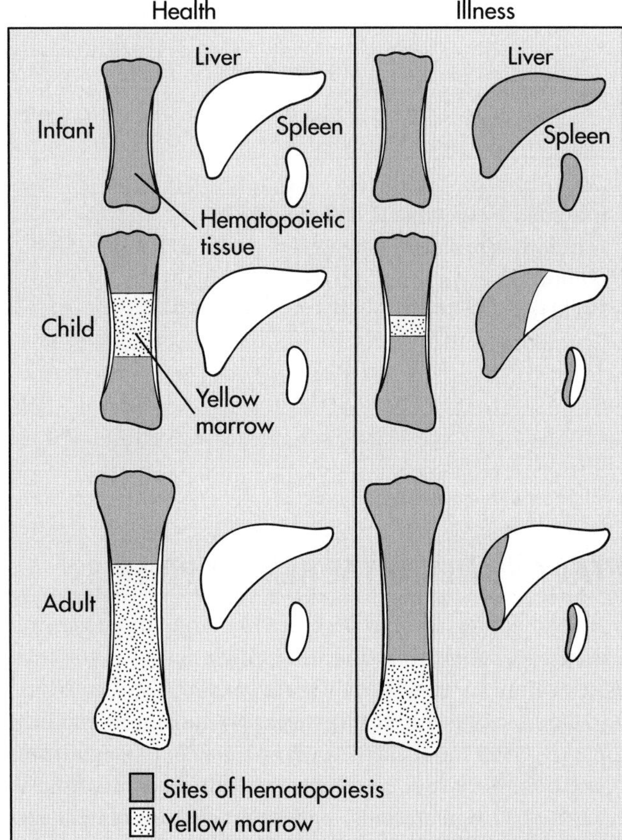

FIGURE 30-1 **Sites of Hematopoiesis in Health and Illness.** With normal maturation, red marrow is partly replaced by yellow marrow in the shafts of the long bones. In adults, red marrow is largely restricted to the proximal ends of the femur and humerus. In response to hemolysis, red marrow replaces yellow marrow in the long bones. In infants, whose long bones already are filled with red marrow, additional hematopoiesis takes place in the liver and spleen. In children and adults, red marrow can replace yellow marrow in response to hemolysis, necessitating less hematopoiesis in the liver and spleen.

The erythrocytes undergo striking changes during gestation, particularly during the first two trimesters, at which time they nearly double in numbers and in hemoglobin content. A proportionate increase in hematocrit also occurs. By the end of gestation the erythrocyte count has more than tripled but the size of each erythrocyte has decreased.

A biochemically distinct type of hemoglobin is synthesized during fetal life. The three **embryonic hemoglobins (Gower 1, Gower 2, and Portland)** and the **fetal hemoglobin (HbF)** are composed of two α- and two γ-chains of polypeptides, whereas the adult hemoglobins (HbA and HbA_2) are composed of two α-chains and two β-chains. (The structure of an adult hemoglobin molecule is illustrated in Figure 27-15, and types of hemoglobin are defined in Table 27-5.) Some unknown regulatory mechanism promotes γ-chain synthesis and inhibits β- and δ-chain synthesis in utero. This results in production of embryonic or fetal hemoglobin. After birth, γ-chain synthesis is inhibited, whereas β- and δ-chain synthesis is facilitated, resulting in production of adult hemoglobins.

Fetal hemoglobin has greater affinity for oxygen than does adult hemoglobin because it interacts less readily with an enzyme (2,3-diphosphoglycerate [DPG]) that inhibits hemoglobin-oxygen binding. The decreased inhibitory effects of 2,3-DPG enable fetal blood to transport oxygen despite the relative lack of oxygen in the uterine environment. The increased affinity for oxygen enables Hb F to bind with maternal oxygen in the placental circulation.

During the first trimester nearly all of the hemoglobin in the fetus is embryonic, but some Hb A can be detected. Therefore, it is possible to identify as early as 16 to 20 weeks of gestation some disorders of adult hemoglobin, such as sickle cell anemia and thalassemia major. In the 6-month fetus, Hb F constitutes 90% of the total. This percentage then begins to decline. At birth, neonatal hemoglobin consists of 70% Hb F, 29% Hb A, and 1% Hb A_2. Between 6 and 12 months of age, normal adult hemoglobin percentages are established (see Chapter 27).

POSTNATAL CHANGES IN THE BLOOD

Blood cell counts tend to rise above adult levels at birth and then decline gradually throughout childhood. Table 30-1 lists normal ranges during infancy and childhood. The immediate rise in values is the result of accelerated hematopoiesis during fetal life, increased numbers of cells that result from the trauma of birth, and cutting of the umbilical cord. These events surrounding the birth also are accompanied by the presence of large numbers of immature erythrocytes and leukocytes (particularly granulocytes) in peripheral blood (see Chapter 27). As the infant develops over the first 2 to 3 months of life, the numbers of these immature blood cells decrease.

Average blood volume in the full-term neonate is 85 ml/kg of body weight. The premature infant has a slightly larger blood volume of 90 ml/kg of body weight, with the mean increasing to 150 mg/kg during the first few days after birth. In full-term and premature infants, blood volume decreases during the first few

TABLE 30-1 HEMATOLOGIC VALUES DURING INFANCY AND CHILDHOOD

AGE	HEMOGLOBIN (g/dl) MEAN	HEMOGLOBIN (g/dl) RANGE	HEMATOCRIT (%) MEAN	HEMATOCRIT (%) RANGE	RETICU-LOCYTES (%)MEAN	MCV (fl) LOWEST	LEUKOCYTES (WBC/mm³) MEAN	LEUKOCYTES (WBC/mm³) RANGE	NEUTROPHILS (%) MEAN	NEUTROPHILS (%) RANGE	LYMPHO-CYTES (%) MEAN*	EOSINO-PHILS (%) MEAN	MONO-CYTES (%) MEAN
Cord blood	16.8	13.7-20.1	55	45-65	5	110	18,000	(9000-30,000)	61	(40-80)	31	2	6
2 wk	16.5	13-20	50	42-66	1		12,000	(5000-21,000)	40		63	3	9
3 mo	12	9.5-14.5	36	31-41	1		12,000	(6000-18,000)	30		48	2	5
6 mo to 6 yr	12	10.5-14	37	33-42	1	70-74	10,000	(6000-15,000)	45		48	2	5
7-12 yr	13	11-16	38	34-40	1	76-80	8,000	(4500-13,500)	55		38	2	5
Adult													
Female	14	12-16	42	37-47	1.6	80	7,500	(5000-10,000)	55	(35-70)	35	3	7
Male	16	14-18	47	42-52		80							

From Behrman R et al, editors: *Nelson textbook of pediatrics,* ed 17th, Philadelphia, 2004, Saunders.
*Relatively wide range.
fl, Femtoliters; *MCV,* mean corpuscular volume; *WBC,* white blood cells.

months. Thereafter the average blood volume is 75 to 77 ml/kg, which is similar to that of older children and adults.

Erythrocytes

The hypoxic intrauterine environment stimulates erythropoietin production in the fetus. This accelerates fetal erythropoiesis, producing polycythemia (excessive proliferation of erythrocyte precursors) of the newborn. After birth the oxygen from the lungs saturates arterial blood, and the amount of oxygen delivered to the tissues increases. In response to the change from a placental to a pulmonary oxygen supply during the first few days of life, levels of erythropoietin and the rate of blood cell formation decrease. The very active rate of fetal erythropoiesis is reflected by the large numbers of immature erythrocytes (reticulocytes) in the peripheral blood of full-term neonates. After birth the number of reticulocytes decreases about 50% every 12 hours, so it is rare to find an elevated reticulocyte count after the first week of life. A decrease in extramedullary hematopoiesis also occurs at this time. In the peripheral blood the erythrocyte count drops for 6 to 8 weeks after birth. During this period of rapid growth the rate of erythrocyte destruction is greater than that in later childhood and adulthood. In full-term infants, normal erythrocyte life span is 60 to 80 days; in premature infants it may be as short as 20 to 30 days; and in children and adolescents, it is the same as that in adults—120 days. (Mechanisms of hemolysis are described in Chapter 27.)

In the premature infant the postnatal fall in hemoglobin and hematocrit values is more marked than in the full-term infant. In the preschool and school-age child, there is a gradual rise in hemoglobin, hematocrit, and red blood cell (RBC) count. Values in males and females first begin to diverge in adolescence. In the female the gradual hemoglobin increase continues into early puberty, at which time it stabilizes. In the male the hemoglobin increase keeps pace with growth and maturation and eventually surpasses that of the female. This higher value of hemoglobin in the mature male is related to androgen secretion.

Metabolic processes within the erythrocytes of neonates differ significantly from those of erythrocytes in the normal adult. The relatively young population of erythrocytes in the newborn consumes greater quantities of glucose than do erythrocytes in adults. Several enzymes that regulate glucose consumption are increased in the erythrocytes of neonates, with a subsequent increase in the rate of glycolysis.

Leukocytes and Platelets

The lymphocytes of children tend to have more cytoplasm and less compact nuclear chromatin than do the lymphocytes of adults. The significance of these differences is unknown. One possible explanation is that children tend to have more frequent viral infections, which are associated with atypical lymphocytes. Even minor infections, in which the child fails to exhibit clinical manifestations of illness, or administration of immunizations may result in lymphocyte changes.[1]

The lymphocyte count is high at birth and continues to rise in some healthy infants during the first year of life. Then a steady decline occurs throughout childhood and adolescence until lower adult values are reached. It is unknown whether these developmental variations are physiologic or are a pathologic response to frequent viral infections and immunizations in children.

At birth the neutrophil count is very high and rises further during the early days of life.[2] After 2 weeks neutrophil counts fall to within or below normal adult ranges. By approximately 4 years of age the neutrophil count is the same as that of an adult. White children have slightly higher counts than black children.[3]

Eosinophil count is high in the first year of life and is higher in children than in teenagers or adults.[4] Monocyte counts are high in the first year of life and then decrease to adult levels. No relationship between age and basophil count has been found. Platelet counts in full-term neonates are comparable to platelet counts in adults and remain so throughout infancy and childhood.[5]

TABLE 30-2 ANEMIAS OF CHILDHOOD

CAUSE	ANEMIC CONDITION
Deficient Erythropoiesis or Hemoglobin Synthesis	
Decreased stem cell population in marrow (congenital or acquired pure red cell aplasia)	Normocytic-normochromic anemia
Decreased erythropoiesis despite normal stem cell population in marrow (infection, inflammation, cancer, chronic renal disease, congenital dyserythropoiesis)	Normocytic-normochromic anemia
Deficiency of a factor or nutrient needed for erythropoiesis	
Cobalamin (vitamin B_{12}), folate	Megaloblastic anemia
Iron	Microcytic-hypochromic anemia
Increased or Premature Hemolysis	
Alloimmune disease (maternal-fetal Rh, ABO, or minor blood group incompatibility)	Hemolytic disease of the newborn (HDN)
Autoimmune disease (idiopathic autoimmune hemolytic anemia, symptomatic systemic lupus erythematosus, lymphoma, drug-induced autoimmune processes)	Autoimmune hemolytic anemia
Inherited defects of plasma membrane structure (spherocytosis, elliptocytosis, stomatocytosis) or cellular size or both (pyknocytosis)	Hemolytic anemia
Infection (bacterial sepsis, congenital syphilis, malaria, cytomegalovirus infection, rubella, toxoplasmosis, disseminated herpes)	Hemolytic anemia
Intrinsic and inherited enzymatic defects (deficiencies of glucose-6-phosphate dehydrogenase [G6PD], pyruvate kinase, 5′-nucleotidase, glucose phosphate isomerase)	Hemolytic anemia
Inherited defects of hemoglobin synthesis	Sickle cell anemia Thalassemia
Disseminated intravascular coagulation (see Chapter 29)	Hemolytic anemia
Galactosemia	Hemolytic anemia
Prolonged or recurrent respiratory or metabolic acidosis	Hemolytic anemia
Blood vessel disorders (cavernous hemangioma, large vessel thrombus, renal artery stenosis, severe coarctation of the aorta) (see Chapter 33)	Hemolytic anemia

DISORDERS OF ERYTHROCYTES

Anemia is the most common blood disorder in children. Like anemia in adults, the anemias of childhood are caused by ineffective erythropoiesis or premature destruction of erythrocytes. The most common cause of insufficient erythropoiesis is iron deficiency, which may result from insufficient dietary intake or chronic loss of iron caused by bleeding. The hemolytic anemias of childhood may be divided into two large categories. The first category consists of disorders that result from premature destruction caused by intrinsic abnormalities of the erythrocytes, and the second category consists of disorders that result from damaging extraerythrocytic factors. The hemolytic anemias are inherited, congenital, or both.

The most dramatic form of acquired congenital hemolytic anemia is **hemolytic disease of the newborn (HDN),** also termed **erythroblastosis fetalis.** HDN is an alloimmune disorder in which maternal blood and fetal blood are antigenically incompatible, causing the mother's immune system to produce antibodies against fetal erythrocytes. Fetal erythrocytes that have been bound to maternal antibodies are recognized as foreign or defective by the fetal mononuclear phagocyte system and are removed from the circulation by phagocytosis, usually in the fetal spleen. (For a complete discussion of HDN, see p. 1059.) Other acquired hemolytic anemias—some of which begin in utero—include those caused by infections or the presence of toxins.

The inherited forms of hemolytic anemia result from intrinsic defects of the child's erythrocytes, any of which can lead to erythrocyte destruction by the mononuclear phagocyte system. Structural defects include abnormal red blood cell size and abnormalities of plasma membrane structure (spherocytosis). Intracellular defects include enzyme deficiencies, the most common of which is G6PD deficiency, and defects of hemoglobin synthesis, which manifest as sickle cell disease or thalassemia, depending on which component of hemoglobin is defective. These and other causes of childhood anemia, some more common than others, are listed in Table 30-2.

Acquired Disorders

Iron Deficiency Anemia

Iron deficiency anemia is the most common blood disorder of infancy and childhood, with the highest incidence occurring between 6 months and 2 years of age. Incidence is not related to gender or race, but socioeconomic factors are important because they affect nutrition, for example, the risk of iron deficiency anemia in children of single, homeless women.[6] However, greater use of iron-fortified products has decreased the prevalence of anemia in low-income infants.[7] Iron deficiency anemia is a common disorder in children because of their extremely high need for iron for normal growth to occur.

Between 4 years of age and the onset of puberty, dietary iron deficiency is uncommon. During adolescence, however, it is relatively common, especially in menstruating females. Rapid growth, together with the average adolescent's dietary habits, causes iron depletion. (Mechanisms of iron depletion are described in Chapter 27.)

PATHOPHYSIOLOGY. Although inadequate intake of iron is the most common cause of iron deficiency anemia during the first few years of life and during adolescence, blood loss is the most common cause in childhood. Chronic iron deficiency anemia from occult (hidden) blood loss may be caused by a gastrointestinal lesion, parasitic infestation, or hemorrhagic disease. Infants and young children who develop severe iron deficiency anemia have chronic intestinal blood loss induced by exposure to a heat-labile protein in cow's milk. Such exposure causes an inflammatory gastrointestinal reaction that damages the mucosa and results in diffuse microhemorrhage.

The amount of iron available for hemoglobin synthesis in the infant depends on maternal iron stores present at birth, rate of growth, the amount of dietary iron absorbed, and physiologic or pathologic loss of iron. During the period of inactive erythropoiesis immediately after birth, iron from erythrocytes that die at the end of their normal life span is stored, as hemosiderin, in bone marrow and liver tissue. This creates an iron reserve that can be used in lieu of dietary intake. The greatest stores are present 4 to 8 weeks after birth. Until erythropoiesis resumes, these iron stores are mobilized. In the premature infant, resumption of erythropoiesis depletes iron stores within 6 to 12 weeks; in the full-term infant, depletion takes longer—about 16 to 20 weeks. Once iron stores have been used, the infant depends on dietary iron.

The amount of dietary iron available for erythropoiesis depends on which foods are consumed. Iron-fortified cereals, green and yellow vegetables, fruits, and milk are common in the average 6-month-old infant's diet and provide iron in the amount of 0.9 to 1.5 mg/kg/day, amounts that satisfy the normal average daily requirement. Iron-fortified formulas are available commercially, and although the amount of iron in breast milk is low, it is easily absorbed.

CLINICAL MANIFESTATIONS. The symptoms of mild anemia—lethargy and listlessness—usually are not present or inconsequential in infants and young children, who are unable to describe these symptoms. Therefore, parents usually do not notice any change in the child's behavior or appearance until moderate anemia has developed. General irritability, decreased activity tolerance, weakness, and lack of interest in play are nonspecific indications of anemia. In mild to moderate iron deficiency anemia (hemoglobin of 6 to 10 g/dl), compensatory mechanisms of tissue oxygenation, such as increased amounts of 2,3-DPG within erythrocytes and a shift of the oxyhemoglobin dissociation curve, may be so effective that few clinical manifestations are apparent. When the hemoglobin falls below 5 g/dl, however, pallor, tachycardia, and systolic murmurs often occur.

Splenomegaly is evident in 10% to 15% of children with iron deficiency anemia, and if the condition is long-standing, the sutures of the skull may be widened. Chronic anemia also may result in decreased physical growth and developmental delays. Some children exhibit pica, a behavior in which nonfood substances are eaten. Weight is not necessarily an indicator of iron deficiency anemia because children may be obese, underweight, or of normal weight.

Iron deficiency anemia may affect neurologic and intellectual function. Decreased iron in the blood may affect attention span, alertness, and learning ability, even when anemia is not severe.

EVALUATION AND TREATMENT. The most definitive test for differentiating iron deficiency from other microcytic anemias is the absence of iron stores in the bone marrow. However, measurement of serum ferritin iron concentration, transferrin saturation, iron-binding capacity, and serum transferrin receptors often is an adequate diagnostic tool and often prevents proceeding to actual bone marrow evaluation. Evaluation and treatment of iron deficiency anemia in children are similar to evaluation and treatment in adults (see Chapter 27). Oral administration of simple ferrous salts usually is satisfactory, and additional vitamin C helps promote absorption.[8] Administration of supplementary trace metals or other vitamins is not necessary. Iron in a liquid form should be administered through a straw because it can stain teeth. If malabsorption is the cause of the anemia (or if oral administration has not been successful), iron dextran is given intravenously. Iron therapy is continued for at least 2 months after erythrocyte indexes have returned to normal in order to replenish iron stores.[9]

Dietary modification is required to prevent recurrences of iron deficiency anemia. Intake of iron-rich foods is increased, and the intake of cow's milk may be restricted, with the exact amount depending on the child's age (from 16 to 32 ounces). Limiting milk intake makes the child hungrier for other iron-rich foods and prevents gastrointestinal blood loss in children whose anemia is aggravated or caused by inflammatory reactions to proteins in cow's milk.

Hemolytic Disease of the Newborn

HDN can occur only if antigens on fetal erythrocytes differ from antigens on maternal erythrocytes. The antigenic properties of erythrocytes are determined genetically: they may be type A, B, or O and may or may not include Rh antigen D. Erythrocytes that express Rh antigen D are Rh-positive; those that do not are Rh-negative. The frequency of Rh negativity is higher in whites (15%) than in blacks (5%), and is rare in Asians. Maternal-fetal incompatibility exists if mother and fetus differ in ABO blood type or if the fetus is Rh-positive and the mother is Rh-negative. (The antigenic properties of erythrocytes are described in Chapter 9.)

ABO incompatibility occurs in about 20% to 25% of all pregnancies, but only 1 in 10 cases of ABO incompatibility results in HDN. Rh incompatibility occurs in less than 10% of pregnancies and rarely causes HDN in the first incompatible fetus. Even after five or more pregnancies, only 5% of women have babies with hemolytic disease. Usually erythrocytes from the first incompatible fetus cause the mother's immune system to produce antibodies that affect the fetuses of subsequent incompatible pregnancies. Only one in three cases of HDN is caused by Rh incompatibility; most cases are caused by ABO incompatibility.

PATHOPHYSIOLOGY. If the mother and fetus have antigenically incompatible erythrocytes, HDN will result if the mother's blood contains preformed antibodies against fetal erythrocytes or produces them on exposure to fetal erythrocytes, if sufficient amounts of antibody (usually immunoglobulin G [IgG]) cross the placenta and enter fetal blood, and if IgG binds with sufficient numbers of fetal erythrocytes to cause widespread antibody-mediated hemolysis or splenic removal. (Antibody-mediated red blood cell destruction is discussed in Chapter 9.)

IgM antibodies are formed against the ABO antigen that a person does not express, the A antigen if the mother is blood type O or B, or the B antigen if the mother is type O or A. These antibodies are produced early in life against gastrointestinal bacteria that make antigens similar to A and B. IgM antibodies do not cross the placenta or cause HDN. Occasionally a mother with blood type O may have also produced IgG against the A or B antigen. If the fetus is blood group A or B, the ABO incompatibility can cause HDN in the first pregnancy. HDN is usually not severe because A and B antigens are expressed on most cells, including the placenta, and much of the IgG against A or B is absorbed before encountering fetal blood cells.

Anti-Rh antibodies, on the other hand, are formed *only* in response to the presence of incompatible (Rh-positive) erythrocytes in the blood of an Rh-negative mother. Sources of exposure include fetal blood that is mixed with the mother's blood at the time of delivery or transfused blood.

The first Rh-incompatible pregnancy usually presents no difficulties because very few fetal erythrocytes cross the placental barrier during gestation. However, when the placenta detaches at birth, large numbers of fetal erythrocytes usually enter the mother's bloodstream. If the mother is Rh-negative and the fetus is Rh-positive, the mother produces anti-Rh antibodies. The capacity of the mother's immune system to produce anti-Rh antibodies depends on many factors, including her genetic capacity to make antibodies against the Rh antigen D, the amount of fetal-to-maternal bleeding, and the occurrence of any bleeding earlier in the pregnancy. Anti-Rh antibodies persist in the bloodstream for a very long time, and if the next offspring is Rh-positive, the mother's anti-Rh antibodies can enter the fetus's bloodstream and destroy the erythrocytes. Antibodies against Rh antigen D are of the IgG class and easily cross the placenta.

IgG-coated fetal erythrocytes are destroyed through extravascular hemolysis, primarily by mononuclear phagocytes in the spleen. As hemolysis progresses, the fetus becomes anemic. Erythropoiesis accelerates, particularly in the liver and spleen, and immature nucleated cells (erythroblasts) are released into the bloodstream, hence the name *erythroblastosis fetalis* (Figure 30-2). The degree of anemia depends on the length of time the antibody has been in the fetal circulation, antibody concentration, and the ability of the fetus to compensate for increased hemolysis. Unconjugated (indirect) bilirubin, which is formed during breakdown of hemoglobin, is transported across the placental barrier into the maternal circulation and is excreted by the mother. **Hyperbilirubinemia** occurs in the neonate after birth because excretion of lipid-soluble unconjugated bilirubin through the placenta no longer is possible.

The pathophysiologic effects of HDN are more severe in Rh incompatibility than in ABO incompatibility. ABO incompatibility may resolve after birth without life-threatening complications. Maternal-fetal incompatibility in which a mother with type O blood has a child with type A or B blood usually is so mild that it does not require treatment.

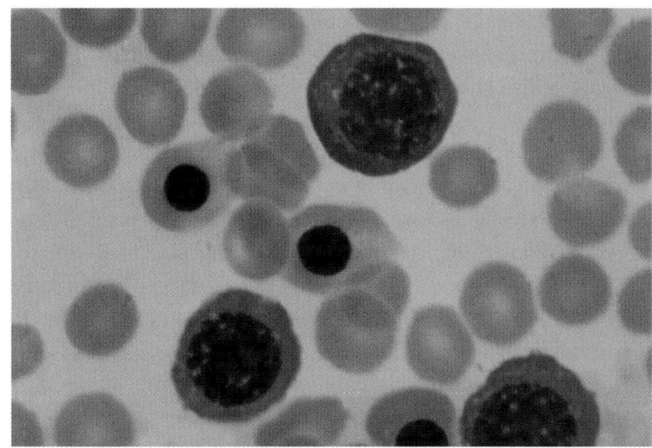

FIGURE 30-2 Rh Incompatibility in Hemolytic Disease of the Newborn. This micrograph shows immature red blood cells not normally found in blood. Large purple cells are erythroblasts; nucleated red blood cells are normoblasts. Normal red blood cells also are shown (× 500). (Copyright Ed Reschke.)

Rh incompatibility is more likely than ABO incompatibility to cause severe or even life-threatening anemia, death in utero, or damage to the central nervous system (CNS). Severe anemia alone can cause death as a result of cardiovascular complications (see Chapter 28). Extensive hemolysis also results in increased levels of unconjugated bilirubin in the circulation. If bilirubin levels exceed the liver's ability to conjugate and excrete bilirubin, some of it is deposited in the brain, causing cellular damage and eventually death, if exchange transfusions are not administered.

Fetuses that do not survive anemia in utero usually are stillborn, exhibiting gross edema throughout the entire body, a condition called **hydrops fetalis.** Death can occur as early as 17 weeks of gestation and results in spontaneous abortion.

CLINICAL MANIFESTATIONS. Neonates with mild HDN may appear healthy or slightly pale, with slight enlargement of the liver and spleen. Pronounced pallor, splenomegaly, and hepatomegaly indicate severe anemia, which predisposes the neonate to cardiovascular failure and shock. Life-threatening Rh incompatibility is rare today, largely because of maternal testing and the routine use of Rh immune globulin.

Because maternal antibodies remain in the neonatal circulation after birth, erythrocyte destruction can continue. This causes hyperbilirubinemia and **icterus neonatorum (neonatal jaundice)** that occurs shortly after birth. Without replacement transfusions, in which the child receives Rh-negative erythrocytes, the bilirubin is deposited in the brain, causing a condition termed **kernicterus.** Kernicterus produces cerebral damage and usually causes death **(icterus gravis neonatorum).** Infants who do not die may have significant developmental delay, cerebral palsy, or high-frequency deafness.

EVALUATION AND TREATMENT. Routine evaluation for HDN includes the Coombs test. The indirect Coombs test measures antibody in the mother's circulation and indicates whether the fetus is at risk for HDN. The direct Coombs test measures antibody already bound to the surfaces of fetal erythrocytes and is used primarily to confirm the diagnosis of antibody-mediated HDN. Determining prior history of fetal hemolytic disease, as well as diagnostic tests, may help predict the severity of the

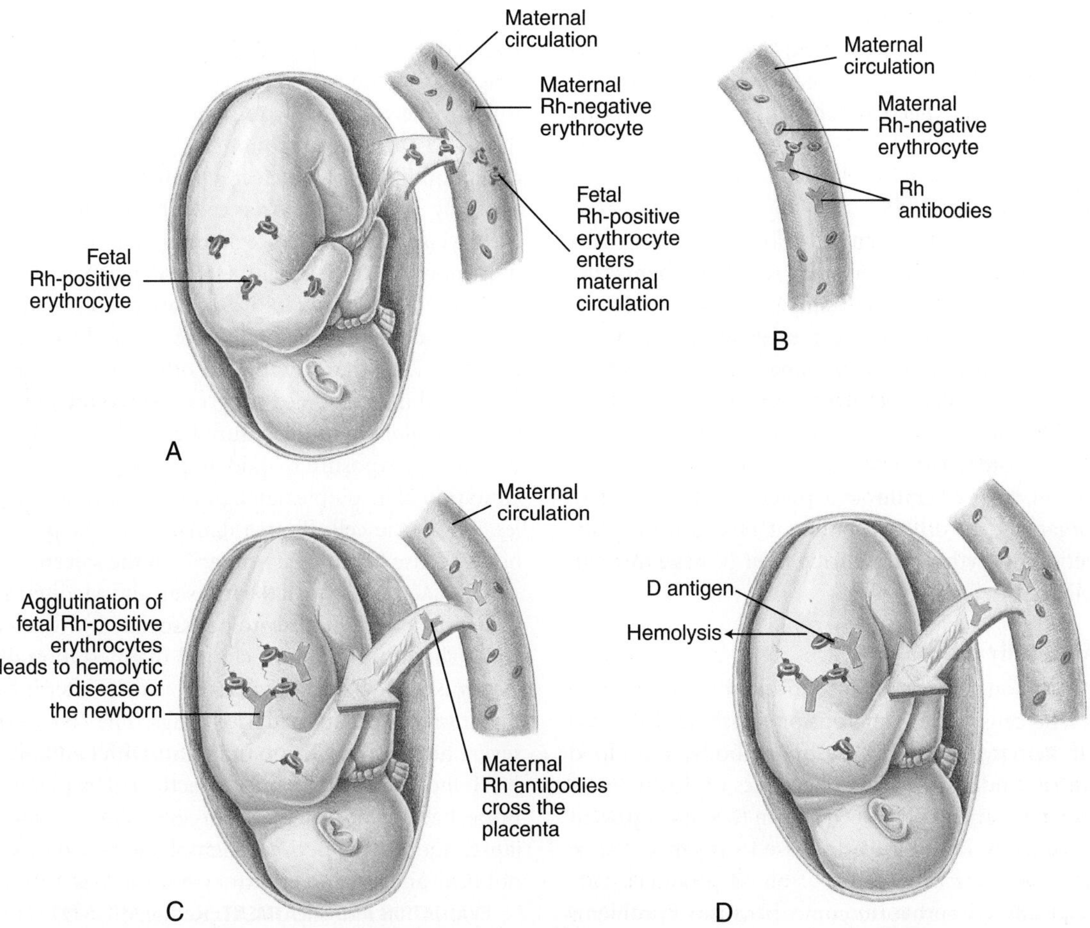

FIGURE 30-3 **Hemolytic Disease of the Newborn (HDN).** **A**, Before or during delivery, Rh-positive erythrocytes from the fetus enter the blood of an Rh-negative woman through a tear in the placenta. **B**, The mother is sensitized to the Rh antigen and produces Rh antibodies. Because this usually happens after delivery, there is no effect on the fetus in the first pregnancy. **C**, During a subsequent pregnancy with an Rh-positive fetus, Rh-positive erythrocytes cross the placenta, enter the maternal circulation, and **(D)** stimulate the mother to produce antibodies against the Rh antigen. The Rh antibodies from the mother cross the placenta, using agglutination and hemolysis of fetal erythrocytes, and HDN develops. (Modified from Seeley RR, Stephens TD, Tate P: *Anatomy and physiology*, ed 3, St Louis, 1995, Mosby.)

disorder. Diagnostic measures include maternal antibody titers, fetal blood sampling, amniotic fluid spectrophotometry, and ultrasound fetal assessment.[10]

The key to treatment of HDN resulting from Rh incompatibility lies in prevention (immunoprophylaxis). Rh immune globulin (RhoGAM), a preparation of antibody against Rh antigen D administered within 72 hours of exposure to Rh-positive erythrocytes, ensures that the mother will not produce antibody against the D antigen, and the next Rh-positive baby will be protected (Figure 30-3). The injected antibodies remain in the mother's bloodstream long enough to prevent her immune system from producing its own anti-Rh antibodies but not long enough to affect subsequent offspring. The mother must be given Rh immune globulin injections after the birth of each Rh-positive baby and after a miscarriage. The mother must be especially careful not to receive a transfusion containing Rh-positive blood, because this would stimulate production of anti-Rh antibodies. In many hospitals Rh immune globulin is given prophylactically at 28 weeks to all pregnant Rh-negative women with Rh-positive partners. Various international recommendations suggest that antenatal anti-D prophylaxis should be administered to unsensitized Rh(D)-negative women as a complement to postpartum prophylaxis.[11]

If antigenic incompatibility of the mother's erythrocytes is not discovered in time to administer Rh immune globulin and a child is born with HDN, treatment consists of exchange transfusions in which the neonate's blood is replaced with new Rh-positive blood that is not contaminated with anti-Rh antibodies. This treatment is instituted during the first 24 hours of extrauterine life to prevent kernicterus. Phototherapy also is used to reduce the toxic effects of unconjugated bilirubin.

Jaundice and indirect hyperbilirubinemia are reduced when the infant is exposed to high-intensity light in the visible spectrum from 420 to 470 nm. Bilirubin in the skin absorbs light energy, which, by photoisomerization, converts the toxic unconjugated bilirubin into conjugated isomers that are excreted in the bile. Phototherapy also causes autosensitization that results in oxidation reactions. Breakdown products from the oxidation reactions are excreted by the liver and kidney without need for conjugation. The therapeutic effect of phototherapy depends on the light energy emitted in the effective wavelengths, the distance between the infant and the light source, and the amount of skin exposed; the rate of hemolysis and the infant's ability to excrete bilirubin also are factors in determining the effectiveness of phototherapy in lowering serum bilirubin levels.

Anemia of Infectious Disease

Infections of the newborn, often initially acquired by the mother and transmitted to the fetus, may result in a hemolytic anemia with clinical manifestations similar to those of HDN. Congenital syphilis, toxoplasmosis, cytomegalic inclusion disease, rubella, coxsackievirus B infection, herpesvirus infection, and bacterial sepsis can cause hemolytic anemia in the neonate.

The exact mechanism of anemia caused by congenital infections is unclear. In some instances it is related to direct injury of erythrocyte membranes or erythrocyte precursors by the infectious microorganism. In other instances it results from traumatic destruction of erythrocytes during their passage through inflamed capillaries.

Anemia in Critically ILL Children

Anemia is a common occurrence in critically ill children (see Chapter 49). The causes are numerous and include decreased erythropoietin activity, poor iron use by the body, and blood loss from diverse conditions and consequences of treatment. A topic of discussion is anemia has been shown to worsen patient outcomes presumably because of decreased oxygen delivery. Controversial is whether transfusion of blood products, particularly packed RBCs, improve outcomes because of problems related to blood storage. New research is ongoing and needed to understand these problems, the development of new blood transfusion strategies, and blood substitutes.[11a]

Inherited Disorders

A number of inherited and intrinsic erythrocyte defects are known to cause increased hemolysis (see Table 30-2). These defects may be associated with enzymatic abnormalities that disrupt metabolic processes and prevent normal biochemical balance within the cell, with alterations of hemoglobin structure or synthesis, or with plasma membrane defects accompanied by changes in erythrocyte size or shape.

Glucose-6-Phosphate Dehydrogenase Deficiency

Glucose-6-phosphate dehydrogenase (G6PD) deficiency is an inherited, X-linked recessive disorder, most fully expressed in homozygous males, although partial expression and a carrier state are possible in heterozygous females. (X-linked inheritance is discussed in Chapter 4.) The deficiency is present in 10% of blacks and tends to occur in Sephardic Jews, Greeks, Iranians, Chinese, Filipinos, and Indonesians, with a frequency ranging from 5% to 40%.

PATHOPHYSIOLOGY. G6PD is an enzyme that normally enables erythrocytes to maintain metabolic processes despite injury, such as the presence of certain drugs (sulfonamides, antimalarial agents, salicylates, or naphthaquinolones); ingestion of fava beans (a dietary staple in some Mediterranean areas); hypoxemia; infection; fever; or acidosis. Therefore, G6PD deficiency is usually asymptomatic unless one of these events occurs. Erythrocyte damage in affected children begins after intense or prolonged exposure to one of these substances or conditions, and it will cease when they are removed. In black males the G6PD defect becomes more pronounced as the erythrocyte ages and in other populations the defect is profound even in young erythrocytes. By ingesting a substance with oxidant properties, such as a salicylate (aspirin), a pregnant woman may cause an episode of hemolysis in a fetus with G6PD deficiency.

In the absence of G6PD, oxidative stressors damage hemoglobin and the plasma membranes of erythrocytes and possibly interfere with the activities of other enzymes within the cell. Hemoglobin is oxidized progressively to methemoglobin, sulfmethemoglobin, and denatured globin-glutathione complexes. Eventually, exposure to oxidating substances results in the precipitation of insoluble hemoglobin inclusions, called *Heinz bodies*, within the cell. Plasma damage and the presence of Heinz bodies cause hemolysis, primarily in the spleen.

CLINICAL MANIFESTATIONS. In Asian and Mediterranean infants, G6PD deficiency is likely to be associated with icterus neonatorum. The most common clinical manifestation of G6PD deficiency is acute hemolytic anemia, usually after infections or the ingestion of certain oxidative drugs. The fava bean produces a severe hemolytic reaction in infants with G6PD deficiency.

Hemolytic episodes are characterized by pallor, icterus, dark urine, back pain, and, in severe cases, shock, cardiovascular collapse, and death. Between hemolytic episodes, the child does not have anemia and erythrocyte survival is normal.

EVALUATION AND TREATMENT. Reduced G6PD activity in erythrocytes is required for diagnosis. Immediately after a hemolytic episode, reticulocytes and young erythrocytes are evident. Because young erythrocytes have significantly higher enzyme activity than do older cells, laboratory evaluation should be performed shortly after a crisis so that a low level of enzyme activity can be demonstrated. G6PD activity that is within the low normal range in the presence of a high reticulocyte count suggests G6PD deficiency. G6PD deficiency also can be detected by electrophoretic analysis.

Prevention of hemolysis is the most important therapeutic measure. Males from high-risk groups (Greeks, southern Italians, Sephardic Jews, Filipinos, Chinese, Africans, Thais) should be tested for the defect before being given drugs known to be oxidative. When hemolysis occurs supportive treatment may include blood transfusions and oral iron therapy. Spontaneous recovery generally follows treatment.

Hereditary Spherocytosis

Hereditary spherocytosis (HS), also known as *congenital hemolytic anemia* or *congenital acholuric jaundice,* is the most common of the hemolytic disorders in which there is no hemoglobin abnormality.

PATHOPHYSIOLOGY. Transmitted as an autosomal dominant trait, HS represents approximately new mutations in about 25% of cases. The defect is believed to be caused by an undefined abnormality in the erythrocyte membrane. Affected cells are overly permeable to sodium and acquire a particular characteristic structure (Figure 30-4). An increased concentration of

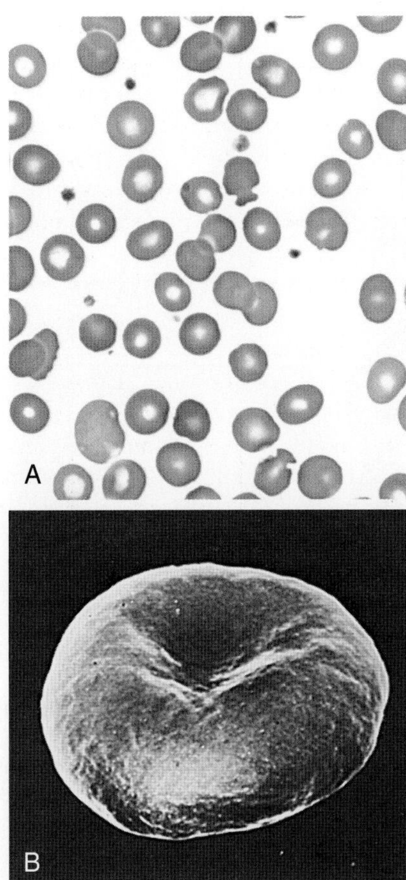

FIGURE 30-4 The Microspherocyte. A, Blood smear from individual with hereditary spherocytosis (Wright stain). **B**, Scanning electron micrograph. (**A** from Hoffbrand AV, Pettit JE, Vyas P: *Color atlas of clinical hematology,* ed 4, Philadelphia, 2009, Mosby. **B** courtesy Dr. M. Bessis. In Miale JB, editor: *Laboratory medicine: hematology,* ed 6, St Louis, 1982, Mosby.)

intracellular sodium is believed to lead to increased use of adenosine triphosphate (ATP) to drive the so-called cation pump. Early aging or destruction of erythrocytes is believed to result from metabolic overwork and loss of erythrocyte membrane.

The spleen is intimately involved in the hemolytic process. The spherocyte is relatively rigid and passes with difficulty through the small openings between the splenic cords and sinuses. Circulation of blood to the spleen creates repeated circulation through a metabolic environment that results in sequestration and destruction of spherocytes.

CLINICAL MANIFESTATIONS. The presenting signs of HS are anemia, jaundice, and splenomegaly. Anemia may be mild or absent in some cases depending on physiologic compensation. If this is the case the reticulocyte count will be elevated. Splenomegaly is usually mild. HS can present at any age, from the neonatal period until older adulthood. More severe types of HS present during the newborn period when the infant develops signs of hemolytic anemia and hyperbilirubinemia.[12] These children therefore may have life-threatening anemia with clinical symptoms ranging from difficulty feeding, circumoral pallor, tachycardia, nasal flaring, diaphoresis, and lethargy. They also are at increased risk for gallstones because of the presence of extra bile pigment. Infection (specifically parvovirus),[13] fever, and stress stimulate the spleen to destroy more red blood cells than usual, leading to a worsening anemia in an already baseline anemic child.

EVALUATION AND TREATMENT. It is important to ascertain family history of spherocytosis. Laboratory findings include spherocytes in the peripheral blood smear, elevated reticulocyte count (with or without anemia), indirect hyperbilirubinemia, and a positive osmotic fragility test. An osmotic fragility test is performed by placing red blood cells in a saline solution for 24 hours. Spherocytes do not tolerate saline solutions, thus causing them to burst more readily than normal red blood cells. Treatment of HS is based on disease severity. Although some children with HS will have severe anemia, blood transfusions are rarely required. Treatment before the age of 5 years consists of daily folic acid supplementation to increase production of healthy red blood cells. In the past, splenectomy was the first line of treatment. Currently, however, splenectomy is only recommended for those children more than 5 years of age with severe disease or those who develop symptomatic gallstones. Partial splenectomy, in which only a portion of the spleen is removed, is being performed on children with HS in an attempt to decrease the risk of postsplenectomy complications.[14]

Sickle Cell Disease

Sickle cell disease (SCD) is a group of disorders characterized by the presence of an abnormal form of hemoglobin—**hemoglobin S (HbS)**—within the erythrocytes. Hb S is formed by a genetic mutation in which one amino acid (valine) replaces another (glutamic acid) (Figure 30-5, *A*). Hb S, also known as sickle hemoglobin, reacts to deoxygenation and dehydration by solidifying and stretching the erythrocyte into an elongated sickle shape. This change causes a variety of pathologic consequences, including hemolytic anemia.

SCD is an inherited autosomal recessive disorder that is expressed as sickle cell anemia, sickle cell–thalassemia disease, or sickle cell–Hb C disease, depending on mode of inheritance (Table 30-3). (See Chapter 4 for a discussion of genetic inheritance of disease.) **Sickle cell anemia,** a homozygous form, is the most severe. **Sickle cell–thalassemia disease** and **sickle cell–Hb C disease** are heterozygous forms in which the child simultaneously inherits another type of abnormal hemoglobin from one parent. **Sickle cell trait,** in which the child inherits Hb S from one parent and normal hemoglobin (Hb A) from the other, is a heterozygous carrier state that rarely has clinical manifestations. All forms of SCD are lifelong conditions. Bone marrow or stem cell transplants can cure sickle cell anemia. However, they are currently not an option for most children because it is often difficult to find well-matched stem cell donors.

SCD tends to occur in people with origins in equatorial countries, particularly central Africa, the Near East, the Mediterranean, and parts of India. In the United States, about 1 out of 500 black children and 1:36,000 Hispanic-American born have sickle cell anemia. Most infants with SCD born in the United States are now identified by routine neonatal screening. Sickle cell trait occurs among about 1:12 blacks and 1:100 Hispanic-Americans. It is estimated that 2.5 million Americans are heterozygous carriers for the sickle cell trait.[15] The sickle cell

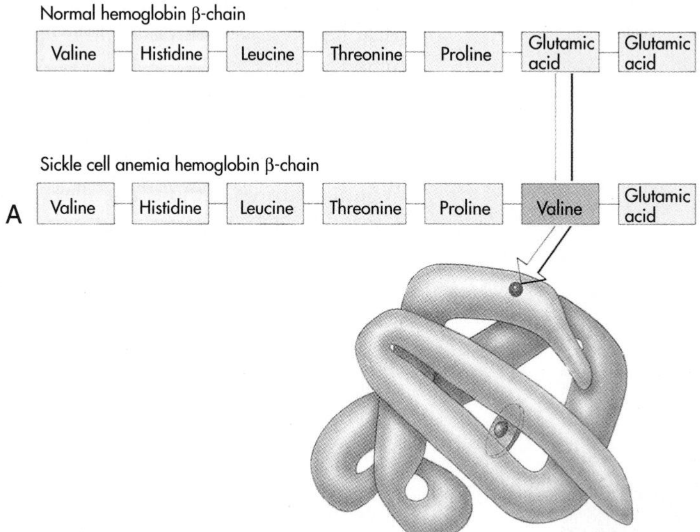

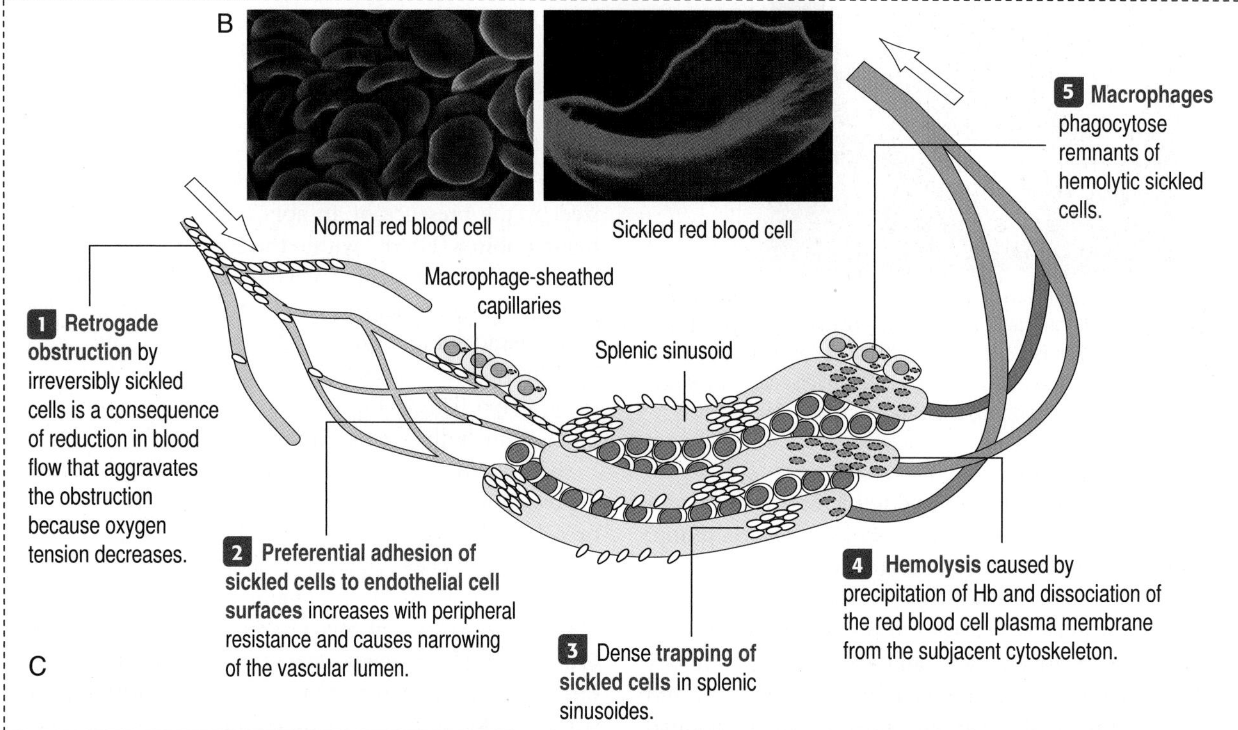

Sickle cell anemia is determined by the substitution of normal hemoglobin (Hb A) by hemoglobin S (Hb S) caused by a point mutation (replacement of the nucleotide triplet CTC coding glutamic acid at the mRNA level [GAG] by the CAC triplet [GUG] coding for valine) that modifies the physicochemical properties of the β-globin chain of hemoglobin. All hemoglobin is abnormal in homozygous individuals for the mutant gene, and red blood cells show a sickling deformity and hemolytic anemia in the presence or absence of normal oxygen tension. Heterozygous individuals contain a mixture of Hb A and Hb S, and sickling and anemia are observed when the tension of oxygen decreases.

Irreversibly sickled red blood cells are trapped within the splenic sinusoids and are destroyed by adjacent macrophages. Hemolysis may also occur in the macrophage-sheathed capillaries of the red pulp.

FIGURE 30-5 **Sickle Cell Hemoglobin.** **A,** Sickle cell hemoglobin is produced by a recessive allele of the gene encoding the β-chain of the protein hemoglobin. It represents a single amino acid change—from glutamic acid to valine at the sixth position on the chain. In this model of a hemoglobin molecule, the position of the mutation can be seen near the end of the upper arm. **B,** Color-enhanced electron micrograph shows normal erythrocytes. **C,** Illustration of the characteristic shape of a red blood cell containing the abnormal hemoglobin. (**A** from Raven PH, Johnson GB: *Biology,* ed 3, St Louis, 1992, Mosby. **B** copyright Dennis Kunkel Microscopy, Inc. **C** from Miale JB: *Laboratory medicine: hematology,* ed 6, St Louis, 1982, Mosby.)

TABLE 30-3 INHERITANCE OF SICKLE CELL DISEASE*

HEMOGLOBIN (Hb) INHERITED FROM FIRST PARENT	HEMOGLOBIN INHERITED FROM SECOND PARENT	FORM OF SICKLE CELL DISEASE IN CHILD
Hb S (an abnormal Hb)	Hb S	Sickle cell anemia: homozygous inheritance in which the child's Hb is mostly Hb S, with the remainder fetal hemoglobin (Hb F)
Hb S	Defective or insufficient α- or β-chains of Hb A (alpha- or beta-thalassemia)	Sickle cell: thalassemia disease (heterozygous inheritance of Hb S and alpha- or beta-thalassemia)
Hb S	Hb C or D (both abnormal Hb)	Sickle cell: Hb C (or D) disease (heterozygous inheritance of Hb S and either Hb C or Hb D)
Hb S	Normal Hb (mostly Hb A)	Sickle cell trait, the carrier state (heterozygous inheritance of Hb S and normal Hb)

*See Chapter 27 for a description of normal fetal and adult hemoglobins.

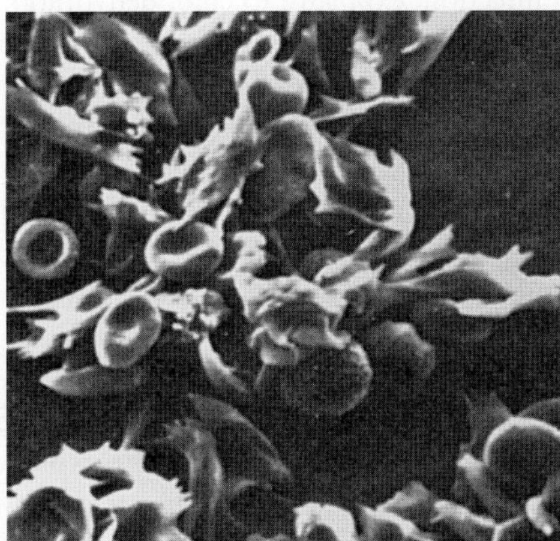

FIGURE 30-6 Normal and Sickle-Shaped Blood Cells. Scanning electron micrograph of normal and sickle-shaped red blood cells. The irregularly shaped cells are the sickle cells; the circular cells are the normal blood cells. (From Raven PH, Johnson GB: *Biology*, ed 3, St Louis, 1992, Mosby.)

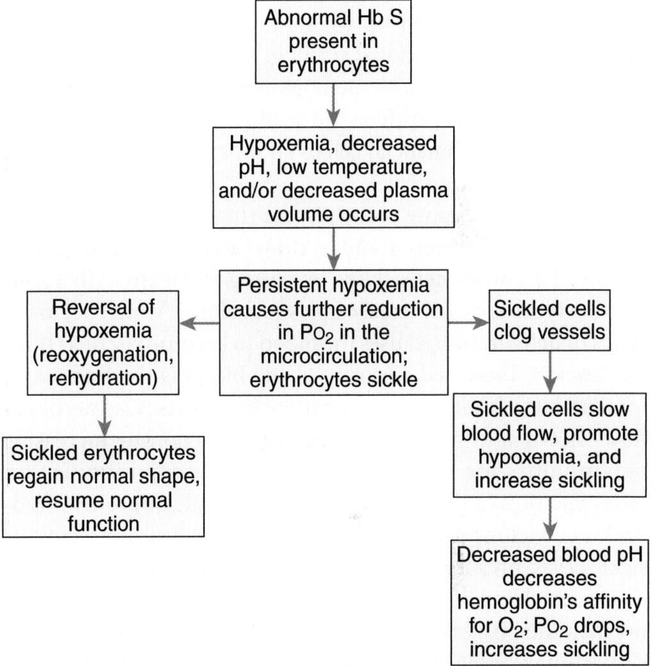

FIGURE 30-7 Sickling of Erythrocytes.

trait may provide protection against lethal forms of malaria, a genetic advantage to carriers who reside in endemic regions for malaria (Mediterranean and African zones) but no advantage to carriers living in the United States.

PATHOPHYSIOLOGY. Deoxygenation is probably the most important variable in determining the occurrence of sickling. The degree of deoxygenation required to produce sickling varies with the percentage of Hb S in the cells. Sickle trait cells will sickle at oxygen tensions of about 15 mmHg, whereas those from an individual with SCD will begin to sickle at about 40 mmHg. Hb S that is not bound with oxygen forms aggregates of semisolid gel that become stacked within the erythrocyte, stretching it into an elongated crescent (see Figure 30-5, *C*; Figure 30-6). Sickled erythrocytes are stiff and cannot change shape as easily as normal cells when they pass through the microcirculation. (The reversible deformability of erythrocytes is described in Chapter 27.) As a result, sickled erythrocytes tend to plug the blood vessels, causing vascular occlusion, pain, and organ infarction. Sickled cells undergo hemolysis in the spleen or become sequestered there, causing blood pooling and infarction of splenic vessels. The anemia that follows triggers erythropoiesis in the marrow and, in extreme cases, in the liver.[16]

Most sickled erythrocytes regain a normal shape after reoxygenation and rehydration. Irreversible sickling is not caused by irreversible hemoglobin changes but rather by irreversible plasma membrane damage caused by sickling. The precise nature of the permanent membrane injury is not known, but it is known that while in the sickled state, the plasma membrane loses some of its capacity for active transport, permitting an influx of calcium ions. (Membrane transport and the effects of calcium influx are described in Chapters 1 and 2.) In people with sickle cell anemia, in which the erythrocytes contain a high percentage of Hb S (75% to 95%), up to 30% of the erythrocytes can become irreversibly sickled. Occasionally, irreversible sickling occurs in SCD but not in children with sickle cell trait.

Sickling is an occasional, intermittent phenomenon that can be triggered or sustained by one or more of the following stressors: decreased oxygen tension (Po_2) of the blood (i.e., hypoxemia), increased hydrogen ion concentration in the blood (decreased pH), increased plasma osmolality, decreased plasma volume, and low temperature (Figure 30-7).

The same decrease in Po_2 will cause the most sickling in persons with sickle cell anemia (high concentrations of Hb S), the second most in children with sickle cell thalassemia, the third most in those with sickle cell–Hb C disease, and the least or none in those with sickle cell trait. The duration of the Po_2 decrease also is important, because sickling tends to occur only after the inciting stimulus has been present for some time.

The level of Po_2 in the microcirculation also affects sickling because hemoglobin releases the oxygen it is carrying to tissues. The Po_2 normally is lower in the microcirculation. The added reduction in Po_2 caused by persistent hypoxemia—induced by stressors—eventually results in sickling in the microcirculation of all cells that contain Hb S in that site (not throughout the body). Sickling within the microcirculation decreases blood flow as sickled cells clog the vessels. Reduced blood flow causes hypoxemia to worsen and perpetuates sickling. Finally, decreased blood pH reduces hemoglobin's affinity for oxygen. As less oxygen is taken up by hemoglobin in the lungs, Po_2 drops, promoting additional sickling.

Polymerization of sickle hemoglobin is central to the disorder. **Polymerization** stiffens the sickled erythrocyte, changing it from a flexible, beneficial cell to an inflexible one that starves and damages tissues.

Increased osmolality of the plasma (increased concentration of solutes; see Chapters 1 and 3) draws water out of the erythrocytes. This promotes sickling by raising the relative Hb S content in erythrocytes. Decreased plasma volume, which occurs in states of dehydration, causes the blood to become viscous (thick and sticky). Increased viscosity of the blood is the final common pathway leading to many pathologic effects. Viscous blood flows slowly and promotes vascular obstruction by increasing opportunities for sickling while decreasing opportunities for reoxygenation in the lungs. This is an example of positive feedback in a vicious cycle of events. Low temperatures precipitate sickle crisis, presumably because of vasoconstriction.[17]

Once sickling begins, it tends to continue until Po_2 returns to normal; then it ceases spontaneously. The extent, severity, and clinical manifestations of sickling depend to a great extent on the percentage of hemoglobin that is Hb S. That is why homozygous inheritance of Hb S produces the severest form of SCD—sickle cell anemia. Heterozygous inheritance of SCD results in less sickling because the individual's erythrocytes contain other forms of abnormal hemoglobin that although defective, do not contribute to sickling to any great degree. Heterozygous inheritance (sickle cell trait), in which abnormal hemoglobin is inherited from one parent and normal hemoglobin from the other, rarely results in sickling because normal Hb F and Hb A do not contribute to sickling at all. Anemia persists because Hb F does not live 120 days.

CLINICAL MANIFESTATIONS. Clinical manifestations of SCD may first be seen at 6 to 12 months of age as fetal hemoglobin is replaced by Hb S. Two characteristics of SCD determine presentation: the first is its nature to be a chronic disease with acute exacerbations; the second is that it is a condition affecting RBCs that supply oxygen to all cells of the body. Therefore, SCD can affect any part of the body. When sickling occurs, the general manifestations of hemolytic anemia—pallor, fatigue, jaundice, and irritability—sometimes are accompanied by acute manifestations called *crises*. Extensive sickling can precipitate four types of crises: (1) vaso-occlusive (or thrombotic) crisis, (2) aplastic crisis, (3) sequestration crisis, or rarely (4) hyperhemolytic crisis. Sites of specific dysfunction are shown in Figure 30-8.

Vaso-occlusive crisis (thrombotic crisis) begins with sickling in the microcirculation. As blood flow is obstructed by tangled masses of rigid, sickled cells, vasospasm occurs and a "log jam" effect brings all blood flow through the vessel to a halt. Unless the process is reversed, thrombosis and infarction (death caused by lack of oxygen) of local tissue follow. Vaso-occlusive crisis is extremely painful and may last for days or even weeks, with an average duration of 4 to 6 days. The frequency of this type of crisis is variable and unpredictable.

Vaso-occlusive crises may develop spontaneously or be precipitated by infection, exposure to cold, dehydration, low Po_2, acidosis (low pH), or localized hypoxemia. Symmetric, painful swelling of the hands and feet (hand-foot syndrome) caused by infarction in the small vessels of the extremities often is the initial manifestation of SCD in infancy. In older children and adults the large joints and surrounding tissue become painful and swollen. Priapism (persistent erection of the penis) may occur if penile veins become obstructed. Severe abdominal pains often are caused by infarction in abdominal structures. Strokes resulting from cerebral occlusion may leave the child with paralysis (usually hemiplegia) or other CNS deficits.

Aplastic crisis, a transient cessation in red blood cell production resulting in acute anemia, occurs as a result of a viral infection, almost always infection with parvovirus B19, which is the virus responsible for the common childhood infection known as fifth disease. The virus causes temporary shutdown of RBC production in the bone marrow. However, hemolysis, the destruction of RBCs, continues. The outcome is a severe drop in hemoglobin with an extremely low reticulocyte count.

In **sequestration crisis** large amounts of blood become pooled in the liver and spleen. This type of crisis is seen only in young children. Because the spleen can hold as much as one fifth of the blood supply at one time, mortality rates up to 50% have been reported, with death caused by cardiovascular collapse. If blood volume and pressure are maintained by hydration and blood transfusion, much of the sequestered blood eventually returns to circulation. Removal of the spleen is the treatment for recurrent sequestration crises and may be performed after the child reaches 5 years of age.[18]

Hyperhemolytic crisis, an accelerated rate of RBC destruction, is unusual but may occur in association with certain drugs or infections. It is characterized by anemia, jaundice, and reticulocytosis. The concomitant presence of G6PD deficiency (see p.1062) contributes to hyperhemolytic episodes, especially when combined with infections.

Acute chest syndrome is the presence of a new pulmonary infiltrate (not atelectasis), involving at least one complete lung segment and chest pain, a temperature of more than 38.5° C (101.3° F) increased respiratory rate (tachypnea), wheezing, or cough. Sickled RBCs attach to the endothelium of the injured, underventilated, and inflamed lung and, as they fail to be reoxygenated, will eventually undergo additional inflammation and lung infarction. The prognosis is poor, and infarction is a

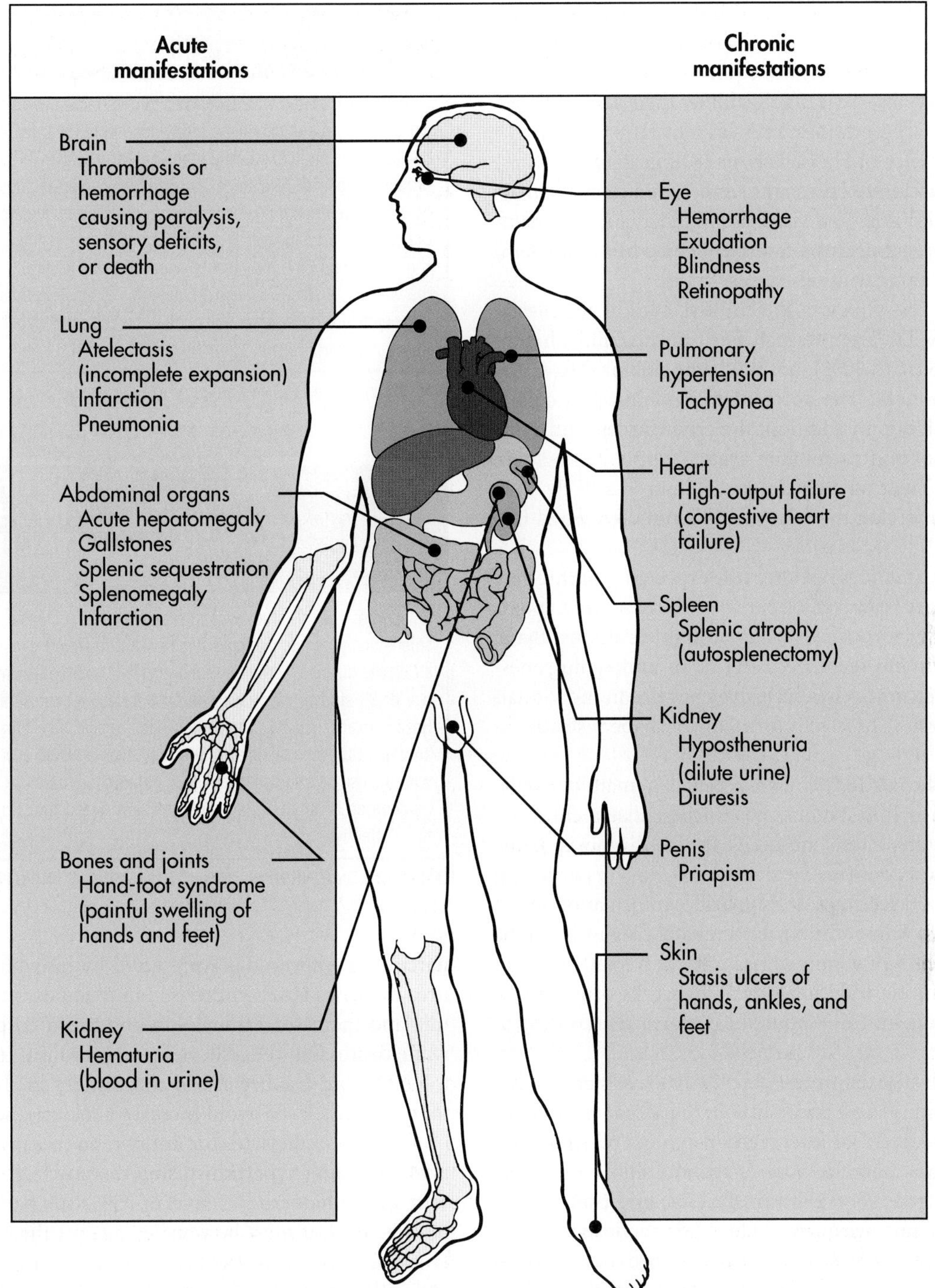

FIGURE 30-8 Clinical Manifestations of Sickle Cell Disease.

leading cause of morbidity. Acute chest syndrome is the cause of death in approximately 25% of all deaths in people with SCD.[19]

Infection is the most common cause of death resulting from SCD. Sepsis and meningitis develop in as many as 10% of children with sickle cell anemia during the first 5 years of life, with a mortality rate of 25%. Survival time is unpredictable, and many young adults die in their 20s.

Glomerular disease, characterized by damage to the glomeruli allowing protein and often red blood cells to leak into the urine, is caused by sickling of red blood cells in the kidneys. Extensive damage to the glomeruli results in nephropathy that may progress to renal failure. The earliest manifestation of SCD in the kidney is hyposthenuria, or the inability of the tubules of the kidneys to concentrate urine. Very low urine specific gravity occurs and in young children this often results in bed-wetting. Proteinuria also is an early manifestation of sickle nephropathy.

Cholecystitis, inflammation of the gallbladder that occurs when a gallstone blocks the cystic duct, can be caused by hemolysis resulting in an increase of bilirubin, which in turn causes the formation of gallstones in the gallbladder. The presence of gallstones can cause right upper quadrant pain, nausea, vomiting, and an elevated white blood cell count and alkaline phosphatase. Cholecystectomy may be required.

Sickle cell–Hb C disease is usually milder than sickle cell anemia. The peripheral blood smear reveals many target cells resulting from the presence of Hb C. The main clinical problems are related to vaso-occlusive crises and are believed to result from higher hematocrit values and viscosity. In older children, sickle cell retinopathy, renal necrosis, and aseptic necrosis of the femoral heads occur along with obstructive crises.

Sickle cell–thalassemia has the mildest clinical manifestations of all the SCDs. Even though most of the child's hemoglobin is Hb S (60% to 90%), normal hemoglobins (Hb A and Hb F) also are present. The normal hemoglobins, particularly Hb F, inhibit sickling. In addition, the erythrocytes tend to be small (microcytic) and to contain relatively little hemoglobin (hypochromic). Their small size makes them less likely than normal-size cells to clog the microcirculation, even when in a sickled state.

The sickle cell trait does not affect life expectancy or interfere with daily activities. However, on rare occasions, severe hypoxia caused by shock, vigorous exercising at high elevations, flying at high altitudes in unpressurized aircraft, or undergoing anesthesia is associated with vaso-occlusive episodes in individuals with sickle cell trait. These cells form an ivy shape instead of a sickle shape.

EVALUATION AND TREATMENT. The parents' hematologic history and clinical manifestations may suggest that a child has SCD, but hematologic tests are necessary for diagnosis. If the sickle solubility test confirms the presence of Hb S in peripheral blood, hemoglobin electrophoresis provides information about the amount of Hb S in erythrocytes. Prenatal diagnosis can be made by chorionic villus sampling as early as 8 to 10 weeks of gestation or amniotic fluid analysis at 15 weeks of gestation. Newborn screening for SCD should be performed according to state law.

Treatment advances since the late 1980s have significantly decreased morbidity and mortality in children with SCD. Aggressive management of fever, early diagnosis of *acute chest syndrome* (hypoxia, anemia, progressive multilobar pneumonia, fat emboli), red blood cell transfusions, and proper pain management can improve quality of life and prognosis for these children. Treatment of SCD consists of supportive care aimed at preventing consequences of anemia and avoiding crises. Crises can be prevented by avoiding fever, infection, acidosis, dehydration, constricting clothes, and exposure to cold. Immediate correction of acidosis and dehydration with appropriate intravenous fluids is imperative. In addition to routine childhood immunizations, children with SCD should receive an annual influenza vaccine and also pneumococcal and meningococcal vaccine series to prevent infection (Box 30-1). Infections require aggressive antibiotic therapy. Oxygen is not needed unless the child becomes hypoxic. Pain associated with SCD is very complex, requiring accurate assessment and multimodal management.[20]

Protocols to implement individual-controlled analgesia in the emergency department shorten the time of initiation of narcotic therapy and are preferred by individuals.[21] Hydroxyurea increases Hb F synthesis in individuals with sickle cell anemia and increases hemoglobin and mean corpuscular volume while decreasing reticulocytes and bilirubin. It is safe and well tolerated and has been used successfully in children for more than 10 years.[22] To avoid increased acidosis, acetaminophen is preferable to salicylates for antipyretic therapy. Blood transfusion, including hypertransfusion therapy (e.g., packed RBCs to raise the hematocrit to a level of 35% for a period of time), can be effective but must be weighed against the risks of hemosiderosis and iron and splenic overload. Oral maintenance therapy with folic acid is needed to meet the increased demands of chronic hemolytic anemia. Laparoscopic splenectomy has been demonstrated to be safe and effective in children with recurrent sequestration crises and is associated with minimal complications, zero mortality, and a short hospital stay. Partial splenectomy has been recently evaluated and appears to be successful in children (Box 30-2). The most definitive approach to the treatment of SCD requires a permanent alteration in the hemoglobin phenotype. This can be accomplished through stem cell transplantation, although well-matched donors are difficult to identify.

Genetic counseling and psychologic support are important for the child and family. Recently, a genetic technique called **preimplantation genetic diagnosis** has been performed on parents

BOX 30-1 PNEUMOCOCCAL VACCINE FOR SICKLE CELL DISEASE

A systematic review was conducted to determine the efficacy of pneumococcal vaccines in preventing morbidity and mortality in patients with sickle cell disease. Two authors searched the Cochrane Cystic Fibrosis and Genetic Disorders Group Trials Register and critically reviewed and determined the quality of randomized and quasi-experimental trials that compared a polysaccharide or conjugate pneumococcal vaccine to a different regimen or no vaccine. Nine trials including 547 participants were included. Overall results suggest that the vaccine is able to induce an immune response in these patients. Clinical outcomes of effectiveness still need to be determined, but the vaccine is safe to use in children.

Data from Davies EG et al: *Cochrane Database Syst Rev* 2012(2), 2012.

BOX 30-2 DIFFERENT TYPES OF SPLENECTOMY IN CHILDREN WITH CONGENITAL HEMOLYTIC ANEMIAS

The purpose of this study was to evaluate the effectiveness of partial or total splenectomy on hematologic function and adverse events in children with sickle cell disease, hereditary spherocytosis, and thalassemias. The methodology of 93 studies was assessed on the basis of the Agency for Healthcare Research and Quality criteria. No hematologic advantage was determined between the types of splenectomy; however, adverse events were minimized with the use of laparoscopy. Results determined there is a need for additional randomized controlled trials, but both partial and total splenectomy appears to be effective.

Data from Rice HE et al: *J Pediatr* 160:684–689, 2012.

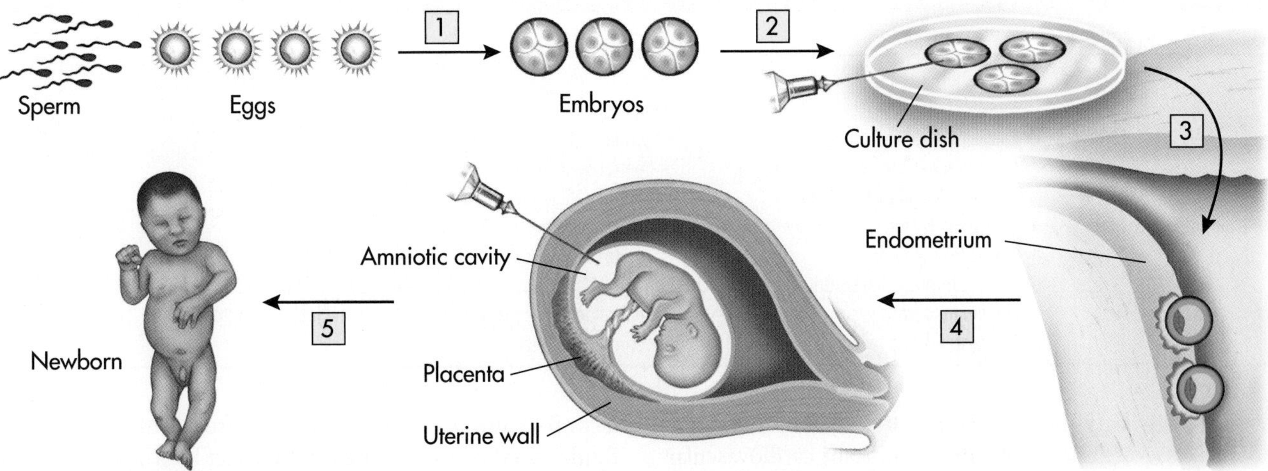

FIGURE 30-9 Prepregnancy sickle cell test. (This technique has potential for other inherited diseases.) **1**, Fertilization produces several embryos. **2**, The embryos are tested for the presence of the gene. **3**, The embryo(s) without the gene are implanted. **4**, Amniocentesis confirms whether the fetus (or fetuses) has the sickle cell gene. **5**, Woman has a normal child.

to diagnose whether their offspring will carry the gene for SCD. Figure 30-9 summarizes this prepregnancy sickle cell test. Genetic counseling enables people with SCD or trait to make informed decisions about transmitting this genetic disorder to their offspring because there is a 25% chance with each pregnancy that a child born to two parents with sickle cell trait will have SCD.

Thalassemias

The alpha- and beta-thalassemias are inherited autosomal recessive disorders that cause an impaired rate of synthesis of one of the two chains—α or β—of Hb A. The disorder was named **thalassemia,** which is derived from the Greek word for *sea,* because it was defined initially in people with origins near the Mediterranean Sea. Beta-thalassemia, in which synthesis of the β-globin chain is slowed or defective, is prevalent among Greeks, Italians, and some Arabs and Sephardic Jews. Alpha-thalassemia, in which the α-chain is affected, is most common among Chinese, Vietnamese, Cambodians, and Laotians. Both alpha- and beta-thalassemia are common among blacks.

Alpha- and beta-thalassemia is characterized as major or minor, depending on how many of the genes that control α- or β-chain synthesis are defective and whether the defects are inherited homozygously (thalassemia major) or heterozygously (thalassemia minor). Pathophysiologic effects range from mild microcytosis to death in utero, depending on the number of defective genes and mode of inheritance. Anemia associated with thalassemia is microcytic-hypochromic hemolytic anemia.

PATHOPHYSIOLOGY. Normally two genes control β-chain synthesis and four genes control α-chain synthesis. The number of genetic defects in the controlling genes determines the severity of the disorder. As in SCD the hemoglobin abnormality usually consists of the substitution of a single amino acid for another amino acid. Other molecular abnormalities that cause thalassemia are two amino acid substitutions, amino acid deletions or fusions, and synthesis of elongated chains.

The fundamental defect in beta-thalassemia is the uncoupling of α- and β-chain synthesis. β-Chain production is depressed—moderately in the heterozygous form, **beta-thalassemia minor,** and severely in the homozygous form, **beta-thalassemia major** (also called **Cooley anemia**). Depression of β-chain synthesis results in erythrocytes having a reduced amount of hemoglobin and accumulations of free α-chains. The free α-chains are unstable and easily precipitate in the cell. Most erythroblasts that contain precipitates are destroyed by mononuclear phagocytes in the marrow, resulting in ineffective erythropoiesis and anemia. Some of the precipitate-carrying cells do mature and enter the bloodstream, but they are destroyed prematurely in the spleen, resulting in mild hemolytic anemia.

There are four forms of alpha-thalassemia:

1. **Alpha trait** (the carrier state), in which a single α-chain–forming gene is defective
2. **Alpha-thalassemia minor,** in which two genes are defective
3. **Hemoglobin H disease,** in which three genes are defective
4. **Alpha-thalassemia major,** a fatal condition in which all four alpha-forming genes are defective; death is inevitable because α-chains are absent and oxygen cannot be released to the tissues

Beta-thalassemia occurs more commonly than does alpha-thalassemia. Occasionally synthesis of γ- or δ-polypeptide chains is defective, resulting in gamma- or delta-thalassemia. (Hemoglobin chains are described in Chapter 27.)

CLINICAL MANIFESTATIONS. Beta-thalassemia minor causes mild to moderate microcytic-hypochromic hemolytic anemia, mild splenomegaly, bronze coloring of the skin, and hyperplasia of the bone marrow. The degree of reticulocytosis depends on the severity of the anemia, resulting in skeletal changes. Hemolysis of immature (and therefore fragile) erythrocytes may cause a slight elevation in serum iron and indirect bilirubin levels. Persons with beta-thalassemia minor usually are asymptomatic.

TABLE 30-4 THE COAGULATION FACTORS

CLOTTING FACTORS	SYNONYM	DISORDER
I	Fibrinogen	Congenital deficiency (afibrinogenemia) and dysfunction (dysfibrinogenemia)
II	Prothrombin	Congenital deficiency or dysfunction
V	Labile factor, proaccelerin	Congenital deficiency (parahemophilia)
VII	Stable factor or proconvertin	Congenital deficiency
VIII	Antihemophilic factor (AHF)	Congenital deficiency is hemophilia A (classic hemophilia)
IX	Christmas factor	Congenital deficiency is hemophilia B
X	Stuart-Power factor	Congenital deficiency
XI	Plasma thromboplastin antecedent	Congenital deficiency, sometimes referred to as hemophilia C
XII	Hageman factor	Congenital deficiency is *not* associated with clinical symptoms
XIII	Fibrin-stabilizing factor	Congenital deficiency

Persons with beta-thalassemia major may become quite ill. Anemia is severe and results in a significant cardiovascular burden, with high-output congestive heart failure. In the past, death resulted from cardiac failure. Today, blood transfusions can increase life span by one to two decades, and death usually is caused by hemochromatosis (from transfusions). (Hemosiderosis and hematochromatosis are described in Chapters 27 and 28.) Liver enlargement occurs as a result of progressive hemosiderosis, whereas enlargement of the spleen is caused by extramedullary hematopoiesis and increased destruction of red blood cells. Spinal impairment that starts in infancy retards linear growth and subsequent upper and lower limb-length discrepancy. Bone marrow hyperplasia causes a characteristic deformity of the facial bones, as the nasal bridge, mandible, and maxilla widen. Osteopenia or osteochondrosis, or both, may develop.

People who inherit the mildest form of alpha-thalassemia, the alpha trait, usually are symptom free, having, at most, mild microcytosis. Alpha-thalassemia minor has clinical manifestations that are virtually identical to those of beta-thalassemia minor: mild microcytic-hypochromic reticulocytosis, bone marrow hyperplasia, increased serum iron concentrations, and moderate splenomegaly.

Signs and symptoms of alpha-thalassemia are similar to those of beta-thalassemia major but milder. Moderate microcytic-hypochromic anemia, enlargement of the liver and spleen, and bone marrow hyperplasia are evident.

Alpha-thalassemia major causes hydrops fetalis and fulminant intrauterine congestive heart failure. In addition to edema and massive ascites, the fetus has a grossly enlarged heart and liver. Diagnosis usually is made postmortem. Prenatal screening for this disorder can be performed by use of chorionic villus sampling. These cells can be analyzed, and a deoxyribonucleic acid (DNA) genetic map can be constructed and evaluated for the characteristic abnormalities associated with hydrops fetalis.

Alpha-thalassemia major and beta-thalassemia major are life threatening. Children with thalassemia major generally are weak, fail to thrive, show poor development, and experience cardiovascular compromise with high-output failure caused by anemia. Untreated, they will die by 5 to 6 years of age.

EVALUATION AND TREATMENT. Diagnosis of thalassemia is based on familial disease history, clinical manifestations, and blood tests. Peripheral blood smears show microcytosis and hemoglobin electrophoresis demonstrates diminished amounts of α- or β-chains. Analysis of fetal DNA from withdrawn amniotic fluid is used as a screening test to detect hydrops fetalis (alpha-thalassemia major). Newborn screening for thalassemia should be done according to state law.

"Silent" carriers or those who have thalassemia minor generally have few if any symptoms and require no specific treatment. Therapies to support and prolong life are necessary, however, for thalassemia major. Prenatal diagnosis and genetic counseling may be the most important therapeutic measures offered.

At present, thalassemia major is treated with the following therapies:

1. Blood transfusions, which can return hemoglobin and hematocrit levels to normal thus alleviating the anemia-induced cardiac failure; iron overload and hemochromatosis are complications of transfusion therapy
2. Iron chelation therapy in combination with hypertransfusion (transfusion to a hematocrit of 35 ml/dl)
3. Splenectomy, which can reduce the need for transfusions by eliminating the site of hemolysis, thus prolonging erythrocyte survival
4. Bone marrow, cord blood, and stem cell transplantation is currently the only cure for thalassemia

DISORDERS OF COAGULATION AND PLATELETS

Inherited Hemorrhagic Disease

Hemophilias

Awareness of a serious bleeding disorder in males was documented nearly 2000 years ago in the Babylonian Talmud, which exempted from the rite of circumcision those boys having male relatives prone to excessive bleeding. In 1803 the first description of this disorder appeared in the medical literature, where it was noted to be X linked and associated with joint bleeding and crippling.

Table 30-4 lists the coagulation factors. Until 1952 the term *hemophilia* was reserved for deficiency of factor VIII (antihemophilic factor). Since then two additional coagulation proteins, factor IX (plasma thromboplastin component [PTC]) and factor XI (plasma thromboplastin antecedent [PTA]), have been identified and their deficiency associated with similar clinical manifestations. Congenital deficiencies of these three plasma clotting factors—VIII, IX, XI—account for 90% to 95% of the hemorrhagic bleeding disorders collectively called *hemophilia.*

Types of Hemophilia. **Hemophilia A (classic hemophilia)** is caused by factor VIII deficiency and occurs in 1 in 5000 male births.[23] It is the most common of the hemophilias—80% to 85% of those with hemophilia have hemophilia A. It is inherited as an X-linked recessive disorder that affects men and is transmitted by women.

Hemophilia B (Christmas disease), caused by factor IX deficiency, also is transmitted as an X-linked recessive trait and is clinically indistinguishable from factor VIII deficiency. It occurs in 1:25,000 male births.[23] Hemophilia A and hemophilia B occur with varying degrees of clinical severity, depending on concentrations of clotting factor VIII or IX in the blood. Severe hemophilia (concentration of clotting factors less than 1% of normal) is associated with spontaneous bleeding. In moderate hemophilia (1% to 5% of normal), bleeding usually occurs only after trauma; in the mild form (5% to 35% of normal), bleeding occurs only after severe trauma or surgery. The severity of hemophilia is similar in all affected members of a family.

Hemophilia C (factor XI deficiency) occurs as an autosomal recessive disease and occurs equally in men and women. Bleeding usually is less severe than in hemophilia A or B.

von Willebrand disease results from an inherited autosomal dominant trait with variable clinical manifestations and hematologic findings. The factor VIII deficiency differs from that of hemophilia A in mode of inheritance and response to treatment. In hemophilia A the deficiency is inherited as an X-linked recessive trait, whereas in von Willebrand disease, it is inherited as an autosomal dominant trait. The most important difference, however, is in responses to the infusion of plasma. In von Willebrand disease, infusion of desmopressin acetate (DDAVP) causes factor VIII activity to increase for several days because infusion of factor VIII temporarily induces endogenous synthesis of factor VIII.

PATHOPHYSIOLOGY. Two types of defects dominate the hereditary defects of hemophilia to date: gene deletions and point mutations. Both types of genetic defects are associated with severe hemophilia A, in which no factor VIII circulates in the blood. Many different gene deletion mutations are associated with factor VIII and factor IX disease. The molecular defect that leads to the deletional mutation is identical among members of a given family.[24]

Point mutations, in which a single base in the DNA is mutated to another base, represent a second type of mutation that causes hemophilia. When a point mutation gives rise to a de novo stop codon (nonsense mutation), translation of the protein ceases and a shortened version of the protein is synthesized. Usually the protein is destroyed intracellularly and never reaches the plasma. This type of defect is associated with severe hemophilia, that is, with coagulant activity levels below 1%. Point mutations in which one amino acid is substituted for another can cause phenotypes of varying severity. The mutation of an important amino acid can destroy protein function, activation, or folding; inhibit intracellular processing; or cause protein clearance.[25] Unlike deletional mutations, point mutations at the same site have been recorded in different families with hemophilia.

Table 30-4 summarizes the types of coagulation disorders. Not all the disorders are discussed in this chapter because some are extremely rare (congenital dysfibrinogenemias) and others have no clinical significance (e.g., Hageman factor deficiency, a condition in which profound laboratory deficiency of factor XII is associated with absolutely no clinical defects).

CLINICAL MANIFESTATIONS. Children with severe hemophilia start to bleed at different ages. Although there is no transfer of maternal clotting factor to the fetus, many boys with hemophilia are circumcised without excessive bleeding. Normal hemostasis is achieved in these infants because clotting is activated through the extrinsic coagulation cascade, which does not involve factors VII, IX, or XI.

During the first year of life spontaneous bleeding often is minimal, but hematoma formation may result from immunizations and from firm holding (e.g., under the arms). Many children are diagnosed around the time they become mobile (i.e., crawling, pulling to stand) and become easily injured (i.e., increased bruising, swelling, redness at joints, mouth bleeding). By 3 to 4 years of age, 90% of children with hemophilia have had episodes of persistent bleeding from relatively minor traumatic lacerations (e.g., to the lip or tongue). This usually is the first clinical manifestation of hemophilia. Hemorrhage into the elbows, knees, and ankles causes pain, limited joint mobility, and predisposes the child to degenerative joint changes. Spontaneous hematuria and epistaxis are troublesome but minor complications.

Recurrent bleeding—spontaneous and after minor trauma—is a lifelong problem. Many affected individuals experience cycles of spontaneous bleeding episodes. Mechanisms that cause this phenomenon are unknown. Intracranial hemorrhage and bleeding into the neck or abdomen are rare but constitute life-threatening emergencies.

EVALUATION AND TREATMENT. Although laboratory tests are of primary value in the diagnosis of hemorrhagic disorders, the history and physical assessment also should be given careful consideration. The three phases of coagulation are assessed individually by simple, reliable tests. In any hemorrhagic condition, the adequacy of phase III should be determined first. Unless adequate fibrinogen is present, the blood is incapable of coagulation; thus other laboratory tests that require formation of a visible clot will be invalid. Phase III can be evaluated by the **thrombin time,** the time required for plasma to clot after the addition of bovine thrombin. Fibrinogen can be measured by chemical or immunologic methods.

Phase II is assessed by the **prothrombin time (PT),** the time required for plasma to clot after the addition of thromboplastin and calcium. If phase III is intact, a prolonged prothrombin time indicates a deficiency involving factors II, V, VII, or X, alone or in combination. Specific assays for each of the factors are available.

Phase I, the most complex part of coagulation, is evaluated by several tests. The **activated partial thromboplastin time (aPTT)** is the time required for clotting of plasma that has been activated by incubation with kaolin when calcium and platelets (or partial thromboplastin) are added. aPTT assesses the adequacy of factors XII, XI, IX, and VII. The **prothrombin consumption time** is a standard prothrombin test of serum instead of plasma. Because prothrombin is used up during coagulation, the serum normally contains little prothrombin and the serum prothrombin time is prolonged. Deficiencies of the phase I factors are associated with poor use of prothrombin. If the serum and plasma prothrombin times are similar, deficiency of a phase I factor is likely. The **thromboplastin generation test** is the most sensitive of all phase I tests. The test can precisely identify deficiencies of factors VIII and IX. If the aPTT, prothrombin consumption, or thromboplastin generation test results are abnormal, the way in which they can be corrected identifies the specific deficiency.

The treatment of hemophilia has changed markedly since the early 1920s. Plasma first was used in the 1920s, and by the 1940s it was used routinely to treat persons with hemophilia. The disadvantages of fresh frozen plasma (FFP), which is low in factor VIII per volume of plasma, led to the development of cryoprecipitate. In 1964 cryoprecipitate (quick-frozen precipitate), which is rich in factor VIII per volume, was used to treat individuals with hemophilia. Although cryoprecipitate advanced the treatment of hemophilia A, it had several disadvantages. The most notable complication was the possibility of transmission of viral diseases, including hepatitis B and C and human immunodeficiency virus (HIV). Factor VIII concentrates were first introduced in 1965. In addition to the predictable factor VIII content, other advantages of the early factor VIII concentrates included greater purity than cryoprecipitate and less contamination with other plasma proteins. The development of recombinant factor VIII resulted in new factor VIII products that minimize the risk of transmission of viral infection (e.g., HIV and hepatitis) and are potentially less expensive than plasma-derived factor VIII.

Recombinant antihemolytic factor plasma/albumin-free method (rAHF-PFM, Advate) is a product used for the prevention and control of bleeding episodes in individuals with hemophilia A, and in the perioperative management of those with hemophilia A. By excluding proteins or raw materials derived from human or animal sources in the final product, the risk of transmission of potentially infectious agents is removed.[26]

Primary prophylaxis consists of regular infusions of factor VIII or IX with the goal of preventing joint bleeding. It is usually given to children with severe hemophilia. A 5-year, multicenter trial found prophylaxis initiated in children between 6 and 30 months of age to be effective in the prevention of joint bleeding, structural joint damage, and frequency of bleeding in boys with factor VIII deficiency.[27]

Congenital Hypercoagulability and Thrombosis

Hereditary bleeding disorders, such as hemophilia, have been recognized and treated for centuries; however, the counterpart of these disorders, **thrombophilia,** has not been recognized until very recently. The inherited thrombophilic conditions generally are caused by defects in the clotting factors that inhibit clot formation; thus the balance between bleeding and clotting is directed toward the clotting aspects of hemostasis. Defects in specific proteins (C and S) and antithrombin (AT), as well as resistance to activated protein C (APC) and hyperhomocystinemia, are the major recognized causes of inherited thrombophilia.

Both proteins C and S are inhibitors of coagulation and depend on vitamin K for synthesis in the hepatocytes of the liver. Decreased levels of either of these proteins interfere with the normal homeostatic balance of procoagulant and anticoagulant activity at the endothelial level. Protein C and S deficiency states predispose affected individuals to thrombosis, especially venous thrombosis of the lower extremities.

Inheritance of **protein C deficiency** is autosomal dominant. Heterozygotes have protein C levels 50% to 60% of normal and may develop superficial thrombophlebitis, deep venous thrombosis, or pulmonary embolism in their late teens and early 20s. The majority of these thrombotic events (75%) occur spontaneously, whereas only 25% are the result of predisposing conditions.[28] Homozygotes have less than 1% of normal levels of protein C and tend to develop thrombosis of the cutaneous vessels with large areas of skin necrosis. It is rare for individuals with protein C deficiency to develop arterial thrombosis.

Protein C deficiency exists in two forms: types I and II. Type I, the more common form, involves a reduction in both biologic and immunologic activity of protein C. Type I is caused by deletion of the entire gene. In type II, the less common form, there is a normal level of protein C antigen but decreased functional levels of activity.

Neonatal purpura fulminans is a fatal syndrome found in neonates who are homozygous or double heterozygous for types I and II protein deficiency. Ecchymosis becomes apparent on the first day of life and develops around the head, trunk, and extremities and often is accompanied by cerebral thrombosis and infarction. The ecchymotic areas often coalesce, and ulceration and necrosis develop. Treatment includes administration of FFP and heparinization, although the infant rarely survives.

Heparin is the treatment for acute episodes of thrombosis caused by protein C deficiency. Long-term therapy is required and consists of either oral warfarin sodium (Coumadin) or subcutaneous heparin. Supplemental protein C concentrates (human) are also available and have been approved for use in children.[29]

Protein S deficiency is similar to protein C deficiency, and the inheritance pattern (autosomal dominant) is also similar. Heterozygotes demonstrate a strong tendency for deep venous thrombosis, with the first incidence often occurring before age 25 years. Other manifestations include superficial thrombophlebitis and pulmonary emboli. There are predisposing conditions for thrombi development in some cases, with evidence of spontaneous thrombi development in most cases.

Protein S deficiency exists in two forms: type I and type II. Type I is identified as a quantitative deficiency and manifests as low levels of protein S antigen and activity, and type II is identified as a qualitative deficiency with low levels of free protein S and normal levels of free and total protein S antigen.[25]

Homozygotes demonstrate severe manifestations of the condition and may develop a form of purpura fulminans in the neonatal period. It also is possible that the homozygous state may lead to uterine death. Treatment with heparin, warfarin (Coumadin), and protein C concentrate is similar to that of protein C deficiency.

Antithrombin III (AT III) deficiency is inherited as an autosomal dominant condition—the heterozygous state is the most common. AT III also exists in two forms, type I and type II, with type I being a quantitative deficiency of the AT III antigen. Type II is characterized as a dysfunctional form: normal levels of AT III are present but with reduced activity.

Individuals with AT III deficiency are at risk for early development of venous thrombosis and pulmonary embolism. These events often occur in the middle to late teens, and can occur as early as 10 years of age. The deep veins of the lower extremities are usually involved, most commonly the iliofemoral vein. Other sites include the mesenteric veins, vena cava, renal veins, and retinal veins. Cerebral thromboses also have been described, and arterial thrombotic events are rare. In some cases thrombosis is precipitated by surgery, trauma, pregnancy, oral contraceptives, and infection.

The treatment of choice for AT III deficiency is heparin. Antiplatelet agents (e.g., aspirin, dipyridamole) may be used, as well as AT III concentrates.

Antibody-Mediated Hemorrhagic Disease

The antibody-mediated hemorrhagic diseases are a group of disorders caused by the immune response. Antibody-mediated destruction of platelets or antibody-mediated inflammatory reactions to allergens damage blood vessels and cause seepage into tissues. The thrombocytopenic purpuras may be intrinsic or idiopathic, or they may be transient phenomena transmitted from mother to fetus. The inflammatory, or "allergic," purpuras occur in response to allergens in the blood. All these disorders first appear during infancy or childhood.

Idiopathic Thrombocytopenic Purpura

Acute **idiopathic thrombocytopenic purpura (ITP) (autoimmune** or **primary thrombocytopenic purpura)** is the most common of the thrombocytopenic purpuras of childhood. It is a disorder of platelet consumption in which antiplatelet antibodies bind to the plasma membranes of platelets, causing platelet sequestration and destruction by mononuclear phagocytes in the spleen and other lymphoid tissues at a rate that exceeds the ability of the bone marrow to produce them.

PATHOPHYSIOLOGY. Platelets have several tissue-specific antigens on their plasma markers that may be targets for antiplatelet antibody. In approximately 70% of cases of ITP, there is an antecedent viral disease (e.g., cytomegalovirus [CMV], Epstein-Barr virus [EBV], HIV, parvovirus, or viral respiratory infection), suggesting that viral sensitization has occurred. The interval between infection and onset of purpura is 1 to 4 weeks. A comparison with purpura seen in adults has identified an immune mechanism as the basis for ITP. High levels of IgG have been found bound to platelets and may represent immune complexes on the platelet surface.[30]

CLINICAL MANIFESTATIONS. One to 4 weeks after a viral infection, bruising and a generalized petechial rash often occur with acute onset. Asymmetric bleeding is typical and is found most often on the legs and trunk. Hemorrhagic bullae of the gums, lips, and other mucous membranes may be prominent. Epistaxis (nosebleed) may be severe and difficult to control. Except for the signs of bleeding, the child appears well. The acute phase of the disease associated with spontaneous hemorrhages lasts 1 to 2 weeks, but thrombocytopenia often persists. Intracranial hemorrhage is the most serious complication of ITP, although the incidence is less than 1%. In some cases the onset is more gradual and clinical manifestations consist of moderate bruising and scattered petechiae.

EVALUATION AND TREATMENT. Laboratory examination reveals a reduced platelet count, and the few platelets observed on a peripheral blood smear are large in size, reflecting increased bone marrow production. Bone marrow aspiration reveals megakaryocytes in normal or increased numbers and normal erythrocytes and granulocytes. The use of bleeding time for diagnosis is not recommended because the results are often confounded by a child who is crying or moving, the depth and direction of the cut, and the device used.

Even without treatment the prognosis for children with ITP is excellent—75% recover completely within 3 months. After the initial acute phase spontaneous clinical manifestations subside. By 6 months after onset, 80% to 90% of affected children have regained normal platelet counts.[27]

Because of the short life span of platelets (10 days), fresh blood or platelet transfusions are only a transient benefit; however, their use is indicated when life-threatening hemorrhage occurs. Corticosteroid therapy reduces the severity and shortens the duration of the initial phase by suppressing the immune attack on platelets. Recent evidence indicates that the use of high-dose methylprednisolone increases bone resorption and may cause osteonecrosis in children with ITP.[28] Intravenous IgG has been demonstrated to increase the platelet count in some children with ITP, but it is quite costly. Anti-D, is a gamma globulin fraction containing a high proportion of antibodies to the $Rh_0(D)$ antigen of the RBCs. Intravenous anti-D is a safe and effective treatment for Rh-positive, nonsplenectomized individuals with ITP. It is an effective treatment for Rh-positive nonsplenectomized children with ITP, although it is associated with side effects including chills, fever, headache, and a decrease in hemoglobin levels. Administration of steroids and antipyretics prior to the anti-D treatment may prevent side effects. Rituximab, a chimeric monoclonal antibody against the protein CD20, has been tested in children with ITP and demonstrated an overall response rate of 69% (see What's New? Clinical Trials of TPO Receptor Agonists for Treatment of Idiopathic Thrombocytopenic Purpura [ITP]). Only mild and self-limited side effects were observed in 18%, and no major infections or long-term toxicities were reported.[31]

WHAT'S NEW?

Clinical Trials of Thrombopoietin (TPO) Receptor Agonists for Treatment of Idiopathic Thrombocytopenic Purpura (ITP)

Rituximab, a chimeric monoclonal antibody against the protein CD20, has been tested in children with ITP. Long-term follow-up at 39.5 months of 49 children with ITP who were treated with rituximab demonstrated an overall response rate of 69%: 21 children had platelet counts of greater than 50,000/mm^3 at 20 months' post-treatment. Only mild and self-limited side effects were observed in 18%, and no major infections or long-term toxicities were reported.

Data from Parodi E et al: *Br J Haematol* 144(14):552–558, 2009.

Parents should be instructed to discourage activities that might cause trauma that could result in bleeding (e.g., contact sports, skateboarding, skiing, bicycle riding). Splenectomy should be reserved for chronic cases that fail to respond to nonsurgical intervention.

Autoimmune Neonatal Thrombocytopenias

Antibody-mediated thrombocytopenic purpura occurs in neonates in either autoimmune or alloimmune form. Both forms are characterized by the immunologic destruction of platelets by antibodies (IgG) against tissue-specific antigens expressed by the platelets (i.e., platelet-specific antigens).

Autoimmune neonatal thrombocytopenia was first noted in the early 1950s, when it was observed that mothers with ITP often delivered infants who were transiently thrombocytopenic. Neonatal thrombocytopenia was observed in approximately 50% of infants at risk and lasted an average of 1 month. As platelet counts returned to normal, a concomitant drop in the level of maternal antiplatelet antibody on the child's platelets occurred. The antibody is directed against antigens common to maternal and neonatal platelets. The prognosis generally is favorable and the frequency of intracranial hemorrhage is rare (1% to 3% of cases). Medical management of affected infants is to prevent the severe thrombocytopenia that can cause significant morbidity by administering intravenous immunoglobulins.

Neonatal alloimmune thrombocytopenic purpura (NATP) is less common, estimated to occur in 1 to 2 per 1000 live births. NATP is caused by maternal immunization against fetal paternally derived platelet-specific antigens (similar to rhesus [Rh] disease). The mother has a normal platelet count, while the fetus can be severely thrombocytopenic.

The diagnosis of NATP is confirmed by detection in the maternal serum of antibody that reacts with platelets from the infant and father but not with platelets from the mother. In approximately 75% to 85% of cases, NATP recurs in subsequent pregnancies. Purpura usually develops in the affected infant shortly after delivery, and intracranial, renal, and gastrointestinal hemorrhages are possible. The mortality rate from intracranial hemorrhage has been estimated at 10% to 15%. Management of the newborn with NATP includes an immediate cranial ultrasound because of the significant risk of intracranial hemorrhage. Severely thrombocytopenic newborns (<10,000/μL) or newborns with intracranial or visceral hemorrhages should receive a matched platelet transfusion (maternal or homozygous human platelet antigen 1b [HPA-1b] donor) as soon as possible. If maternal platelets are used, they must be processed to remove platelet alloantibodies. Newborn thrombocytopenia is difficult to predict because newborn platelet counts do not correlate with maternal platelet counts or antiplatelet antibody titers.[32]

Most of the life-threatening clinical manifestations of transient neonatal thrombocytopenia and NATP can be avoided through cesarean delivery. If the mother has antiplatelet disease, however, surgery can result in hemorrhage and serious maternal morbidity. Maternal morbidity resulting from NATP during pregnancy is low (less than 5%): the principal maternal risk is bleeding from surgical incisions during cesarean delivery. The incidence of transient thrombocytopenia in infants born to mothers with NATP is about 50%. If all deliveries were cesarean, half the mothers would undergo cesarean delivery unnecessarily. Conversely, if all deliveries were vaginal, half the infants—those with thrombocytopenia—would be at risk for intracranial bleeding. Therefore, in the absence of any clear benefit to the neonate (given the low rate of intracranial hemorrhage in infants born to mothers with ITP), cesarean delivery should be reserved for the usual obstetric indications.

Autoimmune Vascular Purpura

Autoimmune vascular purpura (allergic purpura) is caused by antibody-mediated injury of blood vessel walls, typically arterioles and capillaries. The inflammatory reaction is to foreign proteins or chemicals in the blood (microorganisms, drugs, or other chemicals).

Autoimmune vascular purpura usually is seen in young children, with the incidence decreasing in adolescents and adults and occurring only rarely in older adults. The average age at onset is 5 years, with a slightly higher proportion of males affected. Purpura occurs as vessel integrity is disrupted by inflammatory processes, causing effusion of serosanguineous exudate to perivascular tissues.

Clinical manifestations include headache, anorexia, fever, abdominal pain, constipation, arthralgias and urticaria, and erythema that are located symmetrically on the proximal portions of the extremities, particularly on the legs and buttocks, and may be accompanied by itching or paresthesias. Abdominal pain results from hemorrhage into the bowel, which may lead to colic, nausea, and vomiting. These symptoms may precede the appearance of skin lesions. The pain usually is midabdominal but may radiate to other parts of the abdomen. Joint pain and tenderness may be present, but hemarthrosis does not occur. Periarticular swelling and edema of the hands and feet are common and may precede the onset of abdominal pain and purpura. Subacute glomerulonephritis occurs in some cases but usually is reversible.

The characteristic skin lesions (purpura and cutaneous manifestations of allergy), accompanied by a history of joint and abdominal pain, are suspicious for diagnosis. Laboratory test results often reveal no major abnormalities. Attacks may last several weeks and may recur at odd intervals and with changing manifestations with each episode. Treatment, if necessary, consists of symptom management.

LEUKEMIA AND LYMPHOMA

Leukemia, the most common malignancy of childhood, represents approximately 40% of all childhood cancers. Childhood lymphoma is the third most common malignant neoplasm of children in the United States, representing approximately 11% of all childhood cancers. (See Chapter 29 for a discussion of leukemia in adults.)

Leukemia

Of the varieties of childhood leukemia, 75% to 80% of leukemias in children are acute lymphocytic leukemia (ALL) or acute undifferentiated leukemia (AUL). The remaining 20% to 25% are acute nonlymphocytic leukemias (ANLLs) (which include myeloblastic, promyelocytic, monocytic, and myelomonoblastic leukemias) and the very rare red blood cell leukemia, erythroleukemia. Because the vast majority of ANLLs involve the myeloblastic cell, many experts refer to the disease as *acute myelogenous leukemia (AML)*. Leukemia accounts for 25% of cases of cancer in black children and 34% of cases of cancer in white children. Approximately 4100 new cases are diagnosed each year in the United States.[33]

The peak incidence for childhood ALL is between 2 and 6 years of age. ALL affects more white and Hispanic than black children and more males than females. Male predominance is greater in T-cell disease. Incidence of ALL is higher in Western and industrialized nations.[33]

Types of Leukemia

A number of different classifications are used for the leukemias. First, acute leukemia is differentiated from chronic leukemia. Second, the cell line determines whether lymphoid cells or myeloid cells are involved. In acute leukemia this difference separates ALL from AML and vice versa. Within each of these categories, further subdivisions have been developed. (See Chapter 29 for a discussion of leukemias in adults.)

Cytogenic studies of leukemic cells are performed routinely at most major treatment centers during the diagnostic process. Abnormal morphologic characteristics, as well as abnormalities in the number of copies of chromosomes, are found in leukemic cells. Hyperdiploidy (increased number of chromosome copies) is associated with a good prognosis. Common translocations associated with ALL are TEL-AML1, BCR-ABL, and MLL. TEL-AML1 is the most common abnormality (in 20% to 30% of cases) and occurs when the *TEL* gene on chromosome 12p13 fuses with the *AML1* gene on chromosome 21q22. TEL-AML1 is associated with a favorable outcome. MLL arrangement, t(4;11), is located on chromosome 11q23. This translocation, the most common within this subtype, is found in infant ALL and is associated with a poor prognosis despite intensive therapy. Philadelphia chromosome–positive (Ph+) leukemia expresses the BCR-ABL protein and is characterized by the presence of t(9;22)(q34;q11) translocation. Ph+ leukemia can be ALL or chronic myelocytic leukemia (CML), depending where the breakpoint on chromosome 22 occurs. In CML, the translocation can be detected in multiple cell lines. Ph+ ALL occurs in 2% to 3% of cases and responds poorly to conventional chemotherapy. In CML, 99% of cases are characterized by the presence of t(9;22).[34]

Classification of childhood leukemia has become a complex but essential process to determine treatment. Previous classification by the French-American-British Cooperative Group (FAB) was based primarily on the morphologic and biochemical system. A classification scheme developed by the World Health Organization (WHO) is based on a more comprehensive system that uses morphology, immunophenotyping, and cytogenic and clinical features. The three major classifications of childhood leukemia are ALL (75% to 80%), AML (15% to 20%), and CML (less than 5%).

Flow cytometric immunophenotyping has made distinguishing between lymphoblastic and nonlymphoblastic leukemia much easier than in the past, when the degree of immaturity of the cell sometimes made such distinction difficult.

Immunologic classification has been used on identification of various surface markers. Five categories of ALL have been identified on the basis of their presumed origin from thymic cells (T cells) and bursa-equivalent cells (B cells) of normal lymphocytes:

1. T-cell ALL—characterized by the presence of abnormal T lymphocytes and found more commonly in older boys whose diagnosis includes mediastinal masses, high white blood cell counts, and hepatosplenomegaly (20% of ALL)
2. B-cell ALL—characterized by the presence of abnormal B lymphoblasts and associated with a poor prognosis (5% of ALL)
3. Pre—B-cell ALL—characterized by the presence of pre-B lymphoblasts (20% of ALL)
4. Unclassified ALL—also known as null cell (meaning neither T nor B lymphoblasts), and now classified as early B-cell lineage (15% of ALL)
5. Common ALL—characterized by the presence of a specific antigen known as common ALL antigen, or common acute lymphocytic leukemia antigen (CALLA), recently designated cellular differentiation 10 or CD10, in which the actual cell usually is considered to be of the B lineage (39% of ALL)

PATHOGENESIS. The exact cause of childhood leukemia is unclear. Investigations have focused on genetic susceptibility, environmental factors, and viral infections (see Chapter 14). Extraordinary doses of radiation and certain cancer therapies are possible causes (Facts, Spring 2013; Leukemia & Lymphoma Society, White Plains, NY. Accessed June 2013). Repeated exposure to benzene may cause AML. The relationship between childhood cancer and radon[35] and electromagnetic fields has been the focus of many epidemiologic studies, yet no conclusive evidence has been observed. In 2007 a task group of scientific experts convened by WHO reported that it could not confirm the existence of any health consequences from exposure to low-level magnetic fields.[36]

Although not determined to be genetically transmitted, a child who has a sibling with leukemia has a risk for the development of leukemia that is two to four times greater than for children with healthy siblings. The occurrence of leukemia in monozygous twins is estimated as being as high as 25%. In 2006, the Office of the U.S. Surgeon General suggested evidence of a causal relationship between childhood leukemia, lymphoma, and brain tumors and prenatal or postnatal environmental tobacco smoke exposure; the results have suggested an association between parental exposure to pesticides before or during pregnancy.[37] A later study suggested that the risk of leukemia and lymphoma increased when the mother was exposed to pesticides in the prenatal period, and the risk of brain tumors was correlated with paternal exposure (occupational or household use) either before or after birth.[38]

Inherited diseases that predispose a child to leukemia (ALL and AML) include Down syndrome, Fanconi anemia, Bloom syndrome, Diamond-Blackfan anemia, Klinefelter syndrome, Shwachman-Diamond syndrome, and ataxia-telangiectasia. Leukemia also has been associated with known genetic diseases, such as congenital agammaglobulinemia. AML in children sometimes is associated with loss or deletion of chromosome 7.

(see Figure 29-5). AML can develop from preexisting myeloproliferative disorders that also are preleukemia syndromes (i.e., myelodysplastic syndrome).

Childhood exposure to ionizing radiation, drugs, or viruses has been associated with the risk of developing cancer. Retrospective research has shown a significant correlation between radiation-induced malignancies from radiotherapy (as cancer treatment) or from radiation exposure from diagnostic imaging. The relationship between childhood cancer and electromagnetic fields, small appliances, radon, and other sources has been the focus of many epidemiologic studies; however, no conclusive evidence has been observed.[39]

Although chemicals such as benzene have been associated with the development of AML in adults, no evidence suggests a similar chemical or drug association in childhood leukemia. Leukemia (primarily AML) has been reported as a secondary malignancy (development of a second cancer after the first) in children treated for Hodgkin disease and Wilms tumor, although such cases are rare. In most cases the children received chemotherapy (alkylating agents or dactinomycin) and radiation therapy for the primary cancer, perhaps accounting for the subsequent development of another cancer.

Leukemic "clusters" that represent a greater number of leukemia cases occurring in a particular geographic location have raised speculation about environmental factors or infectious patterns of transmission. Careful follow-up, however, has failed to document the abnormal clustering.[40]

The strongest association between viruses and the development of cancer in children has been EBV and Burkitt lymphoma, and nasopharyngeal carcinoma and Hodgkin disease. Children with acquired immunodeficiency syndrome (AIDS) have an increased risk of developing non-Hodgkin lymphoma and Kaposi sarcoma. However, with the use of highly active antiretroviral therapy in the developed world, the incidence of AIDS-related malignancies has declined dramatically. Retroviruses have not been linked with childhood leukemia.

CLINICAL MANIFESTATIONS. Few variations appear in the presenting symptoms of the various cell types of acute leukemias. The onset may be abrupt or insidious, but the most common symptoms reflect the consequence of bone marrow failure, which results in decreased red blood cells and platelets and changes in white blood cells. Pallor, fatigue, petechiae, purpura, bleeding, and fever generally are present. Approximately 45% of children have a hemoglobin level less than 7 g/dl; in contrast to adults, children seem to demonstrate fewer symptoms. If acute blood loss occurs, however, characteristic symptoms of tachycardia, air hunger, restlessness, and thirst may be present. Epistaxis, excessive bruising, and hematuria often occur in children with severe thrombocytopenia. Three quarters of children with ALL have platelet counts less than 100,000/mm^3 at diagnosis, and 28% have platelet counts less than 20,000/mm^3. Half of all children newly diagnosed with AML have platelet counts less than 50,000/mm^3. Disseminated intravascular coagulation occurs more commonly with AML, particularly with promyelocytic leukemia. The granules in the leukemic promyelocytes may then indicate thromboplastin activity.

Fever usually is present as a result of two causes: (1) infection associated with the decrease in functional neutrophils and (2) hypermetabolism associated with the ongoing rapid growth and destruction of leukemic cells. In most children with ALL, the total white blood count is less than 10,000/mm^3, and with AML most have white cell counts less than 50,000/mm^3. In a few children, however, the peripheral white blood count can go well above 100,000/mm^3. White blood cell counts greater than 200,000/mm^3 can cause leukostasis, an intravascular clumping of cells that result in infarction and hemorrhage, usually in the brain and lung. The three most important favorable prognostic factors are age at diagnosis (2 to 10 years), initial leukocyte count (<50,000/mm^3), and initial response to treatment.

Renal failure as a result of hyperuremia (high uric acid levels) can be associated with ALL, particularly at diagnosis. Cell breakdown results as a natural process in the presence of a high white blood cell count or as a result of cellular breakdown caused by chemotherapy. Uric acid levels rise as an end product of purine metabolism from cellular destruction. Because the major excretory pathway is through the kidney, urates can precipitate in renal tubules or ureters and can lead to oliguria and acute renal failure. Renal failure is preventable if uric acid levels are monitored and treatment is aimed at optimal hydration, alkalinization of urine to assist with the excretion of soluble urates, and blockage of further uric acid formation by administration of the drug allopurinol.

Extramedullary invasion with leukemic cells can occur in nearly all body tissue. Most children with ALL have some extramedullary involvement at diagnosis. Leukemic invasion of tissue other than bone marrow is believed to represent metastatic infiltration. Hepatosplenomegaly and lymphadenopathy, resulting from extramedullary hematopoiesis, occur in nearly half of children with ALL, but they are less common in children with AML.

The CNS is a common site of infiltration of extramedullary leukemias, although less than 10% of children with ALL have CNS involvement at diagnosis. CNS infiltration manifests later in the course of the disease. Because successful chemotherapy prolongs the time of remission, the incidence of CNS involvement has increased. The most common symptoms of CNS involvement relate to increased intracranial pressure, causing early morning headaches, nausea, vomiting, irritability, and lethargy. Prophylactic CNS treatment therefore is necessary because systemic treatment with chemotherapy does not cross the blood-brain barrier.

Gonadal involvement, with testicular and ovarian infiltration, has been demonstrated in postmortem examination in 57% and 35% of children, respectively. Clinical detection of gonadal involvement is much less frequent. The incidence of testicular involvement, like CNS involvement, has increased with lengthened duration of remission. Prophylactic treatment has not been successful and currently is not recommended.

Leukemic infiltration into bones and joints is common in children. Reports of bone or joint pain actually lead to the diagnosis of leukemia in some children. In most children bone pain is characterized as migratory, vague, and without areas of

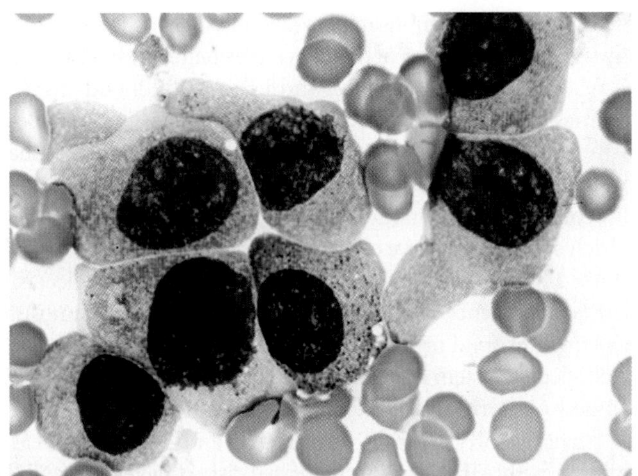

FIGURE 30-10 Monoblasts from Acute Monoblastic Leukemia. Monoblasts in a marrow smear from an individual with acute monoblastic leukemia (M5A). The monoblasts are larger than myeloblasts and usually have abundant cytoplasm, often with delicate scattered azurophilic granules (an element that stains well with blue aniline dyes). (From Damjanov I, Linder J, editors: *Anderson's pathology,* ed 10, St Louis, 1996, Mosby.)

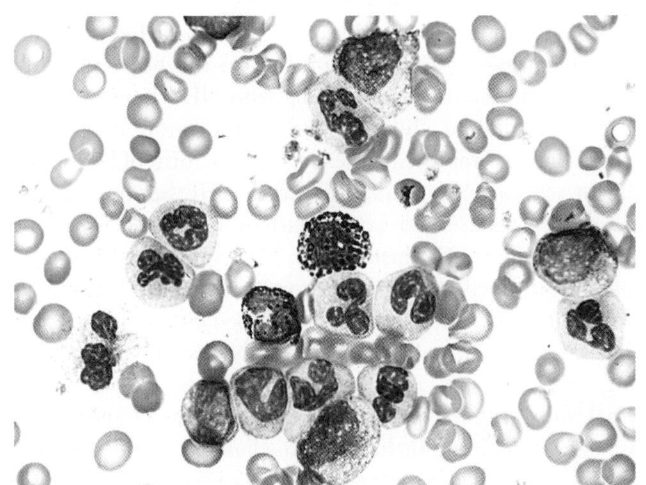

FIGURE 30-11 Leukocytosis and Basophilia in Chronic Myeloid Leukemia. Blood smear from a child with chronic myeloid leukemia (blasts) showing marked leukocytosis and basophilia. Karyotype analysis identified a Philadelphia chromosome (Wright-Giemsa stain). (From Damjanov I, Linder J, editors: *Anderson's pathology,* ed 10, St Louis, 1996, Mosby.)

swelling or inflammation. If joint pain is the primary symptom and some swelling is associated with the pain, however, misdiagnoses of rheumatoid arthritis may occur.

Other organs reported to be sites of leukemic invasion include the kidneys, heart, lungs, thymus, eyes, skin, and gastrointestinal tract. Of these, the kidneys, lungs, and gastrointestinal tract are the most frequently reported sites. Skin involvement is more common in AML than in ALL.

EVALUATION AND TREATMENT. A bone marrow aspiration and biopsy are required to establish the diagnosis. The **blast cell** is the hallmark of acute leukemia (Figure 30-10). The blast cell is a relatively undifferentiated cell characterized by diffusely distributed nuclear chromatin, with one or more nucleoli and basophilic cytoplasm (Figure 30-11).

TABLE 30-5 PROGNOSTIC FACTORS IN ACUTE LYMPHOBLASTIC LEUKEMIA (ALL)

PROGNOSTIC FACTOR	BETTER PROGNOSIS	WORSE PROGNOSIS
Age*		
<2 yr or >10 yr		X
2-7 yr	X	
Gender*		
Male		X
Female	X	
Initial white blood cell count*		
>50,000/mm^3		X
<10,000/mm^3	X	
Race		
Black		X
White	X	
Immunology*		
T- or B-cell ALL		X
Early pre–B-cell or common acute lymphocytic leukemia antigen (CALLA)	X	
Leukemic involvement		
Mediastinal mass		X
Central nervous system involvement at diagnosis		X
Splenic enlargement		X

*The four most reliable prognostic factors. Initial prognostic factors become less effective predictors with increasing length of remission. Age and gender are not significant after 15 months of continuous remission, and white blood cell count is not significant after 24 months of continuous remission.

Healthy children have less than 5% blast cells in the bone marrow and none in the peripheral blood. The bone marrow is categorized on the basis of blast percentage. Normal bone marrow is called M1 marrow; M2 and M3 represent an increased percentage of blasts in the sample. This categorization system should not be confused with the similar terminology used to denote subtypes of AML. In ALL the bone marrow often is replaced by 80% to 100% blast cells, with a reduction in normally developing red blood cells and granulocytes. The marrow, which is considered hypercellular, is composed of a homogeneous population of cells. Occasionally, however, the marrow appears hypocellular, making the diagnosis difficult to differentiate from aplastic anemia. When this occurs, the result of the bone marrow biopsy is necessary to confirm the diagnosis.

Combination chemotherapy, with or without radiation therapy to localized sites, such as the CNS, is the treatment of choice for acute leukemia. In ALL, identification of various risk groups has led to the development of different intensities of drug protocols. Thus treatment is tailored specifically for a particular risk group. (Table 30-5 outlines the various prognostic factors for ALL that are considered in determining the degree of risk.).

Most ALL treatment programs have four distinct phases: (1) induction of remission, (2) preventive therapy for the CNS, (3) intensification (also called *consolidation*), and (4) maintenance. In remission induction, the goal is no clinical evidence of disease and a normal bone marrow biopsy result, which is achieved in 95% of children with ALL. Children with persistent leukemia at the end of 1 month of induction therapy have a dismal prognosis. Prophylactic CNS treatment historically included both chemotherapy and radiation, but therapy, although effective in preventing CNS leukemia, adversely affects neurologic and intellectual function. A marked incidence of learning disabilities has been identified in children previously treated to prevent CNS disease.[41] CNS radiation is no longer given and intrathecal regimens are less toxic. Once remission is achieved, an intensification phase of treatment begins. This treatment is necessary because leukemic cells will continue to be present despite successful remission. Thus the goal of the intensification phase is to further decrease and eliminate the remaining leukemic cells. Intensification therapy often overlaps prophylactic CNS treatment. The final phase of initial treatment is called *maintenance therapy*. The goal of this phase is to maintain disease control. The optimal duration of maintenance therapy is not well defined, but it usually continues for 2.5 to 3 years. During maintenance therapy intermittent "pulses" of new drugs are usually given. Periods of intensified therapy are believed to minimize development of drug-resistant leukemic cells.

An estimated 1310 cancer deaths are expected to occur among children ages 0 to 14 in 2013, about one third from leukemia. However, death rates from childhood cancer have decreased by 66% since 1969 so impressive strides have been made in the treatment of these children.[33] Today, with prompt and appropriate treatment, 80% of children with ALL are cured. Those children with the more favorable early pre–B-cell or CALLA-positive ALL have a survival rate of 90%.[42]

Prognostic factors in AML are not as well defined as they are for ALL because of the small number of affected children and their overall poor prognosis. The goal of treatment for AML is similar to that of ALL except that much more aggressive chemotherapy is administered. With intensive chemotherapy, significant bone marrow suppression is necessary but predisposes children to infection, bleeding, and anemia. The use of colony-stimulating factor (CSF), which stimulates the rapid proliferation of specific blood cell lines, is an advance that shortens this period of bone marrow aplasia (CSFs are discussed in Chapter 27). Although initial remission is achieved relatively easily in all cases of ALL, successful and lasting remission can be achieved in only 70% to 80% of children with AML.[31] If remission is achieved, further treatment, called *continuation therapy*, is required. The specific intensity, timing, and length of continuation therapy are controversial. The use of either a stem cell or bone marrow transplantation (BMT) is an important treatment consideration in AML. Because long-term remission and cure of AML are difficult to achieve with chemotherapy alone, transplant often is recommended after the first remission is achieved. Transplant is the treatment of choice after relapse of AML. The long-term survival rate for children with AML, whether treated with chemotherapy or chemotherapy and BMT, is approximately 50%.[33]

Lymphomas

Non-Hodgkin lymphoma (NHL) and Hodgkin disease make up approximately 15% of all childhood cancer. Approximately 800 cases of childhood lymphoma are diagnosed in the United States annually.[33] Either group of diseases is rare before age 5 years, and the relative incidence increases throughout childhood. NHL is 1.5 times more common than Hodgkin disease in children. Boys are more likely to be diagnosed with a malignant lymphoma than are girls. There is an increased incidence of lymphoma in children with congenital immunodeficiency syndromes such as Wiskott-Aldrich syndrome, severe combined immunodeficiency (SCID), X-linked lymphoproliferative disease, and ataxia-telangiectasia. Increased incidence of NHL also is associated with immunosuppression after solid organ and stem cell transplants, particularly T-cell–depleted stem cell transplantation. The strongest association between viruses and the development of cancer in children has been the EBV, Burkitt lymphoma, and Hodgkin disease. Children with AIDS have an increased risk of developing NHL. However, with the use of highly active antiretroviral therapy in the developed world, the incidence of AIDS-related malignancies has declined dramatically.[43]

Non-Hodgkin Lymphoma

The classification of **non-Hodgkin lymphoma (NHL)** has been confusing because of the heterogeneity of this group of diseases. Generally most classification systems divide NHL into two categories—nodular or diffuse—on the basis of cellular pattern. Whereas half of all adults with NHL have a nodular form of the disease, children rarely demonstrate this pattern. Nodular disease represents a less aggressive form of lymphoma. Almost without exception, childhood NHL becomes evident as a diffuse disease and can be further subdivided into three groups: (1) large cell (histiocytic), (2) lymphoblastic, and (3) small noncleaved cell (Burkitt or non-Burkitt lymphoma). Large-cell NHL often involves chromosomal translocations. Disease sites commonly involve extranodal sites, such as brain, lung, bone, and skin. Lymphoblastic NHL also shows chromosomal translocations, particularly chromosomes 7 and 14. Disease sites commonly include the mediastinum and peripheral lymph nodes. Small noncleaved cell NHL involves chromosome translocations of 8 and 14. It is believed that this translocation triggers the *c-myc* oncogene. Children with small noncleaved cell NHL commonly have intra-abdominal disease at diagnosis.

An area of intensive study concerns the apparent biologic similarities of NHL and ALL in children. These two diseases are cytologically identical, and the histologic distinction between them is indicated by the degree of infiltration in the blood and bone marrow. The more bone marrow involvement and the less nodal and organ infiltration present, the more likely the disease is to be classified as ALL. Childhood NHL also is much more like ALL in its clinical manifestations and much less like Hodgkin disease or adult NHL.

As in ALL, immunophenotyping is an important part of the classification of childhood NHL. Almost 45% of the disease in children originates from T cells; an equal number originates from B cells. The remaining group, which represents 10% of childhood NHLs, is classified as non-T, non-B.

PATHOGENESIS. The origin of NHL in childhood is still elusive. Although defective host immunity is implicated in most children in whom NHL develops, an immune deficit cannot be identified. Viral etiology is suggested, but the role in development of human lymphoma is still unclear. The strongest correlation exists between EBV and African Burkitt lymphoma. This form of NHL is associated with a breakpoint on chromosome 8 that is located near the *c-myc* oncogene.[44] The relationship between EBV infection and Burkitt lymphoma outside Africa is weak, however, even though the tumor is histopathologically and clinically indistinguishable. Chronic immunostimulation also has been suggested as a factor in the development of lymphomas because these diseases are seen more often when chronic persistent antigenic stimulation occurs from infection, such as malaria or intestinal parasites. Genetic susceptibility also may play a role in the process of malignant transformation.

CLINICAL MANIFESTATIONS. In children, NHL has been found to arise from any lymphoid tissue. Signs and symptoms therefore are specific for the site involved. Some children have such widespread involvement that no original site can be determined. Because childhood NHL is a rapidly progressive disease, symptoms generally are present only a few weeks before diagnosis is made. Rapidly enlarging lymphoid tissue and painless lymphadenopathy are common in about one third of children with abdominal sites of involvement, usually representing a gastrointestinal origin for the disease. Symptoms often include abdominal pain and vomiting, but a palpable mass is not always present. Most children with abdominal symptoms have diffuse, small noncleaved cell NHL (Burkitt or non-Burkitt) of B-cell origin. If the tumor recurs, it appears again in the abdomen before distant spread.

The other common site of childhood NHL is the chest region. An anterior mediastinal mass, with or without pleural effusion, often is present. If the mass is large enough, respiratory compromise, tracheal compression, and superior vena cava syndrome may arise, which constitute a medical emergency. Children with anterior mediastinal involvement often are male adolescents and usually have diffuse lymphoblastic lymphoma of T-cell origin. This form of diffuse lymphoblastic lymphoma often evolves into extensive bone marrow involvement and is considered to be an overt leukemic phase (Figure 30-12); therefore, it is referred to as *leukemic transformation.* CNS involvement and testicular infiltration often then occur. CNS involvement occurs in about 30% of individuals with NHL, usually causing multiple deep-seated lesions within the brain parenchyma. In children with AIDS, NHL is the most common mass lesion found in the brain.

Bone marrow involvement is less common than other primary sites, whereas CNS involvement is common. Relatively few children (10% to 20%) with NHL have lymphoid tissue involvement of the head and neck (Waldeyer ring, nasopharynx, sinuses). Signs and symptoms include tonsillitis, sinusitis, and a painless nasopharyngeal mass. In African Burkitt lymphoma, involvement of facial bones, particularly the jaw, is common, although this occurs infrequently in non-African cases.

EVALUATION AND TREATMENT. Diagnosis is made by biopsy of disease sites, usually the involved lymph nodes. Other sites of biopsy include the tonsils, bone marrow, spleen, liver, bowel, or skin. Advances in understanding the disease and progress in treatment strategies have meant that most children with NHL are cured of the disease. The primary therapeutic modality for childhood NHL is chemotherapy, regardless of stage or site(s) of the disease. The tumor responds to many different agents. Many children with NHL receive intrathecal agents (methotrexate [Mexate] or cytarabine [cytosine arabinoside], or both) for CNS prophylaxis. Radiation is not routinely used to treat childhood NHL, with the exception of emergent situations when airway, intestinal, or spinal obstruction requires immediate reduction in tumor size. Cranial radiation therapy (RT) may be used for children with T-cell lymphoblastic lymphoma.

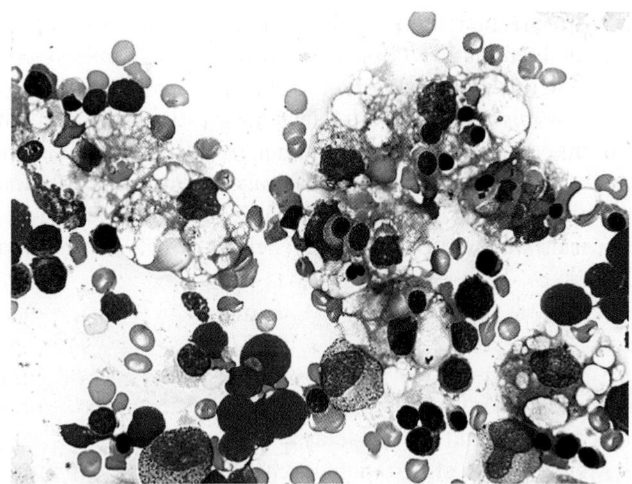

FIGURE 30-12 Bone Marrow Aspirate from a Child with T-Cell Lymphoma in a Lymph Node Biopsy. There is marked histiocytic hyperplasia. Two of the histiocytes contain phagocytosed red cells. The histiocytic hyperplasia regressed with disease remission and recurred with relapse of the lymphoma (Wright-Giemsa stain). (From Damjanov I, Linder J, editors: *Anderson's pathology,* ed 10, St Louis, 1996, Mosby.)

Children with advanced small noncleaved cell lymphoma of the abdomen have the poorest prognosis. Although remission occurs in more than 90% of these children, most experience subsequent relapses. Even in the presence of advanced lymphoblastic lymphoma, however, 70% to 80% of children can be cured. Children with localized disease in more easily treated sites are likely to be cured with prompt and appropriate treatment. Overall, children with localized diseases have a 90% survival rate and those with advanced disease have a 70% to 80% survival rate.[33]

Hodgkin Lymphoma

Hodgkin lymphoma accounts for 6% of all childhood cancers with a significant male-to-female dominance of 4:1 in young children. There is an increased incidence in children with immunologic disorders, whether caused by genetics, infection, or iatrogenic agents. EBV has been associated with Hodgkin lymphoma. Approximately 15% to 25% of adolescents and young adults have EBV-positive Hodgkin lymphoma.[45] Clustering of cases within families may suggest a genetic predisposition to the disease or common exposure to a causative agent.[46]

Hodgkin lymphoma accounts for 6% of all childhood cancers. It occurs infrequently in children younger than 2 years, and few cases are observed before age 5 years. A gradual rise in incidence occurs through age 11 years, with a marked increase through adolescence that continues into the 30s.

Individuals typically have painless supraclavicular or cervical adenopathy. These nodes are firm and rubbery and may be sensitive to palpation if they have grown rapidly. At least two thirds of individuals have mediastinal involvement that may cause symptoms ranging from a nonproductive cough to tracheal or bronchial compression leading to airway obstruction. Systemic symptoms may include fatigue, anorexia, weight loss, fever, drenching night sweats, and pruritus.

The Ann Arbor staging system considers extent and location of disease, as well as substage classifications that consider systemic symptoms (presence of fever of 38° C [100.4° F] for 3 consecutive days, drenching night sweats, or unexplained loss of 10% or more of body weight in the 6 months preceding diagnosis), extranodal, or bulky disease. Combination chemotherapy used in conjunction with involved field low-dose radiation has been shown to be an effective treatment, with long-term cure rates reported from 90% to 95%.[45]

SUMMARY REVIEW

Fetal and Neonatal Hematopoiesis

1. After 2 weeks of gestation, circulating erythrocytes play a major role in delivering oxygen to the tissues.
2. Erythropoiesis in the liver and, to a lesser extent, in the spleen and lymph nodes reaches a peak at about 4 months.
3. By the fifth month of gestation, hematopoiesis begins to occur in the bone marrow, and by the time of delivery it is the only significant site of hematopoiesis.
4. A biochemically distinct type of hemoglobin is synthesized during fetal life, including Gower 1, Gower 2, and Portland.

Postnatal Changes in the Blood

1. Blood cell counts tend to rise above adult levels at birth and then decline gradually throughout childhood.
2. The immediate rise in blood cell counts is the result of increased hematopoiesis during fetal life, trauma of birth, and cutting of the umbilical cord.
3. The active rate of fetal erythropoiesis is observed in the large numbers of reticulocytes in the peripheral blood of the full-term neonate.
4. Erythrocyte values are age dependent, and values in males and females are apparent in adolescence.
5. The lymphocyte count is high at birth, and continues to rise in some healthy infants during the first year of life.
6. Platelet counts in full-term neonates are comparable to platelet counts in children and adults.

Disorders of Erythrocytes

1. Iron deficiency anemia is the most common blood disorder of infancy and childhood; the highest incidence occurs between 6 months and 2 years of age.
2. Hemolytic disease of the newborn (HDN) results from incompatibility between the maternal and the fetal blood, which may involve differences in Rh factors or blood type (ABO). Maternal antibodies enter the fetal circulation and cause hemolysis of fetal erythrocytes. Because the immature liver is unable to conjugate and excrete the excess bilirubin that results from the hemolysis, icterus neonatorum, or kernicterus or both can develop.
3. Kernicterus, which may result from other causes as well, results in increased breakdown of red blood cells or decreased liver output of enzymes.
4. Infections of the newborn, often acquired by the mother and transmitted to the infant, may result in hemolytic anemia.
5. Glucose-6-phosphate dehydrogenase (G6PD) deficiency is an inherited enzyme deficiency in erythrocytes that results in a disruption of a common pathway of glycolysis, shortening erythrocyte life span.
6. Hereditary spherocytosis is the most common of the hereditary hemolytic states in which there is no abnormality of hemoglobin. The basic defect is an undefined abnormality of the proteins or spectrins of the erythrocyte membrane in which affected cells are unduly permeable to sodium and acquire a characteristic structure.
7. Sickle cell disease (SCD) is a genetically determined defect of hemoglobin synthesis, inherited by an autosomal recessive transmission; it causes a change in the shape of a red blood cell that results in decreased oxygen or hydration. This disease is most common among Africans, blacks, and those of Mediterranean descent.
8. The thalassemias are a heterogeneous group of hereditary hypochromic anemias of varying severity. Basic genetic defects include abnormalities of messenger ribonucleic acid (mRNA) processing or deletion of genetic materials, resulting in a decrease in the chains for hemoglobin.

Disorders of Coagulation and Platelets

1. Hemophilia is a condition characterized by impairment of the coagulation of blood and subsequent tendency to bleed. The classic disease is hereditary and limited to males, being transmitted through the female to the second generation. Many similar conditions attributable to the absence of various clotting factors are recognized.
2. von Willebrand disease is a dominantly inherited disease characterized by a vascular abnormality that produces a prolongation of bleeding time and by decreased levels of clotting factor VIII. The platelets in von Willebrand disease have decreased adhesiveness because the plasma factor is absent.
3. Disorders of congenital hypercoagulability and thrombosis include protein C deficiency, protein S deficiency, neonatal purpura fulminans, and antithrombin III deficiency.
4. The acquired antibody-mediated hemorrhagic diseases include idiopathic thrombocytopenic purpura (ITP), autoimmune neonatal thrombocytopenia, and autoimmune vascular purpura.
5. ITP, the most common of the childhood thrombocytopenic purpuras, is a disorder of platelet consumption in which

SUMMARY REVIEW—cont'd

antiplatelet antibodies bind to the plasma membranes of platelets. This results in platelet sequestration and destruction by mononuclear phagocytes at a rate that exceeds the ability of the bone marrow to produce them.

6. Autoimmune neonatal thrombocytopenia is an antibody-mediated disorder that occurs in either autoimmune or alloimmune form.
7. The autoimmune vascular purpuras (allergic purpuras) are caused by the body's responses to allergens in the blood.

Leukemia and Lymphoma

1. The types of childhood leukemia include, in order of their rate of incidence, ALL, AML, and CML.
2. Although the cause of childhood leukemia is not known, it is probably the result of multiple interactions between hereditary or genetic predisposition and environmental influences.
3. Acute lymphoblastic leukemia is a potentially curable disease, with more than 80% of cases cured.
4. The lymphomas of childhood are non-Hodgkin lymphoma and Hodgkin lymphoma.
5. The origin of non-Hodgkin lymphoma is unknown. Factors that have been implicated include defective host immunity, a viral agent, chronic immunostimulation, and genetic predisposition.
6. Non-Hodgkin lymphoma has a favorable prognosis, with a 70% to 80% cure rate.
7. The risk of Hodgkin lymphoma is associated in part with infectious diseases, immune deficits, and genetic susceptibility.
8. Hodgkin lymphoma is a readily curable disease with long-term cure rates of 90% to 95%.

KEY TERMS

Activated partial thromboplastin time (aPTT), 1071
Acute chest syndrome, 1066
Alpha-thalassemia major, 1069
Alpha-thalassemia minor, 1069
Alpha trait, 1069
Antithrombin III (AT III) deficiency, 1073
Aplastic crisis, 1066
Autoimmune neonatal thrombocytopenia, 1074
Autoimmune vascular purpura (allergic purpura), 1074
Beta-thalassemia major (Cooley anemia), 1069
Beta-thalassemia minor, 1069
Blast cell, 1077
Cholecystitis, 1067
Embryonic hemoglobin (Gower 1, Gower 2, Portland), 1056
Fetal hemoglobin (HbF), 1056
Glomerular disease, 1067
Glucose-6-phosphate dehydrogenase (G6PD) deficiency, 1062
Hemoglobin H disease, 1069
Hemoglobin S (HbS), 1063
Hemolytic disease of the newborn (HDN) (erythroblastosis fetalis), 1058
Hemophilia A (classic hemophilia), 1071
Hemophilia B (Christmas disease), 1071
Hemophilia C (factor XI deficiency), 1071
Hereditary spherocytosis (HS), 1062
Hodgkin lymphoma, 1079
Hydrops fetalis, 1060
Hyperbilirubinemia, 1060
Hyperhemolytic crisis, 1066
Icterus gravis neonatorum, 1060
Icterus neonatorum (neonatal jaundice), 1060
Idiopathic thrombocytopenic purpura (ITP) (autoimmune or primary thrombocytopenic purpura), 1073
Kernicterus, 1060
Neonatal alloimmune thrombocytopenic purpura (NATP), 1074
Neonatal purpura fulminans, 1072
Non-Hodgkin lymphoma (NHL), 1078
Polymerization, 1066
Preimplantation genetic diagnosis, 1068
Protein C deficiency, 1072
Protein S deficiency, 1072
Prothrombin consumption time, 1071
Prothrombin time (PT), 1071
Sequestration crisis, 1066
Sickle cell anemia, 1063
Sickle cell disease (SCD), 1063
Sickle cell trait, 1063
Sickle cell–Hb C disease, 1063
Sickle cell–thalassemia disease, 1063
Thalassemia, 1069
Thrombin time, 1071
Thrombophilia, 1072
Thromboplastin generation test, 1072
Vaso-occlusive crisis (thrombotic crisis), 1066
von Willebrand disease, 1071

REFERENCES

1. Nagaoka H: Immunization and infection change the number of recombination activating gene (Rag) expressing B cells in the periphery by altering immature lymphocyte production, *J Exp Med* 191:2113–2120, 2000.
2. Schelonka RL et al: Differentiation of segmented and band neutrophils during the newborn period, *J Pediatr* 127:298–300, 1995.
3. Beutler E, West C: Hematologic differences between African-Americans and whites: the roles of iron deficiency and α-thalassemia on hemoglobin levels and mean corpuscular volume, *Blood* 106:740–745, 2005.
4. Cunningham AS: Eosinophil counts—age and sex differences, *J Pediatr* 87:426–427, 1975.
5. Kühne T, Imbach P: Neonatal platelet physiology and pathophysiology, *Eur J Pediatr* 157:87–94, 1998.
6. Khan JL et al: Persistence and emergence of anemia in children during participation in the Special Supplemental Nutrition Program for Women, Infants, and Children, *Arch Pediatr Adolesc Med* 156(10): 1028–1032, 2002.
7. Bogen DL, Whitaker RC: Anemia screening in the Special Supplemental Nutrition Program for Women, Infants and Children—time for change, *Arch Pediatr Adolesc Med* 156(10):969–970, 2002.
8. Shah M et al: Effect of orange and apple juice on iron absorption in children, *Arch Pediatr Adolesc Med* 157:1232–1236, 2003.
9. De-Regil LM et al: Intermittent iron supplementation for improving nutrition and development in children under 12 years of age, *Cochrane Database Syst Rev* (12):CD009085, 2011.
10. Koelewijn JM et al: Effect of screening for red cell antibodies, other than anti-D, to detect hemolytic disease of the fetus and newborn: a population study in the Netherlands, *Transfusion* 48:941–952, 2008.
11. Liumbruno GM et al: The role of antenatal immunoprophylaxis in the prevention of maternal-fetal anti-Rh(D) alloimmunisation, *Blood Transfus* 8:8–16, 2010.
11a. Sloniewsky D: Anemia and transfusion in critically ill pediatric patients: a review of etiology, management, and outcomes, *Crit Care Clin* 29(2):301–317, 2013.
12. Bolton-Maggs P: *Guidelines for the diagnosis and management of hereditary spherocytosis, The British Committee for Standards in Haematology* Available at www.bcshguidelines.com/documents/HS_BCSH_Sept_2011_final.pdf. Accessed November 29, 2012.
13. Servey JT, Reamy BV, Hodge J: Clinical presentations of parvovirus B19 infection, *Am Fam Physician* 75:373–376, 2007.
14. Buesing KL et al: Partial splenectomy for hereditary spherocytosis: a multi-institutional review, *J Pediatr Surg* 46:178–183, 2011.
15. Centers for Disease Control and Prevention: *Sickle cell disease: data and statistics.* Available at www.cdc.gov/NCBDDD/sicklecell/data.html. Accessed November 8, 2012.

16. Malowany JI, Butany J: Pathology of sickle cell disease, *Sem Diag Path* 29:49–55, 2012.
17. Smith WR et al: Climatic and geographic temporal patterns of pain in the multicenter study of hydroxyurea, *Pain* 146:91–98, 2009.
18. Driscoll CM: Sickle cell disease, *Pediatr Rev* 28:259–268, 2007.
19. Miller ST: How I treat acute chest syndrome in children with sickle cell disease, *Blood* 117(20):5297–5305, 2011.
20. Vijenthira A et al: Benchmarking pain outcomes for children with sickle cell disease hospitalized in a tertiary referral pediatric hospital, *Pain Res Manag* 17:291–296, 2012.
21. Melzer-Lange MD et al: Patient-controlled analgesia for sickle-cell pain crisis in a pediatric emergency department, *Pediatr Emerg Care* 20:2–4, 2004.
22. Platt OS: Hydroxyurea for the treatment of sickle cell anemia, *N Engl J Med* 358:1362–1369, 2008.
23. National Hemophilia Foundation: *Types of bleeding disorders.* Available at www.hemophilia.org/NHFWeb/MainPgs/MainNHF.aspx?menuid=0&;contentid=1. Accessed November 29, 2012.
24. Peyvandi F et al: Genetic diagnosis of haemophilia and other inherited bleeding disorders, *Haemophilia* 12(Suppl 3):82–89, 2006.
25. Bowen DJ: Haemophilia A and haemophilia B: molecular insights, *Mol Pathol* 55:127–144, 2002.
26. Ananyeva N et al: Treating hemophilia A with recombinant blood factors: a comparison, *Exp Opin Pharmacother* 5:1061–1070, 2004.
27. Manco-Johnson MJ et al: Prophylaxis versus episodic treatment to prevent joint disease in boys with severe hemophilia, *N Engl J Med* 357:535–544, 2007.
28. Young G: Diagnosis and treatment of thrombosis in children: general principles, *Pediatr Blood Cancer* 46:540–546, 2006.
29. Goldenberg NA, Manco-Johnson MJ: Protein C deficiency, *Haemophilia* 14(6):1214–1221, 2008.
30. Kubota M et al: Serum immunoglobulin levels at onset: association with the prognosis of childhood idiopathic thrombocytopenic purpura, *Internat J Hematol* 77, 2003. 304–304.
31. Parodi E et al: Long-term follow-up analysis after rituximab therapy in children with refractory symptomatic ITP: identification of factors predictive of a sustained response, *Br J Haematol* 144:552–558, 2009.
32. Sainio S, Jarvenpaa AL, Renlund M: Thrombocytopenia in term infants: a population-based study, *Obstet Gynecol* 95:441–446, 2000.
33. American Cancer Society: *Cancer facts and figures 2013*, Atlanta, 2012, American Cancer Society.
34. Plon SE, Malkin D: Childhood cancer and heredity. In Pizzo PA, Poplack DG, editors: *Principles and practice of pediatric oncology*, ed 6, Philadelphia, 2012, Lippincott Williams & Wilkins, pp 14v37.
35. Tong J et al: Environmental radon exposure and childhood leukemia, *J Toxicol Environ Health B Crit Rev* 15(5):332–347, 2012.
36. Repacholi M: Concern that "EMF" magnetic fields from power lines causes cancer, *Sci Total Environ* 426:454–458, 2012.
37. Clapp RW, Howe GK, Jacobs MM: Environmental and occupational causes of cancer: a call to act on what we know, *Biomed Pharmacother* 61(10):631–639, 2007.
38. Villani A, Malkin D, Tabori U: Syndromes predisposing to pediatric central nervous system tumors: lessons learned and new promises, *Curr Neurol Neurosci Rep* 12(2):153–164, 2012.
39. Buka I, Koranteng S, Osornio-Vargas AR: Trends in childhood cancer incidence: review of environmental linkages, *Pediatr Clin North Am* 54:177–203, 2007.
40. Laurier D et al: Epidemiological studies of leukaemia in children and young adults around nuclear facilities: a critical review, *Radiat Prot Dosimetry* 132:182–190, 2008.
41. National Cancer Institute: *Late effects of the central nervous system, 2012.* Available at www.cancer.gov/cancertopics/pdq/treatment/lateeffects/HealthProfessional/page4. Accessed January 28, 2013.
42. Alvarnez JC et al: Acute lymphoblastic leukemia, *J Natl Comp Canc Netw* 10(7):858–914, 2012.
43. Pajand O et al: Detection of Epstein-Barr virus DNA in plasma and lymph node biopsy samples in pediatric and adult patients with Hodgkin lymphoma, *Pediatr Hematol Oncol* 28(1):10–15, 2011.
44. Gross TG, Perkins SL: Malignant non-Hodgkin lymphomas in children. In Pizzo PA, Poplack DG, editors: *Principles and practice of pediatric oncology*, ed 6, Philadelphia, 2012, Lippincott Williams & Wilkins, pp 722–747.
45. Metzger M et al: Hodgkin lymphoma. In Pizzo PA, Poplack DG, editors: *Principles and practice of pediatric oncology*, ed 6, Philadelphia, 2012, Lippincott Williams & Wilkins, pp 695–721.
46. Oliapuram Jose B et al: Pediatric Hodgkin's disease, *J Ky Med Assoc* 102(3):104–106, 2004.

CHAPTER

31

Structure and Function of the Cardiovascular and Lymphatic Systems

Susanna G. Cunningham, Valentina L. Brashers, and Kathryn L. McCance

evolve WEBSITE

http://evolve.elsevier.com/McCance/
- Review Questions and Answers
- Animations

CHAPTER OUTLINE

The functions of the circulatory system include delivery of oxygen, nutrients, hormones, cells of the immune system, and other substances to body tissues and removal of the waste products of cellular metabolism. Delivery and removal are achieved by a complex array of tubing—the blood and lymphatic vessels—connected to a pump—the heart. The heart continuously pumps blood through the blood vessels in collaboration with other systems, particularly the nervous and endocrine systems, which are intrinsic regulators of the heart and blood vessels. Immune system cells, nutrients, and oxygen are supplied by the immune, digestive, and respiratory systems; gaseous wastes of cellular metabolism are blown off by the lungs; and other wastes are removed by the kidneys and digestive tract.

A critical component of the circulatory system is the vascular endothelium, which is considered by some to be a separate organ. It is a multifunctional tissue whose health is essential to normal vascular and hemostatic physiology and whose dysfunction is an important factor in the pathogenesis of vascular and other diseases.[1]

CIRCULATORY SYSTEM

The heart is comprised of two conjoined pumps that power the movement of blood through two separate circulatory systems, one to the lungs and one to all other parts of the body. Structures on the right side of the heart, or **right heart,** pump blood through the lungs. (This system, termed the **pulmonary circulation,** is described in Chapter 34.) The left side of the heart, or **left heart,** sends blood throughout the **systemic circulation,** which supplies all of the body except the lungs (Figure 31-1).

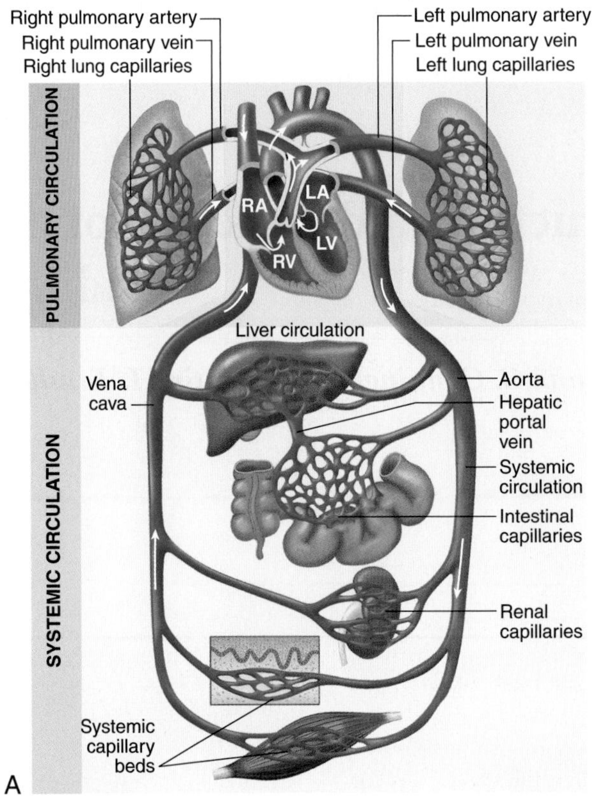

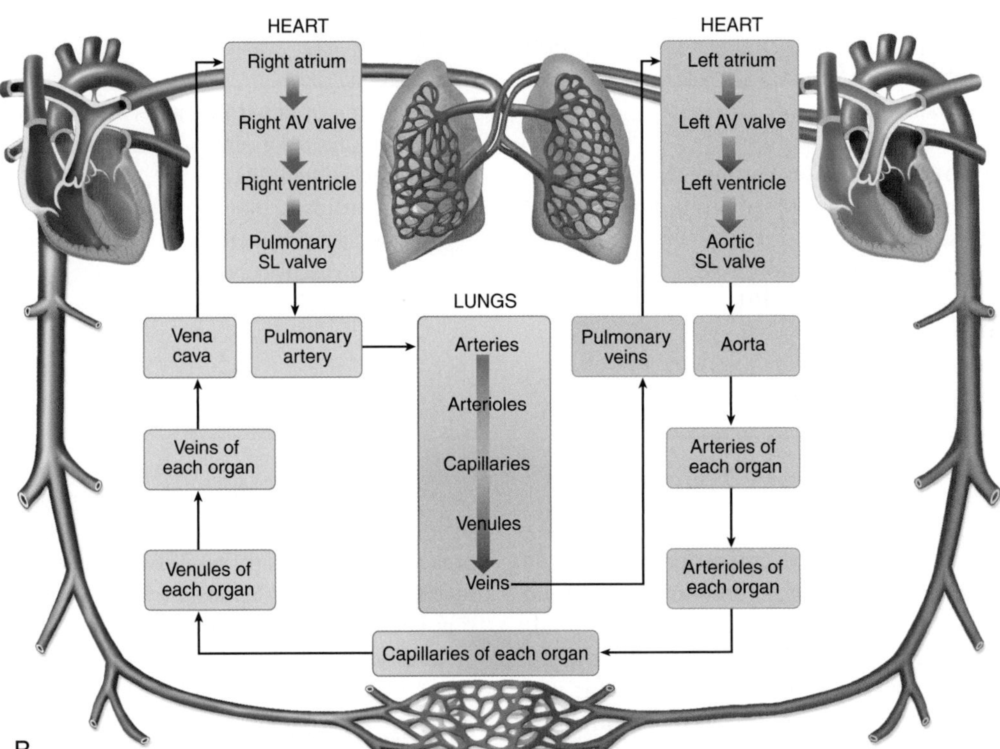

FIGURE 31-1 **Diagram Showing Serially Connected Pulmonary and Systemic Circulatory Systems and How to Trace the Flow of Blood. A,** Right heart chambers propel unoxygenated blood through the pulmonary circulation, and the left heart propels oxygenated blood through the systemic circulation. **B,** The direction of blood flow begins at the left ventricle of the heart; flows to the arteries, arterioles, capillaries of each body organ, venules, veins, right atrium, right ventricle, pulmonary artery, lung capillaries, pulmonary veins, and left atrium; and then returns to the left ventricle. *LA,* Left atrium, *LV,* left ventricle; *RA,* right atrium; *RV,* right ventricle; *SL,* semilunar. (**A** from Patton KT, Thibodeau GA: *Anatomy & physiology,* ed 8, St Louis, 2013, Mosby. **B** from Thibodeau GA, Patton KT: *The human body in health & disease,* ed 6, St Louis, 2014, Mosby.)

These two systems are serially connected so that the output of one pump becomes the input of the other.

Arteries carry blood from the heart to all parts of the body, where they branch into arterioles and even smaller vessels until they become a fine meshwork of capillaries. Capillaries allow the closest contact and exchange between the blood and the interstitial space, or interstitium—the environment in which the cells live. Veins then carry blood from capillaries back to the heart. Some of the plasma or liquid component of the blood passes through the walls of the capillaries into the interstitial space. This fluid, called lymph, is returned to the cardiovascular system by vessels of the lymphatic system. The lymphatic system is also a critical component of the immune system as described in Chapter 8.

THE HEART

The adult heart weighs between 200 and 350 g and is about the size of a fist. It lies obliquely (diagonally) in the **mediastinum,** the area above the diaphragm and between the lungs. Women's hearts are typically about 0.40% of their total body weight whereas men's hearts are about 0.45% of total body weight.[2]

Heart structures can be categorized by function:

1. *Structural support of heart tissues and circulation of pulmonary and systemic blood through the heart.* This category includes the heart wall and fibrous skeleton, which enclose and support the heart and divide it into four chambers; the valves that direct flow through the chambers; and the great vessels that conduct blood to and from the heart.
2. *Maintenance of heart cells.* This category comprises vessels of the coronary circulation—the arteries and veins that serve the metabolic needs of all the heart cells—and the lymphatic vessels of the heart.
3. *Stimulation and control of heart action.* Among these structures are the nerves and specialized muscle cells that direct the rhythmic contraction and relaxation of the heart muscles, propelling blood throughout the pulmonary and systemic circulatory systems.

Structures That Direct Circulation Through the Heart

Heart Wall

The heart wall has three layers—the epicardium, myocardium, and endocardium—and is enclosed in a double-walled membranous sac, the **pericardium** (Figure 31-2). The **pericardial sac** has several functions. It (1) prevents displacement of the heart during gravitational acceleration or deceleration, (2) acts as a physical barrier that protects the heart against infection and inflammation from the lungs and pleural space, and (3) contains pain receptors and mechanoreceptors that can elicit reflex changes in blood pressure and heart rate. The outer layer of the pericardium, the **parietal pericardium,** is composed of a surface layer of mesothelium over a thin layer of connective tissue. The **visceral pericardium,** or **epicardium,** is the inner layer of the pericardium. At one point the visceral pericardium folds back and becomes continuous with the parietal pericardium, allowing the large vessels to enter and leave the heart without breaching the pericardial layers.

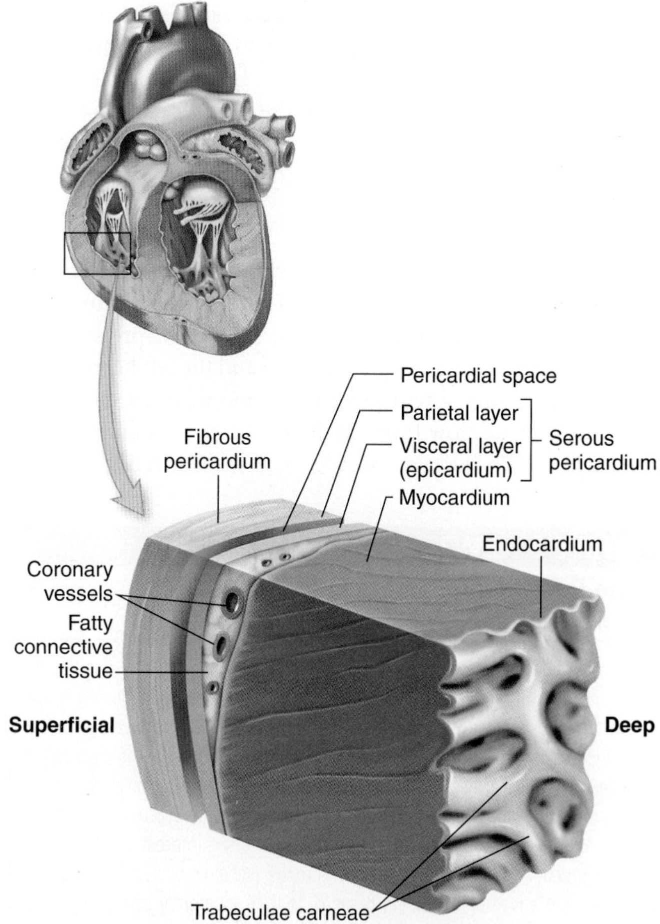

FIGURE 31-2 Wall of the Heart. The cutout section of the heart wall shows the outer fibrous pericardium and the parietal and visceral layers of the serous pericardium (with the pericardial space between them). Note that a layer of fatty connective tissue is located between the visceral layer of the serous pericardium (epicardium) and the myocardium. Note also that the endocardium covers beamlike projections of myocardial muscle tissue, called *trabeculae carneae.* (From Patton KT, Thibodeau GA: *Anatomy & physiology,* ed 8, St Louis, 2013, Mosby.)

The visceral and parietal pericardia are separated by a fluid-containing space called the **pericardial cavity.** The **pericardial fluid** (about 20 ml), which is secreted by cells of the mesothelium, lubricates the membranes that line the pericardial cavity, enabling them to slide over one another with a minimum of friction as the heart beats.[2] The amount and character of the pericardial fluid are altered by inflammation of the pericardium (see Chapter 32).

The outer layer of the heart, the epicardium, provides a smooth surface that allows the heart to contract and relax within the pericardium with a minimal amount of friction. The thickest layer of the heart wall, the **myocardium,** is composed of cardiac muscle and is anchored to the heart's fibrous skeleton. The thickness of the myocardium varies tremendously from one heart chamber to another. Thickness is related to the amount of resistance the muscle must overcome to pump blood from the different chambers. The internal lining of the myocardium is composed of connective tissue and a layer of squamous cells called the **endocardium** (see Figure 31-2). The endocardial lining of the heart is continuous with the endothelium that lines all the arteries, veins, and capillaries of the body, creating a continuous, closed circulatory system (see What's New? The Potential for Using Epicardial Cells in Myocardial Repair).

Chambers of the Heart

The heart has four chambers: the **right atrium, left atrium, right ventricle,** and **left ventricle**. These chambers form two pumps in series: the right heart, which is a low-pressure system pumping blood through the lungs; and the left heart, which is a high-pressure system pumping blood through the rest of the body. (Blood flow through these chambers is illustrated in Figure 31-3.) The atria are smaller than the ventricles and have thinner walls. The walls of the right and left atria are about 1 to 2 mm thick. The ventricles have a thicker myocardial layer and make up much of the bulk of the heart. The wall of the right ventricle is about 4 to 5 mm thick, and that of the left ventricle, the most muscular chamber, is about 12 to 15 mm.[2] The ventricles are formed by a continuum of muscle fibers that originate from the fibrous skeleton at the base of the heart (chiefly around the aortic orifice).

The wall thickness of each cardiac chamber depends on the amount of pressure or resistance it must overcome to eject blood. The two atria have the thinnest walls because they are low-pressure chambers that serve as storage units and conduits for blood that is emptied into the ventricles. Normally, there is little resistance to flow from the atria to the ventricles. The ventricles, on the other hand, must propel blood all the way through the pulmonary or systemic circulation. The ventricular myocardium must be strong enough to pump against pressures in the pulmonary or systemic vessels. The mean pulmonary capillary pressure, the force the right ventricle must overcome, is only 15 mmHg whereas the mean arterial pressure, the force the left ventricle must overcome, is about 92 mmHg. Because the pressure is markedly higher in the systemic circulation, the left ventricle's myocardial wall is several times thicker than that of the right ventricle.

The right ventricle is shaped like a crescent, or triangle, enabling it to function like a bellows and efficiently eject large volumes of blood through the pulmonary semilunar valve into the low-pressure pulmonary system. The left ventricle is larger and bullet shaped, helping it to eject blood through the larger aortic semilunar valve into the high-pressure systemic circulation.

The ventricles are structurally more complex than the atria. Each ventricle contains muscle fibers that divide it roughly into an **inflow tract,** which receives blood from the atrium, and an **outflow tract,** which sends blood to the circulation (see Figure 31-3).

Normally blood does not flow between the chambers of the right side of the heart and the chambers of the left side of the heart except in the fetus before delivery. The adult right and left sides of the heart are separated by intact septal membranes. The atria are separated by the interatrial septum and the ventricles by the interventricular septum. There is an opening between the right and left atria before birth called the foramen ovale; however, this opening closes shortly after birth in most individuals (see Chapter 33). The interventricular septum is an extension of the fibrous skeleton of the heart. Indentations of the endocardium form valves that separate the atria from the ventricles and the ventricles from the aorta and pulmonary arteries.

WHAT'S NEW?

The Potential for Using Epicardial Cells in Myocardial Repair

With cardiovascular disease, including myocardial infarction as one of the leading causes of death and disability, there is great interest in regenerative therapies for the heart muscle. Bone marrow transplants have been tried in an attempt to grow new myocardium but the results are unimpressive. Because studies of heart development in the embryo have shown that both the epicardium and the myocardium develop from a common progenitor, called epicardium-derived cells (EPDCs), there is now great interest in identifying these precursor cells and using them to repair ischemic or dying myocardial tissue. One advantage of using these cells that apparently can be isolated from an adult's heart is that in addition to forming new heart muscle they also will release the appropriate cytokines and growth factors for muscle regeneration and the growth of nourishing blood vessels.

Data from Gittenberger-de Groot AC et al: *Differentiation* 84(1):41–53, 2012; Limana F, Capogrossi MC, Germani A: *Pharmacol Ther* 129(1):82–96, 2011.

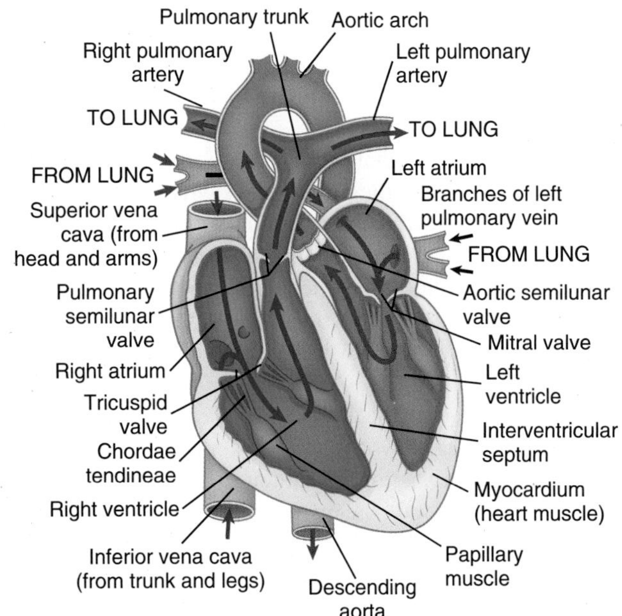

FIGURE 31-3 Structures That Direct Blood Flow Through the Heart. Arrows indicate path of blood flow through chambers, valves, and major vessels.

Fibrous Skeleton of the Heart

Four rings of dense fibrous connective tissue provide a firm anchorage for the attachments of the atrial and ventricular musculature, as well as the valvular tissue. The fibrous rings are adjacent and form a central, fibrous supporting structure collectively termed the annuli fibrosi cordis.

Valves of the Heart

One-way blood flow through the heart is ensured by the four heart valves as well as the pressure gradients that they maintain.

During ventricular relaxation the two **atrioventricular valves** open and blood flows from the relatively higher pressure in the atria to the lower pressure in the relaxed ventricles. With increasing ventricular pressure these valves close and prevent backflow into the atria as the ventricles contract. The **semilunar valves** of the heart open when intraventricular pressure exceeds aortic and pulmonary pressures and blood flows out of the ventricles and into the systemic and pulmonary circulations, respectively. After ventricular contraction and ejection, intraventricular pressure falls and the **pulmonic** and **aortic semilunar valves** close when the pressure in the vessels is greater than the pressure in the ventricles, thus preventing backflow into the right and left ventricles, respectively (Figure 31-4; also see Figure 31-3).

The atrioventricular (AV) (tricuspid and mitral) valve openings are composed of flaps of tissue called *leaflets or cusps* that

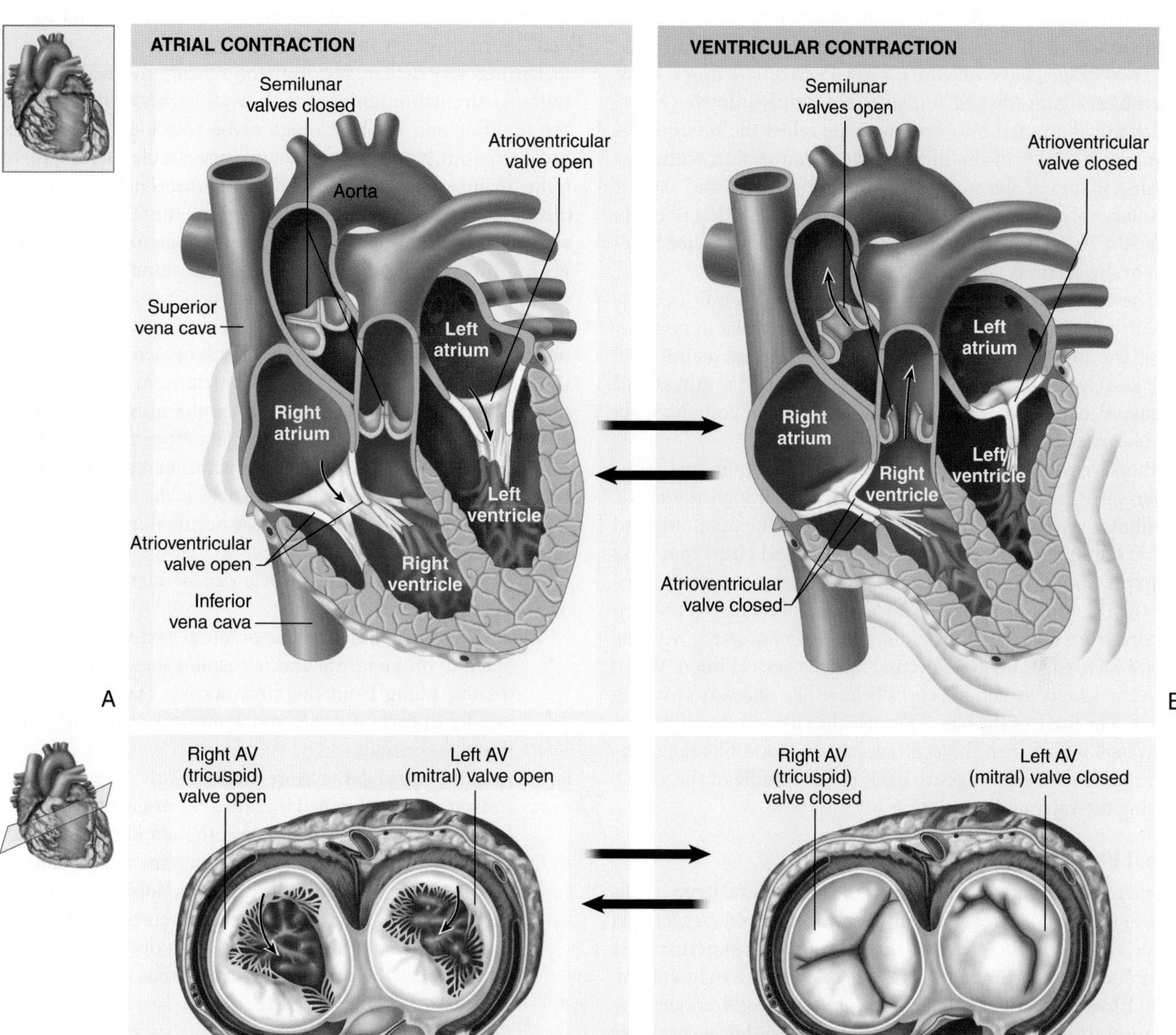

FIGURE 31-4 Chambers and Valves of the Heart. Chambers and valves of the heart. **A,** During atrial contraction cardiac muscle in the atrial wall contracts, forcing blood through the atrioventricular *(AV)* valves and into the ventricles. Bottom illustration shows superior view of all four valves, with semilunar *(SL)* valves closed and AV valves open. **B,** During ventricular contraction that follows, the AV valves close and the blood is forced out of the ventricles through the SL valves and into the arteries. Bottom illustration shows superior view of SL valves open and AV valves closed. (From Patton KT, Thibodeau GA: *Anatomy & physiology,* ed 8, St Louis, 2013, Mosby.)

are attached at the upper end to one of the rings in the fibrous skeleton of the heart and at the lower end to papillary muscles by the **chordae tendineae** (see Figure 31-3). The **papillary muscles** are extensions of the myocardium that help hold the cusps together and downward at the onset of ventricular contraction, thus preventing their backward expulsion, or **prolapse,** into the atria (see p. 1087 for a description of pressure changes and valvular function).

The right AV valve is called the **tricuspid valve** because it has three cusps. The tricuspid opening (orifice) has the largest diameter of all the heart valves. The left AV valve is a bicuspid (two cusps) valve called the **mitral valve.** The mitral valve resembles a cone-shaped funnel that extends into the cusps, which are connected by a fibrous tissue called the *commissure.* The anterior cusp of the mitral valve is continuous with supporting tissues of the aortic semilunar valve cusps and the left coronary valve cusps. (The coronary circulation is described on p. 1090.) Thus damage to this continuous tissue can alter function of the aortic as well as the mitral valves.

The tricuspid and mitral valves function as a unit because the atrium, fibrous rings, valvular tissue, chordae tendineae, papillary muscles, and ventricular walls are all connected. Collectively, these six structures are known as the **mitral and tricuspid complex.** Damage to any one of the complex's six components can alter function significantly.

Blood leaves the right ventricle through the pulmonic semilunar valve, and it leaves the left ventricle through the aortic semilunar valve (see Figures 31-3 and 31-4). The pulmonic and aortic semilunar valves have three cup-shaped cusps that arise from the fibrous skeleton. The pulmonic cusps are slightly thinner than the aortic cusps. The lower edges of each cusp are suspended from the root of the pulmonary artery or aorta, with the upper valve edges freely projecting into the vessel lumen. When the ventricles contract, the cusps behave like one-way swinging doors. The force of the blood propels the cusps outward against the vessel wall. When the ventricles relax, blood fills the cusps and causes their free edges to meet in the middle of the vessel, closing the valve and preventing any backflow.

Great Vessels

Blood moves in and out of the heart through several large vessels (see Figure 31-3). The right heart receives venous deoxygenated blood from the systemic circulation through the **superior vena cava** and the **inferior vena cava,** which enter the right atrium. Blood leaves the right ventricle and enters the pulmonary circulation through the pulmonary artery. The **pulmonary artery** divides into **right** and **left pulmonary arteries** to transport unoxygenated blood from the right heart to the right and left lungs. The pulmonary arteries branch further into the pulmonary capillary bed, where oxygen enters the blood and carbon dioxide leaves it as each gas moves from its higher to lower concentration gradient.

Four **pulmonary veins,** two from the right lung and two from the left lung, carry oxygenated blood from the lungs to the left side of the heart. The oxygenated blood moves through the left atrium and ventricle and out into the **aorta,** which delivers it to systemic vessels that supply the body.

Blood Flow During the Cardiac Cycle

The pumping action of the heart consists of contraction and relaxation of the heart muscle or myocardium. Each ventricular contraction and the relaxation that follows it constitute one **cardiac cycle.** (Blood flow through the heart during a single cardiac cycle is illustrated in Figure 31-4.) During the period of relaxation, termed **diastole,** blood fills the ventricles. The contraction that follows, termed **systole,** propels the blood out of the ventricles and into the pulmonary and systemic circulations. Contraction of the left ventricle occurs slightly earlier than contraction of the right ventricle.

During ventricular systole, blood from the veins of the systemic circulation enters the thin-walled right atrium from the superior and inferior venae cavae (see Figures 31-3 and 31-4). Venous blood from the coronary circulation enters the right atrium through the coronary sinus. The right atrium fills, which, along with the falling right ventricular pressures, allows the right AV (tricuspid) valve to open and fill the right ventricle during ventricular diastole (occasionally called atrial systole). The same sequence of events occurs a split second earlier in the left heart. The four pulmonary veins, two from the right lung and two from the left lung, carry blood from the pulmonary circulation to the left atrium. As the left atrium fills and left ventricular pressure falls, the mitral valve opens and blood flows into the left ventricle. Left atrial contraction, termed "atrial kick," provides significant increases in the volume of blood entering the left ventricle at the end of diastole. Filling of the right and left ventricles occurs during one period of diastole.

Five phases of the cardiac cycle can be identified (Figures 31-5 and 31-6):

Phase 1: Ventricular diastole or atrial systole begins with opening of the mitral and tricuspid valves and then ventricular filling from the atria occurs. The ventricles fill rapidly in early diastole and again in late diastole when the atria contract.

Phase 2: Ventricular systole begins with "isovolumetric contraction," so-called because ventricular volume is constant since both the AV and the semilunar valves are closed. The first detectable rise in ventricular pressure occurs during isovolumetric contraction. This contraction pushes the AV valves shut. Their cusps bulge slightly into the atria but are prevented from opening back into the atria by their anchors, the chordae tendineae (see Figure 31-3).

Phase 3: When ventricular pressure reaches and then slightly exceeds that of the pulmonary artery and aorta, the semilunar valves open and ventricular ejection occurs. Intraventricular pressure and ventricular volume decrease rapidly.

Phase 4: With ventricular relaxation and decreased ventricular pressure, the aortic valve closes and "isovolumetric relaxation" occurs. Again, both the AV and the semilunar valves are closed during this phase.

Phase 5: When left ventricular pressure falls below atrial pressure, the mitral and tricuspid valves open and *passive ventricular filling occurs.*

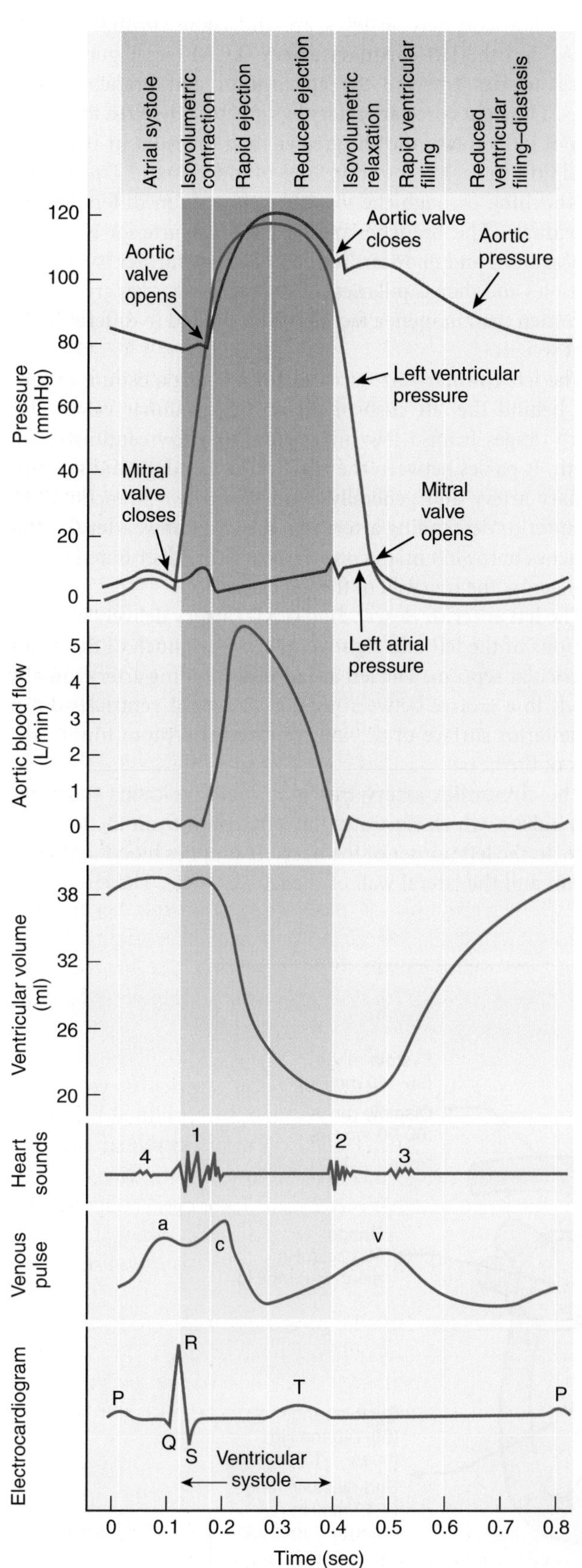

FIGURE 31-5 Composite Chart of Heart Function. This chart is a composite of several diagrams of heart function (blood pressure, blood flow, volume, heart sounds, venous pulse, and electrocardiogram [ECG]), all adjusted to the same time scale.

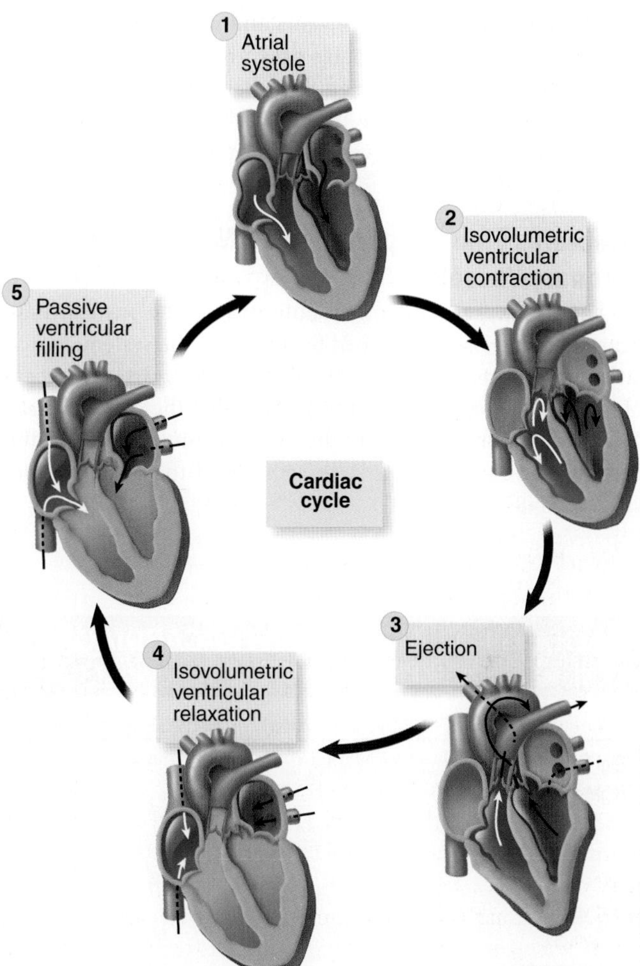

FIGURE 31-6 Phases of the Cardiac Cycle. **1,** Atrial systole. **2,** Isovolumetric ventricular contraction. Ventricular volume remains constant as pressure increases rapidly. **3,** Ejection. **4,** Isovolumetric ventricular relaxation. Both sets of valves are closed, and the ventricles are relaxing. **5,** Passive ventricular filling. The atrioventricular *(AV)* valves are forced open, and the blood rushes into the relaxing ventricles. (From Patton KT, Thibodeau GA: *Anatomy & physiology,* ed 8, St Louis, 2013, Mosby.)

As blood is pushed through the inflow and outflow tracts of the ventricles, it flows around the **crista supraventricularis**—the muscle that separates the inflow from the outflow tracts—and is mixed by passing through the strands of the **trabeculae carneae.**

Normal Intracardiac Pressures

Normal intracardiac pressures are shown in Table 31-1 and Figure 31-7. Atrial pressure (see venous pulse in Figure 31-5) curves are composed of the **a wave,** which is generated by atrial contraction, and the **v wave,** which is an early diastolic peak caused by filling of the atrium from the peripheral veins. A smaller pressure increase, the **c wave,** occurs after the a wave in early systole and may represent bulging of the mitral valve into the left atrium during early systole. Two aspects of falling atrial pressure have also been named. The **x descent** follows the a wave and is produced by the descent of the tricuspid valve ring and by the ejection of blood from both ventricles. The **y descent** that follows the v wave reflects the rapid flow of blood from the great veins and right atrium into the right ventricle. Left ventricular pressures are illustrated by a peak systolic pressure and an end-diastolic pressure, which is the ventricular pressure immediately before the onset of systole. The minimal left ventricular pressure occurs in early diastole.

Structures That Support Cardiac Metabolism: The Coronary Vessels

To supply oxygen and other nutrients to the myocardium, heart structures are nourished by vessels of the systemic circulation, the *coronary circulation.* The coronary arteries receive blood through openings in the aorta, called the *coronary ostia.* The cardiac veins empty into the right atrium through another ostium, the opening of a large vein called the *coronary sinus* (Figure 31-8).

TABLE 31-1 NORMAL INTRACARDIAC PRESSURES

	MEAN (mmHg)	RANGE (mmHg)
Right atrium	4	0-8
Right ventricle		
Systolic	24	15-28
End-diastolic	4	0-8
Left atrium	7	4-12
Left ventricle		
Systolic	130	90-140
End-diastolic	7	4-12

Coronary Arteries

The major coronary arteries are the **right coronary artery (RCA)** and the **left coronary artery (LCA)** (see Figure 31-8). These arteries traverse the epicardium and branch several times. The right coronary artery has greater flow than the left in 70% of individuals, the left greater than the right in 10%, and equal flow in each is found in 20% of individuals.[3] The pattern of branching through the visceral pericardium differs among individuals. The branches of the coronary arteries enter the myocardium and endocardium and branch further to become arterioles and then capillaries. The coronary arteries are smaller in women than in men, a fact that is attributed to differences in heart weight.

The left coronary artery arises from a single ostium (opening) behind the left cusp of the aortic semilunar valve. This artery ranges from a few millimeters to a few centimeters in length. It passes between the left atrial appendage and the pulmonary artery and generally divides into two branches—the left anterior descending artery and the circumflex artery. Other branches of the left main coronary artery are distributed diagonally across the free wall of the left ventricle.

The **left anterior descending (LAD) artery** delivers blood to portions of the left and right ventricles and much of the interventricular septum. The left anterior descending artery initially travels in a groove between the left and right ventricles down the anterior surface of the interventricular septum toward the apex of the heart.

The **circumflex artery** travels in a groove called the **coronary sulcus,** which separates the left atrium from the left ventricle, to the left border of the heart. It supplies blood to the left atrium and the lateral wall of the left ventricle. The circumflex

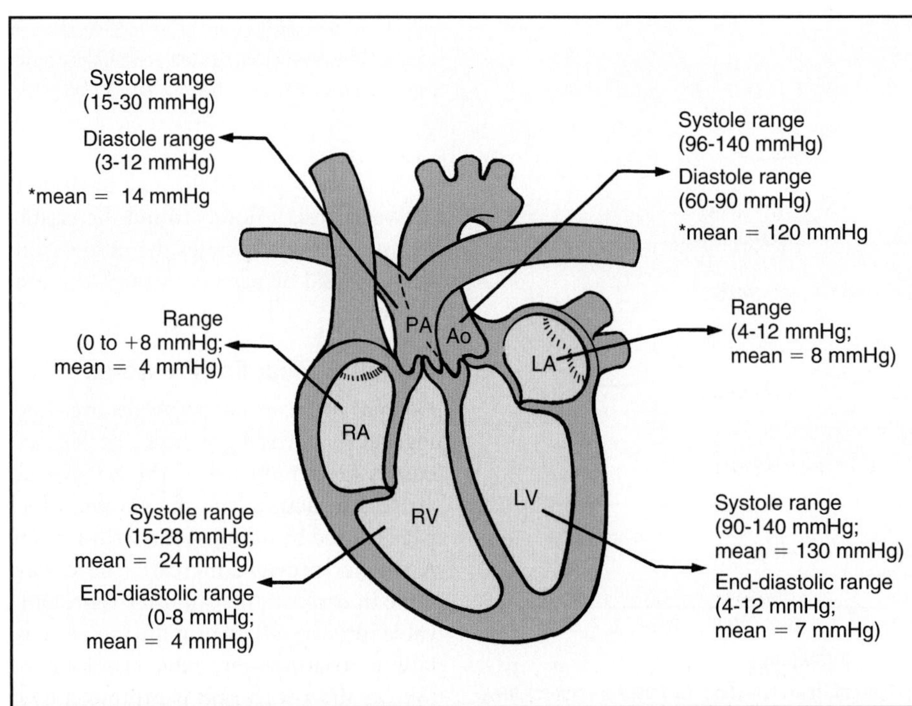

FIGURE 31-7 Normal Intracardiac Pressures. *Ao,* Aorta; *LA,* left atrium; *LV,* left ventricle; *PA,* pulmonary artery; *RA,* right atrium; *RV,* right ventricle. *Main mean pressure.

artery often branches to the posterior surfaces of the left atrium and left ventricle (see Figure 31-8).

The right coronary artery originates from an ostium behind the right aortic cusp, travels behind the pulmonary artery, and extends around the right heart to the heart's posterior surface, where it branches to the right atrium and ventricle. The three major branches of the right coronary artery include the conus, which supplies blood to the upper right ventricle; the right marginal branch, which traverses the right ventricle to the apex; and the posterior descending branch, which lies in the posterior interventricular sulcus and supplies smaller branches to both ventricles.

Collateral Arteries

The **collateral arteries** are connections, or anastomoses, between branches of the same coronary artery or connections of branches of the right coronary artery with branches of the left. They are particularly common within the interventricular and interatrial septa, at the apex of the heart, over the anterior surface of the right ventricle, and around the sinus node. The epicardium contains more collateral vessels than the endocardium.

The functional importance of the collateral circulation is that it protects the heart from ischemia. The collateral circulation is responsible for supplying blood and oxygen to the myocardium that has been deprived of oxygen following narrowing

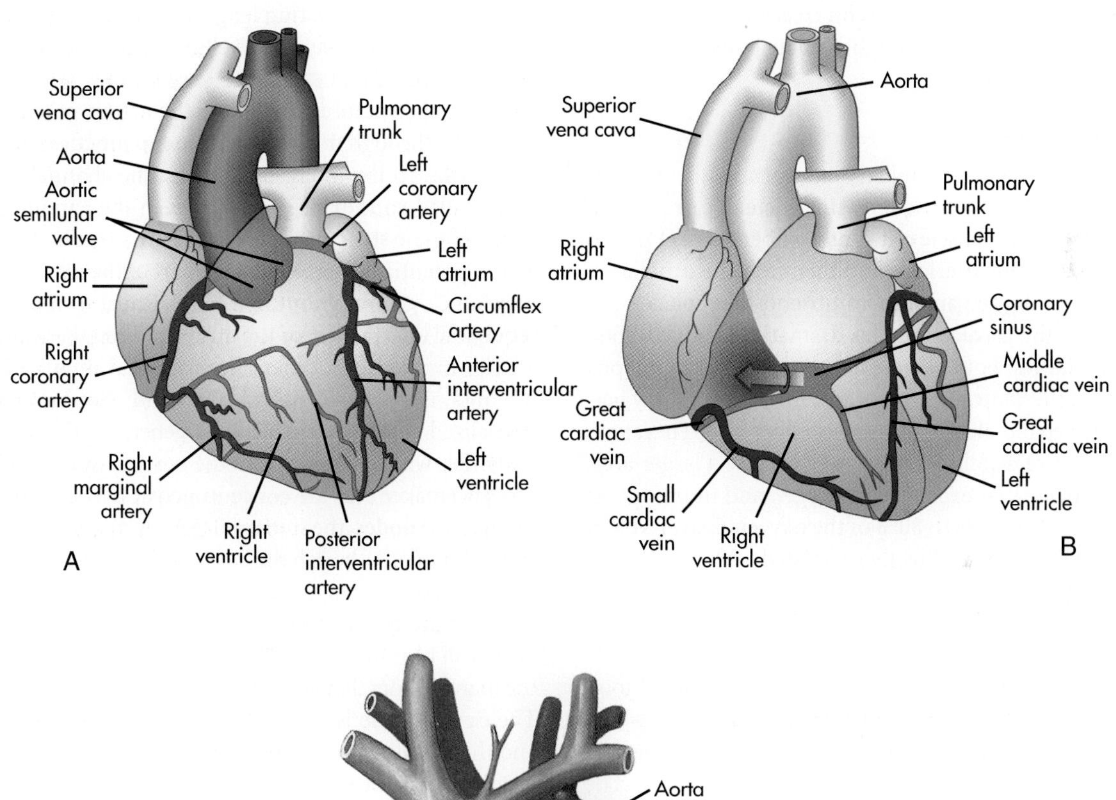

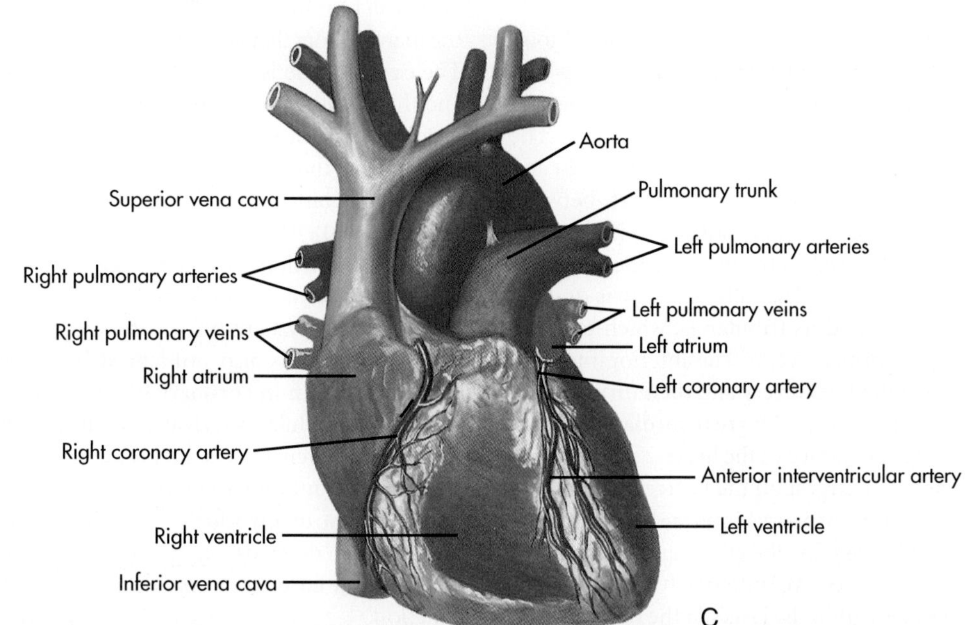

FIGURE 31-8 Coronary Circulation. **A,** Arteries. **B,** Veins. Both **A** and **B** are anterior views of the heart. Vessels near the anterior surface are more darkly colored than vessels of the posterior surface seen through the heart. **C,** View of the anterior (sternocostal) surface. (**A** and **B** modified from Patton KT, Thibodeau GA: *Anatomy & physiology,* ed 8, St Louis, 2013, Mosby. **C** from Seeley RR, Stephens TD, Tate P: *Anatomy & physiology,* ed 3, St Louis, 1995, Mosby.)

of a major coronary artery (coronary artery disease). Gradual coronary occlusion results in the growth of coronary collaterals. New collateral vessels are formed through two processes: **arteriogenesis** (new artery growth branching from pre-existing arteries) and **angiogenesis** (growth of new capillaries within a tissue).[4] A key stimulus to collateral growth is the **shear stress** caused by increased blood flow velocity that occurs close to sites of **stenosis** (narrowing) or occlusion. Shear stress activates the endothelium of the pre-existing arterioles and stimulates the production of growth factors and cytokines, including monocyte chemoattractant protein-1 (MCP-1) and vascular endothelial growth factor (VEGF).[5] Current research is focused on identifying whether some of these factors that stimulate collateral growth might prove to be useful treatments for persons with myocardial ischemia, although to date none have been demonstrated to be effective.[5]

Coronary Capillaries

The heart has an extensive capillary network, with approximately 3300 capillaries per square millimeter (ca/mm^2) or about one capillary per muscle cell (muscle fiber). Blood travels from the arteries to the arterioles and then into the capillaries, where exchange of oxygen and other nutrients takes place.

Alterations of the cardiac muscles dramatically affect blood flow in the capillaries. For example, in ventricular hypertrophy (enlargement of the ventricular myocardium), the capillary network does not expand along with muscle fiber size. Therefore, the same number of capillaries must now perfuse a larger area. This results in decreased exchange of oxygen and nutrients. At rest, the heart extracts 70% to 80% of the oxygen delivered to it and coronary blood flow is directly correlated with myocardial oxygen consumption.[6]

Coronary Veins and Lymphatic Vessels

After passing through the extensive capillary network, blood from the coronary arteries drains into the cardiac veins, which travel alongside the arteries. Most of the venous drainage of the heart occurs through veins in the visceral pericardium. The veins then feed into the great cardiac vein (see Figure 31-8) and coronary sinus on the posterior surface of the heart, between the atria and ventricles, in the coronary sulcus. Venous coronary blood empties into the right atrium from the coronary sinus. Blood from the left ventricular walls generally is drained through the coronary sinus and its tributaries, which together form the largest system of coronary veins. The anterior interventricular vein flows beside the LAD artery and then turns to join the circumflex artery and becomes the **great cardiac vein** that primarily drains the anterior surface of the heart. The **posterior vein of the left ventricle,** the largest on the posterior surface of the heart, branches from the coronary sinus and accompanies the circumflex artery and then joins the great cardiac vein.[3]

The myocardium has an extensive system of lymphatic capillaries and collecting vessels within the layers of the myocardium and also in the valves. With cardiac contraction the lymphatic vessels drain fluid to the paratracheal lymph nodes in the anterior mediastinum and then continue to join the mediastinal lymphatic vessels. Impairment of cardiac lymphatic function has been hypothesized to impact cardiac conduction, protection from infection, and the development of myocardial fibrosis and atherosclerosis.[7]

Structures That Control Heart Action

Our lives depend on the continuous repetition of the cardiac cycle (systole and diastole) that occurs because of the transmission of electrical impulses, termed **cardiac action potentials,** through the myocardium. (Action potentials are described in Chapters 1 and 3.) As an electrical impulse passes from cell to cell (fiber to fiber) in the myocardium, it stimulates an intracellular process that results in fiber shortening—that is, muscular contraction or systole. Between action potentials, the fibers relax and return to their resting length, causing diastole. The muscle fibers of the myocardium are electrically coupled so that action potentials pass from cell to cell very rapidly and efficiently. The myocardial structures that allow the action potentials to move so rapidly through the heart are the gap junctions in the intercalated disks. In the intercalated disks, the channel-forming proteins, called **connexins,** form pores in the gap junctions.[8] As a result of these structures plus the heart's conduction system, an action potential generated in one part of the myocardium passes very quickly throughout the heart, causing rapid, organized, sequential contraction of the atria and then the ventricles.

The myocardium differs from skeletal muscle tissue in that it contains its own pacemakers and **conduction system**—specialized cells that enable it to generate and transmit action potentials without input from the nervous system (Figure 31-9). The pacemaker cells are concentrated at two sites in the myocardium called **nodes,** the sinoatrial (SA) node and the atrioventricular (AV) node. Although the heart is innervated by the autonomic nervous system (sympathetic and parasympathetic fibers), neural impulses are not needed to maintain the cardiac cycle. Thus the heart will beat in the absence of any nervous connection, one of the many factors that allow heart transplantation to be successful. The cardiac cycle is stimulated by the nodes of specialized cells and then adjusted to the physical needs of the body by the autonomic fibers. The sympathetic and parasympathetic nerves affect the speed of the cardiac cycle (**heart rate,** or beats per minute), the force of contraction, and the diameter of the coronary vessels (Figure 31-10). The sympathetic nervous system increases heart rate and conduction through the nodes, the parasympathetic nervous system slows heart rate and prolongs intranodal conduction time, and both systems cause coronary vasodilation.[9]

Heart action is also influenced by substances delivered to the myocardium in coronary blood. Nutrients and oxygen are needed for cellular survival and normal function, and hormones and biochemicals, including medications, can affect the strength and duration of myocardial contraction and the degree and duration of myocardial relaxation. Normal or appropriate function depends on the availability of these substances, which is why coronary artery disease can seriously disrupt heart function.

Conduction System

Normally electrical impulses arise in the **sinoatrial (SA) node (SA node, sinus node),** the usual *pacemaker of the heart.* The SA

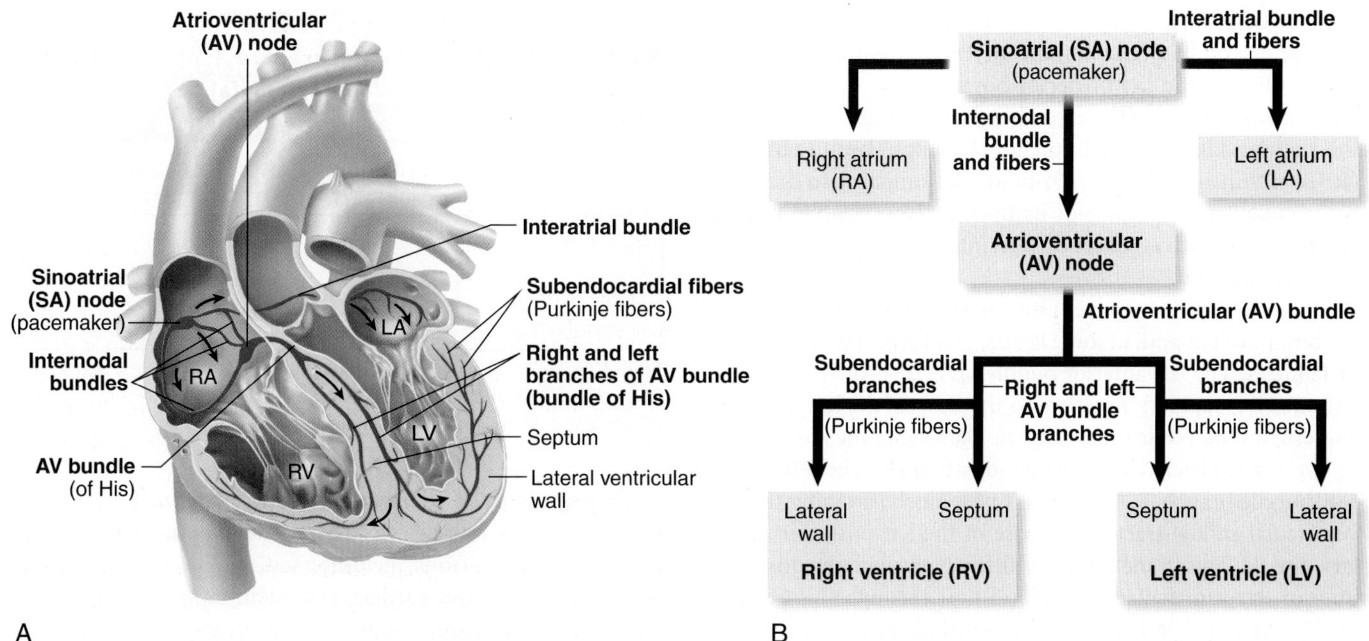

FIGURE 31-9 Conduction System of the Heart. Specialized cardiac muscle cells *(boldface type)* in the wall of the heart rapidly initiate or conduct an electrical impulse throughout the myocardium. Both the sketch of the conduction system **(A)** and the flowchart **(B)** show the origin and path of conduction. The signal is initiated by the SA node (pacemaker) and spreads to the rest of the right atrial myocardium directly, to the left atrial myocardium by way of a bundle of interatrial conducting fibers, and to the AV node by way of three internodal bundles. The AV node then initiates a signal that is conducted through the ventricular myocardium by way of the AV bundle (of His) and subendocardial branches (Purkinje fibers). (From Patton KT, Thibodeau GA: *Anatomy & physiology,* ed 8, St Louis, 2013, Mosby.)

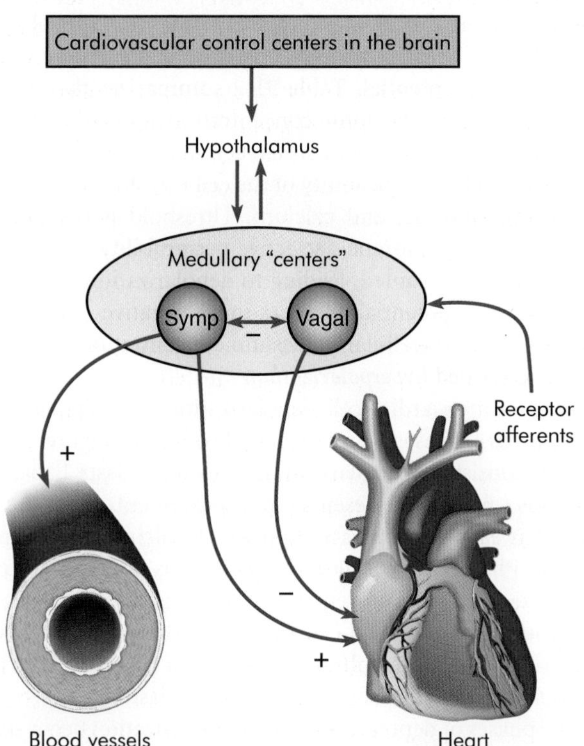

FIGURE 31-10 Autonomic Innervation of Cardiovascular System. *+,* Activation; *–,* inhibition; *Symp,* sympathetic.

node is located at the junction of the right atrium and superior vena cava, just above the tricuspid valve (see Figure 31-9). The SA node sits only about 1 mm beneath the visceral pericardium, making it vulnerable to injury and disease, especially pericardial inflammation. The SA node is nourished by the sinus node artery, which passes through the center of the node. The SA node is heavily innervated by both sympathetic and parasympathetic nerve fibers. Impulse formation is thought to occur in two cell types found in the node—spindle- and spider-shaped cells.[9]

In the resting adult the SA node generates about 60 to 100 action potentials per minute depending on age and physical condition. Each action potential travels rapidly from cell to cell and through special pathways in the atrial myocardium, causing both atria to contract, beginning systole. The action potential is transmitted from the atrial to the ventricular myocardium through fibers of the conduction system, traveling first to the **atrioventricular (AV) node,** then to the **bundle of His (atrioventricular bundle, common bundle),** and finally through the **bundle branches** of the interventricular septum to Purkinje fibers in the heart wall (see Figure 31-9).

The AV node is well situated for mediating conduction between the atria and ventricles. It is located in the right atrial wall above the tricuspid valve and anterior to the ostium of the coronary sinus. There is variability in the size and length of the AV node fibers. Generally the AV node is thicker and shorter in size than the SA node. Behind the AV node are numerous autonomic parasympathetic ganglia. (The nervous systems are described in Chapter 15.)

Conducting fibers from the AV node converge to form the bundle of His. The bundle of His, which is triangular shaped, lies within the posterior border of the interventricular septum. The two lower ends of the triangle give rise to the right and left bundle branches. The **right bundle branch (RBB)** is thin and travels without much branching to the right ventricular apex. Because of its thinness and relative lack of branches, the RBB is susceptible to interruption by damage to the endocardium.

The **left bundle branch (LBB)** arises perpendicularly from the bundle of His and, in some hearts, divides into two branches, or fascicles. The left anterior bundle branch (LABB) passes the left anterior papillary muscle and the base of the left ventricle and crosses the aortic outflow tract. Damage to the aortic valve or the left ventricle can interrupt this branch. The left posterior bundle branch (LPBB) travels posteriorly, crossing the left ventricular inflow tract to the base of the left posterior papillary muscle. This branch spreads diffusely through the posterior inferior left ventricular wall. Blood flow through this portion of the left ventricle is relatively nonturbulent, so the LPBB is somewhat protected from injury caused by wear and tear. The **Purkinje fibers** are the terminal branches of the right and left bundle branches. They extend from the ventricular apexes to the fibrous rings and penetrate the heart wall to the outer myocardium.

Cardiac Excitation. From the SA node the impulse that begins systole spreads throughout the right atrium at a conduction velocity of about 35 cm/sec.[9] Because impulses from the SA node arrive at the AV node very quickly, investigators have proposed that these nodes are connected by internodal pathways, called the anterior, middle, and posterior internodal pathways. However, the existence of these pathways is controversial; not all experts agree that they exist.[9]

The action potential is delayed in the region of the AV node, possibly because of electrophysiologic differences in the cells that comprise the AV region. Conduction velocity within the node is about 10 cm/sec, markedly slower than conduction through the atria.[9] The delay between atrial and ventricular excitation permits an additional boost to ventricular filling by atrial contraction (atrial kick). From the AV node the impulse travels from the AV bundle and through the bundle branches to the Purkinje fibers. Conduction velocities in the AV and Purkinje fibers are the most rapid in the heart.

Ventricular activation occurs sequentially in three phases: (1) septal activation, (2) apical activation, and (3) basal (upper) and posterior activation. The first areas of the ventricles to be excited are portions of the interventricular septum. The septum is activated from both the RBB and the LBB, although the impulse travels from left to right. The extensive network of Purkinje fibers promotes the rapid spread of the impulse to the ventricular apexes. Activation traverses the heart wall from the inside outward (from the endocardium to the epicardium; see Figure 31-2). The basal and posterior portions of the ventricles are the last to be activated. Deactivation, which begins in diastole, occurs in the opposite direction, spreading from the outside inward (epicardium to endocardium). All areas of the ventricle recover at about the same time.

TABLE 31-2 INTRACELLULAR AND EXTRACELLULAR ION CONCENTRATIONS IN THE MYOCARDIUM

ION	INTRACELLULAR CONCENTRATION	EXTRACELLULAR CONCENTRATION
Sodium (Na^+)	15 mM	145 mM
Potassium (K^+)	150 mM	4 mM
Chloride (Cl^-)	5-30 mM	120 mM
Calcium (Ca^{++})	10^{-7} M	2 mM

From Bonow RO et al, editors: *Braunwald's heart disease: a textbook of cardiovascular medicine,* ed 9, Philadelphia, 2012, Elsevier Saunders. *M,* Moles; *mM,* millimoles per kilogram.

Propagation of Cardiac Action Potentials. Electrical activation of the muscle cells, termed **depolarization,** is caused by the movement of ions, including sodium, potassium, calcium, and chloride, across cardiac cell membranes. Deactivation, called **repolarization,** occurs the same way. (Movement of ions across cell membranes is described in Chapter 1; electrical activation of muscle cells is described in Chapter 43.)

Movement of ions into and out of the cell creates an electrical (voltage) difference across the cell membrane called the *membrane potential.* The resting membrane potential of myocardial cells is between −80 and −90 millivolts (mV), whereas the SA node is between −50 and −60 mV and the AV node is between −60 and −70 mV.[9] During depolarization the inside of the cell becomes less negatively charged. In cardiac cells the difference between resting membrane potential (in millivolts) and the decreased negative charge caused by depolarization is the cardiac action potential. Table 31-2 summarizes the intracellular and extracellular ionic concentrations of cardiac muscle. The various phases of the cardiac action potential are related to changes in the permeability of the cell membrane to sodium, potassium, chloride, and calcium. Threshold is the point at which the cell membrane's selective permeability to these ions is temporarily disrupted, leading to depolarization. If the resting membrane potential becomes more negative as a result of a decrease in extracellular potassium concentration (hypokalemia), it is termed *hyperpolarization.*

Normal myocardial cell depolarization and repolarization occur in five phases numbered 0 through 4 (Figure 31-11). Phase 0 consists of depolarization. This phase lasts 1 to 2 milliseconds (ms) and represents rapid sodium entry into the cell. Phase 1 is early repolarization, in which calcium slowly enters the cell. Phase 2, also called the *plateau,* is a continuation of repolarization, with slow entry of calcium and sodium into the cell. Potassium is moved out of the cell during phase 3, with a return to resting membrane potential in phase 4.[9] The time between action potentials corresponds to diastole.

The phases of depolarization and repolarization occur somewhat differently in the SA and AV node cells, a difference that enables these cells to generate cardiac action potentials independently. The cells of the Purkinje fibers, atria, and ventricles begin with a negative resting membrane potential and proceed to a rapid upstroke, or depolarization (phase 0), a rapid early

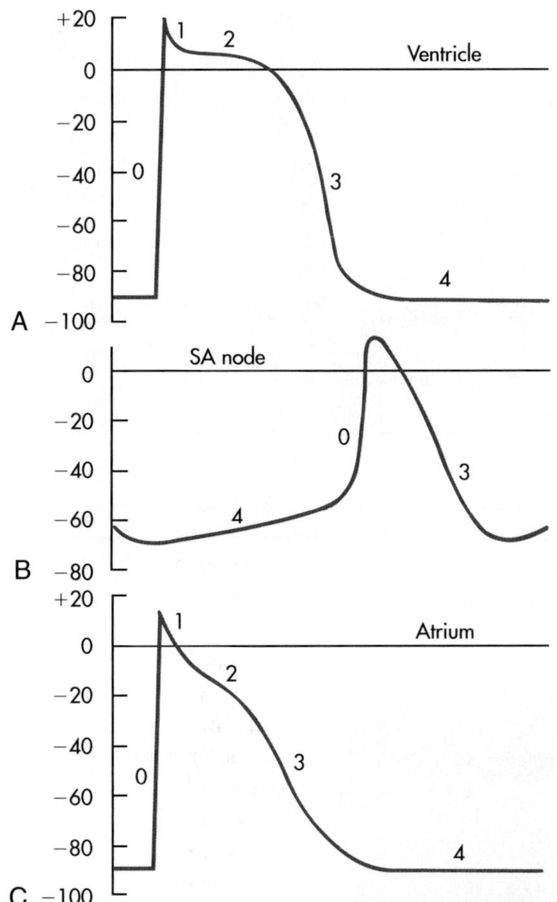

FIGURE 31-11 Cardiac Action Potentials. **A,** Ventricle. **B,** Sinoatrial *(SA)* node. **C,** Atrium. Sweep velocity in **B** is half that in **A** or **C.** (Modified from Koeppen BM, Stanton BA: *Berne and Levy physiology,* ed 6, Philadelphia, 2010, Mosby.)

repolarization (phase 1), a plateau (phase 2), and a rapid later repolarization (phase 3) (see Figure 31-11, *A* and *C*). The fast inward current of phase 0 is mediated by sodium ions flowing through "fast channels" in the cell membrane and causes the rapid upstroke of the action potential in Purkinje fibers, atria, and ventricles. In contrast, the cells of the SA and AV nodes begin with a less negative resting membrane potential, proceed to a slow upstroke (phase 0), and usually lack a plateau (phase 2) (see Figure 31-11, *B*). The slow inward current, mediated by calcium through transient and long-lasting channels and sodium ions flowing through "slow channels" of the cell membrane, is responsible for the action potential of the SA node and the AV node. Hence, drugs that block calcium have profound effects on the slow inward current and can alter heart rate. Slow channel-blocking drugs, such as verapamil, are used to treat a variety of cardiovascular disorders.

A refractory period, during which no new cardiac action potential can be initiated by a stimulus, follows depolarization. This effective or absolute refractory period corresponds to the time needed for the reopening of channels that permit sodium and calcium influx (phase 0 through half of phase 3). A relative refractory period occurs near the end of repolarization, following the effective refractory period. During this time the membrane can be depolarized again but only by a greater than normal stimulus. Abnormal refractory periods as a result of disease can cause abnormal heart rhythms, or dysrhythmias, including ventricular fibrillation and cardiac arrest (see Chapter 32).

Normal Electrocardiogram. The genesis of the normal electrocardiogram is from electrical activity recorded by skin electrodes, that is, the sum of all cardiac action potentials (Figure 31-12). The **P wave** represents atrial depolarization. The **PR interval** is a measure of time from the onset of atrial activation to the onset of ventricular activation; it normally ranges from 0.12 to 0.20 second. The PR interval represents the time necessary to travel from the sinus node through the atrium, AV node, and His-Purkinje system to activate ventricular myocardial cells. The **QRS complex** represents the sum of all ventricular muscle cell depolarizations. The configuration and amplitude of the QRS complex vary considerably among individuals. The duration is normally between 0.06 and 0.10 second. During the **ST interval** the entire ventricular myocardium is depolarized. The **QT interval** is sometimes called the "electrical systole" of the ventricles. It lasts about 0.4 second, but it varies inversely with the heart rate.

Automaticity. Automaticity, or the property of generating spontaneous depolarization to threshold, enables the SA and AV nodes to generate cardiac action potentials without any stimulus. Cells capable of spontaneous depolarization are called **automatic cells.** The automatic cells of the cardiac conduction system can stimulate the heart to beat even when the heart is removed from the body. Spontaneous depolarization is possible in automatic cells because the membrane potential does not "rest" during phase 4. Instead, it slowly creeps toward threshold during the diastolic phase of the cardiac cycle. Because threshold is approached during diastole, phase 4 in automatic cells is called **diastolic depolarization.** The electrical impulse normally begins in the SA node because its cells depolarize more rapidly than other automatic cells. The ionic basis for this diastolic depolarization is the regular rhythmic oscillation of calcium with the automatic cells, a phenomenon known as the "calcium clock."[9]

Rhythmicity. Rhythmicity is the regular generation of an action potential by the heart's conduction system. The SA node sets the pace because normally it has the fastest rate of depolarization, which is why it is called the *natural pacemaker of the heart.* The SA node depolarizes spontaneously 60 to 100 times per minute. If the SA node is damaged, the AV node will become the heart's pacemaker at a rate of about 40 to 60 spontaneous depolarizations per minute. Purkinje fibers also are capable of spontaneous depolarization but at a rate of only 30 to 40 beats/minute; therefore they only function as pacemakers when the SA and AV nodes are diseased or there is interruption to movement of electrical current through the heart.

Cardiac Innervation

Although the heart's nodes and conduction system generate cardiac action potentials independently, the autonomic nervous system influences the rate of impulse generation (firing), depolarization, and repolarization of the myocardium and the strength of atrial and ventricular contraction. Autonomic neural transmission produces changes in the heart and

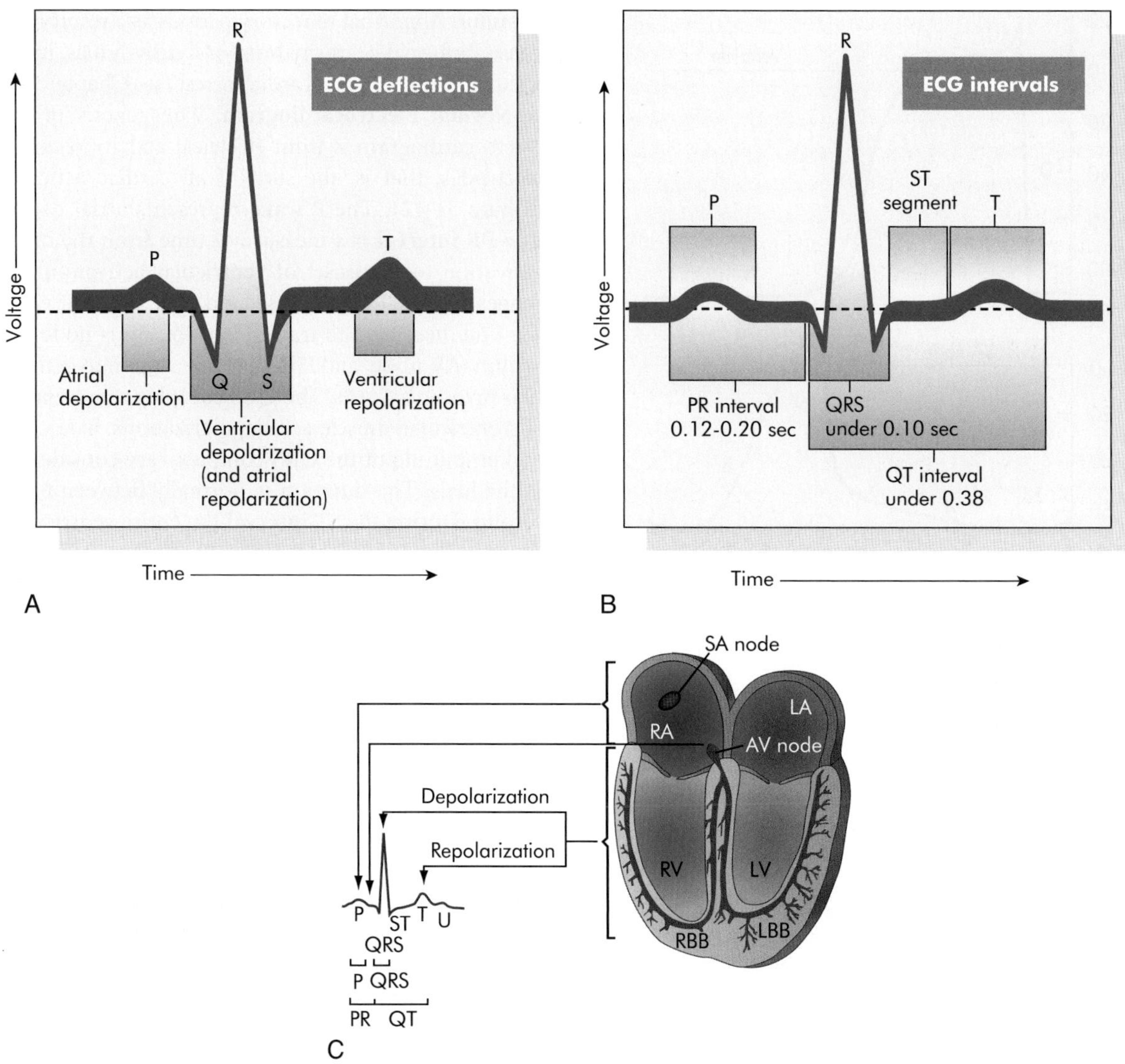

FIGURE 31-12 **Electrocardiogram (ECG) and Cardiac Electrical Activity. A,** Normal ECG. Depolarization and repolarization. **B,** ECG intervals among P, QRS, and T waves. **C,** Schematic representation of ECG and its relationship to cardiac electrical activity. *AV,* Atrioventricular; *LA,* left atrium; *LBB,* left bundle branch; *LV,* left ventricle; *RA,* right atrium; *RBB,* right bundle branch; *RV,* right ventricle. (**A** and **B** from Thibodeau GA, Patton KT: *Anatomy & physiology,* ed 5, St Louis, 2003, Mosby. **C** from Thibodeau GA: *Anatomy & physiology,* St Louis, 1987, Mosby.)

circulatory system faster than metabolic or humoral agents (see Figure 31-10). Speed is important, for example, in stimulating the heart to increase its pumping action during times of stress and fear, the so-called *fight-or-flight response,* or with increased physical activity. Although increased delivery of oxygen, glucose, hormones, and other blood-borne factors sustains increased cardiac activity, the rapid initiation of increased activity depends on the sympathetic and parasympathetic fibers of the autonomic nervous system. (The autonomic nervous system is described and illustrated in Chapter 15.)

Sympathetic and Parasympathetic Nerves. Sympathetic and parasympathetic nerve fibers innervate all parts of the atria and ventricles and the SA and AV nodes. In general, sympathetic stimulation increases electrical conductivity and the strength of myocardial contraction, and vagal parasympathetic nerve activity does the opposite, slowing the conduction of action potentials through the heart and reducing the strength of contraction.

Efferent sympathetic fibers originate in the thoracic spinal cord and branch into the superior middle and inferior cardiac nerves. They join at the **cardiac plexus,** a neural junction located at the root of the aorta in front of the trachea. Sympathetic nervous activity enhances myocardial performance. Catecholamines speed heart rate, shorten the conduction time through the AV node, and increase the rhythmicity of the AV pacemaker fibers. Neurally released norepinephrine or circulating catecholamines interact with β-adrenergic receptors on the cardiac cell membranes. The overall effect is an increased influx of Ca^{++} during the action potential plateau that increases the contractile strength of the heart.

The efferent parasympathetic fibers originate in the medulla oblongata and travel by way of the vagus nerves to join the sympathetic nerves in the cardiac plexus. Parasympathetic (vagal) activity causes the release of acetylcholine. Receptors for these neurotransmitters are found in the myocardium and coronary vessels of the heart. Acetylcholine decreases heart rate, slows conduction through the AV nodes, and reduces myocardial contraction strength.[9]

Adrenergic Receptor Function. Sympathetic neural stimulation of the myocardium and coronary vessels depends on the presence of G-protein–coupled adrenergic receptors, which bind specifically with neurotransmitters of the sympathetic nervous system. (Receptor physiology is discussed in Chapter 1.) The effects of sympathetic stimulation depend on whether (1) the α- or β-adrenergic receptors are most plentiful on cells of the effector tissue, (2) the neurotransmitter is norepinephrine or epinephrine, and (3) the extent to which the individual variations in receptor structure caused by single nucleotide polymorphisms (SNPs) influence receptor responsiveness.[10,11]

There are five types of adrenergic receptors: β_1, β_2, β_3, α_1, and α_2 (see Table 15-7). Each of the α-adrenergic receptors also has three subtypes, so some sources indicate that there are nine types of adrenergic receptors.[11,12] Overall, cardiovascular structures have more β than α receptors; therefore, effects mediated by the β receptors predominate. Norepinephrine is released by postsynaptic sympathetic nerve endings in the heart while epinephrine is mainly released by the adrenal medulla and reaches the heart through the bloodstream.

The β_1 receptors are found mostly in the heart, specifically the conduction system (AV and SA nodes, Purkinje fibers) and the atrial and ventricular myocardium. The β_2 receptors are found in the heart and also on vascular smooth muscle. Stimulation of both the β_1 and β_2 receptors results in an increase in heart rate (chronotropy) and force of myocardial contraction (inotropy).[13] In addition, stimulation of the β_2 receptors results in vasodilation because of the location of the receptors on vascular smooth muscle. Overall β_1 and β_2 stimulation enables the heart to pump more blood and β_2 stimulation also increases coronary blood flow, and β_3 receptors are also found in the myocardium and coronary vessels. In the heart, stimulation of these receptors opposes the effects of β_1- and β_2-receptor stimulation and decreases myocardial contractility (negative inotropic effect).[13] Thus β_3 receptors may provide a "safety mechanism" to prevent overstimulation of the heart by the sympathetic nervous system.

Norepinephrine binding with α_1 receptors, all of which are postsynaptic in the systemic and coronary arteries, causes smooth muscle contraction and thus vasoconstriction. One of the three subtypes of α_2 receptors, α_{2a}, is located on the sympathetic ganglia and nerve terminals. The effect of norepinephrine on these receptors is to inhibit release of more norepinephrine, which promotes vasodilation, thus providing another safety mechanism to prevent excess blood pressure elevation.[13] Dysfunction of α- and β-adrenergic receptors can occur in many conditions (e.g., diabetes, hypertension) and has been implicated in the pathogenesis of many cardiac diseases, including heart failure, myocardial ischemia, and dysrhythmias.[10,11,13]

Myocardial Cells

The cells of cardiac muscle (the myocardium) and of skeletal muscle are nearly identical in structure, function, and microscopic appearance. (The properties of skeletal muscle are described in detail in Chapter 43.) Both types of muscle tissue are composed of long, narrow cells, called *fibers,* that contain basically the same structures: bundles of longitudinally arranged myofibrils; a single nucleus (cardiac muscle) or many nuclei (skeletal muscle); mitochondria; an internal membrane system (the sarcoplasmic reticulum); cytoplasm (sarcoplasm); and a plasma membrane (the sarcolemma), which encloses the cell. Cardiac and skeletal muscle cells also have an "external" membrane system made up of transverse tubules (T tubules) formed by invaginations of the sarcolemma. The sarcoplasmic reticulum forms a network of channels that surround the muscle fiber.

The microscopic appearance of cardiac and skeletal muscle is somewhat similar as well (see Chapter 1, Table 1-8). Because the myofibrils in both types of fibers consist of alternating light and dark bands of protein, the fibers appear striped, or striated. The dark and light bands of the myofibrils comprise longitudinal repeating units called *sarcomeres.* The length of the sarcomeres, normally between 1.6 and 2.2 mm, is important because it determines the limits of myocardial stretch at the end of diastole and subsequently the force of contraction during systole.

Cardiac muscle differs from skeletal muscle in several respects that reflect heart function. Cardiac cells are arranged in branching networks throughout the myocardium, whereas skeletal muscle cells tend to be arranged in parallel throughout the length of the muscle. Cardiac fibers have only one nucleus, whereas skeletal muscle cells have many nuclei. Other differences enable cardiac fibers to (1) transmit action potentials quickly from cell to cell, (2) maintain high levels of energy synthesis, and (3) gain access to more ions, particularly sodium and potassium, in the extracellular environment.

Rapid transmission of electrical impulses from cardiac fiber to cardiac fiber is possible because the network of fibers is connected at specialized intercellular junctions called *intercalated disks.* **Intercalated disks** are thickened portions of the sarcolemma that enable electrical impulses to spread quickly in a continuous cell-to-cell (syncytial) fashion. The intercalated disks contain three junctions: desmosomes, or macula adherens; the fascia adherens, which mechanically attach one cell to another; and gap junctions, also known as tight junctions or the nexus, which allow the electrical impulse to spread from cell to cell (see Chapter 1). Changes in the function of these junctional elements have been associated with an increased risk of dysrhythmias.[9]

Unlike skeletal muscle, the heart cannot rest and is in constant need of energy that is supplied by molecules such as adenosine triphosphate (ATP). Therefore, the cytoplasm surrounding the bundles of myofibrils in each cardiac muscle cell contains a larger number of mitochondria (25% of the cellular volume) than that found in skeletal muscle cells. The large numbers of mitochondria provide the necessary respiratory enzymes for aerobic metabolism and supply quantities of ATP sufficient for the constant action of the myocardium.

The third major difference between cardiac and skeletal muscle cells involves the T tubule system. Cardiac fibers contain more T tubules than skeletal muscle fibers. This increased proximity to the T tubules gives each myofibril in the myocardium faster access to molecules it needs for the continuous

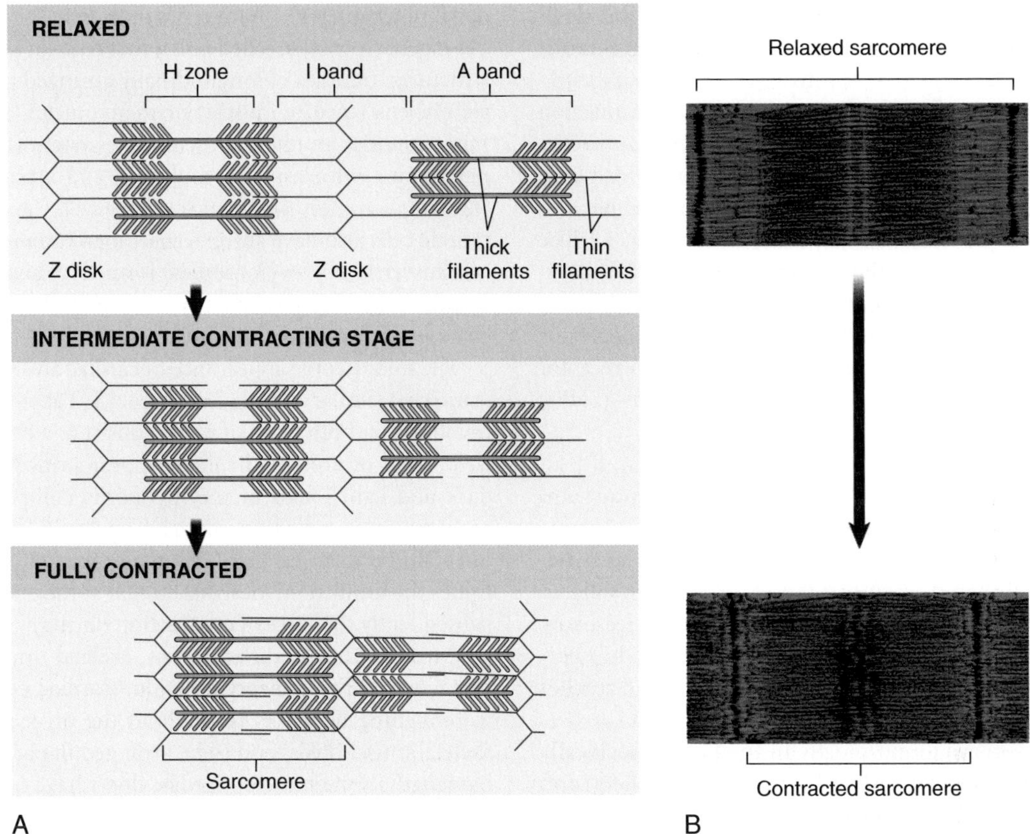

FIGURE 31-13 Sliding-Filament Model. **A,** During contraction, myosin cross-bridges pull the thin filaments toward the center of each sarcomere, thus shortening the myofibril and the entire muscle fiber. **B,** Color-enhanced transmission electron micrographs (TEMs) showing the shortening of a sarcomere caused by the sliding of filaments during muscle contraction. (**A** from Patton KT, Thibodeau GA: *Anatomy & physiology,* ed 8, St Louis, 2013, Mosby. **B** courtesy H.E. Huxley, Brandeis University, Waltham, MA.)

transmission of action potentials, a process that involves transport of sodium and potassium through the walls of the T tubules. (The mechanisms by which sodium and potassium transport causes transmission of cardiac action potentials are described in Chapters 1 and 43.) Because the T tubule system is continuous with the extracellular space and the interstitial fluid, it facilitates the rapid transmission of electrical impulses from the surface of the sarcolemma to the myofibrils inside the fiber. This activates all the myofibrils of one fiber simultaneously. The sarcoplasmic reticulum is located around the myofibrils. When an action potential is transmitted through the T tubules, it induces the sarcoplasmic reticulum to release its stored calcium, which activates the contractile proteins, actin and myosin, within the sarcomere at the same time. T tubule loss, disruption, and dysregulation are associated with heart failure and atrial fibrillation.[14]

Actin, Myosin, Troponin-Tropomyosin Complex, and Titin. Within each myocardial sarcomere the thick filaments of **myosin** constitute the central dark band called the **anisotropic,** or **A, bands** (Figure 31-13). The myosin molecule resembles a golf club with two large bulbous heads protruding from one end of a straight shaft (Figure 31-14). The bilobed heads contain an actin-binding site and a site of ATPase activity. A thick filament called myosin microfilament is composed of about 200 myosin

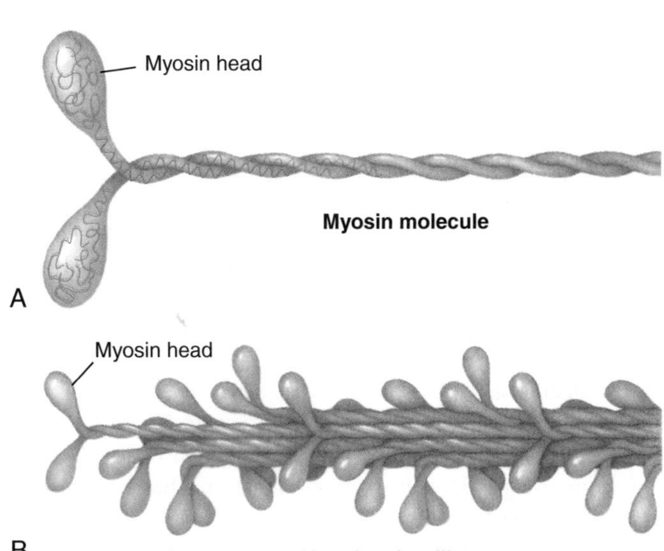

FIGURE 31-14 Structure of Myosin. **A,** Each myosin molecule is a coil of two chains wrapped around each other. At the end of each chain is a globular region, much like a golf club, called the *head.* **B,** Myosin molecules usually are combined into filaments, which are stalks of myosin from which the heads protrude at regular intervals.

molecules bundled together with outward-facing molecule heads called *cross-bridges* because with activation of contraction they will form force-generating bridges with exposed actin molecules (see Figure 31-14, *B*).The actin molecules are part of the thin filaments (Figure 31-15). The light bands are called **isotropic,** or **I, bands** (see Figure 31-13). The thin filaments of actin appear light and extend from the **Z line,** a dense fibrous line that crosses the center of each I band. A sarcomere is the area from one dark Z line to an adjacent Z line with a length that varies from 1.6 to 2.2 mm. In the center of a sarcomere is the H zone, a somewhat less dense region. A thin, dark **M line** travels the center of the H zone. A single tropomyosin molecule (a relaxing protein) lies alongside seven actin molecules. **Troponin,** another relaxing protein, associates with the tropomyosin molecule, forming the **troponin-tropomyosin complex** (see Figure 31-15). The troponin complex itself has three components. **Troponin T** aids in binding of the troponin complex to actin and tropomyosin; **troponin I** inhibits the ATPase of actomyosin; and **troponin C** contains binding sites for the calcium ions involved in contraction. Troponin and tropomyosin are referred to as relaxing proteins because when they cover the myosin-binding sites on the actin, the cross-bridges release and the myocardium relaxes. Also within the sarcomere is a giant elastic protein called **titin** (or connectin), which acts as a spring and is one of the factors responsible for myocardial stiffness and thus impacts diastolic filling of the myocardium.[15]

Myocardial Metabolism. Cardiac muscle, like other muscle tissue, depends on the constant production of ATP for energy. ATP is produced within the mitochondria mainly from glucose, fatty acids, and lactate. If the myocardium is inadequately perfused because of coronary artery disease, anaerobic metabolism must be used as a source of energy (see Chapter 1). The energy produced by metabolic processes is used for muscle contraction and relaxation, electrical excitation, membrane transport, and synthesis of large molecules. Normally, the amount of ATP produced supplies sufficient energy to pump blood systemically.

Cardiac work often is expressed in terms of **myocardial oxygen consumption ($M\dot{V}O_2$).** Because oxidative metabolism is the main process of cardiac energy generation, the rate of oxygen consumption correlates closely with total cardiac energy requirements. $M\dot{V}O_2$ is determined by three major factors: (1) the amount of wall stress during systole, which can be estimated by measuring the systolic blood pressure; (2) the duration of systolic wall tension, which is measured indirectly by the heart rate; and (3) the contractile state of the myocardium, for which no clinical measurement exists.

The oxygen supply to the myocardium is delivered exclusively by the coronary arteries. From 70% to 75% of the oxygen from the coronary arteries is used immediately by cardiac muscle, leaving little oxygen in reserve. Therefore, increased energy needs can be met only by increasing coronary blood flow. Myocardial oxygen consumption can increase several-fold with exercise and decrease moderately under conditions such as hypotension and hypothermia. As myocardial metabolism and consumption of oxygen increases, the concentration of local vasoactive metabolic factors increases. Some of these, such as adenosine, nitric oxide, and prostaglandins, dilate coronary arterioles, thus increasing coronary blood flow.[16]

Myocardial Contraction and Relaxation

Myocardial contractility is a change in developed tension at a given resting fiber length. In functional terms, contractility is the ability of the heart muscle to shorten. On a molecular basis, thin filaments of actin slide over thick filaments of myosin, called the **cross-bridge cycle of muscle contraction.**[17] It is the cycling of cross-bridges that is the molecular basis for myocardial force generation and thus ultimately the heart's ability to pump blood through the circulation. Anatomically, contraction occurs when the sarcomere shortens, causing adjacent Z lines to move closer together (Figure 31-16). The width of the A band, which contains the thick myosin filaments, is unchanged while the I band becomes narrower as the overlap between the thick and thin filaments increases. The degree of shortening of the muscle fibers depends on how much the thin filaments overlap the thick filaments. Maximal contraction occurs when the sarcomere length is 2.2 mm. At 2.2 mm the number of cross-bridge attachments between actin and myosin is maximal.

Cross-Bridge Cycling. The globular head-end of the myosin contains a binding site for actin and a separate enzymatic site that catalyzes the breakdown of ATP to adenosine diphosphate (ADP) and inorganic phosphate (P_i) (see Figure 31-16). This reaction releases the chemical energy stored in ATP. Magnesium is required for the binding of ATP to the myosin site. The splitting of ATP occurs on the myosin molecule before it attaches to actin, but the ADP and inorganic phosphate released remain bound to the active site on myosin. The chemical energy released is transferred to myosin (m), producing a high-energy form of myosin (M):

$$M \bullet ATP \rightarrow M \bullet ADP + P_i$$

The binding of this high-energy myosin-actin form to a cross-bridge releases the energy stored in myosin (e.g., ADP and P_i), producing the force necessary for movement of the cross-bridge. With the attachment of actin to myosin at the cross-bridge, the myosin head molecule undergoes a position change, exerting traction on the rest of the myosin bridge, causing the thin filaments to slide past the thick filaments (see Figure 31-16). During contraction each cross-bridge undergoes several cycles of attachment, movement, and dissociation from the thin filaments.[17]

Calcium and Excitation-Contraction Coupling. **Excitation-contraction coupling** is the process by which an action potential in the plasma membrane of the muscle fiber triggers the cycle of events leading to cross-bridge activity and contraction. Activation of this cycle depends on the availability of calcium.

Calcium is stored in the tubule system and the sarcoplasmic reticulum. It enters the myocardial cell from the interstitial fluid after electrical excitation, which increases the membrane permeability to calcium. Two types of calcium channels (L-type and T-type) are identified in cardiac tissues. The L-type, or long-lasting, channels are the predominant type of calcium channels and are the channels blocked by **calcium channel–blocking drugs** (verapamil, nifedipine, diltiazem). The major

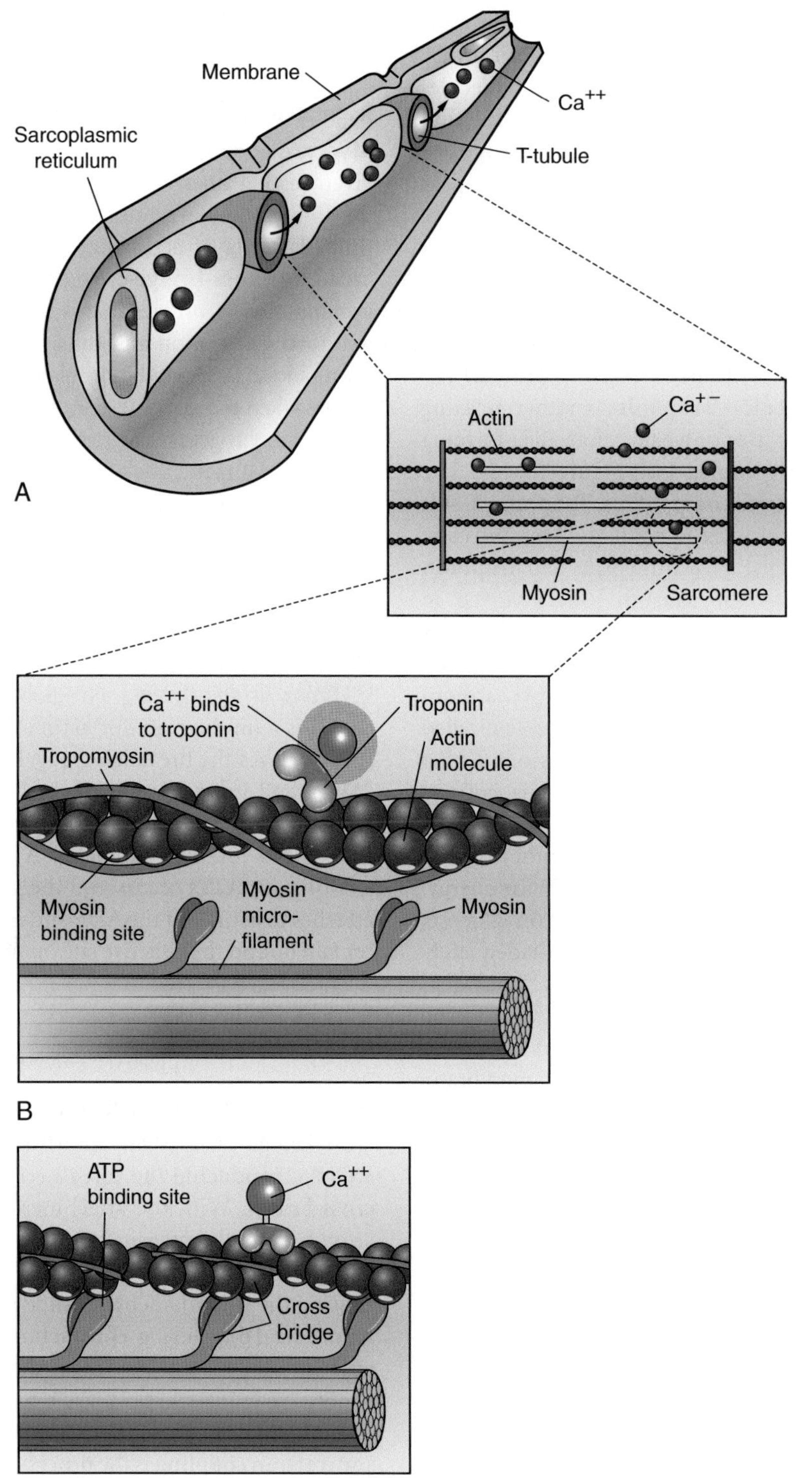

FIGURE 31-15 Myofilaments and Mechanisms of Muscle Contraction. A, Thin and thick myofilaments. In resting muscle, calcium ions are stored in the sarcoplasmic reticulum. When an action potential reaches the muscle cell, the T tubules carry the action potential deep into the sarcoplasm. The action potential causes the sarcoplasmic reticulum to release the store of calcium ions. **B,** In resting muscle the myosin-binding sites are covered by troponin and tropomyosin. The calcium ions released into the sarcoplasm as a result of the action potential bind to the troponin. This binding causes the tropomyosin and troponin to move out of the way of the myosin-binding sites, leaving the myosin heads free to bind to the actin microfilament. **C,** ATP is used as an energy molecule to the myosin cross-bridge. (Adapted from Raven PH, Johnson GB: *Understanding biology,* ed 3, Dubuque, IA, 1995, Brown.)

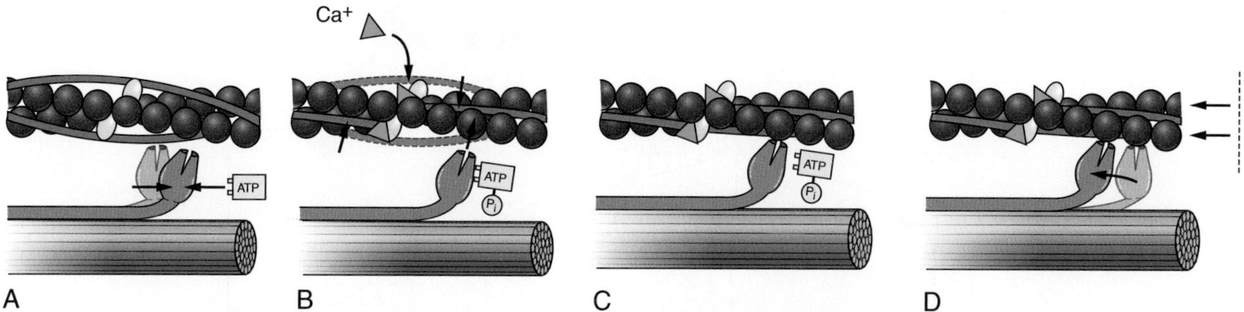

FIGURE 31-16 Cross-Bridge Theory of Muscle Contraction. A, Each myosin cross-bridge in the thick filament moves into a resting position after an adenosine triphosphate (ATP) molecule binds and transfers its energy. **B,** Calcium ions released from the sarcoplasmic reticulum bind to troponin in the thin filament, allowing tropomyosin to shift from its position blocking the active sites of actin molecules. **C,** Each myosin cross-bridge then binds to an active site on a thin filament, displacing the remnants of ATP hydrolysis—adenosine diphosphate (ADP) and inorganic phosphate (P_i). **D,** The release of stored energy from step **A** provides the force needed for each cross-bridge to move back to its original position, pulling actin along with it. Each cross-bridge will remain bound to actin until another ATP molecule binds to it and pulls it back into its resting position **(A).** (Adapted from Thibodeau GA, Patton KT: *Anatomy & physiology,* ed 4, St Louis, 1999, Mosby.)

effect of these medications is to decrease the strength of cardiac contraction. The T-type, or transient, channels are much less abundant in the heart and are not blocked by currently available calcium channel–blocking drugs. Calcium that enters the cell from the interstitial fluid triggers release of calcium from the storage sites. The storage sites most important for contraction are from the sarcoplasmic reticulum. Calcium from these sites diffuses toward the myofibrils, where it binds with troponin.

The calcium-troponin complex facilitates the contraction process. In the resting state, troponin I is bound to actin and the configuration of the tropomyosin molecule is such that it covers the sites where the myosin heads bind to actin, thus preventing interaction between actin and myosin. Calcium binding to troponin inhibits troponin C (which enhances troponin I–actin binding) and results in tropomyosin moving troponin I, which uncovers the binding sites on the myosin heads. Myosin and actin can then form cross-bridges, and ATP can be dephosphorylated to ADP. Sliding of the thick and thin filaments can then occur, and the myocardium contracts.

Myocardial Relaxation

Relaxation is just as vital to optimal cardiac function as contraction, and calcium, troponin, and tropomyosin also facilitate relaxation. After contraction, free calcium ions are actively pumped out of the cell back into the interstitial fluid or taken up again by the sarcoplasmic reticulum and stored. As the concentration of calcium within the sarcomere subsequently falls, troponin releases its bound calcium. The tropomyosin complex blocks the active sites on the actin molecule, preventing cross-bridges with the myosin heads. Each tropomyosin molecule is held in this blocking position by a molecule of troponin. Troponin is bound to both tropomyosin and actin (see Figure 31-15).

Factors Affecting Cardiac Output

Cardiac output is the volume of blood flowing through either the systemic or the pulmonary circuit and is expressed in liters per minute. Cardiac output is calculated by multiplying heart rate in beats per minute by **stroke volume** in liters per beat. Normal adult cardiac output at rest is about 5 L/min. The ventricles do not eject all of the blood they contain with each heartbeat and the amount ejected is called the **ejection fraction.** The ejection fraction is calculated by dividing the stroke volume by the end-diastolic volume. The end-diastolic volume (EDV) of the normal ventricle is about 70 to 80 ml/m^2 and the normal ejection fraction of the resting heart is 55% or higher. Ejection fraction is a valuable clinical indicator of ventricular function.[18]

Four factors affect cardiac output directly: preload, afterload, myocardial contractility, and heart rate (Figure 31-17). **Preload** (pressure generated at the end of diastole) and **afterload** (resistance to ejection during systole) depend on the heart as well as the vascular system. Contractility and heart rate are characteristics of the cardiac tissue per se and are influenced by neural and humoral mechanisms. To understand the role of these factors in cardiac performance, it is first necessary to understand two physical laws that explain the mechanisms of heart action: the Frank-Starling law of the heart and Laplace's law.

Frank-Starling Law of the Heart

Cardiac muscle, like other muscle, increases its strength of contraction when it is stretched. This relationship was described in 1914 by a British physiologist, Ernest Starling, and was based on the earlier work of a German physiologist, Otto Frank. The **Frank-Starling law of the heart,** or the length-tension relationship of cardiac muscle, relates resting sarcomere length, expressed as the volume of blood in the heart at the end of diastole **(end-diastolic volume),** to tension generation, described as development of left ventricular pressure. Thus the volume of blood in the heart at the end of diastole (the length of its muscle fibers) is directly related to the force of contraction during the next systole. Although the change in pressure is related to the volume of the ventricle and, consequently, to the length of the ventricular muscle fibers, preload (i.e., filling pressure) is commonly used as an index of ventricular volume. The length-tension mechanism is the main mechanism by which the normal right and left ventricles maintain equal minute outputs even though their stroke outputs may vary considerably during

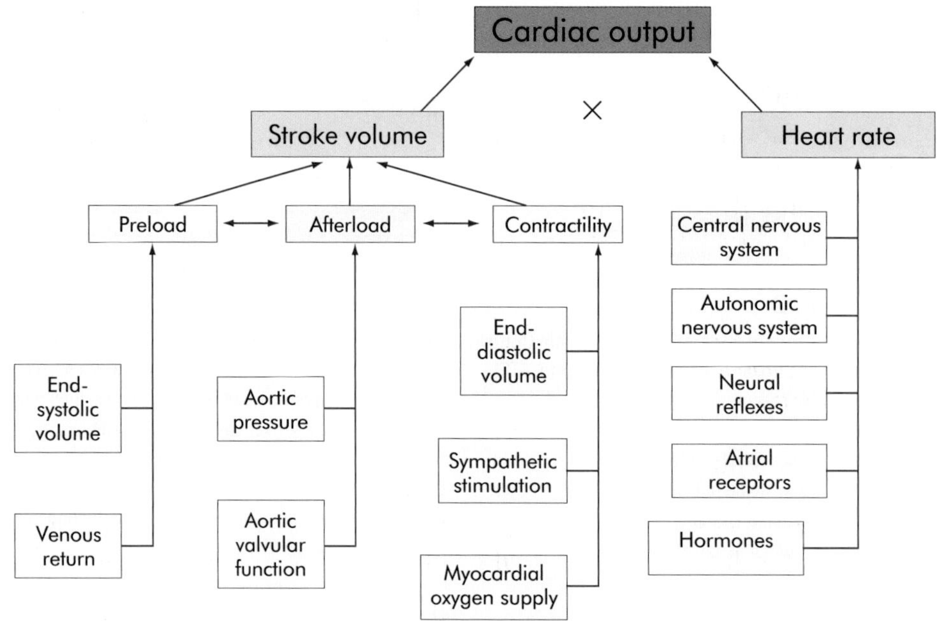

FIGURE 31-17 Factors Affecting Cardiac Performance. Cardiac output, which is the amount of blood (in liters) ejected by the heart per minute, depends on heart rate (beats per minute) and stroke volume (milliliters of blood ejected during ventricular systole).

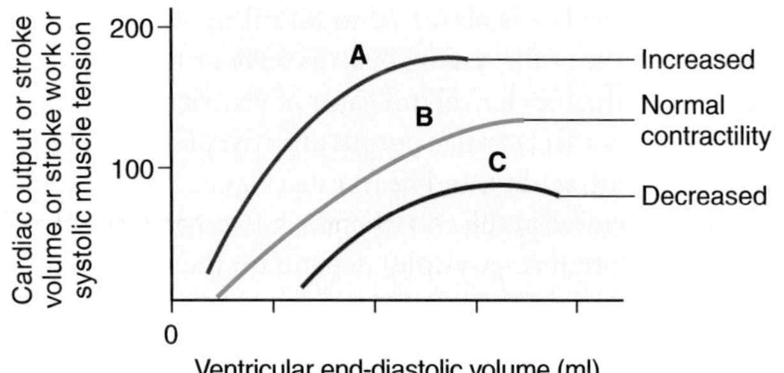

FIGURE 31-18 Frank-Starling Law of the Heart. Relationship between length and tension in the heart. End-diastolic volume determines end-diastolic length of ventricular muscle fibers and is proportional to tension generated during systole, as well as to cardiac output, stroke volume, and stroke work. A change in myocardial contractility causes the heart to perform on a different length-tension curve. *A,* Increased contractility; *B,* normal contractility; *C,* heart failure or decreased contractility. (See text.)

normal respiration. For example, changes in volume occur when an individual assumes a reclining position after being in a standing position; the volume of blood returning to the heart temporarily increases. The right ventricle stretches to accommodate this increase in volume and thereby increases its force of contraction. A larger stroke volume (i.e., the amount of blood ejected per beat) is pumped to the lungs, generating higher pressures. Pulmonary vascular pressure increases, causing a rise in the left ventricular filling pressure or preload. Left ventricular volume and pressure increase. The left ventricle pumps a larger stroke volume, and arterial vascular pressure rises.

The mechanical function of the heart is characterized by a number of length-tension curves (Figure 31-18). Factors that increase contractility (i.e., positive inotropic), such as sympathetic nerve stimulation, cause the heart to operate on a higher length-tension curve (curve *A* in Figure 31-18). A higher tension or increase in ventricular stroke volume is generated without a necessary change in left ventricular end-diastolic volume or fiber length. Heart failure (curve *C* in Figure 31-18) is characterized by a lower length-tension curve (see Chapter 32). The Frank-Starling law of the heart may not apply to dilated or failing hearts because their fibers are already stretched beyond their optimal length. The failing heart responds to increased filling or stretch with a progressive decline in the force of contraction. Thus at the same left ventricular end-diastolic volume as curves *A* and *B* (see Figure 31-18), the force of contraction of stroke volume is decreased.

The cross-bridge arrangement with the sarcomere partially accounts for the length-tension mechanism of cardiac muscle. According to the Frank-Starling law, the longer the initial resting length of the cardiac muscle fiber (optimal length is between 2.2 and 2.4 mm), the greater the strength of contraction. At 2.2 mm an optimal number of active cross-bridges exist between actin and myosin. However, if the fibers are stretched beyond 2.2 to 2.4 mm, the force of contraction decreases because actin and myosin become partially disengaged, disrupting many of the cross-bridges. Excessive stretching, to about 3.65 mm, causes actin and myosin to become completely disengaged so that tension (force of contraction) drops to zero. The relationship between stretch and contraction can be compared with that of a rubber band. Up to a certain point, the more the rubber band is stretched the farther it will fly when one end is released; beyond that point, however, the rubber band will break but, of course, the myocardium does not actually break!

Laplace's Law

Laplace's law states that wall tension is related directly to the product of intraventricular pressure and internal radius and inversely related to the wall thickness as shown in the Laplace equation:

$$T = (p \times r)/\mu m$$

where T = wall tension, p = intraventricular pressure, r = internal radius of the sphere, and µm = wall thickness. In other words, the amount of tension generated in the ventricular wall (or any chamber or vessel) to produce a given intraventricular pressure depends on the size (radius and wall thickness) of the ventricle.

Laplace's law is useful for understanding aneurysm formation, distensibility in blood vessels, and the effects of ventricular dilation on myocardial contraction. Dilation is an important factor in heart failure (see Chapter 32). With a dilated ventricle, myocardial fibers in the wall must develop greater tension to produce a given pressure within the ventricle. The disadvantage of dilation is that the increased force, or tension, in the myocardial fibers required to develop a given pressure inside a dilated ventricle decreases the rate of fiber shortening, thereby decreasing the ability of the ventricle to eject blood.

Preload

Left ventricular preload is the pressure generated in the left ventricle at the end of diastole, or **left ventricular end-diastolic pressure (LVEDP).** It is determined by the **left ventricular end-diastolic volume (LVEDV),** which stretches the cardiac muscle fibers and in turn develops tension, or force, for contraction according to the Frank-Starling law. Preload is determined by two primary factors: (1) the amount of venous return to the ventricle, and (2) the blood left in the ventricle after systole or end-systolic volume (see Figure 31-17). End-systolic volume is dependent on the strength of ventricular contraction and the resistance to ventricular emptying. Within a physiologic range of muscle stretching (2.2 to 2.4 mm), increased preload increases cardiac output. When preload exceeds the physiologic range, further muscle stretching causes a decline in cardiac output (see Frank-Starling law, p. 1101). In monitoring preload the clinician measures indexes of left ventricular end-diastolic pressure. Pressure changes are important because increased left ventricular filling pressures "back up" into the pulmonary circulation, where they force plasma out through vessel walls, causing fluid to accumulate in lung tissues that can cause pulmonary edema (see Chapter 35). Treatment goals in heart failure management are to maintain an end-diastolic volume and pressure that will maintain or increase cardiac output.

Afterload

Ventricular afterload is the resistance to ejection of blood from the ventricle. Aortic systolic pressure is a good index of afterload for the left ventricle. Low aortic pressures (decreased afterload) enable the heart to contract more rapidly, whereas high aortic pressures (increased afterload) slow contraction and cause higher workloads against which the heart must function to eject blood. Pressure in the ventricle must exceed aortic pressure before blood can be pumped out during systole. Increased aortic pressure is usually the result of increased peripheral vascular resistance (PVR), also called total peripheral resistance (TPR). In individuals with hypertension, increased PVR means that afterload is chronically elevated, resulting in increased ventricular workload and hypertrophy of the myocardium. The situation is similar for the right ventricle except the pressures are much lower and the afterload for the right ventricle is pulmonary arterial pressure.

Myocardial Contractility

Stroke volume, or the volume of blood ejected during systole, depends on the force of contraction, which is a function of myocardial contractility, the degree of myocardial fiber shortening. In healthy persons, three major factors determine the force of contraction: (1) changes in the stretching of the ventricular myocardium caused by variations in ventricular volume (preload), (2) alterations in nervous system input to the ventricles, and (3) adequacy of myocardial oxygen supply (see Figure 31-17). As discussed previously, increased blood flow from the veins into the heart distends the ventricle by increasing preload, which, within the physiologic range, increases the stroke volume and, subsequently, cardiac output.

Chemicals affecting contractility are called **inotropic agents.** The most important positive inotropic agents produced by the body are norepinephrine released from the sympathetic nerves supplying the heart and epinephrine released by the adrenal cortex. Other positive inotropes include thyroid hormone and dopamine. The most important negative inotropic agent is acetylcholine released from the vagus nerve. Many medications have positive or negative inotropic properties that can have profound effects on cardiac function.

Myocardial contractility is dependent on oxygen supply with hypoxia contributing to a decrease in contractility. However, because hypoxia also stimulates coronary artery dilation, the impact of hypoxia will vary with activity level and the actual level of hypoxia. Preload, afterload, and contractility all interact with one another to determine stroke volume and cardiac output. Changes in any one of these factors can result in deleterious effects on the others, resulting in heart failure (see Chapter 32). In persons with sepsis, a variety of cytokines, including tumor necrosis factor-alpha (TNF-α), interleukin-beta, lysozyme C and endothelin-1, have been shown to impair myocardial contractility.[19]

Heart Rate

The average heart rate in healthy adults is about 70 beats/min. The average heart rate is significantly greater in children. Heart rate diminishes by 10 to 20 beats/min during sleep and can accelerate to more than 100 beats/min during muscular activity or emotional excitement. In well-conditioned athletes the resting heart rate is about 50 to 60 beats/min. In highly trained or elite athletes the resting heart rate can be less than 50 beats/min. The low resting heart rate is the result of increased vagal stimulation and lower sympathetic stimulation.

Neural factors, including neural reflexes, and hormonal and chemical factors influence the heart rate. Neural control is exerted by the central and autonomic nervous systems. Hormonal factors include the catecholamines (i.e., norepinephrine and epinephrine), thyroid hormones, growth hormones, and endocannabinoids, such as anandamide.[20] (Hormonal function is described in Chapter 21.) Stimulation by the sympathetic nervous system increases the frequency of the cardiac pacemaker (SA node), whereas parasympathetic stimulation has a **bradycardic effect** (heart rate less than 60 beats/min).

Cardiovascular Control Centers in the Brain. The major **cardiovascular control center** is in the brainstem in the medulla with secondary areas in the hypothalamus, the cerebral cortex, the thalamus, and complex networks of exciting or inhibiting interneurons (connecting neurons) throughout the brain. The hypothalamic centers regulate cardiovascular responses to changes in temperature; the cerebral cortex centers adjust cardiac reaction to a variety of emotional states; and the medullary control center regulates heart rate and blood pressure (see page 1114 for blood pressure regulation). The medullary neurons often are classified as cardiac and vasomotor

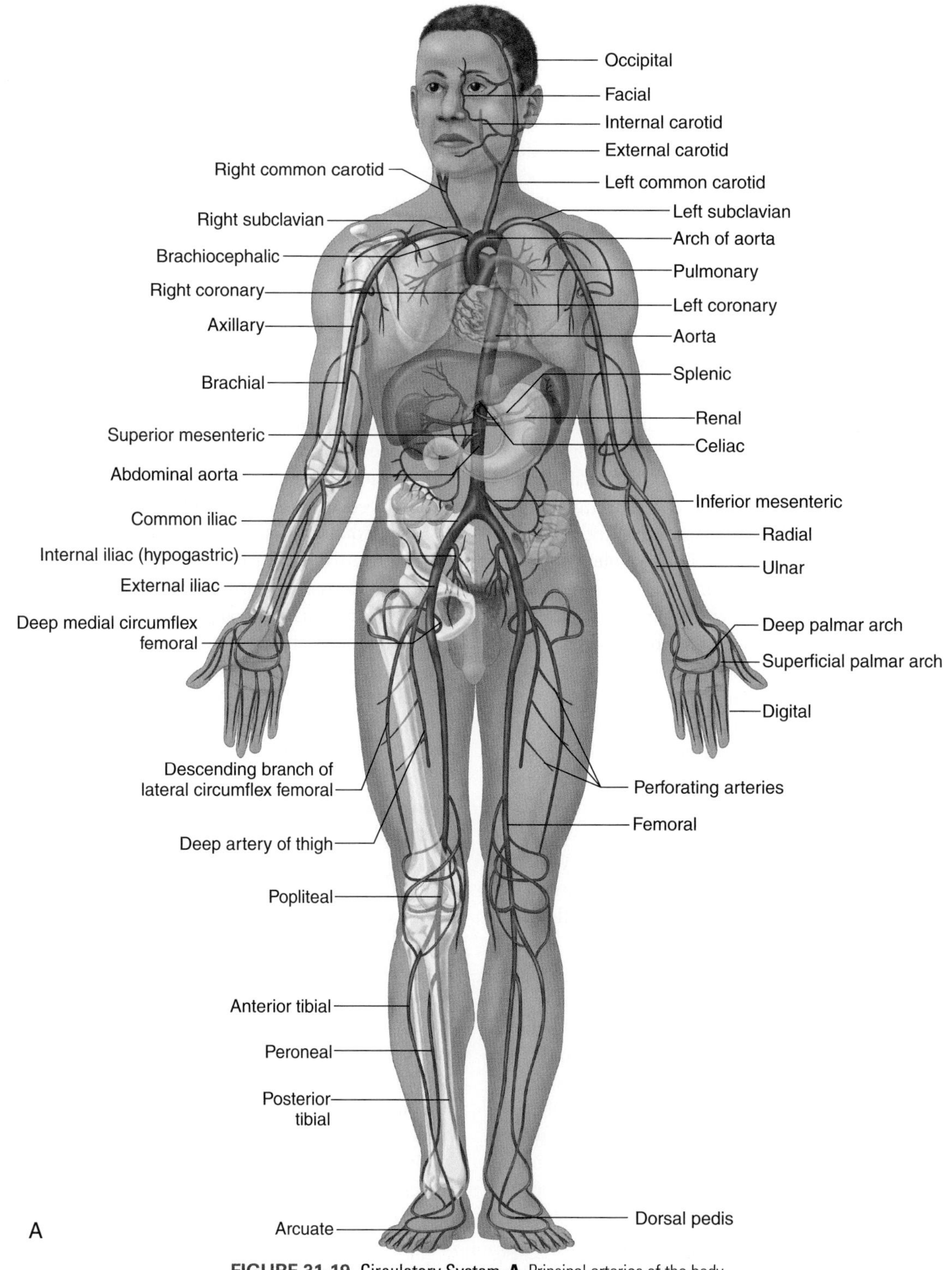

FIGURE 31-19 Circulatory System. **A,** Principal arteries of the body.

(vasoconstrictor or vasodilator) centers; however, because these centers are not discrete anatomic areas and actually constitute diffuse networks of interneurons, it is preferable to call the entire area the cardiovascular control center.

The nerve fibers from the cardiovascular control center synapse with the autonomic neurons (see Chapter 15 and Table 15-7). When the parasympathetic nerves to the heart are stimulated, the sympathetic nerves to the heart, arterioles, and veins usually are inhibited. The opposite also is true: when the sympathetic nerves are stimulated, the parasympathetic nerves usually are inhibited. Because parasympathetic excitation and simultaneous sympathetic inhibition generally depress cardiac function (e.g., decrease the heart rate), these interneurons often are referred to as the **cardioinhibitory center.** Excitation occurs

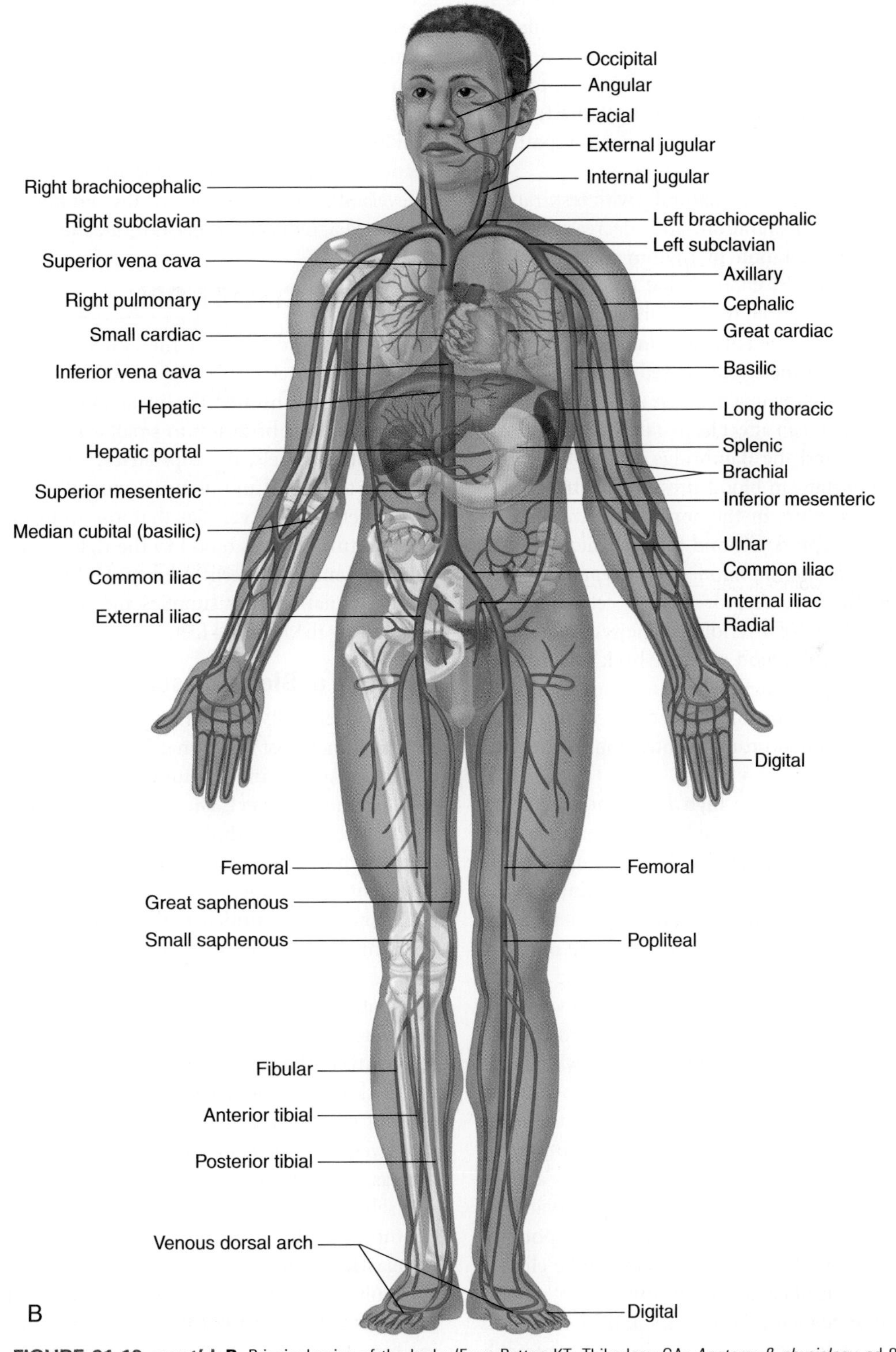

FIGURE 31-19, cont'd B, Principal veins of the body. (From Patton KT, Thibodeau GA: *Anatomy & physiology,* ed 8, St Louis, 2013, Mosby.)

with parasympathetic inhibition and sympathetic stimulation, and these interneurons are collectively called the **cardioexcitatory center.** Therefore, heart rate can be slowed by two simultaneous events that begin in the cardiovascular control center: (1) inhibition of sympathetic stimulation of the SA node, and (2) activation of parasympathetic stimulation of the SA node. Conversely, heart rate can be increased by activation of sympathetic nerves and inhibition of parasympathetic nerves.

The resting heart rate in healthy individuals is primarily under the control of parasympathetic stimulation. While the individual is at rest, parasympathetic effects from the vagus nerves override sympathetic effects in the SA node. Interruption of the vagus nerves causes significant tachycardia (abnormally fast heart rate) because the inhibitory parasympathetic influence is lost.

Neural Reflexes. Heart rate varies naturally with respiration, the rate increasing with inspiration and decreasing with expiration. This normal alteration in rhythm pattern, called **sinus arrhythmia,** is caused by changes that occur within the chest cavity because of respiration. Inspiration results in stretch and an associated increase in firing of the SA node that increases heart rate. With expiration the stretch is reduced and the SA node firing rate slows, resulting in a decrease in heart rate.[21]

Two neural reflexes that can affect heart rate and rhythm are the baroreceptor reflex and the Bainbridge reflex. The **baroreceptor reflex** is important in blood pressure control and is mediated by stretch receptors in the aortic arch and carotid arteries. (Because the receptors respond to mechanical factors, they are also called *aortic and carotid mechanoreceptors.*) When blood pressure falls, the baroreceptor reflex accelerates heart rate and causes constriction of arterioles in the systemic circulation. These responses raise blood pressure back toward normal and are critical to maintaining adequate tissue perfusion. Aging is associated with dysfunction of the baroreceptor reflex (baroreflex) and can result in postural hypotension (orthostatic hypotension, see p. 1140).[22]

The baroreflex also can reduce high blood pressure. The mechanoreceptors increase their rate of discharge when stretched by blood pressure elevations. Neural impulses are then transmitted over the glossopharyngeal nerve (ninth cranial nerve) from the carotid artery and through the vagus nerve from the aorta to the cardiovascular control centers in the medulla. These centers initiate an increase in parasympathetic activity and a decrease in sympathetic activity, causing blood vessels to dilate and heart rate to decrease. Responses to the baroreceptor reflex return the blood pressure to its previous level, which may or may not have been normal.

Bainbridge reflex is the name for the changes in the heart rate that occur after intravenous infusions of blood or other fluids.[23] The change in heart rate is thought to be caused by a reflex mediated by volume receptors in the atria that are innervated by the vagus nerves (volume receptors are thought to respond to increased plasma volume). Although this reflex can be elicited in humans, its relevance is uncertain at this time.[23]

Hormones and Biochemicals. Hormones and biochemicals affect the arteries, arterioles, venules, capillaries, and contractility of the myocardium. Norepinephrine increases heart rate, enhances myocardial contractility, and constricts blood vessels. Epinephrine dilates vessels of the liver and skeletal muscle and causes an increase in myocardial contractility. Some adrenocortical hormones, such as hydrocortisone, potentiate the effects of the catecholamines.

Thyroid hormone, specifically triiodothyronine, causes increases in both heart rate and contractility, resulting in an increase in cardiac output; it also decreases systemic vascular resistance. Triiodothyronine acts directly on the cardiac myocytes to cause gene transcription and cellular changes that result in more calcium release from the sarcoplasmic reticulum.[24] Awareness of these changes helps to understand the cardiovascular changes that occur with thyroid diseases. Growth hormone, working together with insulin-like growth factor 1 (IGF-1), also has been shown to increase myocardial contractility.[25] Decreases in levels of growth hormone or thyroid hormone may result in bradycardia, reduced cardiac output, and low blood pressure.

SYSTEMIC CIRCULATION

The arteries and veins of the systemic circulation are illustrated in Figure 31-19. Oxygenated blood from the left side of the heart flows through the aorta and into the systemic arteries. The **arteries** branch into small **arterioles** that branch into the smallest vessels, the **capillaries,** where nutrient exchange between the blood and tissues occurs. Blood from the capillaries then enters tiny **venules** that join to form the larger **veins,** which return venous blood to the right heart. **Peripheral vascular system** is the term used to describe the part of the systemic circulation that supplies the skin and the extremities, particularly the legs and feet.

Structure of Blood Vessels

Blood vessel walls are composed of three layers: the **tunica intima** (innermost or intimal layer), the tunica media (middle or medial layer), and the tunica externa or adventitia (outermost or external layer). These structures are illustrated in Figure 31-20. The tunica intima is composed of a layer of squamous epithelium or endothelium, a layer of connective tissue, and a basement membrane. (These cellular structures are described in Chapter 1.) The **tunica media** is composed of smooth muscle fibers mixed with elastic fibers. The **tunica externa,** or **adventitia,** is an active layer of connective tissue containing nerves, lymphatic vessels that influences both vessel development, and muscle tone (see What's New? New Roles for the Arterial Adventitia). Blood vessel walls vary in thickness depending on the thickness or absence of one or more of these three layers. Cells of the larger vessels are nourished by the **vasa vasorum,** small vessels located in the tunica externa, and innervated by perivascular nerves. The vasa vasorum arise from the blood vessel itself or from other vessels nearby. In the large elastic vessels the tunica media is separated from the adventitia by the **external elastic lamina.**

Adults are capable of growing new blood vessels through three processes, all of which are important in wound healing but also contribute to tumor growth. The three processes are angiogenesis, arteriogenesis, and vasculogenesis. Both

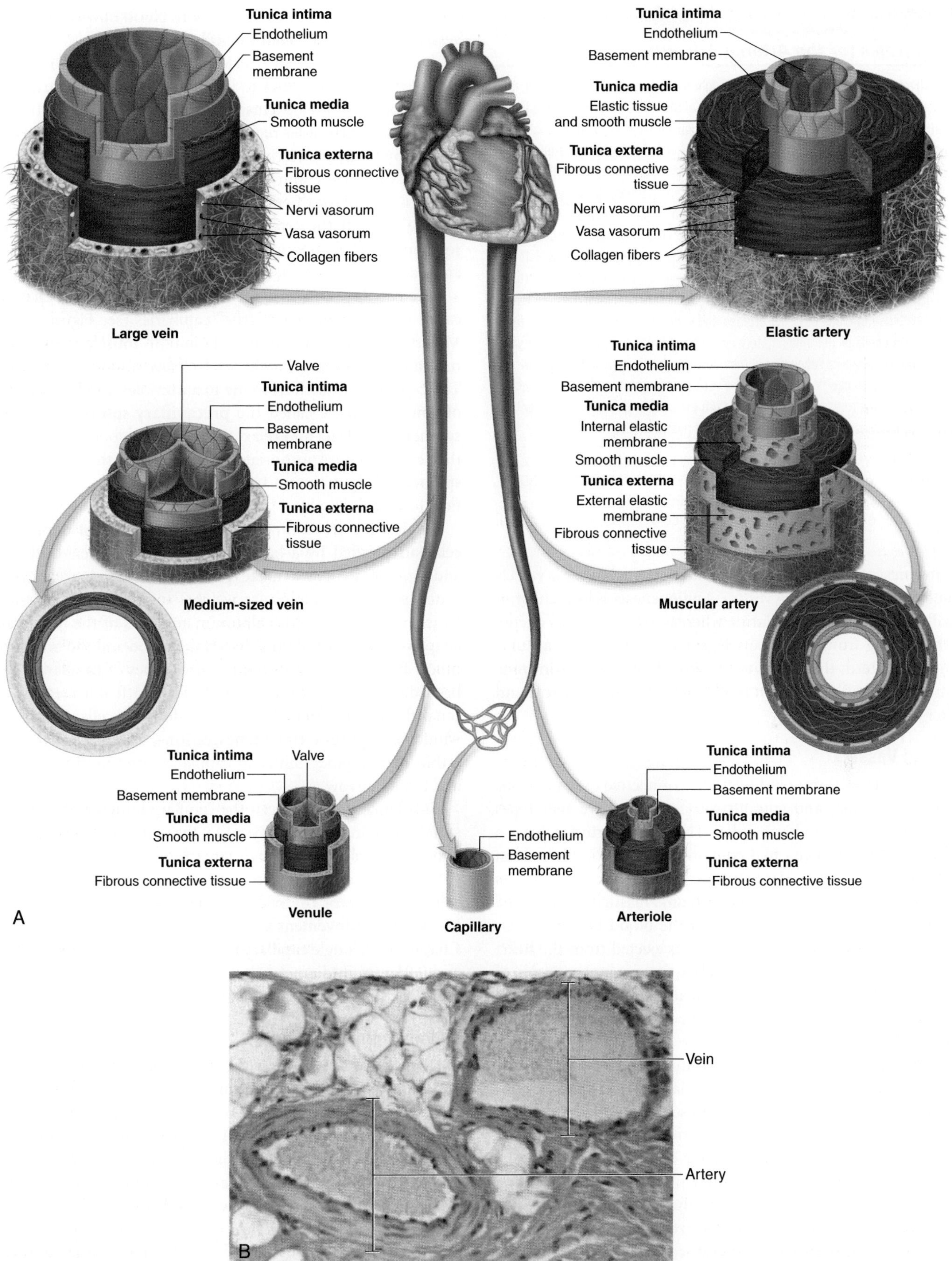

FIGURE 31-20 Structure of Blood Vessels, and an Artery and Vein. A, Structure of blood vessels. The tunica externa of the veins are color-coded blue and the arteries red. **B,** Artery and vein. Light micrograph of a cross section of similar-sized artery *(left)* and vein *(right)*. Notice the thick muscular wall of the artery as compared to the thin-walled vein. (From Patton KT, Thibodeau GA: *Anatomy & physiology*, ed 8, St Louis, 2013, Mosby.)

WHAT'S NEW?

New Roles for the Arterial Adventitia

The adventitia or tunica externa, once thought to be a simple fibrous sheath, is now recognized as a dynamic player in the life of the vessel and the surrounding tissues. The adventitia has roles in vessel response to injury, immune function, and vascular tone. Some of the cell types found include fibroblasts, stem/progenitor cells, mast cells, macrophages, B cells, T cells, and dendritic cells. Other components of this layer include the vasa vasorum, perivascular nerves (nervi vasorum), lymphatic vessels, and extracellular matrix (see Figure 31-20). Studies of labeled cells after arterial injury have shown that new cells migrate from the adventitia into the media and intima to repair and maintain the vessel. It is also possible that, in some cases, these migrating cells may contribute to arterial disease. The vasa vasorum, which forms a miniature circulatory system that supplies blood to walls or larger arteries and veins, also provides a means for transporting cells of the inflammatory response, such as macrophages, across the blood vessel walls. Adventitia fibroblasts have the capacity to become myofibroblasts, which can then influence the vascular tone of the vessel. Research continues on the roles of the adventitia both in health and in a wide variety of vascular diseases such as atherosclerosis and pulmonary hypertension.

Data from Hu Y, Xu Q: *Arterioscler Thromb Vasc Biol* 31(7):1523–1529; Majesky MW et al: *Arterioscler Thromb Vasc Biol* 31(7):1530–1539; Majesky MW et al: *Cells Tissues Organs* 195(1-2):73–81, 2012; Stenmark KR et al: *Ann Rev Physiol* 2012 Dec 3. [Epub ahead of print.].

angiogenesis and arteriogenesis occur by growth of new vessels that branch from existing vessels. **Angiogenesis** is branching of small vessels, such as capillaries, whereas **arteriogenesis** occurs by branching from larger vessels, such as arterioles. **Vasculogenesis** is a term that refers to the growth of vessels from progenitor or stemlike cells that originate in the bone marrow and other body tissues.[26]

Arterial Vessels

Arterial walls are composed of elastic connective tissue, fibrous connective tissue, and smooth muscle. There are two types of arteries: elastic and muscular. The **elastic arteries** have a very thick tunica media that contains more elastic fibers than smooth muscle fibers. Elastic arteries include the aorta and its major branches and the pulmonary trunk. Elasticity enables the vessel to absorb energy imparted to the blood by ventricular contraction and they stretch as blood is ejected from the heart during systole. During diastole, elasticity promotes recoil of the arteries, which is important for maintaining blood pressure within the vessels, and retransfers the energy from the elastic artery walls to the blood.

The **muscular arteries** are medium and small size arteries farther from the heart than the elastic arteries. They contain fewer elastic fibers and more muscle fibers than the elastic arteries and their function is to distribute blood to arterioles throughout the body. Because their smooth muscle can be stimulated to contract or relax, they play a role in controlling blood flow and in directing flow to the parts of the body with the highest need at any time. During exercise more blood is sent to the skeletal muscles, while after a meal more blood is directed to the gut and liver. Contraction narrows the vessel **lumen** (the internal cavity of the vessel), which diminishes flow through the vessel. This condition is termed **vasoconstriction.** When the smooth muscle layer relaxes, more blood flows through the vessel lumen, a state called **vasodilation.**

An artery becomes an arteriole at the point where the diameter of its lumen narrows to less than 0.5 mm. The arterioles are composed almost exclusively of smooth muscle, with little elastic tissue. Arterioles regulate the flow of blood into the capillaries by vasoconstriction, which retards the flow of blood into the capillaries, and vasodilation, which permits blood to enter the capillaries freely (Figure 31-21). The thick, smooth muscle layer of the arterioles is a major determinant of the resistance blood encounters as it flows through the systemic circulation.

The capillary network is composed of connective channels called **metarterioles,** and "true" capillaries (see Figure 31-21). Metarterioles have discontinuous smooth muscle cells in their tunica media whereas capillaries lack any smooth muscle cells. The capillaries branch from the metarterioles, meeting at a ring of smooth muscle called the **precapillary sphincters.** As the sphincters contract and relax, they regulate blood flow through the capillaries. Appropriately stimulated, the precapillary sphincters help maintain arterial pressure and regulate selective flow to vascular beds.

Capillaries are composed solely of a layer of endothelial cells surrounded by a basement membrane. Their thin walls and unique structure make possible the rapid exchange of water; small (low molecular weight) soluble molecules; some larger molecules, such as albumin; and cells of the innate and adaptive immune system between the blood and the interstitial fluid.[1] Based on their structure, three types of capillaries have been described: continuous, sinusoid, and fenestrated. In the renal glomerulus, for example, the endothelial cells contain oval windows or pores termed **fenestrations,** which are covered by a thin diaphragm.[27] Sinusoid capillaries are found in the liver and bone marrow.

Substances pass between the capillary lumen and the interstitial fluid in several ways: (1) through junctions between endothelial cells, (2) through fenestrations in endothelial cells, (3) in vesicles moved by active transport across the endothelial cell membrane, or (4) by diffusion through the endothelial cell membrane. (Movement across cell membranes is described in Chapter 1.) A single capillary may be only 0.5 to 1 mm in length and 0.01 mm in diameter, but the capillaries are so numerous that their total surface area may be more than 600 m^2.

Endothelium

Once thought to be simply the cellular layer lining blood vessels, the vascular **endothelium** is now recognized as important to several body functions and is considered by some to be a separate organ (Figure 31-22). In addition to substance transport, the vascular endothelium has important roles in coagulation, antithrombogenesis, and fibrinolysis; immune system function; tissue growth and wound healing; and **vasomotion,** the contraction and relaxation of vessels. The endothelium performs these vital functions through synthesis and release of vasoactive chemicals. Figures 31-23 and 31-24 and Box 31-1 summarize some of the more important functions. Because of its varying roles, the actual structure

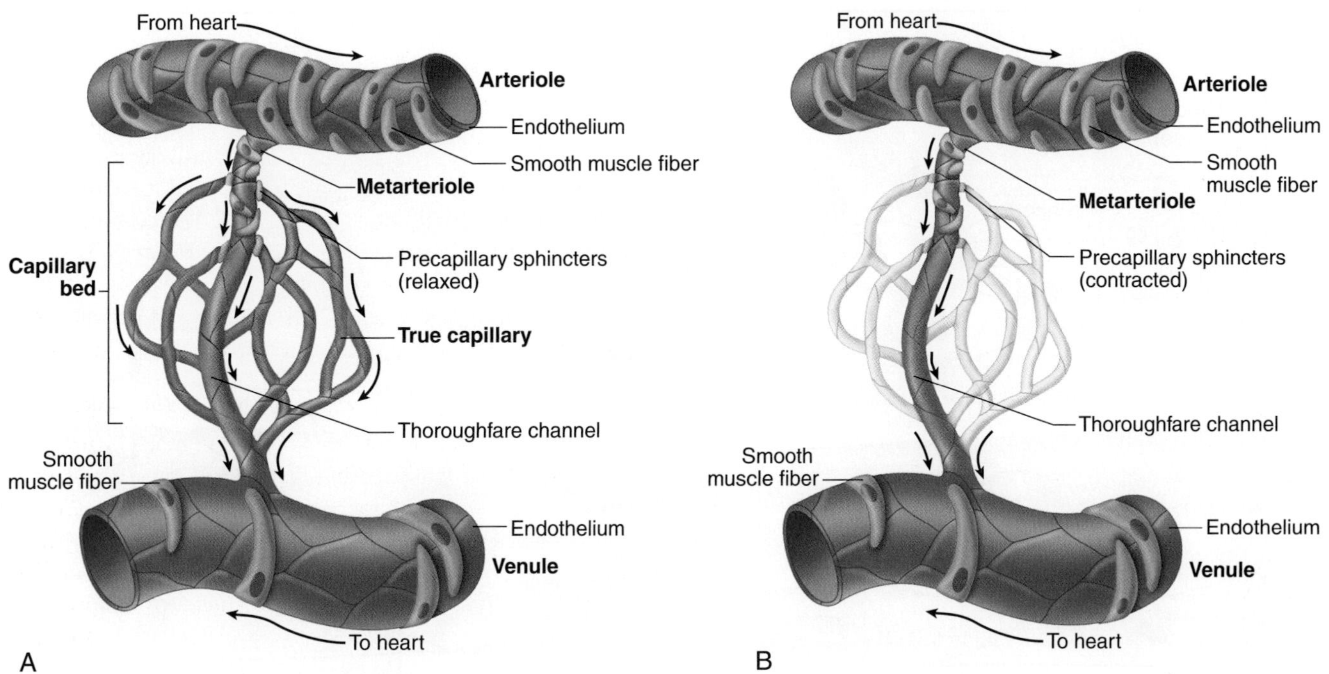

FIGURE 31-21 Capillary Wall and Microcirculation. Control of blood flow through a capillary network is regulated by the relative contraction of precapillary sphincters surrounding arterioles and metarterioles. **A,** Sphincters are relaxed, permitting blood flow to enter the capillary bed. **B,** With sphincters contracted, blood flows from the metarteriole directly into the thoroughfare channel, bypassing the capillary bed. (From Patton KT, Thibodeau GA: *Anatomy & physiology*, ed 8, St Louis, 2013, Mosby.)

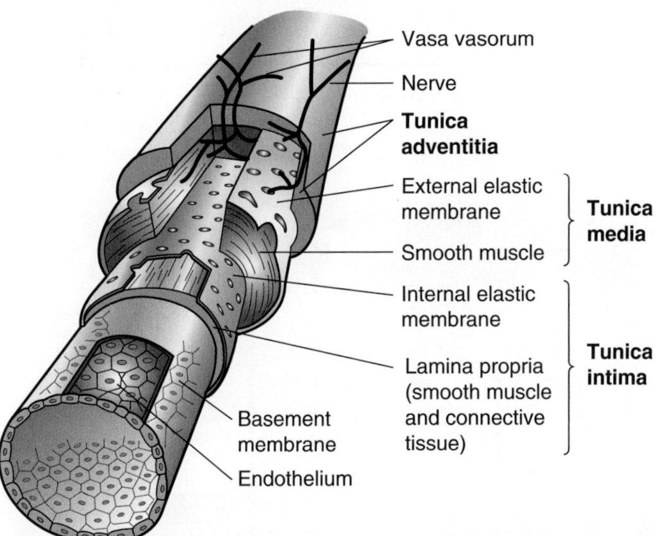

FIGURE 31-22 Endothelium. This schematic shows the endothelium in context with the entire blood vessel. Practically imperceptible, the endothelial cells arrange themselves as a fine lining that has numerous life support functions.

of the endothelium may vary in different vascular beds. For example, within lymph nodes the **endothelial cells** of specialized venules, called "high endothelial venules," are uniquely structured to support the movement of lymphocytes from the blood into the lymph node.[28] Endothelial injury and dysfunction are central processes in many of the most common and serious cardiovascular disorders including hypertension and atherosclerosis (see Chapter 32).

Veins

The smallest venules downstream from the capillaries have an endothelial lining surrounded by fibrous tissue. The largest venules, those farthest from the capillaries, are surrounded by a few smooth muscle fibers comprising a thin tunica media.

Compared with arteries, veins are thin walled and fibrous with a larger diameter (see Figure 31-20). A given vein is larger than the artery that lies within the same sheath. Veins are more numerous than arteries. In veins the tunica externa has less elastic tissue than in arteries, so veins do not recoil after distention as quickly as arteries. Like arteries, veins receive nourishment from the tiny vasa vasorum. Some veins, typically in the legs, contain valves that regulate the one-way flow of blood toward the heart (Figure 31-25). These valves are folds of the tunica intima and are structurally similar to the semilunar valves of the heart. Backflow in veins of the legs is stopped as the flaps of the valves fill with blood and block the vessel. The position of the valves also facilitates blood flow in the proper direction during venous compression. When a person stands up, contraction of the skeletal muscles of the legs compresses the deep veins of the legs and assists the flow of blood toward the heart. This important mechanism of venous return is called the *muscle pump* (see Figure 31-25).

Factors Affecting Blood Flow

Blood flow, the amount of fluid moved per unit of time, is usually expressed as liters or milliliters per minute (ml/min). The factors that influence blood flow include pressure, resistance, velocity, turbulent vs. laminar flow, and compliance.

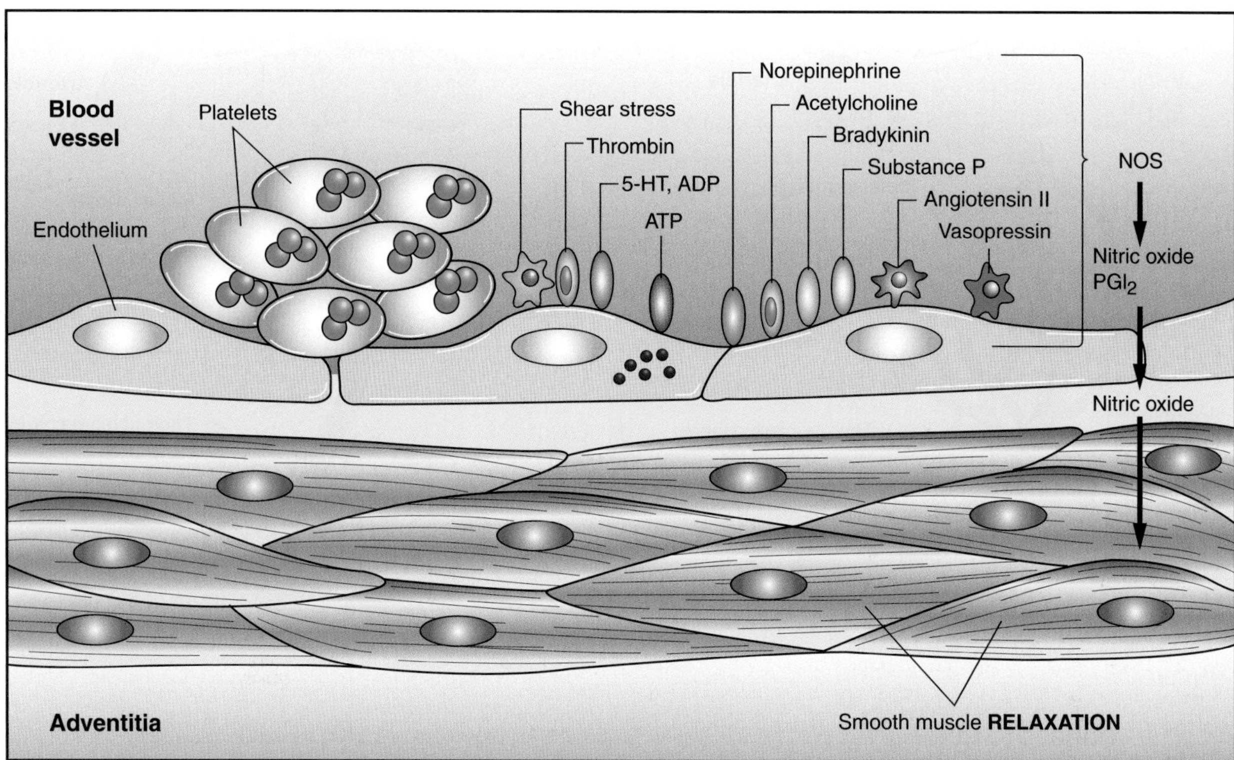

FIGURE 31-23 Factors Causing Endothelium-Dependent Vasodilation. A variety of exogenous pharmacologic substances, platelet-derived factors, and shear stress can promote release of nitric oxide by stimulating nitric oxide synthase (NOS). Prostacyclin (PGI_2) causes relaxation of vascular smooth muscle cells by a cyclic adenosine monophosphate (cAMP)–dependent mechanism, and both nitric oxide and PGI_2 inhibit platelet aggregation. *5-HT,* Serotonin; *ADP,* adenosine diphosphate; *ATP,* adenosine triphosphate.

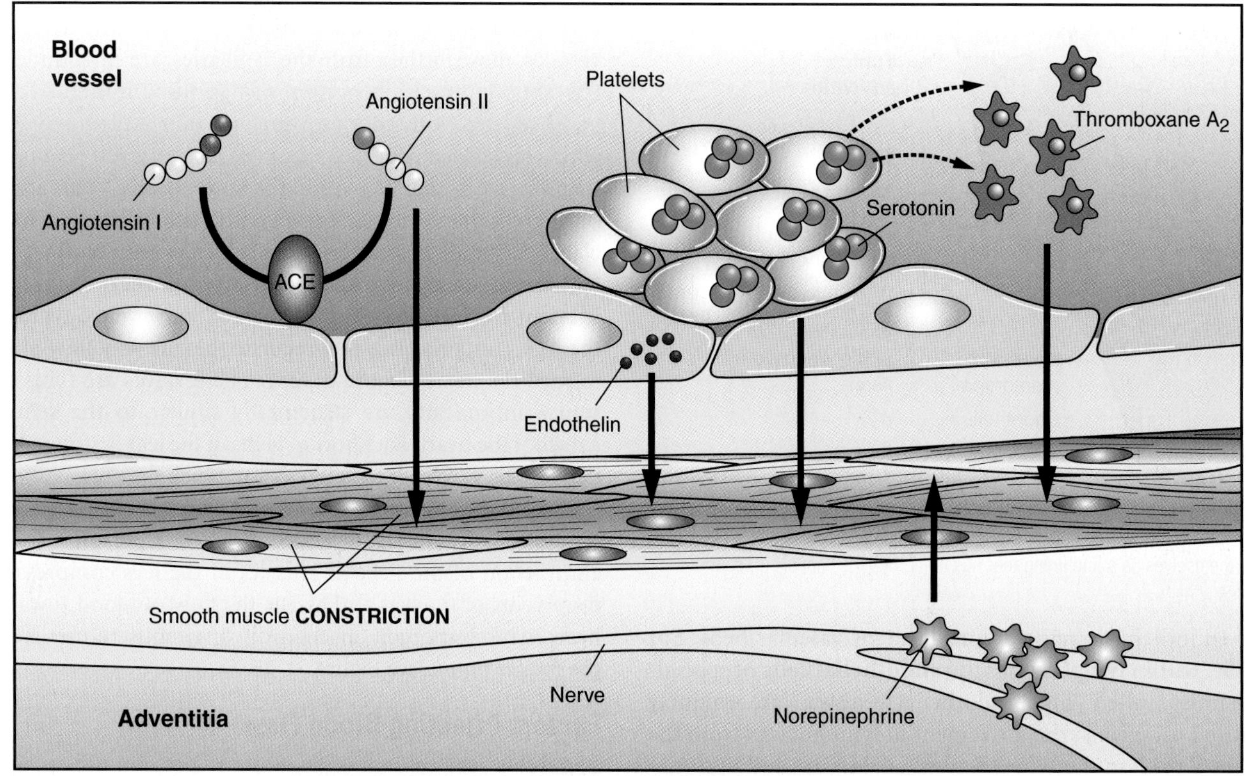

FIGURE 31-24 Endothelium Regulation of Vasomotion (Constriction and Dilation) and Platelet Aggregation by Release of a Variety of Constricting and Dilating Substances. Constricting factors include arachidonic acid and metabolites, such as thromboxane A_2 (which aspirin inhibits), and a potent amino acid peptide called *endothelin.* The endothelium also converts angiotensin I into angiotensin II by the membrane-bound angiotensin-converting enzyme that also metabolizes the endogenous endothelium-dependent vasodilator bradykinin. *ACE,* Angiotensin-converting enzyme.

BOX 31-1 ENDOTHELIUM FUNCTIONS AND VASOACTIVE SUBSTANCES

Dilators

Prostacyclin: A prostaglandin formed from arachidonic acid that can relax vascular smooth muscle through increases in cAMP. The primary function is to inhibit platelet adherence to the endothelium.

Nitric oxide (NO): Bradykinin and shear stress prompt the endothelium to synthesize and release NO, a potent vasodilator. NO is also anti-inflammatory and antithrombotic.

C-type natriuretic hormone: Made throughout the vasculature and works with NO and prostacyclin as a vasodilator.

Insulin: Insulin increases endothelial cell production of nitric oxide.

Estrogen: Triggers enzyme activation and release of NO.

Endothelium-derived relaxing factor: A potent vasodilator made by vascular endothelial cells.

Constrictors

Endothelin: A potent endothelium-derived constrictor.

Urotensin II: Is another potent endothelium-derived constrictor.

Angiotensin II (Ang II): Is a potent vasoconstrictor produced both hormonally via the renin-angiotensin-aldosterone system and locally in vascular tissues. Ang II blocks the release of NO and prostacyclin. Ang II is also proinflammatory: it increases vascular permeability, recruits infiltrating monocytes, increases expression of adhesion molecules, and stimulates release of growth factors.

Thromboxane: Causes vasoconstriction and platelet adhesion.

Prostaglandins: Cause vasoconstriction especially during states of chronic inflammation.

Other Endothelial Functions

Platelet and monocyte adhesion: The endothelium helps regulate clotting and inflammation by modulating the number of platelets and inflammatory cells (monocytes and macrophages) that bind to the vessel wall. Endothelial-derived substances include von Willebrand factor, platelet-activating factor, heparan sulfate, t-PA, thrombomodulin, and others.

Filtration and permeability: The endothelium facilitates movement of large molecules through intercellular junctions and small molecules via vesicles and junctions.

Cell growth and inhibition: NO and prostacyclin inhibit cellular growth; Ang II stimulates growth.

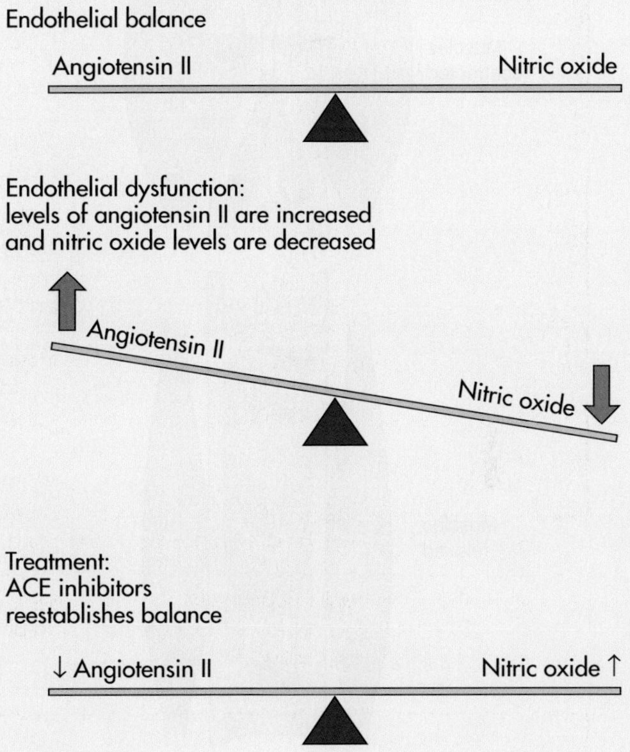

ACE, Angiotensin-converting enzyme; *cAMP,* cyclic adenosine monophosphate; *t-PA,* tissue-type plasminogen activator.
Data from Esper RJ et al: *Adv Cardiol* 45:17–43, 2008; Schafer A, Bauersachs J: *Curr Vasc Pharmacol* 6(1):52–60, 2008; Thijssen DH et al: *J Physiol* 586(2):319–324, 2008. Figure adapted from Rocket JL: *Am J Nurs* 99(10):44, 1999.

Pressure and Resistance

The two main factors influencing blood flow are pressure and resistance, whereas viscosity, type of flow pattern, and compliance have a lesser impact. **Pressure** in a liquid system is the force exerted on the liquid per unit area and is expressed as dynes per square centimeter (dynes/cm^2), millimeters of mercury (mmHg), or torr (1 torr = 1 mmHg). Blood flow to a specific organ depends partly on the pressure difference between the arterial and venous vessels supplying that organ. Fluid moves from the arterial "side" of the capillaries, a region of greater pressure, to the venous side, a region of lesser pressure. Blood flow varies directly with pressure; that is, the greater the pressure differential across a vascular bed, the greater will be the blood flow.

Resistance is the opposition to blood flow. In the cardiovascular system most opposition to blood flow is a result of the diameter and length of the blood vessels. Changes in blood flow through an organ, therefore, result from changes in the vascular resistance within the organ. The major mechanisms causing changes in vascular resistance are increases or decreases in vessel diameter and the opening or closing of vascular channels. The mathematical description of this resistance in a tube is known as the Hagen-Poiseuille equation, sometimes also referred to as Poiseuille's law. This equation indicates that resistance is directly related to tube length and fluid viscosity (blood viscosity) and inversely related to the radius of the tube to the fourth power (r^4). Blood flow is inversely related to resistance so that the greater the resistance in a vascular bed or tissue, the lower the blood flow.

Clinically the most important factor determining resistance in a single vessel is the caliber of the vessel's lumen, which can be measured either as its radius or, as in Figure 31-26, as its diameter. Small changes in the lumen's radius lead to large changes in vascular resistance. Clinically, vasoconstriction will contribute to an increase in resistance whereas vasodilation will cause a decrease that may be reflected by a decrease in blood pressure. Because vessel length is relatively constant and lumen size is quite variable, length is not as important as lumen size in determining flow through a single vessel. Because viscosity is relatively constant, except in the following circumstances,

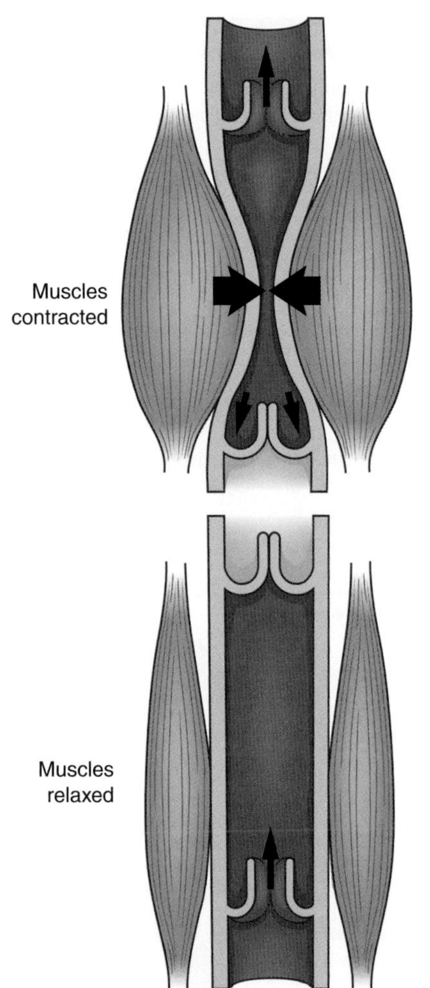

FIGURE 31-25 **Muscle Pump.** As blood returns from downstream and the surrounding muscles contract, the venous valves only allow blood to flow in one direction, back towards the heart.

blood vessel radius is usually the key factor in determining total peripheral resistance.

Generally, resistance to flow is greater in longer tubes because resistance increases with length. That resistance increases with increased length is demonstrated by comparing flow of the same amount of blood under the same pressure through vessels arranged in different configurations. Blood flowing through the distributing arteries, beginning with branches off the aorta and ending at arterioles in the capillary bed, encounters more resistance than blood flowing through the capillary bed itself, where flow is distributed among many short, tiny branches arranged in parallel. This is because the distributing arteries comprise a long system of tubes connected in series (end-to-end), whereas the arterioles and capillaries comprise a short system of many vessels arranged in parallel (side-by-side) (see Figure 31-26). Although the arterioles are arranged in series with the distributing arteries and the capillaries, they are arranged in parallel with other arterioles. Similarly, the capillaries are in series with the metarterioles, but they are in parallel with other capillaries.

Resistance to flow through a system of vessels, or **total resistance,** depends not only on characteristics of individual vessels but also on whether the vessels are arranged in series or in parallel. For vessels arranged in series, total resistance equals the sum obtained by adding all the individual resistances. For vessels arranged in parallel, total resistance equals the sum of the reciprocals *(I/R)* of the individual resistances.

Total resistance is related to the total cross-sectional area of a system of vessels in parallel and to the number of vessels in parallel that make up the total cross-sectional area. The larger the total cross-sectional area, as in the capillary system, the lower the resistance. However, if a cross-sectional area consists of a very large number of parallel vessels, the overall resistance will be greater than it would be if the cross-sectional area were made up of only two or three parallel vessels. Therefore, resistance is greater in smaller vessels than in larger vessels. The total cross-sectional area of the arteriolar system is greater than that of the arterial system (see Figure 31-26); the greater number of arterioles arranged in parallel, however, leads to greater resistance to flow in the arteriolar system. The pressure drop is greatest across the arterioles. Many capillaries arise from each arteriole so that the total cross-sectional area of the capillary bed is very large and resistance is low, despite the fact that the cross-sectional area of each capillary is less (which normally increases resistance) than that of each arteriole. As a result, blood flow becomes quite slow in the capillaries, analogous to water flow in a river. A narrow river whose bed widens flows more slowly through the wide section than through the narrow section. The slow velocity of flow in each vessel is optimal for capillary-tissue exchange.

Both pressure and resistance impact the velocity of the blood within a vessel. **Blood velocity** is the distance blood travels in a unit of time, usually centimeters per second (cm/sec). Blood velocity is directly related to blood flow (amount of blood moved per unit of time) and inversely related to the cross-sectional area of the vessel in which the blood is flowing.

The relationship between velocity and flow can again be understood by thinking of a river. The volume of water flowing in a river is the same whether the river is narrow or wide. Where the river narrows, the water flows quickly; where it widens, the water flows slowly. The volume of water moving between the riverbanks does not change. In the body, as blood moves from the aorta to the capillaries, the total cross-sectional area of the vessels increases and the velocity of flow decreases.

Viscosity

Flow varies inversely with the **viscosity**—thick, sticky consistency of the fluid. Thick fluids move more slowly and cause greater resistance to flow than thin fluids—just think of honey as compared to water. The viscosity of blood depends on red cell content. The greater the percentage of red cells in the blood, the more viscous the blood. This relationship is expressed as the **hematocrit**—the ratio of the volume of red blood cells to the volume of whole blood (see Chapter 27). A high hematocrit value reduces flow through the blood vessels, particularly the microcirculation (arterioles, capillaries, venules). Conditions in which the hematocrit value is elevated, such as a lack of body water, cyanotic congenital heart disease (see Chapter 33), or polycythemia (see Chapter 27), can lead to increased cardiac work as a result of increased vascular resistance.

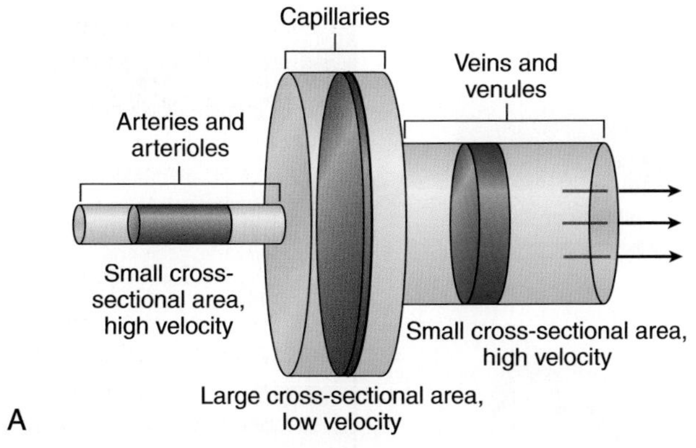

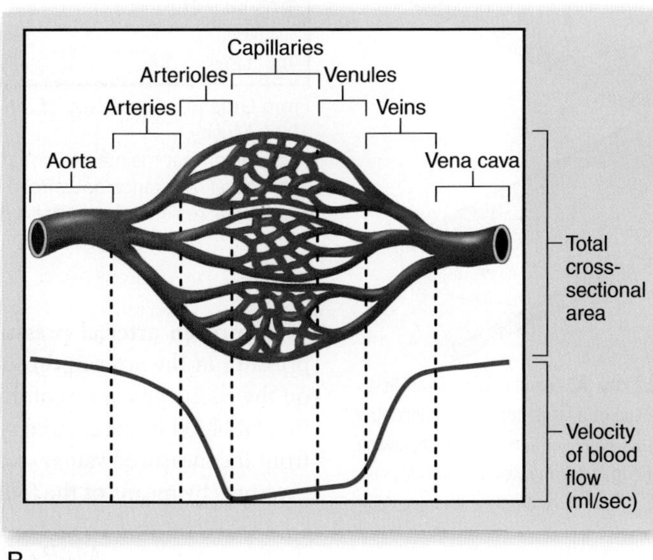

FIGURE 31-26 Relationship Between Cross-Sectional Area and Flow Rate of Blood. As can be seen in the simple diagram **(A)** and the blood vessel chart **(B)**, blood flows with great speed in the large arteries. However, branching of arterial vessels increases the total cross-sectional area of the arterioles and capillaries, reducing the flow rate. When capillaries merge into venules and venules merge into veins, the total cross-sectional area decreases, causing the flow rate to increase. (From Patton KT, Thibodeau GA: *Anatomy & physiology*, ed 8, St Louis, 2013, Mosby.)

Laminar Versus Turbulent Flow

Flow through any tubular system can be either laminar or turbulent. Blood flow through the vessels, except where vessels split or branch, is mainly laminar. In **laminar flow,** concentric layers of molecules move "straight ahead." Each concentric layer flows at a different velocity (Figure 31-27). The cohesive attraction between the fluid and the vessel wall prevents the molecules of blood that are in contact with the wall from moving. The next thin layer of blood is able to slide slowly past the stationary layer and so on until, at the center, the blood velocity is greatest. The centermost concentric layer of fluid is not slowed by friction against the vessel wall. Large vessels have room for a large center layer; therefore, they have less resistance to flow and greater flow and velocity than smaller vessels.

Where flow is obstructed, the vessel turns, or blood flows over rough surfaces, it becomes **turbulent** with whorls or eddy currents that produce noise, causing a murmur to be heard on auscultation, such as occurs during blood pressure measurement with a sphygmomanometer. Resistance increases with turbulence. Arterial areas of turbulence also are places where atherosclerotic plaques are found (see Chapter 32).

Vascular Compliance

Vascular compliance is the increase in volume a vessel is able to accommodate for a given increase in pressure. Compliance depends on the factors related to the nature of a vessel wall, such as the ratio of elastic fibers to muscle fibers in the vessel wall. Elastic arteries are more compliant than muscular arteries; the veins are more compliant than either type of artery because they have less smooth muscle. Because they are more compliant, veins serve as storage areas for the circulatory system.

Compliance determines a vessel's response to pressure changes. For example, with a very small increase in pressure, a large volume of blood can be accommodated by the venous system. In the less compliant arterial system, where smaller volumes and higher pressures are normal, small variations in pressure cause little or no change in the volume of blood within the arterial vessels.

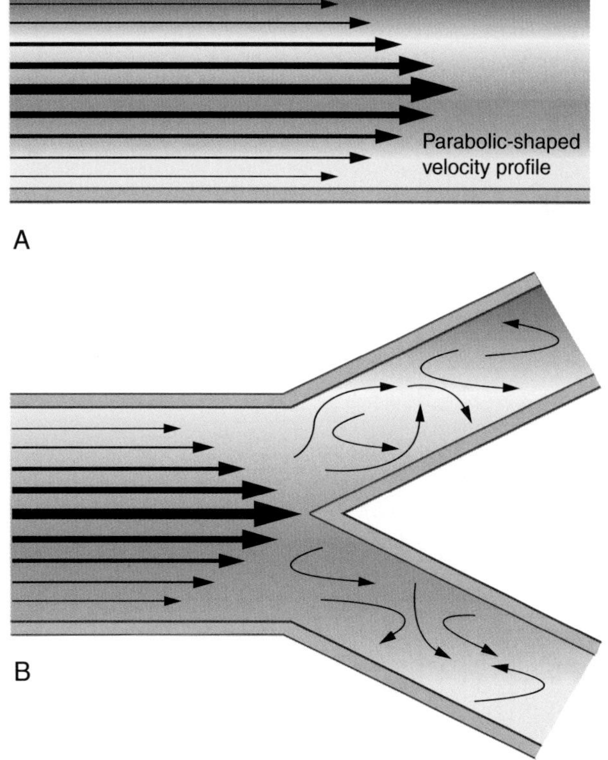

FIGURE 31-27 Laminar and Turbulent Flow. **A,** Laminar flow. Fluid flows in long smooth-walled tubes as if it is composed of a large number of concentric layers. **B,** Turbulent flow is caused by numerous small currents flowing crosswise or oblique to the long axis of the vessel, resulting in flowing whorls and eddy currents. (Adapted from Seeley RR, Stephens TD, Tate P: *Anatomy and physiology,* ed 3, St Louis, 1995, Mosby.)

Stiffness is the opposite of compliance. Several conditions and disorders can increase vascular stiffness, with the most common being aging and arteriosclerosis (see Chapter 32 and section on aging at the end of this chapter). Arteriosclerosis increases the rigidity or stiffness of arterial walls, which in turn increases peak arterial pressure at a given volume of blood.

Regulation of Blood Pressure (Arterial Pressure)

During a wide range of physiologic conditions, including changes in body position, muscular activity, and circulating blood volume, arterial pressure is regulated within a fairly narrow range to maintain tissue **perfusion,** or blood supply to the capillary beds, Systemic arterial blood pressure is a *regulated variable,* which means that the cardiovascular control systems are designed to maintain blood pressure within these limits. Very low pressures are not consistent with survival because body tissues will not be perfused whereas very high pressures increase the risk of stroke and damage to other organs, such as the kidneys, heart, and retinas. Arterial pressure is a function of and varies directly with both cardiac output (heart rate × stroke volume) and peripheral resistance. Increases in one or both will raise arterial pressure, and decreases in one or both will lower the arterial pressure (Table 31-3). The major factors and relationships that regulate arterial blood pressure are summarized in Figure 31-28.

TABLE 31-3 FACTORS THAT AFFECT MEAN ARTERIAL PRESSURE AND CAPILLARY FLOW

	MEAN ARTERIAL PRESSURE	CAPILLARY FLOW
Peripheral Resistance*		
Increased	Increased	Decreased
Decreased	Decreased	Increased
Heart Rate†		
Increased	Increased	Increased
Decreased	Decreased	Decreased
Stroke Volume‡		
Increased	Increased	Increased
Decreased	Decreased	Decreased

From Little RC: *Physiology of the heart and circulation,* ed 3, St Louis, 1985, Mosby.
*Cardiac output maintained constant.
†Peripheral resistance and stroke volume constant.
‡Peripheral resistance and heart rate constant.

The **mean arterial pressure (MAP),** which is the average pressure in the arteries throughout the cardiac cycle, depends on the elastic properties of the arterial walls and the mean volume of blood in the arterial system. MAP can be approximated from the measured values of the systolic *(Ps)* and diastolic *(Pd)* pressures by means of the following formula:

$$MAP = Pd + \frac{1}{3}(Ps\text{-}Pd)$$

The difference between the systolic pressure and diastolic pressure *(Ps – Pd)* is called the **pulse pressure.** Pulse pressure is directly related to arterial wall stiffness and stroke volume.

Effects of Cardiac Output

The cardiac output (minute volume) of the heart can be changed by alterations in heart rate, stroke volume (volume of blood ejected during each ventricular contraction), or both. An increase in cardiac output without a decrease in peripheral resistance will cause mean blood pressure and flow rate to increase. The higher arterial pressure increases blood flow through the arterioles. On the other hand, a decrease in the cardiac output causes an immediate drop in mean arterial blood pressure and flow rate (see Table 31-3).

Effects of Total Peripheral Resistance and Blood Volume

Total resistance in the systemic circulation, often referred to as either systemic vascular resistance (SVR) or *total peripheral resistance (TPR),* is primarily a function of the diameter of the arterioles. If cardiac output remains constant, arteriolar constriction raises mean arterial pressure by reducing the flow of blood into the capillaries and arteriolar dilation has the opposite effect.

Neural Control of Total Peripheral Resistance. Reflex control of cardiac output and peripheral resistance includes: (1) sympathetic stimulation of heart, arterioles, and veins;

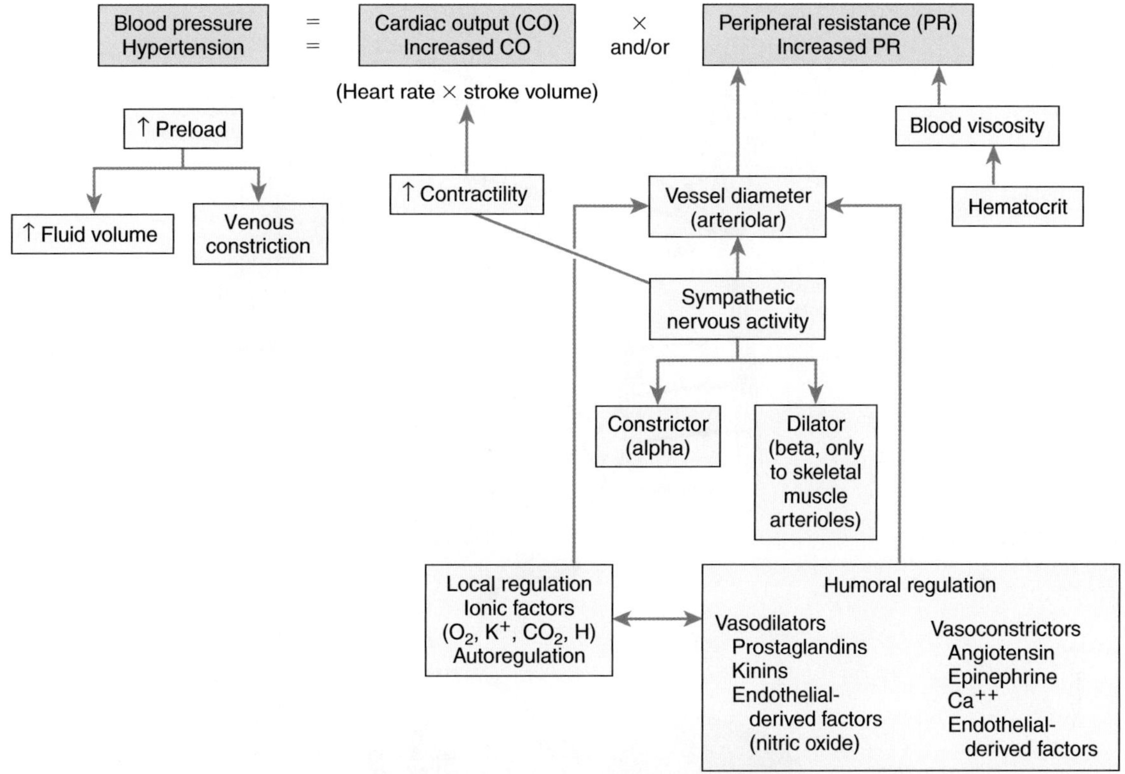

FIGURE 31-28 Factors Regulating Blood Flow.

and (2) parasympathetic stimulation of the heart. The cardiovascular center in the medulla receives input from pressure and blood composition sensors throughout the vascular system and then modifies vagal and sympathetic output to control heart rate and contractility, plus vascular diameter (see Figure 31-10). Another input to the system comes from hypothalamic centers that regulate vascular (and cardiac) responses to changes in temperature. When the body's core temperature exceeds normal, the hypothalamus reflex initiates dilation of arterioles and veins in the skin. This vasodilation shunts blood to the skin, where heat is lost through sweating, radiation, conduction, and/or convection. When body core temperature decreases below normal, surface vessels constrict, shunting blood to the vital organs. Vasoconstriction is regulated by an area of the brainstem that maintains a constant (tonic) output of norepinephrine from sympathetic fibers in the peripheral arterioles. This tonic activity is essential for maintenance of blood pressure.

During exercise and stress, the sympathetic fibers that stimulate vasodilation of skeletal muscle arterioles are thought to be under the direct control of the cerebral cortex and hypothalamus and not the medullary centers. Information about pressure, resistance, and blood composition is sensed by neural receptors (baroreceptors and chemoreceptors) in arterial walls and delivered to the medullary centers.

Baroreceptors. **Baroreceptors** (stretch receptors), located in the aorta, the carotid sinus (Figure 31-29), as well as other locations in the vasculature, influence both heart rate and vascular resistance, and therefore blood pressure. Baroreceptors respond to changes in smooth muscle fiber length by altering their rate of discharge and supply sensory information to the cardiovascular center that regulates blood pressure.[29] (Technically they are mechanoreceptors but they usually are called *baroreceptors* or *pressoreceptors.*) The rate of firing of the baroreceptors increases and decreases with changes in blood pressure. An increase in arterial pressure increases the rate of firing of the carotid sinus and aortic arch baroreceptors. These impulses travel up the afferent nerves to the medulla (e.g., the cardiac control center) and (1) slow heart rate by decreasing sympathetic discharge and increasing parasympathetic discharge (vagus nerve), (2) decrease myocardial contractility by inhibiting sympathetic discharge, and (3) increase arteriolar and venous dilation by decreasing sympathetic discharge to smooth muscle. The net effect of this major blood pressure–regulating reflex is to reduce blood pressure to normal by decreasing cardiac output (heart rate and stroke volume) and peripheral resistance. Conversely, the baroreceptor response to decreased blood pressure results in an increase in heart rate, an increase in myocardial contractility, and peripheral vasoconstriction, thus raising the blood pressure. (Postural changes and the baroreceptor reflex are discussed in Chapter 32.)

Arterial Chemoreceptors. Specialized areas within the medulla oblongata and aortic and carotid arteries are sensitive to concentrations of oxygen (Pao_2), carbon dioxide ($Paco_2$), and hydrogen ions (pH) in the blood. Although these receptors, called *chemoreceptors,* are more important for respiratory control, they also transmit impulses to the medullary cardiovascular centers that regulate blood pressure. A decrease in arterial oxygen concentration or an increase in $Paco_2$ causes

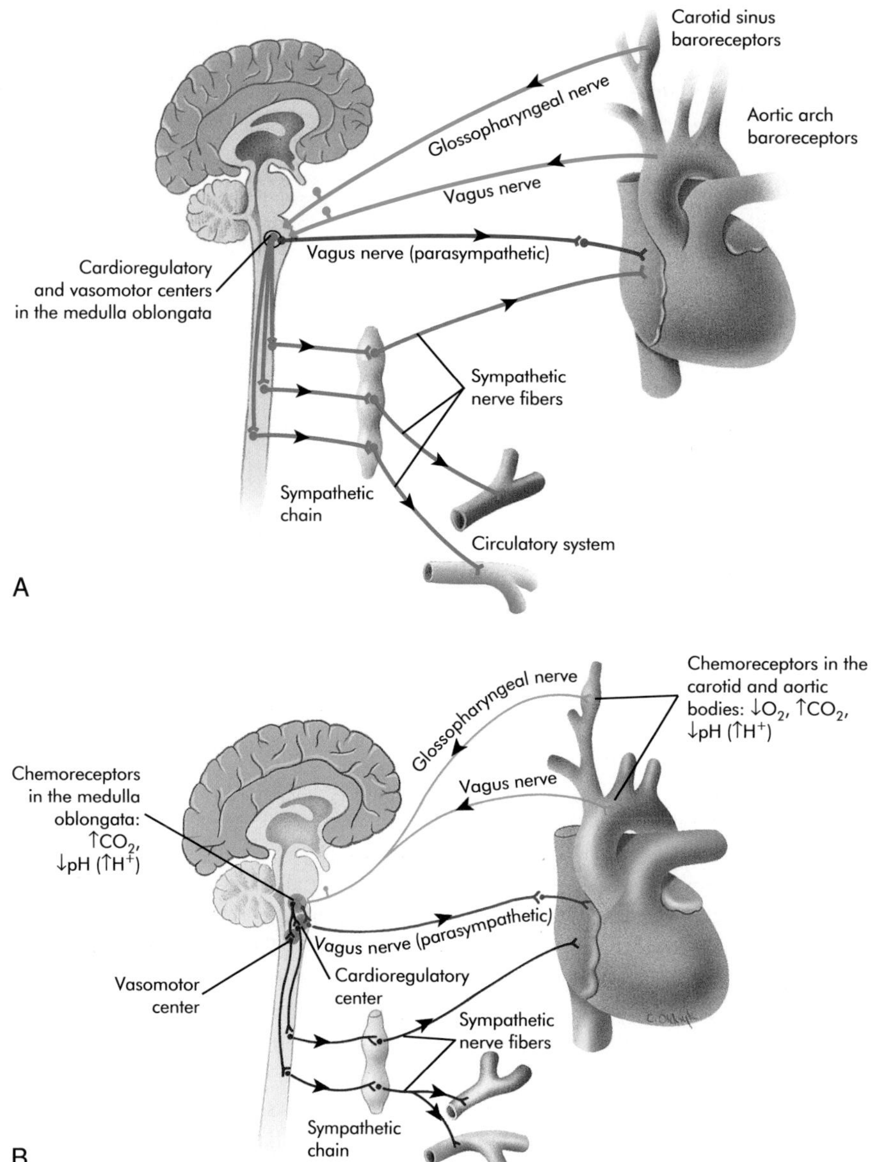

FIGURE 31-29 **Baroreceptor and Chemoreceptor Reflex Control of Blood Pressure. A,** Baroreceptor reflexes. Baroreceptors located in the carotid sinuses and aortic arch detect changes in blood pressure. Action potentials are conducted to the cardioregulatory and vasomotor centers. The heart rate can be decreased by the parasympathetic system; the heart rate and stroke volume can be increased by the sympathetic system. The sympathetic system also can constrict or dilate blood vessels. **B,** Chemoreceptor reflexes. Chemoreceptors located in the medulla oblongata and in the carotid and aortic bodies detect changes in levels of blood oxygen, carbon dioxide, or pH. Action potentials are conducted to the medulla oblongata. In response, the vasomotor center can cause vasoconstriction or dilation of blood vessels by the sympathetic system, and the cardioregulatory center can cause changes in the pumping activity of the heart through the parasympathetic and sympathetic systems. (From Seeley RR, Stephens TD, Tate P: *Anatomy & physiology,* ed 3, St Louis, 1995, Mosby.)

a reflexive increase in heart rate, stroke volume, and blood pressure, whereas an increase in carbon dioxide concentration causes decreases in these variables. The major chemoreceptive reflex is caused by alterations in arterial oxygen concentration. The effects of altered pH or carbon dioxide levels are minor.

Effect of Hyperemia. When metabolic activity is increased in the heart, skeletal muscle, and other muscular organs, it causes an increase in blood flow termed **hyperemia.** For example, the blood flow to exercising skeletal muscle increases in proportion to the activity of the muscle. This condition, known as *active (exercise) hyperemia,* is the result of arteriolar dilation and autoregulation of blood flow within the active organ. *Reactive hyperemia* refers to vasodilation in response to restoration of blood flow after a period of tissue ischemia and results from a buildup of vasodilatory metabolic byproducts in the ischemic tissue. After an infarction in a vascular bed, the subsequent reactive hyperemia that may occur has been associated with damage known as *ischemia reperfusion injury.*[30]

Effects of Hormones. Hormones influence total peripheral resistance and blood volume by changing either vascular tone or blood volume. Certain hormones cause contraction or relaxation of arteriolar smooth muscle. By constricting or dilating arterioles in specific vascular beds, hormones can (1) increase the blood supply to vital organs that require more blood flow in times of stress, (2) redistribute blood volume during hemorrhage or shock, and (3) regulate heat loss.

The **vasoconstrictor hormones** include angiotensin II, vasopressin (also known as antidiuretic hormone), epinephrine, and norepinephrine. **Epinephrine,** the catecholamine hormone released from the adrenal medulla, causes vasoconstriction in most vascular beds except the coronary, liver, and skeletal muscle circulations. **Norepinephrine** mainly acts as a neurotransmitter; however, some is also released from the adrenal medulla and is actually a more potent vasoconstrictor than epinephrine. Both **angiotensin II** and **vasopressin** are vasoconstrictors but they are not thought to have a major role in blood pressure control in normal circumstances.

Both vasopressin and aldosterone influence blood pressure by increasing blood volume through their influence on fluid reabsorption in the kidney and by stimulating thirst. Vasopressin causes the reabsorption of water from tubular fluid in the distal tubule and collecting duct of the nephron. **Aldosterone,** part of the renin-angiotensin-aldosterone system, stimulates the reabsorption of sodium, chloride, and water from the same locations. The natriuretic hormones, which include **brain natriuretic peptide (BNP), C-type natriuretic peptide (CNP),** and **urodilatin,** all cause loss of sodium, chloride, and water through their effects on kidney function.[31]

Adrenomedullin (ADM) is a recently discovered, widely dispersed peptide present in numerous tissues with powerful vasodilatory activity, and is a member of the calcitonin gene–related peptide family. Although it has been found to have numerous cardiovascular effects in animals, including a role in fetal cardiovascular system development and vasodilation, its exact role in adult human cardiovascular function has not been identified. It is likely that it has a role in cardiovascular disease but those links remain to be explored.[32]

Effects of Other Mediators. Several mediators produced by the vascular endothelium have been demonstrated to cause arteriolar vasodilation. These mediators include nitric oxide (NO), prostaglandins, endothelium-derived relaxing factor, and possibly other molecules. The velocity of blood movement within the arterioles causes shear stress at the vascular endothelial surface that in turn is the stimulus that causes the endothelial cells to produce these vasodilator substances. The flow-mediated dilation (FMD) test is used to evaluate endothelial function and to predict the risk of cardiovascular disease. A reduction in FMD is predictive of increased risk.[33]

Venous Pressure

The main determinants of venous blood pressure are: (1) the volume of fluid within the veins, and (2) the compliance (distensibility) of the vessel walls. Veins have much thinner walls than arteries and are more distensible. Typically, the venous system accommodates approximately 66% of the total blood volume with venous pressure averaging less than 10 mmHg. The systemic arteries accommodate about 11% of the total blood volume, with an average arterial pressure (blood pressure) of about 100 mmHg, whereas the rest of the blood volume is within the heart, capillaries, and pulmonary circulation.[18]

The sympathetic nervous system controls compliance. The walls of the veins are highly innervated by sympathetic fibers that control venous smooth muscle. When the sympathetic nerves to the veins fire, the result is an increase in smooth muscle tone rather than vasoconstriction, which would be the result in arterial vessels. This increased smooth muscle tone stiffens the walls of the veins, reducing distensibility and increasing venous blood pressure, thus forcing more blood through the veins and into the right heart.

Two other mechanisms that increase venous pressure and venous return to the heart are: (1) the skeletal muscle pump, and (2) the respiratory pump. During skeletal muscle contraction the veins within the muscles are partially compressed, causing a decrease in venous capacity and increased return to the heart. The respiratory pump acts during inspiration, when the veins of the abdomen are partially compressed by the downward movement of the diaphragm. Increased abdominal pressure moves blood toward the heart.

Regulation of Coronary Circulation

Flow of blood in the coronary circulation, as in all vascular beds, is directly proportional to the perfusion pressure and inversely proportional to the vascular resistance of the bed. **Coronary perfusion pressure** is the difference between pressure in the aorta and pressure in the coronary vessels. Thus aortic pressure is the driving pressure that propels the perfusion of myocardial vessels. Mechanisms of vasodilation and vasoconstriction normally maintain coronary blood flow despite stresses imposed by the constant contraction and relaxation of the heart muscle and despite shifts (within a physiologic range) of coronary perfusion pressure.

Several unique anatomic factors influence coronary blood flow. Because of their location, the aortic valve cusps can obstruct coronary blood flow by pushing against the openings of the coronary arteries during systole. Also during systole, the coronary arteries are compressed by ventricular contraction. These anatomic factors have a **systolic compressive effect,** which is particularly evident in the subendocardial layers of the left ventricular wall and can greatly increase resistance to coronary blood flow. Therefore, most coronary blood flow in the left ventricle occurs during diastole. During the period of systolic compression, when flow is slowed or stopped, oxygen is supplied by **myoglobin,** a protein in heart muscle (also smooth and skeletal muscle) that binds oxygen during contraction, diastole in the heart, and then releases it when blood levels of oxygen fall during relaxation or systole. Myoglobin is structurally different than hemoglobin although both contain a heme group.[34]

Autoregulation

Autoregulation (automatic self-regulation) enables organs to regulate blood flow by altering the resistance in their arterioles. Autoregulation in the coronary circulation maintains the blood flow at a nearly constant rate at perfusion pressures (mean arterial pressure) between 60 and 180 mmHg when

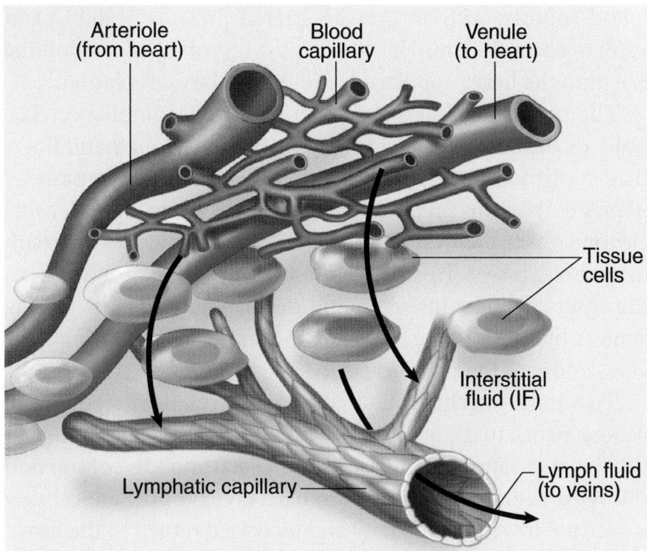

FIGURE 31-30 **Role of the Lymphatic System in Fluid Balance.** Fluid from plasma flowing through the capillaries moves into interstitial spaces. Although *most* of this interstitial fluid is either absorbed by tissue cells or resorbed by blood capillaries, *some* of the fluid tends to accumulate in the interstitial spaces. As this fluid builds up, it usually drains into lymphatic vessels *(green)* that eventually return the fluid to the venous blood. Lymphatic structures are not actually green. Green is used in diagrams to contrast lymphatic structures with nearby blood vessels *(red, blue).* (From Patton KT, Thibodeau GA: *Anatomy & physiology,* ed 8, St Louis, 2013, Mosby.)

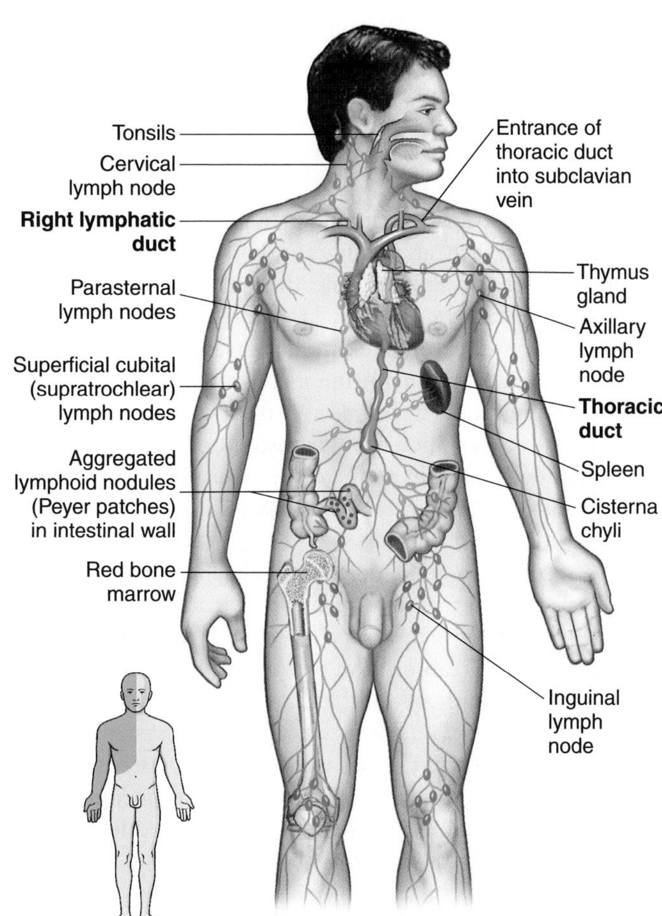

FIGURE 31-31 **Principal Organs of the Lymphatic System.** The inset shows the areas drained by the right lymphatic duct *(green)* and the thoracic duct *(blue).* (From Patton KT, Thibodeau GA: *Anatomy & physiology,* ed 8, St Louis, 2013, Mosby.)

other influencing factors are held constant. Thus autoregulation helps to ensure constant coronary blood flow despite shifts in the perfusion pressure within the stated range. Given that blood flow is directly related to pressure and inversely related to resistance, we know that for flow to stay constant as pressure decreases, resistance also has to decrease; thus the mechanism(s) underlying autoregulation must relate to control of smooth muscle contraction in the arteriolar walls. Although the exact mechanisms underlying autoregulation are not known, some research has indicated that G-protein–coupled receptors that influence calcium release with the myocardium are involved.[35]

LYMPHATIC SYSTEM

The **lymphatic system** is a one-way network of vessels that is important for fluid balance, immune function, and transport of lipids, hormones, and cytokines. Every day about 3 liters of fluid filters out of venous capillaries in body tissues and is not reabsorbed. This fluid becomes the lymph that is carried by the lymphatic vessels to the chest where it enters the venous circulation. The lymphatic vessels run in the same sheaths with the arteries and veins (Figure 31-30). The lymphatic system consists of lymphatic vessels and the lymph nodes (Figure 31-31). (Lymph nodes and lymphoid tissues are described in Chapters 7 and 27.) In this pumpless system a series of valves ensures one-way flow of the excess interstitial fluid (then called *lymph*) toward the heart. The lymphatic capillaries are closed at the distal ends (Figure 31-32).

Lymph consists primarily of water and small amounts of dissolved proteins, mostly albumin, that are too large to be reabsorbed into the less permeable blood capillaries. Lymph also carries two types of cells—lymphocytes and antigen-presenting cells. The antigen-presenting cells are carried to the next lymph node in the system whereas lymphocytes traffic between lymph nodes. Once within the lymphatic system, lymph travels through **lymphatic venules** and **veins** that drain into one of two large ducts in the thorax—the right lymphatic duct and the thoracic duct. The **right lymphatic duct** drains lymph from the right arm and the right side of the head and thorax, whereas the larger thoracic duct receives lymph from the rest of the body (see Figure 31-31). The right lymphatic duct and the **thoracic duct** drain lymph into the right and left subclavian veins, respectively.

The lymphatic veins are thin walled, like the veins of the cardiovascular system. In the larger lymphatic veins, endothelial flaps form valves similar to those in the circulatory veins. The valves permit lymph to flow in only one direction because lymphatic vessels are compressed intermittently by contraction of skeletal muscles, pulsatile expansion of an artery in the same sheath, and contraction of the smooth muscles in the walls of the lymphatic vessel.

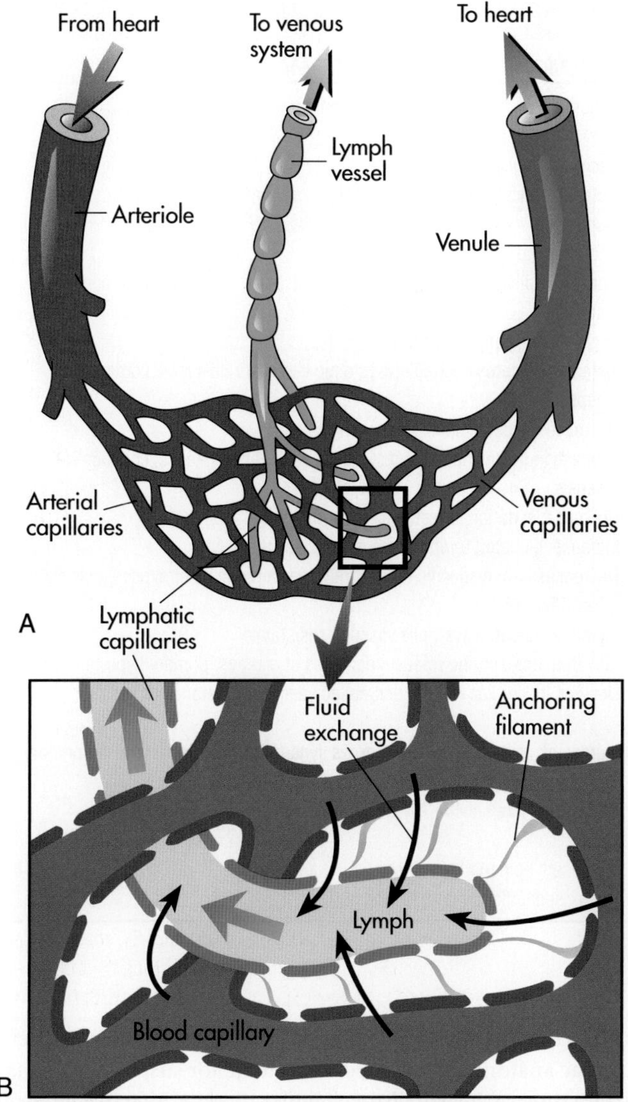

FIGURE 31-32 Lymphatic Capillaries. **A,** Schematic representation of lymphatic capillaries. **B,** Anatomic components of microcirculation.

As lymph is transported toward the heart, it is filtered through thousands of bean-shaped lymph nodes clustered along the lymphatic vessels (see Figure 31-31). Lymph enters the nodes through several **afferent lymphatic vessels,** filters through the sinuses in the nodes, and leaves by way of **efferent lymphatic vessels.** Lymph flows slowly through a node, which facilitates the phagocytosis of foreign substances within the node by antigen-presenting cells and the entry of mature but naïve B and T lymphocytes, which then circulate through the body, moving from one lymph node to the next while waiting for a chance encounter with the antigen to which they are programmed to respond (see What's New? Growth of New Lymphatic Vessels from Macrophages). (Phagocytosis is described in Chapter 7.)

TESTS OF CARDIOVASCULAR FUNCTION

Assessment of the individual with suspected cardiovascular disorders begins with a thorough history for determination of risk factors and symptoms. A careful physical examination looking for evidence of tissue ischemia, pulmonary congestion, and cardiac dysfunction is next. Blood samples are taken and sent for a variety of tests. For many individuals, these basic steps will be complemented with methods that measure heart and vascular function with greater specificity. Cardiac function can be evaluated using indicators calculated from pressures and flow rates in the heart and vessels. Table 31-4 defines the indicators most often used in the clinical setting. The normal values for several testing methods are different for men and women.[36,37] This textbook's inside back cover includes normal blood values for common laboratory tests.

WHAT'S NEW?

Growth of New Lymphatic Vessels from Macrophages

During inflammation and wound healing in adults, new lymphatic vessels sprout from existing vessels in the affected area, a process known as lymphangiogenesis. When inflammation occurs, inflammatory cytokines, such as vascular endothelial growth factors A and C (VEGF-A and VEGF-C), bind to receptors, such as the VEGF receptor 3 (VEGFR-3), on macrophages and stimulate the division of lymphatic endothelial cells and the formation of new lymphatic capillaries that will drain the affected tissue. Some macrophages in the area differentiate into a new subtype, known as a macrophage-derived lymphatic endothelial cell progenitor, that is capable of working with the lymphatic endothelial cells to create the new lymphatic capillaries. Understanding the factors that stimulate and control this growth of new lymphatic vessels may allow treatment of conditions such as lymphedema, as well as some heart conditions, impaired wound healing, and some types of cancer.

Data from Ji R-C: *Cell Mol Life Sci* 69(6):897–914, 2012; Ran S, Montgomery KE: *Cancers (Basel)* 4(3):618–657, 2012.

Cardiac and Coronary Artery Evaluation

Many sophisticated tests are used to evaluate and diagnose cardiac or coronary artery diseases, and new ones are being tested each year. Some of the more commonly used modalities include chest x-ray, electrocardiography, echocardiography, stress testing, computed tomography (CT) and magnetic resonance imaging (MRI), technetium scanning, electrophysiology studies, and catheterization with angiography.

Chest Radiograph Examination

Chest x-rays allow for the examination of the size and contour of the heart and related structures. Evidence of chamber enlargement, pericardial disease, pulmonary edema, valvular calcification, ventricular hypertrophy, and pathology of the great vessels may be visualized. Chest x-ray also is useful to assess for appropriate placement of invasive cardiac conduction devices and for any complications caused by these devices (e.g., pneumothorax or hemothorax; see Chapter 35). A chest x-ray examination is a routine part of a cardiac examination. The most commonly obtained views are posteroanterior (PA) and lateral, with the individual standing upright and the lungs fully expanded. In those individuals confined to bed, an anteroposterior (AP) view may be obtained but is usually of lesser quality than the PA view.

TABLE 31-4 INDICATORS OF CARDIAC FUNCTION

INDICATOR	DEFINITION*	COMMON CAUSE OF ABNORMALITY
Heart rate (HR)	Number of heartbeats (cardiac cycles) per minute Normal adult value: 70 beats/min	Ischemia, electrolyte disturbances, drug toxicity
Cardiac output (CO)	Amount of blood (in L) moved by the heart in 1 min Normal range: 4-8 L/min	Decrease indicates heart failure Increase indicates decreased systemic vascular resistance, common in sepsis
Cardiac index (CI)	Relationship between cardiac output and body surface area (BSA, in m^2) Normal range: 2.8-4.2 L/min/m^2	Decrease indicates heart failure Increase indicates decreased systemic vascular resistance, common in sepsis
Stroke volume (SV)	Amount of blood (in ml) ejected by the left ventricle during systole (i.e., per beat) Normal range: 60-100 ml/beat	Decrease indicates heart failure Increase indicates decreased systemic vascular resistance, common in sepsis
Stroke volume index (SVI)	Relationship between stroke volume and body surface area Normal range: 33-47 ml/beat/m^2	Decrease indicates heart failure Increase indicates decreased systemic vascular resistance, common in sepsis
Oxygen consumption index ($\dot{V}O_2$)	Amount of oxygen (in ml) consumed per minute in relation to BSA	Decrease: sedation, anesthesia, hypothermia Increase: elevated temperature, sepsis, seizures
Stroke work index (SWI)	Amount of work (expressed as done) by the left or right ventricle per systole per square meter of BSA Normal value: 35 g/m^2	Decreases within specific ranges indicate cardiogenic or hypovolemic shock (see Chapter 48) Increase: elevated systemic vascular resistance
Systemic mean arterial pressure (MAP)	Mean blood pressure (in mmHg) in the systemic arteries Normal range: 70-100 mmHg	Elevated: epinephrine release, diseases of arteries, primary hypertension Decreased: cardiac failure, decreased vascular resistance of sepsis
Pulmonary vascular resistance (PVR)	Relationship among cardiac output, preload, and afterload, expressed as units of force of resistance per second per centimeter of water Normal value: less than 250 dynes/sec/cm^{-5}	Increased: acute respiratory distress syndrome (ARDS), pneumonia, primary pulmonary hypertension, congestive heart failure Decreased: late shock
Systemic vascular resistance (SVR)	Same definition as for PVR Normal range: 770-1500 dynes/sec/cm^{-5}	Increased: epinephrine release Decreased: inflammatory response

*Values given are for adults at rest.

Electrocardiography

Electrocardiography, typically a 12-lead electrocardiogram (ECG), gives information about heart rate and rhythm; the effects of activities of daily life, exercise, electrolytes, drugs, and disease on electrical activity in the heart; and the electrical orientation of the cardiac muscle. An ECG provides no direct information about the contractile state or mechanical performance of the heart.

Serial 12-lead ECGs are of primary importance in establishing the presence of myocardial ischemia and infarction or conduction defects and dysrhythmias. This examination has become part of the routine hospital preadmission/admission assessment, even when the admitting diagnosis is not cardiac in nature, because it establishes baseline information about the electrical function of the heart. Also, recent ECGs can be compared with ECGs obtained from the same individual in the past. Changes in the ECG over time assist in determining the cause, amount, or nature of changes in cardiac anatomy and physiology. Ambulatory electrocardiographic or Holter monitoring is used to evaluate rhythm changes that may occur in persons during activities of daily living. Cell phone technology also is rapidly advancing to enable ECG recording and relaying to healthcare providers.

Echocardiography

Echocardiography is the most effective and widely used noninvasive modality for evaluating the structures of the heart. Ultrasound beams reflected by cardiovascular structures produce shapes that can be visualized and allow for recognition of altered cardiac anatomy.[38] It is used to evaluate for suspected coronary artery disease, heart failure, valvular disease, infective endocarditis, cardiomyopathies, pericardial disease, prosthetic valve function, congenital heart disease, and aortic diseases. Through the use of M-mode, two- and three-dimensional techniques with Doppler and color flow imaging, accurate assessments of cardiac output, ejection fraction, and valvular function can be obtained.[38,39] Advances in technology now allow both intracardiac and transesophageal echocardiography for evaluation of the heart anatomy, although anesthesia is required for the transesophageal technique.[40]

Exercise or Stress Testing

Cardiac activity during exercise is examined during a stress test when an intervention is used to increase myocardial work. Stress testing elicits signs and symptoms of heart disease and coronary artery disease that may not appear at rest. Echocardiography or continuous 12-lead ECG and blood pressure measurements are obtained before, during, and after the study. Cardiac stress from exercise is usually induced by having the individual walk on a treadmill. Other, less frequently used forms of exercise include static exercise (hand ergometry or chemical stress), stair climbing (the Stairmaster's double two-step), arm ergometry, and bicycle ergometry. The individual exercises until the maximal heart rate for gender and age is reached or until other subjective or objective indicators of cardiac dysfunction or distress appear. Subjective indicators include chest pain, extreme fatigue, extreme dyspnea, leg pain, or the individual's request to stop the test. Objective criteria are ST-segment elevation or depression, SA node or atrial dysrhythmias, AV node dysrhythmias, ventricular dysrhythmias, elevated or decreased blood pressure, signs of cerebral hypoxia, and signs of circulatory insufficiency. One limitation of this test is that it cannot be used in persons whose capacity for exercise is limited.

Stress testing also may be used to evaluate either fitness for noncardiac surgery or progress in recovery after myocardial infarction or cardiac surgery. Graded exercise in individuals with low- to moderate-risk chest pain evaluated in an emergency department can be used as a prognostic indicator of adverse cardiac events. When a differential diagnosis for chest pain has been difficult to determine, stress testing may help distinguish coronary artery insufficiency from other causes of pain. The risks associated with stress testing include dysrhythmias, myocardial infarction, and death. The risk is greater when the test is performed soon after an acute ischemic event.

Stress testing with ECG monitoring may not be sensitive enough to detect and localize areas of the myocardium at risk for ischemia and infarction. Currently, most stress testing includes the injection of a radiotracer that is absorbed by active heart cells. When the heart is scanned, during and after stress testing, areas where the radiotracer is not taken up by ischemic cells can be seen and those locations indicate areas of myocardial damage.

Single-Photon Emission Computed Tomography

Single-photon emission computed tomography (SPECT) is typically used to evaluate individuals for coronary artery disease and myocardial ischemia during stress testing. A radiotracer (usually thalium-201) is injected intravenously and is absorbed and retained for a while by healthy myocytes.[41] Photons are emitted from the radiotracer in the myocardium in proportion to perfusion of the tissue. A gamma camera visualizes the photons, and views are taken from 360 degrees by CT, which digitizes the information and provides a three-dimensional view of myocardial perfusion. Data about where the myocardium absorbs the tracer normally, slowly, or not at all can be correlated with existing myocardial disease and can help quantify ischemic risk. A new development, high-speed SPECT, has the advantage of taking less time and, thereby, requiring less radiotracer, which decreases radiation exposure for the person being examined.[41]

Computed Tomography (CT) and Magnetic Resonance Imaging (MRI)

Computed tomography (CT) and magnetic resonance imaging (MRI) are used to evaluate cardiac anatomy and physiology. New techniques, including ECG gating (timing of data gathering to the cardiac cycle), electron beam CT, and spiral CT, have improved the ability of tomography to visualize cardiac structures. The high resolution of CT can provide information about calcification of coronary vessels and cardiac valves. Information about coronary artery calcification is being used to improve risk classification for coronary artery disease.[42] It also is a tool for evaluating large-vessel disease. Concerns and debate continue, however, about the radiation risks and use of variable protocols. The International Commission on Radiological Protection (ICRP) recently released a report on radiological protection in cardiology.[43]

MRI is based on the principle that the frequency of energy (resonant frequency) given up by a nucleus is exactly proportional to the surrounding magnetic field (see Chapter 15). The anatomy and physiology of the great blood vessels and myocardium are depicted in three dimensions with excellent resolution. Ventricular function can be evaluated using indexes of ventricular function, such as ejection fraction. Rapidly moving sequences (MRI) can determine regional wall motion and myocardial deformation. Flow direction and velocity also can be quantitatively determined. Stress testing also can be done with MRI using the drug dobutamine to increase the cardiac workload instead of exercise.[44]

Technetium Scanning

Radiopharmaceuticals labeled with ^{99m}technetium preparations, such as sestamibi, teboroxime, and tetrofosmin, are used to image the coronary arteries and myocardium. Technetium pyrophosphate (^{99m}TcPYP) is injected intravenously into a resting individual during a "hot spot" imaging examination. Two hours after injection the distribution pattern of the radioactive solution is recorded by nuclear scan. During the 2-hour delay, the injected material will have been taken up by infarcted areas of the myocardium, particularly 1 to 3 days after the onset of symptoms. This type of scanning also is done with stress testing using exercise or dobutamine.[45] Study results are not definitive during the first 12 hours after an infarct.

Technetium scanning is used when (1) there is a conflicting history for myocardial infarction, (2) there are equivocal ECG abnormalities, or (3) an individual's cardiac enzymes have been elevated because of surgery or trauma. Ongoing research is determining any risks associated with radioactive substances.

Electrophysiology Studies

In-depth evaluation of electrical conduction within the heart can provide important information about the nature and causes of dysrhythmias, such as atrial and ventricular tachycardias and heart block. This evaluation is often referred to as *electrophysiologic mapping* of the myocardium. There are many types of electrophysiology studies that are specific to certain conduction disorders but they have the common goal of documenting abnormal conduction pathways. Furthermore, the techniques used may also allow for ablation of unwanted pathways or the appropriate placement of pacemakers and implantable defibrillators. Mapping can include the use of echocardiography and CT scanning.[46]

One example of an electrophysiology study is AV bundle electrocardiography. Two electrode-tipped catheters are inserted percutaneously into the femoral vein, floated up the inferior vena cava, and positioned in or near the right atrium during AV bundle (His bundle) electrocardiography. AV bundle electrocardiography can detect secondary sites of impulse generation (ectopic foci), as well as accessory pathways of conduction. Other conduction defects and the effects of drugs on conduction also can be illuminated. Risks related to this procedure can be grave and include dysrhythmias, death, vessel or heart perforation, clot or plaque embolization, and kidney failure.

Cardiac Catheterization and Angiography

One or both sides of the heart can be examined using **cardiac catheterization.** This invasive procedure requires the use of fluoroscopy and strict sterile techniques and takes place in a specially equipped catheterization laboratory. Local anesthetic is administered, and a catheter is introduced percutaneously into the vasculature and passed caudally into the atrium and ventricle. For a right-heart catheterization, the catheter is placed in either the jugular, subclavian, brachial, or femoral veins. The femoral artery is commonly used for a left-heart study. Once the catheter has been guided into the heart chambers, pressures are recorded, blood samples are obtained to examine oxygen content, and a contrast medium is injected to visualize chamber function and valve patency.

Cardiac catheterization provides a means to visualize the chambers of the heart continuously, although for a short time. A great deal of information can be obtained about heart structure and function. Pressures in each chamber and across heart valves can be precisely measured, along with timing of events in the cardiac cycle. Of particular value is the ability to compare the oxygen content of blood in each heart chamber. Risks for this procedure that have decreased over time include the development of dysrhythmias. Death can occur secondary to cardiac arrest after ventricular fibrillation.

Fluoroscopic visualization of the coronary arteries and left-heart structures using contrast dye is called **coronary angiography** or arteriography. Like cardiac catheterization, this study takes place in a catheterization laboratory using local anesthesia and a sterile field. A catheter is threaded into the left ventricle through the femoral artery. A ventriculogram generally is performed first. Contrast dye is injected into the apex of the ventricle, and the next few cardiac cycles are visualized and filmed. Like cardiac catheterization, coronary angiography is used to gain information about the structure and function of the ventricles and related valves. After the ventriculogram, catheters are introduced individually into the ostia of the coronary arteries. When the catheter is in position, a small volume of contrast dye is mechanically and rapidly injected into the artery and the results are visualized and filmed. Dye injection is repeated with the individual tilted at various angles to afford views of the artery other than the anteroposterior view.

The risks of for coronary angiography are similar to those of cardiac catheterization, with exceptions. Because the blood supply to the cardiac muscle is briefly interrupted when dye is introduced into the coronary arteries, angina (chest pain) caused by ischemia (lack of oxygen) is much more common. Coronary artery spasms also can occur. Interrupted flow also causes decreased heart rate (bradycardia), as well as some tachydysrhythmias, hypotension, and ST-segment depression.

Systemic Vascular Evaluation

The systemic vascular system can be studied by a variety of techniques in order to evaluate for adequate flow rates, vascular obstruction, and structural defects. These techniques include Doppler ultrasonography, CT and MRI, venography, and arteriography.

Arterial Pressure Pulse Waveform Analysis

Pulsation, described by the flow of blood through an artery during the cardiac cycle, can be drawn as a waveform plotting pressure against time (Figure 31-33). The waveform can be obtained noninvasively by placing a transducer on the skin over the carotid artery while the individual's head is turned slightly away from the transducer. The amplitude and shape of arterial waveforms can provide information about the elasticity of the arterial wall, or its inverse—the stiffness of the wall.

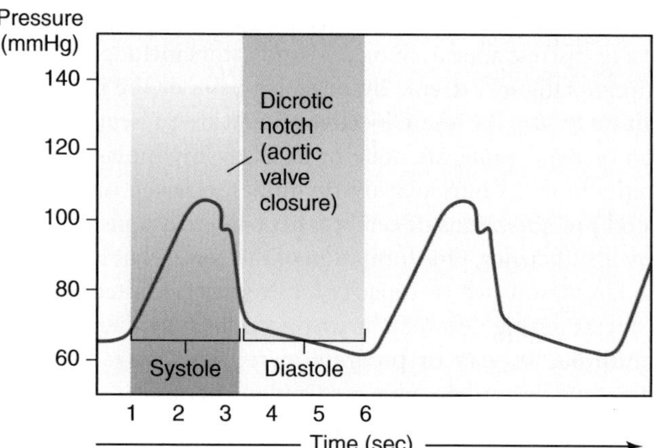

FIGURE 31-33 Arterial Pressure Pulse Waveforms.

Doppler Ultrasonography Studies

A Doppler study is done using a microphone that amplifies and records the sounds made by blood flowing in peripheral vessels. The Doppler microphone is placed over the vessel to be studied, and sounds related to obstructions to flow, vessel wall mobility, and heart murmurs are transmitted through a lubricating gel to the microphone. The audio findings can be digitized into visual findings that can be analyzed for flow velocity and volume. These studies are useful in the evaluation for abnormalities of venous flow (e.g., deep venous thrombosis) and arterial flow (e.g., embolism). Ultrasound also is used to calculate the thickness of arterial walls, yielding a reading called *intimal-medial thickness.* Carotid intimal-medial thickness is used to assess for atherosclerosis.[47] Many people are familiar with ultrasound measurements because they are commonly used to assess fetal growth and development.

Computed Tomography and Magnetic Resonance Imaging

CT and MRI are used to evaluate the systemic circulation, providing information about the structure of the great vessels. Either can be used to evaluate for aneurysms and dissections of the thoracic or abdominal aorta. CT also is used to assess for vessel calcification and provide some insights into the risk for stroke and myocardial infarction through evaluation of the carotid and coronary vessels.

Venography and Arteriography

Radiopaque dye can be injected through intravenous or intra-arterial catheters to allow for visualization of the internal structure, diameter, and patency of veins and arteries. Venography is performed primarily in the lower extremity to assess for the presence of thrombi in the large veins of the leg. Arteriography (angiography) can be used in almost any vascular system,

TABLE 31-5 CARDIOVASCULAR FUNCTION IN OLDER ADULTS

DETERMINANT	RESTING CARDIAC PERFORMANCE	EXERCISE CARDIAC PERFORMANCE
Cardiac index	Unchanged or slightly decreased in women only	Declines because of a decrease in heart rate and stroke volume
Heart rate	Slight decrease	Increases less than in younger people, possibly because of decreased cardiovascular response to catecholamines; overall slight decrease
Stroke volume	Slight increase	Slight increase
Ejection fraction	Unchanged	Increases less from rest to exercise in older people than in younger people
Afterload	Increased	Uncertain
End-diastolic volume	Unchanged	Unchanged
End-systolic volume	Unchanged	Higher in older people than in younger people
Contraction	Increased because of prolonged relaxation	Decreases with vigorous exercise*
Cardiac dilation	No change	Increases at end-diastole and end-systole
O_2 max	Not applicable	Declines because of a decline in skeletal muscle mass and increase in body fat

Data from Najjar SS, Gerstenblith G, Lakatta EG: Aging and the cardiovascular system. In Willerson JT et al, editors: *Cardiovascular medicine*, ed 3, London, 2007, Springer-Verlag.
*As measured by end-systolic volume/systolic blood pressure (ESV/SBP), an index of contractility.

including the great vessels and the pulmonary, coronary (see previously in this chapter), cerebral, mesenteric, renal, hepatic, and peripheral arteries. Risks include rupture, dissection, thrombosis, embolization, or organ infarction involving the arterial system being studied.

AGING AND THE CARDIOVASCULAR SYSTEM

Cardiovascular disease is the most common cause of morbidity and mortality in older adults in Western society and in much of the rest of the world.[48] In addition, age is a key driver of cardiovascular risk, which explains why it is the primary cause of death in persons older than age 65.[49] The most common cardiovascular disease condition is hypertension followed by coronary atherosclerosis for which hypertension is a risk factor.

It is challenging to determine the normal physiologic changes in cardiac function with aging because many pathologic changes are usually present and physical fitness is variable in older people as well. Studies of the effect of age on cardiovascular function must be rigorous in their distinction between persons who are free of disease and those who have disease that may be evident only during testing. There is a wide range in the older population for nearly every cardiovascular variable. These variations are related to an increase in the prevalence of hypertension and coronary disease with advancing age; the growth in the segment of the population older than age 65; and major age-associated changes in lifestyle (e.g., fitness status).[49] The most relevant age-associated physiologic changes in cardiovascular performance include myocardial and blood vessel stiffening, changes in neurogenic control over vascular tone, increased occurrence of atrial fibrillation, and loss of exercise capacity plus left ventricular hypertrophy and fibrosis.[49,50] These changes pose considerable consequences with increased demand for flow, changes in posture, or with disease.

Arterial stiffening occurs with aging even in the absence of clinical hypertension. It can, however, be an important contributor to systolic hypertension and its associated risks for cardiovascular events, dementia, and death. These changes result from alterations within the vascular media, including age-associated changes in cross-linking of collagen, an increase in the amount of collagen, deposition of calcium, and changes in the nature of elastin, the extracellular matrix, inflammatory molecules, endothelial cell function, and reactive oxygen species.[26] The increased arterial stiffness may not be related strictly to an age-associated change in vascular structure but may be caused by changes in baroreceptor activity. Baroreceptor activity may decrease with age, slowing physiologic adjustment to changes in blood pressure, and posture. In persons older than age 60, pulse pressure, which is directly influenced by arterial stiffness, is a better predictor of cardiovascular disease than either diastolic or systolic blood pressure.[51]

Left ventricular hypertrophy and fibrosis also are more common in the aging population, even in the absence of high blood pressure. As the arterial system becomes stiffer the ventricles must work harder to pump blood throughout the body, thus contributing to hypertrophy. Fibrosis, calcification, and increase in stiffness also impact valvular function, particularly the function of the atrioventricular valves. These changes make valvular disease a greater risk for the elderly, along with an increased risk of heart failure related to the left ventricular hypertrophy and stiffness.

The advent of genomic medicine and a deeper exploration of molecular changes with aging continue to enhance our understanding of the myriad changes in our bodies as we age.[49,50] The ongoing hope is that as we better understand the causative factors related to cardiovascular decline with aging, we may be able to develop therapeutics that arrest or slow these changes.

Stress testing is used to uncover functional capacity losses that are not apparent at rest. In contrast to the subtle age effects on resting cardiac tests, more dramatic changes occur during exercise. Table 31-5 summarizes age-associated changes at rest and during exercise. Overall, long-term exercise conditioning in older individuals increases aerobic capacity and decreases arterial stiffness and left ventricular function so that cardiovascular diseases may be prevented or delayed in older adults. Although the risks and benefits of pharmacologic and invasive strategies must always be assessed carefully, many older adults can live longer and healthier lives if appropriate preventive and treatment regimens are offered, even quite late in life.

SUMMARY REVIEW

Circulatory System

1. The circulatory system is the body's transport system and a part of its communication system. It delivers oxygen, nutrients, metabolites, hormones, neurochemicals, proteins, and blood cells, including lymphocytes and leukocytes, throughout the body and carries metabolic wastes to the kidneys and lungs for excretion.
2. The circulatory system consists of the heart, blood vessels, and the lymphatic vessels and is made up of two separate but conjoined, serially connected pump systems: the pulmonary circulation and the systemic circulation, plus the lymphatics.
3. The low-pressure pulmonary circulation is driven by the right side of the heart. The function of the pulmonary circulation is to deliver blood to the lungs for oxygenation.
4. The higher pressure systemic circulation is driven by the left side of the heart, and its function is to move oxygenated blood to body tissues and to deliver waste products to the lungs, kidneys, and liver.
5. The lymphatic vessels collect fluids from the interstitium and return the fluids to the circulatory system. Another important function of the lymphatic system is the movement of lymphocytes and leukocytes between different components of the immune system.

The Heart

1. The heart consists of four chambers (two atria and two ventricles), four valves (two AV valves and two semilunar valves), a muscular wall, a fibrous skeleton, a conduction system, nerve fibers, systemic vessels (the coronary circulation), and openings where the great vessels enter the atria and ventricles.
2. The heart wall, which encloses the heart and divides it into chambers, is made up of three layers: the epicardium (outer layer), the myocardium (muscular layer), and the endocardium (inner lining). The heart is contained within the pericardium, a double-walled sac.
3. The myocardial layer of the two atria, which receive blood entering the heart, is thinner than the myocardial layer of the ventricles, which is stronger because it generates the pressure that causes the blood to circulate through the lungs or the systemic circulation.
4. The right and left sides of the heart are separated by portions of the heart wall called the *interatrial septum* and the *interventricular septum.*
5. Unoxygenated (venous) blood from the systemic circulation enters the right atrium through the superior and inferior venae cavae. From the right atrium the blood passes through the right AV (tricuspid) valve into the right ventricle. In the ventricle the blood flows from the inflow tract to the outflow tract and then through the pulmonic semilunar valve (pulmonary valve) into the pulmonary artery, which delivers it to the lungs for oxygenation.
6. Oxygenated blood from the lungs enters the left atrium through the four pulmonary veins (two from the left lung and two from the right lung). From the left atrium the blood passes through the left AV valve (mitral valve) into the left ventricle. In the ventricle the blood flows from the inflow tract to the outflow tract and then through the aortic semilunar valve (aortic valve) into the aorta, which delivers it to systemic arteries of the entire body.
7. The heart valves that ensure the one-way flow of blood from the atria to the ventricles are called the atrioventricular valves. The valves that ensure one-way flow from the ventricles to either the pulmonary artery or the aorta are called semilunar valves.
8. Oxygenated blood enters the coronary arteries through openings within the semilunar valves at the entrance to the aorta, and deoxygenated blood from the coronary veins enters the right atrium through the coronary sinus.
9. The pumping action of the heart consists of two phases: diastole, during which the myocardium relaxes and the chambers fill with blood; and systole, during which the myocardium contracts, forcing blood out of the ventricles. A cardiac cycle consists of one systolic contraction and the diastolic relaxation that follows it. Each cardiac cycle makes up one heartbeat.
10. The sinoatrial (SA) node generates electrical impulses and the conduction system of the heart transmits these electrical impulses (cardiac action potentials) that stimulate systolic contraction. The autonomic nerves (sympathetic and parasympathetic fibers) can adjust heart rate and systolic force, but they do not stimulate the heart to beat.
11. The normal ECG is the sum of all cardiac action potentials. The P wave represents atrial depolarization; the QRS complex is the sum of all ventricular cell depolarizations. The ST interval occurs when the entire ventricular myocardium is depolarized.
12. Cardiac action potentials are generated by the SA node at the rate of between 60 to 100 impulses per minute. The impulses travel through the conduction system of the heart, stimulating myocardial contraction as they travel.
13. Cells of the cardiac conduction system possess the properties of automaticity and rhythmicity. Automatic cells return to threshold and depolarize rhythmically without an outside stimulus. The cells of the SA node depolarize faster than other automatic cells, making it the natural pacemaker of the heart. If the SA node is disabled, the next fastest pacemaker, the AV node, assumes control.
14. Each cardiac action potential travels from the SA node to the AV node to the bundle of His (AV bundle), through the bundle branches, and finally to the Purkinje fibers and the ventricular myocardium. There the impulse is stopped. It is prevented from reversing its path by the refractory period of cells that have just been polarized. The refractory period ensures that diastole (relaxation) will occur, thereby completing the cardiac cycle.
15. Adrenergic receptor number, type, and function govern autonomic (sympathetic) regulation of heart rate, contractile force, and dilation or constriction of coronary arteries.

SUMMARY REVIEW—cont'd

The presence of specific receptors (α_1, α_2, β_1, β_2, β_3) in the myocardium and coronary vessels determines the effects of the neurotransmitters norepinephrine and epinephrine.

16. Unique features that distinguish myocardial cells from skeletal cells enable myocardial cells to transmit action potentials faster (through intercalated disks), synthesize more ATP (because of a large number of mitochondria), and have readier access to ions in the interstitium (because of an abundance of transverse tubules). These combined differences enable the myocardium to work constantly, which is not required of skeletal muscle.
17. Cross-bridges between actin and myosin enable contraction to occur. Calcium and its interaction with the troponin complex facilitate the contraction process. With troponin release of calcium, myocardial relaxation begins.
18. Cardiac performance is affected by preload, afterload, heart rate, and myocardial contractility.
19. Preload, or pressure generated in the ventricles at the end of diastole, depends on the amount of blood in the ventricle. Afterload is the resistance to ejection of the blood from the ventricle. Afterload depends on pressure in the aorta.
20. Contractility is the potential for myocardial fiber shortening during systole. It is determined by the amount of stretch during diastole (i.e., preload) and by sympathetic stimulation of the ventricles.
21. The Frank-Starling law of the heart states that the myocardial stretch determines the force of myocardial contraction (the greater the stretch, the stronger the contraction).
22. Laplace's law states that the amount of contractile force generated within a chamber depends on the radius of the chamber and the thickness of its wall (the smaller the radius and the thicker the wall, the greater the force of contraction).

Systemic Circulation

1. Blood flows from the left ventricle into the aorta and from the aorta into arteries that eventually branch into arterioles and capillaries, the smallest of the arterial vessels. Oxygen, nutrients, and other substances needed for cellular metabolism pass from the capillaries into the interstitium, where they are available for uptake by the cells. Capillaries also absorb products of cellular metabolism from the interstitium.
2. Venules, the smallest veins, receive capillary blood. From the venules the venous blood flows into larger and larger veins until it reaches the venae cavae, through which it enters the right atrium.
3. Vessel walls consist of three layers: the tunica intima (inner layer), the tunica media (middle layer), and the tunica externa (outer layer).
4. Layers of the vessel wall differ in thickness and composition from vessel to vessel, depending on the vessel's size and location within the circulatory system. In general, the tunica media of arteries close to the heart contains a greater proportion of elastic fibers because these arteries must be able to distend during systole and recoil during diastole. Distributing arteries farther from the heart contain a greater proportion of smooth muscle fibers because these arteries must be able to constrict and dilate to control blood pressure and volume within specific capillary beds.
5. Blood flow into the capillary beds is controlled by the contraction and relaxation of smooth muscle bands (precapillary sphincters) at junctions between metarterioles and capillaries. The endothelium is probably a source of prostaglandins that control vasomotion.
6. Blood flow through the veins is assisted by the contraction of skeletal muscles (the muscle pump), and backwards flow in the lower body is prevented by one-way valves, particularly in the deep veins of the legs.
7. Blood flow is affected by blood pressure; resistance to flow within the vessels; blood consistency (which affects velocity); anatomic features that may cause turbulent or laminar flow; and compliance (distensibility) of the vessels.
8. Poiseuille's law describes the relationship of blood flow, pressure, and resistance as the difference between pressure at the inflow end of the vessel and pressure at the outflow end divided by resistance within the vessel.
9. Resistance to blood flow depends on vessel length and radius and on the viscosity of the blood. The greater a vessel's length and the blood's viscosity and the narrower the radius of the vessel's lumen, the greater the resistance within the vessel.
10. Total peripheral resistance, or the resistance to flow within the entire systemic circulatory system, depends on the combined lengths and radii of all the vessels within the system and on whether the vessels are arranged in series (greater resistance) or in parallel (lesser resistance).
11. Blood flow is influenced also by neural stimulation (of vasoconstriction or vasodilation) and by autonomic features that cause turbulence within the vascular lumen (e.g., protrusions from the vessel wall, twists and turns, bifurcations).
12. Arterial blood pressure is influenced and regulated by factors that affect cardiac output (heart rate and stroke volume), total resistance within the system, and blood volume.
13. Many hormones and other endothelial mediators alter vasomotion including epinephrine, norepinephrine, antidiuretic hormone, renin-angiotensin system, natriuretic peptides, adrenomedullin, nitric oxide, prostaglandins, and endothelium-derived relaxing factor.
14. Venous pressure is influenced by blood volume within the venous system and compliance of the venous walls.
15. Blood flow through the coronary circulation is governed not only by the same principles as flow through other vascular beds but also by two adaptations dictated by cardiac dynamics. First, blood flows into the coronary arteries during diastole rather than systole because during systole, the cusps of the aortic semilunar valve block the openings of the coronary arteries. Second, systolic contraction inhibits coronary artery flow by compressing the coronary arteries.
16. Autoregulation enables the coronary vessels to maintain optimal perfusion pressure despite systolic effects, and

SUMMARY REVIEW—cont'd

myoglobin in heart muscle stores oxygen for use during the systolic phase of the cardiac cycle.

Lymphatic System

1. The vessels of the lymphatic system run in the same sheaths as those of the arteries and veins.
2. Lymph (interstitial fluid plus cells of the immune system) is absorbed by lymphatic venules in the capillary beds and travels through ever larger lymphatic veins until it empties into the right lymphatic duct and the thoracic duct, which drain into the right and left subclavian veins, respectively.
3. As lymph travels toward the thoracic ducts, it passes through lymph nodes clustered around the lymphatic vessels. The lymph nodes are sites of immune function and are ideally placed to sample fluid and cells moving from the periphery into the central circulation.

Tests of Cardiovascular Function

1. The evaluation of an individual with known or suspected cardiovascular disease must include a careful history and physical examination including assessment of risk factors, symptoms, vital signs, level of consciousness, mucous membrane color, and cardiopulmonary functioning.
2. Important tests for cardiac disorders are ECG and Holter monitoring, which detect disturbances of impulse generation or conduction.
3. Stress tests elicit clinical manifestations of cardiovascular disease that might not be present at rest.
4. The sensitivity of stress testing is improved by the use of radiotracer imaging techniques such as SPECT.
5. Echocardiography detects structural and functional cardiac abnormalities over time.
6. Cardiac catheterization is used to measure the oxygen content and pressure of blood in the heart's chambers and to inject contrast media for x-ray examination of the size and shape of the chambers and valves. Injection of contrast medium into the coronary arteries (coronary angiography), on the other hand, permits visualization of the coronary circulation and every tissue perfused by the coronary arteries.
7. Evaluation of the systemic vascular system can include arterial pressure pulse waveform analysis, Doppler ultrasonography, venography, and arteriography.

Aging and the Cardiovascular System

1. Controversy exists regarding the effects of normal aging on the cardiovascular system. Separating the physiologic from the pathologic alterations is difficult because of the wide range of physical fitness in the elderly and the presence of arteriosclerosis in a majority of older adults.
2. Studies have documented no change in cardiac output, a slight decrease in heart rate, and a slight increase in stroke volume in healthy (lack of ischemic heart disease) older adults at rest. No changes were noted at rest in ejection fraction. A slight increase in afterload (e.g., as systolic blood pressure) and prolonged left ventricular relaxation was noted.
3. The most relevant age-associated changes in cardiovascular performance are myocardial and blood vessel stiffening, changes in neurogenic control over vascular tone, and left ventricular hypertrophy and fibrosis.
4. With active risk reduction, physical activity, and disease management, older adults can have markedly improved cardiovascular health.

KEY TERMS

a wave, 1089
Adrenomedullin (ADM), 1117
Afferent lymphatic vessel, 1119
Afterload, 1101
Aldosterone, 1117
Angiogenesis, 1092, 1108
Angiotensin II (Ang II), 1117
Anisotropic band (A band), 1098
Aorta, 1088
Aortic semilunar valve, 1087
Arteriogenesis, 1092, 1108
Arteriole, 1106
Artery, 1106
Atrioventricular (AV) node, 1093
Atrioventricular valve, 1087
Automatic cell, 1095
Automaticity, 1095
Bainbridge reflex, 1106
Baroreceptor, 1115
Baroreceptor reflex, 1106
Blood velocity, 1112
Bradycardic effect, 1104
Brain natriuretic peptide (BNP), 1117
Bundle branch, 1093
Bundle of His (atrioventricular bundle, common bundle), 1093
C-type natriuretic peptide (CNP), 1117
c wave, 1089
Calcium channel–blocking drug, 1099
Capillary, 1106, 1108
Cardiac action potential, 1092
Cardiac catheterization, 1122
Cardiac cycle, 1088
Cardiac output, 1101
Cardiac plexus, 1096
Cardioexcitatory center, 1106
Cardioinhibitory center, 1105
Cardiovascular control center, 1104
Chordae tendineae, 1088
Circumflex artery, 1090
Collateral artery, 1091
Conduction system, 1092
Connexin, 1092
Coronary angiography, 1122
Coronary perfusion pressure, 1117
Coronary sulcus, 1090
Crista supraventricularis, 1089
Cross-bridge cycle of muscle contraction, 1099
Depolarization, 1094
Diastole, 1088
Diastolic depolarization, 1095
Efferent lymphatic vessel, 1119
Ejection fraction, 1101
Elastic artery, 1108
End-diastolic volume, 1101
Endocardium, 1086
Endothelial cell, 1109
Endothelium, 1108
Epinephrine, 1117
Excitation-contraction coupling, 1099
External elastic lamina, 1106
Fenestration, 1108
Frank-Starling law of the heart, 1101
Great cardiac vein, 1092
Heart rate, 1092
Hematocrit, 1112
Hyperemia, 1116
Inferior vena cava, 1088
Inflow tract, 1086
Inotropic agent, 1103
Intercalated disk, 1097
Isotropic band (I band), 1099
Laminar flow, 1113
Left anterior descending (LAD) artery, 1090
Left atrium, 1086
Left bundle branch (LBB), 1094
Left coronary artery (LCA), 1090
Left heart, 1083

KEY TERMS—cont'd

REFERENCES

1. Mehta D, Malik AB: Signaling mechanisms regulating endothelial permeability, *Physiol Rev* 86(1):279–367, 2006.
2. Buja LM: Anatomy of the heart. In Willerson JT et al: *Cardiovascular medicine*, ed 3, London, 2007, Springer.
3. Young PM et al: Cardiac imaging: part 2, normal, variant, and anomalous configurations of the coronary vasculature, *AJR* 197(4):816–826, 2011.
4. Carmeliet P: Angiogenesis in health and disease, *Nat Med* 9(6):653–660, 2003.
5. Fung E, Helisch A: Macrophages in collateral arteriogenesis, *Front Physiol* 3:353, 2012.
6. Bache RJ: Coronary artery disease: regulation of coronary blood flow. In Willerson JT et al: *Cardiovascular medicine*, ed 3, London, 2007, Springer.
7. Loukas M et al: The cardiac lymphatic system, *Clin Anat* 24(6):684–691, 2011.
8. Jansen JA et al: Cardiac connexins and impulse propagation, *J Mol Cell Cardiol* 48(1):76–82, 2010.
9. Rubart M, Zipes DP: Genesis of cardiac arrhythmias: electrophysiologic considerations. In Bonow RO et al: *Braunwald's heart disease: a textbook of cardiovascular medicine*, ed 9, Philadelphia, 2012, Elsevier Saunders.
10. Opie LH, Hasenfuss G: Mechanisms of cardiac contraction and relaxation. In Bonow RO et al: *Braunwald's heart disease: a textbook of cardiovascular medicine*, ed 9, Philadelphia, 2012, Elsevier Saunders.
11. von Homeyer P, Schwinn DA: Pharmacogenomics of β-adrenergic physiology and response to β-blockade, *Anesth Analg* 113(6):1305–1318, 2011.
12. Harmar AJ et al: IUPHAR-DB: the IUPHAR database of G protein-coupled receptors and ion channels, *Nucl Acids Res* 37(Database issue):D680–D685, 2009.
13. Triposkiadis F et al: The sympathetic nervous system in heart failure physiology, pathophysiology and clinical implication, *J Am Coll Cardiol* 54(19):1747–1762, 2009.
14. Ibrahim M et al: The structure and function of cardiac T-tubules in health and disease, *Proc R Soc B* 278(1719):2714–2723, 2011.
15. Granzier HL, Labeit S: The giant protein titin: a major player in myocardial mechanics, signaling, and disease, *Circ Res* 94(3):284–295, 2004.
16. Deussen A et al: Mechanisms of metabolic coronary flow regulation, *J Mol Cell Cardiol* 52(4):794–801, 2012.
17. Stehle R, Iorga B: Kinetics of cardiac sarcomeric processes and rate-limiting steps in contraction and relaxation, *J Mol Cell Cardiol* 48(5):843–850, 2010.
18. Patton KT, Thibodeau GA: *Anatomy & physiology*, ed 8, St Louis, 2013, Mosby.
19. Zanotti-Cavazzoni SL, Hollenberg SM: Cardiac dysfunction in severe sepsis and septic shock, *Curr Opin Crit Care* 15(5):392–397, 2009.
20. Montecucco F, Di Marzo V: At the heart of the matter: the endocannabinoid system in cardiovascular function and dysfunction, *Trends Pharmacol Sci* 33(6):331–340, 2012.
21. Larsen PD et al: Respiratory sinus arrhythmia in conscious humans during spontaneous respiration, *Respir Physiol Neurobiol* 174(1-2):111–118, 2010.
22. Fisher JP et al: Carotid baroreflex control of arterial blood pressure at rest and during dynamic exercise in aging humans, *Am J Physiol Regul Integr Comp Physiol* 299(5):R1241–R1247, 2010.
23. Crystal GJ, Salem MR: The Bainbridge and the "reverse" Bainbridge reflexes: history, physiology, and clinical relevance, *Anesth Analg* 114(3):520–532, 2012.
24. Klein I, Ojamaa K: Thyroid hormone and the cardiovascular system, *N Engl J Med* 344(7):501–509, 2001.
25. Ren J, Samson WK, Sowers JR: Insulin-like growth factor I as a cardiac hormone: physiological and pathophysiological implications in heart disease, *J Mol Cell Cardiol* 31(11):2049–2061, 1999.
26. Lähteenvuo J, Rosenzweig A: Effects of aging on angiogenesis, *Circ Res* 110(9):1252–1263, 2012.
27. Haraldsson B, Nyström J: The glomerular endothelium: new insights on function and structure, *Curr Opin Nephrol Hypertens* 21(3):258–263, 2012.
28. Girard J-P, Moussion C, Förster R: HEVs, lymphatics and homeostatic immune cell trafficking in lymph nodes, *Nat Rev Immunol* 12(11):762–773, 2012.
29. Fadel PJ, Raven PB: Human investigations into the arterial and cardiopulmonary baroreflexes during exercise, *Exp Physiol* 97(1):39–50, 2012.
30. Eltzschig HK, Eckle T: Ischemia and reperfusion—from mechanism to translation, *Nat Med* 17(11):1391–1401, 2011.
31. Nishikimi T, Kuwahara K, Nakao K: Current biochemistry, molecular biology, and clinical relevance of natriuretic peptides, *J Cardiol* 57(2):131–140, 2011.

32. Kuwasako K et al: Shared and separate functions of the RAMP-based adrenomedullin receptors, *Peptides* 32(7):1540–1550, 2011.
33. Stoner L, Sabatier MJ: Use of ultrasound for non-invasive assessment of flow-mediated dilation, *J Atheroscler Thromb* 19(5):407–421, 2012.
34. Kamga C, Krishnamurthy S, Shiva S: Myoglobin and mitochondria: a relationship bound by oxygen and nitric oxide, *Nitric Oxide* 26(4): 251–258, 2012.
35. Kauffenstein G et al: Emerging role of G protein-coupled receptors in microvascular myogenic tone, *Cardiovasc Res* 95(2):223–232, 2012.
36. Lang RM et al: Recommendations for chamber quantification: a report from the American Society of Echocardiography's Guidelines and Standards Committee and the Chamber Quantification Writing Groups, developed in conjunction with the European Association of Echocardiography, a branch of the European Society of Cardiology, *J Am Soc Echo* 18(12):1440–1463, 2005.
37. Salton CJ et al: Gender differences and normal left ventricular anatomy in an adult population free of hypertension. A cardiovascular magnetic resonance study of the Framingham Heart Study Offspring cohort, *J Am Coll Cardiol* 39(6):1055–1060, 2002.
38. Connolly HM, Oh JK: Echocardiography. In Bonow RO et al: *Braunwald's heart disease: a textbook of cardiovascular medicine*, ed 9, Philadelphia, 2012, Elsevier Saunders.
39. Muraru D et al: Mitral valve anatomy and function: new insights from three-dimensional echocardiography, *J Cardiovasc Med* 14(2):91–99, 2013.
40. Ali S et al: Intracardiac echocardiography: clinical utility and application, *Echocardiography* 28(5):582–590, 2011.
41. Udelson JE, Dilsizian V, Bonow RO: Nuclear cardiology. In Bonow RO et al: *Braunwald's heart disease: a textbook of cardiovascular medicine*, ed 9, Philadelphia, 2012, Elsevier Saunders.
42. Polonsky TS et al: Coronary artery calcium score and risk classification for coronary heart disease prediction, *JAMA* 303(16):1610–1616, 2010.
43. Cousins C et al: ICRP publication 120: Radiological protection in cardiology, *Ann ICRP* 42(1):1–125, 2013.
44. Charoenpanichkit C, Hundley WG: The 20 year evolution of dobutamine stress cardiovascular magnetic resonance, *J Cardiovasc Magn Reson* 12:59, 2010.
45. McGhie AE, Gould KL, Willerson JT: Nuclear cardiology. In Willerson JT et al: *Cardiovascular medicine*, ed 3, London, 2007, Springer.
46. Joshi SB et al: CT applications in electrophysiology, *Cardiol Clin* 27(4):619–631, 2009.
47. Crouse JR et al: B-mode ultrasound: a noninvasive method for assessing atherosclerosis. In Willerson JT et al: *Cardiovascular medicine*, ed 3, London, 2007, Springer.
48. Lozano R et al: Global and regional mortality from 235 causes of death for 20 age groups in 1990 and 2010: a systematic analysis for the Global Burden of Disease Study 2010, *Lancet* 380(9859):2095–2128, 2012.
49. North BJ, Sinclair DA: The intersection between aging and cardiovascular disease, *Circ Res* 110(8):1097–1108, 2012.
50. Dai D et al: Cardiac aging: from molecular mechanisms to significance in human health and disease, *Antioxid Redox Signal* 16(12):1492–1526, 2012.
51. Franklin SS et al: Does the relation of blood pressure to coronary heart disease risk change with aging? The Framingham Heart Study, *Circulation* 103(9):1245–1249, 2001.

CHAPTER

32

Alterations of Cardiovascular Function

Valentina L. Brashers

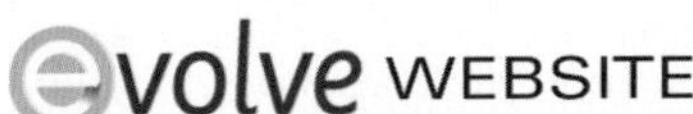

http://evolve.elsevier.com/McCance/
- Review Questions and Answers
- Animations
- Online Course: Module 14

CHAPTER OUTLINE

Cardiovascular disease is the leading cause of death worldwide (Table 32-1).[1] The pathophysiology of heart disease is much more complicated than just structural and hemodynamic changes. Today the focus is on the genetic, neurohumoral, and inflammatory mechanisms that underlie tissue and cellular processes, such as endothelial injury, remodeling, stunning, reperfusion injury, and autoimmune disease.

DISEASES OF THE VEINS

Varicose Veins and Chronic Venous Insufficiency

Varicose veins are a common condition affecting more than 25 million Americans, women nearly twice as often as men.[2] A varicose vein is a superficial vein in which blood has pooled. Varicose veins typically involve the saphenous veins of the legs and are distended, tortuous, and palpable (Figure 32-1). Varicose veins are caused by (1) trauma to the saphenous veins that damages one or more valves, or (2) gradual venous distention caused by the action of gravity on blood in the legs.

Veins are thin-walled, highly distensible vessels. Normally the muscular pump in the legs moves venous blood up toward the heart, and valves prevent backflow and pooling of blood (see Figures 31-35 and 31-31). In individuals who habitually stand for long periods, wear constricting garments, or cross the legs at the knees, distention progresses until the pressure in the vein damages venous valves, rendering the valves incompetent. Damaged valves cannot maintain normal venous pressure, which causes hydrostatic pressure in the vein to increase. As the

TABLE 32-1 DEATH RATES AND PERCENT OF TOTAL DEATHS FOR THE 15 LEADING CAUSES OF DEATH IN THE UNITED STATES ALL RACES, BOTH SEXES, ALL AGES (FINAL DATA REPORT 2010)

RANK ORDER*	CAUSE OF DEATH	RATE†	PERCENT OF TOTAL DEATHS
1	Diseases of the heart	194	24.2
2	Malignant neoplasms	186	23.3
3	Chronic lower respiratory diseases	45	5.6
4	Cerebrovascular diseases	42	5.2
5	Accidents (unintentional injuries)	39	4.9
6	Alzheimer disease	27	3.4
7	Diabetes mellitus	22	2.8
8	Nephritis, nephrotic syndrome, and nephrosis	16	2.2
9	Influenza and pneumonia	16	2.0
10	Intentional self-harm (suicide)	12	1.6
11	Septicemia	11	1.4
12	Chronic liver disease and cirrhosis	10	1.3
13	Essential hypertension and hypertensive disease	9	1.1
14	Parkinson disease	7	0.9
15	Pneumonitis due to solids and liquids	6	0.7

Data from Murphy SL, Xu J, Kochanek KD: Deaths: final data for 2010. National vital statistics reports; vol 61, no 4. Hyattsville, MD: National Center for Health Statistics, 2013. Available at www.cdc.gov/nchs/data/dvs/lcwk1_210.pdf. Accessed July 2, 2013.
*Rank based on number of deaths.
†Rates per 100,000 population.

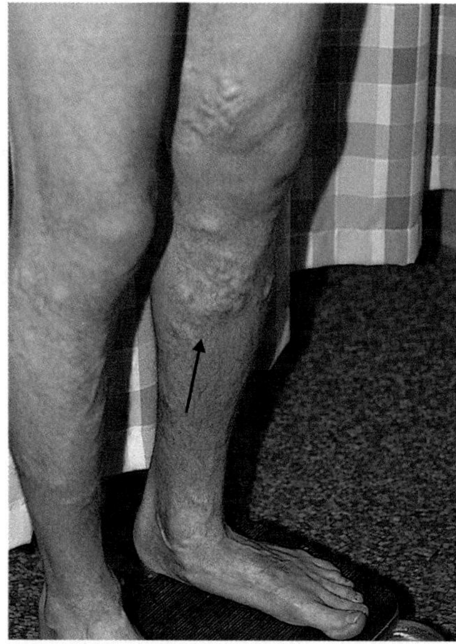

FIGURE 32-1 **Varicose Veins of the Leg** *(arrow).* (Courtesy of Dr. Magruder C. Donaldson, Brigham and Women's Hospital, Boston. From Kumar V et al: *Robbins basic pathology,* ed 8, Philadelphia, 2007, Saunders.)

vein distends further, it becomes tortuous, and edema develops in the extremity.

Evidence has been emerging that varicose veins are not just the result of mechanical pressures. Altered connective tissue proteins, increased proteolytic enzyme activity, and decreased transforming growth factor-beta (TGF-β) in vein walls probably precede the development of valvular damage and the development of varicosities.[2] Inflammatory changes that affect autonomic innervation of veins has also been implicated.[3]

Varicose veins can progress to **chronic venous insufficiency (CVI),** which is defined as sustained inadequate venous return. Venous hypertension, circulatory stasis, and tissue hypoxia lead to an inflammatory reaction in vessels and tissue. This causes fibrosclerotic remodeling of the skin and then ulceration. Symptoms include edema of the lower extremities and hyperpigmentation of the skin of the feet and ankles.

Circulation to the extremities can become so sluggish that the metabolic demands of the cells for oxygen, nutrients, and waste removal are barely met. Any trauma or pressure can therefore lower the oxygen supply and cause cell death and necrosis **(venous stasis ulcers).** Infection can occur because poor circulation impairs the delivery of the cells and biochemicals for the immune and inflammatory responses. This same sluggish circulation makes infection following reparative surgery a significant risk. Treatment of varicose veins and CVI begins conservatively, and wound healing often occurs following noninvasive treatments, such as leg elevation, compression stockings, and physical exercise. New management techniques include endovenous ablation (radiofrequency and laser) and ultrasound-guided foam sclerotherapy. These techniques are as effective and safer than surgical ligation and vein stripping.[4]

Deep Venous Thrombosis

A **thrombus** is a blood clot that remains attached to a vessel wall (Figure 32-2). A detached thrombus is a **thromboembolus.** Venous thrombi are more common than arterial thrombi because flow and pressure are lower in the veins than in the arteries. **Deep venous thrombosis (DVT)** refers to clot formation in the large veins, primarily of the lower extremities and may result in venous thromboembolism (VTE) to the pulmonary circulation. The American Heart Association (AHA) estimates that

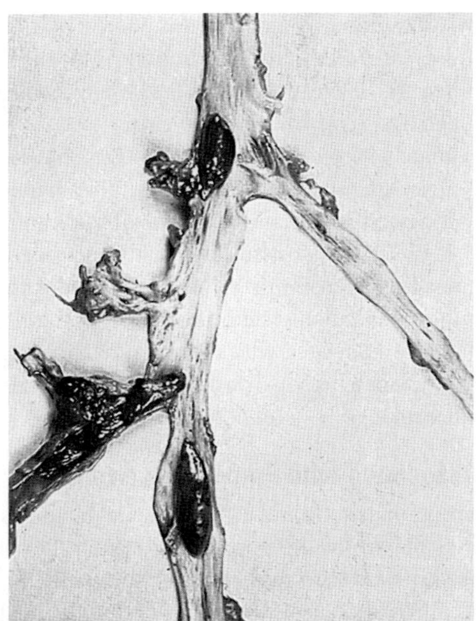

FIGURE 32-2 **Multiple Venous Thrombi.** (From Rosai J: *Ackerman's surgical pathology*, ed 8, vol 2, St Louis, 1996, Mosby.)

more than 900,000 incident or recurrent VTE events occur annually in the United States, of which approximately one third are fatal.[5] Three factors (triad of Virchow) promote venous thrombosis: (1) venous stasis (e.g., immobility, obesity, prolonged leg dependency [e.g., air travel], age, heart failure [HF]), (2) venous endothelial damage (e.g., trauma, medications), and (3) hypercoagulable states (e.g., inherited disorders, malignancy, pregnancy, oral contraceptives, hormone replacement, hyperhomocysteinemia, antiphospholipid syndrome).[6] Virtually everyone who is hospitalized is at significant risk for DVT, especially those with orthopedic trauma or surgery, spinal cord injury, and obstetric/gynecologic conditions. Numerous genetic abnormalities are associated with an increased risk for venous thrombosis primarily related to states of hypercoagulability. These inherited abnormalities include factor V Leiden mutation; prothrombin mutations; and deficiencies of protein C, protein S, and antithrombin. Inherited hypercoagulability states should be suspected in individuals who develop thrombi in the absence of the usual risk factors.[6,7]

Accumulation of clotting factors and platelets leads to thrombus formation in the vein, often near a venous valve. Inflammation around the thrombus promotes further platelet aggregation and the thrombus propagates or grows proximally. This inflammation may cause local symptoms, but because the vein is deep in the leg it is usually not accompanied by clinical symptoms or signs. If the thrombus creates significant obstruction to venous blood flow, increased pressure in the vein behind the clot may lead to edema of the extremity.

Most thrombi eventually dissolve without treatment, but untreated DVT is associated with a high risk of **thromboembolization** of a part of the clot from the leg to the lung (pulmonary embolism) (see Chapter 35).[6] In up to one third of individuals with DVT, persistent venous outflow obstruction may lead to **post-thrombotic syndrome (PTS),** a frequent complication of DVT characterized by chronic, persistent pain; edema; and ulceration of the affected limb.[8]

Because DVT is usually asymptomatic and difficult to detect clinically, prevention for at-risk individuals is crucial. If possible, individuals should be mobilized as soon as possible after illness, injury, or surgery. Prophylactic treatment can include low-molecular-weight heparin, antithrombin agents, warfarin, or pneumatic devices.[9,10] Unfortunately, even these measures may not prevent embolism in high-risk individuals such as those who have undergone hip replacement surgery.[11] In individuals at high risk for pulmonary embolism, but for whom anticoagulation is contraindicated, placement of an inferior vena caval filter may be necessary to prevent pulmonary embolism.

Diagnosis is most often made by combining measurement of serum D-dimer concentration with lower extremity ultrasonography. D-dimer is an indirect measure of the presence of thrombosis that is very sensitive but is not specific. If the D-dimer is negative, DVT is ruled out. If it is positive, the diagnosis must be confirmed with ultrasonography.[6,12] In selected individuals, computed tomography (CT) or magnetic resonance imaging (MRI) may be needed to make the diagnosis. If noninvasive testing is nondiagnostic, a venogram may be indicated.

DVT is treated with low-molecular-weight heparin, unfractionated intravenous heparin, antithrombin agents, or adjusted-dose subcutaneous heparin.[6] Thrombolytic therapy may be used to dissolve the clot more quickly and reduce the risk of postphlebotic syndrome, especially when a large clot is located in a proximal vein.[13] However, bleeding risk is increased, and many people have contraindications to the use of thrombolytics. Pharmacomechanical treatment involves catheter-mediated removal of clots that can be used in selected individuals and so far has a good safety record.[14] DVT has a recurrence rate of 26% 5 years after discontinuation of anticoagulant therapy, especially if it was unprovoked and no identifiable underlying condition can be reversed.[15] In these individuals aspirin therapy can reduce recurrence rates after discontinuation of anticoaglulants.[16]

Superior Vena Cava Syndrome

Superior vena cava syndrome (SVCS) is a progressive occlusion of the superior vena cava (SVC) that leads to venous distention in the upper extremities and head. The leading cause of SVCS is bronchogenic cancer (approximately 70% of cases), followed by lymphomas and metastasis of other cancers.[17] Benign causes of SVCS include thrombosis, histoplasmosis, tuberculosis, mediastinal fibrosis, cystic fibrosis, and benign tumors, such as retrosternal goiter.[18] Invasive therapies, including pacemaker wires, central venous catheters, and pulmonary artery catheters, can lead to acute and chronic SVCS.

The SVC is a relatively low-pressure vessel that lies in the closed thoracic compartment; therefore, tissue expansion can easily compress the SVC. The right mainstem bronchus abuts the SVC so that cancers occurring in this bronchus may press on the vessel and obstruct venous return to the right atrium. Additionally, the SVC is surrounded by lymph nodes and lymph chains that commonly become involved in thoracic cancers and compress the SVC during tumor growth. Because onset of SVCS is slow, collateral venous drainage to the azygos vein usually has time to develop.

Clinical manifestations of SVCS include edema and venous distention in the upper extremities and face, including the ocular beds. Individuals may complain of a feeling of fullness in the head, or tightness of shirt collars, necklaces, and rings. Cerebral and central nervous system (CNS) edema may cause headache, visual disturbance, and impaired consciousness. The skin of the face and arms may become purple and taut, and capillary refill time is prolonged. Respiratory distress may be present because of edema of bronchial structures or compression of the bronchus by a carcinoma.

Diagnosis is made by chest x-ray, Doppler studies, CT, MRI, and ultrasound. With slow onset and the development of collateral venous drainage, SVCS is generally not a vascular emergency but rather an oncologic emergency.[17] Treatment for malignant disorders can include radiation therapy, surgery, chemotherapy, and the administration of diuretics, steroids, and anticoagulants, as necessary. Treatment for nonmalignant causes may include bypass surgery using various grafts, thrombolysis (both locally and systemically), balloon angioplasty, and placement of intravascular stents.[18]

DISEASES OF THE ARTERIES

Hypertension

Hypertension is consistent elevation of systemic arterial blood pressure. Hypertension is the most common primary diagnosis in the United States—approximately 1 in 3 adults greater than 20 years of age has hypertension; this increases to nearly two thirds in those older than age 60. The prevalence of hypertension is nearly equal between men and women. Black adults have among the highest rates of hypertension in the world (44%). Approximately 80% of hypertensive adults are aware of their condition, 71% are using antihypertensive medication, but only 48% of those have their hypertension controlled.[5] Hypertension is defined in the Seventh Report of the Joint National Committee on Prevention, Detection, Evaluation, and Treatment of High Blood Pressure (JNC7)[19] as a sustained systolic blood pressure of 140 mmHg or greater or a diastolic pressure of 90 mmHg or greater (Table 32-2). Normal blood pressure is associated with the lowest cardiovascular risk, whereas those who fall into the prehypertension category (which includes between 25% and 37% of the U.S. population) are at risk for developing hypertension and many associated cardiovascular complications unless lifestyle modification and treatment are instituted.[20]

Some individuals with hypertensive disease have isolated systolic hypertension. **Isolated systolic hypertension (ISH)** is elevated systolic blood pressure accompanied by normal diastolic blood pressure (less than 90 mmHg). ISH is becoming more prevalent in all age groups and is strongly associated with cardiovascular and cerebrovascular events.[21]

TABLE 32-2 CLASSIFICATION OF BLOOD PRESSURE FOR ADULTS AGE 18 YEARS OR OLDER

CATEGORY	SYSTOLIC (mmHg)		DIASTOLIC (mmHg)
Normal	<120	AND	<80
Prehypertension	120-139	OR	80-89
Stage 1 hypertension	140-159	OR	90-99
Stage 2 hypertension	≥160	OR	≥100

Data from the JNC 7 Report, *JAMA* 289(19):2560–2572, 2003.

Approximately 95% of cases of hypertension have no known cause and therefore are diagnosed as primary hypertension.[5] Secondary hypertension accounts for 5% of cases and is caused by altered hemodynamics associated with an underlying primary disease. Hypertension is a complex disorder that affects the entire cardiovascular system, and all types and stages of hypertension are associated with increased risk for target organ disease events, such as myocardial infarction (MI), kidney disease, and stroke.[5]

Factors Associated with Primary Hypertension

A combination of genetic and environmental factors is thought to be responsible for the development of primary hypertension. Genetic predisposition to hypertension is thought to be polygenic. The inherited defects are associated with renal sodium excretion, insulin and insulin sensitivity, activity of the sympathetic nervous system (SNS) and renin-angiotensin-aldosterone system (RAAS), and cell membrane sodium or calcium transport.[22] In blacks, variants of the apolipoprotein L1 *(APOL1)* gene are associated with hypertension and renal disease.[23]

Risk factors associated with primary hypertension include: (1) family history of hypertension; (2) advancing age; (3) gender (men younger than 55 and women older than 70 years); (4) black race; (5) high dietary sodium intake; (6) glucose intolerance (diabetes mellitus); (7) cigarette smoking; (8) obesity; (9) heavy alcohol consumption; and (10) low dietary intake of potassium, calcium, and magnesium.[19] Many of these factors are also risk factors for other cardiovascular disorders. In fact, hypertension, dyslipidemia, and glucose intolerance often are found together in a condition called metabolic syndrome (see Chapter 22).

Although populations with high dietary sodium intake have long been shown to have an increased incidence of hypertension, recent studies indicate that low dietary potassium, calcium, and magnesium intakes are also risk factors because without their intake, sodium is retained. The nicotine in cigarette smoke is a vasoconstrictor that can elevate systolic and diastolic blood pressure acutely. In habitual smokers an individual cigarette may not raise blood pressure, yet habitual smoking is associated with a high incidence of severe hypertension, myocardial hypertrophy, and death resulting from coronary artery disease (CAD). The incidence of hypertension is higher among heavy drinkers of alcohol (more than three drinks per day) than among abstainers, but moderate drinkers (two to four drinks per week) appear to have the lowest average blood pressures and cardiovascular mortality. Obesity is recognized as an important risk factor for hypertension, even in children and adolescents.

PATHOPHYSIOLOGY. Hypertension is caused by increases in cardiac output or total peripheral resistance, or both. (The many factors affecting cardiac output and peripheral resistance are described in Chapter 31.) Cardiac output is increased by any condition that increases heart rate or stroke volume, whereas peripheral resistance is increased by any factor that increases blood viscosity or reduces vessel diameter (vasoconstriction).

Primary Hypertension. **Primary hypertension** is the result of a complicated interaction between genetics and the environment that increase vascular tone (increased peripheral resistance) and blood volume, thus causing sustained increases in blood pressure. Multiple pathophysiologic mechanisms mediate these effects including the sympathetic nervous system (SNS), the RAAS, and natriuretic peptides. Inflammation, endothelial dysfunction, obesity-related hormones, and insulin resistance also contribute to both increased peripheral resistance and increased blood volume. Increased vascular volume is related to a decrease in renal excretion of salt, often referred to as a shift in the **pressure-natriuresis relationship.** This means that for a given blood pressure, individuals with hypertension tend to secrete less salt in their urine. The pathophysiology of primary hypertension is summarized in Figure 32-3.

The SNS contributes to the pathogenesis of hypertension in many people. In the healthy individual the SNS contributes to the maintenance of adequate blood pressure and tissue perfusion by promoting cardiac contractility and heart rate (maintenance of adequate cardiac output) and by inducing arteriolar vasoconstriction (maintenance of adequate peripheral resistance). In individuals with hypertension, overactivity of the SNS can result from increased production of catecholamines (epinephrine and norepinephrine) or from increased receptor reactivity involving these neurotransmitters.[24] Increased SNS activity causes increased heart rate and systemic vasoconstriction, thus raising the blood pressure. Efferent sympathetic outflow stimulates renin release, increases tubular sodium reabsorption, and reduces renal blood flow. Additional mechanisms of SNS-induced hypertension include structural changes in blood vessels (vascular remodeling), insulin resistance, increased renin and angiotensin levels, and procoagulant effects. The SNS is implicated in the cardiovascular and renal complications of hypertension, and new techniques such as renal denervation are being explored to treat hypertension.[25,26] The role of the SNS in the pathogenesis of cardiovascular disease is summarized in Figure 32-4.

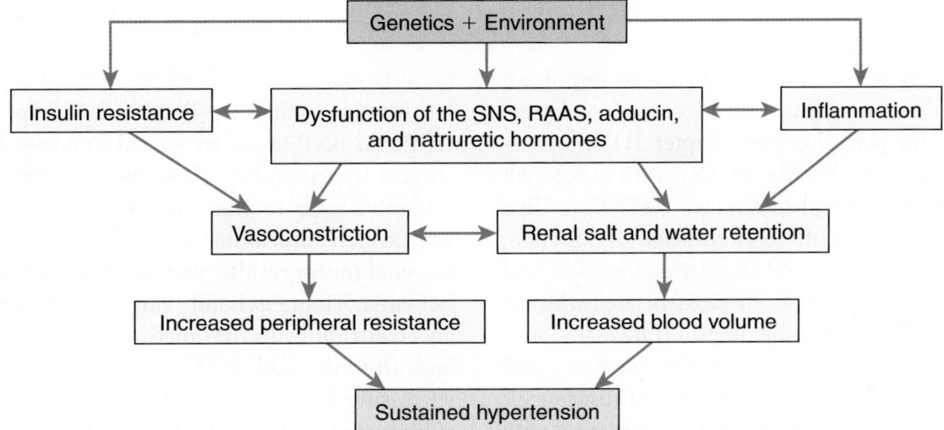

FIGURE 32-3 Pathophysiology of Hypertension. Numerous genetic vulnerabilities have been linked to hypertension and these, in combination with environmental risks, cause neurohumoral dysfunction (sympathetic nervous system [SNS], renin-angiotensin-aldosterone system [RAAS], adducin, and natriuretic hormones) and promote inflammation and insulin resistance. Insulin resistance and neurohumoral dysfunction contribute to sustained systemic vasoconstriction and increased peripheral resistance. Inflammation contributes to renal dysfunction, which, in combination with the neurohumoral alterations, results in renal salt and water retention and increased blood volume. Increased peripheral resistance and increased blood volume are two primary causes of sustained hypertension.

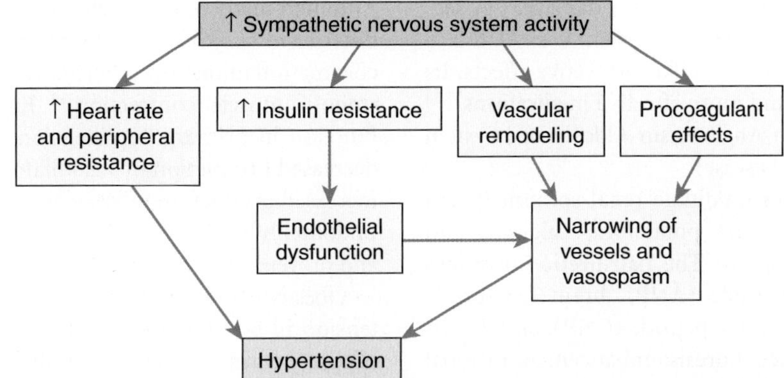

FIGURE 32-4 Role of the Sympathetic Nervous System in the Pathogenesis of Hypertension. Increased activity of the sympathetic nervous system (SNS) not only increases heart rate and peripheral resistance but also causes vascular remodeling with narrowing and vasospasm of arteries. The SNS contributes to insulin resistance, which is associated with endothelial dysfunction and decreased production of vasodilators, such as nitric oxide. The SNS also has procoagulant properties, making vascular spasm and thrombosis more likely. All of these factors contribute to sustained increases in blood pressure.

WHAT'S NEW?

The Renin-Angiotensin-Aldosterone System (RAAS) and Cardiovascular Disease

The RAAS has multiple effects on the cardiovascular system. There are two primary RAA systems. The best known includes the release of renin, the synthesis of angiotensin II (Ang II) through angiotensin-converting enzyme (ACE), stimulation of the AT1 receptor (AT1R), and secretion of aldosterone. Ang II causes systemic vasoconstriction and renal salt and water retention, and stimulates tissue growth and inflammation. When present in abnormal amounts, Ang II contributes to insulin resistance, remodeling of blood vessels, and decreased release of endothelial vasodilators and anticoagulants. In the heart, Ang II and aldosterone contribute to hypertensive hypertrophy and fibrosis of heart muscle, decreased contractility, and an increased susceptibility to arrhythmias and heart failure. In the kidney these hormones cause a shift in the pressure natriuresis curve, inflammation, and glomerular remodeling and are a major contributor to renal failure in individuals with hypertension and diabetes. Drugs that block this RAAS include ACE inhibitors, direct renin inhibitors, Ang II receptor blockers (ARBs), and aldosterone inhibitors. These medications are used widely in managing hypertension, myocardial infarction, and heart failure to lower blood pressure and to protect and improve cardiovascular and renal function. In contrast, the second RAAS serves a counterregulatory system. Activation of a second ACE pathway (ACE2) leads to the synthesis of angiotensin 1-7 from Ang II. Angiotensin 1-7 stimulates Mas receptors in the brain, blood vessels, heart, kidney, gut, pancreas, and inflammatory cells and has vasodilatory, antiproliferative, antifibrotic, and antithrombotic effects. These protective effects lead to lower blood pressure, less vascular inflammation and clotting, and decreased tissue remodeling and damage to target organ tissues. This pathway appears to be especially important in protecting renal tissue in those with diabetes and hypertension. Research is under way to develop genetic and pharmacologic interventions that will stimulate these protective RAAS pathways.

Data from Daien V et al: *Am J Hypertens* 25(1):126–132, 2012; Ferrario CM: ACE2: *Curr Opin Nephrol Hypertens* 20(1):1–6, 2011; Jia L et al: *Front Biosci* 17:221–231, 2012; Patel SK et al: *Am J Hypertens* 25(2):216–222, 2012; Putnam K et al: *Am J Physiol Heart Circ Physiol* 302(6):H1219–H1230, 2012; Souza LL, Costa-Neto CML: *J Cell Physiol* 227(5):2117–2122, 2012; Steckelings UM et al: *Exp Opin Emerging Drugs* 16(4):619–630, 2011; Volpe M: *QJM* 105(1):11–27, 2012

In the healthy individual the RAAS provides an important homeostatic mechanism for maintaining adequate blood pressure and therefore tissue perfusion (see Chapter 31). In hypertensive individuals, overactivity of the RAAS contributes to salt and water retention and increased vascular resistance. High levels of angiotensin II contribute to endothelial dysfunction, insulin resistance, dyslipidemia, and platelet aggregation and play an important role in the complications associated with the metabolic syndrome.[27,28] Further, angiotensin II mediates arteriolar remodeling, which is structural change in the vessel wall that results in permanent increases in peripheral resistance[29] (see Figures 31-28 and 32-5). Angiotensin II is associated with end-organ effects of hypertension, including atherosclerosis, renal disease, and cardiac hypertrophy.[30] Finally, aldosterone not only contributes to sodium retention by the kidney but also has other deleterious effects on the cardiovascular system.[31] Medications, such as angiotensin-converting enzyme (ACE) inhibitors and angiotensin-receptor blockers (ARBs), oppose the activity of the RAAS and are effective in reducing blood pressure and protecting against target organ damage.[32] A second RAAS has also been described. This system uses ACE 2 to create Ang 1-7, which has cardiovascular protective effects. Its discovery may lead to new and more effective medications[33,34] (see What's New? The Renin-Angiotensin-Aldosterone System (RAAS) and Cardiovascular Disease).

The natriuretic hormones modulate renal sodium (Na+) excretion and require adequate potassium, calcium, and magnesium to function properly. The natriuretic hormones include atrial natriuretic peptide (ANP), brain natriuretic peptide (BNP), C-type natriuretic peptide (CNP), and urodilatin. These hormones induce diuresis; enhancement of renal blood flow and glomerular filtration rate, systemic vasodilatation, and suppression of aldosterone; and inhibition of the SNS.[35] Dysfunction of these hormones, along with alterations in the RAA system and the SNS, cause an increase in vascular tone and a shift in the pressure-natriuresis relationship. When there is inadequate natriuretic function, serum levels of the natriuretic peptides are increased. In hypertension, increased ANP and BNP levels are linked to an increased risk for ventricular hypertrophy, atherosclerosis, and heart failure.[36] Salt retention leads to water retention and increased blood volume, which contributes to an increase in blood pressure. Subtle renal injury results, with renal vasoconstriction and tissue ischemia. Tissue ischemia causes inflammation of the kidney and contributes to dysfunction of the glomeruli and tubules and promotes additional sodium retention.[37] In addition to increasing dietary intake of potassium, calcium, and magnesium in order to enhance natriuretic peptide function, a drug that mimics the effect of one of these hormones (nesiritide) is used to treat heart failure.[38] Newer and safer agonists are being studied.[35]

As mentioned, renal inflammation contributes to sodium retention. Inflammation also plays a role in the vascular dysfunction of hypertension. Endothelial injury and tissue ischemia result in the release of vasoactive inflammatory cytokines. Although many of these cytokines (e.g., histamine, prostaglandins) have vasodilatory actions in acute inflammatory injury, chronic inflammation contributes to vascular remodeling and smooth muscle contraction.[39] Endothelial injury and dysfunction in primary hypertension is further characterized by decreased production of vasodilators, such as nitric oxide, and increased production of vasoconstrictors, such as endothelin.[40] Endothelin blockade has been shown to reduce blood pressure and prevent proteinuria.[41]

Obesity is recognized as an important risk factor for hypertension in both adults and children and contributes to many of the neurohumoral, metabolic, renal, and cardiovascular processes that cause hypertension. Obesity causes changes in what are called the adipokines (leptin and adiponectin) and is associated with increased activity of the SNS and the RAAS.[42,43] Obesity is linked to inflammation, small artery remodeling, endothelial dysfunction, and insulin resistance and an increased

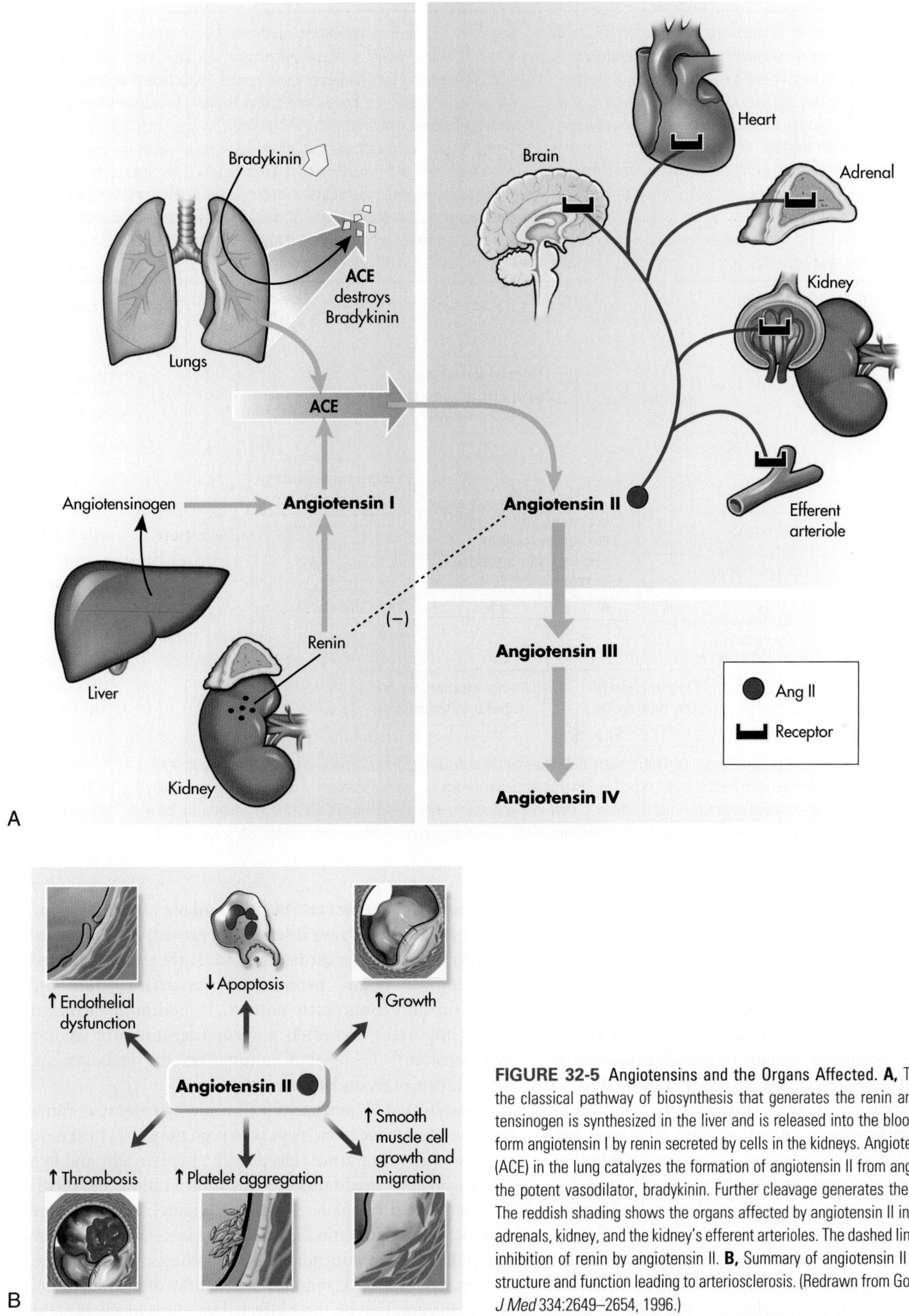

Bradykinin
ACE destroys Bradykinin
Lungs
ACE
Angiotensinogen
Angiotensin I
Liver
Renin
(–)
Kidney
Brain
Heart
Adrenal
Kidney
Angiotensin II
Efferent arteriole
Angiotensin III
Angiotensin IV
Ang II
Receptor
A

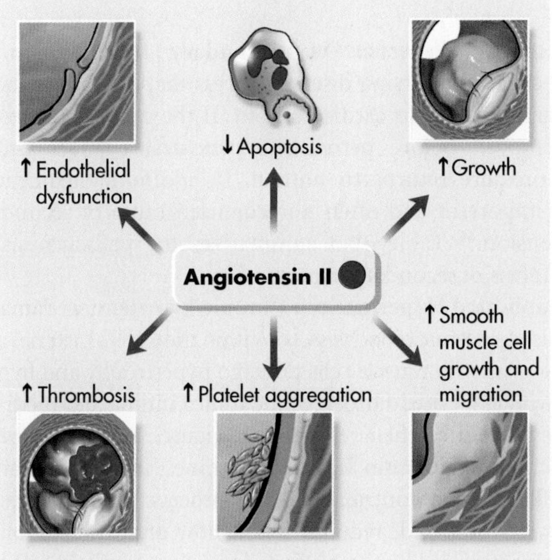

FIGURE 32-5 Angiotensins and the Organs Affected. A, The shaded blue area is the classical pathway of biosynthesis that generates the renin and angiotensin I. Angiotensinogen is synthesized in the liver and is released into the blood where it is cleaved to form angiotensin I by renin secreted by cells in the kidneys. Angiotensin-converting enzyme (ACE) in the lung catalyzes the formation of angiotensin II from angiotensin I, and destroys the potent vasodilator, bradykinin. Further cleavage generates the angiotensins III and IV. The reddish shading shows the organs affected by angiotensin II including the brain, heart, adrenals, kidney, and the kidney's efferent arterioles. The dashed line (on the left) shows the inhibition of renin by angiotensin II. **B,** Summary of angiotensin II effects on blood vessel structure and function leading to arteriosclerosis. (Redrawn from Goodfriend TL et al: *N Engl J Med* 334:2649–2654, 1996.)

WHAT'S NEW?

Obesity and Hypertension

Obesity is a well-known risk factor for hypertension. Adipocytes (fat cells) secrete leptin and adiponectin. Leptin's primary function is to interact with the hypothalamus to control body weight and fat deposition through appetite inhibition and increased metabolic rate. However, chronically high levels of leptin associated with obesity result in resistance to these weight-reducing functions and have been found to increase sympathetic nervous system activity, decrease renal sodium excretion, promote inflammation, and stimulate myocyte hypertrophy. Adiponectin is a protein that is produced by adipose tissue but is reduced in obesity. Decreased adiponectin is associated with insulin resistance, decreased endothelial-derived nitric oxide (vasodilator) production, and activation of the sympathetic nervous and renin-angiotensin-aldosterone systems. Taken together, these obesity-related changes result in vasoconstriction, salt and water retention, and renal dysfunction that may contribute to the development of hypertension. Obese individuals also have been found to have hypertrophic remodeling of subcutaneous small arteries, and endothelial dysfunction in response to acetylcholine. Microvascular dysfunction is linked to both the pathogenesis of hypertension and hypertension-related target organ damage. Obesity also is linked with insulin resistance, which also affects vascular function and contributes to the development of sustained hypertension. Further studies aimed at achieving a better understanding of these mechanisms may lead to new treatments for obesity-related hypertension.

Data from De Boer MP et al: *Microcirculation* 19(1):5–18, 2012; Dorresteijn JA, Visseren FL, Spiering W: *Obesity Rev* 13(1):17–26, 2012; Kalil GZ, Haynes WG: *Hypertens Res* 35(1):4–16, 2012; Rizzoni D et al: *Basic Clin Pharmacol Toxicol* 110(1):56–62, 2012.

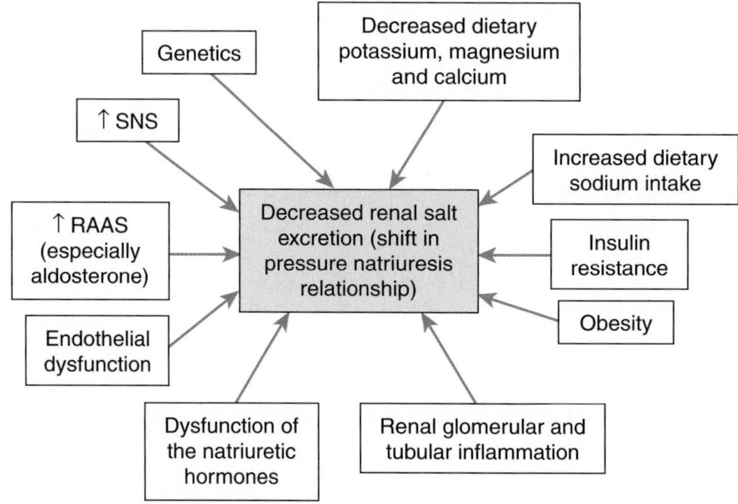

FIGURE 32-6 Shift in the Pressure-Natriuresis Relationship. Numerous factors have been implicated in the pathogenesis of sodium retention in individuals with hypertension. These factors cause less renal excretion of salt than would normally occur with increased blood pressure. This is called a *shift in the pressure-natriuresis relationship* and is believed to be a central process in the pathogenesis of primary hypertension. *RAAS,* Renin-angiotensin-aldosterone system; *SNS,* sympathetic nervous system.

risk for cardiovascular complications from hypertension (see What's New? Obesity and Hypertension).

Finally, insulin resistance is common in hypertension, even in individuals without clinical diabetes. Insulin resistance is associated with decreased endothelial release of nitric oxide and other vasodilators.[44] It also affects renal function and causes renal salt and water retention. Insulin resistance is associated with overactivity of the SNS and the RAAS. It is interesting to note that in many individuals with diabetes treated with drugs that increase insulin sensitivity, blood pressure often declines, even in the absence of antihypertensive drugs. The interactions between obesity, hypertension, insulin resistance, and lipid disorders in the metabolic syndrome result in a high risk of cardiovascular disease.[28]

It is likely that primary hypertension is an interaction between many of these factors leading to sustained increases in blood volume and peripheral resistance. The role of these mechanisms in increasing blood volume in the pathophysiology of primary hypertension is summarized in Figure 32-6.

Secondary Hypertension. **Secondary hypertension** is caused by an underlying disease process that raises peripheral vascular resistance or cardiac output. If the cause is identified and removed before permanent structural changes occur, blood pressure returns to normal. In addition, medications are an important and often unrecognized cause of secondary hypertension.[45] Table 32-3 summarizes the pathogenesis of major forms of secondary hypertension.

Complicated Hypertension. Chronic hypertension damages the walls of systemic blood vessels. Within the walls of arteries and arterioles, smooth muscle cells undergo hypertrophy and hyperplasia with associated fibrosis of the tunica intima and media in a process called vascular remodeling (Figure 32-7). Endothelial dysfunction, angiotensin II, catecholamines, insulin resistance, and inflammation contribute to this process. Once significant fibrosis has occurred, reduced blood flow and dysfunction of the organs perfused by these affected vessels is inevitable. Target organs for hypertension include the kidney, brain, heart, extremities, and eyes (these effects are summarized in Table 32-4).

TABLE 32-3 PATHOGENESIS OF MAJOR FORMS OF SECONDARY HYPERTENSION BY CAUSE

PRIMARY DISEASE	PATHOGENESIS OF HYPERTENSION
Renal Disorders	
Renal parenchymal disease	Disturbances in filtration and reabsorption of serum sodium, potassium, and calcium initiate the hemodynamics of early hypertension
Renovascular disease	Impaired blood flow and renal ischemia invoke the compensatory renin-angiotensin-aldosterone mechanism in an effort to raise the renal perfusion pressure
Renin-producing tumors	Elevated blood renin levels invoke elevations in angiotensin and aldosterone, which causes blood pressure to rise
Renal failure	Disturbances in filtration and reabsorption of serum sodium, potassium, and calcium initiate the hemodynamics of early hypertension
Primary sodium retention	Disturbance in filtration and/or reabsorption of serum sodium initiates the hemodynamics of early hypertension
Endocrine Disorders	
Acromegaly	Excess human growth hormone causes increased peripheral resistance
Hypothyroidism	Mucopolysaccharide deposits in vascular tissue increase resistance
Hypercalcemia	Calcium ion directly affects vascular tonicity; elevated serum calcium levels increase vascular tone and peripheral resistance
Hyperthyroidism	Increased inotropic effect on the heart elevates systolic pressure; diastolic pressure decreases as a result of decreased peripheral resistance
Adrenal disorders Cortical disturbances Cushing syndrome	Glucocorticoids facilitate sodium and water retention, initiating the hemodynamics of early hypertension
Primary aldosteronism	Excess aldosterone promotes sodium retention and initiation of the hemodynamics of early hypertension
Congenital adrenal hyperplasia	Excess production of adrenocortical hormones promotes sodium and water retention
Medullary disturbance: pheochromocytoma	Excess catecholamines raise vascular tone and increase peripheral resistance
Extra-adrenal chromaffin tumors	Excess catecholamines raise vascular tone and increase peripheral resistance
Vascular Disorders	
Coarctation of the aorta	Decreased blood flow in distal areas initiates maximum peripheral resistance as an autoregulatory effort to adjust perfusion pressure
Arteriosclerosis	Loss of elasticity in vessel walls results in increased peripheral resistance
Pregnancy-Induced Hypertension	Pathogenesis unclear
Neurologic Disorders	
Elevated intracranial pressure (brain tumor, encephalitis, respiratory acidosis of pulmonary or central nervous system [CNS] origin)	Higher systemic blood pressure required to maintain adequate cerebral perfusion
Quadriplegia, acute porphyria, familial dysautonomia, lead poisoning, Guillain-Barré syndrome	Interface with neural control of blood pressure initiates increased systemic blood pressure
Acute Stress	
Surgery, psychogenic hyperventilation, hypoglycemia, burns, pancreatitis, alcohol withdrawal, sickle cell crisis, resuscitation, increased intravascular volume	Acute stress precipitates release of catecholamines and glucocorticoids
Drugs and Other Substances	
Oral contraceptives and estrogen	Unknown; possibly caused by sodium retention, plasma retention, weight gain, changes in levels and actions of renin, angiotensin, and aldosterone
Corticosteroids	Same as for Cushing syndrome
Sympathetic stimulants, appetite suppressants, antihistamines	Raises vascular tone and increases vascular resistance
Licorice	Contains glycerrhizic acid, a mineralocorticoid that causes salt and water retention
Monoamine oxidase inhibitors	Hypertension may develop in an individual who routinely takes a monoamine oxidase (MAO) inhibitor with ingestion of a food containing tyramine, such as aged cheese

From Cheng J et al: *PLoS Pathog* May 5(5), 2009. (Epub ahead of print.); Kaplan NM: *Clinical hypertension,* ed 8, Baltimore, 2002, Lippincott Williams & Wilkins.

Cardiovascular complications include left ventricular hypertrophy, angina pectoris, congestive heart failure (left heart failure), CAD, MI, and sudden death. Myocardial hypertrophy in response to hypertension is mediated by several neurohormonal substances, including the SNS and angiotensin II. Hypertrophy is characterized by changes in the myocyte proteins, apoptosis of myocytes, and deposition of collagen in heart muscle, which causes it to become thickened, scarred, and less able to relax during diastole leading to diastolic heart failure.[46] In addition, the increased size of the heart muscle increases demand for oxygen delivery over time, contractility of the heart is impaired, and the individual is at increased risk for systolic heart failure. Vascular complications include the formation, dissection, and rupture of aneurysms (outpouchings in vessel walls); intermittent claudication; and gangrene resulting from vessel occlusion. Renal complications are parenchymal damage, nephrosclerosis, renal arteriosclerosis, and renal insufficiency or failure.[47]

Microalbuminuria (small amounts of protein in the urine) is an early sign of impending renal dysfunction and significantly increased risk for cardiovascular events.[48]

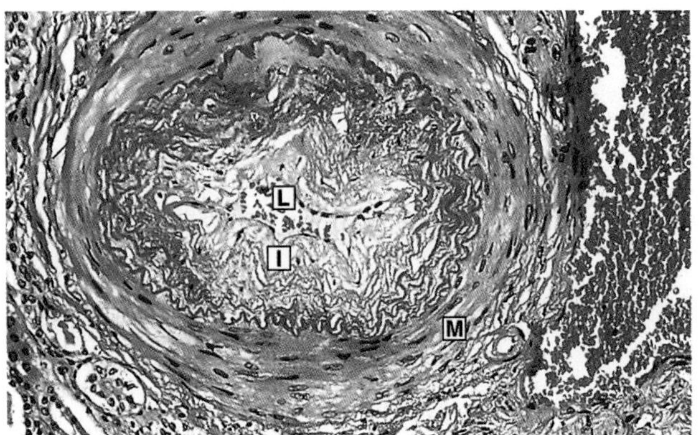

FIGURE 32-7 Dramatic Hypertension Change in Small Arterioles. Fibrous intimal proliferation *(I)* with reduction in lumen vessel caliber (radius) *(L)* and normal media *(M)*. (From Stevens A, Lowe JS, Scott I: *Core pathology*, ed 3, London, 2009, Mosby.)

Changes in the vascular beds can be estimated by viewing the arterioles of the retina. Complications specific to the retina include retinal vascular sclerosis, exudation, and hemorrhage.[49] Cerebrovascular complications are similar to those of other arterial beds and include transient ischemia, stroke, cerebral thrombosis, aneurysm, and hemorrhage. Chronic hypertension also has been linked to cognitive decline with aging.[50-52]

Malignant hypertension (rapidly progressive hypertension in which diastolic pressure is usually greater than 140 mmHg) can cause encephalopathy. Encephalopathy occurs because high arterial pressure renders the cerebral arterioles incapable of regulating blood flow to the cerebral capillary beds. Capillary permeability is increased by high hydrostatic pressures in the capillaries, and vascular fluid exudes into the interstitial space. If blood pressure is not reduced, cerebral edema and cerebral dysfunction increase until death occurs. Organ damage resulting from malignant hypertension is life threatening. Besides encephalopathy, malignant hypertension can cause papilledema, cardiac failure, uremia, retinopathy, and cerebrovascular accident.

CLINICAL MANIFESTATIONS. The early stages of hypertension have no clinical manifestations other than elevated blood pressure. Most important, the lack of signs and symptoms means the individual is unlikely to seek health care; thus hypertension is called a *lanthanic (silent) disease*. The likelihood of developing primary hypertension increases with age, over and above the natural rise in blood pressure associated with aging. Although hypertension usually is thought to be an adult health problem, it is important to remember that hypertension does occur in children and is being diagnosed with increasing frequency. If elevated blood pressure is not detected and treated, it becomes established and may begin to accelerate its effect on tissues when the individual is 30 to 50 years of age. This sets the stage for the complications of hypertension that begin to appear during the fourth, fifth, and sixth decades of life. The clinical manifestations of chronic hypertension tend to be specific for the organs or tissues affected. Evidence of heart disease, renal insufficiency,

TABLE 32-4 PATHOLOGIC EFFECTS OF SUSTAINED, COMPLICATED PRIMARY HYPERTENSION

SITE OF INJURY	MECHANISM OF INJURY	POTENTIAL PATHOLOGIC EFFECT
Heart		
Myocardium	Increased workload combined with diminished blood flow through coronary arteries	Left ventricular hypertrophy, myocardial ischemia, left heart failure
Coronary arteries	Accelerated atherosclerosis (coronary artery disease)	Myocardial ischemia, myocardial infarction, sudden death
Aorta	Weakened vessel wall	Aneurysms, acute aortic syndromes
Kidneys	Renin and aldosterone secretion stimulated by reduced blood flow	Retention of sodium and water, leading to increased blood volume and perpetuation of hypertension
	Inflammation and ischemia	Tissue damage that compromises filtration
	High pressures in renal arterioles	Nephrosclerosis leading to renal failure
Brain	Reduced blood flow and oxygen supply; weakened vessel walls, accelerated atherosclerosis	Transient ischemic attacks, cerebral thrombosis, aneurysm, hemorrhage, acute brain infarction
Eyes (retinas)	Reduced blood flow	Retinal vascular sclerosis
	High arteriolar pressure	Exudation, hemorrhage
Arterial vessels of lower extremities	Reduced blood flow and high pressures in arterioles, accelerated atherosclerosis	Intermittent claudication, arterial thrombosis, gangrene

central nervous system dysfunction, impaired vision, impaired mobility, vascular occlusion, or edema can be caused by sustained hypertension. (See appropriate chapters for specific clinical manifestations of organ dysfunction.)

EVALUATION AND TREATMENT. A single elevated blood pressure reading does not mean that a person has hypertension. Diagnosis requires the measurement of blood pressure on at least two separate occasions averaging two readings at least 2 minutes apart, with the individual seated, the arm supported at heart level, after 5 minutes rest, with no smoking or caffeine intake in the past 30 minutes.[19] Some individuals benefit from 24-hour ambulatory blood pressure monitoring because of better correlation with end-organ damage and the ability to screen out "white coat hypertension" (elevated blood pressure that occurs only in a clinic setting) and "masked hypertension" (normal blood pressure in the clinic setting but elevated elsewhere).[53,54] Ambulatory measurement also detects those who fail to have a nocturnal decrease in blood pressure and who may be at higher cardiovascular risk. It is especially recommended for individuals with drug resistance, hypotensive symptoms with medications, episodic hypertension, and autonomic dysfunction.[54]

Evaluation of the hypertensive individual should include a complete medical history and assessment of lifestyle and other risk factors for hypertension and cardiovascular disease, as well as evidence of possible secondary causes of hypertension. Physical examination should include examination of the optic fundi; calculation of body mass index; auscultation for carotid, abdominal, and femoral bruits; examination of the heart and lungs; palpation of the abdomen; assessment of lower extremity pulses and edema; and neurologic examination. Further routine diagnostic tests for the evaluation of hypertension include hematocrit, urinalysis, biochemical blood profile (fasting glucose, sodium, potassium, calcium, creatinine, total cholesterol, high-density cholesterol, triglycerides), and an electrocardiogram (ECG). Optional tests include urinary albumin excretion or albumin/creatinine ratio. Individuals who have elevated blood pressure are assumed to have primary hypertension unless their history, physical examination, or initial diagnostic screening indicates secondary hypertension.

Treatment of primary hypertension depends on its severity. Figure 32-8 illustrates an overview of the JNC7 recommendations.[19] Treatment begins with reducing or eliminating risk factors. Lifestyle modification can prevent hypertension from developing in those individuals who fall into the prehypertension category, may control the blood pressure in stage I hypertension, and can enhance the effects of drug treatment for those with more significant blood pressure elevation. The usual dietary recommendations are to restrict sodium intake to 2.4 g/day, to increase potassium intake, to restrict saturated fat intake, and to adjust calorie intake as required to maintain optimum weight. The Dietary Approaches to Stop Hypertension (DASH) diet is recommended.[55,56] Although it has been

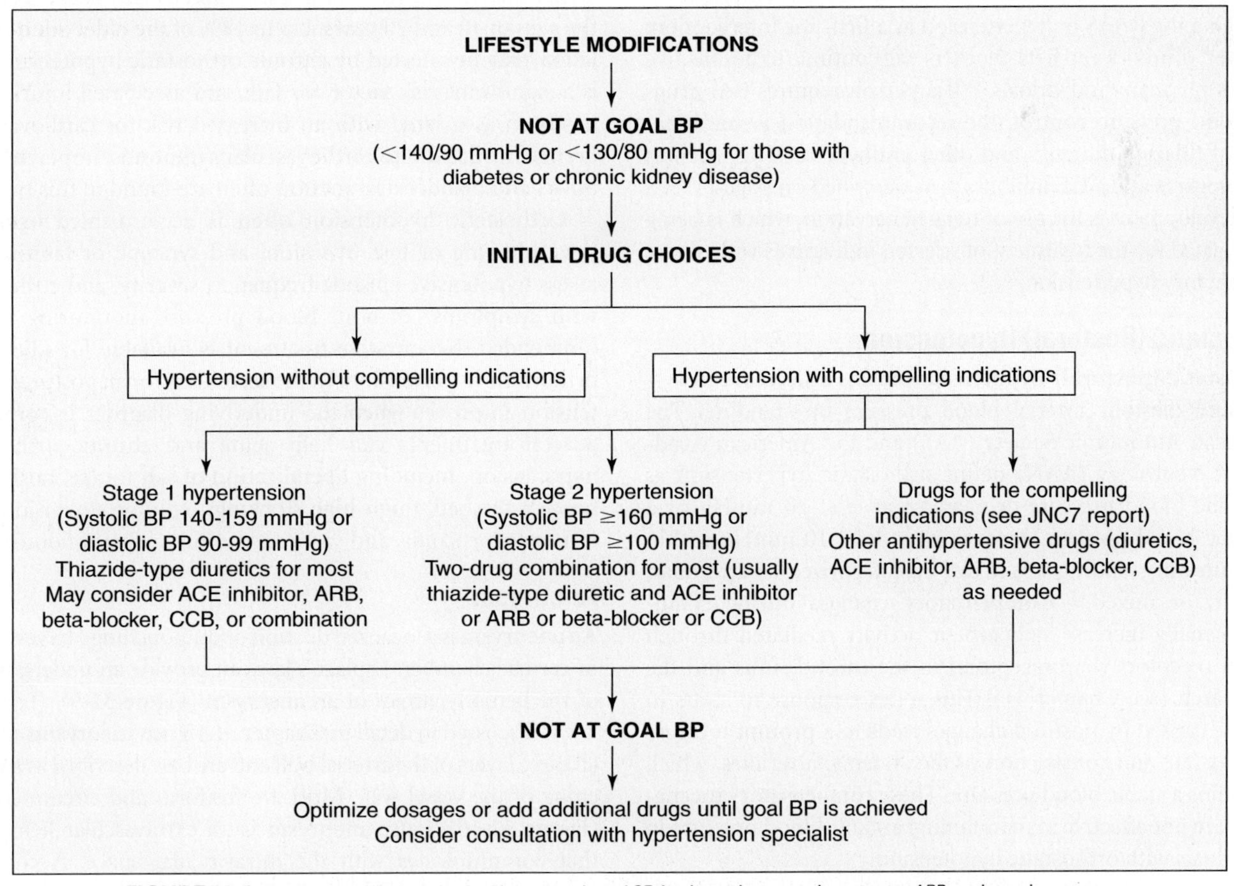

FIGURE 32-8 Summary of Treatment for Hypertension. *ACE,* Angiotensin-converting enzyme; *ARB,* angiotensin-receptor blocker; *BP,* blood pressure; *CCB,* calcium channel blocker. (Data from Chobanian AV et al: *JAMA* 289:2560–2572, 2003.)

widely recommended since 1998, the DASH diet continues to be studied with beneficial effects extending to reduced coronary risks, increased insulin sensitivity, and improved lipid profiles, especially in those with diabetes.[57] An exercise program that promotes endurance and relaxation usually is recommended. Physical training increases stroke volume, which has the effect of lowering heart rate and hence systolic blood pressure, and should consist of regular aerobic physical activity. Relaxation is expected to reduce levels of circulating catecholamines, which has the effect of reducing vascular tone and blood pressure. Individuals are counseled to stop smoking to eliminate vasoconstrictor effects of nicotine.

Pharmacologic treatment of hypertension reduces the risk of end-organ damage and prevents major diseases, such as myocardial ischemia and stroke. Thiazide diuretics and beta-blockers have been shown to be safe and effective medications for lowering blood pressure and preventing the cardiovascular complications of hypertension for many individuals. However, these medications are associated with lipid disorders and glucose intolerance.[58] Many individuals will have "compelling indications" for choosing a particular antihypertensive as a first-line medication. For example, individuals with heart failure or those who have chronic kidney disease, are postmyocardial infarction, or have had recurrent stroke should begin antihypertensive treatment with an ACE inhibitor, ARB, or aldosterone antagonist.[19] It is widely anticipated that the new report from the National Committee on the Prevention, Detection, Evaluation and Treatment of High Blood Pressure (JNC8) will have a greater emphasis on managing the RAAS in hypertension as a first-line intervention; however, diuretics and beta-blockers will continue to be effective choices for many individuals.[59] If a person requires two drugs for blood pressure control, the recommendation is combinations of thiazide diuretics and other antihypertensives, such as beta-blockers and ACE inhibitors. As described on page 1133, a new development is the use of renal denervation, which is being investigated for the treatment of selected individuals with severe or refractory hypertension.[25,60]

Orthostatic (Postural) Hypotension

Orthostatic (postural) hypotension means a decrease in systolic and diastolic arterial blood pressure on standing. The American Autonomic Society (AAS) and the American Academy of Neurology (AAN) define orthostatic hypertension as a systolic blood pressure decrease of at least 20 mmHg or a diastolic blood pressure decrease of at least 10 mmHg within 3 minutes of standing up. It can be categorized as arteriolar, venular, or mixed.[61] Compensatory changes during standing normally increase sympathetic activity mediated through stretch receptors (baroreceptors) in the carotid sinus and the aortic arch (see Chapter 31). This reflex response to shifts in volume caused by postural changes leads to a prompt increase in heart rate and constriction of the systemic arterioles, which maintains a stable blood pressure. These compensatory mechanisms are not effective in maintaining a stable blood pressure in individuals with orthostatic hypotension.

Orthostatic hypotension may be acute or chronic. **Acute orthostatic hypotension** (temporary type) may result from: (1) altered body chemistry, (2) drug action (e.g., antihypertensives or antidepressants), (3) prolonged immobility caused by illness, (4) starvation, (5) physical exhaustion, (6) any condition that produces volume depletion (e.g., massive diuresis, potassium or sodium depletion), and (7) venous pooling (e.g., pregnancy, extensive varicosities of the lower extremities). Older adults are susceptible to this type of orthostatic hypotension, in which postural reflexes are slowed as part of the aging process.

Chronic orthostatic hypotension can be categorized as (1) secondary to a specific disease, and (2) idiopathic or primary. The diseases that cause secondary orthostatic hypotension are endocrine disorders (e.g., adrenal insufficiency, diabetes mellitus), metabolic disorders (e.g., porphyria), or diseases of the central or peripheral nervous system (e.g., intracranial tumors, cerebral infarcts, Wernicke encephalopathy, peripheral neuropathies). Cardiovascular autonomic neuropathy is a common cause of orthostatic hypotension in diabetes and is a serious and often overlooked complication. Severe chronic autonomic failure may result from multiple system atrophy (MSA), in which there are multiple central nervous system degenerative changes, and Parkinson disease. Individuals with these disorders also may exhibit supine hypertension, altered drug sensitivity, hyperresponsiveness of blood pressure to hypo/hyperventilation, sleep apnea, and other neurologic disturbances.[62,63]

Idiopathic, or primary, orthostatic hypotension is the term for hypotension in which there is no known initial cause. It affects men more often than women and usually occurs between the ages of 40 and 70 years. Up to 18% of the older adult population may be affected by chronic orthostatic hypotension.[61] It is a significant risk factor for falls and associated injuries and has been associated with an increased risk for cardiovascular events. In addition to cardiovascular symptoms, impotence and bowel and bladder dysfunction often are found in this type.

Orthostatic hypotension often is accompanied by dizziness, blurring or loss of vision, and syncope or fainting. To assess hypotensive episode frequency, severity, and correlation with symptoms, 24-hour blood pressure monitoring is recommended. No curative treatment is available for idiopathic orthostatic hypertension. In the secondary form, postural hypotension improves when the underlying disorder is corrected. Several treatments can help acute and chronic orthostatic hypotension, including liberalization of salt intake, raising the head of the bed, thigh-high stockings, volume expansion with mineralocorticoids, and vasoconstrictors such as midodrine.[61]

Aneurysm

An **aneurysm** is a localized dilation or outpouching of a vessel wall or cardiac chamber. Laplace's law can provide an understanding of the hemodynamics of an aneurysm (Figure 32-9). (Laplace's law is discussed in detail in Chapter 31.) **True aneurysms** involve all three layers of the arterial wall and are best described as a weakening of the vessel wall. Most are fusiform and circumferential (Figure 32-10). **False aneurysm** is an extravascular hematoma that communicates with the intravascular space. A common cause of this type of lesion is a leak between a vascular graft and a natural artery. Saccular aneurysms are basically spherical.

Arteriosclerosis and hypertension are found in more than half of all individuals with aneurysms. Chronic hypertension results in mechanical and shear forces that contribute to remodeling and weakening of the vessel wall. Atherosclerosis is a common cause of aneurysms because plaque formation erodes the vessel wall. Infections, such as syphilis, collagen disorders (such as Marfan syndrome), and traumatic injury to the chest or abdomen, also can cause aortic aneurysms. Genetic susceptibilities have been identified including gene polymorphisms for the production of growth factors, myosin, and

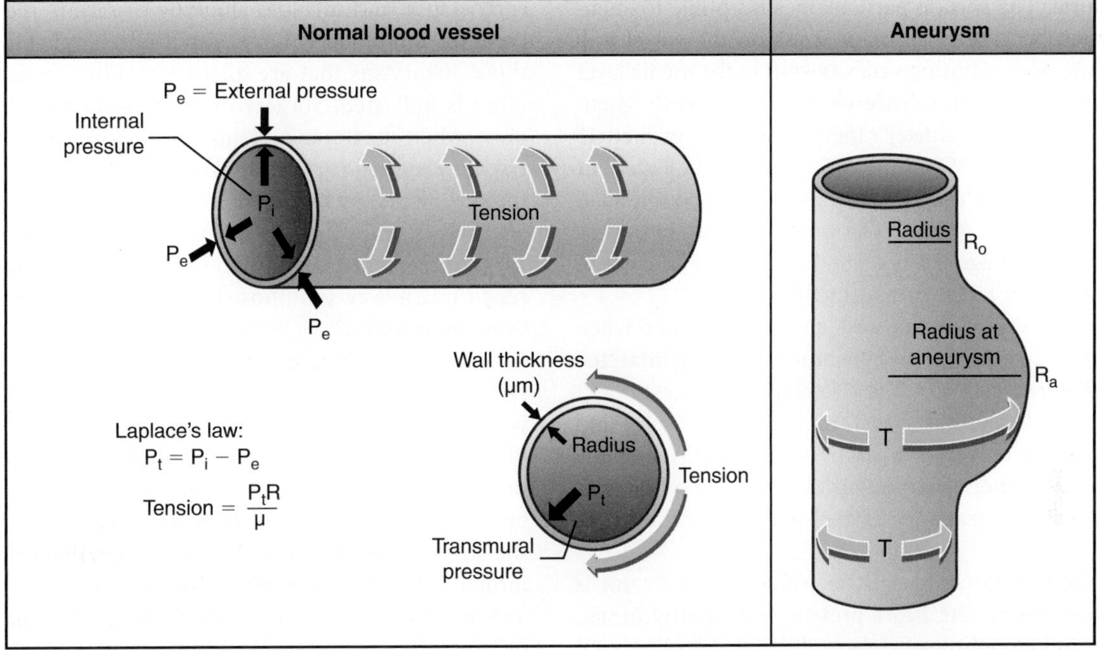

FIGURE 32-9 Pressure-Tension and Wall Thickness Relations in Blood Vessels or Cardiac Chambers (Laplace's Law).

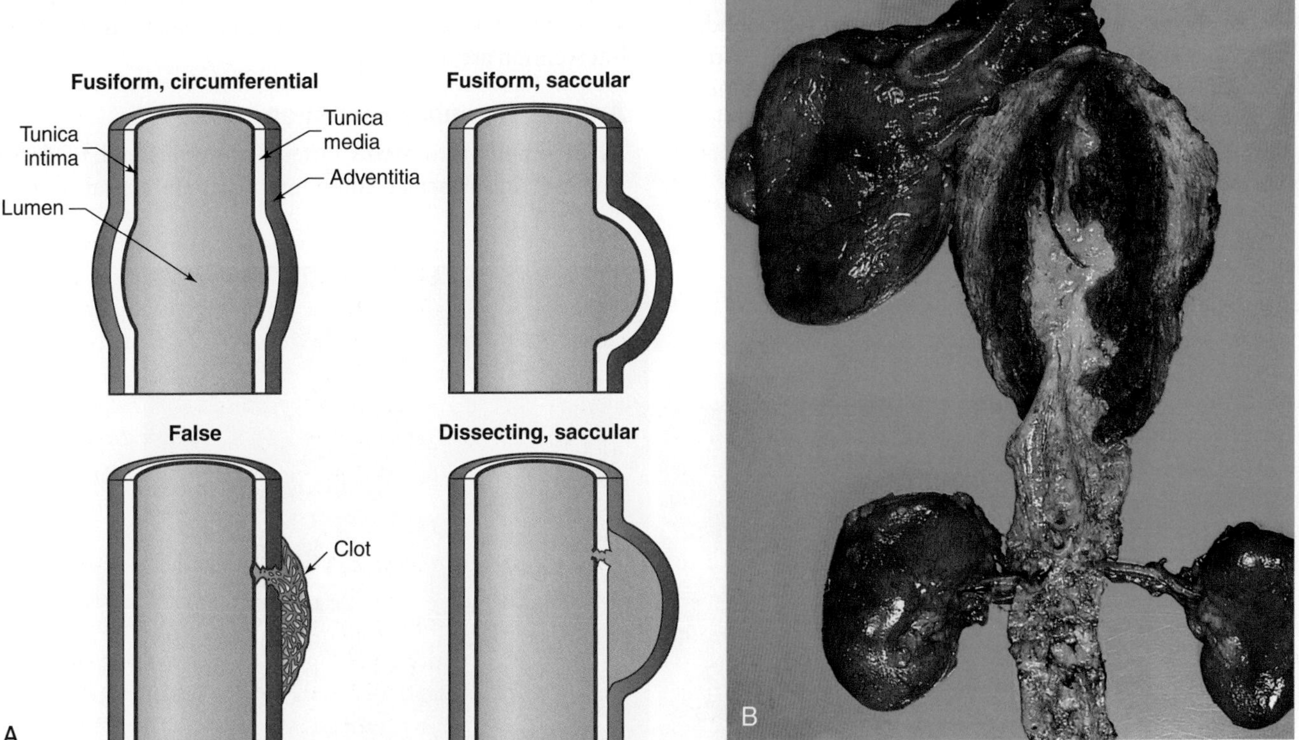

FIGURE 32-10 Longitudinal Sections Showing Types of Aneurysms. **A,** The fusiform circumferential and fusiform saccular aneurysms are true aneurysms, caused by weakening of the vessel wall. False and saccular aneurysms involve a break in the vessel wall, usually caused by trauma. **B,** Dissecting aneurysm of thoracic aorta. (**B** from Damjanov I, Linder J, editors: *Anderson's pathology,* ed 10, St Louis, 1996, Mosby.)

proteases. Inflammation (with the production of toxic oxygen radicals) and changes in cytokines, such as TGF-β, activate matrix degrading proteins and smooth muscle cell apoptosis resulting in loss of medial elastic lamellae and thinning of the tunica media.[64]

Aneurysms most commonly occur in the thoracic or abdominal aorta. The aorta is particularly susceptible to aneurysm formation because of constant stress on the vessel wall and the absence of penetrating vasa vasorum in the media layer (Figure 32-11, *A*). The prevalence of abdominal aortic aneurysms 2.9 to 4.9 cm in diameter ranges from 1.3% in men 45 to 54 years of age to 12.5% in men 75 to 84 years of age. For women, the prevalence ranges from zero in the youngest to 5.2% in the oldest age group.[5] The prevalence of aneurysms has decreased in men ages 65 years and older likely because of improvements in risk factor management.[65]

Formation of a ventricular wall aneurysm occurs when intraventricular tension stretches the noncontracting infarcted muscle (see Figure 32-11, *B*). The stretching produces infarct expansion, a weak and thin layer of necrotic muscle, and fibrous tissue that bulges with each systole. With time the aneurysm becomes more fibrotic but continues to bulge with each systole, thus acting as a "reservoir" for some of the stroke volume.

Clinical manifestations depend on where the aneurysm is located. Aneurysms in the heart present with dysrhythmias, heart failure, and embolism of clots to the brain or other vital organs. Aortic aneurysms often are asymptomatic until they rupture, when they become painful. Symptoms of dysphagia (difficulty in swallowing) and dyspnea (breathlessness) are caused by the pressure of a thoracic aneurysm on surrounding organs. An abdominal aneurysm can impair flow to an extremity and cause symptoms of ischemia. Aneurysms that occur elsewhere in the body have variable symptoms and signs related to the size of the aneurysm and the potential for rupture and hemorrhage.

The diagnosis of an aneurysm is usually confirmed by ultrasonography, CT, MRI, or angiography. The goals of medical treatment of aneurysms are to maintain a low blood volume and low blood pressure to decrease mechanical forces thought to contribute to vessel wall dilation. Medical treatment is indicated for slow-growing aortic aneurysms, particularly in early stages, and includes smoking cessation, reducing blood pressure and blood volume, and β-adrenergic blockage.[64] For those aneurysms that are dilating rapidly, surgical treatment often is indicated. Surgery or endovascular repair should be done when aortic aneurysms reach 5 cm in diameter. The risk for eventual rupture approaches 20% for abdominal aortic aneurysms greater than 5 cm, and greater than 50% for aneurysms more than 7 cm in diameter.[5] New endovascular surgical techniques with placement of a stent make aneurysm repair possible even in those individuals with acute symptoms or complications.[66]

Aortic aneurysms can be complicated by the acute aortic syndromes that include aortic dissection, hemorrhage into the vessel wall, or vessel rupture. **Aortic dissection** is a devastating complication that can involve any part of the aorta (ascending, arch, or descending) and can disrupt flow through arterial branches, thus creating a surgical emergency. Dissection of the layers of the arterial wall occurs when there is a tear in the intima and blood enters the wall of the artery (see Figure 32-10). This occurs most commonly when there is trauma to the aorta or when there is tissue ischemia and necrosis at the edge of an atherosclerotic plaque that weakens the intima. Persistent chronic hypertension and inflammation contribute to further degradation of the vessel wall with fibrotic obstruction of vessels that feed the arterial wall. Emergent evaluation and surgical intervention are indicated.[67]

Arterial Thrombus Formation

As in venous thrombosis, arterial thrombi tend to develop wherever intravascular conditions promote activation of the

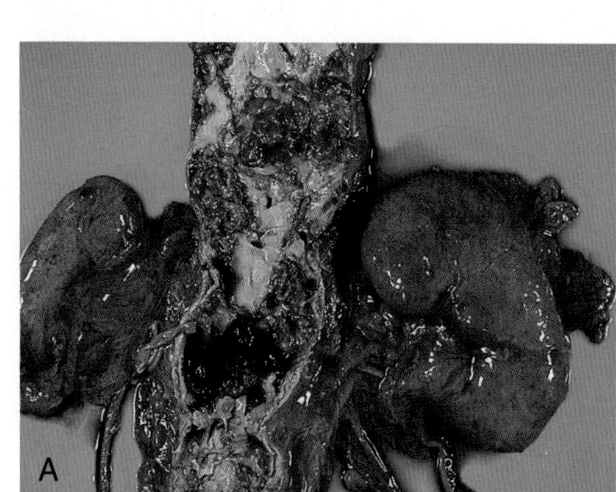

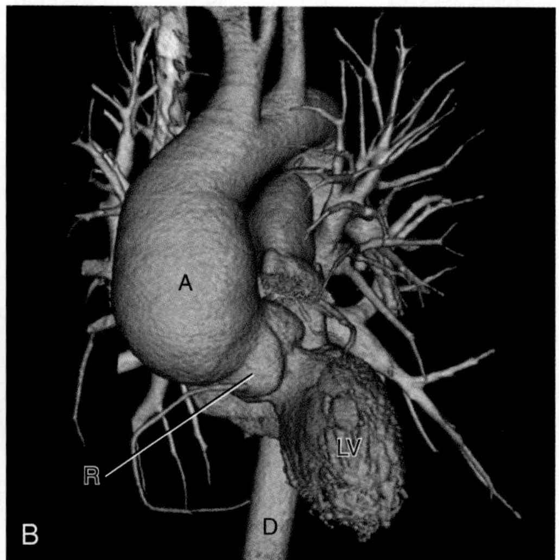

FIGURE 32-11 Aneurysms. A, Abdominal aortic atherosclerotic aneurysm. **B,** A three dimensional CT scan shows the aneurysm. *(A)* involves the ascending thoracic aorta. *D,* descending aorta; *LV,* left ventricle. (**A** from Damjanov I, Linder J, editors: *Anderson's pathology,* ed 10, St Louis, 1996, Mosby.)

coagulation, or clotting, cascade. These conditions include intimal irritation and roughening, inflammation, traumatic injury, infection, and low blood pressures or obstructions that cause blood stasis and pooling within the vessels. (Mechanisms of coagulation are described in Chapter 27.) In the arteries, activation of the coagulation cascade usually is caused by roughening of the tunica intima by atherosclerosis. Invasion of the tunica intima by an infectious agent also roughens the normally smooth lining of the artery, causing platelets to adhere readily. Anatomic changes of an artery (such as an aneurysm) can stimulate thrombus formation, particularly if the change results in pooling of arterial blood. Thrombi form also on heart valves altered by calcification or bacterial vegetation. Valvular thrombi are associated most commonly with inflammation of the endocardium (endocarditis) and rheumatic heart disease.

Widespread arterial thrombus formation can occur in shock, particularly shock resulting from septicemia. In septic shock, systemic inflammation activates the intrinsic and extrinsic pathways of coagulation resulting in microvascular thrombosis throughout the systemic arterial circulation (see Chapters 29 and 48).

Arterial thrombi pose two potential threats to the circulation. First, the thrombus may grow large enough to occlude the artery, causing ischemia in tissue supplied by the artery. Second, the thrombus may dislodge, becoming a thromboembolus that travels through the vascular system until it occludes flow into a distal systemic vascular bed.

Diagnosis of arterial thrombi is usually accomplished through the use of Doppler ultrasonography and angiography. Pharmacologic treatment involves the administration of heparin, warfarin derivatives, thrombin inhibitors, or thrombolytics. A balloon-tipped catheter also can be used to remove or compress an arterial thrombus. Various combinations of drug and catheter therapies are sometimes used concurrently.

Embolism

Embolism is the obstruction of a vessel by an **embolus**—a bolus of matter that is circulating in the bloodstream. The embolus may consist of a dislodged thrombus; an air bubble; an aggregate of amniotic fluid; an aggregate of fat, bacteria, or cancer cells; or a foreign substance. An embolus travels in the bloodstream until it reaches a vessel through which it cannot fit. No matter how tiny it is, an embolus eventually will lodge in a systemic or pulmonary vessel. The source of the embolus determines whether the embolus will lodge in a vessel of the pulmonary or systemic circulation. Pulmonary emboli originate in the venous circulation (mostly from the deep veins of the legs) or in the right heart (see p. 1275). Arterial emboli most commonly originate in the left heart and are associated with thrombi after MI, valvular disease, left heart failure, endocarditis, and dysrhythmias.

Embolism causes ischemia or infarction in tissues distal to the obstruction. A limb that is ischemic because of arterial occlusion is characterized (1) by an almost waxy whiteness of the skin because the vasculature is devoid of erythrocytes, and (2) by numbness and pain resulting from neural ischemia.

Embolism to a central organ causes organ dysfunction and pain. For example, pulmonary artery embolism causes chest pain and dyspnea; renal artery embolism causes abdominal pain and oliguria; and mesenteric artery embolism causes abdominal pain and a paralytic, ischemic bowel. In the coronary, cerebral, and peripheral arterial systems, embolism may occur as a result of rupture or mechanical disruption of an atherosclerotic plaque. This phenomenon is sometimes referred to as cholesterol embolization syndrome or atheroembolism.[68,69] Embolism to a coronary or cerebral artery is an immediate threat to life if the embolus severely obstructs a major vessel. Occlusion of a coronary artery causes an MI (see p. 1157), whereas occlusion of a cerebral artery causes a stroke (see Chapter 18).

Infarction and subsequent necrosis of a central organ are life threatening, not only because of organ dysfunction but also because of sepsis. Necrotic tissue is a rich medium for the growth of bacteria from the lungs, bowel, and occasionally, bladder, and can quickly lead to septicemia.

Thromboembolism

Thromboembolism is a vascular obstruction resulting from a dislodged thrombus. The most common source of arterial thromboemboli to the systemic circulation is the heart. Mitral or aortic valvular disease, especially that associated with abnormal heart rhythms (atrial fibrillation and flutter), causes thrombus formation on roughened vascular surfaces and in atrial blood as a result of stasis. More than half of these thromboemboli lodge in the lower extremities (in the femoral and popliteal arteries). Others lodge in the coronary arteries and the cerebral vasculature. Heart failure also is associated with an increased risk of thrombotic complications, although the mechanism for this increased risk is unclear.

Air Embolism

Room air that enters the circulation through intravenous lines is probably the most common cause of air embolism. Room air is about 70% nitrogen. Although nitrogen dissolves quickly in blood, large amounts of air cannot be dissolved rapidly enough to prevent the displacement of blood in the arterioles and capillary beds. Ischemia and necrosis occur when air totally blocks a vessel.

Air also can be introduced into the bloodstream if trauma to the chest causes air from the lungs to enter the vascular space. For example, gunshot wounds and puncture wounds of the thorax sometimes introduce air emboli. Treatment for air embolism is supportive, including bed rest and supplemental oxygen, once the connection between the source of air and the vascular system is eliminated.

Amniotic Fluid Embolism

The great intra-abdominal pressures generated during labor and delivery may force amniotic fluid into the mother's bloodstream through the highly vascular uterine wall. Amniotic fluid not only displaces blood, reducing oxygen, nutrient, and waste exchange, but also introduces antigens, cells, and protein aggregates that trigger inflammation, coagulation, and the immune response within the bloodstream. Capillary beds usually are affected by amniotic fluid emboli, especially the capillary beds of the lungs and kidneys. Treatment is supportive and may include dialysis, particularly after a cesarean delivery or hysterectomy.

Bacterial Embolism

Isolated bacteria in the bloodstream do not cause embolism, but aggregates of bacteria may be large enough to do so. The most common cause of bacterial embolism is subacute bacterial endocarditis, during which clumps of vegetation are dislodged from infected cardiac valves and ejected into the pulmonary or systemic circulation. A less common cause is erosion of an artery or vein by bacteria at a source of infection, such as an abscess. Treatment for bacterial embolism includes bed rest, supplemental oxygen, and antibiotics to eradicate the source of infection.

Fat Embolism

Trauma to the long bones is associated with fat embolism, particularly in the lungs. Two mechanisms have been proposed to account for the generation of fat emboli after skeletal trauma. The first is that trauma to the bones initiates defective fat metabolism, causing globules of fat to form in the blood. Platelets adhere to these globules until the conglomerate is large enough to lodge in a capillary bed. The second possible explanation is that globules of fat are released from fatty bone marrow exposed by fracture. Again, platelets adhere to the fat globules, and embolism occurs.

Treatment for fat embolism consists of prompt immobilization of fractures and supportive measures that include administration of supplemental oxygen, steroids, and glucose. Steroid administration may decrease the inflammation that occurs with vascular occlusion. Inflammation in the pulmonary bed is especially dangerous because it can cause acute respiratory distress syndrome (ARDS) (see Chapter 35).

Foreign Matter

Foreign matter can enter the bloodstream during trauma or through an intravenous or intra-arterial line. Small particles, such as drug precipitates, small glass shards, or fibers from linen, are sometimes introduced unintentionally into a vessel through intravenous injections or manipulation of monitoring lines. Once in the blood, these small particles initiate the coagulation cascade. The thromboemboli that form around the particles are large enough to occlude a vessel and result in ischemia. Treatment is aimed at preventing thrombus formation around the particle, dissolution of the particle, and supportive measures to alleviate ischemia. If the bolus of foreign matter is relatively large, it usually is removed surgically.

Peripheral Vascular Diseases

Thromboangiitis Obliterans (Buerger Disease)

Thromboangiitis obliterans (Buerger disease) is an inflammatory disease of the peripheral arteries. It is associated with smoking in approximately 95% of cases—the other 5% are related to frostbite, trauma, or the use of sympathomimetic drugs.[70] The incidence of Buerger disease has been steadily declining, presumably because of a decrease in cigarette smoking in men. Inflammatory lesions are accompanied by thrombi and sometimes by vasospasm of arterial segments. The pathogenesis of thromboangiitis obliterans is still being explored. There is evidence of significant T-cell activation and autoimmunity, as well as a lack of appropriate production of endothelial precursor cells in the bone marrow.[71] Inflammation, thrombus formation, and vasospasm eventually can occlude and obliterate portions of small and medium-size arteries. Typically affected are the digital, tibial, and plantar arteries of the feet and the digital, palmar, and ulnar arteries of the hands.

The chief symptoms of thromboangiitis obliterans are pain and tenderness of the affected part. Clinical manifestations are caused by sluggish blood flow and include rubor (redness of the skin), which is caused by dilated capillaries under the skin, and cyanosis, which is caused by blood that remains in the capillaries after its oxygen has diffused into the interstitium. Chronic ischemia causes the skin to thin and become shiny and the nails to become thickened and malformed. In advanced disease, ischemia resulting from vessel obliteration can cause gangrene, which may require amputation.

There are five primary criteria for the diagnosis of Buerger disease: (1) onset before age 50; (2) history of tobacco use; (3) ischemia of the digits; (4) typical arteriographic findings; and (5) exclusion of autoimmune disease, thrombophilia, diabetes, and proximal embolic source.[70] The most important part of treatment is cessation of cigarette smoking. All other measures are aimed at improving circulation to the foot or hand and include exercise and dependent positioning to improve circulation, vasodilators to alleviate vasospasm, and antithrombotics to prevent thrombus formation. If vasospasm persists, sympathectomy may be performed. Newer therapies include immunomodulation, spinal cord stimulation, and bone marrow transplantation.[70,72]

Raynaud Phenomenon and Disease

Raynaud phenomenon and Raynaud disease are characterized by attacks of vasospasm in the small arteries and arterioles of the fingers and, less commonly, the toes. Although the clinical manifestations of the phenomenon and the disease are the same, their causes differ.

Raynaud phenomenon is secondary to systemic diseases, such as collagen vascular disease (e.g., scleroderma), chemotherapy, cocaine use, hypothyroidism, pulmonary hypertension, thoracic outlet syndrome, serum sickness, vasculitis, malignancy, or long-term exposure to environmental conditions, such as cold or vibrating machinery in the workplace. Raynaud phenomenon associated with malignancy can be especially severe and is an important clue to finding a previously undiagnosed cancer.[73]

Raynaud disease is a primary vasospastic disorder of unknown origin. Blood vessels in affected individuals demonstrate endothelial dysfunction with an imbalance in endothelium-derived vasodilators (e.g., nitric oxide) and vasoconstrictors (e.g., endothelin-1). Platelet activation also may play a role. It tends to affect young women and to consist of vasospastic attacks triggered by brief exposure to cold or by emotional stress. Genetic predisposition may play a role in its development.

The clinical manifestations of the vasospastic attacks of either disorder are changes in skin color and sensation caused by ischemia. Vasospasm occurs with varying frequency and severity and causes pallor, numbness, and the sensation of cold in the digits. Attacks tend to be bilateral, and manifestations usually begin at the tips of the digits and progress to the proximal phalanges. Sluggish blood flow resulting in ischemia may cause the skin to appear cyanotic. Rubor follows as vasospasm ends and the capillaries become engorged with oxygenated blood. Rubor often is accompanied by throbbing and paresthesias. Skin color returns to normal after the attack, but frequent, prolonged attacks interfere with cellular metabolism, causing the skin of the fingertips to thicken and the nails to become brittle. In severe, chronic Raynaud phenomenon or disease, ischemia eventually can cause ulceration and gangrene. This outcome is rare, however.

The diagnostic criteria for Raynaud disease include not only the characteristic clinical manifestations described previously but also the absence of necrosis, no detectable underlying cause, normal capillaroscopy findings, normal laboratory tests for inflammation, and negative tests for antinuclear factors.[74]

Treatment for Raynaud phenomenon consists of removing the stimulus or treating the primary disease process. When Raynaud phenomenon is associated with malignancy, surgical removal of the tumor may resolve the ischemia. For Raynaud phenomenon not associated with malignancy, treatment is limited to amelioration of symptoms with arm exercises and medications, such as calcium channel blockers, alpha-blockers, prostaglandin analogs, or endothelin antagonists.[74]

Treatment of Raynaud disease is limited to prevention or alleviation of vasospasm itself, because no underlying disorder has been identified. Stimuli that trigger attacks (e.g., emotional stress, cold) are avoided, and cigarette smoking is stopped to eliminate the vasoconstricting effects of nicotine. Exercises that build centrifugal force in the extremities also are helpful in the early stages of vasospasm. If attacks of vasospasm become frequent or prolonged, pharmacologic management can include calcium channel blockers, nitric oxide agonists, alpha-blockers, prostaglandin analogs, and selective serotonin reuptake inhibitors. Biofeedback may be helpful.[75] Sympathectomy may be recommended in severe cases but is not always effective and has a high rate of recurrence.[76] If ischemia leads to ulceration and gangrene, amputation is necessary.

Atherosclerosis

Atherosclerosis is a form of arteriosclerosis in which thickening and hardening of the vessel are caused by the accumulation of lipid-laden macrophages within the arterial wall, which leads to the formation of a lesion called a **plaque.** Atherosclerosis is not a single disease but rather a pathologic process that can affect vascular systems throughout the body, resulting in ischemic syndromes that can vary widely in their severity and clinical manifestations. It is the leading cause of coronary artery and cerebrovascular disease. (Atherosclerosis of the coronary arteries is described on p. 1148; atherosclerosis of the cerebral arteries is discussed in Chapter 18.)

PATHOPHYSIOLOGY. Atherosclerosis is an inflammatory disease that develops and proceeds in the presence of elevated plasma cholesterol levels.[77] Both innate and adaptive immunity play a role in the development and progression of atherosclerotic lesions.[78] Pathologically, the lesions progress from endothelial injury and dysfunction to fatty streak to fibrotic plaque to complicated lesion (Figures 32-12 and 32-13). Atherosclerosis begins with injury to the endothelial cells that line artery walls. Possible causes of endothelial injury include the common risk factors for atherosclerosis, such as smoking, hypertension, diabetes, increased levels of low-density lipoprotein (LDL), decreased levels of high-density lipoprotein (HDL), and autoimmunity.[79,80] Other causes of endothelial injury include inflammatory factors that are being explored as nontraditional cardiovascular risk factors, such as elevated C-reactive protein (CRP), increased serum fibrinogen, infection, and periodontal disease. These risk factors are discussed in more detail in the following section on coronary artery disease (see p. 1148). Recent evidence indicates that individuals with a defect in the production of precursor endothelial cells in the bone marrow are at greater risk for atherosclerotic disease because these precursor cells are not available to repair injured endothelium.[81]

Once injury has occurred, endothelial dysfunction and inflammation lead to the following pathophysiologic events:

1. Injured endothelial cells become inflamed and cannot make normal amounts of antithrombotic and vasodilating cytokines (see Figure 31-23).
2. Numerous inflammatory cytokines are released, including tumor necrosis factor-alpha (TNF-α), interferon-gamma (IFN-γ), interleukin-1 (IL-1), toxic oxygen radicals, CRP, and heat shock proteins.
3. Macrophages adhere to injured endothelium by way of adhesion molecules, such as vascular cell adhesion molecule-1 (VCAM-1).
4. These macrophages then release enzymes and toxic oxygen radicals that create oxidative stress, oxidize LDL, and further injure the vessel wall.
5. Growth factors also are released, including angiotensin II, fibroblast growth factor, TGF-β, and platelet-derived growth factor, which stimulate smooth muscle cell proliferation in the affected vessel.

LDL penetrates into the subintima of arterial walls, where it is trapped by proteoglycans. Inflammation, oxidative stress, and activation of macrophages cause the aggregated LDL to become oxidized (see Figure 32-13). Diabetes, smoking, and hypertension (especially with increased levels of angiotensin II) contribute to increased LDL oxidation. Oxidized LDL is toxic to endothelial cells and causes smooth muscle proliferation. Oxidized LDL also increases endothelial adhesion molecule expression, which recruits more monocyte/macrophages that penetrate the vessel wall. Several types of receptors on these macrophages (Toll-like receptors [TLRs], LDL receptor-related protein [LRP]) enable detection and engulfment of the LDL, which contributes to activation of additional innate and adaptive immune responses.[82,83] Macrophages filled with oxidized LDL are called **foam cells** (see Figure 32-13).

Once these lipid-laden foam cells accumulate in significant amounts, they form a lesion called a **fatty streak** (see Figure 32-12). These lesions can be found in the walls of arteries of most

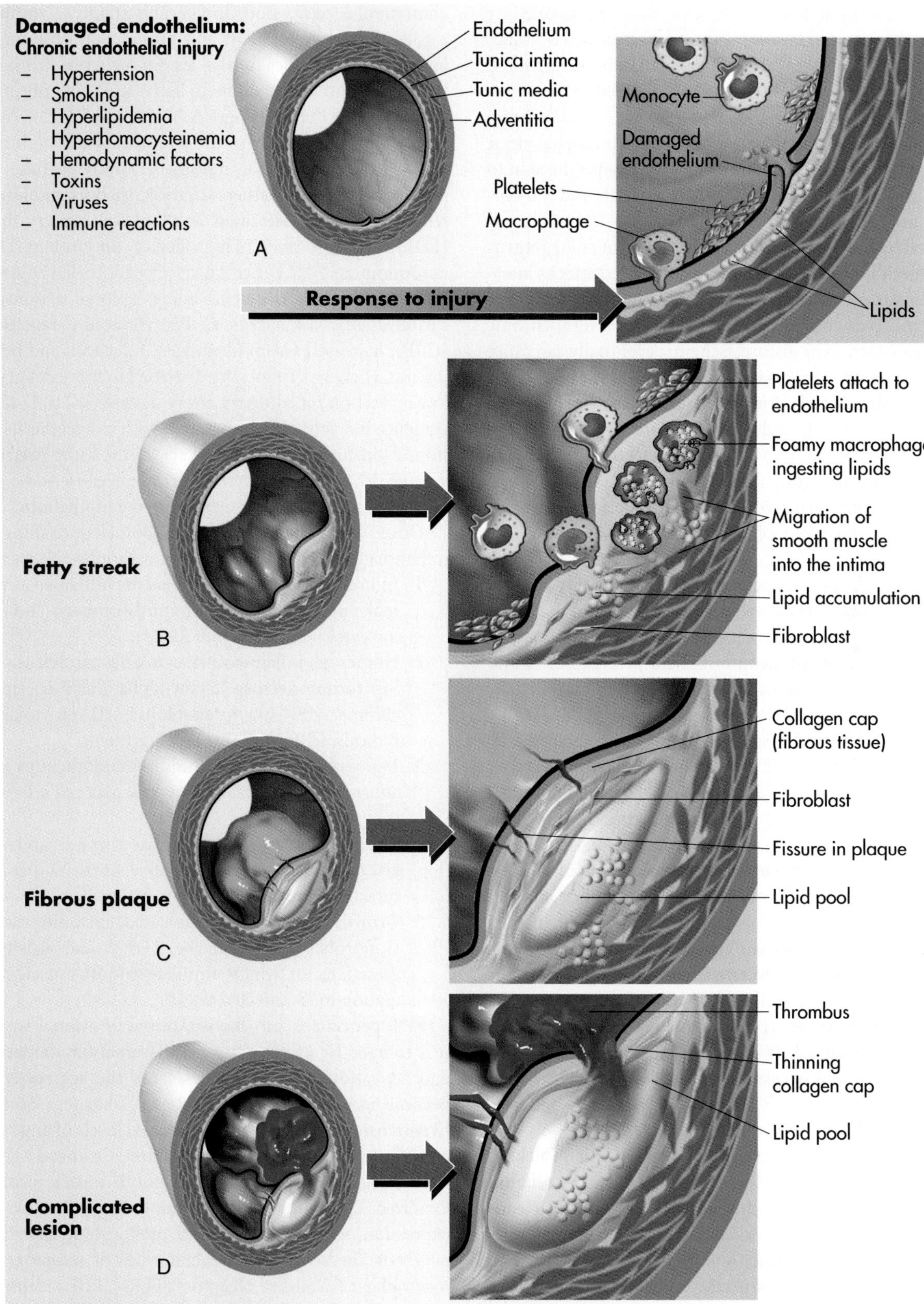

FIGURE 32-12 Progression of Atherosclerosis. **A,** Damaged endothelium. **B,** Diagram of fatty streak and lipid core formation (see Figure 32-13 for a diagram of oxidized low-density lipoprotein [LDL]). **C,** Diagram of fibrous plaque. Raised plaques are visible: some are yellow; others are white. **D,** Diagram of complicated lesion; thrombus is red; collagen is blue. Plaque is complicated by red thrombus deposition.

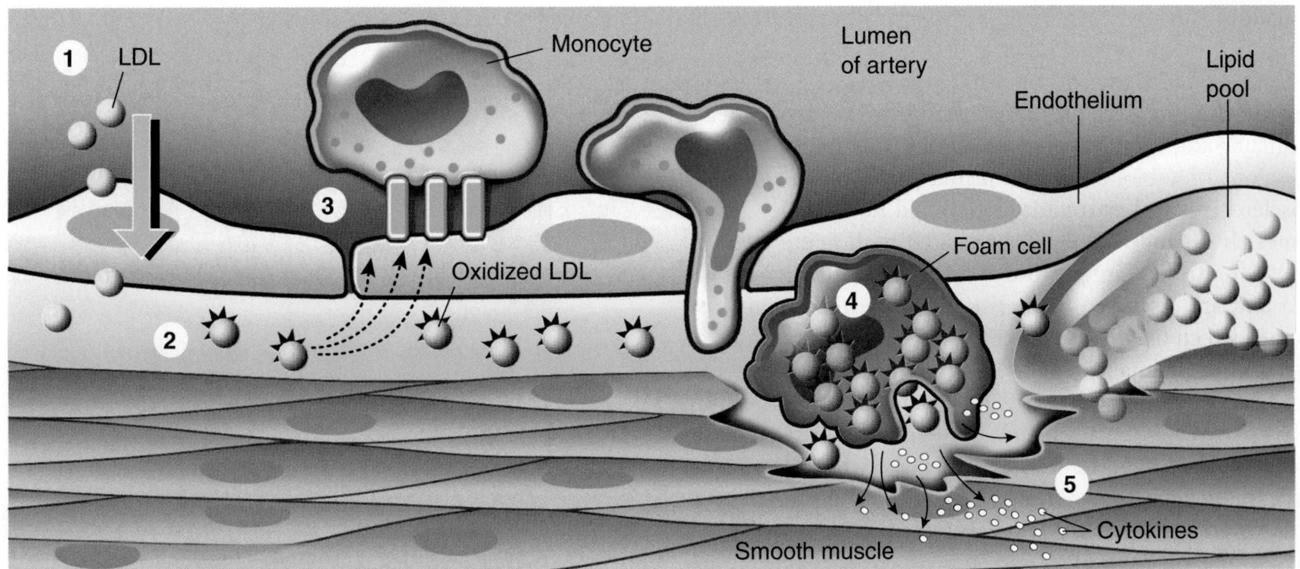

FIGURE 32-13 **Low-Density Lipoprotein Oxidation.** **(1)** Low-density lipoprotein (LDL) enters the arterial intima through an intact endothelium. In hypercholesterolemia, the influx of LDL exceeds the eliminating capacity and an extracellular pool of LDL is formed. This is enhanced by association of LDL with the extracellular matrix. **(2)** Intimal LDL is oxidized through the action of free oxygen radicals formed by enzymatic or nonenzymatic reactions. **(3)** This generates proinflammatory lipids that induce endothelial expression of the adhesion molecule; vascular cell adhesion molecule-1 activates complement and stimulates chemokine secretion. All of these factors cause adhesion and entry of mononuclear leukocytes, particularly monocytes and T lymphocytes. **(4)** Monocytes differentiate into macrophages. Macrophages up-regulate and internalize oxidized LDL and transform into foam cells. Macrophage update of oxidized LDL also leads to presentation of fragments of it to antigen-specific T cells. **(5)** This induces an autoimmune reaction that leads to production of proinflammatory cytokines. Such cytokines include interferon-gamma, tumor necrosis factor-alpha, and interleukin-1, which act on endothelial cells to stimulate expression of adhesion molecules and procoagulant activity; on macrophages to activate proteases, endocytosis, nitric oxide (NO), and cytokines; and on smooth muscle cells (SMCs) to include NO production and inhibit growth, collagen, and actin expression. (Modified from Crawford MH, DiMarco JP, Paulus WJ: *Cardiology, ed 3,* London, 2010, Mosby.)

people, even young children. Once formed, fatty streaks produce more toxic oxygen radicals and cause immunologic and inflammatory changes, resulting in progressive damage to the vessel wall. At this point, smooth muscle cells proliferate, produce collagen, and migrate over the fatty streak forming a **fibrous plaque** (see Figure 32-12). This process is mediated by many inflammatory cytokines, including growth factors (e.g., TGF-β).[84] The fibrous plaque may calcify, protrude into the vessel lumen, and obstruct blood flow to distal tissues, especially during exercise, which may cause symptoms (e.g., angina or intermittent claudication).

Many plaques, however, are "unstable," meaning they are prone to rupture even before they affect blood flow and are clinically silent until they rupture. Plaque rupture occurs because of the inflammatory activation of proteinases (matrix metalloproteinases and cathepsins), apoptosis of cells within the plaque, and bleeding within the lesion (plaque hemorrhage).[85] Plaques that have ruptured are called **complicated plaques** (see Figure 32-12). Once rupture occurs, exposure of underlying tissue results in platelet adhesion, initiation of the clotting cascade, and rapid thrombus formation that may suddenly occlude the affected vessel, resulting in ischemia and infarction. Aspirin or other antithrombotic agents are used to prevent this complication of atherosclerotic disease.

CLINICAL MANIFESTATIONS. Atherosclerosis presents with symptoms and signs that result from inadequate tissue perfusion because of obstruction of the vessels that supply them. Partial vessel obstruction may lead to transient ischemic events, often associated with exercise or stress. Once the lesion becomes complicated, increasing obstruction with superimposed thrombosis may result in tissue infarction. CAD caused by atherosclerosis is the major cause of myocardial ischemia and is one of the most important health issues in the United States. Atherosclerotic obstruction of the vessels supplying the brain is the major cause of stroke. Similarly, any part of the body may become ischemic when its blood supply is compromised by atherosclerotic lesions. Often more than one vessel is involved with this disease process; consequently, an individual may present with symptoms from several ischemic tissues at the same time, and disease in one area may indicate that the individual is at risk for other ischemic complications elsewhere.

EVALUATION AND TREATMENT. In evaluating individuals for the presence of atherosclerosis, a complete health history (including risk factors and symptoms of ischemia) is essential. Physical examination may reveal arterial bruits and evidence of decreased blood flow to tissues. Laboratory tests include measurement of lipids, blood glucose, and high sensitivity CRP (hs-CRP). Judicious use of x-ray films, electrocardiography, ultrasonography, nuclear scanning, CT, MRI, and angiography may be necessary to identify affected vessels, particularly coronary vessels. New modalities aimed at identifying vulnerable plaques before the rupture are being evaluated.[86]

Current management of atherosclerosis is focused on detecting and treating preclinical lesions with drugs aimed at stabilizing and reversing plaques before they rupture.[87] Once a lesion obstructs blood flow, the primary goal in managing atherosclerosis is to restore adequate blood flow to the affected tissues. If an individual has presented with acute ischemia (e.g., MI, stroke), interventions are specific to the diseased area and are discussed further under those topics. In situations in which the disease process does not require immediate intervention, management focuses on reducing risk factors, removing the initial causes of vessel damage, and preventing lesion progression. This includes exercise, smoking cessation, and control of hypertension and diabetes when appropriate while reducing LDL cholesterol by diet or medications or both. (Management of atherosclerotic risk factors is discussed further starting on p. 1154.)

Peripheral Artery Disease

Peripheral artery disease (PAD) refers to atherosclerotic disease of arteries that perfuse the limbs, especially the lower extremities. PAD affects approximately 8 to 12 million Americans, 12% to 20% of whom are 65 years of age or older, and is associated with significant morbidity and mortality. Prevalence increases with age, and PAD disproportionately affects blacks.[5] The risk factors for PAD are the same as those for atherosclerotic disease, and it is especially prevalent in individuals who smoke and those with diabetes. PAD is a significant predictor of systemic atherosclerotic disease such that those with documented PAD have nearly double the risk of coronary artery disease than those without.

Lower-extremity ischemia, resulting from arterial obstruction in PAD, can be gradual or acute. In most individuals gradually increasing obstruction to arterial blood flow to the legs caused by atherosclerosis in the iliofemoral vessels results in pain with ambulation called **intermittent claudication.** However, only 10% of people with PAD have the classic symptom of intermittent claudication, and 40% do not complain of leg pain.[5] If a thrombus forms over the atherosclerotic lesion, perfusion can cease acutely with severe pain, loss of pulses, and skin color changes in the affected extremity.

Evaluation for PAD requires a careful history and physical examination that focuses on looking for evidence of atherosclerotic disease (e.g., bruits), ankle-brachial index, and noninvasive Doppler measurement of blood flow. Treatment includes risk factor reduction (smoking cessation and treatment of diabetes, hypertension, and dyslipidemia) and antiplatelet therapy. Symptomatic PAD should be managed with vasodilators in combination with antiplatelet or antithrombotic medications (aspirin, cilostazol, ticlopidine, or clopidogrel), cholesterol-lowering medications, and exercise rehabilitation.[88] If acute or refractory symptoms occur, emergent percutaneous or surgical revascularization may be indicated. Newer treatment modalities that are being explored include autologous stem cell therapies, gene therapy, and angiogenesis.[89,90]

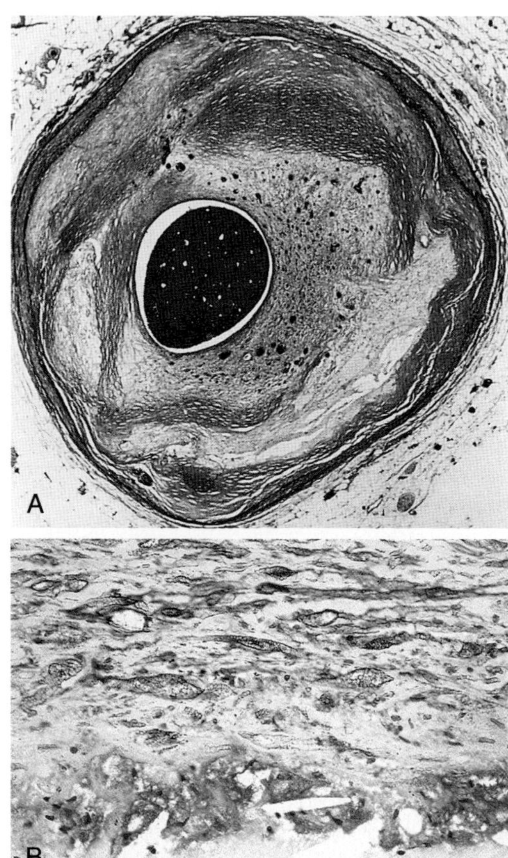

FIGURE 32-14 Atherosclerosis. **A,** Concentric coronary plaque. The lumen is central. Multiple new small blood vessels are shown within the plaque, the late result of disruption. **B,** Cell types in a fibrolipid plaque. The plaque cap (brownish) contains numerous elongated smooth muscle cells; some contain lipid. Macrophages are clustered on the edge of the core. (From Damjanov I, Linder J, editors: *Anderson's pathology,* ed 10, St Louis, 1996, Mosby.)

Coronary Artery Disease, Myocardial Ischemia, and Acute Coronary Syndromes

CAD, myocardial ischemia, and MI form a pathophysiologic continuum that impairs the pumping ability of the heart by depriving the heart muscle of blood-borne oxygen and nutrients. The earliest lesions of the continuum are those of **coronary artery disease (CAD)** which occludes the coronary arteries. By far the most common cause of coronary artery obstruction is atherosclerosis (Figure 32-14). CAD can diminish the myocardial blood supply until deprivation impairs myocardial metabolism enough to cause **ischemia,** a local state in which the cells are temporarily deprived of blood supply. They remain alive but cannot function normally. Persistent ischemia or the complete occlusion of a coronary artery causes **acute coronary syndrome. Infarction** (irreversible myocardial injury) constitutes the often-fatal event known as a *heart attack.*

Development of Coronary Artery Disease

The American Heart Association estimates that approximately 7% of the U.S. population older than age 20 years has CAD, resulting in approximately 610,000 new and 325,000 recurrent heart attacks each year (one every 25 seconds) causing 1 of every 6 deaths.[5]

TABLE 32-5 CRITERIA FOR DYSLIPIDEMIA

	OPTIMAL	NEAR OPTIMAL	DESIRABLE	LOW	BORDERLINE	HIGH	VERY HIGH
Total cholesterol			<200		200-239	≥240	
LDL	<100	100-129			130-159	160-189	≥190
Triglycerides			<150		150-199	200-499	≥500
HDL				<40		≥60	

Data from Expert Panel on Detection, Evaluation, and Treatment of High Blood Cholesterol in Adults, *JAMA* 285:2486-2497, 2001.
HDL, High-density lipoprotein; *LDL,* low-density lipoprotein.

Risk factors for CAD are the same as those for atherosclerosis and can be categorized as conventional (major) versus nontraditional (novel) and modifiable versus nonmodifiable. Much new information has been obtained about the conventional risk factors that has markedly improved the prevention and management of CAD.[91] In addition, the more recently identified nontraditional risk factors have provided insight in to the pathogenesis of CAD and may lead to more effective interventions.

Conventional or major risk factors for CAD that are nonmodifiable include: (1) advanced age, (2) male gender or women after menopause, and (3) family history. Aging and menopause are associated with increased exposure to risk factors and poor endothelial healing. Family history may contribute to CAD through genetics and shared environmental exposures. Many gene polymorphisms have been associated with CAD and its risk factors.[92] Blood type also has been linked to cardiovascular risk, with type O associated with the lowest risk and type AB the highest.[93]

Major modifiable conventional risks include: (1) dyslipidemia, (2) hypertension, (3) cigarette smoking, (4) diabetes and insulin resistance, (5) obesity, (6) sedentary lifestyle, and (7) an atherogenic diet. In individuals with known CAD, the majority have the growing epidemic of obesity in the United States. If individuals receive appropriate preventive care, modification of these factors can significantly reduce the risk for CAD. Of great concern is the finding that exposure to particulate matter air pollution is associated with an increase in myocardial infarction risk and air pollution is a worsening global problem.[94]

Dyslipidemia. The link between CAD and elevated plasma lipoprotein concentrations is well documented.[5] The term **lipoprotein** refers to lipids, phospholipids, cholesterol, and triglycerides bound to carrier proteins. Lipids (cholesterol in particular) are required by most cells for the manufacture and repair of plasma membranes. Cholesterol is also a necessary component for the manufacture of such essential substances as bile acids and steroid hormones. Although cholesterol can easily be obtained from dietary fat intake, most body cells also can manufacture cholesterol.

The cycle of lipid metabolism is complex. Dietary fat is packaged into particles known as **chylomicrons** in the small intestine. Chylomicrons are required for absorption of fat; they function by transporting exogenous lipid from the intestine to the liver and peripheral cells. Chylomicrons are the least dense of the lipoproteins and primarily contain triglyceride. Some of the triglyceride may be removed and either stored by adipose tissue or used by muscle as an energy source. The chylomicron remnants, composed mainly of cholesterol, are taken up by the liver. A series of chemical reactions in the liver results in the production of several lipoproteins that vary in density and function. These include **very-low-density lipoproteins (VLDLs),** primarily triglyceride and protein; **low-density lipoproteins (LDLs),** mostly cholesterol and protein; and **high-density lipoproteins (HDLs),** mainly phospholipids and protein.

Dyslipidemia (or **dyslipoproteinemia**) refers to abnormal concentrations of serum lipoproteins as defined by the Third Report of the National Cholesterol Education Program (Table 32-5).[95] It is estimated that nearly half of the U.S. population has some form of dyslipidemia, especially among white and Asian populations.[5] These abnormalities are the result of a combination of genetic and dietary factors. Primary or familial dyslipoproteinemias result from genetic defects that cause abnormalities in lipid-metabolizing enzymes and abnormal cellular lipid receptors (Table 32-6). Secondary causes of dyslipidemia include several common systemic disorders, such as diabetes, hypothyroidism, pancreatitis, and renal nephrosis, as well as the use of certain medications such as certain diuretics, beta-blockers, glucocorticoids, interferons, and antiretrovirals.

An increased serum concentration of LDL is a strong indicator of coronary risk. LDL is responsible for the delivery of cholesterol to the tissues. Serum levels of LDL are normally controlled by hepatic receptors for LDL that bind LDL and limit liver synthesis of this lipoprotein. High dietary intake of cholesterol and fats, often in combination with a genetic predisposition to accumulations of LDL in the serum (e.g., dysfunction of the hepatic LDL receptor), results in high levels of LDL in the bloodstream. LDL oxidation, migration into the vessel wall, and phagocytosis by macrophages are key steps in the pathogenesis of atherosclerosis (see p. 1145 and Figure 32-13). LDL also plays a role in endothelial injury, inflammation, and immune responses that have been identified as being important in atherogenesis.[79] The term LDL actually describes several types of LDL molecules. Measurement of LDL subfractions allows for better prediction of coronary risk. For example, LDL-C measurements allow for detection of the small dense LDL particles that are the most atherogenic, and apolipoprotein B (structural protein found in both LDL and VLDL) levels are a very strong predictor of future coronary events.[96]

Low levels of HDL cholesterol also are a strong indicator of coronary risk. HDL is responsible for "reverse cholesterol transport," which returns excess cholesterol from the tissues to the liver, where it binds to hepatic receptors (including the LDL receptor) and is processed and eliminated as bile or converted to cholesterol-containing steroids.[97] Recent evidence shows that

HDL can remove excess cholesterol from the arterial wall through several pathways, including mediating the efflux of cholesterol from lipid-laden macrophages (foam cells) through the activation of adenosine triphosphate (ATP)–binding cassette transporter proteins (ABC proteins).[98] This discovery has resulted in the initiation of a whole new area of pharmacologic investigation into optimizing HDL function. HDL also participates in endothelial repair and decreases thrombosis. As HDL cholesterol is transported, it progresses through three subtypes of HDL: pre-β HDL, HDL3, and HDL2. Apolipoprotein (ApoA-I) on the pre-β HDL

TABLE 32-6 FAMILIAL DYSLIPOPROTEINEMIAS

NAME	LABORATORY FINDINGS	CLINICAL FEATURES	THERAPY
Type I: exogenous hyperlipidemia; fat-induced hypertriglyceridemia	Cholesterol normal Triglycerides increased three times Chylomicrons increased	Abdominal pain Hepatosplenomegaly Skin and retinal lipid deposits Usual onset: childhood	Low-fat diet
Type IIa: hypercholesterolemia	Triglycerides normal LDL increased Cholesterol increased	Premature vascular disease Xanthomas of tendons and bony prominences Common Onset: all ages	Low-saturated-fat and low-cholesterol diet Cholestyramine[a] Colestipol[b] Lovastatin[c] Nicotinic acid[d] Neomycin[e] Intestinal bypass
Type IIb: combined hyperlipidemia; carbohydrate-induced hypertriglyceridemia	LDL, VLDL increased Cholesterol increased Triglycerides increased	Same as IIa	Same as IIa; *plus* carbohydrate restriction Clofibrate[f] Gemfibrozil[g] Lovastatin
Type III: dysbetalipoproteinemia	IDL or chylomicron remnants increased Cholesterol increased Triglycerides increased	Premature vascular disease Xanthomas of tendons and bony prominences Uncommon Onset: adulthood	Weight control Low-carbohydrate, low-saturated-fat, and low-cholesterol diet Alcohol restriction Clofibrate Gemfibrozil Lovastatin Nicotinic acid Estrogens[h] Intestinal bypass
Type IV: endogenous hyperlipidemia; carbohydrate-induced hypertriglyceridemia	Glucose intolerance Hyperuricemia Cholesterol normal or increased VLDL increased Triglycerides increased	Premature vascular disease Skin lipid deposits Obesity Hepatomegaly Common onset: adulthood	Weight control Low-carbohydrate diet Alcohol restriction Clofibrate Nicotinic acid Intestinal bypass
Type V: mixed hyperlipidemia; carbohydrate and fat-induced hypertriglyceridemia	Glucose intolerance Hyperuricemia Chylomicrons increased VLDL increased LDL increased Cholesterol increased Triglycerides increased three times	Abdominal pain Hepatosplenomegaly Skin lipid deposits Retinal lipid deposits Onset: childhood	Weight control Low-carbohydrate and low-fat diet Clofibrate Lovastatin Nicotinic acid Progesterone[i] Intestinal bypass

IDL, Intermediate-density lipoprotein; *LDL,* low-density lipoprotein; *VLDL,* very-low-density lipoprotein.
[a]*Cholestyramine* (Questran), anion exchange resin; binds bile acids; enhances cholesterol excretion.
[b]*Colestipol* (Colestid), same as cholestyramine.
[c]*Lovastatin,* 3-hydroxy-3-methylglutaryl coenzyme A (HMG-CoA) reductase inhibitor; decreases cholesterol synthesis in the liver.
[d]*Nicotinic acid* (niacin), decreases release of free fatty acids from adipose tissue; increases lipogenesis in liver; decreases glucagon release; most effective for type V disorder.
[e]*Neomycin,* experimental medication; questionable mode of action; decreases LDLs.
[f]*Clofibrate* (Atromid-S), decreases release of free fatty acids from adipose tissue; decreases hepatic secretion of VLDL and increases catabolism of VLDL.
[g]*Gemfibrozil* (Lopid), similar to clofibrate but increases HDLs more.
[h]*Estrogens,* decrease IDL levels in type III disorders; experimental.
[i]*Progesterone,* decreases plasma triglycerides in type V disorders; experimental.

binds cholesterol where it is converted to cholesteryl ester creating HDL3. HDL3 then increases in size to form HDL2, which is fully loaded with cholesterol. The smaller HDL3 molecule is the most protective in preventing atherosclerosis, and research continues to explore the best approach to increasing this type of HDL.[79]

Despite the wealth of evidence that HDL plays an important role in preventing atherosclerotic coronary disease, studies have suggested that raising overall levels of HDL is not adequate to prevent cardiovascular disease. A study of individuals who have a rare genetic trait that increases their HDL levels dramatically failed to show any reduced cardiovascular risk in that population.[99] Furthermore, niacin and fibrates are drugs that can cause modest increases in HDL, but are not correlated with an improvement in cardiovascular risk in individuals without documented coronary disease (primary prevention) (see What's New? Controversies in the Use of Medications for the Primary Prevention of Cardiovascular Disease). Drugs that are being developed are aimed specifically at increasing HDL and include recombinant apolipoprotein A-I (ApoA-I) mimetics, thiazolidinediones (used to treat diabetes), and cholesteryl ester transfer protein inhibitors, although their effectiveness in preventing heart disease and their safety are still being evaluated.[100] At present, experts recommend exercise, weight loss, fish oil consumption, and moderate alcohol to increase HDL levels.

Other lipoproteins associated with increased cardiovascular risk include elevated serum VLDL (triglycerides) and increased lipoprotein (a). Triglycerides are associated with an increased risk for CAD, especially in combination with other risk factors such as diabetes.[101] Because of this, the measurement of "non-HDL cholesterol" (LDL plus VLDL) is frequently used to assess cardiovascular risk rather than just LDL or HDL levels alone. **Lipoprotein (a) (Lp[a])** is a genetically determined molecular complex between LDL and a serum glycoprotein called apoprotein (a) that has been shown to be an important risk factor for coronary atherosclerosis, especially in women.[102]

Hypertension. Hypertension is responsible for a two- to threefold increased risk of atherosclerotic cardiovascular disease including MI.[103] It contributes to endothelial injury, a key step in atherogenesis (see p. 1145), and causes myocardial hypertrophy, which increases myocardial demand for coronary flow. The overactivity of the SNS and RAAS commonly found in hypertension also contributes to the genesis of coronary artery disease. Drugs that block the effects of the SNS and RAAS to treat hypertension have many positive effects on the vasculature.

Cigarette Smoking. Direct and passive (environmental) smoking increase the risk of CAD. The mechanism by which smoking increases atherosclerosis is uncertain. Nicotine stimulates the release of catecholamines (epinephrine and norepinephrine), which increases heart rate and causes peripheral vascular constriction. As a result blood pressure increases, as do cardiac workload and oxygen demand. Cigarette smoking is associated with an increase in LDL and a decrease in HDL, and contributes to vessel inflammation and thrombosis. The risk of CAD increases with heavy smoking and decreases when smoking is stopped.

Diabetes Mellitus. Diabetes mellitus and insulin resistance are extremely important risk factors for CAD. Insulin resistance, hyperinsulinemia, and hyperglycemia have multiple effects on the cardiovascular system. These effects can include endothelial damage, thickening of the vessel wall, increased inflammation and leukocyte adhesion, increased thrombosis, glycation of vascular proteins, and decreased production of endothelial-derived vasodilators such as nitric oxide[104,105] (diabetes and atherogenesis are described in more detail in Chapter 22). Diabetes is also associated with dyslipidemia because of the resulting alteration of hepatic lipoprotein synthesis and increases triglycerides and in LDL oxidation.[106] Aggressive management of this additional risk factor can significantly improve CAD risk in individuals with diabetes.

Obesity and Sedentary Lifestyle. It is estimated that nearly two thirds of the U.S. adult population is overweight or obese

WHAT'S NEW?

Controversies in the Use of Medications for the Primary Prevention of Cardiovascular Disease

Despite clear evidence for the benefit of the use of medications to improve lipid levels in individuals who already have documented atherosclerotic disease (secondary prevention), primary prevention of cardiovascular disease through pharmacologic modulation of lipid levels remains controversial. Although some clinical trials and meta-analyses have shown a reduction in primary cardiovascular events with the use of the 3-hydroxy-3-methyl-glutaryl-CoA (HMG-CoA) reductase drugs (statins), niacin, and other cholesterol-lowering medications, other studies have provided mixed results, especially in women. In addition, statin use is linked to several significant complications including muscle soreness, elevation in liver enzymes, cognitive impairment, and diabetes. For example, in a recent large study exploring the role of statins in primary prevention, statin therapy lowered low-density lipoprotein (LDL) and C-reactive protein and reduced overall cardiovascular risk by 39% and overall mortality by 17%. But it also increased the risk for diabetes by 28% among individuals with risk factors for diabetes at baseline. Overall, women demonstrate less cardiovascular benefit than men, and have no improvement in mortality with the use of statins for primary prevention. The ability to weigh the risks and benefits of medication use for primary prevention is complicated by these mixed results.

Low levels of high-density lipoprotein (HDL) also have been strongly correlated with increased cardiovascular risk, yet several primary prevention trials in which drugs such as niacin and fibrates raised HDL levels failed to demonstrate benefit. In fact, use of the cholesteryl ester transfer protein (CETP) inhibitor torcetrapib, which is highly effective at increasing HDL levels, actually resulted in an increase in cardiovascular risk. Subsequent clinical studies found that this adverse risk response to torcetrapib was "molecule specific" and independent of its CETP inhibition effect. The other two CETP inhibitors, dalcetrapib and anacetrapib, have so far been well tolerated in phase I and II clinical trials and do not adversely affect blood pressure and aldosterone as torcetrapib did. It is clear from these studies that despite decades of research, there is still much work needed to fully understand the proper role of medications in the prevention of cardiovascular disease.

Data from Badimon L, Vilahur G: *Ann N Y Acad Sci* (1):18–32, 2012; Boden WE et al: *N Engl J Med* 365(24):2255–2267, 2011; Cholesterol Treatment Trialists' (CTT) Collaborators: *Lancet* 380:581–590, 2012; Gutierrez J et al: *Arch Intern Med* 172(12):909–919, 2012; Johns DG et al: *Drugs* 72(4):491–507, 2012; Michos ED et al: *J Am Coll Cardiol* 59(23):2058–2064, 2012; Prasad V, Vandross A: *Arch Intern Med* 172(8):656–659, 2012; Ridker PM et al: *Lancet* 380:565–571, 2012; Sampson UK, Fazio S, Linton MF: *Curr Atheroscler Rep* 14(1):1–10, 2012.

resulting in a much increased risk for CAD and stroke. An estimated 47 million residents have a combination of obesity, dyslipidemia, and hypertension (called **metabolic syndrome**) (see Chapter 22), which is associated with an even higher risk for CAD events.[107] Obesity is caused by genetics, diet, and inadequate physical exercise. Abdominal obesity has the strongest link with increased CAD risk and is related to insulin resistance, decreased HDL, increased blood pressure, and inflammation.[108] Obesity also is associated with changes in the adipokines (see following) that affect cardiovascular risk. A sedentary lifestyle not only increases the risk of obesity but also has an independent effect on increasing CAD risk. Physical activity and weight loss offer substantial reductions in risk factors for CAD. There is emerging evidence that bariatric surgery procedures, such as gastric bypass, can provide sustained improvement in risk factors for cardiovascular disease such as hypertension, dyslipidemia, and diabetes[109,110] (see What's New? Cardiovascular Risk Reduction with Bariatric Surgery).

Nontraditional Risk Factors. Nontraditional, or novel, risk factors for CAD include: (1) increased serum markers for inflammation and thrombosis, (2) troponin I, (3) hyperhomocysteinemia, (4) adipokines, (5) infection, (6) air pollution, and (7) coronary artery calcification and carotid wall thickness. The amount of risk conferred by these relatively newly identified factors is still being explored, although the preponderance of evidence suggests that the traditional risk factors continue to be more predictive of cardiovascular disease and should remain the focus of risk factor reduction efforts.[111]

Markers of Inflammation and Thrombosis. Of the numerous markers of inflammation that have been linked to an increase in CAD risk (hs-CRP, fibrinogen, protein C, plasminogen activator inhibitor), the relationship between serum levels of CRP and CAD has been explored in the greatest depth. **Highly sensitive C-reactive protein (hs-CRP)** is an acute phase reactant or protein mostly synthesized in the liver and is an indirect measure of atherosclerotic plaque-related inflammation. Elevated levels of hs-CRP are associated with numerous other CAD risk factors including smoking, obesity, and diabetes, and have been found to be an independent risk factor for coronary disease. However, as a nonspecific serum marker for inflammation, its utility as a screening tool for cardiovascular risk continues to be debated. A recent study demonstrated that hs-CRP levels can be used to better assign individuals into cardiovascular risk categories that aid in decision-making about pharmacologic interventions for individuals with other risk factors for coronary disease.[112] Other markers of inflammation associated with CAD include erythrocyte sedimentation rate, von Willebrand factor concentration, uric acid, IL-6, IL-18, TNF-α, fibrinogen, and YKL-40 is a 40 kDa (mass) glycoprotein produced by inflammatory cells, cancer cells, and stem cells.

Troponin I. Troponin I (TnI) is a serum protein whose measurement is used as a sensitive and specific diagnostic test to help identify myocardial injury during acute coronary syndromes. Highly sensitive TnI assays are used in individuals without a history of CAD to assess risk for future CHD events, mortality, and heart failure.[96]

Hyperhomocysteinemia. Hyperhomocysteinemia occurs because of a genetic lack of the enzyme that breaks down homocysteine (an amino acid) or because of a nutritional deficiency of folate, cobalamin (vitamin B_{12}), or pyridoxine (vitamin B_6). Although it has not been identified by the AHA as a major risk factor for CAD, hyperhomocysteinemia is associated with increased LDL oxidation, decreased endogenous vasodilators, increased smooth muscle proliferation, and an increased tendency for thrombosis. Elevated levels of homocysteine may interact with other risk factors (such as dyslipidemia and hypertension) in certain populations to further increase coronary risk.[113] Routine serum measurement of homocysteine is not currently recommended, and prevention and management have been focused on increasing the dietary intake of folate and B vitamins. Unfortunately, no controlled treatment study has shown that folic acid supplements reduce the risk of atherosclerosis or that taking these vitamins affects the development or recurrence of cardiovascular disease.

Adipokines. Adipokines are a group of hormones released from adipose cells. The two that are most studied are adiponectin and leptin. Leptin is primarily implicated in obesity, hypertension, and diabetes (see p. 1134) but is also being explored as a factor in autoimmune responses affecting blood vessels.[114] Decreased adiponectin in obese individuals has been linked to a significant increase in cardiovascular risk. Its antiatherogenic effects include

WHAT'S NEW?

Cardiovascular Risk Reduction with Bariatric Surgery

With the devastating increase in obesity-related diabetes and cardiovascular disease, bariatric surgical procedures for weight loss are being used in more and more individuals. Although there are surgery-related risks, including bleeding, leakage at the surgical site, and hernias, the number of bariatric procedures is increasing rapidly, and safer surgical techniques are being developed. Bariatric surgery has been shown to be effective in reversing diabetes, metabolic syndrome, hypertension, and dyslipidemia with associated risk reduction for cardiovascular disease. For example, one large study documented a 72% reversal of diabetes with gastric bypass surgery as compared to 21% of those who underwent medically managed weight loss. Similarly, more than 80% of individuals with dyslipidemia treated with surgery were found to have significant improvements in low-density lipoprotein, high-density lipoprotein, and triglycerides such that they were able to discontinue their drug regimens. These changes have been found to be sustained (over 6 years) in a large proportion of surgically treated individuals. Although approximately 7% of weight is regained, and some individuals have recurrence of their diabetes, overall mortality is reduced after bariatric surgery as compared with medically managed weight loss. The American Heart Association recommends bariatric surgery for individuals who have severe obesity in whom efforts at medical therapy have failed and an acceptable operative risk is present.

Data from Adams TD et al: *JAMA* 308(11):1122–1131, 2012; Apovian CM, Gokce N: *Circulation* 125(9):1178–1182, 2012; Benraouane F, Litwin SE: *Curr Opin Cardiol* 26(6):555–561, 2011; Mingrone G et al: *N Engl J Med* 366(17):1577–1585, 2012; Olbers T, Svensson PA, Carlsson LM: *JAMA* 307(1):56–65, 2012; Poirier P et al: *Circulation* 123(15):1683–1701, 2011; Sjostrom L et al: *N Engl J Med* 366(17):1567–1576, 2012.

anti-inflammatory, insulin-sensitizing enhancement of nitric oxide generation, attenuation of reactive oxygen species production in endothelial cells, and reduced vascular smooth muscle cell proliferation.[115] A more recently described adipokine is resistin, which has been linked to inflammation, endothelial dysfunction, thrombosis, and smooth muscle cell dysfunction.[116] Emerging evidence suggests that adipokine changes occurring in perivascular adipose cells may play a significant role in metabolic and vascular disorders.[117] Weight loss and exercise improve adipokine levels and are correlated with improved cardiovascular risk.

Infection. Infections with various microorganisms, including *Chlamydia pneumoniae, Helicobacter pylori*, and cytomegalovirus, have been linked to an increased risk for CAD, although cause and effect have not been proven. Periodontal disease also has been linked to an increased risk for CAD.[118] One hypothesis is that systemic infection results in increased inflammation of vessels and therefore contributes to vascular disease. Unfortunately, the use of antibiotics for the prevention and treatment of CAD has not yielded consistently positive results.

Air Pollution. Exposure to air pollution, especially roadway exposures, is strongly correlated with coronary risk. It is postulated that toxins in pollution contribute to macrophage activation, oxidation of LDL, thrombosis, and inflammation of vessel walls.[119]

Coronary Artery Calcification (CAC) and Carotid Artery Wall Thickness (*CAWT*). Coronary risk related to changes in vessel walls can be assessed using various types of vascular imaging techniques. CAC, as detected by CT scanning, and CIMT, as detected by ultrasonography, are two important imaging modalities in widespread use for determining coronary heart disease risk.[120,121]

Myocardial Ischemia

PATHOPHYSIOLOGY. The coronary arteries normally supply blood flow sufficient to meet the demands of the myocardium as it labors under varying workloads. Oxygen extraction from these vessels occurs with maximal efficiency. If efficient exchange does not meet myocardial oxygen needs, healthy coronary arteries are able to dilate to increase the flow of oxygenated blood to the myocardium. Narrowing of a major coronary artery by more than 50% impairs blood flow sufficiently to hamper cellular metabolism under conditions of increased myocardial demand (see Figure 32-14).

Myocardial ischemia develops if the supply of coronary blood cannot meet the demand of the myocardium for oxygen and nutrients. Imbalances between myocardial demand and coronary blood supply can result from a number of conditions. Common causes of increased myocardial demand for blood include tachycardia, exercise, hypertension (hypertrophy), and valvular disease. The most common cause of decreased coronary blood flow and resultant myocardial ischemia is the formation of atherosclerotic plaques in the coronary circulation. As the plaque increases in size, it may partially occlude the vessel lumina, thus limiting coronary flow and causing ischemia especially during exercise. Some plaques are "unstable," meaning they are prone to ulceration or rupture (see p. 1156 and Figure 32-20). When this ulceration or rupture occurs, underlying tissues of the vessel wall are exposed, resulting in platelet adhesion and thrombus formation. Thrombus formation can suddenly cut off blood supply to the heart muscle, resulting in acute myocardial ischemia, and if the vessel obstruction cannot be reversed rapidly, ischemia will progress to infarction. Myocardial ischemia also can result from other causes of decreased blood and oxygen delivery to the myocardium, such as coronary spasm, hypotension, dysrhythmias, and decreased oxygen-carrying capacity of the blood (anemia, hypoxemia).

Myocardial cells become ischemic within 10 seconds of coronary occlusion. After several minutes the heart cells lose the ability to contract, and cardiac output decreases. Ischemia also causes conduction abnormalities that lead to changes in the electrocardiogram and may initiate dysrhythmias. Anaerobic processes take over, and lactic acid accumulates. Cardiac cells remain viable for approximately 20 minutes under ischemic conditions. If blood flow is restored, aerobic metabolism resumes, contractility is restored, and cellular repair begins. If the coronary artery occlusion persists beyond 20 minutes, MI occurs (Figure 32-15).

CLINICAL MANIFESTATIONS. Individuals with reversible myocardial ischemia present clinically in several ways. Chronic coronary

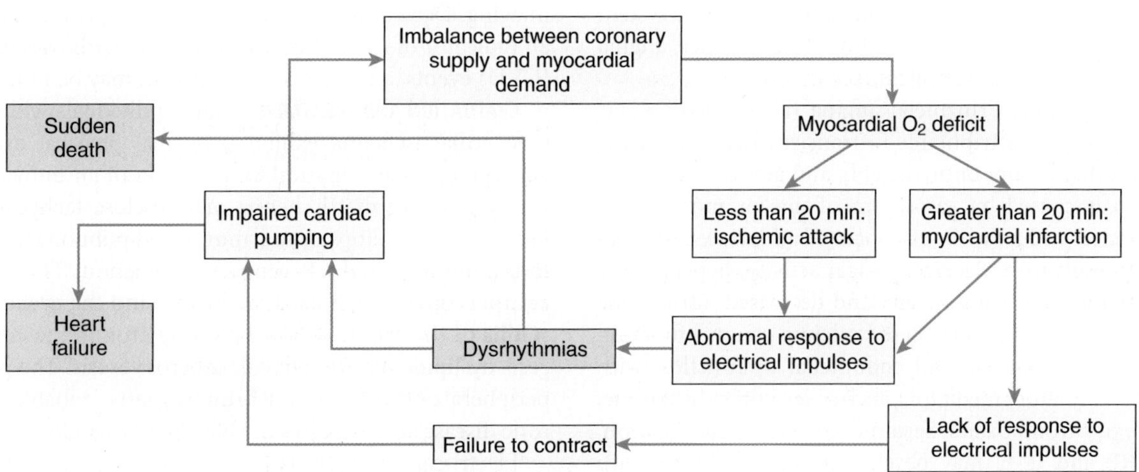

FIGURE 32-15 Cycle of Ischemic Events.

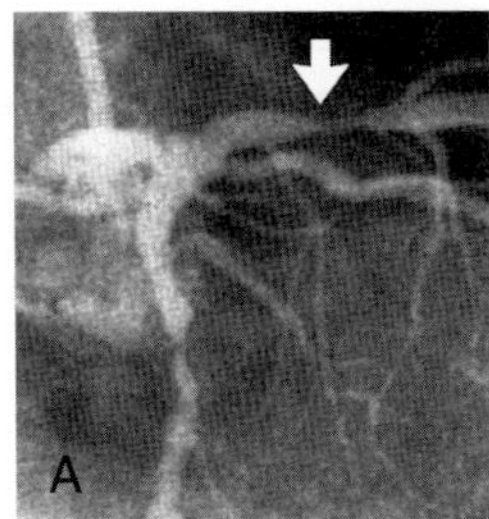

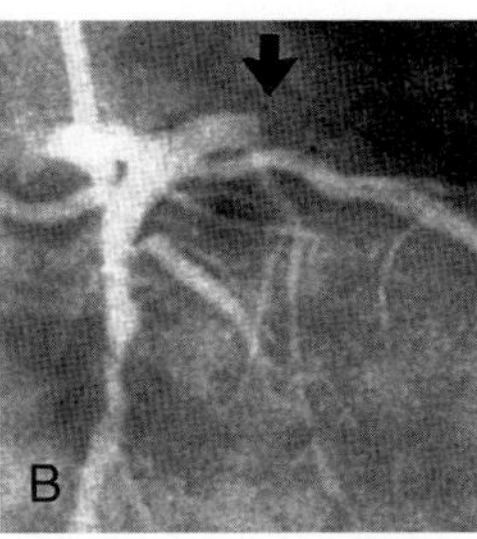

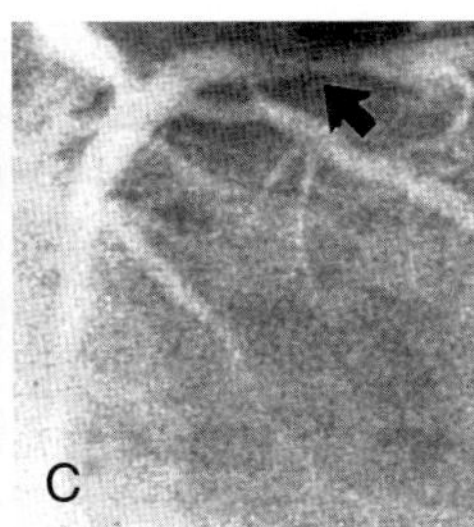

FIGURE 32-16 Angiogram. **A,** Baseline (*arrow* points to narrowing). **B,** Transient total occlusion of left anterior descending branch of the left coronary artery after mental stress *(arrow)*. **C,** After administration of nitrates and nifedipine, artery reopened to same diameter as baseline *(arrow)*. (From Stern S, editor: *Silent myocardial ischemia,* St Louis, 1998, Mosby.)

obstruction usually results in recurrent predictable chest pain called **stable angina.** Abnormal vasospasm of coronary vessels results in unpredictable chest pain called **Prinzmetal angina.** Myocardial ischemia that does not cause detectable symptoms is called **silent ischemia.**

Stable Angina. Angina pectoris is chest pain caused by myocardial ischemia. Stable angina is caused by gradual luminal narrowing and hardening of the arterial walls, so that affected vessels cannot dilate in response to increased myocardial demand associated with physical exertion or emotional stress. If demand is decreased, no necrosis of myocardial cells results. **Angina pectoris** is typically experienced as transient substernal chest discomfort, ranging from a sensation of heaviness or pressure to moderately severe pain. Individuals often describe the sensation by clenching a fist over the left sternal border. The discomfort may be mistaken for indigestion. The pain is caused by the buildup of lactic acid or abnormal stretching of the ischemic myocardium that irritates myocardial nerve fibers. These afferent sympathetic fibers enter the spinal cord from levels C3 to T4, accounting for the variety of locations and radiation patterns of anginal pain. Pain may radiate to the neck, lower jaw, left arm, and left shoulder or occasionally to the back or down the right arm. Pallor, diaphoresis, and dyspnea may be associated with the pain. The pain is usually relieved by rest and nitrates; lack of relief indicates an individual may be developing infarction.

Myocardial ischemia in women may not present with typical anginal pain. Common symptoms in women include atypical chest pain, palpitations, sense of unease, and severe fatigue. Similarly, in individuals who have autonomic nervous system dysfunction, such as older adults or those with diabetes, angina may be mild, atypical, or even silent (see following).

Prinzmetal Angina. Prinzmetal angina (also called variant angina) is chest pain attributable to transient ischemia of the myocardium that occurs unpredictably and almost exclusively at rest. Pain is caused by vasospasm of one or more major coronary arteries with or without associated atherosclerosis. The angina may result from decreased vagal activity, hyperactivity of the sympathetic nervous system, and decreased nitric oxide activity. Other causes include altered calcium channel function in arterial smooth muscle and endothelial dysfunction with release of inflammatory mediators, such as serotonin, histamine, endothelin, or thromboxane. Serum markers of inflammation, such as CRP and IL-6, may be elevated in individuals with this form of angina. The pain often occurs at night during rapid eye movement sleep and may have a cyclic pattern of occurrence. If the spasm persists long enough, infarction or serious dysrhythmias may occur. However, most individuals are successfully treated with vasodilators and overall prognosis is good.[122]

Silent Ischemia and Mental Stress (Induced Ischemia). Myocardial ischemia does not always cause angina and may be associated only with nonspecific symptoms such as fatigue, dyspnea, or feeling of unease. Some individuals only have silent ischemia, whereas episodes of silent myocardial ischemia may occur in individuals who also experience angina. Silent ischemia and atypical symptoms are more common in women, although the pathophysiologic mechanisms are poorly understood.[123] Global or regional abnormalities in left ventricular sympathetic afferent innervation have been implicated in autonomic dysfunction in diabetes mellitus, following surgical denervation during coronary artery bypass grafting (CABG) or cardiac transplantation, or following ischemic local nerve injury by MI.[124] Silent ischemia also may occur in some individuals during mental stress (Figures 32-16 and 32-17). Mental stress has been linked to increased markers of inflammation, such as CRP, decreased activity of vasodilators, such as nitric oxide, and a hypercoagulable state that may contribute to acute ischemic events.[125] Although stress management has been associated with a reduction in CAD events in men, further research into the brain-heart pathways is under way to better elucidate appropriate interventions.

Screening for silent ischemia is based on the presence of risk factors and is most often detected using stress radionucleotide imaging. Detection of silent ischemia is important because it is an indicator of increased risk for serious cardiovascular disease (CVD) events, and aggressive treatment may be indicated.[124]

EVALUATION AND TREATMENT. Many individuals with reversible myocardial ischemia exhibit a normal physical examination between episodes. Physical examination of an individual experiencing myocardial ischemia may disclose tachycardia, extra heart sounds (gallops or murmurs), and pulmonary congestion indicating impaired left ventricular function. The presence of **xanthelasmas** (small fat deposits) around the eyelids or **arcus senilis** of the eyes (a yellow lipid ring around the cornea) suggests dyslipidemia and possible atherosclerosis. The presence of peripheral or carotid arterial bruits suggests probable atherosclerotic disease and increases the likelihood that CAD is present.

Electrocardiography is a critical tool for diagnosing myocardial ischemia. Because many individuals have normal ECGs

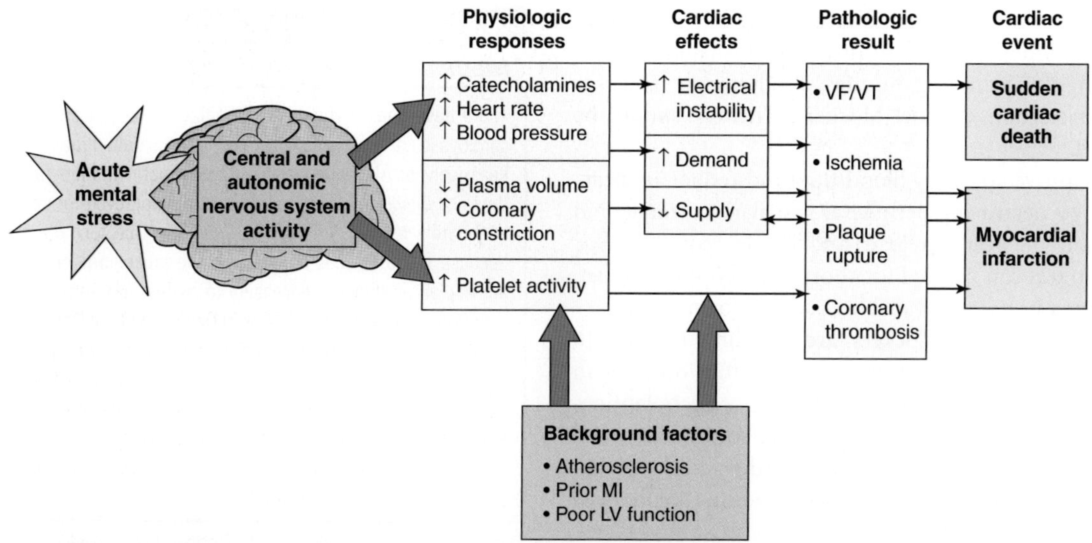

FIGURE 32-17 **Pathophysiologic Model of Acute Stress Effects Triggering Cardiac Clinical Events.** Acting via the central and autonomic nervous systems, stress can produce a cascade of physiologic responses that may lead to myocardial ischemia, potentially fatal dysrhythmia, plaque rupture, or coronary thrombosis. *LV,* Left ventricular; *MI,* myocardial infarction; *VF,* ventricular fibrillation; *VT,* ventricular tachycardia. (From Kranz DS et al: Mental stress as a trigger of myocardial ischemia and infarction. In Deedwania PC, Tofler GH, editors: *Triggers and timing of cardiac events,* ed 2, London, 1996, Saunders.)

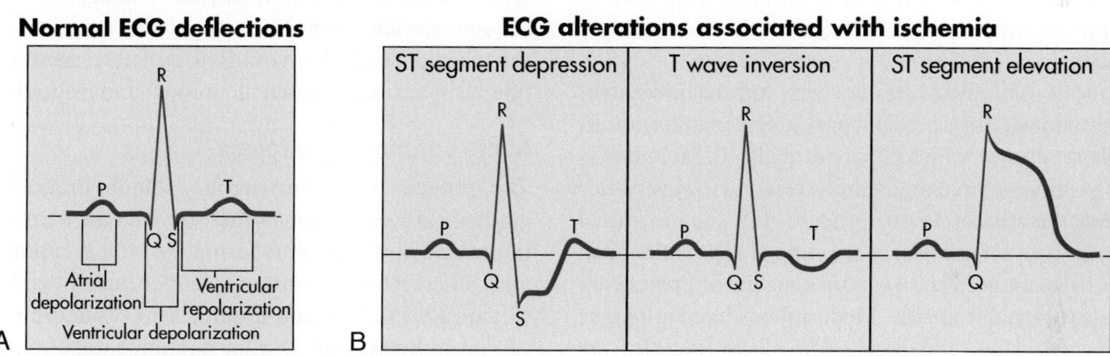

FIGURE 32-18 **Electrocardiogram (ECG) and Ischemia. A,** Normal ECG. **B,** Electrocardiographic alterations associated with ischemia.

in the absence of pain, diagnosis may require that electrocardiography be performed during an attack of angina. Transient ST-segment depression and T-wave inversion are characteristic signs of subendocardial ischemia frequently seen in angina. ST elevation, indicative of transmural ischemia, can be seen in individuals with Prinzmetal angina but is more common in infarction (Figure 32-18). The ECG also can give some indication of which coronary artery is involved. Approximately 30% of individuals with angina have nondiagnostic ECG tracings and require other diagnostic studies.

Stress radionucleotide imaging is indicated to detect ischemic changes in asymptomatic individuals with multiple risk factors for coronary disease, such as diabetes and dyslipidemia, and for older individuals who plan to start vigorous exercise. Stress testing is made more sensitive when radioisotope imaging is added to the ECG as an indicator of myocardial ischemia. Currently, the modality of choice for the diagnosis of myocardial ischemia is single-photon emission computed tomography (SPECT), which is effective at identifying ischemia and estimating risk for coronary events. Radioisotope imaging with thallium-201 and stress echocardiography also are used. Unfortunately, although all of these tests are helpful in documenting coronary obstruction, they cannot detect the presence of unstable plaques, which are the cause of the majority of acute coronary syndromes.

Imaging the coronary arteries for the evaluation of atherosclerotic plaques involves the use of CT with and without angiography, MRI, or intravascular ultrasound. Coronary angiography is useful in determining the anatomic extent of CAD. The procedure is expensive and carries some risk; thus it is used primarily to evaluate for possible percutaneous coronary intervention (PCI) or CABG surgery for individuals whose noninvasive studies suggest severe disease.

The primary aim of therapy for myocardial ischemia and angina is to increase delivery of oxygen by improving coronary artery blood flow and to reduce myocardial oxygen consumption. Recommendations for appropriate diet, exercise, and risk reduction strategies have been widely distributed. Coronary blood flow is improved by reversing vasoconstriction, preventing clotting, and reducing plaque growth and rupture. Myocardial oxygen consumption is reduced by manipulation of blood pressure, heart rate, contractility, and left ventricular volume. Many different classes of drugs are available to manage stable angina, including nitrates, β-adrenergic receptor blockers, and calcium channel blockers. Therapy should be individualized.[126,127]

Nitrates improve coronary blood flow and reduce myocardial demand by decreasing peripheral vascular resistance and venous return to the heart (preload) and thereby reduce cardiac workload. Nitrates can be used for short-term symptom relief, and long acting nitrates are available in several forms.[126]

β-Adrenergic receptor blockers are first-line therapy to reduce the myocardial oxygen requirements that occur with physical exertion. Beta-blockers diminish catecholamine-induced elevations of heart rate, myocardial contractility, and blood pressure. Reduction in heart rate provides additional diastolic filling time for coronary perfusion, leading to enhanced oxygen delivery to the heart.

Calcium channel blockers decrease the influx of calcium into myocardial cells and vascular smooth muscle cells. They also modify the pacemaker activity of the sinoatrial (SA) node and conduction properties of the atrioventricular (AV) node so that myocardial oxygen demand is reduced. However, short-acting formulations should be used with caution because of potentially harmful effects on cardiac contractility and heart rate.[126]

Combinations of nitrates, beta-blockers, and calcium antagonists may provide dramatic relief from clinical manifestations of ischemic heart disease, which improves quality of life and may make more invasive interventions unnecessary. However, they do not reverse the atherosclerotic process; thus the individual remains at risk for persistent or worsening CAD. Antianginal medications have not been shown to prolong life or prevent MI in individuals with stable angina. Medications aimed at plaque stabilization, regression, and prevention of clotting also are indicated in the majority of individuals. These include statins, ACE inhibitors or receptor blockers, and antithrombotics.[126]

Coronary revascularization is indicated for those individuals who do not respond adequately to antianginal drugs or who have high-risk atherosclerotic lesions. **Percutaneous coronary intervention (PCI)** is a procedure whereby stenotic (narrowed) coronary vessels are dilated with a catheter. Several different types of catheters can be used to open the blocked vessel. PCI is most often used to treat single-vessel disease, but it can be effective with multiple-vessel disease or restenosis of a coronary artery bypass graft in selected individuals. Restenosis of the artery is the major complication of the procedure; however, placement of a coronary stent can reduce this risk (see What's New? Medical Devices—Are They Safe and Effective?) Antithrombotic treatment such as aspirin, clopidogrel, or glycoprotein IIb/IIIa receptor antagonists after stenting also can improve outcomes.[128]

Severe CAD can be surgically treated by CABG, usually using the saphenous vein from the lower leg. In selected individuals, a modified CABG procedure called minimally invasive direct coronary artery bypass (MIDCAB) can be used with much less surgical morbidity and more rapid recovery. Investigational therapies for refractory angina that stimulate angiogenesis include transmyocardial laser revascularization (TMR), gene therapy for myocardial angiogenesis, spinal cord stimulation, laser revascularization, and percutaneous in situ coronary venous arterialization. New drugs being evaluated in the medical management of myocardial ischemic syndromes include ranolazine, trimetazidine, nicorandil, and ivabradine.[126]

WHAT'S NEW?

Medical Devices—Are They Safe and Effective?

There have been many medical technology advances for individuals with cardiovascular problems, such as stents, defibrillators, and mechanical heart valves. Although many of these treatments are lifesaving, many of these cardiovascular medical devices are approved for use before they are adequately tested. Although the same is true for numerous new drugs, because these devices require invasive procedures or because once they are implanted they are necessary to sustain life, they are considered high risk. Between January 1, 2000, and December 31, 2011, only 48% of devices were tested using an active control group prior to approval by the U.S. Food and Drug Administration (FDA) and 35% were approved without any control group at all. Thus about half of high-risk cardiac devices were approved without determining if they provide better outcomes than other treatments. As more devices are approved, concern is increasing about the relative risks and benefits of these interventions.

Data from Chen CE, Dhruva SS, Redberg RF: *JAMA* 308(17):1740–1742, 2012; Goldberg NH et al: *JAMA* 305(17):1786–1789, 2011.

Acute Coronary Syndromes

The process of atherosclerotic plaque progression can be gradual. However, when there is sudden coronary obstruction caused by thrombus formation over a ruptured or ulcerated atherosclerotic plaque, acute coronary syndromes result (Figure 32-19). **Unstable angina** is the result of reversible myocardial ischemia and is a harbinger of impending infarction. **Myocardial infarction (MI)** results when prolonged ischemia causes irreversible damage to the heart muscle. MI can be further subdivided into **non–ST-elevation MI (non-STEMI)** and **ST-elevation MI (STEMI).** Sudden cardiac death can occur as a result of any of the acute coronary syndromes.

An atherosclerotic plaque that is prone to rupture is called "unstable" and has a core that is especially rich in deposited oxidized LDL and a thin fibrous cap (Figure 32-20). These unstable plaques may not extend into the lumen of the vessel and may be clinically silent until they rupture. Plaque disruption (ulceration or rupture) occurs because of shear forces, inflammation with release of multiple inflammatory mediators, secretion of macrophage-derived degradative enzymes, and apoptosis of cells at the edges of the lesions. Exposure of the plaque substrate activates the clotting cascade. In addition, platelet activation results in the release of coagulants and exposure of platelet glycoprotein IIb/IIIa surface receptors, resulting in further platelet aggregation and adherence. The resulting thrombus can form very quickly (Figure 32-21, *A*). Vessel obstruction is further exacerbated by the release of vasoconstrictors, such as thromboxane A2 and endothelin. The thrombus may break up before permanent myocyte damage has occurred (unstable angina) or it may cause prolonged ischemia with infarction of the heart muscle (myocardial infarction) (see Figure 32-21, *B*). Diagnostic tests aimed at identifying unstable plaques before they rupture include intravascular ultrasound or MRI, angioscopy, and spectroscopy. Medications such as statins, ACE inhibitors, and beta-blockers can help stabilize plaques and prevent rupture.

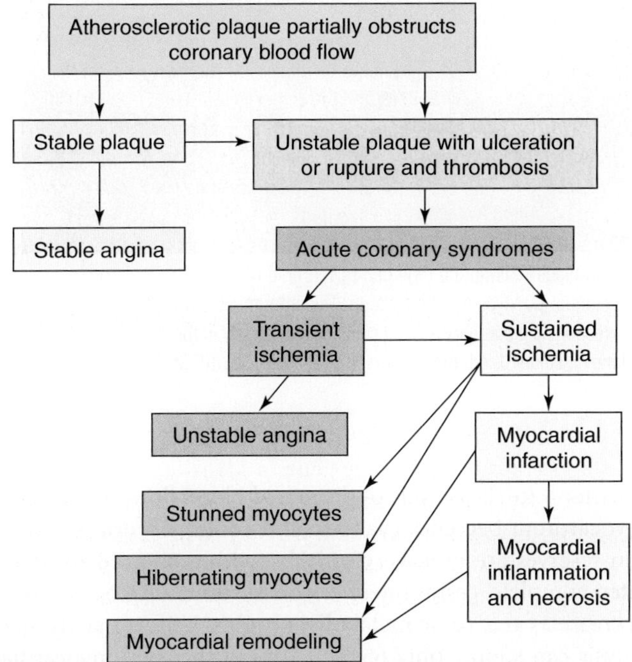

FIGURE 32-19 Pathophysiology of Acute Coronary Syndromes. The atherosclerotic process can lead to stable plaque formation and stable angina or can result in unstable plaques that are prone to rupture and thrombosis. Thrombus formation on a ruptured plaque that disperses in less than 20 minutes leads to transient ischemia and unstable angina. If the vessel obstruction is sustained, myocardial infarction with inflammation and necrosis of the myocardium result. In addition, myocardial infarction is associated with other structural and functional changes, including myocyte stunning and hibernation and myocardial remodeling.

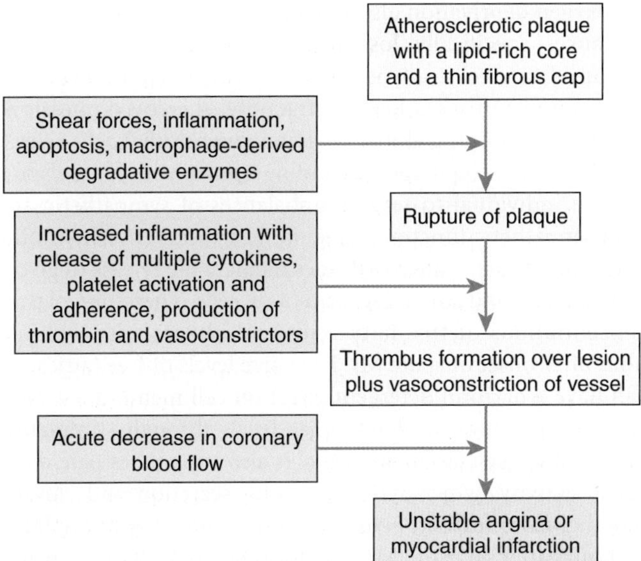

FIGURE 32-20 Pathogenesis of Unstable Plaques and Thrombus Formation.

Unstable Angina. Unstable angina is a form of acute coronary syndrome that results in reversible myocardial ischemia. It is important to recognize this syndrome because it signals that the atherosclerotic plaque has ruptured, and infarction may soon follow.

PATHOPHYSIOLOGY. Unstable angina occurs when fissuring or superficial erosion of the plaque leads to transient episodes of thrombotic vessel occlusion and vasoconstriction at the site of plaque damage. This thrombus is labile and occludes the vessel for no more than 10 to 20 minutes, with return of perfusion before significant myocardial necrosis occurs.

CLINICAL MANIFESTATIONS. Unstable angina presents as new-onset angina, angina that is occurring at rest, or angina that is increasing in severity or frequency (Box 32-1). Individuals may experience increased dyspnea, diaphoresis, and anxiety as the angina worsens.

EVALUATION AND MANAGEMENT. Physical examination may reveal evidence of ischemic myocardial dysfunction such as tachycardia or pulmonary congestion. The ECG most commonly reveals ST-segment depression and T-wave inversion during pain that resolves as the pain is relieved. The serum cardiac biomarkers (troponins, creatine phosphokinase-myocardial bound [CPK-MB] and lactate dehydrogenase [LDH1]) remain normal. Approximately 20% of people with unstable angina progress within hours to days to MI or death. Management of unstable angina requires immediate hospitalization with administration of oxygen, aspirin (if not contraindicated), nitrates, and morphine if pain is still present. Additional antithrombotic therapy with clopidogrel or IIb/IIIa platelet receptor antagonists may be indicated. Beta-blockers and ACE inhibitors also may be used. Anticoagulants, such as low-molecular-weight heparin, or direct thrombin inhibitors (e.g., fondaparinux) also can be given. Individuals with refractory angina and those with electrical or hemodynamic instability require immediate intervention with PCI or CABG.[129,130]

Myocardial Infarction. When coronary blood flow is interrupted for an extended period, myocyte necrosis occurs. This results in MI. In the majority of cases of MI, the decrease in coronary flow is the result of atherosclerotic CAD; other causes include coronary spasm and coronary artery embolism. Pathologically there are two major types of MI: subendocardial infarction and transmural infarction. Clinically, however, MI is categorized as non-STEMI or STEMI.

PATHOPHYSIOLOGY. Plaque progression, disruption, and subsequent clot formation is the same for myocardial infarction as it is for unstable angina (see Figures 32-19, 32-20, and 32-21). In this case, however, the thrombus is less labile and occludes the vessel for a prolonged period, such that myocardial ischemia progresses to myocyte necrosis and death. The duration of ischemia determines the size and character of the infarction.[131] If the thrombus breaks up before complete distal tissue necrosis has occurred, the infarction will involve only the myocardium directly beneath the endocardium (subendocardial MI). This infarction usually presents with ST depression and T-wave inversion and is termed non-STEMI. It is especially important to recognize this form of acute coronary syndrome because recurrent clot formation on the disrupted atherosclerotic

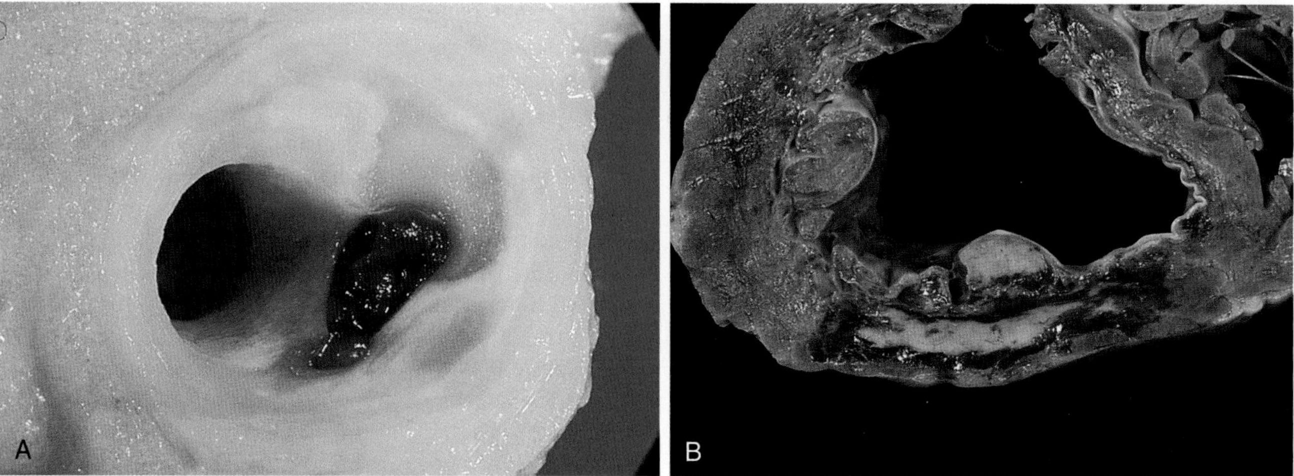

FIGURE 32-21 Plaque Disruption and Myocardial Infarction. A, Plaque disruption. The cap of the lipid-rich plaque has become torn with the formation of a thrombus, mostly inside the plaque. **B,** Myocardial infarction. This infarct is 6 days old. The center is yellow and necrotic with a hemorrhagic red rim. The responsible coronary artery occlusion is probably in the right coronary artery. The infarct is on the posterior wall. (From Damjanov I, Linder J, editors: *Anderson's pathology,* ed 10, St Louis, 1996, Mosby.)

BOX 32-1 THREE PRINCIPAL PRESENTATIONS OF UNSTABLE ANGINA

Rest angina*—angina occurring at rest and prolonged, usually >20 minutes
New-onset angina—new-onset angina of at least Canadian Cardiovascular Society (CCS) class III severity
Increasing angina—previously diagnosed angina that has become distinctly more frequent, longer in duration, or lower in threshold (i.e., increased by ≥1 CCS class to at least CCS class III severity)

From Anderson J et al: *J Am Coll Cardiol* 50:e1–e157, 2007. Originally adapted from Braunwald E: *Circulation* 80:410–414, 1989.
*Individuals with non–ST-elevation myocardial infarction (non-STEMI) usually present with angina at rest.

plaque is likely to occur unless some intervention is undertaken as soon as possible. If the thrombus lodges permanently in the vessel, the infarction will extend through the myocardium all the way from endocardium to epicardium (transmural MI), resulting in severe cardiac dysfunction. Transmural infarction usually causes marked elevations in the ST segments on ECG. Individuals with elevations are categorized as having STEMI. Clinically it is important to identify those with STEMI because they are at highest risk for serious complications and require immediate intervention.

Cellular Injury. Cardiac cells can withstand ischemic conditions for about 20 minutes before cellular death takes place. After only 30 to 60 seconds of hypoxia, ECG changes are visible. Yet even if cells are metabolically altered and nonfunctional, they can remain viable if blood flow returns within 20 minutes. Reports suggest previous recurrent episodes of myocardial ischemia can result in myocyte adaptation to oxygen deprivation and preservation of myocardium. This process, termed **ischemic preconditioning,** is being studied to determine whether it has potential prophylactic or therapeutic uses.[132]

After 8 to 10 seconds of decreased blood flow, the affected myocardium becomes cyanotic and cooler. Myocardial oxygen reserves are used very quickly (within about 8 seconds) after complete cessation of coronary flow. Glycogen stores decrease as anaerobic metabolism begins. Unfortunately, glycolysis can supply only 65% to 70% of the total myocardial energy requirement and produces much less ATP than aerobic processes. Hydrogen ions and lactic acid accumulate. Because myocardial tissues have poor buffering capabilities and myocardial cells are very sensitive to low cellular pH, accumulation of these products further compromises the myocardium. Acidosis may make the myocardium more vulnerable to the damaging effects of lysosomal enzymes and may suppress impulse conduction and contractile function, thereby leading to heart failure.

Oxygen deprivation also is accompanied by electrolyte disturbances, specifically, loss of potassium, calcium, and magnesium from cells. Myocardial cells deprived of necessary oxygen and nutrients lose contractility, thereby diminishing the heart's pumping ability. Ischemic myocardial cells release catecholamines (epinephrine and norepinephrine), predisposing the individual to serious imbalances of sympathetic and parasympathetic function, irregular heartbeats (dysrhythmia), and heart failure. Catecholamines mediate the release of glycogen, glucose, and stored fat from body cells. Therefore, plasma concentrations of free fatty acids and glycerol rise within 1 hour after onset of acute MI. Excessive levels of free fatty acids can have a harmful detergent effect on cell membranes. Norepinephrine elevates blood sugar levels through stimulation of liver and skeletal muscle cells. It also suppresses pancreatic B-cell activity, which reduces insulin secretion and elevates blood glucose further. Hyperglycemia is noted approximately 72 hours after an acute MI and is associated with an increased risk of death; therefore, careful glucose monitoring and control after MI is essential.

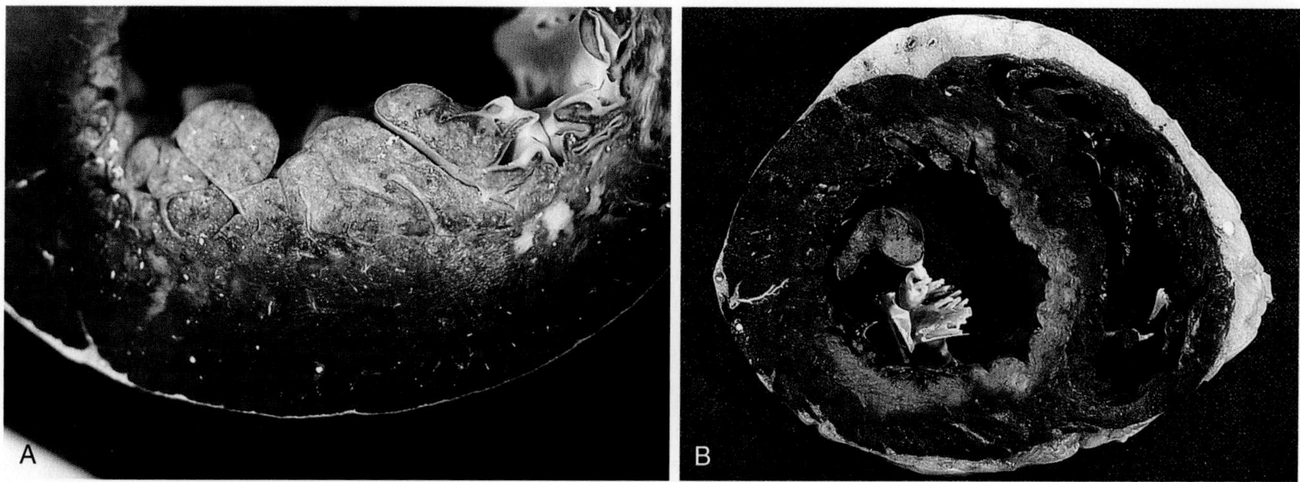

FIGURE 32-22 Myocardial Infarction. **A,** Local infarct confined to one region. **B,** Massive large infarct caused by occlusion of three coronary arteries. (From Damjanov I, Linder J, editors: *Anderson's pathology,* ed 10, St Louis, 1996, Mosby.)

TABLE 32-7 TISSUE CHANGES AFTER MYOCARDIAL INFARCTION

TIME AFTER MYOCARDIAL INFARCTION	TISSUE CHANGES	STAGE OF HEALING PROCESS
6-12 hours	No gross changes; subcellular cyanosis with decreased temperature	Not begun
18-24 hours	Pale to gray-brown; slight pallor	Inflammatory response; intercellular enzyme release
2-4 days	Visible necrosis: yellow-brown in center and hyperemic around edges	Proteolytic enzymes remove debris; catecholamines, lipolysis, and glycogenolysis elevate plasma glucose and increase free fatty acids to assist depleted myocardium recovery from anaerobic state
4-10 days	Area soft, with fatty changes in center, regions of hemorrhage in infarcted area	Debris cleared; collagen matrix laid down
10-14 days	Weak, fibrotic scar tissue with beginning revascularization	Healing continues but area very mushy, vulnerable to stress
6 weeks	Scarring usually complete	Tough inelastic scar replaces necrotic myocardium

Note: Processes of tissue healing are described and illustrated in Chapter 7.

Ischemic injury can be exacerbated by what is termed **reperfusion injury** once blood flow is restored. This process involves the release of toxic oxygen radicals, calcium flux, and pH changes that cause a sustained opening of mitochondrial permeability transition pores (mPTP) and contribute to resultant cellular death. Therapies aimed at reducing reperfusion injury are being explored, including endovascular cooling, adenosine, atrial natriuretic peptide, cyclosporine, nicorandil, and incretins.[131,132]

Angiotensin II is released during myocardial ischemia and contributes to the pathogenesis of MI in several ways. First, it results in the systemic effects of peripheral vasoconstriction and fluid retention. These homeostatic responses are counterproductive in that they increase myocardial work and thus exacerbate the effects of the loss of myocyte contractility. Angiotensin II is also released locally, where it is a growth factor for vascular smooth muscle cells, myocytes, and cardiac fibroblasts; promotes catecholamine release; and causes coronary artery spasm.

Cellular Death. After about 20 minutes of myocardial ischemia, irreversible hypoxic injury causes cellular death and tissue necrosis. (Types of necrosis are described in Chapter 2.) Necrosis of myocardial tissue results in the release of certain intracellular enzymes through the damaged cell membranes into the interstitial spaces. The lymphatics pick up the enzymes and transport them into the bloodstream, where they can be detected by serologic tests. Recent evidence has found that along with necrosis myocardial tissue also is destroyed by the tightly controlled process of apoptosis. An increased understanding of the steps of the apoptotic pathway of MI may lead to new therapies aimed at limiting infarct size.[133]

Structural and Functional Changes. MI results in structural and functional changes of cardiac tissues (Figure 32-22). Table 32-7 outlines the tissue changes that may follow MI. Gross tissue changes in the area of infarction may not become apparent for several hours, despite almost immediate onset (within 30 to 60 seconds) of ECG changes. The infarcted myocardium is surrounded by a zone of hypoxic injury, which may progress to necrosis, undergo remodeling, or return to normal.

Cardiac tissue surrounding the area of infarction also undergoes pathophysiologic changes. **Myocardial stunning,** a temporary loss of contractile function that persists for hours to days after perfusion, has been restored. This pathophysiologic state can occur both with MI and in individuals who suffer ischemia during cardiovascular procedures such as cardiac surgery. Stunning is caused by the alterations in electrolyte pumps, calcium homeostasis, and the release of toxic oxygen radicals. It is characterized by decreased contraction and conduction and can contribute to heart failure, shock, and dysrhythmias. Stunning is less severe in individuals who have experienced ischemic preconditioning. New therapies are being explored that can simulate ischemic preconditioning prior to cardiovascular procedures, or that can be used after ischemic events to reduce the effects of stunning (post-conditioning).[131,134]

Hibernating myocardium refers to tissue that is persistently ischemic and undergoes metabolic adaptation to prolong myocyte survival until perfusion can be restored. Restoring adequate perfusion to the myocardium with revascularization therapies can improve myocardial function.[135]

Myocardial remodeling is a process mediated by angiotensin II, aldosterone, catecholamines, adenosine, oxidative stress, and inflammatory cytokines, which causes myocyte hypertrophy, scarring, and loss of contractile function in the areas of the heart distant from the site of infarction.[136] These changes can be limited and even reversed (reverse remodeling) through rapid restoration of coronary flow and the use of ACE inhibitors, beta-blockers, statins, sequential pacemakers, and ventricular assist devices after MI.[137]

Repair. MI causes a severe inflammatory response that ends with wound repair (see Chapter 7). Repair consists of degradation of damaged cells, proliferation of fibroblasts, and synthesis of scar tissue. Many cell types, hormones, and nutrient substrates must be available for optimal healing to proceed. Within 24 hours, leukocytes infiltrate the necrotic area and proteolytic enzymes from scavenger neutrophils degrade necrotic tissue. A collagen matrix is deposited and is initially weak, mushy, and vulnerable to reinjury. Unfortunately it is at this time in the recovery period (10 to 14 days after infarction) that individuals feel more capable of increasing activities and thus may stress the newly formed scar tissue. After 6 weeks the necrotic area is completely replaced by scar tissue, which is strong but unable to contract and relax like healthy myocardial tissue.

CLINICAL MANIFESTATIONS. The first symptom of acute MI is usually sudden, severe chest pain. It is not possible to distinguish between angina and MI by symptoms alone, although the pain associated with MI tends to be more severe and prolonged. It may be described as heavy and crushing, such as an "elephant sitting on my chest." Radiation to the neck, jaw, back, shoulder, or left arm is common. Some individuals (especially older adults or those with diabetes) experience no pain, thereby having a "silent" infarction. Infarction often simulates a sensation of unrelenting indigestion. Nausea and vomiting may occur because of reflex stimulation of vomiting centers by pain fibers. Vasovagal reflexes from the area of the infarcted myocardium also may affect the gastrointestinal tract. Various cardiovascular changes are found on physical examination:

1. The SNS is reflexively activated to compensate, resulting in a temporary increase in heart rate and blood pressure, although severe myocardial damage may cause hypotension despite elevated catecholamine activity.
2. Abnormal extra heart sounds reflect left ventricular dysfunction.
3. Cardiac murmurs may indicate acute valvular insufficiency.
4. Pulmonary findings of congestion including dullness to percussion and inspiratory crackles at the lung bases can occur if the individual develops heart failure.
5. Peripheral vasoconstriction may cause the skin to become cool and clammy.

EVALUATION AND TREATMENT. The diagnosis of acute MI is made on the basis of history, physical examination, ECG, and serial cardiac biomarker alterations (Box 32-2). It is important to note that nearly half of MIs are not preceded by any previous angina symptoms and up to one-third present with STEMI as the first symptomatic manifestation of coronary disease.[5] MI can occur

BOX 32-2 UNIVERSAL DEFINITION OF MYOCARDIAL INFARCTION

The term *myocardial infarction* should be used when there is evidence of myocardial necrosis in a clinical setting with myocardial ischemia. Under these conditions any one of the following criteria meets the diagnosis for myocardial infarction:

- Detection of rise and/or fall of cardiac biomarkers (preferably troponin) with at least one value above the 99th percentile of the upper reference limit (URL) together with evidence of myocardial ischemia with at least one of the following:
- Symptoms of ischemia
- Electrocardiographic changes indicative of new ischemia (new ST-T changes or new left bundle branch block ([LBBB])
- Development of pathologic Q waves in the electrocardiogram
- Imaging evidence of new loss of viable myocardium or new regional wall motion abnormality
- Sudden, unexpected cardiac death, involving cardiac arrest, often with symptoms suggestive of myocardial ischemia, and accompanied by presumably new ST elevation, or new LBBB, and/or evidence of fresh thrombus by coronary angiography and/or at autopsy; but death occurring before blood samples could be obtained, or at a time before the appearance of cardiac biomarkers in the blood.
- For percutaneous coronary interventions (PCIs) in patients with normal baseline troponin values, elevations of cardiac biomarkers above the 99th percentile URL are indicative of periprocedural myocardial necrosis. By convention, increases of biomarkers greater than 3 × 99th percentile URL have been designated as defining PCI-related myocardial infarction. A subtype related to a documented stent thrombosis is recognized.
- For coronary artery bypass grafting (CABG) in patients with normal baseline troponin values, elevations of cardiac biomarkers above the 99th percentile URL are indicative of periprocedural myocardial necrosis. By convention, increases of biomarkers greater than 5 × 99th percentile URL plus either new pathologic Q waves or new LBBB, or angiographically documented new graft or native coronary artery occlusion, or imaging evidence of new loss of viable myocardium have been designated as defining CABG-related myocardial infarction.
- Pathologic findings of an acute myocardial infarction

Data from Thygesen K, Alpert J, White H: *J Am Coll Cardiol* 50:2173–2195, 2007.

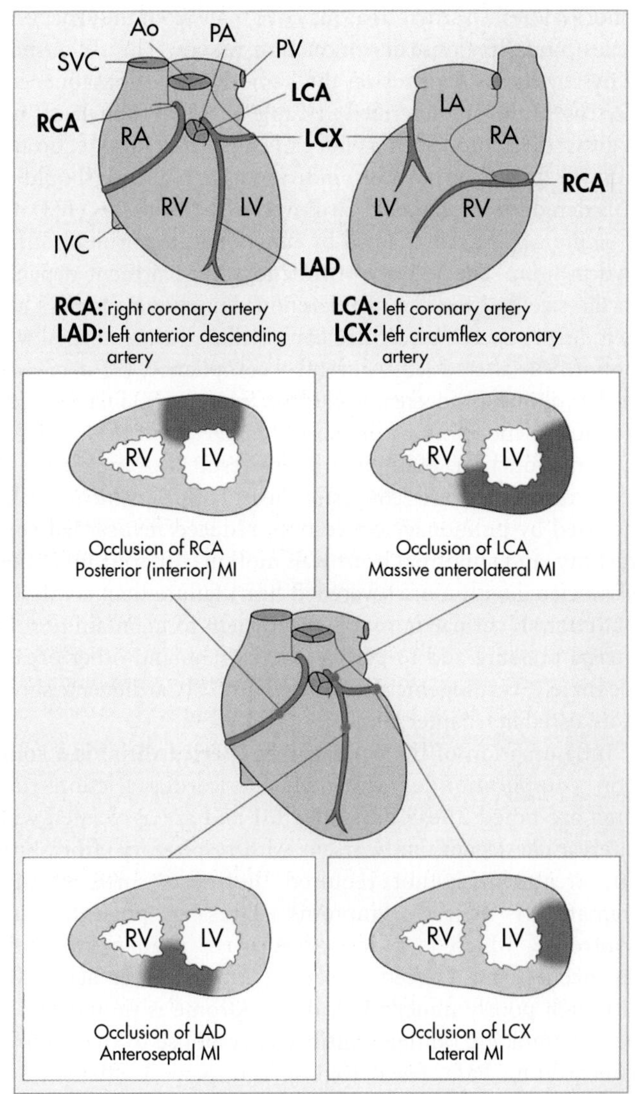

FIGURE 32-23 Site of Myocardial Infarction (MI) and Vessel Involvement. *Ao,* Aorta; *IVC,* inferior vena cava; *LA,* left atrium; *LV,* left ventricle; *PA,* pulmonary artery; *PV,* pulmonary vein; *RA,* right atrium; *RV,* right ventricle; *SVC,* superior vena cava. (From Stevens A, Lowe JS, Scott I: *Core pathology,* ed 3, London, 2009, Mosby.)

in various regions of the heart wall and may be described as anterior, inferior, posterior, lateral, subendocardial, or transmural depending on its location and extent of tissue damage from infarction. Twelve-lead ECGs help localize the affected area through identification of changes in ST segments and T waves (Figure 32-23). The infarcted myocardium is surrounded by a zone of hypoxic injury, which may progress to necrosis or return to normal, and adjacent to this zone of hypoxic injury is a zone of reversible ischemia (Figure 32-24). In STEMI, a characteristic Q wave often develops on ECG some hours later.

Cardiac troponin I (cTnI) is the most specific indicator of MI and should be obtained on admission to the emergency department. cTnI elevation is detectable 2 to 4 hours after onset of symptoms. Additional measurements within 6 to 9 hours and again at 12 to 24 hours are recommended if clinical suspicion is high and previous samples were negative. cTnI has a sensitivity of more than 95% and a negative predictive value of 99% for the diagnosis of acute MI.[138] Troponin levels also can be used to estimate infarct size and therefore the likelihood of complications.[139] Other biomarkers released by myocardial cells include CPK-MB and LDH. These isoenzymes exist in several different active molecular forms called isoenzymes and are present in different amounts within particular tissues. Blood is drawn for troponin and isoenzyme determinations as soon as possible after the onset of symptoms; serial serum levels of these biomarkers are assessed for several days.

Additional laboratory data may reveal leukocytosis and elevated CRP, both of which indicate inflammation. The individual's blood sugar is usually elevated and the glucose tolerance level may remain abnormal for several weeks. Hypoxemia may accompany heart failure.

Acute MI requires admission to the hospital. The individual should be placed on supplemental oxygen and given an aspirin immediately (clopidogrel or prasugrel if intolerant to aspirin). Pain is treated with morphine sulfate. Continuous monitoring of cardiac rhythms and biomarker changes is essential because the first 24 hours after onset of symptoms is the time of highest risk for sudden death. Non-STEMI is treated in the same way as unstable angina including antithrombotics, anticoagulation

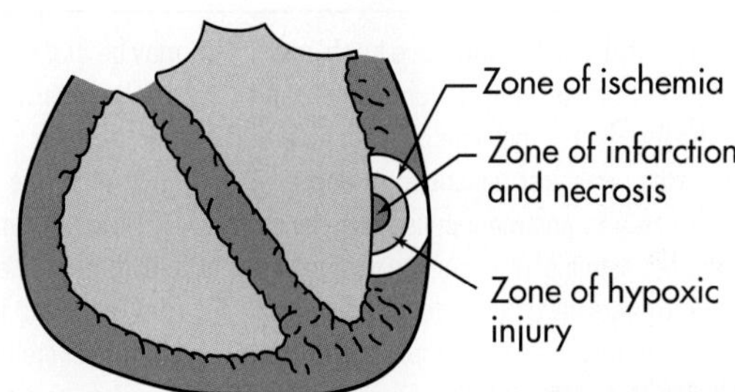

FIGURE 32-24 Electrocardiographic Alterations Associated with the Three Zones of Myocardial Infarction.

or PCI, or both.[130] STEMI is best managed with emergent PCI and antithrombotics.[139a] Thrombolytics may be used if PCI is not readily available. Hyperglycemia is treated with insulin.[140] Once the person is stabilized, further management includes ACE inhibitors, beta-blockers, and statins.[138,141,142] Individuals who are in shock require aggressive fluid resuscitation, inotropic drugs, and possible emergent invasive procedures.[143]

Bed rest, followed by gradual return to activities of daily living, reduces the myocardial oxygen demands of the compromised heart. Individuals not receiving thrombolytic or heparin infusion must receive DVT prophylaxis as long as their activity is significantly limited. Stool softeners are given to eliminate the need for straining, which can precipitate bradycardia and can be followed by increased venous return to the heart, causing possible cardiac overload. Education on diet, caffeine, smoking cessation, exercise, and other aspects of risk factor reduction is crucial for secondary prevention of recurrent myocardial ischemia.

Approximately 1% to 2% of people initially diagnosed with STEMI do not have myocardial infarction, but rather have a stress-induced syndrome known as the *broken heart syndrome* or *Takotsubo cardiomyopathy*. These individuals present with the acute onset of chest pain, ST elevation, elevated troponins, and BNP after emotional stress, but generally do not have coronary artery disease and must be managed differently[144] (see What's New? The Broken Heart Syndrome).

COMPLICATIONS. The number and severity of postinfarction complications depend on the location and extent of necrosis, the individual's physiologic condition before the infarction, and the availability of swift therapeutic intervention.

Dysrhythmias (arrhythmias), which are disturbances of cardiac rhythm, are the most common complication of acute MI. Dysrhythmias can be caused by ischemia, hypoxia, autonomic nervous system (ANS) imbalances, lactic acidosis, electrolyte abnormalities, alterations of impulse conduction pathways or conduction defects, drug toxicity, or hemodynamic abnormalities. Dysrhythmias may originate from the atria, ventricles, nodal regions, or conduction tissues. The seriousness of dysrhythmias depends on the hemodynamic consequences. (Dysrhythmias are described in Table 32-12.) Prophylactic use of antiarrhythmics, such as lidocaine and amiodarone, do not improve mortality; however, individuals at high risk should be considered for implantable cardioverter-defibrillators (ICDs).

Acute MI is accompanied by functional impairment of the myocardium. The severity of functional impairment depends on the size and the site of infarction. Functional changes can include: (1) decreased cardiac contractility with abnormal wall motion, (2) altered left ventricular compliance, (3) decreased stroke volume, (4) decreased ejection fraction, (5) increased left ventricular end-diastolic pressure (LVEDP), and (6) SA or AV node malfunction. Many infarctions result in some degree of left ventricular failure (congestive heart failure), which is characterized by pulmonary congestion, reduced myocardial contractility, and abnormal heart wall motion. Anterior infarction is associated with more severe left heart failure than is inferior infarction. If cardiac output is insufficient to maintain normal arterial pressure and to perfuse the kidneys and other organs adequately, **cardiogenic shock** develops.[143] (Cardiogenic shock is discussed in Chapter 48.)

Inflammation of the pericardium **(pericarditis)** is a common complication of acute MI. Pericardial friction rubs often are noted 2 to 3 days after MI and are associated with anterior chest pain that worsens with respiratory effort. Specific treatment is not required; however, corticosteroids dramatically relieve symptoms. **Dressler postinfarction syndrome,** which is a delayed form of acute pericarditis, can occur from 1 week to several months after acute MI. Although poorly understood, the syndrome is thought to be an immunologic (antigen-antibody) response to the necrotic myocardium. Pain, fever, friction rub, pleural effusion, and arthralgias may accompany this syndrome. Steroids may alleviate symptoms.

WHAT'S NEW?

The Broken Heart Syndrome

Episodes of extreme mental stress, like the loss of a loved one, have been linked to sudden onset of myocardial ischemia, arrhythmias, heart failure, shock, and even death. This has been called the "broken heart syndrome." This phenomenon, now called Takotsubo cardiomyopathy, was first described in Japan in 1991, where it was found to occur most often in postmenopausal women at times of acute stress. Since then it has been found to occur in women and men of all ages, and many other stressful triggers have been identified such as earthquakes, lightning strikes, noncardiac surgery, seizures, trauma, anesthesia, and alcohol withdrawal to name just a few. Although the manifestations are variable, it has been found that many individuals have weakening and ballooning of the left ventricular apex during systole that begins within minutes to hours after the stressful episode. Although the pathophysiology is still being explored, catecholamines play an important role in the pathogenesis causing coronary artery spasm, coronary microvascular abnormalities, direct myocardial damage, and neurogenic myocardial stunning. Postmenopausal women may be especially vulnerable because of estrogen deficiency–mediated effects on the microvasculature. On myocardial biopsy, most people have inflammation without necrosis. People with Takotsubo cardiomyopathy present clinically with the same symptoms as acute ST-elevation myocardial infarction (STEMI), including chest pain, dyspnea, ST-segment elevation, and moderately elevated cardiac biomarkers, such as troponins and brain natriuretic peptide. The American Heart Association/May Criteria for the diagnosis describe transient dyskinesis of the left ventricle in the absence of acute coronary artery disease, acute head trauma, myocarditis, or other forms of cardiomyopathy. Management usually includes aspirin, beta-blockers, angiotensin-converting enzyme inhibitors, and statins, although targeted emotional support and standard psychologic counseling have the greatest effect on recovery and reducing the risk for recurrence. An interprofessional team that includes a social worker, pastor, and mental health care providers has been found beneficial for those suffering from this cardiomyopathy.

Data from Ahmed KA, Madhavan M, Prasad A: *Coron Artery Dis* 23(4):259–264, 2012; Golabchi A, Sarrafzadegan N: *J Res Med Sci* 16(3):340–345, 2011; Neil CJ et al: *Exp Rev Cardiovasc Ther* 10(2):215–221, 2012; Shah RM et al: *Am J Ther* 19(3):e105–e113, 2012.

Organic brain syndrome may occur in acute or chronic form if blood flow to the brain is impaired secondary to MI. Transient ischemic attacks or an outright cerebrovascular accident may result from thromboemboli that have broken loose from the wall of the left ventricle or from cardiac valves.

Cardiac complications of MI can include rupture of heart structures. Tissue necrosis in or around the papillary muscles can cause rupture of these muscles or of the chordae tendineae. Factors that lead to rupture of the free wall of the infarcted ventricle include thinning of the wall, poor collateral flow, shearing effect of muscular contraction against the stiffened necrotic area, marked necrosis at the terminal end of the blood supply, and aging of the myocardium with laceration of the myocardial microstructure. Infarctions around septal structures that separate the heart chambers can lead to septal rupture. Ruptures are associated with audible, harsh cardiac murmurs; increased LVEDP; and decreased systemic blood pressure.

Weakening of the wall of the infarcted ventricle can cause **ventricular aneurysm** formation. According to Laplace's law, with decreased muscle mass at the infarcted site, the wall is weakened and tension stretches the noncontracting infarcted heart muscle, thus producing infarct expansion or aneurysm formation (see p. 1140 for a discussion of aneurysm). Decreased muscle mass causes an increase in the radius of the ventricle, and because the radius is directly proportional to pressure and tension, both increase with time. The wall of the aneurysm becomes more fibrotic but continues to bulge with systole. The bulge results in impaired pump function. Although rare, rupture may occur when the tension becomes too great. Death in individuals with a left ventricular aneurysm is usually related to ventricular tachydysrhythmias and not to ventricular rupture. Left ventricular aneurysm is a late complication of MI, occurring months or years after the acute event.

Thromboembolism is commonly found during postmortem examinations of individuals who have died of MI. Thromboemboli may disseminate from debris and clots that collect inside dilated aneurysmal sacs or from the infarcted endocardium and travel to the pulmonary or systemic vascular systems. Pulmonary emboli also may result from the breaking loose of deep venous thrombi of the legs in individuals who are confined to bed (see p. 1275). Early mobilization and prophylactic anticoagulation therapy are essential to reduce the incidence of this complication.

Sudden death resulting from cardiac arrest is often caused by dysrhythmias, particularly ventricular fibrillation. Other dysrhythmias may be equally lethal. Widespread knowledge of cardiopulmonary resuscitation has increased the probability of survival during the first few hours after cardiac insult. Immediate intervention and careful monitoring also have reduced mortality and have improved chances for long-term survival. Several factors, however, contribute to the risk of death during acute infarction or reduce the chances of long-term survival, despite the best possible treatment. They are: (1) degree of left ventricular dysfunction, (2) degree of left ventricular ischemia, (3) potential for ventricular dysrhythmias, and (4) the individual's age.

DISORDERS OF THE HEART WALL

Disorders of the Pericardium

Pericardial disease is often a manifestation of another disorder, such as infection (bacterial, viral, fungal, rickettsial, parasitic); trauma or surgery; neoplasm; or a metabolic, immunologic, or vascular disorder (uremia, rheumatoid arthritis, systemic lupus erythematosus, periarteritis nodosa). The pericardial response to injury from these diverse causes may consist of acute pericarditis, pericardial effusion, or constrictive pericarditis.

Acute Pericarditis

Acute pericarditis is acute inflammation of the pericardium. The etiology of acute pericarditis is most often idiopathic or caused by viral infection by coxsackievirus, influenza, hepatitis, measles, mumps, or varicella viruses. It also is the most common cardiovascular complication of human immunodeficiency virus (HIV) infection. Other causes include MI, trauma, neoplasm, surgery, uremia, bacterial infection (especially tuberculosis), connective tissue disease (especially systemic lupus erythematosus and rheumatoid arthritis), or radiation therapy.[145] The pericardial membranes become inflamed and roughened, and a pericardial effusion may develop that can be serous, purulent, or fibrinous (Figure 32-25). Possible sequelae of pericarditis include recurrent pericarditis, pericardial constriction, and cardiac tamponade.

Most individuals with acute pericarditis describe several days of fever, myalgias, and malaise followed by the sudden onset of severe chest pain that worsens with respiratory movements and with lying down. Although the pain may radiate to the back, it is generally felt in the anterior chest and may be confused initially with the pain of acute MI. Individuals with acute pericarditis also may report dysphagia, restlessness, irritability, anxiety, and weakness.

Physical examination often discloses low-grade fever and sinus tachycardia. A pericardial friction rub—a short, scratchy, grating sound—may be heard at the cardiac apex and left sternal

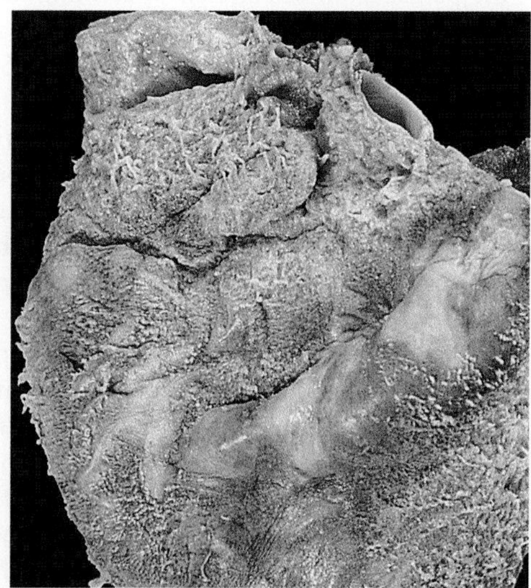

FIGURE 32-25 Acute Pericarditis. Note shaggy coat of fibers covering surface of heart. (From Damjanov I, Linder J: *Pathology: a color atlas,* St Louis, 2000, Mosby.)

border and is highly specific for pericarditis. The rub is caused by the roughened pericardial membranes rubbing against each other. Friction rubs are not always present and may be intermittently heard. ECG changes may reflect inflammatory processes through diffuse ST-segment elevation that is concaved upward without Q waves.[145] The ECG may remain abnormal for days or even weeks. Echocardiography may reveal a pericardial effusion.

Treatment for uncomplicated acute pericarditis consists of relieving symptoms. Rest is helpful during episodes of acute pain. Salicylates and nonsteroidal anti-inflammatory drugs (NSAIDs) reduce inflammation. Combined nonsteroidals and colchicine (prevents fibrosis) is a highly effective regimen.[145] Additional analgesics may be given to relieve pain. Exploring the underlying cause is important. If pericardial effusion develops, aspirating the excessive fluid may be necessary.

Pericardial Effusion

Pericardial effusion, the accumulation of fluid in the pericardial cavity, can occur in all forms of pericarditis. The fluid may be a transudate, such as the serous effusion that develops with left heart failure, overhydration, or hypoproteinemia. More often, however, the fluid is an exudate, which indicates pericardial inflammation like that seen with acute pericarditis, heart surgery, some chemotherapeutic agents, infections, and autoimmune disorders, such as systemic lupus erythematosus.[145,146] (Types of exudate are described in Chapter 7.) If the fluid is serosanguineous, the underlying cause is likely to be tuberculosis, neoplasm, uremia, or radiation. Idiopathic serosanguineous (cause unknown) effusion is possible, however. Effusions of frank blood are generally related to aneurysms, trauma, or coagulation defects. If chyle leaks from the thoracic duct, it may enter the pericardium and lead to cholesterol pericarditis.

Pericardial effusion, even in large amounts, is not necessarily clinically significant, except that it indicates an underlying disorder. The important consideration is whether the fluid creates sufficient pressure to cause cardiac compression, which is a serious condition known as **tamponade.**[145] If an effusion develops gradually, the pericardium can stretch to accommodate large quantities of fluid without compressing the heart. If the fluid accumulates rapidly, however, even a small amount (50 to 100 ml) may cause serious tamponade. The danger is that pressure exerted by the pericardial fluid eventually equals diastolic pressure within the heart chambers, thus preventing chamber filling. The first structures to be affected by tamponade are the right atrium and ventricle, where diastolic pressures are normally lowest. Compression by pericardial fluid interferes with right atrial filling during diastole, resulting in increased venous pressure, systemic venous congestion, and signs and symptoms of right heart failure (distention of the jugular veins, edema, hepatomegaly). Decreased atrial filling leads to decreased ventricular filling, decreased stroke volume, and reduced cardiac output. If the left atrium collapses because of lack of filling, life-threatening circulatory collapse may occur.[145,146] Individuals with cardiac tamponade most often present with dyspnea, tachycardia, jugular venous distention, cardiomegaly, and pulsus paradoxus. Pulsus paradoxus means that the arterial blood pressure during expiration exceeds arterial pressure during inspiration by more than 10 mmHg. This clinical finding reflects impairment of diastolic filling of the left ventricle plus reduction of blood volume within all four cardiac chambers. Presence of a large pericardial effusion or tamponade magnifies the normally insignificant effect of inspiration on intracardiac flow and volume.

Other clinical manifestations of pericardial effusion are distant or muffled heart sounds, poorly palpable apical pulse, dyspnea on exertion, and dull chest pain. A chest x-ray may disclose a "water-bottle" configuration of the cardiac silhouette. An echocardiogram can detect an effusion as small as 20 ml and is considered the most accurate and reliable method of diagnosis, although CT also is commonly used.[146]

Treatment of pericardial effusion or tamponade generally consists of pericardiocentesis (aspiration of excessive pericardial fluid). Pericardiocentesis is diagnostic and therapeutic: the fluid is analyzed to identify the cause of the effusion, and its removal alone may bring dramatic relief from symptoms. Persistent pain may be treated with analgesics, anti-inflammatory medications, or steroids. Surgery may be required if the underlying cause of tamponade is trauma or aneurysm. If an effusion is neoplasm induced, chemotherapeutic agents may be injected into the pericardial space.[146] If the effusion recurs, a pericardial "window" can be created or the individual may require pericardectomy.

Constrictive Pericarditis

Constrictive pericarditis, or **restrictive pericarditis (chronic pericarditis),** was synonymous with tuberculosis years ago, and tuberculosis continues to be an important cause of pericarditis in immunocompromised individuals.[146] In the United States this form of pericardial disease is more often idiopathic or associated with radiation exposure, rheumatoid arthritis, uremia, or CABG. In constrictive pericarditis, fibrous scarring with occasional calcification of the pericardium causes the visceral and parietal pericardial layers to adhere, obliterating the pericardial cavity. The fibrotic lesions encase the heart in a rigid shell (Figure 32-26). Like tamponade, constrictive pericarditis compresses the heart and eventually reduces cardiac output. Unlike tamponade, however, constrictive pericarditis never develops suddenly.

Because the onset of constrictive pericarditis is gradual, clinical manifestations seldom include pulsus paradoxus. Symptoms tend to be exercise intolerance, dyspnea on exertion, fatigue, and anorexia. Clinical assessment shows weight loss, edema, jugular vein distention, and hepatic congestion. Restricted ventricular filling may cause a pericardial knock (early diastolic sound).

ECG findings include T-wave inversions and atrial fibrillation. Chest x-ray often discloses prominent pulmonary vessels and calcification of the pericardium. CT, MRI, and transesophageal echocardiography are used to detect pericardial thickening and constriction. Pericardial biopsy may be needed to determine the etiology.

Initial treatment for constrictive pericarditis consists of dietary sodium restriction, digitalis glycosides, and diuretics to improve cardiac output.[145,146] If these modalities are not successful, surgical excision of the restrictive pericardium is indicated.

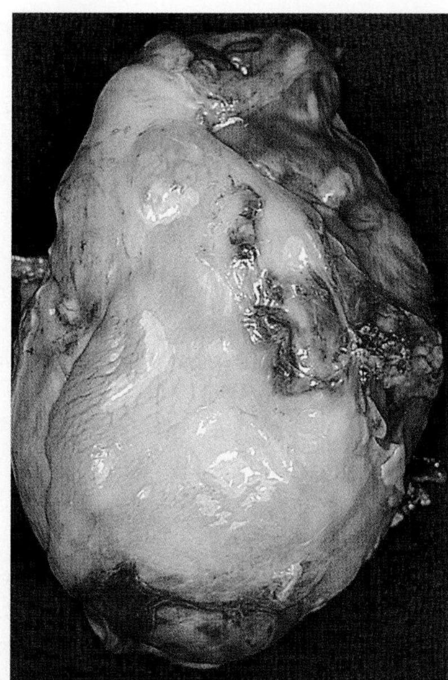

FIGURE 32-26 Constrictive Pericarditis. The fibrotic pericardium encases the heart in a rigid shell. (From Damjanov I, Linder J: *Pathology: a color atlas,* St Louis, 2000, Mosby.)

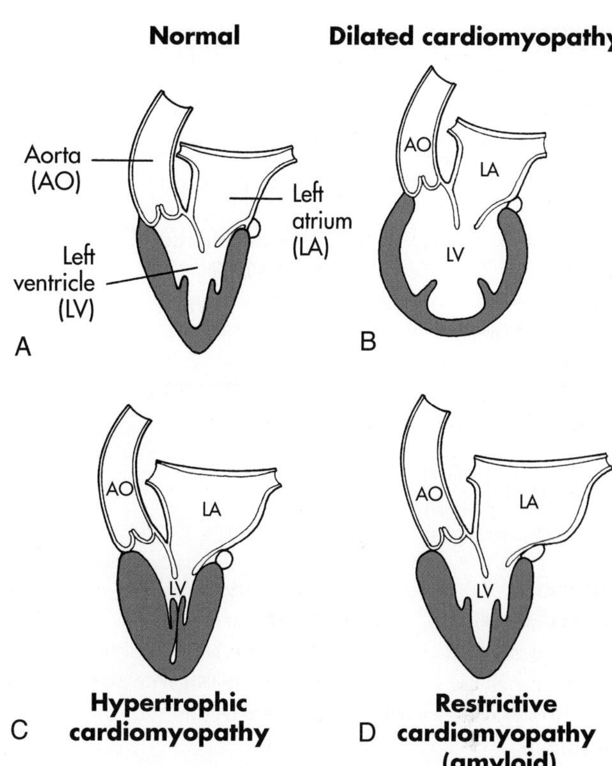

FIGURE 32-27 Diagram Showing Major Distinguishing Pathophysiologic Features of the Types of Cardiomyopathy. **A,** The normal heart. **B,** In the dilated type of cardiomyopathy, the heart has a globular shape, and the largest circumference of the left ventricle is not at its base but midway between apex and base. **C,** In the hypertrophic type of cardiomyopathy the wall of the left ventricle is greatly thickened; the left ventricular cavity is small, but the left atrium may be dilated because of poor diastolic relaxation of the ventricle. **D,** In the restrictive type the left ventricular cavity is of normal size, but again, the left atrium is dilated because of the reduced diastolic compliance of the ventricle. (From Kissane JM, editor: *Anderson's pathology,* ed 9, St Louis, 1990, Mosby.)

Disorders of the Myocardium: The Cardiomyopathies

The **cardiomyopathies** are a diverse group of diseases that affect the myocardium. Most are the result of remodeling caused by the effect of the neurohumoral responses to ischemic heart disease or hypertension on the heart muscle. Cardiomyopathies also can be secondary to inherited disorders, infectious disease, exposure to toxins, systemic connective tissue disease, infiltrative and proliferative disorders, or nutritional deficiencies. Many cases of cardiomyopathy are idiopathic. The cardiomyopathies are categorized as dilated, hypertrophic, or restrictive depending on their tissue characteristics, genomics, and hemodynamic effects (Figure 32-27 and Table 32-8). An individual may display characteristics of more than one type.

Dilated Cardiomyopathy

Dilated cardiomyopathy is characterized by diminished myocardial contractility, which is reflected in diminished systolic performance of the heart. This impaired systolic function leads to increases in intracardiac volume, ventricular dilation, and systolic heart failure (Figure 32-28). This form of cardiomyopathy is usually the result of ischemic heart disease, valvular disease, diabetes, renal failure, hyperthyroidism, alcohol or drug toxicity, peripartum complications, genetic disorder, or infection. Idiopathic dilated cardiomyopathy often has a familial origin with associated alterations in genes coding for contractile proteins, mitochondrial dysfunction, and immune defects.[147,148]

Ischemic cardiomyopathy is the most common and can occur as the direct result of myocardial infarction or can result from repetitive ischemic insults in those with poorly controlled angina.[149] Valvular heart disease causes cardiac chamber volume and pressure overload that can result in long-term myocardial dysfunction. Diabetes and uremia are associated with decreased myocardial contractility and dilated cardiomyopathy. Alcohol can be directly toxic to the myocardium, as can many drugs such as some chemotherapeutic, inotropic, and antidysrhythmic agents. Many nutritional deficiencies can cause cardiomyopathy including niacin, vitamin D, and selenium. Peripartum cardiomyopathy occurs in previously healthy women in the final month of pregnancy and up to 5 months after delivery. Although the incidence is less than 0.1% of pregnancies, morbidity and mortality rates are high at 5% to 32%.[150] Dilated cardiomyopathies also may be the late autoimmune consequences of previous viral infections resulting in myocarditis and subsequent decreases in contractility.[151] Hyperthyroidism may present with atrial fibrillation and dilated cardiomyopathy, which may be reversible with treatment of the thyroid disorder. (Pathophysiologic effects of the cardiomyopathies are summarized in Table 32-8.)

The most common symptoms of dilated cardiomyopathy are dyspnea and fatigue. Pulmonary congestion is expected, although fulminant pulmonary edema is uncommon. Palpitations and associated dysrhythmias may cause dizziness (syncope). Systemic and pulmonary emboli are common complications. Chest pain may be present but it is usually nonspecific and unlike anginal pain.

TABLE 32-8 PATHOPHYSIOLOGIC EFFECTS OF THE CARDIOMYOPATHIES

PATHOPHYSIOLOGY	TYPE OF CARDIOMYOPATHY: DILATED	HYPERTROPHIC	RESTRICTIVE
Major symptoms	Fatigue, weakness, palpitations	Dyspnea, angina pectoris, fatigue, dizziness (syncope), palpitations	Dyspnea, fatigue
Cardiomegaly	Moderate to marked	Mild to moderate	Mild
Hypertrophy	Left ventricular myocardium	Left ventricular myocardium and interventricular septum	Left ventricular myocardium
Alterations of chamber volume	Volume increased	Volume decreased, particularly in left ventricle	Volume normal to decreased
Alterations of chamber compliance	Compliance increased	Compliance decreased, particularly in left ventricle	Compliance decreased, particularly in left ventricle
Alterations of systolic function (myocardial contractility)	Contractility decreased in left ventricle	Contractility normal	None
Conduction defects	Intraventricular	Nonspecific	Atrioventricular
Dysrhythmias	Sinoatrial tachycardia; atrial and ventricular dysrhythmias	Atrial and ventricular dysrhythmias	Tachydysrhythmias
Thromboembolism	Systemic or pulmonary	Systemic or pulmonary	Systemic or pulmonary
Associated conditions	Alcoholism, pregnancy, infection, nutritional deficiency, exposure to toxins	Inherited defect of muscle growth and development or hypertension	Infiltrative disease
Eventual cardiovascular event	Left heart failure	Left heart failure	Right heart failure

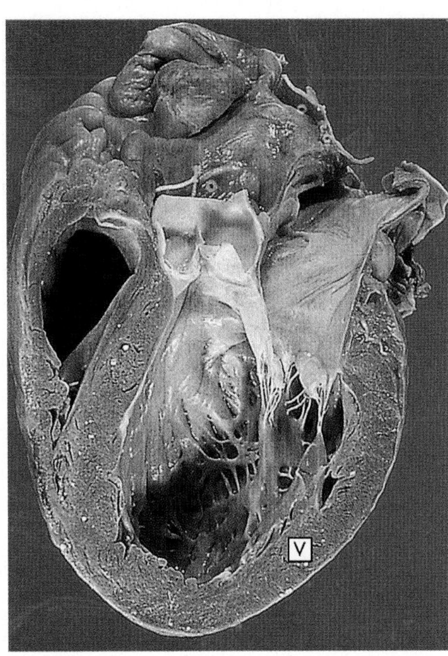

FIGURE 32-28 Dilated Cardiomyopathy. The dilated left ventricle has a thin wall *(V)*. (From Stevens A, Lowe JS, Scott I: *Core pathology*, ed 3, London, 2009, Mosby.)

In the presence of dilated heart failure, blood pressure may be elevated initially; however, hypotension indicates progressive decreases in contractility. Extra heart sounds and cardiac murmurs may be present as well. Echocardiography and MRI can confirm the diagnosis; however, careful evaluation for potentially reversible underlying causes is essential.

General treatment for dilated cardiomyopathy consists of salt restriction and the careful use of vasodilators, diuretics, and inotropic agents. Anticoagulants are given to prevent pulmonary and systemic embolism. Corticosteroids and immunosuppressants can benefit individuals with documented inflammatory disease. Myocardial pacemakers (pacing) can improve cardiac output in many individuals. Cardiac transplantation may be lifesaving. The use of cardiac stem cells to restore myocardial contractility is an area of promising research.[152]

Hypertrophic Cardiomyopathy

Hypertrophic cardiomyopathy refers to two major categories of thickening of the myocardium: (1) hypertrophic obstructive cardiomyopathy (asymmetric septal hypertrophic cardiomyopathy or subaortic stenosis), and (2) hypertensive or valvular hypertrophic cardiomyopathy. These two categories are very different in their etiology, pathophysiology, and clinical presentation.

Hypertrophic obstructive cardiomyopathy is the most common inherited heart defect, occurring in 1 of 500 individuals through autosomal dominant inheritance.[5] It is characterized by thickening of the septal wall (Figure 32-29), which may cause outflow obstruction to the left ventricle outflow tract. Additional changes include abnormalities of collagen deposition and altered contractile proteins in the myocytes.[153] The thickening of the septum results in a hyperdynamic state, especially with exercise. Diastolic relaxation also is impaired and ventricular compliance is decreased. Obstruction of left ventricular outflow can occur when heart rate is increased and intravascular volume is decreased. Individuals complain of angina, syncope, palpitations, and symptoms of MI and left heart failure. Examination may reveal extra heart sounds and murmurs. Echocardiography and cardiac catheterization can confirm the diagnosis.[154] This type of hypertrophic cardiomyopathy is a significant risk for serious ventricular arrhythmias and sudden death. Management includes beta-blockers or verapamil to slow the heart rate, surgical resection of the hypertrophied myocardium, septal ablation, and prophylactic placement of an ICD in high-risk individuals.[155]

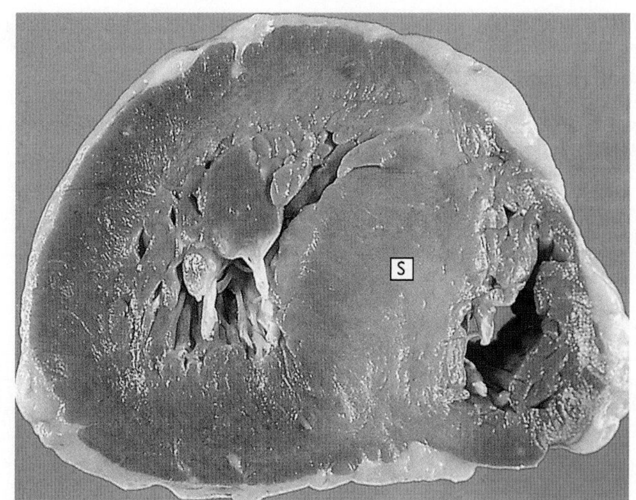

FIGURE 32-29 Hypertrophic Cardiomyopathy. There is marked left ventricular hypertrophy. This often affects the septum *(S)*. (From Stevens A, Lowe JS, Scott I: *Core pathology*, ed 3, London, 2009, Mosby.)

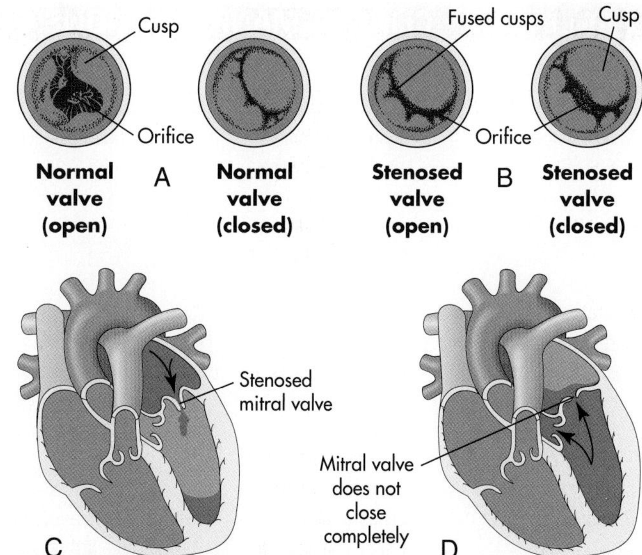

FIGURE 32-30 Valvular Stenosis and Regurgitation. A, Normal position of the valve leaflets, or cusps, when the valve is open and closed. **B,** Open position of a stenosed valve *(left)* and open position of a closed regurgitant valve *(right)*. **C,** Hemodynamic effect of mitral stenosis. The stenosed valve is unable to open sufficiently during left atrial systole, inhibiting left ventricular filling. **D,** Hemodynamic effect of mitral regurgitation. The mitral valve does not close completely during left ventricular systole, permitting blood to reenter the left atrium.

Hypertensive or valvular hypertrophic cardiomyopathy occurs because of increased resistance to ventricular ejection commonly seen in hypertension or in valvular stenosis (usually aortic). In this case, hypertrophy of the myocytes is an attempt to compensate for increased myocardial workload. Long-term dysfunction of the myocytes develops over time, with first diastolic dysfunction leading eventually to systolic dysfunction of the ventricle (see Heart Failure, p. 1175). Individuals with hypertrophic cardiomyopathy may be asymptomatic or may complain of angina, syncope, dyspnea on exertion, and palpitations. Examination may reveal extra heart sounds and murmurs. Echocardiography and cardiac catheterization can confirm the diagnosis.

Restrictive Cardiomyopathies

Restrictive cardiomyopathy is characterized by restrictive filling and reduced diastolic volume of either or both ventricles with normal or near-normal systolic function and wall thickness.[156] It may occur idiopathically or as a cardiac manifestation of systemic diseases, such as scleroderma, amyloidosis, sarcoidosis, lymphoma, and hemochromatosis, or a number of inherited storage diseases. The myocardium becomes rigid and noncompliant, impeding ventricular filling and raising filling pressures during diastole. The overall clinical and hemodynamic picture mimics and may be confused with that of constrictive pericarditis.

The most common clinical manifestation of restrictive cardiomyopathy is right heart failure with systemic venous congestion. Cardiomegaly and dysrhythmias are common. A thorough evaluation for the underlying cause should be initiated (and may include myocardial biopsy).[156] Treatment is aimed at the underlying cause. Death occurs as a result of heart failure or dysrhythmias.

Disorders of the Endocardium

Valvular Dysfunction

Disorders of the endocardium, the innermost lining of the heart wall, all damage the heart valves, which are made up of endocardial tissue. Endocardial damage can be either congenital or acquired. The acquired forms cause inflammatory, ischemic, traumatic, degenerative, or infectious alterations of valvular structure and function. Structural alterations of the heart valves lead to stenosis, incompetence, or both. Although all four heart valves may be affected, those of the left heart (mitral and aortic semilunar valves) are more commonly affected than those of the right heart (tricuspid and pulmonic semilunar valves).

In **valvular stenosis** the valve orifice is constricted and narrowed, impeding the forward flow of blood and increasing the workload of the cardiac chamber proximal to the diseased valve (Figure 32-30). Intraventricular or atrial pressure increases in the chamber to overcome resistance to flow through the valve. Increased pressure causes the myocardium to work harder, causing myocardial hypertrophy. In **valvular regurgitation** (also called *insufficiency* or *incompetence*) the valve leaflets, or cusps, fail to shut completely, permitting blood flow to continue even when the valve is supposed to be closed (see Figure 32-30). During systole or diastole some blood leaks back into the chamber proximal to the incompetent valve. Valvular regurgitation increases the volume of blood the heart must pump and increases the workload of the affected heart chamber. Increased volume leads to chamber dilation, and increased workload leads to hypertrophy.

Valvular dysfunction stimulates chamber dilation and/or myocardial hypertrophy, both of which are compensatory mechanisms intended to increase the pumping capability of the heart. Eventually, myocardial contractility is diminished, the ejection fraction is reduced, diastolic pressure increases, and the affected heart chamber fails from overwork. Depending on the severity of the valvular dysfunction and the capacity of the heart to compensate, valvular alterations cause a range of symptoms and some degree of incapacitation (Table 32-9).

TABLE 32-9 CLINICAL MANIFESTATIONS OF VALVULAR STENOSIS AND REGURGITATION

MANIFESTATION	AORTIC STENOSIS	MITRAL STENOSIS	AORTIC REGURGITATION	MITRAL REGURGITATION	TRICUSPID REGURGITATION
Most common cause	Congenital bicuspid valve, degenerative (calcification) changes with aging, rheumatic fever	Rheumatic heart disease	Infective endocarditis; aortic root disease (connective tissue diseases, Marfan syndrome); dilation of the aortic root due to hypertension and aging	Myxomatous degeneration (mitral valve prolapse)	Congenital
Cardiovascular outcome (untreated)	Left ventricular hypertrophy followed by left heart failure; decreased coronary blood flow with myocardial ischemia	Left atrial hypertrophy and dilation with fibrillation, followed by right ventricular failure	Left ventricular hypertrophy and dilation, followed by heart failure	Left atrial hypertrophy and dilation, followed by left heart failure	Right heart failure
Pulmonary effects	Pulmonary edema: dyspnea on exertion	Pulmonary edema: dyspnea on exertion, orthopnea, paroxysmal, nocturnal dyspnea, predisposition to respiratory infections, hemoptysis, pulmonary hypertension, and edema	Pulmonary edema with dyspnea on exertion	Pulmonary edema with dyspnea on exertion	Dyspnea
Central nervous system effects	Syncope, especially on exertion	Neural deficits only associated with emboli (e.g., hemiparesis)	Syncope	None	None
Pain	Angina pectoris	Atypical chest pain	Angina pectoris	Atypical chest pain	Palpitations
Heart sounds	Systolic murmur heard best at the right parasternal second intercostal space and radiating to the neck	Low rumbling diastolic murmur heard best at the apex and radiating to the axilla, accentuated first heart sound, opening snap	Diastolic murmur heard best at the right parasternal second intercostal space and radiating to the neck	Murmur throughout systole heard best at the apex and radiating to the axilla	Murmur throughout systole heard best at the left lower sternal border

Data from Braunwald E, editor: *Heart disease: a textbook of cardiovascular medicine,* ed 7, Philadelphia, 2005, Saunders; Carabello BA, Paulus WJ: Valvular heart disease. In Crawford MH, DiMarco JP, editors: *Cardiology,* London, 2001, Mosby-Wolfe.

In general, valvular disease is diagnosed by echocardiography, which can be used to assess the severity of valvular obstruction or regurgitation before the onset of symptoms. Management almost always includes careful fluid management, valvular repair, or valve replacement with a prosthetic valve followed by long-term anticoagulation.[157] In the case of mechanical valve replacement, lifelong antibiotic prophylaxis prior to invasive procedures is required.[158]

Stenosis

Aortic Stenosis. Aortic stenosis is the most common valvular abnormality affecting nearly 2% of adults older than 65 years.[5] The three common causes are: (1) congenital bicuspid valve, (2) calcific degeneration related to aging, and (3) inflammatory damage caused by rheumatic heart disease (less than 10% of cases). Numerous gene abnormalities have been associated with aortic stenosis. Aortic stenosis is also associated with many risk factors for coronary artery disease. In the United States, 29% of adults were found to have degenerative sclerotic aortic valves, and approximately 2% to 5% progress to aortic stenosis.[5,159] Aortic valve degeneration with aging is associated with lipoprotein deposition in the tissue with chronic inflammation and leaflet calcification. Evidence suggests that degenerative aortic stenosis is linked to hyperlipidemia and that its prevalence might be decreased by more aggressive lipid lowering in adults. Disorders in calcium transport, apoptosis of endocardial cells, and decreased nitric oxide synthesis also have been implicated. In aortic stenosis from any cause, the orifice of the aortic semilunar valve narrows, causing diminished blood flow from the left ventricle into the aorta (Figures 32-31). Outflow obstruction increases pressure within the left ventricle as it tries to eject blood through the narrowed opening. Left ventricular hypertrophy develops to compensate for the increased workload. Eventually, hypertrophy increases myocardial oxygen demand that the coronary arteries may not be able to supply. If this occurs, ischemia may cause attacks of angina. Untreated aortic stenosis can lead to dysrhythmias, myocardial infarction, and heart failure.

Aortic stenosis tends to develop gradually. The classic manifestations of aortic stenosis are angina, syncope, and heart failure. Clinical manifestations include decreased stroke volume, reduced systolic blood pressure, and narrowed pulse pressure (difference between systolic and diastolic pressure). Heart rate is often slow, and pulses are faint. Resistance to flow through the stenotic valve gives rise to a crescendo-decrescendo systolic heart murmur heard best at the second intercostal space and may radiate to the neck. Echocardiography is used to follow

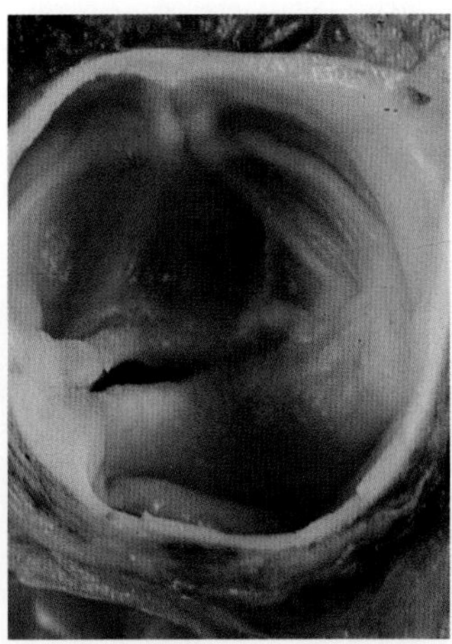

FIGURE 32-31 Aortic Stenosis. Mild stenosis in valve leaflets of a young adult. (From Damjanov I, Linder J: *Pathology: a color atlas,* St Louis, 2000, Mosby.)

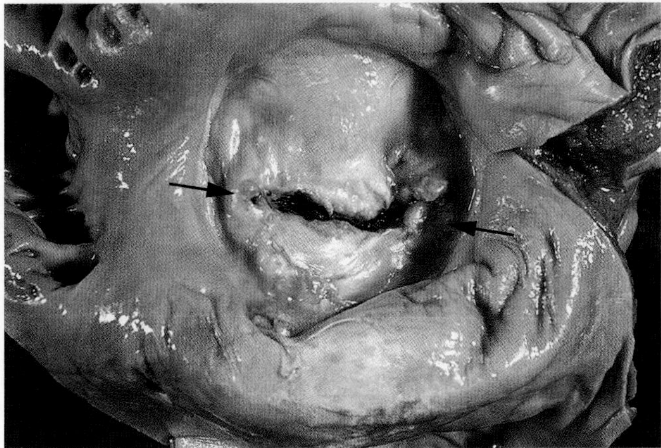

FIGURE 32-32 Mitral Stenosis with Classic "Fish Mouth" (Arrows) Orifice. (From Kumar V, et al: *Robbins & Cotran pathologic basis of disease,* ed 8, St Louis, 2010, Mosby.)

valve orifice and cardiac functioning. Medical management with careful monitoring for complications, such as heart failure and myocardial ischemia, may be indicated for selected individuals, but most require valve repair or replacement with a prosthetic valve followed by long-term anticoagulation.[157] Transcatheter aortic valve implantation is used increasingly to avoid major heart surgery in selected individuals.[160] The prognosis is poor once an individual becomes symptomatic from aortic stenosis.[159]

Mitral Stenosis. Mitral stenosis impairs the flow of blood from the left atrium to the left ventricle. Mitral stenosis is most commonly caused by acute rheumatic fever (see p. 1171) and is two to three times more common in women than in men. Congenital mitral valve stenosis is less common and includes a wide range of anatomic variants.[161] Autoimmunity in response to group A beta-hemolytic streptococcal M protein antigens leads to inflammation and scarring of the valvular leaflets. Scarring causes the leaflets to become fibrous and fused and the chordae tendineae cordis becomes shortened (Figure 32-32).

Clinical manifestations depend on the size of the valvular orifice. Impedance to blood flow results in incomplete emptying of the left atrium and elevated atrial pressure as the chamber tries to force blood through the stenotic valve. Continued increases in left atrial volume and pressure cause chamber dilation and hypertrophy. The risk of developing atrial dysrhythmias (especially fibrillation) and dysrhythmia-induced thrombi is high. As mitral stenosis progresses, symptoms of decreased cardiac output occur, especially during exertion. Continued elevation of left atrial pressure and volume causes pressure to rise in the pulmonary circulation. The outcomes of untreated chronic mitral stenosis are pulmonary hypertension, edema, and right ventricular failure.

Blood flow through the stenotic valve gives rise to a rumbling decrescendo diastolic murmur heard best over the cardiac apex and radiating to the left axilla. If the mitral valve is forced open during diastole, it may make a sharp noise called an *opening snap*. The first heart sound (S_1) is often accentuated and somewhat delayed because of increased left atrial pressure. Other signs and symptoms result from pulmonary congestion and right heart failure. Atrial enlargement is demonstrated by chest x-rays and electrocardiography. Mitral stenosis can often be repaired surgically but may require valve replacement in advanced cases.[157]

Regurgitation

Aortic Regurgitation. Aortic regurgitation results from an inability of the aortic valve leaflets to close properly during diastole resulting from abnormalities of the leaflets or the aortic root, or both. It can be congenital (bicuspid valve) or acquired. Acquired aortic regurgitation can be caused by rheumatic heart disease, bacterial endocarditis, syphilis, hypertension, connective tissue disorders (e.g., Marfan syndrome and ankylosing spondylitis), appetite-suppressing medications, trauma, or atherosclerosis. More than a third of cases of aortic regurgitation are idiopathic. The hemodynamic repercussions depend on the size of the "leak." During systole, blood is ejected from the left ventricle into the aorta. If the aortic semilunar valve fails to close completely, some of the ejected blood flows back into the left ventricle during diastole. Volume overload occurs in the ventricle because it receives blood from the left atrium and the aorta during diastole. Over time, the end-diastolic volume of the left ventricle increases and myocardial fibers stretch to accommodate the extra fluid. Compensatory dilation permits the left ventricle to increase its stroke volume and maintain cardiac output. Ventricular hypertrophy also occurs as an adaptation to the increased volume and increased afterload created by the high stroke volume and resultant systolic hypertension. Ventricular dilation and hypertrophy eventually cease to compensate for aortic incompetence, and heart failure develops.

Clinical manifestations include widened pulse pressure resulting from increased stroke volume and diastolic backflow. Turbulence across the aortic valve during diastole produces a decrescendo murmur heard best in the second, third, or fourth intercostal spaces parasternally and may radiate to the neck. Large stroke volume and rapid runoff of blood from the aorta cause prominent carotid pulsations and bounding peripheral pulses (Corrigan pulse). Other symptoms are usually associated with heart failure that occurs when the ventricle can no longer pump adequately. Dysrhythmias and endocarditis are common complications of aortic regurgitation. The severity of

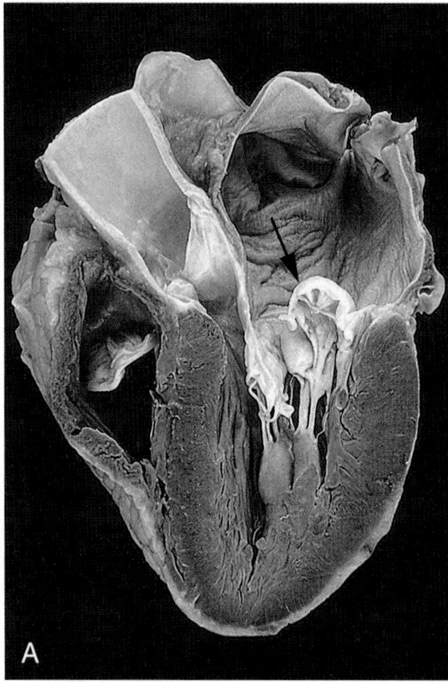

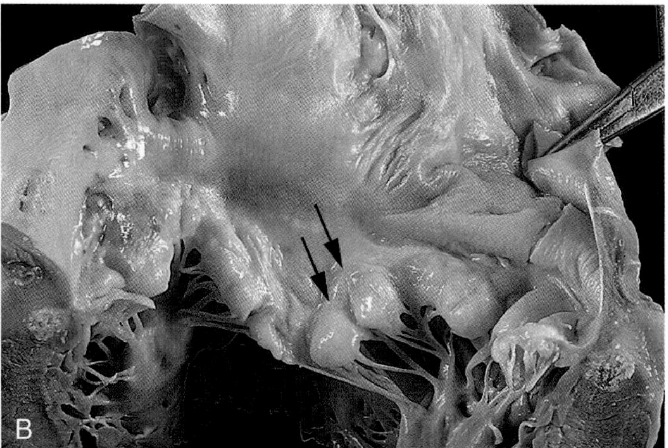

FIGURE 32-33 Mitral Valve Prolapse. **A,** Prolapsed mitral valve. Prolapse permits the valve leaflets to billow back *(arrow)* into the atrium during left ventricular systole. The billowing causes the leaflets to part slightly, permitting regurgitation into the atrium. **B,** Looking down into the mitral valve, the ballooning *(arrows)* of the leaflets is seen. (From Kumar V, et al: *Robbins & Cotran pathologic basis of disease,* ed 8, St Louis, 2010, Mosby.)

regurgitation can be estimated by echocardiography, and valve replacement may be delayed for many years through careful use of vasodilators and inotropic agents.[157]

Mitral Regurgitation. Mitral regurgitation has a variety of causes. The most common are mitral valve prolapse and rheumatic heart disease. Other causes include infective endocarditis, CAD, connective tissue diseases (Marfan syndrome), and congestive cardiomyopathy. Mitral regurgitation permits backflow of blood from the left ventricle into the left atrium during ventricular systole, giving rise to a loud pansystolic (throughout systole) murmur heard best at the apex that radiates into the back and axilla. Because of increased volume in the left atrium that then enters the ventricle, the left ventricle becomes dilated and hypertrophied to maintain adequate cardiac output. The volume of backflow reentering the left atrium gradually increases, causing atrial dilation and associated atrial fibrillation. As the left atrium enlarges, the valve structures stretch and become deformed, leading to further backflow. As mitral valve regurgitation progresses, left ventricular function may become impaired to the point of failure. Eventually, increased atrial pressure also causes pulmonary hypertension and failure of the right ventricle. Mitral incompetence is usually well tolerated—often for years—until ventricular failure occurs. Most clinical manifestations are caused by heart failure. The severity of regurgitation can be estimated by echocardiography, and surgical repair or valve replacement may become necessary.[157,162] In acute mitral regurgitation caused by MI, surgical repair must be done emergently.

Tricuspid Regurgitation. Tricuspid regurgitation is more common than tricuspid stenosis and usually is associated with dilation and failure of the right ventricle secondary to pulmonary hypertension. Rheumatic heart disease and infective endocarditis are less common causes. Tricuspid valve incompetence leads to volume overload in the right atrium and ventricle, increased systemic venous blood pressure, and right heart failure.[163] Pulmonic valve dysfunction can have the same consequences as tricuspid valve dysfunction.

Mitral Valve Prolapse Syndrome. **Mitral valve prolapse syndrome** is a condition in which the anterior and posterior cusps of the mitral valve billow upward (prolapse) into the atrium during systole (Figure 32-33). The most common cause of mitral valve prolapse is myxomatous degeneration of the leaflets in which the cusps are redundant, thickened, and scalloped because of changes in tissue proteoglycans, increased proteinases, and infiltration by myofibroblasts. The chordae tendineae may be elongated, permitting the valve cusps to stretch upward. Mitral regurgitation occurs if the ballooning valve permits blood to leak into the atrium.[164]

Mitral valve prolapse is the most common valve disorder in the United States, with a prevalence estimated at 2.4%.[5] Mitral valve prolapse tends to be most prevalent in young women. Studies suggest an autosomal dominant and X-linked inheritance pattern. Because mitral valve prolapse often is associated with other inherited connective tissue disorders (Marfan syndrome, Ehlers-Danlos syndrome, osteogenesis imperfecta), it is thought to result from a genetic or environmental disruption of valvular development during the fifth or sixth week of gestation. There may be a relationship between symptomatic mitral valve prolapse and hyperthyroidism. Other neuroendocrine abnormalities have been suggested, including polymorphisms of the angiotensin II type 1 (AT_1) receptor and alterations in ANS function.[164]

Many cases of mitral valve prolapse are completely asymptomatic. Cardiac auscultation on routine physical examination may disclose a regurgitant murmur or midsystolic click in an otherwise healthy individual, or echocardiography may demonstrate the condition in the absence of auscultatory findings. Symptomatic mitral valve prolapse can cause palpitations related to dysrhythmias, tachycardia, lightheadedness, syncope, fatigue (especially in the morning), lethargy, weakness, dyspnea, chest tightness, hyperventilation, anxiety, depression, panic attacks, and atypical chest pain. Many symptoms are vague and puzzling and are unrelated to the degree of prolapse. Although severe sequelae—such as chordae rupture, ventricular failure, systemic emboli, and sudden death—are possible, the disorder is actually associated with minimal mortality and morbidity. Most individuals with mitral valve prolapse have an excellent prognosis, do not develop symptoms, and do not require any restriction in activity or medical management. Occasionally, beta-blockers are needed to alleviate syncope, severe chest pain, or palpitations. However, a subset of individuals have an increased risk for complications such as infective endocarditis, cardioembolic stroke, and sudden death. These high-risk individuals can be identified by clinical and echocardiographic findings. If regurgitation is present, medical treatment includes afterload reduction, diuresis, anticoagulation for associated atrial fibrillation, and other medications for heart failure.[164]

Acute Rheumatic Fever and Rheumatic Heart Disease

Rheumatic fever is a systemic, inflammatory disease caused by a delayed immune response to infection by group A beta-hemolytic streptococci.[165] In its acute form rheumatic fever is a febrile illness characterized by inflammation of the joints, skin, nervous system, and heart.[166] If untreated, rheumatic fever can cause scarring and deformity of cardiac structures, resulting in **rheumatic heart disease (RHD).**

The incidence of acute rheumatic fever declined in the United States during the 1960s, 1970s, and early 1980s because of medical and socioeconomic improvements, as well as changes in the virulence of group A streptococci.[167] Because crowding and poor hygiene are environmental risk factors for acute rheumatic fever, the disease continues to be a major cause of death and disability for underprivileged populations.

The acute disease occurs most often in children between 5 and 15 years of age.[165] Because beta-hemolytic streptococcus infection must persist for some time to cause acute rheumatic fever, appropriate antibiotic therapy given within the first 9 days of infection usually prevents rheumatic fever. Initiation of antibiotic therapy 2 weeks after the start of streptococcal infection does not prevent rheumatic fever in susceptible individuals.

Rheumatic fever tends to run in families, lending support to the concept of genetic predisposition, including changes in major histocompatibility antigens.[165] Individuals who have experienced one attack of acute rheumatic fever are more susceptible than the general population to recurrent attacks.

PATHOPHYSIOLOGY. Acute rheumatic fever can develop *only* as a sequel to pharyngeal infection by group A beta-hemolytic streptococci. Streptococcal skin infections do not progress to acute rheumatic fever because the strains of the microorganism that infect the skin do not have the same antigenic molecules in their cell membranes as do those that cause pharyngitis and therefore do not elicit the same kind of immune response. However, both skin infections and pharyngeal infections can cause acute glomerulonephritis.

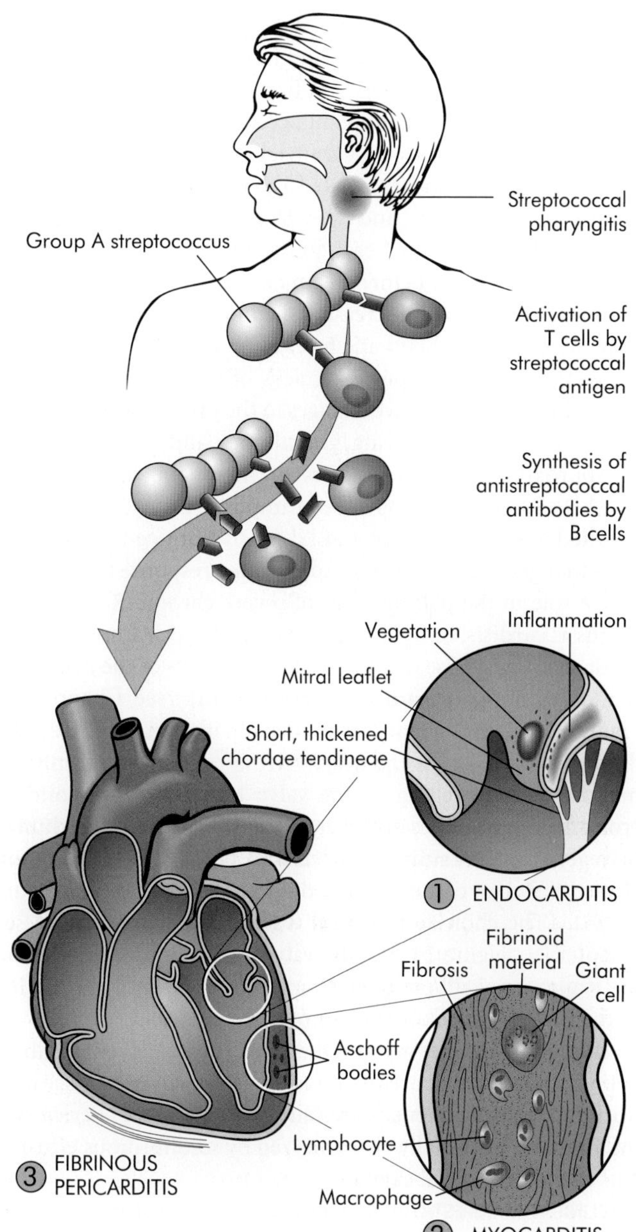

FIGURE 32-34 Pathogenesis and Structural Alterations of Acute Rheumatic Heart Disease. Beginning usually with a sore throat, rheumatic fever can develop only as a sequel to pharyngeal infection by group A beta-hemolytic streptococcus. Suspected as a hypersensitivity reaction, it is proposed that antibodies directed against the M proteins of certain strains of streptococci cross-react with tissue glycoproteins in the heart, joints, and other tissues. The exact nature of cross-reacting antigens has been difficult to define, but it appears that the streptococcal infection causes an autoimmune response against self-antigens. Inflammation is found in various sites including **(1)** endocardium, **(2)** myocardium, and **(3)** pericardium. The most distinctive inflammatory lesions within the heart are called *Aschoff bodies.* The chronic sequelae result from progressive fibrosis because of healing of the inflammatory lesions and the changes induced by valvular deformities. (From Damjanov I: *Pathology for the health professions,* ed 4, Philadelphia, 2012, Saunders.)

Acute rheumatic fever affects the heart, joints, CNS, and skin through an abnormal humoral and cell-mediated immune response to the M proteins on the microorganisms that cross-react with normal tissues (Figure 32-34). Antibodies against a streptococci bacterial wall antigen (GlcNAc) display cross-reactivity against laminin, a protein present in extracellular tissues around heart cells and in the valves. Cardiac myosin is another target antigen. Antibodies also cross-react within neuronal cells triggering dopamine release.[167] These antibodies also affect skin, muscles, and synovial joints.

Autoimmunity and associated intense inflammation result in diffuse, proliferative, and exudative lesions in the connective tissues, especially in the heart, joints, and skin.[167] The inflammation may subside before treatment, leaving behind damage to the heart valves and increasing the individual's susceptibility to recurrent acute rheumatic fever after any subsequent streptococcal infections. Repeated attacks of acute rheumatic fever cause chronic proliferative changes in the previously mentioned organs as a result of scarring, granulomas, and thromboses.[166]

Approximately 10% of cases of rheumatic fever develop RHD.[165] Several genes have been implicated in RHD, including the HLA-DR 1 antigen and HLA-DR 6 antigen, which suggests that genetically determined immune response factors may play a role in the pathogenesis of severe chronic RHD.[5] RHD begins as **carditis,** or inflammation of the heart. Although rheumatic fever can cause carditis in all three layers of the heart wall (endocardium, myocardium, pericardium) (see Chapter 31, Figure 31-2), the primary lesion usually involves the endocardium, which includes the heart valves.[167] Endocardial inflammation causes swelling of the valve leaflets, with secondary erosion along the lines of leaflet contact. Small beadlike clumps of vegetation containing platelets and fibrin are deposited on eroded valvular tissue and on the chordae tendineae (Figure 32-35). (The chordae tendineae anchor the valve leaflets; see Chapter 31, Figure 31-3). The valves lose their elasticity, and the leaflets may adhere to each other. Scarring and shortening of the involved structures occur over time.

If inflammation penetrates the myocardium, localized fibrin deposits develop that are surrounded by areas of necrosis. These fibrinoid necrotic deposits are called *Aschoff bodies.* Pericardial inflammation is usually characterized by serofibrinous effusion within the pericardial cavity.

CLINICAL MANIFESTATIONS. The common symptoms of acute rheumatic fever are fever, lymphadenopathy, arthralgia, nausea, vomiting, epistaxis (nose bleed), abdominal pain, and tachycardia. The major clinical manifestations of acute rheumatic fever (carditis, acute migratory polyarthritis, chorea, and erythema marginatum) usually occur singly or in combination 1 to 5 weeks after streptococcal infection of the pharynx.

Carditis. Carditis occurs a few weeks after the initial infection in about 50% of patients with acute rheumatic fever.[165] The earliest cardiac manifestation of acute rheumatic fever may be a previously undetected murmur caused by mitral or aortic semilunar valve dysfunction. Chest pain is caused by pericardial inflammation. Pericardial effusion produces an audible friction rub. Extra heart sounds, heart block (see p. 1181), atrial fibrillation, and a prolonged PR interval are often associated with chronic rheumatic heart disease. Endocardial inflammation may be manifested years later with serious valvular diseases (stenosis and regurgitation) and recurrent infective endocarditis.

Polyarthritis. Acute migratory polyarthritis (inflammation of more than one joint) occurs in 60% to 80% of individuals with rheumatic fever.[165] Although all of the synovial joints may be involved, the large joints of the extremities are most often affected. Two or more joints are usually involved simultaneously or in succession, with each joint being symptomatic for approximately 2 to 3 days while the overall polyarthritis continues for up to 3 weeks. Exudative synovitis causes heat, redness, swelling, severe pain, and tenderness but no permanent disability. Palpable subcutaneous nodes often develop over bony prominences and along extensor tendons. They do not interfere with joint function and often go unnoticed.

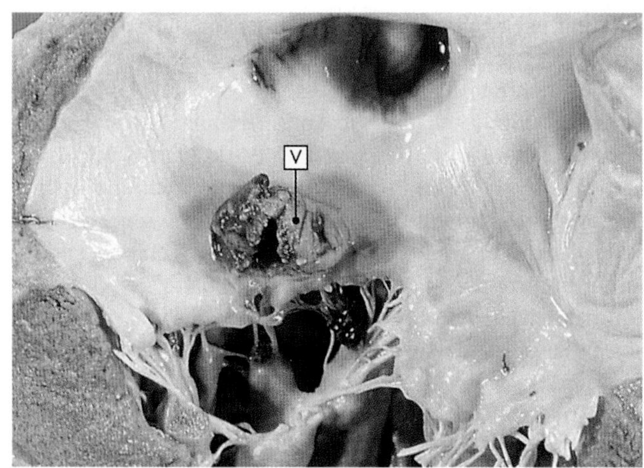

FIGURE 32-35 Valvular Vegetations in Mitral Stenosis. Mitral stenosis and clumps of vegetation *(V)* containing platelets and fibrin. Mitral leaflets are thickened and fused and have clumps of vegetation containing platelets and fibrin. (From Stevens A, Lowe JS, Scott I: *Core pathology,* ed 3, London, 2009, Mosby.)

Chorea. **Sydenham chorea,** or **St. Vitus dance,** is a disorder of the CNS characterized by sudden, aimless, irregular, involuntary movements. (Chorea is described in Chapter 17.) It is the most common acquired chorea in children and is more common in girls than in boys. The chorea is self-limiting, although severe cases may require the use of dopamine receptor blockers and antiepileptic medications. It resolves within 1 to 6 months and has no permanent neural sequelae.

Erythema Marginatum. **Erythema marginatum** is a distinctive truncal rash that often accompanies acute rheumatic fever. It consists of nonpruritic, pink, erythematous macules that never occur on the face or hands. The rash is transitory and may change in appearance within minutes or hours. Heat (e.g., bathing) darkens the rash. The macules may fade in the center and be mistaken for ringworm.

EVALUATION AND TREATMENT. Criteria for the diagnosis of rheumatic fever have been developed and updated by both the AHA and the World Health Organization[168] (Table 32-10). When correlated with findings from physical assessment, laboratory values lend significant support to the diagnosis of acute rheumatic fever. A throat culture positive for group A beta-hemolytic streptococci can be an important finding when associated with certain physical signs. Cultures may be negative when the rheumatic attack begins, however. Most strains of group A beta-hemolytic streptococci produce a hemolytic factor called *streptolysin-O.* Antibodies against this hemolytic factor increase as an individual's immune system fights the disease. A high or rising antistreptolysin-O (ASO) antibody titer is an accurate means of diagnosing the

TABLE 32-10 JONES CRITERIA (REVISED) FOR DIAGNOSIS OF RHEUMATIC FEVER

CRITERIA	DESCRIPTION
Essential	Evidence of streptococcal infection (increased titer of streptococcal antibodies: antistreptolysin-O [ASO]; positive throat culture for group A streptococci; recent scarlet fever)
Major	Carditis, arthritis, chorea, erythema marginatum, subcutaneous nodules
Minor	*Clinical:* arthralgia, fever *Laboratory:* increased C-reactive protein, increased white blood cell count, increased erythrocyte sedimentation rate *Electrocardiographic:* prolonged PR interval

From Dajani AS et al: *Circulation* 87:302–307, 1993.

presence of a streptococcal infection. Several other antibody tests are sensitive indicators of streptococcal infection. These include antideoxyribonucleotidase (anti-DNase B), antihyaluronidase, and antistreptozyme (ASTZ).

Elevated white blood cell count, erythrocyte sedimentation rate, and CRP indicate inflammation. All three are usually increased at the time cardiac or joint symptoms begin to appear. They are more useful in identifying an acute inflammatory process and suggesting prognosis than in diagnosing acute rheumatic fever. The levels of these tests decrease as the inflammatory process resolves.

Therapy for acute rheumatic fever is aimed at eradicating the streptococcal infection using a 10-day regimen of antibiotics. NSAIDs are used as anti-inflammatory agents for rheumatic carditis and arthritis and help relieve symptoms, but do not prevent complications.[167] Unfortunately there is little evidence that anti-inflammatory medications (including corticosteroids) are effective in treating acute carditis.[169] Serious carditis may require that cardiac glycosides, diuretics, and bed rest be added to the regimen. Surgical repair of damaged valves may be necessary in cases of chronic recurrent rheumatic fever or carditis. Active disease is considered resolved when (1) the murmur has disappeared or cardiac status becomes stable, (2) major manifestations are no longer present, (3) the individual is afebrile, and (4) the erythrocyte sedimentation rate is normal or stabilized. This may take 1 to 6 months.

A rheumatic recurrence will develop in 50% to 65% of children with known rheumatic fever if they have another group A streptococcal infection. Recurrence rates decline with the length of time elapsed since the last infection. Continuous prophylactic antibiotic therapy for as long as 5 years is necessary to prevent recurrence of acute rheumatic fever. Several group A streptococcus vaccines are in development.[165]

Infective Endocarditis

Infective endocarditis is a general term used to describe infection and inflammation of the endocardium, especially the cardiac valves. There are approximately 15,000 new cases of infective endocarditis per year in the United States that account for approximately 1 in 1000 admissions to the hospital. Bacteria are the most common cause of infective endocarditis, especially streptococci, staphylococci and enterococci. Other causes include viruses, fungi, rickettsia, and parasites. Infective endocarditis was once a lethal disease, but morbidity and mortality diminished significantly with the advent of antibiotics and improved diagnostic techniques (Box 32-3).

BOX 32-3 RISK FACTORS FOR INFECTIVE ENDOCARDITIS

- Acquired valvular heart disease (especially mitral valve prolapse)
- Implantation of prosthetic heart valves
- Congenital lesions associated with highly turbulent flow (e.g., ventricular septal defect)
- Previous attack of infective endocarditis
- Intravenous drug use
- Long-term indwelling intravenous catheterization (e.g., for pressure monitoring, feeding, hemodialysis)
- Implantable cardiac pacemakers
- Heart transplant with defective valve

PATHOPHYSIOLOGY. The pathogenesis of infective endocarditis requires at least three critical elements (Figure 32-36):

1. Endocardial damage. Trauma, congenital heart disease, valvular heart disease, and the presence of prosthetic valves are the most common risk factors for endocardial damage that leads to infective endocarditis. Turbulent blood caused by these abnormalities usually affects the atrial surface of atrioventricular valves or the ventricular surface of semilunar valves. Endocardial damage exposes the endothelial basement membrane, which contains a type of collagen that attracts platelets and thereby stimulates sterile thrombus formation on the membrane. This causes an inflammatory reaction (nonbacterial thrombotic endocarditis).
2. Blood-borne microorganism adherence to the damaged endocardial surface. Bacteria may enter the bloodstream during injection drug use, trauma, dental procedures that involve manipulation of the gingiva, cardiac surgery, genitourinary procedures and indwelling catheters in the presence of infection, or gastrointestinal instrumentation, or they may spread from uncomplicated upper respiratory or skin infections. Bacteria adhere to the damaged endocardium using adhesins.
3. Formation of infective endocardial vegetations (Figure 32-37). Bacteria infiltrate the sterile thrombi and accelerate fibrin formation by activating the clotting cascade. These vegetative lesions can form anywhere on the endocardium but usually occur on heart valves and surrounding structures. Although endocardial tissue is constantly bathed in antibody-containing blood and is surrounded by scavenging monocytes and polymorphonuclear leukocytes, bacterial colonies are inaccessible to host defenses because they are embedded in the protective fibrin clots. Embolization from these vegetations can lead to abscesses and characteristic skin changes, such as petechiae, splinter hemorrhages, Osler nodes, and Janeway lesions.

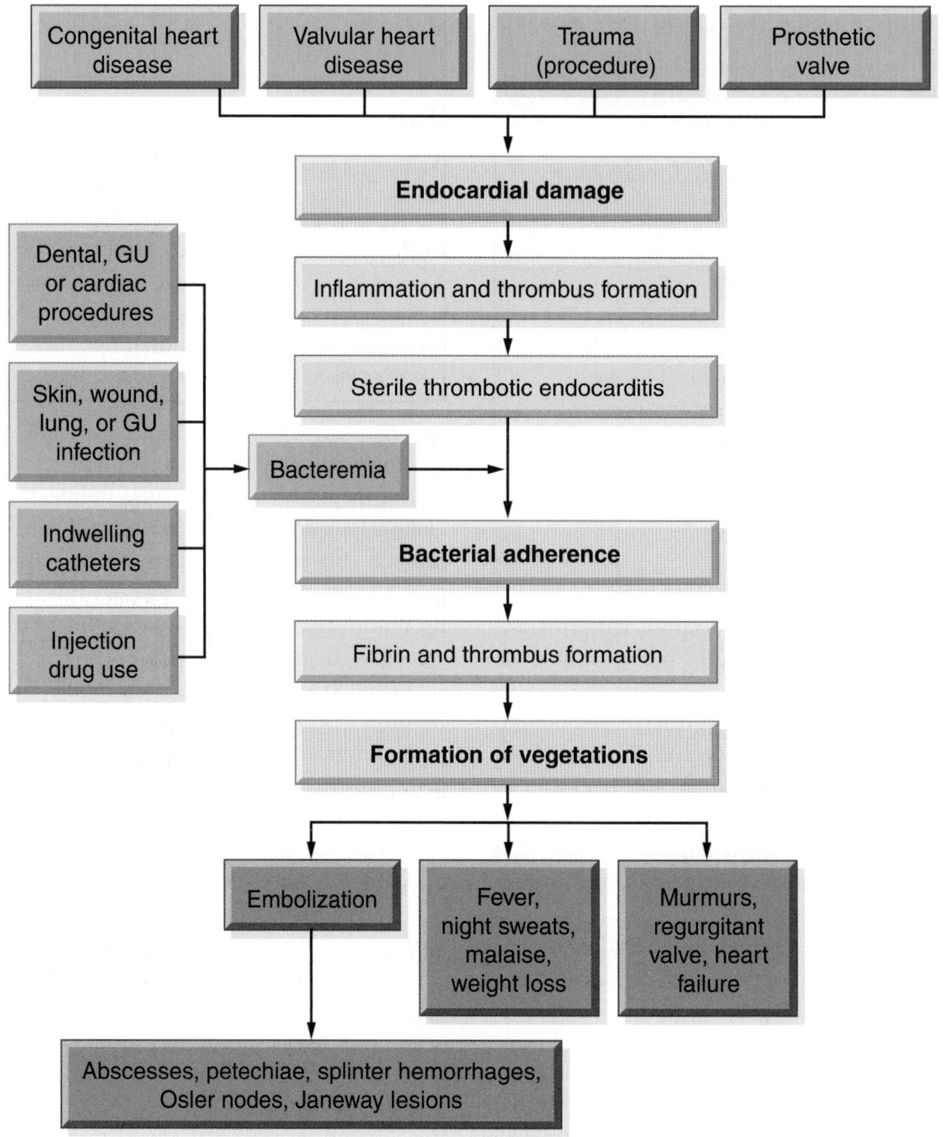

FIGURE 32-36 Pathogenesis of Infective Endocarditis.

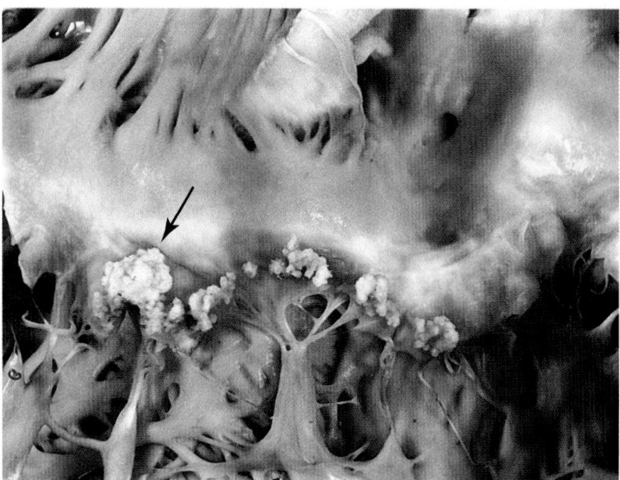

FIGURE 32-37 Bacterial Endocarditis of Mitral Valve. Lesion *(arrow)* in combination with old rheumatic valvulitis. (From Damjanov I, Linder J: *Pathology: a color atlas,* St Louis, 2000, Mosby.)

CLINICAL MANIFESTATIONS. Infective endocarditis may be acute, subacute, or chronic. It causes varying degrees of valvular dysfunction and may be associated with manifestations involving several organ systems (lungs, eyes, kidneys, bones, joints, CNS), making diagnosis exceedingly difficult. Signs and symptoms of infective endocarditis are caused by infection and inflammation, systemic spread of microemboli, and immune complex deposition. The "classic" findings are fever; new or changed cardiac murmur; and petechial lesions of the skin, conjunctiva, and oral mucosa.[170] Characteristic physical findings include Osler nodes (painful erythematous nodules on the pads of the fingers and toes) and Janeway lesions (nonpainful hemorrhagic lesions on the palms and soles). Other manifestations include weight loss, back pain, night sweats, and heart failure. CNS, splenic, renal, pulmonary peripheral arterial, coronary and ocular emboli may lead to a wide variety of signs and symptoms. Sudden onset of severely debilitating symptoms indicates acute disease.

EVALUATION AND TREATMENT. The criteria for the diagnosis of infective endocarditis include persistent bacteremia, new heart murmurs, vascular complications, and appropriate electrocardiographic and echocardiographic findings.[171] If emboli are suggested, organ scans can be performed to confirm their presence. Antimicrobial therapy is generally given for 4 to 6 weeks, beginning with intravenous and ending with oral administration.[170,171] In some cases two different antibiotics are given simultaneously to eliminate the offending microorganism and prevent the development of drug resistance. Other drugs may be necessary to treat left heart failure secondary to valvular dysfunction, and surgical intervention to repair or replace the valve may be required.[171]

In the past, individuals with valvular heart disease received prophylactic antibiotics for dental, genitourinary, or gastrointestinal procedures to prevent infective endocarditis; however, evidence has shown that the risk of endocarditis is low in most individuals. For example, infective endocarditis resulting from dental procedures in individuals with mitral valve prolapse is estimated at only 1 case per 1.1 million dental procedures.[5] In 2008 the recommendations were changed such that only "high risk" individuals (history of infective endocarditis, prosthetic valves, cyanotic congenital heart disease, heart transplant with valvular defect) receive antibiotic prophylaxis, and only in the setting of gingival procedures or in the presence of documented acute gastrointestinal or genitourinary infection.[158]

Cardiac Complications in Acquired Immunodeficiency Syndrome

Individuals infected with HIV and resultant acquired immunodeficiency syndrome (AIDS) are at risk for numerous cardiac complications. Pericardial effusion and left heart failure are the most common complications of HIV infection. Other conditions include cardiomyopathy, myocarditis, tuberculous pericarditis, infective and nonbacterial endocarditis, heart block, pulmonary hypertension, and non-antiretroviral drug-related cardiotoxicity. Malignancies, such as lymphoma and Kaposi sarcoma, are often seen in individuals with AIDS and can affect the heart. Furthermore, treatment with combination antiretroviral therapy (cART) can cause hyperlipidemia and atherosclerotic disease.

MANIFESTATIONS OF HEART DISEASE

Heart Failure

Heart failure is defined as the pathophysiologic condition in which the heart is unable to generate an adequate cardiac output such that there is inadequate perfusion of tissues or increased diastolic filling pressure of the left ventricle, or both, so that pulmonary capillary pressures are increased. It is estimated that nearly 10% of Americans older than age 65 have symptomatic heart failure and approximately 20% of asymptomatic individuals older than age 40 have some evidence of myocardial dysfunction.[5] Ischemic heart disease and hypertension are the most important predisposing risk factors. Other risk factors include age, obesity, diabetes, renal failure, valvular heart disease, cardiomyopathies, myocarditis, congenital heart disease, and excessive alcohol use. Numerous genetic polymorphisms have been linked to an increased risk for heart failure, including genes for cardiomyopathies, myocyte contractility, and neurohumoral receptors. Genetic changes in kinases, phosphatases, and cellular calcium cycling are being explored. Most causes of heart failure result in dysfunction of the left ventricle (systolic and diastolic heart failure). The right ventricle also may be dysfunctional, especially in pulmonary disease (right ventricular failure). Finally, some conditions cause inadequate perfusion despite normal or elevated cardiac output (high-output failure).

Types

Left Heart Failure (Congestive Heart Failure). **Left heart failure,** commonly called **congestive heart failure,** is categorized as heart failure with reduced ejection fraction (systolic heart failure) or heart failure with preserved ejection fraction (diastolic heart failure). These two types of heart failure can occur together in one individual or singly.

Heart Failure with Reduced Ejection Fraction (HFrEF) (Systolic Heart Failure). Heart failure with reduced ejection fraction (systolic heart failure) is defined as an ejection fraction of <40% and an inability of the heart to generate an adequate cardiac output to perfuse vital tissues.[5a] Cardiac output depends on the heart rate and stroke volume. Stroke volume is influenced by three major factors: contractility, preload, and afterload (see Chapter 31). Contractility is reduced by diseases that disrupt myocyte activity. Myocardial infarction is the most common cause of decreased contractility; other causes include myocarditis and cardiomyopathies. Secondary causes of decreased contractility, such as myocardial ischemia and increased myocardial workload, contribute to inflammatory, immune, and neurohumoral changes (activation of the SNS and RAAS) that mediate a process called ventricular remodeling. **Ventricular remodeling** results in disruption of the normal myocardial extracellular structure with resultant dilation of the myocardium and causes progressive myocyte contractile dysfunction over time (Figure 32-38). When contractility is decreased, stroke volume falls, and left ventricular end-diastolic volume (LVEDV) increases. This causes dilation of the heart and an increase in preload.

Preload, or LVEDV, increases with decreased contractility or when there is an excess of plasma volume (intravenous fluid

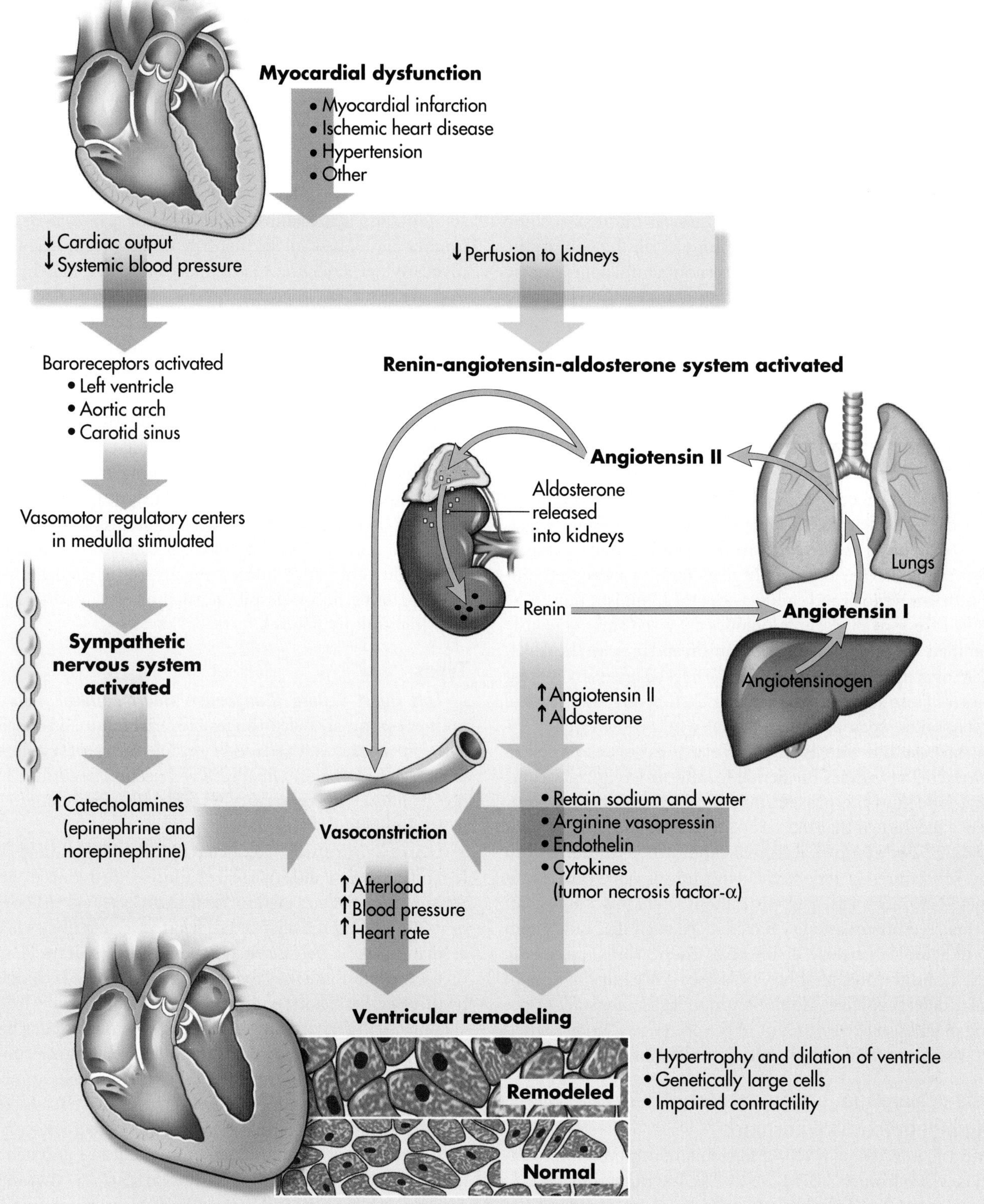

FIGURE 32-38 **Pathophysiology of Ventricular Remodeling.** Myocardial dysfunction activates the renin-angiotensin-aldosterone and sympathetic nervous systems, releasing neurohormones (angiotensin II, aldosterone, catecholamines, and cytokines). These neurohormones contribute to ventricular remodeling. (Redrawn from Carelock J, Clark AP: *Am J Nurs* 101[12]:27, 2001.)

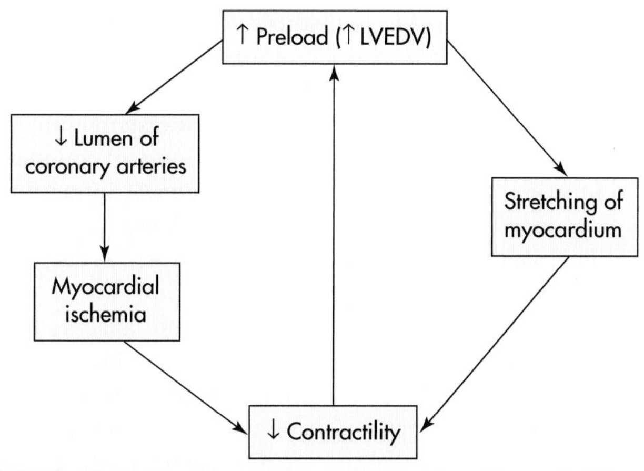

FIGURE 32-39 The Effect of Elevated Preload on Myocardial Oxygen Supply and Demand. *LVEDV*, Left ventricular end-diastolic volume.

administration, renal failure, mitral valvular disease). Increases in LVEDV can actually improve cardiac output up to a certain point, but as preload continues to rise, it causes a stretching of the myocardium that eventually can lead to dysfunction of the sarcomeres and decreased contractility (Figure 32-39).

Increased afterload is most commonly a result of increased peripheral vascular resistance (PVR), such as that seen with hypertension (Figure 32-40). Nearly 75% of cases of heart failure have antecedent hypertension.[5] Although much less common, it also can be the result of aortic valvular disease. With increased PVR, there is resistance to ventricular emptying and more workload for the left ventricle, which responds with hypertrophy of the myocardium. This process differs from the physiologic myocyte response to increased workload (exercise) in which the workload is intermittent rather than sustained, resulting in an increase in muscle mass but no distortion of the cardiac architecture.[172] Sustained afterload leads to pathologic hypertrophy mediated by angiotensin II and catecholamines. This pathologic increase in muscle mass results in an increase in oxygen and energy demand. The myocardium consumes a huge amount of metabolic energy and relies on the efficient production of ATP. This production of ATP depends on the myocytes getting enough fuel, having adequate mitochondrial function, and using an effective creatine kinase system. When demand for energy is greater than the ability of these systems to supply the necessary ATP, contractility of the myocardium is compromised. An energy-starved state develops that further contributes to changes in the myocytes themselves and ventricular remodeling that significantly impairs contractility and therefore ventricular function (see Figure 32-38).[173] Remodeling also results in the deposition of collagen between the myocytes, which can disrupt the integrity of the muscle, decrease contractility, and make the ventricle more likely to dilate and fail.[174] Weakness of the cardiac muscle due to hypertension-induced hypertrophy is called hypertensive hypertrophic cardiomyopathy.

As cardiac output falls, renal perfusion diminishes with activation of the RAAS, which acts to increase PVR and plasma volume, thus increasing afterload and preload further. In addition, baroreceptors in the central circulation detect the decrease in

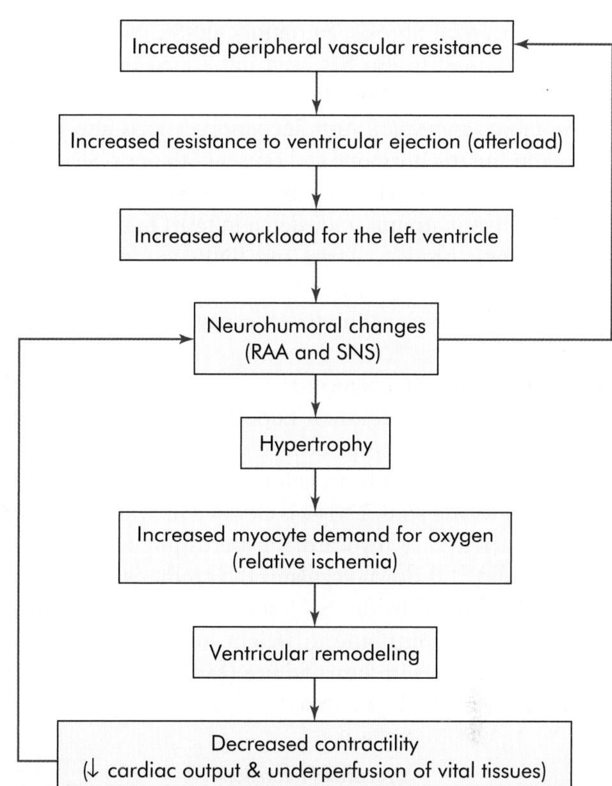

FIGURE 32-40 The Role of Increased Afterload in the Pathogenesis of Heart Failure. *RAA*, Renin angiotensin aldosterone, *SNS*, sympathetic nervous system.

perfusion and stimulate the SNS to cause yet more vasoconstriction and to cause the hypothalamus to produce antidiuretic hormone. This vicious cycle of decreasing contractility, increasing preload, and increasing afterload causes progressive worsening of left heart failure (Figure 32-41).

In addition to these hemodynamic interactions, systolic congestive heart failure is characterized by a complex constellation of neurohumoral, inflammatory, and metabolic processes:

1. *Catecholamines.* Sympathetic nervous system activation initially compensates for a decrease in cardiac output by increasing heart rate and peripheral vascular resistance. However, catecholamines cause numerous deleterious effects on the myocardium, including direct toxicity to myocytes, induction of myocyte apoptosis, myocardial remodeling, down-regulation of adrenergic receptors, facilitation of dysrhythmias, and potentiation of autoimmune effects on the heart muscle.
2. *RAAS*
   a. Angiotensin II (Ang II). Activation of the RAAS causes not only increases in preload and afterload but also direct toxicity to the myocardium (see Figure 32-38). Ang II mediates remodeling of the ventricular wall, contributing to sarcomere death, loss of the normal collagen matrix, and interstitial fibrosis. This leads to decreased contractility, changes in myocardial compliance, and ventricular dilation.
   b. Aldosterone. Aldosterone not only causes salt and water retention by the kidney but also contributes to

myocardial fibrosis, autonomic dysfunction, and dysrhythmias. It also has been implicated in endothelial dysfunction and prothrombotic effects.[175]

3. *Arginine vasopressin.* Arginine vasopressin is also known as antidiuretic hormone and causes both peripheral vasoconstriction and renal fluid retention. These actions exacerbate hyponatremia and edema in heart failure.
4. *Natriuretic peptides.* Atrial and BNPs are increased and may have some protective effect by decreasing preload; however, their compensatory mechanisms are inadequate in heart failure.[176]
5. *Inflammatory cytokines*
   a. Endothelial hormones. Endothelin is a potent vasoconstrictor and is associated with a poor prognosis in individuals with heart failure.
   b. TNF-α and IL-6. TNF-α is elevated in heart failure and contributes to myocardial hypertrophy and remodeling.[177,178] It down-regulates the synthesis of the vasodilator nitric oxide (NO), induces myocyte apoptosis, and may contribute to weight loss and weakness in individuals with heart failure (cardiac cachexia). IL-6 also is elevated in individuals with severe heart failure and cardiogenic shock and may contribute to further deleterious immune activation.

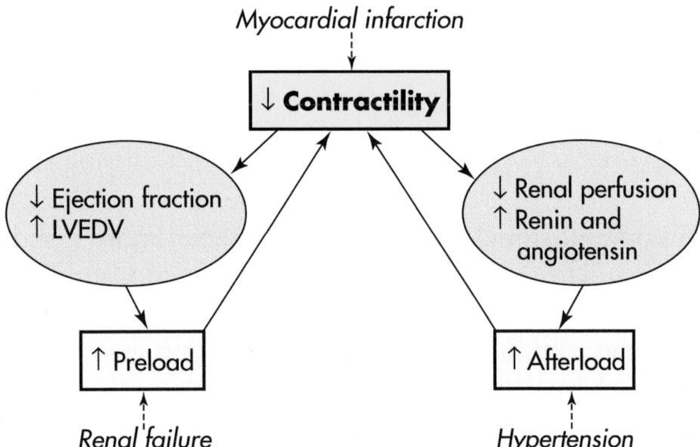

FIGURE 32-41 The Vicious Cycle of Systolic Heart Failure. Although the initial insult may be one of primary decreased contractility (e.g., myocardial infarction), increased preload (e.g., renal failure), or increased afterload (e.g., hypertension), all three factors play a role in the progression of left heart failure. *LVEDV,* Left ventricular end-diastolic volume.

6. *Myocyte calcium transport.* Calcium transport into, out of, and within myocytes is critical to normal contractile function. Changes in calcium ion channels, intracellular transport mechanisms in the sarcoplasmic reticulum, and calcium cycling have all been implicated in decreased myocardial contractility and heart failure.[179]
7. *Insulin resistance and diabetes.* Insulin resistance is a likely contributor to, as well as complication of, heart failure. Insulin resistance causes abnormal myocyte fatty acid metabolism and generation of ATP, which contributes to decreased myocardial contractility and remodeling[180] (see What's New? Metabolic Changes in Heart Failure). Heart failure activates the SNS and RAAS, which contribute to insulin resistance. Diabetes contributes to heart failure through disturbed calcium metabolism, oxidative stress, changes in fatty acid and glucose metabolism, and mitochondrial dysfunction. In addition, receptors on myocytes for damaging advanced glycation end-products (RAGE) (see Chapter 22) are up-regulated in injuries to the heart, including ischemia and reperfusion injury. Measurement of levels of RAGE in plasma or serum may correlate with the degree of heart failure.[181] Unfortunately, many of the new medications used to treat diabetes and insulin resistance have deleterious side effects on cardiac functioning; however, newer agents that modify fatty acid metabolism and insulin activity are being explored.[182]

The interaction of these metabolic, neurohumoral, and inflammatory processes results in a gradual decline in myocardial function. Pathologically, the heart muscle exhibits progressive changes in myocyte myofilaments, decreased contractility, myocyte apoptosis and necrosis, abnormal fibrin deposition in the ventricle wall, myocardial hypertrophy, and changes in the ventricular chamber geometry. These changes reduce myocardial function and cardiac output and lead to increased morbidity and mortality. These discoveries have led to the routine use of ACE inhibitors, aldosterone blockers, and beta-blockers in the management of heart failure, which has

WHAT'S NEW?

Metabolic Changes in Heart Failure

The heart is the largest consumer of energy in the body and relies on the efficient production of adenosine triphosphate (ATP). The heart has very little capacity for energy storage. In the failing heart, increased demand for oxygen and energy is coupled with a decreased ability to use fatty acids as an energy source. As a result, there is activation of several genes that alter the ability of myoctyes to use lipids and glucose as fuel sources, the most studied of which are the peroxisome proliferator-activated receptor (PPAR) family of genes. These genes control fatty acid oxidation and are of particular importance in heart failure associated with insulin resistance and diabetes. Energy starvation and high levels of catecholamines associated with heart failure lead to altered fatty acid oxidation and decreased effective ATP generation and use. This results in decreased myocardial contractility and structural changes in the myocardium (remodeling). Increasing knowledge of these mechanisms has led to the exploration of potential therapies for heart failure. For example, PPAR agonists have been shown to enhance fatty acid oxidation, improve endothelial cell function, and decrease myocardial fibrosis and hypertrophy in animal models of heart failure. Unfortunately currently available PPAR-gamma agonists (thiazolidinediones) are contraindicated in worsening heart failure because of increased fluid retention at the renal tubule. Many new potential pharmacologic interventions are under investigation, including trimetazidine, a partial fatty-acid-oxidation inhibitor that may decrease hospitalization for cardiac causes, improve clinical symptoms and cardiac function, and reduce left ventricular remodeling in people with CHF.

Data from Abel E et al: *Arterioscler Throm Vasc Biol* 32(9):2068–2076, 2012; Ardehali H et al: *Eur J Heart Fail* 14(2):120–129, 2012; Sarma S, Ardehali H, Gheorghiade M: *Heart Fail Rev* 17(1):35–43, 2012; Zhang L et al: *J Am Coll Cardiol* 59(10):913–922, 2012.

WHAT'S NEW?

Brain Natriuretic Peptide and Heart Failure

Brain natriuretic peptide (BNP) is produced and released in response to pressure and volume overload of the cardiac chambers. This occurs in both systolic and diastolic heart failure (HF). BNP causes arterial and venous dilation, natriuresis, and suppression of the renin-angiotensin-aldosterone system and the sympathetic nervous system. BNP inhibits myocardial fibrosis and hypertrophy and enhances diastolic function. There are currently four uses for BNP: three are measures of serum levels of endogenous BNP and one is a therapeutic use for exogenous BNP:

1. *Diagnosis of heart failure:* Significantly elevated serum levels of BNP have a sensitivity ranging from 93% to 98% in diagnosing heart failure in symptomatic patients, and negative predictive values ranging from 92% to 98%, demonstrating BNP ability to rule out heart failure. BNP also can be used to diagnose diastolic heart failure.
2. *Prognosis in HF:* Serum levels of BNP are correlated with the American Heart Association/American College of Cardiology class of heart failure morbidity and mortality, and risk for future acute exacerbations.
3. *Monitoring treatment of HF:* Serum levels of BNP-guided treatment of heart failure reduced total cardiovascular events, mortality, and hospital readmission with heart failure.
4. *Treatment of HF:* Approved in August 2001 by the U.S. Food and Drug Administration, nesiritide is the first of a new class of drugs, human B-type natriuretic peptide (hBNP); it is manufactured from *Escherichia coli* using recombinant deoxyribonucleic acid (DNA) technology. Intravenous administration of nesiritide (recombinant BNP) also improves preload and contractility; however, results of this therapy have been mixed and a new natriuretic peptide (ularitide) is being evaluated. In a limited number of studies, human recombinant ANP (hANP) has been shown to improve pulmonary capillary wedge pressure and cardiac output, but not mortality.

Data from Florea VG, Anand IS: *Heart Fail Clin* 8(2):207–224, 2012; Gassanov N et al: *Eur J Clin Pharmacol* 68(3):223–230, 2012; Januzzi JL Jr: *Arch Cardiovasc Dis* 105(1):40–50, 2012; Kobayashi D et al: *Can J Cardiol* 28(1):102–199, 2012; Richards AM, Troughton RW: *Clin Chem* 58(1):62–71, 2012; Saremi A, Gopal D, Maisel AS: *Exp Rev Cardovasc Ther* 10(2):191–203, 2012; Sato Y, Fujiwara H, Takatsu Y: *J Cardiol* 59(1):1–7, 2012.

resulted in significant decreases in morbidity and mortality.[137] Individuals selected for use of these medications may soon be facilitated through the use of pharmacogenetics that can identify those genotypes most likely to respond favorably to specific treatment options.[183]

EVALUATION. The clinical manifestations of HFrEF are the result of pulmonary vascular congestion and inadequate perfusion of the systemic circulation. Individuals experience dyspnea, orthopnea, cough of frothy sputum, fatigue, decreased urine output, and edema. Physical examination often reveals pulmonary edema (cyanosis, inspiratory crackles, pleural effusions), hypotension or hypertension, an S_3 gallop, and evidence of underlying CAD or hypertension.[184] An ECG and serum troponin should be obtained to evaluate for acute ischemia. A chest x-ray should be obtained to assess heart size and evidence of pulmonary congestion, and echocardiography, to confirm decreased cardiac output and cardiomegaly.[5a] Invasive catheterization to monitor hemodynamics or to document underlying coronary disease may be needed. Serum BNP levels should be measured to assist in diagnosing heart failure and to give some insight into its severity and response to treatment[5a,185] (see What's New? Brain Natriuretic Peptide and Heart Failure). Numerous other biomarkers are emerging that may aid in the diagnosis and management of heart failure.[186]

Management of HFrEF is aimed at interrupting the worsening cycle of decreasing contractility, increasing preload, and increasing afterload, as well as blocking the neurohormonal mediators of myocardial toxicity.[187] The acute onset of left heart failure is most often the result of acute myocardial ischemia and must be managed in conjunction with the underlying coronary disease. Oxygen, nitrates, and morphine administration improve myocardial oxygenation and help relieve coronary spasm while lowering preload through systemic venodilation. Diuretics reduce preload and are the mainstay of therapy. Intravenous inotropic drugs, such as dobutamine and milrinone, increase contractility and can help raise the blood pressure in hypotensive individuals; however, long-term use is associated with a high mortality.[188] Calcium-sensitizing inotropic drugs (e.g., levosimendan) have shown promise for acute heart failure in selected individuals.[189] ACE inhibitors (which reduce preload and afterload) and intravenous beta-blockers (which reduce myocardial demand) have been found to reduce mortality but must be used with caution in hypotensive individuals. Intravenous administration of nesiritide (recombinant BNP) also improves preload and contractility; however, results of this therapy have been mixed and new natriuretic peptides (human recombinant ANP and ularitide) are being evaluated.[190,191] Individuals with severe systolic failure because of myocardial ischemia may benefit from acute coronary bypass or PCI. Those with refractory hypotension may be supported with the intra-aortic balloon pump (IABP) until they can be taken safely to the operating room; the IABP is positioned in the aorta just distal to the aortic valve and is inflated during diastole to improve coronary perfusion and deflated during systole to reduce afterload.

Management of **chronic left heart failure** also relies on increasing contractility and reducing preload and afterload. In all patients with reduced ejection fraction, ACE inhibitors and beta blockers are indicated to reduce mortality.[5a,137] Salt restriction, loop diuretics, and aldosterone-blockers such as spironolactone and eplerenone are effective in reducing preload and improving outcomes.[192,193] ACE inhibitors reduce preload and afterload and have been shown to significantly reduce mortality in chronic left heart failure. ARBs do not improve morbidity or mortality in individuals with heart failure and should be used only in those who do not tolerate ACE inhibitors.[194] Beta-blockers, especially some of the newer drugs, such as bisoprolol, improve symptoms and increase survival.[195] Catheter-based renal sympathetic denervation is

WHAT'S NEW?

Gene Therapy for Heart Failure

The effectiveness and safety of recent gene therapy trials for heart failure have led to an explosion of interest in these innovative methods for restoring cardiac function. The most studied of the potential gene targets include sarcoendoplasmic reticulum calcium ATPase (SERCA2a) and S100A1, which affect intracellular myocyte calcium handling. Another exciting target is adenylyl cyclase 6 (AC6), the enzyme catalyzing cAMP formation and beta-adrenergic receptor function. Other targets include SDF1/CXCR4 complex, which promotes homing of stem cells to infarcted myocardium, microRNAs, and genes that code for critical neurohumoral factors, including insulin-like growth factor-1 (IGF-1), growth hormone, and B-type natriuretic peptide. Gene delivery vectors fall into one of two categories: nonviral or viral. Nonviral gene delivery vectors are safe and have minimal immunogenicity, but do not appear to be efficient at delivering the genes to the tissues. Viral vectors are more efficient at delivering genes to cells, but safety concerns persist. Today the viruses most widely used for cardiovascular gene transfer are adenovirus, sendai virus, and adeno-associated virus (AAV). These viruses exhibit fairly good cardiotropism, and various methods are being explored for delivering these gene vectors most efficiently to the myocardium, including antegrade or retrograde coronary infusion, intravenous infusion, direct myocardial injection, and pericardial injection. It is clear that the future will reveal many new and potentially lifesaving gene therapies for individuals with intractable heart failure.

Data from Hulot JS, Senyei G, Hajjar RJ: *Gene Ther* 19(6):596–599, 2012; Kairouz V et al: *Ann N Y Acad Sci* 1254:42–50, 2012; Ritterhoff J, Most P: *Gene Ther* 19(6):613–621, 2012; Tang T, Gao MH, Hammond HK: *Gene Ther* 19(6):606–612, 2012; Tilemann L et al: *Circ Res* 110(5):777–793, 2012.

TABLE 32-11 COMPARISON OF SYSTOLIC AND DIASTOLIC HEART FAILURE

CHARACTERISTIC	SYSTOLIC HEART FAILURE	DIASTOLIC HEART FAILURE
Gender	Male>female	Female>male
Left ventricular ejection fraction	Decreased	Normal
Left ventricular chamber size	Increased	Decreased
Left ventricular hypertrophy on electrocardiogram	Possible	Probable
Chest radiography	Pulmonary congestion with cardiomegaly	Pulmonary congestion without cardiomegaly
Gallop	S_3	S_4

Adapted from Jessup M, Brozena S: *N Engl J Med* 348(20):2007–2018, 2003.

being explored for heart failure.[196] The inotropic drug digoxin may be considered in some individuals, especially those with atrial fibrillation. Statins are not indicated for the treatment of heart failure unless other comorbid conditions (e.g., CAD) are present. Anticoagulants and antithrombotics may be indicated in selected individuals, particularly those with intracardiac thrombi or atrial fibrillation. Although many individuals with left heart failure die suddenly from dysrhythmias, prophylactic administration of antidysrhythmics has not been shown to improve survival. In individuals with sustained ventricular tachycardia, amiodarone or ICDs are indicated. Cardiac resynchronization therapy is proving to be an important modality in selected individuals.[197] Coronary bypass surgery or PCI may improve perfusion to ischemic myocardium (hibernating myocardium) and improve cardiac output. Other types of surgical intervention that improve ventricular geometry may be considered. Heart transplant may be the only remaining option. Experimental therapies, including gene and stem cell therapies, are being explored[198,199] (see What's New? Gene Therapy for Heart Failure).

Diastolic Heart Failure. Diastolic heart failure (also called heart failure with preserved ejection fraction) can occur singly or along with systolic heart failure. Isolated diastolic heart failure is defined as pulmonary congestion despite a normal stroke volume and cardiac output. It is the cause of approximately 50% of all cases of left heart failure and is more common in women. The major causes of diastolic dysfunction include hypertension-induced myocardial hypertrophy and myocardial ischemia with resultant ventricular remodeling. Hypertrophy and ischemia cause a decreased ability of the myocytes to actively pump calcium from the cytosol, resulting in impaired relaxation. Other causes include aortic valvular disease, mitral valve disease, pericardial diseases, and cardiomyopathies. Diabetes also increases the risk for diastolic dysfunction. Like systolic heart failure, diastolic failure is characterized by sustained activation of the RAAS and the SNS.

Two areas of pathophysiologic changes in the ventricle have been identified in diastolic dysfunction: decreased compliance of the left ventricle and abnormal diastolic relaxation (lusitropy). Decreased ventricular compliance has been linked to changes in myocardial structure such as that seen with molecular alterations in collagen, which forms the extracellular matrix for myocytes. Another recently identified structural change is because of abnormalities in an intracellular protein component of the myocyte cytoskeleton called titin. Abnormal lusitropy is caused by changes in calcium transport from myocytes and may be related to the activity of sarcoplasmic reticulum–calcium adenosine triphosphatase (ATPase).[200] The resultant noncompliant and poorly lusitropic ventricle cannot accept filling with blood without significant resistance and an increase in wall tension. Thus HFpEF occurs because a normal LVEDV is associated with an increased LVEDP. The resultant increase

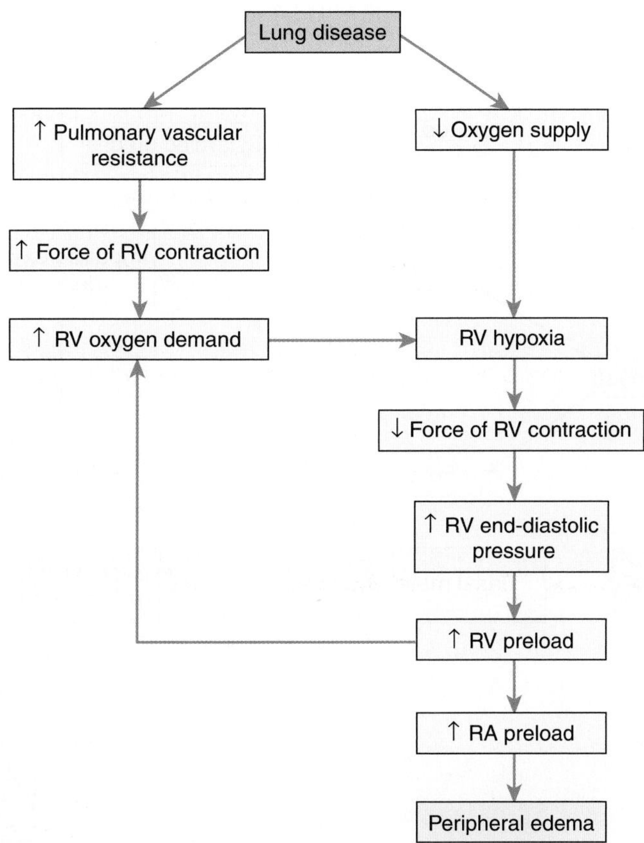

FIGURE 32-42 Right Heart Failure (Cor Pulmonale) Caused By Lung Disease. The presence of peripheral edema in cor pulmonale is caused by lung disease. *RA,* Right atrial; *RV,* right ventricular.

in left atrial pressure is then reflected back into the pulmonary circulation and results in pulmonary edema. The increase in pressure is made worse when ventricular filling is rapid so symptoms worsen with tachycardia (e.g., with exercise).

Individuals with diastolic dysfunction most often present with dyspnea on exertion and fatigue. If diastolic dysfunction is severe, there may be evidence of pulmonary edema (inspiratory crackles on auscultation, pleural effusions). Pulmonary hypertension and right ventricular failure may develop.[201] Late in diastole, atrial contraction with rapid ejection of blood into the noncompliant ventricle may give rise to an S_4 gallop. Electrocardiography often reveals evidence of left ventricular hypertrophy, and chest x-ray shows pulmonary congestion without cardiomegaly (Table 32-11).There also may be evidence of underlying coronary disease, hypertension, or valvular disease. Diagnosis is based on three factors: signs and symptoms of heart failure, normal left ventricular ejection fraction, and evidence of diastolic dysfunction. The diagnosis is initially made by echocardiography, which demonstrates poor ventricular filling with normal ejection fractions.[202] Management is aimed at improving ventricular relaxation and prolonging diastolic filling times to reduce diastolic pressure. Physical training (aerobic and weight training) improves endurance and quality of life.[203] Beta-blockers, ACE inhibitors, ARBs, and aldosterone blockers have been used with varying success,[204,205] however current guidelines focus on treating hypertension or valvular disease.[5a] Inotropic drugs are not indicated in isolated diastolic heart failure because contractility and ejection fraction are not affected. Outcomes for individuals with HFpEF can be as poor as those with systolic heart failure, and there has been little improvement in prognosis despite numerous new treatment trials.

Right Heart Failure. **Right heart failure** is defined as the inability of the right ventricle to provide adequate blood flow into the pulmonary circulation at a normal central venous pressure. It most often results from left heart failure when the increase in left ventricular filling pressure that is reflected back into the pulmonary circulation is severe enough.[206] As pressure in the pulmonary circulation rises, the resistance to right ventricular emptying increases. The right ventricle is poorly prepared to compensate for this increased workload and will dilate and fail. When this happens, pressure will rise in the systemic venous circulation, resulting in jugular venous distention, peripheral edema, and hepatosplenomegaly. Treatment relies on management of the left ventricular dysfunction as just outlined. When right heart failure occurs in the absence of left heart failure, it is caused most commonly by pulmonary hypertension resulting from diffuse hypoxic pulmonary disease such as chronic obstructive pulmonary disease (COPD), cystic fibrosis, and ARDS[207] (Figure 32-42). The mechanisms for this type of right ventricular dysfunction *(cor pulmonale)* are discussed in Chapter 35. Finally, right heart failure can result from right ventricular MI, cardiomyopathies, and pulmonic valvular disease.

High-Output Failure. **High-output failure** is the inability of the heart to adequately supply the body with blood-borne nutrients, despite adequate blood volume and normal or elevated myocardial contractility. In high-output failure the

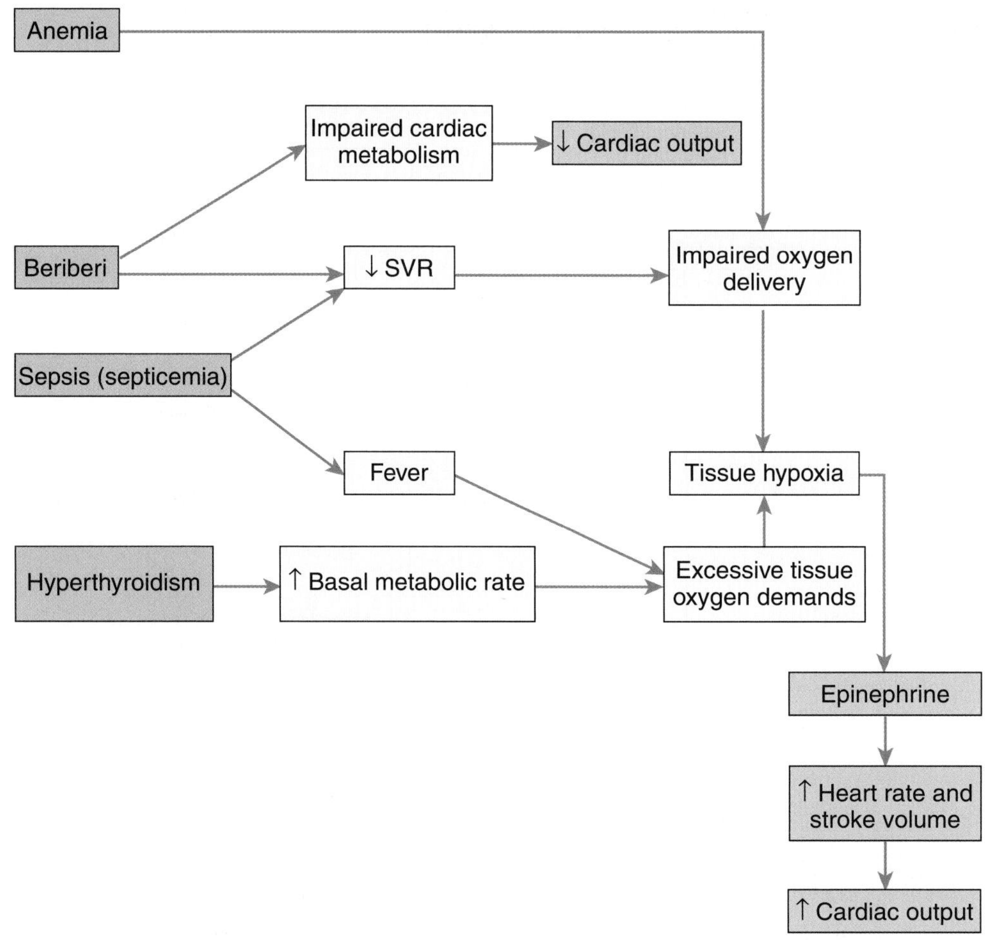

FIGURE 32-43 High-Output Failure. *SVR,* Systemic vascular resistance.

heart increases its output but the body's metabolic needs are still not met. Common causes of high-output failure are anemia, septicemia, hyperthyroidism, and beriberi (Figure 32-43).

Anemia decreases the oxygen-carrying capacity of the blood (see Chapter 28). Metabolic acidosis occurs as the body's cells switch to anaerobic metabolism (see Chapter 3). In response to metabolic acidosis, heart rate and stroke volume increase in an attempt to circulate blood faster. If anemia is severe, however, even maximum cardiac output does not supply the cells with enough oxygen for metabolism.

In septicemia, disturbed metabolism, bacterial toxins, and the inflammatory process cause systemic vasodilation and fever. Faced with a lowered systemic vascular resistance (SVR) and an elevated metabolic rate, cardiac output increases to maintain blood pressure and prevent metabolic acidosis. In overwhelming septicemia, however, the heart may not be able to raise its output enough to compensate for vasodilation. Body tissues show signs of inadequate blood supply despite a very high cardiac output.

Hyperthyroidism accelerates cellular metabolism through the actions of elevated levels of thyroxine from the thyroid gland. This may occur chronically (thyrotoxicosis) or acutely (thyroid storm). Because the body's increased demand for oxygen threatens to cause metabolic acidosis, cardiac output increases. If blood levels of thyroxine are high and the metabolic response to thyroxine is vigorous, even an abnormally elevated cardiac output may be inadequate.

In the United States, beriberi (thiamine deficiency) usually is caused by malnutrition secondary to chronic alcoholism. Beriberi actually causes a mixed type of heart failure. Thiamine deficiency impairs cellular metabolism in all tissues, including the myocardium. In the heart, impaired cardiac metabolism leads to insufficient contractile strength. In blood vessels, thiamine deficiency leads mainly to peripheral vasodilation, which decreases SVR. Heart failure ensues as decreased SVR triggers increased cardiac output, which the impaired myocardium is unable to deliver. The strain of demands for increased output in the face of impaired metabolism may deplete cardiac reserves until low-output failure begins.

Dysrhythmias

A dysrhythmia, or arrhythmia, is a disturbance of heart rhythm. Normal heart rhythms are generated by the SA node and travel through the heart's conduction system, causing the atrial and ventricular myocardium to contract and relax at a regular rate that is appropriate to maintain circulation at various levels of physical activity (see Chapter 31). Dysrhythmias range in severity from occasional "missed" or rapid beats to serious disturbances that impair the pumping ability of the heart, contributing to heart failure and death. Dysrhythmias can be caused by either an abnormal rate of impulse generation (Table 32-12) by the SA node or other pacemaker or the abnormal conduction of impulses (Table 32-13) through the heart's conduction system, including the myocardial cells themselves.

TABLE 32-12 DISORDERS OF IMPULSE FORMATION

TYPE	ELECTROCARDIOGRAM	EFFECT	PATHOPHYSIOLOGY	TREATMENT
Sinus bradycardia	P rate 60 or less PR interval normal QRS for each P	Increased preload Decreased mean arterial pressure	Hyperkalemia: slows depolarization Vagal hyperactivity: unknown Digoxin toxicity common Late hypoxia: lack of adenosine triphosphate (ATP)	If hypotensive, treat cause and support Follow with sympathomimetics, cardiotonics, and pacer Vagolytics
Simple sinus tachycardia	P rate 100-150 PR interval normal QRS for each P	Decreased filling times Decreased mean arterial pressure Increased myocardial demand	Catecholamines; rise in resting potential, calcium influx Fever: unknown Early failure and lung disease: hypoxic cell metabolism Hypercalcemia	Oxygen, bed rest Calcium channel blockers
Premature atrial contractions (PACs) or beats*	Early P waves that may have changed morphology PR interval normal QRS for each P	Occasional decreased filling time and mean arterial pressure	Electrolyte disturbances: decrease in all phases Hypoxia and elevated preload: cell membrane disturbances Hypercalcemia	Treat underlying cause Digoxin
Sinus dysrhythmias	Rate varies P-P regularly irregular, short with inspiration, long with exhalation PR interval normal QRS for each P	Variable filling times Variable mean arterial pressures Variable oxygen demand	Unknown Common in young children and young adults	None
Atrial tachycardia (includes premature atrial tachycardia if onset is abrupt)	P rate 151-250P morphology may differ from sinus PPR interval normal P:QRS ratio variable	Decreased filling time Decreased mean arterial pressure Increased myocardial demand	Same as PACs: leads to increased atrial automaticity, atrial reentry Digoxin toxicity: common	Control ventricular rate Digoxin, calcium channel blockers, vagus stimulation Pace to override
Atrial flutter*	P rate 251-300; morphology may vary from sinus P PR interval usually not observable P:QRS ratio variable	Decreased filling time Decreased mean arterial pressure	Same as atrial tachycardia Aging	Same as atrial tachycardia Synchronous cardioversion
Atrial fibrillation*	P rate >300 and usually not observable No PR interval QRS rate variable and rhythm irregular	Same as atrial flutter	Same as atrial tachycardia Aging	Same as atrial tachycardia
Idiojunctional rhythm	P absent or independent QRS normal, rate 41-59, regular	Decreased cardiac output from loss of atrial contribution to ventricular preload Decreased mean atrial pressure as a result of bradycardia	Atrial and sinus bradycardia, standstill, or block	Same as sinus bradycardia
Junctional bradycardia	P absent or independent QRS normal, rate 40 or less	Same as idiojunctional rhythm	Same as idiojunctional rhythm Vagal hyperactivity	Same as sinus bradycardia
Premature junctional contractions (PJCs) or beats	Early beats without P waves QRS morphology normal	Decreased cardiac output from loss of atrial contribution to ventricular preload for that beat	Hyperkalemia (6-5.4 mEq/L) Hypercalcemia, hypoxia, and elevated preload (see PACs)	Same as PACs
Accelerated junctional rhythm	P absent or independent QRS morphology normal, rate 60-99	Decreased cardiac output from loss of atrial contribution to ventricular preload	Same as PJCs	Same as PACs
Junctional tachycardia	P absent or independent QRS morphology normal, rate 100 or more	Decreased cardiac output from loss of atrial contribution to ventricular preload Increased myocardial demand because of tachycardia	Same as PJCs	Same as PACs
Idioventricular rhythm[†]	P absent or independent QRS >0.11 and rate 20-39	Same as idiojunctional rhythm	Sinus, atrial, and junctional bradycardia, standstill, or block	Same as sinus bradycardia

Continued

TABLE 32-12 **DISORDERS OF IMPULSE FORMATION—cont'd**

TYPE	ELECTROCARDIOGRAM	EFFECT	PATHOPHYSIOLOGY	TREATMENT
Ventricular bradycardia†	P absent or independent QRS >0.11 and rate 60-21	Same as idiojunctional rhythm	Same as idiojunctional rhythm	Same as sinus bradycardia
Agonal rhythm/ electromechanical dissociation†	P absent or independent QRS >0.11 and rate 20 or less	Absent or barely present cardiac output and pulse Not compatible with life	Depolarization and contraction not coupled: electrical activity present with little or no mechanical activity Usually caused by profound hypoxia	Vigorous pharmacology aimed at restoring rate and force Usually ineffective May attempt to pace
Ventricular standstill or asystole†	P absent or independent QRS absent	No cardiac output Not compatible with life	Profound ischemia, hyperkalemia, acidosis	Same as agonal rhythm, including electrical defibrillation
Premature ventricular contractions (PVCs) or depolarizations*	Early beats with P waves QRS occasionally opposite in deflection from usual QRS	Same as PJCs	Same as PJCs, including aging and induction of anesthesia Impulse originates in cell outside normal conduction system and spreads through intercalated disks	Pharmacology to change thresholds, refractory periods; reduce myocardial demand, increase supply Removal of cause
Accelerated ventricular rhythm	P absent or independent QRS >0.11 and rate 41-99	Same as accelerated junctional rhythm	Same as PVCs	Same as PVCs
Ventricular tachycardia†	P absent or independent QRS >0.11 and rate 100 or more	Same as junctional tachycardia	Same as PVCs	Same as PVCs, including electrical cardioversion
Ventricular fibrillation†	P absent QRS >300 and usually not observable	Same as ventricular standstill	Same as PVCs Rapid infusion of potassium	Same as PVCs including electrical defibrillation

*Most common in adults.
†Life threatening in adults.

TABLE 32-13 **DISORDERS OF IMPULSE CONDUCTION**

TYPE	ELECTROCARDIOGRAM	EFFECT	PATHOPHYSIOLOGY	TREATMENT
Sinus block	Occasionally absent P, with loss of QRS for that beat	Occasional decrease in cardiac output Increase in preload for the following beat	Local hypoxia, scarring of intra-atrial conduction pathways, electrolyte imbalances Increased atrial preload	Conservative Usually do not progress in severity Pharmacologic treatment includes vagolytics, sympathomimetics, pacing
First-degree block*	PR interval >0.2	None	Same as sinus block Hyperkalemia (>7 mEq/L) Hypokalemia (<3.5 mEq/L) Formation of myocardial abscesses in endocarditis	Conservative Discovery and correction of cause
Second-degree block, Mobitz I, or Wenckebach*	Progressive prolongation of PR interval until one QRS is dropped Pattern of prolongation resumes	Same as sinus block	Hypokalemia (<3.5 mEq/L) Faulty cell metabolism in atrioventricular (AV) node Severity increases as heart rate increases Supports theory that AV node is fatiguing Digoxin toxicity, beta-blockade Coronary artery disease (CAD), myocardial infarction (MI), hypoxia, increased preload, valvular surgery and disease, diabetes	Same as sinus block
Second-degree block or Mobitz II	Same as sinus block	Same as sinus block	Hypokalemia (<3.5 mEq/L) Faulty cell metabolism below AV node Antidysrhythmics, cyclic antidepressants CAD, MI, hypoxia, increased preload, valvular surgery and disease, diabetes	More aggressively than Mobitz I because block can progress to type III Pacemaker after pharmacologic treatment

TABLE 32-13 **DISORDERS OF IMPULSE CONDUCTION—cont'd**

TYPE	ELECTROCARDIOGRAM	EFFECT	PATHOPHYSIOLOGY	TREATMENT
Third-degree block†	P waves present and independent of QRS No observed relationship between P and QRS Always AV dissociation	Same as idiojunctional rhythm	Hypokalemia (<3.5 mEq/L) Faulty cell metabolism low in bundle of His MI, especially inferior wall, as nodal artery interrupted; results in ischemia of AV node	Pharmacologic until pacemaker inserted Temporary pacing if caused by inferior MI because ischemia usually resolves
Atrioventricular dissociation	P waves present and independent of QRS, but not always because of block (e.g., ventricular tachycardia) AV dissociation not always third-degree block	Decreased cardiac output from loss of atrial contribution to ventricular preload Variable effect on myocardial demand, depending on ventricular rate	May result from third-degree block or accelerated junctional or ventricular rhythm, or be caused by sinus, atrial, and junctional bradycardias	Treat according to cause Pacemaker or reducing rate of AV or ventricular discharge, or increasing rate of sinus or AV node discharge
Ventricular block	QRS >0.11 R-S-R' in V_1, V_2, V_5, V_6	None	Faulty cell metabolism in right and left bundle branches RBBB more common than LBBB because of dual blood supply to left bundle branch Congestive heart failure, mitral regurgitation, especially anterior MI, because of infarct of fascicles Left anterior hemiblock more common than left posterior hemiblock, since posterior fascicles have dual blood supply	Isolated right bundle branch block (RBBB) or left bundle branch block (LBBB) or hemiblock not treated If acute and/or associated with acute anterior MI, treated with permanent pacer and vigorous pharmacology
Aberrant conduction	QRS >0.11	None unless ventricular rate abnormalities present	Conduction of impulse through intercalated disks because conduction system transiently blocked because of hypoxia, electrolyte imbalances, digoxin toxicity, excessively rapid rates of discharge	Correct underlying cause
Preexcitation syndromes (Wolff-Parkinson-White and Lown-Ganong-Levine)	P present with QRS for each P PR interval >0.12 and QRS >0.11 because of presence of delta wave in PR interval	None	Congenital presence of accessory pathways (bundle of Kent and fiber of Mahaim) that conduct very rapidly and bypass the AV node, causing early ventricular depolarization in relation to atrial depolarization Prone (reason unknown) to tachycardias and atrial fibrillation that can result in very rapid ventricular rates	Aimed at lining up refractory periods of accessory pathway and AV node to prevent reentry May slow rate with pharmacology May surgically cut pathways
Ventricular block	QRS >0.11 R-S-R' in V_1, V_2, V_5, V_6	None	Faulty cell metabolism in right and left bundle branches RBBB more common than LBBB because of dual blood supply to left bundle branch Congestive heart failure, mitral regurgitation, especially anterior MI, because of infarct of fascicles Left anterior hemiblock more common than left posterior hemiblock, because posterior fascicles have dual blood supply	Isolated RBBB or LBBB or hemiblock not treated If acute and/or associated with acute anterior MI, treated with permanent pacer and vigorous pharmacology

Continued

TABLE 32-13 **DISORDERS OF IMPULSE CONDUCTION—cont'd**

TYPE	ELECTROCARDIOGRAM	EFFECT	PATHOPHYSIOLOGY	TREATMENT
Aberrant conduction	QRS >0.11	None unless ventricular rate abnormalities present	Conduction of impulse through intercalated disks because conduction system transiently blocked because of hypoxia, electrolyte imbalances, digoxin toxicity, excessively rapid rates of discharge	Correct underlying cause
Preexcitation syndromes (Wolff-Parkinson-White and Lown-Ganong-Levine)	P present with QRS for each P PR interval >0.12 and QRS >0.11 because of presence of delta wave in PR interval	None	Congenital presence of accessory pathways (bundle of Kent and fiber of Mahaim) that conduct very rapidly and bypass the AV node, causing early ventricular depolarization in relation to atrial depolarization Prone (reason unknown) to tachycardias and atrial fibrillation that can result in very rapid ventricular rates	Aimed at lining up refractory periods of accessory pathway and AV node to prevent reentry May slow rate with pharmacology May surgically cut pathways

*Most common in adults.
†Life threatening in adults.

SUMMARY REVIEW

Diseases of the Veins

1. Varicosities are areas of veins in which blood has pooled, usually in the saphenous veins. Varicosities may be caused by damaged valves as a result of trauma to the valve or by chronic venous distention involving gravity and venous constriction.
2. Chronic venous insufficiency is inadequate venous return over a long period that causes pathologic ischemic changes in the vasculature, skin, and supporting tissues.
3. Venous stasis ulcers follow the development of chronic venous insufficiency and probably develop as a result of the borderline metabolic state of the cells in the affected extremities.
4. DVT occurs in individuals who have venous stasis (immobility, age, left heart failure), spinal cord injury, vein wall damage (trauma, intravenous medications), or hypercoagulable states (pregnancy, oral contraceptives, malignancy, genetic coagulopathies).
5. DVT is often asymptomatic but may lead to fatal pulmonary emboli; prevention and careful assessment in individuals at risk are crucial.

Diseases of the Arteries

1. Hypertension is a sustained elevation of the systemic arterial blood pressure resulting from increases in cardiac output or total peripheral resistance, or both. Hypertension can be primary (without known cause) or secondary (caused by disease or drugs). Systolic hypertension is the most significant factor in causing target organ damage.
2. The risk factors for hypertension include a positive family history; male gender; advanced age; black race; obesity; high sodium intake; low potassium, calcium, and magnesium intake; diabetes mellitus; labile blood pressure; cigarette smoking; and heavy alcohol consumption.
3. Primary hypertension is the result of extremely complicated interactions of genetics and the environment mediated by a host of neurohumoral effects. These genes interact with diet, smoking, age, and the other risk factors to cause chronic changes in vasomotor tone and blood volume.
4. The most frequently cited theories of the pathogenesis of primary hypertension include overactivity of the SNS; overactivity of the RAAS; alterations in other neurohumoral mediators of blood volume and vasomotor tone such as ANP, BNP, and adrenomedullin; inflammation; a complex interaction involving insulin resistance and endothelial function; and obesity-related hormonal changes.
5. Clinical manifestations of hypertension result from damage of organs and tissues outside the vascular system. These include heart disease, renal disease, CNS problems, and retinal changes.
6. Hypertension is managed pharmacologically, using diuretics, adrenergic blockers, calcium channel blockers, ACE inhibitors, and Ang II receptor blockers. Nonpharmacologic methods include cessation of smoking, dietary modifications, and exercise.
7. Orthostatic hypotension is a drop in blood pressure that occurs on standing. The compensatory vasoconstriction response to standing is altered by a marked vasodilation and blood pooling in the muscle vasculature.
8. Orthostatic hypotension may be acute or chronic. The acute form is caused by a delay in the normal regulatory mechanisms. The chronic forms are secondary to a specific disease or are idiopathic.

SUMMARY REVIEW—cont'd

9. The clinical manifestations of orthostatic hypotension include fainting and may involve cardiovascular symptoms, as well as impotence and bowel and bladder dysfunction.
10. An aneurysm is a localized dilation of a vessel wall to which the aorta is particularly susceptible.
11. A thrombus is a clot that remains attached to a vascular wall.
12. An embolus is a mobile aggregate of a variety of substances that occludes the vasculature. Sources of emboli include thrombi, air, amniotic fluid, bacteria, fat, and foreign matter.
13. The most common sources of arterial thrombotic emboli from the heart are mitral and aortic valvular disease and atrial fibrillation. Tissues affected include the lower extremities, the brain, and the heart.
14. Emboli to the central organs cause tissue death in lungs, kidneys, and mesentery.
15. The generation of air emboli requires a connection between the vascular compartment and a source of air. These emboli cause ischemia and necrosis when a vessel is totally blocked.
16. Amniotic fluid may be forced into the bloodstream and generate an embolus during the labor and delivery of pregnancy.
17. Aggregates of bacteria in the vasculature may be large enough to form an embolus.
18. Fat emboli are caused mainly by trauma to the long bones, either through defective fat metabolism after trauma or through the release of fat globules from bone marrow exposed by fracture.
19. The introduction of foreign matter into the vasculature can occur with trauma and also can occur in a hospital setting in which intravenous and intra-arterial lines are being used.
20. Vasospastic disorders include Raynaud disease, involving arterioles of the extremities; variant angina, involving coronary arteries; and Buerger disease, involving arteries of the hands and feet.
21. Atherosclerosis is a form of arteriosclerosis and is the leading cause of coronary artery and cerebrovascular disease.
22. Atherosclerosis is an inflammatory disease that begins with endothelial injury and progresses through several stages to become a fibrotic plaque.
23. Traditional risk factors include age, family history, gender, smoking, dyslipidemia, hypertension, and diabetes.
24. Novel risk factors include elevated CRP, increased serum fibrinogen, oxidative stress, infection, and periodontal disease.
25. Once a plaque has formed it can rupture, resulting in thrombosis and vasoconstriction that leads to obstruction of the lumen and inadequate perfusion of distal tissues.
26. PAD is atherosclerosis of arteries that perfuse the limbs, especially the lower extremities.
27. PAD is often asymptomatic but can present with intermittent claudication (pain in leg on walking). Treatment includes risk factor reduction and antiplatelet therapy.
28. CAD is spasm or occlusion of the coronary arteries and is most often the result of atherosclerotic lesions that limit the flow of blood to the heart.
29. Many risk factors contribute to the onset and escalation of CAD, including advanced age, male gender (younger than age 60), hypertension, dyslipidemia (including elevated Lp[a]), diabetes mellitus, smoking, obesity, sedentary lifestyle, psychosocial factors, elevated CRP, and possibly infectious agents.
30. CAD results in an imbalance between coronary supply of blood and myocardial demand for oxygen and nutrients such that reversible myocardial ischemia or irreversible infarction may result.
31. Reversible myocardial ischemia presents clinically in several ways. Chronic coronary obstruction results in recurrent predictable chest pain called *stable angina.* Abnormal vasospasm of coronary vessels results in unpredictable chest pain called *Prinzmetal angina.* Myocardial ischemia that does not cause detectable symptoms is called *silent ischemia.*
32. Stable angina is evaluated by noninvasive techniques of assessing coronary flow with or without exercise (stress ECG, thallium, or SPECT). Management may include lifestyle changes, vasodilators, antithrombotics, PCI, or CABG surgery.
33. When there is sudden coronary obstruction because of thrombosis formation over a ruptured atherosclerotic plaque, the acute coronary syndromes result. Unstable angina causes reversible myocardial ischemia and is a harbinger of impending infarction. MI results when prolonged ischemia causes irreversible damage to the heart muscle. Sudden cardiac death can occur in any of the acute coronary syndromes.
34. Unstable angina occurs because of transient episodes of thrombotic vessel occlusion and vasoconstriction at the site of plaque damage, with return of perfusion before significant myocardial necrosis occurs. This must be managed aggressively with antithrombotic agents to prevent MI.
35. When coronary blood flow is interrupted for an extended period, myocyte necrosis occurs; this is called MI. Pathologically, there are two major types of myocardial infarction: subendocardial infarction and transmural infarction. In addition to myocyte necrosis, other changes in the heart with MI include hibernating, stunning, and remodeling of the myocardium.
36. Acute coronary syndromes are assessed by measuring serum enzymes, such as creatinine kinase and troponins, as well as looking for characteristic changes in the ECG. Those individuals at highest risk for complications present with ST-segment elevations on the ECG (STEMI) and require immediate intervention. Smaller subendocardial infarctions are not associated with ST-segment elevations (non-STEMI) but suggest that additional myocardium is still at risk for recurrent ischemia and infarction. Management may include thrombolytic drugs, antithrombotic drugs, vasodilators, PCI, or immediate surgery.

SUMMARY REVIEW—cont'd

37. Dysrhythmias, congestive heart failure, and sudden death are the most common complications of the acute coronary syndromes.

Disorders of the Heart Wall

1. Inflammation of the pericardium (pericarditis) may result from innumerable sources (infection, drug therapy, tumors). Pericarditis presents with symptoms that are physically troublesome, but in and of themselves they are not life threatening.
2. Fluid may collect within the pericardial sac (pericardial effusion). Cardiac function may be severely impaired if a large volume of fluid accumulates rapidly.
3. Cardiomyopathies are a diverse group of primary myocardial disorders that are poorly understood. The cardiomyopathies are categorized as dilated (congestive), restrictive (rigid and noncompliant), and hypertrophic (asymmetric). Size of the cardiac muscle walls and chambers may increase or decrease, depending on the type of cardiomyopathy, thereby altering contractile activity.
4. Hemodynamic integrity of the cardiovascular system depends to a great extent on properly functioning cardiac valves. Congenital or acquired disorders that result in stenosis or incompetence or both can structurally alter the valves.
5. Characteristic heart sounds, cardiac murmurs, and systemic complaints assist in determining which valve is abnormal. If severely compromised function exists, a prosthetic heart valve may be surgically implanted to replace the faulty one.
6. Mitral valve prolapse is a common finding, especially in young women. Although not grossly abnormal, the mitral valve leaflets do not position themselves properly during systole. Mitral valve prolapse may be a completely asymptomatic condition or it may result in severe subjective symptoms. Afflicted valves may be at greater risk for developing infective endocarditis.
7. Rheumatic fever is an inflammatory disease that results from a delayed autoimmune response to a streptococcal infection. The disorder usually resolves without sequelae if treated early.
8. Severe or untreated cases of rheumatic fever may progress to rheumatic heart disease, a potentially disabling cardiovascular disorder.
9. Infective endocarditis is a general term for infection and inflammation of the endocardium, especially the cardiac valves. A wide range of conditions predisposes one to the development of this disorder. In the mildest cases, valvular function may be slightly impaired by vegetations that collect on the valve leaflets. If infective endocarditis is left unchecked, severe valve abnormalities, chronic bacteremia, and systemic emboli may occur as vegetations break off the valve surface and travel through the bloodstream. Antibiotic therapy can limit the extent of this disease.
10. HIV is associated with cardiac abnormalities, including myocarditis, endocarditis, pericarditis, and cardiomyopathy. Left heart failure is the most common clinical manifestation.

Manifestations of Heart Disease

1. Heart failure is an inability of the heart to supply the metabolism with adequate circulatory volume and pressure.
2. Left heart failure can be categorized as systolic heart failure or diastolic heart failure.
3. Systolic heart failure is defined as an inability of the heart to generate an adequate cardiac output to perfuse vital tissue.
4. Cardiac output depends on the heart rate and stroke volume. Stroke volume is influenced by contractility, preload, and afterload. MI is the most common cause of decreased contractility. Myocardial ischemia results in ventricular remodeling that causes progressive myocyte contractile dysfunction over time.
5. Preload LVEDV is increased when there is decreased contractility or excess plasma volume.
6. Increased afterload is most commonly the result of increased peripheral vascular resistance. This increase in resistance decreases ventricular emptying and makes more workload for the left ventricle, resulting in hypertrophy and ventricular remodeling. The vicious cycle of decreasing contractility, increasing preload, and increasing afterload causes progressive worsening.
7. Neurohumoral mechanisms of CHF include abnormalities in the SNS, RAAS, arginine vasopressin, natriuretic peptides, inflammatory cytokines, and myocyte metabolism.
8. The clinical manifestations of left heart failure are the result of pulmonary vascular congestion and inadequate systemic perfusion.
9. Management of left heart failure relies on increasing contractility and reducing preload and afterload.
10. Diastolic heart failure can occur singly or with systolic heart failure. The major causes of diastolic dysfunction include hypertension-induced myocardial hypertrophy and ischemia with resultant ventricular remodeling.
11. Right heart failure can result from left heart failure and/or diffuse hypoxic pulmonary disease, such as COPD, cystic fibrosis, and ARDS (these mechanisms are discussed in Chapter 35).
12. High output failure is the inability of the heart to adequately supply the body with blood-borne nutrients despite adequate volume and normal or elevated myocardial contractility. Common causes are anemia, septicemia, hyperthyroidism, and beriberi.
13. A dysrhythmia (arrhythmia) is a disturbance of heart rhythm. Dysrhythmias range in severity from occasional missed beats or rapid beats to disturbances that impair myocardial contractility and are life threatening.
14. Dysrhythmias can occur because of an abnormal rate of impulse generation or the abnormal conduction of impulses.

KEY TERMS

Acute coronary syndrome, 1148
Acute orthostatic hypotension, 1140
Acute pericarditis, 1163
Aneurysm, 1140
Angina pectoris, 1154
Aortic dissection, 1142
Aortic regurgitation, 1159
Aortic stenosis, 1168
Arcus senilis, 1154
Atherosclerosis, 1145
Cardiogenic shock, 1162
Cardiomyopathy, 1165
Carditis, 1172
Chronic left heart failure, 1179
Chronic venous insufficiency (CVI), 1130
Chylomicron, 1149
Complicated plaque, 1147
Constrictive pericarditis (restrictive pericarditis, chronic pericarditis), 1164
Coronary artery disease (CAD), 1148
Deep venous thrombosis (DVT), 1130
Diastolic heart failure, 1180
Dilated cardiomyopathy, 1165
Dressler postinfection syndrome, 1162
Dyslipidemia (dyslipoproteinemia), 1149
Dysrhythmia (arrhythmia), 1162
Embolism, 1143
Embolus, 1143
Erythema marginatum, 1172
False aneurysm, 1140
Fatty streak, 1145
Fibrous plaque, 1147
Foam cell, 1145
Heart failure, 1175
Hibernating myocardium, 1160
High-density lipoprotein (HDL), 1149
Highly sensitive C-reactive protein (hs-CRP), 1152
High-output failure, 1181
Hyperhomocysteinemia, 1152
Hypertension, 1132
Hypertrophic cardiomyopathy, 1166
Hypertrophic obstructive cardiomyopathy, 1166
Infarction, 1148
Infective endocarditis, 1173
Intermittent claudication, 1148
Ischemia, 1148
Ischemic preconditioning, 1158
Isolated systolic hypertension (ISH), 1132
Left heart failure (congestive heart failure), 1175
Lipoprotein, 1149
Lipoprotein (a) (Lp[a]), 1151
Low-density lipoprotein (LDL), 1149
Malignant hypertension, 1138
Metabolic syndrome, 1152
Mitral regurgitation, 1170
Mitral stenosis, 1169
Mitral valve prolapse syndrome, 1170
Myocardial infarction (MI), 1156
Myocardial remodeling, 1160
Myocardial stunning, 1159
Non–ST-elevation MI (non-STEMI), 1156
Organic brain syndrome, 1163
Orthostatic (postural) hypotension, 1140
Percutaneous coronary intervention (PCI), 1156
Pericardial effusion, 1164
Pericarditis, 1162
Peripheral artery disease (PAD), 1148
Plaque, 1145
Post-thrombotic syndrome (PTS), 1131
Pressure-natriuresis relationship, 1133
Primary hypertension, 1133
Prinzmetal angina, 1154
Raynaud disease, 1144
Raynaud phenomenon, 1144
Reperfusion injury, 1159
Restrictive cardiomyopathy, 1167
Rheumatic fever, 1171
Rheumatic heart disease (RHD), 1171
Right heart failure, 1181
Secondary hypertension, 1136
Silent ischemia, 1154
Stable angina, 1154
ST-elevation MI (STEMI), 1156
Superior vena cava syndrome (SVCS), 1131
Sydenham chorea (St. Vitus dance), 1172
Systolic heart failure, 1175
Tamponade, 1164
Thromboangiitis obliterans (Buerger disease), 1144
Thromboembolism, 1143
Thromboembolization, 1131
Thromboembolus, 1143
Thrombus, 1130
Tricuspid regurgitation, 1170
True aneurysm, 1140
Unstable angina, 1156
Valvular regurgitation, 1167
Valvular stenosis, 1167
Varicose vein, 1129
Venous stasis ulcer, 1130
Ventricular aneurysm, 1163
Ventricular remodeling, 1175
Very-low-density lipoprotein (VLDL), 1149
Xanthelasma, 1154

REFERENCES

1. World Health Organization: *Global atlas on cardiovascular disease prevention and control*, updated 2013. Available at www.who.int/cardiovascular_diseases/en/. Accessed January 27, 2013.
2. Oklu R et al: Pathogenesis of varicose veins, *J Vasc Intervent Radiol* 23(1):333–339, 2012, quiz 40.
3. Perrin M, Ramelet AA: Pharmacological treatment of primary chronic venous disease: rationale, results and unanswered questions, *Eur J Vasc Endovasc Surg* 41(1):117–125, 2011.
4. Feliciano BA, Dalsing MC: Varicose vein: current management, *Adv Surg* 45:45–62, 2011.
5. Roger VL et al: Heart disease and stroke statistics—2012 update: a report from the American Heart Association, *Circulation* 125:e2–e220, 2012.

5a. Yancy CW et al: 2013 ACCF/AHA Guideline for the Management of Heart Failure: a report of the American College of Cardiology Foundation/American Heart Association Task Force on Practice Guidelines, *Circulation*. Retrieved June 5, 2013, from http://circ.ahajournals.org/content/early/2013/06/03/CIR.0b013e31829e8776.

6. Goldhaber SZ, Bounameaux H: Pulmonary embolism and deep vein thrombosis, *Lancet* 379(9828):1835–1846, 2012.
7. Varga EA, Kujovich JL: Management of inherited thrombophilia: guide for genetics professionals, *Clin Genet* 81(1):7–17, 2012.
8. Kahn SR: The post thrombotic syndrome, *Thromb Res* 127(Suppl 3): S89–S92, 2011.
9. Brunelli A: Deep vein thrombosis/pulmonary embolism: prophylaxis, diagnosis, and management, *Thorac Surg Clin* 22(1):252–258, v, 2012.
10. Kearon C et al: Antithrombotic therapy for VTE disease: antithrombotic therapy and prevention of thrombosis, ed 9, American College of Chest Physicians Evidence-Based Clinical Practice Guidelines, *Chest* 141(2 Suppl):e419S–e494S, 2012.
11. Januel JM et al: Symptomatic in-hospital deep vein thrombosis and pulmonary embolism following hip and knee arthroplasty among patients receiving recommended prophylaxis: a systematic review, *JAMA* 307(3):294–303, 2012.
12. Bates SM et al: Diagnosis of DVT: antithrombotic therapy and prevention of thrombosis, 9th ed, American College of Chest Physicians evidence-based clinical practice guidelines, *Chest* 141(2 Suppl):e351S–e418S, 2012.
13. Comerota AJ: Thrombolysis for deep venous thrombosis, *J Vasc Surg* 55(2):607–611, 2012.
14. Dasari TW, Pappy R, Hennebry TA: Pharmacomechanical thrombolysis of acute and chronic symptomatic deep vein thrombosis: a systematic review of literature, *Angiology* 63(2):138–145, 2012.
15. Labropoulos N et al: Recurrent deep vein thrombosis: long-term incidence and natural history, *Ann Surg* 251(4):749–753, 2010.
16. Becattini C et al: Aspirin for preventing the recurrence of venous thromboembolism, *N Engl J Med* 366(21):1959–1967, 2012.
17. Lepper PM et al: Superior vena cava syndrome in thoracic malignancies, *Resp Care* 56(5):653–666, 2011.
18. Shaheen K, Alraies M: Superior vena cava syndrome, *Clev Clin J Med* 79(6):410–412, 2012.
19. Chobanian AV: The seventh report of the Joint National Committee on Prevention, Detection, Evaluation, and Treatment of High Blood Pressure, JNC report, *JAMA* 289(19):2560–2572, 2003.
20. Gaddam KK, Ventura H, Lavie CJ: Antihypertensive therapy versus alternative therapeutic options for prehypertension: an evidence-based approach, *Future Cardiol* 8(1):115–122, 2012.
21. Grebla RC et al: Prevalence and determinants of isolated systolic hypertension among young adults: the 1999-2004 US National Health and Nutrition Examination Survey, *J Hypertens* 28(1):15–23, 2010.
22. Basson J, Simino J, Rao DC: Between candidate genes and whole genomes: time for alternative approaches in blood pressure genetics, *Curr Hypertens Rep* 14(1):46–61, 2012.

23. Freedman BI, Murea M: Target organ damage in African American hypertension: role of APOL1, *Curr Hypertens Rep* 14(1):21–28, 2012.
24. Currie G et al: Disorders of blood pressure regulation-role of catecholamine biosynthesis, release, and metabolism, *Curr Hypertens Rep* 14(1):38–45, 2012.
25. Cohen DL, Townsend RR: Renal denervation revisited: promising treatment for resistant hypertension? *J Clin Hypertens* 13(12):931–932, 2011.
26. Grassi G, Bertoli S, Seravalle G: Sympathetic nervous system: role in hypertension and in chronic kidney disease, *Curr Opin Nephrol Hypertens* 21(1):46–51, 2012.
27. Kalupahana NS, Moustaid-Moussa N: The renin-angiotensin system: a link between obesity, inflammation and insulin resistance, *Obesity Rev* 13(2):136–149, 2012.
28. Putnam K et al: The renin-angiotensin system: a target of and contributor to dyslipidemias, altered glucose homeostasis, and hypertension of the metabolic syndrome, *Am J Physiol Heart Circ Physiol* 302(6): H1219–H1230, 2012.
29. Volpe M: Should all patients at high cardiovascular risk receive renin-angiotensin system blockers? *QJM* 105(1):11–27, 2012.
30. Jia L et al: Angiotensin II induces inflammation leading to cardiac remodeling, *Front Biosci* 17:221–231, 2012.
31. Nguyen Dinh Cat A, Jaisser F: Extrarenal effects of aldosterone, *Curr Opin Nephrol Hypertens* 21(2):147–156, 2012.
32. Daien V et al: Treatment of hypertension with renin-angiotensin system inhibitors and renal dysfunction: a systematic review and meta-analysis, *Am J Hypertens* 25(1):126–132, 2012.
33. Ferrario CM: ACE2: more of Ang-(1-7) or less Ang II? *Curr Opin Nephrol Hypertens* 20(1):1–6, 2011.
34. Patel SK et al: Association of ACE2 genetic variants with blood pressure, left ventricular mass, and cardiac function in Caucasians with type 2 diabetes, *Am J Hypertens* 25(2):216–222, 2012.
35. McKie PM, Ichiki T, Burnett JC Jr: M-atrial natriuretic peptide: a novel antihypertensive protein therapy, *Curr Hypertens Rep* 14(1):62–69, 2012.
36. Calvieri C, Rubattu S, Volpe M: Molecular mechanisms underlying cardiac antihypertrophic and antifibrotic effects of natriuretic peptides, *J Mol Med* 90(1):5–13, 2012.
37. Rodriguez-Iturbe B et al: Renal inflammation, autoimmunity and salt-sensitive hypertension, *Clin Exp Pharmacol Physiol* 39(1):96–103, 2012.
38. Saremi A, Gopal D, Maisel AS: Brain natriuretic peptide-guided therapy in the inpatient management of decompensated heart failure, *Exp Rev Cardiovasc Ther* 10(2):191–203, 2012.
39. Schiffrin EL: Immune modulation of resistance artery remodeling, *Basic Clin Pharmacol Toxicol* 110(1):70–72, 2012.
40. Rautureau Y, Schiffrin EL: Endothelin in hypertension: an update, *Curr Opin Nephrol Hypertens* 21(2):128–136, 2012.
41. Jandeleit-Dahm KA, Watson AM: The endothelin system and endothelin receptor antagonists, *Curr Opin Nephrol Hypertens* 21(1):66–71, 2012.
42. Dorresteijn JA, Visseren FL, Spiering W: Mechanisms linking obesity to hypertension, *Obesity Rev* 13(1):17–26, 2012.
43. Kalil GZ, Haynes WG: Sympathetic nervous system in obesity-related hypertension: mechanisms and clinical implications, *Hypertens Res* 35(1):4–16, 2012.
44. De Boer MP et al: Microvascular dysfunction: a potential mechanism in the pathogenesis of obesity-associated insulin resistance and hypertension, *Microcirculation* 19(1):5–18, 2012.
45. Grossman E, Messerli FH: Drug-induced hypertension: an unappreciated cause of secondary hypertension, *Am J Med* 125(1):14–22, 2012.
46. Lacchini R et al: Common matrix metalloproteinase 2 gene haplotypes may modulate left ventricular remodelling in hypertensive patients, *J Human Hypertens* 26(3):171–177, 2012.
47. Peralta CA et al: Blood pressure components and end-stage renal disease in persons with chronic kidney disease: the Kidney Early Evaluation Program (KEEP), *Arch Intern Med* 172(1):41–47, 2012.
48. Seeman T et al: Microalbuminuria in children with primary and white-coat hypertension, *Pediatr Nephrol* 27(3):461–467, 2012.
49. Bhargava M, Ikram MK, Wong TY: How does hypertension affect your eyes? *J Human Hypertens* 26(2):71–83, 2012.
50. Joas E et al: Blood pressure trajectories from midlife to late life in relation to dementia in women followed for 37 years, *Hypertens* 59(4):796–801, 2012.
51. Shah NS et al: Midlife blood pressure, plasma beta-amyloid, and the risk for Alzheimer disease: the Honolulu Asia Aging Study, *Hypertens* 59(4):780–786, 2012.
52. Wysocki M et al: Hypertension is associated with cognitive decline in elderly people at high risk for dementia, *Am J Geriatr Psychiatry* 20(2):179–187, 2012.
53. Cuspidi C et al: Masked hypertension and echocardiographic left ventricular hypertrophy: an updated overview, *Blood Press Monit* 17(1): 8–13, 2012.
54. Kanbay M et al: Ambulatory blood pressure monitoring: from old concepts to novel insights, *Int Urol Nephrol* 44(1):173–182, 2012.
55. Frisoli TM et al: Salt and hypertension: is salt dietary reduction worth the effort? *Am J Med* 125(5):433–439, 2012.
56. Graudal NA, Hubeck-Graudal T, Jurgens G: Effects of low-sodium diet vs. high-sodium diet on blood pressure, renin, aldosterone, catecholamines, cholesterol, and triglyceride (Cochrane Review), *Am J Hypertens* 25(1):1–15, 2012.
57. Azadbakht L et al: Effects of the Dietary Approaches to Stop Hypertension (DASH) eating plan on cardiovascular risks among type 2 diabetic patients: a randomized crossover clinical trial, *Diabetes Care* 34(1):55–57, 2011.
58. Deano R, Sorrentino M: Lipid effects of antihypertensive medications, *Curr Atherosclerosis Rep* 14(1):70–77, 2012.
59. *The eighth report of the Joint National Committee on Prevention, Detection, Evaluation, and Treatment of High Blood Pressure (JNC 8)*, updated Oct 2012. Available at www.nhlbi.nih.gov/guidelines/hypertension/jnc8/index.htm. Accessed January 26, 2013.
60. Azizi M et al: Catheter-based radiofrequency renal-nerve ablation in patients with resistant hypertension, *Eur J Vasc Endovasc Surg* 43(3):293–299, 2012.
61. Lanier JB, Mote MB, Clay EC: Evaluation and management of orthostatic hypotension, *Am Fam Physician* 84(5):527–536, 2011.
62. Iodice V et al: Cardiovascular autonomic dysfunction in MSA and Parkinson's disease: similarities and differences, *J Neurol Sci* 310(1-2): 133–138, 2011.
63. Mustafa HI et al: Dysautonomia: perioperative implications, *Anesthesiology* 116(1):205–215, 2012.
64. Muscogiuri G et al: Medical therapy of aortic aneurysms: a pathophysiology-based approach, *Curr Vasc Pharmacol* 9(5):572–584, 2011.
65. Von Allmen RS, Powell JT: The management of ruptured abdominal aortic aneurysms: screening for abdominal aortic aneurysm and incidence of rupture,, *J Cardiovasc Surg* 53(1):69–76, 2012.
66. Guzzardi G et al: Emergency endovascular treatment of acute symptomatic or ruptured abdominal aortic aneurysm: a single-center experience, *Vascular* 20(2):81–87, 2012.
67. Nordon I, Thompson M, Loftus I: Endovascular treatment of acute aortic dissection: indications, techniques and results, *J Cardiovasc Surg* 53(1 Suppl 1):43–51, 2012.
68. Konstantinou DM et al: Cholesterol embolization syndrome following thrombolysis during acute myocardial infarction, *Herz* 37(2):231–233, 2012.
69. Saric M, Kronzon I: Cholesterol embolization syndrome, *Curr Opin Cardiol* 26(6):472–479, 2011.
70. Berryman R, Currie I, McCarthy R: Ischaemia of the extremities in a smoker, *BMJ* 343:d8193, 2011.
71. Katsuki Y et al: Early outgrowth EPCs generation is reduced in patients with Buerger's disease, *Clin Res Cardiol* 100(1):21–27, 2011.
72. Idei N et al: Autologous bone-marrow mononuclear cell implantation reduces long-term major amputation risk in patients with critical limb ischemia: a comparison of atherosclerotic peripheral arterial disease and Buerger disease, *Circ Cardiovasc Interv* 4(1):15–25, 2011.
73. Rugiene R et al: Prevalence of paraneoplastic rheumatic syndromes and their antibody profile among patients with solid tumours, *Clin Rheumatol* 30(3):373–380, 2011.
74. Goundry B et al: Diagnosis and management of Raynaud's phenomenon, *BMJ* 344:e289, 2012.
75. Herrick AL: The pathogenesis, diagnosis and treatment of Raynaud phenomenon, *Nat Rev Rheumatol* 8(8):469–479, 2012.
76. Coveliers HM et al: Thoracic sympathectomy for digital ischemia: a summary of evidence, *J Vasc Surg* 54(1):273–277, 2011.
77. Libby P, Ridker PM, Hansson GK: Progress and challenges in translating the biology of atherosclerosis, *Nature* 473:317–325, 2011.
78. Libby P: Inflammation in atherosclerosis, *Arterioscler Thromb Vasc Biol* 32(9):2045–2051, 2012.
79. Badimon L, Vilahur G: LDL-cholesterol versus HDL-cholesterol in the atherosclerotic plaque: inflammatory resolution versus thrombotic chaos, *Ann N Y Acad Sci* 1254:18–32, 2012.
80. Soehnlein O: Multiple roles for neutrophils in atherosclerosis, *Circ Res* 110(6):875–888, 2012.
81. Devaraj S, Jialal I: Dysfunctional endothelial progenitor cells in metabolic syndrome, *Exp Diabetes Res* 2012:585018, 2012.

82. Campbell KA et al: Lymphocytes and the adventitial immune response in atherosclerosis, *Circ Res* 110(6):889–900, 2012.
83. Monaco C: The tolls and dangers of atherosclerotic disease, *Curr Pharm Biotechnol* 13(1):77–87, 2012.
84. Toma I, McCaffrey TA: Transforming growth factor-beta and atherosclerosis: interwoven atherogenic and atheroprotective aspects, *Cell Tissue Res* 347(1):155–175, 2012.
85. Arbab-Zadeh A et al: Acute coronary events, *Circulation* 125(9): 1147–1156, 2012.
86. Moreno PR: Vulnerable plaque: definition, diagnosis, and treatment, *Cardiol Clin* 28(1):1–30, 2010.
87. Peters SA et al: Improvements in risk stratification for the occurrence of cardiovascular disease by imaging subclinical atherosclerosis: a systematic review, *Heart* 98(3):177–184, 2012.
88. Rooke TW et al: 2011 ACCF/AHA focused update of the guideline for the management of patients with peripheral artery disease (updating the 2005 guideline): a report of the American College of Cardiology Foundation/American Heart Association Task Force on Practice Guidelines: developed in collaboration with the Society for Cardiovascular Angiography and Interventions, Society of Interventional Radiology, Society for Vascular Medicine, and Society for Vascular Surgery, *Catheter Cardiovasc Interv* 79(4):501–531, 2012.
89. Mughal et al: Gene therapy in the treatment of peripheral arterial disease, *Br J Surg* 99(1):6–15, 2012.
90. Ransohoff JD, Wu JC: Imaging stem cell therapy for the treatment of peripheral arterial disease, *Curr Vasc Pharmacol* 10(3):361–373, 2012.
91. deGoma EM et al: The evolution and refinement of traditional risk factors for cardiovascular disease, *Cardiol Rev* 20(3):118–129, 2012.
92. Narula N et al: "My parents died of myocardial infarction: is that my destiny?" *Med Clin North Am* 96:67–86, 2012.
93. He M et al: ABO blood group and risk of coronary heart disease in two prospective cohort studies, *Arterioscler Thromb Vasc Biol* 32(9): 2314–2320, 2012.
94. Mustafic H et al: Main air pollutants and myocardial infarction: a systematic review and meta-analysis, *JAMA* 307(7):713–721, 2012.
95. Expert Panel on Detection: Evaluation and treatment of high blood cholesterol in adults: Executive summary of the third report of the National Cholesterol Education Program (NCEP) Expert Panel on Detection, Evaluation, and Treatment of High Blood Cholesterol in Adults (Adult Treatment Panel III), *JAMA* 285(19):2486–2497, 2001.
96. Wilkins JT, Lloyd-Jones DM: Are novel serum biomarkers informative? *Med Clin North Am* 96(1):1–11, 2012.
97. Baliga RR: HDL-cholesterol: perfection is the enemy of good? *Med Clin North Am* 96(1):27–37, 2012.
98. Rosenson RS et al: Cholesterol efflux and atheroprotection: advancing the concept of reverse cholesterol transport, *Circulation* 125(15): 1905–1919, 2012.
99. Voight BF et al: Plasma HDL cholesterol and risk of myocardial infarction: a mendelian randomisation study, *Lancet* 380:572–580, 2012.
100. Gordon SM, Davidson WS: Apolipoprotein A-I mimetics and high-density lipoprotein function, *Curr Opin Endocrinol Diabetes Obes* 19(2):109–114, 2012.
101. Kohli P, Cannon CP: Triglycerides: how much credit do they deserve? *Med Clin North Am* 96(1):39–55, 2012.
102. Dube JB et al: Lipoprotein(a): more interesting than ever after 50 years, *Curr Opin Lipidol* 23(2):133–140, 2012.
103. Pedrinelli R et al: Hypertension and acute myocardial infarction: an overview, *J Cardiovasc Med* 13(3):194–202, 2012.
104. Miyazawa T et al: Lipid glycation and protein glycation in diabetes and atherosclerosis, *Amino Acids* 42(4):1163–1170, 2012.
105. Rask-Madsen C, Kahn CR: Tissue-specific insulin signaling, metabolic syndrome, and cardiovascular disease, *Arterioscler Thromb Vasc Biol* 32(9):2052–2059, 2012.
106. Sparks JD, Sparks CE, Adeli K: Selective hepatic insulin resistance, VLDL overproduction, and hypertriglyceridemia, *Arterioscler Thromb Vasc Biol* 32(9):2104–2112, 2012.
107. Leroith D: Pathophysiology of the metabolic syndrome: implications for the cardiometabolic risks associated with type 2 diabetes, *Am J Med Sci* 343(1):13–16, 2012.
108. Williams PT: Evidence that obesity risk factor potencies are weight dependent, a phenomenon that may explain accelerated weight gain in western societies, *PloS One* 6(11):e27657, 2011.
109. Adams TD et al: Health benefits of gastric bypass surgery after 6 years, *JAMA* 308(11):1122–1131, 2012.
110. Escalona A et al: Weight loss and metabolic improvement in morbidly obese subjects implanted for 1 year with an endoscopic duodenal-jejunal bypass liner, *Ann Surg* 255(6):1080–1085, 2012.
111. Kavousi M et al: Evaluation of newer risk markers for coronary heart disease risk classification: a cohort study, *Ann Intern Med* 156(6): 438–444, 2012.
112. The Emerging Risk Factors Collaboration: C-reactive protein, fibrinogen, and cardiovascular disease prediction, *N Engl J Med* 367:1310–1320, 2012.
113. Balogh E et al: Interaction between homocysteine and lipoprotein(a) increases the prevalence of coronary artery disease/myocardial infarction in women: a case-control study, *Thromb Res* 129(2):133–138, 2012.
114. Procaccini C, Jirillo E, Matarese G: Leptin as an immunomodulator, *Mol Aspects Med* 33(1):35–45, 2012.
115. Vaiopoulos AG et al: The role of adiponectin in human vascular physiology, *Int J Cardiol* 155(2):188–193, 2012.
116. Jamaluddin MS et al: Resistin: functional roles and therapeutic considerations for cardiovascular disease, *Br J Pharmacol* 165(3):622–632, 2012.
117. Aghamohammadzadeh R et al: Perivascular adipose tissue from human systemic and coronary vessels: the emergence of a new pharmacotherapeutic target, *Br J Pharmacol* 165(3):670–682, 2012.
118. Southerland JH et al: Periodontitis and diabetes associations with measures of atherosclerosis and CHD, *Atherosclerosis* 222(1):196–201, 2012.
119. Campen MJ, Lund A, Rosenfeld M: Mechanisms linking traffic-related air pollution and atherosclerosis, *Curr Opin Pulm Med* 18(2):155–160, 2012.
120. Lorenz MW et al: Carotid intima-media thickness progression to predict cardiovascular events in the general population (the PROG-IMT collaborative project): a meta-analysis of individual participant data, *Lancet* 379(9831):2053–2062, 2012.
121. Yeboah J et al: Comparison of novel risk markers for improvement in cardiovascular risk assessment in intermediate-risk individuals, *JAMA* 308(8):788–795, 2012.
122. Moukarbel GV, Weinrauch LA: Disruption of coronary vasomotor function: the coronary spasm syndrome, *Cardiovasc Ther* 30(2):e66–e73, 2012.
123. Vavas E et al: Noninvasive diagnostic techniques for coronary disease in women, *Clin Cardiol* 35(3):149–155, 2012.
124. Conti CR, Bavry AA, Petersen JW: Silent ischemia: clinical relevance, *J Am Coll Cardiol* 59(5):435–441, 2012.
125. Paine NJ, Bosch JA, Van Zanten JJ: Inflammation and vascular responses to acute mental stress: implications for the triggering of myocardial infarction, *Curr Pharm Des* 18(11):1494–1501, 2012.
126. Chaitman BR, Laddu AA: Stable angina pectoris: antianginal therapies and future directions, *Nat Rev Cardiol* 9(1):40–52, 2012.
127. Fraker TD et al: 2007 chronic angina focused update of the ACC/AHA 2002 guidelines for the management of patients with chronic stable angina: a report of the American College of Cardiology/American Heart Association Task Force on Practice Guidelines Writing Group to develop the focused update of the 2002 Guidelines for the management of patients with chronic stable angina, *Circulation* 116(23):2762–2772, 2007.
128. Lavine GN et al: 2011 ACCF/AHA/SCAI Guideline for Percutaneous Coronary Intervention: executive summary: a report of the American College of Cardiology Foundation/American Heart Association Task Force on Practice Guidelines and the Society for Cardiovascular Angiography and Interventions, *Catheter Cardiovasc Interv* 79(3):453–495, 2012.
129. Braunwald E: Unstable angina and non-ST elevation myocardial infarction, *Am J Resp Crit Care Med* 185(9):924–932, 2012.
130. Jneid H et al: 2012 ACCF/AHA focused update of the guideline for the management of patients with unstable angina/non-ST-elevation myocardial infarction (updating the 2007 guideline and replacing the 2011 focused update): a report of the American College of Cardiology Foundation/American Heart Association Task Force on practice guidelines, *Circulation* 126:875–910, 2012.
131. Sanz-Rosa D, Garcia-Prieto J, Ibanez B: The future: therapy of myocardial protection, *Ann N Y Acad Sci* 1254:90–98, 2012.
132. Gerczuk PZ, Kloner RA: An update on cardioprotection: a review of the latest adjunctive therapies to limit myocardial infarction size in clinical trials, *J Am Coll Cardiol* 59(11):969–978, 2012.
133. Konstantinidis K, Whelan RS, Kitsis RN: Mechanisms of cell death in heart disease, *Arterioscler Throm Vasc Biol* 32(7):1552–1562, 2012.
134. Heusch G: Reduction of infarct size by ischaemic post-conditioning in humans: fact or fiction? *Eur Heart J* 33(1):13–25, 2012.
135. Carluccio E et al: Improvement of myocardial performance (Tei) index closely reflects intrinsic improvement of cardiac function: assessment in revascularized hibernating myocardium, *Echocardiography* 29(3):298–306, 2012.

136. Sovari AA, Shroff A, Kocheril AG: Postinfarct cardiac remodeling and the substrate for sudden cardiac death: role of oxidative stress and myocardial fibrosis, *Exp Rev Cardiovasc Ther* 10(3):267–270, 2012.
137. Koitabashi N, Kass DA: Reverse remodeling in heart failure–mechanisms and therapeutic opportunities, *Nat Rev Cardiol* 9(3):147–157, 2012.
138. Welch TD et al: Modern management of acute myocardial infarction, *Curr Prob Cardiol* 37(7):237–310, 2012.
139. Hallen J: Troponin for the estimation of infarct size: what have we learned? *Cardiology* 121(3):204–212, 2012.
139a. O'Gara PT et al: 2013 ACCF/AHA Guidelines for the management of ST-elevation myocardial infarction: a report of the American College of Cardiology Foundation/American Heart Association Task Force on Practice Guidelines, *Circulation* 127:e362–e425, 2013.
140. Shah B, Amoroso NS, Sedlis SP: Hyperglycemia in nondiabetic patients presenting with acute myocardial infarction, *Am J Med Sci* 343(4):321–326, 2012.
141. Kushner FG et al: 2009 focused updates: ACC/AHA guidelines for the management of patients with ST-elevation myocardial infarction (updating the 2004 guideline and 2007 focused update) and ACC/AHA/SCAI guidelines on percutaneous coronary intervention (updating the 2005 guideline and 2007 focused update): a report of the American College of Cardiology Foundation/American Heart Association Task Force on Practice Guidelines, *Circulation* 120:2271–2306, 2009.
142. Trost JC, Lange RA: Treatment of acute coronary syndrome: part 2: ST-segment elevation myocardial infarction, *Crit Care Med* 40(6):1939–1945, 2012.
143. Westaby S, Kharbanda R, Banning AP: Cardiogenic shock in ACS. Part 1: prediction, presentation and medical therapy, *Nat Rev Cardiol* 9(3):158–171, 2012.
144. Shah RM et al: Fixing the "broken heart": pharmacologic implications, *Am J Ther* 19(3):e105–e113, 2012.
145. Dudzinski DM, Mak GS, Hung JW: Pericardial diseases, *Curr Prob Cardiol* 37(3):75–118, 2012.
146. Imazio M: Contemporary management of pericardial diseases, *Curr Opin Cardiol* 27(3):308–317, 2012.
147. Dandel M et al: Role of beta1-adrenoceptor autoantibodies in the pathogenesis of dilated cardiomyopathy, *Immunobiology* 217(5):511–520, 2012.
148. Limongelli G et al: Mitochondrial diseases and the heart: an overview of molecular basis, diagnosis, treatment and clinical course, *Future Cardiol* 8(1):71–88, 2012.
149. Sanz J: Evolving diagnostic and prognostic imaging of the various cardiomyopathies, *Ann N Y Acad Sci* 1254:123–130, 2012.
150. Johnson-Coyle L et al: Peripartum cardiomyopathy: review and practice guidelines, *Am J Crit Care* 21(2):89–98, 2012.
151. Kindermann I et al: Update on myocarditis, *J Am Coll Cardiol* 59(9):779–792, 2012.
152. Sun N et al: Patient-specific induced pluripotent stem cells as a model for familial dilated cardiomyopathy, *Sci Transl Med* 4(130), 2012.
153. Frey N, Luedde M, Katus HA: Mechanisms of disease: hypertrophic cardiomyopathy, *Nat Rev Cardiol* 9(2):91–100, 2012.
154. Ho CY: Hypertrophic cardiomyopathy in 2012, *Circulation* 125(11):1432–1438, 2012.
155. Gersh BJ et al: 2011 ACCF/AHA guideline for the diagnosis and treatment of hypertrophic cardiomyopathy, *Circulation* 124:e783–e831, 2011.
156. Gupta A et al: Cardiac MRI in restrictive cardiomyopathy, *Clin Radiol* 67(2):95–105, 2012.
157. Bonow RO et al: 2008 Focused update incorporated into the ACC/AHA 2006 guidelines for the management of patients with valvular heart disease: a report of the American College of Cardiology/American Heart Association Task Force on Practice Guidelines (Writing Committee to Revise the 1998 Guidelines for the Management of Patients With Valvular Heart Disease): endorsed by the Society of Cardiovascular Anesthesiologists, Society for Cardiovascular Angiography and Interventions, and Society of Thoracic Surgeons, *Circulation* 118(15):e523–e661, 2008.
158. Nishimura RA et al: ACC/AHA 2008 guideline update on valvular heart disease: focused update on infective endocarditis: a report of the American College of Cardiology/American Heart Association Task Force on Practice Guidelines: endorsed by the Society of Cardiovascular Anesthesiologists, Society for Cardiovascular Angiography and Interventions, and Society of Thoracic Surgeons, *Circulation* 118(8):887–896, 2008.
159. Sawaya F et al: Aortic stenosis: a contemporary review, *Am J Med Sci* 343(6):490–496, 2012.
160. Rodes-Cabau J: Transcatheter aortic valve implantation: current and future approaches, *Nat Rev Cardiol* 9(1):15–29, 2012.
161. del Nido PJ, Baird C: Congenital mitral valve stenosis: anatomic variants and surgical reconstruction, *Semin Thorac Cardiovasc Surg Pediatr Card Surg Annu* 15(1):69–74, 2012.
162. De Bonis M et al: Treatment and management of mitral regurgitation, *Nat Rev Cardiol* 9(3):133–146, 2012.
163. Thapa R, Dawn B, Nath J: Tricuspid regurgitation: pathophysiology and management, *Curr Cardiol Rep* 14(2):190–199, 2012.
164. Guy TS, Hill AC: Mitral valve prolapse, *Annu Rev Med* 63:277–292, 2012.
165. Marijon E et al: Rheumatic heart disease, *Lancet* 379(9819):953–964, 2012.
166. Cunningham MW: Streptococcus and rheumatic fever, *Curr Opin Rheumatol* 24(4):408–416, 2012.
167. Azevedo PM, Pereira RR, Guilherme L: Understanding rheumatic fever, *Rheumatol Int* 32(5):1113–1120, 2012.
168. World Health Organization: *Rheumatic fever and rheumatic heart disease: report of a WHO expert consultation*, Geneva, 2004, Author.
169. Cilliers A et al: Anti-inflammatory treatment for carditis in acute rheumatic fever, *Cochrane Database Syst Rev* 6:CD003176, 2012.
170. Pierce D, Calkins BC, Thornton K: Infectious endocarditis: diagnosis and treatment, *Am Fam Physician* 85(10):981–986, 2012.
171. Thuny F et al: Management of infective endocarditis: challenges and perspectives, *Lancet* 379(9819):965–975, 2012.
172. Prior DL, La Gerche A: The athlete's heart, *Heart* 98(12):947–955, 2012.
173. Savinova OV, Gerdes AM: Myocyte changes in heart failure, *Heart Fail Clin* 8(1):1–6, 2012.
174. Eckhouse SR, Spinale FG: Changes in the myocardial interstitium and contribution to the progression of heart failure, *Heart Fail Clin* 8(1):7–20, 2012.
175. Messaoudi S et al: Aldosterone, mineralocorticoid receptor, and heart failure, *Mol Cell Endocrinol* 350(2):266–272, 2012.
176. Grewal AS et al: The heart as an endocrine system, *Int Anesthesiol Clin* 50(2):111–127, 2012.
177. Kalogeropoulos AP, Georgiopoulou VV, Butler J: From risk factors to structural heart disease: the role of inflammation, *Heart Fail Clin* 8(1):113–123, 2012.
178. Ueland T et al: TNF revisited: osteoprotegerin and TNF-related molecules in heart failure, *Curr Heart Fail Rep* 9(2):92–100, 2012.
179. Swaminathan PD et al: Calmodulin-dependent protein kinase II: linking heart failure and arrhythmias, *Circ Res* 110(12):1661–1677, 2012.
180. Abel E et al: Insulin resistance: metabolic mechanisms and consequences in the heart, *Arterioscler Throm Vasc Biol* 32(9):2068–2076, 2012.
181. Ramasamy R, Schmidt AM: Receptor for advanced glycation end products (RAGE) and implications for the pathophysiology of heart failure, *Curr Heart Fail Rep* 9(2):107–116, 2012.
182. Zhang L et al: Additional use of trimetazidine in patients with chronic heart failure: a meta-analysis, *J Am Coll Cardiol* 59(10):913–922, 2012.
183. Bristow MR: Pharmacogenetic targeting of drugs for heart failure, *Pharmacol Ther* 134(1):107–115, 2012.
184. Ahmed M, Hill J: A rational approach to assess volume status in patients with decompensated heart failure, *Curr Heart Fail Rep* 9(2):139–147, 2012.
185. Januzzi JL Jr: The role of natriuretic peptide testing in guiding chronic heart failure management: review of available data and recommendations for use, *Arch Cardiovasc Dis* 105(1):40–50, 2012.
186. Sato Y, Fujiwara H, Takatsu Y: Biochemical markers in heart failure, *J Cardiol* 59(1):1–7, 2012.
187. Jessup M et al: 2009 Focused update: ACCF/AHA Guidelines for the Diagnosis and Management of Heart Failure in Adults: a report of the American College of Cardiology Foundation/American Heart Association Task Force on Practice Guidelines: developed in collaboration with the International Society for Heart and Lung Transplantation, *Circulation* 119(14):1977–2016, 2009.
188. Tacon CL, McCaffrey J, Delaney A: Dobutamine for patients with severe heart failure: a systematic review and meta-analysis of randomised controlled trials, *Intensive Care Med* 38(3):359–367, 2012.
189. Landoni G et al: Effects of levosimendan on mortality and hospitalization. A meta-analysis of randomized controlled studies, *Crit Care Med* 40(2):634–646, 2012.
190. Gassanov N et al: Natriuretic peptides in therapy for decompensated heart failure, *Eur J Clin Pharmacol* 68(3):223–230, 2012.
191. Kobayashi D et al: Human atrial natriuretic peptide treatment for acute heart failure: a systematic review of efficacy and mortality, *Can J Cardiol* 28(1):102–109, 2012.
192. Faris RF et al: Diuretics for heart failure, *Cochrane Database Syst Rev* 2:CD003838, 2012.

193. Haddad H, Mielniczuk L, Davies RA: Recent advances in the management of chronic heart failure, *Curr Opin Cardiol* 27(2):161–168, 2012.
194. Heran BS et al: Angiotensin receptor blockers for heart failure, *Cochrane Database Syst Rev* 4:CD003040, 2012.
195. Chrysant SG, Chrysant GS: Current status of beta-blockers for the treatment of hypertension: an update, *Drugs Today* 48(5):353–366, 2012.
196. Sobotka PA et al: The role of renal denervation in the treatment of heart failure, *Curr Cardiol Rep* 14(3):285–292, 2012.
197. Nery PB, Keren A, Birnie DH: Cardiac resynchronization therapy: expanding clinical indications and refining patient selection, *Curr Opin Cardiol* 27(2):137–142, 2012.
198. Donndorf P, Strauer BE, Steinhoff G: Update on cardiac stem cell therapy in heart failure, *Curr Opin Cardiol* 27(2):154–160, 2012.
199. Ptaszek LM et al: Towards regenerative therapy for cardiac disease, *Lancet* 379(9819):933–942, 2012.
200. Drazner MH: The progression of hypertensive heart disease, *Circulation* 123(3):327–334, 2011.
201. Ohara T, Ohte N, Little WC: Pulmonary hypertension in heart failure with preserved left ventricular ejection fraction: diagnosis and management, *Curr Opin Cardiol* 27(3):281–287, 2012.
202. Hayley BD, Burwash IG: Heart failure with normal left ventricular ejection fraction: role of echocardiography, *Curr Opin Cardiol* 27(2):169–180, 2012.
203. Haykowsky M, Brubaker P, Kitzman D: Role of physical training in heart failure with preserved ejection fraction, *Curr Heart Fail Rep* 9(2):101–106, 2012.
204. Crouse M et al: Clinical inquiries. Which medications benefit patients with diastolic heart failure? *J Fam Pract* 60(2):101–102, 2011.
205. Oghlakian GO, Sipahi I, Fang JC: Treatment of heart failure with preserved ejection fraction: have we been pursuing the wrong paradigm? *Mayo Clin Proc* 86(6):531–539, 2011.
206. Sayer GT, Semigran MJ: Right ventricular performance in chronic congestive heart failure, *Cardiol Clin* 30(2):271–282, 2012.
207. Rich S: Right ventricular adaptation and maladaptation in chronic pulmonary arterial hypertension, *Cardiol Clin* 30(2):257–269, 2012.

CHAPTER

33

Alterations of Cardiovascular Function in Children

Nancy L. McDaniel

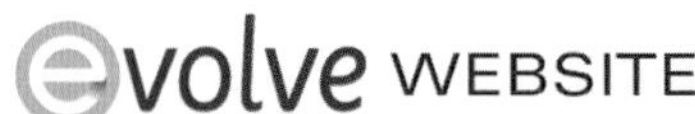

http://evolve.elsevier.com/McCance/
- Review Questions and Answers

CHAPTER OUTLINE

Cardiovascular disease in children can be classified as congenital or acquired heart disease. Congenital heart disease is the most common. The diagnosis and management of congenital heart defects continue to improve with the use of fetal echocardiography, early interventional catheterization, and refined surgical repair. Acquired heart defects in children continue to present challenges to the practitioner; although guidelines for diagnosing acquired defects are available, work is needed in developing standards of treatment and long-term follow-up.

DEVELOPMENT OF THE CARDIOVASCULAR SYSTEM

Developmental Anatomy

Embryology

Cardiogenesis begins at approximately 3 weeks of gestation; however, most cardiovascular development occurs between the fourth and seventh weeks.[1] The heart arises from the mesenchyme and begins development as an enlarged blood vessel with a large lumen and a muscular wall (Figure 33-1, *A*). Initially, two lateral endocardial heart tubes fuse to form a single structure (Figure 33-1, *B*). During the fifth week of gestation, the midsection of this tube begins to grow faster than its ends. This single heart tube elongates and rotates to the right (D-loop formation), creating a bulboventricular loop by approximately the twenty-eighth day[1] (Figure 33-1, *C*). Also at this time the first fetal heart contractions occur. At this stage the primitive heart structures include a common atrium; common ventricle; the sinus venosus, which eventually evolves into the superior and inferior venae cavae; the bulbus cordis, which eventually evolves into the ventricular outflow tracts; and the truncus arteriosus, which eventually yields the main pulmonary artery (PA) and aorta (Figure 33-1, *D*). By the fourth week of gestation, cardiovascular septation, ventricular development, aortic arch evolution, and circulation begin.

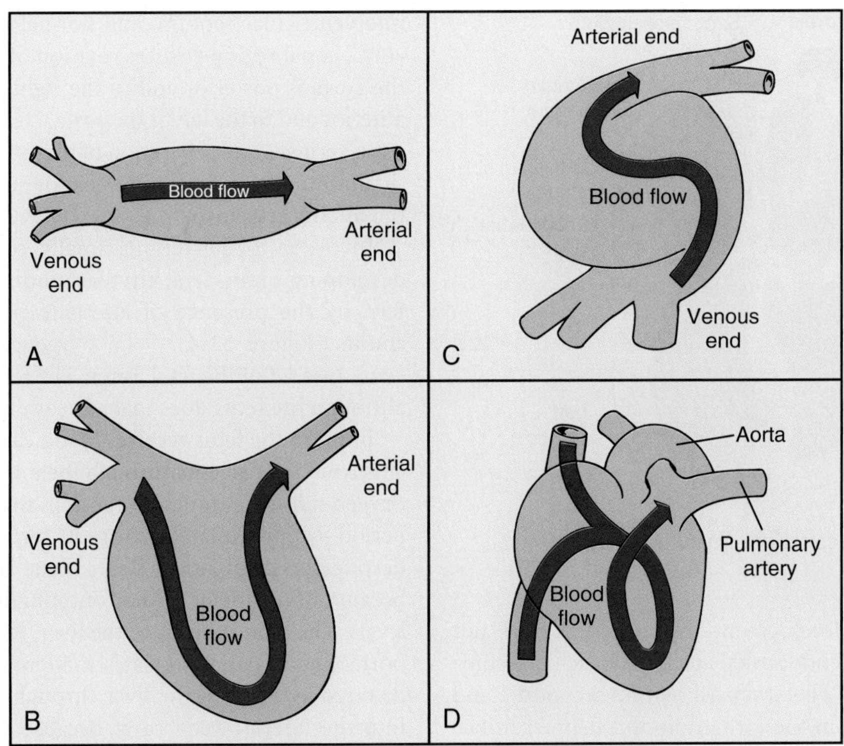

FIGURE 33-1 **Embryologic Development of the Heart.** **A,** The earliest heart structure consists of a muscular tube with a large lumen. About the fifth week of gestation, the tube, **B,** bulges and, **C,** twists until, **D,** the ends come together and fuse.

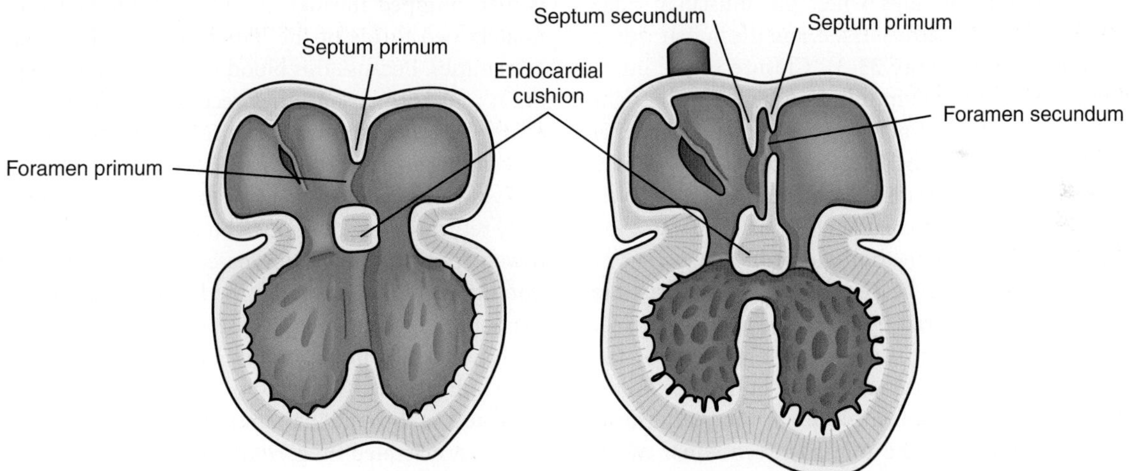

FIGURE 33-2 **Development of the Cardiac Septa.**

Cardiac Septation

Separation first begins when collections of mesenchymal cells cause the endocardial lining of the heart to bulge into the internal lumen. These changes, known as **endocardial cushions,** are instrumental in closing the lower portion of the atrial septum, dividing the atrioventricular (AV) canals into the right and left AV orifices, and forming the upper portion of the interventricular septum. Altered formation of the endocardial cushions can result in ostium primum atrial septal defects, inlet ventricular septal defects (VSDs), malformation of the AV valves, or a complete AV defect (also known as atrioventricular septal defect).[2]

Atrial septation begins when two thin membranelike structures, known as the **septum primum** and the **septum secundum,** grow toward the area of the endocardial cushions (Figure 33-2). The septum primum forms along the posterior wall of the common atrium and grows downward toward the center portion of the heart. The gap between the two structures, known as the **ostium primum,** normally closes by extensions from the endocardial cushions. At the time of closure, fenestrations or openings develop in the superior portion of the septum primum, creating the **ostium secundum.** Failure of the septum primum to fuse with the endocardial cushions results in an ostium primum defect in the atrial septum near the AV valve area.

The septum secundum is also a fenestrated, membranelike structure located anteriorly that grows toward the endocardial

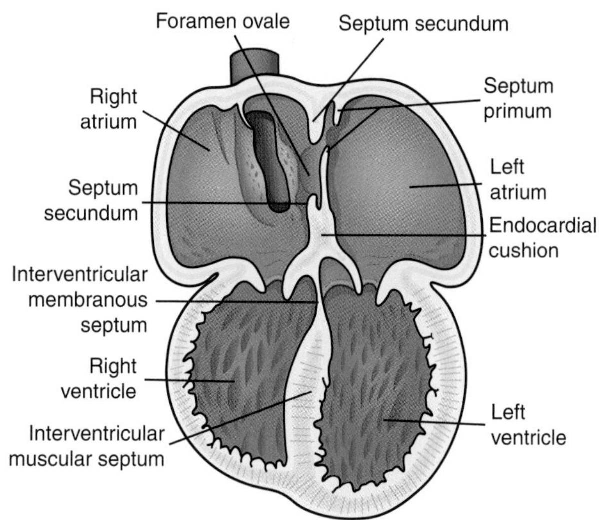

FIGURE 33-3 Septal Development of the Heart.

cushions. During fetal development this structure does not completely fuse with the endocardial cushions to achieve complete atrial septal closure. The nonfused septum secundum and ostium secundum result in the formation of a flapped orifice known as the **foramen ovale,** which allows the right-to-left shunting necessary for fetal circulation. Altered development in any of these structures can lead to an atrial septal defect.

Ventricular septation develops when the muscular ridge located at the apex, the endocardial tissue, and the bulbar ridges in the bulbus cordis fuse (Figure 33-3). Closure of the interventricular septum ensures communication between the right ventricle (RV) and the PA and between the left ventricle (LV) and the aorta. Further evolution of the endocardial tissue gives rise to the membranous ventricular septum and the AV valves. The conal portion of the ventricular septum that separates the aorta from the PA forms from the **bulbus cordis.**

When the single primitive heart tube begins to form the D-loop, the venous and arterial poles of the heart are fixed, resulting in torsion within the anterosuperior region of the loop, known as the *truncus arteriosus*. This torsion creates a spiral ridgelike structure or septum within the truncus arteriosus that divides it into the PA and the aorta. The semilunar valves evolve from tubercles after this division is complete.

Before this division occurs, however, two large arteries form at the distal end of the truncus arteriosus. Over time they give rise to a series of arterial vessels, collectively called the six aortic arches. By the fifth week of gestation, the first two pairs disappear and the third eventually evolves into the common carotid artery, the external carotid artery, and part of the internal carotid artery. The fourth pair of aortic arches will form part of the true aortic arch and the proximal segment of the right subclavian artery. The fifth pair disappears; however, the sixth pair yields the proximal and branch pulmonary arteries within the lung parenchyma and the ductus arteriosus.

Swellings in the conal region at the base of the main trunk separate the right ventricular outflow (pulmonary outflow) tract from the left ventricular outflow (aortic outflow) tract. The conus also contributes to complete closure of the interventricular septum, and normal reabsorption of the subaortic conal region ensures rotation of the great arteries so that the aorta is posterior and to the right of the PA and the PA is anterior and to the left of the aorta. Despite division of the truncus arteriosus and separation of the right and left outflow tracts, a communication exists between the aorta and the PA known as the **ductus arteriosus.**

In order to deliver maximally oxygenated blood to the developing brain, fetal circulation differs from the adult pattern by the presence of alternate pathways known as fetal shunts (Figure 33-4). Fetal oxygenation occurs in the placenta instead of the fetal lungs. The fetal lungs are not aerated, although the fetus does make breathing motions.

In utero the fetus receives blood carrying oxygen and nutrients from the placenta through the umbilical vein. Fetal arterial oxygen tension is much lower than that found in the postnatal period—approximately 20 to 30 torr (mmHg pressure). Yet, despite this hypoxemic state, tissue hypoxia does not occur because of high fetal cardiac output and high fetal hemoglobin levels. The blood travels to the liver, where a portion enters the portal and hepatic circulation; approximately half the flow is diverted away from the liver through the ductus venosus and into the inferior vena cava. Because the blood received from the inferior vena cava yields a higher pressure, blood entering the right atrium (RA) from the inferior vena cava is shunted through the foramen ovale and into the left atrium (LA) and is then pumped through the LV and into the aorta. Approximately two thirds of the blood flows to the head and upper extremities. Because this blood is mainly from the placenta, the brain and coronary arteries receive the blood with the highest oxygen concentration. The remaining blood flows into the descending aorta.

Less-saturated blood, with an oxygen tension of 15 to 19 torr, returns from the upper body, head, neck, and arms and travels from the superior vena cava into the RA. A small portion of this blood flows into the RV and out the PA and enters the nonfunctioning lungs. Most of the blood, however, bypasses the lungs by flowing through the ductus arteriosus and into the descending aorta. Blood from the descending aorta returns to the placenta through two umbilical arteries.[1]

The nonaerated lungs and low oxygen tension induce vasoconstriction, creating high pulmonary vascular resistance. This is transmitted to the right side of the heart and the PAs. Conversely, fetal systemic resistance is low because of the large-volume placenta and ductus arteriosus. Therefore, because blood flow follows the path of least resistance, high pulmonary resistance diverts most of the blood flow into the PA, through the ductus arteriosus, and into the aorta. From there it travels into the low-resistance placenta.

Transitional Circulation

At birth a series of circulatory changes occur that affect blood flow, vascular resistance, and oxygen tension. The most important change that takes place in the circulation is the shift of gas exchange from the placenta to the lungs. In addition, alterations in pressure and volume of blood flowing through the heart chambers functionally close the ductus arteriosus, ductus

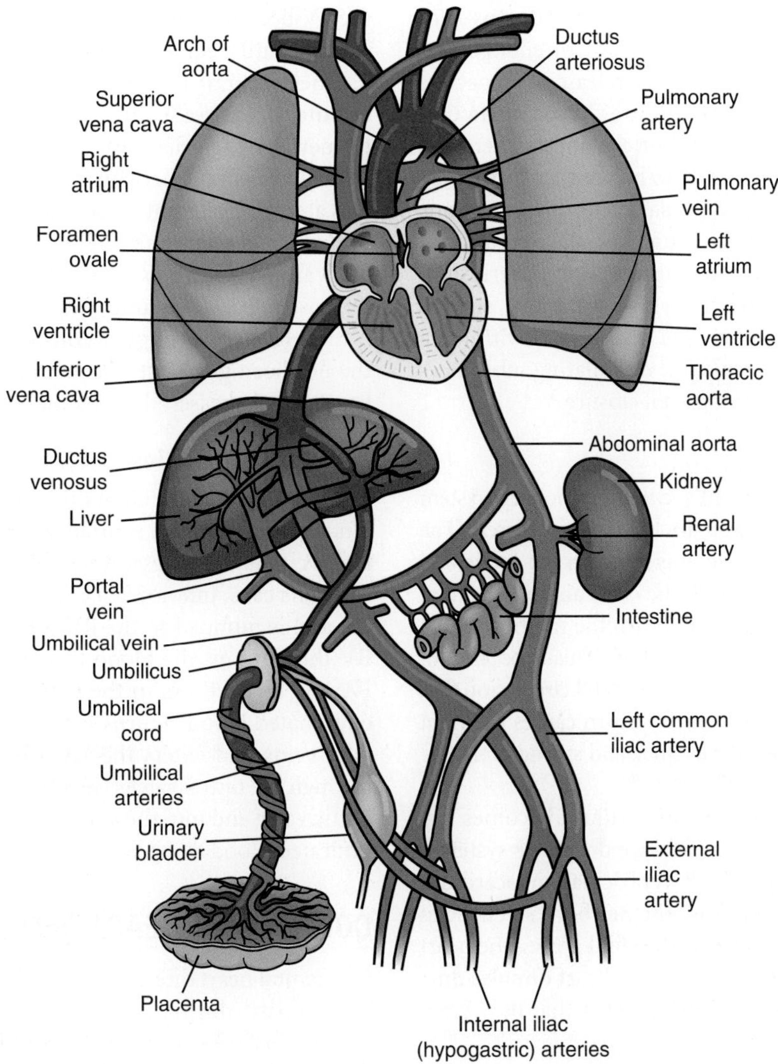

FIGURE 33-4 **Fetal Circulation.** Circulation of the fetus reflects the fact that oxygenation of fetal blood does not take place in the lungs, but rather in the placenta. Therefore, the pulmonary circulatory system is essentially "bypassed." Instead of traveling from the right heart to the lungs, as occurs after birth, most blood entering the right heart passes through the ductus arteriosus and into the systemic circulation.

venosus, and foramen ovale. A decrease of pulmonary vascular resistance and an increase of systemic vascular resistance lead to changes in the size and shape of the heart chambers.

Clamping of the umbilical cord and expansion of the lungs at birth shift gas exchange from the placenta to the lungs. Removal of the low-resistance placenta from circulation also causes an immediate increase in systemic vascular resistance to about twice that before birth. Conversely, pulmonary vascular resistance decreases because of expansion of the lungs, which result from the infant's respirations and exposure to more oxygen-rich blood.

Closure of Fetal Shunts

Once the umbilical cord is clamped, the umbilical arteries and vein, which comprise the cord, vasoconstrict and undergo fibrous changes. Therefore, blood flow through the ductus venosus falls instantly; absence of fetal shunting through this vessel usually occurs within the first 7 days of life. Once the ductus venosus closes, its remnants form the **ligamentum venosum,** or round ligament of the liver.

Increased pulmonary venous return and decreased inferior vena cava return cause functional closure of the foramen ovale within the first month of life. In the fetus the foramen ovale is held open by the blood flow from the higher-pressure right side, reflecting pulmonary vascular resistance, to the lower-pressure area on the left side of the heart, reflecting systemic vascular resistance. At birth the pressure gradients reverse (left atrial pressure exceeds right atrial pressure by a small degree), causing the valve flaps of the foramen ovale to close. Functional closure occurs by the adherence of these flaps to the atrial septum. Anatomic closure occurs within the first month of life after deposition of fibrin tissue and cell products permanently seals the flaps closed. Until this occurs, any condition that stimulates an increase in the right-sided pressures or causes dilation of the RA can reopen the foramen ovale. Conditions in which a patent foramen ovale may continue past the first month of life include pulmonary hypertension, RV failure, and tricuspid atresia.

The ductus arteriosus closes more gradually. Increased oxygen saturation in the systemic arterial blood is thought to be the major stimulus causing vasoconstriction of the ductus arteriosus. In addition, a decrease in the amount of endogenous prostaglandins promoting dilation and the release of vasoactive substances stimulate further ductal closure. Vasoconstriction of the ductal medial smooth muscle shortens and thickens the intima of the ductal wall within 15 to 18 hours after birth. Permanent closure is complete 10 to 21 days after birth. Fibrous tissue adheres to the remaining structure, and the ductus arteriosus eventually evolves into the ligamentum arteriosum. Conditions that involve low arterial oxygen saturations, such as cyanotic heart disease, decreased medial muscle layer within the ductus, or increased levels of circulating vasodilating substances in the blood, may delay or prevent ductal closure.[3]

Postnatal Development

Compared to the adult, the infant's cardiopulmonary system is proportionally larger in relation to body surface area. The infant's heart points at a transverse angle, but as the lungs and heart mature, the heart shifts lower in the chest and is rotated at a more oblique angle. Unlike the adult heart, the newborn heart has RV dominance with a thickened RV wall. This is because of the high pulmonary vascular resistance in the fetal circulation that subjects the RV to high afterload, which in turn causes the right ventricular myocardium to become as thick and strong as the LV myocardium.

After birth the right ventricular myocardium becomes less dominant as pulmonary vascular resistance drops. As systemic vascular resistance increases, the left ventricular myocardium becomes thicker. By 1 month of age, the newborn's ventricles are approximately equal in weight. As the child grows, the heart size increases accordingly. The weight of the heart doubles during the first year of life and increases six times that by 9 years of age.[3]

Postnatal changes involve a rise in arterial oxygen tension and an increase in alveolar oxygenation that stimulates vasodilation, resulting in a decrease in pulmonary vascular resistance. During the first 2 to 9 weeks of life, the inner medial linings of the small pulmonary arterioles become thinner in response to decreased pulmonary arterial pressure. This increased diameter of the pulmonary vessels, along with further development of the pulmonary bed in response to lung growth, results in a decrease in pulmonary vascular resistance. By 2 months of age, pulmonary resistance may approximate adult levels. During the neonatal period the pulmonary vascular bed remains hyperactive. Adverse conditions, such as alveolar hypoxia, acidosis, and hypothermia, may trigger pulmonary vasoconstriction and lead to pulmonary hypertension.

Postnatal Hemodynamics

As stated, systemic vascular resistance begins to rise once the placenta is removed from the circulation. Normal levels in the infant range from approximately 10 to 15 Wood units × body surface area (in square meters) and gradually increase to 15 to 30 Wood units × body surface area (in square meters) by childhood.[4] Likewise, the systolic pressure is low in the full-term newborn (approximately 39 to 59 mmHg), reflecting the low systemic vascular resistance. As the systemic vascular resistance increases, the LV becomes more developed and the systolic pressure rises steadily until it equals adult levels once the child reaches puberty.

The heart rate of the newborn ranges from 100 to 180 beats/minute, which gradually decreases as the child grows. Similarly, the newborn's cardiac output is high, which is a reflection of the fetal circulation described earlier. Oxygen consumption doubles at birth; to maintain adequate oxygen delivery, the cardiac output also remains high. These changes, however, cause minimal cardiac reserve in the newborn. Additional stressors could increase oxygen demands and result in acute deterioration. By 2 months of age, oxygen consumption decreases by half. As the newborn grows, stroke volume steadily increases while the heart rate decreases, thus maintaining cardiac output.[2]

Postnatal Circulation

Postnatal circulation allows the lungs to oxygenate the venous blood and allows fully saturated blood to be delivered to the systemic circulation. Desaturated blood returning from the superior vena cava, inferior vena cava, and coronary veins enters the RA and is pumped to the RV through the tricuspid valve. The RV then pumps the blood through the pulmonic valve to the PA; the blood flows to the lungs, where it is oxygenated. The oxygenated blood returns from the lungs through the pulmonary veins and enters the LA, which pumps blood to the LV through the mitral valve. The LV then pumps blood through the aortic valve and into the aorta. The coronary arteries receive the saturated blood along with delivery to the systemic circulation.

CONGENITAL HEART DEFECTS

Congenital heart disease is the leading cause of death, excluding prematurity, during the first year of life.[5] It is estimated that as many as 35% of deaths caused by congenital heart defects occur in the first year of life and that one third of children born with congenital heart disease will die as a result of their cardiac disease (Box 33-1). There are more than 35 documented types

BOX 33-1 ENDOCARDITIS RISK

Until 2008 it was common to prescribe an antibiotic to be administered before dental, gastrointestinal, or genitourinary procedures for almost all children with congenital heart defects. This practice started in the 1950s and continued until a committee of the American Heart Association (AHA) reviewed all of the major literature related to infectious endocarditis (IE), a serious and sometimes fatal condition in which the heart valves become infected with bacteria. The AHA committee concluded that: (1) IE is more likely to result from bacteremia from daily activities, such as brushing one's teeth, than from procedures; (2) prophylaxis was not effective in preventing IE; (3) there are significant risks to giving antibiotics; and (4) good oral health and hygiene is most important in the prevention of IE. Current recommendations suggest administration of prophylactic antibiotics before dental procedures only to the most high-risk children and adults: those with prosthetic cardiac valves, cyanotic congenital heart disease, repaired heart defects for the first 6 months after the procedure, repaired heart defects with certain residual defects, and those with previous IE. The best thing we as healthcare providers can teach our patients and their parents is to take excellent care of their teeth!

Data from Nishimura RA et al: *Circulation* 118(8):887–896, 2008.

of congenital heart defects, and the frequency of occurrence in the United States is on the rise. Although researchers have not determined the reason for this increase, one explanation is that it may be the result of improved methods of detection.[6]

The underlying cause of congenital heart disease is known in only 10% of cases. Several factors place the fetus at risk for developing congenital heart disease, including prenatal, environmental, and genetic factors. Among the prenatal factors are maternal rubella, maternal insulin-dependent diabetes, maternal alcoholism, maternal age (older than 40 years), maternal phenylketonuria, and maternal hypercalcemia (Table 33-1). The use of some drugs during pregnancy is associated with an above-average incidence of congenital heart disease. Examples of these drugs include thalidomide, lithium, phenytoin (Dilantin), and warfarin. The incidence of heart defects also has been found to be higher in stillbirths, spontaneous abortions, and low-birth-weight or small-for-gestational-age infants.[2] In general, the likelihood of unaffected parents having a child with congenital heart disease is about 1% with a recurrence risk of 2% to 6%.

Genetic factors also have been implicated in the development of congenital heart disease, although the mechanism of causation is often multifactorial. Recent progress, accelerated through the Human Genome Project, has resulted in the rapid identification of some genes causing congenital heart disease.[5]

ETIOLOGY. The etiology of most congenital heart disease is unknown. Early epidemiologic studies report a multifactorial influence to be the cause of up to 90% of cardiac anomalies, with a recurrence rate of 2% to 6%.[2] Associated risk factors include maternal, gestational, and familial conditions. (Maternal risk factors are discussed in the previous section.) Exposure to teratogens in utero also may be a risk factor. Likewise, fetal exposure to active maternal infections, such as rubella, herpesvirus, coxsackievirus B5, and cytomegalovirus, may be a risk.

Chromosomal aberrations account for about 6% of all congenital heart defects (Table 33-2). Many genetic and hereditary diseases are associated with congenital heart defects, although the mechanism of causation is unknown (Table 33-3). As many as 50% of infants with trisomy 21 have a congenital heart defect, either an AV canal defect or a VSD. Extracardiac defects are noted in as many as 35% of infants with cardiac lesions. Prospective studies using chromosomal analysis have suggested that congenital cardiac malformations may be the result of a single gene defect.[5]

Because of improved screening methods, surgical interventions, and management, children with congenital heart defects are now surviving into adulthood and bearing children of their own. Studies report a 5% to 15% incidence of congenital heart disease in offspring of a parent having a congenital heart lesion. If two siblings have a congenital cardiac anomaly, the recurrence risk is 9%, and if three siblings have a congenital cardiac anomaly, the rate jumps to a 50% chance that the next child also will have a cardiovascular malformation.

TABLE 33-1 ENVIRONMENTAL FACTORS AND ASSOCIATED CONGENITAL HEART DEFECTS

CAUSE	TYPE OF CONGENITAL HEART DEFECT
Infection	
Intrauterine	Patent ductus arteriosus (PDA), pulmonary stenosis, coarctation of aorta
Systemic viral	PDA, pulmonary stenosis, coarctation of aorta
Rubella	PDA, pulmonary stenosis, coarctation of aorta
Coxsackie B5	Endocardial fibroelastosis
Herpesvirus	Can infect endothelial cells and vascular endothelium
Cytomegalovirus (HCMV)	
Radiation	Studies of cancer survivors reveal radiation can cause atherosclerosis; myocardial, endocardial, and pericardial disease; conduction disturbances; and endothelial vessel disease
Metabolic Disorders	
Diabetes	Ventricular septal defect (VSD), cardiomegaly, transposition of the great vessels
Phenylketonuria (PKU)	Coarctation of the aorta, PDA
Hypercalcemia	Supravalvular aortic stenosis, pulmonic stenosis; aortic hyperplasia
Drugs	
Thalidomide	No specific lesion
Alcohol	Tetralogy of Fallot, atrial septal defect (ASD), VSD
Lithium	Exact effect not known
Phenytoin	Embryonic dysrhythmia and valvular heart disease
Warfarin	ASD and PDA
Peripheral Conditions	
Increased maternal age	VSD, tetralogy of Fallot (relationship unclear)
Antepartal bleeding	Various defects (relationship unclear)
Prematurity	PDA, VSD
High altitude	PDA, ASD (increased incidence)

Classification of Congenital Heart Defects and Associated Conditions

There are more than 35 different types of congenital anomalies that can be classified into 4 categories based on blood flow pattern: (1) lesions increasing pulmonary blood flow; (2) lesions decreasing pulmonary blood flow; (3) obstructive lesions, in which right- or left-sided outflow tract obstructions curtail or prohibit blood flow out of the heart; and (4) mixing lesions, in which desaturated blood and saturated blood mix within the chambers or great arteries of the heart (Table 33-4). By classifying lesions in this way, the clinical manifestations, as well as associated sequelae, are more predictable.

Associated conditions and their clinical manifestations are lesion dependent. The two most common conditions associated with congenital heart disease are heart failure (HF) and hypoxemia. Lesions increasing pulmonary blood flow include

TABLE 33-2 GENETIC FACTORS AND CONGENITAL HEART DEFECTS

CHROMOSOMAL ABERRATIONS OR SYNDROME	INCIDENCE OF DEFECTS	TYPE OF DEFECT
Trisomy 13	80%	Ventricular septal defect (VSD), atrial septal defect (ASD), patent ductus arteriosus (PDA), anomalous pulmonary venous connection, bicuspid aorta, overriding aorta
Trisomy 18	90%	VSD, PDA, patent foramen ovale, bicuspid aortic valve, dextrocardia
Down syndrome	12-44%	Endocardial cushion defects, VSD, PDA, ASD, transposition of great vessels, tetralogy of Fallot, persistent truncus arteriosus, coarctation of aorta, endocardial fibroelastosis
Cri du chat syndrome	20%	PDA, mixed defects
Turner syndrome	20-40%	Coarctation of aorta, pulmonary stenosis, subaortic and aortic stenosis, PDA, septal defects

Data from Doyle EF, Rutkowski M: *Cardiovasc Clin* 2:1, 1970.

TABLE 33-3 DISORDERS COEXISTENT WITH CONGENITAL HEART DEFECTS

DISORDER	ASSOCIATED CARDIOVASCULAR DEFECT
Connective Tissue Disorders	
Marfan syndrome	Aortic or mitral regurgitation, aortic aneurysm
Hurler syndrome	Pseudoatherosclerosis
Hunter syndrome	Pseudoatherosclerosis, hypertension
Osteogenesis imperfecta	Incompetent aortic valve
Complex Syndromes	
Kartagener syndrome	Dextrocardia
Holt-Oram syndrome	Atrial septal defect (ASD), ventricular septal defect (VSD)
Ellis–van Creveld syndrome	Defect or absence of atrial septum
Laurence-Moon-Biedl syndrome	Tetralogy of Fallot, single ventricle, transposition of aorta
Inborn Errors of Metabolism	
Pompe disease	Cardiomegaly, left heart failure, supraventricular tachycardia
Homocystinuria	Thromboembolic episodes, pulmonic and aortic regurgitation
Phakomatosis	
Neurofibromatosis (von Recklinghausen disease)	Hypertension, pheochromocytoma
von Hippel–Lindau disease	Hypertension, pheochromocytoma
Sturge-Weber-Dimitri disease	Anomalies of carotid and meningeal arteries
Vascular Malformations	
Osler-Weber-Rendu disease (hereditary hemorrhagic telangiectasia)	Atrioventricular fistula, telangiectasia
Milroy disease (lymphedema)	Hypoplasia or lymphatic vessels

Data from Doyle EF, Rutkowski M: *Cardiovasc Clin* 2:1, 1970.

defects that allow blood flow to shunt from the high-pressure left side to the lower-pressure right side, resulting in pulmonary congestion. Lesions that cause decreased pulmonary blood flow are generally complex and result in cyanosis. Obstructive lesions increase the pressure needed to eject the blood from the ventricles. The two types of obstructive lesions are right-sided lesions that may result in hypoxemia and cyanosis, and left-sided lesions that may result in HF. Mixing lesions are variable in their physiology and clinical manifestations.

Heart Failure

Heart failure (HF), sometimes called congestive heart failure (CHF), is classified as an acquired condition. HF occurs when the heart is unable to maintain sufficient cardiac output to meet the metabolic demands of the body. HF can occur as the result of decreased myocardial function or excessive metabolic demands. The most common causes of HF in infancy and childhood are cardiomyopathy or the result of poor ventricular function. Table 33-5 lists the congenital heart defects that cause HF by age. Pulmonary overcirculation from large left-to-right shunts (mixing) is often called CHF but is not usually associated with decreased ventricular function and failure to meet metabolic demands. However, the clinical manifestations are similar, such as failure to thrive (FTT), tachypnea, tachycardia, and respiratory tract infections.

PATHOPHYSIOLOGY. In general, the pathophysiologic mechanisms of HF in infants and children are very similar to those

TABLE 33-4 CLASSIFICATION OF CONGENITAL HEART DEFECTS

CLASSIFICATION	SHUNT DIRECTION	PRESENTATION	SPECIFIC DEFECTS
Lesions increasing pulmonary blood flow	Left to right	Acyanotic congestive heart failure	Patent ductus arteriosus, atrial septal defect, ventricular septal defect, complete atrioventricular canal defect
Lesions decreasing pulmonary blood flow	Right to left	Cyanotic	Tetralogy of Fallot, tricuspid atresia
Obstructive lesions*	None	Low cardiac output Shock	Coarctation of the aorta, hypoplastic left heart syndrome, aortic stenosis, pulmonary stenosis
Mixed lesions†	Variable	Variable	Transposition of the great arteries, total anomalous pulmonary venous connection, truncus arteriosus

*If patent ductus arteriosus closes, newborns with hypoplastic left heart syndrome, coarctation of the aorta, or critical aortic stenosis will present with shock. Newborns with aortic stenosis or pulmonary stenosis may have only mild symptoms depending on severity of stenosis.
†Transposition of the great arteries and truncus arteriosus will present with cyanosis as patent ductus arteriosus closes. Total anomalous pulmonary venous connection usually presents with congestive heart failure.

TABLE 33-5 CONGENITAL HEART DEFECTS CAUSING HEART FAILURE

AGE	CONGENITAL HEART DEFECT
Time of birth	Hypoplastic left heart syndrome Volume overload caused by tricuspid regurgitation (rare) Arteriovenous fistula
Birth to 1 week	Hypoplastic left heart syndrome Aortic atresia Transposition of the great vessels with ventricular septal defect (VSD) Coarctation of the aorta Total anomalous pulmonary venous connection (TAPVC) with obstruction Patent ductus arteriosus (PDA) in premature infants
First 4 weeks	Coarctation of the aorta TAPVC Large left-to-right shunt caused by VSD, PDA in premature infants Tricuspid atresia All previously mentioned defects
4 to 6 weeks	Transposition of the great vessels with VSD Large left-to-right shunt caused by endocardial cushion defect
6 weeks to 6 months	VSD
6 months	Endocardial fibroelastosis Persistent truncus arteriosus with large left-to-right shunt

in adults. The same compensatory mechanisms are activated in the face of inadequate cardiac output. An acute decrease in blood pressure stimulates stretch receptors and baroreceptors in the aorta and carotid arteries, which in turn stimulate the sympathetic nervous system. With the release of catecholamines and the stimulation of β receptors, heart rate and the force of myocardial contraction increase. Venous smooth muscle tone also increases, which increases return of venous blood to the heart. Sympathetic stimulation also decreases blood flow to the kidneys, skin, spleen, and extremities so that maximum flow to the brain, heart, and lungs can be maintained. Decreased blood flow to the kidneys causes the release of renin, angiotensin, and aldosterone. If chronic, this cycle results in retention of sodium and fluid by the kidneys, which in turn increases volume in the circulatory system.

These neurohumoral and hemodynamic changes create abnormal ventricular wall stress and cause the myocardium to hypertrophy. The myocardial fibers also stretch to accommodate the increased volume. Hypertrophy and fiber stretch temporarily increase contractility and hence the force of ventricular contraction. These mechanisms eventually fail to maintain cardiac output as HF progresses. A review of the Frank-Starling law of the heart (see Chapter 31) is useful for an understanding of the cycle of compensation and decompensation that occurs in HF.

CLINICAL MANIFESTATIONS. Symptomatic HF in children has many causes. It is not usually necessary to determine if it is right- or left-sided HF. When assessing a child with HF, a combination of symptoms generally is present. Pulmonary overcirculation is the predominant cause associated with congenital defects.

HF in infants is manifested as poor feeding and sucking, often leading to failure to thrive (FTT). Dyspnea, tachypnea, and diaphoresis may be accompanied by retractions, grunting, and nasal flaring. Wheezing, coughing, and rales are rare even with significant HF. Common skin changes, such as pallor or mottling, are often present.

Hepatomegaly (enlargement of the liver) is atypically attributable to systemic venous congestion. In infants the normal liver is soft, sharp-edged, and palpable 1 to 2 cm below the costal margin. However, the absence of hepatomegaly does not rule out HF.

Periorbital edema and weight gain without caloric increase are uncommon manifestations of right ventricular failure in infants. Peripheral edema, which is a common finding in adults, is rare in infants and young children and more often signifies renal disease rather than cardiac disease. The clinical manifestations of HF are listed in Box 33-2.

EVALUATION AND TREATMENT. A thorough physical examination with an emphasis on cardiac and pulmonary findings often will reveal the degree of HF. Plotting the child's growth (height, weight, head circumference) is an important method for monitoring a child's health. Infants with HF and pulmonary overcirculation usually have low weight with normal length and head

BOX 33-2 CLINICAL MANIFESTATIONS OF HEART FAILURE

IMPAIRED MYOCARDIAL FUNCTION	PULMONARY CONGESTION	SYSTEMIC VENOUS CONGESTION
Tachycardia	Tachypnea	Weight gain
Sweating (inappropriately)	Dyspnea	Hepatomegaly
Decreased urinary output	Retractions (infants)	Peripheral edema (rare)
Fatigue	Flaring nares	Ascites
Weakness	Exercise intolerance	Neck vein distention (rare in children)
Restlessness	Orthopnea	
Anorexia	Cough, hoarseness	
Pale, cool extremities	Cyanosis	
Weak peripheral pulses	Wheezing (rare)	
Decreased blood pressure	Grunting	
Gallop rhythm		
Cardiomegaly		

From Hockenberry MJ, Wilson D: *Wong's nursing care of infants and children,* ed 9, St Louis, 2011, Mosby.

circumference. FTT is usually the result of increased metabolic expenditure relative to caloric intake. An electrocardiogram (ECG) should be performed to determine the presence of dysrhythmias or hypertrophy. A chest radiograph is useful in assessing the presence of cardiomegaly and signs of increased pulmonary circulation.

Treatment is aimed at decreasing cardiac workload and increasing the efficiency of heart function. Medical management initially consists of diuretics, such as furosemide. Depending on the degree of HF, other diuretics can be used in combination with furosemide to counteract potassium losses. Agents that reduce afterload, such as angiotensin-converting enzyme (ACE) inhibitors and beta-blockers, have recently been used to further manage severe HF.[2,3] Caloric supplementation is routinely prescribed.

Hypoxemia

Heart defects that allow desaturated blood to enter the systemic system without passing through the lungs result in hypoxemia and cyanosis. Hypoxemia occurs when arterial oxygen tension is below normal and results in low oxygen arterial saturations and cellular function alteration. **Cyanosis,** a blue discoloration of the mucous membranes and nail beds, results from deoxygenated hemoglobin in a concentration of at least 5 g/dl of blood or from arterial saturations less than 85%.[2,4] Anemia may mask the signs of hypoxemia, whereas children who are polycythemic with a normal arterial saturation may appear cyanotic. Older children who have an unrepaired septal defect with a left-to-right shunt may become cyanotic because of pulmonary vascular changes secondary to increased pulmonary blood flow. Because of these progressive pulmonary vascular changes, pulmonary vascular resistance increases to exceed or equal vascular resistance, resulting in a reversal of shunting known as **Eisenmenger syndrome.** Three types of defects cause hypoxemia and cyanosis:

1. Lesions that cause right ventricular outflow tract obstruction and shunting from the right side of the heart to the left side, as in tetralogy of Fallot (see p. 1207)
2. Defects involving the mixing of saturated and unsaturated blood within the heart chambers, as in a univentricular heart (also referred to as a single ventricle)
3. Defects in children with transposition of the great arteries (see p. 1214), in which two parallel circulations exist and survival depends on the existence of a patent ductus arteriosus or septal defect

CLINICAL MANIFESTATIONS. Infants with mild hypoxemia may show signs of cyanosis only occasionally when stressed; otherwise, they may exhibit near-normal age-projected growth and development. Infants with severe hypoxemia may display signs of feeding intolerance, poor weight gain, tachypnea, and dyspnea. Children with chronic hypoxemia are small for their age, may display cognitive and motor skill delays, experience shortness of breath with exertion, fatigue easily, and have exercise intolerance. Acute, severe hypoxemia will lead to tissue hypoxia, metabolic acidosis, hyperventilation, poor perfusion, and eventually shock.

In response to chronic hypoxemia, polycythemia occurs as the body generates additional red blood cells to increase the oxygen-carrying capacity of the blood. In some infants, however, microcytic anemia may result because of limited stores of iron. Polycythemia and the associated platelet dysfunction also place children at risk for thromboembolic events, especially infants with severe cyanosis and iron deficiency anemia. In addition to the 2% risk of cerebrovascular accidents, there is a small chance that children with right-to-left shunting will develop a brain abscess.[4] Clubbing of the nail beds occurs because of chronic tissue hypoxemia and polycythemia.

Defects Increasing Pulmonary Blood Flow

Cardiac lesions that increase pulmonary blood flow include defects that involve septal abnormalities or communications between the great arteries. These allow the shunting of blood from the high-pressure left side to the lower-pressure right side. Infants with left-to-right shunts are acyanotic and, depending on the degree of shunting, may develop signs and symptoms of CHF. Children with significant left-to-right shunts left untreated are at risk for development of irreversible pulmonary hypertension.

Patent Ductus Arteriosus

The **patent ductus arteriosus (PDA)** is a vessel located between the junction of the main and left pulmonary arteries and the lesser curvature of the descending aorta, usually just distal to the left subclavian artery (Figure 33-5, *A*). During fetal circulation the PDA allows blood to shunt from the PA to the aorta. At birth, once the placenta is removed and the lungs are expanded, the PDA will start to constrict within the first hours of life. Closure of the PDA in full-term infants is usually noted between 15 hours of life and 2 weeks of age.[7] As an isolated defect, PDA occurs in

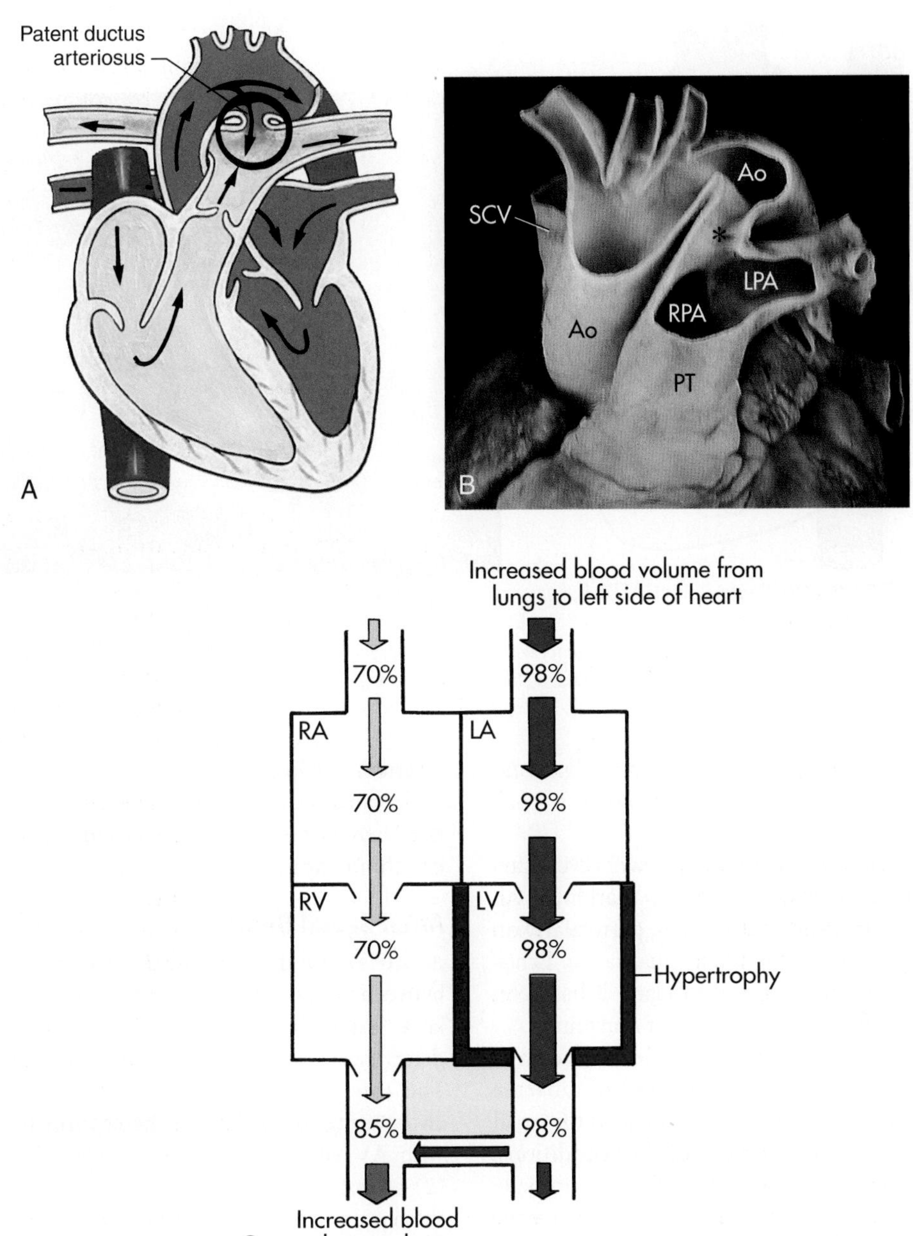

FIGURE 33-5 Patent Ductus Arteriosus (PDA). **A,** PDA with left-to-right shunt. **B,** PDA *(asterisk)* in an adult with pulmonary hypertension. **C,** Changes in oxygen saturation, left ventricular volume, and the myocardium caused by left-to-right shunt through a PDA. *Ao,* Aorta; *LA,* left atrium; *LPA,* left pulmonary artery; *LV,* left ventricle; *PT,* pulmonary trunk; *RA,* right atrium; *RPA,* right pulmonary artery; *RV,* right ventricle; *SCV,* subclavian vein. (**A** from Hockenberry MJ, Wilson D: *Wong's essentials of pediatric nursing,* ed 9, St Louis, 2013, Mosby; **B** from Damjanov I, Linder J, editors: *Anderson's pathology,* ed 10, St Louis, 1996, Mosby.)

5% to 10% of all congenital cardiac defects. Studies have shown that the incidence of PDA is high in premature infants.[8]

PATHOPHYSIOLOGY. Failure of the PDA to close results in persistent patency of the ductus arteriosus. The hemodynamic effects of PDA depend on the size of the lumen and the resistance in the pulmonary and systemic circulations. At birth the pulmonary and systemic vascular resistances are almost equal and are reflected in the PA and aorta, respectively; therefore, shunting is minimal. However, as pulmonary vascular resistance falls, a reversal of fetal shunting occurs. Blood now begins to shunt left to right, from the aorta to the PA. The hemodynamic effect is increased pulmonary blood flow, resulting in increased pulmonary venous return to the LA and LV with increased workload on the left side of the heart. The increased workload is caused by increased pulmonary venous return to the LA and, potentially, an increase in right ventricular pressure if pulmonary vascular changes occur in response to the increased blood flow, leading to an increase in pulmonary vascular pressure (see Figure 33-5, *B*).

CLINICAL MANIFESTATIONS. If pulmonary vascular resistance has fallen, infants with PDA will characteristically have a continuous-machinery type murmur heard best at the left upper sternal border throughout systole and diastole. If the PDA is significant, the infant also will have bounding pulses,

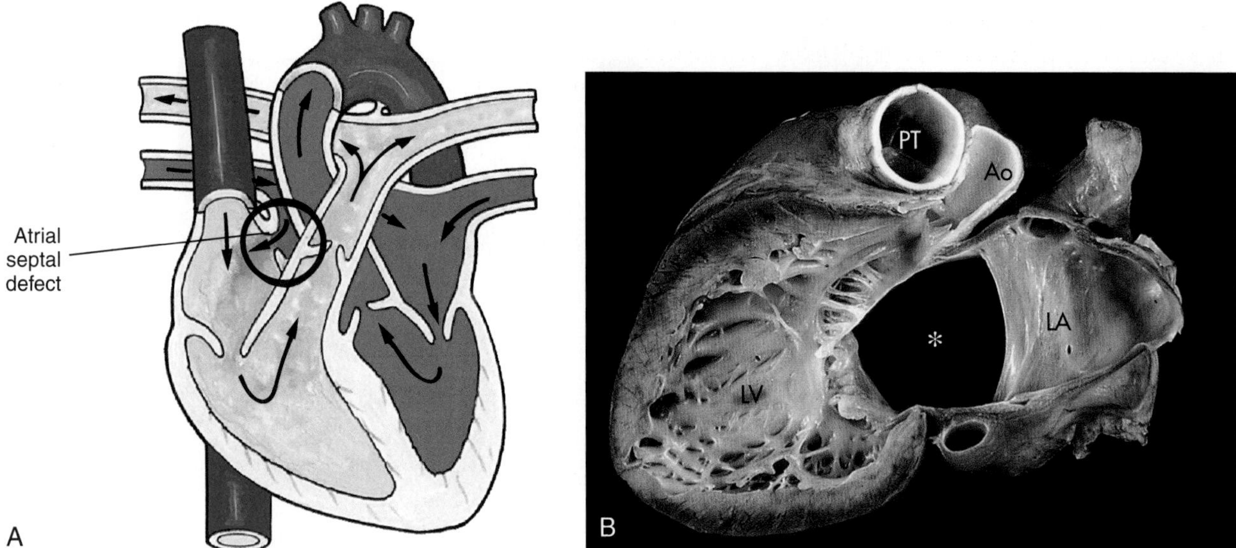

FIGURE 33-6 Atrial Septal Defect (ASD). **A,** Abnormal opening between the atria causing blood from the higher-pressure left atrium to flow into the lower-pressure right atrium. **B,** Complete ASD *(asterisk)* form in children. *Ao,* Aorta; *LA,* left atrium; *LV,* left ventricle; *PT,* pulmonary artery trunk. (**A** from Hockenberry MJ, Wilson D: *Wong's essentials of pediatric nursing,* ed 9, St Louis, 2013, Mosby; **B** from Damjanov I, Linder J, editors: *Anderson's pathology,* ed 10, St Louis, 1996, Mosby.)

an active precordium, a thrill upon palpation, and signs and symptoms of pulmonary overcirculation. Infants with a small PDA will usually remain asymptomatic.

EVALUATION AND TREATMENT. Chest radiograph will reveal cardiomegaly and increased pulmonary vascular markings. An ECG may demonstrate ventricular enlargement, particularly on the left, but in most cases it is within the normal range. Echocardiography and auscultation confirm the diagnosis based on the characteristic continuous-machinery type of murmur.

PDA closure in asymptomatic children with a murmur is recommended by 2 years of age because of the risk of subacute bacterial endocarditis. No treatment is recommended for small PDA in the absence of a murmur or other cardiac conditions. Premature infants who develop respiratory distress are initially given indomethacin, a prostaglandin inhibitor, to close the duct. If this is unsuccessful, surgical ligation and division may be warranted.

Historically the most widely used method for PDA closure is surgical closure involving ligation and division of the ductus with complete closure in nearly 100% of cases. Mortality associated with surgical intervention nears 0%; however, there continues to be some morbidity associated with the approach through a left thoracotomy incision.

Several other options for PDA closure are available depending on the size of the child and the PDA. Many specialists perform interventional closure of the PDA during catheterization. The catheter is advanced into the ductal opening whereby multiple coils or other devices are placed into the lumen that prohibit flow through the duct. The greatest advantages to this procedure are the avoidance of a surgical procedure and thoracotomy pain and a brief observation stay in the hospital.

Another option is closure through video-assisted thoracoscopic surgery. This procedure involves making three small incisions in the left lateral wall, through which a probe is inserted. A clip is then placed around the vessel to occlude it. An advantage of this procedure over open surgical procedures is that there is less associated morbidity because of the avoidance of a thoracotomy incision.[8]

Atrial Septal Defect

An **atrial septal defect (ASD)** is an abnormal communication between the atria (Figure 33-6, *A* and *B*). Although it is an isolated lesion, it is the fourth most common congenital heart defect, occurring in 5% to 10% of all congenital cardiac defects. The three major types are: (1) an ostium primum defect, an opening found low in the septum that may be associated with AV valve abnormalities, especially mitral insufficiency; (2) an ostium secundum defect, an opening in the center of the septum (this is the most common type of atrial defect); and (3) a sinus venosus defect, an opening that occurs high up in the atrial septum near the superior vena cava and RA junction. This defect is often associated with partial anomalous pulmonary venous connection.

PATHOPHYSIOLOGY. Although the pressure difference between the two atria is minimal, the ASD allows blood to be shunted from left to right because of the slightly higher pressure of the left atrial chamber and lower pulmonary vascular resistance as compared with systemic vascular resistance. Right atrial and ventricular enlargement develops as a result of left-to-right shunting. Children with ASD are generally asymptomatic and rarely display signs of pulmonary overcirculation. Moderate to large ASDs allow an increase in pulmonary blood flow and, over time, pulmonary vascular changes can occur that may, although rarely, result in pulmonary hypertension.

CLINICAL MANIFESTATIONS. Because most children with ASD are asymptomatic, diagnosis usually is made during a routine physical examination by the auscultation of a crescendo-decrescendo systolic ejection murmur that reflects increased blood flow through the pulmonary valve. The location of the murmur is between the second and third intercostal spaces along the left sternal border. A wide fixed splitting of the second heart sound is also characteristic of ASD, reflecting volume overload to the RV, causing prolonged ejection time and delay of pulmonic valve closure.

EVALUATION AND TREATMENT. In most cases an echocardiogram is sufficient to confirm the diagnosis of an ASD. A chest radiograph may reveal cardiomegaly and increased pulmonary vascular markings in an asymptomatic child. An ECG may demonstrate right-axis deviation and diastolic overload of the RV manifested as right ventricular hypertrophy.[2]

ASD closure, generally before the child reaches school age, results in improved health later in life. If left unrepaired, right ventricular compliance decreases with age, and pulmonary hypertension and right ventricular hypertrophy may occur, placing the person at risk for the development of HF, atrial dysrhythmias, or embolic events later in life. Surgical closure is one method of closure and involves a pericardial patch or suture closure of the defect, depending on the size of the opening. Repair is done through a midsternal approach with the use of cardiopulmonary bypass. Minimally invasive techniques are being used on near–adult-sized patients. Sinus venosus defects require a slightly different approach that consists of a synthetic patch to close the opening and baffle the anomalous right pulmonary venous drainage to the LA. Operative mortality associated with ASD closure is near 0%, with minimal morbidity.[7,9,10] Device closure performed in the catheterization laboratory is becoming a routine alternative to open surgical procedures.[7]

Ventricular Septal Defect

A **ventricular septal defect (VSD)** is an abnormal communication between the ventricles (Figure 33-7, *A*). VSDs are the most common type of congenital heart lesion and account for 25% to 33% of all congenital heart defects. The four types of VSDs are based on location in the septum. The perimembranous type, which occurs in the outflow tract of the LV immediately below the aortic valve, is the most common type, accounting for up to 80% of all VSDs that require treatment. Muscular VSDs, which occur low or anterior in the ventricular septum between the trabeculae (see Figure 33-7, *B*) are most likely to close spontaneously and are difficult to close surgically because of their location low in the ventricular apex. Most muscular VSDs are hemodynamically insignificant and require no medical or surgical treatment. Supracristal VSDs (also called outlet VSD) occur in the right ventricular outflow tract or infundibulum, below the pulmonary valve. AV canal or inlet VSDs occur posterior and inferior to the membranous system, beneath the septal cusp of the tricuspid valve and inferior to the papillary muscles of the conus.

PATHOPHYSIOLOGY. The direction of shunting in a child with a VSD is from the high-pressure left side to the lower-pressure right side. The amount of shunting depends on the size of the defect and the degree of pulmonary vascular resistance. Small VSDs present increased resistance to shunting and limit blood flow through the defect; thus the degree of pulmonary vascular congestion and ventricular chamber enlargement is minimal (see Figure 33-7, *C*).

After 1 to 2 weeks of life, when pulmonary vascular resistance has decreased, moderate-sized to large VSDs allow a large amount of shunting from left to right. The shunted blood flows directly out the RV outflow tract and into the PA rather than remain in the RV cavity (see Figure 33-7, *D*). Therefore, the main PA, LA, and LV all enlarge. LV hypertrophy occurs to effectively pump the additional volume. Pulmonary overcirculation accounts for the symptoms associated with a large VSD in most cases.

Over time the pulmonary bed also undergoes changes because of increased pulmonary blood flow caused by the left-to-right shunting. The smooth muscle layer in the arteriolar walls thickens and proliferation of the intimal layer occurs. The effect of these changes is a decrease in the diameter of the pulmonary vessels, which increases the resistance to blood flow. If the pulmonary vascular resistance is severely increased these changes eventually become irreversible, and pulmonary vascular resistance continues to rise. In some cases it exceeds systemic vascular resistance, causing the shunt through the VSD to reverse direction. Deoxygenated blood now flows into the systemic circulation, and cyanosis occurs, a phenomenon known as *Eisenmenger syndrome*.

CLINICAL MANIFESTATIONS. Clinical manifestations in children with VSDs depend on the age of the child, size of the defect, and level of pulmonary vascular resistance. Newborns with small VSDs are relatively asymptomatic. Initially no murmur is present because the newborn's high pulmonary vascular resistance causes equalization of the pressures between both ventricles. Once pulmonary vascular resistance has dropped, left-to-right shunting occurs, creating a murmur. Infants with large VSDs display symptoms of HF and poor weight gain. Adults who develop pulmonary vascular obstructive disease as a result of unrepaired VSD will be cyanotic and have clubbing.

On physical examination a loud, harsh, holosystolic murmur and systolic thrill can be detected at the left lower sternal border. The intensity of the murmur reflects the pressure gradient across the VSD. An apical diastolic rumble may be present with a moderate to large defect, reflecting increased flow across the mitral valve.

EVALUATION AND TREATMENT. ECG and chest radiographs reflect the amount of shunting through the defect. The ECG of an individual with a small VSD may be normal, whereas the ECG of an individual with a large VSD may reveal biventricular hypertrophy and LA enlargement. Chest roentgenographic findings are significant for cardiomegaly and increased pulmonary vascular markings; again, the severity is directly related to the magnitude of shunting. An echocardiogram identifies the position, size, direction of shunting, and dimensions of the LA, LV, and RV chambers. It also can provide an estimate of PA and RV pressures. Cardiac catheterization may be performed to determine hemodynamics and, in some instances, the location of other defects and additional VSDs.

Many VSDs spontaneously close during the first year of life.[2] Infants with symptoms of HF and poor weight gain despite medical management should have their VSD corrected as soon as possible. Left-to-right shunting with a pulmonary flow/systemic flow (Q_p/Q_s) ratio of greater than 2:1 or evidence of

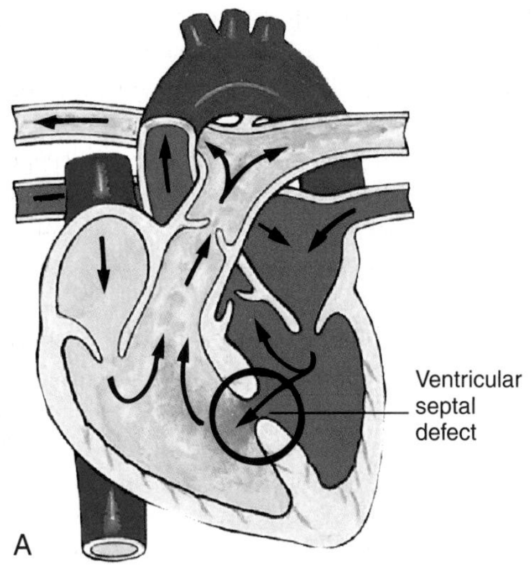

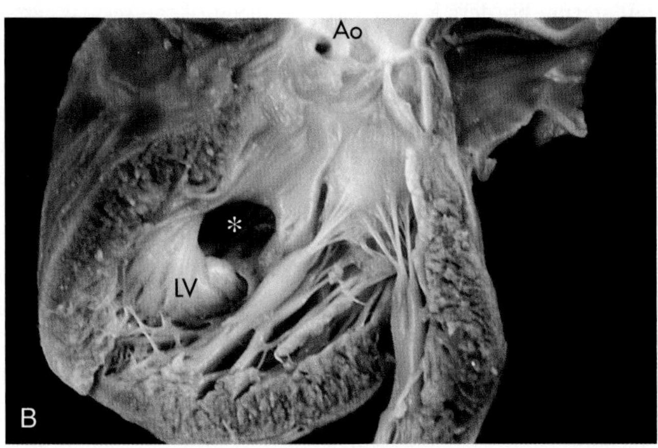

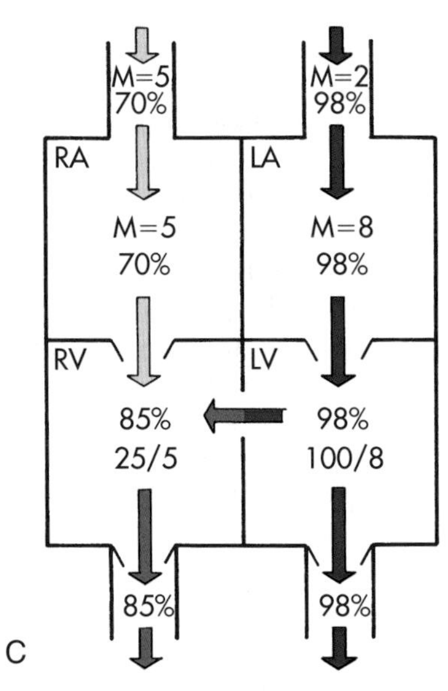

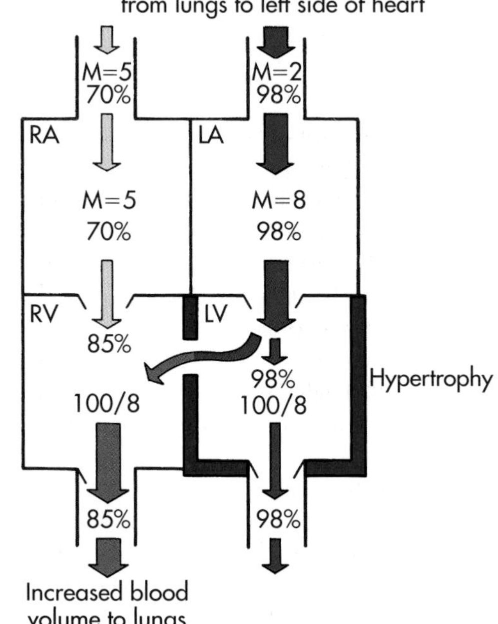

FIGURE 33-7 Ventricular Septal Defects (VSDs). A, VSD with left-to-right shunt. **B,** Muscular *(asterisk)* defect (opened left ventricle). **C,** Hemodynamics of a small VSD with left-to-right shunt. Mean *(M)* indicates mean of pressure; systolic/diastolic pressures are in mmHg; and percentages indicate oxygen saturation. **D,** Hemodynamics of a large VSD with left-to-right shunt. Like the shunting that occurs in preductal coarctation of the aorta, the shunting pictured here causes left ventricular overload and hypertrophy. *Ao,* Aorta; *LA,* left atrium; *LV,* left ventricle; *RA,* right atrium; *RV,* right ventricle. (**A** from Hockenberry MJ, Wilson D: *Wong's essentials of pediatric nursing,* ed 9, St Louis, 2013, Mosby; **B** from Damjanov I, Linder J, editors: *Anderson's pathology,* ed 10, St Louis, 1996, Mosby.)

elevated pulmonary vascular resistance are indications for closure. Closure of the VSD at this time is to prevent the development of pulmonary vascular obstructive disease.

Placement of a PA band to decrease the amount of pulmonary blood flow was initially used as a palliative procedure but is now rarely used unless the presence of an additional lesion makes complete repair difficult. Patch closure, using a synthetic material or pericardium, is accomplished through a sternotomy and with the use of cardiopulmonary bypass. A transatrial approach is preferable to a right ventriculotomy because of the increased incidence of conduction disturbances associated with ventriculotomy. Contraindications for VSD closure include evidence of pulmonary vascular obstructive disease or Eisenmenger syndrome.[2,7] Occlusion devices for VSD closure performed in the cardiac catheterization laboratory are now in early clinical use.[7,11]

Atrioventricular Canal Defect

An **atrioventricular canal (AVC) defect** results from nonfusion of the endocardial cushions during fetal life, yielding abnormalities in both the atrial and ventricular septa and the AV valves

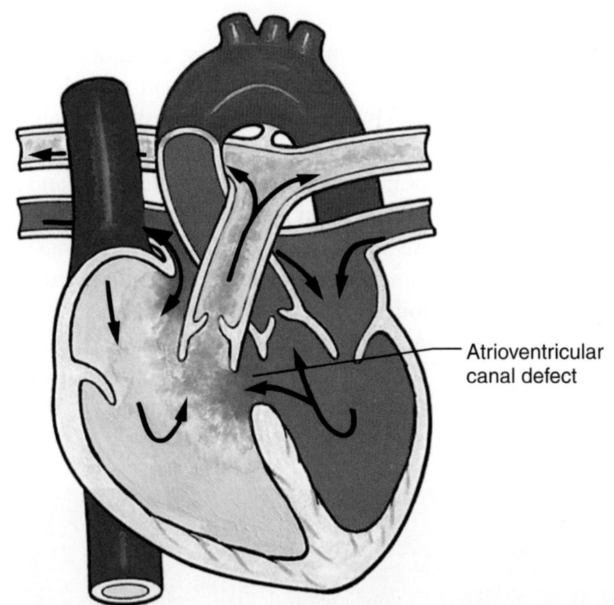

FIGURE 33-8 Atrioventricular Canal Defect. (From Hockenberry MJ, Wilson D: *Wong's essentials of pediatric nursing,* ed 9, St Louis, 2013, Mosby.)

(Figure 33-8). This defect accounts for as many as 5% of all congenital heart defects, and approximately 30% of AVC defects occur in children with Down syndrome.[7] The three types of AVC defects are based on the cardiac components involved. **Complete AVC (CAVC) defects** consist of an inlet VSD, a primum type of ASD, and defects in both the mitral and tricuspid valves. **Partial AVC (PAVC) defects** consist of a primum type of ASD and a cleft in the septal or anterior leaflet of the mitral valve. **Transitional AVC (TAVC) defects** involve partial fusion of the endocardial cushions, resulting in variable AV valve abnormalities.[7]

PATHOPHYSIOLOGY. Hemodynamic abnormalities seen in AVC defects depend on the components of the lesion and the level of pulmonary vascular resistance. Shunting is minimal during the neonatal period when pulmonary vascular resistance is high. However, once pulmonary vascular resistance drops, left-to-right shunting occurs through the septal defects, resulting in increased pulmonary blood flow and HF.

PAVC defects mimic the hemodynamics of secundum ASD in which the left-to-right shunting through the primum ASD causes RA and RV dilation and increased pulmonary blood flow. The mitral regurgitation that occurs, caused by the cleft mitral valve, is usually hemodynamically insignificant.

CAVC defects reflect the hemodynamics of an ASD and a VSD, resulting in biatrial and biventricular enlargement. RA and RV volume overload occurs because of shunting through the primum ASD and tricuspid regurgitation. Likewise, LA and LV volume overload occurs because of shunting through the VSD, increased pulmonary venous return, and mitral regurgitation.

CLINICAL MANIFESTATIONS. Children with PAVC defects are generally asymptomatic. Findings on physical examination are similar to those of secundum ASD with the addition of a holosystolic, regurgitant murmur of mitral regurgitation at the apex. At 4 to 12 weeks of age, when pulmonary vascular resistance drops, children with CAVC defects usually begin to show symptoms of HF. Physical findings are similar to those found in individuals with VSDs with the addition of a holosystolic murmur radiating to the back and apex, reflecting mitral regurgitation. A mid-diastolic rumble at the left lower sternal border or apex reflects relative stenosis of the mitral or tricuspid valve from increased flow. Infants with CAVC may have signs of HF and frequent respiratory tract infections.

EVALUATION AND TREATMENT. The ECG generally demonstrates a superior left-axis deviation (−90 to −180 degrees), first-degree AV block, and RV hypertrophy or right bundle branch block. The ECG of CAVC defects also may show LV hypertrophy. Chest radiograph shows cardiomegaly, increased pulmonary vascular markings, and a prominent main PA. Echocardiography allows visualization of the components of the defect, including continuity between the AV valves, their sizes, and chordal attachments. Cardiac catheterization may be electively performed and can confirm the location of septal defects, AV valve abnormalities, degree of left-to-right shunting, and presence of pulmonary hypertension.

Timing of surgical repair depends on the severity of symptoms, degree of shunting, and level of pulmonary vascular resistance. The trend is to perform complete repair between 3 and 6 months after birth to avoid the development of pulmonary vascular changes. Surgical repair is performed through a mid-sternotomy implementing a one- or two-patch repair to close the septal defects and repair the involved AV valves. Mortality has declined below 10% unless the child is a newborn, has severe AV valve incompetence, or has a small LV (unbalanced AV canal). Postoperative complications include heart block, dysrhythmias, or mitral regurgitation requiring further surgical intervention or valve replacement.[7,12]

Defects Decreasing Pulmonary Blood Flow

Defects decreasing pulmonary blood flow involve obstruction to pulmonary blood flow and septal communications. Because of RV outflow tract obstruction, right-sided pressures exceed left-sided pressures, resulting in right-to-left shunting. Children with these defects have hypoxemia and cyanosis.

Tetralogy of Fallot

Tetralogy of Fallot (TOF) consists of four defects: a large VSD that is high in the septum, an overriding aorta that straddles the VSD, pulmonary stenosis (PS), and RV hypertrophy (Figure 33-9, *A* and *B*). It is the most common cyanotic congenital heart defect and accounts for 10% of all defects.[2]

PATHOPHYSIOLOGY. TOF develops during two phases of embryologic growth: (1) during the division of the truncus arteriosus by the spiral septum in the third or fourth week of gestation, and (2) during the division of the ventricles between the fourth and eighth weeks of gestation. Normally as these events progress, the truncal septum fuses with the bulbar ridges and in turn with the endocardial cushions. The membranous portion of the interventricular septum grows upward to meet the endocardial cushions, and ultimately all of these tissues unite to complete the interventricular septum.

The embryologic error that causes TOF is not definitively known, but two theories have been proposed.[1] The first is that the truncus arteriosus divides unevenly, resulting in great vessels of unequal size. The second theory proposes that infundibular overgrowth in the RV is the major developmental anomaly. Defects in ventricular septation also occur, producing the large VSD, which allows the aorta to override the VSD.

The pathophysiology associated with TOF varies widely, depending primarily on the degree of pulmonary stenosis, the size of the VSD, and the pulmonary and systemic resistance to flow. Because the VSD is usually large, pressures are equal in the RV and LV. Therefore, the major determinant of shunt direction through the VSD is the difference between pulmonary and systemic vascular resistance (see Figure 33-9, *C*). Infants who have little or no right-to-left shunting are acyanotic and are known as "pink tets." They may have a net left-to-right shunt similar to a large VSD. If pulmonary vascular resistance is higher than systemic resistance, the shunt is from right to left. Because many factors can alter the balance between pulmonary and systemic resistance, shunt direction is not necessarily constant.

Pulmonary stenosis decreases blood flow to the lungs and, consequently, the amount of oxygenated blood that returns to the left heart. If blood also shunts from right to left through the VSD, deoxygenated blood mixes with the oxygenated blood returning from the lungs. The result is low oxygen saturation (hypoxemia) in the systemic circulation. The body attempts

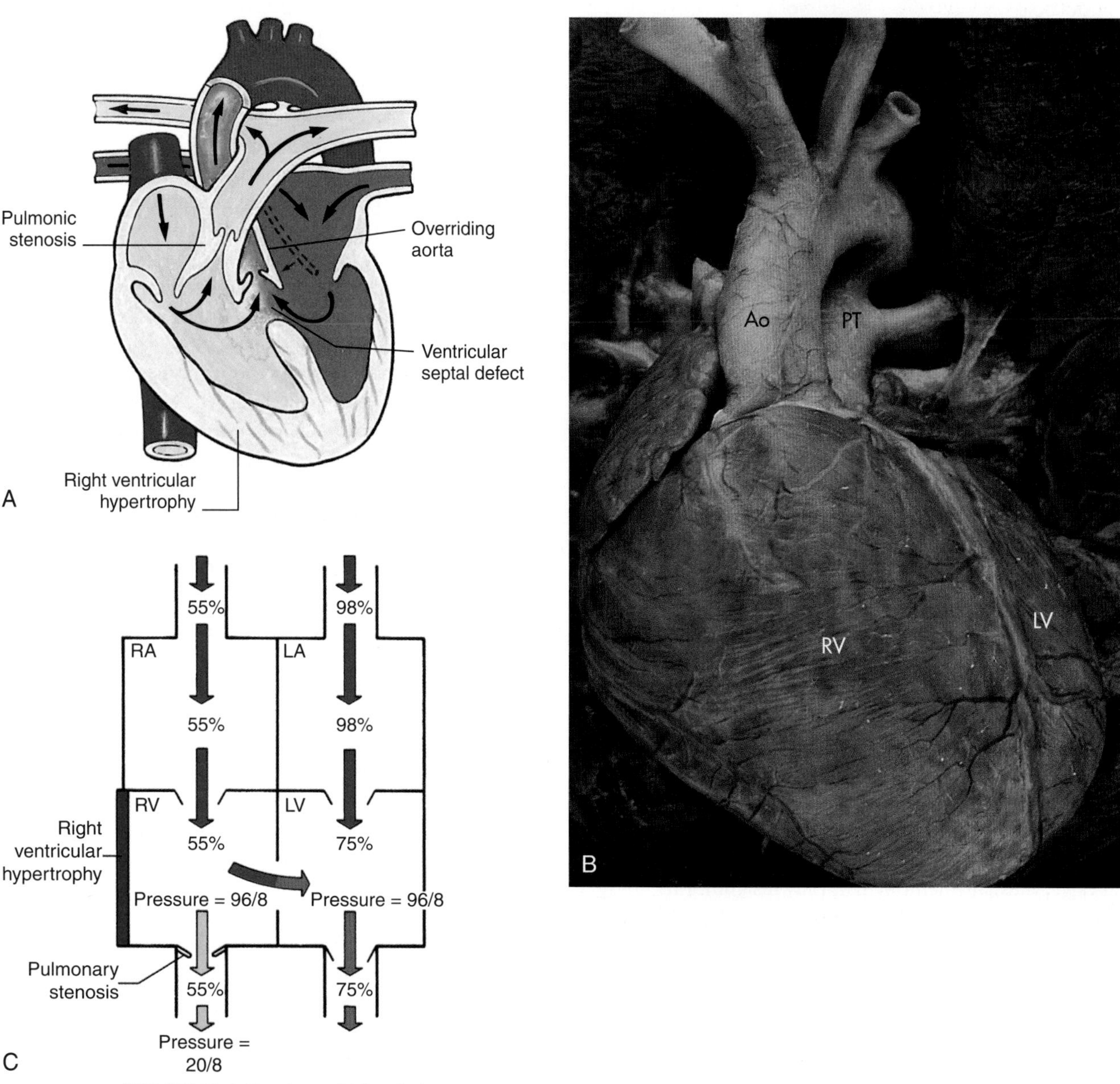

FIGURE 33-9 Tetralogy of Fallot. **A,** Anatomic defects in tetralogy of Fallot. **B,** Complete transposition of the aorta and pulmonary artery. **C,** Hemodynamics of tetralogy of Fallot with right-to-left shunt. *Ao,* Aorta; *LA,* left atrium; *LV,* left ventricle; *PT,* pulmonary artery trunk; *RA,* right atrium; *RV,* right ventricle. (**A** from Hockenberry MJ, Wilson D: *Wong's essentials of pediatric nursing,* ed 9, St Louis, 2013, Mosby; **B** from Damjanov I, Linder J, editors: *Anderson's pathology,* ed 10, St Louis, 1996, Mosby.)

to compensate for chronic hypoxemia by producing more red blood cells (thereby causing polycythemia) and by increasing blood flow to the lungs through collateral bronchial vessels in long-standing cases.

CLINICAL MANIFESTATIONS. In cases with decreased pulmonary flow through the right ventricular outflow tract as long as the ductus arteriosus remains open, the newborn's pulmonary blood flow may be adequate. As the ductus closes, however, cyanosis becomes apparent. Chronic hypoxemia causes clubbing of the fingers and toes (see Chapter 35).

A rare manifestation of TOF is the sudden onset of dyspnea, cyanosis, and restlessness, sometimes called a *hypercyanotic spell* or a *"tet spell,"* that generally occurs with crying and exertion. The cause of these episodes is unknown, but it is theorized that the RV outflow tract goes into spasm or the systemic resistance drops suddenly. In either case the relative or actual increase in pulmonary vascular resistance increases the right-to-left shunt and the cyanosis. Hypercyanotic spells are often the event that initiates surgical intervention. If the spells are frequent or do not terminate spontaneously, they are considered a medical-surgical emergency.[7]

Infants with TOF may have difficulty with feeding because the exertion required increases hypoxia, and therefore they experience slow growth and FTT. Most infants with TOF grow normally.

Squatting is a spontaneous compensatory mechanism used by older children with unrepaired TOF to alleviate hypoxic spells. Squatting and its variants increase systemic resistance while decreasing venous return to the heart from the inferior vena cava. The decrease of systemic return makes relatively more oxygenated blood available to the body. The increase of systemic resistance also reverses the shunt through the VSD to a left-to-right shunt, which has the effect of increasing pulmonary blood flow. Through both of these mechanisms, squatting temporarily decreases the degree of hypoxemia. It is uncommon to witness this because most cases are surgically corrected in early infancy.

The typical heart murmur of TOF is a pulmonary systolic ejection murmur caused by the obstruction in the outflow tract, which creates turbulence during systole. More obstruction to flow (e.g., smaller orifice for the flow of blood) produces a louder murmur. This explains why the murmur often disappears during a hypoxic spell, when obstruction increases and pulmonary blood flow decreases to a minimal amount. The second heart sound seems to be single, but in fact it is not. The pulmonary component is very soft and delayed and usually is not heard, although it is present. The enlarged RV may cause the left side of the chest to be more prominent, and a "heave" also may be palpated.

EVALUATION AND TREATMENT. The ECG indicates RV hypertrophy. Chest radiographic examination shows that the heart is shaped like a boot (upturned apex because of a small main PA) and that pulmonary vascular markings are decreased. Echocardiograms and angiograms enable the clinician to see the size and position of the VSD, the stenotic pulmonary infundibulum or valve, the smaller-than-normal PA, and the overriding aorta. Measurements made during cardiac catheterization (electively done in rare cases) demonstrate equal systemic pressure in the RV and LV, decreased pressure in the PA distal to the obstruction, and low oxygen saturation in the aorta if there is right-to-left shunting.

The current practice is to repair TOF before 1 year of age. Triggers for repair include increasing cyanosis and hypercyanotic spells. Palliative procedures include the placement of a pulmonary-to-systemic artery shunt known as the Blalock-Taussig shunt to increase pulmonary blood flow or a modification of the shunt using prosthetic graft material placed from either the subclavian or the innominate artery to the PA. These shunts may cause PA distortion but may be necessary in a very small symptomatic child. Corrective repair involves patch closure of the VSD, resection of infundibular or valvular stenosis, and patch augmentation of the RV outflow tract. The procedure is done through a median sternotomy while the child is on cardiopulmonary bypass. The operative mortality is less than 5%. Complications include dysrhythmias and occasionally heart block. Many children require further surgery to relieve recurrent pulmonary stenosis or treat severe pulmonary insufficiency.[13]

Tricuspid Atresia

Tricuspid atresia consists of an imperforate tricuspid valve, resulting in no communication between the RA and RV (Figure 33-10). This defect accounts for 2% to 3% of congenital heart defects and is the third most common cyanotic heart defect. Tricuspid atresia is a combination of defects, including the imperforate tricuspid valve as well as a septal defect, hypoplastic or absent RV, enlarged mitral valve and LV, and varying degrees of pulmonic stenosis. Tricuspid atresia also may be associated with transposition of the great vessels. The most common type of tricuspid atresia involves a hypoplastic RA with decreased pulmonary blood flow, ASD, VSD, and normally related great vessels.[2]

PATHOPHYSIOLOGY. Systemic blood returns through the superior and inferior venae cavae to the RA. Venous return flows through the ASD into the LA, mixing with blood returning from the pulmonary circulation. The blood then enters the LV. Most of this blood passes into the systemic circulation through the aorta, but varying amounts flow through the VSD into the hypoplastic RV and to the lungs. Pulmonary circulation depends on the presence of a VSD and the presence of a functioning RV of reasonable capacity. If the RV is absent, the pulmonary valve is usually imperforate as well. If this is the case, a PDA is necessary to ensure that some blood flows into the pulmonary circulation.[7]

Pulmonary circulation also depends on the relationship between pulmonary and systemic vascular resistance. As long as pulmonary resistance is lower than systemic resistance, blood flows through the VSD from left to right, feeding the pulmonary circulation. If pulmonary resistance rises above systemic resistance, pulmonary blood flow will be significantly diminished.

CLINICAL MANIFESTATIONS. Some degree of central cyanosis is common in tricuspid atresia, depending on the amount of pulmonary blood flow. Growth failure also is common. Children experience exertional dyspnea, tachypnea, and hypoxemia. Long-term effects of hypoxia are polycythemia and clubbing.

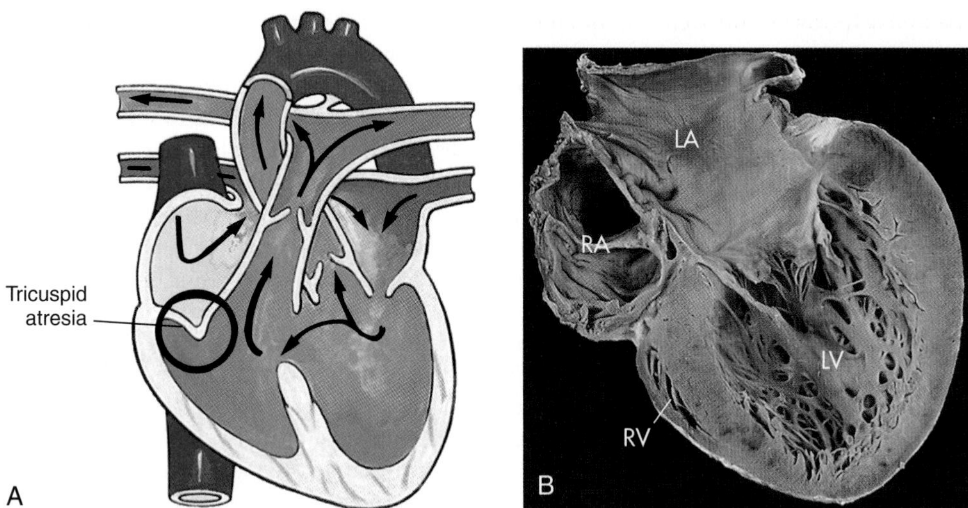

FIGURE 33-10 Tricuspid Atresia. **A,** No communication from the right atrium to the right ventricle. **B,** Tricuspid atresia with absent right atrioventricular connection with a hypoplastic right ventricle (four-chamber view). *LA,* Left atrium; *LV,* left ventricle; *RA,* right atrium; *RV,* right ventricle. (**A** from Hockenberry MJ, Wilson D: *Wong's essentials of pediatric nursing,* ed 9, St Louis, 2013, Mosby; **B** from Damjanov I, Linder J, editors: *Anderson's pathology,* ed 10, St Louis, 1996, Mosby.)

These children also may display hypercyanotic spells. Hepatomegaly may be present if the ASD is restrictive or CHF occurs as a result of increased pulmonary blood flow.

The murmur heard with tricuspid atresia may have several components. The VSD causes a systolic regurgitant murmur; the murmur is likely to be softer and shorter as the VSD enlarges. A narrowly split second heart sound caused by decreased pulmonary blood flow may be present, or the second heart sound may be single if there is pulmonary atresia.

EVALUATION AND TREATMENT. Chest radiographic examination shows a heart size that is normal or slightly increased. ECG usually shows RA, LA, and LV hypertrophy with left-axis deviation. Echocardiography and cardiac catheterization, if performed, depict left-to-right shunting at the ventricular level, inability of blood flow to enter the RV from the absent tricuspid opening, and the presence of associated defects.

Newborns with ductal dependent pulmonary blood flow are immediately given prostaglandins to maintain adequate pulmonary perfusion. Initial surgical intervention involves the placement of a Blalock-Taussig shunt (or its modification). If the ASD is restrictive, a Rashkind procedure (balloon atrial septostomy) may be performed during catheterization. Children who experience increased pulmonary blood flow may require the placement of a PA band. Corrective repair involves closing the septal defects, removing the previous shunts or band, and connecting the superior and inferior venae cavae to the PA to separate the pulmonary systemic circulation (Fontan procedure and its modifications). Postoperative complications include pleural effusions, elevated pulmonary vascular resistance, LV dysfunction, and dysrhythmias.[13]

Obstructive Defects

Obstructive defects are conditions in which anatomic stenosis (narrowing) in either the right or the left outflow tract causes obstruction to blood flow and results in a pressure load on the ventricles. The gradient reflects the severity of the narrowing; the higher the gradient the more obstruction to flow and more afterload on the ventricle. The location is classified according to the location of the narrowing in relation to the valve. Valvular stenosis refers to stenosis of the valve itself; subvalvular indicates that the obstruction is below the valve or in the ventricular outflow tract; and supravalvular is the area above the valve in the great artery. The great vessel itself can be narrowed and the site of obstruction can be the same as that in coarctation of the aorta. The obstructive defects include coarctation of the aorta, aortic stenosis, pulmonary stenosis, and hypoplastic left heart syndrome. Symptoms associated with the defect depend on the site and severity of stenosis.

Coarctation of the Aorta

Coarctation of the aorta (COA) is a narrowing of the lumen of the aorta that impedes blood flow. This defect accounts for 8% to 10% of all congenital heart defects. COA is almost always in a juxtaductal position, although it can occur anywhere between the origin of the aortic arch and the bifurcation of the aorta in the lower abdomen. About 50% of individuals with COA have a bicuspid aortic valve (Figure 33-11).[2]

PATHOPHYSIOLOGY. COA may develop because of abnormal contractile ductal tissue that constricts at the time of ductal closure. COA causes a condition in which there are higher pressures proximal to the site of stenosis and lower pressures distal to the site. In preductal COA the RV acts as a systemic pump, sending unoxygenated blood through the ductus into the descending aorta below the coarctation (Figure 33-12). In postductal COA the RV cannot pump enough blood through the ductus to the descending aorta because of pressure caused by the narrowed aorta. Systolic pressure increases in the ascending aorta and LV and decreases in the descending aorta beyond the COA (Figure 33-13). In long-standing COA, collateral circulation, which involves small arteries arising from the subclavian arteries, joins intercostal arteries that flow into the descending aorta. These collateral vessels bypass the COA and supply blood to the lower extremities. The direction of shunting through the ductus, if present, depends on the pressure difference between the PA and aorta and the location of the ductus. When blood pressure is greater in the aorta than in the PA, blood flow through the ductus will be left to right toward the lungs, resulting in increased pulmonary venous return to the left side of the heart. This may place an additional strain on the LA and LV, leading to increased volume and workload. With time, LV hypertrophy develops because of increased afterload and obstruction to flow caused by the coarctation. HF also may develop.

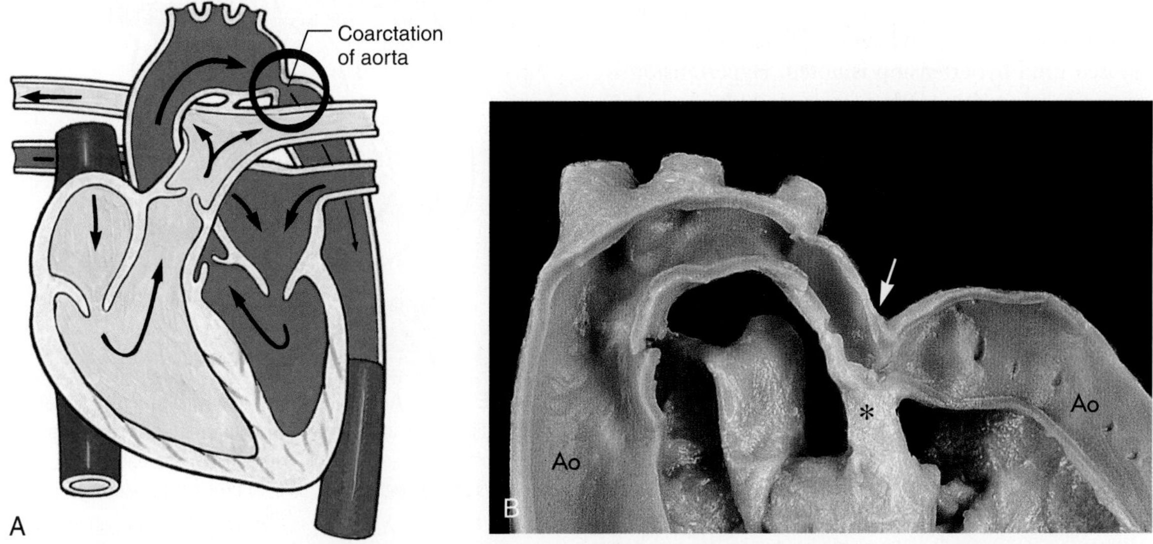

FIGURE 33-11 Postductal and Preductal Coarctation of the Aorta. A, Postductal coarctation occurs distal to ("after") the insertion of the closed ductus arteriosus into the aortic arch. Preductal coarctation occurs proximal to ("before") insertion of the patent ductus arteriosus. The coarctation consists of a flap of tissue that protrudes from the tunica media of the aortic wall. **B,** Coarctation of the aorta with typical indentation of the aortic wall *(arrow)* opposite the ductal arterial ligament *(asterisk). Ao,* Aorta. (**A** from Hockenberry MJ, Wilson D: *Wong's essentials of pediatric nursing,* ed 9, St Louis, 2013, Mosby; **B** from Damjanov I, Linder J, editors: *Anderson's pathology,* ed 10, St Louis, 1996, Mosby.)

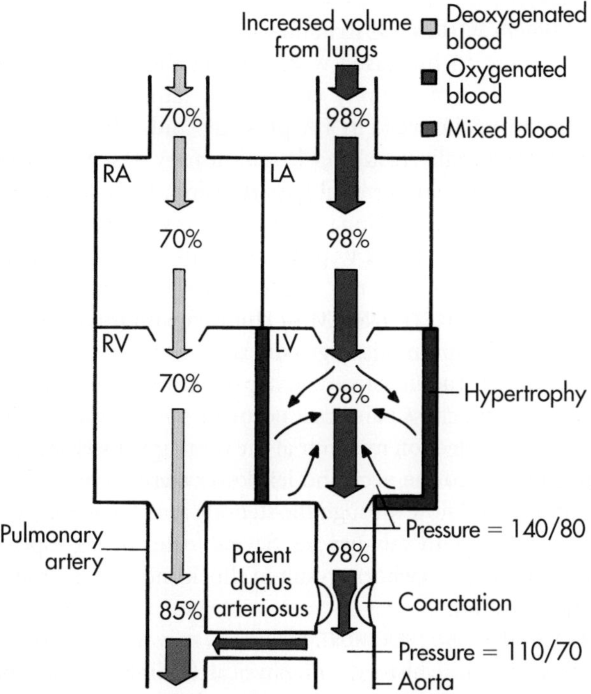

FIGURE 33-12 Hemodynamics of Preductal Coarctation of the Aorta with a Patent Ductus Arteriosus. The left-to-right shunt through the ductus arteriosus increases the volume of blood in the pulmonary circulation. Afterload *(small black arrows)* is increased in the left heart by increased return from the lungs and decreased ventricular outflow caused by the coarctation. The outcome is heart failure. *LA,* Left atrium; *LV,* left ventricle; *RA,* right atrium; *RV,* right ventricle.

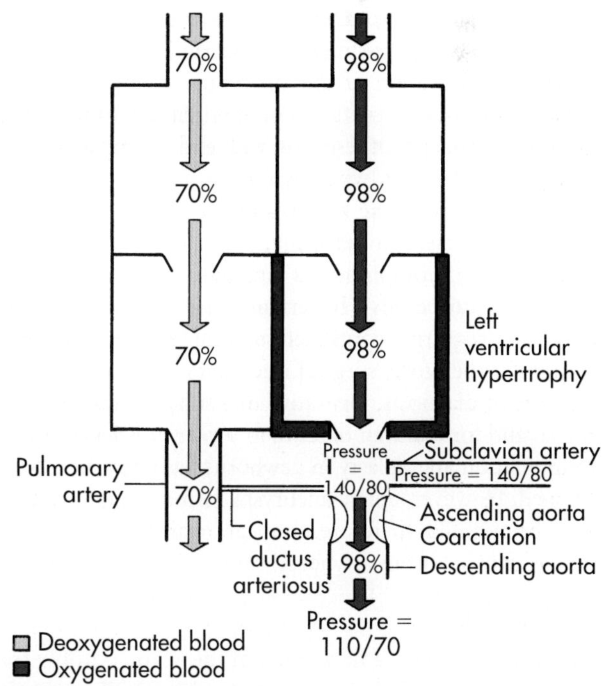

FIGURE 33-13 Hemodynamics of Postductal Coarctation of the Aorta. Blood pressure increases in the ascending aorta and subclavian artery and decreases in the descending aorta. These pressure changes eventually occur in the parts of the systemic circulation served by arteries that branch from the aorta before and after the coarctation.

CLINICAL MANIFESTATIONS. Clinical manifestations vary depending on the severity of the coarctation and age of presentation. In newborns the onset of symptoms depends on the timing of ductal closure after a fall in pulmonary vascular resistance, the location of the COA, and the presence of associated defects. The newborn usually presents with CHF symptoms. Once the ductus closes, these infants will deteriorate rapidly from the development of hypotension, acidosis, and shock. Older children may not be diagnosed until hypertension is noted. Hypertension is noted in the upper extremities with decreased or absent pulses in the lower extremities. Children may have cool, mottled skin and occasionally leg cramps during exercise. A systolic ejection murmur, heard best at the left interscapular area, is caused by rapid blood flow through the narrowed area.

EVALUATION AND TREATMENT. A chest radiograph shows an enlarged heart with congested lung fields in newborns. Rib notching between the fourth and eighth ribs may be seen in children older than 5 years, reflecting erosion of the ribs as a result of enlarged collateral vessels from the ascending aorta to the descending aorta, bypassing the coarctation. An ECG may be normal or reveal LV hypertrophy. An echocardiogram will confirm the diagnosis and rule out other intracardiac defects. Cardiac catheterization and/or magnetic resonance imaging (MRI) is performed only if the echocardiogram is inconclusive.

The first step in treatment of the symptomatic infant is stabilization, which may require prostaglandin administration, mechanical ventilation, and inotropic support to maintain adequate cardiac output. Once this is achieved, surgical intervention is indicated. Surgical repair for infants younger than 1 year consists of either a subclavian flap aortoplasty technique to enlarge the constricted area or a resection with end-to-end anastomosis of the arch segments. Depending on the arch morphology, a modification of this procedure enlarges the aorta beyond the area of constriction. For children older than 1 year, surgical repair consists of resection with end-to-end anastomosis.[13] Cardiopulmonary bypass is not required because of the extracardiac nature of the lesion, and the approach is accomplished through a left thoracotomy.

Postoperative complications include recoarctation and paradoxical postoperative hypertension. Residual permanent hypertension requiring continued medical therapy is related to age at repair; therefore, surgical intervention is recommended at the time of diagnosis. Operative mortality for infants is less than 5%, and for children older than 1 year, it is less than 1%. Balloon dilation angioplasty in newborns has been successfully performed. However, aortic aneurysm formation and restenosis have been noted; therefore, surgical repair remains the correction of choice for the newborn.[13-16]

Aortic Stenosis

Aortic stenosis (AS) is a narrowing of the aortic outflow tract (Figure 33-14). The lesion accounts for 5% of all congenital heart defects.[2] Valvular stenosis is caused by malformation or fusion of the cusps. It is the most common type of AS, tends to be progressive, and, in rare cases, can lead to sudden death as a result of low cardiac output or myocardial ischemia. For children with mild AS, no exercise restrictions may be needed. For those with moderate AS, some exercise limitations may be advised. Severe AS is an indication for limiting exercise until the repair is accomplished. Less common forms of AS are subvalvular stenosis caused by a constricting fibrous ring below the valve and supravalvular stenosis that occurs above the valve.[7]

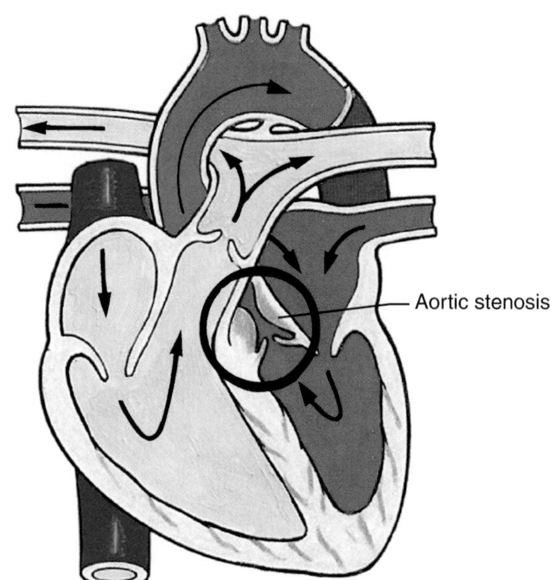

FIGURE 33-14 Aortic Stenosis. Narrowing of the aortic valve causing resistance to blood flow in the left ventricle, decreased cardiac output, left ventricular hypertrophy, and pulmonary congestion. (From Hockenberry MJ, Wilson D: *Wong's essentials of pediatric nursing*, ed 9, St Louis, 2013, Mosby.)

PATHOPHYSIOLOGY. Obstruction to blood flowing out of the aorta causes an increased workload on the LV, resulting in left ventricle hypertrophy (LVH). LV failure may develop, leading to an increase in LA pressure and a backup in the system, eventually resulting in pulmonary vascular congestion and pulmonary arterial hypertension. LVH can decrease coronary artery perfusion, resulting in myocardial ischemia, and it can alter the LV papillary muscle, causing mitral insufficiency.

CLINICAL MANIFESTATIONS. Most children with mild to moderate AS are asymptomatic. Signs of exercise intolerance may not appear until preadolescence. Syncopal episodes, epigastric pain, and exertional chest pain may occur in more severe forms of AS. A systolic ejection murmur at the right upper sternal border that transmits to the neck and left lower sternal border is produced by blood flow through the stenotic area. An ejection click may be heard with valvular AS. Severe forms of AS, especially critical AS in the newborn, result in shock and require immediate intervention.

EVALUATION AND TREATMENT. Diagnosis may be made based on previous medical history and physical findings. Chest radiographic examination may reveal a dilated ascending aorta or LV enlargement. Increased pulmonary vascular markings may be seen in severe forms. In mild cases the ECG is normal. LVH with strain pattern (features of LVH with inverted T waves in the lateral precordial leads) may be seen in severe forms. An

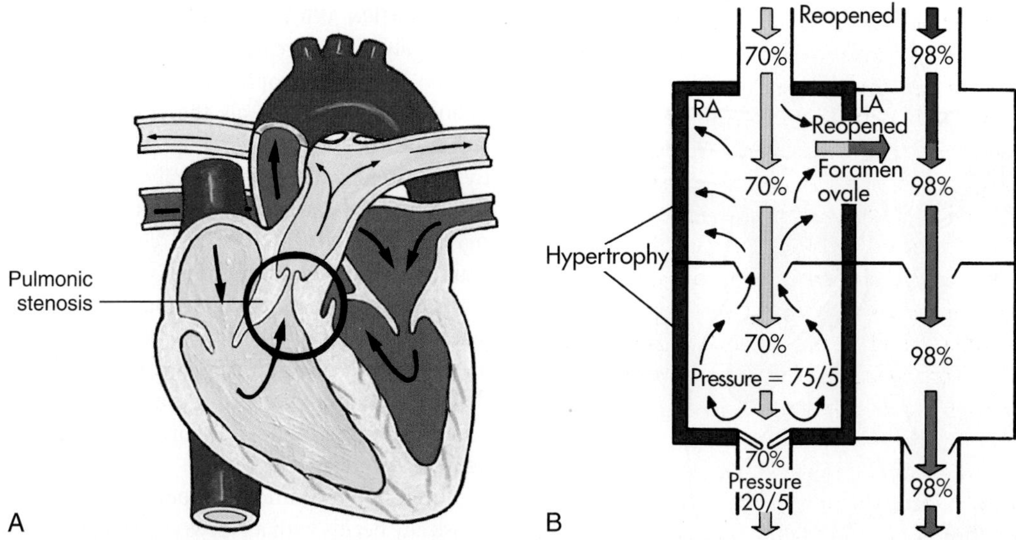

FIGURE 33-15 Pulmonary Stenosis. A, Obstruction of right ventricular outflow caused by pulmonary stenosis. Pressure on the ventricular side of the pulmonic semilunar valve (pulmonary valve) is much greater than that on the pulmonary arterial side. This difference disrupts the normal pressure gradient across the valve. Pulmonary stenosis increases ventricular afterload by decreasing blood flow through the valve, which causes ventricular hypertrophy. **B,** The backup of ventricular afterload into the right atrium reopens the foramen ovale. Venous blood then flows from the area of higher pressure (the right atrium) to the area of lower pressure (the left atrium), causing a right-to-left shunt. Cyanosis occurs if enough venous blood shunts from right to left to reduce oxygen saturation in the systemic circulation by 3% to 5%. *LA,* left atrium; *RA,* right atrium. (**A** from Hockenberry MJ, Wilson D: *Wong's essentials of pediatric nursing,* ed 9, St Louis, 2013, Mosby.)

echocardiogram may reveal a thickened and poorly functioning LV with abnormal structure, opening and closure of the aortic valve. Cardiac catheterization may be performed to augment echocardiographic data or perform intervention.

The presence of ST-segment changes on ECG, manifestation of severe CHF, and evidence of discrete severe stenosis at the aortic outflow tract are indications for intervention. Balloon aortic valvuloplasty is a palliative procedure performed for valvular AS; however, it is associated with complications, including aortic insufficiency and dysrhythmia.[17] Aortic valvotomy, under inflow occlusion or cardiopulmonary bypass, is performed for valvular AS. Operative mortality remains high in infants (up to 20%), although older children have a mortality close to 0%.[13] As many as 25% of individuals require a second surgery within 10 years for restenosis, at which time valve replacement may be the procedure of choice.

Subvalvular AS and supravalvular AS require surgical repair involving excision of the area causing the constriction. For subvalvular AS involving a small LV outflow tract and aortic annulus, a Konno procedure may be done to enlarge the LV outflow tract and aortic annulus with a patch.[13,18]

Pulmonary Stenosis

Pulmonary stenosis (PS) is the narrowing of the pulmonary outflow tract. This may be in the form of abnormal thickening of the valve leaflets or narrowing of the arterial (supravalvular) or ventricular (subvalvular) side of the valve (Figure 33-15, *A*). **Pulmonary atresia** is the severe form of PS and involves complete fusion of the commissures, allowing no blood flow out of the RV to the PA. PS accounts for 5% to 8% of all congenital heart defects.[2]

PATHOPHYSIOLOGY. PS creates resistance to blood flow from the RV to the PA. The narrowed orifice (valve) produces increased resistance (afterload) to ejection. In order for the RV to maintain adequate cardiac output, the myocardium hypertrophies. If the RV outflow tract obstruction is severe, blood may back up into the RA, causing dilation. This may result in reopening of the foramen ovale with resultant unoxygenated blood shunting to the LA, causing cyanosis (see Figure 33-15, *B*).

CLINICAL MANIFESTATIONS. Clinical manifestations depend on the severity of PS. A systolic ejection murmur at the left upper sternal border reflects obstruction to flow through the narrowed pulmonary valve. In some children a variable systolic ejection click is present with valvular stenosis at the upper left sternal border. A thrill also may be palpated at the upper left sternal border. Children with moderate PS may have exertional dyspnea and fatigability because of the inability of the body to increase pulmonary blood flow to meet demands for increased cardiac output. Severe PS will produce cyanosis and HF.

EVALUATION AND TREATMENT. A chest radiograph shows a normal-size heart with a prominent main PA caused by post-stenotic dilation. An ECG is usually normal but may reveal right-axis deviation and RV hypertrophy with moderate PS. Echocardiography confirms the diagnosis and detects associated defects. Cardiac catheterization, if performed for interventional purposes, further demonstrates PA anatomy.

Mild to moderate PS will not likely require intervention but should be observed closely. Most mild PS is not progressive. Treatment is indicated when a significant pressure gradient is detected across the RV outflow tract.

Critical (severe) PS must be addressed immediately. The treatment of choice is balloon angioplasty. This procedure is

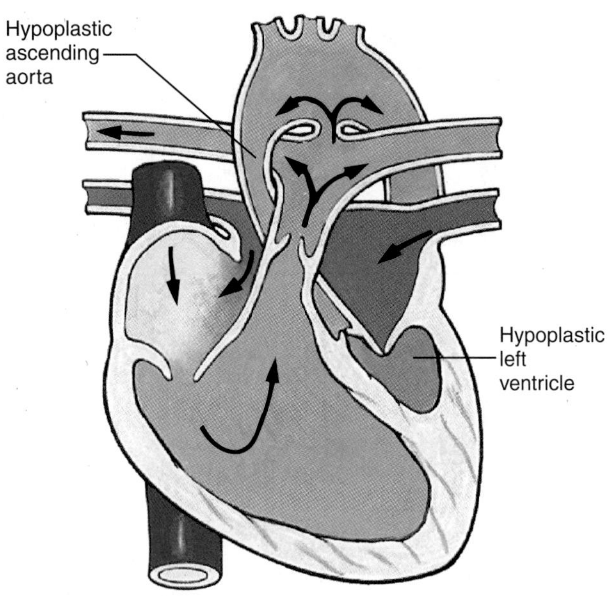

FIGURE 33-16 Hypoplastic Left Heart Syndrome. (From Hockenberry MJ, Wilson D: *Wong's essentials of pediatric nursing,* ed 9, St Louis, 2013, Mosby.)

considered highly effective in decreasing the pressure gradient across the pulmonic valve and is noted to have few associated complications.[19] Surgical correction involves a pulmonary valvotomy incising the fused commissures. Operative mortality is less than 1%.[2] Both valvotomy and balloon angioplasty may result in some pulmonary valve incompetence, and long-term follow-up may reveal the need for further intervention.

Hypoplastic Left Heart Syndrome

Hypoplastic left heart syndrome (HLHS) refers to the abnormal development of the left-sided cardiac structures, resulting in obstruction to blood flow from the LV outflow tract. HLHS involves underdevelopment of the LV, aorta, and aortic arch, as well as mitral atresia or stenosis (Figure 33-16). Therefore, infants with HLHS must have a well-functioning RV and the presence of a PDA and atrial septal communication for survival. HLHS accounts for 1% of all congenital heart defects and is considered the most complex congenital defect.[7]

PATHOPHYSIOLOGY. Because of the high pressures caused by LV outflow tract obstruction, saturated blood enters the LA and mixes with desaturated blood in the RA through an atrial septal communication. Blood flow follows the normal pathways through the right side of the heart. Exiting the PA, the mixed-saturation blood flows through the ductus and to the descending aorta. The amount of blood flow that travels to the pulmonary and systemic circulations depends on vascular resistance in the respective systems. Retrograde blood flow through the hypoplastic ascending aorta provides coronary and cerebral blood flow if there is complete aortic atresia.

CLINICAL MANIFESTATIONS. Newborns with HLHS generally are born full-term and initially appear healthy. As the ductus closes, systemic perfusion is decreased, resulting in hypoxemia, acidosis, and shock. Usually no heart murmur is detected. The second heart sound is loud and single because of aortic atresia.

EVALUATION AND TREATMENT. A chest radiograph shows cardiomegaly and increased pulmonary venous congestion. ECG shows RV hypertrophy and diminished left-sided forces. Echocardiography reveals the components of the defect with a diminutive LV cavity, hypoplastic aortic valve and arch, and hypoplastic or absent mitral valve with an enlarged RV cavity. Interventional cardiac catheterization with balloon septostomy may be necessary if the atrial communication is inadequate. This procedure is very high risk.[7]

Prostaglandin infusion to maintain patency of the ductus arteriosus is essential for newborn infant survival. Immediate correction of acidosis, inotropic support for adequate cardiac output, and ventilatory manipulation to balance systemic and pulmonary blood flow prevent further deterioration and achieve stabilization.

Surgical intervention includes a three-stage approach that classically begins with a Norwood procedure. The Norwood procedure consists of an atrial septectomy, placement of a pulmonary-to-systemic artery shunt to maintain adequate pulmonary blood flow, creation of a permanent communication between the RV and aorta, and patch augmentation of the hypoplastic aorta. The Sano modification utilizes a graft between the RV and the PA to provide stable pulmonary blood flow rather than a pulmonary to systemic arterial shunt.[20] Postoperative complications include imbalance of systemic and pulmonary blood flow, leading to inadequate cardiac output and persistent HF. In most centers, survival after the initial procedure is now averaging greater than 70%.

The second stage is the bidirectional Glenn procedure, which is performed between 2 and 9 months of age, depending on the child's clinical status, pulmonary vascular resistance, and ventricular function. This involves joining the superior vena cava to the PA and take-down of the shunt to the lungs. Complications include superior vena cava obstruction, pleural effusion, and low cardiac output.

The third stage is the Fontan procedure, described earlier, which separates the systemic from the pulmonary circulation. Timing for surgical repair depends on the child's ventricular function, presence of AV valve regurgitation, and pulmonary vascular resistance. Most surgeons perform the Fontan procedure when the child is approximately 2 to 4 years of age.[7,13]

Cardiac transplant also may be an option for these newborns. Most surgical centers offer the three-staged palliative surgeries as an initial approach, with an option for cardiac transplantation later in life.[7,21]

Mixing Defects

Many complex defects are classified as mixing defects because of their dependence on the mixing of pulmonary and systemic circulations for survival during the postnatal period. This mixing results in desaturated systemic blood flow and cyanosis. Pulmonary congestion occurs because of preferential pulmonary blood flow. Clinically each defect has varying degrees of cyanosis and HF depending on the various components of the lesion.

Transposition of the Great Arteries

Transposition of the great arteries (TGA) refers to a condition in which the aorta arises from the RV and the PA from the LV

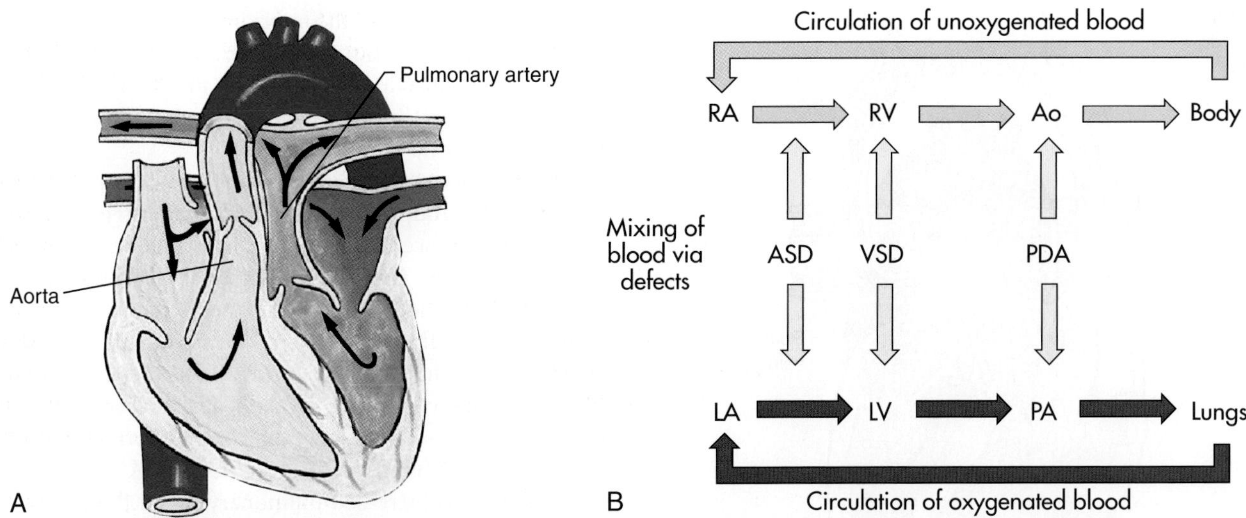

FIGURE 33-17 Hemodynamics in Transposition of the Great Arteries (TGA). **A,** Complete transposition of the great vessels with an intact interventricular septum. The aorta arises from the right ventricle and the pulmonary artery from the left. **B,** Oxygen saturation in the two parallel circuits. *Ao,* Aorta; *ASD,* atrial septal defect; *LA,* left atrium; *LV,* left ventricle; *PA,* pulmonary artery; *PDA,* patent ductus arteriosus; *RA,* right atrium; *RV,* right ventricle; *VSD,* ventricular septal defect. (**A** from Hockenberry MJ, Wilson D: *Wong's essentials of pediatric nursing,* ed 9, St Louis, 2013, Mosby.)

(Figure 33-17, *A*). The result is two separate, parallel circuits in which unoxygenated blood circulates continuously through the systemic circulation and oxygenated blood circulates repeatedly through the pulmonary circulation. This condition is incompatible with extrauterine life unless a communication exists between the two circuits to provide the necessary oxygen to the body. Communication is accomplished by mixing of pulmonary and systemic circulations through a PDA, ASD, or VSD (see Figure 33-17, *B*). Dextro-transposition of the great arteries (D-TGA) is the most common cyanotic congenital heart defect and accounts for 10% of all congenital heart defects; "dextro" refers to the aorta remaining to the right of the PA.[2,7]

Two factors allow newborns with complete transposition to survive long enough to be treated. First, blood from the two closed systems can mix through the ductus arteriosus for a short time after birth if pulmonary vascular resistance remains high. Some mixing also may occur through the foramen ovale. If the child has a VSD, mixing occurs through that opening as well.

PATHOPHYSIOLOGY. It is not known precisely which embryologic events lead to transposition, but researchers have proposed that the fault lies in the development of conal tissue in the fibrous skeleton of the heart.[1] The **conus** is a segment of muscle that separates the AV (tricuspid and mitral) valves from the semilunar (aortic and pulmonic) valves. (The fibrous skeleton and heart valves are described and illustrated in Chapter 31; see Figure 31-4.) The interventricular septum is intact in about 60% of cases of transposition; a VSD is present in the remaining 40%. PS is associated with the transposition in about 4% to 6% of children with intact septa and in 28% to 31% of children with VSDs.[2,7]

The discussion that follows is limited to the pathophysiology of complete transposition with an intact interventricular septum.

CLINICAL MANIFESTATIONS. The degree of mixing permitted by fetal structures determines the type and severity of clinical manifestations. Cyanosis may be mild shortly after birth and worsen during the first day because of functional closure of the ductus arteriosus. Low oxygen levels in the blood (hypoxemia) cause metabolic acidosis, tachycardia, and tachypnea. The presence of a PDA or large ASD allows for more mixing and results in only mild cyanosis, but the infant may develop CHF.

The first heart sound is normal, and the second sound may be heard as a single sound even though both the aortic and pulmonic valves are functioning. The loud single S_2 may occur because transposition places the aortic valve closer to the chest wall than the pulmonic valve. No murmur is noted with transposition of the great arteries with an intact ventricular septum.

EVALUATION AND TREATMENT. On chest radiograph the heart has a characteristic shape—like an egg on its side—and pulmonary vascular markings are increased. The heart may be enlarged if the infant is a few weeks old and has a VSD. ECG findings reveal a right-axis deviation and some RV hypertrophy. Echocardiography confirms the diagnosis of transposition of the great arteries. Cardiac catheterization may be necessary to define the coronary anatomy; measure ventricular ratios; and, if necessary, perform a balloon septostomy. Balloon septostomy is done only if the situation is critical because there are risks involved.[22]

Surgical repair during the newborn period involves the arterial switch operation that moves the great arteries. The coronary arteries are removed from the aorta before the arterial switch is performed and reimplanted without torsion or kinking into the aorta. This establishes normal blood flow with the LV as the systemic pump. Results are approaching 100% survival. Complications include narrowing at the sites of the great artery anastomoses and, rarely, coronary insufficiency.[7,22]

Mustard and Senning operations (the creation of an intra-atrial tunnel to baffle the systemic venous blood flow to the

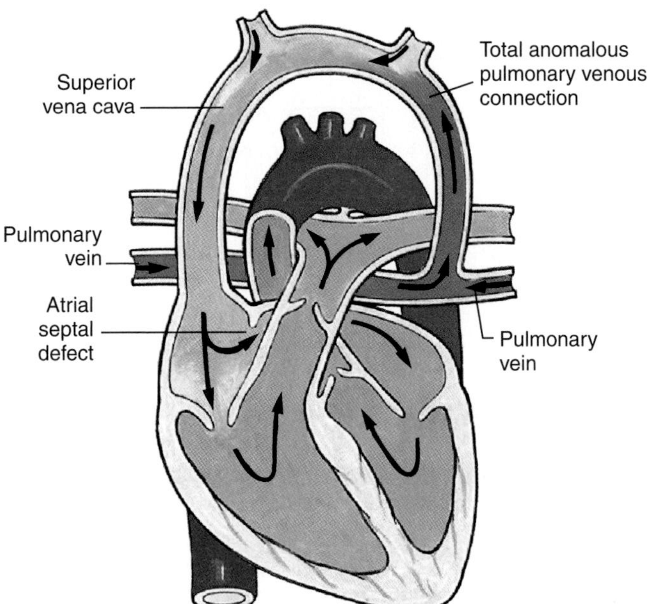

FIGURE 33-18 Hemodynamics of Total Anomalous Pulmonary Venous Connection (TAPVC). In the form of TAPVC represented here, the pulmonary veins enter the left anomalous vertical vein instead of the left atrium. From the left anomalous vertical vein, the mixed blood from the lungs flows into the superior vena cava through an innominate vein (literally, a "vein without a name"). Oxygen saturation within the four heart chambers, the pulmonary artery, and the aorta is the same. Blood pressure in the right heart exceeds that in the left heart because the right heart is receiving blood from both the pulmonary and systemic circulatory systems. (Abnormal vessels are shaded.) (From Hockenberry MJ, Wilson D: *Wong's essentials of pediatric nursing,* ed 9, St Louis, 2013, Mosby.)

mitral valve and the pulmonary venous blood flow to the tricuspid valve) are no longer the procedures of choice because the RV must perform as the systemic pump. Long-term follow-up of children with Mustard and Senning operations revealed significant rates of RV failure and dysrhythmias.[7]

The Rastelli procedure is used in children with transposition, VSD, and severe PS. This procedure involves closing the VSD with a baffle by rerouting LV blood through the VSD to the aorta. The pulmonary valve is closed, and an RV-to-PA prosthetic or homograft valve conduit is placed. This procedure requires prosthetic conduit replacement as the child grows and is associated with ventricular failure and dysrhythmias in the postoperative period.[7]

Total Anomalous Pulmonary Venous Connection

Total anomalous pulmonary venous connection (TAPVC), or total anomalous pulmonary venous return, occurs when the pulmonary veins abnormally connect to the right side of the heart either directly or through one or more systemic veins that drain into the RA (Figure 33-18). An ASD generally is present also. This defect is extremely rare, accounting for only 1% of all congenital heart defects. The four types of TAPVC are based on the site of drainage. Supracardiac TAPVCs are the most common form (50%) and drain to the superior vena cava through the vertical or innominate vein. Cardiac TAPVCs (20%) drain directly into the RA or through the coronary sinus. Infracardiac TAPVCs (20%) traverse the diaphragm and drain into the portal or hepatic vein or the inferior vena cava. Mixed TAPVCs (10%) are a combination of the various types. Partial anomalous venous connection is a condition in which only one or two of the pulmonary veins, usually the right-sided veins, drains into the RA or one of its tributaries.[2]

PATHOPHYSIOLOGY. Physiologically TAPVC can be differentiated into two groups: nonobstructive and obstructive, depending on the absence or presence of obstruction to pulmonary venous drainage. The hemodynamics of the nonobstructive group involve the RA receiving the oxygenated blood that would normally flow into the LA. The amount of blood shunted into the LA vs. the volume entering the RV depends on the size of the ASD and compliance of the RV. Therefore, if the ASD is restrictive and RV compliance approaches normal, more blood will enter the RV than the LA, resulting in RA and RV enlargement, as well as increased pulmonary blood flow. This causes increased pulmonary venous blood return and larger amounts of saturated blood. If the ASD is unrestrictive and the RV does not become thinner to increase compliance, the majority of mixed saturated blood is shunted from the higher-pressure RA to the LA.

The hemodynamics of obstructed TAPVC cause pulmonary venous hypertension because of resistance caused by the obstruction resulting in an elevation in pulmonary vascular and RV pressures. Pulmonary edema occurs from hydrostatic capillary pressure exceeding the osmotic pressure of the blood and eventually contributing to the development of HF. This group has a strong association with the infracardiac type of TAPVC and is a surgical emergency.

CLINICAL MANIFESTATIONS. The predominant clinical manifestation in infants with TAPVC is cyanosis caused by mixture of oxygenated and deoxygenated blood entering the systemic circulation. The degree of cyanosis is inversely related to the amount of pulmonary blood flow. Children with unobstructed TAPVC may be asymptomatic until pulmonary vascular resistance drops, at which time pulmonary blood flow will increase, resulting in signs of pulmonary overcirculation, particularly growth retardation and frequent pulmonary infections, in addition to mild cyanosis. Obstructed TAPVC results in cyanosis and rapid deterioration necessitating immediate surgical correction, or death will occur.

Physical examination may reveal a systolic murmur at the left upper sternal border and a mid-diastolic murmur at the left lower sternal border. A murmur may be absent in obstructed TAPVC. A characteristic quadruple rhythm, consisting of S_1, widely split S_2, and S_3 or S_4, or a gallop rhythm also is present.

EVALUATION AND TREATMENT. The ECG shows a right-axis deviation, RV hypertrophy, and occasionally RA hypertrophy. The chest radiograph of unobstructed TAPVC reveals cardiomegaly, increased pulmonary vascular markings, and a snowman or figure-eight appearance in the supracardiac type. A chest roentgenogram of obstructed TAPVC shows a normal-size heart and a ground-glass appearance of the lung fields, reflecting pulmonary venous congestion or edema. The echocardiogram reveals the abnormal pulmonary venous connections.

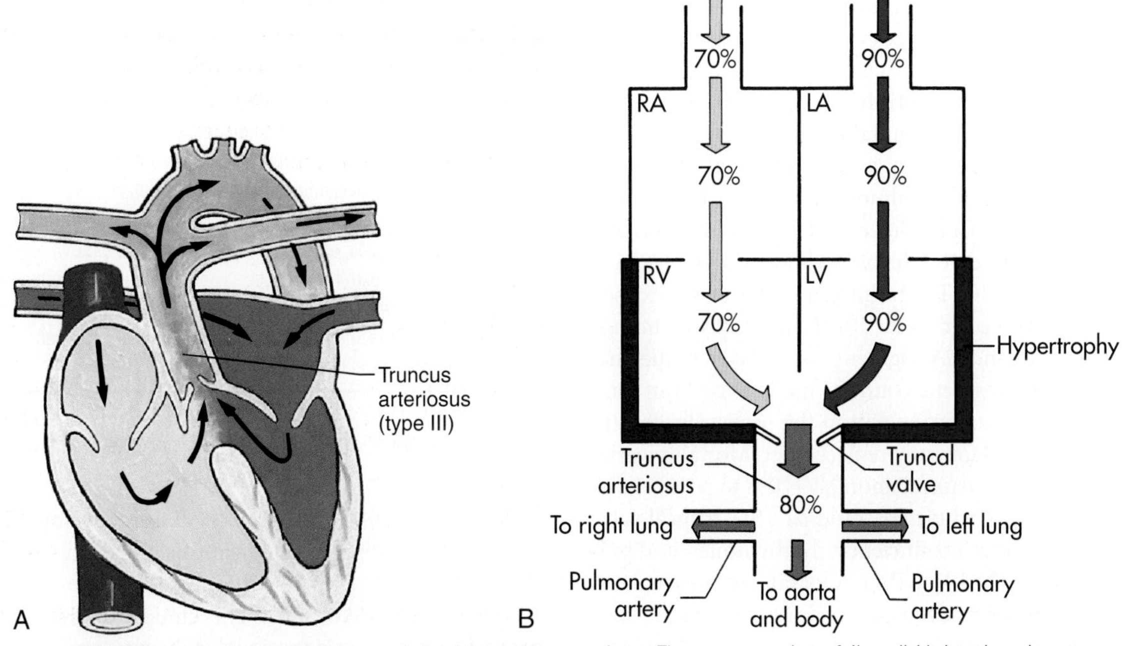

FIGURE 33-19 Truncus Arteriosus. **A,** Persistent truncus arteriosus. The truncus arteriosus fails to divide into the pulmonary artery and aorta, and the interventricular septum fails to close at the top. Blood from both ventricles mixes in the truncus arteriosus and then enters the pulmonary and systemic circuits. **B,** Alterations of hemodynamics and oxygen saturation by persistent truncus arteriosus. *LA,* Left atrium; *LV,* left ventricle; *RA,* right atrium; *RV,* right ventricle. (**A** from Hockenberry MJ, Wilson D: *Wong's essentials of pediatric nursing,* ed 9, St Louis, 2013, Mosby.)

Surgical repair varies with the type of TAPVC and whether the defect is obstructed or unobstructed. Obstructed lesions are repaired at the time of diagnosis, whereas the unobstructed type generally is repaired during infancy. The procedure is performed while the patient is on cardiopulmonary bypass and involves anastomosis of the common pulmonary vein to the LA and closing the ASD, as in the supracardiac and infracardiac types. Repair of the supracardiac type involves baffling the pulmonary venous drainage to the LA. This repair has the highest success rate because of the low technical difficulty, whereas infracardiac repair is associated with a high mortality (up to 25%) and morbidity. Potential complications include reobstruction; atrial dysrhythmias, including sick sinus syndrome; PA hypertension; and LV dysfunction.[13]

Truncus Arteriosus

Truncus arteriosus is the failure of the large embryonic artery, the truncus arteriosus, to divide into the PA and the aorta. This results in a single vessel arising from both ventricles, providing blood flow to the pulmonary and systemic circulations (Figure 33-19, *A*). This common trunk straddles the VSD (always present) and has a single valve with three or four leaflets, which may result in stenosis, regurgitation, or both. The incidence is 2% of all congenital heart defects, and a right aortic arch is present 50% of the time. There are four types of truncus arteriosus. Type I is the most common (60%) and involves the main PA arising from the truncus and then dividing into the right and left PAs. Type II is less common (20%) and involves the PAs arising from the posterior aspect of the truncus. Type III is the least common (10%) and involves the PAs arising from the lateral aspect of the truncus. Type IV, also known as pseudotruncus, is now considered a severe form of TOF with the bronchial arteries arising from the descending aorta to supply the lungs.[2]

PATHOPHYSIOLOGY. Blood flow from the RV and LV is pumped into the main truncus, resulting in mixing of the pulmonary and systemic circulations (see Figure 33-19, *B*). The differential flow out to either the pulmonary bed or the systemic circulation depends on the pulmonary and systemic vascular resistances. Generally the pulmonary vascular resistance is less than the systemic vascular resistance, resulting in the majority of blood flow traveling to the lungs. This may be altered, however, because of PS, small pulmonary arteries, or increased pulmonary vascular resistance. Pulmonary vascular disease develops early with this defect because of increased pulmonary blood flow.

CLINICAL MANIFESTATIONS. Physical findings depend on the amount of pulmonary blood flow and the presence of other cardiac anomalies. If PS is present, a newborn will present with cyanosis, caused by already elevated pulmonary vascular resistance, but no HF. Conversely, if PS is not present, the newborn initially will have mild to moderate cyanosis that worsens with activity. Once pulmonary vascular resistance drops, the pulmonary bed will receive preferential flow and the infant will have signs of HF. A harsh systolic regurgitant murmur is usually present along the left sternal border as a result of the VSD, and a systolic click at the apex and left upper sternal border may be present, reflecting opening of the truncal valve. An apical rumble with or without a gallop rhythm also may be present because of increased pulmonary blood flow. If truncal valve insufficiency exists, an early diastolic, high-pitched decrescendo murmur may be present.

EVALUATION AND TREATMENT. An ECG generally reveals biventricular hypertrophy and occasionally LA enlargement. A chest radiograph reveals cardiomegaly with biventricular and LA enlargement, as well as increased pulmonary vascular markings. When PS is present, the heart size is normal and the pulmonary vascular markings are decreased. Echocardiography and cardiac catheterization, if performed, determine the type of truncal defect, competency of the truncal valve, and differential blood flow.

Surgical repair in early infancy is recommended to prevent the sequelae of severe HF and pulmonary vascular disease. The definitive repair consists of a modified Rastelli procedure involving VSD patch closure to divert the blood flow from the LV outflow tract into the truncus. The pulmonary arteries are excised from the aorta and connected to the RV through a tissue homograft—namely, aortic and PA segments or cadaver tissue that is specially preserved. Synthetic conduits may be used but tend to calcify and develop narrowing within the lumen, leading to obstruction and the need for early replacement. Mortality varies depending on the type of truncal anomaly (20% to 50%). Postoperative complications include HF, residual VSD, truncal valve (now the aorta) stenosis or insufficiency, dysrhythmias, and pulmonary hypertension. The RV to PA homograft requires replacement because it becomes inadequate for somatic growth.[13]

ACQUIRED CARDIOVASCULAR DISORDERS

Acquired heart diseases are those disease processes or abnormalities that occur after birth. They result from various causes, such as infection, genetic disorders, autoimmune processes in response to infection, environmental factors, or autoimmune diseases. Examples of acquired heart diseases include Kawasaki disease, myocarditis, rheumatic heart disease, cardiomyopathy, and systemic hypertension. This chapter discusses Kawasaki disease and systemic hypertension. Myocarditis, rheumatic heart disease, and cardiomyopathy are discussed in Chapter 32.

Kawasaki Disease

Kawasaki disease, formerly known as mucocutaneous lymph node syndrome, is an acute, self-limiting systemic vasculitis that may result in cardiac sequelae. Although Kawasaki disease occurs throughout the world, the greatest number of cases are reported in Japan.

Kawasaki disease is primarily a condition of young children: 80% of cases are seen in children younger than 5 years of age, with the incidence peaking in the toddler age group. Males are affected slightly more than females. Its peak incidence is in winter and spring.

The etiology of Kawasaki disease remains unknown. Theories center on an immunologic response to an infectious, toxic, or antigenic substance (including superantigen).[2,7,23]

PATHOPHYSIOLOGY. Kawasaki disease progresses pathologically and clinically in the following stages:

Stage I (days 1 to 12): Small capillaries, arterioles, and venules become inflamed, as does the heart itself.

Stage II (days 13 to 25): Inflammation spreads to larger vessels, and aneurysms of the coronary arteries develop.

Stage III (days 26 to 40): Medium-size arteries begin the granulation process, causing coronary artery thickening; inflammation resolves in the microcirculation; and there is risk of thrombus formation.

BOX 33-3 DIAGNOSTIC CRITERIA FOR KAWASAKI DISEASE

The child must exhibit five of the following six criteria, including fever:

1. Fever for 5 or more days (often diagnosed with shorter duration of fever if other symptoms are present)
2. Bilateral conjunctival infection without exudation
3. Changes in the oral mucous membranes, such as erythema, dryness, and fissuring of the lips; oropharyngeal reddening; or "strawberry tongue"
4. Changes in the extremities, such as peripheral edema, peripheral erythema, and desquamation of palms and soles, particularly periungual peeling
5. Polymorphous rash, often accentuated in the perineal area
6. Cervical lymphadenopathy

Modified from Hockenberry MJ, Wilson D: *Wong's nursing care of infants and children,* ed 9, St Louis, 2011, Mosby.

Stage IV (day 41 and beyond): Vessels develop scarring, intimal thickening, calcification, and stenosis of coronary arteries.

CLINICAL MANIFESTATIONS. The clinical course of the disease progresses in three stages: acute, subacute, and convalescent. In the acute phase the child has fever, conjunctivitis, oral changes ("strawberry" tongue), rash, and lymphadenopathy and is often irritable. During this phase myocarditis in addition to the vasculitis may develop. The subacute phase begins when the fever ends and continues until the clinical signs have resolved. It is at this time that the child is most at risk for coronary artery aneurysm development. Desquamation of the palms and soles occurs at this time, as well as marked thrombocytosis. The convalescent phase is marked by the continued elevation of the erythrocyte sedimentation rate and platelet count. Arthritis still may be present. This phase continues until all laboratory values return to normal—usually about 6 to 8 weeks after onset.

EVALUATION AND TREATMENT. The diagnosis is based on the diagnostic criteria for Kawasaki disease, which state that the child must exhibit five of six criteria, including fever (Box 33-3). These children usually have leukocytosis, increased erythrocyte sedimentation rates, marked thrombocytosis, and elevated levels of liver enzymes. An echocardiogram is obtained at the time of diagnosis as a baseline to assess for coronary aneurysms or inflammation. Serial echocardiograms are obtained after treatment to assess for future development of coronary aneurysms.

The use of aspirin and intravenous immunoglobulin during the acute phase has decreased the mortality of Kawasaki disease and has reduced the incidence of coronary abnormalities from approximately 20% to less than 2% at 6 to 8 weeks after initiation of therapy. Most children recover completely from Kawasaki disease, including the regression of aneurysms. The most common, although rare, cardiovascular sequela is coronary thrombosis. Studies are investigating long-term results of the disease.[5,23]

Systemic Hypertension

Hypertension (HTN) in children differs from adult HTN in etiology and presentation. Children diagnosed with HTN are often found to have some underlying disease, such as renal disease or COA (Box 33-4). In recent years an increased prevalence

BOX 33-4 CONDITIONS ASSOCIATED WITH SECONDARY HYPERTENSION IN CHILDREN

Renal Disorders

Congenital defects
- Polycystic kidney, ectopic kidney, horseshoe kidney, etc.
- Obstructive anomalies
- Hydronephrosis

Renal tumor
- Wilms tumor
- Retrovascular tumor

Abnormalities of renal arteries

Renal vein thrombosis

Acquired disorders
- Glomerulonephritis—acute or chronic
- Pyelonephritis
- Nephritis associated with collagen disease

Cardiovascular Disease

Coarctation of the aorta

Arteriovenous fistulae

Patent ductus arteriosus

Aortic or mitral insufficiency

Metabolic and Endocrine Diseases

Adrenal tumors
- Adenoma
- Pheochromocytoma
- Neuroblastoma
- Cushing syndrome
- Adrenogenital syndrome
- Hyperthyroidism
- Aldosteronism
- Hypercalcemia
- Diabetes mellitus

Neurologic Disorders

Space-occupying lesions of cranium (increased intracranial pressure)
- Tumors, cysts, hematoma
- Cerebral edema
- Encephalitis (including Guillain-Barré and Reye syndromes)

Miscellaneous Causes

Drugs (corticosteroids, oral contraceptives, pressor agents, amphetamines)

Burns

Genitourinary surgery

Trauma (e.g., stretching of femoral nerve with leg traction)

Insect bites (e.g., scorpion)

Intravascular overload (blood, fluid)

Hypernatremia

Toxemia of pregnancy

Heavy metal poisoning

From Hockenberry MJ, Wilson D: *Wong's essentials of pediatric nursing,* ed 9, St Louis, 2013, Mosby.

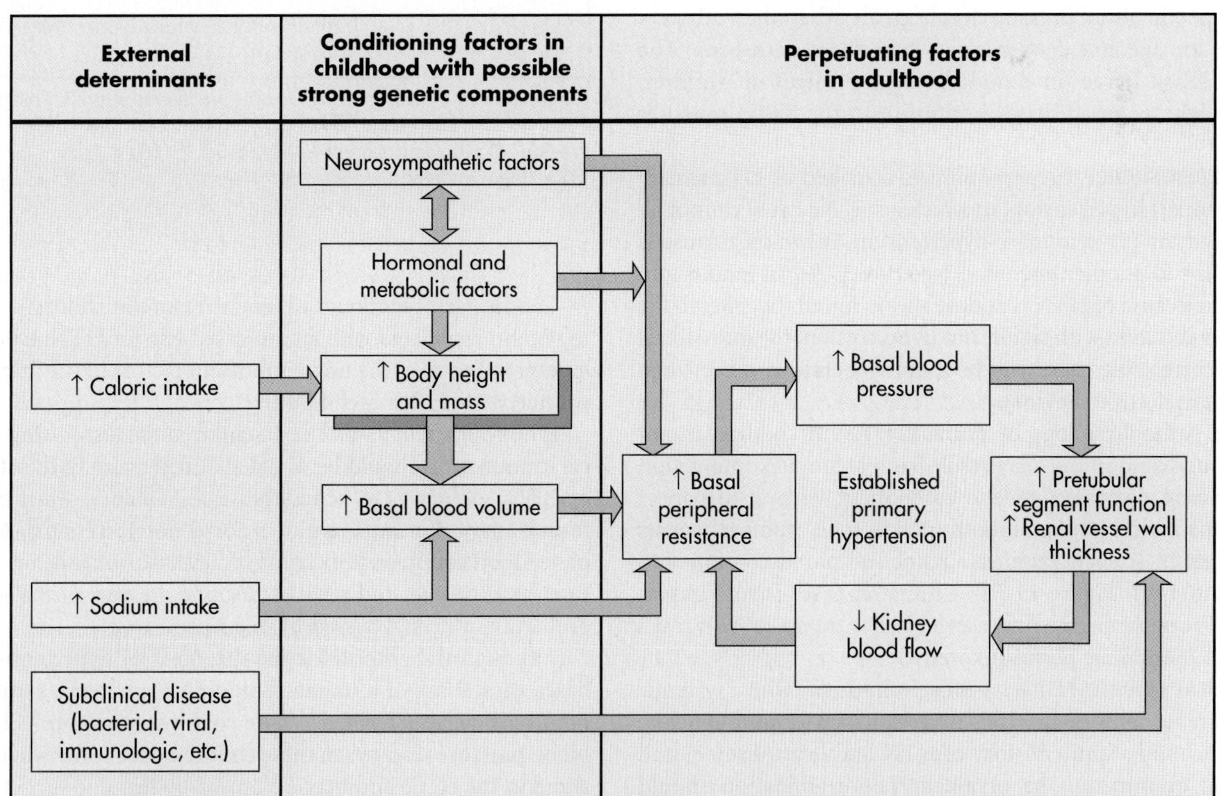

FIGURE 33-20 Mechanisms Believed to Influence Blood Pressure in Children. According to this model, a critical factor in the development of hypertension is obesity during childhood. Increased body mass, coupled with excessive sodium intake, can cause primary hypertension in children or set the stage for its development later in life.

TABLE 33-6 SUGGESTED NORMAL BP VALUES (mmHg) BY AUSCULTATORY METHOD (SYSTOLIC/DIASTOLIC K5)

AGE (YEARS)	MEAN BP LEVELS	90th PERCENTILE	95th PERCENTILE
6-7	104/55	114/73	117/78
8-9	106/58	117/76	120/82
11-11*	108/60	120/77	124/82
12-13*	112/62	124/78	128/83
14-15			
Boys	116/66	132/80	138/86
Girls	112/68	126/80	130/83
16-18			
Boys	121/70	136/82	140/86
Girls	110/68	125/81	127/84

From Park MK: *Pediatric cardiology for practitioners,* ed 4, Philadelphia, 2002, Mosby; modified from Goldring D et al: *J Pediatr* 91:884, 1977; Prineas RJ et al: *Hypertension* 1(Suppl):18, 1980.
*Values for ages 10 to 13 years have been extrapolated from these two studies using age-related increments from other studies.
BP, Blood pressure; *K5,* phase V of Korotkoff sound.

TABLE 33-7 NORMATIVE BP LEVELS (SYSTOLIC/DIASTOLIC [MEAN]) BY DINAMAP/ MONITOR IN CHILDREN 5 YEARS OLD AND YOUNGER

AGE	MEAN BP LEVELS (mmHg)	90th PERCENTILE	95th PERCENTILE
1-3 days	64/41 (50)	75/49 (50)	78/52 (62)
1 month-2 years	95/58 (72)	106/68 (83)	110/71 (86)
2-5 years	101/57 (74)	112/66 (82)	115/68 (85)

From Park MK: *Pediatric cardiology for practitioners,* ed 5, Philadelphia, 2008, Mosby; modified from Park MK, Menard SM: *Am J Dis Child* 143:860, 1989.
BP, Blood pressure.

of primary HTN in older children has been noted. Researchers are now focusing on primary HTN in older children in relation to morbidity and mortality and the presence of early atherosclerotic disease.[2,7,24,25]

Systemic hypertension in children is defined as systolic and diastolic blood pressure levels greater than the 95th percentile for age and gender on at least three occasions. The Fourth Task Force on Blood Pressure Control in Children uses height as an additional criterion to the blood pressure guide.[26]

PATHOPHYSIOLOGY. Hypertension is classified as (1) primary (or essential) hypertension, in which a specific cause cannot be identified; or (2) secondary hypertension, in which a cause is secondary to another alteration (see Box 33-4). In infants and children a cause of HTN is almost always found. In general, the younger the child with significant hypertension, the more likely that a correctable cause can be found. Therefore, a thorough evaluation needs to be done.[27]

The pathophysiology of primary HTN in children is not clearly understood but may result from a complex interaction of a strong disposing genetic component with disturbances in sympathetic vascular smooth muscle tone, humoral agents (angiotensin, catecholamines), renal sodium excretion, and cardiac output (Figure 33-20). Ultimately these factors impair the ability of the peripheral vascular bed to adjust its own resistance to meet tissue perfusion needs.[24]

CLINICAL MANIFESTATIONS. Most children with systemic HTN are asymptomatic. It is necessary that a thorough history (including family history of HTN and heart disease) and physical examination be obtained. The examination should include an accurate blood pressure measurement on three separate occasions using a cuff of appropriate size (Tables 33-6 and 33-7).

TABLE 33-8 MOST COMMON CAUSES OF CHRONIC SUSTAINED HYPERTENSION

AGE GROUP	CAUSES
Newborn	Renal artery thrombosis, renal artery stenosis, congenital renal malformation, COA, bronchopulmonary dysplasia
<6 years	Renal parenchymal disease, COA, renal artery stenosis
6-10 years	Renal artery stenosis, renal parenchymal disease, primary hypertension
>10 years	Primary hypertension, renal parenchymal disease

From Park MK: *Pediatric cardiology for practitioners,* ed 5, Philadelphia, 2008, Mosby; adapted from Report of the Second Task Force on Blood Pressure Control in Children: *Pediatrics* 79:1, 1987.
COA, Coarctation of the aorta.

Certain factors influence blood pressure in children. Smoking is also associated with an increased risk for HTN. Obesity is emerging as one of the most important factors in the increasing prevalence of HTN in children.

EVALUATION AND TREATMENT. In children the history and physical examination should be directed at determining the etiology of HTN, such as COA or renal disease (Table 33-8). If COA is found, surgical or interventional correction is initiated. A complete blood count, serum chemistry levels, urinalysis, urine culture, lipid profile, and renal ultrasound are part of the routine evaluation for renal disease (Table 33-9).

Although the criteria for the diagnosis of hypertension are based on the use of a standard blood pressure cuff, some children have what is termed "white coat hypertension." Elevated blood pressure readings in these children occur only when measured in the clinic and may be caused by fear and anxiety. The use of ambulatory blood pressure monitoring (ABPM) records the blood pressure over a 24-hour period. In addition to identifying children with white coat hypertension, ABPM has been

TABLE 33-9 ROUTINE AND SPECIAL LABORATORY TESTS FOR HYPERTENSION

LABORATORY TEST	SIGNIFICANCE OF ABNORMAL RESULTS
Urinalysis, urine culture, blood urea nitrogen, creatinine, uric acid	Renal parenchymal disease
Serum electrolyte levels (hypokalemia)	Hyperaldosteronism (primary or secondary) Adrenogenital syndrome Renin-producing tumors
ECG, chest x-ray studies, and possibly echocardiography	Cardiac cause of hypertension, also baseline function
Intravenous pyelogram (or ultrasonography, radionuclide studies, computed tomography, or magnetic resonance imaging of the kidneys)	Renal parenchymal disease Renovascular hypertension Tumors (neuroblastoma, Wilms tumor)
Plasma renin activity (peripheral)	High-renin hypertension (renovascular hypertension, renin-producing tumors, some Cushing syndrome, some essential hypertension) Low-renin hypertension (adrenogenital syndrome, primary hyperaldosteronism)
24-hour urine collection for 17-ketosteroids and 17-hydroxycorticosteroids	Cushing syndrome Adrenogenital syndrome
24-hour urine collection for catecholamine levels and vanillylmandelic acid	Pheochromocytoma Neuroblastoma
Aldosterone	Hyperaldosteronism (primary or secondary) Renovascular hypertension Renin-producing tumors
Renal vein plasma renin activity	Unilateral renal parenchymal disease Renovascular hypertension
Abdominal aortogram	Renovascular hypertension Abdominal coarctation of the aorta Unilateral renal parenchymal diseases Pheochromocytoma
Intra-arterial digital subtraction angiography	Renovascular hypertension

From Park MK: *Pediatric cardiology for practitioners*, ed 5, Philadelphia, 2008, Mosby.
ECG, Electrocardiogram.

found to be useful in children with hypertension that is resistant to treatment (see What's New? Ambulatory Blood Pressure Monitoring in Children).[26]

If HTN is found to be essential, or primary, in nature, nonpharmacologic therapy is used initially. Moderate weight loss can decrease systolic and diastolic pressures in many children. Appropriate diet, regular physical activity, and avoidance of smoking have been shown to be effective in reducing blood pressure.[28]

Drug therapy is controversial in children with primary hypertension; however, when nonpharmacologic therapy fails, a staged approach with the use of diuretics and/or beta-blockers and afterload reduction is indicated. The emphasis on preventive cardiology, especially for children, is significant because many investigators believe signs of atherosclerosis and other cardiovascular risk factors are present from childhood.[29-32]

WHAT'S NEW?

Ambulatory Blood Pressure Monitoring in Children

Ambulatory blood pressure monitoring (ABPM) records blood pressure over a 24-hour period. Its use in children was endorsed by the Fourth Report of the National High Blood Pressure Education Program Working Group on High Blood Pressure in Children primarily to help identify those children with "white coat hypertension." Paradoxically, some children have normal blood pressure readings in the clinic but are hypertensive during other parts of the day. This is called "masked hypertension" and also can be identified by ABPM. ABPM is useful in documenting what is called the "BP load," which is the total amount of time the blood pressure (BP) is elevated above normal limits during a 24-hour period. By measuring BP load, ABPM may be able to identify those children who are at greatest risk for target organ damage. It can also help with management of children who suffer hypotensive episodes in response to pharmacologic therapy for their hypertension. Finally, ABPM facilitates medication changes in those with hypertension resistant to medication.

Data from Flynn JT, Urbina EM: *J Clin Hypertens* 14(6):372–382, 2012; National High Blood Pressure Education Program Working Group on High Blood Pressure in Children: *Pediatrics* 114:555–576, 2004.

Childhood Obesity

Childhood obesity is considered an epidemic not only in the United States but also in other countries such as Australia.[33-35] Despite attention from U.S. federal and state initiatives, the prevalence of obesity in children and young adults has steadily increased over the past four decades, with estimates as high as 25% of children considered obese.[33] Although not without controversy, percentile of body mass index (BMI) expressed as weight/height^2 (BMI-kg/m^2) is used to identify overweight and obesity in children and adolescents. The Centers for Disease Control and Prevention (CDC), the supplier of national growth charts and prevalence data, avoids characterizing children and adolescents as "obese"; instead, the CDC suggests two levels of overweight: (1) the 85th percentile, an "at risk" level; and (2) the 95th percentile, the more severe level.[36]

Causes of obesity in young children and adolescents are multivariable and multidimensional. Risk factors associated with developing childhood obesity include race, socioeconomic status, and lack of health insurance. Children of black and Hispanic race are at higher risk, as well as children with no insurance.[34] The presence of parental obesity also is associated with childhood obesity.[37] In addition, early childhood nutrition, level of physical activity, and engagement of sedentary activities, such as watching television and computer use, is associated with the development of overweight and obese children.[38-40]

Similar to obese adults, overweight and obese children are at risk for acquiring numerous other serious and potentially life-threatening illnesses, such as asthma, sleep apnea, hypertension, type 2 diabetes, dyslipidemia, and cardiovascular disease.[7] Researchers also have reported a multitude of social and economic consequences in adolescents as a result of being overweight. Overweight adolescents are more likely to complete fewer years of education, are less likely to marry, and have a lower household income in adulthood, independent of familial socioeconomic status.[41]

As in other acquired diseases, efforts should be focused on prevention. The initial approach is a combined program of physical activity with nutritional improvements. Healthcare professionals play a vital role in recognizing the need for intervention, immediate referral, and support. Successful outcomes for most overweight and obese children require support, change in lifestyle at home, and involvement of family members. Researchers are involving school-based programs in promoting and preventing obesity in the young.[42]

SUMMARY REVIEW

Development of the Cardiovascular System

1. The heart arises from the mesenchyme and begins as an enlarged blood vessel with a large lumen and a muscular wall. By approximately the eighth week of gestation, all structures of the fetal heart and vascular system are present.
2. The endocardial cushions are instrumental in closing the atrial septum, dividing the AV canals into the right and left AV orifices, and closing the septum.
3. In the fetus the pulmonary and systemic circulatory systems are connected by the foramen ovale, an opening between the atria; by the ductus arteriosus, a fetal vessel that joins the PA to the aorta; and by the ductus venosus, a fetal vessel that connects the inferior vena cava to the umbilical vein.
4. Fetal circulation is different from postnatal circulation because of the presence of fetal shunts and altered metabolic needs of the various organs.
5. Fetal blood flow depends on resistance for its distribution through the body. Resistance in the pulmonary circulation is higher than resistance in the systemic circulation, so myocardial thickness is about the same in the right heart and the left heart.
6. After birth, systemic resistance increases and pulmonary resistance decreases.
7. Pulmonary vascular resistance drops suddenly at birth because the lungs expand and the pulmonary vessels dilate. It continues to decrease gradually during the first 6 to 8 weeks after birth. Decreased resistance causes the right myocardium to become thinner.
8. Systemic vascular resistance increases markedly at birth because severance of the umbilical cord removes the low-resistance placenta from the systemic circulation. Increased systemic resistance causes the left myocardium to become dominant and thicken over time.
9. Changes in resistance cause disappearance of the fetal connections between the pulmonary and systemic circulatory systems. The foramen ovale closes functionally at birth and anatomically several months later; the ductus arteriosus closes functionally 15 to 18 hours after birth and anatomically within 10 to 21 days; and the ductus venosus closes within 1 week after birth.
10. At birth a series of circulatory changes occur that affect blood flow, vascular resistance, and oxygen tension. The most important change is the shift of gas exchange from the placenta to the lungs.
11. After birth, significant postnatal changes occur, including thinning of the right ventricular myocardium as the pulmonary vascular resistance drops. As the systemic vascular resistance increases, the left ventricular myocardium becomes thicker and more dominant as it is in the adult heart.

Congenital Heart Defects

1. Most congenital cardiovascular defects have begun to develop by the eighth week of gestation, and most have many causes, both environmental and genetic.
2. Environmental risk factors associated with the incidence of congenital heart defects typically are maternal conditions. Among these are viral infections, diabetes, drug intake, alcohol intake, metabolic disorders, and advanced maternal age.
3. Genetic factors associated with congenital heart defects include but are not limited to Down syndrome, trisomy 13, trisomy 18, cri du chat syndrome, and Turner syndrome. It now appears, however, that most genetic mechanisms of causation are multifactorial.
4. Classification of congenital heart defects is based on whether they: (a) cause blood flow to the lungs to increase or decrease, (b) obstruct ventricular blood flow patterns, or (c) cause mixing of unoxygenated and oxygenated blood.
5. Symptoms of HF are usually the result of congenital heart defects that increase blood volume and pressure in the pulmonary circulation. Clinical manifestations are almost the same as the manifestations of CHF in adults. A unique manifestation in children is FTT.
6. Cyanosis, a bluish discoloration of the skin, indicates that the tissues are not receiving fully adequate oxygenated blood. Cyanosis can be caused by defects that (a) reduce pulmonary blood flow; (b) overload the pulmonary

SUMMARY REVIEW—cont'd

circulation, causing pulmonary hypertension, pulmonary edema, and respiratory difficulty; and (c) cause large amounts of unoxygenated blood to shunt from the pulmonary to the systemic circulation.

7. Congenital defects that maintain or create direct communication between the pulmonary and systemic circulatory systems cause blood to shunt from one system to another, mixing oxygenated and unoxygenated blood and increasing blood volume and pressure on the receiving side of the shunt.
8. The direction of shunting through an abnormal communication depends on differences in pressure and resistance between the two systems. Flow is always from an area of high pressure to an area of low pressure. The resistance to flow determines the volume of the shunting.
9. Acyanotic congenital defects that increase pulmonary blood flow consist of abnormal openings (PDA, ASD, VSD, AVC defect, or truncus arteriosus) that permit blood to shunt from left (systemic circulation) to right (pulmonary circulation). Cyanosis does not occur because the left-to-right shunt does not interfere with the flow of oxygenated blood through the systemic circulation.
10. If the abnormal communication between the left and right circuits is large, volume and pressure overload in the pulmonary circulation leads to CHF.
11. In truncus arteriosus the main trunk fails to divide longitudinally into the aorta and PA. All blood from both ventricles enters the truncus, so that mixed blood is delivered by both circulatory systems, causing varying degrees of cyanosis and HF.
12. In heart defects that decrease pulmonary blood flow (TOF, tricuspid atresia), myocardial hypertrophy cannot compensate for restricted right ventricular outflow. Flow to the lungs decreases, and cyanosis is caused by mixing of systemic and pulmonary venous return.
13. Obstruction of ventricular outflow commonly is caused by PS, AS, COA, interrupted aortic arch, or hypoplastic left heart syndrome.
14. Despite obstruction, ventricular output remains normal for a long time because of compensatory ventricular hypertrophy stimulated by increased afterload and, in postductal COA, development of collateral circulation around the coarctation.
15. Signs of HF can occur with pulmonary overcirculation or myocardial failure.
16. Complex congenital defects that depend on mixing of the pulmonary and systemic circulations for survival during the postnatal period include complete transposition of the great arteries and total anomalous pulmonary venous connection. This mixing results in desaturated systemic blood flow and cyanosis.
17. In complete transposition of the great vessels, the circulatory systems are not connected serially or through a shunt, so that oxygenated blood remains permanently in the pulmonary circulation and unoxygenated blood remains in the systemic circulation. Survival depends on patency of the ductus arteriosus; in the absence of patency, surgical intervention is mandatory.
18. Total anomalous pulmonary venous connection is caused by abnormal pulmonary vein development and the lack of direct pulmonary venous return to the LA. All blood from the pulmonary and systemic circulations enters the RA. Mixed blood enters the LA through an ASD; it then flows into the systemic circulation and causes cyanosis.
19. Treatment for all hemodyamically severe congenital defects is surgical or interventional correction of the anomaly and management of cyanosis and HF.

Acquired Cardiovascular Disorders

1. The most common acquired cardiovascular disorders of childhood are Kawasaki disease, rheumatic heart disease, and hypertension.
2. Kawasaki disease is an acute systemic vasculitis that also may result in the development of coronary artery aneurysms and thrombosis.
3. Essential or primary hypertension in children is the same as that in adults, except that it is more likely to be diagnosed in an early, asymptomatic stage. Most cases of hypertension in young children are secondary to an underlying cause.
4. Obesity in childhood is epidemic in the United States and other countries.
5. Obese children are at risk for acquiring numerous other serious and potentially life-threatening illnesses, such as asthma, sleep apnea, hypertension, type 2 diabetes mellitus, and cardiovascular disease.

KEY TERMS

Aortic stenosis (AS), 1212
Atrial septal defect (ASD), 1204
Atrioventricular canal (AVC) defect, 1206
Bulbus cordis, 1196
Coarctation of the aorta (COA), 1210
Complete AVC (CAVC) defect, 1207
Conus, 1215
Cyanosis, 1202
Ductus arteriosus, 1196
Eisenmenger syndrome, 1202
Endocardial cushion, 1195
Foramen ovale, 1196
Heart failure (HF), 1200
Hypoplastic left heart syndrome (HLHS), 1214
Kawasaki disease, 1218
Ligamentum venosum, 1197
Ostium primum, 1195
Ostium secundum, 1195
Partial AVC (PAVC) defect, 1207
Patent ductus arteriosus (PDA), 1202
Pulmonary atresia, 1213
Pulmonary stenosis (PS), 1213
Septum primum, 1195
Septum secundum, 1195
Systemic hypertension, 1220
Tetralogy of Fallot (TOF), 1207
Total anomalous pulmonary venous connection (TAPVC), 1216
Transitional AVC (TAVC) defect, 1207
Transposition of the great arteries (TGA), 1214
Tricuspid atresia, 1209
Truncus arteriosus, 1217
Ventricular septal defect (VSD), 1205

REFERENCES

1. Clark EB, Nakazawa M, Takao A, editors: *Etiology and morphogenesis of congenital heart disease: twenty years of progress in genetics and developmental biology*, Mount Kisco, NY, 2000, Futura Publishing.
2. Park MK: *Pediatric cardiology for practitioners*, ed 5, Philadelphia, 2008, Mosby.
3. Wilson D, Hockenberry MJ: *Wong's clinical manual of pediatric nursing*, ed 7, St Louis, 2008, Mosby.
4. Hazinski MF: *Manual of pediatric critical care*, ed 2, St Louis, 1999, Mosby.
5. American Heart Association: *Heart disease and stroke statistics, 2013 update*, Dallas, 2012, Author. *Circulation* 2013:e6–e245.
6. Ziegler VL: Congenital heart disease and genetics, *Crit Care Nurs Clin North Am* 20:159–169, 2008.
7. Allen HD: *Moss and Adam's heart disease in infants, children, and adolescents: including the fetus and young adult*, ed 8, Philadelphia, 2013, Wolters Kluwer Health/Lippincott Williams & Wilkins.
8. Mezu-Ndubuisi OJ et al: Patent ductus arteriosus in premature neonates, *Drugs* 72:907–916, 2012.
9. Moake L, Ndinjkat SK: Transcatheter device closure for ASD: safety efficacy, complications and costs, *Crit Care Nurs Clin North Am* 23:339–348, 2011.
10. Moodie DS, Sterba R: Long-term outcomes excellent for atrial septal defect repair in adults, *Cleve Clin J Med* 67(8):591–597, 2000.
11. Minette M, Sahn D: Ventricular septal defects, *Circulation* 114: 2190–2197, 2006.
12. El-Najdawi EK et al: Operation for partial atrioventricular septal defect: a forty-year review, *J Thorac Cardiovasc Surg* 119(5):880–889, 2000.
13. Mavroudis C, Backer CL, editors: *Pediatric cardiac surgery*, ed 3, St Louis, 2003, Mosby.
14. Thanopoulos BD et al: Initial and six-year results of stent implantation for aortic coarctation in children, *Am J Cardiol* 109(10):1499–1503, 2012.
15. Walhout RJ et al: Comparison of surgical repair with balloon angioplasty for native coarctation in patients from 3 months to 16 years of age, *Eur J Cardiothorac Surg* 25(5):722–727, 2004.
16. Tanous D, Benson LN, Horlick EM: Coarctation of the aorta: evaluation and management, *Curr Opin Cardiol* 24(6):509–515, 2009.
17. d'Udekem Y: Aortic valve surgery in children, *Heart* 97(14):1182–1189, 2011.
18. Hrasja V et al: Ross and Ross-Konno procedure in children and adolescents: mid-term results, *Eur J Cardiothorac Surg* 25(5):742–747, 2004.
19. Poon LK, Menahem S: Pulmonary regurgitation after percutaneous balloon valvoplasty for isolated pulmonary valvar stenosis in childhood, *Cardiol Young* 13(5):444–450, 2003.
20. Feinstein JA et al: Hypoplastic left heart syndrome current considerations and expectations, *J Am Coll Cardiol* 59(Suppl 1):S1–S42, 2012.
21. Newburger JW et al: Early developmental outcome in children with hypoplastic left heart syndrome and related anomalies: the single ventricle reconstruction trial, *Circulation* 125(17):2081–2091, 2012.
22. McQuillen PS: Balloon atrial septostomy is associated with preoperative stroke in neonates with transposition of the great arteries, *Circulation* 113(2):280–285, 2006.
23. Rowley AH: Kawasaki disease genetics, pathology, and a need for earlier diagnosis and treatment, *Contemp Pediatr* 29(12):18–24, 2012.
24. Malatesta-Muncher R, Mitsnefes MM: Management of blood pressure in children, *Curr Opin Nephrol Hypertens* 21(3):318–322, 2012.
25. Roley M, Bluhm B: High blood pressure in children and adolescents, *Am Fam Physician* 85(7):693–700, 2012.
26. National High Blood Pressure Education Program Working Group on High Blood Pressure in Children: The fourth report on the diagnosis, evaluation, and treatment of high blood pressure in children and adolescents, *Pediatrics* 114:555–576, 2004.
27. Nguyen M, Mitsnefes M: Evaluation of hypertension by the general pediatrician, *Curr Opin Pediatr* 19(2):165–169, 2007.
28. Garin EH, Araya CE: Treatment of systemic hypertension in children and adolescents, *Curr Opin Pediatr* 21(5):600–604, 2009.
29. Flynn JT, Urbina EM: Pediatric ambulatory blood pressure monitoring: indications and interpretations, *J Clin Hypertens* 14(6):372–382, 2012.
30. Brady TM et al: Racial differences among children with primary hypertension, *Pediatrics* 126(5):931–937, 2010.
31. Meininger JC et al: Overweight and central adiposity in school-age children and links with hypertension, *J Pediatr Nurs* 25(2):119–125, 2010.
32. Din-Dzietham R et al: High blood pressure trends in children and adolescents in national surveys, 1963-2002, *Circulation* 116(13):1488–1496, 2007.
33. Beilin L, Huang RC: Childhood obesity, hypertension, the metabolic syndrome and adult cardiovascular disease, *Clin Exp Pharmacol Physiol* 35(4):409–411, 2008.
34. Ness M et al: Correlates of overweight and obesity among American Indian/Alaska Native and non-Hispanic white children and adolescents: national survey of children's health, *Matern Child Health J* 16(Suppl):268–277, 2012.
35. van Emmerik NM et al: High cardiovascular risk in severely obese young children and adolescents, *Arch Dis Child* 97(9):818–821, 2012.
36. Rudolf MC, Krom AJ, Cole TH: How good are BMI charts for monitoring children's attempts at obesity reduction? *Arch Dis Child* 97(5):418–422, 2012.
37. Liu J, Zhang A, Li L: Sleep duration and overweight/obesity in children: review and implications for pediatric nursing, *J Spec Pediatr Nurs* 17(3):193–204, 2012.
38. Crespo CJ et al: Television watching, energy intake, and obesity in U.S. children: results from the third National Health and Nutrition Examination Study, 1988-1994, *Arch Pediatr Adolesc Med* 155(3):360–365, 2001.
39. Gordon-Larsen P, McMurray RG, Popkin BM: Adolescent physical activity and inactivity vary by ethnicity: The National Longitudinal Study of Adolescent Health, *J Pediatr* 135(3):301–306, 1999.
40. Long JM et al: Overweight and obesity among white, black, and Mexican American children: implications for when to intervene, *J Spec Pediatr Nurs* 17(1):41–50, 2012.
41. Foltz JL et al: Population-level intervention strategies and examples for obesity prevention in children, *Annu Rev Nutr* 32:391–415, 2012.
42. Centers for Disease Control and Prevention: Guidelines for school health programs to promote lifelong healthy eating: Centers for Disease Control, *MMWR Recomm Rep* 45(RR-9):1–41, 1996.

CHAPTER

34

Structure and Function of the Pulmonary System

Valentina L. Brashers

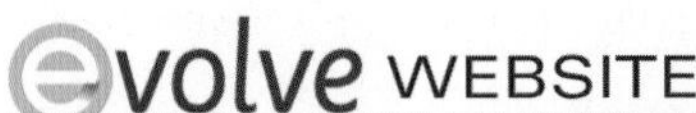

http://evolve.elsevier.com/McCance/

- Review Questions and Answers

CHAPTER OUTLINE

The pulmonary system consists of upper and lower airways, the chest wall, and pulmonary circulation. The primary function of the pulmonary system is the exchange of gases between the environmental air and the blood. There are three steps in this process: (1) ventilation, the movement of air into and out of the lungs; (2) diffusion, the movement of gases between air spaces in the lungs and the bloodstream; and (3) perfusion, the movement of blood into and out of the capillary beds of the lungs to body organs and tissues. The first two functions are carried out by the pulmonary system and the third by the cardiovascular system (see Chapter 31). Normally the pulmonary system functions efficiently under a variety of conditions and with little energy expenditure.

STRUCTURES OF THE PULMONARY SYSTEM

The pulmonary system is made up of the upper airways, two lungs, the lower airways, and the blood vessels that serve them (Figure 34-1); the chest wall, or thoracic cage; and the diaphragm. The lungs are divided into lobes: three in the right lung (upper, middle, lower) and two in the left lung (upper, lower). Each lobe is further divided into segments and lobules. The space between the lungs, which contains the heart, great vessels, and esophagus, is called the *mediastinum.* A set of conducting airways, called bronchi, deliver air to each section of the lung. The lung tissue that surrounds the airways supports them, preventing their distortion or collapse as gas moves in and out during ventilation. The diaphragm is a dome-shaped muscle that separates the thoracic and abdominal cavities and is involved in ventilation.

The lungs are protected from a variety of exogenous contaminants by a series of mechanical and cellular defenses (Table 34-1). These defense mechanisms are so effective that in the healthy individual, contamination of the lung tissue itself is unusual. (Other defense mechanisms are discussed in Chapters 7 and 8.)

Conducting Airways

The conducting airways are the portion of the pulmonary system that provides a passage for the movement of air into and out of the gas-exchange portions of the lung. They consist of upper and lower airways. The **nasopharynx, oropharynx,** and related structures often are called the *upper airway* (Figure 34-2). These structures are lined

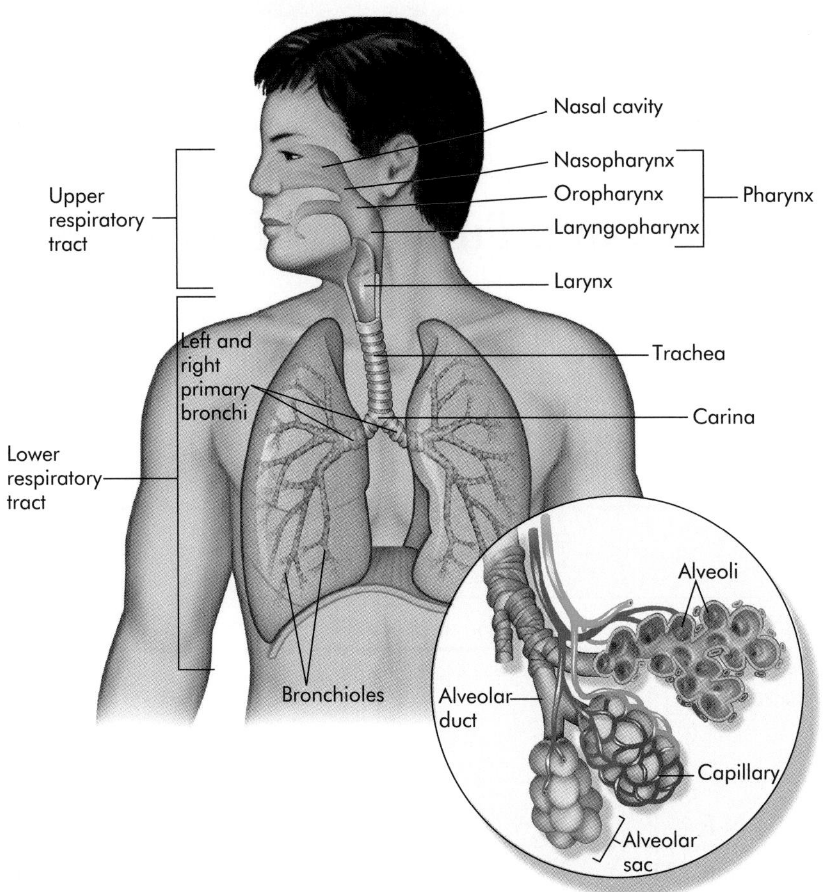

FIGURE 34-1 **Structural Plan of the Respiratory System.** *Inset* shows alveolar sacs where the interchange of oxygen and carbon dioxide takes place through the walls of the grapelike alveoli. Capillaries surround the alveoli. (From Patton KT, Thibodeau GA: *Anatomy & physiology,* ed 8, St Louis, 2013, Mosby.)

TABLE 34-1 PULMONARY DEFENSE MECHANISMS

STRUCTURE OR SUBSTANCE	MECHANISM OF DEFENSE
Upper respiratory tract mucosa	Maintains constant temperature and humidification of gas entering the lungs; traps and removes foreign particles, some bacteria, and noxious gases from inspired air
Nasal hairs and turbinates	Trap and remove foreign particles, some bacteria, and noxious gases from inspired air
Mucous blanket	Protects trachea and bronchi from injury; traps most foreign particles and bacteria that reach the lower airways
Cilia	Propel mucous blanket and entrapped particles toward the oropharynx, where they can be swallowed or expectorated
Alveolar macrophages	Ingest and remove bacteria and other foreign material from alveoli by phagocytosis (see Chapter 7)
Surfactant	Enhance phagocytosis of pathogens and allergens in alveoli; down-regulate inflammatory responses
Irritant receptors in nares (nostrils)	Stimulation by chemical or mechanical irritants triggers sneeze reflex, which results in rapid removal of irritants from nasal passages
Irritant receptors in trachea and large airways	Stimulation by chemical or mechanical irritants triggers cough reflex, which results in removal of irritants from the trachea and large airways

with a ciliated mucosa with a very rich vascular supply. The mucosal lining warms and humidifies inspired air to 100% and removes foreign particles from it as it passes into the lungs. During quiet breathing, gas usually flows through the nose, nasopharynx, and oropharynx to the lower airways. The mouth and oropharynx provide for ventilation when the nose is obstructed or when increased flow is required, such as during exercise. Filtering and humidifying are not as efficient with mouth breathing.

The **larynx** connects the upper and lower airways. The structure of the larynx consists of the endolarynx and its surrounding triangular-shaped bony and cartilaginous structures. The endolarynx is formed by two pairs of folds that form the false vocal cords (supraglottis) and the true vocal cords. The slit-shaped space between the true cords forms the glottis (see Figure 34-2). The vestibule is the space above the false vocal cords. The laryngeal box is formed by three large cartilages—the epiglottis, thyroid, and cricoid—and three smaller

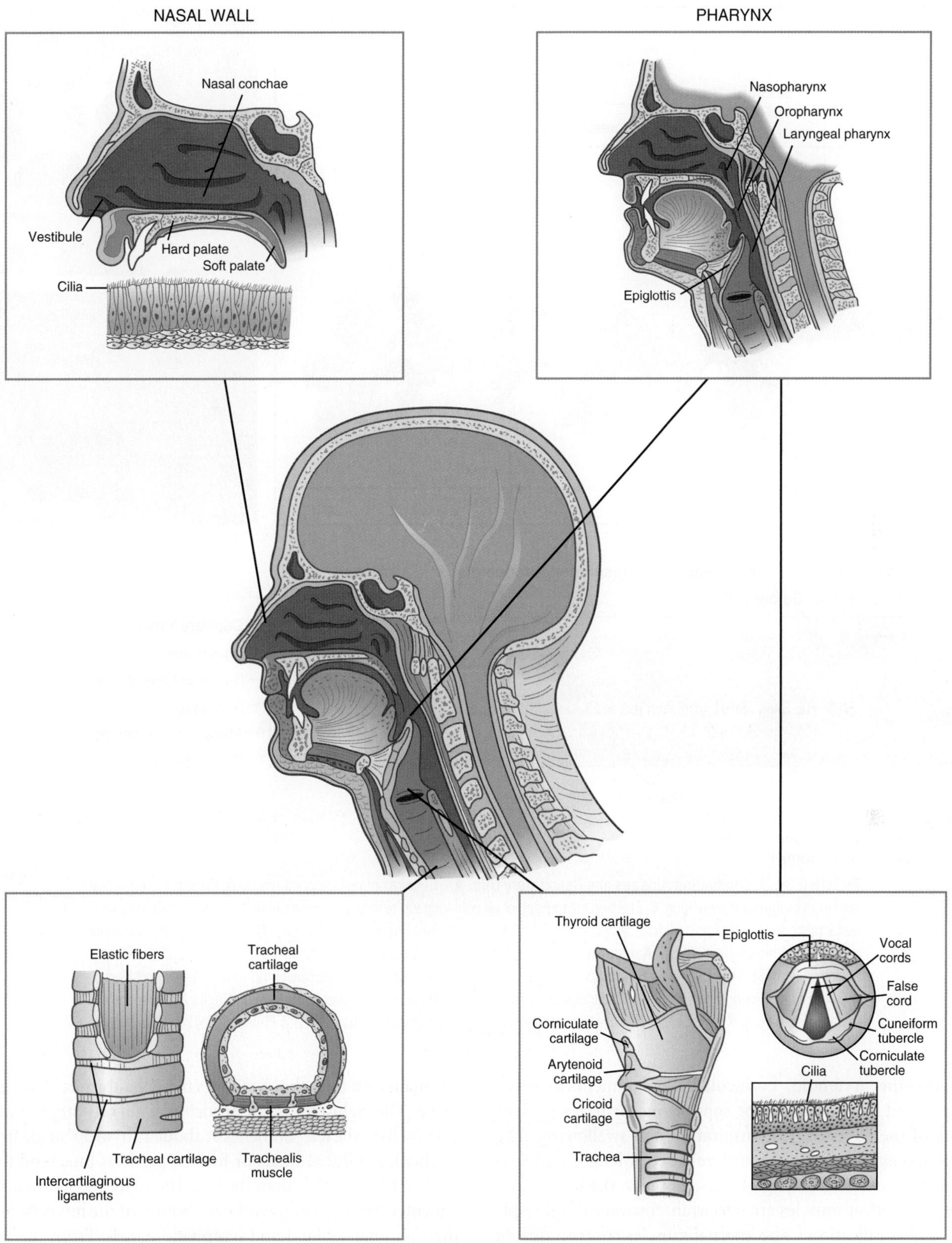

FIGURE 34-2 **Structures of the Upper Airway.** (Redrawn from Thompson JM et al: *Mosby's clinical nursing,* ed 5, St Louis, 2002, Mosby.)

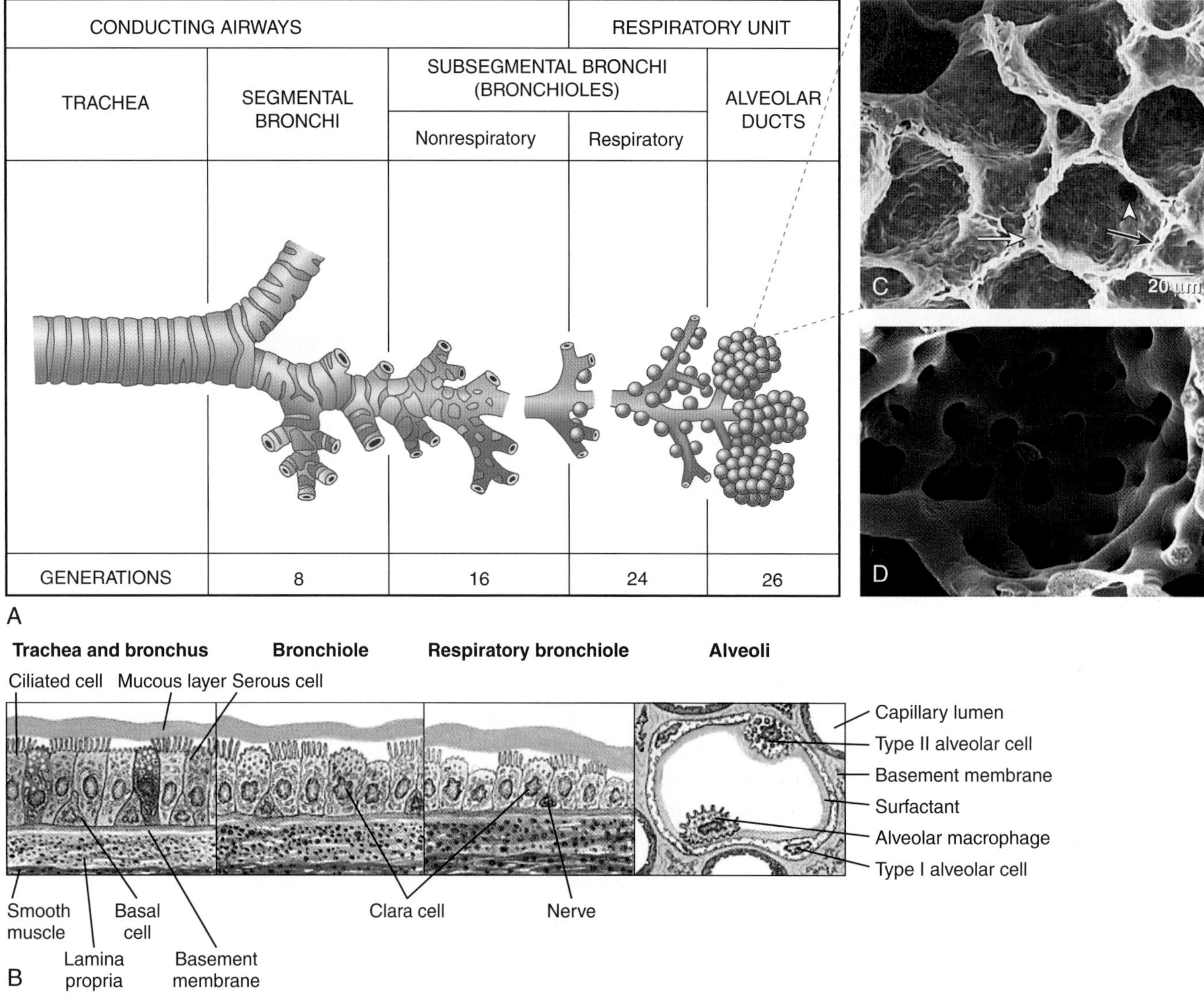

FIGURE 34-3 Conducting Airways and Respiratory Unit. **A,** Structures of respiratory airways. **B,** Changes in bronchial wall with progressive branching. **C,** Electron micrograph of alveoli: long white arrow identifies type II pneumonocyte (secretes surfactant); short white arrow identifies pores of Kohn; red arrow identifies alveolar capillary. **D,** Plastic cast of pulmonary capillaries at high magnification. (**A** redrawn from Thompson JM et al: *Mosby's clinical nursing,* ed 5, St Louis, 2002, Mosby; **B** from Wilson SF, Thompson JM: *Respiratory disorders,* St Louis, 1990, Mosby; **C** from Mason RJ et al: *Murray and Nadel's textbook of respiratory medicine,* ed 5, Philadelphia, 2010, Saunders; **D** courtesy A. Churg, MD, and J. Wright, MD, Vancouver, Canada. From Leslie KO, Wick MR: *Practical pulmonary pathology: a diagnostic approach,* ed 2, Philadelphia, 2011, Saunders.)

cartilages—the arytenoid, corniculate, and cuneiform—that are connected by ligaments. The supporting cartilages prevent collapse of the larynx during inspiration and swallowing. The internal laryngeal muscles control vocal cord length and tension, and the external laryngeal muscles move the larynx as a whole. Both sets of muscles are important to swallowing, respiration, and vocalization.[1] The internal muscles contract during swallowing to prevent aspiration into the trachea and contribute to voice pitch.

The **trachea,** which is supported by U-shaped cartilage, connects the larynx to the **bronchi,** the conducting airways of the lungs. The trachea divides into the two main airways, or bronchi, at the **carina** (see Figure 34-1). This area is very sensitive and when stimulated can cause coughing and airway narrowing. The left mainstem bronchus branches from the trachea at about a 45° angle. The right mainstem bronchus is slightly larger and more vertical than the left (branches at about a 20° to 30° angle from the trachea). Aspirated fluids or foreign particles thus tend to enter the right lung rather than the left. The right and left main bronchi enter the lungs at the **hila,** or "roots" of the lungs, along with the pulmonary blood and lymphatic vessels. From the hila the main bronchi branch into lobar bronchi, then to segmental and subsegmental bronchi, and finally end at the sixteenth division in the smallest of the conducting airways, the terminal **bronchioles** (Figure 34-3). With these multiple divisions, the cross-sectional area of the airways increases to 20 times that of the trachea. This results in decreased velocity of airflow into the gas-exchange portion of the lung and allows for optimal gas diffusion.[2]

The bronchial walls have three layers: an epithelial lining, a smooth muscle layer, and a connective tissue layer. In the large bronchi (to approximately the tenth division), the connective tissue layer contains cartilage. The epithelial lining of the bronchi contains single-celled exocrine glands—the mucus-secreting **goblet cells**—and ciliated cells. High columnar pseudostratified epithelium lines the larger airways, changing to columnar cuboidal epithelium in the bronchioles (types of epithelia are illustrated in Chapter 1). The submucosal glands of the bronchial lining also produce mucus, contributing to the mucous blanket that covers the bronchial epithelium. The ciliated epithelial cells rhythmically beat this mucous blanket toward the trachea and pharynx, where it can be swallowed or expectorated by coughing. Foreign particles and microorganisms that are not expelled by mucociliary clearance and coughing are attacked by cellular components of the inflammatory response and antibodies of the secretory immune system (see Chapter 8).[3] The biochemical mediators released early in inflammation also play a part in antibody-mediated hypersensitivity reactions, such as asthma, because they stimulate bronchial smooth muscles to constrict. With branching, the layers of epithelium that line the bronchi become thinner (see Figure 34-3). Ciliated cells and goblet cells become more sparse, and smooth muscle and connective tissue layers thin toward the terminal bronchioles.[4]

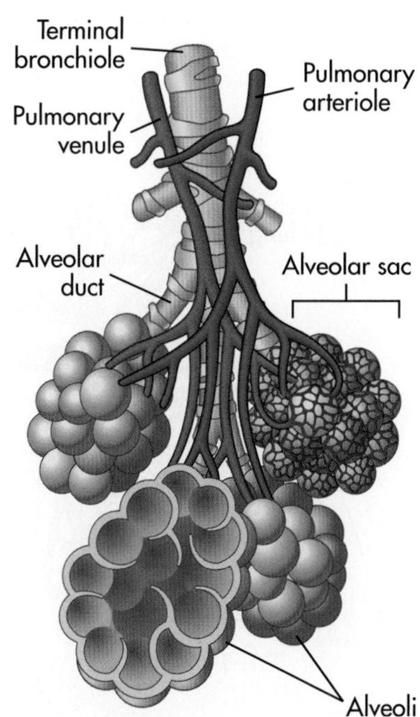

FIGURE 34-4 Alveoli. Bronchioles subdivide to form tiny tubes called *alveolar ducts* that end in clusters of alveoli called *alveolar sacs.* (From Patton KT, Thibodeau GA: *Anatomy & physiology,* ed 8, St Louis, 2013, Mosby.)

Gas-Exchange Airways

The bronchioles terminate in gas-exchange airways, where oxygen (O_2) enters the blood and carbon dioxide (CO_2) is removed from it. The gas-exchange airways consist of **respiratory bronchioles, alveolar ducts,** and **alveoli** (see Figure 34-3). These structures together are sometimes called the **acinus,** and all of them participate in gas exchange.[5]

The bronchioles from the sixteenth through the twenty-third divisions contain increasing numbers of alveoli and are called *respiratory bronchioles.* The walls of the respiratory bronchioles are very thin, consisting of an epithelial layer devoid of cilia and goblet cells, very little smooth muscle fiber, and a very thin and elastic connective tissue layer. These bronchioles end in alveolar ducts, which lead to alveolar sacs made up of numerous alveoli.

The alveoli are the primary gas-exchange units of the lung, where oxygen enters the blood and CO_2 is removed (Figure 34-4). Tiny passages called *pores of Kohn* permit some air to pass through the septa from alveolus to alveolus, promoting collateral ventilation and even distribution of air among the alveoli. The lungs contain approximately 50 million alveoli at birth and about 480 million by adulthood.[4,6]

The alveolar septa consist of an epithelial layer and a thin, elastic basement membrane but no muscle layer (see Figure 34-3). Two major types of epithelial cells appear in the alveolus. Type I alveolar cells provide structure, and type II alveolar cells secrete **surfactant,** a lipoprotein that coats the inner surface of the alveolus and facilitates its expansion during inspiration, lowers alveolar surface tension at end-expiration, and, thereby, prevents lung collapse.[7] Surfactant also contributes to control of lung inflammation and innate and adaptive immunity.[7a]

Like the bronchi, alveoli contain cellular components of inflammation and immunity, particularly the mononuclear phagocytes. The mononuclear phagocytes of the lungs are called *alveolar macrophages.* These cells ingest foreign material that reaches the alveolus and prepare it for removal through the lymphatics.[8] (Phagocytosis and the mononuclear phagocyte system are described in Chapters 7 and 8.)

Pulmonary and Bronchial Circulation

The pulmonary circulation facilitates gas exchange, delivers nutrients to lung tissues, acts as a blood reservoir for the left ventricle, and serves as a filtering system that removes clots, air, and other debris from the circulation (Figure 34-5).

Although the entire cardiac output from the right ventricle goes into the lungs, the pulmonary circulation has a lower pressure and resistance than the systemic circulation. Pulmonary arteries are exposed to about one fifth the pressure of the systemic circulation and have a much thinner muscle layer. (Systemic vessels are described in Chapter 31.) Mean pulmonary artery pressure is 18 mmHg; mean aortic pressure is 90 mmHg. About one third of the pulmonary vessels are filled with blood (perfused) at any given time.[9] More vessels become perfused when right ventricular cardiac output increases. Therefore, increased delivery of blood to the lungs does not normally increase mean pulmonary artery pressure.

The **pulmonary artery** divides and enters the lung at the hilus, travels with each main bronchus, and branches with the bronchus at every division so that every bronchus and bronchiole has an accompanying artery or arteriole. The arterioles, less than 1 mm in diameter, regulate blood flow through their respective capillary beds.[9]

The arterioles divide at the terminal bronchiole to form a network of **pulmonary capillaries** around the acinus. The capillaries are an integral part of the alveolar septa. Capillary walls

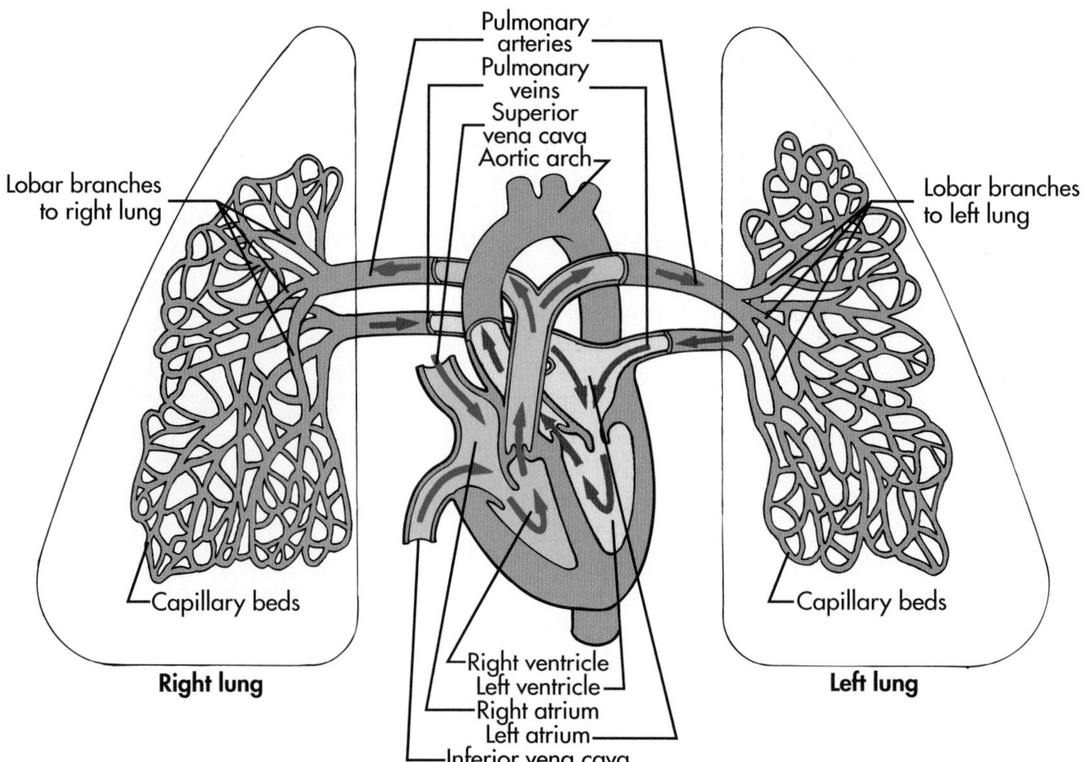

FIGURE 34-5 **The Pulmonary Circulation.** The right and left pulmonary veins and arteries and the branching capillaries are illustrated. Note the pulmonary artery carries venous blood, and the pulmonary vein carries arterial blood.

consist of an endothelial layer and a thin basement membrane, which often fuses with the basement membrane of the alveolar septum (see Figure 34-3). This results in very little separation between blood in the capillary and gas in the alveolus.

The shared alveolar and capillary walls compose the **alveolocapillary membrane,** a very thin membrane made up of the alveolar epithelium, the alveolar basement membrane, an interstitial space, the capillary basement membrane, and the capillary endothelium (Figure 34-6). These extremely thin alveolar walls are easily damaged and can leak plasma and blood into the alveolar space. Gas exchange occurs across the alveolocapillary membrane. With normal perfusion approximately 100 ml of blood in the pulmonary capillary bed is spread very thinly over about 140 m^2 of alveolar surface area.[9] The alveolocapillary membrane efficiently exposes large quantities of blood to gas in the alveoli. Any disorder that thickens the membrane impairs gas exchange.

Each **pulmonary vein** drains several pulmonary capillaries. Unlike the pulmonary arteries, which follow the branching bronchi, pulmonary veins are dispersed randomly throughout the lung and then leave the lung at the hila and enter the left atrium. They are similar to veins in the systemic circulation, but they have no valves.

The bronchial circulation is part of the systemic circulation. It supplies nutrients to the conducting airways, nerves, lymph nodes, large pulmonary vessels, and membranes (pleurae) that surround the lungs and moistens inspired air.[10] The bronchial circulation is unique in that not all of its capillaries drain into its own venous system. Some of the bronchial capillaries empty into the pulmonary vein and contribute to the normal venous admixture (mixing of oxygenated and deoxygenated blood) or right-to-left shunt (right-to-left shunts [ventilation-perfusion abnormalities] are described in Chapter 35). The bronchial circulation does not participate in gas exchange.

Lung vasculature also includes deep and superficial **pulmonary lymphatic capillaries.** The deep lymphatic capillaries begin at the level of the terminal bronchioles; there are no lymphatic structures in the acinus. Fluid and alveolar macrophages migrate from the alveoli to the terminal bronchioles, where they enter the lymphatic system. The superficial lymphatic capillaries drain the membrane that surrounds the lungs. Both deep and superficial lymphatic vessels leave the lung at the hilus through a series of mediastinal lymph nodes. The lymphatic system plays an important role in keeping the lung free of fluid and providing immune defense. (The lymphatic system is described in Chapter 31.)

Control of the Pulmonary Circulation

The caliber of pulmonary artery lumina decreases as smooth muscle in arterial walls contracts. Contraction increases pulmonary artery pressure. Caliber increases as these muscles relax, decreasing blood pressure. Contraction (vasoconstriction) and relaxation (vasodilation) occur in response to local humoral conditions, even though the pulmonary circulation is innervated by the autonomic nervous system (ANS) in the same manner as the systemic circulation.

The most important cause of pulmonary artery constriction is a low alveolar partial pressure of oxygen (P_{AO_2}).

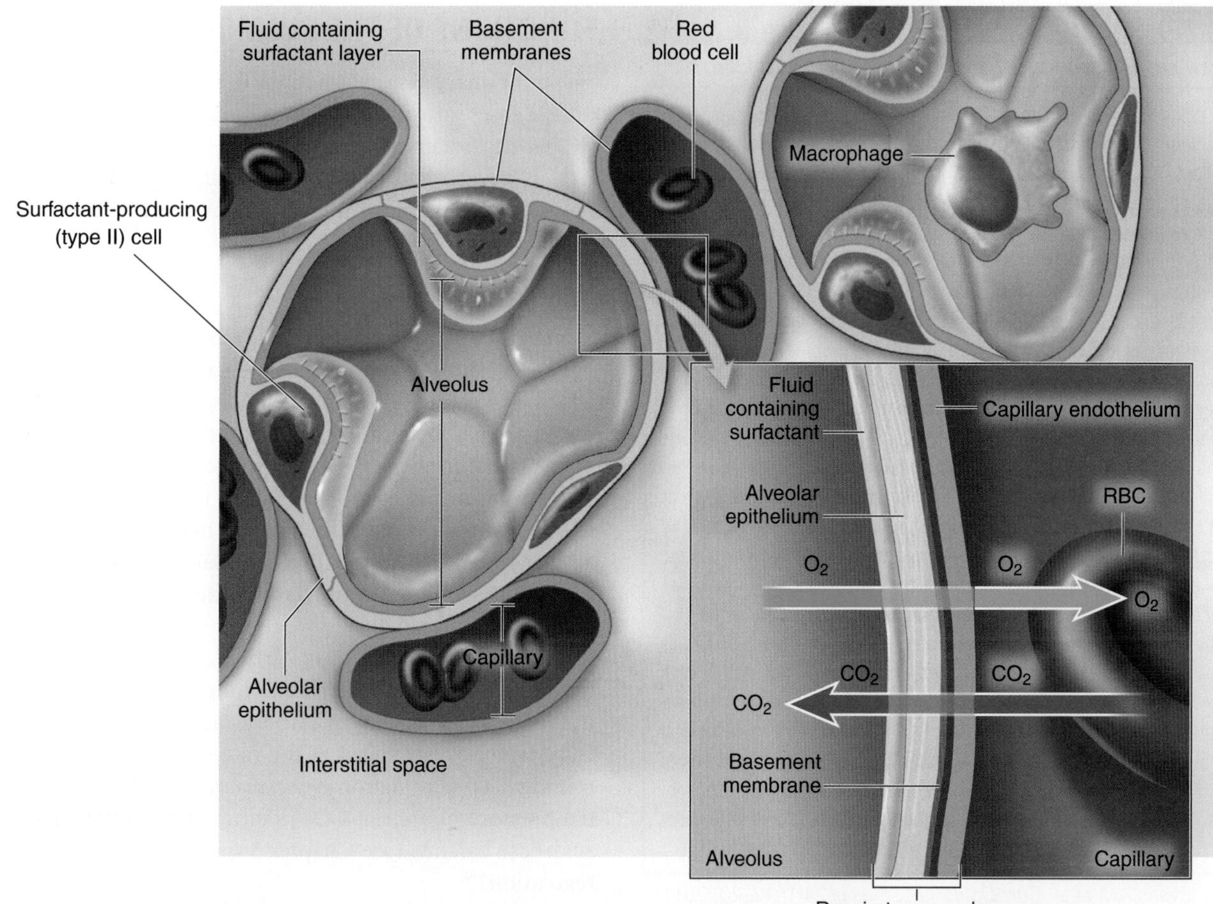

FIGURE 34-6 **Section Through the Alveolar Septum (Gas-Exchange Membrane).** *Inset* shows a magnified view of the respiratory membrane composed of the alveolar wall (fluid containing surfactant, epithelial cells, basement membrane), interstitial space, and wall of a pulmonary capillary (basement membrane, endothelial cells). The gases—carbon dioxide *(CO_2)* and oxygen *(O_2)*—diffuse across the respiratory membrane. (From Patton KT, Thibodeau GA: *Anatomy & physiology,* ed 8, St Louis, 2013, Mosby.)

Vasoconstriction caused by alveolar and pulmonary venous hypoxia, often termed **hypoxic pulmonary vasoconstriction,** can affect only one portion of the lung or the entire lung. If only one segment of the lung is involved, the arterioles to that segment constrict, shunting blood to other, well-ventilated portions of the lung. This reflex improves the lung's efficiency by better matching ventilation and perfusion. If alveolar hypoxia affects all segments of the lung, however, vasoconstriction occurs throughout the pulmonary vasculature, and pulmonary hypertension (elevated pulmonary artery pressure) can result. The pulmonary vasoconstriction caused by low P_{AO_2} is reversible if the P_{AO_2} is corrected. Chronic alveolar hypoxia can result in permanent pulmonary artery hypertension, which eventually leads to cor pulmonale and heart failure (see What's New? Update on Hypoxic Pulmonary Vasoconstriction).[11]

Acidemia also causes pulmonary artery constriction. If the acidemia is corrected, the vasoconstriction is reversed. (Respiratory acidosis and metabolic acidosis are described in Chapter 3.) It is important to note that an elevated Pa_{CO_2} without a drop in pH does not cause pulmonary artery constriction. Other biochemical factors that affect the caliber of vessels in pulmonary circulation are histamine, prostaglandins, endothelin, serotonin, nitric oxide, and bradykinin.

Chest Wall and Pleura

The chest wall (skin, ribs, intercostal muscles) protects the lungs from injury, and its muscles, in conjunction with the **diaphragm,** perform the muscular work of breathing. The **thoracic cavity** is contained by the chest wall and encases the lungs (Figure 34-7). A serous membrane called the **pleura** adheres firmly to the lungs. It then folds over itself and attaches firmly to the chest wall. The membrane covering the lungs is the visceral pleura; that lining the thoracic cavity is the parietal pleura. The area between the two pleurae is called the **pleural space,** or **pleural cavity.** Normally only a thin layer of fluid secreted by the pleura (pleural fluid) fills the pleural space. About 18 ml of fluid is in the pleural space with a pH of about 7.6, a few cells, about 1 g/dl protein, and glucose and electrolyte concentrations that approximate those of the plasma.[9] This lubricates the pleural surfaces, allowing the two layers to slide over each other without separating. Pressure in the pleural space is usually negative or subatmospheric (−4 to −10 mmHg).

WHAT'S NEW?

Update on Hypoxic Pulmonary Vasoconstriction

Hypoxic pulmonary vasoconstriction is a physiologic response to changes in the environment and pulmonary pathologic conditions that affect alveolar oxygen content (P_{AO_2}). Decreases in P_{AO_2} to less than 12% of normal induce a locally controlled constriction of preacinar arteriolar smooth muscle and endothelial cells and therefore decrease blood flow through those vessels. When a pulmonary disorder is characterized by localized areas of acutely decreased alveolar oxygen content, vasoconstriction of the arterioles perfusing those areas is a positive compensatory mechanism that reduces shunt (wasted perfusion). However, in diffuse and chronic lung disorders (e.g., chronic obstructive pulmonary disease [COPD] or cystic fibrosis), widespread and persistent hypoxic pulmonary vasoconstriction creates resistance to pulmonary blood flow and raises the pressure in the pulmonary artery, causing a condition known as *secondary pulmonary artery hypertension*. Pulmonary hypertension can become severe enough to impede right ventricular ejection and eventually cause right heart failure known as *cor pulmonale*. In addition, lung hypoxia activates many hypoxia-dependent genes in pulmonary vascular endothelial cells to produce a variety of chemicals and growth factors. Recent studies have shown that alveolar hypoxia causes the production of reactive oxygen species (toxic oxygen radicals), vasoconstrictors (such as endothelin), and vascular endothelial growth factor that in conjunction with vascular fibroblasts cause deleterious changes in the pulmonary arteriolar walls called *remodeling*. Remodeling is a process by which the vascular wall becomes scarred and thickened, thus resulting in permanent decreases in luminal diameter, increased resistance to blood flow, and permanent pulmonary artery hypertension. Research is in progress to inhibit and potentially reverse this remodeling.

Data from Evans AM et al: *Curr Opin Anaesthesiol* 24(1):13–20, 2011; Kummer W: *Proc Am Thorac Soc* 8(6):471–476, 2011; Orr R, Smith LJ, Cuttica MJ: *Curr Opin Pulm Med* 18(2):138–143, 2012; Pitsiou G, Papakosta D, Bouros D: *Respiration* 82(3):294–304, 2011; Sylvester JT et al: *Physiol Rev* 92(1):367–520, 2012.

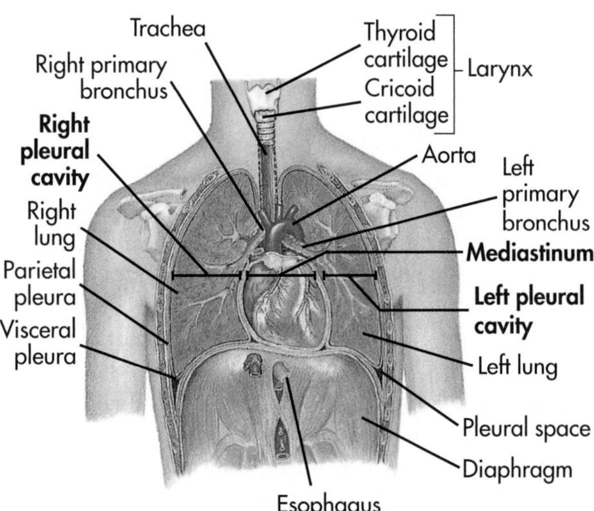

FIGURE 34-7 Thoracic (Chest) Cavity and Related Structures. The thoracic cavity is divided into three subdivisions (left and right pleural divisions and mediastinum) by a partition formed by a serous membrane called the *pleura*. (From Thibodeau GA, Patton KT: *Anatomy & physiology*, ed 3, St Louis, 1996, Mosby.)

FUNCTIONS OF THE PULMONARY SYSTEM

The pulmonary system functions to (1) ventilate the alveoli, (2) diffuse gases into and out of the blood, and (3) perfuse the lungs so that the organs and tissues of the body receive blood that is rich in oxygen and low in CO_2. Each component of the pulmonary system contributes to one or more of these functions (Figure 34-8).

Ventilation

Ventilation is the mechanical movement of gas or air into and out of the lungs. Ventilation often is misnamed **respiration,** which is actually the exchange of O_2 and CO_2 during cellular metabolism. "Respiratory rate" is actually the ventilatory rate, or the number of times gas is inspired and expired per minute. The amount of effective ventilation is calculated by multiplying the ventilatory rate (breaths per minute) by the volume of air per breath (liters per breath, tidal volume). This is called the **minute volume** (or **minute ventilation**) and is expressed in liters per minute.

CO_2, the gaseous form of carbonic acid (H_2CO_3), is a product of cellular metabolism. The lung eliminates about 10,000 milliequivalents (mEq) of carbonic acid per day in the form of CO_2, which is produced at the rate of approximately 200 ml/minute. CO_2 elimination is necessary to maintain a normal partial pressure of arterial CO_2 (Pa_{CO_2}) of 40 mmHg and normal acid-base balance (see Chapter 3 for a discussion of acid-base regulation).[9]

The adequacy of **alveolar ventilation** *cannot* be accurately determined by observation of ventilatory rate, pattern, or effort. If a healthcare professional needs to determine the adequacy of ventilation, an arterial blood gas analysis must be performed to measure Pa_{CO_2}.

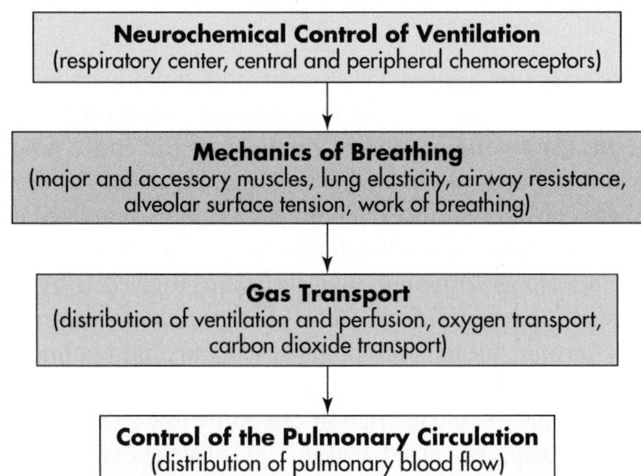

FIGURE 34-8 Functional Components of the Respiratory System. The central nervous system responds to neurochemical stimulation of ventilation and sends signals to the chest wall musculature. The response of the respiratory system to these impulses is influenced by several factors that affect the mechanisms of breathing and therefore affect the adequacy of ventilation. Gas transport between the alveoli and pulmonary capillary blood depends on a variety of physical and chemical activities. The control of the pulmonary circulation plays a role in the appropriate distribution of blood flow.

Neurochemical Control of Ventilation

The mechanisms that control respiration are very complex.[12-14] Breathing is usually involuntary because homeostatic changes in the ventilatory rate and volume are adjusted automatically by the nervous system to maintain normal gas exchange. Voluntary breathing is necessary for talking, singing, laughing, and holding one's breath.

The **respiratory center** in the brainstem controls respiration by transmitting impulses to the respiratory muscles, causing them to contract and relax (Figure 34-9). The respiratory center is composed of several groups of neurons located bilaterally in the brainstem: the dorsal respiratory group (DRG), the ventral respiratory group (VRG), the pneumotaxic center, and the apneustic center.[15] The basic automatic rhythm of respiration is set by the DRG, a cluster of inspiratory nerve cells located in the medulla that sends efferent impulses to the diaphragm and inspiratory intercostal muscles. The DRG also receives afferent impulses from **peripheral chemoreceptors** in the carotid and aortic bodies, which detect the $Paco_2$ and the amount of oxygen in the arterial blood (Pao_2). In addition, several different types of receptors in the lungs stimulate the VRG through afferent nerves. The VRG, also located in the medulla, contains inspiratory and expiratory neurons. It is almost inactive during normal, quiet respiration, becoming active when increased ventilatory effort is required. The pneumotaxic center and apneustic center, situated in the pons, do not generate primary rhythm, but rather act as modifiers of the inspiratory depth and rate established by the medullary centers.[16] Breathing can be modified by input from the cortex, the limbic system, and the hypothalamus, and the pattern of breathing can be influenced by emotion and by disease.

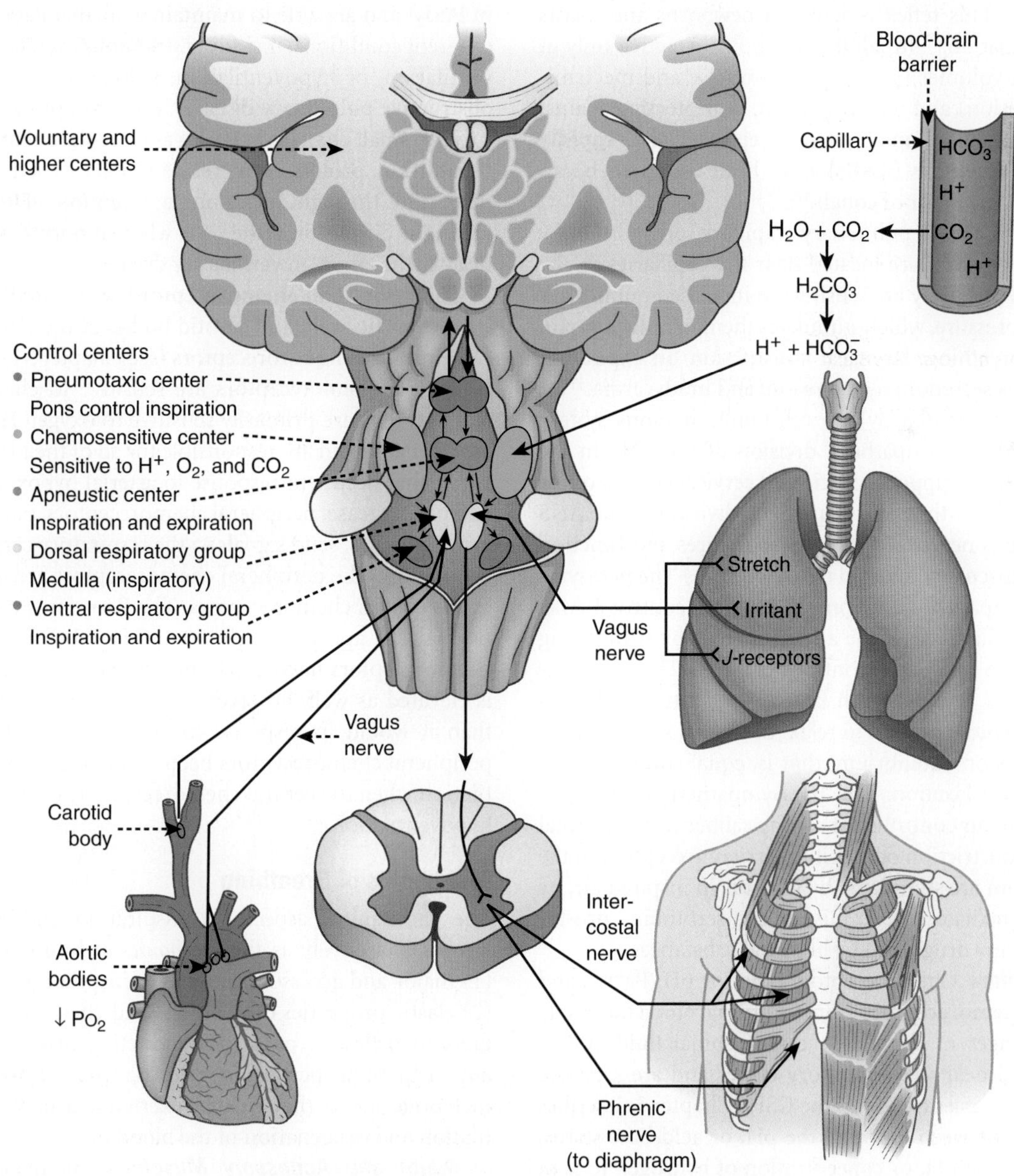

FIGURE 34-9 Neurochemical Respiratory Control System.

Lung Receptors. Three types of lung receptors send impulses from the lungs to the dorsal respiratory group:

1. **Irritant receptors** (rapidly adapting receptors) are found in the epithelium of the conducting airways. They are sensitive to noxious aerosols (vapors), gases, and particulate matter (e.g., inhaled dusts), which cause them to initiate the cough reflex. When stimulated, irritant receptors also cause bronchoconstriction and increased ventilatory rate. These receptors are located primarily in the proximal larger airways and are nearly absent in the distal airways; thus it is possible for secretions to accumulate in the distal respiratory tree without initiating cough.
2. **Stretch receptors** (slowly adapting receptors) are located in the smooth muscles of airways and are sensitive to increases in the size or volume of the lungs. They decrease ventilatory rate and volume when stimulated, an occurrence sometimes referred to as the *Hering-Breuer expiratory reflex.* This reflex is active in newborns and assists with ventilation.[17] In adults, this reflex is active only at high tidal volumes (such as with exercise and mechanical ventilation) and may play a role in protecting against excess lung inflation. Stretch receptors called **rapidly adapting receptors (RARs)** have been found to be an important mediator of cough.[18]
3. ***J*-receptors** (juxta-pulmonary capillary or pulmonary C fiber receptors) are located near the capillaries in the alveolar septa. They are sensitive to increased pulmonary capillary pressure, which stimulates them to initiate rapid, shallow breathing; laryngeal constriction on expiration and mucus secretion; hypotension; and bradycardia.[19]

The lung is innervated by the autonomic nervous system (ANS). Fibers of the sympathetic division of the ANS in the lung branch from the upper thoracic and cervical ganglia of the spinal cord. Fibers of the parasympathetic division of the ANS travel in the vagus nerve to the lung. (Structures and function of the ANS are discussed in detail in Chapter 15.) The parasympathetic and sympathetic divisions of the ANS control airway caliber (interior diameter of the airway lumen) by stimulating bronchial smooth muscle to contract or relax. The parasympathetic receptors cause smooth muscle to contract, whereas sympathetic receptors cause it to relax. Bronchial smooth muscle tone depends on equilibrium, that is, equal stimulation of contraction and relaxation. The parasympathetic division of the ANS is the main controller of airway caliber under normal conditions.[20] Constriction occurs if the irritant receptors in the airway epithelium are stimulated by irritants in inspired air, by inflammatory mediators (e.g., histamine, serotonin, prostaglandins), by many drugs, and by humoral substances.

Chemoreceptors. Chemoreceptors monitor pH, $Paco_2$, and Pao_2. **Central chemoreceptors** monitor arterial blood indirectly by sensing changes in the pH of cerebrospinal fluid (CSF). They are located near the respiratory center and are sensitive to hydrogen ion concentration in the CSF. (Chapter 3 describes the relationship between ions and the pH, or acid-base status, of body fluids.) The pH, or concentration of hydrogen ions in the CSF, reflects $Paco_2$ because, unlike H^+ ions, CO_2 in arterial blood diffuses across the blood-brain barrier (the capillary wall separating blood from cells of the central nervous system) into the CSF until the partial pressure of CO_2 (Pco_2) is equal on both sides. CO_2 that has entered the CSF combines with H_2O to form carbonic acid, which subsequently dissociates into hydrogen ions that are capable of stimulating the central chemoreceptors. In this way $Paco_2$ regulates ventilation through its effect on the pH (hydrogen ion content) of the CSF.[12,13,21]

If alveolar ventilation is inadequate, $Paco_2$ increases. CO_2 diffuses across the blood-brain barrier until Pco_2 in the blood and CSF reaches equilibrium. As the central chemoreceptors sense the resulting decrease in pH (increase in hydrogen ion concentration), they stimulate the respiratory center to increase the depth and rate of ventilation. Increased ventilation causes the $Paco_2$ to decrease below that of the CSF, and CO_2 diffuses back out of the CSF, returning its pH to normal.

The central chemoreceptors are sensitive to very small changes in the pH of CSF (equivalent to a 1 to 2 mmHg change in Pco_2) and are able to maintain a normal $Paco_2$ under many different conditions, including strenuous exercise. If inadequate ventilation, or hypoventilation, is long term (e.g., in chronic obstructive pulmonary disease), these receptors become insensitive to small changes in $Paco_2$ and regulate ventilation poorly. In addition, prolonged increases in $Paco_2$ result in renal compensation through bicarbonate retention. This bicarbonate gradually diffuses into the CSF, where it normalizes the pH and negates the effect on ventilatory drive.[22]

The **peripheral chemoreceptors** are located in aortic bodies, the aortic arch, and carotid bodies at the bifurcation of the carotids, near the baroreceptors (see Chapter 31). Although the peripheral chemoreceptors are sensitive to changes in $Paco_2$ and pH, they are primarily sensitive to oxygen levels in arterial blood (Pao_2) and are responsible for all of the increase in ventilation that occurs in response to arterial hypoxemia.[23] As Pao_2 and pH decrease, peripheral chemoreceptors, particularly in the carotid bodies, send signals to the respiratory center to increase ventilation. The peripheral chemoreceptors are not as sensitive as the central chemoreceptors. The Pao_2 must drop well below normal (to approximately 60 mmHg) before the peripheral chemoreceptors have much influence on ventilation.[9] If $Paco_2$ is elevated as well, however, ventilation increases much more than it would in response to either abnormality alone. The peripheral chemoreceptors become the major stimulus to ventilation when the central chemoreceptors are "reset" by chronic hypoventilation.

Mechanics of Breathing

The mechanical aspects of inspiration and expiration are known collectively as the *mechanics of breathing* and involve: (1) major and accessory muscles of inspiration and expiration, (2) elastic properties of the lungs and chest wall, and (3) resistance to airflow through the conducting airways. Alterations in any of these properties increase the work of breathing, or the metabolic energy that must be exerted to achieve adequate ventilation and oxygenation of the blood.

Major and Accessory Muscles. The major muscles of inspiration are the diaphragm and the external intercostal muscles (muscles between the ribs) (Figure 34-10). The

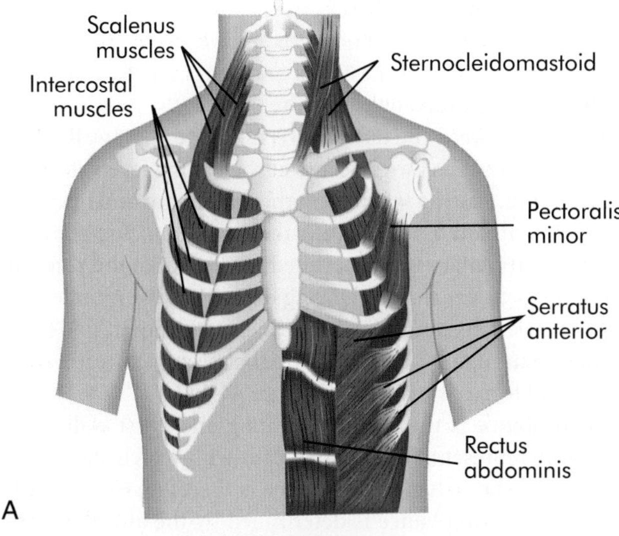

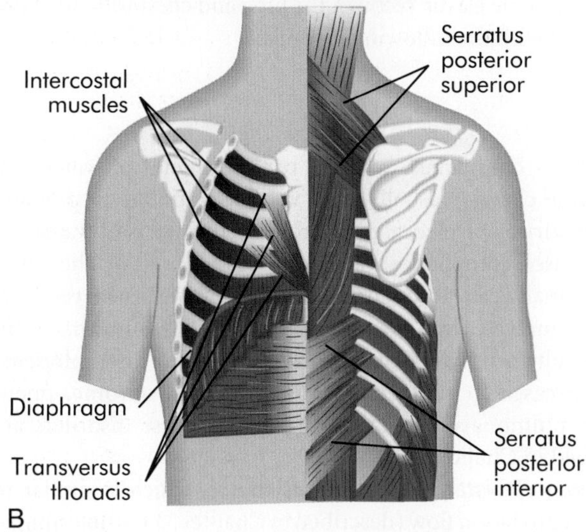

FIGURE 34-10 Muscles of Ventilation. **A,** Anterior view. **B,** Posterior view. (Modified from Thompson JM et al: *Mosby's clinical nursing,* ed 5, St Louis, 2002, Mosby.)

diaphragm is a dome-shaped muscle that separates the abdominal and thoracic cavities. When the diaphragm contracts, it flattens downward, increasing the volume of the thoracic cavity, and creates a negative pressure that draws gas into the lungs through the upper airways and trachea. Contraction of external intercostal muscles elevates the anterior portion of the ribs. This increases the volume of the thoracic cavity by increasing its front-to-back (anteroposterior [AP]) diameter. Although the external intercostal muscles may contract during quiet breathing, inspiration at rest usually is assisted by the diaphragm only.

The accessory muscles of inspiration are the sternocleidomastoid and scalene muscles. Like the external intercostal muscles, these muscles enlarge the thorax by increasing its AP diameter. The accessory muscles of inspiration assist inspiration when the minute volume (volume of air inspired and expired per minute) is very high, such as during strenuous exercise or when the work of breathing is increased because of disease. The accessory muscles do not increase the volume of the thorax as efficiently as the diaphragm does.

There are no major muscles of expiration because normal, relaxed expiration is passive and requires no muscular effort. The accessory muscles of expiration, the abdominal and internal intercostal muscles, assist expiration when minute volume is high, during coughing, or when airway obstruction is present. When the abdominal muscles contract, intra-abdominal pressure increases, pushing up the diaphragm and decreasing the volume of the thorax. The internal intercostal muscles pull down the anterior ribs, decreasing the AP diameter of the thorax.

Alveolar Surface Tension. **Surface tension** occurs at any gas-liquid interface and refers to the tendency for liquid molecules that are exposed to air to adhere to one another. This phenomenon can be seen, for example, in a glass of liquid that is about to overflow or in the way liquids "bead" when splashed on a waterproof surface. In both examples this phenomenon decreases the surface area exposed to the air.

Within a sphere, such as an alveolus, surface tension tends to make expansion difficult. According to the law of Laplace, the pressure *(P)* required to inflate a sphere is equal to two times the surface tension *(2T)* divided by the radius *(r)* of the sphere, or $P = 2T/r$.[9] As the radius of the sphere (or alveolus) becomes smaller, more and more pressure is required to inflate it. If the alveoli were lined with a water-like fluid, taking breaths would be extremely difficult.

Alveolar ventilation, or distention, is made possible by surfactant, which lowers the surface tension by coating the air-liquid interface in the alveoli (see Figure 34-3). Surfactant, a lipoprotein (90% lipids and 10% protein) produced by type II alveolar cells, includes two groups of surfactant proteins. One group (SP-B and SP-C) consists of small hydrophobic molecules that have a detergent-like effect that separates the liquid molecules, thereby decreasing alveolar surface tension. The second group (SP-A and SP-D) consists of large hydrophilic molecules called **collectins** (pattern recognition molecules) that are capable of inhibiting foreign pathogens[7a] (see Chapter 7).

Surfactant lines the alveolar side of the alveolocapillary membrane and, in effect, reverses Laplace's law. As the radius of a surfactant-lined sphere (alveolus) grows smaller, the surface tension *decreases,* and as the radius grows larger, the surface tension *increases.* This occurs because the surfactant molecules have much weaker intermolecular attraction compared with the liquid molecules. The surfactant molecules occupy most of the air-fluid interface and disrupt the intermolecular forces that tend to collapse the alveoli. Therefore, the alveoli are much easier to inflate at low lung volumes (i.e., after expiration) than at high volumes (i.e., after inspiration). The decrease in surface tension caused by surfactant also is responsible for keeping the alveoli free of fluid. If surfactant production is disrupted or surfactant is not produced in adequate quantities, alveolar surface tension increases, causing alveolar collapse, decreased lung expansion, increased work of breathing, and severe gas-exchange abnormalities (see What's New? Update on Surfactant and Immunity).

WHAT'S NEW?

Update on Surfactant and Immunity

Surfactant is produced from alveolar type II cells and is a complex molecule made up of glycophospholipid, cholesterol, and protein. Surfactant's primary role is to form a lipid monolayer between the surface of the alveoli and the inspired air and therefore reduce surface tension, preventing expiratory alveolar collapse. More recent investigations have found multiple roles for surfactant in immune function, preventing infection and acting as an antioxidant both in the alveoli and in extrapulmonary mucosal tissues. The protein component of surfactant includes surfactant proteins A, B, C, and D (SP-A, SP-B, SP-C, SP-D). SP-A and SP-D are *collectins,* which are involved in initiating the immune response and clearing pathogens and allergens. SP-A and SP-D appear to decrease the growth of certain bacteria and viruses. SP-A is also called an *opsonin,* which means it makes microorganisms more vulnerable to phagocytosis, including viruses, bacteria, and fungi. SP-D is postulated to activate macrophages and enhance their recognition of pathogens by increasing their cell surface receptors. Both SP-A and SP-D regulate the inflammatory response in the lung, have antioxidant properties, and down-regulate allergic reactions. These findings are leading to exciting developments in the synthesis of therapeutic forms of surfactant that may be useful in treating a broad range of pulmonary disorders.

Data from Glasser JR, Mallampalli RK: *Microbes Infect* 14(1):17–25, 2012; Nayak A et al: *Front Immunol* 3:131, 2012; Silveyra P, Floros J: *Front Biosci* 17:407–429, 2012.

The decrease in surface tension caused by surfactant is also responsible for keeping the alveoli free of fluid. In the absence of surfactant, the surface tension tends to attract fluid into the alveoli. In addition, surfactant participates in host defense against respiratory pathogens.[25]

Elastic Properties of the Lung and Chest Wall. The lung and chest wall have elastic properties that permit expansion during inspiration and return to resting volume during expiration. The elasticity of the lungs is caused both by elastin fibers in the alveolar walls and surrounding the small airways and pulmonary capillaries and by surface tension at the alveolar air-liquid interface.[9] The elasticity of the chest wall is the result of the configuration of its bones and musculature.

Elastic recoil is the tendency of the lungs to return to the resting state after inspiration. Normal elastic recoil permits passive expiration, eliminating the need for major muscles of expiration. Passive elastic recoil may be insufficient during labored breathing (high minute volume), in which case the accessory muscles of expiration may be needed. The accessory muscles also are used if disease comprises elastic recoil (e.g., in emphysema) or blocks the conducting airways.

Normal elastic recoil depends on an equilibrium between opposing forces of recoil in the lungs and chest wall. Under normal conditions the chest wall tends to recoil by expanding outward. This can be observed readily during open heart surgery. When the sternum is split to open the thoracic cavity, the chest wall moves outward laterally. The tendency of the chest wall to recoil by expanding is balanced by the tendency of the lungs to recoil or collapse around the hila. This reaction is caused by elastic recoil and surface tension in the alveoli. The tendency of the lungs to collapse can be demonstrated if the chest is opened without mechanically ventilating the lungs (e.g., at postmortem examination). As the thorax is opened, the lungs immediately collapse, like inflated balloons that have been released. The opposing forces of the chest wall and lungs create, in part, the small negative intrapleural pressure.

Balance between the outward recoil of the chest wall and the inward recoil of the lungs occurs at the resting level, at the end of expiration. During inspiration the diaphragm and intercostal muscles contract, air flows into the lungs, and the chest wall expands. Muscular effort is needed to overcome the resistance of the lungs to expansion. During expiration the muscles relax and the elastic recoil of the lungs causes the thorax to decrease in volume until, once again, balance between the chest wall and lung recoil forces is reached[26] (Figure 34-11).

Compliance is the measure of lung and chest wall distensibility. It represents the relative ease with which these structures can be stretched. Compliance is therefore the reciprocal of elasticity. Compliance is determined by the alveolar surface tension and the elastic recoil of the lung and chest wall. It can be measured with the following formula:

$$C = \frac{\Delta V}{\Delta P}$$

where C = compliance in liters per centimeter of water, ΔV = volume change (usually tidal volume), and ΔP = pressure change (airway or pleural pressure) in centimeters of water.[9]

Increased compliance indicates that the lungs or chest wall is abnormally easy to inflate and has lost some elastic recoil. A decrease indicates that the lungs or chest wall is abnormally stiff or difficult to inflate. Compliance is increased in emphysema and decreased in acute respiratory distress syndrome, pneumonia, pulmonary edema, and fibrosis. (These disorders are described in Chapter 35.)

Airway Resistance. **Airway resistance,** which is similar to resistance to blood flow (described in Chapter 31), is determined by the length, radius, and cross-sectional area of the airways and by the density, viscosity, and velocity of the gas (Poiseuille's law). Resistance is computed by dividing change in pressure *(P)* by rate of flow *(F)*, or $R = P/F$ (Ohm's law), and can easily be measured in the pulmonary function laboratory.[9]

Airway resistance is normally very low. One half to two thirds of total airway resistance occurs in the nose. The next highest resistance is in the oropharynx and larynx. There is very little resistance in the conducting airways of the lungs because of their large cross-sectional area. Resistance increases as the diameter of the airways (total cross-sectional area) decreases; airway resistance increases when the diameter of the airways decreases. **Bronchoconstriction,** which increases airway resistance, can be caused by stimulation of parasympathetic receptors in the bronchial smooth muscle and by numerous irritants and inflammatory mediators.[27]

Bronchodilation, which decreases resistance to airflow, is caused by β_2-adrenergic receptor stimulation. Airway resistance also can be increased by edema of the bronchial mucosa and by airway obstructions such as mucus, tumors, or foreign bodies.

Work of Breathing. The **work of breathing** is determined by the muscular effort (and therefore oxygen and energy) required for ventilation. The work of breathing is normally very low,

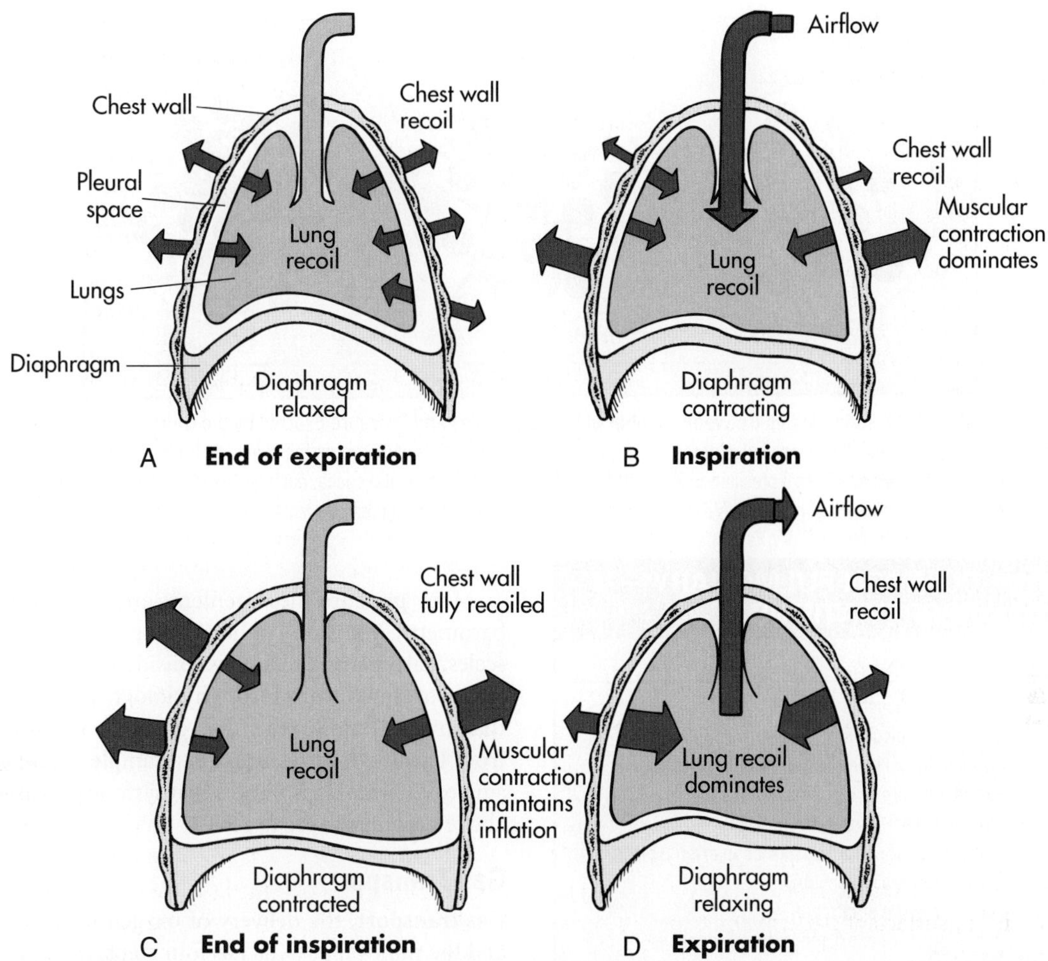

FIGURE 34-11 Interaction of Forces During Inspiration and Expiration. **A,** Outward recoil of the chest wall equals inward recoil of the lungs at the end of expiration. **B,** During inspiration, contraction of respiratory muscles, assisted by chest wall recoil, overcomes tendency of lungs to recoil. **C,** At the end of inspiration, respiratory muscle contraction maintains lung expansion. **D,** During expiration, respiratory muscles relax, allowing elastic recoil of the lungs to deflate the lungs.

but may increase considerably in disease states that disrupt the equilibrium between forces exerted by the lung and chest wall. More muscular effort is required when lung compliance is decreased (e.g., in pulmonary edema), chest wall compliance is decreased (e.g., in spinal deformity or obesity), or airways are obstructed by bronchospasm or mucous plugging (e.g., in asthma or bronchitis).[28] An increase in the work of breathing can result in a marked increase in oxygen consumption and metabolic demand, which can cause significant morbidity in individuals with severe lung disease.

Measurement of Gas Pressure

A gas is made up of millions of molecules moving randomly. As they move, they collide with each other and the wall of the space in which they are contained. These collisions exert pressure. If more molecules are present in the space, the pressure, or number of collisions, increases (Figure 34-12). If the same number of gas molecules is contained in a small and a large container, the pressure is greater in the small container because more collisions occur in the smaller space. Heat increases the speed of the molecules, which increases the number of collisions. Therefore, pressure also increases at higher temperatures.

Barometric pressure (P_B) (atmospheric pressure) is the pressure exerted by gas molecules in air at specific altitudes. At sea level, barometric pressure is 760 mmHg. This number is the sum of the pressure exerted by each gas in the air at sea level. The portion of the total pressure exerted by any individual gas is its **partial pressure** (see Figure 34-12). At sea level the air is made up of oxygen (20.9%), nitrogen (78.1%), and a few other trace gases. The partial pressure of oxygen is equal to the percentage of oxygen in the air (20.9%) times the total pressure (760 mmHg), or 159 mmHg ($760 \times 0.209 = 158.84$). (Symbols used in the measurement of gas pressures and pulmonary ventilation are defined in Table 34-2.)

The amount of water vapor contained in a gas mixture is determined by the temperature of the gas and is unrelated to barometric pressure. Gas that enters the lungs becomes saturated with water vapor (humidified) as it passes through the upper airway. At body temperature (37° C, 98.6° F), water vapor exerts a pressure of 47 mmHg. Because this is true regardless of total (barometric) pressure, the partial pressure of water vapor (always 47 mmHg) must be subtracted from the barometric pressure before the partial pressure of other gases in the mixture can be determined. In saturated

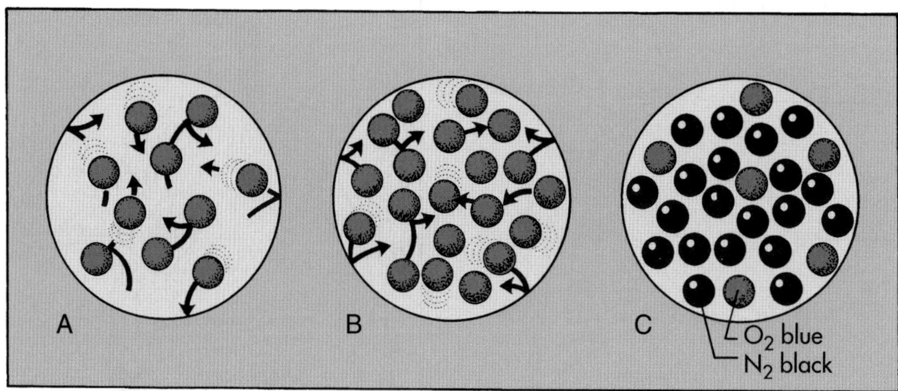

FIGURE 34-12 Relationship Between Number of Gas Molecules and Pressure Exerted by the Gas in an Enclosed Space. A, Theoretically 10 molecules of the same gas exert a total pressure of 10 within the space. **B,** If the number of molecules is increased to 20, total pressure is 20. **C,** If there are different gases in the space, each gas exerts a partial pressure: here the partial pressure of nitrogen *(N_2)* is 18, that of oxygen *(O_2)* is 6, and total pressure is 24.

TABLE 34-2 COMMON PULMONARY ABBREVIATIONS

SYMBOL*	DEFINITION
V	Volume or amount of gas
Q	Perfusion or blood flow
P	Pressure (usually partial pressure) of a gas
Pa_{O_2}	Partial pressure of oxygen in arterial blood
P_{AO_2}	Partial pressure of oxygen in alveolar blood
Pa_{CO_2}	Partial pressure of carbon dioxide in arterial blood
P_{H_2O}	Partial pressure water vapor
P_{N_2}	Partial pressure of nitrogen
$P\bar{v}_{O_2}$	Partial pressure of oxygen in mixed venous or pulmonary artery blood
$P(A-a)_{O_2}$	Difference between alveolar and arterial partial pressure of oxygen (A–a gradient)
P_B	Barometric or atmospheric pressure
Sa_{O_2}	Saturation of hemoglobin (in arterial blood) with oxygen
$S\bar{v}_{O_2}$	Saturation of hemoglobin (in mixed venous blood)
V_A	Alveolar ventilation—effective total lung capacity
V_D	Dead-space ventilation
V_E	Minute capacity
V_T	Tidal volume or average breath
$\dot{V}/\dot{Q}$	Ratio of ventilation to perfusion
Fi_{O_2}	Fraction of inspired oxygen
FRC	Functional residual capacity
FVC	Forced vital capacity
FEV_1	Forced expiratory volume in 1 second
ERV	Expiratory reserve volume
IRC	Inspiratory reserve volume
IC	Inspiratory capacity

From Kacmarek RM, Stoller JK, Jeuer AJ: *Egan's fundamentals of respiratory care,* ed 10, St Louis, 2013, Mosby.
*Subscripts identify the particular gas, volume, or pressure being discussed. A dot, such as above $\dot{V}/\dot{Q}$, means measurement over time, usually 1 minute.

air at sea level, the partial pressure of oxygen is therefore $(760 - 47) \times 0.209 = 149$ mmHg.[9] All pressure and volume measurements made in pulmonary function laboratories specify the temperature and humidity of a gas at the time of measurement.

Many pressure measurements are stated as variations from barometric pressure, rather than percentages of it. On such scales, barometric pressure is considered zero, and pressure varies up or down from zero. Physiologic pressure measurements that involve fluids, rather than gases, are measured as variations from barometric pressure. For example, a systolic blood pressure of 120 mmHg indicates that systolic pressure is 120 mmHg above barometric pressure.

Gas Transport

Gas transport, the delivery of oxygen to the cells of the body and the removal of CO_2, has four steps:

1. Ventilation of the lungs
2. Diffusion of oxygen from the alveoli into the capillary blood
3. Perfusion of systemic capillaries with oxygenated blood
4. Diffusion of oxygen from systemic capillaries into the cells

Steps in the transport of CO_2 occur in reverse order:

1. Diffusion of CO_2 from the cells into the systemic capillaries
2. Perfusion of the pulmonary capillary bed by venous blood
3. Diffusion of CO_2 into the alveoli
4. Removal of CO_2 from the lung by ventilation

If any step in gas transport is impaired by a respiratory or cardiovascular disorder, gas exchange at the cellular level is compromised.

Distribution of Ventilation and Perfusion

Effective gas exchange depends on an approximately even distribution of gas (ventilation) and blood (perfusion) in all portions of the lungs. The lungs are suspended from the hila in the thoracic cavity. When the individual is in an upright position (sitting or standing), gravity pulls the lungs down toward the diaphragm and compresses their lower portions or bases. The alveoli in the upper portions, or apexes, of the lungs contain a greater residual volume of gas and are larger and less numerous than those in the lower portions. Because surface tension increases as the alveoli become larger, the larger alveoli in the upper portions of the lung are more difficult to inflate (less

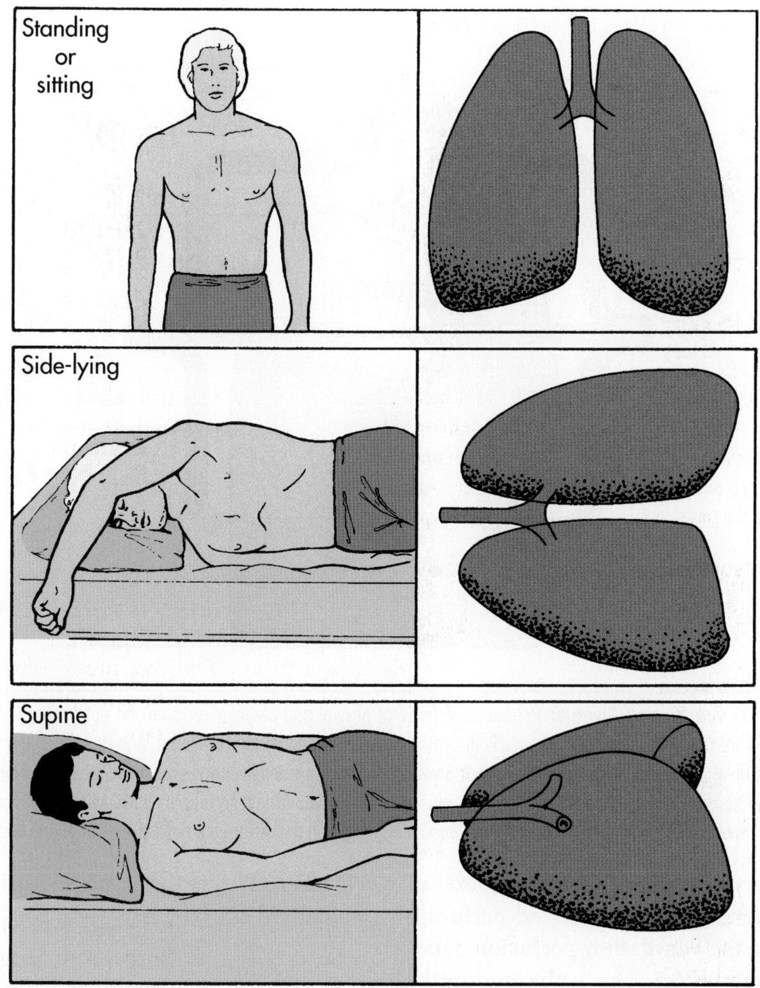

FIGURE 34-13 Pulmonary Blood Flow and Gravity. The greatest volume of pulmonary blood flow will normally occur in the gravity-dependent areas of the lungs. Body position has a significant effect on the distribution of pulmonary blood flow.

compliant) than the smaller alveoli in the lower portions of the lung. Therefore, during ventilation most of the tidal volume is distributed to the bases of the lungs, where compliance is greater.

The heart pumps against gravity to perfuse the pulmonary circulation. As blood is pumped into the lung apexes of a sitting or standing individual, some blood pressure is dissipated in overcoming gravity. As a result, blood pressure at the apexes is lower than that at the bases. Because greater pressure causes greater perfusion, the bases of the lungs are better perfused than the apexes (Figure 34-13). Thus ventilation and perfusion are greatest in the same lung portions: the lower lobes. Ventilation and perfusion depend on body position. If a standing individual assumes a supine or side-lying position, the areas of the lungs that are then most dependent become the best ventilated and perfused.

Distribution of perfusion in the pulmonary circulation also is affected by alveolar pressure (gas pressure in the alveoli). The pulmonary capillary bed differs from the systemic capillary bed in that it is surrounded by gas-containing alveoli. If the gas pressure in the alveoli exceeds the blood pressure in the capillary, the capillary collapses and flow ceases. This is most likely to occur in portions of the lung where blood pressure is lowest and alveolar gas pressure is greatest, that is, the apex of the lung.

The lungs are divided into three zones on the basis of the relationships among all the factors affecting pulmonary blood flow. Alveolar pressure plus the forces of gravity, arterial blood pressure, and venous blood pressure affect the distribution of perfusion (Figure 34-14).

Zone I is where alveolar pressure exceeds pulmonary arterial and venous pressures. The capillary bed collapses, and normal blood flow ceases. Normally zone I is a very small part of the lung at the apex. Zone II is the portion where alveolar pressure is greater than venous pressure, but not greater than arterial pressure. Blood flows through zone II, but it is impeded to a certain extent by alveolar pressure. Zone II is normally above the level of the left atrium. In zone III arterial and venous pressures are greater than alveolar pressure and blood flow is not affected by alveolar pressure. Zone III is in the base of the lung. Blood flow through the pulmonary capillary bed increases in regular increments from the apex to the base.

Although blood flow and ventilation are greater at the base of the lungs than at the apexes, they are not perfectly matched in any of the zones. Perfusion exceeds ventilation in the bases

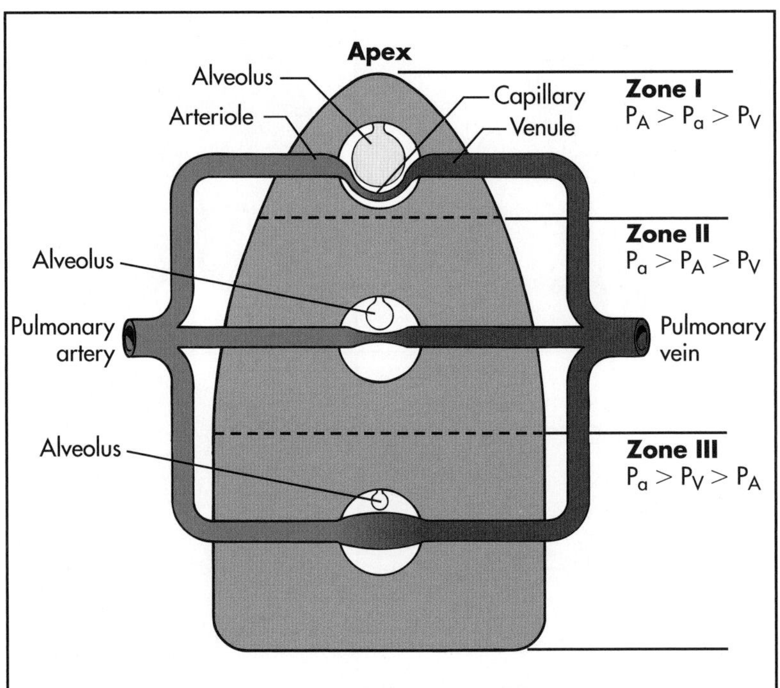

FIGURE 34-14 **Gravity and Alveolar Pressure.** Effects of gravity and alveolar pressure on pulmonary blood flow in the three lung zones. In zone I, alveolar pressure *(P_A)* is greater than arterial and venous pressure, and no blood flow occurs. In zone II, arterial pressure *(P_a)* exceeds alveolar pressure, but alveolar pressure exceeds venous pressure *(P_V)*. Blood flow occurs in this zone, but alveolar pressure compresses the venules (venous ends of the capillaries). In zone III, both arterial and venous pressures are greater than alveolar pressure and blood flow fluctuates, depending on the difference between arterial and venous pressures.

of the lungs, and ventilation exceeds perfusion in the apexes of the lung. The relationship between ventilation and perfusion is expressed as a ratio called the **ventilation-perfusion ratio,** or $\dot{\mathbf{V}}/\dot{\mathbf{Q}}$.[9] The normal $\dot{V}/\dot{Q}$ ratio is 0.8. This is the amount by which perfusion exceeds ventilation under normal conditions.

Oxygen Transport

Approximately 1000 ml (1 L) of oxygen is transported to the cells each minute. Oxygen is transported in the blood in two forms. A small amount dissolves in plasma, and the remainder binds to hemoglobin molecules. Without hemoglobin, oxygen would not reach the cells in amounts sufficient to maintain normal metabolic function. (Hemoglobin is discussed in detail in Chapter 27; cellular metabolism is discussed in Chapter 1.)

Diffusion Across the Alveolocapillary Membrane. The alveolocapillary membrane is the ideal medium for oxygen diffusion, because it has a large total surface area (70 to 100 m^2) and is very thin (0.5 μm). In addition, the partial pressure of oxygen molecules (Po_2) is much greater in alveolar gas than in capillary blood, a condition that promotes rapid diffusion down the concentration gradient from the alveolus into the capillary.[9]

The amount of oxygen in the alveoli (P_{AO_2}) depends on the amount of oxygen in the inspired air and on the amount of air that remains in the alveoli and tracheobronchial tree between breaths (**physiologic dead space**).[9] The P_{AO_2} can be estimated by using the alveolar gas equation:

$$P_{AO_2} = P_{IO_2} - P_{ACO_2}/0.8$$

where P_{IO_2} is the inspired partial pressure of oxygen and is calculated as:

$$P_{IO_2} = (\text{Barometric pressure} - 47) \times F_{IO_2}$$

This value is approximately 104 mmHg at sea level with relaxed breathing; therefore a pressure gradient of approximately 60 mmHg facilitates the diffusion of oxygen from the alveolus into the capillary (Figure 34-15). Different values for P_{AO_2} can be calculated if there are changes in the inspired oxygen content or the $Paco_2$, which are common occurrences in clinical settings.

Blood remains in the pulmonary capillary for about 0.75 second, but only 0.25 second is required for oxygen concentration to equilibrate (equalize) across the alveolocapillary membrane.[9] Therefore, oxygen has ample time to diffuse into the blood, even during increased cardiac output, which speeds blood flow, shortening the time the blood remains in the capillary.

Determinants of Arterial Oxygenation. As oxygen diffuses across the alveolocapillary membrane, it dissolves in the plasma, where it exerts pressure (the partial pressure of oxygen in arterial blood, or Pao_2). As the Pao_2 increases, oxygen moves from the plasma into the red blood cells (erythrocytes) and binds with hemoglobin molecules. Oxygen continues to bind with hemoglobin until the hemoglobin binding sites are filled or saturated. Oxygen then continues to diffuse across the alveolocapillary membrane until the Pao_2 and P_{AO_2} equilibrate, eliminating the pressure gradient across the alveolocapillary membrane. At this point diffusion ceases (see Figure 34-15).

Normally approximately 20 ml of oxygen is transported per 100 ml of blood. Because oxygen is not very soluble in plasma, most of the oxygen molecules bind with hemoglobin. Plasma

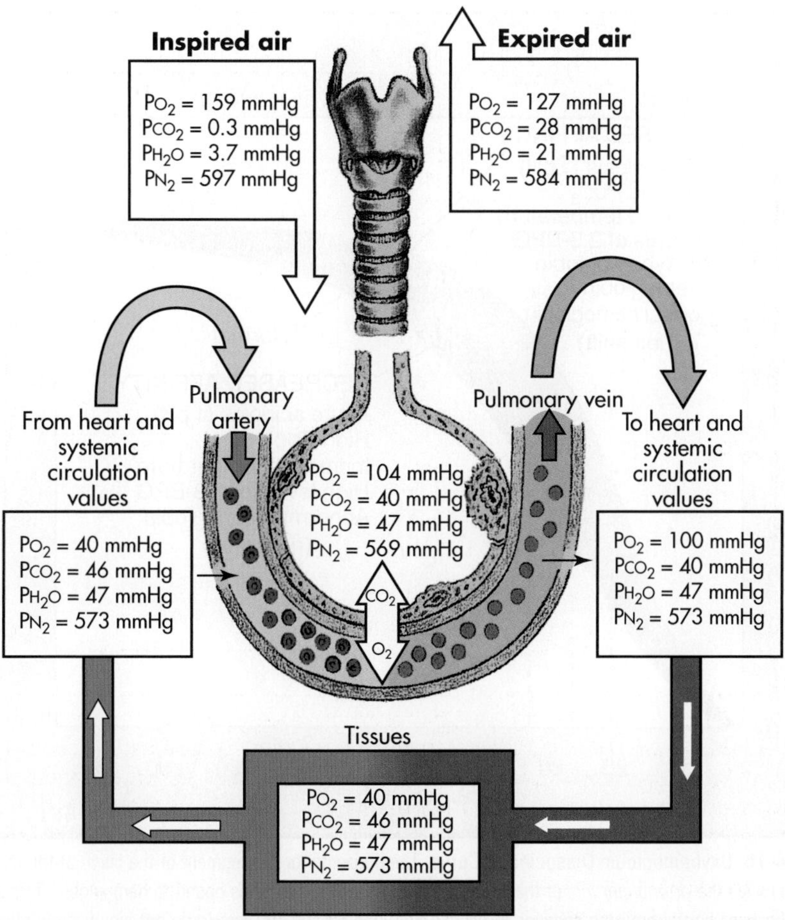

FIGURE 34-15 **Partial Pressure of Respiratory Gases in Normal Respiration.** These are average values. The values of Po_2, Pco_2, and PN_2 fluctuate from breath to breath. *CO_2*, Carbon dioxide; *O_2*, oxygen; *Pco_2*, partial pressure of carbon dioxide; *PH_2O*, partial *pressure* of water; *PN_2*, partial pressure of nitrogen; *Po_2*, partial pressure of oxygen.

level). Although the remaining 19.7 ml is carried by hemoglobin, it is the small amount of oxygen dissolved in plasma that is responsible for oxygen's partial pressure (Pao_2) in the blood.

Although Pao_2 is important in that it provides the driving pressure that loads the hemoglobin with oxygen, it gives little information about the *amount* of oxygen carried in the blood. This amount, which is measured in milliliters per deciliter (1 dl = 100 ml) of blood, is the **oxygen content** of the blood. The total oxygen content of the blood depends on the amount of oxygen chemically combined with hemoglobin, as well as that dissolved in the blood. To calculate the total arterial oxygen content, we must know (1) hemoglobin concentration, or the amount of hemoglobin that is available to bind with oxygen (hemoglobin [Hb] in grams per deciliter); (2) the oxygen saturation or percentage of available hemoglobin that is bound to oxygen (Sao_2); and (3) the partial pressure of oxygen (Pao_2). The maximum amount of oxygen that can be transported by hemoglobin is 1.34 ml/g. The amount of oxygen that can be physically dissolved in blood is 0.003 ml/dl per mmHg. If these specific values are known, the oxygen content of arterial blood can be calculated.[9] To calculate the oxygen content of venous blood, the partial pressure of mixed venous blood (Pvo_2) and venous oxygen saturation (Svo_2) are substituted for the arterial values in the basic formula. Normal venous oxygen content is 15 to 16 ml/dl.

Because hemoglobin transports all but a small fraction of the oxygen carried in arterial blood, increases in hemoglobin concentration affect the oxygen content of the blood. Decreases in hemoglobin concentration below the normal value of 15 ml/dl of blood reduce oxygen content, and increases in hemoglobin concentration may minimize the effect of impaired gas exchange. In fact, an increase in hemoglobin concentration is a major compensatory mechanism in pulmonary diseases that impair gas exchange. For this reason, measurement of hemoglobin concentration is important in assessing individuals with pulmonary disease. If cardiovascular function is normal, the body's initial response to low oxygen content is to accelerate cardiac output. In individuals who also have cardiovascular disease, this compensatory mechanism does not work, making increased hemoglobin concentration an even more important compensatory mechanism. (Hemoglobin structure and function are described in Chapter 27.)

Oxyhemoglobin Association and Dissociation. When hemoglobin molecules bind with oxygen, **oxyhemoglobin (HbO_2)** is formed. Binding occurs in the lungs and is called *oxyhemoglobin association* or *hemoglobin saturation with oxygen*

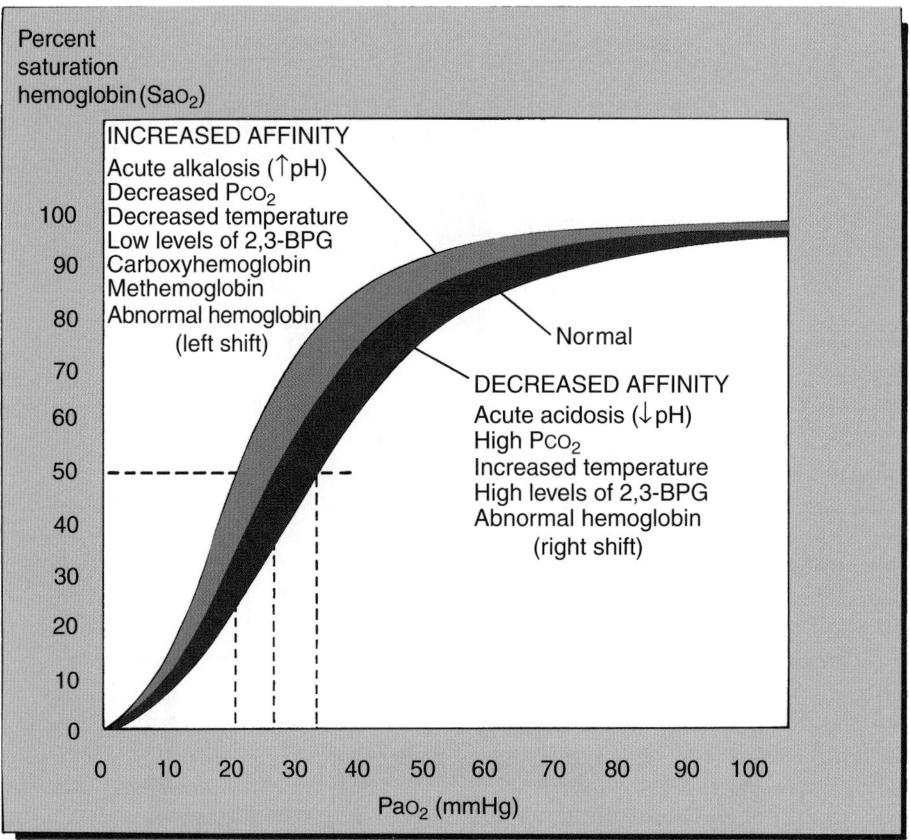

FIGURE 34-16 Oxyhemoglobin Dissociation Curve. The horizontal or flat segment of the curve at the top of the graph is sometimes called the *arterial portion,* or that part of the curve where oxygen is bound to hemoglobin. This portion of the curve is flat because partial pressure changes of oxygen between 60 and 100 mmHg do not significantly alter the percent saturation of hemoglobin with oxygen. The wide range of partial pressures of oxygen (Pao_2 of 60 to 100 mmHg), represented by the flat part of the curve, allows adequate hemoglobin saturation at a variety of *altitudes.* For example, a Pao_2 of 100 mmHg at sea level results in a hemoglobin saturation with oxygen of 98%. At an altitude of 5000 feet the Pao_2 is about 70 mmHg and hemoglobin saturation is 94%, only 4% less than at sea level. If the relationship between Sao_2 and Pao_2 were linear (in a downward-sloping straight line) instead of flat between 60 and 100 mmHg, there would be inadequate saturation of hemoglobin with oxygen. For example, with a Pao_2 of 70 mmHg the saturation would be only 70%, which is equivalent to normal venous oxygen saturation, and life could not be sustained at altitudes much higher than sea level. The steep part of the oxyhemoglobin dissociation curve occurs after the Pao_2 drops below 60 mmHg and represents the rapid dissociation of oxygen from hemoglobin. During this phase oxygen diffuses rapidly from the blood into tissue cells. Conditions associated with altered affinity of hemoglobin for O_2 are listed. P_{50} is the Pao_2 at which hemoglobin is 50% saturated, normally 26.6 mmHg. A lower than normal P_{50} represents increased affinity of hemoglobin for O_2; a high P_{50} is seen with decreased affinity. Note that variation from the normal is associated with decreased (low P_{50}) or increased (high P_{50}) availability of O_2 to tissues *(dashed lines).* The *shaded area* shows the entire oxyhemoglobin dissociation curve under the same circumstances. *2,3-BPG,* 2,3-Biphosphoglycerate. (From Lane EE, Walker JF: *Clinical arterial blood gas analysis,* St Louis, 1987, Mosby.)

(Sao_2). The reverse process, in which oxygen is released from hemoglobin, occurs in the body tissues at the cellular level and is called *hemoglobin desaturation.* When hemoglobin saturation and desaturation are plotted on a graph, the result is a distinctive S-shaped curve known as the **oxyhemoglobin dissociation curve** (Figure 34-16).

Several factors can change the relationship between Pao_2 and Sao_2, causing the oxyhemoglobin dissociation curve to shift to the right or left (see Figure 34-16). A shift to the right depicts hemoglobin's decreased affinity for oxygen or an increase in the ease with which oxyhemoglobin dissociates and oxygen moves into the cells. A shift to the left depicts hemoglobin's increased affinity for oxygen, which promotes association in the lungs and inhibits dissociation in the tissues.

The oxyhemoglobin dissociation curve is shifted to the right by acidosis (low pH) and hypercapnia (increased $Paco_2$). In the tissues the increased levels of CO_2 and hydrogen ions produced by metabolic activity decrease the affinity of hemoglobin for oxygen. The curve is shifted to the left by alkalosis (high pH) and hypocapnia (decreased $Paco_2$). In the lungs, as CO_2 diffuses from the blood into the alveoli, the blood CO_2 level is reduced and the affinity of hemoglobin for oxygen is increased. The shift in the oxyhemoglobin dissociation curve caused by changes in CO_2 and hydrogen ion concentration in the blood is called the **Bohr effect.**[9]

The oxyhemoglobin curve is shifted also by changes in body temperature and increased or decreased levels of 2,3-biphosphoglycerate (2,3-BPG), a substance normally present in erythrocytes. Hyperthermia and increased 2,3-BPG levels shift the curve to the right. Hypothermia and decreased 2,3-BPG levels shift the curve to the left.

Carbon Dioxide Transport

Approximately 200 ml of CO_2 is produced by the tissues per minute as a byproduct of cellular metabolism. This CO_2 equilibrates with carbonic acid ($H_2O + CO_2 \rightleftharpoons H_2CO_3 \rightleftharpoons H + HCO_3^-$) and must be eliminated continuously to prevent acidosis. The elimination of CO_2 by the lungs plays an important role in the regulation of acid-base balance (see Chapter 3).

CO_2 is carried in the blood in three ways: (1) dissolved in plasma, (2) as bicarbonate, and (3) as carbamino compounds. As CO_2 diffuses out of the cells into the blood, it dissolves in the plasma. Approximately 10% of the total CO_2 in venous blood and 5% of the CO_2 in arterial blood are carried dissolved in the plasma. As CO_2 moves into the blood, it diffuses into the red blood cells. Within the red blood cells, CO_2, with the help of the enzyme carbonic anhydrase, combines with water to form carbonic acid and then quickly dissociates into H^+ and HCO_3^-. As carbonic acid dissociates, the H^+ binds to hemoglobin, where it is buffered, and the HCO_3^- moves out of the red blood cell into the plasma. Approximately 60% of the CO_2 in venous blood and 90% of the CO_2 in arterial blood are carried in the form of bicarbonate. The remainder combines with blood proteins, hemoglobin in particular, to form carbamino compounds (see Figure 3-12). Approximately 30% of the CO_2 in venous blood and 5% of the CO_2 in arterial blood are carried as carbamino compounds.[9]

CO_2 is 20 times more soluble than O_2 and diffuses quickly from the tissue cells into the blood.[9] The amount of CO_2 that is able to enter the blood is enhanced by diffusion of oxygen out of the blood and into the cells. Reduced hemoglobin (hemoglobin that is dissociated from oxygen) is able to carry more CO_2 than hemoglobin that is saturated with O_2. Therefore, the drop in Sao_2 at the tissue level increases the ability of hemoglobin to carry CO_2 back to the lung.

The diffusion gradient for CO_2 in the lung is only approximately 6 mmHg (venous $Pvco_2$ = 46 mmHg; alveolar $PACO_2$ = 40 mmHg), yet CO_2 is so soluble in the alveolocapillary membrane that the CO_2 in the blood quickly diffuses into the alveoli, where it is removed from the lung with each expiration.[9] Diffusion of CO_2 in the lung is so efficient that diffusion defects that cause hypoxemia (low oxygen content of the blood) do not cause hypercapnia (excessive CO_2 in the blood).

The diffusion of CO_2 out of the blood also is enhanced by oxygen binding with hemoglobin in the lung. As hemoglobin binds with O_2, the amount of CO_2 carried by the blood is decreased. Thus in the tissue capillaries, O_2 dissociation from hemoglobin facilitates the pickup of CO_2, and the binding of O_2 to hemoglobin in the lungs facilitates the release of CO_2 from the blood. This effect of oxygen on CO_2 transport is called the **Haldane effect** and can have significant clinical implications for the management of lung disease.[29,30]

TESTS OF PULMONARY FUNCTION

Several laboratory tests aid in the diagnosis and evaluation of pulmonary system abnormalities. Most of them are easy to perform at hospitals and clinics. They provide valuable information about the possible cause of a respiratory abnormality and evaluate the progression or resolution of disease.

Spirometry is used to measure forced expiration, which often is affected by diffuse pulmonary disease. Because the pulmonary system has remarkable reserves, disease may become well established before clinical manifestations appear. Spirometry enables clinicians to detect restrictive or obstructive deficits early in the course of disease. Restrictive lung diseases restrict the lungs' volume: the lungs are unable to expand normally, diminishing the amount of gas that can be inspired. Obstructive diseases affect gas flow: airflow into and out of the lungs is obstructed.

Spirometry measures both volume and flow. The test is performed with a spirometer, which is a water-filled cylinder into which an inverted cylinder or bell has been inserted. A length of tubing runs from the inverted bell to a mouthpiece through which a person breathes during testing. The bell is attached to a pen that writes on calibrated paper rotating at a constant speed. As a person performs various breathing maneuvers, the inverted bell moves up and down, causing the pen to move on the calibrated paper. This produces a spirogram, which is a record of the individual's ventilation in relation to time (Figure 34-17). Clinically the most important spirometric tests are the forced vital capacity (FVC) and the forced expiratory volume in 1 second (FEV_1).[31] (These tests and other important measures are described in Table 34-3.)

Lung capacities, such as vital capacity and total lung capacity, are always the sum of two or more volumes. Norms for volumes and capacities are based on age, gender, and height and are referred to as *predicted values.* Changes from predicted or baseline values are taken into account in diagnosing and assessing respiratory disorders.

Diffusing capacity is a measure of the rate of gas diffusion across the alveolocapillary membrane. Oxygen, or more commonly carbon monoxide, is used to measure diffusing capacity. The measurement is made by determining how much carbon monoxide is taken up by the blood and dividing this amount by the pressure gradient across the alveolocapillary membrane. Helium often is added to the gas mixture to obtain a simultaneous measurement of **residual volume (RV), functional reserve capacity (FRC),** and **total lung capacity (TLC).** Individuals are asked to perform ventilatory maneuvers similar to those of spirometry. A decreased diffusing capacity can be the result of an abnormal ventilation-perfusion ratio or an actual diffusion defect. Diffusing capacity is decreased in individuals with emphysema.

Arterial blood gas analysis commonly is performed for individuals with suggested or diagnosed pulmonary disease. Direct analysis of the pH and gas concentrations in arterial blood provides valuable information about an individual's gas exchange and acid-base status. Acidosis (low pH), alkalosis (high pH), ventilatory alterations, and decreased Pao_2 can be diagnosed accurately only by arterial blood gas analysis. A blood gas report may be divided into an acid-base/ventilation portion and an oxygenation portion. (Normal values for arterial blood gases are given in Table 34-4; acid-base alterations are described in Chapter 3.) Oximetry can be used to monitor oxygen saturation

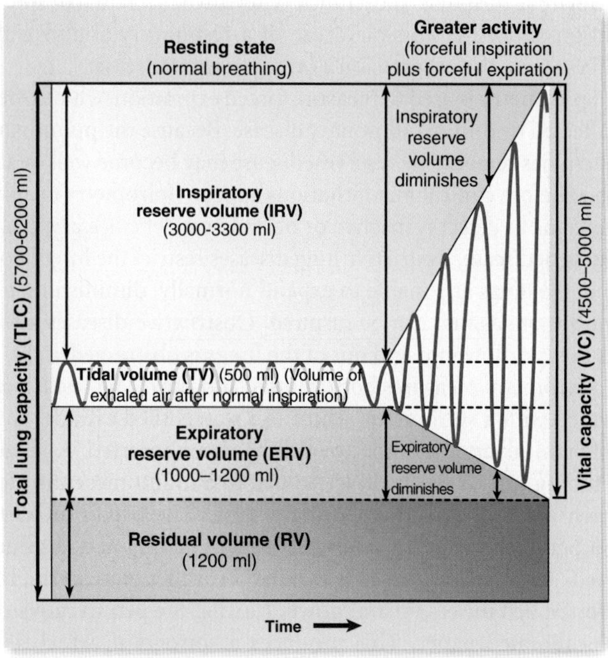

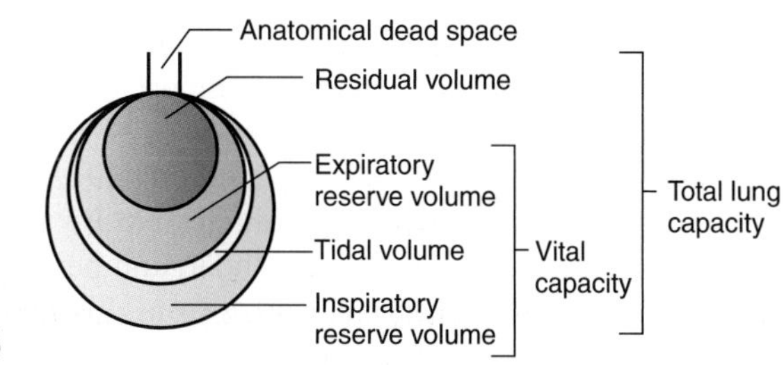

FIGURE 34-17 Pulmonary Ventilation and Lung Capacities. **A,** Spirogram. During normal, quiet respirations the atmosphere and lungs exchange about 500 ml of air (V_T). With a forcible inspiration, about 3300 ml more air can be inhaled *(IRV)*. After a normal inspiration and normal expiration, approximately 1000 ml more air can be forcibly expired *(ERV)*. Vital capacity is the amount of air that can be forcibly expired after a maximal inspiration and indicates, therefore, the largest amount of air that can enter and leave the lungs during respiration. Residual volume *(RV)* is the air that remains trapped in the alveoli. **B,** Lung capacities. (From Patton KT, Thibodeau GA: *Anatomy & physiology*, ed 8, St Louis, 2013, Mosby.)

once the arterial blood gas analysis has accurately measured the $Pa{O_2}$, but it does not measure $Pa{CO_2}$ or pH.

Signs and symptoms of most respiratory abnormalities first appear when the system is stressed during exercise. Therefore, if pulmonary disease is suspected, the individual is evaluated at rest and during exercise. During exercise the usual procedures are spirometry and withdrawal of arterial blood for gas analysis. The exercise usually consists of riding a stationary bicycle or walking on a treadmill. Exercise testing enables clinicians to detect early changes in respiratory function and thus begin treatment. Exercise tests also are used in planning and evaluating exercise and rehabilitation programs.

Chest radiographs are among the most common examinations of the pulmonary system. A few of the abnormalities detected in chest radiographs are air trapping in the alveoli and airways (e.g., in asthma or emphysema), consolidation of lung tissue (e.g., in pneumonia or pulmonary edema), cavities (e.g., abscesses or tuberculosis), and nodules (e.g., lung cancer). Often pulmonary abnormalities are detected in routine chest radiographs of asymptomatic individuals. Various radiographic techniques are available for the diagnosis and evaluation of respiratory disorders.

TABLE 34-3 VALUES MEASURED BY SPIROMETRY

SYMBOL	VENTILATORY PROPERTY MEASURED
FVC	Forced vital capacity: maximum amount of gas that can be displaced from the lung during a forced expiration
FEV_1	Forced expiratory volume in 1 second: maximum amount of air that can be expired from the lung in 1 second
FEV_1/FVC	Percentage of maximum inspiration that is expired in 1 second, usually 80% of FVC
FEV_3	Forced expiratory volume in 3 seconds; maximum amount of gas that can be expired in 3 seconds
FEV_3/FVC	Percentage of FVC that is expired in 3 seconds; usually 95% of FVC
$FEF_{25\%-75\%}$	Forced expiratory flow rate during the middle 50% of expiration; sometimes reported as maximum midexpiratory flow rate (MMFR)

AGING AND THE PULMONARY SYSTEM

Most knowledge about pulmonary structure and function is based on norms for the middle years. Less is known about structure and function in the very young (see Chapter 36) and older adults, but a few normal physiologic (developmental and degenerative) changes are known to occur from birth to old age. An understanding of these changes is needed to provide appropriate care and to differentiate between normal alterations and disease. Normal alterations include: (1) loss of elastic recoil, (2) stiffening of the chest wall, (3) changes in gas exchange, and (4) increases in flow resistance (Figure 34-18). These changes are gradual and usually without adverse consequences in healthy individuals. They are influenced by environmental and sociocultural factors, nutritional status, respiratory disease, body size, gender, and race.[32-34]

During adulthood and as age advances, the alveoli tend to lose alveoli wall tissue and capillaries. This process diminishes alveolar surface area available for gas diffusion and decreases airway support provided by normal lung tissues. Mechanical changes involve elastic properties of the lungs and chest wall. Chest wall compliance decreases with age, because the ribs become ossified (less flexible) and joints become stiffer. As a result the chest wall loses some of its ability to expand. In addition, respiratory muscle strength and endurance decrease by up to 20% by age 70.[33] These mechanical changes in the lung and chest wall, along with structural changes in the alveoli, reduce ventilatory capacity in older adults.[35] Vital capacity decreases and residual volume increases; however, total lung capacity remains unchanged. These changes decrease ventilatory reserves and lead to decreased ventilation-perfusion ratios. With advancing

TABLE 34-4 NORMAL RANGES FOR ARTERIAL AND MIXED VENOUS BLOOD GASES

MEASUREMENT	ARTERIAL BLOOD	MIXED VENOUS BLOOD*	CLINICAL NOTES
Acid-base status (pH)	7.35-7.45	7.33-7.43	Most important acid-base value; detects acidosis or alkalosis
Partial pressure of carbon dioxide (Pco_2)	35-45 mmHg	41-57 mmHg	Measures adequacy of ventilation and respiratory contribution of acid-base abnormality (respiratory acidosis)
Bicarbonate (HCO^-_3)	22-26 mEq/L	24-28 mEq/L	Measures metabolic contribution to acid-base abnormality (metabolic acidosis); calculated from pH and Pco_2
Base excess (BE)	−2 to +2	0 to +4	Reflects deviation of bicarbonate concentration from normal
Partial pressure of oxygen (Po_2) (sea level)	80-100 mmHg	35-40 mmHg	Indicates driving pressure that causes oxyhemoglobin binding; varies with age and barometric pressure
Saturation of hemoglobin with oxygen (So_2)	96-98%	70-75%	Indicates abnormalities of oxyhemoglobin association and dissociation; may be measured directly or calculated from Pco_2, pH, and body temperature
Concentration of hemoglobin in the blood	15 g/dl	15 g/dl	Detects alterations of gas transport caused by anemia

*Mixed venous (pulmonary artery) blood is analyzed for critically ill individuals and those undergoing cardiac catheterization (it is not practical to withdraw samples except from a pulmonary artery catheter). Mixed venous blood gas analysis, in conjunction with arterial analysis, provides important information about the adequacy of cardiac output and tissue oxygenation.

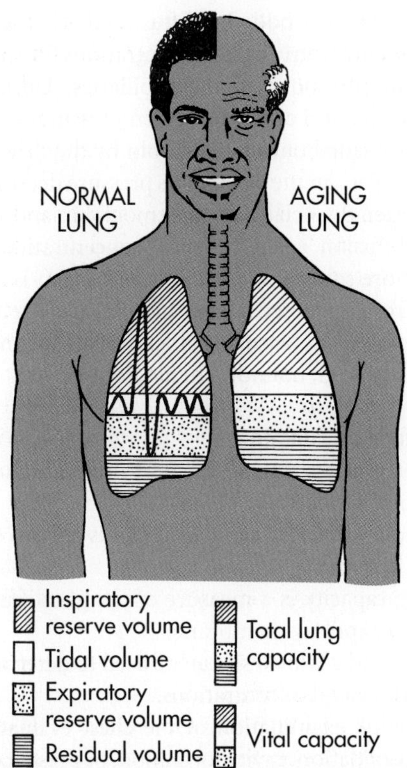

FIGURE 34-18 Changes in Lung Volumes with Aging. With aging, note particularly the decrease in vital capacity and the increase in residual volume.

age there is also increased immune dysregulation, asymptomatic low-grade inflammation, and increased risk of infection.[33,36-39]

Alterations in gas exchange are reflected by blood gas analysis. With advancing age, pH and $Paco_2$ do not change much, even though it has been documented that the chemoreceptors become less sensitive to gas partial pressures with age.[40] Older adults have a decreased compensatory response to hypercapnia and hypoxemia; however, the perception of dyspnea remains intact and is even enhanced. Pao_2 declines with age as a result of structural and mechanical changes, such as loss of alveolar surface area and increased ventilation-perfusion mismatch. The maximum Pao_2 in an older adult at sea level can be estimated by multiplying the person's age by 0.3 and subtracting the product from 100. For example, an 80-year-old individual would have an estimated maximum Pao_2 of 76 mmHg ($0.3 \times 80 = 24$; $100 - 24 = 76$).[41] There is also a decrease in the capillary network.

The decrease in Pao_2 and diminished ventilatory reserve in an older adult lead to a decrease in exercise tolerance. Respiratory muscle strength and endurance decrease with age.[39] Furthermore, older adults are at greater risk for respiratory depression caused by medications. Changes in respiratory structure and function can vary considerably from person to person, however. Changes also are affected by activity and fitness earlier in life. A very active, physically fit individual will, all else being equal, have fewer changes in function at any age than one who has been sedentary.

SUMMARY REVIEW

Structures of the Pulmonary System

1. The pulmonary system consists of the lungs, airways, chest wall, diaphragm, and pulmonary and bronchial circulation.
2. Air is inspired and expired through the conducting airways, which include the nasopharynx, oropharynx, trachea, bronchi, and bronchioles to the sixteenth division.
3. Gas exchange occurs in structures beyond the sixteenth division: the respiratory bronchioles, alveolar ducts, and alveoli. Together these structures comprise the acinus.
4. The chief gas-exchange units of the lungs are the alveoli. The membrane that surrounds each alveolus and contains the pulmonary capillaries is called the *alveolocapillary membrane.*

SUMMARY REVIEW—cont'd

5. The gas-exchange airways are served by the pulmonary circulation, a separate division of the circulatory system. The bronchi and other lung structures are served by a branch of the systemic circulation called the *bronchial circulation.*
6. The pulmonary circulation is innervated by the ANS, but vasodilation and vasoconstriction are controlled mainly by local and humoral factors, particularly arterial oxygenation and acid-base status.
7. Vasoconstriction of the pulmonary arterial system is caused by alveolar hypoxia, acidemia, and inflammatory mediators (histamine, serotonin, prostaglandins, and bradykinin).
8. The chest wall, which contains and protects the contents of the thoracic cavity, consists of the skin, ribs, and intercostal muscles, which lie between the ribs.
9. The chest wall is lined by a serous membrane called the *parietal pleura;* the lungs are encased in a separate membrane called the *visceral pleura.* The area where these two pleurae come into contact and slide over each another is called the *pleural space.*

Functions of the Pulmonary System

1. The pulmonary system enables oxygen to diffuse into the blood and CO_2 to diffuse out of the blood.
2. Ventilation is the process by which air flows into and out of the gas-exchange airways.
3. Ventilation is involuntary most of the time. It is controlled by the respiratory center in the brainstem and by the sympathetic and parasympathetic divisions of the ANS, which adjust airway caliber (by causing bronchial smooth muscle to contract or relax) and control the rate and depth of ventilation.
4. Neuroreceptors in the lungs (lung receptors) monitor the mechanical aspects of ventilation. Irritant receptors sense the need to expel unwanted substances, stretch receptors sense lung volume (lung expansion), and *J*-receptors sense alveolar size.
5. Chemoreceptors in the circulatory system and brainstem sense the effectiveness of ventilation by monitoring the pH status of cerebrospinal fluid and the oxygen content of arterial blood (Pao_2).
6. Successful ventilation involves the mechanics of breathing: the interaction of forces and counterforces involving the muscles of inspiration and expiration, alveolar surface tension, elastic properties of the lungs and chest wall, and resistance to airflow.
7. The major muscle of inspiration is the diaphragm. When the diaphragm contracts, it moves downward in the thoracic cavity, creating a vacuum that causes air to flow into the lungs.
8. The alveoli produce surfactant, produced by type II alveolar cells. It is a lipoprotein that lines the alveoli. Surfactant reduces alveolar surface tension and permits the alveoli to expand more easily with air intake.
9. Compliance is the ability of the lungs and chest wall to expand during inspiration. Lung compliance is ensured by adequate production of surfactant; chest wall expansion depends on flexibility.
10. Elastic recoil is the tendency of the lungs and chest wall to return to their resting state after inspiration. The elastic recoil forces of the lungs and chest wall are in opposition and pull on each other, creating the normally negative pressure of the pleural space.
11. Gas transport depends on ventilation of the alveoli, diffusion across the alveolocapillary membrane, perfusion of the pulmonary and systemic capillaries, and diffusion between systemic capillaries and tissue cells.
12. Efficient gas exchange depends on an even distribution of ventilation and perfusion within the lungs. Ventilation and perfusion are greatest in the bases of the lungs because the alveoli in the bases are more compliant (their resting volume is low), and perfusion is greater in the bases as a result of gravity.
13. Almost all of the oxygen that diffuses into pulmonary capillary blood is transported by hemoglobin, a protein contained within red blood cells. The remainder of the oxygen is transported dissolved in plasma.
14. Oxygen enters the body by diffusing down the concentration gradient, from high concentrations in the alveoli to lower concentrations in the capillaries. Diffusion ceases when alveolar and capillary oxygen pressures equilibrate.
15. Oxygen is loaded onto hemoglobin by the driving pressure exerted by Pao_2 in the plasma. As pressure decreases at tissue level, oxygen dissociates from hemoglobin and enters tissue cells by diffusion, again down the concentration gradient.
16. CO_2 is more soluble in plasma than oxygen is and diffuses readily from tissue cells into plasma. CO_2 returns to the lungs dissolved in plasma, as bicarbonate, or in carbamino compounds (e.g., bound to hemoglobin).

Tests of Pulmonary Function

1. Spirometry measures volume and flow rate during forced expiration.
2. The alveolar-arterial oxygen gradient is used to evaluate the cause of hypoxia.
3. Diffusing capacity is a measure of the gas diffusion rate at the alveolocapillary membrane.
4. Arterial blood gas analysis can be used to determine pH and oxygen and CO_2 concentrations.
5. Radiographic examination of the chest evaluates air trapping, consolidation, cavity formation, or presence of tumors.

Aging and the Pulmonary System

1. Aging affects the mechanical aspects of ventilation by decreasing chest wall compliance and elastic recoil of the lungs. Changes in these elastic properties reduce ventilatory reserve.
2. Aging causes the Pao_2 to decrease but does not affect the $Paco_2$.

KEY TERMS

Acinus, 1229
Airway resistance, 1236
Alveolar duct, 1229
Alveolar ventilation, 1232
Alveoli (*sing.*, alveolus), 1229
Alveolocapillary membrane, 1230
Arterial blood gas analysis, 1243
Bohr effect, 1242
Bronchiole, 1228
Bronchoconstriction, 1236
Bronchodilation, 1236
Bronchus (*pl.*, bronchi), 1228
Carina, 1228
Central chemoreceptor, 1234
Chest radiograph, 1244
Collectin, 1235
Compliance, 1236
Diaphragm, 1231
Diffusing capacity, 1243
Elastic recoil, 1236
Functional reserve capacity (FRC), 1243
Gas transport, 1238
Goblet cell, 1229
Haldane effect, 1243
Hilus (*pl.*, hila), 1228
Hypoxic pulmonary vasoconstriction, 1231
Irritant receptor, 1234
J-receptor, 1234
Larynx, 1226
Minute volume (minute ventilation), 1232
Nasopharynx, 1225
Oropharynx, 1225
Oxygen content, 1241
Oxyhemoglobin (HbO_2), 1241
Oxyhemoglobin dissociation curve, 1242
Partial pressure (of a gas), 1237
Peripheral chemoreceptor, 1233, 1234
Physiologic dead space, 1240
Pleura (*pl.*, pleurae), 1231
Pleural space (pleural cavity), 1231
Pulmonary artery, 1229
Pulmonary capillary, 1229
Pulmonary lymphatic capillary, 1230
Pulmonary vein, 1230
Rapidly adapting receptor (RAR), 1234
Residual volume (RV), 1243
Respiration, 1232
Respiratory bronchiole, 1229
Respiratory center, 1233
Spirometry, 1243
Stretch receptor, 1234
Surface tension, 1235
Surfactant, 1229
Thoracic cavity, 1231
Total lung capacity (TLC), 1243
Trachea, 1228
Ventilation, 1232
Ventilation-perfusion ratio ($\dot{V}/\dot{Q}$), 1240
Work of breathing, 1236

REFERENCES

1. McCulloch TM, Van Daele D, Ciucci MR: Otolaryngology head and neck surgery: an integrative view of the larynx, *Head Neck* 33(Suppl 1):S46–S53, 2011.
2. Barash PG et al: *Clinical anesthesia*, ed 6, Philadelphia, 2009, Lippincott Williams & Wilkins.
3. Vareille M et al: The airway epithelium: soldier in the fight against respiratory viruses, *Clin Microbiol Rev* 24(1):210–229, 2011.
4. Barrett KE et al: *Ganong's review of medical physiology*, ed 24, Philadelphia, 2012, McGraw-Hill.
5. Corrin B, Nicholson A: *Pathology of the lungs*, ed 3, London, 2011, Churchill Livingstone.
6. Ochs MD et al: The number of alveoli in the human lung, *Am J Respir Crit Care Med* 169:120–124, 2004.
7. Raghavendran K, Willson D, Notter RH: Surfactant therapy for acute lung injury and acute respiratory distress syndrome, *Crit Care Clin* 27(3):525–559, 2011.

7a. Nayak A et al: An insight into the diverse roles of surfactant proteins, SP-A and SP-D in innate and adaptive immunity, *Front Immunol* 3:131, 2012.

8. Miyata R, van Eeden SF: The innate and adaptive immune response induced by alveolar macrophages exposed to ambient particulate matter, *Toxicol Appl Pharmacol* 257(2):209–226, 2011.
9. Kacmarek RM, Stoller JK, Jeuer AJ: *Egan's fundamentals of respiratory care*, ed 10, St Louis, 2013, Mosby.
10. Osiro S et al: A friend to the airways: a review of the emerging clinical importance of the bronchial arterial circulation, *Surg Radiol Anat* 34(9):791–798, 2012.
11. Sylvester JT et al: Hypoxic pulmonary vasoconstriction, *Physiol Rev* 92(1):367–520, 2012.
12. Housley GD: Recent insights into the regulation of breathing, *Auton Neurosci* 164(1-2):3–5, 2011.
13. Moreira TS et al: Central chemoreceptors and neural mechanisms of cardiorespiratory control, *Braz J Med Biol Res* 44(9):883–889, 2011.
14. Ramirez JM et al: The role of spiking and bursting pacemakers in the neuronal control of breathing, *J Biol Phys* 37(3):241–261, 2011.
15. Smith JC et al: Structural and functional architecture of respiratory networks in the mammalian brainstem, *Philos Trans R Soc Lond B Biol Sci* 364(1529):2577–2587, 2009.
16. Spyer KM, Gourine AV: Chemosensory pathways in the brainstem controlling cardiorespiratory activity, *Philos Trans R Soc Lond B Biol Sci* 364(1529):2603–2610, 2009.
17. Landolfo F et al: Hering-Breuer reflex, lung volume and position in prematurely born infants, *Pediatr Pulmonol* 43(8):767–771, 2008.
18. Canning BJ: Anatomy and neurophysiology of the cough reflex, *Chest* 129:33s–47s, 2006.
19. Anand A, Srivastava N, Raj H: Effect of sublingual nitrate on respiratory reflexes arising from stimulation of juxta-pulmonary capillary (J) receptors by i.v. lobeline and short duration exercise, *Respir Physiol Neurobiol* 181(3):259–266, 2012.
20. Meurs H et al: Muscarinic receptors on airway mesenchymal cells: novel findings for an ancient target, *Pulm Pharmacol Ther* 26(1):145–155, 2013.
21. Guyenet PG, Stornetta RL, Bayliss DA: Central respiratory chemoreception, *J Comp Neurol* 518(19):3883–3906, 2010.
22. Madias NE: Renal acidification responses to respiratory acid-base disorders, *J Nephrol* 23(Suppl 16):S85–S91, 2010.
23. Forster HV, Smith CA: Contributions of central and peripheral chemoreceptors to the ventilatory response to CO_2/H^+, *J Appl Physiol* 108(4):989–994, 2010.
24. Deleted in proofs.
25. Glasser JR, Mallampalli RK: Surfactant and its role in the pathobiology of pulmonary infection, *Microbes Infect* 14(1):17–25, 2012.
26. Lumb AB: *Nunn's applied respiratory physiology*, ed 7, St Louis, 2010, Elsevier.
27. Chitano P: Models to understand contractile function in the airways, *Pulm Pharmacol Ther* 24(5):444–451, 2011.
28. Des Jardins T, Burton GC: *Clinical manifestations and assessment of respiratory disease*, ed 6, St Louis, 2011, Mosby.
29. Cavaliere F et al: Comparison of two methods to assess blood CO_2 equilibration curve in mechanically ventilated patients, *Resp Physiol Neurobiol* 146(1):77–83, 2005.
30. Chien JW et al: Uncontrolled oxygen administration and respiratory failure in acute asthma, *Chest* 117(3):728–733, 2000.
31. Mason RJ et al: *Murray and Nadel's textbook of respiratory medicine*, ed 5, St Louis, 2010, Elsevier.
32. Becklake MR, Kauffmann F: Gender differences in airway behaviour over the human life span, *Thorax* 54(12):1119–1138, 1999.
33. Sharma G, Goodwin J: Effect of aging on respiratory system physiology and immunology, *Clin Interven Aging* 1(3):253–260, 2006.
34. Vaz Fragoso CA, Gill TM: Respiratory impairment and the aging lung: a novel paradigm for assessing pulmonary function, *J Gerontol A Biol Sci Med Sci* 67(3):264–275, 2012.
35. Miller MR: Structural and physiological age-associated changes in aging lungs, *Semin Respir Crit Care Med* 31(5):521–527, 2010.
36. Dyer C: The interaction of ageing and lung disease, *Chron Respir Dis* 9(1):63–67, 2012.
37. Ely KH et al: Aging and CD8+ T cell immunity to respiratory virus infections, *Exp Gerontol* 42(5):427–431, 2007.
38. Haas CF, Loik PS, Gay SE: Airway clearance applications in the elderly and in patients with neurologic or neuromuscular compromise, *Respir Care* 52(10):1362–1381, 2007. discussion 1381.
39. Taylor BJ, Johnson BD: The pulmonary circulation and exercise responses in the elderly, *Semin Respir Crit Care Med* 31(5):528–558, 2010.
40. Dyer C: The interaction of ageing and lung disease, *Chron Respir Dis* 9(1):63–67, 2012.
41. Hardie JA et al: Reference values for arterial blood gases in the elderly, *Chest* 125(6):2053–2060, 2004.

CHAPTER

35

Alterations of Pulmonary Function

Valentina L. Brashers and Sue E. Huether

evolve WEBSITE

http://evolve.elsevier.com/McCance/

- Review Questions and Answers
- Animations
- Online Course: Module 15

CHAPTER OUTLINE

Pulmonary disease is often classified as acute or chronic, obstructive or restrictive, and infectious or noninfectious. Because skillful and knowledgeable care plays a major role in decreasing respiratory morbidity and mortality, the clinician with a clear understanding of the pathophysiology of common respiratory problems can greatly affect the outcome for each individual.

CLINICAL MANIFESTATIONS OF PULMONARY ALTERATIONS

Signs and Symptoms of Pulmonary Disease

Pulmonary disease is associated with many signs and symptoms and their specific characteristics often help in identifying the underlying disorder. The most common are dyspnea and cough. Others include abnormal sputum, hemoptysis, altered breathing patterns, hypoventilation and hyperventilation, cyanosis, clubbing of the digits, and chest pain.

Dyspnea

Dyspnea is a subjective experience of breathing discomfort that is comprised of qualitatively distinct sensations that vary in intensity. The experience derives from interactions among multiple physiologic, psychologic, social, and environmental factors, and it may induce secondary physiologic and behavioral responses. It is often described as breathlessness, air hunger, shortness of breath, increased work of breathing, chest tightness, and preoccupation with breathing.[1] Dyspnea may be the result of pulmonary disease or many other conditions, such as pain, heart disease, trauma, and anxiety.

The severity of the experience of dyspnea may not directly correlate with the severity of underlying disease.[2,3] Either diffuse or focal disturbances of ventilation, gas exchange, or ventilation-perfusion relationships can cause dyspnea, as can increased work of breathing or diseases that damage lung tissue (lung parenchyma). One proposed mechanism involves an impaired sense of effort where the perceived work of breathing is greater than the actual motor response generated. Stimulation of many receptors can contribute to the sensation of dyspnea including mechanoreceptors (the stretch receptors, irritant receptors, and *J*-receptors), upper airway receptors, and central and peripheral chemoreceptors that interact with the sensory and motor cortex.[4,5]

The more severe signs of dyspnea include flaring of the nostrils, use of accessory muscles of respiration, and retraction (pulling back) of the intercostal spaces. In dyspnea caused by parenchymal disease (e.g., pneumonia), retractions of tissue between the ribs (subcostal and intercostal retractions) are observed more often than supercostal retractions (retractions of tissues above the ribs), which predominate in upper airway obstruction. Retractions of any type are more commonly seen in children or in adults who are thin and have poorly developed thoracic musculature. Dyspnea can be quantified by the use of ordinal rating scales or visual analog scales.[3]

Dyspnea can occur transiently or can become chronic. The first episode commonly occurs with exercise and is called **dyspnea on exertion. Orthopnea** is dyspnea that occurs when an individual lies flat and is common in individuals with heart failure. The recumbent position redistributes body water, causes the abdominal contents to exert pressure on the diaphragm, and decreases the efficiency of the respiratory muscles. Sitting in a forward-leaning posture or supporting the upper body on several pillows generally relieves orthopnea. **Paroxysmal nocturnal dyspnea (PND)** occurs when individuals with heart failure or lung disease wake up at night gasping for air and must sit up or stand to relieve the dyspnea.

Cough

Cough is a protective reflex that helps clear the airways by an explosive expiration. Inhaled particles, accumulated mucus, inflammation, or the presence of a foreign body initiates the cough reflex by stimulating irritant receptors in the airway. There are few such receptors in the most distal bronchi and the alveoli; thus it is possible for significant amounts of secretions to accumulate in the distal respiratory tree without cough being initiated. The cough reflex consists of inspiration, closure of the glottis and vocal cords, contraction of the expiratory muscles, and reopening of the glottis, causing a sudden, forceful expiration that removes the offending matter. The effectiveness of the cough depends on the depth of the inspiration and the degree to which the airways narrow, increasing the velocity of expiratory gas flow. Stimulation of cough receptors is transmitted centrally through the vagus nerve, and central modulation of the cough reflex can be influenced by opiates and serotonergic agents.[6,7] Cough occurs frequently in healthy individuals; however, those with an inability to cough effectively are at greater risk for pneumonia.

Acute cough is cough that resolves within 2 to 3 weeks of the onset of illness or resolves with treatment of the underlying condition. It is most commonly the result of upper respiratory tract infections, allergic rhinitis, acute bronchitis, pneumonia, congestive heart failure, pulmonary embolus, or aspiration. **Chronic cough** is defined as cough that has persisted for more than 3 weeks, although some researchers have suggested that 7 or 8 weeks is a more appropriate timeframe because acute cough and bronchial hyperreactivity can be prolonged in some cases of viral infection. In nonsmokers, chronic cough is commonly caused by postnasal drainage syndrome, nonasthmatic eosinophilic bronchitis, asthma, gastroesophageal reflux disease, or heightened cough reflex sensitivity.[8] In smokers, chronic bronchitis is the most common cause of chronic cough, although lung cancer must always be considered. Individuals taking angiotensin-converting enzyme inhibitors for hypertension may develop chronic cough that resolves with discontinuation of the drug.

Abnormal Sputum

Changes in the amount, consistency, color, and odor of **sputum** provide information about progression of disease and effectiveness of therapy. The gross and microscopic appearances of sputum enable the clinician to identify cellular debris or microorganisms that aid in diagnosis and choice of therapy.

Hemoptysis is the coughing up of blood or bloody secretions. This is sometimes confused with hematemesis, which is the vomiting of blood. Blood that is coughed up is usually bright red, has an alkaline pH, and is mixed with frothy sputum. Blood that is vomited is dark, has an acidic pH, and is mixed with food particles.

Hemoptysis usually indicates infection or inflammation that damages the bronchi (bronchitis, bronchiectasis) or the lung parenchyma (pneumonia, tuberculosis, lung abscess). Other causes include cancer and pulmonary infarction. The amount and duration of bleeding provide important clues about its source. Bronchoscopy, combined with chest computed tomography (CT), is used to confirm the site of bleeding.[9]

Abnormal Breathing Patterns

Normal breathing (eupnea) is rhythmic and effortless. Ventilatory rate is 8 to 16 breaths per minute, and tidal volume ranges from 400 to 800 ml. A short expiratory pause occurs with each breath, and the individual takes an occasional deeper breath or sigh. Sigh breaths, which help maintain normal lung function, are usually 1.5 to 2 times the normal tidal volume and occur approximately 10 to 12 times per hour.

The rate, depth, regularity, and effort of breathing undergo characteristic alterations in response to physiologic and pathophysiologic conditions. Patterns of breathing automatically adjust to minimize the work of respiratory muscles. Strenuous exercise or metabolic acidosis induces **Kussmaul respirations (hyperpnea).** Kussmaul respirations are characterized by a slightly increased ventilatory rate, very large tidal volume, and no expiratory pause.

Labored breathing occurs whenever there is an increased work of breathing, especially if the airways are obstructed, as in chronic obstructive pulmonary disease (COPD). If the large airways are obstructed, a slow ventilatory rate, increased effort, prolonged inspiration or expiration, and stridor (high-pitched sounds made during inspiration) or audible wheezing (whistling sounds on expiration) are typical. In small airway obstruction, like that seen in asthma and chronic obstructive pulmonary disease, a rapid ventilatory rate, small tidal volume, increased effort, prolonged expiration, and wheezing are often present.

Restricted breathing is commonly caused by disorders such as pulmonary fibrosis that stiffen the lungs or chest wall and decrease compliance. Restricted breathing is characterized by small tidal volumes and rapid ventilatory rate (tachypnea).

Shock and severe cerebral hypoxia (insufficient oxygen in the brain) contribute to gasping respirations that consist of irregular, quick inspirations with an expiratory pause. Anxiety can cause sighing respirations that consist of irregular breathing characterized by frequent, deep sighing inspirations.

Cheyne-Stokes respirations are characterized by alternating periods of deep and shallow breathing. Apnea lasting 15 to 60 seconds is followed by ventilations that increase in volume until a peak is reached, after which ventilation (tidal volume) decreases again to apnea. Cheyne-Stokes respirations result from any condition that slows the blood flow to the brainstem, which in turn slows impulses sending information to the respiratory centers of the brainstem. Neurologic impairment above the brainstem is also a contributing factor (see Table 17-4 and Figure 17-1).

Hypoventilation and Hyperventilation

Hypoventilation is inadequate alveolar ventilation in relation to metabolic demands. It is caused by alterations in pulmonary mechanics or in the neurologic control of breathing such that minute volume (tidal volume × respiratory rate) is reduced. When alveolar ventilation is normal, carbon dioxide (CO_2) is removed from the lungs at the same rate at which it is produced by cellular metabolism. This maintains arterial CO_2 pressure ($Paco_2$) at normal levels (40 mmHg). With hypoventilation, CO_2 removal does not keep up with CO_2 production and $Paco_2$ increases, causing hypercapnia ($Paco_2$ greater than 44 mmHg). (Table 34-2 contains the definition of gas partial pressure and other pulmonary abbreviations.) This results in an increase in hydrogen ion in the blood, termed respiratory acidosis, which can affect the function of many tissues throughout the body.

Hypoventilation is often overlooked until it is severe because breathing pattern and ventilatory rate may appear normal. Blood gas analysis (i.e., measurement of the $Paco_2$ of arterial blood) reveals the hypercapnia. Pronounced hypoventilation can cause somnolence or disorientation. In addition, alveolar hypoventilation with hypercapnia results in secondary hypoxemia because the accumulation of alveolar CO_2 displaces oxygen (see Hypercapnia, p. 1251).

Hyperventilation is alveolar ventilation that exceeds metabolic demands. The lungs remove CO_2 at a faster rate than it is produced by cellular metabolism, resulting in decreased $Paco_2$ or **hypocapnia** ($Paco_2$ less than 36 mmHg). Hypocapnia results in a respiratory alkalosis that also can interfere with tissue function. Like hypoventilation, hyperventilation can be determined only by arterial blood gas analysis. Hyperventilation commonly occurs with severe anxiety, acute head injury, and conditions that cause insufficient oxygenation of the blood.

Cyanosis

Cyanosis is a bluish discoloration of the skin and mucous membranes caused by increasing amounts of desaturated or reduced hemoglobin (which is bluish) in the blood. It generally develops when 5 g of hemoglobin is desaturated, regardless of hemoglobin concentration. For example, if total hemoglobin concentration is 15 g/dl of blood, 5 g/dl must be desaturated to cause cyanosis. If total hemoglobin level is 11 g/dl, 5 g/dl must still be desaturated for cyanosis to occur.

Peripheral cyanosis (slow blood circulation in fingers and toes) is most often caused by poor circulation resulting from intense peripheral vasoconstriction, like that seen in Raynaud's disease, cold environments, or severe stress. Peripheral cyanosis is best seen in the nail beds. *Central cyanosis* is caused by decreased arterial oxygenation (low Pao_2) from pulmonary diseases or pulmonary or cardiac right-to-left shunts. Central cyanosis is best seen in buccal mucous membranes and lips.

Lack of cyanosis does not necessarily indicate that oxygenation is normal. In adults, cyanosis is not evident until severe hypoxemia is present and, therefore, is an insensitive indication of respiratory failure. For example, severe anemia (inadequate hemoglobin concentration) and carbon monoxide poisoning (in which hemoglobin binds to carbon monoxide instead of binding to oxygen) can result in inadequate oxygenation of tissues without causing cyanosis. Individuals with polycythemia (an abnormal increase in numbers of red blood cells), however, may have cyanosis when tissue oxygenation is adequate. Because polycythemia causes hemoglobin concentration to be greater than normal, 5 g/dl can be desaturated, causing cyanosis, without having much effect on oxygenation. Therefore, the significance of cyanosis as a clinical finding must be interpreted in relation to the underlying pathophysiology. If cyanosis is suggested, the Pao_2 should be measured.

Clubbing

Clubbing is the selective bulbous enlargement of the end (distal segment) of a digit (finger or toe) (Figure 35-1) whose severity can be graded from 1 to 5 based on the extent of nail bed hypertrophy and the amount of changes in the nails themselves. It is usually painless. Clubbing is commonly associated with diseases that interfere with oxygenation, such as bronchiectasis, cystic fibrosis, pulmonary fibrosis, lung abscess, and congenital heart disease. It is rarely reversible with treatment of the underlying pulmonary condition. It can sometimes be seen in individuals with lung cancer even without hypoxemia, because of the effects of inflammatory cytokines and growth factors *(hypertrophic osteoarthropathy)*.[10]

Pain

Pain caused by pulmonary disorders originates in the pleurae, airways, or chest wall.[11] Pleural pain is the most common pain caused by pulmonary disease and is usually sharp or stabbing in character. Infection and inflammation of the parietal pleura (pleuritis or pleurisy) cause pain when the pleurae stretch

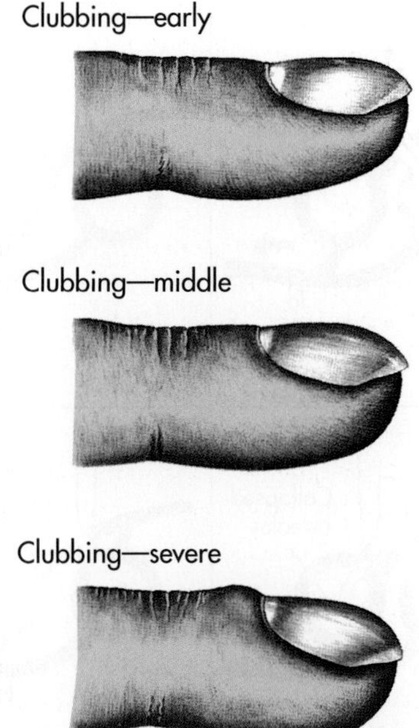

FIGURE 35-1 Clubbing of Fingers Caused by Chronic Hypoxemia. (From Seidel HM et al: *Mosby's guide to physical examination,* ed 6, St Louis, 2006, Mosby.)

during inspiration. The pain is usually localized to a portion of the chest wall, where a unique breath sound called a *pleural friction rub* may be heard over the painful area. Laughing or coughing makes pleural pain worse. Pleural pain is also common with pulmonary infarction (tissue death) caused by pulmonary embolism and emanates from the area around the infarction.

Pulmonary pain can be central chest pain that is pronounced after coughing and occurs in individuals with infection and inflammation of the trachea or bronchi (tracheitis or tracheobronchitis). Central chest pain can be difficult to differentiate from cardiac pain (see Chapter 32). High blood pressure in the pulmonary circulation (pulmonary hypertension) can cause pain during exercise that is often mistaken for cardiac pain (angina pectoris).

Pain in the chest wall is muscle pain or rib pain. The common causes of chest wall pain are rib fractures and excessive coughing, which make the muscles sore. Inflammation of the costochondral junction (costochondritis) also can cause chest wall pain. Chest wall pain can often be reproduced by pressing on the sternum or ribs.

Conditions Caused by Pulmonary Disease or Injury

Hypercapnia

Hypercapnia, or increased CO_2 concentration in the arterial blood (increased $Paco_2$), is caused by hypoventilation of the alveoli.[12] As discussed in Chapter 34, CO_2 is easily diffused from the blood into the alveolar space; thus minute volume (respiratory rate × tidal volume) determines not only alveolar ventilation, but also $Paco_2$. Hypoventilation is often overlooked because breathing pattern and ventilatory rate may appear normal; it is important to obtain blood gas analysis to determine the severity of hypercapnia and resultant respiratory acidosis (acid-base balance is described in Chapter 3).

There are many causes of hypercapnia.[13] Most are a result of a decreased drive to breathe or an inadequate ability to respond to ventilatory stimulation. Causes include: (1) depression of the respiratory center by drugs; (2) diseases of the medulla, including infections of the central nervous system or trauma; (3) abnormalities of the spinal conducting pathways, as in spinal cord disruption or poliomyelitis; (4) diseases of the neuromuscular junction or of the respiratory muscles themselves, as in myasthenia gravis or muscular dystrophy; (5) thoracic cage abnormalities, as in chest injury or congenital deformity; (6) large airway obstruction, as in tumors or sleep apnea; and (7) increased work of breathing or physiologic dead space, as in emphysema.

Hypercapnia and the associated respiratory acidosis can result in several important clinical manifestations. Of greatest concern are electrolyte abnormalities that occur in response to the low pH that may cause dysrhythmias. Individuals also may have somnolence and even be in a coma because of changes in intracranial pressure associated with high levels of arterial carbon dioxide, which causes cerebral vasodilation. Alveolar hypoventilation with increased alveolar carbon dioxide limits the amount of alveolar oxygen available for diffusion into the blood, leading to secondary hypoxemia.

Hypoxemia

Hypoxemia, or reduced oxygenation of arterial blood (reduced Pao_2), is caused by respiratory alterations, whereas **hypoxia,** or reduced oxygenation of cells in tissues, may be caused by alterations of other systems as well. Although hypoxemia can lead to tissue hypoxia, tissue hypoxia can result from other abnormalities, such as low cardiac output or cyanide poisoning.

Hypoxemia results from problems with one or more of the major mechanisms of oxygenation:

1. Oxygen delivery to the alveoli
    a. Oxygen content of the inspired air (Fio_2)
2. Ventilation of the alveoli
3. Diffusion of oxygen from the alveoli into the blood
    a. Balance between alveolar ventilation and perfusion ($\dot{V}/\dot{Q}$ mismatch)
    b. Diffusion of oxygen across the alveolocapillary membrane
4. Perfusion of pulmonary capillaries

Table 35-1 lists some of the common clinical causes of these problems.

The amount of oxygen in the alveoli is called the P_{AO_2} and is dependent on two factors. The first factor is the presence of adequate oxygen content of the inspired air. The amount of oxygen in inspired air is expressed as the percentage or fraction of air that is composed of oxygen, called the Fio_2. The Fio_2 of air at sea level is approximately 21% or 0.21. Anything that decreases the Fio_2 (such as high altitude) decreases the P_{AO_2}. The second factor is the amount of alveolar minute ventilation (tidal volume × respiratory rate). Hypoventilation results in an increase in P_{ACO_2} and a decrease in P_{AO_2} such that there is less oxygen available in the alveoli for diffusion into the blood. This type of hypoxemia can be completely corrected if alveolar ventilation is improved by increases in the rate and depth of breathing. Hypoventilation causes hypoxemia in unconscious persons; in

TABLE 35-1 CAUSES OF HYPOXEMIA

MECHANISM	COMMON CLINICAL CAUSES
Decrease in inspired oxygen (decreased FiO_2)	High altitude Low oxygen content of gas mixture Enclosed breathing spaces (suffocation)
Hypoventilation of the alveoli	Lack of neurologic stimulation of the respiratory center (oversedation, drug overdose, neurologic damage) Defects in chest wall mechanics (neuromuscular disease, trauma, chest deformity, air trapping) Large airway obstruction (laryngospasm, foreign body aspiration, neoplasm) Increased work of breathing (emphysema, severe asthma)
Ventilation-perfusion mismatch	Asthma Chronic bronchitis Pneumonia Acute respiratory distress syndrome Atelectasis Pulmonary embolism
Alveolocapillary diffusion abnormality	Edema Fibrosis Emphysema
Decreased pulmonary capillary perfusion	Intracardiac defects Intrapulmonary arteriovenous malformations

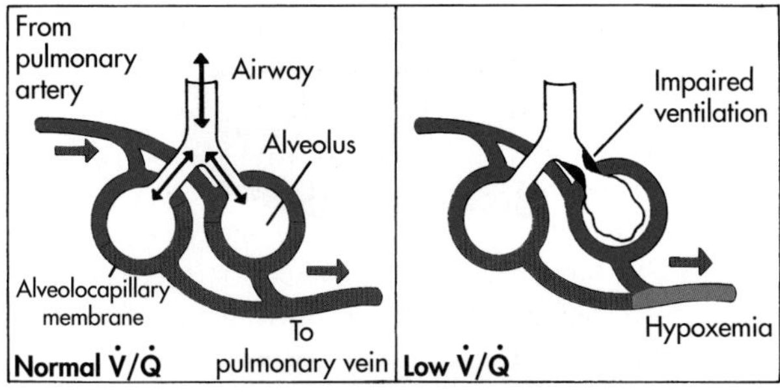

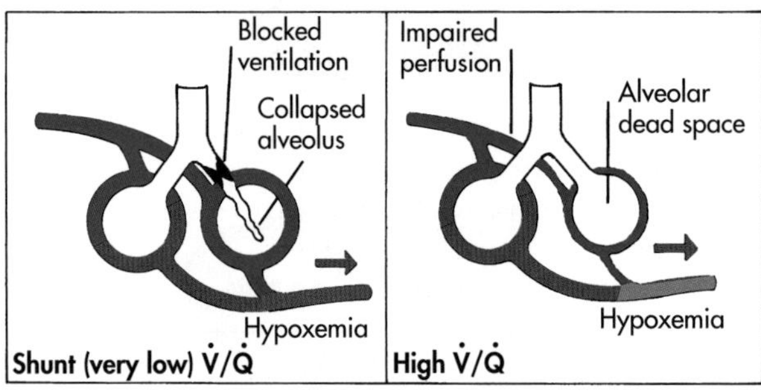

FIGURE 35-2 Ventilation-Perfusion Abnormalities. (Data from Glenny RW: *Adv Physiol Educ* 32[3]:192–195, 2008.)

people with neurologic, muscular, or bone diseases that restrict chest expansion; and in individuals who have COPD.

Diffusion of oxygen from the alveoli into the blood is also dependent on two factors. The first is the balance between the amount of air getting into alveoli ($\dot{V}$) and the amount of blood perfusing the capillaries around the alveoli ($\dot{Q}$). An abnormal ventilation-perfusion ratio ($\dot{V}/\dot{Q}$) is the most common cause of hypoxemia (Figure 35-2). Normally, alveolocapillary lung units receive almost equal amounts of ventilation and perfusion. The normal $\dot{V}/\dot{Q}$ is 0.8 to 0.9 because perfusion is somewhat greater than ventilation in the lung bases and because some blood is normally shunted to the bronchial circulation. $\dot{V}/\dot{Q}$ mismatch refers to an abnormal distribution of ventilation and perfusion. Hypoxemia can be caused by inadequate ventilation of well-perfused areas of the lung (low $\dot{V}/\dot{Q}$). Mismatching of this type, called **shunting,** occurs in atelectasis, in asthma as a result of bronchoconstriction, and in pulmonary edema and pneumonia when alveoli are filled with fluid. When blood passes through portions of the pulmonary capillary bed that receive no ventilation, right-to-left shunt occurs, resulting in decreased systemic PaO_2 and hypoxemia. Hypoxemia also can be caused by poor perfusion of well-ventilated portions of the lung (high $\dot{V}/\dot{Q}$), resulting in wasted ventilation. The most common cause of high $\dot{V}/\dot{Q}$ is a pulmonary embolus that impairs blood flow to a segment of the lung. An area where alveoli are ventilated but not perfused is termed **alveolar dead space.**

The second factor affecting diffusion of oxygen from the alveoli into the blood is the alveolocapillary barrier. Diffusion of oxygen through the alveolocapillary membrane is impaired if the alveolocapillary membrane is thickened or the surface area available for diffusion is decreased. Abnormal thickness, as occurs with edema (tissue swelling) and fibrosis (formation of fibrous lesions), increases the time required for diffusion across the alveolocapillary membrane. If diffusion is slowed enough, the oxygen in the alveolar gas (P_AO_2) and capillary blood does not have time to equilibrate during the fraction of a second that blood remains in the capillary. Destruction of alveoli, such as that which occurs in emphysema, decreases the surface area available for diffusion. Hypercapnia is rarely produced by impaired diffusion, because carbon dioxide diffuses so easily from capillary to alveolus that the individual with impaired diffusion would die from hypoxemia before hypercapnia could occur.

Hypoxemia most often is associated with a compensatory hyperventilation and resultant respiratory alkalosis (i.e., decreased $PaCO_2$ and increased pH). However, in individuals with associated ventilatory difficulties, hypoxemia may be complicated by hypercapnia and respiratory acidosis. Hypoxemia results in widespread tissue dysfunction and, when severe, can lead to organ infarction. In addition, hypoxic pulmonary vasoconstriction can contribute to increased pressures in the pulmonary artery (pulmonary artery hypertension) and lead to right-sided heart failure and cor pulmonale (see p. 1276). Clinical manifestations of acute hypoxemia may include cyanosis, confusion, tachycardia, edema, and decreased renal output.

Acute Respiratory Failure

Respiratory (lung) failure is defined as inadequate gas exchange, that is, hypoxemia, in which PaO_2 is ≤50 mmHg, or hypercapnia, in which $PaCO_2$ is ≥50 mmHg with a pH of ≤7.25. Respiratory failure can result from direct injury to the lungs, airways, or chest wall or indirectly because of injury to another body system, such as the brain or liver.[14] It can occur in individuals who have an otherwise normal respiratory system or in those with underlying chronic pulmonary disease. Most pulmonary diseases can cause episodes of acute respiratory failure. If the respiratory failure is primarily hypercapnic, it is the result of inadequate alveolar ventilation (see Hypercapnia, p. 1251) and the individual must receive ventilatory support, such as with a bag-valve mask, noninvasive positive pressure ventilation, or intubation and placement on mechanical ventilation. If the respiratory failure is primarily hypoxemic, it is the result of inadequate exchange of oxygen between the alveoli and the capillaries (see Hypoxemia, p. 1251) and the individual must receive supplemental oxygen therapy. Many individuals have a combined hypercapnic and hypoxemic respiratory failure and require both kinds of support.

Respiratory failure is an important potential complication of any major surgical procedure, especially those that involve the central nervous system, thorax, or upper abdomen. Smokers are at risk, particularly if they have preexisting lung disease. Limited cardiac reserve, chronic renal failure, chronic hepatic disease, and infection also increase the tendency to develop postoperative respiratory failure. The most common postoperative pulmonary problems are atelectasis, pneumonia, pulmonary edema, and pulmonary emboli (these conditions are discussed later in this chapter).

Prevention of postoperative respiratory failure includes frequent turning and position changes, deep breathing exercises, and early ambulation to prevent atelectasis and accumulation of secretions. Humidification of inspired air can help loosen secretions. Incentive spirometry gives individuals immediate feedback about tidal volumes, which encourages them to breathe deeply. Supplemental oxygen is given for hypoxemia, and antibiotics are given as appropriate to treat infection. If respiratory failure develops, the individual may require conventional mechanical ventilation, high-frequency ventilation, or extracorporeal membrane oxygenation.[15]

DISORDERS OF THE CHEST WALL AND PLEURA

There are many conditions that can affect the chest wall and/or pleura and impact the function of the respiratory system. Chest wall disorders primarily affect tidal volume and therefore result in hypercapnia. Pleural diseases affect ventilation and oxygenation.

Disorders of the Chest Wall

Chest Wall Restriction

If the chest wall is deformed, traumatized, immobilized, or made heavy by fat, the work of breathing is increased and ventilation may be compromised because of a decrease in tidal volume. The degree of ventilatory impairment depends on the severity of the chest wall abnormality. Grossly obese individuals are often dyspneic on exertion or when recumbent. Individuals with severe kyphoscoliosis (lateral bending and rotation of the spinal column with distortion of the thoracic cage) often have dyspnea on exertion that can progress to respiratory failure. Such individuals also are susceptible to lower respiratory tract infections. Obesity and kyphoscoliosis are risk factors for respiratory disease in individuals admitted to a hospital for other problems, particularly those who require surgery. Other

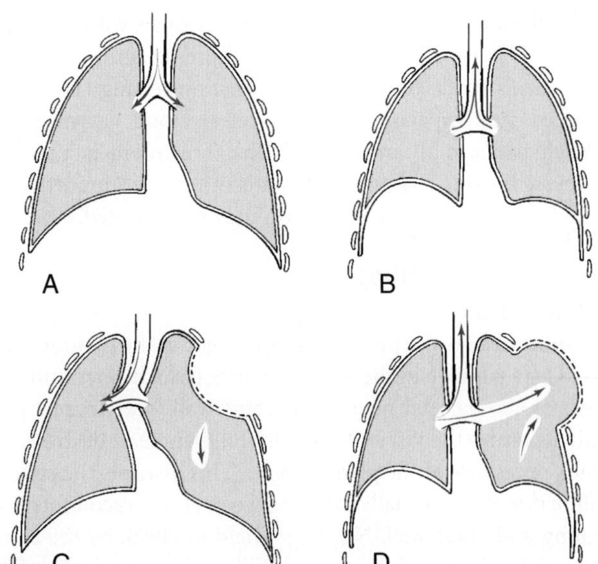

FIGURE 35-3 Flail chest. Normal respiration: **A,** inspiration; **B,** expiration. Paradoxical motion: **C,** inspiration, area of lung underlying unstable chest wall sucks in on inspiration; **D,** expiration, unstable area balloons out. Note movement of mediastinum toward opposite lung during inspiration.

musculoskeletal abnormalities that can impair ventilation are ankylosing spondylitis and pectus excavatum (a deformity characterized by depression of the sternum) (see Chapters 44 and 45, respectively). Pain from chest wall injury, surgery, or disease is also an important cause of restriction and decreased tidal volume. This can cause significant hypoventilation, especially in those with underlying lung disease.

Impairment of respiratory muscle function caused by neuromuscular disease also can restrict the chest wall or impair pulmonary function. Muscle weakness can result in hypoventilation and hypercapnia, inability to remove secretions, and hypoxemia. The most common cause of hospital admission for individuals with neuromuscular diseases, such as muscular dystrophy, myasthenia gravis, and Guillain-Barré syndrome, is respiratory difficulty. (See Unit V for a more complete discussion of these disorders.)

Trauma to the thorax or upper abdomen can restrict chest expansion because of pain. Trauma to the chest also can cause structural and mechanical changes that impair the ability of the chest to expand normally. **Flail chest** results from the fracture of several consecutive ribs in more than one place, or the fracture of the sternum and several consecutive ribs. These multiple fractures result in instability of a portion of the chest wall, causing paradoxical movement of the chest with breathing. During the negative intrathoracic pressure of inspiration, the unstable portion of the chest wall moves inward and during expiration it moves outward, impairing movement of gas in and out of the lungs (Figure 35-3). Flail chest is usually associated with significant underlying lung contusion. The clinical manifestations of flail chest are pain, dyspnea, unequal chest expansion, hypoventilation, and hypoxemia. Treatment is internal fixation by controlled mechanical ventilation until the chest wall has stabilized.

Chest wall restriction results in decreased tidal volume. An increase in respiratory rate can temporarily compensate and restore minute ventilation, but many individuals will eventually progress to hypercapnic respiratory failure. Diagnosis of chest restriction is made by pulmonary function testing (reduction in forced vital capacity [FVC]), arterial blood gas measurement (hypercapnia), and radiographs. Treatment is aimed at any reversible underlying cause, but is otherwise supportive. In severe cases, mechanical ventilation may be indicated.

Pleural Abnormalities

Pneumothorax

Pneumothorax is the presence of air or gas in the pleural space caused by a rupture in the visceral pleura (which surrounds the lungs) or the parietal pleura and chest wall (see Chapter 34). As air separates the visceral and parietal pleurae, it destroys the negative pressure of the pleural space. This disrupts the state of equilibrium that normally exists between elastic recoil forces of the lung and chest wall. No longer held in check by the recoil forces of the chest wall, the lung fulfills its tendency to recoil by collapsing toward the hilum.

Primary (spontaneous) pneumothorax, which occurs unexpectedly in healthy individuals (usually men) between ages 20 and 40 years, is most often caused by the spontaneous rupture of blebs (blister-like formations) on the visceral pleura, although there may be underlying pleural disease with emphysema-like changes.[16] Approximately 10% of affected individuals have a significant family history of primary pneumothorax that has been linked to mutations in the folliculin gene (Birt-Hogg-Dubé syndrome), which influences cell–cell adhesion.[17] Bleb rupture can occur during sleep, rest, or exercise. The ruptured bleb or blebs are usually located in the apexes of the lungs. **Secondary (traumatic) pneumothorax** can be caused by chest trauma, such as a rib fracture, stab or bullet wounds, or a surgical procedure that tears the pleura; rupture of a bleb or bulla (larger vesicle) as occurs in COPD; or mechanical ventilation, particularly if it includes positive end-expiratory pressure (PEEP).[18] **Iatrogenic pneumothorax** is most commonly caused by transthoracic needle aspiration.[19]

Spontaneous and traumatic pneumothorax can present as either open or tension. In **open pneumothorax (communicating pneumothorax),** air pressure in the pleural space equals barometric pressure because air that is drawn into the pleural space during inspiration (through the damaged chest wall and parietal pleura or through the lungs and damaged visceral pleura) is forced back out during expiration. In **tension pneumothorax,** however, the site of pleural rupture acts as a one-way valve, permitting air to enter on inspiration, but preventing its escape by closing during expiration. As more and more air enters the pleural space, air pressure in the pneumothorax begins to exceed barometric pressure. The pathophysiologic effects of tension pneumothorax are life threatening. Air pressure in the pleural space pushes against the already recoiled lung, causing compression atelectasis, and against the mediastinum, compressing and displacing the heart and great vessels (Figure 35-4).

Clinical manifestations of spontaneous or secondary pneumothorax begin with sudden pleural pain, tachypnea, and possibly mild dyspnea. Manifestations depend on the size of the pneumothorax. Physical examination may reveal absent or decreased breath sounds and hyperresonance to percussion on the affected side. Diagnosis of pneumothorax is made with chest radiographs, ultrasound, and CT. Tension pneumothorax may be complicated by severe hypoxemia, tracheal deviation away from the affected lung, and hypotension (low blood pressure). Deterioration occurs rapidly and immediate treatment is required. Pneumothorax is treated with insertion of a chest tube that is attached to a water-seal drainage system with suction. After the pneumothorax is evacuated and the pleural rupture is healed, the chest tube is removed. For individuals with persistent air leaks, other interventions may be needed including surgery, pleurodesis (instillation of a caustic substance, such as talc, into the pleural space), or thoracoscopic surgical techniques.[20]

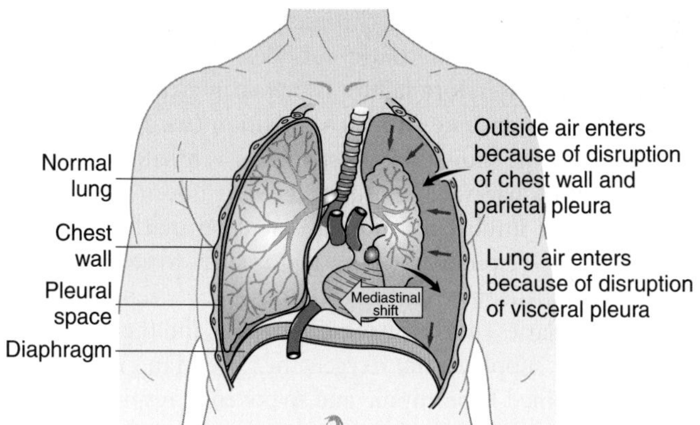

FIGURE 35-4 Tension Pneumothorax. Air in the pleural space causes the lung to collapse around the hilus and may shift trachea and mediastinal contents (heart and great vessels) toward the other lung.

Pleural Effusion

Pleural effusion is the presence of fluid in the pleural space. The source of the fluid is usually blood vessels or lymphatic vessels lying beneath either pleura, but occasionally an abscess or other lesion may drain into the pleural space. Because the pleura is a relatively permeable membrane, fluids that accumulate in the lung can cross into the pleural space. Pleural effusions that enter the pleural space from the intact blood vessels can be transudative or exudative. In **transudative effusion,** the fluid, or transudate, is watery and diffuses out of the capillaries as a result of disorders that increase intravascular hydrostatic pressure or decrease capillary oncotic pressure. Examples are congestive heart failure, in which venous and left atrial pressures are increased, and liver or kidney disorders that cause hypoproteinemia. Hypoproteinemia decreases capillary oncotic pressure, which promotes diffusion of water out of the capillaries. (This mechanism is discussed in Chapter 3).

Exudative effusion is less watery and contains high concentrations of white blood cells and plasma proteins. Exudative effusion occurs in response to inflammation, infection, or malignancy and involves inflammatory processes that increase capillary permeability (see Chapter 7). When stimulated by biochemical mediators of inflammation, junctions in the capillary endothelium separate slightly, enabling leukocytes and plasma proteins to migrate out into affected tissues. Other

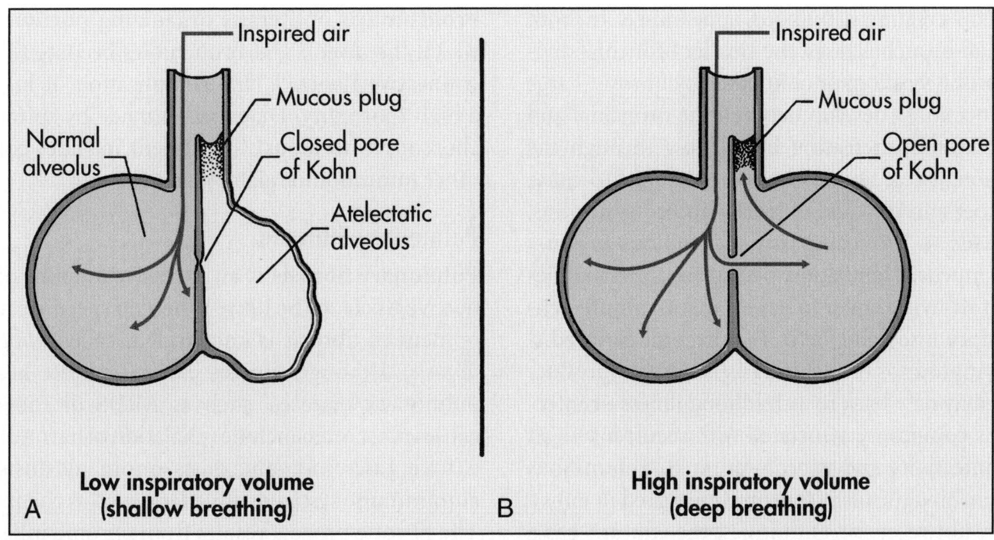

FIGURE 35-5 Pores of Kohn. **A,** Absorption atelectasis caused by lack of collateral ventilation through pores of Kohn. **B,** Restoration of collateral ventilation during deep breathing.

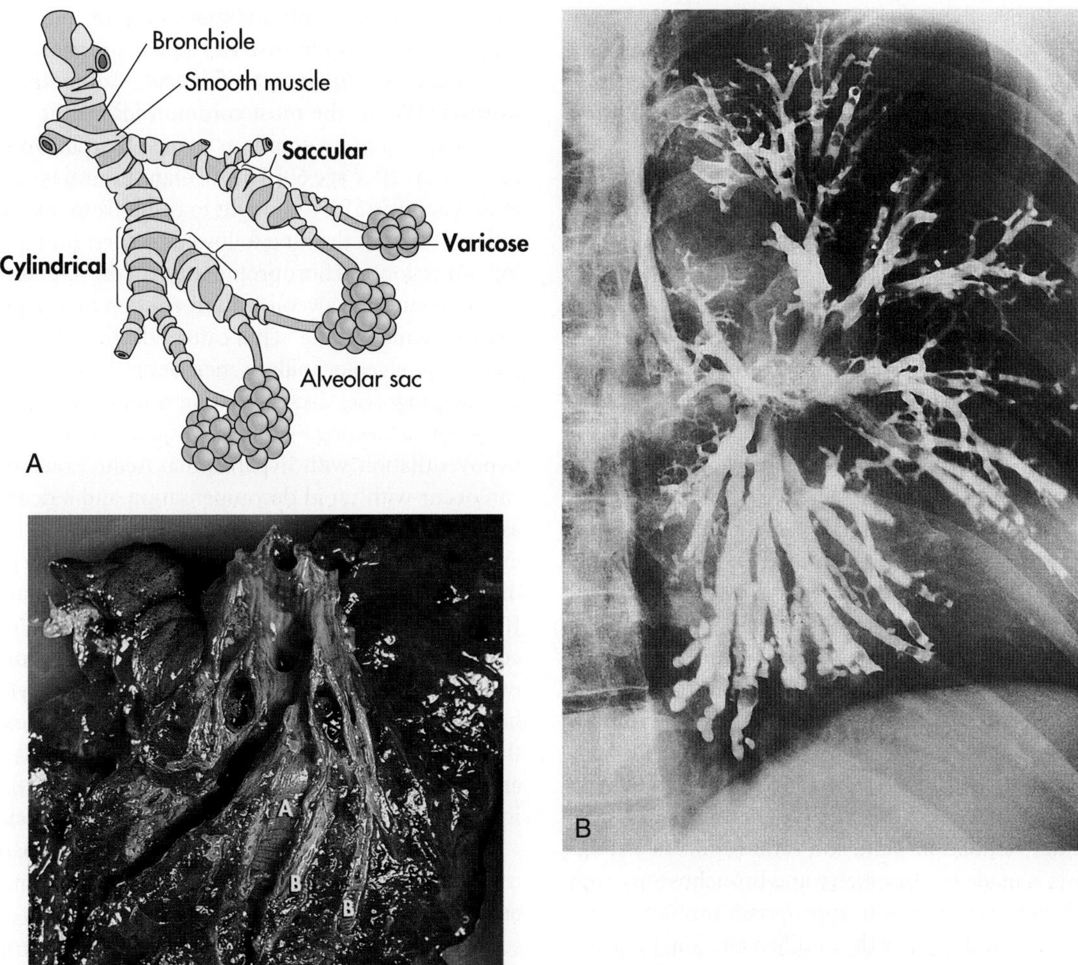

FIGURE 35-6 Bronchiectasis. **A,** Types of bronchiectasis. **B,** Left posterior oblique projection of a left bronchogram showing cylindrical bronchiectasis affecting the entire lower lobe except for the superior segment. Few side branches fill. The basal airways are crowded together, indicating volume loss of the lower lobe, a common feature in bronchiectasis. **C,** Cylindrical bronchiectasis. The dilated bronchi *(A)* and bronchioles *(B)* can be dissected almost to the pleural surface. (**B** from Hansell: *Imaging of diseases of the chest,* ed 5, St Louis, 2009, Mosby; **C** from Damjanov I, Linder J, editors: *Anderson's pathology,* ed 10, St Louis, 1996, Mosby.)

deform the bronchi, creating a bulbous appearance. In both varicose and saccular bronchiectases, the smaller bronchial divisions are plugged with secretions or obliterated by fibrosis. Large anastomoses (connections) develop between the bronchial and pulmonary blood vessels, increasing blood flow through the bronchial circulation. These anastomoses are thought to cause the hemoptysis experienced by individuals with bronchiectasis. Airway damage leads to bronchospasm and copious production of purulent mucus. Ventilation-perfusion abnormalities develop and result in hypoxemia. In severe cases, minute ventilation is also compromised and $Paco_2$ may become elevated.

The primary symptom of bronchiectasis is chronic productive cough, which may date back to a childhood illness or infection. The disease is commonly associated with recurrent lower respiratory tract infections and expectoration of voluminous amounts of foul-smelling purulent sputum (measured in cups). If the individual is not receiving antibiotics, the sputum has a foul odor. Clubbing of the fingers from chronic hypoxemia is common. Hemoptysis can occur from mucosal inflammation and necrosis and, in some instances, can be massive. Pulmonary function studies show decreases in FVC and expiratory flow rates. Diagnosis is usually confirmed by the use of high-resolution CT. Bronchiectasis is treated with sputum culture antibiotics, bronchodilators, anti-inflammatory drugs, chest physiotherapy, and supplemental oxygen. In selected individuals with localized areas of involvement, surgery may be indicated to remove the affected portion of the lung.[28]

Bronchiolitis

Bronchiolitis is diffuse inflammation of the small airways or bronchioles. It is most common in children (see Chapter 36). In adults it usually occurs with chronic bronchitis, but can occur in otherwise healthy individuals in association with an upper or lower airway viral infection (e.g., respiratory syncytial virus [RSV]), or with inhalation of toxic gases. Atelectasis or emphysematous destruction of the alveoli may develop distal to the inflammatory lesion. Bronchiolitis is usually diffuse. The resulting decrease in the ventilation-perfusion ratio results in hypoxemia. A decrease in minute ventilation with resulting carbon dioxide retention also may occur as lung restriction worsens.

Clinical manifestations include a rapid ventilatory rate; marked use of accessory muscles; low-grade fever; dry, nonproductive cough; and hyperinflated chest. If bronchiolitis is caused by an inhalation injury, pulmonary edema occurs rapidly. Respiratory distress can develop within 24 to 72 hours with severe hypoxia. Infiltrates can be seen on chest radiographs.[29] A decrease in the ventilation-perfusion ratio results in hypoxemia. Diagnosis is made by spirometry and bronchoscopy with biopsy. Bronchiolitis is treated with appropriate antibiotics, steroids, and chest physical therapy (humidified air, coughing and deep breathing, postural drainage).

Bronchiolitis obliterans is a late-stage fibrotic process that occludes the airways and causes permanent scarring of the lungs. This process can occur in all causes of bronchiolitis, but is most common after lung transplantation and is associated with acute rejection and infection. Bronchiolitis obliterans can be further complicated by the development of pneumonia (called **bronchiolitis obliterans organizing pneumonia** [**BOOP**]) in which the alveoli and bronchioles become filled with plugs of connective tissue.[30] This complication of lung transplant has a high morbidity. Diagnosis is made by spirometry and bronchoscopy with biopsy. Treatment includes corticosteroids and other immunomodulatory agents.[31]

Pulmonary Fibrosis

Pulmonary fibrosis is an excessive amount of fibrous or connective tissue in the lung. When no specific cause for the development of fibrosis is known, it is called *idiopathic pulmonary fibrosis.* Although fibrosis can complicate healing after active pulmonary diseases, such as ARDS or tuberculosis, specific causes most often include inhalation of harmful substances, such as toxic gases, inorganic dusts, or organic dusts, and underlying autoimmune systemic disorders, such as rheumatologic disease. The fibrotic process results from chronic inflammation, alveolar epithelialization, and myofibroblast proliferation. Fibrosis causes a marked loss of lung compliance. The lung becomes stiff and difficult to ventilate, and the diffusing capacity of the alveolocapillary membrane may decrease, causing hypoxemia. Diffuse pulmonary fibrosis has a poor prognosis.

Idiopathic Pulmonary Fibrosis. **Idiopathic pulmonary fibrosis (IPF)** is the most common idiopathic interstitial lung disorder. It is more common in men than in women and most cases occur after age 60. The median survival is only 2 to 4 years after diagnosis. IPF is thought to result from multiple injuries at different sites of the lung followed by aberrant repair.[32] Chronic inflammation and fibroproliferation of the interstitial lung tissue occur around the alveoli with disruption of the alveolocapillary basement membrane. This causes decreased oxygen diffusion across the alveolocapillary membrane and hypoxemia. As the disease progresses decreased lung compliance leads to increased work of breathing, decreased tidal volume, and resultant hypoventilation with hypercapnia. Acute exacerbations of IPF can occur with rapid decompensation and a death rate as high as 50%.[33] The primary symptom of IPF is increasing dyspnea on exertion; examination reveals diffuse inspiratory crackles and diagnosis is confirmed by pulmonary function testing (decreased FVC), high-resolution CT, and lung biopsy. Treatment with corticosteroids alone causes remission in approximately 50% of individuals. Combined treatment with cytotoxic drugs has a higher success rate, but also higher toxicity. Newer therapies include antifibrotic drugs (such as *N*-acetylcysteine and pirfenidone), interferon, and anticoagulation. Selected individuals may benefit from lung transplantation.[34]

Exposure to Toxic Gases. Inhalation of gaseous irritants can cause significant respiratory dysfunction. Commonly encountered toxic gases include ammonia, hydrogen chloride, sulfur dioxide, chlorine, phosgene, and nitrogen dioxide. Inhalation injuries in burns can include toxic gases from household or industrial combustants, heat, and smoke particles. Inhaled toxic particles cause damage to the airway epithelium, cilia, and alveoli. There is increased mucus secretion, promotion of inflammation, and mucosal and pulmonary edema. Surfactant and other protective buffers and antioxidants are inactivated.[35] The cellular effects of toxic gases are described in

Chapter 2. Acute toxic inhalation is frequently complicated by the development of ARDS and pneumonia. Initial symptoms include burning of the eyes, nose, and throat; coughing; chest tightness; and dyspnea. Hypoxemia is common. Treatment includes supplemental oxygen, mechanical ventilation with PEEP, and support of the cardiovascular system. Corticosteroids sometimes are used, although their effectiveness has not been well documented. Most individuals respond quickly to therapy. Some, however, may improve initially and then deteriorate as a result of bronchiectasis or bronchiolitis.

Prolonged exposure to high concentrations of supplemental oxygen can result in a relatively rare iatrogenic condition known as **oxygen toxicity.** The basic underlying mechanism of injury is a severe inflammatory response mediated primarily by oxygen free radicals. The result is damage to alveolocapillary membranes, disruption of surfactant production, interstitial and alveolar edema, and decrease in compliance.[36] Treatment involves ventilatory support and reduction of inspired oxygen concentration to less than 60%, as soon as tolerated.

Pneumoconiosis. **Pneumoconiosis** represents any change in the lung caused by inhalation of inorganic dust particles, which usually occurs in the workplace. As in all cases of environmentally acquired lung disease, the individual's history of exposure is important in determining the diagnosis. Pneumoconiosis often occurs after years of exposure to the offending dust with progressive fibrosis of lung tissue.

The dusts of silica, asbestos, and coal are the most common causes of pneumoconiosis. Others include talc, fiberglass, clays, mica, slate, cement, cadmium, beryllium, tungsten, cobalt, aluminum, and iron. Deposition of these materials in the lungs cause the release of proinflammatory cytokines (e.g., interleukin-1-beta). This leads to chronic inflammation with scarring of the alveolocapillary membrane, resulting in pulmonary fibrosis and progressive pulmonary deterioration. Clinical manifestations with advancement of disease may include cough, sputum production, dyspnea, decreased lung volumes, and hypoxemia. In most cases, diagnosis is made by performing chest x-ray or CT and by obtaining careful occupational history.[37] Treatment is usually palliative and focuses on preventing further exposure and improving working conditions, along with pulmonary rehabilitation and management of associated hypoxemia and bronchospasm.

Silicosis is a type of pneumoconiosis resulting from the inhalation of free silica (silicon dioxide) and silica-containing compounds as occurs in mining and industries involved with the extraction and processing of ores; preparation and use of sand; and manufacture of pipe, building, and roofing materials. Silica exposure activates innate and adaptive immune mechanisms, and triggers inflammation with subsequent fibrosis.[38] Acute inflammation contributes to bronchospasm and wheezing. Release of proteolytic enzymes and toxic oxygen free radicals increases the risk for lung cancer. Exposed individuals may remain asymptomatic long after the nodules are visible on chest radiography. When clinical manifestations do appear, they include cough and dyspnea. There is no curative treatment for the disease, although corticosteroids may produce some improvement in the early, more acute stages.

Coal worker pneumoconiosis (coal miner lung, black lung) is caused by coal dust deposits in the lung. Although coal dust itself is relatively well tolerated by the lung, it is frequently inhaled as a mixture of coal, silica, and quartz, which is strongly inflammatory. Its mild form is asymptomatic, except for possible chronic bronchitis. Its advanced form manifests as severe pulmonary fibrosis. Individuals usually are seen with a productive cough and wheezing. Symptoms are more severe with advanced disease and mimic those of chronic bronchitis and emphysema.[39] Diagnosis is made by obtaining a history of exposure and observing chest radiographs for characteristic signs. There is no specific treatment for coal worker pneumoconiosis. Individuals with the mild form of the disease usually have a favorable prognosis. Those with more complicated forms often develop marked cardiopulmonary dysfunction.

Asbestos exposure affects not only factory workers but also individuals who live in areas of asbestos emission. Asbestos exposure can result in a type of pulmonary fibrosis called **asbestosis,** but can also cause lung cancer, mesothelioma (cancer of the pleura), or pleural plaques, especially in those also exposed to cigarette smoke.[40]

Asbestosis is caused by inhalation of hydrous silicates of various metals in fibrous form. Asbestos fibers cause inflammation and alveolitis. Activated macrophages release toxic oxygen free radicals and cause cellular apoptosis, leading to both fibrosis and malignancy. The most prominent clinical manifestations of asbestosis with fibrosis are dyspnea on exertion, a nonproductive cough, diffuse inspiratory crackles on examination, hypoxemia, and decreased lung volume. Progressive disease may take years and leads to respiratory failure and cardiac complications. Diagnosis is made by chest x-ray, pulmonary function testing, and CT. Therapy is supportive.

Hypersensitivity Pneumonitis. **Hypersensitivity pneumonitis (extrinsic allergic alveolitis)** is an allergic, inflammatory disease of the lungs caused by inhalation of organic particles or fumes. Many allergens (antigens) can cause this disorder, including grains, silage, bird droppings or feathers, wood dust (particularly redwood and maple), cork dust, animal pelts, coffee beans, fish meal, mushroom compost, grain molds, mists from standing water, and fumes from paints and resins. A type III immune response (see Chapter 9) is initiated by alveolar macrophages and results in immunoglobulin G (IgG) antibody production. Continued exposure results in a type IV cellular immune activation. The inflammatory response causes pneumonitis.[41] Granuloma formation is common. Lung capacity and alveolocapillary diffusion are reduced. A genetic predisposition may increase the risk for this disease.

Allergic alveolitis can be acute, subacute, or chronic. The acute form causes a fever, cough, dyspnea, and chills a few hours after exposure that resolve without treatment in 1 to 3 days. With continued exposure, the disease becomes chronic and pulmonary fibrosis develops. (The mechanisms of hypersensitivity reactions are discussed in Chapter 9.) Chronic allergic alveolitis causes weight loss, fever, fatigue, and gradually progressive respiratory failure. Diagnosis is made by obtaining a history of allergen exposure and by performing serum antibody testing,

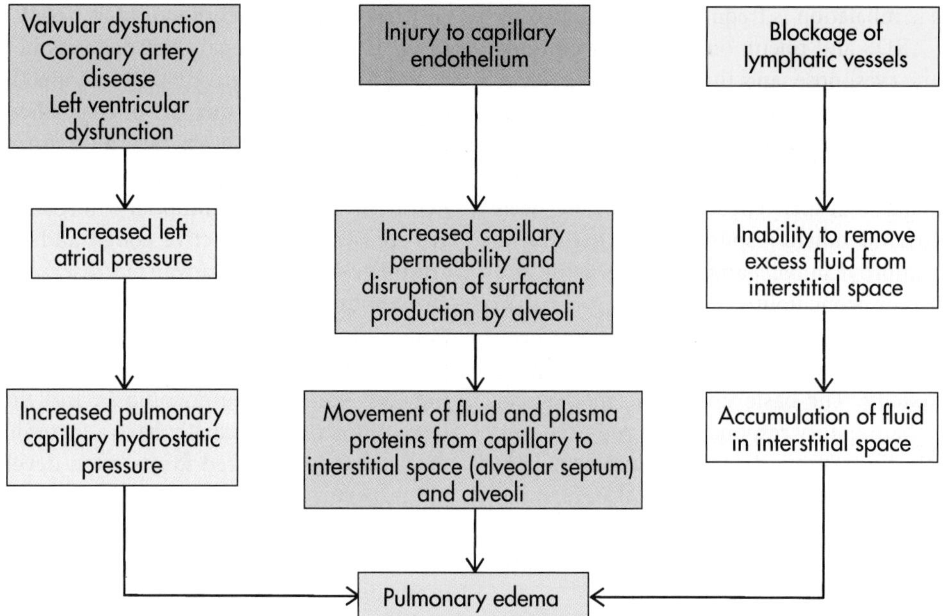

FIGURE 35-7 Pathogenesis of Pulmonary Edema.

chest x-ray, bronchoscopy, CT, and in some cases lung biopsy.[42] Treatment consists of avoidance of the offending agent and corticosteroid administration.

Systemic Disorders and the Lungs

Several systemic diseases affect the airways, pleurae, or lung parenchyma, causing fibrosis, vasculitis, pulmonary hemorrhage, or granuloma formation. Clinical manifestations of lung involvement are usually nonspecific, and the diagnosis is based on involvement of other organs. There is usually no specific treatment, although corticosteroids often are used. Some of the systemic diseases affecting the lung are granulomatous disorders such as sarcoidosis, Wegener granulomatosis, lymphomatoid granulomatosis, and eosinophilic granuloma; connective tissue diseases such as rheumatoid arthritis, systemic lupus erythematosus, scleroderma, polymyositis or dermatomyositis, Sjögren syndrome, and polyarteritis nodosa; angioimmunoblastic or immunoblastic lymphadenopathy (a disease of the lymph nodes); cystic fibrosis (see Chapter 36); and Goodpasture syndrome (a pulmonary and renal disorder).

Pulmonary Edema

Pulmonary edema is excess water in the lung. The normal lung contains very little fluid. It is kept dry by lymphatic drainage and a balance among capillary hydrostatic pressure, capillary oncotic pressure, and capillary permeability. In addition, surfactant lining the alveoli repels water, keeping fluid from entering the alveoli. Predisposing factors for pulmonary edema include heart disease, ARDS, and inhalation of toxic gases. The pathogenesis of pulmonary edema is illustrated in Figure 35-7.

The most common cause of pulmonary edema is left-sided heart disease (see Chapter 32). When the left ventricle fails, filling pressures on the left side of the heart increase and cause a concomitant increase in pulmonary capillary hydrostatic pressure. When the hydrostatic pressure exceeds oncotic pressure, fluid moves into the interstitium, or interstitial space (the space within the alveolar septum between alveolus and capillary). Fluid moves to the lymphatic vessels and is then removed from the lung. When the flow of fluid out of the capillaries exceeds the lymphatic system's ability to remove it, pulmonary edema develops. Pulmonary edema usually begins to develop at a pulmonary capillary wedge pressure or left atrial pressure of 20 mmHg. If the capillary oncotic pressure is decreased for any reason (e.g., anemia or decreased levels of plasma proteins), pulmonary edema develops at a lower hydrostatic pressure.

Another cause of pulmonary edema is capillary injury that increases capillary permeability. Capillary injury causes edema in cases of adult respiratory distress syndrome (ARDS) or inhalation of toxic gases, such as ammonia. Capillary injury causes water and plasma proteins to leak out of the capillary and move into the interstitium. When plasma proteins move into the lung interstitium, they increase the interstitial oncotic pressure, which is usually very low. As the interstitial oncotic pressure begins to equal capillary oncotic pressure, water moves out of the capillary and into the lung. (Mechanisms of edema are discussed in Chapter 3.)

Pulmonary edema also can result from obstruction of the lymphatic system. Drainage can be blocked by compression of lymphatic vessels caused by edema, tumors, and fibrotic tissue or by increased systemic venous pressure that elevates the hydrostatic pressure of the large pulmonary veins into which the pulmonary lymphatic system drains. This can happen in left-sided heart failure.

Postobstructive pulmonary edema (POPE, or **negative pressure pulmonary edema)** is a rare life-threatening complication that can occur after relief of upper airway obstruction (e.g., postextubation laryngospasm after anesthesia, epiglottitis, laryngeal tumor, or obstructive tonsils). Attempted inspiration against an occluded airway creates excessive intrathoracic negative pressure, causing increased venous return and blood flow to the right side of the heart and decreased outflow from the left side of the heart from the increased afterload. This combination of events causes increased pulmonary blood volume and venous pressure and leads to pulmonary edema.[43]

Clinical manifestations of pulmonary edema include dyspnea, orthopnea, hypoxemia, and increased work of breathing. Physical examination may reveal inspiratory crackles (rales), dullness to percussion over the lung bases, and evidence of ventricular dilation (S_3 gallop and cardiomegaly). In severe edema, pink, frothy sputum is expectorated, hypoxemia worsens, and hypoventilation with hypercapnia may develop.

The treatment of pulmonary edema depends on its cause. If the edema is caused by increased hydrostatic pressure resulting from heart failure, therapy is geared toward improving cardiac output and volume status with diuretics, vasodilators, and drugs that improve the contraction of the heart muscle. If edema is the result of increased capillary permeability resulting from injury, the treatment is focused on removing the offending agent and supportive therapy to maintain adequate oxygenation, ventilation, and circulation. POPE is treated with positive end-expiratory pressure ventilation. Individuals with any type of pulmonary edema require supplemental oxygen. Mechanical ventilation may be needed if edema significantly impairs ventilation and oxygenation.

Acute Lung Injury/Acute Respiratory Distress Syndrome

Acute lung injury (ALI)/acute respiratory distress syndrome (ARDS) represents a spectrum of acute lung inflammation and diffuse alveolocapillary injury. In the United States, ALI/ARDS is estimated at 64 to 78 cases per 100,000 people.[44] Advances in therapy have decreased the overall death rate to approximately 42% to 47%, although older people and those who have severe infections or are immunocompromised continue to have a much higher mortality.[45] Most survivors have almost normal lung function 1 year after the acute illness, but may have other health problems, including neurocognitive disorders up to 5 years later.[46] The most common predisposing factors for ARDS are genetic factors, sepsis, and multiple trauma (especially when multiple transfusions are received); however, there are many other causes, including pneumonia, burns, aspiration, cardiopulmonary bypass surgery, pancreatitis, drug overdose, smoke or noxious gas inhalation, oxygen toxicity, radiation therapy, and disseminated intravascular coagulation.[47,48]

PATHOPHYSIOLOGY. All disorders that result in ARDS cause acute injury to the alveolocapillary membrane producing massive pulmonary inflammation, increased capillary permeability, severe pulmonary edema, shunting, $\dot{V}/\dot{Q}$ mismatch, and hypoxemia. The alveolocapillary injury can occur directly, as with the aspiration of highly acidic gastric contents or the inhalation of toxic gases; or indirectly, as from circulating inflammatory mediators released in response to systemic disorders, such as sepsis and trauma. Lung inflammation and injury damages the alveolar epithelium and the vascular endothelium. Because the pulmonary edema is not secondary to heart failure, ARDS is often referred to as *noncardiogenic pulmonary edema.* ARDS progresses through three overlapping phases characterized by histologic changes in the lung: exudative (inflammatory), proliferative, and fibrotic (Figure 35-8).

Exudative (Inflammatory) Phase (Within 72 Hours). The initial lung injury damages the alveolocapillary membrane. Lung injury activates neutrophils, platelets, macrophages, lung epithelial and endothelial cells, and uncontrolled inflammation. Inflammatory mediators include complement, cytokines, arachidonic acid metabolites, platelet-activating factor, reactive oxygen species, and other mediators (specifically tumor necrosis factor [TNF], interleukin-1 [IL-1], and IL-6).[49] Activated complement factors and platelet aggregation result in intravascular microthrombus formation and further damage to lung capillaries.[50] In ARDS caused by sepsis, bacterial toxins are recognized by the CD14 receptors on macrophages and lead to chemotaxis of large numbers of neutrophils to the lungs. A cascade of inflammatory mediators is released by the macrophages, including TNF, IL-1, alpha and beta chemokines, and other interleukins.

The role of neutrophils is central to the development and progression of ARDS. Activated neutrophils release a battery of harmful inflammatory mediators, among them proteolytic enzymes, oxygen free radicals (superoxide radicals, hydrogen peroxide, hydroxyl radicals), arachidonic acid metabolites (prostaglandins, thromboxanes, leukotrienes), and platelet-activating factor. These mediators cause extensive damage to the alveolocapillary membrane and greatly increase capillary membrane permeability. Increased capillary permeability, a hallmark of ARDS, allows fluids, proteins, and blood cells to leak from the capillary bed into the pulmonary interstitium and alveoli (hemorrhagic exudate). The resulting pulmonary edema and hemorrhage severely reduce lung compliance and impair alveolar ventilation (Figure 35-9).

Mediators released by neutrophils, and to a certain extent by macrophages, also cause pulmonary vasoconstriction. Because vasoconstriction occurs more in some vascular beds than others, blood flow to selected areas of the lungs is decreased, resulting in $\dot{V}/\dot{Q}$ mismatching. Pulmonary hypertension occurs early in the course of the disease secondary to vasoconstriction. Thrombi composed of aggregated neutrophils, macrophages, platelets, and fibrin are formed.

Surfactant is inactivated, and its production by type II alveolar cells is impaired as alveoli and respiratory bronchioles fill with fluid or collapse.[51] The lungs become less compliant, the work of breathing increases, ventilation of alveoli decreases, and hypercapnia develops.

Proliferative Phase (4 to 21 Days). Within 1 to 3 weeks after the initial lung injury, there is resolution of the pulmonary edema and proliferation of type II pneumocytes, fibroblasts, and myofibroblasts. The intra-alveolar hemorrhagic exudate becomes a cellular granulation tissue appearing as hyaline membranes and there is progressive hypoxemia.

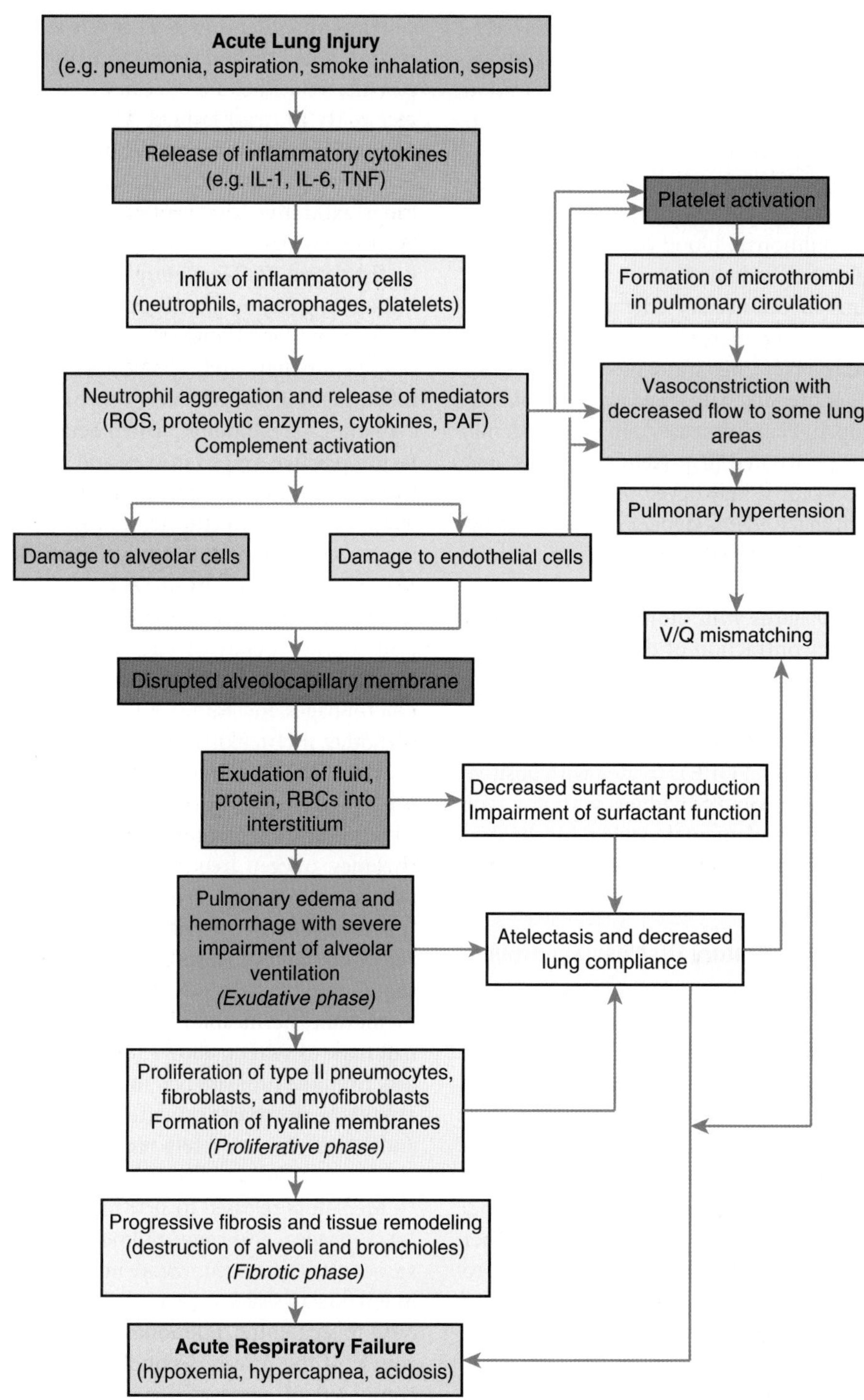

FIGURE 35-8 Pathogenesis of Acute Respiratory Distress Syndrome (ARDS). *IL-1,* Interleukin-1; *IL-6,* interleukin-6; *PAF,* platelet-activating factor; *RBCs,* red blood cells; *ROS,* reactive oxygen species; *TNF,* tumor necrosis factor.

Fibrotic Phase (14 to 21 Days). About 2 to 3 weeks after the initial injury, remodeling and fibrosis occur. The fibrosis progressively obliterates the alveoli, respiratory bronchioles, and interstitium, leading to a decrease in functional residual capacity (FRC) and continuing $\dot{V}/\dot{Q}$ mismatch with severe right-to-left shunt. The result of this overwhelming inflammatory response by the lungs is acute respiratory failure.

The same chemical mediators responsible for the alveolocapillary damage of ARDS often cause inflammation, endothelial damage, and capillary permeability throughout the body, resulting in the systemic inflammatory response syndrome (SIRS). SIRS then leads to multiple organ dysfunction syndrome (MODS). In fact, death may not be caused by respiratory failure alone, but by MODS associated with ARDS. (MODS is discussed in Chapter 48.)

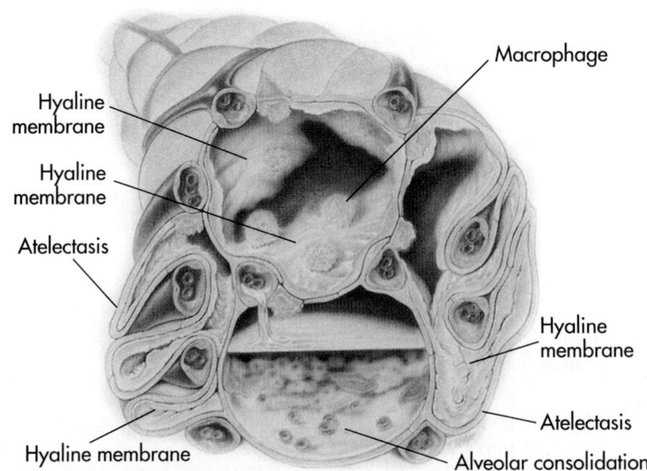

FIGURE 35-9 Acute Respiratory Distress Syndrome (ARDS). Cross-sectional view of alveoli in ARDS. (Modified from Des Jardins T, Burton GG: *Clinical manifestations and assessment of respiratory disease,* ed 3, St Louis, 1995, Mosby.)

CLINICAL MANIFESTATIONS. The clinical manifestations of ARDS are progressive as follows:

Dyspnea and hypoxemia with poor response to oxygen supplementation
↓
Hyperventilation and respiratory alkalosis
↓
Decreased tissue perfusion, metabolic acidosis, and organ dysfunction
↓
Increased work of breathing, decreased tidal volume, and hypoventilation
↓
Hypercapnia, respiratory acidosis, and worsening hypoxemia
↓
Decreased cardiac output, hypotension, and death

The new Berlin definition of ARDS provides categories of severity based on hypoxemia: mild (200 mmHg $< PaO_2/FIO_2 \leq$ 300 mmHg), moderate (100 mmHg $< PaO_2/FIO_2 \leq$ 200 mmHg), and severe ($PaO_2/FIO_2 \leq$ 100 mm Hg).[51a]

Worsening hypoxemia and hypercapnia lead to respiratory failure. Decreased oxygen delivery to tissues results in metabolic acidosis and organ dysfunction (e.g., decreased urine output and a decline in cognitive functioning). Decreased cardiac output and hypotension eventually lead to death.

EVALUATION AND TREATMENT. Diagnosis is made on the basis of a history of lung injury, physical examination, analysis of arterial blood gases, and chest radiographs. ALI/ARDS is defined as: (1) the acute onset of bilateral infiltrates on chest radiograph, (2) a low ratio of partial pressure of arterial oxygen to the fraction of inhaled oxygen, and (3) the absence of clinical evidence of left atrial hypertension.[52] Initial physical examination may show fine inspiratory crackles. Over the first 24 to 48 hours after injury, interstitial and alveolar infiltrates appear on chest radiographs. Serum biomarkers, such as TNF, brain natriuretic peptide (BNP), IL-6 and IL-8, and surfactant proteins, are being studied.[53]

Treatment strategies include early detection and management of contributing etiologies, supportive therapy to prevent progression of lung injury, and prevention of complications such as pneumonia and stress ulcer.[54,55] Traditional therapy includes mechanical ventilation with PEEP and high oxygen concentrations. Alternative modalities of ventilation are being evaluated, including low-volume ventilation, noninvasive positive-pressure ventilation, permissive hypercapnia, prone positioning, extracorporeal gas exchange, and partial liquid ventilation; some of these methods have shown reductions in death rates.[44]

Many studies are investigating new ways to prevent or treat ARDS.[56] Although recombinant human activated protein C was initially found to improve outcomes in individuals with shock and ARDS, more recent reviews found it to have no effect on mortality and the drug was removed from the market.[57] Prophylactic immunotherapy, antibodies against endotoxins, antioxidants, surfactant replacement, nitric oxide inhalation, and inhibition of various inflammatory mediators are among other possibilities being tested. High-dose corticosteroid administration is no longer recommended, but low-dose therapy improves outcomes.[58]

Obstructive Pulmonary Disease

Obstructive pulmonary disease is characterized by airway obstruction that is worse with expiration. More force (i.e., use of accessory muscles of expiration) or more time is required to expire a given volume of air and emptying of the lungs is slowed. The unifying symptom of obstructive pulmonary disease is dyspnea; the unifying sign is wheezing. Individuals have an increased work of breathing, ventilation-perfusion mismatching, and a decreased forced expiratory volume in one second (FEV_1). The most common obstructive diseases are asthma, chronic bronchitis, and emphysema. Because many individuals have chronic bronchitis with emphysema, these diseases together are often called COPD.

Asthma

Asthma is a chronic inflammatory disorder of the bronchial mucosa that causes bronchial hyperresponsiveness, constriction of the airways, and variable airflow obstruction that is reversible.[59] Asthma occurs at all ages, with approximately half of all cases developing during childhood (see Chapter 36) and another third before age 40. In the United States, it is estimated that 24.6 million people have asthma and the prevalence continues to increase. Death rates are highest for adult females, black persons, and adults older than 65.[60]

Asthma is most commonly a familial disorder and more than 100 genes have been identified that may play a role in the susceptibility and pathogenesis of asthma, including those that influence the production of IL-4, IL-5, and IL-13; IgE; eosinophils; mast cells; adrenergic receptors; leukotrienes; nitric oxide; and transmembrane proteins in the endoplasmic reticulum.[61] Specific gene expression may impart associated phenotypes, such as inflammation, sensitization to allergens, airway fibroblasts, airway remodeling, and responsiveness to asthma therapies[62,63] (see Chapter 36, p. 1309, for What's New? Asthma Phenotypes). Other risk factors include allergen exposure; urban residence; exposure to air pollution, tobacco smoke, and environmental tobacco smoke; recurrent respiratory tract viral infections; esophageal reflux; and obesity.[59,64] These factors cause epigenetic changes that influence the function of asthma susceptibility genes.[65-67] Exposure to high levels of certain allergens during childhood increases the risk for asthma. Furthermore, decreased exposure to certain infectious organisms appears to create an immunologic imbalance that favors the development of allergy and asthma in some individuals. This complex relationship has been called the *hygiene hypothesis* (see the Asthma section on p. 1308 in Chapter 36 for more detail).[68]

PATHOPHYSIOLOGY. Airway epithelial exposure to antigen initiates both an innate and an adaptive immune response in sensitized individuals (see Chapter 9).[69] Many cells and cellular elements contribute to the persistent inflammation of the bronchial mucosa and hyperresponsiveness of the airways, including macrophages (dendritic cells), T helper 2 (Th2) lymphocytes, B lymphocytes, mast cells, neutrophils, eosinophils, and basophils. There is both an immediate (early asthmatic response) and a late (delayed) response.

During the *early asthmatic response,* antigen exposure to the bronchial mucosa activates dendritic cells (antigen-presenting cells) to present the antigen to CD4+ T cells, which differentiate into Th2 cells (see Chapter 9). These Th2 cells release numerous cytokines including IL-4, IL-5, IL-8, IL-13, IL-17, and IL-22. IL-4 stimulates B-cell activation, proliferation, and production of antigen-specific IgE. IL-5 stimulates the activation, migration, and proliferation of eosinophils, which cause direct tissue injury and release of toxic neuropeptides that contribute to increased bronchial hyperresponsiveness, fibroblast proliferation, epithelial injury, and airway scarring. IL-8 activates neutrophils that contribute to a more exaggerated inflammatory response. IL-13 impairs mucociliary clearance, enhances fibroblast secretion, and contributes to bronchoconstriction and airway remodeling.[70] IL-17 increases neutrophilic inflammation and IL-22 stimulates airway epithelial cells, which play an important role in stimulating further innate and adaptive immune responses.[71,72]

The Fc portion of preformed IgE binds to receptors on the surface of mast cells. Once bound to antigen, the IgE causes the mast cells to degranulate, releasing a large number of inflammatory mediators[73] (see Figure 7-11 for additional details regarding mast cells). Together these mediators cause vasodilation, increased capillary permeability, mucosal edema, bronchial smooth muscle contraction (bronchospasm), and tenacious mucus secretion from mucosal goblet cells with narrowing of the airways and obstruction to airflow[69] (Figures 35-10, 35-11, and 35-12).

The *late asthmatic response* begins 4 to 8 hours after the early response. Chemotactic recruitment of lymphocytes, eosinophils, and neutrophils during the acute response causes a latent release of inflammatory mediators, again inciting bronchospasm, edema, and mucus secretion with obstruction to airflow. Synthesis of leukotrienes contributes to prolonged smooth muscle contraction. Eosinophil mediators cause direct tissue injury with fibroblast proliferation and airway scarring. Release of toxic neuropeptides contribute to increased bronchial hyperresponsiveness. Damage to ciliated epithelial cells contributes

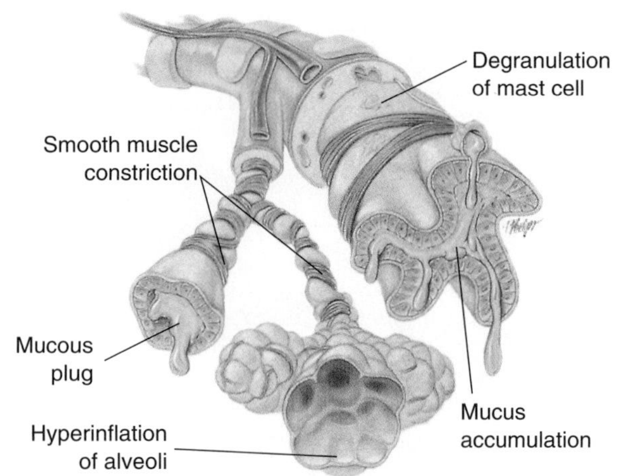

FIGURE 35-10 Bronchial Asthma. Thick mucus, mucosal edema, and smooth muscle spasm cause obstruction of small airways; breathing becomes labored and expiration is difficult. (Modified from Des Jardins T, Burton GG: *Clinical manifestations and assessment of respiratory disease,* ed 3, St Louis, 1995, Mosby.)

to impaired mucociliary function with accumulation of mucus and cellular debris forming plugs in the airways (increased synthesis of nitric oxide contributes to oxidative injury and chronic inflammation).[74] A decrease in the number or function of T regulatory (Treg) cells are associated with asthma.[69] Untreated inflammation can lead to long-term airway damage that is irreversible, known as *airway remodeling* (subepithelial fibrosis, smooth muscle and mucous gland hypertrophy).[75]

Airway obstruction increases resistance to airflow and decreases flow rates, especially expiratory flow. Impaired expiration causes air trapping, hyperinflation distal to obstructions and increased work of breathing. Changes in resistance to airflow are not uniform throughout the lungs and the distribution of inspired air is uneven, with more air flowing to the less resistant portions. Continued air trapping increases intrapleural and alveolar gas pressures and causes decreased perfusion of the alveoli. Increased alveolar gas pressure, decreased ventilation, and decreased perfusion lead to variable and uneven ventilation-perfusion relationships within different lung segments. Hyperventilation is triggered by lung receptors responding to increased lung volume and obstruction. The result is early hypoxemia without CO_2 retention. Hypoxemia further increases hyperventilation through stimulation of the respiratory center, causing $Paco_2$ to decrease and pH to increase (respiratory alkalosis). With progressive obstruction of expiratory airflow, air trapping becomes more severe and the lungs and thorax become hyperexpanded, putting the respiratory muscles at a mechanical disadvantage. This leads to a fall in tidal volume with increasing CO_2 retention and respiratory acidosis. Respiratory acidosis signals respiratory failure, especially when left ventricular filling and, thus, cardiac output become compromised because of severe hyperinflation.

CLINICAL MANIFESTATIONS. Individuals are asymptomatic between attacks and pulmonary function tests are normal. No clinical symptoms are present during partial remission, but pulmonary function tests are abnormal. At the beginning of an attack, the individual experiences chest constriction, expiratory

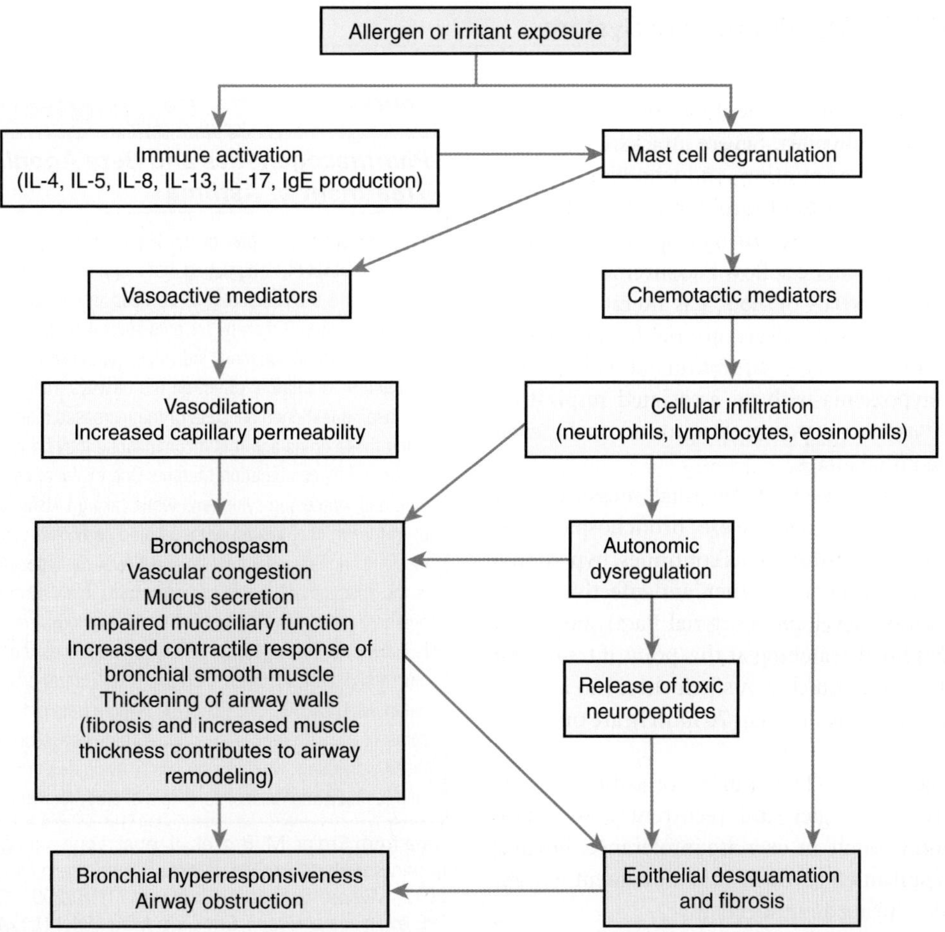

FIGURE 35-11 Pathophysiology of Asthma. Allergen or irritant exposure results in a cascade of inflammatory events leading to acute and chronic airway dysfunction. *IgE,* Immunoglobulin E; *IL,* interleukin.

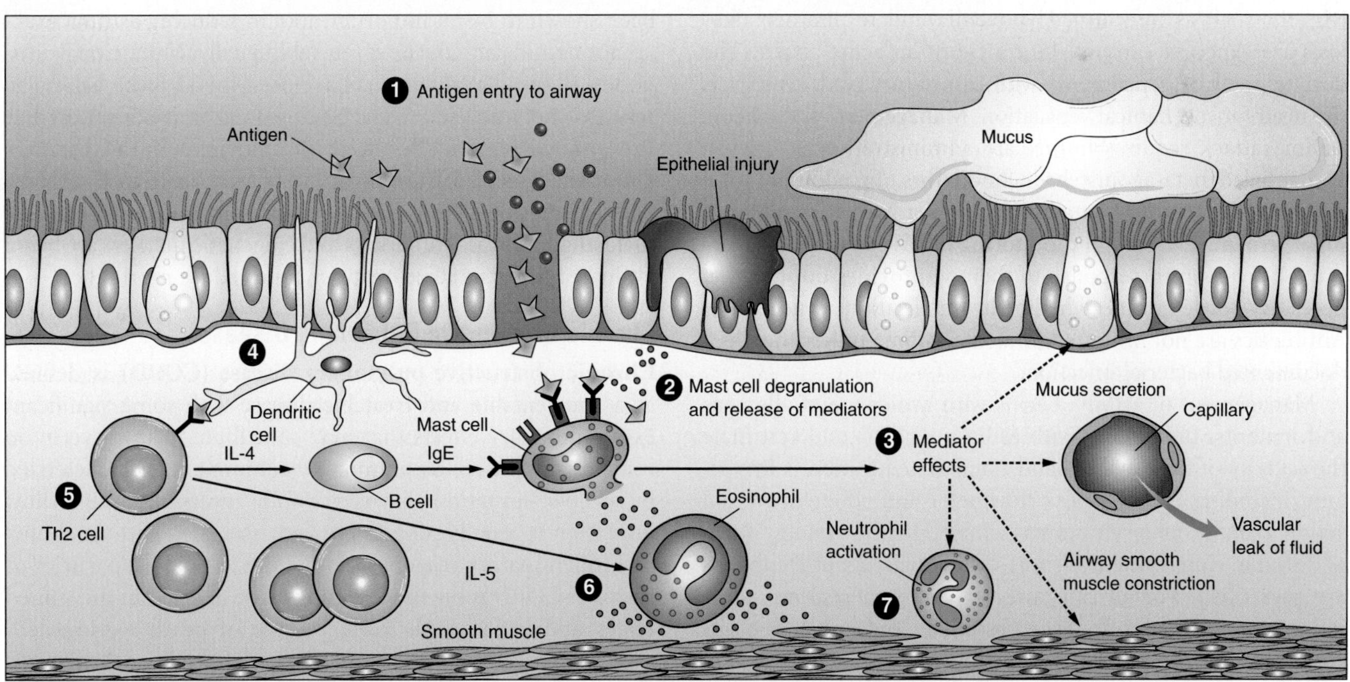

FIGURE 35-12 Acute Asthmatic Responses. Inhaled antigen **(1)** binds to mast cells covered with preformed IgE. Mast cells degranulate **(2)** and release inflammatory mediators such as histamine, bradykinins, leukotrienes, prostaglandins, platelet-activating factor, and interleukins. Secreted mediators **(3)** induce active bronchospasm (airway smooth muscle constriction), edema from increased capillary permeability, and airway mucus secretion from goblet cells. At the same time, antigen is detected by **(4)** dendritic cells that process and present it to Th2 cells **(5),** which produce interleukin-4 *(IL-4)* and many other interleukins (see text). IL-4 promotes switching of B cells to favor immunoglobulin E *(IgE)* production. Th2 cells also produce IL-5 **(6),** which activates eosinophils. Eosinophil products, such as major basic protein and eosinophilic cationic protein, damage the respiratory epithelium. Many inflammatory cells, including neutrophils **(7),** also contribute to the inflammatory process. *IgE,* Immunoglobulin E.

wheezing, dyspnea, nonproductive coughing, prolonged expiration, tachycardia, and tachypnea. Severe attacks involve the use of accessory muscles of respiration, and wheezing is heard during both inspiration and expiration. A **pulsus paradoxus** (decrease in systolic blood pressure during inspiration of more than 10 mmHg) may be noted. Peak flow measurements should be obtained. Because the severity of blood gas alterations is difficult to evaluate by clinical signs alone, arterial blood gas tensions should be measured if oxygen saturation falls below 90%. Usual findings are hypoxemia with an associated respiratory alkalosis. In the *late asthma response,* symptoms can be even more severe than the initial attack.

If bronchospasm is not reversed by usual measures, the individual is considered to have severe bronchospasm or **status asthmaticus.** If status asthmaticus continues, hypoxemia worsens, expiratory flows decrease further, and effective ventilation decreases. Acidosis develops as arterial $Paco_2$ begins to rise. Asthma becomes life threatening at this point if treatment does not reverse this process quickly. A silent chest (no audible air movement) and a $Paco_2$ greater than 70 mmHg are ominous signs of impending death.

EVALUATION AND TREATMENT. The diagnosis of asthma is supported by a history of allergies and recurrent episodes of wheezing, dyspnea and cough, or exercise intolerance. Further evaluation includes spirometry, which may document reversible decreases in FEV_1 during an induced attack.

The evaluation of an acute asthma attack requires the rapid assessment of arterial blood gases and expiratory flow rates (using a peak flowmeter) and a search for underlying triggers, such as infection. Hypoxemia and respiratory alkalosis are expected early in the course of an acute attack. The development of hypercapnia with respiratory acidosis signals the need for mechanical ventilation. Management of the acute asthma attack requires immediate administration of oxygen and inhaled beta-agonist bronchodilators. In addition, oral corticosteroids should be administered early in the course of management.[59,76] Careful monitoring of gas exchange and airway obstruction in response to therapy provides information necessary to determine whether hospitalization is necessary. Antibiotics are not indicated for acute asthma unless there is a documented bacterial infection.

Management of asthma begins with avoidance of allergens and irritants. Individuals with asthma tend to underestimate the severity of their asthma and extensive education is important, including use of a peak flowmeter and adherence to an action plan should symptoms worsen. In the mildest form of asthma (intermittent), short-acting beta-agonist inhalers are prescribed. For all categories of persistent asthma, anti-inflammatory medications are essential and inhaled corticosteroids are the mainstay of therapy. In individuals whose symptoms are not adequately controlled using inhaled corticosteroids, leukotriene antagonists can be considered. In more severe asthma, long-acting beta agonists can be used to control persistent bronchospasm; however, these agonists can actually worsen asthma in some individuals with certain genetic polymorphisms (see What's New? Pharmacogenetics and Beta Agonists in the Treatment of Asthma). Immunotherapy has been shown to be an important tool in reducing asthma exacerbations and can now be given sublingually. Monoclonal antibodies to IgE (omalizumab) have been found to be helpful in selected individuals.[77,78] The National Asthma Education and Prevention Program offers stepwise guidelines for the diagnosis and management of chronic asthma based on clinical severity, and they may be reviewed at www.nhlbi.nih.gov/guidelines/asthma/asthgdln.htm. Biomarkers and epigenetic markers are being evaluated to personalize treatment and reduce mortality.[79]

WHAT'S NEW?

Pharmacogenetics and Beta Agonists in the Treatment of Asthma

In the recent third report of the National Asthma Education and Prevention Program (NAEPP), long-acting beta agonists (LABAs) (salmeterol and formoterol) are recommended to be used in conjunction with inhaled corticosteroids as step 3 therapy for persistent asthma. LABAs have been found to improve symptoms in many individuals, and exert a long-term bronchodilatory and anti-inflammatory effect on the airways. However, the safety of LABAs has been questioned because of the increased mortality in some populations using these drugs and it is recommended they be withdrawn once asthma is controlled by combination therapy. One explanation is that those individuals who had worsening symptoms while taking LABAs were using them instead of (rather in conjunction with) inhaled corticosteroids and thus were simply masking ongoing inflammation and airway damage. LABAs should not be used in the absence of inhaled corticosteroids. New evidence suggests that some persons have a polymorphism of the β-adrenergic receptor gene *(ADRβ2).* This is known as the Arg16Arg genotype and places those individuals at risk for worsening bronchospasm, increased hospitalizations, and increased mortality when using LABAs. This genotype is more frequent in blacks and may explain some of the differences in asthma treatment response and mortality among these individuals. Studies continue to evaluate other genes and their relationship to medication response, a field of study known as pharmacogenetics.

Data from Erdinç M, Brozek JL et al: Long-acting β2-agonist step-off in patients with controlled asthma, *Arch Intern Med* 172(18):1365-1375, 2012; Mysore S, Ruffin RE: *Drugs* 71(16):2091–2097, 2011; Wechsler ME et al: *Am J Respir Crit Care Med* 184(11):1247–1253, 2011; Wells KE et al: *J Allergy Clin Immunol* 129(5):1274–1279, 2012.

Chronic Obstructive Pulmonary Disease

Chronic obstructive pulmonary disease (COPD) is defined as a "preventable and treatable disease with some significant extrapulmonary effects that may contribute to the severity in individual patients. Its pulmonary component is characterized by airflow limitation that is not fully reversible. The airflow limitation is usually progressive and associated with an abnormal inflammatory response of the lung to noxious particles or gases."[80] COPD is the third leading cause of death in the United States and is the sixth leading cause of death worldwide.[80] Overall mortality from COPD has increased in the United States over the past 30 years; however, mortality in women has increased more than twice that much.[81] Risk factors for COPD include tobacco smoke (cigarette, pipe, cigar, and environmental tobacco smoke), occupational dusts and chemicals (vapors, irritants, and fumes), indoor air pollution from biomass fuel used for cooking and heating (in poorly vented dwellings), outdoor air pollution, and any factor that affects lung growth

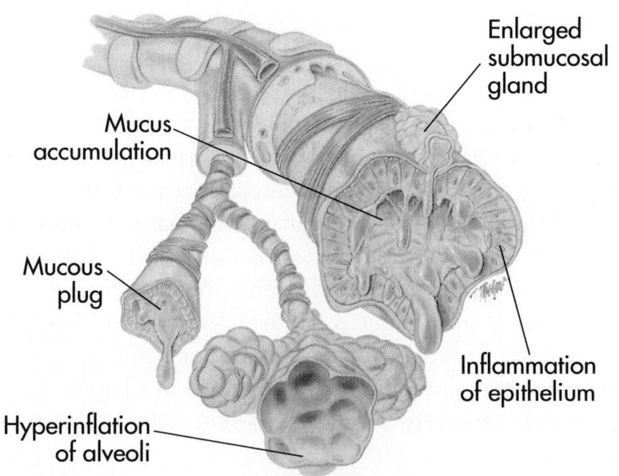

FIGURE 35-13 Chronic Bronchitis. Inflammation and thickening of mucous membrane with accumulation of mucus and pus leading to obstruction characterized by productive cough. (Modified from Des Jardins T, Burton GG: *Clinical manifestations and assessment of respiratory disease,* ed 3, St Louis, 1995, Mosby.)

during gestation and childhood (low birth weight, respiratory tract infections).[80] Genetic susceptibilities have been identified, including polymorphisms of genes that code for tumor necrosis factor, surfactant, proteases, antiproteases, and risks for lung cancer. The clinical phenotypes of COPD are chronic bronchitis and emphysema.[82] An inherited mutation in the α_1-antitrypsin gene results in the development of COPD (emphysema) at an early age, even in nonsmokers.[83,84]

The pathologic changes of COPD occur in large central airways, small peripheral airways, and the lung parenchyma, the dominant features of chronic bronchitis and emphysema. Chronic irritant exposure recruits macrophages, neutrophils, and lymphocytes to the lung, resulting in progressive damage from oxidative stress, inflammation, extracellular matrix proteolysis, and apoptotic and autophagic cell death.[85,86] Systemic abnormalities, such as renal and hormonal abnormalities, malnutrition, muscle wasting, osteoporosis, and anemia, are associated with COPD.[87]

Chronic Bronchitis. **Chronic bronchitis** is defined as hypersecretion of mucus and chronic productive cough that continues for at least 3 months of the year (usually the winter months) for at least 2 consecutive years.

PATHOPHYSIOLOGY. Inspired irritants result in airway inflammation with infiltration of neutrophils, macrophages, and lymphocytes into the bronchial wall. Tobacco smoke directly injures airway epithelial cells. Continual bronchial inflammation causes bronchial edema and increases the size and number of mucous glands and goblet cells in the airway epithelium. Thick, tenacious mucus is produced and cannot be cleared because of impaired ciliary function (Figure 35-13). The lung's defense mechanisms are, therefore, compromised, increasing susceptibility to pulmonary infection, which contributes to airway injury.[88] Frequent infectious exacerbations are complicated by bronchospasm with dyspnea and productive cough.[89] The pathogenesis of chronic bronchitis is shown in Figure 35-14.

Initially chronic bronchitis affects only the larger bronchi, but eventually all airways are involved. The thick mucus and hypertrophied bronchial smooth muscle narrow the airways and lead to obstruction, particularly during expiration when the airways are constricted. Obstruction eventually leads to ventilation-perfusion mismatch with hypoxemia. The airways collapse early in expiration, trapping gas in the distal portions of the lung (Figure 35-15). Air trapping expands the thorax, putting the respiratory muscles at a mechanical disadvantage. This leads to decreased tidal volume, hypoventilation, and hypercapnia.

CLINICAL MANIFESTATIONS. The common symptoms of chronic bronchitis include decreased exercise tolerance, wheezing, and shortness of breath. Individuals usually have a productive cough ("smoker's cough"), and evidence of airway obstruction (decreased FEV_1) is shown by spirometry. Hypoxemia may occur with exercise. As the disease progresses, copious amounts of sputum are produced, accompanied by frequent pulmonary infections.[90] FVC and FEV_1 values become markedly reduced, and FRC and residual volume (RV) measurements are increased as airway obstruction and air trapping become more pronounced.

Airway obstruction results in decreased alveolar ventilation and increased $Paco_2$. Marked hypoxemia leads to polycythemia (overproduction of erythrocytes) and cyanosis. If not reversed, hypoxemia leads to pulmonary hypertension and eventually results in cor pulmonale (see p. 1278) and can lead to severe disability or death. (Table 35-3 lists the common clinical manifestations of chronic bronchitis.)

EVALUATION AND TREATMENT. Diagnosis is based on history of symptoms, physical examination, chest radiograph, pulmonary function tests, and blood gas analyses; these tests reflect the progressive nature of the disease. Prevention of chronic bronchitis is the best treatment because pathologic changes are not reversible. By the time an individual seeks medical care for symptoms, considerable airway damage is present. If the individual stops smoking, disease progression can be halted.

Bronchodilators (long-acting inhaled anticholinergics or long-acting inhaled beta agonists for symptomatic persons with COPD and FEV_1 <60% predicted) and expectorants are prescribed to reduce dyspnea and control cough. Chest physical therapy may be helpful and includes deep breathing and postural drainage. During acute exacerbations (infection and bronchospasm), individuals require treatment with antibiotics and corticosteroids and may need mechanical ventilation. Chronic oral corticosteroids may be needed late in the course of the disease, but should be considered a last resort. Individuals with severe hypoxemia will require continuous oxygen therapy. Teaching includes nutritional counseling, respiratory hygiene, recognition of the early signs of infection, and techniques that relieve dyspnea, such as pursed-lip breathing, all of which may be useful in the treatment of chronic bronchitis in selected individuals.[91,92] (see Nutrition & Disease: Chronic Obstructive Pulmonary Disease). Oxygen is administered with care to individuals with severe hypoxemia and CO_2 retention. Chronic elevation of $Paco_2$ diminishes the sensitivity of central chemoreceptors and they no longer act as the primary stimulus for breathing. (Chemoreceptors are described in Chapter 34.) This role is taken over by the peripheral chemoreceptors, which are sensitive to changes in Pao_2. Peripheral chemoreceptors do not stimulate breathing if the Pa_{O_2} is much more than 60 mmHg. Therefore, if oxygen therapy causes Pa_{O_2} to exceed 60 mmHg, the stimulus to breathe decreases, Pa_{CO_2} increases, and apnea results. However, severe hypoxemia must be reversed, especially if there are comorbidities (e.g., heart disease, tissue injury) that require adequate tissue oxygenation. If titration of oxygen therapy cannot be achieved without causing respiratory depression, the individual's lungs must be mechanically ventilated.[93]

Emphysema. **Emphysema** is abnormal permanent enlargement of gas-exchange airways (acini) accompanied by destruction of alveolar walls without obvious fibrosis. The major mechanism of airflow limitation in emphysema is loss of elastic recoil. Some degree of emphysema is considered normal in older adults, but results in a slow and predictable decline in lung function with aging.

Primary emphysema, which accounts for 1% to 3% of all cases of emphysema, is commonly linked to an inherited deficiency of the enzyme α_1-antitrypsin.[94] Normally α_1-antitrypsin inhibits the action of many proteolytic enzymes (enzymes that break down proteins). Individuals who have α_1-antitrypsin deficiency (an autosomal recessive trait) have an increased likelihood of developing emphysema, because proteolysis in lung tissues is not inhibited. Homozygous individuals have a 70% to 80% likelihood of developing lung disease. (Mechanisms of genetic inheritance are described in Chapter 4.) Persons with α_1-antitrypsin deficiency who smoke are even more

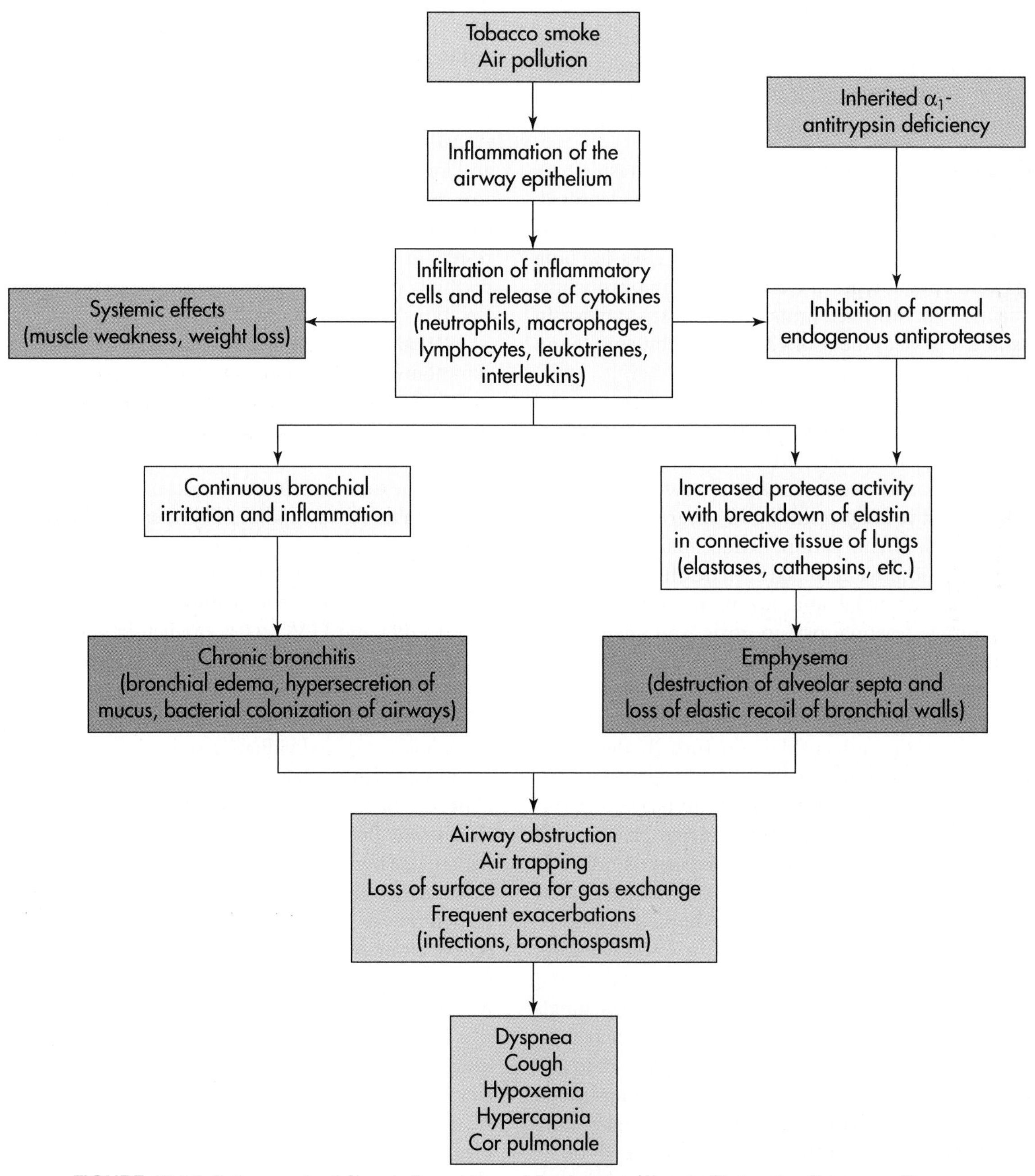

FIGURE 35-14 Pathogenesis of Chronic Bronchitis and Emphysema (Chronic Obstructive Pulmonary Disease [COPD]).

susceptible to emphysema than those with the deficiency alone. α_1-Antitrypsin deficiency is suggested in nonsmokers and individuals who develop emphysema before age 40 years (or in their early forties).

The major cause of secondary emphysema is the inhalation of cigarette smoke, although air pollution, occupational exposures, and childhood respiratory tract infections are known to be contributing factors. Not all smokers develop emphysema, but approximately 15% to 20% are especially susceptible and develop significant lung damage, if they continue to smoke.[95]

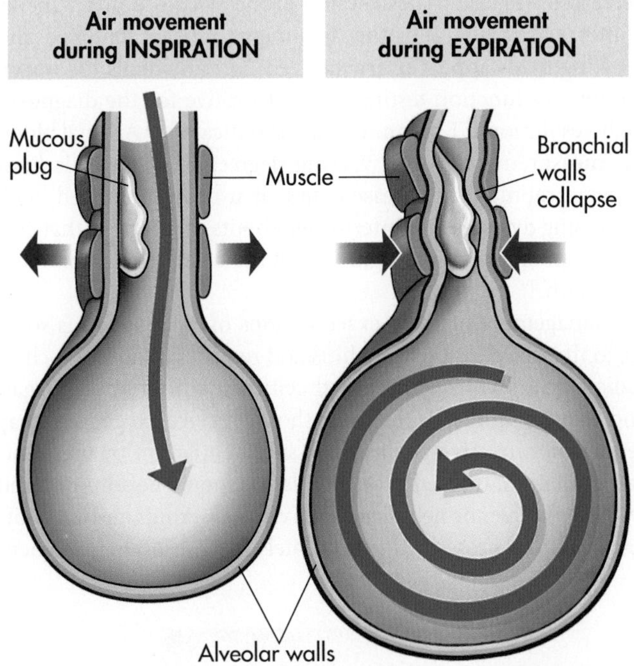

FIGURE 35-15 Mechanisms of Air Trapping in Chronic Obstructive Pulmonary Disease (COPD). Mucous plugs and narrowed airways cause air trapping and hyperinflation on expiration. During inspiration the airways are pulled open, allowing gas to flow past the obstruction. During expiration decreased elastic recoil of the bronchial walls results in collapse of the airways and prevents normal expiratory airflow.

TABLE 35-3 CLINICAL MANIFESTATIONS OF CHRONIC PULMONARY DISEASE

CLINICAL MANIFESTATIONS	CHRONIC BRONCHITIS	EMPHYSEMA
Productive cough	Classic sign	Late in course with infection
Dyspnea	Late in course	Common
Wheezing	Intermittent	Minimal
History of smoking	Common	Common
Barrel chest	Occasionally	Classic
Prolonged expiration	Always present	Always present
Cyanosis	Common	Uncommon
Chronic hypoventilation	Common	Late in course
Polycythemia	Common	Late in course
Cor pulmonale	Common	Late in course

PATHOPHYSIOLOGY. Emphysema is characterized by destruction of alveoli through the breakdown of elastin within the septa by an imbalance between proteases and antiproteases, oxidative stress, and apoptosis of lung structural cells[87,96] (see Figure 35-14). Cellular apoptosis and early cellular senescence contribute to loss of alveolar cells and reduced surface area for gas exchange. Alveolar destruction also produces large air spaces within the lung parenchyma (bullae) and air spaces adjacent to pleurae (blebs). Bullae and blebs are not effective in gas exchange and combined with loss of portions of the pulmonary capillary bed, there is significant ventilation-perfusion ($\dot{V}/\dot{Q}$) mismatching and hypoxemia. Expiration becomes difficult because loss of elastic recoil reduces the volume of air that can be expired passively and air is trapped in the lungs (see Figure 35-15). **Air trapping** causes hyperexpansion of the chest, which puts the muscles of respiration at a mechanical disadvantage. This results in increased work of breathing, so that many individuals will develop hypoventilation and hypercapnia late in the course of the disease. Persistent inflammation in the airways can result in hyperreactivity of the bronchi with bronchoconstriction, which may be partially reversible with bronchodilators. Chronic inflammation also can have significant systemic effects including weight loss, muscle weakness, and increased susceptibility to comorbidities, such as infection.

Emphysema can be centriacinar (centrilobular) or panacinar (panlobular) (Figure 35-16), depending on the site of involvement. In **centriacinar emphysema** septal destruction occurs in the respiratory bronchioles and alveolar ducts, usually in the upper lobes of the lung. The alveolar sac (alveoli distal to the respiratory bronchiole) remains intact. It tends to occur

NUTRITION & DISEASE

Chronic Obstructive Pulmonary Disease

Malnutrition occurs in up to one third of individuals with chronic obstructive pulmonary disease (COPD) and is a major concern because these individuals have increased work of breathing and energy expenditure, decreased energy intake, and impaired oxygenation. The disproportionate muscle wasting is similar to what occurs with other chronic diseases, such as cancer, heart failure, and acquired immunodeficiency syndrome (AIDS). Systemic inflammatory mediators may impair appetite and contribute to hypermetabolism. Malnutrition (1) adversely affects exercise tolerance by limiting skeletal and respiratory muscle strength and aerobic capacity, (2) limits surfactant production, (3) reduces cell-mediated immune responses, (4) decreases protein synthesis, and (5) increases morbidity and mortality. The medical nutrition therapy goal is to maintain an acceptable and stable weight for the person. This can be accomplished through high-energy foods, oral nutritional support, frequent snacking, soft foods and beverages, assistance with shopping, and meal preparation. Reducing the amount of carbohydrates while providing adequate protein and lipids may improve carbon dioxide balance. Increasing omega-3 fatty acids and antioxidant intake may modulate the effects of systemic inflammation. Vitamin D and calcium supplementation is indicated to improve bone health. Serum phosphate levels also should be monitored to prevent hypophosphatemia, which can contribute to muscle weakness.

Data from Collins PF, Stratton RJ, Elia M: *Am J Clin Nutr* 95(6):1385–1395, 2012; Criner GJ et al: *Am J Respir Crit Care Med* 184(7):763–770, 2011; Kelly RJ, Giaccone G: *Cancer J* 17(5):302–308, 2011; Raguso CA, Luthy C: *Nutrition* 27(2):138–143, 2011.

in smokers with chronic bronchitis. **Panacinar emphysema** involves the entire acinus, with damage more randomly distributed and involving the lower lobes of the lung (Figure 35-17). It tends to occur in older adults and in those with α_1-antitrypsin deficiency.[97]

CLINICAL MANIFESTATIONS. Dyspnea on exertion that later progresses to marked dyspnea, even at rest, is the most common symptom of emphysema (see Table 35-3). Little coughing and very little sputum are produced. Often the individual is thin, has tachypnea with prolonged expiration, and must use accessory muscles for ventilation. The anteroposterior diameter of the chest is increased (barrel chest), and the chest has a hyperresonant sound with percussion. To increase lung capacity, the individual often leans forward with arms extended and braced on knees when sitting. In addition, people with emphysema often exhale through pursed lips which helps prevent expiratory airway collapse.

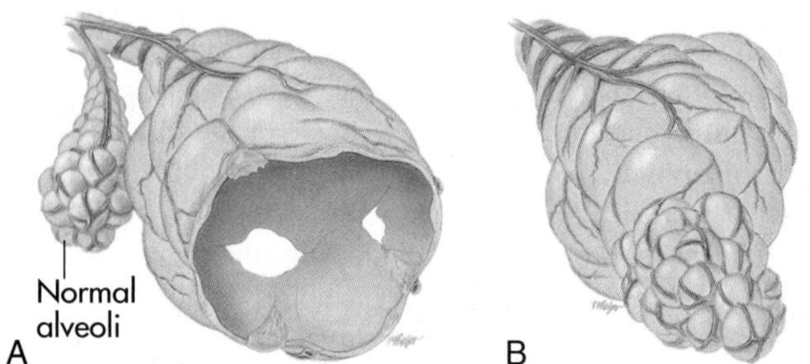

FIGURE 35-16 Emphysema. Enlargement and destruction of alveolar walls with loss of elasticity and trapping of air. **A,** Panlobular emphysema showing abnormal weakening and enlargement of all air spaces distal to the terminal bronchioles (normal alveoli shown for comparison only); **B,** centrilobular emphysema showing abnormal weakening and enlargement of the respiratory bronchioles in the proximal portion of the acinus. (Modified from Des Jardins T, Burton GG: *Clinical manifestations and assessment of respiratory disease,* ed 3, St Louis, 1995, Mosby.)

EVALUATION AND TREATMENT. Emphysema is usually diagnosed and staged by pulmonary function measures. In COPD, pulmonary function tests indicate obstruction to gas flow during expiration with a marked decrease in FEV_1. Airway collapse and air trapping in distal portions of the lung lead to a decrease in FVC (but less so than FEV_1) and an increase in FRC, residual volume (RV), and total lung capacity (TLC). Diffusing capacity is decreased because of destruction of the alveolocapillary membranes. On radiographs the diaphragm appears flattened and the lung fields appear overdistended. In individuals for whom pulmonary function testing is not definitive for the diagnosis, high-resolution CT scanning may be indicated.[98] Arterial blood gas measurements reveal varying degrees of hypoxemia and/or hypercapnia. The disease course is usually prolonged, with increasing dyspnea and intermittent bouts of infection that culminate in failure of the right side of the heart (cor pulmonale) and death.[99]

Management of acute exacerbations of emphysema is similar to that for chronic bronchitis and requires obtaining a chest radiograph, serum white blood cell count, arterial blood gas, and sputum sample. Individuals should receive oxygen and may require noninvasive positive-pressure ventilation or mechanical ventilation. Inhaled bronchodilators should be administered by either inhaler or nebulizer. Oral corticosteroids and antibiotics should be prescribed immediately.[87] Chronic management

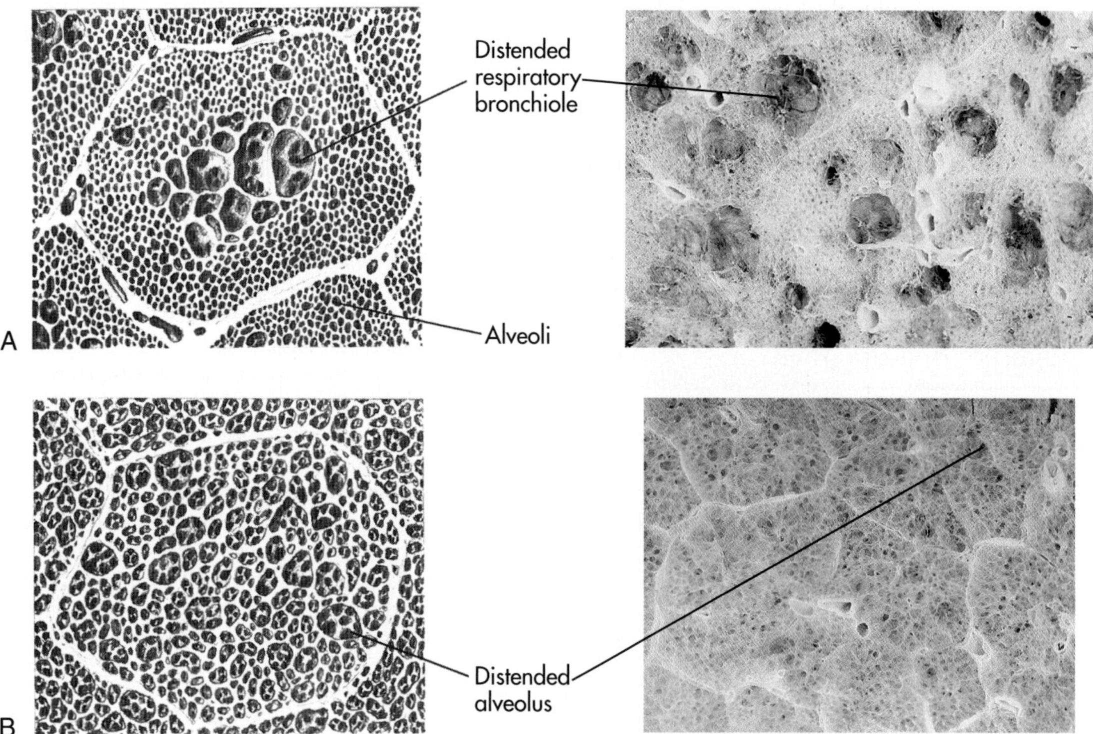

FIGURE 35-17 Micrographs of Types of Emphysema. **A,** Centriacinar emphysema. **B,** Panacinar emphysema. (Micrographs from Damjanov I, Linder J, editors: *Anderson's pathology,* ed 10, St Louis, 1996, Mosby.)

of emphysema begins with smoking cessation. Pharmacologic management is based on clinical severity, defined by the Global Initiative for Chronic Obstructive Lung Disease (GOLD), as mild, moderate, severe, or very severe. Inhaled anticholinergic agents and beta agonists should be prescribed. Inhaled corticosteroids added to long-acting anticholinergics of beta agonists diminish the number of acute exacerbations, slow the rate of decline in quality of life, and reduce the rate of decline in FEV_1; however, their use must be weighed against the potential side effects (oropharyngeal candidiasis and hoarseness, and risk of pneumonia).[100] Long-term therapy with oral corticosteroids should be avoided, if possible. Pulmonary rehabilitation, improved nutrition, and breathing techniques can all improve symptoms. Oxygen therapy is indicated in chronic hypoxemia, but must be administered with care. Progressive pulmonary dysfunction with hypoxemia and hypercapnia may require long-term oxygen therapy and ventilation, if indicated.[101] In selected patients, lung volume reduction surgery or transplantation can be considered.[102] The recently approved phosphodiesterase E4 (PDE4) inhibitor roflumilast reduces airway inflammation and is proving to be effective in selected individuals with severe COPD.[103] α_1-Antitrypsin augmentation may be indicated for primary emphysema.[91,104]

Respiratory Tract Infections

Respiratory tract infections are the most common cause of short-term disability in the United States. Most of these infections—the common cold, pharyngitis (sore throat), and laryngitis—involve only the upper airways. Although the lungs have direct contact with the atmosphere, they remain sterile under most circumstances. Infections of the lower respiratory tract occur most often in the very young, the very old, or individuals with impaired immunity or underlying disease. In all cases the body's normal defense mechanisms are impaired.

Pneumonia

Pneumonia is infection of the lower respiratory tract caused by bacteria, viruses, fungi, protozoa, or parasites. It is the sixth leading cause of death in the United States and is responsible for more disease and death than any other infection.[105] More than half of those hospitalized for pneumonia are older than age 65; mortality from pneumonia is highest in older adults. Risk factors for pneumonia include advanced age, immunocompromised status, underlying lung disease (especially COPD), alcoholism, altered consciousness, impaired swallowing, smoking, endotracheal intubation, malnutrition, immobilization, underlying cardiac or liver disease, and residence in a nursing home.

Pneumonia can be categorized as community-acquired (CAP), healthcare-associated (HCAP), hospital-acquired (HAP), or ventilator-associated (VAP). CAP is one of the most common reasons for hospitalization in the United States. HCAP is defined as occurring in individuals with recent hospitalization, residence in a nursing home or extended care facility, home infusion therapy, chronic dialysis, or home wound care. It is estimated that nearly one third of all hospital admissions for pneumonia are now considered HCAP. HAP is the second most common nosocomial infection (urinary tract infection [UTI] most common), but has the greatest mortality (overall 20% to 50% mortality). VAP occurs in 9% to 27% of individuals who require intubation and mechanical ventilation.[106-108] The microorganisms that most commonly cause CAP are different from those infections that cause HCAP, HAP, and VAP (Box 35-1). In addition, the characteristics of the individual are important in determining which etiologic microorganism is likely; for example, immunocompromised persons tend to be susceptible to opportunistic infections that are uncommon in normal adults (see Box 35-1).

PATHOPHYSIOLOGY. Aspiration of oropharyngeal secretions is the most common route of lower respiratory tract infection; thus the nasopharynx and oropharynx constitute the first line of defense for most infectious agents. Another route of infection is through the inhalation of microorganisms that have been released into the air when an infected individual coughs, sneezes, or talks, or from aerosolized water, such as that from contaminated respiratory therapy equipment. This route of infection is most important in viral and mycobacterial pneumonias and in *Legionella* outbreaks. Endotracheal tubes become colonized with bacteria that form biofilms (protected colonies of bacteria that are resistant to host defenses and treatment with antibiotics) and can seed the lung with microorganisms, especially during endotracheal suctioning.[109] Pneumonia also can occur when bacteria are spread to the lungs in the blood from bacteremia that can result from infection elsewhere in the body or from intravenous drug use.

In healthy individuals, pathogens that reach the lungs are expelled or held in check by mechanisms of self-defense (see Chapters 7, 8, and 34). If a microorganism enters the upper airway defense mechanisms, such as the cough reflex and mucociliary clearance, the next line of defense is the airway epithelial

BOX 35-1 ETIOLOGIC MICROORGANISMS FOR PNEUMONIA IN ADULTS

CAP	HCAP/HAP/VAP	IMMUNOCOMPROMISED INDIVIDUALS
Streptococcus pneumoniae	*Pseudomonas aeruginosa*	*Pneumocystis jiroveci* (formerly *P. carinii*)
Haemophilus influenzae	*Staphylococcus aureus* (including methicillin-resistant strains)	*Mycobacterium tuberculosis*
Staphylococcus aureus	*Klebsiella pneumoniae*	Atypical mycobacteria
Mycoplasma pneumoniae	*Enterobacter* species	Respiratory viruses
Chlamydia pneumoniae		Protozoa
Moraxella catarrhalis		Parasites
Legionella pneumophila		
Influenza		
Rhinovirus		
Coronavirus		

CAP, Community-acquired pneumonia; *HAP,* hospital-acquired pneumonia; *HCAP,* healthcare-associated pneumonia; *VAP,* ventilator-associated pneumonia.

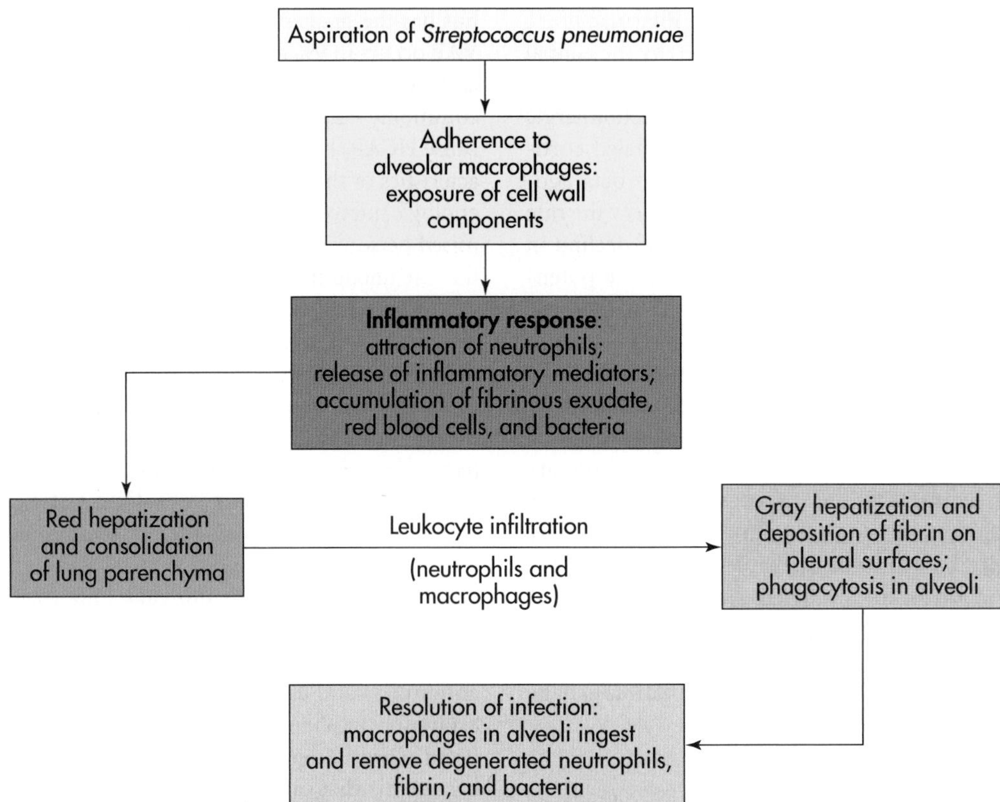

FIGURE 35-18 Pathophysiologic Course of Pneumococcal Pneumonia *(Streptococcus pneumoniae).*

cell. Airway epithelial cells can recognize some pathogens directly (e.g., *Pseudomonas aeruginosa* and *Staphylococcus aureus*). However, the most important guardian cell of the lower respiratory tract is the alveolar macrophage and it recognizes pathogens through its pattern-recognition receptors (e.g., Toll like receptors). Macrophages present infectious antigens to the adaptive immune system, activating T cells and B cells with the induction of cellular and humoral immunity. Release of TNF-α and IL-1 from macrophages and chemokines and chemotactic signals from mast cells and fibroblasts contributes to widespread inflammation in the lung with recruitment of neutrophils from the capillaries of the lungs into the alveoli. Neutrophils are critical phagocytes that kill microbes through the formation of phagolysosomes filled with degradative enzymes, antimicrobial proteins, and toxic oxygen free radicals.[110]

Neutrophils have also been found to extrude a meshwork of proteins called a neutrophil extracellular trap (NET) that can capture any bacteria that have not yet been phagocytosed. Unfortunately, many pathogens, such as the pneumococcus, can release a DNase that cleaves the NET and thus escape neutrophil defense.[111] The release of inflammatory mediators and immune complexes can damage bronchial mucous membranes and alveolocapillary membranes, causing the acini and terminal bronchioles to fill with infectious debris and exudate. In addition, some microorganisms release toxins from their cell walls that can cause further lung damage. The accumulation of exudate in the acinus leads to dyspnea and to $\dot{V}/\dot{Q}$ mismatching and hypoxemia.

Pneumococcal Pneumonia. The pathogenesis of pneumococcal pneumonia *(Streptococcus pneumoniae)* has been well documented and serves as a model for understanding other forms of bacterial pneumonia (Figure 35-18). *S. pneumoniae* microorganisms initiate innate and adaptive immune responses (see Chapters 7 and 8). The immune response includes complement activation and the production of antibodies, which are crucial for opsonizing the encapsulated bacterium. Rapid lysis of pneumococcal bacteria (as occurs with antibiotic treatment) results in the release of intracellular bacterial proteins that can be toxic. The best known of these proteins is pneumolysin, which is cytotoxic to virtually every cell in the lung and is partially responsible for the worsening in clinical symptoms sometimes seen in individuals immediately after they begin antibiotic treatment.[112] Inflammatory cytokines and cells are released that cause alveolar edema. Edema creates a medium for the multiplication of bacteria and aids in the spread of infection into adjacent portions of the lung. The involved lobe undergoes consolidation, which alveoli fill with blood cells, fibrin, edematous fluid, and pneumococci, giving lung tissue a red appearance. This passes into the stage in which affected tissues become gray because of fibrin deposition over the pleural surfaces and the presence of fibrin and neutrophils in the consolidated alveoli, where phagocytosis is rapidly taking place. With resolution, increasing numbers of macrophages appear in the alveolar spaces, the neutrophils degenerate, and the fibrin threads and remaining bacteria are digested by macrophages and removed by lymphatic vessels. Usually infection is limited to one or two lobes.

Viral Pneumonia

Viral pneumonia is seasonal, usually mild and self-limiting, but it can set the stage for a secondary bacterial infection (especially by *S. aureus* and *Streptococcus pneumoniae*) by providing an ideal environment for bacterial growth and by damaging ciliated epithelial cells, which normally prevent pathogens from reaching the lower airways.[113] Viral pneumonia can be a primary infection (e.g., influenza pneumonia) or a complication of another viral illness (e.g., chickenpox, measles). Influenza virus is the most common viral cause of pneumonia. The virus not only destroys the ciliated epithelial cells, but also invades the goblet cells and bronchial mucous glands. Sloughing of destroyed bronchial epithelium occurs throughout the respiratory tract, preventing mucociliary clearance. Bronchial walls become edematous and infiltrated with leukocytes.[114]

Some forms of viral pneumonia can progress to severe systemic illness with many complications and a high morbidity and mortality. Severe viral pneumonia can include common types of influenza that can be fatal, especially in older adults.[115] Other severe viral infections are considered opportunistic infections, such as cytomegalovirus pneumonia in immunocompromised individuals. New or atypical forms of viral infection, such as swine influenza A (H1N1) virus, avian influenza A (H5N1) virus, and the coronavirus that causes severe acute respiratory syndrome (SARS), are affecting previously healthy populations and pose a considerable threat for pandemics.[116,117]

CLINICAL MANIFESTATIONS. Most cases of pneumonia are preceded by an upper respiratory tract infection, which is usually viral. This is then followed by the onset of cough, dyspnea, and fever. The cough is often productive, but may be nonproductive, especially in viral pneumonia. Other symptoms include chills, malaise, and pleuritic chest pain. Physical examination may reveal signs of pulmonary consolidation, such as inspiratory crackles, increased tactile fremitus, egophony, and whispered pectoriloquy. Individuals also may demonstrate symptoms and signs of underlying systemic disease or sepsis.

EVALUATION AND TREATMENT. Diagnosis is made on the basis of history, physical examination (tachypnea, tachycardia, crackles, bronchial breath sounds, and findings of pleural effusion), white blood cell count, chest x-ray, stains and cultures of blood, and cultures of respiratory secretions. The white blood cell count is usually elevated, although it may be low if the individual is debilitated, immunocompromised, or has overwhelming infection.[118] Chest radiographs show infiltrates that may involve a single lobe of the lung or may be more diffuse. Once the diagnosis of pneumonia has been made, the pathogen is identified by means of sputum characteristics (Gram stain, color, odor) and cultures or, if sputum is absent, blood cultures. Because many pathogens exist in the normal oropharyngeal flora, the specimen may be contaminated with pathogens from oral secretions. If sputum studies fail to identify the pathogen, the individual is immunocompromised, or the individual's condition worsens, further diagnostic studies may include molecular testing of blood or urine, bronchoscopy, or lung biopsy.[119,120]

Prevention of pneumonia includes prevention of aspiration, respiratory isolation of immunocompromised individuals, vaccination for appropriate populations, and reduction of ventilator-associated pulmonary infections through a variety of dental and endotracheal tube interventions.[109,121,122] The first step in the management of pneumonia is establishing adequate ventilation and oxygenation. Most individuals have hypoxemia and a respiratory alkalosis, although persons with underlying lung disease may require ventilation. Adequate hydration and good pulmonary hygiene (e.g., deep breathing, coughing, chest physical therapy) are also important.

Antibiotics are used to treat bacterial pneumonia; however, resistant strains of *Pneumococcus* are becoming more prevalent.[123] In individuals for whom a specific microorganism is not identified, empirical antibiotics are chosen based on the likely causative microorganism.[124,125] Viral pneumonia is usually treated with supportive therapy alone (unless secondary bacterial infection is present); however, antivirals may be needed in severe cases. Infections with opportunistic microorganisms may be polymicrobial and require multiple drugs, including antifungals.

Tuberculosis

Tuberculosis (TB) is an infection caused by *Mycobacterium tuberculosis,* an acid-fast bacillus that usually affects the lungs, but may invade other body systems. TB is the leading cause of death from a curable infectious disease throughout the world. TB cases increased greatly during the mid-1990s because of AIDS. Individuals with AIDS are highly susceptible to respiratory tract infections, including multidrug-resistant TB.[126] Many ambitious programs for prevention and treatment have been initiated worldwide and the World Health Organization (WHO) *2011 Global Tuberculosis Control Report* indicates that global TB incidence and prevalence have declined in most regions of the world in recent years.[127] In the United States, the incidence of TB has reached its lowest level since 1953, but the rate of decline has begun to slow with more than half of new cases of TB occurring in foreign-born individuals, especially among non-Hispanic Asians, non-Hispanic blacks, and Hispanics.[128]

PATHOPHYSIOLOGY. TB is highly contagious and is transmitted from person-to-person in airborne droplets. Host susceptibility to infection is influenced by host and parasite genetic polymorphisms, including those that affect macrophages, tumor necrosis factor, and interleukins.[129] In immunocompetent individuals, the microorganism usually is contained by the inflammatory and immune response systems, and latent TB infection (LTBI) develops with no clinical evidence of disease.[130] Microorganisms lodge in the lung periphery, usually in the upper lobe. Once the bacilli are inspired into the lung, they multiply and cause nonspecific pneumonitis (lung inflammation). Some bacilli migrate through the lymphatics and become lodged in the lymph nodes, where they encounter lymphocytes and initiate the immune response. Inflammation in the lung causes neutrophils and macrophages to migrate to the area. These cells are phagocytes that engulf the bacilli and begin the process by which the body's defense mechanisms isolate the bacilli, preventing their spread. However, the bacterium is successful as a pathogen because it can survive within macrophages, resist lysosomal killing, multiply within the cell, form well-organized granulomas creating a confined environment, terminate its own central metabolism, stop replication, and transit into a stage of dormancy rendering itself extremely resistant to host defense and drug treatment.[131,132] In defense, macrophages and lymphocytes release interferon, which inhibits the replication of the microorganisms and stimulates more macrophages to attack the bacterium. Apoptotic infected macrophages also can activate cytotoxic T cells (CD8). Neutrophils, lymphocytes, and macrophages seal off the colonies of bacilli, forming a granulomatous lesion called a *tubercle*.[133] Infected tissues within the tubercle die, forming cheeselike material called *caseation necrosis*. (Necrosis is described in Chapter 2.) Collagenous scar tissue then grows around the tubercle, completing isolation of the bacilli. The immune response is complete after about 10 days, preventing further multiplication of the bacilli.

Once the bacilli are isolated in tubercles and immunity develops, TB may remain dormant for life.[134] If the immune system is impaired, progressive active disease occurs and may spread through the blood and lymphatics to other organs. Infection with human immunodeficiency virus (HIV) is the single greatest risk factor for reactivation of tuberculosis infection. Cancer, immunosuppressive medications, poor nutritional status, renal failure, and other debilitating diseases can reactivate disease.

CLINICAL MANIFESTATIONS. Latent TB infection is asymptomatic. Symptoms of active disease develop so gradually that they are not noticed until the disease is advanced. However, symptoms can appear in immunosuppressed individuals within weeks of exposure to the bacillus. Common clinical manifestations include fatigue, weight loss, lethargy, anorexia (loss of appetite), a low-grade fever that usually occurs in the afternoon, and night sweats. (These are common signs and symptoms of all chronic infections.) A cough that produces purulent sputum develops slowly and becomes more frequent over several weeks or months. Dyspnea, chest pain, and hemoptysis also may occur as the disease progresses. Extrapulmonary TB disease is common in HIV-infected individuals and may cause neurologic deficits, meningitis symptoms, bone pain, and urinary symptoms.

EVALUATION AND TREATMENT. TB is diagnosed by a positive tuberculin skin test (TST; purified protein derivative [PPD]), sputum culture, immunoassays, and chest radiographs.[135,136] A positive tuberculin skin test indicates the need for yearly chest radiographs to detect active disease. The skin test does not differentiate between past, latent, or active forms of the disease. In addition, those individuals who have received the TB vaccine with bacille Calmette-Guérin (BCG) will have a positive TST even if they have never had TB. When active pulmonary disease is present, the tubercle bacillus can be cultured from the sputum and may be seen with an acid-fast stain. However, sputum culture can take up to 6 weeks to become positive. Chest radiographs of individuals with current or previous active disease demonstrate characteristic changes. Nodules, calcifications, cavities, and hilar enlargement (enlarged mediastinal lymph nodes) commonly are seen in the upper lobes. Two immunoassays (enzyme-linked immunospot and quantitative blood interferon-gamma assay) are available. These new tests are more sensitive and specific for the diagnosis of latent TB and are not confounded by previous BCG vaccination. However, they are often not available in high poverty populations and new techniques need to be developed for cost-effective and simple to use diagnostic tests.[137] Prevention of tuberculosis infection is a complex challenge. Isolating individuals with active tuberculosis, limiting use of immunosuppressive medications, and treating underlying immunocompromising diseases, such as AIDS, are all critical steps. Development of an effective TB vaccine has been elusive and vaccines are currently in clinical development.[138]

Treatment consists of combinations of antibiotics (isoniazid, rifampin, pyrazinamide, and ethambutol) to control active disease or prevent reactivation of latent TB infection. The choice of drugs and the duration of treatment depend on the individual's health history, the likelihood of bacterial resistance to certain drugs, and the presence of active disease. The waxy coat of *M. tuberculosis* renders it impermeable to many common drugs. For drug-resistant bacilli, the recommended treatment is administration for an 18-month timeframe of a combination of at least four drugs to which the microorganism is susceptible, including a review of drug effectiveness at 6 months.[139] New drugs and drug combinations are being tested to overcome drug resistance, including immune amplifiers.[140,141]

Abscess Formation and Cavitation

An **abscess** is a circumscribed area of suppuration and destruction of lung parenchyma. Abscess formation follows **consolidation** of lung tissue, in which inflammation causes alveoli to fill with fluid, pus, and microorganisms. Necrosis (death and decay) of consolidated tissue may progress proximally until it communicates with a bronchus. If this occurs, the abscess empties into the bronchus, leaving a cavity that has a radiographic appearance similar to that of a lesion of tuberculosis.

Pneumonia caused by aspiration or by exposure to *Klebsiella* or *Staphylococcus* is the most common cause of abscess formation. Aspiration abscess is usually associated with alcohol abuse, seizure disorders, general anesthesia, and swallowing disorders. Immunocompromised individuals also are at greater risk for lung abscesses and may be infected with opportunistic microorganisms, such as fungi and mycobacteria. The clinical manifestations of abscess formation are similar to those of pneumonitis: fever, cough, chills, excessive sputum production, and pleural pain. Abscess communication with a bronchus causes a severe cough, copious amounts of often foul-smelling sputum, and occasionally hemoptysis. **Cavitation** is the process of abscess emptying and cavity formation. Diagnosis is made by radiography. Treatment includes the administration of appropriate antibiotics and chest physical therapy, including chest percussion and postural drainage. Bronchoscopy may be performed to drain the abscess.[142]

Acute Bronchitis

Acute bronchitis is acute infection or inflammation of the airways or bronchi. The vast majority of cases of acute bronchitis are caused by viruses. Many of the clinical manifestations are similar to those of pneumonia (i.e., cough, fever, chills, malaise), but physical examination does not reveal signs of pulmonary consolidation and chest radiographs do not show

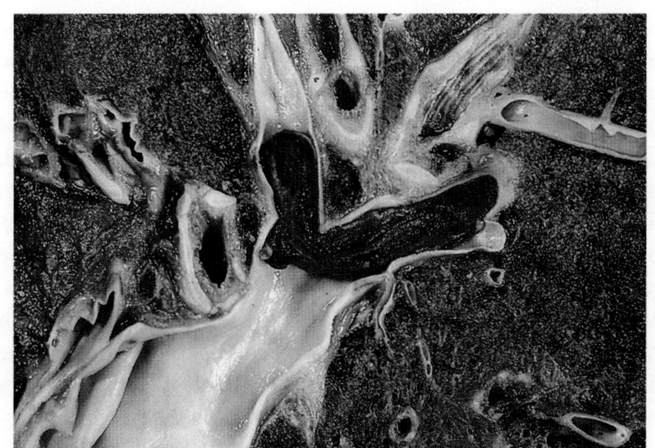

FIGURE 35-19 **Pulmonary Embolus.** The embolus extends into major branches of the pulmonary artery. (From Kumar V et al: *Robbins & Cotran pathologic basis of disease,* ed 8, Philadelphia, 2010, Saunders.)

infiltrates. Individuals with viral bronchitis usually have a nonproductive cough that occurs in paroxysms and is aggravated by cold, dry, or dusty air. However, purulent sputum may be produced with some viral infections. Chest pain often develops from the effort of coughing. Treatment consists of rest, aspirin, humidity, and a cough suppressant, such as codeine.

Individuals with bacterial bronchitis have a productive cough, fever, and pain behind the sternum (breast bone) that is aggravated by coughing. It is rare in previously healthy adults except after viral infection, but is common in those with COPD. Bacterial bronchitis is treated with rest, aspirin, humidity, and antibiotics.[143]

Pulmonary Vascular Disease

Blood flow through the lungs can be disrupted by a number of disorders that result in occlusion of the vessels, an increase in pulmonary vascular resistance, or destruction of the vascular bed. The consequences of altered pulmonary blood flow may be of no functional significance or can result in severe and life-threatening changes in ventilation-perfusion ratios. Major disorders that result from pulmonary vascular diseases include pulmonary embolism, pulmonary hypertension, and cor pulmonale.

Pulmonary Embolism

Pulmonary embolism (PE) is occlusion or partial occlusion of the pulmonary artery or its branches by an embolus. PE most commonly results from embolization of a clot from deep venous thrombosis involving the lower leg (see Chapter 32). Other less common nonthrombotic emboli include tissue fragments, lipids (fats), a foreign body, or an air bubble (Figure 35-19). Risk factors for PE include conditions and disorders that promote blood clotting as a result of *venous stasis* (immobilization, heart failure), *hypercoagulability* (inherited coagulation disorders, malignancy, hormone replacement, oral contraceptives, pregnancy), and *endothelial injury* to the cells that line the vessels (trauma, caustic intravenous infusions). Increased risk for thrombosis associated with hemodynamic stasis, hypercoagulability, and endothelial injury is known as Virchow's triad[144] (see Chapter 32). Genetic risks include factor V Leiden mutation (activated protein C resistance), antithrombin II deficiency, protein S deficiency, protein C deficiency, and prothrombin *20210* gene mutations. No matter its source, a blood clot becomes an embolus when all or part of it breaks away from the site of formation and begins to travel in the bloodstream.[145,146] Thromboembolism is described further in Chapter 32.

PATHOPHYSIOLOGY. The effect of the embolus depends on the extent of pulmonary blood flow obstruction, the size of the affected vessels, the nature of the embolus, and the secondary effects.[147] Pulmonary emboli can result in any of the following:

1. Embolus with infarction: an embolus that causes infarction (death) of a portion of lung tissue
2. Embolus without infarction: an embolus that does not cause permanent lung injury (perfusion of the affected lung segment is maintained by the bronchial circulation)
3. Massive occlusion: an embolus that occludes a major portion of the pulmonary circulation (i.e., main pulmonary artery embolus)
4. Multiple pulmonary emboli: multiple emboli may be chronic or recurrent

As a result of the thrombus lodging in the pulmonary circulation, there is a release both of neurohumoral substances, such as serotonin, histamine, catecholamines, and angiotensin II, and of inflammatory mediators, such as endothelin, leukotrienes, thromboxanes, and toxic oxygen free radicals. This causes widespread vasoconstriction that further impedes blood flow to the lung. Hemodynamically, this results in increased pulmonary artery pressures and can lead to right heart failure.[148] Absent blood flow to a lung segment causes a ventilation-perfusion mismatch (increased dead space) and a decrease in surfactant production. The resulting atelectasis of the affected lung segments further contributes to hypoxemia. If the thrombus is large enough, infarction of lung tissue, dysrhythmias, decreased cardiac output, shock, and death are possible.[149] The pathogenesis of venous thromboembolism is summarized in Figure 35-20.

If the embolus does not cause infarction, the clot is dissolved by the fibrinolytic system (see Chapter 27) and pulmonary function returns to normal. If pulmonary infarction occurs, shrinking and scarring develop in the affected area of the lung. The risk of recurrent venous thromboembolism is 30% over the next 10 years, and is much higher in those individuals who have irreversible risk factors for the disease.[150]

CLINICAL MANIFESTATIONS. In most cases the clinical manifestations of PE are nonspecific; therefore, evaluation of risk factors and predisposing factors is an important aspect of diagnosis. Consequently, the recognition of individuals at high risk for PE is crucial to assessing the clinical presentation. A list of an individual's predisposing factors for venous thromboembolism can be inserted into one of several clinical prediction models (e.g., Wells Prediction Rule model) to obtain a prediction score that helps determine risk probability.[151] In suspected PE, assessment for DVT may indicate the presence of a lower extremity source for the thromboembolism. Calf pain and tenderness, along with calf asymmetry when documented with a tape measure, are some of the most important findings in DVT. Unfortunately, DVT is often asymptomatic and clinical examination has low

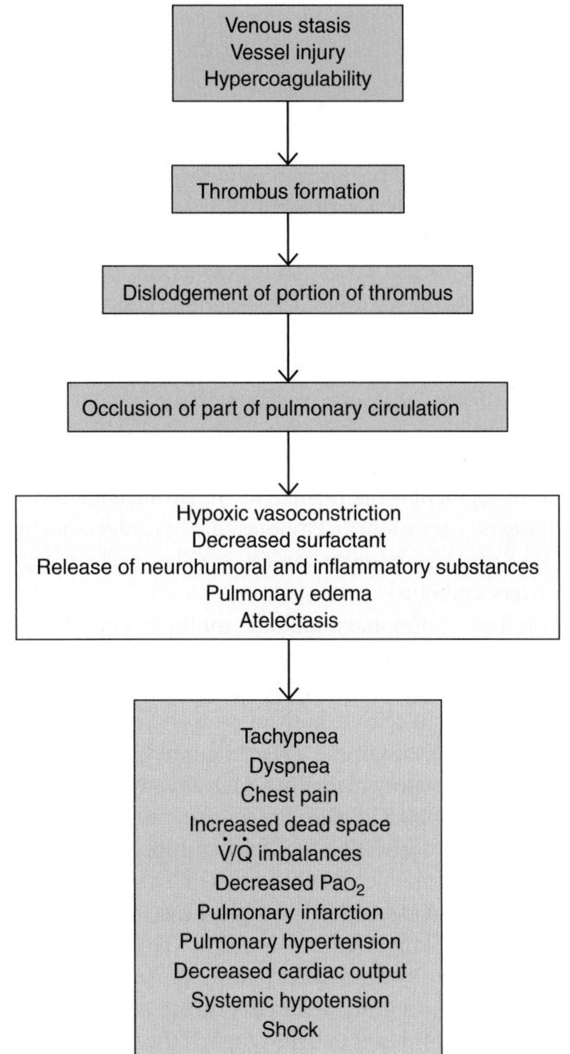

FIGURE 35-20 Pathogenesis of Massive Pulmonary Embolism Caused by a Thrombus (Pulmonary Thromboembolism).

sensitivity for the presence of a clot, especially in the thigh and pelvis. Therefore, the lack of clinical indicators for DVT does not rule out the possibility for PE.

An individual with PE usually presents with the sudden onset of pleuritic chest pain, dyspnea, tachypnea, tachycardia, and unexplained anxiety. Occasionally syncope (fainting) or hemoptysis occurs. With large emboli, a pleural friction rub, pleural effusion, fever, and leukocytosis may be noted. Recurrent pulmonary emboli occur in individuals with a history of previous emboli. Recurrent small emboli may not be detected until progressive incapacitation, precordial pain, anxiety, dyspnea, and right ventricular enlargement are exhibited. Massive occlusion causes profound shock, hypotension, tachypnea, tachycardia, severe pulmonary hypertension, and chest pain.

EVALUATION AND TREATMENT. When an individual is suspected of having a PE based on the presence of risk factors, symptoms, and physical findings, a chest x-ray, arterial blood gas, and electrocardiogram (ECG) are obtained immediately. Chest x-ray findings are nonspecific in PE and often can be normal for the first 24 hours until atelectasis occurs in the lung. The arterial blood gas results commonly reveal hypoxemia with a respiratory alkalosis (most individuals will hyperventilate in response to PE). The ECG may show evidence of strain on the right side of the heart. The serum D-dimer level measures a product of thrombus degradation by the fibrinolytic system and, if normal, makes the presence of a PE highly unlikely. Further evaluation is conducted using single or multidetector spiral CT arteriography.[152,153] This highly sensitive and specific test has replaced the radionucleotide ventilation-perfusion scan in most hospitals. Magnetic resonance imaging (MRI) is used in some centers. In rare cases, a pulmonary angiogram is necessary to confirm the diagnosis of PE. Recently, the measurement of elevated serum troponin I levels has been useful in stratifying the risk and severity of PE because it increases with right ventricular strain or failure.[154] Diagnostic algorithms guide diagnosis and treatment.[153]

The ideal treatment of PE is prevention through risk factor recognition and elimination of predisposing factors. Venous stasis in hospitalized individuals is minimized by bed exercises, frequent position changes, early ambulation, and pneumatic calf compression.[155] Most at-risk individuals also will receive prophylactic anticoagulation with unfractionated heparin, low-molecular-weight heparin, warfarin, or fondaparinux.[156] In individuals who have contraindications to anticoagulation, the placement of a filter in the inferior vena cava can prevent emboli from reaching the lungs.[157]

Management of PE begins with administration of oxygen and hemodynamic stabilization with fluids, if needed, followed by rapid administration of anticoagulation, usually unfractionated or low-molecular-weight heparin and factor Xa inhibitors (fondaparinux, idraparinux, rivaroxaban, and apixaban).[155,157] If a massive life-threatening embolism occurs, a fibrinolytic agent, such as streptokinase, can be used and may be infused through a pulmonary artery catheter. Some individuals require emergent percutaneous or surgical embolectomy.[158] Reversal of the underlying cause of the thrombus is important in preventing recurrent venous thromboembolism.

Pulmonary Artery Hypertension

Pulmonary artery hypertension (PAH) is defined as a mean pulmonary artery pressure greater than 25 mmHg at rest.[159] Pulmonary artery pressure is lower than systemic arterial pressure and is normally 15 to 18 mmHg. Box 35-2 contains the WHO clinical categories for PAH. Idiopathic PAH (IPAH) is rare and usually occurs in women between the ages of 20 and 40 years.[159,160] Familial PAH (FPAH) is caused by mutations in the gene encoding the bone morphogenetic protein receptor type II (BMPR2).[160,161] Associated PAH (APAH) is a leading cause of mortality in many connective tissue disorders (e.g., scleroderma) and affects up to 1 in 200 individuals infected with HIV.[160] Diet drugs, amphetamines, and cocaine also have been linked to an increased risk for PAH. Pulmonary artery hypertension associated with left heart failure or valvular disease is caused by increased pulmonary venous pressure and is discussed in Chapter 32. COPD is the most common lung disease associated with PAH, but any condition that causes chronic hypoxemia can result in pulmonary hypertension. Recurrent pulmonary embolism may be subclinical in

BOX 35-2 CLASSIFICATION OF PULMONARY HYPERTENSION (DANA POINT, 2008)

1. Pulmonary artery hypertension (PAH)
   - 1.1 Idiopathic (IPAH)
   - 1.2 Heritable
     - 1.2.1 BMPR2
     - 1.2.2 ALK1, endoglin (with or without hereditary hemorrhagic telangiectasia)
     - 1.2.3 Unknown
   - 1.3 Drug and toxin induced
   - 1.4 Associated with (APAH)
     - 1.4.1 Connective tissue disease
     - 1.4.2 HIV infection
     - 1.4.3 Portal hypertension
     - 1.4.4 Congenital heart disease
     - 1.4.5 Schistosomiasis
     - 1.4.6 Chronic hemolytic anemia
   - 1.5 Persistent pulmonary hypertension of the newborn

1′. Pulmonary veno-occlusive disease (PVOD) and/or pulmonary capillary hemangiomatosis (PCH)

2. Pulmonary hypertension associated with left-sided heart diseases
   - 2.1 Systolic dysfunction
   - 2.2 Diastolic dysfunction
   - 2.3 Valvular disease
3. Pulmonary hypertension associated with lung diseases and/or hypoxia
   - 3.1 Chronic obstructive pulmonary disease
   - 3.2 Interstitial lung disease
   - 3.3 Other pulmonary diseases with mixed restrictive and obstructive pattern
   - 3.4 Sleep-disordered breathing
   - 3.5 Alveolar hypoventilation disorders
   - 3.6 Chronic exposure to high altitude
   - 3.7 Developmental abnormalities
4. Chronic thromboembolic pulmonary hypertension
5. Pulmonary hypertension with unclear multifactorial mechanisms
   - 5.1 Hematologic disorders: myeloproliferative disorders, splenectomy
   - 5.2 Systemic disorders: sarcoidosis, pulmonary Langerhans cell histiocytosis, lymphangioleiomyomatosis, neurofibromatosis, vasculitis
   - 5.3 Metabolic disorders: glycogen storage disease, Gaucher disease, thyroid disorders
   - 5.4 Others: tumoral obstruction, fibrosing mediastinitis, chronic renal failure on dialysis

Data from Simonneau G et al: *J Am Coll Cardiol* 54(1 Suppl):S43–S54, 2009.
HIV, Human immunodeficiency virus.

its presentation and unrecognized until the signs and symptoms of PAH are detected.

PATHOPHYSIOLOGY. Idiopathic PAH is characterized by endothelial dysfunction with overproduction of vasoconstrictors (e.g., thromboxane and endothelin) and decreased production of vasodilators (e.g., nitric oxide and prostacyclin).[159,160] Release of growth factors causes proliferation of endothelial cells, smooth muscle cells, and fibroblasts, resulting in patchy changes in precapillary pulmonary arteries (resistance vessels). This process results in luminal narrowing and abnormal vasoconstriction and is called *remodeling.*[162] Increased cytosolic calcium (vasoconstriction), phosphodiesterases (modulate cellular proliferation),

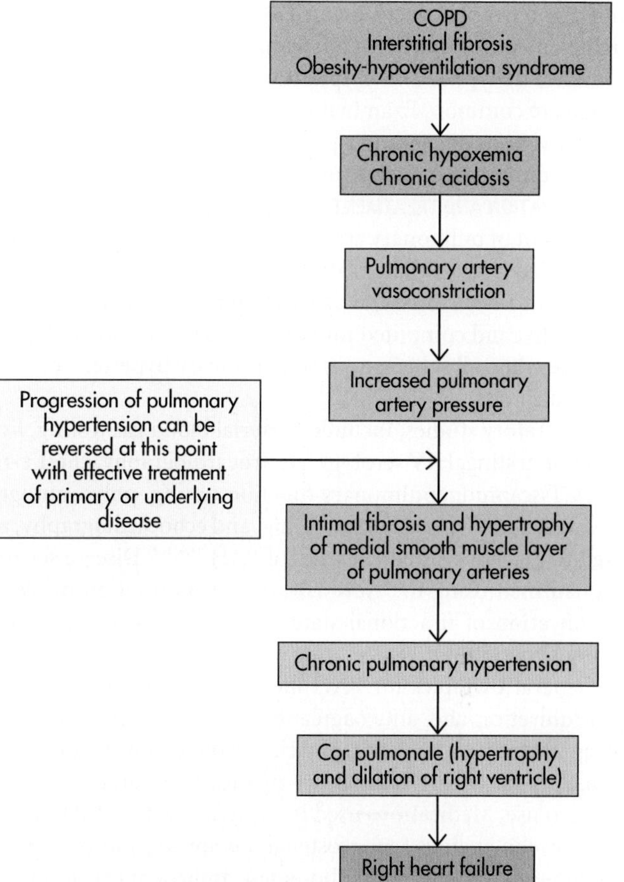

FIGURE 35-21 **Pathogenesis of Pulmonary Hypertension and Cor Pulmonale Caused by Disease of the Respiratory System or Hypoxia.** *COPD,* Chronic obstructive pulmonary disease.

serotonin (vasoconstrictor), and adrenomedullin (vasodilator) also play a role in the pathogenesis of this disorder. These combined changes cause resistance to pulmonary artery blood flow, thus increasing the pressure in the pulmonary arteries. As resistance and pressure increase, the workload of the right ventricle increases and subsequent right ventricular hypertrophy, followed by failure, may occur (cor pulmonale). Gas exchange is reduced with restriction in lung volumes. In individuals with *BMPR2* gene mutations, intracellular signaling abnormalities result in vascular proliferation. Eventually death results in most individuals with PAH. The pathogenesis of pulmonary artery hypertension and cor pulmonale, resulting from disease of the respiratory system or hypoxia, is shown in Figure 35-21.

Pulmonary hypertension associated with lung respiratory disease or hypoxia, or both, is a serious complication of many acute and chronic pulmonary disorders, such as COPD and hypoventilation associated with obesity. These conditions are complicated by hypoxic pulmonary vasoconstriction, which further increases pulmonary artery pressures.[163]

CLINICAL MANIFESTATIONS. Pulmonary artery hypertension may not be detected until it is quite severe. The symptoms are often masked by primary pulmonary or cardiovascular disease. The first indication of pulmonary hypertension is often an abnormality seen on a chest radiograph (enlarged pulmonary arteries and right heart border) or an electrocardiogram that shows right ventricular hypertrophy. Symptoms of fatigue, chest discomfort, tachypnea and dyspnea on exertion, palpitations, and cough are common. Examination may reveal peripheral edema, jugular venous distention, a precordial heave, and accentuation of the pulmonary compartment of the second heart sound.[164]

EVALUATION AND TREATMENT. Definitive diagnosis and accurate assessment of pulmonary artery pressure can be made only with right-sided heart catheterization. Common diagnostic modalities used to determine the cause include chest x-ray, echocardiography, and computed tomography. The diagnosis of IPAH is made when all other causes of pulmonary hypertension have been ruled out.

Laboratory studies, including arterial blood gas testing, liver function testing, HIV serology, electrocardiography, chest x-ray and CT scanning, pulmonary function testing, polysomnography, ventilation-perfusion scanning, and echocardiography, are used to detect underlying causes of PAH.[159,160] Disease severity is quantified using the New York Heart Association or WHO classification of functional status of patients with pulmonary artery hypertension.[165]

General therapies for PAH include administration of oxygen, diuretics, and anticoagulants and avoidance of contributing factors such as air travel, decongestant medications, nonsteroidal anti-inflammatory medications, pregnancy, and tobacco use. Medications used in the treatment of PAH include prostacyclin analogs (epoprostenol, beraprost, iloprost), endothelin receptor antagonists (bosentan, ambrisentan), and phosphodiesterase-5 inhibitors.[166] Those who fail medical therapy may be candidates for lung transplantation.

The most effective treatment for secondary pulmonary artery hypertension is treatment of the primary disorder. However, once pulmonary hypertension has persisted long enough for hypertrophy of the medial smooth muscle layer to develop (as it does with chronic hypoxemia), it is no longer reversible. Treatment relies on the use of supplemental oxygen to reverse hypoxic vasoconstriction.

Cor Pulmonale

Cor pulmonale is secondary to pulmonary artery hypertension and consists of right ventricular enlargement (hypertrophy, dilation, or both).[167]

PATHOPHYSIOLOGY. Cor pulmonale develops as pulmonary artery hypertension creates chronic pressure overload in the right ventricle similar to that created in the left ventricle by systemic hypertension. (Systemic hypertension is discussed in Chapter 32.) Pressure overload increases the work of the right ventricle, causes hypertrophy of the normally thin-walled heart muscle, and compromises right ventricular myocardial perfusion. Acute hypoxemia, such as might occur with pneumonia, can exaggerate pulmonary hypertension and dilate the ventricle as well. Right ventricular filling pressures are normal until failure occurs. The right ventricle usually fails when pulmonary artery pressure equals systemic blood pressure.

CLINICAL MANIFESTATIONS. The clinical manifestations of cor pulmonale may be obscured by primary respiratory disease and appear only during exercise testing. The heart appears normal at rest, but with exercise, cardiac output falls. The electrocardiogram shows right ventricular hypertrophy. Chest pain is common. The pulmonary component of the second heart sound, which represents closure of the pulmonic valve, may be accentuated, and a pulmonic valve murmur also may be present. Tricuspid valve murmur may accompany the development of right ventricular failure. Peripheral edema, hepatic congestion, and jugular venous distention often may be detected.

EVALUATION AND TREATMENT. Diagnosis is made on the basis of physical examination, radiologic examination, and electrocardiogram or echocardiogram, or both. The goal of treatment for cor pulmonale is to decrease the workload of the right ventricle by lowering pulmonary artery pressure. Treatment is the same as for pulmonary artery hypertension, and its success depends on reversal of the underlying lung disease.

Malignancies of the Respiratory Tract

Laryngeal Cancer

Cancer of the larynx represents approximately 2% to 3% of all cancers in the United States. There were an estimated 12,260 new cases and 3630 deaths in 2013.[168]

The risk of **laryngeal cancer** is increased by the amount of tobacco smoked; risk is further heightened with the combination of smoking and alcohol consumption. Gastroesophageal reflux disease is also a risk factor.[169] The human papillomavirus (HPV) has been linked to both benign and malignant disease of the larynx.[170] The highest incidence is in men between 50 and 75 years of age.

PATHOPHYSIOLOGY. Carcinoma of the true vocal cords (glottis) is more common than that of the supraglottic structures (epiglottis, aryepiglottic folds, arytenoids, and false cords). Tumors of the subglottic area are rare. Squamous cell carcinoma is the most common cell type, although small cell carcinomas also occur (Figure 35-22). Laryngeal dysplasia has a high risk of progressing to malignancy. Metastasis develops by spreading to the draining lymph nodes, and distant metastasis, usually to the lung, is rare.

CLINICAL MANIFESTATIONS. The presenting symptoms of laryngeal cancer include hoarseness, dyspnea, and cough. Progressive hoarseness is the most significant symptom and can result in voice loss. Dyspnea is rare in the case of supraglottic tumors, but can be severe in subglottic tumors. Cough occurs less commonly and may follow swallowing. Laryngeal pain or a sore throat is likely to be present with supraglottic lesions.

EVALUATION AND TREATMENT. Evaluation of the larynx includes external inspection and palpation of the larynx and the lymph nodes in the neck. Indirect laryngoscopy provides a stereoscopic view of the structure and movement of the larynx. A biopsy also can be obtained during this procedure. Direct laryngoscopy provides specific visualization of the tumor. Plain films of the larynx and CT facilitate the identification of tumor boundaries and the degree of extension to surrounding tissue. Magnetic resonance imaging (MRI) and positron-emission tomography (PET) can be used for staging.

Combined chemotherapy and radiation can result in cure in selected cases; however, sequelae such as swallowing and speech difficulties may result.[171] Photodynamic therapy improves

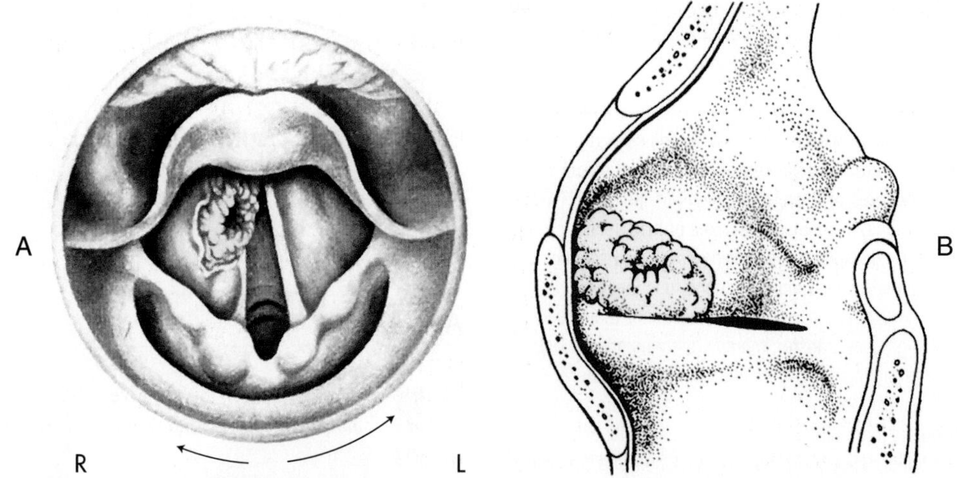

FIGURE 35-22 Laryngeal Cancer. **A,** Mirror view of carcinoma of right false cord partially hiding true cord. **B,** Lateral view. (From del Regato JA, Spjut HJ, Cox JD: *Ackerman and del Regato's cancer,* ed 2, St Louis, 1985, Mosby.)

outcomes while preserving function in many individuals with early stage disease. Partial laryngectomies are the preferred treatment for small supraglottic and subglottic malignancies. Total laryngectomy is required when lesions are extensive and involve the cartilage.[172,173] Swallowing and speech therapy after treatment can significantly improve recovery.

Lung Cancer

Lung cancers (bronchogenic carcinomas) arise from the epithelium of the respiratory tract. As such, the term *lung cancer* excludes other pulmonary tumors, including sarcomas, lymphomas, blastomas, hematomas, and mesotheliomas. Important trends in lung cancer are summarized in Box 35-3. The most common cause of lung cancer is tobacco smoking, and approximately 10% to 15% of active smokers will develop lung cancer. About 10% to 25% of lung cancers occur in never-smokers and it is estimated that one fourth of lung cancer cases among never-smokers could be attributed to exposure to passive tobacco smoke.[174] Tobacco smoke contains several organ-specific carcinogens, and smoking has been causally related to carcinogenesis at several sites, including the larynx, oral cavity, esophagus, and urinary bladder. Many genetic mechanisms have been implicated in the risk for lung cancer including gene mutations, gene amplification, increases in protein expression, losses in protein expression, tumor-suppressing alterations, tumor-acquired DNA methylation, and chromosomal aberrations[175] (see What's New? Genetic and Immunologic Breakthroughs in Lung Cancer Treatment). Theories of carcinogenesis are discussed in Chapter 12. Currently there are no specific tools for predicting risk for or rate of progression of lung cancer.[176]

Environmental or occupational risk factors associated with lung cancer include benzopyrene, radon gas, metals (chromium, cadmium, arsenic), asbestos fibers, diesel exhaust, nitrogen mustard gases, nickel, silica, vinyl chloride, and chloromethyl methyl ether.[168] Primary lung cancers arise from cells that line the bronchi within the lungs and are therefore called *bronchogenic carcinomas.* It is now believed that most of these

BOX 35-3 IMPORTANT TRENDS FOR LUNG CANCER

Incidence

An estimated 22,190 new cases in 2013: 118,080 in men and 110,100 in women.

Mortality

An estimated 159,480 deaths in 2012: 87,260 in men and 72,200 in women. The death rate in men is declining but continues to rise for women, and lung cancer remains by far the greatest cancer killer of men and women.

Risk Factors

Cigarette smoking is the number one risk factor. Environmental smoke exposure (exposure to someone else's cigarette smoke) increases the risk of lung cancer. Occupational risk factors include exposure to asbestos dust, arsenic, chromium, nickel, ionizing radiation, chloromethyl methyl ether, coal products, mustard gas, and vinyl chloride.

Warning Signs

A persistent cough, sputum streaked with blood, chest pain, recurring attacks of pneumonia or bronchitis, weight loss, hard nodes in neck or axilla.

Early Detection and Prevention

Lung cancer is very difficult to detect early. Periodic chest x-ray films, sputum cytologic analysis, and computed tomography can detect presymptomatic, early stage lung cancers, particularly of the squamous cell type; however, no conclusive evidence of reduction in lung cancer mortality as a consequence of screening has been found.

Treatment

Surgical resection of the entire tumor is the only treatment that results in cure; however, the disease is often too advanced by the time of diagnosis for surgery to be indicated. Radiation therapy and chemotherapy can be used as adjunctive or palliative treatment modalities. New treatments include gene and immunotherapies.

Survival

Although the stage of cancer progression at the time of diagnosis greatly affects prognosis, overall only 20% of individuals live 5 or more years after diagnosis.

Data from American Cancer Society: *Cancer facts and figures 2013.* Available at www.cancer.org/research/cancerfactsfigures/cancerfactsfigures/cancer-facts-figures-2013.

WHAT'S NEW?

Genetic and Immunologic Breakthroughs in Lung Cancer Treatment

New chemotherapeutic agents have slightly improved outcomes in the management of lung cancer, but overall survival rates for advanced stage disease remain poor and the toxicities of these regimens limit their use. New understandings of the genetic and immunologic features of lung cancer cells have led to new treatments. Gene therapy is emerging as a way of inducing tumor apoptosis, restoring normal tumor-suppressor gene function (e.g., *p53*), promoting tumor-suicide gene expression, and increasing tumor responsiveness to chemoradiation through gene transfer, thereby restoring normal DNA methylation patterns and altering microRNA function. Immunologic therapies include vaccines that stimulate tumor-specific antibodies, antibodies to epidermal growth factor receptors (erlotinib, gefitinib, and cetuximab), and antiangiogenesis drugs; direct tumor delivery of activating cytokines; and blocking tumor immunosuppression. The effectiveness of these strategies, the timing of delivery, optimal drug combinations and their side effects are still being evaluated, but new knowledge is leading to new opportunities for treatment.

Data from Amos SM et al: *Blood* 118(3):499–509, 2011; Gonzalez Marinello GM, Santos ES, Raez LE: *Expert Rev Anticancer Ther* 12(4): 439–445, 2012; Kelly RJ, Giaccone G: *Cancer J* 17(5):302–308, 2011; Vachani A et al: *Clin Chest Med* 32(4):865–885, 2011; Zarogoulidis P et al: *Cancer Gene Ther* 19(9):593–600, 2012.

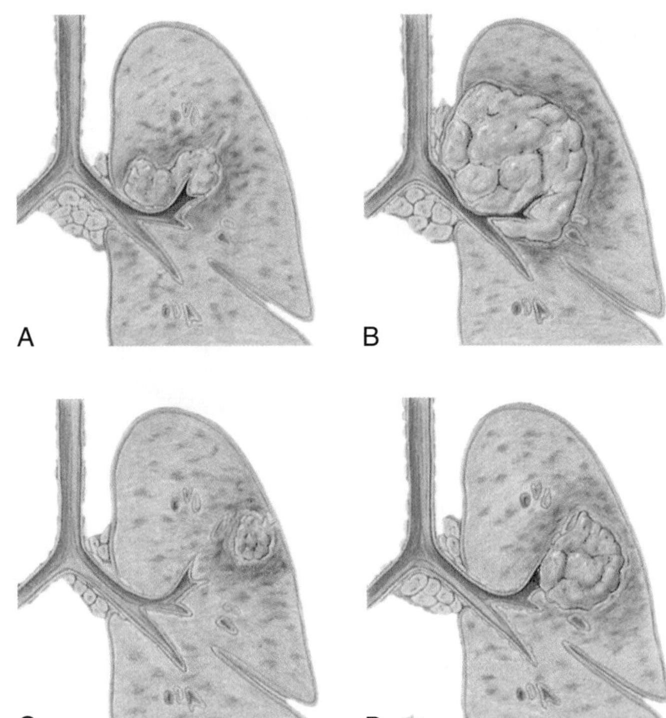

FIGURE 35-23 **Cancer of the Lung. A,** Squamous (epidermoid) cell carcinoma. **B,** Small cell (oat cell) carcinoma. **C,** Adenocarcinoma. **D,** Large cell carcinoma. (From Des Jardins T, Burton GG: *Clinical manifestations and assessment of respiratory disease,* ed 3, St Louis, 1995, Mosby.)

cancers arise from mutated epithelial stem cells. Although there are many types of lung cancer, they are divided into two major categories based on cell histology: non–small cell lung carcinoma (NSCLC, about 85% of all lung cancers) and neuroendocrine tumors (about 14% of all lung cancers). NSCLC can be subdivided into three common types of lung cancer: squamous cell carcinoma, adenocarcinoma, and large cell undifferentiated carcinoma, and they each have cellular subtypes.[177] Neuroendocrine tumors of the lung can be divided into small cell carcinoma, large cell neuroendocrine carcinoma, typical carcinoid tumors, and atypical carcinoid tumors. Small cell carcinoma is the most common of these neuroendocrine tumors. The clinical and pathologic features that most commonly characterize these cancer types are illustrated in Figure 35-23 and described in Table 35-4. Many cancers that arise in other organs of the body metastasize to the lungs; however, these are not considered lung cancers and are categorized by their primary site of origin.

Non–Small Cell Lung Cancer (NSCLC)

Squamous Cell Carcinoma. Squamous cell carcinoma (SCC) accounts for about 30% of bronchogenic carcinomas, representing a sharp decline in incidence in the past two decades. SCC has the strongest association with smoking. Smokers with COPD have a higher incidence of this tumor type.[178] The tumors are typically located centrally near the hila and project into bronchi. Because of this central location, nonproductive cough or hemoptysis is common. Pneumonia and atelectasis are often associated with squamous cell carcinoma (Figure 35-24, *A*). Chest pain is a late symptom associated with large tumors. These tumors can remain fairly well localized and tend not to metastasize until late in the course of the disease.

Adenocarcinoma. Adenocarcinoma (tumor arising from glands) of the lung constitutes 35% to 40% of all bronchogenic carcinomas (Figure 35-24, *B*). Adenocarcinoma occurs more frequently in women, in non-smokers, and in Asians. Environmental tobacco smoke, occupational carcinogens, viruses, hormones, and positive family history are associated with this tumor type.[179] *Epidermal growth factor receptor (EGFR)* mutations are also common in this type of lung cancer.[180] These tumors, which are usually smaller than 4 cm, more commonly arise in the peripheral regions of the pulmonary parenchyma. Pulmonary adenocarcinoma develops in a stepwise fashion through atypical adenomatous hyperplasia, adenocarcinoma in situ, and minimally invasive adenocarcinoma to invasive carcinoma. They may be asymptomatic and discovered by routine chest roentgenogram in the early stages, or the individual may seek treatment for pleuritic chest pain and shortness of breath from pleural involvement by the tumor.

Included in the category of adenocarcinoma is bronchoalveolar cell carcinoma. These tumors tend to arise from the terminal bronchioles and alveoli. They are slow-growing tumors with an unpredictable pattern of metastasis. Metastasis occurs through the pulmonary arterial system and mediastinal lymph nodes. This cell type has the weakest association with smoking.[181]

Diagnosis of NSCLC requires cytologic analysis from biopsy, and therapy is based on histologic and molecular markers (e.g., EGFR tyrosine kinase inhibitors for adenocarcinoma) for a targeted approach to therapy. Surgical resection is possible in a high proportion of adenocarcinoma cases, but because metastasis occurs early (70% of lung cancers present in advanced stages), the 5-year survival rate remains below 15%.[182] Clinical trials are in progress to develop immunotherapies/vaccines for NSCLC.[183]

TABLE 35-4 **CHARACTERISTICS OF LUNG CANCERS**

TUMOR TYPE	GROWTH RATE	METASTASIS	MEANS OF DIAGNOSIS	CLINICAL MANIFESTATIONS AND TREATMENT
Squamous cell carcinoma	Slow	Late; mostly to hilar lymph nodes	Biopsy, sputum analysis, bronchoscopy, electron microscopy, immunohistochemistry	Cough, sputum production, airway obstruction; treated surgically, chemotherapy adjunctive
Adenocarcinoma	Moderate	Early	Radiography, fiberoptic bronchoscopy, electron microscopy	Pleural effusion; treated surgically, chemotherapy adjunctive
Large cell carcinoma	Rapid	Early and widespread	Sputum analysis, bronchoscopy, electron microscopy (by exclusion of other cell types)	Chest wall pain, pleural effusion, cough, sputum production, hemoptysis, airway obstruction resulting in pneumonia (if airways involved); treated surgically
Small cell (oat cell) carcinoma	Very rapid	Very early; to mediastinum or distally in lung	Radiography, sputum analysis, bronchoscopy, electron microscopy, immunohistochemistry, and clinical manifestations (cough, chest pain, dyspnea, hemoptysis, localized wheezing)	Airway obstruction, signs and symptoms of excessive hormone secretion; treated by chemotherapy and ionizing radiation to thorax and central nervous system

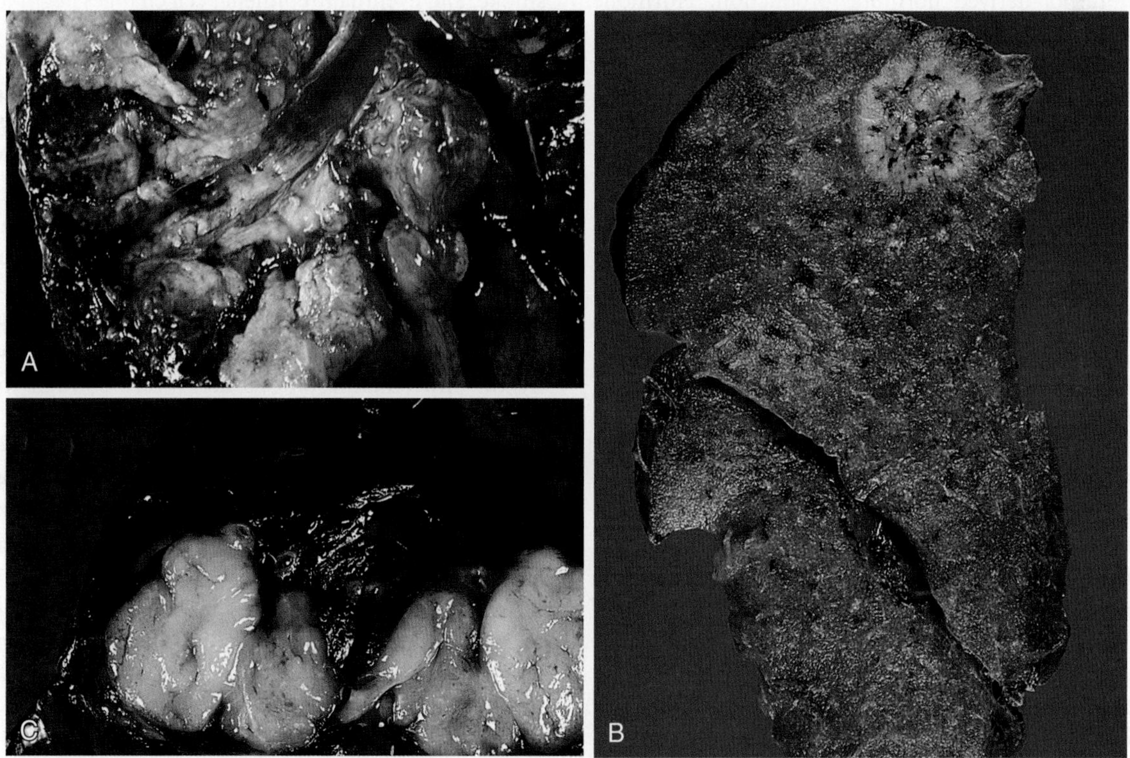

FIGURE 35-24 Lung Cancer. **A,** Squamous cell carcinoma. This hilar tumor originates from the main bronchus. **B,** Peripheral adenocarcinoma. The tumor shows prominent black pigmentation, suggestive of having evolved in an anthracotic scar. **C,** Small cell carcinoma. The tumor forms confluent nodules. On cross sectioning, the nodules have an encephaloid (like brain tissue) appearance. (From Damjanov I, Linder J, editors: *Anderson's pathology,* ed 10, St Louis, 1996, Mosby.)

Large Cell Carcinoma (Undifferentiated). **Large cell carcinomas** constitute 10% to 15% of bronchogenic carcinomas. This cell type has lost all evidence of differentiation and is therefore commonly referred to as **undifferentiated large cell anaplastic cancer.** Because large cell carcinomas show none of the histologic findings of squamous cell carcinoma or adenocarcinoma, they are diagnosed by a process of exclusion. The cells are generally larger than leukocytes and contain large, darkly stained nuclei. These tumors commonly arise peripherally but are found centrally and can grow to distort the trachea and cause widening of the carina.

Once metastasis has occurred, surgical therapy is limited to palliative procedures (comfort measures) designed to relieve obstructive pneumonitis or prevent recurrence of pleural effusion. Neither radiation therapy nor chemotherapy has been successful in increasing survival.

Neuroendocrine Lung Tumors

Small Cell (Oat Cell) Carcinoma. Small cell lung carcinomas (SCLCs) are the most common type of neuroendocrine lung tumors and constitute about 14% of bronchogenic carcinomas, but cause 25% of lung cancer deaths.[184] Most tumors arise from the central part of the lung (see Figures 35-23 and 35-24, *C*). Cell sizes range from 6 to 8 μm. This cell type has the strongest correlation with tobacco smoking. Because these tumors show a rapid rate of growth and tend to metastasize early and widely, this type of carcinoma has the worst prognosis of all lung cancers. Staging for small cell carcinoma is divided into only two categories: limited disease (TNM stages I to III: 20% to 30%) and extensive disease (TNM stage IV: 70% to 80%).[185] Survival time for untreated small cell carcinoma is less than 5% at 5 years.[186]

Small cell carcinoma arises from neuroendocrine cells that contain neurosecretory granules and exist throughout the tracheobronchial tree. Thus small cell carcinoma is often associated with tumor-derived hormone production. Hormone production is important to the clinician because resulting signs and symptoms (called *paraneoplastic syndromes*) may be the first manifestation of the underlying cancer. Examples include hyponatremia (antidiuretic hormone), Cushing syndrome (adrenocorticotropic hormone), hypocalcemia (calcitonin), gynecomastia (gonadotropins), and carcinoid syndrome (serotonin).[187]

Bronchial Carcinoid Tumors. Bronchial carcinoid tumors are rare, represent about 1% of all lung tumors, are not related to smoking, are slow growing, and have a low potential to metastasize. Carcinoid tumors can occur from childhood through older age. They arise more commonly in the main or segmental bronchi, are easily visualized bronchoscopically, and are found on routine chest radiographs. The tumor cells have dense granules containing neuroendocrine-like hormones, but they rarely produce endocrine symptoms. Cells are not recovered from bronchial washings, because the tumor is covered with normal mucosa. Fifty percent of individuals with bronchial carcinoid tumors are asymptomatic. Local surgical resection is curative if metastasis has not occurred; this can often be done by bronchoscopic resection.[188,189]

Other Lung Cancers. **Adenocystic tumors (cylindromas)** and **mucoepidermoid carcinomas** are rare bronchial gland tumors. They arise predominantly in the trachea or large airways and cause obstruction. They can be malignant and metastasize early, although distal pulmonary metastases are usually slow growing. Thus it is not unusual for an individual to survive 10 to 15 years after diagnosis.

Mesotheliomas are rare tumors associated with asbestos exposure (80%). Most tumors are aggressive malignant tumors arising from mesothelial cells that line the pleural cavities. A long latent interval between exposure to asbestos and appearance of mesothelioma usually occurs, and onset of symptoms may take 20 to 40 years. Clinical manifestations include dyspnea and chest pain that result from tumor-derived pleural fluid and invasion of the chest wall. Early detection is difficult because radiologic studies do not reveal the tumor at an early stage. Diagnosis is made by chest x-ray, CT scan, and thoracentesis with cytologic examination of the pleural fluid. Thoracoscopy also may be used for biopsy. Osteopontin and mesothelin are being explored as potential tumor markers for early diagnosis. Current management of malignant mesothelioma includes a combination of pleuropneumonectomy, chemotherapy, radiation, and hyperthermia.[190,191]

PATHOGENESIS. Environmental carcinogens found in tobacco smoke and asbestos are associated with malignant transformations. Tobacco smoke contains as many as 30 lung carcinogens and is responsible for the vast majority of lung cancers. These carcinogens, along with inherited genetic predisposition to cancers, result in tumor development.[192] Once lung cancer is initiated by these carcinogen-induced mutations, further tumor development is promoted by growth factors that alter cell growth and differentiation, such as epidermal growth factor, and by production of inflammatory mediators, such as toxic oxygen free radicals. The bronchial mucosa suffers multiple carcinogenic "hits" because of repetitive exposure to tobacco smoke, and eventually epithelial cell changes begin to be visible on biopsy. These changes progress from metaplasia to carcinoma in situ and finally to invasive carcinoma.[193] Tumor progression includes invasion of surrounding tissues and, finally, metastasis to distant sites, including the brain, bone marrow, and liver.

CLINICAL MANIFESTATIONS. Symptoms of early stage, localized disease are nonspecific and are likely to be attributed by the individual to the effects of smoking. The clinical manifestations are ambiguous and insidious; they include coughing, chest pain, excessive sputum production, hemoptysis, pneumonia, airway obstruction, pleural effusions, and weight loss. By the time manifestations are severe enough to motivate the individual to seek medical advice, the disease is usually advanced. Symptoms and signs of metastatic disease (e.g., neurologic deficits, bone pain) or paraneoplastic syndromes may be evident.[194]

EVALUATION AND TREATMENT. Although it is clear that diagnosing and treating lung cancer early in its development are crucial for long-term survival, screening for the presence of asymptomatic tumors in high-risk individuals remains controversial. The latest guidelines state that the evidence remains insufficient to recommend screening of asymptomatic individuals with sputum cytologic examination, chest x-ray, or spiral CT. However, many clinicians and researchers continue to examine these and other modalities in an effort to find more effective ways of catching this deadly disease when it is still curable. Screening using low-dose spiral CT scans decreases risk of dying from lung cancer in heavy smokers.[195]

The diagnosis of lung cancer relies on the history of risk factors and symptoms, a careful physical examination, and a constellation of diagnostic tests including sputum cytology, chest x-ray, low-dose CT scanning in high-risk individuals, PET scanning, bronchoscopy, biopsy, testing for epidermal growth factor mutations and other molecular markers, and search for potential metastatic disease.[196] The goal of these evaluations is to (1) establish the presence of a primary lung cancer,

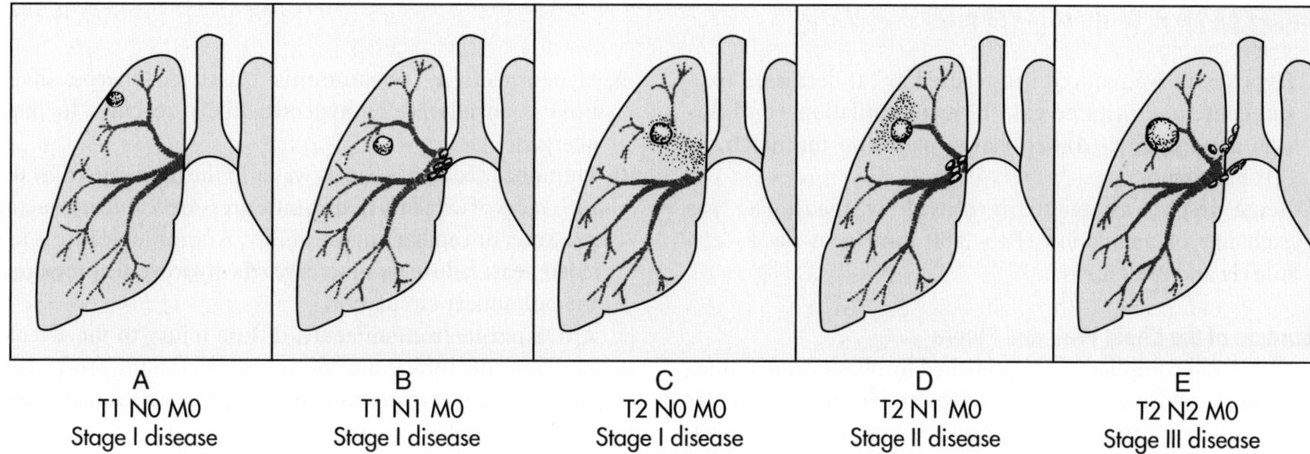

FIGURE 35-25 Staging of Lung Cancer by the TNM Classification System. **A, B,** Stage I disease includes tumors classified as T1, with or without metastasis to the lymph nodes in the ipsilateral hilar region. **C,** Also included in stage I are tumors classified as T2 but having no nodal or distant metastases. **D,** Stage II disease includes those tumors classified as T2, with metastasis only to the ipsilateral hilar lymph nodes. **E,** Stage III includes all tumors more extensive than T2 or any tumor with metastasis to the lymph nodes in the mediastinum or adjacent organs. Stage IV (not shown) involves spread to other organs.

(2) determine its cell type, and (3) stage the tumor. As stated, SCLC is staged as either limited or extensive. The staging of NSCLC uses the **TNM classification system** in which *T* denotes the extent of the primary tumor, *N* indicates nodal involvement, and *M* describes the extent of metastasis, and is illustrated in Figure 35-25.[197] The use of biomarkers is advancing as an approach to early detection and staging of lung cancer and targeted therapies.[198]

For all types of early stage lung carcinoma, the preferred treatment is surgical resection. Once metastasis has taken place, total surgical resection is more difficult and survival rates dramatically decrease. NSCLC is less responsive to chemotherapy than is small cell carcinoma, but chemotherapy (e.g., platinum) and radiation are commonly used as adjuvant or palliative care.[199-201] Small cell carcinoma is usually widely metastasized by the time of diagnosis. Palliative chemotherapy or radiation can improve survival.[202] New treatment modalities, such as dose-intensified radiation radiofrequency ablation, microwave ablation, cryotherapy, and brachytherapy, may be available as primary or palliative treatment for those for whom surgical removal is not an option.[203,204] New and exciting treatments for lung cancer are under investigation, including antiangiogenic therapy, targeting of growth factor receptors, tumor sensitizing agents, gene therapy, and immunotherapy.[205,206] Prevention of lung cancer relies primarily on reduction of exposure to carcinogens. For most individuals this means smoking cessation, and numerous governmental and private organizations are working toward the complete end of cigarette smoking. Other forms of prevention also are being explored, including chemoprevention in the form of dietary supplements and pharmaceuticals.[192,207] Work is in progress to establish the best methods for screening and early detection.[208,209]

SUMMARY REVIEW

Clinical Manifestations of Pulmonary Alterations

1. Dyspnea is a feeling of breathlessness and increased respiratory effort. Orthopnea is dyspnea when a person lies flat. Paroxysmal nocturnal dyspnea occurs at night and requires the person to sit or stand for relief.
2. Coughing is a protective reflex that expels secretions and irritants from the lower airways.
3. Abnormal sputum is a change in the amount, consistency, color, and odor of sputum.
4. Hemoptysis is expectoration of bloody mucus that can be caused by bronchitis, TB, abscess, neoplasms, and other conditions that cause hemorrhage from damaged vessels.
5. Abnormal breathing patterns are adjustments made by the body to minimize the work of respiratory muscles. They include Kussmaul, obstructed, restricted, gasping, and/or Cheyne-Stokes respirations, and sighing.
6. Hypoventilation is decreased alveolar ventilation caused by airway obstruction, chest wall restriction, or altered neurologic control of breathing. Hypoventilation causes increased Pa_{CO_2}.
7. Hyperventilation is increased alveolar ventilation produced by anxiety, head injury, or severe hypoxemia. Hyperventilation causes decreased Pa_{CO_2}.
8. Cyanosis is a bluish discoloration of the skin caused by desaturation of hemoglobin, polycythemia, or peripheral vasoconstriction.
9. Clubbing of the fingertips is associated with diseases that interfere with oxygenation of the tissues.
10. Chest pain can result from inflamed pleurae, trachea, bronchi, or respiratory muscles.
11. Hypercapnia is increased Pa_{CO_2} caused by a decrease in minute volume (respiratory rate × tidal volume).

SUMMARY REVIEW—cont'd

12. Hypoxemia is a reduced $Pa{O_2}$ caused by (a) decreased oxygen content of inspired gas, (b) hypoventilation, (c) diffusion abnormality, (d) ventilation-perfusion mismatch, or (e) shunting.
13. Acute respiratory failure is caused by inadequate gas exchange or ventilation ($Pa{O_2}$ ≤50 mmHg or $Pa{CO_2}$ ≥50 mmHg and pH ≥7.25).

Disorders of the Chest Wall and Pleura

1. Chest wall compliance is diminished by obesity and kyphoscoliosis, which compress the lungs, and by neuromuscular diseases that impair chest wall muscle function.
2. Flail chest results from rib or sternal fractures that disrupt the mechanics of breathing.
3. Pneumothorax is the accumulation of air in the pleural space. It can be caused by spontaneous rupture of weakened areas of the pleura or can be secondary to pleural damage caused by disease, trauma, or mechanical ventilation.
4. Tension pneumothorax is a life-threatening condition caused by trapping of air in the pleural space.
5. Pleural effusion is the accumulation of fluid in the pleural space, usually resulting from disorders that promote transudation or exudation from capillaries underlying the pleura but occasionally resulting from blockage or injury that causes lymphatic vessels to drain into the pleural space.
6. Empyema is the presence of pus in the pleural space (infected pleural effusion). The source of the pus is usually lymphatic drainage from sites of bacterial pneumonia.

Pulmonary Disorders

1. Aspiration is passage of fluid and solid particles into the lung, usually from impaired swallowing and coughing. It frequently results in pneumonitis and pulmonary infection.
2. Atelectasis is the collapse of alveoli resulting from compression of the lung tissue or absorption of gas from obstructed alveoli.
3. Bronchiectasis is abnormal dilation of the bronchi secondary to another pulmonary disorder, usually infection or inflammation.
4. Bronchiolitis is the inflammatory obstruction of small airways. It is most common in children.
5. Pulmonary fibrosis is an excessive amount of connective tissue in the lung. It diminishes lung compliance and may be idiopathic or caused by disease.
6. Inhalation of noxious gases or prolonged exposure to high concentrations of oxygen can damage the bronchial mucosa or alveolocapillary membrane and cause inflammation or acute respiratory failure.
7. Pneumoconiosis, which is caused by inhalation of dust particles in the workplace, including coal dust, silica, and asbestos, can cause chronic inflammation, pulmonary fibrosis, and susceptibility to lower airway infection and tumor formation.
8. Silicosis is a type of pneumoconiosis caused by inhalation of silica.
9. Hypersensitivity pneumonitis (extrinsic allergic alveolitis) is an allergic or hypersensitivity reaction to many allergens.
10. Pulmonary edema is excess water in the lung caused by disturbances of capillary hydrostatic pressure, capillary oncotic pressure, or capillary permeability. A common cause is left-sided heart failure that increases the hydrostatic pressure in the pulmonary circulation.
11. ARDS results from an acute, diffuse injury to the alveolocapillary membrane and decreased surfactant production, which increases membrane permeability and causes edema and atelectasis.
12. Obstructive pulmonary disease is characterized by airway obstruction that causes difficult expiration. Obstructive disease can be acute or chronic and includes asthma, chronic bronchitis, and emphysema.
13. Asthma is a chronic inflammatory disorder of the bronchial mucosa that causes bronchial hyperresponsiveness, mucosal edema, airway constriction, and variable obstruction to airflow. Obstruction is caused by episodic attacks of bronchospasm, bronchial inflammation, mucosal edema, and increased mucus production.
14. COPD is the coexistence of chronic bronchitis and emphysema.
15. Chronic bronchitis is a chronic inflammation of the bronchi that causes airway obstruction resulting from bronchial smooth muscle hypertrophy and production of thick, tenacious mucus.
16. Emphysema results from destruction of the alveolar septa and loss of passive elastic recoil, leading to airway collapse and obstruction to gas flow during expiration and air trapping.
17. Emphysema in which septal deterioration is caused by α_1-antitrypsin deficiency or old age tends to be panacinar.
18. Emphysema in which septal deterioration results from smoking tends to be centriacinar.
19. Upper respiratory tract infections are the most common cause of short-term disability in the United States and include rhinitis (the common cold), pharyngitis, and laryngitis.
20. Serious lower respiratory tract infections, which occur most often in older adults and individuals with impaired immunity or underlying disease, include pneumonia and tuberculosis.
21. Pneumonia can be categorized as community-acquired (CAP), healthcare-associated (HCAP), hospital-acquired (HAP), or ventilator-associated (VAP).
22. Pneumococcal pneumonia is an acute lung infection resulting in an inflammatory response with four phases: (a) consolidation, (b) red hepatization, (c) gray hepatization, and (d) resolution.
23. Viral pneumonia is an acute, self-limiting lung infection usually caused by the influenza virus.
24. TB is a lung infection caused by *M. tuberculosis* (tubercle bacillus).

SUMMARY REVIEW—cont'd

25. In TB the inflammatory response isolates colonies of bacilli by enclosing them in tubercles and surrounding the tubercles with scar tissue.
26. Bacilli may remain dormant within the tubercles for life, or if the immune system becomes compromised, they may cause recurrence of active disease.
27. Abscesses are circumscribed areas of destruction of lung parenchyma with suppuration usually resulting from aspiration pneumonia.
28. Acute bronchitis is acute infection or inflammation of the airways or bronchi usually caused by a virus.
29. Pulmonary vascular diseases are caused by embolism or hypertension in the pulmonary circulation.
30. PE is occlusion of a portion of the pulmonary vascular bed by a thrombus (most common), a tissue fragment, or an air bubble. Depending on its size and location, the embolus can cause hypoxic vasoconstriction, pulmonary edema, atelectasis, pulmonary hypertension, shock, and even death.
31. Pulmonary artery hypertension (pulmonary artery pressure 5 to 10 mmHg greater than normal) is caused by (a) elevated left ventricular pressure, (b) increased blood flow through the pulmonary circulation, (c) obliteration or obstruction of the vascular bed, or (d) active constriction of the vascular bed produced by hypoxemia or acidosis.
32. Cor pulmonale is right ventricular enlargement caused by chronic pulmonary hypertension. Cor pulmonale progresses to right ventricular failure if the pulmonary hypertension is not reversed.
33. Laryngeal cancer occurs primarily in men and represents 2% to 3% of all cancers. Squamous cell carcinoma of the true vocal cords is most common and manifests with a clinical symptom of progressive hoarseness.
34. Lung cancer, the most frequent cause of cancer death in the United States, is commonly caused by cigarette tobacco smoking.
35. Cancer cell types include non–small cell lung cancer (squamous cell carcinoma, adenocarcinoma, large cell undifferentiated carcinoma) and neuroendocrine tumors (small cell carcinoma and bronchial carcinoid tumors). Other tumors include small cell (oat cell) carcinoma, bronchial adenoma, adenocystic tumors (cylindromas), mucoepidermoid carcinomas (bronchial tumors), and mesothelioma. Each type arises in a characteristic site or type of tissue, causes distinctive clinical manifestations, and differs in likelihood of metastasis and prognosis.

KEY TERMS

Abscess, 1274
Absorption atelectasis, 1256
Acute cough, 1249
Acute lung injury (ALI), 1261
Acute respiratory distress syndrome (ARDS), 1261
Adenocarcinoma, 1280
Adenocystic tumor (cylindroma), 1282
Air trapping, 1269
Alveolar dead space, 1252
Asbestosis, 1256
Asbestos exposure, 1259
Aspiration, 1255
Asthma, 1263
Atelectasis, 1256
Bronchial carcinoid tumor, 1282
Bronchiectasis, 1256
Bronchiolitis, 1258
Bronchiolitis obliterans, 1258
Bronchiolitis obliterans organizing pneumonia (BOOP), 1258
Cavitation, 1274
Centriacinar emphysema, 1269
Cheyne-Stokes respiration, 1250
Chronic bronchitis, 1267
Chronic cough, 1249
Chronic obstructive pulmonary disease (COPD), 1266
Chylothorax, 1255
Clubbing, 1250
Coal worker pneumoconiosis (coal miner lung, black lung), 1259
Compression atelectasis, 1256
Consolidation, 1274
Cor pulmonale, 1278
Cough, 1249
Cyanosis, 1250
Cylindrical bronchiectasis, 1256
Dyspnea, 1248
Dyspnea on exertion, 1249
Emphysema, 1268
Empyema (infected pleural effusion), 1255
Exudative effusion, 1254
Flail chest, 1253
Hemoptysis, 1249
Hemothorax, 1255
Hypercapnia, 1251
Hypersensitivity pneumonitis (extrinsic allergic alveolitis), 1259
Hyperventilation, 1250
Hypocapnia, 1250
Hypoventilation, 1250
Hypoxemia, 1251
Hypoxia, 1251
Iatrogenic pneumothorax, 1254
Idiopathic pulmonary fibrosis (IPF), 1258
Kussmaul respiration (hyperpnea), 1249
Large cell carcinoma, 1281
Laryngeal cancer, 1278
Lung cancer, 1279
Mesothelioma, 1282
Mucoepidermoid carcinoma, 1282
Obstructive pulmonary disease, 1263
Open pneumothorax (communicating pneumothorax), 1254
Orthopnea, 1249
Oxygen toxicity, 1259
Pain, 1250
Panacinar emphysema, 1270
Paroxysmal nocturnal dyspnea (PND), 1249
Pleural effusion, 1254
Pneumoconiosis, 1259
Pneumonia, 1271
Pneumothorax, 1254
Postobstructive pulmonary edema (POPE), or negative pressure pulmonary edema, 1260
Primary (spontaneous) pneumothorax, 1254
Pulmonary artery hypertension (PAH), 1276
Pulmonary edema, 1260
Pulmonary embolism (PE), 1275
Pulmonary fibrosis, 1258
Pulsus paradoxus, 1266
Respiratory (lung) failure, 1252
Saccular bronchiectasis, 1256
Secondary (traumatic) pneumothorax, 1254
Shunting, 1252
Silicosis, 1259
Small cell (oat cell) lung carcinoma (SCLC), 1282
Sputum, 1249
Status asthmaticus, 1266
Surfactant impairment, 1256
Tension pneumothorax, 1254
TNM classification system, 1283
Transudative effusion, 1254
Tuberculosis (TB), 1273
Undifferentiated large cell anaplastic cancer, 1281
Varicose bronchiectasis, 1256

REFERENCES

1. Nishino T: Dyspnoea: underlying mechanisms and treatment, *Br J Anaesth* 106(4):463–474, 2011.
2. Parshall MB et al: American Thoracic Society Committee on Dyspnea: An official American Thoracic Society statement: update on the mechanisms, assessment, and management of dyspnea, *Am J Respir Crit Care Med* 185(4):435–452, 2012.
3. Spector N et al: Dyspnea: applying research to bedside practice, *AACN Adv Crit Care* 18(1):45–58, quiz 59-60, 2007.
4. Boulet LP: Future directions in the clinical management of cough: ACCP evidence-based clinical practice guidelines, *Chest* 129:287S–292S, 2006.
5. Scano G, Innocenti-Bruni G, Stendardi L: Do obstructive and restrictive lung diseases share common underlying mechanisms of breathlessness? *Respir Med* 104(7):925–933, 2010.
6. Canning BJ: Afferent nerves regulating the cough reflex: mechanisms and mediators of cough in disease, *Otolaryngol Clin North Am* 43(1): 15–25, vii, 2010.
7. Canning BJ: Functional implications of the multiple afferent pathways regulating cough, *Pulm Pharmacol Ther* 24(3):295–299, 2011.
8. Birring SS: Controversies in the evaluation and management of chronic cough, *Am J Respir Crit Care Med* 183(6):708–715, 2011.
9. Hurt K, Bilton D: Haemoptysis: diagnosis and treatment, *Acute Med* 11(1):39–45, 2012.
10. Nguyen S, Hojjati M: Review of current therapies for secondary hypertrophic pulmonary osteoarthropathy, *Clin Rheumatol* 30(1):7–13, 2011.
11. Brims FJ, Davies HE, Lee YC: Respiratory chest pain: diagnosis and treatment, *Med Clin North Am* 94(2):217–232, 2010.
12. Chebbo A, Tfaili A, Jones SF: Hypoventilation syndromes, *Med Clin North Am* 95(6):1189–1202, 2011.
13. Curley G, Kavanagh B: Bench-to-bedside review: carbon dioxide, *Crit Care* 14(2):220, 2010.
14. Mac Sweeney R, McAuley DF, Matthay MA: Acute lung failure, *Semin Respir Crit Care Med* 32(5):607–625, 2011.
15. Sud S et al: High-frequency ventilation versus conventional ventilation for treatment of acute lung injury and acute respiratory distress syndrome, *Cochrane Database Syst Rev* (2):CD004085, 2013.
16. Grundy S, Bentley A, Tschopp JM: Primary spontaneous pneumothorax: a diffuse disease of the pleura, *Respiration* 83(3):185–189, 2012.
17. Furuya M, Nakatani Y: Birt-Hogg-Dube syndrome: clinicopathological features of the lung, *J Clin Pathol* 66(3):178–186, 2013.
18. Lin YC et al: Pigtail catheter for the management of pneumothorax in mechanically ventilated patients, *Am J Emerg Med* 28(4):466–471, 2010.
19. Haynes D, Baumann MH: Management of pneumothorax, *Semin Respir Crit Care Med* 31(6):769–780, 2010.
20. Weldon E, Williams J: Pleural disease in the emergency department, *Emerg Med Clin North Am* 30(2):475–499, ix–x, 2012.
21. Bhatnagar R, Maskell NA: Treatment of complicated pleural effusions in 2013, *Clin Chest Med* 34(1):47–62, 2013.
22. Huggins JT, Doelken P, Sahn SA: Intrapleural therapy, *Respirology* 16(6):891–899, 2011.
23. Metheny NA, Stewart BJ, McClave SA: Relationship between feeding tube site and respiratory outcomes, *JPEN J Parenter Enteral Nutr* 35(3):346–355, 2011.
24. Marik PE: Pulmonary aspiration syndromes, *Curr Opin Pulm Med* 17(3):148–154, 2011.
25. Hedenstierna G, Edmark L: Mechanisms of atelectasis in the perioperative period, *Best Pract Res Clin Anaesthesiol* 24(2):157–169, 2010.
26. Sachdev G, Napolitano LM: Postoperative pulmonary complications: pneumonia and acute respiratory failure, *Surg Clin North Am* 92(2):321–344, ix, 2012.
27. Truong T: The overlap of bronchiectasis and immunodeficiency with asthma, *Immunol Allergy Clin North Am* 33(1):61–78, 2013.
28. Feldman C: Bronchiectasis: new approaches to diagnosis and management, *Clin Chest Med* 32(3):535–546, 2011.
29. Mosier MJ et al: Predictive value of bronchoscopy in assessing the severity of inhalation injury, *J Burn Care Res* 33(1):65–73, 2012.
30. Epler GR: Bronchiolitis obliterans organizing pneumonia, 25 years: a variety of causes, but what are the treatment options? *Exp Rev Respir Med* 5(3):353–361, 2011.
31. Hayes D Jr: A review of bronchiolitis obliterans syndrome and therapeutic strategies, *J Cardiothorac Surg* 18(6):92, 2011.
32. Margaritopoulos GA et al: Recent advances in the pathogenesis and clinical evaluation of pulmonary fibrosis, *Eur Respir Rev* 21(123):48–56, 2012.
33. Song JW et al: Acute exacerbation of idiopathic pulmonary fibrosis: incidence, risk factors and outcome, *Eur Respir J* 37(2):356–363, 2011.
34. Adamali HI, Maher TM: Current and novel drug therapies for idiopathic pulmonary fibrosis, *Drug Des Devel Ther* 6:261–272, 2012.
35. Bessac BF, Jordt SE: Sensory detection and responses to toxic gases: mechanisms, health effects, and countermeasures, *Proc Am Thorac Soc* 7(4):269–277, 2010.
36. Gore A et al: Hyperoxia sensing: from molecular mechanisms to significance in disease, *J Immunotoxicol* 7(4):239–254, 2010.
37. Chong S et al: Pneumoconiosis: comparison of imaging and pathologic findings, *Radiograph* 26(1):59–77, 2006.
38. Leung CC, Yu IT, Chen W: Silicosis, *Lancet* 379(9830):2008–2018, 2011.
39. Santo Tomas LH: Emphysema and chronic obstructive pulmonary disease in coal miners, *Curr Opin Pulm Med* 17(2):123–125, 2011.
40. Mossman BT et al: Pulmonary endpoints (lung carcinomas and asbestosis) following inhalation exposure to asbestos, *J Toxicol Environ Health B Crit Rev* 14(1-4):76–121, 2011.
41. Blatman KH, Grammer LC: Chapter 19: hypersensitivity pneumonitis, *Allergy Asthma Proc* 33(Suppl 1):64–66, 2012.
42. Myers JL: Hypersensitivity pneumonia: the role of lung biopsy in diagnosis and management, *Mod Pathol* 25(Suppl 1):S58–S67, 2012.
43. Udeshi A, Cantie SM, Pierre E: Postobstructive pulmonary edema, *J Crit Care* 25(3):508.e1–508.e5, 2010.
44. Walkey AJ et al: Acute respiratory distress syndrome: epidemiology and management approaches, *Clin Epidemiol* 4:159–169, 2012.
45. Villar J et al: ALIEN Network: the ALIEN study: incidence and outcome of acute respiratory distress syndrome in the era of lung protective ventilation, *Intensive Care Med* 37(12):1932–1941, 2011.
46. Herridge MS et al: Canadian Critical Care Trials Group. Functional disability 5 years after acute respiratory distress syndrome, *N Engl J Med* 364(14):1293–1304, 2011.
47. Dushianthan A et al: Acute respiratory distress syndrome and acute lung injury, *Postgrad Med J* 87(1031):612–622, 2011.
48. Garcia JG: Genomic investigations into acute inflammatory lung injury, *Proc Am Thorac Soc* 8(2):167–172, 2011.
49. Pierrakos C et al: Acute respiratory distress syndrome: pathophysiology and therapeutic options, *J Clin Med Res* 4(1):7–16, 2012.
50. Grommes J, Soehnlein O: Contribution of neutrophils to acute lung injury, *Mol Med* 17(3-4):293–307, 2011.
51. Raghavendran K, Willson D, Notter RH: Surfactant therapy for acute lung injury and acute respiratory distress syndrome, *Crit Care Clin* 27(3):525–559, 2011.

51a. ARDS Definition Task Force, Ranieri VM et al: Acute respiratory distress syndrome: the Berlin Definition, *JAMA* 307(23):2526–2533, 2012.

52. Bernard GR et al: The American-European Consensus Conference on ARDS. Definitions, mechanisms, relevant outcomes, and clinical trial coordination, *Am J Respir Crit Care Med* 149:818–824, 1994.
53. Bhargava M, Wendt CH: Biomarkers in acute lung injury, *Transl Res* 159(4):205–217, 2012.
54. Pierrakos C et al: Acute respiratory distress syndrome: pathophysiology and therapeutic options, *J Clin Med Res* 4(1):7–16, 2012.
55. Saguil A, Fargo M: Acute respiratory distress syndrome: diagnosis and management, *Am Fam Physician* 85(4):352–358, 2012.
56. Yamashita CM, Lewis JF: Emerging therapies for treatment of acute lung injury and acute respiratory distress syndrome, *Exp Opin Emerg Drugs* 17(1):1–4, 2012.
57. Marti-Carvajal AJ et al: Human recombinant activated protein C for severe sepsis, *Cochrane Database Syst Rev* 3:004388, 2012.
58. Patel GP, Balk RA: Systemic steroids in severe sepsis and septic shock, *Am J Resp Crit Care Med* 185(2):133–139, 2012.
59. National Heart, Lung, and Blood Institute: *National Asthma Education and Prevention Program Expert Panel report 3: guidelines for the diagnosis and management of asthma, 2007*. Available at www.ncbi.nlm.nih.gov/books/NBK7223. Accessed May 14, 2013.
60. Akinbami LJ et al: Trends in asthma prevalence, health care use, and mortality in the United States, 2001–2010. *NCHS data brief, no 94*, Hyattsville, MD, 2012, National Center for Health Statistics. Available at www.cdc.gov/nchs/data/databriefs/db94.htm.
61. Slager RE et al: Genetics of asthma susceptibility and severity, *Clin Chest Med* 33(3):431–443, 2012.
62. Antó JM: Recent advances in the epidemiologic investigation of risk factors for asthma: a review of the 2011 literature, *Curr Allergy Asthma Rep* 12(3):192–200, 2012.
63. Ingram JL et al: Airway fibroblasts in asthma manifest an invasive phenotype, *Am J Respir Crit Care Med* 183:1625–1632, 2011.

64. Effros RM, Nagaraj H: Asthma: new developments concerning immune mechanisms, diagnosis and treatment, *Curr Opin Pulm Med* 13(1): 37–43, 2007.
65. Ober C, Yao TC: The genetics of asthma and allergic disease: a 21st century perspective, *Immunol Rev* 242(1):10–30, 2011.
66. Rigoli L et al: Gene-environment interaction in childhood asthma, *Int J Immunopathol Pharmacol* 24(Suppl 4):41–47, 2011.
67. Wenzel SE: Asthma phenotypes: the evolution from clinical to molecular approaches, *Nat Med* 18(5):716–725, 2012.
68. Fishbein AB, Fuleihan RL: The hygiene hypothesis revisited: does exposure to infectious agents protect us from allergy? *Curr Opin Pediatr* 24(1):98–102, 2012.
69. Holgate ST: Innate and adaptive immune responses in asthma, *Nat Med* 18(5):673–683, 2012.
70. Schmidt-Weber CB: Anti-IL-4 as a new strategy in allergy, *Chem Immunol Allergy* 96:120–125, 2012.
71. Lambrecht BN, Hammad H: The airway epithelium in asthma, *Nat Med* 18(5):684–692, 2012.
72. Silverpil E, Linden A: IL-17 in human asthma, *Exp Rev Resp Med* 6(2):173–186, 2012.
73. Amin K: The role of mast cells in allergic inflammation, *Resp Med* 106(1):9–14, 2012.
74. Ghosh S, Erzurum SC: Nitric oxide metabolism in asthma pathophysiology, *Biochim Biophys Acta* 1810(11):1008–1016, 2011.
75. Brightling CE et al: Lung damage and airway remodelling in severe asthma, *Clin Exp Allergy* 42(5):638–649, 2012.
76. Nair P: Early interventions with inhaled corticosteroids in asthma: benefits and risks, *Curr Opin Pulm Med* 17(1):12–15, 2011.
77. Barnes PJ: Severe asthma: advances in current management and future therapy, *J Allergy Clin Immunol* 129(1):48–59, 2012.
78. Murata A, Ling PM: Asthma diagnosis and management, *Emerg Med Clin North Am* 30(2):203–222, vii, 2012.
79. Szefler SJ: Advancing asthma care: the glass is only half-full! *J Allergy Clin Immunol* 128(3):485–494, 2011.
80. Global Strategy for the Diagnosis: *Management and Prevention of COPD (updated 2013)*. Available at http://www.goldcopd.org/guidelines-global-strategy-for-diagnosis-management.html. Accessed May 14, 2013.
81. Ben-Zaken Cohen S et al: The growing burden of chronic obstructive pulmonary disease and lung cancer in women: examining sex differences in cigarette smoke metabolism, *Am J Respir Crit Care Med* 176(2):113–120, 2007.
82. Miravitlles M, Calle M, Soler-Cataluña JJ: Clinical phenotypes of COPD: identification, definition and implications for guidelines, *Arch Bronconeumol* 48(3):86–98, 2012.
83. Nakamura H: Genetics of COPD, *Allergol Int* 60(3):253–258, 2011.
84. Serapinas D, Sakalauskas R: Sensitivity of alpha-1 antitrypsin level for inherited deficiency detection in COPD patients, *Pneumologia* 61(1):34–36, 2012.
85. Kheradmand F et al: Autoimmunity in chronic obstructive pulmonary disease: clinical and experimental evidence, *Exp Rev Clin Immunol* 8(3):285–292, 2012.
86. Tuder RM, Petrache I: Pathogenesis of chronic obstructive pulmonary disease, *J Clin Invest* 122(8):2749–2755, 2012.
87. Decramer M, Janssens W, Miravitlles M: Chronic obstructive pulmonary disease, *Lancet* 379(9823):1341–1351, 2012.
88. Tam A, Sin DD: Pathobiologic mechanisms of chronic obstructive pulmonary disease, *Med Clin North Am* 96(4):681–698, 2012.
89. Wenzel RP, Fowler AA 3rd, Edmond MB: Antibiotic prevention of acute exacerbations of COPD, *N Engl J Med* 367(4):340–347, 2012.
90. Kim V et al: The chronic bronchitic phenotype of COPD: an analysis of the COPD Gene Study, *Chest* 140(3):626–633, 2011.
91. Qaseem A et al: Diagnosis and management of stable chronic obstructive pulmonary disease: a clinical practice guideline update from the American College of Physicians, American College of Chest Physicians, American Thoracic Society, and European Respiratory Society, *Ann Intern Med* 155(3):179–191, 2011.
92. Gold PM: The 2007 GOLD Guidelines: a comprehensive care framework, *Respir Care* 54(8):1040–1049, 2009. Review. Erratum in *Respir Care* 54(11):1501, 2009.
93. Kent BD, Mitchell PD, McNicholas WT: Hypoxemia in patients with COPD: cause, effects, and disease progression, *Int J Chron Obstruct Pulmon Dis* 6:199–208, 2011.
94. Tuder RM, Janciauskiene SM, Petrache I: Lung disease associated with alpha1-antitrypsin deficiency, *Proc Am Thorac Soc* 7(6):381–386, 2010.
95. El-Zein RA et al: Genetic predisposition to chronic obstructive pulmonary disease and/or lung cancer: important considerations when evaluating risk, *Cancer Prev Res (Phila)* 5(4):522–527, 2012.
96. Min T et al: Critical role of proteostasis-imbalance in pathogenesis of COPD and severe emphysema, *J Mol Med (Berl)* 89(6):577–593, 2011.
97. Mets OM et al: Quantitative computed tomography in COPD: possibilities and limitations, *Lung* 190(2):133–145, 2012.
98. Washko GR: The role and potential of imaging in COPD, *Med Clin North Am* 96(4):729–743, 2012.
99. Minai OA, Benditt J, Martinez FJ: Natural history of emphysema, *Proc Am Thorac Soc* 5(4):468–474, 2008.
100. Yang IA et al: Inhaled corticosteroids for stable chronic obstructive pulmonary disease, *Cochrane Database Sys Rev* 7:002991, 2012.
101. Make B et al: Oxygen therapy in advanced COPD: in whom does it work? *Semin Respir Crit Care Med* 31(3):334–342, 2010.
102. Criner GJ et al: The National Emphysema Treatment Trial (NETT): Part I: lessons learned about emphysema, *Am J Respir Crit Care Med* 184(7):763–770, 2011.
103. Pinner NA et al: Roflumilast: a phosphodiesterase-4 inhibitor for the treatment of severe chronic obstructive pulmonary disease, *Clin Ther* 34(1):56–66, 2012.
104. Stoller JK, Aboussouan LS: A review of α1-antitrypsin deficiency, *Am J Respir Crit Care Med* 185(3):246–259, 2012.
105. Mizgerd JP: Acute lower respiratory tract infection, *N Engl J Med* 358(7):716–727, 2008.
106. Ashraf M, Ostrosky-Zeichner L: Ventilator-associated pneumonia: a review, *Hosp Pract (Minneap)* 40(1):93, 2012.
107. Lobdell KW, Stamou S, Sanchez JA: Hospital-acquired infections, *Surg Clin North Am* 92(1):65–77, 2012.
108. Patterson CM, Loebinger MR: Community acquired pneumonia: assessment and treatment, *Clin Med* 12(3):283–286, 2012.
109. Bouadma L, Wolff M, Lucet JC: Ventilator-associated pneumonia and its prevention, *Curr Opin Infect Dis* 25(4):395–404, 2012.
110. Rigby KM, DeLeo FR: Neutrophils in innate host defense against *Staphylococcus aureus* infections, *Semin Immunopathol* 34(2):237–259, 2012.
111. Hirose T et al: Dynamic changes in the expression of neutrophil extracellular traps in acute respiratory infections, *Am J Resp Crit Care Med* 185(10):1130–1131, 2012.
112. Calbo E, Garau J: Factors affecting the development of systemic inflammatory response syndrome in pneumococcal infections, *Curr Opin Infect Dis* 24(3):241–247, 2011.
113. Short KR et al: Interactions between *Streptococcus pneumoniae* and influenza virus: a mutually beneficial relationship? *Future Microbiol* 7(5):609–624, 2012.
114. Almond MH et al: Influenza-related pneumonia, *Clin Med* 12(1):67–70, 2012.
115. Lee N, Ison MG: Diagnosis, management and outcomes of adults hospitalized with influenza, *Antiviral Ther* 17(1 Pt B):143–157, 2012.
116. Fukuyama S, Kawaoka Y: The pathogenesis of influenza virus infections: the contributions of virus and host factors, *Curr Opin Immunol* 23(4):481–486, 2011.
117. Ruuskanen O et al: Viral pneumonia, *Lancet* 377(9773):1264–1275, 2011.
118. Nair GB, Niederman MS: Community-acquired pneumonia: an unfinished battle, *Med Clin North Am* 95(6):1143–1161, 2011.
119. Haessler S, Schimmel JJ: Managing community-acquired pneumonia during flu season, *Cleve Clin J Med* 79(1):67–78, 2012.
120. Krüger S, Welte T: Biomarkers in community-acquired pneumonia, *Exp Rev Respir Med* 6(2):203–214, 2012.
121. Jefferies JM et al: 13-valent pneumococcal conjugate vaccine (PCV13), *Hum Vaccin* 7(10):1012–1018, 2011.
122. Ramirez P, Bassi GL, Torres A: Measures to prevent nosocomial infections during mechanical ventilation, *Curr Opin Crit Care* 18(1):86–92, 2012.
123. Rivera AM, Boucher HW: Current concepts in antimicrobial therapy against select gram-positive organisms: methicillin-resistant *Staphy lococcus aureus*, penicillin-resistant *Pneumococci*, and vancomycin-resistant *Enterococci*, *Mayo Clin Proc* 86(12):1230–1243, 2011.
124. American Thoracic Society: Guidelines for the management of adults with hospital-acquired, ventilator-associated, and healthcare-associated pneumonia, *Am J Respir Crit Care Med* 171:388–416, 2005.
125. Patterson CM, Loebinger MR: Community acquired pneumonia: assessment and treatment, *Clin Med* 12(3):283–286, 2012.
126. Pawlowski A et al: Tuberculosis and HIV co-infection, *PLoS Pathogens* 8(2):e1002464, 2012.
127. World Health Organization: *Global tuberculosis control 2011*. Available at www.who.int/tb/publications/global_report/en/.
128. Centers for Disease Control and Prevention: Trends in tuberculosis–United States, 2011, *MMWR* 61(11):181–185, 2012.

129. Forrellad MA et al: Virulence factors of the *Mycobacterium* tuberculosis complex, *Virulence* 4(1):3–66, 2013.
130. Druszczyńska M et al: Latent *M. tuberculosis* infection—pathogenesis, diagnosis, treatment and prevention strategies, *Pol J Microbiol* 61(1):3–10, 2012.
131. Ernst JD: The immunological life cycle of tuberculosis, *Nat Rev Immunol* 12(8):581–591, 2012.
132. Gengenbacher M, Kaufmann SH: Mycobacterium tuberculosis: success through dormancy, *FEMS Microbiol Rev* 36(3):514–532, 2012.
133. Russell DG: Who puts the tubercle in tuberculosis? *Nat Rev Microbiol* 5(1):39–47, 2007.
134. Cardona PJ: New insights on the nature of latent tuberculosis infection and its treatment, *Inflamm Allergy Drug Targets* 6(1):27–39, 2007.
135. Lalvani A: Diagnosing tuberculosis infection in the 21st century: new tools to tackle an old enemy, *Chest* 131(6):1898–1906, 2007.
136. Yew WW, Leung CC: Update in tuberculosis 2007, *Am J Respir Crit Care Med* 177(5):479–485, 2008.
137. Lawn SD et al: Advances in tuberculosis diagnostics: the Xpert MTB/RIF assay and future prospects for a point-of-care test, *Lancet Infect Dis* 13(4):349–361, 2013.
138. Lienhardt C, Fruth U, Greco M: The blueprint for vaccine research & development: walking the path for better TB vaccines, *Tuberculosis (Edinb)* 92(Suppl 1):S33–S35, 2012.
139. Chhabra N et al: Pharmacotherapy for multidrug resistant tuberculosis, *J Pharmacol Pharmacother* 3(2):98–104, 2012.
140. Lauzardo M, Peloquin CA: Antituberculosis therapy for 2012 and beyond, *Exp Opin Pharmacother* 13(4):511–526, 2012.
141. Uhlin M et al: Adjunct immunotherapies for tuberculosis, *J Infect Dis* 205(Suppl 2):S325–S334, 2012.
142. Schweigert M et al: Modern history of surgical management of lung abscess: from Harold Neuhof to current concepts, *Ann Thorac Surg* 92(6):2293–2297, 2011.
143. Albert RH: Diagnosis and treatment of acute bronchitis, *Am Fam Physician* 82(11):1345–1350, 2010.
144. Wolberg AS et al: Procoagulant activity in hemostasis and thrombosis: Virchow's triad revisited, *Anesth Analg* 114(2):275–285, 2012.
145. Hunt JM, Bull TM: Clinical review of pulmonary embolism: diagnosis, prognosis, and treatment, *Med Clin North Am* 95(6):1203–1222, 2011.
146. Khashper A et al: Nonthrombotic pulmonary embolism, *AJR Am J Roentgenol* 198(2):W152–W159, 2012.
147. Goldhaber SZ, Bounameaux H: Pulmonary embolism and deep vein thrombosis, *Lancet* 379(9828):1835–1846, 2012.
148. Castillo C, Tapson VF: Right ventricular responses to massive and submassive embolism, *Cardiol Clin* 30(2):233–241, 2012.
149. Wood KE: Major pulmonary embolism, *Crit Care Clin* 27(4):885–906, vi–vii, 2011.
150. Tapson VF: Acute pulmonary embolism, *N Engl J Med* 358(10):1037–1052, 2008.
151. Adams AG, Awsare BK: Review for hospitalists: acute pulmonary embolism, *Hosp Pract (Minneap)* 39(4):55–62, 2011.
152. Fesmire FM et al: Critical issues in the evaluation and management of adult patients presenting to the emergency department with suspected pulmonary embolism, *Ann Emerg Med* 57(6):628–652, e75, 2011.
153. Ouellette DW, Patocka C: Pulmonary embolism, *Emerg Med Clin North Am* 30(2):329–375, viii, 2012.
154. Ferrari E et al: Timing of troponin I measurement in pulmonary embolism, *Heart* 98(9):732–735, 2012.
155. Brunelli A: Deep vein thrombosis/pulmonary embolism: prophylaxis, diagnosis, and management, *Thorac Surg Clin* 22(1):25–28, v, 2012.
156. Abunasser J, Tejada JP, Foley RJ: The diagnosis and management of pulmonary embolism, *Conn Med* 76(1):5–14, 2012.
157. Geske JB et al: Care of patients with acute pulmonary emboli: a clinical review with cardiovascular focus, *Expert Rev Cardiovasc Ther* 10(2): 235–250, 2012.
158. Stein PD, Matta F: Thrombolytic therapy in unstable patients with acute pulmonary embolism: saves lives but underused, *Am J Med* 125(5):465–470, 2012.
159. Highland KB: Pulmonary arterial hypertension, *Am J Med Sci* 335(1):40–45, 2008.
160. Heresi GA, Dweik RA: Pulmonary hypertension: evaluation and management, *Comprehen Ther* 33(3):150–161, 2007.
161. Wilkins MR: Pulmonary hypertension: the science behind the disease spectrum, *Eur Respir Rev* 21(123):19–26, 2012.
162. Rabinovitch M: Molecular pathogenesis of pulmonary arterial hypertension, *J Clin Invest* 122(12):4306–4313, 2012.
162a. Kuhr FK et al: New mechanisms of pulmonary arterial hypertension: role of Ca^{2+} signaling, *Am J Physiol Heart Circ Physiol* 302(8): H1546–1562, 2012.
163. Zakynthinos E et al: Pulmonary hypertension in COPD: pathophysiology and therapeutic targets, *Curr Drug Targets* 12(4):501–513, 2011.
164. McLaughlin VV, Davis M, Cornwell W: Pulmonary arterial hypertension, *Curr Probl Cardiol* 36(12):461–517, 2011.
165. Rubin LJ: Diagnosis and management of pulmonary arterial hypertension: ACCP Evidence-Based Clinical Practice Guidelines. Introduction, *Chest* 126:7S–10S, 2004.
166. Agarwal R, Gomberg-Maitland M: Current therapeutics and practical management strategies for pulmonary arterial hypertension, *Am Heart J* 162(2):201–213, 2011.
167. Rich S: Right ventricular adaptation and maladaptation in chronic pulmonary arterial hypertension, *Cardiol Clin* 30(2):257–269, 2012.
168. American Cancer Society: *Cancer facts and figures 2013*. Available at www.cancer.org/research/cancerfactsfigures/cancerfactsfigures/cancer-facts-figures-2013.
169. Karamanolis G, Sifrim D: Developments in pathogenesis and diagnosis of gastroesophageal reflux disease, *Curr Opin Gastroenterol* 23(4): 428–433, 2007.
170. Torrente MC et al: Human papillomavirus infections in laryngeal cancer, *Head Neck* 33(4):581–586, 2011.
171. Hutcheson KA, Lewin JS: Functional outcomes after chemoradiotherapy of laryngeal and pharyngeal cancers, *Curr Oncol Rep* 14(2):158–165, 2012.
172. Mostafa BE, Youssef AM: Conservation surgery for early laryngeal carcinoma, *ORL J Otorhinolaryngol Relat Spec* 72(4):220–224, 2010.
173. Nhembe F et al: Subglottic carcinoma treated with surgery and adjuvant photodynamic therapy, *Photodiagnosis Photodyn Ther* 7(4):284–287, 2010.
174. Dubey S, Powell CA: Update in lung cancer 2008, *Am J Respir Crit Care Med* 179(10):860–868, 2009.
175. Toyooka S et al: Molecular oncology of lung cancer, *Gen Thorac Cardiovasc Surg* 59(8):527–537, 2011.
176. Brody JS, Steiling K: Interaction of cigarette exposure and airway epithelial cell gene expression, *Annu Rev Physiol* 73:437–456, 2011.
177. Travis WD et al: International Association for the Study of Lung Cancer/American Thoracic Society/European Respiratory Society international multidisciplinary classification of lung adenocarcinoma, *J Thorac Oncol* 6(2):244–285, 2011.
178. Caramori G et al: Mechanisms involved in lung cancer development in COPD, *Int J Biochem Cell Biol* 43(7):1030–1044, 2011.
179. Torok S et al: Lung cancer in never smokers, *Future Oncol* 7(10): 1195–1211, 2011.
180. Brandao GD, Brega EF, Spatz A: The role of molecular pathology in non-small-cell lung carcinoma—now and in the future, *Curr Oncol* 19(Suppl 1), S24–3S2, 2012.
181. Garfield DH, Cadranel J, West HL: Bronchioloalveolar carcinoma: the case for two diseases, *Clin Lung Cancer* 9(1):24–29, 2008.
182. Travis WD: Pathology of lung cancer, *Clin Chest Med* 32(4):669–692, 2011.
183. Villaflor VM, Salgia R: Targeted agents in non-small cell lung cancer therapy: What is there on the horizon? *J Carcinog* 12:7, 2013.
184. Sher T, Dy GK, Adjei AA: Small cell lung cancer, *Mayo Clin Proc* 83(3):355–367, 2008.
185. van Meerbeeck JP, Fennell DA, De Ruysscher DK: Small-cell lung cancer, *Lancet* 378(9804):1741–1755, 2011.
186. Stovold R et al: Biomarkers for small cell lung cancer: neuroendocrine, epithelial and circulating tumour cells, *Lung Cancer* 76(3):263–268, 2012.
187. Yeung SC, Habra MA, Thosani SN: Lung cancer-induced paraneoplastic syndromes, *Curr Opin Pulm Med* 17(4):260–268, 2011.
188. Cakir M, Grossman A: The molecular pathogenesis and management of bronchial carcinoids, *Exp Opin Ther Targets* 15(4):457–491, 2011.
189. Detterbeck FC: Management of carcinoid tumors, *Ann Thorac Surg* 89(3):998–1005, 2010.
190. Rascoe PA et al: Molecular pathogenesis of malignant mesothelioma, *Exp Rev Mol Med* 14:e12, 2012.
191. Rodríguez Portal JA: Asbestos-related disease: screening and diagnosis, *Adv Clin Chem* 57:163–185, 2012.
192. Marshall AL, Christiani DC: Genetic susceptibility to lung cancer–light at the end of the tunnel? *Carcinogenesis* 34(3):487–502, 2013.
193. Maitra A, Kumar V: The lung. In Kumar V et al: *Robbins basic pathology*, ed 8, Philadelphia, 2007, Saunders.
194. Yeung SC, Habra MA, Thosani SN: Lung cancer-induced paraneoplastic syndromes, *Curr Opin Pulm Med* 17(4):260–268, 2011.

195. National Cancer Institute: *Screening and testing to detect cancer: lung cancer*. Available at www.cancer.gov/cancertopics/screening/lung. Accessed June 28, 2013.
196. Sawaya GF, Tice JA: Evidence at the point of practice change, *Arch Intern Med* 10:1–3, 2012.
197. Kalemkerian GP: Staging and imaging of small cell lung cancer, *Cancer Imaging* 11:253–258, 2012.
198. Cheng L et al: Molecular pathology of lung cancer: key to personalized medicine, *Mod Pathol* 25(3):347–369, 2012.
199. Koh PK et al: Targeted agents in non-small cell lung cancer (NSCLC): clinical developments and rationale for the combination with thoracic radiotherapy, *Cancer Treat Rev* 38(6):626–640, 2012.
200. Saintigny P, Burger JA: Recent advances in non-small cell lung cancer biology and clinical management, *Discov Med* 13(71):287–297, 2012.
201. Sibille A, Wauters I, Vansteenkiste J: Maintenance therapy for advanced non-small-cell lung cancer: ready for clinical practice? *Exp Rev Anticancer Ther* 12(4):529–539, 2012.
202. Joshi M, Ayoola A, Belani CP: Small-cell lung cancer: an update on targeted therapies, *Adv Exp Med Biol* 779:385–404, 2013.
203. Carrafiello G et al: Complications of microwave and radiofrequency lung ablation: personal experience and review of the literature, *Radiol Med* 117(2):201–213, 2012.
204. Kawamura H et al: Long-term results of curative intraluminal high dose rate brachytherapy for endobronchial carcinoma, *Radiat Oncol* 7:112, 2012.
205. Bearz A et al: Target therapies in lung cancer, *J Biomed Biotechnol* 2011:921231, 2011.
206. Reckamp KL: Antiangiogenic agents as second-line therapy for advanced non-small cell lung cancer, *Cancer Lett* 321(2):101–109, 2012.
207. Hodkinson PS, Sethi T: Advances in the prevention and treatment of lung cancer, *J R Coll Physicians (Edinb)* 41(2):142–149, 2011.
208. Wender R et al: American Cancer Society lung cancer screening guidelines, *CA Cancer J Clin* 63(2):107–117, 2013.
209. Arenberg D, Kazerooni EA: Setting up a lung cancer screening program, *J Natl Compr Canc Netw* 10(2):277–285, 2012.

CHAPTER

36

Alterations of Pulmonary Function in Children

Valentina L. Brashers and Sue E. Huether

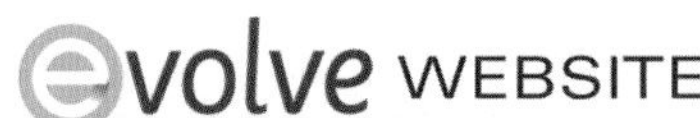

http://evolve.elsevier.com/McCance/
- Review Questions and Answers
- Animations

CHAPTER OUTLINE

Alterations of respiratory function in children are influenced by age, development, gender, race, genetic dominance, and environmental conditions. Newborns, premature newborns in particular, are especially vulnerable to a variety of upper and lower airway infections caused by immaturity of the airways, circulation, chest wall, and the immune system. Structural differences in infants and children also render them less competent to tolerate conditions that cause increased work of breathing. Access to health care and timeliness of immunizations influence the incidence and severity of pulmonary disorders.

STRUCTURE AND FUNCTION

A number of structural characteristics of the pulmonary system influence the way in which infants and children respond to respiratory disturbances. These include structural characteristics of the upper and lower respiratory tracts, chest wall and lung dynamics, metabolic requirements, immunologic immaturity, and physiologic control of respiration.

Upper Airway

All conducting airways (the portions of airway that do not participate in gas exchange) are present at birth and change only in size throughout childhood. Branching of the bronchial tree is in fact complete by the sixteenth week of fetal life.

Because infants and children naturally have smaller-diameter airways than adults, they suffer more obstruction for a given degree of mucosal edema or secretion accumulation. The relative sizes of tonsils, adenoids, and epiglottis likewise are proportionately greater in the young child and with swelling can impose a significant site of obstruction. Infants up to 2 to 3 months of age are "obligatory nose breathers" and are unable to breathe in through their mouths. Nasal congestion is therefore a serious threat to a young infant.

Lower Airways and Lung Parenchyma

During fetal development the lung is transformed from a somewhat dense organ to one that is more delicately structured to facilitate air exchange. Beginning in the second trimester, there is loss of interstitial (mesenchymal) tissue with concomitant expansion of the future air spaces. Capillaries grow into the distal respiratory units that keep subdividing (alveolarization) to maximize surface area for gas exchange. The number of alveoli continues to increase during the first 5 to 8 years of life, after which the alveoli increase in size and complexity. In addition to the structural development of the lung in utero, there is accompanying functional maturation during which specialized cell types, such as type II cells, manifest. (Figure 36-1 contains a summary of alveolar development and stages of fetal lung development.)

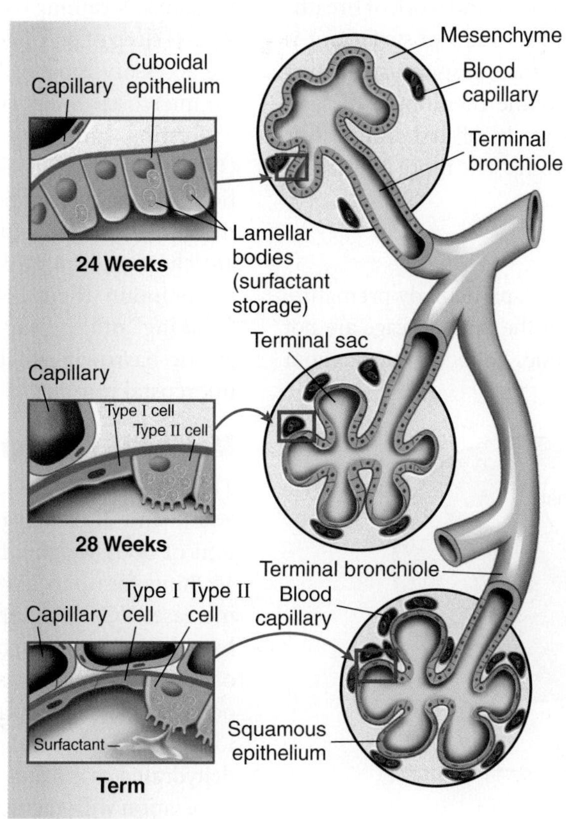

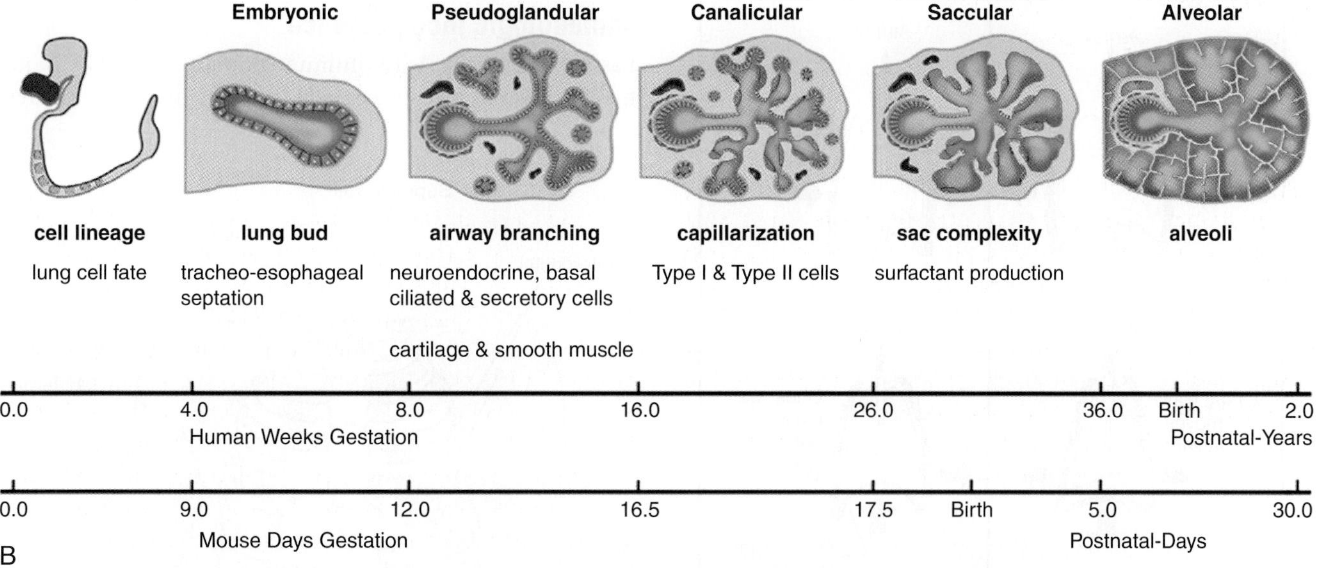

FIGURE 36-1 **Prenatal Development of the Alveolar Unit and Stages of Lung Development. A,** Epithelial cells differentiate into type II and type I cells. Mature type II cells are cuboidal, have apical microvilli, and contain lamellar bodies for surfactant storage and secretion. Type I cells are derived from type II cells and consist of flattened epithelium overlying capillaries, thus forming part of the desired thin air-blood barrier. During fetal development the pulmonary capillaries initially are randomly distributed in mesenchyme. They progressively arrange around the epithelial tubes and establish close contacts to the lining epithelium. Overall the volume of mesenchyme decreases and that of the potential air space increases. **B,** Stages of fetal lung development. (**B** adapted from Gleason CA, Devaskar S: *Avery's diseases of the newborn,* ed 9, Philadelphia, 2012, Saunders.)

Surfactant is a lipid-protein mix that is produced by type II alveolar cells and is critical for maintaining alveolar expansion (thus allowing normal gas exchange). It lines alveoli and reduces surface tension, preventing alveolar collapse at the end of each exhalation. Without surfactant the alveoli tend to stay closed, demanding greater inspiratory force and work of breathing to reexpand on the next breath. Deficiency of surfactant is often seen in premature infants and causes respiratory distress syndrome (RDS), also known as hyaline membrane disease. Surfactant is produced by 20 to 24 weeks of gestation and is secreted into the fetal airways by 30 weeks. The more premature the infant, the higher the risk of RDS.

Chest Wall Dynamics

Chest wall compliance is high in infants, particularly premature infants. The cartilaginous structures of the thoracic cage are not yet well ossified (ossification continues to occur throughout childhood), and the chest wall is easily collapsible. During inspiration in the young child, air is drawn in by the downward movement of the diaphragm, but the resulting negative pressure causes the "soft" chest wall to be drawn *inward* (Figure 36-2); this produces so-called *paradoxic breathing,* or *diaphragmatic breathing.* Paradoxic breathing is especially seen during rapid eye movement (REM) sleep of premature infants. With pulmonary compromise the accessory muscles are drawn inward, creating retraction of the intercostal and supraclavicular spaces (Figure 36-3).

Resting lung volume, or **functional residual capacity (FRC),** represents the balance point between the natural elastic recoil of the lungs (to collapse) and the elastic recoil of the chest wall (to expand). In the face of an overly compliant chest wall, infants up to about 1 year of age are thought to maintain their FRC and avoid atelectasis by muscular "braking" of their expiration. This may occur either by active glottic narrowing or by increased activity of the inspiratory intercostal muscles.

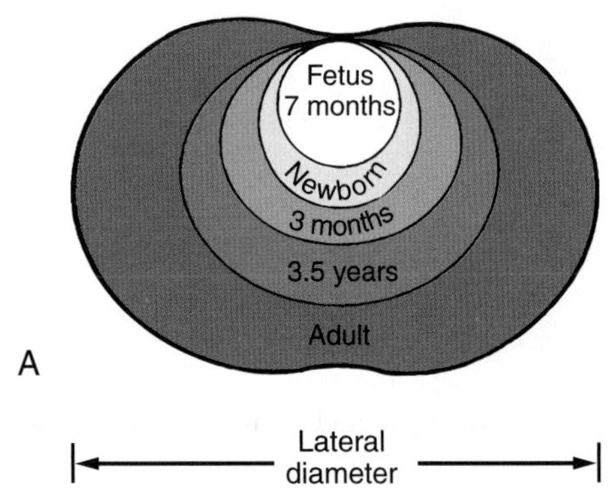

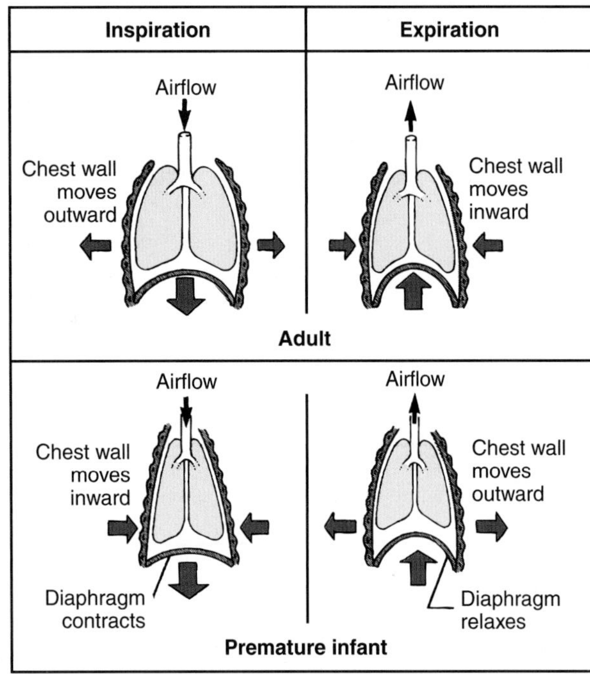

FIGURE 36-2 Developmental Differences in the Chest Wall and Lung Mechanics. **A,** Changes in chest wall shape with age. **B,** Differences in lung mechanics caused by differences in chest wall compliance (degree of rigidity) in premature infants and adults. (Arrows indicate direction of airflow, chest wall movement, and diaphragm movement.)

Metabolic Characteristics

The basal metabolic rate of a child is greater than that of an adult, and thus oxygen consumption (VO_2) is greater per unit of body weight. The VO_2 of the child's normal breathing accounts for up to 25% of the total VO_2. The work of breathing increases VO_2 exponentially with respiratory distress. Children have less muscle glycogen reserve, which limits the efficiency of accessory muscles, such that fatigue with lactic acidosis can occur quickly. Children also have a high proportion of extracellular fluid and therefore more quickly lose fluid and become dehydrated as a result of fever, from environmental heat, or in association with tachypnea (which causes evaporation from the respiratory tract).

Immunologic Incompetence

Passive immunity with immunoglobulin G (IgG) is normally conveyed transplacentally from the mother to the fetus

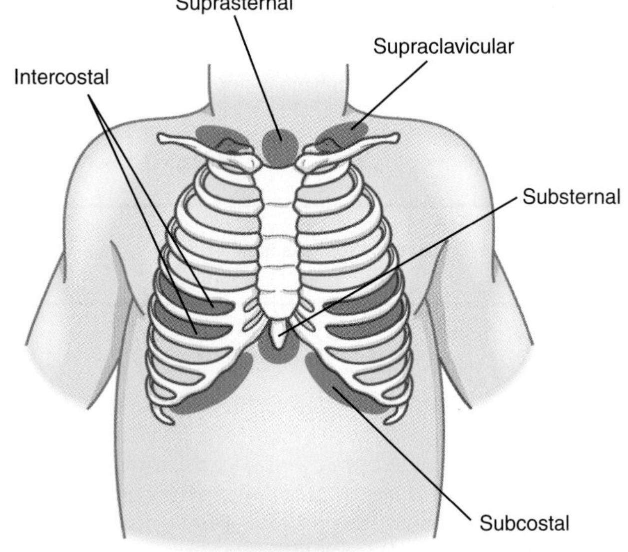

FIGURE 36-3 Areas of Chest Muscle Retraction.

beginning at 20 weeks of gestation; thus IgG levels are lower in preterm than term infants. Breast-feeding allows transfer of secretory IgA, IgG, and IgM after birth. Because IgG has a half-life of approximately 21 days, the placentally transferred antibodies are depleted after just a few months. Infants are able to synthesize IgG, IgM, and IgA, and the levels of these immunoglobulins increase slowly with age. Cell-mediated immunity is also not fully developed in the neonate, which creates a situation of enhanced susceptibility to viral and fungal infections.

Physiologic Control of Respiration

For up to 3 weeks of age, the newborn has a blunted ventilatory response to hypoxia compared with older children and adults. The mechanisms for this are not well understood but may reflect reduced activity of the peripheral chemoreceptors (in the carotid body) and nonadaptive responses in the respiratory center (in the brainstem). Ventilatory response to hypercarbia is normal in term infants but may be reduced in premature infants. Congenital or acquired lesions of the central nervous system may cause hypoventilation or apnea. Exposure to maternal smoking both during and after fetal development can have significant deleterious effects on lung development and subsequent susceptibility to pulmonary disorders (see What's New? Maternal Smoking: Fetal Lung Development and Lung Disease).

DISORDERS OF THE UPPER AIRWAYS

Pulmonary dysfunction can be categorized into disorders of either the upper airway or the lower airway. Signs of acute respiratory failure are the same regardless of etiology. These include the following:

- Increased respiratory effort with retractions (see Figure 36-3) or gasping (apnea in some conditions)
- Cyanosis or pallor
- Agitation
- Decreased level of consciousness
- Cardiovascular signs: tachycardia, mottled color, or bradycardia
- Physiologic compromise reflected by hemoglobin desaturation, hypoxemia, hypercarbia, and acidosis

WHAT'S NEW?

Maternal Smoking: Fetal Lung Development and Lung Disease

Maternal smoking during pregnancy is a risk factor for several adverse developmental outcomes, including abnormal fetal lung development. Lung development is most critical during late fetal and early postnatal life—the saccular and alveolar developmental phases. Abnormalities occurring during these stages can have long-term effects on lung function, contributing to the development of asthma in children and lung disease in adults. Maternal smoking and altered fetal pulmonary structure are related to nicotine that crosses the placenta and is expressed in breast milk. There is up-regulation of nicotinic acetylcholine receptors in the fetal lung. Animal models have demonstrated alterations in lung structure including decreased alveolarization, thickening of the alveolocapillary membrane, decreased synthesis of surfactant, decreased airway diameter, decreased vessel density, and increased airway hyperresponsiveness. Smoke exposure also changes the genetics that control lung growth and maintenance of lung structure, and accelerates lung aging. Prevention of maternal smoking during pregnancy and lactation is required and nicotine replacement therapy is not advised for these women.

Data from Abbott LC, Winzer-Serhan UH: *Crit Rev Toxicol* 42(4):279–303, 2012; Harding R, Maritz G: *Semin Fetal Neonatal Med* 17(2):67–72, 2012; Kajeka R: *Pharmacol Ther* 114:129–145, 2007; Maritz GS, Harding R: *Int J Environ Res Public Health* 8(3):875–898, 2011; Wongtrakool C et al: *Am J Respir Cell Mol Biol* 46(5):695–702, 2012.

Upper Airway Obstruction

The crucial issue in the upper airways is patency. The most common causes of *acute-onset* **upper airway obstruction (UAO)** in children are infections, foreign body aspiration, angioedema, obstructive sleep apnea, and trauma. *Chronic UAO* has many etiologies, including congenital malformations affecting the airway, cartilaginous weakness, vocal cord paralysis, and subglottic stenosis. Chronic upper airway symptoms should prompt referral to a pediatric pulmonologist or an otolaryngologist because specialized diagnostic studies may be needed. A list of causes of pediatric UAO can be found in Box 36-1.

The site and nature of the obstruction are often discernible by assessing the noise associated with breathing, the quality of the voice or cry, and the presence of feeding difficulties. This assessment often can be made without even touching the child. Likewise, the severity of the problem often can be judged by visual observation of signs, including retractions, nasal flaring, gasping or obstructed breaths, anxiety, restlessness, or need to maintain a specific head or body position. Agitation should be regarded as a likely sign of hypoxemia or obstruction. In acute UAO, increasing the child's anxiety by excessive physical examination can worsen the condition. The child should be kept as calm as possible. The clinician should never attempt a pharyngeal examination if there is any suspicion of epiglottitis or retropharyngeal abscess because this maneuver may precipitate acute obstruction of the airway.

The sounds of the child's breathing can provide key clues (Figure 36-4). A sonorous, snoring noise is typical for nasopharyngeal obstruction, such as adenotonsillar hypertrophy. A common sign of pediatric UAO is **stridor,** a harsh, vibratory sound of variable pitch caused by turbulent flow through the partially obstructed airway. A diagnostic approach to stridor is outlined in Figure 36-5. Whether it is present in inspiration, expiration, or both reflects the site of the problem. In general, *inspiratory* stridor is generated with obstruction of the *extrathoracic* airway (above the thoracic inlet), which includes the supraglottic structures, the larynx, the subglottic space, and the upper trachea. *Expiratory* stridor or a monophonic wheeze may be generated by an obstruction in the *intrathoracic* airway (the middle to lower trachea and central bronchi). Biphasic stridor typically reflects obstruction at the glottis (e.g., vocal cord paralysis) itself or a *fixed* rather than a *dynamic* lesion in the subglottic space (e.g., hemangioma or subglottic stenosis). Biphasic noise may sometimes mean abnormalities of both the extrathoracic and intrathoracic trachea (long-segment stenosis or malacia).

BOX 36-1 CAUSES OF UPPER AIRWAY OBSTRUCTION IN CHILDREN ACCORDING TO SITE OF OBSTRUCTION

Nose and Pharynx
Choanal atresia
Lingual thyroid or thyroglossal cyst
Macroglossia
Micrognathia
Hypertrophic tonsils/adenoids
Retropharyngeal or peritonsillar abscess

Larynx
Laryngomalacia
Laryngeal web, cyst, or laryngocele
Laryngotracheobronchitis (viral croup)
Acute spasmodic laryngitis (spasmodic croup)
Epiglottitis
Vocal cord paralysis
Laryngotracheal stenosis
Intubation
Foreign body
Cystic hygroma
Subglottic hemangioma
Laryngeal papilloma
Angioneurotic edema
Laryngospasm (hypocalcemic tetany)
Psychogenic stridor

Trachea
Tracheal stenosis
Tracheomalacia
Bacterial tracheitis
External compression

Adapted with permission from Diagnosis of Stridor in Children, November 15, 1999, *American Family Physician*.

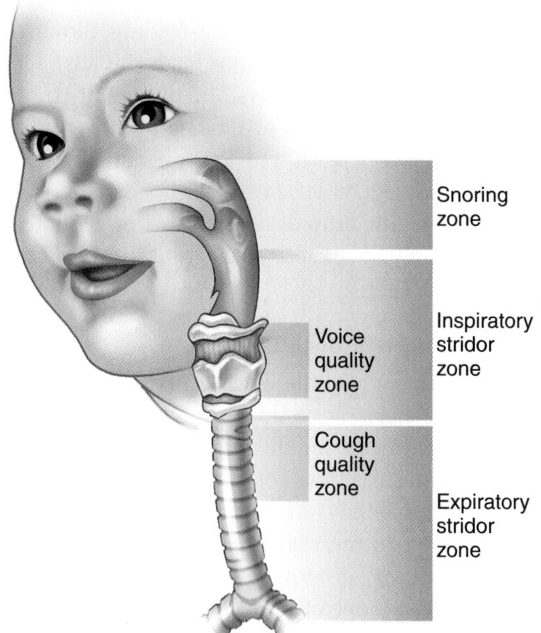

FIGURE 36-4 Listening Can Help Locate the Site of Airway Obstruction. A loud, gasping snore suggests enlarged tonsils or adenoids. Stridor during inspiration suggests the airway is compromised at the level of the supralaryngeal structures (epiglottis and arytenoid cartilages), vocal cords, subglottic region, or upper trachea. With forced inspiration, intrathoracic pressure becomes quite negative and is less than atmospheric pressure, promoting collapse at or just above the site of obstruction. Expiratory stridor or central wheeze results from narrowing or collapse of the lower trachea or bronchi. During forced exhalation, rising pleural pressure may exceed intratracheal pressure. Airway noise during both inspiration and expiration often represents a fixed obstruction of the vocal cords or subglottic space. Hoarseness or a weak cry is a byproduct of obstruction at the vocal cords. If a cough is croupy or low pitched, suspect tracheal pathology. (Redrawn from Eavey RD: *Contemp Pediatr* 3[6]:78, 1986; used with permission; original illustration by Paul Singh-Roy.)

Abnormalities of voice or cry (weak or hoarse) suggest problems at the larynx, such as vocal cord paralysis. Muffling of the voice, especially in an acute condition, suggests supralaryngeal obstruction, such as epiglottitis or retropharyngeal abscess. Pronounced cough may be an irritative symptom, such as that produced by an aspirated foreign body, or may be a sign of tracheal obstruction. The cough associated with croup or tracheal foreign body is usually harsh and barking.

Airway obstruction occurs sooner in infants than in older children. Obviously, airway luminal size is smaller in accordance with smaller body size, but any decrease in luminal diameter will be much more significant. This is because airway resistance is proportional to the inverse of the *fourth* power of the radius; thus a decrease to half the original diameter increases resistance 16-fold. Furthermore, an infant's cartilaginous structures are more collapsible and thus are prone to creating or contributing to a situation of UAO.

Infections

Infections of the upper airway (Table 36-1) are common in children; some have the potential to cause life-threatening emergencies. Recognition and rapid evaluation of these problems are crucial pediatric care skills.

Croup. Croup illnesses can be divided into two categories: (1) acute laryngotracheobronchitis (croup) and (2) spasmodic croup. Diphtheria can be considered a croup illness but is now rare because of vaccinations. Croup illnesses are all characterized by infection and obstruction of the upper airways.[1]

Croup is an acute **laryngotracheobronchitis** and most commonly occurs in children from 6 months to 3 years of age, with peak incidence at 2 years of age.[2] In 85% of cases, croup is caused by a virus, most commonly parainfluenza; however, other viruses such as influenza A virus, respiratory syncytial virus (RSV), rhinovirus, adenovirus, and rubella virus (measles) as well as the atypical bacterium *Mycoplasma pneumoniae* has been associated with causation. The incidence of croup is highest in late autumn and winter, corresponding to the parainfluenza and RSV seasons, respectively. Croup is more common in boys than girls. In a significant portion of affected children, croup is a recurrent problem during childhood, and there is a family history of croup in about 15% of cases. **Spasmodic croup** is characterized by similar hoarseness, barking cough, and stridor, but is of sudden onset, usually at night and without viral

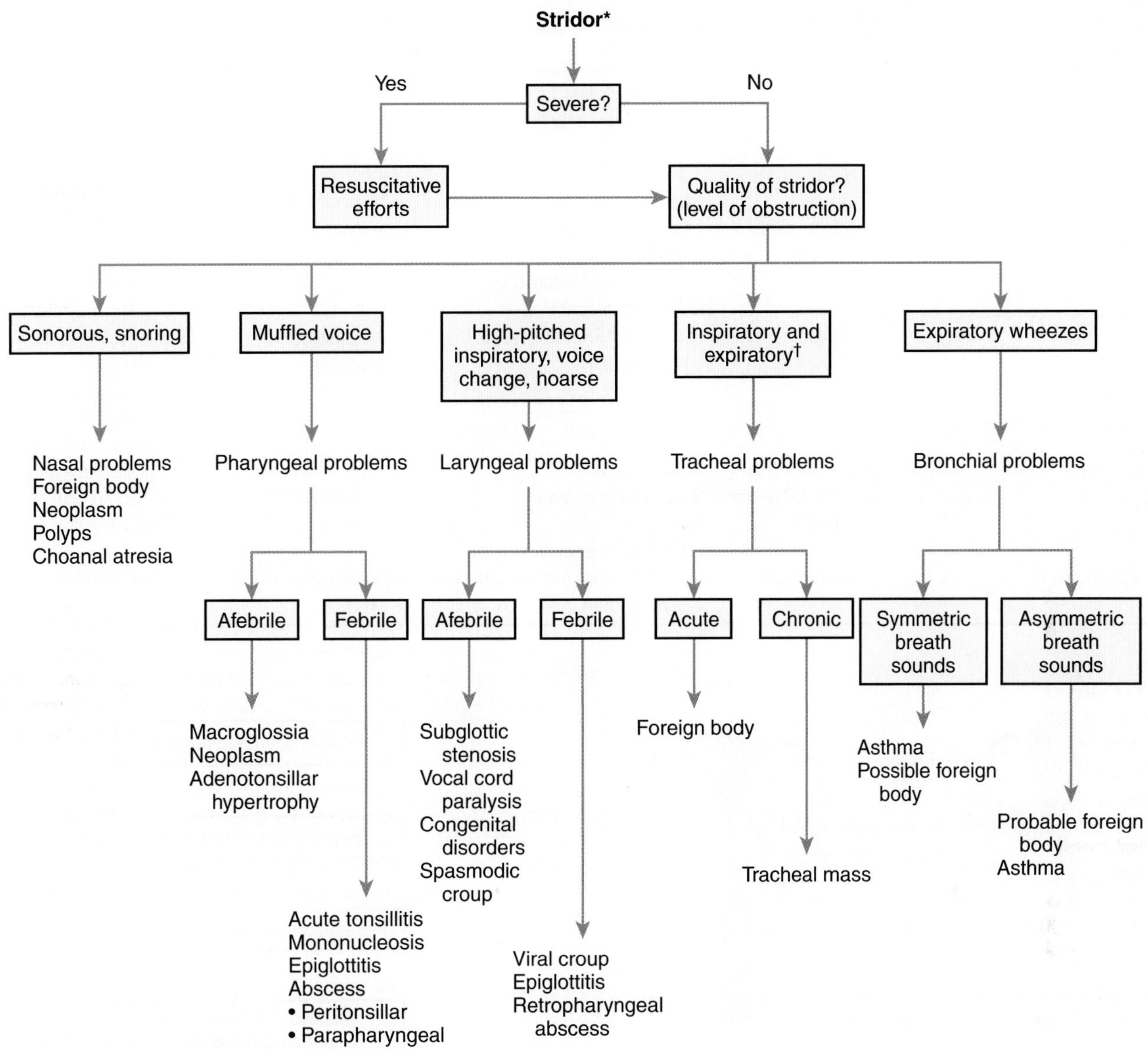

FIGURE 36-5 Diagnostic Approach to Stridor. (Adapted from Handler SD: Stridor. In Fleisher GR, Ludwig S, editors: *Textbook of pediatric emergency medicine,* Baltimore, 1993, Williams & Wilkins.)

prodrome. It often resolves as quickly as it develops and usually occurs in older children. The etiology is unknown although association with viruses, allergies, asthma, and gastroesophageal reflux disease (GERD) is being investigated.[3]

PATHOPHYSIOLOGY. The pathophysiology of viral croup is caused primarily by subglottic edema from the infection. The mucous membranes of the larynx are tightly adherent to the underlying cartilage, whereas those of the subglottic space are looser and thus allow accumulation of mucosal and submucosal edema (Figure 36-6). Furthermore, the cricoid cartilage is structurally the narrowest point of the airway, making edema in this area critical. As illustrated in Figure 36-7, increased resistance to airflow leads to increased work of breathing, which generates more negative intrathoracic pressure, which in turn may exacerbate dynamic collapse of the upper airway.

CLINICAL MANIFESTATIONS. Typically there is a prodrome of rhinorrhea, sore throat, and low-grade fever for a few days. The child then develops the characteristic harsh (seal-like) barking cough, hoarse voice, and inspiratory stridor. Most cases are mild and resolve spontaneously after several more days. Occasionally, however, UAO becomes severe and requires urgent management.

EVALUATION AND TREATMENT. The degree of symptoms determines the level of treatment. Most children have a barking cough and viral symptoms and may need no specific treatment. However, the presence of stridor (especially at rest), retractions, or agitation suggests a sicker child. The tool most often used for estimating croup severity is the Westley croup score, which provides a cumulative score for the degree of stridor, retractions, air entry, cyanosis, dyspnea, and level of consciousness in the child.[4]

TABLE 36-1 COMPARISON OF UPPER AIRWAY INFECTIONS

CONDITION	AGE	ONSET	ETIOLOGY	PATHOPHYSIOLOGY	SYMPTOMS
Acute laryngotracheobronchitis (croup)	6 mo-3 yr	Usually gradual	Viral (parainfluenza 1 and 3, influenza A, respiratory syncytial virus)	Inflammation from vocal cords to bronchial lumina	Harsh cough; stridor; low-grade fever; may have nasal discharge, conjunctivitis
Acute tracheitis	1-12 yr	Abrupt or following viral illness	*Staphylococcus aureus*/methicillin-resistant *Staphylococcus aureus* (MRSA) *Haemophilus influenzae* type B Group A streptococci	Inflammation of upper trachea	High fever; toxic appearance; thick harsh cough; purulent secretions; may prefer head elevation
Epiglottitis	2-6 yr	Abrupt	*Haemophilus influenzae* type B (Hib) Group A streptococci	Inflammation of supraglottic structures	Severe sore throat; high fever; toxic appearance; muffled voice; may drool; sits erect and quietly
Retropharyngeal abscess	>6 yr	Gradual, 2-5 days; may follow oral trauma	*S. aureus*/MRSA *Streptococcus pyogenes* Anaerobes Group A beta-hemolytic streptococci	Abscess in posterior pharyngeal wall	Similar to epiglottitis
Peritonsillar abscess	>9 yr	May be abrupt	Group A beta-hemolytic streptococci *S. aureus*/MRSA	Abscess within or around tonsil	Similar to epiglottitis; may have trismus

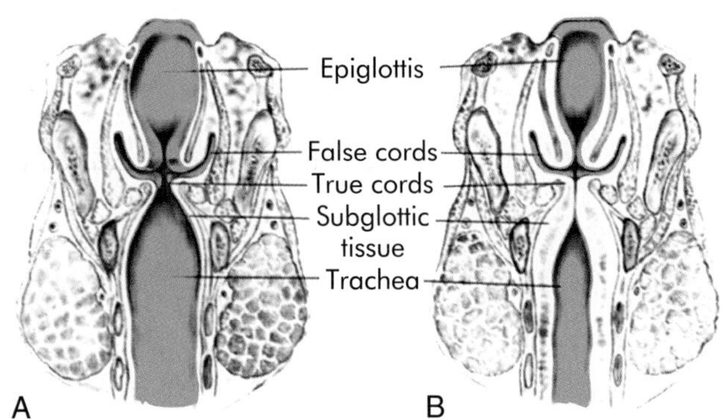

FIGURE 36-6 The Larynx and Subglottic Trachea. **A,** Normal. **B,** Narrowing and obstruction from edema caused by croup. (From Hockenberry MJ, Wilson D: *Wong's nursing care of infants and children,* ed 9, St Louis, 2011, Mosby.)

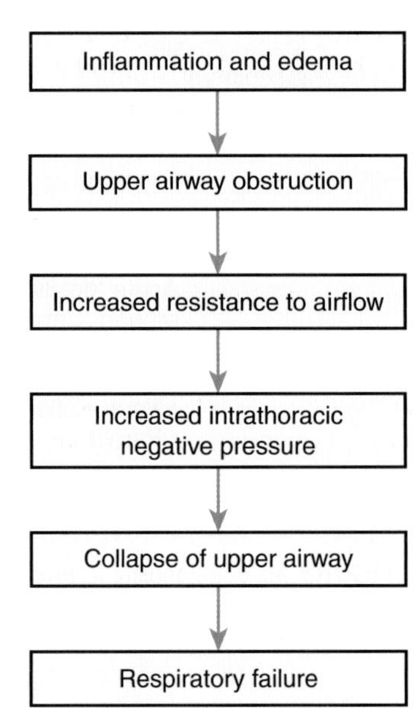

FIGURE 36-7 Upper Airway Obstruction with Croup.

Severity also is classified as mild, moderate, and severe. Most children with croup require no treatment. Inhalation of humidified air does not improve symptoms in mild to moderate croup.[5] Glucocorticoids, either injected or oral (dexamethasone) or nebulized (budesonide), have been shown to improve symptoms within 6 hours. Less sleep is lost by children, less stress is experienced by parents, and fewer children have a need for return healthcare visits or hospitalization when corticosteroids are used.[6] The use of nebulized racemic epinephrine improves outcomes with moderate to severe croup.[2,7] Epinephrine stimulates α- and β-adrenergic receptors and is thought to decrease airway secretions and mucosal edema. It is a temporizing measure until concomitantly given corticosteroids begin to take effect. Thus children who are given nebulized epinephrine should be closely observed for 2 to 3 hours to ensure that they will remain stable. Oxygen also should be administered. Heliox (helium-oxygen mixture of 80:20 or 70:30) may be used for severe cases of croup, although there is lack of scientific evidence to establish use in routine clinical practice.[8]

Acute Epiglottitis. Historically, **acute epiglottitis** was caused by *Haemophilus influenzae* type B (Hib). Since the advent of Hib immunization, the overall incidence of acute epiglottitis in children has decreased significantly, although Hib still accounts for approximately 25% of the cases seen in children. Infants less than 1 year of age are at greater risk.[9] Current pediatric cases usually represent Hib vaccine failures or are caused by alternative pathogens, such as groups A, B, C, F, and

G streptococci, *Streptococcus pneumoniae, Candida* species, *Staphylococcus aureus,* and viral pathogens. Thermal injuries, trauma, and posttransplant lymphoproliferative disorder also have been reported as causes of epiglottitis.[10]

PATHOPHYSIOLOGY. The epiglottis arises from the posterior tongue base and covers the laryngeal inlet during swallowing. It has a rich blood and lymphatic circulation. Bacterial invasion of the mucosa with associated inflammation leads to the rapid development of edema causing severe, life-threatening obstruction of the upper airway.[10]

CLINICAL MANIFESTATIONS. In the classic form of the disease, a child between 2 and 6 years of age suddenly develops high fever, irritability, sore throat, a "hot potato voice," inspiratory stridor, and severe respiratory distress. The child appears ill and classically will adopt a forward-leaning position (tripod position) with drooling and dysphagia (inability to swallow). Examination of the throat may trigger laryngospasm and cause respiratory collapse. Death may occur in a few hours. Pneumonia, cervical lymph node inflammation, otitis, and, rarely, meningitis or septic arthritis may occur during the course of epiglottitis.

EVALUATION AND TREATMENT. Acute epiglottitis is a life-threatening emergency. The essentials are early recognition, avoidance of disturbing the child (which could worsen the obstruction), and securing the airway. Examination of the throat should not be attempted because it may trigger laryngospasm and cause respiratory collapse. Tracheal intubation should be accomplished by the most experienced personnel (usually an anesthesiologist and/or otolaryngologist) using fiberoptic laryngoscopy. Subsequent culture of the airway is obtained and intravenous broad-spectrum antibiotics are administered promptly. Therapy is reevaluated after culture results return. Corticosteroids also are generally used in treatment regimens although there are no published randomized trials to support this practice.[10-12] Despite the severe presentation of epiglottitis, resolution with treatment is usually rapid, with intubation rarely needed for more than a couple of days. When Hib epiglottitis is diagnosed, the American Academy of Pediatrics (AAP) recommends that postexposure prophylaxis with rifampin be administered to household contacts (specific to certain ages of children present).[12] When caused by microorganisms other than *H. influenzae,* as is now the usual situation, epiglottitis may present in ages outside the typical range and with more gradual rather than fulminant onset, thus making diagnosis less obvious. Such cases also may respond more slowly to treatment.

Tonsillar Infections. Tonsillar infections (tonsillitis) are occasionally severe enough to cause UAO.[13] As with other infections of the upper airway, the incidence of tonsillitis secondary to group A beta-hemolytic *Streptococci* (GABHS) and methicillin-resistant *S. aureus* (MRSA) has risen notably in the past 15 years.[14] Significant swelling of the tonsils and pharynx occurs, and a tenacious membrane may cover the mucosa. UAO because of tonsillitis is a well-known complication of infectious mononucleosis, especially in a young child. The development of UAO in tonsillar infections requires the use of appropriately selected antibiotics and may require the use of corticosteroids, especially in the case of mononucleosis.[15] Some children with recurrent tonsillitis benefit from tonsillectomy.

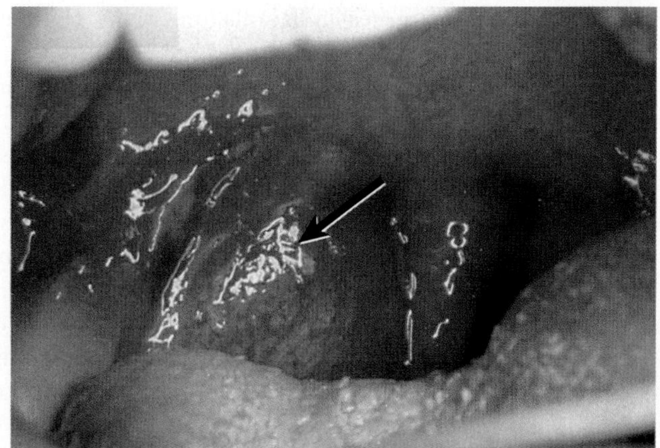

FIGURE 36-8 Peritonsillar Abscess. Unilateral bulging of the tonsillar region is evident. (From Whiting JL, Chow AW: *J Crit Ill* 2[7]:36, 1987.)

Peritonsillar abscess is usually unilateral and is most often a complication of acute tonsillitis.[16] The most common causative microorganism is GABHS. Children have fever, sore throat, dysphagia, trismus, pooling of saliva, and muffled voice. Peritonsillar bulging (Figure 36-8) and cervical adenopathy on the same side are usually visible. The abscess must be drained and the child given antibiotics.[17] Death can occur from spontaneous abscess rupture with aspiration or airway obstruction.[18]

Bacterial Tracheitis. **Bacterial tracheitis** is the most common potentially life-threatening upper airway infection in children. It is most often caused by *Staphylococcus aureus (S. aureus)* (including methicillin-resistant [MRSA] strains), *H. influenzae,* group A beta-hemolytic *Streptococcus* (GABHS [*Streptococcus pyogenes*]), or *Moraxella catarrhalis.*[19] It accounts for 5% to 14% of UAOs in children requiring intensive care.[20] A virus or a fungus is more likely to be seen as the source of tracheitis in immunocompromised children.[21] Treatment of viral croup with corticosteroids has increased the risk for serious bacterial tracheitis (especially by GABHS), resulting in death rates between 18% and 40%.[20] The presence of airway edema and copious purulent secretions leads to airway obstruction that can be worsened by the formation of a tracheal pseudomembrane and mucosal sloughing. Increased morbidity can occur because of respiratory and cardiopulmonary arrest, respiratory failure, pneumonia, septic shock, toxic shock syndrome, acute respiratory distress syndrome (ARDS), and multiple organ dysfunction syndrome (MODS). The onset of symptoms may be sudden or may be preceded by a pre-existing viral upper respiratory tract infection or croup. The acute clinical presentation frequently includes tachypnea, stridor, hoarse voice, fever, cough, and/or increased secretions from the mouth and nose. There may be evidence of concurrent infections, such as sinusitis, otitis, pneumonia, or pharyngitis.[22] Children with chronic gastroesophageal reflux are more likely to experience difficulty with these types of concurrent infections. Management requires the rapid administration of broad-spectrum intravenous antibiotics. The majority of children with tracheitis require endotracheal intubation in order to prevent airway obstruction. Corticosteroids (parenteral and inhaled) are used to decrease tracheal inflammation. Many children recover adequately to be extubated within 72 to 96 hours.[23]

Retropharyngeal Abscess. **Retropharyngeal abscess** can be caused by aerobic, anaerobic, or polymicrobial infection. A decrease in retropharyngeal abscess has been noted in the past several years that is likely related to the use of corticosteroids in the treatment of influenza and croup. There also has been an increase in GABHS strains associated with this condition, and the emergence of MRSA as the offending microorganism is increasingly noted.[24]

Retropharyngeal abscess usually occurs more commonly in male children about 4 years of age and as a consequence of either nasopharyngeal infection or penetrating local injury.[25] Clinical signs include fever, dysphagia, drooling, stridor, respiratory distress, and stiff neck. This condition requires intravenous antibiotics targeted at the suspected microorganism, and sometimes incision and drainage.[26]

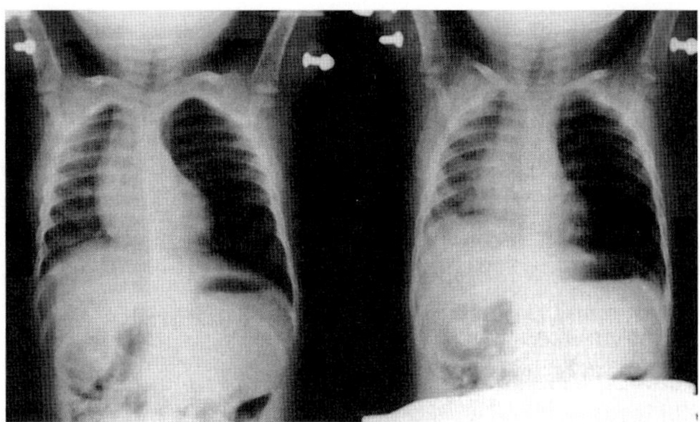

FIGURE 36-9 Foreign Body Aspiration. Inspiratory *(left)* and expiratory *(right)* chest radiographs of a child who aspirated a portion of a potato into the left mainstem bronchus. Left lung field is hyperaerated and the mediastinum is shifted to the right on expiration because of left-sided obstructive emphysema. (From Kenna MA, Bluestone CD: *Pediatr Rev* 10[1]:25, 1988.)

Aspiration of Foreign Bodies

Most children who aspirate a foreign object (**foreign body aspiration**) are between 1 and 3 years of age. More than 100,000 cases occur each year.[27] Often the aspiration either is not witnessed or does not seem significant to the parent; thus medical care is often not pursued until after the first 24 hours. At the time of aspiration, the child may cough, choke, gag, or wheeze, and stridor or cyanosis occasionally occurs. This may be followed by a quiescent interval of minutes to even weeks or months before symptoms reappear from resulting local irritation, granulation, bronchial obstruction, or infection (pneumonia or bronchiectasis). Pronounced inspiratory stridor, cough, and wheezing are typical symptoms that prompt the parents to seek medical attention. Examples of common aspirated objects include nuts, sunflower seeds, hot dog chunks, popcorn, coins, and small toys or toy parts. Meat or food impactions are more common in adolescents. Items of particular concern are batteries and multiple magnets. In general, foreign bodies require early intervention secondary to their propensity to cause respiratory symptoms and complications, including esophageal erosions or aortoesophageal fistula (rare).

The symptom history is often the most critical aid in diagnosis.[28] Symptoms are determined by the size of the object and the site in which it is located, as well as the child's age and size (see Figure 36-4). Foreign bodies lodged in the upper trachea typically produce inspiratory stridor, whereas those located in the lower intrathoracic airways more commonly produce wheezing. About 75% of aspirated foreign bodies lodge in a bronchus. Children with an unexplained persistent cough and refractory parenchymal infiltrates also should be considered for unrecognized foreign body aspiration.[29] Many objects are not radiopaque; however, if the object has completely occluded a lung segment, atelectasis will be visible on a chest radiograph. Occasionally, air will accumulate distal to the obstruction if the object is causing a ball-valve effect. This effect can sometimes be documented by inspiratory and expiratory chest films (Figure 36-9). In a younger child, bilateral decubitus films may show failure to compress the obstructed lung when in the "down" position.

Most foreign bodies can be removed by bronchoscopy and only rarely is a pulmonary lobectomy required. Soft particles such as food, as well as hard objects, must be removed because infectious processes will otherwise occur.[30] Objects lodged in the laryngeal or subglottic regions are particularly dangerous because of their potential for complete or near-complete airway occlusion.

Angioedema

Angioedema is a localized edema involving the deep, subcutaneous layers of skin or mucous membranes. Generally, angioedema causes facial swelling first, particularly around the eyes and lips, and may progress to airway swelling.[31] Angioedema is usually secondary to allergic phenomena (e.g., allergy to peanuts, cow's milk, chicken eggs).[32] If airway compromise is apparent, standard treatment includes epinephrine (subcutaneous), antihistamines, and corticosteroids. An occasional cause of pediatric angioedema is use of angiotensin-converting enzyme inhibitors for treatment of hypertension or heart disease. Increased levels of bradykinin appear to mediate this adverse effect by causing vasodilation, increased vascular permeability, and histamine release.[33]

An inherited deficiency of the plasma protein C-1 inhibitor (C-1 INH) causes *hereditary angioneurotic edema* (HAE), a rare but serious problem in children. About 50% of cases occur during childhood.[34] The mean age of onset of initial symptoms is 8 to 12 years but it also may occur as early as the first year of life. This condition is characterized by recurring attacks of angioedema involving subcutaneous tissues (especially limbs, genitalia, and face); abdominal and pelvic viscera; and, much less often, the airway. Laryngeal attacks in these individuals may be life threatening and do not respond reliably to standard measures for airway edema. Complement studies usually provide an accurate diagnosis.[34] The mortality of undiagnosed HAE can be as high as 50%. The mainstays of supportive care are airway monitoring, hydration, pain relief, and control of nausea. Concentrates of C-1 INH appear to produce rapid improvement within 15 to 60 minutes. Short- and long-term prophylaxis can be instituted using antifibrinolytic agents, attenuated androgens, and C-1 INH concentrates.[35]

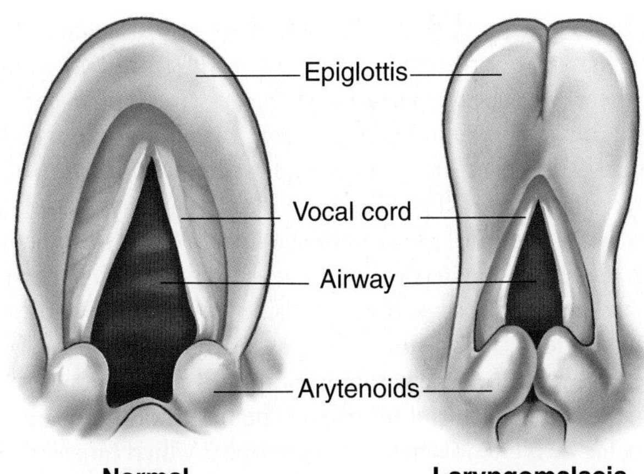

FIGURE 36-10 Laryngomalacia. In the normal larynx *(left),* supralaryngeal structures maintain their upright orientation during inspiration. In contrast, in infants with laryngomalacia *(right),* there is inward prolapse of the arytenoid masses, which include the prominent cuneiform tubercles and the arytenoid cartilages. The glottis becomes partially covered, and airflow is impeded. Sometimes the edges of the epiglottis curl inward, further exacerbating the obstruction. In expiration, these structures are "blown" aside passively.

Congenital Malformations

Congenital malformations can occur at multiple sites from the nasal openings to the subglottis. Anatomic or functional obstruction can cause severe respiratory distress.

Laryngomalacia and Tracheomalacia. **Laryngomalacia** results from abnormally soft laryngeal cartilages and is the most common cause of chronic stridor in infants. Boys are twice as likely as girls to present with symptoms. In laryngomalacia, the epiglottis or arytenoids, or both, fold inward with inspiration, partially covering the glottis (Figure 36-10). The pathophysiology of these abnormalities is still not completely understood. Two primary hypotheses are anatomic or neuromuscular.[36] Anatomically there may be foreshortened or tight aryepiglottic folds or there may be redundant soft tissue in the supraglottis.[37] The neuromuscular hypothesis suggests that there is an abnormality of the sensorimotor integrative function of the brainstem and peripheral reflexes are responsible for laryngeal tone and airway patency.[38] Laryngeal nerve hypertrophy also has been documented.[39] Gastroesophageal reflux disease (GERD) and other comorbidities are associated with laryngomalacia.[40]

Typical signs of laryngomalacia include inspiratory stridor beginning in the first days or weeks of life, accentuated with activity, and sometimes with positional changes (worse in supine or head-flexed positions). Feeding difficulties may be noted, but they are usually mild. Cry is normal. Laryngoscopy is used to confirm the diagnosis. Laryngomalacia is usually mild and improves spontaneously over the first year of life as the supralaryngeal cartilage structures stiffen; thus most cases are managed with watchful waiting. A late-onset variant of this disease has been noted in the literature and should be suspected if the following occurs: potential cause of feeding difficulties in toddlers, sleep apnea in children, and exercise intolerance in teenagers.[41,42]

In **tracheomalacia,** or **tracheobronchomalacia,** the tracheobronchial cartilages are flaccid and tend to collapse during the expiratory cycle, causing stridor. This may be classified as primary (idiopathic) or secondary. When malacia is caused by a secondary source, it is usually related to extrinsic compression of the trachea from a vascular malformation (congenital tracheomalacia). Tracheobronchomalacia presents clinically as a spectrum of respiratory illnesses that range from life-threatening conditions to chronic cough and wheeze conditions. In some cases symptoms may be more subtle than in laryngomalacia. Low-pitched inspiratory stridor may be a sign of malacia of the upper trachea or centrally located, single-pitch (monophonic) wheeze may be present in malacia of the middle to distal trachea. Tracheomalacia can be suspected clinically and confirmed by bronchoscopy. Depending on the type and severity of the lesion, surgical approaches for repair may be indicated.[43]

Vocal Cord Paralysis. Vocal cord paralysis is second to laryngomalacias as a cause of stridor and is a relatively uncommon congenital disorder. The vocal cords should move apart to facilitate inspiration and move together to facilitate vocalization. Paralysis of one or both vocal cords may affect breathing, swallowing, and speech. The etiology of the congenital abnormality is unclear but may be caused by immaturity of the vagus nerve or brainstem, or both. Iatrogenic injury is frequently cited as the major secondary cause of vocal cord paralysis, such as surgical trauma to the recurrent laryngeal nerve during cardiac surgery. Other secondary causes include Arnold-Chiari malformation (the region of the brainstem in which the nucleus ambiguus acts as the "relay station" for laryngeal function), cerebral palsy, hydrocephalus, myelomeningocele, spina bifida, or hypoxia.[44] Other associations include infectious and neoplastic causes, trauma, and inflammatory conditions.[45] In older children and adolescents, exercise has been known to precipitate vocal cord dysfunction (VCD).[46]

Clinical findings of vocal cord paralysis in children less than 1 year include dysphonia, glottic incompetence, GERD, and stridor.[45] It sometimes resolves spontaneously (most often during the first year of life) or with correction of the underlying problem. Flexible laryngoscopy and chest x-ray are common evaluative tools that may help determine the cause. In some individuals, VCD may be misdiagnosed as asthma.[47] Medical therapy may include use of corticosteroids, proton pump inhibitors, and speech therapy. Recurrent pulmonary infections secondary to aspiration may occur and require treatment until the cords are repaired.[48] Severe cases may necessitate endotracheal intubation and tracheostomy. Tracheostomy may be used until the vocal cords are surgically repaired or can be used as a permanent measure for bilateral vocal cord paralysis.[48]

Subglottic Stenosis. Congenital **subglottic stenosis** is the third most common laryngeal anomaly and is defined as a subglottic airway diameter of less than 4 mm at the cricoid region in a full-term infant, and less than 3 mm in a premature infant.[48] Incomplete recanalization of the laryngotracheal tube during the third month of gestation results in this defect. Subglottic stenosis also is associated with eosinophilic esophagitis, Wegener granulomatosis, and neurofibromatosis.[49-51] Traumatic injury to the upper airway with development of subglottic stenosis is a well-described complication of endotracheal intubation.[52] Factors that contribute to subglottic stenosis include utilization of long-term assisted ventilation, use of an endotracheal tube that is too large, excessive movement of the tube, and susceptibility of the individual.[53] Neonates can tolerate long periods of endotracheal intubation; the overall rate of symptomatic subglottic stenosis in neonates is 0.2%.[53] The occurrence of subglottic stenosis can be minimized by ensuring that the tube size allows a small air leak during inspiration (at a peak inspiratory force of approximately 25 mmHg) and that the tube is securely taped. Sedation is generally required to reduce head movement for children who are intubated. Because of the rapid growth of the lumen of the trachea and cricoid cartilage in the first year (which triples in size), infants may outgrow the obstruction, particularly if mild or moderate.[54] Serial balloon dilation can be effective.[55] For severe subglottic stenosis, laryngotracheal reconstruction (LTR) along with cricotracheal resection and thyrotracheal anastomosis may be required.[56]

Other Congenital Malformations. Congenital malformations of the upper airways, trachea, and bronchial tree are rare and cause airway obstruction. Lesions include coanal atresia; laryngeal atresias, webs, cysts, clefts, and subglottic hemangiomas; and tracheal stenosis. **Coanal atresia** can be unilateral or bilateral and causes lack of patency of the nasal cavity within the nasopharynx. Bilateral coanal atresia can be life threatening in newborns because they are obligate nasal breathers.[57] **Laryngeal atresias** and webs are caused by failure of the larynx to recanalize during embryogenesis. Most of these disorders are in the area of the glottis with extension into the subglottis.[48] **Tracheal stenosis** is a rare malformation characterized by inspiratory and expiratory stridor within the first few weeks of birth. It is usually associated with pulmonary, cardiovascular, and gastrointestinal malformations.[58] Structural abnormalities such as pectus excavatum or abnormalities involving the great vessels also can result in tracheal compression. For example, absent pulmonary valve syndrome dilates the pulmonary artery, which can compress the trachea and bronchi.[59] Tracheal or bronchial compression results in airway symptoms or feeding difficulties, or both, ranging from dysphagia, recurrent respiratory tract infections, wheezing, and stridor to acute respiratory distress or "dying spells." Many older children are first thought to have gastroesophageal reflux or asthma as the principal problem. Surgical management is usually required for these conditions, and some infants may require mechanical ventilation while awaiting surgery.[59]

Obstructive Sleep Apnea Syndrome

Obstructive sleep apnea syndrome (OSAS) is a breathing disorder defined by prolonged partial and/or intermittent complete UAO during sleep with disruption of normal ventilation and normal sleep patterns. Childhood OSAS is common with an estimated prevalence of 2% to 3% among middle-school children and as many as 13% of children ages 3 to 6 years. Prevalence is estimated to be two to four times higher in vulnerable populations (blacks, Hispanics, and preterm infants).[60] Unlike adults, OSAS in children occurs equally among males and females. Infants are at risk because they have both anatomic and physiologic predispositions toward airway obstruction and gas-exchange abnormalities, including a superiorly placed larynx, increased chest wall compliance, ventilation-perfusion mismatching, and ventilatory control instability. Congenital abnormalities of the airway, as described previously in this chapter, may have adverse effects on airway patency. Neck flexion, airway secretions, gastroesophageal reflux, and sleep deprivation can be associated with airway obstruction. Obstructive sleep apnea in infants has been associated with failure to thrive, behavioral deficits, and sudden infant death.[61]

PATHOPHYSIOLOGY. The pathophysiology of childhood OSAS is likely to be multifactorial in origin. The most common predisposing factor is adenotonsillar hypertrophy, which causes physical impingement on the nasopharyngeal airway. OSAS often occurs more frequently in overweight or obese children, as well as in those with orthodontic/craniofacial anomalies, neurologic disorders, allergy, asthma, abnormalities in the motor tone of the upper airways (frequently an issue in neurologically impaired children), abnormal arousal mechanisms, and genetic susceptibility.[62] Recent studies have documented that children with sleep disordered breathing (SDB) have increased inflammation in the upper airway and elevated serum levels of C-reactive protein, particularly in obese children.[63] Activation of inflammatory pathways contributes to end-organ injury with cardiovascular and metabolic morbidities.[64]

CLINICAL MANIFESTATIONS. Common manifestations of OSAS include snoring and labored breathing, restlessness, and sweating during sleep, which can be continuous or intermittent. There may be episodes of increased respiratory effort, but no audible airflow, often terminated by snorting, gasping, repositioning, or arousal. Affected children are often chronic mouth breathers and have large tonsils. They also may exhibit nocturnal enuresis.[65] It appears that there also may be a correlation between OSAS and elevated blood pressure similar to adults.[66] This is further linked to increased body mass index (BMI) and episodes of desaturation and apnea/hypopnea.[67]

OSAS can result in chronic hypoxemia and hypercapnia affecting multiple organ systems. Significant morbidity is associated with OSAS including cognitive problems, neurobehavioral impairment (e.g., inattention, hyperactivity, aggression, conduct problems, attention-deficit/hyperactivity disorder [ADHD]/emotional [mood]), excessive daytime sleepiness, impaired school performance, and poor quality of life.[68] Left untreated it also can cause cardiovascular disease, particularly left ventricular hypertrophy, and insulin resistance, as well as pulmonary complications (upper and lower respiratory tract infections) and reduced somatic growth.[69-71]

EVALUATION AND TREATMENT. All parents should be asked if their child exhibits snoring, a symptom that is often not spontaneously reported to a healthcare provider. The history and physical examination are the most effective means of diagnosis. Screening tools and sleep questionnaires may be helpful in evaluating the presence of SDB.[72] Radiographic images of the upper airway may reveal upper airway narrowing caused by adenoidal hypertrophy, and magnetic resonance imaging (MRI) and acoustic reflectometry may detect reduced upper airway dimensions.[73] The most definitive evaluation ("gold standard") is the polysomnographic sleep study, which documents obstructed breathing and physiologic impairment and may be combined with nocturnal oximetry studies. If obstructive sleep apnea caused by tonsillar enlargement is documented or strongly suspected clinically, children are most often referred for tonsillectomy and adenoidectomy (T&A). For severely affected children who do not respond to T&A or who have different problems, such as obesity that cannot be rapidly remedied, continuous positive airway pressure (CPAP) delivered through a tight-fitting nasal mask may be used during sleep. Treatment is important to prevent associated morbidities. Successful medical or surgical treatment results in improvement in physical, behavioral, and emotional difficulties as well as quality of life.[74-76]

DISORDERS OF THE LOWER AIRWAYS

Lower airway disease is one of the leading causes of morbidity in the first year of life and continues to be an important component of other illnesses. Pulmonary disorders commonly observed include perinatal conditions, such as neonatal RDS, congenital malformations, asthma, cystic fibrosis, infections, aspiration syndrome, and ARDS.

Respiratory Distress Syndrome of the Newborn

Respiratory distress syndrome (RDS) of the newborn (previously known as **hyaline membrane disease [HMD]**) is a major cause of neonatal morbidity and mortality. It occurs almost exclusively in premature infants and the incidence has increased in the United States over the past two decades. Preterm births account for about 12% of all births. Black mothers have 1.5 times the risk of preterm birth and 3.4 times the risk of preterm-related mortality.[77] RDS occurs in 50% to 60% of infants born at 29 weeks of gestation and decreases significantly by 36 weeks. Infants of diabetic mothers and those with cesarean delivery (especially elective C-section) are more likely to develop RDS because the labor-associated catecholamine and steroid surge do not occur, causing decreased pulmonary surfactant release.[78] It is more common in boys than girls and in one cohort it was more common in black infants.[79,80] Death rates have declined significantly since the introduction of antenatal steroid therapy and postnatal surfactant therapy. The major predisposing factor is prematurity because the immature lung is not well structured for gas exchange and has not yet developed adequate surfactant production and secretion. Death rates have declined significantly since the introduction of antenatal steroid therapy and postnatal surfactant therapy. The epidemiology, pathophysiology, and clinical presentation of RDS are outlined in Box 36-2.

PATHOPHYSIOLOGY. RDS is caused by surfactant deficiency, which decreases the alveolar surface area available for gas exchange. Surfactant lipoproteins have a detergent-like effect that separates the liquid molecules inside the alveoli, thereby decreasing alveolar surface tension. Without surfactant, alveoli collapse at the end of each exhalation.[81] Surfactant normally is not secreted by the alveolar cells until approximately 20 to 24 weeks of gestation (see Figure 36-1). Premature infants also are born with underdeveloped and small alveoli that are difficult to inflate. Additionally, the alveoli have thick walls and an inadequate capillary blood supply such that gas exchange is significantly impaired. The infant's chest wall is weak and highly compliant and, thus, the rib cage tends to collapse inward with respiratory effort. The net effect is *atelectasis* (Figure 36-11), resulting in significant hypoxemia. Atelectasis is difficult for the neonate to overcome because it requires a significant negative inspiratory pressure to open the alveoli with each breath. The increased work of breathing and a decrease in tidal volume cause alveolar hypoventilation and hypercapnia. Hypoxia and hypercapnia cause pulmonary vasoconstriction, which increases intrapulmonary resistance and shunting. Increased pulmonary vascular resistance causes a partial return to fetal circulation, with right-to-left shunting of blood through the ductus arteriosus and foramen ovale further compromising pulmonary perfusion. There is decreased surfactant production with inadequate pulmonary perfusion and alveolar ventilation.

Prolonged hypoxemia and inadequate tissue perfusion activates anaerobic glycolysis, producing lactic acid and thus causing metabolic acidosis. Alveolar hypoventilation causes respiratory acidosis. Inadequate alveolar ventilation can be further complicated by increased pulmonary capillary permeability. Additionally, many premature infants with RDS require positive pressure mechanical ventilation with high oxygen content, which damages the alveolar epithelium (e.g., barotrauma and oxygen toxicity). Together these conditions result in the leakage of plasma proteins into the alveoli and pulmonary edema. Fibrin deposits in the air spaces create the appearance of *hyaline membranes* for which the disorder was originally named. The plasma proteins leaked into the air space have the additional adverse effect of inactivating any surfactant that may be present. The pathogenesis of RDS is summarized in Figures 36-11 and 36-12.

CLINICAL MANIFESTATIONS. Signs of RDS appear within minutes of birth. Some neonates require immediate resuscitation because of asphyxia or initial severe respiratory distress. Characteristic signs are tachypnea (respiratory rate more than 60 breaths per minute), expiratory grunting, intercostal and subcostal retractions, nasal flaring, and cyanosis. The natural course is characterized by progressive hypoxemia and dyspnea with severity progressing over the first 2 days of life. Apnea and irregular respirations occur as the infant tires. The severity of the hypoxemia and the difficulty in providing adequate supplemental oxygenation result in the Vermont Oxford Neonatal Network definition of RDS as a Pa_{O_2} less than 50 mmHg in room air, central cyanosis in room air, or a need for supplemental oxygen to maintain Pa_{O_2} greater than 50 mmHg, as well as the classic chest film appearance.[82] Typically, a chest radiograph shows diffuse, fine granular densities within the first 6 hours of life. This "ground glass" appearance is associated with alveolar flooding. In most cases the clinical manifestations reach a peak within 3 days, after which there is gradual improvement with appropriate treatment.

EVALUATION AND TREATMENT. Diagnosis is made on the basis of clinical manifestations, chest radiographs, and, if needed, analysis of amniotic fluid or tracheal aspirates to estimate lung maturity (lecithin/sphingomyelin ratio [L/S ratio]). The

BOX 36-2 NEWBORN RESPIRATORY DISTRESS SYNDROME

Epidemiology
Worldwide
Prematurity predisposes
Cesarean section without labor predisposes
Perinatal asphyxia predisposes
Male > female
White > black
Second-born twin at greater risk
PROM spares
IUGR spares
Maternal stress spares
Maternal diabetes predisposes if less than 37 weeks
Maternal hemorrhage predisposes

Clinical Signs
Onset near the time of birth
Tachypnea
Increased work of breathing:
- Nasal flaring
- Retractions of respiratory muscles

Expiratory grunt
Cyanosis
Systemic hypotension
Characteristic chest film
Course to death or improvement in 3 to 5 days
Fine inspiratory rales
Hypothermia
Peripheral edema
Pulmonary edema

Pathophysiology
Reduced lung compliance
Reduced FRC
Poor lung distensibility
Poor alveolar stability
Right-to-left shunts
Reduced effective pulmonary blood flow
If hypotensive and hypoxic, poor peripheral perfusion, poor renal perfusion, myocardial malfunction
Patent ductus arteriosus contributes

Pathobiochemistry
Respiratory acidosis
Decreased saturated phospholipids
Low amniotic fluid L/S ratio
Low surfactant-associated proteins
Decreased total serum proteins
Decreased fibrinolysis
Low thyroxine levels

Pathology
Atelectasis
Injury to epithelial cells, edema
Membrane contains fibrin and cellular products
No tubular myelin
Osmiophilic lamellar bodies decreased early, increased later

Etiology
Surfactant deficiency during disease
Probable inadequate hormonal (corticoid) stimulus in utero
DPL synthesis impaired and/or destruction increased
Autonomic dysfunction

Prevention
Prenatal glucocorticoids for more than 24 hours
Prevention of asphyxia
Surfactant replacement:
- Prophylactically—within 15 minutes after birth
- Early rescue—within 60 minutes after birth
- Established RDS—within 12 hours after birth

Continuous positive airway pressure

From Jackson JC: Respiratory distress in the preterm infant. In Gleason CA, Devaskar SU, editors: *Avery's diseases of the newborn,* ed 9, Philadelphia, 2011, Saunders.
DPL, Dipalmitoyl lecithin; *FRC,* functional residual capacity; *IUGR,* intrauterine growth restriction; *L/S,* lecithin/sphingomyelin; *PROM,* prolonged rupture of membranes (>16 hours).

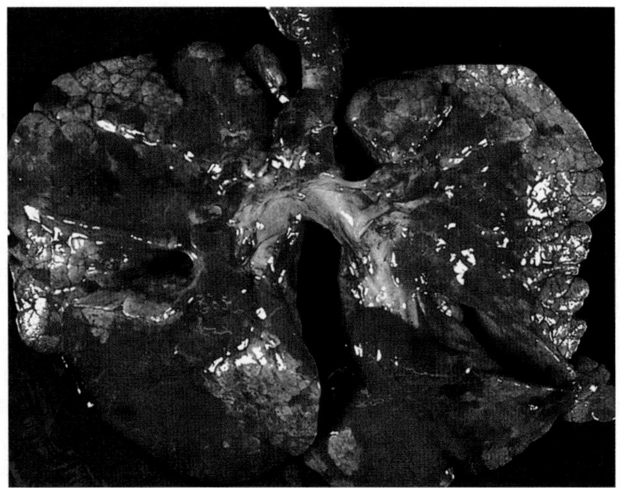

FIGURE 36-11 Patchy Atelectasis of Neonatal Lungs with Respiratory Distress Syndrome (RDS). (From Damjanov I, Linder J, editors: *Anderson's pathology,* ed 10, St Louis, 1996, Mosby.)

ultimate treatment for RDS would be prevention of premature birth. For women in preterm labor, antenatal treatment with glucocorticoids induces a significant and rapid acceleration of lung maturation and stimulation of surfactant production in the fetus. There is extensive evidence that when there is risk of preterm labor antenatal corticosteroid therapy given between 26 and 34 weeks of gestation reduces the incidence of RDS and death. Repeated courses of corticosteroids may be safe in this setting.[83,84] Glucocorticoids induce a significant and rapid acceleration of lung maturation and stimulation of surfactant production in the fetus. There is extensive evidence that maternal steroid therapy significantly reduces the incidence of RDS, central nervous system hemorrhage, and neonatal mortality.[85,86] Glucocorticoids may not significantly affect respiratory outcomes when given after 34 weeks of gestation.[87,88]

Current recommendations for infants weighing less than 1000 g include prophylaxis beginning within 15 to 30 minutes of birth by administration of exogenous surfactant (either

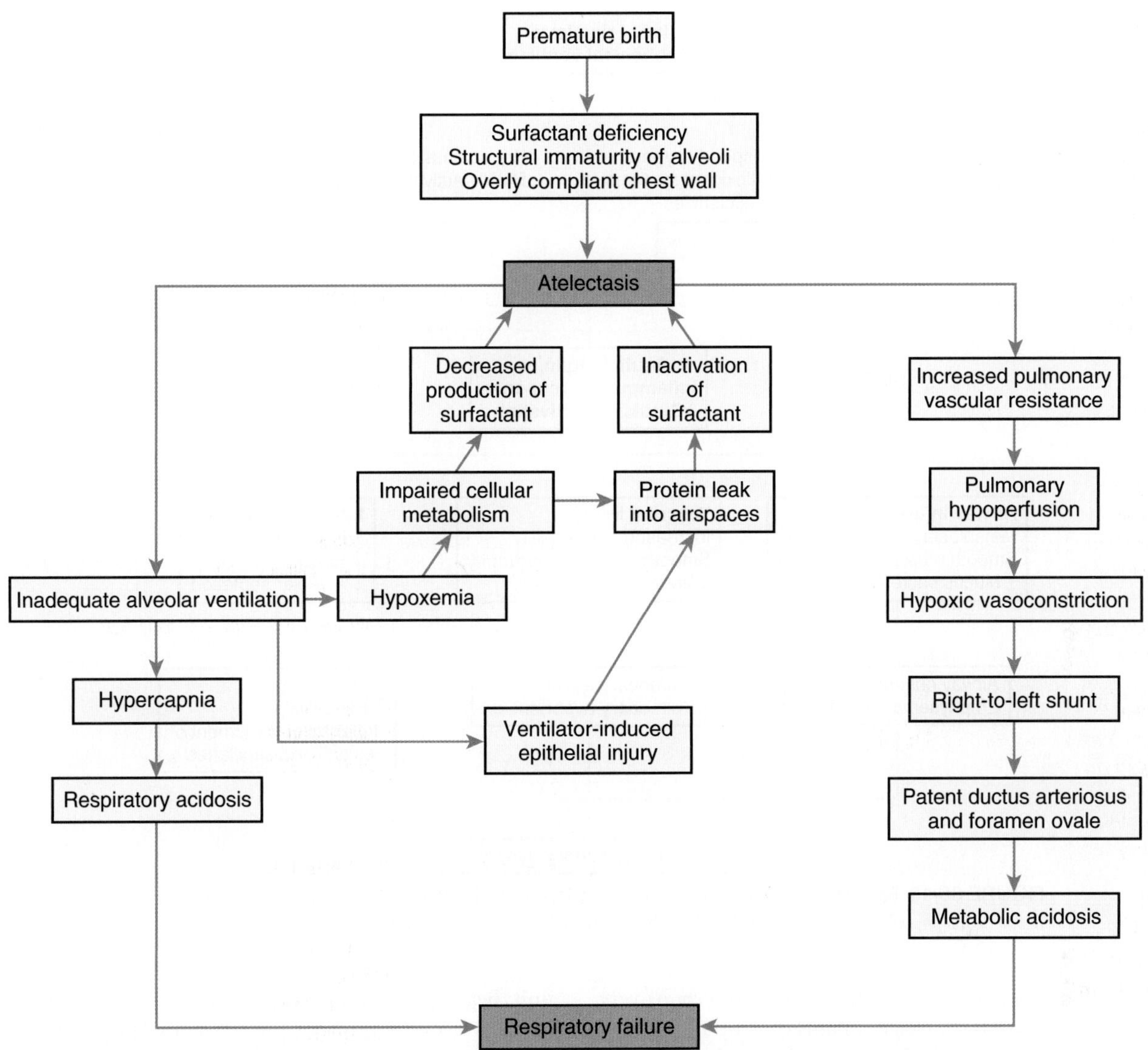

FIGURE 36-12 Pathogenesis of Respiratory Distress Syndrome (RDS) of the Newborn. RDS is also known as hyaline membrane disease.

synthetic or natural) through a nebulizer or nasal continuous positive airway pressure (CPAP) ventilation.[81] Repeat doses are given every 12 hours for the first few days. There is usually a dramatic improvement in oxygenation, as well as a decreased incidence of RDS death, pneumothorax, and pulmonary interstitial emphysema.[89,90] For infants weighing more than 1000 g, surfactant replacement is based on clinical need. Surfactant therapy should be considered complementary to antenatal glucocorticoids. The two therapies together appear to have an additive effect on improving lung function.[91] Supplemental inositol also may promote maturation of surfactant and prevent adverse neonatal outcomes.[92]

Supportive care includes oxygen administration and mechanical ventilation. Mechanical ventilation can result in a proinflammatory state that may contribute to the development of chronic lung disease, such as bronchopulmonary dysplasia (BPD). Strategies that are lung protective, such as greater reliance on nasal continuous positive airway pressure (NCPAP) to prevent lung injury, permissive hypercapnia, lower oxygen saturation targets, modulation of tidal volume (V_t) settings, and use of high-frequency oscillation, are being evaluated.[93,94] Mechanical ventilation with mixtures of oxygen and nitric oxide or helium may improve gas exchange and reduce airflow resistance and have improved outcomes.[95-97] Most infants survive RDS and, in many cases, recovery may be complete within 10 to 14 days. However, the incidence of subsequent chronic lung disease is significant among very low birth weight infants.[98,99]

Bronchopulmonary Dysplasia

Bronchopulmonary dysplasia (BPD), also known as *chronic lung disease of prematurity,* is the major cause of pulmonary disease in infants. It is associated with premature birth (usually before 28 weeks of gestation), perinatal supplemental oxygen, and positive pressure ventilation. There are approximately 60,000 infants born weighing less than 1500 g in the

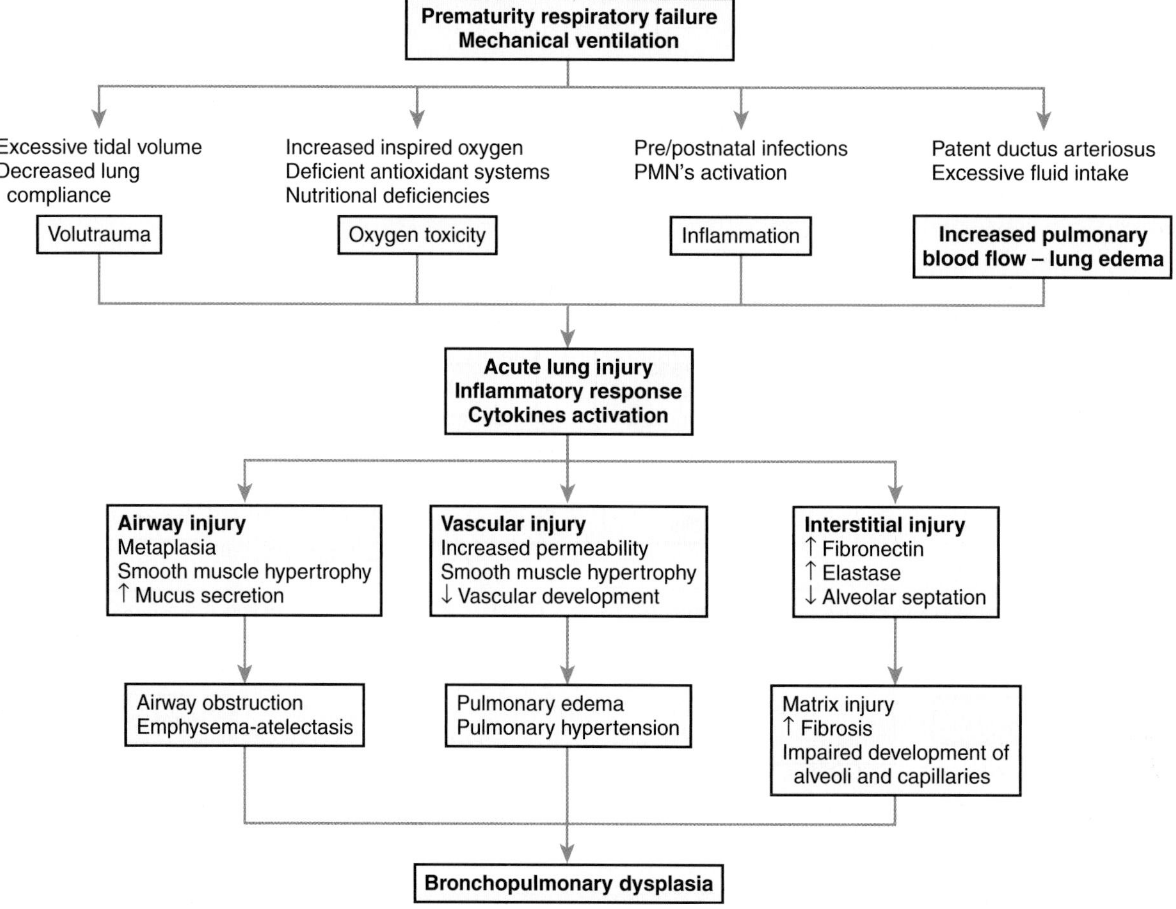

FIGURE 36-13 Pathophysiology of Bronchopulmonary Dysplasia (BPD). (From Polin RA, Fox WW, Abman SH: *Fetal and neonatal physiology,* ed 4, Philadelphia, 2011, Philadelphia.)

United States on an annual basis. About 20% to 30% of very low and extremely low birth weight infants develop BPD.[100,101]

In the current era of neonatology, the widespread use of antenatal glucocorticoids, postnatal surfactant, and NCPAP has lessened the incidence and severity of RDS and thus also reduced the incidence of BPD. Surprisingly, some of the tiny infants who develop BPD have shown few or no clinical signs of RDS at birth or have initially received only low levels of supplemental oxygen or ventilatory support for apnea.[102] The presence of antenatal chorioamnionitis, postnatal sepsis, a patent ductus arteriosus, and genetic susceptibility confer additive risk of developing BPD.[103]

BPD is a multisystem condition and is associated with developmental disorders in other systems, such as growth retardation, pulmonary hypertension, neurodevelopmental delays (e.g., cerebral palsy), hearing defects, and retinopathy of prematurity.[100]

PATHOPHYSIOLOGY. Lung immaturity and inflammation contributes to the development of BPD. In preterm infants born at less than 28 weeks of gestation, the fetal lung is in the *canalicular stage* of development (16 to 28 weeks), a critical period during which type II epithelial cells appear, capillaries grow into the future distal alveolar regions, and the interstitium begins to condense (see Figure 36-1). Ultimately the alveoli must have a very thin interface between the air space and the capillary for appropriate gas exchange. The extensive network of alveoli develops by septation within the terminal respiratory unit, beginning in the *saccular stage,* starting at approximately 26 to 28 weeks. The alveoli are vulnerable to inflammation and impaired growth during this stage.[104]

Before the widespread use of surfactant therapy, BPD was a disease characterized by airway injury, inflammation, and parenchymal fibrosis *(classic BPD).* Now, after the initiation of surfactant therapy, what is called *new BPD* is most often a form of arrested lung development with poor formation of the alveolar architecture. Alveoli are large and fewer in number, thereby presenting decreased surface area for gas exchange. There is abnormal vascular endothelial growth factor that results in abnormal pulmonary capillary development and mild fibrosis accompanied by persistent inflammation contributing to perfusion mismatch and pulmonary hypertension.[105] Genetic influences on surfactant proteins and inflammatory regulation have been documented in association with the "new BPD."[106]

Levels of proinflammatory cytokines, such as tumor necrosis factor-alpha (TNF-α), interleukin 1 (IL-1), interleukin 6 (IL-6), and interleukin 8 (IL-8), are all elevated in the amniotic fluid or tracheal aspirates, or both, of preterm infants who later develop BPD. Inflammation invites neutrophils and macrophages to release reactive oxygen species and proteolytic enzymes. Interestingly, the predominant mediators of *new BPD* are profibrotic and angiogenic cytokines rather than proinflammatory cytokines.[104,107] Figure 36-13 illustrates the pathophysiology of BPD.

CLINICAL MANIFESTATIONS. The current clinical definition of BPD includes the need for supplemental oxygen at 36 weeks of postmenstrual age (estimated time of conception to birth plus weeks since birth) and for at least 28 days after birth, with a graded severity dependent on required respiratory support at term (divided into mild, moderate, and severe based on oxygen requirements and ventilatory needs). Clinically, the infant exhibits hypoxemia caused by ventilation-perfusion mismatch and diffusion defects. Work of breathing is elevated, resulting in hypercapnia. The ability to feed may be impaired. Intermittent bronchospasm with wheezing, mucus plugging, and pulmonary hypertension characterizes the clinical course of the most severely affected babies.

EVALUATION AND TREATMENT. Infants with severe BPD require prolonged, assisted ventilation with cautious weaning. Prevention of lung damage with "gentle ventilation" (see lung protective strategies of ventilation in RDS section, p. 1303) or early nasal CPAP, or both, is used in clinical situations when permitted. Use of CPAP prevents airway collapse and results in fewer days of oxygen and ventilator requirement by reducing the amount of lung injury as compared with mechanical ventilation.[108] Additionally, oxygen supplementation at lower than previously accepted values (89% to 94% saturations) is a means to reduce oxidant injury to the lungs and retinal vasculature. Diuretics are used to control pulmonary edema, bronchodilators reduce airway resistance, and inhaled corticosteroids improve the rate of extubation and reduce the time that mechanical ventilation is required. Caffeine citrate is used to prevent apnea and for neuroprotection.[109] Supplementation with vitamin A provides antioxidant protection and stimulates lung growth and surfactant production.[110] Careful nutritional and fluid and electrolyte support is routinely used and has resulted in improved outcomes.

Respiratory Tract Infections

Infections may be localized to the bronchioles, bronchi, alveoli, interstitium, or pleura. The cause and site of infections are related to the age of the child, seasonal variables, and environmental exposures. Infants and young children tend to have more viral infections, especially during late autumn to early spring. Environmental factors may play a role, such as the presence of siblings and daycare exposure.

Bronchiolitis

Bronchiolitis is a common viral-induced lower respiratory tract infection of the small airways that occurs in children younger than 2 years of age. The most common associated pathogen is RSV, but it also may be associated with adenovirus, rhinovirus (older children), influenza, parainfluenza virus (PIV), and human metapneumovirus.[1] Bronchiolitis has a peak incidence during winter (late December) and a spike in February, and then tapers off in the spring, paralleling the RSV season. There are distinct regional differences in the United States depending on variation in the viral season based on geography. It is a major reason for hospital admission of children younger than 1 year, particularly children of lower socioeconomic status.[111] Healthy infants usually make a full recovery from RSV bronchiolitis, but infants who are premature (birth weight <2500 g) or who have underlying lung disease, heart disease, or immune deficiency may have a much more severe or even deadly course. Bronchiolitis has been linked to an increased risk for asthma later in childhood.[112,113] Bronchiolitis has a worldwide annual death rate between 160,000 and 600,000 deaths.[114]

PATHOPHYSIOLOGY. Viral infection causes inflammation and necrosis of the bronchial epithelium and destruction of ciliated epithelial cells. There is infiltration with lymphocytes around the bronchioles and a cell-mediated hypersensitivity to viral antigens with release of lymphokines causing inflammation, as well as activation of eosinophils, neutrophils, and monocytes. The submucosa becomes edematous, and cellular debris and fibrin form plugs within the bronchioles. Edema of the bronchiolar wall, accumulation of mucus and cellular debris, and possibly bronchospasm narrow or occlude many peripheral airways. Areas of atelectasis and uneven ventilation lead to ventilation-perfusion mismatch and hypoxemia.

The mechanics of breathing are disrupted by bronchiolitis. Airway narrowing causes obstruction of airflow that is worse with expiration. This leads to air trapping, hyperinflation, and an increase in FRC. Airway resistance and hyperinflation result in decreased lung compliance and increased work of breathing and may cause hypercapnia in severe cases.

CLINICAL MANIFESTATIONS. Symptoms usually begin with significant rhinorrhea followed by a tight cough over the next several days, along with systemic signs of decreased appetite, lethargy, and fever. Infants may have tachypnea, expiratory wheezing, cough, rhinorrhea, mild fever, varying degrees of respiratory distress, and abnormal auscultatory findings of the chest. In severe cases, chest radiographs reveal hyperexpanded lungs, patchy or peribronchial infiltrates, and atelectasis. Severely affected infants appear anxious and distressed because of dyspnea or hypoxemia. The thoracic cage is overexpanded, particularly in its anteroposterior diameter. The infant takes rapid, short breaths, and wheezing and rales are often heard on auscultation. With overexpansion of the lungs, the diaphragm is flattened, causing downward displacement of the liver and spleen. Abdominal distention results from air swallowing. Genetic tendencies have been noted that correlate RSV bronchiolitis with asthma.[115]

EVALUATION AND TREATMENT. Diagnosis of bronchiolitis is made by review of signs and symptoms (e.g., rhinitis, cough, wheezing, crackles, chest retractions and/or hyperinflation, tachypnea) and radiologic examination. Nasal washings/swabbings may be tested for specific viral agents, such as RSV. RSV swabs are positive in 70% of cases of bronchiolitis. In severe cases, chest imaging may be required for diagnosis and follow-up. Ultrasound is a reliable option without risk of irradiation.[116]

Treatment is determined by the severity of the disease and the age of the child.[117] Most cases are mild and are managed at home with supportive care. In more severe cases, supplemental oxygen and increased hydration are commonly used. Inhaled hypertonic saline has been found to decrease clinical severity and length of hospital stay.[67] Inhaled bronchodilators or bronchodilators and corticosteroids benefit infants with underlying lung disease or wheezing.[118-120] Mechanical ventilation is occasionally necessary and clinical indicators for CPAP are being evaluated.[121,122] Preventive treatment with RSV-specific monoclonal antibody, provided as a monthly injection through the RSV season, is recommended for high-risk infants less than 2 years old who meet specific criteria (e.g., bronchopulmonary dysplasia, recurrent aspiration pneumonitis, cystic fibrosis, or pulmonary malformation). Development of other immunotherapies and a RSV vaccine is in progress.[123,124]

Pneumonia

Pneumonia is infection and inflammation in the terminal airways and alveoli. **Community-acquired pneumonia (CAP)** is one of the most common global infections in the pediatric age group and the leading cause of morbidity and mortality in infants.[125] The incidence of viral and bacterial pneumonia varies according to age, time of year, and geographic location. Viral pneumonias are most common in young children and infections occur most often in winter to early spring. Mortality from respiratory viruses in developed countries is rare but morbidity is significant. In less developed countries, viral pneumonia results in nearly 5 million deaths annually in children younger than the age of 5.[126] Bacterial pneumonias are less common and occur across all age groups. Fungal and anaerobic pneumonias are rare in children.[127] Risk factors for developing CAP include age younger than 2 years, overcrowded living conditions, winter season, recent antibiotic treatment, attendance at daycare centers, and passive smoke exposure. Nutritional status, age, and underlying disease process influence morbidity and mortality related to CAP.

PATHOPHYSIOLOGY. Viral pneumonia is two to three times more likely in children than in adults. Viral-bacterial co-infections are common. The most common cause in infants and young children is respiratory syncytial virus (RSV). A number of other viruses are important, including parainfluenza, *Haemophilus influenzae* types A and B, coronaviruses, rhinoviruses, enteroviruses, human metapneumovirus (hMPV), bocavirus, and adenoviruses.

Viral infection is acquired by direct contact, droplet transmission, or aerosol transmission. Viral infection of the lower respiratory tract results in destruction of ciliated epithelium of the distal airway, with sloughing of cellular material. A mononuclear-predominant inflammatory response occurs first in the interstitium and may later involve the alveoli. Certain serotypes of adenovirus can cause necrotizing disease, sometimes leading to obliterative bronchiolitis and significant lung disability.

Early in the course of illness, it is often difficult to determine whether the pneumonia is of viral or bacterial origin. In bacterial pneumonia, the degree of elevated temperature, absolute neutrophil counts, and percent of bands are consistently higher than in those cases of viral etiology.[128] Diagnosis of a viral etiology requires laboratory confirmation (immunofluorescence tests). Development of safe agents to treat and prevent viral pneumonias continues to be a priority, as is development of more effective vaccines.[129]

Bacterial pneumonia beyond the neonatal period is most commonly the result of infection with streptococcal and staphylococcal microorganisms (Table 36-2). Pneumococcal *(S. pneumoniae)* pneumonia is the most common cause of bacterial pneumonia; other causative microorganisms include *Staphylococcus aureus* group A streptococci and atypical bacteria. Bacterial pneumonia most often presents acutely and with variable severity. Pneumococci have specific virulence factors (such as capsules) that increase their survival and proliferation while causing insult to the host.[130] A polyvariant pneumococcal conjugate vaccine (PCV7 or PCV13) is incorporated into routine childhood immunizations and appears to have lessened the incidence of pneumococcal pneumonia in children younger than 2 years of age.[131]

Bacterial pneumonia usually begins with aspiration of one's own nasopharyngeal bacteria into the trachea. A preceding viral infection sometimes sets the stage for bacterial infection by causing epithelial damage and reduced mucociliary clearance in the trachea and major bronchi. Colonization of the trachea then ensues, with the microorganism, host, and environment all playing a role in the development of pneumonia. Once in the alveolar region, bacteria encounter local host defenses, such as antibodies, complement, phagocytes, and cytokines, that prepare bacteria for ingestion by alveolar macrophages.

If these mechanisms fail, neutrophils will be recruited and an intense cytokine-mediated inflammation will ensue. Vascular engorgement, edema, and a fibrinopurulent exudate with tissue damage occur. Alveolar filling precludes gas exchange and, if extensive, can lead to respiratory failure. If sepsis occurs at the same time, shock and end-organ hypoperfusion may develop. Staphylococcal and group A streptococcal pneumonia can be particularly fulminant and necrotizing, with a high incidence of accompanying empyema, pneumatoceles, and sepsis. Empyema is increasingly associated with pneumococcal infections and antibiotic-resistant microorganisms.[132,133]

The clinical presentation of bacterial pneumonia, particularly pneumococcal, may include a preceding viral illness followed by fever with chills and rigors, shortness of breath, and an increasingly productive cough. Occasionally there is blood streaking of the sputum. Respiratory rate and oxygen saturation are important clinical indicators. Auscultation usually reveals such abnormalities as crackles or decreased breath sounds. Other less specific findings may include malaise, emesis, abdominal pain, and chest pain. Chest film will usually present with a lobar pattern in older children and adolescents but may appear patchier with a bronchopneumonic pattern in younger children.[134]

Atypical pneumonia *(Mycoplasma pneumoniae, Chlamydophila pneumoniae)* is the most common cause of CAP for school-age children (ages 5 and older) and young adults.[127] *Chlamydophila* pneumonia is clinically indistinguishable from and is typically grouped with *Mycoplasma* as "atypical pneumonia." Transmission is from person-to-person with a 2- to 3-week incubation period.

Mycoplasma is known to cause a wide spectrum of disease and has more extensive complications than previously recognized. Studies reveal that macrolide-resistant *Mycoplasma pneumoniae* is seen increasingly in infants and younger children.[135,136] Children experiencing recurrent respiratory tract

TABLE 36-2 **COMMON TYPES OF PNEUMONIA IN CHILDREN**

TYPE	CAUSAL AGENT	AGE	ONSET	SIGNS/SYMPTOMS	PATHOPHYSIOLOGY
Viral pneumonia	Respiratory syncytial virus (RSV), influenza (A and B), adenovirus, parainfluenza, human metapneumovirus (hMPV)	Infants for RSV All ages for others	Acute or gradual, winter and early spring	Mild to high fever, cough, rhinorrhea, malaise, rales, rhonchi, or wheezing; variable radiographic pattern	Edema, increased mucus, and interstitial pneumonia
Pneumococcal pneumonia	Pneumococci *(Streptococcus pneumoniae)*	1-4 yr	Acute, follows an upper respiratory tract infection, winter and early spring	High fever, productive cough, pleuritic pain, increased respiratory rate, decreased breath sounds in area of consolidation; lobar pattern or "round pneumonia" on radiograph	Inflammation of bronchial mucosa, alveolar exudate *Early:* red hepatization with WBCs, RBCs, and fibrin consolidation *Late:* gray hepatization with fibrin and neutrophils in alveoli *Resolution:* many phagocytic macrophages
Staphylococcal pneumonia	*Staphylococcus aureus* Methicillin-resistant *Staphylococcus aureus* (MRSA)	1 wk-2 yr	Acute, winter months	High fever, cough, respiratory distress, toxic appearance, sepsis, empyema, pneumatoceles are common; multilobar consolidation	Necrotizing patterns may occur in severe cases
Streptococcal pneumonia	Group A streptococci	All ages	Acute, any season	High fever, chills, respiratory distress, sepsis or shock; empyema, pneumatoceles	Tracheobronchitis, interstitial pneumonia with ulcers, exudate edema, and localized hemorrhage
Mycoplasma and *Chlamydophila pneumonia*	*M. pneumoniae* *C. pneumoniae*	School age and adolescents	Gradual	Low-grade fever; cough	Inflammation of bronchi with lymphocyte and chlamydia neutrophil recruitment

RBCs, Red blood cells; *WBCs,* white blood cells.

infections often have been found to be infected with atypical bacteria.

Mycoplasma microorganisms lack cell walls but have a limiting membrane and a specialized tip for attaching to ciliated respiratory epithelial cells. Local sloughing of cells occurs. Peribronchial lymphocytic infiltration develops, along with neutrophil recruitment to the airway lumen. The pattern resembles bronchitis or bronchopneumonia.

Onset of symptoms is usually gradual, resembling a typical upper respiratory tract infection with low-grade fever and prominent cough. There may be accompanying sore throat, myalgia, and headache. Cases are not usually clinically severe, and full recovery should be expected without complications. When complications do occur, they can include bronchopneumonia, parapneumonic effusions, and necrotizing pneumonitis.[137]

EVALUATION AND TREATMENT. Diagnosis of pneumonia is based on clinical, laboratory, and chest radiograph findings. Guidelines have been developed to improve and aid assessment and management of pediatric pneumonia.[138] Identifying etiologic pathogens can be very difficult in children, especially because there is often overlap between bacterial and viral pathogens. Biomarkers facilitate more rapid diagnosis and procalcitonin is most specific to bacterial infection and can guide antibiotic therapy. The highly sensitive C-reactive protein (hs-CRP) is less specific and elevated in both viral and bacterial infections.[139] Other laboratory tests that may be helpful include a white cell–granulocyte count or erythrocyte sedimentation rate (ESR) but do not indicate a specific etiology. Several microbiologic tests are available including polymerase chain reaction (PCR) and nucleic acid amplification tests (NAATs). On chest radiography, a bacterial pneumonia initially produces an alveolar infiltrate and later causes a segmental or lobar disease. A viral infection is more likely to be associated with an interstitial pattern.

Most pneumonias may be treated on an outpatient basis; however, some children require oxygen supplementation and, occasionally, assisted ventilation. This is particularly true with infants who have a viral interstitial pneumonia, such as RSV. In addition, adequate hydration, nutrition, and supportive pulmonary therapy are required to reduce the duration and severity of illness. Many hospitalized infants are markedly tachypneic and unable to coordinate their breathing with swallowing such that they may require enteral feeding. Aspiration is always a risk with infants in respiratory distress.

Appropriate antibiotic administration, whether oral or intravenous (IV), for bacterial pneumonias is dependent on age and severity assessment. Hospitalized children require antibiotic therapy.[140] Local patterns of drug resistance must be considered.[140] Both pneumococcal and mycoplasma pneumonia present some unique treatment obstacles and often need a multifaceted approach to care, including vaccine antigens, antibiotic combinations, and immunoadjuvant therapies.[141] Children should be vaccinated against influenza and pneumococcus.[142]

Aspiration Pneumonitis

Aspiration pneumonitis is caused by a foreign substance, such as food, meconium, secretions (saliva or gastric secretions), or environmental compounds entering the lung and causing inflammation of lung tissue. The aspiration of meconium from amniotic fluid can occur at birth. Meconium contains bile salts from the fetal intestinal tract that cause inflammation. Neurologically compromised children or children with chronic lung disease may have chronic pulmonary aspiration (CPA) because of failure of protective reflexes. This can cause progressive lung disease, bronchiectasis, and respiratory failure and is the leading cause of death in children who are neurologically compromised.[143,144] Children undergoing sedation or anesthesia also may aspirate oral secretions contaminated with anaerobic bacteria or stomach contents, which may be acidic.

The severity of lung injury after an acute aspiration incident is determined by the volume of material aspirated, the pH of the aspirated material, and the presence of pathogenic bacteria. Very low pH or very high pH causes a significant inflammatory response. With hydrocarbon ingestions, lung injury is determined by the volatility and viscosity of the aspirated substance. A low-viscosity substance, such as gasoline or lighter fluid, is the most toxic; high-viscosity hydrocarbons, such as petroleum jelly or mineral oil, are much less likely to cause pneumonitis. Treatment for aspiration pneumonitis depends on the material aspirated but generally includes broad-spectrum antibiotic therapy. Children with CPA and a large amount of upper respiratory tract secretions may benefit from salivary gland injection with botulinum toxin A (BTX-A) to suppress secretion.[145]

Bronchiolitis Obliterans

Bronchiolitis obliterans (BO) is fibrotic obstruction of the respiratory bronchioles and alveolar ducts secondary to intense inflammation. It is relatively rare in children. Two types are noted in the literature—proliferative and constrictive—with the latter being the more common form. Most cases of BO in children are associated with viral pulmonary infections, such as adenovirus (most common), influenza, pertussis (whooping cough), measles, parainfluenza, RSV, human immunodeficiency virus (HIV), or *M. pneumoniae*. BO may occur after allograft transplantation (lung, heart-lung, and bone marrow) as a manifestation of graft-versus-host disease. It also is associated with collagen vascular disease, toxic fume inhalation, chronic hypersensitivity pneumonitis, Crohn disease, and Stevens-Johnson syndrome.[146,147] Initially, cough, respiratory distress, and cyanosis occur, followed by a brief period of improvement. The progression of disease is then reflected by tachypnea, sputum production, increased anterior/posterior diameter, crackles, wheezing, and hypoxemia.[148]

There is no specific treatment for BO and, because it is so rare, there have been no randomized clinical trials. Therapeutic options include inhaled corticosteroids, bronchodilators, antibiotics, and oxygen supplementation. Mechanical ventilation may contribute to the progression of the disease. Use of antiviral agents may be warranted in managing those with viral infection. For transplant recipients, augmentation of immunosuppressive therapies and treatment with anti-inflammatory agents are showing promise in reducing airway inflammation, thus improving pulmonary function.[149] Clinical progression can be quite variable depending on the predisposing condition. Some children experience partial recovery, whereas others follow a course of steady decline in lung function. Lung transplantation may be considered.[147]

Asthma

Asthma is a chronic inflammatory disease characterized by sensitization to allergens, bronchial hyperreactivity, and reversible airway obstruction. It is the most prevalent chronic disease in childhood, affecting about 10% of U.S. children between 5 and 17 years of age, with boys more often affected than girls. Asthma prevalence is increasing, especially among non-Hispanic blacks,[150] obese children,[151] and children from urban and low-income populations.[152] The overall asthma-related death rate is decreasing[153] and asthma-related deaths almost always occur outside the hospital setting.

The severity and persistence of asthma are influenced by age at disease onset, genetics, behavior, atopy, air pollution, level of allergen exposure, environmental tobacco smoke, gastroesophageal reflux, and respiratory tract infections.[154] Additional confounding variables that affect disparity in asthma morbidity and therapy are social stress in the home (e.g., violence and depressed housing conditions), lack of health insurance, poor access to asthma specialists, inappropriate utilization of health-care resources, and inadequate medical care.[153,155]

The wide spectrum of clinical disease in asthma and differential responses to standard treatment reflects a complex interaction between environmental factors and genetic susceptibility. *Environmental factors* include early exposure to allergens (e.g., air pollution, dust mites, cockroach antigen, cat exposure, tobacco smoke, and dietary factors); infections, particularly viral respiratory tract infections (e.g., rhinovirus and RSV); and stress.[156,157] Vitamin D insufficiency may be a risk factor for wheezing in children since vitamin D suppresses Th2-mediated allergic disease.[158] Environmental exposures interact with an individual's genetic vulnerabilities to induce the onset of clinical asthma and epigenetic mechanisms are being studied.[154,159,159a]

The *genetics of asthma* are complex. Genetic studies have led to the identification of many candidate genes or chromosomal regions that are associated with asthma.[160-163] Included in the long list of asthma-associated genes are those that code for increased levels of immune and inflammatory mediators (e.g., IL-4, IL-5, IL-13, IgE, and leukotrienes), adrenergic receptors, nitric oxide, and transmembrane proteins in the endoplasmic reticulum.[163,164] In addition, specific gene expression may impart associated phenotypes, such as bronchial hyperresponsiveness (BHR), inflammation, sensitization to allergens, airway fibroblasts, airway remodeling, and responsiveness to asthma therapies.[165] Linking specific genes to specific asthma phenotypes is leading to targeted therapies and personalized approaches to asthma treatment (see What's New? Asthma Phenotypes).

WHAT'S NEW?

Asthma Phenotypes

The severity and clinical course of asthma in children can vary from mild and transient to severe and lifelong. Research is now emerging that suggests genetically influenced differences in inflammatory and immune mechanisms may explain much of this variability. The majority of asthmatic children have the well-described allergic (type I hypersensitivity) form of asthma that is characterized by high levels of Th2 cytokines, IgE synthesis, and activation of eosinophils (therefore also called *eosinophilic asthma*), resulting in episodic bronchospasm that is responsive to inhaled bronchodilators and anti-inflammatory medications. Other mechanisms have been implicated in children whose asthma phenotype is characterized by more severe symptoms and relative unresponsiveness to treatment with inhaled steroids. One of these mechanisms is called *neutrophilic asthma* in which Th1 cytokines and activation of large numbers of polymorphonucleocytes appear to dominate lung injury. Neutrophilic asthma especially involves the cytokines TNF-α, interferon-gamma (IFN-γ), IL-17, and IL-27. Other genotypic changes can lead to diverse asthma phenotypes. For example, variability in the response to inhaled glucocorticoids may be related to the role of IL-13. Another example involves a specific polymorphism in the gene for the β-adrenergic receptor that is prevalent in black children and is associated with poor response to β-adrenergic inhaled medication. Variability of response to leukotriene receptor 1 antagonist is related to variation in leukotriene pathway candidate genes. Finally, genetic factors also have been identified that are important to the development of airway remodeling. Increased understanding of these asthma phenotypes is leading to new therapies that may provide significant improvements in personalized management of severe and drug-resistant asthma.

Data from Carolan BJ, Sutherland ER: *J Allergy Clin Immunol* 131(3):627-634, 2013; Corren J et al: *N Engl J Med* 365:1088–1098, 2011; Cowan K, Guilbert TW: *Curr Opin Pediatr* 24:344–351, 2012; Ducharme FM, Krajinovic M: *Pediatr Resp Rev* 12:170–176, 2011; Kotani H et al: *J Clin Pharm Ther* 37(1):112–116, 2012; Siroux V, Garcia-Aymerich J: *Curr Opin Allergy Clin Immunol* 11:393–399, 2012; Thomson NC, Patel M, Smith AD: *Biologics* 6:329–335, 2012; Wenzel S: *Nat Med* 18:716–725, 2012.

One hypothesis for the high prevalence of asthma in westernized cultures is called the "hygiene hypothesis." Allergen exposure shifts the immune system toward Th2-predominant phenotype with resultant increase in the production of antibodies, including IgE. This effect is normally balanced by exposure to numerous siblings, daycare, farming, endotoxin, and certain microorganisms (e.g., *Toxoplasma gondii*, hepatitis A virus, and *Helicobacter pylori*). It is proposed that children exposed to a highly hygienic environment and who receive vaccinations to prevent infections lack adequate exposure to common pathogens and therefore do not achieve a proper balance of their immune systems.[166,167] Asthma develops because the Th2 response (in which CD4 T-helper [Th] cells produce specific cytokines, such as IL-4, IL-5, and IL-13) promotes an atopic/allergic inflammatory response in the airways.[164] IL-4 and IL-13 are particularly important for B-cell switching to favor IgE production, and IL-5 is crucial for local differentiation and enhanced survival of eosinophils within the airways. This theory about the origins of asthma is consistent with many of the epidemiologic and pathophysiologic features of childhood asthma but is not yet proved.[168]

PATHOPHYSIOLOGY. The pathophysiology of asthma in children is similar to that for adults and is described in Chapter 35 (p. 1264). Asthma is initiated by a type I hypersensitivity reaction primarily mediated by IgE (see Figures 35-10, 35-11, and 35-12, pp. 1264-1265). As in adults, inflammation, bronchospasm, and mucus production in the airways lead to ventilation and perfusion mismatch with hypoxemia and expiratory airway obstruction with air trapping and increased work of breathing. In young children, airway obstruction can be more severe because of the smaller diameter of their airways.

CLINICAL MANIFESTATIONS. In a typical acute asthma attack in children, the major complaints are coughing, wheezing, and shortness of breath. About 70% to 80% of acute wheezing episodes are associated with viral respiratory tract infections. As a result, there may be signs of a preceding upper respiratory tract infection, such as rhinorrhea, or low-grade fever. In infants and toddlers younger than 2 years old, the most common of these is RSV.[169] In older children and adults, the major viral trigger is rhinovirus.[170]

There is expiratory wheezing that is often described as high pitched and musical, along with prolongation of the expiratory phase of the respiratory cycle. Breath sounds may become faint when air movement is poor. Sometimes hyperinflation (barrel chest) is visible. Respiratory and heart rates are elevated. Nasal flaring and accessory muscle use are evident, with retractions in the substernal, subcostal, intercostal, suprasternal, or sternocleidomastoid areas. Infants may appear to be "head bobbing" because of sternocleidomastoid muscle use. Pulsus paradoxus (decrease in systolic blood pressure of more than 10 mmHg during inspiration) may be present. The child may appear anxious or diaphoretic, important signs of respiratory compromise. The child may speak in clipped sentences or not at all because of dyspnea.

Findings in chronic asthma may include hyperinflation of the thorax (barrel chest) or pectus excavatum. Clubbing should not be seen in those with asthma and, if present, should trigger evaluation for other conditions, such as cystic fibrosis. Exercise intolerance may indicate underlying asthma.

EVALUATION AND TREATMENT. Asthma is often underdiagnosed and untreated, especially in preschool-age children because asthma symptoms overlap with other respiratory illness, such as bronchitis or upper respiratory tract infections. Diagnosis is based on symptom patterns (episodes of wheezing), presence of risk factors, and therapeutic responses. The major historical and physical factors that contribute to the diagnosis of asthma in children are parental history of asthma, physician-diagnosed atopic dermatitis, evidence of sensitization to aeroallergens, increased IgE and eosinophil levels, and reversible airflow obstruction on lung function.[171]

The modified asthma predictive index (API) can be used to help with asthma diagnosis and is recommended by the National Institutes of Health (NIH) guidelines.[171] Many children with less severe asthma outgrow the disease by adulthood.[172]

Confirmation of the diagnosis of asthma relies on pulmonary function testing using spirometry, which can be accomplished only after the child is 5 to 6 years of age. Characteristic abnormalities of spirometry would be reduced expiratory flow rates that are reversible in response to an inhaled bronchodilator. For younger children, an empirical trial of asthma medications is commonly initiated.

The goal of asthma therapy is to achieve long-term control by reduction in impairment and risk.[154] Management of asthma medications in children is often difficult because fluctuations in severity of symptoms is common. Care providers must periodically assess asthma control in children to decide if a "step up" (increase) or "step down" (decrease) is indicated in their asthma therapy. Algorithms can help assess asthma control and offer information about how to adjust therapy accordingly. Before therapy is increased, care providers need to assess medication administration techniques, environmental controls, comorbidities, and educational needs. For a reduction in therapy, the child's asthma should be well controlled for a minimum of 3 months.[154] The pharmacologic treatment of asthma in children is essentially the same as that for adults and is initiated in a stepwise sequence based on asthma severity and response to treatment (see Chapter 35).

Acute Lung Injury/Acute Respiratory Distress Syndrome

Acute lung injury (ALI)/acute respiratory distress syndrome (ARDS) occurs in children of all ages. ALI precedes the development of ARDS and can result either from a direct or indirect injury, such as pneumonia, aspiration, near-drowning, and smoke inhalation, or from a systemic insult, such as sepsis, multiple trauma, or burns. ARDS is characterized by progressive respiratory distress, severe hypoxemia refractory to treatment with supplemental oxygen, decreased pulmonary compliance, bilateral infiltrates on chest x-ray, and no evidence of heart failure.[173]

The overall mortality in children is less than that experienced by the adult population but can be as high as 40%, depending on age and associated conditions and complications.[174] Children younger than 5 years appear to have diminished mortality compared with those older than 5 years of age. Children with underlying disease processes, such as Down syndrome[175] or systemic lupus erythematosus, and those who have undergone lung transplantation have decreased survival.

PATHOPHYSIOLOGY. The pathophysiology of ARDS in children is the same as that described for adults in Chapter 35 (see p. 1261 and Figure 35-8).

CLINICAL MANIFESTATIONS. ARDS develops acutely after the initial insult, usually within 24 hours (although occasionally it is delayed up to a few days). There is progressive respiratory distress and severe hypoxemia with poor response to oxygen supplementation. Initially, hyperventilation occurs, but CO_2 retention may ultimately develop because of inadequate functional air space, atelectasis, decreased pulmonary compliance, and respiratory muscle fatigue. Severity of the clinical course is modified by the cause of lung injury, comorbid factors (such as the presence of sepsis or multisystem organ failure), and the development of complications (such as nosocomial pneumonia). Some children who recover have residual pulmonary abnormalities.

EVALUATION AND TREATMENT. ARDS in older children and adolescents is similar to that in adults. However, infants have more compliant chest walls, lower hematocrit levels, higher baseline airway resistance, and lower functional residual capacity. The maturing lung may be at greater risk for ventilator-induced lung injury.[176,177] These factors have implications for management strategies that are different than those for older children and adolescents. There are few randomized controlled trials that have been completed to guide clinical management of ALI/ARDS in infants and very young children.

Treatment of ARDS remains supportive in nature and definitive studies related to infants and children are limited.[176,177] The goals of therapy are to preserve and restore oxygen delivery, minimize acute lung injury, and decrease morbidity and mortality by avoiding iatrogenic pulmonary complications. Most individuals with ARDS require oxygen administration with mechanical ventilation and relatively high levels of positive end-expiratory pressure to promote alveolar recruitment, stabilization, and redistribution of alveolar edema fluid into the interstitium. Lung-protective ventilation strategies may be used for ARDS, such as low tidal volumes, positive end-expiratory pressure (PEEP) ventilation, prone positioning, inverse inspiratory/expiratory ratio, high-frequency oscillatory ventilation, and airway pressure release ventilation.[178-180] Use of corticosteroids in children with ARDS is controversial and remains at the discretion of the clinician. There have been no randomized clinical trials regarding this treatment. Surfactant therapy appears to improve oxygenation and increase survival time in children 1 week to 21 years of age, particularly in cases of direct lung injury.[174,181] Extracorporeal membrane oxygenation (ECMO) has improved survival in some centers.[182,183]

Cystic Fibrosis

Cystic fibrosis (CF) is an autosomal recessive inherited disorder that is associated with defective epithelial chloride ion transport. The CF gene is located on chromosome 7. There are more than 1900 known mutations of this gene[184] divided into 6 classes with varying severity of disease expression. Classes 1 through 3 are associated with more severe disease and classes 4 through 6 with milder pulmonary disease (generally pancreatic sufficient). Death rates correlate respectively with the classes noted in the previous sentence.[185] CF affects primarily whites (approximately 1 in 3200) and is one of the most common lethal genetic diseases in this ethnic group. Approximately 30,000 individuals in the United States and 70,000 worldwide manifest the disease. The incidence in blacks is 1:15,000 and in Asian Americans is 1:31,000.[186] Estimated symptomless carrier frequency is higher, affecting 10 million or 1 in 29 whites in the United States. Approximately 1000 new cases of CF are diagnosed each year, and the median age at diagnosis is 6 months; 75% of cases are diagnosed by 1 year of age. Approximately 10% of cases are not diagnosed until after age 10; however, these cases usually have milder symptoms. The median age of survival in the United States is 37 years of age (2008 data).[186]

PATHOPHYSIOLOGY. CF is characterized by abnormal secretions that cause obstructive problems within the respiratory, digestive, and reproductive tracts. However, research suggests that there may be additional CF-associated primary defects, such as an intrinsic proinflammatory state and abnormal local immune defenses in the lungs. The *cystic fibrosis transmembrane conductance regulator (CFTCR) gene* mutation results in the abnormal expression of **cystic fibrosis transmembrane conductance regulator (CFTCR) protein,** which is a cyclic adenosine monophosphate (cAMP)–activated chloride channel present on the surface of many types of epithelial cells, including those lining airways, bile ducts, the pancreas, sweat ducts, and the vas deferens. Despite knowing that chloride transport is a fundamental abnormality, the exact disease mechanisms in CF have still not been clearly defined at the cellular and end-organ levels.[187]

Although CF is a multiorgan disease, the lungs are the most critical site of involvement, and respiratory failure is almost always the cause of death. The typical features of CF lung disease are mucus plugging, chronic inflammation, and infection of the small airways.[188] The disease process causes progressive bronchiectasis that becomes widespread. Parenchymal involvement occurs much later and includes microabscess formation, patchy consolidation and pneumonia, peribronchial fibrosis, and cyst formation (Figure 36-14). The pathophysiology for these changes is outlined in Figure 36-15. Airway obstruction and weakening of the airway wall can lead to the development of peripheral bullae, which may rupture and cause pneumothorax. Hemoptysis, sometimes life threatening, may occur because of erosion of enlarged bronchial arteries that develop in response to the inflammation associated with bronchiectasis. Over a long period of time, pulmonary vascular remodeling occurs because of localized hypoxia and arteriolar vasoconstriction; pulmonary hypertension and cor pulmonale may develop with end-stage disease.

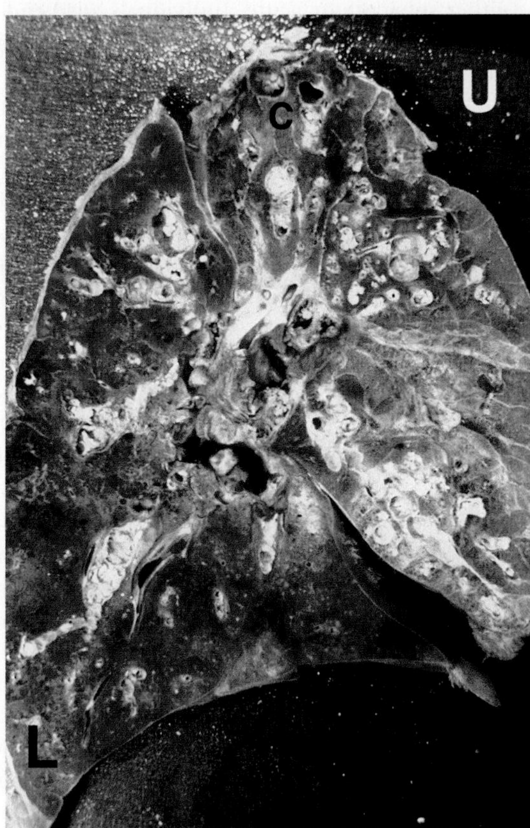

FIGURE 36-14 Pathology of the Lung in End-Stage Cystic Fibrosis. Key features are widespread mucous impaction of airways and bronchiectasis (especially in upper lobe, *U*), with hemorrhagic pneumonia in the lower lobe *(L)*. Small cysts *(C)* are present at the apex of the lung. (From Kleinerman J, Vauthy P: *Pathology of the lung in cystic fibrosis,* Atlanta, 1976, Cystic Fibrosis Foundation.)

The mucus plugging seen in CF probably results from the combination of increased production of mucus, altered physicochemical properties of the mucus, and reduced mucociliary clearance.[189] Mucus-secreting airway cells (goblet cells and submucosal glands) are increased in number and size. It has been postulated that the CFTCR protein mutation results in dysregulation of the airway epithelial sodium channel (ENaC), although this relationship has recently been called into question.[190] What is clear is that abnormal chloride excretion and exaggerated sodium absorption with depletion of the airway surface liquid volume result in dehydration of airway mucus.[191] This facilitates adherence of mucus to the epithelium, subsequent impairment of ciliary mobility, and retention of bacteria that can then form biofilms. Finally, after secretion, CF mucus becomes even more viscous because of deoxyribonucleic acid (DNA) and filamentous (F) actin released from the high number of degraded neutrophils present in CF airways.

There are abnormal cytokine profiles in CF airway fluids, including deficient levels of IL-10 and excessive amounts of IL-1, IL-8, and TNF-α, all changes conducive to promoting inflammation. Neutrophils are present in great excess in CF airways and play a critical role in long-term damage[192] in large measure because of their release of damaging oxidants,

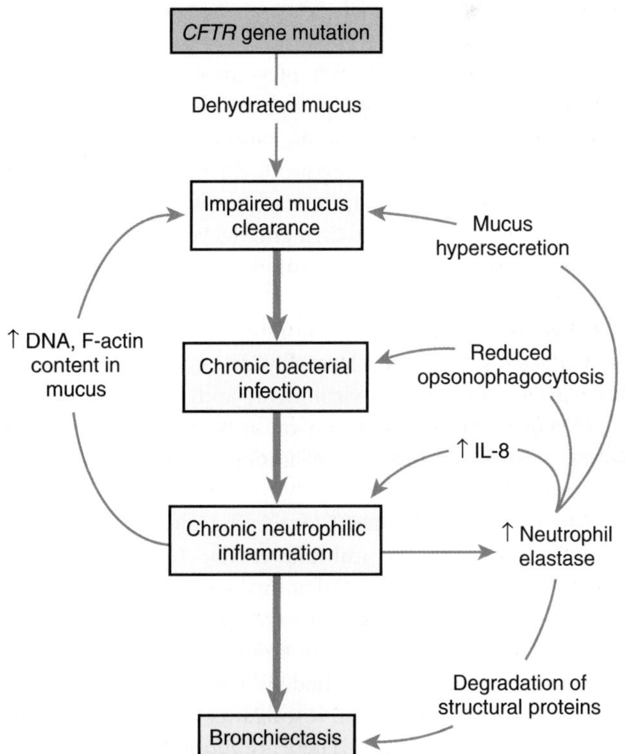

FIGURE 36-15 Pathogenesis of Cystic Fibrosis Lung Disease. *CFTR,* Cystic fibrosis transmembrane conductance regulator; *IL-8,* interleukin-8.

such as myeloperoxidase[193] and proteases, in massive amounts that overwhelm local antiprotease defenses. The mutant CFTR channel does not transport antioxidants to counteract neutrophil-associated oxidative stress.[194] One protease in particular, *neutrophil elastase,* has the following detrimental effects: (1) direct damage to lung structural proteins, such as elastin; (2) induction of airway cells to produce IL-8, a strong attractant for neutrophils and thus a means for augmenting a local "vicious cycle" of inflammation; (3) destruction of IgG and complement components important for opsonization and phagocytosis of pathogens; and (4) direct stimulation of mucus secretion by mucus-producing cells.

The majority of children with CF have chronic endobronchial infection. It is likely that local factors in the CF airway microenvironment favor bacterial colonization because no systemic immune defect has been found. Several bacteria colonize the CF lung including *Staphylococcus aureus* and *Burkholderia cepacia.*[195] However, *Pseudomonas aeruginosa* ultimately colonizes airways in 75% of children with CF. Infecting colonies of *Pseudomonas* adopt a mucoid phenotype and organize themselves into adherent biofilms, making it difficult for antibiotics and local defenses to reach them.[196] Their biofilm resists beta-lactam antibiotics and their rapid mutation makes them antibiotic resistant.[197] Persistence of infection incites chronic local inflammation, airway damage, bronchiectasis, microabscess formation, and foci of hemorrhagic pneumonia. There is progressive damage to the normal architecture of the lung with decline in pulmonary function.[198,199]

CLINICAL MANIFESTATIONS. The most common manifestations are respiratory and gastrointestinal (also see Chapter 42). Respiratory symptoms include persistent cough or wheeze, sputum production, and recurrent or severe pneumonia. More subtle respiratory tract presentations of CF include chronic sinusitis and nasal polyps. With appropriate treatment, cough, sputum production, and exercise limitation do not usually reach debilitating levels during childhood. Digital clubbing may appear quite early even in the absence of significant pulmonary impairment. Development of barrel chest or persistent crackles occurs much later in the course of the disease.

The overall severity of CF lung disease is highly variable. Even affected siblings may have disparate courses despite identical *CFTR* mutations, environment, and treatment strategy. We now know that some genetic variants significantly influence disease progression and survival among children with the same mutations.[200,201]

EVALUATION AND TREATMENT. Screening algorithms for cystic fibrosis include the immunoreactive trypsinogen (IRT) blood test, which is performed at birth (may be repeated) and is elevated in CF. This test can have false positives and negatives. Genotyping for *CFTR* mutations also is available as a supplemental diagnostic method.[202] The sweat test is a standard method of diagnosis and reveals sweat chloride concentration in excess of 60 mEq/L. There are more than 1900 specific mutations, but most standard laboratory panels include fewer than 100 mutations.[186] Newborn screening for CF is universal in the United States.[203] Genetic counseling of CF gene carriers is important so they understand risk assessment in relation to disease.[204]

Treatment is primarily focused on pulmonary health and nutrition. Because the pulmonary decline in CF is slow and insidious, and because of the early onset of chronic inflammation and infection, treatment strategies begin immediately at diagnosis and are modified over time as disease progresses. Pulmonary therapies include techniques to promote mucus clearance, such as chest physical therapy and related equipment (such as the high-frequency chest wall oscillation vest) and an assortment of handheld positive expiratory pressure (PEP) devices. Aerosol therapy includes antibiotics, bronchodilators, and nebulized deoxyribonuclease (DNase). DNase acts to liquefy mucus and may even have anti-inflammatory effects.[205,206]

Antibiotic practices vary, with prophylactic and treatment strategies being used. Increasing emphasis has been placed on delaying and controlling microbe colonization, particularly *Pseudomonas,* such as the maintenance use of inhaled antibiotics.[207] Inhaled hypertonic saline also has proven beneficial to improve airway surface water, thus improving mucus viscosity and airway clearance.[208] Azithromycin, ibuprofen, and corticosteroids can reduce airway inflammation and improve lung function.[209] Intravenous antibiotics are used to treat major exacerbations of pulmonary infection, which may be either subacute or acute. Individuals with end-stage lung disease may consider double lung transplant as a life-lengthening measure.[210]

Nutritional problems are extremely common in CF and poor nutrition is correlated with worse outcomes including progression of lung disease; onset of additional complications, such as decreased bone mineral density; and growth failure.[211,212] Elements of aggressive nutritional support include meticulous monitoring of growth parameters, controlling fat malabsorption, ensuring adequate caloric intake, and keeping overall health stable. Approximately 90% of children with CF have pancreatic insufficiency. This is the result of abnormal ion transport causing decreased fluid and bicarbonate secretion from the pancreatic acinar cells, which leads to thickened secretions plugging the smaller pancreatic ducts, and eventual autodigestion or atrophy of the acinar cells. Therefore, patients must take exogenous pancreatic enzymes with meals and snacks in order to absorb nutrients and control malabsorptive symptoms. Fat-soluble vitamins (A, D, E, and K) must be supplemented.[213] Caloric needs are high, especially with advancing lung disease, and high-calorie supplements or even gastrostomy feeding may be warranted (see Nutrition & Disease: Cystic Fibrosis [CF]).

Future treatments for CF in trial phases are aimed at improving inhaled antibiotic therapy, developing a vaccine against *Pseudomonas,* and incorporating growth hormone in the treatment regimen. Newer approaches to gene therapy are being developed, including mutation-specific diagnosis and treatment.[214]

There is a growing contingent of adults with CF living into their forties and fifties. Care for these individuals shifts away

NUTRITION & DISEASE

Cystic Fibrosis (CF)

Chronic inflammation, pancreatic enzyme deficiency, and undernutrition contribute to growth failure and poor clinical outcomes in CF. Energy needs to meet normal growth and weight gain in CF require a diet composed of 35% to 40% of calories from fat. Breast-feeding for the first 4 to 6 months has shown to be protective for the infant with CF, and then supplemental formula fortified with additional fat increases energy content. Oral pancreatic enzyme replacement is important in maintaining adequate nutritional status, particularly for fat absorption. The Food and Drug Administration now requires approval for the marketing of these products. Selection of dose and preparations is based on weight gain and individual response. High doses of lipase can be associated with fibrosing colonopathy and new products are being tested in clinical trials. Fecal pancreatic elastase-1 is a common diagnostic test for evaluating pancreatic insufficiency. Yearly monitoring of fat-soluble vitamins (A, D, E, and K) is recommended with supplementation as needed. Vitamin D supplements are needed to maintain serum concentrations at 30 ng/ml. Current recommendations are to follow the Cystic Fibrosis Foundation nutrition care guidelines available at www.cff.org/treatments/CFCareGuidelines/Nutrition/. The management of CF-related diabetes mellitus is a particular challenge and guidelines have been published by the American Diabetes Association. Nutritional counseling is a necessary component of care for all individuals with CF.

Data from Kalnins D, Wilschanski M: *Drug Des Dev Ther* 6:151–161, 2012; Moran A et al: *Diabetes Care* 33(12):2697–2708, 2010; Nakajima K et al: *Core Evid* 7:77–91, 2012; Tangpricha V et al: *J Clin Endocrinol Metab* 97(4):1082–1093, 2012; Wier HA, Kuhn RJ: *Curr Opin Pediatr* 23(5):541–544, 2011.

from a pediatric focus because their care needs are unique and often extremely complex.[215] Challenges noted in this specialty area are pregnancy and details about balancing disease management and adult life issues.[216]

SUDDEN INFANT DEATH SYNDROME

Sudden infant death syndrome (SIDS) remains a disease of unknown cause and is the most common cause of unexplained infant death in Western countries.[217,218] It is defined as "sudden death of an infant under 1 year of age which remains unexplained after a thorough case investigation, including performance of a complete autopsy, examination of the death scene, and review of the clinical history."[217]

The incidence of SIDS is low during the first month of life but sharply increases in the second month of life, peaks at 2 to 4 months of age, and is unusual after 6 months of age. The incidence of SIDS in the United States is 0.54 per 1000 live births.[219] It is more common in male infants (60%) than female (40%) infants and among American Indian/Alaskan Natives and blacks.[220] It almost always occurs during nighttime sleep, when infants are least likely to be observed. A seasonal variation has been noted, with higher frequencies during the winter months. This has been related to a higher rate of respiratory tract infection during those months, and such infections are often reported to have preceded the death.

Clinical risk groups include babies who were preterm or low birth weight, multiple births, and siblings of prior SIDS victims (fourfold to sixfold increased risk). SIDS is more prevalent among infants of low or adverse socioeconomic status and occurs more frequently when family size is larger.[221] Nevertheless, about 75% of all SIDS victims have no known predisposing clinical risk factor. Maternal factors that predict increased SIDS risk are maternal smoking, young maternal age (younger than 20 years), unmarried mother, less prenatal care, poverty, and illicit drug use or binge-drinking.[222] Avoidable risk factors that relate to the baby's sleeping situation are prone positioning (and to a lesser extent, side sleeping), sleeping on soft bedding, overheating (environmental or overwrapping), and bed sharing with an adult (particularly one who smokes).[223] Epidemiologic studies have shown that SIDS rates decreased where massive public campaigns warned against prone sleeping for infants (e.g., the Back-to-Sleep campaign).[224]

The etiology of SIDS remains unknown, but probably involves a combination of predisposing factors including a vulnerable infant, environmental stressors, a critical developmental period for homeostatic control, and altered cardiorespiratory, circulatory, and arousal characteristics.[225,226] There has been long-standing interest in hypotheses involving impaired autonomic regulation and failure of cardiovascular, ventilatory, and arousal responses (particularly those regulated by the hypoglossal nucleus [HGN]) to hypoxemia or hypercarbia.[227] Alternative theories involve airway obstruction events, such as control of tongue movements related to inspiratory activity; increased vagal tone; sudden intrapulmonary shunting because of abnormalities of surfactant or pulmonary vessels; or exaggerated inflammation, eosinophil degranulation, and massive cytokine release causing pulmonary edema in response to either bacterial pathogens from the nasopharynx or viral respiratory tract infections.[228,229]

Finally, there is growing evidence that genetic factors may predispose certain individuals to SIDS. The most important risk factor genes include those involved in the regulation of the immune system, cardiac function, and the serotonergic network related to brainstem function.[230,231] It is estimated that 10% to 20% of SIDS cases may be caused by genetic variation in either ion channel or ion channel–associated proteins associated with primary electrical heart disease (e.g., long-QT and short-QT syndrome).[232]

Currently, the best strategy to reduce SIDS is avoidance of all the controllable risk factors. Recommendations include supine positioning; use of a firm sleep surface; room-sharing without bed-sharing; routine immunization; consideration of a pacifier; and avoidance of soft bedding, overheating, and exposure to tobacco smoke, alcohol, and illicit drugs.[233] Breast-feeding has been identified as a specific risk reduction measure.[234] Parents of infants with clinical risk should be taught cardiopulmonary resuscitation as a precaution. Home monitoring has not been proven to decrease the incidence of SIDS and more research is needed.[235] Some at-risk infants may warrant cardiorespiratory monitoring after careful consideration of the individual situation.

SUMMARY REVIEW

Structure and Function

1. The airways of infants and children are narrower than those of adults, thus making them more prone to obstruction.
2. Infants and young children continue to form new alveoli for several years after birth.
3. Surfactant production is an important marker of developmental maturity of the fetal lung and is secreted into the airways by 30 weeks of gestation.
4. The immature chest wall is soft and compliant, contributing to inefficient mechanisms of breathing.
5. Children have greater oxygen consumption than adults per unit of body weight.
6. Immune mechanisms are not fully developed at birth, making young infants more susceptible to infection.
7. Physiologic control of breathing may be impaired during the first few weeks of life.

Pulmonary Disorders

1. Physical examination can provide important clues in assessing the location and nature of UAO.
2. Upper airway infections can pose serious threats because of inflammatory edema and airway obstruction, including bacterial tracheitis, retropharyngeal abscess, and peritonsillar infections. Recognition and rapid evaluation are crucial.
3. Viral croup (laryngotracheobronchitis) is the most common cause of acute upper airway obstruction in children and usually affects children ages 6 months to 5 years. Subglottic edema may be mild to severe. Parainfluenza is the most common cause.
4. Acute epiglottitis is a life-threatening emergency that is now rarely seen because of vaccination against *H. influenzae,* which had been the primary causative microorganism. Current cases usually represent vaccine failure or are caused by other bacteria, such as group A streptococci.
5. Aspiration of a foreign body should be considered whenever there is a sudden onset of stridor, coughing, wheezing, or hoarseness. This usually occurs in 1- to 3-year-olds. Occasionally diagnosis is delayed and symptoms may be attributed to asthma, bronchitis, or pneumonia without recognition of the underlying cause.
6. Chronic UAO may be manifested by stridor, abnormal cry, wheezing, or dyspnea. The most common cause of stridor in infants is laryngomalacia. Other causes include subglottic stenosis, vocal cord paralysis, and vascular rings.
7. Obstructive sleep apnea usually occurs in older children rather than infants and is underdiagnosed. Typical symptoms are snoring, gasping, and restless sleep. The most common cause in children is adenotonsillar hypertrophy.
8. RDS of the newborn usually occurs in premature infants who are born before surfactant production and alveolocapillary development are complete. Atelectasis and hypoventilation cause shunting, hypoxemia, and hypercapnia.
9. BPD is a chronic lung disease of infancy that is usually the consequence of acute respiratory disease in premature infants who required oxygen and positive pressure ventilatory support. Contributing factors include structural immaturity, inflammation, and disordered lung repair processes.
10. Bronchiolitis occurs in infants and toddlers, usually in the winter and early spring. It is caused by viruses, most commonly RSV. There is extensive edema, inflammation, and damage to the bronchiolar epithelium. Injections of monoclonal antibody against RSV are recommended as a preventive measure for high-risk infants.
11. Childhood pneumonia can be caused by viruses (most common), bacteria, or *Mycoplasma.* Lobar pneumonia is usually bacterial. Certain bacteria, such as *S. aureus* and group A streptococci, can cause particularly fulminant disease, as well as abscesses and empyema.
12. Aspiration pneumonitis can occur because of lung inflammation from entry of any foreign substance, including food, drink, or chemicals. Aspiration of oropharyngeal bacteria can occur because of loss of protective reflexes in neurologically impaired children, or during induction of anesthesia.
13. Asthma is an obstructive airway disease with episodes of acute respiratory symptoms (cough, wheeze, dyspnea) and intermittent or chronic subacute symptoms. It is the most common chronic condition in children. It is a disease of local airway inflammation, with exacerbation in response to triggers, such as infections or allergens. Inflammatory cell infiltration, mucosal edema, mucus plugging of airways, and epithelial damage cause obstruction to airflow, and there is evidence of long-term remodeling of airways.
14. ARDS is an acute life-threatening condition characterized by severe hypoxemia, poor lung compliance, and diffuse densities on chest radiograph. It can be triggered by acute pulmonary insults or major systemic illness (e.g., sepsis) or trauma. High-level ventilatory support is required, and mortality is significant.
15. CF is an autosomal recessive disease characterized by thick, tenacious mucus, plugging of airways, chronic pulmonary infection, and bronchiectasis related to airway epithelial chloride and sodium transport. The other major manifestations are digestive and nutritional, related to pancreatic insufficiency. Median survival is currently 37 years, with mortality primarily related to lung disease.

Sudden Infant Death Syndrome

1. SIDS is a diagnosis of exclusion after thorough investigation and autopsy following sudden death of an infant less than 6 months of age. Usually the event occurs during nighttime sleep.
2. The cause is unknown. However, some known risk factors are avoidable, such as maternal smoking, prone sleeping, soft bedding surfaces, and overheating. The incidence of SIDS has decreased significantly since public health campaigns have encouraged the supine sleeping position for babies.

KEY TERMS

Acute epiglottitis, 1296
Acute lung injury (ALI), 1310
Acute respiratory distress syndrome (ARDS), 1310
Angioedema, 1298
Aspiration pneumonitis, 1308
Asthma, 1308
Atypical pneumonia *(Mycoplasma pneumoniae, Chlamydophila pneumoniae)*, 1306
Bacterial pneumonia, 1306
Bacterial tracheitis, 1297
Bronchiolitis, 1305
Bronchiolitis obliterans (BO), 1308
Bronchopulmonary dysplasia (BPD), 1303
Coanal atresia, 1300
Community-acquired pneumonia (CAP), 1306
Croup, 1294
Cystic fibrosis (CF), 1310
Cystic fibrosis transmembrane conductance regulator (CFTCR) protein, 1311
Foreign body aspiration, 1298
Functional residual capacity (FRC), 1292
Hyaline membrane disease (HMD), 1301
Laryngeal atresia, 1300
Laryngomalacia, 1299
Laryngotracheobronchitis, 1294
Obstructive sleep apnea syndrome (OSAS), 1300
Peritonsillar abscess, 1297
Pneumonia, 1306
Respiratory distress syndrome (RDS) of the newborn, 1301
Retropharyngeal abscess, 1298
Spasmodic croup, 1294
Stridor, 1293
Subglottic stenosis, 1299
Sudden infant death syndrome (SIDS), 1313
Surfactant, 1292
Tracheal stenosis, 1300
Tracheomalacia (tracheobronchomalacia), 1299
Upper airway obstruction (UAO), 1293
Viral pneumonia, 1306

REFERENCES

1. Choi J, Lee GL: Common pediatric respiratory emergencies, *Emerg Med Clin North Am* 30(2):529–563, x, 2012.
2. Zoorob R, Sidani M, Murray J: Croup: an overview, *Am Fam Physician* 83(9):1067–1073, 2011.
3. Wall SR et al: The viral aetiology of croup and recurrent croup, *Arch Dis Child* 94:359–360, 2009.
4. Westley CR, Cotton ED, Brooks JG: Nebulized racemic epinephrine by IPPB for the treatment of croup, *Am J Dis Child* 132:484–487, 1978.
5. Pitluk JD, Uman H, Safranek S: Clinical inquiries. What's best for croup? *J Fam Pract* 60(11):680–681, 2011.
6. Dobrovoljac M, Geelhoed GC: How fast does oral dexamethasone work in mild to moderately severe croup? A randomized double-blinded clinical trial, *Emerg Med Australas* 24(1):79–85, 2012.
7. Bjornson C et al: Nebulized epinephrine for croup in children, *Cochrane Database Syst Rev* (2):CD006619, 2011.
8. Vorwerk C, Coats T: Heliox for croup in children, *Cochrane Database Syst Rev* (2):CD006822, 2010.
9. Shah RK, Stocks C: Epiglottitis in the United States: national trends, variances, prognosis, and management, *Laryngoscope* 120(6):1256–1262, 2010.
10. Sobol SE, Zapata S: Epiglottitis and croup, *Otolaryngol Clin North Am* 41(3):551–566, ix, 2008.
11. Glynn F, Fenton J: Diagnosis and management of supraglottitis (epiglottitis), *Curr Infect Dis Rep* 10:200–204, 2008.
12. Alcaide M, Bisno A: Pharyngitis and epiglottitis, *Infect Dis Clin North Am* 21:449–469, 2007.
13. Sidell D, Shapiro NL: Acute tonsillitis, *Infect Disord Drug Targets* 12(4):271–276, 2012.
14. Calò L et al: Role of biofilms in chronic inflammatory diseases of the upper airways, *Adv Otorhinolaryngol* 72:93–96, 2011.
15. Thompson SK, Doerr TD, Hengerer AS: Infectious mononucleosis and corticosteroids: management practices and outcomes, *Arch Otolaryngol Head Neck Surg* 131(10):900–904, 2005.
16. Kordeluk S et al: Relation between peritonsillar infection and acute tonsillitis: myth or reality? *Otolaryngol Head Neck Surg* 145(6):940–945, 2011.
17. Powell J, Wilson JA: An evidence-based review of peritonsillar abscess, *Clin Otolaryngol* 37(2):136–145, 2012.
18. Byard RW: Tonsillitis and sudden childhood death, *J Forensic Leg Med* 15(8):516–518, 2008.
19. Bjornson CL, Johnson DW: Croup, *Lancet* 371(9609):329–339, 2008.
20. Hopkins A et al: Changing epidemiology of life-threatening upper airway infections: the reemergence of bacterial tracheitis, *Pediatrics* 118(4):1418–1421, 2006.
21. Graf J, Stein F: Tracheitis in pediatric patients, *Semin Pediatr Infect Dis* 17:11–13, 2006.
22. Miranda AD, Valdez TA, Pereira KD: Bacterial tracheitis: a varied entity, *Pediatr Emerg Care* 27(10):950–953, 2011.
23. Balfour-Lynn IM, Davies JC: Acute infections that produce upper airway obstruction. In Wilmott RW et al: *Kendig and Cherick's disorders of the respiratory tract in children*, ed 8, Philadelphia, 2012, Saunders, pp 424–436.
24. Abdel-Haq N, Quezada M, Asmar BI: Retropharyngeal abscess in children: the rising incidence of methicillin-resistant *Staphylococcus aureus*, *Pediatr Infect Dis J* 31(7):696–699, 2012.
25. Grisaru-Soen G et al: Retropharyngeal and parapharyngeal abscess in children—epidemiology, clinical features and treatment, *Int J Pediatr Otorhinolaryngol* 74(9):1016–1020, 2010.
26. Hoffmann C et al: Retropharyngeal infections in children. Treatment strategies and outcomes, *Int J Pediatr Otorhinolaryngol* 75(9):1099–1103, 2011.
27. Kay M, Wyllie R: Pediatric foreign bodies and their management, *Curr Gastroenterol Rep* 7(3):212–218, 2005.
28. Rizk H, Rassi S: Foreign body inhalation in the pediatric population: lessons learned from 106 cases, *Eur Ann Otorhinolaryngol Head Neck Dis* 128(4):169–174, 2011.
29. Shlizerman L et al: Foreign body aspiration in children: the effects of delayed diagnosis, *Am J Otolaryngol* 31(5):320–324, 2010.
30. Hitter A et al: Diagnostic value of various investigations in children with suspected foreign body aspiration: review, *Eur Ann Otorhinolaryngol Head Neck Dis* 128(5):248–252, 2011.
31. Farkas H: Management of hereditary angioedema in pediatric patients, *Pediatrics* 120(3):e713–e722, 2007.
32. Ferrari GG, Eng PA: IgE-mediated food allergies in Swiss infants and children, *Swiss Med Wkly* 141:w13269, 2011.
33. Zuran BL: Current and future therapy for hereditary angioedema, *Clin Immunol* 114(1):10–16, 2005.
34. Farkas H: Pediatric hereditary angioedema due to C1-inhibitor deficiency, *Allergy Asthma Clin Immunol* 6(1):18, 2010.
35. Papadopoulou-Alataki E: Upper airway considerations in hereditary angioedema, *Curr Opin Allergy Clin Immunol* 10(1):20–25, 2010.
36. Smith JL et al: State-dependent laryngomalacia in sleeping children, *Ann Otol Rhinol Laryngol* 114(2):111–114, 2005.
37. Zainal A, Goh BS, Mohamed AS: Supraglottoplasty for laryngomalacia: who will benefit? *Asian J Surg* 34(2):92–96, 2011.
38. Thompson DM: Abnormal sensorimotor integrative function of the larynx in congenital laryngomalacia: a new theory of etiology, *Laryngoscope* 117(6 Pt 2, Suppl 114):1–33, 2007.
39. Munson PD et al: Submucosal nerve hypertrophy in congenital laryngomalacia, *Laryngoscope* 121(3):627–629, 2011.
40. Thompson DM: Laryngomalacia: factors that influence disease severity and outcomes of management, *Curr Opin Otolaryngol Head Neck Surg* 18(6):564–570, 2010.
41. Revell SM, Clark WD: Late-onset laryngomalacia: a cause of pediatric obstructive sleep apnea, *Int J Pediatr Otorhinolaryngol* 75(2):231–238, 2011.
42. Wright CT, Goudy SL: Congenital laryngomalacia: symptom duration and need for surgical intervention, *Ann Otol Rhinol Laryngol* 121(1):57–60, 2012.
43. Gaissert HA, Burns J: The compromised airway: tumors, strictures, and tracheomalacia, *Surg Clin North Am* 90(5):1065–1089, 2010.
44. Ada M, Isildak H, Saritzali G: Congenital vocal cord paralysis, *J Craniofac Surg* 21(1):273–274, 2010.
45. Ishman S et al: Management of vocal paralysis: a comparison of adult and pediatric practices, *Otolaryngol Head Neck Surg* 135:590–594, 2006.
46. Doshi D, Weinberger M: Long-term outcome of vocal cord dysfunction, *Ann Allergy Asthma Immunol* 96:794–799, 2006.
47. Kennedy JL, Heymann PW, Platts-Mills TA: The role of allergy in severe asthma, *Clin Exp Allergy* 42(5):659–669, 2012.
48. Daniel S: The upper airway: congenital malformations, *Paediatr Respir Rev* 7S:S260–S263, 2006.
49. Alvarez-Neri H et al: Primary cricotracheal resection with thyrotracheal anastomosis for the treatment of severe subglottic stenosis in children and adolescents, *Ann Otol Rhinol Laryngol* 114(1 Pt 1):2–6, 2005.
50. Dauer EH et al: Airway manifestations of pediatric eosinophilic esophagitis: a clinical and histopathologic report of an emerging association, *Ann Otol Rhinol Laryngol* 155(7):507–517, 2006.

51. Erickson VR, Hwang PH: Wegener's granulomatosis: current trends in diagnosis and management, *Curr Opin Otolaryngol Head Neck Surg* 15(3):170–176, 2007.
52. Wei JL, Bond J: Management and prevention of endotracheal intubation injury in neonates, *Curr Opin Otolaryngol Head Neck Surg* 19(6):474–477, 2011.
53. Sidman J, Jaguan A, Couser R: Tracheotomy and decannulation rates in a level 3 neonatal intensive care unit: a 12 year study, *Laryngoscope* 116:136–139, 2006.
54. Bluestone C: Humans are born too soon: impact on pediatric otolaryngology, *Int J Pediatr Otorhinolaryngol* 69:1–8, 2005.
55. Maturo SC, Hartnick CJ: Pediatric airway balloon dilation, *Adv Otorhinolaryngol* 73:112–115, 2012.
56. Gallagher TQ, Hartnick CJ: Laryngotracheal reconstruction, *Adv Otorhinolaryngol* 73:31–38, 2012.
57. Cedin AC et al: Surgery for congenital choanal atresia, *Cochrane Database Syst Rev* (2):CD008993, 2012.
58. Koltai PJ: Pediatric tracheal stenosis, *Otolaryngol Clin North Am* 41(5):999–1021, 2008.
59. Ywakim R, El-Hakim H: Congenital tracheal stenosis managed conservatively: systematic review of the literature, *J Otolaryngol Head Neck Surg* 41(4):288–302, 2012.
60. Ievers-Landis C, Redline S: Pediatric sleep apnea, *Am J Respir Crit Care Med* 175:436–441, 2007.
61. Katz ES, Mitchell RB, D'Ambrosio CM: Obstructive sleep apnea in infants, *Am J Respir Crit Care Med* 185(8):805–816, 2012.
62. Katz ES, D'Ambrosio CM: Pediatric obstructive sleep apnea syndrome, *Clin Chest Med* 31(2):221–234, 2010.
63. Gozal D et al: C-reactive protein and obstructive sleep apnea syndrome in children, *Front Biosci (Elite Ed)* 4:2410–2422, 2012.
64. Kim J et al: Inflammatory pathways in children with insufficient or disordered sleep, *Respir Physiol Neurobiol* 178(3):465–474, 2011.
65. Jeyakumar A et al: The association between sleep-disordered breathing and enuresis in children, *Laryngoscope* 122(8):1873–1877, 2012.
66. Horne RS et al: Elevated blood pressure during sleep and wake in children with sleep-disordered breathing, *Pediatrics* 128(1):e85–e92, 2011.
67. Leung L et al: Twenty-four-hour ambulatory BP in snoring children with obstructive sleep apnea syndrome, *Chest* 130:1009–1017, 2006.
68. Lal C, Strange C, Bachman D: Neurocognitive impairment in obstructive sleep apnea, *Chest* 141(6):1601–1610, 2012.
69. Brown KA: Outcome, risk, and error and the child with obstructive sleep apnea, *Paediatr Anaesth* 21(7):771–780, 2011.
70. O'Driscoll DM et al: Increased sympathetic activity in children with obstructive sleep apnea: cardiovascular implications, *Sleep Med* 12(5):483–488, 2011.
71. Tatlipinar A et al: The effects of obstructive sleep apnea syndrome due to adenotonsillar hypertrophy on the cardiovascular system in children, *Turk J Pediatr* 53(4):359–363, 2011.
72. Gasparini G et al: Clinical evaluation of obstructive sleep apnea in children, *J Craniofac Surg* 23(2):387–391, 2012.
73. Donnelly LF: Magnetic resonance sleep studies in the evaluation of children with obstructive sleep apnea, *Semin Ultrasound CT MR* 31(2):107–115, 2010.
74. Church GD: The role of polysomnography in diagnosing and treating obstructive sleep apnea in pediatric patients, *Curr Probl Pediatr Adolesc Health Care* 42(1):2–25, 2012.
75. Kaditis A, Kheirandish-Gozal L, Gozal D: Algorithm for the diagnosis and treatment of pediatric OSA: a proposal of two pediatric sleep centers, *Sleep Med* 13(3):217–227, 2012.
76. Shott SR: Evaluation and management of pediatric obstructive sleep apnea beyond tonsillectomy and adenoidectomy, *Curr Opin Otolaryngol Head Neck Surg* 19(6):449–454, 2011.
77. Shapiro-Mendoza CK, Lackritz EM: Epidemiology of late and moderate preterm birth, *Semin Fetal Neonatal Med* 17(3):120–125, 2012.
78. Raju TN: Developmental physiology of late and moderate prematurity, *Semin Fetal Neonatal Med* 17(3):126–131, 2012.
79. Colin A, McEvoy C, Castile R: Respiratory morbidity and lung function in preterm infants of 32 to 36 weeks' gestational age, *Pediatrics* 126:115–128, 2010.
80. Teune MJ et al: A systematic review of severe morbidity in infants born late preterm, *Am J Obstet Gynecol* 205(4):374.e1–374.e9, 2011.
81. Bersani I, Speer CP, Kunzmann S: Surfactant proteins A and D in pulmonary diseases of preterm infants, *Expert Rev Anti Infect Ther* 10(5):573–584, 2012.
82. Sweet D et al: European consensus guidelines on the management of neonatal respiratory distress syndrome, *J Perinatal Med* 35:175–186, 2007.
83. Bonanno C, Wapner RJ: Antenatal corticosteroids in the management of preterm birth: are we back where we started? *Obstet Gynecol Clin North Am* 39(1):47–63, 2012.
84. McKinlay CJ et al: Repeat antenatal glucocorticoids for women at risk of preterm birth: a Cochrane Systematic Review, *Am J Obstet Gynecol* 206(3):187–941, 2012.
85. Carlo WA et al: Association of antenatal corticosteroids with mortality and neurodevelopmental outcomes among infants born at 22 to 25 weeks' gestation, *J Am Med Assoc* 306(21):2348–2358, 2011.
86. Smith PB et al: Approach to infants born at 22 to 24 weeks' gestation: relationship to outcomes of more-mature infants, *Pediatrics* 129(6):e1508–e1516, 2012.
87. Gyamfi-Bannerman C et al: Effect of antenatal corticosteroids on respiratory morbidity in singletons after late-preterm birth, *Obstet Gynecol* 119(3):555–559, 2012.
88. Kamath-Rayne BD, DeFranco EA, Marcotte MP: Antenatal steroids for treatment of fetal lung immaturity after 34 weeks of gestation: an evaluation of neonatal outcomes, *Obstet Gynecol* 119(5):909–916, 2012.
89. Engle WA: American Academy of Pediatrics Committee on Fetus and Newborn: Surfactant-replacement therapy for respiratory distress in the preterm and term neonate, *Pediatrics* 121(2):419–432, 2008.
90. Verder H et al: Nasal CPAP and surfactant for treatment of respiratory distress syndrome and prevention of bronchopulmonary dysplasia, *Acta Paediatr* 98(9):1400–1408, 2009.
91. Rojas-Reyes MX, Morley CJ, Soll R: Prophylactic versus selective use of surfactant in preventing morbidity and mortality in preterm infants, *Cochrane Database Syst Rev* (3):CD000510, 2012.
92. Howlett A, Ohlsson A, Plakkal N: Inositol for respiratory distress syndrome in preterm infants, *Cochrane Database Syst Rev* (3):CD000366, 2012.
93. Mahmoud RA, Roehr CC, Schmalisch G: Current methods of non-invasive ventilatory support for neonates, *Paediatr Respir Rev* 12(3): 196–205, 2011.
94. Rocha G et al: Respiratory support strategies for the preterm newborn—national survey 2008, *Rev Port Pneumol* 15(6):1043–1071, 2009.
95. Colnaghi M et al: Nasal continuous positive airway pressure with heliox in preterm infants with respiratory distress syndrome, *Pediatrics* 129(2):e333–e338, 2012.
96. Migliori C et al: The effects of helium/oxygen mixture (heliox) before and after extubation in long-term mechanically ventilated very low birth weight infants, *Pediatrics* 123(6):1524–1528, 2009.
97. Patrianakos-Hoobler AI et al: Safety and efficacy of inhaled nitric oxide treatment for premature infants with respiratory distress syndrome: follow-up evaluation at early school age, *Acta Paediatr* 100(4):524–528, 2011.
98. Jobe AH: Lung maturation: the survival miracle of very low birth weight infants, *Pediatr Neonatol* 51(1):7–13, 2010.
99. Landry JS, Menzies D: Occurrence and severity of bronchopulmonary dysplasia and respiratory distress syndrome after a preterm birth, *Paediatr Child Health* 16(7):399–403, 2011.
100. Groothuis JR, Makari D: Definition and outpatient management of the very low-birth-weight infant with bronchopulmonary dysplasia, *Adv Ther* 29(4):297–311, 2012.
101. Van Marter LJ: Epidemiology of bronchopulmonary dysplasia, *Semin Fetal Neonatal Med* 14(6):358–366, 2009.
102. Bancalari E, Claure N, Sosenko IRS: Bronchopulmonary dysplasia: changes in pathogenesis, epidemiology, and definition, *Semin Neonatol* 8(1):63–71, 2003.
103. Trembath A, Laughon MM: Predictors of bronchopulmonary dysplasia, *Clin Perinatol* 39(3):585–601, 2012.
104. Viscardi RM: Perinatal inflammation and lung injury, *Semin Fetal Neonatal Med* 17(1):30–35, 2012.
105. Jobe AH: The new bronchopulmonary dysplasia, *Curr Opin Pediatr* 23:167–172, 201, 2011.
106. Somaschini M et al: Genetic susceptibility to neonatal lung diseases, *Acta Biomed* 83(Suppl 1):10–14, 2012.
107. De Paepe ME, Greco D, Mao Q: Angiogenesis-related gene expression profiling in ventilated preterm human lungs, *Exp Lung Res* 36(7):399–410, 2010.
108. Pfister RH, Soll RF: Initial respiratory support of preterm infants: the role of CPAP, the INSURE method, and noninvasive ventilation, *Clin Perinatol* 39(3):459–481, 2012.
109. Picone S, Bedetta M, Paolillo P: Caffeine citrate: when and for how long. A literature review, *J Matern Fetal Neonatal Med* 25(Suppl 3):11–14, 2012.
110. Guimarães H et al: Vitamin A in prevention of bronchopulmonary dysplasia, *Curr Pharm Des* 18(21):3101–3113, 2012.
111. Robinson RF: Impact of respiratory syncytial virus in the United States, *Am J Health Syst Pharm* 65(23 Suppl 8):S3–S6, 2008.

112. Bacharier LB et al: Determinants of asthma after severe respiratory syncytial virus bronchiolitis, *J Allergy Clin Immunol* 130(1):91–100, 2012.
113. Jartti T, Korppi M: Rhinovirus-induced bronchiolitis and asthma development, *Pediatr Allergy Immunol* 22(4):350–355, 2011.
114. Krilov LR: Respiratory syncytial virus disease: update on treatment and prevention, *Expert Rev Anti Infect Ther* 9(1):27–32, 2011.
115. Faber TE et al: IL1RL1 gene variants and nasopharyngeal IL1R1-a levels are associated with severe RSV bronchiolitis: a multicenter cohort study, *PLoS One* 7(5):e34364, 2012.
116. Caiulo VA et al: Lung ultrasound in bronchiolitis: comparison with chest X-ray, *Eur J Pediatr* 170(11):1427–1433, 2011.
117. American Academy of Pediatrics Subcommittee on Diagnosis and Management of Bronchiolitis: Diagnosis and management of bronchiolitis, *Pediatrics* 118:1774–1793, 2006.
118. Gadomski AM, Brower M: Bronchodilators for bronchiolitis, *Cochrane Database Syst Rev* (12):CD001266, 2010.
119. Hartling L et al: Epinephrine for bronchiolitis, *Cochrane Database Syst Rev* (6):CD003123, 2011.
120. Hartling L et al: Steroids and bronchodilators for acute bronchiolitis in the first two years of life: systematic review and meta-analysis, *Br Med J* 342:d1714, 2011.
121. Evans J, Marlais M, Abrahamson E: Clinical predictors of nasal continuous positive airway pressure requirement in acute bronchiolitis, *Pediatr Pulmonol* 47(4):381–385, 2012.
122. Donlan M, Fontela PS, Puligandla PS: Use of continuous positive airway pressure (CPAP) in acute viral bronchiolitis: a systematic review, *Pediatr Pulmonol* 46(8):736–746, 2011.
123. Costello HM et al: Targeting RSV with vaccines and small molecule drugs, *Infect Disord Drug Targets* 12(2):110–128, 2012.
124. Geevarghese B, Simões EA: Antibodies for prevention and treatment of respiratory syncytial virus infections in children, *Antivir Ther* 17(1 Pt B): 201–211, 2012.
125. Falade AG, Ayede AI: Epidemiology, aetiology and management of childhood acute community-acquired pneumonia in developing countries—a review, *Afr J Med Sci* 40(4):293–308, 2011.
126. Kesson A: Respiratory virus infections, *Paediatr Respir Rev* 8:240–248, 2007.
127. Stuckey-Schrock K, Hayes BL, George CM: Community-acquired pneumonia in children, *Am Fam Physician* 86(7):661–667, 2012.
128. Moreno L et al: Development and validation of a clinical predication rule to distinguish bacterial from viral pneumonia in children, *Pediatr Pulmonol* 41:331–337, 2006.
129. Graham BS: Biological challenges and technological opportunities for respiratory syncytial virus vaccine development, *Immunol Rev* 239(1):149–166, 2011.
130. Tam PY: Approach to common bacterial infections: community-acquired pneumonia, *Pediatr Clin North Am* 60(2):437–453, 2013.
131. Alicino C et al: The dangerous synergism between influenza and *Streptococcus pneumoniae* and innovative perspectives of vaccine prevention, *J Prev Med Hyg* 52(3):102–106, 2011.
132. Grijalva CG et al: Increasing incidence of empyema complicating childhood community-acquired pneumonia in the United States, *Clin Infect Dis* 50(6):805–813, 2010.
133. Hersh AL et al: Variability in pediatric infectious disease consultants' recommendations for management of community-acquired pneumonia, *PLoS One* 6(5):e20325, 2011.
134. Wolf J, Daly A: Microbiological aspects of bacterial lower respiratory tract illness in children: typical pathogens, *Paediatr Respir Rev* 8:204–211, 2007.
135. Bébéar C, Pereyre S, Peuchant O: *Mycoplasma pneumoniae*: susceptibility and resistance to antibiotics, *Future Microbiol* 6(4):423–431, 2011.
136. Yamada M et al: Rising rates of macrolide-resistant *Mycoplasma pneumoniae* in the central United States, *Pediatr Infect Dis J* 31(4):409–410, 2012.
137. Bradley J et al: Comparative study of levofloxacin in the treatment of children with community-acquired pneumonia, *Pediatr Infect Dis J* 26(10):868–878, 2007.
138. Bradley JS et al: The management of community acquired pneumonia in infants and children older than 3 months of age: clinical practice guidelines by the Pediatric Infectious Diseases Society and the Infectious Diseases Society of America, *Clin Infect Dis* (7):617–630, 2011.
139. Krüger S, Welte T: Biomarkers in community-acquired pneumonia, *Expert Rev Respir Med* 6(2):203–214, 2012.
140. Nascimento-Carvalho CM: Pharmacotherapy of childhood pneumonia, *Exp Opin Pharmacother* 11(2):225–231, 2010.
141. Mulholland S, Gavranich JB, Chang AB: Antibiotics for community-acquired lower respiratory tract infections secondary to *Mycoplasma pneumoniae* in children, *Cochrane Database Syst Rev* (7):CD004875, 2010.
142. Nair GB, Niederman MS: Community-acquired pneumonia: an unfinished battle, *Med Clin North Am* 95(6):1143–1161, 2011.
143. Boesch RP et al: Advances in the diagnosis and management of chronic pulmonary aspiration in children, *Eur Respir J* 28:847–861, 2006.
144. Trinick R et al: Reflux aspiration in children with neurodisability—a significant problem, but can we measure it? *J Pediatr Surg* 47(2): 291–298, 2012.
145. Khan WU et al: Botulinum toxin A for treatment of sialorrhea in children: an effective, minimally invasive approach, *Arch Otolaryngol Head Neck Surg* 137(4):339–344, 2011.
146. Kurland G, Michelson P: Bronchiolitis obliterans in children, *Pediatr Pulmonol* 39:193–208, 2005.
147. Fischer GB et al: Post infectious bronchiolitis obliterans in children, *Paediatr Respir Rev* 11(4):233–239, 2010.
148. Colom A et al: Risk factors for the development of bronchiolitis obliterans in children with bronchiolitis, *Thorax* 61:503–506, 2006.
149. Verleden G et al: Azithromycin reduces airway neutrophilia and interleukin-8 in patients with bronchiolitis obliterans syndrome, *Am J Respir Crit Care Med* 174:566–570, 2006.
150. Centers for Disease Control and Prevention: *Asthma in the U.S. growing every year,* updated May 4, 2011. Available at www.cdc.gov/VitalSigns/Asthma/index.html. Accessed October 22, 2012.
151. Jensen ME, Wood LG, Gibson PG: Obesity and childhood asthma—mechanisms and manifestations, *Curr Opin Allergy Clin Immunol* 12(2):186–192, 2012.
152. Hines AB: Asthma: a health disparity among African American children: the impact and implications for pediatric nurses, *J Pediatr Nurs* 26(1):25–33, 2011.
153. Akinbami LJ et al: Trends in asthma prevalence, health care use, and mortality in the United States, 2001-2010, *NCHS Data Brief* (94):1–8, 2012.
154. National Heart, Lung, and Blood Institute: *National Asthma Education and Prevention Program Expert Panel report 3: guidelines for the diagnosis and management of asthma*, 2007. Available at www.nhlbi.nih.gov/guidelines/asthma/index.htm.
155. Ungar WJ et al: Relationship of asthma management, socioeconomic status, and medication insurance characteristics to exacerbation frequency in children with asthma, *Ann Allergy Asthma Immunol* 106(1):17–23, 2011.
156. Bijanzadeh M, Mahesh PA, Ramachandra NB: An understanding of the genetic basis of asthma, *Indian J Med Res* 134:149–161, 2011.
157. Gern JE: The Urban Environment and Childhood Asthma study, *J Allergy Clin Immunol* 125(3):545–549, 2010.
158. Luong KV, Nguyen LT: The role of vitamin D in asthma, *Pulm Pharmacol Ther* 25(2):137–143, 2012.
159. Rigoli L et al: Gene-environment interaction in childhood asthma, *Int J Immunopathol Pharmacol* 24(Suppl 4):41–47, 2011.
159a. Yang IV, Schwartz DA: Epigenetic mechanisms and the development of asthma, *J Allergy Clin Immunol* 130(6):1243–1255, 2012.
160. Barnes KC: Genetic studies of the etiology of asthma, *Proc Am Thorac Soc* 8(2):143–148, 2011.
161. Torgerson DG et al: Meta-analysis of genome-wide association studies of asthma in ethnically diverse North American populations, *Nat Genet* 43(9):887–892, 2011.
162. Postma DS et al: Asthma and chronic obstructive pulmonary disease: common genes, common environments? *Am J Respir Crit Care Med* 183(12):1588–1594, 2011.
163. Slager RE et al: Genetics of asthma susceptibility and severity, *Clin Chest Med* 33(3):431–443, 2012.
164. Mukherjee AB, Zhang Z: Allergic asthma: influence of genetic and environmental factors, *J Biol Chem* 286(38):32883–32889, 2011.
165. Ingram JL et al: Airway fibroblasts in asthma manifest an invasive phenotype, *Am J Respir Crit Care Med* 183:1625–1632, 2011.
166. Fishbein AB, Fuleihan RL: The hygiene hypothesis revisited: does exposure to infectious agents protect us from allergy? *Curr Opin Pediatr* 24(1):98–102, 2012.
167. Lluis A, Schaub B: Lesson from the farm environment, *Curr Opin Allergy Clin Immunol* 12(2):158–163, 2012.
168. Matricardi PM: 99th Dahlem conference on infection, inflammation and chronic inflammatory disorders: controversial aspects of the 'hygiene hypothesis', *Clin Exp Immunol* 160(1):98–105, 2010.
169. Wu P, Hartert TV: Evidence for a causal relationship between respiratory syncytial virus infection and asthma, *Expert Rev Anti Infect Ther* 9(9):731–745, 2011.
170. Proud D: Role of rhinovirus infections in asthma, *Asian Pac J Allergy Immunol* 29(3):201–208, 2011.
171. Bacharier LB, Guilbert TW: Diagnosis and management of early asthma in preschool-aged children, *J Allergy Clin Immunol* 130(2):287–296, 2012.

172. Bisgaard H, Bønnelykke K: Long-term studies of the natural history of asthma in childhood, *J Allergy Clin Immunol* 126(2):187–197, 2010.
173. Bernard GR et al: The American-European Consensus Conference on ARDS: definitions, mechanisms, relevant outcomes, and clinical trial coordination, *Am J Respir Crit Care Med* 149:818–824, 1994.
174. Willson DF, Chess PR, Notter RH: Surfactant for pediatric acute lung injury, *Pediatr Clin North Am* 55(3):545–575, ix, 2008.
175. Bruijn M et al: High incidence of acute lung injury in children with Down syndrome, *Intensive Care Med* 33(12):2179–2182, 2007.
176. Cheifetz IM: Management of acute lung injury: sharing data between adults and children, *Respir Care* 56(9):1258–1268, 2011. discussion 1268–1272.
177. Cheifetz IM: Pediatric acute respiratory distress syndrome, *Respir Care* 56(10):1589–1599, 2011.
178. Pierrakos C et al: Acute respiratory distress syndrome: pathophysiology and therapeutic options, *J Clin Med Res* 4(1):7–16, 2012.
179. Prabhakaran P: Acute respiratory distress syndrome, *Indian Pediatr* 47(10):861–868, 2010.
180. Saguil A, Fargo M: Acute respiratory distress syndrome: diagnosis and management, *Am Fam Physician* 85(4):352–358, 2012.
181. Raghavendran K, Willson D, Notter RH: Surfactant therapy for acute lung injury and acute respiratory distress syndrome, *Crit Care Clin* 27(3):525–559, 2011.
182. Goto T et al: The impact of extracorporeal membrane oxygenation on survival in pediatric patients with respiratory and heart failure: review of our experience, *Artif Organs* 35(11):1002–1009, 2011.
183. Peng CC et al: Clinical experience of extracorporeal membrane oxygenation for acute respiratory distress syndrome associated with pneumonia in children, *J Formos Med Assoc* 111(3):147–152, 2012.
184. Cystic Fibrosis Center at the Hospital for Sick Children in Toronto: *Cystic fibrosis mutation database.* Available at www.genet.sickkids.on.ca/cftr/StatisticsPage.html. Accessed May 15, 2013.
185. Kreindler JL: Cystic fibrosis: exploiting its genetic basis in the hunt for new therapies, *Pharmacol Ther* 125(2):219–229, 2010.
186. Salvatore D et al: An overview of international literature from cystic fibrosis registries. Part 4: update 2011, *J Cyst Fibros* 11(6):480–493, 2012.
187. Gillen AE, Harris A: Transcriptional regulation of CFTR gene expression, *Front Biosci (Elite Ed)* 4:587–592, 2012.
188. Tiddens HA et al: Cystic fibrosis lung disease starts in the small airways: can we treat it more effectively? *Pediatr Pulmonol* 45(2):107–117, 2010.
189. Rogers DF: Physiology of airway mucus secretion and pathophysiology of hypersecretion, *Respir Care* 52(9):1134–1146, 2007. discussion 1146–1149.
190. Collawn JF et al: The CFTR and ENaC debate: how important is ENaC in CF lung disease? *Am J Physiol Lung Cell Mol Physiol* 302(11):L1141–L1146, 2012.
191. Donaldson SH, Boucher RC: Sodium channels and cystic fibrosis, *Chest* 132(5):1631–1636, 2007.
192. Hayes E et al: The cystic fibrosis neutrophil: a specialized yet potentially defective cell, *Arch Immunol Ther Exp (Warsz)* 59(2):97–112, 2011.
193. Chapman AL et al: Myeloperoxidase-dependent oxidative metabolism of nitric oxide in the cystic fibrosis airway, *J Cyst Fibros* 9(2):84–92, 2010.
194. Cohen TS, Prince A: Cystic fibrosis: a mucosal immunodeficiency syndrome, *Nat Med* 18(4):509–519, 2012.
195. Zemanick ET, Sagel SD, Harris JK: The airway microbiome in cystic fibrosis and implications for treatment, *Curr Opin Pediatr* 23(3): 319–324, 2011.
196. Elkin S, Geddes D: Pseudomonal infection in cystic fibrosis: the battle continues, *Expert Rev Anti Infect Ther* 1(4):609–618, 2003.
197. Ciofu O et al: Phenotypes selected during chronic lung infection in cystic fibrosis patients: implications for the treatment of *Pseudomonas aeruginosa* biofilm infections, *FEMS Immunol Med Microbiol* 65(2): 215–225, 2012.
198. Zemanick ET et al: Inflammation and airway microbiota during cystic fibrosis pulmonary exacerbations, *PLoS One* 8(4):e62917, 2013.
199. Regamey N et al: Increased airway smooth muscle mass in children with asthma, cystic fibrosis and non-cystic fibrosis bronchiectasis, *Am J Respir Crit Care Med* 177:837–843, 2008.
200. Becq F: Cystic fibrosis transmembrane conductance regulator modulators for personalized drug treatment of cystic fibrosis: progress to date, *Drugs* 70(3):241–259, 2010.
201. Sosnay PR et al: Evaluation of the disease liability of CFTR variants, *Methods Mol Biol* 742:355–372, 2011.
202. Therrell BL Jr et al: Immunoreactive trypsinogen (IRT) as a biomarker for cystic fibrosis: challenges in newborn dried blood spot screening, *Mol Genet Metab* 106(1):1–6, 2012.
203. Wagener JS, Zemanick ET, Sontag MK: Newborn screening for cystic fibrosis, *Curr Opin Pediatr* 24(3):329–335, 2012.
204. Dungan JS: Carrier screening for cystic fibrosis, *Obstet Gynecol Clin North Am* 37(1):47–59, 2010.
205. Dentice R, Elkins M: Timing of dornase alfa inhalation for cystic fibrosis, *Cochrane Database Syst Rev* (5):CD007923, 2011.
206. Ryan G, Singh M, Dwan K: Inhaled antibiotics for long-term therapy in cystic fibrosis, *Cochrane Database Syst Rev* (3):CD001021, 2011.
207. Hofmann T: New developments in inhaled antibiotics for the treatment of *Pseudomonas aeruginosa, Curr Pharm Des* 18(5):683–695, 2012.
208. Elkins M, Dentice R: Timing of hypertonic saline inhalation for cystic fibrosis, *Cochrane Database Syst Rev* (2):CD008816, 2012.
209. Pressler T: Targeting airway inflammation in cystic fibrosis in children: past, present, and future, *Paediatr Drugs* 13(3):141–147, 2011.
210. Braun AT, Merlo CA: Cystic fibrosis lung transplantation, *Curr Opin Pulm Med* 17(6):467–472, 2011.
211. Munck A: Nutritional considerations in patients with cystic fibrosis, *Exp Rev Respir Med* 4(1):47–56, 2010.
212. Scaparrotta A et al: Growth failure in children with cystic fibrosis, *J Pediatr Endocrinol Metab* 25(5–6):393–405, 2012.
213. Alicandro G et al: Insulin secretion, nutritional status and respiratory function in cystic fibrosis patients with normal glucose tolerance, *Clin Nutr* 31(1):118–123, 2012.
214. Dorfman R: Modifier gene studies to identify new therapeutic targets in cystic fibrosis, *Curr Pharm Des* 18(5):674–682, 2012.
215. Parkins MD et al: Changing epidemiology and clinical issues arising in an ageing cystic fibrosis population, *Ther Adv Respir Dis* 5(2):105–119, 2011.
216. McArdle JR: Pregnancy in cystic fibrosis, *Clin Chest Med* 32(1):111–120, ix, 2011.
217. American Academy of Pediatrics Task Force on Sudden Infant Death Syndrome: The changing concept of sudden infant death syndrome: diagnostic coding shifts, controversies regarding the sleeping environment, and new variables to consider in reducing risk, *Pediatrics* 116(5):1245, 2005.
218. Centers for Disease Control and Prevention: *Sudden infant death syndrome.* Updated October 1, 2012. Available at www.cdc.gov/Features/SidsAwarenessMonth/.
219. Poetsch M et al: Impact of sodium/proton exchanger 3 gene variants on sudden infant death syndrome, *J Pediatr* 156(1):44–48, 2010.
220. National SUID/SIDS Resource Center: Statistics, updated February 2013. Available at www.sidscenter.org/Statistics.html.
221. Blair P, Fleming P: Recurrence risk of sudden infant death syndrome, *Arch Dis Child* 93(4):269–270, 2008.
222. McDonnell-Naughton M et al: Maternal smoking and alcohol consumption during pregnancy as risk factors for sudden infant death, *Ir Med J* 105(4):105–108, 2012.
223. Schnitzer PG, Covington TM, Dykstra HK: Sudden unexpected infant deaths: sleep environment and circumstances, *Am J Public Health* 102(6):1204–1212, 2012.
224. Trachtenberg FL et al: Risk factor changes for sudden infant death syndrome after initiation of Back-to-Sleep campaign, *Pediatrics* 129(4):630–638, 2012.
225. Horne RS et al: Cardiovascular control during sleep in infants: implications for Sudden Infant Death Syndrome, *Sleep Med* 11(7):615–621, 2010.
226. Ostfeld BM et al: Concurrent risks in sudden infant death syndrome, *Pediatrics* 125(3):447–453, 2010.
227. Lavezzi AM et al: Study of the human hypoglossal nucleus: normal development and morpho-functional alterations in sudden unexplained late fetal and infant death, *Brain Develop* 32:275–284, 2010.
228. Vennemann MM et al: Cytokines and sudden infant death, *Int J Legal Med* 126(2):279–284, 2012.
229. Weber MA et al: Virological investigations in sudden unexpected deaths in infancy (SUDI), *Forensic Sci Med Pathol* 6(4):261–267, 2010.
230. Opdal SH, Rognum TO: Gene variants predisposing to SIDS: current knowledge, *Forensic Sci Med Pathol* 7(1):26–36, 2011.
231. Waters K: Serotonin in the sudden infant death syndrome, *Drug News Perspect* 23(9):537–548, 2010.
232. Tfelt-Hansen J et al: Cardiac channelopathies and sudden infant death syndrome, *Cardiology* 119(1):21–33, 2011.
233. Task Force on Sudden Infant Death Syndrome, Moon RY: SIDS and other sleep-related infant deaths: expansion of recommendations for a safe infant sleeping environment, *Pediatrics* 128(5): e1341–e1367, 2011.
234. Young J et al: Responding to evidence: breastfeed baby if you can—the sixth public health recommendation to reduce the risk of sudden and unexpected death in infancy, *Breastfeed Rev* 20(1):7–15, 2012.
235. Strehle EM et al: Can home monitoring reduce mortality in infants at increased risk of sudden infant death syndrome? A systematic review, *Acta Paediatr* 101(1):8–13, 2012.

CHAPTER

37

Structure and Function of the Renal and Urologic Systems

Alexa K. Doig and Sue E. Huether

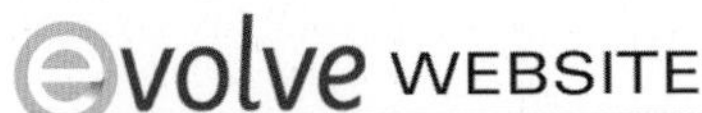

http://evolve.elsevier.com/McCance/

- Review Questions and Answers

CHAPTER OUTLINE

The primary function of the kidney is to maintain a stable internal environment for optimal cell and tissue metabolism. The kidneys accomplish these life-sustaining tasks by balancing solute and water transport, excreting metabolic waste products, conserving nutrients, and regulating acids and bases. The kidney also has an endocrine function, secreting the hormones renin, erythropoietin, and 1,25-dihydroxy-vitamin D_3 for regulation of blood pressure, erythrocyte production, and calcium metabolism, respectively. The kidney also can synthesize glucose from amino acids, performing the process of gluconeogenesis (see What's New? The Kidney and Glucose Regulation). The formation of urine is achieved through the processes of filtration, reabsorption, and secretion by the glomeruli and tubules within the kidney. The bladder stores the urine that it receives from the kidney by way of the ureters. Urine is then removed from the body through the urethra.

STRUCTURES OF THE RENAL SYSTEM

Structures of the Kidney

The **kidneys** are paired organs located in the posterior region of the abdominal cavity behind the peritoneum (Figure 37-1). They lie on either side of the vertebral column with their upper and lower poles extending from approximately the twelfth thoracic to the third lumbar vertebrae. The right kidney is slightly lower than the left and is displaced downward by the overlying liver. Each kidney is approximately 11 cm long, 5 to 6 cm wide, and 3 to 4 cm thick. A tightly adhering capsule (the **renal capsule**) surrounds each kidney, and the kidney then is embedded in a mass of fat. The capsule and fatty layer are covered with a double layer of **renal fascia,** fibrous tissue that attaches the kidney to the posterior abdominal wall.

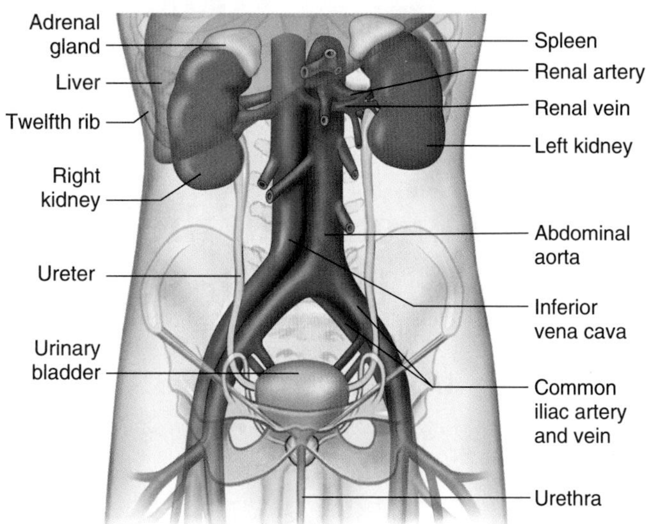

FIGURE 37-1 Organs of the Urinary System. (From Patton KT, Thibodeau GA: *Anatomy & physiology,* ed 8, St Louis, 2013, Mosby.)

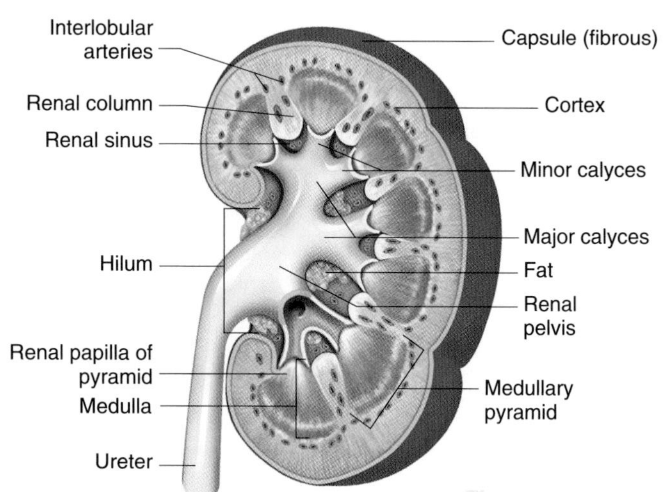

FIGURE 37-2 Kidney Structure. (From Patton KT, Thibodeau GA: *Anatomy & physiology,* ed 8, St Louis, 2013, Mosby.)

WHAT'S NEW?

The Kidney and Glucose Regulation

The human kidney contributes to the regulation of glucose concentration by making glucose through gluconeogenesis, by taking up glucose from the circulation, and by reabsorbing glucose from the glomerular filtrate. The human liver and kidneys release approximately equal amounts of glucose through gluconeogenesis in the postabsorptive state (4 to 12 hours after meal ingestion). Other tissues lack the enzyme necessary for gluconeogenesis (glucose-6-phosphatase) and cannot participate in gluconeogenesis. In the postprandial state (up to 4 hours after meal ingestion), although overall endogenous glucose release decreases substantially, renal gluconeogenesis increases by approximately twofold.

About 180 grams of glucose are normally filtered each day by the kidneys. Almost all of this is actively reabsorbed by means of sodium-glucose cotransporter 2 (SGLT2), a transmembrane protein expressed in the luminal border of the proximal tubule. This ensures sufficient energy is available during fasting periods. When plasma glucose concentrations exceed a threshold, the SGLT2 becomes saturated and glucose appears in the urine. Individuals with diabetes mellitus have an increased transport maximum (T_M) for glucose from enhanced expression of SGLT2 and this contributes to hyperglycemia when there is poor glucose control. SGLT2 inhibitors are being evaluated for reducing hyperglycemia associated with diabetes mellitus.

Renal glucose release is stimulated by epinephrine and is inhibited by insulin. Insulin suppresses glucose release in both the liver and the kidney. The kidneys do not synthesize glycogen and, therefore, do not release glucose through glycogenolysis. In the postabsorptive state, the kidneys utilize about 10% of all glucose used by the body. When there is hypoglycemia, the liver initially releases glucose through glycogenolysis and then increases gluconeogenesis. The kidney also counter-regulates hypoglycemia through gluconeogenesis, which may explain in part why individuals with renal failure tend to develop hypoglycemia.

Data from DeFronzo RA, Davidson JA, Del Prato S: *Diabetes Obes Metab* 14(1):5–14, 2012; Gerich JE: *Diabet Med* 27(2):136–142, 2010; Mather A, Pollock C: *Kidney Int Suppl* (120):S1–S6, 2011; Mitrakou A: *Diabetes Res Clin Pract* 93(Suppl 1):S66–S72, 2011.

The cushion of fat and the position of the kidney between the abdominal organs and muscles of the back protect it from trauma. A medial indentation (the **hilum**) is where the renal blood vessels, nerves, lymphatic vessels, and ureter enter and exit the kidney.

The structures of the kidney are summarized in Figure 37-2. The outer layer of the kidney is called the **cortex** and contains all of the glomeruli, most of the proximal tubules, and some segments of the distal tubule. The **medulla** forms the inner part of the kidney and consists of regions called the **pyramids. Renal columns** extend from the cortex down between the renal pyramids. The apexes of the pyramids project into **minor calyces** (cup-shaped cavities) that unite to form **major calyces.** The minor calyces receive urine from the collecting ducts through the renal papilla. The major calyces join to form the **renal pelvis,** which connects with the proximal end of the ureter. The walls of the calyces, pelvis, and ureter are lined with epithelial cells and contain smooth muscle cells that contract to move urine to the bladder.

The structural unit of the kidney is the lobe. Each lobe is composed of a pyramid and the overlying cortex. On average, there are 14 lobes in each kidney.

Nephron

The **nephron** is the functional unit of the kidney. Each kidney contains approximately 1.2 million nephrons. The nephron is a tubular structure with subunits that include the renal corpuscle, proximal convoluted tubule, loop of Henle (nephron ansa), distal convoluted tubule, and collecting duct, all of which contribute to the formation of urine (Figure 37-3). The different epithelial cells lining various segments of the tubule facilitate the special functions of reabsorption and secretion (Figure 37-4).

The kidney has three kinds of nephrons: (1) **superficial cortical nephrons** (85% of all nephrons), which extend partially into the medulla; (2) **midcortical nephrons** with short or long loops; and (3) **juxtamedullary nephrons,** which lie close to and extend deep into the medulla and are important for the process

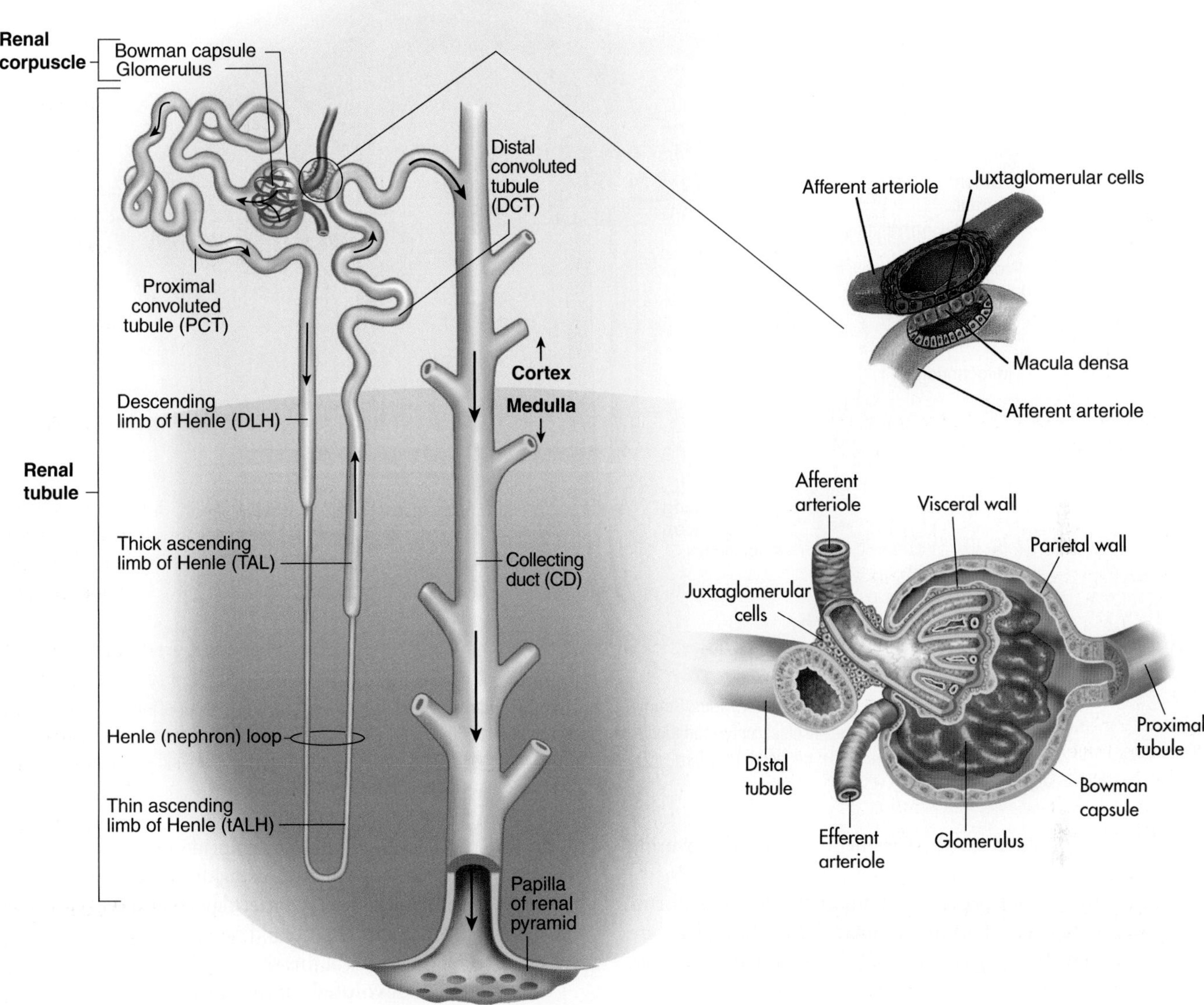

FIGURE 37-3 Components of the Nephron. (From Patton KT, Thibodeau GA: *Anatomy & physiology,* ed 8, St Louis, 2013, Mosby; Damjanov I: *Pathology for health professions,* ed 4, St Louis, 2012, Mosby.)

of concentrating urine (Figure 37-5). The **glomerulus** (Figure 37-6; see also Figure 37-3) is a tuft of capillaries that loop into the circular **Bowman glomerular capsule (Bowman space),** like fingers pushed into bread dough. **Mesangial cells** and the **mesangial matrix,** secreted by mesangial cells, lie between and support the glomerular capillaries. Different mesangial cells contract like smooth muscle cells to regulate glomerular capillary blood flow. They also have phagocytic properties similar to monocytes and release inflammatory cytokines and growth factors.[1] Together, the glomerulus, Bowman capsule, and mesangial cells are called the **renal corpuscle.**

The **glomerular filtration membrane** filters selected blood components through its three layers: (1) the inner layer is the glomerular endothelium, (2) the middle layer is the glomerular basement membrane (GBM), and (3) the outer layer is the visceral epithelium, which forms the inner layer of Bowman capsule. Each layer has unique structural properties that allow all components of the blood to be filtered, with the exception of blood cells and plasma proteins with a molecular weight greater than 70,000 (Figure 37-7; see also Figure 37-6).

Glomerular endothelial cells synthesize nitric oxide (a vasodilator) and endothelin-1 (a vasoconstrictor) that help regulate glomerular blood flow. The **glomerular endothelium** is perforated by many small openings or windows, called *fenestrae.* The fenestrae are maintained by vascular epithelial growth factor (VEGF) produced by the visceral epithelium. The middle basement membrane is composed of a selectively permeable network of proteoglycans (type IV collagen) secreted and maintained by the epithelial cells.[2] The **visceral epithelium** of the Bowman capsule is composed of cells called **podocytes** (foot-like processes)[3]

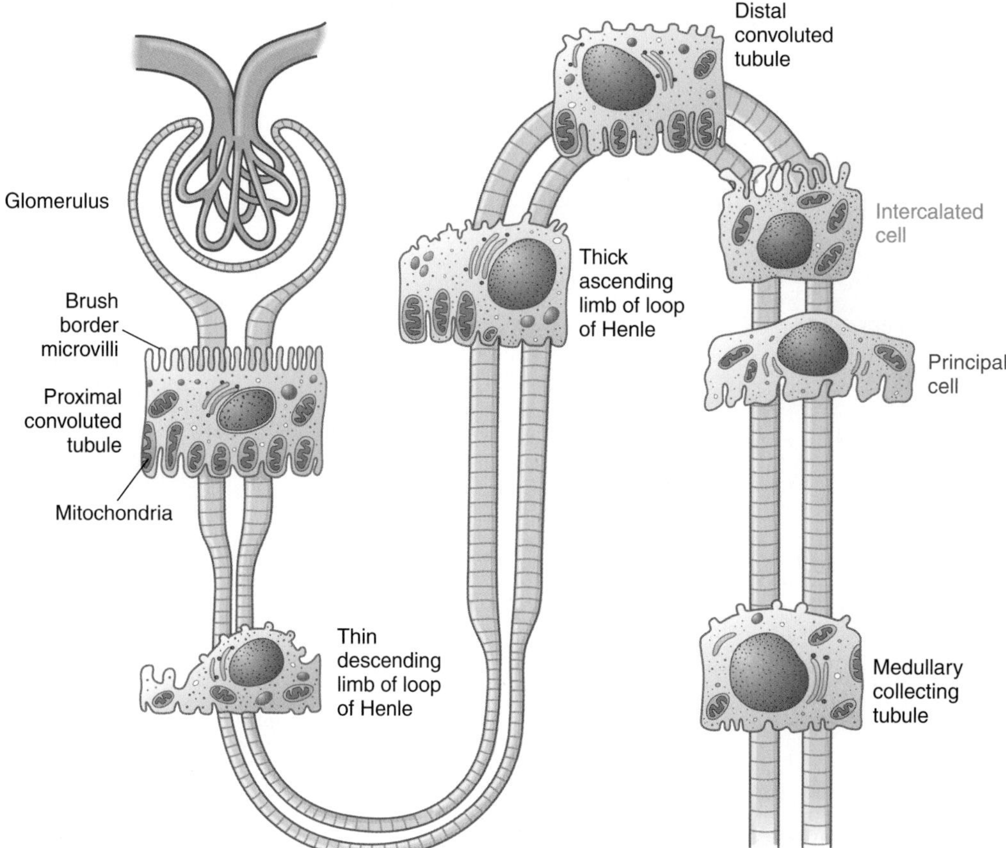

FIGURE 37-4 Epithelial Cells of the Various Segments of Nephron Tubules. The brush border and high number of mitochondria in the cells of the proximal convoluted tubule permit reabsorption of 60% of the glomerular filtrate. *Intercalated cells (blue text)* secrete either H^+ (reabsorb HCO_3^-) or HCO_3^- and reabsorb K^+. *Principal cells (magenta text)* reabsorb Na^+ and water and secrete K^+.

that radiate and adhere to the basement membrane covering the glomerular capillaries. The foot processes of one podocyte interlock with the foot processes of adjacent podocytes, forming an elaborate network of intercellular clefts. These clefts are called **filtration slits** (see Figure 37-7) and modulate filtration. *Nephrin, podocin, CD2-associated protein,* and other protein molecules ensure proper function of the fenestrae.[4]

The podocytes are endocytic, which allow molecules to enter the cell without passing through the cell membrane, and they prevent leakage of proteins into the urine. The visceral epithelium is reflected back at the vascular pole to become the **parietal epithelium.** The space between the visceral and parietal epithelia is the **Bowman (urinary) space,** which is continuous with the lumen of the renal tubules.

Glomerular filtration occurs when plasma filtrate from the glomerulus passes through the three layers of the glomerular membrane into Bowman space to form the primary urine. The endothelium, basement membrane, and podocytes are covered with protein molecules bearing anionic (negative) charges that retard the filtration of anionic proteins and prevent proteinuria.

The glomerulus is supplied by the afferent arteriole and drained by the efferent arteriole. A group of specialized cells known as **juxtaglomerular cells** are located around the afferent arteriole where it enters the glomerulus (see Figures 37-3 and 37-6). Between the afferent and efferent arterioles is a portion of the distal convoluted tubule with specialized sodium- and chloride-sensing cells known as the **macula densa.** Together the juxtaglomerular cells and macula densa cells form the **juxtaglomerular apparatus (JGA)** (see Figure 37-6). Control of renal blood flow, glomerular filtration, and renin secretion occurs at this site.

The **proximal convoluted tubule** continues from the Bowman capsule and has an initial convoluted segment (pars convoluta) and then a straight segment (pars recta) that descends toward the medulla (see Figure 37-3). The wall of the tubule consists of one layer of cuboidal epithelial cells with a surface layer of microvilli (a brush border) that increases reabsorptive surface area. This is the only surface inside the nephron where the cells are covered with microvilli (see Figure 37-4). The proximal convoluted tubule joins the hairpin-shaped **loop of Henle**. The loop is composed of a thin descending segment, thin ascending segment and a thick ascending segment. The thin descending segment is composed of squamous cells, and is highly permeable to water but less permeable to ions. It has no active transport functions. The thin ascending segment is permeable to ions but not to water. The thick ascending segment actively transports ions into the interstitium and passes urine into the distal convoluted tubule (see Figure 37-14).

The more numerous cortical nephrons have glomeruli originating close to the surface of the cortex or in the midcortex, unlike the juxtamedullary nephrons, whose glomeruli are

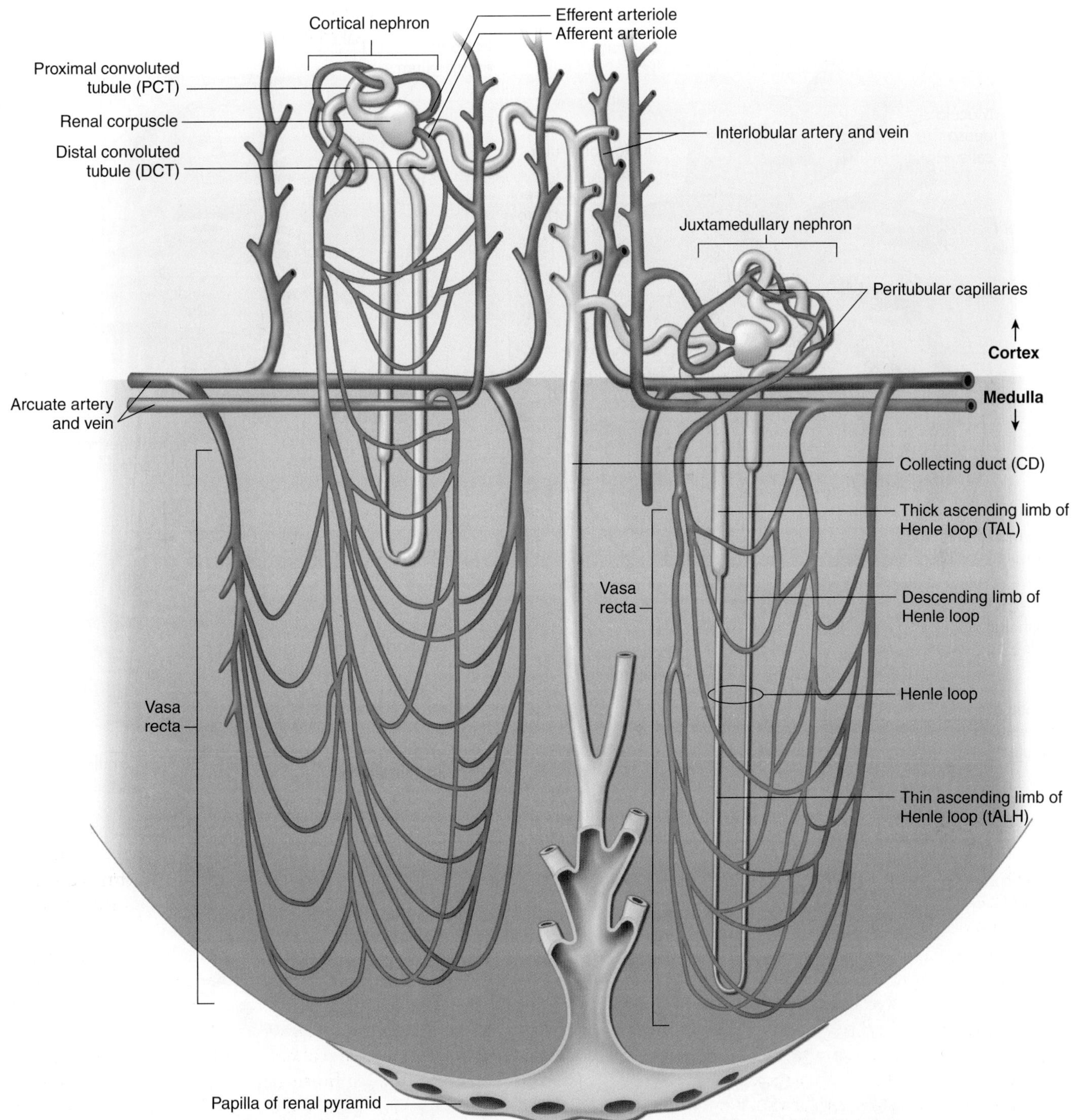

FIGURE 37-5 The Nephron Unit with Its Blood Vessels. Blood flows through nephron vessels as follows: interlobular artery, afferent arteriole, glomerulus, efferent arteriole, peritubular capillaries (around the tubules), venules, interlobular vein. (From Patton KT, Thibodeau GA: *Anatomy & physiology*, ed 8, St Louis, 2013, Mosby.)

located deep in the cortex close to the medulla. The major structural difference between the glomeruli in the two types of nephrons is the length of the loop of Henle. In cortical nephrons the loop is short and may not extend into the medulla. The loop of Henle for the juxtamedullary nephrons, however, may extend the whole length of the medulla (40 mm). Juxtamedullary nephrons represent about 12% of the total number of nephrons and are important for the concentration and dilution of urine.

The **distal convoluted tubule** extends from the distal portion of the loop of Henley to the **collecting duct.** The collecting duct is a large tubule that descends down the cortex through the renal pyramids of the inner and outer medullae, draining urine into the minor calyx. The collecting duct is composed of two epithelial cell types: **principal cells** that reabsorb sodium and water and secrete potassium, and **intercalated cells** that secrete hydrogen and reabsorb potassium (see Figure 34-4).

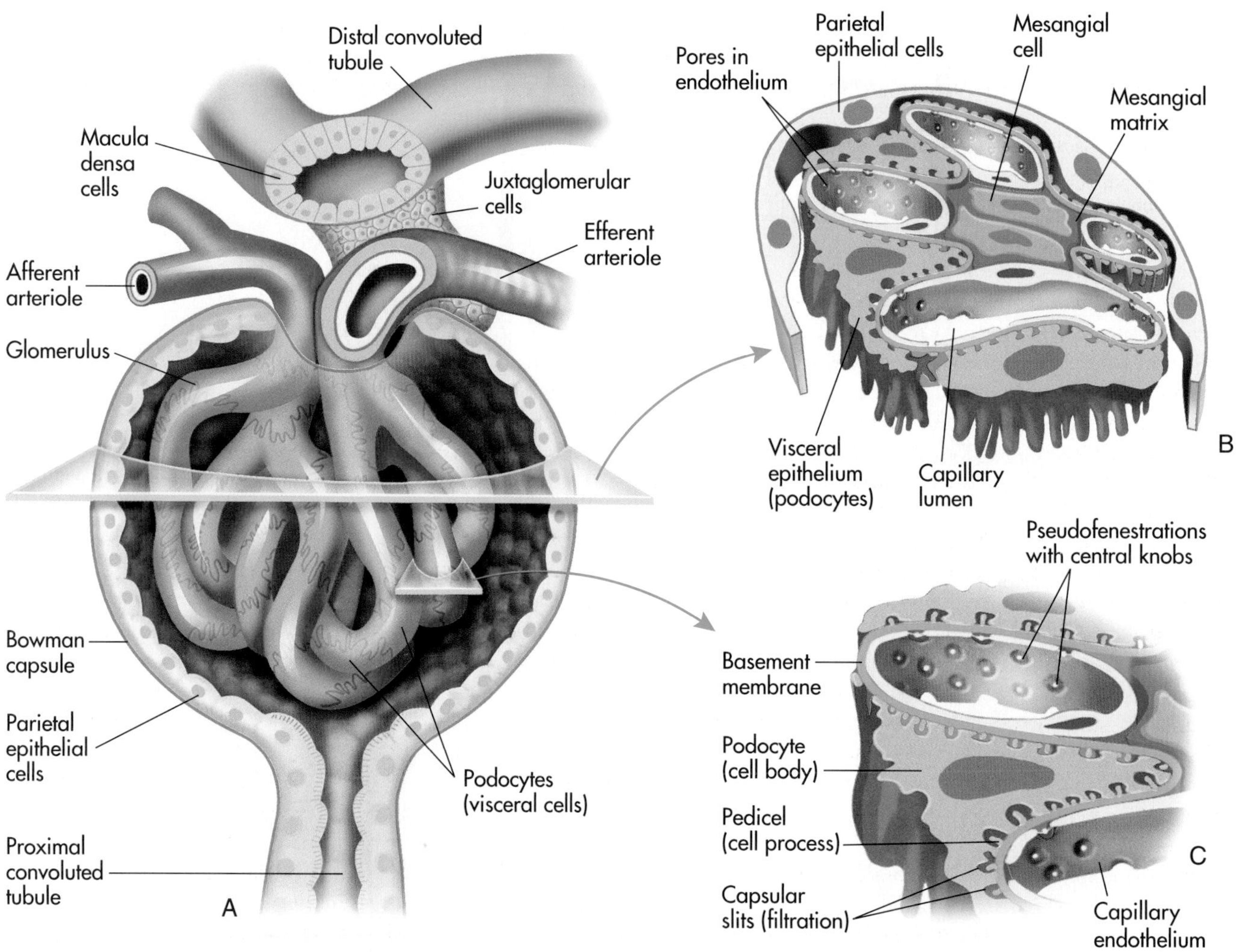

FIGURE 37-6 Anatomy of the Glomerulus and Juxtaglomerular Apparatus. **A,** Longitudinal cross section of glomerulus and juxtaglomerular apparatus. **B,** Horizontal cross section of glomerulus. **C,** Enlargement of glomerular capillary filtration membrane.

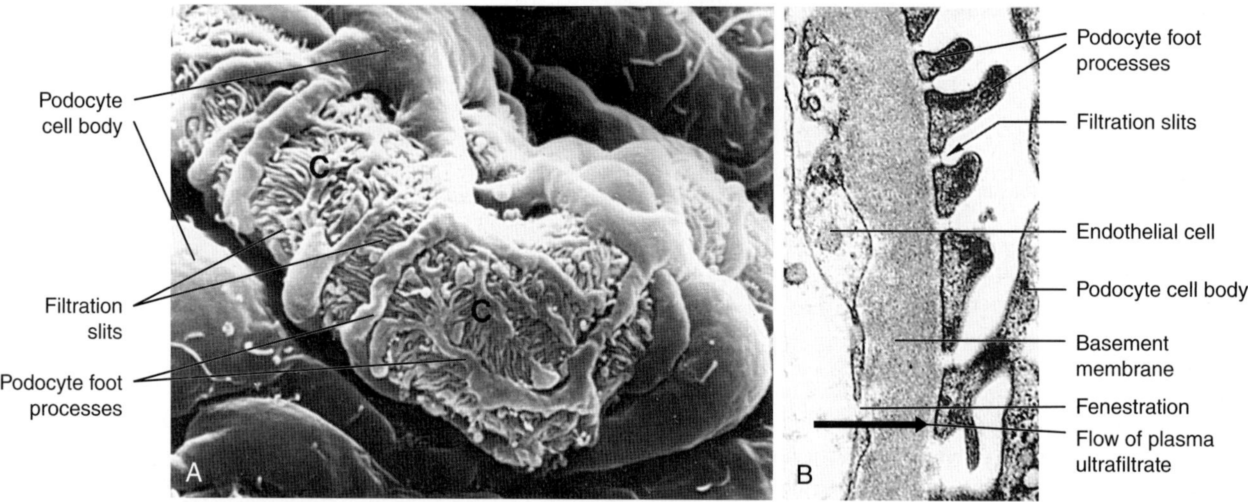

FIGURE 37-7 Glomerular Capillary. **A,** Scanning electron micrograph of normal glomerular capillary *(C).* **B,** Glomerular capillary wall (filtration membrane) (× 40,000). Black arrow indicates direction of urine flow. (From Kissane JM, editor: *Anderson's pathology,* ed 9, St Louis, 1990, Mosby.)

Blood Vessels

The blood vessels of the kidney closely parallel nephron structure. The **renal arteries** arise from the abdominal aorta at the first lumbar vertebra and supply approximately 20% of the cardiac output to the kidneys. At the renal hilum they divide into anterior and posterior branches and then subdivide into lobar arteries that supply blood to the lower, middle, and upper portions of the kidney. The **interlobar arteries** are further subdivisions that travel down the renal columns and between the pyramids. At the cortical-medullary junction, interlobar arteries branch into the **arcuate arteries** that arch over the base of the pyramids and run parallel to the surface of the kidney. The interlobular arteries arise from the arcuate arteries and extend through the cortex toward the periphery of the kidney and supply the afferent glomerular arterioles (see Figure 37-5).

The afferent arterioles subdivide into the glomerulus, a fistlike structure of four to eight **glomerular capillaries** (see Figure 37-6). The glomerular capillaries feed into the efferent arteriole, which conveys blood to a second capillary bed, the peritubular capillaries. This is the only place in the body where an arteriole is positioned between two capillary beds. Increases or decreases in the resistance of the afferent and efferent arterioles increase or decrease glomerular filtration. The **peritubular capillaries** surround the the proximal and distal convoluted tubules and the loop of Henle (see Figure 37-5). The peritubular capillaries are adapted differently for the cortical and juxtamedullary nephrons. The peritubular capillaries surrounding the tubules of the cortical nephrons are similar to capillaries in other tissues. For the juxtamedullary nephrons a network of capillaries called the **vasa recta** forms loops and closely follows the loops of Henle. The capillaries of the vasa recta are the only blood supply to the medulla. They influence the osmolar concentration of the medullary extracellular fluid, which is important to the formation of concentrated urine. All capillaries then drain into the venous system. The renal veins follow the arterial path in a reverse direction and have the same names as the arteries. The renal vein empties into the inferior vena cava. The lymphatic vessels tend also to follow the distribution of the blood vessels.

Urinary Structures

Ureters

The urine formed by the nephrons flows from the distal tubules and collecting ducts through the duct of Bellini and the **renal papillae** (projections of the ducts) into the calyces, where it is collected in the renal pelvis (see Figure 37-2) and then funneled into the **ureters.** Each adult ureter is approximately 30 cm long and is composed of long, intertwining smooth muscle bundles. The lower ends of the ureters pass obliquely through the posterior aspect of the bladder wall. The close approximation of smooth muscle cells permits the direct transmission of electrical stimulation from one cell to another. The resulting downward peristaltic activity propels urine into the bladder. Contraction of the bladder during **micturition** (urination) compresses the lower end of the ureter, preventing reflux. Peristalsis is maintained even when the ureter is denervated, so ureters can be transplanted.

Sensory innervation for the upper part of the ureter arises from the tenth thoracic nerve roots, with referred pain to the umbilicus. The innervation of lower segments arises from the sacral nerves with referred pain to the vulva or penis. The ureters have a rich blood supply. The primary arteries come from the kidney with contributions from the lumbar and superior vesical arteries.

Bladder and Urethra

The **bladder** is a bag composed of a basket weave of smooth muscle fibers that forms the **detrusor muscle** and its smooth lining of **transitional epithelium (uroepithelium).** As the bladder fills with urine, it distends and the layers of transitional epithelial cells within the lining slide past each other and become thinner as the volume of the bladder increases. The transitional epithelium forms the interface between the urinary space and underlying vasculature, connective, nervous, and muscle tissue. It senses and transduces information about luminal pressure and urine composition within the urinary tract.[5] The **trigone** is a smooth triangular area lying between the openings of the two ureters and the urethra (Figure 37-8). The position of the bladder varies with age and gender. In infants and young children the bladder rises above the symphysis pubis, providing easy access for percutaneous aspiration. In adults it lies in the true pelvis, in front of the rectum and in front of the uterus in women. Inferiorly, the bladder sits on the prostate in men and on the anterior vagina in women. The bladder has a profuse blood supply, accounting for the bleeding that readily occurs with trauma, surgery, or inflammation.

The **urethra** extends from the inferior side of the bladder to the outside of the body. Two muscles called *sphincters* control excretion of urine from the bladder through the urethra. A ring of smooth muscle forms the **internal urethral sphincter** at the junction of the urethra and bladder. The **external urethral sphincter** is composed of striated skeletal muscle and is under voluntary control. The entire urethra is lined with mucus-secreting glands. The female urethra is short (3 to 4 cm). The male urethra is long (18 to 20 cm) and has three main segments: prostatic, membranous, and penile. The prostatic urethra is

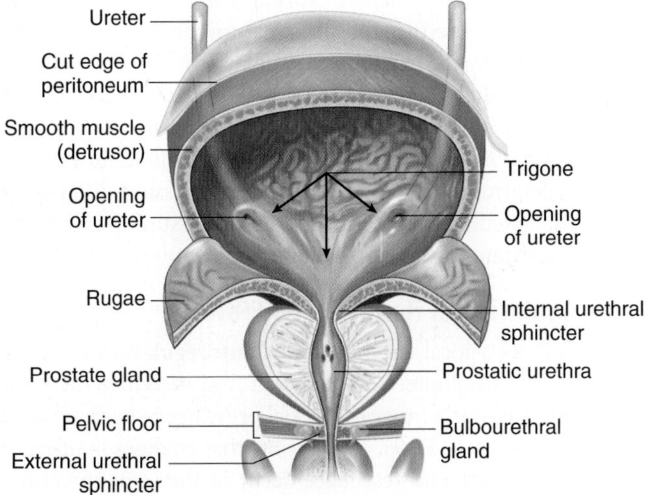

FIGURE 37-8 **Structure and Location of the Urinary Bladder.** Frontal view of a dissected urinary bladder (male) in a fully distended position. (From Patton KT, Thibodeau GA: *Anatomy & physiology*, ed 8, St Louis, 2013, Mosby.)

closest to the bladder. It passes through the prostate gland and contains the openings of the ejaculatory ducts. The membranous urethra is the segment that passes through the floor of the pelvis. The penile segment forms the remainder of the tube. The penile segment is surrounded by the corpus spongiosum erectile tissue and contains the openings of the bulbourethral glands.

The innervation of the bladder and internal urethral sphincter is supplied by parasympathetic fibers of the autonomic nervous system that arise from the sacral levels of the spinal cord (S2 to S4). Sensory fibers from the bladder and urethra may extend as high as the T6 portion of the spinal cord. Skeletal motor neurons in the pudendal nerve innervate the external urethral sphincter. The reflex arc required for micturition is stimulated by mechanoreceptors that respond to stretching of tissue. The mechanoreceptors sense bladder fullness and send impulses to the sacral level of the spinal cord with bladder filling. When the bladder accumulates 250 to 300 ml of urine, the bladder contracts and the internal urethral sphincter relaxes through activation of the spinal reflex arc (known as the *micturition reflex*). At this time a person feels the urge to void. In older children and adults, the reflex can be inhibited or facilitated by impulses coming from the brain, resulting in voluntary control of micturition.

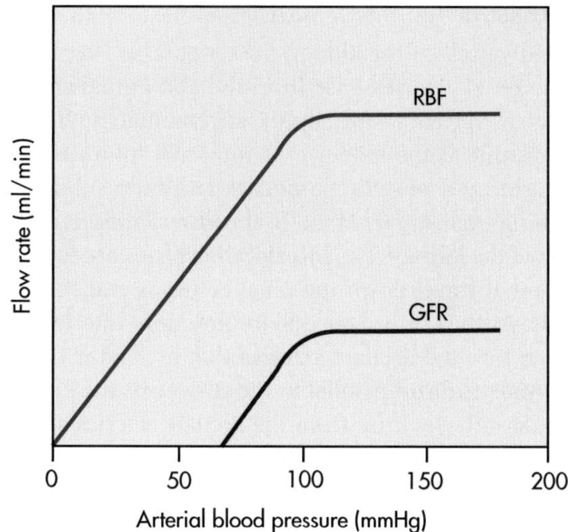

FIGURE 37-9 Autoregulation of Renal Blood Flow. Blood flow and glomerular filtration rate are stabilized with changes in mean arterial pressure between about 80 and 180 mmHg. (From Berne RM, Levy MN, editors: *Principles of physiology,* ed 4, St Louis, 2006, Mosby.) *GFR,* Glomerular filtration rate; *RBF,* renal blood flow.

RENAL BLOOD FLOW

The kidneys are highly vascular organs and receive about 20% to 25% of the cardiac output, which in adults is equivalent to 1000 to 1200 ml of blood per minute. With a normal hematocrit of 45%, about 600 to 700 ml of blood flowing through the kidney per minute is plasma. From the renal plasma flow (RPF), 20% (approximately 120 to 140 ml/minute) is filtered at the glomerulus and passes into the Bowman capsule. The filtration of the plasma per unit of time is known as the **glomerular filtration rate (GFR),** which is directly related to the perfusion pressure in the glomerular capillaries.

The remaining 80% (about 480 ml/minute) of plasma flows through the efferent arterioles to the peritubular capillaries. The ratio of glomerular filtrate to RPF per minute (120/600 = 0.20) is called the *filtration fraction.* Normally all but 1 to 2 ml per minute of the glomerular filtrate is reabsorbed and returned to the circulation by the peritubular capillaries.

The GFR is directly related to renal blood flow (RBF), which is regulated by intrinsic autoregulatory mechanisms, neural regulation, and hormonal regulation. In general, blood flow to any organ is determined by the arteriovenous pressure differences across the vascular bed. If mean arterial pressure decreases or vascular resistance increases, renal blood flow decreases.

Autoregulation of Renal Blood Flow

In the kidney a local mechanism of **autoregulation** tends to keep the rate of glomerular perfusion and therefore the GFR fairly constant over a range of arterial pressures between 80 and 180 mmHg (Figure 37-9). This means that changes in afferent arteriolar pressure and resistance occur in the same direction. For example, as systemic blood pressure increases, the afferent arterioles constrict, preventing an increase in filtration pressure. Opposite processes occur with a decrease in systemic blood pressure. Therefore, renal blood flow and GFR are relatively constant. The purpose of renal autoregulation is to prevent wide fluctuations in systemic arterial pressure from being transmitted to the glomerular capillaries. In this way, large fluctuations in GFR are prevented and solute and water excretion is constantly maintained despite arterial pressure changes.[6] Autoregulation may also protect the kidney from damage by hypertension.

One mechanism responsible for the autoregulatory response in the kidney is a **myogenic mechanism.** As arterial pressure declines, the stretch on the afferent arteriolar smooth muscle decreases and the arteriole relaxes, causing an increase in glomerular perfusion; an increase in arteriolar pressure causes the arteriole smooth muscle to contract and decreases glomerular perfusion. **Tubuloglomerular feedback** is a second mechanism for keeping renal blood flow and GFR constant and stable. As the GFR in an individual nephron increases or decreases, the macula densa cells in the distal tubule sense the increasing or decreasing amounts of filtered sodium. When sodium filtration increases, the macula densa cells stimulate afferent arteriolar vasoconstriction to decrease GFR. The opposite occurs with decreases in sodium filtration at the macula densa.[7] A third unknown mechanism also contributes to autoregulation.[8]

Neural Regulation

The blood vessels of the kidney are innervated by sympathetic adrenergic/noradrenergic fibers that cause arteriolar vasoconstriction to reduce renal blood flow. The innervation of the kidney comes primarily from the celiac ganglion and greater splanchnic nerve (see Figure 15-25). The afferent and efferent arterioles are richly innervated, but nerves have not been observed in the glomerular capillaries.

Renal blood flow is reflexively related to the systemic arterial pressure. When systemic arterial pressure decreases, increased sympathetic nerve activity is mediated reflexively through feedback from the baroreceptors of the carotid sinus and aortic arch. This is achieved through the baroreceptor reflex, which stimulates vasoconstriction of the afferent arterioles with activation of α_1-adrenoreceptors. This decreases glomerular perfusion and GFR, although autoregulatory processes dampen the response. Decreased GFR diminishes excretion of sodium and water, promoting an increase in blood volume and thus an increase in blood pressure.

Exercise, body position, and hypoxia also influence renal blood flow. Exercise and change of body position activate renal sympathetic neurons and cause mild vasoconstriction. Severe hypoxia stimulates the chemoreceptors of the carotid and aortic bodies and decreases renal blood flow by means of sympathetic stimulation.

Hormones and Other Factors

Hormonal factors and many mediators can alter the resistance of the renal vasculature by stimulating vasodilation or vasoconstriction. A major hormonal regulator of renal blood flow is the renin-angiotensin-aldosterone system (RAAS), which can increase systemic arterial pressure and increase sodium reabsorption. Renin is an enzyme formed and stored in granular cells of the afferent arterioles of the JGA (see Figure 37-3). The release of renin is principally triggered by decreased blood pressure in the afferent arterioles, which reduces stretch of the juxtaglomerular cells; decreased sodium chloride concentrations in the distal convoluted tubule; sympathetic nerve stimulation of β-adrenergic receptors on the juxtaglomerular cells; and release of prostaglandins.[9]

When renin is released, it cleaves an α-globulin (angiotensinogen produced by liver hepatocytes) in the plasma to form angiotensin I, which is physiologically inactive. In the presence of angiotensin-converting enzyme (ACE) produced from the pulmonary and renal endothelium, angiotensin I is converted to angiotensin II. **Angiotensin II** stimulates secretion of aldosterone by the adrenal cortex (see Chapter 21), is a potent vasoconstrictor, and stimulates antidiuretic hormone (ADH) secretion and thirst. Vitamin D_3 is a potent negative endocrine regulator of renin gene expression.[10] Numerous physiologic effects of the RAAS serve the purpose of stabilizing systemic blood pressure and preserving the extracellular fluid volume during hypotension or hypovolemia, including sodium reabsorption, potassium excretion, systemic vasoconstriction, sympathetic nerve stimulation, thirst stimulation, and drinking. (The combined effects of the RAAS are summarized in Figure 37-10.) ACE inhibitors are a class of drugs that reduce blood pressure by inhibiting the formation of angiotensin II and aldosterone.

Natriuretic peptides are a group of peptide hormones, including **atrial natriuretic peptide (ANP),** secreted from myocardial cells in the atria and **brain natriuretic peptide (BNP)** secreted from myocardial cells in the cardiac ventricles. When the heart dilates during volume expansion or heart failure, ANP and BNP inhibit sodium and water absorption by kidney tubules, inhibit secretion of renin and aldosterone, vasodilate the afferent arterioles, and constrict the efferent arterioles. The result is increased urine formation leading to decreased blood volume and blood pressure.[11] **C-type natriuretic peptide** is secreted from vascular endothelium and in the nephron and causes vasodilation.[12] **Urodilatin** is secreted by the distal convoluted tubules and collecting ducts and causes vasodilation and natriuretic and diuretic effects. Other hormones and mediators that influence renal blood flow are summarized in Table 37-1.

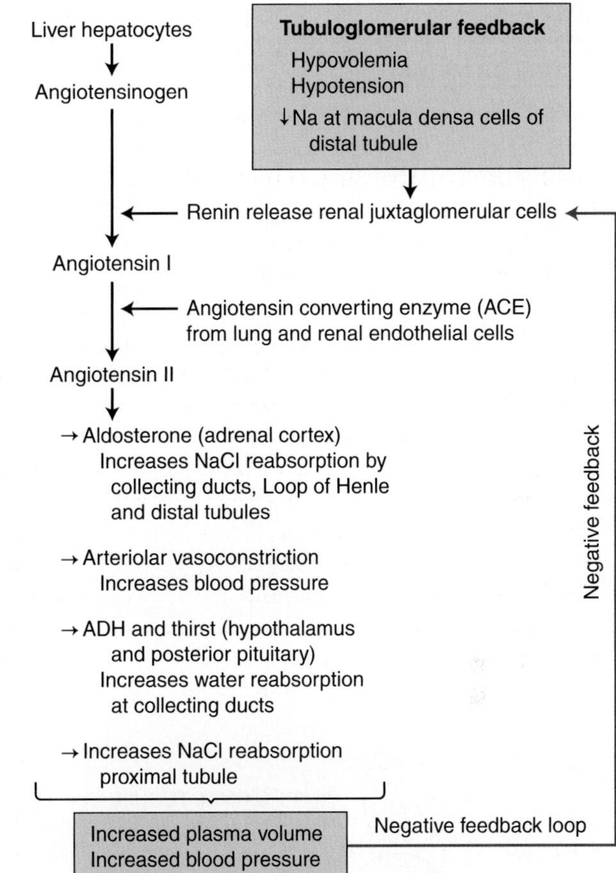

FIGURE 37-10 Renin-Angiotensin-Aldosterone System. Activation of tubuloglomerular feedback mechanisms stimulates the release of renin with activation of the renin-angiotensin-aldosterone system. Plasma volume and blood pressure are increased with the reabsorption of sodium chloride and water from the renal tubules. The restoration of plasma volume and blood pressure then decrease the release of renin, forming a negative feedback loop. *ADH,* Antidiuretic hormone.

KIDNEY FUNCTION

The major function of the kidney is urine formation and involves the processes of filtration, reabsorption, and secretion. These processes are the function of the nephrons. Fluid is filtered at the glomerulus. Substances are reabsorbed from the filtrate or secreted into the filtrate by the renal tubules. The final urine flows into the minor and major calyces, and then is propelled by the ureters to the bladder for storage and elimination.

Nephron Function

The nephron can perform many functions simultaneously. It filters the plasma at the glomerulus and reabsorbs and secretes different substances at various parts of its tubular structure (Figure 37-11). The function of the nephron is to form a filtrate

TABLE 37-1 HORMONES, MEDIATORS, AND RENAL BLOOD FLOW

HORMONE OR MEDIATOR	EFFECT ON RENAL BLOOD FLOW
Adenosine	Produced within kidney; causes vasoconstriction of afferent arteriole; decreases RBF and GFR
Angiotensin II	Produced systemically and within kidneys; constricts afferent and efferent arterioles; decreases RBF and GFR
Atrial and brain natriuretic peptides	Produced by atria and ventricles of the heart with hypertension and increased blood volume; causes vasodilation of afferent arteriole and vasoconstriction of efferent arteriole; modest increase in GFR with little change in RBF
Bradykinin	Produced in kidney from kininogen and causes vasodilation by release of nitric oxide and prostaglandins; increases RBF and GFR
Dopamine	Produced by the proximal tubule; increases RBF; inhibits renin secretion
Endothelin	Produced by renal vessel endothelial cells, mesangial cells, and distal tubule cells in response to bradykinin, angiotensin II, epinephrine, and stretch; most active with renal disease; profound vasoconstriction of afferent and efferent arterioles; decreases RBF and GFR
Histamine	Produced locally within the kidney; modulates RBF in basal state and during inflammation; increases RBF by decreasing afferent and efferent arteriolar resistance and does not decrease GFR
Nitric oxide	Produced by renal vessel endothelial cells with increased stretch and by stimulation of acetylcholine, histamine, bradykinin, ATP; increases vasodilation of afferent and efferent arterioles
Prostaglandins, PGI_2, PGE_2	Produced locally within kidney with decreased RBF; dampen vasoconstriction caused by sympathetic nerves and angiotensin II; prevent harmful vasoconstriction and renal ischemia
Urodilatin (a natriuretic peptide)	Produced by distal tubule and collecting duct when there is increased circulating volume and increased blood pressure; inhibits sodium and water reabsorption from medullary part of collecting duct, thereby producing diuresis

GFR, Glomerular filtration rate; *RBF,* renal blood flow.

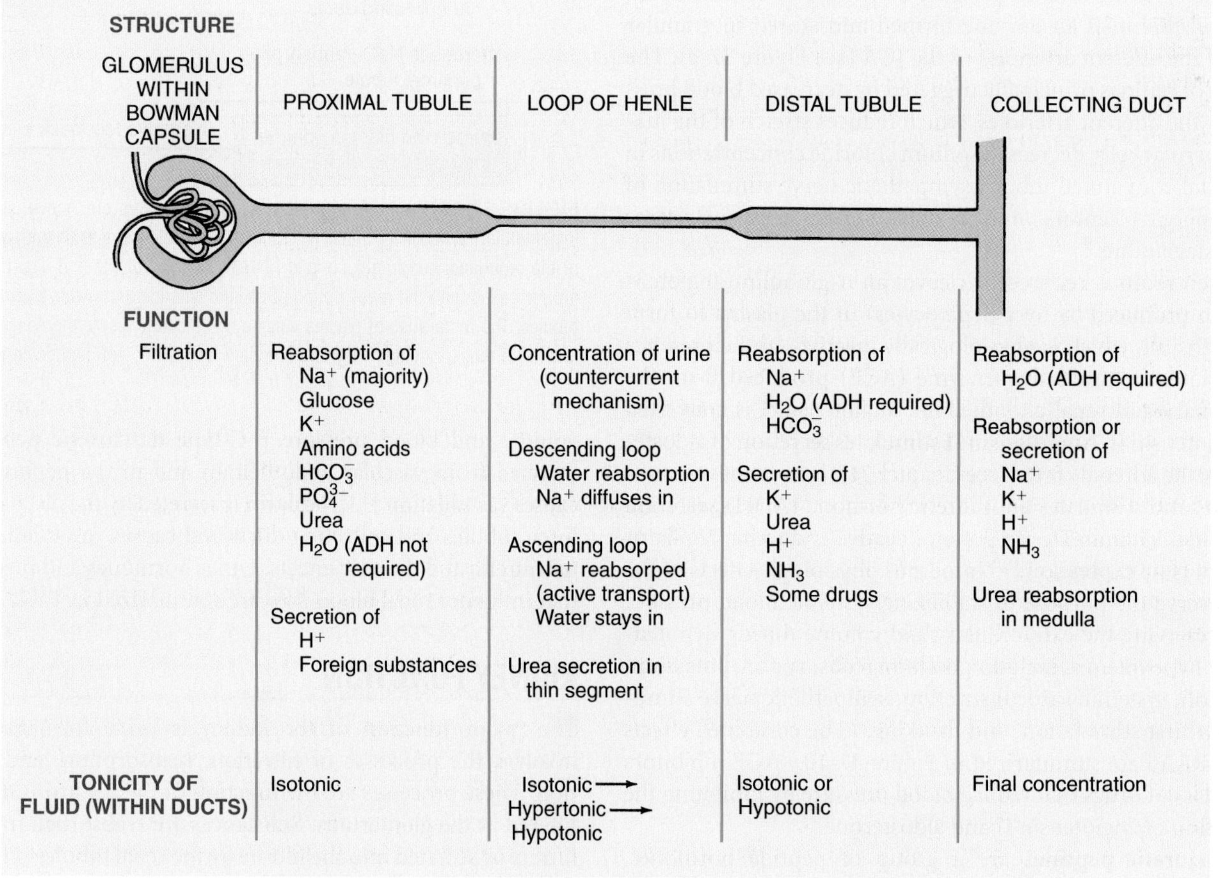

FIGURE 37-11 Major Functions of Nephron Segments. *ADH,* Antidiuretic hormone. (Modified from Hockenberry MJ: *Wong's nursing care of infants and children,* ed 8, St Louis, 2007, Mosby.)

of protein-free plasma. This process, known as **ultrafiltration,** occurs across the glomerular membrane. The nephron then regulates the filtrate to maintain body fluid volume, electrolyte composition, and pH within narrow limits.

Regulation of the filtrate occurs through two processes: tubular reabsorption and tubular secretion. **Tubular reabsorption** is the movement of fluids and solutes from the tubular lumen to the peritubular capillary plasma. Transfer of substances from the plasma of the peritubular capillary to the tubular lumen is **tubular secretion.** The mechanisms involve active as well as passive transport. **Excretion** is the elimination of a substance in the final urine (Figure 37-12).

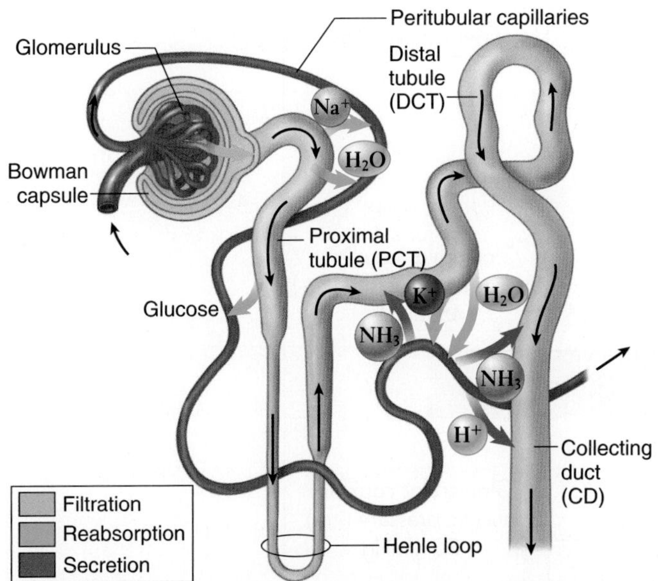

FIGURE 37-12 **Urine Formation: Glomerular Filtration, Tubular Reabsorption, and Tubular Secretion.** The three processes by which the kidneys excrete urine. Water, electrolytes, glucose, and organic molecules are filtered at the glomerulus. Sodium and glucose are reabsorbed into peritubular capillaries by active transport from the proximal convoluted tubules and water reabsorption follows by osmosis. Sodium is reabsorbed by active transport from distal convoluted tubules; more sodium is conserved when aldosterone is secreted. Osmotic reabsorption of water from them occurs when ADH is present. Secretion of ammonia (NH_3), hydrogen, and potassium occurs from peritubular capillaries into distal tubules by active transport. (From Patton KT, Thibodeau GA: *Anatomy & physiology*, ed 8, St Louis, 2013, Mosby.)

Glomerular Filtration

The fluid filtered by the glomerular capillary filtration membrane is protein free but contains electrolytes such as sodium, chloride, and potassium and organic molecules such as creatinine, urea, and glucose in the same concentrations as in plasma. Like other capillary membranes, the glomerulus is freely permeable to water and relatively impermeable to large colloids such as plasma proteins. The size of the molecules and their electrical charge are important factors affecting the permeability of substances crossing the glomerulus. The small size of the filtration slits in the glomerular epithelium restricts the passage of proteins and other macromolecules. The negative charge along the filtration membrane further impedes the passage of negatively charged macromolecules (because like forces repel each other). Positively charged macromolecules therefore permeate the membrane more readily than neutrally charged particles.

Capillary pressures also affect glomerular filtration. The hydrostatic pressure within the capillary is the major force for inducing water and solute movement across the filtration membrane into Bowman capsule. This pressure is determined by the systemic arterial pressure and the resistances to blood flow in the afferent and efferent arterioles. Two forces oppose the filtration effects of the glomerular capillary hydrostatic pressure (P_{GC}): (1) the hydrostatic pressure in Bowman space (P_{BC}), and (2) the effective oncotic pressure of the glomerular capillary blood (π_{GC}). (As explained in Chapter 3, hydrostatic pressure is a pushing force in relation to water, and oncotic pressure is a pulling force.) Because the fluid in Bowman space normally contains only minute amounts of protein, it usually does not have an oncotic influence on the plasma of the glomerular capillary (Figure 37-13).

The combined effect of forces favoring and forces opposing filtration determines the filtration pressure. The **net filtration pressure (NFP)** is the sum of forces favoring and opposing filtration and is expressed by the following equation:

$$\text{NFP} = (P_{GC} + \pi_{BC}) \text{ (forces favoring filtration)} - (P_{BC} + \pi_{GC}) \text{ (forces opposing filtration)}$$

The estimated values contributing to the forces of net filtration are presented in Figure 37-13.

As the protein-free fluid is filtered into Bowman capsule, the plasma oncotic pressure increases and the hydrostatic pressure decreases. The increase in glomerular capillary oncotic pressure is great enough to reduce the net filtration pressure to zero at the efferent end of the capillary and to stop the filtration process effectively. The low hydrostatic pressure and increased oncotic pressure in the efferent arteriole then are transferred to the peritubular capillaries and facilitate reabsorption of fluid from the proximal convoluted tubules.

Filtration Rate. The total volume of fluid filtered by the glomeruli averages 180 L/day, or approximately 120 ml/minute, a phenomenal amount considering the size of the kidneys. Because only 1 to 2 L of urine is excreted per day, 99% of the filtrate is reabsorbed into the peritubular capillaries and thus is returned to the blood. The factors determining the GFR are directly related to the pressures that favor or oppose filtration. Any changes in afferent or efferent arteriolar resistance will alter glomerular capillary hydrostatic pressure and GFR. Vasoconstriction of one or the other of these two arterioles produces opposite effects on glomerular pressure. For example, if the afferent arteriole constricts, blood flow decreases, with a corresponding drop in glomerular pressure. The GFR then decreases, and body fluids are conserved. Conversely, constriction of the efferent arteriole increases the net filtration pressure, and the GFR increases. When both afferent and efferent arterioles constrict, little change occurs in filtration pressure, but renal blood flow is reduced and so is the GFR.

Obstruction to the outflow of urine (caused by strictures, stones, or tumors along the urinary tract) can cause a retrograde increase in pressure at Bowman capsule and a decrease in GFR. Low levels of plasma protein in the blood from severe malnutrition or liver disease result in a decrease in π_{GC}, which increases GFR. Excessive loss of protein-free fluid from vomiting, diarrhea, use of diuretics, or excessive sweating can increase glomerular capillary oncotic pressure and decrease the GFR. Renal disease also can cause changes in pressure relationships by altering capillary permeability and the surface area available for filtration (see Chapter 38).

Tubular Transport. By the time the filtrate reaches the end of the proximal convoluted tubule, approximately 60% to 70% of filtered sodium and water and about 50% of urea have been reabsorbed, along with 90% or more of potassium, glucose, bicarbonate, calcium, phosphate, amino acids, and uric acid. All this occurs by active transport. Chloride, water, and urea are reabsorbed passively but are linked to the active transport of

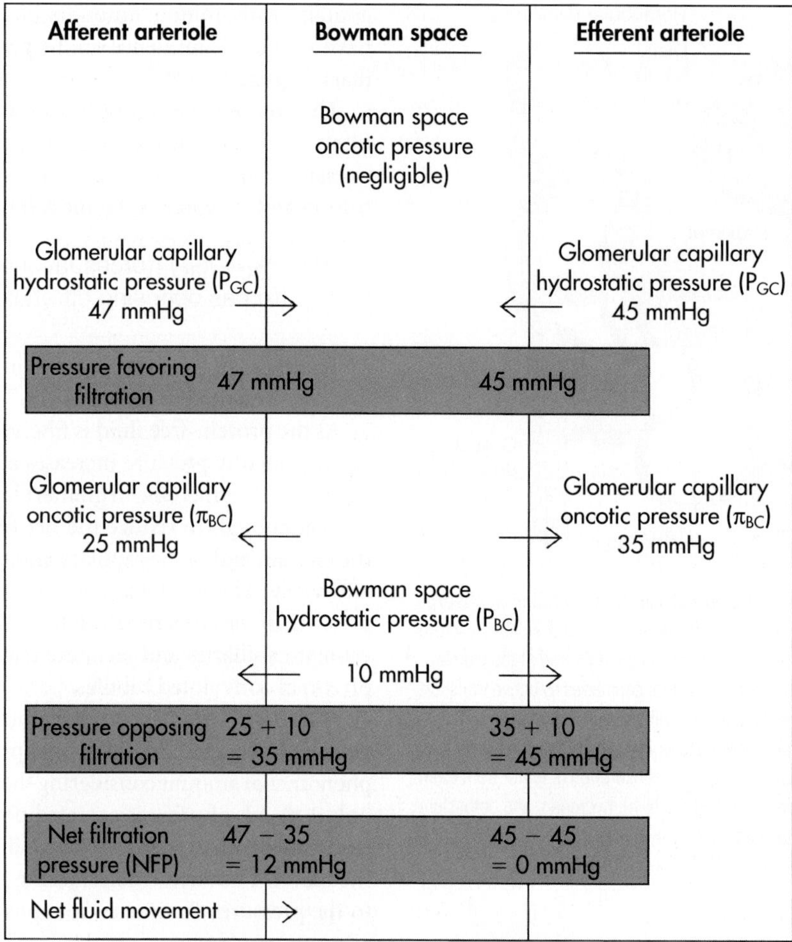

FIGURE 37-13 Glomerular Filtration Pressures.

sodium (a cotransport mechanism). For some molecules, active transport in the renal tubules is limited as carrier molecules become saturated, a phenomenon known as **transport maximum (T_m).** The reabsorption of glucose is an important example. Glucose reabsorption in the proximal convoluted tubule is coupled to sodium transport and has a maximal transport capacity, or renal threshold. This means that when the carrier molecules for glucose become saturated, what is not reabsorbed is excreted in the urine. Normally the plasma level and filtered glucose load are not high enough to saturate the carrier mechanism. When the plasma glucose concentration reaches 180 mg/dl, however, as occurs in the individual with uncontrolled diabetes mellitus, the renal threshold for glucose is achieved. Any further increase in the plasma level causes loss of glucose in the urine.

Proximal Convoluted Tubule. Active reabsorption of sodium is the primary function of the proximal convoluted tubule. Water, most other electrolytes, and organic substances are cotransported with sodium. The osmotic force generated by active sodium transport promotes the passive diffusion of water out of the tubular lumen and into the peritubular capillaries. Passive transport of water is further enhanced by the elevated oncotic pressure of the blood in the peritubular capillaries. The reabsorption of water leaves an increased concentration of urea within the tubular lumen, creating a gradient for its passive diffusion to the peritubular plasma.

As the positively charged sodium ions leave the tubular lumen, negatively charged chloride ions passively follow to maintain electroneutrality. Because the inner membrane of the proximal tubular cell has a limited permeability to chloride, chloride reabsorption lags behind sodium.

Hydrogen ions are actively exchanged for sodium ions in the tubular lumen. The hydrogen ions (H^+) then combine with bicarbonate (HCO_3^-) in the tubular lumen to form carbonic acid (H_2CO_3). The carbonic acid rapidly breaks down, or dissociates, to carbon dioxide (CO_2) and water (H_2O), which then diffuse into the tubular cell where carbonic anhydrase catalyzes the reaction between CO_2 and H_2O to form HCO_3^- and H^+. HCO_3^- combines with sodium and is transported (reabsorbed) to the peritubular capillary blood. The H^+ is not excreted but is again exchanged for sodium and reenters the lumen to recombine with HCO_3^-. Thus, in the proximal convoluted tubule, for every H^+ ion secreted into the tubular lumen, a HCO_3^- ion enters the blood (see Figure 3-13, p. 126).

Bicarbonate is freely filtered at the glomerulus, but is not readily reabsorbed because the peritubular capillary membrane is not highly permeable to the molecule. As described previously, HCO_3^- combines with H^+ in the tubular cell and is eventually reabsorbed as CO_2 and H_2O. One of the unusual aspects of this process is that the bicarbonate molecule filtered at the glomerulus is not the same molecule that is reabsorbed

BOX 37-1 SUBSTANCES TRANSPORTED BY RENAL TUBULES

REABSORPTION	SECRETION
Albumin	Choline
Ascorbate	Creatinine
Fructose	Histamine
Galactose	Methyl guanidine
Glucose	*para*-Aminohippurate
Glutamate	Penicillin
Phosphate	Steroid glucuronides
Sulfate	Thiamine
Xylose	

(because it dissociates) and the hydrogen ion secreted by the proximal tubule is not excreted in the urine. Bicarbonate is thus conserved, and in this exchange, bicarbonate and hydrogen normally do not contribute to the urinary excretion of acid or the addition of acid to the blood. In the form of CO_2 and H_2O, approximately 90% of filtered bicarbonate is reabsorbed by the proximal tubules.

In addition to the proximal tubular secretion of hydrogen ions, secretory transport maximums (T_m) exist for creatinine, other organic bases, and endogenous and exogenous organic acids, including *para*-aminohippurate (PAH) and penicillin (Box 37-1). These secretory mechanisms are important for eliminating drugs and other exogenous chemical products from the body. Frequently, exogenous substances are conjugated with sulfate and glucuronic acid by the liver and then actively secreted by the renal tubules. This has important clinical implications because many drugs and their metabolites are eliminated from the body in this way. When the renal tubules are damaged, metabolic byproducts and drugs may accumulate, causing toxic levels in the body.

Loop of Henle and Distal Convoluted Tubule. The filtrate entering and leaving the proximal convoluted tubule is essentially isosmotic with the plasma and has a concentration of about 285 mOsm. Although approximately 65% of salt and water is reabsorbed along the proximal tubule, they are reabsorbed in equal amounts, causing only minor changes in the osmotic and electrolyte concentrations of the fluid flowing into the loop of Henle. Therefore, any concentration or dilution of urine occurs at more distal sites of the nephron, principally in the medullary loop of Henle and collecting ducts. Near the top of the renal pyramids, the interstitial osmolality reaches 1200 mOsm/L.

These quantitative changes taking place in the loop of Henle are related to the length of the loop and its depth of penetration into the medulla. The structural features of the medullary hairpin loops provide the kidney with the ability to concentrate urine and conserve water for the body. The transition of the filtrate into urine is a function of the concentrating ability of the loops and final adjustments in urine composition made by the distal tubule and collecting duct.

The primary function of the loop of Henle is to establish a hyperosmotic state within the medullary interstitial fluid. This is achieved by reabsorbing more solute than water into the interstitium. The fluid leaving the ascending limb of the loop is therefore hypoosmotic, or more dilute than the fluid that entered. This dilution allows the distal tubule and collecting duct to make final adjustments in the concentration or dilution of the excreted urine according to body needs. The vasa recta act to maintain the high osmotic gradient established by the loop of Henle (see Figure 37-14, p. 1332).

Different transport or permeability functions of the loop of Henle are important for dilution and concentration of urine. The thin, descending segment of the loop of Henle is highly permeable to water and moderately permeable to sodium, urea, and other solutes. The thin, ascending segment is more permeable to solutes and almost impermeable to water. The thick portion of the ascending segment is highly permeable to sodium, potassium, and chloride and significantly less permeable to water and urea. *Tamm-Horsfall glycoprotein,* also known as uromodulin, is formed on the epithelial surface of the thick ascending segment and the first segment of the distal tubule. It is the most abundant urinary protein and protects against bacterial adhesion and urolithiasis, and is a ligand for lymphokines.[13]

The convoluted portion of the distal tubule has limited permeability to water but readily absorbs ions and contributes to the dilution of the tubular fluid. The later, straight segment of the distal tubule and the collecting duct are permeable to water as controlled by ADH. Sodium is readily absorbed by the later segment of the distal tubule and collecting duct under the regulation of the hormone aldosterone (see Chapter 21). Potassium is actively secreted by principal cells and is reabsorbed in lesser amounts by intercalated cells in these segments. Potassium secretion is controlled by aldosterone and other factors related to the concentration of potassium in body fluids.[14]

Hydrogen is also secreted by the distal tubule and combines with non–bicarbonate buffers (ammonium and phosphate) for the elimination of excess acids in the urine. The distal tubule thus contributes to the regulation of acid-base balance by excreting hydrogen ions into the urine and by adding new bicarbonate to the plasma (see Figure 3-13, p. 126). The mechanism is similar to the conservation of bicarbonate by the proximal tubule, except that the hydrogen ion is excreted in the urine. (The specific mechanisms of acid-base balance and acid excretion are described in Chapter 3.)

Glomerulotubular Balance. Normally, 99% of the glomerular filtrate is reabsorbed. When the GFR spontaneously decreases or increases, the renal tubules and, primarily the proximal tubules, automatically adjust their rate of reabsorption of sodium and water to balance the change in GFR. Thus a constant fraction of filtered sodium and water is reabsorbed from the proximal tubule. This prevents wide fluctuations in sodium and water excretion into the urine and maintains sodium and water balance.[15]

Concentration and Dilution of Urine

The production of concentrated urine involves a **countercurrent exchange system,** in which fluid flows in opposite directions through parallel tubes. A concentration gradient causes fluid to be exchanged across the parallel pathways. In the nephron the fluid moves up and down the parallel sides of the hairpin loop of Henle in the medulla. The longer the loop, the greater the concentration gradient because the concentration gradient increases from the cortex to the tip of the medulla. The loops of Henle therefore serve as multipliers of the concentration

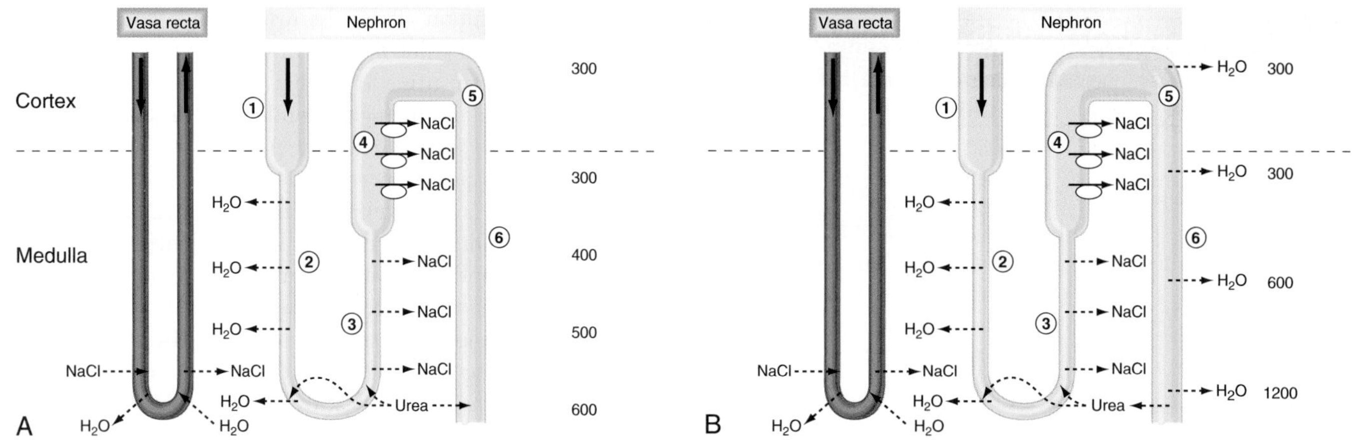

FIGURE 37-14 **Countercurrent Mechanism for Concentrating and Diluting Urine. A,** Urine dilution; **B,** urine concentration. **1,** Filtrate isotonic to plasma. **2,** Descending thin limb permeable to water. **3,** Ascending thin limb impermeable to water; permeable to ions. **4,** Ascending thick limb actively transports NaCl; impermeable to water and urea. **5,** DT actively resorbs NaCl; resorbs water in presence of ADH. **6,** Medullary CD actively resorbs NaCl, and slightly permeable to water and urea. (**NOTE:** Numbers on illustration represent milliosmols [mOsm]). (From: Koeppen BM, Stanton BA: *Berne and Levy Physiology* (updated), ed 6, St Louis, 2010, Mosby.). *ADH,* Antidiuretic hormone; *CD,* collecting duct, *NaCl,* sodium chloride, *H_2O,* water. See text for details.

gradient, and the vasa recta act as a countercurrent exchanger for maintaining the gradient.[16]

Water, Sodium, and Chloride

The process is initiated in the thick ascending limb of the loop of Henle with the active transport of sodium chloride out of the tubular lumen and into the medullary interstitium (Figure 37-14). Because the lumen of the ascending limb is impermeable to water, water cannot follow the sodium/chloride transport. This lack of luminal permeability causes the ascending tubular fluid to become hypoosmotic and the medullary interstitium to become hyperosmotic. The descending thin limb of the loop, which receives fluid from the proximal tubule, is highly permeable to water, but it is the only place in the nephron that does not actively transport either sodium or chloride. Sodium and chloride may, however, diffuse into the descending tubule from the interstitium. The hyperosmotic interstitium causes water to move out of the descending thin limb, and the remaining fluid in the descending tubule becomes increasingly concentrated as it flows toward the tip of the medulla. As the tubular fluid rounds the loop and enters the ascending thin limb, sodium and chloride are removed and water is retained. The fluid then becomes more and more dilute as it encounters the distal tubule. The data tubule resorbs water in the presence of antidiuretic hormone.

The slow rate of blood flow and the hairpin structure of the vasa recta allow blood to flow through the medullary tissue without disturbing the osmotic gradient. As blood flows into the descending limb of the vasa recta, it encounters the increasing osmotic concentration gradient of the medullary interstitium. Water moves out, and sodium and chloride diffuse into the descending vasa recta. The plasma becomes increasingly concentrated as it flows toward the tip of the medulla.

As the blood flow passes into the ascending limb and back toward the cortex, the surrounding interstitial fluid becomes comparatively more dilute. Water then moves back into the vasa recta, and sodium and chloride diffuse out. The net result is a preservation of the medullary osmotic gradient. If blood were to flow rapidly through the vasa recta, as occurs in some renal diseases, the medullary concentration gradient would be washed away and the ability to concentrate urine and conserve water would be lost. The efficiency of water conservation is related to the length of the loops: the longer the loops, the greater the ability to concentrate the urine. Many desert animals have very long loops and can reabsorb water so efficiently that they rarely need to drink.

Urea

Urea is an end product of protein metabolism and is the major constituent of urine along with water. The glomerulus freely filters urea. Tubular reabsorption depends on urine flow rate with less reabsorption occurring at higher flow rates. Approximately 50% of urea is excreted in the urine, and 50% is recycled within the kidney. The recycling of urea from the tubules and collecting ducts contributes to the osmotic gradient within the medulla and is necessary for the concentration and dilution of urine. Because urea is an end product of protein metabolism, individuals with protein deprivation cannot maximally concentrate their urine.

Catecholamines

In response to hemorrhage or extracellular fluid depletion, sympathetic neurons release norepinephrine, and the adrenal medulla releases epinephrine and norepinephrine. Norepinephrine and epinephrine promote afferent arteriolar vasoconstriction and decrease GFR and RBF. **Renalase** is a hormone produced by the kidney that degrades catecholamines and regulates blood pressure.[17]

Antidiuretic Hormone

The distal tubule in the cortex receives the hypoosmotic urine from the ascending limb of the loop of Henle. The concentration

TABLE 37-2 ACTION OF DIURETICS

DIURETIC	SITE OF ACTION	ACTION	SIDE EFFECTS
Osmotic Diuretic			
Mannitol Glycerol Urea	Proximal tubule	Freely filtered but not reabsorbed; osmotically attracts water and diminishes sodium reabsorption	Hypokalemia, dehydration
Carbonic Anhydrase Inhibitors			
Acetazolamide	Proximal tubule	Inhibits carbonic anhydrase; blocks hydrogen ion secretion and reabsorption of sodium and bicarbonate	Hypokalemia, systemic acidosis, alkaline urine
Inhibitors of Sodium/Chloride Reabsorption			
Thiazides	Between end of ascending loop and beginning of distal tubule	Blocks sodium and chloride reabsorption; mildly suppresses carbonic anhydrase	Hypokalemia, metabolic alkalosis
Furosemide Ethacrynic acid Torsemide	Thick ascending limb of Henle loop	Blocks active transport of chloride, sodium, and potassium	Hypokalemia, uric acid retention
Bumetanide	Cortical vasodilation	Increased rate of urine formation	Hypokalemia, uric acid retention
Potassium Sparing			
Spironolactone Eplerenone	Distal tubule	Inhibits aldosterone, blocks sodium reabsorption, and results in potassium retention	Hyperkalemia, nausea, confusion, gynecomastia
Triamterene Amiloride	Distal tubule	Blocks sodium reabsorption and inhibits potassium excretion	Nausea, vomiting, headache, and amiloride granulocytopenia, skin rash
Aquaretics			
Vasopressin (V2 receptor) blockers (i.e., conivaptan)	Distal tubule and collecting ducts	Blocks action of antidiuretic hormone	Dehydration

of the final urine is controlled by **antidiuretic hormone (ADH),** which is secreted from the posterior pituitary, or neurohypophysis. ADH increases water permeability in the last segment of the distal tubule and along the entire length of the collecting ducts, which pass through the inner and outer zones of the medulla.

In the presence of ADH, water reabsorption is high. Most of the water is reabsorbed in the medullary collecting ducts because of the high osmotic gradient in the medullary interstitium. The water diffuses into the ascending limb of the vasa recta and returns to the systemic circulation. The excreted urine can have a high osmotic concentration, up to 1400 mOsm. The volume is normally reduced to about 1% of the amount that was filtered at the glomerulus.

Excess ADH secretion is therefore one cause of **oliguria,** or diminished excretion of urine, clinically defined as less than 400 ml/day or 30 ml/hr. The syndrome of inappropriate secretion of ADH occurs when the posterior pituitary hypersecretes ADH, resulting in excess water reabsorption and water excess in the plasma (see Chapters 3 and 22).

Inadequate secretion of ADH occurs in diabetes insipidus, and causes the distal tubules and collecting ducts to become impermeable to water. Water remains in the tubular lumen and is excreted as a dilute and large volume of urine. (The mechanism for the regulation of ADH and plasma osmolality is described in Chapter 3 and 21.)

Natriuretic Peptides

The natriuretic peptides (urodilatin, atrial natriuretic peptide [ANP], and brain natriuretic peptide [BNP]) promote diuresis and were described on p. 1327.

Diuretics as a Factor in Urine Flow

A **diuretic** is any agent that enhances the flow of urine. Clinically, diuretics interfere with renal sodium reabsorption and reduce extracellular fluid volume. Diuretics are commonly used to treat hypertension and edema caused by heart failure, cirrhosis, and nephrotic syndrome.

Different diuretics affect different sites of tubular function and may produce side effects that alter acid-base and electrolyte balance. Therefore, health professionals need to understand their indications for use, mechanisms of action, and toxic side effects. Diuretics are divided into five general categories: (1) osmotic diuretics, (2) carbonic anhydrase inhibitors (inhibitors of urinary acidification), (3) inhibitors of loop sodium or chloride transport, (4) aldosterone antagonists, and (5) aquaretics. (The physiologic mechanism related to each category is summarized in Table 37-2.)

Renal Hormones

The kidneys activate or synthesize a series of hormones that have significant systemic effects and include the active form of vitamin D, erythropoietin, renin-angiotensin-aldosterone and natriuretic hormones (see p. 1327).

Vitamin D

Vitamin D is a hormone that can be obtained in the diet or synthesized by the action of ultraviolet radiation on cholesterol in the skin. These forms of vitamin D (cholecalciferol) are inactive and require two hydroxylations to establish a metabolically active form. The first step occurs in the liver with hydroxylation at carbon-25 (calcifediol), and the second hydroxylation occurs at the first carbon position in the kidneys and is stimulated by parathyroid hormone. The end product is 1,25-dihydroxycholecalciferol, or 1,25-dihydroxy-vitamin D_3 (1,25-OH_2D_3) (calcitriol), the active form of vitamin D.

Calcitriol (vitamin D_3) is necessary for the absorption of calcium and phosphate by the small intestine. A decreased plasma calcium level (less than 10 mg/dl) stimulates the secretion of parathyroid hormone. Parathyroid hormone then stimulates a sequence of events that help restore plasma calcium level back toward normal including:

- Calcium mobilization from bone
- Absorption of calcium and phosphate from the intestine by stimulating renal activation of vitamin D
- Increased renal calcium and phosphate reabsorption and decreased secretion

Serum phosphate level fluctuations also influence the renal hydroxylation of vitamin D. Decreased levels stimulate active 1,25-OH_2D_3 formation, and increased levels inhibit formation. This results in compensatory changes in phosphate absorption from bone and the intestine. The clinical significance of the role of the kidney in calcium and phosphate metabolism is evident in renal disease. Patients with renal disease have a deficiency of 1,25-OH_2D_3 and manifest symptoms of disturbed calcium and phosphate balance[18](see Chapter 38).

Erythropoietin

Erythropoietin is produced by the fetal liver and the adult kidney and is essential for normal erythropoiesis. In response to renal tissue hypoxia, peritubular fibroblasts in the kidneys release erythropoietin, which stimulates the bone marrow to increase the rate of red blood cell production (see Chapter 27). Individuals with chronic renal failure develop anemia related to reduced erythropoietin secretion. The anemia of chronic renal failure and cancer chemotherapy is treated with recombinant human erythropoietin (r-HuEPO). Erythropoietin also affects the endothelium and promotes angiogenesis, mitogenesis, and anti-apoptosis and is neurotrophic.[19]

TESTS OF RENAL FUNCTION

The Concept of Clearance

A number of specific renal functions can be measured by renal clearance. Renal clearance techniques determine how much of a substance can be cleared from the blood by the kidneys per given unit of time. The application of this principle permits an indirect measure of GFR, tubular secretion, tubular reabsorption, and renal blood flow.

Clearance and Glomerular Filtration Rate

The GFR provides the best estimate of functioning renal tissue. Damage to the glomerular membrane or loss of nephrons leads to a corresponding decrease in GFR. The measurement of GFR requires use of a substance that has a stable plasma concentration, is not protein bound, is freely filtered at the glomerulus, does not influence GFR, and is not secreted, reabsorbed, or metabolized by the tubules. *Inulin* (a fructose polysaccharide) is one substance that meets the criteria for measurement of GFR.

The kidney "clears" inulin from the plasma by filtering it at the glomerulus, reabsorbing nearly all of the fluid, and excreting the inulin left behind in the urine. The amount of inulin filtered is equal to the volume of plasma filtered (GFR) multiplied by the plasma concentration of inulin (P_{IN}). The amount of inulin in the urine is equal to a volume of urine per unit of time ($\dot{V}$) (usually 24 hours) multiplied by the inulin concentration of urine (U_{IN}). Because all the inulin filtered is excreted in the urine,

$$GFR \times P_{IN} = U_{IN} \times \dot{V}$$

GFR can be calculated by rearranging the formula:

$$GFR\ (ml/min) = \frac{U_{IN} \times \dot{V}}{P_{IN}}$$

The accurate determination of **insulin clearance** requires constant infusion to maintain a stable plasma level. This is time consuming, inconvenient, and prone to error. Therefore, the clearance of *creatinine,* a natural substance produced by muscle and released into the blood at a relatively constant rate, is commonly used clinically. It is freely filtered at the glomerulus and is not reabsorbed by the renal tubules, but a small amount is secreted by the renal tubules. Therefore, creatinine clearance overestimates the GFR but within tolerable limits. **Creatinine clearance** provides a good estimate of GFR because only one blood sample is required in addition to a 24-hour volume of urine. The GFR estimated by creatinine clearance is calculated as follows:

$$GFR\ (ml/min) = \frac{U_{CR} \times \dot{V}}{P_{CR}}$$

Numerous formulas have been developed for estimating GFR using creatinine and other indicators such as cystatin C.[20]

Clearance and Renal Blood Flow

The standard clearance formula also can be used to estimate renal plasma flow (RPF) and RBF using a molecule called *para*-aminohippuric acid (PAH). Some PAH is filtered at the glomerulus, and most of the remainder is secreted into the tubules in one circulation through the kidney. If all the PAH were removed from the plasma during a single pass through the kidney, total RPF could be determined. Because the supporting and nonsecreting structures of the kidney receive 10%

to 15% of **effective renal blood flow (ERBF)**, clearance of PAH measures only what is known as the **effective renal plasma flow (ERPF)**, which is 85% to 90% of the true renal plasma flow:

$$\text{ERPF} = \frac{U_{PAH} \times \dot{V}}{P_{PAH}}$$

where U_{PAH} = concentration of PAH in urine, and P_{PAH} = concentration of PAH in plasma.

The estimation of ERBF can then be calculated by considering the hematocrit in the following formula:

$$\text{ERBF} = \text{ERPF} \quad \frac{}{\substack{\text{1-Hematocrit} \\ (1.0\text{-}0.45)}}$$

Blood Tests

Evaluation of the biochemical components of the blood and plasma provides valuable information regarding renal function.

Plasma Creatinine Concentration

A long-term decline in GFR over weeks or months is reflected in the **plasma creatinine (P_{CR}) concentration** (normal value = 0.7 to 1.2 mg/dl). The P_{CR} concentration has a stable value when the GFR is stable because creatinine has a constant rate of production as a product of muscle metabolism. The amount filtered is approximately equal to the amount excreted. When the GFR declines, the P_{CR} increases proportionately. Thus the GFR and P_{CR} are inversely related. If the GFR were to decrease by 50%, the filtration and excretion of creatinine would be reduced by 50% and creatinine would accumulate in plasma to twice the normal value. Therefore, elevated P_{CR} values represent decreasing GFR. In the new steady-state, however, the total amount of creatinine excreted in the urine would remain the same because of the proportionate decrease in GFR and increase in P_{CR}.

The application of this principle is simple and useful for monitoring progressive changes in renal function. The test is most valuable for monitoring the progress of chronic rather than acute renal disease because it takes 7 to 10 days for the plasma creatinine level to stabilize when GFR declines. Serial measures can be obtained over a long time and plotted as a curve of glomerular function. Normal P_{CR} value decreases with advanced age, since older adults experience a decrease in lean muscle mass. The P_{CR} value becomes elevated during trauma or breakdown of muscle tissue. In such instances the value is then not useful for estimating GFR.

Plasma Cystatin C Concentration

Serum concentrations of **cystatin C** (a plasma protein freely filtered at the glomerulus) have been proposed for estimations of GFR.[21] The reciprocal of the serum concentrations of cystatin C can be used as estimates of changes in GFR similar to measures of plasma creatinine concentration. The National Kidney Foundation publishes calculators for estimating GFR for monitoring renal failure.[22]

Blood Urea Nitrogen

The concentration of urea nitrogen in the blood reflects glomerular filtration and urine-concentrating capacity. Because urea is filtered at the glomerulus, **blood urea nitrogen (BUN)** levels increase as glomerular filtration drops. Because urea is reabsorbed by the blood through the permeable tubules, the BUN value rises in states of dehydration and acute and chronic renal failure when passage of fluid through the tubules is slowed. BUN value also varies as a result of altered protein intake and protein catabolism and therefore is a poor measure of GFR. The normal range for BUN value in the adult is 10 to 20 mg/dl of blood.

Urinalysis

Urinalysis is a noninvasive and relatively inexpensive diagnostic procedure. The best results are obtained from a fresh, cleanly voided specimen because decay permits changes in the composition of urine. Urinalysis includes evaluation of color, turbidity, protein, pH, specific gravity, sediment, and supernatant.

Urine color is normally a clear, light yellow because of urochrome and other pigments. When formed substances (crystals, blood cells, or casts) are in the urine, it appears turbid. Protein in the urine creates marked foaming when shaken, and the foam is yellow or orange when the urine contains bile pigments. Urine does not normally contain protein or bile.

Urine pH normally ranges between 5 and 6.5, but it may vary from 4.5 to 8. Urine is more alkaline after eating and then becomes less alkaline before the next meal. Because sleep is accompanied by intermittent hypoventilation, urine is more acidic on awakening.

Specific gravity is an estimated measure of the solute concentration of the urine. The specific gravity of any solution is measured by comparing the weight of the solution with an equal volume of distilled water. Hence specific gravity is not a true measure of the number or concentration of particles, but it correlates well with osmolality and is a useful clinical tool. Specific gravity usually is measured with a hydrometer in a cylinder of urine; the normal value is 1.016 to 1.022. Dipstick evaluations may be falsely high when urine pH is less than 6 and falsely low when the pH is more than 7.

The final urine osmolality is primarily a function of ADH, which controls water reabsorption in the collecting ducts. If the kidney is unable to concentrate or dilute urine, given a stimulus, the cause is usually a malfunction of the renal tubules or inappropriate ADH secretion by the posterior pituitary gland. The state of hydration also affects the urine specific gravity, so hydration status should be evaluated before making a diagnosis. This determination is helpful for differentiating oliguria caused by intrinsic renal disease from hypovolemia as a result of dehydration.

Urine Sediment

The urine sediment is examined microscopically and may contain cells, casts, crystals, and bacteria. Epithelial cells may be seen in the microscopic field because they are shed naturally throughout the urinary tract.

Red Blood Cells. Normal urine contains few or no red blood cells. If a large number of red cells are present, this is known as **hematuria,** and the sediment may be red. An alkaline or hypotonic urine causes lysis of red cells, however, so that the cells will not be seen. Urine then will be positive for hemoglobin, and the specific gravity will be elevated. Hematuria can occur with the administration of anticoagulants and with several renal diseases.

Casts. **Casts** (accumulations of cellular precipitates) originate in the renal tubules, from which they take their shape. They are cylindrical with distinct borders. All casts have a precipitated microprotein matrix and arise primarily from the ascending limb of the distal tubule. Red cell casts indicate bleeding into the tubules; white cell casts are associated with an inflammatory process. Epithelial cell casts indicate degeneration of the tubular lumen or necrosis of the renal tubules. The type of cast identified suggests the disease process occurring in the kidney.

Crystals. Numerous kinds of **crystals** can be observed in the urine. They may be composed of cystine, uric acid, calcium oxalate, or phosphate. They may not be initially observable, but as the urine cools, crystals will form. Crystals tend to form in a concentrated acidic or alkaline urine. Generally they are not clinically significant. Crystal formation is diagnostically significant, usually indicating inflammation, infection, or a metabolic disorder.

White Blood Cells. White blood cells (WBCs) in the urine (a condition termed **pyuria**) are indicative of urinary tract infection, particularly when bacteria are present. Glomerulonephritis and nephrotic syndrome also may demonstrate pyuria but usually in combination with proteinuria, red cells, and casts. The finding of WBC casts reflects a kidney infection because these casts are not formed in the bladder or prostate. If WBCs are present in the urine, a culture should be done for specific identification of bacteria and sensitivity of bacteria to antibiotics.

Other Measures

Dipsticks and reagent strips are available for detecting other substances in the urine, including glucose, bilirubin, urobilinogen, leukocyte esterase and nitrates, ketones, proteins, hemoglobin, and myoglobin.

AGING AND RENAL FUNCTION

Throughout life the kidney responds to an increased workload by compensatory hypertrophy. This hypertrophy is marked in individuals who have donated a kidney for transplant or have lost functioning nephrons from trauma or disease. The glomeruli increase in diameter, and the tubules enlarge effectively to maintain the regulatory functions of the kidney. Hypertrophy occurs more rapidly and with a larger size increase in younger individuals and in those with high protein intake.

Changes in the kidneys occur throughout life, resulting in a reduction in size and a linear decrease in renal blood flow and GFR; however, it is less pronounced in healthy individuals.[23] The number of nephrons decreases with aging, possibly related to oxidative stress, inflammation, and associated clinical conditions (e.g., hypertension and diabetes mellitus).[24,25] The primary mechanism appears to be a change in the renal vasculature and perfusion pattern, which leads to a reduction in numbers of nephrons. The rate of nephron loss accelerates between 40 and 80 years of age. By 75 years of age the nephron population is reduced by 30% to 50%, with loss of renal mass occurring primarily in the cortex. Degenerative changes within nephrons also occur with aging. The glomerular capillaries become sclerotic and remaining glomeruli become hypertrophic.[26] The glomeruli may disappear completely. The arcuate and interlobular arteries become tortuous, contributing to ischemia. The loss of the glomerular tuft may cause a shunt between the afferent and efferent arterioles. Although loss of juxtaglomerular nephrons still allows the vasa recta to be perfused, the combination of events contributes to a reduced ability to excrete a concentrated urine.[27] Thus the specific gravity of the urine in older individuals tends to be on the low side of normal.

Tubular transport changes with aging, although under normal conditions the tubules function adequately. Adaptation to stressful conditions is more difficult. Glucose, bicarbonate, and sodium are not as efficiently reabsorbed, and hyperkalemia is more common because of decreased secretion. Response to acid or base loads is delayed and prolonged. Sudden or large changes in pH or fluid load may lead to serious imbalances with increased risk of hypervolemia or hypovolemia. Acute losses or chronic fluid deficits can lead to renal insufficiency in the older adult. Administration of drugs eliminated by renal processes may require dose modifications and more astute observations for toxic side effects.[28]

The T_m for glucose reabsorption decreases with age, contributing to a greater amount of glucose in the urine. This is an important consideration when glycosuria is used for screening or monitoring the process of diabetes mellitus in older adults. These changes occur independently of disease, however, indicating a normal process of aging. An age-related decline in renal activation of vitamin D decreases intestinal absorption of calcium, and older adults need more vitamin D to overcome diminishing renal function.[29] Previous or concurrent renal disease or urinary tract obstruction may amplify age-related changes in function.

Bladder symptoms are common among older adults and include frequency, urgency, and nocturia. Neurogenic and myogenic changes in bladder structure and function may contribute to some symptoms as well as influences outside the urinary tract. Changes in neurotransmission influence the micturition reflex and may lead to an overactive or underactive bladder.[30] Obstruction related to prostate hypertrophy may lead to urine retention with frequency, urgency, nocturia, and slow or intermittent urinary stream.

SUMMARY REVIEW

Structures of the Renal System

1. The kidneys are paired structures lying bilaterally between the twelfth thoracic and third lumbar vertebrae.
2. The kidney is composed of an outer cortex containing the glomeruli and an inner medulla containing the tubules and collecting ducts that drain into the calyces.
3. The calyces join to form the renal pelvis and are continuous with the upper end of the ureter.
4. The nephron is the urine-forming unit of the kidney and is composed of the glomerulus, proximal tubule, hairpin loops of Henle, distal tubule, and collecting duct.
5. The glomerulus contains loops of capillaries that loop in the Bowman capsule. The capillary walls serve as a filtration membrane for the formation of the primary urine. The layers of the glomerular capillary include the endothelium, basement membrane, and epithelium. The epithelium is composed of podocytes that interlock to provide filtration slits.
6. Mesangial cells and matrix lie between and support the glomerular capillaries in the Bowman capsule.
7. Juxtaglomerular cells secrete renin and are located around the afferent arteriole. They are contiguous with the sodium-sensing macula densa cells of the distal convoluted tubule.
8. The Bowman capsule is the space between the visceral and parietal epithelium.
9. The proximal tubule is lined with microvilli to increase surface area and enhance reabsorption.
10. The hairpin-shaped loops of Henle selectively transport solutes and water, contributing to the hypertonic state of the medulla.
11. The distal tubule adjusts acid-base balance by excreting acid into the urine and forming new bicarbonate ions.
12. The collecting duct contains principal cells that resorb sodium and water and excrete potassium and intercalated cells that secrete hydrogen or bicarbonate and potassium.
13. The ureters extend from the renal pelvis to the posterior wall of the bladder. Urine flows through the ureters by means of peristaltic contraction of the ureteral muscles.
14. The bladder is a bag composed of the detrusor and trigone muscles and innervated by parasympathetic fibers. When accumulation of urine reaches 250 to 300 ml, mechanoreceptors, which respond to stretching of tissue, stimulate the micturition reflex.

Renal Blood Flow

1. Renal blood flows at about 1000 to 1200 ml/min, or 20% to 25% of the cardiac output.
2. Blood flow through the glomerular capillaries is maintained at a constant rate in spite of a wide range of arterial pressures (autoregulation).
3. The GFR is the filtration of plasma per unit of time and is directly related to the perfusion pressure of renal blood flow.
4. Autoregulation of RBF and sympathetic neural regulation of vasoconstriction maintain a constant GFR.
5. The renal blood vessels are innervated by the sympathetic noradrenergic nerves that regulate vasoconstriction.
6. Renin is an enzyme secreted from the juxtaglomerular apparatus; it causes the generation of angiotensin I, which is converted to angiotensin II by the action of ACE. Angiotensin II is a potent vasoconstrictor and also stimulates release of aldosterone from the adrenal cortex. Thus the renin-angiotensin-aldosterone system is a regulator of renal blood flow and blood pressure.
7. Natriuretic peptides promote sodium and water loss by inhibiting aldosterone and increasing sodium chloride excretion.

Kidney Function

1. The major function of the nephron is urine formation, which involves the processes of glomerular filtration, tubular reabsorption, and tubular secretion and excretion.
2. Glomerular filtration is favored by capillary hydrostatic pressure and opposed by oncotic pressure in the capillary and hydrostatic pressure in the Bowman capsule. The balance of favoring and opposing filtration forces is the net filtration pressure (NFP).
3. The GFR is approximately 120 ml/minute, and 99% of the filtrate is reabsorbed.
4. The proximal convoluted tubule reabsorbs about 60% to 70% of the filtered sodium and water and 90% of other electrolytes.
5. Because most molecules are reabsorbed by active transport, the carrier mechanism can become saturated at the T_m. Molecules not reabsorbed are excreted with the urine.
6. The distal tubules actively reabsorb sodium and water and secrete potassium and hydrogen for the regulation of fluid, electrolyte, and acid-base balance.
7. The concentration of the final urine is a function of the level of ADH that stimulates the distal tubules and collecting ducts to reabsorb water. The countercurrent exchange system of the long loops of Henle and their accompanying capillaries establishes a concentration gradient within the renal medulla to facilitate the reabsorption of water from the collecting duct.
8. The distal nephron regulates acid-base balance by excreting hydrogen ions and forming new bicarbonate.
9. The kidney secretes or activates a number of hormones that have systemic effects, including vitamin D_3 (1,25-OH_2D_3) and erythropoietin, which stimulates erythropoiesis when there is hypoxia.

Tests of Renal Function

1. Tests that measure renal clearance indicate how much of a substance can be cleared from the blood by the kidneys per given amount of time.
2. Creatinine, a substance produced by muscle, is measured in plasma and urine to calculate a commonly used clinical measurement of GFR (creatinine clearance).
3. The plasma creatinine concentration, cystatin C plasma concentration, and BUN levels indicate glomerular function.

SUMMARY REVIEW—cont'd

Plasma creatinine and cystatin C are measured to monitor progressive renal dysfunction; BUN is an indicator of hydration status.

4. PAH clearance is used to determine renal plasma flow and blood flow.
5. Urinalysis involves evaluation of color, turbidity, protein, pH, specific gravity, sediment, and supernatant.
6. Presence of bacteria, red blood cells, white blood cells, casts, or crystals in the urine sediment may indicate a renal disorder.

Aging and Renal Function

1. As a person ages, a decrease occurs in the number of nephrons. Renal blood flow and glomerular filtration rate decline.
2. Tubular transport and reabsorption decrease with age. Response to acid-base changes and reabsorption of glucose are delayed. Drugs eliminated by the kidney can accumulate in the plasma, causing toxic reactions.
3. Neurogenic and myogenic changes in the bladder may lead to symptoms of urgency and frequency.

KEY TERMS

Angiotensin II, 1327
Antidiuretic hormone (ADH), 1333
Arcuate artery, 1325
Atrial natriuretic peptide (ANP), 1327
Autoregulation, 1326
Bladder, 1325
Blood urea nitrogen (BUN), 1335
Bowman glomerular capsule (Bowman space), 1321
Bowman (urinary) space, 1322
Brain natriuretic peptide (BNP), 1327
Calcitriol (vitamin D_3), 1334
Cast, 1336
Collecting duct, 1323
Cortex, 1320
Countercurrent exchange system, 1331
Creatinine clearance, 1334
Crystal, 1336
C-type natriuretic peptide, 1327
Cystatin C, 1335
Detrusor muscle, 1325
Distal convoluted tubule, 1323
Diuretic, 1333
Effective renal blood flow (ERBF), 1335
Effective renal plasma flow (ERPF), 1335
Excretion, 1328
External urethral sphincter, 1325
Filtration slit, 1322
Glomerular capillary, 1325
Glomerular endothelium, 1321
Glomerular filtration membrane, 1321
Glomerular filtration rate (GFR), 1326
Glomerulus, 1321
Hematuria, 1336
Hilum, 1320
Insulin clearance, 1334
Intercalated cell, 1323
Interlobar artery, 1325
Internal urethral sphincter, 1325
Juxtaglomerular apparatus (JGA), 1322
Juxtaglomerular cell, 1322
Juxtamedullary nephron, 1320
Kidney, 1319
Loop of Henle, 1322
Macula densa, 1322
Major calyx, 1320
Medulla, 1320
Mesangial cell, 1321
Mesangial matrix, 1321
Micturition, 1325
Midcortical nephron, 1320
Minor calyx, 1320
Myogenic mechanism, 1326
Natriuretic peptide, 1327
Nephron, 1320
Net filtration pressure (NFP), 1329
Oliguria, 1333
Parietal epithelium, 1322
Peritubular capillary, 1325
Plasma creatinine (P_{CR}) concentration, 1335
Podocyte, 1321
Principal cell, 1323
Proximal convoluted tubule, 1322
Pyramid, 1320
Pyuria, 1336
Renal artery, 1325
Renalase, 1332
Renal capsule, 1319
Renal column, 1320
Renal corpuscle, 1321
Renal fascia, 1319
Renal papillae, 1325
Renal pelvis, 1320
Specific gravity, 1335
Superficial cortical nephron, 1320
Transitional epithelium (uroepithelium), 1325
Transport maximum (T_m), 1330
Trigone, 1325
Tubular reabsorption, 1328
Tubular secretion, 1328
Tubuloglomerular feedback, 1326
Ultrafiltration, 1328
Urea, 1332
Ureter, 1325
Urethra, 1325
Urinalysis, 1335
Urine color, 1335
Urine pH, 1335
Urodilatin, 1327
Vasa recta, 1325
Visceral epithelium, 1321
Vitamin D, 1334

REFERENCES

1. Abboud HE: Mesangial cell biology, *Exp Cell Res* 318(9):979–985, 2012.
2. Miner JH: The glomerular basement membrane, *Exp Cell Res* 318(9): 973–978, 2012.
3. Greka A, Mundel P: Cell biology and pathology of podocytes, *Annu Rev Physiol* 74:299–323, 2012.
4. Garg P, Holzman LB: Podocytes: gaining a foothold, *Exp Cell Res* 318(9):955–963, 2012.
5. Birder LA et al: How does the urothelium affect bladder function in health and disease? ICI-RS 2011, *Neurourol Urodyn* 31(3):293–299, 2012.
6. Just A: Mechanisms of renal blood flow autoregulation: dynamics and contributions, *Am J Physiol Regul Integr Comp Physiol* 292(1):R1–R17, 2007.
7. Singh P, Thomson SC: Renal homeostasis and tubuloglomerular feedback, *Curr Opin Nephrol Hypertens* 19(1):59–64, 2010.
8. Seeliger E et al: The renin-angiotensin system and the third mechanism of renal blood flow autoregulation, *Am J Physiol Renal Physiol* 296:F1334–F1345, 2009.
9. Schweda F et al: Renin release, *Physiology (Bethesda)* 22:310–319, 2007.
10. Vaidya A, Williams JS: The relationship between vitamin D and the renin-angiotensin system in the pathophysiology of hypertension, kidney disease, and diabetes, *Metabolism* 61(4):450–458, 2012.
11. Gassanov N et al: Natriuretic peptides in therapy for decompensated heart failure, *Eur J Clin Pharmacol* 68(3):223–230, 2012.
12. Kalra PR et al: C-type natriuretic peptide production by the human kidney is blunted in chronic heart failure, *Clin Sci (Lond)* 118(1):71–77, 2009.
13. El-Achkar TM, Wu XR: Uromodulin in kidney injury: an instigator, bystander, or protector? *Am J Kidney Dis* 59(3):452–461, 2012.
14. Rodan AR, Cheng CJ, Huang CL: Recent advances in distal tubular potassium handling, *Am J Physiol Renal Physiol* 300(4):F821–F827, 2011.
15. Thomson SC, Blantz RC: Glomerulotubular balance, tubuloglomerular feedback, and salt homeostasis, *J Am Soc Nephrol* 19(12):2272–2275, 2008.

16. Sands JM, Layton HE, Fenton RA: Chapter 10: Urine concentration and dilution. In Taal MW et al: *Brenner and Rector's the kidney*, ed 9, Philadelphia, 2011, Saunders, pp 332–333.
17. Desir G: Novel insights into the physiology of renalase and its role in hypertension and heart disease, *Pediatr Nephrol* 27(5):719–725, 2012.
18. Dusso AS, Tokumoto M: Defective renal maintenance of the vitamin D endocrine system impairs vitamin D renoprotection: a downward spiral in kidney disease, *Kidney Int* 79(7):715–729, 2011.
19. Ponce LL et al: Erythropoietin neuroprotection with traumatic brain injury, *Pathophysiology* 20(1):31–38, 2013.
20. Stevens LA, Padala S, Levey AS: Advances in glomerular filtration rate-estimating equations, *Curr Opin Nephrol Hypertens* 19(3):298–307, 2010.
21. Odutayo A, Cherney D: Cystatin C and acute changes in glomerular filtration rate, *Clin Nephrol* 78(1):64–75, 2012.
22. National Kidney Foundation: *Calculators for health care professionals.* Available at www.kidney.org/professionals/kdoqi/gfr_calculator.cfm. Accessed October 16, 2012.
23. Esposito C, Dal Canton A: Functional changes in the aging kidney, *J Nephrol* 23(Suppl 15):S41–S45, 2010.
24. Choudhury D, Levi M: Kidney aging—inevitable or preventable? *Nat Rev Nephrol* 7(12):706–717, 2011.
25. Pannarale G et al: The aging kidney: structural changes, *J Nephrol* 23(Suppl 15):S37–S40, 2010.
26. Stojanovic VR et al: Morphometric analysis of nonsclerosed glomeruli size and connective tissue content during the aging process, *Scientific-World Journal* 2012:845046, 2012.
27. Sands JM: Urine concentrating and diluting ability during aging, *J Gerontol A Biol Sci Med Sci* 67(12):1352–1357, 2012.
28. Corsonello A, Pedone C, Incalzi RA: Age-related pharmacokinetic and pharmacodynamic changes and related risk of adverse drug reactions, *Curr Med Chem* 17(6):571–584, 2010.
29. Vieth R, Ladak Y, Walfish PG: Age-related changes in the 25-hydroxyvitamin D versus parathyroid hormone relationship suggest a different reason why older adults require more vitamin D, *J Clin Endocrinol Metab* 88(1):185–191, 2003.
30. Smith PP: Aging and the underactive detrusor: a failure of activity or activation? *Neurourol Urodyn* 29(3):408–412, 2010.

CHAPTER

38

Alterations of Renal and Urinary Tract Function

Alexa K. Doig and Sue E. Huether

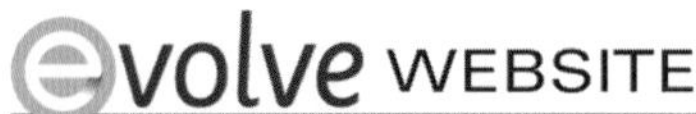

http://evolve.elsevier.com/McCance/

- Review Questions and Answers
- Animations
- Online Course: Module 16

CHAPTER OUTLINE

Renal and urinary function can be affected by a variety of disorders. The most common type of urinary dysfunction is infection. Stones, tumors, or inflammation also can obstruct the urinary tract. Renal function can be impaired by disorders of the kidney itself or by many other systemic diseases and ultimately may result in acute kidney injury or chronic kidney disease. Because the kidney filters the blood, it is directly linked to every other organ system. Renal failure, whether acute or chronic, is life-threatening.

URINARY TRACT OBSTRUCTION

Urinary tract obstruction is an interference with the flow of urine at any site along the urinary tract (Figure 38-1). An obstruction may be anatomic or functional. It impedes flow proximal to the obstruction, dilates structures distal to the obstruction, increases risk for infection, and compromises renal function. Anatomic changes in the urinary system caused by obstruction are referred to as **obstructive uropathy.** The severity of an obstructive uropathy is determined by: (1) the location of the obstructive lesion, (2) the involvement of one or both upper urinary tracts (ureters and renal pelvis), (3) the completeness of the obstruction, (4) the duration of the obstruction, and (5) the nature of the obstructive lesion.[1,2] Obstructions may be relieved or partially alleviated by correction of the obstruction, although permanent impairments occur if a complete or partial obstruction persists over weeks to months or longer.

Upper Urinary Tract Obstruction

Common causes of upper urinary tract obstruction include stricture or congenital compression of a calyx or the ureteropelvic or ureterovesical junction (e.g., stones [calculi]); ureteral compression from an aberrant vessel, tumor, or abdominal inflammation and scarring (retroperitoneal fibrosis); or

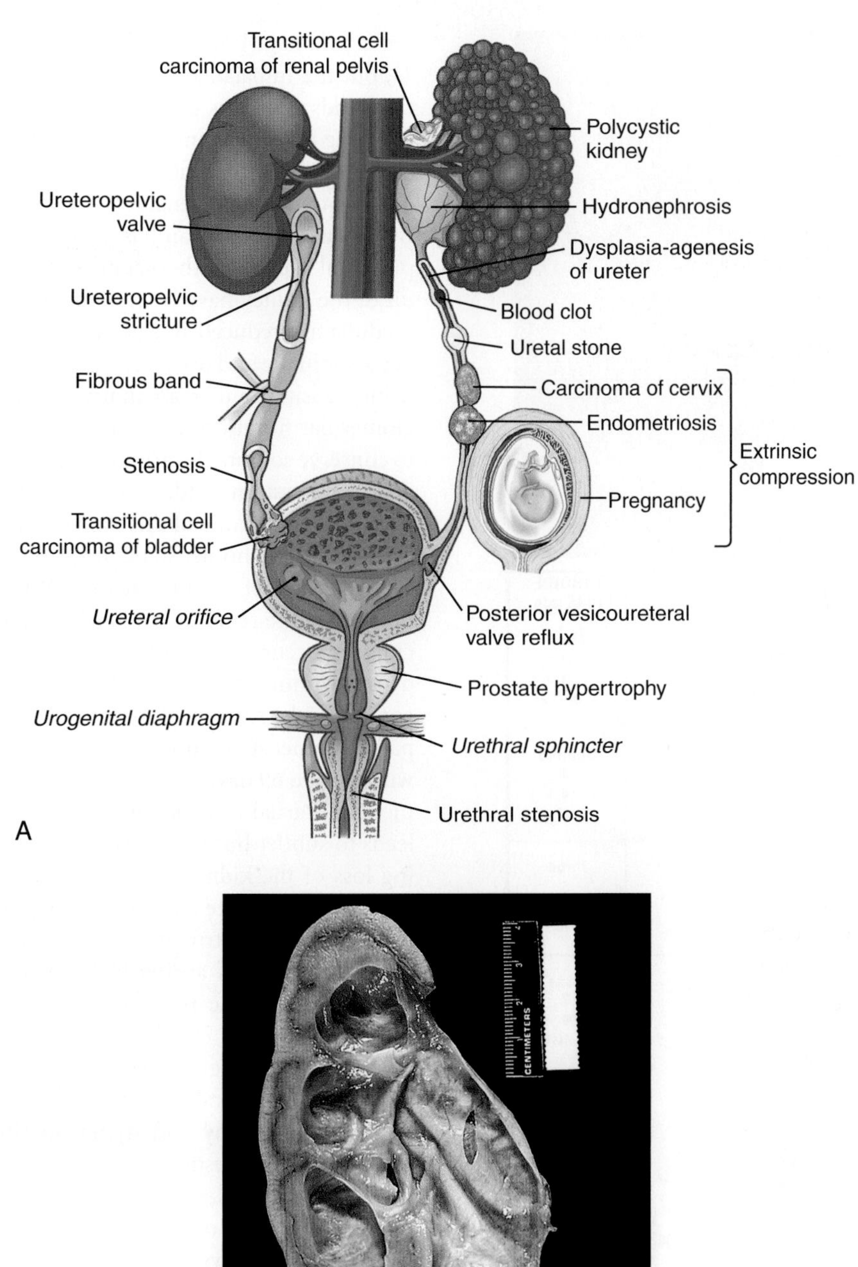

FIGURE 38-1 Urinary Tract Obstruction and Hydronephrosis. **A,** Causes of urinary tract obstruction. Terms in italics are normal structures. **B,** Hydronephrosis, marked dilation of renal pelvis and calyces with thinning of parenchyma.

ureteral blockage from stones or a malignancy of the renal pelvis or ureter.

Obstruction of the upper urinary tract causes dilation of the ureter, renal pelvis, calyces, and renal parenchyma proximal to the site of urinary blockage. Dilation of the ureter is referred to as **hydroureter** (accumulation of urine in the ureter), and dilation of the renal pelvis and calyces proximal to a blockage leads to **hydronephrosis** (enlargement of the renal pelvis and calyces) or **ureterohydronephrosis** (dilation of both the ureter and the pelvicaliceal system) (Figure 38-2). Dilation of the upper urinary tract is an early response to obstruction and reflects smooth muscle hypertrophy and accumulation of urine above the level of blockage (urinary stasis/retention). The increased pressure is transmitted to the glomerulus, which decreases filtration. Unless the obstruction is relieved, this dilation leads to enlargement with tubulointerstitial fibrosis and apoptosis affecting the distal nephron and renal function. **Tubulointerstitial fibrosis** is the deposition of excessive amounts of extracellular matrix

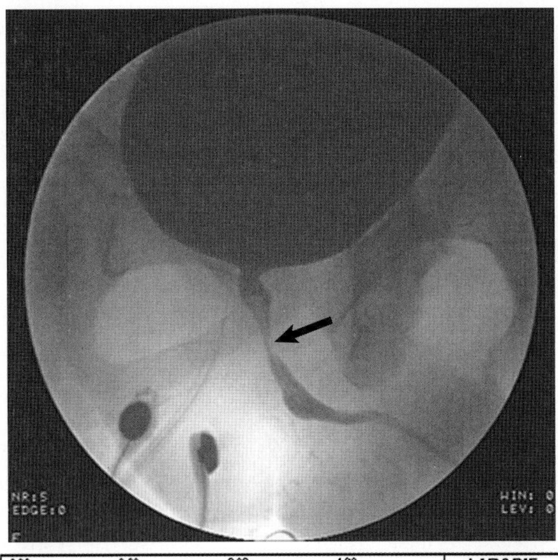

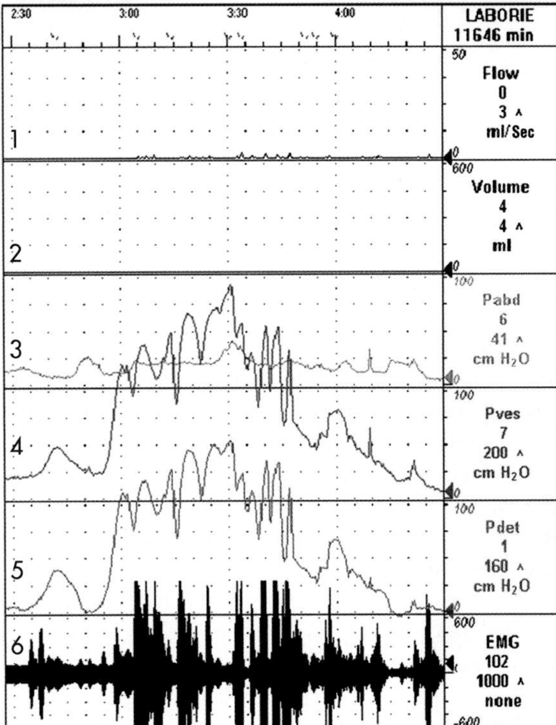

FIGURE 38-2 Neurogenic Detrusor Overactivity with Vesicosphincter. The arrow indicates narrowing of the striated sphincter consistent with electromyographic activity *(Line 6)* noted on the urodynamic tracing. Note the characteristic poor flow pattern *(Line 1)* with elevated voiding pressures *(Lines 4 and 5)* indicating obstruction. *Line 1* = Urine flow rate; *Line 2* = urine volume; *Line 3* = abdominal pressure *(Pabd); Line 4* = intravesicular (inside bladder) pressure *(Pves); Line 5* = detrusor muscle pressure *(Pdet); Line 6* = bladder electromyelogram *(EMG).*

(collagen and other proteins). Deposition of extracellular matrix is a normal process of organ repair and maintenance, and the deposition of extracellular matrix is balanced by its breakdown under the influence of metalloproteinases. Multiple cytokines and growth factors have been implicated in the process of tubulointerstitial fibrosis and irreversible loss of kidney function, including transforming growth factor-beta-1 (TGF-β1), angiotensin II, aldosterone, and various tumor necrosis factors. **Apoptosis** is a normal process that the body uses to replace damaged or senescent cells with new ones (see Chapter 1), but the imbalance in growth factors provoked by obstruction leads to excess cellular destruction and death, ultimately resulting in loss of functioning nephrons and kidney damage.

Tubulointerstitial fibrosis and apoptosis result in detectable damage to the distal renal tubules within approximately 7 days. By 14 days, obstruction has adversely affected both distal and proximal aspects of the nephron. Within 28 days the glomeruli of the kidney have been damaged and the renal cortex and medulla are reduced in size (thinned). Distal tubular damage occurs initially and decreases the kidney's ability to concentrate urine, causing an increase in urine volume despite a decrease in glomerular filtration rate (GFR). The affected kidney is unable to conserve sodium, bicarbonate, and water or to excrete hydrogen or potassium, leading to metabolic acidosis and dehydration. The magnitude of this damage, and the kidney's ability to recover normal homeostatic function, is affected by the severity and duration of the obstruction. With complete obstruction, damage to the renal tubules and compression of the renal vasculature occurs in a matter of hours, and irreversible damage occurs within 3 to 4 weeks. Nevertheless, even in the face of a complete obstruction, the human kidney may recover at least partial homeostatic function provided the blockage is removed within 56 to 69 days.[3,3a] This recovery requires approximately 4 months. Partial obstruction, in the absence of renal infection, leads to subtler but ultimately permanent impairments including loss of the kidney's ability to concentrate urine, reabsorb bicarbonate, excrete ammonia, or regulate metabolic acid-base balance if the obstruction is not relieved. Complete bilateral obstruction causes anuria because the retrograde increase in tubular hydrostatic pressure completely opposes glomerular filtration.

The body is able to partially counteract the negative consequences of unilateral obstruction by a process called **compensatory hypertrophy** and **hyperfunction.**[4] The compensatory response is the result of two growth processes: **obligatory growth** occurs under the influence of somatomedins, and **compensatory growth** occurs under the influence of a hormone or hormones that have not yet been identified. These processes cause the contralateral (unobstructed) kidney to increase the size of individual glomeruli and tubules but not the total number of functioning nephrons. The ability of the body to engage in compensatory hypertrophy and hyperfunction diminishes with age, and the process is reversible when relief of obstruction results in recovery of function by the obstructed kidney. Unilateral obstruction may remain silent for a long time.

Relief of bilateral, partial urinary tract obstruction or complete obstruction of one kidney is usually followed by a brief period of diuresis (commonly called **postobstructive diuresis**).[5] It is a physiologic response and is typically mild, representing a restoration of fluid and electrolyte imbalance caused by the obstructive uropathy. Alterations in tubular transport and water reabsorption and volume expansion contribute to the diuresis. Occasionally relief of obstruction will cause rapid excretion of large volumes of water, sodium, or other electrolytes, resulting in a urine output of 10 L/day or more (minimal normal daily urine output is approximately 720 ml/day). Rapid postobstructive diuresis causes dehydration and fluid and electrolyte imbalances if not promptly corrected. Risk factors for severe postobstructive diuresis include bilateral obstruction, impairment of one or both kidneys' ability to concentrate urine or reabsorb sodium *(nephrogenic diabetes insipidus),* hypertension, edema and weight gain, congestive heart failure, and uremic encephalopathy.

Kidney Stones

Calculi, or **urinary stones (urolithiasis),** are masses of crystals, protein, or other substances that are a common cause of urinary tract obstruction in adults. They can be located in the kidneys, ureters, and urinary bladder. The prevalence of stones in the United States is approximately 6% in women and 15% in men, and is more common in whites.[6] The recurrence rate is approximately 30% to 50% within 5 years.[7] The risk of urinary calculi formation is influenced by a number of factors, including age, gender, race, geographic location, seasonal factors, fluid intake, diet, occupation, genetic predisposition, and other conditions including urinary tract infection, hypertension, atherosclerosis, metabolic syndrome, obesity, and diabetes.[8] Most persons develop their first stone before age 50 years. Geographic location influences the risk of stone formation because of indirect factors, including average temperature, humidity, and rain fall, and their influence on fluid and dietary patterns. Persons who regularly consume an adequate volume of water and those who are physically active are at reduced risk when compared with people who are inactive or consume lower volumes of fluid. Most kidney stones are unilateral and are a risk factor for chronic kidney disease and an increased risk for myocardial infarction.[9,10]

Urinary calculi can be classified according to the primary minerals (salts) that comprise the stones. The most common stone types include calcium oxalate or phosphate (70% to 80%), struvite (magnesium, ammonium, and phosphate) (15%), and uric acid (7%). Cystine stones are rare, less than 1%. Less common stone elements include cystine, 2,8-dihydroxyadeninuria (a rare genetic disorder that increases risk of xanthine stones), triamterene (a diuretic), and indinavir (a protease inhibitor used in management of human immunodeficiency virus [HIV] infection). Urinary calculi also can be classified according to location and size. *Staghorn calculi* are large and fill the minor and major calyces. *Non-staghorn calculi* are of variable size and are located in the calyces, in the renal pelvis, or at different sites along the ureter.

PATHOPHYSIOLOGY. Renal calculus formation is complex and related to: (1) supersaturation of one or more salts in the urine, (2) precipitation of the salts from a liquid to a solid state (crystals), (3) growth through crystallization or agglomeration (sometimes called aggregation), and (4) the presence or absence of stone inhibitors.[11] *Supersaturation* is the presence of a higher concentration of a salt within a fluid (in this case, the urine) than the volume is able to dissolve to maintain equilibrium. Human urine contains many positively and negatively charged ions capable of *precipitating* from solution and forming a variety of salts. The salts form crystals that are retained and grow into stones. *Crystallization* is the process by which crystals grow from a small *nidus* or nucleus to larger stones in the presence of supersaturated urine. Although supersaturation is essential for free stone formation, the urine need not remain continuously supersaturated for a calculus to grow once its nidus has precipitated from solution. Intermittent periods of supersaturation after the ingestion of a meal or during times of dehydration are sufficient for stone growth in many individuals. In addition, the apical papillae have interstitial sites where hydroxyapatite deposits (Randall plaque) become exposed and serve as sites for calcium oxalate stone formation (but not calcium phosphate stone formation).[12] *Matrix* is an organic material (i.e., mucoprotein) in which the components of a kidney stone are embedded.[11]

The pH of the urine also influences the risk of precipitation and calculus formation. An alkaline urinary pH significantly increases the risk of calcium phosphate stone formation, whereas acidic urine increases the risk of a uric acid stone. Cystine and xanthine precipitate more readily in acidic urine.

Stone or *crystal growth inhibiting substances,* including potassium citrate, pyrophosphate, and magnesium, are capable of crystal growth inhibition, thereby reducing the risk of calcium phosphate or calcium oxalate precipitation in the urine and preventing subsequent stone formation.

Retention of *crystal particles* occurs primarily at the papillary collecting ducts. Although most crystals are flushed from the tract through antegrade urine flow, urinary stasis, anatomic abnormalities, or inflamed epithelium within the urinary tract may prevent prompt flushing of crystals from the system, thus increasing the risk of calculus formation.

The size of a stone determines the likelihood that it will pass through the urinary tract and be excreted through micturition.[13] Stones smaller than 5 mm have about a 50% chance of spontaneous passage, whereas stones that are 1 cm have almost no chance of spontaneous passage. Nevertheless, the person with ureteral dilation from the previous passage of a stone may be able to excrete larger stones when compared with the person experiencing an initial obstructing calculus.

Calcium stones (urolithiasis) account for 70% to 80% of all stones requiring treatment. Calcium oxalate accounts for about 80% of these stones and calcium phosphate about 15%.[14] Both genetic and environmental factors may increase susceptibility. Most affected individuals have *idiopathic calcium oxalate urolithiasis (ICOU),* a condition whose exact etiology has not yet been defined. Stones can form freely in supersaturated urine or detach from interstitial sites of formation.[15] Hypercalciuria, hyperoxaluria, hyperuricosuria, hypocitraturia, mild renal tubular acidosis, crystal growth inhibitor deficiencies, and alkaline urine are associated with calcium stone formation.[16,17] Hypercalciuria and hyperoxaluria are usually attributable to intestinal hyperabsorption and less commonly to a defect in renal calcium reabsorption. Hyperparathyroidism and bone demineralization associated with prolonged immobilization are also known to cause hypercalciuria.

Struvite stones primarily contain magnesium-ammonium-phosphate as well as varying levels of matrix. Matrix forms in an alkaline urine and during infection with a urease-producing

TABLE 38-1 TYPES OF INCONTINENCE

TYPE	DESCRIPTION
Urge incontinence (most common in older adults)	Involuntary loss of urine associated with an abrupt and strong desire to void (urgency). Often associated with involuntary contractions of the detrusor. When associated with a neurologic disorder this is called detrusor hyperreflexia. When no neurologic disorder exists this is called detrusor instability. May be associated with decreased bladder wall compliance.
Stress incontinence (most common in women younger than 60 years and men who have had prostate surgery)	Involuntary loss of urine during coughing, sneezing, laughing, or other physical activity associated with increased abdominal pressure.
Overflow incontinence	Involuntary loss of urine with overdistention of the bladder. Associated with neurologic lesions below S1, polyneuropathies, and urethral obstruction (i.e., an enlarged prostate).
Mixed incontinence (most common in older women)	A combination of stress and urge incontinence.
Functional incontinence	Involuntary loss of urine caused by dementia or immobility.

Data from Agency for Healthcare Research and Quality: *Overview: urinary incontinence in adults, clinical practice guideline update,* Rockville, MD, 1996, Author. Available at www.ahrq.gov/clinic/uiovervw.htm.

bacterial pathogen, such as a *Proteus, Klebsiella,* or *Pseudomonas.* Struvite calculi may grow quite large and branch into a staghorn configuration (**staghorn calculus**) that approximates the pelvicaliceal collecting system. Women are at greater risk for struvite stones because they have an increased incidence of urinary tract infection (see p. 1349).

Uric acid is primarily a product of biosynthesis of endogenous purines and is secondarily affected by consumption of purines in the diet. Persons who excrete excessive uric acid in the urine, such as those with gouty arthritis, are at particular risk for **uric acid stones.** A consistently acidic urine greatly increases this risk. Cystine and xanthine are amino acids that precipitate more readily in acidic urine. *Cystinuria* and *xanthinuria* are genetic disorders of amino acid metabolism, and their excess in urine can cause **cystinuric,** or **xanthine, stone** formation in the presence of a low urine pH of 5.5 or less.

CLINICAL MANIFESTATIONS. **Renal colic,** described as moderate to severe pain often originating in the posterior hypochondrium (flank) and radiating to the groin, usually indicates obstruction of the renal pelvis or proximal ureter. Colic that radiates to the lateral flank or lower abdomen typically indicates obstruction in the midureter, and bothersome lower urinary tract symptoms (urgency, frequent voiding, urge incontinence) indicate obstruction of the lower ureter or ureterovesical junction. The pain can be severe and incapacitating and may be accompanied by nausea and vomiting. Gross (visible blood in the urine) or microscopic hematuria (three or more red blood cells per high power microscopic field) may be present.[18]

EVALUATION AND TREATMENT. The evaluation and diagnosis of urinary calculi are based on presenting symptoms and history combined with a focused physical assessment, imaging studies, and possibly a functional study of renal pelvic and ureteral pressures.[16] The history queries dietary habits; the age of the first stone episode; stone analysis; and presence of complicating factors, including recurrent urinary tract infection, hyperparathyroidism, or recent gastrointestinal or genitourinary surgery. Urinalysis (including pH) is obtained and a 24-hour urine is completed to identify calcium oxalate, citrate, and other significant constituents. In addition, every effort is made to retrieve and analyze calculi that are passed spontaneously or retrieved through aggressive intervention. Additional tests are obtained in selected individuals, such as those with suspected hyperparathyroidism or cystine or uric acid stones, in order to diagnose and manage underlying metabolic disorders. Imaging of kidney stones includes plain abdominal radiography, ultrasound, intravenous pyelogram, computed tomography, and magnetic resonance imaging.[19]

The goals of treatment are to manage acute pain, promote stone passage, reduce the size of stones already formed, and prevent new stone formation. The components of treatment include: (1) administering parenteral and/or oral analgesics for acute pain, (2) providing medical therapy to promote stone passage (alpha antagonists or calcium channel blockers), (3) reducing the concentration of stone-forming substances by increasing urine flow rate with high fluid intake, (4) decreasing the amount of stone-forming substances in the urine by decreasing dietary intake or endogenous production or by altering urine pH,[20] and (5) removing stones using percutaneous nephrolithotomy, ureteroscopy, or ultrasonic or laser lithotripsy to fragment stones for excretion in the urine.[21,22] Obstructing kidney stones with a suspected proximal urinary tract infection are urologic emergencies requiring emergent decompression and antibiotics.[23]

Lower Urinary Tract Obstruction

Obstructive disorders of the lower urinary tract (LUT) are primarily related to storage of urine in the bladder or emptying of urine through the bladder outlet. The causes of the obstruction include neurogenic and anatomic alterations or, in some instances, a combination of both. Incontinence is a common symptom. Types of incontinence are reviewed in Table 38-1.

Neurogenic Bladder

Neurogenic bladder is a general term for bladder dysfunction caused by neurologic disorders. The types of dysfunction are related to the sites in the nervous system that control sensory and motor bladder function (Figure 38-3). Lesions that develop in upper motor neurons of the brain and spinal cord result in **dyssynergia** (loss of coordinated neuromuscular contraction) and overactive or hyperreflexive bladder function. Lesions in

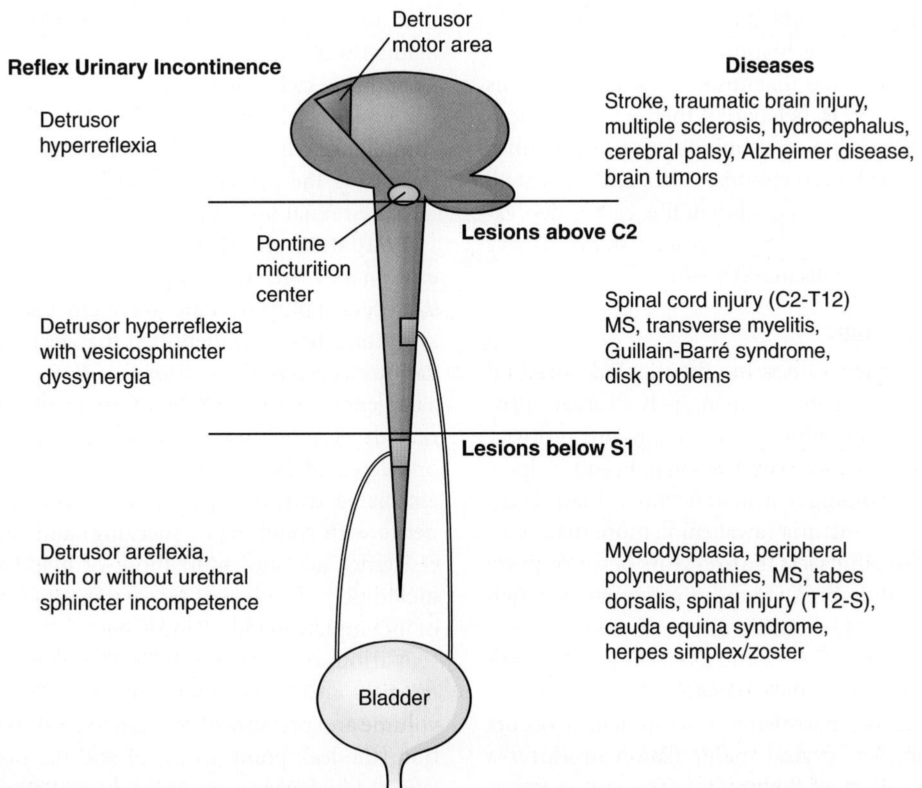

FIGURE 38-3 Causes of Neurogenic Bladder and Reflex Incontinence. (Adapted from Doughty DB, editor: *Urinary and fecal incontinence: current management concepts,* ed 3, Philadelphia, 2006, Mosby.)

the sacral area of the spinal cord or peripheral nerves result in underactive, hypotonic, or atonic (flaccid) bladder function, often with loss of bladder sensation.

Neurologic disorders that develop above the pontine micturition center result in **detrusor hyperreflexia,** also known as an uninhibited or reflex bladder. This is an upper motor neuron disorder in which the bladder empties automatically when it becomes full and the external sphincter functions normally. Because the pontine micturition center remains intact, there is coordination between detrusor muscle contraction and the relaxation of the urethral sphincter. Stroke, traumatic brain injury, dementia, and brain tumors are examples of disorders that result in detrusor hyperreflexia. Symptoms include urine leakage and incontinence.

Neurologic lesions that occur below the pontine micturition center but above the sacral micturition center (between C2 and S1) are also upper motor neuron lesions and result in **detrusor hyperreflexia with vesicosphincter (detrusor sphincter) dyssynergia.** There is loss of pontine coordination of detrusor muscle contraction and external sphincter relaxation, so both the bladder and the sphincter are contracting at the same time, causing a functional obstruction of the bladder outlet.[24] Spinal cord injury, multiple sclerosis, Guillain-Barré syndrome, and intervertebral disk problems are causes of this disorder. There is diminished bladder relaxation during storage with small urine volumes and high intravesicular (inside the bladder) pressures. This results in an overactive bladder syndrome with symptoms of urgency, frequency, urge incontinence, and increased risk for urethral turbulence and urinary tract infection.

Lesions that involve the sacral micturition center (below S1; may also be termed *cauda equina syndrome*) or peripheral nerve lesions result in **detrusor areflexia** (acontractile detrusor), a lower motor neuron disorder. The result is an acontractile detrusor or atonic bladder with retention of urine and distention. If the sensory innervation of the bladder is intact, the full bladder will be sensed but the detrusor may not contract. This is an *underactive bladder syndrome* and may have symptoms of stress and overflow incontinence. Myelodysplasia, multiple sclerosis, tabes dorsalis, and peripheral polyneuropathies are associated with this disorder.

Overactive Bladder Syndrome

Overactive bladder syndrome (OAB) is a chronic syndrome of detrusor overactivity in the absence of infection. It is estimated that 29.8 million adults over the age of 40 have bothersome OAB symptoms.[25] OAB is characterized by urgency with involuntary detrusor contractions during the bladder filling phase. The contraction may be spontaneous or provoked and associated with hyperexcitable nerves or involuntary reflexes.[26] There is coordination between the contracting bladder and the external sphincter, but the detrusor is too weak to empty the bladder, resulting in urinary retention with overflow or stress incontinence. Overactive bladder is defined by the International Continence Society as a *symptom syndrome* of urgency, with or without urge incontinence and usually associated with frequency and nocturia.[27] Overactive bladder syndrome affects millions of men, women, and children; adults are often reluctant to discuss this syndrome with their healthcare provider.

Sexual dysfunction and bowel problems often accompany OAB. Diagnosis is usually made by evaluation of symptoms. Urodynamic evaluation confirms the diagnosis. Treatment options include lifestyle modifications, behavioral therapy, pharmacotherapy (e.g., antimuscarinics), neuromodulation, botulinum toxin therapy, and surgical interventions. When left untreated, OAB is costly, impairs health and quality of life, causes depression, and leads to social isolation.[28,29] OAB is a risk for urinary tract infection and a risk for falls in older adults.[30]

Obstructions to Urine Flow

Anatomic causes of resistance to urine flow include urethral stricture, prostatic enlargement in men, pelvic organ prolapse in women, and tumor compression. Symptoms of lower urinary tract obstruction are more common in men and include: (1) frequent daytime voiding (urination more than every 2 hours while awake); (2) nocturia (awakening more than once each night to urinate for adults less than 65 years of age or more than twice for older adults); (3) bothersome urgency, often combined with hesitancy; (4) dysuria; (5) poor force of stream; (6) intermittency of urinary stream; and (7) feelings of incomplete bladder emptying despite micturition.

A **urethral stricture** is a narrowing of its lumen. It occurs when infection, injury, or surgical manipulation produces a scar that reduces the caliber of the urethra. The vast majority of urethral strictures occur in men; they are rare in women.[31,32] The severity of obstruction is influenced by its location within the urethra, its length, and the minimum caliber of urethral lumen within the stricture. Specifically, proximal urethral strictures cause more severe obstruction than do strictures of the distal urethra, longer strictures tend to be more obstructive, and the magnitude of blockage is in *reverse* proportion to the urethral caliber.[33]

Prostate enlargement is caused by acute inflammation, benign prostatic hyperplasia, or prostate cancer (see Chapter 25). Each of these disorders can cause encroachment on the urethra with obstruction to urine flow and the symptoms summarized previously.

Severe **pelvic organ prolapse** (see Chapter 24) in a woman causes bladder outlet obstruction when, most commonly, a cystocele (the downward protrusion of the bladder into the vagina) descends below the level of the urethral outlet.[34] Cystoceles (see Figure 24-11) that reach or protrude beyond the vaginal introitus create the greatest risk for obstruction, particularly if the bladder neck (in females the bladder neck and proximal urethra constitute the internal sphincter of the bladder) has been surgically repaired without simultaneous repair of the cystocele.[35] In men the bladder may rarely herniate into the scrotum, causing a similar type of obstruction.

Partial obstruction of the bladder outlet or urethra initially causes an increase in the force of detrusor contraction. If the blockage persists, afferent nerves within the bladder wall are adversely affected, leading to urinary urgency and, in some cases, overactive detrusor contractions (a myogenic cause of overactive bladder). When obstruction persists, there is an increased deposition of collagen within the smooth muscle bundles of the detrusor muscle *(trabeculation)*, possibly in an attempt to increase the force of its contraction strength. Ultimately, the bladder wall loses its ability to stretch and accommodate urine, a condition called **low bladder wall compliance,** and the detrusor loses its ability to contract efficiently. Low bladder wall compliance chronically elevates intravesicular pressure, greatly increasing the problems of hydroureter, hydronephrosis, and impaired renal function.

EVALUATION AND TREATMENT. Although the history and physical examination are critical to the evaluation of lower urinary tract disorders, it must be remembered that no symptom or cluster of symptoms has been identified that accurately differentiates the various causes of these disorders. For example, symptoms such as urgency, urge incontinence, frequent urination, and nocturia may develop because of overactive bladder or either increased or decreased bladder outlet resistance. Reduced resistance is associated with the symptom of stress incontinence (incontinence with coughing or sneezing) and symptoms of increased resistance are similar to those of bladder outlet obstruction, including poor force of urinary stream, hesitancy, and feelings of incomplete bladder emptying.

Various diagnostic tests assist with evaluation. A *cystometric test* uses a catheter and manometer to evaluate bladder urine volume and pressure in relation to involuntary bladder contraction (the leak point pressure) and the urge to void. The *postvoid residual urine* is measured by catheterization within 5 to 15 minutes of urination or through a bladder ultrasound machine that measures bladder height and width to provide an approximation of urine within the vesicle. This measurement may be combined with *uroflowmetry,* a graphic representation of the force of the urinary stream expressed as milliliters voided per second. Each of these measurements assesses the lower urinary tract's efficiency in evacuating urine through micturition but neither differentiates poor detrusor contraction strength from obstruction as a cause of urinary retention. Instead, *multichannel urodynamic testing* is used to identify obstruction, quantify its severity, and measure detrusor contraction strength (see Figure 38-2). *Video-urodynamic recordings* can also demonstrate overactive bladder and detrusor sphincter dyssynergia. An evaluation of renal function, including functional imaging studies and measurement of serum creatinine level, is completed particularly when obstruction is severe and associated with elevated residuals or urinary tract infection. *Electromyography* measures electrical activity in the bladder neck using surface or needle electrodes.

Because the bladder neck consists of circular smooth muscle with adrenergic innervation, detrusor sphincter dyssynergia may be managed by α-adrenergic blocking (antimuscarinic) medications or botulinum toxin.[36] Obstruction that is not adequately managed by pharmacotherapy may require bladder neck incision. Detrusor sphincter dyssynergia may be managed by intermittent catheterization in combination with higher dose antimuscarinic drugs to prevent overactive detrusor contractions and associated dyssynergia while ensuring regular, complete bladder evacuation through catheterization. Alternatively, men with dyssynergia may be managed by condom catheter containment, supplemented by an α-adrenergic blocking drug or transurethral sphincterotomy (surgical incision of the striated sphincter) in order to relieve obstruction. Low bladder wall compliance may be managed by antimuscarinic drugs and intermittent catheterization; however, more severe cases may require augmentation enterocystoplasty (enlargement of the low compliant bladder wall using a detubularized piece of small bowel), urinary diversion, or long-term indwelling catheterization.[37] Prostate enlargement is managed by treating the underlying cause of the prostate enlargement with medication or surgery. Acute prostatitis is initially managed by broad-spectrum antibiotics until the results of a urine culture are obtained. Urinary retention may require transient placement of a suprapubic catheter. The management of benign prostatic hyperplasia and treatment options for prostate cancer are presented in Chapter 25.

Urethral stricture is treated with urethral dilation accomplished by using a steel instrument shaped like a catheter (urethral sound) or a series of incrementally increasing diameter catheter-like tubes (filiforms and followers). Long, dense strictures typically require surgical urethroplasty to prevent recurrence.

A pessary (rubber or silicone device designed to compensate for vaginal wall prolapse) may be inserted to mechanically reverse severe pelvic organ (bladder, uterus, or rectum) prolapse. Depending on the device, the woman may be able to remove, cleanse, and replace the pessary, or it may be changed during a clinic visit. Intravaginal hormone replacement therapy and regular follow-up visits are critical to the long-term success of a pessary.[38] Alternatively, pelvic organ prolapse may be repaired surgically; the procedure may be combined with a urethral suspension to correct stress urinary incontinence or rectocele repair.[39]

Tumors

Renal Tumors

Renal tumors account for about 65,150 (3.9%) new cancer cases and 13,680 (2.3%) deaths in 2013.[40] There are a number of different types of kidney tumors. **Renal adenomas** (benign tumors) are uncommon but are increasing in number. The tumors are solid and encapsulated and are usually located near the cortex of the kidney. Because they can become malignant, they are usually surgically removed. **Renal transitional cell carcinoma (RTCC)** is rare and primarily arises in the renal parenchyma and renal pelvis. **Renal cell carcinoma (RCC)** is the most common renal neoplasm (85% to 90% of all renal neoplasms) (Figure 38-4). Renal cell carcinoma usually occurs in men (two times more often than in women) between 50 and 60 years of age and the incidence is increasing. Blacks have a higher incidence and mortality. Risk factors include cigarette smoking, obesity, hypertension, and advanced stage chronic renal failure (CRF).[41,42] Five-year survival for all stages is about 50% and about 10% for stage IV cancer (metastatic disease).[43]

PATHOGENESIS. Renal cell carcinomas are adenocarcinomas and the etiology is unknown. They are classified according to cell type and extent of metastasis. *Clear cell tumors,* the most common, are dominated by mutations of the von Hippel-Lindau *(VHL)* gene located on chromosome 3p in 90% of cases. They present a better prognosis than papillary (10%),

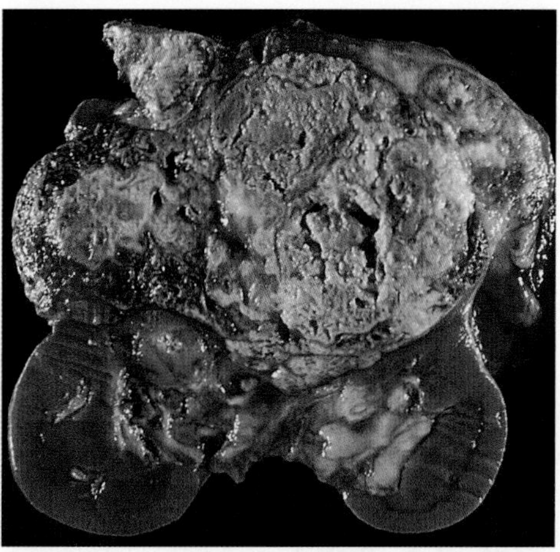

FIGURE 38-4 **Renal Cell Carcinoma.** Renal cell carcinomas usually are spheroidal masses composed of yellow tissue mottled with hemorrhage, necrosis, and fibrosis. (From Damjanov I, Linder J, editors: *Anderson's pathology,* ed 10, St Louis, 1996, Mosby.)

chromophobe (5%), oncocytoma (3% to 4%), collecting duct tumors (1%), or unclassified (rare) tumors.[44] Clear cell and papillary tumors arise from proximal tubular epithelium. Chromophobe, oncocytoma, and collecting duct tumors are believed to arise from the distal nephron epithelium. Confinement within the renal capsule, together with treatment, is associated with a better survival rate. The tumors usually occur unilaterally (see Figure 38-4). About 25% to 30% of individuals with RCC present with metastasis (stage IV).[45,46] The most common sites of distant metastasis are the lung, lymph nodes, liver, bone, thyroid, and central nervous system.[47,48]

CLINICAL MANIFESTATIONS. The classic clinical manifestations of renal tumors are hematuria, dull and aching flank pain, and palpable flank mass in thinner individuals. Systemic manifestations usually represent an advanced stage of disease and include weight loss, fatigue, intermittent fever from tumor cytokines, anemia from hematuria and lack of erythropoietin, polycythemia from tumor secretion of erythropoietin, hypertension from elevated renin levels, and alterations in liver function tests. All of these symptoms occur in less than 10% of cases. Further, they represent an advanced stage of disease, whereas earlier stages are often silent.

EVALUATION AND TREATMENT. Diagnosis is based on the clinical symptoms, plain x-ray films of the abdomen, intravenous pyelography, renal angiography, and computed tomography (CT). (Staging of renal cell carcinoma is presented in Table 38-2.) Staging systems using molecular tumor markers (measurable biologic molecules released from a tumor or the host tissues that distinguish a malignancy) are rapidly advancing.[49] Treatment for localized disease is surgical removal of the affected kidney (radical nephrectomy) or partial nephron sparing nephrectomy for smaller tumors. Surgery is combined with the use of chemotherapeutic agents, although RCC is resistant to conventional chemotherapy.[50] Use of traditional cytokine therapy, specifically high-dose interleukin-2, is limited by significant toxicity (hypotension requiring vasopressor support, oliguria, pulmonary congestion, arrhythmias, and neurologic toxicity).[51] Agents targeting the vascular endothelial

TABLE 38-2 STAGING OF RENAL CELL CARCINOMA (TNM SYSTEM)

STAGE	METASTASIS
I	Tumor confined within kidney capsule ≤7 cm in size.
II	Invasion through renal capsule and renal vein but within surrounding fascia ≥7 cm in size.
III	Involvement of adrenal glands and vena cava and one nearby lymph node:
	T3a-T3c, N0, M0: The main tumor has reached the adrenal gland, the fatty tissue around the kidney, the renal vein, and/or the large vein (vena cava) leading from the kidney to the heart. It has not spread beyond Gerota's fascia. There is no spread to lymph nodes or distant organs.
	T1a-T3c, N1, M0: The main tumor can be any size and may be outside the kidney, but it has not spread beyond Gerota's fascia. The cancer has spread to one nearby lymph node but has not spread to distant lymph nodes or other organs.
IV	Distant metastases (e.g., liver, lung, bones, brain) and more than one lymph node:
	T4, N0-N1, M0: The main tumor has invaded beyond Gerota's fascia. It has spread to no more than one nearby lymph node. It has not spread to distant lymph nodes or other organs.
	Any T, N2, M0: The main tumor can be any size and may be outside the kidney. The cancer has spread to more than one nearby lymph node but has not spread to distant lymph nodes or other organs.
	Any T, Any N, M1: The main tumor can be any size and may be outside the kidney. It has spread to distant lymph nodes and/or other organs.

Adapted from American Cancer Society: *Kidney cancer (adult)—renal cell carcinoma,* 2013. Available at www.cancer.org/cancer/kidneycancer/detailedguide/kidney-cancer-adult-staging. Accessed April 2013.
T, Tumor; *N,* node; *M,* metastasis.

growth factor pathway and the mammalian target of rapamycin (mTOR) have shown efficacy in randomized clinical trials for treatment of metastatic disease.[52,53] There is ongoing research to identify molecular tumor markers that predict individual response to targeted molecular therapies.[54] Radiation therapy may be used for palliation, and new techniques using stereotactic radiofrequency ablation, cryoablation, and laparoscopy are promising. Tumor obstruction is relieved by placement of ureteral catheters or nephrostomy tubes or by completion of urinary diversion procedures. Survival is related to tumor grade, tumor cell type, and extent of metastasis.

Bladder Tumors

Bladder tumors represent about 4.5% of all malignant tumors and are the fourth most common malignancy in men. Approximately 72,570 people developed bladder cancer with 15,210 deaths (2.5% of all cancer deaths) in 2013.[40] The development of bladder cancer is most common in men older than 60 years. **Urothelial (transitional cell) carcinoma** is the most common bladder malignancy, appearing on the inner lining of the bladder.

PATHOGENESIS. The risk of primary bladder cancer is greater among people who smoke or are exposed to any of the following: metabolites of aniline dyes or other aromatic amines or chemicals, high levels of arsenic in drinking water, or heavy consumption of phenacetin.[55] Oncogenes of the *ras* gene family and tumor-suppressor genes including *TP53* mutations and inactivation of *retinoblastoma gene (pRb)* are implicated in bladder cancer. Loss of heterozygosity at chromosome 9 has been found in all stages of urothelial cell carcinoma.[56] The tumor is usually composed of uroepithelial cells (cells lining the bladder, ureters, urethra, and renal pelvis), most have a papillary growth pattern (a tuftlike lesion attached to a stalk), and they rarely progress to invasive disease (Figure 38-5). Nonpapillary tumors (10% to 30% of bladder tumors) are not as common as papillary tumors, but they tend to be more invasive and have a poorer prognosis. Carcinoma in situ can present with papillary

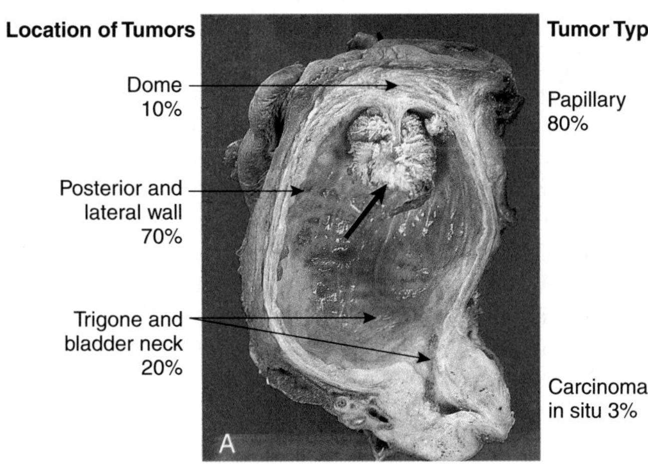

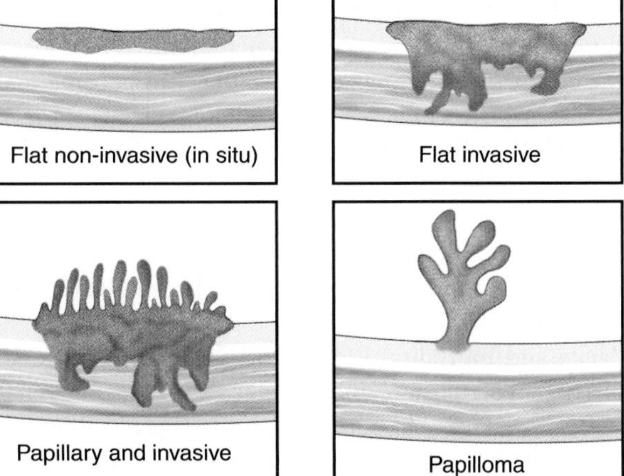

FIGURE 38-5 Carcinoma of the Bladder. A, Papillary transitional cell carcinoma arising in the dome of the bladder as a cauliflower-like lesion *(black arrow);* location and frequency of bladder tumor types noted. **B,** Bladder cancer with morphologic patterns of most common tumors. (**A** from Stevens A, Lowe J, Scott I, editors: *Core pathology,* ed 3, London, 2009, Mosby; **B** from Kissane JM, editor: *Anderson's pathology,* ed 9, St Louis, 1990, Mosby.)

TABLE 38-3 STAGING OF BLADDER CARCINOMA (TNM SYSTEM)

STAGE	DESCRIPTION
Primary Tumor	
T0	No primary tumor identified
Ta	Noninvasive papillary carcinoma—not in bladder muscle
Tis	Carcinoma in situ (CIS)
T1	Tumor invades connective tissue
T2	Tumor invades detrusor muscle
T3	Invasion of fatty tissue around bladder
T4	Tumor has invaded adjacent structures
Region of Lymph Nodes	
N0	No lymph node involvement
N1 to N3	Lymph node metastasis to pelvic or adjacent region
Distant Metastasis	
M0	No metastasis
M1	Distant metastasis

Adapted from American Cancer Society: *Bladder cancer,* 2013. Available at www.cancer.org/cancer/bladdercancer/detailedguide/bladder-cancer-staging. Accessed April 2013.
T, Tumor; *N,* node; *M,* metastasis.

tumors.[57] Worldwide, renal squamous cell carcinoma is the most prevalent and certain forms present at a higher stage and with a poorer prognosis.[58] Metastasis is usually to lymph nodes, liver, bones, lungs, and adrenal glands. Staging for bladder carcinoma is presented in Table 38-3. Secondary bladder cancer develops by invasion of cancer from bordering organs, such as cervical carcinoma in women or prostatic carcinoma in men.

CLINICAL MANIFESTATIONS. Gross painless microscopic hematuria is the archetypal clinical manifestation of bladder cancer. Episodes of hematuria tend to recur, and they are often accompanied by bothersome lower urinary tract symptoms including daytime voiding frequency, nocturia, urgency, and urge urinary incontinence. Flank pain may occur if tumor growth obstructs one or both ureterovesical junctions. Bothersome lower urinary tract symptoms are particularly intense in individuals with carcinoma in situ. Metastasis is the cause of death from bladder cancer, usually from high-grade muscle-invasive tumors.[59]

EVALUATION AND TREATMENT. Urinalysis for evidence of hematuria in the absence of infection provides a useful screening tool for high-risk patients. Urine cytology (pathologic analysis of sloughed cells within the urine) is completed in individuals with evidence of hematuria from unknown causes; cystoscopy or fluorescence cystoscopy with tissue biopsy can confirm the diagnosis. Biologic markers for the diagnosis and prognosis of bladder cancer are under investigation (e.g., cadherins, cyclooxygenase-2 [COX-2] protein, karyopherin-α2 [KPNA2], tyrosine kinase HER2 [RTOG-0524], and epidermal growth factor receptor [EGFR)]).[60,61]

Newer magnetic resonance techniques are helpful for local staging and whole-body computed tomography detects metastasis.[62] Transurethral resection or laser ablation, combined with intravesical chemotherapy or immunotherapy, is effective for superficial tumors. Radical cystectomy with urinary diversion and adjuvant chemotherapy is required for locally invasive tumors, and radiation therapy may be used to support palliative or adjuvant treatment for muscle-invasive tumors.[63-65]

URINARY TRACT INFECTION

Causes of Urinary Tract Infection

A **urinary tract infection (UTI)** is an inflammation of the urinary epithelium usually caused by bacteria from gut flora. A UTI can occur anywhere along the urinary tract including the urethra, bladder, ureter, or kidney. At risk are premature newborns; prepubertal children; sexually active and pregnant women; women treated with antibiotics that disrupt vaginal flora; spermicide users; estrogen-deficient postmenopausal women; individuals with indwelling catheters; and persons with diabetes mellitus, neurogenic bladder, or urinary tract obstruction (see What's New? Catheter-Associated Urinary Tract Infections). UTIs are commonly classified by their location or complicating factors: *cystitis* (bladder inflammation), *pyelonephritis* (inflammation of upper urinary tract), *uncomplicated UTI* (occur in a normally functioning urinary system), and *complicated UTI* (occur with defects in the urinary system

WHAT'S NEW?

Catheter-Associated Urinary Tract Infections

Catheter-associated urinary tract infections are the most common healthcare-associated infection worldwide, and most individuals are asymptomatic. Appropriate indications for use of catheters include acute urinary retention or obstruction; perioperative applications in select procedures; and the frequent, accurate measurement of urine output in critically ill individuals. Other uses include sacral or perineal wound healing with incontinence and immobilization from unstable spine or pelvic fractures. The smallest bore catheter should be used and inserted under aseptic conditions and removed as soon as possible. Some reviews recommended the use of silver alloy or antimicrobial-impregnated catheters. The system is maintained using a closed-drainage system that is replaced if the system is disconnected. The drainage bag is kept below the level of the bladder. Prophylactic antibiotics are not recommended except in special cases (e.g., before traumatic urinary tract interventions). Bacteriuria develops in several ways: periurethral microorganisms may be introduced at the time of catheterization; contaminated urine from the drainage bag or tubing may reflux back into the bladder; and microorganisms can be introduced when there is a break in the closed system. Additionally, bacterial biofilm develops along the inside and outside of the tubing, providing an environment that allows for bacterial colonization and spread with protection against host defenses and antibiotics. *Proteus mirabilis* and *Providencia stuartii* are known to produce greater amounts of biofilm and their adhesion factors and motility allow them to ascend more rapidly in the urinary tract. *E. coli* is the most common pathogen associated with short-term catheterization.

Data from Agency for Healthcare Research and Quality National Guideline Clearinghouse: Catheter-associated UTIs. In *Guidelines on urological infections,* updated December 23, 2011, available at www.guideline.gov/content.aspx?id=34100; Tambyah PA, Oon J: *Curr Opin Infect Dis* 25(4):365–370, 2012; Beattie M, Taylor J: *J Clin Nurs* 20(15-16):2098–2108, 2011; Conway LJ, Larson EL: *Heart Lung* 41(3):271–283, 2012; Nicolle LE: *Infect Dis Clin North Am* 26(1):13–27, 2012; Chenoweth C, Saint S: *Crit Care Clin* 29(1):19-32, 2013.

or in individuals with health problems that compromise host defenses or response to treatment).

Host Defense Mechanisms and Urinary Tract Infection

Host defense mechanisms maintain a sterile posterior urethra and bladder in a healthy individual. Even if bacteria manage to enter the bladder, these defense mechanisms prevent it from clinging to the walls of the bladder or ascending to the upper urinary tracts.[66] Several factors normally combine to protect against UTI. Most bacteria are washed out of the urethra during micturition. The low pH and high osmolality of urea, the presence of Tamm-Horsfall protein, and the presence of secretions from the uroepithelium provide a bactericidal effect. The ureterovesical junction closes during bladder contraction, preventing reflux of urine to the ureters and kidneys. Periurethral mucus-secreting glands surround the distal two thirds of the female urethra. Mucus from these glands traps bacteria before it can ascend from the proximal urethra to the bladder. In men, the length of the male urethra and secretions from the prostate and accessory periurethral glands combine to form a protective barrier against infection. In addition, the urethral sphincter mechanism acts as a mechanical barrier to bacterial ascent from the distal urethra.

Bacteria that successfully ascend the urethra face detection and destruction by components of the body's immune system provided they come into contact with the bladder wall. Protective uroepithelial immune responses include Toll-like receptor (e.g., TLR4) recognition of pathogen-associated molecular patterns on the bacteria, neutrophil and macrophage recruitment and phagocytosis, and the presence of antimicrobial proteins (defensins, cathelicidin, and Tamm-Horsfall protein). Susceptibility to infection also is influence by genetic variation in the host immune response to bacterial virulence and to the virulence of the pathogen.[67] Unfortunately, time is required for the immune system to respond to the potential threat, and this period may provide adequate time for bacteria or other pathogens to reproduce several times.

The efficiency of the bladder's defenses is also influenced by the person's Lewis blood group.[68] This taxonomy is based on recognition of inherited antigens associated with the ABO blood factors. Individuals with certain Lewis blood groups are more prone to UTIs because they secrete fewer antigens capable of resisting bacterial adherence by pili formation.

Most people are able to rapidly rid the urinary tract of invading bacteria, but some show evidence of bacteria in the urine that does not provoke an infection. This condition, called **asymptomatic bacteriuria,** does not harm urinary function or require intervention except in pregnant women.[69] A UTI occurs when a pathogen circumvents or overwhelms the host's defense mechanisms and rapidly reproduces.

Virulence of Uropathogens. **Virulence** is a pathogen's ability to evade or overwhelm the host defense mechanisms and cause disease in a host (see Chapter 10). Several factors contribute to bacterial virulence within the urinary tract, including the ability of uropathic bacteria to adhere (attach) to the uroepithelium. Uropathic strains of *Escherichia coli* have *type-1 pili.* Type-1 pili have adhesins that allow them to bind to mucosal cellular receptors and enter uroepithelial cells and resist flushing during normal micturition. Once inside the cell, they can persist quiescently for long periods and cause recurrent infection or multiply rapidly, safe from host defenses and protected from antibiotic therapy.[70] Additionally, uropathic strains have pyelonephritis-associated fimbriae *(P. fimbriae)* that bind to the uroepithelial P-blood group antigen (present in most of the human population) and readily ascend the urinary tract. Strains of *E. coli* also produce *siderophores* for acquiring nutrient iron, are resistant to bactericidal effects of complement, and express toxins including *cytotoxin necrotizing factor-1* and *hemolysins.* Certain bacterial species also enhance their virulence by acting together to form a biofilm that enhances colonization and resists efficiency of innate host defense mechanisms and antimicrobial therapy, particularly in catheter-associated UTI.[71,72]

Types of Urinary Tract Infection

Acute Cystitis

Acute cystitis is an inflammation of the bladder and is the most common site of UTI. Cystitis is more common in women because of the shorter urethra and the closeness of the urethra to the vagina and anus (increasing the possibility of bacterial contamination).[73]

The morphologic appearance of the bladder through cystoscopy describes different types of cystitis. With mild inflammation, the mucosa is hyperemic (red). More advanced cases may show diffuse hemorrhage (termed *hemorrhagic cystitis*), pus formation, or suppurative exudates (termed *suppurative cystitis*) on the epithelial surface of the bladder. Prolonged infection may lead to sloughing of the bladder mucosa with ulcer formation (termed *ulcerative cystitis*). The most severe infections may cause necrosis of the bladder wall (termed *gangrenous cystitis*). Generally, infections are mild, without complications, and occur in individuals with a normal urinary tract. Acute cystitis may occur alone or in association with pyelonephritis, prostatitis, or kidney stones.

PATHOPHYSIOLOGY. Two factors account for the presence of a UTI: the efficiency of defense mechanisms within the host (individual) and the virulence of the pathogen (bacterium, fungus, or parasite). The most common infecting microorganisms are uropathic strains of *E. coli* (80% to 85%) and the second most common is *Staphylococcus saprophyticus* (10%). Less common microorganisms include *Klebsiella, Proteus, Pseudomonas,* fungi, viruses, parasites, or tubercular bacilli. Bacterial contamination of the normally sterile urine usually occurs by retrograde movement of gram-negative bacilli into the urethra and bladder and then to the ureter and kidney. Some women may be genetically susceptible to certain strains of *E. coli* attachment and may harbor pathogenic strains in their vaginal flora.[73] In rare instances bloodstream infections (sepsis) can spread to the bladder tissue.

Fungal infections are comparatively uncommon. The most common pathogen is *Candida,* but multiple fungal species may colonize the urinary tract or urinary catheters and produce symptomatic UTIs, particularly in those who are immunosuppressed.[74]

Infection initiates an inflammatory response and the symptoms of cystitis. The inflammatory edema in the bladder wall stimulates discharge of stretch receptors, initiating symptoms of bladder fullness with small volumes of urine and producing the urgency and frequency of urination associated with cystitis.

Schistosomiasis haematobium is the most common cause of parasitic invasion of the urinary tract on a global basis; it infects more than 200 million people.[75] Although rare among people living in the United States, the parasite dwells in waters of the various rivers of fresh water bodies in Africa, South America, and Pacific Rim countries. It usually enters the human by swimming up the urethra while the host swims or is partly submerged in an infected body of water. The parasite burrows into the walls of the urinary tract, causing inflammation and scarring of the urinary tract, and an increased risk for urothelial malignancies or renal failure.[76]

CLINICAL MANIFESTATIONS. Many individuals with bacteriuria are asymptomatic. Clinical manifestations of cystitis are related to the host inflammatory response and usually include frequency, urgency, dysuria (painful urination), and suprapubic and low back pain. Hematuria, cloudy and foul-smelling urine, and flank pain are more serious symptoms. Approximately 10% of individuals with bacteriuria have no symptoms and have low TLR4 levels,[77] and 30% of individuals with symptoms are abacteriuric. Older adults with cystitis may be asymptomatic or demonstrate confusion or vague abdominal discomfort. Older adults with recurrent UTI and other concurrent illness have a higher risk of morbidity and mortality.[78]

EVALUATION AND TREATMENT. Infections are diagnosed by urine culture of specific microorganisms with counts of 10,000/ml or more from freshly voided urine. Dipstick urinalysis and microscopy are adequate to diagnose an uncomplicated UTI, but urine culture is critical for complicated infections.[79] Risk factors, such as a urinary tract obstruction, which are associated with a complicated UTI, should be identified and treated. Increased fluid intake and analgesics can relieve symptoms. Evidence of bacteria from urine culture and antibiotic sensitivity warrants treatment with a microorganism-specific antibiotic to eradicate the underlying pathogen. A single large dose of antibiotic or a 3-day course may be effective when symptoms are of short duration and there are no complications. A treatment period of 3 to 7 days is most common depending on antimicrobial selection; older adults with obstructive disorders may require 7 to 14 days of treatment. Frequent, recurrent, acute uncomplicated UTI requires low-dose antimicrobial therapy from 6 months to 2 years or prophylactic treatment, depending on frequency and individual responses.[80] Follow-up urine cultures should be obtained 1 week after initiation of treatment and at monthly intervals for 3 months. Clinical symptoms are frequently relieved, but bacteriuria may still be present, particularly with the development of antimicrobial-resistant bacterial strains. Repeat cultures should be obtained every 3 to 4 months until 1 year after treatment for evaluation of recurrent infection. Urosepsis and septic shock are medical emergencies that usually demand parenteral, broad-spectrum antibiotic therapy and may require hospitalization. A UTI caused by *Schistosomiasis* is treated with praziquantel, and vaccines are under development.[81]

Painful Bladder Syndrome/Interstitial Cystitis

Painful bladder syndrome/interstitial cystitis (PBS/IC) is a condition that includes **nonbacterial infectious cystitis** (viral, mycobacterial, chlamydial, fungal) and **noninfectious cystitis** (radiation, chemical, autoimmune, hypersensitivity).[82] It occurs most commonly in women ages 20 to 40 years who have symptoms of cystitis, such as frequency, urgency, dysuria, and nocturia, for more than 6 weeks duration but with negative urine cultures and no other known etiology. Nonbacterial infectious cystitis is most common among those who are immunocompromised. Noninfectious cystitis is associated with radiation or chemotherapy treatment for pelvic and urogenital cancers.

The cause of PBS/IC is unknown, but an autoimmune reaction may be responsible for the inflammatory response, which includes mast cell activation, altered epithelial permeability, neuroinflammation, and increased sensory nerve sensitivity.[83] The inflammation is associated with a derangement of the glycosaminoglycan layer of the bladder mucosa that makes it more susceptible to penetration by bacteria and noxious urinary solutes. Inflammation and fibrosis of the bladder wall are accompanied by the presence of hemorrhagic ulcers (Hunner ulcers) and bladder volume may decrease as a result of fibrosis, particularly in older individuals.[84] More recently, the identification of antiproliferative factor (APF), a protein expressed by the bladder uroepithelium in those with IC, is important. APF appears to block the normal growth of cells that line the inside wall of the bladder and indirectly increases bladder sensation.[85] Characteristic symptoms of IC include bladder fullness, frequency (including nocturia), small urine volume, and chronic pelvic pain with symptoms lasting longer than 9 months. Chronic pain and sleep deprivation can lead to depression. Diagnosis of IC requires the exclusion of other diagnoses, and extensive evaluations are completed.[86] No single treatment is effective. Oral and intravesical therapies, sacral nerve stimulation, and onabotulinumtoxinA are used for symptom relief. Surgery is used in refractory cases.[87] More research is needed to understand the pathogenesis and treatment of this disease.

Acute Pyelonephritis

Pyelonephritis is an infection of one or both upper urinary tracts (ureter, renal pelvis, and kidney interstitium). Common causes are summarized in Table 38-4. Urinary obstruction and reflux of urine from the bladder (vesicoureteral reflux) are the most common underlying risk factors. Most cases occur in young adult women.

PATHOPHYSIOLOGY. Microorganisms usually associated with acute pyelonephritis include *E. coli, Proteus,* or *Pseudomonas.* The latter two microorganisms are more commonly associated with infections after urethral instrumentation or urinary tract surgery. These microorganisms also split urea into ammonia, making alkaline urine that increases the risk of stone formation. The infection is probably spread by ascending uropathic

TABLE 38-4 COMMON CAUSES OF PYELONEPHRITIS

PREDISPOSING FACTORS	PATHOLOGIC MECHANISMS
Kidney stones	Obstruction and stasis of urine contributing to bacteriuria and hydronephrosis; irritation of epithelial lining with entrapment of bacteria
Vesicoureteral reflux	Chronic reflux of urine up the ureter and into kidney during micturition, contributing to bacterial infection
Pregnancy	Dilation and relaxation of ureter with hydroureter and hydronephrosis; partly caused by obstruction from enlarged uterus and partly from ureteral relaxation caused by higher progesterone levels
Neurogenic bladder	Neurologic impairment interfering with normal bladder and urethral sphincter contraction with residual urine and ascending infection
Instrumentation	Introduction of organisms into urethra and bladder by catheters and endoscopes introduced into the urinary tract for diagnostic purposes
Female sexual trauma	Movement of organisms from the urethra into the bladder with infection and retrograde spread to kidney

microorganisms along the ureters, but dissemination also may occur by way of the bloodstream. The inflammatory process is usually focal and irregular, primarily affecting the pelvis, calyces, and medulla. The infection causes medullary infiltration of white blood cells with renal inflammation, renal edema, and purulent urine. In severe infections, localized abscesses may form in the medulla and extend to the cortex. Primarily affected are the renal tubules; the glomeruli usually are spared. Necrosis of renal papillae can develop. After the acute phase, healing occurs with deposition of scar tissue, fibrosis, and atrophy of affected tubules (Figure 38-6). Acute pyelonephritis rarely causes renal failure.[88]

CLINICAL MANIFESTATIONS. The onset of symptoms is usually acute, with fever, chills, and flank or groin pain. Symptoms characteristic of a UTI, including frequency, dysuria, and costovertebral tenderness, may precede systemic signs and symptoms. Older adults may have nonspecific symptoms, such as low-grade fever and malaise.

EVALUATION AND TREATMENT. Differentiating symptoms of cystitis from those of pyelonephritis by clinical assessment alone is difficult. The specific diagnosis is established by urine culture, urinalysis, and clinical signs and symptoms. White blood cell casts indicate pyelonephritis, but they are not always present in the urine. Complicated pyelonephritis requires blood cultures and urinary tract imaging.[89]

Uncomplicated acute pyelonephritis responds well to 2 to 3 weeks of microorganism-specific antibiotic therapy. Follow-up urine cultures are obtained at 1 and 4 weeks after treatment if symptoms recur. Antibiotic-resistant microorganisms or reinfection may occur in cases of urinary tract obstruction or reflux.[90] Intravenous pyelography and voiding cystourethrography identify surgically correctable lesions.

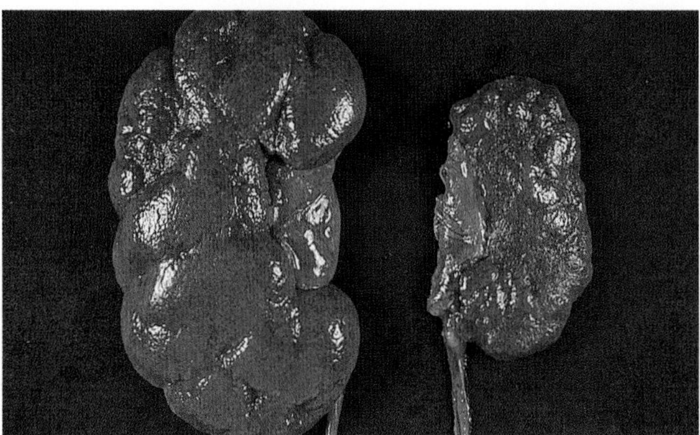

FIGURE 38-6 Pyelonephritis. *(Right)* Small, shrunken, irregularly scarred kidney of an individual with chronic pyelonephritis. *(Left)* Kidney is of normal size but also shows scarring on the upper pole. (From Damjanov I: *Pathology for the health professions,* ed 4, Philadelphia, 2012, Saunders.)

Chronic Pyelonephritis

Chronic pyelonephritis is a persistent or recurrent infection of the kidney leading to scarring of the kidney. One or both kidneys may be involved. The specific cause of chronic pyelonephritis may be unknown (idiopathic) or associated with vesicoureteral reflux or renal stones. Recurrent infections from acute pyelonephritis may be associated with chronic pyelonephritis. Causes other than chronic pyelonephritis include drug toxicity from analgesics such as nonsteroidal anti-inflammatory drugs, ischemia, irradiation, and immune-complex diseases.

PATHOPHYSIOLOGY. Chronic urinary tract obstruction prevents elimination of bacteria and starts a process of progressive inflammation, alterations of the renal pelvis and calyces, destruction of the tubules, atrophy or dilation and diffuse scarring, and, finally, impaired urine-concentrating ability, leading to chronic kidney failure. The lesions of chronic pyelonephritis are sometimes termed *chronic interstitial nephritis* because the inflammation and fibrosis are located in the interstitial spaces between the tubules (see Figure 38-6).

CLINICAL MANIFESTATIONS. The early symptoms of chronic pyelonephritis are often minimal and commonly include frequency, dysuria, and flank pain, and may include hypertension. Progression of disease leads to renal failure, particularly in the presence of other risk factors (i.e., obstructive uropathy or diabetes mellitus). There is an inability to conserve sodium with loss of tubular function, and development of hyperkalemia and metabolic acidosis. Risk for dehydration must be considered if there is loss of the ability to concentrate the urine.

EVALUATION AND TREATMENT. Urinalysis, intravenous pyelography, and ultrasound are used diagnostically. Treatment is related to the underlying cause. Obstruction must be relieved. Antibiotics may be given, with prolonged antibiotic therapy for recurrent infection.

GLOMERULAR DISORDERS

Glomerulonephritis

Glomerulonephritis is an inflammation of the glomerulus caused by *primary glomerular injury,* including immunologic responses, ischemia, free radicals, drugs, toxins, vascular disorders, and infection. *Secondary glomerular injury* is a consequence of systemic diseases, including diabetes mellitus, systemic lupus erythematosus, and, less commonly, congestive heart failure and HIV-related kidney disease. Glomerular disease is a significant cause of chronic kidney disease and end-stage renal failure worldwide.[91,92]

Acute Glomerulonephritis

Acute glomerulonephritis includes renal diseases in which glomerular inflammation is caused by immune mechanisms that damage the glomerular capillary filtration membrane including the endothelium, basement membrane, and epithelium (podocytes). Mesangial expansion can be a component of the disease. The classic symptoms include sudden onset of hematuria including red blood cell casts and proteinuria, and in more severe cases, these symptoms are also accompanied by edema, hypertension, and impaired renal function. Nonimmune acute glomerular injury is related to ischemia, toxin exposure, drugs, vascular disorders, and infection with direct injury to glomerular cells.

PATHOPHYSIOLOGY. Immune mechanisms and inflammation are a major cause of injury for both primary and secondary types of acute glomerulonephritis (Figure 38-7). Immune injury includes: (1) deposition of circulating antigen-antibody immune complexes on the glomerulus (type III hypersensitivity reaction); (2) antibodies reacting in situ against planted antigens within the glomerulus (type III hypersensitivity); (3) action of antibodies directed against the glomerular capillary wall (antiglomerular basement membrane antibodies), the least common and most severe form of immune injury (type II hypersensitivity); and (4) cell-mediated immune injury (type IV hypersensitivity) (Table 38-5). In nearly all types of acute glomerulonephritis, the epithelial or podocyte layer of the glomerular capillary membrane is disturbed with loss of negative charges and changes in membrane permeability; the mesangial matrix may be expanded or the basement membrane thickened (see Figure 38-7). Different causes of injury may result in more than one type of glomerular lesion; thus lesions are not necessarily disease specific (Table 38-6). Many types of acute glomerulonephritis occur, most often in children or young adults, including acute postinfectious glomerulonephritis, Henoch-Schönlein purpura nephritis, and minimal change nephropathy (lipoid nephrosis) associated with nephrotic syndrome. Details of these diseases are presented in Chapter 39. The types, causes, and histopathology of acute glomerulonephritis are summarized in Table 38-7. The mechanisms of acute glomerulonephritis are presented next and include IgA nephropathy, membranous glomerulonephritis, crescentic or rapidly progressive glomerulonephritis, mesangial proliferative glomerulonephritis, and membranous proliferative glomerulonephritis.

IgA nephropathy (Berger disease) is the most common form of idiopathic acute glomerulonephritis in developed countries, especially Asia. The cause is unknown and more commonly affects children and young adults aged 20 to 30 years. It occurs almost twice as often in males as in females and is rare in blacks. Henoch-Schönlein purpura is a milder systemic form of the disease that presents with hematuria and occurs more often in children (see Chapter 39). Abnormal glycosylated IgA-1 (galactose-deficient IgA-1) is produced by the bone marrow. Glycan-specific IgG and IgA antibodies are formed against abnormal IgA-1, can activate complement, and bind to glomerular mesangial cells, stimulating them to proliferate, secrete extracellular matrix proteins, and release inflammatory cytokines and chemokines (interleukin-6, tumor necrosis factor-alpha, and transforming growth factor-beta 1) that cause injury. The immune response contributes to diffuse mesangioproliferative glomerular injury and glomerulosclerosis, which is reversible.[93] A genetic factor may promote the overproduction of IgA-1.[94] B cells that respond to mucosal infections, particularly tonsillitis, might produce the nephritogenic IgA-1 molecule.[95]

The disease manifests with gross or microscopic (30% to 40%) hematuria 24 to 48 hours after an upper respiratory or gastrointestinal tract viral infection. Proteinuria, edema, and hypertension are more severe symptoms and must be treated to prevent future loss of kidney function.[96] Diagnosis is made by renal biopsy. Treatment includes angiotensin-converting enzyme (ACE) inhibitors as first-line therapy, with glucocorticoids added when severe proteinuria is present.[97] The disease is more mild in children than in adults.[98] Tonsillectomy combined with steroid-pulse therapy has promoted clinical remission among individuals with the disease in Japan.[99,100] The prognosis is variable, with 20% to 40% of cases progressing to renal failure over a period of years. Long-term follow-up consists of evaluating blood pressure, urinalysis, proteinuria levels, and renal function every 6 to 12 months.[101,102]

Membranous nephropathy, also known as **membranous glomerulonephritis,** is one of the most common causes of acute glomerulonephritis. Primary membranous nephropathy is caused by subepithelial deposition of circulating antibodies or antibodies (IgG4 subclass) formed in situ to antigens (M-type phospholipase A_2 receptor [PLA2R] protein) located on glomerular podocytes. The antigen-antibody complexes activate C5b-C9 fragments of complement (the membrane attack complex) with injury and release of inflammatory mediators by mesangial and epithelial cells, resulting in increased membrane permeability, thickening of the glomerular membrane, and ultimately glomerular sclerosis. Secondary membranous nephropathy is associated with various disorders including infections (e.g., hepatitis), systemic lupus erythematosus, drugs, and some cancers. Proteinuria and nephrotic syndrome are common manifestations.[103,104]

Rapidly progressive (crescentic) glomerulonephritis (RPGN), also known as subacute or extracapillary glomerulonephritis, develops over days to weeks. The disease affects primarily adults in their fifties and sixties and may be idiopathic or associated with a proliferative glomerular disease (diffuse proliferation of extracapillary cells), such as lupus or poststreptococcal glomerulonephritis. Antiglomerular basement membrane antibodies and antineutrophil cytoplasmic antibodies are associated with glomerular injury.[105,106] There is accumulation of T

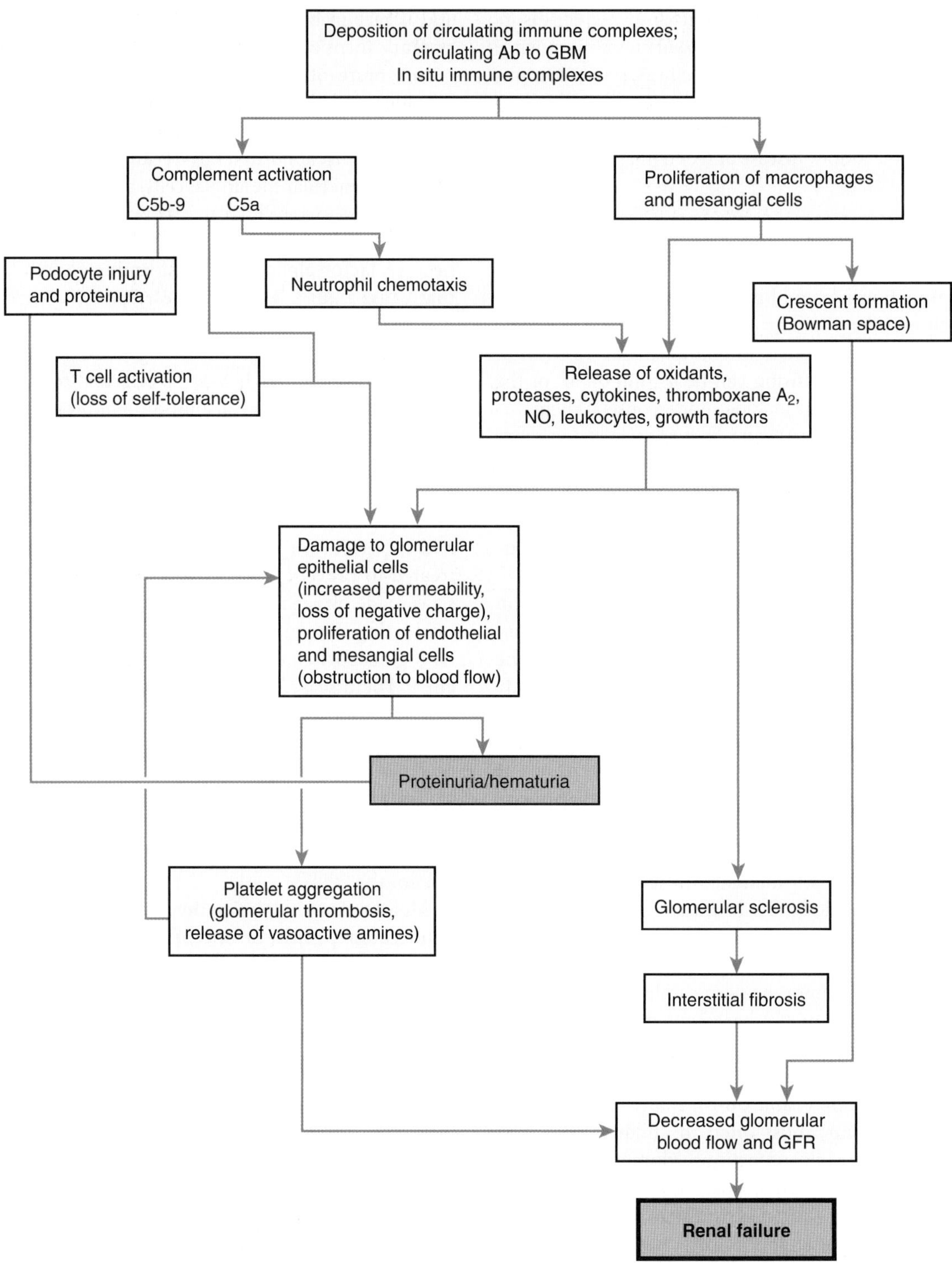

FIGURE 38-7 Mechanisms of Glomerular Injury. *Ab,* Antibody; *GBM,* glomerular basement membrane; *GFR,* glomerular filtration rate; *NO,* nitric oxide.

cells and macrophages with extensive proliferation of glomerular epithelial cells into the Bowman space. The accumulation of cells promotes crescent formation (the shape of the Bowman capsule). Heparin-binding epidermal growth factor–like growth factor (HB-EGF) released from glomerular epithelial cells is associated with the proliferation.[107] Typically the glomerular injury is accompanied by a rapid decline in glomerular function, progressing to renal failure in a few weeks or months. Hematuria is common and may or may not be accompanied by proteinuria, edema, or hypertension. There are three types of RPGN distinguished by immunofluorescence and electron microscopic study of the renal biopsy (Figure 38-8).[108] They are summarized in Table 38-7.

RPGN has a relatively poor prognosis if not diagnosed and treated early. Anticoagulants may be of some benefit in reducing the fibrin component of crescent formation. Plasmapheresis

TABLE 38-5 IMMUNOLOGIC PATHOGENESIS OF GLOMERULONEPHRITIS

GLOMERULAR INJURY	MECHANISM
Soluble immune-complex glomerulonephritis (90%)	Formation of antibodies stimulated by the presence of endogenous or exogenous antigens results in circulating soluble antigen-antibody complexes, which are deposited in glomerular capillaries, or the in situ formation of immune complexes to planted antigens or to structural components within the glomerulus; glomerular injury occurring with complement deposition and activation and release of immunologic substances that lyse cells and increase membrane permeability; immune deposits with a microscopic appearance that fluoresce in a *granular pattern* when stained with fluorescein and viewed under ultraviolet light; severity of glomerular injury related to the number of complexes formed; a type III hypersensitivity reaction
Antiglomerular basement membrane glomerulonephritis (5%)	Antibodies are formed and act directly against the glomerular basement membrane; immune response that causes crescent formation and a *linear pattern* of immunofluorescence; generally associated with rapidly progressive renal failure such as Goodpasture syndrome (type II hypersensitivity reaction)
Alternative complement pathway	A relatively obscure mechanism associated with low levels of complement and membranoproliferative glomerulonephritis
Cell-mediated immunity	A delayed hypersensitivity response that damages the glomerulus; actual cellular mechanism not clearly understood but may involve cytokine secretion, activation of effector cells such as macrophages or by inducing autoantibodies or immune complexes; cytotoxic CD8+ T-cell responses and failure of regulatory T cells may represent two additional types of antirenal hypersensitivity*

*Data from Kurts C et al: *Semin Immunopathol* 29(4):317–335, 2007.

TABLE 38-6 CLASSIFICATION OF GLOMERULAR LESIONS

LESION	DISTRIBUTION WHEN MANY GLOMERULI CONSIDERED
Diffuse	Relatively uniform involvement of most (>50%) or all glomeruli; most common form of glomerulonephritis
Focal	Changes in only some glomeruli (>50%), whereas others are normal
LESION	**DISTRIBUTION WHEN SINGLE GLOMERULI CONSIDERED**
Global	A lesion involving the entire glomerulus
Segmental-local	Changes in one part of the glomerulus with other parts unaffected
LESION	**LESION CHARACTERISTICS**
Mesangial	Deposits of immunoglobulins in the mesangial matrix; mesangial cell proliferation
Membranous	Thickening of the glomerular capillary wall with immune deposits (i.e., IgG and C3)
Proliferative	Increase in the number of glomerular cells: endothelial, epithelial, mesangial
Sclerotic	Glomerular scarring from previous glomerular injury
Crescentic	Accumulation of proliferating cells within Bowman space, making the appearance of a crescent
Interstitial fibrosis	Scarring between the glomerulus and the tubules

is usually combined with corticosteroids and immunosuppression therapy. Dialysis or transplantation is required when failure is irreversible.[109-111]

Mesangial proliferative glomerulonephritis is usually idiopathic and involves deposits of immune complex in the mesangium with mesangial cell proliferation. It can be associated with IgA nephropathy, lupus nephritis, or early diabetic nephropathy. Mesangial expansion reduces blood flow and alters filtration membrane permeability with development of hematuria, proteinuria, hypertension, and uremia (nephritic syndrome).

Membranoproliferative glomerulonephritis (MPGN) is usually idiopathic and involves proliferation of mesangial cells and formation of crescents related to the deposition of complement (C3 component) and inflammatory injury. This disease is rare and occurs more commonly in children and young adults. Hypocomplementemia is associated with all types of MPGN and they are differentiated by light microscopy. All three types stain positive for complement component C3. The subtypes are summarized in Table 38-7. Injury to the glomerular capillary wall in all types of MPGN can cause proteinuria, hematuria, nephrotic syndrome, and acute or chronic kidney failure.[112,113]

The immune injury of acute glomerulonephritis is caused by activation of biochemical mediators of inflammation (i.e., complement cytokines from leukocytes and fibrin) and begins after the antibody or antigen-antibody complexes have deposited or formed in the glomerular capillary wall. Complement is deposited with the antibodies, and its activation can cause cell lysis or serve as a chemotactic stimulus for attraction of neutrophils, monocytes, and T lymphocytes.[114] Activated platelets can further the inflammatory reaction by releasing lysosomal enzymes, reactive oxygen species, and cytokines. These inflammatory mediators injure the glomerular filtration membrane, including endothelial cells, glomerular basement membrane, and epithelial cells (podocytes). The injury increases glomerular membrane permeability and reduces glomerular membrane surface area (podocyte injury). There also may be swelling and proliferation of mesangial cells and expansion of the extracellular matrix in the Bowman space, contributing to crescent

TABLE 38-7 TYPE, CAUSE, AND HISTOPATHOPHYSIOLOGY OF ACUTE GLOMERULONEPHRITIS

TYPE AND CAUSE	HISTOPATHOPHYSIOLOGY
Associated with Nephritic Syndrome	
Acute postinfectious glomerulonephritis (PIGN) (e.g., group A beta-hemolytic streptococci [more common in children]; staphylococcus [more common in older adults])	Subepithelial deposits of IgG and complement complexes; infiltration of neutrophils and monocytes; proliferation of mesangial and epithelial cells with occlusion of glomerular capillary blood flow and decreased glomerular filtration; usually diffuse lesions
Rapidly progressive or crescentic glomerulonephritis (a clinical syndrome): *Type I:* Formation of IgG antibodies against pulmonary capillary and glomerular basement membrane (Goodpasture syndrome); activation of complement and neutrophils; more common in young men; causes pulmonary hemorrhage and renal failure *Type II:* Mesangial immune complex deposition (PIGN, SLE, IgA nephropathy) *Type III:* Pauci-immune, lack of anti-GBM antibodies or immune complexes; presence of serum antineutrophil cytoplasmic (ANC) antibodies associated with systemic vasculitides (usually idiopathic); nonspecific response to glomerular injury; can occur in any severe glomerular disease	Accumulation of fibrin, macrophages, and epithelial cell proliferation into the Bowman space forms crescents and occludes glomerular capillary blood flow decreasing glomerular filtration; antiglomerular basement membrane antibodies lead to necrotizing, proliferative glomerulonephritis, and renal failure; diffuse lesions
Mesangial proliferative glomerulonephritis Can be associated with IgA nephropathy or lupus nephritis	Deposits of immune complexes in the mesangium with mesangial cell proliferation; results in decreased glomerular blood flow and glomerular filtration; leads to hematuria/proteinuria and nephrotic syndrome
Associated with Nephrotic Syndrome	
Minimal change nephropathy (lipoid nephrosis) Glomerular basement membrane appears normal Most common cause of nephrotic syndrome in children (see Chapter 39) Usually idiopathic	Glomeruli look normal under light microscopy; electron microscopy reveals uniform diffuse effacement of epithelial (podocyte) foot processes; loss of negative charge in basement membrane and increased permeability lead to severe proteinuria and nephrotic syndrome
Focal segmental glomerulosclerosis Usually idiopathic Can be associated with HIV infection, IgA nephropathy	Focal proliferation of endothelial and mesangial cells and glomerulosclerosis from hyaline deposits in segmental parts of the glomerular membrane; there is effacement (thinning or deletion) of epithelial podocytes, with a significant increase in pore size resulting in proteinuria and nephrotic syndrome; can progress to involve entire glomerulus and development of tubulointerstitial fibrosis
Membranous nephropathy (autoimmune response to unknown renal antigen) Usually idiopathic; can be associated with systemic diseases (i.e., hepatitis B virus, hepatitis C virus, systemic lupus erythematosus, solid malignant tumors)	Diffuse thickening of glomerular basement membrane and capillary wall from deposits of antibody, complement, and release of inflammatory cytokines; increased permeability with proteinuria and leading cause of nephrotic syndrome in white adults
Membranoproliferative (MPGN) Usually idiopathic; associated with hypocomplementemia *Type I:* Activation of classical complement pathway with nephrotic syndrome (hepatitides B and C, SLE) *Type II:* Activation of alternate complement pathway with hematuria (idiopathic); no circulating immune complexes *Type III:* Activation of alternative complement pathway with nephrotic syndrome; can be familial	Mesangial cell proliferation; thickening of basement membrane; subendothelial deposits of immune complex occlude glomerular capillary blood flow and decrease glomerular filtration; diffuse lesions
IgA nephropathy (Berger disease) Usually idiopathic (can be associated with cirrhosis and minimal change disease); elevated IgA plasma levels (also see Henoch-Schönlein purpura nephritis in Chapter 39)	Mesangial proliferation with deposition of IgA; release of inflammatory mediators with cellular proliferation; crescent formation, glomerulosclerosis, interstitial fibrosis, decreased GFR and hematuria; usually focal, some diffuse lesions

GBM, Glomerular basement membrane; *GFR,* glomerular filtration rate; *HIV,* human immunodeficiency virus; *IgA,* immunoglobulin A; *IgG,* immunoglobulin G; *SLE,* systemic lupus erythematosus.

formation (deposition of substances in the Bowman space forming the shape of a crescent moon) and decreased glomerular blood flow.[115] The result is decreased driving hydrostatic pressure, decreased GFR, and alterations in microcirculatory blood flow within the renal cortex (hypoxic injury).[116]

Loss of the negative electrical charge across the glomerular filtration membrane and increase in filtration pore size enhance movement of proteins into the urine. Proteins are normally repelled because they also have a negative charge. Red blood cells also escape if pore size is large enough. Proteinuria (excess protein in the urine, usually albumin) or hematuria (blood in the urine), or both, develop. The severity of glomerular damage and decline in glomerular function is related to the size, number, and location (focal or diffuse) of cells injured, the

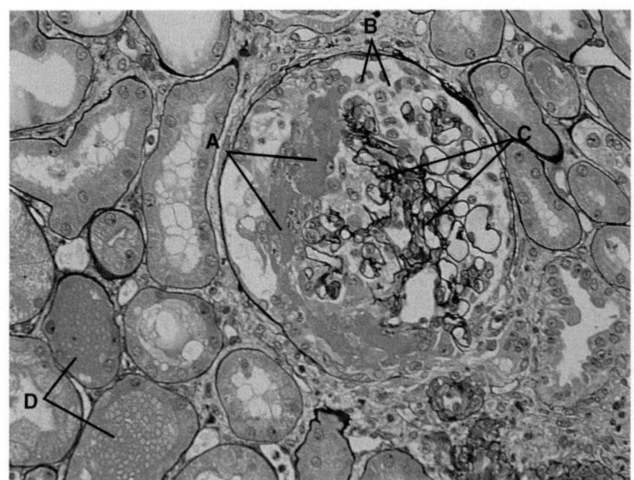

FIGURE 38-8 Antiglomerular Basement Membrane Nephritis. Glomerulus with a fresh crescent consisting of fibrin and cells in the Bowman space *(A)*. There is disruption of the basement membrane of the Bowman capsule, with migration of cells from the interstitium into the Bowman space *(B)*. The capillary tufts *(C)* are distorted and compressed because of the crescent. Note the free erythrocytes in tubular lumina *(D)*. The interstitium is mildly edematous. (Periodic acid–methenamine silver stain.) (Modified from Damjanov I, Linder J, editors: *Anderson's pathology,* ed 10, St Louis, 1996, Mosby.)

duration of antigen exposure, and the type of antigen-antibody complexes.

CLINICAL MANIFESTATIONS. The onset of glomerular disease may be sudden or insidious and significant loss of nephron function can occur before symptoms develop. Acute glomerulonephritis may be silent, mild, moderate, or severe in symptom presentation.

Two major symptoms distinctive of more severe glomerulonephritis are: (1) hematuria with red blood cell casts, and (2) proteinuria exceeding 3 g/day to 5 g/day with albumin (macroalbuminuria) as the major protein. Nephrotic syndrome is associated with gross proteinuria (see p. 1358). Red blood cells escaping through the glomerular membrane produce a smoky, brown-tinged urine; red blood cell casts; and an accompanying proteinuria, which is associated with nephritic syndrome (see p. 1358). Glomerular bleeding provides prolonged contact with the acidic urine and transforms hemoglobin to methemoglobin, which has a brownish color and no blood clots. In comparison, bleeding from sites lower in the urinary tract produces a pink- or red-colored urine.

Different types of glomerulonephritis may be associated with different patterns of urinary sediment. Urine with **nephrotic sediment** contains massive amounts of protein and lipids and either a microscopic amount of blood or no blood. Urine in diseases associated with a **nephritic sediment** is characterized by the presence of blood in the urine with red cell casts, white cell casts, and varying degrees of protein, which usually is not severe. The sediment of chronic glomerular disease has waxy casts, granular casts, and less protein and blood than found in nephrotic or nephritic sediment.

Severe or progressive glomerular disease causes oliguria (urine output of 30 ml/hour or less), hypertension, and renal failure. Focal lesions tend to produce less severe clinical symptoms. Salt and water are reabsorbed, contributing to fluid volume expansion, edema, and hypertension.

EVALUATION AND TREATMENT. The diagnosis of glomerular disease is confirmed by the progressive development of clinical manifestations and laboratory findings of abnormal urinalysis with proteinuria, red blood cells, white blood cells, and casts. Reduced GFR during glomerulonephritis is evidenced by elevated plasma urea, cystatin C, and creatinine concentrations, or by reduced renal creatinine clearance (see Chapter 37). Renal biopsy provides a specific determination of renal injury and type of pathologic condition. Patterns of antigen-antibody complex deposition or formation within the glomerular capillary filtration membrane have been established using light, electron, and immunofluorescent microscopy. Electron microscopy differentiates morphologic changes within the glomerular capillary wall (e.g., subendothelial and mesangial electron-dense deposits, increased mesangial matrix, mesangialization of capillary loops, and foot process fusion). Staining with fluorescein identifies different antibodies (i.e., immunoglobulin G [IgG] or IgA) and their configurations when viewed under ultraviolet light with light microscopy (see Figure 39-5, *C,* p. 1382).

Management principles for treating glomerulonephritis are related to treating the primary cause; preventing or minimizing immune responses; and correcting accompanying problems, such as edema and hypertension. Specific treatment regimens are necessary for particular types of glomerulonephritis. Antibiotic therapy is essential for the management of underlying infections that may be contributing to ongoing antigen-antibody responses. Corticosteroids decrease antibody synthesis and suppress inflammatory responses. Cytotoxic agents (e.g., cyclophosphamide) may be used to suppress the immune response in corticosteroid-resistant cases. Anticoagulants may be useful for controlling fibrin crescent formation in rapidly progressive glomerulonephritis.

Chronic Glomerulonephritis

Chronic glomerulonephritis encompasses glomerular diseases with a progressive course leading to chronic kidney disease (see p. 1364). There may be no history of renal disease before the diagnosis. Proteinuria and hypercholesterolemia have been associated with progressive glomerulosclerosis, tubulointerstitial fibrosis, and tubular atrophy.[117] The primary cause may be difficult to establish because advanced pathologic changes may obscure specific disease characteristics (Figure 38-9). Renal insufficiency usually begins to develop after 10 to 20 years, followed by nephrotic syndrome and an accelerated progression to end-stage kidney failure. Symptom patterns vary depending on the underlying cause. Corticosteroids usually do not change the course of chronic glomerular disease, and dialysis or kidney transplantation ultimately may be needed. Diabetes mellitus and systemic lupus erythematosus are common secondary causes of chronic glomerular injury.

Diabetic nephropathy develops from metabolic (advanced glycosylated end products), inflammatory (transforming growth factor-beta and protein kinase C), and microvascular complications related to chronic hyperglycemia (see Chapter 22). Changes in the glomerulus are characterized by podocyte

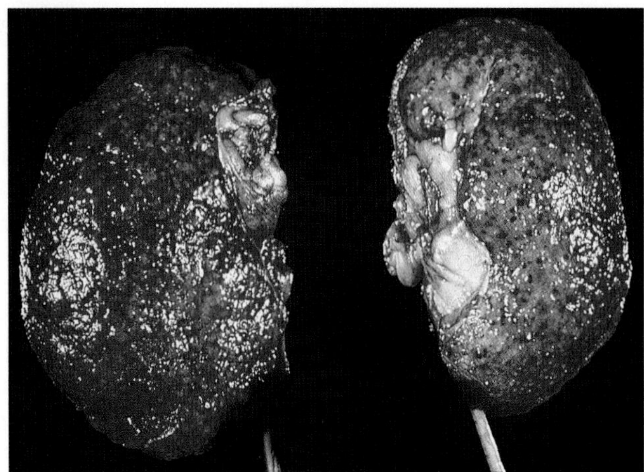

FIGURE 38-9 Chronic Glomerulonephritis. The kidneys appear small, are uniformly shrunken, and have a finely granular external surface. (From Damjanov I: *Pathology for the health professions,* ed 4, Philadelphia, 2012, Saunders.)

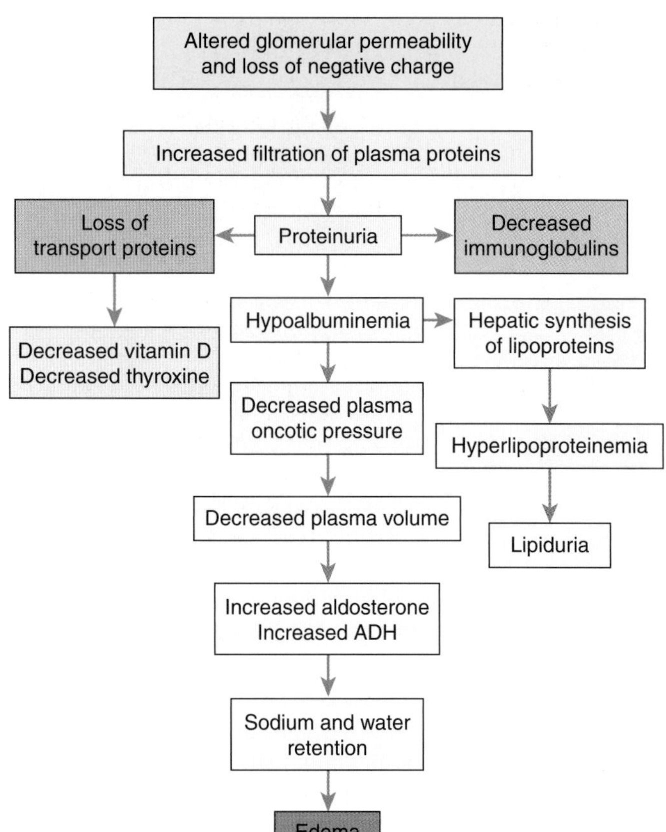

FIGURE 38-10 Pathophysiology of Nephrotic Syndrome.

injury, progressive thickening and fibrosis of the glomerular basement membrane, and expansion of the mesangial matrix (diffuse diabetic glomerulosclerosis) with proteinuria and progression to chronic renal failure.[118] Diabetic nephropathy is the most common cause of chronic kidney disease and end-stage renal failure, but has been declining since 1995.[119-121]

Lupus nephritis is an inflammatory complication of the chronic autoimmune syndrome systemic lupus erythematosus (see Chapter 9). The renal component of the disease is caused by the formation of autoantibodies against double-stranded DNA and nucleosomes with glomerular deposition of the immune complexes triggering of alpha-interferon dependent antiviral immune responses.[121a] There is complement activation and a cascade of inflammatory events results in damage to the glomerular membrane with mesangial expansion (see Chapter 8). Different glomerular lesion patterns are identifiable on biopsy including membranous, mesangial, membranoproliferative, and diffuse proliferative glomerulonephritis; and tubular fibrosis can be present (see Table 38-6).[122,123] Symptom presentation is variable depending on lesion involvement and can include proteinuria, microscopic hematuria, edema, and other signs of nephrotic syndrome. Disease progression may be silent or may progress to end-stage kidney failure over a period of years. Treatment includes the use of immunosuppressive agents.[123a]

Nephrotic and Nephritic Syndromes

Nephrotic syndrome is the excretion of 3.0 g or more of protein in the urine per day, hypoalbuminemia (less than 3.0 g/dl), and peripheral edema. Nephrotic syndrome is characteristic of glomerular injury. *Primary causes of nephrotic syndrome* include minimal change disease (lipoid nephrosis), membranous glomerulonephritis, and focal segmental glomerulosclerosis (see Table 38-7). *Secondary forms of nephrotic syndrome* occur in systemic diseases including diabetes mellitus, amyloidosis, systemic lupus erythematosus, and Henoch-Schönlein purpura (see Chapter 39). Nephrotic syndrome also is seen with certain drugs, infections, malignancies, and vascular disorders. Familial forms of nephrotic syndrome result from genetic defects that affect the function and composition of the glomerular capillary wall (i.e., Alport syndrome with alterations in basement membrane type IV collagen).[124] It often signifies a more serious prognosis when present as a secondary complication. Nephrotic syndrome is more common in children than in adults (see Chapter 39).

In **nephritic syndrome,** the presenting symptom is hematuria (usually microscopic) and red blood cell casts are present in the urine in addition to proteinuria, which is not severe. This syndrome is caused by increased permeability of the glomerular filtration membrane with pore sizes large enough to allow the passage of red blood cells and protein. Nephritic syndrome is associated with postinfectious glomerulonephritis, rapidly progressive (crescentic) glomerulonephritis, IgA nephropathy (see Chapter 8 for types of immunoglobulins), lupus nephritis, and diabetic nephropathy (see Table 38-7). The pathophysiology is related to immune injury of the glomerulus as previously described and can occur simultaneously with nephrotic syndrome. Hypertension, uremia, and oliguria occur in advanced stages of disease. The symptoms and treatment are similar to those for nephrotic syndrome.[125]

PATHOPHYSIOLOGY. Disturbances in the glomerular basement membrane (GBM) and podocyte injury lead to increased permeability to protein and loss of electrical negative charge (see Chapter 37).[126] Loss of plasma proteins, particularly albumin and some immunoglobulins, occurs across the injured glomerular filtration membrane (Figure 38-10). Sustained proteinuria can result in the release of inflammatory mediators and

TABLE 38-8 CLINICAL MANIFESTATIONS OF NEPHROTIC SYNDROME

MANIFESTATIONS	CONTRIBUTING FACTORS	RESULT
Proteinuria	Increased glomerular permeability, decreased proximal tubule reabsorption	Edema, increased susceptibility to infection from loss of immunoglobulins
Hypoalbuminemia	Increased urinary losses of protein	Edema
Edema	Hypoalbuminemia (decreased oncotic pressure, sodium and water retention, increased aldosterone and antidiuretic hormone [ADH] secretion), unresponsiveness to atrial natriuretic peptides	Soft, pitting, generalized edema
Hyperlipidemia	Decreased serum albumin; increased hepatic synthesis of very-low-density lipoproteins; increased cholesterol, phospholipids, triglycerides	Increased atherogenesis
Lipiduria	Sloughing of tubular cells containing fat (oval fat bodies); free fat from hyperlipidemia	Fat droplets that may float in urine
Decreased vitamin D	The globulin to which 1,25-dihydroxy-vitamin D_3 is attached for transport passes through the glomerulus and is lost in the urine	Decreased absorption of calcium from gut Risk for osteodystrophies
Hypothyroidism	Loss of thyroid-binding globulin and other thyroid hormone transport proteins in the urine	May have no symptoms; may have elevated thyroid-stimulating hormone

cytokines by tubular cells with influx of leukocytes resulting in progressive glomerulosclerosis and renal fibrosis.[127] Hypoalbuminemia results from urinary loss of albumin combined with a diminished synthesis of replacement albumin by the liver. Albumin is lost in the greatest quantity because of its high plasma concentration and low molecular weight. Decreased dietary intake of protein from anorexia or malnutrition or accompanying liver disease may also contribute to lower levels of plasma albumin. Loss of albumin stimulates lipoprotein synthesis by the liver and hyperlipidemia. Loss of immunoglobulins may increase susceptibility to infections. Sodium retention also is associated with nephrotic syndrome contributing to the development of edema and ascites. The exact mechanism is unknown but the site of retention is the distal tubules and collecting ducts.[128]

CLINICAL MANIFESTATIONS. Many clinical manifestations of nephrotic syndrome are related to loss of serum proteins (Table 38-8) and retention of sodium. They include edema, hyperlipidemia, lipiduria, vitamin D deficiency, and hypothyroidism.[129,130] Vitamin D deficiency is related to loss of serum transport proteins and decreased vitamin D activation by the kidney. Hypothyroidism can result from urinary loss of thyroid-binding protein and thyroxine but there may be no symptoms. Alterations in coagulation factors cause hypercoagulability and may lead to thromboembolic events, particularly in young adults.[131]

EVALUATION AND TREATMENT. Nephrotic syndrome is diagnosed when the protein level in a 24-hour urine collection is greater than 3.0 g. Serum albumin level decreases (to less than 3 g/dl), and concentrations of serum cholesterol, phospholipids, and triglycerides increase. Fat bodies may be present in the urine. The specific pathologic condition is identified by renal biopsy.

Nephrotic syndrome is commonly treated with a normal-protein (i.e., 1 g/kg body weight/day) low-fat diet, salt restriction, diuretics, immunosuppression, and heparinoids. When diuretics are used, care must be taken to observe for hypovolemia and hypokalemia or potassium toxicity in the presence of renal insufficiency. Aldactone may be combined with loop diuretics to suppress aldosterone activity to conserve potassium. Corticosteroids or cyclophosphamide may be particularly effective for the initial treatment of steroid-dependent nephrotic syndrome in children. Immunosuppressive drugs and angiotensin-converting enzyme inhibitors are used with steroid-resistant nephrotic syndrome.[132,133]

ACUTE KIDNEY INJURY

Classification of Kidney Dysfunction

Kidney injury may be acute and rapidly progressive (within hours), and the process may be reversible. Kidney failure also can be chronic, progressing to end-stage kidney failure over a period of months or years. The terms *renal insufficiency, renal failure, uremia,* and *azotemia* are associated with decreasing renal function but are not specific in relation to cause of kidney disease. Often they are used synonymously, although with some distinctions. Generally, **renal insufficiency** refers to a decline in renal function to about 25% of normal or a GFR of 25 to 30 ml/minute. Levels of serum creatinine and urea are mildly elevated. **Renal failure** refers to significant loss of renal function. When less than 10% of renal function remains, this is termed **end-stage kidney disease (ESKD).** Specific criteria for acute renal dysfunction are discussed in the next section. **Uremia** is a syndrome of renal failure and includes elevated blood urea and creatinine levels accompanied by fatigue, anorexia, nausea, vomiting, pruritus, and neurologic changes. Uremia represents numerous consequences related to renal failure, including retention of toxic wastes, deficiency states, electrolyte disorders, and immune activation promoting a proinflammatory state. **Azotemia** is characterized by increased serum urea levels and frequently increased creatinine levels as well. Renal insufficiency or renal failure causes azotemia. Both azotemia and uremia indicate an accumulation of nitrogenous waste products in the blood, a common characteristic that explains the overlap in definitions of terms.

TABLE 38-9 **RIFLE CRITERIA FOR ACUTE RENAL DYSFUNCTION/FAILURE**

CATEGORY	GFR CRITERIA	URINE OUTPUT (UO) CRITERIA
Risk	Increased creatinine × 1.5 or GFR decrease >25%	UO <0.5 ml/kg/hr × 6 hr
Injury	Increased creatinine × 2 or GFR decrease >50%	UO <0.5 ml/kg/hr × 12 hr
Failure	Increased creatinine × 3 or GFR decrease >75%	UO <0.3 ml/kg/hr × 24 hr or anuria
Loss	Persistent ARF: complete loss of kidney function >4 weeks	
ESKD	End-stage kidney disease: complete loss of kidney function >3 months	
AKIN 1	Increased S_{Creat} by 1.5-2 × above baseline or by 0.3 mg/dl	UO <0.5 ml/kg/hr × 6 hr
AKIN 2	Increased S_{Creat} by 2-3 × above baseline	UO <0.5 ml/kg/hr × 12 hr
AKIN 3	Increased S_{Creat} by >3 × above baseline or by ≥0.3 mg/dl in patients with baseline S_{Creat} >4 mg/dl	UO <0.3 ml/kg/hr × 24 hr or anuria for 12 hr

From Crowley ST, Peixoto AJ: *Clin Chest Med* 30(1):29–43, vii–viii, 2009.
AKIN, Acute Kidney Injury Network ESKD stages; *ARF,* acute renal failure; *GFR,* glomerular filtration rate; S_{Creat}, serum creatinine level; *UO,* urine output.

Acute Kidney Injury

Acute kidney injury (AKI) affects about 5% of hospitalized individuals and has a mortality of 50% to 80%.[134] AKI is a sudden decline in kidney function with a decrease in glomerular filtration and accumulation of nitrogenous waste products in the blood as demonstrated by an elevation in plasma creatinine and blood urea nitrogen levels. The term *acute kidney injury* is preferred to the term **acute renal failure** because it captures the diverse nature of this syndrome, ranging from minimal or subtle changes in renal function to complete renal failure requiring renal replacement therapy. Classification criteria have been developed to guide the diagnosis of renal injury described by the acronym RIFLE (*R* = risk, *I* = injury, *F* = failure, *L* = loss, and *E* = end-stage kidney disease [ESKD]) representing renal dysfunction of increasing severity (Table 38-9).[135,136]

PATHOPHYSIOLOGY. AKI commonly results from extracellular volume depletion, decreased renal blood flow, or toxic/inflammatory injury to kidney cells that results in alterations in renal function that may be minimal or severe. Even small changes in renal function may be associated with significant morbidity and mortality. The etiologies of AKI can be described considering three categories of injury: (1) renal hypoperfusion (prerenal AKI); (2) disorders involving the renal parenchymal or interstitial tissue (intrarenal or intrinsic AKI); and (3) disorders associated with acute urinary tract obstruction (postrenal AKI) (Table 38-10). Most types of AKI are reversible if diagnosed and treated early.

TABLE 38-10 **CLASSIFICATION OF ACUTE KIDNEY INJURY**

AREA OF DYSFUNCTION	POSSIBLE CAUSES
Prerenal	Hypovolemia
	Hemorrhagic blood loss (trauma, gastrointestinal bleeding, complications of childbirth)
	Loss of plasma volume (burns, peritonitis)
	Water and electrolyte losses (severe vomiting or diarrhea, intestinal obstruction, uncontrolled diabetes mellitus, inappropriate use of diuretics)
	Systemic hypotension or hypoperfusion
	Septic shock systemic inflammation
	Cardiac failure or shock
	Massive pulmonary embolism
	Stenosis or clamping of renal artery
	Increased intra-abdominal pressure (abdominal compartment syndrome)
Intrarenal	Acute tubular necrosis (postischemic or nephrotoxic)
	Glomerulopathies
	Acute interstitial necrosis (tumors or toxins)
	Vascular damage
	Malignant hypertension, vasculitis
	Coagulation defects
	Renal artery/vein occlusion
	Bilateral acute pyelonephritis
Postrenal	Obstructive uropathies (usually bilateral—fibrosis)
	Ureteral destruction (edema, tumors, stones, clots)
	Bladder neck obstruction (enlarged prostate)
	Neurogenic bladder

Prerenal acute kidney injury is the most common cause of AKI. Reduced effective arterial blood volume causes renal hypoperfusion that occurs rapidly over a period of hours with elevation of BUN and plasma creatinine levels. During the early phases of hypoperfusion protective autoregulatory mechanisms maintain GFR at a relatively constant level through afferent arteriolar dilation and efferent arteriolar vasoconstriction (mediated by angiotensin II). Tubuloglomerular feedback mechanisms also maintain GFR and distal tubular nephron flow (see Chapter 37). The GFR ultimately declines because of the decrease in filtration pressure. Poor perfusion can result from renal artery thromobosis, hypotension related to hypovolemia (dehydration, diarrhea, fluid shifts) or hemorrhage, renal vasoconstriction and alterations in renal regional blood flow, microthrombi, or kidney edema that restricts arterial blood flow.[137] Sepsis/septic shock and cardiogenic shock following cardiac surgery are the most common causes of AKI in the intensive care unit.[138] AKI may occur during chronic kidney failure if a sudden stress is imposed on already marginally functioning kidneys, hastening the progression to end-stage kidney disease. Failure to restore blood volume or blood pressure and oxygen delivery can cause cell injury and acute tubular necrosis and apoptosis or acute interstitial necrosis, a more severe form of AKI.

Intrarenal (intrinsic) acute kidney injury (AKI) may result from ischemic acute tubular necrosis (ATN), nephrotoxic ATN (i.e., exposure to radiocontrast media or antibiotics), acute glomerulonephritis, vascular disease (malignant hypertension, disseminated intravascular coagulation, and renal vasculitis), allograft rejection, or interstitial disease (drug allergy, infection, tumor growth). **Acute tubular necrosis (ATN)** caused by ischemia is the most common cause of intrarenal AKI. It occurs most often after surgery (40% to 50% of cases) but is also associated with severe sepsis; obstetric complications; and severe trauma, including severe burns; or small vessel vasculitis. A combination of events and predisposing factors leads to the greatest risk for acute renal failure. The terms *acute tubular necrosis* and *acute kidney injury* are sometimes used interchangeably, but the conditions are not the same because acute kidney injury can occur without ATN. ATN is generally described as postischemic or nephrotoxic or it can be a combination of both. Postischemic ATN involves persistent hypotension, hypoperfusion, and hypoxemia, producing ischemia and reduced levels of ATP and generating toxic oxygen-free radicals with loss of antioxidant protection that causes cell swelling, injury, and necrosis. Activation of inflammatory cells (e.g., neutrophils, macrophages, and lymphocytes) and complement and release of inflammatory cytokines contribute to tubular injury.[139] Transport of sodium and other molecules is disrupted with damage primarily to the proximal tubular epithelium and shedding of the brush border with the appearance of tubular granular casts in the urine. Ischemic necrosis tends to be patchy and may be distributed along any part of the nephron tubules. Injury is most severe in the outer medulla with scattered necrosis in the cortex and loss of cells along the tubular epithelium.[140] Severe disease of the glomeruli (i.e., acute or rapidly progressive glomerulonephritis) or renal microvascular disorders can also cause intrinsic kidney injury. Oliguria is common (urine output less than 30 ml/hour) with intrarenal AKI, but anuria is rare. Creatinine values in septic renal injury may not reflect renal injury because sepsis decreases production of creatinine without major alterations in body weight, hematocrit level, or amount of extracellular fluid. Creatinine level usually increases with decreased renal blood flow and decreased GFR. However, in sepsis-induced AKI, creatinine values can remain within normal ranges and may be related to alterations in intrarenal microcirculatory blood flow that are different from the kidney ischemia that develops related to systemic hypotension and hypoperfusion of nonseptic AKI.[141,142]

Nephrotoxic ATN can be produced by numerous antibiotics, but the aminoglycosides (gentamicin, tobramycin) are the major culprits. The drugs tend to accumulate in the renal cortex and may not cause renal failure until after treatment is complete. Radiocontrast media (x-ray media) and cisplatin also may be nephrotoxic. Dehydration, advanced age, concurrent renal insufficiency, and diabetes mellitus tend to enhance nephrotoxicity from either aminoglycosides or radiocontrast media. Other substances such as carbon tetrachloride, heavy metals (mercury, arsenic), methoxyflurane anesthesia, or bacterial toxins may promote renal failure. Endogenous substances toxic to renal tubules are excessive myoglobin (oxygen-transporting substance in muscles) and hemoglobin. Necrosis and tubular cell apoptosis caused by nephrotoxins are usually uniform and limited to the proximal tubules. The high surface area of the brush border (microvilli) of the proximal tubular cells and the reabsorption properties of epithelial cells make them more vulnerable to toxic injury.[143]

Postrenal acute kidney injury is rare and usually occurs with urinary tract obstruction that affects the kidneys bilaterally (e.g., bilateral ureteral obstruction, bladder outlet obstruction–prostatic hypertrophy, tumors or neurogenic bladder, and urethral obstruction). The obstruction causes an increase in intraluminal pressure upstream from the site of obstruction with a gradual decrease in GFR. A pattern of several hours of anuria with flank pain followed by polyuria is a characteristic finding. This type of AKI can occur after diagnostic catheterization of the ureters, a procedure that may cause edema with obstruction of the tubular lumen.

Oliguria (less than 400 ml of urine output per day) can occur in AKI, and three mechanisms have been proposed to account for the decrease in urine output. All three mechanisms probably contribute to oliguria in varying combinations and degrees throughout the course of the disease (Figure 38-11). These mechanisms are as follows[144]:

1. *Alterations in renal blood flow.* Efferent arteriolar vasoconstriction may be produced by intrarenal release of angiotensin II or by redistribution of blood flow from the cortex to the medulla. Autoregulation of blood flow may be impaired, resulting in decreased GFR. Changes in glomerular permeability and decreased GFR also may result from the ischemia.
2. *Tubular obstruction.* Advanced injury with necrosis of the tubules causes sloughing of cells, cast formation, or ischemic edema that results in tubular obstruction, which in turn causes a retrograde increase in pressure and reduces the GFR. Renal failure can occur within 24 hours.
3. *Backleak.* Glomerular filtration remains normal, but tubular reabsorption or "leak" of filtrate is accelerated as a result of permeability caused by ischemia and increased tubular pressure from obstruction.

CLINICAL MANIFESTATIONS. The clinical progression of acute kidney injury, particularly acute tubular necrosis, occurs in three phases: initiation phase, maintenance phase, and recovery phase. The *initiation phase* is the phase of reduced perfusion or toxicity in which renal injury is evolving, usually lasting 24 to 36 hours. Prevention of injury is possible during this phase. The *maintenance* or *oliguric phase* is the period of established renal injury and dysfunction after the initiating event has been resolved and may last from weeks to months. Urine output is lowest during this phase, and serum creatinine, blood urea nitrogen, and serum potassium levels increase; metabolic acidosis develops; and there is salt and water overload. The *recovery phase* is the interval when renal injury is repaired and normal renal function is reestablished. GFR returns toward normal but the regenerating tubules cannot concentrate the filtrate. Diuresis is common during this phase, with a decline in serum creatinine and urea levels and an increase in creatinine clearance. Polyuria can result in excessive loss of sodium, potassium, and water. Fluid and electrolyte balance requires careful maintenance.

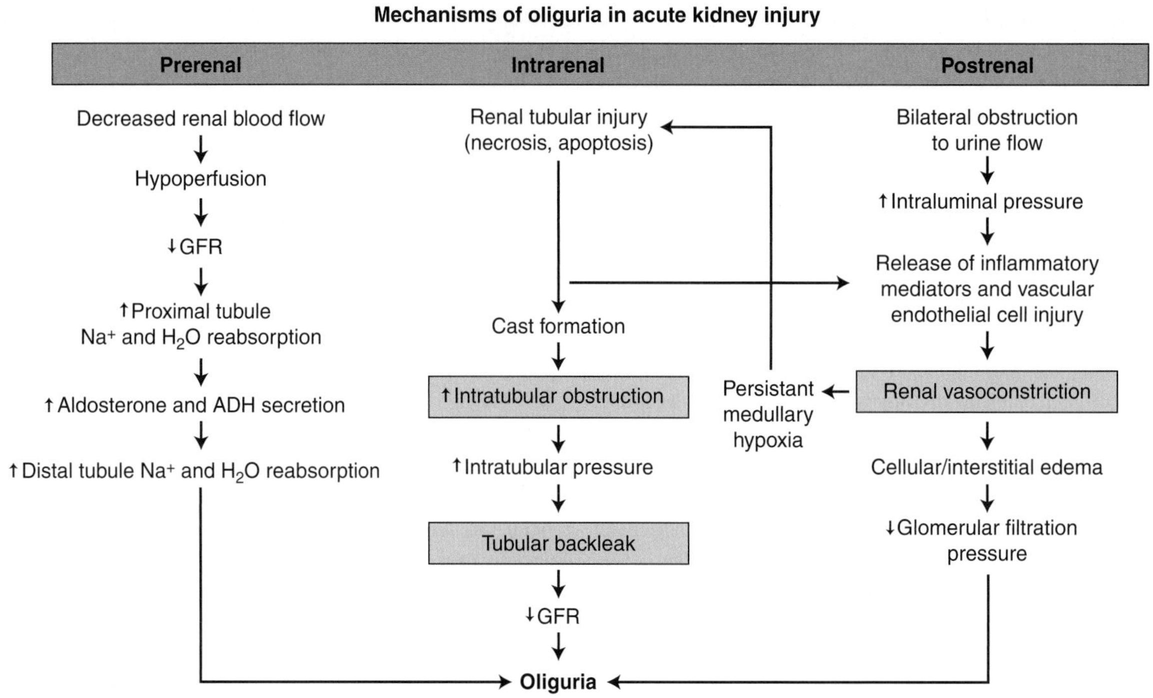

Mechanisms of oliguria in acute kidney injury

Prerenal	Intrarenal	Postrenal
Decreased renal blood flow ↓ Hypoperfusion ↓ ↓GFR ↓ ↑Proximal tubule Na^+ and H_2O reabsorption ↓ ↑Aldosterone and ADH secretion ↓ ↑Distal tubule Na^+ and H_2O reabsorption → Oliguria	Renal tubular injury (necrosis, apoptosis) ↓ Cast formation ↓ ↑Intratubular obstruction ↓ ↑Intratubular pressure ↓ Tubular backleak ↓ ↓GFR ↓ Oliguria	Bilateral obstruction to urine flow ↓ ↑Intraluminal pressure ↓ Release of inflammatory mediators and vascular endothelial cell injury ↓ Renal vasoconstriction ↓ Cellular/interstitial edema ↓ ↓Glomerular filtration pressure → Oliguria

Renal tubular injury → Release of inflammatory mediators and vascular endothelial cell injury; Renal vasoconstriction → Persistant medullary hypoxia → Renal tubular injury

FIGURE 38-11 Acute Kidney Injury and Mechanisms of Oliguria. *ADH,* Antidiuretic hormone; *GFR,* glomerular filtration rate.

Oliguria begins within 1 day after a hypotensive event and lasts for 1 to 3 weeks, but it may regress in several hours or extend for several weeks, depending on the duration of ischemia or severity of toxic injury and the initiation of treatment. **Anuria** (urine output less than 50 ml/day) is uncommon in ATN, and 10% to 20% of cases have nonoliguric failure. Anuria involves both kidneys and suggests bilateral renal artery occlusion, obstructive uropathy, or acute cortical necrosis. **Nonoliguric renal failure** usually represents less severe injury and is associated with toxin exposure or drug toxicity. The renal tubules have impaired reabsorption and concentration and dilution function. The urine output may be greater than 2 L per day, but the BUN and plasma creatinine concentrations increase.

Other early manifestations depend on the underlying cause of renal failure. Individuals who have experienced trauma or surgery or people in a catabolic state may have more rapid elevations in BUN level. They are prone to hyperkalemia and metabolic acidosis related to decreased potassium level and hydrogen excretion. Renal phosphate excretion is decreased, causing hyperphosphatemia. Fluid retention may cause edema. Symptoms of congestive heart failure develop in persons with cardiac disease. Nausea, vomiting, and fatigue accompany uremia and electrolyte imbalances. Wound healing is delayed, and the risk of infection, particularly pneumonia, is greater. Nonoliguric renal failure generally has a better prognosis because of fewer complications and regeneration of the tubular epithelium. Individuals with oliguria may require maintenance dialysis to attenuate symptoms of renal failure.

As renal function improves during the recovery phase, increase in urine volume (diuresis) is progressive. During the early diuretic phase the tubules are still recovering secretory and reabsorptive function. Sodium and potassium are lost in the urine, and the risk for hypokalemia is greater. Volume depletion may ensue, with fluid losses of 3 to 4 L/day. Fluid and electrolyte balance must be carefully monitored and excessive urinary losses replaced. Return to normal status may take 3 to 12 months. Approximately 30% of individuals do not have full recovery of a normal GFR or tubular function and progress to end-stage kidney disease.[145]

EVALUATION AND TREATMENT. The diagnosis of AKI is related to the cause of the disease. The history can help distinguish the different etiologies of AKI. Prerenal causes are associated with a history of blood volume depletion or other causes of poor kidney perfusion (e.g., shock, heart failure, renal artery thrombi). Intrinsic causes include exposure to nephrotoxins and infection. Postrenal causes are associated with obstructive uropathies (e.g., an enlarged prostate or stones). The diagnostic challenge is to differentiate prerenal acute renal injury from acute tubular necrosis. Urine composition may provide helpful diagnostic clues to changes in tubular function (Table 38-11).

The ratios of the BUN to plasma creatinine concentration and fractional excretion of sodium (the ratio of filtered sodium to excreted sodium) are helpful diagnostic indicators because the tests reflect renal tubular reabsorption ability. In prerenal AKI, tubular function is maintained and salt, water, and urea are reabsorbed. With ATN, reabsorption and urinary concentration abilities are compromised. Other causes of renal failure also may exhibit similar clinical findings. *Cystatin C,* a serum protein constantly produced by nucleated cells, is freely filtered by the glomerulus, and its concentration can serve as a measure of GFR and may be useful for detecting early changes in glomerular filtration rate.[146] Serial measurements of plasma creatinine concentration provide an index of renal function during

TABLE 38-11 URINE CHARACTERISTICS OF PRERENAL AND INTRINSIC ACUTE KIDNEY INJURY

DIAGNOSTIC INDEX	PRERENAL	ATN
Urine volume	<400 ml	<400 ml
Urine specificity	1.016-1.020	1.010-1.012
Urine osmolality	>500 mOsm	<300 mOsm
Urine sodium	<10 mEq/L	>30 mEq/L
BUN/plasma	>15:1	<15:1 creatinine
FE_{Na}	<1% (also seen in acute glomerulonephritis	>1% (also seen in urinary tract obstruction and renal parenchymal disease)
Urine sediment	Usually no cells, some hyaline casts	Brown granular casts, epithelial cells

ATN, Acute tubular necrosis; *BUN*, blood urea nitrogen; FE_{Na}, fractional excretion of sodium.

the recovery phase. However, changes in serum creatinine level occur only if more than 50% of glomerular filtration is lost and are often delayed by more than 24 hours. Such diagnostic delays make the implementation of early therapy very difficult, contributing to disease progression and mortality. Advances are being made in the use of biomarkers that allow assessment of kidney injury before elevation of serum creatinine level (see What's New? Biomarkers and Acute Kidney Injury).

Prevention of AKI and maintenance of renal perfusion involve maintenance of fluid volume before and after surgery or diagnostic procedures or when nephrotoxic drugs or contrast agents are in use. There is no specific treatment for acute renal failure. The primary goal of therapy, once AKI has occurred, is to maintain the individual's life until renal function has recovered. Management principles directly related to physiologic alterations generally include (1) correcting fluid and electrolyte disturbances, (2) managing blood pressure, (3) preventing and treating infections, (4) maintaining nutrition, and (5) remembering that certain drugs or their metabolites are not excreted and can be toxic. Fluid and electrolyte replacement must be carefully calculated with consideration of urine losses, insensible losses (up to 1000 ml/day), and production of endogenous water by oxidation (450 ml/day). Overhydration of patients dilutes their plasma sodium concentration. Metabolic acidosis is usually not treated until serum bicarbonate concentration is less than 15 mEq/L.[147]

Hyperkalemia can be managed by restricting dietary sources of potassium, using non–potassium-sparing diuretics, or using cation ion exchange resins, which may be administered orally or rectally. These resins exchange potassium for another cation, such as sodium in the bowel, and the potassium is then excreted attached to the resin. With severe hyperkalemia (more than 6.5 mEq/L), dialysis may be required or potassium can be driven back temporarily into the cells by administering glucose and insulin or by infusing sodium bicarbonate or albuterol. Glucose metabolism causes potassium to move to the intracellular fluid, and insulin infusions therefore can be effective in shifting potassium from the extracellular to intracellular space, along with the transport of glucose, within 30 minutes. (Glucose metabolism is discussed in Chapter 1 and Chapter 21.) Using sodium bicarbonate to cause alkalemia also shifts potassium into cells in exchange for hydrogen ions. However, use of sodium bicarbonate in AKI is controversial.[148] Careful monitoring of the electrocardiogram for peaking T waves is essential

WHAT'S NEW?

Biomarkers and Acute Kidney Injury

Rising serum creatinine concentrations and urine output have conventionally determined evolving acute kidney injury (AKI). However, these changes may occur 2 to 3 days after the initiating renal insult and delay potentially effective therapies that are limited to the early stage of injury. New biomarkers are under investigation that would enhance the differential diagnosis of kidney injury and dysfunction and provide guidance for very early treatment before a rise in serum creatinine level. Candidate molecules include neutrophil gelatinase–associated lipocalin, urinary cystatin C, kidney injury molecule-1, IL-18, renal vanin-1 protein, and hematopoietic growth factor–inducible neurokinin 1. A recent multicenter prospective study in the emergency department found levels of urinary neutrophil gelatinase–associated lipocalin and urinary kidney injury molecule-1 more predictive than serum creatinine level in identifying risk for AKI. Future research is necessary to clarify whether serial measurements of a specific biomarker or the use of a panel of biomarkers may be more useful for diagnosis and predicting severity and duration of AKI.

Data from Ferguson MA, Waikar SS: *Clin Chem* 58(4):680–689, 2012; Nickolas TL et al: *J Am Coll Cardiol* 59(3):246–255, 2012; Schiffl H, Lang SM: *Mol Diagn Ther* 16(4):199–207, 2012; Slocum JL, Heung M, Pennathur S: *Transl Res* 159(4):277–289, 2012; Vanmassenhove J et al: *Nephrol Dial Transplant* 28(2):254–273, 2013.

for individuals with hyperkalemia. Intravenous infusion of calcium is the most rapid method of treating cardiac effects of hyperkalemia. Calcium decreases the threshold potential and reduces the membrane excitability caused by hyperkalemia (see Chapter 3). Calcium should be used only in emergencies, however, because hypercalcemia also may cause cardiac arrest.

Azotemia is generally controlled and nutrition maintained with a low-protein, high-carbohydrate diet. Essential amino acid replacement can be given orally or parenterally. Adequate carbohydrate intake slows protein catabolism and helps prevent release of potassium from cellular breakdown. Because sepsis is a common serious and potentially fatal complication of renal failure, observation for signs of infection and early treatment with antibiotics are necessary. Drug dosage levels may require adjustment if they are metabolized or excreted by the kidneys. Recovery may take up to 1 year.

Continuous renal replacement therapy (CRRT [hemodialysis]) (mechanical removal of water, electrolytes, and toxins from the blood) is indicated for uncontrollable hyperkalemia or acidosis or severe fluid overload. CRRT is particularly promising in critically ill people with multiple organ dysfunction or

TABLE 38-12 **STAGES OF CHRONIC KIDNEY DISEASE**

STAGE	SEVERITY*	GFR (ml/min)	PROGRESSION	SYMPTOMS
1	Kidney damage: normal or increased GFR	≥90	None apparent	Usually none Hypertension common
2	Kidney damage: mild ↓ GFR	60-89	Increasing PTH Early bone disease Increasing plasma creatinine and urea	Subtle hypertension
3	Moderate: ↓ GFR	30-59	Erythropoietin deficiency, anemia Increased plasma creatinine and urea	Mild hypertension
4	Severe: ↓ GFR	15-29	Increased triglycerides Metabolic acidosis Hyperkalemia Salt/water retention Increasing plasma creatinine and urea	Moderate hypertension Hyperphosphatemia Anemia
5	End-stage kidney disease; kidney failure	<15	Uremia	Severe hypertension Hyperphosphatemia Anemia

Adapted from National Kidney Foundation: *Chronic Kidney Disease 2006: a guide to select NKF KDOQI guidelines and recommendations,* 2006. Available at www.kidney.org/professionals/kls/pdf/Pharmacist_CPG.pdf.
*Normal glomerular filtration rate in a 70-kg male is about 120 ml/min.
GFR, Glomerular filtration rate; *PTH,* parathyroid hormone.

sepsis. The timing and optimal dose-response relationships for CRRT are under investigation.[149,150]

CHRONIC KIDNEY DISEASE

Chronic kidney disease (CKD) is the progressive loss of renal function associated with systemic diseases such as hypertension, diabetes mellitus, systemic lupus erythematosus, or intrinsic kidney disease, including kidney stones, acute kidney injury, chronic glomerulonephritis, chronic pyelonephritis, obstructive uropathies, or vascular disorders. The National Kidney Foundation (www.kidney.org/professionals/) defines kidney damage as a GFR less than 60 ml/min/1.73 m^2 for 3 months or more, irrespective of cause. *Chronic kidney disease* is the preferred terminology and is referenced to declining GFR. The terms *renal insufficiency* and *chronic renal failure* are still often used to describe declining renal function, but they do not have the specificity of the stages recommended by the National Kidney Foundation (Table 38-12). CKD decreases filtration and tubular functions with consequences manifested throughout all organ systems (Table 38-13).

PATHOPHYSIOLOGY. The kidneys have a remarkable ability to adapt to loss of nephron mass. Symptomatic changes resulting from increased levels of creatinine, urea, and potassium and alterations in salt and water balance usually do not become apparent until renal function declines to less than 25% of normal when adaptive renal reserves have been exhausted.

Different theories have been proposed to account for the adaptation to loss of renal function. The *intact nephron hypothesis* proposes that loss of nephron mass with progressive kidney damage causes the surviving nephrons to sustain normal kidney function. These nephrons are capable of a compensatory hypertrophy and expansion or hyperfunction in their rates of filtration, reabsorption, and secretion and can maintain adaptive changes in solute and water regulation in the presence of overall declining GFR. Although the urine of an individual with chronic kidney failure may contain abnormal amounts of protein and red and white blood cells or casts, the major end products of excretion are similar to those of normally functioning kidneys until the advanced stages of renal failure when there is a significant reduction of functioning nephrons.[151] With severe or repeated injury, epithelial cells have an impaired proliferative response resulting in interstitial capillary loss and fibroblast proliferation. The progressive process of glomerulosclerosis and tubulointerstitial fibrosis contributes to end-stage kidney disease.[152] The *particular location of kidney damage* also can influence loss of kidney function. For example, tubular interstitial diseases damage primarily the tubular or medullary parts of the nephron, producing problems such as renal tubular acidosis, salt wasting, and difficulty diluting or concentrating the urine. When the damage is primarily vascular or glomerular, proteinuria, hematuria, and nephrotic syndrome are more prominent. A summary of factors involved in the progression of chronic kidney disease is outlined in Table 38-14 and Figure 38-12.

The factors that contribute to the pathogenesis of CKD are complex and involve the interaction of many cells, cytokines, and structural alterations. Two factors that have consistently been recognized to advance renal disease are proteinuria and angiotensin II activity. Glomerular hyperfiltration and increased glomerular capillary permeability lead to proteinuria. Proteinuria contributes to tubulointerstitial injury by accumulating in the interstitial space and activating complement proteins and other mediators and cells, such as macrophages, that promote inflammation and progressive fibrosis.[153] Angiotensin II activity is elevated with progressive nephron injury. **Angiotensin II** promotes glomerular hypertension and hyperfiltration caused by efferent arteriolar vasoconstriction and also promotes systemic hypertension. The chronically high intraglomerular pressure increases glomerular capillary permeability, contributing to proteinuria. Angiotensin II also may promote the activity of

TABLE 38-13 SYSTEMIC EFFECTS OF CHRONIC KIDNEY DISEASE AND UREMIA

SYSTEM	MANIFESTATIONS	MECHANISMS	TREATMENT
Skeletal	Spontaneous fractures and bone pain Deformities of long bones	Chronic kidney disease-mineral bone disorder: bone inflammation with fibrous degeneration related to hyperparathyroidism; bone resorption associated with vitamin D and calcium deficiency	Control of hyperphosphatemia to reduce hyperparathyroidism; administration of calcium and aluminum hydroxide antacids, which bind phosphate in the gut, together with a phosphate-restricted diet; vitamin D replacement; avoidance of magnesium antacids because of impaired magnesium excretion
Cardiopulmonary	Pulmonary edema, Kussmaul respirations	Fluid overload associated with pulmonary edema and metabolic acidosis leading to Kussmaul respirations	ACE inhibitors; combination of propranolol, hydralazine, and minoxidil for those with high levels of renin; bilateral nephrectomy with dialysis or transplantation
Cardiovascular	Left ventricular hypertrophy, cardiomyopathy, and ischemic heart disease; hypertension, dysrhythmias, accelerated atherosclerosis; pericarditis with fever, chest pain, and pericardial friction rub	Extracellular volume expansion and hypersecretion of renin associated with hypertension; anemia increases cardiac workload; hyperlipidemia promotes atherosclerosis; toxins precipitate into pericardium	Volume reduction with diuretics that are not potassium sparing (to avoid hyperkalemia); lipid lowering drugs; blood pressure–lowering strategies; dialysis
Neurologic	Encephalopathy (fatigue, loss of attention, difficulty with problem solving); peripheral neuropathy (pain and burning in the legs and feet, loss of vibration sense and deep tendon reflexes); loss of motor coordination, twitching, fasciculations, stupor, and coma with advanced uremia	Progressive accumulation of uremic toxins associated with end-stage renal disease Stroke or intracerebral hemorrhage associated with chronic dialysis	Dialysis or successful kidney transplantation
Endocrine	Restricted growth in children Higher incidence of goiter Osteomalacia	Elevated parathyroid hormone levels Decreased thyroid hormone	Endogenous recombinant human growth hormone; thyroid hormone replacement Same as skeletal above
Hematologic	Anemia, usually normochromic normocytic; platelet disorders with prolonged bleeding times	Reduced erythropoietin secretion and reduced red cell production; uremic toxins shorten red blood cell survival and alter platelet function	Dialysis; recombinant human erythropoietin (controversial) and iron supplementation; conjugated estrogens; DDAVP (1-deamino-[8-c-arginine] vasopressin); transfusion
Gastrointestinal	Anorexia, nausea, vomiting; mouth ulcers, stomatitis, urinous breath (uremic factor), hiccups, peptic ulcers, gastrointestinal bleeding, and pancreatitis associated with end-stage renal failure	Retention of metabolic acids and other metabolic waste products	Protein-restricted diet for relief of nausea and vomiting; Na^+-based alkali or alkali-inducing food
Integumentary	Abnormal pigmentation and pruritus	Retention of urochromes, contributing to sallow, yellow color; high plasma calcium levels and neuropathy associated with pruritus	Dialysis with control of serum calcium and phosphate levels
Immunologic	Increased risk of infection that can cause death; increased risk of carcinoma	Suppression of cell-mediated immunity; reduction in number and function of lymphocytes, diminished phagocytosis	Routine dialysis
Reproductive	Sexual dysfunction: menorrhagia, amenorrhea, infertility, and decreased libido in women; decreased testosterone levels, infertility, and decreased libido in men	Dysfunction of ovaries and testes; presence of neuropathies	No specific treatment

TABLE 38-14 FACTORS REPRESENTING PROGRESSION OF CHRONIC KIDNEY DISEASE

FACTOR	CHARACTERISTICS
Proteinuria	Glomerular hyperfiltration of protein contributes to tubular intestinal injury by accumulating in the interstitial space and promoting inflammation and progressive fibrosis.
Creatinine and urea clearance	In chronic renal failure, the GFR falls and the plasma creatinine concentration increases by a reciprocal amount; because there is no regulatory adjustment for creatinine, plasma levels continue to rise and serve as an index of changing glomerular function.
	As GFR declines, urea clearance increases. (**Note:** Urea is filtered and reabsorbed and varies with the state of hydration.)
Sodium and water balance	In chronic renal failure, sodium load delivered to nephrons exceeds normal, so excretion must increase; thus less is reabsorbed. Obligatory loss occurs, leading to sodium deficits and volume depletion. As GFR is reduced, ability to concentrate and dilute urine diminishes.
Phosphate and calcium balance	Changes in acid-base balance affect phosphate and calcium balance. The major disorders associated with chronic renal failure are reduced renal phosphate excretion, decreased renal synthesis of 1,25-$(OH)_2$-vitamin D_3, and hypocalcemia.
	Hypocalcemia leads to secondary hyperparathyroidism, GFR falls, and progressive hyperphosphatemia, hypocalcemia, and dissolution of bone result.
Hematocrit	Lack of erythropoietin and anemia accompany chronic renal failure. Lethargy, dizziness, and low hematocrit are common.
Potassium balance	In chronic renal failure, tubular secretion of potassium increases until oliguria develops. Use of potassium-sparing diuretics also may precipitate elevated serum potassium levels. As disease progresses, total body potassium levels can rise to life-threatening levels and dialysis is required.
Acid-base balance	In early renal insufficiency, acid excretion and bicarbonate reabsorption are increased to maintain normal pH. Metabolic acidosis begins when GFR reaches 30% to 40%. Metabolic acidosis and hyperkalemia may be severe enough to require dialysis when end-stage renal failure develops.
Dyslipidemia	Chronic hyperlipidemia may induce glomerular and tubulointerstitial injury contributing to the progression of chronic kidney disease.

GFR, Glomerular filtration rate.

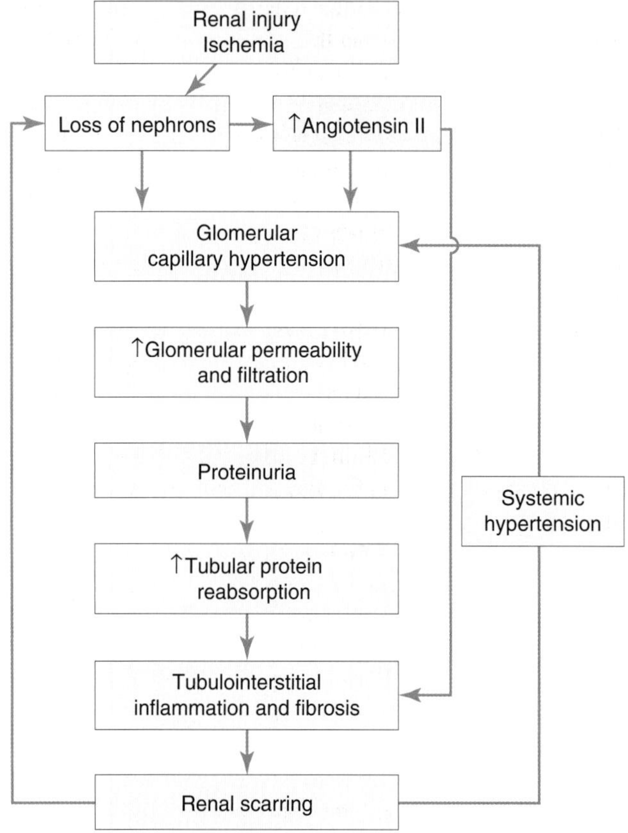

FIGURE 38-12 Mechanisms Related to the Progression of Chronic Kidney Disease.

inflammatory cells and growth factors that participate in tubulointerstitial fibrosis and scarring (see Figure 38-12).[154]

CLINICAL MANIFESTATIONS. The clinical manifestations of chronic kidney disease are often described using the terms azotemia and uremia. Azotemia is manifested by increased levels of serum urea, serum creatinine, and other nitrogenous compounds related to decreasing kidney function. Uremia is a proinflammatory state with many systemic effects known as **uremic syndrome**[155] and is associated with the accumulation of urea and other nitrogenous compounds and toxins. Sources of toxins include the accumulation of end products of protein metabolism, alterations in fluid and electrolytes, metabolic acidosis, intestinal absorption of toxins produced by gut bacteria, and results of altered renal hormone synthesis (i.e., anemia, hyperphosphatemia, and hypocalcemia). Generally, the symptoms include hypertension, anorexia, nausea, vomiting, diarrhea or constipation, malnutrition and weight loss, pruritus, edema, anemia, and neurologic, cardiovascular disease, and skeletal changes. The many systemic manifestations associated with uremia are summarized in Table 38-13, p. 1365, and Figure 38-13.

Creatinine and Urea Clearance

Creatinine is constantly released from muscle and excreted primarily by glomerular filtration. In CKD, as the GFR declines, the plasma creatinine level increases by a reciprocal amount to maintain a constant rate of excretion (Figure 38-14). Because no significant tubular adjustment occurs for creatinine (i.e., tubular secretion), the plasma levels continue to increase as the GFR decreases. Therefore, measures of plasma creatinine can serve as an index of changing glomerular function. The clearance of *urea* follows a similar pattern, but urea is filtered

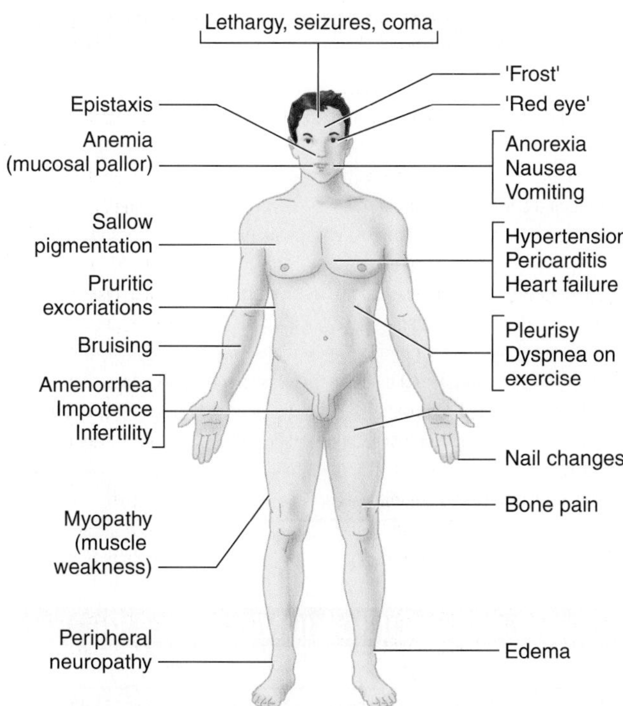

FIGURE 38-13 Common Signs and Symptoms of Kidney Dysfunction (See Text for Reference Site). (From Goldman L, Schafer AI: *Goldman's Cecil medicine,* ed 24, Philadelphia, 2012, Saunders; redrawn from Forbes CD, Jackson WF: *Color atlas and text of clinical medicine,* ed 3, London, 2003, Mosby.)

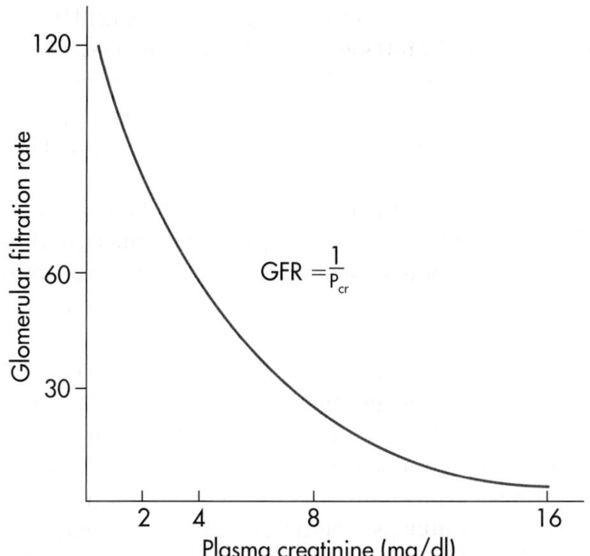

FIGURE 38-14 Plasma Creatinine (P_{cr}) and Glomerular Filtration Rate (GFR).

as well as reabsorbed and varies with the state of hydration; it is not a good index of GFR. However, as the GFR decreases, plasma urea concentration also increases.[156]

Fluid and Electrolyte Balance

Fluid and electrolyte and acid-base balances are significantly disturbed with chronic kidney disease. A summary of electrolyte and acid-base balance alterations is presented in Table 38-15.

Levels of *sodium* must be regulated within narrow limits because sodium is the major extracellular solute. In CKD sodium and water balance is maintained very close to normal until the development of stage V ESKD. This occurs because of the increased fractional excretion of sodium, particularly in the distal nephron, in relation to decreasing GFR. Hormones including aldosterone, prostaglandins, and natriuretic peptides also modulate sodium excretion and their levels are elevated with progressive renal failure. Individual variation in the underlying pathology of CKD must be considered in the management of sodium intake or restriction. Sodium wasting may be present with tubulointerstitial causes of CKD and there may also be extra renal losses of sodium from vomiting, diarrhea, or fever. Sodium retention is more likely in ESKD particularly in the presence of nephrotic syndrome or heart failure. Sodium retention contributes to hypertension, edema, heart failure, and mortality. Management of salt and water balance requires individual assessment, and both hyponatremia and hypernatremia require management.[157]

The regulation of *water balance* and osmolality is normally achieved by urinary concentration mediated by antidiuretic hormone (ADH). As GFR is reduced, ability to concentrate and dilute the urine diminishes. In earlier stages of renal failure, this may be caused by osmotic diuresis produced by increased fractional excretion of solutes by the remaining nephrons or by a decreased tubular response to ADH. Individual nephrons can maintain water balance until severe renal failure occurs and GFR declines to 15% to 20% of normal with extensive loss of nephron and tubular function. At this stage the urinary concentration becomes fixed and approaches that of the plasma at 285 mOsm/L with a specific gravity of about 1.010.

Urinary excretion of *potassium* is related primarily to distal tubular secretion mediated by aldosterone and sodium-potassium adenosine triphosphatase (see Chapter 3). In renal failure there is increased tubular secretion that provides effective regulation until the onset of oliguria. With hyperkalemia larger amounts of potassium can be eliminated through the bowel.[158]

Although nonoliguric patients can maintain potassium excretion with normal dietary intake, they are more prone to develop hyperkalemia with increased loading (i.e., use of salt substitutes). Use of potassium-sparing diuretics, such as spironolactone (aldactone), volume depletion, acute infection, severe acidosis, or marked hyperglycemia also may precipitate elevated levels of serum potassium.[159] With progression of disease to end-stage renal failure (ESRF), total body potassium can increase to life-threatening levels and must be controlled by dietary restriction, loop diuretics, cation exchange resins, and dialysis. Severe acute hyperkalemia is treated with intravenous calcium gluconate, intravenous dextrose and insulin, and nebulized or intravenous salbutamol (sympathetic beta$_2$ agonist, promotes Na^+-K^+-ATPase pump and intracellular movement of potassium). Renal replacement therapy may be required (support of renal function using hemodialysis or peritoneal dialysis).[160]

The intake of a normal diet produces 50 to 100 mEq of hydrogen per day. These ions are secreted from the renal tubules and excreted in the urine combined with phosphate and ammonia buffers (buffering is described in Chapter 3). *Metabolic acidosis* (Chapter 3) develops when GFR decreases to less than 20% to 25%

TABLE 38-15 ELECTROLYTE AND ACID-BASE ALTERATIONS OF CHRONIC KIDNEY DISEASE

FACTOR	CHARACTERISTICS
Sodium and water balance	In chronic renal failure, sodium load delivered to nephrons exceeds normal, so excretion must increase; thus less is reabsorbed. Obligatory loss occurs, leading to sodium deficits and volume depletion. As GFR is reduced, ability to concentrate and dilute urine diminishes.
Phosphate and calcium balance	Changes in acid-base balance affect phosphate and calcium balance. The major disorders associated with chronic renal failure are reduced renal phosphate excretion, decreased renal synthesis of 1,25-$(OH)_2$-vitamin D_3 (calcitriol), and hypocalcemia. Hypocalcemia leads to secondary hyperparathyroidism, GFR falls, and progressive hyperphosphatemia, hypocalcemia, and dissolution of bone result.
Potassium balance	In chronic renal failure, tubular secretion of potassium increases until oliguria develops. Use of potassium-sparing diuretics also may precipitate elevated serum potassium levels. As disease progresses, total body potassium levels can rise to life-threatening levels and dialysis is required.
Acid-base balance	In early renal insufficiency, acid excretion and bicarbonate reabsorption are increased to maintain normal pH. Metabolic acidosis begins to develop when GFR decreases to 30% to 40% of normal. When end-stage renal failure develops, the metabolic acidosis may be severe enough to require dialysis.

GFR, Glomerular filtration rate.

TABLE 38-16 CALCIUM AND PHOSPHATE METABOLISM IN CHRONIC KIDNEY DISEASE

KIDNEY	PLASMA	BONE
Decreased renal production of vitamin D_3	Decreased calcium absorption from gut Decreased ionized calcium Increased PTH secretion (secondary hyperparathyroidism)	Decreased calcium deposition
Decreased phosphate excretion	Elevated phosphate Formation of $CaHPO_4$	Release of calcium and phosphate Osteitis fibrosa, osteomalacia, calcium deposits in soft tissue (occurs when kidney fails to respond to PTH secretion because of loss of renal mass and calcium and phosphate continues to be absorbed from bone)

$CaHPO_4$, Calcium hydrogen phosphate; *PTH,* parathyroid hormone.

of normal. The causes of acidosis are primarily related to decreased hydrogen ion elimination and decreased bicarbonate reabsorption. With end-stage renal failure, metabolic acidosis may be severe enough to require alkali therapy and dialysis. Bicarbonate levels should be maintained at about 22 mEq/L.[161]

Calcium, Phosphate, and Bone

Bone and skeletal changes develop with alterations in **calcium** and **phosphate metabolism** (Table 38-16). These changes begin when the GFR decreases to 25% or less. *Hypocalcemia* is accelerated by impaired renal synthesis of 1,25-dihydroxy-vitamin D_3 (calcitriol) with decreased intestinal absorption of calcium. Renal phosphate excretion also decreases and the increased serum phosphate binds calcium, further contributing to hypocalcemia. Acidosis also contributes to a negative calcium balance. Decreased serum calcium level stimulates parathyroid hormone secretion with mobilization of calcium from bone and may cause calcium levels to approach normal. The combined effect of *hyperparathyroidism* and *vitamin D deficiency* can result in renal osteodystrophies (i.e., *osteomalacia* and *osteitis fibrosa* with increased risk for fractures) (see Chapter 44).[162] Other consequences of secondary hyperparathyroidism include soft tissue and vascular calcification, cardiovascular disease, and, less commonly, calcific uremic arteriolopathy.[163]

Protein, Carbohydrate, and Fat Metabolism

Protein, carbohydrate, and fat metabolism are altered in chronic kidney disease (CKD). *Proteinuria* and a catabolic state contribute to a negative nitrogen balance. Levels of serum proteins diminish, including albumin, complement, and transferrin, and there is loss of muscle mass. Proteinuria may independently cause renal damage by promoting tubular inflammation and fibrosis.[153] The amount of proteinuria is also related to the extent of renal injury and predicts disease progression.[164] Monitoring of proteinuria using the albumin to creatinine ratio among all individuals with CKD who are not receiving chronic dialysis therapy has been recommended as a quality performance measure for improving patient outcomes.[165]

Hyperinsulinemia and glucose intolerance related to insulin resistance are common and may be related to alterations in adipokines that interfere with insulin action and oxidative stress that contribute to renal tubular and vascular injury in both nondiabetic and diabetic CKD.[166] Hyperparathyroidism also decreases insulin sensitivity and impairs glucose tolerance. High levels of adiponectin have been associated with increased mortality in CKD.[167]

Dyslipidemia is common among individuals with CKD. There is a high ratio of low-density lipoprotein (LDL) to high-density lipoprotein (HDL), high levels of triglycerides, and accumulation of LDL particles with accelerated atherosclerosis and vascular calcification. Uremia causes a deficiency in lipoprotein lipase and decreased hepatic triglyceride lipase. Decreased lipolytic activity results in a reduction in HDL level. Apolipoprotein B concentration is also elevated, thereby accelerating atherogenesis.[168,169]

Cardiovascular System

Cardiovascular disease (Chapter 32) is a major cause of morbidity and mortality in CKD. Proinflammatory mediators, oxidative stress, altered vitamin D metabolism, and metabolic derangements are significant contributors. Declining erythropoietin production causes anemia, which reduces oxygen delivery to the myocardium. Elevated renin level stimulates the secretion of aldosterone, increasing sodium and water reabsorption. *Hypertension* is the result of excess sodium and fluid volume. *Dyslipidemia* occurs early in CKD. Arterial wall thickness increases with decreased elastic fibers and increased extracellular matrix. Atheromatous plaque and arterial calcification contribute to loss of vessel elasticity and obstruction and are accelerated by the oxidative stress of CKD. Macrovascular disease is responsible for increased risk for ischemic heart disease, left ventricular hypertrophy, congestive heart failure, stroke, and peripheral vascular disease in individuals with uremia.[170] Endothelial cell dysfunction and calcium deposits lead to a loss of vessel elasticity and vascular calcification.[171] The resulting vascular disease increases the risk for *ischemic heart disease, left ventricular hypertrophy, congestive heart failure, stroke,* and *peripheral vascular disease* in individuals with uremia. *Pericarditis* can develop from inflammation caused by the presence of uremic toxins. Accumulation of fluid in the pericardial space can compromise ventricular filling and cardiac output.

Pulmonary System

Pulmonary edema results from fluid overload and congestive heart failure. *Dyspnea* is common in ESKD. Metabolic acidosis can cause Kussmaul respirations.

Hematologic System

Hematologic alterations include *normochromic normocytic anemia, impaired platelet function,* and *hypercoagulability*. Inadequate production of erythropoietin decreases red blood cell production and is the most significant factor in contributing to anemia. Chronic inflammation, iron deficiency, and decreased half-life of erythrocytes are also contributing factors. Anemia contributes to decreased tissue oxygenation and contributes to progression of kidney disease. Low levels of hemoglobin and symptoms of anemia, such as lethargy, weakness, and dizziness, are common findings. Treatment of anemia includes erythropoiesis stimulating agents (i.e., recombinant human erythropoietin) and intravenous iron.[172]

Disorders of hemostasis in CKD are primarily related to defective platelet aggregation and impaired adhesion of platelets to the vascular endothelium. The consequence is an increased bleeding tendency manifested by bruising, epistaxis and other mucosal bleeding, gastrointestinal bleeding, and cerebrovascular hemorrhage.[173,174] Adequate dialysis improves platelet function. Alterations of individual clotting factors, fibrin, thrombin, and fibrinolysis contribute to alterations of blood coagulation and can promote a hypercoagulable state and thrombosis with increased risk for myocardial infarction and stroke.[175,176]

Immune System

Immune system dysregulation with immune suppression, deficient response to vaccination, and increased risk for infection develops with CKD. Chemotaxis, phagocytosis, antibody production, and cell-mediated immune responses are suppressed.[177] Malnutrition, metabolic acidosis, hyperglycemia, or effects of hemodialysis may amplify immunosuppression.

Neurologic System

Neurologic symptoms are common and progressive with CKD and are related to uremic toxicity, chronic hyperkalemic depolarization, and anemia.[178] Symptoms may include headache, drowsiness, pain, sleep disorders, impaired concentration, memory loss, and impaired judgment. Neuromuscular irritation can cause hiccups, muscle cramps, and muscle twitching. In advanced stages of renal failure, symptoms may progress to seizures and coma. Peripheral neuropathies also develop with impaired sensations, decreased tendon reflexes, muscle weakness, and muscle atrophy, most commonly in the lower extremities.

Gastrointestinal System

Gastrointestinal complications are common in individuals with CKD. Uremic gastroenteritis can cause bleeding ulcer and significant blood loss. Nonspecific symptoms include anorexia, nausea, vomiting, and constipation or diarrhea. Uremic fetor is a form of bad breath caused by the breakdown of urea by salivary enzymes. Malnutrition is common.

Endocrine and Reproductive Systems

Endocrine and reproductive alterations develop with progression of CKD. Males and females have a decrease in the levels of circulating sex steroid hormones. Males often experience a reduction in testosterone levels and may be impotent. Oligospermia and germinal cell dysplasia can result in infertility. Females have reduced estrogen levels, amenorrhea, and difficulty maintaining a pregnancy to term. A decrease in libido occurs in both genders.[179,180]

Insulin resistance is common in uremia. Low-grade systemic inflammation and oxidative stress may be contributing factors with increased risk for cardiovascular disease. As CKD progresses the ability of the kidney to degrade insulin is reduced, and the half-life of insulin is prolonged. Individuals with diabetes mellitus and CKD need to carefully manage their insulin dosages. Low-protein diets and renal replacement therapy improve insulin sensitivity.[181,182]

CKD also causes alterations in thyroid hormone metabolism and low thyroid hormone levels and is known as nonthyroidal illness syndrome (euthyroid sick syndrome). Low-grade inflammation and oxidative stress may be contributing factors.[183] Uremia also reduces conversion of T_3 to T_4.[183] A low-protein, low-phosphorus diet may improve thyroid hormone function.[184]

Integumentary System

Skin changes are associated with other complications that develop with CKD. Anemia can cause pallor and bleeding into the skin and results in hematomas and ecchymosis. Retained urochromes manifest as a sallow skin color. Hyperparathyroidism and uremic skin residues (known as uremic frost) are associated with irritation and pruritus with scratching, excoriation, and increased risk for infection.[185]

EVALUATION AND TREATMENT. Early screening and evaluation of CKD are based on risk factors, history, presenting signs and symptoms, and diagnostic testing.[186] Prediction equations are used for estimating GFR from serum creatinine values or creatinine clearance may be completed. Markers of kidney damage include urine protein, particularly albumin, and examination of urine sediment. New biomarkers for predicting progression of CKD are being evaluated.[187] Ultrasound, CT scan, or plain x-ray films will show small kidney size. Renal biopsy confirms the diagnosis.

Management involves dietary control, including management of protein intake, vitamin D supplementation, sodium and fluid maintenance, potassium restriction, adequate caloric intake, management of dyslipidemias, and erythropoietin as needed[188,189] (see Nutrition & Disease: Chronic Kidney Disease). ACE inhibitors or receptor blockers are often used to control systemic hypertension and provide renoprotection, particularly in the presence of diabetes mellitus.[190,191] ESKD related to diabetic nephropathy can be significantly reduced with control of hyperglycemia, hypertension, and hyperlipidemia.[121,192] ESKD is treated with dialysis, supportive therapy, and renal transplantation.

NUTRITION & DISEASE

Chronic Kidney Disease

The malnutrition-inflammation complex syndrome or protein-energy wasting is a common condition associated with renal failure and leads to accelerated atherosclerosis and cardiovascular disease and increased mortality for individuals on maintenance dialysis. Elevated levels of leptin, ghrelin, and inflammatory cytokines, including interleukin-6, tumor necrosis factor-alpha, and interferon, suppress appetite and cause muscle proteolysis, decreased protein assimilation, and hypoalbuminemia. Reduced renal function, oxidative stress, decreased levels of antioxidants, infection, exposure to dialysis tubing and membranes during hemodialysis, and back-filtration of contaminants during hemodialysis contribute to inflammation. Acidosis also acts synergistically with inflammatory cytokines and insulin resistance to promote mitochondrial dysfunction and protein catabolism. The provision of nutrients, including adequate calories along with protein supplementation that includes amino acids, in the form of intradialytic parenteral nutrition or enteral feeding during dialysis, assists a person to meet the metabolic requirements. Dietary supplements of antioxidants, such as vitamins A and C, selenium, and carotinoids, are required. Low-protein, low-phosphorous, and low-sodium diets assist with reducing proteinuria, preventing hyperphosphatemia and secondary hyperparathyroidism, and lowering blood pressure. The vegetarian nature of renal diets may improve lipid profiles. Adequate nutritional support promotes renal recovery and may prevent consequences of muscle weakness and immune dysfunction.

Data from Aparicio M et al: *J Ren Nutr* 22(2 Suppl):S1–S21, 2012; Garibotto G, Bonanni A, Verzola D: *Curr Opin Clin Nutr Metab Care* 15(1):78–84, 2012; Guarnieri G, Barazzoni R: *J Ren Nutr* 21(1):2–6, 2011; Oner-Iyidogan Y et al: *J Ren Nutr* 21(4):316–321, 2011.

SUMMARY REVIEW

Urinary Tract Obstruction

1. Obstruction can occur anywhere in the urinary tract, and may be anatomic or functional, including renal stones, tumors, an enlarged prostate gland, or urethral strictures. The most serious complications are hydronephrosis, hydroureter, ureterohydronephrosis, and infection caused by the accumulation of urine behind the obstruction.
2. Compensatory hypertrophy and hyperfunction of the opposite kidney compensate for loss of function of the kidney with obstructive disease.
3. Relief of obstruction is usually followed by postobstructive diuresis and may cause fluid and electrolyte imbalance.
4. Kidney stones are caused by supersaturation of the urine with precipitation of stone-forming substances, changes in urine pH, or urinary tract infection. Most stones are unilateral.
5. The most common kidney stone is formed from calcium oxalate and most often causes obstruction by lodging in the ureter.
6. Obstructions of the bladder are a consequence of neurogenic or anatomic alteration of the bladder or both.
7. A neurogenic bladder is caused by a neural lesion that interrupts innervation of the bladder.
8. Upper motor neuron lesions above the pontine micturition center result in detrusor hyperreflexia and uninhibited or reflex bladder.
9. Upper motor neuron lesions between C2 and S1 result in overactive or hyperreflexive bladder function and vesicosphincter dyssynergia (lack of coordinated neuromuscular contraction).
10. Lower motor neuron lesions below S1 result in detrusor areflexia with underactive, hypotonic, or atonic bladder function.
11. OAB syndrome is an uncontrollable or premature contraction of the bladder that results in urgency with or without incontinence, frequency, and nocturia.
12. Anatomic obstructions to urine flow include prostatic enlargement, urethral stricture, and pelvic organ prolapse in women.
13. Partial obstruction of the bladder can result in overactive bladder contractions with urgency. There is deposition of collagen in the bladder wall over time, resulting in decreased bladder wall compliance and ineffective detrusor muscle contraction.
14. Renal cell carcinoma is the most common renal neoplasm. The larger neoplasms tend to metastasize to the lung, liver, and bone.
15. Bladder tumors are commonly composed of transitional cells with a papillary appearance and a high rate of recurrence.

Urinary Tract Infection

1. UTIs are commonly caused by the retrograde movement of bacteria into the urethra and bladder. UTIs are uncomplicated when the urinary system is normal or complicated when there is a defect or abnormality.

SUMMARY REVIEW—cont'd

2. Host defenses that protect against urinary tract infection include high osmolality and acidic pH of urine, mucus, Tamm-Horsfall and other antimicrobial proteins that activate the immune response, sphincters that prevent reflux, and urine flow that washes out bacteria.
3. Virulent uropathogens have pili or fimbriae, or both, that promote binding to the uroepithelium. Formation of biofilms enhances colonization and resists host defenses and antimicrobial therapy.
4. Cystitis is an inflammation of the bladder commonly caused by bacteria and may be acute or chronic. Manifestations of frequency, urgency, and dysuria are caused by inflammation.
5. Painful bladder syndrome/interstitial cystitis includes nonbacterial infectious cystitis (viral, mycobacterial, chlamydial, fungal), noninfectious cystitis (i.e., radiation injury), and interstitial cystitis, which is probably related to autoimmune injury.
6. Pyelonephritis is an acute or chronic inflammation of the renal pelvis often related to ascending infection and obstructive uropathies and may cause abscess formation and scarring with an alteration in renal function.

Glomerular Disorders

1. Glomerular disorders are a group of related diseases of the glomerulus that can be primary and are caused by immune injury, infection, ischemia, toxins or drugs, or vascular disorders or, secondarily, caused by systemic diseases.
2. Acute glomerulonephritis commonly results from inflammatory damage to the glomerulus as a consequence of immune reactions including deposition of circulating immune complexes, antibodies reacting in situ to planted antigens, and antibodies directed against the glomerular basement membrane.
3. The urine sediment may contain large amounts of protein (nephrotic sediment) or have red and white blood cells and protein (nephritic sediment).
4. Acute postinfectious glomerulonephritis is commonly associated with immune complex deposition in the glomerulus or in situ formation.
5. Lupus nephritis is caused by the formation of autoantibodies against double-stranded DNA (dsDNA) and nucleosomes in the glomerulus, causing inflammation and injury.
6. IgA nephropathy is the binding of abnormal IgA to mesangial cells in the glomerulus resulting in injury and mesangial proliferation.
7. Membranous nephropathy is complement-mediated glomerular injury with increased glomerular permeability and glomerulosclerosis.
8. RPGN is associated with injury that results in the proliferation of glomerular capillary endothelial cells and a rapid loss of renal function.
9. Membranous nephropathy is complement-mediated glomerular injury with increased glomerular permeability and glomerulosclerosis.
10. Membranoproliferative glomerulonephritis involves mesangial cell proliferation, complement deposition, and crescent formation.
11. Chronic glomerulonephritis is related to a variety of diseases that cause deterioration of the glomerulus and a progressive loss of renal function over a period of months to years, including diabetic nephropathy and lupus nephritis.
12. Diabetic nephropathy develops from metabolic, inflammatory, and microvascular complications associated with chronic hyperglycemia.
13. Lupus nephritis is caused by the formation of autoantibodies against dsDNA and nucleosomes in the glomerulus, causing inflammation and injury.
14. Nephrotic syndrome is the excretion of at least 3.5 g of protein (primarily albumin) in the urine per day primarily because of glomerular injury with increased capillary permeability and loss of membrane negative charge. The principal signs are hypoproteinemia, hyperlipidemia, and edema. The liver cannot produce enough protein to adequately compensate for urinary loss.

Acute Kidney Injury

1. AKI is the sudden decline in kidney function with decreased glomerular filtration and an increase in serum creatinine and BUN levels.
2. AKI is considered in three categories as prerenal, intrarenal, or postrenal and is usually accompanied by oliguria with elevated plasma BUN and plasma creatinine levels.
3. Prerenal acute renal failure is caused by decreased renal perfusion with a decreased GFR, ischemia, and tubular necrosis.
4. Intrarenal acute renal failure is associated with several systemic diseases but is commonly related to ATN.
5. Postrenal acute renal failure is associated with diseases that obstruct the flow of urine from the kidneys.
6. Oliguria is a urine output of less than 400 ml per day and can be caused by alterations in renal blood flow, tubular obstruction, or tubular fluid backleak, or by a combination of these events.

Chronic Kidney Disease

1. Chronic kidney disease is a progressive loss of renal function. Plasma creatinine levels gradually become elevated as GFR declines, sodium is lost in the urine, potassium is retained, acidosis develops, calcium metabolism and phosphate metabolism are altered, and erythropoietin production is diminished. All organs systems are affected by CRF.
2. Symptomatic changes usually do not become evident until renal function declines to less than 25%.
3. Glomerular hypertension, hyperfiltration, and tubulointerstitial inflammation and fibrosis contribute to the progression of chronic kidney disease. Proteinuria and angiotensin II promote the pathologic changes of chronic renal injury.
4. Uremic syndrome is a proinflammatory state with the accumulation of urea and other nitrogenous compounds as well as toxins and alterations in fluid, electrolyte, and acid-base balance that result from chronic kidney failure. All organ systems are affected and contribute to disease symptoms.

KEY TERMS

Acute cystitis, 1350
Acute kidney injury (AKI), 1360
Acute renal failure, 1360
Acute tubular necrosis (ATN), 1361
Angiotensin II, 1364
Anuria, 1362
Apoptosis, 1342
Asymptomatic bacteriuria, 1350
Azotemia, 1359
Calcium metabolism, 1368
Calcium stone (urolithiasis), 1343
Calculus (*pl.,* calculi) (urinary stone [urolithiasis]), 1343
Chronic glomerulonephritis, 1357
Chronic kidney disease (CKD), 1364
Chronic pyelonephritis, 1352
Compensatory growth, 1342
Compensatory hypertrophy, 1342
Continuous renal replacement therapy (CRRT [hemodialysis]), 1363
Cystinuric (xanthine) stone, 1344
Detrusor areflexia, 1345
Detrusor hyperreflexia, 1345
Detrusor hyperreflexia with vesicosphincter (detrusor sphincter) dyssynergia, 1345
Diabetic nephropathy, 1357
Dyssynergia, 1344
End-stage kidney disease (ESKD), 1359
Glomerulonephritis, 1352
Hydronephrosis, 1341
Hydroureter, 1341
Hyperfunction, 1342
IgA nephropathy (Berger disease), 1353
Intrarenal (intrinsic) acute kidney injury (AKI), 1360
Low bladder wall compliance, 1346
Lupus nephritis, 1358
Membranoproliferative glomerulonephritis (MPGN), 1355
Membranous nephropathy (membranous glomerulonephritis), 1353
Mesangial proliferative glomerulonephritis, 1355
Nephritic sediment, 1357
Nephritic syndrome, 1358
Nephrotic sediment, 1357
Nephrotic syndrome, 1358
Neurogenic bladder, 1344
Nonbacterial infectious cystitis, 1351
Noninfectious cystitis, 1351
Nonoliguric renal failure, 1362
Obligatory growth, 1342
Obstructive uropathy, 1340
Oliguria, 1361
Overactive bladder syndrome (OAB), 1345
Painful bladder syndrome/interstitial cystitis (PBS/IC), 1351
Partial obstruction of the bladder outlet or urethra, 1346
Pelvic organ prolapse, 1346
Phosphate metabolism, 1368
Postobstructive diuresis, 1342
Postrenal acute kidney injury, 1361
Prerenal acute kidney injury, 1360
Prostate enlargement, 1346
Pyelonephritis, 1351
Rapidly progressive (crescentic) glomerulonephritis (RPGN), 1353
Renal adenoma, 1347
Renal cell carcinoma (RCC), 1347
Renal colic, 1344
Renal failure, 1359
Renal insufficiency, 1359
Renal transitional cell carcinoma (RTCC), 1347
Staghorn calculus, 1344
Struvite stone, 1343
Tubulointerstitial fibrosis, 1341
Uremia, 1359
Uremic syndrome, 1366
Ureterohydronephrosis, 1341
Urethral stricture, 1346
Uric acid stone, 1344
Urinary tract infection (UTI), 1349
Urothelial (transitional cell) carcinoma, 1348
Virulence, 1350

REFERENCES

1. Siddiqui MM, McDougal WS: Urologic assessment of decreasing renal function, *Med Clin North Am* 95(1):161–168, 2011.
2. Tseng TY, Stoller ML: Obstructive uropathy, *Clin Geriatr Med* 25(3):437–443, 2009.
3. Gillenwater JY: Hydronephrosis. In Gillenwater JY et al: *Adult and pediatric urology*, ed 4, Philadelphia, 2002, Lippincott Williams & Wilkins.

3a. López-Novoa JM et al: Common pathophysiological mechanisms of chronic kidney disease: therapeutic perspectives, *Pharmacol Ther* 128(1):61–81, 2010.

4. Helal I et al: Glomerular hyperfiltration: definitions, mechanisms and clinical implications, *Nat Rev Nephrol* 8(5):293–300, 2012.
5. Frokiaer J, Zeidel ML: Chapter 37: Urinary tract obstruction. In Taal MW et al: *Brenner and Rector's the kidney*, ed 9, Philadelphia, 2012, Saunders, pp 1394–1402.
6. Curhan GC: Epidemiology of stone disease, *Urol Clin North Am* 34(3):287–293, 2007.
7. Chandhoke PS: Evaluation of the recurrent stone former, *Urol Clin North Am* 34(3):315–322, 2007.
8. Sas DJ: An update on the changing epidemiology and metabolic risk factors in pediatric kidney stone disease, *Clin J Am Soc Nephrol* 6(8):2062–2068, 2011.
9. Rule AD et al: Kidney stones associate with increased risk for myocardial infarction, *J Am Soc Nephrol* 21(10):1641–1644, 2010.
10. Rule AD, Krambeck AE, Lieske JC: Chronic kidney disease in kidney stone formers, *Clin J Am Soc Nephrol* 6(8):2069–2075, 2011.
11. Evan AP: Physiopathology and etiology of stone formation in the kidney and the urinary tract, *Pediatr Nephrol* 25(5):831–841, 2010.
12. Bagga HS et al: New insights into the pathogenesis of renal calculi, *Urol Clin North Am* 40(1):1–12, 2013.
13. Lingeman JE, Lifshitz DA, Evan AP: Surgical management of urinary lithiasis. In Walsh PC et al: *Campbell's urology*, ed 8, Philadelphia, 2002, Saunders.
14. Coe FL, Evan A, Worcester E: Pathophysiology-based treatment of idiopathic calcium kidney stones, *Clin J Am Soc Nephrol* 6(8):2083–2092, 2011.
15. Tiselius HG: A hypothesis of calcium stone formation: an interpretation of stone research during the past decades, *Urol Res* 39(4):231–243, 2011.
16. Sakhaee K, Maalouf NM, Sinnott B: Clinical review. Kidney stones 2012: pathogenesis, diagnosis, and management, *J Clin Endocrinol Metab* 97(6):1847–1860, 2012.
17. Wagner CA, Mohebbi N: Urinary pH and stone formation, *J Nephrol* 23(Suppl 16):S165–S169, 2010.
18. Xavier A, Maxwell AP: Which patients with renal colic should be referred? *Practitioner* 255(1737):15–17, 2011. 2.
19. Mandeville JA, Gnessin E, Lingeman JE: Imaging evaluation in the patient with renal stone disease, *Semin Nephrol* 31(3):254–258, 2011.
20. Ortiz-Alvarado O et al: Impact of dietary counseling on urinary stone risk parameters in recurrent stone formers, *J Endourol* 25(3):535–540, 2011.
21. Aboumarzouk OM et al: Extracorporeal shock wave lithotripsy (ESWL) versus ureteroscopic management for ureteric calculi, *Cochrane Database Syst Rev* 5:CD006029, 2012.
22. Amer T et al: Standard versus tubeless percutaneous nephrolithotomy: a systematic review, *Urol Int* 88(4):373–382, 2012.
23. Graham A, Luber S, Wolfson AB: Urolithiasis in the emergency department, *Emerg Med Clin North Am* 29(3):519–538, 2011.
24. Bacsu CD, Chan L, Tse VL: Diagnosing detrusor sphincter dyssynergia in the neurological patient, *BJU Int* 109(Suppl 3):31–34, 2012.
25. Coyne KS et al: National community prevalence of overactive bladder in the United States stratified by sex and age, *Urology* 77(5):1081–1087, 2011.
26. Chapple C: Pathophysiology of the lower urinary tract and CNS, *Can Urol Assoc J* 5(Suppl 2):S126–S127, 2011.
27. Abrams P et al: The standardisation of terminology of lower urinary tract function: report from the Standardisation Sub-committee of the International Continence Society, *Am J Obstet Gynecol* 187(1):116–126, 2002.
28. Allahdin S, Oo N: An overview of treatment of overactive bladder syndrome in women, *J Obstet Gynaecol* 32(3):217–221, 2012.
29. Milsom I et al: Effect of bothersome overactive bladder symptoms on health-related quality of life, anxiety, depression, and treatment seeking in the United States: results from EpiLUTS, *Urology* 80(1):90–96, 2012.
30. Walsh CA, Moore KH: Overactive bladder in women: does low-count bacteriuria matter? A review, *Neurourol Urodyn* 30(1):32–37, 2011.
31. Keegan KA, Nanigian DK, Stone AR: Female urethral stricture disease, *Curr Urol Rep* 9(5):419–423, 2008.
32. Lumen N et al: Etiology of urethral stricture disease in the 21st century, *J Urol* 182(3):983–987, 2009.
33. Rourke K, Hickle J: The clinical spectrum of the presenting signs and symptoms of anterior urethral stricture: detailed analysis of a single institutional cohort, *Urology* 79(5):1163–1167, 2012.

34. Ahmed F, Sotelo T: Management of pelvic organ prolapse, *Can J Urol* 18(6):6050–6053, 2011.
35. Anger JU, Raz S, Rodriguez LV: Severe cystocele: optimizing results, *Curr Urol Rep* 8(5):394–398, 2007.
36. Mahfouz W, Corcos J: Management of detrusor external sphincter dyssynergia in neurogenic bladder, *Eur J Phys Rehabil Med* 47(4):639–650, 2011.
37. Escudero RM et al: Bladder augmentation using the gastrointestinal tract. Indication, follow up and complications, *Arch Esp Urol* 64(10):953–959, 2011.
38. Culligan PJ: Nonsurgical management of pelvic organ prolapse, *Obstet Gynecol* 119(4):852–860, 2012.
39. Machin SE, Mukhopadhyay S: Pelvic organ prolapse: review of the aetiology, presentation, diagnosis and management, *Menopause Int* 17(4):132–136, 2011.
40. American Cancer Society: *Cancer facts & figures 2013.* Available at http://www.cancer.org/research/cancerfactsfigures/cancerfactsfigures/cancer-facts-figures-2013. Accessed May 13, 2013.
41. Lipworth L, Tarone RE, McLaughlin JK: Renal cell cancer among African Americans: an epidemiologic review, *BMC Cancer* 11:133, 2011.
42. Navai N, Wood CG: Environmental and modifiable risk factors in renal cell carcinoma, *Urol Oncol* 30(2):220–224, 2012.
43. Cho E, Adami HO, Lindblad P: Epidemiology of renal cell cancer, *Hematol Oncol Clin North Am* 25(4):651–665, 2011.
44. Audenet F et al: Genetic pathways involved in carcinogenesis of clear cell renal cell carcinoma: genomics towards personalized medicine, *BJU Int* 109(12):1864–1870, 2012.
45. Cairns P: Renal cell carcinoma, *Cancer Biomark* 9(1–6):461–473, 2010.
46. Deng FM, Melamed J: Histologic variants of renal cell carcinoma: does tumor type influence outcome? *Urol Clin North Am* 39(2):119–132, 2012. v.
47. Corgna E et al: Renal cancer, *Crit Rev Oncol Hematol* 64(3):247–262, 2007.
48. Sountoulides P, Metaxa L, Cindolo L: Atypical presentations and rare metastatic sites of renal cell carcinoma: a review of case reports, *J Med Case Rep* 5:429, 2011.
49. Sun M et al: Prognostic factors and predictive models in renal cell carcinoma: a contemporary review, *Eur Urol* 60(4):644–661, 2011.
50. Dutcher JP, Mourad WF, Ennis RD: Integrating innovative therapeutic strategies into the management of renal cell carcinoma, *Oncology (Williston Park)* 26(6):526–530, 532, 534, 2012.
51. Eisengart LJ, MacVicar GR, Yang XJ: Predictors of response to targeted therapy in renal cell carcinoma, *Arch Pathol Lab Med* 136(5):490–495, 2012.
52. Hu B, Lara PN Jr, Evans CP: Defining an individualized treatment strategy for metastatic renal cancer, *Urol Clin North Am* 39(2):233–249, vii. 2012.
53. Pécuchet N, Fournier LS, Oudard S: New insights into the management of renal cell cancer, *Oncology* 84(1):22–31, 2013.
54. Singer EA et al: Evolving therapeutic targets in renal cell carcinoma, *Curr Opin Oncol* 25(3):273–280, 2013.
55. Kiriluk KJ et al: Bladder cancer risk from occupational and environmental exposures, *Urol Oncol* 30(2):199–211, 2012.
56. Volanis D et al: Molecular mechanisms in urinary bladder carcinogenesis, *J BUON* 16(4):589–601, 2011.
57. Kamat AM, Mathew P: Bladder cancer: imperatives for personalized medicine, *Oncology (Williston Park)* 25(10):951–958, 960, 2011.
58. Pons F et al: Variant forms of bladder cancer: basic considerations on treatment approaches, *Curr Oncol Rep* 13(3):216–221, 2011.
59. Gorin MA, Ayyathurai R, Soloway MS: Diagnosis and treatment of bladder cancer: how can we improve? *Postgrad Med* 124(3):28–36, 2012.
60. Netto GJ, Cheng L: Emerging critical role of molecular testing in diagnostic genitourinary pathology, *Arch Pathol Lab Med* 136(4):372–390, 2012.
61. Ru Y, Dancik GM, Theodorescu D: Biomarkers for prognosis and treatment selection in advanced bladder cancer patients, *Curr Opin Urol* 21(5):420–427, 2011.
62. Verma S et al: Urinary bladder cancer: role of MR imaging, *Radiographics* 32(2):371–387, 2012.
63. Costantini C, Millard F: Update on chemotherapy in the treatment of urothelial carcinoma, *ScientificWorldJournal 1981–1994*, 2011.
64. Jones G et al: Intravesical gemcitabine for non-muscle invasive bladder cancer, *Cochrane Database Syst Rev* 1:CD009294, 2012.
65. Kim JJ: Recent advances in treatment of advanced urothelial carcinoma, *Curr Urol Rep* 13(2):147–152, 2012.
66. Hladunewich M, Rosenthal MH: Pathophysiology and management of renal insufficiency in the perioperative and critically ill patient, *Anesthesiol Clin North Am* 18(4):773–789, 2000.
67. Ragnarsdottir B, Svanborg C: Susceptibility to acute pyelonephritis or asymptomatic bacteriuria: host-pathogen interaction in urinary tract infection, *Pediatr Nephrol* 27(11):2017–2019, 2012.
68. Sakallioglu O, Sakallioglu AE: The effect of ABO-Rh blood group determinants on urinary tract infections, *Int Urol Nephrol* 39(2):577–579, 2007.
69. Schnarr J, Smaill F: Asymptomatic bacteriuria and symptomatic urinary tract infections in pregnancy, *Eur J Clin Invest* 38(Suppl 2):50–57, 2008.
70. Hannan TJ et al: Host-pathogen checkpoints and population bottlenecks in persistent and intracellular uropathogenic *Escherichia coli* bladder infection, *FEMS Microbiol Rev* 36(3):616–648, 2012.
71. Agarwal J, Srivastava S, Singh M: Pathogenomics of uropathogenic, *Escherichia coli, Indian J Med Microbiol* 30(2):141–149, 2012.
72. Spurbeck RR et al: Fimbrial profiles predict virulence of uropathogenic *Escherichia coli* strains: contribution of ygi and yad fimbriae, *Infect Immun* 79(12):4753–4763, 2011.
73. Dielubanza EJ, Schaeffer AJ: Urinary tract infections in women, *Med Clin North Am* 95(1):27–41, 2011.
74. Kauffman CA et al: Candida urinary tract infections—diagnosis, *Clin Infect Dis* 52(Suppl 6):S452–S456, 2011.
75. Salem S et al: Successful control of schistosomiasis and the changing epidemiology of bladder cancer in Egypt, *BJU Int* 107(2):206–211, 2011.
76. Khalaf I, Shokeir A, Shalaby M: Urologic complications of genitourinary schistosomiasis, *World J Urol* 30(1):31–38, 2012.
77. Nielubowicz GR, Mobley HL: Host-pathogen interactions in urinary tract infection, *Nat Rev Urol* 7(8):430–441, 2010.
78. Guzzo TJ, Drach GW: Major urologic problems in geriatrics: assessment and management, *Med Clin North Am* 95(1):253–264, 2011.
79. Colgan R, Williams M: Diagnosis and treatment of acute uncomplicated cystitis, *Am Fam Physician* 84(7):771–776, 2011.
80. Nosseir SB, Lind LR, Winkler HA: Recurrent uncomplicated urinary tract infections in women: a review, *J Womens Health (Larchmt)* 21(3):347–354, 2012.
81. Riveau G et al: Safety and immunogenicity of rSh28GST antigen in humans: phase 1 randomized clinical study of a vaccine candidate against urinary schistosomiasis, *PLoS Negl Trop Dis* 6(7):e1704, 2012.
82. van de Merwe JP et al: Diagnostic criteria, classification, and nomenclature for painful bladder syndrome/interstitial cystitis: an ISSIC proposal, *Eur Urol* 53(1):60–67, 2008.
83. Butrick CW, Howard FM, Sand PK: Diagnosis and treatment of interstitial cystitis/painful bladder syndrome: a review, *J Womens Health (Larchmt)* 19(6):1185–1193, 2010.
84. Rais-Bahrami S et al: Symptom profile variability of interstitial cystitis/painful bladder syndrome by age, *BJU Int* 109(9):1356–1359, 2012.
85. Keay S et al: Normalization of proliferation and tight junction formation in bladder epithelial cells from patients with interstitial cystitis/painful bladder syndrome by D-proline and D-pipecolic acid derivatives of antiproliferative factor, *Chem Biol Drug Des* 77(6):421–430, 2011.
86. French LM, Bhambore N: Interstitial cystitis/painful bladder syndrome, *Am Fam Physician* 83(10):1175–1181, 2011.
87. Quillin RB, Erickson DR: Management of interstitial cystitis/bladder pain syndrome: a urology perspective, *Urol Clin North Am* 39(3):389–396, 2012.
88. Funfstuck R, Ott U, Naber KG: The interaction of urinary tract infection and renal insufficiency, *Int J Antimicrob Agents* 28(Suppl 1):S72–S77, 2006.
89. Colgan R, Williams M, Johnson JR: Diagnosis and treatment of acute pyelonephritis in women, *Am Fam Physician* 84(5):519–526, 2011.
90. Gupta K et al: International clinical practice guidelines for the treatment of acute uncomplicated cystitis and pyelonephritis in women: a 2010 update by the Infectious Diseases Society of America and the European Society for Microbiology and Infectious Diseases, *Clin Infect Dis* 52(5):e103–e120, 2011.
91. Barsoum RS: Glomerulonephritis in disadvantaged populations, *Clin Nephrol* 74(Suppl 1):S44–S50, 2010.
92. Segelmark M, Hellmark T: Autoimmune kidney diseases, *Autoimmun Rev* 9(5):A366–A371, 2010.
93. Mestecky J et al: IgA nephropathy: molecular mechanisms of the disease, *Annu Rev Pathol* 8:217–240, 2013.
94. Lai KN: Pathogenesis of IgA nephropathy, *Nat Rev Nephrol* 8(5):275–283, 2012.

95. Boyd JK et al: An update on the pathogenesis and treatment of IgA nephropathy, *Kidney Int* 81(9):833–843, 2012.
96. Barbour SJ, Reich HN: Risk stratification of patients with IgA nephropathy, *Am J Kidney Dis* 59(6):865–873, 2012.
97. Rosselli JL et al: Treatment of IgA nephropathy: an update, *Ann Pharmacother* 45(10):1284–1296, 2011.
98. Wang T et al: Comparison of clinicopathological features between children and adults with IgA nephropathy, *Pediatr Nephrol* 27(8): 1293–1300, 2012.
99. Komatsu H, Fujimoto S: Tonsillectomy combined with steroid pulse therapy induces clinical remission of IgA nephropathy, *Adv Otorhinolaryngol* 72:57–59, 2011.
100. Nakagawa N et al: Retrospective comparison of the efficacy of tonsillectomy with and without steroid-pulse therapy in IgA nephropathy patients, *Intern Med* 51(11):1323–1328, 2012.
101. Hogg RJ: Idiopathic immunoglobulin A nephropathy in children and adolescents, *Pediatr Nephrol* 25(5):823–829, 2010.
102. Le W et al: Long-term renal survival and related risk factors in patients with IgA nephropathy: results from a cohort of 1155 cases in a Chinese adult population, *Nephrol Dial Transplant* 27(4):1479–1485, 2012.
103. Glassock RJ: The pathogenesis of membranous nephropathy: evolution and revolution, *Curr Opin Nephrol Hypertens* 21(3):235–242, 2012.
104. Ronco P, Debiec H: Pathogenesis of membranous nephropathy: recent advances and future challenges, *Nat Rev Nephrol* 8(4):203–213, 2012.
105. Bajema IM: Pathological classification of anti-neutrophil cytoplasmic antibody (ANCA)-associated glomerulonephritis, *Clin Exp Immunol* 164(Suppl 1):14–16, 2011.
106. Cui Z, Zhao MH: Advances in human antiglomerular basement membrane disease, *Nat Rev Nephrol* 7(12):697–705, 2011.
107. Flamant M et al: Epidermal growth factor: a new therapeutic target in glomerular disease, *Nephrol Dial Transplant* 27(4):1297–1304, 2012.
108. Kambham N: Crescentic glomerulonephritis: an update on Pauci-immune and anti-GBM diseases, *Adv Anat Pathol* 19(2):111–124, 2012.
109. Pedchenko V, Vanacore R, Hudson B: Goodpasture's disease: molecular architecture of the autoantigen provides clues to etiology and pathogenesis, *Curr Opin Nephrol Hypertens* 20(3):290–296, 2011.
110. Chan AL et al: Cutting edge issues in Goodpasture's disease, *Clin Rev Allergy Immunol* 41(2):151–162, 2011.
111. Rutgers A et al: Pauci-immune necrotizing glomerulonephritis, *Rheum Dis Clin North Am* 36(3):559–572, 2010.
112. Sethi S, Fervenza FC: Membranoproliferative glomerulonephritis: pathogenetic heterogeneity and proposal for a new classification, *Semin Nephrol* 31(4):341–348, 2011.
113. Sethi S, Nester CM, Smith RJ: Membranoproliferative glomerulonephritis and C3 glomerulopathy: resolving the confusion, *Kidney Int* 81(5):434–441, 2012.
114. Berger SP, Daha MR: Complement in glomerular injury, *Semin Immunopathol* 29(4):375–384, 2007.
115. Lizakowski S et al: Plasma tissue factor and tissue factor pathway inhibitor in patients with primarily glomerulonephritis, *Scand J Urol Nephrol* 41(3):237–242, 2007.
116. Norman JT, Fine LG: Intrarenal oxygenation in chronic renal failure, *Clin Exp Pharmacol Physiol* 33(10):989–996, 2006.
117. Gyebi L, Soltani Z, Reisin E: Lipid nephrotoxicity: new concept for an old disease, *Curr Hypertens Rep* 14(2):177–181, 2012.
118. Fioretto P, Mauer M: Histopathology of diabetic nephropathy, *Semin Nephrol* 27(2):195–207, 2007.
119. Centers for Disease Control and Prevention: Incidence of end-stage renal disease among persons with diabetes—United States, 1990–2002, *MMWR Morb Mortal Wkly Rep* 54(43):1097–1100, 2005.
120. Najafian B, Alpers CE, Fogo AB: Pathology of human diabetic nephropathy, *Contrib Nephrol* 170:36–47, 2011.
121. Pyram R et al: Chronic kidney disease and diabetes, *Maturitas* 71(2): 94–103, 2012.
121a. Borchers AT et al: Lupus nephritis: a critical review, *Autoimmun Rev* 12(2):174–194, 2012.
122. Giannakakis K, Faraggiana T: Histopathology of lupus nephritis, *Clin Rev Allergy Immunol* 40(3):170–180, 2011.
123. Yung S, Chan TM: Autoantibodies and resident renal cells in the pathogenesis of lupus nephritis: getting to know the unknown, *Clin Dev Immunol* 2012:139365, 2012.
123a. Henderson L et al: Treatment for lupus nephritis, *Cochrane Database Syst Rev* 12:CD002922, 2012.
124. Cosgrove D: Glomerular pathology in Alport syndrome: a molecular perspective, *Pediatr Nephrol* 27(6):885–890, 2012.
125. Khanna R: Clinical presentation & management of glomerular diseases: hematuria, nephritic & nephrotic syndrome, *Mol Med* 108(1):33–36, 2011.
126. Galle P, Labejof L: In nephrotic syndromes podocytes synthesize and excrete proteins into the tubular fluid: an electron and ion microscopic study, *C R Biol* 334(10):713–719, 2011.
127. Siddall EC, Radhakrishnan J: The pathophysiology of edema formation in the nephrotic syndrome, *Kidney Int* 82(6):635–642, 2012.
128. Svenningsen P, Skøtt O, Jensen BL: Proteinuric diseases with sodium retention: is plasmin the link? *Clin Exp Pharmacol Physiol* 39(1): 117–124, 2012.
129. de Seigneux S, Martin PY: Management of patients with nephrotic syndrome, *Swiss Med Wkly* 139(29-30):416–422, 2009.
130. Iglesias P, Díez JJ: Thyroid dysfunction and kidney disease, *Eur J Endocrinol* 160(4):503–515, 2009.
131. Kerlin BA, Ayoob R, Smoyer WE: Epidemiology and pathophysiology of nephrotic syndrome-associated thromboembolic disease, *Clin J Am Soc Nephrol* 7(3):513–520, 2012.
132. Lombel RM et al: Treatment of steroid-resistant nephrotic syndrome in children: new guidelines from KDIGO, *Pediatr Nephrol* 28(3):409–414, 2013.
133. Ulinski T, Aoun B: New treatment strategies in idiopathic nephrotic syndrome, *Minerva Pediatr* 64(2):135–143, 2012.
134. Hofmann RM: Preventing harm during treatment of acute kidney injury: what do we really know? *Adv Chronic Kidney Dis* 19(3):142–148, 2012.
135. Bellomo R et al: Acute Dialysis Quality Initiative Workgroup. Acute renal failure—definition, outcome measures, animal models, fluid therapy and information technology needs: the Second International Consensus Conference of the Acute Dialysis Quality Initiative (ADQI) Group, *Crit Care* 8(4):R204–R212, 2004.
136. Cruz DN et al: Acute kidney injury: classification and staging, *Contrib Nephrol* 164:24–32, 2010.
137. Bouglé A, Duranteau J: Pathophysiology of sepsis-induced acute kidney injury: the role of global renal blood flow and renal vascular resistance, *Contrib Nephrol* 174:89–97, 2011.
138. Bellomo R et al: Acute kidney injury, *Lancet 25* 380(9843):756–766, 2012.
139. Lee DW, Faubel S, Edelstein CL: Cytokines in acute kidney injury (AKI), *Clin Nephrol* 76(3):165–173, 2011.
140. Bonventre JV, Yang L: Cellular pathophysiology of ischemic acute kidney injury, *J Clin Invest* 121(11):4210–4221, 2011.
141. Honore PM et al: Septic AKI in ICU patients. Diagnosis, pathophysiology, and treatment type, dosing, and timing: a comprehensive review of recent and future developments, *Ann Intensive Care* 1(1):32, 2011.
142. Zarjou A, Agarwal A: Sepsis and acute kidney injury, *J Am Soc Nephrol* 22(6):999–1006, 2011.
143. Ortiz A et al: Targeting apoptosis in acute tubular injury, *Biochem Pharmacol* 66(8):1589–1594, 2003.
144. Clarkson MR et al: Acute kidney injury. In Brenner BM, editor: *Brenner and Rector's the kidney*, ed 8, Philadelphia, 2007, Saunders.
145. Coca SG, Singanamala S, Parikh CR: Chronic kidney disease after acute kidney injury: a systematic review and meta-analysis, *Kidney Int* 81(5):442–448, 2012.
146. Odutayo A, Cherney D: Cystatin C and acute changes in glomerular filtration rate, *Clin Nephrol* 78(1):64–75, 2012.
147. Sharfuddin AA et al: Chapter 30: Acute kidney injury. In Taal MW et al: *Brenner & Rector's the kidney*, ed 9, Philadelphia, 2012, Saunders, p 1081.
148. Hewitt J et al: Sodium bicarbonate supplements for treating acute kidney injury, *Cochrane Database Syst Rev* 6:CD009204, 2012.
149. Joannidis M, Forni LG: Clinical review: timing of renal replacement therapy, *Crit Care* 15(3):223, 2011.
150. Palevsky PM: Renal replacement therapy in acute kidney injury, *Adv Chronic Kidney Dis* 20(1):76–84, 2013.
151. Yang L, Humphreys BD, Bonventre JV: Pathophysiology of acute kidney injury to chronic kidney disease: maladaptive repair, *Contrib Nephrol* 174:149–155, 2011.
152. Grgic I et al: Targeted proximal tubule injury triggers interstitial fibrosis and glomerulosclerosis, *Kidney Int* 82(2):172–183, 2012.
153. Gorriz JL, Martinez-Castelao A: Proteinuria: detection and role in native renal disease progression, *Transplant Rev (Orlando)* 26(1):3–13, 2012.
154. Rüster C, Wolf G: Angiotensin II as a morphogenic cytokine stimulating renal fibrogenesis, *J Am Soc Nephrol* 22(7):1189–1199, 2011.
155. Libetta C et al: Oxidative stress and inflammation: implications in uremia and hemodialysis, *Clin Biochem* 44(14–15):1189–1198, 2011.

156. Ferguson MA, Waikar SS: Established and emerging markers of kidney function, *Clin Chem* 58(4):680–689, 2012.
157. Kovesdy CP: Significance of hypo- and hypernatremia in chronic kidney disease, *Nephrol Dial Transplant* 27(3):891–898, 2012.
158. Sorensen MV et al: Colonic potassium handling, *Pflugers Arch* 459(5):645–656, 2010.
159. Lehnhardt A, Kemper MJ: Pathogenesis, diagnosis and management of hyperkalemia, *Pediatr Nephrol* 26(3):377–384, 2011.
160. Fleming GM: Renal replacement therapy review: past, present and future, *Organogenesis* 7(1):2–12, 2011.
161. Kraut JA, Madias NE: Consequences and therapy of the metabolic acidosis of chronic kidney disease, *Pediatr Nephrol* 26(1):19–28, 2011.
162. Ott SM: Bone disease in CKD, *Curr Opin Nephrol Hypertens* 21(4): 376–381, 2012.
163. Mejía N et al: Chronic kidney disease—mineral and bone disorder: a complex scenario, *Nefrologia* 31(5):514–519, 2011.
164. Viswanathan G, Upadhyay A: Assessment of proteinuria, *Adv Chronic Kidney Dis* 18(4):243–248, 2011.
165. Thorp ML et al: Proteinuria among patients with chronic kidney disease: a performance measure for improving patient outcomes, *Jt Comm J Qual Patient Saf* 38(6):277–282, 2012.
166. Ikee R et al: Glucose metabolism, insulin resistance and renal pathology in non-diabetic chronic kidney disease, *Nephron Clin Pract* 108(2): c163–c168, 2008.
167. Jia T et al: The complex role of adiponectin in chronic kidney disease, *Biochimie* 94(10):2150–2156, 2012.
168. Navab KD et al: Chronic inflammatory disorders and accelerated atherosclerosis: chronic kidney disease, *Curr Pharm Des* 17(1):17–20, 2011.
169. Bakris GL: Lipid disorders in uremia and dialysis, *Contrib Nephrol* 178:100–105, 2012.
170. Bhandari S: Risk factors and metabolic mechanisms in the pathogenesis of uraemic cardiac disease, *Front Biosci* 16:1364–1387, 2011.
171. Briet M, Burns KD: Chronic kidney disease and vascular remodelling: molecular mechanisms and clinical implications, *Clin Sci (Lond)* 123(7):399–416, 2012.
172. Locatelli F, Del Vecchio L: New erythropoiesis-stimulating agents and new iron formulations, *Contrib Nephrol* 171:255–260, 2011.
173. Kaw D, Malhotra D: Platelet dysfunction and end-stage renal disease, *Semin Dial* 19(4):317–322, 2006.
174. Saeed F et al: Lower gastrointestinal bleeding in chronic hemodialysis patients, *Int J Nephrol* 2011:272535, 2011.
175. Fabbian F et al: Stroke and renal dysfunction: are we always conscious of this relationship? *Clin Appl Thromb Hemost* 18(3):305–311, 2012.
176. McCullough PA et al: Cardiovascular disease in chronic kidney disease: data from the Kidney Early Evaluation Program (KEEP), *Curr Diab Rep* 11(1):47–55, 2011.
177. Vaziri ND et al: Effect of uremia on structure and function of immune system, *J Ren Nutr* 22(1):149–156, 2012.
178. Krishnan AV, Kiernan MC: Uremic neuropathy: clinical features and new pathophysiological insights, *Muscle Nerve* 35(3):273–290, 2007.
179. Iglesias P, Carrero JJ, Díez JJ: Gonadal dysfunction in men with chronic kidney disease: clinical features, prognostic implications and therapeutic options, *J Nephrol* 25(1):31–42, 2012.
180. Nevis IF et al: Pregnancy outcomes in women with chronic kidney disease: a systematic review, *Clin J Am Soc Nephrol* 6(11):2587–2598, 2011.
181. Chauveau P, Aparicio M: Benefits in nutritional interventions in patients with CKD stage 3-4, *J Ren Nutr* 21(1):20–22, 2011.
182. Garg R, Williams ME: Diabetes management in the kidney patient, *Med Clin North Am* 97(1):135–156, 2013.
183. Adler S, Wartofsky L: The nonthyroidal illness syndrome, *Endocrinol Metab Clin North Am* 36(3):657–672, 2007.
184. Rosolowska-Huszcz D, Kozlowska L, Rydzewski A: Influence of low protein diet on nonthyroidal illness syndrome in chronic renal failure, *Endocrine* 27(3):283–288, 2005.
185. Manenti L, Tansinda P, Vaglio A: Uraemic pruritus: clinical characteristics, pathophysiology and treatment, *Drugs* 69(3):251–263, 2009.
186. Fink HA et al: *Chronic kidney disease stages 1-3: screening, monitoring, and treatment* [internet], Rockville, MD, 2012, Agency for Healthcare Research and Quality. Available at www.ncbi.nlm.nih.gov/books/NBK84564/.
187. Fassett RG et al: Biomarkers in chronic kidney disease: a review, *Kidney Int* 80(8):806–821, 2011.
188. Fouque D et al: Nutrition and chronic kidney disease, *Kidney Int* 80(4):348–357, 2011.
189. Prabhu MV et al: Maximizing the erythropoietin response: iron strategies, *Contrib Nephrol* 178:95–99, 2012.
190. Nicholas SB et al: What should be the blood pressure target for patients with chronic kidney disease? *Curr Opin Cardiol* 28(4):439–445, 2013.
191. Van Buren PN, Inrig JK: Hypertension and hemodialysis: pathophysiology and outcomes in adult and pediatric populations, *Pediatr Nephrol* 27(3):339–350, 2012.
192. O'Toole SM et al: Managing diabetes in dialysis patients, *Postgrad Med J* 88(1037):160–166, 2012.

CHAPTER

39

Alterations of Renal and Urinary Tract Function in Children

Patti Ring and Sue E. Huether

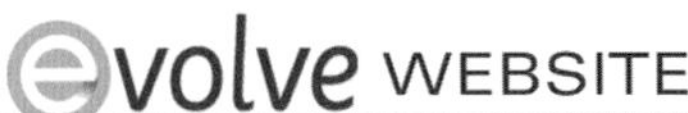

http://evolve.elsevier.com/McCance/

- Review Questions and Answers

CHAPTER OUTLINE

Renal and urinary disorders occur in children as well as adults. In childhood, however, the kidney and genitourinary structures are continuing to develop, so renal dysfunction may be associated with mechanisms and manifestations that are different from those in adults. In addition, some renal and urinary disorders are congenital and involve structural anomalies of the kidney and urinary drainage system.

STRUCTURE AND FUNCTION OF THE URINARY SYSTEM IN CHILDREN

Development of the Urinary System

The embryonic urinary system develops as three sets of sequentially replaced organs: the pronephros, mesonephros, and metanephros. The **pronephros** is a nonfunctional structure that arises at the level of the cervical and upper thoracic regions during the third fetal week and connects the primitive wolffian duct to the cloaca as the foundation for male sexual development (Figure 39-1). The development of the **mesonephros** and **metanephros** is described in Figure 39-1. The Wilms tumor 1 *(WT1)* gene plays an important role at all stages of kidney development and maintenance of kidney function. The wingless type signaling (WNT signaling) transduction pathway also is important for mesenchyme growth and differentiation.[1,2]

After glomeruli and tubules form, the tissues organize and progressively differentiate over approximately 30 days. Initial glomerular development is staggered, so there are glomeruli in various stages. In fact, a few of the first glomeruli formed degenerate and disappear during the later stages of fetal development. Progressive development continues into the ninth fetal month, when all metanephrogenic tissue then disappears.

As the embryo develops and the vertebral column straightens, the kidneys appear to ascend to the sacral area at about 6 weeks, to the third lumbar area by the third month, and to the first lumbar area at term. The kidneys rotate 90 degrees as they ascend so that renal tissue is lateral and the collecting system is medial.

While the kidneys mature, the *cloaca* becomes the urogenital sinus. It then differentiates into the vesicourethral canal, which forms the bladder and the upper urethra, and the urogenital sinus, which forms the main part of the urethra.

At birth the kidneys occupy a large portion of the posterior abdominal wall, and the ureters are proportionately shorter than those of an adult. All the nephrons are present at birth, and their number does not increase as the kidney grows and

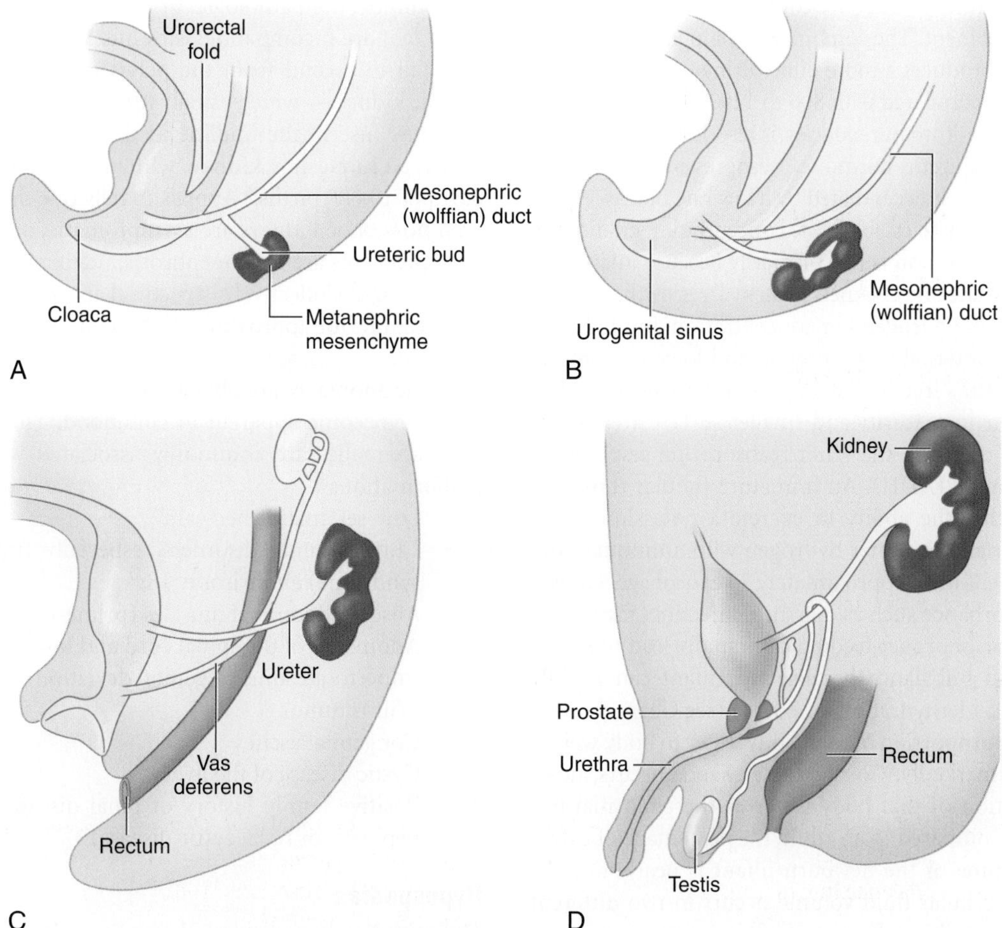

FIGURE 39-1 Embryonic Development of the Kidneys. The mesonephros begins development more caudally about the fourth fetal week and begins excretory function in the sixth week. Most of the mesonephros degenerates and disappears by the end of the embryonic period. The metanephros, the permanent kidney, arises distal to the bifurcation of the aorta and develops from two different sources: (1) the *ureteric bud* (metanephric duct) forms as an outgrowth of the mesonephritic (wolffian) duct and grows dorsocranially and starts subdividing to become the collecting system for the kidneys by forming the ureter, renal pelvis, and calyces; by the fifth fetal month it will have progressively branched into the collecting ducts; and (2) the *metanephrogenic mesenchyme* sits atop the terminal branches of the collecting ducts and develops into primitive glomeruli and uriniferous tubules **(A).** Genetic information from the metanephrogenic mesenchyme guides the development of the ureteric bud. Establishing the connection between the uriniferous tubules and the collecting ducts is a vital part of kidney development; errors in this stage can result in polycystic kidneys. As the embryo grows, the definitive kidneys migrate from the caudal position to the lumbar region and the ureters connect with the bladder **(B-D).** In the 8-week male embryo, the wolffian duct begins to give rise to the epididymis, the seminal vesicles, and the caudal part of the vas deferens **(C).** The external genitalia develop between 8 and 16 weeks, and testicular descent begins in month 7 of gestation **(D).** (From Goldman L, Schafer AI: *Goldman's Cecil medicine,* ed 24, Philadelphia, 2012, Saunders.)

matures. The kidney reaches adult size by adolescence and, because of maturation of the tubular system, increases in weight 10-fold from the time of birth.

Urine formation and excretion begin by the third month of gestation, contributing to the amniotic fluid. In infancy the bladder lies close to the abdominal wall, making urinary bladder aspiration for diagnostic purposes a relatively simple procedure. The bladder descends into the pelvis with growth, changing from a cylindrical organ to the adult pyramidal shape. Although small amounts of urine are found in the bladder at birth, the newborn may not void for 12 to 24 hours.

Immediately at birth the renal blood flow and glomerular filtration rate (GFR) increase because of a decrease in vascular resistance and the need to perform excretory functions no longer performed by the placenta. Renal vascular resistance remains higher in newborns and infants, however, which may be attributed to increased levels of circulating renin. The resistance progressively declines during the first year of development, with an increasing fraction of the cardiac output going to the kidney. The GFR continues to increase, achieving adult levels by 2 years of age.

Fluid and Electrolyte Balance in Children

Because the kidney develops from the center toward the periphery, renal distribution of blood flow during the newborn period is primarily to the renal medulla. The result is a preferential flow to the medullary nephrons, which have comparatively short loops at this stage of development. The combination of higher blood flow and shorter loops produces a more dilute urine—approximately 600 to 700 mOsm (compared with 800 to 1200 mOsm in adults) (see Chapter 3). The immature kidney is also less responsive to the actions of antidiuretic hormone (vasopressin) (see Figure 3-5).[3] The dilute urine is accentuated by a low rate of urea excretion, which is necessary to establish the concentration gradient in the medulla. Urea excretion is low primarily because infants are in a high anabolic state and use their protein for growth.

Because of a high hydrogen ion concentration, limited ability to regulate the internal environment, and lowered osmotic pressure, the infant's renal system has a narrow chemical safety margin. The immaturity and smaller surface area of the tubules also may diminish the water reabsorption response to antidiuretic hormone (ADH). An immature tubular transport capacity means that the ability to excrete a potassium load, reabsorb bicarbonate, or buffer hydrogen with ammonia does not become efficient until approximately 2 years of age. Consequently, any disturbance such as diarrhea, infection, fasting for diagnostic tests, or improper feeding can rapidly lead to severe acidosis and fluid imbalance because the infant can rapidly develop over- or underhydration, or edema (see Chapter 3).[4]

After birth the proportion of total body water to body weight does not change markedly. Considerable change occurs, however, in the location of that body water as the child matures (see Chapter 3). Compared to an adult, the percentage of extracellular fluid volume of the newborn infant is nearly double. Decrease in extracellular fluid volume occurs in two different periods of rapid growth—infancy and adolescence.

An infant has not only a greater content of extracellular fluid but also a greater rate of fluid exchange. The adult consumes and excretes approximately 2000 ml of water daily, representing 5% of the total body fluid and 14% of the extracellular fluid. In contrast, the infant's daily exchange of 600 to 700 ml represents about 20% of the total body water or nearly 60% of the extracellular volume, making control of dehydration and overhydration more difficult.

The composition of body fluids differs slightly with age. The total electrolyte concentration in extracellular fluids is greater in the newborn than in the adult. The concentrations of sodium, chloride, phosphates, and organic acids are also greater. The concentration of bicarbonate ions is lower in the infant than in the older child, with a mild acidosis evidenced by a lowered pH. These variations, combined with a lowered plasma protein level, cause a reduced oncotic pressure of the vascular compartment and favor accumulation of fluid in the tissue spaces and an increased GFR. In the healthy child these differences remain for a few weeks or months. The premature infant and the normal newborn infant are usually in a state of well-compensated acidosis and potential edema.

ALTERATIONS IN RENAL AND BLADDER FUNCTION IN CHILDREN

Congenital Abnormalities

Congenital abnormalities of the kidney and urinary tract occur in about 1 out of 500 newborns.[5] Structural abnormalities range from minor, nonpathologic, or easily correctable anomalies to those that are incompatible with life. For example, the kidneys may fail to ascend from the pelvis to the abdomen, causing ectopic kidneys—which usually function normally. The kidneys also may fuse in the midline as they ascend, causing a single U-shaped **horseshoe kidney,** with an incidence rate of 0.25 to 0.61 per 10,000 births.[6] Approximately one third of individuals with horseshoe kidneys are asymptomatic, and the most common problems are hydronephrosis, infection, stone formation, and tumors.[7] Collectively, structural anomalies of the renal system account for approximately 45% of cases of renal failure in children.

Some anomalies are obvious at birth, whereas others remain silent or become apparent in childhood. The following structural anomalies are commonly associated with urinary tract malformations[8]:

- Low-set, malformed ears
- Chromosomal disorders, especially trisomy 13 (Patau syndrome) and trisomy 18
- Absent abdominal muscles (prune-belly syndrome)
- Anomalies of the spinal cord and lower extremities
- Imperforate anus or genital deviation
- Wilms tumor
- Congenital ascites
- Cystic disease of the liver
- Positive family history of renal disease (e.g., hereditary nephritis or renal cystic disease)

Hypospadias

Hypospadias is a congenital condition in which the urethral meatus is located on the ventral side or undersurface of the penis. The meatus can be located anywhere on the glans, the penile shaft, the base of the penis, the penoscrotal junction, or the perineum (Figure 39-2). This is the most common anomaly of the penis and occurs in about 1 in 125 infant boys. The etiology is multifactorial and related to disruptions in male hormones, including testosterone biosynthesis defects, steroid 5α-reductase type 2 mutations, genes associated with penile and urethral development, hormones administered for in vitro fertilization, advanced maternal age, and other environmental factors.[9] **Chordee,** or penile torsion, may accompany hypospadias. In chordee a shortage of skin on the ventral surface causes the penis to bend or to "bow" ventrally (Figure 39-3). *Penile torsion* is a counterclockwise twist of the penile shaft. Partial absence of the foreskin, inguinal hernia, and cryptorchidism (undescended testes; see Chapter 25) are associated with the anomaly.[10]

The goals for corrective surgery on the child with hypospadias are: (1) a straight penis when erect to facilitate sexual intercourse as an adult, (2) a uniform urethra of adequate caliber to prevent spraying during urinations, (3) a cosmetic appearance satisfactory to the individual, and (4) repair completed in as few procedures as possible. Formerly performed in two or more stages, hypospadias repairs are now done in one stage. Improvements in microsurgical techniques have enhanced outcomes and decreased complications and the need for follow-up surgery. Surgery is usually performed between 4 and 12 months of age.[11]

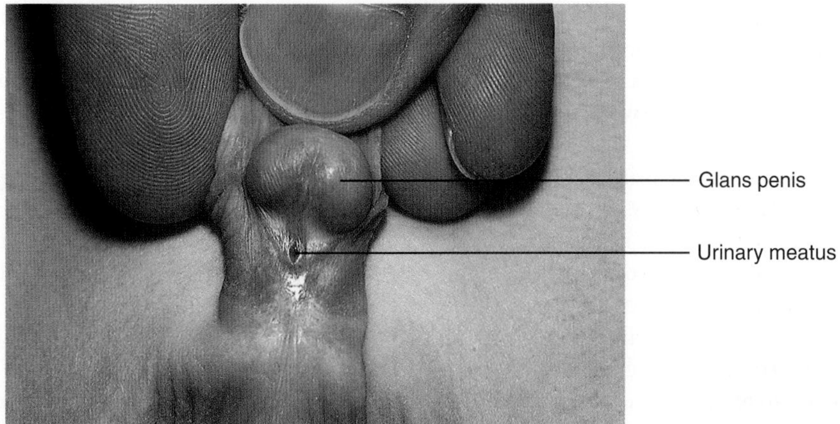

FIGURE 39-2 Hypospadias. (Courtesy H. Gil Rushton, MD, Children's National Medical Center, Washington, DC; from Hockenberry MJ, Wilson D: *Wong's nursing care of infants and children,* ed 9, St Louis, 2011, Mosby.)

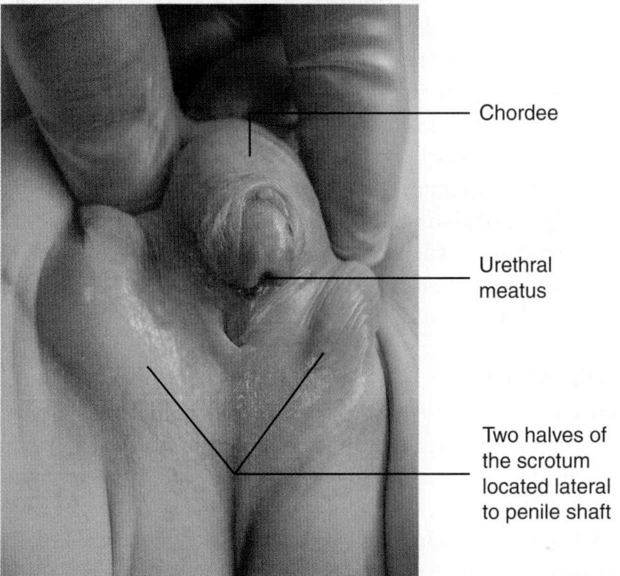

FIGURE 39-3 Perineal Hypospadias with Chordee and Partial Penoscrotal Transposition. (From Kliegman RM et al, editors: *Nelson textbook of pediatrics,* ed 19, Philadelphia, 2011, Saunders.)

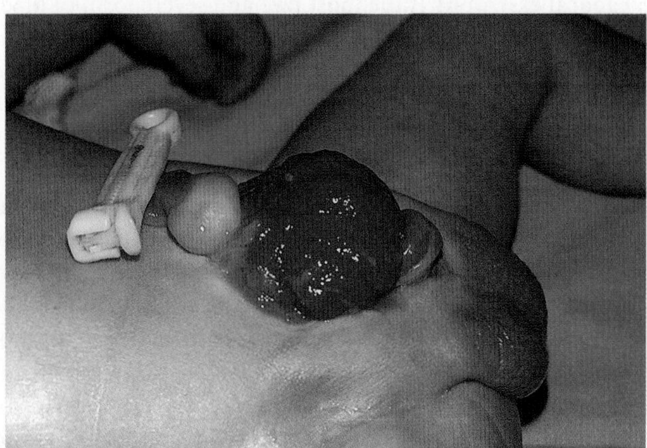

FIGURE 39-4 Exstrophy of Bladder. (Courtesy H. Gil Rushton, MD, Children's National Medical Center, Washington, DC; from Hockenberry MJ, Wilson D: *Wong's nursing care of infants and children,* ed 9, St Louis, 2011, Mosby.)

Epispadias

Epispadias and exstrophy of the bladder are the same congenital defect but expressed to a different degree. The dorsal urethra is not fused in epispadias and has failed to form into a tube. In male epispadias the urethral opening is on the dorsal surface of the penis. In females a cleft along the ventral urethra usually extends to the bladder neck. The incidence of epispadias is about 1 in 40,000 to 118,000 births. About twice as many boys as girls present with this defect.

In boys the urethral opening may be small and situated behind the glans (anterior epispadias), or a fissure may extend the entire length of the penis and into the bladder neck (posterior epispadias). The majority of children with epispadias can achieve urinary continence, although surgical intervention may be necessary.[12]

Exstrophy of the Bladder

Exstrophy of the bladder is a rare extensive congenital anomaly of herniation of the bladder through the abdominal wall with failure of the abdominal muscles, pelvic ring, and pelvic floor musculature to fuse in the midline (Figure 39-4). The posterior portion of the bladder mucosa is exposed and appears bright red. The prevalence of exstrophy of the bladder is about 2.07 in 100,000 live births. Boys are predominant with a ratio of about 2:1 and this complication is more common in whites.[13]

Exstrophy of the bladder is caused by intrauterine failure of the abdominal wall and the mesoderm of the anterior bladder to fuse. Urine seeps onto the abdominal wall from the ureters, causing a constant odor of urine and excoriation of the surrounding skin. The rectus muscles below the umbilicus are separated, and the pubic rami (bony projections of the pubic bone) are not joined. The clitoris in girls is divided into two halves with the urethra between them. The penis in boys is epispadic. In addition, the posterior aspect of the pelvis is externally rotated, which retroverts the acetabula and causes external rotation of the feet. This causes a waddling gait when the child first learns to walk, but most children quickly learn to compensate. Surgical intervention may be required.[14] Because the exposed bladder mucosa becomes hyperemic and edematous, it bleeds easily and is painful. It should be covered with Silastic or a plastic dressing (e.g., kitchen plastic wrap) for protection from diaper irritation while permitting urine drainage. The unrepaired exstrophic bladder is cosmetically unacceptable and prone to cancerous changes as soon as 1 year after birth. Ideally the bladder and pubic defect should be closed before the infant is 72 hours old. Surgical reconstruction is usually performed within the first year either as a complete primary repair or as staged procedures. Staged procedures may include bladder augmentation and bladder neck and epispadias repair.[15] Objectives of management include preservation of renal function, attainment of urinary control, prevention of infection, reconstructive repair of the defect, and improvement of sexual function and quality of life.

Cloacal exstrophy is the most rare and severe form of bladder exstrophy. The intestines, genitourinary tract, and spine may be involved, and reconstruction with restored urine and fecal control is difficult.

Ureteropelvic Junction Obstruction

Ureteropelvic junction (UPJ) obstruction is a blockage of the tapered point where the renal pelvis transitions into the ureter.[16] An intrinsic malformation of smooth muscle hypertrophy and fibrosis produces obstruction in 90% of cases.[17] It is the most common cause of hydronephrosis in neonates.[18] Diagnosis is made by ultrasound. Open or endoscopic surgery to relieve the obstruction occurs if there is decline of renal drainage or function.[19] During infancy or childhood, **secondary ureteropelvic junction obstruction** is caused by kinking or secondary scarring in the presence of high-grade vesicoureteral reflux. Children with UPJ obstruction have an increased risk of vesicoureteral reflux. Other defects are sometimes associated with ureteral duplication including complete ureteral duplication (abnormal growth of two ureters and ureteral orifices draining a single kidney), incomplete duplication (bifurcation of the ureter terminates into one ureteral orifice and serves a single kidney), and ureterocele (cystic dilation of the intravesical ureter). Obstruction of the distant ureter (ureterovesical junction obstruction) causes dilation of the entire ureter, renal pelvis, and calyceal system (megaureter). Megaureter can occur when a short acontractile segment of the ureter develops just above the ureterovesical junction or from ureteral reflux.[20]

Bladder Outlet Obstruction

Congenital causes of bladder outlet obstruction are rare and include urethral valves, urethral polyps, and urethral atresia. A **urethral valve** is a thin membrane that occludes the urethral lumen and obstructs urinary outflow in males. It is the most common cause of congenital lower urinary tract obstruction and renal failure. Most valves occur in the posterior urethra, although a few arise from the embryologically distinct anterior urethra.[21] **Urethral polyps** arising from the prostatic urethra are rare. Symptoms of polyps may include hematuria; voiding issues, such as urinary retention or straining to void; and dilation of the upper tracts.[22] **Urethral atresia** is absence of the urethra and is rare.

Congenital urethral valves or polyps can be diagnosed with prenatal ultrasound and treated with prenatal bladder shunting or with resection during the first days of life.[23] Infants with significant renal (and pulmonary) hypoplasia who are unable to undergo primary resection may be managed with a vesicostomy, a small opening created between the bladder wall and the abdomen.[24]

Hypoplastic or Dysplastic Kidneys

During embryologic development the ureteric duct grows into the metanephric tissue, triggering the formation of the kidneys. If this growth does not occur, the kidney is absent—a condition called **renal aplasia.** A **hypoplastic kidney** is small with a decreased number of nephrons. These conditions may be unilateral or bilateral; the occurrence may be incidental or familial.[24] Bilateral hypoplastic kidneys are a common cause of chronic renal failure in children. Segmental hypoplasia (the Ask-Upmark kidney) may be congenital or secondary to vesicoureteral reflux.[25]

Renal dysplasia usually results from abnormal differentiation of the renal tissues; for example, primitive glomeruli and tubules, cysts, and nonrenal tissue (such as cartilage) are found in the dysplastic kidney. Dysplasia may be secondary to antenatal obstruction of the urinary tract from ureteroceles, posterior urethral valves, or prune-belly syndrome (congenital absence of abdominal muscles).

Renal Agenesis

Renal agenesis (the absence of one or both kidneys) may be unilateral or bilateral, and may occur randomly or be hereditary. It may be an isolated entity or associated with anomalies in other organs.[26]

Unilateral renal agenesis occurs in approximately 1 of 1000 live births in the United States. Males are more often affected, and it is usually the left kidney that is absent. The single kidney is often completely normal so that the child can expect a normal, healthy life. The normal solitary kidney grows because of compensatory hypertrophy before[27] and after birth. By the time the child is several years older, the volume of this kidney may approach twice the normal size. In some instances the single kidney is abnormally formed and associated with abnormalities of its collecting system.[28] Extrarenal congenital abnormalities are relatively more common with unilateral renal agenesis.

Bilateral renal agenesis (also called **Potter syndrome**) is a rare disorder incompatible with extrauterine life.[29] Approximately 75% of affected infants are male. Bilateral renal agenesis results from either an abnormal development of the normal progression from pronephros to mesonephros to metanephros or an isolated bilateral failure of development of the ureteral buds. The term *Potter syndrome* refers to the association with a specific group of facial anomalies (wide-set eyes, parrot-beak nose, low-set ears, and receding chin). Oligohydramnios (low amount of amniotic fluid) leads to underdeveloped lungs. Affected infants rarely live more than a few hours because of pulmonary insufficiency. Approximately 40% of affected infants are stillborn. Renal agenesis can be detected prenatally by ultrasound.

Polycystic Kidneys

Autosomal dominant polycystic kidney disease (ADPKD) is an inherited disorder that occurs in about 1 in 1000 live births in the United States. Mutations of two genes, *PKD-1* (chromosome 16) and *PKD-2* (chromosome 4), account for the disease most often presenting in late childhood or adulthood. The gene products (polycystins) regulate growth and differentiation of the tubular epithelium.[30] Defects in the formation of epithelial cells and their cilium result in cyst formation and obstruction accompanied by destruction of renal parenchyma, interstitial fibrosis, and loss of functional nephrons. Cysts may occur in other organs including the liver, ovaries, and pancreas. Hypertension, heart valve defects, and cerebral and aortic aneurysms may develop. Urinary tract infection, hematuria, and flank pain may occur. Diagnosis is usually confirmed by ultrasound. Individuals may live for decades before developing symptoms of renal disease and not all progress to end-stage disease.[31] Autosomal recessive PKD *(ARPKD)* with cystic changes in the kidney and liver is often first suspected on a prenatal ultrasound. The gene mutation for *ARPKD (PKHD1)* encodes a protein important to maintaining structural integrity and cellular function of the kidneys and liver. Renal replacement therapy is usually required during childhood or adolescence. Biomarkers and therapies to slow the progression of cyst development and renal failure are being studied.[32]

Glomerular Disorders

The most common glomerular disorders in children are glomerulonephritis, nephrotic syndrome, and hemolytic uremic syndrome. Most glomerular diseases are acquired and immunologically mediated. The disease can be acute or chronic. The likelihood of developing renal failure depends on the specific condition. The most common glomerular disorders in children are presented below.

Glomerulonephritis

Acute glomerulonephritis includes a number of renal disorders in which proliferation and inflammation of the glomeruli are secondary to an immune mechanism (Table 39-1). (The major glomerulopathies and their histologic characteristics can be reviewed in Chapter 38 and Table 38-7.) The symptoms usually include the sudden onset of hematuria with red blood cell casts and proteinuria, and can be accompanied by renal salt and water retention, edema, hypertension, and in severe cases azotemia (i.e., decreased glomerular filtration rate). Chronic glomerulonephritis is the causative factor for 30% to 50% of renal failure in children and is the condition responsible for most school-age and teenage children requiring dialysis and kidney transplantation.

Acute Poststreptococcal Glomerulonephritis. **Acute poststreptococcal glomerulonephritis** (PSGN) is one of the most common immune complex–mediated renal diseases in children ages 5 to 15 years and it is representative of acute glomerulonephritis. It most commonly occurs after a throat (pharyngitis) or skin (impetigo) infection with nephritogenic strains of group A beta-hemolytic streptococci, although other bacteria (e.g., Staphylococcus) and viruses also may be responsible. Sporadic occurrences of infectious glomerulonephritis have been observed after bacterial endocarditis, which may be associated with streptococcal or staphylococcal microorganisms, or after viral diseases, such as varicella and hepatitides B and C. Glomerulonephritis develops with the deposition of antigen-antibody complexes (immunoglobulin G [IgG], IgA, and C_3 complement) (see Chapter 8) in the glomerulus or the antigen may be trapped within the glomerulus and immune complexes formed in situ.[33] The exact mechanism of immune complex formation is unknown. The immune complexes initiate inflammation and glomerular injury. Immunofluorescence microscopy shows lumpy deposits of immunoglobulin (IgG) and complement (C3) on the glomerular basement membrane (Figure 39-5). The thickened glomerular membrane contributes to decreased GFR. Activated complement, inflammatory cytokines, oxidants, proteases, and growth factors attack epithelial cells, alter membrane permeability, and cause hematuria and proteinuria. More severe renal disease is observed after a prolonged infection and before antibiotic therapy. Hypertension occurs primarily because of fluid retention.[34]

Symptoms usually begin 1 to 2 weeks after an upper respiratory tract infection (more common during cold weather) and up to 6 weeks after skin infections, such as impetigo (more common during warm, humid weather). The onset of symptoms in the child is abrupt, varying with disease severity. The urine is usually smoky brown or cola colored because of the presence of red blood cells. The child may complain of flank or midabdominal pain, irritability, general malaise, and fever. Acute hypertension may cause headache, vomiting,

TABLE 39-1 PRIMARY GLOMERULONEPHRITIS IN CHILDREN

CLASSIFICATION	FINDINGS
Cause	Poststreptococcal infection Related to other bacterial or viral infection Unknown
Immunologic mechanism	Antigen-antibody complex deposition Planted antigens with immune complex formed in situ Formation of antiglomerular basement membrane antibodies (rare) No immunologic cause established
Histopathology	No lesion Diffuse, focal, or segmented Membranous, proliferative, or combination of types Lobular, exudative, necrotizing, and other types Chronic with glomerular proliferation
Clinical manifestations of disease	Acute glomerulonephritis Persistent (chronic) glomerulonephritis Idiopathic nephrotic syndrome

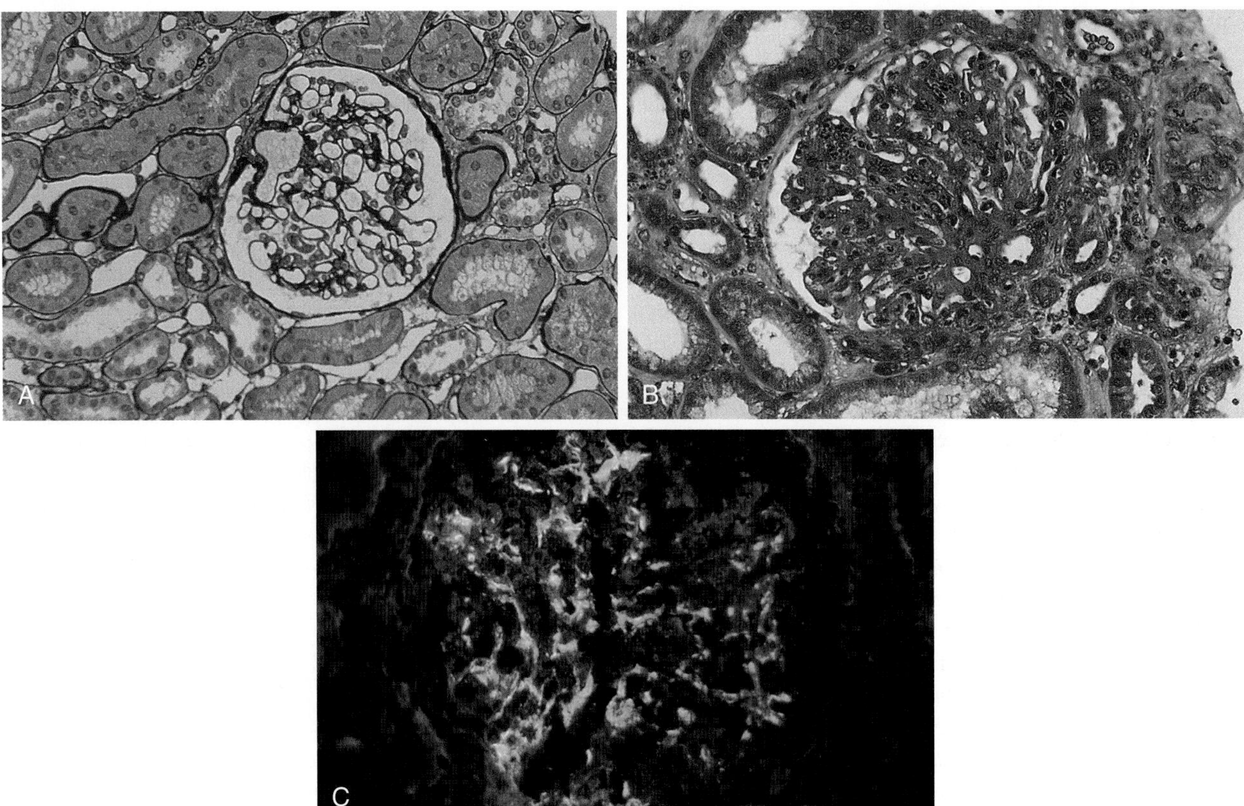

FIGURE 39-5 Glomerulonephritis. **A,** Normal glomerulus; note single-contoured walls, patent capillaries, inconspicuous mesangium, and degree of cellularity. (Periodic acid–methenamine silver stain.) **B,** Acute postinfectious glomerulonephritis. There is considerable increase in cellularity, mainly because of accumulation of numerous polymorphonuclear leukocytes in capillary lumina. Note numerous subepithelial hump-shaped fuchsinophilic deposits in many capillary walls. Protein precipitates (hyalinization) are in the arteriole. (Masson trichrome stain.) **C,** Postinfectious glomerulonephritis. Irregular mesangial and capillary wall immunostaining for C3. (From Damjanov I, Linder J, editors: *Anderson's pathology,* ed 10, St Louis, 1996, Mosby.)

somnolence, and other central nervous system (CNS) manifestations, including seizures. Cardiovascular symptoms are related to circulatory overload and are compounded by hypertension. These include dyspnea, tachypnea, and an enlarged, tender liver. The most severely affected children develop acute renal failure with oliguria. As many as half the children affected are asymptomatic. The disease is usually mild and runs its course in 1 month, but urine abnormalities may be found up to 1 year after the onset. Less than 5% of children become oliguric or develop rapidly progressive glomerulonephritis, or progress to chronic glomerulonephritis. Prolonged proteinuria and abnormal GFR indicate an unfavorable prognosis. More than 95% recover completely.

Acute glomerulonephritis (AGN) may be accompanied by a positive throat or skin culture for *Streptococcus.* Antistreptolysin-O titers confirm a recent streptococcal infection. Antihyaluronidase, antideoxyribonuclease B, and antistreptokinase antibody are other diagnostic markers. Serum complement level is decreased, and serum creatinine concentration and blood urea nitrogen level are elevated. The urine usually contains red blood cells and proteins. Treatment is supportive and symptom specific. For severe disease oliguria and hypertension are common, and fluid, sodium, and potassium intakes are restricted. Antihypertensive medication and diuretic agents may be indicated during the acute phase.

Henoch-Schönlein Purpura Nephritis. **Henoch-Schönlein purpura (HSP) nephritis (anaphylactoid purpura)** is an immune-mediated IgA vasculitis that affects glomerular blood vessels, causing inflammation and damage to the vessel wall (see Chapter 38 for the pathophysiology of IgA nephropathy). The disease also involves small vessels in the skin and gut. Classic symptoms of HSP include palpable purpura, arthritis, abdominal pain, and renal disease characterized by gross or microscopic hematuria with mild or no proteinuria. Kidney biopsy demonstrates IgA deposition in the mesangium[35] (see Table 38-7 in Chapter 38). The development of interstitial fibrosis and crescent formation from subepithelial immune deposits along the glomeruli increases the risk of chronic renal failure.[36] Most children recover with supportive care, although some progress to kidney failure. Severe symptoms require corticosteroids and other immunosuppressant drugs.[37]

Hemolytic Uremic Syndrome

Hemolytic uremic syndrome (HUS) is an acute disorder characterized by microangiopathic hemolytic anemia, thrombocytopenia, and renal impairment. It is the most common community-acquired cause of acute renal failure in young children. The disease occurs most frequently in infants and children younger than 4 years of age. The prognosis has improved dramatically in recent years, with more than 90% of children surviving and most regaining normal renal function.

PATHOPHYSIOLOGY. HUS has been associated with both bacterial and viral agents, as well as endotoxins, especially those from *Escherichia coli* 0157:H7 and recently *Escherichia coli* 0104:H4 (Shiga toxins).[38] Potential sources of exposure include animals, unpasteurized beverages, and contaminated meat and vegetables. The disease also occurs with cancer and use of chemotherapeutic agents.[39] In HUS, verotoxin (Shiga toxin) from *E. coli* is absorbed from the intestines into the blood, binds to polymorphonuclear leukocytes, and is transported to the kidney, causing a cascade of effects, including lysis of glomerular capillary endothelial cells, separation of endothelial cells from the basement membrane, activation and aggregation of platelets, and activation of the coagulation cascade. The glomerular arterioles become swollen and occluded with platelets and fibrin clots. There is decreased glomerular filtration, and the damaged glomerular membrane results in hematuria and proteinuria. Oliguria with renal failure occurs in up to 50% of children. Narrowed vessels damage passing erythrocytes. These damaged red blood cells, identified as burr cells, helmet cells, and fragmented red blood cells, are removed by the spleen, causing acute hemolytic anemia. Fibrinolysis, the process of dissolution of a clot, acts on precipitated fibrin, causing the fibrin split products to appear in serum and urine. The platelet clustering within damaged vessels, combined with the damage and removal of platelets, produces thrombocytopenia. Fibrin-rich thrombi can be found throughout the microcirculation.[40] Other tissues, including the brain, liver, heart, and intestines, are often involved, which portends a poorer prognosis.

CLINICAL MANIFESTATIONS. Typical HUS is preceded by a prodromal gastrointestinal (GI) illness with diarrhea (usually caused by Shiga toxin–producing *E. coli*) and is known as D+ HUS. Less frequently atypical or sporadic HUS is preceded by an unknown event or an upper respiratory tract infection and is known as D− HUS. A rare familial form is associated with mutations in complement proteins. P-hemolytic-uremic syndrome is associated with *Streptococcus pneumoniae* respiratory tract infection and is mediated by neuraminidase that injures glomerular epithelial cells. It occurs without diarrhea. The onset of D+ HUS occurs about 1 to 2 weeks after a GI illness with a symptom-free 1- to 5-day period. There is sudden onset of pallor, bruising or purpura, irritability, and oliguria. Slight fever, anorexia, vomiting, diarrhea (with the stool characteristically watery and blood stained—hemorrhagic diarrhea), abdominal pain, mild jaundice, and circulatory overload are accompanying symptoms. Seizures and lethargy indicate CNS involvement. Renal failure is apparent within 2 days to 2 weeks of onset. The renal failure causes metabolic acidosis, uremia, hyperkalemia, and often hypertension.

EVALUATION AND TREATMENT. Clinical evaluation includes history of preexisting illness, presenting symptoms, and urine and blood analysis. Antibiotics are not used in the initial treatment because they increase Shiga toxin release and increase the risk of HUS. Management consists of maintaining nutrition and hydration (to dilute toxins) and controlling hypertension, hyperkalemia, and seizures.[41] When renal failure occurs, dialysis is indicated. Blood transfusions with packed red blood cells are needed to maintain reasonable hemoglobin levels. Most children recover; however, some will develop hypertension, proteinuria, or renal insufficiency or failure. Death usually occurs from complications related to CNS or myocardial involvement.[42] Preventing Shiga toxin–producing bacterial infection (i.e., *E. coli*) prevents HUS.

Nephrotic Syndrome

Nephrotic syndrome is a term used to describe a symptom complex characterized by proteinuria, hypoalbuminemia, hyperlipidemia, and edema. The syndrome is more common in children than adults. When no identifiable cause is found, the condition is termed **primary (idiopathic) nephrotic syndrome.** If it results from a systemic disease or other causes (e.g., drugs, toxins, diabetes mellitus, lupus nephritis) it is called **secondary nephrotic syndrome.** Primary nephrotic syndrome is usually described by histopathologic results (i.e., minimal change nephropathy [MCN], focal segmental glomerulosclerosis [FSGS], membranous nephropathy [MN], or membranoproliferative glomerulonephritis [MPGN]) (see Table 38-7). Secondary nephrotic syndrome has the same patterns of histopathology but is associated with an underlying cause.

Approximately 95% of cases of nephrotic syndrome in children occur in the absence of systemic or preexisting renal disease. Primary nephrotic syndrome is found predominantly in preschool children, with a peak incidence of onset between 2 and 3 years of age. Onset is rare after 8 years of age. Boys are affected more often than girls. No prevalent racial or geographic distributions are evident. The incidence is approximately 2 to 3 per 100,000 children per year.[43]

PATHOPHYSIOLOGY. The cause of nephrotic syndrome in children is usually idiopathic and includes minimal change nephropathy (85%), FSGS (10%), and mesangial proliferative nephropathy (MPN) (5%) (see Chapter 38, Table 38-7).[44] Secondary nephrotic syndrome may develop during the course of several different renal or systemic diseases. The pathophysiology (see Figure 38-10) and common clinical manifestations of nephrotic syndrome in adults are described in Chapter 38 (Table 38-8), and are similar in children. The most common causes of nephrotic syndrome in children are presented here.

Minimal change nephropathy (MCN), also known as *lipoid nephrosis,* is the most common cause of nephrotic syndrome in children ages 2 to 6 years. A systemic immune mechanism is a likely cause of the disease, but the true etiology is unknown. The mechanism of increased glomerular permeability is unknown but is related, in part, to release of permeability factors from abnormal circulating T cells that injure the glomerular epithelial cells. The glomeruli appear normal by light microscopy, and immunoglobulin deposition is usually absent. The only change is *fusion of epithelial cell podocyte foot processes.*[44] There are few other renal structural abnormalities. Loss of the electrical negative charge and increased permeability within the glomerular capillary wall lead to albuminuria.[45] Hyperlipidemia leads to hyperlipiduria and primarily results from increased hepatic lipid synthesis and decreased plasma lipid catabolism.[46]

Focal segmental glomerulosclerosis (FSGS) is present in approximately 10% to 15% of children with nephrotic syndrome and is more common in blacks. The frequency of FSGS is increasing in children and adults.[47] The primary injury is effacement (thinning or deletion) of epithelial podocytes, with a significant increase in pore size leading to impairment of size selectivity and proteinuria. Progressive disease results in proliferation of endothelial and mesangial cells with occlusion and sclerosis of glomerular capillaries. The more severe the proteinuria, the more likely that end-stage renal disease will occur.[48]

Edema is the classic symptom of nephrotic syndrome. Several factors contribute to edema formation with hypoalbuminemia (decreased plasma oncotic pressure) and sodium retention as major contributors. The movement of fluid from the vascular to the interstitial space can decrease blood volume and increase the activity of aldosterone and antidiuretic hormone (vasopressin), and decrease atrial natriuretic peptide concentration, all of which promote fluid retention.[49]

Hyperlipidemia occurs in inverse proportion to the decrease in plasma proteins, particularly albumin. There are high concentrations of triglycerides, low-density lipoprotein (LDL), and very-low-density lipoprotein (VLDL) cholesterol. High-density lipoprotein (HDL) cholesterol concentration is decreased. Hypoalbuminemia leads to a deficiency in the carrier protein for the transport of fatty acids, and they remain elevated in the serum. There is hepatic compensation for hypoalbuminemia with increased synthesis of lipoproteins to maintain plasma oncotic pressure. Hypoalbuminemia also leads to an increased hepatic stimulus for synthesis of LDL and VLDL cholesterol by the liver. Serum lipids may remain elevated from 1 to 3 months after remission of proteinuria.

Hypercoagulation with risk for arterial or venous thrombosis results from abnormalities in the coagulation pathways during nephrotic syndrome. Although rare, thrombosis can occur in the brain or lung. Family history and predisposing risk factors should be evaluated. Anticoagulants may be required.[50]

Congenital, or **infantile, nephrotic syndrome (Finnish type)** is caused by an autosomal recessive mutation of the *NPHS1* gene that encodes an immunoglobulin-like protein, nephrin, at the podocyte slit membrane. Lack of nephrin causes heavy proteinuria.[51] The disease usually manifests within the first 3 to 12 months of life, and these infants do not respond to corticosteroid treatment.[52]

CLINICAL MANIFESTATIONS. Onset of nephrotic syndrome is often insidious, with periorbital edema as the first sign. The edema is most noticeable in the morning but subsides during the day as fluid shifts to the abdomen and lower extremities (Figure 39-6). Parents may notice diminished, frothy, or foamy urine output; when edema becomes pronounced with ascites, respiratory difficulty from pleural effusion and labial or scrotal swelling may develop.

Edema of the intestinal mucosa may cause diarrhea, anorexia, and poor absorption. Edema often masks the malnutrition caused by malabsorption and protein loss. Because of protein deficiency, changes in the quality of hair indicate a malnourished state. Pallor, with shiny skin and prominent veins, may be present. Blood pressure is usually normal. The child has an increased susceptibility to infection, especially pneumonia, peritonitis, cellulitis, and septicemia. Irritability, fatigue, and lethargy are common. Infants born with congenital nephrotic syndrome have large fontanels and separated cranial sutures.

EVALUATION AND TREATMENT. The diagnosis of nephrotic syndrome is evident from the clinical presentation and findings of proteinuria, hyperlipidemia, and edema. Several diagnostic tests, including kidney biopsy, may be required to determine whether the cause is an intrinsic renal disease or a consequence of systemic disease.

The goals of treatment are to reduce the excretion of protein and to maintain protein-free urine. Prevention or treatment of infection, control of edema, establishment of a balanced nutritional state, and restoration of normal metabolic processes also are important in managing the disorder and avoiding adverse aspects of treatment. Basic management of nephrotic syndrome includes administering glucocorticosteroids (prednisone); adhering to a low-sodium, well-balanced diet; performing good skin care; and, if edema becomes problematic, administering diuretics (furosemide, metolazone).[53] Angiotensin-converting enzyme (ACE) inhibitors inhibit formation of

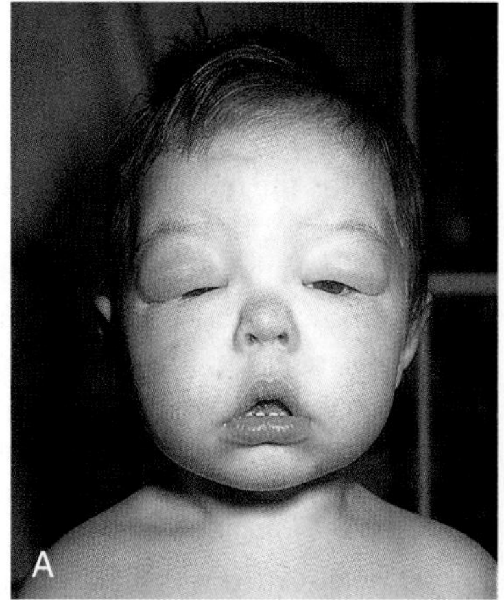

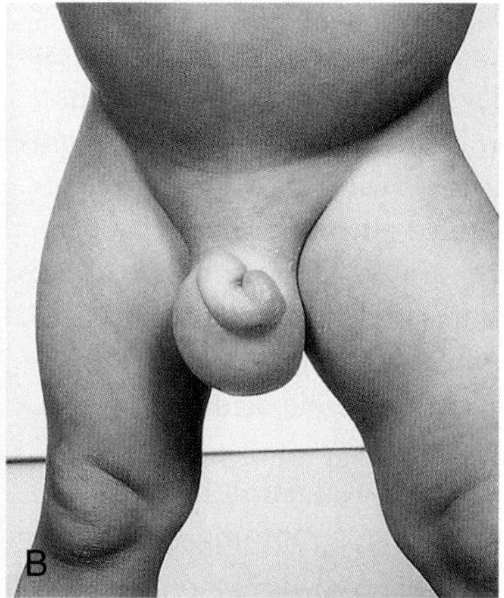

FIGURE 39-6 Nephrotic Syndrome. **A,** Facial edema. **B,** Gross edema of scrotum and legs with abdominal distention from ascites. (From Lissauer T, Clayden G: *Illustrated textbook of paediatrics,* ed 4, London, 2012, Mosby.)

angiotensin II and aldosterone, resulting in decreased blood pressure and decreased renal sodium reabsorption. Nephrotic syndrome is often described by the response to steroid therapy (Table 39-2). **Steroid-sensitive nephrotic syndrome** usually results in complete remission without serious adverse effects. **Steroid-resistant nephrotic syndrome** is described for children (usually infants 3 to 12 months of age or adolescents) who fail to respond to prednisone within 8 weeks. They may be treated with noncorticosteroid immunosuppressive agents (i.e., cyclophosphamide) or combinations of corticosteroids and noncorticosteroid immunosuppressives to prolong remission.[54,55] Children with minimal change disease tend to have a very favorable prognosis, whereas those with other conditions, such as FSGS, may develop end-stage kidney disease.[56]

Kidney Injury

Kidney injury, either acute or chronic, is rare in children. The pathophysiology (see Figure 38-11) and management are similar to those for kidney injury in adults. A modification of the RIFLE criteria (*R* = risk, *I* = injury, *F* = failure, *L* = loss, and *E* = end-stage kidney disease [ESKD]) that was proposed to standardize the definition of acute kidney injury in adults has been used in critically ill children (pRIFLE criteria) (Table 39-3).[57]

TABLE 39-2 CORTICOSTEROID RESPONSE IN CHILDREN WITH NEPHROTIC SYNDROME

RESPONSE TO CORTICOSTEROID	OUTCOMES
Steroid sensitive	May have just one or recurrent episodes.
Steroid dependent (frequently relapsing)	May require low-dose prednisone or treatment with other immunosuppressive agents to prevent recurrence
Steroid resistant	Treatment with immunosuppressive and nonimmunosuppressive medications; risk for development of end-stage kidney disease

Data from Gipson DS et al: *Pediatrics* 124(2):747–757, 2009.

TABLE 39-3 PEDIATRIC-MODIFIED RIFLE (pRIFLE) CRITERIA

RISK CATEGORY	ESTIMATED CCL-GFR CRITERIA	URINE OUTPUT CRITERIA
Risk	eCCl decrease by 25%	<0.5 ml/kg/hr for 8 hr
Injury	eCCl decrease by 50%	<0.5 ml/kg/hr for 16 hr
Failure	eCCl decrease by 75% or eCCl <35 ml/min/1.73 m^2	<0.3 ml/kg/hr for 24 hr or anuric for 12 hr
Loss (of kidney function)	Persistent failure >4 weeks	
End-stage	End-stage renal disease (persistent failure >3 months)	

Data from Akcan-Arikan A et al: *Kidney Int* 71(10):1028–1035, 2007.
eCCl, Estimated creatinine clearance; *GFR,* glomerular filtration rate; *pRIFLE,* pediatric risk, injury, failure, loss, and end-stage renal disease.

The most common causes of *prerenal acute kidney injury* are dehydration, hemorrhage, and sepsis. Glomerulonephritis, hemolytic uremic syndrome, and hypersensitivity reactions to drugs or infectious agents are the most common causes of *intrinsic acute kidney injury*. Obstructive uropathies, such as posterior urethral valves and obstruction of the ureteropelvic junction, are associated with *postrenal acute kidney injury*.[58] Chronic kidney failure in very young children is commonly associated with congenital renal structural abnormalities. In older children the most common cause is glomerulonephropathies.[59,60] Renal replacement modalities available for children with end-stage renal disease include peritoneal and hemodialysis and kidney transplant.[61,62] The use of growth hormone before and after transplant has contributed to normal growth and development, particularly in prepubertal children.[63]

Wilms Tumor

Wilms tumor is an embryonal tumor of the kidney arising from epigenetic and genetic changes that lead to abnormal proliferation of renal stem cells (metanephric blastema). It is also known by the histologic name of **nephroblastoma** and is the most common solid tumor occurring in children.

The incidence of Wilms tumor remains constant in the United States, with approximately 650 children diagnosed each year. Most children are between 1 and 5 years of age when they are diagnosed. The peak incidence occurs between 2 and 3 years of age. Wilms tumor is slightly more common in females and in black than in white children, and is less common in Asian children.[64,65]

Microscopically, Wilms tumor is composed of three cellular components: stromal, epithelial, and blastemic. This occurs because blastemic cells, which are primitive and undifferentiated, may have partially developed into epithelial or stromal tissue. With each of these three cellular components, varying stages of differentiation may be evident within the tumor.

PATHOGENESIS. Wilms tumor (nephroblastoma) has sporadic and inherited origins. The sporadic form occurs in children with no known genetic predisposition. Inherited cases, which are relatively rare (1% to 2% of cases), are transmitted in an autosomal dominant fashion.

A "two-hit" hypothesis for the development of Wilms tumor has been proposed wherein children who inherit a mutation in one allele of a tumor-suppression gene require just one more somatic mutation for a tumor to form[66] (see Figure 16-18). This hypothesis may not apply to all Wilms tumors, however, because a number of genetic abnormalities have been identified in Wilms tumors.[67,68] Wilms tumor-suppressor genes *WT1* and *WT2* are located on chromosome 11. Chromosomal abnormalities, including gains, losses, and rearrangements, are often present in Wilms tumors. Gains in chromosomes 6, 7, 8, 12, 13, and 18 and losses in chromosomes 11, 16, 22, and X are among the most common findings, although multiple other chromosomal abnormalities also have been identified.[69] *WTX* is a tumor-suppressor gene located on the X chromosome.[67] Approximately 10%

of children who have Wilms tumor also have loss of other important genes and therefore have a number of congenital anomalies. These anomalies include aniridia (lack of an iris in the eye), hemihypertrophy (an asymmetry of the body), and genitourinary malformations (i.e., horseshoe kidneys, hypospadias, ureteral duplication, polycystic kidneys, uterine abnormalities).[70,71] Children with congenital anomalies as well as Wilms tumor are more likely to have the inherited bilateral form of the disease.

CLINICAL MANIFESTATIONS. Most Wilms tumors (90%) present as an enlarging asymptomatic upper abdominal mass in a healthy, thriving child. Other presenting complaints include vague abdominal pain, hematuria, fever, and hypertension.[72]

EVALUATION AND TREATMENT. On physical examination the tumor feels firm, nontender, and smooth, and generally is a solitary mass of varying size confined to one side of the abdomen. Diagnostic imaging demonstrates a solid intrarenal mass.

Diagnosis is based on surgical biopsy. Additional laboratory and radiologic studies are used to evaluate the presence or absence of metastasis. The most common sites of metastasis are regional lymph nodes and the lungs and less commonly liver, brain, and bone.

Staging systems for Wilms tumor have been developed and serve as guides to treatment. The most widely accepted system was developed by the National Wilms Tumor Study Group (Table 39-4). The system is based on surgical findings and the extent of disease at diagnosis.[73] Children are further classified as either high or low risk according to favorable or unfavorable histologic presentation (anaplasia).

Primary treatment is usually (1) surgical exploration and resection, or (2) chemotherapy followed by surgical resection. In bilateral disease, surgical intervention may include heminephrectomy of the less involved kidney and nephrectomy of the other. Radiation therapy has been found to be most effective if begun 1 to 3 days after surgery for stages III and IV disease and metastases. Chemotherapy is specific to histologic presentation and stage of disease.[74]

The overall cure rate is as high as 95% for children with stage I through stage III disease (Table 39-5). Prognosis is improving for children with metastases, and this is one of the few tumors for which lung metastases have been cured. Recurrent disease is treated aggressively in children with favorable histologic results.

TABLE 39-4 STAGING OF WILMS TUMOR

STAGE*	TUMOR CHARACTERISTICS
Stage I (40% to 45%)	Tumor limited to the kidney, completely resected
Stage II (20% to 25%)	Tumor ascending beyond the kidney or into vessels of renal sinus, but appearing to be totally resected
Stage III (20% to 25%)	Residual nonhematogenous tumor confined to the abdomen, positive lymph nodes in renal hila
Stage IV (10%)	Hematogenous metastases (e.g., lung, liver, bone, brain)
Stage V (5%)	Bilateral disease either at diagnosis or later, but need to stage each kidney

Data from American Cancer Society: *Wilms tumor,* 2013. Available at www.cancer.org/cancer/wilmstumor/detailedguide/wilms-tumor-staging. Accessed April 2013.

***Note:** Staging system of the Third National Wilms Tumor Study Group (NWTS-3).

Bladder Disorders

Urinary Tract Infections

Urinary tract infection (UTI) is the colonization of a pathogen anywhere along the urinary tract (urethra, bladder, ureter, kidney) and occurs commonly in children.[75] The incidence of UTI is greater in boys up to 1 year of age, particularly among those not circumcised.[76] Girls have a greater incidence after 1 year of age with an increasing incidence at adolescence. UTIs in girls occur as a result of perineal bacteria, especially *E. coli,* ascending the urethra, which lies close to the anus. The incidence of UTI in neonates and infants is low, but the risk is increased because of an immature immune system.

The pathophysiology of UTIs in children is similar to that of adults (see Chapter 38). Although nephrolithiasis can be associated with UTI in adults, nephrolithiasis in children is rare, but is increasing in incidence (see What's New? Kidney Stones in Children). UTIs in children are often clinically categorized as first or recurrent infection. Individual susceptibility, bacterial virulence, and the host's anatomy (presence of reflux, obstruction, stasis, stones, or structural anomalies of the urinary tract) affect the severity of the disease. The recurrence rate is approximately 30% to 40%[77] and is highest in females. Sexually active female adolescents are at increased risk to have a UTI. Similar to adult women, susceptibility is increased when genetically controlled blood group antigens (P1 and Lewis blood group nonsecretor) are present on surface uroepithelial cells and act as receptors for bacterial attachment.[78]

TABLE 39-5 NATIONAL WILMS TUMOR STUDY 4-YEAR SURVIVAL RATES

TUMOR STAGE	FAVORABLE HISTOLOGY	UNFAVORABLE HISTOLOGY (ANAPLASTIC WILMS TUMOR)
I	99%	83%
II	98%	81%
III	94%	72%
IV	86%	38%
V	87%	55%

From American Cancer Society: *Wilms tumor,* 2013. Available at www.cancer.org/Cancer/WilmsTumor/DetailedGuide/wilms-tumor-survival-rates. Accessed April 2013.

WHAT'S NEW?

Kidney Stones in Children

Nephrolithiasis in children is rare although the incidence of calcium stones among children is increasing, particularly in adolescents. There are limited data available regarding the pathogenesis of kidney stones in children, but the mechanisms appear different compared to those of adults. Epidemiologic data indicate nephrolithiasis in children is more common in non-Hispanic white adolescent females between ages 13 and 18 years (male to female ratio 1:1.4). Proposed risk factors include obesity; diets high in salt, protein, or fructose, or low in water or calcium; and use of certain antiseizure, diuretic, vitamin, or antibiotic medications. Kidney stones also can be associated with urinary tract malformations (reflux disease and megaureter). Calcium stones are the most common stone type (72% to 88%). Children who form stones have higher supersaturation of calcium oxalate; however, the significance to stone formation is unknown. The most common symptom presentation is pain and gross hematuria. Prevention and treatment are individualized and any metabolic cause needs to be evaluated. Stone inhibitors, magnesium, and citrate have been effective in some groups. Surgical methods include extracorporeal shock wave lithotripsy, ureteroscopy, and percutaneous nephrolithotomy.

Data from Ayoob R, Wang W, Schwaderer A: *Pediatr Nephrol* 26(12):2173–2178, 2011; Bergsland KJ et al: *Kidney Int* 81(11): 1140–1148, 2012; Chahed J et al: *Afr J Paediatr Surg* 8(2):168–171, 2011; Dwyer ME et al: *J Urol* 188(1):247–252, 2012; Granberg CF, Baker LA: *Pediatr Clin North Am* 59(4):897–908, 2012; Sas DJ: *Clin J Am Soc Nephrol* 6(8):2062–2068, 2011; Schissel BL, Johnson BK: *Pediatr Emerg Care.* 27(7):676–681, 2011.

Cystitis, or infection of the bladder, results in mucosal inflammation and congestion. This causes detrusor muscle hyperactivity and a resulting decrease in the bladder capacity. It also can lead to transient reflux of urine up the ureters, sending bacteria all the way to the kidney, causing acute or chronic pyelonephritis and renal abscesses or scarring.

Symptoms of UTI in children are nonspecific, and differentiating whether an infection is in the bladder or kidneys is difficult based on symptoms alone. Infants usually develop vomiting, diarrhea, or jaundice. Infants and young children may present only with fever of undetermined origin and others may present with urinary tract symptoms of frequency; urgency; enuresis or incontinence in a previously dry child; abdominal, flank, or back pain; foul-smelling urine; and sometimes hematuria. **Acute pyelonephritis** usually causes chills, fever, and flank or abdominal pain along with enlarged kidney(s) caused by edema. **Chronic pyelonephritis** may be asymptomatic.

Diagnosis of UTIs is by urine culture of a pathogen before antimicrobial treatment. An accompanying urinalysis can show pyuria, nitrites, and hematuria. The presence of casts in the urine can indicate pyelonephritis. Ultrasound, voiding cystourethrography (VCUG) or radionuclide cystography, or computed tomography (CT) scan may be necessary to rule out obstructions, abscesses, or reflux, particularly in young children who do not respond to antimicrobial therapy.

With treatment, UTI symptoms are usually relieved in 1 to 2 days and the urine becomes sterile. A 2- to 4-day course of oral antibiotics is effective for uncomplicated UTI.[79] Longer treatment may be required if the child has a recurrent UTI, has a complicated UTI including congenital abnormalities of the urinary tract, or is immunosuppressed. Imaging of children after a first UTI is controversial.[80,81] The age of the child and seriousness of the infection should be considered when making imaging decisions. Repeat urine cultures are not needed if a child has responded to treatment.[82]

Management of constipation, promotion of adequate fluid intake, and elimination of dysfunctional voiding patterns are the cornerstones of minimizing the risk of recurrence.[83] Prophylactic antibiotics may be helpful for some children. Educating families about signs and symptoms of UTI allows for early identification and treatment. Surgical correction of vesicoureteral reflux or obstruction may be necessary.

Vesicoureteral Reflux

Vesicoureteral reflux (VUR) is the retrograde flow of bladder urine into the kidney or ureters, or both. Reflux allows infected urine from the bladder to reach the kidneys. Reflux perpetuates infection by preventing complete emptying of the bladder as refluxed urine drains back into the bladder at the end of each void. In addition, the reflux allows the maximal intravesical pressure to be transmitted to the renal calyces and pyramids. The combination of reflux and infection is an important cause of pyelonephritis, especially in children younger than 5 years.

Vesicoureteral reflux occurs more often in girls by a ratio of 10:1 and is less common in blacks. Its incidence is approximately 1 in 1000 children, and siblings of those affected have an approximately 30% chance of developing reflux.[84] Reflux nephropathy in males is associated with congenitally abnormal kidneys.[85] The shortness of the submucosal segment of the ureter during infancy and childhood renders the antireflux mechanism relatively inefficient and delicate. Thus reflux is seen commonly in association with infections during early childhood but rarely in older children and adults. (Among adults with UTIs, the incidence of reflux is approximately 5%.) Reflux may be unilateral or bilateral, and it can be classified or graded (Figure 39-7) for comparative purposes:

Grade I—Reflux into a nondilated distal ureter

Grade II—Reflux into the upper collecting system without dilation

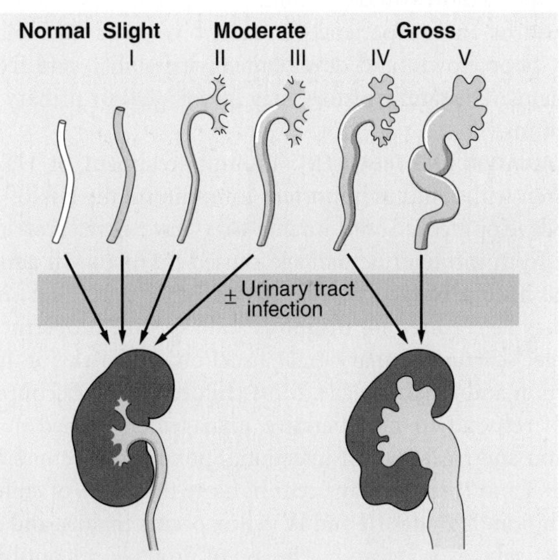

FIGURE 39-7 Grades of Reflux. (From Feehally J, Floege J, Johnson RJ: *Comprehensive clinical nephrology*, ed 3, Philadelphia, 2008, Mosby.)

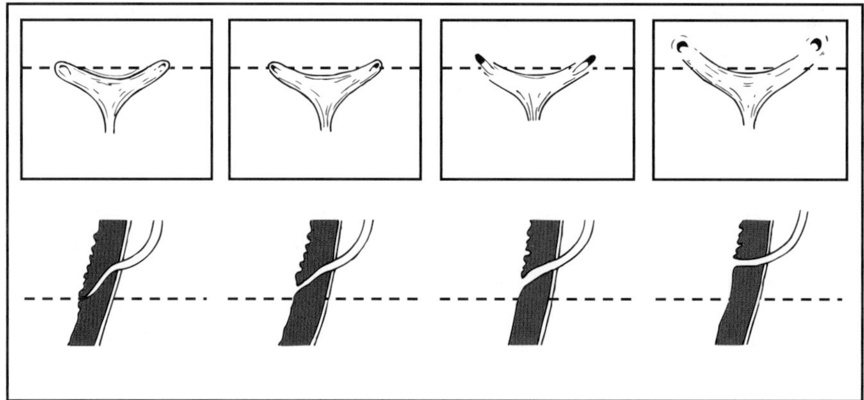

FIGURE 39-8 Normal and Abnormal Configuration of the Ureteral Orifices. *Left to right:* Progressive lateral displacement of the ureteral orifices and shortening of the intramural tunnels. *Top row:* Endoscopic appearance. *Bottom row:* Sagittal view through the intramural ureter. (From Kliegman RM et al, editors: *Nelson textbook of pediatrics,* ed 19, Philadelphia, 2011, Saunders.)

Grade III—Reflux into dilated ureter or blunting of calyceal fornices

Grade IV—Reflux into a grossly dilated ureter

Grade V—Massive reflux with ureteral dilation and tortuosity and effacement of the calyceal details; occurs almost exclusively in male infants[86]

PATHOPHYSIOLOGY. Primary reflux results from a congenitally abnormal or ectopic insertion of the ureter into the bladder. In some infants VUR may be related to inadequate relaxation of the external urethral sphincter.[87] Occasionally the condition is hereditary. Secondary reflux may be transient or persistent. It develops in association with infection, malformations of the ureterovesical (UV) junction, increased intravesical pressures, voiding disorders, or surgery on the UV junction (Figure 39-8). Urinary tract infection associated with VUR may lead to permanent renal scarring, particularly when there is pyelonephritis.[88] The actual cause of renal cell damage and scarring is unknown but contributing factors include inflammatory cytokines activated by bacterial virulence factors.[89]

CLINICAL MANIFESTATIONS. Children with reflux may be asymptomatic or may experience recurrent UTIs or unexplained fever, poor growth and development, irritability, and feeding problems. The family history may reveal VUR or urinary tract infections.

EVALUATION AND TREATMENT. Prompt treatment of UTIs in children with reflux is important to minimize the risk of renal scar development. Some infants may have renal scarring at birth from intrauterine damage caused by reflux. In addition to the history of recurrent UTIs and other symptoms, imaging may be required for diagnosis and assessment of structural change, scarring, urinary tract function, and risk for future infection and renal damage. Most children with vesicoureteral reflux respond to nonoperative management aimed at prevention and treatment of infection. Spontaneous remission of grades I and II reflux may occur in more than 80% of children. Resolution of grades III and IV reflux occurs in 46% and 30%, respectively, over 5 years.[90] The use of prophylactic antibiotics for these children is controversial with concerns regarding efficacy and the development of antibiotic resistance.[91] Recurrent infection or high-grade reflux are possible indications for surgical intervention or endoscopic injection of biomaterials into the bladder wall below the ureteral orifice. Surgical repair of reflux has been shown to decrease the incidence of pyelonephritis but does not decrease the risk of the development or progression of renal damage.[92] The value of screening asymptomatic siblings of children with vesicoureteral reflux is debatable. One current recommendation is to perform a renal ultrasound and consider a VCUG only in children with scarring or otherwise abnormal appearing kidneys.[84]

Urinary Incontinence

Urinary incontinence refers to the involuntary passage of urine by a child who is beyond the age when voluntary bladder control should have been acquired. Nighttime wetting is called **enuresis.** Bladder control is accomplished by most children before the age of 5 years, although this is largely influenced by cultural beliefs and parental toilet training practices. **Functional incontinence** is urinary incontinence in which no structural or neurologic abnormality can be identified. The underlying mechanism may include disorders of both the storage and voiding phases of the bladder cycle. A child may have daytime incontinence or enuresis, or both.

The incidence of incontinence is difficult to determine because it is not a problem that parents readily share with others and because definitions vary according to cultural norms and family practices. The incidence of enuresis in children older than 5 years ranges from 15% to 20%. Boys are more enuretic than girls by a ratio of 2:1. Less than 2% of adults experience enuresis. Daytime incontinence occurs in up to 9% of early school age children.[93]

PATHOGENESIS. Multiple factors are likely responsible for incontinence. All or part of each one might be operating in a given child. A reasonable approach is to eliminate organic, behavioral, or physiologic causes before exploring the psychologic ones.

Organic causes of incontinence account for 2% to 10% of cases. The causes include urinary tract infections; neurologic disturbances; congenital defects of the meatus, urethra, and bladder neck; allergies; constipation;[94] obesity;[95] or alteration in renal tubular ion and water transport related to prostaglandin secretion. Disorders that increase the normal output of urine, such as diabetes mellitus and diabetes insipidus, or disorders that impair the concentrating ability of the kidney must be considered in the evaluation of enuresis.[96] Enuresis in children may be associated with a maturational lag. Studies have demonstrated that some children with enuresis have smaller functional bladder capacities than nonenuretic children.[97] Children who do not have the normal nocturnal elevation of vasopressin produce a higher volume of urine with a lower osmolality than controls.[98] A number of children experience bladder overactivity with elevated intravesical pressure and spikelike detrusor contractions during bladder filling. Incontinence often spontaneously disappears in children as they get older.

Genetic factors as a cause of enuresis are being investigated. Linkages have been proposed between nocturnal enuresis and chromosomes 8, 12, 13, and 22.[99] Bed-wetting occurs with high frequency among parents, siblings, and other near relatives of symptomatic children. These observations are further supported by a high concordance rate in enuretic monozygotic twins.

Multiple studies have examined the role of sleep architecture on enuresis. Findings have ranged from elevated arousal thresholds[100] to increased light sleep with frequent cortical arousal without complete awakening.[101] Enuresis may be associated with obstructive sleep apnea. Inspiratory effort against a closed airway increases intrathoracic negative pressure, causing cardiac distention and release of atrial natriuretic hormone and decreased levels of vasopressin and renin-angiotensin-aldosterone complex.[102]

A variety of psychosocial factors also have been postulated as explanations of enuresis. Enuresis has been associated with attention-deficit/hyperactivity disorders, anxiety disorders, depression, and opposition defiant disorders.[103,104]

CLINICAL MANIFESTATIONS. **Primary incontinence** refers to a condition in which the child has never been continent. **Secondary incontinence** occurs when a child who has experienced a period of dryness of at least 6 months after toilet training becomes incontinent again. Secondary enuresis may be diurnal, nocturnal, or a combination of both. (Types of incontinence are defined in Table 39-6.)

TABLE 39-6 CLASSIFICATION OF INCONTINENCE

TYPES OF INCONTINENCE	DEFINITION
Daytime voiding frequency	Decreased: 3 or fewer voids per day Increased: 8 or more voids per day
Dysfunctional voiding	Habitual contraction of the urethral sphincter during voiding; observed by uroflow
Enuresis	Intermittent incontinence of urine while sleeping
Incontinence, intermittent	Leakage of urine in discrete episodes during the day and/or night
Incontinence, stress	Leakage of small amounts of urine with exertion or raised intra-abdominal pressure
Urgency	Sudden, unexpected, immediate need to void
Overactive bladder	Child has urgency with or without frequency or incontinence
Underactive bladder	Decreased voiding frequency with use of raised intra-abdominal pressure to void

Data from Nevéus T et al: *J Urol* 176(1):312–324, 2006.

EVALUATION AND TREATMENT. Evaluation of incontinence includes use of questionnaires, drinking and voiding charts, physical examination, and urinalysis. Underlying pathology, including kidney disease, vesicoureteral reflux, urinary tract infection, or neurogenic bladder, is excluded. Radiologic and urodynamic evaluation may be required.[105,106]

Therapeutic management of incontinence or enuresis begins with education. If the child and family understand the probable etiology of the child's condition, they are better able to choose and participate in therapies that are most likely to succeed. Treatment of daytime incontinence includes behavioral therapy, including timed voiding; fluid management; treatment of constipation, urinary tract infections, and other coexisting conditions if present; and medication (anticholinergic, alpha-blocker).[107,108] Enuresis treatment also may include enuresis alarms or other medications (desmopressin acetate tablets).[109,110]

SUMMARY REVIEW

Structure and Function of the Urinary System in Children

1. The Wilms tumor 1 gene and *WNT* signaling are important for kidney development, growth, and differentiation.
2. The kidney develops from three sets of structures: the pronephros (nonfunctional by the end of the embryonic period), mesonephros (nonfunctional), and metanephros (the functional kidney).
3. All nephrons are present at birth. The number does not increase with maturation, but they do increase in weight and function.
4. Urine formation begins by the third gestational month and contributes to the amniotic fluid.
5. Infants have a narrow chemical safety margin because of high hydrogen ion concentration, limited ability to regulate the internal environment, and lowered osmotic pressure.
6. Any disturbance, such as diarrhea, infection, fasting, or feeding alterations, can lead rapidly to severe acidosis and fluid imbalance in infants.
7. The composition of body fluids differs with age, thus making children more vulnerable to pathophysiologic changes.
8. Because the kidney develops from the medulla to the cortex, blood flow to the medullary nephrons is limited in infancy, and infants thus have limited urine-concentrating capacity.

SUMMARY REVIEW—cont'd

Alterations in Renal and Bladder Function in Children

1. Congenital renal disorders affect about 1 out of 500 newborns. These disorders range in severity from minor, easily correctable anomalies to those incompatible with life.
2. Horseshoe kidney is a single U-shaped kidney that develops from fusion of the kidneys as they descend from the midline. The kidney may be asymptomatic or associated with hydronephrosis, stone formation, or infection.
3. Hypospadias is a congenital condition in which the urethral meatus is located on the undersurface of the penis; epispadias is a congenital condition in which the urethral opening is located on the dorsal surface of the penis.
4. Exstrophy of the bladder is a congenital malformation in which the pubic bones are separated, the lower portion of the abdominal wall and anterior wall of the bladder are missing, and the back wall of the bladder is everted through the opening.
5. Ureteropelvic junction obstruction is blockage where the renal pelvis joins the ureter and is often caused by smooth muscle or urothelial malformation or scarring that leads to hydronephrosis.
6. Bladder outlet obstruction is usually caused by urethral valves or polyps.
7. A dysplastic kidney is the result of abnormal differentiation of renal tissues. The hypoplastic kidney is a very small but otherwise normal kidney.
8. Renal agenesis is the failure of a kidney to grow or develop. The condition may be unilateral or bilateral and may occur as an isolated entity or in association with other disorders.
9. Polycystic kidney disease is an autosomal dominant or recessive disorder in which the renal tubule or epithelium proliferates; excessive fluid transport causes cyst formation and obstruction.
10. Glomerulonephritis is an inflammation of the glomeruli secondary to immune mechanisms characterized by hematuria, edema, and hypertension. Poststreptococcal glomerulonephritis may occur after infection, especially of the upper respiratory tract.
11. IgA nephropathies result from deposition of IgA immunoglobulins and other immune products in the mesangium of the glomerular capillaries. It is the most common type of childhood glomerulonephritis.
12. Henoch-Schönlein nephritis is an IgA nephropathy that affects glomerular blood vessels.
13. Hemolytic uremic syndrome is an acute disorder characterized by hemolytic anemia, acute renal failure, and thrombocytopenia and can be associated with *E. coli* verotoxin.
14. Nephrotic syndrome is a term used to describe a symptom complex characterized by proteinuria, hypoalbuminemia, hyperlipidemia, and edema. Metabolic, biochemical, or physiochemical disturbance in the glomerular basement membrane leads to increased permeability to protein. The most common form is minimal change nephropathy.
15. Acute or chronic renal injury is rare in children and the most common cause is prerenal acute renal failure related to dehydration, sepsis, or hemorrhage.
16. Wilms tumor is an embryonal tumor of the kidney that usually presents between birth and 5 years of age as an inherited (5% to 10%) or sporadic form. The tumor can be successfully treated by surgery, with a combination of drugs, and, sometimes, with radiation therapy.
17. Urinary tract infections can result from general sepsis in the newborn but are usually caused by bacteria ascending the urethra in older children. The bladder alone is infected in cystitis. The infection ascends to the kidney or kidneys in pyelonephritis. Urinary tract anomalies may need surgical correction to prevent frequent recurrent infections.
18. Vesicoureteral reflux, which refers to the retrograde flow of bladder urine into the kidney and/or ureters, provides mechanisms for bladder infection in children whose ureters are shorter than those of adults. It can be unilateral or bilateral.
19. Urinary incontinence refers to the involuntary passage of urine beyond the age when normal continence should have occurred. This may occur during the day (incontinence) or night (enuresis). These disorders can have a variety of organic and psychologic causes.

KEY TERMS

REFERENCES

1. Fanni D et al: Expression of WT1 during normal human kidney development, *J Matern Fetal Neonatal Med* 24(Suppl 2):44–47, 2011.
2. Hendry C et al: Defining and redefining the nephron progenitor population, *Pediatr Nephrol* 26(9):1395–1406, 2011.
3. Bonilla-Felix M: Development of water transport in the collecting duct, *Am J Physiol Renal Physiol* 287(6):F1093–F1101, 2004.
4. Quigley R: Developmental changes in renal function, *Curr Opin Pediatr* 24(12):184–190, 2012.
5. Song R, Yosypiv IV: Genetics of congenital anomalies of the kidney and urinary tract, *Pediatr Nephrol* 26(3):353–364, 2011.
6. Harris J, Robert E, Källén B: Epidemiologic characteristics of kidney malformations, *Eur J Epidemiol* 16(11):985–992, 2000.
7. Allen RC: *Horseshoe kidney*. Available at www.medscape.com/article/441510-overview. Retrieved May 23, 2013.
8. Casas KA, Kamil ES, Rimoin DL: Congenital disorders of the urinary tract. In Rimon KD et al: *Principles and practice of medical genetics*, ed 5, vol 2, Philadelphia, 2007, Churchill Livingstone, Elsevier.
9. Blaschko SD, Cunha GR, Baskin LS: Molecular mechanisms of external genitalia development, *Differentiation* 84(3):261–268, 2012.
10. Montag S, Palmer LS: Abnormalities of penile curvature: chordee and penile torsion, *ScientificWorldJournal* 11:1470–1478, 2011.
11. Macedo A Jr et al: Long-term results with a one-stage complex primary hypospadias repair strategy (the three-in-one technique), *J Pediatr Urol* 7(3):299–304, 2011.
12. Chalmers D, Ferrer F: Continent urinary diversion in the epispadias-exstrophy complex, *Semin Pediatr Surg* 20(2):102–108, 2011.
13. Siffel C et al: Bladder exstrophy: an epidemiologic study from the International Clearinghouse for Birth Defects Surveillance and Research, and an overview of the literature, *Am J Med Genet C* 157(4):321–332, 2011.
14. Wild AT et al: The role of osteotomy in surgical repair of bladder exstrophy, *Semin Pediatr Surg* 20(2):71–78, 2011.
15. Purves JT: Modern approaches in primary exstrophy closure, *Semin Pediatr Surg* 20(2):79–84, 2011.
16. Alberti C: Congenital ureteropelvic junction obstruction: physiopathology, decoupling of tout court pelvic dilatation-obstruction semantic connection, biomarkers to predict renal damage evolution, *Eur Rev Med Pharmacol* 16(2):213–219, 2012.
17. Rosen S et al: The kidney in congenital ureteropelvic junction obstruction: a spectrum from normal to nephrectomy, *J Urol* 179(4):1257–1263, 2008.
18. Hashim H, Woodhouse C: Ureteropelvic junction obstruction, *Eur Urol Suppl* 11(2):25–32, 2012.
19. Heinlen JE et al: Operative versus nonoperative management of ureteropelvic junction obstruction in children, *Urology* 73(3):521–525, 2009.
20. Hodges SJ et al: Megaureter, *ScientificWorldJournal* 10:603–612, 2012.
21. Krishnan A et al: The anatomy and embryology of posterior urethral valves, *J Urol* 175(4):1214–1220, 2006.
22. Eziyi AK et al: Management of male urethral polyps in children: experience with four cases, *Afr J Paediatr Surg* 6(1):49–51, 2011.
23. Morris RK, Kilby MD: Long-term renal and neurodevelopmental outcome in infants with LUTO, with and without fetal intervention, *Early Hum Dev* 87(9):607–610, 2011.
24. Woolf AS: Renal hypoplasia and dysplasia: starting to put the puzzle together, *J Am Soc Nephrol* 17(10):2647–2649, 2006.
25. Babin J et al: The Ask-Upmark kidney: a curable cause of hypertension in young patients, *J Hum Hypertens* 19(4):315–316, 2005.
26. Dursan H et al: Associated anomalies in children with congenital solitary functioning kidney, *Pediatr Surg Int* 21(6):456–459, 2005.
27. Van Vuuren SH et al: Compensatory enlargement of a solitary functioning kidney during fetal development, *Ultrasound Obstet Gynecol* 40(6):665–668, 2012.
28. Calisti A et al: The risk of associated urological abnormalities in children with pre- and postnatal occasional diagnosis of solitary, small or ectopic kidney: is a complete urological screening always necessary? *World J Urol* 26(3):281–284, 2008.
29. Stojanovic J et al: Prevalence and 1 year outcome of severe congenital renal anomalies, *Arch Dis Child-Fetal* 96(Suppl 1):Fa18–Fa19, 2011.
30. Taklar V, Caplan MJ: Polycystic kidney disease: pathogenesis and potential therapies, *BBA-Mol Basis Dis* 1812(10):1337–1343, 2011.
31. Grantham JJ, Mulamalla S, Swenson-Fields KI: Why kidneys fail in autosomal dominant polycystic kidney disease, *Nat Rev Nephrol* 7(10):556–566, 2011.
32. Steinman TI: Polycystic kidney disease: a 2011 update, *Curr Opin Nephrol Hypertens* 21(2):189–194, 2012.
33. Kambham N: Postinfectious glomerulonephritis, *Adv Anat Pathol* 19(5):338–347, 2012.
34. Ahn S, Ingulli E: Acute poststreptococcal glomerulonephritis: an update, *Curr Opin Pediatr* 20(2):157–162, 2008.
35. Kamath N, Rao S: Henoch-Schonlein purpura: an update, *Indian J Rheum* 7(Suppl 1):92–98, 2012.
36. Coppo R, Amore A: Henoch-Schoenlein purpura. In Avner E et al: *Pediatric nephrology*, ed 6, Berlin Heidelberg, 2009, Springer.
37. Ninchoji T et al: Treatment strategies for Henoch-Schönlein purpura nephritis by histological and clinical severity, *Pediatr Nephrol* 26(4): 563–569, 2011.
38. Kemper MJ: Outbreak of hemolytic uremic syndrome caused by *E. coli* O104:H4 in Germany: a pediatric perspective, *Pediatr Nephrol* 27(2):161–164, 2012.
39. Scheiring J, Rosales A, Zimmerhackl LB: Today's understanding of the haemolytic uraemic syndrome, *Eur J Pediatr* 169(1):7–13, 2010.
40. Petruzziello-Pellegrini TN, Marsden PA: Shiga toxin-associated hemolytic uremic syndrome: advances in pathogenesis and therapeutics, *Curr Opin Nephrol Hypertens* 21(4):433–440, 2012.
41. Bitzan M, Schaefer F, Reymond D: Treatment of typical (enteropathic) hemolytic uremic syndrome, *Semin Thromb Hemost* 36(6):594–610, 2010.
42. Scheiring J, Andreoli SP, Zimmerhackl LB: Treatment and outcome of Shiga-toxin-associated hemolytic uremic syndrome (HUS), *Pediatr Nephrol* 23(10):1749–1760, 2008.
43. Spencer JD et al: Has the incidence of childhood steroid sensitive nephrotic syndrome changed? *Clin Nephrol* 78(2):112–115, 2012.
44. Gordillo R, Spitzer A: The nephrotic syndrome, *Pediatr Rev* 30(3): 94–104, 2009.
45. Lane JC, Kaskel FJ: Pediatric nephrotic syndrome: from the simple to the complex, *Semin Nephrol* 29(4):389–398, 2009.
46. Lacquaniti A et al: Alterations of lipid metabolism in chronic nephropathies: mechanisms, diagnosis and treatment, *Kidney Blood Press Res* 33(2):100–110, 2010.
47. Woo K et al: Global evolutionary trend of the prevalence of primary glomerulonephritis over the past three decades, *Nephron Clin Pract* 116(4):c337–c346, 2010.
48. D'Agati VD et al: Focal segmental glomerulosclerosis, *N Engl J Med* 365(25):2398–2411, 2011.
49. Siddall EJ, Radhakrishnan J: The pathophysiology of edema formation in the nephrotic syndrome, *Kidney Int* 82(6):635–642, 2012.
50. Kerlin BA, Ayoob R, Smoyer WE: Epidemiology and pathophysiology of nephrotic syndrome-associated thromboembolic disease, *Clin J Am Soc Nephrol* 7(3):513–520, 2012.
51. Simons M, Huber TB: It's not all about nephrin, *Kidney Int* 73(6): 697–704, 2008.
52. Jalanko H: Congenital nephrotic syndrome, *Pediatr Nephrol* 24(11):2121–2128, 2009.
53. Gipson DS et al: Management of childhood onset nephrotic syndrome, *Pediatrics* 124(2):747–757, 2009.
54. Greenbaum LA, Benndorf R, Smoyer WE: Childhood nephrotic syndrome—current and future therapies, *Nat Rev Nephrol* 8(8): 445–458, 2012.
55. Van Husen M, Kemper MJ: New therapies in steroid-sensitive and steroid-resistant idiopathic nephrotic syndrome, *Pediatr Nephrol* 26(6):881–892, 2011.
56. Crosson JT: Focal segmental glomerulosclerosis and renal transplantation, *Transplant Proc* 39(3):737–743, 2007.
57. Akcan-Arikan A et al: Modified RIFLE criteria in critically ill children with acute kidney injury, *Kidney Int* 71(10):1028–1035, 2007.
58. Andreoli SP: Acute kidney injury in children, *Pediatr Nephrol* 24(2):253–263, 2009.
59. Harambat J et al: Epidemiology of chronic kidney disease in children, *Pediatr Nephrol* 27(3):363–373, 2012.
60. Mong Hiep TT et al: Clinical characteristics and outcomes of children with stage 3-5 chronic kidney disease, *Pediatr Nephrol* 25(5):935–940, 2010.
61. LaRosa C, Jorge Baluarte H, Meyers K: Outcomes in pediatric solid-organ transplantation, *Pediatr Transplant* 15(2):1228–1241, 2011.
62. Neu AM, Frankenfield DL: Clinical outcomes in pediatric hemodialysis patients in the USA: lessons from CMS' ESRD CPM Project, *Pediatr Nephrol* 24(7):1287–1295, 2009.
63. Fine R: Etiology and treatment of growth retardation in children with chronic kidney disease and end-stage renal disease: a historical perspective, *Pediatr Nephrol* 25(4):725–732, 2010.
64. Davidoff AM: Wilms tumor, *Adv Pediatr* 59(1):247–267, 2012.

65. Axt J et al: Race disparities in Wilms tumor incidence and biology, *J Surg Res* 170(1):112–119, 2011.
66. Knudson AG Jr, Strong LC: Mutation and cancer: a model for Wilms' tumor of the kidney, *J Natl Cancer Inst* 48(2):313–324, 1972.
67. Md Zin R, Murch A, Charles A: Pathology, genetics and cytogenetics of Wilm's tumour, *Pathology* 43(4):302–312, 2011.
68. Aune GJ: Wilms tumor, *Pediatr Rev* 29(4):142–143, 2008.
69. Md Zin R, Murch A, Charles A: Cytogenetic findings in Wilms' tumour: a single institute study, *Pathology* 42(7):643–649, 2010.
70. Varan A: Wilms' tumor in children: an overview, *Nephron Clin Pract* 108(2):c83–c90, 2008.
71. Ko EY, Ritchey ML: Current management of Wilms' tumor in children, *J Pediatr Urol* 5(1):56–65, 2009.
72. Ganesh S, Vennila JJ, Scholz H: An overview and perspectives of Wilm's tumor, *Int J Cancer Res* 7(1):1–7, 2011.
73. Kaste SC et al: Wilms tumour: prognostic factors, staging, therapy and late effects, *Pediatr Radiol* 38(1):2–17, 2008.
74. Green DM: The evolution of treatment for Wilms tumor, *J Pediatr Surg* 48(1):14–19, 2013.
75. Bhat RG, Katy TA, Place FC: Pediatric urinary tract infections, *Emerg Med Clin North Am* 29(3):637–653, 2011.
76. Sadeh SA, Mattoo TK: Managing urinary tract infections, *Pediatr Nephrol* 26(11):1967–1976, 2011.
77. Brandström P et al: The Swedish Reflux Trial in Children: III. Urinary tract infection pattern, *J Urol* 184(1):286–291, 2010.
78. Khunda A, Elneil S: Recurrent urinary tract infections associated with gynecological disorders, *Curr Bladder Dysfunct Rep* 7(2):131–140, 2012.
79. Michael M et al: Short versus standard duration oral antibiotic therapy for acute urinary tract infection in children, *Cochrane Database Syst Rev* (1):CD003966, 2003.
80. Newman TB: The new American Academy of Pediatrics urinary tract infection guideline, *Pediatrics* 128(3):572–575, 2011.
81. Wan J et al: Section on urology response to new guidelines for the diagnosis and management of UTI, *Pediatrics* 129(4):e1051–e1053, 2012.
82. Park KH et al: The clinical usefulness of a repeat urine culture 48 hours after microbial treatment in anatomically normal and abnormal urinary tract infection, *J Korean Soc Pediatr Nephrol* 13(1):49–55, 2009.
83. Yang SS et al: Advances in non-surgical treatments for urinary tract infections in children, *World J Urol* 30(1):69–75, 2012.
84. Skoog SJ et al: Pediatric Vesicoureteral Reflux Guidelines Panel summary report: clinical practice guidelines for screening siblings of children with vesicoureteral reflux and neonates/infants with prenatal hydronephrosis, *J Urol* 184(3):1145–1151, 2010.
85. Blumenthal I: Vesicoureteric reflux and urinary tract infection in children, *Postgrad Med J* 82(963):31–35, 2006.
86. Sung J, Skoog S: Surgical management of vesicoureteral reflux in children, *Pediatr Nephrol* 27(4):551–561, 2012.
87. Sjöström S et al: Change in urodynamic patterns in infants with dilating vesicoureteral reflux: 3-year follow-up, *J Urol* 182(5):2446–2454, 2009.
88. Peters C, Rushton HG: Vesicoureteral reflux associated renal damage: congenital reflux nephropathy and acquired renal scarring, *J Urol* 184(1):265–273, 2010.
89. Tramma D et al: Interleukin-6 and interleukin-8 levels in the urine of children with renal scarring, *Pediatr Nephrol* 27(9):1525–1530, 2012.
90. Coleman R: Early management and long-term outcomes in primary vesico-ureteric reflux, *BJUI* 108(Suppl 2):3–8, 2011.
91. Peters CA et al: Summary of the AUA Guideline on Management of Primary Vesicoureteral Reflux in Children, *J Urol* 184(3):1134–1144, 2010.
92. Fonseca FF, Tanno FY, Nguyen HT: Current options in the management of primary vesicoureteral reflux in children, *Pediatr Clin North Am* 59(4):819–834, 2012.
93. Buckley BS, Lapitan MC: Prevalence of urinary incontinence in men, women, and children—current evidence: findings of the Fourth International Consultation on Incontinence, *Urology* 76(2):265–271, 2010.
94. Nurko S, Scott SM: Coexistence of constipation and incontinence in children and adults, *Best Pract Res Clin Gastroenterol* 25(1):29–41, 2011.
95. Guven A, Giramonti K, Kogan BA: The effect of obesity on treatment efficacy in children with nocturnal enuresis and voiding dysfuntion, *J Urol* 178(4):1458–1462, 2007.
96. Nevéus T: Nocturnal enuresis—theoretic background and practical guidelines, *Pediatr Nephrol* 26(8):1207–1214, 2011.
97. Kim J: Diagnostic value of functional bladder capacity, urine osmolality, and daytime storage symptoms for severity of nocturnal enuresis, *Korean J Urol* 53(2):114–119, 2012.
98. Chang J et al: Clinical characteristics, nocturnal antidiuretic hormone levels, and responsiveness to DDAVP of school children with primary nocturnal enuresis, *World J Urol* 30(4):567–571, 2012.
99. von Gontard A et al: Molecular genetics of nocturnal enuresis: linkage to a locus on chromosome 22, *Scand J Urol Nephrol Suppl* 202:76–80, 1999.
100. Gozmen S, Keskin S, Akil I: Enuresis nocturna and sleep quality, *Pediatr Nephrol* 23(2):1293–1296, 2008.
101. Yeung CD, Diao M, Sreedhar B: Cortical arousal in children with severe enuresis, *N Engl J Med* 358(22):2414–2515, 2008.
102. Su MS et al: Nocturnal enuresis in children: prevalence, correlates, and relationship with obstructive sleep apnea, *J Pediatr* 159(2):238–242, 2011.
103. von Gontard A: Does psychological stress affect LUT function in children? ICI-RS 2011, *Neurourol Urodynam* 31(3):344–348, 2012.
104. Yang T et al: Correlation between symptoms of voiding dysfunction and attention deficit disorder with hyperactivity in children with lower urinary tract symptoms, *J Urol* 187(2):656–663, 2012.
105. Franco I: Functional bladder problems in children: pathophysiology, diagnosis, and treatment, *Pediatr Clinic North Am* 59(4):783–817, 2012.
106. Deshpande AV et al: Management of daytime urinary incontinence and lower urinary tract symptoms in children, *J Paediatr Child Health* 48(2):e44–e52, 2012.
107. Thom M et al: Management of lower urinary tract dysfunction: a stepwise approach, *J Pediatr Urol* 8(1):20–24, 2012.
108. Vande Walle J et al: Practical consensus guidelines for the management of enuresis, *Eur J Pediatr* 171(6):971–983, 2012.
109. Alloussi SH et al: Desmopressin treatment regimens in monosymptomatic and nonmonosymptomatic enuresis: a review from a clinical perspective, *J Pediatr Urol* 7(1):10–20, 2011.
110. Brown ML, Pope AW, Brown EJ: Treatment of primary nocturnal enuresis in children: a review, *Child Care Hlth Dev* 37(2):153–160, 2011.

CHAPTER

40

Structure and Function of the Digestive System

Alexa K. Doig and Sue E. Huether

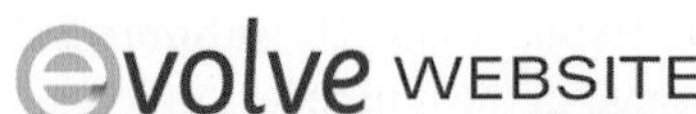

http://evolve.elsevier.com/McCance/

- Review Questions and Answers
- Animations

CHAPTER OUTLINE

The digestive system breaks down ingested food, prepares it for uptake by the body's cells, provides body water, and eliminates wastes. This system consists of the gastrointestinal tract and accessory organs of digestion: the liver, gallbladder, and exocrine pancreas.

Food breakdown begins in the mouth with chewing and continues in the stomach, where food is churned and mixed with acid, mucus, enzymes, and other secretions. From the stomach, the fluid and partially digested food pass into the small intestine, where biochemicals and enzymes secreted by the liver, exocrine pancreas, and small intestinal epithelium break it down into absorbable components of proteins, carbohydrates, and fats. These nutrients pass through the small intestinal epithelium into underlying blood vessels and lymphatics that carry them to the liver via the hepatic portal circulation for further processing and storage.

Ingested substances and secretions that are not absorbed in the small intestine pass into the large intestine, where fluid continues to be absorbed. Solid wastes pass into the rectum and are eliminated from the body through the anus.

Except for chewing, swallowing, and defecation of solid wastes, the activities of the digestive system are controlled by hormones and the autonomic nervous system. As ingested substances move through the gastrointestinal tract, they trigger the release of hormones that stimulate or inhibit (1) the muscular contractions (gastrointestinal motility) that mix and propel food from the esophagus to the anus, and (2) the timely secretion of substances that aid in digestion. The autonomic innervation, sympathetic and parasympathetic, is controlled by centers in the brain and by local stimuli that are mediated by neural plexuses within the gastrointestinal walls.

THE GASTROINTESTINAL TRACT

The **gastrointestinal tract (alimentary canal)** consists of the mouth, esophagus, stomach, small intestine, large intestine,

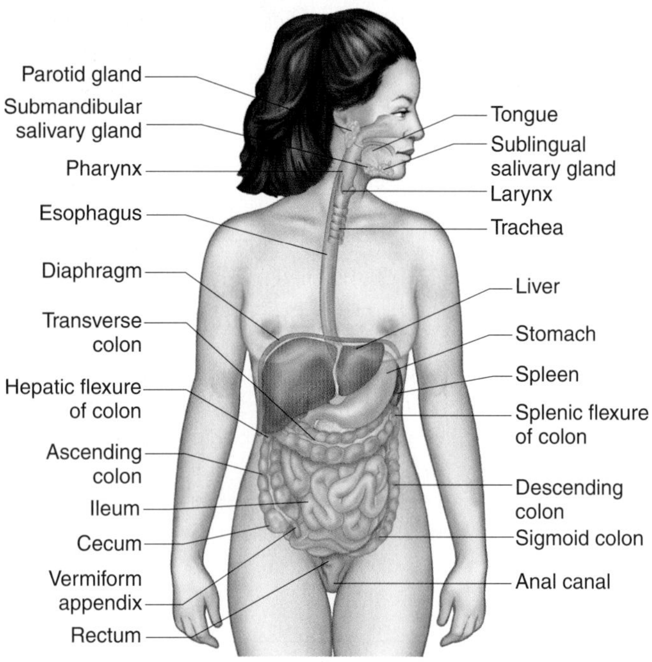

FIGURE 40-1 Structures of the Digestive System.

rectum, and anus (Figure 40-1). It carries out the following digestive processes:

1. Ingestion of food
2. Propulsion of food and wastes from the mouth to the anus
3. Secretion of mucus, water, and enzymes
4. Mechanical digestion of food particles
5. Chemical digestion of food particles
6. Absorption of digested food
7. Elimination of waste products by defecation

Histologically, the gastrointestinal tract consists of four layers. From the inside out, they are the mucosa, submucosa, muscularis, and serosa or adventitia (esophagus only). These concentric layers vary in thickness, and each layer has sublayers (Figure 40-2). Neurons forming the **enteric nervous system** are located solely within the gastrointestinal tract and are controlled by local and autonomic nervous system stimuli. The enteric nervous system comprises three nerve plexuses located in different layers of the gastrointestinal walls. The **submucosal plexus (Meissner plexus)** is located in the muscularis mucosae, the **myenteric plexus (Auerbach plexus)** between the inner circular and outer longitudinal muscle layers in the muscularis, and the **subserosal plexus** just beneath the serosa. The enteric (intramural) plexus neurons regulate motility reflexes, blood flow, absorption, secretions, and immune response.[1]

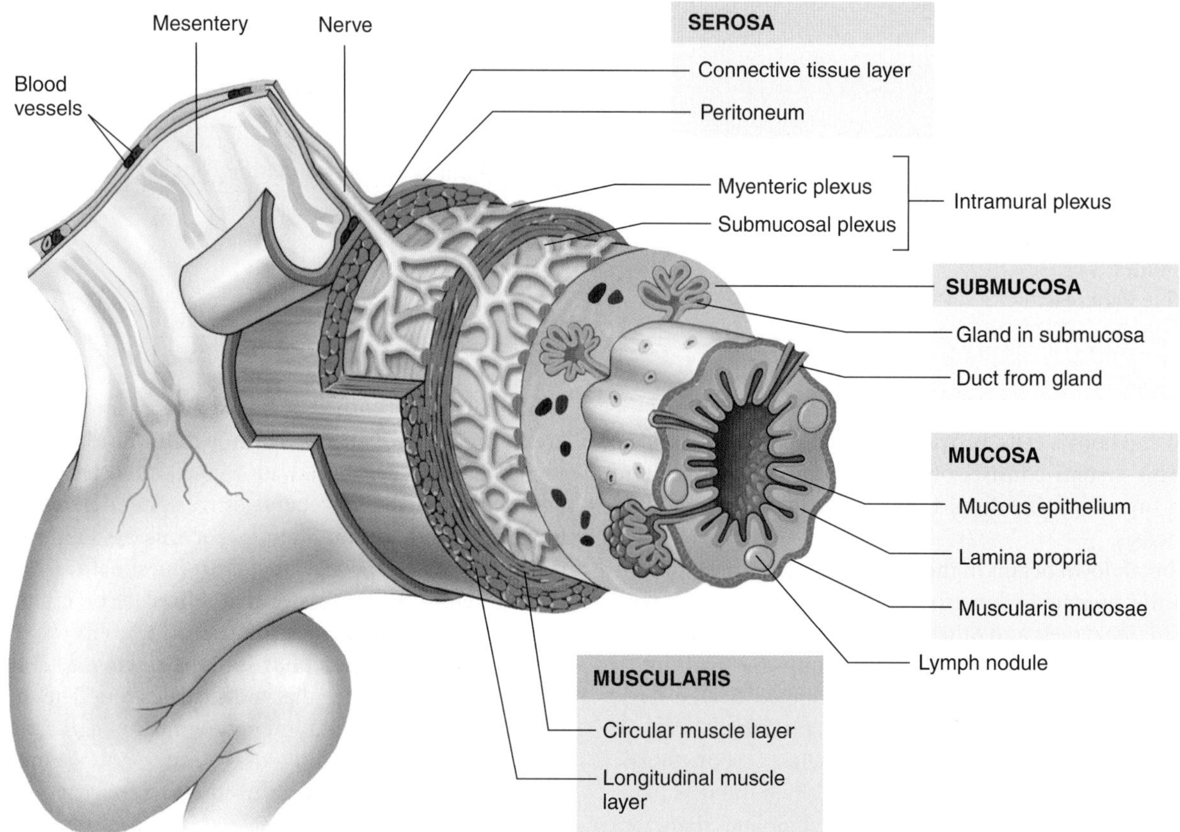

FIGURE 40-2 Wall of the Gastrointestinal (GI) Tract. The wall of the GI tract is made up of four layers with a network of nerves between the layers. Shown here is a generalized diagram of a segment of the GI tract. Note that the serosa is continuous with a fold of serous membrane called a *mesentery.* Note also that digestive glands may empty their products into the lumen of the GI tract by way of ducts. (From Patton KT, Thibodeau GA: *Anatomy & physiology,* ed 8, St Louis, 2013, Mosby.)

Mouth and Esophagus

The **mouth** is a reservoir for the chewing and mixing of food with saliva. As food particles become smaller and move around in the mouth, the taste buds and olfactory nerves are continuously stimulated, adding to the satisfaction of eating. The tongue's surface and soft palate contains thousands of chemoreceptors, or taste buds, that can distinguish salty, sour, bitter, umami, and sweet tastes. Tastes and food odors help initiate salivation and the secretion of gastric juice in the stomach. There are 32 permanent teeth in the adult mouth, and they are important for speech and mastication.

Salivation

The three pairs of **salivary glands** (the submandibular, sublingual, and parotid glands) (Figure 40-3) secrete about 1 L of saliva per day. **Saliva** consists mostly of water that contains varying amounts of mucus, sodium, bicarbonate, chloride, potassium, and **salivary α-amylase (ptyalin),** an enzyme that initiates carbohydrate digestion in the mouth and stomach.

The sympathetic and parasympathetic divisions of the autonomic nervous system control salivation. Because cholinergic parasympathetic fibers stimulate the salivary glands, atropine (an anticholinergic agent) inhibits salivation and makes the mouth dry. β-Adrenergic stimulation from sympathetic fibers also increases salivary secretion. The salivary glands are not regulated by hormones, although hormones are found in saliva.[1a]

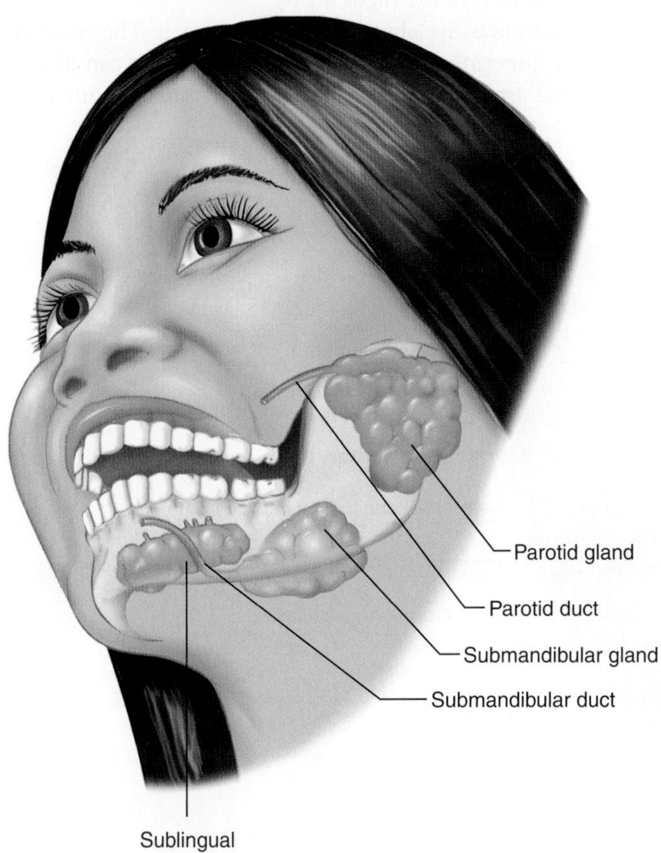

FIGURE 40-3 Salivary Glands. (From Patton KT, Thibodeau GA: *Anatomy & physiology*, ed 8, St Louis, 2013, Mosby.)

The composition of saliva depends on the rate of secretion. Aldosterone can decrease the rate of secretion by increasing an exchange of sodium for potassium. Sodium and water are conserved and potassium is excreted. The bicarbonate concentration of saliva sustains a pH of about 7.4, which neutralizes bacterial acids and prevents tooth decay. Saliva also contains immunoglobulin A (IgA), which helps prevent infection. Exogenous fluoride (e.g., fluoride in drinking water) is absorbed and then secreted in the saliva, providing additional protection against tooth decay.

Swallowing

The **esophagus** is a hollow muscular tube approximately 25 cm long that conducts substances from the oropharynx to the stomach (see Figure 40-1). The pharynx and upper third of the esophagus contain striated muscle that is directly innervated by skeletal motor neurons that control swallowing. The middle third contains a mix of striated and smooth muscle, and the lower third is smooth muscle that is innervated by preganglionic cholinergic fibers from the vagus nerve. Peristalsis is stimulated when afferent fibers distributed along the length of the esophagus sense changes in wall tension caused by stretching as food passes. The greater the tension, the greater the intensity of esophageal contraction. Occasionally, intense contractions cause pain similar to "heartburn" or angina.

Each end of the esophagus is opened and closed by a sphincter. The **upper esophageal sphincter (cricopharyngeal muscle)** prevents entry of air into the esophagus during respiration.[2] The **lower esophageal sphincter (cardiac sphincter)** prevents regurgitation from the stomach. The lower esophageal sphincter is located near the esophageal hiatus—the opening in the diaphragm where the esophagus ends at the stomach.[3]

Swallowing is a complex event mediated by the trigeminal nucleus, nucleus tractus solitarius, and reticular formation of the brainstem and also involves other brain regions, including the insula/claustrum and cerebellum.[4]

Swallowing occurs in two phases: the oropharyngeal (voluntary) phase and the esophageal (involuntary) phase. During the **oral** and **pharyngeal phases of swallowing,** food is segmented into a bolus by the tongue and forced posteriorly toward the pharynx as the tongue pushes upward against the hard palate. The superior constrictor muscle of the pharynx contracts, preventing movement of food into the nasopharynx. At the same time, respiration is inhibited and the epiglottis folds downward to prevent the bolus from entering the larynx and trachea. The movements of the tongue and pharyngeal constrictors propel the food into the esophagus in a series of coordinated events, taking less than 1 or 2 seconds.

During the **esophageal phase of swallowing,** the bolus is transported to the stomach by the coordinated sequential contraction and relaxation of outer longitudinal and inner circular layers of smooth muscle. The wave of relaxation reduces resistance and allows food to pass, after which the wave of contraction pushes food farther along. The terminal 1 to 2 cm portion of the musculature forms the lower esophageal sphincter, which relaxes just before the arrival of a peristaltic wave. The sphincter muscles return to their resting tone after the bolus of food passes into the stomach. The esophageal phase of swallowing takes 5 to 10 seconds, with the bolus moving 2 to 6 cm/second. Throughout swallowing, the sphincters and esophagus work in concert with the peristaltic wave that moves food from the mouth to the stomach.

Peristalsis that immediately follows the oropharyngeal phase of swallowing is called **primary peristalsis.** If a bolus of food becomes stuck in the esophageal lumen, the distention of the esophageal wall stimulates **secondary peristalsis,** a wave of contraction and relaxation that is independent of voluntary swallowing. This is in response to stretch receptors that are stimulated by increased wall tension, causing an increase in impulses from the swallowing center of the brain.

When it is closed, the lower esophageal sphincter serves as a barrier between the stomach and esophagus. Cholinergic vagal stimulation and the digestive hormone gastrin increase sphincter tone. Nonadrenergic, noncholinergic vagal impulses relax the lower esophageal sphincter, as do the hormones progesterone, secretin, and glucagon. Relaxation during swallowing is mediated by the vagus nerve.[5]

Stomach

The **stomach** is a hollow muscular organ that stores food during eating, secretes digestive juices, mixes food with these juices, and propels partially digested food, called **chyme,** into the duodenum of the small intestine. The anatomy of the stomach is presented in Figure 40-4. Its major anatomic boundaries are the lower esophageal sphincter, where food passes through the **cardiac orifice** at the gastroduodenal junction into the stomach, and the **pyloric sphincter,** which relaxes as food is propelled into the duodenum. Functional areas of the stomach are the **fundus** (upper portion), **body** (middle portion), and **antrum** (lower portion).

The stomach has three layers of smooth muscle: an outer, longitudinal layer; a middle, circular layer; and an inner, oblique layer (the most prominent) (see Figure 40-4). These layers become progressively thicker in the body and antrum, where food is mixed, churned, and pushed into the duodenum. The circular layer is most prominent and the oblique layer is the least complete; the longitudinal layer is absent on the anterior and posterior surfaces. The glandular epithelium is discussed in the section about secretory functions of the stomach (see p. 1398).

Blood is supplied to the stomach by branches of the celiac artery. The blood supply is so abundant that nearly all arterial vessels must be occluded before ischemic changes occur in the stomach wall. A series of small veins (short gastric, left and right gastric, and left and right gastro-omental) drain blood from the stomach towards the hepatic portal vein.

The stomach is innervated by sympathetic and parasympathetic divisions of the autonomic nervous system. Some of the autonomic nerves are extrinsic; that is, they originate in the central nervous system and are controlled by nerve centers in the brain. The vagus nerve provides parasympathetic innervation and branches of the celiac plexus innervate the stomach sympathetically. Other neurons are intrinsic; that is, they originate within the stomach and respond to local stimuli and are components of the enteric nervous system. Extrinsic sympathetic fibers reach the stomach through the celiac plexus (solar plexus), whereas extrinsic parasympathetic fibers enter through the gastric branch of the vagus nerve.

Few substances are absorbed in the stomach. The stomach mucosa is impermeable to water, but the stomach can absorb alcohol and aspirin and other nonsteroidal anti-inflammatory agents.

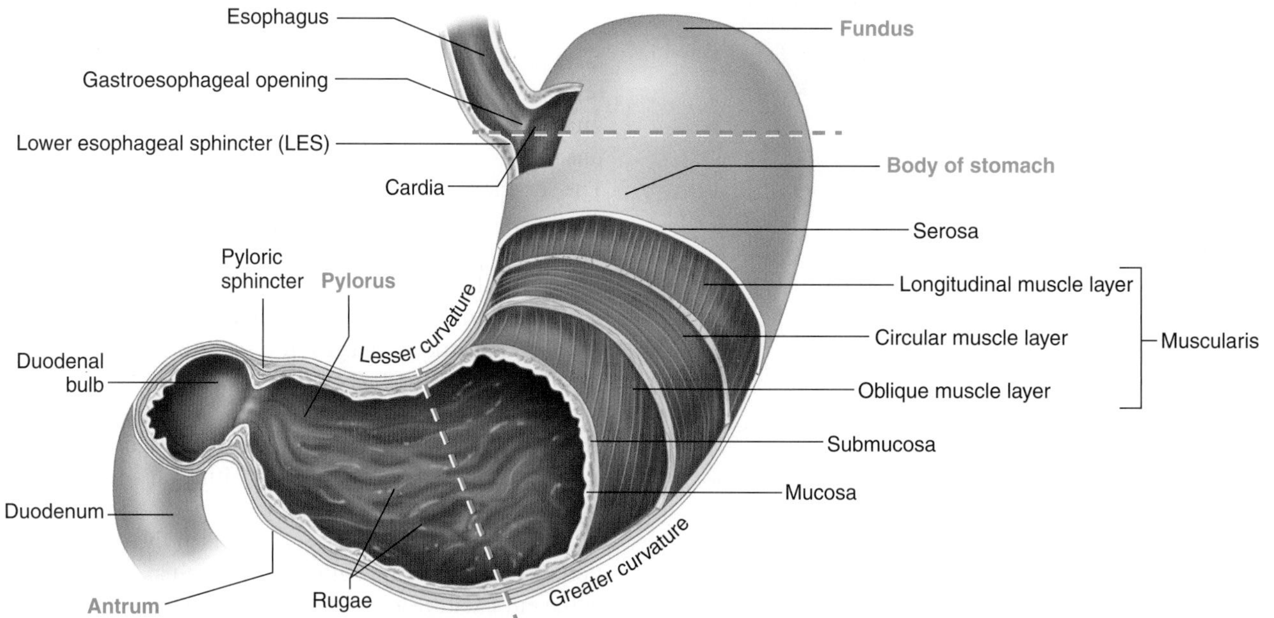

FIGURE 40-4 **Stomach.** A portion of the anterior wall has been cut away to reveal the muscle layers of the stomach wall. Note that the mucosa lining the stomach forms folds called *rugae.* The dashed lines distinguish the fundus, body, and antrum of the stomach. (Modified from Patton KT, Thibodeau GA: *Anatomy & physiology,* ed 8, St Louis, 2013, Mosby.)

Gastric Motility

In its resting state the stomach is small and contains about 50 ml of fluid. There is little wall tension, and the muscle layers in the fundus contract very little. Swallowing causes the fundus to relax (receptive relaxation) to receive a bolus of food from the esophagus. Relaxation is coordinated by efferent, nonadrenergic, noncholinergic vagal fibers and is facilitated by gastrin and cholecystokinin, two polypeptide hormones secreted by the gastrointestinal mucosa. (The actions of digestive hormones are summarized in Table 40-1.) Food is stored in vertical or oblique layers as it arrives in the fundus, whereas fluids flow relatively quickly down to the antrum.

Gastric (stomach) motility increases with the initiation of peristaltic waves, which sweep over the body of the stomach toward the antrum. The rate of peristaltic contractions is approximately three per minute and is influenced by neural and hormonal activity. **Gastrin** and **motilin** (small intestine hormones) and the vagus nerve increase contraction by making the threshold potential of muscle fibers less negative. (The neural and biochemical mechanisms of muscle contraction are described in Chapter 43.) Sympathetic activity and **secretin** (another small intestine hormone) are inhibitory and make the threshold potential more negative. The rate of peristalsis is mediated by pacemaker cells that initiate a wave of depolarization (basic electrical rhythm), which moves from the upper part of the stomach to the pylorus.

Gastric mixing and subsequent emptying of gastric contents (chyme) from the stomach take several hours (3 to 6 hours depending on the composition and volume of food intake). Mixing occurs as food is propelled toward the antrum. As food approaches the pylorus, the velocity of the peristaltic wave increases, forcing the contents back toward the body of the stomach. This **retropulsion** effectively mixes food with digestive juices, and the oscillating motion breaks down large food particles. With each peristaltic wave a small portion of the chyme passes through the pylorus and into the duodenum. The pyloric sphincter is about 1.5 cm long and is always open about 2 mm. It opens wider during antral contraction. Normally there is no regurgitation from the duodenum into the antrum.

The rate of **gastric emptying** (movement of gastric contents into the duodenum) depends on the volume, osmotic pressure, and chemical composition of the gastric contents. Larger volumes of food increase gastric pressure, peristalsis, and rate of emptying. Solids, fats, and nonisotonic solutions delay gastric emptying.[6] (Osmotic pressure and tonicity are described in Chapters 1 and 3.) Products of fat digestion, which are formed

TABLE 40-1 SELECTED HORMONES AND NEUROTRANSMITTERS OF THE DIGESTIVE SYSTEM*

SOURCE	HORMONE†	STIMULUS FOR SECRETION	ACTION
Mucosa of the stomach	Gastrin	Presence of partially digested proteins in the stomach	Stimulates gastric glands to secrete hydrochloric acid and pepsinogen; growth of gastric mucosa; promotes gastric motility
	Histamine	Gastrin	Stimulates acid secretion
	Somatostatin	Acid in the stomach	Inhibits acid and pepsinogen secretion and release of gastrin
	Acetylcholine	Vagus and local nerves in stomach	Stimulates release of pepsinogen and acid secretion
	Gastrin-releasing peptide (bombesin)	Vagus and local nerves in stomach	Stimulates gastrin and release of pepsinogen and acid secretion
Mucosa of the small intestine	Motilin	Presence of acid and fat in the duodenum	Increases gastrointestinal motility
	Secretin	Presence of chyme (acid, partially digested proteins, fats) in the duodenum	Stimulates pancreas to secrete alkaline pancreatic juice and liver to secrete bile; decreases gastrointestinal motility; inhibits gastrin and gastric acid secretion
	Cholecystokinin	Presence of chyme (acid, partially digested proteins, fats) in the duodenum	Stimulates gallbladder to eject bile and pancreas to secrete alkaline fluid; decreases gastric motility; constricts pyloric sphincter; inhibits gastrin; delays gastric emptying
	Enteroglucagon	Intraluminal fats and carbohydrates	Weakly inhibits gastric and pancreatic secretion and enhances insulin release, lipolysis, ketogenesis, and glycogenolysis; delays gastric emptying
	Entero-oxyntin	Presence of chyme in duodenum	Delays gastric emptying
	Gastric inhibitory peptide (GIP)	Fat and glucose in small intestine	Inhibits gastric secretion and gastric emptying, stimulates insulin release; inhibits intestinal motility
	Peptide YY	Intraluminal fat and bile acids	Inhibits postprandial gastric acid and pancreatic secretion and delays gastric and small bowel emptying
	Pancreatic polypeptide	Protein, fat, and glucose in small intestine	Decreases pancreatic and enzyme secretion
	Vasoactive intestinal peptide	Intestinal mucosa and muscle	Relaxes intestinal smooth muscle, increases blood flow

Modified from Johnson LR: *Gastrointestinal physiology,* ed 7, St Louis, 2007, Mosby.
*Data from Schubert ML, Peura DA: *Gastroenterology* 134(7):1842–1860, 2008; Wren AM, Bloom SR: *Gastroenterology* 132(6):2116–2130, 2007.
†NOTE: The digestive hormones are not secreted into the gastrointestinal lumen but rather into the bloodstream, in which they travel to target tissues. There are more than 30 peptide hormone genes expressed in the gastrointestinal tract and more than 100 hormonally active peptides.

in the duodenum by the action of bile from the liver and enzymes from the pancreas, stimulate the secretion of **cholecystokinin.**[7] This hormone inhibits food intake, reduces gastric motility, and decreases gastric emptying so that fats are not emptied into the duodenum at a rate that exceeds the rate of bile and enzyme secretion. Osmoreceptors in the wall of the duodenum are sensitive to the osmotic pressure of duodenal contents. The arrival of hypertonic or hypotonic gastric contents activates the osmoreceptors, which delays gastric emptying to facilitate formation of an isosmotic duodenal environment. The rate at which acid enters the duodenum also influences gastric emptying. Secretions from the pancreas, liver, and duodenal mucosa neutralize gastric hydrochloric acid in the duodenum. The rate of emptying is adjusted to the duodenum's ability to neutralize the incoming acidity. Peristaltic activity in the stomach is also affected by blood glucose levels. Low blood glucose levels stimulate the vagus nerve and gastric smooth muscles, increasing the rate of contraction.[8]

Gastric Secretion

Stimulated by eating, the stomach produces large volumes of gastric secretions. Specialized cells located throughout the gastric mucosa produce mucus, acid, enzymes, hormones, intrinsic factor, and gastroferrin. Intrinsic factor is necessary for the intestinal absorption of vitamin B_{12} and gastroferrin facilitates small intestinal absorption of iron. The hormones are secreted into the blood and travel to target tissues in the bloodstream. The other gastric secretions are released directly into the stomach lumen under neural and hormonal regulation.[9] Mucus covering the entire mucosa, intercellular tight junctions, bicarbonate secretion, and submucosal acid sensors form a protective barrier against acid and proteolytic enzymes, which otherwise would damage the gastric lining.[10]

In the fundus and body of the stomach the **gastric glands** of the mucosa are the primary secretory units (Figure 40-5). Several of these glands (three to seven) empty into a common duct known as the **gastric pit.** The **parietal cells (oxyntic cells)** within the glands secrete hydrochloric acid, intrinsic factor, and gastroferrin. The **chief cells** within the glands secrete **pepsinogen,** an enzyme precursor that is readily converted to **pepsin** (a proteolytic enzyme) in the gastric fluid. The pyloric gland mucosa in the antrum synthesizes and releases the hormone gastrin from **G cells. Enterochromaffin-like cells** secrete **histamine,** and **D cells** secrete **somatostatin.**

The composition of gastric fluid depends on volume and flow rate (Figure 40-6). Potassium level remains relatively constant, but its concentration is greater in gastric secretions than in plasma. The rate of secretion varies with the time of day; lower in the morning and higher in the afternoon and evening. Loss of gastric secretions through vomiting, drainage, or suction may decrease body stores of sodium, potassium, hydrogen, and chloride.

Acid. The major functions of **gastric hydrochloric acid** are to dissolve food fibers, act as a bactericide against swallowed organisms, and convert pepsinogen to pepsin. The production of acid by the parietal cells requires the transport of hydrogen and chloride from the parietal cells to the stomach lumen. Acid is formed in the parietal cells, primarily through the hydrolysis of water (Figure 40-7). At a high rate of gastric secretion, bicarbonate moves into the plasma, producing an "alkaline tide" in the venous blood, which also may result in a more alkaline urine.[11]

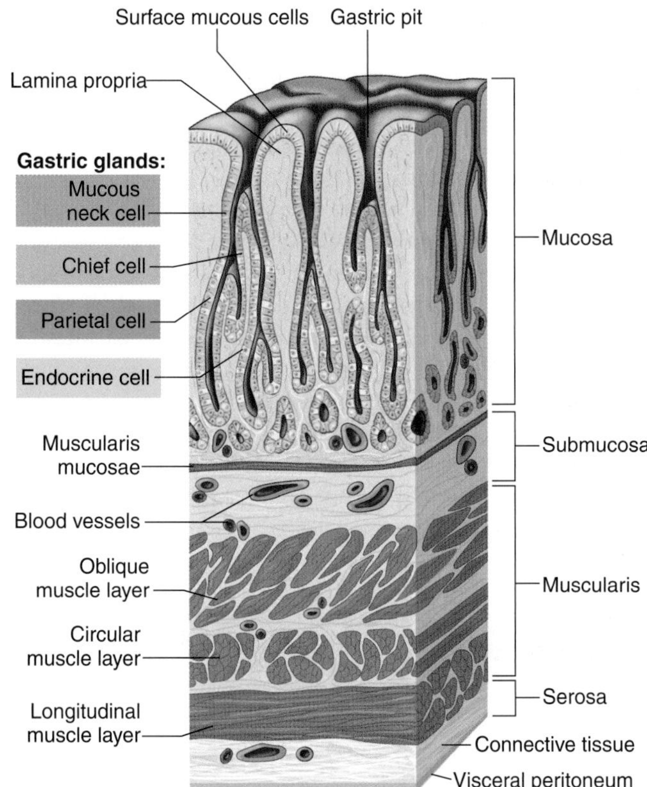

FIGURE 40-5 Gastric Pits and Gastric Glands. Gastric pits are depressions in the epithelial lining of the stomach. At the bottom of each pit is one or more tubular gastric glands. Chief cells produce the enzymes of gastric juice, and parietal cells produce stomach acid. (From Patton KT, Thibodeau GA: *Anatomy & physiology,* ed 8, St Louis, 2013, Mosby.)

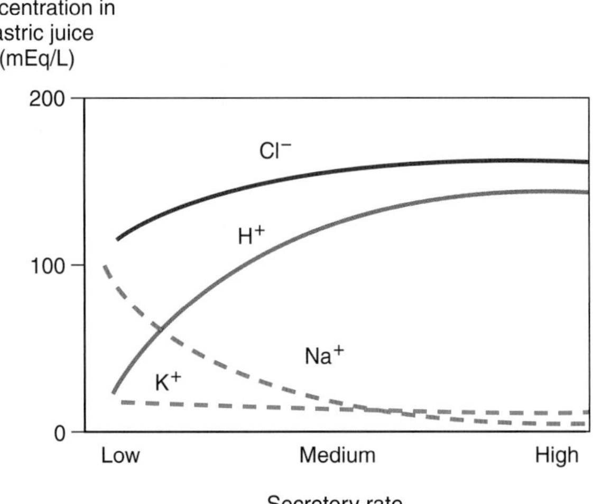

FIGURE 40-6 Relationship Between Secretory Rate and Electrolyte Composition of the Gastric Secretions. Sodium *(Na^+)* concentration is lower in the gastric secretions than in the plasma, whereas hydrogen *(H^+),* potassium *(K^+),* and chloride *(Cl^-)* concentrations are higher. Gastric secretions are close to isotonic. Secretory rate increases during the cephalic and gastric phases of digestion.

Acid secretion by parietal cells is stimulated by acetylcholine (ACh) (a neurotransmitter), gastrin (a hormone), and histamine (a biochemical mediator). The vagus nerve releases ACh and stimulates the secretion of histamine and gastrin-releasing peptide (GRP), which stimulates release of gastrin.[12] Histamine secretion is also stimulated by gastrin. Histamine is stored in enterochromaffin cells (mast cells; see Chapter 7) in the gastric mucosa. Histamine receptors in the gastric mucosa are H2 receptors (unlike those in the bronchial mucosa, which are H1 receptors). Gastric lipase is produced by glands in the fundus of the stomach and is most effective in an acidic environment. Caffeine stimulates acid secretion, as does calcium. Prostaglandins, enterogastrones (such as gastric inhibitory peptide), somatostatin, and secretin inhibit acid secretion.[13]

Pepsin. Acetylcholine, through vagal stimulation during the cephalic and gastric phases, is the strongest stimulation for pepsin secretion. The precursor pepsinogen is quickly converted to pepsin at a pH of 2. Acid also stimulates a local cholinergic reflex and stimulates chief cells to secrete pepsin. Gastrin and secretin are weaker pepsinogen secretagogues. **Pepsin** is a proteolytic enzyme that breaks down protein-forming polypeptides in the stomach. Once chyme has entered the duodenum, the alkaline environment of the duodenum inactivates pepsin.

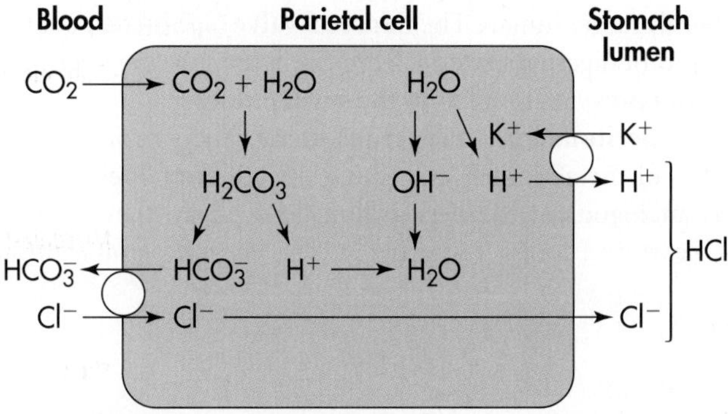

FIGURE 40-7 Hydrochloric Acid Secretion by Parietal Cell.

Mucus. The gastric mucosa is protected from the digestive actions of acid and pepsin by a coating of mucus called the **mucosal barrier.** Gastric mucosal blood flow is important to maintaining mucosal barrier function.[14]

The quality and quantity of mucus and the tight junctions between epithelial cells make gastric mucosa relatively impermeable to acid. Prostaglandins and nitric oxide protect the mucosal barrier by stimulating the secretion of mucus and bicarbonate and by inhibiting the secretion of acid. A break in the protective barrier may occur because of exposure to aspirin or other nonsteroidal anti-inflammatory drugs, *Helicobacter pylori,* ethanol, regurgitated bile, or ischemia. Breaks cause inflammation and ulceration.

Intrinsic factor (IF), a mucoprotein produced by parietal cells, combines with vitamin B_{12} in the stomach. It is required for the absorption of vitamin B_{12} by the ileum. Atrophic gastritis and failure to absorb vitamin B_{12} result in pernicious anemia (see Chapter 28).

Phases of Gastric Secretion. The secretion of gastric juice is influenced by numerous stimuli that together facilitate the process of digestion. The **phases of gastric secretion** are the cephalic phase, gastric phase, and intestinal phase (Figure 40-8).

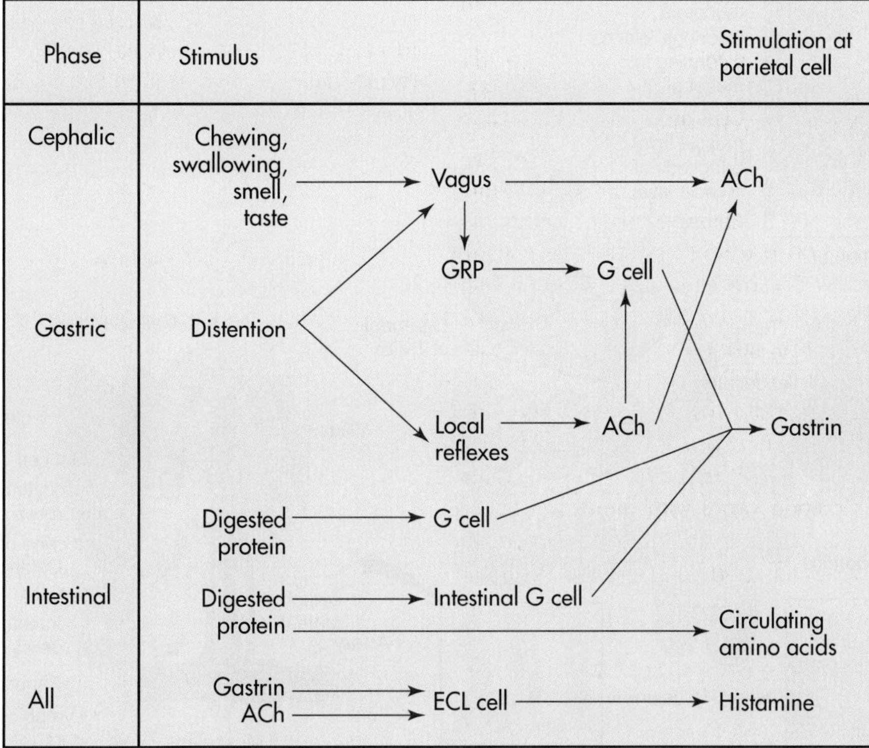

FIGURE 40-8 Mechanisms for Stimulating Acid Secretion. *ACh,* Acetylcholine; *ECL,* enterochromaffin-like cell; *GRP,* gastrin-releasing peptide. (From Johnson LR: *Gastrointestinal physiology,* ed 7, St Louis, 2007, Mosby.)

Cephalic Phase. The anticipatory and sensory experiences of smelling, seeing, tasting, chewing, and swallowing food contribute to the **cephalic phase of secretion.**[15] The cephalic phase of gastric secretion is mediated by the vagus nerve through the myenteric plexus. Acetylcholine stimulates the parietal and chief cells to secrete acid and pepsinogen, respectively. The G cells in the antrum release gastrin, which circulates through the bloodstream to the gastric glands and stimulates acid and pepsinogen secretion.

Insulin secretion by the endocrine pancreas, stimulated by hyperglycemia, also is a strong stimulus for gastric secretion and is mediated by the vagus nerve through sensors located in the hypothalamus. Maintenance of steady serum glucose levels suppresses the gastric response to insulin.

Gastric Phase. The **gastric phase of secretion** begins with the arrival of food in the stomach. Two major stimuli have a secretory effect: (1) distention of the stomach, and (2) the presence of digested protein. The vagus and enteric nerve plexuses are stimulated by distention and contribute to gastric secretion through a local reflex. Both neural reflexes are mediated by ACh and can be blocked by atropine. As digestion proceeds, products of protein break down, stimulating the release of more gastrin from G cells.

Intestinal Phase. The movement of chyme from the stomach into the duodenum initiates the **intestinal phase of secretion.** This phase represents a deceleration of the gastric secretory response; however, the presence of digested protein and amino acids in the duodenum continues to stimulate some gastric secretion.

Concurrently, in response to low duodenal pH and the presence of lipids, inhibitory vagal and enteric reflexes decrease gastric motility when chyme enters the duodenum. The release of secretin and cholecystokinin stimulate pancreatic secretions and inhibit gastric secretions.

Small Intestine

The **small intestine** is about 5 to 6 m long and is functionally divided into three segments: the duodenum, jejunum, and ileum (Figure 40-9). The **duodenum** begins at the pylorus and ends where it joins the **jejunum** at a suspensory ligament called the *Treitz ligament*. The end of the jejunum and beginning of the **ileum** are not distinguished by an anatomic marker. These structures are not grossly different, but the jejunum has a slightly larger lumen. The **ileocecal valve (sphincter)** controls the flow of digested material from the ileum into the large intestine and prevents reflux into the small intestine.

The **peritoneum** is the serous membrane surrounding the organs of the abdomen and lining the abdominopelvic cavity. It is analogous to the pericardium and pleura that surround the heart and lungs, respectively. The *visceral peritoneum* lies

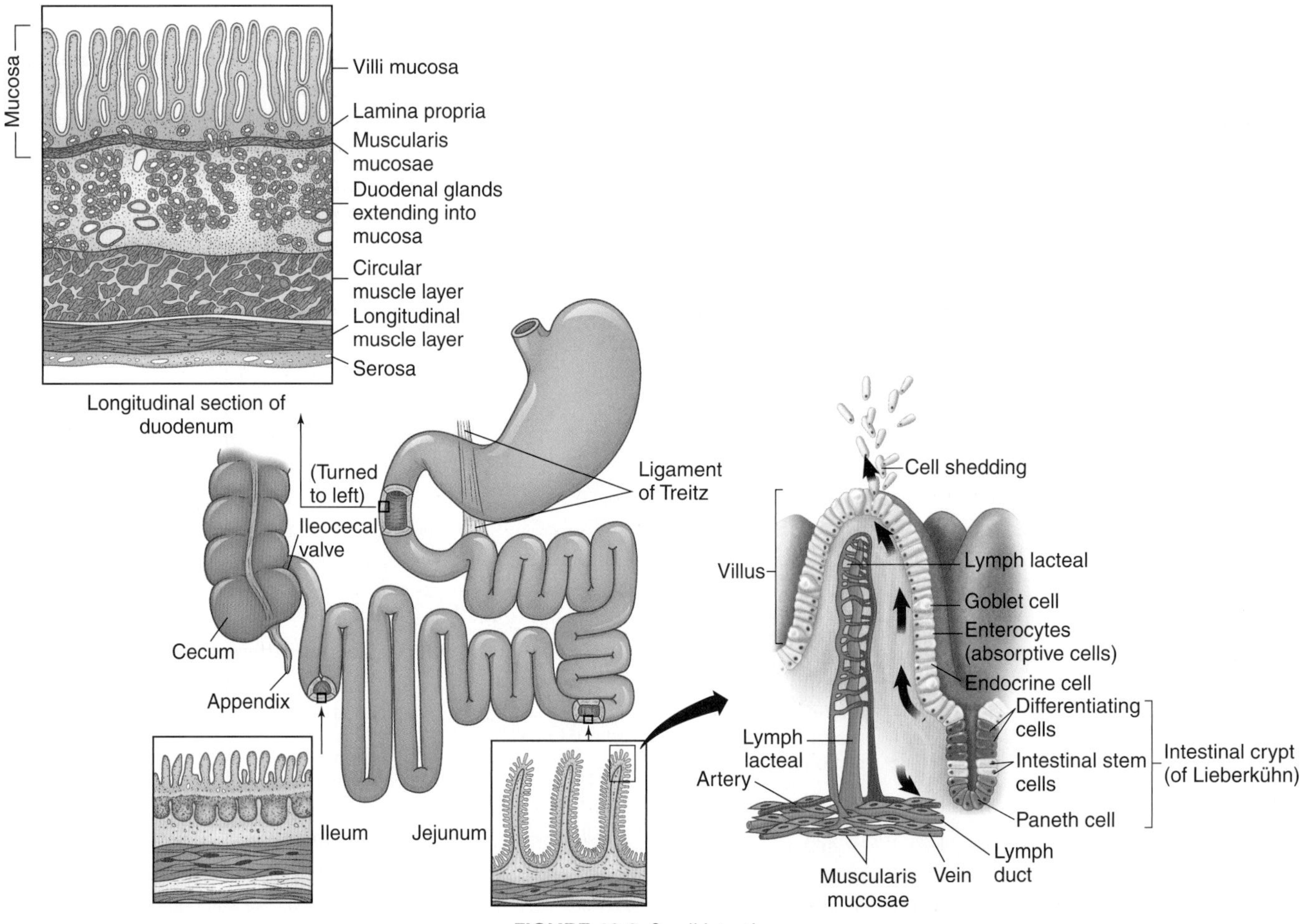

FIGURE 40-9 Small Intestine.

on the surface of the organs, and the *parietal peritoneum* lines the wall of the body cavity. The space between these two layers is called the **peritoneal cavity.** This cavity normally contains just enough fluid to lubricate the two layers and prevent friction during organ movement. Inflammation of the peritoneum, called *peritonitis,* may occur with perforation of the intestine or after abdominal surgery. As the inflammatory process resolves, scar tissue adhesions may form and cause intestinal obstruction.

The duodenum lies behind the peritoneum, or retroperitoneally, and has an essential role in mixing food with digestive juices from the liver and pancreas. The ileum and jejunum are suspended from the posterior abdominal wall by a component of the peritoneum called the **mesentery.** The loose folds of the mesentery facilitate intestinal motility and support blood vessels, nerves, and lymphatics.

The arterial supply to the duodenum arises primarily from the gastroduodenal artery, a small branch of the celiac artery. The jejunum and ileum are supplied by branches of the superior mesenteric artery. Blood flow increases significantly during digestion. The superior mesenteric vein drains blood from the entire small intestine and empties into the hepatic portal circulation. The regional lymphatics drain into the thoracic duct. Both divisions of the autonomic nervous system innervate the small intestine. Secretion, motility, and intestinal reflexes (e.g., relaxation of the lower esophageal sphincter) are mediated parasympathetically by the vagus nerve. Sympathetic activity inhibits motility and produces vasoconstriction. Intrinsic reflexive activity is mediated by the myenteric plexus (Auerbach plexus) and the submucosal plexus (Meissner plexus) of the enteric nervous system.

The smooth muscles of the small intestine are arranged in two layers: a longitudinal, outer layer; and a thicker, inner circular layer (see Figure 40-9). Circular folds of the small intestine mucosa slow the passage of food, thereby providing more time for digestion and absorption. The folds are most numerous and prominent in the jejunum and upper ileum.

Absorption occurs through **villi,** which cover the circular folds and are the functional units of the intestine (see Figure 40-9). A villus is composed of absorptive columnar epithelial cells (enterocytes) and mucus-secreting goblet cells of the mucosa. Each villus secretes some of the enzymes necessary for digestion and absorbs nutrients. Near the surface, columnar cells closely adhere to each other at sites called *tight junctions.* Water and electrolytes are absorbed through these intercellular spaces. The surface of each columnar epithelial cell on the villus contains tiny projections called **microvilli** (see Figure 40-9). Together the microvilli create a mucosal surface known as the **brush border.** The villi and microvilli greatly increase the surface area available for absorption. Coating the brush border is an "unstirred" layer of fluid that is important for the absorption of substances other than water and electrolytes. The **lamina propria** (a connective tissue layer of the mucosa) lies beneath the epithelial cells of the villi and contains lymphocytes; plasma cells, which produce immunoglobulins; and macrophages.

Central arterioles ascend within each villus and branch into a capillary array that extends around the base of the columnar cells and cascades down to the venules that lead to the hepatic portal circulation. The opposing ascending and descending blood flow provides a countercurrent exchange system for absorbed substances and blood gases. A central **lacteal,** or lymphatic capillary, is also contained within each villus and is important for the absorption and transport of fat molecules. Contents of the lacteals flow to regional nodes and channels that eventually drain into the thoracic duct[16] (see Figure 40-9).

Between the bases of the villi are the **crypts of Lieberkühn** (intestinal glands), which extend to the submucosal layer. Undifferentiated (**stem cells**) and secretory cells and Paneth epithelial cells are located here. The stem cells are precursors of columnar epithelial and goblet cells. These premature cells produce alkaline fluids containing electrolytes, mucus, and water. These cells arise from the base of the crypt and move toward the tip of the villus, maturing in shape and function as they progress. After becoming columnar cells and completing their migration to the tip of the villus, they function for a few days and then are shed into the intestinal lumen and digested. The entire epithelial population is replaced about every 4 to 7 days. Many factors can influence this process of cellular proliferation. Starvation, vitamin B_{12} deficiency, and cytotoxic drugs or irradiation suppress cell division and shorten the villi. The decreased absorption that results can cause diarrhea and malnutrition. Nutrient intake and intestinal resection stimulate cell production. The **Paneth cells** located at the base of the crypts produce defensins and other antibiotic peptides and proteins.[17] Other secretory cells produce digestive enzymes.

Intestinal Digestion and Absorption

The process of intestinal digestion is initiated in the stomach by the actions of gastric hydrochloric acid and pepsin, which break down food fibers and proteins. The chyme that passes into the duodenum is a liquid that contains small particles of undigested food. Digestion is continued in the proximal portion of the small intestine by the action of pancreatic enzymes, intestinal brush-border enzymes, and bile salts (Box 40-1). Here carbohydrates are broken down to monosaccharides and disaccharides; proteins are degraded further to amino acids and peptides; and fats are emulsified and reduced to fatty acids and monoglycerides (Figure 40-10). These nutrients, along with water, vitamins, and electrolytes, are absorbed across the intestinal mucosa and into the blood by active transport, diffusion, or facilitated diffusion. Products of carbohydrate and protein breakdown move into villus capillaries and then to the liver through the hepatic portal vein. Digested fats move into the lacteals and eventually reach the liver through the systemic circulation. Intestinal motility exposes nutrients to a large mucosal surface area by mixing chyme and moving it through the lumen. Different segments of the gastrointestinal tract absorb different nutrients. Digestion and absorption of all major nutrients occur in the small intestine. Sites of absorption are shown in Figure 40-11.

Water and Electrolyte Transport by the Small Intestine. The epithelial cell membranes of the small intestine are formed of lipids and therefore are hydrophobic, or tend to repel water. (The properties of cell membranes are described in Chapter 1.) Therefore, water and electrolytes are transported in both directions (toward the capillary blood or toward the intestinal lumen) through the tight junctions and intercellular spaces

BOX 40-1 SOURCES OF DIGESTIVE ENZYMES

Salivary Glands
Amylase
Lingual lipase

Stomach
Pepsin
Gastric lipase

Pancreas
Amylase
Trypsin
Chymotrypsin
Carboxypeptidase
Elastase
Lipase-colipase
Phospholipase A_2
Cholesterol esterase–nonspecific lipase

Small Intestine
Enterokinase
Disaccharidases
  Maltase
  Sucrase
  Lactase
  α,α-Trehalase
Isomaltase
Peptidases
  Amino-oligopeptidase
  Dipeptidase

From Johnson LR: *Gastrointestinal physiology,* ed 7, St Louis, 2007, Mosby.

rather than across cell membranes. Water diffuses passively across hydrostatic pressure and osmotic gradients established by the active transport of sodium and other substances. Approximately 85% to 90% of the water that enters the gastrointestinal tract each day is absorbed in the small intestine. The remaining water and electrolytes are absorbed at a constant rate in the large intestine.[18] Sodium passes through the tight junctions and is actively transported across cell membranes. Sodium and glucose share a common active transport carrier (sodium-glucose ligand transporter1 [SGLT1]) so that sodium absorption is enhanced by glucose transport[18a] (Figure 40-12). Potassium moves passively across the tight junctions with changes in the electrochemical gradient. Chloride is actively secreted throughout the large and small intestines.

Carbohydrates. Carbohydrate (starch, table sugar [sucrose], milk sugar [lactose], cereal sugar [maltose]) accounts for at least 50% of the American diet. Because only monosaccharides (ribose, galactose, glucose, fructose) are absorbed by the intestinal mucosa, the complex carbohydrates (polysaccharides and oligosaccharides) must be hydrolyzed to their simplest form (see Figure 40-10). Salivary and pancreatic amylases break down starches to oligosaccharides by splitting α-1,4-glucosidic linkages of long-chain molecules. The major disaccharides are sucrose (glucose-fructose), maltose (glucose-glucose), and lactose (glucose-galactose). Approximately half of starch hydrolysis occurs in the stomach and about half in the duodenum. In the small intestine, disaccharides are hydrolyzed by brush-border enzymes (sucrase, maltase, and lactase) to their respective monosaccharides.

The sugars are absorbed primarily in the duodenum and upper jejunum. The monosaccharides pass through the unstirred layer by diffusion. At the cell membrane, glucose and galactose are actively transported with a sodium carrier (SGLT1) and fructose absorption is facilitated by glucose transporter 5 (GLUT5) and GLUT7.[19] Transport of all three monosaccharides from the cytosol to the bloodstream is facilitated by GLUT2[20] (see Figure 40-12). Insulin facilitates glucose transport into fat and muscle cells via glucose transporter 4 (GLUT4).

Insulin is not required for the intestinal absorption of glucose. Cellulose is a glucose polysaccharide found in plants. Humans lack enzymes to digest cellulose, and the undigested fiber contributes to stool volume and stimulates large intestine motility.

Proteins. Adults require 44 to 56 g of protein per day. Approximately 20 to 30 g of protein is derived endogenously from shed epithelial cells and small amounts of plasma proteins. Most ingested protein is absorbed; only 5% to 10% is eliminated in the stool.

The site of digestion of protein depends on the source of the protein. For example, casein from bovine milk precipitates in the stomach and is digested by gastric pepsin and acid, whereas the soluble proteins whey and soy pass rapidly through the stomach and are digested by pancreatic enzymes.[21] Major protein hydrolysis is accomplished in the small intestine by the pancreatic enzymes trypsin, chymotrypsin, and carboxypeptidase (see Figure 40-10). **Trypsin** and **chymotrypsin** (endopeptidase) hydrolyze the interior bonds of the large molecules, and **carboxypeptidases** cleave the end amino acids (exopeptidase). Hydrolysis of proteins is also carried out by the brush-border enzymes and enzymes in the epithelial cytosol (intracellular fluid). The brush-border enzymes hydrolyze the large oligopeptides (proteins composed of three to six amino acids) into smaller peptides, which can cross cell membranes. Enzymes in the cytosol then break them down to amino acids. Amino acids are actively transported from the cytosol into the bloodstream by a sodium-dependent carrier in the basolateral membrane. There also are free amino acids that can be absorbed directly from the intestinal lumen using a membrane transport protein. Like the sugars, proteins are absorbed primarily in the proximal area of the small intestine.

Fats

Approximately 90 to 100 g of fat is consumed daily by the average American. **Fat** is an important source of calories and is a primary structural component of cell membranes and organelles. Sources of dietary fat are reviewed in Box 40-2. Although triglycerides are the major dietary lipids, cholesterol, phospholipids, and fat-soluble vitamins also have nutritional importance. The digestion and absorption of fat occur in four phases: (1) emulsification and lipolysis, (2) micelle formation, (3) fat absorption, and (4) resynthesis of triglycerides and phospholipids.

The mechanical action of the stomach and small intestine disperses the triglyceride droplets into small particles.

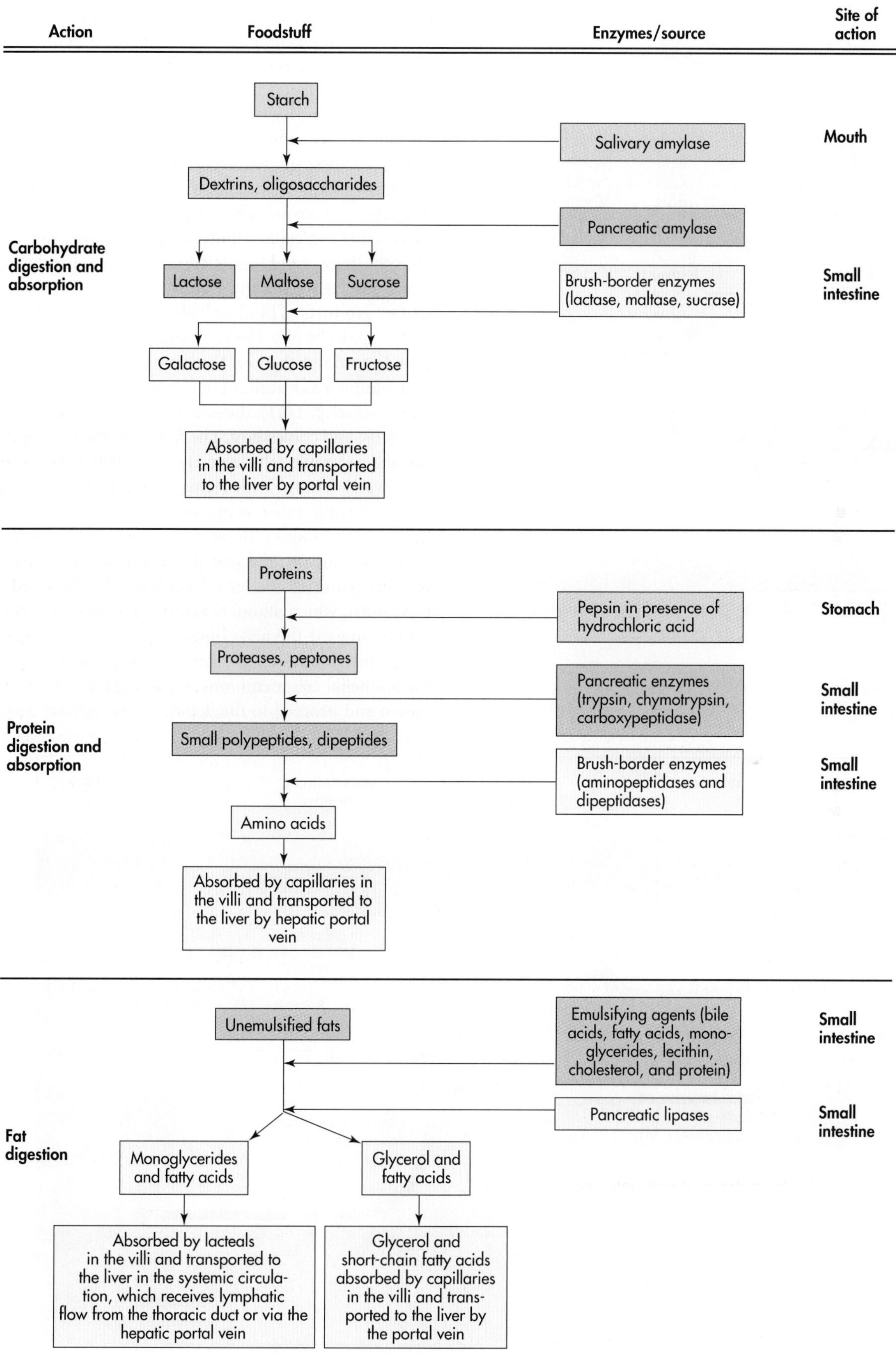

FIGURE 40-10 Digestion and Absorption of Foodstuffs.

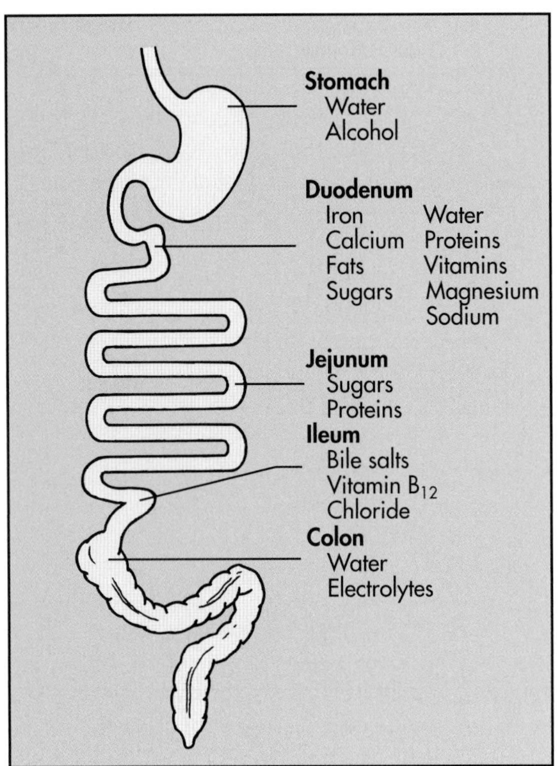

FIGURE 40-11 Sites of Absorption of Major Nutrients.

Emulsification is the process by which emulsifying agents (fatty acids, monoglycerides, lecithin, cholesterol, protein, bile salts) in the small intestinal lumen cover the small fat particles and prevent them from re-forming into fat droplets. Emulsified fat is then ready for **lipolysis** (lipid hydrolysis) by pancreatic lipase, phospholipase, and hydrolase. **Lipase** breaks down triglycerides to diglycerides, monoglycerides, free fatty acids, and glycerol (see Figure 40-10). The action of lipase requires the presence of **colipase,** a pancreatic enzyme that allows lipase to penetrate the triglyceride molecule. **Phospholipase** cleaves fatty acids from phospholipids, and **cholesterol esterase** breaks cholesterol esters into fatty acids and glycerol.

The products of lipid hydrolysis must be made water soluble if they are to be absorbed efficiently from the intestinal lumen. This is accomplished by the formation of water-soluble molecules known as **micelles** (Figure 40-13). Micelles are formed of bile salts (see p. 1411), the products of fat hydrolysis, fat-soluble vitamins, and cholesterol. The fats form the core of the micelle, and the polar bile salts form an outer shell, with the hydrophobic ("water-hating") side facing the interior and the hydrophilic ("water-loving") side facing the aqueous (water-like) content of the intestinal lumen. Because the unstirred layer of the brush border is aqueous, the micelles readily diffuse through it. The micelles maintain the fat molecules in the dissolved or solubilized form, which allows them to move more rapidly from the micelle toward the absorbing surface of the intestinal epithelium. The fat products of the micelle then readily diffuse through the epithelial cell membrane, while the bile salts remain in the lumen and proceed to the ileum, where they are absorbed into

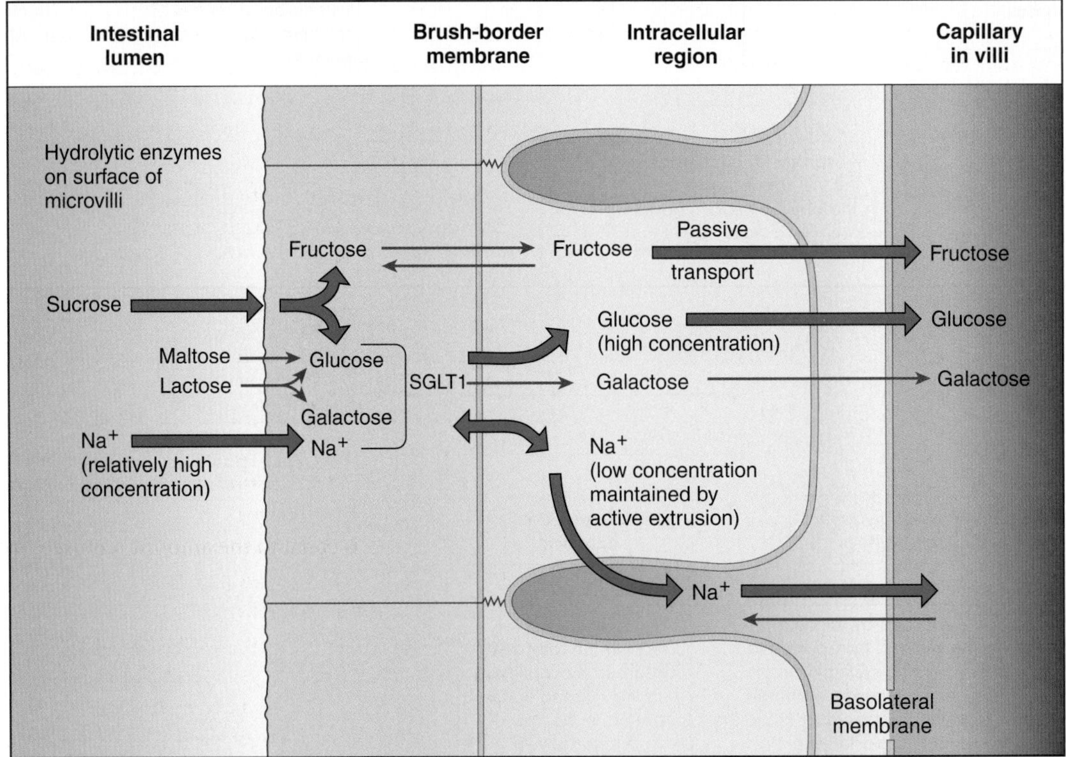

FIGURE 40-12 **Monosaccharides and Sodium Transport.** Schematic showing monosaccharides and sodium *(Na^+)* transport through the small intestinal epithelium. Glucose, galactose, and sodium are transported into the epithelial cell by sodium-glucose ligand transporter 1 *(SGLT1)*. See text for details.

BOX 40-2 DIETARY FAT

Saturated Fatty Acid (Palmitic Acid [$C_{16}H_{32}O_2$])

Each carbon atom in the chain is linked by single bonds to adjacent carbon and hydrogen atoms; atoms are solid at room temperature and found in animal fat and tropical oils (coconut and palm oils); they increase low-density lipoprotein (LDL) cholesterol ("bad" cholesterol) blood levels and increase the risk of coronary artery disease.

Unsaturated Fatty Acid

Unsaturated fatty acids are soft or liquid at room temperature; omega-6 fatty acids are found in plants and vegetables (olive, canola, and peanut oils), and omega-3 fatty acids are found in fish and shellfish.

1. Monounsaturated fatty acids (e.g., oleic acid [$C_{18}H_{34}O_2$]): Contain one double bond in the carbon chain and are found in plants and animals; may be beneficial in reducing blood cholesterol, glucose levels, and systolic blood pressure; do not lower high-density lipoprotein (HDL) cholesterol ("good" cholesterol) level; low HDL levels have been associated with coronary heart disease.
2. Polyunsaturated fatty acids (e.g., linoleic acid [$C_{18}H_{32}O_2$]): Contain two or more double bonds in the carbon chain and are found in plants and fish oils; omega-6 fatty acids lower total and LDL cholesterol blood levels; high levels of polyunsaturated fatty acids may lower LDL level; omega-3 fatty acids lower blood triglyceride levels, reduce platelet aggregation and blood-clotting tendency, are necessary for growth and development, and may prevent coronary artery disease, hypertension, cancer, and inflammatory and immune disorders.

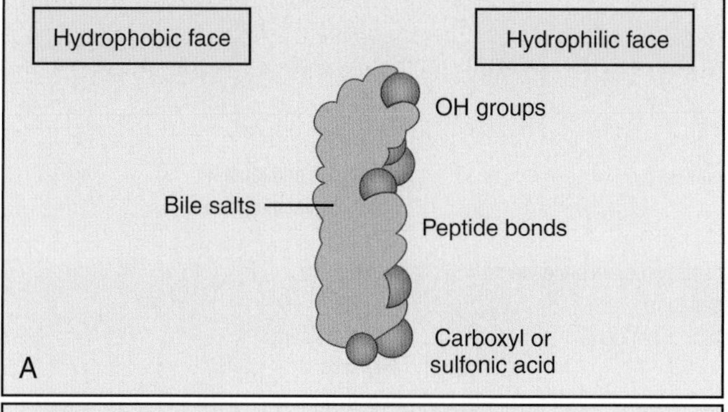

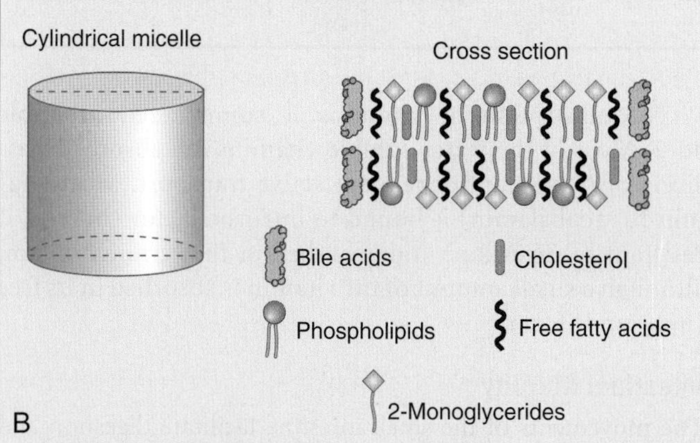

FIGURE 40-13 Structure of Bile Acid and Micelle. **A,** A bile salt molecule in solution. The molecule is amphipathic in that it has a hydrophilic face and a hydrophobic face. The amphipathic structure is key in the ability of the bile salts to emulsify lipids and form micelles. **B,** A model of the structure of a bile salt–lipid mixed micelle, an emulsified fat. (From Levy MN, Koeppen BM, Stanton BA: *Principles of physiology,* ed 4, St Louis, 2006, Mosby.)

the circulation and returned to the liver via the enterohepatic circulation (Figure 40-14 and Figure 40-20, p. 1411). Almost all of the bile salts are recycled in this way.

When the fat products reach the inside of the epithelial cell, they are resynthesized into triglycerides and phospholipids. The triglycerides are covered with phospholipids, lipoproteins, and cholesterol to become particles called **chylomicrons.** The chylomicrons travel to the basolateral membrane of the columnar epithelial cells, where they are extruded into the intercellular spaces of the villus. From here they enter the lacteals and lymphatic channels and, eventually, the systemic circulation.

Minerals and Vitamins. The recommended intake of calcium ranges from 1000 to 1500 mg/day. Between 500 and 600 mg is secreted or shed into the lumen with desquamated epithelial cells. Not all of this calcium is absorbed. Daily absorption of **calcium** is approximately 600 mg. This amount increases with increased intake. When its concentration in the lumen is greater than 5 mmol/L, calcium is absorbed by passive diffusion. At concentrations less than 5 mmol/L, calcium is transported actively across cell membranes, bound to a carrier protein. The carrier formation requires the presence of the active form of vitamin D_3 (1,25-dihydroxy-vitamin D). The calcium-protein complex moves into the epithelial cell, where the calcium binds to proteins or other substances. Then these complexes move through the basolateral membrane to the interstitial fluid by diffusion or active transport. Calcium is absorbed throughout the small intestine, but primarily in the ileum. Increased serum calcium concentration inhibits parathyroid hormone, which in turn decreases the formation of vitamin D_3 by the kidney, thus regulating calcium absorption.

Increased demand for calcium results in increased uptake, as evidenced by the fact that calcium is absorbed more rapidly in children and pregnant or lactating women. Bile salts enhance calcium absorption indirectly by facilitating the absorption of vitamin D, which is fat soluble. In addition, bile salts promote the absorption of free fatty acids that, at high concentrations, bind calcium and form soaps in the intestinal lumen. In older individuals calcium is absorbed less readily because of inadequate amounts of the active form of vitamin D.[22]

The recommended intake of **magnesium** for adults is 300 to 350 mg/day. Approximately 50% of it is absorbed by active transport or passive diffusion in the jejunum and ileum. **Phosphate** is also absorbed in the small intestine by passive diffusion and active transport.

The levels of **iron** in the body are regulated primarily by intestinal absorption and secretion. The average intake ranges from 15 to 30 mg/day. Of this amount, menstruating women absorb 1 to 1.5 mg and men absorb 0.15 to 1 mg. Generally the amount of iron absorbed is equal to the amount required. Iron is absorbed more rapidly if a deficiency exists. A primary source of iron is heme from animal protein. This iron is rapidly absorbed by the epithelial cells primarily in the duodenum. Inorganic iron (e.g., iron in fruits, cereals, eggs, vegetables) is also readily absorbed. The presence of vitamin C reduces ferric iron to ferrous iron, which is the form more easily absorbed. Calcium phosphate and phosphoproteins (milk and antacids) in the intestinal lumen bind iron and reduce absorption. Tea also binds iron and inhibits its absorption by forming iron tannate complexes.

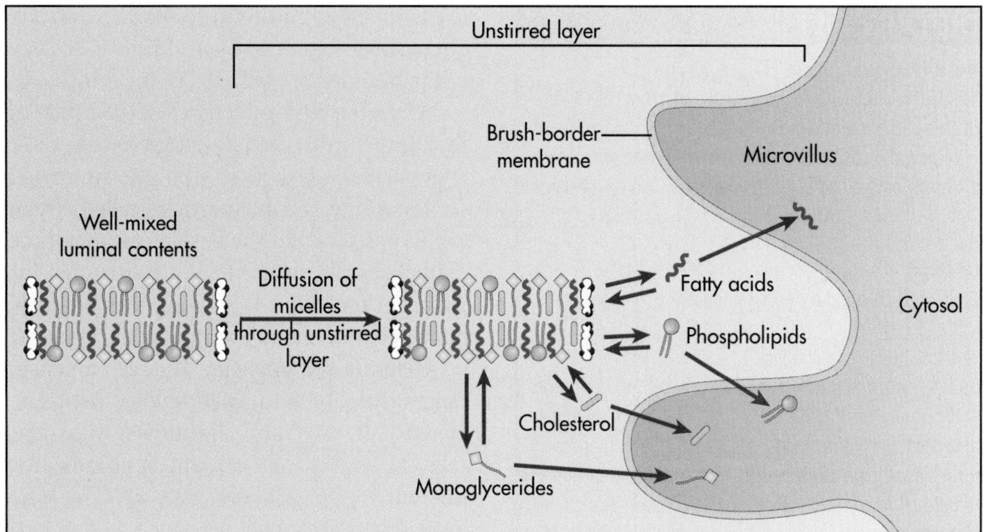

FIGURE 40-14 **Lipid Absorption in the Small Intestine.** Micelles of bile salts and products of lipid digestion diffuse through the unstirred layer and among the microvilli. As digestive products are absorbed from free solution by epithelial cells of the villi, more digestive products dissociate from the micelles. (From Levy MN, Koeppen BM, Stanton BA: *Principles of physiology,* ed 4, St Louis, 2006, Mosby.)

TABLE 40-2 INTESTINAL ABSORPTION OF VITAMINS

VITAMIN	MECHANISMS OF ABSORPTION	SITE OF ABSORPTION
Fat-Soluble Vitamins	Micelle formation with bile salts; lipid diffusion	Ileum
A (retinal)		
D_3 (1,25-dihydroxy-vitamin D)		
E (α-tocopherol)		
K		
Water-Soluble Vitamins		
B_1 (thiamine)	Active transport (sodium dependent)	Duodenum and jejunum
B_2 (riboflavin)	Unknown	Duodenum and jejunum
Niacin (nicotinic acid)	Passive diffusion	Jejunum
C (ascorbic acid)	Passive diffusion; active transport (sodium dependent)	Ileum
Folic acid	Active transport (sodium dependent)	Jejunum
B_{12} (cobalamin)	Active transport (intrinsic factor dependent)	Terminal ileum
B_6 (pyridoxine, pyridoxamine, pyridoxal phosphate)	Passive diffusion	Jejunum
Pantothenic acid	Passive diffusion	Duodenum and jejunum
Biotin	Unknown	Unknown

Iron is bound to *intestinal transferrin* in the lumen and is absorbed and bound to the protein *ferritin* and to amino acid chelates in the cytosol of the enterocytes. Transport of iron across the basolateral membrane is determined by the amount of iron in the circulation. It is transported in the blood by *plasma transferrin,* a glycoprotein, and is carried to body tissues. When there is less need for iron, it remains in the enterocyte as ferritin and is carried into the lumen when the cell is sloughed from the end of the villus. Following hemorrhage, the intestinal cells require 3 days to increase their rate of iron absorption. This is because the need for iron is perceived by the precursor stem cells in the crypts of Lieberkühn, and they take 3 days to mature and migrate to the tips of the villi, where they absorb more iron. **Hepcidin** is a protein synthesized by the liver that inhibits apical uptake of iron by enterocytes and modulates iron trafficking.[23]

The absorption of **vitamins** is summarized in Table 40-2. Most of the water-soluble vitamins are absorbed passively or by sodium-dependent active transport. Most vitamin B_{12} (cobalamin) is bound to intrinsic factor (making it resistant to digestion) and absorbed in the terminal ileum, although a small amount of the vitamin is absorbed in its free (unbound) form.

Intestinal Motility

The movements of the small intestine facilitate digestion and absorption. Chyme coming from the stomach stimulates intestinal movements that mix in secretions from the liver, pancreas, and intestinal glands. A churning motion brings the luminal content into contact with the absorbing cells of the villi. Propulsive movements then advance the chyme toward the large intestine.

Intestinal motility is regulated by the enteric nervous system, vagal stimulation, and hormones (see Table 40-1). Two movements promote motility: segmentation and peristalsis. **Segmentation** consists of localized rhythmic contractions of the circular smooth muscles and occurs more frequently than peristalsis.[24] The contraction waves occur at different rates in different parts of the small intestine in segments of 1 to 4 cm. Frequency is greatest (12 per minute) in the upper small intestine and least (8 per minute) in the distal part of the ileum. Segmentation divides and mixes the chyme, bringing it into contact with the absorbent mucosal surface. It also helps to propel the chyme toward the large intestine. The frequency of the segmentation is regulated intrinsically by the frequency of the basic electrical rhythm (BER), which arises in the myenteric plexus of longitudinal smooth muscle and is controlled by the interstitial cells of Cajal, the pacemaker cells of the gastrointestinal (GI) tract. Although the basic rate of contraction is controlled intrinsically, the force of contraction can be enhanced extrinsically by vagal stimulation.[25]

Intestinal peristalsis involves short segments (about 10 cm) of longitudinal smooth muscle and propels chyme through the intestine. The wave of contraction moves slowly (1 to 2 cm/second) to allow time for digestion and absorption.

Peptide hormones, including motilin, gastrin, secretin, and cholecystokinin, facilitate intestinal motility. Neural reflexes along the length of the small intestine facilitate motility, digestion, and absorption. Through reflex action, receptors in one part of the intestine transmit signals that influence the function of another part. The **ileogastric reflex** inhibits gastric motility when the ileum becomes distended. This prevents the continued movement of chyme into an already distended intestine. The **intestinointestinal reflex** inhibits intestinal motility when one part of the intestine is overdistended. Both of these reflexes require extrinsic innervation. The **gastroileal reflex,** which is activated by an increase in gastric motility and secretion, stimulates an increase in ileal motility and relaxation of the ileocecal sphincter. This empties the ileum and prepares it to receive more chyme. The gastroileal reflex is probably regulated by the hormones gastrin and cholecystokinin or through the autonomic nerves.

During prolonged fasting or between meals, particularly overnight, slow waves sweep along the entire length of the intestinal tract from the stomach to the terminal ileum. This is known as the *interdigestive myoelectric complex,* and it appears to propel residual gastric and intestinal contents, including bacteria, into the colon.

The intestinal villi move with contractions of the muscularis mucosae, a very thin layer of muscle that separates the mucosa and submucosa. Absorption is promoted by the swaying of villi in the luminal contents. Contractile activity also helps to empty the central lacteals, which contain products of fat digestion.

The **ileocecal valve (sphincter)** marks the junction between the terminal ileum and the large intestine. This valve is intrinsically regulated and is normally closed. The arrival of peristaltic waves from the last few centimeters of the ileum causes the ileocecal valve to open, allowing a small amount of chyme to pass through. Distention of the upper large intestine causes the sphincter to constrict, preventing further distention or retrograde flow of intestinal contents.

Large Intestine

The **large intestine** is approximately 1.5 m long and consists of the cecum, appendix, colon, rectum, and anal canal (Figure 40-15). The **cecum** is a pouch that receives chyme from the ileum. Attached to the cecum is the **vermiform appendix,** an appendage having little or no physiologic function. From the cecum, chyme enters the **colon,** a four-part length of intestine that loops upward, traverses the abdominal cavity, and descends to the anal canal. The four parts of the colon are the **ascending colon, transverse colon, descending colon,** and **sigmoid colon.** Two sphincters control the flow of intestinal contents through the cecum and colon: the ileocecal valve, which admits chyme from the ileum to the cecum, and the **rectosigmoid (O'Beirne) sphincter,** which controls the movement of wastes from the sigmoid colon into the rectum. A thick (2.5 to 3 cm) portion of smooth muscle surrounds the anal canal, forming the **internal anal sphincter.** Overlapping it distally is the striated skeletal muscle of the **external anal sphincter.**

In the cecum and colon the longitudinal muscle layer consists of three longitudinal bands called **teniae coli** (see Figure 40-15). The teniae coli are shorter than the colon, giving the colon its "gathered" appearance. The circular muscles of the colon separate the gathers into outpouchings called **haustra.** The haustra become more or less prominent with the contractions and relaxations of the circular muscles. The mucosal surface of the colon has rugae (folds), particularly between the haustra, and Lieberkühn crypts but no villi. Columnar epithelial cells and mucus-secreting goblet cells form the mucosa throughout the large intestine. The columnar epithelium absorbs fluid and electrolytes, and the mucus-secreting cells lubricate the mucosa.

The enteric nervous system regulates motor and secretory activity independently of extrinsic nervous system control. Extrinsic parasympathetic innervation occurs through the vagus nerve and extends from the cecum up to the first part of the transverse colon. Vagal stimulation increases rhythmic contraction of the proximal colon. Extrinsic parasympathetic fibers reach the distal colon through the sacral parasympathetic splanchnic nerves. The internal anal sphincter is usually in a state of contraction, and its reflex response is to relax when the rectum is distended. The myenteric plexus provides the major innervation of the internal anal sphincter, but responds to sympathetic stimulation to maintain contraction and parasympathetic stimulation that facilitates relaxation when the rectum is full. Sympathetic innervation of this sphincter arises from the celiac and superior mesenteric ganglia and the sphincter nerve. The external anal sphincter is innervated by the pudendal nerve arising from sacral levels of the spinal cord. Voluntary control of the external anal sphincter is paralyzed after injury of the lower spinal cord, but the internal sphincter is still functional. Sympathetic activity in the entire large intestine modulates intestinal reflexes, conveys somatic sensations of fullness and pain, participates in the defecation reflex, and constricts blood vessels. The blood supply of the large intestine and rectum is derived primarily from branches of the superior and inferior mesenteric artery.[26]

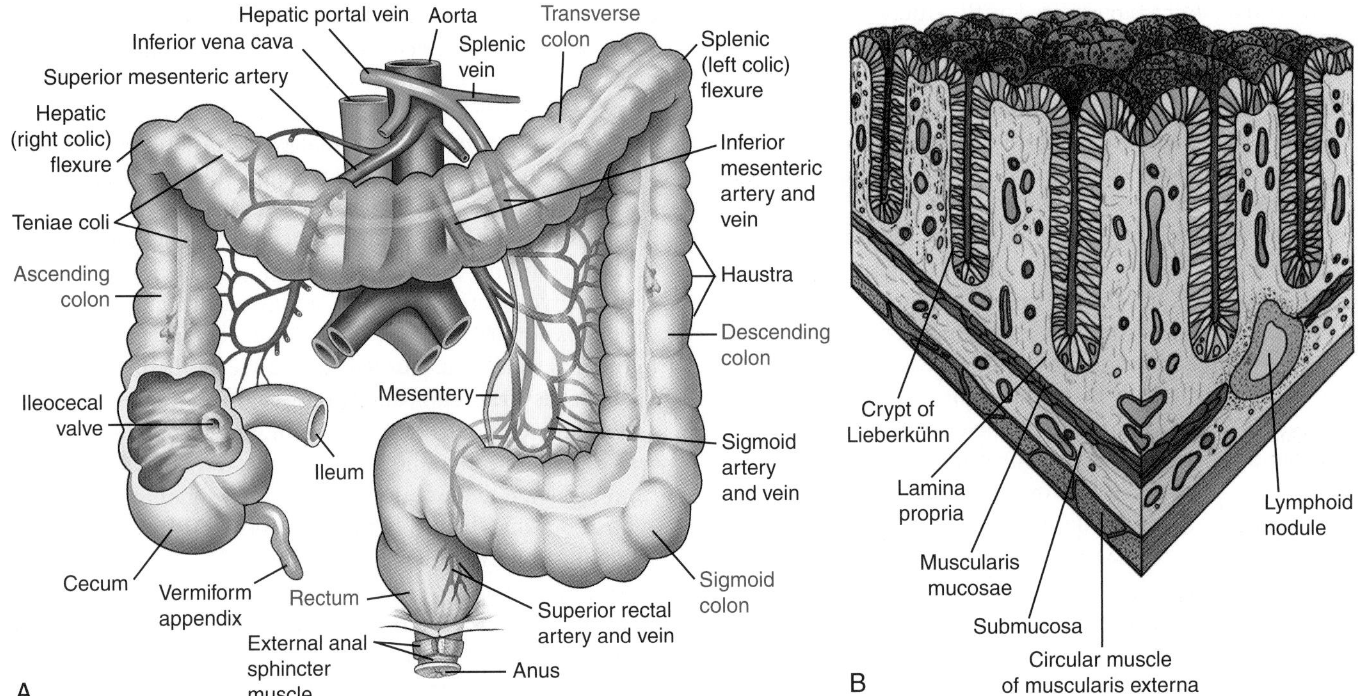

FIGURE 40-15 Large Intestine. **A,** Structure of the large intestine. **B,** Microscopic cross section illustrating cellular structures of the large intestine. The wall of the large intestine is lined with columnar epithelium in contrast to the villi characteristics of the small intestine. The longitudinal layer of muscularis is reduced to become the teniae coli. (**A** modified from Patton KT, Thibodeau GA: *Anatomy & physiology,* ed 8, St Louis, 2013, Mosby; **B** from Gartner LP, Hiatt JL: *Color textbook of histology,* Philadelphia, 2007, Saunders.)

The primary type of colonic movement is segmental. The circular muscles contract and relax at different sites, shuttling the intestinal contents back and forth between the contracting and relaxing haustra. The movements massage the intestinal contents, then called the **fecal mass,** and facilitate the absorption of water. Propulsive movement occurs with the proximal-to-distal contraction of several haustral units. **Peristaltic movements** also occur and promote the emptying of the colon. The **gastrocolic reflex** initiates propulsion in the entire colon, usually during or immediately after eating, when chyme enters from the ileum. The gastrocolic reflex causes the fecal mass to pass rapidly into the sigmoid colon and rectum, stimulating defecation. Gastrin and cholecystokinin participate in stimulating this reflex. Epinephrine inhibits contractile activity.

Approximately 500 to 700 ml of chyme flows from the ileum to the cecum per day. Most of the water is absorbed in the colon by diffusion and active transport. The electrochemical gradient established by sodium movement enhances the diffusion of serum potassium from the capillaries in the lumen. Aldosterone increases colon membrane permeability to sodium, thereby increasing both the diffusion of sodium into the cell and the active transport of sodium across the basolateral membrane to the interstitial fluid. (See Chapters 3, 21, and 37 for a discussion of aldosterone secretion.) This increases the cell-to-lumen diffusion gradient for potassium. Potassium moves outward, and chloride is absorbed with sodium as the complementary anion. Chloride also enters the cell in exchange for bicarbonate.

By the time the fecal mass enters the sigmoid colon, the mass consists entirely of wastes and is called the feces. **Feces,** or excrement, consists of food residue, unabsorbed gastrointestinal secretions, shed epithelial cells, and bacteria. The movement of feces into the sigmoid colon and rectum stimulates the **defecation reflex (rectosphincteric reflex).** The rectal wall stretches and the tonically constricted internal anal sphincter relaxes, creating the urge to defecate. The defecation reflex can be overridden voluntarily by contraction of the external anal sphincter and muscles of the pelvic floor. The rectal wall gradually relaxes, reducing tension, and the urge to defecate passes. Retrograde contraction of the rectum may displace the feces out of the rectal vault until a more convenient time for evacuation. Pain or fear of pain associated with defecation (e.g., rectal fissures or hemorrhoids) can inhibit the defecation reflex. The defecation reflex is regulated by parasympathetic and cholinergic fibers. Voluntary inhibition or facilitation of defecation is mediated from cortical projections onto the medulla and down to sacral segments of the cord.

Defecation is facilitated by squatting or sitting because these positions straighten the angle between the rectum and anal canal and increase the efficiency of straining (increasing intra-abdominal pressure). Intra-abdominal pressure is increased by initiating the **Valsalva maneuver.** This maneuver consists of inhaling and forcing the diaphragm and chest muscles against the closed glottis. This increases both intrathoracic and intra-abdominal pressure, which is transmitted to the rectum.

Intestinal Bacteria

The type and number of bacterial flora vary greatly throughout the normal gastrointestinal tract, with an increasing number

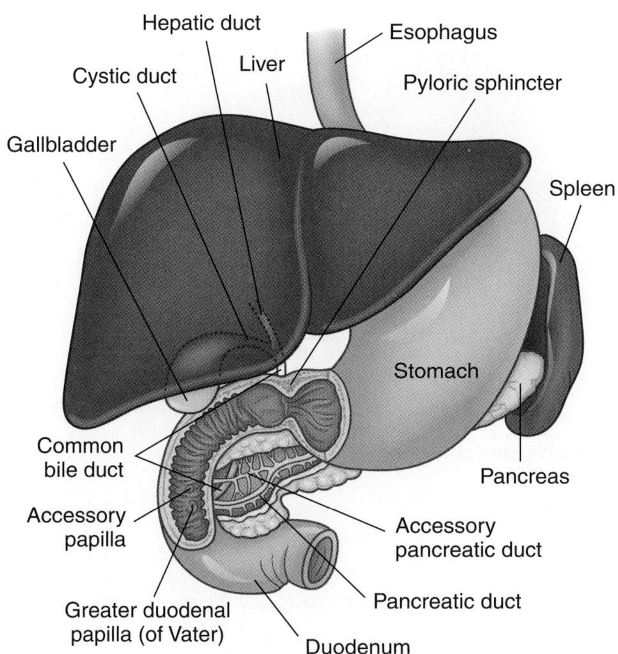

FIGURE 40-16 Locations of the Liver, Gallbladder, and Exocrine Pancreas, Which Are the Accessory Organs of Digestion.

of bacteria from the stomach to the distal colon. The stomach is relatively sterile because of the secretion of acid that kills ingested pathogens or inhibits bacterial growth. Bile acid secretion, intestinal motility, and antibody production suppress bacterial growth in the duodenum, and in the duodenum and jejunum there is a low concentration of aerobes (10^{-1} to 10^{-4}/ml), primarily streptococci, lactobacilli, staphylococci, enterobacteria, and *Bacteroides.* Anaerobes are only found distal to the ileocecal valve. They constitute about 95% of the fecal flora in the colon and contribute one third of the solid bulk of feces. *Bacteroides,* clostridia, anaerobic lactobacilli, and coliforms are the most common microorganisms from the ileum to the cecum.[27]

The intestinal tract is sterile at birth but becomes colonized with *Escherichia coli, Clostridium welchii,* and *Streptococcus* within a few hours. Within 3 to 4 weeks after birth, the normal flora are established. The normal flora do not have the virulence factors associated with pathogenic microorganisms, thus permitting immune tolerances. The intestinal mucosal environment also produces a broad spectrum of protective antimicrobial agents.[28] The intestinal bacteria play a role in the metabolism of bile salts (contributing to the intestinal reabsorption of bile and the elimination of toxic bile metabolites); the metabolism of estrogens, androgens, and lipids and conversion of unabsorbed carbohydrates to absorbable organic acids; the synthesis of vitamin K_2 and B vitamins; and the metabolism of various nitrogenous substances and drugs.[29]

ACCESSORY ORGANS OF DIGESTION

The liver, gallbladder, and exocrine pancreas all secrete substances necessary for the digestion of chyme. These secretions are delivered to the duodenum through ducts (Figure 40-16). The liver produces bile, which contains salts necessary for fat digestion and absorption. Between meals bile is stored in the gallbladder. The exocrine pancreas produces enzymes needed for the complete digestion of carbohydrates, proteins, and fats. The exocrine pancreas also produces an alkaline fluid that neutralizes chyme, creating a duodenal pH that supports enzymatic action. The liver receives nutrients absorbed by the small intestine and metabolizes or synthesizes these nutrients into forms that can be absorbed by the body's cells. It then releases the nutrients into the bloodstream or stores them for later use.

Liver

The **liver,** which weighs 1200 to 1600 g, is the largest solid organ in the body. It is located under the right diaphragm and is divided into right and left lobes. The larger, right lobe is divided further into the caudate and quadrate lobes (Figure 40-17). The *falciform ligament* separates the right and left lobes and attaches the liver to the anterior abdominal wall. A fibrous cord called the *round ligament (ligamentum teres)* extends along the free edge of the falciform ligament. The round ligament is the remnant of the umbilical vein and extends from the umbilicus to the inferior surface of the liver. The *coronary ligament* branches from the falciform ligament and extends over the superior surface of the right and left lobes, adhering the liver to the inferior surface of the diaphragm. The liver is covered by a fibroelastic capsule called the *Glisson capsule.* When the liver is diseased or swollen, distention of the capsule causes pain because it is innervated by afferent neurons.

The metabolic functions of the liver require a large amount of blood. The liver receives blood from both arterial and venous sources. The **hepatic artery** branches from the celiac artery and provides oxygenated blood at the rate of 400 to 500 ml/minute (about 25% of the cardiac output). The **hepatic portal vein,** which receives deoxygenated blood from the inferior and superior mesenteric veins and the splenic vein, delivers about 1000 to 1200 ml/minute of blood to the liver. The hepatic portal vein, which carries 70% of the blood supply to the liver, is rich in nutrients that have been absorbed from the digestive tract (Figure 40-18).

Within the liver lobes are multiple, smaller anatomic units called **liver lobules** (Figure 40-19). The lobules are formed of cords or plates of **hepatocytes,** which are the functional cells of the liver. These cells are capable of regeneration; therefore, damaged or resected liver tissue can regrow. Hepatocytes secrete electrolytes, lipids, lecithin, bile acids, and cholesterol into the canaliculi. Plasma proteins are also synthesized and released into the bloodstream. **Lipocytes** are star-shaped cells that store lipids, including vitamin A. Small capillaries, or **sinusoids,** are located between the plates of hepatocytes. The sinusoids receive a mixture of venous and arterial blood from branches of the hepatic artery and hepatic portal vein. Blood from the sinusoids drains into a central vein in the middle of each liver lobule. Venous blood from all the lobules then flows into the **hepatic vein,** which empties into the inferior vena cava. The sinusoids of the liver lobules are lined with highly permeable endothelium. This permeability enhances the transport of nutrients from the sinusoids into the hepatocytes, where they are metabolized.[30] The sinusoids are also lined with phagocytic

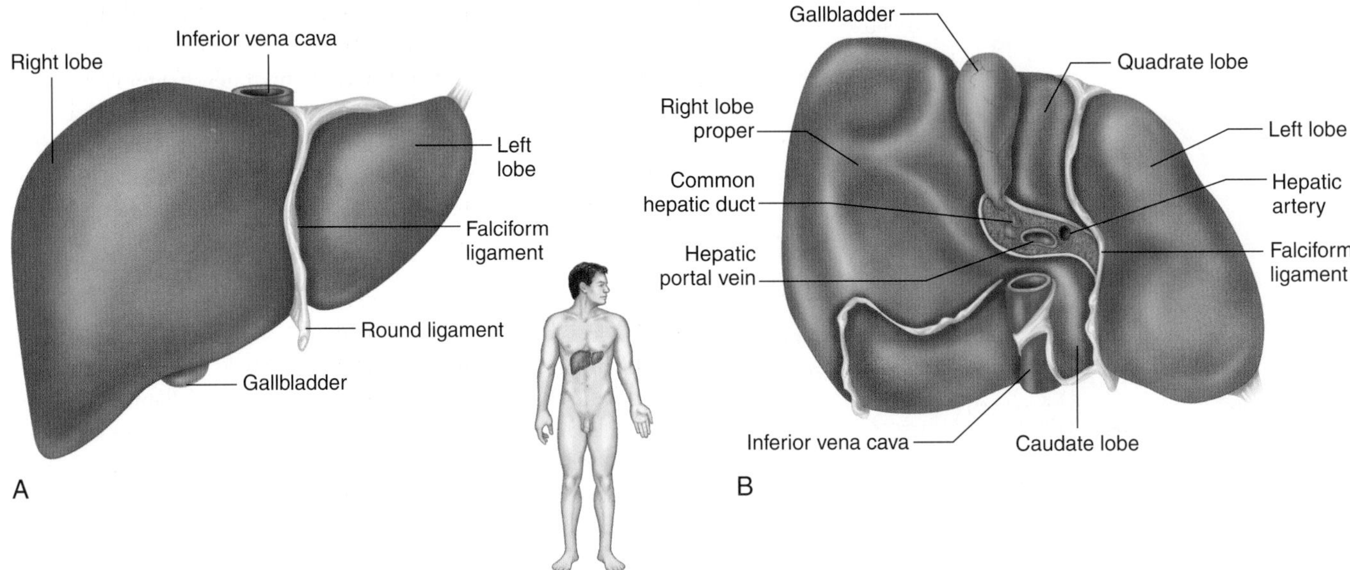

FIGURE 40-17 Gross Structure of the Liver. **A,** Anterior view. **B,** Inferior view. (From Patton KT, Thibodeau GA: *Anatomy & physiology,* ed 8, St Louis, 2013, Mosby.)

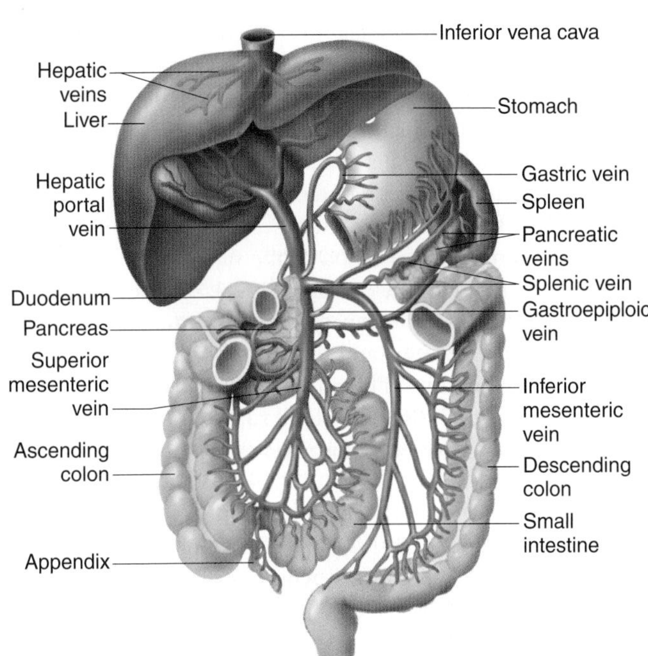

FIGURE 40-18 Hepatic Portal Circulation. In this unusual circulatory route, a vein is located between two capillary beds. The hepatic portal vein collects blood from capillaries in visceral structures located in the abdomen and empties into the liver for distribution to the hepatic capillaries. Hepatic veins return blood to the inferior vena cava. (Organs are not drawn to scale.) (From Patton KT, Thibodeau GA: *Anatomy & physiology,* ed 8, St Louis, 2013, Mosby.)

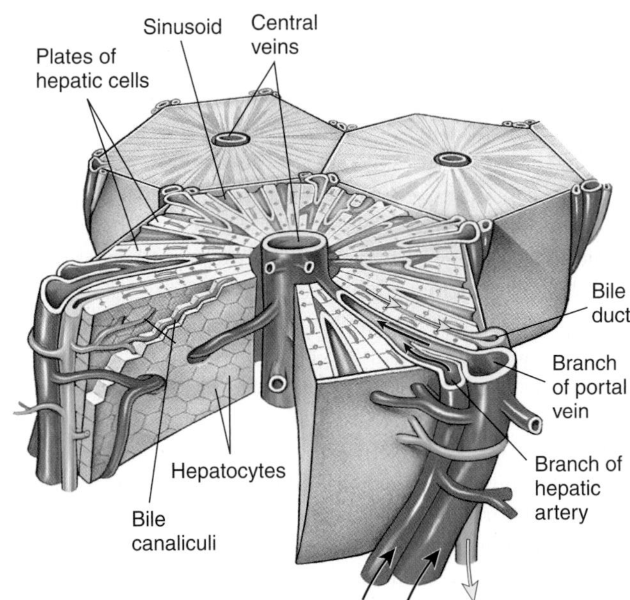

FIGURE 40-19 Diagrammatic Representation of a Liver Lobule. A central vein is located in the center of the lobule, with plates of hepatocytes disposed radially. Branches of the portal vein and hepatic artery are located on the periphery of the lobule, and blood from both vessels perfuses the sinusoids. Peripherally located bile ducts drain the bile canaliculi that run between the hepatocytes. (Modified from Patton KT, Thibodeau GA: *Anatomy & physiology,* ed 8, St Louis, 2013, Mosby.)

cells, known as **Kupffer cells,** which are part of the mononuclear phagocyte system (see Chapters 7 and 27) and are the largest population of tissue macrophages in the body. They are bactericidal and central to innate immunity.[31] **Stellate cells** contain retinoids (vitamin A), are contractile in liver injury, regulate sinusoidal blood flow, may proliferate into myofibroblasts, and participate in liver fibrosis.[32] They remove foreign substances from the blood and trap bacteria. **Pit cells** are natural killer cells found in the sinusoidal lumen; they produce interferon-γ and are important in tumor defense.[33] Between the endothelial lining of the sinusoid and the hepatocyte is the **Disse space,** which drains interstitial fluid into the hepatic lymph system.

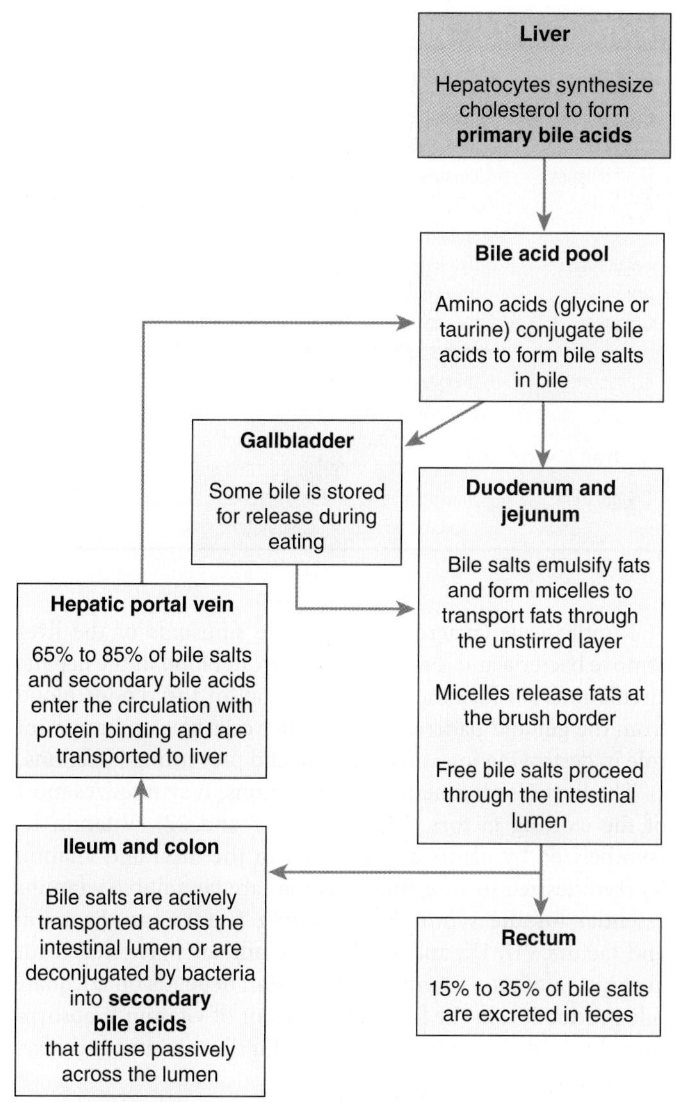

FIGURE 40-20 The Enterohepatic Circulation of Bile Salts.

Secretion of Bile

The liver assists intestinal digestion by secreting 700 to 1200 ml of bile per day. **Bile** is an alkaline, bitter-tasting yellowish green fluid that contains bile salts (conjugated bile acids), cholesterol, bilirubin (a pigment), electrolytes, and water. It is formed by hepatocytes and secreted into the canaliculi, which are small channels adjacent to hepatocytes. **Bile salts,** which are conjugated bile acids, are required for the intestinal emulsification and absorption of fats. The **bile canaliculi** empty into hepatic bile ducts and eventually drain into the **common bile duct** (see Figure 40-19). The union of the common bile duct and pancreatic duct is at the papilla or **ampulla of Vater,** which empties into the duodenum through an opening called the **major duodenal papilla** and is surrounded by the **sphincter of Oddi.**[34] Having facilitated fat emulsification and absorption in the small intestine, most bile salts are actively absorbed in the terminal ileum and returned to the liver through the portal circulation for resecretion. The pathway for recycling of bile salts is termed the **enterohepatic circulation** (Figure 40-20).[35]

Bile has two fractional components: the acid-dependent fraction and the acid-independent fraction. Hepatocytes secrete the **bile acid–dependent fraction** of the bile. This fraction consists of bile acids, cholesterol, lecithin (a phospholipid), and bilirubin (a bile pigment). The **bile acid–independent fraction** of the bile, which is secreted by the hepatocytes and epithelial cells of the bile canaliculi, is a bicarbonate-rich aqueous fluid that gives bile its alkaline pH.

Bile salts are conjugated in the liver from primary and secondary bile acids. The **primary bile acids** are cholic acid and chenodeoxycholic (chenic acid or chenodiol) acid. These acids are synthesized from cholesterol by the hepatocytes. The **secondary bile acids** are deoxycholic acid and lithocholic acid. These acids are formed in the small intestine by the action of intestinal bacteria, after which they are absorbed and flow to the liver (see Figure 40-20). Both forms of bile acids are conjugated with amino acids (glycine or taurine) in the liver to form bile salts. Conjugation makes the bile acids more water soluble, thus restricting their diffusion from the duodenum and ileum. The primary and secondary bile acids together form the **bile acid pool.**

Bile secretion is called **choleresis.** A **choleretic agent** is a substance that stimulates the liver to secrete bile. One strong stimulus is a high concentration of bile salts. Other choleretics include secretin, which increases the rate of bile flow by promoting the secretion of bicarbonate from canaliculi and other intrahepatic bile ducts; cholecystokinin; and vagal stimulation.

Metabolism of Bilirubin

Bilirubin is a byproduct of destruction of aged red blood cells. It gives bile a greenish black color and produces the yellow tinge of jaundice. Aged red blood cells are taken up and destroyed by macrophages of the mononuclear phagocyte system, primarily in the spleen and liver. (In the liver these macrophages are Kupffer cells.) Within these cells, hemoglobin is separated into its component parts—heme and globin (Figure 40-21). The globin component is further degraded into its constituent amino acids, which are recycled to form new protein. The heme moiety is converted to **biliverdin** by the enzymatic (heme oxygenase) cleavage of iron. The iron attaches to transferrin in the plasma and can be stored in the liver or used by the bone marrow to make new red blood cells. The biliverdin is enzymatically converted to bilirubin in the macrophage of the mononuclear phagocytic system and then is released into the plasma. In the plasma, bilirubin binds to albumin and is known as **unconjugated bilirubin,** or free bilirubin, which is lipid soluble. Bilirubin also may have a role as an antioxidant and provide cytoprotection.[36,37]

In the liver, unconjugated bilirubin moves from plasma in the sinusoids into the hepatocyte. Within hepatocytes it joins with glucuronic acid to form **conjugated bilirubin,** which is water soluble. Conjugation transforms bilirubin from a lipid-soluble substance that can cross biologic membranes to a water-soluble substance that can be excreted in the bile. When conjugated bilirubin reaches the distal ileum and colon, it is deconjugated by bacteria and converted to

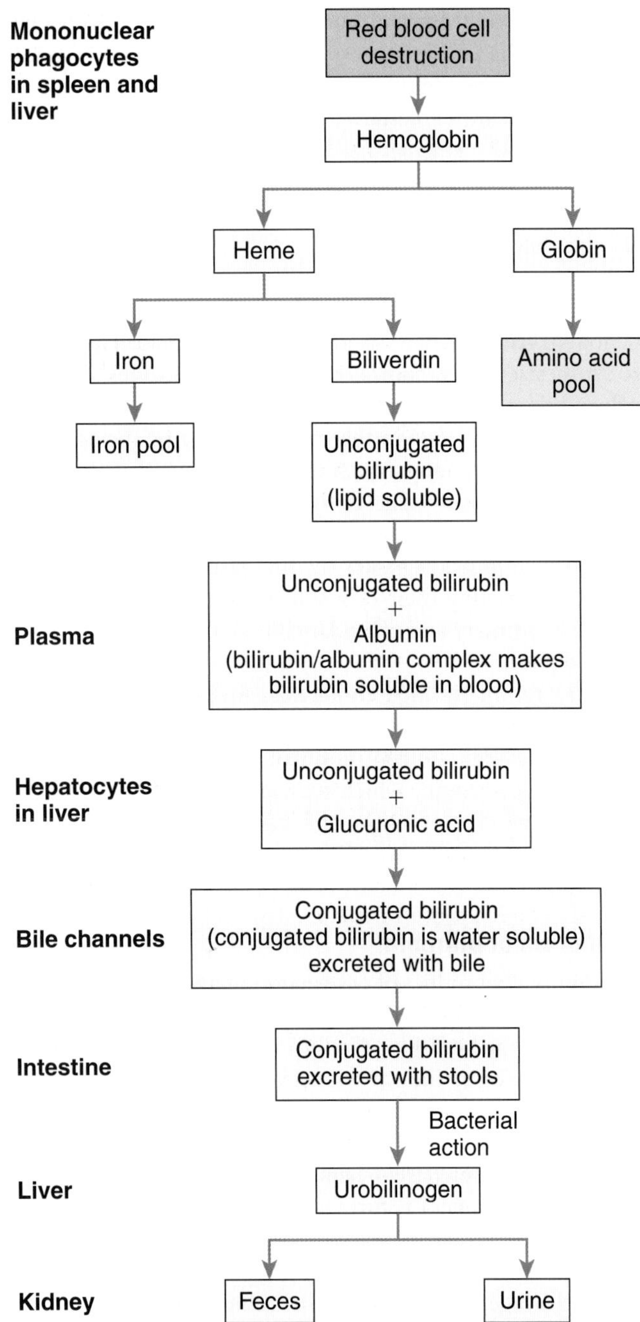

FIGURE 40-21 Bilirubin Metabolism. See text for further explanation.

urobilinogen. Urobilinogen is then reabsorbed in the intestines and transported to the kidney where it is excreted in the urine as urobilin, giving urine its yellow color. A small amount of urobilin is recirculated back into the liver and eliminated in feces as stercobilin, which contributes to the stool's brown pigmentation.

Vascular and Hematologic Functions

Because of its extensive vascular network, the liver can store a large volume of blood. The amount stored at any one time depends on pressure relationships in the arteries and veins. The liver also can release blood to maintain systemic circulatory volume in the event of hemorrhage.

TABLE 40-3 PROTEINS IN THE BODY

ROLE	EXAMPLE
Contraction	Actin and myosin enable muscle contraction.
Energy	Proteins can be metabolized for energy.
Fluid balance	Albumin is a major source of plasma oncotic pressure.
Protection	Antibodies and complement protect against infection and foreign substances.
Regulation	Enzymes control chemical reactions; hormones regulate many physiologic processes.
Structure	Collagen fibers provide structural support to many parts of the body; keratin strengthens skin, hair, and nails.
Transport	Hemoglobin transports oxygen and carbon dioxide in the blood; plasma proteins serve as transport molecules; proteins in cell membranes control movement of materials into and out of cells.
Coagulation	Hemostasis is regulated by proteins that balance coagulation and anticoagulation.

Kupffer cells (macrophages) in the sinusoids of the liver remove bacteria and foreign particles from blood in the hepatic circulation. Because the liver receives all of the venous blood from the gut and pancreas, the Kupffer cells play an important role in destroying intestinal bacteria and preventing infections.

The liver also has hemostatic functions. It synthesizes most of the clotting factors (see Chapters 7 and 27). Vitamin K_1 (synthesized by plants and ingested in the diet) and vitamin K_2 (synthesized by intestinal bacteria) are fat-soluble vitamins essential for the synthesis of clotting factors (prothrombin and factors VII, IX, and X). Because bile salts are needed for absorption of fats, vitamin K absorption depends on adequate bile production in the liver. Impairment of vitamin K absorption diminishes production of clotting factors and increases risk of bleeding.

Metabolism of Nutrients

Fats. Ingested fat absorbed by lacteals in the intestinal villi enters the liver through the lymphatics, primarily as triglycerides. In the liver the triglycerides can be hydrolyzed to glycerol and free fatty acids and used to produce metabolic energy (ATP), or they can be released into the bloodstream bound to proteins (lipoproteins). The lipoproteins are carried by the blood to adipose cells for storage. The liver also synthesizes phospholipids and cholesterol, which are needed for the hepatic production of bile salts, steroid hormones, components of plasma membranes, and other special molecules.

Proteins. Protein synthesis requires the presence of all the essential amino acids (obtained only from food), as well as nonessential amino acids. Proteins perform many important roles in the body and are summarized in Table 40-3.

Within hepatocytes, amino acids are converted to carbohydrates by the removal of ammonia (NH_3), a process known as **deamination.** The ammonia is converted to urea by the liver and passes into the blood to be excreted by the kidneys. The plasma proteins, including albumins and globulins (with the exception of gamma globulin, which is formed in lymph nodes and lymphoid tissue), are synthesized by the liver. The liver also synthesizes several nonessential amino acids and serum enzymes that become elevated with liver injury (and other diseases):

- **Aspartate aminotransferase (AST)** (previously called serum glutamate-oxaloacetate transaminase [SGOT]): also present in red blood cells and skeletal muscle; AST transfers an α-amino group between aspartate and glutamate.
- **Alanine aminotransferase (ALT)** (previously called serum glutamate-pyruvate transaminase [SGPT]): also present in small amounts in the kidneys, heart, skeletal muscle, and pancreas; ALT transfers an amino group from alanine to α-ketoglutarate to form pyruvate and glutamate.
- **Lactate dehydrogenase (LDH):** catalyzes the conversion of lactate to pyruvate; LDH is widely distributed throughout the body and different isoenzymes are found in different tissues.
- **Alkaline phosphatase:** removes phosphate groups, particularly in an alkaline environment.
- **Gamma-glutamyltransferase:** transfers the gamma-glutamyl moiety of glutathione to an acceptor to form glutamate and is a pro-oxidant.

Reference values for the above enzymes can be reviewed in Table 40-6 and are summarized on the inside back book cover.

Carbohydrates. The liver contributes to the stability of blood glucose levels by releasing glucose during states of hypoglycemia (low blood glucose levels) and taking up glucose during states of hyperglycemia (high blood glucose levels) and storing it as glycogen (glyconeogenesis) or converting it to fat. When all glycogen stores have been used, the liver can convert amino acids and glycerol to glucose.

Metabolic Detoxification

The liver alters exogenous and endogenous chemicals (e.g., drugs), foreign molecules, and hormones to make them less toxic or less biologically active. This process, called **metabolic detoxification (biotransformation),** diminishes intestinal or renal tubular reabsorption of potentially toxic substances and facilitates their intestinal and renal excretion. In this way alcohol, barbiturates, amphetamines, steroids, and hormones (including estrogens, aldosterone, antidiuretic hormone, and testosterone) are metabolized or detoxified, preventing excessive accumulation and adverse effects.

Although metabolic detoxification is usually protective, sometimes the end products of metabolic detoxification become toxins. Those of alcohol metabolism, for example, are acetaldehyde and hydrogen. Excessive intake of alcohol over a prolonged period causes these end products to damage hepatocytes. Acetaldehyde damages cellular mitochondria, and the excess hydrogen promotes fat accumulation. This is how alcohol impairs the liver's ability to function (see Chapter 2).

Storage of Minerals and Vitamins

The liver stores certain vitamins and minerals, including iron and copper, in times of excessive intake and releases them in times of need. The liver can store vitamins B_{12} and D for several months and vitamin A for several years. The liver also stores vitamins E and K. Iron is stored in the liver as ferritin, an iron-protein complex, and is released as needed for red blood cell production.

Gallbladder

The **gallbladder** is a saclike organ that lies on the inferior surface of the liver (Figures 40-17 and 40-22). The wall of the gallbladder is composed of the mucous membrane, muscularis, and serosa. The primary function of the gallbladder is to store and concentrate bile between meals. During the interdigestive period, bile flows from the liver through the right or left hepatic duct into the common bile duct and meets resistance at the closed **sphincter of Oddi,** which controls flow into the duodenum and prevents reflux of duodenal contents into the pancreatobiliary system. Bile then flows into the gallbladder through the **cystic duct** where it is concentrated and stored. The mucosa of the gallbladder wall readily absorbs water and electrolytes, leaving a high concentration of bile salts, bile pigments, and cholesterol. The gallbladder holds about 90 ml of bile.

Within 30 minutes after eating, the gallbladder begins to contract, forcing stored bile through the cystic duct and into the common bile duct. The sphincter of Oddi relaxes, and bile flows into the duodenum through the major duodenal papilla. During the cephalic and gastric phases of digestion, gallbladder contraction is mediated by cholinergic branches of the vagus nerve. Hormonal regulation of gallbladder contraction is derived primarily from the release of *cholecystokinin* secreted by the duodenal and jejunal mucosa in the presence of fat. Vasoactive intestinal peptide, pancreatic polypeptide, and sympathetic nerve stimulation relax the gallbladder.

Exocrine Pancreas

The **pancreas** is approximately 20 cm long, with its head tucked into the curve of the duodenum and its tail touching the spleen. The body of the pancreas lies deep in the abdomen, behind the stomach (see Figure 40-16). The pancreas is unique in that it has endocrine as well as exocrine functions. The endocrine pancreas secretes insulin, glucagon, somatostatin, and pancreatic polypeptide (see Chapter 21).

The **exocrine pancreas** is composed of acinar cells that secrete enzymes and networks of ducts that secrete alkaline fluids with important digestive functions. The acinar cells are organized into spherical lobules (acini) around small secretory ducts (see Figure 40-22). Secretions drain into a system of ducts that leads to the **pancreatic duct (Wirsung duct),** which empties into the common bile duct at the **ampulla of Vater** and then through the duodenal papilla into the duodenum. In some individuals an accessory duct (the duct of Santorini) branches off the pancreatic duct and drains directly into the duodenum at an opening called the *minor duodenal papilla* (see Figure 40-22).

Arterial blood is supplied to the pancreas by branches of the celiac and superior mesenteric arteries. Venous blood leaves the head of the pancreas through the tributaries to the hepatic portal vein, with the body and tail being drained through the splenic vein. All hormonal pancreatic secretions also pass through the hepatic portal vein into the liver.

Pancreatic innervation arises from parasympathetic neurons of the vagus nerve, which stimulate enzymatic and hormonal

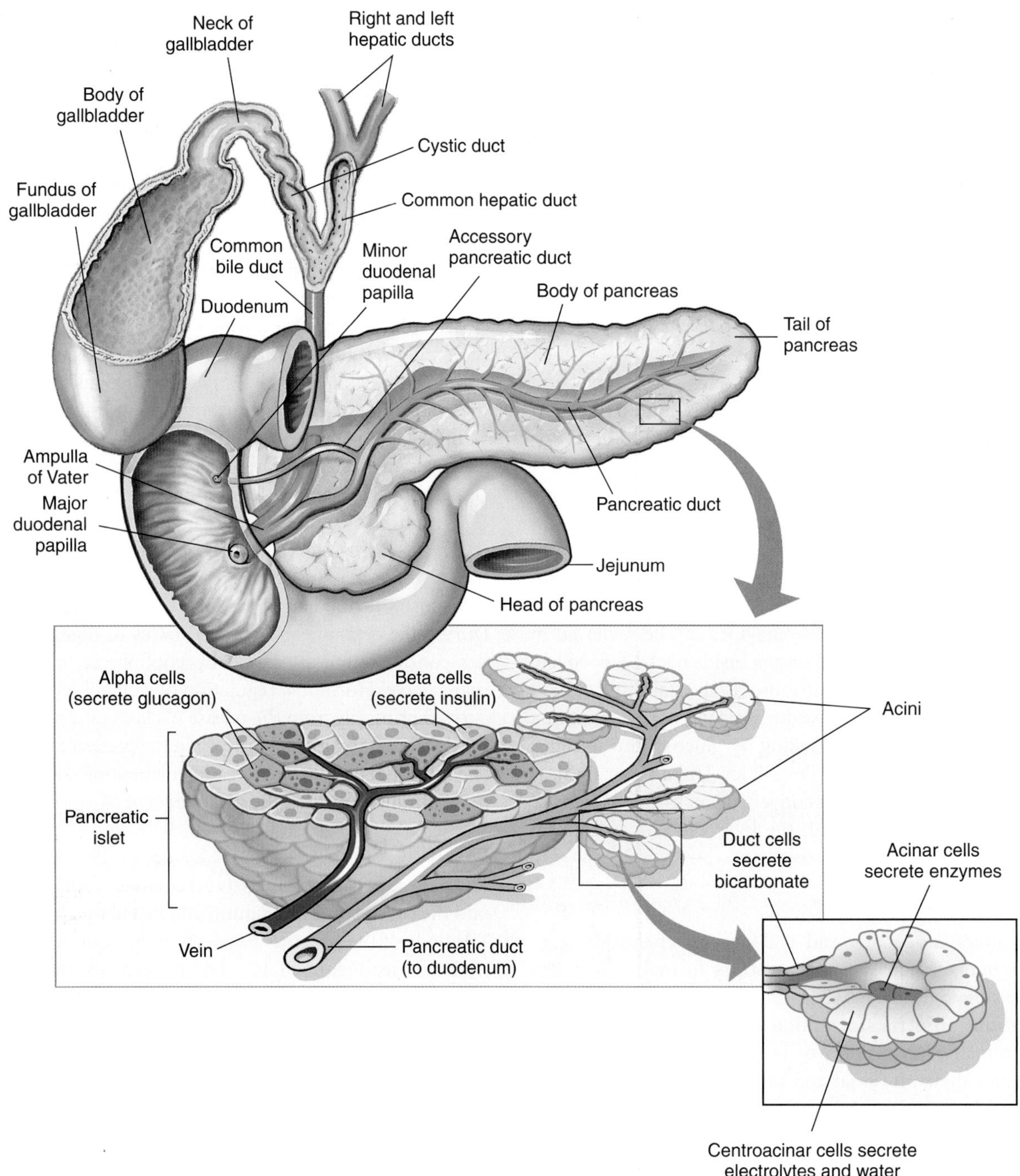

FIGURE 40-22 **Associated Structures of the Gallbladder, Pancreas, and Pancreatic Acinar Cells and Duct.** (Modified from Patton KT, Thibodeau GA: *Anatomy & physiology,* ed 6, St Louis, 2007, Mosby.)

secretion. Sympathetic postganglionic fibers from the celiac and superior mesenteric plexuses innervate the blood vessels and cause vasoconstriction and inhibit pancreatic secretion.[38]

The aqueous secretions of the exocrine pancreas are isotonic and contain potassium, sodium, bicarbonate, magnesium, calcium, and chloride. Sodium and potassium concentrations are about equal to those in the plasma. The concentration of bicarbonate in pancreatic juice varies directly with the secretory flow rate. As bicarbonate secretion increases, chloride secretion decreases to maintain a constant anionic concentration. The highly alkaline pancreatic juice neutralizes the acidic chyme that enters the duodenum from the stomach and provides the alkaline medium needed for the actions of digestive enzymes and the absorption of fat in the intestine.

In the pancreas, transport of water and electrolytes through the ductal epithelium involves active and passive mechanisms. The ductal cells actively transport hydrogen into the blood and bicarbonate into the duct lumen. Potassium and chloride are secreted by diffusion according to changes in electrochemical potential gradients. As the secretion flows down the duct, water is osmotically transported into the juice until it becomes isosmotic. At low flow rates, bicarbonate is exchanged passively for chloride, but at higher flow rates there is less time for this exchange and bicarbonate concentration increases. Because

TABLE 40-4 SELECTED STUDIES OF GASTROINTESTINAL STRUCTURE

TEST	DESCRIPTION	APPLICATION
Plain roentgenograms	Use of high-energy electromagnetic radiation to evaluate tissue structure by radiopacity or radiolucency	Visualization of the position, size, and structure of abdominal contents
Air or barium contrast roentgenograms	Introduction of radiopaque substances into the upper or lower gastrointestinal tract	Enhanced visualization of the contours, position, and size of the gastrointestinal tract to detect umbilical hernia, ulcers, diverticula, congenital anomalies, polyps, tumors, strictures, obstructions
Endoscopy Esophagoscopy (esophagus) Gastroscopy (stomach) Duodenoscopy (duodenum) Colonoscopy (large intestine) Sigmoidoscopy (sigmoid colon)	Passage of rigid or flexible (fiberoptic) endoscope into the gastrointestinal tract for visualization or biopsy	Visualization or biopsy of inflamed hernias, polyps, ulcers, strictures, varices, tumors, sites of bleeding, mucosal or neoplastic lesions and for culture of *Helicobacter pylori* from stomach
Ultrasound	Use of piezoelectric crystal to generate sound waves that are reflected from tissue interfaces to provide an image	Imaging of abdominal organs (gallbladder, liver, pancreas, spleen), masses, stones, abscesses, structural abnormalities
Computed tomography (CT)	Use of a computer to integrate differences in absorption of a large number of x-rays to produce a cross-sectional image; may be done with contrast agents	Imaging of gallbladder, liver, pancreas, spleen, cysts, hematomas, abscesses, stones, extrahepatic bile ducts, and portal vein
Magnetic resonance imaging (MRI)	Projection of differences in magnetic properties of molecules within different cells and tissues, using the field of a large magnet	Same applications as CT scan; also can detect blood flow and vessel patency

eating stimulates the flow of pancreatic juice, the juice is most alkaline when it needs to be—during digestion. Secretion of the aqueous and enzymatic components of pancreatic juice is controlled by hormonal and vagal stimuli.

The *pancreatic enzymes* hydrolyze proteins (proteases), carbohydrates (amylases), and fats (lipases). The proteases include trypsin, chymotrypsin, carboxypeptidase, and elastase. These enzymes are secreted in their inactive forms—that is, as trypsinogen, chymotrypsinogen, and procarboxypeptidase—to protect the pancreas from the digestive effects of its own enzymes. For further protection the pancreas produces **trypsin inhibitor,** which prevents the activation of proteolytic enzymes while they are in the pancreas. Once in the duodenum, the inactive forms (proenzymes) are activated by **enterokinase,** an enzyme secreted by the duodenal mucosa. Trypsinogen is the first proenzyme to be activated. Its conversion to trypsin stimulates the conversion of chymotrypsinogen to chymotrypsin and procarboxypeptidase to carboxypeptidase. Each of these enzymes cleaves specific peptide bonds to reduce polypeptides to smaller peptides.

Pancreatic α-amylase is secreted in active form and digests intestinal carbohydrate by cleaving interior α-1,4-glucosidic bonds to yield glucose and maltose at an optimum pH of approximately 6.9. **Pancreatic lipases** hydrolyze triglycerides, cholesterol, and phospholipids to free fatty acids in the intestine. *Secretin* stimulates the acinar and duct cells to secrete the bicarbonate-rich fluid that neutralizes chyme and prepares it for enzymatic digestion. As chyme enters the duodenum, its acidity (pH of 4.5 or less) stimulates the **S cells** of the duodenum to release secretin, which is absorbed by the intestine and delivered to the pancreas in the bloodstream. In the pancreas, secretin causes ductal and acinar cells to release alkaline fluid. Secretin also inhibits the actions of gastrin, thereby decreasing gastric hydrochloric acid secretion and motility. The overall effect is to neutralize the contents of the duodenum.

Enzymatic secretion follows, stimulated by **cholecystokinin,** which activates ACh from the vagus nerve and release of ACh from pancreatic stellate cells.[39] Cholecystokinin is released in the duodenum in response to the essential amino acids and fatty acids already present in chyme. Once in the small intestine, activated pancreatic enzymes inhibit the release of more cholecystokinin and ACh. This feedback mechanism inhibits the secretion of more pancreatic enzymes. Pancreatic polypeptide is released after eating and inhibits postprandial pancreatic exocrine secretion. (Table 40-1 summarizes hormonal stimulation of pancreatic secretions.)

TESTS OF DIGESTIVE FUNCTION

Gastrointestinal Tract

Although important diagnostic information can be obtained from the patient's medical history and presenting symptoms, numerous disease-specific tests must be performed to evaluate the structure and function of the gastrointestinal tract. A description of selected studies is presented in Tables 40-4 and 40-5. Radiography and imaging techniques—including radionuclide, positron emission tomography (PET), magnetic resonance (MR), computed tomography (CT) scanning, and ultrasound—are procedures for evaluating structure and function. Plain radiographs using contrast media such as barium- or iodine-containing compounds can be used to outline the gastrointestinal lumen, biliary tree and pancreatic ducts, fistulae, and arteriovenous systems. CT scanning is particularly useful for diagnosis of intestinal lesions and pancreatic or hepatic tumors or cysts. Ultrasonic scanning is a safe, simple, and relatively inexpensive technique used to detect gallstones and intra-abdominal masses, particularly abscesses.

TABLE 40-5 SELECTED TESTS OF GASTROINTESTINAL FUNCTION

TEST	NORMAL FINDINGS	CLINICAL SIGNIFICANCE OF ABNORMAL FINDINGS
Stool studies	Resident microorganisms: clostridia, enterococci, *Pseudomonas,* a few yeasts	Detection of *Salmonella typhi* (typhoid fever), *Shigella* (dysentery), *Vibrio cholerae* (cholera), *Yersinia* (enterocolitis), *Escherichia coli* (gastroenteritis), *Staphylococcus aureus* (food poisoning), *Clostridium botulinum* (food poisoning), *Clostridium perfringens* (food poisoning), *Aeromonas* (gastroenteritis)
	Fat: 2-6 g/24 hr	Steatorrhea (increased values) can result from intestinal malabsorption or pancreatic insufficiency
	Pus: none	Large amounts of pus are associated with chronic ulcerative colitis, abscesses, and anorectal fistula
	Occult blood: none (orthotolidine or guaiac test)	Positive tests associated with bleeding
	Ova and parasites: none	Detection of *Entamoeba histolytica* (amebiasis), *Giardia lamblia* (giardiasis), and worms
D-Xylose absorption	5-hr urinary excretion: 4.5 g/L Peak blood level: >30 mg/dl	Differentiation of pancreatic steatorrhea (normal D-xylose absorption) from intestinal steatorrhea (impaired D-xylose absorption)
Gastric acid stimulation	11-20 mEq/hr after stimulation	Detection of duodenal ulcers, Zollinger-Ellison syndrome (increased values), gastric atrophy, gastric carcinoma (decreased values)
Manometry (use of water-filled catheters connected to pressure transducers passed into the esophagus, stomach, colon, or rectum to evaluate contractility)	Values vary at different levels of the intestine	Inadequate swallowing, motility, sphincter function
Culture and sensitivity of duodenal contents	No pathogens	Detection of *Salmonella typhi* (typhoid fever)
Breath tests		
Glucose or D-xylose breath test	Negative for hydrogen or CO_2	May indicate intestinal bacterial overgrowth
Urea breath test	Negative for isotopically labeled CO_2	Presence of *Helicobacter pylori* infection
Lactose breath test	Negative for exhaled hydrogen	Lactose intolerance

Fiberoptic endoscopy, using flexible endoscopes, allows direct visualization of the gastrointestinal tract. A biopsy channel allows tissue sampling, and suction can be applied to remove gastrointestinal secretions or blood. Analysis of stool, gastric secretions, tissue, and plasma provides important clues to infection, malabsorption syndromes, ulcerative lesions, and tumor growth.

Liver

A variety of diagnostic tests can be performed to evaluate liver function[40,41] (Table 40-6). Imaging techniques similar to those described for the gastrointestinal tract also are useful for evaluating liver structure and function. Nuclear imaging is useful after liver transplant.[42] Elevated plasma levels of liver enzymes are associated with many liver diseases because of the release of cytoplasmic enzymes into the circulation when there is damage to the hepatocyte. Of particular importance are elevations of aminotransferases and lactate dehydrogenase (LDH). Obstruction of bile canaliculi or ducts results in regurgitation of bile back into the hepatic sinusoids and into the circulation, manifesting with elevation of conjugated bilirubin levels. Prothrombin times (a measure of clotting tendency) are often prolonged with both hepatitis and chronic liver disease. In severe disease, other plasma proteins, such as albumin and globulins, may be diminished as a result of hepatocyte damage. Liver biopsies are often performed to evaluate the extent of liver involvement or degeneration with cirrhosis, hepatitis, or fatty liver disease.

Gallbladder

Evaluation of structural alterations in the gallbladder may be achieved by the use of various imaging techniques. Table 40-7 summarizes these techniques. Obstruction of the bile ducts from stones, tumors, or inflammation prevents the flow of bile from the liver and gallbladder from reaching the gastrointestinal tract. Both the conjugated and total serum bilirubin values are elevated, urine urobilinogen level is increased, stools are clay colored, and jaundice develops. Fat absorption can be impaired and the prothrombin time prolonged if vitamin K is not absorbed. With inflammation of the gallbladder, the white cell count is elevated.

Exocrine Pancreas

Tests of pancreatic function are summarized in Table 40-8. Evaluation of serum lipase and urinary amylase provides particularly significant measures of pancreatic injury. Inflammation or obstruction of the pancreas results in an early increase in serum amylase levels. Serum lipase level remains elevated after serum amylase has returned to normal levels and provides greater sensitivity with delayed presentation of pancreatitis. Elevation of urine amylase level also occurs later (after 48 hours) when serum amylase may have returned to normal levels. Urinary trypsinogen 2 (available as dipstick) is used to diagnose acute pancreatitis and is comparable to serum amylase and lipase.[43] Increased stool fat can reflect pancreatic insufficiency caused by decreased lipase secretion when biliary function is normal.

TABLE 40-6 COMMON LIVER FUNCTION TESTS

TEST	NORMAL VALUE	INTERPRETATION
Serum Enzymes		
Alkaline phosphatase	13-39 units/L	Increases with biliary obstruction and cholestatic hepatitis
Gamma-glutamyltranspeptidase (GGT)	Male 12-38 units/L Female 9-31 units/L	Increases with biliary obstruction and cholestatic hepatitis
Aspartate aminotransferase (AST; previously serum glutamate-oxaloacetate transaminase [SGOT])	5-40 units/L	Increases with hepatocellular injury (and injury in other tissues, i.e., skeletal and cardiac muscle)
Alanine aminotransferase (ALT; previously serum glutamate-pyruvate transaminase [SGPT])	5-35 units/L	Increases with hepatocellular injury and necrosis
Lactate dehydrogenase (LDH)	90-220 units/L	Isoenzyme LD_5 is elevated with hypoxic and primary liver injury
5′-Nucleotidase	2-11 units/L	Increases with increase in alkaline phosphatase and cholestatic disorders
Bilirubin Metabolism		
Serum bilirubin		
Unconjugated (indirect)	<0.8 mg/dl	Increases with hemolysis (lysis of red blood cells)
Conjugated (direct)	0.2-0.4 mg/dl	Increases with hepatocellular injury or obstruction
TOTAL	<1.0 mg/dl	Increases with biliary obstruction
Urine bilirubin	0	Increases with biliary obstruction
Urine urobilinogen	0-4 mg/24 hr	Increases with hemolysis or shunting of portal blood flow
Serum Proteins		
Albumin	3.5-5.5 g/dl	Reduced with hepatocellular injury
Globulin	2.5-3.5 g/dl	Increases with hepatitis
TOTAL	6-7 g/dl	
Albumin/globulin (A/G) ratio	1.5:1 to 2.5:1	Ratio reverses with chronic hepatitis or other chronic liver disease
Transferrin	250-300 mcg/dl	Liver damage with decreased values, iron deficiency with increased values
Alpha fetoprotein (AFP)	6-20 ng/ml	Elevated values in primary hepatocellular carcinoma
Blood-Clotting Functions		
Prothrombin time (PT)	11.5-14 sec or 90-100% of control	Increases with chronic liver disease (cirrhosis) or vitamin K deficiency
Partial thromboplastin time (PTT)	25-40 sec	Increases with severe liver disease or heparin therapy
Bromsulphthalein (BSP) excretion	<6% retention in 45 min	Increased retention with hepatocellular injury

TABLE 40-7 DIAGNOSTIC EVALUATION OF THE GALLBLADDER

TEST	APPLICATION
Plain roentgenogram of the abdomen	Visualization of calcified gallstones
Oral cholecystogram (use of an oral contrast medium such as iopanoic acid, which is excreted with bile and concentrated in the gallbladder for visualization by radiography; may be administered as a double dose)	Visualization of gallstones; evaluation of filling and emptying of gallbladder
Intravenous cholangiography (use of intravenous contrast agents for visualization of gallbladder and bile ducts)	Diagnosis of acute gallbladder inflammation (cholecystitis) or disease of bile ducts
Cholecystography (ultrasound imaging of gallbladder and bile ducts)	Preferred method for detecting gallstones; differentiation of hepatic disease from biliary obstruction; diagnosis of chronic cholecystitis
Cholescintigraphy (radioisotope imaging of gallbladder)	Diagnosis of cholecystitis in individuals allergic to iodine-containing contrast agents; diagnosis of cystic duct obstruction
Endoscopic retrograde cholangiography (instillation of contrast medium through cannulation of ampulla of Vater with a duodenoscope)	Differentiation of intrahepatic or extrahepatic obstructive jaundice
Computed tomography (CT)	Diagnosis of biliary obstruction or malignancy when ultrasound is not successful

AGING AND THE GASTROINTESTINAL SYSTEM

Age-related changes in gastrointestinal function can begin to occur before 50 years of age.[44] Tooth enamel and dentin wear down, making the teeth vulnerable to cavities. Teeth are lost, often as a result of periodontal (gum) disease, recession of the gums, osteoporotic bone changes, and more brittle roots that fracture easily. Taste buds decline in number, and the sense of smell diminishes.[45] Together these losses decrease the sense of taste. Salivary secretion decreases and contributes to dry mouth and loss of taste.[46] In very old adults these oral and sensory changes make eating less pleasurable and reduce appetite. Food may not be chewed or lubricated sufficiently, making

TABLE 40-8 SELECTED TESTS OF PANCREATIC FUNCTION

TEST	NORMAL VALUE	CLINICAL SIGNIFICANCE
Serum amylase	60-180 Somogyi units/ml	Elevated levels with pancreatic inflammation
Serum lipase	1.5 Somogyi units/ml	Elevated levels with pancreatic inflammation (may be elevated with other conditions; differentiates with amylase isoenzyme study)
Urine amylase	35-260 Somogyi units/hr	Elevated levels with pancreatic inflammation
Secretin test	Volume 1.8 ml/kg/hr Bicarbonate concentration: >80 mEq/L Bicarbonate output: >10 mEq/L/30 sec	Decreased volume with pancreatic disease as secretin stimulates pancreatic secretion
Stool fat	2-5 g/24 hr	Measures fatty acids; decreased pancreatic lipase increases stool fat

swallowing difficult. The esophagus develops decreased motility, and changes in the upper esophageal sphincter, history of stroke, and dementia may affect swallowing and contribute to gastroesophageal reflux.[47]

Age also diminishes gastric motility and volume, including secretion of bicarbonate and gastric mucus in some individuals. Acid content of gastric juice is related to gastric atrophy, which results in hypochlorhydria (insufficient hydrochloric acid), delayed gastric emptying, and compromise of the gastric mucosal barrier.[48] Decreased production of intrinsic factor leads to inadequate small intestinal absorption of vitamin B_{12} and pernicious anemia.[49] Aging may be associated with a change in the composition of the intestinal microflora and increased susceptibility to disease.[50] The ileal villi of the small intestine may become broader and shorter, perhaps because of a decrease in cell turnover. Intestinal absorption, motility, and blood flow decrease, impairing nutrient absorption.[51] Proteins, fats, minerals (including iron and calcium), and vitamins are absorbed more slowly and in lesser amounts, and absorption of carbohydrates is decreased. Intestinal transit time is delayed. Constipation is often described as a condition of old age, but it is probably caused by lifestyle factors (e.g., diet, lack of fluid intake) rather than physiologic decline although studies demonstrate there can be alterations in intestinal innervation.[52]

The rate of liver regeneration decreases with advancing age but the volume of the liver can be maintained.[53] Alterations in liver function in older individuals are usually a sign of a pathologic condition. Liver blood flow and enzyme activity decrease with age and can influence the efficiency of drug and alcohol metabolism.[54] However, liver function test results often remain within relatively normal ranges. Alterations in liver function in older individuals are usually a sign of a pathologic condition. The pancreas undergoes structural changes, such as fibrosis, fatty acid deposits, and atrophy. Pancreatic secretion decreases, but there is usually no observable dysfunction.[55] Aging does not cause apparent changes in the structure and function of the gallbladder and bile ducts, but the incidence of gallstones increases.[56]

SUMMARY REVIEW

The Gastrointestinal Tract

1. The major functions of the gastrointestinal tract are the mechanical and chemical breakdown of food and the absorption of digested nutrients.
2. The gastrointestinal tract is a hollow tube that extends from the mouth to the anus.
3. The walls of the gastrointestinal tract have several layers: mucosa, muscularis mucosa, submucosa, muscularis (circular muscle and longitudinal muscle), and serosa (adventitia in the esophagus).
4. Except for swallowing and defecation, which are controlled voluntarily, the functions of the gastrointestinal tract are controlled by extrinsic autonomic nerves (vagus, parasympathetic splanchnic, and sympathetic nerves) and intrinsic autonomic nerves (enteric nervous system) and intestinal hormones.
5. Digestion begins in the mouth, with chewing and salivation. The digestive component of saliva is α-amylase, which initiates carbohydrate digestion.
6. The esophagus is a muscular tube that transports food from the mouth to the stomach. The muscularis in the upper part of the esophagus is striated muscle, and that in the lower part is smooth muscle.
7. Swallowing is controlled by the swallowing center in the reticular formation of the brain. The two phases of swallowing are the oropharyngeal phase (voluntary swallowing) and the esophageal phase (involuntary swallowing).
8. Food is propelled through the gastrointestinal tract by peristalsis: waves of sequential relaxations and contractions of the muscularis.
9. The lower esophageal sphincter opens to admit swallowed food into the stomach and then closes to prevent regurgitation of food back into the esophagus.
10. The stomach is a baglike structure that secretes digestive juices, mixes and stores food, and propels partially digested food (chyme) into the duodenum. The smooth muscles of the stomach include the outer longitudinal, middle circular, and internal oblique.
11. The vagus nerve stimulates gastric (stomach) secretion and motility.
12. The hormones gastrin and motilin stimulate gastric emptying; the hormones secretin and cholecystokinin delay gastric emptying.
13. Gastric glands in the fundus and body of the stomach secrete intrinsic factor, which is needed for vitamin B_{12} absorption,

SUMMARY REVIEW—cont'd

and hydrochloric acid, which dissolves food fibers, kills microorganisms, and activates the enzyme pepsin.

14. Chief cells in the stomach secrete pepsinogen, which is converted to pepsin in the acidic environment created by hydrochloric acid.
15. Acid secretion is stimulated by the vagus nerve, gastrin, and histamine and inhibited by sympathetic stimulation and cholecystokinin. Acetylcholine stimulates pepsin secretion.
16. Mucus is secreted throughout the stomach and protects the stomach wall from acid and digestive enzymes.
17. The three phases of acid secretion by the stomach are the cephalic phase (anticipation and swallowing), the gastric phase (food in the stomach), and the intestinal phase (chyme in the intestine).
18. The small intestine is 5 m long and has three segments: the duodenum, jejunum, and ileum. Digestion and absorption of all major nutrients and most ingested water occur in the small intestine.
19. The peritoneum is a double layer of membranous tissue. The visceral layer covers the abdominal organs, and the parietal layer extends along the abdominal wall.
20. Blood flow to the small intestine is primarily provided by the superior mesenteric artery.
21. The duodenum receives chyme from the stomach through the pyloric valve. The presence of chyme stimulates the liver and gallbladder to deliver bile and the pancreas to deliver digestive enzymes and alkaline secretions. Bile and enzymes flow through an opening guarded by the sphincter of Oddi.
22. Bile is produced by the liver and is necessary for fat digestion and absorption. Bile's alkalinity helps neutralize chyme, thereby creating a pH that enables the pancreatic enzymes to digest proteins, carbohydrates, and sugars.
23. Enzymes secreted by the small intestine (maltase, sucrase, lactase), pancreatic enzymes (proteases, amylase, and lipase), and bile salts act in the small intestine to digest proteins, carbohydrates, and fats.
24. Digested substances are absorbed across the intestinal wall and then transported to the liver through the hepatic portal vein, where they are metabolized further.
25. The ileocecal valve connects the small and large intestines and prevents reflux into the small intestine.
26. Villi are small fingerlike projections that extend from the small intestinal mucosa and increase its absorptive surface area.
27. Carbohydrates, amino acids, and fats are absorbed primarily by the duodenum and jejunum; bile salts and vitamin B_{12} are absorbed by the ileum. Vitamin B_{12} absorption requires the presence of intrinsic factor.
28. Bile salts emulsify and hydrolyze fats and incorporate them into water-soluble micelles that transport them through the unstirred layer to the brush border of the intestinal mucosa. The fat content of the micelles readily diffuses through the epithelium into lacteals (lymphatic ducts) in the villi. From there fats flow into the lymphatics and into the systemic circulation, which delivers them to the liver.
29. Minerals and water-soluble vitamins are absorbed by active and passive transport throughout the small intestine.
30. Peristaltic movements created by longitudinal muscles propel the chyme along the intestinal tract, whereas contractions of the circular muscles (segmentation) mix the chyme and promote digestion.
31. The ileogastric reflex inhibits gastric motility when the ileum is distended.
32. The intestinointestinal reflex inhibits intestinal motility when one intestinal segment is overdistended.
33. The gastroileal reflex increases intestinal motility when gastric motility increases.
34. The large intestine consists of the cecum, appendix, colon (ascending, transverse, descending, and sigmoid), rectum, and anal canal.
35. The teniae coli are three bands of longitudinal muscle that extend the length of the colon.
36. Haustra are pouches of colon that are formed with alternating contraction and relaxation of the circular muscles.
37. The mucosa of the large intestine contains mucus-secreting cells and mucosal folds, but no villi.
38. The large intestine massages the fecal mass and absorbs water and electrolytes.
39. Distention of the ileum with chyme causes the gastrocolic reflex, or the mass propulsion of feces to the rectum.
40. Defecation is stimulated when the rectum is distended with feces. The conically contracted internal anal sphincter relaxes and, if the voluntarily regulated external sphincter relaxes, defecation occurs.
41. The largest numbers of intestinal bacteria are in the colon. They are anaerobes consisting of *Bacteroides,* clostridia, coliforms, and lactobacilli.
42. The intestinal tract is sterile at birth and becomes totally colonized within 3 to 4 weeks.
43. Endogenous infections of the gastrointestinal tract occur by excessive proliferation of bacteria, perforation of the intestine, or contamination from neighboring structures.

Accessory Organs of Digestion

1. The liver is the largest organ in the body. It has digestive, metabolic, hematologic, vascular, and immunologic functions.
2. The liver is divided into the right and left lobes and is supported by the falciform, round, and coronary ligaments.
3. Liver lobules consist of plates of hepatocytes, which are the functional cells of the liver.
4. The hepatic artery supplies blood to the liver. The portal vein receives blood from the inferior and superior mesenteric veins.
5. Hepatocytes synthesize 700 to 1200 ml of bile per day and secrete it into the bile canaliculi, which are small channels between the hepatocytes. The bile canaliculi drain bile into the common bile duct and then into the duodenum through an opening called the *major duodenal papilla (sphincter of Oddi).*

SUMMARY REVIEW—cont'd

6. Sinusoids are capillaries located between the plates of hepatocytes. Blood from the hepatic portal vein and hepatic artery flows through the sinusoids to a central vein in each lobule and then into the hepatic vein and inferior vena cava.
7. Kupffer cells, which are part of the mononuclear phagocyte system, line the sinusoids and destroy microorganisms in sinusoidal blood.
8. The primary bile acids are synthesized from cholesterol by the hepatocytes. The primary acids are then conjugated to form bile salts. The secondary bile acids are the product of bile salt deconjugation by bacteria in the intestinal lumen.
9. Most bile salts and acids are recycled. The absorption of bile salts and acids from the terminal ileum and their return to the liver are known as the enterohepatic circulation of bile.
10. Bilirubin is a pigment liberated by the lysis of aged red blood cells in the liver and spleen. Unconjugated bilirubin is fat soluble and can cross cell membranes. Unconjugated bilirubin is converted to water-soluble, conjugated bilirubin by hepatocytes and is secreted with bile.
11. Fats are synthesized by the liver from protein and carbohydrates and include glycerol, free fatty acids, phospholipids, and cholesterol. Fat absorbed by intestinal lacteals is primarily triglyceride, which is hydrolyzed to glycerol and free fatty acid.
12. Protein synthesis by the liver requires all essential amino acids. The liver synthesizes albumin, globulin, and several serum enzymes and can convert amino acids to carbohydrates by removal of ammonia.
13. Carbohydrates can be released as glucose, stored as glycogen, or converted to fat.
14. The liver performs many metabolic functions including detoxification of exogenous and endogenous chemicals and hormones.
15. The gallbladder is a saclike organ located in the inferior surface of the liver. The gallbladder stores bile between meals and ejects it when chyme enters the duodenum.
16. Stimulated by cholecystokinin, the gallbladder contracts and forces bile through the cystic duct and into the common bile duct. The sphincter of Oddi relaxes, enabling bile to flow through the major duodenal papilla into the duodenum.
17. The pancreas is a gland located behind the stomach. The endocrine pancreas produces hormones (glucagon and insulin) that facilitate the formation and cellular uptake of glucose. The exocrine pancreas secretes an alkaline solution and the enzymes (trypsin, chymotrypsin, carboxypeptidase, α-amylase, lipase) that digest proteins, carbohydrates, and fats.
18. Secretin stimulates pancreatic secretion of alkaline fluid, and cholecystokinin and ACh stimulate secretion of enzymes. Pancreatic secretions originate in acini and ducts of the pancreas and empty into the duodenum through the common bile duct or an accessory duct that opens directly into the duodenum.

Tests of Digestive Function

1. Numerous diagnostic tests can evaluate structure and function (digestion, secretion, absorption) of the gastrointestinal tract. Radiographs and scans are most commonly used to evaluate structure, in addition to direct observation by endoscopy. Gastric and stool analysis and blood studies provide important information about digestion, absorption, and secretion.
2. Plasma chemistry levels and imaging procedures are commonly used to diagnose alterations in liver function. Of particular importance are the enzymes LDH, AST, and ALT. Plasma bilirubin levels reflect alterations in bilirubin and bile metabolism, and prothrombin times are prolonged in hepatitis and chronic liver disease.
3. Obstructive diseases of the gallbladder are evident by elevated serum bilirubin levels, elevated urine urobilinogen levels, and increased stool fat. The serum leukocyte levels become elevated with inflammation of the gallbladder.
4. The most significant indicators of pancreatic dysfunction are serum amylase and stool fat. Both values are increased with diseases of the pancreas.

Aging and the Gastrointestinal System

1. Advancing age is often associated with the loss or deterioration of teeth, diminished senses of taste and smell, and diminished salivary secretions, all of which may make eating difficult and reduce appetite.
2. Aging reduces gastric motility and secretions, particularly of hydrochloric acid. These changes slow gastric digestion and emptying.
3. Intestinal motility and absorption of carbohydrates, proteins, fats, and minerals decrease with age.
4. Efficiency of drug and alcohol metabolism decreases with age and can be related to decreased liver perfusion and decreased liver enzymes.

KEY TERMS

Alanine aminotransferase (ALT), 1413
Alkaline phosphatase, 1413
Ampulla of Vater, 1411, 1413
Antrum of stomach, 1396
Ascending colon, 1407
Aspartate aminotransferase (AST), 1413
Bile, 1411
Bile acid–dependent fraction, 1411
Bile acid–independent fraction, 1411
Bile acid pool, 1411
Bile canaliculi, 1411
Bile salt, 1411
Bilirubin, 1411
Biliverdin, 1411
Body of stomach, 1396
Brush border, 1401
Calcium, 1405
Carboxypeptidase, 1402
Cardiac orifice, 1396
Cecum, 1407
Cephalic phase of secretion, 1400
Chief cell, 1398
Cholecystokinin, 1398, 1415
Choleresis, 1411
Choleretic agent, 1411
Cholesterol esterase, 1404
Chylomicron, 1405
Chyme, 1396
Chymotrypsin, 1402
Colipase, 1404
Colon, 1407
Common bile duct, 1411
Conjugated bilirubin, 1411

KEY TERMS—cont'd

Crypts of Lieberkühn, 1401
Cystic duct, 1413
D cell, 1398
Deamination, 1412
Defecation reflex (rectosphincteric reflex), 1408
Descending colon, 1407
Disse space, 1410
Duodenum, 1400
Emulsification, 1404
Enteric nervous system, 1394
Enterochromaffin-like cell, 1398
Enterohepatic circulation, 1411
Enterokinase, 1415
Esophageal phase of swallowing, 1395
Esophagus, 1395
Exocrine pancreas, 1413
External anal sphincter, 1407
Fat, 1402
Fecal mass, 1408
Feces, 1408
Fundus of stomach, 1396
G cell, 1398
Gallbladder, 1413
Gamma-glutamyltransferase, 1413
Gastric emptying, 1397
Gastric gland, 1398
Gastric hydrochloric acid, 1398
Gastric phase of secretion, 1400
Gastric pit, 1398
Gastrin, 1397
Gastrocolic reflex, 1408
Gastroileal reflex, 1407
Gastrointestinal tract (alimentary canal), 1393
Haustrum (*pl.*, haustra), 1407
Hepatic artery, 1409
Hepatic portal vein, 1409
Hepatic vein, 1409
Hepatocyte, 1409
Hepcidin, 1406
Histamine, 1398
Ileocecal valve (sphincter), 1400, 1407
Ileogastric reflex, 1407
Ileum, 1400
Internal anal sphincter, 1407
Intestinal peristalsis, 1407
Intestinal phase of secretion, 1400
Intestinointestinal reflex, 1407
Intrinsic factor (IF), 1399
Iron, 1405
Jejunum, 1400
Kupffer cell, 1410
Lactate dehydrogenase (LDH), 1413
Lacteal, 1401
Lamina propria, 1401
Large intestine, 1407
Lipase, 1404
Lipocyte, 1409
Lipolysis, 1404
Liver, 1409
Liver lobule, 1409
Lower esophageal sphincter (cardiac sphincter), 1395
Magnesium, 1405
Major duodenal papilla, 1411
Mesentery, 1401
Metabolic detoxification (biotransformation), 1413
Micelle, 1404
Microvillus (*pl.*, microvilli), 1401
Motilin, 1397
Mouth, 1395
Mucosal barrier, 1399
Myenteric plexus (Auerbach plexus), 1394
Oral phase of swallowing, 1395
Pancreas, 1413
Pancreatic α-amylase, 1415
Pancreatic duct (Wirsung duct), 1413
Pancreatic lipase, 1415
Paneth cell, 1401
Parietal cell (oxyntic cell), 1398
Pepsin, 1398, 1399
Pepsinogen, 1398
Peristaltic movement, 1408
Peritoneal cavity, 1401
Peritoneum, 1400
Pharyngeal phase of swallowing, 1395
Phases of gastric secretion, 1399
Phosphate, 1405
Phospholipase, 1404
Pit cell, 1410
Primary bile acid, 1411
Primary peristalsis, 1396
Pyloric sphincter, 1396
Rectosigmoid (O'Beirne) sphincter, 1407
Retropulsion, 1397
S cell, 1415
Saliva, 1395
Salivary α-amylase (ptyalin), 1395
Salivary gland, 1395
Secondary bile acid, 1411
Secondary peristalsis, 1396
Secretin, 1397
Segmentation, 1407
Sigmoid colon, 1407
Sinusoid, 1409
Small intestine, 1400
Somatostatin, 1398
Sphincter of Oddi, 1411, 1413
Stellate cell, 1410
Stem cell, 1401
Stomach, 1396
Submucosal plexus (Meissner plexus), 1394
Subserosal plexus, 1394
Swallowing, 1395
Teniae coli, 1407
Transverse colon, 1407
Trypsin, 1402
Trypsin inhibitor, 1415
Unconjugated bilirubin, 1411
Upper esophageal sphincter (cricopharyngeal muscle), 1395
Urobilinogen, 1412
Valsalva maneuver, 1408
Vermiform appendix, 1407
Villus (*pl.*, villi), 1401
Vitamin, 1406

REFERENCES

1. Furness JB: The enteric nervous system and neurogastroenterology, *Nat Rev Gastroenterol Hepatol* 9(5):286–294, 2012.
1a. Gröschl M: The physiological role of hormones in saliva, *Bioessays* 31(8):843–852, 2009.
2. Lang IM, Shaker R: An overview of the upper esophageal sphincter, *Curr Gastroenterol Rep* 2(3):185–190, 2000.
3. Hershcovici T, Mashimo H, Fass R: The lower esophageal sphincter, *Neurogastroenterol Motil 2011* 23(9):819–830, 2011.
4. Lang IM: Brain stem control of the phases of swallowing, *Dysphagia* 24(3):333–348, 2009.
5. Goyal RK, Chaudhury A: Physiology of normal esophageal motility, *J Clin Gastroentrol* 42(5):610–619, 2008.
6. Hellström PM, Grybäck P, Jacobsson H: The physiology of gastric emptying, *Best Pract Res Clin Anaesthesiol* 20(3):397–407, 2006.
7. Dockray GJ: Cholecystokinin, *Curr Opin Endocrinol Diabetes Obes* 19(1):8–12, 2012.
8. Middleton SJ, Balan K: Idiopathic accelerated gastric emptying presenting in adults with post-prandial diarrhea and reactive hypoglycemia: a case series, *J Med Case Rep* 6(1):132, 2012.
9. Chu S, Schubert ML: Gastric secretion, *Curr Opin Gastroenterol* 28(6):587–593, 2012.
10. Palileo C, Kaunitz JD: Gastrointestinal defense mechanisms, *Curr Opin Gastroenterol* 27(6):543–548, 2011.
11. Longkumer T et al: Assessment of vagotomy status with postprandial urinary alkaline tide, *Trop Gastroenterol* 30(2):91–94, 2009.
12. Ramsay PT, Carr A: Gastric acid and digestive physiology, *Surg Clin North Am* 91(5):977–982, 2011.
13. Schubert ML: Hormonal regulation of gastric acid secretion, *Curr Gastroenterol Rep* 10(6):523–527, 2008.
14. Tarnawski AS, Ahluwalia A, Jones MK: The mechanisms of gastric mucosal injury: focus on microvascular endothelium as a key target, *Curr Med Chem* 19(1):4–15, 2012.
15. Zafra MA, Molina F, Puerto A: The neural/cephalic phase reflexes in the physiology of nutrition, *Neurosci Biobehav Rev* 30(7):1032–1044, 2006.
16. Miller MJ, McDole JR, Newberry RD: Microanatomy of the intestinal lymphatic system, *Ann N Y Acad Sci* 1207(Suppl 1):E21–E28, 2010.
17. Santaolalla R, Abreu MT: Innate immunity in the small intestine, *Curr Opin Gastroenterol* 28(2):124–129, 2012.
18. Ashton KA et al: Basal and meal-stimulated colonic absorption, *Dis Colon Rectum* 39(8):865–870, 1996.
18a. Wright EM, Loo DD, Hirayama BA: Biology of human sodium glucose transporters, *Physiol Rev* 91(2):733–794, 2011.
19. Cheeseman C: GLUT7: a new intestinal facilitated hexose transporter, *Am J Physiol Endocrinol Metab* 295(2):E238–E241, 2008.
20. Leturque A, Brot-Laroche E, Le Gall M: GLUT2 mutations, translocation, and receptor function in diet sugar managing, *Am J Physiol Endocrinol Metab* 296(5):E985–E992, 2009.
21. Jahan-Mihan A et al: Dietary proteins as determinants of metabolic and physiologic functions of the gastrointestinal tract, *Nutrients* 3(5):574–603, 2011.
22. Christakos S et al: Vitamin D and intestinal calcium absorption, *Mol Cell Endocrinol* 347(1-2):25–29, 2011.
23. Drakesmith H, Prentice AM: Hepcidin and the iron-infection axis, *Science* 338(6108):768–772, 2012.
24. Husebye E: The patterns of small bowel motility: physiology and implications in organic disease and functional disorders, *Neurogastroenterol Motil* 11(3):141–161, 1999.

25. Lubbers T, Buurman W, Luyer M: Controlling postoperative ileus by vagal activation, *World J Gastroenterol* 16(14):1683–1687, 2010.
26. Byard RW: Acute mesenteric ischaemia and unexpected death, *J Forensic Leg Med* 19(4):185–190, 2012.
27. Manson JM, Rauch M, Gilmore MS: The commensal microbiology of the gastrointestinal tract, *Adv Exp Med Biol* 635:15–28, 2008.
28. Abraham C, Medzhitov R: Interactions between the host innate immune system and microbes in inflammatory bowel disease, *Gastroenterology* 140(6):1729–1737, 2011.
29. Resta SC: Effects of probiotics and commensals on intestinal epithelial physiology: implications for nutrient handling, *J Physiol* 587(Pt 17): 4169–4174, 2009.
30. Yokomori H et al: Recent advances in liver sinusoidal endothelial ultrastructure and fine structure immunocytochemistry, *Micron* 43(2-3): 129–134, 2012.
31. Yang Q et al: The evolving story of macrophages in acute liver failure, *Immunol Lett* 147(1-2):1–9, 2012.
32. Tacke F, Weiskirchen R: Update on hepatic stellate cells: pathogenic role in liver fibrosis and novel isolation techniques, *Expert Rev Gastroenterol Hepatol* 6(1):67–80, 2012.
33. Tian Z et al: Natural killer cells in liver disease, *Hepatol* 57(4):1654–1662, 2013.
34. Horiguchi S, Kamisawa T: Major duodenal papilla and its normal anatomy, *Dig Surg* 27(2):90–93, 2010.
35. Hofmann AF: The enterohepatic circulation of bile acids in mammals: form and functions, *Front Biosci* 14:2584–2598, 2009.
36. Jansen T et al: Conversion of biliverdin to bilirubin by biliverdin reductase contributes to endothelial cell protection by heme oxygenase-1—evidence for direct and indirect antioxidant actions of bilirubin, *J Mol Cell Cardiol* 49(2):186–195, 2010.
37. Jirásková A et al: Association of serum bilirubin and promoter variations in HMOX1 and UGT1A1 genes with sporadic colorectal cancer, *Int J Cancer* 131(7):1549–1555, 2012.
38. Rodriguez-Diaz R et al: Innervation patterns of autonomic axons in the human endocrine pancreas, *Cell Metab* 14(1):45–54, 2011.
39. Chandra R, Liddle RA: Recent advances in pancreatic endocrine and exocrine secretion, *Curr Opin Gastroenterol* 27(5):439–443, 2011.
40. Aranda-Michel J, Sherman KE: Tests of the liver: use and misuse, *Gastroenterologist* 6(1):34–43, 1998.
41. Johnston DE: Special considerations in interpreting liver function tests, *Am Fam Physician* 59(8):2223–2230, 1999.
42. Hoekstra LT et al: Physiological and biochemical basis of clinical liver function tests: a review, *Ann Surg* 257(1):27–36, 2013.
43. Mayumi T et al: Validity of the urinary trypsinogen-2 test in the diagnosis of acute pancreatitis, *Pancreas* 41(6):869–875, 2012.
44. Grassi M et al: Changes, functional disorders, and diseases in the gastrointestinal tract of elderly, *Nutr Hosp* 26(4):659–668, 2011.
45. Gaines AD: Anosmia and hyposmia, *Allergy Asthma Proc* 31(3):185–189, 2010.
46. Gupta A, Epstein JB, Sroussi H: Hyposalivation in elderly patients, *J Can Dent Assoc* 72(9):841–846, 2006.
47. Sura L et al: Dysphagia in the elderly: management and nutritional considerations, *Clin Interv Aging* 7:287–298, 2012.
48. Salles N: Is stomach spontaneously ageing? Pathophysiology of the ageing stomach, *Best Pract Res Clin Gastroenterol* 23(6):805–819, 2009.
49. Patel KV: Epidemiology of anemia in older adults, *Semin Hematol* 45(4):210–217, 2008.
50. Tiihonen K, Ouwehand AC, Rautonen N: Human intestinal microbiota and healthy ageing, *Ageing Res Rev* 9(2):107–116, 2010.
51. Drozdowski L, Thomson AB: Aging and the intestine, *World J Gastroenterol* 12(47):7578–7584, 2006.
52. Rayner CK, Horowitz M: Physiology of the ageing gut, *Curr Opin Clin Nutr Metab Care* 16(1):33–38, 2013.
53. Schmucker DL, Sanchez H: Liver regeneration and aging: a current perspective, *Curr Gerontol Geriatr Res* 2011:526379, 2011.
54. McLachlan AJ, Pont LG: Drug metabolism in older people—a key consideration in achieving optimal outcomes with medicines, *J Gerontol A Biol Sci Med Sci* 67(2):175–180, 2012.
55. Herzig KH et al: Fecal pancreatic elastase-1 levels in older individuals without known gastrointestinal diseases or diabetes mellitus, *BMC Geriatr* 11:4, 2011.
56. Stinton LM, Shaffer EA: Epidemiology of gallbladder disease: cholelithiasis and cancer, *Gut Liver* 6(2):172–187, 2012.

CHAPTER

41

Alterations of Digestive Function

Alexa K. Doig and Sue E. Huether

evolve WEBSITE

http://evolve.elsevier.com/McCance/

- Review Questions and Answers
- Animations
- Online Course: Module 17

CHAPTER OUTLINE

Disorders of the gastrointestinal tract disrupt one or more of its functions. Structural and neural abnormalities can slow, obstruct, or accelerate the movement of intestinal content at any level of the gastrointestinal tract. Inflammatory and ulcerative conditions of the gastrointestinal wall disrupt secretion, motility, and absorption. Inflammation or obstruction of the liver, pancreas, or gallbladder can alter metabolism and result in local or systemic symptoms, or both. Many clinical manifestations of gastrointestinal tract disorders are nonspecific and can be caused by a variety of impairments. These manifestations are described in the section below.

DISORDERS OF THE GASTROINTESTINAL TRACT

Clinical Manifestations of Gastrointestinal Dysfunction

Anorexia

Anorexia is lack of a desire to eat despite physiologic stimuli that would normally produce hunger. Anorexia is a nonspecific symptom that is often associated with nausea, abdominal pain, diarrhea, and psychologic distress. Side effects of drugs and disorders of other organ systems, including cancer, heart disease, and renal disease, are often accompanied by anorexia.

Vomiting

Vomiting is the forceful emptying of stomach and intestinal contents through the mouth. The vomiting center lies in the medulla oblongata and includes the reticular formation and tractus solitarius nucleus. Stimulation of the vomiting center occurs directly by irritants or indirectly. Indirect stimulation includes the cerebral cortex and thalamus (anxiety and pain); the vestibular system through the eighth cranial nerve (motion sickness); several types of intestinal, vagal, or sympathetic input, including the presence of ipecac or copper salts in the duodenum; side effects of many drugs; distention of the stomach or duodenum; or torsion or trauma affecting the ovaries, testes, uterus, bladder, or kidney. Serotonin (5-hydroxytryptamine [5-HT]) stimulates the vomiting center and appears to be released from enterochromaffin cells in the intestinal wall, which activate vagal afferents leading to the chemoreceptor trigger zone (CTZ).[1] Activation of the CTZ, which lies in the area postrema between the medulla and floor of the fourth ventricle, leads to vomiting by triggering receptors for substances such as dopamine (D_2), opioids, acetylcholine, substance P, serotonin (5-hydroxytryptamine type 3), and neurokinin-1. Serotonin and neurokinin-1 antagonists are effective antiemetics and have been used to treat nausea and vomiting associated with postoperative vomiting and cancer chemotherapy. Apomorphine, levodopa, and bromocriptine are dopamine D_2 agonists that cause nausea and vomiting. Metoclopramide, domperidone, and haloperidol are D_2 antagonists and are effective antiemetics.[2]

Nausea and retching usually precede vomiting although they are distinct entities. **Nausea** is a subjective experience that is associated with many different conditions, including visceral pain, labyrinthine stimulation (i.e., motion), and use of opiate medications. Specific neural pathways have not been identified for nausea. Hypersalivation and tachycardia are common associated symptoms.

With vomiting, the duodenum and antrum of the stomach produce retrograde peristalsis while the body of the stomach and the esophagus relax. When the stomach is full of gastric contents, the diaphragm is forced high into the thoracic cavity by strong contractions of the abdominal muscles. The higher intrathoracic pressure forces the upper esophageal sphincter to open, and chyme is expelled from the mouth. Then the stomach relaxes and the upper part of the esophagus contracts, forcing the remaining chyme back into the stomach. The lower esophageal sphincter then closes. The cycle is repeated if there is a volume of chyme remaining in the stomach.

Retching is the muscular event of vomiting without the expulsion of vomitus. Retching begins with deep inspiration. The glottis then closes, intrathoracic pressure falls, and the esophagus becomes distended. Simultaneously, the abdominal muscles contract creating a pressure gradient from abdomen to thorax. The lower esophageal sphincter and body of the stomach relax, but the duodenum and antrum of the stomach spasm. The reverse peristalsis and pressure gradient force chyme from the stomach and duodenum up into the esophagus. Because the upper esophageal sphincter is closed, chyme does not enter the mouth. As the abdominal muscles relax, the contents of the esophagus drop back into the stomach. This process may be repeated several times before vomiting occurs. A diffuse sympathetic discharge causes the tachycardia, tachypnea, and sweating that accompany retching and vomiting. The parasympathetic system mediates copious salivation, increased gastric motility, and relaxation of the upper and lower esophageal sphincters.

Projectile vomiting is spontaneous vomiting that is not preceded by nausea or retching. Projectile vomiting is caused by direct stimulation of the vomiting center by neurologic lesions (e.g., increased intracranial pressure, tumors, or aneurysms involving the brainstem [see Chapters 17 and 20]). The metabolic consequences of vomiting are fluid, electrolyte, and acid-base disturbances, including hyponatremia, hypokalemia, hypochloremia, and metabolic alkalosis (see Chapter 3).

Constipation

Constipation is difficult or infrequent defecation and is estimated to affect 2% to 28% of the population. Constipation must be individually defined because patterns of bowel evacuation differ greatly among individuals. Normal bowel habits range from two or three evacuations per day to one per week. Constipation is not significant until it causes health risks (e.g., severe abdominal distention or fecal impaction) or impairs quality of life.[3]

PATHOPHYSIOLOGY. Primary constipation is generally classified into three categories. *Normal transit (functional) constipation* involves a normal rate of stool passage but there is difficulty with stool evacuation. Functional constipation is most common and is associated with low-residue diet (the habitual consumption of highly refined foods) or low fluid intake, which decreases the volume and number of stools and can contribute to constipation. Physical activity stimulates peristalsis; therefore, a sedentary lifestyle and lack of regular exercise are common causes of constipation. Lack of access to toilet facilities, consistent suppression of the urge to empty the bowel, and dehydration are other causes. *Slow-transit constipation* involves impaired colonic motor activity with infrequent bowel movements, straining to defecate, mild abdominal distention, and palpable stool in the sigmoid colon. *Pelvic floor dysfunction* (pelvic floor dyssynergia-anismus) is difficulty expelling stool because of failure of the pelvic floor muscles or anal sphincter to relax with defecation.

Secondary constipation can be caused by neurogenic disorders (e.g., stroke, Parkinson disease, spinal cord injury, multiple sclerosis) in which neurotransmitters are altered or neural pathways are diseased or degenerated, resulting in delayed colon transit time. Opiates, particularly codeine, antacids containing calcium carbonate or aluminum hydroxide; anticholinergics; iron; and bismuth tend to inhibit bowel motility. Endocrine or metabolic disorders associated with constipation include hypothyroidism, diabetes mellitus, hypokalemia, and hypercalcemia. Pelvic hiatal hernia (herniation of the bowel through the floor of the pelvis), diverticuli, irritable bowel syndrome–constipation predominant, and pregnancy also can be associated with constipation. Aging can result in constipation caused from decreased motility related to the degeneration of neurons in the myenteric plexus, decreased neurotransmitter function, use of medications, and comorbid medical conditions.[4] Constipation as a notable change in bowel habits can be an indication of colorectal cancer.

Many mechanical conditions can slow intestinal transit time. The abdominal muscles are normally used to create the intra-abdominal pressure required to evacuate the rectum. Weakness or pain can interfere with the generation of adequate intra-abdominal pressure. Lesions of the anus, such as inflamed hemorrhoids, fissures, or fistulae, make defecation painful because of stretching. With the urge to defecate, the sphincter becomes hypertonic and the stool is not eliminated. Depression often impairs bowel evacuation, partly because depressed individuals tend to be sedentary and lack the motivation to eat a healthy diet. The problem is made worse if antidepressant drugs (e.g., anticholinergics) are used to treat the depression.

CLINICAL MANIFESTATIONS. Indicators of constipation include two of the following for at least 3 months: (1) straining with defecation at least 25% of the time, (2) lumpy or hard stools at least 25% of the time, (3) sensation of incomplete emptying at least 25% of the time, (4) manual maneuvers to facilitate stool evacuation for at least 25% of defecations, and (5) fewer than three bowel movements per week.[5] Changes in bowel evacuation patterns, such as less frequent defecation, smaller stool volume, hard stools, difficulty passing stools (straining), or a feeling of bowel fullness and discomfort or blood in the stools, require investigation. Fecal impaction (hard, dry stool retained in the rectum) is associated with rectal bleeding, abdominal or cramping pain, nausea and vomiting, weight loss, and episodes of diarrhea. Straining to evacuate stool may cause engorgement of the hemorrhoidal veins and hemorrhoidal disease or thrombosis with rectal pain, bleeding, and itching. Passage of hard stools can cause painful anal fissures.

EVALUATION AND TREATMENT. The history, current use of medications, physical examination, and stool diaries provide precise clues regarding the nature of constipation. Sudden-onset constipation can accompany the development of colorectal cancer and requires careful evaluation. The individual's description of frequency, stool consistency, associated pain, and presence of blood or whether evacuation was stimulated by enemas or cathartics (laxatives) is significant. Cramping abdominal pain may be symptomatic of partial bowel obstruction. Palpation discloses colonic distention, masses, and tenderness. Blood may be caused by bleeding hemorrhoids or a neoplastic lesion of the colon.

Digital examination of the rectum and anorectal manometry are performed to assess sphincter tone and detect anal lesions. Proctosigmoidoscopy and colonoscopy are used to visualize the lumen directly. Colonic transit studies and imaging techniques can assist in identifying the etiology of constipation.

The treatment for constipation is to manage the underlying cause or disease for each individual. Management usually consists of bowel retraining, in which the individual establishes a satisfactory bowel evacuation routine without becoming preoccupied with bowel movements. Moderate exercise, increased fluid and fiber intake, stool softeners, and laxative agents are useful for some individuals. Enemas can be used to establish bowel routine, but they should not be used habitually. Biofeedback training can be effective for dyssynergic defecation.[6] Drugs used to treat constipation include the colonic secretagogues lubiprostone and plecanatide and the 5-HT_4 agonist prucalopride. Methylnaltrexone is a peripherally acting μ-opioid receptor antagonist approved for opioid-induced constipation in terminally ill individuals.[7]

Diarrhea

Diarrhea is an increase in the frequency of defecation and the fluid content, volume, and weight of feces. Three or more loose or liquid stools per day or more frequently than is normal for the individual are considered abnormal.[8] Many factors determine stool volume and consistency, including the water content of the colon and the presence of unabsorbed food, unabsorbable material, and intestinal secretions. Stool volume in the normal adult averages less than 200 g/day. Stool volume in children depends on age and size. An infant may pass up to 100 g/day. The adult intestine processes approximately 9 L of luminal contents per day; 2 L is ingested, and the remaining 7 L consists of intestinal secretions. Of this volume, 99% of the fluid is absorbed—90% (7 to 8 L) in the small intestine and 9% (1 to 2 L) in the colon. Normally, approximately 150 ml of water is excreted daily in the stool.

PATHOPHYSIOLOGY. Diarrhea in which the volume of feces is increased is called *large-volume diarrhea.* Large-volume diarrhea generally is caused by excessive amounts of water or secretions, or both, in the intestines. *Small-volume diarrhea,* in which the volume of feces is not increased, usually results from excessive intestinal motility. The three major mechanisms of diarrhea are osmotic, secretory, and motility.[9] (Specific mechanisms of diarrhea in children are described in Chapter 42.)

In **osmotic diarrhea,** a nonabsorbable substance in the intestine draws water into the lumen by osmosis. The excess water and the nonabsorbable substance cause large-volume diarrhea. Large oral doses of poorly absorbed ions, such as magnesium, sulfate, and phosphate, can increase intraluminal osmotic pressure. Excessive ingestion of synthetic, nonabsorbable sugars (e.g., sorbitol); introduction of full-strength tube feeding formulas; and dumping syndrome associated with gastric resection draw water into the intestinal lumen (see p. 1440). Osmotic diarrhea disappears when ingestion of the osmotic substance stops. Malabsorption related to lactase deficiency, pancreatic enzyme or bile salt deficiency, small intestine bacterial overgrowth, and celiac disease also cause diarrhea.

Secretory diarrhea is a form of large-volume diarrhea caused by excessive mucosal secretion of chloride- or bicarbonate-rich fluid or inhibition of net sodium absorption. Infectious causes include viruses (e.g., rotavirus), bacterial enterotoxins (e.g., *Escherichia coli* and *Vibrio cholerae*), or exotoxins from overgrowth of *Clostridium difficile* following antibiotic therapy. These infections cause secretion of transmitters from enteroendocrine cells (e.g., 5-HT) and activation of afferent neurons that stimulate submucosal secretomotor neurons and altered sodium and chloride transport resulting in decreased water absorption.[10,11] Neoplasms (such as gastrinoma or thyroid carcinoma) produce hormones that stimulate intestinal secretion causing diarrhea.

Small-volume diarrhea usually is caused by an inflammatory disorder of the intestine, such as ulcerative colitis, Crohn disease, or microscopic colitis. Inflammation of the colon causes smooth muscle contraction, cramping pain, urgency, and frequency. Small-volume diarrhea also can be caused by fecal impaction, a severe form of constipation. This diarrhea consists of secretions (mucus and fluid) produced by the colon to lubricate the impacted feces and move it toward the anal canal. These secretions flow around the impaction and cause low-volume, secretory diarrhea.

Motility diarrhea is caused by resection of the small intestine (short bowel syndrome), surgical bypass of an area of the intestine, fistula formation between loops of intestine, irritable bowel syndrome–diarrhea predominant, diabetic neuropathy, hyperthyroidism, and laxative abuse. Excessive motility decreases transit time, mucosal surface contact, and opportunities for fluid absorption, resulting in diarrhea.

CLINICAL MANIFESTATIONS. Diarrhea can be acute or chronic, depending on its cause. Systemic effects of prolonged diarrhea are dehydration, electrolyte imbalance (hyponatremia, hypokalemia), metabolic acidosis, and weight loss. Manifestations of acute bacterial or viral infection include fever, with or without cramping pain. Fever, cramping pain, and bloody stools accompany diarrhea caused by inflammatory bowel disease. Steatorrhea (fat in the stools) and diarrhea are common signs of malabsorption syndromes. Anal and perineal skin irritation can occur.

EVALUATION AND TREATMENT. A thorough history is taken to document the onset, frequency, and volume of stools. Exposure to contaminated food or water is indicated if the individual has traveled in foreign countries or areas where drinking water might be contaminated. Iatrogenic diarrhea is suggested if the individual has undergone abdominal radiation therapy, intestinal resection, or treatment with selected drugs (e.g., antibiotics, diuretics, antihypertensives, laxatives). Physical examination helps the clinician to identify underlying systemic disease. Stool culture, examination of stool specimens for blood, abdominal roentgenograms, endoscopy, and intestinal biopsies provide more specific data.[12]

Treatment for diarrhea includes restoration of fluid and electrolyte balance, antimotility (e.g., loperamide [an opiate] or Lomotil [atropine]) and/or water-absorbent (e.g., attapulgite and polycarbophil) medications, and treatment of causal factors. Nutritional deficiencies need to be corrected in cases of chronic diarrhea or malabsorption. Natural bran and commercial preparations of psyllium are inexpensive and effective treatments for mild diarrhea. Probiotics can be useful for treating *Clostridium difficile*–associated diarrhea as an approach to restoring normal microflora in addition to antibiotic therapy.[13] Fecal transplantation can be used for cases that are resistant to conventional therapies.[14]

Abdominal Pain

Abdominal pain is the presenting symptom of a number of gastrointestinal (GI) diseases and can be acute or chronic. The causal mechanisms are *mechanical, inflammatory,* or *ischemic.* (The physiology of pain is described in Chapter 16.) Abdominal pain may be generalized to the abdomen or localized to a particular abdominal quadrant. The pain is often described as sharp, dull, or colicky. Generally the abdominal organs are not sensitive to mechanical stimuli, such as cutting, tearing, or crushing. These organs are, however, sensitive to stretching and distention, which activate nerve endings in both hollow and solid structures. The onset of pain is associated with rapid distention; gradual distention causes little pain. Traction on the peritoneum caused by adhesions, distention of the common bile duct, or forceful peristalsis resulting from intestinal obstruction causes pain because of increased tension. Capsules that surround solid organs, such as the liver and gallbladder, contain pain fibers that are stimulated by stretching if these organs swell.

Biochemical mediators of the inflammatory response, such as histamine, bradykinin, and serotonin, stimulate pain nerve endings and produce abdominal pain. The edema and vascular congestion that accompany chemical, bacterial, or viral inflammation also cause painful stretching. Obstruction of blood flow from the distention of bowel obstruction or mesenteric vessel thrombosis produces the pain of ischemia, and increased concentrations of tissue metabolites stimulate pain receptors.

Abdominal pain can be parietal (somatic), visceral, or referred. **Parietal pain** arises from the parietal peritoneum. This pain is more localized and intense than visceral pain, which arises from the organs themselves. Nerve fibers from the parietal peritoneum travel with peripheral nerves to the spinal cord, and the sensation of pain corresponds to skin dermatomes T6 and L1. Parietal pain lateralizes because, at any particular point, the parietal peritoneum is innervated from only one side of the nervous system.

Visceral pain arises from a stimulus (distention, inflammation, ischemia) acting on an abdominal organ. Chronic low-grade inflammation can cause pain hypersensitivity with involvement of neurokinins, serotonin, and voltage-gated ion channels.[15,16] Pain is usually felt near the midline in the epigastrium, midabdomen, or lower abdomen. The pain is poorly localized, is dull rather than sharp, and is difficult to describe. Visceral pain is diffuse and vague because nerve endings in abdominal organs are sparse and multisegmented. Pain arising from the stomach, for example, is experienced as a sensation of fullness, cramping, or gnawing in the midepigastric area. **Referred pain** is visceral pain felt at some distance from a diseased or an affected organ. Referred pain is usually well localized and is felt in the skin dermatomes or deeper tissues that share a central afferent pathway with the affected organ. Gallbladder pain is, for example, referred to the right shoulder or scapulae.

Gastrointestinal Bleeding

Upper gastrointestinal (GI) bleeding is bleeding in the esophagus, stomach, or duodenum and is characterized by frank, bright red bleeding in emesis or dark, grainy digested blood ("coffee grounds") in stool. Upper GI bleeding is caused by esophageal or gastric varices, a Mallory-Weiss tear at the esophageal-gastric junction from severe retching, cancer, angiodysplasias, or peptic ulcers.[17] **Lower gastrointestinal (GI) bleeding,** bleeding from the small intestine (jejunum or ileum), colon, or rectum, can be caused by polyps, inflammatory bowel disease, diverticulosis, cancer, vascular ectasias, or hemorrhoids.[18] **Occult bleeding** is usually caused by slow, chronic blood loss that is not obvious and results in iron deficiency anemia as iron stores in the bone marrow are slowly depleted. Acute, severe GI bleeding is life threatening depending on the volume and rate of blood loss, associated disease, age, and effectiveness of treatment.

Physiologic response to gastrointestinal bleeding depends on the amount and rate of the loss (Figure 41-1). Changes in blood pressure and heart rate are the best indicators of massive blood loss in the gastrointestinal tract. Blood losses of 1000 ml or more over a short time cause a decrease in blood pressure and a corresponding increase in heart rate. With losses of 1000 ml or more, the heart rate is greater than 100 beats/minute and

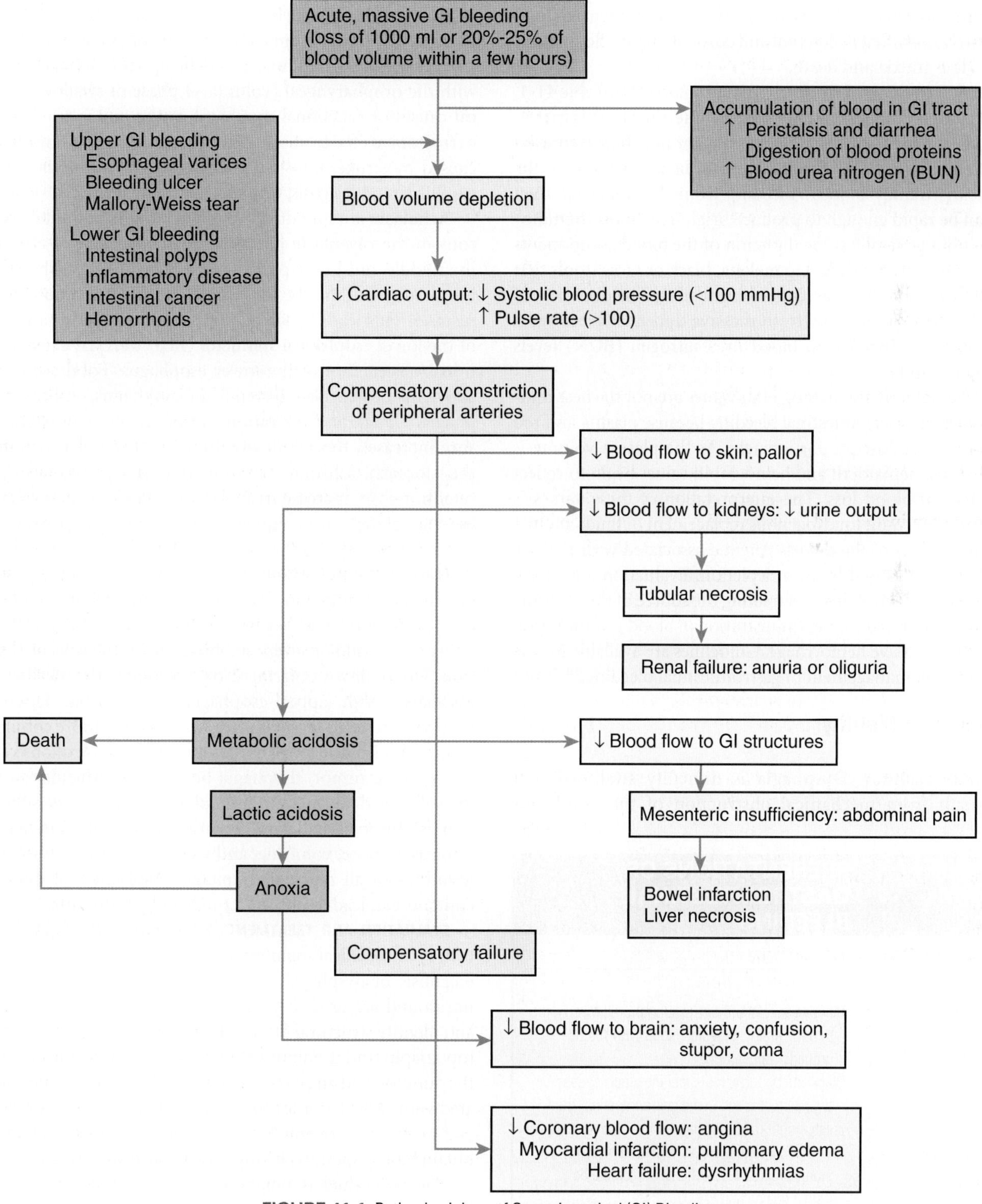

FIGURE 41-1 Pathophysiology of Gastrointestinal (GI) Bleeding.

systolic blood pressure is less than 100 mmHg. During the early stages of blood volume depletion, the peripheral arteries and arterioles constrict to shunt blood to vital organs, including the brain (see Chapters 32 and 48). Signs of large-volume blood loss are postural hypotension (a drop in blood pressure that occurs with a change from the recumbent position to a sitting or upright position), lightheadedness, and loss of vision. If blood loss continues, hypovolemic shock develops. Diminished blood flow to the kidneys causes decreased urine output and may lead to oliguria (low urine output), tubular necrosis, and renal failure. Ultimately, insufficient cerebral and coronary blood flow causes irreversible anoxia and death.

The presentation of GI bleeding is summarized in Table 41-1. The accumulation of blood in the gastrointestinal tract is irritating and increases peristalsis, causing vomiting **(hematemesis)** or diarrhea, or both. If bleeding is from the lower GI tract, the diarrhea is frankly bloody. Bleeding from the upper GI tract also can be rapid enough to produce bright red stools **(hematochezia),** but generally some digestion of the blood components will have occurred, producing **melena,** black or tarry stools that are sticky and have a characteristic foul odor. The digestion of blood proteins originating from massive upper GI bleeding is reflected by an increase in blood urea nitrogen (BUN) levels (see Figure 41-1).

The hematocrit and hemoglobin values are not the best indicators of acute gastrointestinal bleeding because plasma and red cell volume are lost proportionately. As the plasma volume is replaced, the hematocrit and hemoglobin values begin to reflect the extent of blood loss. The interpretation of these values is modified to account for exogenous replacement of fluids and the hydration status of the tissues. Anemia associated with chronic GI bleeding is caused by iron depletion. Evaluation and treatment involves identifying and treating the source of the bleeding and replacing iron losses. Administration of blood products may be used for massive hemorrhage. Guidelines are available for the diagnosis and management of gastrointestinal bleeding.[19-21]

Disorders of Motility

Dysphagia

PATHOPHYSIOLOGY. **Dysphagia** is difficulty swallowing. It can result from mechanical obstruction of the esophagus or a functional disorder that impairs esophageal motility. *Mechanical obstructions* can be intrinsic or extrinsic. Intrinsic obstructions originate in the wall of the esophageal lumen. Tumors, strictures, and diverticular herniations (outpouchings) are all causes of intrinsic mechanical obstruction. Extrinsic mechanical obstructions originate outside the esophageal lumen and narrow the esophagus by pressing inward on the esophageal wall. The most common cause of extrinsic mechanical obstruction is tumor.

Functional dysphagia is caused by neural or muscular disorders that interfere with voluntary swallowing or peristalsis. Disorders that affect the striated muscles of the upper esophagus interfere with the oropharyngeal (voluntary) phase of swallowing. Typical causes of functional dysphagia in the upper esophagus are dermatomyositis (a muscle disease) and neurologic impairments caused by stroke, multiple sclerosis, Parkinson disease, amyotrophic lateral sclerosis, or myasthenia gravis.[22]

Achalasia is a rare disorder related to loss of inhibitory neurons in the myenteric plexus with smooth muscle atrophy in the middle and lower portions of the esophagus. The etiology is unknown but may be related to viral or autoimmune mechanisms.[23] This leads to altered esophageal peristalsis and failure of the lower esophageal sphincter (LES) to relax, causing functional obstruction of the lower esophagus. Food accumulates above the obstruction, distends the esophagus, and causes dysphagia. Cough and aspiration can occur. As hydrostatic pressure increases, food is slowly forced past the obstruction into the stomach. Chronic inflammation from esophageal food retention can increase risk for esophageal cancer. Chronic esophageal distention requires dilation or surgical myomotomy of the lower esophageal sphincter (LES).[24]

CLINICAL MANIFESTATIONS. Clinical manifestations of dysphagia vary according to the location of the obstruction. Distention and spasm of the esophageal muscles during eating or drinking may cause a mild or severe stabbing pain at the level of obstruction. Discomfort occurring 2 to 4 seconds after swallowing is associated with upper esophageal obstruction. Discomfort occurring 10 to 15 seconds after swallowing is more common in obstructions of the lower esophagus. If the cause of obstruction is a growing tumor, dysphagia begins with difficulty swallowing solids and advances to difficulty swallowing semisolids and liquids. Retrosternal pain, regurgitation of undigested food, unpleasant taste, vomiting, and weight loss are common manifestations of all types of dysphagia. Aspiration of esophageal contents can lead to chronic cough and pneumonia.

EVALUATION AND TREATMENT. Knowledge of the individual's history and clinical manifestations contributes significantly to a diagnosis of dysphagia. Videofluoroscopy and high-frequency ultrasound are used to visualize the contours of the esophagus and identify structural defects. High-resolution manometry with topography and intraluminal impedance monitoring documents the duration and amplitude of abnormal pressure changes associated with obstruction or loss of neural regulation.[25] Esophageal endoscopy is performed to examine the esophageal mucosa, obtain biopsy specimens, or perform corrective surgery.

The individual is taught to manage symptoms by eating slowly, eating small meals, taking fluid with meals, and sleeping

TABLE 41-1 PRESENTATIONS OF GASTROINTESTINAL BLEEDING

PRESENTATION	DEFINITION
Acute bleeding	
Hematemesis	Bloody vomitus; either fresh, bright red blood or dark, grainy, digested blood with "coffee grounds" appearance
Melena	Black, sticky, tarry, foul-smelling stools caused by digestion of blood in the gastrointestinal tract
Hematochezia	Fresh, bright red blood passed from the rectum
Occult bleeding	Trace amounts of blood in normal-appearing stools or gastric secretions; detectable only with a guaiac test

with the head elevated to prevent regurgitation and aspiration. Oral medications may need to be formulated so they can be swallowed.[26] Tube feedings may be required for some individuals, particularly following stroke.[27] Anticholinergic drugs may alleviate symptoms. Definitive treatments include mechanical dilation of the esophageal sphincter and surgical separation of the lower esophageal muscles with a longitudinal incision (myotomy) widening the passage into the stomach.[28]

Gastroesophageal Reflux Disease

Gastroesophageal reflux disease (GERD) is the reflux of acid and pepsin from the stomach to the esophagus that causes **esophagitis.** Risk factors for GERD include obesity, hiatal hernia, and drugs or chemicals that relax the LES (anticholinergics, nitrates, calcium channel blockers, nicotine).[29] GERD may be a trigger for asthma or chronic cough.[30] Gastroesophageal reflux that does not cause symptoms is known as *physiologic reflux.* In *nonerosive reflux disease (NERD),* individuals have symptoms of reflux disease but no visible esophageal mucosal injury (functional heartburn).[31]

PATHOPHYSIOLOGY. The resting tone of the LES tends to be lower than normal from either transient relaxation or weakness of the sphincter in those who develop GERD. Vomiting, coughing, lifting, bending, or obesity increases abdominal pressure, contributing to the development of reflux esophagitis. Delayed gastric emptying contributes to reflux esophagitis by: (1) lengthening the period during which reflux is possible and (2) increasing the acid content of chyme. Disorders that delay emptying include gastric or duodenal ulcers, which can cause pyloric edema; strictures that narrow the pylorus; and hiatal hernia, which can weaken the LES.[32]

GERD causes inflammatory responses in the esophageal wall resulting in hyperemia, edema, tissue fragility, erosion, and ulcerations (Figure 41-2). Severity of inflammation is related to composition of gastric contents and length of exposure time.[33] Fibrosis, basal cell hyperplasia, and elongation of papillae are common.

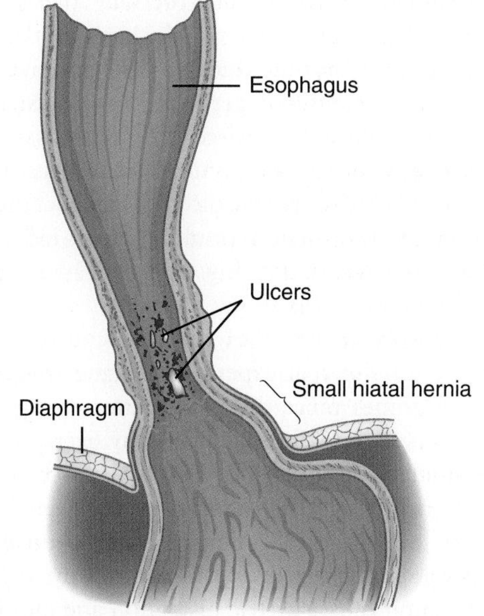

FIGURE 41-2 Esophagitis with Esophageal Ulcerations.

Precancerous lesions (Barrett esophagus, see p. 1466) with progression to adenocarcinoma can be a long-term consequence.[33,34]

CLINICAL MANIFESTATIONS. The clinical manifestations of reflux esophagitis are heartburn from acid regurgitation, chronic cough, asthma attacks (see Chapter 35), and laryngitis.[30] Upper abdominal pain usually occurs within 1 hour of eating and can be relapsing and remitting. Symptoms can worsen if the individual lies down or if intra-abdominal pressure increases (e.g., as a result of coughing, vomiting, or straining at stool). Symptoms may be present when no acid is in the esophagus.[35] Heartburn also may be experienced as chest pain, which requires ruling out cardiac ischemia. Edema, fibrosis (strictures), esophageal spasm, or decreased esophageal motility may result in dysphagia. Alcohol or acid-containing foods, such as citrus fruits, can cause discomfort during swallowing.

EVALUATION AND TREATMENT. Diagnosis of reflux esophagitis is based on the history and clinical manifestations. Esophageal endoscopy shows hyperemia, edema, erosion, and strictures. Dysplastic changes (Barrett esophagus) can be identified by tissue biopsy. Impedance/pH monitoring measures the movement of stomach contents upward into the esophagus and the acidity of the refluxate.

Proton pump inhibitors are the most effective monotherapy. Other therapies include histamine-2 (H2) receptor antagonists, prokinetics, and antacids. Pain medication may be used in resistant cases. Elevation of the head of the bed 6 inches prevents reflux. Weight reduction and cessation of smoking also help to alleviate symptoms. Laparoscopic fundoplication is the most common surgical intervention when medical treatment fails.[36,37]

Eosinophilic esophagitis is a rare, idiopathic inflammatory disease of the esophagus characterized by esophageal infiltration of eosinophils associated with atopic disease, including asthma and food allergies. It occurs in adults and children. Dysphagia, food impaction, vomiting, and weight loss are common symptoms. Endoscopy with biopsy identifies the eosinophilc infiltration and differentiation from GERD. Treatment is symptomatic including elimination diets, proton pump inhibitors, and immunosuppression.[38]

Hiatal Hernia

PATHOPHYSIOLOGY. Hiatal hernia is the protrusion (herniation) of the upper part of the stomach through the diaphragm and into the thorax.[39] There are four types: sliding (type I); paraesophageal (type II); mixed (type III), which include elements of types I and II (Figure 41-3).[40] In type IV the entire stomach and other abdominal organs slide into the thorax.

In type I, **sliding hiatal hernia** (the most common type, 90%), the proximal portion of the stomach moves into the thoracic cavity through the esophageal hiatus, an opening in the diaphragm for the esophagus and vagus nerves. A congenitally short esophagus, fibrosis or excessive vagal nerve stimulation, or weakening of the diaphragmatic muscles at the gastroesophageal junction contributes to the hernia. While the individual is in the supine position, the lower esophagus and stomach are pulled into the thorax. Standing causes the organs to "slide" back into the abdomen. Sliding hiatal hernia is exacerbated by factors that increase intra-abdominal pressure, such as coughing, bending, wearing tight clothing, ascites, obesity, or pregnancy. This type of hernia is associated with gastroesophageal reflux because the hernia diminishes the resting pressure of the LES. In pregnant women with sliding hiatal hernia, progesterone and estrogen may lower the resting pressure of the LES further.

In type II, **paraesophageal hiatal hernia** (rolling hiatal hernia), herniation of the greater curvature of the stomach is through a secondary opening in the diaphragm (see Figure 41-3). A giant paraesophageal hiatal hernia develops when 30% to 60% of the stomach moves into the thorax. As the stomach protrudes through the opening into the thorax, it lies alongside the esophagus. The gastroesophageal junction remains below the diaphragm. With paraesophageal hernia, reflux is uncommon. The position of a portion of the stomach above the diaphragm, however, causes congestion of mucosal blood flow and can lead to gastritis and ulcer formation. A mechanical strangulation of the hernia is a major complication, and surgical correction is required. Strangulation occludes blood vessels and causes vascular engorgement, edema, ischemia, and hemorrhage. Type III, mixed hiatal hernia, is a combination of both types I and II and tends to occur in conjunction with several other diseases, including gastroesophageal reflux, peptic ulcer, cholecystitis (gallbladder inflammation), cholelithiasis (gallstones), chronic pancreatitis, and diverticulosis. Type IV is an aggravated form of type III.

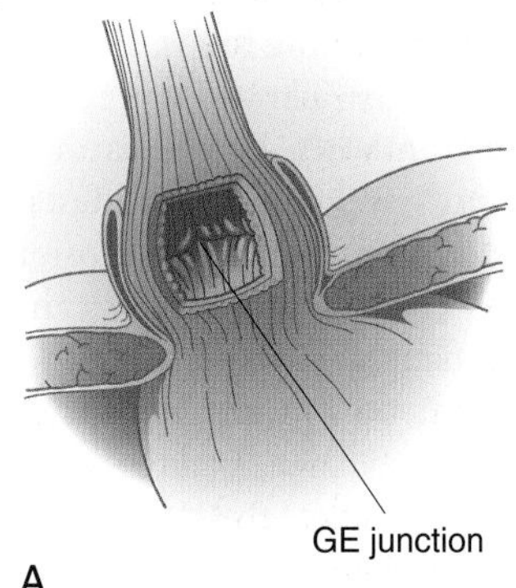

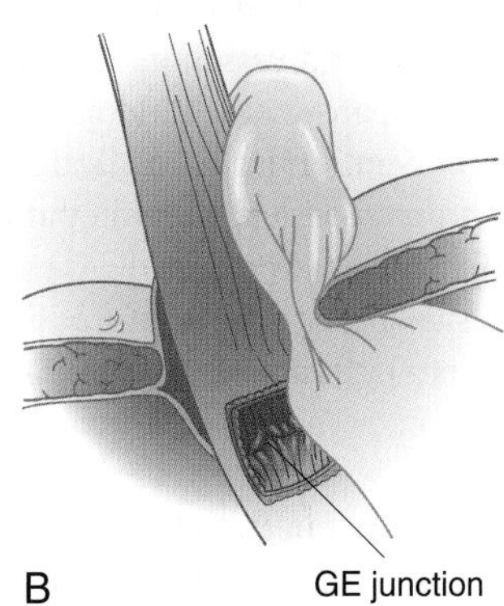

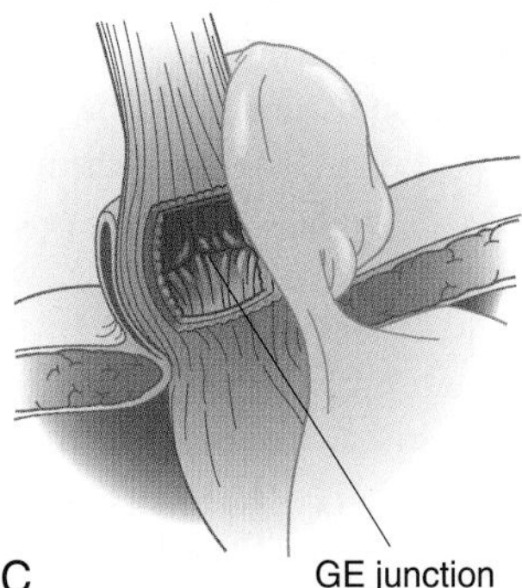

FIGURE 41-3 The Three Types of Hiatal Hernia. **A,** Type I—*sliding hernia.* The visceral peritoneum remains intact and restrains the size of the hernia in sliding hiatal hernia. **B,** Type II—*paraesophageal* or *rolling hernia.* The membrane becomes thinner or defective in paraesophageal hernia, allowing a true peritoneal sac to protrude into the posterior mediastinum where negative intrathoracic pressure causes it to enlarge. **C,** Type III—*mixed hernia. GE,* Gastroesophageal. (From Townsend CM et al: *Sabiston textbook of surgery,* ed 19, Philadelphia, 2012, Saunders.) **Note:** Type IV-complex paraesophageal hernia is not shown.

CLINICAL MANIFESTATIONS. Hiatal hernias are often asymptomatic. Generally, a wide variety of symptoms develop later in life and are associated with other gastrointestinal disorders, including GERD. Manifestations of the various types of hiatal hernia are difficult to distinguish. Symptoms include heartburn, regurgitation, dysphagia, and epigastric pain.[41] Ischemia from hernia strangulation causes acute, severe chest or epigastric pain, nausea, vomiting, and GI bleeding.

EVALUATION AND TREATMENT. Diagnostic procedures include chest x-ray with oral barium and endoscopy. A chest x-ray often will show the protrusion of the stomach into the thorax, indicating paraesophageal hiatal hernia.

Treatment for sliding hiatal hernia is usually conservative. The individual can diminish reflux by eating small, frequent meals and avoiding the recumbent position after eating. Abdominal supports and tight clothing are avoided, and weight control is recommended for obese individuals. Antacids alleviate reflux esophagitis. Drugs that relax the LES (anticholinergic, nitrates, calcium channel blockers) are contraindicated because they delay gastric emptying. Laparoscopic surgery (i.e., fundoplication) may be performed for paraesophageal hiatal hernia or if medical management fails to control symptoms.[42]

Pyloric Obstruction

PATHOPHYSIOLOGY. Pyloric obstruction (gastric outlet obstruction) is the narrowing or blocking of the opening between the stomach and the duodenum. This condition can be congenital (i.e., infantile hypertrophic pyloric stenosis, see Chapter 42) or acquired. Acquired obstruction is caused by peptic ulcer disease or carcinoma near the pylorus. Duodenal ulcers are more likely than gastric ulcers to obstruct the pylorus. Ulceration causes obstruction resulting from inflammation, edema, spasm, fibrosis, or scarring. Tumors cause obstruction by growing into the pylorus.[43]

CLINICAL MANIFESTATIONS. Early in the course of pyloric obstruction, the individual experiences vague epigastric fullness, which becomes more distressing after eating and later in the day. Nausea and epigastric pain may occur as the muscles of the stomach contract in attempts to force chyme past the obstruction. These symptoms disappear when the chyme finally moves into the duodenum. As obstruction progresses anorexia develops sometimes accompanied by weight loss. Severe obstruction causes gastric distention and atony (lack of muscle tone and gastric motility). Gastric distention stimulates gastric secretion, which increases the feeling of fullness. Rolling or jarring of the abdomen produces a sloshing sound called the *succussion splash.* At this stage, vomiting is a cardinal sign of obstruction. It is usually copious and occurs several hours after eating. The vomitus contains undigested food but no bile. Prolonged vomiting leads to dehydration, which is accompanied by a hypokalemic and hypochloremic metabolic alkalosis caused by the respective loss of gastric potassium and acid. Because food does not enter the intestine, stools are infrequent and small. Prolonged pyloric obstruction causes severe malnutrition and dehydration.

EVALUATION AND TREATMENT. Diagnosis is based on clinical manifestations, a history of peptic ulcer disease, and examination of residual gastric contents. Endoscopy for the purpose of biopsy is performed if gastric carcinoma is the suggested cause of pyloric obstruction. Barium studies are contraindicated because the barium may harden and be retained in the stomach.

Obstructions resulting from ulceration often resolve with conservative management. Gastric drainage is used to decompress the stomach and restore normal motility. Gastric secretions that contribute to inflammation and edema can be suppressed with proton pump inhibitors or histamine-2 (H2) receptor antagonists. Fluids and electrolytes (sodium chloride and potassium) are given intravenously to effect rehydration and correct hypochloremia, alkalosis, and hypokalemia (see Chapter 3). Severely malnourished individuals may require parenteral hyperalimentation (intravenous nutrition). Surgery or stenting may be required to treat gastric carcinoma or persistent obstruction caused by fibrosis and scarring.[44]

Intestinal Obstruction and Ileus

Intestinal obstruction can be caused by any condition that prevents the normal flow of chyme through the intestinal lumen or failure of normal intestinal motility in the absence of an obstructing lesion (ileus). The small intestine is more commonly obstructed because of its narrower lumen. Common causes of intestinal obstruction are summarized in Table 41-2. Criteria for classifying intestinal obstruction are summarized in Table 41-3. Intestinal obstruction is classified by cause as simple or functional. *Simple obstruction* is mechanical blockage of the lumen by a lesion and is the most common type of intestinal obstruction. **Paralytic ileus,** or *functional obstruction*, is a failure of motility after gastrointestinal or abdominal surgery. Anesthetic agents, local inflammatory reactions, use of opioid analgesia, and hyperactivity of the sympathetic nervous system contribute to postoperative ileus.

Simple obstruction of the small intestine from fibrous adhesions is the most common type of intestinal obstruction.[45] Acute obstructions usually have mechanical causes, such as adhesions or hernias (Figure 41-4). Chronic or partial obstructions are more often associated with tumors or inflammatory disorders, particularly of the large intestine. Intussusception is rare in adults compared with the more frequent occurrence in infants. The most common causes of large bowel obstruction are colorectal cancer, volvulus (twisting), and strictures related to diverticulitis. Common causes of intestinal obstruction in children are presented in Chapter 42.

PATHOPHYSIOLOGY. The consequences of intestinal obstruction are related to its onset and location, the length of intestinal tract proximal to the obstruction, and the presence and severity of ischemia. The major pathophysiologic alterations are presented in Figure 41-5. Postoperative paralytic ileus results from inhibitory neural reflexes associated with inflammatory mediators, and the influence of exogenous (meperidine) and endogenous opioids (endorphins) that affect the entire GI tract, including the stomach.[46,47] **Small intestine obstruction** leads to accumulation of fluid and gas inside the lumen proximal to the obstruction. Fluids accumulate from impaired water and electrolyte absorption and enhanced secretion with net movement of fluid from the vascular space to the intestinal lumen. Gas from swallowed air, and to a lesser extent from bacterial overgrowth, contributes to the distention. Distention begins almost immediately, as gases and fluids accumulate proximal to the obstruction. Distention decreases the intestine's ability to absorb water and electrolytes and increases the net secretion of these substances into the lumen. Within 24 hours, up to 8 L of fluid and electrolytes enters the lumen in the form of saliva, gastric juice, bile, pancreatic juice, and intestinal secretions. Copious vomiting or sequestration of fluids in the intestinal lumen prevents their reabsorption and produces severe fluid

TABLE 41-2 COMMON CAUSES OF INTESTINAL OBSTRUCTION

CAUSE	PATHOPHYSIOLOGY
Herniation	Protrusion of the intestine through a weakness in the abdominal muscles or through the inguinal ring
Intussusception	Telescoping of one part of the intestine into another; this usually causes strangulation of the blood supply; more common in the ileocecal area in infants 10 to 15 months of age than in adults
Torsion (volvulus)	Twisting of the intestine on its mesenteric pedicle, with occlusion of the blood supply; often associated with fibrous adhesions in the small intestine; occurs most often in the large intestine in older adults
Diverticulosis	Inflamed saccular herniations (diverticula) of the mucosa and submucosa through the tunica muscularis of the colon; diverticula are interspersed between thick, circular, fibrous bands; most common in obese individuals older than 60 years
Tumor	Tumor growth into the intestinal lumen; adenocarcinoma of the colon and rectum is the most common tumoral obstruction; most common in individuals older than 60 years
Paralytic (adynamic) ileus	Loss of peristaltic motor activity in the intestine; associated with abdominal surgery, peritonitis, hypokalemia, ischemic bowel, spinal trauma, pneumonia, neuropathies, or myopathies; affects small and large intestines
Fibrous adhesions	Peritoneal irritation from surgery or trauma leads to formation of fibrin and adhesions that attach to intestine, omentum, or peritoneum and can cause traction and obstruction; most common in small intestine

TABLE 41-3 CLASSIFICATION OF INTESTINAL OBSTRUCTION

CRITERIA FOR CLASSIFICATION	DEFINITION
Onset	
Acute	Sudden onset; often caused by torsion, intussusception, or herniation
Chronic	Protracted onset; more commonly from tumor growth or progressive formation of strictures
Extent of Obstruction	
Partial	Incomplete obstruction of intestinal lumen
Complete	Complete obstruction of intestinal lumen
Location of Obstructing Lesion	
Intrinsic	Obstruction develops within intestinal lumen; examples: luminal edema or hemorrhage, foreign bodies (gallstones), tumors, or intraluminal fibrosis
Extrinsic	Obstruction originates outside the intestine; examples: tumors, torsion, fibrosis, hernia, intussusception
Effects on Intestinal Wall	
Simple	Luminal obstruction without impairment of blood supply
Strangulated	Luminal obstruction with occlusion of blood supply
Closed loop	Obstruction at each end of a segment of the intestine
Causal Factors	
Mechanical	Blockage of the intestinal lumen by intrinsic or extrinsic lesions; usually treated surgically
Functional (paralytic ileus)	Paralysis of the intestinal musculature as a result of accidental or surgical trauma, peritonitis, electrolyte imbalances, or spasmolytic agents; usually treated medically

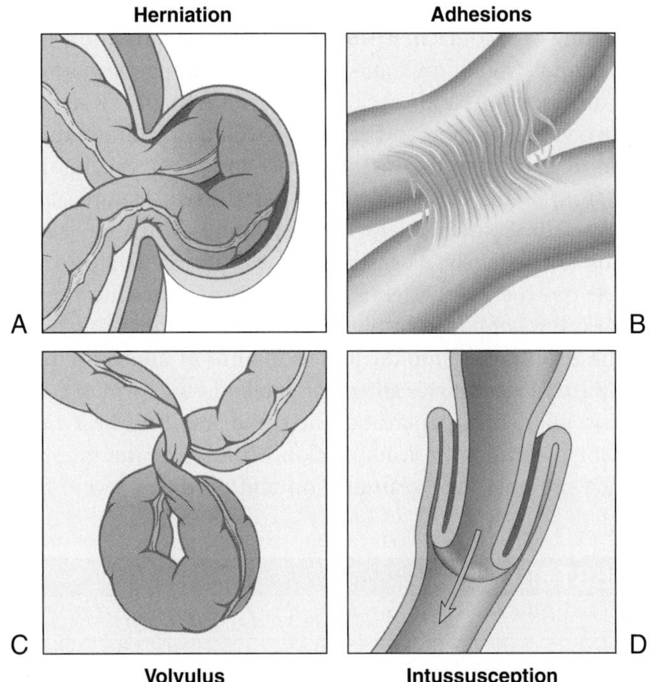

FIGURE 41-4 Intestinal Obstructions. **A,** Hernia. **B,** Constriction from adhesions. **C,** Volvulus. **D,** Intussusception. (From Kumar V, Abbas AK, Aster J: *Robbins basic pathology,* ed 9, Philadelphia, 2013, Saunders.)

and electrolyte disturbances. Extracellular fluid volume and plasma volume decrease, causing dehydration. Hemoconcentration (decreased plasma volume) elevates hematocrit level and causes hypotension and tachycardia. Severe dehydration leads to hypovolemic shock.

If the obstruction is at the pylorus or high in the small intestine, metabolic alkalosis develops initially as a result of excessive loss of hydrogen ions that normally would be reabsorbed from the gastric juice. With prolonged obstruction or obstruction lower in the intestine, metabolic acidosis is more likely to occur because bicarbonate from pancreatic secretions and bile cannot be reabsorbed. Hypokalemia from vomiting and decreased potassium absorption can be extreme, promoting acidosis and atony of the intestinal wall. Metabolic acidosis also may be accentuated by ketosis, the result of declining carbohydrate stores caused by starvation. Lack of circulation permits the buildup of significant amounts of lactic acid, which worsen the metabolic acidosis. If pressure from the distention is severe enough, it occludes the arterial circulation and causes ischemia, necrosis, perforation, and peritonitis. Fever and leukocytosis are often associated with overgrowth of bacteria, ischemia, and bowel necrosis. Bacterial proliferation and translocation across the mucosa to the mesenteric lymph nodes or systemic circulation cause sepsis. The release of inflammatory mediators into the circulation causes remote organ failure (see Chapter 48).

Consequences of **large bowel obstruction** are related to the competence of the ileocecal valve, which normally prevents reflux of colonic contents into the small intestine. When the ileocecal valve is competent, the cecum cannot decompress into the small intestine, resulting in distention. Ischemia occurs when the intraluminal pressure exceeds the capillary pressure in the lumen. **Acute colonic pseudo-obstruction** (Ogilvie syndrome) is a massive dilation of the large bowel that occurs in critically ill patients and immobilized older adults. It is characterized by significant dilation of the cecum and absence of mechanical obstruction, and is related to excessive sympathetic motor input or decreased parasympathetic motor input.

CLINICAL MANIFESTATIONS. Signs and symptoms of *small intestine obstruction* are consistent with the pathophysiology.

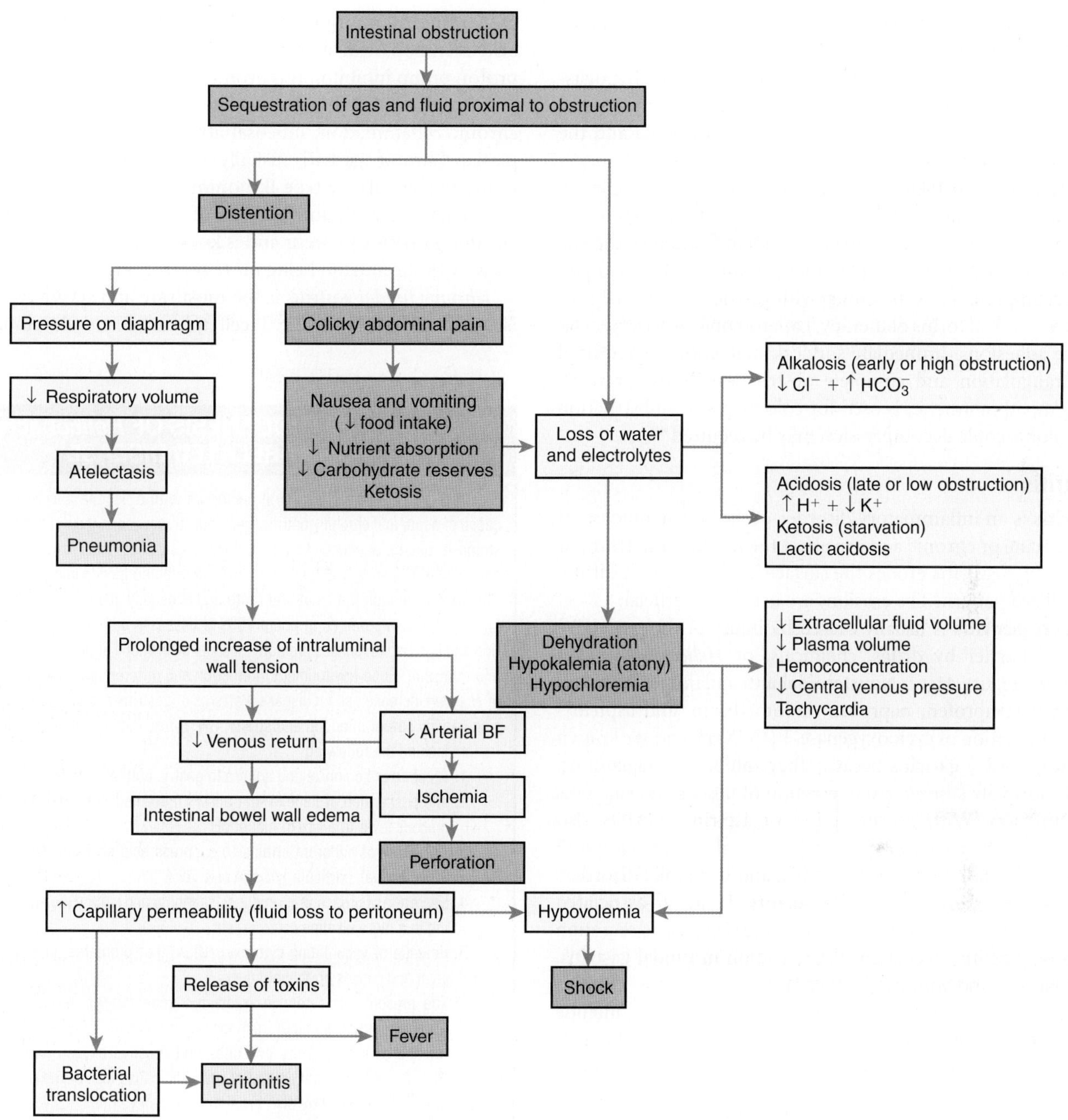

FIGURE 41-5 Pathophysiology of Intestinal Obstruction. *BF,* Blood flow.

Colicky pains caused by intestinal distention followed by nausea and vomiting are the cardinal symptoms. Typically the pain occurs intermittently. Pain intensifies for seconds or minutes as a peristaltic wave of muscle contraction meets the obstruction. The passing of the wave is followed by a pain-free interval. Pain may be continuous with severe distention and then diminish in intensity. If ischemia occurs, the pain loses its colicky character, becoming more constant and severe. Sweating and tachycardia occur as a sympathetic nervous system response to hypotension. Fever, severe leukocytosis, abdominal distention, and rebound tenderness develop as ischemia progresses to necrosis, perforation, and peritonitis.

Vomiting and abdominal distention vary, depending on the level and completion of the obstruction. Obstruction at the pylorus causes early, profuse vomiting of clear gastric fluid. Obstruction in the proximal small intestine causes mild distention and vomiting of bile-stained fluid. Obstruction in the distal small intestine causes more pronounced distention because a greater length of intestine is proximal to the obstruction. In this case, vomiting may not occur or may occur later and contain fecal material. Partial obstruction can cause diarrhea or constipation, but complete obstruction usually causes constipation only. Complete obstruction increases the number of bowel sounds, which may be tinkly and accompanied by peristaltic rushes and crampy, abdominal pain. Signs of hypovolemia and metabolic acidosis (see Chapter 3) may be observed as early as 24 hours after the occurrence of complete obstruction. Distention may be severe enough to push against the diaphragm and decrease lung volume. This can lead to atelectasis and pneumonia, particularly in debilitated individuals.

Large intestine obstruction usually presents with hypogastric pain and abdominal distention. Pain can vary from vague to excruciating, depending on the degree of ischemia and the development of peritonitis.

EVALUATION AND TREATMENT. Evaluation is based on clinical manifestations and includes ultrasound and radiography.[48] Successful management requires early identification of the site and type of obstruction. Replacement of fluid and electrolytes and decompression of the lumen with gastric or intestinal suction are essential forms of therapy. Laparoscopic procedures can release adhesions. Immediate surgical intervention is required for strangulation and complete obstruction. Neostigmine, a parasympathomimetic, is used for colonic pseudo-obstruction and colonoscopic decompression may be required.[49]

Gastritis

Gastritis is an inflammatory disorder of the gastric mucosa. It can be acute or chronic and can affect the fundus or antrum, or both. Acute gastritis erodes the surface epithelium in a diffuse or localized pattern. The erosions are usually superficial.

Acute gastritis is usually caused by injury of the protective mucosal barrier by drugs, chemicals, or *Helicobacter pylori* infection (Figure 41-6). Nonsteroidal anti-inflammatory drugs (NSAIDs [ibuprofen, naproxen, indomethacin, and aspirin]) inhibit the action of cyclooxygenase-1 (COX-1), and are known to cause erosive gastritis because they inhibit prostaglandins, which normally stimulate the secretion of mucus and suppress inflammation. With the exception of aspirin, NSAIDs also cause gastric hypermotility, causing mucosal compression and injury.[50] Alcohol, histamine, digitalis, and metabolic disorders such as uremia are contributing factors. *H. pylori*–associated acute gastritis causes inflammation, increased gastric secretion in antral gastritis, decreased gastric section in fundal gastritis, pain, nausea, and vomiting[51] (Box 41-1).

The clinical manifestations of acute gastritis can include vague abdominal discomfort, epigastric tenderness, and bleeding. Healing usually occurs spontaneously within a few days.

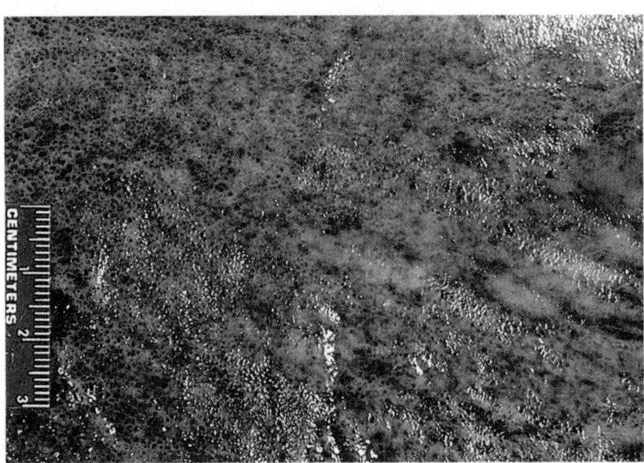

FIGURE 41-6 Acute Erosive Gastritis. Acute erosive gastritis is shown in the opened stomach. The mucosa appears hyperemic, and the foci of superficial ulceration are manifested as scattered, small, red areas termed erosions. (From Kumar V et al: *Pathologic basis of disease*, ed 7, Philadelphia, 2006, Saunders.)

Discontinuing injurious drugs, using antacids, or decreasing acid secretion with a histamine H2-receptor antagonist and proton pump inhibitor also promote healing.

Chronic gastritis tends to occur in older adults and causes chronic inflammation, mucosal atrophy, and epithelial metaplasia. Chronic gastritis usually is classified as type A, or immune (fundal), or type B, nonimmune (antral), depending on the pathogenesis and location of the lesions. Both types of chronic gastritis can occur and is known as type AB, or pangastritis, with the antrum being more severely involved.

Chronic fundal gastritis is the most rare and severe type and is associated with loss of T-cell tolerance and development

BOX 41-1 PATHOGENESIS OF *Helicobacter pylori*–RELATED DISEASE

H. pylori is a gram-negative spiral bacterium with a flagella and is a major cause of acute and chronic gastritis, peptic ulcer disease in the duodenum and stomach, gastric adenocarcinoma, and gastric mucosa–associated lymphoid tissue (MALT) (see p. 1467) in about 20% of infected individuals. *H. pylori* is transmitted through the fecal-oral route and is usually acquired in childhood. Infection is asymptomatic in about 70% of cases. In other cases, inflammation and immune responses promote mucosal ulcerations or prevent healing of injured tissue. Gene-environment interaction and different pathogenic strains of *H. pylori* increase risk for disease. Patterns of gastritis and disease progression vary by site of infection and strain of *H. pylori*. Pathogenic and virulence factors include the following:

1. An ability to colonize and adhere to gastric epithelial cells
2. The possession of flagella that allows movement through the luminal mucous layer to a site of higher pH
3. An ability of adherent strains to suppress acid secretion to improve their survival, particularly *CagA* and *VacA*
4. Secretion of urease that produces ammonia and carbon dioxide, resulting in a more alkaline environment
5. Release of vacuolating cytotoxin *(VacA)* that promotes bacterial survival and causes epithelial injury
6. The presence of cytotoxin-associated gene *(CagA)* strains that can escape normal immune responses and cause inflammation with release of inflammatory cytokines and reactive oxygen metabolites that damage mucosal epithelial cells and cause loss of the protective mucosal barrier; they also promote tumor development by degrading *p53* tumor suppression
7. Recruitment and activation of neutrophils, macrophages, and mast cells with release of inflammatory cytokines (tumor necrosis factor-alpha [TNF-α], interleukin-1 [IL-1], IL-6, IL-8, histamine) that promote cellular injury
8. Down-regulation of antral somatostatin leading to increased gastrin, increased acid, impaired mucosal bicarbonate production, and increased mucosal exposure to acid and pepsin
9. Activation or inhibition of T- and B-cell immune responses that may contribute to mucosal injury
10. Release of cytokines and chemokines that promote gastric epithelial cell death (apoptosis) and cell proliferation that can result in atrophy, ulcers, or malignant growth

Data from Costa AM et al: *FEBS Lett* 587(3):259–265, 2013; Peek RM Jr, Fiske C, Wilson KT: *Physiol Rev* 90(3):831–858, 2010; Ruggiero P: *Curr Opin Infect Dis* 25(3):337–344, 2012; Suzuki R, Shiota S, Yamaoka Y: *Infect Genet Evol* 12(2):203–213, 2012; Varbanova M, Malfertheiner P: *Dig Dis* 29(6):592–599, 2011.

of autoantibodies to gastric H^+-K^+ ATPase. Infection with *H. pylori* can trigger the immune response through molecular mimicry.[52] The gastric mucosa degenerates extensively in the body and fundus of the stomach, leading to gastric atrophy. Loss of parietal cells diminishes secretion of hydrochloric acid and intrinsic factor. Because acid secretion is insufficient, the feedback mechanism that normally inhibits gastrin secretion is impaired, causing elevated plasma levels of gastrin. *Chronic antral gastritis* generally involves the antrum only and is more common than fundal gastritis. It is caused by *H. pylori* bacteria or chronic use of alcohol, tobacco, and nonsteroidal anti-inflammatory drugs. There are high levels of hydrochloric acid secretion with an increased risk of duodenal ulcers. *H. pylori* can also progress to autoimmune atrophic gastritis and involve the fundus, thus becoming pangastritis. In these cases there is greater risk for the development of gastric cancer.[53]

Signs and symptoms of chronic gastritis often do not correlate with the severity of the disease. Gastroscopic examination and biopsy may show a long-standing inflammatory process and gastric atrophy in an individual with no history of abdominal distress. The presence of antiparietal cell antibody and elevated plasma ghrelin level are specific for atrophic gastritis.[54]

H. pylori infection is evidence for *H. pylori* gastritis. In chronic fundal gastritis, failure to stimulate acid secretion confirms achlorhydria (diminished secretion of hydrochloric acid). The gastric secretions also can be evaluated for the presence of intrinsic factor. Pernicious anemia can develop because intrinsic factor is less available to facilitate vitamin B_{12} absorption. Individuals may report vague symptoms, including anorexia, fullness, nausea, vomiting, and epigastric pain. Gastric bleeding may be the only clinical manifestation of gastritis. Evaluation for gastric carcinoma is completed with chronic *H. pylori* infection.[55] Symptoms can usually be managed with consumption of smaller meals, including a soft, bland diet; and avoidance of alcohol and NSAIDs. Combination antibiotics are used to treat *H. pylori,* and the emergence of antimicrobial resistance is a concern.[56] Vitamin B_{12} is administered to correct pernicious anemia (see Chapter 28).[57]

Alkaline reflux gastritis is a stomach inflammation caused by reflux of bile and alkaline pancreatic secretions that contain proteolytic enzymes and disrupt the mucosal barrier in the remnant stomach. This form of gastritis occurs in 5% to 20% of individuals who have undergone gastrectomy or pyloroplasty. Clinical manifestations include nausea, bilious vomiting (vomiting in which the vomitus contains bile), and sustained epigastric pain that worsens after eating and is not relieved by antacids. Endoscopy shows a hemorrhagic and friable gastric mucosa. Antacids do not consistently improve symptoms. Avoidance of aspirin and alcohol may decrease gastric irritation, and a low-fat diet may limit bile secretion. Surgical correction may ultimately be required.[58]

Peptic Ulcer Disease

A **peptic ulcer** is a break, or ulceration, in the protective mucosal lining of the lower esophagus, stomach, or duodenum. It is estimated that 10% to 17% of the population have peptic ulcer disease; however, the true incidence is unkown.[59]

Risk factors for peptic ulcer disease include genetic predisposition, *H. pylori* infection of the gastric mucosa (see Box 41-1), and habitual use of NSAIDs. Additional factors include excessive use of alcohol, smoking, acute pancreatitis, chronic obstructive pulmonary disease, obesity, cirrhosis, and age greater than 65 years.[60,61] Psychologic stress may be a risk factor for peptic ulcer disease but the exact mechanism of causation is not known.[62,63]

Peptic ulcers can be acute or chronic, and superficial or deep. Superficial ulcerations are called *erosions* because they erode the mucosa but do not penetrate the muscularis mucosae (Figure 41-7). True ulcers extend through the muscularis mucosae and damage blood vessels, causing hemorrhage or perforating the gastrointestinal wall.

Chronic use of NSAIDs suppresses mucosal prostaglandin synthesis, resulting in decreased bicarbonate secretion and mucin (a component of the gut barrier) production and increased secretion of hydrochloric acid. The interaction of NSAIDs and *H. pylori* can contribute to the pathogenesis of peptic ulcer.[64] Disruption of the mucosa exposes submucosal areas to gastric secretions and autodigestion causing erosion and ulceration.

Duodenal Ulcers

Duodenal ulcers occur with greater frequency than other types of peptic ulcers. Idiopathic duodenal ulcers are rare and can be associated with altered mucosal defenses, rapid gastric emptying, elevated serum gastrin levels, or acid production stimulated by smoking.

PATHOPHYSIOLOGY. Causative factors, singly or in combination, cause acid and pepsin concentrations in the duodenum to penetrate the mucosal barrier and lead to ulceration[65] (Figure 41-8).

CLINICAL MANIFESTATIONS. The characteristic manifestation of a duodenal ulcer is chronic intermittent pain in the epigastric area. The pain begins 30 minutes to 2 hours after eating, when the stomach is empty. It is not unusual for pain to occur in the middle of the night and disappear by morning. The pain results from sensorineural stimulation by acid or muscle spasm, or both. Pain is relieved rapidly by ingestion of food or antacids, creating

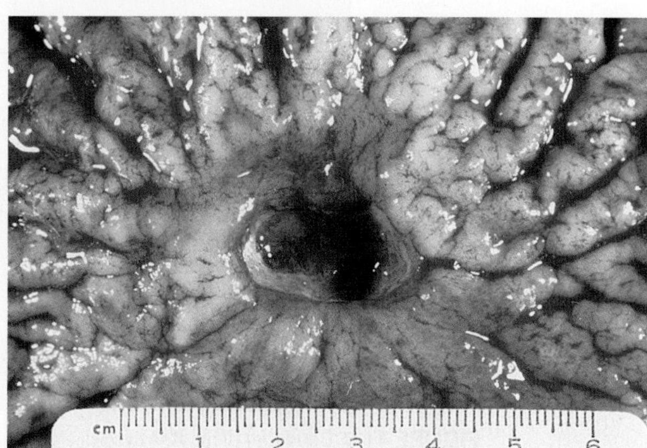

FIGURE 41-7 Chronic Peptic Ulcer. Gross photograph of a chronic peptic ulcer located in the lesser curvature, straddling the antrum and corpus of the stomach. (From Damjanov I, Linder J, editors: *Anderson's pathology,* ed 10, St Louis, 1996, Mosby.)

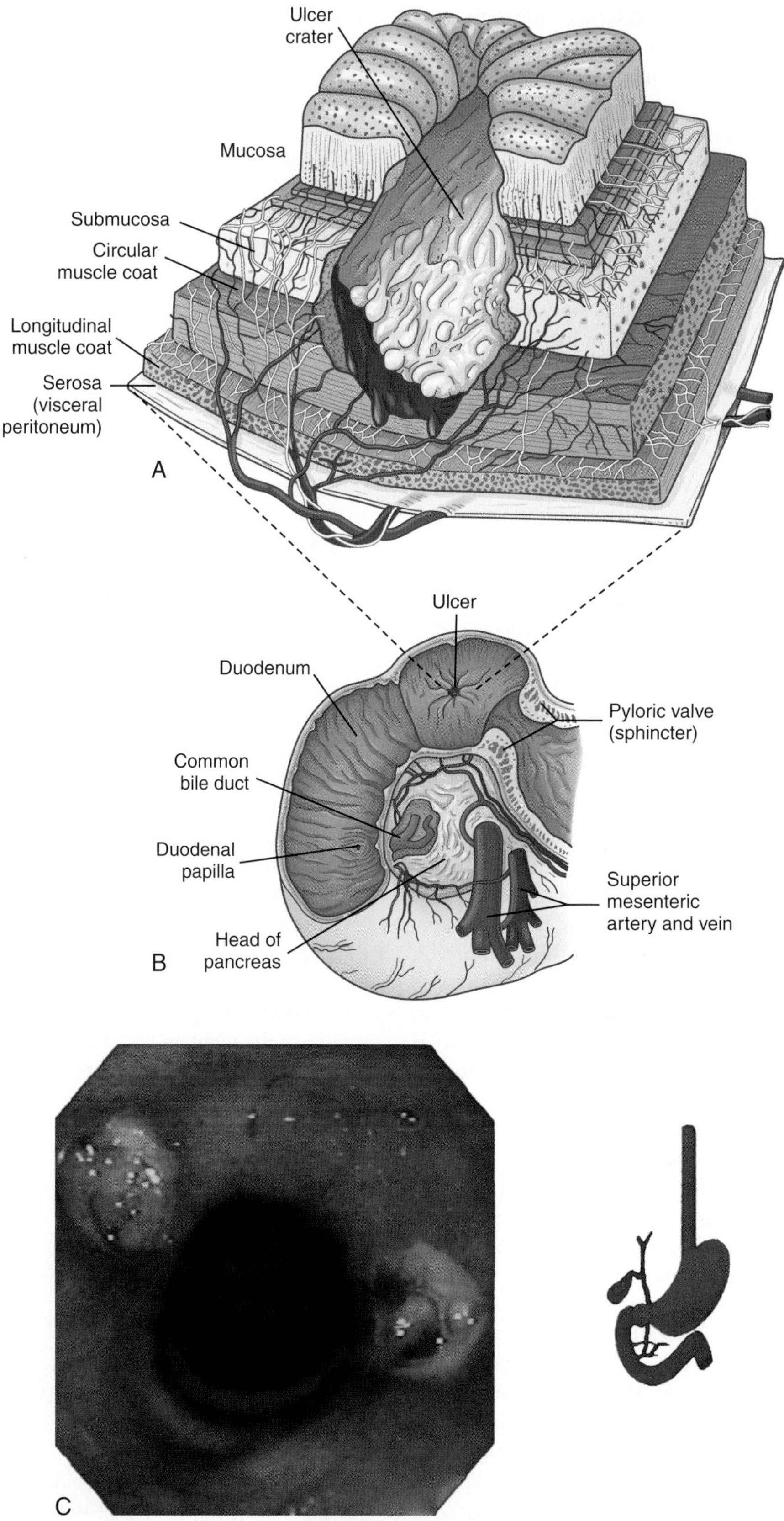

FIGURE 41-8 Duodenal Ulcer. A, A deep ulceration in the duodenal wall extending as a crater through the entire mucosa and into the muscle layers. **B,** Duodenal ulcer. **C,** Bilateral (kissing) duodenal ulcers in a person using nonsteroidal anti-inflammatory drugs (NSAIDs). (**C** courtesy David Bjorkman, MD, Department of Gastroenterology, University of Utah School of Medicine, Salt Lake City, UT.)

TABLE 41-4 CHARACTERISTICS OF GASTRIC AND DUODENAL ULCERS

CHARACTERISTICS	GASTRIC ULCER	DUODENAL ULCER
Incidence		
Age at onset	50-70 years	20-50 years
Family history	Usually negative	Positive
Gender (prevalence)	Equal in women and men	Equal in women and men
Stress factors	Increased	Average
Ulcerogenic drugs	Normal use	Increased use
Cancer risk	Increased	Not increased
Pathophysiology		
Helicobacter pylori infection	Often present (60-80%)	Often present (95-100%)
Abnormal mucus	May be present	May be present
Parietal cell mass	Normal or decreased	Increased
Acid production	Normal or decreased	Increased
Serum gastrin	Increased	Normal
Serum pepsinogen	Normal	Increased
Associated gastritis	More common	Usually not present
Clinical Manifestations		
Pain	Located in upper abdomen Intermittent Pain-antacid-relief pattern Food-pain pattern	Located in upper abdomen Intermittent Pain-antacid or food-relief pattern Nocturnal pain common
Clinical course	Chronic ulcer without pattern of remission and exacerbation	Pattern of remissions and exacerbations for years

a typical "pain-food-relief" pattern. Some individuals with duodenal ulcer have no symptoms, particularly older adults; the first manifestation may be hemorrhage or perforation, particularly with a history of NSAID or anticoagulant use. Healing is accompanied by relief of pain. Constant, unremitting pain may be caused by complications, such as intestinal obstruction or perforation. Bleeding from duodenal ulcers causes hematemesis or melena. It is not clear why individuals infected with *H. pylori* duodenal ulcers are negatively associated with gastric cancer.[66]

EVALUATION AND TREATMENT. Several diagnostic approaches are used to differentiate duodenal ulcers from gastric ulcers or gastric carcinoma. Endoscopic evaluation allows visualization of lesions and biopsy. Radioimmune assays of gastrin levels are evaluated to identify ulcers associated with gastric carcinomas. A urea breath test; measurement of levels of serum antibodies, stool, and serum antigen; and findings from gastric biopsy are used to detect *H. pylori* infection.[67]

Management of duodenal ulcers is aimed at relieving the causes and effects of hyperacidity and preventing complications. Antacids neutralize gastric contents, elevate pH, inactivate pepsin, relieve pain, and are cytoprotective.[67a] Acid secretion can be suppressed with drugs that block H2 receptors and inhibit the secretion of acid. Proton pump inhibitors inhibit acid production. Eradication of *H. pylori* with bismuth and combinations of antibiotics supplemented with vitamin C usually prevents relapse, although there is increasing drug resistance.[68,69] Ulcer-coating agents, such as sucralfate and colloidal bismuth, promote healing. Anticholinergic drugs may be used to inhibit gastric secretion, suppress gastric motility, and delay gastric emptying. Surgical resection may be required for complications including bleeding, perforation, obstruction, or peritonitis.[70] Risk of duodenal ulcer may be reduced with a diet high in vitamin A and fiber.[71] Development of a vaccine against *H. pylori* is progressing slowly.[72]

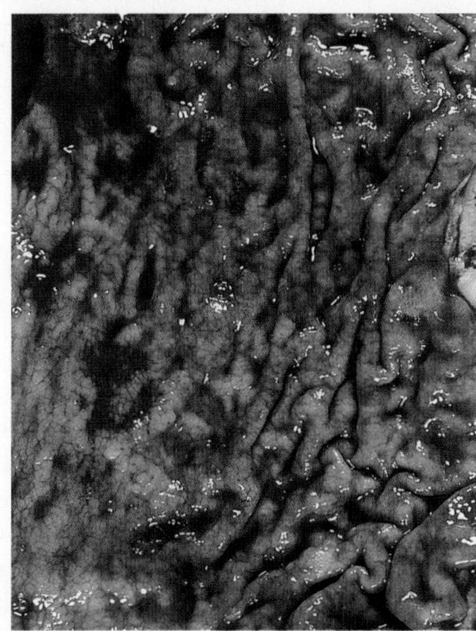

FIGURE 41-9 Macroscopic Appearance of Benign Gastric Ulcers. (From Damjanov I, Linder J, editors: *Anderson's pathology*, ed 10, St Louis, 1996, Mosby.)

Gastric Ulcers

Gastric ulcers are ulcers of the stomach. They usually occur between the ages of 55 and 65 years, and are about one fourth as common as duodenal ulcers (Table 41-4 and Figure 41-9).

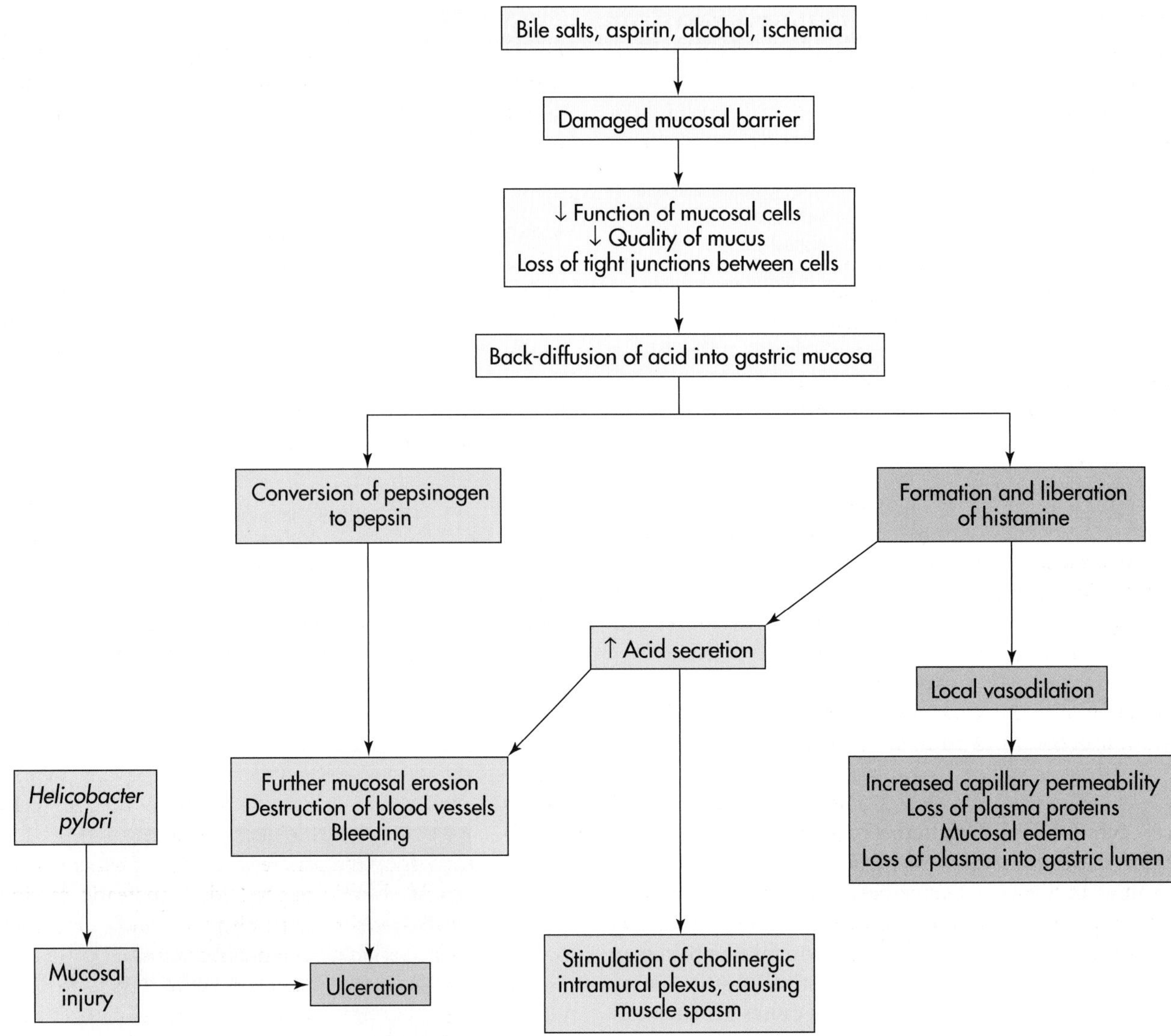

FIGURE 41-10 Pathophysiology of Gastric Ulcer Formation.

PATHOPHYSIOLOGY. Generally gastric ulcers develop in the antral region, adjacent to the acid-secreting mucosa of the body, and are frequently caused by *H. pylori* (see Box 41-1). The primary defect is an abnormality that increases the mucosal barrier's permeability to hydrogen ions. Gastric secretion may be normal or less than normal and there may be a decreased mass of parietal cells. Chronic pangastritis is often associated with development of gastric ulcers and may precipitate ulcer formation by limiting the mucosa's ability to secrete a protective layer of mucus (Figure 41-10).[73]

Duodenal reflux of bile is associated with gastric ulcer (alkaline reflux gastritis, p. 1435) and may occur after cholecystectomy, pyloroplasty, or gastrojejunostomy. The pyloric sphincter also may fail to respond to stimuli that normally increase resting tone, such as entry of acid, protein, and fat into the duodenum, allowing reflux of bile and pancreatic enzymes to damage the gastric mucosa. The damaged mucosal barrier permits hydrogen ions to diffuse into the mucosa, where they disrupt permeability and cellular structure. A vicious cycle can be established as the damaged mucosa liberates histamine, which stimulates the increase of acid and pepsinogen production, blood flow, and capillary permeability. The disrupted mucosa becomes edematous and loses plasma proteins. Destruction of small vessels causes bleeding.

Zollinger-Ellison syndrome is associated with peptic ulcers related to increased secretion of gastrin, which causes excess secretion of gastric acid. A gastrinoma (a gastrin-secreting neuroendocrine tumor or multiple tumors) of the pancreas or duodenum stimulates a proliferation of gastric parietal cells and chronic secretion of gastric acid. The resulting excess acid causes gastric and duodenal ulcers, gastroesophageal reflux with abdominal pain, and diarrhea. Diagnosis includes secretin- or calcium-stimulated measures of gastrin levels, gastric pH levels less than 2, and symptomatic evidence of peptic ulcer disease. Proton pump inhibitors reduce gastric acid secretion, and surgical removal of tumors limits metastasis.[74,75]

CLINICAL MANIFESTATIONS. The clinical manifestations of gastric ulcers are similar to those of duodenal ulcers (see Table 41-4). The pattern of pain, food, and relief is common, but the pain of gastric ulcers also occurs immediately after eating. Gastric ulcers also tend to be chronic rather than alternate between periods of remission and exacerbation and cause more anorexia, vomiting, and weight loss than duodenal ulcers.

EVALUATION AND TREATMENT. The evaluation and treatment of gastric ulcers are similar to the evaluation and treatment of duodenal ulcers (see p. 1437).

Stress-Related Mucosal Disease

A **stress ulcer (stress-related mucosal disease)** is an acute form of peptic ulcer that tends to accompany the physiologic stress of severe illness; multisystem organ failure; or major trauma, including severe burns or head injury. Usually, multiple sites of ulceration are distributed within the stomach or duodenum. Stress ulcers may be classified as ischemic ulcers or Cushing ulcers.

Ischemic ulcers develop within hours of an event—such as hemorrhage, multisystem trauma, severe burns, heart failure, or sepsis—that causes ischemia of the stomach and duodenal mucosa. Stress ulcers that develop as a result of burn injury are often called **Curling ulcers.**

Cushing ulcer is a stress ulcer associated with severe head trauma or brain surgery. This ulcer results from decreased mucosal blood flow and hypersecretion of acid caused by overstimulation of the vagal nuclei. Excessive acid damages the mucosal barrier, initiating the processes summarized in Figure 41-10.

The primary clinical manifestation of stress-related mucosal disease is bleeding that occurs more readily with the presence of coagulopathy.[76] Other symptoms may not be present. The bleeding may be slight or, if a small vessel is perforated, amount to hundreds of milliliters. Prophylactic treatment regimens are used to prevent this disease.[77,78] Stress ulcers seldom become chronic.

Surgical Treatment of Ulcer

Advances in the medical treatment of peptic ulcer disease with proton pump inhibitors and eradication of *H. pylori,* and laparoscopic and endoscopic repair techniques have significantly reduced the number of cases requiring open surgery.[79] The indications for ulcer surgery are recurrent or uncontrolled bleeding and complicated perforation of the stomach or duodenum.[80]

Weight loss often follows gastric resection but stabilizes within 3 months. Inadequate food intake is a common cause because many individuals cannot tolerate the osmotic effect of carbohydrates or a normal-size meal. Foods may be poorly absorbed because the stomach is less able to mix, churn, and break down food particles. Abdominal pain, vomiting, diarrhea, and malabsorption of fats also contribute to weight loss. In the case of bariatric surgery for extreme obesity, weight loss is the intended outcome.

Acute complications of gastrectomy or anastomosis, such as poor wound healing, abscess formation, or suture failure, are relatively uncommon except in the debilitated person. Chronic complications, however, occur more often and are likely to develop if a large portion of the stomach has been removed. These complications and their pathophysiologic mechanisms are described in the next section.

Postgastrectomy Syndromes

Postgastrectomy syndromes are a group of signs and symptoms that occur after gastric resection. They are caused by changes in motor and control functions of the stomach and upper small intestine.[81]

Malabsorption Syndromes

Malabsorption syndromes interfere with nutrient absorption. Historically malabsorption disorders have been classified as maldigestion or malabsorption. **Maldigestion** is failure of the chemical processes of digestion that take place in the intestinal lumen or at the brush border of the intestinal mucosa of the small intestine. **Malabsorption** is the failure of the intestinal mucosa to absorb (transport) the digested nutrients. Often maldigestion and malabsorption are interrelated or occur together, making classification difficult. Generally, however, maldigestion is caused by deficiencies of enzymes, such as pancreatic lipase or intestinal lactase, which are necessary for digestion. Inadequate secretion of bile salts and inadequate reabsorption of bile in the ileum also contribute to maldigestion. Malabsorption is the result of mucosal disruption caused by gastric or intestinal resection, vascular disorders, or intestinal disease.

Pancreatic Insufficiency

The pancreatic enzymes (lipase, amylase, trypsin, chymotrypsin) are required for the digestion of proteins, carbohydrates, and fats. **Pancreatic insufficiency** is the deficient production of these enzymes by the pancreas. Causes of pancreatic insufficiency include chronic pancreatitis, pancreatic carcinoma, pancreatic resection, and cystic fibrosis. Significant damage to or loss of pancreatic tissue must occur before enzyme levels decrease sufficiently to cause maldigestion. Although pancreatic insufficiency causes poor digestion of all nutrients, fat maldigestion is the chief problem. Salivary amylase and enzymes secreted by the intestinal brush border assist in carbohydrate and protein digestion, but these enzymes do not digest fats. Absence of pancreatic bicarbonate in the duodenum and jejunum causes an acidic pH that worsens maldigestion by preventing activation of pancreatic enzymes that are present. A large amount of fat in the stool (steatorrhea) and weight loss are the most common signs of pancreatic insufficiency. Lipase supplementation is usually successful.[82]

Lactase Deficiency

Deficiency of disaccharidase at the villus brush border of the small intestine is caused by a congenital defect in the lactase gene. **Lactase deficiency** inhibits the breakdown of lactose (milk sugar) into monosaccharides and therefore prevents lactose digestion and absorption across the intestinal wall. Lactase deficiency is most common in blacks. Congenital lactase deficiency causes watery diarrhea in breast milk or lactose-containing formulas in infants. Lactase expression is lost before adulthood in adult-type lactose intolerance.[83] Secondary (acquired) lactase deficiency can be caused by several diseases of the intestine, including gluten-sensitive enteropathy (see Chapter 42), enteritis, and bacterial overgrowth.

The undigested lactose remains in the intestine, where bacterial fermentation causes gases to form. Undigested lactose also increases the osmotic gradient in the intestine, causing irritation and osmotic diarrhea. Clinical manifestations of lactose consumption with lactase deficiency are bloating, crampy pain, diarrhea, and flatulence. The disorder is diagnosed by genetic testing, a lactose-hydrogen breath test, dietary lactose withdrawal, or rarely small intestinal biopsy.[84] Avoiding milk products and adhering to a lactose-free diet relieve symptoms. Maintaining an adequate calcium intake with restricted intake of milk products decreases risk of osteoporosis.

Bile Salt Deficiency

Conjugated bile acids (bile salts) are necessary for the digestion and absorption of fats. Bile salts are conjugated in the bile that is synthesized from cholesterol and secreted from the liver.[85] When bile enters the duodenum, the bile salts aggregate with fatty acids and monoglycerides to form micelles. Micelle formation makes fat molecules more soluble and allows them to pass through the unstirred layer at the brush border of the small intestinal villi (see Chapter 40). A minimum concentration of bile salts, termed the *critical micelle concentration,* is required to allow micelles to form. Therefore, conditions that decrease the production or secretion of bile result in decreased micelle formation and fat malabsorption. These conditions include advanced liver disease, which decreases production of bile salts; obstruction of the common bile duct, which decreases flow of bile into the duodenum; intestinal stasis (lack of motility), which permits overgrowth of intestinal bacteria that deconjugate bile salts; and diseases of the ileum, which prevent the reabsorption and recycling of bile salts (enterohepatic circulation).[86]

Clinical manifestations of bile salt deficiency are related to poor intestinal absorption of fat and fat-soluble vitamins (A, D, E, and K). Increased fat in the stools (steatorrhea) leads to diarrhea and decreased plasma proteins. The losses of fat-soluble vitamins and their effects include the following:

1. Vitamin A deficiency results in night blindness.
2. Vitamin D deficiency results in decreased calcium absorption with bone demineralization (osteoporosis), bone pain, and fractures.
3. Vitamin K deficiency prolongs prothrombin time, leading to spontaneous development of purpura (bruising) and petechiae.
4. Vitamin E deficiency has uncertain effects but may cause testicular atrophy and neurologic defects in children.

The most effective treatment for fat-soluble vitamin deficiency is to increase the amount of medium-chain triglycerides in the diet, for example, by using coconut oil for cooking. Vitamins A, D, and K are given parenterally.

Dumping Syndrome

Dumping syndrome is the rapid emptying of hypertonic chyme from the surgically created, residual stomach into the small intestine 10 to 20 minutes after eating (early dumping syndrome). It occurs with varying severity in 5% to 10% of individuals who have undergone partial gastrectomy, bariatric surgical procedures, or pyloroplasty.[81,87] It is not as common in individuals who have undergone a Billroth II anastomosis (gastrojejunostomy) accompanied by vagotomy. Factors that promote *early dumping syndrome* include: (1) loss of gastric capacity, (2) loss of emptying control when the pylorus is removed, and (3) loss of feedback control by the duodenum when it is removed. Rapid gastric emptying and creation of a nonphysiologic, high osmotic gradient within the small intestine cause a sudden shift of fluid from the vascular compartment to the intestinal lumen. Plasma volume decreases, causing vasomotor responses, such as increased pulse rate, hypotension, weakness, pallor, sweating, and dizziness. Rapid distention of the intestine produces a feeling of epigastric fullness, cramping, nausea, and vomiting. Diarrhea can accompany dumping syndrome or occur as a solitary symptom. Diarrhea can occur as frequent, persistent elimination of liquid stool or as intermittent, precipitous, and unpredictable elimination of a large volume of stool. Both types can be either mild or severe.

A less common form of dumping syndrome, *late dumping syndrome* occurs 1 to 3 hours after eating. The symptoms include weakness, diaphoresis, and confusion but they cannot be explained by rapid gastric emptying. After a high-carbohydrate meal, individuals who have undergone gastrectomy may develop hypoglycemia, which causes the symptoms. The hypoglycemia is caused by an increase in insulin secretion stimulated by the hyperglycemia that follows eating. Other hormonal responses also may participate in the development of hypoglycemia.

Most cases of dumping syndrome respond well to dietary management.[88] Frequent small meals that are high in protein and low in carbohydrates relieve symptoms. Other measures include drinking fluids between meals instead of at mealtime and reclining on the left side after eating. Some cases require surgical intervention, including reconstruction of the pylorus or a gastrojejunostomy. Octreotide reduces abdominal and vasomotor symptoms of dumping syndrome by inhibiting insulin and gut hormone release, slowing intestinal transit time, and inhibiting food-induced circulatory changes.[89]

Inflammatory Bowel Disease

Ulcerative colitis and Crohn disease are chronic, relapsing inflammatory bowel diseases (IBDs) of unknown origin. The incidence of IBD is increasing around the world and varies from 3 to 300 per 100,000 persons.[90] Both diseases are associated with genetic factors, alterations in epithelial cell barrier functions, immunopathology related to abnormal T-cell reactions to commensal microflora and other luminal antigens, and varying phenotypes.[91] **Microscopic colitis** is increasing in prevalence and is reviewed in What's New? Microscopic Colitis.

Ulcerative Colitis

Ulcerative colitis (UC) is a chronic inflammatory disease that causes ulceration of the colonic mucosa and extends proximally from the rectum into the colon (Figure 41-11). The lesions appear in susceptible individuals between 20 and 40 years of age. Risk factors include family history of disease or Jewish descent, and the disease is more prevalent among white populations and Northern Europeans. UC is less common in smokers.[92]

Although the cause of UC is unknown, dietary, infectious, genetic, and immunologic factors are all suggested causes.[93] Inflammation may be caused by commensal or pathogenic enteric microorganisms with increased mucosal adherence and invasion and persistent activation of T cells. The familial tendency to develop ulcerative colitis and the occurrence of disease in identical twins support a genetic theory of causation. Perhaps most significant are the humoral and cellular immunologic factors associated with the disease. Colonic epithelial antibodies of the immunoglobulin G (IgG) class have been identified in the sera of individuals with ulcerative colitis and a large number of plasma cells are found in the inflamed colon. Lymphocytes (T cells) in individuals with ulcerative colitis may have cytotoxic effects on the epithelial cells of the colon, as well as damage caused by inflammatory cytokines (interleukin-1 [IL-1], IL-2, IL-6, IL-8, IL-10, tumor necrosis factor-alpha [TNF-α]), toxic oxygen free radicals, and interferon-gamma (IFN-γ).[94] Furthermore, autoimmune disorders, such as systemic lupus erythematosus and erythema nodosum, may accompany ulcerative colitis.

WHAT'S NEW?

Microscopic Colitis

Microscopic colitis is a relatively common cause of diarrhea and occurs primarily in females and older adults. There are two histologic forms: lymphocytic and collagenous. The symptoms of frequent chronic daily watery diarrhea are the same for both types and can be accompanied by abdominal pain and weight loss. The cause is unknown and the prevalence is increasing. There are associations with numerous drugs and celiac disease. Autoantibodies have been found in some individuals including intestinal goblet cells, antinuclear antibodies (ANAs), antineutrophil cytoplasmic antibodies, and anti–*Saccharomyces cerevisiae* antibody (ASCA). The colon mucosa appears normal on endoscopy. Biopsy reveals histopathologic descriptions. Lymphocytic colitis shows an increase in intraepithelial lymphocytes of more than 20 lymphocytes per 100 surface colonocytes. Collagenous colitis is characterized by a thickened subepithelial collagen layer of more than 10 μm, alteration of the vascular mucosal pattern, and mucosal nodularity. Antidiarrheal agents and budesonide (an anti-inflammatory steroid) are the best documented short-term treatments and new immunosuppressive agents are being evaluated. An optimal long-term strategy is yet to be identified. The disease is negatively associated with colorectal cancer.

Data from Gentile NM et al: *Am J Gastroenterol* 108(2):256–259, 2013; Ianiro G et al: *World J Gastroenterol* 18(43):6206–6215, 2012; Koulaouzidis A, Saeed AA: *World J Gastroenterol* 17(37):4157–4165, 2011; Mahajan D et al: *Adv Anat Pathol* 19(1):28–38, 2012; Yen EF et al: *Dig Dis Sci* 57(1):161–169, 2012.

PATHOPHYSIOLOGY. The primary lesions of UC are continuous with no skip lesions, are limited to the mucosa, and are not transmural. The mucous layer is thinner than normal and there is impairment of the epithelial barrier. The rectum is almost always involved. Inflammation begins at the base of the crypt of Lieberkühn in the large intestine, primarily the left colon, with infiltration and release of inflammatory cytokines from neutrophils, lymphocytes, plasma cells, macrophages, eosinophils, and mast cells. Activated macrophages also contribute cytokines that cause fever and the acute phase response. The inflammation damages the epithelial mucosal barrier with leak of fluids into the gut.[95] The disease is most severe in the rectum and sigmoid colon. With milder inflammation, the mucosa is hyperemic and edematous, and may appear dark red and velvety (Figure 41-12). In more severe inflammation, the mucosa becomes hemorrhagic, and small erosions form and coalesce into ulcers. Abscess formation occurs in the crypts. Necrosis and ragged ulceration of the mucosa ensue. Edema and thickening of the muscularis mucosae may narrow the lumen of the involved colon. In chronic disease, inflammatory polyps (pseudopolyps) develop in the colon from rapidly regenerating epithelium.

CLINICAL MANIFESTATIONS. The course of UC consists of intermittent periods of remission and exacerbation. Clinical

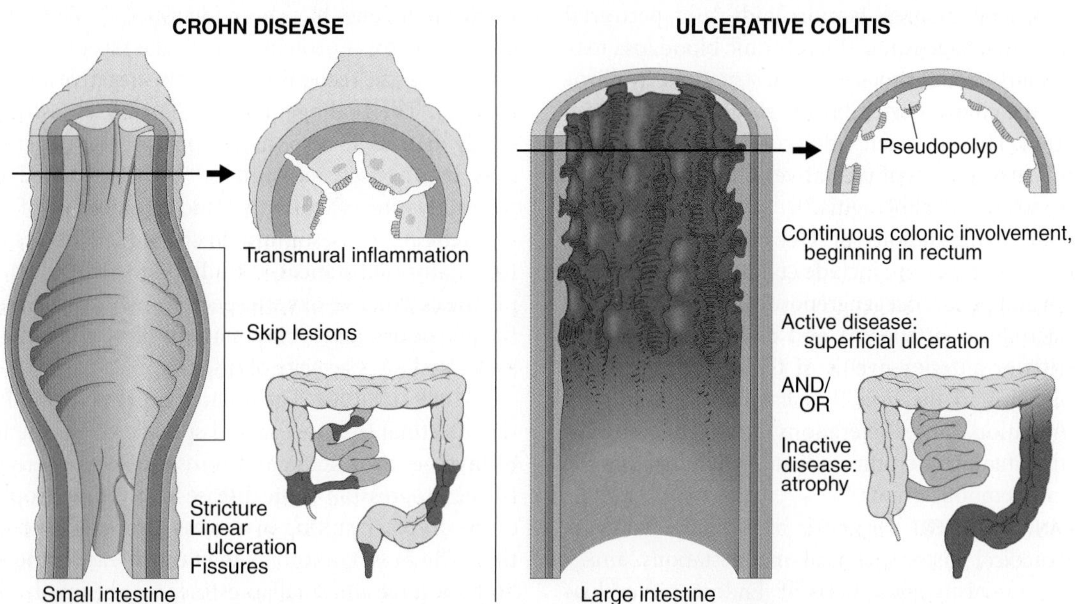

FIGURE 41-11 Distribution Patterns of Crohn Disease and Ulcerative Colitis. Comparison of distribution patterns of Crohn disease and ulcerative colitis as well as different conformations of ulcers and wall thickenings. (From Kumar V et al: *Robbins basic pathology*, ed 8, St Louis, 2008, Mosby.)

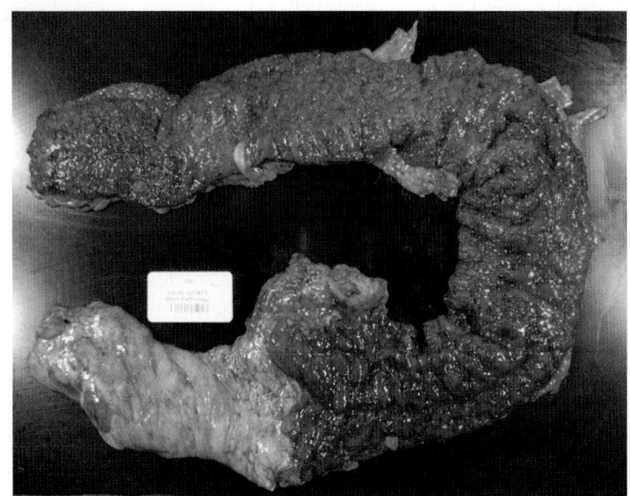

FIGURE 41-12 Acute Ulcerative Colitis. A gross specimen of subtotal ulcerative colitis showing diffuse continuous disease starting from the distal rectum and continuing up to the midportion of the ascending colon. (From Odze RD, Goldblum JR, editors: *Surgical pathology of the GI tract, liver, biliary tract, and pancreas,* ed 2, Philadelphia, 2009, Saunders.)

manifestations vary with the severity and extent of disease. Loss of the absorptive mucosal surface and decreased colonic transit time can cause large volumes of watery diarrhea. Mucosal destruction causes bleeding, cramping pain, and an urge to defecate. There is frequent bloody diarrhea with passage of purulent mucus.[96] Mild UC involves less mucosa and may be limited to proctitis, so that frequency of bowel movements, bleeding, and pain is minimal. Severe forms may involve the entire colon (pancolitis) and are characterized by fever, elevated pulse rate, frequent diarrhea (10 to 20 movements per day), urgency, obviously bloody stools, and continuous crampy pain. Dehydration, weight loss, anemia, and fever result from fluid loss, bleeding, and inflammation. Complications include toxic megacolon, anal fissures, hemorrhoids, and perirectal abscess. Severe hemorrhage is rare, but chronic blood loss may precipitate hypotension and shock. Edema, strictures, or fibrosis can obstruct the colon. Perforation is an unusual but possible complication. The risk of left-sided colon cancer increases significantly after many years of ulcerative colitis and the presence of primary sclerosing cholangitis.[97]

Extraintestinal manifestations of UC and Crohn disease occur in about 30% of cases and include cutaneous lesions (erythema nodosum and pyoderma gangrenosum), migratory polyarthritis and sacroiliitis, osteopenia and osteoporosis, mouth ulcers, episcleritis or anterior uveitis of the eye, and primary sclerosing cholangitis in the liver.[98] Gallstones are common. Chronic inflammation causes alterations in coagulation and can cause life-threatening microthrombi, deep vein thrombosis, and other thromboembolic events.[99]

EVALUATION AND TREATMENT. Diagnosis of ulcerative colitis is based on the medical history, clinical manifestations, imaging procedures, and histologic criteria.[100] Endoscopic evaluation shows an inflamed and hemorrhagic mucosa. Radiologic assessment may show loss of haustra, ulceration, and irregular mucosa. The laboratory data include low hemoglobin values, hypoalbuminemia, and low serum potassium levels. Infectious causes are ruled out by stool culture. The symptoms of ulcerative colitis can be very similar to those of Crohn disease, and serological markers may be used for differential diagnosis.[101]

Treatment depends on the severity of symptoms and the extent of mucosal involvement. First-line therapy is 5-aminosalicylic acid (mesalazine). Corticosteroids and salicylates suppress the inflammatory response and help alleviate the cramping pain. Immunosuppressive agents (e.g., 6-mercaptopurine or azathioprine), cyclosporine, tacrolimus, and infliximab (a monoclonal anti–TNF-α antibody) are used for chronic active disease.[102] Broad-spectrum antibiotics may induce remission.[103] For unknown reasons, nicotine may have a protective effect in ulcerative colitis but not in Crohn disease.[104] Severe, unremitting disease can require hospital admission and administration of intravenous fluids. Extreme malnutrition may require intravenous hyperalimentation. Surgical resection of the colon or a colostomy may be performed if other forms of therapy are unsuccessful.[105] *Pouchitis* is a complication of restorative proctocolectomy with ileal pouch–anal anastomosis performed as surgical treatment for both UC and Crohn disease. Antibiotic treatment is usually successful.[106]

Crohn Disease

Crohn disease (CD) (granulomatous colitis, ileocolitis, or regional enteritis) is an idiopathic inflammatory disorder that affects any part of the gastrointestinal tract from the mouth to the anus. The distal small intestine and proximal large colon are most commonly affected by the disease. In a small percentage of cases, CD is difficult to differentiate from ulcerative colitis (Table 41-5). Risk factors include family history, smoking, Jewish ethnicity, urban residency, age less than 40 years, and a slight predominance in women.[107] The *CARD15/NOD2* (nucleotide-binding-oligomerization-domains) gene mutations have the strongest association with CD (35% to 45% of cases) although many other genes have been identified.[108] The *CARD15 /NOD2* genes code for a protein (a Toll-like receptor; see Chapter 10) involved in the recognition of gram-negative and gram-positive bacteria. The pathogenesis of CD may be associated with an overly aggressive response to normal flora bacteria in genetically predisposed individuals.[109] Th1-mediated inflammation with activation of leukocytes and cytokines (TNF-α, IFN-γ, and interleukins) causes injury. Recruited leukocytes release proinflammatory substances, including prostaglandins, leukotrienes, proteases, reactive oxygen species, and nitric oxide, which cause further injury and inflammation. Elevations in IgG levels are associated with severity of disease.[110]

PATHOPHYSIOLOGY. The inflammatory process of CD begins in the intestinal submucosa and spreads across the intestinal wall to involve the mucosa and serosa in areas overlying lymphoid tissue. Progression of the disease involves neutrophil infiltration of the crypts, resulting in abscess formation and crypt destruction. The most common site of the disease is the ileocolon, but both the large and small intestines may be involved. The inflammation can affect some haustral segments but not others, creating a pattern called *skip lesions.* One side of the intestinal wall may be affected but not the other.

TABLE 41-5 FEATURES OF ULCERATIVE COLITIS AND CROHN DISEASE

FEATURE	ULCERATIVE COLITIS	CROHN DISEASE
Incidence		
Age at onset	Any age; 10-40 years most common	Any age; 10-30 years most common
Family history	Less common	More common
Gender (prevalence)	Equal in women and men	About equal in women and men
Cancer risk	Increased	Increased
Pathophysiology		
Location of lesions	Colon and rectum, no "skip" lesions	All of GI tract: mouth to anus, "skip" lesions common
Inflammation and ulceration	Mucosal layer involved	Entire intestinal wall involved
Granulomas	Rare	Common
Friable mucosa	Common	Less common
Fistulae and abscesses	Rare	Common
Strictures and possible obstruction	Rare	Common
Clinical Manifestations		
Abdominal pain	Occasional	Common
Diarrhea	Common	Common
Bloody stools	Common	Less common
Abdominal mass	Rare	Common
Small intestinal malabsorption	Rare	Common
Steatorrhea	Rare	Common
Potential for malignancy	Common	Common
Antineutrophil cytoplasmic antibodies	Common	Rare
Anti–*Saccharomyces cerevisiae* antibodies	Rare	Common
Clinical course	Remissions and exacerbations	Remissions and exacerbations

GI, Gastrointestinal.

The ulcerations of CD produce longitudinal and transverse fissures that extend inflammation into lymphoid tissue. The typical chronic lesion is a granuloma having cobblestone projections of inflamed tissue surrounded by areas of ulceration (Figure 41-13). (Granulomas are described in Chapter 7.) The lumen can narrow with inflammation, edema, and fibrotic strictures. Fistulae may form in the perianal area between loops of intestine or extend into the bladder.

CLINICAL MANIFESTATIONS. Individuals with CD may have no specific symptoms other than an "irritable bowel" for several years. Symptoms vary and are associated with disease location. Abdominal pain and diarrhea are the most common signs (more than five stools per day), with passage of blood and mucus. Diarrhea can result from decreased colonic absorption, bypass fistulae, medications, bacterial overgrowth, and the presence of bile in the colon that inhibits water absorption. Other manifestations are related to the location and extent of intestinal involvement. Inflammation of the ileum, for example, causes tenderness in the lower right side of the abdomen. If the ileum is involved, the individual may be anemic as a result of malabsorption of vitamin B_{12}. There also may be deficiencies in folic acid, vitamin D absorption, and calcium leading to bone disease. Proteins may be lost, leading to hypoalbuminemia. Weight loss is common. Anal manifestations occur in about 30% of cases, including anal fissure, perianal abscess, and fistula.[111] Individuals with CD of long duration are also at risk for intestinal adenocarcinoma.[112] Complications include obstruction, fistulae, abscess formation, and chronic blood loss. Extraintestinal manifestations are similar to those described for UC.

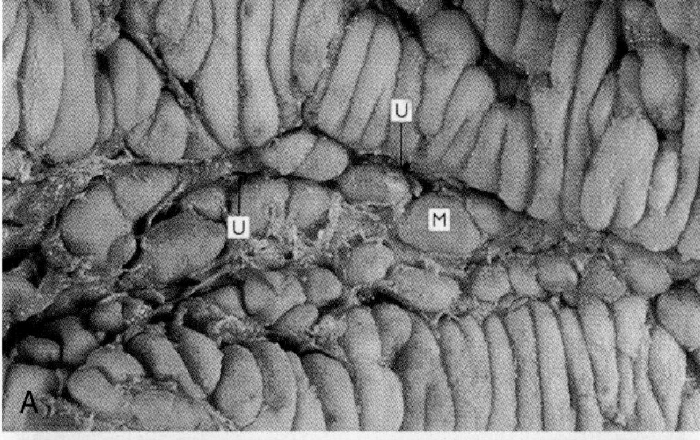

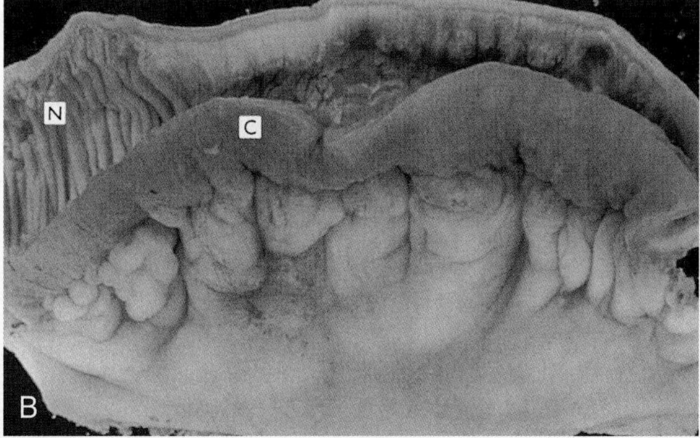

FIGURE 41-13 Crohn Disease. A, The mucosa in Crohn disease demonstrates a cobblestone pattern as a result of fissured ulcers *(U)* with intervening areas of edematous mucosa *(M).* **B,** Compared with normal small bowel wall *(N),* the Crohn segment *(C)* shows wall thickening that has caused a stenosis. (From Kumar V et al: *Pathologic basis of disease,* ed 7, Philadelphia, 2006, Saunders.)

EVALUATION AND TREATMENT. The diagnosis and treatment of CD are similar to the diagnosis and treatment of ulcerative colitis. Treatment with immunomodulatory agents can be effective. TNF-α–blocking agents are used for treatment of fistulae and to maintain remission.[113] Surgery is generally performed to manage complications such as strictures, fistulae, abscesses, and perforation, or to relieve obstruction.[114] When treatment involves surgical resection of small intestinal segments, complications related to **short bowel syndrome** can occur, including malabsorption, diarrhea, and nutritional deficiencies. Symptoms are related to the extent and location of resection.[115]

Diverticular Disease of the Colon

Diverticula are herniations or saclike outpouchings of mucosa through the muscle layers of the colon wall. **Diverticulosis** is asymptomatic diverticular disease. **Diverticulitis** represents inflammation. The cause of diverticular disease is unknown but is associated with age greater than 60 years, decreased dietary fiber, increased intracolonic pressure, abnormal neuromuscular function, and alterations in intestinal motility.[116]

PATHOPHYSIOLOGY. Diverticula can occur anywhere in the gastrointestinal tract but the most common site is the left colon. They rarely occur in the small intestine.[117] The diverticula form at weak points in the colon wall, usually where arteries penetrate the tunica muscularis to nourish the mucosal layer. The colonic mucosa herniates through the smooth muscle layers (Figure 41-14). A common associated finding is thickening of the circular and longitudinal (teniae coli) muscles surrounding the diverticula. Hypertrophy and contraction of these muscles increase intraluminal pressure and degree of herniation. Habitual consumption of a low-residue diet reduces fecal bulk, thus reducing the diameter of the colon. According to Laplace's law (see Chapter 31), wall pressure increases as the diameter of a cylindrical structure decreases. Therefore, pressure within the narrow lumen can increase enough to rupture the diverticula. Insoluble dietary fiber deficiency also may change the intestinal microflora, decreasing the immune response and levels of inflammatory cytokines in the colon.[118,119] Diverticulitis can cause abscess formation, fistula formation, peritonitis, or obstruction.[120]

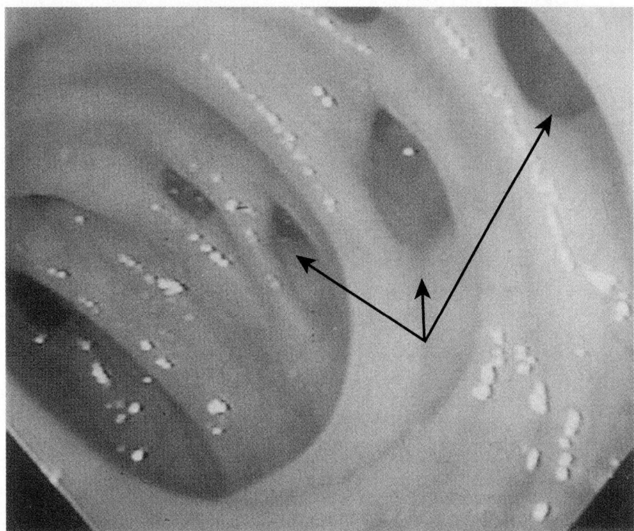

FIGURE 41-14 Diverticular Disease. In diverticular disease, the outpouches *(arrows)* of mucosa seen in the sigmoid colon appear as slitlike openings from the mucosal surface of the opened bowel. (From Townsend CM et al: *Sabiston textbook of surgery,* ed 19, Philadelphia 2012, Saunders.)

CLINICAL MANIFESTATIONS. Symptoms of diverticular disease are usually vague or absent and about 30% of individuals develop specific symptoms. Cramping pain of the lower abdomen can accompany constriction of the hypertrophied colonic muscles. Diarrhea, constipation, distention, or flatulence may occur. Diverticula with an obstructed opening become inflamed or abscesses form, and the individual develops fever, leukocytosis (increased white blood cell count), and tenderness of the lower left quadrant. Right lower quadrant pain and severe complications, such as hemorrhage, perforation with peritonitis, bowel obstruction, and fistula formation, are rare.[120]

EVALUATION AND TREATMENT. Diverticula are often discovered during diagnostic procedures performed for other problems. Ultrasound, sigmoidoscopy, or barium enema is used for diagnosis of uncomplicated diverticula. Abdominal computed tomography (CT) is used for complicated cases.

An increase of dietary fiber intake increases stool weight, lowers colonic pressures, improves transit times, and often relieves symptoms (see Nutrition & Disease: Diverticular Disease and Diet). Uncomplicated diverticular disease is treated with bowel rest and antibiotics.[121] Surgical resection may be required if there are severe complications, including hemorrhage, bowel stenosis, obstruction, abscesses, fistulae, bowel perforation, and peritonitis.[122]

NUTRITION & DISEASE
Diverticular Disease and Diet

Daily consumption of fiber-enriched foods is recommended for the prevention of diverticula. A high-fiber diet increases fecal bulk, decreases transit time, lowers intracolonic pressures, and eases stool elimination. The recommendation for fiber is 20 to 35 g/day. Some examples of high-fiber choices are whole wheat bread and other grain products, baked potato with skin, fresh fruit with skins, raw vegetables, beans, peas, legumes, wheat bran, and brown rice. Side effects may include flatulence, intestinal rumbling, cramps, and diarrhea. A gradual increase in dietary fiber over 1 or 2 months helps to avoid these problems. Other potential problems with an excessively high-fiber diet (greater than 40 to 45 g) might include a decrease in nutrient absorption because of the increased volume of intestinal contents, which in turn decreases the ability of the digestive enzymes to come into contact with the food. An increase of water intake (eight 8-ounce glasses) is important so intestinal blockage will not occur. For small children and older adults, a high-fiber diet increases the volume of food needed to meet energy requirements, and that increase may be difficult to obtain. Although some physicians recommend restricting nuts, seeds, and foods containing seeds such as berries, kiwi, and tomatoes that might lodge in the pouches, there is no evidence that this happens. If the diverticula become inflamed, a low-fiber, low-residue (no milk products), or elemental diet, or in complicated cases total parenteral nutrition (TPN), is required to prevent continued irritation of the inflamed tissue. Controlled clinical trials are needed to evaluate the effectiveness of high-fiber diets in preventing diverticular disease.

Data from Crowe FL et al: *BMJ* 343:d4131, 2011; Strate LL: *Dig Dis* 30(1):35–45, 2012; Ünlü C et al: *Int J Colorectal Dis* 27(4):419–427, 2012; Wick JY: *Consult Pharm* 27(9):613–618, 2012.

Appendicitis

Appendicitis is an inflammation of the vermiform appendix, which is a projection from the apex of the cecum. It is the most common surgical emergency of the abdomen and usually occurs between 20 and 30 years of age, although it may develop at any age.[123]

PATHOPHYSIOLOGY. The exact cause of appendicitis is controversial. Obstruction of the lumen with stool, tumors, or foreign bodies with consequent increased intraluminal pressure, ischemia, bacterial infection, and inflammation is a common theory. The obstructed lumen does not allow drainage of the appendix, and as mucosal secretion continues, intraluminal pressure increases. The resultant increased pressure decreases mucosal blood flow, and the appendix becomes hypoxic. The mucosa ulcerates, promoting bacterial or other microbial invasion with further inflammation and edema. Inflammation may involve the distal or entire appendix. Gangrene develops from thrombosis of the luminal blood vessels, followed by perforation.

CLINICAL MANIFESTATIONS. Epigastric or periumbilical pain is the typical symptom of an inflamed appendix. The pain may be vague at first, increasing in intensity over 3 to 4 hours. It may subside and then recur with a shift of location to the right lower quadrant with rebound tenderness. Right lower quadrant pain is associated with extension of the inflammation to the surrounding tissues. Nausea, vomiting, and anorexia follow the onset of pain, and fever is common. Diarrhea occurs in some individuals, particularly children; others have a sensation of constipation. Perforation, peritonitis, and abscess formation are the most serious complications of appendicitis.[124]

EVALUATION AND TREATMENT. In addition to clinical manifestations, the clinician can usually locate the painful site with one finger. Rebound tenderness is usually referred to the right lower quadrant. The white blood cell count ranges from 10,000 to 16,000 cells/mm^3 with elevations in the levels of neutrophils, C-reactive protein.[125] Abdominal CT scans and ultrasound assist diagnostic accuracy. The combined information provides the best discriminating diagnosis.[126]

Antibiotics and appendectomy is the treatment for simple or perforated appendicitis. Laparoscopic surgery provides quick recovery for simple appendicitis. Recovery is more complicated in cases of perforation or abscess formation and in individuals of older age.[127,128]

Irritable Bowel Syndrome

Irritable bowel syndrome (IBS) is a functional gastrointestinal disorder characterized by abdominal pain and altered bowel habits that affects about 10% of individuals throughout the world and is more common in women, with a higher prevalence in youth and middle age. Individuals with IBS are more likely to have anxiety and depression.[129]

PATHOPHYSIOLOGY. There are no specific structural or biochemical alterations as a cause of IBS but there is increasing evidence to explain the varying symptom presentations and they are summarized as follows:

1. *Visceral hypersensitivity or hyperalgesia,* particularly with distention of the rectum but also other areas of the gut: This occurs in about 30% to 40% of those with IBS. The cause is unknown; it may originate in either the peripheral or the central nervous system. The mechanism may be related to pain and a dysregulation of the "brain-gut axis" (alterations in gut or central nervous system processing of gut nociceptive information), increased permeability that stimulates nociceptors, the role of serotonin in the enteric nervous system of the gut, infiltration and activation of mast cells and T lymphocytes, or alterations in the autonomic nervous system.[130]
2. *Abnormal gastrointestinal permeability, motility, and secretion:* Individuals with diarrhea-type IBS have more rapid colonic transit times and increased intestinal permeability, whereas those with bloating and constipation have delayed transit times and decreased intestinal permeability. The mechanisms may be related to visceral hypersensitivity and dysregulation of the brain-gut axis or to the role of serotonin in the function of the enteric nervous system and to activity of mast cells.[131]
3. *Postinfectious IBS:* Two or more of the following symptoms are present: fever, vomiting, diarrhea, and a positive stool culture Intestinal infection (bacterial enteritis) has been associated with symptoms of IBS and may be related to altered gut microbiota, ongoing low-grade inflammation, and an abnormal immune response in gut tissues.[132]
4. *Overgrowth of intestinal flora:* Small intestinal overgrowth of normal gut bacteria may precipitate IBS symptoms and it is proposed that methane gas may slow intestinal transit time, resulting in constipation and bloating.[133,134]
5. *Food allergy or food intolerance:* Food antigens may activate the mucosal immune system, mediating hypersensitivity reactions and IBS symptoms. Individualized food elimination approaches are helpful in some cases because different foods alter neural and hormonal small intestinal responses. Allergic conditions, including rhinitis and asthma, have been associated with IBS.[135]
6. *Psychosocial factors:* Psychosocial factors including emotional stress influence brain-gut interaction including neuroendocrine, neuroimmune, autonomic nervous system, and pain modulatory responses contributing to the symptoms of IBS.[136]

CLINICAL MANIFESTATIONS. IBS is characterized by lower abdominal pain, diarrhea-predominant, constipation-predominant, or alternating diarrhea/constipation (mixed), gas, bloating, and nausea. Individuals may also describe fecal urgency and incomplete evacuation. Symptoms are usually relieved with defecation and usually do not interfere with sleep.

EVALUATION AND TREATMENT. The diagnosis of IBS is based on signs and symptoms and includes the exclusion of structural or biochemical causes of disease. In the absence of "alarm symptoms" such as fever, weight loss, gastrointestinal bleeding, anemia, or abdominal mass, only limited diagnostic tests are needed. The individual may be evaluated for food allergies, lactose intolerance, parasites, or bacterial growth. The Rome III criteria for diagnosing IBS have been released to guide evaluation (Box 41-2).

There is no cure for IBS, and treatment is individualized. Treatment of symptoms may include laxatives and dietary

BOX 41-2 DIAGNOSTIC CRITERIA FOR IRRITABLE BOWEL SYNDROME

Rome III Criteria

For a disorder to be diagnosed as irritable bowel syndrome, at least two or more of the following conditions will have existed for at least 3 months, with onset occurring at least 6 months before the beginning of the recurrent abdominal pain or discomfort:

1. Improvement with defecation
2. Onset associated with a change in stool frequency
3. Onset associated with a change in form (appearance) of stool

Manning Criteria

1. Onset of pain linked to more frequent bowel movements
2. Looser stools associated with onset of pain
3. Pain relieved by passage of stool
4. Noticeable abdominal bloating
5. Sensation of incomplete evacuation more than 25% of the time
6. Diarrhea with mucus more than 25% of the time

Modified from Longstreth GF et al: *Gastroenterology* 130(5):1480–1491, 2006; Suares NC, Ford AC: *Discov Med* 11(60):425–433, 2011; Whitehead WE, Drossman DA: *Am J Gastroenterol* 105(4):814–820, 2010.

fiber, antidiarrheals, antispasmodics, low-dose antidepressants, and serotonin agonists or antagonists. For severe constipation, 5-hydroxytryptamine-4 agonists (e.g., tegaserod) may be used (not approved for use in North America since 2007 because of cardiac ischemic events) or CIC-2 chloride channel activators (e.g., lubiprostone). For severe diarrhea, 5-hydroxytryptamine-3 receptor antagonists (e.g., alosetron) or rifaximin (an antibiotic) may be used to normalize bowel habits. Low-dose tricyclic antidepressants and selective serotonin reuptake inhibitors (SSRIs) have been used for severe pain. Alternative therapies including prebiotics (stimulate growth of healthy gut bacteria), probiotics, selected herbal treatments (e.g., peppermint oil), hypnosis, and psychotherapy are treatment options. Research continues to advance the management of this complex syndrome.[137,138]

Intestinal Vascular Insufficiency

The stomach and intestines are supplied by three branches of the abdominal aorta: the celiac artery and the superior and inferior mesenteric arteries. Atherosclerotic lesions, thrombi, and emboli can develop in these vessels, occluding blood flow and causing ischemia or necrosis in the gastrointestinal tract.

Mesenteric venous thrombosis is the least common of the causes of mesenteric vascular insufficiency. Malignancies, right-sided heart failure, and deep vein thrombosis are risk factors.

Acute mesenteric ischemia caused by acute occlusion of the mesenteric artery results in a significant reduction in mucosal blood flow to the large and small intestines. Dissecting aortic aneurysms, arterial thrombi, or emboli can be causes. Embolic obstruction is associated with atrial fibrillation, mitral valve disease, heart valve prostheses, or myocardial infarction. The superior mesenteric artery has a more direct line of flow from the aorta; therefore, emboli enter it more readily than they enter the inferior branch, causing ischemia and necrosis of the small intestine. Ischemia and necrosis alter membrane permeability. There is initially increased motility, nausea and vomiting, urgent bowel evacuation, and severe abdominal pain. Ischemia leads to decreased motility and distention. The damaged intestinal mucosa cannot produce enough mucus to protect itself from digestive enzymes. Mucosal alteration causes fluid to move from the blood vessels into the bowel wall and peritoneum. Fluid loss causes hypovolemia and further decreases in intestinal blood flow. As intestinal infarction progresses, shock, fever, bloody diarrhea, and leukocytosis develop. Bacteria invade the necrotic intestinal wall, causing gangrene and peritonitis.[139,140]

Chronic mesenteric ischemia is rare. It can develop secondary to atherosclerosis (most common), congestive heart failure, dysrhythmias, hemorrhage, thrombus formation, aortic aneurysm, or any condition that decreases arterial blood flow. Chronic occlusion is often accompanied by formation of collateral circulation that may be able to nourish the resting intestine. After eating, however, when the intestine requires more blood, the arterial supply may be insufficient. Ischemia develops, causing a cramping abdominal pain, called *abdominal angina,* after meals. Progressive vascular obstruction eventually causes continuous abdominal pain and necrosis of the intestinal tissue. Reperfusion injury related to reactive oxygen metabolites and inflammatory mediators contributes to further tissue damage.

Colicky abdominal pain after eating is a cardinal symptom of chronic mesenteric insufficiency. Some individuals suffer significant weight loss because they stop eating to control the pain.

Diagnosis of acute and chronic mesenteric ischemia is based on clinical manifestations, laboratory findings, and imaging studies. Bruit often can be heard over a partially occluded artery. Medical management includes antibiotics, anticoagulation, vasodilators, and inhibitors of reperfusion injury. Surgery is required to remove necrotic tissue, repair sclerosed vessels, and revascularize tissue. Acute occlusion is a surgical emergency and mortality is high (50% to 90%). Early diagnosis and aggressive treatment result in the best survival rates.[141,142]

Disorders of Nutrition

Obesity

Obesity is an increase in body fat mass and a metabolic disorder that has become an epidemic worldwide. The incidence is rapidly increasing among children and adolescents and they tend to become obese adults.[143,144]

Obesity is defined as a body mass index (BMI) that exceeds 30 kg/m^2 and generally develops when caloric intake exceeds caloric expenditure in genetically susceptible individuals.[145] Obesity is a major risk factor for morbidity, death, and high healthcare cost in the United States and worldwide.[146] Three leading causes of death in the United States are associated with obesity: cardiovascular disease, type 2 diabetes mellitus, and cancer (colorectal, breast in postmenopausal women, endometrial, prostate, renal, and esophageal).[147] Obesity is also a risk factor for hypertension, stroke, hyperlipidemia, gallstones, nonalcoholic steatohepatitis, gastroesophageal reflux, osteoarthritis, infectious disease, asthma, and obstructive sleep apnea. However, some studies have shown that a BMI between 25 and 34 in older individuals is associated with lower mortality.[148,149]

The causes and consequences of obesity are multiple and complex and there is rapidly advancing research regarding

BOX 41-3 HORMONES AND ADIPOKINES SECRETED BY ADIPOSE TISSUE

Leptin
Satiety (hunger/appetite suppression) and regulation of eating behavior by hypothalamus
Sympathoactivation
Insulin sensitizing
Modulating role in reproduction, angiogenesis, immune response, blood pressure control, and osteogenesis

Adiponectin
Insulin sensitizing
Anti-inflammatory
Anti-atherogenic

Resistin
Promotes insulin resistance and increased blood glucose levels
Inhibits adipocyte differentiation and may function as a feedback regulator of adipogenesis

Apelin
Regulates glucose homeostasis and lowers serum glucose level; vasodilation

Visfatin (from Visceral Fat)
Mimics insulin and binds to insulin receptors in rats

Vaspin—May Be Insulin Sensitizing, Reduces Food Intake
Insulin sensitizing
Anti-inflammatory action

Retinol-Binding Protein 4 (RBP4)
Promotes insulin resistance, promotes fat deposition

Regulators of Lipoprotein Metabolism
Lipoprotein lipase
Lipotransin
Apolipoprotein E
Cholesterol ester transfer protein

Inflammatory Cytokines
Prostaglandins
Tumor necrosis factor-alpha
Interleukins (IL-1β, IL-6, IL-8, IL-10)
Plasminogen activator inhibitor 1
Monocyte chemoattractant protein 1

Other Hormones and Cytokines
Acylation stimulating protein
Adipocyte relaxing factor—decreased in obesity
Adipophilin
AdipoQ
Agouti protein
Angiotensinogen
Chemerin—adipocyte differentiation and lipolysis
Dipeptidyl peptidase IV (DPP-IV)
Estrogen
FABP4 (fatty acid binding protein 4)—suppresses cardiomyocyte contraction
Insulin-like growth factor
Monobutyrin
Nitric oxide synthase
Tissue factor
Transforming growth factor-beta

Data from Blüher M: *Diabetes Metab J* 36(5):317–327, 2012; Maenhaut N, Van de Voorde J: *BMC Med* 16(9):25, 2011.

causal mechanisms, complications, and treatment. Genotype and gene-envirnonment interactions are important predisposing factors.[150] Single-gene defects are rare and obesity is usually polygenic and associated with other phenotypes such as endocrine disorders (i.e., diabetes and hypothyroidism) and mental retardation (i.e., Down and Prader-Willi syndromes). Single-gene defects include the melanocortin-4 receptor gene (decreases appetite), leptin gene (also known as the *obesity gene*), and leptin-receptor gene. All single-gene defects are directly or indirectly related to leptin and melanocortin pathways.[151] Metabolic abnormalities contributing to obesity include Cushing syndrome, Cushing disease, polycystic ovary syndrome, hypothyroidism, and hypothalamic injury. Environmental factors include culture, socioeconomic status, food intake, and exercise. Obesity is associated with adverse social and psychologic consequences.[152,153]

PATHOPHYSIOLOGY. The pathophysiology of obesity is complex and involves the interaction of numerous cytokines, hormones, and neurotransmitters. Mechanisms contributing to the imbalance of energy intake in relation to energy expenditure and the multiple pathogenic effects of excess adipose tissue are not completely understood. The adipocyte is the cellular basis of obesity. Adipocytes secrete a number of hormones and cytokines known as adipokines[154] (Box 41-3). Adipokines participate in regulation of food intake, lipid storage and metabolism, insulin sensitivity, the alternative complement system, vascular homeostasis, blood pressure regulation, angiogenesis, the inflammatory and immune responses, female reproduction, and regulation of energy metabolism. Visceral fat accumulation causes dysfunction of adipocytes and results in alterations in the regulation and interaction of these hormones. Macrophages infiltrate excess adipocytes with increased expression of inflammatory cytokines (e.g., TNF-α and IL-1β). The low-grade inflammation and alterations in adipokines, and other hormones and neurotransmitters contributes to the causes and complications of obesity, particularly cardiovascular disease and type 2 diabetes mellitus.[155]

Regulation of appetite and satiety occurs through neuroendocrine regulation of eating behavior, energy metabolism, and body fat mass. The system is complex and controlled by a dynamic circuit of signaling molecules from the periphery acting on central controls including the brainstem, hypothalamus, and autonomic nervous system. An imbalance in this system is usually associated with excessive caloric intake in relation to exercise with the consequence of weight gain and obesity.

The arcuate nucleus (ARC) in the hypothalamus has two sets of neurons with opposing effects that interact to regulate

BOX 41-4 EXAMPLES OF HORMONES AND NEUROPEPTIDES THAT INFLUENCE EATING BEHAVIOR

Orexins (Appetite Stimulants)
Neuropeptide Y (NPY)
Melanin-concentrating hormone (MCH)
Agouti-related protein (AGRP)
Ghrelin
Galanin
Orexins A and B
Peptide YY (PYY)
Endocannabinoids
Cortisol

Anorexins (Appetite Suppressants)
Leptin
Insulin
Cholecystokinin (CCK)
Glucagon-like peptide 1 (GLP1)
Corticotropin-releasing factor (CRF)
Urocortin (a CRF satiety signaling hormone)
Cocaine- and amphetamine-regulated transcript (CART)
Alpha-melanocyte–stimulating hormone (α-MSH)
Bombesin
Serotonin
Calcitonin

and balance food intake and energy metabolism. One set of neurons produces neuropeptide Y (NPY) and agouti-related protein (AGRP), which promotes appetite, stimulates eating, and decreases metabolism (anabolic). Another set of neurons synthesizes pro-opiomelanocortin (POMC)–producing peptide and cocaine-and-amphetamine–regulated transcript (CART), collectively known as POMC/CART neurons, which suppress appetite, inhibit eating, and increase metabolism (catabolic).

Molecules that stimulate eating are called *orexins* (i.e., hypocretins [from the hypothalamus], a peptide family that act as neurotransmitters for stimulating eating). Molecules that inhibit eating are called *anorexins* (Box 41-4). Peripheral effects of these signaling pathways are transmitted through the autonomic nervous and endocrine systems to regulate appetite, food intake, and energy metabolism.[156]

Many different hormones also control appetite, satiety, and body weight. Their sources include ghrelin from the stomach; peptide YY, cholecystokinin (CCK), and glucagon-like peptide 1 (GLP-1) from the intestines; insulin from pancreatic beta cells; leptin, adiponectin, and retinol-binding protein 4 (RBP4) from adipose tissue; and endocannabinoids (arachidonic acid based lipids) from brain and peripheral nerves. These hormones circulate in the blood at concentrations that increase or decrease in relation to body fat mass, and serve as *peripheral signals* to the ARC in the hypothalamus, where appetite (food intake) and metabolism (energy expenditure) are regulated. Leptin and insulin normally decrease appetite by inhibiting NPY/AGRP neurons (anabolic circuits) and stimulating POMC/CART neurons (catabolic circuits). Ghrelin and other hormones stimulate appetite by activating NPY/AGRP-expressing neurons. Intestinal peptide YY (PYY), CCK, endocannabinoids, and other hormones decrease appetite. Other peripheral hormones and neurotransmitters also can influence the hypothalamus and affect appetite and energy expenditure (see Box 41-4). Obesity is associated with increased circulating plasma levels of leptin (leptin resistance), retinol-binding protein 4, insulin (insulin resistance), and ghrelin. There are decreased levels of adiponectin and peptide YY. Interaction among these hormones and adipokines at the level of the hypothalamus and in the periphery may be important determinants of excessive fat mass. Leptin resistance, decreased adiponectin levels, increased ghrelin levels, insulin resistance, and inflammation are particularly important in the complications of obesity.

Leptin, a product of the obesity gene (*Ob* gene) and expressed primarily by adipocytes, acts on the hypothalamus to suppress appetite and regulates body weight within a fairly narrow range. Low leptin levels during fasting normally stimulate food intake and reduce energy expenditure and high leptin levels in the fed state inhibit food intake and increase energy expenditure. Leptin secretion increases as adipocytes increase in size or number (hyperleptinemia). The high levels of leptin in obesity are ineffective at decreasing appetite and increasing energy expenditure—this is known as decreased leptin sensitivity or **leptin resistance.** Leptin resistance disrupts hypothalamic satiety signaling, promotes overeating and excessive weight gain, and is a factor in the development of obesity.[157]

The cause of leptin resistance is unknown. It may be related to a defect in leptin transport, an inability of leptin to cross the blood-brain barrier; an alteration in the permissive effect of leptin on urocortin (a satiety-signaling molecule); or a defect in the leptin receptor. *Hyperleptinemia* also stimulates the sympathetic nervous system, chronic inflammation, oxidative stress, and ventricular hypertrophy and may contribute to the pathogenesis of hypertension, atherosclerosis, and cardiovascular disease associated with obesity.[158-160]

Adiponectin, produced primarily by visceral adipose tissue, has insulin-sensitizing properties and plasma levels decrease with visceral obesity, contributing to insulin resistance and type 2 diabetes mellitus. Decreased levels of adiponectin are associated with complications of obesity, including increased risk for coronary artery disease resulting from hyperlipidemia, hypertension, and factors that promote thrombosis and inflammation[161] (see Chapter 32). Decreased adiponectin levels are associated with increased hepatic gluconeogenesis, decreased skeletal muscle glucose uptake, and increased levels of inflammatory markers, such as IL-6 and TNF-α. Adiponectin may serve as an anti-inflammatory and anti-atherogenic plasma protein and has an important role in vascular remodeling that is limited with obesity.[162,163]

Insulin resistance is associated with obesity. The mechanisms are not clear but there is an association between hyperlipidemia and fat storage, macrophages and inflammation, and alterations in adipokines. Leptin resistance and decreased adiponectin contribute to insulin resistance.[164] Retinol-binding protein 4 is an adipokine that is increased in visceral adiposity and contributes to insulin resistance in liver and muscle.[165] Insulin resistance results in hyperglycemia and predisposition to type 2 diabetes mellitus.

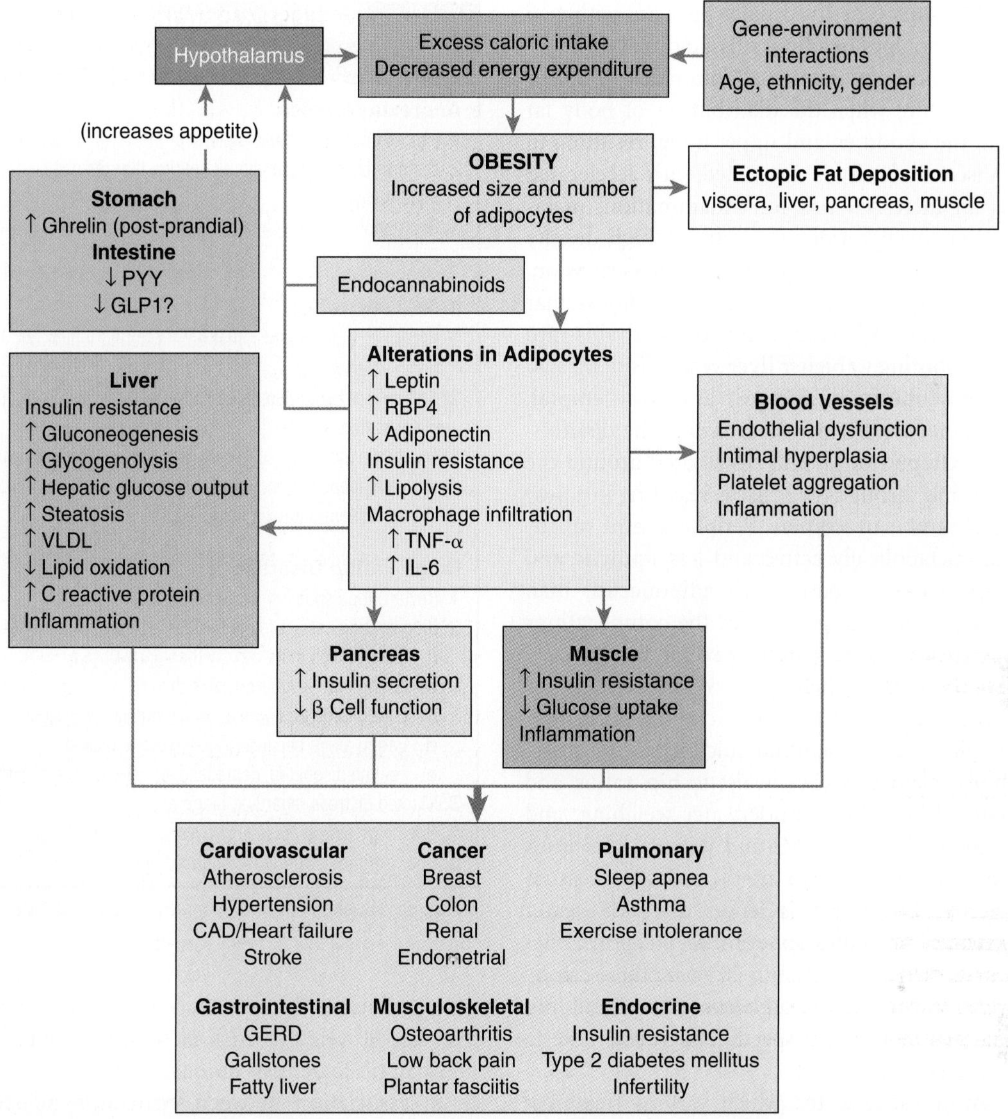

FIGURE 41-15 **Pathophysiology and Common Complications of Obesity.** See text for details. *CAD,* Coronary artery disease; *GERD,* gastroesophageal reflux disease; *GLP1,* glucagon-like peptide 1; *IL-6,* interleukin-6; *PYY,* intestinal peptide YY; *RBP4,* retinol-binding protein 4; *TNF-α,* tumor necrosis factor-alpha; *VLDL,* very-low-density lipoprotein.

Ghrelin is produced by the stomach in response to hunger and stimulates food intake through activation of the ghrelin receptor (GHS-R) located on neuropeptide Y (NPY)/agouti-related peptide (AGRP) neurons in the hypothalamus. Ghrelin induces metabolic changes leading to an increase in body weight and body fat mass. Ghrelin also stimulates release of growth hormone (GH) from anterior pituitary cells, release of gastric acid, gastrointestinal motility, and pancreatic functions. It has satiety, vasodilatory, cardioprotective, and antiproliferative effects.[166]

Leptin and ghrelin are complementary, yet antagonistic signals reflecting acute and chronic changes in energy balance, the effects of which are mediated by hypothalamic neuropeptides, such as NPY and AGRP. In obesity, plasma ghrelin level does not decrease after eating and its role in contributing to obesity is yet to be defined. Endocrine and vagal afferent pathways are also involved in the actions of ghrelin and leptin, adding to the complexity of mechanisms that can affect obesity.[167]

Glucose-like peptide 1 is an incretin secreted from intestinal endocrine cells when nutrients enter the small intestine. GLP-1 stimulates pancreatic glucose-dependent insulin secretion, delays gastric emptying, and suppresses appetite. GLP-1 levels may be decreased in obese individuals.[168]

Peptide YY (PYY) is released from intestinal endocrine cells in response to nutrients entering the intestine and inhibits gastric motility and decreases appetite. The level of PYY decreases with increases in adiposity and decreased PYY level is associated with obesity.[169]

Endocannabinoids (i.e., anandamide) are expressed in both the brain and peripheral nerve tissues and have effects on endocannabinoid receptors in orexigenic pathways. They increase appetite, enhance nutrient absorption, stimulate lipogenesis, and increase adipose tissue accumulation by acting at both central (CB1 receptor) and peripheral sites (CB2 receptor). An increase in endocannabinoids is proposed to be associated with obesity.[170] Figure 41-15 summarizes the pathophysiology and complications of obesity.

CLINICAL MANIFESTATIONS. Obesity usually presents with two different forms or phenotypes of adipose tissue distribution.[171] **Visceral obesity** (also known as intra-abdominal, central, or masculine obesity) occurs when the distribution of body fat is localized around the abdomen and upper body, resulting in an apple shape. Visceral obesity is associated with accelerated lipolysis and has an increased risk for inflammation, metabolic syndrome (hypertriglyceridemia, reduced high-density lipoprotein, increased low-density lipoproteins, hypertension, and insulin resistance), type 2 diabetes mellitus, cardiovascular complications, and cancer. Visceral venous blood drains into the portal vein, contributing to higher liver synthesis of plasma lipids.[172,173] **Peripheral obesity** (also known as gluteal-femoral, feminine, or subcutaneous obesity) occurs when the distribution of body fat is extraperitoneal and distributed around the thighs and buttocks and through the muscle, resulting in a pear shape; it is more common in women. Peripheral and subcutaneous fat is less metabolically active and less lipolytic and releases fewer adipocytokines (particularly adiponectin) than visceral fat. Risk factors are still present for the complications of obesity but they are less severe than for visceral obesity.[174]

EVALUATION AND TREATMENT. There are several methods for measuring or estimating body fat mass, including anthropometric measurements, such as skinfold thickness, circumferences, various body diameters (i.e., waist-to-hip ratios and waist circumference, BMI tables), underwater weighing, and bioimpedance analysis.[175,176] The BMI and waist-to-hip ratios are most commonly used because they are the easiest to measure and most cost-effective. Overweight is defined as a BMI greater than 25 kg/m^2 and obesity is a BMI greater than 30 kg/m^2. BMI charts are available for children ages 2 to 20 years; these can be used for comparison during adulthood because obese children generally become obese adults. No specific diagnostic criteria for obesity have been established.[177]

Obesity is a chronic disease for which various treatment approaches have been used, including correction of metabolic abnormalities, individually tailored weight-reduction diets, and exercise programs.[178] A combination of weight reduction and exercise is the most effective. Self-motivation and support systems are critical aspects of treatment.[179] Additional treatments include psychotherapy, behavioral modification, and anti-obesity drugs.[180] Bariatric surgical procedures (i.e., the Roux-en-Y gastric bypass, gastric banding, or sleeve gastrectomy) also are prescribed and when successful result in a significant reduction in weight, reduction in comorbidities, and a decrease in insulin resistance. Unraveling the causes of obesity will lead to more specific prevention and pharmacotherapies.[181-183]

Anorexia Nervosa, Bulimia Nervosa, and Binge Eating Disorder

Many young adults and adolescents—as many as 1% of women and adolescent girls in the United States—are affected by complex and related eating disorders: anorexia nervosa, bulimia nervosa, and binge eating. These disorders are included in the proposed *DMS-5* classification of eating disorders by the American Psychiatric Association (Box 41-5). They rarely occur in black women, and only 5% to 10% of cases are men.[184] Onset may occur in children and women over age 50 years.[185] Risk factors include genetic, epigenetic, familial, biologic, psychologic, and social factors.[186,187] There is an association between posttraumatic stress and sexual assault history and eating disorders.[188] An increasing number of children, young men, and older adult women are experiencing eating disorders, often with an associated depression, anxiety, or personality disorder.[189,190] The death rate is highest among women with anorexia nervosa.[191]

BOX 41-5 CLASSIFICATION OF EATING DISORDERS

Anorexia Nervosa

1. Fear of becoming obese despite progressive weight loss
2. Distorted body image: the perception that the body is fat when it is actually underweight
3. Restriction of energy intake leading to significantly low body weight
4. Behavioral resistance to gaining weight

Bulimia Nervosa

1. Recurrent episodes of binge eating during which the individual fears not being able to stop
2. Self-induced vomiting, use of laxatives, or fasting to oppose the effect of binge eating
3. One binge eating episode per week for at least 3 months
4. Undue influence of body shape or weight on self-evaluation
5. Does not meet anorexia nervosa criteria

Binge Eating Disorder

1. Recurrent episodes of binge eating
2. Binge eating associated with three or more of the following:
   a. Eating much more rapidly than normal
   b. Eating until uncomfortably full
   c. Eating large amounts of food when not physically hungry
   d. Eating alone because of being embarrassed
   e. Feeling disgusted, depressed, or very guilty after overeating
3. Marked distress regarding binge eating
4. One binge eating episode per week for at least 3 months
5. Does not meet criteria for anorexia nervosa or bulimia nervosa

Data from: Sysko R et al: *Psychiatry Res* 196(2):302–308, 2012.

Starvation

Malnutrition is lack of nourishment from inadequate amounts of calories, protein, vitamins, or minerals and is caused by improper diet, alterations in digestion or absorption, chronic disease, or a combination of these factors. **Starvation** is a reduction in energy intake leading to weight loss. Short-term starvation and long-term starvation have different effects. Therapeutic short-term starvation is part of many weight-reduction programs because it causes an initial rapid weight loss that reinforces the individual's motivation to diet. Therapeutic long-term starvation is used in medically controlled environments to facilitate rapid weight loss in morbidly obese individuals. Pathologic long-term starvation can be caused by poverty; chronic diseases of the cardiovascular, pulmonary, hepatic, and digestive systems; malabsorption syndromes; human immunodeficiency virus (HIV) infection; and cancer.[192]

Short-term starvation, or extended fasting, consists of several days of total dietary abstinence or deprivation. The body responds with protective mechanisms. For 4 to 6 hours after the last meal, the body is in a well-fed state and its energy requirements are supplied by glucose from recently ingested carbohydrates. Once all available energy has been absorbed from the intestine, glycogen in the liver is converted to glucose through **glycogenolysis,** the splitting of glycogen into glucose. This process peaks within 4 to 8 hours, and gluconeogenesis begins. **Gluconeogenesis** is the formation of glucose from noncarbohydrate molecules: lactate, pyruvate, amino acids, and the glycerol portion of fats. Like glycogenolysis, gluconeogenesis takes place within the liver. Both of these processes deplete stored nutrients and thus cannot meet the body's energy needs indefinitely. Proteins continue to be catabolized to a minimal degree, providing carbon for the synthesis of glucose.[193]

Long-term starvation begins after several days of dietary abstinence and eventually causes death. Absolute deprivation of food causes **marasmus** or protein-energy malnutrition (loss of muscle mass and body fat depletion). Protein deprivation in the presence of carbohydrate intake is called **kwashiorkor** (loss of muscle mass with sustained body fat). Marasmic kwashiorkor (edematous, severe childhood malnutrition) is a combination of chronic energy deficiency and chronic or acute protein deficiency and inadequate micronutrients.[194] Anorexia nervosa is a psychologic cause of long-term starvation (see Box 41-5). **Cachexia** (also known as cytokine-induced malnutrition) is physical wasting with loss of weight and muscle atrophy, fatigue, and weakness. Inflammatory mediators (i.e., TNF-α, interferon-γ, IL-1, IL-6) and a blunted response to ghrelin and adiponectin are associated with the cachexia of advanced cancer.[195] Cancer, AIDS, tuberculosis, and other major chronic progressive diseases contribute to cachexia. Anorexia and cachexia often occur together. Cachexia is not the same as food deprivation starvation. A healthy person's body can adjust to starvation by slowing metabolism; however, in cachexia, the body does not make this adjustment.

The major characteristic of long-term starvation is a decreased dependence on gluconeogenesis and an increased use of ketone bodies (products of lipid and pyruvate metabolism) as a cellular energy source. During long-term starvation, depressed insulin levels and increased levels of glucagon, cortisone, epinephrine, and growth hormones promote lipolysis in adipose tissue. Lipolysis liberates fatty acids, which supply energy to cardiac and skeletal muscle cells, and ketone bodies, which sustain brain tissue. Fatty acid, or ketone body, oxidation meets most of the energy needs of the cells. (Some glucose is still needed as fuel for brain tissue.) Once the supply of adipose tissue is depleted, proteolysis begins. The breakdown of muscle and visceral protein is the last process the body engages to supply energy for life. Death results from severe alterations in electrolyte balance and loss of renal, pulmonary, and cardiac function.[196]

Adequate ingestion of appropriate nutrients is the obvious treatment for starvation. In medically induced starvation the body is maintained in a ketotic state until the desired amount of adipose tissue has been lysed. Starvation imposed by chronic disease, long-term illness, or malabsorption is treated with enteral or parenteral nutrition and there is the potential to develop refeeding syndrome. Perioperative or critical care management of nutrition is necessary to prevent unnecessary starvation.[197] Care must be taken to prevent **refeeding syndrome** during the treatment of long-term starvation (see What's New? Refeeding Syndrome).

WHAT'S NEW?

Refeeding Syndrome

Refeeding syndrome occurs in severely malnourished individuals when parenteral or enteral nutritional therapy is initiated. During starvation, loss of body minerals causes the movement of phosphate, magnesium, and potassium ions out of the cells and into the plasma. When refeeding starts, an increase in insulin levels stimulates the movement of glucose and these ions back into the cells, and the plasma concentrations can decrease to dangerously low levels, causing hypophosphatemia, hypomagnesemia, hypokalemia, hyponatremia, hypocalcemia, and vitamin deficiency. Rapid expansion of the extracellular fluid volume also can occur with carbohydrate refeeding and may cause fluid overload. Hypophosphatemia contributes to alterations in red blood cell shape and function contributing to tissue hypoxia and increased respiratory drive. The consequence of these alterations includes life-threatening dysrhythmias, congestive heart failure, muscle weakness (including respiratory muscles), and death. Individuals at greatest risk are those with starvation from any cause including anorexia nervosa, chronic alcoholism, morbid obesity with massive weight loss, and prolonged fasting. Refeeding syndrome is prevented by slowly reinstituting feeding (about 20 kcal/kg/day for the first few days) and monitoring plasma levels of phosphate, potassium, magnesium, and calcium.

Data from Byrnes MC, Stangenes J: *Curr Opin Clin Nutr Metab Care* 14(2):186–192, 2011; Kohn MR, Madden S, Clarke SD: *Curr Opin Pediatr* 23(4):390–394, 2011; Skipper A: *Nutr Clin Pract* 27(1):34–40, 2012.

DISORDERS OF THE ACCESSORY ORGANS OF DIGESTION

The accessory organs of digestion (liver, gallbladder, pancreas) secrete substances necessary for digestion and, in the case of the liver, carry out metabolic functions needed to maintain life.

Common Complications of Liver Disorders

Of all the accessory organ disorders, acute or chronic liver disease leads to the most systemic, life-threatening complications. Complications of chronic liver disorders include portal hypertension, ascites, hepatic encephalopathy, jaundice, and hepatorenal syndrome.

Acute Liver Failure

Acute liver failure (fulminant liver failure) is a rare clinical syndrome (2000 cases in the United States annually)[198] resulting from severe impairment or necrosis of liver cells without preexisting liver disease or cirrhosis. Acetaminophen overdose is the leading cause of acute liver failure in the United States[199] (see What's New? Acetaminophen and Acute Liver Failure). It also may occur as a complication of viral hepatitis, particularly heptatitis B virus (HBV) infection compounded by infection with the delta virus, as well as metabolic liver disorders.

WHAT'S NEW?

Acetaminophen and Acute Liver Failure

Acetaminophen (paracetamol) toxicity from chronic use or intentional overdose is the leading cause of acute liver failure in the United States and Great Britain. Liver injury may occur with doses of 4 to 10 g and hepatotoxicity with mitochondrial injury and hepatocyte necrosis should be suspected when doses exceed 4 g/day. The onset is sudden and unpredictable accompanied by coagulopathy and encephalopathy. Elevated serum aminotransferase levels (may be up to 400 times normal) accompanied by hypoprothrombinemia, metabolic acidosis, and renal failure support a diagnosis of acute liver failure caused by acetaminophen. Complications of cerebral edema and infection are difficult to diagnose and treat and may lead to multiorgan failure and irreversible brain damage. Early treatment with correct dosing with *N*-acetylcysteine provides a 66% chance of recovery and there is 70% survival at 1 year after liver transplant.

Data from Hodgman MJ, Garrard AR: *Crit Care Clin* 28(4):499–516, 2012; Jaeschke H, McGill MR, Ramachandran A: *Drug Metab Rev* 44(1):88–106, 2012; Khandelwal N et al: *Hepatology* 53(2):567–576, 2011.

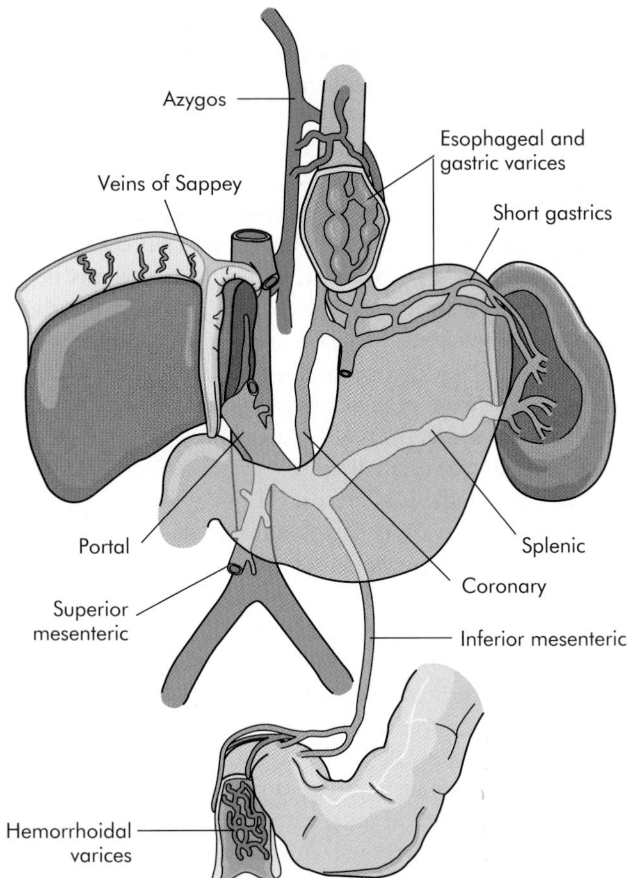

FIGURE 41-16 Varices Related to Portal Hypertension. Portal vein, its major tributaries, and the most important shunts (collateral veins) between the portal and caval systems. (From Monahan FD et al: *Phipps' medical-surgical nursing: concepts and clinical practice,* ed 8, St Louis, 2007, Mosby.)

Pathogenic mechanisms of acute liver failure are poorly understood. Hepatocytes become edematous, and patchy areas of necrosis and inflammatory cell infiltrates disrupt the parenchyma. The hepatic necrosis is irreversible.

Acute liver failure usually develops 6 to 8 weeks after the initial symptoms of viral hepatitis or a metabolic liver disorder (e.g., Wilson disease). Anorexia, vomiting, abdominal pain, and progressive jaundice are initial signs, followed by ascites and gastrointestinal bleeding. Coagulopathy and encephalopathy occur in individuals without preexisting liver disease and can cause cerebral edema manifested as lethargy, altered motor functions, coma, and death. Liver function tests show elevations the levels of both conjugated and unconjugated serum bilirubin, serum transaminases, and blood ammonia. Prothrombin time is prolonged.[198] Treatment of acute liver failure requires rapid evaluation and critical care. *N*-Acetylcysteine is used for acetaminophen poisoning; antiviral therapy appears to improve survival in cases of viral hepatitis; and lowering blood ammonia levels may improve prognosis. Liver transplantation may be lifesaving but needs to be performed early and obtaining a liver for transplant can be difficult.[200] Artificial liver support systems and use of hepatic stem cells are still in experimental stages of development.[198,201] Survivors usually do not develop cirrhosis or chronic liver disease.

Portal Hypertension

Portal hypertension is abnormally high blood pressure in the portal venous system primarily caused by resistance to portal blood flow. Pressure in this system is normally 3 mmHg; portal hypertension is an increase to at least 10 mmHg.

PATHOPHYSIOLOGY. Portal hypertension is caused by disorders that obstruct or impede blood flow through any component of the hepatic portal system. *Intrahepatic* causes result from vascular remodeling with intrahepatic shunts, thrombosis, inflammation, or fibrosis, as occurs in cirrhosis of the liver, viral hepatitis, or schistosomiasis (a parasitic infection). *Posthepatic* causes occur from hepatic vein thrombosis or cardiac disorders that impair the pumping ability of the right side of the heart (i.e., right-sided heart failure).[202] This causes blood to back up and increase pressure in the portal system. Thrombosis or narrowing of the hepatic portal vein is the major *prehepatic* cause. Long-term portal hypertension causes several pathophysiologic problems that are difficult to treat and can be fatal. These problems include varices, splenomegaly, hepatopulmonary syndrome, ascites, and hepatic encephalopathy.

Varices are distended, tortuous, collateral veins. Prolonged elevation of pressure in the hepatic portal vein causes collateral veins to open between the portal vein and systemic veins and their transformation into varices, particularly in the lower esophagus and stomach but also over the abdominal wall (known as the caput medusae [Medusa head]) and rectum (hemorrhoidal varices) (Figure 41-16). Rupture of varices can cause life-threatening hemorrhage.[203,204]

Splenomegaly is an enlargement of the spleen. Portal hypertension contributes to congestive splenomegaly caused by increased pressure in the splenic vein, a tributary to the hepatic portal vein. Thrombocytopenia from platelet sequestration is the most common manifestation and can contribute to an increased bleeding tendency. Splenomegaly also can be predictive of esophageal varices severity.[205]

Hepatopulmonary syndrome (intrapulmonary vasodilation, intrapulmonary shunting, and hypoxia)[206] and **portopulmonary hypertension** (pulmonary vasoconstriction and vascular remodeling)[206] are common respiratory complications of advanced liver disease and portal hypertension. Hyperdynamic (high-flow) state, increased pulmonary venous congestion, and vascular constriction or obstruction of the pulmonary arterial bed are contributing factors.[207] There are no specific clinical manifestations, although dyspnea, cyanosis, and digital clubbing may occur. Diagnosis is made by contrast echocardiography and right heart catheterization. In portopulmonary hypertension, pulmonary artery pressure is greater than 25 mmHg. Treatment may include systemic vasodilators and endothelin receptor antagonists, which can reduce pulmonary and portal hypertension.[208]

CLINICAL MANIFESTATIONS. The most common clinical manifestation of portal hypertension is vomiting of blood from bleeding **esophageal varices.**[204,209] Bleeding is usually from varices that have developed slowly over a period of years. Slow, chronic bleeding from varices causes anemia or melena.

Acute rupture of esophageal varices causes hemorrhage and voluminous vomiting of dark blood. The ruptured varices are usually painless. Rupture is caused by a combination of erosion by gastric acid and elevated venous pressure. Mortality from ruptured esophageal varices ranges from 15% to 20%. Hemorrhoidal varices present as hematochezia and copious rectal bleeding. Recurrent bleeding of esophageal or gastric varices indicates a poor prognosis. Most individuals die within 1 year.

EVALUATION AND TREATMENT. Diagnosis of portal hypertension is often made at the time of variceal bleeding and confirmed by endoscopy and evaluation of portal venous pressure. Distended collateral veins may radiate over the abdomen, giving rise to caput medusae (Medusa's head) from opening of the paraumbilical veins. The individual usually has a history of hepatitis or alcoholism.

Beta-blockers can be effective in preventing variceal bleeding. Emergency management of bleeding varices includes fluid resuscitation, prophylactic antibiotics, vasoactive drugs (e.g., nonselective β-receptor antagonists and terlipressin, a vasopressin derivative), endoscopic variceal band ligation, compression of the varices with an inflatable tube or balloon, and injection of a sclerosing agent. Surgical construction of a transjugular intrahepatic portosystemic shunt (TIPS) (anastomosis of the portal vein to the inferior vena cava) may decompress the varices, but this treatment can precipitate encephalopathy or liver failure resulting from reduced hepatic blood flow. There is no definitive treatment for portal hypertension.[204] Liver transplant is the most successful option for liver failure.[210]

Ascites

Ascites is the accumulation of fluid in the peritoneal cavity and is a complication of portal hypertension. Ascites traps body fluid in the peritoneal cavity from which it cannot escape. The effect reduces the amount of fluid available for normal physiologic functions. Cirrhosis is the most common cause of ascites; ascites is the most common complication of cirrhosis. Other diseases associated with ascites include right heart failure, abdominal malignancies, nephrotic syndrome, and malnutrition. Twenty-five percent of individuals who develop ascites caused by cirrhosis die within 1 year. Continued heavy drinking of alcohol is associated with this mortality because of increased risk for cirrhosis.

PATHOPHYSIOLOGY. Several factors contribute to the development of ascites, including portal hypertension, splanchnic vasodilation, hypoalbuminemia, and sodium and water retention. The *overflow theory* proposes that renal sodium retention is stimulated by portal hypertension with intravascular hypervolemia and overflow into the peritoneal cavity (transudative effusion). Portal hypertension also increases capillary hydrostatic pressures in the intestinal wall, which causes fluid to "weep" into the peritoneal cavity. Reduced capillary oncotic pressure adds to the fluid shift. The *underfill theory* proposes an increase in hepatic sinusoidal hydrostatic pressure and decreased plasma oncotic pressure with weeping of lymph fluid from the surface of the liver. The resulting decrease in effective circulating plasma volume activates the renin-angiotensin-aldosterone system, stimulating the kidney to retain more sodium and water and leading to intravascular volume overload. The *peripheral arterial vasodilation theory,* or *forward theory,* is a synthesis of the overflow and underfill theories and the most accepted theory. This theory proposes that circulating nitric oxide and carbon monoxide causes splanchnic vasodilation. The decrease in systemic vascular resistance overcomes compensatory cardiac output. Stimulation of baroreceptors activates renal sodium retention through activation of the renin-angiotensin-aldosterone system, increased sympathetic tone, secretion of antidiuretic hormones, and fluid retention. Combined portal hypertension and splanchnic vasodilation causes fluid transudation and lymph formation producing ascites. The release of endotoxin from translocation of intestinal bacteria also can trigger arterial vasodilation of the splanchnic organs.[211] Ascites can be complicated by bacterial peritonitis. Figure 41-17 summarizes the mechanisms by which cirrhosis of the liver causes ascites.

CLINICAL MANIFESTATIONS. The accumulation of ascitic fluid causes abdominal distention, increased abdominal girth, and weight gain (Figure 41-18). Large volumes of fluid (10 to 20 L) displace the diaphragm and cause dyspnea by decreasing lung capacity. Respiratory rate increases, and the individual assumes a semi-Fowler position to relieve the dyspnea. Some peripheral edema is usually present. Dilutional hyponatremia is a consequence of excess fluid volume. Approximately 10% of individuals with ascites develop bacterial peritonitis, either spontaneously or as a result of paracentesis (needle aspiration of ascitic fluid). Peritonitis causes fever, chills, abdominal pain, decreased bowel sounds, and cloudy ascitic fluid.

EVALUATION AND TREATMENT. Diagnosis of ascites is usually based on clinical manifestations and identification of liver disease. The serum-ascites albumin gradient (SAAG) is the most specific diagnostic indicator for portal hypertension–related ascites. Chest and abdominal x-rays, ultrasonography, or CT scans are used to evaluate the cause and extent of the ascites, and complications such as peritonitis. The goal of treatment is to relieve discomfort. If the restoration of liver function is possible (e.g., in ascites caused by viral hepatitis), the ascites diminishes spontaneously. In the meantime, dietary salt restriction

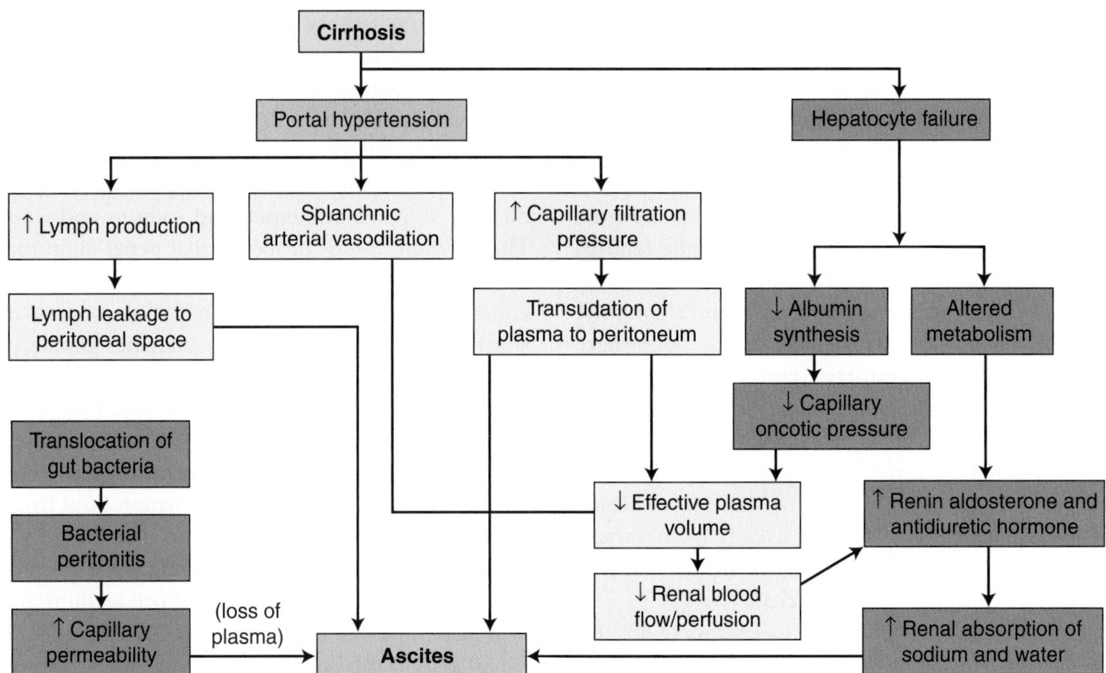

FIGURE 41-17 Mechanisms of Ascites Caused by Cirrhosis.

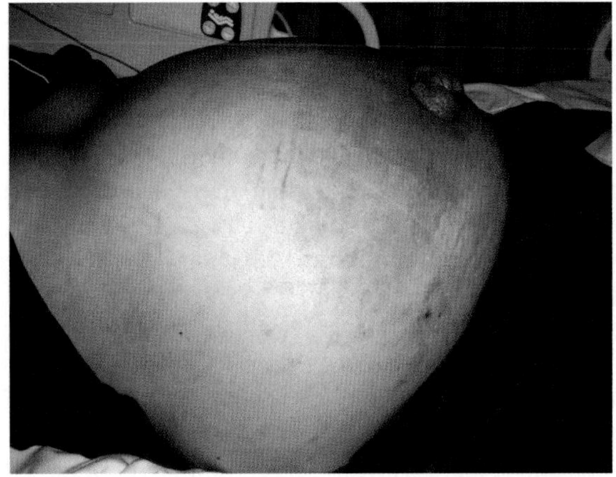

FIGURE 41-18 Massive Ascites in an Individual with Cirrhosis. Distended abdomen, dilated upper abdominal veins, and everted umbilicus are classic manifestations. (From Goldman L, Schafer AI: *Goldman's Cecil medicine*, ed 24, Philadelphia, 2012, Saunders.)

and potassium-sparing diuretics can reduce ascites. Strong diuretics, such as furosemide or ethacrynic acid, may be used and vasopressin receptor-2 antagonists are effective for dilutional hyponatremia. Albumin may be given.[212] Serum electrolyte levels are monitored carefully because the individual is at risk for hyponatremia and hypokalemia.[213]

Palliative measures include paracentesis to remove 1 or 2 L of ascitic fluid and relieve respiratory distress. This procedure can have serious complications, however. The removal of too much fluid too fast relieves pressure on blood vessels, causing arteriolar vasodilation, which carries the risk of hypotension, shock, or death. Despite repeated paracentesis, ascitic fluid reaccumulates in individuals with irreversible disease, drawing more albumin and electrolytes out of the vascular compartment. Paracentesis is also likely to cause peritonitis. Peritonitis is treated with long-term antibiotics. A transjugular intrahepatic portosystemic shunt or peritoneovenous shunt may be used to treat refractory ascites. Individuals with ascites and portal hypertension have a poor prognosis, and liver transplant is the best treatment option.[214]

Hepatic Encephalopathy

Hepatic encephalopathy (portosystemic encephalopathy) is a complex neurologic syndrome characterized by impaired cognitive function, flapping tremor (asterixis), and electroencephalogram (EEG) changes. The syndrome may develop rapidly during acute fulminant hepatitis (type A) in association with portosystemic bypass and in the absence of intrinsic liver disease (type B); or slowly during the course of chronic liver disease (type C: episodic, persistent, or covert).[215] Risk factors in the presence of advanced liver disease include gastrointestinal bleeding, increased dietary protein, electrolyte imbalance, and hypoxia.

PATHOPHYSIOLOGY. Hepatic encephalopathy results from a combination of biochemical alterations that affect neurotransmission. Liver dysfunction and collateral vessels that shunt blood around the liver to the systemic circulation permit neurotoxins and other harmful substances absorbed from the gastrointestinal tract to accumulate and circulate freely to the brain. Substances include inflammatory cytokines, short-chain fatty acids, serotonin, tryptophan, and false neurotransmitters. The most hazardous substances are end-products of intestinal protein digestion, particularly ammonia, which cannot be converted to urea by the diseased liver. The digestion of blood from leaking or ruptured varices adds to the amount of ammonia present in systemic blood, as does the action of ammonia-forming bacteria in the colon. Ammonia

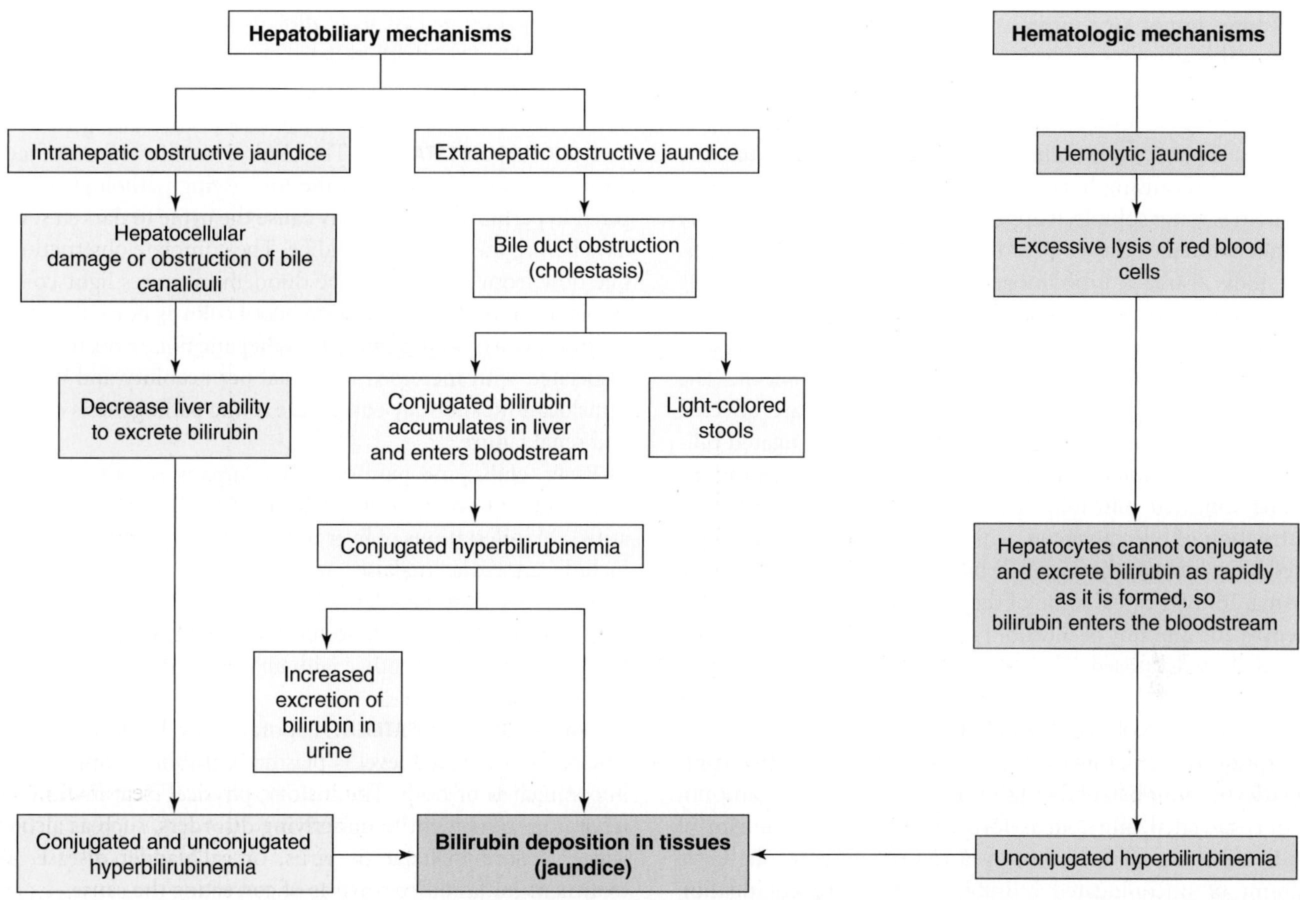

FIGURE 41-19 Mechanisms of Jaundice.

that reaches the brain is metabolized to glutamine with osmotic disturbances and alterations in cerebral blood flow that interfere with neurotransmitters and cause astrocyte edema (cytotoxic edema) and oxidation. Permeability of the blood-brain barrier also may be increased (vasogenic edema), contributing to brain edema and intracranial hypertension.[216,217] Excessive amounts of gamma-aminobutyric acid (GABA), an inhibitory neurotransmitter, may contribute to reduced levels of consciousness. Infection, hemorrhage, inflammation, electrolyte imbalance, sedatives, and analgesics also can precipitate stupor and coma in the presence of liver disease.[218,219]

CLINICAL MANIFESTATIONS. Subtle changes in personality, memory loss, irritability, lethargy, and sleep disturbances are common initial manifestations of hepatic encephalopathy and can be invisible (minimal hepatic encephalopathy). In acute liver failure, symptom onset can be rapid with confusion, flapping tremor of the hands, stupor, convulsions, and coma. Coma is usually a sign of severe liver dysfunction and ultimately results in death.[220]

EVALUATION AND TREATMENT. There is no specific diagnostic test of hepatic encephalopathy. Diagnosis is based on a history of liver disease, clinical manifestations, and psychometric testing. Electroencephalography and blood chemistry tests, including blood ammonia levels, provide supportive data. Tracking levels of serum ammonia assesses treatment effectiveness and liver function.

Correction of fluid and electrolyte imbalances and withdrawal of depressant drugs metabolized by the liver are the first steps in the treatment of hepatic encephalopathy. Reduction of blood ammonia levels is a major objective. This is accomplished by restricting dietary protein intake and eliminating intestinal bacteria. Neomycin is effective in sterilizing the bowel, but it can be nephrotoxic. Lactulose may be administered to prevent ammonia absorption in the colon.[221] Rifaximin decreases intestinal production and absorption of ammonia by altering gastrointestinal flora and is minimally absorbed. Sodium benzoate and L-ornithine-L-aspartate also detoxify ammonia and lactulose enemas promote ammonia excretion.[222]

Jaundice

Jaundice (icterus) is a yellow or greenish pigmentation of the skin caused by **hyperbilirubinemia** (total plasma bilirubin concentrations greater than 2.5 to 3 mg/dl). Hyperbilirubinemia and jaundice can result from (1) extrahepatic obstruction to bile flow (gallstones), (2) intrahepatic obstruction (hepatocellular disease such as cirrhosis or hepatitis), or (3) excessive production of bilirubin (excessive hemolysis of red blood cells)[223] (Figure 41-19). Jaundice in newborns is caused by impaired bilirubin uptake and conjugation (see Chapter 42).

PATHOPHYSIOLOGY. **Obstructive jaundice** can result from extrahepatic or intrahepatic obstruction.[224] *Extrahepatic obstructive jaundice* develops if the common bile duct is occluded by a gallstone, tumor, or compression from edema of pancreatitis. Because the bile duct is obstructed, bilirubin is conjugated by the hepatocytes but cannot flow into the duodenum. (Conjugated bilirubin is soluble in water and is then soluble in aqueous bile.) Therefore, it accumulates in the liver and enters the bloodstream, causing hyperbilirubinemia. Because conjugated bilirubin is water soluble, it appears in the urine. The stools may be light colored or clay colored because they lack bile pigments. The stools also lack urobilinogen because bile is not available for conversion to urobilinogen.

Intrahepatic obstructive jaundice involves disturbances in hepatocyte function and obstruction of *bile canaliculi*. The uptake, conjugation, and excretion of bilirubin are affected with elevated levels of both conjugated and unconjugated bilirubin. Hepatocellular damage increases plasma concentrations of unconjugated bilirubin. The major disorder, however, is obstruction of bile canaliculi, which diminishes flow of conjugated bilirubin into the common bile duct with elevations in the plasma. In mild cases, some of the bile canaliculi open. Consequently, the amount of bilirubin in the intestinal tract may be only slightly decreased. The stools may appear normal or light colored.

Excessive hemolysis (breakdown) of red blood cells or absorption of hematoma can cause **hemolytic jaundice (prehepatic** or **nonobstructive jaundice).** An increased amount of unconjugated bilirubin is formed through metabolism of the heme component of destroyed red blood cells. The extra amount of unconjugated bilirubin exceeds the conjugation ability of the liver, causing blood levels of unconjugated bilirubin to rise. Because unconjugated bilirubin is not water soluble, it is not excreted in the urine. The reserve conjugation ability of the liver usually prevents long-term unconjugated hyperbilirubinemia greater than 4 to 5 mg/dl. If unconjugated hyperbilirubinemia exceeds 5 mg/dl, both hemolytic and liver disorders are indicated.

Hyperbilirubinemia and jaundice can be caused also by metabolic defects that impair the uptake or conjugation of unconjugated bilirubin in the liver. *Gilbert disease,* for example, causes an elevation of unconjugated bilirubin level in the plasma but no other symptoms of liver disease. Gilbert disease is probably caused by an inherited deficiency of glucuronyl transferase enzyme, which is required for the hepatic uptake of unconjugated bilirubin. The causes of jaundice are summarized in Table 41-6.

CLINICAL MANIFESTATIONS. The clinical manifestations of jaundice vary and are related to the underlying pathology. Conjugated hyperbilirubinemia may cause the urine to darken several days before the onset of jaundice. The complete obstruction of bile flow from the liver to the duodenum causes light-colored stools. With partial obstruction, stool color is normal and bilirubin is present in the urine. Extrahepatic biliary obstruction is associated with increased intestinal permeability and bacterial translocation, and may contribute to the pathogenesis of sepsis and renal failure.[225]

Fever, chills, and pain often accompany jaundice resulting from viral or bacterial inflammation of the liver (e.g., viral hepatitis). Manifestations of liver injury from any cause commonly include anorexia, malaise, and fatigue. Yellow discoloration may first occur in the sclera of the eye and then progress to the skin. Skin xanthomas (cholesterol deposits) and pruritus commonly accompany jaundice with an elevation of serum alkaline phosphatase level.[226]

EVALUATION AND TREATMENT. Laboratory evaluation establishes whether the elevated level is plasma bilirubin is conjugated or unconjugated or both. The history, physical examination, and laboratory tests identify underlying disorders, such as alcoholism, exposure to hepatitis virus, or gallbladder disease. The treatment for jaundice consists of correcting the cause.

Hepatorenal Syndrome

Hepatorenal syndrome (HRS) is functional renal failure; it develops as a complication of advanced liver disease that tends to occur with ascites. Renal disorders associated with liver disease can have numerous causes but HRS is usually associated with alcoholic cirrhosis. The renal failure is not caused by primary renal disease or other extrinsic factors, but rather by arterial vasodilation of the splanchnic vasculature, reduced effective blood volume, and renal vasoconstriction.[227] There are two types of HRS: type 1 involves rapid and progressive renal failure

TABLE 41-6 THREE COMMON TYPES OF JAUNDICE

TYPE	MECHANISM	CAUSES
Hemolytic jaundice (predominantly unconjugated bilirubin)	Excessive destruction of erythrocytes	Membrane defect of erythrocytes Hemolytic anemias Immune reaction Severe infection Toxic substances in the circulation (e.g., snake venom) Transfusion of incompatible blood
Obstructive (cholestatic) jaundice (predominantly conjugated bilirubin)	Obstruction to passage of conjugated bilirubin from liver to intestine	Obstruction of bile duct by gallstones or tumor (extrahepatic obstructive jaundice) Obstruction of bile flow through the liver (intrahepatic obstructive jaundice) Drugs
Hepatocellular jaundice (both conjugated and unconjugated bilirubin)	Failure of liver cells (hepatocytes) to conjugate bilirubin and of bilirubin to pass from liver to intestine	Genetic defect of hepatocyte (decreased enzymes), such as occurs in premature infants (see Chapter 42) Hepatitis or biliary cirrhosis

related to severe reduction in blood volume and decreased cardiac output; type 2 is slower, is more stable, and is accompanied by refractory ascites.[228]

PATHOPHYSIOLOGY. Hepatorenal syndrome generally accompanies a sudden decrease in blood volume secondary to massive gastrointestinal or variceal bleeding and hypotension caused by bleeding and splanchnic vasodilation associated with failing liver function. Hypotension also can be caused by the excessive use of diuretics to treat ascites. The decrease in blood volume and hypotension result in decreased renal perfusion, decreased glomerular filtration, and oliguria (see Chapter 39). The ability to concentrate and dilute urine is usually maintained. Intrarenal vasoconstriction may result from the selective effects of vasoactive substances that accumulate in the blood because of liver failure. The diseased liver fails to remove excessive angiotensin, vasopressin, prostaglandins, and catecholamines from the blood, which travel to the kidneys and cause vasoconstriction. Vasoconstriction also may be a compensatory response to portal hypotension and vasodilation in the splanchnic circulation. The exact reason for the renal vasoconstriction is unknown but is related to vasoconstrictive mediators and sympathetic nerve stimulation.[229]

CLINICAL MANIFESTATIONS. The onset of hepatorenal manifestations may be gradual or acute. Oliguria and complications of advanced liver disease, including jaundice, ascites, and gastrointestinal bleeding, are usually present. Systolic blood pressure is usually less than 100 mmHg. Nonspecific symptoms of hepatorenal syndrome include anorexia, weakness, and fatigue.

EVALUATION AND TREATMENT. Diagnosis of HRS is made by excluding all other causes of renal failure. Despite decreased glomerular filtration, serum potassium levels do not become dangerously elevated until the terminal stages of the hepatorenal syndrome. Serum creatinine values increase rapidly (within 2 weeks) in type 1 HRS and slowly or not at all in type 2 HRS. Urine osmolality is increased, but urine sodium concentrations are below normal (unlike acute tubular necrosis). Urine specific gravity is greater than 1.015. The prognosis for hepatorenal syndrome is usually poor and is related to liver function. Secondary problems, including fluid and electrolyte disorders, bleeding, infections, and encephalopathy, are vigorously treated. Treatments to increase renal perfusion include systemic vasoconstrictors (α-adrenergic agonists and telepressin) and albumin, which are effective in 50% of individuals with type 1 HRS. Vasoconstrictors also may be combined with TIPS as a bridge to liver transplant. Liver transplant reverses symptoms in most individuals and it may be combined with kidney transplantation.[230-232]

Disorders of the Liver

Autoimmune Hepatitis

Autoimmune hepatitis is a rare chronic, progressive T-cell–mediated inflammatory liver disease that affects females, both adults and children. Serologically, there is hypergammaglobulinemia and an association with human leukocyte antigens DR3 or DR4 and absence of viral hepatitis. Biopsy shows interface (parenchymal–connective tissue interface) hepatitis. Aspartate and alanine aminotransferase levels are elevated. There may be no symptoms or jaundice, fatigue, loss of appetite, and amenorrhea. Most individuals respond to immunosuppressive drug therapy (e.g., corticosteroids or in combination with azathioprine) with remission within 24 months. Relapses are common with treatment withdrawal. About 10% of cases require liver transplant.[233-235]

Viral Hepatitis

Viral hepatitis is a relatively common systemic disease that affects primarily the liver. Different strains of viruses cause different types of hepatitis: hepatitis A virus (HAV), hepatitis B virus (HBV), hepatitis D virus (HDV) associated with HBV, hepatitis C virus (HCV), and hepatitis E virus (HEV) (Table 41-7). Hepatitis A was previously known as infectious hepatitis, and hepatitis B as serum hepatitis. Coinfection of HBV, HCV, HDV,

TABLE 41-7 CHARACTERISTICS OF VIRAL HEPATITIS

CHARACTERISTIC	HEPATITIS A	HEPATITIS B	HEPATITIS D	HEPATITIS C	HEPATITIS E
Size of virus	27-nm RNA virus	47-nm DNA virus	36-nm RNA virus, defective virus with HBsAg coat	30- to 60-nm RNA virus	32-nm RNA virus
Incubation phase	30 days	60-180 days	30-180 days; dependent on HBV for multiplication	35-72 days	15-60 days
Route of transmission	Fecal-oral, parenteral, sexual	Parenteral, sexual	Parenteral, fecal-oral, sexual	Parenteral	Fecal-oral
Onset	Acute with fever	Insidious	Insidious	Insidious	Acute
Carrier state	Negative	Positive	Positive	Positive	Negative
Severity	Mild	Severe; may be prolonged or chronic	Severe	Mild to severe	Severe in pregnant women
Chronic hepatitis	No	Yes	Yes	Yes	No
Age-group affected	Children and young adults	Any	Any	Any	Children and young adults
Prophylaxis	Hygiene, immune serum globulin, HAV vaccine	Hygiene, HBV vaccine	Hygiene, HBV vaccine	Hygiene, screening blood, interferon-alpha or combined with ribavirin	Hygiene, safe water and meat

DNA, Deoxyribonucleic acid; *HBsAg,* hepatitis B surface antigen; *HBV,* hepatitis B virus; *RNA,* ribonucleic acid.

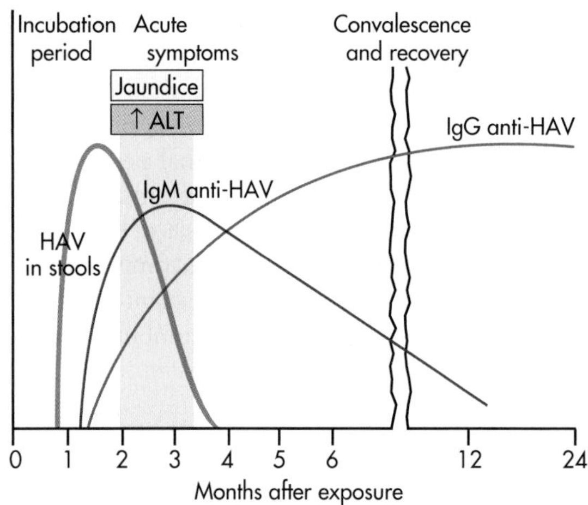

FIGURE 41-20 Course of Infection with the Hepatitis A Virus (HAV). *ALT,* Alanine transaminase; *IgG,* immunoglobulin G; *IgM,* immunoglobulin M.

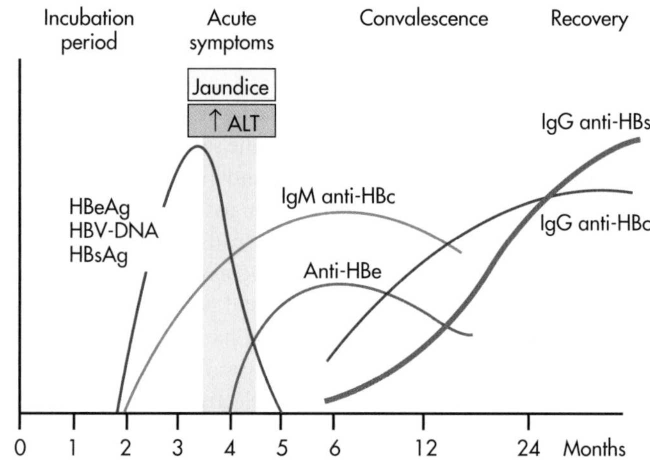

FIGURE 41-21 Course of Infection with the Hepatitis B Virus (HBV). *ALT,* Alanine transaminase; *anti-HBe,* antibody to HBeAg; *HBV-DNA,* hepatitis B virus deoxyribonucleic acid; *IgG,* immunoglobulin G; *IgM,* immunoglobulin M; *HBsAg,* hepatitis B surface antigen; *IgG anti-HBs,* antibody to HBsAg; *HBeAg,* hepatitis B e-antigen; *IgM anti-HBc,* antibody to hepatitis B core antigen.

and HIV occurs because these viruses share the same routes of transmission (contact between infected body fluids, broken skin or mucous membranes, or intravenously). Progression of liver disease is more rapid in these cases.[236] Characteristics of the various types of hepatitis are presented in Table 41-7.

Hepatitis A Virus (HAV). HAV can be recovered from the feces, bile, and sera of infected individuals. The usual mode of transmission is the fecal-oral route (contaminated food or water), but the virus can be spread also by the transfusion of infected blood. Approximately 45% of adults in urban areas have HAV antibodies in their blood. The disease spreads readily in crowded, unsanitary conditions, usually through contaminated food or water. Person-to-person spread is more likely to occur in institutional care settings where there is contact between clients and caregivers who are not vaccinated.

The incubation period (the time between exposure and onset of symptoms) for HAV is 4 to 6 weeks (Figure 41-20). Fecal shedding of the virus is greatest for 10 to 14 days before the onset of symptoms and during the first week of symptoms and up to 3 months after onset of symptoms. The disease is most contagious during this time. Antibodies to HAV (anti-HAV) develop about 4 weeks after infection. The serum immunoglobulin M (IgM) concentration increases initially and is followed by an increase of serum IgG, whose levels remain elevated for several years after infection, creating immunity to the disease. (See Chapters 7 and 8 for a description of immune functions.) The administration of immunoglobulin before exposure or early in the incubation period can prevent hepatitis A. HAV vaccine and combined HAV and HBV vaccines are available and effective in preventing the disease and confer long-term immunity.[237] Transmission of HAV is prevented by handwashing and use of gloves when disposing fecal matter. Molecular procedures are available for direct surveillance of HAV in food and water.[238]

Hepatitis B Virus (HBV). HBV is transmitted through blood-blood contact and the sexual route. People who are immunosuppressed; receive hemodialysis, multiple blood transfusions, or immunosuppressive drugs; have multiple sex partners; or share needles, syringes, or other drug equipment or infants born to infected mothers have a greater risk of exposure or less resistance to HBV coinfection with HCV, HDV. HIV is common because these viruses share the same routes of transmission.[239,240]

Mother-infant transmission of HBV occurs if the mother becomes infected during the third trimester of pregnancy. In women who are seropositive for both hepatitis B surface antigen (HBsAg) and hepatitis B e antigen (HBeAg), vertical transmission is approximately 90%.[241,242] Transmission among homosexual men may be by oral or genital contact with bleeding lesions in the rectal mucosa. Up to 400 million people worldwide carry the hepatitis B surface antigen (HBsAg) marker for active HBV. HBV is a major cause of chronic hepatitis, cirrhosis, and hepatocellular carcinoma.[243]

Three types of viral particles are involved in HBV infection. The larger (47 nm) Dane particle probably represents the intact HBV. The Dane particle has a double-layered outer coat and carries HBsAg, which was originally called the *Australia antigen.* HBsAg can be identified in the serum by radioimmunoassay. Hepatitis B core antigen (HBcAg) usually is not detected in the serum. The HBeAg is a derivative of HBcAg and is a marker of HBV replication. The HBV has an incubation period of 6 to 8 weeks. The initial serologic change is a transient increase in IgM levels. Levels of IgG antibodies to HBsAg rise more slowly and remain elevated for years (Figure 41-21). Chronic infection develops in 15% to 30% of those with acute infection. HBV DNA measures viral load and the efficacy of drug treatment. Persistent liver cell injury and deregulation of cellular growth control genes lead to increased risk for cirrhosis and hepatocellular carcinoma.[244] Antiviral and immunomodulatory treatment for chronic hepatitis B includes monotherapy, combination therapy, and prevention of drug resistance. Vaccine prevents transmission of hepatitis B, the development of acute or chronic hepatitis B, and reduction of hepatocellular carcinoma, particularly in high-risk populations. Mutant strains can develop with escape from vaccine protection or diagnosis with HBsAg.[245] Hepatitis B immunoglobulin provides postexposure prophylaxis against HBV after contact with blood or body fluids of individuals infected with hepatitis B.[246] HBV vaccine or a combined vaccine for HAV and HBV provides protective immunity.

Hepatitis C Virus (HCV). HCV (previously known as non-A, non-B hepatitis) is a parenterally transmitted flavivirus with six genotypes. About 40% of HCV cases involve intravenous drug users, who also have a high incidence of HIV infection.[247] Coinfection with HBV also is prevalent. Approximately 80% of cases develop chronic liver disease.[248] HCV is diagnosed through detection of anti-HCV IgG.[249] Persistent infection with recurring acute symptoms and elevated aminotransferase levels represent the clinical presentation. Antiviral drug therapy is available.[250] Progression of disease to cirrhosis or hepatocellular carcinoma is greatest among individuals with HIV or coexisting liver disease.[251] The variants of HCV make vaccine development difficult and resistance to drug therapy is common.[252] There is no vaccine for HCV. The Centers for Disease Control and Prevention have recommended that all persons born from 1945 through 1965 be screened for HCV infection.[253]

Hepatitis D Virus (HDV). HDV occurs in individuals with hepatitis B. The delta virus depends on the HBV for its replication because the viral coat consists of HBsAg molecules that are on the surface of HBV. Hepatitis D has been shown to suppress replication of HBV. Parenteral drug users have a high incidence of HDV infection. HDV symptoms can be mild or severe with progression to fulminant liver failure. HDV is diagnosed by the presence of antibodies directed against HDAg (anti-HD) and HDV RNA in serum. Treatment for chronic HDV includes pegylated interferon alpha and it is effective in about 25% of individuals. New treatments are in clinical development.[254,255]

Hepatitis E Virus (HEV). HEV is most common in Asian and African countries and is transmitted by the fecal-oral route, usually by way of contaminated water or uncooked meat. It is also found in developed countries and must be differentiated from drug-induced liver injury. Animal reservoirs of HEV include domestic pigs, wild boars, deer, and rodents. It is more prevalent among adults and has the highest mortality in pregnant women. Clinically, it resembles HAV and is diagnosed based on detection of anti-HEV IgM. A vaccine for HEV has been approved in China but not in other countries.[256,257]

PATHOPHYSIOLOGY. The pathologic lesions of hepatitis are similar to those caused by other viral infection. Hepatic cell necrosis, scarring, Kupffer cell hyperplasia, and infiltration by mononuclear phagocytes occur with varying severity. Cellular injury is promoted by cell-mediated immune mechanisms (i.e., cytotoxic T cells, T regulatory cells, and natural killer cells).[258] Regeneration of hepatic cells begins within 48 hours of injury. The inflammatory process can damage and obstruct bile canaliculi, leading to cholestasis and obstructive jaundice. In milder cases the liver parenchyma is not damaged. Damage tends to be most severe in cases of hepatitis B and hepatitis C. Hepatitis B is also associated with *acute fulminating hepatitis,* a rare form of the disease that is characterized by massive hepatic necrosis. Acute fulminating hepatitis causes severe encephalopathy, which is manifested as confusion, stupor, and coma. Liver failure can occur, leading to GI bleeding, cardiorespiratory insufficiency, and hepatorenal syndrome. Mortality is high, but recovery can be complete.

CLINICAL MANIFESTATIONS. The clinical manifestations of the various types of hepatitis are very similar. The spectrum of manifestations ranges from absence of symptoms to fulminating hepatitis, with rapid onset of liver failure and coma. Acute viral hepatitis causes abnormal liver function test results. The serum aminotransferase values, aspartate transaminase (AST) and alanine transaminase (ALT), are elevated, but their elevation may not be consistent with the extent of cellular damage. The clinical course of hepatitis usually consists of four phases: incubation, prodromal, icteric, and recovery phases. The **incubation phase** and manifestations vary depending on the virus (see Table 41-7).

Prodromal Phase. The **prodromal (preicteric) phase** of hepatitis begins about 2 weeks after exposure and ends with the appearance of jaundice. Fatigue, anorexia, malaise, nausea, vomiting, headache, hyperalgia, cough, and low-grade fever are prodromal symptoms that precede the onset of jaundice. About 10% of individuals may develop extrahepatic symptoms including rash, arthralgias, and purpura. HBV and HCV may cause nephritis related to glomerular immune complex deposition.[259,260] Infection with HCV may have no symptoms. Right upper abdominal pain is common, and a weight loss of 2 to 4 kg is not unusual. The infection is highly transmissible during this phase.

Icteric Phase (Jaundice). The **icteric phase** begins about 1 to 2 weeks after the prodromal phase and lasts 2 to 6 weeks. Individuals who develop chronic HBV infection do not become jaundiced and may not be diagnosed.[261] Hepatocellular destruction and intrahepatic bile stasis cause jaundice (icterus). The urine may be dark and the stools clay colored before the onset of jaundice from conjugated hyperbilirubinemia. The icteric phase is the actual phase of illness. The liver is enlarged, smooth, and tender, and percussion over the liver causes pain. During the icteric phase, gastrointestinal and respiratory symptoms subside, but fatigue and abdominal pain may persist or become more severe. The stools may be lighter in color as a result of cholestasis. Serum bilirubin levels range from 5 to 10 mg/dl, with conjugated bilirubin fraction increasing. The jaundice may last 2 to 6 weeks or longer. Mild and transient itching often accompanies jaundice. The prothrombin time may be prolonged in individuals with more serious forms of the disease.

Recovery Phase. The posticteric or **recovery phase** begins with resolution of jaundice, about 6 to 8 weeks after exposure. Although the liver may still be enlarged and tender, symptoms diminish. In most cases, liver function test results return to normal within 2 to 12 weeks after the onset of jaundice.

Chronic hepatitis may begin at this point and is associated with HBV, HCV, and HDV infection. **Chronic active hepatitis** is the persistence of clinical manifestations and liver inflammation after the acute stages. Liver function tests remain abnormal

BOX 41-6 CAUSES OF CIRRHOSIS

Hepatitis virus—B and C (common)
Excessive alcohol intake (common)
Idiopathic (common)
Nonalcoholic fatty liver disease (NAFLD), also known as nonalcoholic steatohepatitis (NASH)
Autoimmune disorders
- Autoimmune hepatitis
- Primary biliary cirrhosis
- Primary sclerosing cholangitis

Hereditary metabolic disorder
- α_1-Antitrypsin deficiency
- Hemochromatosis
- Wilson disease
- Glycogen or lipid storage diseases

Prolonged exposure to chemicals (e.g., carbon tetrachloride, cleaning and industrial solvents, copper salts)
Hepatic venous outflow obstruction
- Budd-Chiari syndrome
- Right sided heart failure

for longer than 6 months, and HBsAg persists. Chronic, active HBV and HBC is a predisposition to cirrhosis and primary hepatocellular carcinoma. Chronic active hepatitis constitutes a carrier state, and HBV and HCV can be transmitted from mothers to infants.[262]

EVALUATION AND TREATMENT. Diagnosis and treatment were previously described for the different types of hepatitis viruses. Physical activity may be restricted. A low-fat, high-carbohydrate diet is beneficial if bile flow is obstructed.

There should be no direct contact with blood or body fluids of individuals with hepatitis B or hepatitis C. A combined vaccine for HAV and HBV is available. Hepatitis B immunoglobulin provides passive prophylactic immunity against HBV. Prophylaxis is recommended for healthcare workers, liver transplant recipients, and others who are at risk for contact with infected body fluids.[263]

Cirrhosis

Cirrhosis is an irreversible inflammatory, fibrotic liver disease and the twelfth leading cause of death in the United States. Many disorders can cause cirrhosis and are summarized in Box 41-6. Alcohol abuse and viral hepatitis are the most common causes.[264] The process of cellular injury depends on the cause of cirrhosis; however, not all causes are clearly understood. Structural changes result from injury (alcoholism, viruses, steatosis, chemicals) and fibrosis. Fibrosis is a consequence of Kupffer cell (liver macrophages) activation with release of inflammatory mediators, reactive oxygen species, and growth factors and activation of fibrogenic fibroblasts.[265] Chaotic fibrosis alters or obstructs biliary channels and blood flow, producing jaundice and portal hypertension. New vascular channels form shunts, and blood from the portal vein bypasses the liver, contributing to portal hypertension, metabolic alterations, and toxin accumulation. The process of regeneration is disrupted by hypoxia, necrosis, atrophy, and (ultimately) liver failure. The formation of fibrous bands and regenerating nodules distorts the architecture of the liver parenchyma and gives the liver a cobbly appearance.[266] The liver may be larger or smaller than normal and is usually firm or hard when palpated. Cirrhosis develops slowly over a period of years. Its severity and rate of progression depend on the cause.

If alcohol is involved, the rate of cell death and the severity of inflammation depend on the amount of alcohol present.[267] Removal of alcohol slows the progression of liver damage and enhances the process of regeneration.

Alcoholic Liver Disease. Abuse of any type of alcoholic beverage can cause alcoholic liver disease and the severity of disease is related to the amount and duration of alcohol consumed and formation of acetaldehyde (see Chapter 2 and Figure 2-15).[267] The incidence of alcoholic cirrhosis is greatest in middle-aged men; however, women develop more severe liver injury than men.[268] In the United States, mortality resulting from cirrhosis is highest among Hispanic white males and females; however, the death rates for all groups are declining.[269] Malnutrition may add to the risk of cirrhosis in alcohol abusers. Many alcoholics are malnourished and the liver cannot regenerate without adequate nutrition. The spectrum of alcoholic liver disease includes steatosis, alcoholic hepatitis, and alcoholic cirrhosis (fibrosis).[270]

PATHOPHYSIOLOGY. **Alcoholic fatty liver (steatosis)** is the mildest form of alcoholic liver disease. It can be caused by chronic ingestion of relatively small amounts of alcohol (more than one alcoholic drink [14 grams of alcohol] per day for women and two alcoholic drinks [28 grams of alcohol] per day for men), may be asymptomatic, and is reversible with cessation of drinking.[271,272] Fat deposition (deposition of triglycerides) within the liver is caused primarily by increased lipogenesis and decreased fatty acid oxidation and fat metabolism by hepatocytes. Lipids mobilized from adipose tissue or dietary fat intake may contribute to fat accumulation.

Alcoholic hepatitis (steatohepatitis) is a precursor of cirrhosis characterized by inflammation; degeneration and necrosis of hepatocytes; infiltration of neutrophils, macrophages, and lymphocytes; immunologic alterations; and lipid peroxidation. The injured hepatocytes contain Mallory bodies (hyaline endoplasmic reticulum), indicating the onset of fibrosis. Neutrophils infiltrate and surround degenerating hepatocytes. The mechanism of hepatocyte injury is not clearly understood, but inflammatory mediators, acetaldehyde, reactive oxygen and nitrogen species, and genetic factors are involved.[273,274] Alcohol also increases gut permeability, and translocation of bacteria-derived lipopolysaccharide contributes to inflammation, oxidative stress, and the severity of alcoholic liver disease.[275] Serum IgA level is often elevated in individuals with alcoholic hepatitis, and liver antigens and antibodies have been identified in persons with progressive alcoholic liver disease.[276] The inflammation and necrosis caused by alcoholic hepatitis stimulate the fibrosis characteristic of the cirrhotic stage of disease. Corticosteroids and pentoxifylline are used for treatment.[277]

Alcoholic cirrhosis is caused by the toxic effects of alcohol metabolism on the liver, immunologic alterations, oxidative stress from lipid peroxidation, and malnutrition.[278] Alcoholic cirrhosis is more severe when associated with HCV.[279]

Although alcoholic cirrhosis is the most prevalent of the various types of cirrhosis, the occurrence of cirrhosis among persons with alcoholism is relatively low (approximately 35%). Alcohol is transformed to acetaldehyde. Excessive amounts of acetaldehyde are toxic and induce lipid peroxidation and oxidative stress and disrupt cytoskeletal and membrane function. Acetaldehyde inhibits export of proteins from the liver, alters metabolism of vitamins and minerals, promotes liver fibrosis, and contributes to malnutrition.[280] Mitochondrial function is impaired, decreasing oxidation of fatty acid. Enzyme and protein synthesis may be depressed or altered, and hormone and ammonia degradation is diminished. Alcohol also may stimulate the formation of autoantibodies specific to hepatic cells.[270] Alcohol also increases gut permeability, and translocation of bacteria-derived endotoxin from the intestine contributes to progressive injury and inflammation.[275] Cellular damage initiates an inflammatory response. Inflammatory cytokines, including TNF-α and IL-6, IL-8, and IL-18, and activation of complement are associated with alcoholic liver disease. Inflammation and necrosis result in excessive collagen formation. Transforming growth factor-beta (TGF-β) contributes to fibrosis and is produced in part by activated Kupffer cells. TGF-β activates hepatic stellate cells to produce excess collagen. Dense bands of fibrosis surround regenerative hepatocellular nodules. Fibrosis and scarring alter the structure of the liver and obstruct biliary and vascular channels and hepatocytes lose their ability to regenerate.[270] There is increased risk for hepatocellular carcinoma. Examples of liver damage are shown in Figure 41-22.

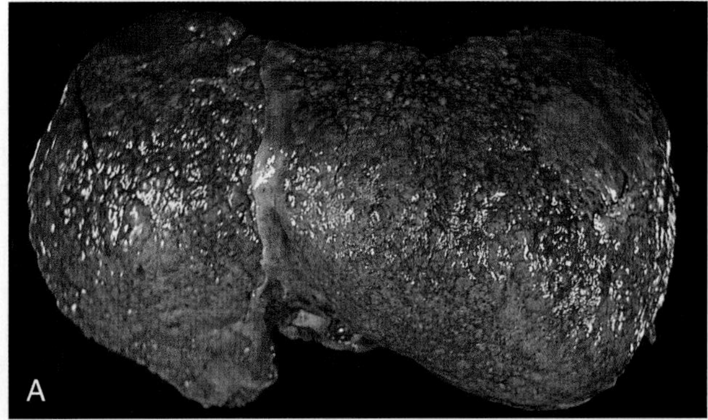

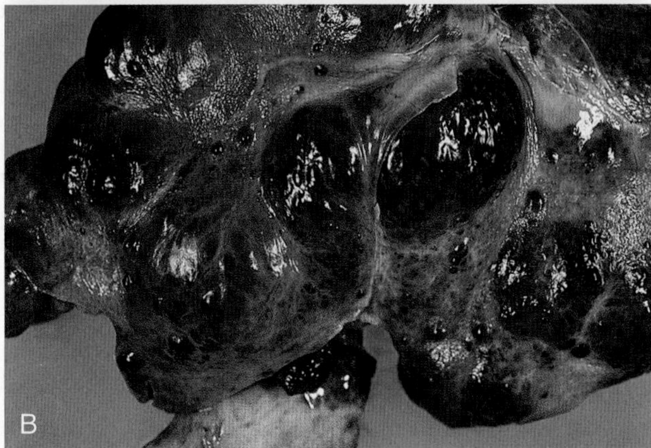

FIGURE 41-22 Cirrhosis. **A,** Micronodular cirrhosis. The nodular appearance develops from regeneration of hepatocytes projecting through fibrous bands of tissue. **B,** Macronodular cirrhosis. (From Damjanov I, Linder J, editors: *Anderson's pathology,* ed 10, St Louis, 1996, Mosby.)

CLINICAL MANIFESTATIONS. Fatty infiltration causes no specific symptoms or abnormal liver function test results. The liver is usually enlarged, however, and the individual has a history of continuous alcohol intake during the previous weeks or months. The clinical manifestations of alcoholic hepatitis can be mild or severe. Nonspecific symptoms include fatigue, weight loss, and anorexia. Manifestations of acute illness include nausea, anorexia, fever, abdominal pain, and jaundice.[281] Toxic effects of alcohol also can cause gynecomastia, testicular atrophy, reduced libido, azoospermia, and decreased testosterone level in men.[282] Cirrhosis is a multiple-system disease and causes hepatomegaly, splenomegaly, ascites, gastrointestinal hemorrhage, portal hypertension, hepatic encephalopathy, and esophageal varices. Anemia results from blood loss, malnutrition, and hypersplenism. Hepatorenal syndrome is usually a late complication. Risk for infection is greater, in part because of innate immune dysfunction.[283] The presence of numerous and severe manifestations increases the risk of death. The clinical features of alcoholic cirrhosis depend on the duration of the disease and the severity of liver damage (Figure 41-23).

EVALUATION AND TREATMENT. The diagnosis of alcoholic hepatitis is based on the individual's history and clinical manifestations. The results of liver function tests are abnormal, and serologic studies show elevated levels of serum enzymes and bilirubin and decreased serum albumin levels. Prolonged prothrombin time cannot easily be corrected with vitamin K therapy. Liver biopsy can confirm the diagnosis of cirrhosis, but biopsy is not necessary if clinical manifestations of cirrhosis are evident.

There is no specific treatment for alcoholic liver disease, but many of the complications are treatable. Rest, a nutritious diet, corticosteroids, antioxidants, drugs that slow fibrosis, and management of complications such as ascites, gastrointestinal bleeding, infection, and encephalopathy slow disease progression.[284] Cessation of alcohol consumption slows the progression of liver damage, improves clinical symptoms, and prolongs life. Although the liver damage is irreversible, measures that halt the inflammation and destruction of liver cells prolong life. Liver transplant is the treatment for liver failure and artificial liver support systems are being developed.[285,286]

Nonalcoholic Fatty Liver Disease and Nonalcoholic Steatohepatitis. **Nonalcoholic fatty liver disease (NAFLD)** is infiltration of hepatocytes with fat, primarily in the form of triglycerides, but it occurs in the absence of alcohol intake. It is associated with obesity (including obese children), high levels of cholesterol and triglycerides, metabolic syndrome, and type 2 diabetes mellitus, and is the most common chronic liver disease in the United States. Some individuals with NAFLD will develop **nonalcoholic steatohepatitis (NASH)** with hepatocellular injury, inflammation, and fibrosis; this condition is difficult to distinguish from alcohol-induced liver fibrosis.[272] NAFLD is usually asymptomatic and may remain undetected for years. The most severe forms of NASH progress to cirrhosis, end-stage liver disease, and an increased risk for hepatocellular carcinoma.[287]

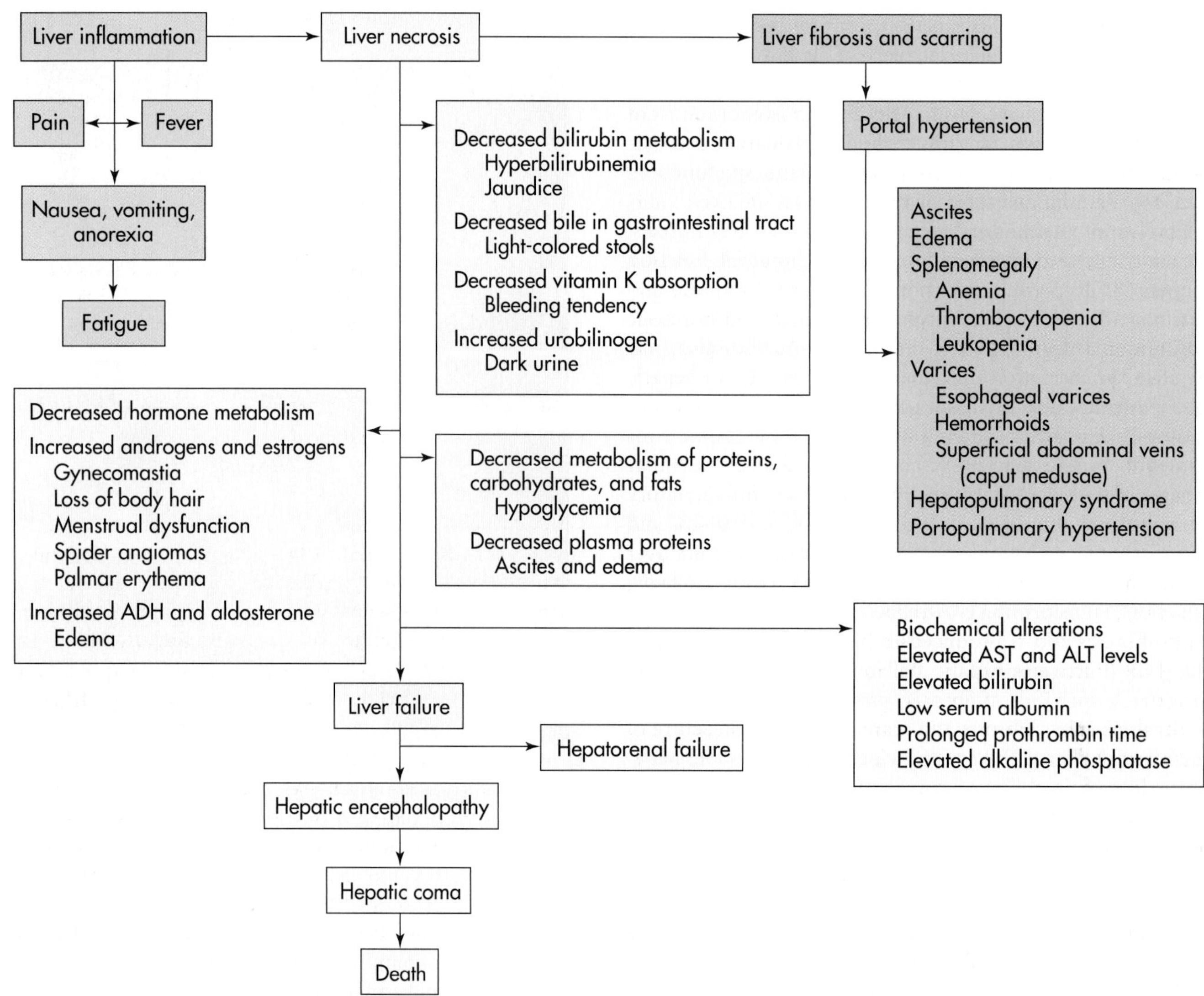

FIGURE 41-23 Clinical Manifestations of Cirrhosis. *ADH,* Antidiuretic hormone; *ALT,* alanine transaminase; *AST,* aspartate transaminase.

Biliary Cirrhosis. **Biliary cirrhosis** differs from alcoholic cirrhosis in that the damage and inflammation leading to cirrhosis begin in bile canaliculi and bile ducts, rather than in the hepatocytes. The two types of biliary cirrhosis are *primary* and *secondary*. Although both involve bile duct pathology, they differ with respect to cause, risk factors, and mechanisms of obstruction and inflammation.

Primary Biliary Cirrhosis. Primary biliary cirrhosis (PBC) is a T lymphocyte- and antibody-mediated destruction of the small intrahepatic bile ducts. The disease is thought to be caused by superimposed environmental antigens (e.g., infectious agents) in genetically susceptible individuals. Women are affected more commonly (90%) than men. Symptoms rarely develop before the age of 30 years. Primary biliary cirrhosis often accompanies other autoimmune diseases.[288]

PBC develops insidiously. Antimitochondrial antibody is the hallmark of the disease and 30% to 50% of individuals have antinuclear antibodies. Expression of glycoprotein 210 (gp210) antibodies and anticentromere antibodies confers different risks for disease progression with anti-gp210 causing the most severe disease.[289] Pathogenesis includes inflammation, destruction, fibrosis, and obstruction of the intrahepatic bile ducts. Nodular regeneration, cirrhosis, and portal hypertension can develop during later stages of the disease.

Diagnosis is based on two of the following three criteria: (1) biochemical evidence of cholestatic liver disease for at least 6-month's duration, (2) antimitochondrial antibody (AMA) positivity, and (3) histologic features of PBC on liver biopsy.[290] Serologic tests show elevated levels of alkaline phosphatase and γ-glutamyl transpeptidase, hyperbilirubinemia, and hyperlipidemia with or without other clinical manifestations. Most individuals have a circulating IgG antimitochondrial antibody that is not found in other types of liver disease. Biopsy shows cholangitis and excludes other inflammatory liver diseases. Evaluation involves ruling out biliary obstruction caused by gallstones, tumor, or inflammation of the common bile duct (i.e., secondary biliary cirrhosis).

Individuals with primary biliary cirrhosis may be asymptomatic or symptomatic at diagnosis and may have minimal disease or rapid progression to cirrhosis and liver failure. The earliest manifestations are pruritus, fatigue, and abdominal pain. Jaundice and light-colored stools are symptoms of advanced disease. These symptoms are caused by intrahepatic obstruction of bile flow. Steatorrhea and fat-soluble vitamin deficiencies are present in some cases. The malabsorption can lead to osteomalacia and osteoporosis. Cirrhosis, symptoms of portal hypertension, encephalopathy, and ultimately liver failure develop in untreated individuals.

Long-term treatment with ursodeoxycholic acid is highly effective.[288] The distressing pruritus may be relieved by cholestyramine, which binds bile salts in the intestine. Intramuscular injections of vitamins D and K alleviate the vitamin deficiency. The other symptoms of cirrhosis are managed as they develop. Liver transplant is the only option for those with progressive disease not responding to medical treatment.[291]

Secondary Biliary Cirrhosis. Secondary biliary cirrhosis develops when there is prolonged partial or complete obstruction of the common bile duct or its branches. The obstruction may be caused by gallstones, tumors, fibrotic strictures, or chronic pancreatitis. Biliary atresia and cystic fibrosis cause secondary biliary cirrhosis in children.

Chronic obstruction to bile flow increases pressure in the hepatic bile duct and results in the accumulation of bile in the centrilobular spaces. Necrotic areas develop and are followed by proliferation and inflammation of the portal ducts that result in edema and fibrosis. Pools of bile form when the portal ducts rupture into surrounding necrotic areas. Injury is accompanied by regeneration of hepatic cells with the development of finely nodular cirrhosis.

Clinical manifestations are similar to those of primary biliary cirrhosis, with jaundice and pruritus the most distressing symptoms. Right upper quadrant pain is common, and a low-grade fever may be present from bile duct inflammation (cholangitis).

Cholangiography provides the most definitive diagnosis. Laboratory tests usually show elevated conjugated bilirubin and alkaline phosphatase levels. Aminotransferase level increases if there is an accompanying cholangitis. Surgery or endoscopy relieves obstruction, prolongs survival, and diminishes or resolves symptoms. Continued obstruction leads to advanced cirrhosis and liver failure.

Primary Sclerosing Cholangitis. Primary sclerosing cholangitis (PSC) is a chronic inflammatory fibrotic disease of the hepatic bile ducts that leads to secondary biliary cirrhosis. The disease is immune-mediated but the exact mechanism is unknown. PSC is associated with inflammatory bowel disease (75%) and primarily affects genetically susceptible males. There is no effective sustaining medical or surgical therapy and liver transplant is required for liver failure.[292,293]

Disorders of the Gallbladder

Obstruction and inflammation are the most common disorders of the gallbladder. Obstruction is caused by **gallstones** (cholelithiasis), which are aggregates of substances in the bile. The gallstones may remain in the gallbladder or be ejected, with bile, into the cystic duct. Gallstones that become lodged in the cystic duct obstruct the flow of bile into and out of the gallbladder and cause inflammation. Gallstone formation is termed *cholelithiasis.* Inflammation of the gallbladder or cystic duct is known as *cholecystitis.*

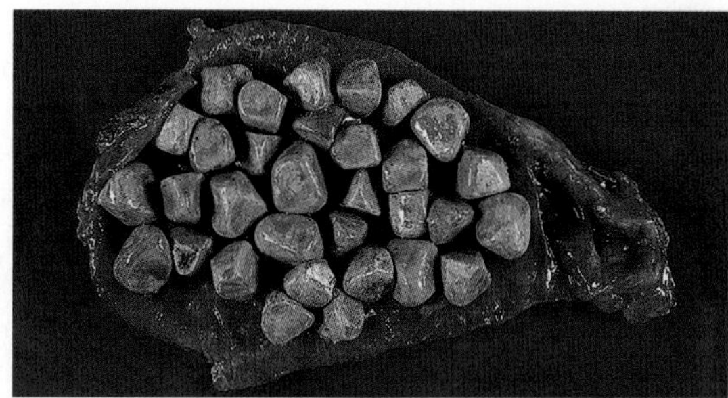

FIGURE 41-24 Resected Gallbladder Containing Mixed Gallstones. (From Kissane JM, editor: *Anderson's pathology,* ed 9, St Louis, 1990, Mosby.)

Cholelithiasis (Gallstones)

Cholelithiasis is a prevalent disorder in developed countries, where the incidence is 10% to 15%. The actual incidence is unknown because many individuals who have gallstones are asymptomatic. Risk factors include obesity; rapid weight loss in obese individuals; middle age; female gender; use of oral contraceptives; American Indian ancestry; gallbladder, pancreatic, or ileal disease; low HDL cholesterol level and hypertriglyceridemia; and gene-environmental interactions.[294]

PATHOPHYSIOLOGY. Gallstones are commonly of two types: cholesterol and pigmented. Cholesterol stones are the most common. *Cholesterol gallstones* form in bile that is supersaturated with cholesterol produced by the liver. Supersaturation sets the stage for cholesterol crystal formation, or the formation of "microstones." More crystals then aggregate on the microstones, which grow to form "macrostones" within a mucin matrix. This process usually occurs in the gallbladder. The stones may lie "silent" or become lodged in the cystic or common duct, causing pain and cholecystitis. Gallstone formation may be such that the stones accumulate and fill the entire gallbladder (Figure 41-24).

It is not known why the hepatocytes secrete bile that is supersaturated with cholesterol. Proposed mechanisms include: (1) an enzymatic defect that increases the hepatocytes' synthesis of cholesterol; (2) diminished secretion of bile acids, which normally promote cholesterol solubility; (3) decreased resorption of bile salts from the ileum, which decrease the bile acid pool; (4) gallbladder smooth muscle hypomotility and stasis; (5) genetic predisposition; and (6) some combination of these mechanisms.[295] In obese individuals the mechanism appears to involve cholesterol synthesis, whereas in nonobese individuals, it appears to involve decreased secretion of bile acids.

Pigmented stones are black (hard) or brown (soft). Black pigmented stones are formed in a sterile environment and consist primarily of calcium bilirubinate polymer. They are associated with hyperbilirubinbilia (biliary hypersecretion of bilirubin conjugates) and hemolytic diseases, such as sickle cell anemia and Gilbert syndrome (hereditary hyperbilirubinemia). The formation of brown stones is associated with bacterial infection of the bile ducts with formation of stone composed of calcium soaps, unconjugated bilirubin, cholesterol, fatty acids, and mucin. They are more common in East Asia.[296]

CLINICAL MANIFESTATIONS. Epigastric and right hypochondrium pain and intolerance to fatty foods are the cardinal manifestations of cholelithiasis. Vague symptoms include heartburn, flatulence, epigastric discomfort, pruritus, jaundice, and food intolerances, particularly to fats and cabbage. The pain, often called *biliary colic,* is most characteristic and is caused by the lodging of one or more gallstones in the cystic or common duct.[297] The pain can be intermittent or steady. It usually is located in the right upper quadrant and radiates to the mid-upper back. Jaundice indicates that the stone is located in the common bile duct. Abdominal tenderness and fever indicate cholecystitis. Complications can include pancreatitis from obstruction of the pancreatic duct.

EVALUATION AND TREATMENT. Diagnosis is based on the individual's medical history, physical examination, and imaging evaluation. An oral cholecystogram usually outlines the stones. Intravenous cholangiography is used to differentiate cholelithiasis from other causes of extrahepatic biliary obstruction if the cholecystogram is negative. Endoscopic or percutaneous cholangiography and endoscopic or transabdominal ultrasonography are diagnostic options.[298]

Laparoscopic cholecystectomy is the preferred treatment for gallstones that cause obstruction or inflammation. Use of transluminal endoscopic surgery is advancing rapidly. Endoscopic retrograde cholangiopancreatography and sphincterotomy with stone retrieval is used for the treatment of bile duct stones. Large stones may be managed with lithotripsy.[299,300] An alternative treatment is the administration of drugs that dissolve smaller stones. For example, the bile acid chenodeoxycholic acid (CDCA) can completely or partially dissolve cholesterol gallstones. Ursodeoxycholic acid (UDCA), which is structurally similar to CDCA, is also effective, is less toxic to hepatocytes, and does not cause fatty diarrhea, as does CDCA.

Cholecystitis

Cholecystitis can be acute or chronic. Both forms are almost always caused by the lodging of a gallstone in the cystic duct. Obstruction causes the gallbladder to become distended and inflamed. The pain is similar to that caused by gallstones. Pressure against the distended wall of the gallbladder decreases blood flow. Ischemia, necrosis, and perforation of the gallbladder are possible. Fever, leukocytosis, rebound tenderness, and abdominal muscle guarding are common findings. Serum bilirubin and alkaline phosphatase levels may be elevated. Nevertheless, the acute abdominal pain of cholecystitis must be differentiated from the pain caused by other disorders, such as pancreatitis, intestinal vascular insufficiency, and acute pyelonephritis of the right kidney. Cholescintigraphy tracks the production and flow of bile from the liver to the gallbladder and small intestine and shows if bile is blocked at any point along the way; it has the highest diagnostic accuracy but involves the use of ionizing radiation. Ultrasound and magnetic resonance imaging have a substantial margin of error but can demonstrate nonspecific morphologic changes.[301]

Treatment includes pain control, replacement of fluid and electrolytes, and fasting. Antibiotics are often prescribed to manage bacterial infection in severe cases. Immediate cholecystectomy is required for complications such as peritonitis from gallbladder perforation. Persistent symptoms or development of chronic cholecystitis punctuated by recurrent acute attacks usually requires cholecystectomy.[302]

Disorders of the Pancreas

Pancreatitis, or inflammation of the pancreas, is a relatively rare (about 17 cases per 100,000 people in the United States)[303] and a potentially serious disorder. Incidence is about equal in men and women and is more common between 50 and 60 years of age. Risk factors include alcoholism, obstructive biliary tract disease (particularly cholelithiasis), peptic ulcers, abdominal trauma, hyperlipidemia, certain drugs, and genetic factors (hereditary pancreatitis, cystic fibrosis). The cause is unknown in 15% to 25% of cases.[304] Pancreatitis can be acute or chronic.

Acute Pancreatitis

Acute pancreatitis is usually a mild disease and resolves spontaneously, but about 20% of those with the disease develop a severe acute pancreatitis requiring hospitalization. Pancreatitis develops because of obstruction to the outflow of pancreatic digestive enzymes caused by bile duct or pancreatic duct obstruction (e.g., gallstones). Chronic alcohol use may also cause spasm of the sphincter of Oddi and formation of protein plugs in pancreatic ducts, resulting in obstruction. Acute pancreatitis can also result from direct cellular injury from drugs or viral infection.[305]

PATHOPHYSIOLOGY. In obstructive disease, the backup of pancreatic secretions causes activation and release of enzymes (activated trypsin activates chymotrypsin, lipase, and elastase) within the pancreatic acinar cells. The activated enzymes cause autodigestion (e.g., proteolysis, lipolysis) of pancreatic cells and tissues, resulting in inflammation. The autodigestion causes vascular damage, coagulative necrosis, fat necrosis (see Chapter 2), and formation of pseudocysts (walled-off collections of pancreatic secretions).[306] Edema within the pancreatic capsule leads to ischemia and can contribute to necrosis.

Systemic effects are associated with severe acute pancreatitis. Proinflammatory cytokines (e.g., interleukin-6, tumor necrosis factor-alpha, transforming growth factor-beta, and platelet-activating factor) and vasoactive peptides are released into the bloodstream. Activation of leukocytes, injury to vessel walls, and coagulation abnormalities with development of vasodilation, hypotension, and shock occur.[307] These systemic effects can lead to acute respiratory distress syndrome (ARDS), heart failure, renal failure, coagulopathies, and the systemic inflammatory response syndrome (SIRS) (see Chapter 48) (Figures 41-25 and 41-26). Translocation of intestinal bacteria to the bloodstream may cause peritonitis or sepsis. Anti-inflammatory cytokines and specific cytokine inhibitors are produced in response to the systemic inflammatory response and may increase risk of infection.[308] As the pancreatitis progresses, pancreatic stellate cells become activated, causing pancreatic fibrosis, strictures, and duct obstruction and leading to chronic pancreatitis.

CLINICAL MANIFESTATIONS. Epigastric or midabdominal pain is the cardinal symptom of acute pancreatitis. The pain may radiate to the back because of the retroperitoneal location of

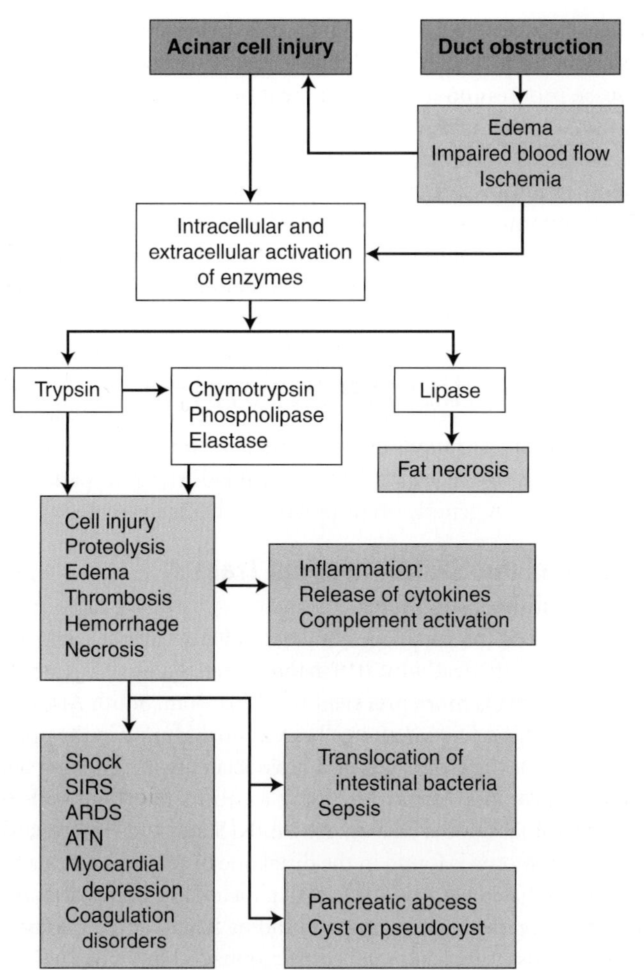

FIGURE 41-25 Pathophysiology of Acute Pancreatitis. *ARDS,* Acute respiratory distress syndrome; *ATN,* acute tubular necrosis; *SIRS,* systemic inflammatory response syndrome.

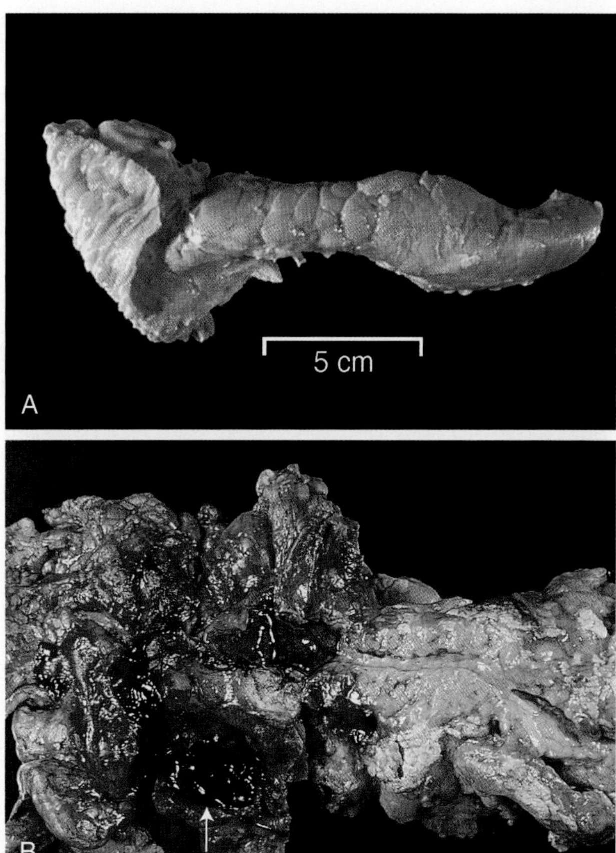

FIGURE 41-26 Acute Severe Pancreatitis with Hemorrhage. **A,** Normal pancreas. **B,** Acute hemorrhagic pancreatitis. The pancreas has hemorrhage, fat necrosis *(white patches),* and a pseudocyst filled with blood *(white arrow).* (**A** from Klatt EC, editor: *Robbins and Cotran atlas of pathology,* Philadelphia, 2006, Saunders. **B** from Damjanov I, Linder J, editors: *Pathology: a color atlas,* St Louis, 2000, Mosby.)

the pancreas. The pain is caused by edema, which distends the pancreatic ducts and capsule; chemical irritation and inflammation of the peritoneum; and irritation or obstruction of the biliary tract. Fever and leukocytosis accompany the inflammatory response. Nausea and vomiting are caused by hypermotility or paralytic ileus secondary to the pancreatitis or peritonitis.

Abdominal distention accompanies bowel hypermotility or paralytic ileus and the accumulation of fluids in the peritoneal cavity (ascites). Hypotension and shock occur with hypovolemia and SIRS.[309] Tachypnea and hypoxemia are indicative of ascites, diaphragmatic irritation, or respiratory complications.[310] In severe cases, hypovolemia decreases renal blood flow sufficiently to impair renal function.[311-313] Transient hyperglycemia also can occur if glucagon is released from damaged A cells in the pancreatic islets. SIRS and multiple organ failure account for most deaths with severe pancreatitis.[307] In severe acute pancreatitis, some individuals develop flank or periumbilical ecchymosis, a sign of poor prognosis.

EVALUATION AND TREATMENT. Diagnosis of pancreatitis is based on clinical findings, identification of associated disorders, laboratory studies, and imaging techniques (CT scan, MRI, and ultrasonography). Elevated serum lipase level is the primary diagnostic marker for acute pancreatitis. Serum lipase levels increase within 4 to 8 hours of clinical symptom onset and decrease within 8 to 14 days. Serum amylase level is elevated but is not diagnostic of severity or specificity of disease. Serum trypsin levels are very specific for pancreatitis but the test is not widely available.[314] C-reactive protein, procalcitonin, blood urea nitrogen, and Bedside Index of Severity in Acute Pancreatitis are predictors of severity.[315,316]

Acute pancreatitis is difficult to diagnose because several other disorders can cause similar clinical and laboratory findings (e.g., perforating duodenal ulcer, acute cholecystitis, and kidney stones). Intra-abdominal pressure monitoring assesses risk for abdominal compartment syndrome[317] (see What's New? Abdominal Compartment Syndrome).

There is no specific treatment for acute pancreatitis. The goal of treatment is to stop the process of autodigestion and prevent systemic complications. Hemodynamic monitoring and parenteral fluids are essential to restore blood volume and prevent hypotension and shock, particularly in the first 24 hours. Narcotic medications may be needed to relieve pain. Meperidine hydrochloride (Demerol) is used instead of morphine because it causes less spasm of the sphincter of Oddi than morphine. Nasogastric suction may not be necessary with mild pancreatitis but may help relieve pain and prevent

WHAT'S NEW?

Abdominal Compartment Syndrome

Abdominal compartment syndrome (ACS), also known as *intra-abdominal hypertension,* develops when there is abnormally high intra-abdominal pressure associated with organ dysfunction. It occurs in 20% to 40% of intensive care unit patients. ACS is associated with abdominal injury, including trauma, ruptured aortic aneurysm, acute pancreatitis, sepsis, significant thermal injury, liver failure with ascites, and massive fluid volume replacement with mechanical ventilation. Increased intra-abdominal pressure increases intrathoracic, intracardiac, and intracranial filling pressures and results in decreased cardiac output, atelectasis, pulmonary edema, oliguria, compromise of splanchnic and hepatic blood flow, and translocation of bacteria from the gut. The end consequence is multiple organ failure.

Normally intra-abdominal pressure is slightly greater than atmospheric pressure (5 to 7 mmHg, up to 12 mmHg). Organ dysfunction develops at pressures greater than 20 mmHg that last for more than 6 hours. ACS is difficult to detect from physical diagnosis alone. Automated serial or continuous monitoring of pressure inside the bladder provides a reliable estimate of intra-abdominal pressure. Gastric monitoring is not always feasible and inferior vena cava monitoring is more invasive. Treatment is tiered medical management and decompressive laparotomy, which may be performed at the bedside if the individual is too unstable to move. Elevating the head of the bed to 30 degrees is helpful for some individuals.

Data from Luckianow GM et al: *Crit Care Res Pract* 2012:908169, 2012; Starkopf J, Tamme K, Blaser AR: *Ann Intensive Care* 2(Suppl 1):S9, 2012; Yi M et al: *J Crit Care* 27(2):222.e1e–6, 2012.

paralytic ileus in individuals who are nauseated and vomiting. Feeding is usually initiated within 24 to 48 hours if ileus is not present. In severe acute pancreatitis, enteral nutrition with use of jejunal tube feeding is usually well tolerated and may decrease pancreatic enzyme secretion, prevent gut bacterial overgrowth, and maintain gut barrier function. Parenteral hyperalimentation should be initiated only when enteral feeding is not tolerated. Drugs that decrease gastric acid production (e.g., H2 receptor antagonists) can decrease stimulation of the pancreas by secretin. Necrotizing pancreatitis requires surgical resection, and antibiotics may control infection. The risk of mortality increases significantly with the development of pulmonary, cardiac, and renal complications.[318]

Chronic Pancreatitis

Chronic alcohol abuse is the most common cause of **chronic pancreatitis** because repeated exacerbations of acute pancreatitis can lead to chronic changes. Obstruction from gallstones, autoimmune disease, gene mutations, smoking, occupational chemical exposure, and obesity are associated with chronic pancreatitis. The disease is idiopathic in about 25% of cases. Toxic metabolites and chronic release of inflammatory cytokines contribute to the destruction of acinar cells and islets of Langerhans. The pancreatic parenchyma is destroyed and replaced by fibrous tissues, strictures, calcification, ductal obstruction, and pancreatic cysts. The cysts are walled-off areas or pockets of pancreatic juice, necrotic debris, or blood within or adjacent to the pancreas. Continuous or intermittent abdominal pain is the classic symptom. Pain is associated with increased intraductal pressure, increased tissue pressure, ischemia, neuritis, ongoing injury, and changes in central pain perception. Weight loss and, less commonly, steatorrhea and diabetes mellitus accompany disease progression and require treatment with oral lipase and insulin. Autoimmune chronic pancreatitis is treated with corticosteroids. Preventing disease progression includes lifestyle modification to stop alcohol use and smoking. Pain management is complex with use of analgesics, endoscopic therapy, nerve block, and surgical drainage of cysts or partial resection of the pancreas.[319-321] Chronic pancreatitis is a risk factor for pancreatic cancer.[322]

CANCER OF THE DIGESTIVE SYSTEM

Cancer occurs throughout the alimentary tract and the accessory organs of digestion (liver, gallbladder, and pancreas) (Table 41-8). A genetic predisposition is being evaluated.[323]

Cancer of the Gastrointestinal Tract

Cancer of the Esophagus

Carcinoma of the esophagus is a rare disease with 17,990 new cases and 15,210 deaths in 2013 in the United States.[324] Squamous cell carcinoma is more prevalent in China, Iran, South America, and South Africa. Squamous cell carcinoma is found in the upper two thirds of the esophagus and is associated with smoking and alcohol ingestion. Adenocarcinoma accounts for about 58% of esophageal carcinoma cases in the United States and is increasing. Adenocarcinoma is found in the distal one third of the esophagus and is associated with risk factors that include smoking, abdominal obesity, reflux esophagitis, and sliding hiatal hernia. Carcinomas are most common at the gastroesophageal junction.[325]

PATHOGENESIS. The pathogenesis of esophageal carcinoma is facilitated by (1) chronic inflammation, metaplasia, and dysplasia caused by gastroesophageal reflux **(Barrett esophagus);** and (2) long-term exposure to irritants, such as alcohol and tobacco, that cause neoplastic transformation (see Chapter 12). Both genomic and epigenomic events are associated with Barrett esophagus and mutation of the *TP53* gene is an early event.[326,327] The *CagA*-positive strain of *H. pylori* may be a protection against esophageal adenocarcinoma.[328]

CLINICAL MANIFESTATIONS. Early stages of esophageal carcinoma are asymptomatic. The two main manifestations of esophageal carcinoma are chest pain and dysphagia. The most common type of pain is heartburn (pyrosis). It is initiated by eating spicy or highly seasoned foods and by lying down. Dysphagia (pain on swallowing), another common symptom, is usually pressure-like and may radiate posteriorly between the scapulae. Some individuals with esophageal cancer complain of a constant retrosternal pain that radiates to the back. Dysphagia usually progresses rapidly.

EVALUATION AND TREATMENT. Individuals who present with dysphagia undergo endoscopy so that specimens can be examined for neoplastic change and type of carcinoma. CT studies of the thorax also are used for diagnosis. Treatment of gastroesophageal reflux is essential for the prevention of Barrett esophagus. Barrett esophagus with high-grade dysplasia is treated with endoscopic radiofrequency ablation, cryotherapy, or resection.[329]

TABLE 41-8 CANCER OF THE GUT, LIVER, AND PANCREAS*

ORGAN	PERCENTAGE OF DEATHS OF ALL CANCERS	RISKS	CELL TYPE	COMMON MANIFESTATIONS
Esophagus	2	Malnutrition Alcohol Tobacco Chronic reflux	Squamous cell Adenocarcinoma	Chest pain Dysphagia
Stomach	2	Salty food Nitrates and nitrosamines Gastric atrophy	Adenocarcinoma Squamous cell	Anorexia Malaise Weight loss Upper abdominal pain Vomiting Occult blood
Colorectal	9	Polyps Ulcerative colitis Diverticulitis High–refined-carbohydrate, low-fiber, high-fat diet	Adenocarcinoma (left colon grows in ring; right colon grows as mass)	Pain Mass Anemia Bloody stool Obstruction Distention
Liver	3	Hepatitis B, C, and D viruses Cirrhosis Intestinal parasite Aflatoxin from moldy peanuts	Hepatomas Cholangiomas	Pain Anorexia Bloating Weight loss Portal hypertension Ascites ± jaundice
Pancreas	6	Chronic pancreatitis Cigarette smoking Alcohol (?) Diabetic women	Adenocarcinoma (exocrine part of gland, ductal epithelium)	

Amended with permission from the American Cancer Society: *Cancer facts and figures, 2009*, Atlanta, GA, 2009, Author.
***Note:** Esophageal (men), colorectal, liver, and pancreatic cancers are within the top 10 causes of death from cancer.

Untreated esophageal cancer metastasizes rapidly and has a poor prognosis. At the time of diagnosis, 50% of esophageal cancers present with metastatic disease. The lymphatic vessels of the esophagus are continuous with vital mediastinal structures (trachea, heart, and great vessels) and drain to the celiac lymph nodes, making it impossible to remove all the lymph nodes with the tumor. Removal of the primary lesion and the local lymph nodes, however, can benefit the individual with esophageal cancer and cure is likely if there is no metastasis. If spread has occurred, treatment is combined radiation, chemotherapy, and palliative care (e.g., self-expanding metal stents).[330]

Cancer of the Stomach

Although the incidence of gastric cancer has declined in the United States, it still represents about 2% (21,600 cases) of all new cancer cases and 10,990 deaths in 2013.[324] The majority of cases are adenocarcinoma. The incidence of gastric cancer is greater in men than in women. In countries such as Eastern Asia, Eastern Europe, and South America, the incidence of stomach cancer has remained consistently high.[331] Nonenvironmental risk factors include a family history of gastric adenocarcinoma; blood type (blood group A); type A atrophic gastritis; and pernicious anemia, which is associated with atrophy of the gastric mucosa in the same locations where gastric tumors arise.[332-334]

The most important environmental risk factors in causing gastric cancer are: (1) infection with *H. pylori* that carries the *CagA* gene product cytotoxin-associated antigen A (80% of cases); (2) dietary factors, such as salt added to food, food additives (e.g., nitrates) in pickled or salted foods (e.g., bacon), and low intake of fruits and vegetables; and (3) lifestyle, such as alcohol consumption and cigarette smoking. Infection with *H. pylori* and severe chronic gastritis change the mucosal cell proliferation pattern, destroy cell junctions, inhibit cell proliferation, and promote cell invasive ability, increasing the risk for gastric and duodenal carcinoma.[335-337]

H. pylori also is causatively linked to **mucosa-associated lymphoid tissue (MALT) lymphoma** (a low-grade B-cell lymphoma) that can originate in the stomach. Dietary salt enhances the conversion of nitrates to carcinogenic nitrosamines in the stomach. Salt is also caustic to the stomach and can cause chronic atrophic gastritis. Hypertonic salt solutions delay gastric emptying. Delayed emptying increases the time during which carcinogenic nitrosamines can exert their effects on the stomach mucosa. Nitrates interact with amino acids in the stomach to form nitrosamines. The conversion of these carcinogenic nitrosamines is enhanced at a low pH by iodides and thiocyanates. Nitrates are thought to be active only when converted to nitrites and to cause stomach cancer once atrophic gastritis has occurred. Smoking decreases the production of prostaglandins that maintain gastric mucosal integrity, and smokers have a higher incidence of *H. pylori* infection.[338]

PATHOGENESIS. Gastric adenocarcinoma usually begins in the glands of the stomach mucosa. Approximately 50% of all gastric cancers develop in the prepyloric antrum (Figure 41-27). Atrophic gastritis and intestinal metaplasia are strongly linked to the development of gastric cancer. Insufficient acid secretion by the atrophic mucosa creates a relatively alkaline environment that permits bacteria to multiply and act on nitrates. The resulting increase in nitrosoamines damages the deoxyribonucleic acid (DNA) of mucosal cells further, promoting metaplasia and neoplasia. Duodenal reflux also may contribute to intestinal metaplasia. The reflux contains caustic bile salts that destroy the mucosal barrier that normally protects the stomach. Epigenetic alterations (DNA methylation, histone methylation, and histone acetylation) and multiple genes are involved in gastric cancer including oncogenes, tumor-suppressor genes, DNA repair genes, and cell cycle regulator genes. Genetics also can distinguish well-differentiated (intestinal) from undifferentiated (diffuse) gastric adenocarcinomas. About 10% to 15% of gastric cancers are familial.[339,340]

CLINICAL MANIFESTATIONS. The early stages of gastric cancer are generally asymptomatic or produce vague symptoms such as loss of appetite (especially for meat), malaise, and unexplained weight loss. Later manifestations include upper abdominal pain, vomiting, change in bowel habits, and anemia caused by persistent occult bleeding. The prognosis is poor because symptoms usually do not occur until the tumor has penetrated the muscle layers of the stomach, spread to surrounding tissues, and entered the draining lymph nodes and veins, causing distant metastases. Generally the first manifestations of carcinoma are caused by distant metastases.

EVALUATION AND TREATMENT. The choice of diagnostic tests depends on the clinical manifestations at the time of presentation. Most symptoms suggest a problem in the upper gastrointestinal tract. Direct endoscopic visualization and biopsy usually establish the diagnosis, or microscopic examination of exfoliated cells obtained by lavage during endoscopy.

Surgery is the treatment for gastric cancer. Staging is determined by pathologic findings after resection. Chemotherapy combined with chemoradiotherapy may provide the best postoperative outcomes. Five-year survival is less than 20%. Screening and eradication of *H. pylori* infection is the best preventive approach to gastric cancer and remission of gastric MALT lymphoma.[341] Dietary modifications include high intake of fruits and vegetables, vitamin C, carotenoids, and fiber and reduced intake of salt, salted food, and red meat.[342]

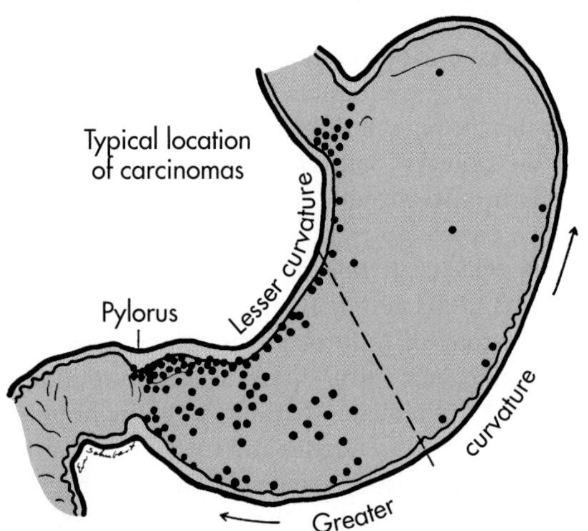

FIGURE 41-27 Typical Sites of Stomach Cancer. (From del Regato JA, Spjut HJ, Cox JD: *Cancer: diagnosis, treatment, and prognosis,* ed 2, St Louis, 1985, Mosby.)

Cancer of the Small Intestine

Small intestine carcinoma is rare and represents less than 3% of gastrointestinal cancers (8810 estimated new cases and 1170 deaths in 2013).[324] Adenocarcinoma is the most common tumor type followed by carcinoid (neuroendocrine) tumors.[343] Carcinoma occurs more frequently in familial adenomatous polyposis and Crohn disease.[344] Long-term management includes frequent screening and endoscopic surveillance.[345]

Cancer of the Colon and Rectum

Cancer of the lower intestinal tract (colon [78%], rectum [28%]) is the third most common cause of cancer death in the United States for men and women. Colon and rectal cancer (CRC) accounted for an estimated 102,480 colon and 40,340 rectal new cancer cases, and 50,830 deaths (colon and rectal combined) in 2013. The median age at diagnosis was 69 years in 2009. It is more common in blacks[324] worldwide, and the prevalence of colorectal cancer is highest in populations with high socioeconomic standards.[346,347] CRC develops in individuals with an acquired or inherited genetic predisposition who are exposed to a combination of environmental risk factors (Box 41-7).

BOX 41-7 SELECTED RISK FACTORS AND COLORECTAL CANCER

Higher Risk

Family history of colorectal cancer
Familial adenomatous polyposis
Inflammatory bowel disease
Smoking or chewing tobacco
Obesity
Alcohol consumption
Red meat consumption
Type 2 diabetes mellitus
High-fat, low-fiber diet

Lower Risk

Diets high in cereal grains, vegetables, milk; fish; folic acid, calcium, and vitamin D; magnesium and selenium
Postmenopausal estrogen use
Physical activity
Use of NSAIDs

Data from Aune D et al: *Ann Oncol* 23(1):37–45, 2012; Aune D et al: *BMJ* 343:d6617, 2011; Avivi D et al: *Exp Opin Ther Targets* 16(Suppl 1): S51–S62, 2012; Bardou M et al: *Gut* 62(6):933–947, 2013; Kennedy DA et al: *Cancer Epidemiol* 35(1):2–10, 2011; Méplan C, Hesketh J: *Mutagenesis* 27(2):177–186, 2012; Meyerhardt JA: *Semin Oncol* 38(4):533–541, 2011; Schrör K: *Best Pract Res Clin Gastroenterol* 25(4-5):473–484, 2011; Wu S et al: *Am J Med* 125(6):551–559, 2012; Yuhara H et al: *Am J Gastroenterol* 106(11):1911–1921, 2011; Zhang X, Giovannucci E: *Best Pract Res Clin Gastroenterol* 25(4-5):485–494, 2011.

PATHOGENESIS. Genetic and environmental factors (epigenetics, see Chapter 6)[348] are associated with the development of CRC (Figure 41-28). CRC can develop through molecular pathways, gene mutations, and genomic instability (the cell cycle loses control of the gene mutation rate). Gene mutations may be inherited or acquired after birth (somatic mutations). Family history of CRC occurs in about 25% of cases but only 5% to 6% of these are related to highly penetrating gene mutations, mostly autosomal dominant (e.g., familial adenomatous polyposis [FAP] and hereditary nonpolyposis colorectal cancer

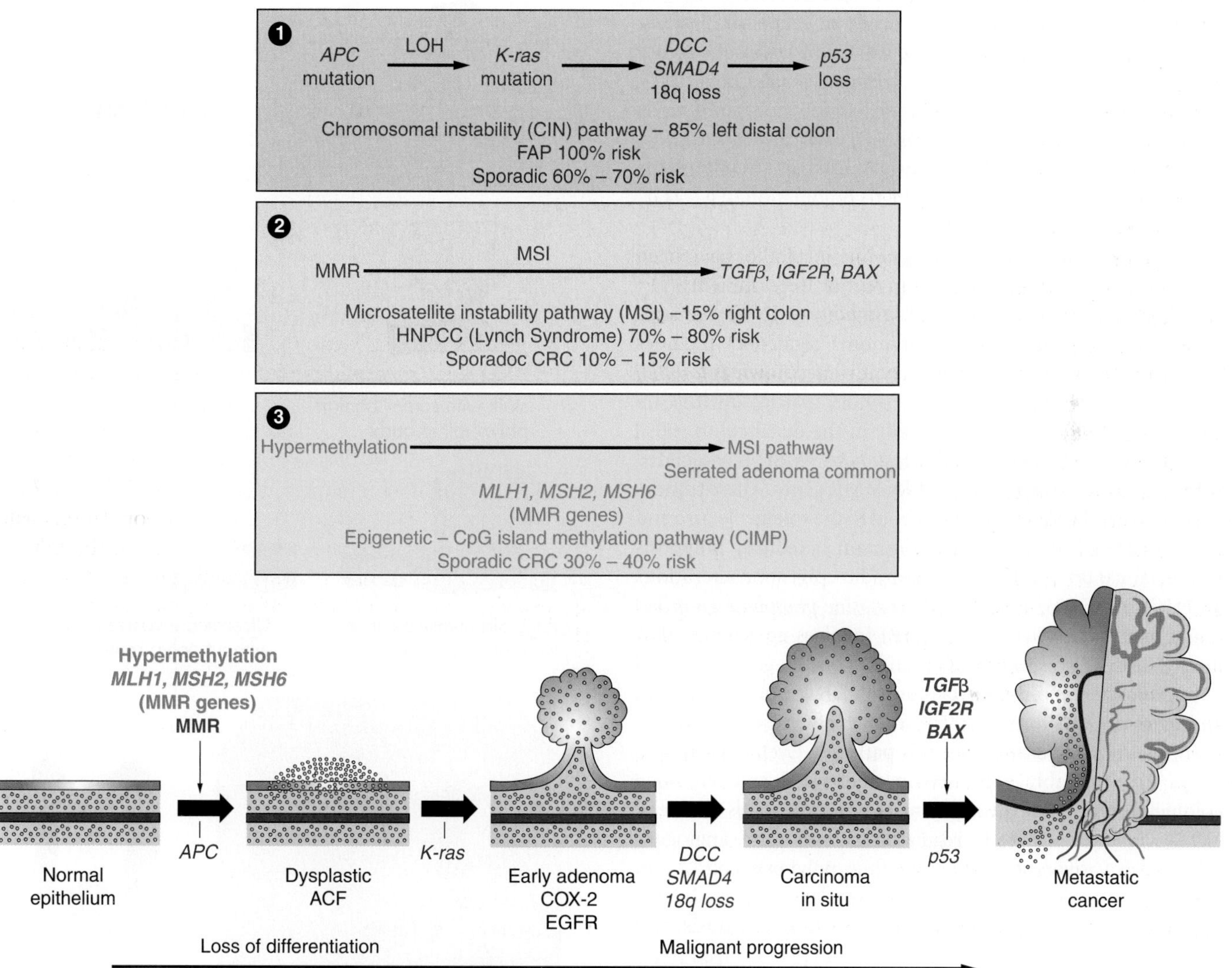

FIGURE 41-28 Multistage Development of Colonic Cancer. Colorectal carcinoma develops from the sequential progression of genetic abnormalities in different pathways. These pathways overlap in many tumors. **1,** Most CRC arises in the CIN pathway with imbalances in chromosomal numbers (aneuploidy) and loss of heterozygosity. Abnormalities in oncogenes and tumor-suppressor genes activate the pathways for CRC initiation and progression. Mutations in the *APC* gene are the earliest known event and inactivation of *APC* accelerates cell cycle progression. *K-ras* overexpression leads to loss of *p53* and transforms an adenoma into a metastatic carcinoma. *p53* loss occurs in ≈75% of colorectal carcinomas, but occurs infrequently in benign lesions. Growth factors COX-2 and EGFR promote tumor growth and angiogenesis in response to inflammatory cytokines and proto-oncogenes. **2,** The microsatellite instability *(MSI)* pathway involves the epigenetic mutation of DNA mismatch repair genes *(MMR)* that encode key molecules that repair DNA, resulting in replication errors and deactivation of proteins from other downstream mutations (*TGFβ, IGF2R, BAX*). **3,** The epigenetic pathway, CpG island methylator phenotype *(CIMP),* involves early hypermethylation of DNA with gene silencing of *MMR* genes that then transform into the MSI pathway. *ACF,* Aberrant crypt foci; *APC, APC* gene (a tumor-suppressor gene); *BAX,* Bcl-2-associated X protein (apoptosis-related protein); *CIN,* chromosomal instability; *COX-2,* cyclooxygenase-2; *CpG,* cytosine-phosphodiester bond-guanine DNA region; *CRC,* colorectal cancer; *DCC,* deleted in colorectal cancer (located at chromosome 18q); *EGFR,* epidermal growth factor receptor; *FAP,* familial adenomatous polyposis; *HNPCC,* hereditary nonpolyposis colorectal cancer; *IGF2R,* insulin growth factor type II receptor; *K-ras,* a proto-oncogene (promotes cell growth); *LOH,* loss of heterozygosity; *MLH1, MSH2, MSH6,* deoxyribonucleic acid (DNA) mismatch repair genes; *MMR,* mutation mismatch repair; *MSI,* microsatellite instability; *p53,* protein 53 or tumor protein 53 (a tumor-suppressor protein); *SMAD4,* a tumor-suppressor gene; *TGFβ,* transforming growth factor-beta.

[HNPCC or Lynch syndrome]). The remainder of inherited CRCs are related to less penetrant genes, and environmental interactions increase risk.[349] About 75% of CRC is sporadic (nonhereditary or acquired) and the environment contributes to multiple somatic mutations.

Most CRCs arise from epithelial tissue in the form of adenomatous polyps. Progression from polyps to colon cancer (adenocarcinoma) involves a multistep cascade of genetic mutations. The gene mutations include: (1) activation of proto-oncogenes (promote cell growth; e.g., *K*-ras [retrovirus-associated DNA sequence] and *BRAF*); (2) loss of tumor-suppressor gene activity (inhibit cell growth [e.g., *APC, TP53, TFTB* and *SMAD4, DCC*]); and (3) abnormalities in DNA mismatch repair (MMR) genes (fix errors in DNA replication and recombination, e.g., *TGF, EGFR, hMSH1, hMSH2, hMSH6*).

Three molecular subtypes of genomic instability have been recognized and they can overlap in tumor development[350-352] (see Figure 41-28). *Chromosomal instability* (CIN or the suppressor pathway or adenoma-carcinoma sequence) includes the autosomal dominant inherited syndrome known as *familial adenomatous polyposis (FAP)* coli. Tumors associated with CIN are primarily located on the left side in the distal colon (50% to 85% of tumors). *Microsatellite instability* (MSI) is associated with epigenetic methylation of DNA MMR genes. These tumors are located in the right colon proximal to the splenic flexure and are associated with autosomal dominant hereditary polyposis colorectal cancer (HNPCC) or sporadic epigenetic alterations in 15% to 20% of CRCs. *CpG (cytosine-phosphate-guanine) island methylator phenotype* (CIMP) involves epigenetic DNA methylation of promoter CpG islands silencing genes involved in tumor suppression, cell cycle control, DNA repair, apoptosis, and invasion. It is found in 35% to 40% of CRCs and serrated adenomas are associated with this pathway. Cyclooxygenase-2 (COX-2) is variably expressed in right-sided and left-sided colorectal cancer, but the mechanism of expression is not clear. COX-2 may participate in regulation of apoptosis, angiogenesis, and invasiveness of adenomatous polyposis coli[353] (see Figure 41-28). Understanding the molecular events associated with CRC is allowing more targeted detection, diagnosis, and prognosis prediction, and more specific and personalized treatment approaches.[354,355]

Most CRC develops from adenomatous polyps (Figure 41-29). A **polyp** is a mass or fingerlike projection arising from the intestinal mucosal epithelium. Most polyps are benign. Grossly, they are described as pedunculated (with a stalk) or sessile (flat, without a stalk). Histologically, they are classified as tubular with branched tubular glands (the most prevalent), villous with fingerlike projections of the epithelium (more related to CRC), or tubulovillous adenomas. Sessile serrated polyps have a serrated crypt and include hyperplastic polyps. They generally lack atypia but when they are large (greater than 1 cm), numerous (more than 20), and located in the right colon they are associated with cancer (Figure 41-30). The adenomatous polyp forms in an area of epithelial cell hyperproliferation and crypt dysplasia. Once the adenoma traverses the muscularis mucosae, it becomes invasive and highly malignant. Adenomas can be detected early, however, and the submucosa may not be penetrated for several years. The larger the polyp and the greater the degree of dysplasia, the greater the risk of CRC. Thus, screening colonoscopy with polypectomy is important when polyps are found. Table 41-9 gives other conditions commonly confused with colorectal cancer.

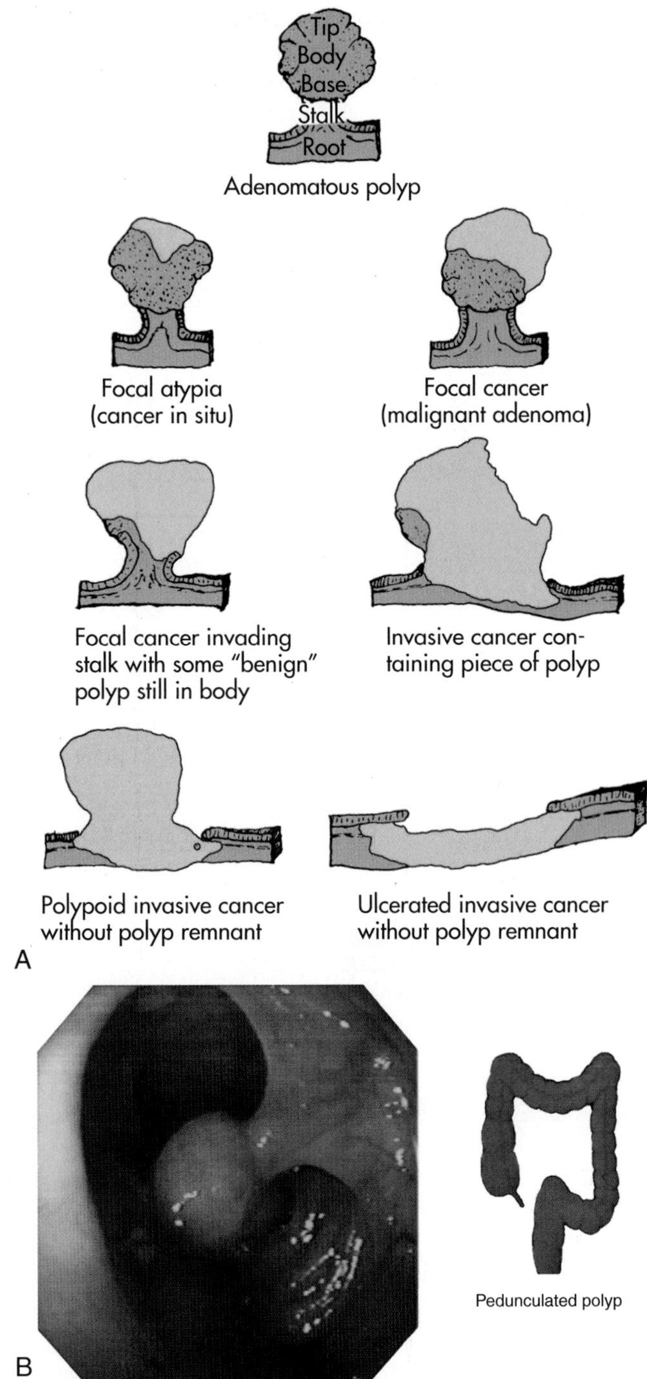

FIGURE 41-29 Development of Cancer of the Colon from Adenomatous Polyps. A, The tumor becomes invasive if it penetrates the muscularis mucosae and enters the submucosal layer. **B,** Endoscopic image of pedunculated polyp in descending colon. (**A** from del Regato JA, Spjut HJ, Cox JD: *Cancer: diagnosis, treatment, and prognosis,* ed 2, St Louis, 1985, Mosby. **B** courtesy David Bjorkman, MD, Department of Gastroenterology, University of Utah School of Medicine, Salt Lake City, UT.)

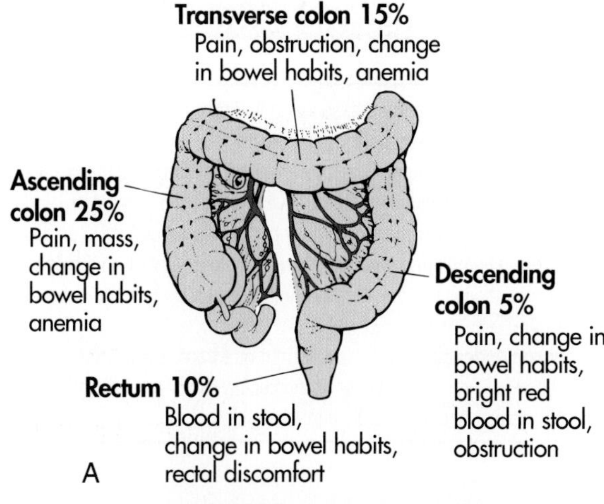

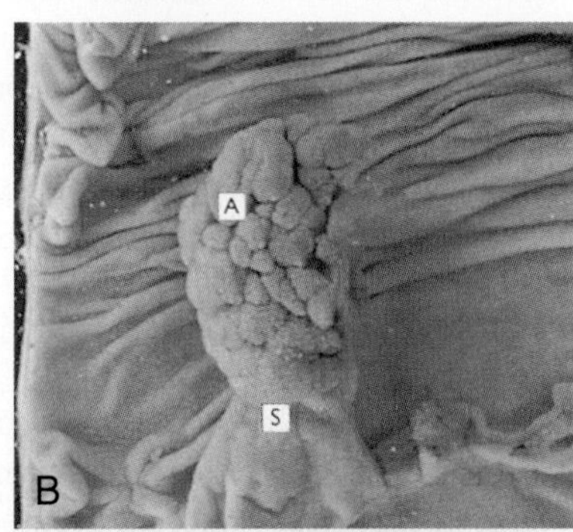

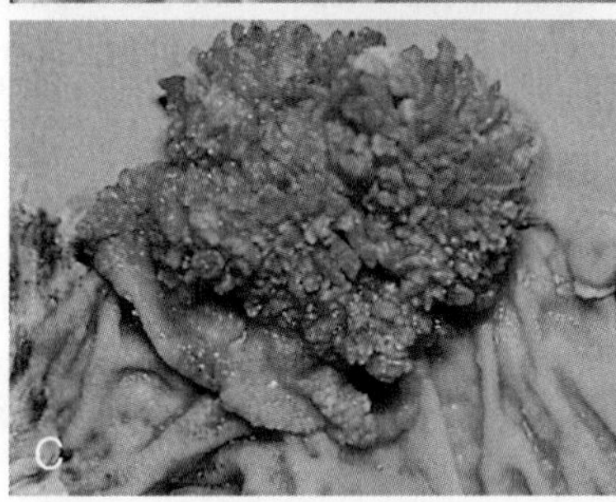

FIGURE 41-30 Signs and Symptoms of Colorectal Cancer by Location of Primary Lesion. **A,** Clinical manifestations are listed in order of frequency for each region (lymphatics of colon also shown). **B,** Tubular adenomas *(A)* are rounded lesions 0.5 to 2 cm in size that are generally red and sit on a stalk *(S)* of normal mucosa that has been dragged up by traction of the polyp in the bowel lumen. **C,** Villous adenomas are frondlike lesions about 0.6 cm thick that occupy a broad area of mucosa generally 1 to 5 cm in diameter. (**B** and **C** from Stevens A, Lowe JS, Scott I: *Core pathology,* ed 3, London, 2009, Mosby.)

Most colorectal cancers are moderately differentiated adenocarcinomas. These tumors have a long preinvasive phase, and when they invade they tend to grow slowly (10 to 15 years). Because the lymphatic channels are located underneath the muscularis mucosae, the lesions must traverse this layer before metastasis can occur. Systemic lymphatic spread occurs along the aorta to the mesenteric and pancreatic lymph nodes. Liver metastasis follows invasion of the mesenteric veins (left colon) or superior veins (right colon), which drain into the portal circulation.

Rectal carcinomas are defined as tumors occurring up to 15 cm from the anal opening. Tumors of the rectum can spread through the rectal wall to nearby structures: the prostate in men and the vagina in women. Penetration occurs more readily in the lower third of the rectum because it has no serosal covering. Systemic and pulmonary metastases occur through the hemorrhoidal plexus, which drains into the vena cava.

CLINICAL MANIFESTATIONS. Symptoms of colorectal cancer depend on the location, size, shape, and metastasis of the lesion. Tumors of the right (ascending) and left (descending) colon evolve into two distinct types. On the right side the lesions are polypoid and extend along one wall of the cecum and ascending colon. These tumors may be silent, evolving to pain, with a palpable mass in the lower right quadrant, anemia, fatigue, and dark red or mahogany-colored blood mixed with the stool (see Figure 41-30). These tumors can become large and bulky with necrosis and ulceration, contributing to persistent blood loss and anemia. Obstruction is unusual because the growth does not encircle the colon.

Tumors of the left, or descending, colon are small, elevated, button-like masses. This type grows circumferentially, encircling the entire bowel wall, and eventually ulcerating in the middle as the tumor penetrates the blood supply. Obstruction is common but occurs slowly and stools become narrow and pencil shaped. Manifestations include progressive abdominal distention, pain, vomiting, constipation, need for laxatives, cramps, and bright blood on the surface of the stool. In 8% to 29% of cases, bowel obstruction is the primary symptom at diagnosis.[356] Other symptoms can develop related to distant organ metastasis.

EVALUATION AND TREATMENT. Individuals with hereditary polyposis or a strong family history of CRC should begin screening at an early age (10 to 12 years) using colonoscopy and biopsy with a consideration of prophylactic surgery.[357] Fecal immunochemical testing (FIT) may be more accurate than stool occult blood testing.[358,359] Screening for nonhereditary CRC in asymptomatic individuals older than age 50 years includes fecal occult blood and immunochemical tests, stool DNA and sigmoidoscopy, colonoscopy, virtual colonoscopy, or double-contrast barium enema.[360,361]

The staging of colorectal cancer involves preoperative testing and operative exploration. Preoperative testing begins with physical examination of the abdomen to detect liver enlargement and ascites and palpation of appropriate lymph nodes. Elevations in the level of carcinoembryonic antigen (CEA) are often detected in the sera of individuals with colorectal carcinoma. The amount of CEA in the serum is a function of the stage of the disease and the type of tumor. Operative staging consists of careful exploration during surgery and biopsy of possible metastases. The National Cancer Institute[362] classification is widely used for staging of colorectal cancer and is as follows:

Stage 0 (carcinoma in situ): involves only the mucosal lining; also known as carcinoma in situ

Stage I: extension of cancer to the middle layers of the colon wall, no spread to lymph nodes; stage I colon cancer is sometimes called Dukes' A colon cancer

Stage II: extension beyond the colon wall to nearby tissues around the colon or *rectum,* and/or through the *peritoneum*; stage II colon cancer is sometimes called Dukes' B colon cancer

TABLE 41-9 CONDITIONS COMMONLY CONFUSED WITH COLORECTAL CANCER

CONDITION	SIGNIFICANT CHARACTERISTICS
Diverticulitis	Left-sided pain similar to that of appendicitis; tender lower left quadrant; associated findings: nausea, vomiting, fever, obstruction, anorexia, and leukocytosis; mucosa is intact, and perforation, peritonitis, and abscesses occur more often than in cancer; ultrasound, CT scan, MRI, and proctosigmoidoscopy are used to distinguish from cancer
Ulcerative colitis	Younger people with chronic attacks of bloody diarrhea, crampy abdominal pain, fever, malnutrition, and dehydration; usually involves the left colon and rectum; endoscopy, barium enema, and biopsy performed for definitive diagnosis
Crohn disease (granulomatous colitis)	Generally involves the right colon; chronic diarrhea with abdominal cramps, fever, weight loss, and often a palpable abdominal mass; difficult at times to distinguish Crohn disease from ulcerative colitis; endoscopic examination and CT scan used to distinguish from cancer
Appendicitis	Vague abdominal symptoms, often with a tender or nontender mass in the lower right quadrant; associated symptoms: mild fever and leukocytosis; CT scan used to distinguish cancer of the cecum from appendiceal abscess
Thrombosed hemorrhoids	Examination shows a tender, swollen, bluish painful mass in the anus; individual has a history of hemorrhoids

Stage III: spread beyond the colon into lymph nodes and nearby organs and/or through the *peritoneum;* stage III colon cancer is sometimes called Dukes' C colon cancer

Stage IV: spread to nearby *lymph nodes* and has spread to other parts of the body, such as the *liver* or *lungs;* stage IV colon cancer is sometimes called Dukes' D colon cancer

Treatment for cancer of the colon is always surgical. The location and amount of colon resected depend on the site of the cancer. Resection and anastomosis can be performed for early stage tumors and is usually curative. These surgeries are performed using laparoscopic techniques or through abdominal incisions, and natural defecation is preserved. Growths in the lower portion of the rectum require removal of the entire rectum with formation of a permanent colostomy. Prognosis after surgery depends on the stage and location of the tumor. TNM classifications are available from the National Cancer Institute.[363]

Radiation therapy is often given before surgery in the hope that it will shrink the tumor, alter the malignant cells, or both so that these cells will not survive after surgery. Adjuvant chemoradiotherapy is used to treat metastatic disease and cases with a high risk of recurrence. Monoclonal antibody therapy may be added.[364-366] Vaccines for colon cancer are in clinical trials.[367,368] Treatment of rectal cancer includes preoperative chemoradiotherapy, total mesorectal excision surgery, and adjuvant chemotherapy with fluorouracil.[369]

Anal carcinoma is rare (estimated 7060 cases and 880 deaths in 2013).[324] The most common tumor type is squamous cell carcinoma, about 80%; other anal cancers are adenocarcinoma, lymphoma, or sarcoma. The most common risk factor is infection with human papillomavirus (93%) and less commonly anal involvement in Crohn disease.[370] Squamous cell anal carcinoma is more common among the human immunodeficiency virus–infected population.[371]

Cancer of the Accessory Organs of Digestion

Cancer of the Liver

Hepatocellular carcinoma represented about 2% of new cancers (30,640) and 3.6% of cancer deaths (21,670) in 2013. The overall 5-year survival rate is 14%.[324] Blacks and Hispanics are almost twice as likely to develop these cancers as whites.[372] In the United States, the incidence of primary hepatocellular carcinoma is increasing as a result of chronic hepatitis C infection. Liver cancer is common in densely populated parts of Southeast Asia and sub-Saharan Africa where hepatitis B virus infection is endemic.[324] Primary liver cancer is rare before the age of 40 years and most common during the sixth decade. Cancer in the liver is usually caused by metastatic spread from a primary site elsewhere in the body.

Risk factors for primary liver cancer include the following[373-376]:

1. Infection with HBV, HCV, and HDV, particularly in conjunction with cirrhosis, acts either as a carcinogen or as a co-carcinogen in chronically infected hepatocytes[377]
2. Chronic alcoholic liver disease and nonalcoholic liver disease that results in cirrhosis
3. Exposure to mycotoxins; the most significant mycotoxins are the aflatoxins, particularly those produced by *Aspergillus flavus,* a mold found on spoiled corn, peanuts, and grain; aflatoxins cause mutation of the *TP53* suppressor gene and activation of WNT signal transduction pathway
4. Long duration of heavy smoking (greater than 20 years)
5. Nonalcoholic fatty liver disease
6. Hepatic iron overload

PATHOGENESIS. Primary carcinomas of the liver are hepatocellular or cholangiocellular. Hepatocellular carcinoma develops in the hepatocytes, whereas cholangiocellular carcinoma (cholangiocarcinoma) develops in the bile ducts. **Hepatocellular carcinoma (hepatocarcinoma) (HCC)** can be nodular (consisting of multiple, discrete nodules), massive (consisting of a large tumor mass having satellite nodules), or diffuse (consisting of very small nodules distributed throughout most of the liver). HCC is the type of primary liver cancer that is closely associated with cirrhosis (Figure 41-31). Chronic hepatitis B and hepatitis C and cirrhosis give rise to HCC repetitive cellular proliferation that occurs in the inflamed liver in response to growth factor and cytokine stimulation and oxidative stress–induced DNA damage. Numerous genetic and epigenetic alterations, including activation of oncogenes, failure of tumor-suppressor genes, and signaling pathways, combine to promote carcinogenesis.[378] Because carcinoma of the liver invades the hepatic and portal veins, it often spreads to the heart and lungs. Other sites of metastases are the brain, kidney, and spleen.

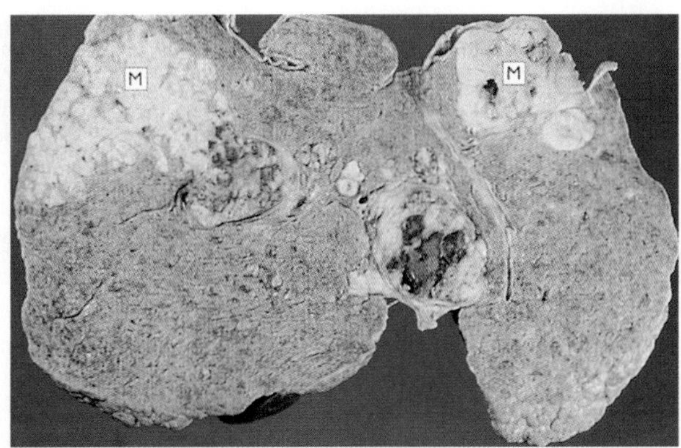

FIGURE 41-31 **Hepatocellular Carcinoma.** Macroscopically, hepatocellular carcinomas may be single or multifocal. They usually develop in a liver already affected by cirrhosis. Tumor appears as an abnormal mass *(M)* within the liver. (From Stevens A, Lowe JS, Scott I: *Core pathology,* ed 3, London, 2009, Mosby.)

Cholangiocellular carcinomas (cholangiocarcinoma) occur less often than hepatocellular carcinomas in the United States and represent about 10% to 25% of hepatobiliary malignancies. The disease predominates in men. Incidence demonstrates geographic variation and is common in Southeast Asia where liver fluke infestation is prevalent. The mechanism by which fluke infestation causes cholangiocellular carcinoma is multifactorial and includes parasite secretions, immunopathology, and mechanical damage. Other risk factors include primary sclerosing cholangitis, hepatolithiasis, and choledochal cysts.[379] Intrahepatic cholangiocellular carcinoma also is associated with cirrhosis, HBV and HCV infection, obesity, and diabetes. However, most individuals diagnosed with cholangiocellular carcinoma do not have an identifiable risk factor except age.[380,381] Cholangiocellular carcinoma can occur anywhere along the bile duct, both within and outside the liver, and usually is a solitary lesion. It is difficult to distinguish an invasion of cholangiocellular carcinoma from a metastatic adenocarcinoma except by neoplastic changes found in nearby ducts.

CLINICAL MANIFESTATIONS. The clinical presentation of liver cancer in adults is characterized by vague abdominal symptoms, such as nausea and vomiting, fullness, pressure, dull ache in the right hypochondrium, and weight loss. Manifestations of hepatocellular carcinoma can occur slowly or abruptly. In individuals with cirrhosis, deepening jaundice or abrupt lack of appetite is a sign of hepatocellular carcinoma. Obstruction by the tumor can cause sudden worsening of portal hypertension and development of ascites. As the tumor enlarges, it causes pain. Cholangiocellular carcinoma more commonly presents insidiously as pain, loss of appetite, weight loss, and gradual onset of jaundice. Some carcinomas of the liver rupture spontaneously, causing hemorrhage. Others are discovered accidentally during evaluation of a bone fracture or surgical exploration.

EVALUATION AND TREATMENT. There is no specific test for the diagnosis of liver cancer. For HCC high-risk individuals, alpha fetoprotein and abdominal ultrasound are common screening tools and can be used for screening in individuals with cirrhosis.[382] Additional serum markers are being evaluated.[383] The diagnosis is based on additional laboratory findings, radiologic examination, biopsy findings, and exploratory laparotomy. Serum levels of alkaline phosphatase, aspartate aminotransferase (AST), and alanine aminotransferase (ALT) are commonly elevated in individuals with HCC.

Staging of HCC is important to guiding treatment but does not accurately predict postoperative outcome. Surgical resection is possible with solitary tumors and the absence of portal hypertension.[384] Radiofrequency (thermal) ablation has emerged as the most effective method for local tumor destruction. Tyrosine kinase inhibitors (e.g., sorafenib) and monoclonal antibodies are improving survival; many new therapies are in clinical trials.[385] Transarterial embolization and radiation is used for management of pain and to reduce tumor size.[384] Surgical resection or liver transplantation is the only alternative for cure; however, very early stage HCC is difficult to diagnose.[382] Primary prevention of HCC is vaccination against HBV and antiviral therapy for HCV.[386]

Cholangiocarcinoma causes duct obstruction, and radiotherapy, chemotherapy, photodynamic therapy, and stenting can temporarily relieve the blockage for unresectable disease.[387-390]

Cancer of the Gallbladder

Cancer of the gallbladder and biliary tract is a rare but lethal disease. An estimated 10,310 new cases and 3230 deaths were recorded in 2013.[324] It rarely occurs before age 40 and is most common between the ages of 50 and 60 years. Risk factors include gallstones, advancing age, female gender (2:1), anomalous pancreaticobiliary ductal junction, and obesity. Native populations in North and South America have greater risk of gallbladder cancer, and it is more common in Chile, Poland, India, Japan, and Israel.[391-394] Most cancerous tumors in the gallbladder are caused by metastasis.

PATHOGENESIS. Most primary cancers of the gallbladder are adenocarcinomas and, less commonly, squamous cell carcinomas. The mechanisms of tumorigenesis are not clear. Multiple genes and oncogenes are involved in the initiation and progression of gallbladder cancer. Research is in progress to target these genes for diagnosis and treatment.[395] Infiltrative tumors are associated with gallstones, and invasion of the liver and lymph nodes occurs early. Spreading extends to the pancreas and retroperitoneal lymph nodes. Direct invasion of the stomach and the duodenum can cause pyloric obstruction. Infection often accompanies cancer of the gallbladder. Generalized peritonitis, gangrene, perforation, and liver abscesses are potential complications of infection.

CLINICAL MANIFESTATIONS. Early stages of gallbladder carcinoma are asymptomatic. A typical presentation is steady upper right quadrant pain for about 2 months. Other symptoms mimic benign gallbladder disease, including diarrhea, belching, weakness, loss of appetite, weight loss, and vomiting. Obstructive jaundice can occur if an enlarging tumor presses on the extrahepatic ducts.

EVALUATION AND TREATMENT. Early diagnosis of gallbladder cancer is rare and the disease is often found incidentally when removing gallstones or when an individual presents with an advanced stage of disease.[396] Individuals with gallstones, especially older women, are evaluated carefully. Inflammatory disorders, such as cholangitis (bile duct inflammation) and peritonitis, often obscure an underlying malignancy. The most specific diagnostic procedures include ultrasonography, CT, and MRI.

Complete surgical resection of the gallbladder is the only effective treatment. Because advanced malignancies cannot be resected, gallbladders containing stones are removed as a preventive measure. Palliative chemotherapy or chemoradiation provides symptom improvement but does not improve survival.[397] The prognosis of gallbladder cancer is extremely poor; most individuals die within 1 to 2 years after surgery.[398,399]

Cancer of the Pancreas

Pancreatic cancer represents about 2.6% of all new cancers. There are 45,220 new cases and 38,460 deaths estimated for 2013.[324] The incidence of pancreatic cancer rises steadily with age. Men are affected slightly more often than women and blacks more often than whites.[324] Mortality is about 95% within 12 months. Risk factors include cigarette smoking, heavy alcohol use, family history of pancreatic cancer, and non-O blood group.[400] Chronic pancreatitis is associated with about 4% to 5% of pancreatic cancers.[401,402]

PATHOGENESIS. Cancer of the pancreas can arise from exocrine or endocrine cells. Most pancreatic tumors arise from exocrine cells in the ducts and are called *ductal adenocarcinomas.* Tumors arising in small ducts invade nearby glandular tissue, penetrate the covering of the pancreas, and extend into surrounding tissues.[403] Pancreatic cancer is a disease of inherited and acquired mutations in cancer-related genes associated with chronic inflammation.[403a] A *K-ras* mutation is the most common genetic alteration; tumor-suppressor gene alterations are also found, including *TP53, CDKN2A, SMAD4, BRCA2,* and *PALB2.*[404] Growth factors are overexpressed in ductal cancer.[405,406]

Ductal adenocarcinomas are the most common tumor and can occur in the head, body, or tail of the pancreas. Tumors of the head quickly spread to obstruct the common bile duct and portal vein (Figure 41-32). These tumors can then infiltrate the superior mesenteric artery, the vena cava, and the aorta. Cancer cells that enter the blood vessels can form emboli. Tumors of the body and tail infiltrate the posterior abdominal wall. Lymphatic invasion occurs early and rapidly and involves local and regional lymph nodes. Venous invasion causes metastases to the liver. Tumor implants on the peritoneal surface can obstruct veins and promote development of ascites.

Ductal adenocarcinomas arising in the head of the pancreas cause biliary obstruction somewhat early in the disease. Individuals with such tumors survive slightly longer than those with cancer of the body and tail, presumably because they seek medical attention earlier.

Tumors of the endocrine pancreas are rare neoplasms of the islets of Langerhans known as *apudomas.* The first four letters in *apudoma* derive from *amine precursor uptake* and *decarboxylation.* The apudomas are so named because they contain neurosecretory granules. Endocrine neoplasms secrete abnormal amounts of hormones, such as insulin.

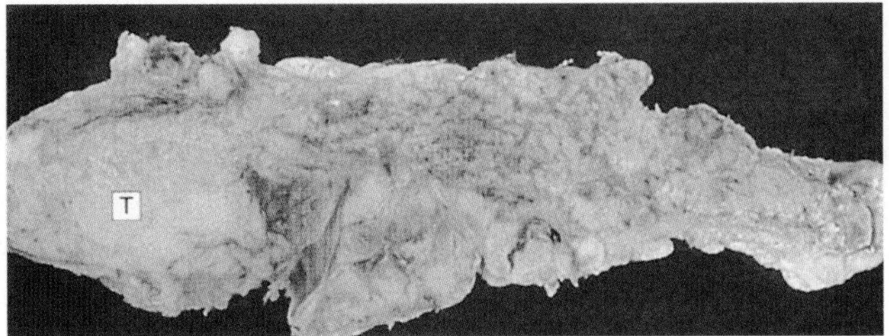

FIGURE 41-32 Pancreatic Carcinoma. Tumors appear as gritty, gray, hard nodules *(T)* irregularly invading the adjacent gland and local structures. (From Stevens A, Lowe JS, Scott I: *Core pathology,* ed 3, London, 2009, Mosby.)

CLINICAL MANIFESTATIONS. Cancer of the body and tail of the pancreas is generally asymptomatic until there is intraductal obstruction or the tumor invades adjacent tissue. Often vague, abdominal or mid-back pain is an initial symptom.[407] Jaundice develops in most cases, usually caused by obstruction of the bile duct. Because obstruction impairs enzyme secretion and flow to the duodenum, pancreatic cancer causes fat and protein malabsorption, resulting in weight loss. Some individuals develop diabetes mellitus. Distant metastases are found in the cervical lymph nodes, the lungs, and the brain. Most individuals die of hepatic failure, malnutrition, or systemic complications.

EVALUATION AND TREATMENT. Pancreatic cancer is usually diagnosed at an advanced stage and has a poor prognosis. The most effective screening method for those at risk is endoscopic ultrasound because it detects small lesions; the search for biomarkers is continuing.[408] *Autoimmune pancreatitis* is a rare, fibroinflammatory disorder of the pancreas that mimics and must be differentiated from pancreatic cancer.[409] Contrast CT scans, contrast MRI, and abdominal and endoscopic ultrasound (EUS) are used for initial diagnosis. EUS also provides opportunity for biopsy, or CT-guided fine needle aspiration can confirm diagnosis although this is not necessary when cancer suspicion is high.[410] Laparotomy is used to establish a definitive diagnosis, evaluate the extent of disease, and determine whether palliative bypass surgery (i.e., cholecystojejunostomy and gastrojejunostomy) is needed.

Individuals with small tumors and complete resection have the best possibility of cure (15% to 20% of cases). Pancreaticoduodenectomy (Whipple procedure) is the most common procedure and portal or superior mesenteric vein resection and reconstruction may be performed. Some surgeons recommend a total pancreatectomy because cancer of the pancreas seldom consists of a single lesion.[411] The dense stromal structure of the tumor impairs chemotherapeutic drug delivery, resulting in poor response to chemotherapy.[412] Adjuvant chemotherapy is used for curative attempts in resected low-grade tumors. Chemoradiation therapy is used for advanced disease in some centers. Treatments with molecular targets are in clinical trials.[413-415] Palliative care, including pain management and nutrition, are important.[416]

SUMMARY REVIEW

Disorders of the Gastrointestinal Tract

1. Anorexia (loss of appetite), vomiting, constipation, diarrhea, abdominal pain, and evidence of gastrointestinal bleeding are clinical manifestations of many disorders of the gastrointestinal tract.
2. Vomiting is the forceful emptying of the stomach effected by gastrointestinal contraction and reverse peristalsis of the esophagus. It is usually preceded by nausea and retching with the exception of projectile vomiting, which is associated with direct stimulation of the vomiting center in the brain.
3. Primary constipation is defined in three categories: functional, associated with low-residue, low-fluid diet; slow-transit, related to impaired colonic motor function; and pelvic floor dyssynergia-anismus. Secondary constipation results from a neurogenic disease, drugs that decrease intestinal motility, endocrine or metabolic disorders, or obstruction.
4. Diarrhea can be caused by excessive fluid drawn into the intestinal lumen by osmosis (osmotic diarrhea), excessive secretion of fluids by the intestinal mucosa (secretory diarrhea), or excessive gastrointestinal motility.
5. Abdominal pain is caused by stretching, inflammation, or ischemia and originates in the peritoneum (parietal pain) or in the organs themselves (visceral pain). Visceral pain is often referred to the back.
6. Gastrointestinal bleeding can occur in the upper or lower gastrointestinal tract. Obvious manifestations of gastrointestinal bleeding are hematemesis (vomiting of blood), melena (dark, tarry stools), and hematochezia (frank bleeding from the rectum). Occult bleeding can be detected only by testing stools or vomitus for the presence of blood.
7. Dysphagia is difficulty in swallowing. It can be caused by a mechanical or functional obstruction of the esophagus. Functional obstruction is an impairment of esophageal motility.
8. Achalasia is a form of functional dysphagia caused by loss of esophageal innervation or relaxation of the lower esophageal sphincter.
9. Gastroesophageal reflux disease is the regurgitation of chyme from the stomach into the esophagus, causing esophagitis from repeated exposure to acids and enzymes in the regurgitated gastric contents.
10. Hiatal hernia is the protrusion of the upper part of the stomach through the hiatus (esophageal opening in the diaphragm) at the gastroesophageal junction. Hiatal hernia can be sliding, paraesophageal, or mixed.
11. Pyloric obstruction is the narrowing or blockage of the pylorus, which is the opening between the stomach and the duodenum. It can be caused by a congenital defect, inflammation and scarring secondary to a gastric ulcer, or tumor growth.
12. Intestinal obstruction prevents the normal movement of chyme through the intestinal tract. It is usually mechanical—that is, caused by torsion, herniation, or tumor. Functional obstruction is caused by paralytic ileus.
13. The most severe consequences of intestinal obstruction are fluid and electrolyte losses, hypovolemia, shock, intestinal necrosis, and perforation of the intestinal wall.
14. Gastritis is an acute or a chronic inflammation of the gastric mucosa.
15. Regurgitation of bile, use of anti-inflammatory drugs or alcohol, *H. pylori* infection, and some systemic diseases are associated with gastritis.
16. Chronic fundal gastritis is rare and associated with autoantibodies to parietal cells and intrinsic factor, resulting in gastric atrophy and causing pernicious anemia.
17. Chronic antral gastritis is the most common and is associated with *H. pylori* and NSAIDs.
18. Alkaline reflux gastritis is stomach inflammation caused by the reflux of bile and pancreatic secretions from the duodenum into the stomach. These substances disrupt the mucosal barrier and cause inflammation.
19. A peptic ulcer is a circumscribed area of mucosal inflammation and ulceration caused by excessive secretion of gastric acid, disruption of the protective mucosal barrier, or both.
20. The three types of peptic ulcers are duodenal, gastric, and stress ulcers and they are usually caused by *H. pylori* infection or NSAIDs.
21. Duodenal ulcers, the most common peptic ulcers, are associated with increased numbers of parietal (acid-secreting) cells in the stomach, elevated gastrin levels, and rapid gastric emptying. Pain occurs when the stomach is empty, and pain is relieved with food or antacids. Duodenal ulcers tend to heal spontaneously and recur frequently.
22. Gastric ulcers develop near parietal cells, generally in the antrum, and tend to become chronic. Gastric secretions may be normal or decreased, and pain may occur after eating.
23. Zollinger-Ellison syndrome is associated with a gastrinoma, chronic secretion of gastric acid, and gastric and duodenal ulcers.
24. Stress ulcer (stress-related mucosal disease) is an acute form of peptic ulcer associated with severe illness or extensive trauma.
25. Ischemic stress ulcers develop suddenly after severe illness, systemic trauma, neural injury, or burns (Curling ulcer). Ulceration follows mucosal damage caused by ischemia (decreased blood flow to the gastric mucosa).
26. Cushing ulcer is a stress ulcer caused by head trauma. Ulceration follows hypersecretion of hydrochloric acid caused by overstimulation of the vagal nuclei.
27. Malabsorption syndromes result in impaired digestion or absorption of nutrients.
28. Pancreatic insufficiency causes malabsorption associated with insufficient amounts of the enzymes that digest protein, carbohydrates, and fats into components that can be absorbed by the intestine.
29. Deficient lactase production in the brush border of the small intestine inhibits the breakdown of lactose. This prevents lactose absorption and causes osmotic diarrhea.
30. Bile salt deficiency causes fat malabsorption, including fat-soluble vitamins, and steatorrhea (fatty stools). Bile salt deficiency can result from inadequate secretion of bile, excessive bacterial deconjugation of bile, or impaired reabsorption of bile salts caused by ileal disease.

SUMMARY REVIEW—cont'd

31. Dumping syndrome causes malabsorption by the rapid emptying of hypertonic chyme from the surgically created residual stomach into the small intestine. It causes an osmotic shift of fluid from the vascular compartment to the intestinal lumen, which decreases plasma volume.
32. Ulcerative colitis is an inflammatory bowel disease that causes ulceration, abscess formation, and necrosis of the colonic and rectal mucosa. Cramping pain, bleeding, frequent diarrhea, dehydration, and weight loss accompany severe forms of the disease. A course of frequent remissions and exacerbations is common.
33. Crohn disease is similar to ulcerative colitis, but it affects the large and small intestines, and ulceration tends to involve all the layers of the lumen. "Skip lesion" fissures and granulomas are characteristic of Crohn disease. Abdominal tenderness, nonbloody diarrhea, and weight loss are the usual symptoms.
34. Diverticula are outpouchings of colonic mucosa through the muscle layers of the colon wall. Diverticulosis is the presence of these outpouchings; diverticulitis is inflammation of the diverticula.
35. Appendicitis is the most common surgical emergency of the abdomen. Obstruction of the lumen leads to increased pressure, ischemia, and inflammation of the appendix. Without surgical resection, inflammation may progress to gangrene, perforation, and peritonitis.
36. Vascular insufficiency in the intestine is associated most often with acute or chronic occlusion or obstruction of the mesenteric vessels or insufficient mesenteric arterial blood flow. The resulting ischemia and necrosis produce abdominal pain, fever, bloody diarrhea, hypovolemia, and shock.
37. Obesity is defined as a BMI greater than 30 kg/m^2 and usually results from energy intake exceeding expenditure.
38. Single-gene and polygenetic disorders are associated with obesity, as well as social, cultural, economic, exercise, and metabolic factors.
39. Increases in body fat mass are associated with macrophage infiltration of adipocytes with release of inflammatory mediators, increased adipocyte lipolysis, increased leptin (leptin resistance) and RBP4 levels, and decreased adiponectin level. Insulin resistance may develop. Increased levels of ghrelin and endocannabinoids and decreased levels of PYY and GLP1 are associated with obesity. Alterations in the expression of these hormones and neurotransmitters affect appetite and metabolic rate at the level of the hypothalamus.
40. The eating disorders include anorexia nervosa, bulimia nervosa, and binge eating disorder. They are psychogenic disorders that can lead to malnutrition. Anorexia nervosa is the most serious and can be fatal.
41. Short-term starvation, or lack of dietary intake for 3 or 4 days, stimulates mobilization of stored glucose by two metabolic processes: glycogenolysis (splitting of glycogen into glucose) and gluconeogenesis (formation of glucose from noncarbohydrate molecules).
42. Long-term starvation triggers the breakdown of ketone bodies and fatty acids. Eventually proteolysis (protein breakdown) begins, and death ensues if nutrition is not restored.

Disorders of the Accessory Organs of Digestion

1. Portal hypertension, ascites, hepatic encephalopathy, jaundice, and hepatorenal syndrome are complications of many liver disorders.
2. Portal hypertension is an elevation of portal venous pressure to at least 10 mmHg. It is caused by increased resistance to venous flow in the portal vein and its tributaries, including the sinusoids and hepatic vein.
3. Portal hypertension is the most serious complication of liver disease because it can cause fatal complications, such as bleeding varices, ascites, hepatic encephalopathy, and renal failure.
4. Varices are distended, tortuous, collateral veins associated with portal hypertension.
5. Splenomegaly is an enlargement of the spleen resulting from increased splenic vein pressure caused by portal hypertension.
6. Hepatopulmonary syndrome is pulmonary hypertension related to the release of vasodilators that effect pulmonary arterioles and is associated with portal hypertension and severe liver disease.
7. Ascites is the accumulation and sequestration of fluid in the peritoneal cavity, often as a result of portal hypertension, decreased concentrations of plasma proteins, and sodium retention.
8. Hepatic encephalopathy (portosystemic encephalopathy) is impaired cerebral function caused by blood-borne toxins (particularly ammonia) not metabolized by the liver.
9. Jaundice (icterus) is a yellow or greenish pigmentation of the skin or sclera of the eyes caused by increases in plasma bilirubin concentration (hyperbilirubinemia).
10. Obstructive jaundice is caused by obstructed bile canaliculi (intrahepatic obstructive jaundice) or obstructed bile ducts outside the liver (extrahepatic obstructive jaundice). Bilirubin accumulates proximal to sites of obstruction, enters the bloodstream, and is deposited in the skin and other connective tissues.
11. Hemolytic jaundice is caused by destruction of red blood cells at a rate that exceeds the liver's ability to metabolize unconjugated bilirubin.
12. Hepatorenal syndrome is functional renal failure caused by advanced liver disease, particularly cirrhosis with portal hypertension. Renal failure is caused by a sudden decrease in blood flow to the kidneys, usually as a result of massive gastrointestinal hemorrhage or liver failure. Its chief clinical manifestation is oliguria.
13. Autoimmune hepatitis is T cell mediated with hypergammaglobulinemia and absence of viral hepatitis.
14. Viral hepatitis is an infection of the liver caused by strains of the hepatitis virus: HAV, HBV, HCV, HDV, and HEV. HAV and HEV are transmitted via the fecal-oral route. The hepatitis viruses are blood-borne and can cause hepatic cell necrosis, Kupffer cell hyperplasia, and infiltration of liver tissue by mononuclear phagocytes. These changes obstruct bile flow and impair hepatocyte function.

SUMMARY REVIEW—cont'd

15. The clinical manifestations of viral hepatitis depend on the stage of infection. Fever, malaise, anorexia, and liver enlargement and tenderness characterize the prodromal phase (stage 1). Jaundice and hyperbilirubinemia mark the icteric phase (stage 2). During the recovery phase (stage 3), symptoms resolve. Recovery takes several weeks.
16. Chronic active hepatitis can occur with HBV and HCV with predisposition to cirrhosis and hepatocellular carcinoma.
17. Fulminant hepatitis is a complication of hepatitis B (with or without hepatitis D infection) or hepatitis C. It causes widespread hepatic necrosis and is often fatal.
18. Cirrhosis is an irreversible inflammatory disease of the liver that causes disorganization of lobular structure, fibrosis, and nodular regeneration. Bile obstruction causes jaundice. Vascular obstruction causes portal hypertension, shunting, and varices. Cirrhosis can result from hepatitis or exposure to toxins, such as acetaldehyde (a product of alcohol metabolism). The disease causes progressive irreversible liver damage, usually over a period of years.
19. Alcoholic liver disease impairs the hepatocytes' ability to oxidize fatty acids, synthesize enzymes and proteins, degrade hormones, and clear portal blood of ammonia and toxins. The disease is progressive and includes steatosis, steatohepatitis, and alcoholic cirrhosis.
20. Nonalcoholic fatty liver disease is fat infiltration of hepatocytes associated with obesity.
21. Primary biliary cirrhosis is an autoimmune disease with inflammatory destruction of intrahepatic bile ducts. Mitochondrial autoantibodies are found in this disease.
22. Secondary biliary cirrhosis develops from prolonged obstruction of bile flow (e.g., gallstones) with increased pressure in the hepatic bile ducts that causes pooling of bile and necrosis of tissue. Relief of obstruction alleviates symptoms of jaundice and pruritus. Continued obstruction causes cirrhosis and liver failure.
23. Primary sclerosing cholangitis is a fibrotic disease of medium and large sized bile ducts outside the liver.
24. Cholelithiasis (the formation of gallstones) is a result of bile aggregation of cholesterol crystals (cholesterol stones) or precipitates of unconjugated bilirubin (pigmented stones). Gallstones that fill the gallbladder or obstruct the cystic, or common, bile duct cause abdominal pain and jaundice.
25. Cholecystitis is an inflammation of the gallbladder. It is usually associated with obstruction of the cystic duct by gallstones.
26. Acute pancreatitis (pancreatic inflammation) is a serious but relatively rare disorder associated with biliary obstruction and alcoholism. Injury permits leakage of digestive enzymes into pancreatic tissue, where they become activated and begin the process of autodigestion, inflammation, and destruction of tissues. Release of pancreatic enzymes into the bloodstream or abdominal cavity causes damage to other organs.
27. Chronic pancreatitis results from structural or functional impairment of the pancreas usually related to alcoholism or recurrent acute pancreatitis. It causes recurrent abdominal pain and digestive disorders.

Cancer of the Digestive System

1. Cancer of the esophagus is rare and tends to occur in people older than 60 years. Alcohol and tobacco use, reflux esophagitis, radiation exposure, and nutritional deficiencies are associated with esophageal carcinoma.
2. Dysphagia and chest pain are the primary manifestations of esophageal cancer. Early treatment of tumors that have not spread into the mediastinum or lymph nodes results in a good prognosis.
3. Gastric carcinoma is associated with *H. pylori (CagA)*, high salt intake, food preservatives (nitrates and nitrites), and atrophic gastritis.
4. Approximately 50% of all gastric cancers are located in the prepyloric antrum. Clinical manifestations (weight loss, upper abdominal pain, vomiting, hematemesis, anemia) develop only after the tumor has penetrated the wall of the stomach.
5. Cancer of the colon and rectum (colorectal cancer) is the second most common type of cancer death in the United States. Small intestinal cancers are rare. Familial adenomatous polyposis coli is an inherited form of colon cancer. Preexisting large and numerous polyps are highly associated with sporadic adenocarcinoma of the colon.
6. Tumors of the right (ascending) colon are usually large and bulky; tumors of the left (descending, sigmoid) colon develop as small button-like masses. Manifestations of colon tumors include pain, bloody stools, and change in bowel habits.
7. Rectal carcinoma is located up to 15 cm from the opening of the anus. The tumor spreads transmurally to the vagina in women or to the prostate in men.
8. Metastatic invasion of the liver is more common than primary cancer of the liver.
9. Primary liver cancers are associated with chronic liver disease (cirrhosis and hepatitides B and C). Hepatocellular carcinomas arise from the hepatocytes, whereas cholangiocellular carcinomas arise from the bile ducts. Primary liver cancer spreads to the heart, lungs, brain, kidney, and spleen through the circulation.
10. Cancer of the gallbladder is relatively rare and tends to occur in women older than 50 years. Adenocarcinoma is most common. Because clinical manifestations occur late in the disease, metastases to lymph channels have usually occurred by the time of diagnosis, and the prognosis is poor.
11. Cancer of the pancreas ranks fifth as a cause of cancer deaths. The one known risk factor is heavy cigarette smoking. Most tumors are adenocarcinomas that arise in the exocrine cells of ducts in the head, body, or tail of the pancreas. Symptoms may not be evident until the tumor has spread to surrounding tissues. Treatment is palliative, and mortality is nearly 100%.

KEY TERMS

Achalasia, 1428
Acute colonic pseudo-obstruction, 1432
Acute gastritis, 1434
Acute liver failure (fulminant liver failure), 1451
Acute mesenteric ischemia, 1446
Acute pancreatitis, 1464
Adiponectin, 1448
Alcoholic cirrhosis, 1460
Alcoholic fatty liver (steatosis), 1460
Alcoholic hepatitis (steatohepatitis), 1460
Alkaline reflux gastritis, 1435
Anal carcinoma, 1472
Anorexia, 1423
Appendicitis, 1445
Ascites, 1453
Barrett esophagus, 1466
Biliary cirrhosis, 1462
Cachexia, 1451
Cholangiocellular carcinoma (cholangiocarcinoma), 1473
Cholecystitis, 1464
Cholelithiasis, 1463
Chronic active hepatitis, 1459
Chronic gastritis, 1434
Chronic mesenteric ischemia, 1446
Chronic pancreatitis, 1466
Cirrhosis, 1460
Constipation, 1424
Crohn disease (CD), 1442
Curling ulcer, 1439
Cushing ulcer, 1439
Diarrhea, 1425
Diverticula (*sing.*, diverticulum), 1444
Diverticulitis, 1444
Diverticulosis, 1444
Dumping syndrome, 1440
Duodenal ulcer, 1435
Dysphagia, 1428
Endocannabinoid, 1449
Eosinophilic esophagitis, 1429
Esophageal varices, 1453
Esophagitis, 1429
Gallstone, 1463
Gastric ulcer, 1437
Gastritis, 1434
Gastroesophageal reflux disease (GERD), 1429
Ghrelin, 1449
Gluconeogenesis, 1451
Glucose-like peptide 1, 1449
Glycogenolysis, 1451
Hematemesis, 1428
Hematochezia, 1428
Hemolytic jaundice (prehepatic jaundice, nonobstructive jaundice), 1456
Hepatic encephalopathy, 1454
Hepatocellular carcinoma (hepatocarcinoma; HCC), 1472
Hepatopulmonary syndrome, 1453
Hepatorenal syndrome (HRS), 1456
Hiatal hernia, 1429
Hyperbilirubinemia, 1455
Icteric phase (jaundice), 1459
Incubation phase, 1459
Insulin resistance, 1448
Intestinal obstruction, 1431
Irritable bowel syndrome (IBS), 1445
Ischemic ulcer, 1439
Jaundice (icterus), 1455
Kwashiorkor, 1451
Lactase deficiency, 1439
Large bowel obstruction, 1432
Leptin, 1448
Leptin resistance, 1448
Long-term starvation, 1451
Lower gastrointestinal (GI) bleeding, 1426
Malabsorption, 1439
Maldigestion, 1439
Malnutrition, 1450
Marasmus, 1451
Melena, 1428
Mesenteric venous thrombosis, 1446
Microscopic colitis, 1440
Motility diarrhea, 1426
Mucosa-associated lymphoid tissue (MALT) lymphoma, 1467
Nausea, 1424
Nonalcoholic fatty liver disease (NAFLD), 1461
Nonalcoholic steatohepatitis (NASH), 1461
Obesity, 1446
Obstructive jaundice, 1455
Occult bleeding, 1427
Osmotic diarrhea, 1425
Pancreatic insufficiency, 1439
Pancreatitis, 1464
Paraesophageal hiatal hernia, 1430
Paralytic ileus, 1431
Parietal pain, 1426
Peptic ulcer, 1435
Peptide YY (PYY), 1449
Peripheral obesity, 1450
Polyp, 1470
Portal hypertension, 1452
Portopulmonary hypertension, 1453
Primary biliary cirrhosis, 1462
Prodromal (preicteric) phase, 1459
Projectile vomiting, 1424
Pyloric obstruction (gastric outlet obstruction), 1430
Recovery phase, 1459
Rectal carcinoma, 1471
Refeeding syndrome, 1451
Referred pain, 1426
Retching, 1424
Secondary biliary cirrhosis, 1463
Secretory diarrhea, 1425
Short bowel syndrome, 1444
Short-term starvation, 1451
Sliding hiatal hernia, 1429
Small intestine carcinoma, 1468
Small intestine obstruction, 1431
Splenomegaly, 1452
Starvation, 1450
Stress ulcer (stress-related mucosal disease), 1439
Ulcerative colitis (UC), 1440
Upper gastrointestinal (GI) bleeding, 1426
Varices, 1452
Viral hepatitis, 1457
Visceral obesity, 1450
Visceral pain, 1426
Vomiting, 1424
Zollinger-Ellison syndrome, 1438

REFERENCES

1. Feyer P, Jordan K: Update and new trends in antiemetic therapy: the continuing need for novel therapies, *Ann Oncol* 22(1):30–38, 2011.
2. Becker DE: Nausea, vomiting, and hiccups: a review of mechanisms and treatment, *Anesth Prog* 57(4):150–156, 2010.
3. Andrews CN, Storr M: The pathophysiology of chronic constipation, *Can J Gastroenterol* 25(Suppl B):16B–21B, 2011.
4. Grassi M et al: Changes, functional disorders, and diseases in the gastrointestinal tract of elderly, *Nutr Hosp* 26(4):659–668, 2011.
5. Lacy BE, Levenick JM, Crowell M: Chronic constipation: new diagnostic and treatment approaches, *Therap Adv Gastroenterol* 5(4):233–247, 2012.
6. Rao SS: Biofeedback therapy for constipation in adults, *Best Pract Res Clin Gastroenterol* 25(1):159–166, 2011.
7. Tack J: Current and future therapies for chronic constipation, *Best Pract Res Clin Gastroenterol* 25(1):151–158, 2011.
8. World Health Organization: *Diarrhoea*. Available at www.who.int/topics/diarrhoea/en/. Accessed March 15, 2013.
9. Corinaldesi R et al: Clinical approach to diarrhea, *Intern Emerg Med* 7(Suppl 3):S255–S262, 2012.
10. Camilleri M, Nullens S, Nelsen T: Enteroendocrine and neuronal mechanisms in pathophysiology of acute infectious diarrhea, *Dig Dis Sci* 57(1):19–27, 2012.
11. Sandle GI: Infective and inflammatory diarrhoea: mechanisms and opportunities for novel therapies, *Curr Opin Pharmacol* 11(6):634–639, 2011.
12. Juckett G, Trivedi R: Evaluation of chronic diarrhea, *Am Fam Physician* 84(10):1119–1126, 2011.
13. Bradley C et al: Probiotics for the prevention of *Clostridium difficile*–associated diarrhea: a systematic review and meta-analysis, *Ann Intern Med* 157(12):878–888, 2012.
14. Kassam Z et al: Fecal microbiota transplantation for *Clostridium difficile* infection: systematic review and meta-analysis, *Am J Gastroenterol* 108(4):500–508, 2013.
15. Makharia GK: Understanding and treating abdominal pain and spasms in organic gastrointestinal diseases: inflammatory bowel disease and biliary diseases, *J Clin Gastroenterol* 45(Suppl):S89–S93, 2011.
16. Vergnolle N: Postinflammatory visceral sensitivity and pain mechanisms, *Neurogastroenterol Motil* 20(Suppl 1):73–80, 2008.
17. DiMaio CJ, Stevens PD: Nonvariceal upper gastrointestinal bleeding, *Gastrointest Endosc Clin North Am* 17(2):253–272, 2007.
18. Edelman DA, Sugawa C: Lower gastrointestinal bleeding: a review, *Surg Endosc* 21(4):514–520, 2007.
19. Laine L, Jensen DM: Management of patients with ulcer bleeding, *Am J Gastroenterol* 107:345, 2012.
20. Raju GS et al: American Gastroenterological Association (AGA) Institute medical position statement on obscure gastrointestinal bleeding, *Gastroenterology* 133:1694, 2007.
21. Srygley FD et al: Does this patient have a severe upper gastrointestinal bleed? *J Am Med Assoc* 307:1072, 2012.
22. Cook IJ: Diagnostic evaluation of dysphagia, *Nat Clin Pract Gastroenterol Hepatol* 5(7):393–403, 2008.

23. Chuah SK et al: 2011 update on esophageal achalasia, *World J Gastroenterol* 18(14):1573–1578, 2012.
24. Stavropoulos SN, Modayil R, Friedel D: Achalasia, *Gastrointest Endosc Clin N Am* 23(1):53–75, 2013.
25. Kuo P, Holloway RH, Nguyen NQ: Current and future techniques in the evaluation of dysphagia, *J Gastroenterol Hepatol* 27(5):873–881, 2012.
26. Stegemann S, Gosch M, Breitkreutz J: Swallowing dysfunction and dysphagia is an unrecognized challenge for oral drug therapy, *Int J Pharm* 430(1-2):197–206, 2012.
27. Foley N et al: Dysphagia treatment poststroke: a systematic review of randomised controlled trials, *Age Ageing* 37(3):258–264, 2008.
28. Cecconi E, Di Piero V: Dysphagia—pathophysiology, diagnosis and treatment, *Front Neurol Neurosci* 30:86–89, 2012.
29. Richter JE: Gastrooesophageal reflux disease, *Best Pract Res Clin Gastroenterol* 21(4):609–631, 2007.
30. Saritas Yuksel E, Vaezi MF: Extraesophageal manifestations of gastroesophageal reflux disease: cough, asthma, laryngitis, chest pain, *Swiss Med Wkly* 142:w13544, 2012.
31. Zerbib F et al: Functional heartburn: definition and management strategies, *Curr Gastroenterol Rep* 14(3):181–188, 2012.
32. Herbella FA, Patti MG: Gastroesophageal reflux disease: from pathophysiology to treatment, *World J Gastroenterol* 16(30):3745–3749, 2010.
33. Tytgat GN: Recent developments in gastroesophageal reflux disease and Barrett's esophagus: ANNO, 2012, *J Dig Dis* 13(6):291–295, 2012.
34. Poehlmann A et al: Inflammation and Barrett's carcinogenesis, *Pathol Res Pract* 208(5):269–280, 2012.
35. Haggitt RC: Histopathology of reflux-induced esophageal and supraesophageal injuries, *Am J Med* 108(Suppl 4a):109S, 2000.
36. Fass R: Therapeutic options for refractory gastroesophageal reflux disease, *J Gastroenterol Hepatol* 27(Suppl 3):3–7, 2012.
37. Bredenoord AJ, Pandolfino JE, Smout AJ: Gastro-oesophageal reflux diseases, *Lancet* 381(9881):1933–1942, 2013.
38. Redd M, Schey R: Eosinophilic esophagitis: current treatment, *Dig Dis Sci* 58(3):613–620, 2013.
39. Weber C et al: Hiatal hernias: a review of the pathophysiologic theories and implication for research, *Surg Endosc* 25(10):3149–3153, 2011.
40. Hyun JJ, Bak YT: Clinical significance of hiatal hernia, *Gut Liver* 5(3):267–277, 2011.
41. Boushey RP et al: Laparoscopic repair of paraesophageal hernias: a Canadian experience, *Can J Surg* 51(5):355–360, 2008.
42. Khanna A, Finch G: Paraoesophageal herniation: a review, *Surgeon* 9(2):104–111, 2011.
43. Appasani S et al: Benign gastric outlet obstruction—spectrum and management, *Trop Gastroenterol* 32(4):259–266, 2011.
44. Alonso-Lárraga JO et al: Self-expanding metal stents versus antrectomy for the palliative treatment of obstructive adenocarcinoma of the gastric antrum, *Rev Esp Enferm Dig* 104(4):185–189, 2012.
45. Attard JA, MacLean AR: Adhesive small bowel obstruction: epidemiology, biology and prevention, *Can J Surg* 50(4):291–300, 2007.
46. Wehner S et al: Immune mediators of postoperative ileus, *Langenbecks Arch Surg* 397(4):591–601, 2012.
47. Scott FI et al: Secular trends in small-bowel obstruction and adhesiolysis in the United States: 1988-2007, *Am J Surg* 204(3):315–320, 2012.
48. Masselli G, Gualdi G: MR imaging of the small bowel, *Radiology* 264(2):333–348, 2012.
49. De Giorgio R, Knowles CH: Acute colonic pseudo-obstruction, *Br J Surg* 96(3):229–239, 2009.
50. Takeuchi K: Pathogenesis of NSAID-induced gastric damage: importance of cyclooxygenase inhibition and gastric hypermotility, *World J Gastroenterol* 18(18):2147–2160, 2012.
51. Malfertheiner P: The intriguing relationship of *Helicobacter pylori* infection and acid secretion in peptic ulcer disease and gastric cancer, *Dig Dis* 29(5):459–464, 2011.
52. Toh BH et al: Cutting edge issues in autoimmune gastritis, *Clin Rev Allergy Immunol* 42(3):269–278, 2012.
53. Smolka AJ, Backert S: How *Helicobacter pylori* infection controls gastric acid secretion, *J Gastroenterol* 47(6):609–618, 2012.
54. di Mario F, Cavallaro LG: Non-invasive tests in gastric diseases, *Dig Liver Dis* 40(7):523–530, 2008.
55. Nagini S: Carcinoma of the stomach: a review of epidemiology, pathogenesis, molecular genetics and chemoprevention, *World J Gastrointest Oncol* 4(7):156–169, 2012.
56. Malfertheiner P, Selgrad M, Bornschein J: *Helicobacter pylori:* clinical management, *Curr Opin Gastroenterol* 28(6):608–614, 2012.
57. Erkurt MA et al: Effects of cyanocobalamin on immunity in patients with pernicious anemia, *Med Princ Pract* 17(2):131–135, 2008.
58. Zobolas B et al: Alkaline reflux gastritis: early and late results of surgery, *World J Surg* 30(6):1043–1049, 2006.
59. Sobieraj DM, Coleman SM, Coleman CI: US prevalence of upper gastrointestinal symptoms: a systematic literature review, *Am J Manag Care* 17(11):e449–e458, 2011.
60. Lee KM et al: Association between acute pancreatitis and peptic ulcer disease, *World J Gastroenterol* 17(8):1058–1062, 2011.
61. Yeomans ND: The ulcer sleuths: the search for the cause of peptic ulcers, *J Gastroenterol Hepatol* 26(Suppl 1):35–41, 2011.
62. Fink G: Stress controversies: post-traumatic stress disorder, hippocampal volume, gastroduodenal ulceration, *J Neuroendocrinol* 23(2):107–117, 2011.
63. Fuller-Thomson E et al: Is childhood physical abuse associated with peptic ulcer disease? Findings from a population-based study, *J Interpers Violence* 26(16):3225–3247, 2011.
64. Musumba C et al: The relative contribution of NSAIDs and *Helicobacter pylori* to the aetiology of endoscopically-diagnosed peptic ulcer disease: observations from a tertiary referral hospital in the UK between 2005 and 2010, *Aliment Pharmacol Ther* 36(1):48–56, 2012.
65. Gisbert JP, Calvet X: Review article: *Helicobacter pylori*-negative duodenal ulcer disease, *Aliment Pharmacol Ther* 30(8):791–815, 2009.
66. Ubukata H et al: Why is the coexistence of gastric cancer and duodenal ulcer rare? Examination of factors related to both gastric cancer and duodenal ulcer, *Gastric Cancer* 14(1):4–12, 2011.
67. Hirschi AM, Makristathis A: Methods to detect *Helicobacter pylori*: from culture to molecular biology, *Helicobacter* 12(Suppl 2):6–11, 2007.
67a. Tarnawski A, Ahluwalia A, Jones MK: Gastric cytoprotection beyond prostaglandins: cellular and molecular mechanisms of gastroprotective and ulcer healing actions of antacids, *Curr Pharm Des* 19(1):126–132, 2013.
68. Khan A et al: Antibiotic resistance and *cagA* gene correlation: a looming crisis of *Helicobacter pylori*, *World J Gastroenterol* 18(18):2245–2252, 2012.
69. Georgopoulos SD, Papastergiou V, Karatapanis S: Current options for the treatment of *Helicobacter pylori*, *Expert Opin Pharmacother* 14(2):211–223, 2013.
70. Milosavljevic T et al: Complications of peptic ulcer disease, *Dig Dis* 29(5):491–493, 2011.
71. Ryan-Harshman M, Aldoori W: How diet and lifestyle affect duodenal ulcers. Review of the evidence, *Can Fam Physician* 50:727–732, 2004.
72. Czinn SJ, Blanchard T: Vaccinating against *Helicobacter pylori* infection, *Nat Rev Gastroenterol Hepatol* 8(3):133–140, 2011.
73. Holle GE: Pathophysiology and modern treatment of ulcer disease, *Int J Mol Med* 25(4):483–491, 2010.
74. Rehfeld JF et al: The Zollinger-Ellison syndrome and mismeasurement of gastrin, *Gastroenterol* 140(5):1444–1453, 2011.
75. Wilcox CM et al: Zollinger-Ellison syndrome: presentation, response to therapy, and outcome, *Dig Liver Dis* 43(6):439–443, 2011.
76. Gross AK, Norman J, Cook AM: Contemporary pharmacologic issues in the management of traumatic brain injury, *J Pharm Pract* 23(5): 425–440, 2010.
77. Barkun AN et al: Proton pump inhibitors vs. histamine 2 receptor antagonists for stress-related mucosal bleeding prophylaxis in critically ill patients: a meta-analysis, *Am J Gastroenterol* 107(4):507–520, 2012.
78. Pilkington KB, Wagstaff MJ, Greenwood JE: Prevention of gastrointestinal bleeding due to stress ulceration: a review of current literature, *Anaesth Intensive Care* 40(2):253–259, 2012.
79. Holster IL, Kuipers EJ: Management of acute nonvariceal upper gastrointestinal bleeding: current policies and future perspectives, *World J Gastroenterol* 18(11):1202–1207, 2012.
80. Aga H et al: Fall in peptic ulcer mortality associated with increased consultant input, prompt surgery and use of high dependency care identified through peer-review audit, *BMJ Open* 2(1):e000271, 2012.
81. Bolton JS, Conway WC II: Postgastrectomy syndromes, *Surg Clin North Am* 91(15):1105–1122, 2011.
82. Nakajima K et al: Pancrelipase: an evidence-based review of its use for treating pancreatic exocrine insufficiency, *Core Evid* 7:77–91, 2012.
83. Järvelä I, Torniainen S, Kolho KL: Molecular genetics of human lactase deficiencies, *Ann Med* 41(8):568–575, 2009.
84. Pohl D et al: Excellent agreement between genetic and hydrogen breath tests for lactase deficiency and the role of extended symptom assessment, *Br J Nutr* 104(6):900–907, 2010.
85. Norlin M, Wikvall K: Enzymes in the conversion of cholesterol into bile acids, *Curr Mol Med* 7(2):199–218, 2007.
86. Johnston I et al: New insights into bile acid malabsorption, *Curr Gastroenterol Rep* 13(5):418–425, 2011.
87. Hammer HF: Medical complications of bariatric surgery: focus on malabsorption and dumping syndrome, *Dig Dis* 30(2):182–186, 2012.

88. Rogers C: Postgastrectomy nutrition, *Nutr Clin Pract* 26(2):126–136, 2011.
89. Didden P, Penning C, Masclee AA: Octreotide therapy in dumping syndrome: analysis of long-term results, *Aliment Pharmacol Ther* 24(9):1367–1375, 2006.
90. Molodecky NA et al: Increasing incidence and prevalence of the inflammatory bowel diseases with time, based on systematic review, *Gastroenterol* 142(1):46–54, 2012.
91. Vermeire S, Van Assche G, Rutgeerts P: Classification of inflammatory bowel disease: the old and the new, *Curr Opin Gastroenterol* 28(4):321–326, 2012.
92. Bastida G, Beltrán B: Ulcerative colitis in smokers, non-smokers and ex-smokers, *World J Gastroenterol* 17(22):2740–2747, 2011.
93. Packey CD, Sartor RB: Interplay of commensal and pathogenic bacteria, genetic mutations, and immunoregulatory defects in the pathogenesis of inflammatory bowel diseases, *J Intern Med* 263(6):597–606, 2008.
94. Zhong W et al: Chemokines orchestrate leukocyte trafficking in inflammatory bowel disease, *Front Biosci* 13:1654–1664, 2008.
95. Hering NA, Fromm M, Schulzke JD: Determinants of colonic barrier function in inflammatory bowel disease and potential therapeutics, *J Physiol* 590(Pt 5):1035–1044, 2012.
96. Ordás I et al: Ulcerative colitis, *Lancet* 380(9853):1606–1619, 2012.
97. Ekmektzoglou KA et al: Genomic instability in ulcerative colitis: a prerequisite for cancer in the inflammatory colon? *Acta Gastroenterol Belg* 75(3):293–299, 2012.
98. Veloso FT: Extraintestinal manifestations of inflammatory bowel disease: do they influence treatment and outcome? *World J Gastroenterol* 17(22):2702–2707, 2011.
99. Scaldaferri F et al: Haemostatic system in inflammatory bowel diseases: new players in gut inflammation, *World J Gastroenterol* 17(5):594–608, 2011.
100. Vucelic B: Inflammatory bowel diseases: controversies in the use of diagnostic procedures, *Dig Dis* 27(3):269–277, 2009.
101. Sandborn WJ: The future of inflammatory bowel disease therapy: where do we go from here? *Dig Dis* 30(Suppl 3):140–144, 2012.
102. Di Sabatino A et al: Recent advances in understanding ulcerative colitis, *Intern Emerg Med* 7(2):103–111, 2012.
103. Khan KJ et al: Antibiotic therapy in inflammatory bowel disease: a systematic review and meta-analysis, *Am J Gastroenterol* 106(4):661–673, 2011.
104. Lakhan SE, Kirchgessner A: Anti-inflammatory effects of nicotine in obesity and ulcerative colitis, *J Transl Med* 9:129, 2011.
105. Biondi A et al: Surgical treatment of ulcerative colitis in the biologic therapy era, *World J Gastroenterol* 18(16):1861–1870, 2012.
106. Shen B: Acute and chronic pouchitis—pathogenesis, diagnosis and treatment, *Nat Rev Gastroenterol Hepatol* 9(6):323–333, 2012.
107. Hovde Ø, Moum BA: Epidemiology and clinical course of Crohn's disease: results from observational studies, *World J Gastroenterol* 18(15):1723–1731, 2012.
108. Tsianos EV, Katsanos KH, Tsianos VE: Role of genetics in the diagnosis and prognosis of Crohn's disease, *World J Gastroenterol* 17(48):5246–5259, 2011.
109. Keita AV, Söderholm JD: Barrier dysfunction and bacterial uptake in the follicle-associated epithelium of ileal Crohn's disease, *Ann N Y Acad Sci* 1258:125–134, 2012.
110. Harmsen HJ et al: Crohn's disease patients have more IgG-binding fecal bacteria than controls, *Clin Vaccine Immunol* 19(4):515–521, 2012.
111. Lewis RT, Maron DJ: Anorectal Crohn's disease, *Surg Clin North Am* 90(1):83–97, 2010.
112. Schmidt C et al: Surveillance strategies in inflammatory bowel disease, *Minerva Gastroenterol Dietol* 56(2):189–201, 2010.
113. Cheifetz AS: Management of active Crohn disease, *JAMA* 309(20):2150–2158, 2013.
114. Kosmidis C, Anthimidis G: Emergency and elective surgery for small bowel Crohn's disease, *Tech Coloproctol* 15(Suppl 1):S1–S4, 2011.
115. Uchino M et al: Risk factors for short bowel syndrome in patients with Crohn's disease, *Surg Today* 42(5):447–452, 2012.
116. Böttner M, Wedel T: Abnormalities of neuromuscular anatomy in diverticular disease, *Dig Dis* 30(1):19–23, 2012.
117. Ferreira-Aparicio FE et al: Diverticular disease of the small bowel, *Case Rep Gastroenterol* 6(3):668–676, 2012.
118. Chuang SC et al: The intake of grain fibers modulates cytokine levels in blood, *Biomarkers* 16(6):504–510, 2011.
119. Yen CH et al: Long-term supplementation of isomalto-oligosaccharides improved colonic microflora profile, bowel function, and blood cholesterol levels in constipated elderly people—a placebo-controlled, diet-controlled trial, *Nutrition* 27(4):445–450, 2011.
120. Wilkins T, Embry K, George R: Diagnosis and management of acute diverticulitis, *Am Fam Physician* (9)612–620, 2013.
121. Weizman AV, Nguyen GC: Diverticular disease: epidemiology and management, *Can J Gastroenterol* 25(7):385–389, 2011.
122. Psarras K et al: Current management of diverticular disease complications, *Tech Coloproctol* 15(Suppl 1):S9–S12, 2011.
123. Cole MA, Maldonado N: Evidence-based management of suspected appendicitis in the emergency department, *Emerg Med Pract* 13(10):1–29, 2011.
124. Chan L et al: Pathologic continuum of acute appendicitis: sonographic findings and clinical management implications, *Ultrasound Q* 27(2):71–79, 2011.
125. Yu CW et al: Systematic review and meta-analysis of the diagnostic accuracy of procalcitonin, C-reactive protein and white blood cell count for suspected acute appendicitis, *Br J Surg* 100(3):322–329, 2013.
126. Hennelly KE, Bachur R: Appendicitis update, *Curr Opin Pediatr* 23(3):281–285, 2011.
127. Dhupar R et al: Outcomes of operative management of appendicitis, *Surg Infect (Larchmt)* 13(3):141–146, 2012.
128. Liu K, Fogg L: Use of antibiotics alone for treatment of uncomplicated acute appendicitis: a systematic review and meta-analysis, *Surgery* 150(4):673–683, 2011.
129. Choung RS, Locke GR III: Epidemiology of IBS, *Gastroenterol Clin North Am* 40(1):1–10, 2011.
130. Zhou Q, Verne GN: New insights into visceral hypersensitivity—clinical implications in IBS, *Nat Rev Gastroenterol Hepatol* 8(6):349–355, 2011.
131. Gecse K et al: Leaky gut in patients with diarrhea-predominant irritable bowel syndrome and inactive ulcerative colitis, *Digestion* 85(1):40–46, 2012.
132. Ghoshal UC, Ranjan P: Post-infectious irritable bowel syndrome: the past, the present and the future, *J Gastroenterol Hepatol* 26(Suppl 3):94–101, 2011.
133. Furnari M et al: Reassessment of the role of methane production between irritable bowel syndrome and functional constipation, *J Gastrointestin Liver Dis* 21(2):157–163, 2012.
134. Spiegel BM: Questioning the bacterial overgrowth hypothesis of irritable bowel syndrome: an epidemiologic and evolutionary perspective, *Clin Gastroenterol Hepatol* 9(6):461–469, 2011.
135. Eswaran S, Tack J, Chey WD: Food: the forgotten factor in the irritable bowel syndrome, *Gastroenterol Clin North Am* 40(1):141–162, 2011.
136. Surdea-Blaga T, Băban A, Dumitrascu DL: Psychosocial determinants of irritable bowel syndrome, *World J Gastroenterol* 18(7):616–626, 2012.
137. Magge S, Lembo A: Complementary and alternative medicine for the irritable bowel syndrome, *Gastroenterol Clin North Am* 40(1):245–253, 2011.
138. Suares NC, Ford AC: Diagnosis and treatment of irritable bowel syndrome, *Discov Med* 11(60):425–433, 2011.
139. Klar E et al: Acute mesenteric ischemia: a vascular emergency, *Dtsch Arztebl Int* 109(14):249–256, 2012.
140. Stamatakos M et al: Mesenteric ischemia: still a deadly puzzle for the medical community, *Tohoku J Exp Med* 216(3):197–204, 2008.
141. White CJ: Chronic mesenteric ischemia: diagnosis and management, *Prog Cardiovasc Dis* 54(1):36–40, 2011.
142. Pecoraro F et al: Chronic mesenteric ischemia: critical review and guidelines for management, *Ann Vasc Surg* 27(1):113–122, 2013.
143. Holterman MJ, Le Holterman AX, Browne AF: Pediatric obesity, *Surg Clin North Am* 92(3):559–582, viii, 2012.
144. Thompson AL: Developmental origins of obesity: early feeding environments, infant growth, and the intestinal microbiome, *Am J Hum Biol* 24(3):350–360, 2012.
145. National Heart, Lung, and Blood Institute, National Institutes of Health: *Clinical guidelines on the identification, evaluation, and treatment of overweight and obesity in adults—executive summary*, 1998. Available at www.nhlbi.nih.gov/guidelines/obesity/sum_intr.htm.
146. Thorpe KE, Philyaw M: The medicalization of chronic disease and costs, *Annu Rev Public Health* 33:409–423, 2012.
147. Feneberg A, Malfertheiner P: Epidemic trends of obesity with impact on metabolism and digestive diseases, *Dig Dis* 30(2):143–147, 2012.
148. Chang SH et al: A systematic review of body fat distribution and mortality in older people, *Maturitas* 72(3):175–191, 2012.
149. Donini LM et al: A systematic review of the literature concerning the relationship between obesity and mortality in the elderly, *J Nutr Health Aging* 16(1):89–98, 2012.
150. Herrera BM, Keildson S, Lindgren CM: Genetics and epigenetics of obesity, *Maturitas* 69(1):41–49, 2011.

151. Cheung WW, Mao P: Recent advances in obesity: genetics and beyond, *ISRN Endocrinol* 2012:536905, 2012.
152. Ali MM, Amialchuk A, Rizzo JA: The influence of body weight on social network ties among adolescents, *Econ Hum Biol* 10(1):20–34, 2012.
153. Karasu SR: Of mind and matter: psychological dimensions in obesity, *Am J Psychother* 66(2):111–128, 2012.
154. Blüher M: Clinical relevance of adipokines, *Diabetes Metab J* 36(5):317–327, 2012.
155. Harwood HJ Jr: The adipocyte as an endocrine organ in the regulation of metabolic homeostasis, *Neuropharmacol* 63(1):57–75, 2012.
156. Yu JH, Kim MS: Molecular mechanisms of appetite regulation, *Diabetes Metab J* 36(6):391–398, 2012.
157. Myers MG Jr et al: Challenges and opportunities of defining clinical leptin resistance, *Cell Metab* 15(2):150–156, 2012.
158. Coppari R, Björbæk C: Leptin revisited: its mechanism of action and potential for treating diabetes, *Nat Rev Drug Discov* 11(9):692–708, 2012.
159. Hou N, Luo JD: Leptin and cardiovascular diseases, *Clin Exp Pharmacol Physiol* 38(12):905–913, 2011.
160. Wauman J, Tavernier J: Leptin receptor signaling: pathways to leptin resistance, *Front Biosci* 16:2771–2793, 2011.
161. Shehzad A et al: Adiponectin: regulation of its production and its role in human diseases, *Hormones (Athens)* 11(1):8–20, 2012.
162. Stears A et al: Metabolic insights from extreme human insulin resistance phenotypes, *Best Pract Res Clin Endocrinol Metab* 26(2):145–157, 2012.
163. Vaiopoulos AG et al: The role of adiponectin in human vascular physiology, *Int J Cardiol* 155(2):188–193, 2012.
164. Rabe K et al: Adipokines and insulin resistance, *Mol Med* 14(11-12): 741–751, 2008.
165. Kotnik P et al: RBP4: a controversial adipokine, *Eur J Endocrinol* 165(5):703–711, 2011.
166. Perello M et al: Functional implications of limited leptin receptor and ghrelin receptor coexpression in the brain, *J Comp Neurol* 520(2): 281–294, 2012.
167. McKenney RL, Short DK: Tipping the balance: the pathophysiology of obesity and type 2 diabetes mellitus, *Surg Clin North Am* 91(6): 1139–1148, vii, 2011.
168. Deacon CF, Ahrén B: Physiology of incretins in health and disease, *Rev Diabet Stud* 8(3):293–306, 2011.
169. Karra E, Chandarana K, Batterham RL: The role of peptide YY in appetite regulation and obesity, *J Physiol* 587(Pt 1):19–25, 2009.
170. Quarta C et al: Energy balance regulation by endocannabinoids at central and peripheral levels, *Trends Mol Med* 17(9):518–526, 2011.
171. Ibrahim MM: Subcutaneous and visceral adipose tissue: structural and functional differences, *Obes Rev* 11(1):11–18, 2010.
172. de Heredia FP, Gómez-Martínez S, Marcos A: Obesity, inflammation and the immune system, *Proc Nutr Soc* 71(2):332–338, 2012.
173. Tchernof A, Després JP: Pathophysiology of human visceral obesity: an update, *Physiol Rev* 93(1):359–404, 2013.
174. Shuster A et al: The clinical importance of visceral adiposity: a critical review of methods for visceral adipose tissue analysis, *Br J Radiol* 85(1009):1–10, 2012.
175. Sweeting HN: Measurement and definitions of obesity in childhood and adolescence: a field guide for the uninitiated, *Nutr J* 6:32, 2007.
176. Thibault R, Pichard C: The evaluation of body composition: a useful tool for clinical practice, *Ann Nutr Metab* 60(1):6–16, 2012.
177. Pi-Sunyer FX: Obesity: criteria and classification, *Proc Nutr Soc* 59(4):505–509, 2000.
178. Xiao J, Yang W: Weight loss is still an essential intervention in obesity and its complications: a review, *J Obes* 2012:369097, 2012.
179. Jacob JJ, Isaac R: Behavioral therapy for management of obesity, *Indian J Endocrinol Metab* 16(1):28–32, 2012.
180. Kim GW et al: Regulation of appetite to treat obesity, *Exp Rev Clin Pharmacol* 4(2):243–259, 2011.
181. Nguyen N et al: A review of unmet needs in obesity management, *Obes Surg* 22(6):956–966, 2012.
182. Rodgers RJ, Tschöp MH, Wilding JP: Anti-obesity drugs: past, present and future, *Dis Model Mech* 5(5):621–626, 2012.
183. Noria SF, Grantcharov T: Biological effects of bariatric surgery on obesity-related comorbidities, *Can J Surg* 56(1):47–57, 2013.
184. Smink FR, van Hoeken D, Hoek HW: Epidemiology of eating disorders: incidence, prevalence and mortality rates, *Curr Psychiatry Rep* 14(4):406–414, 2012.
185. Lapid MI et al: Eating disorders in the elderly, *Int Psychogeriatr* 22(4):523–536, 2010.
186. Helder SG, Collier DA: The genetics of eating disorders, *Curr Top Behav Neurosci* 6:157–175, 2011.
187. Pjetri E et al: Epigenetics and eating disorders, *Curr Opin Clin Nutr Metab Care* 15(4):330–335, 2012.
188. Dubosc A et al: Early adult sexual assault and disordered eating: the mediating role of posttraumatic stress symptoms, *J Trauma Stress* 25(1):50–56, 2012.
189. Fischer S, Stojek M, Hartzell E: Effects of multiple forms of childhood abuse and adult sexual assault on current eating disorder symptoms, *Eat Behav* 11(3):190–192, 2010.
190. Reyes-Rodríguez ML et al: Posttraumatic stress disorder in anorexia nervosa, *Psychosom Med* 73(6):491–497, 2011.
191. Smink FR, van Hoeken D, Hoek HW: Epidemiology of eating disorders: incidence, prevalence and mortality rates, *Curr Psychiatry Rep*(4): 406–414, 2012.
192. Jensen GL, Wheeler D: A new approach to defining and diagnosing malnutrition in adult critical illness, *Curr Opin Crit Care* 18(2):206–211, 2012.
193. Finn PF, Dice JF: Proteolytic and lipolytic responses to starvation, *Nutrition* 22(7-8):830–844, 2006.
194. Tierney EP, Sage RJ, Shwayder T: Kwashiorkor from a severe dietary restriction in an 8-month infant in suburban Detroit, Michigan: case report and review of the literature, *Int J Dermatol* 49(5):500–506, 2010.
195. Kim HJ et al: Pathophysiological role of hormones and cytokines in cancer cachexia, *J Korean Med Sci* 27(2):128–134, 2012.
196. Berkley JA et al: Prognostic indicators of early and late death in children admitted to district hospital in Kenya: cohort study, *BMJ* 326(7385):361, 2003.
197. Hiesmayr M: Nutrition risk assessment in the ICU, *Curr Opin Clin Nutr Metab Care* 15(2):174–180, 2012.
198. Lee WM: Acute liver failure, *Semin Respir Crit Care Med* 33(1):36–45, 2012.
199. Ichai P, Samuel D: Epidemiology of liver failure, *Clin Res Hepatol Gastroenterol* 35(10):610–617, 2011.
200. Tillmann HL, Zachou K, Dalekos GN: Management of severe acute to fulminant hepatitis B: to treat or not to treat or when to treat? *Liver Int* 32(4):544–553, 2012.
201. Hassanein TI, Schade RR, Hepburn IS: Acute-on-chronic liver failure: extracorporeal liver assist devices, *Curr Opin Crit Care* 17(2):195–203, 2011.
201a. Berzigotti A et al: Assessing portal hypertension in liver diseases, *Expert Rev Gastroenterol Hepatol* 7(2):141–155, 2013.
202. Bari K, Garcia-Tsao G: Treatment of portal hypertension, *World J Gastroenterol* 18(11):1166–1175, 2012.
203. Maruyama H, Yokosuka O: Pathophysiology of portal hypertension and esophageal varices, *Int J Hepatol* 2012:895787, 2012.
204. García-Pagán JC et al: Acute variceal bleeding, *Semin Respir Crit Care Med* 33(1):46–54, 2012.
205. Poordad F: Review article: thrombocytopenia in chronic disease, *Aliment Pharmacol Ther* 26(Suppl 1):5–11, 2007.
206. Machicao VI, Fallon MB: Hepatopulmonary syndrome, *Semin Respir Crit Care Med* 33(1):11–16, 2012.
207. Krowka MJ: Portopulmonary hypertension, *Semin Respir Crit Care Med* 33(1):17–25, 2012.
208. Giusca S et al: Portopulmonary hypertension: from diagnosis to treatment, *Eur J Intern Med* 22(5):441–447, 2011.
209. Habib A, Sanyal AJ: Acute variceal hemorrhage, *Gastrointest Endosc Clin North Am* 17(2):223–252, 2007.
210. Bachir NM, Larson AM: Adult liver transplantation in the United States, *Am J Med Sci* 343(6):462–469, 2012.
211. Gordon FD: Ascites, *Clin Liver Dis* 16(2):285–299, 2012.
212. Lee JS: Albumin for end-stage liver disease, *Korean J Intern Med* 27(1):13–19, 2012.
213. Wong F: Management of ascites in cirrhosis, *J Gastroenterol Hepatol* 27(1):11–20, 2012.
214. Singhal S et al: Management of refractory ascites, *Am J Ther* 19(2): 121–132, 2012.
215. Mullen KD, Prakash RK: New perspectives in hepatic encephalopathy, *Clin Liver Dis* 16(1):1–5, 2012.
216. Shawcross DL, Wendon JA: The neurological manifestations of acute liver failure, *Neurochem Int* 60(7):662–671, 2012.
217. Thumburu KK et al: Neuropathology of acute liver failure, *Neurochem Int* 60(7):672–675, 2012.
218. Bismuth M et al: Hepatic encephalopathy: from pathophysiology to therapeutic management, *Eur J Gastroenterol Hepatol* 23(1):8–22, 2011.
219. Häussinger D: Hepatic encephalopathy, *Acta Gastroenterol Belg* 73(4):457–464, 2010.

220. Patel D et al: Hepatic encephalopathy, *Br J Hosp Med (Lond)* 73(2): 79–85, 2012.
221. Av SP: Hepatic encephalopathy: pathophysiology and advances in therapy, *Trop Gastroenterol* 28(1):4–10, 2007.
222. Khungar V, Poordad F: Hepatic encephalopathy, *Clin Liver Dis* 16(2):301–320, 2012.
223. Winger J, Michelfelder A: Diagnostic approach to the patient with jaundice, *Prim Care* 38(3):469–482, viii, 2011.
224. Roche SP, Kobos R: Jaundice in the adult patient, *Am Fam Physician* 69(2):299–304, 2004.
225. Assimakopoulos SF, Scopa CD, Vagianos CE: Pathophysiology of increased intestinal permeability in obstructive jaundice, *World J Gastroenterol* 13(48):6458–6464, 2008.
226. Raiford DS: Pruritus of chronic cholestasis, *QJM* 88(9):603, 1995.
227. Wadei HM: Hepatorenal syndrome: a critical update, *Semin Respir Crit Care Med* 33(1):55–69, 2012.
228. Angeli P et al: Hepatorenal syndrome, *Contrib Nephrol* 174:46–55, 2011.
229. Guevara M, Arroyo V: Hepatorenal syndrome, *Exp Opin Pharmacother* 12(9):1405–1417, 2011.
230. Davenport A et al: Medical management of hepatorenal syndrome, *Nephrol Dial Transplant* 27(1):34–41, 2012.
231. Fong TL et al: Combined liver-kidney transplantation is preferable to liver transplant alone for cirrhotic patients with renal failure, *Transplantation* 94(4):411–416, 2012.
232. Leung W, Wong F: Hepatorenal syndrome: do the vasoconstrictors work? *Gastroenterol Clin North Am* 40(3):581–598, 2011.
233. Czaja AJ: Acute and acute severe (fulminant) autoimmune hepatitis, *Dig Dis Sci* 58(4):897–914, 2013.
234. Lata J: Diagnosis and treatment of autoimmune hepatitis, *Dig Dis* 30(2):212–215, 2012.
235. Liberal R et al: Pathogenesis of autoimmune hepatitis, *Best Pract Res Clin Gastroenterol* 25(6):653–664, 2012.
236. Sukowski MS: Viral hepatitis and HIV coinfection, *J Hepatol* 48(2): 353–367, 2008.
237. Irving GJ et al: Hepatitis A immunisation in persons not previously exposed to hepatitis A, *Cochrane Database Syst Rev* 7:CD009051, 2012.
238. Blaise-Boisseau S et al: Duplex real-time qRT-PCR for the detection of hepatitis A virus in water and raspberries using the MS2 bacteriophage as a process control, *J Virol Methods* 166(1-2):48–53, 2010.
239. Calle Serrano B, Manns MP: Wedemeyer H: Hepatitis delta and HIV infection, *Semin Liver Dis* 32(2):120–129, 2012.
240. Lacombe K, Rockstroh J: HIV and viral hepatitis coinfections: advances and challenges, *Gut* 61(Suppl 1):i47–i58, 2012.
241. American College of Obstetricians and Gynecologists: ACOG practice bulletin No. 86: viral hepatitis in pregnancy, *Obstet Gynecol* 110(4): 941–956, 2007.
242. Kumar A: Hepatitis B virus infection and pregnancy: a practical approach, *Indian J Gastroenterol* 31(2):43–54, 2012.
243. Kuo A, Gish R: Chronic hepatitis B infection, *Clin Liver Dis* 16(2): 347–369, 2012.
244. Chisari FV, Isogawa M, Wieland SF: Pathogenesis of hepatitis B virus infection, *Pathol Biol (Paris)* 58(4):258–266, 2010.
245. Alavian SM, Miri SM, Jazayeri SM: Hepatitis B vaccine: prophylactic, therapeutic, and diagnostic dilemma, *Minerva Gastroenterol Dietol* 58(2):167–178, 2012.
246. Congly SE, Burak KW, Coffin CS: Hepatitis B immunoglobulin for prevention of hepatitis B virus infection and recurrence after liver transplantation, *Exp Rev Clin Immunol* 7(4):429–436, 2011.
247. Lambotin M et al: Challenges for HCV vaccine development in HIV-HCV coinfection, *Exp Rev Vaccines* 11(7):791–804, 2012.
248. Tarr AW, Urbanowicz RA, Ball JK: The role of humoral innate immunity in hepatitis C virus infection, *Viruses* 4(1):1–27, 2012.
249. Kamili S et al: Laboratory diagnostics for hepatitis C virus infection, *Clin Infect Dis* 55(Suppl 1):S43–S48, 2012.
250. De Clercq E: A cutting-edge view on the current state of antiviral drug development, *Med Res Rev*, 2013 Mar 11. [Epub ahead of print.].
251. Pol S et al: Hepatitis C: epidemiology, diagnosis, natural history and therapy, *Contrib Nephrol* 176:1–9, 2012.
252. Feinstone SM, Hu DJ, Major ME: Prospects for prophylactic and therapeutic vaccines against hepatitis C virus, *Clin Infect Dis* 55(Suppl 1): S25–S32, 2012.
253. Smith BD et al: Recommendations for the identification of chronic hepatitis C virus infection among persons born during 1945-1965, *MMWR Recomm Rep* 61(RR-4):1–32, 2012.
254. Rizzetto M: Current management of delta hepatitis, *Liver Int* 33(Suppl 1): 195–197, 2013.
255. Wedemeyer H: Hepatitis D revival, *Liver Int* 31(Suppl 1):140–144, 2011.
256. Aggarwal R, Jameel S: Hepatitis E, *Hepatology* 54(6):2218–2226, 2011.
257. Wedemeyer H, Pischke S, Manns MP: Pathogenesis and treatment of hepatitis e virus infection, *Gastroenterology* 142(6):1388–1397, 2012.
258. Tian Z, Chen Y, Gao B: Natural killer cells in liver disease, *Hepatology* 57(4):1654–1662, 2013.
259. Elewa U et al: Treatment of hepatitis B virus-associated nephropathy, *Nephron Clin Pract* 119(1):c41–c49, 2011.
260. Morales JM, Kamar N, Rostaing L: Hepatitis C and renal disease: epidemiology, diagnosis, pathogenesis and therapy, *Contrib Nephrol* 176:10–23, 2012.
261. Shiffman ML: Management of acute hepatitis B, *Clin Liver Dis* 14(1): 75–91, 2010.
262. Panda B, Panda A, Riley LE: Selected viral infections in pregnancy, *Obstet Gynecol Clin North Am* 37(2):321–331, 2010.
263. Aspinall EJ et al: Hepatitis B prevention, diagnosis, treatment and care: a review, *Occup Med (Lond)* 61(8):531–540, 2011.
264. Starr SP, Raines D: Cirrhosis: diagnosis, management, and prevention, *Am Fam Physician* 84(12):1353–1359, 2011.
265. Mormone E, George J, Nieto N: Molecular pathogenesis of hepatic fibrosis and current therapeutic approaches, *Chem Biol Interact* 193(3):225–231, 2011.
266. Schuppan D, Afdhal NH: Liver cirrhosis, *Lancet* 371(9615):838–851, 2008.
267. Hill DB, Kugelmas M: Alcoholic liver disease: treatment strategies for the potentially reversible stages, *Postgrad Med* 103(4):261, 1998.
268. Eagon PK: Alcoholic liver injury: influence of gender and hormones, *World J Gastroenterol* 16(11):1377–1384, 2010.
269. Yoon Y-H, Yi H: *Surveillance report #93: liver cirrhosis mortality in the United States, 1970-2009*, Arlington, VA, 2012, U.S. Department of Health and Human Services. Available at http://pubs.niaaa.nih.gov/publications/Surveillance93/Cirr09.htm.
270. Gao B, Bataller R: Alcoholic liver disease: pathogenesis and new therapeutic targets, *Gastroenterology* 141(5):1572–1585, 2011.
271. Division of Population Health, National Center for Chronic Disease Prevention and Health Promotion: *Alcohol and public health*, Atlanta, GA, 2012, Centers for Disease Control and Prevention.
272. Völzke H: Multicausality in fatty liver disease: is there a rationale to distinguish between alcoholic and non-alcoholic origin? *World J Gastroenterol* 18(27):3492–3501, 2012.
273. Sakaguchi S et al: Progression of alcoholic and non-alcoholic steatohepatitis: common metabolic aspects of innate immune system and oxidative stress, *Drug Metab Pharmacokinet* 26(1):30–46, 2011.
274. Bradbury MW, Berk PD: Lipid metabolism in hepatic steatosis, *Clin Liver Dis* 8(3):639–671, 2004.
275. Yan AW, Schnabl B: Bacterial translocation and changes in the intestinal microbiome associated with alcoholic liver disease, *World J Hepatol* 4(4):110–118, 2012.
276. Tissandié E et al: Both IgA nephropathy and alcoholic cirrhosis feature abnormally glycosylated IgA1 and soluble CD89-IgA and IgG-IgA complexes: common mechanisms for distinct diseases, *Kidney Int* 80(12):1352–1363, 2011.
277. Singal AK, Shah VH: Alcoholic hepatitis: prognostic models and treatment, *Gastroenterol Clin North Am* 40(3):611–639, 2011.
278. Crawford JM: Histologic findings in alcoholic liver disease, *Clin Liver Dis* 16(4):699–716, 2012.
279. McCartney EM, Beard MR: Impact of alcohol on hepatitis C virus replication and interferon signaling, *World J Gastroenterol* 16(11):1337–1343, 2010.
280. Mello T et al: Alcohol induced hepatic fibrosis: role of acetaldehyde, *Mol Aspects Med* 29(1-2):17–21, 2008.
281. Choi G, Runyon BA: Alcoholic hepatitis: a clinician's guide, *Clin Liver Dis* 16(2):371–385, 2012.
282. Yurci A et al: Effects of testosterone gel treatment in hypogonadal men with liver cirrhosis, *Clin Res Hepatol Gastroenterol* 35(12):845–854, 2011.
283. Leber B, Spindelboeck W, Stadlbauer V: Infectious complications of acute and chronic liver disease, *Semin Respir Crit Care Med* 33(1):80–95, 2012.
284. Beier JI, Arteel GE, McClain CJ: Advances in alcoholic liver disease, *Curr Gastroenterol Rep* 13(1):56–64, 2011.
285. Dom G, Francque S, Michielsen P: Risk for relapse of alcohol use after liver transplantation for alcoholic liver disease: a review and proposal of a set of risk assessment criteria, *Acta Gastroenterol Belg* 73(2):247–251, 2010.

286. Tritto G, Davies NA, Jalan R: Liver replacement therapy, *Semin Respir Crit Care Med* 33(1):70–79, 2012.
287. Lomonaco R et al: Nonalcoholic fatty liver disease: current issues and novel treatment approaches, *Drugs* 73(1):1–14, 2013.
288. Bhandari BM, Bayat H, Rothstein KD: Primary biliary cirrhosis, *Gastroenterol Clin North Am* 40(2):373–386, viii, 2011.
289. Ishibashi H et al: Risk factors and prediction of long-term outcome in primary biliary cirrhosis, *Intern Med* 50(1):1–10, 2011.
290. Nguyen DL, Juran BD, Lazaridis KN: Primary biliary cirrhosis, *Best Pract Res Clin Gastroenterol* 24(5):647–654, 2010.
291. Ilyas JA, O'Mahony CA, Vierling JM: Liver transplantation in autoimmune liver diseases, *Best Pract Res Clin Gastroenterol* 25(6):765–782, 2011.
292. Imam MH, Talwalkar JA, Lindor KD: An update on primary sclerosing cholangitis: from pathogenesis to treatment, *Minerva Gastroenterol Dietol* 59(1):49-58, 2013.
293. Tabibian JH, Lindor KD: Primary sclerosing cholangitis: a review and update on therapeutic developments, *Expert Rev Gastroenterol Hepatol* 7(2):103–114, 2013.
294. Stinton LM, Shaffer EA: Epidemiology of gallbladder disease: cholelithiasis and cancer, *Gut Liver* 6(2):172–187, 2012.
295. Venneman NG, van Erpecum KJ: Pathogenesis of gallstones, *Gastroenterol Clin North Am* 39(2):171–183, vii, 2010.
296. Vítek L, Carey MC: New pathophysiological concepts underlying pathogenesis of pigment gallstones, *Clin Res Hepatol Gastroenterol* 36(2): 122–129, 2012.
297. Berger MY et al: Abdominal symptoms: do they predict gallstones? A systemic review, *Scand J Gastroenterol* 35(1):70, 2000.
298. Petrov MS, Savides TJ: Systematic review of endoscopic ultrasonography versus endoscopic retrograde cholangiopancreatography for suspected choledocholithiasis, *Br J Surg* 96(9):967–974, 2009.
299. Itoi T, Wang HP: Endoscopic management of bile duct stones, *Dig Endosc* 22(Suppl 1):S69–S75, 2010.
300. Tandan M, Reddy DN: Extracorporeal shock wave lithotripsy for pancreatic and large common bile duct stones, *World J Gastroenterol* 17(39):4365–4371, 2011.
301. Kiewiet JJ et al: A systematic review and meta-analysis of diagnostic performance of imaging in acute cholecystitis, *Radiology* 264(3):708–720, 2012.
302. Sasaki K et al: Original single-incision laparoscopic cholecystectomy for acute inflammation of the gallbladder, *World J Gastroenterol* 18(9): 944–951, 2012.
303. Brown A et al: Are health related outcomes in acute pancreatitis improving? An analysis of national trends in the U.S. from 1997 to 2003, *J Pancreas* 9(4):408–414, 2008.
304. Yadav D, Lowenfels AB: The epidemiology of pancreatitis and pancreatic cancer, *Gastroenterology* 144(6):1252–1261, 2013.
305. Lowenfels AB, Maisonneuve P, Sullivan T: The changing character of acute pancreatitis: epidemiology, etiology, and prognosis, *Curr Gastroenterol Rep* 11(2):97–103, 2009.
306. Cruz-Santamaría DM, Taxonera C, Giner M: Update on pathogenesis and clinical management of acute pancreatitis, *World J Gastrointest Pathophysiol* 3(3):60–70, 2012.
307. Mayerle J et al: Differential roles of inflammatory cells in pancreatitis, *J Gastroenterol Hepatol* 27(Suppl 2):47–51, 2012.
308. Kylänpää ML, Repo H, Puolakkainen PA: Inflammation and immunosuppression in severe acute pancreatitis, *World J Gastroenterol* 16(23):2867–2872, 2010.
309. Yegneswaran B, Kostis JB, Pitchumoni CS: Cardiovascular manifestations of acute pancreatitis, *J Crit Care* 26(2):225, e11–e18, 2011.
310. Elder AS, Saccone GT, Dixon DL: Lung injury in acute pancreatitis: mechanisms underlying augmented secondary injury, *Pancreatology* 12(1):49–56, 2012.
311. Lin HY et al: Acute renal failure in severe pancreatitis: A population-based study, *Ups J Med Sci* 116(2):155–159, 2011.
312. Zhang XP, Tian H: Pathogenesis of pancreatic encephalopathy in severe acute pancreatitis, *Hepatobiliary Pancreat Dis Int* 6(2):134–140, 2007.
313. Zhu R et al: Utility of clot formation and lysis assay to monitor global coagulation state of patients with severe acute pancreatitis, *Dig Dis Sci* 57(5):1399–1403, 2012.
314. Lippi G, Valentino M, Cervellin G: Laboratory diagnosis of acute pancreatitis: in search of the Holy Grail, *Crit Rev Clin Lab Sci* 49(1):18–31, 2012.
315. Bezmarević M et al: Procalcitonin and BISAP score versus C-reactive protein and APACHE II score in early assessment of severity and outcome of acute pancreatitis, *Vojnosanit Pregl* 69(5):425–431, 2012.
316. Gardner TB: BUN level as a marker of severity in acute pancreatitis: simple, universal, and accurate: comment on "Blood urea nitrogen in the early assessment of acute pancreatitis," *Arch Intern Med* 171(7):676–677, 2011.
317. Ke L et al: Risk factors and outcome of intra-abdominal hypertension in patients with severe acute pancreatitis, *World J Surg* 36(1):171–178, 2012.
318. Wu BU, Banks PA: Clinical management of patients with acute pancreatitis, *Gastroenterology* 144(6):1272–1281, 2013.
319. Braganza JM et al: Chronic pancreatitis, *Lancet* 377(9772):1184–1197, 2011.
320. Forsmark CE: Management of chronic pancreatitis, *Gastroenterology* 144(6):1282–1291, e3, 2013.
321. Trikudanathan G, Navaneethan U, Vege SS: Modern treatment of patients with chronic pancreatitis, *Gastroenterol Clin North Am* 41(1):63–76, 2012.
322. Kudo Y et al: Incidence of and risk factors for developing pancreatic cancer in patients with chronic pancreatitis, *Hepatogastroenterology* 58(106):609–611, 2011.
323. Robertson EV, Jankowski JA: Genetics of gastroesophageal cancer: paradigms, paradoxes, and prognostic utility, *Am J Gastroenterol* 103(2): 443–449, 2008.
324. American Cancer Society: *Cancer facts and figures, 2013*. Available at www.cancer.org/research/cancerfactsfigures/cancerfactsfigures/cancer-facts-figures-2013.
325. Mawhinney MR, Glasgow RE: Current treatment options for the management of esophageal cancer, *Cancer Manag Res* 4:367–377, 2012.
326. Kaz AM et al: Aberrantly methylated PKP1 in the progression of Barrett's esophagus to esophageal adenocarcinoma, *Genes Chromosomes Cancer* 51(4):384–393, 2012.
327. Reid BJ, Kostadinov R, Maley CC: New strategies in Barrett's esophagus: integrating clonal evolutionary theory with clinical management, *Clin Cancer Res* 17(11):3512–3519, 2011.
328. Islami F, Kamangar F: *Helicobacter pylori* and esophageal cancer risk: a meta-analysis, *Cancer Prev Res (Phila)* 1(5):329–338, 2008.
329. Gaddam S, Wani S: Endoscopic therapy of Barrett esophagus, *Gastrointest Endosc Clin N Am* 23(1):1–16, 2013.
330. Sgourakis G et al: Survival after chemotherapy and/or radiotherapy versus self-expanding metal stent insertion in the setting of inoperable esophageal cancer: a case-control study, *BMC Cancer* 12:70, 2012.
331. Nagini S: Carcinoma of the stomach: a review of epidemiology, pathogenesis, molecular genetics and chemoprevention, *World J Gastrointest Oncol* 4(7):156–169, 2012.
332. Dhalla F et al: Review of gastric cancer risk factors in patients with common variable immunodeficiency disorders, resulting in a proposal for a surveillance programme, *Clin Exp Immunol* 165(1):1–7, 2011.
333. Edgren G et al: Risk of gastric cancer and peptic ulcers in relation to ABO blood type: a cohort study, *Am J Epidemiol* 172(11):1280–1285, 2010.
334. Vannella L, Lahner E, Annibale B: Risk for gastric neoplasias in patients with chronic atrophic gastritis: a critical reappraisal, *World J Gastroenterol* 18(12):1279–1285, 2012.
335. Bornschein J et al: Gastric cancer: clinical aspects, epidemiology and molecular background, *Helicobacter* 16(Suppl 1):45–52, 2011.
336. Compare D, Rocco A, Nardone G: Risk factors in gastric cancer, *Eur Rev Med Pharmacol Sci* 14(4):302–308, 2010.
337. Wang P et al: Effects of *Helicobacter pylori* on biological characteristics of gastric epithelial cells, *Histol Histopathol* 27(8):1079–1091, 2012.
338. González CA, López-Carrillo L: *Helicobacter pylori*, nutrition and smoking interactions: their impact in gastric carcinogenesis, *Scand J Gastroenterol* 45:6–14, 2010.
339. Gigek CO et al: Epigenetic mechanisms in gastric cancer, *Epigenomics* 4(3):279–294, 2012.
340. Van Ness M et al: Genetics and molecular pathology of gastric malignancy: development of targeted therapies in the era of personalized medicine, *J Gastrointest Oncol* 3(3):243–251, 2012.
341. Yahalom J: Patients with *H pylori*-independent MALT lymphoma are curable with radiotherapy, *Oncology (Williston Park)* 25(12):1147–1149, 2011.
342. Gonzalez CA, Riboli E: Diet and cancer prevention: contributions from the European Prospective Investigation into Cancer and Nutrition (EPIC) study, *Eur J Cancer* 46(14):2555–2562, 2010.

343. Gore RM et al: Diagnosis and staging of small bowel tumours, *Cancer Imaging* 6:209–212, 2006.
344. Widmar M et al: Small bowel adenocarcinoma in Crohn's disease, *J Gastrointest Surg* 15(5):797–802, 2011.
345. Will OC et al: Familial adenomatous polyposis and the small bowel: a loco-regional review and current management strategies, *Pathol Res Pract* 204(7):449–458, 2008.
346. Pufulete M: Intake of dairy products and risk of colorectal neoplasia, *Nutr Res Rev* 21(1):56–67, 2008.
347. Sharma S, O'Keefe SJ: Environmental influences on the high mortality from colorectal cancer in African Americans, *Postgrad Med J* 83(983):583–589, 2007.
348. Goel A, Boland CR: Epigenetics of colorectal cancer, *Gastroenterology* 143(6):1442–1460, 2012.
349. Lin OS: Colorectal cancer screening in patients at moderately increased risk due to family history, *World J Gastrointest Oncol* 4(6):125–130, 2012.
350. Al-Sohaily S et al: Molecular pathways in colorectal cancer, *J Gastroenterol Hepatol* 27(9):1423–1431, 2012.
351. Armaghany T et al: Genetic alterations in colorectal cancer, *Gastrointest Cancer Res* 5(1):19–27, 2012.
352. Kanthan R, Senger JL, Kanthan SC: Molecular events in primary and metastatic colorectal carcinoma: a review, *Patholog Res Int* 2012:597497, 2012.
353. Dixon DA et al: Mechanistic aspects of COX-2 expression in colorectal neoplasia, *Recent Results Cancer Res* 191:7–37, 2013.
354. Carethers JM: Proteomics, genomics, and molecular biology in the personalized treatment of colorectal cancer, *J Gastrointest Surg* 16(9): 1648–1650, 2012.
355. Jasmine F et al: A genome-wide study of cytogenetic changes in colorectal cancer using SNP microarrays: opportunities for future personalized treatment, *PLoS One* 7(2):e31968, 2012.
356. De Salvo GL et al: Curative surgery for obstruction from primary left colorectal carcinoma: primary or staged resection? *Cochrane Database Syst Rev* (2):CD002101, 2004.
357. Al-Sukhni W, Aronson M, Gallinger S: Hereditary colorectal cancer syndromes: familial adenomatous polyposis and Lynch syndrome, *Surg Clin North Am* 88(4):819–844, 2008.
358. de Wijkerslooth TR et al: Immunochemical fecal occult blood testing is equally sensitive for proximal and distal advanced neoplasia, *Am J Gastroenterol* 107(10):1570–1578, 2012.
359. Legolvan MP, Taliano RJ, Resnick MB: Application of molecular techniques in the diagnosis, prognosis and management of patients with colorectal cancer: a practical approach, *Hum Pathol* 43(8):1157–1168, 2012.
360. National Cancer Institute: *Colorectal cancer screening,(PDQ®)*, updated May 23, 2013. Available at http://www.cancer.gov/cancertopics/pdq/screening/colorectal/HealthProfessional.
361. Logan RF: A single FIT (≥50 ng Hb/mL) detected 38% of screen-detected advanced colorectal neoplasia, *Ann Intern Med* 157(10): JC5–JC10, 2012.
362. National Cancer Institute: *Stages of colon cancer, 5/16/2013*. Available at http://www.cancer.gov/cancertopics/pdq/treatment/colon/Patient/page2.
363. National Cancer Institute: *SEER stat fact sheets: small intestine*. Available at http://seer.cancer.gov/statfacts/html/smint.html. Accessed May 30, 2013.
364. Edwards MS et al: A systematic review of treatment guidelines for metastatic colorectal cancer, *Colorectal Dis* 14(2):e31–e47, 2012.
365. Marin JJ et al: Chemoprevention, chemotherapy, and chemoresistance in colorectal cancer, *Drug Metab Rev* 44(2):148–172, 2012.
366. Toomey PG et al: Immunotheraphy for gastrointestinal malignancies, *Cancer Control* 20(1):32–42, 2013.
367. Arlen M et al: The use of specific monoclonal antibodies to target immunogenic tumor membrane proteins in patients with recurrent pancreatic and colon cancer, *Curr Drug Deliv* 9(1):52–56, 2012.
368. Okuno K et al: Recent advances in active specific cancer vaccine treatment for colorectal cancer, *Curr Pharm Biotechnol* 13(8):1439–1445, 2013.
369. Rödel C et al: Preoperative chemoradiotherapy and postoperative chemotherapy with fluorouracil and oxaliplatin versus fluorouracil alone in locally advanced rectal cancer: initial results of the German CAO/ARO/AIO-04 randomised phase 3 trial, *Lancet Oncol* 13(7):679–687, 2012.
370. Iesalnieks I et al: Fistula-associated anal adenocarcinoma in Crohn's disease, *Inflamm Bowel Dis* 16(10):1643–1648, 2010.
371. Gervaz P et al: Squamous cell carcinoma of the anus—an opportunistic cancer in HIV-positive male homosexuals, *World J Gastroenterol* 17(25), 2987–2991, 2011.
372. National Cancer Institute: *A snapshot of liver and bile duct cancers*. Available at www.cancer.gov/researchandfunding/snapshots/liverandbileduct. Accessed May 30, 2013.
373. Blonski W, Kotlyar DS, Forde KA: Non-viral causes of hepatocellular carcinoma, *World J Gastroenterol* 16(29):3603–3615, 2010.
374. El-Serag HV: Hepatocellular carcinoma, *N Engl J Med* 365:1118–1127, 2011.
375. McGlynn KA, London WT: The global epidemiology of hepatocellular carcinoma: present and future, *Clin Liver Dis* 15(2):223–243, 2011.
376. Trichopoulos D et al: Hepatocellular carcinoma risk factors and disease burden in a European cohort: a nested case-control study, *J Natl Cancer Inst* 103(22):1686–1695, 2011.
377. Arzumanyan A, Reis HM, Feitelson MA: Pathogenic mechanisms in HBV- and HCV-associated hepatocellular carcinoma, *Nat Rev Cancer* 13(2):123–135, 2013.
378. Herceg Z, Paliwal A: Epigenetic mechanisms in hepatocellular carcinoma: how environmental factors influence the epigenome, *Mutat Res* 727(3):55–61, 2011.
379. Tyson GL, El-Serag HB: Risk factors for cholangiocarcinoma, *Hepatology* 54(1):173–184, 2011.
380. Ben-Menachem T: Risk factors for cholangiocarcinoma, *Eur J Gastroenterol Hepatol* 19(8):615–617, 2007.
381. Palmer WC, Patel T: Are common factors involved in the pathogenesis of primary liver cancers? A meta-analysis of risk factors for intrahepatic cholangiocarcinoma, *J Hepatol* 57(1):69–76, 2012.
382. Forner A, Llovet JM, Bruix J: Hepatocellular carcinoma, *Lancet* 379(9822):1245–1255, 2012.
383. Masuzaki R, Karp SJ, Omata M: New serum markers of hepatocellular carcinoma, *Semin Oncol* 39(4):434–439, 2012.
384. Lencioni R: Chemoembolization for hepatocellular carcinoma, *Semin Oncol* 39(4):503–509, 2012.
385. Carr BI: Some new approaches to the management of hepatocellular carcinoma, *Semin Oncol* 39(4):369–373, 2012.
386. Cabibbo G et al: Causes of and prevention strategies for hepatocellular carcinoma, *Semin Oncol* 39(4):374–383, 2012.
387. Leyva-Illades D et al: Cholangiocarcinoma pathogenesis: role of the tumor microenvironment, *Transl Gastrointest Cancer* 1(1):71–80, 2012.
388. Singh MK, Facciuto ME: Current management of cholangiocarcinoma, *Mt Sinai J Med* 79(2):232–245, 2012.
389. Tyson GL, El-Serag HB: Risk factors for cholangiocarcinoma, *Hepatology* 54(1):173–184, 2011.
390. Wijaya I, Abdullah M: Diagnosis and treatment update: cholangiocarcinoma, *Acta Med Indones* 43(3):212–215, 2011.
391. Dutta U: Gallbladder cancer: can newer insights improve the outcome? *J Gastroenterol Hepatol* 27(4):642–653, 2012.
392. Lowenfels AB et al: Epidemiology of gallbladder cancer, *Hepatogastroenterology* 46(27):1529, 1999.
393. Pandy M: Risk factors for gallbladder cancer: a reappraisal, *Eur J Cancer Prev* 12(1):15–24, 2003.
394. Wang F, Wang B, Qiao L: Association between obesity and gallbladder cancer, *Front Biosci* 17:2550–2558, 2012.
395. Andrén-Sandberg A: Molecular biology of gallbladder cancer: potential clinical implications, *N Am J Med Sci* 4(10):435–441, 2012.
396. Fuks D et al: Incidental gallbladder cancer by the AFC-GBC-2009 Study Group, *World J Surg* 35(8):1887–1897, 2011.
397. Thomas MB: Targeted therapies for cancer of the gallbladder, *Curr Opin Gastroenterol* 24(3):372–376, 2008.
398. Gore RM, Shelhamer RP: Biliary tract neoplasms: diagnosis and staging, *Cancer Imaging* 7(Spec No A):S15–S23, 2007.
399. Marsh Rde W et al: Comprehensive review of the diagnosis and treatment of biliary tract cancer 2012. Part I: diagnosis-clinical staging and pathology, *J Surg Oncol* 106(3):332–338, 2012.
400. Duell EJ: Epidemiology and potential mechanisms of tobacco smoking and heavy alcohol consumption in pancreatic cancer, *Mol Carcinog* 51(1):40–52, 2012.
401. Kudo Y et al: Incidence of and risk factors for developing pancreatic cancer in patients with chronic pancreatitis, *Hepatogastroenterology* 58(106):609–611, 2011.
402. Raimondi S et al: Pancreatic cancer in chronic pancreatitis; aetiology, incidence, and early detection, *Best Pract Res Clin Gastroenterol* 24(3):349–358, 2010.

403. Kloppel G, Luttges J: The pathology of ductal-type pancreatic carcinomas and pancreatic intraepithelial neoplasia: insights for clinicians, *Curr Gastroenterol Rep* 6(2):111–118, 2004.
403a. Momi N et al: Discovering the route from inflammation to pancreatic cancer, *Minerva Gastroenterol Dietol* 58(4):283–297, 2012.
404. Klein AP: Genetic susceptibility to pancreatic cancer, *Mol Carcinog* 51(1):14–24, 2012.
405. Macgregor-Das AM, Iacobuzio-Donahue CA: Molecular pathways in pancreatic carcinogenesis, *J Surg Oncol* 107(1):8–14, 2013.
406. Birnbaum D, Mamessier E, Birnbaum D: The emerging role of the TGFβ tumor suppressor pathway in pancreatic cancer, *Cell Cycle* 11(4), 2012.
407. Lomberk G: Pain management, *Pancreatology* 8(6):542–543, 2008.
408. Stoita A, Penman ID, Williams DB: Review of screening for pancreatic cancer in high risk individuals, *World J Gastroenterol* 17(19):2365–2371, 2011.
409. Sugumar A: Diagnosis and management of autoimmune pancreatitis, *Gastroenterol Clin North Am* 41(1):9–22, 2012.
410. Tummala P, Junaidi O, Agarwal B: Imaging of pancreatic cancer: an overview, *J Gastrointest Oncol* 2(3):168–174, 2011.
411. Casadei R et al: Total pancreatectomy: indications, operative technique, and results: a single centre experience and review of literature, *Updates Surg* 62(1):41–46, 2010.
412. Corbo V, Tortora G, Scarpa A: Molecular pathology of pancreatic cancer: from bench-to-bedside translation, *Curr Drug Targets* 13(6):744–752, 2012.
413. Herreros-Villanueva M et al: Adjuvant and neoadjuvant treatment in pancreatic cancer, *World J Gastroenterol* 18(14):1565–1572, 2012.
414. Yee NS: Toward the goal of personalized therapy in pancreatic cancer by targeting the molecular phenotype, *Adv Exp Med Biol* 779:91–143, 2013.
415. Vincent A et al: Pancreatic cancer, *Lancet* 378(9791):607–620, 2011.
416. Saif MW: Palliative care of pancreatic cancer. Highlights from the "2011 ASCO Annual Meeting." Chicago, IL, USA; June 3-7, 2011, *JOP* 12(4):355–357, 2011.

CHAPTER

42

Alterations of Digestive Function in Children

Sue E. Huether

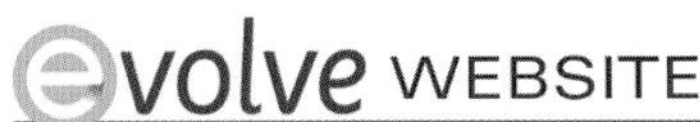

http://evolve.elsevier.com/McCance/
- Review Questions and Answers
- Animations

CHAPTER OUTLINE

Disorders of the gastrointestinal tract, liver, and pancreas in children include congenital anomalies with structural and functional alterations, enzyme deficiencies, and infections. These disorders lead to impairment of motility, digestion, nutrition, and normal growth and development.

DISORDERS OF THE GASTROINTESTINAL TRACT

Congenital Impairment of Motility

Cleft Lip and Cleft Palate

Cleft lip (harelip) and cleft palate (CLP) are developmental anomalies of the first branchial arch (Figure 42-1). The incidence of CLP is estimated at 1 in 1000 live births in the United States.[1] Incidence is lower in black populations and higher in Asian populations.[2] Cleft lip, with or without cleft palate, is more common in males and isolated cleft palate is more common in females. Both anomalies can be unilateral or bilateral, partial or complete and may also be associated with other malformations. *Nonsyndromic (isolated) CLP* is a malformation with an incomplete separation between nasal and oral cavities without any associated anomaly. Syndromic CLP is associated with other malformations (e.g., Crouzon syndrome [craniofacial dysostosis], Treacher Collins syndrome [mandibulofacial dysostosis], hemifacial microsomia).[3]

In most cases, cleft lip and cleft palate are caused by multiple gene-environmental interactions, including maternal deficiency of B vitamins (B_6, folic acid, and B_{12}), maternal smoking and alcohol use, maternal hyperhomocysteinemia, and maternal diabetes mellitus as well as genetic variations of interferon regulatory factor-6, fibroblast growth factor, tumor growth factor-alpha, and other growth factors.[4] (This phenomenon, called *multifactorial inheritance,* is discussed in Chapter 4.) Together these factors reduce the amount of neural crest mesenchyme that migrates into the area that will develop into the face of the embryo.[5]

PATHOPHYSIOLOGY. Cleft lip (harelip) is caused by the incomplete fusion of the nasomedial and intermaxillary processes beginning during the fourth week of embryonic development,[6] a period of rapid fetal growth. The cleft causes structures of the face and mouth to develop without the normal restraints of encircling lip muscles. The facial cleft may affect not only

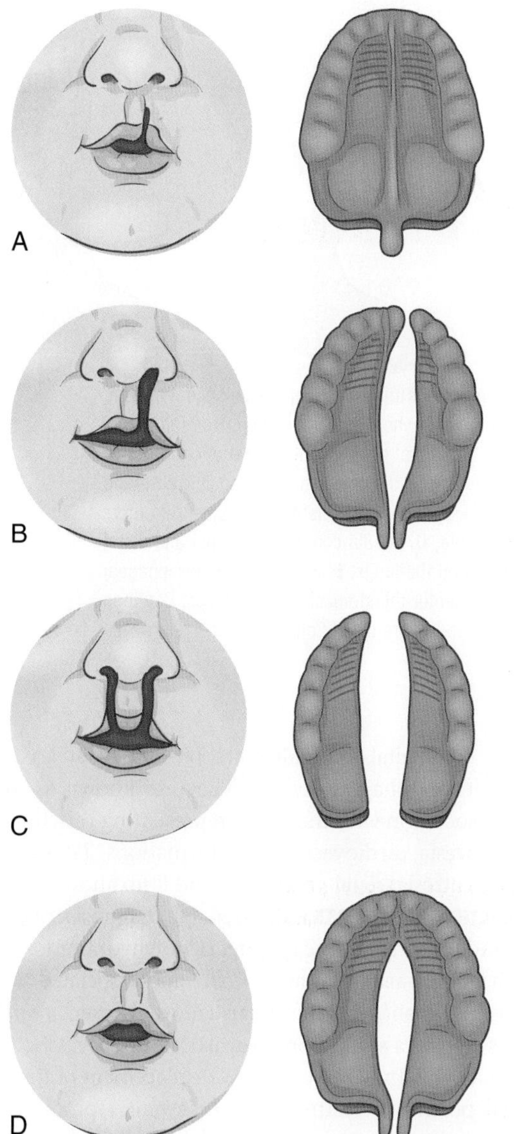

FIGURE 42-1 Variations in Clefts of the Lip and Palate. **A,** Notch in vermilion border. **B,** Unilateral cleft lip and palate. **C,** Bilateral cleft lip and cleft palate. **D,** Cleft palate.

the lip but also the external nose, the nasal cartilages, the nasal septum, and the alveolar processes (bony ridge of maxilla that contains the tooth sockets).

The cleft is usually just beneath the center of one nostril. The defect may occur bilaterally and may be symmetric or asymmetric. The cleft can range in severity from a slight indentation of the lip to a fissure that extends to the nostril, causing a sagging and flattening of the nose. The failure of lip fusion by 35 days of gestation may impair closure of the palatal shelves. The more complete the cleft lip, the greater the chance that teeth in the line of the cleft will be missing or malformed.

Cleft palate is often associated with cleft lip but may occur without it. Cleft palate results from the failure of the primary palatal shelves, or processes, to fuse during the third month of gestation. The fissure may affect only the uvula and soft palate, or it may extend forward to the nostril and involve the hard palate and the maxillary alveolar ridge. It may be unilateral or bilateral, with the cleft occupying the midline posteriorly and as far forward as the alveolar process, where it deviates to the involved side. Clefts involving the palate only are usually but not necessarily in the midline. In some cases the vomer and nasal septum are partly or completely undeveloped. When these facial bones are involved, the nasal cavity may freely communicate with the oral cavity. Teeth in the cleft palate area may be missing or deformed.[7]

CLINICAL MANIFESTATIONS. Feeding the infant with cleft lip usually presents no difficulty if the cleft lip is simple and the palate intact. Nursing at breast or bottle depends on suction developed by pressing the nipple against the hard palate with the tongue. Closure of the lips is not necessary, but the tongue must work harder if the lips cannot be pursed. A baby with cleft palate usually requires large, soft nipples with cross-cut openings and better tolerates feeding when in an upright position to prevent milk escaping through the nose. Although most infants with cleft palate can be successfully breast-fed, it may be impossible for some because of an unproductive suck and difficulty swallowing.[8] An orthodontic prosthesis for the roof of the mouth may facilitate sucking for some infants.[9]

EVALUATION AND TREATMENT. Prenatal diagnosis is made by ultrasound; facial x-ray films confirm the extent of bone deformity. Soft tissue alterations are evaluated by history and physical examination.[10] The nature and extent of the cleft, the infant's condition, and the method of surgical correction proposed determine the course of treatment. Surgical correction is planned as soon as possible and may be in stages.[11] The aim of surgery is to obtain an airtight closure of the palatal cleft and to preserve the mobility and length of the soft palate without compromising mid-facial growth.[12] Children with cleft palate tend to have repeated infections of the paranasal sinuses and middle ear both before and after surgery, which require treatment. The child should be evaluated for hearing loss.[13] Excessive dental decay is not unusual. Speech training and special attention by a prosthodontist and orthodontist are almost always required.[14] Periconceptual B vitamins, folate, and folic acid intake and reduced tobacco and alcohol use may prevent orofacial clefts.[5] Surgical correction facilitates feeding and normal growth and development.[15]

Esophageal Malformations

Congenital malformations of the esophagus are rare and occur in about 1 in 3000 live births, depending on geographic region.[16] **Esophageal atresia** is a condition in which the esophagus ends in a blind pouch and is usually accompanied by a fistula between the esophagus and the trachea. This connection is called a **tracheoesophageal fistula (TEF).** Either defect can occur alone or in association with other defects (Figure 42-2). Many genes have been implicated.[17]

PATHOPHYSIOLOGY. The pathogenesis of esophageal abnormalities is unknown. They are thought to arise from defective differentiation as the trachea separates from the esophagus during the fourth to sixth weeks of embryonic development. Defective growth of endodermal cells leads to atresia. Incomplete fusion of the lateral walls of the foregut leads to incomplete closure of the laryngotracheal tube and fistula formation.[18]

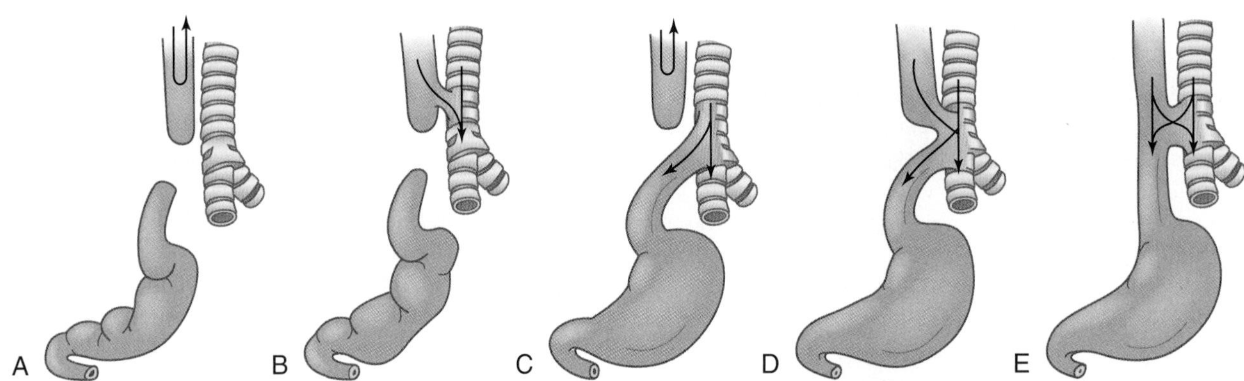

FIGURE 42-2 Five Types of Esophageal Atresia and Tracheoesophageal Fistulae. A, Simple esophageal atresia. Proximal esophagus and distal esophagus end in blind pouches, and there is no tracheal communication. Nothing enters the stomach; regurgitated food and fluid may enter the lungs. **B,** Proximal and distal esophageal segments end in blind pouches, and a fistula connects the proximal esophagus to the trachea. Nothing enters the stomach; food and fluid enter the lungs. **C,** Proximal esophagus ends in a blind pouch, and a fistula connects the trachea to the distal esophagus. Air enters the stomach; regurgitated gastric secretions enter the lungs through the fistula. **D,** Fistula connects proximal and distal esophageal segments to the trachea. Air, food, and fluid enter the stomach and the lungs. **E,** Simple tracheoesophageal fistula between otherwise normal esophagus and trachea. Air, food, and fluid enter the stomach and the lungs. Between 85% and 90% of esophageal anomalies are type C; 6% to 8% are type A; 3% to 5% are type E; and less than 1% are type B or D. **NOTE:** Type F, esophageal stenosis, is not shown.

CLINICAL MANIFESTATIONS. Polyhydramnios (excessive amniotic fluid) is reported to occur in 14% to 90% of mothers of affected infants.[19] The blind end of the proximal esophagus has a capacity of only a few milliliters. Normally swallowed amniotic fluid is absorbed into the placental circulation, and it accumulates in the uterus if the fetus cannot swallow. As the infant with esophageal atresia swallows oral secretions, the pouch fills and overflows into the pharynx, resulting in drooling and occasionally in aspiration (see Figure 42-2, *A* and *C*).

If a fistula connects the trachea with the distal esophagus, the abdomen fills with air and becomes distended. The distention may be great enough to interfere with breathing (see Figure 42-2, *C* to *E*). If the fistula connects the proximal esophagus to the trachea, the first feeding after birth will be problematic (see Figure 42-2, *B, D,* and *E*). As the infant drinks, the blind end of the esophagus and the mouth fill with fluid. When the infant tries to take a breath, the fluid is aspirated into the lungs, which triggers protective cough and choke reflexes. Intermittent cyanosis may result. Plain water or glucose is recommended for the initial feeding to minimize the dangers associated with aspiration. If an abnormality of the esophagus is indicated, oral feedings are withheld until a diagnosis is confirmed.

Pulmonary complications are compounded by reflux of air and gastric secretions into the tracheobronchial tree through the fistula (see Figure 42-2, *D* and *E*), causing severe chemical irritation. The upper lobe of the right lung is most commonly involved because of its proximity to the tracheoesophageal (TE) fistula. Infants with esophageal atresia but no fistula have a scaphoid (boat-shaped), gasless abdomen. In fistula without atresia (see Figure 42-2, *E*), the usual symptoms are recurrent aspiration, pneumonia, and atelectasis that remains "silent" for days or even months. Late complications of esophageal atresia or tracheal esophageal fistula include stricture, reflux, dysphagia, chronic cough, and dyspnea on exertion.[20]

Other congenital anomalies are present in at least 50% of infants with esophageal defects. They are known as the VACTERAL association with the letters representing *v*ertebral anomalies, *a*nal atresia, *c*ardiovascular malformations, *TE* fistula and/or esophageal atresia, *r*enal *a*nomalies, and *l*imb anomalies.[21]

EVALUATION AND TREATMENT. Prenatal diagnosis may include ultrasound imaging but the findings of polyhydramnios and small stomach bubble are often nonspecific and associated with other problems.[22] Esophageal atresia is usually diagnosed at birth, when attempts to pass a small-bore orogastric or nasogastric tube into the stomach fail. Imaging will show displacement of the tube.[23]

Initial postnatal treatment is to prevent aspiration. Surgery restores esophageal continuity, and the fistula is eliminated. Surgery is usually undertaken after birth, sometimes in stages. The child may continue to have problems with aspiration, gastroesophageal reflux, and esophagitis after surgical repair. The overall survival rate for infants with esophageal defects exceeds 90%.[24]

Pyloric Stenosis

Pyloric stenosis is an obstruction of the pyloric sphincter caused by hypertrophy of the sphincter muscle. It is one of the most common disorders of early infancy and affects infants between the ages of either 1 and 2 weeks or 3 and 4 months.[25] The incidence of pyloric stenosis among males is approximately 5 in 1000, whereas among females it is only 1 in 1000.[26] Whites are affected more often than blacks or Asians, and full-term infants are affected more often than premature infants. The cause is unknown but increased gastrin secretion by the mother in the last trimester of pregnancy raises the likelihood of pyloric stenosis in the infant. The overproduction of gastric secretions in the infant may be caused by stress-related factors in the mother. Exogenous administration of prostaglandin E is associated with an increased incidence of pyloric stenosis. There is an increased incidence of pyloric stenosis in those children who have a family member with pyloric stenosis, suggesting a genetic predisposition.[27]

PATHOPHYSIOLOGY. The circular muscle of the pylorus is grossly enlarged because of an increase in cell size (hypertrophy) and an increase in cell number (hyperplasia).[27] The mucosal lining of the pyloric opening is folded and the lumen is narrowed by the encroaching muscle. Because of the extra peristaltic effort necessary to force the gastric contents through the narrow pylorus, the muscle layers of the stomach may become hypertrophied as well.

CLINICAL MANIFESTATIONS. Between 2 and 3 weeks after birth, an infant who is fed well and gained weight begins to vomit without apparent reason and the vomiting becomes more forceful. The forceful, or projectile, vomiting usually occurs immediately after eating, and the vomitus consists of the bulk of the feeding plus some food retained from previous feedings but is almost always free of bile. Usually infants are hungry and want to eat again after vomiting.

Prolonged retention of food in the stomach is a characteristic feature of pyloric stenosis and food is present after 4 hours unless vomiting has occurred. Constipation is the rule because most food does not reach the intestine.

In severe untreated cases, increased gastric peristalsis and vomiting lead to severe fluid and electrolyte imbalances (hypokalemic, hypochloremic metabolic alkalosis), chronic malnutrition, and weight loss that can be fatal within 4 to 6 weeks. Infants with pyloric stenosis are irritable because of hunger, and they may have esophageal discomfort caused by repeated vomiting and esophagitis. The vomitus may be blood streaked because of rupture of gastric and esophageal vessels.

EVALUATION AND TREATMENT. Diagnosis is based on the history of clinical manifestations. Occasionally, gastric peristalsis is observable over the abdomen. A firm, small, movable mass, approximately the size of an olive, is felt in the right upper quadrant in 70% to 90% of infants with pyloric stenosis. A visible gastric peristaltic wave after eating is observed in some infants. Ultrasound clearly shows the hypertrophied pyloric muscles and narrowed pyloric channel.

The standard treatment for hypertrophic pyloric stenosis is a pyloromyotomy, in which the muscles of the pylorus are split and separated. The procedure can be completed with an open technique or with laparoscopy. The mortality associated with surgical correction is less than 0.5%. Fluid and electrolyte losses are managed before surgical intervention and children usually can tolerate feeding several hours after surgery.[28]

Intestinal Malrotation

During the tenth week of embryonic development, the emerging ileum and cecum normally rotate, so that the cecum moves into the lower right quadrant of the abdomen and is fixed there by the mesentery. **Intestinal malrotation** is a condition in which rotation does not occur and the colon remains in the upper right quadrant, where an abnormal membrane or band may press on and obstruct the duodenum. The obstructing band over the duodenum, called a **periduodenal band (Ladd's band),** is one of the most significant findings in malrotation (Figure 42-3). Genetic factors associated with malrotation are being identified and most occur with other malformations or abnormalities.[29]

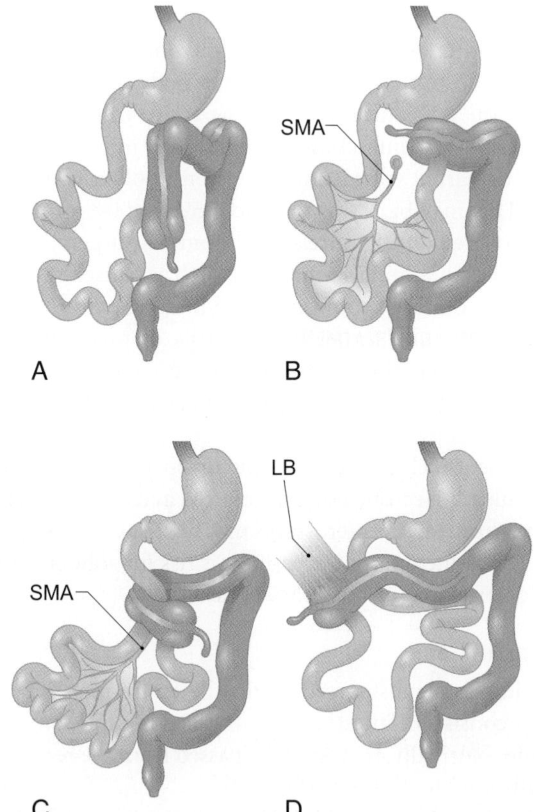

FIGURE 42-3 Variations of Intestinal Malrotation. **A,** Nonrotation. **B,** Incomplete rotation. **C,** Midgut volvulus with duodenal obstruction and obstruction of superior mesenteric artery blood flow. **D,** Incomplete rotation with Ladd's bands extending from the lateral and posterior abdominal wall to the subhepatic cecum. *LB,* Ladd's band; *SMA,* superior mesenteric artery. (From Gilbert-Barness E et al: *Potter's pathology of the fetus, infant and child,* ed 2, Philadelphia, 2007, Mosby.)

Associated abnormalities include 50% of children with duodenal atresia and 33% of those with jejunal atresia, as well as biliary or pancreatic malformations and heart defects.[30]

PATHOPHYSIOLOGY. The small intestine lacks a normal posterior fixation in malrotation because it has only a rudimentary attachment near the origin of the superior mesenteric artery. Therefore, the entire mass can twist when the mobile loops of intestine from the duodenojejunal junction to the middle of the transverse colon twist on themselves. The twisting is termed *volvulus.* Intestinal twisting around the rudimentary mesentery angulates and obstructs the intestinal lumen and partly or completely occludes the superior mesenteric artery, causing infarction and necrosis of the entire midgut.

CLINICAL MANIFESTATIONS. Although most cases of malrotation-associated volvulus and infarction develop during the neonatal period or infancy (younger than 1 year), some develop during childhood or even adulthood. In one study, 48% of individuals first diagnosed with malrotation were adults.[31] In infants the obstruction causes intermittent or persistent bile-stained vomiting after feedings. Abdominal distention is limited initially to the epigastrium because only the stomach and duodenum are dilated. The degree of distention depends on the pressure of swallowed air and the degree of obstruction caused by the volvulus. Dehydration and electrolyte imbalance may occur rapidly because large amounts of pancreatic juice, bile, and gastric secretions are lost through vomiting. Fever usually ensues. Pain, scanty stools, diarrhea, bloody stools, and severe dehydration are associated with progressive volvulus, vascular compression, and infarction of the intestine in infants.[32] Intermittent or partial volvulus may be seen in older children and adults. This may be asymptomatic (25% to 50% of the time) and discovered during unrelated abdominal surgery, or it may cause minor abdominal complaints, such as nausea after meals, recurrent episodes of vomiting, or abdominal pain.[33]

EVALUATION AND TREATMENT. Diagnosis of malrotation with volvulus and infarction is based on a review of the clinical manifestations, upper gastrointestinal contrast imaging, and explorative laparoscopy.[34]

Treatment includes laparoscopic or open surgery to reduce the volvulus.[35] Necrotic bowel is resected and a primary anastomosis performed. An enterostomy may be created. Most children have a good outcome; however, there is risk for adhesion-related bowel obstruction in about 15% of cases.[36]

Meconium Ileus

Meconium is a substance that fills the entire intestine before birth. It consists of intestinal gland secretions and some amniotic fluid. Normally, meconium is passed from the rectum during the first 12 to 72 hours after birth.

Meconium ileus (MI) is intestinal obstruction caused by meconium formed in utero that is abnormally sticky and adheres firmly to the mucosa of the small intestine, resisting passage beyond the terminal ileum. The cause is usually a lack of digestive enzymes during fetal life. This meconium is also found to contain albumin, which is not normally found in meconium. MI is associated with cystic fibrosis.[37] In the cases *not* associated with cystic fibrosis, genes other than *CFTR* mutations have been identified.[38] The cause usually is unknown. Partial aplasia of the pancreas is an associated factor, however, and one fifth of infants with meconium ileus are premature or have a history of maternal hydramnios (excessive amniotic fluid). After intestinal atresia and malrotation with volvulus, meconium ileus is the most common cause of small intestinal obstruction in newborns.

PATHOPHYSIOLOGY. The terminal ileum is plugged with thick, viscous meconium resulting from the formation of an insoluble, calcium-glycoprotein compound in abnormal mucus. The segment of the ileum proximal to the obstruction is distended with liquid contents, and its walls may be hypertrophied. The segment distal to the obstruction is collapsed and filled with small pellets of pale-colored stool. Meconium in the obstructed segment has the consistency of thick syrup or glue. Peristalsis fails to propel this viscous material through the ileum, so it becomes impacted. Volvulus, atresia, or perforation of the bowel sometimes accompanies meconium ileus.

CLINICAL MANIFESTATIONS. Abdominal distention usually develops during the first few days after birth. The infant does not pass meconium and begins to vomit within hours or days of birth. Infants with cystic fibrosis may have signs of pulmonary involvement, such as tachypnea, intercostal retractions, and grunting respirations. The distended abdomen shows patterns of dilated intestinal loops that feel doughlike when palpated. Some of the loops contain scattered, firm, movable masses. Despite hyperactive peristalsis, the rectal ampulla is empty.

EVALUATION AND TREATMENT. All women of reproductive age should be offered preconception and prenatal cystic fibrosis (CF) carrier screening. Prenatal diagnosis of MI can be made by ultrasound. Radiologic imaging is used to confirm the presence of MI.[39] The sweat test is performed to detect or rule out cystic fibrosis. It is considered the "gold standard" and is accurate in 90% of infants. The treatment of choice for cases not complicated by volvulus or perforation is a hyperosmolar enema (e.g., metglutamine diatrizoate [Gastrografin]) performed under fluoroscopy. The fluid is drawn into the meconium mass, hydrating and softening it. Transient osmotic diarrhea follows. A warm saline enema containing 4% *N*-acetylcysteine may be given to help complete the evacuation. Surgical management includes tube enterostomy (a percutaneous drain), open enterostomy, or resection to remove the meconium mass. Survival of infants with meconium ileus is improving, with survival rates approaching 100%.[40] The mortality increases if obstruction is complicated by peritonitis.[41]

Distal Intestinal Obstruction Syndrome

Distal intestinal obstruction syndrome (DIOS), formerly called *meconium ileus equivalent,* affects approximately 15% of children and adults with cystic fibrosis.[42] DIOS is the partial or complete obstruction of the colon or the terminal ileum by abnormally viscous intestinal contents, particularly after episodes of dehydration or lack of pancreatic enzymes. It can occur in children or adults. The child displays signs and symptoms of intestinal obstruction. In most cases the obstruction is relieved by hypertonic enemas.[43]

Obstructions of the Duodenum, Jejunum, and Ileum

Congenital obstruction of the duodenum can be caused by intrinsic malformations (atresia or stenosis) or external pressure. The obstruction may be partial or complete and usually is located at or near the major duodenal papilla. Extrinsic obstructions can be caused by peritoneal bands that constrict the duodenum. The duodenum can be obstructed by an annular pancreas—a defect in which the head of the pancreas surrounds part of the duodenum. Congenital obstructions of the jejunum and ileum can be attributable to atresia, stenosis, meconium ileus, megacolon (Hirschsprung disease), intussusception, Meckel diverticulum, intestinal duplication, or strangulated hernia.

In **ileal atresia** or **jejunal atresia**, the intestine ends blindly proximal and distal to an interruption in its continuity, with or without a gap in the mesentery. Stenosis (narrowing of the lumen) causes dilation proximal to the obstruction and luminal collapse distal to it.

Meckel Diverticulum

Meckel diverticulum is an outpouching of all layers of the small intestinal wall (usually in the ileum) and is the most common congenital malformation of the gastrointestinal tract. The rules of 2 are cited in association with Meckel diverticulum: it occurs in about 2% of the population, 2% develop complications usually before 2 years of age, there are 2 types of common ectopic tissue (gastric and pancreatic), and it is located within 2 feet of the ileocecal valve. Meckel diverticulum develops when there is failure to obliterate the omphalomesenteric duct, which normally leaves a fibrous band that connects the small intestine to the umbilicus during the first months of fetal development. Ectopic gastric mucosal cells are contained in the diverticuli and may cause peptic ulcer. Although most Meckel diverticuli are asymptomatic, the most common symptom is painless rectal bleeding. Intestinal obstruction, intussusception, and volvulus occur more commonly in adults. Diagnosis is made by symptom presentation and radionucleotide scintingraphy. The scan shows the gastric mucosal cells in the diverticuli. Treatment in those with symptoms is surgical resection.[44]

Congenital Aganglionic Megacolon

Congenital aganglionic megacolon (Hirschsprung disease) is a functional obstruction of the colon caused by the absence of the enteric ganglia along a variable length of the colon with inadequate motility. The incidence is approximately 1 in 5000 live births with an increased incidence in males, siblings of children with Hirschsprung disease, and children with Down syndrome or other congenital malformations.[45] The exact cause is unknown but multiple interacting factors and a complex inheritance pattern with mutations in multiple genes are involved.[46]

PATHOPHYSIOLOGY. Congenital aganglionic megacolon is caused by a malformation of the parasympathetic nervous system. It is characterized by abnormalities of the basement membrane and extracellular matrix and absence of the intramural ganglion cells in the enteric nerve plexuses (Meissner and Auerbach plexuses) along variable lengths of the colon, and there may be skipped segments. Lacking neural stimulation, the muscle layers of the colon wall fail to propel feces through the colon, leading to functional obstruction. In 80% of cases the aganglionic segment is limited to the rectosigmoid region (short-segment); in 3% the entire colon lacks ganglion cells and the ileum may be involved. The abnormally innervated colon impairs fecal movements, causing the proximal colon to become distended, hence the term *megacolon* (Figure 42-4).

The ganglia normally develop from an advancing neural crest between the muscle layers (tunica muscularis) in the submucosal area (muscularis mucosae) of the intestinal wall. In cases of congenital megacolon, neurologic development is blocked and large, nonmyelinated fibers develop in place of these ganglion cells. The segment of colon that lacks ganglion cells has a relatively normal lumen caliber and wall thickness. In the segment of the colon proximal to it, the lumen is dilated and the muscle hypertrophied. Therefore, the abnormal portion of the colon appears to be normal and the normal portion appears to be diseased.[47]

CLINICAL MANIFESTATIONS. The extent of the aganglionic portion of the colon determines the severity of the symptoms of congenital aganglionic megacolon. The most distal part of the rectum is always involved. This is the extent of the aganglionic portion in some children, and the child is said to have "ultrashort-segment" Hirschsprung disease and generally has only mild constipation as a symptom. These individuals may not be diagnosed until adulthood. Symptoms of chronic constipation, poor feeding, poor weight gain, and progressive abdominal distention increase in severity as the aganglionic portion extends proximally. Diarrhea may be the first sign, however, because only water can travel around the impacted feces.

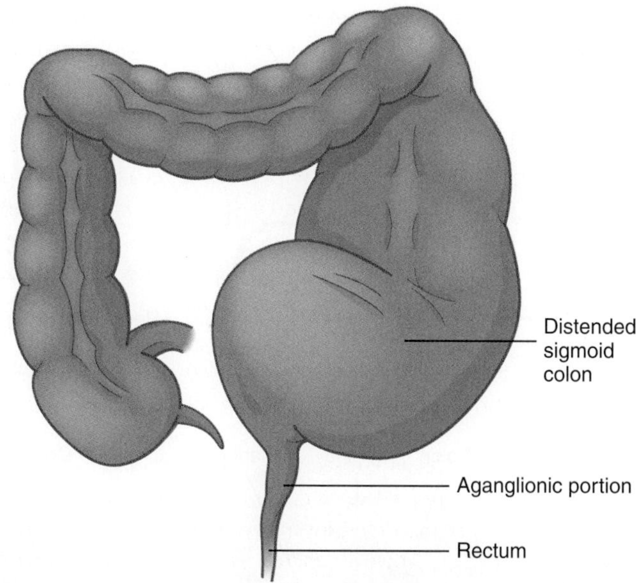

FIGURE 42-4 Congenital Aganglionic Megacolon (Hirschsprung Disease).

In the neonate there is delayed passage of meconium and abdominal distention, with or without bilious vomiting. Bowel dilation stretches and partly occludes the encircling blood and lymphatic vessels, causing edema, ischemia, infarction of the mucosa, and significant outflow of fluid into the bowel lumen. Copious, liquid stools result. In severe cases infarction and destruction of the mucosa enable enteric microorganisms to penetrate the bowel wall. Frequently, gram-negative sepsis occurs, accompanied by fever and vomiting. Severe and rapid electrolyte changes may take place, causing collapse and rapid death.[48]

EVALUATION AND TREATMENT. Hirschsprung disease in usually diagnosed in the newborn period and should be suspected with failure to pass meconium within 24 to 48 hours after birth. Radiocontrast enema, anorectal manometry, and rectal suction biopsy are screening tools for the diagnosis of Hirschsprung disease. Serial manometry measurements may be required in neonates.[49] This test has uncovered ultrashort-segment Hirschsprung disease in older children with a history of constipation.[50] The definitive diagnosis is made by rectal suction biopsy showing an absence of ganglion cells in the submucosa of the colon.[51]

The involved segment is usually resected within the first few months of life using a "pull-through" procedure that anastomoses the proximal and distal segments of remaining bowel or rectum. Laparoscopic or open approaches may be used. In skipped segment disease, the area of normal bowel may be preserved.[52] For children with short-segment Hirschsprung disease, enemas are given to relieve impaction, and laxatives with a dietary and bowel training program are used in preference to surgical intervention.[50] The child is not treated for diarrhea.

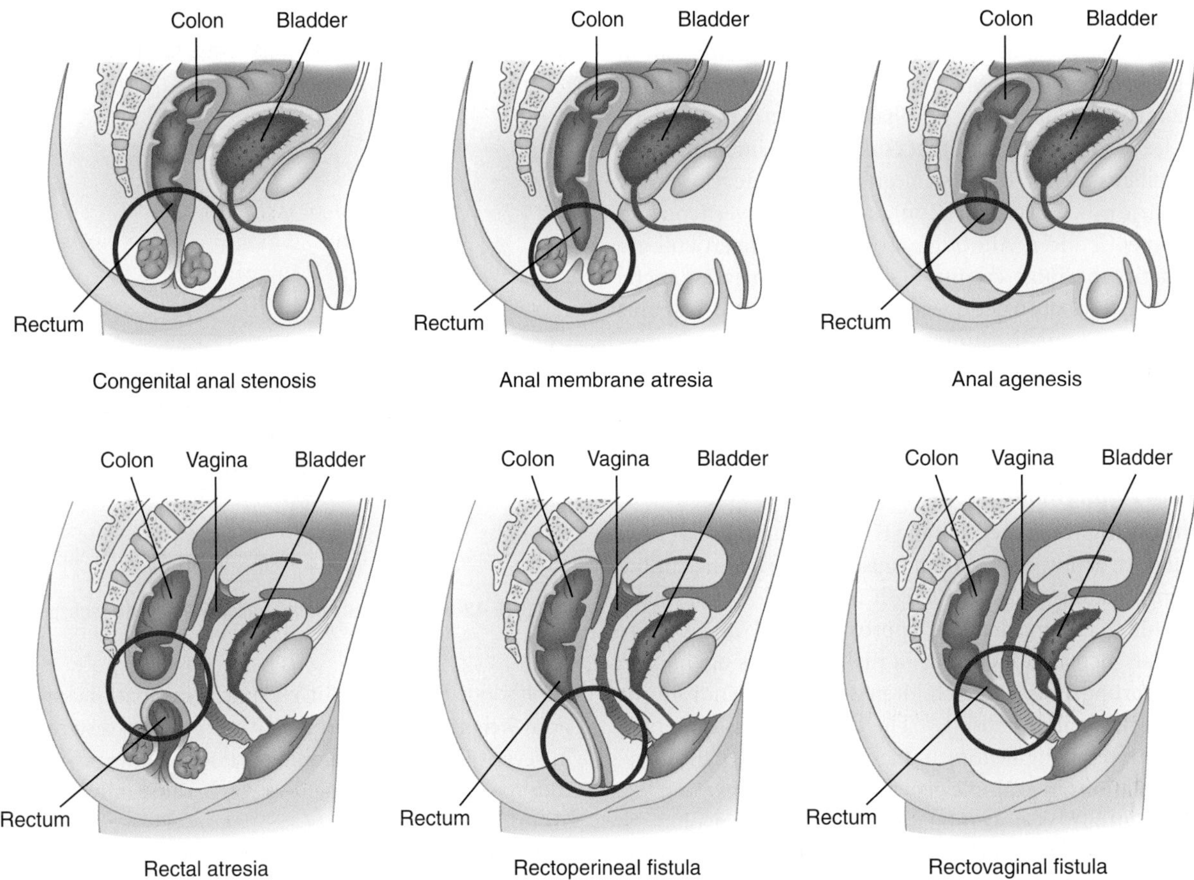

FIGURE 42-5 Anorectal Stenosis and Imperforate Anus.

Hirschsprung-associated enterocolitis is a postsurgical complication that sometimes recurs. If postoperative enterocolitis is allowed to persist, pseudopolyps may appear. Because these are essentially identical to the lesions of ulcerative colitis, they have malignant potential. Therefore, a colectomy is indicated if pseudopolyps develop.

In general, the prognosis of congenital megacolon is satisfactory for children who undergo surgical treatment. Bowel training may be prolonged; however, most children achieve bowel continence before puberty whereas others have long-term constipation or fecal incontinence.[53]

Anorectal Malformations

Congenital anorectal malformations (ARMs) are rare birth defects of unknown etiology that range from mild anal stenosis, which is corrected by simple dilation, to complex deformities, such as anal or rectal agenesis, atresia, and rectourethral fistula (Figure 42-5). Deformities that cause complete obstruction are known collectively as **imperforate anus.** The cause is unknown.[54] ARM occurs in approximately 1 in 2500 to 1 in 5000 newborn babies.[55]

Approximately 40% of infants with ARMs have other developmental anomalies, including Down syndrome, congenital heart disease, renal and urologic abnormalities, cryptorchidism, esophageal atresia, and malformations of the spine.[56] Imperforate anus may not be obvious. It can be detected by gentle insertion of a rectal tube; x-ray films show dilations throughout the intestinal tract. Anal stenosis can be treated by dilations, but all other anorectal malformations require surgical correction. The overall death rate is approximately 10%. More than 90% of children with a low (anal) anomaly and intact sacrum achieve bowel continence with stenosis as a common complication. Children with very high anomalies or anomalies associated with genitourinary fistulae have more difficulty achieving continence.[57,58]

Acquired Impairment of Motility

Intussusception

Intussusception is the telescoping or invagination of one portion of the intestine into another. It is the most common cause of acquired intestinal obstruction in infants between 5 and 10 months of age, although it can occur at any age. The ileum usually invaginates the cecum and part of the ascending colon by collapsing through the ileocecal valve (ileocolic intussusception). It can occur anywhere from the duodenum to the rectum. Intussusception is more common in males and can be idiopathic, can be associated with lead points (polyps or tumors, Meckel diverticulum, intestinal adhesions) or cystic fibrosis, or can develop immediately after abdominal surgery.[59]

PATHOPHYSIOLOGY. Most commonly, the proximal portion of the intestine, the intussusceptum, collapses into the distal portion, the intussuscipiens, in the direction of peristaltic flow (Figure 42-6). As this occurs, the intussusceptum drags its mesentery into the enveloping lumen. Initially, the mesentery

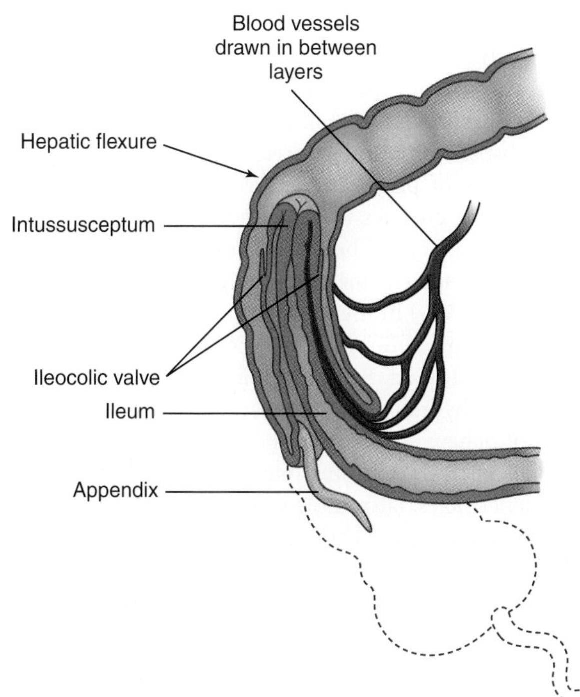

FIGURE 42-6 Ileocolic Intussusception.

is constricted, obstructing venous return. Compression of the mesenteric vessels between the two layers of intestinal wall and at the U-shaped angle at either end of the intussusceptum leads within hours to venous stasis, engorgement, edema, exudation, and further vascular compression. Unless the intussusception is treated, bleeding, necrosis, bowel perforation, and gangrene ensue. The tension of the mesentery on the intussusceptum tends to arch the bowel in a curve with its center at the mesenteric root. Edema and compression obstruct the flow of chyme through the intestine.

CLINICAL MANIFESTATIONS. The affected infant suddenly develops *abdominal pain,* becomes irritable (colicky), and flexes the knees. *Vomiting* occurs soon afterward. A single normal stool may be passed, evacuating the colon distal to the apex of the intussusception. Following the passage of normal stool, 60% of infants pass *"currant jelly" stools,* which appear dark and gelatinous because of their blood and mucus content. In one study, less than one third of children had this clinical triad of vomiting, colicky abdominal pain, and bloody stools.[60] Most infants have a tender, sausage-shaped *abdominal mass.* Abdominal tenderness and distention develop as intestinal obstruction becomes more acute.

EVALUATION AND TREATMENT. Diagnosis is based on clinical manifestations and onset of symptoms. Ultrasound of the abdomen, computed tomography (CT), and magnetic resonance imaging (MRI) are commonly completed for diagnosis.[61] More than 82% of children have positive ultrasound results in ileocolic and jejunointestinal intussusception. Reduction is an emergency procedure involving hydrostatic pressure generated by an air or a barium enema given using fluoroscopic guidance. This technique is successful most of the time with about a 10% to 13% recurrence rate. Surgical reduction is done on children who fail or, in rare cases, have perforation.[62,63] Untreated intussusception in infants is nearly always fatal. Most infants recover if the intussusception is reduced within 24 hours. Spontaneous reduction of intussusception may occur in symptomatic or asymptomatic children.[64]

Gastroesophageal Reflux Disease

Gastroesophageal reflux (GER) is the return of stomach contents into the esophagus because of relaxation or incompetence of the lower esophageal sphincter. In newborns, gastroesophageal reflux is normal (physiologic reflux) because neuromuscular control of the gastroesophageal sphincter is not fully developed. The frequency of reflux is highest in premature infants and decreases during the first 6 to 12 months of life. Children usually outgrow their reflux. **Gastroesophageal reflux disease (GERD)** occurs when protective mechanisms are ineffective and persistent reflux results in complications such as mucosal erosion, bleeding, dysphagia, or failure to thrive.

PATHOPHYSIOLOGY. GERD in children may be related to delayed maturation of the lower esophageal sphincter or impaired hormonal or neurotransmitter response mechanisms (i.e., vasoactive intestinal peptide and nitric oxide). Factors that maintain lower esophageal sphincter integrity in children include location of the gastroesophageal junction in a high-pressure zone within the abdomen, mucosal gathering within the sphincter, and the angle at which the esophagus is inserted into the stomach. Reflux persists if any of these pressure-maintaining factors is altered. Irritation of the mucosa by acidic gastric contents results in inflammation of the esophageal epithelium (esophagitis) and stimulation of the vomiting reflex.[65]

GERD may be a factor in the stimulation of reactive airway disease and otitis media with effusion in some children but the exact relationships are yet to be defined.[66,67] The relationship between apnea of prematurity caused by GERD and laryngospasm is controversial.[68]

Eosinophilic esophagitis is differentiated from GERD (see Chapter 41) and can occur in children. It is thought to be an atopic disease involving immediate as well as delayed hypersensitivity reactions to food ingestion. A mast cell, eosinophil, and T lymphocyte infiltrate are associated with inflammation of the entire esophagus that is nonresponsive to acid-suppression therapy. Eosinophilic inflammation may lead to *progressive subepithelial fibrosis* with esophageal strictures, narrowing, and dysphagia. The esophageal mucosa can appear normal in children at endoscopy. Dysphagia, food impaction, and vomiting are common symptoms and other atopic diseases, such as asthma and eczema, may be present. Treatment includes elimination diets and oral corticosteroids.[69,70]

CLINICAL MANIFESTATIONS. The signs and symptoms of GERD are caused by exposure of the esophageal epithelium to refluxed gastric contents; 85% of affected infants vomit excessively during the first week of life and usually have other symptoms by 6 weeks, including feeding difficulty, feeding refusal, and failure to thrive.

Vomiting may be forceful and must be differentiated from pyloric stenosis. Aspiration pneumonia develops in one third of infants with gastroesophageal reflux (GER). In cases that persist into childhood, chronic cough, wheezing, hoarseness, and recurrent pneumonia are common.[71,72] Repeated vomiting leads to inadequate retention of nutrients, adversely affecting growth and weight gain. Esophagitis from exposure of the esophageal mucosa to acidic gastric contents is manifested by pain, bleeding, and eventually stricture formation and abnormal motility. Approximately 10% to 25% of children with GERD also have iron deficiency anemia caused by frank or occult blood loss.[73]

EVALUATION AND TREATMENT. The clinical manifestations are often adequate to confirm a diagnosis of GERD. However, irritability, crying, feeding refusal, and regurgitation can be common problems in infants and not specific to GERD. Esophageal pH monitoring with a probe for 24 hours and endoscopy with biopsy are routinely used for diagnosis.[74-76] Mild GER resolves without treatment. Thickened feedings may help some infants[77]; however, this has not been shown to be consistently helpful. Techniques for managing infant reflux include small, frequent feedings; prolonged feeding duration and slower flow rate; and frequent burping.[78,79]

Medications are used to treat erosive esophagitis and prokinetic agents must be used with caution.[80] If no improvement is seen with medical management or the child has life-threatening events with reflux, an antireflux surgical procedure, including gastropexy and fundoplication, is performed. A fundoplication recreates a valve by wrapping the fundus of the stomach around the lower esophagus and can be completed using laparoscopic techniques.[65, 81]

Impairment of Digestion, Absorption, and Nutrition

Cystic Fibrosis

Classic gastrointestinal manifestations of cystic fibrosis include meconium ileus at birth, which is usually pathognomonic for cystic fibrosis (CF). Approximately 15% to 20% of individuals with CF present with this symptom. Rectal prolapse is an occasional presenting sign that should always prompt testing for CF. About 10% of CF patients do not experience gastrointestinal problems and are termed "pancreatic sufficient." Several specific *CFTR* mutations are predictive of this milder phenotype. Males with CF are typically infertile (98%).

Cystic fibrosis of the pancreas, which is also called *mucoviscidosis* or *fibrocystic disease* of the pancreas, is a genetically transmitted disease (mutation of the long arm of chromosome 7) that involves many organs and systems and usually causes death in childhood or young adulthood. It is the most common cause of chronic suppurative lung disease in children and is the most common life-threatening inherited disease in the white population. This section focuses on the deficiency of pancreatic enzymes. (Chapter 36 discusses the pulmonary consequences of cystic fibrosis.)

PATHOPHYSIOLOGY. The pathophysiologic triad that is the hallmark of CF includes: (1) pancreatic enzyme deficiency, which causes maldigestion; (2) overproduction of mucus in the respiratory tract and inability to clear secretions, which cause progressive chronic obstructive pulmonary disease; and (3) abnormally elevated sodium and chloride concentrations in sweat. Exocrine secretions tend to be abnormally thick and precipitate in the glandular ducts, obstructing flow. Almost all clinical manifestations of CF are a result of overproduction of extremely viscous mucus and pancreatic enzyme deficiency. The full spectrum of involvement is summarized in Table 42-1.

Pancreatic function may range from normal to completely ablated. Approximately 85% of patients have pancreatic insufficiency. Obstruction of the pancreatic ducts with thick mucus blocks the flow of pancreatic enzymes and causes degenerative and fibrotic changes in the pancreas. Pancreatic damage eventually can affect the beta cells, resulting in diabetes mellitus (10% to 25%). The incidence of diabetes mellitus and cirrhosis (13% to 17%) in this population has increased as larger numbers of people with cystic fibrosis have moved into young and middle adulthood. Severe problems with maldigestion of proteins, carbohydrates, and fats occur because of insufficient secretion of pancreatic enzymes. Failure to thrive, growth failure, malabsorptive symptoms, metabolic abnormalities, trace element deficiencies, fat-soluble vitamin alterations, electrolyte imbalances, and decreased bone mineral density can occur early in the disease.[82-84]

CLINICAL MANIFESTATIONS. Clinical manifestations are presented in Table 42-1.

EVALUATION AND TREATMENT. To determine the extent of pancreatic function 72-hour stool fat measurements are used. Stools also may be examined for absence of pancreatic enzymes, particularly fecal elastase, trypsin, and chymotrypsin. To optimize treatment, the carbon-13 (^{13}C) mixed triglyceride breath test offers a simple, noninvasive way of assessing the need for pancreatic enzyme supplementation in children with cystic fibrosis.[85] Pancreatic replacement enzymes are administered before or with meals and high-calorie, high-protein diets with frequent snacks and vitamin supplements are used to treat malnutrition.[86] However, anorexia is not uncommon in this group secondary to pulmonary disease and frequently large sputum output. To combat the worsening problem of growth failure in children with cystic fibrosis, nasogastric or gastrostomy tube feedings are used to supplement oral intake and promote weight gain. Monitoring of growth and body mass index is critical to treatment evaluation.[87,88]

Gluten-Sensitive Enteropathy

Gluten-sensitive enteropathy, formerly called *celiac sprue* or *celiac disease,* is an autoimmune disease of the small intestinal villous epithelium when there is ingestion of the cereal protein gluten (gliadin) found in wheat, rye, barley, and oats in genetically susceptible individuals. The disease has a prevalence of about 1% worldwide and about 0.71% in the United States; many cases are undiagnosed.[89] Although gluten-sensitive enteropathy is widely perceived as a malabsorption syndrome of childhood, the diagnosis is usually made in adulthood. It is not known why disease presentation varies so widely.[90] Numerous genes have been identified and other autoimmune diseases can be associated with the autoantibodies of gluten-sensitive enteropathy, including type 1 diabetes mellitus, autoimmune thyroiditis, and Addison disease.[91]

PATHOPHYSIOLOGY. The disease is complex and involves the interaction of genetic, immune, and environmental factors. Both cellular immunity and humoral immunity are implicated.[92] The major pathophysiologic characteristic is T-cell–mediated

TABLE 42-1 PATHOPHYSIOLOGY, CLINICAL MANIFESTATIONS, AND COMPLICATIONS OF CYSTIC FIBROSIS

ORGAN INVOLVED	SECRETORY DYSFUNCTION	CLINICAL MANIFESTATIONS	COMPLICATIONS
Sweat glands	Elevated concentrations of sodium and chloride in sweat	Hyponatremia; hypochloremia	Heat prostration; shock
Intestine			
Newborn	Viscid meconium	Meconium ileus with intestinal obstruction	Meconium peritonitis
Older child and adult	Inspissated (dried out) mucofecal masses (intestinal sludging)	Partial intestinal obstruction with severe cramping pains	Gastroesophageal reflux Volvulus (obstruction), intussusception (prolapse) Distal intestinal obstruction syndrome
Pancreas (enzyme deficiency)	Inspissation and precipitation of pancreatic secretions, causing obstruction of pancreatic ducts	Absence of pancreatic enzymes, causing malabsorption of food; fatty, bulky stools	Hypoproteinemia; iron deficiency anemia; malnutrition
		Decreased vitamins A, D, E, and K absorption	Vitamins A, D, E, and K deficiency and rectal prolapse
		Growth failure	Decreased bone density and risk of fractures in adolescents and adults
	Insulin deficiency	Glucose intolerance	Diabetes mellitus
Liver	Inspissation and precipitation of bile in biliary system	Focal biliary cirrhosis; shrunken, "hobnail" liver	Portal hypertension with esophageal varices, hematemesis and hypersplenism Steatorrhea from lack of bile salts
Salivary glands	Inspissation and precipitation of secretions in small ducts of submaxillary and sublingual salivary glands	Mild patchy fibrosis of salivary glands	None
Paranasal structures	Viscid mucus	Retention of mucus; clouding seen on sinus roentgenograms	Mucopyoceles (pus accumulations) with nasal deformity or orbital cavity extension
Nose	Nasal polyps	Obstruction of nasal airflow	None
Lungs	Viscid mucus in bronchioles and bronchi	Obstruction of bronchioles causing bronchiolectasis, bronchiectasis, and chronic lung infection	Hemoptysis; pneumothorax; cor pulmonale; atelectasis; chronic bacterial infection; respiratory failure
Reproductive tract			
Male	Viscid genital tract secretions during embryologic development, causing failure of formation of normal vas deferens	Sterility	None
Female	Distention of endocervical epithelial cells with cytoplasmic mucin	Decreased fertility	Polypoid cervicitis (cervical inflammation) while taking oral contraceptives

Data from Gelfond D, Borowitz D: *Clin Gastroenterol Hepatol* 11(4):333–342, 2013; Javier RM, Jacquot J: *Joint Bone Spine* (5):445–450, 2011; Rudolph CD et al: *Rudolph's pediatrics,* ed 21, New York, 2003, McGraw-Hill.

autoimmune injury to the intestinal epithelial cells.[91] Transglutaminase 2 (TG2) and endomysial autoantibodies closely correlate with the acute phase of the disease in the presence of gluten.[93] T-cell infiltration results in mucosal cell destruction with inflammation, atrophy, and flattening of villi in the upper small intestine (Figures 42-7 and 42-8). The atrophy is caused by accelerated shedding of epithelial cells from the villi. To compensate for this loss, epithelial cell production increases, causing hypertrophy of the crypts of Lieberkühn. Increased cell production is not sufficient to keep pace with cell loss, and the cells are not mature enough to sustain absorptive functions. The microvilli and brush border disappear, leaving patches of bald mucosa. The loss of mucosal surface area and brush-border enzymes leads to severe malabsorption. The pathologic process is most pronounced in the duodenum and jejunum. The ileum may be spared. The severity of disease correlates with the length of the small intestinal mucosa involved.[94,95]

Damage to the mucosa of the duodenum and jejunum has secondary effects that exacerbate malabsorption. The secretion of intestinal hormones, such as secretin and cholecystokinin, may be diminished. Because these chemical messengers are scarce, secretion of pancreatic enzymes and expulsion of bile from the gallbladder decrease.

Destruction of mucosal cells causes inflammation, and water and electrolytes are secreted, leading to watery diarrhea. In addition, absorption that normally occurs by sodium-dependent

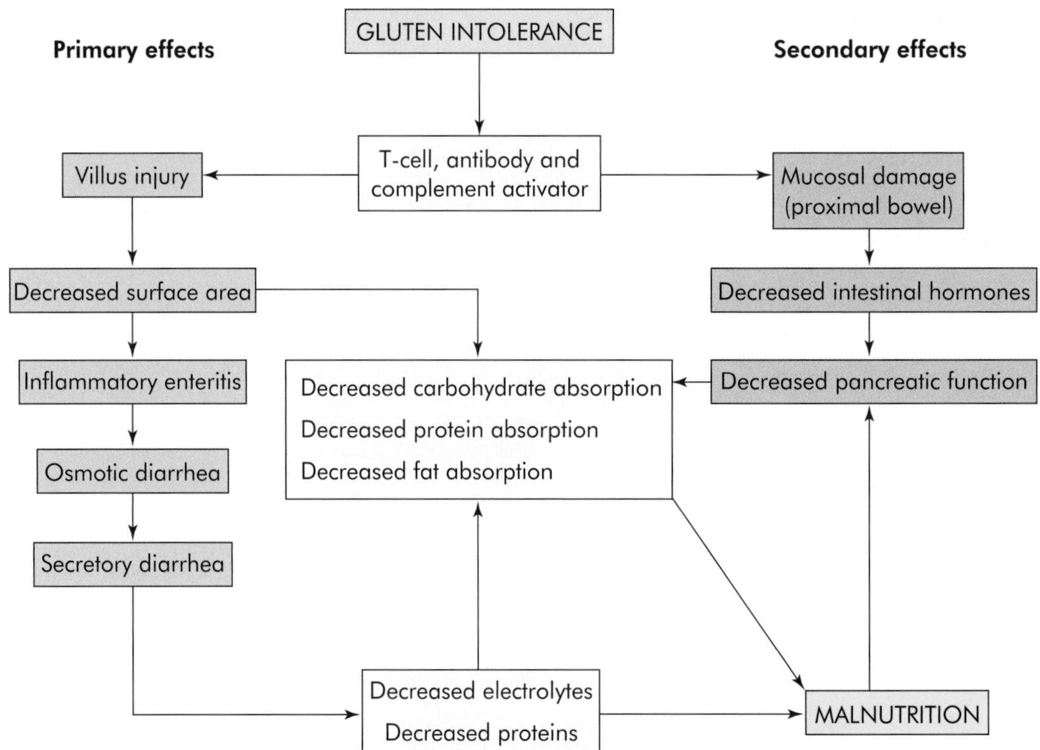

FIGURE 42-7 Pathophysiology of Gluten-Sensitive Enteropathy.

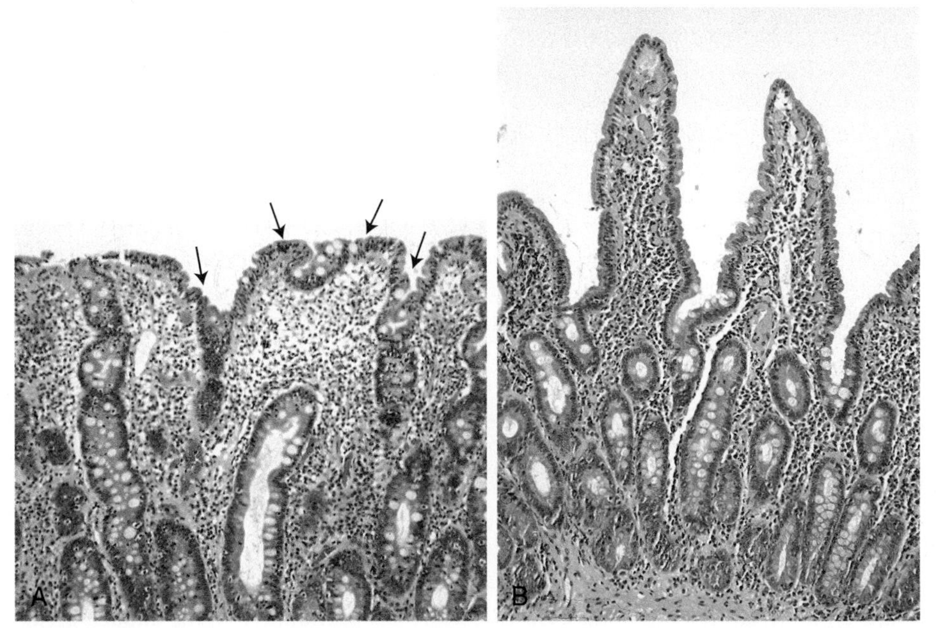

FIGURE 42-8 Gluten-Sensitive Enteropathy. **A,** Atrophy of villi and elongation of crypts that result in malabsorption *(arrows)*. **B,** Recovery of normal villus structure after 6 months of gluten-free diet. (From Damjanov I, Linder J: *Pathology: a color atlas,* St Louis, 2000, Mosby.)

active transport or facilitated diffusion is impaired. Carbohydrates, amino acids, dipeptides, water-soluble vitamins, bile salts, and cations are not absorbed from the intestinal lumen. Potassium loss, which is more severe than sodium loss, leads to muscle weakness. Magnesium and calcium malabsorption can cause seizures or tetany. Unabsorbed fatty acids combine with calcium, and secondary hyperparathyroidism increases phosphorus excretion, resulting in bone reabsorption. Calcium is no longer available to bind oxalate in the intestine and is absorbed, which causes hyperoxaluria. Gallbladder function may be abnormal, and bile salt conjugation may be decreased.

Fat malabsorption in the jejunum is the major cause of steatorrhea (fatty stools). Malabsorption may be mild early in the disease. Fecal nitrogen level is elevated because peptidase deficiencies impair protein absorption. Pancreatic function is decreased, not only because of decreased hormonal levels but also because of malnutrition.

Deficiencies of fat-soluble vitamins are common in children with gluten-sensitive enteropathy. Vitamin K malabsorption leads to hypoprothrombinemia. In one third of cases, iron and folic acid malabsorption is manifested as cheilosis; anemia; and a smooth, red tongue. Vitamin B_{12} absorption is impaired in those with extensive ileal disease. Because the absorption of folate and iron is greatest in the proximal small intestine, deficiencies of these substances are common.

Dermatitis herpetiformis is a cutaneous manifestation of gluten-sensitive enteropathy that involves transglutaminase 3 IgA autoantibodies. They circulate to the skin and interact with antigens produced by keratinocytes. The antigen-antibody complex activates neutrophils in the papillary dermis, causing blister formation. The lesions present with a symmetric distribution on the extensor surfaces of the elbows (90%), knees (30%), shoulders, middle line of the back, or buttocks. The sacral region, scalp, nuchal area, face, and groin also may be involved.[96]

CLINICAL MANIFESTATIONS. The onset of clinical manifestations of gluten-sensitive enteropathy depends on the age of the infant when gluten-containing substances are added to the diet. In 50% of affected children, onset occurs by 18 months of age, with latent intervals varying from months to years. Severity of symptoms can vary tremendously, and children older than 3 years of age can present with mild to severe gastrointestinal symptoms.[97]

Diarrhea is an early sign in most infants accompanied by failure to thrive and anemia. The stools are pale, bulky, greasy, and foul smelling, and may contain oil droplets. Three to five such movements occur daily. As early as 3 or 4 months of age, growth failure, anorexia, and constipation can begin. In older children constipation is occasionally seen despite steatorrhea. Vomiting and abdominal pain are prominent in infants but unusual in older children. Anorexia is prevalent. The classic physical manifestations of organic failure to thrive, such as abdominal protuberance, wasted buttocks and limbs, and hypotonia, occur in less than 50% of infants with gluten-sensitive enteropathy. Growth is usually diminished.[98]

Manifestations of malabsorption, such as rickets, tetany, frank or occult bleeding, or anemia, may be obvious. Some children urinate more at night. The tongue is smooth and red, and the child may bruise and bleed easily. Hypomagnesemia and hypocalcemia cause irritability, tremor, convulsions, tetany, bone pain, osteomalacia, and dental abnormalities. If vitamin D deficiency is prolonged, rickets and clubbing of the terminal phalanges are likely. Eighty-six percent of older children have fingerprint changes (ridge atrophy). In older children, delayed puberty and infertility may be a manifestation of otherwise subtle gluten-sensitive enteropathy.[99]

EVALUATION AND TREATMENT. Diagnosis includes confirmation with serologic antiendomysial and antitransglutaminase IgA antibodies and HLA-type DQ2 or DQ8 (human leukocyte antigen class II haplotypes that regulate immunity). Intestinal biopsy detects the classic mucosal changes caused by gluten-sensitive enteropathy and confirms the diagnosis. The initial biopsy may be followed by a second intestinal biopsy to demonstrate regeneration of intestinal villi after treatment with a gluten-free diet.[100] Most children with celiac disease remain undiagnosed.

Treatment consists of the immediate and permanent institution of a gluten-free diet. Lactose (milk sugar) intolerance is presumed because of damage to the villi; therefore, lactose is excluded from the diet. With removal of gluten and healing of the mucosa, lactose may be reintroduced at a later point.[101] Infants are routinely given vitamin D, iron, and folic acid supplements to treat deficiencies. Breast-feeding at the time of gluten introduction in the diet delays the appearance of celiac disease.[102]

Most children have complete remission of symptoms with clearing of serologic markers and an excellent prognosis. Approximately 25% of children experience recurrent relapses that interfere with growth. There is an increased incidence of malignant disease, particularly T-cell lymphoma, in individuals who fail to respond to gluten-free diets.[103]

Severe Acute Malnutrition

Kwashiorkor (nutritional edema) and marasmus, or a combination of both, are the most common types of malnutrition in children. These disorders are known collectively as **severe acute malnutrition (SAM),** previously known as **protein-energy malnutrition (PEM).** Both are states of starvation associated with food shortages (see Chapter 41). **Kwashiorkor** is severe protein deficiency, and **marasmus** is severe deficiency of all nutrients. Kwashiorkor is a widespread nutritional problem among children in developing countries and economically destitute populations particularly when associated with human immunodeficiency virus (HIV) infection.[104] The disease usually occurs in infants or children from 1 to 4 years of age who have been weaned from breast milk to a high-starch, protein-deficient diet.

Marasmus can occur at any age, but it is common in children younger than 1 year. In marasmus, starvation is attributable to lack of protein and carbohydrates. One third of the world's children suffer from PEM, with the highest concentrations in Asia, Africa, Latin America, and the Carribbean.[105]

The mortality risk for children in developing countries has been found to be inversely related to anthropometric indicators (height, weight, head circumference, skinfold thickness, midarm muscle circumference). There is elevated risk even in the mild to moderate range of malnutrition.[106] Poor sanitation, early weaning of breast-fed infants, use of overdiluted commercial formulas, and infection (measles, malaria, pneumonia, HIV, tuberculosis, and diarrheal disease) are major risk factors for SAM.

SAM is a complication of some diseases, such as chronic fever, malignancy, digestive and malabsorptive disorders, and psychogenic illness. Radiation therapy, chemotherapy and long-term dialysis also can contribute to SAM. Acute and chronic malnutrition is common in hospitalized children.[107]

PATHOPHYSIOLOGY. In kwashiorkor, the deficit of dietary amino acids reduces protein synthesis in all tissues. Physical growth and mental growth are stunted, and maintenance of minimal life processes is in jeopardy. The lack of sufficient plasma proteins, particularly albumin, causes systemic pressure changes that result in generalized edema. The volume of total body water and extracellular fluid increases. Life-threatening hypokalemia, hyponatremia, and hypophosphatemia can occur.[108] The liver swells with stored fat because no hepatic proteins are synthesized to form and release lipoproteins. Pancreatic atrophy and fibrosis may be present. Kwashiorkor also causes malabsorption, reduced bone density, and impaired renal function. If the condition is not reversed, the prognosis is very poor.

Because the intake of all dietary nutrients is reduced to a minimum in marasmus, metabolic processes, including liver function, are preserved but growth is severely retarded. Caloric intake is too low to support protein synthesis for growth or the storage of fat. If more protein is needed than is ingested, muscle wasting occurs. Fat wasting and anemia are common and can be severe. The volume of total body water is high. Serum triglyceride and phospholipid levels increase with increasing severity of malnutrition, but other serum values, such as cholesterol, are normal or slightly reduced. High fasting phospholipid and triglyceride concentrations are predictive of a poor prognosis for these children.[109] Severe vitamin A deficiency contributes to blindness.[110]

CLINICAL MANIFESTATIONS. Retarded physical, mental, and psychologic development; muscle wasting; diarrhea; dermatosis; low hemoglobin level; and infection characterize marasmus. The presence of subcutaneous fat, hepatomegaly, and fatty liver distinguishes kwashiorkor from marasmus. These manifestations are missing in marasmus because caloric intake is not sufficient to support fat synthesis and storage.[111]

EVALUATION AND TREATMENT. Evaluation of SAM is based on nutritional history and clinical manifestations. Providing deficient nutrients resolves clinical symptoms in 4 to 6 weeks. Physical and mental retardation may not be reversible, however. Nutritional rehabilitation with appropriate environmental stimulation for infants and young children resolves or improves cerebral shrinkage, physical growth, and psychomotor development.[112,113] Advances are being made in the local preparation of ready-to-use therapeutic food for both home- and community-based malnutrition management.[114] Breast-feeding needs to be encouraged and some infants and children require intensive inpatient treatment.[115] High morbidity and mortality occur in some regions of the world.[116] Routine use of antibiotics for uncomplicated SAM needs investigation.[116a]

Failure to Thrive

Failure to thrive (FTT) is the inadequate intake, insufficient absorption, or excessive expenditure of calories. It is manifested as a deceleration in weight gain, a low weight/height ratio, or a low weight/height/head circumference ratio. FTT is a common problem and can present at any time in childhood.

PATHOPHYSIOLOGY. Organic FTT has a pathophysiologic cause, such as GERD, pyloric stenosis, gastroenteritis, cystic fibrosis, malabsorption syndromes, infection by intestinal parasites, congenital anomalies, very low birth weight, or chronic diseases of major body systems. All these factors either reduce the availability of nutrients for maintenance and growth or increase nutrient requirements, particularly when there is chronic infection. A chronic disease or congenital anomaly that causes weakness or reduced stature can create developmental, psychosocial, and emotional problems for the child.

Nonorganic FTT occurs in the absence of any gastrointestinal, endocrine, or other chronic diseases. It is usually associated with psychosocial deprivation, although behavioral problems may contribute to its occurrence in the absence of maternal pathologic findings. Behavioral and psychosocial problems may be compounded by inadequate economic resources and lack of knowledge. Generally the problem in nonorganic FTT is ineffective nurturing or neglect by parents and primary caregivers. A variety of parental stressors may be involved and include the following:

- Lack of nurturance in the parents' own childhood
- Unwanted pregnancy
- Inability to bond with the infant because of health or other problems
- Postpartum or maternal depression
- Family crisis, such as a death or marital problems
- Stress caused by single parenthood or social isolation
- Mental, emotional, or physical illness

The first few postnatal months appear to be a sensitive period in the relationship between growth and mental development, suggesting a critical need for early diagnosis and aggressive interventions.[117-119]

CLINICAL MANIFESTATIONS. Clinical manifestations of organic FTT are delayed growth accompanied by manifestations of the underlying disease (e.g., diarrhea). Manifestations of nonorganic FTT are delayed growth plus reduced energy level, reduced responsiveness and interaction with the environment, social isolation, spasticity or rigidity when held or touched, inability to make eye contact or smile, refusal to eat, and rejection of foods. Weight loss and decelerated growth are accompanied by restricted development in many areas. Nonorganic FTT is a complex syndrome involving psychosocial, emotional, and parent-child problems that compound the pathophysiologic abnormalities.[120,121] Children with primarily organic FTT have been found to have lower developmental skills, and their parents have been found to have higher emotional distress. Infant stress, vomiting, feeding disorders, and psychosocial factors have been noted in children with organic and inorganic FTT, making the distinction between the two complex.[122]

EVALUATION AND TREATMENT. Failure to thrive is suggested if a child falls below the third percentile on the growth curve or is lagging in a previously established growth curve. Organic FTT is manifested in infancy by weight, height, and head circumference growth that may be parallel to but below the normal ranges. If no genetic, endocrine, or other systemic disorder is identified and if the physical and laboratory examinations show no abnormalities other than delayed growth, an environmental cause is indicated.[123]

Hospital admission is recommended if the diagnosis is unclear or the child is in nutritional or emotional jeopardy. Eating patterns, food preferences, caloric intake, and family interactions can be assessed during the hospital stay. If the cause is environmental, the hospitalized child with FTT usually begins to gain weight. Organic and nonorganic FTT can coexist, making the distinction between them more difficult.

If an organic problem has been identified, management of FTT consists of treating the cause. Management of nonorganic FTT involves the immediate total care of the child and measures to address: (1) the psychosocial and emotional problems of the caregivers, (2) parent-child interactions, and (3) access to adequate nutritional resources. Counseling, parental modeling, and long-term family support are sometimes required. Clinical manifestations of organic FTT have inorganic components in the majority of children. The most successful interventions not only treat the underlying organic cause but also address ways to assist parents with feeding practices and management of psychosocial symptoms.[124,125]

Necrotizing Enterocolitis

Necrotizing enterocolitis (NEC) is an ischemic, inflammatory condition that causes bowel necrosis and perforation, and infant death if untreated. It is the most common gastrointestinal emergency in the newborn. The overall death rate is between 12% and 30% and is higher for infants requiring surgery.[126] The incidence of NEC is increasing, causing 1500 to 2000 infant deaths every year in the United States.[127] NEC primarily occurs in premature very low birth weight infants.[128] The risk of NEC decreases as the gastrointestinal tract matures.

PATHOPHYSIOLOGY. The exact etiology of NEC is unclear. Multiple factors contribute to the development of NEC including premature birth (<28 weeks), low birth weight, immature immunity, immature intestinal motility and barrier function, abnormal bacterial colonization, infections, maternal age greater than 35 years, maternal hypertensive disease of pregnancy, perinatal stress and low Apgar scores, effects of medications, enteral feeding, and genetic predisposition.[129,130] The immature mucosal barrier delays digestion and motility is slower, allowing for the accumulation of noxious substances that damage the intestine and increase permeability and increase the risk for infection. Translocation of intestinal bacteria and other substances contributes to injury, inflammation, and development of systemic inflammatory disease. Immature intestinal innate immunity and an unfavorable balance between normal and pathogenic bacteria promote intestinal inflammation and release of proinflammatory mediators.[131] Accumulation of gas in the intestine can cause pressure that decreases blood flow and an imbalance between vasodilator and vasoconstrictor inputs in the immature gut may lead to vasoconstriction, promoting ischemia, necrosis, and perforation. Injury to Paneth cells located in the intestinal crypts has also been proposed.[131a] The terminal ileum and proximal colon are most often involved.[132,133]

CLINICAL MANIFESTATIONS. Manifestations of NEC appear suddenly and usually within 2 weeks of birth after introduction of enteral feeding. Symptoms may appear earlier in full-term infants (5.3 days compared with 15.3 days in premature infants).[134] They range from mild abdominal distention to bowel perforation, sepsis, and death. Abdominal pain, unstable temperature, bradycardia, and apnea are nonspecific signs. Affected infants have abdominal distention, occult or grossly bloody stools, retained gastric contents, and septicemia with elevated white blood cell and falling platelet counts. The more premature the infant, the greater the incidence of NEC and related diseases of prematurity, such as respiratory distress syndrome and immunocompromised status.

EVALUATION AND TREATMENT. Diagnosis is based on clinical manifestations, laboratory results, and plain films of the abdomen that show gas accumulation in the intestine. Preventive strategies include following written feeding guidelines; encouraging feeding with breast milk; ensuring judicious fluid management to prevent patent ductus arteriosus; and administering arginine, glutamine, and lactoferrin supplements, epidermal growth factor to support intestinal epithelial cell growth, and enteral prebiotics and probiotics to support commensal gut bacteria.[135-137] Treatments include cessation of feeding formula milk, avoidance of H2-receptor antagonists, use of gastric suction to decompress the intestines, maintenance of fluid and electrolyte balance, and administration of antibiotics to control sepsis.[138-140] Enteral feeding should be started as soon as possible.[141,142]

Surgical resection is the treatment of choice for intestinal perforation, and the mortality is high at about 60%, particularly for small bowel resection.[143] For very ill infants peritoneal drainage may be used as an adjunct to laparotomy.[144] Following treatment of NEC, infants treated by medical and surgical management are at risk for the following complications: intestinal obstruction related to the development of strictures, short bowel syndrome, and neurodevelopmental delay.[145] Infants who have extensive resection of necrotic bowel may develop short bowel syndrome, requiring chronic total parenteral nutrition. Preserving bowel length with stents and intestinal transplantation are available as a lifesaving option for these children.[146,147]

Diarrhea

Diarrhea is an increase in the water content, volume, or frequency of stools and can be acute or chronic. Diarrhea is a common gastrointestinal problem during infancy and early childhood, and infectious diarrhea is the leading cause of death in young children, particularly in developing countries. Severe diarrhea occurs one to three times during the first 3 years of life. Most episodes are self-limiting and resolve within 72 hours.

The pathophysiologic mechanisms of diarrhea in children are similar to those for adults, including osmotic, secretory, or increased motility (see Chapter 41). Prolonged diarrhea is more dangerous in children, because they have much smaller fluid reserves than those of adults. Therefore, dehydration can develop rapidly if any disturbance increases fluid secretion into the gastrointestinal lumen (secretory diarrhea), draws fluid into the lumen by osmosis (osmotic diarrhea), or increases motility and prevents fluid absorption in the intestine.

Infant diarrhea is of special concern because its cause may be a congenital or metabolic anomaly. Common causes of acute diarrhea in infants include infections, congenital aganglionic megacolon, milk-protein allergies, and NEC. Less common causes are adrenogenital syndrome, impaired chloride-bicarbonate exchange, congenital lactase deficiency, glucose-galactose malabsorption, and sucrase-isomaltase deficiency. Infants have low fluid reserves and relatively rapid peristalsis and metabolism. Therefore, the danger of dehydration is great. Causes of diarrhea in young children are unknown in about 40% of cases.[148]

Acute and Chronic Diarrhea in Infants and Children

Acute infectious diarrhea in infants and young children is usually associated with acute viral or bacterial gastroenteritis. Viral causes of diarrhea include rotaviruses, noroviruses, astroviruses, and certain types of adenoviruses. **Rotavirus** is the leading cause of severe diarrhea in infants and young children worldwide. Rotavirus invades enterocytes of the intestinal mucosa and releases an enterotoxin that damages these cells. Damage decreases viable absorptive surface area, causing an imbalance of secretion and absorption, and increases motility, resulting in diarrhea and dehydration. Recovery from mucosal damage may take several weeks. Rotavirus is transmitted by the fecal-oral route among humans. Rotavirus vaccine is an effective preventive strategy and is reducing disease burden in both developed and developing countries. Monitoring is ongoing to evaluate resistant strains.[149] By 5 years of age most children have developed resistance to rotavirus infection. Viral gastroenteritis tends to be self-limiting.

Bacterial causes of diarrhea include *Escherichia coli, Klebsiella,* staphylococci, *Salmonella, Shigella,* and *Vibrio cholerae. Giardia intestinalis, Cryptosporidium parvum* or *hominis,* and *Strongyloides stercoralis* are parasites that cause diarrhea in tropical areas. Infectious diarrhea has a rapid onset, and acidosis and shock can occur quickly. *Clostridium difficile* is often associated with previous antibiotic therapy and can cause acute, profuse, watery diarrhea, and symptoms of colitis (pseudomembranous colitis). The symptoms are more severe in immunosuppressed children. Use of probiotics can be helpful in preventing *C. difficile*–associated diarrhea.[150,151]

Bacterial gastroenteritis is treated with antibiotics if the causal pathogen can be identified. Other causes of acute diarrhea in the older child include antibiotic therapy, appendicitis, chemotherapy, inflammatory bowel disease, parasitic infestation, and ingestion of toxic substances. Children with acute gastroenteritis often remain mildly symptomatic for up to 2 weeks; therefore, diarrhea that persists longer than 2 weeks is considered to be chronic.

Causes of **chronic diarrhea in children** include persistent infectious diarrhea (viral, bacterial, or parasitic), chronic osmotic diarrhea (lactose intolerance or ingestion of large amounts of poorly absorbable sugars), and disease that impairs absorption (e.g., celiac disease, pancreatic insufficiency, or inflammatory bowel disease). Persistent diarrhea is a significant factor in causing malnutrition and growth failure.

Treatment of diarrhea requires rehydration with fluids, electrolytes, and glucose; maintenance of nutrition; and treatment of associated conditions and antibiotics as indicated. Intravenous solutions are used only when oral rehydration solutions are not tolerated. Antiemetics can facilitate oral rehydration.[152] Zinc supplements (not used in children less than 6 months of age), yogurt-based or amino acid–based diets, and probiotics may accelerate recovery[153-155] (see What's New? Pediatric Inflammatory Bowel Disease).

WHAT'S NEW?

Pediatric Inflammatory Bowel Disease

Pediatric inflammatory bowel disease (IBD) includes both Crohn disease (CD) and ulcerative colitis (UC) (see Chapter 41). The incidence in children is unknown, but CD appears to be increasing across the world. It is often diagnosed in late childhood or during adolescence. The etiology is unknown, but there are suspected genetic, epigenetic, and environmental factors involved, and children with IBD are more likely to have parents with the disease. Male children more commonly develop CD; the disease is more extensive and progressive than in adults, involving both the ileum and the colon; growth failure is common and associated with corticosteroid treatment; there are higher rates of hospitalizations and surgery; and growth failure is more common. A recent large population-based study of IBD in children reported an increased risk associated with any antianaerobic antibiotic exposure in a dose-response manner, further emphasizing the need for caution in prescribing antibiotics for children. Fecal calprotectin (FC) level is elevated in IBD and can be used as a marker for IBD diagnosis in children. Treatment for childhood IBD is currently the same as that for adults, but new treatment approaches are needed. Nutritional management is required to maintain normal growth and development. The risk of cancer and death is low in children with IBD.

Data from Abraham BP, Mehta S, El-Serag HB: *J Clin Gastroenterol* 46(7):581–589, 2012; Benchimol EI et al: *Inflamm Bowel Dis* 17(1): 423–439, 2011; Henderson P et al: *Am J Gastroenterol* 107(6):941–949, 2012; Kronman MP et al: *Pediatrics* 130(4):e794–e803, 2012; Sauer CG, Kugathasan S: *Gastroenterol Clin North Am* 38(4):611–628, 2009; Sherlock ME, Griffiths AM: *Curr Gastroenterol Rep* 14(2):166–173, 2012; Tsang J et al: *BMC Pediatr* 12:162, 2012.

Primary Lactose Intolerance. **Lactose intolerance** is the inability to digest lactose (milk sugar). It is caused by inadequate production of lactase and is a common cause of diarrhea in children, particularly nonwhite children younger than 7 years of age. The malabsorption of lactose results in osmotic diarrhea, in which fluids move by osmosis from the vascular compartment into the intestinal lumen. The undigested sugar is processed by the colonic bacteria, and intestinal gas is produced. The diarrhea is accompanied by abdominal pain, bloating, and flatulence. Diagnosis includes elimination of dietary lactose or hydrogen breath testing. Treatment consists of using lactase-treated dairy products or lactase supplements or reducing dairy product consumption. Other sources of dietary calcium or supplements need to be provided if dairy products are eliminated. Some children can tolerate lactose in fermented forms, such as cheese and yogurt.[156-158]

DISORDERS OF THE LIVER

Disorders of Biliary Metabolism and Transport

Neonatal Jaundice

Physiologic jaundice (hyperbilirubinemia) of the newborn is usually a transient, benign icterus that occurs during the first week of life in otherwise healthy full-term infants. It is caused by mild unconjugated (indirect-reacting) hyperbilirubinemia. **Pathologic jaundice** appears within 24 hours after birth with total serum bilirubin level greater than 20 mg/dl or an indirect bilirubin level greater than 15 mg/dl. Risk factors include fetal-maternal blood type incompatibility (ABO and Rh incompatibility), prematurity, exclusive breast-feeding, maternal age greater than or equal to 25 years, an infant of male gender, delayed meconium passage, and excessive birth trauma such as bruising or cephalhematomas.[159] Prediction tools for hyperbilirubinemia are available to reduce risk associated with early hospital discharge (within 48 hours) when hyperbilirubinemia may not yet be evident.

PATHOPHYSIOLOGY. Pathologic jaundice results from the complex interaction of factors that cause: (1) increased bilirubin production (e.g., hemolysis), (2) impaired hepatic uptake or excretion of unconjugated bilirubin, and (3) delayed maturation of liver conjugating mechanisms.[160] The most common cause is hemolytic disease of the newborn, also known as erythroblastosis fetalis (ABO blood incompatibility; see Chapters 9 and 30). Unconjugated bilirubin (indirect bilirubin) is lipid soluble, bound to albumin in the blood, and in the free form readily crosses the blood-brain barrier in infants. Chronic bilirubin encephalopathy **(kernicterus)** is caused by the deposition of toxic, unconjugated bilirubin in brain cells and usually does not occur in healthy full-term infants.[161] Elevated level of conjugated bilirubin is a sign of underlying disease. A late rising indirect bilirubin level also may be a manifestation of **glucose-6-phosphate dehydrogenase** (an enzyme important in red blood cell metabolism) **deficiency,** a hereditary X-linked genetic defect.[162,163] Elevated unconjugated bilirubin levels also can cause hemolysis, further increasing neonatal jaundice.[164]

CLINICAL MANIFESTATIONS. Physiologic jaundice develops during the second or third day after birth and usually subsides in 1 to 2 weeks in full-term infants and in 2 to 4 weeks in premature infants. After this, increasing bilirubin values and persistent jaundice indicate pathologic hyperbilirubinemia. Manifestations include yellowing skin, dark urine, light-colored stools, and weight loss. Premature infants with respiratory distress, acidosis, or sepsis are at greater risk for encephalopathy. The resulting disabilities include athetoid cerebral palsy and speech and hearing impairment.[165]

EVALUATION AND TREATMENT. Total and direct (conjugated) bilirubin levels are monitored and the bilirubin/albumin ratio is being evaluated as a corollary to unbound serum bilirubin level for predicting neurotoxicity.[166] Pathologic jaundice should be suspected with serum bilirubin values that increase greater than 5 mg/dl per day, persistent jaundice (more than 7 to 10 days in the full-term infant), or conjugated bilirubin values greater than 2 mg/dl. Other causes of jaundice must be eliminated to confirm physiologic jaundice.

Treatment depends on the degree of hyperbilirubinemia. Physiologic jaundice is usually treated by phototherapy (ultraviolet light) with good eye protection. Phototherapy produces isomers of bilirubin that are water soluble, can be more rapidly excreted in the stools and urine, and do not cross the blood-brain barrier. Pathologic jaundice requires high-intensity phototherapy, exchange transfusion, and treatment of the underlying cause. Advances are being made to improve transcutaneous bilirubin monitoring and use of drugs to reduce serum bilirubin levels.[167-169]

Biliary Atresia

Biliary atresia is a rare congenital or acquired (perinatal) malformation characterized by the absence or obstruction of intrahepatic or extrahepatic bile ducts. Extrahepatic ducts may end in a blind pouch. The cause is unknown. The congenital form may be related to a chromosomal abnormality. The acquired form may be related to a viral infection (cytomegalovirus), chronic inflammatory disease, or autoimmune injury to bile duct epithelium.[170] The points of destruction are influenced by the stage of intrauterine development in which injury occurs. The atresia or progressive destruction leads to inflammation, fibrosis, and plugging of the bile canaliculi and extrahepatic biliary tree with obstruction to bile flow. Progressive obstruction may lead to biliary cirrhosis and portal hypertension (see Chapter 41), which can develop within a few weeks after birth. Liver failure can lead to death within 2 years without treatment.[171,172]

Jaundice is the primary clinical manifestation of biliary atresia. Other signs are hepatomegaly and acholic (clay-colored) stools. Fat absorption is impaired because of the lack of bile salts, and the infant may fail to gain weight and requires nutritional support.[173] Early diagnosis of biliary atresia is mandatory and is based on clinical manifestations and liver biopsy. Liver function test results are abnormal. Serum transaminase and alkaline phosphatase values are elevated and conjugated (direct) serum bilirubin levels rise progressively.

Extrahepatic atresia can be relieved by surgical drainage and correction in approximately 10% of cases. Some infants benefit from the Kasai portoenterostomy, in which a hepatic duct remnant is anastomosed to the jejunum or a jejunal segment is anastomosed to the porta hepatis if the patent hepatic duct remnant is not available (Figure 42-9). Even with initial restoration of bile flow, however, fibrosis and obliteration of intrahepatic bile ducts can continue, resulting in cirrhosis.

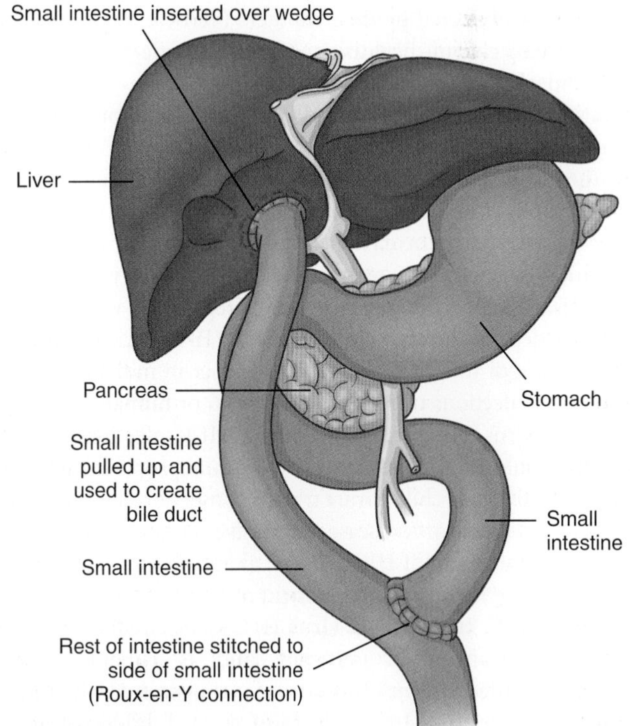

FIGURE 42-9 **Kasai Procedure.** Surgical correction for extrahepatic biliary atresia. The jejunal segment between the liver and the bowel may be externalized, creating a double-barrel portoenterostomy.

Liver transplantation is the long-term therapy when surgery fails. Approximately 40% of children with biliary atresia are immediate candidates for transplantation. Approximately 90% of children who receive transplants for biliary atresia become long-term survivors with good physical and mental development.[174] The use of reduced and split livers from living, related donors has increased the number of children who survive after transplantation.[175]

Inflammatory Disorders

Hepatitis

The pathophysiology of viral and fulminant hepatitis is described in Chapter 41 (see Table 41-7).

Hepatitis A. Approximately one third to one half of the reported cases of **hepatitis A virus (HAV)** occur in children.[176] Incidence is highest among young children of preschool age. Outbreaks tend to occur in daycare centers with large numbers of children who are not toilet trained and staff members who practice poor handwashing techniques.[177] HAV replicates in the liver and is excreted through the biliary system into the stool. HAV in young children is usually mild and asymptomatic. Clinical manifestations, however, may include nausea, vomiting, and diarrhea. Because jaundice is absent, infected children appear to have the "flu." Almost all children recover from hepatitis A without residual liver damage.[178] Vaccination for hepatitis A should begin at 12 to 23 months of age.[179]

Hepatitis B. Risk factors for **hepatitis B virus (HBV)** infection include infants of mothers who are chronic **hepatitis B surface antigen (HBsAg)** carriers, hemophiliacs who receive frequent blood transfusions, children who abuse parenteral drugs, and children who live in residences for the mentally handicapped. Of newborns infected by their mothers (vertical transmission), most develop chronic hepatitis and become carriers.[180] Hepatitis B is endemic in China and other parts of Asia where most infections occur in infants and children as a result of maternal-neonatal transmission.[181]

Chronic hepatitis may develop more often in young children because of their immature immune systems. Infected infants and children are at risk for cirrhosis and hepatocellular carcinoma. The most serious consequence of HBV infection is fulminant hepatitis, which occurs in 1% of cases. Hepatitis D virus (HDV) infection depends on active infection with HBV. There is evidence that the risk of fulminant hepatitis is higher in individuals with combined infections of HBV, HDV, HCV, or human immunodeficiency virus (HIV) than in those with HBV infection alone.[182] Infants should receive passive-active immunoprophylactic treatment at birth. Most children are treated conservatively and antivirals are used for chronic disease. Aggressive vaccination programs reduce the incidence of HBV. Maternal antiviral therapy during pregnancy and lactation is a treatment option.[183,184]

Hepatitis C. **Hepatitis C virus (HCV)** in children is most commonly transmitted vertically and is enhanced with maternal coinfection with HIV. It also is transmitted with blood transfusions. Between 10% and 50% of affected children develop chronic liver disease. Antivirals are effective in the treatment of hepatitis C and liver transplant is required for liver failure.[185] There is currently no vaccination available for hepatitis C.

Chronic Hepatitis. Hepatitis B (HBV) and hepatitis C (HCV) are the main causes of chronic hepatitis in children. Manifestations of chronic hepatitis include malaise, anorexia, fever, gastrointestinal bleeding, hepatomegaly, edema, and transient joint pain. Often there are no symptoms. Serum transaminase and bilirubin levels are elevated. There may be evidence of impairment of synthetic functions of the liver: prolonged prothrombin time and hypoalbuminemia. Diagnosis is based on the clinical manifestations and liver biopsy. There is no curative therapy for chronic HBV or chronic HCV and children are treated with antiviral drugs and should continue to be monitored. There also is an autoimmune form of chronic hepatitis that is treated with immunosuppression therapy.[186] Liver transplant may ultimately be required for chronic hepatitis.[187,188]

Cirrhosis

Cirrhosis is fibrotic scarring of the liver in response to inflammation and tissue damage (see Chapter 41). Most forms of chronic liver diseases in children can progress to cirrhosis, but they seldom do. Causes include cystic fibrosis, biliary atresia, infectious hepatitis, and Wilson disease. Nonalcoholic fatty liver disease (steatohepatitis) is increasing in children in correlation with an increase in childhood obesity and it can progress to cirrhosis and liver cancer.[189]

The complications of cirrhosis in children are the same as those in adults: portal hypertension, the opening of collateral vessels between the portal and systemic veins, and varices. In addition, children with cirrhosis experience growth failure caused by nutritional deficits and developmental delay, particularly in gross motor function because of ascites and weakness. The cause of cirrhosis may influence its severity and course. Some types of cirrhosis can be stabilized if the cause is identified and treated early.

Portal Hypertension

The two basic causes of **portal hypertension** in children are: (1) increased resistance to blood flow within the portal system, and (2) increased volume of portal blood flow. Increased resistance to flow can occur anywhere in the portal circulatory system. Portal hypertension can accompany cirrhosis, intra-abdominal infections, portal vein thrombosis, congenital anomalies of the portal vein, and congenital hepatic fibrosis.

Types of Portal Hypertension

Extrahepatic Portal Hypertension. **Extrahepatic (prehepatic) portal venous obstruction** causes 50% to 70% of extrahepatic portal hypertension in children. For at least half of these children, no specific cause can be found. Obstruction is almost always in the portal vein and is usually caused by thrombosis. Umbilical infection with or without a history of catheterization of the umbilical vein may be a cause in neonates. Portal vein thrombosis can occur as a complication of intra-abdominal infections, pancreatitis, and blunt abdominal trauma. It also has been associated with neonatal dehydration, inflammatory bowel disease, and hypercoagulable states, such as protein C and protein S deficiencies.[190] Life-threatening variceal bleeding can require banding or sclerotherapy. Mesoportal bypass (anastomosis of mesenteric vein to portal vein) restores normal physiologic portal flow to the liver and corrects portal hypertension.[191]

Intrahepatic Portal Hypertension. Cirrhosis is the primary cause of **intrahepatic portal hypertension.** The most common finding is cirrhosis and congenital hepatic fibrosis, which increases resistance to portal blood flow by constricting and reducing the compliance of the hepatic sinusoids. No underlying cause is found in half of cases.[192]

CLINICAL MANIFESTATIONS. The clinical manifestations of portal hypertension are: (1) splenomegaly, (2) upper gastrointestinal bleeding, (3) ascites, and (4) hepatic encephalopathy (see Chapter 41). Severe liver disease is characterized by hypoalbuminemia, prolonged prothrombin times, hyperbilirubinemia, electrolyte imbalance, and hypoglycemia. **Splenomegaly** is the most common sign of portal hypertension in children. The spleen may be firm or hard, depending on the duration of portal hypertension. In children, most episodes of **gastrointestinal bleeding** are caused by rupture of esophageal varices. Hematemesis, possibly associated with abdominal pain, often accompanies sudden pallor. Melena is observed, either at the time of hematemesis or soon afterward. Clotting abnormalities caused by altered liver function promote the bleeding. If plasma volume is increased, esophageal varices readily rupture during activities that increase blood pressure, such as coughing. Acetylsalicylic acid (aspirin), which should not be administered to children, can trigger bleeding. Severe bleeding episodes can cause hypovolemic shock and death. Symptoms of **ascites** include weight gain, protruding abdomen, and reduced tidal volumes if the ascites is severe. **Hepatic encephalopathy** in children can be acute or chronic. Acute encephalopathy is characterized by major disorders of consciousness, which may progress to coma. This may follow an acute episode of variceal bleeding as the impaired liver attempts to metabolize the large protein (nitrogenous) load from the blood. Chronic, or minimal, encephalopathy is characterized by emotional or psychiatric disorders, decreased intellectual functioning, personality disorders caused by minimal brain dysfunction, and spatial disorientation.

EVALUATION AND TREATMENT. Assessment of portal hypertension in children must be thorough because the cause dictates the management. The objectives of the clinical investigation are to locate the site of the venous block and identify the disease responsible for the portal hypertension. Thorough physical examination, laboratory tests of liver function, imaging procedures, and biopsy may be included in the diagnostic evaluation (see Chapter 40). Sclerotherapy, banding, and transjugular intrahepatic portosystemic shunt (TIPS procedure) are treatments for severe esophageal varices in children.[191,193]

The indications for surgical shunting include gastrointestinal hemorrhage not responsive to sclerotherapy. Portosystemic shunts are rarely performed in children but it can be a bridge to liver transplant.[194] The outcome of portal hypertension depends almost entirely on its cause. Children with extrahepatic disease are expected to recover with little morbidity. For children with intrahepatic disease, the prognosis varies.

Metabolic Disorders

More than 5000 genetically determined metabolic pathways have been identified in liver tissue. The earliest possible identification of metabolic disorders is essential because: (1) early treatment may prevent permanent damage to vital organs, such as the liver or brain; (2) precise genetic counseling may be possible with prenatal diagnosis; and (3) complications can be minimized, even if cure is not possible. Galactosemia,[195] fructosemia, and Wilson disease are rare treatable metabolic disorders that have hepatic clinical manifestations. These disorders are summarized in Table 42-2; Wilson disease is discussed next.

TABLE 42-2 GALACTOSEMIA, FRUCTOSEMIA, AND WILSON DISEASE

	GALACTOSEMIA	FRUCTOSEMIA	WILSON DISEASE
Mechanism of disease	Deficiency of galactose and phosphate, uridyl transferase An autosomal recessive trait Cannot convert galactose to glucose Toxic accumulation of galactose in body tissues, liver, and brain	Deficiency of fructose-1-phosphate aldolase An autosomal recessive trait Cannot metabolize fructose, sucrose, or honey; occurs when breast milk is replaced with cow's milk Toxic accumulation of fructose in body tissues	Autosomal recessive: *ATP7B* gene mutation on chromosome 13 Defect in copper excretion by liver Impaired transport of copper in blood caused by diminished transport protein (ceruloplasmin) Toxic accumulations of copper in liver, brain, kidney, corneas
Clinical manifestations	High levels of blood galactose Vomiting Hypoglycemia May have failure to thrive Symptoms of cirrhosis at 2 to 6 months—jaundice Mental retardation if not treated Cataracts if not treated	High levels of blood fructose Vomiting Hypoglycemia May have failure to thrive Hepatomegaly Jaundice Seizures	Intention tremors Indistinct speech Dystonia Greenish yellow rings in cornea Hepatomegaly Jaundice Anorexia Renal tubular defects
Evaluation	Presence of reducing substances in urine when infant is receiving lactose	Detailed dietary history Liver or intestinal mucosa biopsy	Low plasma ceruloplasmin
Treatment	Galactose-free diet	Fructose-, sucrose-, honey-free diet Vitamin C supplementation	Chelation therapy to remove copper from body Decreased dietary intake of copper Liver transplant

Wilson Disease

Wilson disease (hepatolenticular degeneration) is an autosomal recessive defect of copper metabolism related to loss of *ATP7B* gene expression that causes toxic amounts of copper to accumulate in the liver, brain, kidneys, and corneas. *ATP7B* is localized on chromosome 13 and encodes copper-transporting P-type adenosinetriphosphatase (ATPase) membrane-spanning protein. It is highly expressed in the liver, kidney, and placenta and is expressed in lower levels in the brain, heart, muscle, and pancreas.[196] This defect in the uptake and excretion of copper by hepatocytes is an important cause of progressive liver disease in children and young adults. Wilson disease is very rare, with an incidence of 1 in 30,000 live births worldwide.[197] Between 1 in 200 and 1 in 500 persons are carriers.[190]

PATHOPHYSIOLOGY. Two major abnormalities in copper metabolism have been identified: (1) diminished biliary excretion of copper, and (2) failure to insert copper into ceruloplasmin (a glycoprotein that transports copper in the blood). A positive copper balance is present from birth in children with Wilson disease, despite increased excretion of copper in the urine. Copper toxicity with accumulation in the liver and brain is the major abnormality. Excesses of copper generate free radicals that disrupt cellular organelles, deoxyribonucleic acid (DNA), microtubules, enzymes, and proteins. Copper overload is related to impaired biliary excretion of copper and may be related to failure of hepatocyte lysosomes to eliminate copper by exocytosis.[198]

Early in the disease, intestinal absorption of copper is normal, as is hepatic clearance of albumin-bound absorbed copper. As copper-binding proteins in the liver become saturated, hepatic uptake of copper diminishes, with elevated serum copper levels and biochemical and clinical evidence of liver damage caused by copper accumulation. In later stages of the disease, copper accumulates in extrahepatic tissues, including the eyes, brain, and kidneys.

When cerebral copper-binding proteins become saturated, a characteristic pattern of brain damage develops, particularly in the basal ganglia. Neural effects include intention tremor, unsteady gait, dystonia, and behavioral changes. Manifestations of renal tubular injury usually appear simultaneously. The uptake of copper by red blood cells is thought to cause hemolytic anemia, a condition sometimes seen early in the clinical course of Wilson disease.

CLINICAL MANIFESTATIONS. The clinical manifestations of Wilson disease may begin as young as 4 years of age, when control mechanisms responsible for copper homeostasis and biliary excretion should have matured. The classic clinical presentation of Wilson disease is a triad of neuromuscular abnormalities, intention tremors, dysarthria (indistinct speech), and dystonia (disordered muscular tonicity): (1) Kayser-Fleischer rings (accumulation of copper in the limbus of the cornea, causing a greenish yellow ring), (2) cirrhosis associated with elevated serum copper levels, and (3) low ceruloplasmin levels.[199] Initial symptoms vary from malaise and abdominal pain to jaundice. Changes in mental and motor performance may develop at age 6 years or into adult life. The earliest signs of liver involvement include enlargement of the liver and spleen, jaundice, and anorexia. Edema and ascites may develop suddenly, or gastrointestinal hemorrhage may be the initial sign of the disease. Occasionally Wilson disease begins with a hemolytic crisis caused by the toxic effects of copper on the red blood cells. Cirrhosis develops in all untreated cases. Copper deposition in the kidneys causes a proximal renal tubular defect that results in losses of glucose, amino acids, phosphate, and uric acid in the urine and renal tubular acidosis. All untreated individuals will develop behavioral or psychiatric disorders.

EVALUATION AND TREATMENT. Because Wilson disease is rare and has broad clinical manifestations, it may not be diagnosed until older childhood or adulthood. The mean age at diagnosis in one large study was 15.5 years.[200] Laboratory tests detect a serum ceruloplasmin concentration less than 30 mg/dl. Serum copper values may be normal or high, and urine copper values are elevated. Liver biopsy is used to assess structural changes and measure copper concentrations. *ATP7B* gene sequencing can avoid the need for liver biopsy.[201] The goal of therapy is to decrease copper accumulation by decreasing dietary copper intake and intestinal copper absorption, and increasing renal excretion of copper. Medical treatments include D-penicillamine, trientine, zinc (reduces intestinal copper absorption), and ammonium tetrathiomolybdate.[202] Liver transplantation is the only therapy for Wilson disease and gene therapy and hepatocyte cell transplantation are being investigated.[203]

SUMMARY REVIEW

Disorders of the Gastrointestinal Tract

1. Most alterations of digestive function in children are caused by congenital anomalies of the intestinal tract; disorders of digestion, absorption, or nutrition; or liver disease.
2. Cleft lip (harelip) and cleft palate (failure of the bony palate to fuse in the midline) may occur separately or together, and both defects are associated with multiple gene-environmental interactions and deficiency of B vitamins. The fissure may affect the uvula, soft palate, hard palate, nostril, and maxillary alveolar ridge.
3. Esophageal atresia, a condition in which the esophagus ends in a blind pouch, may occur with or without tracheoesophageal fistula, a connection between the esophagus and the trachea. As the infant swallows oral secretions or ingests milk, the pouch fills, causing either drooling or aspiration into the lungs.
4. Pyloric stenosis, an obstruction of the pyloric outlet caused by hypertrophy and hyperplasia of circular muscles in the pyloric sphincter, is more common in male infants and may require surgical correction.
5. Intestinal malrotation occurs with failure of the colon to rotate during fetal development and an obstructing band or volvulus (twisting of the bowel on itself) may partly or completely occlude the gastrointestinal tract and its blood vessels.

SUMMARY REVIEW—cont'd

6. Meconium ileus is a condition in the newborn in which intestinal secretions and amniotic waste products produce a thick tarry plug that obstructs the intestine, usually from lack of fetal digestive enzymes. From 10% to 15% of neonates with CF have meconium ileus as neonates.
7. DIOS, formerly called *meconium ileus equivalent,* can occur when intestinal contents become abnormally thick and obstruct the intestinal lumen. CF, pancreatic enzyme deficiency, and dehydration are common causes.
8. Duodenal, jejunal, and ileal obstructions can be caused by meconium ileus, atresia, peritoneal bands, or acquired obstructive disorders.
9. Meckel diverticulum is an outpouching of all layers of the small intestine caused by failure of the fibrous band that connects the small intestine to the umbilicus.
10. Congenital aganglionic megacolon (Hirschsprung disease) is caused by an absence of enteric ganglia and malformation of the parasympathetic nervous system in a segment of the colon, resulting in inadequate colon motility and functional obstruction.
11. Malformations of the anus and rectum range from mild congenital stenosis of the anus to complex deformities, all of which are classified as imperforate anus.
12. The most common cause of acquired intestinal obstruction in infants is intussusception, a condition in which one portion of the bowel telescopes or invaginates into another. It occurs most commonly in the area of the ileocecal junction.
13. GERD is caused by the relaxation or incompetence of the lower esophageal sphincter. Infants are susceptible to reflux because the sphincter is not fully mature, their diet consists of liquids, and they are seldom in an upright position.
14. Eosinophilic esophagitis involves an eosinophilic inflammation of the esophagus with dysphagia and vomiting that can be associated with asthma and eczema.
15. CF is an inherited disease with a pathophysiologic triad that includes pancreatic enzyme deficiency (which causes maldigestion), overproduction of mucus in the respiratory tract, and abnormally elevated sodium and chloride concentrations in sweat.
16. Gluten-sensitive enteropathy is an immune-mediated lifelong disease characterized by the loss of mature villous epithelium in the presence of a gluten-containing diet. It results in malabsorption and growth failure.
17. Severe acute malnutrition is a group of disorders resulting from a severe dietary deficiency of proteins (kwashiorkor), carbohydrates, or both (marasmus). Starvation causes stunted mental and physical development. Kwashiorkor occurs most often in toddlers who have stopped breast-feeding and subsist on a high-carbohydrate diet.
18. Failure to thrive is inadequate physical growth of a child. Organic failure to thrive is caused by genetic, anatomic, or pathophysiologic factors that restrict normal growth and development. Nonorganic failure to thrive is caused by nutritional deficits associated with inadequate nurturing.
19. Necrotizing enterocolitis is a disorder in neonates, particularly low birth weight or premature infants, thought to result from stress and anoxia of an immature bowel wall. Bacteria invade the mucosa and can result in colitis, necrosis, intestinal perforation, sepsis, and death.
20. Acute diarrhea in infants and children is often caused by infection and can rapidly cause dehydration and electrolyte imbalances because fluid reserves are relatively small. The most common cause of acute diarrhea in children is bacterial or viral enterocolitis.
21. Chronic diarrhea (diarrhea persisting longer than 4 weeks) can be caused by a wide variety of underlying conditions and often leads to growth failure and delayed development.
22. Lactose intolerance causes diarrhea when failure to produce lactase results in osmotic diarrhea with ingestion of lactose-containing dairy products.

Disorders of the Liver

1. Physiologic jaundice of the newborn is caused by mild hyperbilirubinemia that subsides in 1 to 2 weeks. Pathologic jaundice is caused by severe hyperbilirubinemia and can cause brain damage (**kernicterus**).
2. Biliary atresia is a congenital malformation of the bile ducts that obstructs bile flow. Atresia causes jaundice, cirrhosis, and liver failure. Biliary atresia is the most common reason for liver transplantation in children.
3. Acute hepatitis has the same clinical course in children and adults but children have milder cases of the disease. Hepatitis A is the most common form of childhood hepatitis.
4. Young children more readily develop chronic HBV or HCV hepatitis because of their immature immune system.
5. Cirrhosis is fibrotic scarring of the liver and is rare in children but can develop from most forms of chronic liver disease.
6. Portal hypertension in children usually is caused by extrahepatic obstruction. Thrombosis of the portal vein is the most common cause of portal hypertension in children and splenomegaly is the most common sign.
7. The three most common metabolic disorders that cause liver damage in children are galactosemia, fructosemia, and Wilson disease. All are rare, inherited as genetic traits, and permit the accumulation of toxins in the liver.
8. Wilson disease causes defective copper uptake and metabolism. Unexcreted copper accumulates in the liver, brain, kidney, and corneal cells. Damage from accumulated copper is gradual; the disease is usually not diagnosed before age 4 or 5 years.

KEY TERMS

Acute infectious diarrhea, 1500
Ascites, 1503
Biliary atresia, 1501
Chronic diarrhea in children, 1500
Cirrhosis, 1502
Cleft lip (harelip), 1486
Cleft palate, 1487
Congenital aganglionic megacolon (Hirschsprung disease), 1491
Dermatitis herpetiformis, 1497
Diarrhea, 1499
Distal intestinal obstruction syndrome (DIOS), 1490
Eosinophilic esophagitis, 1493
Esophageal atresia, 1487
Extrahepatic (prehepatic) portal venous obstruction, 1502
Failure to thrive (FTT), 1498
Gastroesophageal reflux (GER), 1493
Gastroesophageal reflux disease (GERD), 1493
Gastrointestinal bleeding, 1503
Glucose-6-phosphate dehydrogenase deficiency, 1501
Gluten-sensitive enteropathy, 1494
Hepatic encephalopathy, 1503
Hepatitis A virus (HAV), 1502
Hepatitis B surface antigen (HBsAg), 1502
Hepatitis B virus (HBV), 1502
Hepatitis C virus (HCV), 1502
Ileal or jejunal atresia, 1490
Imperforate anus, 1492
Infant diarrhea, 1499
Intestinal malrotation, 1489
Intrahepatic portal hypertension, 1503
Intussusception, 1492
Kernicterus, 1501
Kwashiorkor, 1497
Lactose intolerance, 1500
Marasmus, 1497
Meckel diverticulum, 1490
Meconium, 1490
Meconium ileus (MI), 1490
Necrotizing enterocolitis (NEC), 1499
Nonorganic FTT, 1498
Organic FTT, 1498
Pathologic jaundice, 1500
Periduodenal band (Ladd's band), 1489
Physiologic jaundice (hyperbilirubinemia) of the newborn, 1500
Portal hypertension, 1502
Protein-energy malnutrition (PEM), 1497
Pyloric stenosis, 1488
Rotavirus, 1500
Severe acute malnutrition (SAM), 1497
Splenomegaly, 1503
Tracheoesophageal fistula (TEF), 1487
Wilson disease, 1504

REFERENCES

1. National Institute of Dental and Craniofacial Research: *Prevalence (number of cases) of cleft lip and palate,* updated October 13, 2011. Available at www.nidcr.nih.gov/DataStatistics/FindDataByTopic/Craniofacial BirthDefects/PrevalenceCleft+LipCleftPalate.htm.
2. Cooper ME, Tatay JS, Marazita ML: Asian oral-facial cleft birth prevalence, *Cleft Palate Craniofac J* 43(5):580–589, 2006.
3. Stuppia L et al: Genetics of syndromic and nonsyndromic cleft lip and palate, *J Craniofac Surg* 22(5):1722–1726, 2011.
4. Dixon MJ et al: Cleft lip and palate: understanding genetic and environmental influences, *Nat Rev Genet* 12(3):167–178, 2011.
5. Mossey PA et al: Cleft lip and palate, *Lancet* 374(9703):1773–1785, 2009.
6. Arosarena OA: Cleft lip and palate, *Otolaryngol Clin North Am* 4(1): 27–60, 2007.
7. Qureshi WA, Beiraghi S, Leon-Salazar V: Dental anomalies associated with unilateral and bilateral cleft lip and palate, *J Dent Child (Chic)* 79(2):69–73, 2012.
8. Miller CK: Feeding issues and interventions in infants and children with clefts and craniofacial syndromes, *Semin Speech Lang* 32(2):115–126, 2011.
9. Turner L et al: The effects of lactation education and a prosthetic obturator appliance of feeding efficiency in infants with cleft lip and palate, *Cleft Palate Craniofac J* 38(5):519–524, 2001.
10. To WW: Prenatal diagnosis and assessment of facial clefts: where are we now? *Hong Kong Med J* 18(2):146–152, 2012.
11. Yang IY, Liao YF: The effect of 1-stage versus 2-stage palate repair on facial growth in patients with cleft lip and palate: a review, *Int J Oral Maxillofac Surg* 39(10):945–950, 2010.
12. Jayaram R, Huppa C: Surgical correction of cleft lip and palate, *Front Oral Biol* 16:101–110, 2012.
13. Rajion ZA et al: The nasopharynx in infants with cleft lip and palate, *Int J Pediatr Otorhinolaryngol* 76(2):227–234, 2012.
14. Cash AC: Orthodontic treatment in the management of cleft lip and palate, *Front Oral Biol* 16:111–123, 2012.
15. McHeik JN, Levard G: Growth in infants in the first two years of life after neonatal repair for unilateral cleft lip and palate, *Int J Pediatr Otorhinolaryngol* 74(5):465–468, 2010.
16. Pedersen RN et al: Oesophageal atresia: prevalence, prenatal diagnosis and associated anomalies in 23 European regions, *Arch Dis Child* 97(3):227–232, 2012.
17. Jacobs IJ, Ku WY, Que J: Genetic and cellular mechanisms regulating anterior foregut and esophageal development, *Dev Biol* 369(1):54–64, 2012.
18. El-Gohary Y, Gittes GK, Tovar JA: Congenital anomalies of the esophagus, *Semin Pediatr Surg* 19(3):186–193, 2010.
19. Langer JC et al: Prenatal diagnosis of esophageal atresia using sonography and magnetic resonance imaging, *J Pediatr Surg* 36(5):804–807, 2001.
20. Legrand C et al: Long-term outcome of children with oesophageal atresia type III, *Arch Dis Child* 97(9):808–811, 2012.
21. Solomon BD: VACTERL/VATER Association, *Orphanet J Rare Dis* 6:56, 2011.
22. de Jong EM et al: Pre- and postnatal diagnosis and outcome of fetuses and neonates with esophageal atresia and tracheoesophageal fistula, *Prenat Diagn* 30(3):274–279, 2010.
23. Pinheiro PF et al: Current knowledge on esophageal atresia, *World J Gastroenterol* 18(28):3662–3672, 2012.
24. Alberti D et al: Esophageal atresia: pre and post-operative management, *J Matern Fetal Neonatal Med* 24(Suppl 1):4–6, 2011.
25. Hernanz-Schulman M: Infantile hypertrophic pyloric stenosis, *Radiology* 227(2):319–331, 2003.
26. Krogh C et al: Pre- and perinatal risk factors for pyloric stenosis and their influence on the male predominance, *Am J Epidemiol* 176(1): 24–31, 2012.
27. Pandya S, Heiss K: Pyloric stenosis in pediatric surgery: an evidence-based review, *Surg Clin North Am* 92(3):527–539, vii–viii, 2012.
28. Ranells JD, Carver JD, Kirby RS: Infantile hypertrophic pyloric stenosis: epidemiology, genetics, and clinical update, *Adv Pediatr* 58(1):195–206, 2011.
29. Martin V, Shaw-Smith C: Review of genetic factors in intestinal malrotation, *Pediatr Surg Int* 26(8):769–781, 2010.
30. Sweeney B, Surana R, Puri P: Jejunoileal atresia and associated malformations: correlation with the timing of in utero insult, *J Pediatr Surg* 36(5):774–776, 2001.
31. Nehra D, Goldstein AM: Intestinal malrotation: varied clinical presentation from infancy through adulthood, *Surgery* 149(3):386–393, 2011.
32. Lin YP et al: Risk factors for intestinal gangrene in children with small-bowel volvulus, *J Pediatr Gastroenterol Nutr* 53(4):417–422, 2011.
33. Cohen Z et al: How much of a misnomer is "asymptomatic" intestinal malrotation? *Israel Med Assoc J* 5(3):172–174, 2003.
34. Hsiao M, Langer JC: Value of laparoscopy in children with a suspected rotation abnormality on imaging, *J Pediatr Surg* 46(7):1347–1352, 2011.
35. Hagendoorn J et al: Laparoscopic treatment of intestinal malrotation in neonates and infants: retrospective study, *Surg Endosc* 25(1):217–220, 2011.
36. El-Gohary Y, Alagtal M, Gillick J: Long-term complications following operative intervention for intestinal malrotation: a 10-year review, *Pediatr Surg Int* 26(2):203–206, 2010.
37. Efrati O et al: Meconium ileus in patients with cystic fibrosis is not a risk factor for clinical deterioration and survival: the Israeli Multicenter Study, *J Pediatr Gastroenterol Nutr* 50(2):173–178, 2010.
38. Romi H et al: Meconium ileus caused by mutations in GUCY2C, encoding the CFTR-activating guanylate cyclase 2C, *Am J Hum Genet* 90(5):893–899, 2010.
39. McAlister WH, Kronemer KA: Emergency gastrointestinal radiology of the newborn, *Radiol Clin North Am* 34(4):819–844, 1996.
40. Carlyle BE, Borowitz DS, Glick PL: A review of pathophysiology and management of fetuses and neonates with meconium ileus for the pediatric surgeon, *J Pediatr Surg* 47(4):772–781, 2012.
41. Karimi A et al: Issues in the management of simple and complex meconium ileus, *Pediatr Surg Int* 27(9):963–968, 2011.

42. Dray X et al: Distal intestinal obstruction syndrome in adults with cystic fibrosis, *Clin Gastroenterol Hepatol* 2(6):498–502, 2004.
43. Colombo C et al: Guidelines for the diagnosis and management of distal intestinal obstruction syndrome in cystic fibrosis patients, *J Cyst Fibros* 10(Suppl 2):S24–S28, 2011.
44. Uppal K et al: Meckel's diverticulum: a review, *Clin Anat* 24(4):416–422, 2011.
45. Travassos D, van Herwaarden-Lindeboom M, van der Zee DC: Hirschsprung's disease in children with Down syndrome: a comparative study, *Eur J Pediatr Surg* 21(4):220–223, 2011.
46. Wallace AS, Anderson RB: Genetic interactions and modifier genes in Hirschsprung's disease, *World J Gastroenterol* 17(45):4937–4944, 2011.
47. Kenny SE, Tam PK, Garcia-Barcelo M: Hirschsprung's disease, *Semin Pediatr Surg* 19(3):194–200, 2010.
48. Doodnath R, Puri P: A systematic review and meta-analysis of Hirschsprung's disease presenting after childhood, *Pediatr Surg Int* 26(11):1107–1110, 2010.
49. Gourlay DM: Colorectal considerations in pediatric patients, *Surg Clin North Am* 93(1):251–272, 2013.
50. Khan AR, Vujanic GM, Huddart S: The constipated child: how likely is Hirschsprung disease? *Pediatr Surg Int* 19(6):439–442, 2003.
51. Noviello C et al: Diagnosis of Hirschsprung's disease: an age-related approach in children below or above one year, *Colorectal Dis* 12(10):1044–1048, 2010.
52. O'Donnell AM, Puri P: Skip segment Hirschsprung's disease: a systematic review, *Pediatr Surg Int* 26(11):1065–1069, 2010.
53. Chumpitazi BP, Nurko S: Defecation disorders in children after surgery for Hirschsprung disease, *J Pediatr Gastroenterol Nutr* 53(1):75–79, 2011.
54. Marcelis C, de Blaauw I, Brunner H: Chromosomal anomalies in the etiology of anorectal malformations: a review, *Am J Med Genet A* 155A(11):2692–2704, 2011.
55. Forrester MB, Merz RD: Risk of selected birth defects with prenatal illicit drug use, Hawaii, 1986-2002, *J Toxicol Environ Health A* 70:7–18, 2007.
56. Levitt MA, Pena A: Anorectal malformations, *Orphanet J Rare Dis* 2:33, 2007.
57. England RJ et al: Laparoscopic repair of anorectal malformations at the Red Cross War Memorial Children's Hospital: taking stock, *J Pediatr Surg* 47(3):565–570, 2012.
58. Mirza B et al: Anorectal malformations in neonates, *Afr J Paediatr Surg* 8(2):151–154, 2011.
59. Pepper VK, Stanfill AB, Pearl RH: Diagnosis and management of pediatric appendicitis, intussusception, and Meckel diverticulum, *Surg Clin North Am* 92(3):505–526, vii, 2012.
60. Fischer TK et al: Intussusception in early childhood: a cohort study of 1.7 million children, *Pediatrics* 114:782–785, 2004.
61. Byrne AT et al: The imaging of intussusception, *Clin Radiol* 60(3):412, 2005.
62. Gilmore AW, Reed M, Tenenbein M: Management of childhood intussusception after reduction by enema, *Am J Emerg Med* 29(9):1136–1140, 2011.
63. Justice FA et al: Recurrent intussusception in infants, *J Paediatr Child Health* 47(11):802–805, 2011.
64. Parikh M et al: Does all small bowel intussusception need exploration? *Afr J Paediatr Surg* 7(1):30–32, 2010.
65. Blanco FC, Davenport KP, Kane TD: Pediatric gastroesophageal reflux disease, *Surg Clin North Am* 92(3):541–558, viii, 2012.
66. Fletcher KC et al: Significance and degree of reflux in patients with primary extraesophageal symptoms, *Laryngoscope* 121(12):2561–2565, 2011.
67. McCoul ED et al: A prospective study of the effect of gastroesophageal reflux disease treatment on children with otitis media, *Arch Otolaryngol Head Neck Surg* 137(1):35–41, 2011.
68. Praud JP: Upper airway reflexes in response to gastric reflux, *Paediatr Respir Rev* 11(4):208–212, 2010.
69. Sridhara S et al: Increased numbers of eosinophils, rather than only etiology, predict histologic changes in patients with esophageal eosinophilia, *Clin Gastroenterol Hepatol* 10(7):735–741, 2012.
70. Blatman KH, Ditto AM: Chapter 26: Eosinophilic esophagitis, *Allergy Asthma Proc* 33(Suppl 1):S88–S90, 2012.
71. Ciorba A et al: Gastroesophageal reflux and its possible role in the pathogenesis of upper aerodigestive tract disorders, *Minerva Gastroenterol Dietol* 53(2):171–180, 2007.
72. Rohen R, Nurko S: The importance of multichannel intraluminal impedence in the evaluation of children with persistent respiratory symptoms, *Am J Gastroenterol* 99(12):2452–2458, 2004.
73. McGovern MC, Smith MB: Causes of apparent life threatening events in infants: a systematic review, *Arch Dis Child* 89(11):1043–1048, 2004.
74. Fike FB et al: Diagnosis of gastroesophageal reflux disease in infants, *Pediatr Surg Int* 27(8):791–797, 2011.
75. Goldani HA, Nunes DL, Ferreira CT: Managing gastroesophageal reflux disease in children: the role of endoscopy, *World J Gastrointest Endosc* 4(8):339–346, 2012.
76. Loots CM, Benninga MA, Omari TI: Gastroesophageal reflux in pediatrics; (patho)physiology and new insights in diagnostics and treatment, *Minerva Pediatr* 64(1):101–119, 2012.
77. Craig WR et al: Metoclopramide, thickened feedings, and positioning for gastro-oesophageal reflux in children under two years, *Cochrane Database Syst Rev* (4):CDC003502, 2004.
78. Czinn SJ, Blanchard S: Gastroesophageal reflux disease in neonates and infants: when and how to treat, *Paediatr Drugs* 15(1):19–27, 2013.
79. Jadcherla SR et al: Impact of feeding strategies on the frequency and clearance of acid and nonacid gastroesophageal reflux events in dysphagic neonates, *JPEN J Parenter Enteral Nutr* 36(4):449–455, 2012.
80. Lightdale JR, Gremse DA: Gastroesophageal reflux: management guidance for the pediatrician, *Pediatrics* 131(5):e1684–1695, 2013.
81. Mauritz FA et al: The effects and efficacy of antireflux surgery in children with gastroesophageal reflux disease: a systematic review, *J Gastrointest Surg* 15(10):1872–1878, 2011.
82. Herrmann U, Dockter G, Lammert F: Cystic fibrosis-associated liver disease, *Best Pract Res Clin Gastroenterol* 24(5):585–592, 2010.
83. Javier RM, Jacquot J: Bone disease in cystic fibrosis: what's new? *Joint Bone Spine* 78(5):445–450, 2011.
84. Scaparrotta A et al: Growth failure in children with cystic fibrosis, *J Pediatr Endocrinol Metab* 25(5-6):393–405, 2012.
85. Domínguez-Muñoz JE: Pancreatic exocrine insufficiency: diagnosis and treatment, *J Gastroenterol Hepatol* 26(Suppl 2):12–16, 2011.
86. Borowitz D et al: Liprotamase long-term safety and support of nutritional status in pancreatic-insufficient cystic fibrosis, *J Pediatr Gastroenterol Nutr* 54(2):248–257, 2012.
87. Bradley GM et al: Nutritional outcomes following gastrostomy in children with cystic fibrosis, *Pediatr Pulmonol* 47(8):743–748, 2012.
88. Conway SP, Morton A, Wolfe S: Enteral tube feeding for cystic fibrosis, *Cochrane Database Syst Rev* (2):CD001198, 2008.
89. Rubio-Tapia A et al: The prevalence of celiac disease in the United States, *Am J Gastroenterol* 107(10):1538–1544, 2012.
90. Rubio-Tapia A, Murray JA: Celiac disease, *Curr Opin Gastroenterol* 26(2):116–122, 2010.
91. Miśkiewicz P, Kępczyńska-Nyk A, Bednarczuk T: Coeliac disease in endocrine diseases of autoimmune origin, *Endokrynol Pol* 63(3): 240–249, 2012.
92. Cianci R et al: New insights on the role of T cells in the pathogenesis of celiac disease, *J Biol Regul Homeost Agents* 26(2):171–179, 2012.
93. Di Sabatino A et al: The function of tissue transglutaminase in celiac disease, *Autoimmun Rev* 11(10):746–753, 2012.
94. Lionetti E, Catassi C: New clues in celiac disease epidemiology, pathogenesis, clinical manifestations, and treatment, *Int Rev Immunol* 30(4):219–231, 2011.
95. Mubarak A, Houwen RH, Wolters VM: Celiac disease: an overview from pathophysiology to treatment, *Minerva Pediatr* 64(3):271–287, 2012.
96. Bonciolini V et al: Newly described clinical and immunopathological feature of dermatitis herpetiformis, *Clin Dev Immunol* 2012:967974, 2012.
97. Kneepkens CM, von Blomberg BM: Clinical practice: coeliac disease, *Eur J Pediatr* 171(7):1011–1021, 2012.
98. Catassi C, Fasano A: Celiac disease as a cause of growth retardation in children, *Curr Opin Pediatr* 16(4):445–449, 2004.
99. Larussa T et al: Bone mineralization in celiac disease, *Gastroenterol Res Pract* 2012:198025, 2012.
100. Ravelli A, Villanacci V: Tricks of the trade: how to avoid histological pitfalls in celiac disease, *Pathol Res Pract* 208(4):197–202, 2012.
101. Ojetti V et al: Regression of lactose malabsorption in celiac patients after receiving a gluten-free diet, *Scand J Gastroenterol* 43(2):174–177, 2008.
102. Guandalini S: The influence of gluten: weaning recommendations for healthy children and children at risk for celiac disease, *Nestle Nutr Workshop Ser Pediatr Program* 60:139–151, 2007.
103. Leslie LA et al: Incidence of lymphoproliferative disorders in patients with celiac disease, *Am J Hematol* 87(8):754–759, 2012.
104. Musoke PM, Fergusson P: Severe malnutrition and metabolic complications of HIV-infected children in the antiretroviral era: clinical care and management in resource-limited settings, *Am J Clin Nutr* 94(6): 1716S–1720S, 2011.

105. Imdad A, Sadiq K, Bhutta ZA: Evidence-based prevention of childhood malnutrition, *Curr Opin Clin Nutr Metab Care* 14(3):276–285, 2011.
106. Pelletier DL: The relationship between child anthropometry and mortality in developing countries: implications for policy, programs and future research, *J Nutr* 123(Suppl 10):2047S–2081S, 1994.
107. Prieto MB, Cid JL: Malnutrition in the critically ill child: the importance of enteral nutrition, *Int J Environ Res Public Health* 8(11):4353–4366, 2011.
108. Manary MJ, Brewster DR: Intensive nursing care of kwashiorkor in Malawi, *Acta Paediatr* 89(2):203–207, 2000.
109. Ogumkeye OO, Ighogboja IS: Increase in total serum triglyceride and phospholipids in kwashiorkor, *Ann Trop Pediatr* 12(4):463–466, 1992.
110. Maida JM, Mathers K, Alley CL: Pediatric ophthalmology in the developing world, *Curr Opin Ophthalmol* 19(5):403–408, 2008.
111. Latham MC: The dermatosis of kwashiorkor in young children, *Semin Dermatol* 10(4):270–272, 1991.
112. Ahmed T et al: Management of severe malnutrition and diarrhea, *Indian J Pediatr* 68(1):45–51, 2001.
113. Greco L et al: Effect of a low-cost food on the recovery and death rate of malnourished children, *J Pediatr Gastroenterol Nutr* 43(4):512–517, 2006.
114. Thakur G, Singh HP, Patel C: Locally-prepared ready-to-use therapeutic food for children with severe acute malnutrition: a controlled trial, *Indian Pediatr*, 2012 Oct 5. [Epub ahead of print.].
115. Vygen SB et al: Treatment of severe acute malnutrition in infants aged <6 months in Niger, *J Pediatr*, 2012 Oct 20. [Epub ahead of print.].
116. Picot J et al: The effectiveness of interventions to treat severe acute malnutrition in young children: a systematic review, *Health Technol Assess* 16(19):1–316, 2012.
116a. Alcoba G et al: Do children with uncomplicated severe acute malnutrition need antibiotics? A systematic review and meta-analysis, *PLoS One* 8(1):e53184, 2013.
117. Atalay A, McCord M: Characteristics of failure to thrive in a referral population: implications for treatment, *Clin Pediatr (Phila)* 51(3): 219–225, 2012.
118. Levy Y et al: Diagnostic clues for identification of nonorganic vs organic causes of food refusal and poor feeding, *J Pediatr Gastroenterol Nutr* 48(3):355–362, 2009.
119. Nützenadel W: Failure to thrive in childhood, *Dtsch Arztebl Int* 108(38):642–649, 2011.
120. Piazza CC et al: Functional analysis of inappropriate mealtime behaviors, *J Appl Behav Anal* 36(2):187–204, 2003.
121. Steward DK: Behavioral characteristics of infants with nonorganic failure to thrive during a play interaction, *MCN Am J Matern Child Nurs* 26(2):79–85, 2001.
122. Bergman P, Graham J: An approach to "failure to thrive, " *Aust Fam Physician* 34(9):725–729, 2005.
123. Mash C et al: Development of a risk-stratification tool for medical child abuse in failure to thrive, *Pediatrics* 128(6):e1467–e1473, 2011.
124. Black MM et al: Early intervention and recovery among children with failure to thrive: follow-up at age 8, *Pediatrics* 120(1):59–69, 2007.
125. Silverman AH: Interdisciplinary care for feeding problems in children, *Nutr Clin Pract* 25(2):160–165, 2010.
126. Lin PW, Stoll BJ: Necrotizing enterocolitis, *Lancet* 368(9543):1271–1283, 2006.
127. Lee JS, Polin RA: Treatment and prevention of necrotizing enterocolitis, *Semin Neonatol* 8(6):449–459, 2003.
128. Lambert DK et al: Necrotizing enterocolitis in term neonates: data from a multihospital health-care system, *J Perinatol* 27(7):437–443, 2007.
129. Berman L, Moss RL: Necrotizing enterocolitis: an update, *Semin Fetal Neonatal Med* 16(3):145–150, 2011.
130. Thompson AM, Bizzarro MJ: Necrotizing enterocolitis in newborns: pathogenesis, prevention and management, *Drugs* 68(9):1227–1238, 2008.
131. Emami CN et al: Role of the host defense system and intestinal microbial flora in the pathogenesis of necrotizing enterocolitis, *Surg Infect (Larchmt)* 10(5):407–417, 2009.
131a. McElroy SJ, Underwood MA, Sherman MP: Paneth cells and necrotizing enterocolitis: a novel hypothesis for disease pathogenesis, *Neonatology*(1)10–20, 2013.
132. Lee JH: An update on necrotizing enterocolitis: pathogenesis and preventive strategies, *Korean J Pediatr* 54(9):368–372, 2011.
133. Patel BK, Shah JS: Necrotizing enterocolitis in very low birth weight infants: a systemic review, *ISRN Gastroenterol* 2012:562594, 2012.
134. Kabeer A, Gunnlaugsson S, Coren C: Neonatal necrotizing enterocolitis: a 12-year review at a county hospital, *Dis Colon Rectum* 38(8):866–872, 1995.
135. Alfaleh K, Bassler D: Probiotics for prevention of necrotizing enterocolitis in preterm infants, *Cochrane Database Syst Rev* (1):CD005496, 2008.
136. Christensen RD, Gordon PV, Besner GE: Can we cut the incidence of necrotizing enterocolitis in half today? *Fetal Pediatr Pathol* 29(4): 185–198, 2010.
137. Siggers RH et al: Nutritional modulation of the gut microbiota and immune system in preterm neonates susceptible to necrotizing enterocolitis, *J Nutr Biochem* 22(6):511–521, 2011.
138. Mihatsch WA et al: Critical systematic review of the level of evidence for routine use of probiotics for reduction of mortality and prevention of necrotizing enterocolitis and sepsis in preterm infants, *Clin Nutr* 31(1):6–15, 2012.
139. Morgan JA, Young L, McGuire W: Pathogenesis and prevention of necrotizing enterocolitis, *Curr Opin Infect Dis* 24(3):183–189, 2011.
140. Shah D, Sinn JK: Antibiotic regimens for the empirical treatment of newborn infants with necrotising enterocolitis, *Cochrane Database Syst Rev* (8):CD007448, 2012.
141. Lee JH: An update on necrotizing enterocolitis: pathogenesis and preventive strategies, *Korean J Pediatr* 54(9):368–372, 2011.
142. Morgan J, Young L, McGuire W: Delayed introduction of progressive enteral feeds to prevent necrotising enterocolitis in very low birth weight infants, *Cochrane Database Syst Rev* (3):CD001970, 2011.
143. Dominguez KM, Moss RL: Necrotizing enterocolitis, *Clin Perinatol* 39(2):387–401, 2012.
144. Choo S et al: Outcomes analysis after percutaneous abdominal drainage and exploratory laparotomy for necrotizing enterocolitis in 4657 infants, *Pediatr Surg Int* 27(7):747–753, 2011.
145. Pike K et al: Outcomes at 7 years for babies who developed neonatal necrotising enterocolitis: the ORACLE Children Study, *Arch Dis Child Fetal Neonatal Ed* 97(5):F318–F322, 2012.
146. Lao OB et al: Outcomes in children after intestinal transplant, *Pediatrics* 125(3):e550–e558, 2010.
147. Romão RL et al: Preserving bowel length with a transluminal stent in neonates with multiple intestinal anastomoses: a case series and review of the literature, *J Pediatr Surg* 46(7):1368–1372, 2011.
148. Finkbeiner SR et al: Metagenomic analysis of human diarrhea: vial detection and discovery, *PLoS Pathol* 4(2):e1000011, 2008.
149. Dennehy PH: Rotavirus infection: an update on management and prevention, *Adv Pediatr* 59(1):47–74, 2012.
150. Enoch DA et al: *Clostridium difficile* in children: colonisation and disease, *J Infect* 63(2):105–113, 2011.
151. Johnston BC et al: Probiotics for the prevention of *Clostridium difficile*–associated diarrhea: a systematic review and meta-analysis, *Ann Intern Med*, 2012 Nov 13. [E-pub ahead of print.].
152. Colletti JE et al: The management of children with gastroenteritis and dehydration in the emergency department, *J Emerg Med* 38(5):686–698, 2010.
153. Lazzerini M, Ronfani L: Oral zinc for treating diarrhoea in children, *Cochrane Database Syst Rev* (6):CD005436, 2012.
154. Moore SR: Update on prolonged and persistent diarrhea in children, *Curr Opin Gastroenterol* 27(1):19–23, 2011.
155. Patel A et al: Therapeutic value of zinc supplementation in acute and persistent diarrhea: a systematic review, *PLoS One* 5(4):e10386, 2010.
156. He T et al: Effects of yogurt and bifidobacteria supplementation on the colonic microbiota in lactose-intolerant subjects, *J Appl Microbiol* 104(2):595–604, 2008.
157. National Medical Association: Lactose intolerance and African Americans: implications for the consumption of appropriate intake levels of key nutrients, *J Natl Med Assoc* 101(Suppl 10):5S–23S, 2009.
158. Teitelbaum JE, Ubhrani D: Triple sugar screen breath hydrogen test for sugar intolerance in children with functional abdominal symptoms, *Indian J Gastroenterol* 29(5):196–200, 2010.
159. Chou SC et al: Management of hyperbilirubinemia in newborns: measuring performance by using a benchmarking model, *Pediatrics* 112(6):1264–1273, 2003.
160. Colletti JE et al: An emergency medicine approach to neonatal hyperbilirubinemia, *Emerg Med Clin North Am* 25(4):1117–1135, 2007. vii.
161. Gazzin S, Tiribelli C: Bilirubin-induced neurological damage, *J Matern Fetal Neonatal Med* 24(Suppl 1):154–155, 2011.
162. Cappellini MD, Fiorelli G: Glucose-6-phosphate dehydrogenase deficiency, *Lancet* 371(9606):64–74, 2008.
163. Kaplan M, Hammerman C: Neonatal screening for glucose-6-phosphate dehydrogenase deficiency: biochemical versus genetic technologies, *Semin Perinatol* 35(3):155–161, 2011.
164. Alexandra Brito M, Silva RF: Brites D: Bilirubin toxicity to human erythrocytes: a review, *Clin Chim Acta* 374(1-2):46–56, 2006.
165. Shapiro SM: Chronic bilirubin encephalopathy: diagnosis and outcome, *Semin Fetal Neonatal Med* 15(3):157–163, 2010.

166. Sato Y et al: Is bilirubin/albumin ratio correlated with unbound bilirubin concentration? *Pediatr Int* 54(1):81–85, 2012.
167. American Academy of Pediatrics: Management of hyperbilirubinemia in the newborn infant 35 or more weeks of gestation, *Pediatrics* 114(1):297–316, 2004. Available at http://aappolicy.aappublications.org/cgi/content/full/pediatrics;114/1/297.
168. Hansen TW: Prevention of neurodevelopmental sequelae of jaundice in the newborn, *Dev Med Child Neurol* 53(Suppl 4):24–28, 2011.
169. Schwartz HP, Haberman BE, Ruddy RM: Hyperbilirubinemia: current guidelines and emerging therapies, *Pediatr Emerg Care* 27(9):884–889, 2011.
170. Bessho K, Bezerra JA: Biliary atresia: will blocking inflammation tame the disease? *Ann Rev Med* 62:171–185, 2011.
171. Feldman AG, Mack CL: Biliary atresia: cellular dynamics and immune dysregulation, *Semin Pediatr Surg* 21(3):192–200, 2012.
172. Haafiz AB: Liver fibrosis in biliary atresia, *Exp Rev Gastroenterol Hepatol* 4(3):335–343, 2010.
173. De Bruyne R et al: Clinical practice: neonatal cholestasis, *Eur J Pediatr* 170(3):279–284, 2011.
174. Pakarinen MP, Rintala RJ: Surgery of biliary atresia, *Scand J Surg* 100(1):49–53, 2011.
175. Lacaille F: Liver transplantation and liver cell transplantation, *Clin Res Hepatol Gastroenterol* 36(3):304–307, 2012.
176. Armstrong GL, Bell BP: Hepatitis A virus infections in the United States: model-based estimates and implications for childhood immunizations, *Pediatrics* 109(5):839–845, 2002.
177. Muecke CJ et al: Hepatitis A seroprevalence and risk factors among day care educators, *Clin Invest Med* 27(5):259–264, 2004.
178. Koslap-Petraco MB, Shub M, Judelsohn R: Hepatitis A: disease burden and current childhood vaccination strategies in the United States, *J Pediatr Health Care* 22(1):3–11, 2008.
179. Centers for Disease Control and Prevention: Prevention of hepatitis A through active or passive immunization: recommendations of the Advisory Committee on Immunizations Practices, *MMWR* 55(RR-7):1–23, 2006.
180. Ni YH: Natural history of hepatitis B virus infection: pediatric perspective, *J Gastroenterol* 46(1):1–8, 2011.
181. World Health Organization: *Hepatitis B fact sheet no. 204, July 2012*. Available at www.who.int/mediacentre/factsheets/fs204/en/.
182. Rapti IN, Hadziyannis SJ: Treatment of special populations with chronic hepatitis B infection, *Exp Rev Gastroenterol Hepatol* 5(3):323–339, 2011.
183. Tran TT, Hepatitis B: treatment to prevent perinatal transmission, *Clin Obstet Gynecol* 55(2):541–549, 2012.
184. Yousef Y et al: Predictive factors of lamivudine treatment success in a hepatitis B virus-infected pediatric cohort: a 10-year study, *Can J Gastroenterol* 26(7):429–435, 2012.
185. Robinson JL, Doucette K: The natural history of hepatitis C virus infection acquired during childhood, *Liver Int* 32(2):258–270, 2012.
186. Roberts EA: Autoimmune hepatitis from the paediatric perspective, *Liver Int* 31(10):1424–1431, 2011.
187. Jonas MM et al: Treatment of children with chronic hepatitis B virus infection in the United States: patient selection and therapeutic options, *Hepatology* 52(6):2192–2205, 2010.
188. Porto AF, Tormey L, Lim JK: Management of chronic hepatitis C infection in children, *Curr Opin Pediatr* 24(1):113–120, 2012.
189. Sinatra FR: Nonalcoholic fatty liver disease in pediatric patients, *JPEN J Parenter Enteral Nutr* 36(Suppl 1):43S–48S, 2012.
190. Behrman RE, Kliegman R, Jenson HB: *Nelson textbook of pediatrics*, ed 18, Philadelphia, 2007, Saunders.
191. Poddar U, Borkar V: Management of extra hepatic portal venous obstruction (EHPVO): current strategies, *Trop Gastroenterol* 32(2):94–102, 2011.
192. Grimaldi C et al: Portal hypertension in children, *Clin Res Hepatol Gastroenterol* 36(3):260–261, 2012.
193. Gugig R, Rosenthal P: Management of portal hypertension in children, *World J Gastroenterol* 18(11):1176–1184, 2012.
194. Lillegard JB et al: A single-institution review of portosystemic shunts in children: an ongoing discussion, *HPB Surg*, 2010:964597, 2010.
195. Berry GT: Galactosemia and amenorrhea in the adolescent, *Ann N Y Acad Sci* 1135:112–117, 2008.
196. Ala A et al: Wilson's disease, *Lancet* 369(9559):397–408, 2008.
197. Brewer GJ: Recognition, diagnosis, and management of Wilson disease, *Proc Soc Exp Biol Med* 233(1):39–46, 2000.
198. Rosencrantz R, Schilsky M: Wilson disease: pathogenesis and clinical considerations in diagnosis and treatment, *Semin Liver Dis* 31(3):245–259, 2011.
199. Mak CM, Lam CW: Diagnosis of Wilson's disease: a comprehensive review, *Crit Rev Clin Lab Sci* 45(3):263–290, 2008.
200. Stremmel W et al: Wilson disease: clinical presentation, treatment, and survival, *Ann Intern Med* 115(9):720–726, 1991.
201. Bennett J, Hahn SH: Clinical molecular diagnosis of Wilson disease, *Semin Liver Dis* 31(3):233–238, 2011.
202. Purchase R: The treatment of Wilson's disease, a rare genetic disorder of copper metabolism, *Sci Prog* 96(Pt 1):19–32, 2013.
203. Catana AM, Medici V: Liver transplantation for Wilson disease, *World J Hepatol* 4(1):5–10, 2010.

CHAPTER

43

Structure and Function of the Musculoskeletal System

Christy L. Crowther-Radulewicz

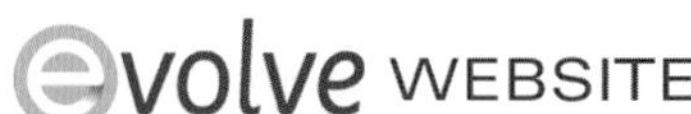

http://evolve.elsevier.com/McCance/

- Review Questions and Answers

CHAPTER OUTLINE

The way an individual functions in daily life, moves about, or manipulates objects physically depends on the integrity of the musculoskeletal system. The musculoskeletal system is actually composed of two systems: (1) the skeleton proper, which is composed of bones and joints; and (2) skeletal muscles. Each of the systems contributes to mobility. The skeleton supports the body and provides leverage to the skeletal muscles so that movement of various parts of the body is possible. This movement is accomplished by contraction of the skeletal muscles and bending or rotation at the joints.

STRUCTURE AND FUNCTION OF BONES

Bones give form to the body, support tissues, and permit movement by providing points of attachment for muscles. Many bones meet in movable joints that determine the type and extent of movement possible. Bones also protect many of the body's vital organs. For example, the bones of the skull, thorax, and pelvis are hard exterior shields that protect the brain, heart, lungs, and reproductive and urinary organs.

Bone marrow is one of the sources of **mesenchymal stem cells (MSCs)** (Figure 43-1). These nonhematopoietic stem cells consist of a small proportion of the stromal cell population in the bone marrow, and can generate bone, cartilage, fat, cells that support the formation of blood, and fibrous connective tissue. Within certain bones, the marrow cavities also serve as storage site for the hematopoietic stem cells that form both blood and immune cells. In adults, blood cells originate exclusively in the marrow cavities of the skull, vertebrae, ribs, sternum, scapulae, and pelvis. Bones also have a crucial role in mineral homeostasis, and storing and releasing minerals (i.e., calcium, phosphate, carbonate, magnesium) that are essential for the proper working of many delicate cellular mechanisms.

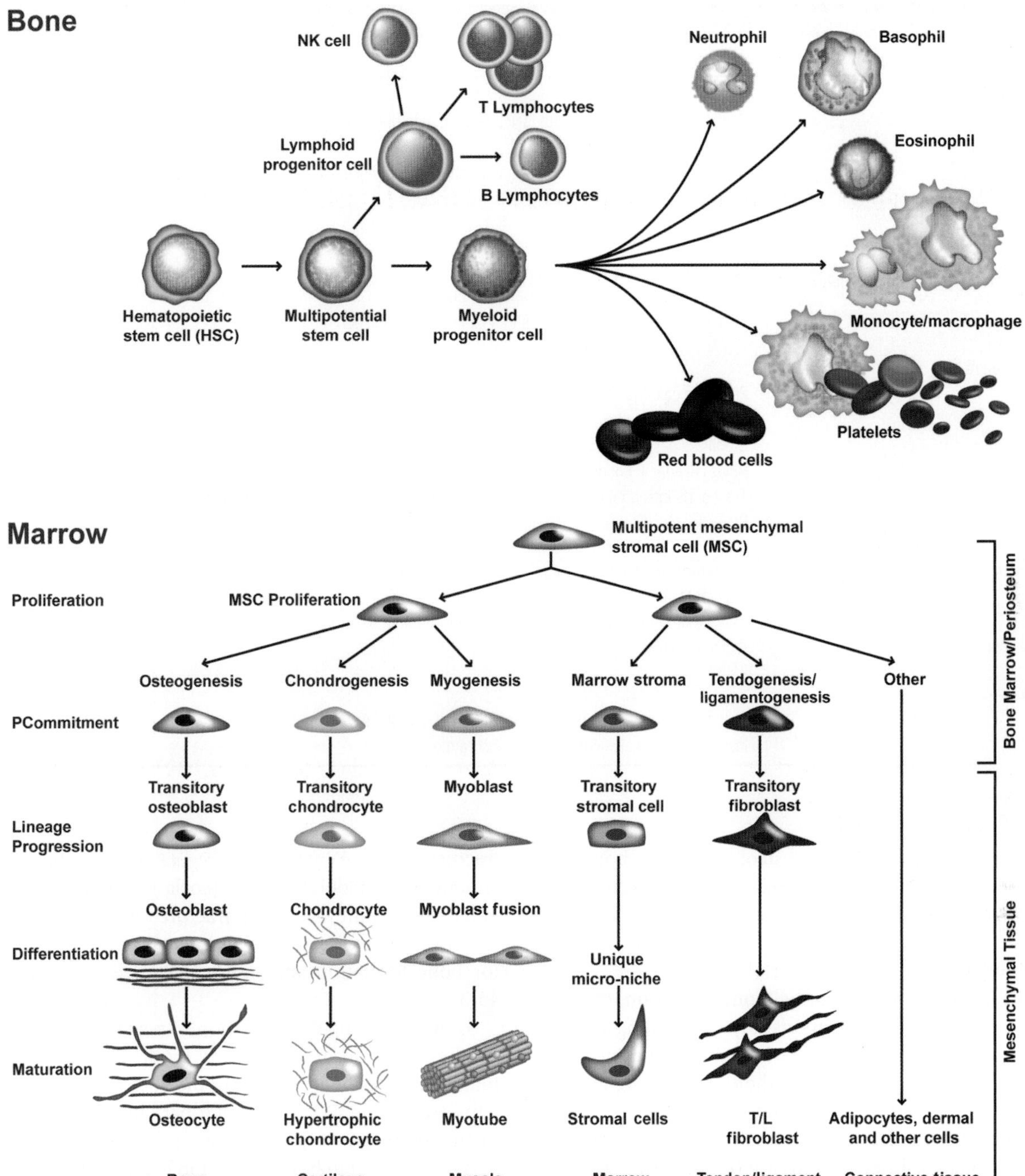

FIGURE 43-1 Hematopoietic and Mesenchymal Stromal Cell Differentiation. Undifferentiated hematopoietic and mesenchymal multipotential cells give rise to a variety of cell types with distinct functions. (Adapted from abcam.com.)

Elements of Bone Tissue

Mature bone is a rigid yet flexible connective tissue consisting of cells, fibers, a gelatinous material termed **ground substance,** and large amounts of crystallized minerals, mainly calcium, that give bone its rigidity. The structural elements of bone are summarized in Table 43-1.

Bone cells enable bone to grow, repair itself, change shape, and continuously synthesize new bone tissue and resorb (dissolve or digest) old tissue. The fibers in bone are made of collagen, which gives bone its tensile strength (the ability to hold itself together). Ground substance acts as a medium for the diffusion of nutrients, oxygen, metabolic wastes, biochemicals, and minerals between bone tissue and blood vessels.

Bone formation arises during embryonic development when mesenchymal stem cells begin differentiating into either chondrocytes or preosteoblasts. Endochondral ossification and intramembranous bone formation are the two major mechanisms responsible for normal bone development.

Endochondral ossification occurs when mesenchymal (**mesenchyme,** or loose tissue found during embryonic development) stem cells begin differentiating into chondrocytes (see Figure 43-1), which in turn develop a mineralized cartilage

TABLE 43-1 STRUCTURAL ELEMENTS OF BONE

STRUCTURAL ELEMENT	FUNCTION
Bone Cells	
Osteoblasts	Synthesize collagen and proteoglycans; stimulate bone formation and are also involved in some osteoclast resorptive activity
Osteocytes	Maintain bone matrix; act as mechanoreceptors; influence osteoblasts and osteoclasts
Osteoclasts	Resorb bone; major role in mineral homeostasis
Bone Matrix	
Collagen fibers	Lend support and tensile strength
Proteoglycans	Control transport of ionized materials through matrix
Bone morphogenic proteins (BMPs)*	Induce cartilage, bone, tendon, and ligament formation and repair
Glycoproteins	
Sialoprotein	Promotes calcification
Osteocalcin	Inhibits calcium-phosphate precipitation; promotes bone resorption
Laminin	Stabilizes basement membranes in bones
Osteonectin	Binds calcium in bones
Albumin	Transports essential elements to matrix; maintains osmotic pressure of bone fluid
α-Glycoprotein	Promotes calcification
Minerals (Elements)	Crystallizes to lend rigidity and compressive strength
Calcium	Regulates vitamin D and thereby promotes mineralization
Phosphate	Balance of organic and inorganic phosphate required for proper bone mineralization; regulates vitamin D
Alkaline phosphatase	Promotes mineralization
Vitamins	
Vitamin D	Assists with differentiation, mineralization of osteoblasts
Vitamin K	Increases bone calcification; reduces serum osteocalcin

*See Table 43-2 for BMP functions.

scaffold that allows formation of osteoblasts. Most bone elements are formed this way. With the second mechanism, **intramembranous bone formation,** mesenchymal stem cells differentiate into a preosteoblast line that then forms osteoblasts without any cartilage framework.[1,2]

Multiple factors influence normal bone formation, maintenance, and remodeling. The superfamily of signaling factors, containing more than 40 members including bone morphogenic proteins (BMPs), is known as the **transforming growth factor-beta (TGF-β)** family. This group is primarily responsible for initiation, differentiation, and commitment of precursor cells into osteoblasts. TGF-β signals are transmitted across the plasma membrane, combine with certain proteins that act as transcription factors (Smads), and then form specific receptors known as R-Smads. These receptors, in turn, initiate intracellular signaling, interact with other transcription factors, and regulate other factors that are important in osteoblast formation, function, and maintenance.[3] Crosstalk between signaling pathways (including TGF-β, BMPs, FGF, Wnt, Notch, MAPK, and Hedgehog) is critical in regulating osteoblasts.

BMPs have multiple crucial functions in the skeletal system. BMP activities are regulated at different molecular levels. Table 43-2 summarizes the role of several important BMPs.

Wnt genes belong to a large family of protein-signaling factors that are required for the development of body systems, including the musculoskeletal system. They play a significant role in forming bone, developing bone mass, remodeling, and fracture healing. Wnt signaling regulates production and differentiation of osteoblasts and osteoclasts, and affects bone mass and density, joint formation, fracture repair, bone remodeling, and some bone diseases. Other important elements responsible for bone formation and homeostasis are presented in Table 43-3.

In mature bone the formation of new tissue begins with the production of an organic matrix by the bone cells. This **bone matrix** consists of ground substances, collagen, and other proteins (see Table 43-1) that take part in bone formation and maintenance.

The next step in bone formation is **calcification,** when minerals are deposited and crystallize. Minerals bind tightly to collagen fibers, producing tensile and compressional strength in bone, and withstand pressure and weightbearing.

Bone Cells

Bone contains three types of cells: osteoblasts, osteocytes, and osteoclasts (Figure 43-2). Osteoblasts are the bone-forming cells, whose primary function is to lay down new bone. Once this function is complete, osteoblasts become osteocytes that are imbedded in bone. Comprising 90% to 95% of bone cells, osteocytes develop dendritic processes that extend to either the bone surface or the bone's vascular space.[4] They help maintain bone by signaling osteoblasts and osteoclasts to form and resorb bone.[5] Osteoclasts are the major bone-resorbing cells responsible for remodeling.

TABLE 43-2 BONE MORPHOGENIC PROTEINS (BMPs) AND THEIR KNOWN FUNCTIONS

BMP	KNOWN FUNCTION
BMP1	Cartilage development; is actually a metalloprotease; key role in extracellular matrix (ECM) formation
BMP2	Induces bone and cartilage formation, osteoblast differentiation, bone healing
BMP3 (osteogenin)	Induces bone formation
BMP4	Regulates formation of teeth, limbs, and bone
BMP5	Involved in cartilage development
BMP6	Found in osteoblasts; helps maintain adult joint integrity; accelerates bone repair
BMP7	Major role in osteoblast differentiation, chondrocyte formation, fracture healing; important in renal development and repair
BMP8a	Bone and cartilage development; up-regulated in fracture nonunion
BMP9	Induces osteogenesis in mature osteoblasts
BMP10	Plays role in development of the heart
BMP12 (cartilage-derived morphogenic protein-3; CDMP-3)	Tendon and ligament formation
BMP13	Cartilage development; tendon and ligament repair
BMP14	Assists in bone and tendon healing; cartilage formation

Data from Caetano-Lopes J, Canhão H, Fonseca JE: *Arthritis Res Ther* 9(Suppl 1):S1, 2007; Hojo H et al: *J Bone Miner Metab* 28(5):489–502, 2010; Fajardo M, Liu C-J, Egol K: *Clin Orthop Relat Res* 467(12):3071–3078, 2009; Li Y et al: *Zhong Nan Da Xue Xue Bao Yi Xue Ban* 37(1):1–5, 2012.

TABLE 43-3 SELECTED FACTORS AFFECTING BONE FORMATION AND HOMEOSTASIS

FACTOR	FUNCTION
Transforming growth factor-beta (TGF-β)	Superfamily of polypeptides; regulates bone formation, many other cellular processes though signaling
Platelet-derived growth factor (PDGF)	Increases number of osteoblasts
Fibroblast growth factor-2 (FGF)	FGF-2 increases osteoblast population, but not function; inhibits alkaline phosphatase activity, osteocalcin, type 1 collagen, and osteopontin
Insulin-like growth factor (IGF)	
IGF-1	Increases peak bone mass during adolescence; decreases osteoblast apoptosis; maintains bone matrix
IGF-2	Increases BMP-9–induced endochondral ossification
Smad proteins	Mediate the signaling cascade of transforming growth factor-beta (TGF-β), especially in embryonic bone development; play a role in crosstalk between BMP/TGF-β and Wnt signaling pathways
Bone morphogenic proteins (BMPs)	Members of transforming growth factor-beta (TGF-β) superfamily of polypeptides; have many functions outside skeletal system; stimulate endochondral bone and cartilage formation and function, promote osteoblast maturation; augment bone remodeling by affecting both osteoblasts and osteoclasts
Tumor necrosis factors (TNFs)	Superfamily of cytokines; play major role in regulating bone metabolism, especially osteoclast function
Osteoprotegerin (OPG)	Inhibits bone remodeling/resorption; produced by several cells, including osteoblasts; is a decoy receptor for RANKL (binds to RANKL, inhibiting RANK/RANKL interactions, suppressing osteoclast formation and bone resorption)
Receptor activator of nuclear factor κβ (RANK)	Stimulates differentiation of osteoclast precursors; activates mature osteoclasts
Bone morphogenic protein antagonists	Prevent BMP signaling
Noggin	Binds BMP-2 and BMP-4, reducing osteoblast function
Gremlin	Multiple effects in and out of skeletal system, but also binds BMP-2, -4, and -7; may play a role in development of osteoporosis
Twisted gastrulation	Acts as either a BMP agonist or an antagonist
Activin (a BMP-related protein)	Affects both osteoblasts and osteoclasts; may promote bone formation and fracture healing; expressed by both osteoblasts and chondrocytes; helps regulate bone mass
Inhibin	Dominant over activin and BMPs; helps regulate bone mass and strength by affecting formation of osteoblasts and osteoclasts
Leptin	Plays role in bone formation and resorption
Wnt (a signaling pathway)	Important in differentiating osteoblasts and bone formation; has overlapping effects with BMPs; helps regulate bone formation and remodeling
Wnt antagonists	
Dickkopf family (Dkk)	Disrupt Wnt signaling, leading to reduced bone mass
Sclerostin	Protein secreted by osteocytes, osteoblasts, and osteoclasts; binds to BMP-6 and BMP-7; interferes with Wnt signaling pathway, inhibiting bone formation by osteoblasts

Continued

TABLE 43-3 SELECTED FACTORS AFFECTING BONE FORMATION AND HOMEOSTASIS—cont'd

FACTOR	FUNCTION
Transcription Factors	
Nuclear factor of activated κβ cells (NF-κβ)	Affects embryonic osteoclastogenesis; plays a role in certain osteoclast, osteoblast, and chondroblast functions
Matrix metalloproteinases (MMPs)	
Family of endopeptidases (enzymes) that includes collagenases, gelatinases, stromelysins, matrilysins	Help maintain equilibrium of extracellular matrix (ECM); break down almost all components of ECM
A disintegrin and metalloproteinase (ADAM)	Proteolytic enzymes; also have cell-signaling functions, usually linked to cell membrane
A disintegrin and metalloproteinase with thrombospondin motifs (ADAMTS)	Similar to ADAMs but are secreted into circulation, are found around cells; various subgroups affect multiple tissues
Cysteine Protease	
Cathepsin	K-expressed by osteoclasts; assists in bone remodeling by cleaving proteins, such as collagen type I, collagen type II, and osteonectin
MMP Inhibitors	
Tetracyclines (especially doxycycline), bisphosphonates	Block enzymatic function of MMPs
Tissue inhibitors of metalloproteinases (TIMPs)	Balance effect of MMPs in maintaining ECM equilibrium

From Boyce GC, Zhenqiang, Zing L: *Ann N Y Acad Sci* 1192:367–375, 2010; Canalis E: *J Cell Biol* 108(4):769–777, 2009; Kim Y-S et al: *J Korean Med Sci* 25:985–991, 2010; Moester MJ et al: *Calcif Tissue Int* 87(2):99–107, 2010; Nicks KN et al: *Mol Cell Endocrinol* 310(1-2):11–20, 2009; Pasternak B, Aspenberg P: *Acta Orthopaedica* 80(6):693–703, 2009; Stewart A, Guan H, Yang K: *J Cell Physiol* 223(3):658–666, 2010; Tat SK et al: *Keio Med J* 58(1):29–40, 2009.

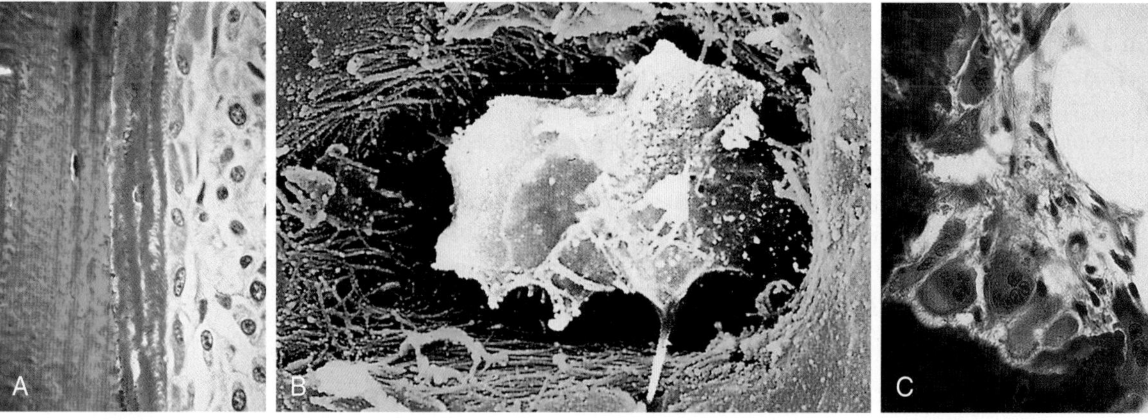

FIGURE 43-2 Bone Cells. **A,** Osteoblasts are responsible for the production of collagenous and noncollagenous proteins that compose osteoid. Active osteoblasts are lined up on the osteoid. Note the eccentrically located nuclei. **B,** Osteocyte. Scanning electron micrograph showing an osteocyte within a lacuna. The cell is surrounded by collagen fibers and mineralized bone. **C,** Osteoclasts actively resorb mineralized tissue. The scalloped surface in which the multinucleated osteoclasts rest is termed the *Howship lacuna.* (**A** and **C** from Damjanov I, Linder J, editors: *Anderson's pathology,* ed 10, St Louis, 1996, Mosby. **B** from Erlandsen S, Magney J: *Color atlas of histology,* St Louis, 1992, Mosby.)

Osteoblasts. **Osteoblasts** are cells derived from mesenchymal stem cells. Osteoblasts produce several substances, including osteocalcin, TGF-β, macrophage colony-stimulating factor, **receptor activator of nuclear factor κβ ligand (RANKL), osteoprotegerin (OPG),** and bone matrix[6] and osteocalcin when stimulated by 1,25-dihydroxy-vitamin D. Osteoblasts are active on the outer surface of bones, where they form a single layer of cells. They initiate the formation of new bone by their synthesis of **osteoid** (nonmineralized bone matrix). The mechanism of osteoblast stimulation is reported to be the production of so-called coupling factors generated during the resorption process. Osteoblasts cause the formation of new bone and the orderly mineralization of bone matrix by concentrating some of the plasma proteins (growth factors) found in the bone matrix and by facilitating the deposit and exchange of calcium and other ions at the site. Osteoblasts alter levels of RANKL and OPG; the balance of these two cytokines determines overall osteoclast formation[7] (see Figure 44-11). As new bone is formed, it is shaped and remodeled through TGF-β, as well as other plasma proteins (growth factors) found in the bone marrow (Table 43-4).

Osteocytes. An **osteocyte** is a transformed osteoblast that is trapped or surrounded in osteoid as it hardens from minerals that enter during ossification (see Figure 43-2, *B*). It is the final differentiation stage for an osteoblast. The osteocyte is within a space in the hardened bone matrix called a **lacuna.** Each osteocyte has a high nucleus/cytoplasm ratio with a thin layer of nonmineralized osteoid around it, similar to the egg white surrounding an egg yolk.

TABLE 43-4 EFFECTS OF SELECTED CYTOKINES (GROWTH FACTORS) ON SKELETAL TISSUES

CYTOKINE (GROWTH FACTOR)	TARGET TISSUE	FORMATION	RESORPTION
Transforming growth factor-beta	Bone	+, –	+, –
	Cartilage	+, –	–
Transforming growth factor-alpha or epidermal growth factor	Bone	+, –	+
	Cartilage	+	0
Insulin-like growth factor	Bone	–	?
	Cartilage	–	0
Fibroblast growth factor	Bone	+, –	?
	Cartilage	–	0
Platelet-derived growth factor	Bone	0	+
	Cartilage		
Colony-stimulating factors	Bone	?	?
	Cartilage	–	–
Interferon-gamma	Bone	–	?
	Cartilage	–	+
Tumor necrosis factor	Bone	–	+
	Cartilage	+, –	+
Interleukins 1, 3, and 6	Bone	–	+
	Cartilage		

+, –, Both stimulatory and inhibitory properties on the specific cell listed; *0,* no effects presently known; *?,* possible effects on cell listed.

The cells of the osteoblastic lineage (osteoblasts and osteocytes) form a network of cells in bone that sense the shape and structure of bone (mechanoreceptors) and determine the appropriate locations for bone formation or resorption, according to Wolff's law (bone is shaped according to its function).

Osteocytes communicate with other bone cells and instruct both osteoblasts and osteoclasts about when and where to form and resorb bone; concentrate nutrients in the matrix; regulate bone mass and minerals (especially calcium and phosphorus); and secrete other proteins, such as sclerostin and fibroblast growth factor-23 (FGF-23), that influence mineral metabolism.[3,4,8,9] Sclerostin inhibits osteoblasts, thus reducing bone formation. Additionally, osteocytes seem to function as endocrine receptors in regulating bone metabolism and are prime target cells of parathyroid hormone (PTH).[9-11] Through exchanges between these cells, hormone catalysts, and minerals, optimal levels of calcium, phosphorus, and other minerals are maintained in blood plasma. The osteocyte also aids in modifying bone matrix through release of enzymes to dissolve the mineralized walls of the lacunae to prepare the bone for remodeling. (Remodeling is described on p. 1519.)

Osteoclasts. **Osteoclasts** are large, multinucleated bone cells derived from hematopoietic stem cells in the bone marrow stroma and are the major resorptive cells of bone. Considered to be the major remodelers of bone, osteoclasts contain lysosomes (digestive vacuoles) filled with hydrolytic enzymes. Fine projections, or microvilli, fan out from the osteoclast cell's surface and are known as **ruffled borders;** these projections result from extensive infoldings of the cell membrane adjacent to the resorptive surface.[12] Osteoclasts in regions of bone resorption lie in pits called *Howship lacunae,* where the infolded, ruffled borders of the osteoclasts greatly increase the surface area of the plasma membrane. The infolds end in numerous channels and vesicles in the cell cytoplasm, permitting them to resorb the bone under their ruffled, infolded borders.

Osteoclasts bind to the bone surface of cell attachment proteins called **integrins.**[12] In contact with bone mineral, osteoclasts use adhesive structures, called *podosomes,* to attach themselves to the bone surface. They then seal their cytoplasm with the underlying bone and dissolve the bone and matrix while protecting the surrounding tissue.[13] They effect resorption of bone by secretion of hydrochloric acid (HCl) and cathepsin K (a protease enzyme), which help dissolve bone minerals and collagenase, thereby aiding the digestion of collagen along with the action of cytokines (see Table 43-4). Matrix metalloproteinases (MMPs), a group of proteolytic enzymes, help control osteoclast-matrix interactions necessary for bone resorption. Once resorption is completed, the osteoclast disappears by degeneration, either by reverting to its parent cell or by leaving the site through the process of cell mobility, wherein the osteoclast then becomes an inactive, or "resting," osteoclast. Overall, bone homeostasis is the result of crosstalk between osteoclasts, osteoblasts, and osteocytes.[14] Recent evidence has indicated that osteoclasts also may play a role in the body's immune system.[15-17]

Bone Matrix

Bone matrix is made of the extracellular elements of bone tissue, composed of about 35% organic and 65% inorganic materials. The major organic components are collagen fibers, and the major inorganic components are the calcium and phosphate minerals. Other parts of the bone matrix are the proteins, carbohydrate-protein complexes, and ground substances. Water comprises 5% to 8% of the matrix. Within the matrix are small particles known as matrix vesicles that "bud" from chondrocytes, osteoblasts, and odontoblasts. These vesicles are the initial sites for calcification in skeletal tissues.[18] Calcification begins as extracellular calcium enters the matrix vesicles and forms hydroxyapatite crystals.

TABLE 43-5 TYPES OF COLLAGEN IN MUSCULOSKELETAL TISSUES

TYPE OF COLLAGEN	DISTRIBUTION IN MUSCULOSKELETAL TISSUES
I	Bone, tendon, ligament, intervertebral disk, muscle*
II	Cartilage, intervertebral disk
III	Skin, muscle, often with type I
IV	Basement cell membrane, muscle
V	Codistributed with type I muscle, most interstitial tissues
VI	Ubiquitous, muscle
IX	Codistributed with type II muscle
X	Cartilage growth plate
XI	Cartilage, muscle
XII	Codistributed with types I and III muscle
XIII	Molecule has not been isolated in connective tissues to date
XIV	Codistributed with type I muscle
XV	Muscle; contains heparin sulfate proteoglycans (HSPGs)
XVII	Muscle; contains HSPGs

*Refers specifically to skeletal muscle.

Collagen Fibers. **Collagen fibers** are the major organic component of bone matrix. The fibers are approximately 90% type I collagen, are essential for bone strength, and are synthesized and secreted by osteoblasts. Once secreted, collagen molecules assemble into thin chains called *α-chains,* which combine in groups of 3 to form **fibrils.** The fibrils form a staggered pattern, overlapping nearby fibrils by approximately one fourth their length. This staggered, overlapping pattern creates regular gaps, called *hole zones,* into which mineral crystals are deposited.[18] After mineral deposition, the fibrils link together and twist to form ropelike fibers. Collagen fibers then join to form a framework that gives bone its tensile strength and enables it to bear weight.

Collagen is the most abundant macromolecule in the body, accounting for approximately one third of all protein and providing the structural framework for nearly all tissues. Collagen is one of the extracellular components, along with proteoglycans and noncollagenous matrix proteins, of articular cartilage. To date, more than 20 types of collagen have been identified, though all their functions are not yet known. Cartilage-specific collagens include types II (the principal component), VI, IX, X, and XI. Type IX collagen is thought to be the "glue" that holds together the type II collagen scaffold of articular cartilage, helps maintain the structural integrity of cartilage, and resists tensile forces on the joint cartilage. Type XI regulates the fibril diameter of type II cartilage. Degradation of type IX collagen by proteolytic enzymes has been seen in the early stages of osteoarthritis and rheumatoid arthritis. Researchers have proposed that this degradation, or "unplugging," may be the mechanism for the degenerative changes seen in osteoarthritic and rheumatoid cartilage. Table 43-5 gives the musculoskeletal distribution of other types of collagen.

Proteoglycans. **Proteoglycans** are large complexes of numerous polysaccharides attached to a common protein core. Hyaline cartilage is primarily composed of the glycosaminoglycans chondroitin sulfate and keratin sulfate. They strengthen bone by forming compression-resistant networks between the collagen fibrils. Proteoglycans also control the transport and distribution of electrically charged particles (ions), particularly calcium, through the bone matrix, thereby playing a role in bone calcium deposition and calcification.

Glycoproteins. **Glycoproteins** are also carbohydrate-protein complexes of bone. Glycoproteins control the collagen interactions that lead to fibril formation. They also play a role in calcification.

Some of the glycoproteins in bone matrix include bone sialoprotein, osteocalcin, osteonectin, laminin, albumin, and α-glycoprotein. Other proteins found in bone matrix are the compounds currently called **bone morphogenic proteins (BMPs)** (see Table 43-2). **Sialoprotein (osteopontin)** comprises about 8% of the noncollagenous matrix of bone and easily binds with calcium.

Osteocalcin is also a calcium-binding protein that binds preferentially to calcium that has already crystallized. The roles of osteocalcin may be to inhibit calcium phosphate precipitation and to play a part in bone resorption by recruiting osteoclasts.

Osteonectin is a bone-specific protein that binds selectively to both hydroxyapatite and collagen in the bone matrix. **Laminin** is an abundant bone matrix protein in humans that stabilizes basement membranes in bones and is important in neurite and axon growth.

Bone albumin is identical to serum albumin. In calcified matrix, bone albumin is permanently fixed to bone mineral crystals and remains so until the bone is resorbed. Bone albumin transports essential elements such as hormones, ions, and other metabolites to and from the bone cells and maintains the osmotic pressure of **bone fluid** (fluid surrounding mineral crystals and osteoblasts).

Bone Minerals

Mineralization is the final step in bone formation, after collagen synthesis and fiber formation. Mineralization has two distinct phases: (1) formation of the initial mineral deposit (initiation), and (2) proliferation or accretion of additional mineral crystals on the initial mineral deposits (growth).[12] The majority of the mineral content in the body is an analog of the naturally occurring mineral *hydroxyapatite.*

Table 43-6 lists the sequence in which calcium and phosphate form amorphous (fluid) calcium phosphate compounds that are converted, in stages, to solid hexagonal crystals of **hydroxyapatite (HAP).** As the calcium and phosphorous concentrations increase in the bone matrix, the first precipitate to form is dicalcium phosphate dihydrate (DCPD). Once DCPD precipitation begins, the remaining phases of bone crystal formation proceed until insoluble HAP is produced, with approximately 80% to 90% of the HAP being incorporated into the collagen fibers. Amorphous calcium phosphate is distributed throughout the bone matrix.

TABLE 43-6 SEQUENCE OF CALCIUM AND PHOSPHATE COMPOUND FORMATION AND CRYSTALLIZATION

FORMULA	NAME	ABBREVIATION
$Ca(HPO_4) \times 2H_2O$	Dicalcium phosphate dehydrate	DCPD
$Ca_4H(PO_4)_3$	Octacalcium phosphate	OCP
$Ca_9(PO_4)_6$ (var.)	Amorphous calcium phosphate	ACP
$Ca_3(PO_4)_2$	Tricalcium phosphate	TCP
$Ca_5(PO_4)_3OH$	Hydroxyapatite	HAP

NOTE: Compounds are listed in order in which precipitation and crystal formation occur.

Types of Bone Tissue

Bone consists of two types of bony (osseous) tissue: **compact bone (cortical bone)** and **spongy bone (cancellous bone)** (Figure 43-3). Compact bone constitutes approximately 85% of the skeleton; spongy bone comprises the remaining 15%. Both types of bone tissue contain the same structural elements, and, with a few exceptions, both compact tissue and spongy tissue are present in every bone. The major difference between the two types of tissue is the organization of the elements.

Compact bone is highly organized, solid, and extremely strong. The basic structural unit in compact bone is the haversian system (Figure 43-4). Each **haversian system** is made up of the following:

1. A central canal called the **haversian canal**
2. Concentric layers of bone matrix called **lamellae**
3. Tiny spaces (lacunae) between the lamellae
4. Bone cells (osteocytes) within the lacunae
5. Small channels or canals called **canaliculi**

Each haversian system is a separate cylindrical entity that looks like a set of concentric rings. In the center of the haversian system is the haversian canal that runs through the long axis of bone and contains one or two blood vessels and nerve fibers. The blood vessels in the canal communicate with blood vessels in the periosteum (surface cover) and marrow cavity to transport nutrients and wastes to and from the osteocytes contained within the lacunae. Surrounding each haversian canal are the concentric lamellae. Between the lamellae are the lacunae, each of which contains one osteocyte. The lacunae are connected to each other and to the haversian canal by the canaliculi, which run parallel to the horizontal axis of the bone. Each canaliculus encloses a small extension (cytoplasmic process) from the osteocyte contained in the lacuna. The canaliculi transport both nourishment and molecular signals into the lacunae, a mechanism essential for osteocyte survival.

Spongy bone is less complex and lacks haversian systems. In spongy bone the lamellae are not arranged in concentric layers but in plates or bars termed **trabeculae** that branch and unite with one another to form an irregular meshwork. The pattern of the meshwork is determined by the direction of stress on the particular bone. The spaces between the trabeculae are filled with red bone marrow. The osteocyte-containing lacunae are distributed between the trabeculae and interconnected by canaliculi. Capillaries pass through the marrow to nourish the osteocytes.

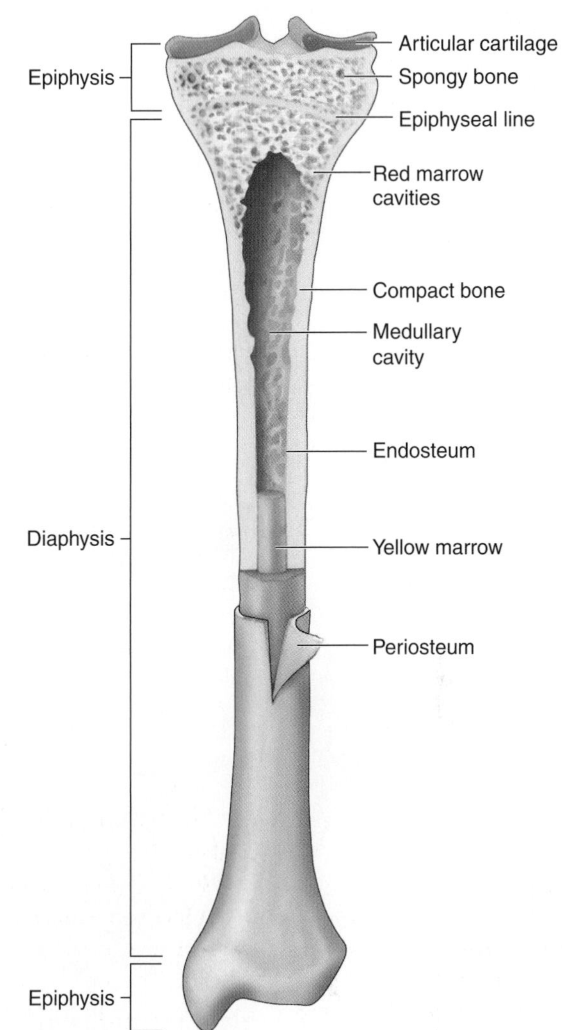

FIGURE 43-3 Cross Section of Bone. Longitudinal section of long bone (tibia) showing cancellous and compact bone. (From Patton KT, Thibodeau GA: *Anatomy & physiology,* ed 8, St Louis, 2013, Mosby.)

All bones are covered with a double-layered connective tissue called the **periosteum.** The outer layer of the periosteum contains blood vessels and nerves, some of which penetrate to the inner structures of the bone through channels called Volkmann canals (see Figure 43-4). The inner layer of the periosteum is anchored to the bone by collagenous fibers (Sharpey fibers) that penetrate the bone. Sharpey fibers also help hold or attach tendons and ligaments to the periosteum of bones.[12]

Characteristics of Bone

The human skeleton consists of 206 bones that constitute the axial skeleton and the appendicular skeleton (Figure 43-5). The **axial skeleton** consists of 80 bones that make up the skull, vertebral column, and thorax. The **appendicular skeleton** consists of 126 bones that make up the upper and lower extremities, the shoulder girdle (pectoral girdle), and the pelvic girdle. The skeleton contributes about 14% of the weight of the adult body.

Bones can be classified by shape as long, flat, short (cuboidal), or irregular. **Long bones** are longer than they are wide and consist of a narrow tubular midportion (**diaphysis**) that merges

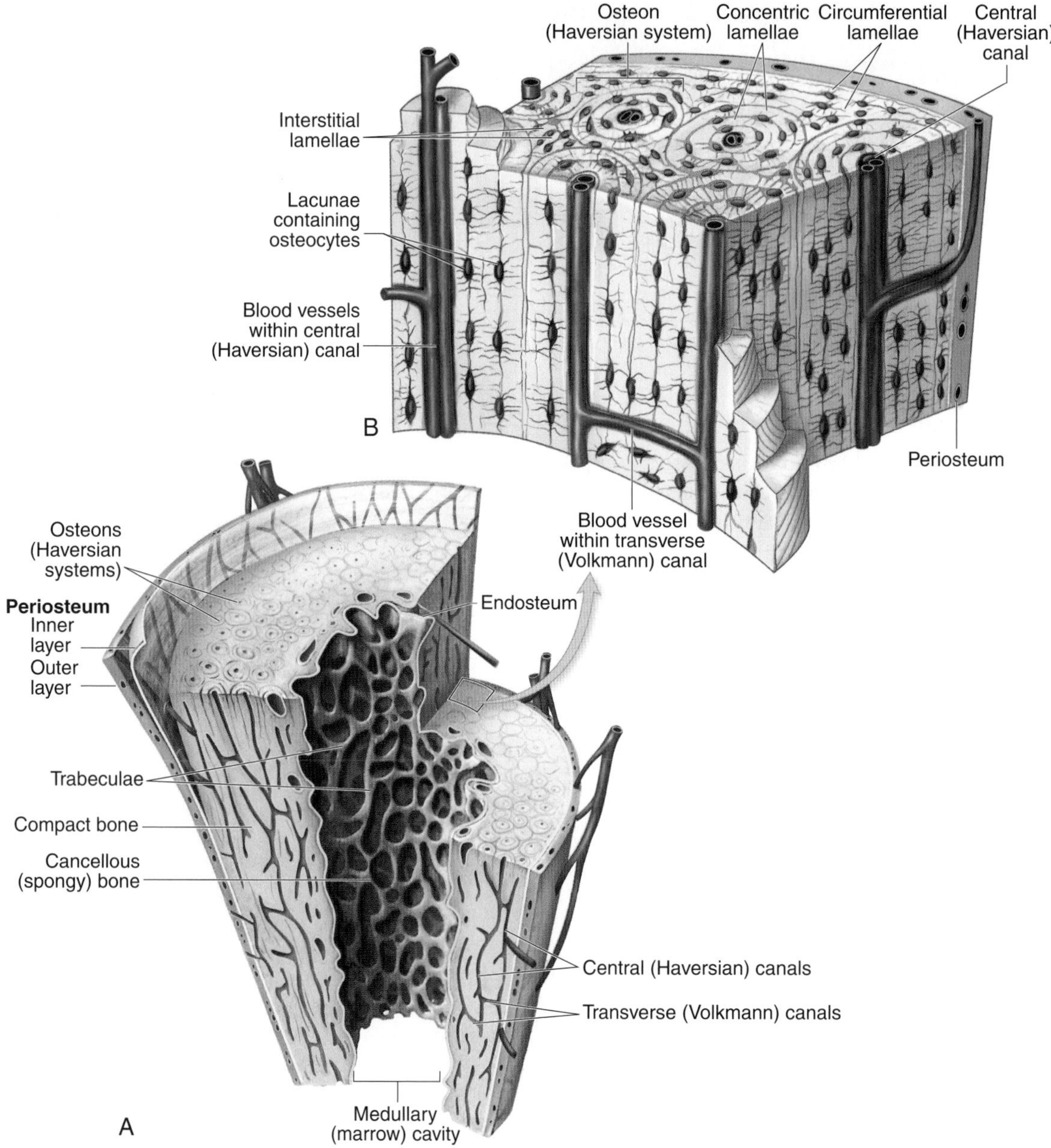

FIGURE 43-4 Structure of Compact and Cancellous Bone. **A,** Longitudinal section of a long bone showing cancellous and compact bone. **B,** A magnified view of compact bone. (From Patton KT, Thibodeau GA: *Anatomy & physiology,* ed 8, St Louis, 2013, Mosby.)

into a broader neck (**metaphysis**) and a broad end (**epiphysis**) (see Figure 43-3).

The diaphysis consists of a shaft of thick, rigid compact bone that can tolerate bending forces. Contained within the diaphysis is the elongated marrow (medullary) cavity. The marrow cavity of the diaphysis contains primarily fatty tissue, which is referred to as *yellow marrow.* The yellow marrow assists red bone marrow in hematopoiesis only during times of stress. The yellow marrow cavity of the diaphysis is continuous with marrow cavities in the spongy bone of the metaphysis and diaphysis. The marrow contained within the epiphysis is red because it contains primarily blood-forming tissue (see Chapter 27). A layer of connective tissue, the **endosteum,** lines the outer surfaces of both types of marrow cavity.

The broadness of the epiphysis allows weightbearing to be distributed over a wide area. The epiphysis is made up of spongy bone covered by a very thin layer of compact bone. In a child the epiphysis is separated from the metaphysis by a cartilaginous **growth plate,** the **epiphyseal plate.** After puberty the epiphyseal plate calcifies and the epiphysis and metaphysis merge. By adulthood the line of demarcation between the epiphysis and metaphysis is undetectable.

In **flat bones,** such as the ribs or scapulae, two plates of compact bone are roughly parallel to each other. Between the compact bone plates is a layer of spongy bone. **Short bones (cuboidal bones),** such as the bones of the wrist or ankle, are often cuboidal in shape. They consist of spongy bone covered by a thin layer of compact bone.

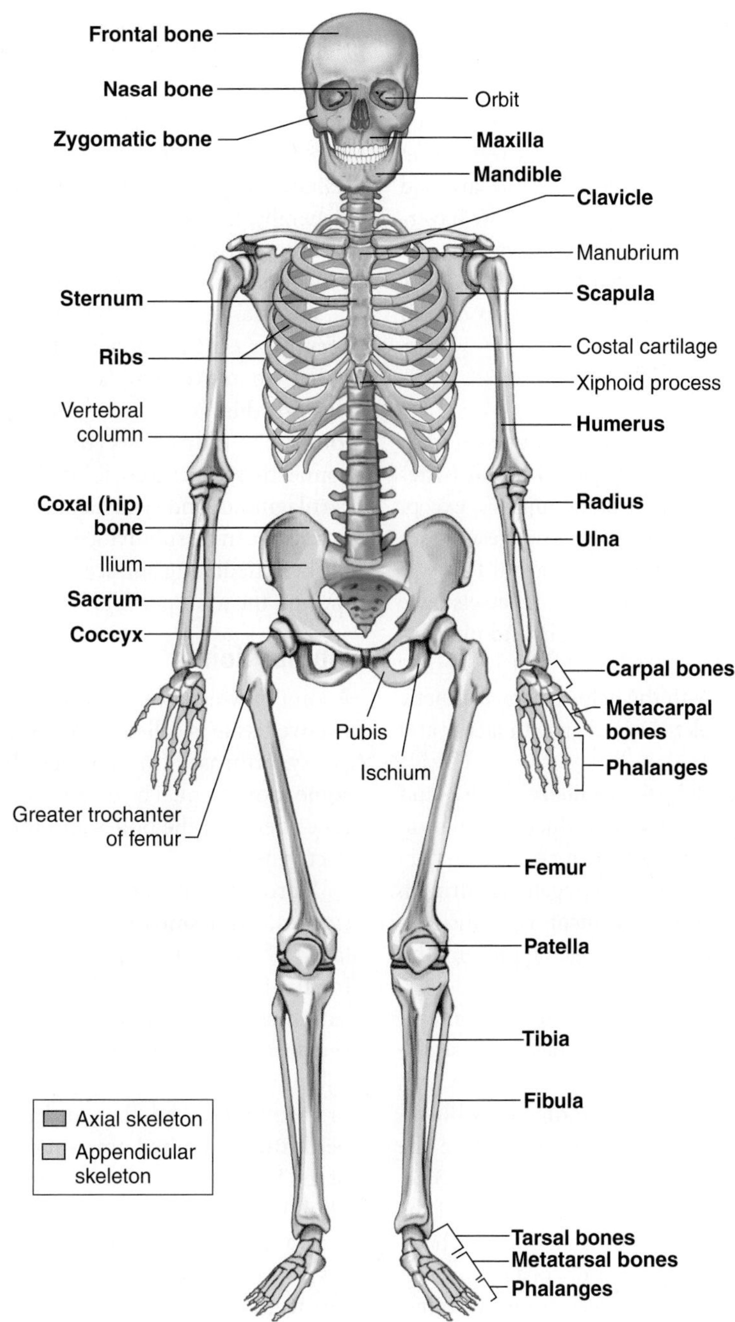

FIGURE 43-5 Anterior View of Skeleton. (From Patton KT, Thibodeau GA: *Anatomy & physiology,* ed 8, St Louis, 2013, Mosby.)

Irregular bones, such as the vertebrae, mandibles, or other facial bones, have various shapes that include thin and thick segments. The thin part of an irregular bone consists of two plates of compact bone with spongy bone between the plates. The thick part consists of spongy bone surrounded by a layer of compact bone.

Maintenance of Bone Integrity

Remodeling

Clusters of bone cells, termed bone-remodeling units, are responsible for maintaining the structure of bone by **remodeling,** a three-phase process in which existing bone is resorbed and new bone is laid down to replace it. The **bone-remodeling units** are made up of bone precursor cells that differentiate into osteoclasts and osteoblasts. Precursor cells are located on the free surfaces of bones and along the vascular channels (especially the marrow cavities).

In phase 1 (activation) of the remodeling cycle, a stimulus (e.g., hormone, drug, vitamin, physical stressor) activates programmed osteocyte cell death (apoptosis). The distribution of these apoptotic osteocytes provides osteoclasts with information about where to begin resorbing damaged bone. In phase 2 (resorption), the osteoclasts form a "cutting cone," which gradually resorbs bone, leaving behind an elongated cavity termed a *resorption cavity.* The resorption cavity in compact bone follows the longitudinal axis of the haversian system, and the resorption cavity in spongy bone parallels the surface of the trabeculae.

Phase 3 (formation) is the laying down of new bone, termed *secondary bone,* by osteoblasts lining the walls of the resorption cavity. Successive layers (lamellae) in compact bone are laid down until the resorption cavity is reduced to a narrow haversian canal around a blood vessel. In this way, old haversian systems are destroyed and new haversian systems are formed. New trabeculae are formed in spongy bone. The entire process of remodeling takes about 3 to 4 months.

Repair

The remodeling process can repair microscopic bone injuries, but gross injuries, such as fractures and surgical wounds (osteotomies), heal by the same stages as soft tissue injuries, except that new bone, instead of scar tissue, is the final result (see Chapter 7). In bone the stages of wound healing are as follows:

1. *Hematoma formation:* This process occurs if vessels have been damaged, causing hemorrhage. Fibrin and platelets within the hematoma form a meshwork that is the initial framework for healing with the help of hematopoietic growth factors such as platelet-derived growth factor and TGF-β (see Table 43-3).
2. *Procallus formation:* Fibroblasts, capillary buds, and osteoblasts move into the wound to produce granulation tissue called **procallus.** Cartilage is formed as a precursor of bone, and types I, II, and III collagen are formed. Enzymes and growth factors, such as insulin and insulin-like growth factors, plus bone morphogenic protein and osteogenin, aid in this stage of healing.
3. *Callus formation:* Osteoblasts in the procallus form membranous or **woven bone (callus).** Enzymes increase the phosphate content and permit the phosphate to join with calcium to be deposited as mineral to harden the callus.
4. *Callus replacement:* Osteoblasts continue to replace the callus with lamellar bone or trabecular bone (Figure 43-6).
5. *Remodeling:* The periosteal and endosteal surfaces of the bone are remodeled to the size and shape of the bone before injury. Synthesis of other types of collagen recedes in favor of type I, which is the collagen found in bone. This final stage of healing, or remodeling, is vital because bone that has not been remodeled does not have good mechanical properties for weightbearing and mobility.

The speed with which bone heals depends on the severity of the bone disruption; the type and amount of bone tissue that must be replaced (spongy bone heals faster); the blood supply and oxygen content at the site; the presence of growth and thyroid hormones, insulin, vitamins, and other nutrients; the presence of systemic disease; the effects of aging; and the effectiveness of treatment, including immobilization and the prevention of complications such as infection. In general, however, hematoma formation occurs within hours of fracture or surgery; formation of procallus by osteoblasts occurs within days; callus formation occurs within weeks; and replacement and contour modeling occur within years—up to 4 years in some cases.

STRUCTURE AND FUNCTION OF JOINTS

The site where two or more bones meet is called a **joint (articulation)** (Figure 43-7). The primary function of joints is to provide stability and mobility to the skeleton. Whether a joint provides stability or mobility depends on its location and its structure. Generally, joints that stabilize the skeleton have a simpler structure than those that enable movement of the skeleton. Most joints provide stability and mobility to some degree (Figure 43-8).

Joints are classified based on the degree of movement they permit or on the connecting tissues that hold them together. Based on movement, a joint is classified as a **synarthrosis (immovable joint),** an **amphiarthrosis (slightly movable joint),** or a **diarthrosis (freely movable joint).** On the basis of connective structures, joints are classified broadly as fibrous, cartilaginous, and synovial. Each of these three structural classifications can be subdivided according to the shape and contour of the articulating surfaces (ends) of the bones and the type of motion the joint permits.

Fibrous Joints

A joint in which bone is united directly to bone by fibrous connective tissue is called a **fibrous joint.** Generally, fibrous joints are synarthroses (immovable), but many fibrous joints allow some movement. The degree of movement depends on the distance between the bones and the flexibility of the fibrous connective tissue.

Fibrous joints are further subdivided into three types: sutures, syndesmoses, and gomphoses. A **suture** has a thin layer of dense fibrous tissue that binds together interlocking flat bones in the skulls of young children. Sutures form an extremely tight union that permits no motion. By adulthood the fibrous tissue has been replaced by bone. A **syndesmosis** is a joint in which the two bony surfaces are united by a ligament or membrane. The fibers of ligaments are flexible and stretch, permitting a limited amount of movement. The paired bones of the lower arm (radius and ulna) and the lower leg (tibia and fibula) and their ligaments are syndesmotic joints. A **gomphosis** is a special type of fibrous joint in which a conical projection fits into a complementary socket and is held there by a ligament. The teeth held in the maxilla or mandible are gomphosis joints.

Cartilaginous Joints

The two types of cartilaginous joints are symphyses and synchondroses. A **symphysis** is a cartilaginous joint in which bones are united by a pad or disk of fibrocartilage. A thin layer of hyaline cartilage usually covers the articulating surfaces of the two bones, and the thick pad of fibrocartilage acts as a shock absorber and stabilizer. Examples of symphyses are the symphysis pubis, which joins the two pubic bones, and the intervertebral disks, which join the bodies of the vertebrae. A **synchondrosis** is a joint in which hyaline cartilage, rather than fibrocartilage, connects the two bones. The joints between the ribs and the sternum are synchondroses. The hyaline cartilage of these joints is called *costal cartilage.* Slight movement at the synchondroses between the ribs and the sternum allows the chest to move outward and upward during breathing.

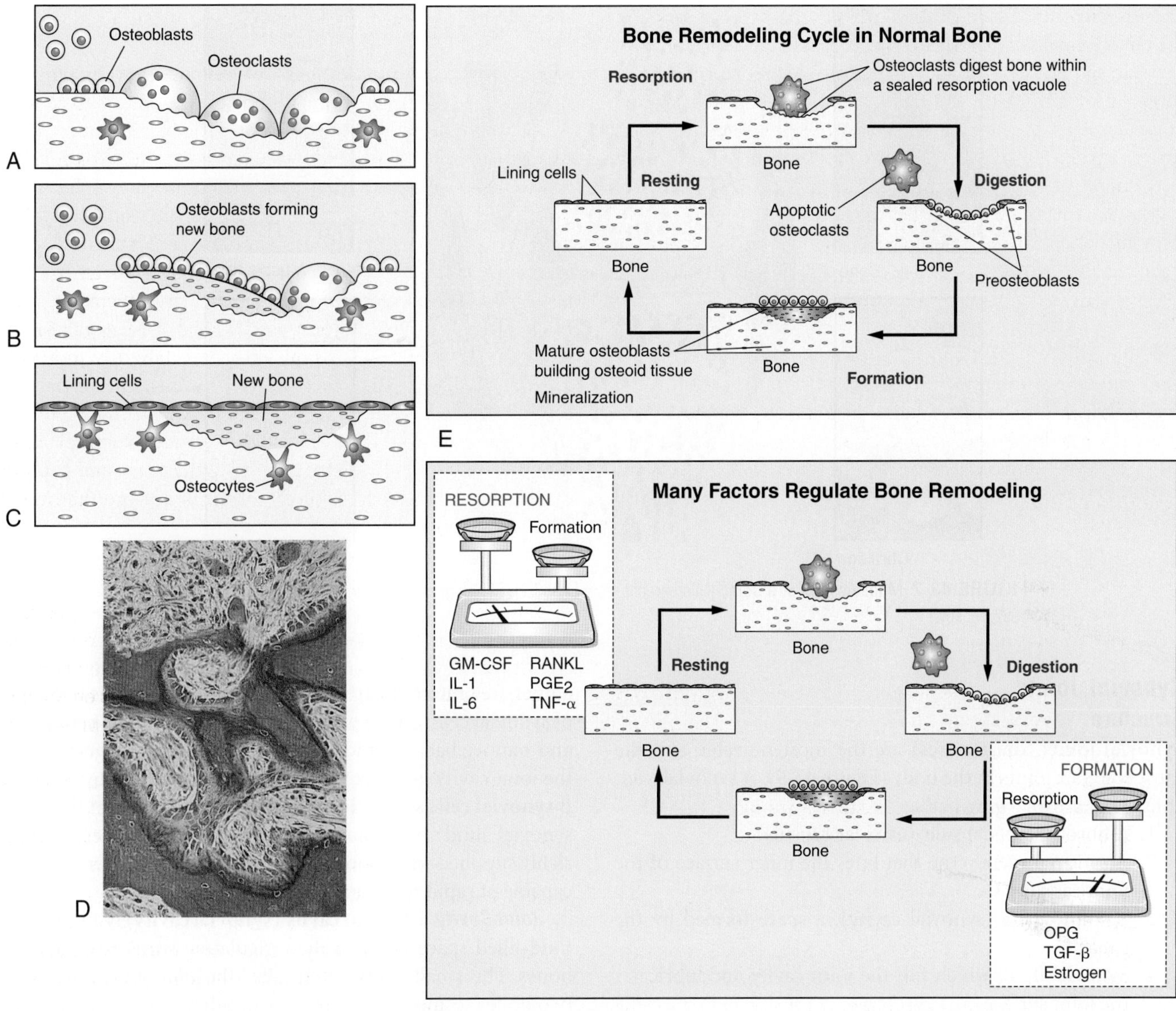

FIGURE 43-6 **Bone Remodeling.** All bone cells participate in bone remodeling. In the remodeling sequence bone sections are removed by bone-resorbing cells (osteoclasts) and replaced with a new section laid down by bone-forming cells (osteoblasts). Bone remodeling is necessary because it allows the skeleton to respond to mechanical loading, maintains quality control (repair and prevent microdamage), and allows the skeleton to release growth factors and minerals (calcium and phosphate) stored in bone matrix to the circulation. The cells work in response to signals generated in the environment (see **F**). Only the osteoclastic cells mediate the first phase of remodeling. They are activated, scoop out bone **(A)**, and resorb it; then the work of the osteoblasts begins **(B)**. They form new bone that replaces bone removed by the resorption process **(C)**. The sequence takes 4 to 6 months. **D,** Micrograph of active bone remodeling seen in the settings of primary or secondary hyperparathyroidism. Note the active osteoblasts surmounted on red-stained osteoid. Marrow fibrosis is present. **E,** Bone remodeling cycle in normal bone **(F)**. Numerous signaling factors are necessary for remodeling. Factors most important for resorption include granulocyte macrophage-colony-stimulating factor *(GM-CSF)*, interleukins-1 and -6 *(IL-1* and *IL-6)*, receptor activator for nuclear factor κβ ligand *(RANKL)*, prostaglandin E_2 *(PGE_2)*, and tumor necrosis factor-alpha *(TNF-α)*. Important factors for bone formation include osteoprotegerin *(OPG)*, transforming growth factor-beta *(TGF-β)*, and estrogen. (Adapted from Nucleus Medical Art. **D** from Damjananov I, Linder J, editors: *Anderson's pathology*, ed 10, St Louis, 1996, Mosby.)

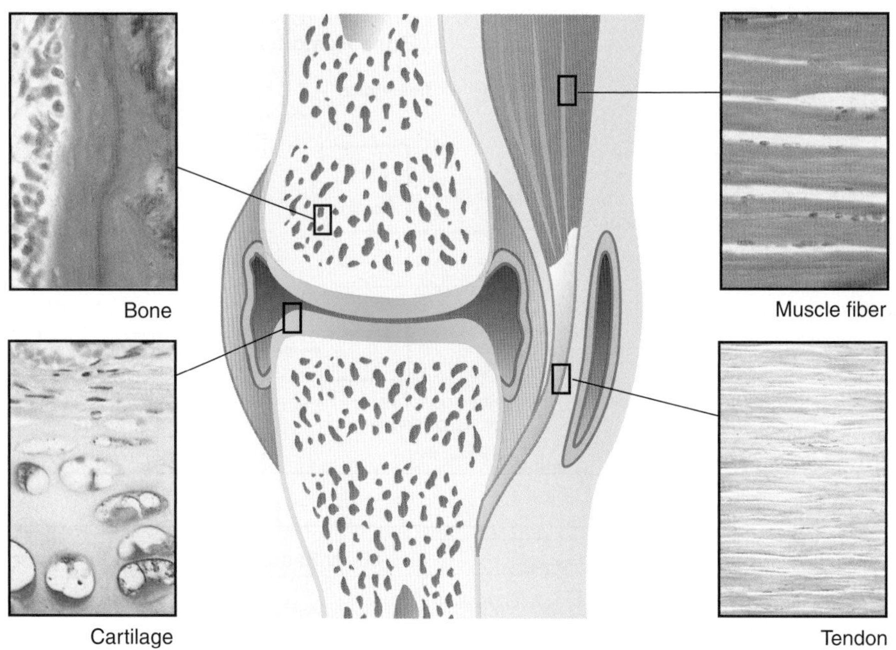

FIGURE 43-7 Main Tissues of a Joint. (Micrographs from Erlandsen SL, Magney JE: *Color atlas of histology,* St Louis, 1992, Mosby.)

Synovial Joints

Structure

Synovial joints (diarthroses) are the most movable and the most complex joints in the body (Figure 43-9). A synovial joint consists of the following parts:

1. A fibrous joint capsule (articular capsule)
2. A synovial membrane that lines the inner surface of the joint capsule
3. A joint cavity (synovial cavity), a space formed by the capsule
4. Synovial fluid, which fills the joint cavity and lubricates the joint surface
5. Articular cartilage, which covers and pads the articulating bony surfaces

Joint Capsule. The fibrous **joint capsule (articular capsule)** is connective tissue that covers the ends of the bones where they meet in the joint. Sharpey fibers firmly attach the proximal and distal capsules to the periosteum and ligaments and tendons, which also reinforce the capsule. The joint capsule consists of parallel, interlacing bundles of dense, white fibrous tissue. It is richly supplied with nerves, blood vessels, and lymphatic vessels. The nerves in and around the joint capsule are sensitive to the rate and direction of motion, compression, tension, vibration, and pain.

Synovial Membrane. The **synovial membrane (synovium)** is the smooth, delicate inner lining of the joint capsule (Figure 43-10). It lines the nonarticular portion of the synovial joint and any ligaments or tendons that traverse the joint cavity. It is made up of two layers—a vascular layer (**subintima**) and a thin cellular layer (**intima**). The vascular subintima merges with the fibrous joint capsule and is composed of loose fibrous connective tissue, elastin fibers, fat cells, fibroblasts, macrophages, and mast cells. The intima consists of rows of synovial cells embedded in a fiber-free intercellular matrix. The intima contains two types of synovial cells: type A and type B. **Type A synovial cells** ingest and remove bacteria and particles of debris by phagocytosis in the joint cavity. (Phagocytosis is described in Chapter 7.) **Type B synovial cells** secrete **hyaluronate,** a binding agent that gives synovial fluid its viscous quality. The synovial membrane is richly supplied with blood and lymphatic vessels; therefore, it is capable of rapid repair and regeneration.

Joint Cavity. The **joint cavity (synovial cavity)** is an enclosed fluid-filled space between the articulating surfaces of the two bones. This small cavity, often called the *joint space,* enables the two bones to move "against" one another. The synovial cavity is surrounded by the synovial membrane and filled with a clear, viscous, slick fluid called the *synovial fluid.*

Synovial Fluid. **Synovial fluid** is superfiltrated plasma from blood vessels in the synovial membrane. Synovial fluid lubricates the joint surfaces, nourishes the pad of the articular cartilage that covers the ends of the bones, and contains free-floating synovial cells and various leukocytes that phagocytize joint debris and microorganisms. Loss of synovial fluid leads to rapid deterioration of articular cartilage.

Articular Cartilage. **Articular cartilage** is a layer of hyaline cartilage that covers the end of each bone (Figure 43-11). It ranges from 2 to 5 mm thick, depending on the size of the joint, the fit of the two bone ends, and the amount of weight and shearing force the joint normally withstands. Cartilage strength and its biologic properties are due to an extensive network of cross-linked collagen fibers. Figure 43-12 illustrates how collagen cross-links from cartilage. The function of articular cartilage is to reduce friction in the joint and to distribute the forces of weightbearing. Articular cartilage is composed of **chondrocytes** (cartilage cells) (making up about 2% of the tissue) and an intercellular matrix made up of collagen (making

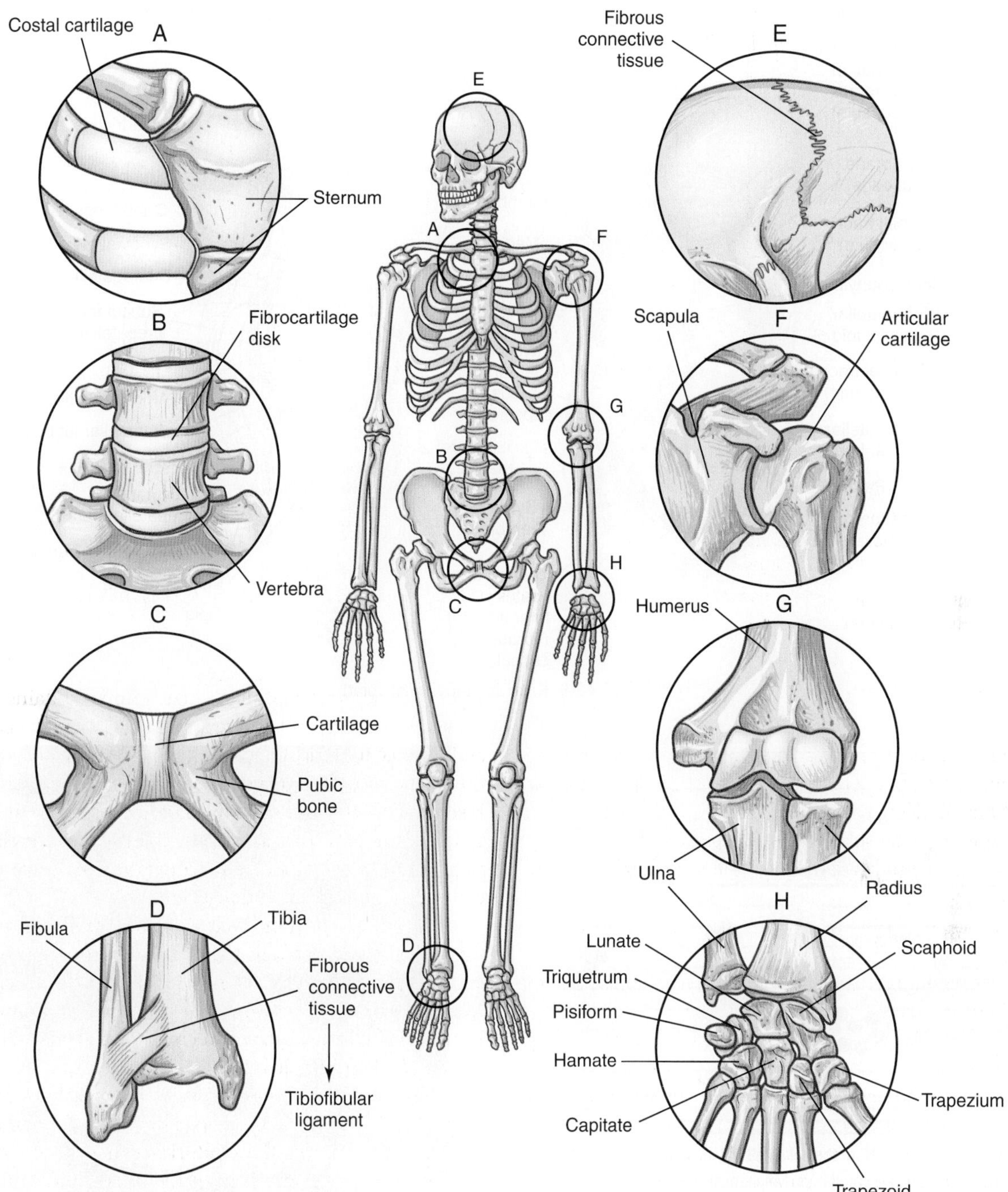

FIGURE 43-8 **Types of Joints.** Cartilaginous (amphiarthrodial) joints, which are slightly movable, include **(A)** a synchondrosis that attaches ribs to costal cartilage; **(B)** a symphysis that connects vertebrae; and **(C)** the symphysis that connects the two pubic bones. Fibrous (synarthrodial) joints, which are immovable, include **(D)** the syndesmosis between the tibia and fibula; **(E)** sutures that connect the skull bones; and the gomphosis (not shown), which holds teeth in their sockets. The synovial joints include **(F)** the spheroid type at the shoulder; **(G)** the hinge type at the elbow; and **(H)** the gliding joints of the hand.

up about 10% to 30% of weight), protein polysaccharides (making up 5% to 10% of weight), and water. The water content ranges from 60% to almost 80% of the net weight of the cartilage, and individual molecules rapidly enter or exit the articular cartilage to contribute to the resiliency of the tissue.

The intercellular matrix is produced by the chondrocytes, which synthesize and extrude collagen that, like the collagen produced by bone cells, is distributed throughout the cartilage in a highly organized system of fibers. Collagen fibers in cartilage are made up of many fine fibrils that, like bone fibrils, are assembled in an orderly fashion that makes them resistant to physical, metabolic, or chemical breakdown. The main differences between bone collagen and cartilage collagen are the amino acid content of the α-chains and the composition of the fibrils. Bone collagen fibrils are made up of two type I chains and one type II chain. Approximately 90% of the cartilage collagen fibrils is made up of three identical type II chains, with the remaining 10% consisting of types V, VI, IX, X, and XI.

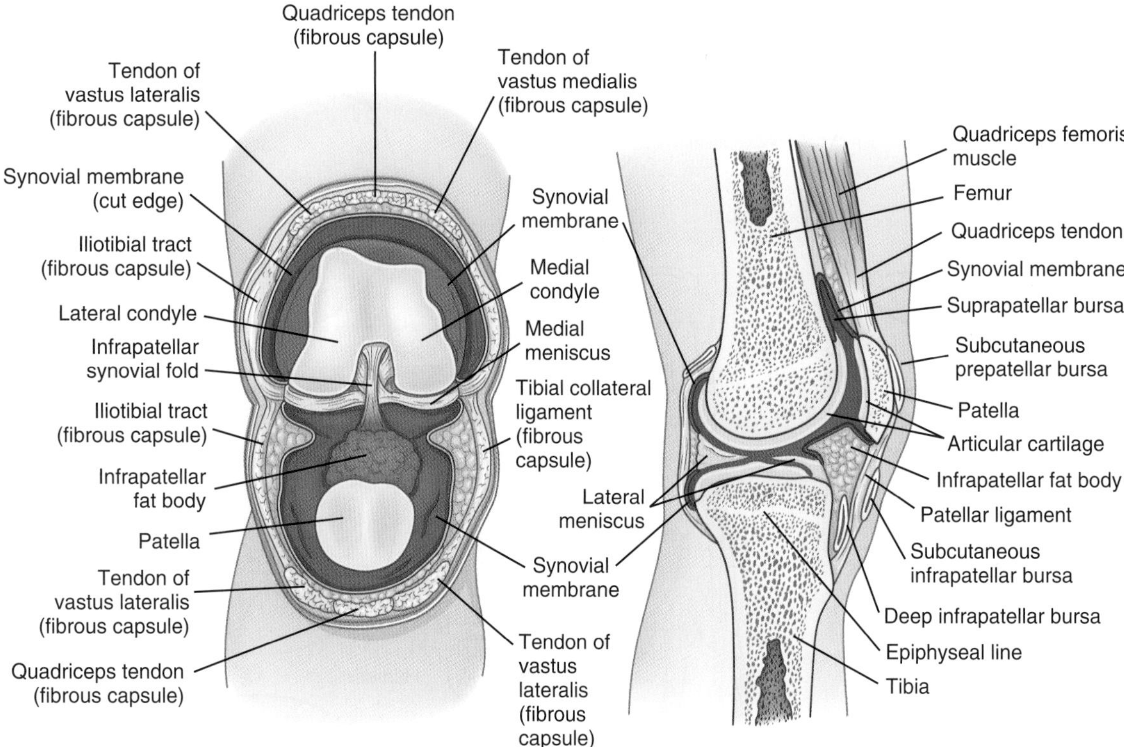

FIGURE 43-9 Knee Joint (Synovial Joint).

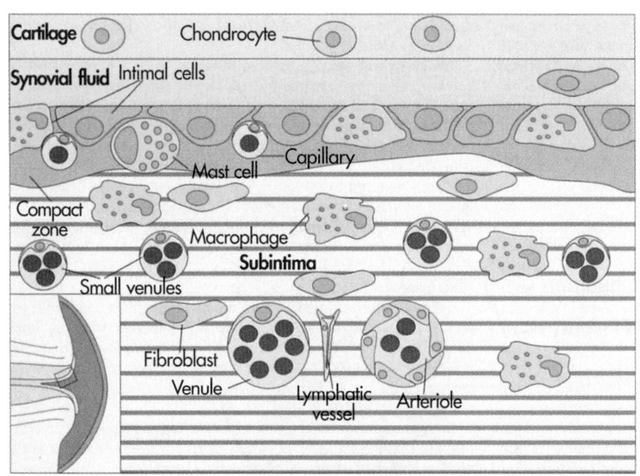

FIGURE 43-10 Synovium. Note the delicate synovial lining resting on a fibroadipose subintimal lining rich in capillaries, lymphatics, and nerve endings. (Modified from Hochberg MC et al: *Rheumatology,* ed 4, Philadelphia, 2008, Mosby.)

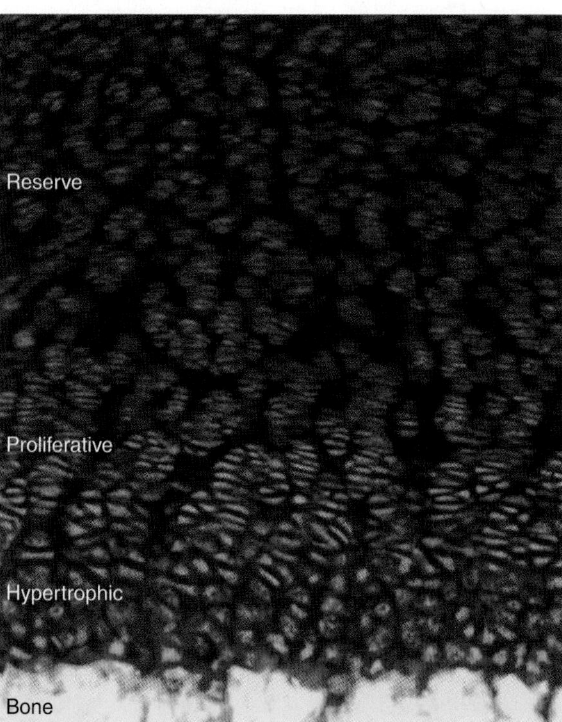

FIGURE 43-11 Collagen Zones. The three collagen zones (reserve, proliferative, and hypertrophic) are distinctly shown in a growth plate. (From Hjorten R et al: *Bone* 41[4]:535, 2007.)

At the surface of articular cartilage, the collagen fibers run parallel to the joint surface and are closely compacted into a dense, protective mat. (Loss of this dense, compacted configuration at the surface subjects the underlying fibers to splitting and thinning, in which case the cartilage is unable to tolerate weightbearing.) In the middle layer (the proliferative zone) of the cartilage, the fibers are arranged tangential to the surface, which allows them to deform and absorb some of the force of weightbearing (see Figure 43-11). In the bottom layer (the hypertrophic zone) of the cartilage, the fibers are perpendicular to the joint surface, allowing them to resist shear forces, and are embedded in a calcified layer of cartilage called the **tidemark.** The tidemark anchors the collagen fibers to the underlying (subchondral) bone and represents the zone between calcified and uncalcified cartilage. Collagen fibers are important components of the cartilage matrix because they account for approximately 60% of the dry weight and because they (1) anchor the cartilage securely to underlying bone, (2) provide a taut framework for the cartilage, (3) control

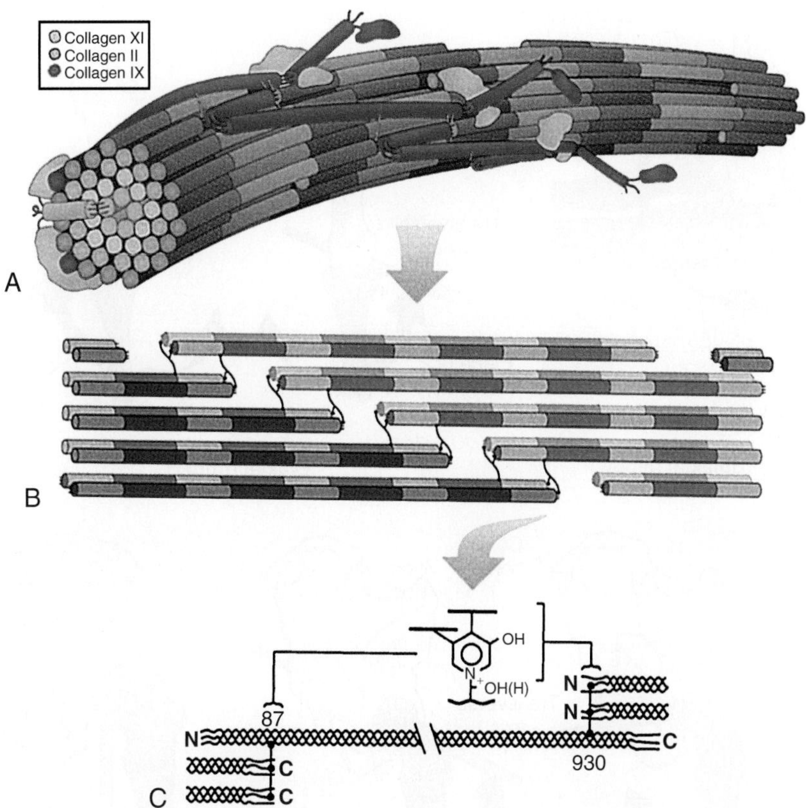

FIGURE 43-12 Heterotypic Collagen Fibril. Hierarchical depiction of heterotypic collagen fibril, emphasizing the internal axial relationships required for mature cross-link formation. **A,** Three-dimensional concept of the type II/IX/XI heterotypic fibril of developing cartilage matrix. **B,** Detail illustrating required nearest neighbor axial relationships for trifunctional intermolecular cross-links to form in collagens of cartilage, bone, and other high-tensile strength tissue matrices. The exact 3D spatial pattern of cross-linking bonds is still unclear for any tissue. **C,** Detail of the axial stagger of individual collagen molecules required for pyridinoline cross-linking. (From Eyre DA, Weiss MA, Wu JJ: *Methods* 4[1]:65, 2008.)

the loss of fluid from the cartilage, and (4) prevent the escape of protein polysaccharides (proteoglycans) from the cartilage.

The proteoglycans are macromolecules consisting of proteins, carbohydrates **(glycosaminoglycans),** and hyaluronic acid. One subgroup of proteoglycans, known as heparin sulfate proteoglycans (HSPGs), binds to many proteins involved in musculoskeletal development and homeostasis, including FGF, BMPs, Wnts, chemokines, interleukins, and extracellular matrix (ECM) proteins.[19] The glycosaminoglycans (keratin sulfate and chondroitin sulfate) are attached to the **protein core,** and several protein cores (with their attached glycosaminoglycans) are bound to a hyaluronic acid chain by a special protein called **link protein.** The proteoglycans give articular cartilage its stiff quality and regulate the movement of synovial fluid through the cartilage. Without proteoglycans, normal weightbearing would rapidly and completely press all the synovial fluid out of the cartilage. Proteoglycans act as a pump, permitting enough fluid to be pressed out to ensure that a fluid film is always present on the surface of the cartilage, even after hours of weightbearing. The pumping action of proteoglycans also draws synovial fluid back into the cartilage after a weightbearing load is released. Mobility and weightbearing are necessary for the pumping action of proteoglycans to occur. Nonuse of a joint quickly reduces the pumping action, which changes the composition of the matrix and interferes with the nutrition of the chondrocytes.

Normal articular cartilage has no blood vessels, lymph vessels, or nerves. Therefore, it is insensitive to pain and regenerates slowly and minimally after injury.[20,21] Regeneration occurs primarily at sites where the articular cartilage meets the synovial membrane, where blood vessels and nutrients are available. In general, it has been difficult to enhance cartilage repair, but that may be changing (see What's New? Progress in Rebuilding Cartilage).

WHAT'S NEW?

Progress in Rebuilding Cartilage

Efforts to repair damaged cartilage have been difficult because of the poor vascularity of cartilage. Currently available techniques, such as autologous chondrocyte transplantation, have not consistently produced good results. Developments in tissue engineering have been aided by maintaining improved biologic control of cell growth, differentiation, and metabolic activity. One persistent challenge is developing material with increased amounts of collagen to allow proper mechanical function of engineered cartilage.

Techniques known as "functional tissue engineering" not only should provide a network of chondrocyte cell growth but also should greatly improve the biomechanical properties of engineered cartilage. By more closely resembling native cartilage, these technologies show great promise for clinically improved outcomes in cartilage repair and replacement.

Data from Kock L, van Donkelaar CC, Ito K: *Cell Tissue Res* 347(3):613–627, 2012.

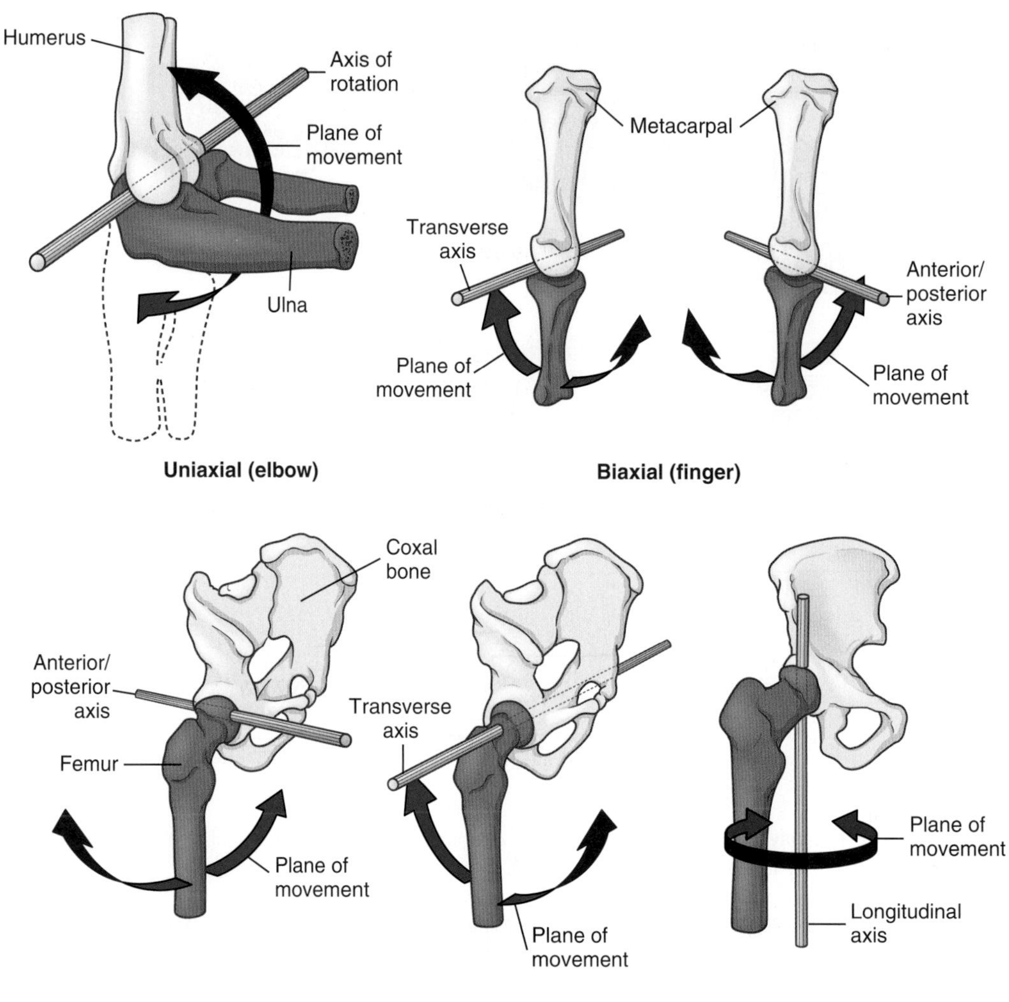

FIGURE 43-13 Movements of Synovial (Diarthrodial) Joints.

Movement

Synovial joints are described as uniaxial, biaxial, or multiaxial according to the shapes of the bone ends and the type of movement occurring at the joint (Figure 43-13). Usually one of the bones is stable and serves as an axis for the motion of the other bone. The body movements made possible by various synovial joints are either circular or angular (Figure 43-14).

STRUCTURE AND FUNCTION OF SKELETAL MUSCLES

Skeletal muscles arise from mesodermal progenitor cells; the most numerous are the somites. Actual formation of skeletal muscle is a complex process controlled by multiple signaling factors. A critical component of successful embryonic muscle formation (myogenesis) is protein kinase, an enzyme that adds phosphate groups to substrate proteins, thereby directing cell processes.[22] In muscle, these factors direct formation of myoblasts. Once myoblasts are formed, they fuse with other myoblasts and form myotubes, eventually developing into muscle fibers. At birth, the muscle fibers have completed development from myoblasts. Final muscle type is determined by transcription factors that regulate both pre- and postnatal muscle development.[23]

All **voluntary muscles** are derived from the mesodermal layer of the embryo. Genetic transcription factors, most notably myoblast determination protein (MyoD), induce skeletal muscle differentiation. Myoblasts are the main cells responsible for muscle growth and regeneration. Myoblasts are termed *satellite cells* when in a dormant state and are crucial in muscle growth, maintenance, repair, and regeneration. Once muscle is injured, satellite cells become activated and increase the number of transcriptional factors necessary to form myoblasts and assist in repair.

Skeletal muscles are made up of millions of individual fibers that by the process of contraction and relaxation do the work necessary to complete movements as varied as a ballerina's pirouette or an artist's deft stroke (Figure 43-15). Muscle constitutes 40% of adults' body weight and 50% of children's body weight. Muscle is 75% water, 20% protein, and 5% organic and inorganic compounds; 32% of all protein stores for energy and metabolism is contained in muscle.

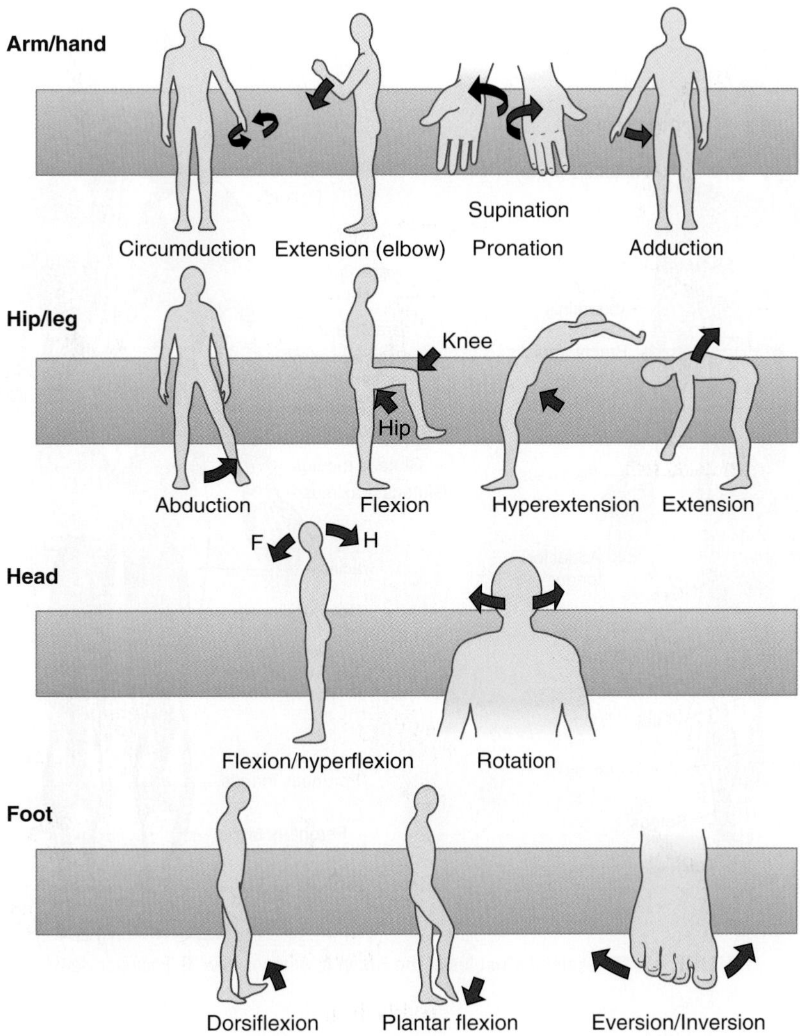

FIGURE 43-14 Body Movements Provided by Synovial (Diarthrodial) Joints.

Whole Muscle

There are more than 350 named muscles; almost all are paired. The body's muscles vary dramatically; they range from 2 to 60 cm in length and are shaped according to function.[24] **Fusiform muscles** are elongated muscles shaped like straps and can run from one joint to another. **Pennate muscles** are broad, flat, and slightly fan shaped, with fibers running obliquely to the muscle's long axis. The multipennate deltoid muscle, which flexes and extends the arm, is a good example of a muscle shaped according to its function.

Each skeletal muscle is a separate organ encased in a three-part connective tissue framework called **fascia.** The layers of connective tissue protect the muscle fibers, attach the muscle to bony prominences, and provide a structure for a network of nerve fibers, blood vessels, and lymphatic channels.

The outermost layer, the **epimysium,** is located on the surface of the muscle and tapers at each end to form the **tendon** (Figure 43-16). Tendons allow a short muscle to exert power on a distant joint, whereas a thick muscle interferes with joint mobility. The next layer, the **perimysium,** further subdivides the muscle fibers into bundles of connective tissue, or **fascicles.** The **endomysium** surrounds the muscle fascicles, the smallest unit of muscle fibers visible without a microscope. The ligaments, tendons, and fascia are made up of connective tissue that also serves to buffer the limbs from the effects of sudden strains or changes in speed. The rapid recovery necessary for strenuous exercise is supported by the elastic property of muscle and its connective tissue.

Skeletal muscle is described, almost interchangeably, as **voluntary, striated,** or **extrafusal.** "Voluntary" indicates that the muscle is controlled directly by the central nervous system. "Striated" describes the striated, or striped, pattern of skeletal muscle viewed under a light microscope. The striations result from the organization of the muscle fibers into the contractile units called *sarcomeres.* "Extrafusal" distinguishes the skeletal muscle fibers from other contractile fibers located within the sensory organs of the muscle.

Other components that are visible on gross inspection of the whole muscle include the motor and sensory nerve fibers. These function together with the muscle, innervating portions of it and providing the electrical impulses needed for motor function.

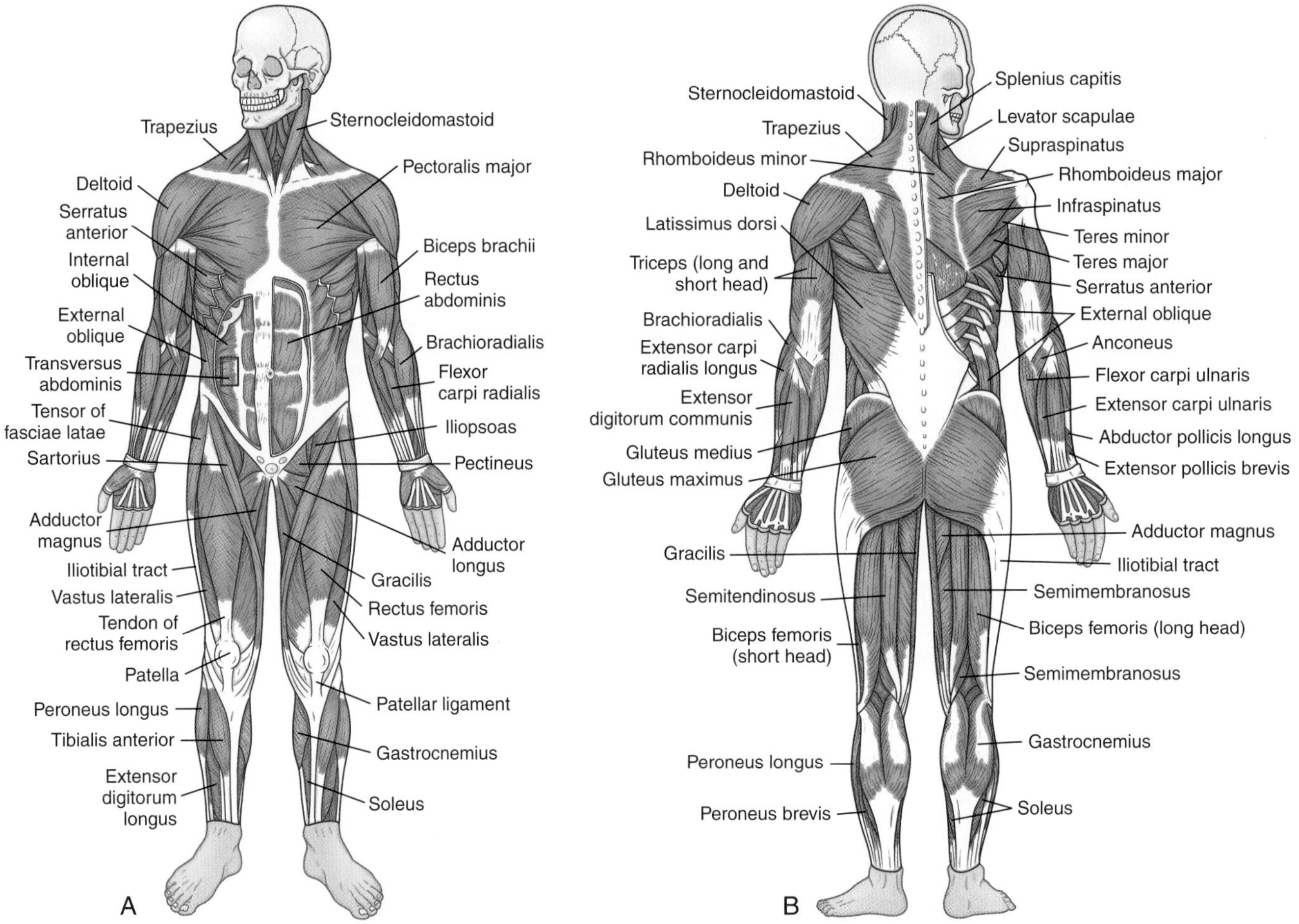

FIGURE 43-15 Skeletal Muscles of the Body. **A,** Anterior view. **B,** Posterior view.

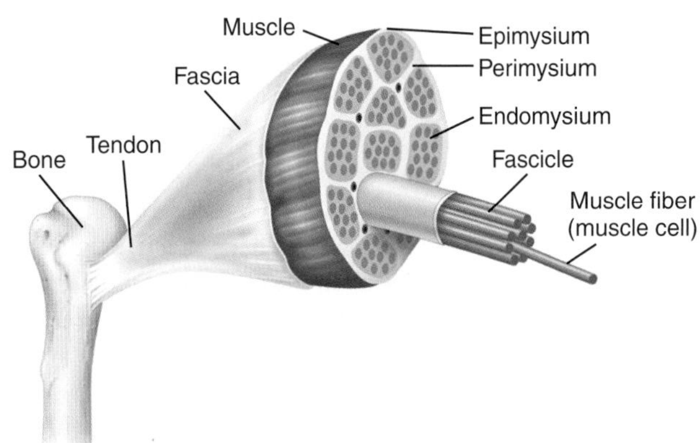

FIGURE 43-16 Cross Section of Skeletal Muscle Showing Muscle Fibers and Their Coverings. (From Thibodeau GA, Patton KT: *Anatomy & physiology,* ed 5, St Louis, 2003, Mosby.)

Motor Unit

From the anterior horn cell of the spinal cord, the axons of motor nerves branch out to innervate a specific group of muscle fibers. Each anterior horn cell, its axon (part of a lower motor neuron; see Chapter 15), and the muscle fibers innervated by it are called a **motor unit** (Figure 43-17). The motor units are composed of lower motor neurons, which extend to skeletal muscles. Often termed the *functional unit* of the neuromuscular system, the motor unit behaves as a single entity and contracts as a whole when it receives an electrical impulse.

The whole muscle may be controlled by several motor nerve axons. These branch to innervate many motor units within the muscle. The whole muscle then may consist of many motor units. The number of motor units per individual muscle varies greatly. In the calf, for example, 1 motor axon will innervate approximately 2000 muscle fibers, out of a total of 1,200,000 muscle fibers. This is a high innervation ratio of muscle fibers to axons, and it contrasts markedly with the low innervation ratio in the laryngeal muscles. There, two or three muscle fibers constitute each motor unit, and the innervation ratio can be of great functional significance. The greater the innervation ratio of a particular organ, the greater its endurance. Higher innervation ratios prevent fatigue, and lower innervation ratios allow for precision of movement.

Sensory Receptors. Although muscles function as effector organs, they also contain sensory receptors and are involved in sending different signals to the central nervous system. Among these are the muscle spindles and Golgi tendon organs. **Spindles** are mechanoreceptors that lie parallel to muscle fibers and respond to muscle stretching. **Golgi tendon organs** are dendrites that terminate and branch to tendons near the neuromuscular junction. Motor and sensory neurons secrete a proteoglycan called *neuroregulin (NRG)* that increases the

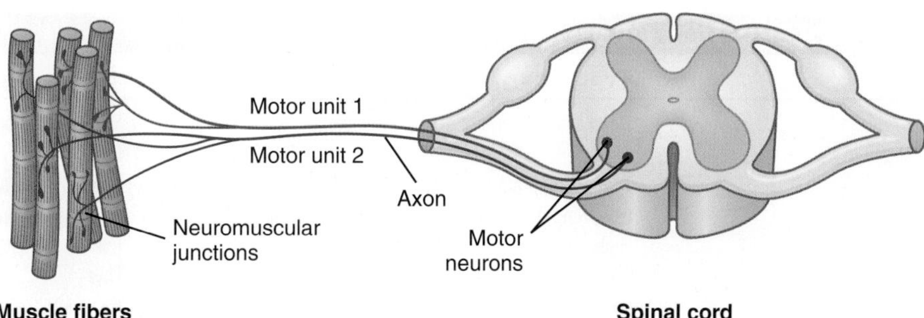

FIGURE 43-17 Motor Units of a Muscle. Each motor unit consists of a somatic motor neuron and all the muscle fibers (cells) supplied by the neuron and its axon branches.

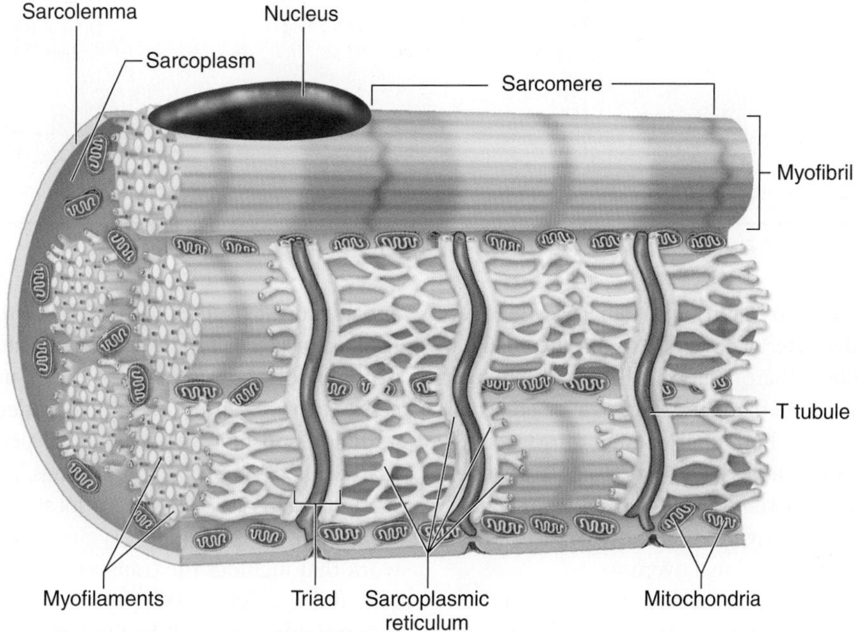

FIGURE 43-18 Myofibrils of a Skeletal Muscle Fiber (Cell) and Overall Organization of Skeletal Muscle. (From Patton KT, Thibodeau GA: *Anatomy & physiology,* ed 8, St Louis, 2013, Mosby.)

number of acetylcholine receptors and helps in the formation of muscle spindle fibers. Muscle spindles, Golgi tendon organs, and free nerve endings provide a means of reporting changes in length, tension, velocity, and tone in the muscle. This system of afferent signals is responsible for the muscle stretch response and maintenance of normal muscle tone.

Muscle Fibers. Each **muscle fiber** is a single **muscle cell.** This long cell is cylindrical and surrounded by a membrane capable of excitation and impulse propagation. The muscle fiber contains bundles of **myofibrils,** the fiber's functional subunits, in a parallel arrangement along the longitudinal axis of the muscle (Figure 43-18). At birth the muscle fibers have completed development from precursor cells called **myoblasts.** All voluntary muscles are derived from the mesodermal layer of the embryo.

The type of peripheral nerve influences the muscle fiber and motor unit considerably. Whether motor nerves are fast or slow determines the type of muscle fibers in the motor unit. Type II fibers, also called *white fast-motor fibers,* are innervated by relatively large type II alpha motor neurons with fast conduction velocities. These fibers rely on a short-term anaerobic glycolytic system for rapid energy transfer, whereas type I fibers depend on aerobic oxidative metabolism. Histochemical stains are now routinely used to describe the structure of muscle fibers and contractile elements of muscle biopsy specimens. White muscle **(type II fibers)** stains dark in the enzyme stain adenosinetriphosphatase (ATPase) at a pH of 9.4. Red muscle **(type I fibers)** appears lightly stained.

The overlap of muscle fibers that appear with staining gives the checkerboard appearance of muscle biopsy specimens and provides an equal distribution of fiber types throughout the muscle. This overlap also helps compensate for muscle fiber loss and fatigue of individual motor units during activity. In spite of this, some muscles contain proportionally more of one fiber type than another. The postural muscles have more type I fibers, allowing them the high resistance to fatigue that is necessary to maintain the same position for extended periods. Ocular muscles have more type II muscle fibers, allowing them to respond rapidly to visual changes. (Table 43-7 describes the specific characteristics of type I and type II fibers.)

The number of muscle fibers varies according to location. Large muscles, such as the gastrocnemius, have more fibers (1,200,000) than smaller muscles, such as the lumbrical muscles in the hand (10,000). The diameter of muscle fibers also varies. The closely

TABLE 43-7 **CHARACTERISTICS OF MUSCLE FIBERS**

CHARACTERISTIC	TYPE I (RED)	TYPE II (WHITE)
Anatomic location	Deep axial portion of surface muscle	Surface portion of surface muscle
Contraction speed	Slow	Fast
Motor neuron type	Type I, small alpha	Type II, large alpha
Firing frequency	Low, long duration	Rapid, short duration
Resistance to fatigue	High	Low
Myoglobin	High	Low
Capillary supply	Profuse	Intermediate to sparse
Metabolism	Oxidative	Glycolysis
Mitochondria	Many	Few
Enzymes	Lactate dehydrogenase, types 1 to 3	Lactate dehydrogenase, types 4 and 5
Creatine kinase	Cardiac type	Fast, skeletal
Example (most muscles are mixed)	Greater proportion of slow-contracting fibers in soleus	Greater proportion of fast-contracting fibers in laryngeal and ocular muscles
Glycogen content	Low	High
Intensity of contraction	Low	High
Aerobic metabolic capacity	High	Low
Fiber diameter	Small	Large
Myosin-adenosinetriphosphatase (ATPase) activity	Low	High

From Spence AP, Mason EE: *Human anatomy and physiology,* ed 4, St Paul, MN, 1992, West Publishing.

packed polygons are small (10 to 20 μm) until puberty, when they attain the normal adult diameter of 40 to 80 μm. Women usually have smaller-diameter fibers than men. Small muscles, such as the ocular muscles, are 15 μm in diameter; larger, more proximal muscles are 40 μm in diameter. Both fiber size and muscle length have functional significance. Studies have shown that larger fiber diameter is associated with generation of greater forces. Fiber diameter can be increased by activities that cause hypertrophied muscle, such as exercise or occupational overuse.

The major components of the muscle fiber include the muscle membrane, myofibrils, sarcotubular system, sarcoplasm, and mitochondria (see Figure 43-18). The **muscle membrane** is a two-part membrane. It includes the **sarcolemma,** which contains the plasma membrane of the muscle cell, and the cell's **basement membrane.** The sarcolemma is 7.5 μm thick and is capable of propagating electrical impulses to initiate contraction. At the motor nerve end plate, where the nerve impulse is transmitted, the sarcolemma forms the highly convoluted synaptic cleft. The sarcolemma is comprised of lipid molecules and protein systems. The protein systems perform special functions, such as transport of nutrients and protein synthesis. They also provide the sodium-potassium pump and include the cell's cholinergic receptor. The basement membrane is 50 μm thick and is composed primarily of proteins and polysaccharides. It serves as the cell's microskeleton and maintains the shape of the muscle cell. The basement membrane also may function in some way to restrict further diffusion of electrolytes once they have crossed the sarcolemma.

The **sarcoplasm** is the cytoplasm of the muscle cell and contains the intracellular components that are common to all cells (see Chapter 1). The sarcoplasm is an aqueous substance that provides a matrix that surrounds the myofibrils. It contains numerous enzymes and proteins that are responsible for the cell's energy production, protein synthesis, and oxygen storage. The mitochondria house enzyme systems for energy production, particularly those that regulate such processes as the citric acid cycle and adenosine triphosphate (ATP) formation. Many other structures are present in the sarcoplasm. The ribosomes are composed primarily of ribonucleic acid (RNA) and participate in the process of protein synthesis. The cell nucleus, satellite cells, glycogen granules, and lipid droplets are suspended in the sarcoplasmic matrix. Blood vessels, nerve endings, muscle spindles, and Golgi tendon organs are also directly located within this structure.

Unique to the muscle is the **sarcotubular system,** a network that includes the transverse tubules and the sarcoplasmic reticulum, which crosses the interior of the cell. The **sarcoplasmic reticulum** is made in the same manner as the endoplasmic reticulum in other cells. In the muscle cells the sarcoplasmic reticulum is involved in calcium transport, which initiates muscle contraction at the **sarcomere,** a portion of the myofibril. The sarcoplasmic reticulum is composed of tubules that run parallel to the myofibrils. The longitudinal tubules are termed **sarcotubules.** The **transverse tubules,** which are closely associated with the sarcotubules, run across the sarcoplasm and communicate with the extracellular space. Together, the tubules of this membrane system allow for intracellular calcium uptake, regulation, and release during muscle contraction, and for the storage of calcium during muscle relaxation.

Myofibrils. Myofibrils, the most abundant subcellular muscle components, are the functional units of muscle contraction. Each myofibril contains sarcomeres, which, in turn, consist of repeating protein filaments[25] (see Figure 43-18). Sarcomeres are chiefly composed of the proteins **actin, myosin, titin,** and **nebulin.** The sarcomere is responsible for converting chemical energy into movement.

On cross section they are irregular polygons with a mean diameter of less than 1 μm. Each myofibril is composed of serially repeating sarcomeres, separated by Z lines that give the muscle its striped, cross-striated appearance. Each sarcomere has a dark A band and is flanked by two light I bands (Figure 43-19). Titin functions as a molecular spring that plays a

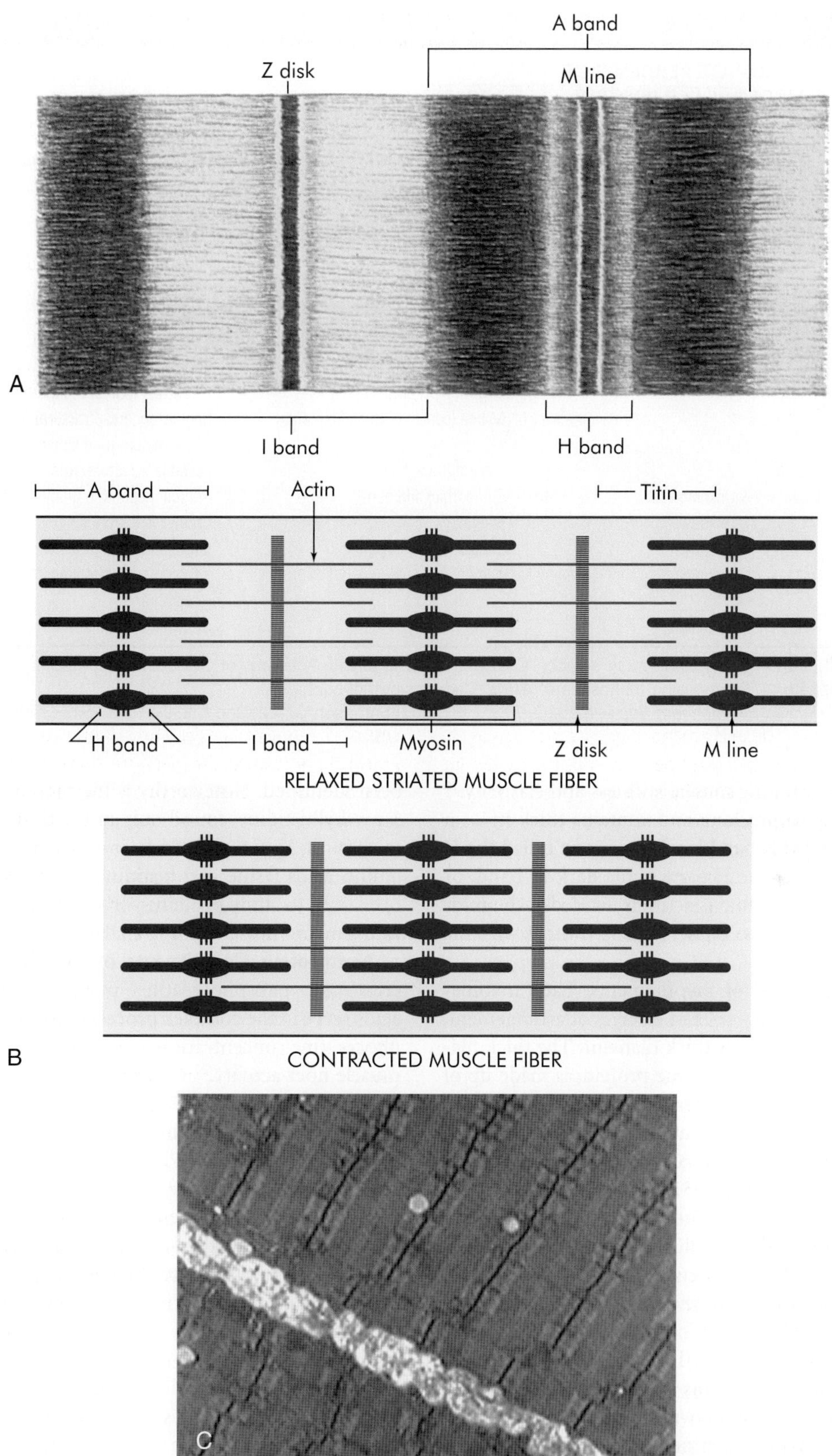

FIGURE 43-19 Muscle Fibers. A, The Z disks define the end of an individual sarcomere. The M line (which lies within the H band) is made of cross-connecting elements of the cytoskeleton. **B,** Actin is the primary protein of the I band (thin filament). Nebulin (not shown) also extends along the I band and contains binding sites for actin and myosin. Myosin (thick filament) extends through the A band. Titin extends from the Z disk to the M line, binding with myosin; strong titin anchoring within the I band is necessary for proper muscle function. During contraction, the I bands and H bands shorten, moving the Z disks closer together. **C,** Electron photomicrograph of human muscle tissue corresponding to schematics in **A** and **B.** (**A** modified from Thompson JM et al: *Mosby's clinical nursing,* ed 5, St Louis, 2002, Mosby; **C** courtesy Louisa Howard.)

TABLE 43-8 CONTRACTILE PROTEINS OF SKELETAL MUSCLE FIBRILS

NAME	APPROXIMATE PERCENTAGE OF MYOFIBRILLAR PROTEIN	LOCATION	FUNCTION
Myosin	55	A band (thick filament)	Contraction; hydrolyzes ATP and develops tension
Actin	20	I band (thin filament)	Contraction; activates myosin ATPase and interacts with myosin
Troponin	7	Thin filament	Regulatory protein; in presence of Ca^{++}, promotes actin-myosin activation
Tropomyosin	5-7	Thin filament	Regulatory and structural function; links filaments, controls filament length
Alpha (α) actin	10	Z band	Regulatory and structural function; links filaments, controls filament length
Beta (β) actin	2	Z band	Regulatory and structural function; links filaments, controls filament length
M protein	2	M line (center of thick filaments)	Regulatory and structural function; provides enzyme creatine kinase
C protein	2	A band (thick filaments)	Possible structural role
Titin	Unknown	Z line (thick filament)	Interconnects thin filaments in Z line
Creatine kinase	Unknown	M line	Catalyzes the phosphorylation of ADP to form ATP
Desmin	Unknown	Z line	Interconnects thin filaments in Z line
Filamin*	Unknown	Z line	Interconnects thin filaments in Z line; stabilizes membrane
Nebulin*	Unknown	Z line	Determines filament length

Modified from Simon SR, editor: *Orthopaedic basic science,* Chicago, 1994, American Academy of Orthopaedic Surgeons.
ADP, Adenosine diphosphate; *ATP,* adenosine triphosphate; *ATPase,* adenosinetriphosphatase.
*Data from Ma K, Wang K: *Fed Eur Biochem Soc Lett* 532(3):273–278, 2002; Sampson LJ, Leyland ML, Dart D: *J Biol Chem* 278(43):41988–41997, 2003.

significant role in determining muscle stiffness and elasticity.[26] The A band is 1.5 to 1.6 μm long and contains thick myosin filaments. Included in the A band is a lighter zone called the H band, and in the center of the H band is the dark M band, or M line. The I band, which contains actin, is divided at the midpoint of each sarcomere by the Z line. Its length varies with the start of muscle contraction.

Myofibrils are composed of myofilaments. Each myofilament is structured in a closely packed hexagonal arrangement, with two thin filaments for every thick filament. The thick filament, along with C protein and M line protein, is made up of myosin. Myosin has two subunits, heavy and light meromyosin, which resemble twisted golf club shafts. The thin filaments are twisted double strands made up of actin, troponin, and tropomyosin (see Chapter 31 and Figure 31-15).

Muscle Proteins. Table 43-8 summarizes muscle protein distribution, location, and possible functional significance. The contractile and regulatory functions of actin, myosin, and the troponin-tropomyosin complex (associated with actin) are the most commonly known. They also account for most of the protein found in the myofibril. The structural and regulatory processes of muscle proteins are less well understood. Alpha actin and beta actin are known to link the filaments. M protein contains the enzyme creatine kinase (CK). Creatine is released when muscle cells are damaged, making serum creatine value an important measurement of pathologic conditions of muscles.

The most abundant proteins, actin and myosin, are also found in other cells, particularly motile cells such as platelets. The complete amino acid sequences of actin and myosin have been identified. Noteworthy is the presence of the amino acid 3-methylhistidine, found only in the thin filament, actin; 85% to 90% of 3-methylhistidine is found in skeletal muscle. The amino acids lysine and histidine, in addition to leucine, have been used to study protein synthesis by means of stable isotope infusion and muscle biopsy analysis.

Nonprotein Constituents of Muscle. Nitrogen, creatine, creatinine, phosphocreatine, purines, uric acid, and amino acids serve in the complex process of muscle metabolism. Phosphocreatine concentration is an extremely sensitive indicator of muscle fiber activity.[27] Glycogen and its derivatives are present as energy sources.

Creatine and creatinine metabolism have been used to measure muscle mass. Plasma creatine is taken up by muscle and converted into the high-energy phosphate compound *phosphocreatine* by the enzyme **creatine kinase.** Creatinine is formed in muscle from creatine at a constant rate of 2% per day. (Tests for plasma creatine are discussed in Chapter 37.) Creatine excretion is increased in muscle wasting. This change reflects the reduction in total body creatine stores and loss of muscle mass.

Inorganic compounds, anions (phosphate, chloride), and cations (calcium, magnesium, sodium, potassium) are important in regulating protein synthesis, muscle contraction, enzyme systems, and membrane stabilization. Intracellular calcium levels influence the force and duration of muscle contraction. Total body potassium (TBK), measured by the K_{40} method, has been used to measure muscle mass, also called *lean body mass.* TBK levels reflect changes in muscle mass seen during growth, malnutrition, and muscle wasting.

TABLE 43-9 ENERGY SOURCES FOR MUSCULAR ACTIVITY

SOURCES	REACTIONS
Short-term (anaerobic) sources	Adenosine triphosphate (ATP) → Adenosine diphosphate (ADP) + Inorganic phosphate (Pi) + Energy
	Phosphocreatine + ADP ⇌ Creatine + ATP
	Glycogen/glucose + Pi + ADP → Lactate + ATP
Long-term (aerobic) sources	Glycogen/glucose + ADP + Pi + O_2 → H_2O + CO_2 + ATP
	Free fatty acids + ADP + Pi + O_2 → H_2O + CO_2 + ATP
	Creatine kinase catalyzes the reversible reaction of ATP to ADP: Creatine phosphate + ADP $\xrightleftharpoons[\text{kinase}]{\text{Creatine}}$ Creatine + ATP

From Spence AP, Mason EE: *Human anatomy and physiology,* ed 4, St Paul, MN, 1992, West Publishing.

Components of Muscle Function

The ultimate function of muscle is to accomplish work. Although variously expressed in such measures as foot-pounds or kilogram-meters, work usually refers to the amount of energy liberated or force exerted over a distance (work = force × distance). Muscles usually contract or tense while doing work. Muscle contraction occurs on the molecular level and leads to the observable phenomenon of muscle movement.

Muscle Contraction at the Molecular Level

Muscle contraction is a four-step process: excitation, coupling, contraction, and relaxation. The initial contraction process is the excitation-contraction coupling (ECC) series, which involves the electrical properties of all cells and the movement of ions across the plasma membrane (see Chapter 1). At rest an electrical charge of −90 mV is continually maintained across the muscle sarcolemma. This resting potential, generated by the separation of positive and negative charges on either side of the membrane, creates an electrochemical equilibrium caused by the selective permeability of the sarcolemma to electrolytes in the intracellular and extracellular fluids, particularly potassium and sodium.

Specific intracellular receptors within skeletal muscle sarcoplasmic reticulum, called **ryanodine receptors (RyRs),** are the primary ion channels that control calcium release. RyRs are the largest known ion channels, allowing for rapid movement of calcium. Three RyRs have been identified: RyR1 is predominantly found in skeletal muscle; RyR2 is found mostly in cardiac muscle; and RyR3 is in the diaphragm, smooth muscle, and brain.[28-30]

Excitation, the first step of muscle contraction, begins with the spread of an action potential from the nerve terminal to the neuromuscular junction. The rapid depolarization of the membrane initiates an electrical impulse in the muscle fiber membrane called the **muscle fiber action potential.** As the action potential advances along the sarcolemmal membrane, it spreads to the transverse tubules (T-tubules). (The velocity of conduction is much slower in muscle fibers than in myelinated nerve fibers—only 3 to 5 m/second compared with 54 to 90 m/second in nerve fibers.)

The generated action potential then triggers voltage-sensitive receptors in the T-tubule wall; in turn, these receptors open the RyR channels, causing release of calcium from the sarcoplasmic reticulum.[28]

Following depolarization of the T-tubules, the second stage, **coupling,** occurs. This stage consists of the migration of calcium ions to the myofilaments. Calcium affects troponin and tropomyosin, muscle proteins that bind with actin when the muscle is at rest. In the presence of calcium, however, both of these proteins are attracted to calcium ions, leaving the actin free to bind with myosin.

Contraction begins as the calcium ions combine with troponin, a reaction that overcomes the inhibitory function of the troponin-tropomyosin system. The thin filament *actin* then slides toward the thick filament *myosin.* The two ends of the myofibril shorten after contraction when the myosin heads attach to the actin molecules, forming a cross-bridge that constitutes an actin-myosin complex. ATP, located on the actin-myosin complex, is released when the cross-bridges attach. This is the **sliding filament theory** and was first described by A.F. Huxley in the 1950s; however, it is now called the **cross-bridge theory** because of the formation of the actin-myosin cross-bridges. The process is so named because the actin actually slides onto the myosin, causing the sarcomere to shorten. The useful distance of contraction of a skeletal muscle is approximately 25% to 35% of the muscle's length. When actin and myosin filaments have maximum interactions, the muscle generates maximum force.[24]

The last step, **relaxation,** begins as the sarcoplasmic reticulum absorbs the calcium molecules, removing them from interaction with troponin. Calcium is pumped back into the sarcoplasmic reticulum by means of an active transport process. The cross-bridges detach, and the sarcomere lengthens. (The cross-bridge theory of muscle contraction is discussed in Chapter 31.)

Muscle Metabolism

Skeletal muscle requires a constant supply of ATP and phosphocreatine. These substances are necessary to fuel the complex processes of muscle contraction, driving the cross-bridges of actin and myosin together and transporting calcium from the sarcoplasmic reticulum to the myofibril. Other internal processes of the muscular system that require ATP include protein synthesis, which replenishes muscle constituents and accommodates growth and repair. The rate of protein synthesis is related to hormone levels (particularly insulin), amino acid substrates, and overall nutritional status. At rest the rate of ATP formation by oxidation of glucose or acetoacetate is sufficient to maintain internal processes, given normal nutritional status. During activity the need for ATP increases 100-fold. The metabolic pathways for muscle activity in Table 43-9 show reactions to the immediate need for increased ATP caused by contraction. Activity lasting longer than 5 seconds expends the available stored ATP and phosphocreatine.

Stored glycogen and blood glucose are converted anaerobically to sustain brief activity without increasing the demand for oxygen. Anaerobic glycolysis is much less efficient than aerobic glycolysis, using six to eight times more glycogen to produce the same amount of ATP. With increased activity, such as intense exercise, or ischemia, an increase in the level of lactic acid occurs because of the breakdown of glycogen, thus causing a shift in muscle pH (see Table 43-9). This short-term mechanism "buys time" by allowing ATP formation in spite of inadequate energy stores or oxygen supply. When the anaerobic threshold is reached and more oxygen is required, physiologic changes occur, including an increase in lactic acid concentration and increases in oxygen consumption, heart rate, respiratory rate, and muscle blood flow.

Strenuous exercise requires oxygen, which activates the aerobic glycogen pathway for ATP formation. During maximal exercise, free fatty acid mobilization and the aerobic glycogen pathways provide ATP over an extended time. These pathways require oxygen to maintain maximal activity and return the muscle to the resting state. Maximal exercise increases oxygen uptake 15 to 30 times over the resting state.[31] When this system becomes exhausted or unable to respond to the need for ATP, fatigue and weakness finally force the muscle to reduce activity, with a resultant buildup of lactic acid in muscle fibers.

The ability to sustain maximal muscular activity leads to the accumulation of oxygen debt. **Oxygen debt** is the amount of oxygen needed to convert the buildup of lactic acid to glucose and replenish ATP and phosphocreatine stores. For example, after running at maximal speed for 10 seconds, the average person has consumed 1 L of oxygen. At rest, oxygen consumption for the same period is approximately 40 ml. As the person recovers, the measured oxygen debt is 4 L greater than the amount used during activity.

Oxygen consumption is measured to calculate the metabolic cost of activity in normal and diseased muscle. It is an indirect measure of energy expenditure, along with timed tests of activity, heart rate, and respiratory quotient (ratio of carbon dioxide to expired oxygen consumed). Energy expenditure is measured directly by heat production because heat is released whenever work is accomplished.

Another factor that changes energy requirements is muscle fiber type. Type II fibers rely on anaerobic glycolytic metabolism and fatigue readily. Type I fibers can resist fatigue for longer periods because of their capacity for oxidative metabolism.

Muscle Mechanics

Muscle contraction cannot be viewed in isolation. Several factors determine how force is transmitted from the cross-bridges on individual muscle fibers to accomplish whole-muscle contraction. First, when a motor unit responds to a single nerve stimulus, it develops a phasic contraction, also called *twitch.* Because the motor unit contracts in an "all or nothing" manner, the contraction that is generated will be a maximal contraction. The central nervous system smoothly grades the force generated by "recruiting" additional motor units and varying the discharge frequency of each active motor unit. This adding of motor units within the muscle is called **repetitive discharge.**

Recruitment and repetitive discharge of motor units allow the muscle to activate the number of motor units needed to generate the desired force. The total force developed is the sum of the force generated by each motor unit. As the strength, speed, and duration of stimuli increase, the summation of contractions reaches a critical frequency called **tetanus.** When tetanus is reached, no further increase in force can be achieved.

Other variables, such as fiber type, innervation ratio, muscle temperature, and muscle shape, influence the efficiency of muscular contraction. The two muscle fiber types differ in their responses to electrical activity. Tetanus and duration of phasic contractions, which take microseconds to accomplish, are achieved more rapidly in type II than in type I muscle fibers. Low-innervation ratios promote control and coordination, whereas high ratios promote strength and endurance. Muscles work best at normal body temperature, 37° C (98.6° F). Finally, muscles with a large cross-sectional area, such as the fan-shaped pennate muscles, develop greater contractile forces than smaller-diameter muscles. The initial length of a muscle and the range of shortening that occur when the muscle contracts also determine the forces it can generate. The long fusiform muscles have a greater range of shortening and can contract up to 57% of their resting length. A certain amount of elongation is necessary to generate sufficient tension and muscular force. The elongation that occurs during the swing of a golf club or tennis racquet is an example of how stretch improves contractile force.

Types of Muscle Contraction

During **isometric contraction (static or holding contraction),** the muscle maintains constant length as tension is increased. Isometric contraction occurs, for example, when the arm or leg is pushed against an immovable object. The muscle contracts, but the limb does not move.

During **isotonic contraction (lengthening or shortening contraction),** the muscle maintains a constant tension as it moves. The terms "eccentric" for lengthening and "concentric" for shortening are technically inaccurate descriptions of muscle movement; the respective terms "lengthening" and "shortening" are more precise. Positive work is accomplished during shortening, and energy is released to exert force or lift a weight. In contrast, during lengthening the muscle lengthens and absorbs energy. Negative work is accomplished on the muscle by the load. Lengthening requires less energy to accomplish and may result in the development of pain and stiffness after unaccustomed exercise.

Movement of Muscle Groups

Muscles do not act alone but rather in groups, often under automatic control. When a muscle contracts it acts as a "prime mover," or **agonist,** and its reciprocal muscle, or **antagonist,** relaxes. This is easily tested by holding the right arm in the horizontal position in front of the body and then bending the elbow while feeling the upper arm, biceps in the front and the triceps in the back, with the other hand. The biceps is firm, and the triceps is soft. As the arm is extended, the muscles change. When the elbow is completely extended, the biceps is soft and the triceps firm. Completing this movement causes the agonist and antagonist to change automatically; only the movement is commanded, not the alternate contraction and relaxation of the specific muscle groups.

Other associated actions may be seen during walking; as the foot leaves the ground, the paravertebral and gluteal muscles on the opposite sides of the body contract to maintain balance. One notices the loss of the associated muscle's action when paralysis offsets this process and decreases balance. If a person is paralyzed, difficulty in maintaining balance is noticeable.

TESTS OF MUSCULOSKELETAL FUNCTION

Tests of Bone Function

Diagnostic procedures to evaluate bone function include gait analysis, measurement of serum calcium and phosphorus levels, and imaging studies. Most imaging techniques provide morphologic rather than functional information about bone. Plain radiographs (x-rays) remain the standard initial imaging tool for bone evaluation because bone absorbs x-ray beams better than soft tissue. Computed tomography (CT) provides multiple images that are then processed into single (2-dimensional) or multiple images taken around a single axis to form (3-dimensional) pictures. Dual-energy computed tomography (DECT) utilizes x-ray beams at two different energy levels to determine different chemical composition of tissues, thereby expanding CT imaging to include soft tissues, bone marrow, and crystals.[32] Advances in CT technology allow for detailed visualization of bone microstructure.[33]

Magnetic resonance imaging (MRI) provides detailed anatomic information and is useful for evaluating primary or metastatic bone lesions, infection, marrow edema, bony erosions, osteonecrosis, fractures, and other pathologic changes of bone. Magnetic resonance arthrography (MRa) involves injection of a contrast agent into the area of interest but allows better visualization of small abnormalities. Detailed functional imaging of bone can be attained with positron emission tomography (PET) scanning. A relatively new technology, MRI-PET combines MRI with functional imaging of molecular events seen with PET.

Nuclear medicine studies also provide imaging about metabolic activity in bone and soft tissue. After a small amount of radioactive tracer is injected, a special camera is used to identify bone absorption of the tracer. Bone scanning is very sensitive, but not specific about the cause of increased metabolic activity.

Dual-photon absorptiometry (DXA) is often used to measure the density of bones in the extremities and the fracture risk of vertebral bodies, femoral neck, and distal radius (DXA). Dual-photon absorptiometry allows the soft tissue components to be subtracted. New technology promises more accurate evaluation of bone.

Serum bone-specific alkaline phosphatase (BAP) is a marker of bone formation. Bone resorption is evaluated with urinary and serum measurements of cross-linked N-terminal telopeptides (NTx), a product of osteoclast bone resorption. NTx is specific for bone because the cross-links assessed are characteristic of bone collagen alone. Urine NTx is a more sensitive and specific biochemical marker of bone resorption than serum NTx.[34,35]

Tests of Joint Function

Procedures used to diagnose joint function include arthrography, arthroscopy, magnetic resonance imaging, and synovial fluid analysis. **Arthrography** (the injection of dye into the joint) is particularly useful to diagnose tears in the fibrocartilage of the knee (meniscus) and the rotator cuff of the shoulder. **Arthroscopy** is the direct visualization of a joint through an arthroscope. **Magnetic resonance imaging (MRI)** produces images of body tissues through the use of electromagnetic (radio) waves that alter the atoms (hydrogen ions) in the nuclei of cells being examined. When the polarized radiowaves are stopped, the nuclear atoms return to their original positions, emitting energy as signals as they move back. The signals produce visible images for examination and diagnosis. MRI produces excellent contrast of soft tissues for evaluation of musculoskeletal conditions. Magnetic resonance arthroscopy (MRa) is injection of contrast into a joint, followed by MRI evaluation.

Analysis of synovial fluid may reveal inflammatory, septic, and noninflammatory joint diseases, which cause characteristic changes in the color, clarity, viscosity, and cellular elements of the fluid. The presence of blood in the joint fluid (hemarthrosis) usually indicates joint trauma. Normal synovial fluid is sterile, so the presence of bacteria in the fluid always indicates disease. Cell fragments and fibrous tissue in the fluid are the result of inflammation or wear-and-tear on the articular surfaces.

Tests of Muscular Function

When the individual's history and physical examination disclose abnormalities, such as weakness, atrophy, muscle tenderness, cramps, and stiffness, specific tests of muscle function are in order. One of the most useful tests is the serum creatine kinase (CK) concentration. CK is found in large quantities in the muscle fibers, and when these are diseased or damaged, CK leaks into the serum. Myoglobin is also detectable in the urine after acute muscle damage caused by crush injury, ischemic disorders, extreme exertion, and some inherited diseases.

Because the muscle membrane tissue is excitable and carries an electrical charge, its capacity to function can be assessed by electromyography. Using sensitive needle electrodes, the **electromyogram (EMG)** records the summation of action potentials of the muscle fibers in each motor unit. The EMG is often compared with the electrocardiogram (ECG), but the activity recorded on the EMG is on a much smaller scale. The amplitude of the ECG is measured in volts, the duration of impulse is recorded in seconds, and both are recorded as the heart rate (e.g., 80 V/60 seconds). EMG amplitude is recorded in millivolts and the duration is measured in milliseconds, with a frequency of about 5 to 50 action potentials per second. Motor unit potentials are measured to determine rate of firing, duration, and amplitude. Abnormalities in EMG and nerve conduction velocities help differentiate muscle diseases (myopathy) from peripheral nerve (neuropathy) and neuromuscular junction disorders. The muscle biopsy (using histologic, histochemical, and electron microscopic studies) is used to further define the presence of myopathic and neuropathic disorders, many of which can be diagnosed only by muscle biopsy. Complex myography, a relatively new technique, allows a noninvasive way to gather information on the mechanical characteristics of muscle.

A new area of evaluation is genetics. Recent advances in molecular genetics, deoxyribonucleic acid (DNA) libraries, genetic probes, and gene localization techniques have enhanced our knowledge of neuromuscular diseases, including types of muscular dystrophy, Charcot-Marie-Tooth disease, and familial amyotrophic lateral sclerosis.

AGING AND THE MUSCULOSKELETAL SYSTEM

Aging of Bones

Aging is accompanied by the loss of bone tissue. Bones become less stiff, less strong, and more brittle with aging. The bone remodeling cycle takes longer to complete, and the rate of mineralization also decelerates. Studies have shown that an individual's bone mass at the end of their growth period helps determine the significance of bone loss as they age. With aging, women experience loss of bone density, accelerated by rapid bone loss during early menopause from increased osteoclastic bone resorption.[36] By age 70, susceptible women have lost an average of 50% of their peripheral cortical bone mass. Extensive loss of bone mass leads to deformity, pain, stiffness, and a high risk for fractures. Asymptomatic vertebral fractures can cause loss of height. Men also experience bone loss but at later ages and much slower rates than women. Also, peak bone mass in men is higher than that in women.[37] In general, age-related bone loss is caused by genetics, hormonal factors (decreased estrogen and estradiol levels), decreased bone formation, vitamin and mineral deficiencies (vitamin D, magnesium, and calcium), underlying conditions (malignancy, autoimmune diseases, hyperthyroidism), and lifestyle choices (physical inactivity, smoking, certain medications, and alcohol intake). Men's peak bone mass is related to race, heredity, hormonal factors (testosterone and estradiol levels), physical activity, and calcium intake during childhood.[38]

Bone mass can be gained in healthy young women up to the third decade through physical activity and intake of dietary calcium and magnesium. In addition to the positive effects of exercise on bone mineral density (BMD), exercise has been shown to improve balance, coordination, muscle strength, lean body mass, and mobility, all of which may decrease the incidence of falls[39,40] (also see Figure 2-22, p. 85).

Aging of Joints

With aging, cartilage becomes more rigid, fragile, and susceptible to fibrillation because of increasing cross-linking of collagen and elastin, decreasing water content in the cartilage ground substance, and decreasing concentrations of glycosaminoglycans. Changes in collagen result in cartilage calcification and muscle stiffness. Decreased range of motion of the joint is related to the changes in ligaments and muscles. Bones in joints develop evidence of osteoporosis with fewer trabeculae and thinner, less dense bones, making them prone to fractures. Intervertebral disk spaces decrease in height.

Aging of Muscles

The function of skeletal muscle depends on many factors that are affected by aging, including the nervous, vascular, and endocrine systems. Mitochondrial dysfunction within cells contributes to oxidative stress and results in increased bone resorption and apoptosis of muscle cells.[41,42] In the young child, development of muscle tissue is highly dependent on continuing neurodevelopmental maturation. Muscle function remains trainable even into advanced age. Muscle diseases have a definite association with specific age groups. Muscular dystrophies occur in children, and muscle disabilities related to rheumatic diseases usually occur in advancing age.

Age-related loss in skeletal muscle is referred to as **sarcopenia** and is a direct cause of the age-related decrease in muscle strength. As the body ages, muscle bulk and strength decline slowly, beginning as early as age 50, with loss of about 1% per year thereafter. Muscle strength declines faster than muscle mass.[42] Type II fibers decrease to a greater extent than the slower acting type I fibers. Loss of satellite cells appears to play a major role in the development of sarcopenia. Although muscle's regenerative function remains largely intact, satellite cell numbers are decreased.[43] The reduced RNA synthesis, loss of mitochondrial volume, shortening of telomeres, and reduction in the size of motor units contribute to sarcopenia. As much as 30% to 40% of skeletal muscle mass and strength may be lost from the third to ninth decades.

Maximal oxygen intake decreases with age. Reduced basal metabolic rate and decreased lean body mass are also seen in the older adult population.

SUMMARY REVIEW

Structure and Function of Bones

1. Bones provide support and protection for the body's tissues and organs and are important sources of minerals and blood cells.
2. Bone formation begins in utero with the differentiation of mesenchymal cells into either chondrocytes or osteoblasts. Bone minerals then either crystallize on a cartilage framework or become bone-forming cells without cartilage.
3. Bone tissue is continuously being resorbed and synthesized by bone-remodeling units of osteoclasts and osteoblasts.
4. RANKL induces osteoclast activation and bone resorption. OPG, a protein, binds to a protein called OPG ligand. This attachment serves as a decoy receptor for RANKL and blocks osteoclast activity, thus decreasing bone resorption. The balance between RANKL and OPG determines the quality of bone.
5. Bones in the body are made up of compact bone tissue and spongy bone tissue. Compact bone is highly organized into haversian systems that consist of concentric layers of crystallized matrix surrounding a central canal that contains

SUMMARY REVIEW—cont'd

blood vessels and nerves. Dispersed throughout the concentric layers of crystallized matrix are small spaces containing osteocytes. Smaller canals, called *canaliculi,* interconnect the osteocyte-containing spaces. The crystallized matrix in spongy bone is arranged in bars or plates. Spaces containing osteocytes are dispersed between the bars or plates and interconnected by canaliculi.

6. BMPs are part of the TGF-β superfamily and involved in nearly all aspects of bone formation.
7. There are 206 bones in the body, divided into the axial skeleton and the appendicular skeleton. Bones are classified by shape as long, short, flat, or irregular. Long bones have a broad end (epiphysis), broad neck (metaphysis), and narrow midportion (diaphysis) that contains the medullary cavity.
8. Bone injuries are repaired in stages. Hematoma formation provides the fibrin framework for formation and organization of granulation tissue. Granulation tissue provides a cartilage model for the formation and crystallization of bone matrix. Remodeling restores the original shape and size to the injured bone.

Structure and Function of Joints

1. A joint is the site of attachment of two or more bones. Joints provide stability and mobility to the skeleton.
2. Joints are classified as synarthroses, amphiarthroses, or diarthroses, depending on the degree of movement they allow. Joints also can be classified by the type of connecting tissue holding them together. Fibrous joints are connected by dense fibrous tissue, ligaments, or membranes. Cartilaginous joints are connected by fibrocartilage or hyaline cartilage. Synovial joints are connected by a fibrous joint capsule. Within the capsule is a small fluid-filled space. The fluid in the space nourishes the articular cartilage that covers the ends of the bones meeting in the synovial joint.
3. Articular cartilage is a highly organized system of collagen fibers and proteoglycans. The fibers firmly anchor the cartilage to the bone, and the proteoglycans control the loss of fluid from the cartilage.
4. Joints help move bones and muscle.

Structure and Function of Skeletal Muscles

1. Skeletal muscle is the largest organ in the body and is made up of millions of individual fibers.
2. Whole muscles vary in size (2 to 60 cm) and shape (fusiform and pennate). They are encased in a three-part connective tissue framework. The fundamental concept of muscle function is the *motor unit,* defined as all muscle fibers innervated by a single motor nerve.
3. Muscle fibers contain bundles of myofibrils arranged in parallel along the longitudinal axis and include the muscle membrane, myofibrils, sarcotubular system, aqueous sarcoplasm, and mitochondria. There are two types of muscle fibers, type I and type II, determined by motor nerve innervation.
4. Myofibrils and myofilaments contain the major muscle proteins actin and myosin, which interact to form cross-bridges during muscle contraction. The nonprotein muscle constituents provide an energy source for contraction and regulate protein synthesis, enzyme systems, and membrane stabilization.
5. Muscle contraction includes excitation, coupling, contraction, and relaxation.
6. Muscle strength is graded by the "all or nothing" phenomenon and recruitment. Speed of contraction is affected by several factors: muscle fiber type, temperature, stretch, and weight of the load.
7. The two types of muscle contraction are isometric and isotonic. Muscle shortening occurs during contraction but can be seen also during pathologic and physiologic contracture.
8. Actin and myosin filaments form cross-bridges that cause the sarcomere to shorten, a process now known as the *cross-bridge theory of muscle contraction.*
9. Skeletal muscle requires a constant supply of ATP and phosphocreatine to fuel muscle contraction and for growth and repair. ATP and phosphocreatine can be generated aerobically or anaerobically. Phosphocreatine concentration is an extremely sensitive indicator of muscle fiber activity.
10. Several factors determine how force is transmitted from the actin-myosin cross-bridges on individual muscle fibers to accomplish whole-muscle contraction. When a motor unit responds to a single nerve stimulus, it develops a phasic contraction. The central nervous system smoothly grades the force generated by "recruiting" additional motor units and varying the discharge frequency of each active motor unit.

Tests of Musculoskeletal Function

1. Various diagnostic procedures are used to evaluate bone function, including urinary markers, serum calcium and phosphorus levels, x-ray films, angiography, bone scanning, and MRI.
2. Procedures used to evaluate joint function include arthrography, arthroscopy, MRI, and synovial fluid analysis.
3. Genetic evaluation is useful in detecting, diagnosing, and developing specific treatment for certain inheritable muscle diseases such as muscular dystrophy.

Aging and the Musculoskeletal System

1. Muscle bulk and strength slowly decline with aging, although not to a pathologic degree. The bone remodeling cycle takes longer to complete, and the rate of mineralization slows.
2. Exercise in older adults improves muscle strength, helps increase bone mineral density, and improves balance, coordination, lean body mass, and mobility.
3. Age-related loss in skeletal muscle is referred to as sarcopenia. Loss of satellite cells appears to play a major role in the development of sarcopenia.

KEY TERMS

Actin, 1530
Agonist, 1534
Amphiarthrosis (slightly movable joint), 1520
Antagonist, 1534
Appendicular skeleton, 1517
Arthrography, 1535
Arthroscopy, 1535
Articular cartilage, 1522
Axial skeleton, 1517
Basement membrane, 1530
Bone albumin, 1516
Bone fluid, 1516
Bone matrix, 1512
Bone morphogenic protein (BMP), 1516
Bone-remodeling unit, 1519
Calcification, 1512
Canaliculus (*pl.*, canaliculi), 1517
Chondrocyte, 1522
Collagen fiber, 1516
Compact bone (cortical bone), 1517
Contraction, 1533
Coupling, 1533
Creatine, 1532
Creatine kinase, 1532
Cross-bridge theory, 1533
Diaphysis, 1517
Diarthrosis (freely movable joint), 1520
Electromyogram (EMG), 1535
Endochondral ossification, 1511
Endomysium, 1527
Endosteum, 1518
Epimysium, 1527
Epiphyseal plate (growth plate), 1518
Epiphysis, 1518
Excitation, 1533
Fascia, 1527
Fascicle, 1527
Fibril, 1516
Fibrous joint, 1520
Flat bone, 1518
Fusiform muscle, 1527
Glycoprotein, 1516
Glycosaminoglycan, 1525
Golgi tendon organ, 1528
Gomphosis, 1520
Ground substance, 1511
Haversian canal, 1517
Haversian system, 1517
Hyaluronate, 1522
Hydroxyapatite (HAP), 1516
Integrin, 1515
Intima, 1522
Intramembraneous bone formation, 1512
Irregular bone, 1519
Isometric contraction (static or holding contraction), 1534
Isotonic contraction (lengthening or shortening contraction), 1534
Joint (articulation), 1520
Joint capsule (articular capsule), 1522
Joint cavity (synovial cavity), 1522
Lacuna, 1514
Lamellae, 1517
Laminin, 1516
Link protein, 1527
Long bone, 1517
Magnetic resonance imaging (MRI), 1535
Mesenchymal stem cell (MSC), 1510
Mesenchyme, 1511
Metaphysis, 1518
Motor unit, 1528
Muscle cell, 1529
Muscle fiber, 1529
Muscle fiber action potential, 1533
Muscle membrane, 1530
Myoblast, 1529
Myofibril, 1529
Myosin, 1530
Nebulin, 1530
Osteoblast, 1514
Osteocalcin, 1516
Osteoclast, 1515
Osteocyte, 1514
Osteoid, 1514
Osteonectin, 1516
Osteoprotegerin (OPG), 1514
Oxygen debt, 1534
Pennate muscle, 1527
Perimysium, 1527
Periosteum, 1517
Procallus, 1520
Protein core, 1525
Proteoglycan, 1516
Receptor activator of nuclear factor κβ ligand (RANKL), 1514
Relaxation, 1533
Remodeling, 1519
Repetitive discharge, 1534
Ruffled border, 1515
Ryanodine receptor (RyR), 1533
Sarcolemma, 1530
Sarcomere, 1530
Sarcopenia, 1536
Sarcoplasm, 1530
Sarcoplasmic reticulum, 1530
Sarcotubular system, 1530
Sarcotubule, 1530
Short bone (cuboidal bone), 1518
Sialoprotein (osteopontin), 1516
Skeletal (voluntary, striated, or extrafusal) muscle, 1527
Sliding filament theory, 1533
Spindle, 1528
Spongy bone (cancellous bone), 1517
Subintima, 1522
Suture, 1520
Symphysis, 1520
Synarthrosis (immovable joint), 1520
Synchondrosis, 1520
Syndesmosis, 1520
Synovial fluid, 1522
Synovial joint (diarthrosis), 1522
Synovial membrane (synovium), 1522
Tendon, 1527
Tetanus, 1534
Tidemark, 1524
Titin, 1530
Trabecula (*pl.*, trabeculae), 1517
Transforming growth factor-beta (TGF-β), 1512
Transverse tubule, 1530
Type A synovial cell, 1522
Type B synovial cell, 1522
Type I fiber, 1529
Type II fiber, 1529
Voluntary muscle, 1526
Wnt genes, 1512
Woven bone (callus), 1520

REFERENCES

1. Hojo H et al: Coordination of chondrogenesis and osteogenesis by hypertrophic chondrocytes in enchondral bone development, *J Bone Miner Metab* 28(5):489–502, 2010.
2. Shapiro F: Bone development and its relation to fracture repair. The role of mesenchymal osteoblasts and surface osteoblasts, *Eur Cell Mater* 15:53, 2008.
3. Chen G, Deng C, Li Y- P: TGF-β and BMP signaling in osteoblast differentiation and bone formation, *Int J Biol Sci* 8:272–288, 2012.
4. Bonewald LF: The amazing osteocyte, *J Bone Miner Res* 26(2):229–238, 2012.
5. Caetano-Lopes J, Canhão H, Fonesca JE: Osteoblasts and bone formation, *Acta Reum Port* 32:103, 2007.
6. Yavropoulou MR, Yovos JG: The role of the Wnt signaling pathway in osteoblast commitment and differentiation, *Hormones* 6(4):279, 2008.
7. Zaudi M et al: Osteoclastogenesis, bone resorption, and osteoclast-based therapeutics, *J Bone Miner Res* 18(4):599–609, 2003.
8. Kennedy OD, Schaffler MB: The roles of osteocyte signaling in bone, *J Am Acad Orthop Surg* 20(10):670–671, 2012.
9. Quarles LD: Skeletal secretion of FGF-23 regulates phosphate and vitamin D metabolism, *Nat Rev Endocrinol* 8(5):276–286, 2012.
10. Bellido T, Saini V, Pajevic PD: Effects of PTH on osteocyte function, *Bone* 12:1245–1248, 2012.
11. Schaffler MB, Kennedy OD: Osteocyte signaling in bone, *Curr Osteoporos Rep* 10(2):118–125, 2012.
12. Buckwalter JA, Einhorn TA, Simon SR, editors: *Orthopaedic basic science*, Rosemont, IL, 1999, American Academy of Orthopaedic Surgeons.
13. Boyce BF, Xing L: Biology of RANK, RANKL, and osteoprotegerin, *Arthritis Res Ther* 9(Suppl 1):S1, 2007.
14. Del Fattore A, Teti A, Rucci N: Bone cells and the mechanisms of bone remodeling, *Front Biosci (Elite Ed)* 4:2302–2321, 2012.
15. Boyce BF, Yao Z, Xing L: Osteoclasts have multiple roles in bone in addition to bone resorption, *Crit Rev Eukaryot Gene Expr* 19(3):171–180, 2009.
16. Jones D, Glimcher LH, Aliprantis AO: Osteoimmunology at the nexus of arthritis, osteoporosis, cancer, and infection, *J Clin Invest* 121(7): 2534–2542, 2011.
17. Nakashima T, Takayanagi H: Osteoclasts and the immune system, *J Bone Miner Metab* 27:519–529, 2009.
18. Golub EE: Biomineralization and matrix vesicles in biology and pathology, *Semin Immunopathol* 33(5):409–417, 2011.
19. Bishop JR, Schuksz M, Esko JD: Heparan sulphate proteoglycans fine-tune mammalian physiology, *Nature* 446(7139):1030–1037, 2007.
20. Kock L, van Donkelaar CC, Ito K: Tissue engineering of functional articular cartilage: the current status, *Cell Tissue Res* 347(3):613–627, 2012.

21. Pesesse L, Sanchez C, Henrotin Y: Osteochondral plate angiogenesis: a new treatment target in osteoarthritis, *Joint Bone Spine* 78(2):144–149, 2011.
22. Knight JD, Kothary R: The myogenic kinome: protein kinases critical to mammalian skeletal myogenesis, *Skeletal Muscle* 1:29–46, 2011.
23. Braun T, Gautel M: Transcriptional mechanisms regulating skeletal muscle differentiation, growth and homeostasis, *Nat Rev Mol Cell Biol* 12:349–361, 2011.
24. Lieber RL, Ward SR: Skeletal muscle design to meet functional demands, *Philos Trans R Soc Lond B Biol Sci* 366(1570):1466–1476, 2011.
25. Myhre JL, Pilgrim DB: At the start of the sarcomere: a previously unrecognized role for myosin chaperones and associated proteins during early myofibrillogenesis, *Biochem Res Int* 2012:712315, 2012.
26. Labiet D et al: Calcium-dependent molecular spring elements in the giant protein titin, *Proc Natl Acad Sci U S A* 100(23):13716–13721, 2003.
27. Sargeant AJ: Structural and functional determinants of human muscle power, *Exp Physiol* 92(2):323, 2007.
28. Capes EM, Loaiza R, Valdivia HH: Ryanodine receptors, *Skelet Muscle* 1(1):18, 2011.
29. Hamilton SL, Serysheva II: Ryanodine receptor structure: progress and challenges, *J Biol Chem* 284(7):4047–4051, 2009.
30. Lanner JT: Ryanodine receptor physiology and its role in disease, *Adv Exp Med Biol* 1(74):217–234, 2012.
31. Richardson RS: Oxygen transport and utilization: an integration of the muscle systems, *Adv Physiol Educ* 27(1-4):183–191, 2003.
32. Nicolaou S et al: Dual-energy CT: a promising new technique for assessment of the musculoskeletal system, *AJR Am J Roentgenol* 199(Suppl 5): S78–S86, 2012.
33. Ito M: Recent progress in bone imaging for osteoporosis research, *J Bone Miner Metab* 29:131–140, 2011.
34. Abe Y, Ishikawa H, Fukao A: Higher efficacy of urinary bone resorption marker measurements in assessing response to treatment for osteoporosis in postmenopausal women, *Tohoku J Exp Med* 214(1):51, 2008.
35. Ulrich-Vinther M et al: Articular cartilage biology, *J Am Acad Orthoped Surg* 11(6):421–430, 2003.
36. Clarke BL, Khosla S: Physiology of bone loss, *Radiol Clin North Am* 48(3):483–495, 2010.
37. Zanatta M et al: Runx-2 gene expression is associated with age-related changes of bone mineral density in the healthy young-adult population, *J Bone Miner Metab*, 2012 Aug 18. [Epub ahead of print.].
38. Adler RA: Osteoporosis in men: insights for the clinician, *Ther Adv Musculoskel Dis* 3(4):191–200, 2011.
39. Bergmann P et al: Loading and skeletal development and maintenance, *J Osteoporos* 2011:786752, 2011.
40. Body JJ et al: Non-pharmacological management of osteoporosis: a consensus of the Belgian Bone Club, *Osteoporos Int* 22:2769–2788, 2011.
41. Karasik D, Cohen-Zinder M: The genetic pleiotropy of musculoskeletal aging, *Front Physiol* 3:303, 2012.
42. Peterson CM, Johannsen DL, Ravussin E: Skeletal mitochondria and aging: a review, *J Aging Res* 194821, 2012.
43. Shadrach JL, Wagers AJ: Stem cells for skeletal muscle repair, *Philos Trans R Soc Lond B Biol Sci* 366(1575):2297–2306, 2011.

CHAPTER

44

Alterations of Musculoskeletal Function

Christy L. Crowther-Radulewicz and Kathryn L. McCance

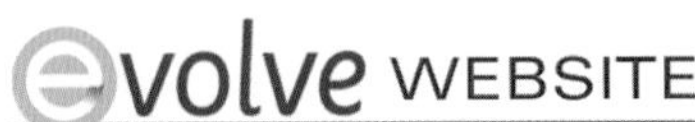

http://evolve.elsevier.com/McCance/

- Review Questions and Answers
- Online Course: Module 18

CHAPTER OUTLINE

Musculoskeletal injuries include fractures, dislocations, sprains, and strains. Alterations in bones, joints, and muscles may be caused by trauma, metabolic disorders, infections, inflammatory or noninflammatory diseases, or tumors. Trauma is the leading cause of death of people ages 1 to 44 years of all races and socioeconomic levels.

MUSCULOSKELETAL INJURIES

Skeletal muscles can withstand many penetrating injuries without permanent loss of function. For example, studies of soldiers with severe combat injuries showed that muscle function was preserved after the removal of large portions of muscle tissue. Successful regeneration of skeletal muscle fibers depends primarily on the extent of injury, the preservation of vascular supply (and source of nutrition), and the availability of satellite cells and terminal axons for reinnervation.

Skeletal Trauma

Fractures

A **fracture** is a break in the continuity of a bone. A break occurs when force is applied that exceeds the tensile or compressive strength of the bone. The highest incidence of fractures occurs in young males (between ages 15 and 24 years) and in adults 65 years of age and older, and varies for individual bones according to age, gender, and possibly race. In a study of more than 158,000 people, fractures were most prevalent among black males younger than age 65, whereas fractures in whites were highest in those age 65 and older.[1] Fractures of healthy bones, particularly the tibia, clavicle, and lower humerus, tend to occur in young persons and are often the result of trauma. Fractures of the hands and feet are usually caused by accidents in the workplace. The incidence of fractures of the upper femur, upper humerus, vertebrae, and pelvis is highest in older or older adults and is often associated with osteoporosis (see p. 1550). In

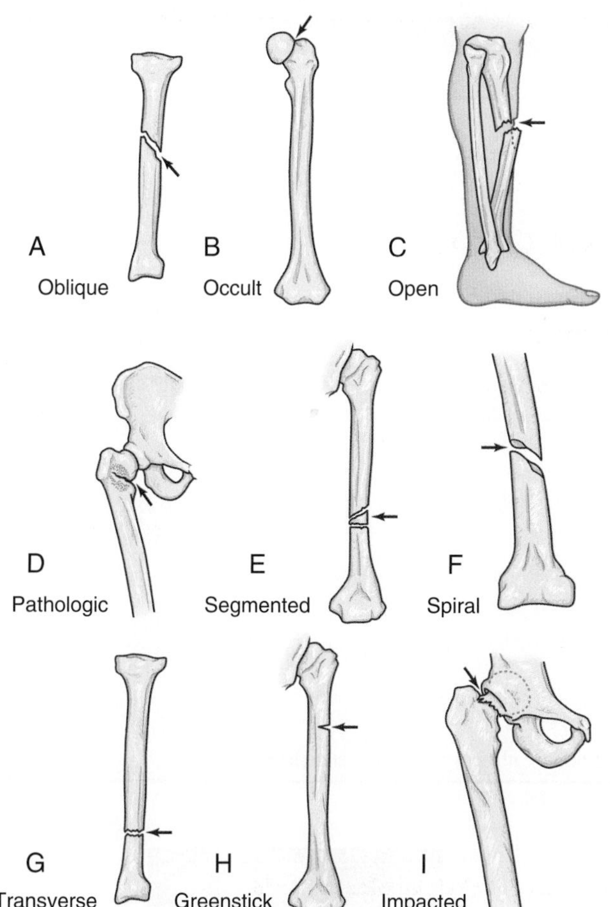

FIGURE 44-1 Examples of Types of Bone Fractures. **A,** *Oblique:* fracture at oblique angle across both cortices. *Cause:* direct or indirect energy, with angulation and some compression. **B,** *Occult:* fracture that is hidden or not readily discernible. *Cause:* minor force or energy. **C,** *Open:* skin broken over fracture; possible soft tissue trauma. *Cause:* moderate to severe energy that is continuous and exceeds tissue tolerances. **D,** *Pathologic:* transverse, oblique, or spiral fracture of bone weakened by tumor pressure or presence. *Cause:* minor energy or force, which may be direct or indirect. **E,** *Segmented:* fracture with two or more pieces or segments. *Cause:* direct or indirect moderate to severe force. **F,** *Spiral:* fracture that curves around cortices and may become displaced by twist. *Cause:* direct or indirect twisting energy or force with distal part held or unable to move. **G,** *Transverse:* horizontal break through bone. *Cause:* direct or indirect energy toward bone. **H,** *Greenstick:* break in only one cortex of bone. *Cause:* minor direct or indirect energy. **I,** *Impacted:* fracture with one end wedged into opposite end of inside fractured fragment. *Cause:* compressive axial energy or force directly to distal fragment. (Redrawn from Mourad L: Musculoskeletal system. In Thompson JM et al, editors: *Mosby's clinical nursing,* ed 7, St Louis, 2002, Mosby.)

1990, an estimated 1.66 million hip fractures occurred worldwide; that number is expected to increase to 6.3 million by the year 2050.[2]

Classification. Fractures can be classified as complete or incomplete and open or closed (Figure 44-1). In a **complete fracture** the bone is broken all the way through, whereas in an **incomplete fracture** the bone is damaged but still in one piece. Complete or incomplete fractures also can be classified as **open** (formerly referred to as *compound*) if the skin is broken or as **closed** (formerly called *simple*) if it is not. A fracture in which a bone breaks into more than two fragments is termed a **comminuted fracture.** Fractures are classified also according to the direction of the fracture line. A **linear fracture** runs parallel to the long axis of the bone. An **oblique fracture** is a slanted fracture of the shaft of the bone. A **spiral fracture** encircles the bone, and a **transverse fracture** occurs straight across the bone.

Incomplete fractures tend to occur in the more flexible, growing bones of children. The three main types of incomplete fractures are greenstick, buckle or torus, and bowing. A **greenstick fracture** perforates one cortex and splinters the spongy bone and is relatively unstable.[3] The name is derived from the damage sustained by a young tree branch (a green stick) when it is bent sharply. The outer surface is disrupted, but the inner surface remains intact. Greenstick fractures typically occur in the metaphysis or diaphysis of the tibia, radius, and ulna. In a buckle or **torus fracture,** the cortex buckles but does not break; this is a relatively stable fracture. **Bowing fractures** usually occur when longitudinal force is applied to bone. This type of fracture is common in children and usually involves the paired radius-ulna or fibula-tibia. A complete diaphyseal fracture occurs in one of the bones of the pair, which disperses the stress sufficiently to prevent a complete fracture of the second bone, which bows. A bowing fracture resists correction (reduction) because the force necessary to reduce it must be equal to the force that bowed it. Treatment of bowing fractures is difficult also because the bowed bone interferes with reduction of the fractured bone. A fracture that results from a low-level trauma (one that would not normally cause a fracture) is called a **fragility fracture,** which is often seen in osteoporosis. Types of fractures are summarized in Table 44-1.

Fractures may be further classified by cause as pathologic, stress, or transchondral. A **pathologic fracture** is a break at the site of a preexisting abnormality (such as a tumor), usually by force that would not fracture a normal bone. Any disease process that weakens a bone (especially the cortex) predisposes the bone to pathologic fracture, commonly associated with tumors, osteoporosis, infections, and metabolic bone disorders.

Stress fractures occur in normal or abnormal bone that is subjected to repeated forces, such as occurs during athletics. **Fatigue fractures** are caused by abnormal stress or torque applied to a bone with normal ability to deform and recover (e.g., joggers, dancers, military recruits) and are a type of stress fracture. **Insufficiency fractures** include fragility fractures of osteoporosis and osteomalacia, and occur in bones lacking normal ability to deform and recover (i.e., normal weightbearing or activity fractures the bone).

A **transchondral fracture** consists of fragmentation and separation of a portion of the articular cartilage that covers the end of a bone at a joint. (Joint structures are defined in Chapter 43.) The fragments may consist of cartilage alone or cartilage and bone. Typical sites of transchondral fracture are the distal femur, the ankle, the kneecap, the elbow, and the wrist. Transchondral fractures are most prevalent in adolescents.

PATHOPHYSIOLOGY. When a bone is broken the periosteum and blood vessels in the cortex, marrow, and surrounding soft tissues are disrupted. Bleeding occurs from the damaged ends of the bone and from the neighboring soft tissue. A clot (hematoma) forms within the medullary canal, between the

TABLE 44-1 TYPES OF FRACTURES

TYPE	DEFINITION
Typical Complete Fractures	
Closed fracture	The skin overlying the bone is intact
Open fracture	Communicating wound between bone and skin
Comminuted fracture	Multiple bone fragments
Linear fracture	Fracture line parallel to long axis of bone
Oblique fracture	Fracture line at an angle to long axis of bone
Spiral fracture	Fracture line encircling bone (as a spiral staircase)
Transverse fracture	Fracture line perpendicular to long axis of bone
Impacted	Fracture fragments are pushed into each other
Pathologic	Fracture occurs at a point in the bone weakened by disease (e.g., bones with tumors or osteoporosis)
Avulsion	A fragment of bone connected to a ligament or tendon breaks off from the main bone
Compression	Fracture is wedged or squeezed together on one side of bone
Displaced	Fracture with one, both, or all fragments out of normal alignment
Extracapsular	Fragment is close to the joint but remains outside the joint capsule
Intracapsular	Fragment extends into or is within the joint capsule
Fragility	Fracture caused by low-level trauma
Typical Incomplete Fractures	
Greenstick fracture	Break on one cortex of bone with splintering of inner bone surface (commonly occurs in children and older adults)
Torus fracture	Buckling of cortex
Bowing fracture	Bending of the bone
Stress fracture	Microfracture
Transchondral fracture	Separation of cartilaginous joint surface (articular cartilage) from main shaft of bone

fractured ends of the bone, and beneath the periosteum. Bone tissue immediately adjacent to the fracture dies. This necrotic tissue (along with any debris in the fracture area) stimulates an intense inflammatory response characterized by vasodilation, exudation of plasma and leukocytes, and infiltration by inflammatory leukocytes and mast cells. Cytokines, including transforming growth factor-beta (TGF-β), platelet-derived growth factor (PDGF), prostaglandins, and other factors that promote healing are released. Within 48 hours after the injury, vascular tissue invades the fracture area from surrounding soft tissue and the marrow cavity, and blood flow to the entire bone is increased. Bone-forming cells in the periosteum, endosteum, and marrow are activated to produce subperiosteal procallus along the outer surface of the shaft and over the broken ends of the bone (Figure 44-2). Healing generally occurs in three overlapping phases. The initial inflammatory phase of healing lasts 3 to 4 days. During the next few days, the repair phase begins and capillary ingrowth, together with mononuclear cells and fibroblasts, begins the transformation of a hematoma into granulation tissue. Osteoblasts within the procallus synthesize collagen and matrix, which becomes mineralized to form callus. As the repair process continues, remodeling occurs, during which unnecessary callus is resorbed and trabeculae are formed along lines of stress; at the end of this stage, bone can withstand normal stresses. The last phase, remodeling, lasts for months to years. Except for the liver, bone is unique among all body tissues in that after a fracture it will heal with normal, not scar, tissue.

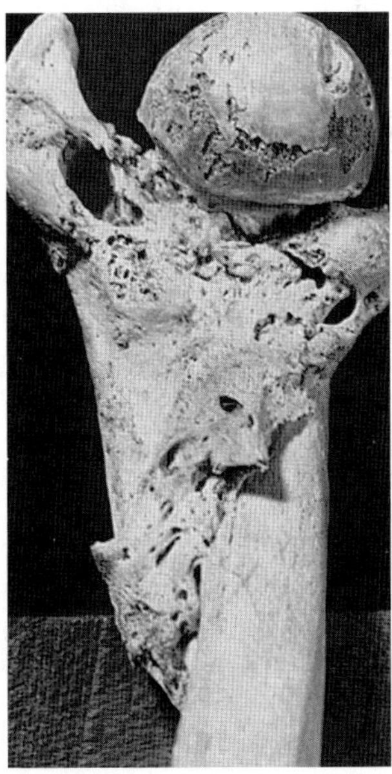

FIGURE 44-2 Exuberant Callus Formation Following Fracture. (From Rosai J: *Ackerman's surgical pathology*, ed 8, St Louis, 1996, Mosby.)

CLINICAL MANIFESTATIONS. The clinical manifestations of a fracture vary according to the type of fracture, site of the fracture, and associated soft tissue injury. In general, the signs and symptoms of a fracture include impaired function, unnatural alignment (deformity), swelling, muscle spasm, tenderness, pain, and impaired sensation. The position of the bone segments is determined by the pull of attached muscles, gravity, and the direction and magnitude of the force that caused the fracture. One or both segments may be rotated inward or outward on the bone's long axis (rotation), be misaligned at an angle (angulation), slide over the other segment (overriding), or be out of normal position (displaced).

The immediate pain of a fracture is severe and usually caused by trauma. Subsequent pain may be produced by muscle spasm, overriding of the fracture segments, or damage to adjacent soft tissues. Numbness is common and is caused by swelling, pinching or severing of a nerve, trauma, or by bone fragments. Pathologic fractures can cause angular deformity, painless swelling, or generalized bone pain. Stress fractures are painful, not because of trauma, but because of accelerated remodeling. The pain occurs during activity and is usually relieved by rest. Stress fractures also cause local tenderness and soft tissue swelling. Transchondral fractures may be entirely asymptomatic or painful during movement. Range of motion in the joint is limited, and movement may evoke audible clicking sounds (crepitus).

EVALUATION AND TREATMENT. Treatment of a displaced fracture involves realigning the bone fragments (reduction) to their normal or anatomic position and holding the fragments in place (immobilization) so that bone union can occur. Several methods are available to reduce a fracture: closed manipulation, traction, and open reduction. Many fractures heal without manipulation—they require only adequate immobilization. A fracture that is malaligned, however, requires more aggressive treatment.

Many fractures can be reduced by closed manipulation: the skin is not opened, and the bone is moved or manipulated into place. Closed manipulation is used when the contour of the bone is in fair alignment and can be maintained well with immobilization.

Traction is used to accomplish or maintain reduction. When bone fragments are displaced (not in their anatomic position), weights are used to apply firm, steady traction (pull) and countertraction to the long axis of the bone. Traction stretches and fatigues muscles that pull the bone fragments out of place, allowing the distal fragment to align with the proximal fragment. Traction can be applied to the skin (skin traction), directly to the involved bone, or distal to the involved bone (skeletal traction). Skin traction is used when only a few pounds of pulling force are needed to realign the fragments or when the traction will be used for brief times only, such as before surgery or, for children with femoral fractures, for 3 to 7 days before applying a cast. In skeletal traction, a pin or wire is drilled through the bone below the fracture site, and a traction bow, rope, and weights are attached to the pin or wire to apply tension and to provide the pulling force needed to overcome the muscle spasm and help realign the fracture fragments.

External fixation can be used to reduce and immobilize significantly displaced open fractures. Pins are placed in the bone proximal and distal to the break and then stabilized by an external frame of clamps and rods (Figure 44-3).

Open reduction is a surgical procedure that exposes the fracture site; the fragments are brought into alignment under direct visualization. Some form of prosthesis, screw, plate, nail, or wire usually is used to maintain the reduction (internal fixation).

Splints and casts are used to immobilize and hold a reduction in place. Improper reduction or immobilization of a fractured bone may result in nonunion, delayed union, or malunion. **Nonunion** is failure of the bone ends to grow together (Figure 44-4). The gap between the broken ends of the bone fills with dense fibrous and fibrocartilaginous tissue instead of new bone. Occasionally the fibrous tissue contains a fluid-filled space that resembles a joint and is termed a *false joint,* or *pseudarthrosis.* **Delayed union** is union that does not occur until approximately 8 to 9 months after a fracture. **Malunion** is the healing of a bone in a nonanatomic position. Treatment of delayed union and nonunion includes use of various modalities designed to stimulate new bone formation. Physical modalities, such as implantable or external electric current devices, electromagnetic field generations, and low-density ultrasound, have been effective in stimulating bone formation.[4] Stem cells and gene therapy also show promise in promoting formation of new bone.[5,6] Large defects in bone can be filled with bone graft or synthetic materials, such as calcium phosphate cement.

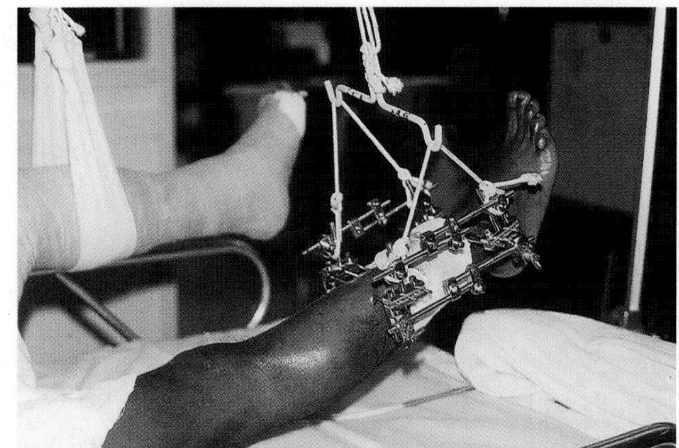

FIGURE 44-3 Example of an External Fixation Device on the Right Leg. The left leg is in a splint.

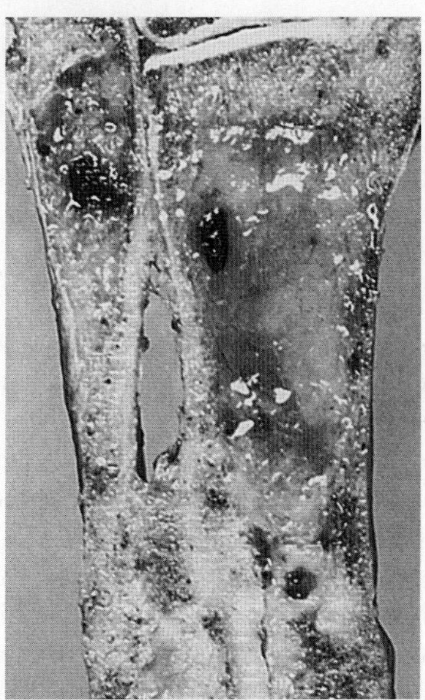

FIGURE 44-4 Nonunion of Old Fracture of Tibia and Fibula in a 53-Year-Old Man. Multiple fractures had occurred in 2 years previous and necessitated bone grafting. (From Rosai J: *Ackerman's surgical pathology,* ed 8, St Louis, 1996, Mosby.)

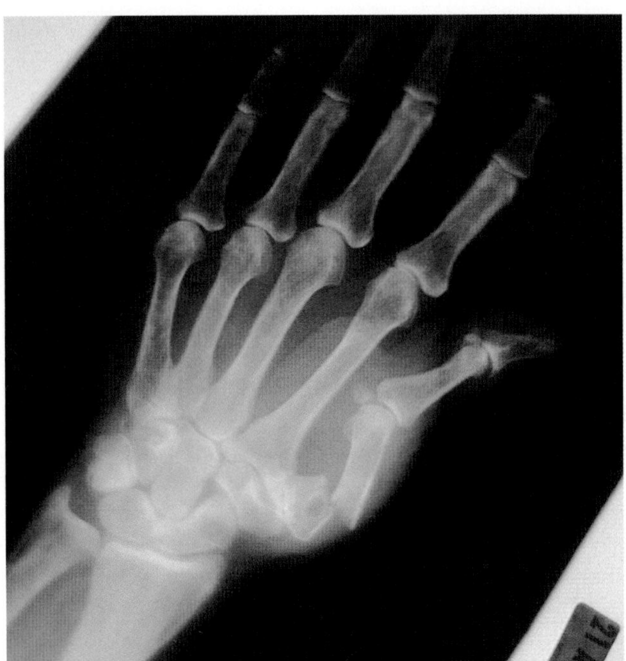

FIGURE 44-5 Displaced Fracture. An x-ray showing a displaced fracture of the base of the first metacarpal, also known as a Bennett fracture.

Dislocation and Subluxation

Dislocation and subluxation are usually caused by trauma but can also be due to ligamentous laxity, nerve injury, rheumatoid disease, or genetic problems. **Dislocation** is the temporary displacement of a bone from its normal position in a joint. If a dislocation does not involve a fracture, it is considered a simple dislocation; if there is an associated fracture, it becomes a complex dislocation. If the contact between the two joint surfaces is only partially lost, the injury is called a **subluxation.**

Dislocation and subluxation are most common in persons younger than 20 years and are generally associated with fractures. Dislocation and subluxation, however, may result from congenital or acquired disorders that cause (1) muscular imbalance, as occurs with congenital hip dislocation or neurologic disorders; (2) incongruities in the articulating surfaces of the bones, such as with rheumatoid arthritis (see p. 1568); or (3) joint instability.

Most often dislocated or subluxated are the joints of the shoulder, elbow, wrist, finger, hip, and knee (Figure 44-5). The shoulder's glenohumeral joint is a relatively unstable joint because the articular surface of the glenoid cavity is only one third as large as the surface of the humeral head. As a result, the glenohumeral joint is often injured. Physical trauma to the shoulder can cause anterior, posterior, superior, or inferior dislocation. Anterior dislocation is the most common and is usually the result of an indirect force that places the shoulder in extreme external rotation. Posterior dislocations usually occur as a result of trauma. A superior dislocation is rare and usually the result of an extreme forward and upward force on an adducted arm. Inferior displacement is often seen in persons with neurologic injuries of the brachial plexus and is believed to be caused by stretching of the supporting muscles or by joint effusion.

Traumatic dislocation of the elbow joint is common in the immature skeleton. In adults an elbow dislocation is usually associated with a fracture of the ulna or head of the radius. Posterior dislocations occur when the individual falls on an outstretched hand with the elbow extended. Anterior dislocations are usually the result of a direct blow to the flexed elbow.

Traumatic dislocation of the wrist usually involves the distal ulna and carpal bones. Any one of the eight carpal bones can be dislocated after an injury. The most common cause is a fall on the hyperextended hand.

Dislocation in the hand usually involves the metacarpophalangeal and interphalangeal joints. Dislocation of the metacarpophalangeal joint is often the result of a fall on the outstretched hand that forces the joint into hyperextension. Dislocation of the interphalangeal joint occurs as a result of injury to the fingers in a hyperextended position.

Considerable trauma is needed to dislocate the hip. Anterior hip dislocation is rather rare and is caused by forced abduction, for example, when an individual lands on the feet from a high fall. Posterior dislocation of the hip can occur in an automobile accident in which the flexed knee strikes the dashboard.

The knee is a relatively unstable joint that depends heavily on the soft tissue structures around it for support. Because the knee is an unstable weightbearing joint exposed to many different types of motion (flexion, extension, rotation), it is one of the most commonly injured joints. A knee dislocation can be anterior, posterior, lateral, medial, or rotary. It is often the result of a hyperextension injury that occurs during sports activities.

PATHOPHYSIOLOGY. Dislocations and subluxations are often accompanied by fracture because stress is placed on areas of bone not normally subjected to stress. In addition, as the bone separates from the joint, it may bruise or tear adjacent nerves, blood vessels, ligaments, supporting structures, and soft tissue. Dislocation of the shoulder may damage the shoulder capsule and the axillary nerve. Damage to the axillary nerve causes anesthesia in the sensory distribution of the nerve and paralysis of the deltoid muscle. Torn periosteum, ligaments, and muscle frequently accompany elbow dislocations. Bleeding from the damaged periosteum and muscle puts pressure on adjacent arteries that stop circulation to and from the forearm and hand. If the pressure is not promptly relieved, ischemic paralysis develops. Dislocations of the hand often result in permanent disability because of damage to the tendons and intricate mechanisms that allow smooth gliding in the joints. In the hip, avascular necrosis of the femoral head is a complication seen with dislocations. Knee dislocation usually tears both the collateral and cruciate ligaments.

CLINICAL MANIFESTATIONS. Signs and symptoms of dislocations or subluxations include pain, swelling, limitation of motion, and joint deformity. Pain may be caused by effusion of inflammatory exudate into the joint or associated tendon and ligament injury. Joint deformity is usually caused by muscle contractions that exert pull on the dislocated or subluxated joint or fluid within the joint. Limitation of motion may be a result of effusion into the joint or the displacement of bones.

Tenderness and deformity are prominent in dislocations of the fingers. Unusual muscle pull and pain often result in abnormal posturing of the fingers; for example, the fingers or thumb may be abnormally flexed. A dislocated elbow is often held in a flexed position, and the joint resists active or passive movement. Pain is the key symptom of shoulder injuries. Attempts to lift the arm aggravate the pain. In most shoulder dislocations, the ability to elevate the arm is minimal and the individual supports the injured arm with the opposite hand. Pain and an abnormal gait or limp or inability to bear full weight usually accompanies traumatic dislocation of the hip. The pain is constant and severe and is often felt in the inguinal region or thigh. The thigh and leg may assume a position of inward rotation, adduction, or flexion and appear shortened. In a rare anterior dislocation, the limb is not shortened and the joint is fixed in abduction, outward rotation, and flexion.

EVALUATION AND TREATMENT. Evaluation of dislocations and subluxations is based on clinical manifestations and roentgenograms. Treatment consists of reduction and immobilization for 2 to 6 weeks and exercises to maintain normal range of motion in the joint. Depending on the joint, healing is usually complete within months to years.

Support Structure Trauma

Sprains and Strains of Tendons and Ligaments

Tendon and ligament injuries can accompany fractures and dislocations. A **tendon** is fibrous connective tissue that attaches skeletal muscle to bone. A **ligament** is a band of fibrous connective tissue that connects bones where they meet at a joint. Tendons and ligaments support the bones and joints and either facilitate or limit motion. Tendons and ligaments can be torn, ruptured, or completely separated from bone at their points of attachment.

A tear in a tendon is commonly known as a **strain.** Major trauma can tear or rupture a tendon at any site in the body. Most often injured are the tendons of the hands and feet, the knee (patellar), the upper arm (biceps and triceps), the thigh (quadriceps), the ankle, and the heel (Achilles). Lifting excessive weight with the arms can cause traumatic rupture of the biceps tendon. Rupture of the Achilles tendon occurs when forced dorsiflexion is applied to the foot when it is in plantar flexion. Spontaneous tendon ruptures can occur in individuals receiving local corticosteroid injections or fluoroquinolones and in persons with rheumatoid arthritis or systemic lupus erythematosus.

Ligament tears are commonly known as **sprains.** Ligament tears and ruptures can occur at any joint but are most common in the wrist, ankle, elbow, and knee joints. A complete separation of a tendon or ligament from its bony attachment site is known as an **avulsion.** An avulsion is the result of abnormal stress on the ligament or tendon and is commonly seen in young athletes, especially sprinters, hurdlers, and runners.

Strains and sprains are classified as first degree (least severe), second degree, and third degree (most severe).

PATHOPHYSIOLOGY. When a tendon or ligament is torn, an extensive cascade of inflammatory processes begins. An inflammatory exudate develops between the torn ends. Later, granulation tissue containing macrophages, fibroblasts, and capillary buds grows inward from the surrounding soft tissue and cartilage to begin the repair process. Within 3 to 4 days after the injury, collagen formation begins. At first, collagen formation is random and disorganized. As the collagen fibers interweave and connect with pre-existing tendon fibers, they become organized parallel to the lines of stress. Eventually vascular fibrous tissue fuses the new and surrounding tissues into a single mass. As reorganization takes place, the healing tendon or ligament separates from the surrounding soft tissue. Usually a healing tendon or ligament lacks sufficient strength to withstand strong pull for 4 to 5 weeks after the injury. If strong muscle pull does occur during this time, the tendon or ligament ends may separate again, which causes the tendon or ligament to heal in a lengthened shape with an excessive amount of scar tissue that renders the tendon or ligament functionless. Scar remodeling may take months to years before it is complete.[7]

CLINICAL MANIFESTATIONS. Tendon and ligament injuries are painful and are usually accompanied by soft tissue swelling, changes in tendon or ligament contour, and dislocation or subluxation of bones. The pain is generally sharp and localized, and tenderness persists over the distribution of the tendon or ligament. Painful joint swelling usually can be seen in finger and elbow sprains. Flexion deformities of the fingers and thumb occur in injuries to the extensor tendons. Crepitus may accompany tendon injury in the wrist. Pain in the elbow may be accentuated by flexion, supination, and extension of the elbow or by extension of the wrist. Lifting small objects requires extension of the wrist and therefore aggravates the pain. Tendon injuries in the upper arm cause weakness when the individual tries to flex the forearm. Pain is often the key symptom of shoulder injuries. It may be referred to the deltoid muscle or extend down the arm and is aggravated by attempts to actively raise the arms. Depending on the ligament or tendon involved, tendon and ligament injuries in the knee may produce pronounced immobility, absence of lateral movement, instability when walking down stairs, flexion deformity, crepitus, or an upward or downward shift of the patella.

EVALUATION AND TREATMENT. Evaluation is based on clinical manifestations, stress radiography, arthroscopy, or arthrography. When possible, treatment consists of protection of the involved structures (splinting), promotion of early motion, and rehabilitation. Suturing the tendon or ligament ends in close approximation may be necessary to treat complete rupture. If this is not possible because of the extent of damage, tendon or ligament grafting may be necessary. Prolonged rehabilitation exercises help ensure that the individual regains nearly normal functions.

Tendinopathy and Bursitis

Trauma and repetitive stress can cause painful degradation of collagen fibers **(tendinosis),** inflammation of tendons **(tendinitis),** or inflammation in bursal sacs **(bursitis).** The term *tendinopathy* includes tendinitis, tendinosis, and paratendinitis. Studies have shown that vascular ingrowth in tendinopathy (neovascularization) is accompanied with nerve ingrowth, facilitating pain transmission in Achilles and patellar tendinopathies.[8] Other causes of tendinopathy include crystal deposits, postural misalignment, and hypermobility in a joint. Table 44-2 summarizes classes of tendinopathies.

TABLE 44-2 HISTOPATHOLOGIC CLASSIFICATION OF TENDON DISORDERS

PATHOLOGIC DIAGNOSIS	MACROSCOPIC PATHOLOGY	HISTOPATHOLOGIC FINDINGS
Tendinosis	Intratendinous degeneration (commonly due to aging, microtrauma, muscular compromise)	Collagen disorientation, disorganization, and fiber separation by an increase in mucoid ground substance, increased preponderance of cells and vascular spaces with or without neovascularization and focal necrosis or calcification
Tendinitis	Symptomatic degeneration of the tendon with vascular disruption and inflammatory repair response	Degenerative changes as noted above with superimposed evidence of tear, including fibroblastic and myofibroblastic proliferation, hemorrhage, and organizing granulation tissue
Paratenonitis	"Inflammation" of the outer layer of the tendon (paratenon) alone, whether or not the paratenon is lined by synovium	Mucoid degeneration if the areolar tissue is seen; a scattered mild mononuclear infiltrate with or without focal fibrin deposition and fibrinous exudate
Paratenonitis with tendinosis	Paratenonitis associated with intratendinous degeneration	Degenerative changes as noted in tendinosis with mucoid degeneration with or without fibrous and scattered inflammatory cells in the paratenon alveolar tissue

From Maffulli N, Wong J, Almekinders LC: *Clin Sports Med* 22(4):675–692, 2003.

Epicondylitis is inflammation of a tendon where it attaches to a bone (at its origin). Most tendon pathology, however, is caused by tissue degeneration rather than inflammation.[9] Epicondylar areas of the humerus, radius, or ulna and the area around the knee are most often involved. **Lateral epicondylopathy,** commonly called **tennis elbow,** is the result of tissue degeneration or irritation of the extensor carpi radialis brevis tendon at its origin. **Medial epicondylopathy,** referred to as **golfer's elbow,** is a degenerative process of the pronator teres, flexor carpi radialis, and palmaris longus tendons at the medial humeral condyle (Figure 44-6). Epicondylopathy is also related to smoking, obesity, and work activities that involve forceful or repetitive cyclic flexion and extension of the elbow, or cyclic pronation, supination, extension, and flexion of the wrist that generates loads to the elbow and forearm region.

Bursae are small sacs lined with synovial membrane and filled with synovial fluid; they are located between tendons, muscles, and bony prominences. Their primary function is to separate, lubricate, and cushion these structures. When irritated or injured, these sacs become inflamed and swell. Because most bursae lie outside joints, joint movement is rarely compromised with bursitis. Acute bursitis occurs primarily in the middle years and is often caused by trauma; repetitive irritation can cause chronic bursitis. Septic bursitis is caused by wound infection or bacterial infection of the skin overlying the bursae. Bursitis commonly occurs in the shoulder, hip, knee, and elbow.

PATHOPHYSIOLOGY. In tendinitis, inflammatory fluid accumulates causing swelling of the tendon and its enclosing sheath. Inflammatory changes cause thickening of the sheath, which limits movements and causes pain. Microtears cause bleeding, edema, and pain in the involved tendons or surrounding structures. At times, after repeated inflammations, calcium may be deposited in the tendon origin area, causing a calcific tendinitis.

The typical bursitis is an inflammation that is reactive to overuse or excessive pressure. The inflamed bursal sac becomes engorged, and the inflammation can spread to adjacent tissues (Figure 44-7). The inflammation may decrease with rest, heat, and aspiration of the fluid. (Inflammation is discussed in Chapter 7.)

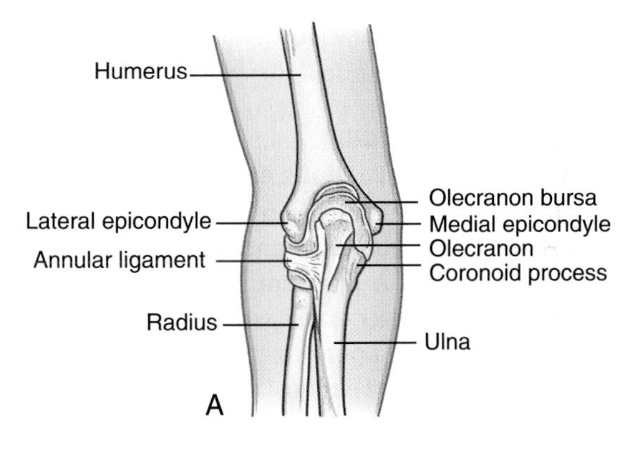

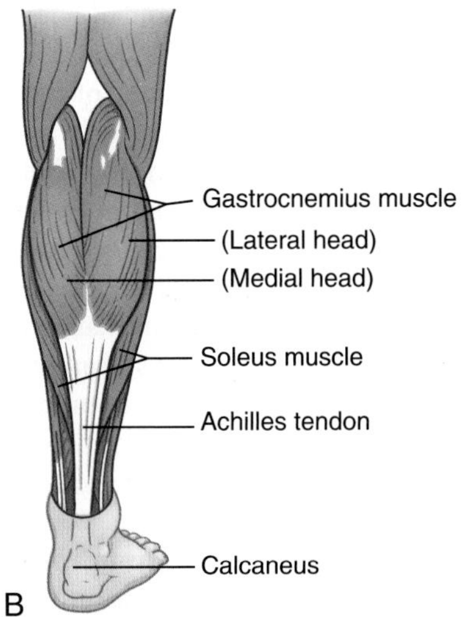

FIGURE 44-6 **Tendinitis and Epicondylitis. A,** Medial or lateral epicondyles of humerus, site of epicondylitis. **B,** Achilles tendon, site of commonly occurring tendinitis.

CLINICAL MANIFESTATIONS. Tendinopathy may be asymptomatic, but generally there is localized pain that worsens with active more than passive motion. With symptomatic tendinopathy, the pain is localized over the involved tendon and movement in the affected joint is limited. In bursitis, onset of pain may be

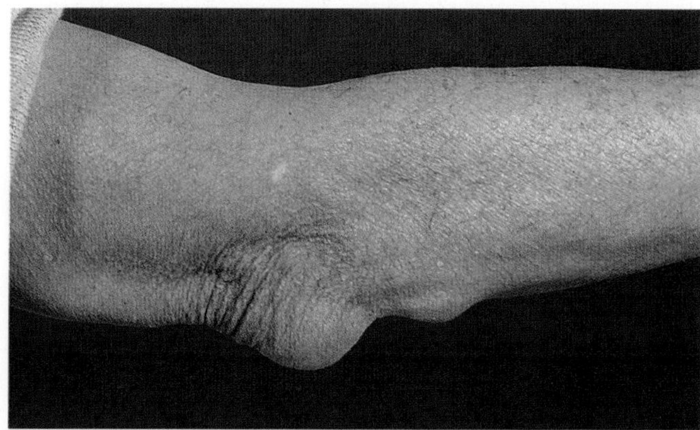

FIGURE 44-7 Olecranon Bursa. A case of olecranon bursitis in a patient with rheumatoid arthritis. A rheumatoid nodule is also shown. (From Hochberg MC et al: *Rheumatology,* ed 5, London, 2011, Mosby.)

TABLE 44-3 COMMON SITES AND CAUSES OF BURSITIS

SITE	COMMON CAUSES
Shoulder (subacromial)	Repetitive overhead activities
Elbow (olecranon)	Rheumatoid arthritis (RA), gout, tuberculosis, leaning on elbow
Hip (greater trochanter)	Acute trauma, chronic stress
Ischial (weaver's bottom)	Overuse (runner, ballet dancers), lumbosacral disease, RA, osteoarthritis (OA)
Knee	
Prepatellar (housemaid's knee)	Trauma, frequent kneeling, infection
Pes anserine (medial knee)	Obesity, long-distance runner, OA, type 2 diabetes
Heel (calcaneal)	Poorly fitting footwear, Achilles tendinitis

gradual or sudden, but movement of the joint itself is normal. Shoulder bursitis impairs arm abduction because of pain and swelling of the bursa. Bursitis in the knee produces pain when climbing stairs, and crossing the legs is painful in bursitis of the hip. Lying on the side of an inflamed trochanteric bursa is also very painful. Table 44-3 summarizes common sites of bursitis. Signs of infectious bursitis may include the presence of a puncture site, prior corticosteroid injection, severe inflammation, or an adjacent source of infection.

EVALUATION AND TREATMENT. Evaluation of tendinopathy, epicondylopathy, and bursitis is based on clinical manifestations, physical examination, arthroscopy, arthrography, ultrasound, and possibly magnetic resonance imaging (MRI). Treatment includes administration of systemic analgesics, application of ice or heat, or local injection of an anesthetic and a corticosteroid to reduce inflammation. Bursitis may require aspiration to drain excess fluid. Physical therapy to prevent loss of function begins after acute symptoms subside.

Muscle Strains

Mild injury such as **muscle strain** is usually seen after traumatic or sports injuries. *Muscle strain* is a general term for local muscle damage. It is often the result of sudden, forced motion causing the muscle to become stretched beyond normal capacity. Strains often involve the tendon as well. Muscles are ruptured more often than tendons in young people; the opposite is true in older adults. Muscle strain may be chronic when the muscle is repeatedly stretched beyond its usual capacity. There is evidence of tissue disruption with subsequent signs of muscle regeneration and connective tissue repair when a biopsy is performed. Hemorrhage into the surrounding tissue and signs of inflammation also may be present. Knife and gunshot wounds also cause traumatic rupture. Regardless of the cause of trauma, muscle cells usually can regenerate. Regeneration may take up to 6 weeks, and the affected muscle should be protected during this time. Types of muscle strain, together with their manifestations and treatment, are summarized in Table 44-4.

A late complication of localized muscle injury is abnormal bone formation in soft tissue, often called **myositis ossificans** or **heterotopic ossification (HO).** Its exact pathophysiology remains unknown, but the basic problem seems to be the inability of mesenchymal cells to differentiate into osteoblastic stem cells and the improper development of fibroblasts into bone-forming cells. Though uncommon, HO is associated with burns, joint surgery, and trauma to the musculoskeletal system or central nervous system. HO may involve muscle or tendons, ligaments, or bones near a muscle.[10] Examples include "rider's bone," in which the adductor muscle of the thigh of equestrians becomes calcified, as well as in football players after muscle injury to thigh muscles; and "drill bone," in which the same complication is seen in the deltoid and pectoral muscles of fencers and infantry soldiers.

Rhabdomyolysis

Once used interchangeably with the term *myoglobinuria,* **rhabdomyolysis** is the rapid breakdown of muscle that causes the release of intracellular contents, including protein pigment myoglobin, into the extracellular space and bloodstream. Physical interruptions in the sarcolemmal membrane, called delta lesions, suggest that the sarcolemmal membrane is the route through which muscle constituents are released. Myoglobinuria, first described in victims of crush injuries in London during World War II, refers to the presence of the muscle protein myoglobin in the urine. More recently, myoglobinuria has been reported in individuals found unresponsive and immobile for long periods, such as drug and alcohol overdoses.

PATHOPHYSIOLOGY. Rhabdomyolysis is sometimes incorrectly used interchangeably with *crush injury* (a description of injuries resulting from crushing of a body part), *compartment syndrome* (the consequences of increased intracompartmental pressures of a muscle), or *crush syndrome* (the pathophysiologic events caused by rhabdomyolysis, primarily involving the kidneys and coagulation syndrome).[11] Although relatively rare, rhabdomyolysis has many causes (Box 44-1) and can result in serious complications, including hyperkalemia (because of the release of intracellular potassium into the circulation), metabolic acidosis (from liberation of intracellular phosphorus and sulfate), acute renal failure (myoglobin precipitates in the tubules, obstructing flow through the nephron and producing injury),

TABLE 44-4 MUSCLE STRAIN

TYPE	MANIFESTATIONS	TREATMENT
First degree (e.g., bench press in untrained athlete)	Muscle overstretched, painful	Ice should be applied 5 or 6 times in the first 24-48 hours; complete rest for up to 2 weeks, followed by weightbearing 3 times per week and range of motion daily
Second degree (e.g., any muscle strain with bruising and pain)	Muscle intact with some tearing pain, mild bruising; fascia is intact	Treatment similar to that for first-degree strains, with added mild analgesia; cryokinetics (a treatment system of alternating applications of cold with progressive exercise)
Third degree (e.g., traumatic injury)	Caused by tearing of fascia; muscle rupture palpable, bleeding present	Surgery to approximate ruptured edges; immobilization and rest for 6 weeks, followed by an individualized rehabilitation regimen of strengthening exercises

BOX 44-1 SELECTED CAUSES OF RHABDOMYOLYSIS

Medications and Toxic Substances That Increase the Risk of Rhabdomyolysis

Direct Myotoxicity

HMG-CoA reductase inhibitors (statins), especially in combination with fibrate-derived lipid-lowering agents such as niacin (nicotinic acid; Nicolar)
Cyclosporine (Sandimmune)
Itraconazole (Sporanox)
Erythromycin
Colchicine
Zidovudine (Retrovir)
Corticosteroids

Other Medications and Toxins

Amphetamines
Anesthetic and paralytic agents (halothane, propofol, succinylcholine—malignant hyperthermia syndrome)
Antihistamines (diphenhydramine, doxylamine)
Anti-hyperlipidemic agents (statins, clofibrate, bezafibrate)
Antipsychotics and antidepressants (amitriptyline, doxepine, fluoxetine, haloperidol, lithium, protriptyline, perphenazine, promethazine, chlorpromazine, trifluoperazine)
Caffeine
Cocaine
HIV integrase inhibitor (raltegravir)
Hypnotics and sedatives (benzodiazepines, barbiturates)
Heroin
LSD
Methamphetamine
Methadone
Methylenedioxymethamphetamine (MDMA; "ecstasy")
Miscellaneous medications (amphotericin B, azathioprine, epsilon-aminocaproic acid, quinidine, penicillamine, salicylates, theophylline, terbutaline, thiazides, vasopressin)
Phencyclidine
Protease inhibitors

Indirect Muscle Damage

Alcohol
Central nervous system depressants
Cocaine
Amphetamines
Ecstasy (MDMA)
LSD
Neuromuscular-blocking agents

Traumatic, Heat-Related, Ischemic, and Exertional Causes

Traumatic Causes

Direct trauma
Lightning strike
Immobilization
Extensive third-degree burn
Crush injury

Heat-Related Causes

Heat stroke
Malignant hyperthermia
Neuroleptic malignant syndrome

Ischemic Causes

Ischemic limb injury

Exertional Causes

Marathon running
Physical overexertion in untrained athletes
Pathologic muscle exertion
Severe dystonia
Tetanus
Status epilepticus
Delirium tremens
Heat dissipation impairment
Physical overexertion in persons with sickle cell disease

Genetic Causes

Lipid Metabolism

Carnitine palmitoyltransferase deficiency
Carnitine deficiency
Short-chain and long-chain acetyl-coenzyme A dehydrogenase deficiency

Carbohydrate Metabolism

Myophosphorylase deficiency (McArdle disease)
Phosphorylase kinase deficiency
Phosphofructokinase deficiency
Phosphoglycerate mutase deficiency
Lactate dehydrogenase deficiency (characteristic elevation of creatine kinase level with normal lactate dehydrogenase level)

Purine Metabolism

Myoadenylate deaminase deficiency
Duchenne muscular dystrophy

BOX 44-1 SELECTED CAUSES OF RHABDOMYOLYSIS—cont'd

Infectious, Inflammatory, Metabolic, and Endocrinologic Causes

Infectious Causes

Viruses: influenza virus B, parainfluenza virus, adenovirus, coxsackievirus, echovirus, herpes simplex virus, cytomegalovirus, Epstein-Barr virus, human immunodeficiency virus

Bacteria: *Streptococcus, Salmonella, Legionella, Staphylococcus,* and *Listeria* species

Inflammatory Causes

Polymyositis

Dermatomyositis

Capillary leak syndrome

Snake bites (mostly in South America, Asia, and Africa)

Metabolic and Endocrinologic Causes

Electrolyte imbalances: hyponatremia, hypernatremia, hypokalemia, hypophosphatemia, hypocalcemia

Hypothyroidism

Thyrotoxicosis

Diabetic ketoacidosis

Nonketotic hyperosmolar syndrome

Herbal Supplements

Red yeast rice (monascus, purpureus)

Compounds containing ma huang, guarana, and garcinia cambogia

Ephedra-based compounds, especially weight-loss supplements

Data from Acharya S et al: *Ann Indian Acad Neurol* 13(3):221–222, 2010; Cervellin G, Comelli I, Lippi G: *Clin Chem Lab Med* 48(6):749–756, 2010; Croce F et al: *Int J STD AIDS* 21(11):783–785, 2010; Halpern P et al: *Hum Exp Toxicol* 29(5):259–266, 2010; Mammen AL, Amato AA: *Curr Opin Rheumatol* 22(6):644–650, 2010; Sauret JM, Narinides G, Wang GK: *Am Fam Physician* 65(3):907, 2002.

HMG-CoA, 3-Hydroxy-3-methylglutaryl coenzyme A; *LSD*, lysergic acid diethylamide; *MDMA*, 3,4-methylenedioxymethamphetamine.

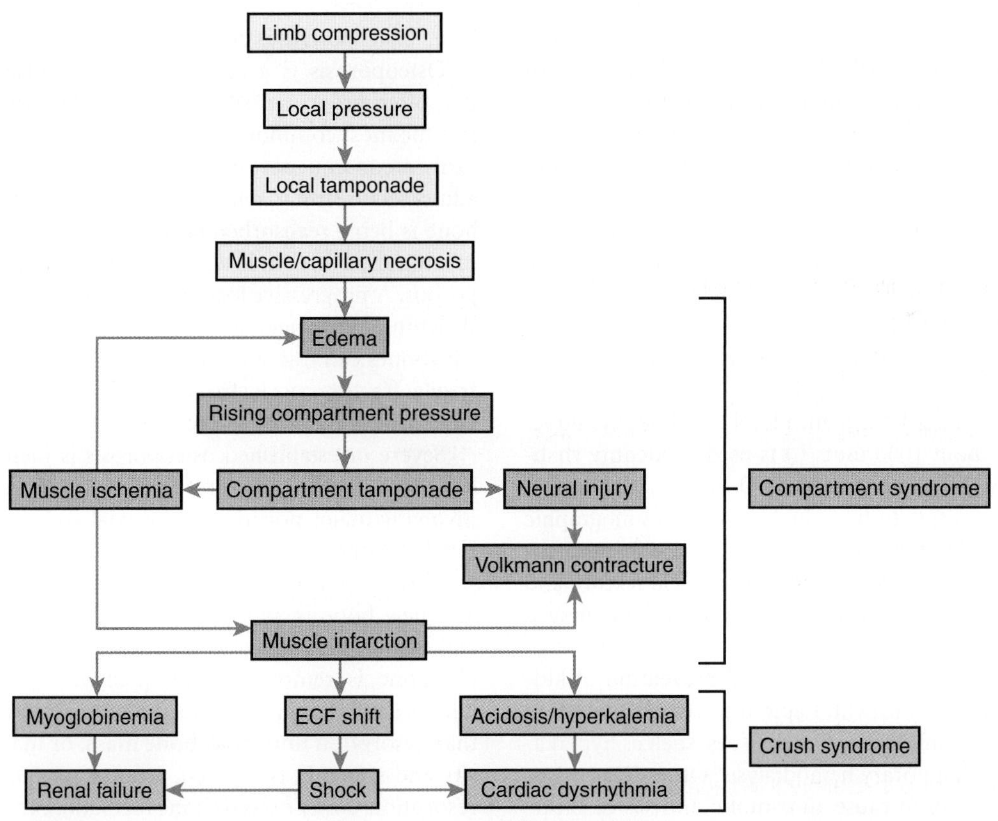

FIGURE 44-8 Pathogenesis of Compartment Syndrome and Crush Syndrome Caused by Prolonged Muscle Compression. *ECF,* Extracellular fluid.

and even disseminated intravascular coagulation (DIC) (likely caused by activation of the clotting cascade by sarcolemma damage and release of intracellular components from the damaged muscles). Even the weight of a limp extremity can generate enough pressure to produce muscle ischemia (Figure 44-8).

Malignant hyperthermia (MH) is a potentially life-threatening hereditary disorder of skeletal muscle ryanodine receptors (RyR1), allowing large quantities of calcium to be released from the sarcoplasmic reticulum (SR) after exposure to certain volatile anesthetics. The sustained elevation of calcium concentration allows excessive stimulation of aerobic and anaerobic glycolytic metabolism, causing a hypermetabolic state resulting in respiratory and metabolic acidosis, muscle rigidity, altered cell permeability, and hyperkalemia.[12] Dantrolene, a skeletal muscle relaxant, inhibits calcium release from the SR and is used to reverse the effects of MH.

Compartment syndromes occur when blood flow to the affected area is compromised because of increased venous pressure, leading to decreased arterial inflow, ischemia, and edema. Emergency treatment may be required to save an affected limb. Classic symptoms of compartment syndrome are: (1) pain out of proportion to the injury, (2) paresthesia, (3) pallor, (4) pulselessness (uncommon), and (5) paralysis (a late finding). Of these symptoms, pain is the most sensitive clinical sign.[13]

When clinical evaluation is inconclusive, the rising compartment pressure can be directly measured by inserting a wick catheter, needle, or slit catheter into the muscle. Immediate fasciotomy and débridement are advocated for reducing elevated intracompartmental pressures.[13] Compartments frequently affected are the compartments of the leg, the volar compartment of the hand, the abdomen, and the gluteal compartments.

CLINICAL MANIFESTATIONS. A *classic triad* of muscle pain, weakness, and dark urine is considered typical of rhabdomyolysis, but those affected may have no complaint of pain or muscle weakness.[11] Abnormally dark urine caused by myoglobinuria may be the first and only symptom. The renal threshold for myoglobin is low (approximately 0.5 mg/dl of urine), so only 200 g of muscle need to be damaged to cause visible changes in the urine. Myoglobin is rapidly cleared and levels may return to normal within 24 hours of injury. Along with the release of myoglobin, creatine kinase (CK) and other serum enzymes are released in massive quantities. The efflux of proteins and enzymes also includes loss of potassium, phosphate, nucleotides, creatinine, and creatine. Serum hypocalcemia is seen early in the course of myoglobinuria and is followed by late hypercalcemia.

EVALUATION AND TREATMENT. The most important and clinically useful measurement in rhabdomyolysis is serum creatine kinase (CK) level. With normal CK serum levels of 5 to 25 units/L for women and 5 to 35 units/L for men, a level five times the upper limit of normal (about 1000 units/L) is used to identify rhabdomyolysis. Once CK levels exceed 5000 units/L, acute renal failure is likely. A recent study evaluated the ultrasonographic appearance of rhabdomyolysis in damaged muscle from earthquake victims and found abnormalities in muscle texture and subcutaneous tissue, as well as areas of liquid in the damaged tissue.[14]

Maintaining adequate urinary flow and prevention of kidney failure are goals of treatment. Rapid intravenous hydration maintains adequate kidney flow. Other issues, such as hyperkalemia, may require temporary hemodialysis. Other treatments, such as using mannitol to cause an osmotic diuresis or bicarbonate to alkalinize the urine, have not been shown to consistently improve outcomes.

DISORDERS OF BONES

Metabolic Bone Diseases

Metabolic bone disease is characterized by abnormal bone structure that is caused by altered or inadequate biochemical reactions resulting in disorders of bone strength. Abnormalities include genetic, mineral, vitamin, and structural abnormalities.

Osteoporosis

Osteoporosis, or porous bone, is a disease in which bone tissue is normally mineralized but the mass—*density of bone*—is decreased and the structural integrity of trabecular bone is impaired. Two types of osteoporosis are generally considered. *Postmenopausal, or primary, osteoporosis* is most common. *Secondary osteoporosis* is osteoporosis caused by other conditions, including hormonal imbalances (endocrine disease, diabetes, hyperparathyroidism, hyperthyroidism), medications (such as heparin, corticosteroids, phenytoin, barbiturates, lithium), and other substances (including tobacco and ethanol). Other conditions, including rheumatoid disease, human immunodeficiency virus (HIV), malignancies, malabsorption syndromes, liver or kidney disease, also increase the risk for developing osteoporosis (Box 44-2). Cortical bone becomes more porous and thinner, making bone weaker and prone to fractures (Figure 44-9). The World Health Organization (WHO) has defined osteoporosis based on bone density:

1. Normal bone mass is greater than 833 mg/cm^2.
2. **Osteopenia,** or decreased bone mass, is 833 to 648 mg/cm^2.
3. Osteoporosis is bone mass less than 648 mg/cm^2.

Osteoporosis is a complex, multifactorial chronic disease that often progresses silently for decades until fractures occur. It is the most common disease that affects bone. It is not necessarily a consequence of the aging process because some older adults retain strong, relatively dense bones. In osteoporosis, old bone is being reabsorbed faster than new bone is being made, causing the bones to lose density, becoming thinner and more porous. A progressive loss of bone mass may continue until the skeleton is no longer strong enough to support itself. Eventually, bones can fracture spontaneously. As bone becomes more fragile, fractures occur from falls or bumps that would not previously have caused fracture.

Severe or established osteoporosis is identified when there has been a fragility fracture. The disease can be (1) generalized, involving major portions of the axial skeleton, or (2) regional, involving one segment of the appendicular skeleton.

Throughout a lifetime, old bone is removed (resorption) and new bone is added (formation) to the skeleton. During childhood and teenage years, new bone is added faster than old bone is removed. Consequently, bones become larger, heavier, and denser. Bone formation continues at a pace faster than resorption until **peak bone mass,** or maximum bone density and strength, is reached, around age 30, after which bone resorption slowly exceeds bone formation. In women, bone loss begins before menopause, and is most rapid in the first years after menopause but persists throughout the postmenopausal years. Though osteoporosis is most common in women, it is estimated that one in five men will experience an osteoporosis-related fracture at some point in his lifetime.[15] In adults over age 50, the prevalence of osteoporosis at either the spine or the femoral neck by age ranges from 3% to 10% in men and from 7% to 35% in women. One study showed that in men the prevalence of osteoporosis did not increase with age until age 80 years and older, but in women it increased for each decade after age 50 years.[16]

BOX 44-2 RISK FACTORS FOR OSTEOPOROSIS

Genetic
Family history of osteoporosis
White/Asian race
Increased age
Female gender

Anthropometric
Small stature
Fair or pale skinned
Thin build

Hormonal and Metabolic
Early menopause (natural or surgical)
Late menarche
Nulliparity
Obesity
Hypogonadism
Gaucher disease
Cushing syndrome
Weight below healthy range
Acidosis

Dietary
Low dietary calcium and vitamin D
Low endogenous magnesium
Excessive protein*
Excessive sodium intake
High caffeine intake
Anorexia
Malabsorption

Lifestyle
Sedentary
Smoker
Alcohol consumption (excessive)

Concurrent
Hyperparathyroidism

Illness and Trauma
Renal insufficiency, hypocalciuria
Rheumatoid arthritis
Spinal cord injury
Systemic lupus erythematosus

Liver Disease
Marrow disease (myeloma, mastocytosis, thalassemia)

Drugs
Corticosteroids
Dilantin
Gonadotropin-releasing hormone agonists
Loop diuretics
Methotrexate
Thyroid
Heparin
Cyclosporine
Depo-medroxyprogesterone acetate
Retinoids

*Low levels of protein intake also have been reported.

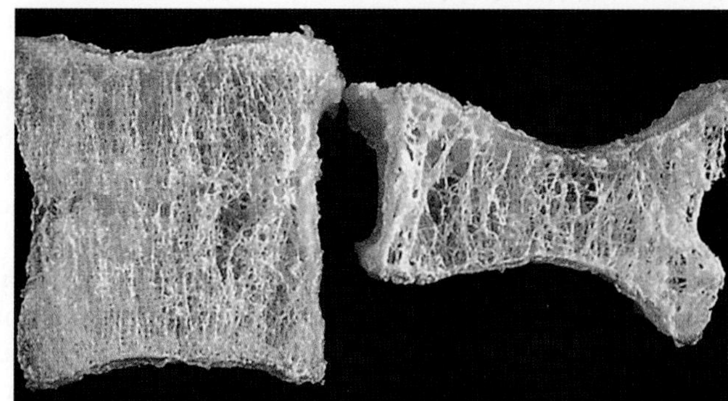

FIGURE 44-9 Vertebral Body. Osteoporotic vertebra *(right)* shortened by compression fractures compared with normal vertebral body *(left)*. Note that the osteoporotic vertebra has characteristic loss of horizontal trabeculae and thickened vertebral trabeculae. (From Kumar V et al: *Robbins & Cotran pathologic basis of disease,* ed 8, Philadelphia, 2010, Saunders.)

Approximately 52 million people in the United States are affected by osteoporosis or low bone density.[17] The major risks for persons with osteoporosis are fractures. Men lose bone density with aging but because they begin with a higher bone density, they reach osteoporotic levels at an older age than do women.[18] Osteoporotic fractures affect 1 in 2 women and 1 in 5 men older than the age of 50.[18] In 2011 the United States Preventive Services Task Force (USPSTF) issued a recommendation that women age 65 and older be routinely screened for osteoporosis.[19] Hip fractures, in particular, can have devastating effects on an individual's life. In addition to direct medical costs, studies have shown decreased quality of life as well as excess loss of life-years for those experiencing hip or osteoporotic fractures.[20,21]

Vertebral fractures are the most common osteoporotic fracture but may be asymptomatic. Even if the fracture does not cause pain, vertebral fractures can cause deformity, reduced pulmonary function, and loss of height. The degree of compression necessary to define a vertebral fracture has not been standardized.

Osteoporosis affects all races and both sexes. Recent data from the National Health and Nutrition Examination Survey (NHANES) showed that Mexican-Americans had higher risk for osteoporosis, whereas non-Hispanic black persons had lower risk of osteopenia or osteoporosis at the lumbar spine or femoral neck.[16] Multiple genetic factors also influence development of osteoporosis.[22]

Whites are more susceptible than other races to osteoporosis caused by loss of bone density with age. Blacks have only about half the fractures found in whites, probably related to their higher peak bone mass, but black women remain at a high risk because of factors such as decreased dietary calcium intake, a high percentage of lactose intolerance, and increased prevalence of diseases, such as sickle cell disease and lupus, that increases the risk of developing osteoporosis.[23] Both black women and black men have generally been undertreated for osteoporosis.[24] Decreased bone strength with aging is partly due to lower bone mass, but other factors such as deterioration of type I collagen likely contribute to increased fracture risk.[25]

Measuring bone mineral density (BMD) by using dual x-ray absorptiometry (DXA) continues to be the most common method of estimating bone mass. Bone quality relates not just to bone mass (as measured by bone density) but also to the microarchitecture of the bone. Other variables include crystal size and shape, brittleness, vitality of the bone cells, structure of the bone proteins, water volume, integrity of the trabecular network, vascular supply, and the ability to repair tiny cracks.[26]

Because bone density relates to *quantity* of bone, bone *quality* is not accurately identified by bone density testing. Therefore, bone density testing may or may not accurately identify individuals with increased fracture risk. An online tool called FRAX incorporates clinical risk factors with BMD at the femoral neck to predict an individual's 10-year probability of fracture. This tool is available at www.shef.ac.uk/FRAX/. **Postmenopausal osteoporosis** occurs in middle-aged and older women. It can occur because of estrogen deficiency as well as estrogen-independent age-related mechanisms (e.g., secondary causes such as hyperparathyroidism and decreased mechanical stimulation). Recent studies indicate that increased oxidative stress (OS) and increased intracellular reactive oxygen species (ROS) play a significant role in the development of age-related bone loss, as well as other age-related changes in the body.[26] Hormonal deficiency also can increase with stress, excessive exercise, and low body weight. Postmenopausal changes include a substantial increase in bone turnover—that is, an imbalance between the remodeling activity of osteoclasts and osteoblasts. Increased formation and longevity of osteoclasts results in increased bone resorption and is associated with a cascade of proinflammatory cytokines. Increased cytokine activation, especially tumor necrosis factor (TNF), can occur with declining estrogen levels.[26] In addition, estrogen helps protect against the effects of OS and osteoclast apoptosis. Biologically, these processes involve the receptor activator nuclear factor κβ ligand (RANKL), transcription factors such as forkhead proteins, the Wnt and osteoprotegerin (OPG) signaling pathways (see the following Pathophysiology section), and insulin-like growth factor (IGF). Other causes may include a combination of inadequate dietary calcium intake and lack of vitamin D, possibly decreased magnesium level, lack of exercise, low body mass, and family history. IGF is known to help in fracture healing and collagen synthesis and improves conditions for bone mineralization. IGF levels significantly decline by age 60.

Sex hormones, especially estrogen and testosterone, are significant in premenopausal bone maintenance; however, when estrogen levels drop after menopause, it appears that circulating androgens become significant effectors on bone metabolism. In clinical studies of women, data have suggested that serum androgens influence bone density in pre-, peri-, and postmenopausal women. Androgens (i.e., testosterone and dihydrotestosterone) have long been recognized to stimulate bone formation. Other risk factors are identified in Box 44-2.

Poor nutrition and insufficient intake or malabsorption of dietary minerals, particularly calcium, are factors in the development of osteoporosis. Calcium absorption from the intestine decreases with age, and studies of individuals with osteoporosis show that their calcium intake is lower than that of age-matched controls. Deficiencies of vitamins, particularly vitamins C, D, E, and K, also contribute to bone loss.[27]

Skeletal homeostasis depends on a very narrow range of plasma calcium and phosphate concentrations, which are maintained by the endocrine system.[28] Therefore, endocrine dysfunction ultimately can cause metabolic bone disease. In addition to declining levels of sex steroids, the hormones most commonly associated with osteoporosis are parathyroid hormone, cortisol, thyroid hormone, and growth hormone. Excessive intakes of caffeine, alcohol, and nicotine along with low body fat have been considered risk factors. In addition, significant differences in the levels of trace elements (zinc, copper, manganese) were noted in the bones and hair of unaffected individuals compared with those with osteoporosis. Development of selective androgen receptor modulators (SARMs) promises novel treatment for osteoporosis through increasing bone formation and building more muscle mass. In theory, selectively affecting bone, muscle mass, and other desired sites while not affecting lipid or estrogen levels or blood pressure, side effects can be controlled but since the direct effects of SARMs on bone are not yet known, this remains a clinical challenge.[29,30]

Secondary osteoporosis sometimes develops temporarily in individuals receiving large doses of heparin, perhaps because heparin promotes bone resorption by decreasing collagen synthesis or by increasing collagen breakdown. Osteoporosis caused by heparin therapy usually resolves when therapy ceases. Treatment with other medications may lead to the development of osteoporosis, such as the use of glucocorticoid treatment for rheumatoid arthritis. Other medications increasing the risk of osteoporosis include lithium, methotrexate, anticonvulsants, cyclophosphamide, and cyclosporine.

One form, transient osteoporosis of the hip, is associated with the third trimester of pregnancy or the immediate postpartum period. However, most transient osteoporosis is a typically self-limiting syndrome affecting the lower extremity joints of middle-aged men. The etiology is unknown and although most cases spontaneously resolve, some occurrences of bone demineralization may be related to osteonecrosis.[31]

Regional osteoporosis—osteoporosis confined to a region or segment of the appendicular skeleton—usually has a known cause. Transient regional osteoporosis has no known etiology, is characterized by bone marrow edema, and can cause severe pain. The lower extremity is most often affected, but other areas also may be involved.[32] Fortunately, it is usually self-limited. It tends to occur in middle-aged men and women in their late second or third trimester of pregnancy.[33] It is characterized by bone marrow edema, seen on magnetic resonance imaging (MRI), and areas of localized bone demineralization are seen on plain radiographs. Treatment is primarily symptomatic and the condition usually resolves spontaneously over 3 to 6 months, with no long-term adverse effects.

Classic regional osteoporosis is associated with disuse or immobilization of a limb because of fractures, motor paralysis, or bone or joint inflammation (see Figure 44-13, p. 1555). A negative calcium balance develops early and continues throughout the period of immobilization. After 8 weeks of immobilization, significant osteoporosis is present, although it may develop earlier in persons younger than 20 years or older than 50 years. A uniform distribution of osteoporosis also has been observed in astronauts and in individuals treated with air suspension therapy as a result of weightlessness and lack of mechanical strain.

PATHOPHYSIOLOGY. Whatever the cause, osteoporosis develops when the remodeling cycle—the process of bone resorption and bone formation—is disrupted, leading to an imbalance in the coupling process. The explosion of new information in the field of bone biology has led to new understanding of the roles of hormones, growth, and signaling factors, and cellular biology in osteoporosis. Although hormonal influences remain important in maintaining bone health, genetic factors and the role of oxidative stress are receiving increased attention as critical determinants of bone homeostasis.[22,26] Reactive oxygen species are normal byproducts of aerobic metabolism, and although they can cause cell damage, at levels below which they cause OS, ROS serve as signaling molecules for many cell types, including osteocytes, osteoblasts, and osteoclasts. When excess ROS accumulate, OS occurs and can result in loss of bone mass and bone strength.[26]

The osteoclast differentiation pathway is directed by a series of processes that include proliferation, differentiation, fusion, and activation. These processes are controlled by hormones, cytokines, and paracrine stromal-cell microenvironment interactions. Thus the intercellular communication in bone and the key molecular regulators are necessary for bone homeostasis. Certain transcription factors, known as Forkhead box (FoxO), help protect against the effects of OS by preventing excess accumulation of ROS and regulating certain genes that affect DNA repair and cell life span. FoxOs help remove damaged and abnormal cells by inducing apoptosis.[26]

Interleukins (IL-1, IL-4, IL-6, IL-7, IL-11, IL-17), tumor necrosis factor-alpha (TNF-α), transforming growth factor-beta (TGF-β), prostaglandin E_2, and hormones interact to control osteoclasts[34] (Figure 44-10). Normal bone homeostasis is dependent on the balance between the cytokine **receptor activator of nuclear factor κβ ligand (RANKL),** its receptor **RANK,** and its decoy receptor **osteoprotegerin (OPG);** understanding this has led to a tremendously increased knowledge of osteoclast biology and pathogenesis of bone loss.[35]

RANKL, a member of the TNF family, is expressed by osteoblasts and their immature precursors and is necessary for osteoclast development. RANKL activates the receptor RANK, which is expressed on osteoclasts and their precursors and suppresses apoptosis, which leads to activation and prolongation of osteoclast survival.[36] The effects of RANKL are blocked by OPG, a glycoprotein that acts as a decoy receptor for RANKL that prevents it from binding and activating RANK (see Figure 44-10). Cytokines and hormones regulate the balance between RANKL and OPG. Alterations of the RANKL/RANK/OPG system can lead to dysregulation and pathologic conditions including osteoporosis, immune-mediated bone diseases, malignant bone disorders, and inherited skeletal diseases (see Figure 44-10).

Postmenopausal osteoporosis is characterized by increased bone resorption relative to the rate of bone formation, leading to sustained bone loss resulting from estrogen deficiency. Bone loss resulting from estrogen deficiency also contributes to osteoporosis in men.[37,38]

Increased bone resorption results from enhanced development of osteoclasts and decreased osteoclast apoptosis (see Figure 44-10). Estrogen stimulates OPG secretion and downregulates RANKL; drugs known as selective estrogen response modifiers (SERMs) also stimulate OPG production. In estrogen deficiency, the exact role of OPG is less clear.[34] Postmenopausal women express higher levels of RANKL on bone marrow stromal cells, T cells, and B cells than premenopausal women. Importantly, RANKL expression is increased when estrogen levels are decreased, leading to increased formation of osteoclasts while reducing osteoclast apoptosis.[18] Other factors, such as sclerostin (SOST), a glycoprotein secreted by osteocytes, are powerful inhibitors of osteoblast formation by binding to low-density lipoprotein (LDL) receptor–related protein 5 (LRP5) and prevent binding with frizzled protein and Wnt signaling, important factors in osteoblast and bone formation.[34]

Sex steroids (e.g., estrogens) exert anti-apoptotic effects on osteoblasts but exert pro-apoptotic effects on osteoclasts; in both scenarios this is accomplished by activating the **extracellular signal regulated kinases (ERKs).** Estrogen activates ERKs outside the nucleus; ERKs then accumulate in the nucleus and activate downstream transcription factors.[39] This confusing and complicated data eventually revealed that the important determinant of whether pro-apoptosis or anti-apoptosis was exhibited was the *length of time* that the phosphorylated ERKs remained in the nucleus. Prolonged nuclear accumulation of activated ERKs converted the anti-apoptotic effect of estradiol to pro-apoptotic. In addition to ERKs, RANKL promotes the anti-apoptotic effects on osteoclasts, thus increasing their life span.[40] Wnt signaling induces a biochemical series of events that increases osteoblast and bone formation. Alterations in Wnt signaling account for critical pathophysiologic changes in most acquired metabolic bone diseases including postmenopausal osteoporosis, aging effects, and glucocorticoid (i.e., cortisone) excess. Agents such as parathyroid hormone and bisphosphonates, used for treatment of bone loss, exert their positive effects by altering the formation of osteoblasts or osteoclasts or by inducing osteoclast apoptosis.

Glucocorticoid (e.g., cortisone)-induced osteoporosis is characterized by increased bone resorption and decreased bone formation. Glucocorticoids increase RANKL expression and inhibit OPG production by osteoblasts (see Figure 44-10). The use of immunosuppressive drugs (e.g., cyclosporine A) to reduce rejection of transplanted organs also alters the OPG/RANKL/RANK system and can lead to posttransplantation osteoporosis. Other conditions affected by OPG/RANKL/RANK include rheumatoid arthritis, myeloma, vascular diseases, and skeletal metastases from neoplastic disorders.

Age-related bone loss begins in the third to fourth decade. The cause remains unclear, but it is known that decreased serum growth hormone (GH) and IGF levels along with increased

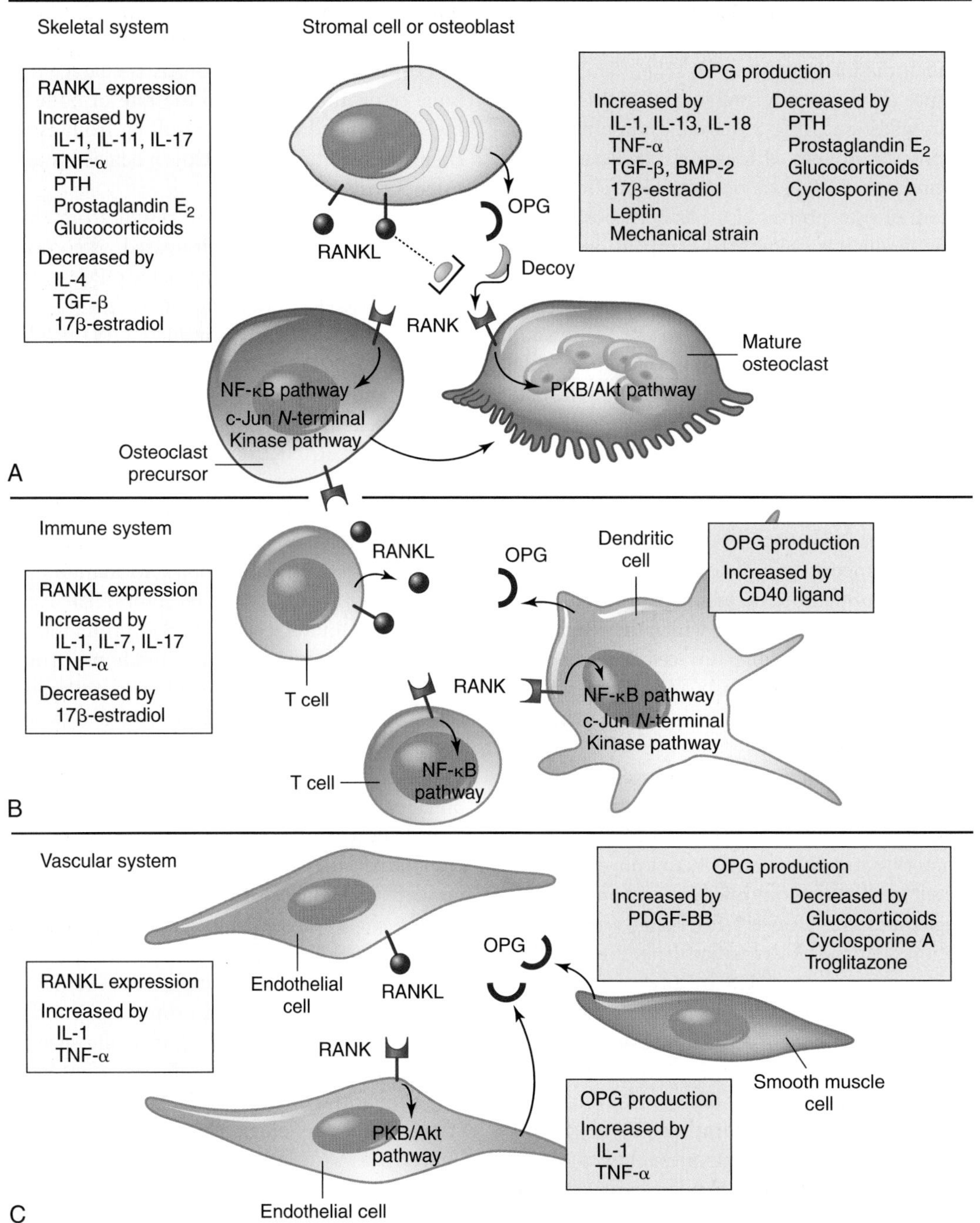

FIGURE 44-10 OPG/RANKL/RANK System. Receptor activator of nuclear factor κβ ligand *(RANKL),* a cytokine and part of the tumor necrosis factor *(TNF)* family, expression and osteoprotegerin *(OPG),* a glycoprotein receptor antagonist, are modulated by various cytokines, hormones, drugs, and mechanical strains (*see inserts*). **A,** In bone, RANKL is expressed by both stromal cells and osteoblasts. RANKL stimulates the receptor RANK on osteoclast precursor cells and mature osteoclasts, and activates intracellular signaling pathways to promote osteoclast differentiation and activation and cytoskeletal reorganization and survival *(PKB/Akt pathway)* that increases resorption and bone loss. OPG, secreted by stromal cells and osteoblasts, acts as a "decoy" receptor and blocks RANKL binding to and activation of RANK. **B,** In the immune system, RANKL is expressed and secreted by T cells. T-cell–derived RANKL also can activate RANK on osteoclasts, T cells, and dendritic cells (antigen-presenting cells), which enhances bone loss that occurs in inflammatory bone diseases such as rheumatoid arthritis. Dendritic cells may regulate these processes by secreting OPG. **C,** In the vascular system, endothelial cells express RANKL and the RANK receptor. RANKL/RANK interactions contribute to endothelial and smooth muscle cells and can block RANKL binding. The physiologic significance of the OPG/RANKL/RANK system in endothelial and smooth muscle cells is being studied. *BMP-2,* Bone morphogenic protein 2; *IL,* interleukin, *PDGF-BP,* platelet-derived growth factor-beta polypeptide; *PTH,* parathyroid hormone; *TGF-α,* tumor necrosis factor-alpha; *TGF-β,* transforming growth factor-beta. (Adapted from Hofbauer LC, Schoppet M: *JAMA* 292[4]:490–495, 2004.)

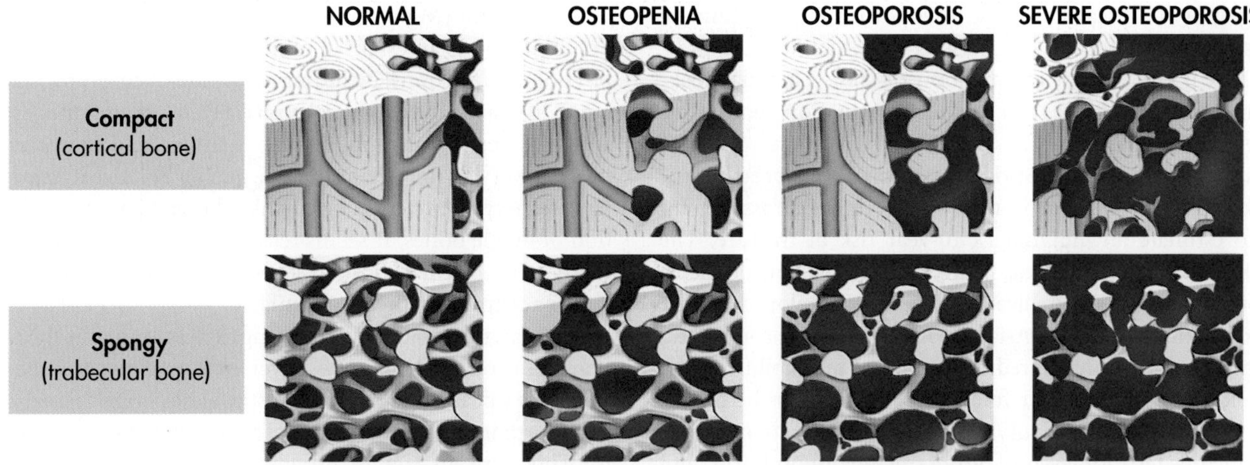

FIGURE 44-11 Osteoporosis in Cortical and Trabecular Bone.

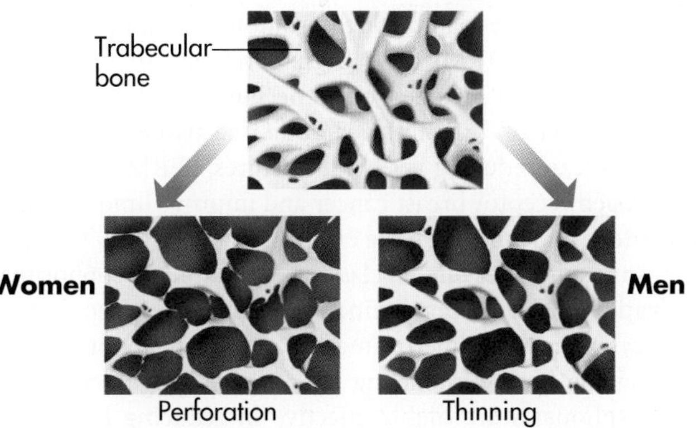

FIGURE 44-12 Mechanism of Loss of Trabecular Bone in Women and Trabecular Thinning in Men. Bone thinning predominates in men because of reduced bone formation. Loss of connectivity and complete trabecular loss predominates in women.

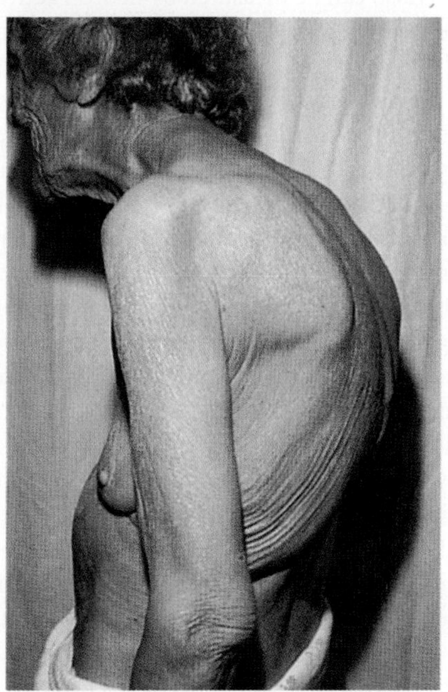

FIGURE 44-13 Kyphosis. This older adult woman's condition was caused by a combination of spinal osteoporotic vertebral collapse and chronic degenerative changes in the vertebral column. (From Kamal A, Brocklehurst JC: *Color atlas of geriatric medicine,* ed 2, St Louis, 1992, Mosby.)

binding of RANKL and decreased OPG affect osteoblast and osteoclast function. Loss of trabecular bone in men proceeds in a linear fashion, with thinning of trabecular bone rather than complete loss as is noted in women (Figure 44-11). Men have approximately 30% more bone mass than women, which may be a factor in their later involvement with osteoporosis (Figure 44-12). Androgens promote osteoprotegerin production, thus inhibiting the osteoclastic effect of RANKL.[41] Reduction in physical activity in older persons also may be a major factor in the degree of bone loss because preservation of bone mass depends on skeletal stress (mechanical) through muscle contraction and weightbearing.[34]

CLINICAL MANIFESTATIONS. The specific clinical manifestations of osteoporosis depend on the bones involved. The most common manifestation, however, is bone deformity. Pain tends to occur only when there is a fragility fracture. Fractures are likely to occur because the trabeculae of spongy bone become thin and sparse and compact bone becomes porous. As the bones lose volume, they become brittle and weak and may collapse or become misshapen. Vertebral collapse causes kyphosis (hunchback) and diminished height (Figure 44-13). Fractures of the long bones (particularly the femur and humerus), distal radius, ribs, and vertebrae are most common. The most serious fractures associated with osteoporosis are hip fractures because of their resultant chronic pain, disability, diminished quality of life, and premature death. Fracture of the neck of the femur (intertrochanteric fracture) tends to occur in older adult women with osteoporosis.[42] Fatal complications of fractures include fat or pulmonary embolism, hemorrhage, and shock. Approximately 20% of persons with a hip fracture die as a result of surgical complications.

EVALUATION AND TREATMENT. Generally, osteoporosis is detected radiographically as increased radiolucency of bone. By the time abnormalities are detected by x-ray examination, as much as 25% to 30% of bone tissue may have been lost.

Types of radiologic examinations include single- or dual-photon absorptiometry (SXA, DXA) and computed tomography (CT) scans. Because osteoporosis is asymptomatic unless a fracture occurs, diagnosis is often delayed. At present, DXA is the current examination of choice for diagnosis. Unfortunately, DXA does not provide information about bone strength or fracture risk.

Because fractures are the primary complication of osteoporosis, the World Health Organization has developed an assessment tool to estimate an individual's 10-year risk of fracture. The WHO's Fracture Risk Assessment (FRAX) is a downloadable computer-drive questionnaire that has been developed for use in Europe, North America, Asia, and Australia. Once completed, the imbedded algorithms predict the 10-year probability of hip, spine, forearm, or shoulder fractures. This tool can be downloaded from www.shef.ac.uk/FRAX. Other evaluation procedures include tests for levels of serum calcium, phosphorus, and alkaline phosphatase as well as protein electrophoresis. Body calcium levels also can be measured by neuron activation analysis, a procedure involving use of radioactive calcium-49, whose gamma activity can be measured with a whole-body counter.

Though prevention of osteoporosis is paramount, treatment is more common and is focused on preventing fractures and maintaining optimal bone function. The role of calcium intake to prevent and treat osteoporosis is controversial. It is well accepted that oral calcium intake sufficient to maintain normal calcium balance is necessary during adolescence to ensure development of peak bone mass, and that calcium-deficient diets can aggravate bone loss associated with menopause and aging. Although recommendations have been established for young women of 1000 mg of calcium daily (particularly from dietary sources) and for postmenopausal women of 1500 mg daily (with vitamin D), it has been difficult to translate these recommendations into clear-cut clinical outcomes (see Nutrition & Disease: Postmenopausal Women Should Not Take Calcium and Vitamin D to Prevent Fractures). A significant relationship has been observed between an individual's lifetime history of calcium intake and peak bone mineral density. Diets with higher fruit and vegetable intake seem to correlate with higher BMD.[43] Other nutrients that appear to have a positive impact on bone health include magnesium, vitamin K_2, and docosahexaenoic acid or DHA (from purified fish oil).[44]

NUTRITION & DISEASE

Postmenopausal Women Should Not Take Calcium and Vitamin D to Prevent Fractures

The beneficial effects of vitamin D on fracture risk are attributed to two explanations: (1) the decrease in bone loss in older adults, and (2) the increase in muscle strength and balance mediated through vitamin D receptors in muscle tissue. Vitamin D alone, however, does not appear to reduce fracture risk. In fact, the U.S. Preventive Services Task Force (USPSTF) has made the recommendation that postmenopausal women should not take supplementary calcium (1000 mg or less) and vitamin D (400 IU or less) because, at these doses, it appears that it does not prevent primary fracture risk and poses a small increased risk for renal stones. The USPSTF also concluded there is not enough evidence either supporting or opposing the use of higher doses of calcium and vitamin D for men or premenopausal women.

Data from Moyer V: *Ann Intern Med* Feb 2013 [online].

Magnesium (Mg^{++}), another mineral important for skeletal development, is an essential mineral in many biochemical and physiologic functions, including activation of enzymes, involvement in adenosine triphosphate (ATP) synthesis and protein synthesis, regulation of membrane channels, and contraction of muscle. Mg^{++} is important to bone quality because it helps control hydroxyapatite crystal growth and thereby prevents formation of brittle bones. It seems reasonable that Mg^{++} is required for normal calcium (Ca^{++}) absorption because severe Mg^{++} deficiency results in hypocalcemia.

Regular, moderate weightbearing exercise can slow the rate of bone loss and, in some cases, reverse demineralization because the mechanical stress of exercise stimulates bone formation. It is important to reduce the risk of falls and enhance bone quality. Therefore, an exercise program to enhance muscle strength is advised. Important new findings suggest that estrogen may prevent excessive bone loss before and after menopause by limiting osteoclast life span through promotion of apoptosis.

SERMs and SARMs have been developed to provide the positive effects of estrogen on bone but minimize estrogen's negative effect on breast and endometrial tissues. As a result, in addition to reducing vertebral fractures, SERMs reduce risk of estrogen receptor breast cancer and improve lipid profiles.[45] Raloxifene and tamoxifen are examples of SERMs.

Bisphosphonates are a class of inorganic pyrophosphate derivatives that bind bone mineral and improve osteoblast and osteocyte survival while promoting osteoclast apoptosis, thus slowing the bone remodeling process.[46] Nitrogen-containing bisphosphonates are highly effective in reducing both vertebral and nonvertebral osteoporotic fractures; because of this, bisphosphonates are the mainstay of osteoporosis treatment. Side effects include alterations in TGF-β signaling that may cause osteonecrosis of the jaw.[47] There also is a small risk of atypical femoral fractures, atrial fibrillation, and possibly esophageal cancer associated with bisphosphonates.[48-51] The optimal length of treatment with bisphosphonates has not yet been determined.[52]

One of the most promising treatments for osteoporosis is denosumab, a monoclonal antibody that that binds the cytokine receptor activator of NF-κβ ligand (RANKL). RANKL inhibition blocks the maturation, function, and survival of osteoclasts, thus reducing bone resorption.[53]

Teriparatide, also called PTH 1-34, is a biosynthetic form of parathormone and contains the first 34 amino acids of parathyroid hormone; PTH 1-84 is a recombinant PTH that contains all 84 amino acids of naturally occurring PTH. Both work by stimulating osteoblasts when administered intermittently.[54] Given by subcutaneous injection, PTH reduces vertebral fractures but use is limited to a period of 24 months because of the risk of developing osteosarcoma. A recent large meta-analysis of osteoporosis treatment found improved BMD and reduced fractures with bisphosphonates, SERMs, and denosumab, though each regimen has potential adverse effects.[55] Restoration of a balanced RANKL/OPG ratio (see p. 1553) or inhibition of RANK responsiveness is known to prevent osteoclast activation and bone resorption. Anti-RANKL therapy significantly reduces bone resorption. Other biologic agents under investigation include cathepsin K inhibitors, antisclerostin, and anti-dickkopf antibodies that affect the Wnt/β-catenin signaling pathway in osteoblasts.[56]

Osteomalacia

Osteomalacia is a metabolic disease characterized by inadequate and delayed mineralization of osteoid in mature compact and spongy bone. In osteomalacia the remodeling cycle proceeds normally through osteoid formation, but mineral calcification (hydroxyapatite formation) does not occur. Bone volume remains unchanged, but the replaced bone consists of soft osteoid instead of rigid bone. The result is abnormal bone matrix mineralization. Rickets is similar to osteomalacia in pathogenesis, but it occurs in the growing bones of children, whereas osteomalacia occurs in adult bone. Chronically low serum phosphate levels can be caused by tumors resulting in osteomalacia.[57] Fibroblast growth factor-23 (FGF-23) plays a significant role in maintaining normal serum phosphate levels. Primarily produced by osteocytes, FGF-23 functions to inhibit reabsorption of phosphate in the renal proximal tubule.[58] (Rickets is described in Chapter 45.)

Osteomalacia and rickets are rare in the United States and Western Europe but are significant health problems in Great Britain, Ethiopia, Pakistan, Iran, and India. In the United States these diseases occur in older adults, in premature infants of very low birth weight, and in individuals adhering to rigid macrobiotic vegetarian diets. Breast-fed black infants who do not receive vitamin D supplementation have been shown to be at risk for developing nutritional rickets.[59,60]

Many factors contribute to the development of osteomalacia, but the most important is a deficiency of vitamin D. The major causes of vitamin D deficiency are diets deficient in vitamin D, decreased endogenous production of vitamin D, intestinal malabsorption of vitamin D, renal tubular diseases, and anticonvulsant therapy. Classic vitamin D deficiency is rare in the United States because of the addition of synthetic vitamin D to dairy products and bread. Still, disorders of the small bowel, kidneys, hepatobiliary system, and pancreas do cause vitamin D deficiency in the United States. In malabsorptive disease of the small bowel, vitamin D and calcium absorption are decreased, so vitamin D is lost in feces. Liver disease interferes with the metabolism of vitamin D to its more active form, and diseases of the pancreas and biliary system cause a deficiency of bile salts, which are necessary for normal intestinal absorption of vitamin D.

The mechanism by which anticonvulsant drug therapy results in decreased bone mineral density is not completely understood, but appears to be from direct impact on bone or effects on other regulators of bone metabolism such as calcium, vitamin D, and parathyroid hormone.[61] The anticonvulsants phenobarbital and phenytoin interfere with calcium absorption and increase degradation of vitamin D metabolism in the liver through activation of the cytochrome P-450 pathway.[62]

PATHOPHYSIOLOGY. Crystallization of minerals in osteoid requires adequate concentrations of calcium and phosphate. When the concentrations are too low, crystallization (and hence ossification) does not proceed normally.

Vitamin D deficiency disrupts mineralization because vitamin D normally regulates and enhances the absorption of calcium ions from the intestine. A lack of vitamin D causes the plasma calcium concentrations to fall. Low plasma calcium levels stimulate increased synthesis and secretion of parathyroid hormone (PTH). Although the increase in the level of circulating PTH raises the plasma calcium concentration, it also stimulates increased renal clearance of phosphate. When the concentration of phosphate in the bone decreases below a critical level, mineralization cannot proceed normally.

Abnormalities occur in spongy as well as compact bone. Trabeculae in spongy bone become thinner and fewer, whereas haversian systems in compact bone develop large channels and become irregular. Because osteoid continues to be produced but not mineralized, abnormal quantities of osteoid accumulate, coating the trabeculae and the linings of the haversian canals. Excessive osteoid also can accumulate in areas beneath the periosteum. The excess of osteoid leads to gross deformities of the long bones, spine, pelvis, and skull.

CLINICAL MANIFESTATIONS. Osteomalacia causes varying degrees of diffuse skeletal pain and tenderness. Bone pain is typically between joints, rather than within them.[59] Pain is noted particularly in the hips, and the individual may be hesitant to walk. Muscular weakness, particularly of the proximal muscles, is common and may contribute to a waddling gait. Facial deformities and bowed knees, or "knock-knees," may be present. Bone fractures and vertebral collapse occur with minimal trauma. Low back pain may be an early complaint, but pain also may involve ribs, feet, other areas of the vertebral column, and other sites. Uremia may be present in renal osteodystrophy.

EVALUATION AND TREATMENT. Laboratory data may include elevated blood urea nitrogen (BUN) and creatinine levels, normal or low serum calcium levels, and a serum inorganic phosphate level that is usually higher than 5.5 mg. Alkaline phosphatase and PTH levels are usually elevated. Radiographic findings show pseudofractures and radiolucent bands perpendicular to the surface of involved bones. Bone biopsy is useful in determining bone structure and remodeling.[63] Diagnosis of certain types of osteomalacia is becoming easier because of the ability to measure an individual's serum FGF-23 level. Elevated FGF-23 levels are common in X-linked hypophosphatemic and tumor-induced osteomalacia.[64]

Treatment of osteomalacia includes the following:

1. Adjusting serum calcium and phosphorous levels to normal
2. Suppressing secondary hyperthyroidism
3. Chelating bone aluminum if needed
4. Administering calcium carbonate to decrease hyperphosphatemia
5. Adding dietary supplements of vitamin D
6. Performing renal dialysis
7. Considering renal transplant for renal osteodystrophy

Paget Disease

Paget disease of bone (PDB or **osteitis deformans)** is a state of increased metabolic activity in bone characterized by abnormal and excessive bone resorption and formation (remodeling).

Genetic manipulations involving the RANK-NF-κβ signaling pathways are significant in the development of Paget disease, resulting in increased osteoclast activity.[65] Chronic accelerated remodeling eventually enlarges and softens the affected bones. Classic PDB arises as a consequence of disorderly bone resorption and formation.

PDB most often affects the axial skeleton, especially the vertebrae, skull, sacrum, sternum, pelvis, and femur. The disease process may occur in one or more bones without causing significant clinical manifestations.

The disease is seldom found before age 40 years, but its incidence almost doubles each decade from age 50. It affects men more than women in a proportion of 1.8:1. Because it is often symptomless and can be diagnosed only by invasive procedures, few epidemiologic data are available. Autopsy data from England and Germany indicate that approximately 3% to 4% of persons older than 40 years have Paget disease. It is most prevalent in Australia, Great Britain, New Zealand, and the United States.

The cause of PDB is unknown; however, studies have implicated both genetic and environmental factors. About 10% to 30% of individuals with PDB have mutations of a specific gene, sequestosome-1.[66-68] Even viral etiologies have been proposed.[65]

PATHOPHYSIOLOGY. Paget disease begins with excessive resorption of spongy bone and deposition of disorganized bone. The trabeculae diminish, and bone marrow is replaced by extremely vascular fibrous tissue. The resorption phase of Paget disease is followed by the formation of abnormal new bone at an accelerated rate. The collagen fibers are disorganized, and glycoprotein levels in the matrix decrease. Mineralization may extend into the bone marrow. Bone formation is excessive around partially resorbed trabeculae, causing them to thicken and enlarge. Eventually, Paget disease progresses to an inactive phase, in which abnormal remodeling is minimal or absent. Osteoclasts of individuals with Paget disease have increased responses to RANKL.[65]

CLINICAL MANIFESTATIONS. In the skull, abnormal remodeling is first evident in the frontal or occipital regions, and then encroaches on the outer and inner surfaces of the entire skull. The skull thickens and assumes an asymmetric shape (Figure 44-14). Thickened segments of the skull may compress areas of the brain, producing altered mentality and dementia. Impingement of new bone on cranial nerves causes sensory abnormalities, impaired motor function, deafness, atrophy of the optic nerve, and obstruction of the lacrimal duct. Headache is commonly noted.

Extensive alterations of the facial bones are rare except in the jaw, where sclerosis and thickening of the maxilla and mandible displace teeth and produce malocclusion. In long bones, resorption begins in the subchondral regions of the epiphysis and extends into the metaphysis and diaphysis. Warmth over the affected area, bone and joint pain, and bone deformity may occur. Occasionally, Paget disease affects both ends of a long bone. In the femur, PDB produces an exaggerated lateral curvature. In the tibia, anterior curvature is also exaggerated. Stress fractures are common in the lower extremities.

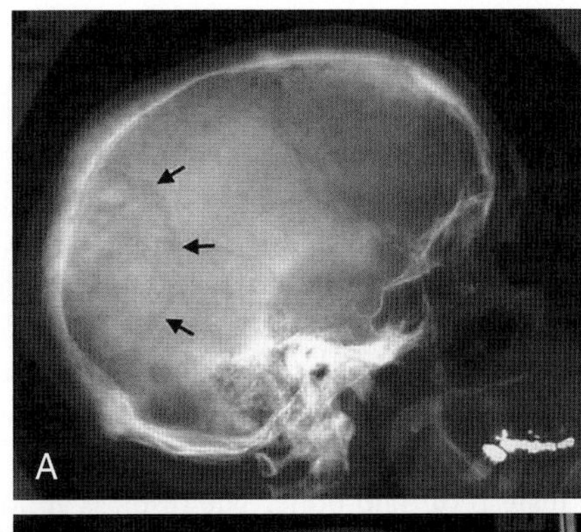

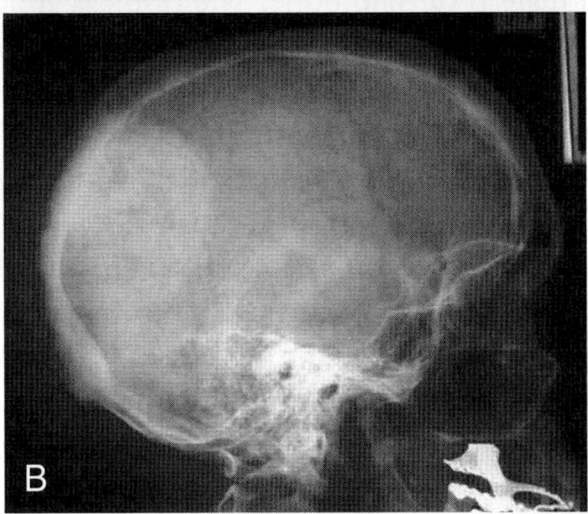

FIGURE 44-14 Paget disease of the skull A, Active Paget disease of the skull, with marked cortical thickening and an area of osteoporosis circumscripta *(arrows).* **B,** The same individual several years later (after bisphosphonate treatment), with the lytic lesion largely replaced by sclerotic bone. (From Walsh JP: *Med J Aust* 181[5]:263, 2004.)

Clinical manifestations of PDB in the vertebral column depend on the level of involvement and are caused by compression of adjacent structures. In the cervical spine, cord compression can lead to spastic quadriplegia. Approximately 1% of persons with PDB develop osteogenic sarcoma. Paget-related sarcoma has a poor prognosis.

EVALUATION AND TREATMENT. Evaluation of PDB is made on the basis of radiographic findings of irregular bone trabeculae with a thickened and disorganized pattern. A typical V-shaped lesion in long bones and rounded areas of thinning bone in the skull are often seen on plain x-ray. Bone scanning can more readily detect early disease as well as extent of PDB through increased uptake of bone radionuclides. Serum total alkaline phosphatase and urinary hydroxyproline levels are elevated.[69]

Most individuals require no treatment because the disease is localized and does not cause symptoms. Treatment during active disease is for pain relief, prevention of deformity, or fracture. Bisphosphonates (alendronate, risedronate, and pamidronate) and calcitonin (salmon and human) are the mainstays of treatment. Surgery is indicated if there are neurologic complications or severe bony deformities.

Infectious Bone Disease: Osteomyelitis

Osteomyelitis is a bone infection most often caused by bacteria; however, fungi, mycobacteria, parasites, and viruses also can infect bone (Figure 44-15). Exogenous osteomyelitis is an infection that enters from outside the body, for example, through

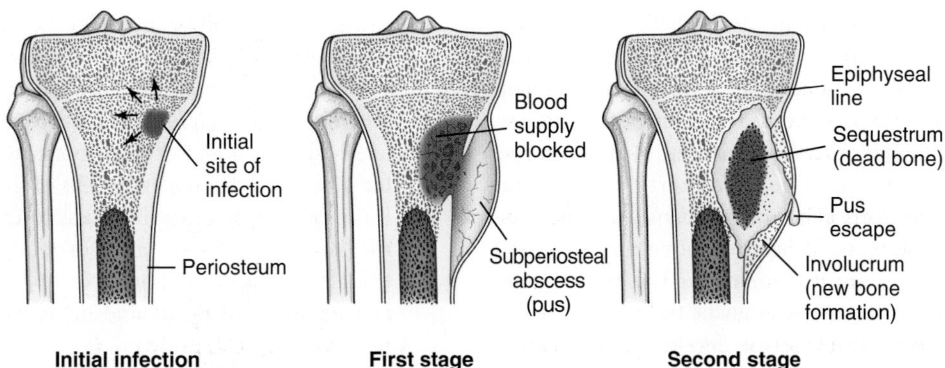

FIGURE 44-15 Osteomyelitis Showing Sequestration and Involucrum.

open fractures, penetrating wounds, or surgical procedures. In exogenous osteomyelitis, infection spreads from soft tissues into adjacent bone. Endogenous osteomyelitis is caused by pathogens carried in the blood from sites of infection elsewhere in the body. In hematogenous osteomyelitis, infection spreads from bone to adjacent soft tissues. Hematogenous osteomyelitis is commonly found in infants, children, and older adults. (Osteomyelitis in children is discussed in Chapter 45.) In infants, incidence rates among males and females are approximately equal. In children and older adults, however, males are most commonly affected. Osteomyelitis is a common complication of sickle cell anemia and low oxygen tension.

Staphylococcus aureus (including methicillin-resistant *Staphylococcus aureus* [MRSA]) is the primary cause of hematogenous osteomyelitis.[70] Other microorganisms include group B streptococci, *Haemophilus influenzae, Salmonella,* and gram-negative bacteria. Group B streptococci and *H. influenzae* tend to infect young children; *Salmonella* infection is associated with sickle cell anemia; and gram-negative infections are most common in older adults and individuals with impaired immunity. Mycobacterial and fungal infections occur in immunocompromised individuals.

Cutaneous, sinus, ear, and dental infections are the primary sources of bacteria in hematogenous bone infections. Soft tissue infections, disorders of the gastrointestinal tract, infections of the genitourinary system, and respiratory tract infections are also sources of bacterial contamination. In addition, infections contracted after total joint replacement surgeries can be causes of osteomyelitis. The vulnerability of specific bone depends on the anatomy of its vascular supply. In adults, hematogenous osteomyelitis is more common in the spine, pelvis, and small bones.

Microorganisms reach the vertebrae through arteries, veins, or lymphatic vessels. The spread of infection from pelvic organs to the vertebrae is well documented. Vaginal, uterine, ovarian, bladder, and intestinal infections can lead to iliac or sacral osteomyelitis.

Exogenous osteomyelitis can be caused by human bites or fist blows to the mouth. Superficial animal or human bites inoculate local soft tissue with bacteria that later spread to underlying bone. Deep bites can introduce microorganisms directly onto bone. The most common infecting organism in human bites is *S. aureus.* In animal bites the most common infecting organism is *Pasteurella multocida,* which is part of the normal mouth flora of cats and dogs.

Direct contamination of bones with bacteria also can occur in open fractures or dislocations with an overlying skin wound. Intervertebral disk surgery and operative procedures involving implantation of large foreign objects, such as metallic plates or artificial joints, are associated with exogenous osteomyelitis. Local injections and venous punctures are significant causes of exogenous osteomyelitis. Exogenous osteomyelitis of the arm and hand bones tends to occur in drug abusers. *S. aureus* is the most common pathogen. In general, persons who are chronically ill, have diabetes or alcoholism, or are receiving large doses of corticosteroids or immunosuppressive drugs are particularly susceptible to exogenous osteomyelitis or recurring episodes of this disease.

PATHOPHYSIOLOGY. Regardless of the source of the pathogen, the pathologic features of bone infection are similar to those in any other body tissue (see Chapter 10). First, the invading pathogen provokes an intense inflammatory response. Inflammation in bone is characterized by vascular engorgement, edema, leukocyte activity, small blood vessel thrombosis, and abscess formation.[71] Once inflammation is initiated, the small terminal vessels thrombose and exudate seals the bone's canaliculi. Inflammatory exudate extends into the metaphysis and the marrow cavity and through small metaphyseal openings into the cortex. In children, exudate that reaches the outer surface of the cortex forms abscesses that lift the periosteum off underlying bone. Lifting of the periosteum disrupts blood vessels that enter bone through the periosteum, which deprives underlying bone of its blood supply; this leads to necrosis and death of the area of bone infected, producing **sequestrum,** an area of devitalized bone (see Figure 44-15). Lifting of the periosteum also stimulates an intense osteoblastic response. Osteoblasts lay down new bone that can partially or completely surround the infected bone. This layer of new bone surrounding the infected bone is called an **involucrum.** Openings in the involucrum allow the exudate to escape into surrounding soft tissue and ultimately through the skin by way of sinus tracts. Involucrum in adults is rare because the periosteum is firmly attached to the cortex and resists displacement. Instead, infection disrupts and weakens the cortex, which predisposes the bone to pathologic fracture.

CLINICAL MANIFESTATIONS. Clinical manifestations of osteomyelitis vary with the age of the individual, site of involvement, initiating event, infecting organism, and whether the infection is acute, subacute, or chronic. Acute osteomyelitis causes an abrupt onset of inflammation. If an acute infection is not completely eliminated, the disease may become subacute or chronic. In subacute osteomyelitis, signs and symptoms are usually vague. In the chronic stage, infection is indolent or silent between exacerbations. The microorganisms persist in small abscesses or fragments of necrotic bone and produce occasional flare-ups of acute osteomyelitis. The progression from acute to subacute osteomyelitis may be the result of inadequate or inappropriate therapy or the development of drug-resistant microorganisms.

In the adult, hematogenous osteomyelitis has an insidious onset. The symptoms are usually vague and include fever, malaise, anorexia, and weight loss. Recent infection (urinary, respiratory, skin) or instrumentation (catheterization, cystoscopy, myelography, diskography) usually precedes onset of symptoms.

Back pain is the primary symptom in vertebral osteomyelitis. Pain may be intermittent or constant, aggravated by motion, and throbbing at rest. It may radiate in a radicular distribution and is commonly accompanied by spinal tenderness and rigidity. Hip contracture can occur in the presence of soft tissue inflammation as a result of irritation of the psoas muscle.[72]

Signs and symptoms of sacroiliac osteomyelitis are generally severe and include local pain, tenderness, and a limp. The pain may radiate to the buttock or the abdomen.

Single or multiple abscesses (Brodie abscesses) characterize subacute or chronic osteomyelitis. Brodie abscesses are painless, circumscribed lesions 1 to 4 cm in diameter, usually in the ends of long bones, and surrounded by dense ossified bone matrix. The abscesses are thought to develop when the infectious microorganism has become less virulent or the individual's immune system is resisting the infection somewhat successfully.

In exogenous osteomyelitis, signs and symptoms of soft tissue infection predominate. Inflammatory exudate in the soft tissues disrupts muscles and supporting structures and forms abscesses. Low-grade fever, lymphadenopathy, local pain, and swelling usually occur within days of contamination by a puncture wound. Osteomyelitis in the hand causes exquisite tenderness over the course of tendon sheaths. The fingers are usually in a semiflexed position, and extension usually causes severe pain. Palmar swelling or symmetric swelling of the fingers may be present.

EVALUATION AND TREATMENT. Laboratory data show an elevated white cell count. Radiographic studies include radionuclide bone scanning, CT, and MRI. MRI is especially useful in detecting early bone changes associated with infection.[73]

Infectious bone disease is expensive and difficult to treat and often culminates in extensive physical disability. The following factors contribute to the difficulty in treating bone infection:

1. Bone contains multiple microscopic channels that are impermeable to the cells and biochemicals of the body's natural defenses. Once bacteria gain access to these channels, they are able to proliferate unimpeded.
2. The microcirculation of bone is highly vulnerable to damage and destruction by bacterial toxins. Vessel damage causes local thrombosis (blockage) of the small vessels, which leads to ischemic necrosis (death) of bone.
3. Bone cells have a limited capacity to replace bone destroyed by infections. Initially, osteoclasts are stimulated by infection to resorb bone, which opens up isolated bone channels so that cells of the inflammatory and immune system can gain access to the infected bone. At the same time, however, resorption weakens the structural integrity of the bone. New bone formation usually lags behind resorption, and the haversian systems in the new bone are incomplete.

Treatment of osteomyelitis includes surgical débridement with bone biopsy and culture before or as soon after initiating antibiotics as possible. Initial antibiotic therapy should be intravenous. Chronic conditions may require surgical removal of the inflammatory exudate followed by continuous wound irrigation with antibiotic solutions in addition to systemic treatment with antibiotics. **Hyperbaric oxygen therapy** of 100% oxygen, given at 2 atmospheres of pressure for 2 hours' duration per day for 30 treatments, is also beneficial for chronic refractory osteomyelitis. Implanted hardware may require removal to more thoroughly treat an infected joint.

Bone Tumors

Primary bone cancer is rare but metastatic disease commonly affects bone. Many different types of tumors involve the skeleton. Based on the tissue of origin, bone tumors are classified as osteogenic, chondrogenic, collagenic, or myelogenic. Each of the four types arises from one of the four stem cells that are ultimately derived from the primitive mesoderm (Figure 44-16). In addition, bone tumors may be classified as being of histiocytic, notochordal, lipogenic, and neurogenic origins (Box 44-3).

The mesoderm contributes the primitive fibroblast and reticulum cells. The fibroblast is the progenitor of the osteoblast and the chondroblast. Each cell synthesizes a specific type of intercellular ground substance, and the type of ground substance produced by the cell generally characterizes the tumor derived from the cell. For example, osteogenic tumors usually contain cells that have the appearance of osteoblasts and produce an intercellular substance that can be recognized as osteoid. Chondrogenic tumors contain chondroblasts and produce an intercellular substance similar to chondroid (cartilage). Collagenic tumors contain fibrous tissue cells and produce an intercellular substance similar to the type of collagen found in fibrous connective tissue.

Tumors are also classified as benign or malignant. The criteria used to identify tumor cells as malignant are: (1) an increased nuclear/cytoplasmic ratio, (2) an irregular nuclear border, (3) an excess of chromatin, (4) a prominent nucleolus, and (5) an increase in the number of cells undergoing mitosis. However, many young, rapidly growing, normal cells and cells subjected to inflammation and change in their blood supply also exhibit many of these same characteristics. (Tumor characteristics in general are described in Chapter 12.)

Epidemiology

The incidence of bone tumors varies with age. Osteosarcoma is the most common primary malignant bone tumor in children

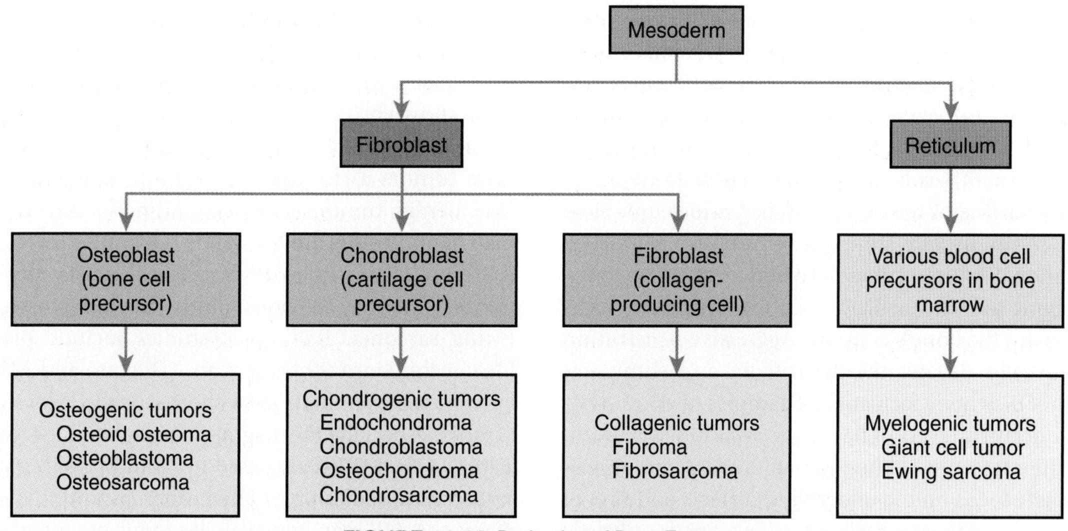

FIGURE 44-16 Derivation of Bone Tumors.

BOX 44-3 WORLD HEALTH ORGANIZATION (WHO) CLASSIFICATION OF BONE TUMORS

Cartilage Tumors
Chondrosarcoma (M)
Chondroma (B)
Osteochondroma (B; but may become malignant)
Chondroblastoma (B)

Osteogenic Tumors
Osteoblastoma (B)
Osteoid osteoma (B)
Osteosarcoma (M)

Fibrogenic Tumors (Often Produce Collagen; Do Not Have a Mineralizing Matrix)
Fibrosarcoma (M)

Fibrohistiocytic Tumors (Comprised of Fibroblasts)
Benign fibrous histiocytoma (B)
Malignant fibrous histiocytoma (M)

Ewing Sarcoma
Ewing sarcoma (M)

Hematopoietic Tumors
Plasma cell myeloma (M)
Malignant lymphoma (M)

Giant Cell Tumor
Giant cell tumor (B, but can grow aggressively)
Malignancy in giant cell tumor (M; very rare tumor)

Smooth Muscle Tumors
Leiomyoma (B)
Leiomyosarcoma (M)

Miscellaneous Tumors
Adamantinoma (M; almost exclusively found in tibia)
Metastatic malignancy (M; most common skeletal malignancy)

Miscellaneous Lesions
Aneurysmal bone cyst (B)
Simple cyst (B)
Fibrous dysplasia (B; rarely can become malignant)
Osteofibrous dysplasia (B)
Langerhans cell histiocytosis (B, but can aggressively grow)
Chest wall hamartoma (B; is excessive growth of mesenchymal tissue [mostly cartilage])

Joint Lesions
Synovial chondromatosis (B; rarely becomes M)

Data from Dorfman HD et al: WHO classification of tumours of bone: introduction. In Christopher DM et al, editors: *World Health Organization classification of tumours, International Agency for Research on Cancer (IARC) pathology and genetics of tumours of soft tissue and bone,* p 226, Lyon, France, 2002, IARC Press.
B, Benign lesion; *M,* malignant lesion.

and young adults.[74-76] Adolescents have the highest incidence of bone tumors, and adults between 30 and 35 years of age have the lowest incidence. After age 35, the incidence slowly increases until, at age 60, it equals the incidence in adolescents, primarily related to metastatic tumors.

Patterns of Bone Destruction

The general pathologic features of bone tumors include bone destruction, erosion or expansion of the cortex, and periosteal response to changes in underlying bone. The least amount of pathologic damage occurs with benign bone tumors that push against neighboring tissue. Because they usually have a symmetric, controlled growth pattern, benign bone tumors tend to compress and displace neighboring normal bone tissue, which weakens the bone's structure until it is incapable of withstanding the stress of ordinary use, leading to pathologic fracture. Other tumors invade and destroy adjacent normal bone tissue by producing substances that promote resorption by increasing osteoclast activity or by interfering with a bone's blood supply. Three patterns of bone destruction by bone tumors have been identified: (1) the geographic pattern, (2) the moth-eaten pattern, and (3) the permeative pattern (Table 44-5).

Tumors that erode the cortex of the bone usually stimulate a periosteal response, that is, new bone formation at the interface between the surface of the bone and the periosteum. Slow erosion of the cortex usually stimulates a uniform periosteal response. Additional layers of bone are added to the exterior surface of the bone to buttress the cortex. Eventually the additional layers expand the bone's contour. Aggressive penetration of the cortex usually elevates the periosteum and stimulates erratic patterns of new bone formation. Examples of erratic patterns include concentric layers of new bone; a sunburst pattern, in which delicate rays of new bone radiate toward the periosteum from a single focus on the underlying surface; and rays of new bone that grow perpendicularly, creating a brush or bristle pattern.

Diagnosis

Malignant bone tumors account for less than 0.2% of all cancers.[76] A tumor must be identified early to allow survival of the individual and the preservation of the affected limb. However, individuals often have only vague symptoms that may be attributed to minor trauma, degenerative changes, or inflammatory conditions. In addition, other conditions may obscure the diagnosis.

Thorough diagnostic studies are needed to determine the exact type and extent of bone tumor present, which also helps determine the optimal treatment regimen. Staging of any bone tumor is critical to determine future treatment and results. The American Joint Committee on Cancer (AJCC) staging system (also known as Enneking or TNM Staging System) is the most commonly used arrangement (Table 44-6). This system classifies tumors as to grade (G), tumor site (T), and metastasis (M). Benign tumors are given a numeric value of zero, whereas malignant tumors are low grade (G_1) or high grade (G_2).

Serum alkaline phosphatase levels are elevated in bone lytic tumors, and they are significantly elevated in osteosarcoma and Ewing sarcoma. Radiologic studies include plain radiologic film, technetium-99 bone scan, CT scan, and MRI, which has become the examination of choice for the local staging of bone tumors, especially the staging of peripheral osteosarcomas (see Table 44-5). MRI is also used to monitor the response of osteosarcomas to radiation or chemotherapy and to detect recurrent disease. A CT scan can evaluate involvement of osteosarcoma in flat bones when the tumor is not well defined on a plain film, can assist in differentiating the tumor, and can locate pulmonary metastases. Radionucleotide bone scans show an increased uptake at the tumor site. Before any surgical procedure, bone biopsy or core needle biopsy should be performed. Core needle biopsy has less risk of tumor seeding.[76]

Additional diagnostic studies performed for specific bone tumors include a complete blood count and erythrocyte sedimentation rate (to rule out infection, myeloma, or Ewing sarcoma) and measurement of serum levels of calcium and phosphorus to detect hypercalcemia. Serum glucose levels may be elevated in chondrosarcoma. Acid phosphatase level may be moderately elevated in bone metastases, multiple myeloma, and advanced Paget disease. Serum protein electrophoresis and immunoelectrophoresis are done to rule out multiple myeloma. Fine-needle biopsy is done, usually at the time of surgery, to determine the exact tumor type.

TABLE 44-5 PATTERNS OF BONE DESTRUCTION BY BONE TUMORS

TYPE OF DESTRUCTION	PATTERN SEEN
Geographic	Well-defined margins separated from surrounding normal bone; well-defined lytic area in affected bone
Moth-eaten	Less-defined margin not easily separated from normal bone; areas of partially destroyed bone adjacent to completely lytic areas
Permeative	Poorly demarcated margins; abnormal lytic bone merges imperceptibly with surrounding normal bone

Types

A very large number of lesions are classified as bone tumors. The bone tumors most representative of the four derivative types (see Figure 44-16)—osteogenic, chondrogenic, collagenic, and myelogenic tumors—are described here.

Osteogenic Tumors: Osteosarcoma. **Osteogenic (bone-forming) tumors** are characterized by the formation of bone or osteoid tissue with a sarcomatous tissue. The tissue can have the appearance of compact or spongy bone. The most common malignant primary bone tumor is osteosarcoma.

TABLE 44-6 THE ENNEKING SURGICAL STAGING SYSTEM FOR MALIGNANT BONE TUMORS

STAGE	GRADE	SITE (T)	METASTASIS (M)
IA	Low (G_1)	Intracompartmental (T_1)	None (M_0)
IB	Low (G_1)	Extracompartmental (T_2)	None (M_0)
IIA	High (G_2)	Intracompartmental (T_1)	None (M_0)
IIB	High (G_2)	Extracompartmental (T_2)	None (M_0)
IIIA	Low (G_1)	Intracompartmental or extracompartmental (T_1 or T_2)	Regional or distant (M_1)
IIIB	High (G_2)	Intracompartmental or extracompartmental (T_1 or T_2)	Regional or distant (M_1)

Data from National Comprehensive Cancer Network: *Recent updates to NCCN clinical practice guidelines in oncology: bone cancer, National Comprehensive Cancer Network,* Version 1, Fort Washington, PA, 2013, Author.

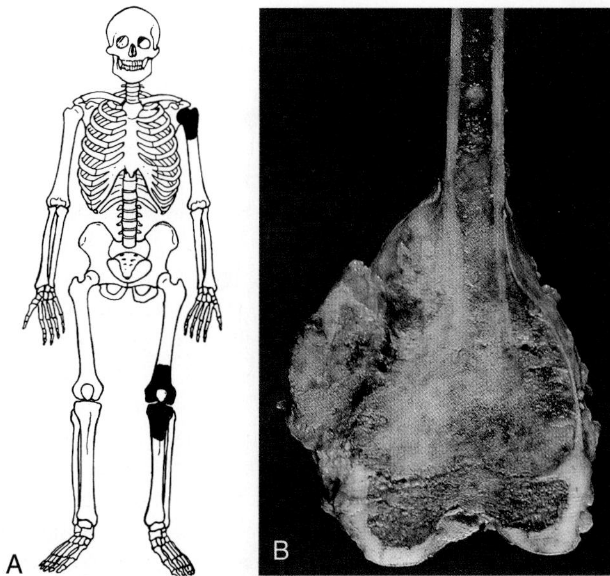

FIGURE 44-17 Osteosarcoma. **A,** Common locations of osteosarcoma. **B,** Femur has a large mass involving the metaphysis of the bone; the tumor has destroyed the cortex, forming a soft tissue component. (From Damjanov I, Linder J, editors: *Anderson's pathology,* ed 10, St Louis, 1996, Mosby.)

Osteosarcomas account for 38% of bone tumors. The male/female ratio is 3:2, and osteosarcoma occurs predominantly in adolescents and young adults; 60% of osteosarcomas occur in persons younger than 20 years. A secondary peak incidence for osteosarcoma occurs in the 60 and older age group, primarily in individuals with a history of radiation therapy several years previously for pelvic or other malignancies (Figure 44-17).

An osteosarcoma is a malignant bone-forming tumor. It is aggressive and most often found in bone marrow; it has a moth-eaten pattern of bone destruction. The borders of the tumor are indistinct and merge into adjacent normal bone. Osteosarcomas always contain osteoid and callus (osteoblastic sarcoma) produced by anaplastic stromal cells, which are atypical, abnormal cells not seen in normal developing bone; they are neither normal nor embryonal. The osteosarcoma also may contain chondroid (cartilage) (chondroblastic sarcoma) and fibrinoid tissue (fibroblastic sarcoma) that may form the bulk of the tumor. The osteoid is deposited in thick masses or "streamers" between the trabeculae of callus, which infiltrate the normal compact bone, destroy it, and replace it with dense callus and masses of osteoid. Demonstrating the presence of osteoid aids in the diagnosis of osteosarcoma. Bone tissue produced by osteosarcomas never matures to compact bone.

Ninety percent of osteosarcomas are located in the metaphyses of long bones, especially the distal femur and proximal tibia, with 50% around the knee area. The tumor typically breaks through the cortex, lifts the periosteum, and forms a soft tissue mass that is *not* covered by a smooth shell of new bone. Lifting of the periosteum stimulates bizarre patterns of new bone formation called a *periosteal reaction.* Distinct osteosarcomas occur on the surface of long bones, called parosteal, periosteal, or high-grade surface osteosarcomas; dedifferentiated parosteal and central osteosarcomas also occur.

The most common initial symptoms are pain and swelling. Initially the pain is slight and intermittent, but within a short time it increases in severity and duration. Pain is usually worse at night and gradually requires medication. Systemic symptoms are uncommon. Usually a coincidental history of trauma is noted. Occasionally the individual may have a pathologic fracture.

Systemic chemotherapy and surgery are the treatments of choice, with the location of the tumor and its size, malignancy grade, and evidence of metastasis dictating the type and extent of surgery. Preoperative chemotherapy has greatly increased the number of individuals qualifying for limb salvage surgery. Limb salvaging procedures have been made possible by advances in reconstructive techniques and endoprosthetics. Limb salvage ultimately may be successful in as many as 80% of persons. Individuals must have achieved most of their bone growth to be candidates for limb salvage procedures, which are preferred to amputation. Skeletally immature individuals may have a limb salvage operation, referred to as a *rotationplasty,* in which the major portions of the thigh, the tumor, and contaminated knee are resected while preserving the nerve supply (sciatic) to the leg and foot. The proximal tibia is internally fixed to the stump of the proximal femur after it has been rotated 180 degrees. The foot is positioned at a desired spot or direction, allowing the ankle joint to function as a knee joint with the foot supplying the traditional role of the tibial stump in a below-knee amputation.

If an amputation is done, individuals are monitored closely with chest roentgenograms and CT. Pulmonary metastases are surgically resected, and chemotherapy is now a common therapy given both before and after surgery, using combinations of chemotherapeutic agents. Promising agents under investigation include monoclonal antibodies, hormone antagonists, gene therapy, and other biologic agents that may dramatically improve survival.[77,78]

Chondrogenic Tumors: Chondrosarcoma. **Chondrogenic (cartilage-forming) tumors** produce cartilage or **chondroid,** a primitive cartilage or cartilage-like substance. The most common chondrogenic tumor is chondrosarcoma, accounting for 20% of bone tumors.

Chondrosarcoma, the second most common primary malignant bone tumor, is a tumor of middle-age and older adults; incidence peaks in the sixth decade of life.[79] The tumor is found more commonly in men than in women. Pre-existing chondral lesions, such as osteochondromas, can give rise to secondary chondrosarcoma, which, generally, has a fairly good prognosis.[80]

A chondrosarcoma is a large ill-defined malignant tumor that infiltrates trabeculae in spongy bone. It produces cartilage-forming cells but there is no ossification, as in normal endochondral bone formation.[81] It occurs most often in the metaphysis or diaphysis of long bones, especially the femur, and in the bones of the pelvis (Figure 44-18). The tumor contains large lobules of hyaline cartilage that are separated by bands of fibrous tissue and anaplastic cells. Chondrosarcomas typically implant in surrounding tissue ("seeding").

Symptoms associated with chondrosarcoma have an insidious onset. Local swelling and pain are the usual symptoms that cause a person to seek treatment. At first the pain is dull and

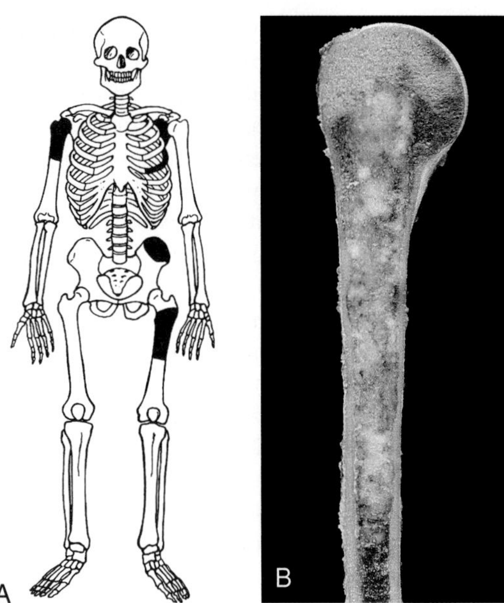

FIGURE 44-18 Chondrosarcoma. **A,** Common locations of chondrosarcoma. **B,** Chondrosarcoma of humerus. (From Damjanov I, Linder J, editors: *Anderson's pathology,* ed 10, St Louis, 1996, Mosby.)

intermittent, then gradually intensifies and becomes constant. It may awaken the person at night.

Diagnostic studies include radiographs, which must be reviewed carefully for an accurate diagnosis. Biopsy is done at the time of surgery. (If biopsy is done before scheduled surgical incision, seeding of tumor cells could occur.) Sufficient tumor material must be obtained to facilitate an accurate diagnosis.

Wide surgical excision is generally regarded as the treatment of choice because chemotherapy and radiation seem to have little effect.[81] Many surgically treated individuals demonstrate recurrences, however, so amputation is becoming one treatment of choice. Therefore, individuals with tumors located in the limbs have a better prognosis than those with pelvic lesions.

Collagenic Tumors: Fibrosarcoma. **Collagenic (collagen-forming) tumors** produce fibrous connective tissue. The most typical collagenic tumor is the fibrosarcoma.

Fibrosarcomas come from fibroblasts that originate from mesenchymal stem cells and represent 4% of primary malignant bone tumors, with a broad age distribution. They may occur at any age but are most common in adults between 30 and 50 years of age. Fibrosarcoma also may be a secondary complication of radiation therapy, Paget disease, and long-standing osteomyelitis; secondary fibrosarcoma tends to be more aggressive, with poorer outcome.

Fibrosarcoma is a solitary tumor that most often affects the metaphyseal region of the femur or tibia. The tumor is composed of a firm fibrous mass of tissue that contains collagen, malignant fibroblasts, and occasional osteoclast-like giant cells.

The tumor begins in the marrow cavity of the bone and infiltrates the trabeculae. It demonstrates a permeative growth pattern, destroys the cortex, and extends into the soft tissue. Metastasis to the lung is common.

Symptoms associated with the tumor have an insidious onset, which delays diagnosis. Pain and swelling, the usual symptoms

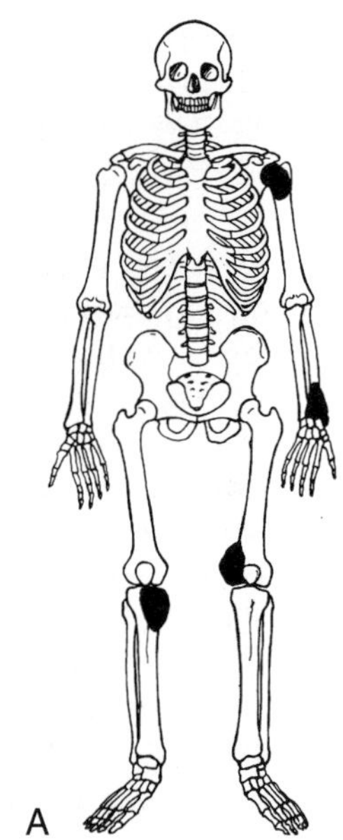

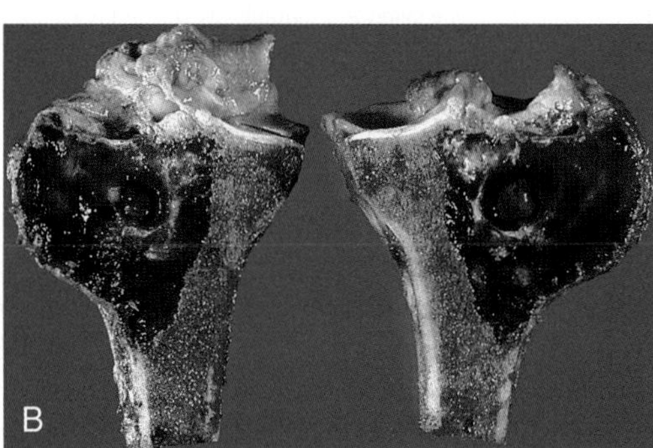

FIGURE 44-19 Giant Cell Tumor of Bone. **A,** Common skeletal locations. **B,** Gross picture of cell tumor of bone (epimetaphysis). (From Damjanov I, Linder J, editors: *Anderson's pathology,* ed 10, St Louis, 1996, Mosby.)

that cause the individual to seek treatment, usually indicate that the tumor has broken through the cortex. Local tenderness, the presence of a palpable mass, and limitation of motion also may be present. A pathologic fracture in the affected bone is often the reason for seeking medical help. Diagnostic studies include radiographs and MRI.

Radical surgery and amputation are the treatments of choice for fibrosarcoma. Radiation therapy is generally considered ineffective treatment for this tumor.

Myelogenic Tumors. **Myelogenic tumors** originate from various bone marrow cells. Two types of myelogenic tumors are giant cell tumor and myeloma. Myeloma is discussed in Chapter 29.

Giant Cell Tumor. Giant cell tumor is the sixth most common of the primary bone tumors, accounting for 4% to 5% of bone tumors. Giant cell tumors have a wide age distribution; however, they are rare in persons younger than 10 years or older than 70 years. Most giant cell tumors are found in persons between 20 and 40 years of age. Unlike most other bone tumors, giant cell tumors affect females more often than males.[82]

Giant cell tumors are generally benign, solitary, circumscribed tumors that cause extensive bone resorption because of their osteoclastic origin (Figure 44-19). There is a high rate of recurrence but metastasis is rare. The tumor is rich in osteoclast-like giant cells and anaplastic stromal cells. It also may contain osteoid, callus, and collagen. Overexpression of several genes, including osteoprotegerin ligand (OPGL), occurs in giant cell tumors. The giant cell tumor is typically located in the center of the epiphysis in the femur, tibia, radius, or humerus. The tumor has a slow, relentless growth rate and is usually contained within the original contour of the affected bone. Tumors are often associated with pathologic fractures because of aggressive bone resorption.[83] It may, however, extend into the articular cartilage. When the tumor extends, it is usually covered by periosteum or periosteal bone growth.

The most common symptoms associated with giant cell tumor are pain, local swelling, and limitation of movement. Diagnostic studies include radiographs, CT, and MRI. Cryosurgery and resection of the tumor with the use of adjuvant polymethylmethacrylate (PMMA) for bone grafts decrease recurrence and are more successful treatments than curettage and radiation.[84] Amputation may be necessary but is not common.

DISORDERS OF JOINTS

The American College of Rheumatology (ACR) recognizes 13 groups of joint disease—**arthropathies.** Most of these disorders can be placed into two major categories: noninflammatory joint disease and inflammatory joint disease. With recent improvements in detection methods, conditions such as osteoarthritis that were previously classified as noninflammatory have now had inflammatory pathways identified.

Osteoarthritis

Osteoarthritis (OA) is a common age-related disorder of synovial joints. It is characterized by local areas of loss and damage of articular cartilage, new bone formation of joint margins (osteophytosis), subchondral bone changes, variable degrees of mild synovitis, and thickening of the joint capsule (Figure 44-20). OA has been commonly classified as **noninflammatory joint disease.** However, it is clear that specific markers of inflammation are present in OA and inflammation is an important feature of OA. The use of MRI and arthroscopy has made it clear that osteoarthritic changes are not defined by changes noted on x-ray films alone.

The exact cause of OA is uncertain; however, pathology centers on load-bearing areas. Advancing disease reveals narrowing of the joint space because of cartilage loss, bone spurs **(osteophytes),** and sometimes changes in the subchondral bone. It is uncommon in people younger than 40 years but rises in incidence with age. Low-grade inflammation, calcification of articular cartilage, genetic alterations, and metabolic disorders combined with the interaction of transcription factors, cytokines, growth factors, matrix molecules, and enzymes affect development and progression of OA.[85,86] OA is generally distributed throughout the peripheral and central joints of the body (hips, hands, knees, and spine). With aging, the quality and quantity of the proteoglycans in cartilage decrease in direct proportion to the severity of OA.

OA can be caused by any condition that damages cartilage directly; subjects the joint surfaces or underlying bone to chronic, excessive, or abnormal forces; or causes instability in the joint. Specific risk factors include the following:

1. Trauma, particularly sprains, strains, joint dislocations, and fractures
2. Long-term mechanical stress associated with athletics, ballet dancing, or repetitive physical tasks worsened by obesity
3. The presence of inflammation in joint structures, during which inflammatory cells release enzymes capable of digesting cartilage cells
4. Joint instability caused by damage to supporting structures, such as the joint capsule, ligaments, or tendons
5. Neurologic disorders (e.g., diabetic neuropathy, Charcot neuropathic joint) in which pain and proprioceptive reflexes are diminished or lost, increasing the tendency for abnormal movement, positioning, or weightbearing
6. Congenital or acquired skeletal deformities
7. Hematologic or endocrine disorders, such as hemophilia, which causes chronic bleeding into the joints, or hyperparathyroidism, which causes bone to lose calcium
8. Drugs (e.g., colchicine, indomethacin, steroids) that stimulate the activity of collagen-digesting enzymes in the synovial membrane
9. Obesity

All of these factors alter articular cartilage in some way and accelerate the rate of cartilage loss.

PATHOPHYSIOLOGY. The primary defect in OA is loss of articular cartilage. Early in the disease, the articular cartilage loses its glistening appearance, becoming yellow-gray or brownish gray. As the disease progresses, surface areas of the articular cartilage flake off and deeper layers develop longitudinal fissures (fibrillation). The cartilage becomes thin and may be absent over some areas, leaving the underlying bone (subchondral bone) unprotected. Consequently, the unprotected subchondral bone becomes sclerotic (dense and hard). Cysts sometimes develop within the subchondral bone and communicate with the longitudinal fissures in the cartilage. Pressure builds in the cysts until the cystic contents are forced into the synovial cavity, breaking through the articular cartilage on the way. As the articular cartilage erodes, cartilage-coated osteophytes may grow outward from the underlying bone and alter the bone contours and joint anatomy. These spur-like bony projections enlarge until small pieces, called *joint mice,* break off into the synovial cavity. If osteophyte fragments irritate the synovial membrane, synovitis and joint effusion result. The joint capsule also becomes thickened and at times adheres to the deformed underlying bone, which may contribute to the limitation of movement (see Figure 44-20).

Articular cartilage is lost through a cascade of cytokine and anabolic growth factor pathways.[87] Enzymatic processes, particularly those involving matrix metalloproteinases, break down the macromolecules of proteoglycans, glycosaminoglycans, and collagen into large, diffusible fragments. The fragments are then taken up by the cartilage cells (chondrocytes) and digested by the cell's own lysosomal enzymes. (Processes of cellular uptake and lysosomal digestion are described in Chapter 1.) The loss of

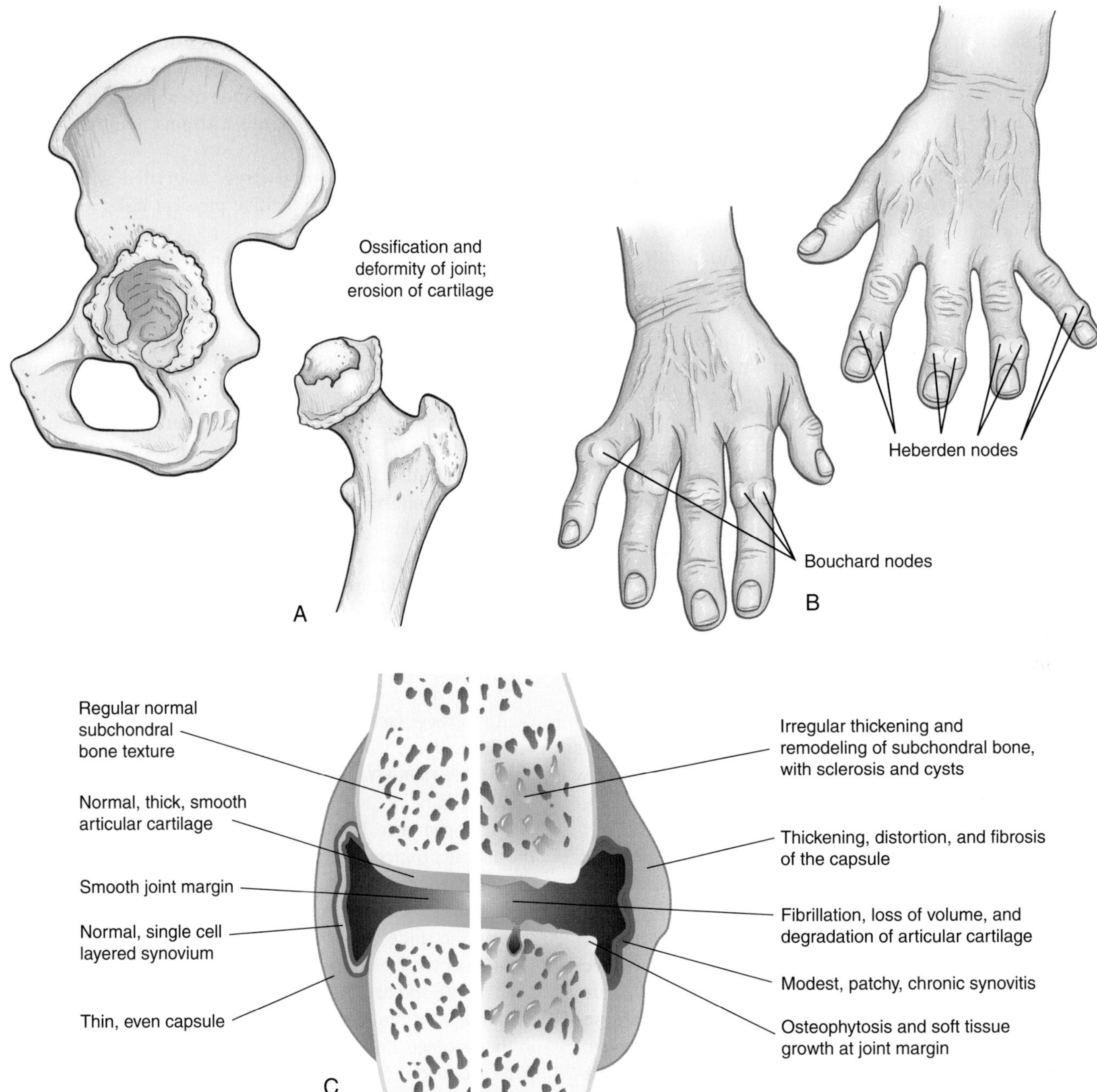

FIGURE 44-20 Osteoarthritis (OA). **A,** Cartilage and degeneration of the hip joint resulting from osteoarthritis. **B,** Heberden nodes and Bouchard nodes. **C,** Characteristics of OA. Normal vs. osteoarthritic synovial joint.

proteoglycans from articular cartilage is a hallmark of the osteoarthritic process.

Enzymatic destruction of articular cartilage begins in the matrix, with destruction of proteoglycans and collagen fibers. Enzymes, particularly stromelysin and matrix metalloproteinases (collagenase), affect proteoglycans by interfering with assembly of the proteoglycan subunit or the proteoglycan aggregate (see Chapter 43); levels of these enzymes are markedly elevated in OA. Changes in the conformation of proteoglycans disrupt the pumping action that regulates movement of water and synovial fluid into and out of the cartilage. Without the regulatory action of the proteoglycan pump, cartilage absorbs too much fluid and becomes less able to withstand the stresses of weightbearing. Also with aging, the proteoglycan content is decreased and the water content in cartilage can be increased by as much as 8%, affecting the strength of the cartilage. Persons with OA, even those with fairly extensive cartilage destruction, have elevated levels of proteoglycans or fragments of proteoglycans in their synovial fluid, perhaps indicative of a more pronounced reparative phase. Inflammatory cytokines, such as IL-1 and TNF (see Chapter 8 for a discussion of cytokines), play a major role in cartilage degradation in part through induction of nitric oxide synthase (iNOS) and nitric oxide (NO) increased generation. Cytokines release and activate proteolytic and collagenolytic enzymes, causing an imbalance of cell responses to growth factor activity.[87]

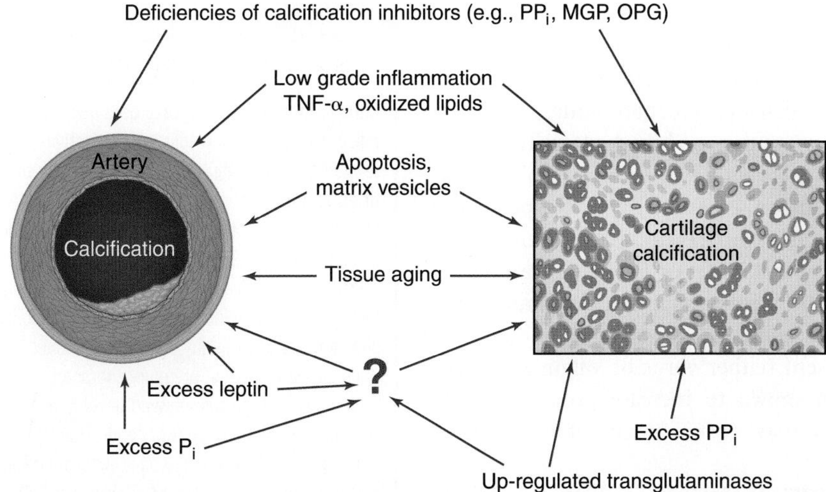

FIGURE 44-21 **Possible Mechanisms Driving Artery and Cartilage Calcification.** All specified factors have been demonstrated to promote calcification in either arteries and/or cartilage (see text). *MGP,* Matrix GLA-protein; *OPG,* osteoprotegerin; *Pi,* inorganic phosphate; *PPi,* inorganic pyrophosphate. (From Rutsch F, Terkeltaub R: *Joint Bone Spine* 72:110–118, 2005.)

Crosstalk between signaling pathways contributes to the development and progression of OA.[88] Some of the enzymes that degrade collagen (e.g., chemokines and metalloproteinases) are produced by the synovium. Chondrocyte apoptosis is increased in OA cartilage and is directly correlated with hydroxyapatite crystal deposition. Nitric oxide (NO) stimulates apoptosis in chondrocytes. The resultant cartilage destruction initiates the IL-1β and TNF-α pathways of inflammation. Genetic deficiencies of inhibitors of calcification also may contribute to "run away" calcification (Figure 44-21). Collagen breakdown destroys the fibrils that give articular cartilage its tensile strength and exposes the chondrocytes to mechanical stress and enzyme attack. Thus a cycle of destruction begins that involves all the components of articular cartilage—proteoglycans, collagen fibers, and chondrocytes.

CLINICAL MANIFESTATIONS. Clinical manifestations of OA typically appear during the fifth or sixth decade of life, although asymptomatic articular surface changes are common after age 40. Pain and stiffness in one or more joints, usually weightbearing or load-bearing joints, are the first symptoms of the disease. Use-related joint pain relieved by rest is a key feature. Examination usually shows general involvement of peripheral and central joints. Peripheral joints most often involved are in the hands, wrists, knees, and feet. Central joints most often affected are in the lower cervical spine, lumbosacral spine, shoulders, and hips.

Pain and stiffness are the predominant symptoms of OA; others include swelling, tenderness, or enlargement/deformity of joints. Symptoms are usually aggravated by weightbearing or use of the joint and relieved by resting the joint. Sometimes pain is referred to another part of the body. For example, osteoarthritis of the lumbosacral spine may mimic sciatica, causing severe pain in the back of the thigh along the course of the sciatic nerve. OA in the lower cervical spine may cause brachial neuralgia (pain in the arm) aggravated by movement of the neck. Osteoarthritic conditions in the hip cause pain that may be referred to the lower thigh and knee area.

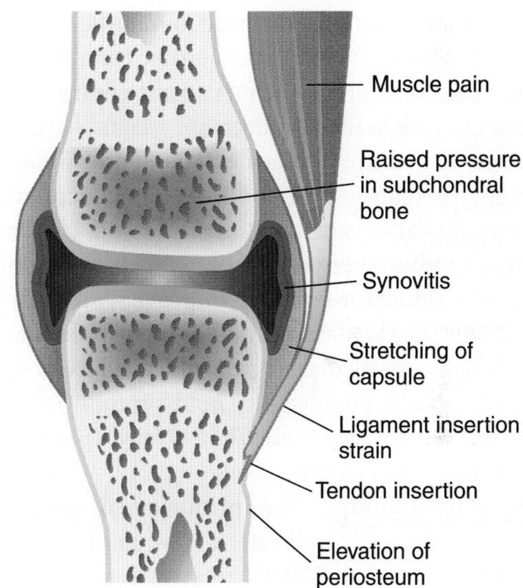

FIGURE 44-22 **Possible Causes of Pain in Osteoarthritis.**

The actual mechanisms of joint pain are complex and poorly understood, but several explanations are possible. Subchondral bone changes, weightbearing stress, and inflammatory mediators may be sources of joint pain in OA.[89,90] Nonetheless, there is little correlation between radiologic appearance of OA and an affected person's pain level.[91] Articular distention and stretching of the fibrous joint capsule, which has an abundant nerve supply may also contribute to pain. In addition, inflammation of the joint capsule causes fibrous shrinking, so that movement of the joint in any direction causes painful stretching (Figure 44-22).

The origin of joint stiffness is unknown. **Joint stiffness** is generally defined as difficulty in initiating joint movement, immobility, or a loss of range of motion. The extent of cartilage degeneration also limits range of motion to some degree. The stiffness usually occurs as joint movement begins and dissipates within 30 minutes. Enlargement and bulging of joint contour, commonly described as swelling, may be caused by bone enlargement or the proliferation of osteophytes around the margins of the joint. These types of typical joint swelling in the fingers are termed Heberden and Bouchard nodes. Swelling also occurs if inflammatory exudate or blood enters the joint cavity, thereby increasing the volume of synovial fluid. This condition, termed **joint effusion,** is caused by (1) the presence of osteophyte fragments in the synovial cavity, (2) drainage of cysts from diseased subchondral bone, or (3) acute trauma to joint structures, resulting in hemorrhage and inflammatory exudation into the synovial cavity.

Abnormal knee alignment (either varus or valgus of more than 5 degrees) has been shown to increase progression of OA.[92] Gait abnormalities may ensue attributable to knee malalignment.

EVALUATION AND TREATMENT. Evaluation consists of clinical assessment and radiologic studies, CT scan, arthroscopy, and MRI. Treatment is based on severity of symptoms. Research is ongoing to evaluate the use of specific biomarkers to allow earlier detection of OA and monitor its progress.[93] Conservative treatment includes rest of the involved joint until inflammation, if present, subsides; participation in aerobic exercise and range-of-motion exercise to prevent joint capsule contraction; use of a cane, crutches, or walker to decrease weightbearing; weight loss if obesity is present; and analgesic and anti-inflammatory drug therapy to reduce pain and swelling. Glucosamine and chondroitin, so-called nutraceuticals, are not currently recommended.[94] Other alternative therapies, including magnetic bracelets and acupuncture, seem to improve symptoms in some people as do intra-articular injection of high-molecular-weight viscosupplements, particularly hyaluronic acid. New technologies, including tissue engineering, hold promise for reversing degenerative joint changes (see What's New? Tissue Engineering for Cartilage and Tendon).

Surgery is used to improve joint movement, correct deformity or malalignment, or create a new joint with artificial implants. There are nearly 250,000 total hip replacements yearly in the United States, most of which are related to OA.

Classic Inflammatory Joint Disease

Inflammatory joint disease commonly is called *arthritis.* Inflammatory joint disease is characterized by damage or destruction in the synovial membrane or articular cartilage and by systemic signs of inflammation (fever, leukocytosis, malaise, anorexia, hyperfibrinogenemia).

Inflammatory joint disease can be infectious or noninfectious. In infectious inflammatory joint disease, inflammation is caused by invasion of the joint by bacteria, mycoplasmas, viruses, fungi, or protozoa. These agents can invade the joint through a traumatic wound, surgical incision, or contaminated needle, or they can be delivered by the bloodstream from sites of infection elsewhere in the body, typically bones, heart valves, or blood vessels. In noninfectious inflammatory joint disease, inflammation is caused by the deposition of crystals of monosodium urate in and around the joint (gout) or by immune reactions (rheumatoid arthritis and ankylosing spondylitis).

WHAT'S NEW?

Tissue Engineering for Cartilage and Tendon

Chronic musculoskeletal disorders involving joints and soft tissue cause significant disability and loss of productivity. Articular cartilage degeneration related to osteoarthritis affects a majority of people over the age of 65 and often results in chronic pain and disability. After laceration or rupture of a tendon, healing can take months to occur and return of normal function is often limited.

Efforts to surgically repair or replace damaged cartilage and tendon have been frustrated by inferior mechanical and functional qualities of repaired tissue compared to healthy, noninjured tissue. New techniques, however, promise improved return of preinjury characteristics.

Nanotechnology has allowed development of a scaffold for cartilage repair that mimics the body's natural endochondral framework for cartilage and bone development. This biomimetic structure has been used to treat osteochondral cartilage defects in a recent clinical trial. Future nanocomposites that mimic bone are also under exploration.

Tendon scaffolds using nanofibers are being investigated. In soft tissue such as tendon, use of scaffolds for implanting mesenchymal stem cells (MCSs) and growth factors can increase tendon strength and improve biomechanical properties of healing tissue. Other ongoing research is focusing on combining MCSs, type I collagen sponges, and constructs treated with mechanical stimulation to improve mechanical and cellular properties of tissue.

Data from Grande DA et al: *J Am Acad Orthop Surg* 19:59–62, 2011; Hogan MV et al: *J Am Acad Orthop Surg* 19:134–142, 2011; Kock L, van Donkelaar CC, Ito K: *Cell Tissue Res* 347:613–627, 2012; Pleshko N, Grande DA, Myers KR: *J Am Acad Orthop Surg* 20:60–62, 2012.

Rheumatoid Arthritis

Rheumatoid arthritis (RA) is a chronic, systemic inflammatory autoimmune disease distinguished by joint swelling and tenderness and destruction of synovial joints, leading to disability and premature death.[95] (Autoimmune disease is described in Chapter 9.) The first joint tissue to be affected is the synovial membrane, which lines the joint cavity (see Chapter 43 and Figure 43-9). Multiple immunoregulatory cytokines (such as interleukins, B cells, and matrix metalloproteinases) contribute to joint damage. Eventually, inflammation may spread to the articular cartilage, fibrous joint capsule, and surrounding ligaments and tendons, causing pain, joint deformity, and loss of function (Figure 44-23). The joints most commonly affected are in the fingers, feet, wrists, elbows, ankles, and knees, but the shoulders, hips, and cervical spine also may be involved, as well as the tissues of the lungs, heart, kidneys, and skin.

Over the past five decades, the incidence and prevalence of RA have decreased, and RA now affects between 0.5% and 1% of the adult population in developed countries.[96] The frequency of RA increases with age. Besides inflammation of the joints, RA can cause fever, malaise, rash, lymph node or spleen enlargement, and Raynaud phenomenon (transient lack of circulation to the fingertips and toes).

Despite intensive research, the cause of RA remains obscure. It is likely a combination of genetic factors interacting with inflammatory meditators. The intricate interplay of chemokines (powerful mediators of inflammation) is largely responsible for RA's chronic inflammatory characteristics. Ligand/receptor chemokines attract T cells and produce inflammatory changes.[97]

A key genetic element has been localized to the human leukocyte antigen-death receptor 4 *(HLA-DR4), HLA-DRB1* (death receptor beta), and *HLA-DP* genes of the major histocompatibility complex in all ethnic groups. A surprising new discovery is the presence of T-cell abnormalities in individuals with RA, indicating a defect in telomere repair that may result in faster aging of telomeres with subsequent loss of efficient immune function.[97] Types of infectious arthritis are summarized in Table 44-7. With long-term or intensive exposure to the antigen, normal antibodies (immunoglobulins [Igs]) become autoantibodies—antibodies that attack host tissues (self-antigens). Because they are usually present in individuals with rheumatoid arthritis, the altered antibodies are termed **rheumatoid factors (RFs).** RFs usually consist of two classes of immunoglobulin antibodies (antibodies for IgM and IgG) but occasionally involve antibodies for IgA. Their main antigenic targets are portions of the immunoglobulin molecules. RFs bind with their target self-antigens in blood and synovial membrane, forming immune complexes (antigen-antibody complexes) (see Chapter 8).

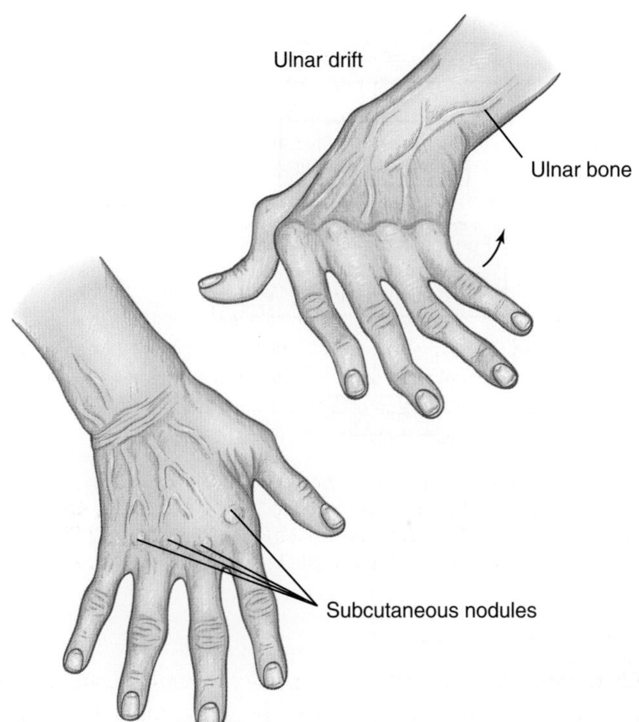

FIGURE 44-23 Rheumatoid Arthritis of the Hand. Note swelling from chronic synovitis of metacarpophalangeal joints, marked ulnar drift, subcutaneous nodules, and subluxation of metacarpophalangeal joints with extension of proximal interphalangeal joints and flexion of distal joints. Note also deformed position of thumb. Hand has wasted appearance. (From Mourad L: *Orthopedic disorders*, St Louis, 1991, Mosby.)

Environmental factors including geographic area of birth, length of breast-feeding, socioeconomic status, and especially smoking have been identified as risk factors for developing RA.[98] RA and other autoimmune diseases have a higher prevalence among women.[99] The reasons for this are unclear, but hormones and genetics play a role as shown by RA symptom improvement during pregnancy and flares with breast-feeding.

PATHOPHYSIOLOGY. Although no specific events (such as trauma, illness, or environmental conditions) have been identified that would cause immune abnormalities to develop into localized tissue and joint inflammation, the pathology of RA is fairly well understood. During inflammation, arginine (an α-amino acid) can be enzymatically modified into another α-amino acid, citrulline. This process (citrullination) changes the structure and function of the protein. Other proteins, like fibrin and vimentin, can become citrullinated during cell death and tissue inflammation.[100] In turn, the citrullinated proteins can be seen as antigens by the body's immune system. Thus, both T and B cells play a role in the autoimmune response. T cells express receptor activator of nuclear factor κβ ligand (RANKL), which promotes osteoclast formation, causing bony erosion.[97]

Inflammatory cytokines, particularly tumor necrosis factor-alpha (TNF-α), interleukin-1 beta (IL-1β), interleukin-6

TABLE 44-7 TYPES OF INFECTIOUS ARTHRITIS

TYPE AND MICROORGANISM	COMMENTS
Lyme arthritis	Initial infection of skin followed by spreading to other sites including joints in days or weeks
Spirochete *Borrelia burgdorferi* Transmitted via ticks *(Ixodes scapularis* or *I. pacificus)*	Arthritis is a predominant feature involving mainly large joints; possibly caused by immune reactions against *Borrelia* antigens (such as Osp A) that cross-react with tissue antigens in joints
Tuberculous arthritis	Weightbearing joints most susceptible
Complication of osteomyelitis or visceral, usually pulmonary, infection	Fibrous ankylosis and destruction of joint space; onset is insidious and gradual
Suppurative arthritis	Classic is a sudden onset of symptoms—painful, hot, swollen joint with decreased range of motion
Bacterial infections with *Gonococcus, Staphylococcus, Streptococcus, Haemophilus influenzae,* and gram-negative bacilli; *H. influenzae* arthritis more common in children younger than 2 years; *S. aureus* in older children and adults	Prompt therapy prevents joint destruction
Viral arthritis	Symptoms vary from acute to subacute
Many viruses including parvovirus B19, rubella, hepatitis C virus, human immunodeficiency virus	Unclear if effects are from direct invasion of the virus or an autoimmune reaction

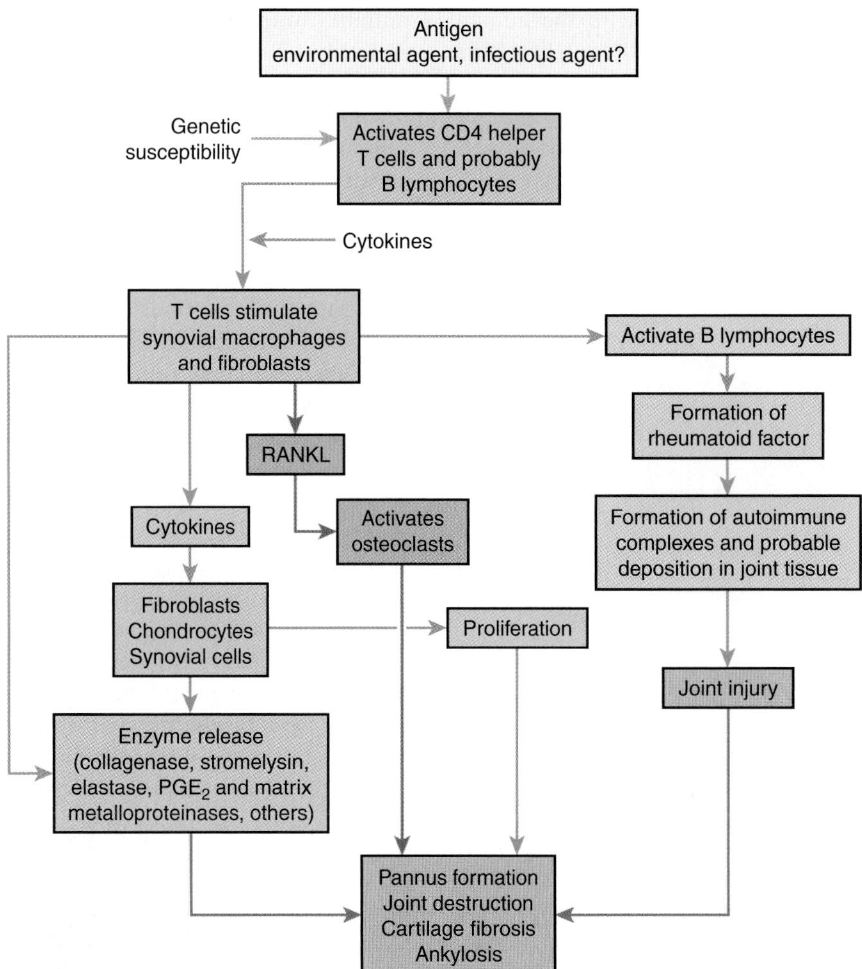

FIGURE 44-24 **Emerging Model of Pathogenesis of Rheumatoid Arthritis.** Rheumatoid arthritis is an autoimmune disease of a genetically susceptible host triggered by an unknown antigenic agent. Chronic autoimmune reaction with activation of CD4+ helper T cells and possibly other lymphocytes and the local release of inflammatory cytokines and mediators eventually destroys the joint. T cells stimulate cells in the joint to produce cytokines that are key mediators of synovial damage. Apparently immune complex deposition also plays a role. Tumor necrosis factor *(TNF)* and interleukin-1 *(IL-1)*, as well as some other cytokines, stimulate synovial cells to proliferate and produce other mediators of inflammation, such as prostaglandin E_2 *(PGE_2)*, matrix metalloproteinases, and enzymes, which all contribute to destruction of cartilage. Activated T cells and synovial fibroblasts also produce receptor activator of nuclear factor κβ ligand *(RANKL)*, which activates the osteoclasts and promotes bone destruction. Pannus is a mass of synovium and synovial stroma with inflammatory cells, granulation tissue, and fibroblasts that grows over the articular surface and causes its destruction.

(IL-6), interleukin-7 (IL-7), and interleukin-21 (IL-21), that induce enzymatic (metalloproteinase) breakdown of cartilage and bone and T cells also interact with synovial fibroblasts (synoviocytes) through TNF-α, converting synovium into a thick, abnormal layer of granulation tissue known as **pannus** (see Figures 44-25 and 44-26, *A*). Composed of these macrophages, plus osteoclasts and fibroblast-like synoviocytes, the pannus acts like a locally invasive tumor.[101,102] Macrophages, components of pannus (Figure 44-24), stimulate the release of IL-1, platelet-derived growth factor (PDGF), and fibronectin. The pathogenesis of rheumatoid arthritis is summarized in Figure 44-24.

Several types of leukocytes are attracted out of the circulation and into the synovial membrane. The phagocytes of inflammation (neutrophils and macrophages) ingest the immune complexes and, in the process of doing so, release powerful enzymes that degrade synovial tissue and articular cartilage (Figure 44-25). The immune system's B and T lymphocytes are also activated. The B lymphocytes are stimulated to produce more RFs, and the T lymphocytes eventually cause release of enzymes that amplify and perpetuate the inflammatory response. Cartilage destruction is mediated by matrix metalloproteinases (MMPs) that activate the synoviocytes to invade and attack the synovium and matrix.[103] In addition, RANKL is expressed by various cells in the synovium and induces osteoclast maturation and activation, thus producing increased bone resorption (see p. 1553).

Inflammatory and immune processes have several damaging effects on the synovial membrane. Along with the swelling caused by leukocyte infiltration, the synovial membrane undergoes hyperplastic thickening as its cells proliferate and become

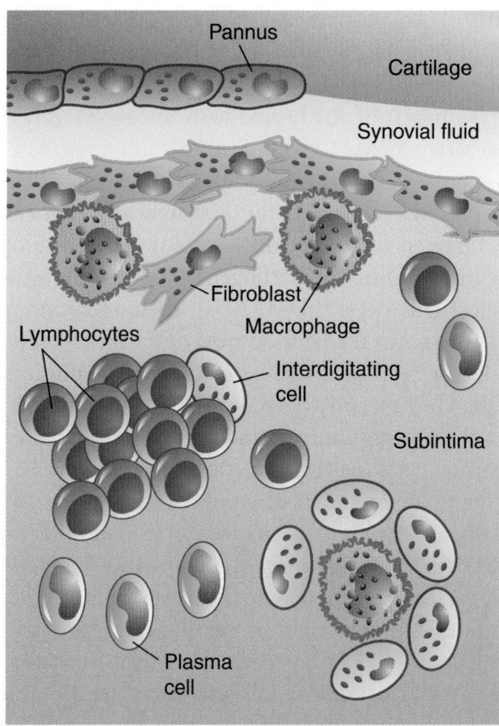

FIGURE 44-25 **Synovitis.** Inflamed synovium showing typical arrangements of macrophages and fibroblastic cells.

abnormally large. As synovial inflammation progresses to involve its blood vessels, small venules become occluded by the hypertrophied endothelial cells, fibrin, platelets, and inflammatory cells, which decrease vascular flow to the synovial tissue. Compromised circulation, coupled with increased metabolic needs because of hypertrophy and hyperplasia, causes hypoxia and metabolic acidosis. Acidosis stimulates the release of hydrolytic enzymes from synovial cells into the surrounding tissue, initiating erosion of the articular cartilage and inflammation in the supporting ligaments and tendons. Inflammation causes hemorrhage, coagulation, and fibrin deposition on the synovial membrane, in the intracellular matrix, and in the synovial fluid. (Figure 44-26, *A* and *B*).

CLINICAL MANIFESTATIONS. The onset of RA is usually insidious, although as many as 15% of cases have an acute onset. RA begins with general systemic manifestations of inflammation, including fever, fatigue, weakness, anorexia, weight loss, and generalized aching and stiffness. Local manifestations also appear gradually over weeks or months. Typically the joints become painful, tender, and stiff. Pain early in the disease is caused by pressure from swelling; later it is caused by sclerosis of subchondral bone and new bone formation. Stiffness usually lasts for about 1 hour after arising in the morning and may be caused by synovitis. Initially most commonly involved joints are the metacarpophalangeal (MCP), proximal interphalangeal (PIP), and wrists, with later involvement of larger weightbearing joints.

Widespread and symmetric joint swelling is caused by increasing amounts of inflammatory exudate (leukocytes, plasma, plasma proteins) in the synovial membrane, hyperplasia of inflamed tissues, and formation of new bone. On

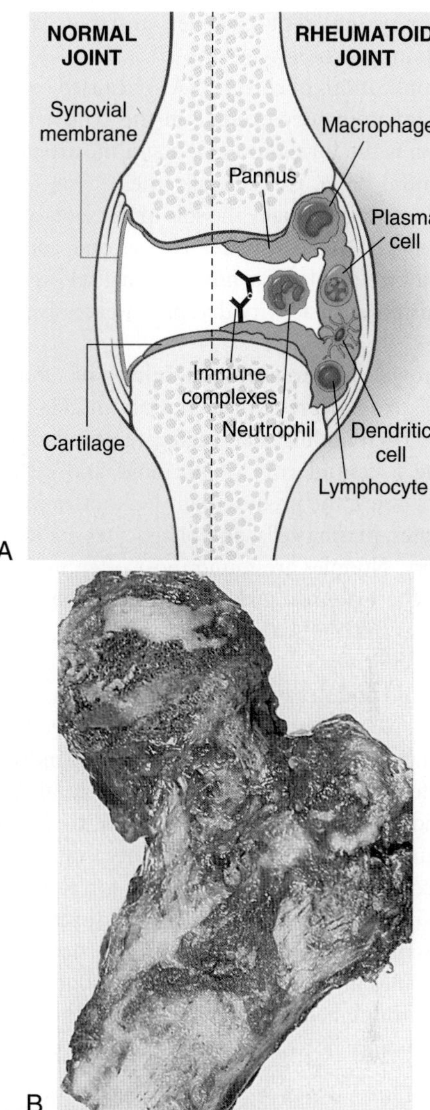

FIGURE 44-26 **Rheumatoid Arthritis. A,** Schematic view of the joint lesion. **B,** Advanced rheumatoid arthritis involving femur. There is prominent proliferation of synovium and almost complete destruction of overlying articular cartilage. (**A** modified from Feldmann M: *Nat Rev Immunol* 2:364, 2002; **B** from Rosai J: *Ackerman's surgical pathology,* ed 10, Philadelphia, 2011, Mosby.)

palpation, the swollen joint feels warm and the synovial membrane feels "boggy." The skin over the joint may have a ruddy or cyanotic hue and may look thin and shiny.

An inflamed joint may lose some of its mobility; even mild synovitis can lead to loss of range of motion. Extension becomes limited and is eventually lost if flexion contractures form. Chronic synovitis weakens ligamentous structures leading to deformities of the fingers, toes, and limbs, including ulnar deviation of the hands, boutonnière and swan-neck deformities of the finger joints,[104] plantar subluxation of the metatarsal heads of the foot, and hallux valgus (angulation of the great toe toward the other toes). Flexion contractures of the knees and hips are also common.

Joint deformities cause the physical limitations experienced by persons with RA. Loss of joint motion is quickly followed by secondary atrophy of the surrounding muscles. With secondary muscle atrophy the joint becomes unstable, which further aggravates joint pathology.

Two complications of chronic RA are caused by an excessive amount of inflammatory exudate in the synovial cavity. One complication is the formation of cysts in the articular cartilage or subchondral bone. Occasionally these cysts communicate with the skin surface (usually the sole of the foot) and can drain through passages called fistulae. The second complication is rupture of a cyst or of the synovial joint itself, usually caused by strenuous physical activity that places excessive pressure on the joint.

Extrasynovial **rheumatoid nodules,** or swellings, are observed in areas of pressure or trauma in 20% of individuals with RA. Each nodule is an aggregate of inflammatory cells surrounding a central core of fibrinoid and cellular debris. T lymphocytes are the predominant leukocytes in the nodule; B lymphocytes, plasma cells, and phagocytes are found around the periphery. Nodules are found most often in subcutaneous tissue over the extensor surfaces of elbows and fingers. Less common sites are the scalp, back, feet, hands, buttocks, and knees.

Rheumatoid nodules also may invade the skin, cardiac valves, pericardium, pleura, lung parenchyma, and spleen. These nodules are identical to those encountered in some individuals with rheumatic fever and are characterized by central tissue necrosis surrounded by proliferating connective tissue. Also noted are large numbers of lymphocytes and occasional plasma cells. Acute glaucoma may result, with nodules forming on the sclera. Pulmonary involvement may result in diffuse pleuritis or multiple intraparenchymal nodules. Together, the occurrence of pulmonary nodules and pneumoconiosis (chronic inflammation of the lungs from inhalation of dust) creates **Caplan syndrome.** Diffuse pulmonary fibrosis may occur because of immunologically mediated immune complex deposition.

Rheumatoid nodules within the heart may cause valvular deformities, particularly of the aortic valve leaflets. Pericardial effusion or other pericardial problems occur in almost 50% of individuals with RA. Lymphadenopathy of the nodes close to the affected joints may develop. Rheumatoid nodules within the spleen result in splenomegaly. Involvement of blood vessels results in an acute necrotizing vasculitis, characteristic of that noted in other immunologic/inflammatory states. Thromboses of such involved vessels may give rise to myocardial infarctions, cerebrovascular occlusions, mesenteric infarction, kidney damage, and vascular insufficiency in the hands and fingers (Raynaud phenomenon). Vascular changes are noted primarily in individuals receiving corticosteroid therapy; thus there is some concern that the therapy may play a role in initiating these lesions. Changes in skeletal muscle are often noted in the form of nonspecific atrophy secondary to joint dysfunction.

EVALUATION AND TREATMENT. The autoantibodies rheumatoid factor (RF) and the much more specific serum marker anti–citrullinated protein antibody (ACPA) can be present for years to decades before synovial or radiographic changes become apparent.[95,100,105] Early, aggressive treatment of RA can prevent disability and joint destruction. In 2010 the American College of Rheumatology (ACR) and the European League Against Rheumatism (EULAR) revised their classification criteria to better identify early stages of RA.[95] Box 44-4 summarizes the criteria for diagnosing RA.

Early treatment of RA begins with disease-modifying antirheumatic drugs (DMARDs) such as methotrexate (MTX), azathioprine, sulfasalazine, hydroxychloroquine, leflunomide, and cyclosporine. MTX remains the first line of treatment. More recently, targeted treatment of RA has involved use of agents aimed at interrupting the pathogenesis of the disease. Known as biological DMARDs (bDMARDs), these medications affect specific processes in the development of RA and include tumor necrosis factor inhibitors such as etanercept, adalimumab, and infliximab. They recently have been augmented by the monoclonal antibodies golimumab and certolizumab. Other agents interfere with cytokine function (anakinra inhibits IL-1 function; tocilizumab targets IL-6), inhibit T-cell activation (abatacept), or deplete B cells (rituximab). Combination therapy with a DMARD and a biologic agent, such as infliximab (a TNF inhibitor), is more effective than using a single agent.[106]

Education is fundamental in treating RA. Other treatments and therapies include nonsteroidal anti-inflammatory drugs (NSAIDs), glucocorticoids, intra-articular steroid injections, physical and occupational therapy with therapeutic exercise, and use of assistive devices. Surgery is used to treat deformities or mechanical deficiencies of joints and can include synovectomy or joint replacement.

Ankylosing Spondylitis

Ankylosing spondylitis (AS) is the most common of a group of inflammatory arthropathies known as spondyloarthropathies. It is a chronic inflammatory joint disease characterized by stiffening and fusion (ankylosis) of the spine and sacroiliac joints. The exact cause of AS is unknown but its high association with the histocompatibility antigen human leukocyte antigen (HLA-B27) has been known for decades. New research has shown that misfolding of HLA-B27 occurs in the endoplasmic reticulum (ER). As misfolded proteins accumulate, it results in a stress response of the ER and increased production of interleukin-23 (IL-23), a potent cytokine that may also act on T-helper 17 cells, promoting their survival.[107] Th17 cells, in turn, produce the inflammatory cytokine IL-17.

Although inflammation is the primary pathologic process in both RA and AS, the two diseases possibly differ in the primary site of inflammation and the end result. In RA the primary site of inflammation is the synovial membrane, resulting in the destruction and instability of synovial joints. In AS, the primary pathologic problem is uncontrolled bone formation, rather than bone destruction seen with most other types of arthritis.[108] The end results of AS are fibrosis, ossification, and fusion of the joint, primarily the sacroiliac joints and the vertebral column. MRI studies demonstrate changes in the sacroiliac joints before they become clinically apparent or visible on plain radiographs.[109]

The prevalence of AS in the United States is approximately 0.5% to 1% among whites, 3% to 4% among blacks, and 18% to 50% in various nations of American Indians. Worldwide, the disease appears to be most prevalent in whites. The prevalence

BOX 44-4 THE 2010 AMERICAN COLLEGE OF RHEUMATOLOGY/EUROPEAN LEAGUE AGAINST RHEUMATISM CLASSIFICATION CRITERIA FOR RHEUMATOID ARTHRITIS

Target population (Who should be tested?) Individuals:

1. who have at least one joint with definite clinical synovitis (swelling)*
2. who have synovitis not better explained by another disease†

Classification criteria for RA (score-based algorithm: add scores of categories A to D; a score of ≥6/10 is needed for classification of a patient as having definite RA)‡

Clinical Finding	Score
A. Joint involvement§	
1 large joint¶	0
2-10 large joints	1
1-3 small joints (with or without involvement of large joints)#	2
4-10 small joints (with or without involvement of large joints)	3
>10 joints (at least 1 small joint)**	5

Clinical Finding	Score
B. Serology (at least 1 test result is needed for classification)††	
Negative RF *and* negative ACPA	0
Low-positive RF *or* low-positive ACPA	2
High-positive RF *or* high-positive ACPA	3
C. Acute-phase reactants (at least 1 test result is needed for classification)‡‡	
Normal CRP *and* normal ESR	0
Abnormal CRP *or* abnormal ESR	1
D. Duration of symptoms§§	
<6 weeks	0
≥6 weeks	1

Data from Aletaha D: *Arthritis Rheum* 62(9):2574, 2010.

*The criteria are aimed at classification of newly presenting patients. In addition, patients with erosive disease typical of rheumatoid arthritis (RA) with a history compatible of prior fulfillment of the 2010 criteria should be classified as having RA. Patients with longstanding disease, including those whose disease is inactive (with or without treatment), who, based on retrospectively available data, have previously fulfilled the 2010 criteria should be classified as having RA.

†Differential diagnoses vary among patients with different presentations, but may include conditions such as systemic lupus erythematosus, psoriatic arthritis, and gout. If it is unclear about the relevant differential diagnoses to consider, an expert rheumatologist should be consulted.

‡Although patients with a score ≥6/10 are not classifiable as having RA, their status can be reassessed and the criteria might be fulfilled cumulatively over time.

§Joint involvement refers to any swollen or tender joint on examination, which may be confirmed by imaging evidence of synovitis. Distal interphalangeal joints, first metacarpophalangeal joints, and first metatarsophalangeal joints are excluded from assessment. Categories of joint distribution are classified according to the location and number of involved joints, with placement into the highest category possible based on the pattern of joint involvement.

¶"Large joints" refer to shoulders, elbows, hips, knees, and ankles.

#"Small joints" refer to the metacarpophalangeal joints, proximal interphalangeal joints, second through fifth metatarsophalangeal joints, thumb interphalangeal joints, and wrists.

**In this category, at least 1 of the involved joints must be a small joint; the others can include any combination of large and additional small joints, as well as other joints not specifically listed elsewhere (e.g., temporomandibular, acromioclavicular, sternoclavicular, etc.).

††Negative refers to IU values that are less than or equal to the upper limit of normal (ULN) for the laboratory and assay; low-positive refers to values that are higher than the ULN but ≤3 times the ULN for the laboratory and assay; high-positive refers to IU values that are >3 times the ULN for the laboratory and assay. Where rheumatoid factor (RF) information is only available as positive or negative, a positive result should be scored as low-positive for RF. *ACPA,* Anti-citrullinated protein antibody.

‡‡Normal/abnormal is determined by local laboratory standards. *CRP,* C-reactive protein; *ESR,* erythrocyte sedimentation rate.

§§Duration of symptoms refers to patient self-report of the duration of signs and symptoms of synovitis (e.g., pain, swelling, tenderness) of joints that are clinically involved at the time of assessment, regardless of treatment status.

of AS in males is at least 10 times greater than previously considered. It affects men three times as often as women. In women, AS may affect the peripheral joints of the appendicular skeleton rather than the axial skeleton, progress less rapidly, and cause less dramatic spinal changes. Many individuals with AS remain undiagnosed.

Primary AS usually develops in late adolescence or young adulthood, with peak incidence at about 20 years of age. Secondary AS affects older age groups and is often associated with other inflammatory diseases (e.g., psoriatic arthropathy, inflammatory bowel disease, Reiter syndrome).

PATHOPHYSIOLOGY. AS has a strong association with the histocompatibility antigen HLA-B27. Several hypotheses have been suggested to explain this association including the arthritogenic peptide theory that proposes that certain HLA-B27 alleles bind certain arthritogenic peptides because of their specific anchoring proteins. Cartilage antigens are proposed as the targets for the immune response and the presentation of such antigens to CD8+ T cells. In the early phases of AS, T cells and macrophages invade and cause erosion of the cartilage at different sites. Based on these observations, it is thought that the cartilage is the primary target for the immune response. **Aggrecan,** a proteoglycan, forms a major part of the extracellular matrix of cartilage and helps maintain its stability. A specific CD4+ T-cell response to proteins derived from aggrecan has been found in animals and humans. Although these T cells have been found in AS, their role as a causative agent in AS remains unclear and necessitates future study.

AS involves inflammation of fibrocartilage in cartilaginous joints, primarily the vertebrae. The fibrous tissue of the joint capsule, the cartilage that surrounds intervertebral disks, the entheses, and the periosteum are infiltrated by inflammatory cells. As inflammatory cells (chiefly macrophages) and lymphocytes infiltrate and erode bone and fibrocartilage in joint structures, repair begins. Repair of cartilaginous structures begins with the proliferation of fibroblasts. Fibroblasts synthesize and

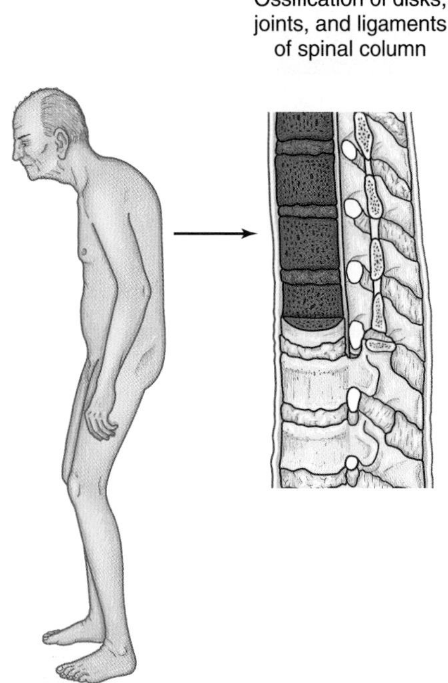

FIGURE 44-27 Ankylosing Spondylitis. Characteristic posture and primary pathologic sites of inflammation and resulting damage.

secrete collagen. The collagen becomes organized into fibrous scar tissue that eventually undergoes calcification and ossification. With time, all the cartilaginous structures of the joint are replaced by ossified scar tissue, causing the joint to fuse, or lose flexibility.

Repair of eroded bone begins with osteoblast activation and proliferation. Osteoblasts lay down new bone (callus), which is remodeled and replaced by compact, lamellar bone. Bone repair changes the contour of the bone's surface because the new bone grows outward to form a new enthesis with the end of the eroded ligament. The new enthesis, which forms on top of the old one, is called a **syndesmophyte.** As calcification of the spinal ligaments progresses, the vertebral bodies lose their concave anterior contour and appear square. On radiographs the spine assumes the classic "bamboo spine" appearance of AS.

CLINICAL MANIFESTATIONS. The most common signs and symptoms of early AS are low back pain and stiffness. Typically the individual with primary disease develops low back pain during the early twenties. The pain is at first insidious but progressively becomes persistent. It is often worse after prolonged rest and is alleviated by physical activity. Early morning stiffness usually accompanies the low back pain, and the individual typically has difficulty sitting up or twisting the spine. Forward flexion, rotation, and lateral flexion of the spine are restricted and painful. Early pain and resultant loss of motion are caused by the underlying inflammation and reflex muscle spasm rather than by soft tissue or bony fusion.

As the disease progresses, the normal convex curve of the lower spine (lumbar lordosis) diminishes and concavity of the upper spine (kyphosis) increases. The individual becomes increasingly stooped. The thoracic spine becomes rounded, the head and neck are held forward on the shoulders, and the hips are flexed (Figure 44-27).

Inflammation in the tendon insertions of the many costosternal and costovertebral muscles can cause pleuritic chest pain and restricted chest movement. The pain is usually worse on inspiration. Movement in the diaphragm is normal and full. Pressure on the anterior chest wall over the sternum, ribs, and costal cartilages may cause tenderness. Tenderness over the pelvic brim may cause discomfort at night and interfere with sleep because turning onto the iliac crests causes pain. Tenderness over the ischial tuberosities may make sitting on hard seats unbearable. Tenderness in the heels may contribute to a limp or the cautious placement of the feet during walking.

Along with low back pain, many individuals have peripheral joint involvement, uveitis, fibrotic changes in the lungs, cardiomegaly, aortic incompetence, amyloidosis, and Achilles tendinitis. Symptoms may include fatigue, weight loss, low-grade fever, hypochromic anemia, and an increased erythrocyte sedimentation rate.

EVALUATION AND TREATMENT. Diagnosis of AS is made on the basis of both clinical and radiologic findings. Low back pain and stiffness lasting more than 3 months that improves with exercise but is not relieved by rest, limited spine range of motion (ROM) in both frontal and sagittal planes, and limited chest expansion relative to normal values for age and gender are the classic clinical criteria. Radiologic changes at the sacroiliac joint are graded according to severity of abnormality; abnormalities include sclerosis, widening, narrowing, or ankylosis.[110] Laboratory tests, including serum analysis for the presence of the histocompatibility antigen HLA-B27, elevated erythrocyte sedimentation rate (ESR) (normal is 0 to 9 mm/hr in males, 0 to 2 mm/hr in females), and elevated alkaline phosphatase levels, can be used to help monitor the course of the disease.

Treatment of individuals with AS consists of a multidisciplinary approach: physical therapy to maintain skeletal mobility and prevent the natural progression of contractures, support groups, nonsteroidal anti-inflammatory drugs (NSAIDs) to provide relief of symptoms, analgesic medications to suppress some of the pain and stiffness and to facilitate exercise, and corticosteroid injections to locally inflamed joints. The medications do not prevent disease progression, but they do provide relief from symptoms. DMARDs such as gold, methotrexate, and sulfasalazine have little or no effect in AS. Three TNF inhibitors (etanercept, infliximab, and adalimumab) have been approved for severe AS. Surgery can help if there is severe disabling deformity.[110]

Gout

Gout is a syndrome caused by an inflammatory response to uric acid production or excretion resulting in high levels of uric acid in the blood (hyperuricemia) and in other body fluids, including synovial fluid. Although hyperuricemia is essential for the development of gout, it is not the only factor. Other factors include age (rare before 30 years), genetic predisposition (X-linked alteration of the enzyme hypoxanthine-guanine phosphoribosyltransferase [HGPRT]), excessive alcohol consumption, obesity, certain drugs (especially thiazides), and lead toxicity. When the uric acid concentration is >6.8 mg/dl in fluids, it crystallizes and forms insoluble precipitates of

TABLE 44-8 MEAN URATE CONCENTRATIONS BY AGE AND GENDER

CHARACTERISTIC	MEAN URATE LEVELS
Prepuberty	3.5 mg/dl
Males (at puberty)	Steep rise to 5.2 mg/dl
Females (puberty to premenopause)	Slow rise to ≅4 mg/dl
Females (after menopause)	4.7 mg/dl
Hyperuricemia	
Men	7 mg/dl
Women	6 mg/dl

monosodium urate (MSU) that are deposited in connective tissues throughout the body. Crystallization in synovial fluid causes acute, painful inflammation of the joint, and triggers an inflammatory response by macrophages. When macrophages phagocytize MSU crystals, they form a protein scaffold known as an inflammasome. Inflammasomes then convert inactive interleukins of IL-1β and IL-18 into their active forms.[111,112] Prolonged accumulation results in joint damage, a condition known as **gouty arthritis.** With time, crystal deposition in subcutaneous tissues causes the formation of small, white nodules, or **tophi,** that are visible through the skin. Crystal aggregates deposited in the kidneys can form urate renal stones and lead to renal failure.

In classic gouty arthritis, monosodium urate crystals form and cause joint inflammation. **Pseudogout** is caused by the formation of calcium pyrophosphate dihydrate (CPPD) crystals. The effect of either crystal is the same—the onset of a cytokine-mediated acute inflammatory response (see Chapter 7).

Gout is rare in children and premenopausal women and is uncommon in males younger than 30 years. The peak age of onset in males is between 40 and 50 years, whereas it is somewhat later in females. The risk of developing gouty arthritis is similar in males and females for a particular urate concentration. The plasma urate concentration is an important determinant of the risk of developing gout (Table 44-8).

Uric acid (UA) is a byproduct of protein metabolism that normally assists with removal of nitrogen waste from the body. At lower levels, UA is an important antioxidant but at higher levels it acts as a pro-oxidant where it increases levels of free radicals and causes other inflammatory changes.[113] When ionized, uric acid can form salts with various cations but 98% of extracellular uric acid is in the form of monosodium urate (uric acid salt). At any time the proportion of uric acid or urate is pH dependent, so the ratio of these two forms varies considerably in urine (Figure 44-28).

The solubility of urate and uric acid is critical to the development of crystals. Urate is more soluble in plasma, synovial fluid, and urine than in aqueous solutions; solubility in urine rises dramatically as the pH increases to more than 4. There is little change, however, in the solubility of urate within the normal pH range that exists in the plasma, synovial fluid, and other tissues. Decreasing temperatures cause both urate and uric acid solubility to fall. The pathways of production of uric acid are shown in Figure 44-29.

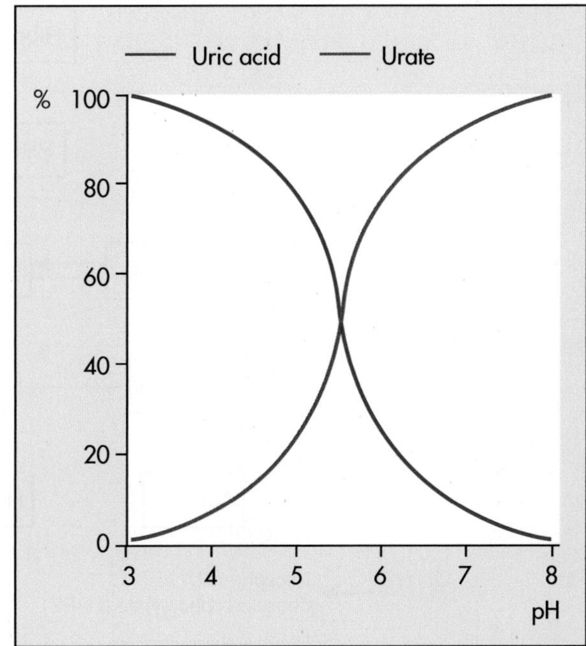

FIGURE 44-28 Effect of pH on Uric Acid and Urate Equilibrium. At pH 5.7, equal amounts of uric acid and urate are present in the solution. (Redrawn from Klippel JH, Dieppe PA, editors: *Rheumatology,* ed 2, London, 1998, Mosby-Wolfe.)

PATHOPHYSIOLOGY. The pathophysiology of gout is closely linked to purine metabolism and kidney function. At the cellular level, purines are synthesized to purine nucleotides, which are used in the synthesis of nucleic acids, adenosine triphosphate, cyclic adenosine monophosphate (cAMP), and cyclic guanosine monophosphate (GMP). Uric acid is a breakdown product of purine nucleotides (uric acid synthesis and elimination are illustrated in Figure 44-30). Some individuals with gout have an accelerated rate of purine synthesis accompanied by an overproduction of uric acid. Other individuals break down purine nucleotides at an accelerated rate that also results in an overproduction of uric acid. A deficiency of the enzyme HGPRT (see earlier) can lead to an increased production of uric acid. A complete absence of HGPRT is uncommon but can occur in the X-linked Lesch-Nyhan syndrome, with males at risk for hyperuricemia, neurologic alterations, and sometimes gouty arthritis. The majority of individuals with gout, however, have an unknown metabolic defect, which is referred to as **primary gout.** When the etiology is known, it is referred to as **secondary gout.**

Most uric acid is eliminated from the body through the kidneys. Urate is filtered at the glomerulus and undergoes reabsorption and excretion within the proximal renal tubules. In primary gout, urate excretion by the kidneys is sluggish; this may be the result of a decrease in glomerular filtration of urate or acceleration in urate reabsorption. In addition, MSU crystals deposited in renal tubules can cause acute nephropathy.[113] (Kidney function is described in Chapter 37.)

Monosodium urate crystals can stimulate and perpetuate the inflammatory response (Figure 44-31). The presence of MSU crystals triggers the acute inflammatory response. Initiation of the complement system activates cytokines and produces other

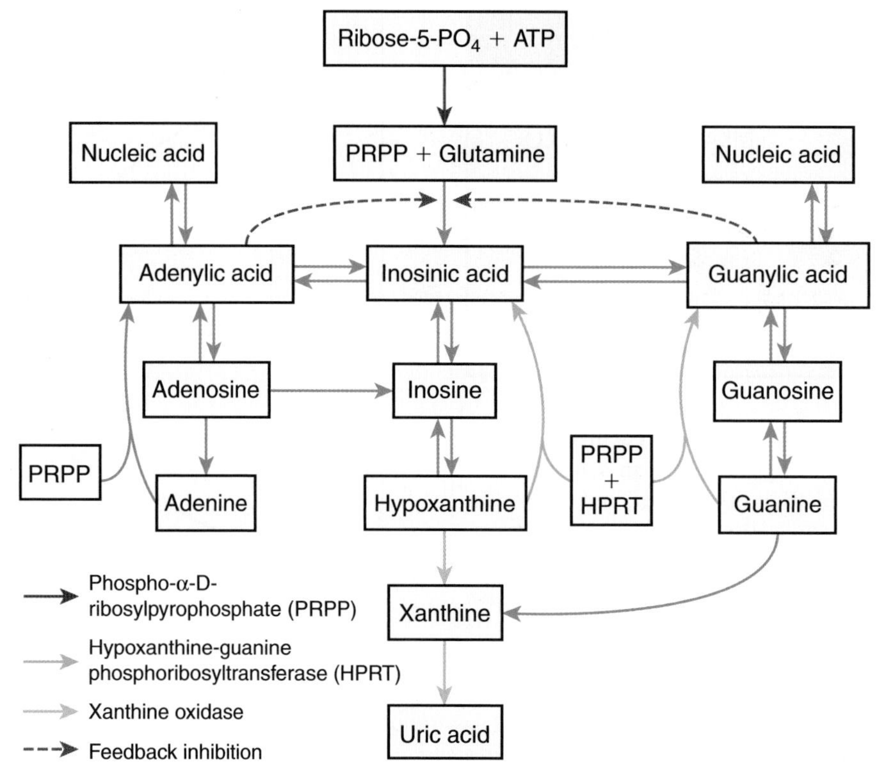

FIGURE 44-29 Production of Uric Acid. The major pathways involved in purine nucleotide synthesis. (Redrawn from Klippel JH, Dieppe PA, editors: *Rheumatology,* ed 2, London, 1998, Mosby-Wolfe.)

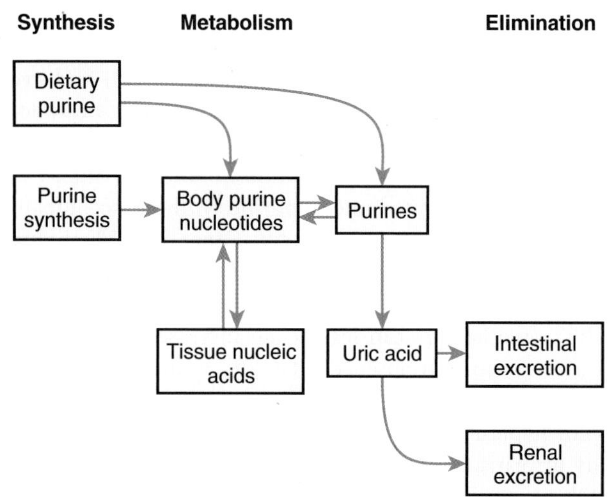

FIGURE 44-30 Uric Acid Synthesis and Elimination. Uric acid is derived from ingested purines or synthesized from ingested foods, as well as being recycled following cell breakdown. Uric acid is then eliminated through the kidneys and gastrointestinal tract. (Redrawn from Klippel JH, Dieppe PA, editors: *Rheumatology,* ed 2, London, 1998, Mosby-Wolfe.)

substances, called chemoattractants, that draw neutrophils out of the circulation to begin phagocytizing (ingesting) the crystals.

A variety of inflammatory mediators are released during the crystal/cell response, of which IL-1β appears to be of prime importance. Other factors including chemotactic factors, lysosomal enzymes, eicosanoids, prostaglandin E (PGE_2), reactive oxygen species, and collagenase also are released (see Figure 44-31, *B*). Some of these mediators stimulate the influx of neutrophils, monocytes, and lymphocytes. (Acute inflammation and phagocytosis are described in Chapter 7.)

Within the joint fluid, urate crystals react particularly with neutrophils and monocytes. Tissue damage begins to occur, principally when the neutrophils release the contents of their phagolysosomes. These contents also perpetuate inflammation. At an early phase of an acute gouty attack, synovial microtophi have been demonstrated. As the process continues, numerous microtophi may be present on the synovial membrane (see Figure 44-31, *C*).

CLINICAL MANIFESTATIONS. Gout is manifested by (1) an increase in serum urate concentration (hyperuricemia); (2) recurrent attacks of monoarticular arthritis (inflammation of a single joint); (3) deposits of monosodium urate monohydrate (tophi) in and around the joints; (4) renal disease involving glomerular, tubular, and interstitial tissues and blood vessels; and (5) the formation of renal stones. These manifestations appear in three clinical stages:

1. **Asymptomatic hyperuricemia:** The serum urate level is elevated but arthritic symptoms, tophi, and renal stones are not present; may persist throughout life.
2. **Acute gouty arthritis:** Attacks develop with increased serum urate concentrations; tends to occur with sudden or sustained increases of hyperuricemia but also can be triggered by trauma, drugs, and alcohol.
3. **Tophaceous gout:** The third and chronic stage of disease; can begin as early as 3 years or as late as 40 years after the initial attack of gouty arthritis. Progressive inability to excrete uric acid expands the urate pool until urate crystal deposits (tophi) appear in cartilage, synovial membranes, tendons, and soft tissue.

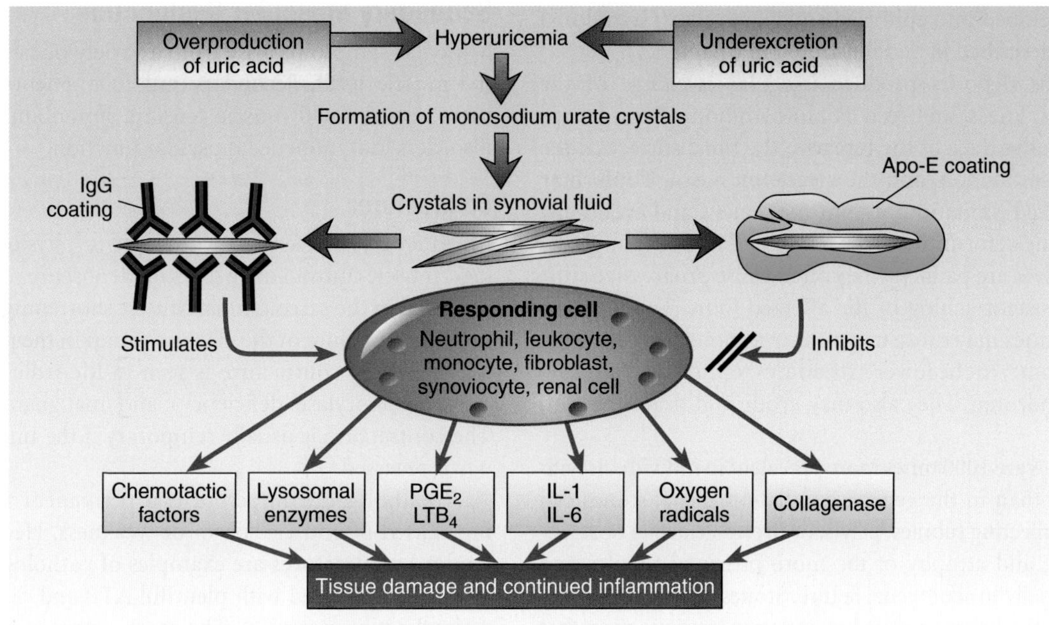

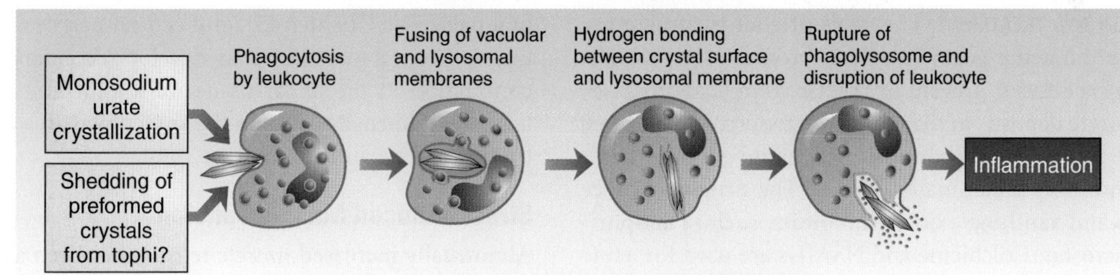

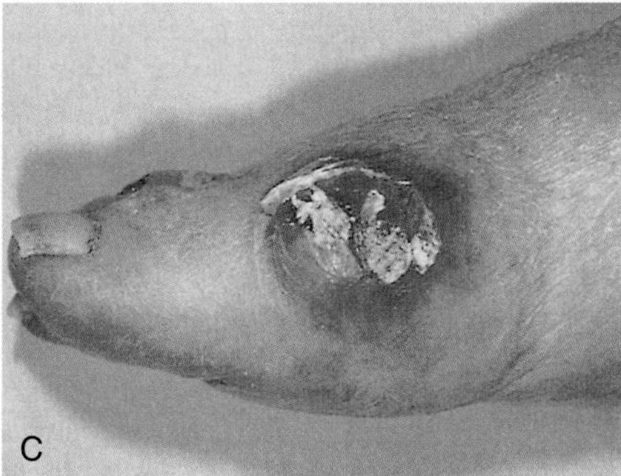

FIGURE 44-31 Pathogenesis of Acute Gouty Arthritis. **A,** Depending on the urate crystal coating, a variety of cells may be stimulated to produce a wide range of inflammatory mediators. **B,** Sequence of events in the production of inflammatory response to urate crystals. **C,** Gouty tophus on right foot. *Apo-E,* Apolipoprotein E; *IgG,* immunoglobulin G; *IL,* interleukin; *LTB_4,* leukotriene B_4; *PGE,* prostaglandin E. (**C** from Dieppe P et al: *Arthritis and rheumatism in practice,* London, 1991, Gower.)

Attacks of gouty arthritis occur abruptly, usually in a peripheral joint. The primary symptom is severe pain. Approximately 50% of the initial attacks occur in the metatarsophalangeal joint of the great toe. The other 50% involve the heel, ankle, and instep of the foot; knee; wrist; or elbow. The pain is usually noticed at night. Within a few hours the affected joint becomes hot, red, and extremely tender and may be slightly swollen. Lymphangitis and systemic signs of inflammation (leukocytosis, fever, elevated sedimentation rate) occasionally are present. Untreated, mild attacks usually subside in several hours but may persist for 1 or 2 days. Severe attacks may persist for several days or weeks. After recovery, the symptoms resolve completely. Intervals between acute attacks of gouty arthritis are called *intercritical periods.* Some individuals never have a second attack; others experience subsequent attacks within days to as long as 5 to 10 years after the first.

The helix of the ear is the most common site of tophi, which are the characteristic diagnostic lesions of chronic gout. Each tophus consists of a deposit of urate crystals, surrounded by a granuloma made up of mononuclear phagocytes (macrophages) that have developed into epithelial and giant cells. (Granuloma formation is described in and illustrated in Chapter 7.)

Tophaceous deposits produce irregular swellings of the fingers, hands, knees, and feet. Tophi commonly form lumps along the ulnar surface of the forearm, the tibial surface of the leg, the Achilles tendon, and the olecranon bursa. Tophi may produce marked limitation of joint movement and eventually cause grotesque deformities of the hands and feet. Although the tophi themselves are painless, they often cause progressive stiffness and persistent aching of the affected joint. Tophi in the upper extremities may cause nerve compressions such as carpal tunnel syndrome; in the lower extremities tophi may cause tarsal tunnel syndrome. They also may erode and drain through the skin.

Renal stones are 1000 times more prevalent in individuals with primary gout than in the general population. Renal stones can form in the collecting tubules, pelvis, or ureters, causing obstruction, dilation, and atrophy of the more proximal tubules and leading eventually to acute renal failure. Stones deposited directly in renal interstitial tissue initiate an inflammatory reaction that leads to chronic renal disease and progressive renal failure.

EVALUATION AND TREATMENT. The goals of gout treatment are to terminate the acute gouty attack as promptly as possible; avoid recurring attacks; prevent or reverse complications associated with urate deposits in the joints, soft tissues, and kidneys; and prevent formation of kidney stones. Acute gouty arthritis is treated with anti-inflammatory drugs. The drugs of choice are NSAIDs and xanthine oxidase inhibitors, such as allopurinol and febuxostat. Colchicine and NSAIDs are used for acute episodes of gout. Hydrocortisone may be injected into the joint to relieve pain. Drugs that block IL-1 have shown promise and investigation into certain plant-based extracts may lead to new therapies.[111,114,115] Ice also may relieve some of the inflammation of the joint. Weightbearing on the involved joint is avoided until the acute attack subsides. Reducing body weight, avoiding alcohol, and increasing consumption of low-fat dairy products, cherries, soybeans, and vegetable sources of protein may reduce recurrent gouty episodes.[112]

DISORDERS OF SKELETAL MUSCLE

Common symptoms of disorders of skeletal muscle are weakness and fatigue. In many cases, neural, traumatic, and psychogenic causes provide an adequate explanation for the failure to generate force (weakness) or sustain force (fatigue) seen in myopathies. The pathophysiologic mechanisms in some of the metabolic and inflammatory muscle diseases have been explored, but the cause of many of the myopathies remains obscure. Recognition and improved understanding of ryanodine receptor (RyR1) function has allowed identification of therapeutic targets in treating central core disease (CCD). The term CCD refers to the mitochondrial lack of oxidative enzyme activity in the central cytoplasmic area of the muscle caused by a genetic abnormality on chromosome 19. Complex interactions between muscles and nerves affect muscular function as well. Only inherited and acquired disorders of skeletal muscles are discussed here.

Secondary Muscular Dysfunction

Muscular symptoms arise from a variety of causes unrelated to the muscle itself. Secondary muscular phenomena (contracture, stress-related muscle tension, immobility) are common disorders that influence muscular function.

Contractures

Contractures are termed pathologic or physiologic. A physiologic muscle contracture occurs in the absence of a muscle action potential in the sarcolemma. Muscle shortening is explained on the basis of failure of the calcium pump in the presence of ATP. A physiologic contracture is seen in McArdle disease (muscle myophosphorylase deficiency) and malignant hyperthermia. The contracture is usually temporary if the underlying pathology is reversed.

A pathologic contracture is a permanent muscle shortening caused by muscle spasm or weakness. Heel cord (Achilles tendon) contractures are examples of pathologic contractures. They are associated with plentiful ATP and occur in spite of a normal action potential. The most common form of contracture is seen in such conditions as muscular dystrophy, cerebral palsy (see Chapter 45), and central nervous system (CNS) injury. Contractures also may develop secondary to scar tissue contraction in the flexor tissues of a joint, for example, contracture of burned tissues in the antecubital area of the forearm leading to a flexion contracture.

Stress-Induced Muscle Tension

Abnormally increased muscle tension has been associated with chronic anxiety, as well as a variety of stress-related muscular symptoms, including neck stiffness, back pain, and headache.[116] Abnormalities in the CNS, reticular activating system, and autonomic nervous system (ANS) have been implicated. The underlying pathophysiology may be related to the fact that as a muscle contracts, the muscle spindle is activated. This gamma-feedback system produces a series of impulses that are transmitted to the brain by the sensitive 1A afferent fibers. Unconscious tension is thought to increase the activity of the reticular activating system as well. This influences increasing firing of the efferent loop of the gamma fibers and produces further muscle contraction and increases muscle tension. ANS function that regulates increased blood flow to the muscle during sympathetic activity may be related to increased muscle contraction tension.

Various forms of treatment have been used to reduce the muscle tension associated with stress. Progressive relaxation training, yoga, meditation, and biofeedback are examples of stress reduction therapies. **Biofeedback** uses an integrated electromyogram (EMG) to make recordings from the skin surface. The goal is to teach the individual to control tension that has been functioning maladaptively. It is particularly useful in individuals who have a connection between skeletal muscle tension and pain.

Progressive relaxation training emphasizes the individual's ability to perceive the difference between tension and relaxation. This technique involves sequential tensing and a relaxing environment. The individual is taught to practice this routine daily, often with the use of audiotaped instructions. By teaching the

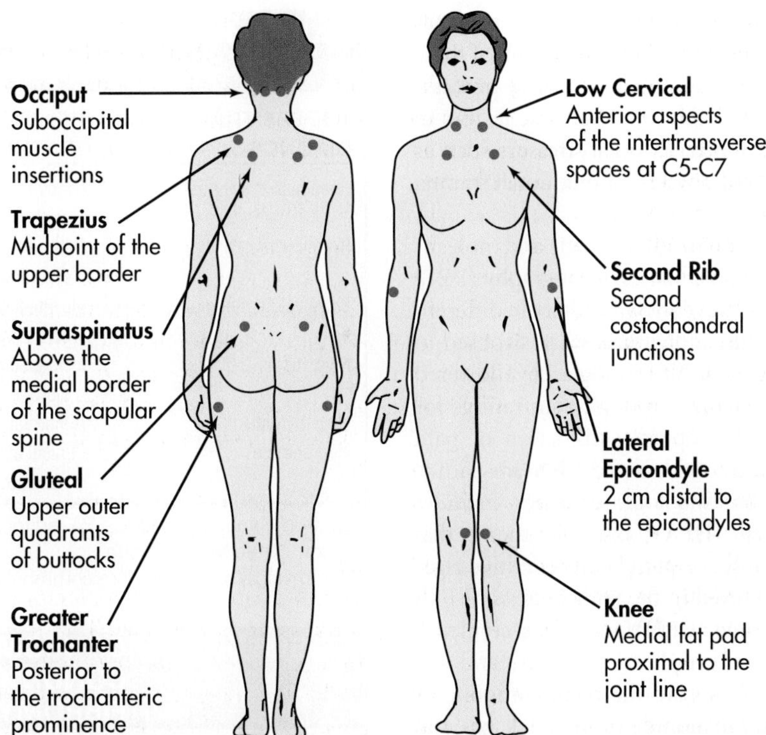

FIGURE 44-32 Location of Specific Tender Points for Diagnostic Classification of Fibromyalgia. (Redrawn from Freundlich B, Leventhal L: The fibromyalgia syndrome. In Schumacher HR Jr, Klippel JH, Koopman WJ, editors: *Primer on the rheumatic diseases,* ed 11, Atlanta, 1997, Arthritis Foundation. Copyright ©1997. Reprinted with permission of the Arthritis Foundation.)

individual to recognize excessive contraction of skeletal muscle, one hopes to enhance the ability to relax specific muscle groups to relieve tension and thus reduce CNS as well as ANS arousal.

Fibromyalgia

Fibromyalgia (FM) is a chronic musculoskeletal syndrome characterized by widespread joint and muscle pain, fatigue, and tender points. Increased sensitivity to touch (i.e., tender points); the absence of systemic or localized inflammation, fatigue, and nonrestorative sleep; and anxiety and depression are common. FM and its symptoms are viewed as the result of CNS dysfunction, where pain transmission and interpretation are amplified, a condition known as central sensitization. In the past, a common misdiagnosis has been chronic fatigue syndrome and there is overlap of symptoms between these two conditions. From 80% to 90% of individuals affected are women, and the peak age is 30 to 50 years. Although the incidence is unknown, the prevalence is reported to be 2% to almost 6% and increases with age. The ACR classification criteria include diffuse soft tissue pain of at least 3 months' duration and pain on palpation of at least 11 of 18 tender points (Figure 44-32). It is more common than RA, but its cause is still unknown.

The etiology of fibromyalgia has been debated for more than a century. It is unlikely that it is caused by a single factor. The most common precipitating factors include the following:

- Flulike viral illness
- Chronic fatigue syndrome
- Human immunodeficiency virus (HIV) infection
- Lyme disease
- Physical trauma
- Emotional trauma
- Medications, especially steroid withdrawal

Certain rheumatic diseases, such as RA or systemic lupus erythematosus, may coexist if not initially manifested with fibromyalgia. In addition, fibromyalgia may overlap with myofascial pain syndromes[117] (Table 44-9).

PATHOPHYSIOLOGY. Fibromyalgia as a chronic pain syndrome is defined by subjective symptoms and not unique pathophysiologic characteristics. Altered circadian activity of several neuroendocrine axes and ANS dysfunction have been reported.[118,119] Genetic factors are increasingly being suggested as important in developing FM. Aggregation of fibromyalgia within families and other coexisting conditions, such as irritable bowel syndrome, chronic fatigue, and mood disorders, suggest a major role for neuroendocrine and stress-response alterations (see Chapter 11).

TABLE 44-9 COMPARISON OF FIBROMYALGIA AND MYOFASCIAL PAIN SYNDROMES

VARIABLE	FIBROMYALGIA	MYOFASCIAL PAIN
Location	Generalized	Regional
Examination	Tender points	Trigger points
Response to local therapy	Not sustained	Curative
Gender	Female/male ratio: 10:1	Equal or unknown
Systemic features	Characteristic	Unknown

Studies of genetic factors have implicated alterations in genes affecting serotonin, catecholamines, and dopamine—all of these substances are involved in stress response and sensory processing.[120,121] In spite of these studies, the role of genetic factors in FM has not yet been fully identified. External stressors such as infection, psychosocial stress, and physical or emotional trauma may precipitate onset of FM.

Functional magnetic resonance imaging (fMRI) and molecular imaging techniques of positron emission tomography (PET) of the brains of persons with FM have shown activity in different areas of the brain than in healthy individuals when exposed to painful stimuli.[122] Individuals with fibromyalgia have lowered mechanical and thermal pain thresholds, high pain ratings for provoking stimuli, and altered temporal summation of pain stimuli. Functional abnormalities within the CNS are shown in Figure 44-32. Other pathophysiologic evidence includes hypothalamic-pituitary-adrenal (HPA) axis alterations that demonstrate abnormal response to pain;[123] recent investigations suggest cytokines are involved in the pathogenesis of FM. Corticotropin-releasing hormone (CRH) and locus ceruleus–norepinephrine (LC/NE), their peripheral effectors, and the hypothalamic-pituitary-adrenal axis are the main components of the stress system. Impaired functioning of the HPA axis and LC/NE system may be associated with fibromyalgia.

CLINICAL MANIFESTATIONS. The prominent symptom of fibromyalgia is diffuse, chronic pain. The locations of nine pairs of tender points for diagnostic classification of fibromyalgia are shown in Figure 44-32. Along with a history of diffuse pain, tenderness in 11 of these 18 points is necessary for diagnosis. Tender points must include areas on both sides of the spine as well as above and below the waist. In an effort to simplify and more accurately diagnose FM, the American College of Rheumatology (ACR) recently expanded the diagnostic criteria to include a widespread pain index (WPI) as "axial pain, left- and right-sided pain, and upper and lower segment pain."[124] Pain often begins in one location, especially the neck and shoulders, but then becomes more generalized. Some investigators have found that the majority of women experienced pain and fatigue for more than 90% of their time awake. Fatigue is most notable when arising from sleep and during the midafternoon. Headaches, symptoms of irritable bowel syndrome, and excess sensitivity to cold (Raynaud-like) are reported in 50% of individuals.

Almost 25% of individuals seek psychologic support for depression. Anxiety, particularly in regard to their diagnosis and future, is almost universal. Again, the only reliable finding on examination is the presence of multiple tender points.

EVALUATION AND TREATMENT. Because the manifestations of chronic, generalized pain and fatigue are present in many musculoskeletal (e.g., rheumatic) disorders, these disorders should be considered in the diagnosis of fibromyalgia (Tables 44-10 and 44-11).

No single regimen of medication has proved successful for fibromyalgia. Medications that improve sleep may be helpful as well as vitamin D supplementation. Anti-inflammatories have been used despite the fact there is no evidence of tissue inflammation, but these medications have not been effective. Certain CNS-active medications, most notably pregabalin, were better than placebo in controlled trials.[125] Probably the best approach is a combination of modalities, including education, medication, exercise, and cognitive-behavioral therapy.[126] Box 44-5 lists some of these modalities.

TABLE 44-10 DIFFERENTIAL DIAGNOSIS OF FIBROMYALGIA

DIFFERENTIAL DIAGNOSIS	HELPFUL DIFFERENTIAL FEATURES
Rheumatoid arthritis*	Synovitis, serologic tests, elevated erythrocyte sedimentation rate (ESR)
Systemic lupus erythematosus,*	Dermatitis, serositis (renal, central nervous system, etc.)
Polymyalgia rheumatic*	Elevated ESR, older adults, response to corticosteroids
Myositis	Increased muscle enzymes, weakness more than pain
Hypothyroidism*	Abnormal thyroid function tests
Neuropathies	Clinical and electrophysiologic evidence of neuropathy

Data from Klippel JH, Dieppe PA, editors: *Rheumatology,* ed 2, London, 1998, Mosby-Wolfe.
*Fibromyalgia may also more commonly coexist with these conditions.

TABLE 44-11 CONCOMITANT CONDITIONS WITH FIBROMYALGIA

CONCOMITANT CONDITION	RELATIONSHIP TO FIBROMYALGIA
Depression	Present in 25-60% of fibromyalgia cases
Irritable bowel	Present in 50-80% of fibromyalgia cases
Migraine	Present in 50% of fibromyalgia cases
Chronic fatigue syndrome (CFS)	70% of CFS cases meet criteria for fibromyalgia
Myofascial pain	May be a localized form of fibromyalgia

Data from Klippel JH, Dieppe PA, editors: *Rheumatology,* ed 2, London, 1998, Mosby-Wolfe.

Chronic Fatigue Syndrome

Chronic fatigue syndrome (CFS), also known as myalgic encephalomyelitis (ME), is a debilitating and complex disorder characterized by profound fatigue, neurologic energy production, and immune impairments. Though controversy about its etiology persists, recent evidence indicates symptoms are the result of central nervous system dysregulation, cardiovascular and immune system abnormalities, and dysfunction of cellular energy metabolism and ion transport.[127] As a result, CFS/ME is less a musculoskeletal disorder than one related to hypersensitivity of the central nervous system, a condition also known as central sensitization. Although individuals with CFS have widespread pain and fatigue, they do not have the tender points associated with fibromyalgia.[128]

PATHOPHYSIOLOGY. A recent International Consensus Criteria have recommended use of the term myalgic encephalomyelitis (ME) rather than chronic fatigue syndrome, because ME indicates an underlying pathophysiology.[127] In support of this,

BOX 44-5 EDUCATION AND REASSURANCE FOR INDIVIDUALS WITH FIBROMYALGIA

- Stress that the illness is real, not imagined.
- Explain that fibromyalgia is not a deforming or deteriorating condition.
- Explain that fibromyalgia is neither life threatening nor markedly debilitating, although it is an irritating presence.
- Discuss the role of sleep disturbances and the relationship of neurohormones to pain, fatigue, abnormal sleep, and mood.
- Reassure that although the cause is unknown, some information is known about the physiologic changes responsible for the symptoms.
- Use muscle "spasms" and perhaps low muscle blood flow to lay the groundwork for exercise recommendations.
- Assist individual to use aerobic exercise to reduce stress and increase rapid eye movement (REM) sleep.

functional MRI (fMRI) has shown lower blood perfusion to the brainstem in individuals affected by CFS.[128] Other researchers have shown apparent central nervous system abnormalities, immunologic dysregulation, and higher-than-normal levels of proinflammatory cytokines. Certain points in skeletal muscle may be affected by oxidative stress reactions (see Chapter 2), accounting for the muscle pain and fatigue associated with CFS; but other research implicates central sensitization of the CNS.[129]

CLINICAL MANIFESTATIONS. Unrestful sleep is a hallmark of CFS. Defining symptoms include debilitating fatigue made worse by physical or mental exercise (postexertional fatigue), muscle pain, noninflammatory joint pain, headaches, flu-like symptoms, and memory or concentration problems. Other common symptoms include bloating, morning joint stiffness, chest or jaw pain, chills and night sweats, visual disturbances, sore throat, and tender axillary or cervical lymph nodes. Symptoms and their consequences can be severe.

EVALUATION AND TREATMENT. Diagnosis of CFS is often delayed or missed because there is no biologic marker or specific laboratory test for CFS, many CFS symptoms are shared with other illnesses, individuals with CFS do not necessarily look sick, and symptoms typically have a variable course. Currently, the CDC recommends considering a diagnosis of CFS if the following two criteria are met[130]:

1. Unexplained, persistent fatigue is not due to ongoing exertion, is not substantially relieved by rest, is of new onset (not lifelong), and results in a significant reduction of previous levels of activity.
2. Four or more of the following symptoms are present for 6 months or more:
   - Impaired memory or concentration
   - Postexertional malaise (extreme, prolonged exhaustion and exacerbation of symptoms following physical or mental exertion)
   - Unrefreshing sleep
   - Muscle pain
   - Multijoint pain without swelling or redness (adults)
   - Headaches of a new type or severity
   - Sore throat that is frequent or recurring
   - Tender cervical or axillary lymph nodes

Treatment of CFS is primarily based on the person's individual needs and involves consideration of psychosocial factors as well as symptomatic and supportive care. Acknowledging the validity of the person's symptoms is important. Collaborative decision-making between the individual and healthcare provider with regard to treatment, professional counseling, medication, diet, and activity helps CFS sufferers deal with the limitations imposed by the disease. Alternative therapies such as acupuncture, massage, and therapeutic touch can relieve anxiety.

Disuse Atrophy

The term **disuse atrophy** describes the pathologic reduction in normal size of muscle fibers after prolonged inactivity from bed rest, trauma (casting), or local nerve damage. The effects of muscular deconditioning associated with lack of physical activity may be apparent in a matter of days. Oxidative stress from lack of muscle activity causes decreased protein synthesis and increased proteolysis, leading to muscle atrophy.[131] The normal individual on bed rest loses muscle strength from baseline levels at a rate of 3% per day. Bed rest also is associated with cardiovascular, skeletal, and other organ system changes. As muscles age, they lose strength and mass, a condition known as sarcopenia.

Certain genes and transcription factors play a role in muscle atrophy.[132,133] Measures to prevent atrophy include adequate nutrition, frequent forceful isometric muscle contractions, and passive lengthening exercises. If reuse is not restored within 1 year, regeneration of muscle fibers becomes impaired.

Muscle Membrane Abnormalities

Two defects of the muscle membrane (plasma membrane of the muscle fiber) have been linked to clinical syndromes: the hyperexcitable membrane seen in the myotonic disorders and the intermittently unresponsive membrane seen in periodic paralyses. Although these are infrequent disorders, research into the pathologic processes has led to an improved understanding of the cell membrane.

Skeletal Muscle Channelopathies

Generally speaking, skeletal muscle channelopathies can be divided into two primary groups: those presenting with myotonia (nondystrophic myotonias) and those associated with episodes of weakness (periodic paralysis). In **myotonic channelopathies,** muscle relaxation is delayed after voluntary contractions such as handgrip or eye closure. With periodic paralysis, depolarization of the sarcolemma is severe enough that the muscle cannot be "fired" again, resulting in paralysis.[134] (Ion channels are discussed in Chapter 1.)

Myotonia can be reproduced by removing extracellular chloride, thus reducing chloride conductance across the plasma membrane. The delicate balance in which sodium diffuses into the intracellular fluid, potassium diffuses out of the intracellular fluid, and chloride is in flux is thus interrupted. Because the normal diffusion processes (described in Chapter 3) stabilize the membrane, the shift in chloride ions is thought to increase membrane excitability. The chloride abnormality may explain the resting membrane hyperexcitability, but it does not explain the delayed relaxation present in myotonia and has not been detected in human myotonia.

Myotonia is seen in several disorders: myotonia congenita, paramyotonia congenita, myotonic muscular dystrophy, and some forms of periodic paralysis. Most are inherited disorders and are mild in symptomatology, with the exception of myotonic muscular dystrophy (see Chapter 45). Myotonia is treated by drugs that reduce muscle fiber excitability, such as procaine, procainamide, and phenytoin. Other treatments include the carbonic anhydrase inhibitors acetazolamide and dichlorphenamide.

Central core disease (CCD) is another inherited channelopathy that involves mutations in ryanodine receptors (RyR1) and affects calcium channels. In CCD, RyR1 channels are defective and either too much or too little calcium is released from the cell's sarcoplasmic reticulum. Classified as a neuromuscular disorder, CCD typically manifests during infancy as decreased muscle tone, delayed motor development, muscle weakness (particularly around the hip girdle), and other skeletal deformities, such as scoliosis.[135] Associated malignant hyperthermia susceptibility is common. Thought to be the most common congenital myopathy, pathology relates to the lack of "cores" within skeletal myofibers that do not contain mitochondria and their oxidative enzymes.[12]

Periodic Paralysis

Periodic paralysis (PP) is caused by autosomal dominant inherited mutations of skeletal muscle sodium, calcium, or potassium channels.[136] During an attack of PP the muscle membrane is unresponsive to neural stimuli and the resting membrane potential is reduced from −90 to −45 mV. Periodic paralysis can be either hyper- or hypokalemic. As the name implies, PP is usually transient.

The paralysis, which leaves the individual flaccid and weak, does not affect the respiratory muscles. In most cases the weakness is accompanied by a change in serum potassium level, although in some individuals the change may be negligible. Cardiac dysrhythmias have been present during attacks.

Hypokalemic periodic paralysis is most often triggered by thyrotoxicosis caused by alterations in potassium ion channels that are regulated by triiodothyronine (T_3).[137] (The effect of potassium on the resting membrane potential is discussed in Chapter 3.) Glucose and insulin infusions and oral potassium loading are used as provocative tests; oral and intravenous potassium can relieve acute attacks. Treatment includes potassium-sparing diuretics and a high-salt diet. Acetazolamide, dichlorphenamide, and a low-salt diet are useful for long-term therapy. **Hyperkalemic periodic paralysis** is caused by a genetic mutation of sodium channels. Attacks are usually less severe than the hypokalemic form. Treatment includes small carbohydrate-rich meals, light exercise, and intravenous calcium gluconate.

Metabolic Muscle Diseases

Disorders in muscle metabolism can be caused by endocrine abnormalities or diseases of energy metabolism, such as glycogen storage disease, enzyme deficiencies, and abnormalities in lipid metabolism and mitochondrial function.

Endocrine Disorders

Often the systemic effects of hormonal imbalance overshadow the individual's muscular symptoms. For example, individuals with thyrotoxicosis may have signs of proximal weakness, paresis of the extraocular muscles (exophthalmic ophthalmoplegia), and, rarely, hypokalemic periodic paralysis. Hypothyroidism is often associated with a decrease in muscle mass and strength, with weak, flabby skeletal muscles and sluggish movements. Thyroid hormone is believed to regulate muscle protein synthesis and electrolyte balance. Changes in muscle protein synthesis and electrolyte balance may therefore explain the changes in muscle mass and contractility seen in endocrine disorders. The muscle symptoms subside with appropriate treatment of the primary hormonal disorder.

Familial hypomagnesemia is an autosomal recessive disease that primarily affects the renal system, causing hypomagnesemia and secondary hypocalcemia and can result in tetany and convulsions.[138] Other endocrine disorders affecting the musculoskeletal system include Dent disease, a syndrome that causes bone deformities, rickets or osteomalacia, and elevated urine calcium levels. Osteopetrosis (also known as Albers-Schönberg disease), caused by failure of osteoclasts to resorb bone, results in increased bone mass but increased bone fragility; growth abnormalities; and in the infantile form, bone marrow failure as bone marrow is replaced by bone.[139]

Diseases of Energy Metabolism

Muscle relies on carbohydrates, such as glycogen and lipids (free fatty acids), for energy. When stored glycogen or lipids cannot be used because of a lack of the enzyme necessary to convert energy for contraction, the individual experiences cramps, fatigue, and exercise intolerance. Disorders of muscle metabolism can be self-limiting, such as is seen in McArdle disease and some lipid disorders, or cause widespread irreparable muscle destruction, as in acid maltase deficiency.

McArdle Disease. **McArdle disease,** or glycogen myophosphorylase deficiency, was the first myopathy in which a single enzyme defect was identified (Figure 44-33). Individuals with McArdle disease lack muscle phosphorylase, which is responsible for the breakdown of glycogen in muscle. Normally after the body uses the short-term ATP and phosphocreatine stores, intramuscular lactic acid accumulates as glycogen is used (see Chapter 43). The individual with McArdle disease is not able to break down glycogen or produce lactic acid.

The altered energy production manifests itself in exercise intolerance, fatigue, and painful muscle cramps. When exercise is carried to an extreme, painful muscle contracture and myoglobinuria develop. Some individuals describe a "second wind" phenomenon, in which exercise tolerance increases if they slow their pace once the initial sensation of fatigue commences. This is caused by the use of free fatty acids as a secondary source of energy.[140] As the disease progresses, some individuals have pronounced muscle weakness and wasting. Other organs are not involved because the absence of phosphorylase is limited to muscle. Generally, individuals with McArdle disease learn to adapt their daily routine to avoid muscle symptoms. Usually the diagnosis of McArdle disease is made by the histochemical

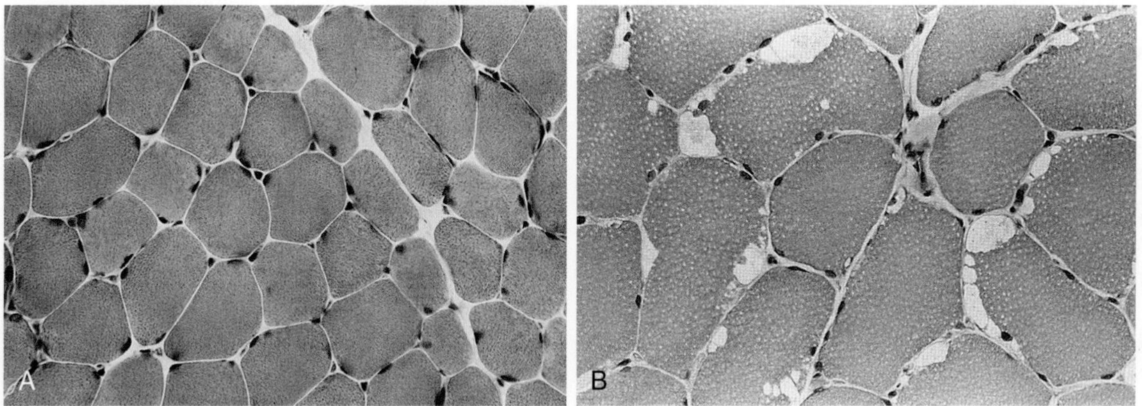

FIGURE 44-33 McArdle Disease. **A,** Normal muscle fibers. **B,** Muscle fibers of McArdle disease. Note the enlarged *(white)* peripheral vacuoles. (From Damjanov I, Linder J, editors: *Anderson's pathology,* ed 10, St Louis, 1996, Mosby.)

evaluation of myophosphorylase activity in frozen sections. There is no staining of myofibrils in affected individuals.

Acid Maltase Deficiency. **Acid maltase deficiency** is an uncommon glycogen storage disease associated with an accumulation of glycogen in the lysosomes of muscle and other tissue cells. The usual pathways of glycogen degradation are preserved. The absence of the enzyme acid maltase is responsible for the abnormality in glycogen metabolism, although the exact mechanism is unknown. It is an autosomal recessive disorder, with the gene located on the long arm of chromosome 17.

The infantile form, **Pompe disease,** is an autosomal recessive disease that causes lysosomal glycogen accumulation. The adult form tends to be less dramatic than the infantile type. The infantile form is recognized shortly after birth by hypotonia, dysreflexia, and an enlarged heart, tongue, and liver. Hypertrophy of these tissues is thought to be the result of glycogen deposition. Until recently, children often died of cardiac or respiratory failure before age 2; now enzyme replacement therapy (ERT) with recombinant human acid α-glucosidase and physical therapy can markedly improve symptoms.[141] The adult variety becomes evident subacutely and muscular symptoms resemble those of muscular dystrophy or polymyositis. A distinguishing feature in adults may be severe respiratory muscle weakness.

Myoadenylate Deaminase Deficiency. **Myoadenylate deaminase deficiency** (**MDD**) is a fairly common enzyme deficiency that causes changes in skeletal muscles and is associated with exercise intolerance. Because these individuals lack myoadenylate deaminase, they have a poor capacity for sustained energy production. Myoadenylate deaminase is the catalytic enzyme that forms phosphocreatine and ATP during exercise through a metabolic pathway that binds the purine and phosphate molecules that constitute ATP. Persons with MDD differ from those with McArdle disease in that during the ischemic exercise test, lactate production is normal when ATP and phosphocreatine are synthesized. Symptoms range from minimal complaints to exercise-induced muscle pain, to rhabdomyolysis.[142]

Lipid Deficiencies. Inherited disorders of lipid metabolism are uncommon but account for severe changes in muscle metabolism. The lipid content of muscle cells consists of free fatty acids, which are oxidized in the mitochondria. These acids require carnitine and the enzyme carnitine palmitoyltransferase (CPT); there are two CPT enzymes, I and II. Both are necessary to transport long-chain fatty acids to the mitochondria. Individuals with CPT deficiency often have mild muscular symptoms but can experience bouts of renal failure caused by rhabdomyolysis. Individuals with a deficiency of carnitine alone have progressive muscle weakness and can experience sudden exacerbations.

Measuring the CPT and carnitine content in muscle aids in the diagnosis. Cells in the muscle biopsy show vacuoles and lipid deposits. Treatments with riboflavin, medium-chain triglycerides, oral carnitine, and prednisone have been suggested.[143]

Inflammatory Muscle Diseases: Myositis

Viral, Bacterial, and Parasitic Myositis

Viral, bacterial, and parasitic infections of varying severity are known to produce inflammatory changes in skeletal muscle, a group of conditions collectively described by the term **myositis.** In tuberculosis and sarcoidosis, chronic inflammatory changes and granulomas are found in muscle, as well as in other affected tissues. In trichinellosis, *Trichinella* larvae reside in infected pork and, after ingestion, migrate to the intestinal mucosa and from there to the lymphatics. Symptoms include severe pain, rash, and muscle stiffness. Treatment includes administration of corticosteroids and antiparasitic agents, such as mebendazole or albendazole. Unfortunately, once trichinella larvae are established they may reside for years in the muscles. Toxoplasmosis, a common parasitic infection, is also associated with a generalized polymyositis that responds rapidly to therapy.

In the tropics, more prevalent disorders include bacterial infections with *Staphylococcus aureus* and parasites such as cysticercus, the larva of the tapeworm *Taenia solium.* Viral infections can be associated with an acute myositis. Muscle pain, tenderness, signs of inflammation, and elevation of CK level are common manifestations of viral myositis. The self-limiting symptoms of muscle aches and pains during a bout of influenza may actually be a subacute form of viral myopathy.

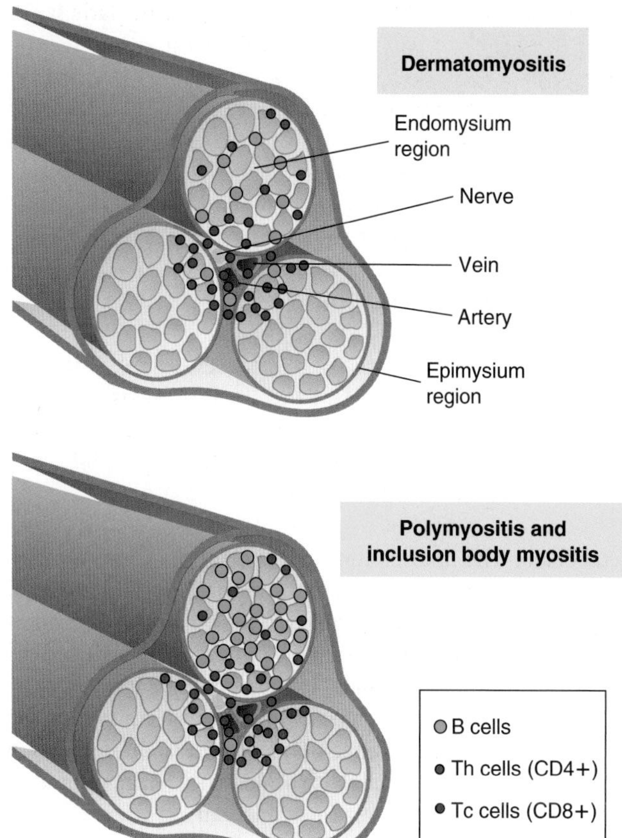

FIGURE 44-34 **Distribution of CD4+ and CD8+ Lymphocytes in Different Types of Myositis.** Dermatomyositis shows perivascular and CD4+ T cells (helper T cells). Polymyositis shows mostly CD8+ T cells (cytotoxic T cells).

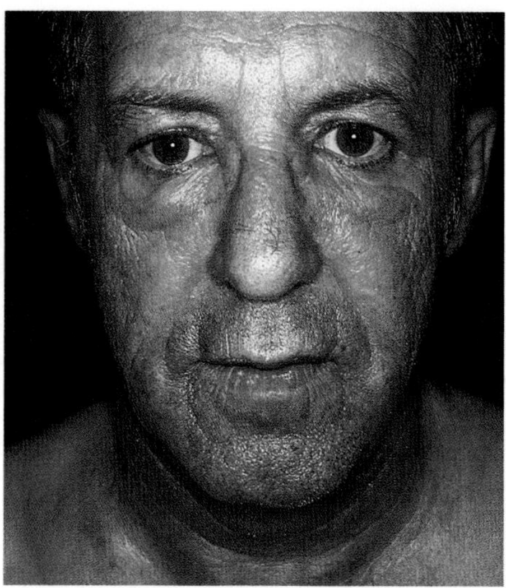

FIGURE 44-35 **Dermatomyositis.** Heliotrope (violaceous) discoloration around the eyes and periorbital edema. (From Habif TP: *Clinical dermatology,* ed 3, St Louis, 1996, Mosby.)

Polymyositis, Dermatomyositis, and Inclusion-Body Myositis

Idiopathic inflammatory myopathies (IIMs) are a group of autoimmune diseases that target skeletal muscle. IIMs are characterized by symmetric proximal muscle (pelvic and shoulder girdle) weakness and myalgia that develops over weeks to months. The three principle types are polymyositis (PM), dermatomyositis (DM), and inclusion-body myositis (IBM). Non-white women over age 50 are most often affected by IIM; however, DM includes a juvenile form (JDM). Interstitial lung disease is common in both PM and DM. The incidence of IIM appears to be increasing, but this may simply reflect improved diagnosis.

PATHOPHYSIOLOGY. Polymyositis and dermatomyositis are characterized by inflammation of connective tissue and muscle fibers. Polymyositis is mediated by T cells, whereas dermatomyositis is humorally-mediated.[144] $CD8^+$ T cells and macrophages are typically found in PM-affected muscles. Figure 44-34 shows the distribution of CD4+ and CD8+ lymphocytes in myositis. Innate and adaptive immune responses are activated in these myopathies, including myositis-specific antibodies and cytokines.[145] Inflammatory cells, including T cells, macrophages, and plasma cells, surround, displace, and even invade muscle fibers in PM. Perimysial and perivascular sites are selectively enriched in B cells and helper T cells in those with DM. DM is thought to be a microvascular disorder that includes deposits of complement in capillaries; however, recent research also has shown up-regulation of interferon signaling in muscle, blood, and skin of people with DM.[146] Ability to demonstrate elevated interferon levels can aid in both diagnosis and determination of targets to treat these diseases.

CLINICAL MANIFESTATIONS. The acute symptoms include many of those seen in any inflammatory process: malaise, fever, muscle swelling, pain and tenderness, lethargy, and listlessness. In adults, weakness of the shoulder and pelvic girdle muscles is a primary manifestation of PM. Both PM and DM often are associated with symmetric proximal muscle weakness and initially can be confused with other myopathies. A thorough evaluation is required to exclude other disorders. Clinical features common to both are dysphagia, reduced esophageal motility, vasculitis, Raynaud phenomenon, cardiomyopathy, and interstitial pulmonary fibrosis. Some individuals have other coexisting collagen vascular disorders, such as RA, systemic lupus erythematosus (SLE), and progressive systemic sclerosis (formerly called *scleroderma*).

Although PM and DM have similar histories of onset, DM includes cutaneous manifestations. The two most classic signs of skin involvement are rashes: (1) a heliotrope (reddish purple) rash that generally covers the eyelids and periorbital area (Figure 44-35), and often includes the chest; and (2) erythematous, scaly lesions (Gottron lesions) that cover joints, such as the knees and elbows. DM is slightly more common in children and older adults, with onset before age 15 or after age 50. The adult with DM occasionally has underlying malignancies.

IBM differs from both PM and DM in several important ways. Muscle biopsy and histopathologic studies of IBM show degenerative changes of muscle, accumulation of multiple proteins within muscle fibers, and evidence of endoplasmic reticular stress with misfolding of proteins.[147,148] Clinically, IBM may show weakness of the wrist and finger flexors as well as asymmetric atrophy and quadriceps weakness.[149]

EVALUATION AND TREATMENT. Muscle biopsy is striking in DM, with most individuals showing inflammatory cells grouped around blood vessels and atrophy of cells in muscle fascicles. This change, perifascicular atrophy, is absent in PM. Creatine kinase (CK) and other muscle enzymes, including aspartate transaminase (AST), lactate dehydrogenase (LDH), and alanine transaminase (ALT), and sedimentation rate are often extremely elevated in both disorders. The presence of serum antinuclear antibodies also may be helpful in diagnosing DM. EMG abnormalities include signs of muscle irritability and myopathic changes—usually large numbers of low-amplitude action potentials of brief duration. The EMG also shows a typical "myopathic" pattern, with short, low-amplitude polyphasic potentials, as well as signs of marked muscle irritability. Muscle biopsy is indispensable for determining a diagnosis of polymyositis or dermatomyositis as opposed to other myotonic diseases. MRI reveals inflammation and edema of the muscles.

Treatment primarily includes immunosuppressive drugs, although they are not always successful if uniformly applied. Most clinicians choose corticosteroids initially, though their utility has recently come into question.[150] High-dose intravenous immunoglobulin administration is sometimes used during active disease. Successful treatment with azathioprine and methotrexate has been reported. Creatine supplements and physical therapy may improve muscle strength.

Myopathy

Myopathy is the term applied to a primary muscle disorder. Many pathologic processes affect muscles and cause loss of functional muscle cells. Myopathies affect muscle strength, tone, and bulk. Primary muscle disease is invariably associated with weakness—usually marked weakness. The distribution of the weakness in myopathy is usually symmetric and proximal, although occasionally the weakness is predominantly distal, such as in myotonic dystrophy. The weakness is associated with mild fatigue. Tone is decreased, as are the tendon reflexes. Atrophy may be present. Some myopathies are associated with muscle hypertrophy as in cretinism and the familial progressive muscular dystrophies of childhood, in which hypertrophied muscles are rubbery and weak. Fasciculations are not present with myopathy because no denervation is present. No sensory changes are found. (Specific neurologic-associated myopathies are discussed in Chapter 17.)

Toxic Myopathies

A number of agents, including corticosteroids, chloroquine, alcohol, phenytoin, azathioprine, organophosphates, and reverse transcriptase inhibitors, have been shown to cause **toxic myopathy.** Alcohol remains the most common cause of toxic myopathy. The incidence of acute alcoholic myopathy has been estimated at up to 20% of individuals admitted with acute alcoholic withdrawal.

The mechanisms by which alcohol affects the muscle include disturbances of energy cell turnover, gene dysregulation, and initiation of apoptosis. Pathologic abnormalities include necrosis of individual muscle fibers, particularly type II fibers; whole segments can be found in the same stage of degeneration.

Acute alcoholic myopathy can range from benign cramps and pain resolving in a matter of hours to severe weakness and markedly increased CK level associated with myoglobinuria and renal failure. Individuals are prone to repeated attacks following recovery. The only treatment is abstinence from alcohol and improved nutrition. An individual with chronic alcoholic myopathy often has a coexisting peripheral neuropathy that complicates the diagnosis.

Repeated intramuscular injections have been associated also with changes in muscle fibers. Local necrosis of muscle fiber and elevated CK concentration have been reported after intramuscular injections of certain cephalosporins, lidocaine, diazepam, and digoxin; these effects were not produced with injections of saline. When drugs are injected over long periods, a chronic focal myopathy develops. Proliferation of connective tissue both in the muscle fiber and in the overlying skin and subcutaneous tissue has been reported. Over time, segments of the muscles, particularly the deltoid and quadriceps, are converted into fibrotic bands. Pathophysiologic mechanisms for these changes include repeated needle trauma and infection, along with the nonphysiologic acidity and alkalinity of the injected material. Box 44-6 lists some of the causes of toxic myopathy.

Muscle Tumors

Rhabdomyoma

Rhabdomyoma is an extremely rare benign tumor of striated muscle that generally occurs in the tongue, neck muscles, larynx, uvula, nasal cavity, axilla, vulva, and heart. These tumors are usually treated by surgical excision and do not recur.

Rhabdomyosarcoma

A rare malignant tumor of striated muscle is called **rhabdomyosarcoma,** which is a subgroup of sarcoma. These tumors are highly malignant, with rapid metastasis. They are located in the muscle tissue of the head, neck, and genitourinary tract in 75% of cases. The remaining 25% of these tumors are located in the trunk and extremities. Rhabdomyosarcomas are the most common soft tissue tumors in children and young adults.

Three types of rhabdomyosarcoma are differentiated on pathologic section: pleomorphic, embryonal, and alveolar. The pleomorphic, or spindle cell, type is considered to be one of the most highly malignant tumors of the extremities seen in adulthood, but has a better outcome in children. Embryonal tumors are most commonly seen in childhood and appear on biopsy to be shaped like a tadpole or tennis racquet. Alveolar-type tumors, which appear lattice-like and look like lung tissue alveoli, have the poorest outcome.[151]

The diagnosis of rhabdomyosarcoma is made by history, physical examination, serologic testing, CT, and MRI, and is confirmed by incisional biopsy and examination of the specimen by a pathologist. On electron microscopy the tissue demonstrates myofilaments and Z-band material; CT scan helps

BOX 44-6 AGENTS THAT CAN CAUSE TOXIC MYOPATHY

Drug-Induced
Alcohol
Amiodarone (and others that inhibit CYP3A4 when combined with simvastatin)
Amphotericin B
Azathioprine
AZT (zidovudine)
Chloroquine
Clofibrate
Cocaine
Colchicine
Ethanol
Ipecac (withdrawn from U.S. markets)
3,4-Methylenedioxymethamphetamine (MDMA, "ecstasy")
Pentachlorophenol (PCP)
Statins
Steroids (especially with prolonged high doses; doses >25 mg/day; fluorinated steroids)

Endocrine Disorders
Adrenal disorders (Addison disease, Cushing disease)
Hyperparathyroidism
Hyperthyroidism (CK may be normal)
Hypothyroidism (CK may be mildly elevated)

Infectious
Coxsackie A and B viruses
Human immunodeficiency virus (HIV)
Influenza
Lyme disease
Staphylococcus aureus muscle infection (frequent cause of pyomyositis)
Toxoplasmosis
Trichinosis

Miscellaneous
Licorice
Certain edible wild mushrooms
Lead poisoning
Organophosphates
Red yeast rice
European migratory quail (quail eat toxic hemlock, hellebore seeds)
Any medication that alters serum concentrations of sodium, potassium, calcium, phosphorus, or magnesium

Data from Kuncl RW: *Curr Opin Neurol* 22(5):506–515, 2009; Valiyil R, Christopher-Stine L: *Curr Rheumatol Rep* 12(3):213–220, 2010.

define the tissue borders. Staging is based on pathologic grade of the tumor and is helpful in determining prognosis and treatment.

Treatment consists of a combination of surgical excision, radiation therapy, and systemic chemotherapy. Overall survival of childhood rhabdomyosarcoma has improved over the past decades but adult survival remains poor (see Chapter 45).

Other Tumors

Metastatic muscle tumors are rare in spite of the extensive vascular supply of skeletal muscles. It is suggested that local pH or metabolic changes discourage metastatic involvement from other tumors. When adjacent carcinomas do cause muscle damage, it is usually related to the compression of tissue and resultant muscle atrophy.

SUMMARY REVIEW

Musculoskeletal Injuries

1. The most common skeletal injury is a fracture. A bone can be completely or incompletely fractured. A closed fracture leaves the skin intact. An open fracture has an overlying skin wound. The direction of the fracture line can be linear, oblique, spiral, or transverse. Greenstick, torus, and bowing fractures are examples of incomplete fractures that occur in children. Stress fractures occur in normal or abnormal bone that is subjected to repeated stress. Fatigue fractures occur in normal bone subjected to abnormal stress. Normal weight-bearing can cause an insufficiency fracture in abnormal bone.
2. Dislocation is complete loss of contact between the surfaces of two bones. Subluxation is partial loss of contact between two bones. As a bone separates from a joint, it may damage adjacent nerves, blood vessels, ligaments, tendons, and muscle.
3. Tendon tears are called *strains,* and ligament tears are called *sprains.* A complete separation of a tendon or ligament from its attachment is called an *avulsion.*
4. Epicondylopathy is degeneration of a tendon where it attaches to a bone. Bursitis is inflammation of the bursae (small sacs lined with synovial membrane and filled with synovial fluid). Bursitis can be inflammatory, septic, or hemorrhagic.
5. Muscle strain can range from mild injury to severe damage that can result in loss of muscle function.
6. Rhabdomyolysis can be a life-threatening complication of severe muscle trauma wherein muscle cell contents are released into the circulation. It may result in myoglobinuria, the presence of myoglobin in the urine, and is often associated with acute renal failure.

Disorders of Bones

1. Metabolic bone diseases are characterized by abnormal bone structure. In osteoporosis bone tissue is normally mineralized, but the density or mass of bone is reduced because the bone remodeling cycle is disrupted. Osteoporosis is a complex, multifactorial, chronic disease that often progresses silently for decades until fractures occur. It is the most common bone disease. Multiple factors are involved including alteration in the OPG/RANKL/RANK system.
2. Postmenopausal osteoporosis occurs in middle-aged and older women and is caused by increased osteoclast activity, probably caused by changes in osteoprotegerin, IGF, a combination of inadequate dietary calcium intake and lack of vitamin D, possibly decreased levels of magnesium, lack of exercise, decreased levels of estrogen, and family history.
3. Glucocorticoids increase RANKL expression and inhibit OPG production by osteoblasts, thus leading to lower bone density.

SUMMARY REVIEW—cont'd

4. Osteomalacia is a metabolic bone disease characterized by inadequate bone mineralization.
5. Excessive and abnormal bone remodeling occurs in Paget disease. Sporadic Paget disease involves overexpression of RANKL.
6. Osteomyelitis is a bone infection caused most often by bacteria (e.g., *S. aureus*) that can enter bone from outside the body (exogenous osteomyelitis) or from infection sites within the body (hematogenous osteomyelitis).
7. Bone tumors originate from bone cells, cartilage cells, fibrous tissue cells, or vascular marrow cells. Each cell produces a specific type of ground substance that is used to classify the tumor as osteogenic (bone cell), chondrogenic (cartilage cell), collagenic (fibrous tissue cell), or myelogenic (vascular marrow cell). Malignant bone tumors are large, aggressively destroy surrounding bone, invade surrounding tissue, and initiate independent growth outside the site of origin. Benign bone tumors are less destructive, limit their growth to the anatomic confines of the bone, and have a well-demarcated border.

Disorders of Joints

1. Noninflammatory joint disease is differentiated from inflammatory joint disease by the absence of synovial membrane inflammation, the absence of systemic signs and symptoms, and the presence of normal synovial fluid.
2. OA is now considered an inflammatory joint disease and is characterized by the degeneration and loss of articular cartilage, sclerosis of underlying bone, and formation of bone spurs (osteophytes).
3. RA is an inflammatory joint disease characterized by inflammatory destruction of the synovial membrane, articular cartilage, joint capsule, and surrounding ligaments and tendons. RA involves an aberrant immune response and the transformed antibodies are called *rheumatoid factors.* The OPG/RANKL/RANK system is also involved. Rheumatoid nodules may also invade the skin, lung, and spleen and involve small and large arteries. RA is a systemic disease that affects the heart, lungs, kidneys, and skin, as well as the joints.
4. AS is a chronic inflammatory joint disease characterized by stiffening and fusion of the spine and sacroiliac joints. Recent data show that synovitis and bone marrow inflammation, rather than solely enthesis involvement, explain the alteration in sacroiliac joints.
5. Gout is a metabolic disorder associated with high levels of uric acid in the blood and body fluids. Uric acid crystallizes in the connective tissue of a joint, where it initiates inflammatory destruction of the joint.

Disorders of Skeletal Muscle

1. A pathologic contracture is permanent muscle shortening caused by muscle spasticity, as seen in CNS injury or severe muscle weakness.
2. Stress-induced muscle tension is presumably caused by increased activity in the reticular activating system and gamma loop in the muscle fiber. Progressive relaxation training and biofeedback have been advocated to reduce muscle tension.
3. Fibromyalgia is a chronic musculoskeletal syndrome characterized by diffuse pain and tender points. It is unknown but suspected that muscle is the end organ responsible for the pain and fatigue of the disease. Comorbidities (e.g., irritable bowel syndrome, mood disorders, and chronic fatigue) suggest a major role for neuroendocrine and stress-response alterations.
4. Chronic fatigue syndrome (CFS) is a debilitating and complex disorder with profound fatigue not improved by bed rest. The actual cause of CFS is unknown and hypotheses include central nervous system alterations, immunologic disruptions, and chronic proinflammatory cytokines.
5. Atrophy of muscle fibers and overall diminished size of the muscle are seen after prolonged inactivity. Isometric contractions and passive lengthening exercises decrease atrophy to some degree in immobilized persons.
6. Hyperexcitable membranes cause the physical and electrical phenomenon of myotonia. The disorder is treated with drugs that reduce fiber excitability. Periodic paralysis is caused by an unresponsive muscle membrane and is accompanied by changes in the level of serum potassium. The biochemical defect is possibly related to changes in the muscle membrane and sarcoplasmic reticulum.
7. Metabolic muscle diseases are caused by endocrine disorders, glycogen storage disease, enzyme deficiencies, and abnormal lipid function. The muscle depends on a complex system of carbohydrates and fats converted by enzymes to produce energy for the muscle cell. Abnormalities in these pathways can inhibit function or cause damage to the muscle fiber. These illnesses are rare, yet they account for significant functional abnormalities.
8. Viral, bacterial, and parasitic infections of muscles produce the characteristic clinical and pathologic changes associated with inflammation. These are usually treatable and self-limiting disorders.
9. Polymyositis (generalized muscle inflammation) and dermatomyositis (polymyositis accompanied with skin rash) are characterized by inflammation of connective tissue and muscle fibers, and muscle fiber necrosis. Cell-mediated and humoral immune factors have been implicated. Treatment with immunosuppressive agents is effective in many cases.
10. Primary disorders with weakness and atrophy are known as myopathies.
11. The most common toxic myopathy is caused by alcohol abuse. Direct toxic effects of alcohol-producing necrosis of muscle fibers and nutritional deficiency have been suggested. The only treatment is abstinence and improved nutrition. The toxic effects of many drugs on muscle fibers cause local trauma to the muscle fibers from direct effects of the needle, secondary infection, and changes caused by nonphysiologic acidity and alkalinity in the fibers.
12. Sarcomas of muscle tissue are rare. Rhabdomyosarcoma has a uniformly poor prognosis because of an aggressive invasion and early, widespread dissemination. The usual treatment includes surgical excision, radiation therapy, and systemic chemotherapy.

KEY TERMS

Acid maltase deficiency, 1583
Acute gouty arthritis, 1576
Age-related bone loss, 1553
Aggrecan, 1573
Ankylosing spondylitis (AS), 1572
Arthropathy, 1565
Asymptomatic hyperuricemia, 1576
Avulsion, 1545
Biofeedback, 1578
Bowing fracture, 1541
Bursae, 1546
Bursitis, 1545
Caplan syndrome, 1572
Central core disease (CCD), 1582
Chondrogenic (cartilage-forming) tumor, 1563
Chondroid, 1563
Chondrosarcoma, 1563
Closed (simple) fracture, 1541
Collagenic (collagen-forming) tumor, 1564
Comminuted fracture, 1541
Complete fracture, 1541
Contracture, 1578
Delayed union, 1543
Dislocation, 1544
Disuse atrophy, 1581
Epicondylitis, 1546
Extracellular signal regulated kinases (ERKs), 1553
Fatigue fracture, 1541
Fibromyalgia, 1579
Fibrosarcoma, 1569
Fracture, 1540
Fragility fracture, 1541
Glucocorticoid (e.g., cortisone)-induced osteoporosis, 1553
Gout, 1574
Gouty arthritis, 1574
Greenstick fracture, 1541
Heterotopic ossification (HO), 1547
Hyperbaric oxygen therapy, 1560
Hyperkalemic periodic paralysis, 1582
Hypokalemic periodic paralysis, 1582
Idiopathic inflammatory myopathy (IIM), 1584
Incomplete fracture, 1541
Inflammatory joint disease (arthritis), 1568
Insufficiency fracture, 1541
Involucrum, 1559
Joint effusion, 1568
Joint stiffness, 1567
Lateral epicondylopathy (tennis elbow), 1546
Ligament, 1545
Linear fracture, 1541
Malunion, 1543
McArdle disease, 1582
Medial epicondylopathy (golfer's elbow), 1546
Muscle strain, 1547
Myelogenic tumor, 1564
Myoadenylate deaminase deficiency (MDD), 1583
Myopathy, 1585
Myositis, 1583
Myositis ossificans, 1547
Myotonic channelopathy, 1581
Noninflammatory joint disease, 1565
Nonunion, 1543
Oblique fracture, 1541
Open (compound) fracture, 1541
Osteoarthritis (OA), 1565
Osteogenic (bone-forming) tumor, 1562
Osteomalacia, 1557
Osteomyelitis, 1558
Osteopenia, 1550
Osteophyte, 1565
Osteoporosis, 1550
Osteoprotegerin (OPG), 1553
Osteosarcoma, 1563
Paget disease of bone (PDB) (osteitis deformans), 1557
Pannus, 1570
Pathologic fracture, 1541
Peak bone mass, 1550
Periodic paralysis (PP), 1582
Pompe disease, 1583
Postmenopausal osteoporosis, 1552
Primary gout, 1575
Progressive relaxation training, 1578
Pseudogout, 1575
RANK, 1553
Receptor activator of nuclear factor κβ ligand (RANKL), 1553
Regional osteoporosis, 1552
Rhabdomyolysis, 1547
Rhabdomyosarcoma, 1586
Rheumatoid arthritis (RA), 1568
Rheumatoid factor (RF), 1569
Rheumatoid nodule, 1572
Secondary gout, 1575
Sequestrum, 1559
Spiral fracture, 1541
Sprain, 1545
Strain, 1545
Stress fracture, 1541
Subluxation, 1544
Syndesmophyte, 1574
Tendinitis, 1545
Tendinosis, 1545
Tendon, 1545
Tophaceous gout, 1576
Tophus (*pl.*, tophi), 1575
Torus fracture, 1541
Toxic myopathy, 1585
Transchondral fracture, 1541
Transverse fracture, 1541

REFERENCES

1. Pressley JC et al: The epidemiology of bone fracture across the age span in blacks and whites, *J Trauma* 71(5 Suppl 2):S541–S548, 2011.
2. Cooper C et al: Secular trends in the incidence of hip and other osteoporotic fractures, *Osteoporos Int* 22(5):1277–1288, 2011.
3. Randsborg P-H, Sivertsen EA: Distal radius fractures in children: substantial difference in stability between buckle and greenstick fractures, *Acta Orthop* 80(5):585–589, 2009.
4. Assiotis A, Sachinis NP, Chalidis BE: Pulsed electromagnetic fields for the treatment of tibial delayed unions and nonunions. A prospective clinical study and review of the literature, *J Orthop Surg Res* 7:24, 2012.
5. Shenaq DS et al: Mesenchymal progenitor cells and their orthopedic applications: forging a path towards clinical trials, *Stem Cells Int* 2010:519028, 2010.
6. Virk MS et al: "Same day" *ex-vivo* regional gene therapy: a novel strategy to enhance bone repair, *Mol Ther*(5):960–968, 2011.
7. Sakabe T, Sakai T: Musculoskeletal diseases—tendon, *Br Med Bull* 99(1):211–225, 2011.
8. Knobloch K: The role of tendon microcirculation in Achilles and patellar tendinopathy, *J Orthop Surg Res* 3:18, 2008.
9. Abate M et al: Pathogenesis of tendinopathies: inflammation or degeneration? *Arthritis Res Ther* 11(3):235–250, 2009.
10. Baird EO, Kang QK: Prophylaxis of heterotopic ossification–an updated review, *J Orthop Surg Res* 4:12, 2009.
11. Cervellin G, Comelli I, Lippi G: Rhabdomyolysis: historical background, clinical, diagnostic, and therapeutic features, *Clin Chem Lab Med* 48(6):749–756, 2010.
12. Capes EM, Loaiza R, Valdiva HH: Ryanodine receptors, *Skelet Muscle* 1:18, 2011.
13. Frink M et al: Compartment syndrome of the lower leg and foot, *Clin Orthop Relat Res* 468(4):940–950, 2010.
14. Su B-H et al: Ultrasonic appearance of rhabdomyolysis in patients with crush injury in the Wenchuan earthquake, *Chin Med J* 122(16):1872–1876, 2009.
15. National Osteoporosis Foundation: *Clinician's guide to prevention and treatment of osteoporosis*, Washington, DC, 2010, Author.
16. Looker AC et al: *Osteoporosis or low bone mass at the femur neck or lumbar spine in older adults: United States, 2005-2008*, Washington, DC, 2012, National Center for Health Statistics.
17. Crandall CJ et al: *Treatment to prevent fractures in men and women with low bone density or osteoporosis: update of a 2007 report*, Rockville, MD, 2012, Agency for Healthcare Research and Quality.
18. Clarke BL, Khosla S: Physiology of bone loss, *Radiol Clin North Am* 48(3):483–495, 2010.
19. Nordin C: Screening for osteoporosis: U.S. Preventive Services Task Force recommendation statement, *Ann Intern Med* 155(4):276–277, 2011.
20. Adachi JD et al: Impact of prevalent fractures on quality of life: baseline results from the global longitudinal study of osteoporosis in women, *Mayo Clin Proc* 85(9):806–813, 2010.
21. Vestergaard P, Rejnmark L, Mosekilde L: Loss of life years after a hip fracture: effects of age and sex, *Acta Orthop* 80(5):525–530, 2009.
22. Estrada K et al: Genome-wide meta-analysis identifies 56 bone mineral density loci and reveals 14 loci associated with risk of fracture, *Nat Genet* 44(5):491–501, 2012.
23. Osteoporosis NIH, Bone Related: *Diseases National Resource Center: Osteoporosis and African American women, June 2010.* Available at www.niams.nih.gov/Health_Info/Bone/Osteoporosis/Background/default.asp. Accessed January 20, 2011.
24. Curtis JR et al: Population-based fracture risk assessment and osteoporosis treatment disparities by race and gender, *J Gen Intern Med* 24(8):856–962, 2009.
25. Manolagas SC, Parfitt AM: What old means to bone, *Trends Endocrinol Metab* 21(6):369–374, 2010.
26. Manolagas SC: From estrogen-centric to aging and oxidative stress: a revised perspective of the pathogenesis of osteoporosis, *Endocr Rev* 31(3):266–300, 2010.
27. Ahmadie H, Arabi A: Vitamins and bone health: beyond calcium and vitamin D, *Nutr Rev* 69(10):584–598, 2011.

28. Bonjour JP: Calcium and phosphate: a duet of ions playing for bone health, *J Am Coll Nutr* 30(5 Suppl 1):438S–448S, 2011.
29. Khosla S: Update in male osteoporosis, *J Clin Endocrinol Metab* 85(1):3–10, 2010.
30. Krum SA: Direct transcriptional targets of sex steroid hormones in bone, *J Cell Biochem* 112(2):401–408, 2011.
31. Mahadevan S, Kumaravel V, Bharath R: Calcium and bone disorders in pregnancy, *Indian J Endocrinol Metab* 16(3):358–363, 2012.
32. Grey A, Dalbeth N, Doyle A: Clinical images: transient regional osteoporosis, *Arthritis Rheum* 60(10):3145, 2009.
33. Rocchietti March M et al: Transient osteoporosis of the hip, *Hip Int* 20(3):297–300, 2010.
34. Demontiero O, Vidal C, Duque G: Aging and bone loss: new insights for the clinician, *Ther Adv Musculoskel Dis* 4(2):61–76, 2012.
35. Trouvin A-P, Goëb V: Receptor activator of nuclear factor-κB ligand and osteoprotegerin: maintaining the balance to prevent bone loss, *Clin Interven Aging* 5:345–354, 2010.
36. Silva I, Branco JA: Rank/Rankl/opg: literature review, *Acta Rheumatol Port* 36(3):209–218, 2011.
37. Chin KY, Ima-Nirwana S: Sex steroids and bone health status in men, *Int J Endocrinol*, 2012 Oct 24. [Epub ahead of print.].
38. Oury F: A crosstalk between bone and gonads, *Ann N Y Acad Sci* 1260:1–7, 2012.
39. Plotkin LI et al: Bisphosphonates and estrogens inhibit osteocyte apoptosis via distinct molecular mechanisms downstream of extracellular signal-regulated kinase activation, *J Biol Chem* 280(8):7317–7325, 2005.
40. Cicek M et al: TGF-β inducible early gene 1 regulates osteoclast differentiation and survival by mediating the NFATc1, AKT, and MEK/ERK signaling pathways, *PLoS One* 6(3):e17522, 2011.
41. Žofková I: Hormonal aspects of the muscle-bone unit, *Physiol Res* 57(Suppl 1):S159, 2008.
42. Tanner DA et al: Hip fractures in men and women change differently with age, *BMC Geriatrics* 10:12, 2010.
43. Nieves JW: Skeletal effects of nutrients and nutraceuticals, beyond calcium and vitamin D, *Osteoporos Int*, 2012 Nov 14. [E-pub ahead of print.].
44. Genius SJ, Bouchard T: Combination micronutrients for bone (COMB) study: bone density after micronutrient intervention, *J Environ Public Health*, 2012 Jan 15. [Published online.].
45. Güerri-Fernádez RC, Diez-Perez A: Is there a future for selective estrogen-receptor modulators in osteoporosis? *Ther Adv Musculoskelet Dis* 4(2):55–59, 2012.
46. Bellido T, Plotkin LI: Novel actions of bisphosphonates in bone: preservation of osteoblast and osteocyte viability, *Bone* 49(1):50–55, 2011.
47. Wehrhan F et al: Bisphosphonate-associated osteonecrosis of the jaw is linked to suppressed TGFβ1-signaling and increased Galectin-3 expression: a histological study on biopsies, *J Transl Med* 9:102–113, 2011.
48. Alshahrani F, Kendler D: Femoral fractures in osteoporotic patients on bisphosphonates: a case report, *J Clin Densitom* 15(3):380–384, 2012.
49. Kennel KA, Drake MT: Adverse effects of bisphosphonates: implications for osteoporosis management, *Mayo Clin Proc* 84(7):632–639, 2009.
50. Khosla S et al: Benefits and risks of bisphosphonate therapy for osteoporosis, *J Clin Endocrinol Metabol* 97(7):2272–2282, 2012.
51. Salari P, Abdollahi M: Long term bisphosphonate use in osteoporotic patients: a step forward, two steps back, *J Pharm Sci* 15(2):305–317, 2012.
52. Black DM et al: Continuing bisphosphonate treatment for osteoporosis—for whom and for how long? *N Engl J Med* 366(22):2015–2053, 2012.
53. Hanley DA et al: Denosumab: mechanism of action and clinical outcomes, *Int J Clin Pract* 66(12):1139–1146, 2012.
54. Vescini F, Grimaldi F: PTH 1-84: bone rebuilding as a target for the therapy of severe osteoporosis, *Clin Cases Miner Bone Metab* 9(1):31–36, 2012.
55. Crandall CJ et al: *Treatment to prevent fractures in men and women with low bone density or osteoporosis: update of a 2007 report [Internet], comparative effectiveness reviews, no. 53*, Rockville, MD, 2012, Agency for Healthcare Research and Quality.
56. Lim V, Clarke BL: New therapeutic targets for osteoporosis: beyond denosumab, *Maturitas* 73(3):269–272, 2012.
57. Penido MG, Alon US: Phosphate homeostasis and its role in bone health, *Pediatr Nephrol* 27(11):2039–2048, 2012.
58. Shimada T, Fukumoto S: FGF23 as a novel therapeutic target, *Adv Exp Med Biol* 728:158–170, 2012.
59. Thacher TD, Clarke BL: Vitamin D deficiency, *Mayo Clin Proc* 86(1): 50–60, 2011.
60. Unuvar T, Buyukgebiz A: Nutritional rickets and vitamin D deficiency in infants, children and adolescents, *Pediatr Endocrinol Rev* 7(3): 283–291, 2011.
61. Jain SK et al: Unusual presentation of altered bone metabolism with long-term antiepileptic therapy: pathological fracture of neck of femur due to brown tumor at calcer, *Musculoskelet Surg* 95(3):265–268, 2011.
62. Jones AN, Hansen KE: Recognizing the musculoskeletal manifestations of vitamin D deficiency, *J Musculoskelet Med* 26(10):389–396, 2009.
63. Kulak CA, Dempster DW: Bone histomorphometry: a concise review for endocrinologists and clinicians, *Arq Bras Endocrinol Metabol* 54(2): 87–98, 2010.
64. Bergwitz C, Jüppner H: Phosphate sensing, *Adv Chronic Kidney Dis* 18(2):132–144, 2011.
65. Shaker JL: Paget's disease of bone: a review of epidemiology, pathophysiology, and management, *Ther Adv Musculoskelet Dis* 1(2):107–125, 2009.
66. Albagha OME et al: Genome wide association study identifies variants at *CSF1, OPTN* and *TNFRSF11A* as genetic risk factors for Paget's disease of bone, *Nat Genet* 42(6):520–524, 2010.
67. Roodman GD: Insights into the pathogenesis of Paget's disease, *Ann N Y Acad Sci* 1192:176–180, 2010.
68. Visconti MR et al: Mutations of SQSTM1 are associated with severity and clinical outcome in Paget disease of bone, *J Bone Miner Res* 25(11):2368–2373, 2010.
69. Michou L, Brown JP: Emerging strategies and therapies for treatment of Paget's disease of bone, *Drug Design Develop Ther* 5:225–239, 2011.
70. Harik NS, Smeltzer MS: Management of acute hematogenous osteomyelitis in children, *Expert Rev Anti Infect Ther* 8(2):175–181, 2010.
71. Calhoun JH, Manring MM, Shirtliff M: Osteomyelitis of the long bones, *Semin Plast Surg* 23(2):59–72, 2009.
72. Hernigou P et al: Septic arthritis in adults with sickle cell disease often is associated with osteomyelitis or osteonecrosis, *Clin Orthop Relat Res* 468:1676–1681, 2010.
73. Kapoor A et al: Magnetic resonance imaging for diagnosing foot osteomyelitis: a meta-analysis, *Arch Intern Med* 167(2):125, 2007.
74. Franchi A: Epidemiology and classification of bone tumors, *Clin Cases Miner Bone Metab* 9(2):92–95, 2012.
75. Martin JW, Squire JA, Zielenska M: The genetics of osteosarcoma, *Sarcoma* 2012:627254, 2012.
76. National Comprehensive Cancer Network (NCCN): *Recent updates to NCCN clinical practice guidelines in oncology: bone cancer, National Comprehensive Cancer Network, Version 1*, Fort Washington, PA, 2013, Author.
77. Buddingh EP et al: Intact interferon signaling in peripheral blood leukocytes of high-grade osteosarcoma patients, *Cancer Immunol Immunother* 61(6):941–947, 2012.
78. Sadikovic B et al: Expression analysis of genes associated with human osteosarcoma tumors shows correlation of RUNX2 overexpression with poor response to chemotherapy, *BMC Cancer* 10:202, 2010.
79. Wesolowski R, Budd GT: Use of chemotherapy for patients with bone and soft-tissue sarcomas, *Clev Clin J Med* 77(Suppl 1):S23–S26, 2010.
80. Lin PP, Moussallem CD, Deavers MT: Secondary chondrosarcoma, *J Am Acad Orthop Surg* 18(10):608–615, 2010.
81. Onishi AC, Hincker AM, Lee FY: Surmounting chemotherapy and radioresistance in chondrosarcoma: molecular mechanisms and therapeutic targets, *Sarcoma* 2011:381654, 2011.
82. Karpik M: Giant cell tumor (tumor gigantocellularis, osteoclastoma)—epidemiology, diagnosis, treatment, *Orthop Traumatol Rehabil* 12(3): 207–215, 2010.
83. Cowan RW, Singh G: Giant cell tumor of bone: a basic science perspective, *Bone* 52(1):238–246, 2013.
84. Kivioja AH et al: Cement is recommended in intralesional surgery of giant cell tumors: a Scandinavian Sarcoma Group study of 294 patients followed for a median time of 5 years, *Acta Orthop* 9(2):86, 2008.
85. Evangelou E et al: Translation research in Europe applied technologies for osteoarthritis (TreatOA): meta-analysis of genome-wide association studies confirms a susceptibility locus for knee osteoarthritis on chromosome 7q22, *Ann Rheum Dis* 70(2):349–355, 2011.
86. Heinegård D, Saxne T: The role of cartilage matrix in osteoarthritis, *Nat Rev Rheumatol* 7(1):50–56, 2010.
87. Kapoor M et al: Role of proinflammatory cytokines in the pathophysiology of osteoarthritis, *Nat Rev Rheumatol* 7:33–42, 2011.
88. Wu L et al: Insights on biology and pathology of HIF-1α/2α, TGFβ/BMP, Wnt/β-catenin, and NF-κB pathways in osteoarthritis, *Curr Pharm Des* 18(22):3293–3312, 2012.
89. Neogi T: Clinical significance of bone changes in osteoarthritis, *Ther Adv Musculoskelet Dis* 4(4):259–267, 2012.
90. Yusuf E et al: Do knee abnormalities visualized in MRI explain knee pain in knee osteoarthritis? A systematic review, *Ann Rheum Dis* 70(1):60–67, 2011.

91. Schiphof D et al: Factors for pain in patients with different grades of knee osteoarthritis, *Arthritis Care Res (Hoboken)*, 2012 Nov 30. [Epub ahead of print.].
92. Tanamas S et al: Does knee malalignment increase the risk of development and progression of knee osteoarthritis? A systematic review, *Arthritis Rheum* 61(4):459–466, 2009.
93. JCh Rousseau: Ganrero P: Biological markers in osteoarthritis, *Bone* 51(2):265–277, 2012.
94. Hochberg MC et al: American College of Rheumatology 2012 recommendations for the use of nonpharmacologic and pharmacologic therapies in osteoarthritis of the hand, hip, and knee, *Arthritis Care Res* 64(4):465–474, 2012.
95. Aletaha D et al: The 2010 American College of Rheumatology/European League Against Rheumatism classification criteria for rheumatoid arthritis: an American College of Rheumatology/European League Against Rheumatism collaborative initiative, *Arthritis Rheum* 62(9):2569–2581, 2010.
96. Gabriel SE, Michaud K: Epidemiological studies in incidence, prevalence, mortality, and comorbidity of the rheumatic diseases, *Arthritis Res Ther* 11(3):229, 2009.
97. Goronzy JJ, Weyand CM: Developments in the scientific understanding of rheumatoid arthritis, *Arthritis Res Ther* 11(5):249, 2009.
98. Liao KP, Alfredsson L, Karlson EW: Environmental influences on risk for rheumatoid arthritis, *Curr Opin Rheumatol* 21(3):279–283, 2009.
99. Oliver JE, Silman AJ: Why are women predisposed to autoimmune rheumatic diseases? *Arthritis Res Ther* 11(5):252, 2009.
100. Song YW, Kang EH: Autoantibodies in rheumatoid arthritis: rheumatoid factors and anticitrullinated protein antibodies, *Q J Med* 103(3):139–146, 2010.
101. Bartok B, Firestein GS: Fibroblast-like synoviocytes: key effector cells in rheumatoid arthritis, *Immunol Rev* 233(1):233–255, 2010.
102. Laragione T, Shah A, Gulko PS: The vitamin D receptor regulates rheumatoid arthritis synovial fibroblast invasion and morphology, *Mol Med* 18(1):194–200, 2012.
103. Sabeh F, Fox D, Weiss SJ: Membrane-type I matrix metalloproteinase-dependent regulation of rheumatoid arthritis synoviocytes function, *J Immunol* 184:6396–6406, 2010.
104. Chung KC, Pushman AG: Current concepts in the management of the rheumatoid hand, *J Hand Surg Am* 36(4):736–747, 2011.
105. Pruijn GJ, Wiik A, van Venrooij WJ: The use of citrullinated peptides and proteins for the diagnosis of rheumatoid arthritis, *Arthritis Res Ther* 12(1):203, 2010.
106. Breedveld FC, Combe B: Understanding emerging treatment paradigms in rheumatoid arthritis, *Arthritis Res Ther* 13(Suppl 1):S3–S10, 2011.
107. Colbert RA et al: From HLA-B27 to spondyloarthritis: a journey through the ER, *Immunol Rev* 233(1):181–202, 2010.
108. Thomas GP, Brown MA: Genomics of ankylosing spondylitis, *Discovery Med* 10(52):263–271, 2010.
109. Østergaard M, Lambert RG: Imaging in ankylosing spondylitis, *Ther Adv Musculoskelet Dis* 4(4):301–311, 2012.
110. Braun J et al: 2010 update of the ASAS/EULAR recommendations for the management of ankylosing spondylitis, *Ann Rheum Dis* 70(6): 896–904, 2011.
111. Crittenden DB, Pillinger MH: The year in gout 2010-2011, *Bull NYU Hosp Joint Dis* 69(3):257–263, 2011.
112. Gonzales EB: An update on the pathology and clinical management of gouty arthritis, *Clin Rheumatol* 31:13–21, 2012.
113. Álvarez-Lario B, Macarrón-Vicente J: Is there anything good in uric acid? *QJM* 104(12):1015–1024, 2011.
114. Jordan KM: Up-to-date management of gout, *Curr Opin Rheumatol* 24(2):145–151, 2012.
115. Spanou C et al: Flavonoid glycosides isolated from unique legume plant extracts as novel inhibitors of xanthine oxidase, *PLoS One* 7(3):e32214.
116. Sjörs A et al: Physiological responses to low-force work and psychosocial stress in women with chronic trapezius myalgia, *BMC Musculoskelet Disord* 10:63–79, 2009.
117. Bennett R: Myofascial pain syndromes and their evaluation, *Best Pract Res Clin Rheumatol* 21(3):427, 2007.
118. De Franco M et al: Autonomic dysfunction and neuropeptide Y in fibromyalgia, *Clin Exp Rheumatol* 27(5 Suppl 56):S75–S78, 2009.
119. Chalaye P et al: Comparing pain modulation and autonomic responses in fibromyalgia and irritable bowel syndrome patients, *Clin J Pain* 28(6):519–526, 2012.
120. Branco JC: State-of-the-art on fibromyalgia mechanism, *Acta Rheumatol Port* 35:10–15, 2009.
121. Buskila D: Developments in the scientific and clinical understanding of fibromyalgia, *Arthritis Res Ther* 11(5):242, 2009.
122. Nebel MB, Gracely RH: Neuroimaging of fibromyalgia, *Rheum Dis Clin North Am* 35(2):313–327, 2009.
123. Xiao Y, He W, Russell IJ: Genetic polymorphisms β2-adrenergic receptor relate to guanosine protein-coupled stimulator receptor dysfunction in fibromyalgia syndrome, *J Rheumatol* 38(6):1095–1103, 2011.
124. Wolfe et al: The American College of Rheumatology preliminary diagnostic criteria for fibromyalgia and measurement of symptom severity, *Arthritis Care Res (Hoboken)* 62(5):600–610, 2010.
125. Smith MT, Moore BJ: Pregabalin for the treatment of fibromyalgia, *Expert Opin Pharmacother* 13(10):1527–1533, 2012.
126. Hassett AL, Williams DA: Non-pharmacological treatment of chronic widespread musculoskeletal pain, *Best Pract Res Clin Rheumatol* 25(2):299–309, 2011.
127. Carruthers BM et al: Myalgic encephalomyelitis: international consensus criteria, *J Intern Med* 270:327–338, 2011.
128. Nijs J et al: Pain in patients with chronic fatigue syndrome: time for specific pain treatment? *Pain Physician* 15(5):E677–E686, 2012.
129. Medow MS et al: Modulation of the axon-reflex response to local heat by reactive oxygen species (ROS) in subjects with chronic fatigue syndrome, *J Appl Physiol*, 2012 Nov 8. [Epub ahead of print.].
130. Centers for Disease Control and Prevention: *Toolkit: fact sheets for healthcare professionals: basic CFS overview*. Available at www.cdc.gov/cfs/toolkit.htm. Accessed June 6, 2009.
131. Calvani R et al: Mitochondrial pathways in sarcopenia of aging and disuse muscle atrophy, *Biol Chem*, 2012 Nov 21. [Epub ahead of print.].
132. Fanzani A et al: Molecular and cellular mechanisms of skeletal muscle atrophy: an update, *J Cachexia Sarcopenia Muscle* 3(3):163–179, 2012.
133. Goldspink G: Age-related loss of muscle mass and strength, *J Aging Res* 2012:158279, 2012.
134. Tan SV et al: Refined exercise testing can aid DNA-based diagnosis in muscle channelopathies, *Ann Neurol* 69(2):328–340, 2011.
135. Lanner JT: Ryanodine receptor physiology and its role in disease, *Adv Exp Med Biol* 740:217–234, 2012.
136. Tricarico D, Camerino DC: Recent advances in the pathogenesis and drug action in periodic paralyses and related channelopathies, *Front Pharmacol* 2:8, 2011.
137. Lin SH, Huang CL: Mechanism of thyrotoxic periodic paralysis, *J Am Soc Nephrol* 23(6):985–988, 2012.
138. Guran T et al: Clinical and molecular characterization of Turkish patients with familial hypomagnesaemia: novel mutations in TRPM6 and CLDN16 genes, *Nephrol Dial Transplant* 27(2):667–673, 2012.
139. Rolim AL et al: Ion channelopathies in endocrinology: recent genetic findings and pathophysiological insights, *Arq Bras Endocrinol Metabol* 54(8):673–681, 2010.
140. Angelini C: State of the art in muscle glycogenoses, *Acta Myologica* 29:339–342, 2010.
141. Kishnani PS, Beckemeyer AA, Mendelsohn NJ: The new era of Pompe disease: advances in the detection, understanding of the phenotypic spectrum, pathophysiology, and management, *Am J Med Genet C Semin Med Genet* 160(1):1–7, 2012.
142. Landau ME et al: Exertional rhabdomyolysis: a clinical review with a focus on genetic influences, *J Clin Neuromuscul Dis* 13(3):122–136, 2012.
143. Liang WC, Nishino I: State of the art in muscle lipid diseases, *Acta Myol* 29(2):351–356, 2010.
144. Raychaudhuri SP, Mitra A: Polymyositis and dermatomyositis: disease spectrum and classification, *Indian J Dermatol*(5):366–370, 2012.
145. Kim G-T et al: Expression of TLR2, TLR4, and TLR9 in dermatomyositis and polymyositis, *Clin Rheumatol* 29(3):273–279, 2010.
146. Greenberg SA: Dermatomyositis and type 1 interferons, *Curr Rheumatol Rep* 12(3):198–203, 2010.
147. Askanas V, Engel WK, Nogalska A: Inclusion body myositis: a degenerative muscle disease associated with intra-muscle fiber multi-protein aggregates, proteasome inhibition, endoplasmic reticulum stress and decreased lysosomal degradation, *Brain Pathol* 19(3):493–506, 2009.
148. Weihl CC, Pestronk A: Sporadic inclusion body myositis: possible pathogenesis inferred from biomarkers, *Curr Opin Neurol* 23(5): 482–488, 2010.
149. Amato AA, Barohn RJ: Inclusion body myositis: old and new concepts, *J Neurol Neurosurg Psychiatry* 80(11):1186–1193, 2009.
150. Schiopu E et al: Predictors of survival in a cohort of patients with polymyositis and dermatomyositis: effect of corticosteroids, methotrexate and azathioprine, *Arthritis Res Ther* 14(1):R22, 2012.
151. Gosiengfiao Y, Reichek J, Walterhouse D: What is new in rhabdomyosarcoma management in children? *Paediat Drugs* 14(6):389–400, 2012.

CHAPTER

45

Alterations of Musculoskeletal Function in Children

Kristen Lee Carroll and Lynne M. Kerr

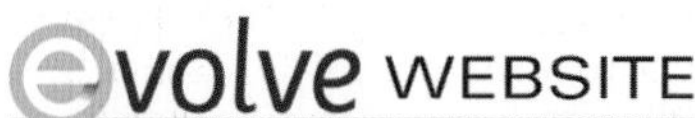

http://evolve.elsevier.com/McCance/

- Review Questions and Answers

CHAPTER OUTLINE

Musculoskeletal alterations in children are very common. They may be congenital, such as clubfoot; hereditary, such as muscular dystrophy; or acquired, such as Legg-Calvé-Perthes disease. Some of these disorders are acute, and the child will recover completely; other disorders are chronic or, in some cases, terminal. An understanding of the pathophysiology of these alterations will aid in providing the best care possible for these children.

MUSCULOSKELETAL DEVELOPMENT IN CHILDREN

Bone Formation

Bone formation, which begins at about the sixth week of gestation, involves two phases: (1) the delivery of bone cell precursors to sites of bone formation and (2) the aggregation of these cells at **primary centers of ossification,** where they mature and begin to secrete osteoid (see Chapter 43). Some of the bone cell precursors are present in fetal connective tissues, whereas others migrate in blood to sites of bone formation after blood vessels have grown into the tissue.

Cellular aggregation and maturation occur in two types of fetal tissue, depending on which bones are being formed. The cranium, facial bones, clavicles, and parts of the jawbone (classically called "flatbones") arise from a fetal membrane termed the *mesenchyme.* Bones that develop on or within the mesenchyme grow by the process of **intramembranous formation of bone.** As the mesenchyme becomes vascularized, the immature bone cells aggregate and mature into osteoblasts, which form the centers of ossification and create solid bone or osteoid.

Endochondral formation of bone is the development of new bone from cartilage (Figure 45-1). First, mesenchymal tissue forms a **cartilage anlage,** which defines the shape of the bone. This is usually found by 6 weeks of gestation. Blood vessel invasion to inside the anlage brings osteoprogenitor cells leading to primary centers of calcification by 8 weeks. Endochondral bone formation begins in the outer layer of the cartilage model, which consists of a layer of dense connective tissue called **perichondrium.** The perichondrium contains cells that develop into osteoblasts, forming a collar of bone, termed the **periosteal collar,** around the cartilage model. Cartilage enclosed within the periosteal collar degenerates, and capillaries from outside the

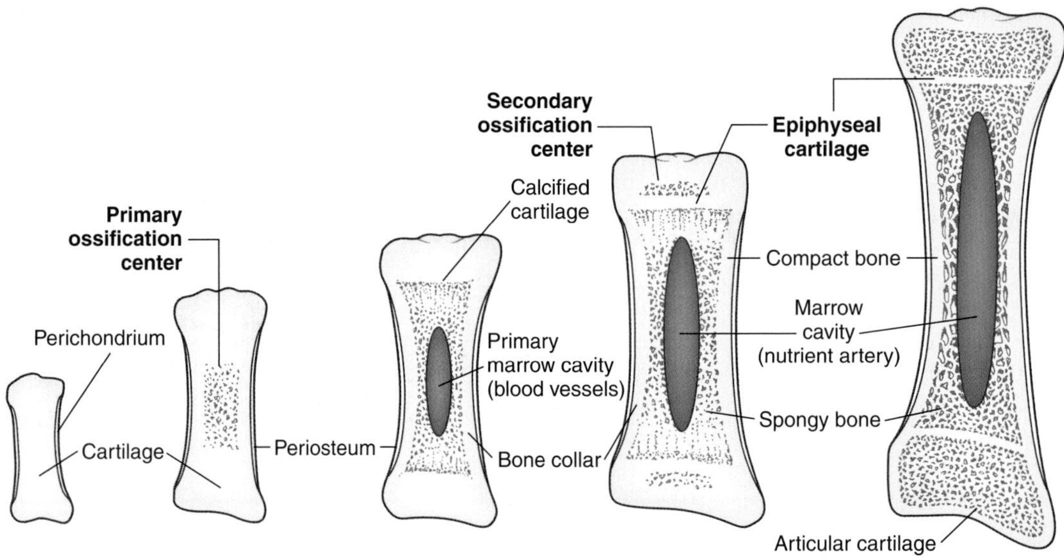

FIGURE 45-1 Stages of Endochondral Bone Formation and Centers of Ossification in Long Bone.

perichondrium invade the degenerating cartilage cells, carrying with them osteoblast precursors from the inner layer of the perichondrium and osteoclast precursors from the blood itself.

Endochondral bone formation progresses at the primary center of ossification in the middle of the cartilage model and extends toward either end of the developing bone. At the same time, the periosteal collar thickens and becomes wider toward the epiphyses. By the end of gestation **secondary centers of ossification** (i.e., the epiphyseal centers) begin to lay down bone at both ends of the cartilage model. Here, too, cartilage within the periosteal collar degenerates, and blood vessels grow inward, delivering bone cell precursors. Once the osteoblasts begin to secrete osteoid, ossification spreads from the secondary centers in all directions until all the cartilage within the model is replaced by bone.

Two regions of cartilage remain at the ends of long bones: (1) articular cartilage over the free ends of the bone, and (2) the physeal plate, a layer of cartilage between the metaphysis and epiphysis. (These structures are described and illustrated in Chapter 43; see Figure 43-3.) The physeal plate retains the ability to form and calcify new cartilage and deposit bone until the skeleton matures approximately 1 year after sexual maturity (11 to 15 years of age in females, 15 to 18 in males).

Bone Growth

Until adult stature is reached, growth in the length of long bones occurs at the physeal plate through endochondral ossification. Cartilage cells at the epiphyseal side of the physeal plate multiply and enlarge. As rapidly as new cartilage cells form, cartilage cells at the metaphyseal side of the plate are destroyed and replaced by bone.

In the shaft of new bone, where growth is relatively slow, the bone produced by accretion is compact and dense. The compact bone is thickest where it has to withstand the maximal stresses, which generally occur in the middle of the shaft.

The two physes of the long bone often have varying activity rates. For example, the distal physis in the femur contributes 80% of the overall length, whereas the proximal physis at the hip contributes only 20%. The more active of the two has more power to remodel deformity but also can be more sensitive to injury. The architecture of the physis also dictates its sensitivity to injury. The distal femur, for example, has an undulating pattern that increases its resistance to sheer force; when injured, however, growth disturbance is highly likely, whereas the distal radius, which contributes 80% of overall radial length, is a flat, smooth physis that is far more resistant to traumatic injury.

Growth in the diameter of bone occurs by deposition of new bone on an existing bone surface. Bone matrix is laid down by osteoblasts on the periosteal surface and subsequently becomes calcified. At the same time, bone resorption occurs on the endosteal surface. Endosteal resorption increases the diameter of the medullary cavity, which contains marrow and spongy bone.

Many factors affect the development, physiology, and rate of growth of the epiphyseal plate. Growth hormone must be secreted by the pituitary gland at a constant rate to stimulate the growth plate consistently. Other known factors affecting growth include peptide regulatory factors (e.g., fibroblast growth factor [FGF]); changes in cell-to-cell interactions through cell adhesion molecules (CAMs) and cell junctions; and complex interactions or changes in the extracellular matrix (ECM), nutrition, general health, and other hormones (e.g., thyroid hormone, adrenal and gonadal androgens, estrogens). When these factors are poorly controlled, skeletal dysplasias, such as achondroplasia, can occur.

Even after physeal closure at skeletal maturity, bone is constantly being destroyed and re-formed (see Chapter 43). This is a rapid process in young children, allowing them to heal bone injury more quickly than adults. By adulthood, however, bone turnover, or remodeling, occurs at a relatively slow rate. Peak bone mass is achieved by the middle to late twenties and slowly decreases throughout life; therefore, ensuring appropriate levels of calcium and phosphorous intake, performing weight-bearing lifting and exercise, and minimizing caffeine intake are especially important for a young female if she is to avoid osteoporosis in later life. Recently, the importance of vitamin D levels also has been emphasized. In one study, nearly 70% of American children had low levels of vitamin D.[1]

Skeletal Development

The axial skeleton changes shape with growth. (The axial skeleton and appendicular skeleton are described and illustrated in Chapter 43; see Figure 43-5). In a newborn the entire spine is concave anteriorly, or **kyphosed.** In the first 3 months of life, with the infant's ability to control the head, the upper (cervical) spine begins to arch, or become **lordotic.** The normal lordotic curve of the lower (lumbar) spine begins to develop with sitting.

The appendicular skeleton (the extremities) grows faster during childhood than does the axial skeleton (see Figure 43-5). The newborn has a relatively large head and long spine with disproportionately shorter limbs than an adult. By 1 year of age, 50% of the total growth of the spine has occurred and is more than 70% complete by age 8.[2] Therefore, failure of the spine to grow (e.g., spinal fusion) does not limit eventual height as much as the premature fusion of the growth plates of the lower extremities. In children with congenital curvature of the spine, growth tends to worsen the deformity rather than to increase the length of the spine.

Besides getting longer, growing bones of the extremities undergo changes in rotation and alignment. In the newborn the proximal femur is rotated forward up to 40 degrees and the tibia is rotated inward. With growth the femur assumes its normal alignment (by 12 years of age) and tibial rotation neutralizes at 8 years of age.[3] Bowlegs and knock knees can be normal at certain stages of growth. At birth the newborn's legs are bowed because of stresses in utero. **Genu varum (bowleg)** reaches a peak by 30 months of age, whereas **genu valgum (knock knee)** maximizes by 5 to 6 years of age. If genu varum or genu valgum persists past these ages, a pathologic process rather than a physiologic phase may be present. Pathologic causes of genu varum are Blount disease, rickets, skeletal dysplasias (such as achondroplastic dwarfism), and traumatic injury. Genu valgum may persist also as a result of skeletal dysplasia or genetic predisposition.

Muscle Growth

The composition and size of muscles vary with age. In the fetus, muscle tissue contains a large amount of water and much intercellular matrix. After birth, both are reduced considerably as the muscle fibers (cells) enlarge by accumulating cytoplasm. Little information is available about the numbers of fibers in a given muscle at various ages, but the total mass of muscle in the body can be estimated from the amount of creatinine excreted in the urine, because the conversion of creatine to creatinine takes place only in muscle (see Chapter 43). Between birth and maturity the number of muscle nuclei in the body increases 14 times in boys and 10 times in girls. Muscle fibers reach their maximal size in girls at approximately 10 years of age and in boys by 14 years. Growth in length occurs at the ends of muscles, and the increase in length is accompanied by an increase in number of nuclei in the fibers. Muscle fibers increase in diameter as the fibrils become more numerous. The fibrils themselves do not increase in diameter. Connective tissue components of muscle grow where the tendon and muscle meet.

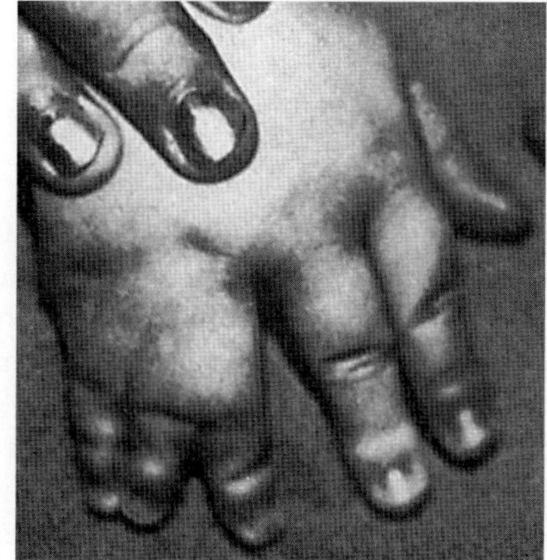

FIGURE 45-2 Syndactyly with Polydactyly.

A potent stimulus to the growth of a muscle is the separation of its attachments as the skeleton grows. The length of a muscle fiber is the direct consequence of its intended range of movement. The stimulus for the formation of a tendon is probably the pull of the muscle rudiment on undifferentiated connective tissue. If the normal opponents of a muscle are paralyzed, the muscle fails to grow properly and can result in contracture of a joint.

Muscle growth during adolescence is a major factor in weight gain. Gender differences in muscle size and weight are minor in childhood but become considerable with the onset of puberty.

In the infant, muscle accounts for approximately 25% of total body weight, compared with 40% in the adult. In the adult, approximately 55% of muscle weight is in the lower limb muscles, whereas in the infant the majority of the weight is axial musculature. The respiratory and facial muscles are well developed at birth so that the infant can perform the vital functions of breathing and sucking. Other muscle groups, such as the pelvic muscles, take several years to develop fully. Throughout life the weight of the skeletal muscles can be increased by exercise.

MUSCULOSKELETAL ALTERATIONS IN CHILDREN

Congenital Defects

Syndactyly

The most common congenital defect of the upper extremity is **syndactyly,** or webbing of the fingers (Figure 45-2). Simple webbing involves the soft tissue envelope alone and is best released surgically when the child is 6 months to 1 year of age. Complex syndactyly involves fusion of the bones and nails as well as the soft tissues; it may be associated with absence or anomaly of bony or neurovascular units. The primary goal in surgical correction of these defects is to achieve maximal function and appearance. Ideally, corrective surgery is deferred until the child is 1 to 2 years old and completed before the child enters school. **Vestigial tabs,** such as an extra digit, however, are best removed during the immediate neonatal period. Anomalies on the radial aspect of the arm, such as a foreshortened or absent radius, are often associated with abnormalities of blood, heart, or kidneys. Lateral or ulnar-sided defects are less often associated with systemic anomalies and are far more rare.

Developmental Dysplasia of the Hip

Developmental dysplasia of the hip (DDH), formerly known as congenital dislocation of the hip, is an abnormality in the development of the proximal femur, acetabulum, or both (Figure 45-3). Although most often present at birth, it may occur at any time in the newborn or infant period.

The incidence of true dislocation of the hip or a dislocatable hip is 1 in 1000 live births. Some degree of instability of the hip is present in approximately 10 per 1000 live births. The left hip is affected in 60% of cases, whereas the right hip alone is affected only 20% of the time. Bilateral DDH occurs 20% of the time.

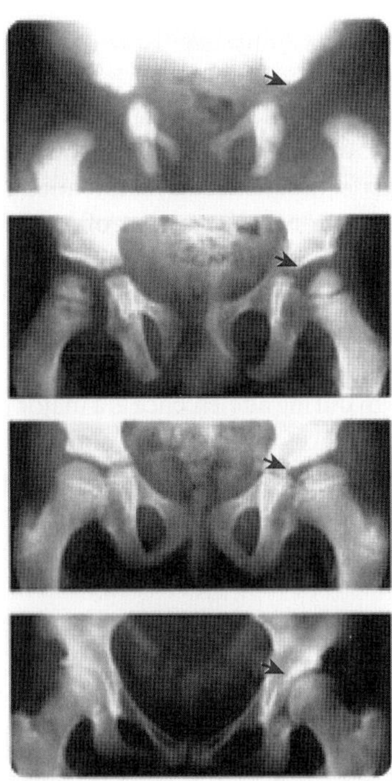

FIGURE 45-3 **Hip Dysplasia in Children.** Developmental dysplasia of the hip (DDH) with residual acetabular dysplasia. Radiographs at birth, 3, 10, and 19 years (top to bottom) show persisting dysplasia.

Risk factors for DDH include family history, female gender (6:1), metatarsus adductus (20%), torticollis (10%), oligohydramnios, first pregnancy, and breech presentation. First pregnancies and oligohydramnios (deficient volume of amniotic fluid) are thought to limit fetal movement, and breech presentation not only limits movement but also places the hips in a position of flexion and adduction, which creates a more shallow socket, or acetabulum. Although only 2% of births have breech history, as many as 40% of infants with DDH had a breech birth. Maternal hormones that reportedly increase joint laxity also have an effect on DDH, although the exact mechanism is unknown. DDH also is more common in whites and those cultures that swaddle infants with the hips in extension and adduction. It is almost unknown in African cultures where infants are carried, with legs abducted, on the back.

PATHOPHYSIOLOGY. The hip can be described as subluxated (partial contact only), dislocated (no contact between femoral head and acetabulum), and acetabular dysplasia (the femoral head is located properly but the acetabulum is shallow) (Figure 45-4). The **subluxated hip** maintains contact with the acetabulum but is not well seated within the hip joint. The acetabulum is often dysplastic (or shallow) although the femur is often normal. The **dislocatable hip** is sometimes located but can be dislocated easily. The dislocated hip has no contact between the femoral head and the acetabulum. Some degree of **acetabular dysplasia** is present in almost all cases. Typically the acetabulum is shallow or sloping rather than cup shaped.

By approximately 10 weeks of gestation, the femur, acetabulum, and hip joint capsule are well developed. It appears that most dysplasias occur within the second and third trimesters and are often the result of positioning factors. Experimentally, DDH can be produced in laboratory animals by placing the developing hip in adduction and extension, replicating the breech position. There is, however, a genetic component that is poorly understood. In addition, 2% of DDH cases are teratologic or caused by a systemic syndrome, such as arthrogryposis or spina bifida, in which muscle contracture or imbalance leads to DDH.

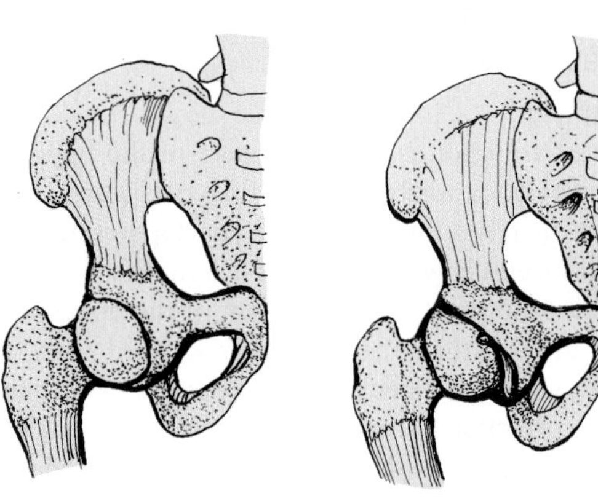

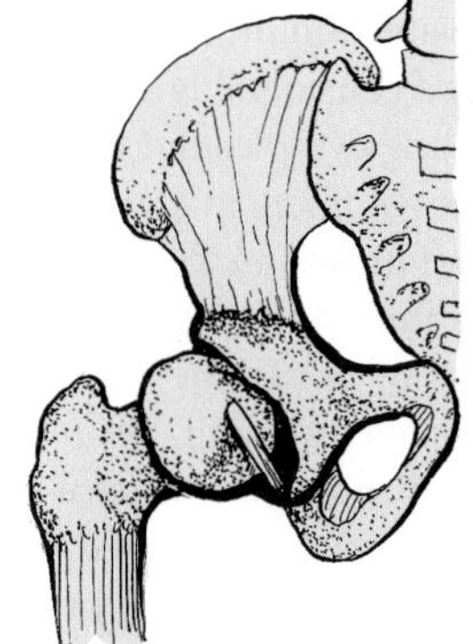

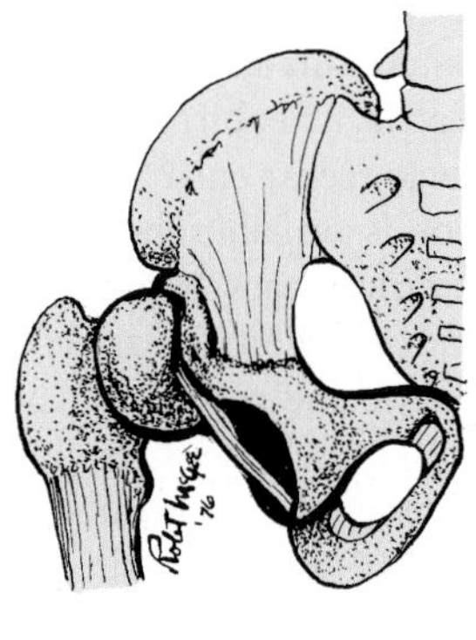

FIGURE 45-4 **Configuration and Relationship of Structures in Developmental Dysplasia of the Hip.** (From Hockenberry MJ, Wilson D: *Wong's nursing care of infants and children,* ed 9, St Louis, 2011, Mosby.)

If DDH is left untreated in the growing child, secondary changes occur. If the hip remains subluxated or dislocated, the acetabulum becomes increasingly shallow and the soft tissues shorten around the proximal femur. Subluxation leads to early osteoarthritis (OA), and it is now estimated that at least 60% of all OA of the hip is related to DDH. If the hip is dislocated, the bone acetabulum fills with soft tissue and a false acetabulum forms where the femoral head contacts the iliac crest. An apparent limb length inequity and hip muscle weakness occurs, leading to a waddling gait. Back pain and hip pain develop in adulthood. Adult reconstruction of a dislocated hip, even with an artificial hip, is very difficult.[4]

CLINICAL MANIFESTATIONS. The clinical manifestations of DDH vary with the severity of the condition and the age of the child. Signs and symptoms that should be noted include the following:

1. Asymmetry of gluteal or thigh folds
2. Limb length discrepancy (Galeazzi sign)
3. Limitation of hip abduction
4. Positive Barlow maneuver (hip reduced, but dislocatable) (Figure 45-5, *A*)
5. Positive Ortolani sign (hip dislocated, but reducible) (Figure 45-5, *B*)
6. Positive Trendelenburg gait (waddling)
7. Pain (very late)

The child also should be examined for other anomalies, such as torticollis or metatarsus adductus, which can be associated with DDH.

EVALUATION AND TREATMENT. In the newborn period clinical examination is the most important diagnostic tool. Real-time ultrasound, in which the hip is examined while the ultrasound is performed, also is extremely valuable in the newborn period, especially in high-risk infants. The use of ultrasound allows visualization of the cartilaginous structures of the hip (the femoral head and the outer lip of the acetabulum), which are not seen on plain roentgenogram. Radiographs are used after age 6 months when the ossific nucleus of the femoral head appears.[5]

Treatment depends on the age of the child, severity of dysplasia, and duration of dysplasia. The earlier that treatment is begun, the better the result. In children less than 4 months of age, a Pavlik harness can brace the hip in abduction and flexion, and the acetabulum will remodel as the femoral head rests centered in the socket (Figure 45-6). With this treatment, up to 98% of children will have an excellent result. A "closed" reduction (without opening the joint) followed by spica or body casting for up to 3 months can be done in children up to 12 months of age. After 12 months, surgical intervention—including opening the joint and cutting and realigning the femur and/or acetabulum—may be required. As the child ages, the percentage of good outcomes decreases. Up to 70% of children treated surgically for DDH after age 3 develop early osteoarthritis.[6] Early intervention before age 1 is critical for a good outcome; therefore, vigilance for this problem within the first year is essential.

Deformities of the Foot

Congenital Deformity. Congenital foot deformity is found in approximately 4% of all newborns, and metatarsus adductus

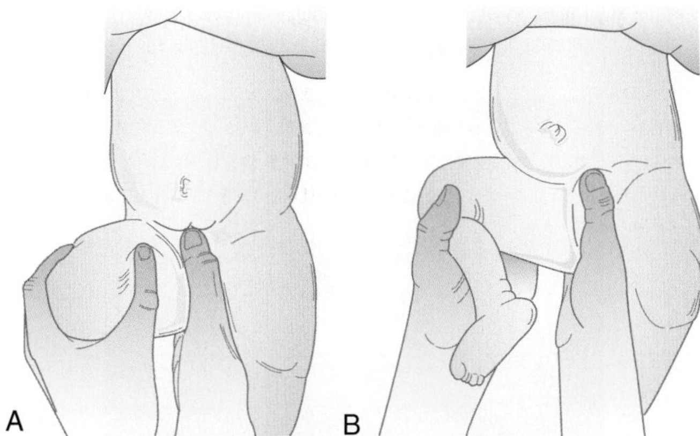

FIGURE 45-5 Congenital Dislocation of the Hip. A, Barlow maneuver. With one hand pressing the symphysis in front and the sacral spine in back, lateral pressure is applied to the thigh with the thumb of the other hand while pressure is applied with the palm to the knee on the side being examined. The hip that has been flexed to 90 degrees is then adducted. A positive sign is a sensation of abnormal movement, indicating dislocation of the femoral head from the acetabulum. The hands are reversed for examining the other hip. This sign and Ortolani sign may be found only in the first weeks of life. **B,** Ortolani maneuver. Sign of jerking into correct position. After the Barlow maneuver **(A),** the hip should be abducted to about 80 degrees while the femur is lifted anteriorly with the fingers along the thigh. A positive sign is a sensation of a jerk or snap with reduction into the joint socket. (Adapted from Specht EE: *Am Fam Physician* 9:88–96, 1974.)

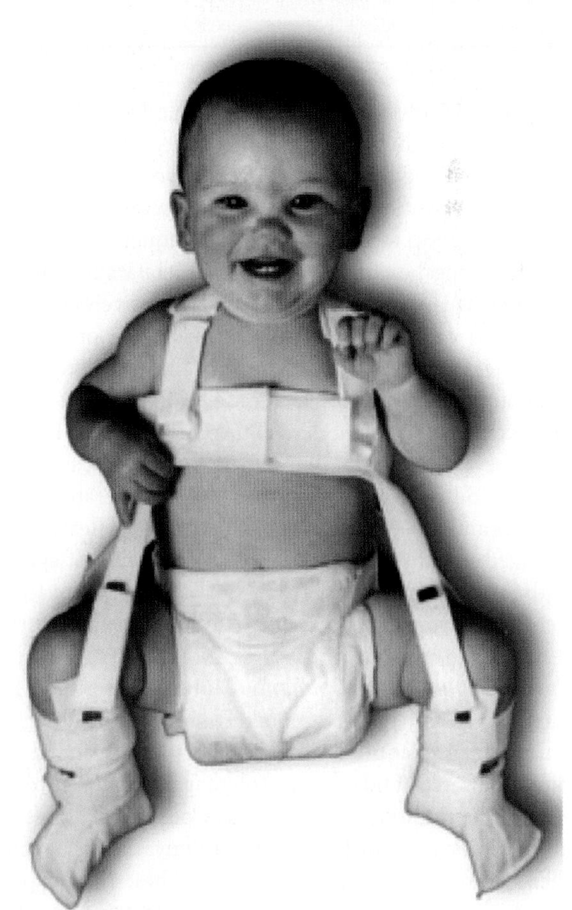

FIGURE 45-6 Pavlik Harness for Bilateral Hip Dislocation. (From Wheaton Brace Co.)

TABLE 45-1 TERMS USED TO DESCRIBE FOOT ABNORMALITIES

TERM	DEFINITION
Position	
Abduction	Lateral deviation away from the midline of the body
Adduction	Lateral deviation toward the midline of the body
Eversion	Twisting of the foot outward along its long axis
Inversion	Twisting of the foot inward on its long axis
Dorsiflexion	Bending the foot upward and backward
Plantar flexion	Bending of the foot downward and forward
Abnormality	
Talipes	Congenital abnormality of the foot (clubfoot)
Pes	Acquired deformity of the foot
Varus	Inversion and adduction of the heel and forefoot
Valgus	Eversion and abduction of the heel and forefoot
Equinus	Plantar flexion of the foot in which the heel is lower than the toes
Calcaneus	Dorsiflexion of the foot in which the heel is lower than the toes
Planus	Flattening of the medial longitudinal arch of the foot (flatfoot)
Cavus	Elevation of the medial longitudinal arch of the foot (high arch)
Equinovarus	Coexistent equinus and varus deformities
Calcaneovarus	Coexistent calcaneus and varus deformities
Equinovalgus	Coexistent equinus and valgus deformities
Calcaneovalgus	Coexistent calcaneus and valgus deformities

accounts for 75% of these deformities (Table 45-1). **Metatarsus adductus** is a forefoot adduction deformity associated with a normal, plantigrade hindfoot and is believed to be secondary to intrauterine positioning. It is associated with developmental dysplasia of the hip in 20% of cases; consequently, the hips of these infants must be carefully evaluated. Metatarsus adductus is usually classified by two criteria: flexibility (passively correctable or rigid) and degree of deformity. The degree of deformity (mild, moderate, severe) is ascertained by the heel bisection line. A mild deformity is one in which the heel bisection line passes medial to the third toe; moderate, through the third or fourth toes; and severe, lateral to the fourth toe. Serial casts during the first 6 months of life are suggested for moderate to severe deformities and those deformities that appear less flexible. Casts are changed weekly for 6 to 12 weeks. By 6 years of age, 87% of children usually correct spontaneously, and 95% by 15 years of age. Even in those children with some residual deformity, functional symptoms are rare.

Clubfoot: Equinovarus Deformity. **Clubfoot** describes a range of foot deformities in which the foot turns inward and downward. Technically called **equinovarus,** the heel is positioned varus (inwardly deviated) and equinus (plantar flexed) (Figures 45-7 and 45-8). The clubfoot deformity can be positional (correctable passively), idiopathic, or teratologic equinovarus (as a result of another syndrome, such as spina bifida). These three types are discussed in the following sections. Overall, the true positional equinovarus lends itself to rapid correction by application of serial casts. The idiopathic variety is treated by attempting

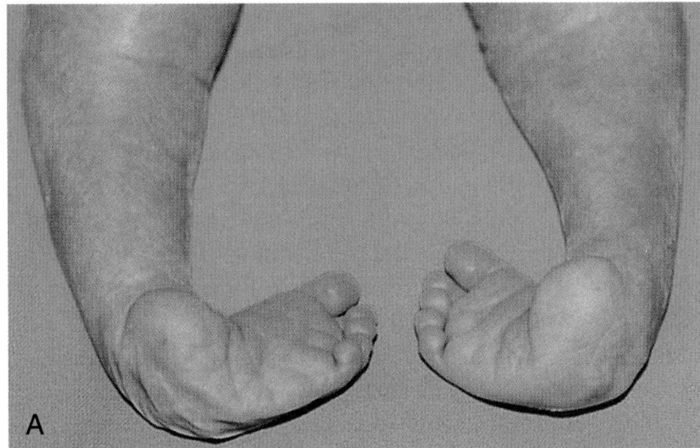

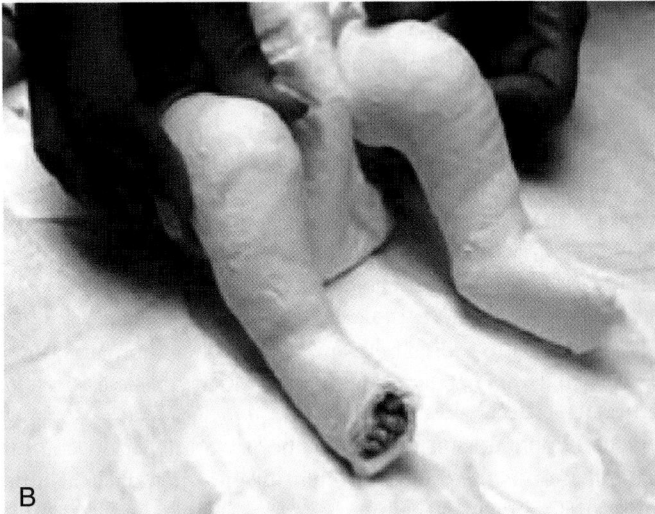

FIGURE 45-7 Bilateral Clubfoot. A, Infant with bilateral congenital talipes equinovarus. **B,** Ponseti casting. (**A** courtesy of Dr. a.E. Chudley, Section of Genetics and Metabolism, Department of Pediatrics and Child Health, Children's Hospital and University of Manitoba, Winnipeg, Manitoba, Canada. In Moore KL, et al: *The developing human,* ed 9, Philadelphia, 2013, Saunders.)

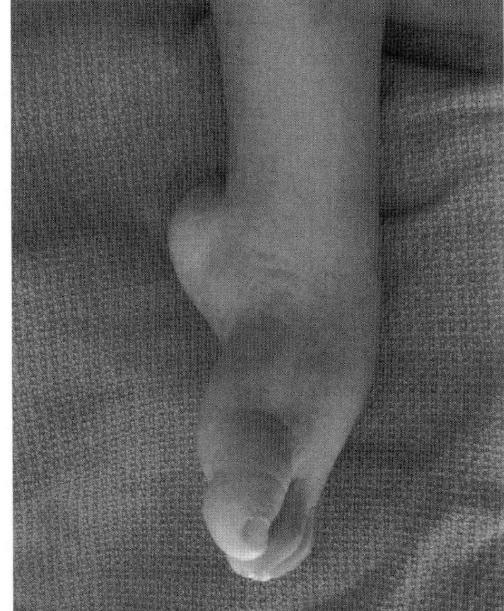

FIGURE 45-8 Idiopathic Clubfoot. Idiopathic clubfoot displaying forefoot adduction (toward midline of body) and supination (upturning) and hindfoot equinus (pointed downward). Note skin creases along arch and back of heal.

cast correction, followed by surgical intervention of resistant deformities. Teratologic equinovarus nearly always requires surgical correction and/or muscle balancing procedures.

Positional Equinovarus. Positional equinovarus is a deformity in which an infant's foot is in equinovarus position but does have flexibility without deep creases at the posterior ankle or midfoot. The Achilles tendon is still flexible. The foot can be passively brought to a plantigrade position and is amenable to casting. In general, 1 to 3 months of serial above-knee casting corrects this foot without the need for surgical intervention or lengthy bracing.

Idiopathic Congenital Equinovarus. The etiology of idiopathic equinovarus (clubfoot) is unknown. In one human fetal study, all clubfeet were associated with identifiable anterior horn cell changes in L5 and S1. Muscle biopsies of both the anterior tibialis long flexors and the peroneus brevis muscles in clubfoot reveal that at least 50% of cases show a decreased number of muscle fibers and/or abnormal fiber histology. The soleus often has an increase in type 1 fibers, whereas the peroneus brevis has a fiber type disproportion. The more abnormal the histopathology, the more severe the deformity, and the greater the chance of recurrent deformity after treatment. The genetic component is unclear and studies are ongoing.

Idiopathic equinovarus occurs in approximately 1 of every 1000 live births, with males being affected twice as often as females. Historically, these deformities were treated by posteromedial release, a surgical procedure that lengthened all tight structures and opened the capsule of all tight joints in the foot. However, since 1998 the casting technique developed by Ignacio Ponseti (see Figure 45-7, *B*) has been used; the technique involves six to eight above-knee casts, left on for 5 to 7 days each, followed by a percutaneous tendoachilles lengthening procedure performed with local anesthesia. The child then uses special braces at night until 3 years of age. Noncompliance with braces leads to increased recurrence and need for additional casting or surgery. Nearly 30% of children may need an anterior tibialis transfer around age 3.[7] Studies comparing operative posteromedial release with Ponseti techniques show better long-term results with less invasive Ponseti method[8] (Box 45-1).

Teratologic Equinovarus. The most common causes of **teratologic equinovarus** are either neuromuscular (such as spina bifida) or syndromic, as in arthrogryposis or osteochondrodysplasia (such as diastrophic dwarfism). The teratologic clubfoot, unlike the idiopathic type, more often fails to be corrected with Ponseti casting and may require operative intervention. The surgery is often more extensive than that for an idiopathic clubfoot, and revision surgery is also more common (Box 45-1).

Pes Planus (Flatfoot) Deformity. Pes planus (flatfoot) commonly raises parental concern. Despite medical evidence to the contrary, it can be very difficult to convince families that a flexible flatfoot is often as functional as one with a "normal" arch. The majority of babies are born with flat (or "fat") feet, with the arch becoming more apparent with age. The relatively benign natural history, however, should not overshadow the importance of accurate diagnosis. Significant ankle valgus, vertical talus, tarsal coalition, and skewfoot must be accurately differentiated from flexible pes planus.

BOX 45-1 PONSETI CASTING

Ponseti casting implements toe-to-groin casts changed weekly for 6 weeks. Casting begins as early as possible after birth and culminates in a percutaneous tendoachilles lengthening in the clinic, followed by a final cast worn for 3 weeks. In recalcitrant cases, a full surgical posteromedial release (PMR) still may be required. The need for PMR in idiopathic clubfoot has decreased from 90% to less than 20% of infants when this casting technique is used. Long-term results, presumably because of less scarring and more long-term flexibility, are better with Ponseti casting than the PMR method.

Flexible flatfoot deformity appears to be familial, with occasional association of generalized ligamentous laxity. Careful evaluation of possible occult Achilles contracture is done by holding the hindfoot in varus position and dorsiflexing the ankle. Achilles contracture can signify a more severe flatfoot variant. The flexibility of the hindfoot is evaluated by having the child stand on his or her toes facing away from the examiner. In flexible pes planus, the hindfoot swings into a varus position as the planter fascia tightens in toe raise. In rigid pes planus, the hindfoot stays in valgus and the child has more difficulty going up onto tip-toe.

The surgical or orthotic treatment of *asymptomatic* flexible pes planus is unnecessary. Custom orthotics, Helfet heelcups, and corrective orthopedic shoes have no influence over the natural history (clinically or radiographically) of flat feet. Adult studies on army recruits have shown that soldiers with flat feet perform just as well as their counterparts without "fallen" arches.

There is a small subset of children with painful flexible flat feet. For these children careful attention to the possibility of Achilles contracture or tarsal coalition (congenital union of the hindfoot bones) must be made. This group of children is best treated with inexpensive shoe inserts and then expectantly watched. If pain continues into adolescence, requiring more aggressive treatment, calcaneal lengthening will correct the pes planus without decreasing hindfoot motion. In rigid flat feet, a computed tomographic (CT) scan often will reveal a coalition, a bony or cartilaginous connection between the bones—if painful, this can be resected. Heel cord contractures can be surgically lengthened if stretching alone is inadequate. All surgery carries risk; if a foot is flat but nonpainful, treatment is not required. The painless flatfoot should be viewed as a variation of normal feet.

Abnormal Density or Modeling of the Skeleton

Osteogenesis Imperfecta

Osteogenesis imperfecta (OI) (brittle bone disease) is a spectrum of disease caused by genetic mutation in the gene that codes for type I collagen, the main component of bone and blood vessels. The disorder was first described in 1840 as a syndrome in newborns that consisted of osteoporosis with fractures and skeletal deformities. The Sillence classification is based on both models of inheritance and clinical findings (Table 45-2). In the most severe form of this disorder, the child is usually stillborn or dies soon after birth, although some survive into childhood. OI in its more severe forms is evident at birth because fractures and deformity have occurred in utero. The less severe forms may not become evident until the child begins to walk.

TABLE 45-2 SILLENCE CLASSIFICATION OF OSTEOGENESIS IMPERFECTA SYNDROMES

TYPE	TRANSMISSION	MAIN BIOCHEMICAL DEFECT	ORTHOPEDIC	MISCELLANEOUS
IA	AD	Decreased production of type I collagen	Mild to moderate bone fragility, osteoporosis, normal stature	Blue sclera, hearing loss, easy bruising, dentinogenesis imperfecta absent
IB	AD		Short stature	More severe in IA with dentinogenesis imperfecta
II	AD, AR, and mosaic	Substitutions of glycyl residue in X1 or X2 chains in triple helix	Multiple intrauterine fractures, extreme bone fragility	Usually lethal in perinatal period, delayed ossification of skull, intrauterine growth restriction
IIA			Long bones broad, crumpled; ribs broad with continuous beading	
IIB			Long bones broad, crumpled; ribs discontinuous or beading	
IIC			Long bones thin, fractured; ribs thin, beaded	
IID			Severely osteoporotic with generally well-formed skeleton; normal-shaped vertebrae and pelvis	
III	AD and AR	Abnormal type I collagen	Progressive deforming phenotype, severe bone fragility with fractures	Hearing loss, short stature, blue sclerae becoming less blue with age, shortened life expectancy, dentinogenesis imperfecta, relative macrocephaly with triangular facies
IVA	AD	Shortened pro-α (I)-chains	Mild to moderate bone fragility, osteoporosis, bowing of long bones, scoliosis	Light sclerae, normal hearing, normal dentition, dentinogenesis imperfecta absent
IVB	AD			Dentinogenesis imperfecta present

AD, Autosomal dominant; *AR,* autosomal recessive.

Some children with this milder form then experience numerous fractures and can be mistaken for nonaccidental trauma until the diagnosis is made.

The prevalence rate of the most common form is about 1 in 30,000. Inheritance is usually autosomal dominant but can be autosomal recessive. At least four syndromes have been identified that have various clinical manifestations and prognoses (see Table 45-2).

PATHOPHYSIOLOGY. The major errors in OI lie in the synthesis of collagen, a triple helix with two matching alpha chains and one beta chain. Collagen is present in bone, cartilage, eye tissue, skin, and the vascular system. The severity of the OI phenotype and the related anomalies of the eye, dentition, or vascular system are all dependent on the severity of the genetic anomaly and the part of the triple helix that is affected.[9] (Genes are discussed in Chapter 4.)

A number of metabolic abnormalities are associated with OI. Some individuals have increased serum thyroxine levels, suggesting hyperthyroidism. This is consistent with the findings of increased sweating, heat intolerance, increased body temperature, a resting tachycardia, and tachypnea. Studies of leukocyte metabolism suggest an uncoupling of oxidative phosphorylation. Reports of alterations of platelet function with defects in adhesion and clot retraction also exist.

CLINICAL MANIFESTATIONS. The classic clinical manifestations of OI are osteoporosis and increased rate of fractures, possible bony deformation, triangular facies, possible vascular weakness (i.e., aortic aneurysm), possible blue sclerae, and poor dentition. The Sillence classification designated types I through IV on the basis of severity. The most severe, types II and III, are comparable to *osteogenesis imperfecta congenita.* These two types are characterized by autosomal recessive inheritance and early onset of manifestations. Both can cause stillbirth or severe neonatal deformity and a short life expectancy. Less severe are types I and IV, which are comparable to *osteogenesis imperfecta tarda.* Type I is slightly more common than types II and III, and type IV is quite rare. Types I and IV are inherited as autosomal dominant traits and vary in age of onset from birth to adulthood. Type IV, especially when the sclerae are white, is the least deforming type and is often confused with nonaccidental trauma (child abuse).

EVALUATION AND TREATMENT. Evaluation of OI is based primarily on clinical manifestations. Serum alkaline phosphatase level is elevated in all forms of the disease. OI can be diagnosed prenatally by ultrasound or chorionic villi sampling. Quantitative analysis of cultured skin fibroblast collagen by electrophoresis shows a decreased quantity of collagen in 95% of individuals.

Type II OI is often terminal in the perinatal period, and therefore little is known about appropriate treatment for the few children who survive. For other types of OI, careful positioning and handling of the newborn help prevent fractures. Beyond the neonatal period, various orthopedic measures are

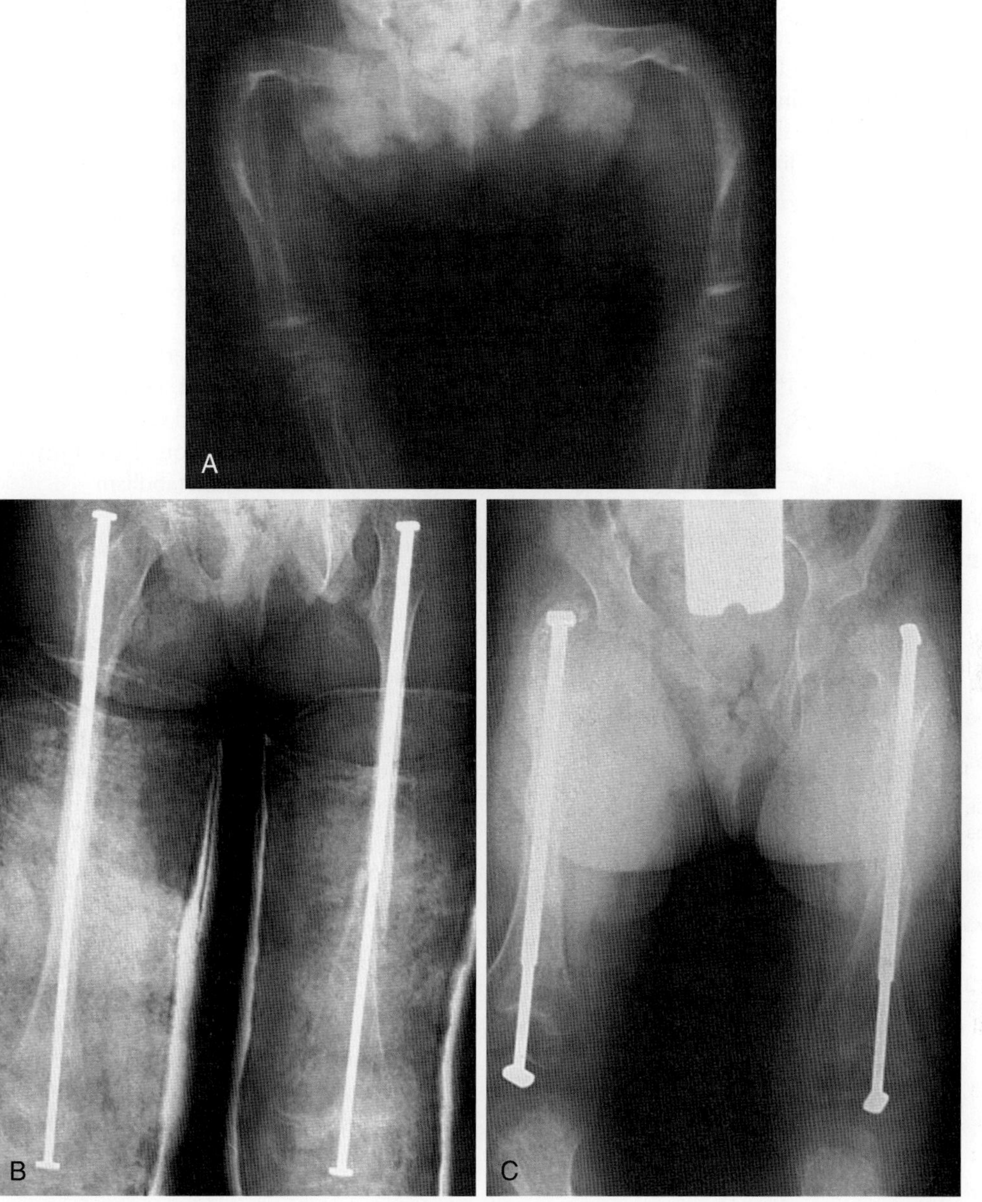

FIGURE 45-9 Osteogenesis Imperfecta Treated with Osteotomies and Telescoping Medullary Rods. **A,** Severe deformity of both femurs. **B,** Same individual after multiple osteotomies with telescoping medullary rod fixation. **C,** Same individual 4 years later demonstrating growth of femurs, no recurrence of deformity, and elongation of rods. (Plaster casts are in place for immobilization of tibial osteotomies.) (From Crenshaw AH, editor: *Campbell's operative orthopaedics,* ed 8, vol 3, St Louis, 1992, Mosby.)

applied, such as prompt splinting of fractures and correction of deformities arising from the progressive bowing or bending of the skeleton by intramedullary rodding of the bones (Figure 45-9). Newer, telescoping rods, which grow with the child, have been shown to reduce the reoperative rate by 30%.[10] Scoliosis is present in up to 50% of Sillence III cases and often requires surgery. A multicenter study of a bisphosphonate therapy showed promising results in type III OI, with marked improvements of bone density (up to 30%). Despite these results, there is concern that the healing of fractures and surgical intervention can be more difficult. More study is needed to address the efficacy and safety of these types of drugs. Genetic counseling for affected families should aim at primary prevention.

Rickets

Rickets is a disorder in which growing bone fails to become mineralized (ossified), resulting in "soft" bones and skeletal deformity (Figure 45-10). Rickets results from either insufficient vitamin D, insensitivity to vitamin D, wasting of vitamin D by the kidney, or inability to absorb vitamin D and calcium in the gut. The most common form is X-linked hypophosphatemic rickets in industrialized nations. In addition to the severe form of metabolic rickets, dietary and lifestyle changes in the United States have led to widespread vitamin D deficiency in children.[11] Although unprotected exposure to ultraviolet rays is not suggested, children still need 15 to 20 minutes per week of true sun exposure to activate vitamin D, the mineral necessary for absorption and metabolism of calcium and phosphate. In one recent study up to 90% of *normal* American children had a low vitamin D level, especially children of color. This can lead to early fracture or slow bone healing after fracture.[12]

Severe metabolic rickets in the immature skeleton leads to short stature and bowing of the limbs with broad, irregular growth plates. The rows of cells in the growth plate that are intended to ossify fail to do so as they reach the metaphysis since calcification is impeded.

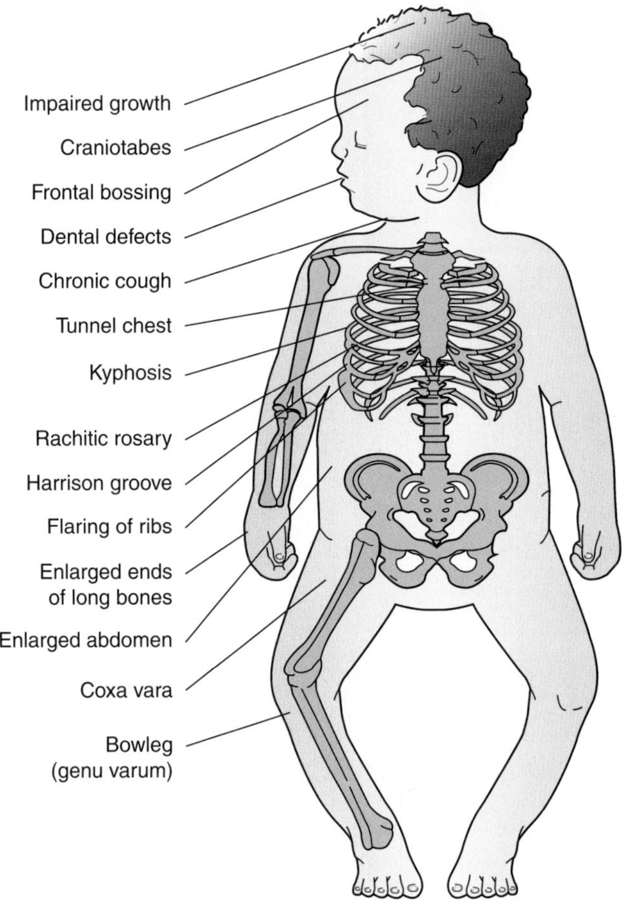

FIGURE 45-10 Rickets.

Children with rickets are often listless and irritable. They have hypotonia and muscle weakness and may be unable to walk without support. Abnormal parietal flattening and frontal bossing occur in the skull. The calvaria become soft, and the sutures may widen. Cartilaginous attachments of the ribs become prominent, and the long bones of the extremities (tibia, femur, radius, ulna) may be bowed. Growth is restricted, and fractures are common.

Like osteogenesis imperfecta, surgical treatment of bony deformity can be required. However, medical management of calcium, phosphorous, and vitamin D levels must be optimized before surgical intervention. Deformity often improves with normalization of bone metabolism.

Scoliosis

Scoliosis is a rotational curvature of the spine most obvious in the anteroposterior plane (Figure 45-11). It can be classified as nonstructural or structural. **Nonstructural scoliosis** results from a cause other than the spine itself, such as posture, leg length discrepancy, or pain. **Structural scoliosis** is curvature of the spine associated with vertebral rotation. Nonstructural scoliosis can become structural if the underlying cause is not found and treated.

Structural scoliosis can be caused by a great variety of conditions. It can result from congenital skeletal abnormalities (15%), neuromuscular diseases (15%), trauma, extraspinal contractures, bone infections that involve the vertebrae, metabolic bone disorders (e.g., rickets, osteoporosis, osteogenesis imperfecta), joint disease, and tumors. Most cases of structural scoliosis, however, have no known cause, although genetic factors are suggested. Structural scoliosis with no known cause, termed **idiopathic scoliosis,** accounts for at least 70% of cases.

Idiopathic scoliosis is classified as infantile, juvenile, or adolescent, depending on the child's age at the time of onset. In infantile scoliosis, spinal curvature develops during the first

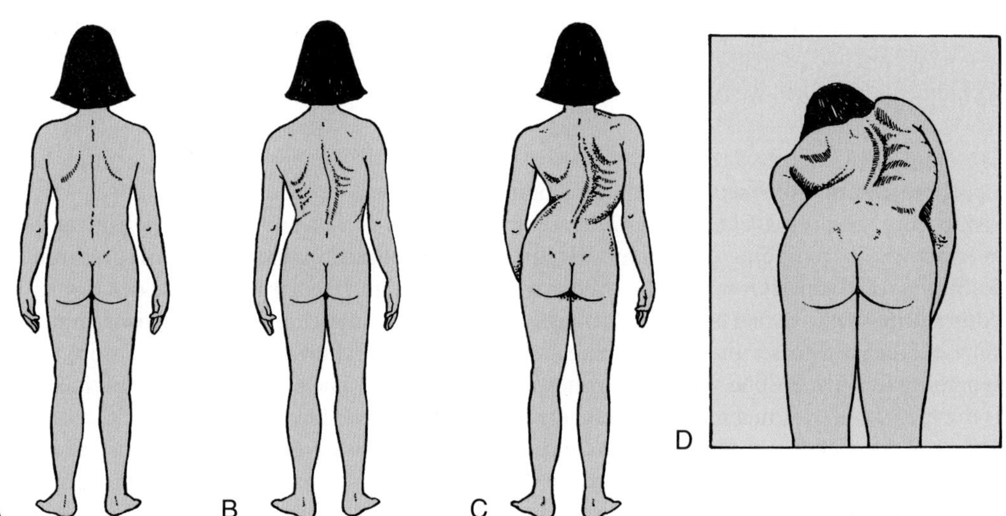

FIGURE 45-11 Scoliosis in Children. Normal spinal alignment and abnormal spinal curvatures associated with scoliosis. **A,** Normal. **B,** Mild. **C,** Severe. **D,** Rotation and curvature of scoliosis.

3 years of life; in juvenile scoliosis, curvature develops between the skeletal age of 4 years and the onset of adolescence; and in adolescent scoliosis, it develops after the skeletal age of 10. Adolescent idiopathic scoliosis is the most common. Scoliosis in its milder forms occurs equally in boys and girls; once curves measure more than 15 degrees, however, girls are five times more likely to have scoliosis than boys.

PATHOPHYSIOLOGY. It has been hypothesized that in individuals with adolescent scoliosis, there is an abnormality of the central nervous system involving the balance mechanism (reticular system) in the midbrain. A genetic component is also suggested because 30% occur within families.

Experimentally it also has been shown that individuals with adolescent idiopathic scoliosis have an abnormality in the function of the posterior columns of the spinal cord. This results in abnormal proprioception and is not evident clinically except in the presence of scoliosis. The exact cause of scoliosis, however, remains elusive.[13]

The earliest pathologic changes, which are probably secondary changes, occur in the soft tissues. The muscles, ligaments, and other soft tissues become shortened on the concave side of the curve. Vertebral deformity occurs as asymmetric forces are applied to the epiphyseal center of the ossification by shortened and tight soft tissues on the concave side of the curve. True curves involve not only bending but also twisting of the torso leading to the "rib hump" seen when the child bends forward.

The curves increase most rapidly during periods of rapid skeletal growth. If the curve is less than 40 degrees at skeletal maturity, the risk of progression is quite small. In curves greater than 50 degrees, the spine is biomechanically unstable, and the curve usually progresses even after the cessation of growth. Curves in the thoracic spine greater than 80 degrees result in decreased pulmonary function, whereas the most common complication of large curves in the lumbar spine is back pain.

CLINICAL MANIFESTATIONS. The clinical manifestations of nonstructural scoliosis are mild spinal curvature with prominence of one hip or rounded shoulders. The curvature disappears with forward flexion of the spine, lying down, or traction of the head. Treatment for nonstructural scoliosis is correction of the underlying disorder. The clinical manifestations of structural scoliosis include asymmetry of hip height, asymmetry of shoulder height, shoulder and scapular (shoulder blade) prominence, and rib prominence.

EVALUATION AND TREATMENT. Spinal curvature is usually visible or palpable, and muscles on one side of the lower back (the convex side) may be prominent or bulging. Most cases of idiopathic scoliosis are noticed during school screening programs. In girls the deformity may be noticed because clothing does not "hang" properly on the body. Diagnosis is made by roentgenographic examinations.

Treatment of curves greater than 20 degrees in the skeletally immature child is with bracing. In most cases a low-profile thoracolumbar brace is used. Low-profile braces are worn for 22 hours per day until skeletal maturity. Bracing will only prevent progression of the curve; it will not correct the curvature. Bracing is not effective in large curves or in skeletally mature individuals; the most effective time for bracing is in growing prepubescents with a small curve.[14] Extensive chiropractic manipulations and electrical stimulation have not been shown to change natural history. Surgical treatment with spinal fusion with instrumentation is recommended for curves greater than 40 to 50 degrees. If surgery is indicated, it is better performed during the adolescent years while there is greater flexibility of the curves and less risk of complications.

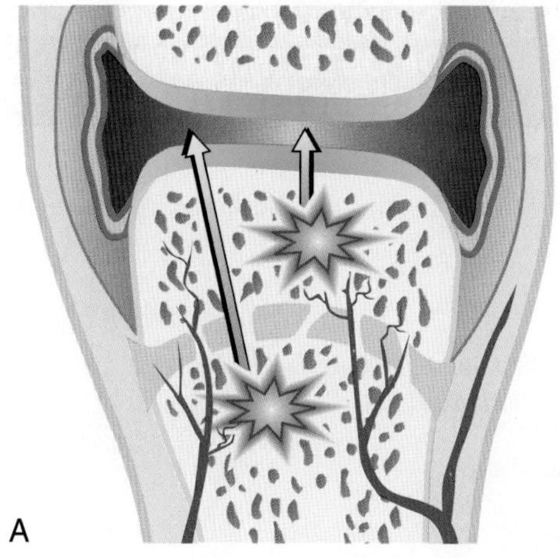

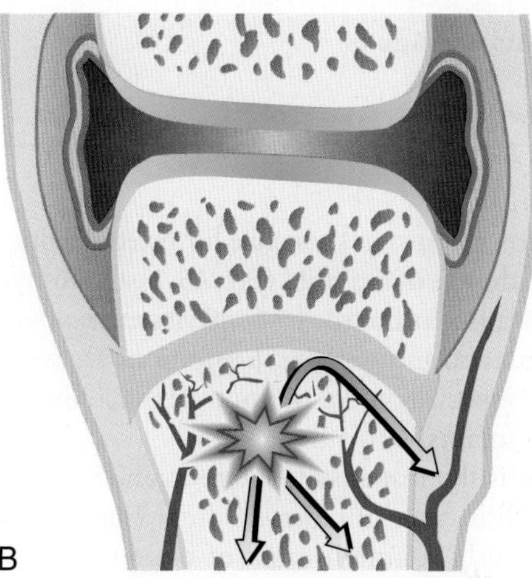

FIGURE 45-12 Pathogenesis of Acute Osteomyelitis Differs with Age. **A,** In infants younger than 1 year the epiphysis is nourished by penetrating arteries through the physis, allowing development of the condition within the epiphysis. **B,** In children up to 15 years of age the infection is restricted to below the physis because of interruption of the vessels.

Bone Infection: Osteomyelitis

Osteomyelitis is an infection of the bone. Occurring twice as often in males as females, acute osteomyelitis may affect infants and children of any age, but it occurs most often between 3 and 12 years of age.

Bacteria enter the bone through the bloodstream and lodge in the medullary cavity, where a rich phagocytic mechanism often prevents most of the bacteria from establishing an infectious state. In some cases, however, the bacteria may lodge at the end of the venous loops beneath the epiphyseal plate, and infection then develops because there are no phagocytic cells present to remove the bacteria[15-17] (Figure 45-12).

BOX 45-2 CAUSATIVE MICROORGANISMS OF OSTEOMYELITIS ACCORDING TO AGE

Newborns
Staphylococcus aureus
Group B streptococcus
Gram-negative enteric rods

Infants
S. aureus (MSSA 70, MRSA 30)
Haemophilus influenzae

Older Children
Staphylococcus aureus
Pseudomonas
Salmonella
Neisseria gonorrhoeae

Adolescents and Adults
Pseudomonas
Mycobacterium tuberculosis

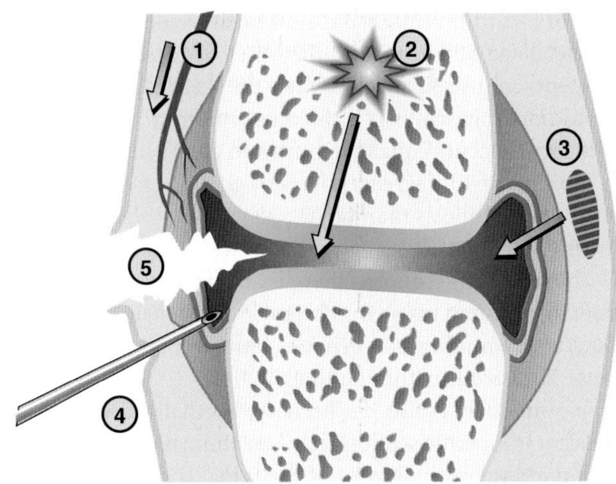

FIGURE 45-13 Routes of Infection to the Joint. **(1)** The hematogenous route; **(2)** dissemination from osteomyelitis; **(3)** spread from an adjacent soft tissue infection; **(4)** diagnostic or therapeutic measures; **(5)** penetrating damage by puncture of cutting.

The microorganism responsible for osteomyelitis varies and is related to the age of the child (Box 45-2). Osteomyelitis in the newborn is caused primarily by *Staphylococcus aureus.* Group B streptococcus and *Escherichia coli* infections are responsible for some cases, especially those of multiple bone involvement and in high-risk infants.[17]

S. aureus is the responsible microorganism in 80% to 90% of osteomyelitis cases in older children. *Haemophilus influenzae,* a previously common cause of osteomyelitis in children less than 5 years of age, has become rare with the improvements in immunization. However, cases of methicillin-resistant *Staphylococcus aureus* (MRSA) have risen alarmingly in the past 5 years. Once an infrequent cause of childhood osteomyelitis, MRSA now causes up to 30% of new cases.[18] Gram-negative microorganisms account for an increasing number of infections of the vertebrae,[19,20] whereas *Salmonella* infections are associated with sickle cell disease.

Factors that predispose an individual to the development of osteomyelitis include impetigo, furunculosis, infected lesions of varicella (chickenpox), infected burns, cerebral abscesses, immunization with bacille Calmette-Guérin (BCG) vaccine, prolonged intravenous or central parenteral alimentation, drug addiction, and direct trauma to the area adjacent to the site of osteomyelitis.

PATHOPHYSIOLOGY. Osteomyelitis usually begins as a bloody abscess in the metaphysis of the bone. The abscess ruptures under the periosteum and spreads along the bone shaft or into the bone marrow cavity if untreated. Infection rarely spreads down the medullary cavity of the bone but rather first gains entrance to the subperiosteal space in the metaphysis. The bone cortex in this area is porous, allowing easier entry for the bacteria than the shaft of the bone.[21] Because of the accumulation of debris caused by the infection, the periosteum may separate and form a shell of new bone around the infected portion of the shaft. Because the periosteum is separated from an adequate blood supply, sections of the bone die; these pieces of dead bone are called **sequestra.** The periosteum that maintains a blood supply generates new bone and is responsible for the appearance of the periosteal new bone, or **involucrum.** The presence of the sequestra and involucrum indicates that the disease is highly aggressive or established.

In cases in which the infection in the metaphysis occurs near the joint, the accumulating pus (bacteria, white blood cells, fluid) creates increasing pressure that may cause a rupture into the joint cavity. If rupture into the joint occurs, the pus causes inflammation and a condition called **secondary septic arthritis.**[19] Studies show that up to 40% of children will have adjacent joint involvement with osteomyelitis. The most common joint to be affected is the knee. Osteomyelitis is most commonly caused by bacteria that reach the metaphysis through the bloodstream but may occur through secondary inoculation of microorganisms caused by trauma or contagious spread of infection from cellulitis in adjacent soft tissue.

Osteomyelitis in infants is often associated with septic arthritis because the infant's bone has blood vessels that perforate the growth plate. Because of the unique nature of the blood supply to an infant's bones, the occurrence of osteomyelitis and septic arthritis in combination is higher than 50%. Normal anatomic variations in infants allow infection to spread directly to the epiphysis, which causes both joint disease and permanent injury to the growth plate. Multiple sites of osteomyelitis are also common in children younger than 2 years of age. Other areas of osteomyelitis and possibly septic arthritis must be evaluated through a bone scan of the entire skeleton.[22]

Children are susceptible to joint involvement for several reasons (Figure 45-13). In the immature infant, there is no epiphyseal plate or an ossific nucleus at the end of the bone and the cartilage precursor of bone is penetrated by vascular channels.

In these infants the infection begins in the vulnerable cartilage precursor of the end bone itself and results in rapid destruction of the joint and arrested growth of the bone. For this reason the early detection and treatment of osteomyelitis are crucial if the infant's joint is to be saved from destruction. As the child matures and the epiphyseal, or growth, plate forms, a temporary barrier is established against infection because the arterioles end beneath the epiphyseal plate.[21]

In children older than 2 years, the epiphyseal plate prevents the spread of a metaphyseal abscess into the epiphysis and the cortex of the metaphysis is thicker. These anatomic differences increase the likelihood that the metaphyseal abscess will extend into the diaphysis, and the blood supply of the bone will be disrupted. The periosteum is also more difficult to perforate in older children; this may lead to a larger subperiosteal abscess that could endanger the periosteal blood supply as well. This process results in extensive sequestrum formation and chronic osteomyelitis.[21]

Osteomyelitis is much less common after the physeal plates are closed, except in the vertebral body. Infection may develop in any part of a bone, and abscesses spread slowly. Destruction of the cortex in a localized area may result in a pathologic fracture.[19,20]

Spread of infection to contiguous joints is related to the child's age. Metaphyseal infection may spread to contiguous joints if the fibrous joint capsule includes the metaphysis and epiphysis. This special situation exists at the hip joint, distal femur, proximal humerus and radius, and lateral ankle. Careful clinical vigilance helps protect children with osteomyelitis from suffering permanent joint injury. Unlike bone, the articular cartilage of joints is unable to repair itself after injury from infection.[22]

CLINICAL MANIFESTATIONS. The clinical manifestations of osteomyelitis are age dependent and are related to the differing vascular patterns found in the skeletal system at various ages. Three distinct groups may be identified: (1) infants younger than 1 year, (2) children from 1 year of age to puberty, and (3) adolescents after cessation of bone growth and adults.

Infants

Osteomyelitis may be an acute illness characterized by fever and failure to move the affected limb (pseudoparalysis). Infantile osteomyelitis is characterized by involvement of multiple sites within the same bone or in multiple bones. If untreated, involvement of the adjacent growth plate can result in growth arrest.

Children

Osteomyelitis in children between the ages of 1 year and puberty is characterized by fever and systemic signs of toxicity. The illness is sometimes subacute, with the child complaining of swelling, fever, tenderness, and decreasing ability to bear weight on or move the affected area. Onset can be abrupt. Osteomyelitis during childhood most often affects the long bones but also may be found in the pelvis and spine. Clinical manifestations are usually accompanied by elevated white blood cell counts and elevated erythrocyte sedimentation rates. When the level of C-reactive protein (CRP) is elevated, it a sensitive sign of osteomyelitis and can rapidly decrease with appropriate treatment. Evidence of infection using roentgenograms can be delayed but bone scan is positive within 48 hours.

Adolescents and Adults

In addition to the sites previously mentioned, osteomyelitis in adolescents and adults may involve the vertebrae. Back pain, with a duration of several weeks, may be the only clinical complaint. This age group is less often affected than younger populations.

EVALUATION AND TREATMENT. White blood cell counts and erythrocyte sedimentation rates are sometimes elevated, but this is not a consistent finding. Monitoring of erythrocyte sedimentation rates is an indication of response to management but can be delayed. CRP is more quickly responsive to appropriate treatment. Blood cultures (positive in 30% to 40%) and aspiration of the soft tissue or bone, or both, should be done to identify the causative microorganism. Appropriate antibiotics should be prescribed *after* culture and sensitivity studies have been completed. A tuberculin test also is administered because *Mycobacterium tuberculosis* is sometimes responsible and has had a slight resurgence in incidence. Bone scans can be quite helpful with diagnosis and in children younger than 1 year are absolutely required to define whether multiple sites are involved.

Treatment includes intravenous (IV) antibiotics or, in highly reliable children and families, a combination of IV and oral antibiotics for 6 weeks. Drainage and margination of bone is required if changes are present on radiographs signifying abscess. Immobilization may help with pain control. If a joint is also infected (termed "septic arthritis"), the situation becomes a *surgical emergency;* surgery on the affected joint can help prevent damage to the articular cartilage by lysozymes released from the involved neutrophils.

Death is rare, but serious sequelae may occur. The course of the disease and prognosis depend on the age of the child, the rapidity with which the diagnosis is established, the initiation of early treatment, and maintenance of treatment for an adequate time. The most serious complications are growth arrest, osseous necrosis, and recurrence. Recurrence with presently available antibiotic regimens is less than 10%.

Juvenile Idiopathic Arthritis

The rheumatic diseases are a group of diverse conditions having in common the inflammation of connective tissues. They include juvenile idiopathic arthritis (JIA, formerly known as juvenile rheumatoid arthritis), systemic lupus erythematosus, dermatomyositis, and progressive systemic sclerosis (formerly called scleroderma). The incidence of these disorders in children is estimated in Table 45-3.

Juvenile idiopathic arthritis (JIA) is the childhood form of rheumatoid arthritis (RA) (see Chapter 43). Like adult-onset RA, JIA is a syndrome that is often accompanied by systemic manifestations. Approximately 5% of all cases of RA begin in childhood. An estimated 250,000 children in the United States have JIA.

TABLE 45-3 INCIDENCE OF CONNECTIVE TISSUE DISEASES IN CHILDREN

DISEASE	ANNUAL RATE/10^5	GENDER RATIO (FEMALE/MALE)	RACE RATIO (WHITE/BLACK)	PEAK AGE GROUP AT RISK (yr)	CHILDHOOD ONSET (%)
Rheumatoid arthritis	40	3:1	Equal	Increases with age (20-50)	5
Systemic lupus erythematosus	6	8:1	1:4	15-45	18
Dermatomyositis	0.8	2:1	1:3	45-65	20
Progressive systemic sclerosis	0.4	3:1	Equal	Increases with age (30-50)	3
Polyarteritis	0.2	1:3	Equal	Midadult	Rare

Data from Hollingworth P. In Klippel JH, Dieppe PA, editors: *Rheumatology,* St Louis, 1994, Mosby.

The basic pathophysiology of JIA is the same as that of adult RA. The clinical manifestations of JIA may differ, however, beginning with mode of onset. Unlike adult RA, which begins insidiously with systemic signs of inflammation and generalized aches, JIA has three distinct modes of onset: arthritis in fewer than five joints (pauciarticular arthritis), arthritis in more than five joints (polyarticular arthritis), and systemic or Still disease. JIA differs from the adult form in the following respects[23,24]:

1. Predominantly the large joints are affected.
2. Subluxation and ankylosis of the cervical spine are common if the disease progresses.
3. Joint pain may not be severe, as in the adult type.
4. Serologic tests often detect antinuclear antibody (ANA).
5. Chronic uveitis is common, especially if ANA positive.
6. Serologic tests seldom detect rheumatoid factor.
7. Rheumatoid nodules are not limited to subcutaneous tissue but are found in the heart, lungs, eyes, and other organs.
8. Cyclic citrullinated peptide antibody is often positive.

Treatment for children with JIA is supportive but not curative. Many children with pauciarticular arthritis who are seronegative for ANA will resolve their symptoms over time. However, with systemic onset (Still disease) or seropositivity, JIA may progress to true adult RA. The aims of treatment are to control inflammation and other clinical manifestations of the disease and to minimize deformity.

Avascular Diseases of the Bone: Osteochondrosis

The avascular diseases of the bone, collectively termed **osteochondroses,** are caused by insufficient blood supply to growing bones. Disturbances of blood supply to primary and secondary centers of ossification during periods of rapid bone growth result in a variety of skeletal abnormalities.

The cause of the osteochondroses remains obscure. In the past, infection, nutritional deficiencies, and hormonal imbalances were blamed, but these causes have been largely disproved. Currently, vascular impairment and trauma, coupled with an underlying developmental or genetic predisposition, have been identified as probable causes of osteochondroses. The most common osteochondroses are Osgood-Schlatter disease (tibial tubercle), Sinding-Larsen-Johansson syndrome (distal patellar pole), Panner disease (radial head), Kohler disease (the navicular bone of the foot), and Sever disease (calcaneus). All are associated with activity-related pain of the affected region that improves with rest. All are more common in boys than girls and in athletes more than nonathletes.

The osteochondroses involve areas of significant tensile or compressing stress that undergo partial osseous necrosis, progressive bony weakness, and then microfracture. Most of these are associated with trauma and overuse and improve with rest. Use of anti-inflammatories, modification of activities, and even immobilization of the affected area are used during active stages of the disease. Reparative correction by revascularization is the rule, although this may be a lengthy process.

Legg-Calvé-Perthes Disease

Legg-Calvé-Perthes (LCP) disease, commonly called Perthes disease, is classically thought to be an osteochondrosis like those previously described. This self-limited disease of the hip is presumably produced by recurrent interruption of the blood supply to the femoral head. The ossification center first becomes necrotic and collapses and then is gradually remodeled by live bone.

LCP disease is relatively common (1 in 5000 children), usually occurring in children between 3 and 10 years of age, with a peak incidence at 6 years. It is more common in boys than in girls by a ratio of about 5:1. The condition is bilateral in approximately 10% of affected children; however, bilateral cases are temporally separated. If LCP disease appears at identical stages and the femoral heads show matched radiographic involvement, then another diagnosis, such as an epiphyseal dysplasia, should be considered.

The cause of decreased blood supply to the head of the femur is unknown. Several theories have been proposed, including trauma, infection, and protein C and S deficiencies, which cause a hypercoagulable state or vascular anomolies.[25] A plausible theory is that acute synovitis (infection of the synovial membrane) and increased hydrostatic pressure in the hip joint compress blood vessels that supply the femoral head.

Constitutional factors definitely play a role. Skeletal maturation is delayed an average of 2 years in children with LCP disease, and affected children are between 2.5 and 7 cm shorter than unaffected children of the same age. Familial occurrence is 30% to 40%. The disease is rare in blacks, and it is frequent in children of Japanese and central European ancestry.

PATHOPHYSIOLOGY. LCP disease runs its natural course in 2 to 5 years. In the initial stage the soft tissues of the hip (synovial membrane and joint capsule) are swollen, edematous, and hyperemic, often with fluid present in the joint (Figure 45-14). The joint space widens, and the joint capsule bulges. The first stage lasts only a few weeks. In the second stage, called

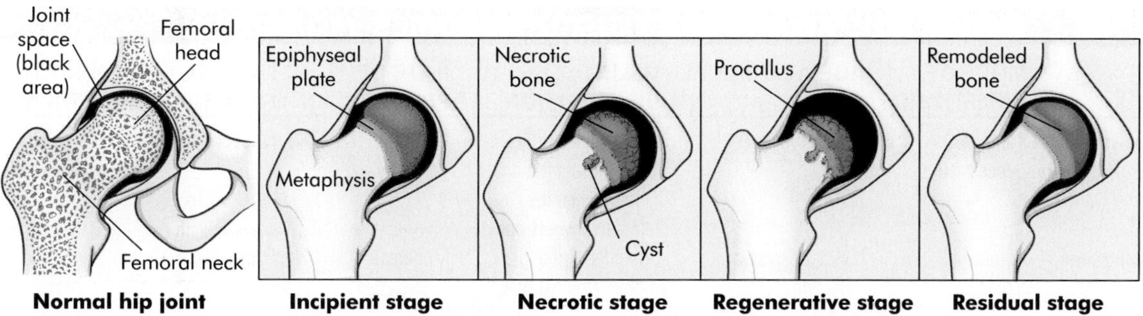

FIGURE 45-14 Stages of Legg-Calvé-Perthes Disease, a Form of Osteochondrosis.

fragmentation, the entire epiphysis or the anterior half of the epiphysis of the femoral head loses blood supply and the metaphyseal bone at the junction of the femoral neck and capital epiphyseal plate is softened because of decalcification. Soon granulation tissue (procallus) and blood vessels invade the dead bone. This stage lasts several months to 1 year.

The third (or regenerative healing) stage ordinarily lasts 2 to 3 years. The dead femoral head is replaced by procallus, and new bone is laid down. Collapse and flattening of the femoral head occur, and the femoral neck becomes short and wide (see Figure 45-14).

In the fourth (or healed) stage, remodeling takes place and the newly formed bone is organized into a live spongy bone. Children less than 6 years of age at onset have more time to remodel the damage LCP has caused and have the best outcome. Recent multicenter studies, using the Herring "lateral pillar" classification,[26] have shown that hips younger than 6 years with *no* involvement of the lateral femoral head (type A) do better than those with involvement of the lateral femoral head. Those children with complete collapse of the lateral femoral head (type C) have the worst prognosis. Long-term studies of type C hips show that 70% to 90% progress to osteoarthritis by 40 years of age.[27]

CLINICAL MANIFESTATIONS. Injury or trauma precedes the onset of clinical manifestations in approximately one third of children with LCP disease. Onset of symptoms is insidious unless trauma aggravates the disease process. The pain often is referred to the knee and can lead to misdiagnosis as a knee injury. The inner thigh and groin also can be painful. In some children, pain may be absent or minimal. If pain is present, it is usually aggravated by activity and relieved by rest.

The typical physical findings include spasm on inward rotation of the hip and a limitation of internal rotation flexion and abduction. If the child is walking, an abnormal gait, termed a Trendelenburg gait or abductor lurch, is apparent. The child dips the trunk toward the affected side with stance to compensate for weak abductor musculature. If the hip pain or limp has been present for a prolonged period, muscles of the hip and thigh atrophy. A limb length inequity may be present if the proximal femoral physis is involved.

EVALUATION AND TREATMENT. Diagnosis is confirmed by radiographic examination. Principles of treatment are *containment* (keeping the ball completely in the socket) and *motion* to maintain the articular cartilage. In the past, children were treated with bed rest and a variety of braces. Most children can be managed with anti-inflammatory medications and crutches for episodes of synovitis and with activity modification (avoidance of jumping activities that place increased stress on the hip) during the active phase of the disease. Serial roentgenograms monitor the progress of the disease and ensure that the hip remains congruent. Surgery may be necessary if the femoral head becomes subluxated or incongruent with the acetabulum before the reparative process. The ball must be congruent to take on the shape of the socket as remodeling occurs. Newer treatments, such as intra-articular injection of bisphosphonates (that reduce the function of osteoclasts), are being studied.[28]

Factors affecting the outcome of LCP disease are the age of the child at onset, the extent of necrosis, and the congruence of the joint at skeletal maturity. Recent studies have shown that girls, despite earlier skeletal maturity, do as well as boys. Outcome is 70% satisfactory with Herring stage A; for Herring stages B and C or age greater than 8 years, outcome is guarded. Present prospective studies are evaluating more aggressive early treatment (i.e., osteotomy of the femur or pelvis) on the more involved hips to change long-term outcome.

Osgood-Schlatter Disease

Osgood-Schlatter disease consists of tendinitis of the anterior patellar tendon, within which the patella (kneecap) is embedded, and associated osteochondrosis of the tubercle of the tibia. Osgood-Schlatter disease occurs most often in preadolescents and adolescents who participate in sports. The incidence is higher in boys than in girls, many of whom have increased outward tibial fusion compared to controls.[29]

PATHOPHYSIOLOGY. The severity of the lesion varies from mild tendinitis to a complete separation of the anterior extension of the tibial epiphysis, which is the part of the epiphysis that contributes to growth of the tibial tubercle. The underlying pathologic alterations also vary. The mildest form of Osgood-Schlatter disease causes ischemic (avascular) necrosis in the region of the bony tibial tubercle, with hypertrophic cartilage formation during the stages of repair. In more severe cases the abnormality involves a true epiphyseal separation of the tibial tubercle.

CLINICAL MANIFESTATIONS. The child experiences pain and swelling in the region of the patellar tendon and tibial tubercle, which becomes prominent and is tender to direct pressure. The pain is most severe after physical activity that involves vigorous

TABLE 45-4 MAJOR MUSCULAR DYSTROPHY SYNDROMES

DISEASE	MODE OF INHERITANCE	AGE AT CLINICAL ONSET	USUAL DISTRIBUTION	RATE OF PROGRESSION	MENTAL RETARDATION	DISTINGUISHING FINDINGS
Duchenne muscular dystrophy (DMD)	X-linked recessive	About 3 years	Hips and shoulders, quadriceps femoris, gastrocnemius (pseudohypertrophy)	Rapid	Frequent	Elevated serum enzymes (CPK, LDH, SGOT, aldolase)
Facioscapulohumeral dystrophy	Autosomal dominant	In first or second decade	Shoulder girdle, neck, face, pelvic girdle (late)	Moderate	Occasional	Several distinct muscle pathologic findings
Limb girdle (LG) dystrophy	Poorly defined or recessive	Variable	Pelvic and shoulder girdles	Variable	Variable	Collection of several diseases
Myotonic dystrophy (MyD)	Autosomal dominant	Variable—birth to fifth decades	Distal extensor muscle, eyelids, face, neck, hands, pharynx	Slow, related to age at clinical onset, faster with younger patients	Frequent	Percussion myotonia, cataracts, diabetic GTT despite increased insulin, testicular atrophy, decreased IgG

quadriceps contraction or direct local trauma to the tibial tubercle area. Often the child experiences sudden acute discomfort referable to the affected region. Sudden onset of pain can represent a pathologic fracture through an area of ischemic necrosis.

EVALUATION AND TREATMENT. Diagnosis is confirmed by roentgenographic examination. The goal of treatment for Osgood-Schlatter disease is to decrease the stress at the tubercle. Often a period of 4 to 8 weeks of restriction from strenuous physical activity is sufficient. If pain relief is not achieved, a cast or brace is required to immobilize the knee, a situation that is particularly difficult if the condition is bilateral.

Gradual resumption of activity is permitted after 8 weeks, but return to unrestricted athletic participation requires an additional 8 weeks to allow for revascularization, healing, and ossification of the tibial tubercle. All types of osteochondroses resolve once skeletal maturity is reached.

Cerebral Palsy

Cerebral palsy (CP) is a general term that refers to nonprogressive disorders of movement and posture resulting from injury or malformation of the developing central nervous system. The resulting disability may be mild, manifesting as a stiff-legged gait; or severe, where the child is in a wheelchair and needs lifelong help eating, ambulating, and communicating. There often are associated conditions, such as intellectual disability, seizures, scoliosis, and hearing or vision, or both, defects, especially in children with more severe forms. The overall incidence is 3% to 5%; this number has stayed approximately the same although changes in prenatal and newborn care have been associated with shifts in the etiologies of CP.[30,31]

EVALUATION AND DIAGNOSIS. The diagnosis of CP is often made when gross motor milestones are not met by predicted ages. In some infants, diagnosis is made at birth because the child has an underlying diagnosis, such as a major brain malformation, that is known to be associated with CP, or as early as 4 months in children with more severe forms.[32] There are classic patterns: hemiplegia involves one side of the body, diplegia usually involves the lower extremities only, and quadriplegia involves all four extremities. All children with CP should receive speech/language therapy with trials of augmentative communication devices so that underlying cognitive abilities, which may not be apparent because of motor problems, are given a chance to manifest.

TREATMENT. Treatment of CP is multifaceted and undergoing constant evolution. Physical and occupational treatments, orthotics, spasticity reduction (by selected dorsal rhizotomy, oral, or intrathecal baclofen), botulinum-A (Botox) toxin injections, and surgery are often used to maximize a child's function. In many centers, a multispecialty approach at "CP clinics" occurs so that a family may, within one clinic visit, see neurology, pediatrics, orthotics, orthopedic surgery, and rehabilitation clinicians.

Children with CP should be carefully followed and given all possible opportunities to flourish. Although CP is a static disorder, progressive deformity because of increased muscle tone can occur. Monitoring these children as they grow with a multispecialty approach is essential to their optimal outcome.

Muscular Dystrophy

The **muscular dystrophies** are a group of inherited disorders that cause progressive muscle fiber loss leading to weakness, mostly of the voluntary muscles. The muscular dystrophies are the most prevalent of the muscle diseases in childhood with increasing disability and deformity, although severity depends on the type of dystrophy (Table 45-4).

Although previous classification of the muscular dystrophies was based on age of onset, rate of progression, distribution of muscular involvement, and patterns of inheritance, increasingly the molecular mechanism or gene, or both, for the condition is used for diagnosis. Examples include Duchenne/Becker muscular dystrophy, both caused by mutations in the gene for the muscle protein dystrophin; myotonic muscular dystrophy, because of a genetic mutation in a protein kinase gene; and

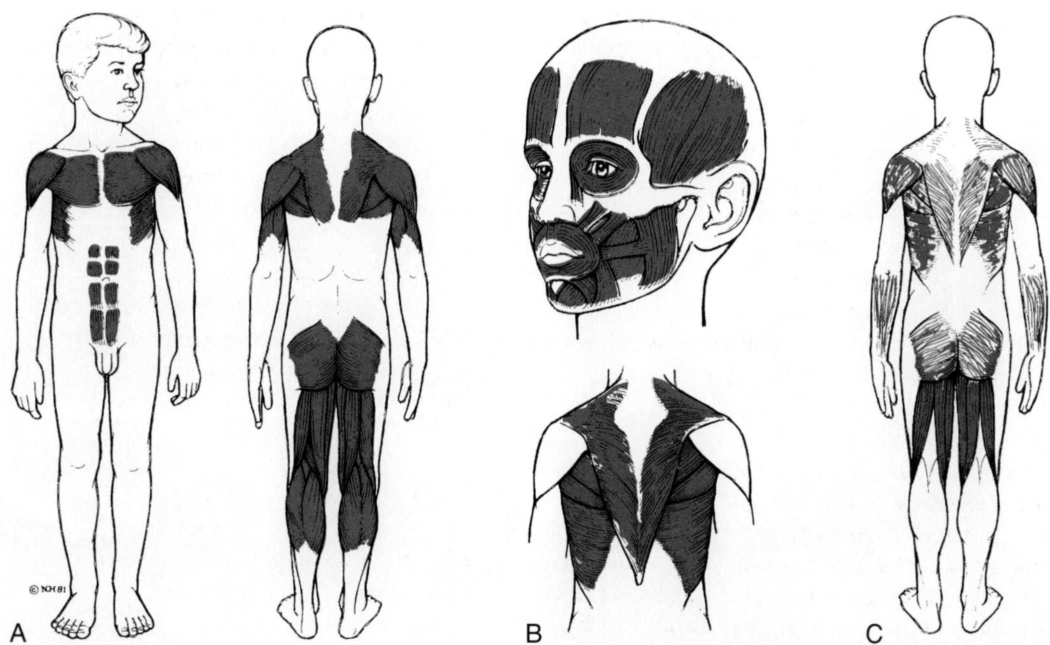

FIGURE 45-15 Initial Muscle Groups Involved in Three Types of Muscular Dystrophy. **A,** Pseudohypertrophic. **B,** Facioscapulohumeral. **C,** Limb girdle. (From Hockenberry MJ, Wilson D: *Wong's nursing care of infants and children,* ed 9, St Louis, 2011, Mosby.)

facioscapulohumeral muscular dystrophy, for which the mutation is still not well understood, although we know that the responsible gene is on chromosome 4 (Figure 45-15).

Duchenne Muscular Dystrophy

In 1868 the French neurologist G.B.A. Duchenne described progressive weakness associated with large calf muscles said to be **pseudohypertrophic,** because they consisted of fat and connective tissue rather than muscle. Today this form of muscular dystrophy, called **Duchenne muscular dystrophy,** is the most common of the muscular dystrophies. Its incidence is approximately 1 in 3500 male births.[33] Classic Duchenne muscular dystrophy occurs only in boys and has a history of X-linked inheritance in half of the cases.

PATHOPHYSIOLOGY. The X-linked inherited type of Duchenne muscular dystrophy is thought to be caused by deletion of a segment of deoxyribonucleic acid (DNA)[33] or a single-gene defect on the short arm of the X chromosome. A protein encoded by the Duchenne muscular dystrophy gene, called **dystrophin,** has been identified.

Dystrophin is present in normal muscle cells and absent in Duchenne muscular dystrophy (it is present in reduced amounts in Becker dystrophy). Dystrophin mediates anchorage of the actin cytoskeleton of skeletal muscle fibers to the basement membrane through a membrane glycoprotein complex. The complete lack of dystrophin in severe Duchenne dystrophy means that poorly anchored fibers tear themselves apart under the repeated stress of contraction. Free calcium then enters the muscle cells, causing cell death and fiber necrosis[34] (Figure 45-16).

Over time, as muscles degenerate, there is increased endomysial connective tissue and fat; loss of striations; and concomitant hyaline, granular, and fatty degeneration of fibers. Disorganization of tendinous insertions is associated with fat accumulation in these areas. Although fibers regenerate in the younger child, regeneration is not able to keep up with muscle cell death.

CLINICAL MANIFESTATIONS. Duchenne muscular dystrophy is usually identified in children at approximately 3 years of age, when the parents first notice slow motor development with progressive weakness and muscle wasting. Sitting, standing, and walking are delayed, and the child is clumsy, falls frequently, and has difficulty climbing stairs.

Muscular weakness begins in the pelvic girdle, causing a "waddling" gait. Hypertrophy of the calf muscles is apparent in 80% of cases. The method of rising from the floor by "climbing up the legs" (Gower sign) is characteristic and is caused by weakness of the lumbar and gluteal muscles. The foot assumes an equinovarus position (see Figure 45-7), and the child tends to walk on the toes because of weakness of the anterior tibial and peroneal muscles. Within 3 to 5 years, muscles of the shoulder girdle become involved. Contractures and wasting of the muscles contribute to muscular atrophy and deformity of the skeleton.

Duchenne muscular dystrophy has serious complications, although these are decreased by treatment with oral corticosteroids at diagnosis. The recent addition of oral corticosteroids early in the disease has dramatically improved outcome. Children are able to walk an additional 2 to 5 years and life expectancy has increased.[35] Complications, such as compromised pulmonary function and kyphoscoliosis ("humped" upper spine combined with scoliosis), are delayed. Full-scale IQ is 85, which is significantly lower than the average IQ of 100, although studies suggest this decrease may be caused by specific learning

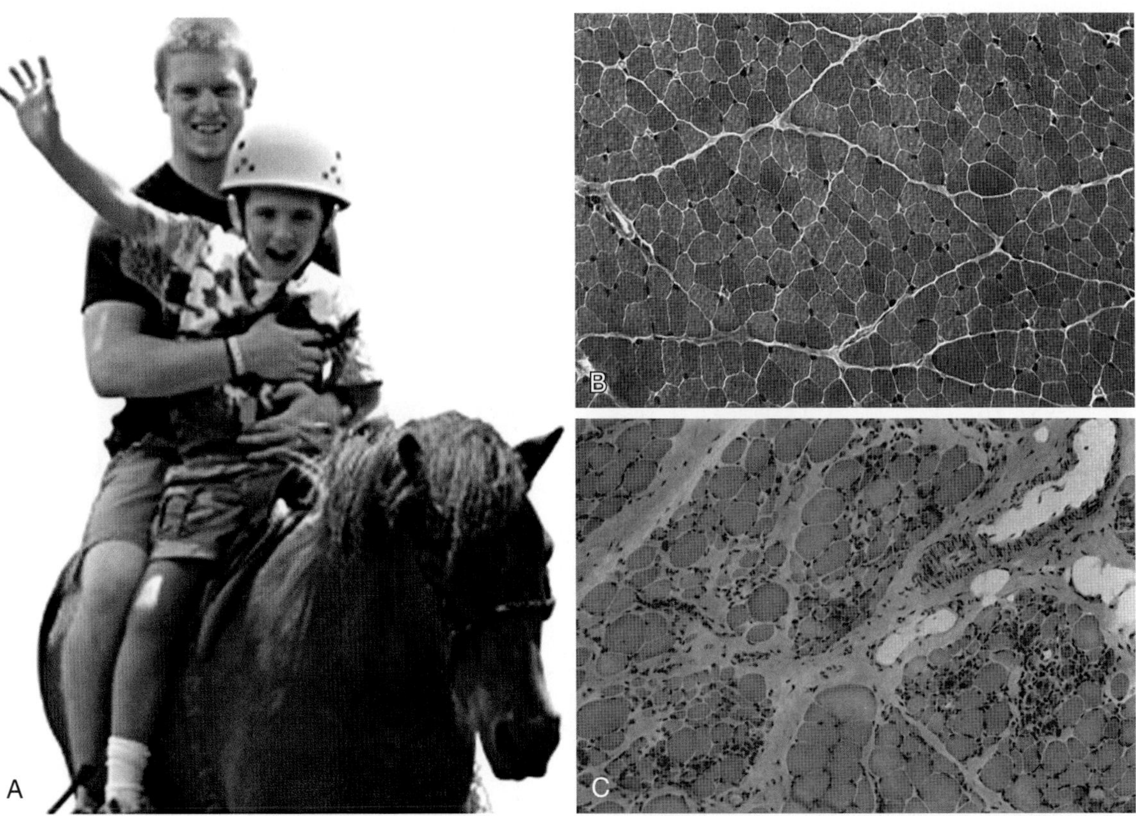

FIGURE 45-16 Duchenne Muscular Dystrophy. **A,** Young boy with Duchenne muscular dystrophy but on horseback. **B,** Transverse section of gastrocnemius muscle from a healthy boy. **C,** Transverse section of gastrocnemius muscle from a boy with Duchenne muscular dystrophy. Normal muscle fiber is replaced with fat and connective tissue. (**C** from Jorde LB, Carey JC, Bamshad MJ: *Medical genetics,* ed 4, Philadelphia, 2010, Mosby.)

disabilities rather than a true decreased intelligence. As the condition develops, constipation and incontinence of urine and stool may develop, possibly because of smooth muscle involvement. Although the life expectancy of boys with Duchenne continues to increase, death usually occurs from respiratory tract infection and a compromised respiratory system, with the majority living into their middle twenties. Some individuals who have chosen ventilatory support live a decade or more longer.

EVALUATION AND TREATMENT. Diagnosis is confirmed by genetic testing, which is informative in 95% of cases. Levels of serum enzymes, especially creatine phosphokinase (CPK), are increased to more than 10 times normal, even during infancy and before the onset of weakness. This test may be done as a screening test before gene testing. Electrodiagnostic testing and biopsy are rarely necessary.

Genetic counseling is recommended for all families who have children with DMD. With X-linked inheritance, male siblings of an affected child have a 50% chance of being affected and female siblings have a 50% chance of being carriers. Prenatal diagnosis is now possible and female carriers can be identified, especially if there is a known genetic defect in a son with muscular dystrophy. However, a negative carrier test cannot exclude the female being a carrier since the female's germ cells (her eggs) may be of two different types: one with Duchenne and one without (mosaicism). About one third of the time, the mutation in a boy with DMD is sporadic; that is, the boy is the first person in the family to develop the mutation causing DMD. Various strategies to develop gene therapy are currently in development for children with DMD.

Maintaining function in unaffected muscle groups for as long as possible is the primary goal. Although activity fosters maintenance of muscle function, very strenuous exercise may hasten the breakdown of muscle fibers. Range-of-motion exercises, bracing, and surgical release of contracture deformities are used to maintain normal function as long as possible. To prolong respiratory function or walking ability, or both, surgery for scoliosis is suggested when curves reach greater than 20 degrees. Children with DMD require a multidisciplinary approach to care, including attention to heart and breathing problems, weight loss/gain, constipation, rehabilitative/developmental problems, psychosocial needs, neurologic issues, and orthopedic problems (Figure 45-17).

Becker Muscular Dystrophy

Becker muscular dystrophy is caused by the same mutation in the gene coding for the muscle structural protein dystrophin; therefore, it shares the X-linked inheritance pattern and has similar but milder clinical features. Clinical symptoms often begin between 5 and 15 years of age. Children with Becker muscular dystrophy remain ambulatory into their teens and early twenties Heart failure is infrequent but can be a cause of premature death and disability.

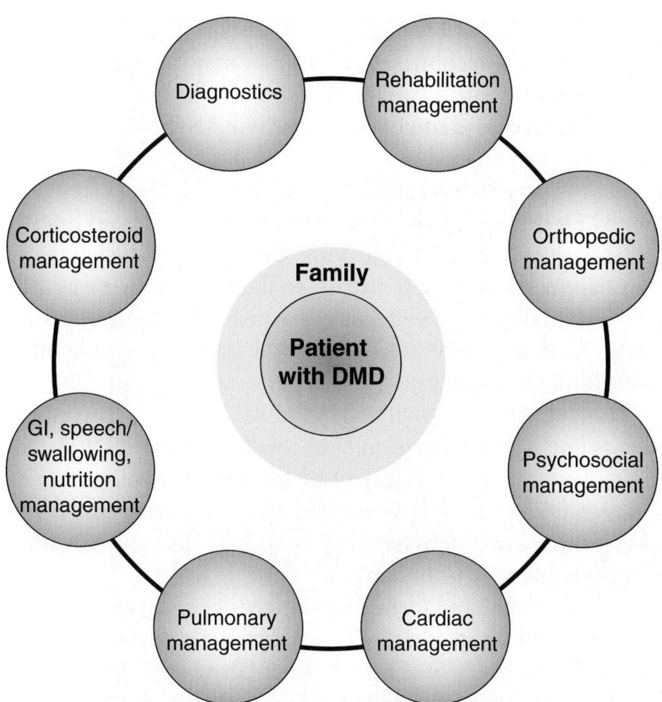

FIGURE 45-17 Multisystem Approach for Evaluation and Treatment of Duchenne Muscular Dystrophy. (Adapted from Bushby K: *Diagnosis and management of Duchenne muscular dystrophy part 1: diagnosis and pharmacological and psychosocial management,* 2009; Bushby K: *Diagnosis and management of Duchenne muscular dystrophy part 2: implementation of multidisciplinary care,* 2009. Available at www.thelancet.com/neurology. Published online November 30, 2009. [doi: 10.1016/S1474-4422(0970271].)

Maintaining ambulation and ensuring careful follow-up examinations for evidence of cardiopulmonary complications are essential for long-term care. If the affected individual marries and has children, all daughters will be carriers of this X-linked recessive disorder; however, male children will be unaffected. Genetic counseling should be offered to the mother, female siblings, offspring, and any maternal relatives.

Facioscapulohumeral Muscular Dystrophy

Facioscapulohumeral muscular dystrophy (FSHD) is a mild form of progressive, autosomal dominant muscular dystrophy. Age at onset varies from early childhood to adulthood, and the disease affects males and females equally. As the name implies, clinical manifestations begin with weakness and atrophy of facial and shoulder girdle (scapulohumeral) muscles. The illness progresses slowly. Inability to close the eyes completely may be noted from early childhood. The face is expressionless, and pouting of the lips makes whistling impossible. The first symptoms usually include drooping of the shoulders with difficulty in raising the arms above the head. Onset of weakness in the lower limbs often is delayed for 20 to 30 years, and pseudohypertrophy of muscles is rare. Contractures and skeletal deformities develop less often and are less prominent than in Duchenne muscular dystrophy. FSHD is rare compared to the other dystrophies in that it often manifests asymmetrically.

Treatment includes supportive physiotherapy to prevent contractures and prolong ambulation. Lightweight plastic ankle-foot orthoses (AFOs) for footdrop are extremely helpful. Shoulder pain is often present and figure-of-eight bracing or surgery to stabilize the shoulder is sometimes advised.

Musculoskeletal Tumors in Children

Bone Tumors

Bone tumors are uncommon childhood tumors and comprise less than 5% of all childhood malignancies. Of the malignant tumors, osteosarcoma and Ewing sarcoma are the most common. Fortunately, the majority of pediatric tumors are benign, most commonly nonossifying fibroma, osteochondroma, simple bone cyst, aneurysmal bone cyst, osteoid osteoma, and fibrous dysplasia.

Benign Bone Tumors

Nonossifying Fibroma. Nonossifying fibromas are sharply demarcated, cortically based lesions of fibrocytes that have replaced normal bone. These fibromas constitute about 50% of benign bone tumors. Most fibrous cortical defects are metaphyseal and resolve spontaneously or are obliterated by reparative ossification or remodeling. In some cases, however, the nonossifying fibroma persists and proliferates, affecting the structural integrity of the bone.

Nonossifying fibromas are usually asymptomatic and found incidentally on radiographs. In the 1950s, when fluoride was added to drinking water, random skeletal surveys were done on hundreds of children. Nonossifying fibromas were discovered in 20% to 30% of children and were distributed in nearly every bone of the body.

Nonossifying fibroma is not treated until it occupies more than 50% of the diameter of the bone or extends more than 3 to 4 cm into the cortex. When the tumor grows to this size, a pathologic fracture may occur, and curettage and bone grafting of the defect is undertaken. Quantitative CT scans help define a large lesion clearly and are used for preoperative planning.

Osteochondroma. Osteochondroma (or **exostosis**) is a very common benign tumor that results in a bony protuberance of bone growing near the growth plate. They can occur as a solitary lesion or as an inherited syndrome of **hereditary multiple exostoses (HMEs).** Osteochondromas are covered with a cartilage cap that, very rarely, can degenerate into malignant chondrosarcoma. Osteochondromas can occur on any bone and mature while a child is growing. They are the most commonly removed bony tumor.

Hereditary multiple exostosis (HME) occurs in about 1 of every 50,000 live births and results in multiple osteochondroma. It is autosomal dominant and caused by inactivation of EXT1 and EXT2 mutations on chromosomes 8 and 11, respectively. Multiple surgeries are common in affected individuals because the lesions lead to angulation of the bones, pain from pressure on nerves or tendons, and growth abnormalities. The malignant transformation rate is higher, reaching 5%. All affected children should be screened with a spinal MRI to discover if the cord is at risk of injury by spinal exostosis. Involvement of the spine in children with multiple hereditary exostoses is common.[36]

Simple Bone Cyst. Simple bone cysts (SBCs) are cystic lesions of the central region of the metaphyseal area in children.

With growth these lesions may appear within the diaphysis. Affected children are usually asymptomatic until pathologic fracture or incidental discovery occurs. Lesions often heal after a fracture, but large lesions may require treatment. A large prospective, randomized study compared steroid injection (the classic treatment for these lesions) with bone marrow injection for treatment. Both treatment modalities were found to have comparable healing rates if the pseudolining of the lesion was scraped from the cyst wall.[37] Very large lesions in weightbearing areas may require internal fixation and bone grafting.

Aneurysmal Bone Cyst. Aneurysmal bone cysts (ABCs) are typically eccentric, metaphyseal lesions that occur in a slightly older population than SBCs. The etiology remains controversial; many consider ABC a lesion secondary to another process, such as giant cell tumor. This lesion must be differentiated from malignant telangiectatic osteosarcoma; thus biopsy is necessary. Recent findings of genetic aberration in chromosome band 17p13 suggest a neoplastic basis for ABC.[38] Once diagnosed, curettage with complete removal of the "pseudolining" must be done with chemical cautery or electrocautery to minimize recurrence. Bone graft is placed in the defect. Even with modern techniques, recurrence can be as high as 21%.[39]

Osteoid Osteoma. Osteoid osteoma, or the larger counterpart osteoblastoma, presents as painful lesions of the diaphysis or metadiaphysis of long bones. Involvement of the posterior elements of the spine—with resultant "splinting" scoliosis—can occur. Night pain is common, as is relief from symptoms with nonsteroidal anti-inflammatory drugs (NSAIDs), because these tumors release prostaglandins. When pain is too extreme to be controlled medically, resection of the "nidus," or central portion, of the lesion is uniformly successful. CT guidance to the lesion is often used and, if possible, CT-guided laser ablation can be done. When present in the spine, surgical resection must be used since the heat of laser ablation can injure the spinal cord.

Fibrous Dysplasia. Fibrous dysplasia (FD) is a disease that causes thinning of the bone or the formation of growths or lesions that can occur in one bone (monostotic) or in multiple bones (polyostotic). **Albright syndrome** is a triad of polyostotic FD, precocious puberty, and cutaneous pigmentation. Although any bone can be affected, the long bones, ribs, and skull are the most common. A radiographic "ground glass" appearance is present primarily in the metaphyseal or metadiaphyseal areas. Deformity can be marked and necessitate operative intervention. When Albright syndrome is present, endocrine abnormalities also must be addressed.

Malignant Bone Tumors

Osteosarcoma. Osteosarcoma is the most common malignant bone tumor that occurs during childhood; it originates from bone-producing mesenchymal cells. It accounts for 60% of all malignant bone tumors and strikes between the ages of 10 and 18.

Molecular analysis has demonstrated deletion of genetic material on the long arm of chromosome 13, leading to the identification of a tumor-suppressor gene as part of the mechanism for tumor development. The oncogene *src* also has been associated with osteosarcoma.

PATHOPHYSIOLOGY. Osteosarcoma occurs mainly in the metaphyses of long bones. Most tumors arise in bones involved with the knee joint at the distal end of the femur or proximal end of the tibia. As a tumor of mesenchymal cells, osteosarcoma makes osteoid tissue.

Osteosarcoma is a bulky tumor that extends beyond the bone into the soft tissues. It may encircle the bone and destroy the trabeculae of the diseased bone. Osteosarcoma disseminates through the bloodstream, usually to the lung. As many as 25% of children diagnosed with osteosarcoma exhibit lung metastases at diagnosis. Other sites of metastatic spread include other bones and visceral organs.

CLINICAL MANIFESTATIONS. The most common presenting complaint is pain. There may be swelling, warmth, and redness caused by the vascularity of the tumor. Symptoms also may include cough, dyspnea, and chest pain if lung metastasis is present. If a lower extremity is involved, a limp or even pathologic fracture may be present.

Initial evaluation includes roentgenographic examination that shows the osteosarcoma's characteristic osteoblastic and osteolytic changes. "Staging" studies to determine not only the local extent of the tumor but also possible metastatic spread must be done. These include bone scan (to assess bony spread), magnetic resonance imaging (MRI) of the lesion (to plan surgical resection and to compare with postchemotherapy studies), and chest roentgenograms or CT, or both. The chest roentgenogram must be done *before* biopsy because the general anesthetic required for biopsy can give false-positive results on the roentgenogram.

EVALUATION AND TREATMENT. Tissue biopsy confirms the diagnosis, although needle biopsy is often sufficient to establish the diagnosis. There are five histologic types of osteosarcoma, each determined by the predominant cell type. The tumor is then graded according to degree of malignancy; the higher the number, the worse the prognosis.

Surgery and multiagent chemotherapy are the primary treatments for osteosarcoma. Radiation is occasionally used. The 5-year survival rate with modern protocols is 70% to 80%.[40]

Chemotherapy is used preoperatively to shrink the size of the tumor and minimize metastatic growth. Following chemotherapy, the child is given a short "rest period" to regain strength for surgery. Following adjunctive chemotherapy, the majority of children undergo "limb salvage" rather than amputation procedures. The long-term survival rate of children treated with limb salvage and chemotherapy is now nearly equal to amputation in 5- and 10-year survival.[41]

Ewing Sarcoma. Ewing sarcoma is a malignant round cell tumor of bone and soft tissue that has a poor prognosis. It is the second most common and most lethal malignant bone tumor that can occur during childhood. The peak incidence is 10 to 20 years. Like osteosarcoma, Ewing sarcoma is slightly more common in males than females and is linked with periods of rapid bone growth. The incidence of Ewing sarcoma is less than 2% in blacks.[42]

PATHOPHYSIOLOGY. Ewing sarcoma commonly occurs in the diaphysis of long bones or in flat bones. The most common sites include the pelvis, femur, and tibia (Figure 45-18). The femur

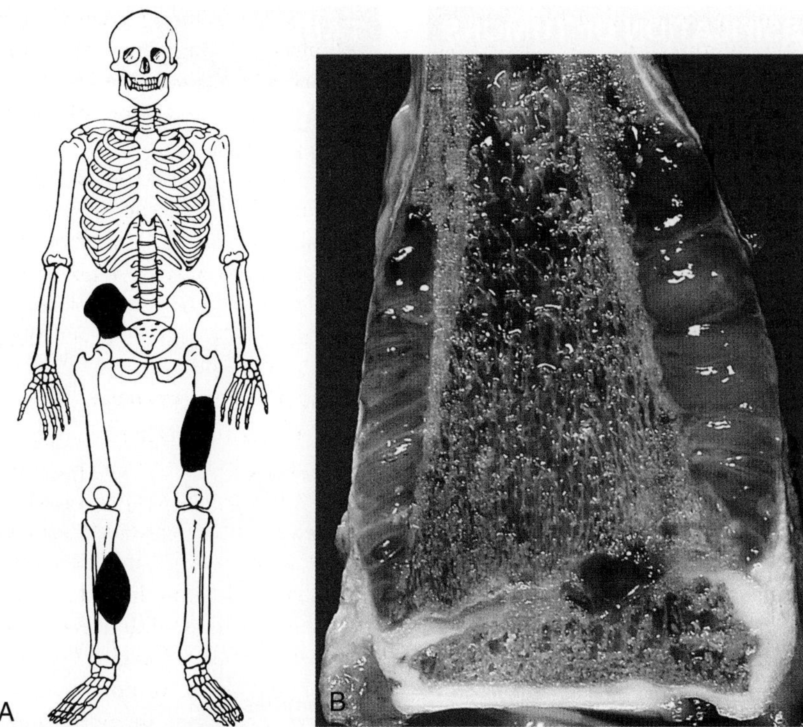

FIGURE 45-18 Ewing Sarcoma. **A,** Most common anatomic sites. **B,** Close-up view of Ewing sarcoma of the distal end of the tibia. Tumor extends into the soft tissue. (From Damjanov I, Linder J, editors: *Anderson's pathology,* ed 10, St Louis, 1996, Mosby.)

is involved in most cases, with the pelvis being the second most common site. It can occur in any bone.

Arising from bone marrow, Ewing sarcoma can break through the cortex of the bone to form a soft tissue mass. It does not form bone, but abundant reactive bone may be present in an attempt to contain this quickly growing lesion. Metastasis occurs early and is usually apparent at diagnosis or within 1 year. The most common sites are the lung, other bones, lymph nodes, bone marrow, liver, spleen, and central nervous system, although invasion of any organ is possible.

CLINICAL MANIFESTATIONS. Like osteosarcoma, the most common complaint is pain. A soft tissue mass is often present. Additional symptoms may include fever, malaise, and anorexia. Known as "the great imitator," Ewing sarcoma can appear radiographically identical to infection or even benign lesions such as Langerhans cell granulomatosis. Any pervasive diaphyseal or rib lesion must be regarded with a high index of suspicion.

EVALUATION AND TREATMENT. In addition to plain roentgenogram, CT and MRI are needed to help establish the diagnosis and extent of the tumor. Bone scan, chest roentgenogram, and chest CT scan are also used to detect metastases. No specific laboratory test is diagnostic; however, the sedimentation rate will be elevated and lactic dehydrogenase (LDH) level often is elevated. An elevated LDH level is a poor prognostic sign. Biopsy is used to conclusively establish the diagnosis. The identification of an 11:22 chromosomal translocation within the tumor cells confirms the diagnosis of Ewing sarcoma.

The use of multidrug chemotherapy has improved survival rates. Treatment protocols call for preoperative chemotherapy followed by radiation or surgical resection or both, with continuation of chemotherapy for 12 to 18 months afterward. Surgical resection is essential.

Historically, Ewing sarcoma had a dismal prognosis with 5-year survival rates no better than 5% to 10%. Combinations of aggressive radiation, chemotherapy, and surgical resection have improved the survival rate for extremity disease to 65% to 75%.[43] Disease of the trunk or pelvis continues to have a 5-year survival of only 40%. The major predictor of prognosis appears to be the location of the primary tumor and the presence of metastases at diagnosis.

Muscle Tumors

Most soft tissue tumors in children are benign. Only two malignant soft tissue tumors occur with any frequency—rhabdomyosarcoma in the younger child and synovial cell sarcoma in the teenager. Both of these occur rarely. The annual incidence is 8 cases per million for white children and 7.7 per million for black children. About 230 U.S. children are diagnosed with a soft tissue tumor each year. Soft tissue tumors originate from the primitive mesenchymal cells that normally give rise to muscle, tendons, blood vessels, lymphatic structures, fibrous and connective tissue, and bursa and fascia. Table 45-5 identifies the classification of soft tissue tumors according to origin. All malignant soft tissue tumors are characterized as highly aggressive tumors that invade surrounding structures and metastasize early.

Rhabdomyosarcoma (RMS) is the most common soft tissue sarcoma of childhood and accounts for more than 50% of soft tissue tumors but less than 3% of all childhood cancers. RMS arises from embryonal rhabdomyoblasts that normally differentiate into mature striated muscle.

TABLE 45-5 CLASSIFICATION OF TUMORS BY ORIGIN

TISSUE	TUMOR
Muscle	
Striated	Rhabdomyosarcoma
Smooth	Leiomyosarcoma
Adipose	Liposarcoma
Fibrous	Fibrosarcoma
Synovial mesothelium	Synovial sarcoma
Lymphatic structures	Lymphangiosarcoma
Blood vessels	Hemangiopericytoma
Nerve sheath	Neurogenic sarcoma

RMS can develop anywhere striated muscle is located. The primary locations and percentage range of incidence are the head and neck (including the orbit), 36% to 61%; the trunk, 8% to 33%; the extremities, 14% to 24%; and the genitourinary tract, 10% to 17%. Two age ranges (2 to 6 years and 15 to 19 years) are associated with RMS. More than two thirds of children with RMS are diagnosed by 10 years of age, and RMS is slightly more common in males than females.

Recent studies demonstrate an association between *TP53* (a tumor-suppressor gene) mutations and sporadic rhabdomyosarcoma.[44] Three oncogenes *(src, ras,* and *c-myb)* have been associated with this tumor.[45]

PATHOPHYSIOLOGY. RMS generally appears as a firm, fleshy, grayish white mass. RMS has various appearances, depending on the phase of differentiation of the rhabdomyoblast. The cells may be round, spindle shaped, tadpole shaped, or multinucleated giant cells.

At least 20% of children with RMS have metastatic disease at diagnosis. The preferred sites of metastases include the lungs, lymph nodes, bone marrow, liver, brain, and bone. Another 30% have disease that is unresectable, although not widely spread.

CLINICAL MANIFESTATIONS. The signs and symptoms of RMS depend on the anatomic location of the primary tumor and the presence of symptomatic metastases. The tumors are usually painless, and early detection of RMS is facilitated by the presence of a palpable or visible mass. Deep-seated tumors may cause functional impairment but can be silent until they are very large. The clinical manifestations of RMS are outlined in Table 45-6.

EVALUATION AND TREATMENT. Diagnostic studies during the pretreatment phase are used to determine the extent of the primary tumor and metastases. Specific diagnostic studies depend on the primary site, but a combination of radiographic, nuclear, and CT scanning or MRI technology and blood studies is used. A biopsy of the primary tumor is necessary to confirm the diagnosis.

RMS is treated by a combination of surgery, radiation, and chemotherapy. Complete surgical resection combined with multiagent chemotherapy has increased the overall survival rate to 70%. If surgical resection leads to serious disfigurement or functional disability (e.g., enucleation for orbital tumors or cystectomy for bladder tumors), chemotherapy and radiation serve as the primary treatment, and surgery is avoided or minimized.

TABLE 45-6 CLINICAL MANIFESTATIONS OF RHABDOMYOSARCOMA

LOCATION	MANIFESTATION
Head and Neck	
Orbit	Ptosis
	Exophthalmos
	Proptosis
Paranasal sinuses	Nasal obstruction
	Epistaxis
	Swelling
	Chronic sinusitis
Nasopharynx	Hypernasal speech
	Nasal discharge
	Visible polypoid mass
Oropharyngeal	Dysphagia
	Painful mastication
Middle ear	Chronic serous otitis media
	Discharge from affected ear
	Facial nerve palsy
	Conduction hearing loss
	Visible polypoid mass
Extremities	
All locations	Deep-seated, fixed palpable mass
Retroperitoneal	
All locations	Usually asymptomatic
	May have vague abdominal pain
	Bowel or genitourinary obstruction (late)
	Possible palpable mass
Genitourinary	
Vaginal	Abnormal vaginal bleeding
	Protruding polypoid mass
Prostate	Urinary tract obstruction
Bladder	Urinary retention
	Straining to void
	Hematuria
Paratesticular	Mass in scrotum that may be painful

The primary prognostic factor in RMS is the degree of residual disease after surgical resection. Children with localized disease (stages I and II) have long-term survival rates of 70% to 80%. With widespread disease, long-term survival rates drop to 20%. Orbital tumors have an overall favorable prognosis, probably because of the lack of lymphatics in the area and early physical signs of disease.

NONACCIDENTAL TRAUMA

Abuse is estimated to occur in more than 1.5 million U.S. children per year. The maltreatment may be psychologic, sexual, or physical. Of children who suffer physical abuse, 30% are initially seen by an orthopedist. Accurate and appropriate referrals to child protection services are not only legally mandated but also essential for the well-being of the child; an abused child who returns unmonitored to an abusive situation has a 15% chance of mortality.

ETIOLOGY. Children who are not yet ambulatory and present with a long bone fracture have a greater than 75% chance of that fracture being caused by nonaccidental trauma. **"Corner" metaphyseal fractures,** caused by a twisting force, are *nearly pathognomonic* of abuse but occur only 25% of the time (Figure 45-19). Fractures at multiple stages of healing are also suggestive; however, osteogenesis imperfecta must be ruled out. The most common presentation is a transverse tibia fracture.[46] After walking age, only 2% of long bone fractures are the result of nonaccidental trauma.[47]

EVALUATION. If suspected, nonaccidental trauma necessitates early consultation with child protective services. The child should undergo skeletal radiographic survey, especially if less than 2 years of age, and have a complete physical examination to evaluate for patterned bruising, burns, or multiple soft tissue injuries. Ophthalmologic examination and brain CT should be used to evaluate for retinal or brain hemorrhage caused by shaking. A thorough history must be obtained for all identified injuries. Bone scan can be helpful in diagnosing subtle injuries, especially rib fractures. Posterior rib fractures are especially likely to be caused by abuse. It is important to remember that social isolation can lead to increased likelihood of abuse, but no social stratum is immune.

TREATMENT. A nonjudgmental attitude on the part of the treating healthcare provider is essential. The child and family involved in nonaccidental trauma are delicate and require not only physical but also emotional care. Social workers need to be involved early to ensure appropriate medical care to the child. Fortunately, fractures heal quickly in young children; neurologic injury and social disease, however, are much more difficult to cure.

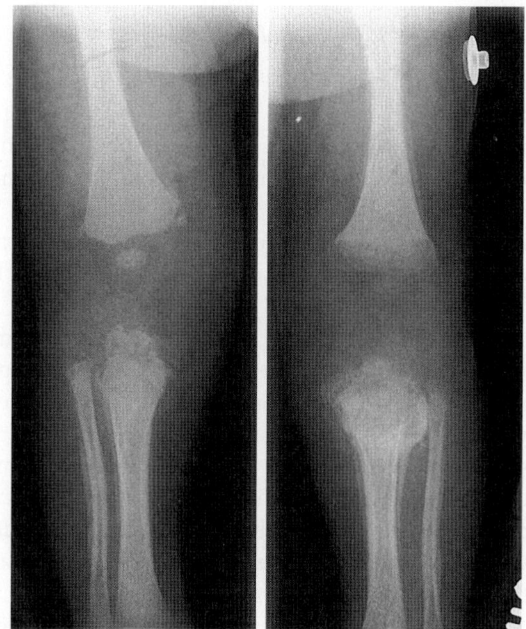

FIGURE 45-19 Corner Fracture. Bilateral knee radiograph showing healing corner fractures of bilateral proximal tibias and distal femurs. Note the varying amount of callus formation signifying fractures at different stages of healing.

SUMMARY REVIEW

Musculoskeletal Development in Children

1. Skeletal growth and development consists of two phases: (a) delivery of bone cell precursors to sites of bone formation, and (b) the aggregation of these cells at primary centers of ossification where they mature to secrete osteoid.
2. Ossification takes place in two centers in long bones: (a) the primary center, or the diaphysis (the long, central portion of the bone); and (b) the secondary center, or the epiphysis (the end portions of the bone).
3. Peak bone mass is achieved by the middle to late twenties.
4. By 1 year of age 50% of the total growth of the spine has occurred, and most children have achieved 50% of their adult height by 2 years of age.
5. The appendicular skeleton (extremities) grows faster during childhood than does the axial skeleton.
6. Muscle fibers reach their maximal size in females at 10 years of age and at 14 years of age in males.

Musculoskeletal Alterations in Children

1. The most common congenital defect of the upper extremities is syndactyly (webbing of the fingers).
2. Developmental dysplasia of the hip (DDH) is an abnormality in the development of the femoral head, acetabulum, or both. It is a serious and disabling condition in children if not diagnosed and treated early, preferably in infancy.
3. Clubfoot (equinovarus) is a common deformity in which the foot is twisted out of its normal shape or position. Clubfoot can be positional, idiopathic, or teratologic.
4. Congenital muscle disorders (myopathies) include absence of muscles, hypoplasia, hyperplasia, and faulty intrinsic development.
5. Osteogenesis imperfecta (brittle bone disease) is a genetic disorder of collagen that affects primarily bones and results in fractures of many bones.
6. Rickets is a condition caused by deficiencies in vitamin D, calcium, and usually phosphorus that is characterized by the failure of bones to become mineralized (ossified) and results in skeletal deformity.
7. Scoliosis is a lateral curvature of the spinal column that can be caused by congenital malformations of the spine, neuromuscular disease, trauma, extraspinal contractures, bone infections, metabolic bone disorders, joint disease, and tumors.
8. Osteomyelitis is a local or generalized bacterial infection of bone and bone marrow. Bacteria are usually introduced by direct extension from a nearby infection, through the bloodstream, or by trauma. Septic arthritis (bacteria within

SUMMARY REVIEW—cont'd

the joint) may be associated with osteomyelitis and is a surgical emergency.

9. Juvenile idiopathic arthritis is an inflammatory joint disorder characterized by pain and swelling. Large joints are most commonly affected.
10. Avascular diseases of the bone are collectively referred to as osteochondroses and are caused by an insufficient blood supply to growing bones.
11. Legg-Calvé-Perthes disease is one of the most common osteochondroses. This disorder is characterized by epiphyseal necrosis or degeneration of the head of the femur followed by regeneration or recalcification.
12. Osgood-Schlatter disease is characterized by inflammation or partial separation of the tibial tubercle caused by chronic irritation, usually as a result of overuse of the quadriceps muscles. The condition is seen primarily in muscular, athletic adolescent males.
13. The muscular dystrophies are a group of genetically transmitted diseases characterized by progressive atrophy of symmetric groups of skeletal muscles without evidence of involvement or degeneration of neural tissue. There is an insidious loss of strength in all forms of the disorder with increasing disability and deformity.
14. The two most common forms of benign bone tumors include nonossifying fibroma and osteochondroma. Other benign bone tumors include simple bone cysts, aneurysmal bone cysts, osteoid osteoma, and fibrous dysplasia.
15. The two main types of malignant childhood bone tumors are osteosarcoma and Ewing sarcoma.
16. Osteosarcoma, the most common malignant childhood bone tumor, originates in bone-producing mesenchymal cells and is most often located in the distal end of the femur or proximal end of the tibia.
17. Most childhood osteosarcoma tumors occur between the ages of 10 and 18 years.
18. Ewing sarcoma originates from cells within the bone marrow space and is located most often in the midshaft of long bones, in ribs, or in flat bones.
19. Ewing sarcoma is more common in males and is diagnosed most often between the ages of 5 and 15 years.
20. Pain is the usual presenting symptom for either osteosarcoma or Ewing sarcoma.
21. The primary treatments for osteosarcoma are surgery and chemotherapy. The primary treatment for Ewing sarcoma is a combination of chemotherapy, radiation, and surgery.
22. The most common type of childhood soft tissue tumor is rhabdomyosarcoma.
23. Rhabdomyosarcoma originates from embryonal rhabdomyoblasts that normally differentiate into mature striated muscle.
24. Clinical manifestations of rhabdomyosarcoma depend on the anatomic location; superficial tumors exhibit a painless palpable mass, whereas deep-seated tumors cause functional impairment.
25. Rhabdomyosarcoma is treated with a combination of surgery, radiation, and chemotherapy.

Nonaccidental Trauma

1. Nonaccidental trauma must be considered with any long bone injury in a preambulatory child.
2. Evidence of soft tissue injury, corner fractures, and fractures at different stages of healing are extremely helpful in making a diagnosis of nonaccidental trauma.
3. When nonaccidental trauma is suspected, a child must be evaluated radiographically for other fractures, head trauma, and retinal hemorrhage.
4. All social strata are at risk.
5. The healthcare provider is legally responsible to report suspected nonaccidental trauma.

KEY TERMS

REFERENCES

1. Misra M et al: Vitamin D deficiency in children and its management: review of current knowledge and recommendations, *Pediatrics* 122(2):398–417, 2007.
2. Simkin P: The musculoskeletal system. In Klippel JH, Dieppe PA, editors: *Rheumatology*, ed 2, London, 1998, Mosby-Wolfe.
3. Sankar WN, Laird CT, Baldwin KD: Hip range of motion in children: what is the norm? *J Pediatr Orthop* 32(4):399–405, 2012.
4. Weinstein SL: Congenital hip dislocation: long range problems, residual signs, and symptoms after successful treatments, *Clin Orthop Relat Res Aug* (281):69–74, 1992.
5. Weintroub S, Grill F: Ultrasonography in developmental dysplasia of the hip, *J Bone Joint Surg Am* 82A(7):1004–1018, 2000.
6. Holman J et al: Long term follow-up of open reduction surgery for DDH, *J Pediatr Orthop* 32(2):121–124, 2012.
7. Ippolito E et al: Long-term comparative results in patients with congenital clubfoot treated with two different protocols, *Arch Gynecol Obstet* 268(4):331–332, 2003.
8. Zionts LE et al: Treatment of idiopathic clubfoot: experience with the Mitchell-Ponseti brace, *J Pediatr Orthop* 32(7):706–713, 2012.
9. Zaleske DJ, Doppelt SH, Mankin HJ: Endocrine abnormalities of the immature skeleton. In Lovell WW, Winter RB, editors: *Pediatric orthopedics*, ed 2, Philadelphia, 1986, Lippincott.
10. Zeitlin L, Fassier F, Glorieux FH: Modern approach to children with osteogenesis imperfecta, *J Pediatr Orthop B* 12(2):77–87, 2003.
11. Wharton B, Bishop N: Rickets, *Lancet* 362(9393):1389–1400, 2003.
12. Parry J, Sullivan E, Scott AC: Vitamin D sufficiency screening in preoperative pediatric orthopaedic patients, *J Pediatr Orthop* 31(3):331–333, 2011.
13. Barrack R et al: Vibratory hypersensitivity in idiopathic sclerosis, *J Pediatr Orthop* 8(4):389, 1988.
14. Vijermans V et al: Factors determining the final outcome of treatment of idiopathic scoliosis with the Boston brace: a longitudinal study, *J Pediatr Orthop B* 13(3):143–149, 2004.
15. Caksen H et al: Septic arthritis in childhood, *Pediatr Int* 42(5):534, 2000.
16. Gillespie WJ et al: Aspects of the microbe:host relationship in staphylococcal hematogenous osteomyelitis, *Orthopedics* 10(3):475, 1987.
17. Hedström SA, Lidgren L: Septic arthritis and osteomyelitis. In Klippel JH, Dieppe PA, editors: *Rheumatology*, ed 2, London, 1998, Mosby-Wolfe.
18. Stanitski C: Changes in pediatric acute hematogenous osteomyelitis management, *J Pediatr Orthop* 24(4):444–445, 2004.
19. Przybylski GJ, Sharan AD: Single-stage autogenous bone grafting and internal fixation in the surgical management of pyogenic discitis and vertebral osteomyelitis, *J Neurosurg* 94(Suppl 1):1, 2001.
20. Ray NJ, Basset RL: Pyogenic vertebral osteomyelitis, *Orthopedics* 8(4):504, 1985.
21. Mader JT et al: The host and skeletal infection: classification and pathogenesis of acute bacterial bone and joint sepsis, *Baillieres Best Pract Res Clin Rheumatol* 13(1):1, 1999.
22. Perlman M et al: The incidence of joint involvement of adjacent osteomyelitis in pediatric patients, *J Pediatr Orthop* 20(1):40, 2000.
23. Cassidy JT: *Textbook of pediatric rheumatology*, New York, 1982, Wiley & Sons.
24. Hollingworth P: Juvenile chronic arthritis. In Klippel JH, Dieppe PA, editors: *Rheumatology*, ed 2, London, 1998, Mosby-Wolfe.
25. Glueck CJ et al: Association of antithrombotic factor deficiencies and hypofibrinolysis with Legg-Perthes disease, *J Bone Joint Surg Am* 78(1):3–13, 1996.
26. Herring JA et al: The lateral pillar classification of Legg-Calvé-Perthes disease, *J Pediatr Orthop* 12(2):143–150, 1992.
27. Schoenecker PL et al: Legg-Perthes disease in children under 6 years old, *Orthop Rev* 22:201, 1993.
28. Little DG et al: Potential for bisphosphonate treatment in Legg-Calve-Perthes disease, *J Pediatr Orthop* 31(Suppl 2):S182–S188, 2011.
29. Gigante A et al: What is the best treatment for Osgood-Schlatter disease? *J Fam Pract* 53(2):153–156, 2004.
30. Himmelmann K et al: The changing panorama of cerebral palsy in Sweden. IX. Prevalence and origin in the birth-year period 1995-1998, *Acta Paediatr* 94(3):287–294, 2005.
31. Hagberg B et al: The changing panorama of cerebral palsy in Sweden. V. The birth year period 1979-82, *Acta Pediatr Scand* 78(2):283–290, 1989.
32. Swanson MW et al: Identification of neurodevelopmental abnormality at 4 and 8 months by the movement assessment of infants, *Dev Med Child Neurol* 34(4):321–337, 1992.
33. Scott MO et al: Duchenne muscular dystrophy gene expression in normal and diseased human muscle, *Science* 239:1418, 1988.
34. Stevens A, Lowe J: *Pathology*, London, 1995, Mosby-Wolfe.
35. Moxley RT 3rd et al: Practice parameter: corticosteroid treatment of Duchenne dystrophy: report of the Quality Standards Subcommittee of the American Academy of Neurology and the Practice Committee of the Child Neurology Society, *Neurology* 64(1):13–20, 2005.
36. Roach JW, Klatt JW, Faulkner ND: Involvement of the spine in patients with multiple hereditary exostoses, *J Bone Joint Surg Am* 91(8): 1942–1948, 2009.
37. Wright JG et al: A randomized clinical trial comparing intralesional bone marrow and steroid injections for simple bone cysts, *J Bone Joint Surg Am* 90:722–730, 2008.
38. Oliveira AM et al: Aneurismal bone cyst variant translocations upregulate USP6, *Oncogene* 24(21):3410–3426, 2005.
39. Dorman JP et al: Surgical treatment and recurrence rate of aneurismal bone cysts in children, *Clin Orthop* 421:205–211, 2004.
40. Glasser DB et al: Survival, prognosis, and therapeutic response in osteogenic sarcoma: the Memorial Hospital experience, *Cancer* 69(3):698–708, 1992.
41. Bielack SS et al: Prognostic factors in high-grade osteochondromas of the extremity and trunk: an analysis of 1702 patients treated on neoadjuvant cooperative osteosarcoma study group protocols, *J Clin Oncol* 20(3):776–790, 2002.
42. Ayala AG, Ro JY, Raymond AK: Bone tumors. In Damjanov I, Linder J, editors: *Anderson's pathology*, ed 10, St Louis, 1996, Mosby.
43. Ruyman FB, Grovas AC: Progress in the diagnosis and treatment of rhabdomyosarcoma and related soft tissue sarcomas, *Cancer Invest* 18(3):223, 2000.
44. Lugo-Vicente H: Molecular biology and genetics affecting pediatric solid tumors, *Bol Asoc Med P R* 92(4-8):72–82, 2000.
45. Israel MA: Molecular and cellular biology in pediatric malignancies. In Pizzo PA, editor: *Principles and practice of pediatric oncology*, Philadelphia, 1989, Lippincott.
46. King J et al: Analysis of 429 fractures in 189 battered children, *J Pediatr Orthop* 8(5):585–589, 1988.
47. Thomas SA et al: Long-bone fracture in young children: distinguishing accidental injuries from child abuse, *Pediatrics* 88(3):471–476, 1991.

CHAPTER

46

Structure, Function, and Disorders of the Integument

Sue Ann McCann and Sue E. Huether

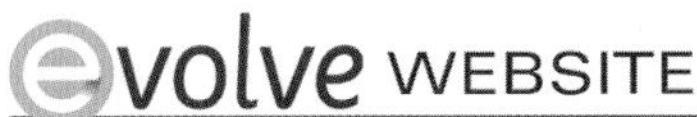

http://evolve.elsevier.com/McCance/
- Review Questions and Answers
- Animations

CHAPTER OUTLINE

The skin covers the entire body and is the body's largest organ, accounting for approximately 20% of the body's weight. Combined with the accessory structures of hair, nails, and glands, it forms the *integumentary system.* The primary function of the skin is to protect the body from the environment by serving as a barrier against microorganisms, ultraviolet (UV) radiation, loss of body fluids, and the stress of mechanical forces. The skin also regulates body temperature within a very narrow range, and is involved in immune surveillance and the activation of vitamin D. Touch and pressure receptors provide important protective functions and pleasurable sensations. The commensal (normal) microorganisms of the skin protect against pathologic bacteria.

STRUCTURE AND FUNCTION OF THE SKIN

Layers of the Skin

The skin is formed of two major layers: (1) a superficial or outer layer of **epidermis,** and (2) a deeper layer of **dermis** (the true skin) (Figure 46-1). The subcutaneous layer **(hypodermis)** is the lowest lying layer of connective tissue that contains macrophages, fibroblasts, fat cells, nerves, fine muscles, blood vessels, lymphatics, and hair follicle roots. Each skin layer contains cells that represent progressive stages of skin cell differentiation and function as the skin grows. These are summarized in Table 46-1.

Epidermis

The **epidermis** is a defensive barrier that continually renews itself by shedding the superficial layer of **stratum corneum.** It is formed primarily of keratinocytes embedded in a lipid matrix. These cells are named for the substances they produce. **Keratinocytes** produce **keratin,** a scleroprotein that provides protection from mechanical stress. Keratin is the main constituent of skin, hair, and nail cells. The thickness of the epidermis varies from 0.3 mm on the eyelids to 1.5 mm on the palms of the hands and soles of the feet. New cells (keratinocytes) formed in the **basal layer (stratum basale)** move upward and differentiate, forming

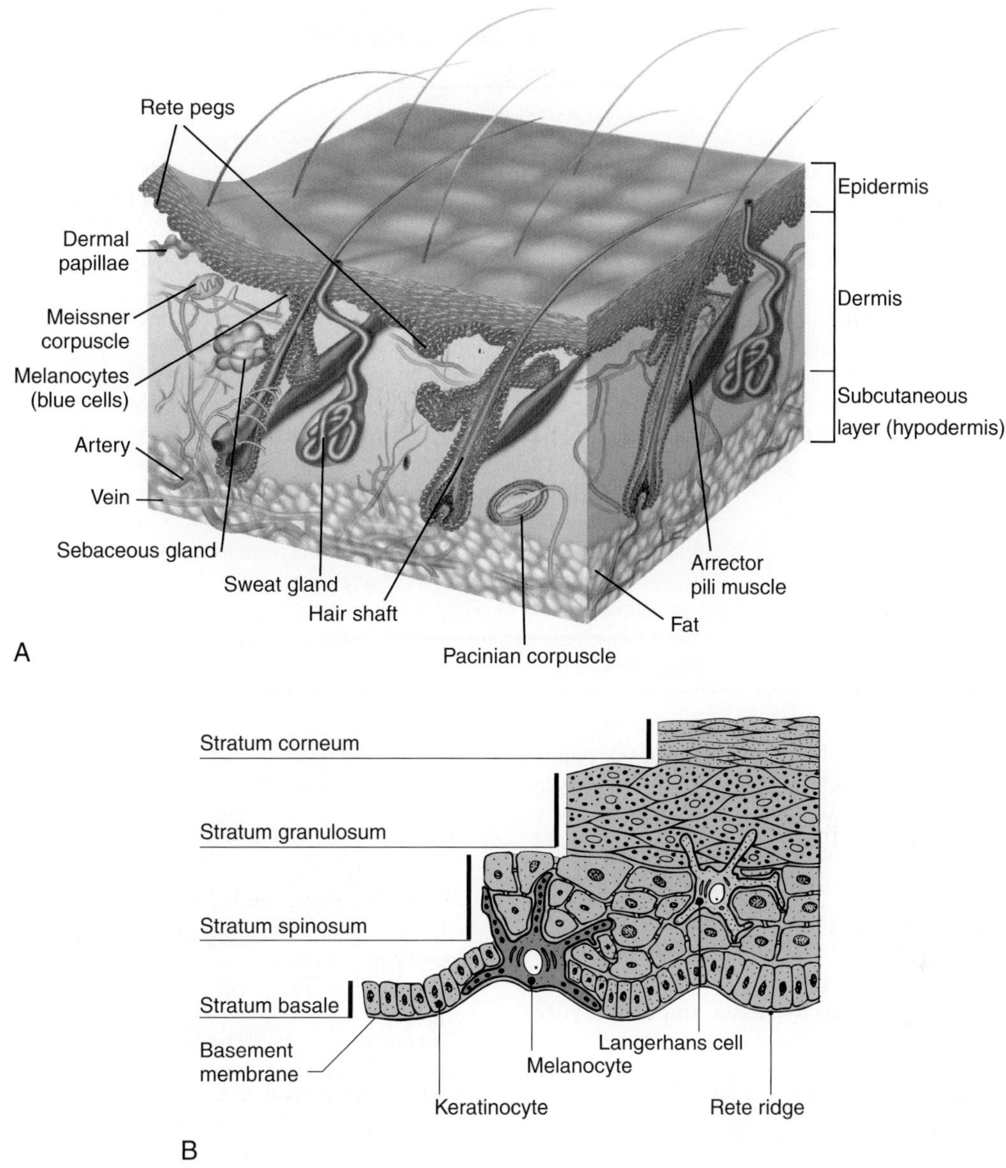

FIGURE 46-1 Structure of the Skin. **A,** Cross section showing major skin structures. **B,** Layers of the epidermis. (**A** from Kumar V et al: *Robbins & Cotran pathologic basis of disease,* ed 8, St Louis, 2009, Saunders; **B** from Gawkrodger D, Ardern-Jones MR: *Dermatology,* ed 5, Philadelphia, 2012, Churchill Livingstone.)

the **spinous layer (stratum spinosum).** Together they form the **germinative layer (stratum germinativum)** and ensure continual renewal of the skin. The cells enlarge and then become flattened, stacked, and cornified (stratum corneum) as they ascend to the skin surface. Cornification, or keratinization, prevents dehydration of deeper skin layers and loss of body water. The average turnover of the epidermis is about 30 days.

The epidermis has three additional types of cells that facilitate its functional characteristics: melanocytes, Langerhans cells, and Merkel cells. The **melanocytes** are usually located near the base of the epidermis. They synthesize and secrete the pigment melanin with exposure to UV light in response to melanocyte-stimulating hormone (MSH). Melanin in the epidermis provides a shield against UV radiation and determines skin color. **Vitiligo** is an autoimmune-related loss of melanocytes resulting in the depigmentation of patches of skin (see "Patch" in Table 44-3, p. 1547). **Langerhans cells** migrate to the epidermis from the bone marrow. Langerhans cells (a type of dendritic cell) and dermal dendritic cells initiate an immune response by presenting processed antigen to T cells, thus providing a defense against environmental antigens.[1] **Merkel cells** are associated with touch receptors and function as slowly adapting mechanoreceptors when stimulated by deformation of the epidermis.

Dermis

The **dermis** is 1 to 4 mm thick and is composed of three types of connective tissue: (1) collagen, (2) elastin and reticulin, and (3) a gel-like ground substance. The haphazard arrangement of connective tissue allows the skin to be mobile and to stretch and contract with body movement. Hair follicles, sebaceous glands, sweat glands, blood vessels, lymphatic vessels, and nerves are

TABLE 46-1 **LAYERS OF THE SKIN**

LAYER	CELL TYPES	CHARACTERISTICS
Epidermis		Most important layer of skin; normally very thin (0.12 mm) but can thicken and form corns or calluses with constant pressure or friction; includes rete pegs that extend into papillary layer of dermis
Stratum corneum	Keratinocytes	Tough superficial sheets of cornified cells
Stratum lucidum	Keratinocytes	Clear layers of cells containing eleidin, which becomes keratin as cells move up to the corneum layer; *found only in palmoplantar skin*
Stratum granulosum	Keratinocytes	Lose their nuclei Keratohyalin gives a granular appearance to this layer
Stratum spinosum	Keratinocytes	Polygonal-shaped with spinous processes projecting between adjacent keratinocytes
	Langerhans cells	Cells with dendritic processes and immune function
Stratum basale (germinativum)	Keratinocytes	Basal layer where keratinocytes divide and move upward to replace cells shed from the surface
	Melanocytes	Originate in neural crest and migrate to stratum basale and produce melanin
	Merkel cells	The function of Merkel cells is not clearly known—have role in light touch
Dermis	Macrophages	Irregular connective tissue layer with rich blood, lymphatic, and nerve supply; contains sensory receptors and sweat glands (apocrine, eccrine, sebaceous); macrophages (phagocytic and important for wound healing) and mast cells (release histamine) have immune functions (see Chapter 7)
Papillary layer (thin)	Mast cells	
Reticular layer (thick)	Histiocytes	Histiocytes are wandering macrophages that collect pigments and inflammatory debris
	Fibroblasts	Generate connective tissue; imported for wound healing
Subcutaneous (Hypodermis)		Subcutaneous tissue or superficial fascia of varying thickness that connects the overlying dermis to underlying muscle; contains macrophages, fibroblasts, fat cells, nerves, blood vessels, lymphatics, and hair follicle roots

contained in the dermis. The conelike projections of the papillary dermis interface with the epidermis. The papillae provide texture to the surface of the skin by forming *rete pegs.*

The cells of the dermis include fibroblasts, mast cells, and macrophages. Fibroblasts secrete the connective tissue matrix and collagen. Mast cells release histamine and play a role in hypersensitivity reactions in the skin. Macrophages are phagocytic and participate in immune responses. Histiocytes are macrophages that reside in loose connective tissue and phagocytize pigments and the debris of inflammation.

Subcutaneous Layer

The third layer of the skin is subcutaneous tissue and consists of fat cells or adipocytes. The lobules are separated by fibrous walls (septa) of collagen and large blood vessels. Dermal collagen is continuous with the collagen found in the subcutaneous tissue.

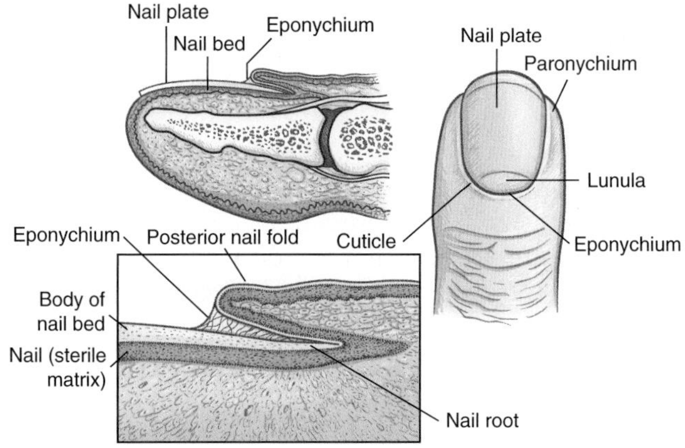

FIGURE 46-2 **Structures of the Nail.** (Redrawn from Thompson JM et al: *Mosby's clinical nursing,* ed 5, St Louis, 2002, Mosby.)

Dermal Appendages

The **dermal appendages** include the nails, hair, sebaceous glands, and the eccrine and apocrine sweat glands. The **nails** are protective keratinized plates composed of four structural units: (1) the proximal nail fold, (2) the matrix from which the nail grows, (3) the hyponychium (nail bed), and (4) the nail plate (Figure 46-2). Nail growth is continuous throughout life at a rate of 1 mm or less per day.

Hair follicles and sebaceous glands are integrated units (see Figure 46-1). Hair color, density, grain, and pattern of distribution have considerable variability and depend on age, gender, and race. **Hair follicles** arise from the matrix (or bulb) located deep in the dermis. They extend from the dermis at an angle and have an erector pili muscle attached near the mid-dermis that straightens the follicle when contracted, causing the hair to stand up. Hair growth begins in the bulb, with cellular differentiation of stem cells occurring as the hair progresses up the follicle.[2] Hair color is determined by melanin-secreting follicular melanocytes. Hair is fully hardened, or cornified, by the time it emerges at the skin surface. Hair growth is cyclic, with periods of growth and rest that vary over different body surfaces.

The **sebaceous glands** open onto the surface of the skin through a canal. They are found in greatest numbers on the face, chest, and back; modified glands are found on the eyelids, lips, nipple, glans penis, and prepuce. Sebaceous glands secrete sebum, composed primarily of lipids, that oils the skin and hair and prevents drying. Growth of sebaceous glands is stimulated by androgens, and their enlargement is one of the early signs of puberty.

The **eccrine sweat glands** are distributed over the body, with the greatest numbers in the palms of the hands, soles of the feet, and forehead. These secretions are important in thermoregulation and cooling of the body through evaporation. The **apocrine sweat glands** are fewer in number and are located in the axillae, scalp, face, abdomen, and genital area and have very limited proven function.

TABLE 46-2 SUMMARY OF SKIN DIAGNOSTIC PROCEDURES

TEST	PURPOSE
Dermoscopy	Magnified illumination of the skin using a liquid medium and transparent plate to examine skin lesions
Skin biopsy	Histologic examination of tissue to determine differential diagnosis of cellular structure (i.e., benign growths vs. carcinoma, chronic infections, blistering diseases, and vasculitis)
Microscopic immunofluorescence	Identification of antibodies, immunoglobulins, and complement components for diseases such as pemphigus, vasculitis, and discoid lupus erythematosus using fluorescent light on slide-mounted biopsy specimens
Gram stain	Differentiation of gram-positive from gram-negative bacteria according to stain absorption
Culture	Identification of chronic bacterial and fungal infections by incubating skin specimens in culture media
Wood lamp examination	Examination of skin or hair to identify fungus that fluoresces bright yellow-green under ultraviolet light
Patch and scratch tests	Application of suspected allergens to skin by patch or scratch for evaluation of immune system responses to known allergens and evaluation of cell-mediated immune function (*Candida albicans*, skin fungus, chemicals, aeroallergens, and foods)
Skin scrapings	Application of potassium hydroxide and low heat to skin scrapings on a glass slide to identify dermatophytes and *C. albicans*
Side lighting	Indirect lighting of the skin using light to the side of the lesions to evaluate patterns of depression and elevation of skin lesions
Diascopy	Use of glass or clear plastic pressed on the skin to differentiate erythema caused by dilated capillaries (blanching) from extravasation of blood (no blanching)
Tzanck smear	A microscopic examination of cellular material from skin lesions to help diagnose vesicular diseases, including herpes simplex virus and varicella-zoster virus

Blood Supply and Innervation

The blood supply to the skin is limited to the **papillary capillaries,** or plexus, of the dermis. These capillary loops arise from a subpapillary plexus that is supplied by a deeper horizontal cutaneous arterial plexus. Branches from the deep plexus supply hair follicles and sweat glands. A subpapillary network of veins drains the capillary loops. Arteriovenous anastomoses in the dermis facilitate the regulation of body temperature. Heat loss can be regulated by varying blood flow through the skin by opening and closing the arteriovenous anastomoses in conjunction with evaporative heat loss of sweat. The sympathetic nervous system regulates vasoconstriction and vasodilation through α-adrenergic receptors. The lymphatic vessels arise in the papillary dermis and drain into larger subcutaneous trunks, removing cells, proteins, and immunologic mediators.

AGING AND SKIN INTEGRITY

Many age-associated changes in the skin are generalized and readily observable. Genetics and cumulative environmental factors, including UV radiation from sun exposure (photoaging), inflammatory responses, tobacco smoke, and gravity contribute to cutaneous changes with aging.[3,4] Structurally the skin becomes thinner, less elastic, drier, and wrinkled with a change in pigmentation. The cellular alterations contributing to the changes include a flattening of the dermoepidermal junction with a shortening and decrease in the number of capillary loops. There are fewer melanocytes, resulting in decreased protection against UV radiation. A significant decrease in the number of Langerhans cells reduces the skin's immune response with aging. The thickness of the dermis also decreases and accounts for the translucent, paper-thin quality of the skin. Loss of the rete pegs gives the skin a smooth, shiny appearance.[5]

The decreased vasculature and lymphatic drainage contribute to loss of barrier protection and the atrophy of eccrine, apocrine, and sebaceous glands, all of which promote dry skin. Loss of elastin fibers is associated with wrinkling. Collagen fibers become fragmented, and fibroblasts decrease in number, resulting in a decreased ability of the skin to stretch and regain shape. Decreased cell proliferation, diminished blood supply, and depressed immune responses also delay wound healing in aging skin. Changes in hair color and distribution also occur. Graying is caused by loss of melanocytes from hair bulbs, and thinning occurs from a gradual decline in the number of hair follicles and growth of finer hair.[6]

Epidermal cells change shape, and the barrier function of the stratum corneum is reduced. There is increased permeability and decreased clearance of toxic oxidative substances from the dermis. The accumulation of such substances is related to decreased vascularity and can cause skin irritation. Temperature regulation is compromised in older adults, with an increased risk for heat stroke and hypothermia. Loss of cutaneous vasomotion and subcutaneous fat, reduced vascularity, and decreased eccrine sweat production are contributing factors.[7] The pressure and touch receptors and free nerve endings decrease in number and reduce sensory perception. With aging many of the protective functions of the skin decrease, whereas the likelihood of infection and delay in wound healing increase.[8]

Tests of Skin Function

Diagnostic evaluations of skin disorders often can be completed by gathering historical information, performing a physical examination, and observing the distribution and characteristics of the presenting lesions. Additional diagnostic studies are summarized in Table 46-2.

Clinical Manifestations of Skin Dysfunction

Lesions

Lesions of the skin are readily observable and easily assessed for distribution and structure. Identification of the morphologic structure, including a differentiation between the primary and secondary lesions, and the general appearance of the skin is critical. The physical exam, in combination with a thorough health history, is essential to identify the underlying pathophysiology. Table 46-3 describes and illustrates the primary lesions of the skin and Table 46-4 describes and illustrates the

Text continued on p. 1625

TABLE 46-3 PRIMARY SKIN LESIONS

LESIONS	EXAMPLES
Macule A flat, circumscribed area that is a change in the color of the skin; less than 1 cm in diameter	Freckles, flat moles (nevi), petechiae, measles, scarlet fever
Papule An elevated, firm, circumscribed area less than 1 cm in diameter	Wart (verruca), elevated moles, lichen planus, fibroma, insect bite
Patch A flat, nonpalpable, irregular-shaped macule more than 1 cm in diameter	Vitiligo, port-wine stains, mongolian spots, café-au-lait spots
Plaque Elevated, firm, and rough lesion with flat top surface greater than 1 cm in diameter	Psoriasis, seborrheic and actinic keratoses

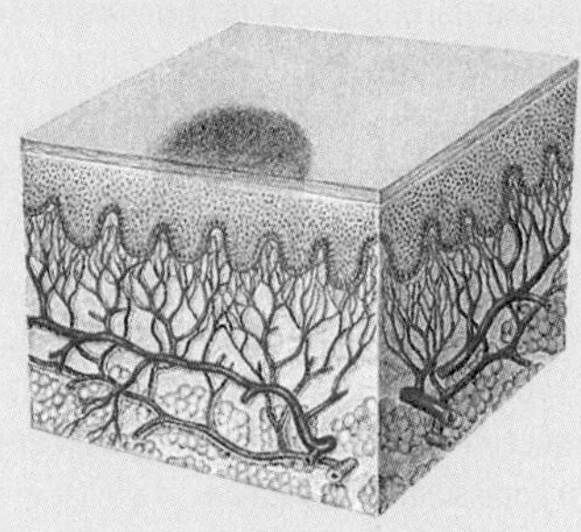

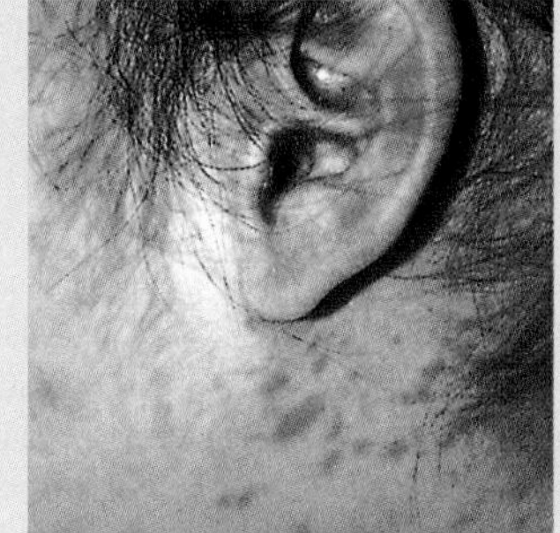

Macules[a]

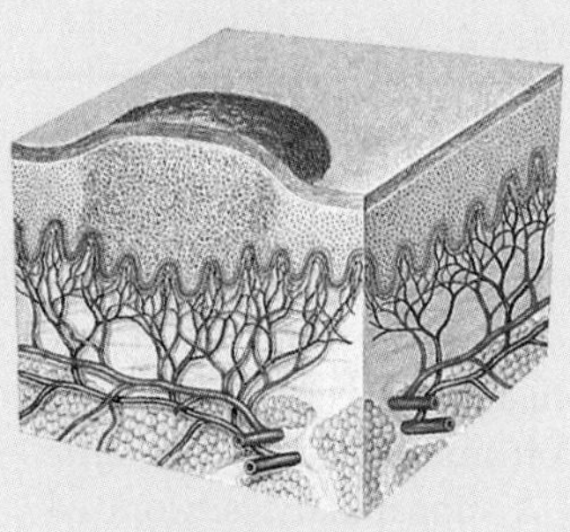

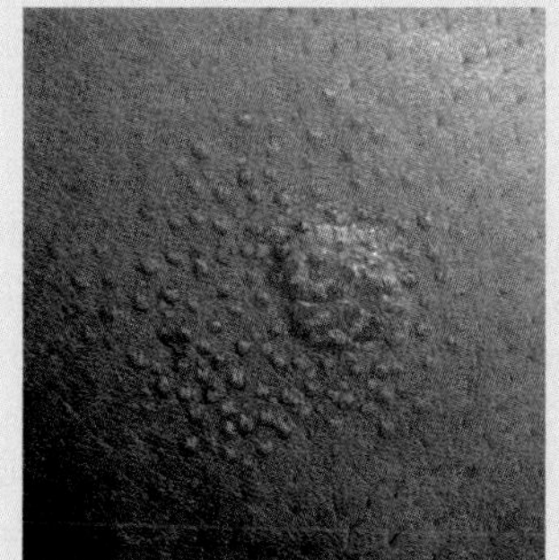

Lichen planus[b]

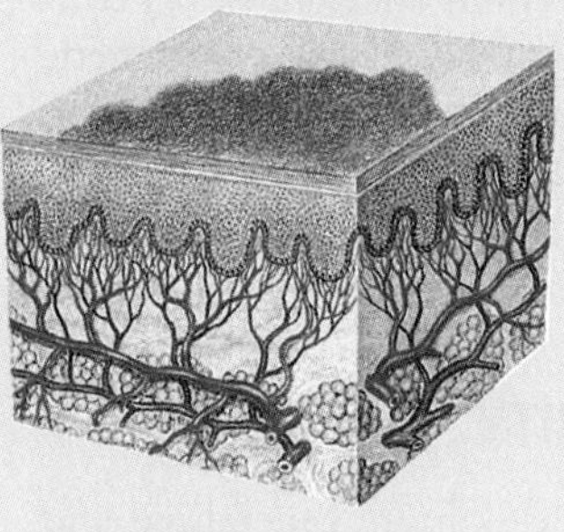

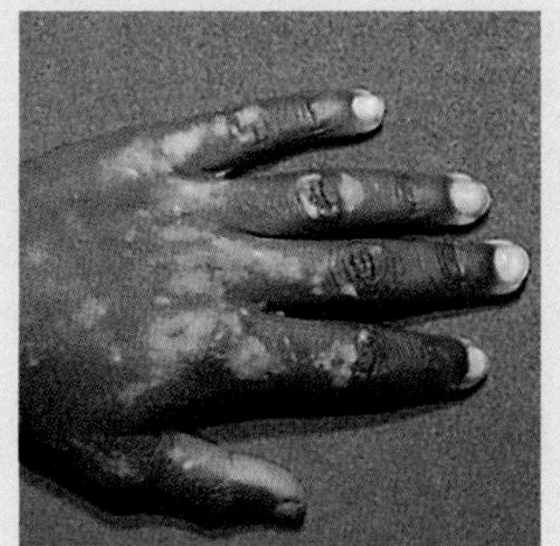

Vitiligo[c]

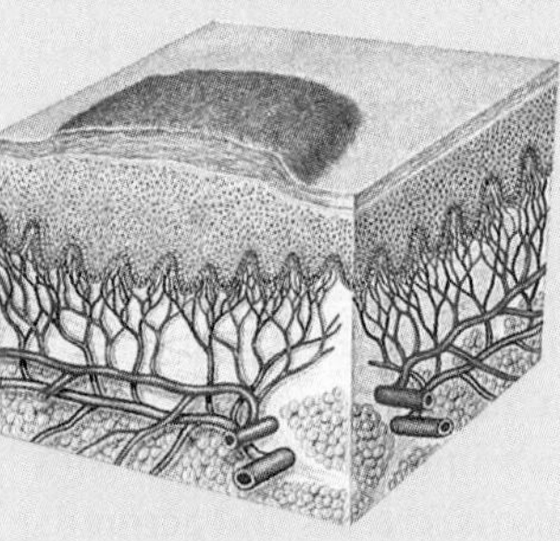

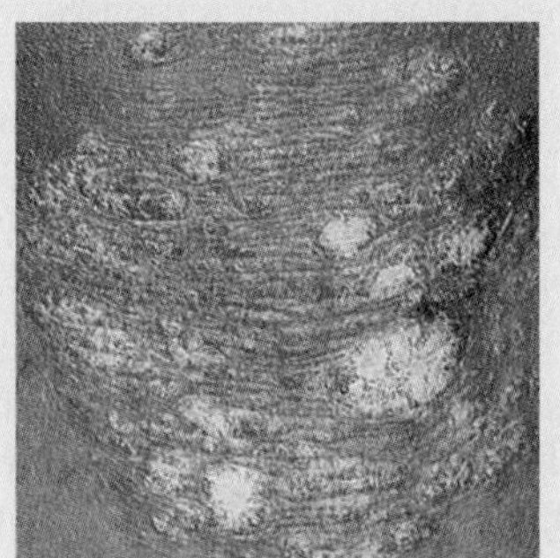

Plaque[d]

TABLE 46-3 PRIMARY SKIN LESIONS—cont'd

LESIONS	EXAMPLES
Wheal Elevated, irregular-shaped area of cutaneous edema; solid, transient; variable diameter	Insect bites, urticaria, allergic reaction

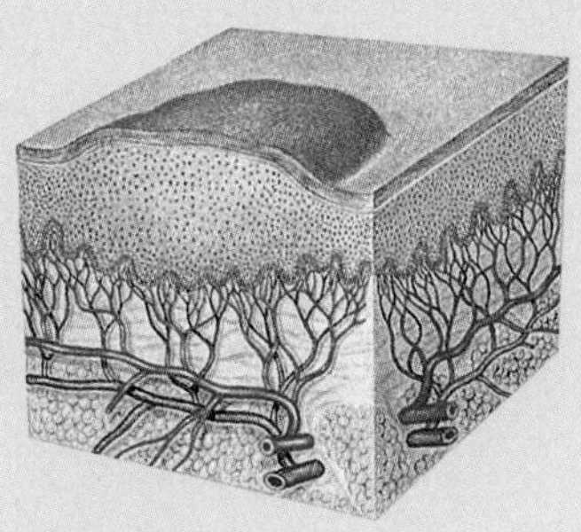
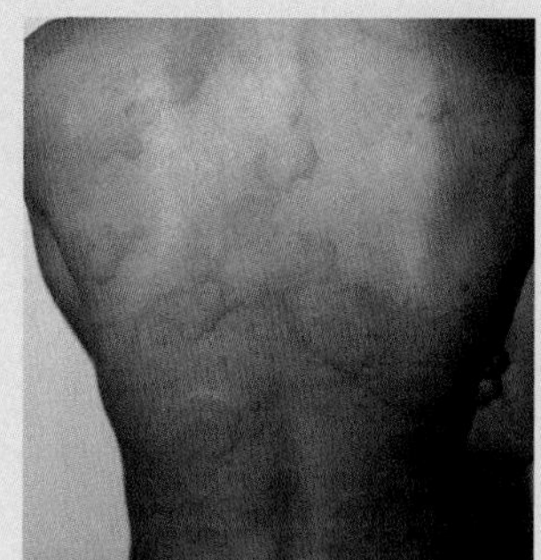

Wheal[e]

LESIONS	EXAMPLES
Nodule Elevated, firm, circumscribed lesion; deeper in dermis than a papule; 1-2 cm in diameter	Erythema nodosum, lipomas

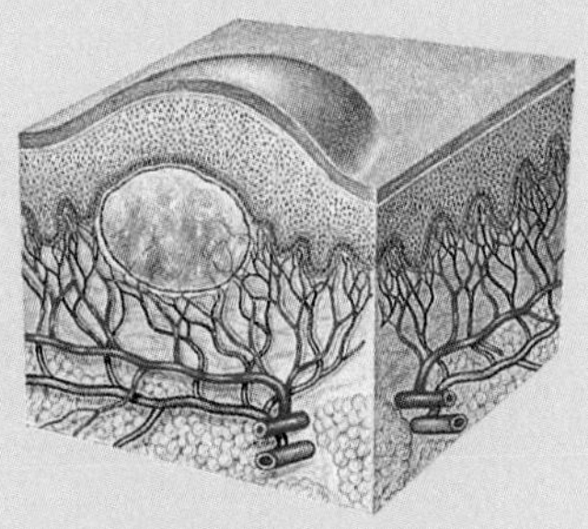
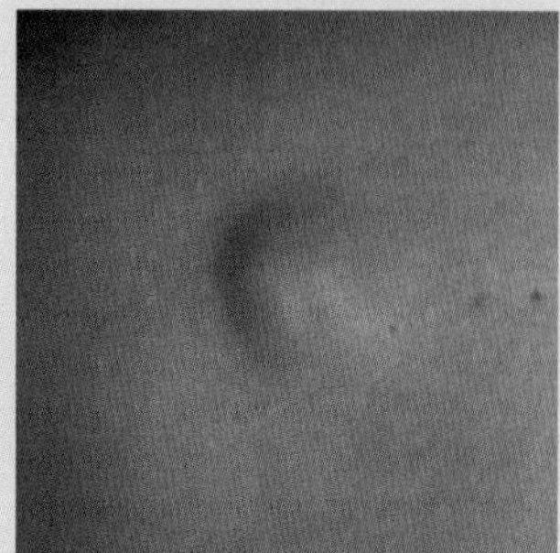

Lipoma[f]

LESIONS	EXAMPLES
Tumor Elevated, solid lesion; may be clearly demarcated; deeper in dermis; greater than 2 cm in diameter	Neoplasms, benign tumor, lipoma, neurofibroma, hemangioma

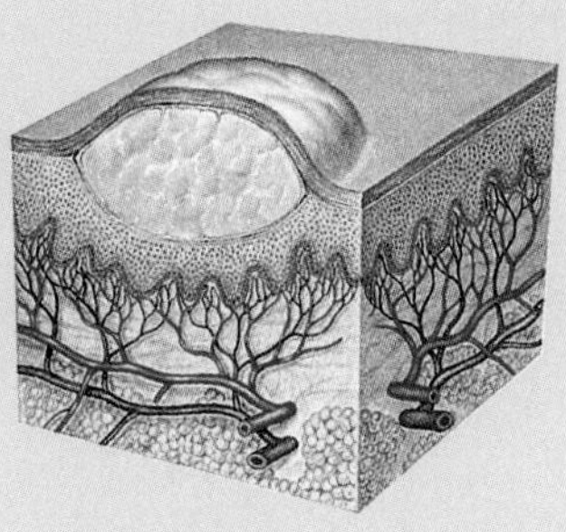
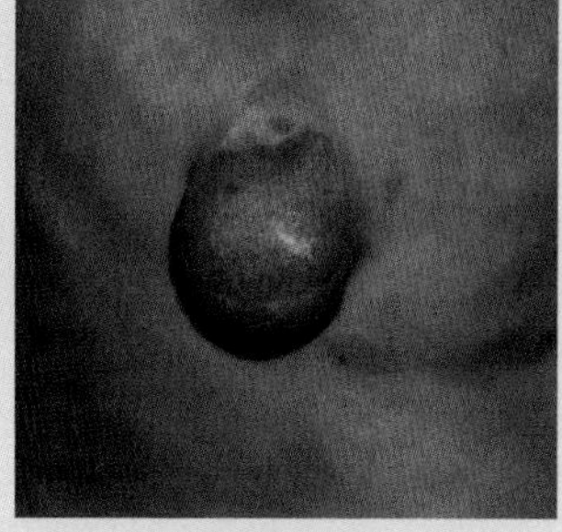

Neurofibroma[f]

LESIONS	EXAMPLES
Vesicle Elevated, circumscribed, superficial, does not extend into dermis; filled with serous fluid; less than 1 cm in diameter	Varicella (chickenpox), herpes zoster (shingles), herpes simplex

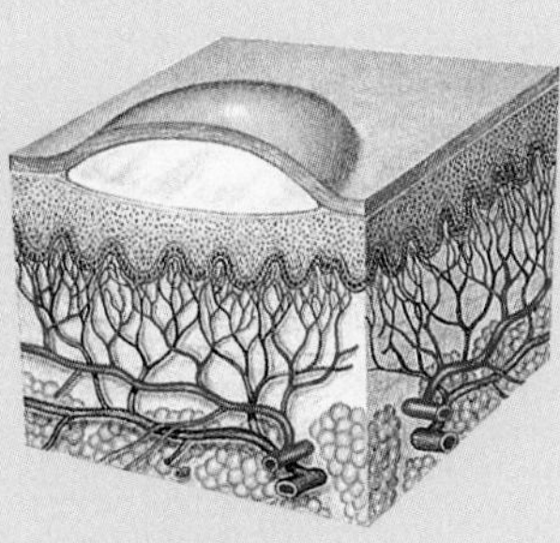
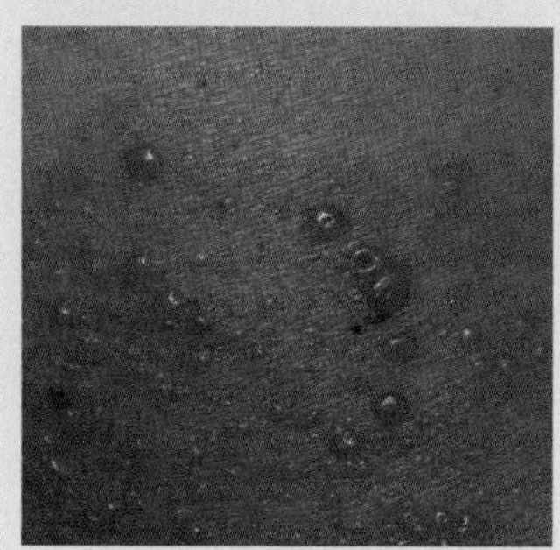

Vesicles[g]

Continued

TABLE 46-3 **PRIMARY SKIN LESIONS—cont'd**

LESIONS	EXAMPLES
Bulla Vesicle greater than 1 cm in diameter	Blister, pemphigus vulgaris
Pustule Elevated, superficial lesion; similar to a vesicle but filled with purulent fluid	Impetigo, acne
Cyst Elevated, circumscribed, encapsulated lesion; in dermis or subcutaneous layer; filled with liquid or semisolid material	Sebaceous cyst, cystic acne
Telangiectasia Fine (0.5-1.0 mm), irregular red lines produced by capillary dilation; can be associated with acne rosacea (face), venous hypertension (spider veins in legs), systemic sclerosis, or developmental abnormalities (port-wine birthmarks)	Telangiectasia in rosacea

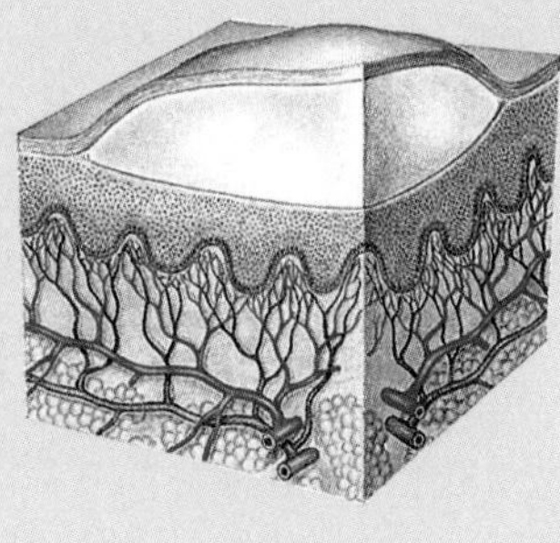

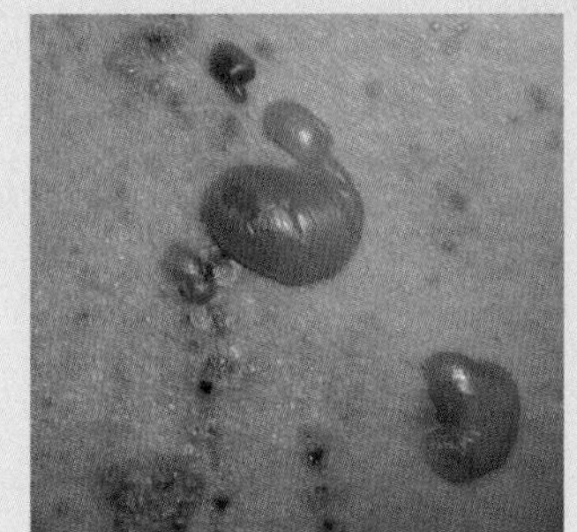

Bullae[h]

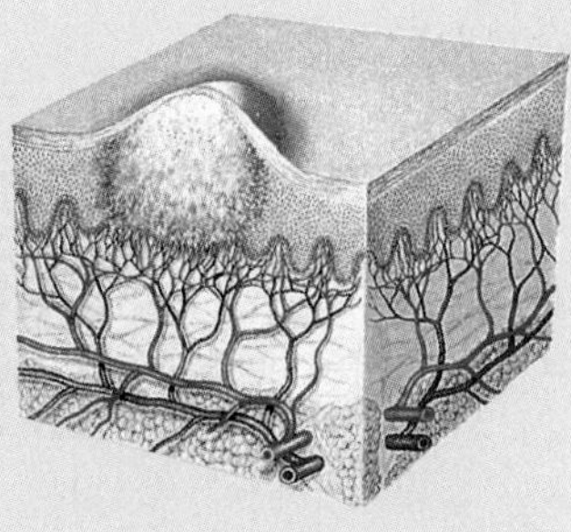

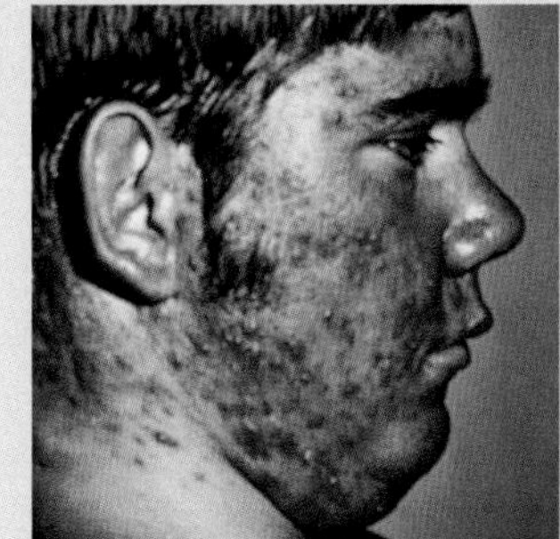

Acne[c]

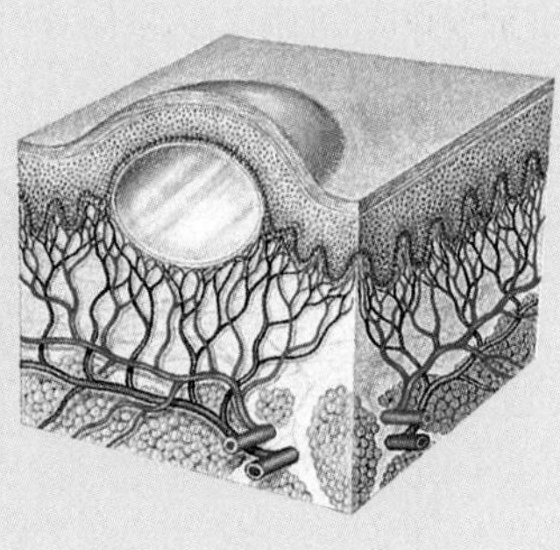

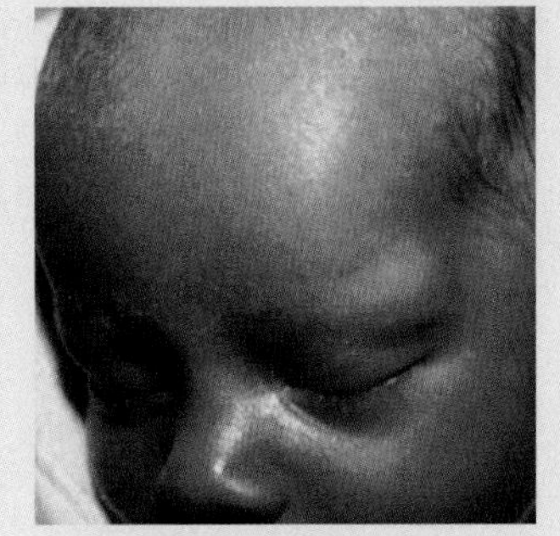

Sebaceous cyst[c]

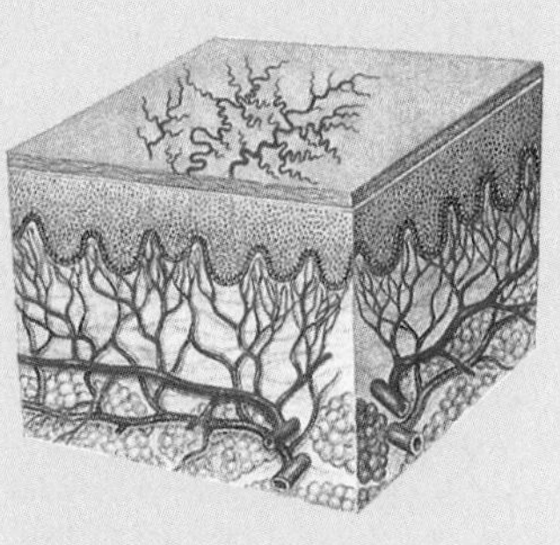

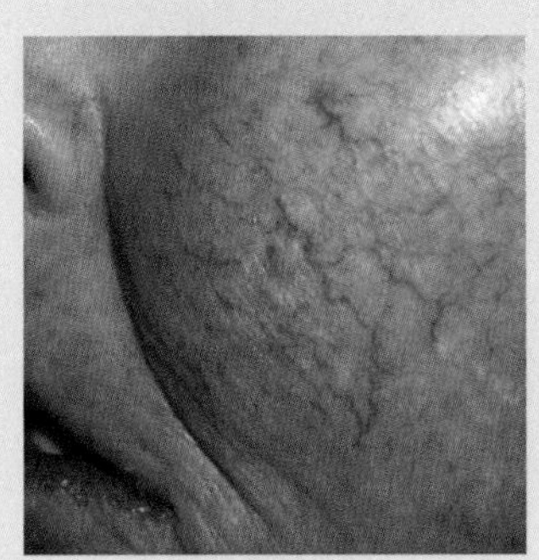

Telangiectasia[e]

[a]Farrar WE et al: *Infectious diseases,* ed 2, London, 1992, Gower.
[b]James WD, Berger T, Elston DMD: *Andrews' diseases of the skin,* ed 11, Philadelphia, 2011, Saunders.
[c]Weston WL, Lane AT: *Color textbook of pediatric dermatology,* ed 3, Philadelphia, 2002, Mosby.
[d]Habif TP: *Clinical dermatology: a color guide to diagnosis and therapy,* ed 5, Philadelphia, 2010, Mosby.
[e]Bolognia JL, Jorizzo JL, Schaffer JV: *Dermatology,* ed 3, Philadelphia, 2012, Saunders.
[f]Weston WL, Lane AT, Morelli JG: *Color textbook of pediatric dermatology,* ed 4, Philadelphia, 2007, Mosby.
[g]Black MM et al: *Obstetric and gynecologic dermatology,* ed 3, Philadelphia, 2008, Mosby.
[h]Marks JG, Miller JJ: *Lookingbill & Marks' principles of dermatology,* ed 4, London, 2006, Saunders.

TABLE 46-4 SECONDARY SKIN LESIONS

LESIONS	EXAMPLES		
Scale Heaped-up, keratinized cells; flaky skin; irregular-shape; thick or thin; dry or oily; variation in size	Flaking of skin with seborrheic dermatitis following scarlet fever, or flaking of skin following a drug reaction; dry skin	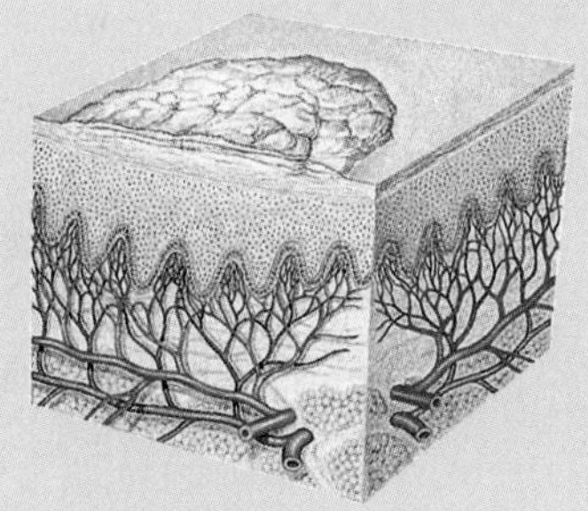	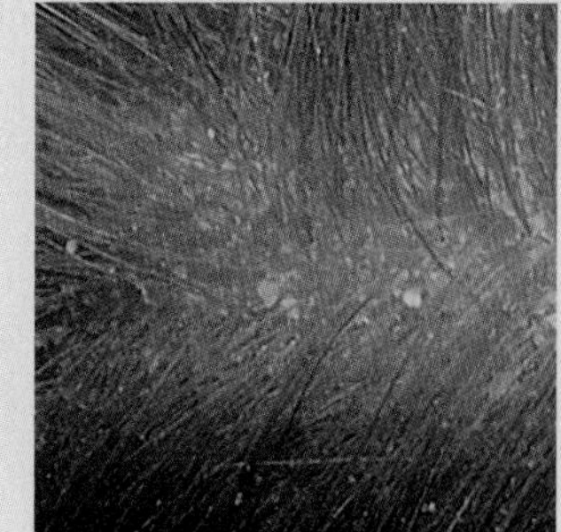 Fine scaling[a]
Lichenification Rough, thickened epidermis secondary to persistent rubbing, itching, or skin irritation; often involves flexor surface of extremity	Chronic dermatitis	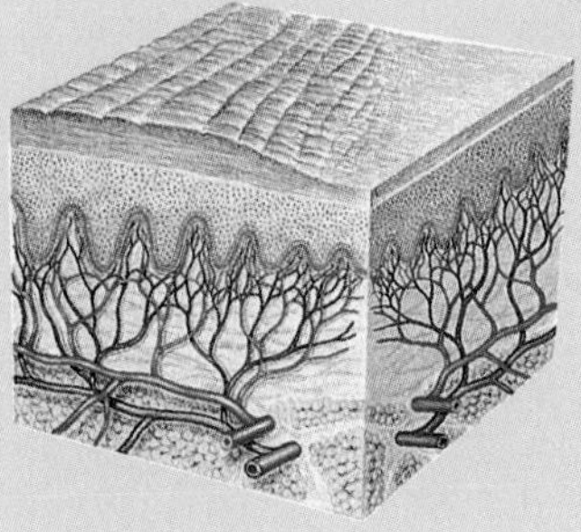	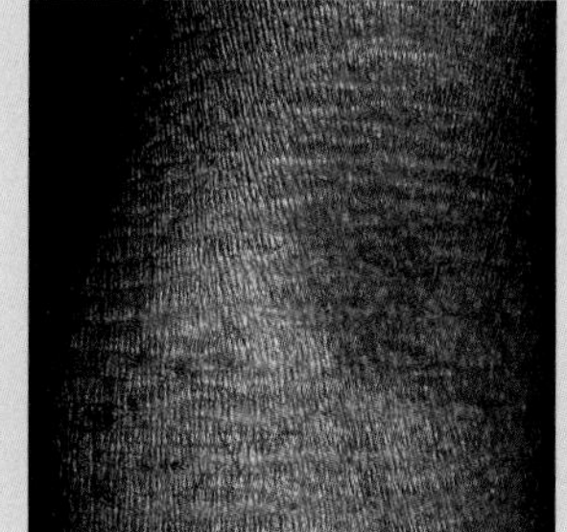 Atopic dermatitis of arm[b]
Keloid Irregular-shaped, elevated, progressively enlarging scar; grows beyond the boundaries of the wound; caused by excessive collagen formation during healing	Keloid formation following surgery	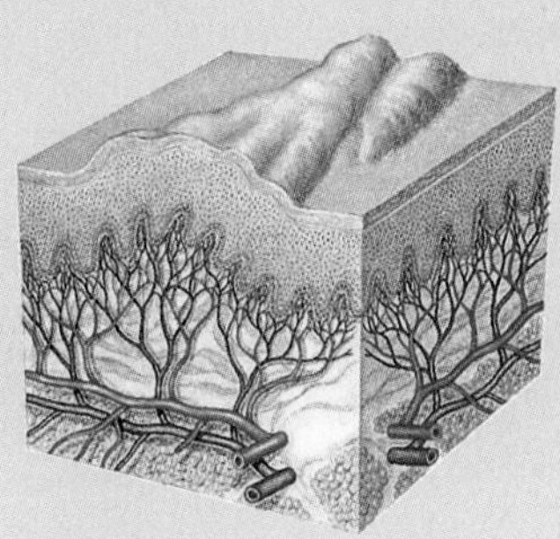	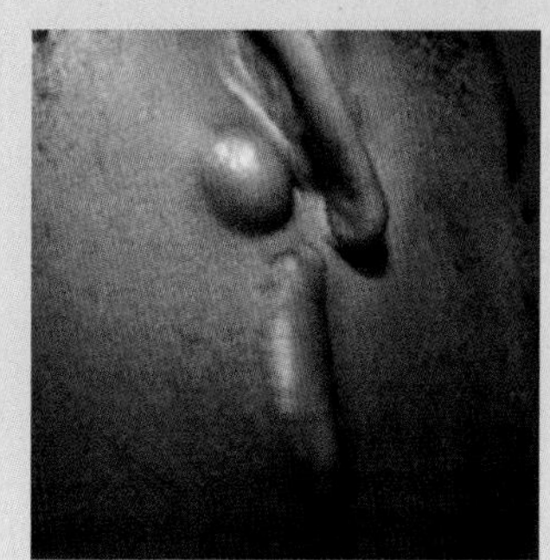 Keloid[c]
Scar Thin to thick fibrous tissue that replaces normal skin following injury or laceration to the dermis	Healed wound or surgical incision	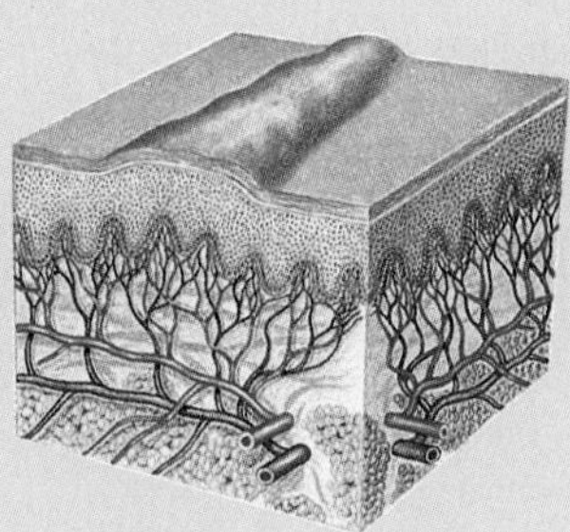	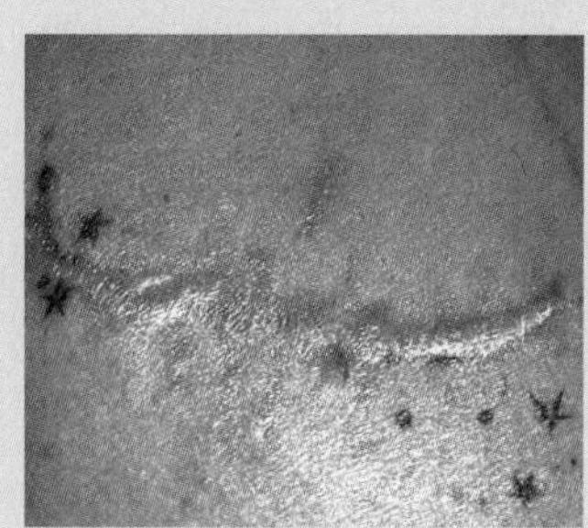 Hypertrophic scar[d]

Continued

TABLE 46-4 SECONDARY SKIN LESIONS—cont'd

LESIONS	EXAMPLES		
Excoriation Loss of the epidermis; linear, hollowed-out, crusted area	Abrasion or scratch, scabies	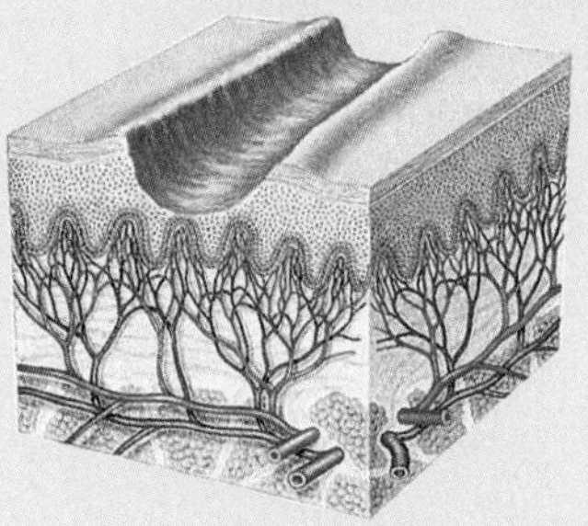	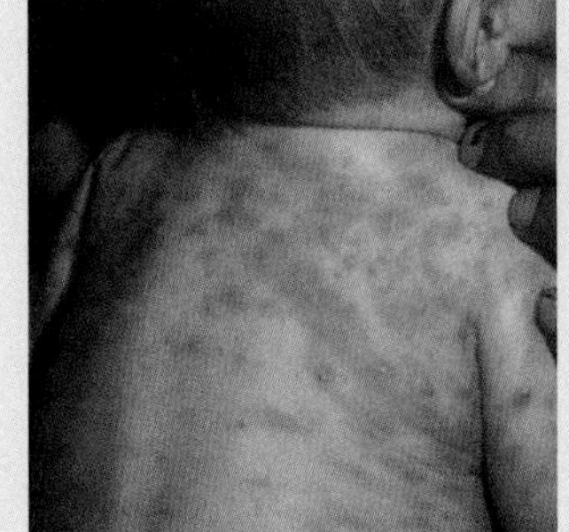 Scabies[c]
Fissure Linear crack or break from the epidermis to the dermis; may be moist or dry	Athlete's foot, cracks at the corner of the mouth, anal fissure, dermatitis	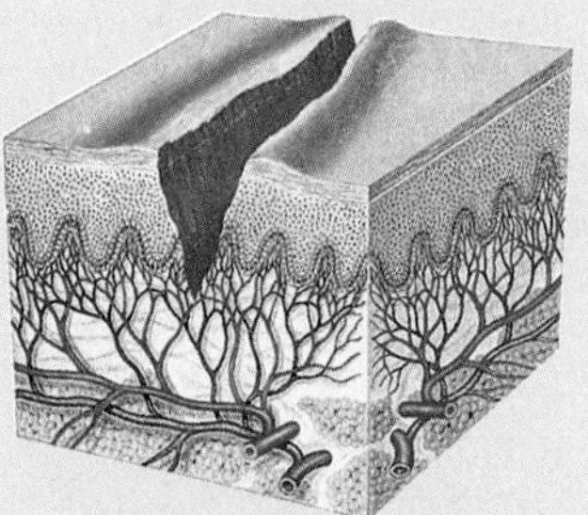	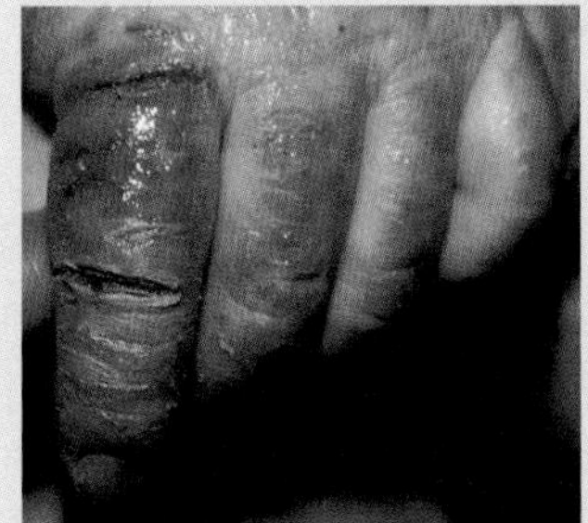 Fissures from infected dermatitis[c]
Erosion Loss of part of the epidermis; depressed, moist, glistening; follows rupture of a vesicle or bulla or chemical injury	Chemical injury	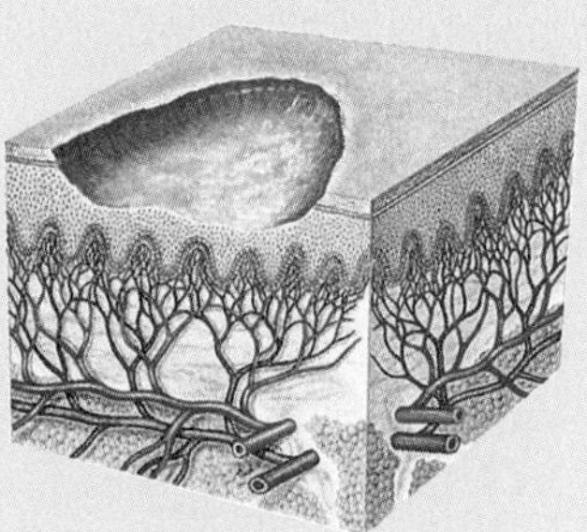	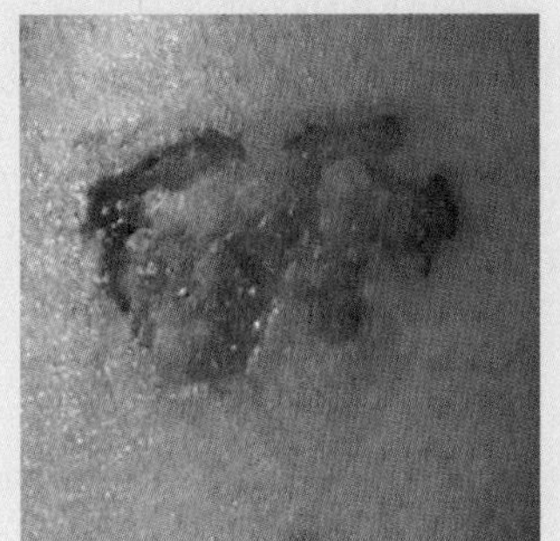 Erosion on leg[e]
Ulcer Loss of epidermis and dermis; concave; varies in size	Pressure ulcer, stasis ulcers	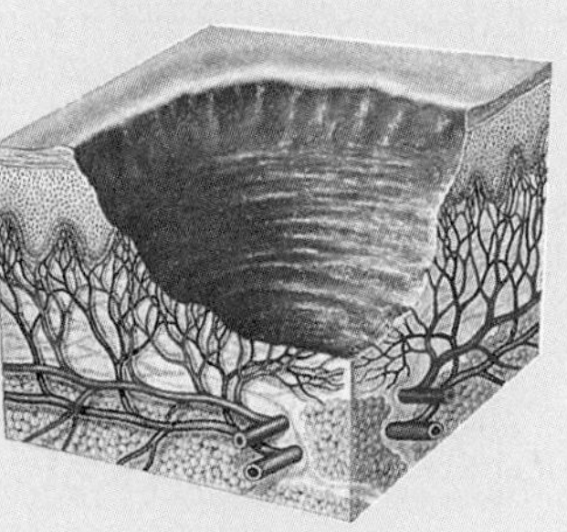	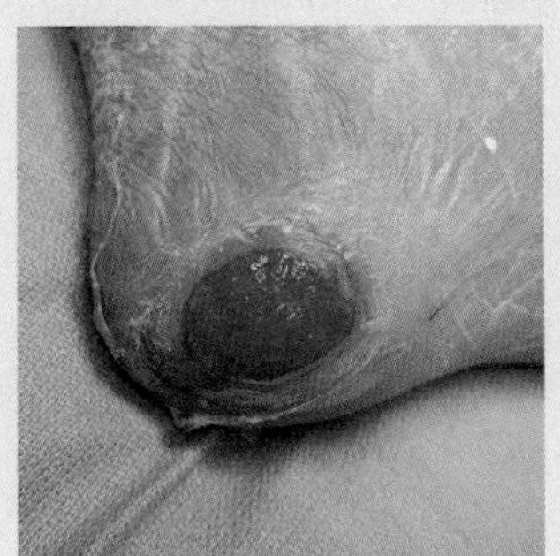 Pressure ulcer on heel[f]

TABLE 46-4 SECONDARY SKIN LESIONS—cont'd

LESIONS	EXAMPLES
Atrophy	
Thinning of the skin surface and loss of skin markings	Aged skin, striae

Aged skin[g]

[a]Baran R, Dawber RR, Levene GM: *Color atlas of the hair, scalp, and nails,* St Louis, 1991, Mosby.
[b]James WD, Berger T, Elston DMD: *Andrews' diseases of the skin,* ed 11, Philadelphia, 2011, Saunders.
[c]Weston WL, Lane AT, Morelli JG: *Color textbook of pediatric dermatology,* ed 4, Philadelphia, 2007, Mosby.
[d]Nouri K, Leal-Khouri S: *Techniques in dermatologic surgery,* Philadelphia, 2003, Mosby.
[e]Bolognia JL, Jorizzo JL, Schaffer JV: *Dermatology,* ed 3, Philadelphia, 2012, Saunders.
[f]Robinson JK et al: *Surgery of the skin,* ed 2, Philadelphia, 2010, Mosby.
[g]Seidel HM et al: *Mosby's guide to physical examination,* ed 7, St Louis, 2011, Mosby.

TABLE 46-5 SPECIAL SKIN LESIONS

TYPE	CLINICAL MANIFESTATIONS
Comedone	A plug of sebaceous and keratin material lodged in the opening of a hair follicle; an open comedone has a dilated orifice (blackhead), and a closed comedone has a narrow opening (whitehead)
Burrow	A narrow, raised, irregular channel caused by a parasite
Petechiae	A circumscribed area of blood less than 0.5 cm in diameter
Purpura	A circumscribed area of blood greater than 0.5 cm in diameter

secondary lesions of the skin. Special skin lesions are described in Table 46-5.

Pressure Ulcers. Pressure ulcers are ischemic ulcers resulting from unrelieved pressure, shearing forces, friction, and moisture. Pressure that consistently interrupts arterial and venous blood flow to and from the skin or deeper tissue is the most significant cause.[9] The term *decubitus ulcer* refers to an ulcer or pressure sore that results when an individual lies or sits in one position for a long time. The more general terms of *pressure sore* or *ulcer* are used here. Risk factors for pressure ulcers are summarized in Box 46-1.

Most individuals with darkly pigmented skin are at greater risk for developing pressure ulcers because early signs of skin damage may not be clearly visible.[10] Pressure sores usually develop over bony prominences: the sacrum, heels, ischia, and greater trochanters are the most common sites. Continuous pressure on tissue between the bony prominence and a resistant outside surface distort capillaries and occlude the blood flow and oxygen supply. Several scales are available for predicting pressure sore risk; the Braden Scale is one of those most frequently used.[11-13] One classification of pressure ulcer grades or stages is summarized as follows[14]:

I. Nonblanchable erythema of intact skin usually over bony prominence; darkly pigmented skin may not have visible blanching
II. Partial-thickness skin loss (erosion or blistering) involving epidermis or dermis presenting as a shallow open ulcer with a red-pink wound bed, without slough
III. Full-thickness skin loss involving damage or necrosis of subcutaneous tissue that may extend to, but not through, underlying fascia
IV. Full-thickness tissue loss with exposure of muscle, bone, or supporting structures (tendons or joint capsules); can include undermining and tunneling

Suspected deep tissue injury is localized in an area of purple or maroon discolored intact skin or blood-filled blister caused by underlying soft tissue damage from pressure and/or shear.

Unstageable is full-thickness tissue loss with base of ulcer covered by slough or eschar, or both, in the wound bed.

Superficial damage results in a layer of dead tissue that appears as a blister, erosion, or nonblanchable red/darkened skin or as a reddish blue discoloration when there is deeper tissue damage. Superficial sores are more common on the sacrum as a result of shearing or friction forces (forces parallel to the skin). Deep sores develop closer to the bone as a result of tissue distortion and vascular occlusion from pressure that is perpendicular to the tissue (over the heels, trochanter, and ischia) (Figure 46-3).

The primary goal for those at risk for pressure ulcers is prevention, including frequent skin assessment with repositioning and turning; use of pressure reduction surfaces and specialty beds; elimination of incontinence, moisture, and drainage; and maintenance of fluid, protein, and caloric intakes.[15,16]

BOX 46-1 PRESSURE ULCER RISK FACTORS

Prolonged Pressure/Immobilization

Lying in bed or sitting in chair or wheelchair without changing position or relieving pressure over an extended period
- Lying for hours on hard x-ray and operating tables
- Neurologic disorders (coma, spinal cord injuries, cognitive impairment, or cerebrovascular disease)
- Fractures or contractures
- Debilitation: elderly persons in hospitals and nursing homes
- Pain
- Sedation

Shearing forces
- Turning by dragging on coarse bed sheets

Disease/Tissue Factors

Impaired perfusion; ischemia
Fecal or urinary incontinence; prolonged exposure to moisture
Malnutrition, dehydration
Chronic diseases accompanied by anemia, edema, renal failure, malnutrition, peripheral vascular disease, or sepsis
Previous history of pressure ulcers

Additional Risk Factors for the Critically Ill

Norepinephrine infusion
Acute Physiology and Chronic Health Evaluation (APACHE II) score
Anemia
Age greater than 40 years
Multiple organ system disease or comorbid complications
Length of hospital stay

Data from Alderden J et al: *Crit Care Nurse* 31(4):30–43, 2011; Coleman S et al: *Int J Nurs Stud* 50(7):974–1003, 2013; Cowan LJ et al: *Wound Repair Regen* 20(2):137–148, 2012; Guihan M, Bombardier CH: *J Spinal Cord Med* 35(4):240–250, 2012; Jaul E: *Drugs Aging* 27(4):311–325, 2010; Thomas DR: *J Am Med Dir Assoc* 11(6):397–405, 2010; White-Chu EF et al: *Clin Geriatr Med* 27(2):241–258, 2011.

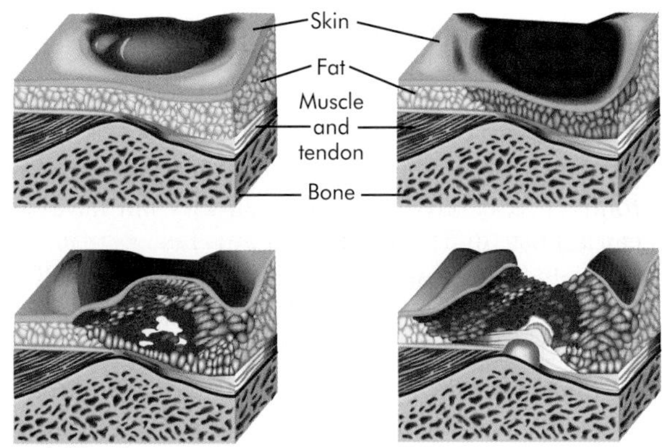

FIGURE 46-3 Progression of Decubitus Ulcer. Sustained pressure over a bony prominence compresses the tissue and reduces blood flow, resulting in progressive ischemia and necrosis of tissue.

Superficial ulcers should be covered with flat, moisture-retaining dressings that cannot wrinkle and cause increased pressure or friction; multiple options are available.[17] Successful healing requires continued adequate relief of pressure; débridement of dead tissue; use of specialty wound care products (dressings, foams, gels, cleansers); and repair with skin flaps for large, deep ulcers. Negative pressure wound healing is a useful technology in the treatment of stage III/IV pressure ulcers.[18,19] Infection requires treatment with antibiotics and pain should be controlled.[20] Randomized controlled trials are needed to determine the best methods for treating pressure ulcers.[21,22]

Keloids and Hypertrophic Scars. **Keloids** are rounded, firm, elevated scars with irregular clawlike margins that extend beyond the original site of injury. **Hypertrophic scars** are elevated erythematous fibrous lesions that do not expand beyond the border of injury. Both lesions are genetically influenced and caused by abnormal wound healing with excessive fibroblast activity and collagen formation during dermal connective tissue repair.[23,24] A familial tendency for keloid formation has been found and both autosomal recessive and autosomal dominant inheritance patterns have been reported.[25] Genes regulating fibroblasts may be up- or down-regulated in keloid tissue.[26]

Keloids are most common in darkly pigmented skin types and burn scars (see Chapter 48). Excessive or poorly aligned tension on a wound, introduction of foreign material into the skin, and the occurrence of certain types of trauma (e.g., burns) are provocative factors. At risk are the shoulders, back, chin, ears, and lower legs. Keloids can appear within weeks to months after a stable scar has formed. Individuals 10 to 30 years of age develop lesions much more commonly than do children before puberty or older adults. Hypertrophic scars usually regress within a year.

The amount of type III collagen is increased with keloids. The increased synthesis of collagen is associated with interleukin-6 (IL-6) signaling and dermal fibroblasts that have high metabolic and mitotic rates. There is aberrant expression of transforming growth factor-beta (TGF-β) and platelet-derived growth factor (PDGF).[27]

Myofibroblasts, cells with characteristics of fibroblasts and smooth muscle cells, are the principal cells in keloids. Collagenase activity in keloids is normal or increased, but the collagen may be protected from degradation by **proteoglycan,** a glycoprotein present in connective tissue that serves as a binding (cementing) material, and by specific inhibitors of proteolytic enzymes.[28] Keloids first appear as pink or red, firm, well-defined rubbery plaques that persist for several months after trauma. Later, uncontrolled overgrowth causes extension beyond the site of the original wound and the tumor becomes smoother, irregularly shaped, hyperpigmented, and harder with **clawlike prolongations** (Figure 46-4).

Keloids are the most extreme example of cutaneous scarring and the most difficult to treat. Preventive measures such as avoidance of unnecessary elective surgeries, recognition of familial tendency, and early detection are of paramount

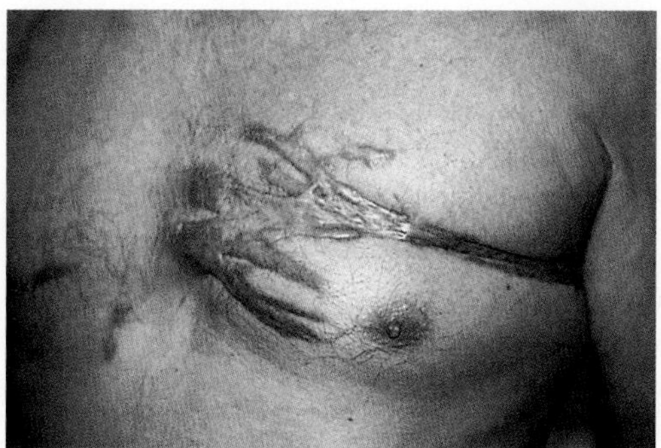

FIGURE 46-4 **Keloid.** (Courtesy Department of Dermatology, School of Medicine, University of Utah.)

importance. Standard management of keloids and hypertrophic scars includes intralesional corticosteroids, cryotherapy, radiotherapy, and surgical/laser procedures whereas intralesional injections of interferon, bleomycin, and 5-fluorouracil (5-FU) are emerging treatments.[29] There remains a need for research to improve treatment outcome.[30,31]

Pruritus

Pruritus, or itching, is the most common symptom associated with many primary skin disorders, such as eczema, psoriasis, or lice infestations, or it can be a manifestation of systemic disease (e.g., xerosis, chronic renal failure, cholestatic liver disease, thyroid disorders, iron deficiency, neuropathies, or malignancy) or drug reactions. Pruritus may be acute (e.g., mosquito bite) or chronic, and may be localized or generalized and migratory.

Multiple stimuli can produce itching and there is interaction between itch and pain sensations. Peripheral pruritogenic (itch) mediators include histamine, neuropeptides, serotonin, prostaglandins, bradykinin, substance P, opioids, acetylcholine, interleukin-31, and nerve growth factor. Itch sensation is thought to be carried by specific unmyelinated C nerve fibers and thinly myelinated Aδ nerve fibers. Specific spinal pathways carry itch sensations through the spinal cord to the brain.[32] These nerve fibers also may interact with dermal eosinophils, lymphocytes, and mast cells.[33]

Central nervous system mechanisms also can modulate itching, which is less perceptible when the mind is distracted by other stimuli. How the central nervous system influences the itch sensation is unclear. *Neuropathic itch* (itch without pruritogenic stimuli) is related to pathology along an afferent pathway (i.e., postherpetic neuropathy).[34] *Psychogenic itch* is associated with psychologic disorders (e.g., depression and obsessive-compulsive disorder).[35]

Chronic itching is an unpleasant sensation that may or may not be relieved by scratching—often done so intensely that trauma to the skin occurs, resulting in infection, skin thickening (lichenification), and scarring. Both central and peripheral sensitization occurs.[35] Some individuals become so distraught with the constant irritation that they apply heat and/or ice with enough intensity and duration to produce skin injury. Management of itching is challenging and depends on the cause; the primary condition must be treated. Both topical and systemic therapies are used.[36,37]

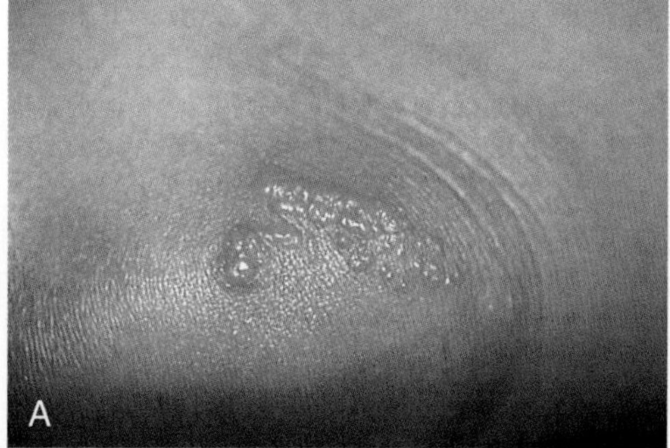

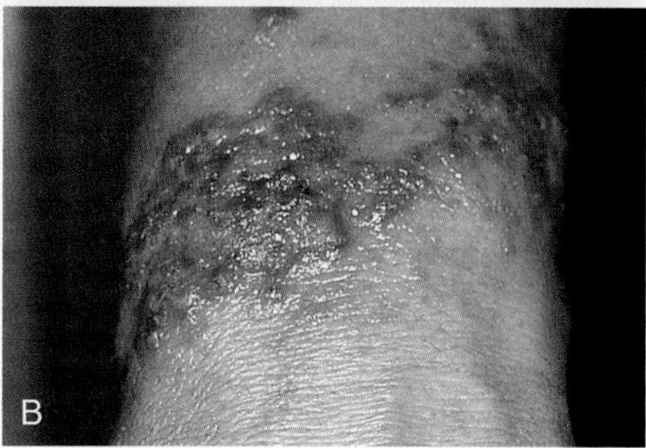

FIGURE 46-5 **Poison Ivy. A,** Poison ivy on knee. **B,** Poison ivy dermatitis. (Courtesy Department of Dermatology, School of Medicine, University of Utah.)

DISORDERS OF THE SKIN

Disruptions in skin integrity may be precipitated by trauma, abnormal cellular function, infection and inflammation, and systemic diseases. Many skin disorders are benign and self-limiting, whereas others are severe and life threatening.

Inflammatory Disorders

The most common inflammatory disorder of the skin is **eczema,** or dermatitis. Eczema and dermatitis are general terms that describe a particular type of inflammatory response in the skin—the terms can be used interchangeably. Eczematous disorders are generally characterized by pruritus, lesions with indistinct borders, and epidermal changes. These lesions either can appear as erythema, papules, or scales or can present in an acute, subacute, or chronic phase. Edema, serous discharge, and crusting occur with continued irritation and scratching. In chronic eczema the skin becomes thickened, leathery, and hyperpigmented from recurrent irritation and scratching. The location of eczema is related to the underlying cause. Eczematous inflammations need to be differentiated from other dermatoses, particularly psoriasis.

Allergic Contact Dermatitis

Allergic contact dermatitis is a common form of T-cell–mediated or delayed hypersensitivity (type IV).[38] (See Chapter 9 for various types of allergic responses.) Genetic susceptibility involves several genes including loss-of-function mutations in the gene encoding the epidermal protein filaggrin.[39] Allergens (e.g., microorganisms, chemicals, foreign proteins, drugs, metals, latex) can form the sensitizing antigen; contact with poison ivy is a common example (Figure 46-5). The response is a reaction to irritants with release of cytokines, chemokines, and cytotoxins from keratinocytes, dendritic cells (Langerhans cells), and natural killer cells. When the allergen comes into contact with the skin the allergen is bound to a carrier protein, forming a hapten-specific sensitizing antigen. Langerhans cells process the antigen and carry it to T cells that then become sensitized to the antigen, releasing cytokines and chemokines and leading to leukocyte infiltration and inflammation.[40] Latex allergy can be either a type IV hypersensitivity reaction to chemicals used in latex rubber processing or a type I immediate hypersensitivity reaction with IgE antibodies formed in response to latex rubber protein.[41]

In delayed hypersensitivity, several hours pass before an immunologic response is apparent. The T cells play an important role because they differentiate and secrete lymphokines that affect macrophage movement and aggregation, coagulation, and other inflammatory responses (see Chapter 9). Sensitization usually develops with first exposure to the antigen, and symptoms of dermatitis occur with reexposure.

The manifestations of allergic contact dermatitis include erythema and swelling with pruritic (itching) vesicular lesions in the areas of allergen contact. The pattern of distribution provides clues to the source of the antigen (e.g., hands exposed to chemical solutions or boundaries from rings and bracelets). Patch tests with specific antigens may assist with diagnosis. Removal of the allergen is necessary for resolution of the inflammatory response and tissue repair. Topical or systemic steroids, as well as other symptomatic treatment, may be required depending on the severity of the lesion.[42]

Irritant Contact Dermatitis

Irritant contact dermatitis is a common nonimmunologically-mediated inflammation of the skin. The intensity of the inflammation is related to the concentration of the irritant, exposure time, disruption of the skin barrier, and age.[43] Irritation can occur from almost anything, especially if the epidermal barrier is compromised in any way (Box 46-2). The skin lesions are similar in appearance to allergic contact dermatitis. Removing the source of irritation and using topical agents (i.e., corticosteroids and petroleum-based emollients) and nonirritating soaps constitute effective treatment.

Atopic Dermatitis

Atopic dermatitis (allergic dermatitis) is more common in infancy and childhood; however, some individuals are affected throughout life. See Chapter 47 for details.[44]

Stasis Dermatitis

Stasis dermatitis usually occurs on the legs as a result of venous stasis and edema. The disorder is associated with varicosities (incompetent venous valves), phlebitis, and vascular trauma. Pooling of venous blood traps leukocytes that may release proteolytic enzymes. Increased venous pressure widens interendothelial pores with deposition of red blood cells, fibrin, and other macromolecules, making them unavailable for repair and promoting inflammation.[45] Edema evolves to erythema and pruritus with progression to scaling, petechiae, and hyperpigmentation. Progressive lesions become ulcerated (stasis ulcers), particularly around the ankles and tibia (Figure 46-6).

Treatment includes elevating the legs as often as possible, refraining from wearing tight clothes around the legs, and avoiding standing for long periods. Defined infections are treated with antibiotics. Chronic lesions with ulceration are treated with moist dressings, external compression garments, and vein ablation surgery.[46]

BOX 46-2 SUBSTANCES KNOWN TO CAUSE CONTACT DERMATITIS*

- Alkalis
  - Soaps
  - Detergents
  - Ammonia preparations
  - Lye
  - Drainpipe cleaners
  - Toilet bowl cleaners
  - Oven cleaners
- Acids
- Metal salts
  - Cyanides of calcium, copper, mercury, nickel, silver, zinc
  - Chlorides of calcium and zinc
- Bromine, chlorine, iodine, fluorine
- Insecticides
- Herbicides
- Dusts of lime, zinc, arsenic
- Dyes and fragrances
- Wood dust from teak, cinchona bark, quinine, pyrethrum
- Tobacco dust from cigars
- Explosive powders
- Hydrocarbons
  - Crude petroleum, lubricating oil, cutting oil
  - Paraffins, mineral oils
  - Asphalt, other tar products
- Soot, peat
- Preservatives

*For chemicals that cause occupational allergic contact dermatitis see National Library of Medicine: Haz-map Table 1: Chemicals that cause occupational allergic contact dermatitis, Bethesda, MD, last updated April 2013. Available at www.hax-map.com/allergic.htm.

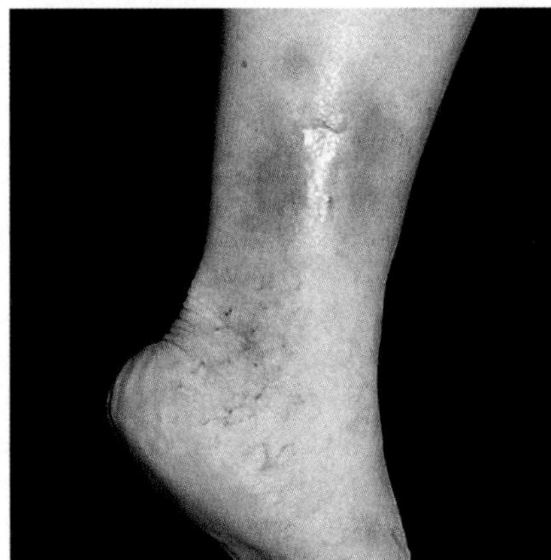

FIGURE 46-6 Stasis Ulcer. (Courtesy Department of Dermatology, School of Medicine, University of Utah.)

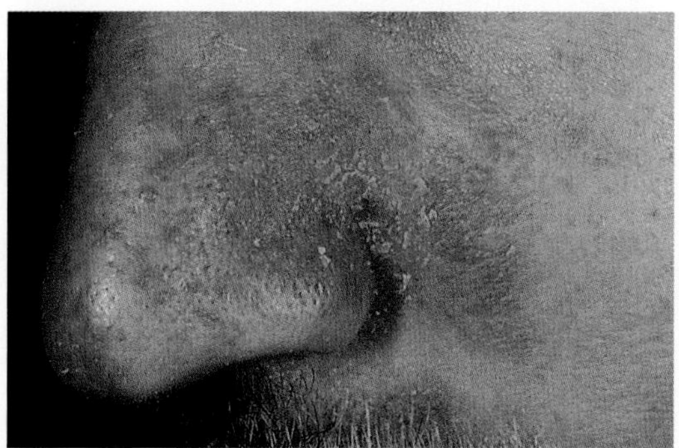

FIGURE 46-7 Seborrheic Dermatitis. (Courtesy Department of Dermatology, School of Medicine, University of Utah.)

Seborrheic Dermatitis

Seborrheic dermatitis is a common chronic inflammation of the skin involving the scalp, eyebrows, eyelids, ear canals, nasolabial folds, axillae, chest, and back (Figure 46-7). In infants it is known as *cradle cap.* The cause is unknown, but genetic predisposition, the production of specific phospholipases from the presence of *Malassezia yeasts, and immune responses* are implicated.[47,48] The lesions appear from infancy to old age, with periods of remission and exacerbation. The lesions appear as greasy, scaly, white, or yellowish inflammatory plaques in sebaceous areas with mild pruritus. Mild cases are treated with shampoos containing sulfur, salicylic acid, or tar. Ketoconazole has antifungal and anti-inflammatory effects and has been used with success along with topical calcineurin inhibitors. Corticosteroid applications are useful for suppression of severe symptoms but should not be used for maintenance therapy.[49]

Papulosquamous Disorders

Psoriasis, pityriasis rosea, and lichen planus are inflammatory disorders characterized by papules, scales, plaques, and erythema. Collectively they are described as **papulosquamous disorders.**

Psoriasis

Psoriasis is a chronic, relapsing, proliferative, inflammatory disorder that involves the skin, scalp, and nails and can occur at any age. The disease affects about 1% to 8% of the world population and is more common in countries north of the equator.[50] The onset is generally established by 20 years of age. A family history of psoriasis is common. The genetic mechanisms are complex and the human leukocyte antigen (HLA)-Cw6 allele *(PSORS1)* is a major susceptibility gene that affects skin barrier function and innate immune responses.[51] Psoriasis is a T helper (Th) cell–mediated autoimmune disease. The interleukin (IL)-23/T helper (Th) 17 cell axis plays an important role in the pathogenesis of psoriasis.[52] Inflammatory cytokines involved include tumor necrosis factor-alpha (TNF-α), interferon-gamma (IFN-γ), IL-6, IL-12, IL-15, IL-17, IL-20, IL-21, and IL-22 derived from activated T cells, B cells, dendritic cells, and macrophages.[53]

The dermis and epidermis are thickened with keratinocyte hyperproliferation, altered keratinocyte differentiation, expanded dermal vasculature, infiltration of neutrophils and lymphocytes, and inflammation.[54] The turnover time for shedding the epidermis is decreased from the normal 26 to 30 days to 3 to 4 days. There are increased numbers of germinative cells and an increase in transit time of cells through the dermis. The rapid cellular proliferation does not allow time for cell maturation and keratinization to occur, resulting in a thickened epidermis and plaque formation. The loosely cohesive keratin gives the lesion a silvery, scaly appearance. There is often capillary dilation and increased vascularization to accommodate the increased cell metabolism. The increased vascularity causes erythema.

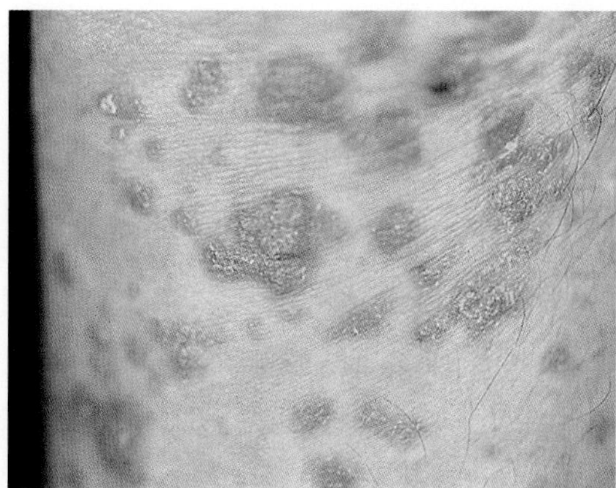

FIGURE 46-8 Psoriasis. Typical oval plaques with well-defined borders and silvery scale. (Courtesy Department of Dermatology, School of Medicine, University of Utah.)

The types of psoriasis include plaque (psoriasis vulgaris), inverse, guttate, pustular, and erythrodermic. **Plaque psoriasis** is the most common and affects 80% to 90% of individuals with psoriasis. The disease can be mild, moderate, or severe, depending on the size, distribution, and inflammation of the lesions. Early onset psoriasis is an inflammatory lesion with epidermal hyperproliferation and the presence of activated T lymphocytes. The typical lesion of plaque psoriasis is a well-demarcated, thick, silvery, scaly, erythematous plaque surrounded by normal skin (Figure 46-8). Initial lesions usually develop insidiously as small erythematous papules that enlarge and coalesce into larger inflammatory lesions that can be painful. The lesions are commonly located on the scalp, elbows, and knees and at sites of trauma. The scales are usually loosely adherent and may cause small bleeding points when removed. **Inverse psoriasis** is rare and involves lesions that develop in skinfolds (i.e., axilla or groin). They are large, smooth, dry, and deep red. The clinical course of psoriasis is characterized by remissions and exacerbations. Psoriasis may be triggered by drugs including antimalarials, lithium, nonsteroidal anti-inflammatories, and beta-blockers.[55]

In **guttate psoriasis,** small papules (1 to 10 mm) appear suddenly on the trunk and extremities (Figure 46-9). The lesions may appear a few weeks after a streptococcal respiratory tract infection and are more common in children. Guttate psoriasis may resolve spontaneously in weeks or months. **Pustular psoriasis** appears as blisters of noninfectious pus (collections of neutrophils) that develop over areas of plaque psoriasis.

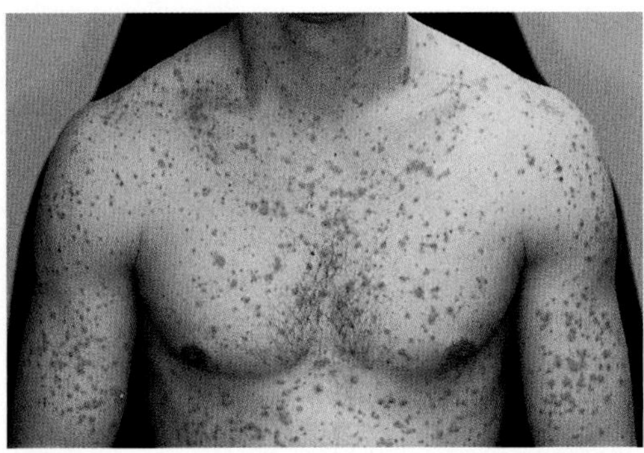

FIGURE 46-9 Guttate Psoriasis after Streptococcal Infection. Numerous uniformly small lesions may abruptly occur after streptococcal pharyngitis. (Courtesy Department of Dermatology, School of Medicine, University of Utah.)

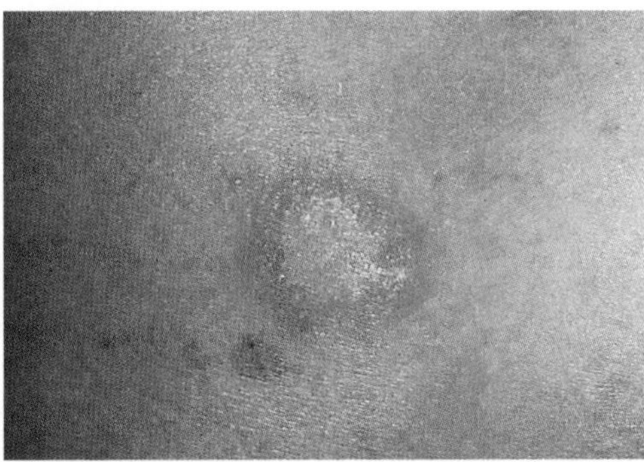

FIGURE 46-10 Pityriasis Rosea Herald Patch. A collarette pattern has formed around the margins. (Courtesy Department of Dermatology, School of Medicine, University of Utah.)

Erythrodermic (exfoliative) psoriasis is characterized by widespread red, scaling lesions that cover a large body surface area (BSA) and is often accompanied by itching or pain associated with constitutional symptoms (fever, chills, fatigue) and skin infections.

Psoriatic arthritis (PsA) and ankylosing spondylitis are associated with the proinflammatory cytokines that cause psoriatic skin lesions. Joints of the hands, feet, knees, and ankles are involved, and 5% to 50% of individuals with psoriasis have seronegative joint involvement. Psoriatic arthritis mutilans involves pronounced bone destruction and there is greater risk of cardiovascular disease with PsA.[56,57] **Psoriatic nail disease** can occur in all psoriasis subtypes with pitting, onycholysis, subungual hyperkeratosis, and nail plate dystrophy. Psoriasis also is a risk factor for a number of comorbidities including inflammatory bowel disease; metabolic syndrome, including hypertension insulin resistance, dyslipidemias, and abdominal obesity; and increased risk for atherosclerosis and cardiovascular disease that is independent of traditional risk factors for these diseases.[58,59]

Treatment is individualized and related to maintaining skin moisture, reducing epidermal cell turnover and itching, and improving immunomodulation. Mild lesions are usually treated with emollients, keratolytic agents, and corticosteroids. Moderate lesions may respond to UVB light, tar preparations, or a combination of both, and to methotrexate, cyclosporine A, and acitretin. Moderate to severe disease is responsive to the photosensitizing agent oral psoralen in combination with UVA light (PUVA), although skin cancer risk (melanoma and squamous cell) with cumulative dose remains a valid concern.[60] Vitamin D_3 (calcitriol) is used to reduce epidermal proliferation. Moderate to severe disease is the indication for biologic treatment including TNF-α blockers (adalimumab, etanercept, infliximab) and interleukin (IL)-12/-23 inhibitors (ustekinumab). Clinical trials are evaluating new agents.[61,62]

Pityriasis Rosea

Pityriasis rosea is a benign self-limiting inflammatory disorder that occurs more often in young adults, with seasonal peaks in the spring and fall. This is a benign disorder except when contracted during pregnancy, when risks are increased for miscarriage and premature delivery.[63] The cause is unknown but is thought to be associated with a virus (e.g., human herpesvirus 6 [HHV-6] and HHV-7) because of the timing and clustering of the outbreaks.[64] Pityriasis rosea begins as a single lesion known as a **herald patch** (Figure 46-10) that is circular, demarcated, and salmon-pink; is approximately 3 to 4 cm in diameter; and is usually located on the trunk. Early lesions are macular and papular; secondary lesions develop within 14 to 21 days and extend over the trunk and upper part of the extremities. Lesions are rarely located on the face. They emerge as small erythematous papules that expand into characteristic oval lesions. There may be few or hundreds of lesions. The pattern of distribution follows the skin lines around the trunk and resembles a drooping pine tree. As scales flake off from the margin of the lesions, a collarette pattern is formed. Itching is the most common symptom. Headache, fatigue, or sore throat may precede the development of the lesions.

The diagnosis of pityriasis rosea is made by the clinical appearance of the lesion. Secondary syphilis, psoriasis, drug eruption, nummular eczema, and seborrheic dermatitis are among the differential diagnosis considerations. The disorder is usually self-limiting and resolves in a few months with symptomatic treatment for pruritus or cosmetic concerns. UV light (with some risk for hyperpigmentation), antihistamines, or topical corticosteroids may be used to control itching. Erythromycin and acyclovir also may be used for treatment.[65]

Lichen Planus

Lichen planus (LP) is a benign, autoimmune inflammatory disorder of the skin and mucous membranes with multiple clinical variations. The cause is unknown, but T cells, adhesion molecules, inflammatory cytokines, perforin, and antigen-presenting cells are involved.[66] The infiltrate of T cells mediates immunoreactivity against basal layer keratinocytes, which have altered surface antigens and adhesion molecules.[67] LP is also linked to hepatitis C virus. Some individuals develop lichenoid lesions after exposure to drugs or film-processing chemicals. The age of onset is usually between 30 and 70 years. The disorder begins with flat purple, polygonal, pruritic, nonscaling papules 2 to 4 mm in size, usually located on the wrists, ankles, lower legs, and genitalia (Figure 46-11). New lesions are pale pink and evolve into a dark violet. Persistent lesions may be thickened and red, forming hypertrophic LP. Oral lesions

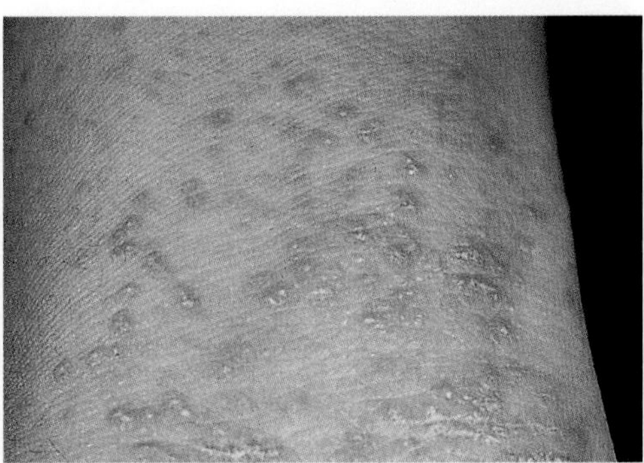

FIGURE 46-11 Hypertrophic Lichen Planus on Arms. (Courtesy Department of Dermatology, School of Medicine, University of Utah.)

(oral lichen planus) appear as lacy white rings that must be differentiated from leukoplakia or oral candidiasis and they may be precancerous lesions.[68] Fine white lines, known as Wickham striae, can be seen throughout the oral lesions on magnification. These lesions also can develop on the penis and vulvovaginal area. More commonly, oral lesions do not ulcerate, but localized or extensive painful ulcerations do, and frequently, occur. Chronic ulcerated lesions become malignant in 1% of individuals with the disease. Thinning and splitting of nails are common, and part or all of the nail may be shed.

Pruritus is the most distressing symptom. The lesions are self-limiting and may last for months or years, with an average duration of 6 to 18 months. Postinflammatory hyperpigmentation is a common consequence of the lesion. Approximately 20% of individuals have a recurrence. Diagnosis is commonly made by the clinical appearance of the lesion; however, histopathologic diagnosis is recommended. For cutaneous LP, treatment is individualized and includes topical, intralesional, or systemic corticosteroids (second line for resistant LP), and systemic acitretin with/without adjuvant light therapy. Antihistamines are given for itching, and topical or systemic corticosteroids may be used to control inflammation. Short-term systemic glucocorticoids are indicated if oral lesions are severe or for LP involving three or more nails. Mucous membrane lesions are treated with potent topical steroids, topical retinoids, and systemic glucocorticoids.[69-71]

Acne Vulgaris

Acne vulgaris is an inflammatory disorder of the pilosebaceous follicle (the sebaceous gland contiguous with a hair follicle). It occurs most commonly during adolescence. Details of this disorder are presented in Chapter 47. Hidradenitis suppurativa (inverse acne) is summarized in What's New? Hidradenitis Suppurativa (Inverse Acne).

Acne Rosacea

Acne rosacea is a chronic, readily exacerbated, inflammatory skin disease with varied presentations and extent of involvement that develops primarily in middle-age adults. There are four types of lesions: erythematotelangiectatic, papulopustular, phymatous, and ocular.[72] They occur in the middle third of the face, including the forehead, nose, cheeks, and chin (Figure 46-12). The cause is unknown, but immune-mediated inflammation may be a factor. The lesions are associated with chronic,

WHAT'S NEW?

Hidradenitis Suppurativa (Inverse Acne)

Hidradenitis suppurativa (inverse acne) is a chronic, inflammatory, recurring, scarring disease of the pilosebaceous follicular ducts involving areas of skin where there are folds, hair follicles, and apocrine (sweat) glands (i.e., axillary, inguinal, inframammary, genital, buttocks, and perineal areas of the body) (see figure). The incidence is unknown but estimated at 1% to 4% of the population and is more common in females. The pathogenesis of the disease is complex and includes a combination of genetic, hormonal, immune, and environmental factors. Aggravating factors include tight clothing, heat and perspiration, obesity, stress, and smoking. Follicular hyperkeratosis and occlusion obstructs the pilosebaceous unit, causing perifolliculitis, abscess formation, sinus tracts, and scarring. Bacterial infection is a secondary event. The lesions present as deep, firm, painful subcutaneous nodules that track and rupture horizontally under the skin. They are differentiated from "boils" (carbuncles) because boils extend vertically and discharge onto the skin. Diagnosis can be difficult, delaying effective treatment. Treatment can include administering systemic medications, performing incision and drainage of nodules, obtaining a culture of the exudate, and giving antibiotics, with concern about the presence of methicillin-resistant *Staphylococcus aureus* (MRSA), topical or intralesional corticosteroids, and retinoids. Lesions often require surgical excision and skin grafting. Complete, spontaneous resolution is rare. Deterrence includes avoiding heat and perspiration, losing weight if obese, wearing loose clothing, refraining from shaving affected areas, stopping smoking, and using zinc gluconate supplements to reduce inflammation.

The disease can recur for years with negative effects on quality of life. Clinical trials are needed to identify the best treatment options.

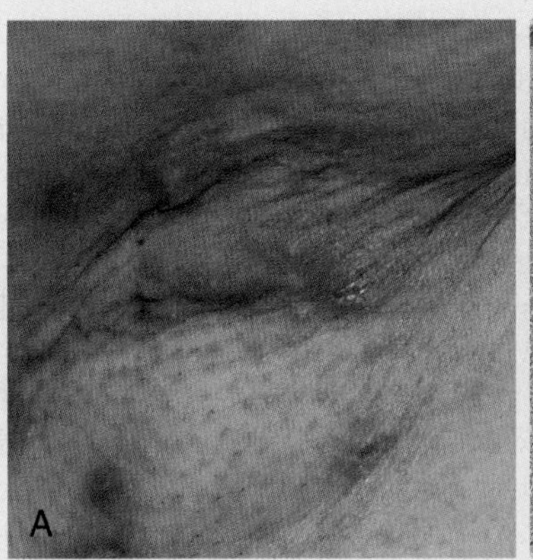

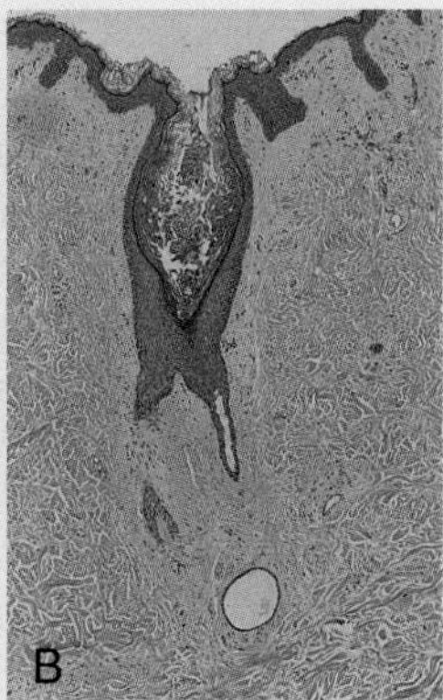

A, Characteristic painful pustules and draining sinus tracts. **B,** Histology shows follicular plugging and connection to a dilated apocrine duct. (**A** courtesy Kalman Watsky, MD; from Bolognia JL, Jorizzo JL, Schaffer JV: *Dermatology,* ed 3, Philadelphia, 2012, Saunders. **B** from Bolognia JL, Jorizzo JL, Rapini RP: *Dermatology,* ed 2, Philadelphia, 2008, Saunders.)

Data from Alikhan A, Lynch PJ, Eisen DB: *J Am Acad Dermatol* 60(4):539–561, 2009; Bieniek A et al: *Dermatol Surg* 36(12):1998–2004, 2010; Danby FW, Margesson LJ: *Dermatol Clin* 28(4):779–793, 2010; Danby FW et al: *Br J Dermatol* 168(5):1034-1039, 2013; Yazdanyar S, Jemec GB: *Curr Opin Infect Dis* 24(2):118–123, 2011.

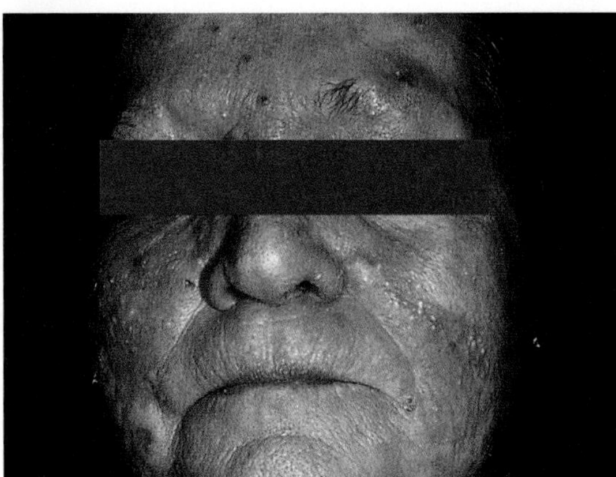

FIGURE 46-12 Rosacea. Pustules and erythema occur on the forehead, cheeks, and nose. (Courtesy Department of Dermatology, School of Medicine, University of Utah.)

inappropriate vasodilation resulting in flushing and sensitivity to the sun. Sebaceous hypertrophy, fibrosis, and telangiectasia may be severe enough to produce an irreversible bulbous appearance of the nose, known as *rhinophyma.* The vascular abnormalities induce local production of transforming growth factor-β1 (TGF-β1) capable of creating fibrosis and, therefore, cutaneous thickening.[73] *Demodex folliculorum* (mites) infection may be a contributing factor.[74] Disorders of the eye often accompany rosacea, particularly conjunctivitis and, more rarely, keratitis, which can result in visual impairment.[75] Facial application of fluorinated topical steroids may precipitate rosacea-like lesions that are difficult to treat.

Hot drinks or alcohol should be taken cautiously because the heat and vasodilation accentuate erythema. Daily use of photoprotection, including sunscreens, is recommended; both topical (metronidazole, azelaic acid) and oral drugs (tetracyclines) may be effective.[76] Surgical excision of excessive tissue may be required for rhinophyma.

Lupus Erythematosus

Lupus erythematosus is an inflammatory, autoimmune, systemic disease with cutaneous manifestations. Discoid (or cutaneous) lupus erythematosus (DLE) is limited to the skin and can progress to systemic lupus erythematosus (SLE). DLE may be described as a subset of SLE, with cutaneous manifestations as the only symptom[77] (Figure 46-13). (SLE, a diffuse, multisystem disease that also has cutaneous manifestations, is discussed in Chapter 9.)

Discoid (Cutaneous) Lupus Erythematosus. **Discoid (cutaneous) lupus erythematosus (DLE)** usually occurs in genetically susceptible adults, particularly in women in their late thirties or early forties. There are three forms of the disease: acute, subacute, and chronic. The lesions may be single or multiple and of various sizes. Often the lesions are located on light-exposed areas of the skin, and photosensitivity is common. The face is the most common site of lesion involvement. The characteristic manifestations of the different categories of DLE are summarized in Table 46-6.

The cause is unknown but thought to be related to genetic and environmental factors and an altered immune response to

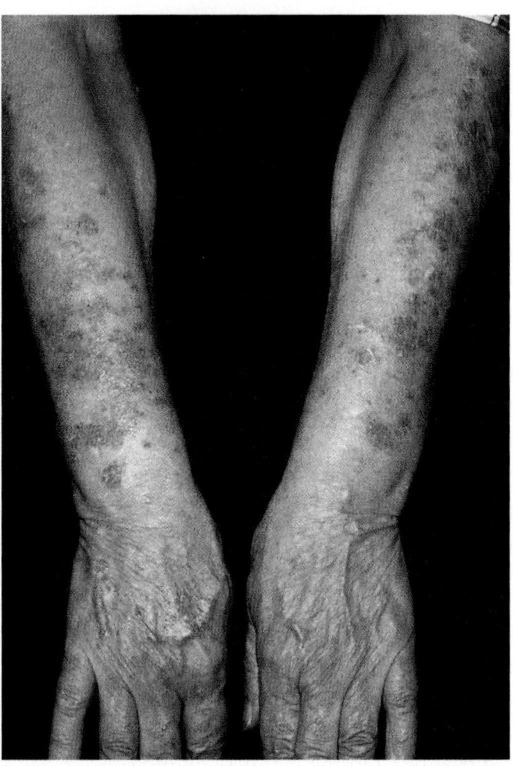

FIGURE 46-13 Subacute Cutaneous Lupus (Discoid Lupus Erythematosus). (Courtesy Department of Dermatology, School of Medicine, University of Utah.)

an unknown antigen or response to UV wavelengths with the development of self-reactive T and B cells, decreased number of regulatory T cells, and increased proinflammatory cytokines. Autoantibodies and immune complexes cause tissue damage.[78]

Diagnosis of DLE is made from the presenting symptoms, biopsy of skin lesions with direct immunofluorescence, as well as histologic results. Skin biopsy with immunofluorescent observation reveals lumpy deposits of immunoglobulins, especially IgM and C3.[79] DLE can progress to systemic lupus erythematosus and individuals with SLE should be regularly screened for this progression.[80]

Individuals with DLE must use sunscreen and sun protection because direct sun exposure initiates or exacerbates lesions. Treatment options include topical steroids, calcineurin inhibitors, antimalarial drugs (e.g., hydroxychloroquine sulfate), and immunosuppressors. These medications must be used with caution to prevent serious side effects.[81]

Vesiculobullous Disorders

Vesiculobullous skin diseases share a common characteristic of vesicle, or blister, formation. Two such diseases are pemphigus and erythema multiforme.

Pemphigus

Pemphigus (meaning to blister or bubble) is a rare autoimmune blistering disease of the skin and oral mucous membranes caused by circulating autoantibodies directed against the cell surface adhesion molecule desmoglein at the desmosomal cell junction in the suprabasal layer of the epidermis. Pemphigus

TABLE 46-6 CATEGORIES AND MANIFESTATIONS OF DISCOID LUPUS ERYTHEMATOSUS (DLE)

CATEGORY OF DLE	CLINICAL MANIFESTATIONS
Acute	
Localized	Butterfly pattern of erythema over bridge of nose and malar areas of face (malar rash); may have fine surface scales and underlying edema; scalp areas may develop alopecia; lasts for hours to days
Generalized	Diffuse or papular erythema of face, upper trunk, or extremities; develops quickly and lasts hours to days
Subacute	Erythematous macules and papules that evolve into *papulosquamous* or *annular* plaques developing on sun-exposed areas of the upper body (V area of neck, upper chest, back, shoulders, extensor surface of arms and hands); can be associated with reaction to drugs; may be accompanied by mild systemic disease
Chronic	Classic discoid lupus erythematosus is the most common form; lesions are red to purple macules or papules with a superficial brownish scale; scale can penetrate hair follicle leaving a carpet-tack appearance when removed; may have residual scarring, dermal atrophy hypopigmentation, alopecia, and telangiectasia; Raynaud phenomenon occurs in some individuals

Data from Kuhn A, Biji M: *Lupus* 17(5):389–393, 2008; Rothfield N, Sontheimer RD, Bernstein M: *Clin Dermatol* 24(5):348–362, 2006; Uva L et al: *Autoimmune Dis* 2012:834291, 2012.

can occur in all age groups but is more prevalent between 40 and 50 years of age. There is a genetic predisposition as well as environmental triggers, most of which are unknown.[82] Pemphigus presents in varying forms:

- **Pemphigus vulgaris** is the most common form with acantholysis at the suprabasal level. Immunoglobulin G (IgG) autoantibodies and C3 complement bind to the desmoglein adhesion molecules, resulting in the destruction of cell-to-cell adhesion (acantholysis) in the epidermis with fluid accumulation and the resulting symptom of blister formation.[83] Oral lesions precede the onset of skin blistering, which is more prominent on the face, scalp, and axilla. The blisters rupture easily because of the thin, fragile overlying portion of epidermis, resulting in painful erosions. *Pemphigus vegetans* is a rare variant of pemphigus vulgaris with large blisters that progress to hypertrophic granulomas with tissue erosion and pustules (vegetating plaques). They usually occur in tissue folds.
- **Pemphigus foliaceus** is a milder form of the disease and involves acantholysis at the subcorneal level with blistering, erosions, scaling, crusting, and erythema usually of the face and chest. Oral mucous membranes are rarely involved. *Pemphigus erythematosus* is a subset of pemphigus foliaceus often associated with systemic lupus erythematosus with positive antinuclear antibodies. The lesions are generally less widely distributed.
- **Paraneoplastic pemphigus** is the most severe form of pemphigus and is associated with lymphoproliferative neoplasms. Internal organs, including lungs, thyroid, kidney, smooth muscle, and the gastrointestinal tract, also are involved, leading to the term *paraneoplastic autoimmune multiorgan syndrome.* In contrast to pemphigus vulgaris, the lesions develop from inflammatory papules or macules rather than normal skin.[84]
- **IgA pemphigus** is the most benign form of pemphigus characterized by tissue-bound and circulating IgA antibodies targeting desmosomal or nondesmosomal cell surface components in the basement membrane of the epidermis. Acantholysis is not as severe as that in pemphigus vulgaris but there is still blister formation.[85]

The diagnosis of pemphigus is made from the clinical manifestations and histologic examination of the skin. Immunofluorescence demonstrates the presence of antibodies at the site of blister formation. The clinical course of the disease may range from rapidly fatal to relatively benign. The primary treatment for pemphigus is systemic corticosteroids in combination with adjuvant immunosuppressants and, in difficult cases, adjuvant protein A immunoadsorption intravenous immunoglobulins, plasmapheresis, and anti-CD20 monoclonal antibody therapy. Newer methods of treatment and a clearer understanding of the pathogenesis have improved the prognosis and decreased mortality.[86]

Bullous Pemphigoid

Bullous pemphigoid (BP) is a more benign autoimmune disease than pemphigus vulgaris, with blistering of the subepidermal skin layer. Autoantibodies (IgG and IgE) to hemidesmosomal proteins designated BP 180 and BP 230 have been found. There are numerous triggers, including drugs and skin trauma. The autoantibodies activate complement with inflammatory infiltration of neutrophils, eosinophils, and lymphocytes. Loss of dermal-epidermal adhesion is caused by inflammatory cytokines.[87,88] The lesions of pemphigoid begin with localized erythema or as pruritic plaques that extend and become edematous. The plaques turn reddish purple by 2 to 3 weeks, with vesicles and bullae emerging on the surface (Figure 46-14). Oral lesions can occur. The bullae do not extend with pressure. The blisters rupture within 1 week and heal rapidly. BP occurs more commonly after 60 years of age.

Diagnosis is by skin biopsy and immunofluorescent examination. The presence of subepidermal blistering and eosinophils distinguishes pemphigoid from pemphigus. Treatment usually includes hydroxyzine (Atarax) for itching and topical or systemic corticosteroids. Adjuvant immunosuppressive drugs may be prescribed. Relapse may occur with discontinuation of treatment.[89,90]

Erythema Multiforme

Erythema multiforme is not a single disease but rather a syndrome characterized by inflammation of skin and mucous

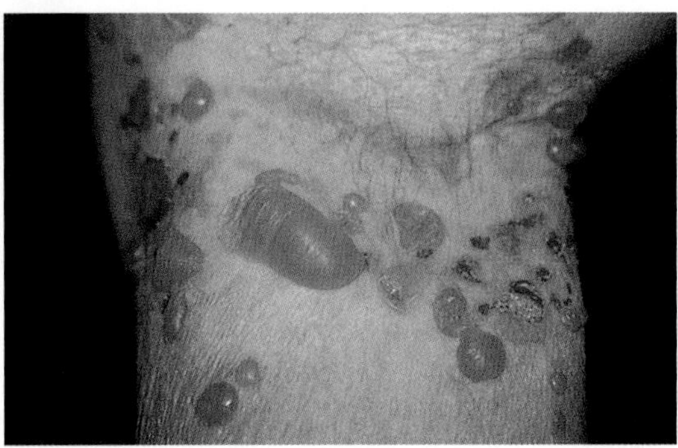

FIGURE 46-14 Bullous Pemphigoid. Generalized eruption with blisters arising from an edematous, erythematous annular base. (Courtesy Department of Dermatology, School of Medicine, University of Utah.)

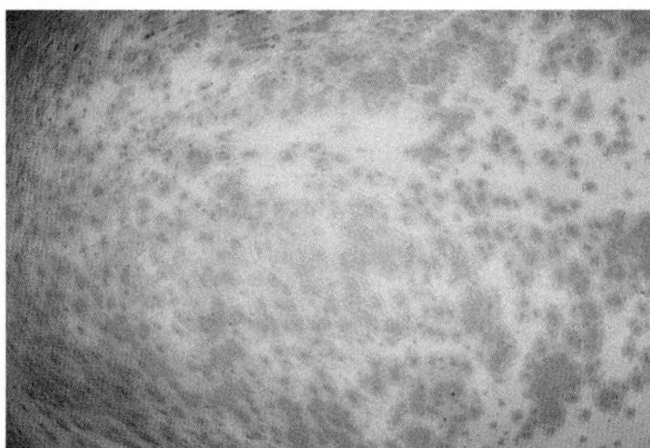

FIGURE 46-15 Erythema Multiforme Caused by Doxepin. (Courtesy Department of Dermatology, School of Medicine, University of Utah.)

membranes. It often is associated with a T-cell–mediated immunologic reaction to microorganisms (e.g., herpes simplex virus, *Mycoplasma pneumoniae*) or a toxic reaction to drugs in which TNF-α causes tissue damage.[91] Overall, it is relatively rare and can occur at any age but is more common between 20 and 40 years of age. Immune complex formation and deposition of complement (C3), IgM, and fibrinogen around the superficial dermal blood vessels, basement membrane, and keratinocytes are found in most individuals with erythema multiforme. Edema develops in the superficial dermis, leading to the formation of vesicles and bullae. The lesions vary in clinical presentation and may involve the skin or mucous membranes, or both. The characteristic "bull's-eye" or "target" lesions occur on the skin surface with a central dusky region surrounded by concentric rings or alternating edema and inflammation.[92,93] The lesions usually occur suddenly in groups over 2 to 3 weeks. Urticarial plaques, 1 to 2 cm in diameter, can develop without the target lesion. A vesiculobullous form is characterized by mucous membrane lesions and erythematous plaques over elbows and knees. Single or multiple vesicles or bullae may arise on a part of the plaque, accompanied by pruritus and burning. In the minor form, there may be tens to hundreds of lesions.[94] The lesions heal within 3 to 4 weeks (Figure 46-15).

Prodromal symptoms of erythema multiform include fever, headache, malaise, sore throat, and cough in approximately one third of cases. The bullous lesions form erosions and crusts when ruptured. The mouth, air passages, esophagus, urethra, and conjunctiva may be involved when mucous membranes are affected. Blindness can result from corneal ulcerations. Difficulty with eating, breathing, and urinating may develop with severe manifestations. Severe forms of the disease can be fatal.

Diagnosis is made by medication history, by recognition of the target lesion, or by skin biopsy to establish the diagnosis. Mild, acute forms of the disease last 10 to 14 days, are usually self-limiting, and require no treatment. Any ongoing drug therapy should be withdrawn or reevaluated and underlying infections treated. Treatment is individualized according to severity.[93] Antiviral prophylaxis may be required. Fluid and electrolyte balance should be monitored in severe forms of the disease, and mucous membranes must be carefully managed with a bland diet, warm saline eyewashes, topical anesthetics, or corticosteroids to maintain comfort and prevent infection. Use of systemic steroids is controversial. Cutaneous blisters can be treated with wet compresses of nanocrystalline silver. Ophthalmic, kidney, and lung involvement requires special care. Resolution occurs in 8 to 10 days, usually without scarring. Mucosal lesions may take 6 weeks to heal.[93]

Infections

Cutaneous infections are common forms of skin disease. They generally remain localized; however, serious complications can develop with systemic involvement. The types of skin infection include bacterial, viral, and fungal. Most infections occur superficially; however, systemic signs and symptoms occasionally develop and rarely become life threatening. Aerobes, yeast, and anaerobes comprise the normal flora of the skin and often provide protection against pathogens that cause skin infections, including *Staphylococcus* and *Streptococcus.*

Bacterial Infections

Most bacterial infections of the skin are caused by local invasion of pathogens. Coagulase-positive *Staphylococcus aureus* and, less often, beta-hemolytic *Streptococci* are the common causative microorganisms. Community-acquired methicillin-resistant *Staphylococcus aureus* (CA-MRSA) is also a cause of serious skin infection (Box 46-3).

Folliculitis. **Folliculitis** is an infection of the hair follicle and can be caused by bacteria, viruses, or fungi. *S. aureus* is a common causative microorganism.[95] The infection develops from proliferation of the microorganism around the opening of the follicle and then spreads into the follicle. Inflammation is caused by the release of chemotactic factors and enzymes from the bacteria. The lesions appear as pustules with a surrounding area of erythema. They are most prominent on the scalp and extremities and rarely cause systemic symptoms. Prolonged skin moisture, occlusive clothing, topical agents, skin trauma (e.g., shaving facial hair), and poor hygiene are associated contributing factors to the development of folliculitis. Cleaning with soap and water and topical application of antibiotics are effective forms of treatment.

Furuncles and Carbuncles. A **furuncle,** or "boil," is an inflammation of the hair follicles that may develop from a preceding folliculitis and spread through the follicular wall into the surrounding dermis. The invading microorganism is

BOX 46-3 COMMUNITY-ACQUIRED METHICILLIN-RESISTANT *Staphylococcus aureus* (CA-MRSA)

CA-MRSA is a serious skin and soft tissue infection that includes abscesses, cellulitis, and necrotizing fasciitis, and can serve as a source for bloodstream infections. Infections are documented among healthy individuals who have no known risk factors, that is, no recent hospitalization, surgical procedures, or prolonged antibiotic treatment. Outbreaks have been documented among athletic teams, among prisoners, and in daycare centers. CA-MRSA strains are epidemiologically and clonally different from hospital- or nursing home–acquired MRSA. The most common tests involve genotyping for the staphylococcal chromosomal cassette mec (SCCmec) type IV and Panton-Valentine leukocidin genes. The USA300-0114 strain has been epidemic in the United States. It also has caused life-threatening pneumonia, osteomyelitis, and septic arthritis and is spreading internationally. CA-MRSAs are more sensitive to antibiotic treatment and there is a wider choice of antibiotic treatment options for CA-MRSA compared with hospital-acquired MRSA. CA-MRSA is usually susceptible to a variety of oral non–beta-lactam antibiotics, including trimethoprim-sulfamethoxazole, clindamycin, tetracyclines, and linezolid. Parenteral therapy with vancomycin or daptomycin also can be considered. Ceftaroline has been effective for both skin and systemic infections. Mupirocin may be used to clear MRSA from nasal secretions if cultures show contamination in the nose. New drugs are under investigation. Preventive measures include practicing good hand hygiene, applying antiseptics and covering cuts and abrasions, using antibacterial soaps for showers after contact sports, avoiding sharing towels and razors, and frequently washing towels.

Data from Casapao AM et al: *Expert Opin Pharmacother* 13(8):1177–1186, 2010; Nimmo GR: *Clin Microbiol Infect* 18(8):725–734, 2012; Tattevin P et al: *Clin Infect Dis* 55(6):781–788, 2012; Tonn K, Ryan TJ: *J Environ Health* 75(6):44–49, 2013; Watkins RR, David MZ, Salata RA: *J Med Microbiol* 61(Pt 9):1179–1193, 2012.

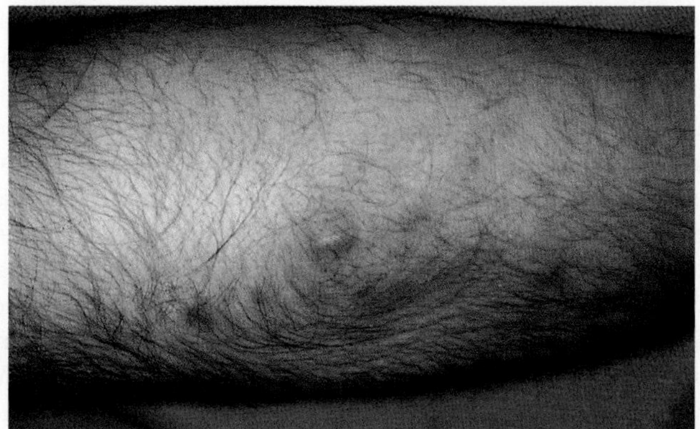

FIGURE 46-16 Furuncle on the Forearm. (Courtesy Department of Dermatology, School of Medicine, University of Utah.)

usually *S. aureus,* including community-associated methicillin-resistant *S. aureus* (CA-MSRA). The infecting strain may spread to the skin from the anterior nares. Any skin area with hair can be infected, and one or several lesions may be present. The precipitating events are similar to those for folliculitis. The initial lesion is a deep, firm, red, painful nodule 1 to 5 cm in diameter (Figure 46-16). Within a few days the initial erythematous nodule changes to a large fluctuant and tender cystic nodule that may be accompanied by cellulitis. No systemic symptoms are present, and the lesion may drain large amounts of pus and necrotic tissue.[96]

A **carbuncle** is a collection of infected hair follicles occurring most often on the back of the neck, the upper back, and the lateral thighs. The lesion begins in the subcutaneous tissue and lower dermis as a firm mass that evolves into an erythematous, painful, swollen mass that drains through many openings. Abscesses may develop. Chills, fever, and malaise are systemic symptoms that can occur during the early stages of lesion development.

Furuncles and carbuncles are treated with warm compresses to provide comfort and promote localization and spontaneous drainage. Abscess formation requires incision and drainage and recurrent infections, extensive lesions, or those associated with cellulitis or systemic symptoms are treated with systemic antibiotics.

Cellulitis. **Cellulitis** is an infection of the dermis and subcutaneous tissue usually caused by *Staphylococcus,* CA-MRSA, or group B streptococci. Cellulitis can occur as an extension of a skin wound, of an ulcer, or from furuncles or carbuncles. It can be associated with chronic venous insufficiency and stasis dermatitis. Risk factors include diabetes mellitus, edema, peripheral vascular disease, tinea pedis, insect bites, and immune suppression. The infected area is erythematous, warm, swollen, and painful and can extend to lymph nodes and the blood. Initial systemic treatment with antibiotics should cover both *Staphylococci* and *Streptococci,* and Burrow soaks can be used to relieve pain. Corticosteroids are used for adjuvant therapy.[97]

Cellulitis must be differentiated from **necrotizing fasciitis.** Necrotizing fasciitis is a rare, rapidly spreading inflammation starting in the fascia, muscles, and subcutaneous fat with subsequent necrosis of the overlying skin; it is treated with antibiotics and often requires surgical débridement.[98]

Erysipelas. **Erysipelas** is an acute superficial infection of the upper dermis (a superficial form of cellulitis) most often caused by *Streptococcus pyogenes,* beta-hemolytic streptococci, and *Staphylococcus aureus.* The face, ears, and lower legs are common sites of involvement, and the site of initial infection may not be identified. Chills, fever, and malaise precede the onset of lesions by 4 hours to 20 days. The initial lesions appear as firm, red spots that enlarge and coalesce to form a clearly circumscribed, advancing edge, bright red, hot lesion with a raised border. Vesicles may appear over the lesion and at the border, producing a bullous form of the disease. Itching, burning, and tenderness accompany the development of the lesion. Cold compresses provide symptomatic relief, and systemic antibiotics are required to arrest the infection.[99]

Impetigo. **Impetigo,** most common in children, is a superficial lesion of the skin caused by coagulase-positive *Staphylococcus aureus* or alpha-hemolytic streptococci[100] (see Chapter 47).

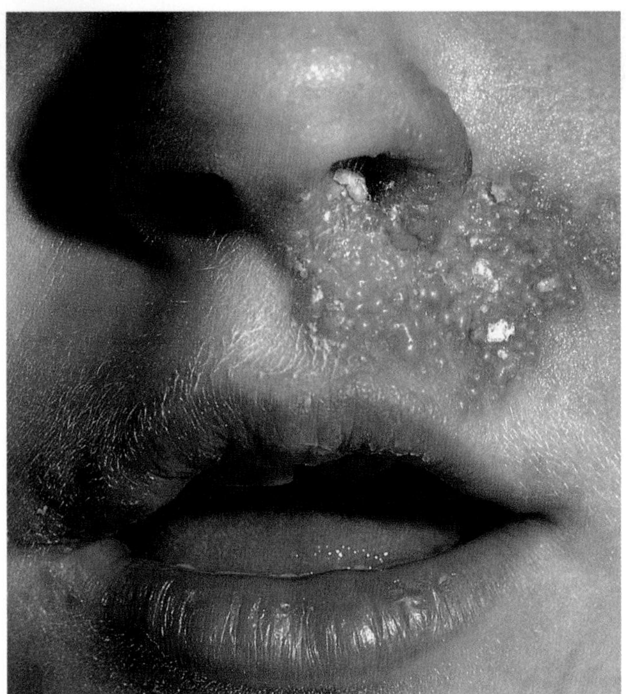

FIGURE 46-17 **Herpes Simplex.** Typical presentation with tense vesicles involving the nasal mucosa and extending onto the skin. (From Habif TP: *Clinical dermatology: a color guide to diagnosis and therapy,* ed 4, Philadelphia, 2004, Mosby.)

Viral Infections

Herpes Simplex Virus. Skin infections with **herpes simplex virus (HSV)** are commonly caused by two types: HSV-1 and HSV-2. Either type can occur in different parts of the body, including oral and genital locations. Their differences are distinguished by laboratory tests. HSV-1 is generally associated with oral infections (cold sore or fever blister) or infection of the cornea (herpes keratitis) but it also can cause genital herpes.[101] HSV-1 is usually transmitted by contact with infected saliva. With primary infection, the virus infects epithelial cells and moves by retrograde axonal transport to the dorsal root ganglion, where the virus develops lifelong latency. The incubation period ranges from 2 to 14 days. During the secondary phase, the lesions occur at the same site from reactivation of the virus. The virus travels down the peripheral nerve to the site of the original infection, where it is shed. Exposure to ultraviolet light, skin irritation, fever, fatigue, or stress may cause reactivation.

The lesions for HSV-1 appear as a rash or clusters of inflamed and painful vesicles (e.g., within the mouth, over the tongue, on the lips, within and/or around the nose) (Figure 46-17). Increased sensitivity, paresthesias, and mild burning often occur before onset of the lesions. The vesicles rupture, forming a crust. Lesions may last from 2 to 6 weeks. Treatment is symptomatic and includes topical antiviral agents; lesions usually resolve within 2 weeks. Oral antivirals may be indicated at the time of acute infection or through daily suppressive dosing to prevent acute infections.[102]

Genital infections are more commonly caused by HSV-2. The virus is spread by skin-to-skin mucous membrane contact during viral shedding. Risk of infection is high after sexual contact with infected individuals and for those who are immunosuppressed and there is increased risk for human immunodeficiency virus (HIV) infection. Vertical transmission from mother to neonate is associated with significant neonatal neurologic morbidity and mortality.[103] The primary infection is asymptomatic. With recurrent exposure, the lesions begin as small vesicles that progress to ulceration within 3 to 4 days with pain, itching, and weeping. Treatment is symptomatic and includes topical or oral antiviral agents. Efforts are in progress to develop prophylactic vaccines.[104]

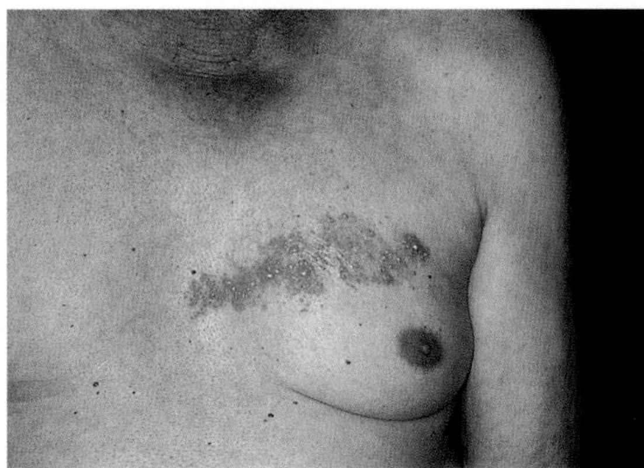

FIGURE 46-18 **Herpes Zoster.** Diffuse involvement of a dermatome. (Courtesy Department of Dermatology, School of Medicine, University of Utah.)

Herpes Zoster and Varicella. **Herpes zoster** (shingles) and **herpes varicella** (chickenpox, see Chapter 47) are caused by the same herpes virus—varicella-zoster virus (VZV). VZV is the primary infection followed years later by herpes zoster (shingles) from reactivation of the virus, particularly among those who are immunosuppressed.[105] It can cause severe disease in nonimmune pregnant women. Following the primary infection the virus remains latent in trigeminal and dorsal root ganglia.

Herpes zoster has initial symptoms of pain and paresthesia localized to the affected dermatome (the cutaneous area innervated by a single spinal nerve; see Chapter 15), followed by vesicular eruptions along a facial, cervical, or thoracic lumbar dermatome (Figure 46-18). Some individuals have vesicles scattered outside the area of the dermatome but lesions do not usually cross the midline. Local symptoms are alleviated with compresses, calamine lotion, or baking soda. Persistent pain may last for weeks or months and is a debilitating complication, particularly in older adults, and requires treatment. Approximately 15% to 20% of individuals experience postherpetic neuralgias.[106] There is no cure for herpes zoster. Antiviral drugs are useful if used within the first 72 hours.[107] Treatment includes a topical lidocaine patch, anticonvulsant medication, controlled-release narcotics, tricyclic antidepressants, and topical capsaicin.[108] Because older adults are at increased risk due to declining immunocompetence, the live-attenuated varicella vaccine is recommended for those older than age 60 as it is well tolerated and effective and may boost humoral and cellular immunity.[109,110]

Warts. **Warts** (verrucae) are benign lesions of the skin caused by the many different types of **human papillomavirus (HPV)** that infect the stratified epithelium of skin and mucous

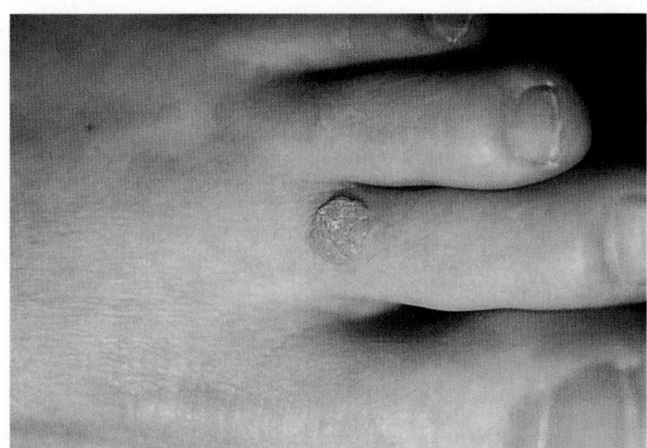

FIGURE 46-19 Verruca Vulgaris. (Courtesy Department of Dermatology, School of Medicine, University of Utah.)

membranes. Specific viruses are associated with specific kinds and locations of lesions.[111] The lesions are round and elevated with a rough, grayish surface; can occur anywhere on the skin; and are transmitted by touch. *Common warts* (verrucae vulgaris) occur most often in children and are usually on the fingers, although they may be located on any skin surface or mucous membrane. Warts vary in shape, size (flat, round, or fusiform), and location (Figure 46-19). Plantar warts are usually located at pressure points on the bottom of the feet.

Diagnosis of warts is by visualization. Treatment considers age of the individual and size and location of the lesion. Warts can be removed by freezing with liquid nitrogen, electrocauterization, vaporization with lasers, application of keratolytics, or application of irritants and corrosives such as salicylic acid, formaldehyde, interferons, or podophyllum.[112] Recalcitrant warts may benefit from application of topicals such as imiquimod 5% cream (immunomodulatory) or 5-fluorouracil, by intralesional injections of bleomycin or *Candida* (immunoreactive antigen), or by more aggressive surgical procedures.[113] Many warts resolve spontaneously but often recur.

Condylomata acuminata (venereal warts) are highly contagious and sexually transmitted. The cauliflower-like lesions occur in moist areas along the glans of the penis, vulva, and anus (see Chapter 26). Oncogenic HPV (e.g., types 16 and 18) is a primary cause of cervical cancer (see Chapter 24).

Fungal Infections

The fungi causing superficial skin infections are called *dermatophytes,* and they thrive on keratin (stratum corneum, hair, nails). Fungal disorders are known as *mycoses;* when caused by dermatophytes, the mycoses are termed *tinea* (dermatophytosis or ringworm).

Tinea Infections. **Tinea infections** are fungal infections of the skin and are classified according to their location on the body.[114] The most common sites are summarized in Table 46-7. These infections are common in children (see Chapter 47). **Tinea unguium (onychomycosis)** is a fungal infection of the nails and is discussed on p. 1647. **Tinea pedis** is a chronic, superficial fungal infection of the skin of the foot common in adults (Figure 46-20). In prepubertal children, most scaling disorders of the toes and feet are eczema. **Tinea corporis** **(ringworm)** and **tinea capitis** (a fungal infection of the scalp) are much more common in children than adults. (See Chapter 47 for a discussion of fungal infections in children.)

Tinea is diagnosed by culture, microscopic examination of skin scrapings prepared with potassium hydroxide wet mount, or observation of the skin with a UV light (Wood lamp).

TABLE 46-7 COMMON SITES OF TINEA INFECTIONS

SITE	CLINICAL MANIFESTATIONS
Tinea capitis (scalp)	Scaly, pruritic scalp with bald areas; hair breaks easily
Tinea corporis (skin areas, excluding scalp, face, hands, feet, groin)	Circular, clearly circumscribed, mildly erythematous scaly patches with a slightly elevated ringlike border; some forms are dry and macular, and other forms are moist and vesicular
Tinea cruris (groin, also known as "jock itch")	Small erythematous and scaling vesicular patches with a well-defined border that spreads over the inner and upper surfaces of the thighs; occurs with heat and high humidity
Tinea pedis (foot, also known as "athlete's foot")	Occurs between the toes and may spread to the soles of the feet, nails, and skin of toes; slight scaling, macerated painful skin, occasionally with fissures and vesiculation
Tinea manus (hand)	Dry, scaly, erythematous lesions, or moist vesicular lesions that begin with clusters of intensely itching, clear vesicles; often associated with fungal infection of the feet
Tinea unguium or onychomycosis (nails)	A superficial or deep inflammation of the nail that develops yellow-brown accumulations of brittle keratin over all or portions of the nail

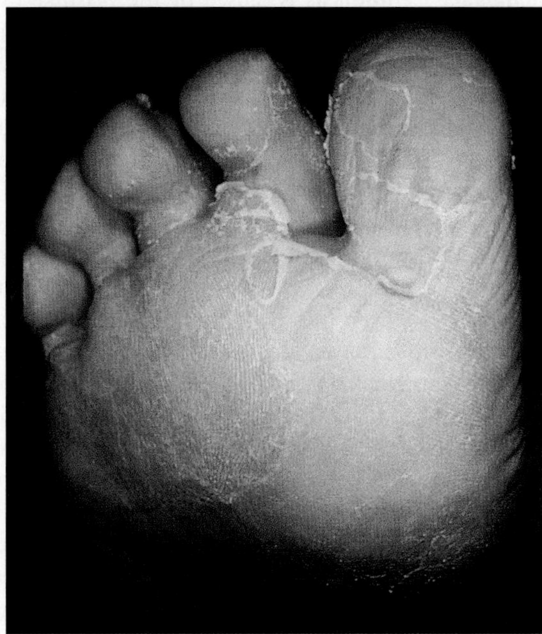

FIGURE 46-20 Tinea Pedis. Inflammation has extended from the web area onto the dorsum of the foot. (Courtesy Department of Dermatology, School of Medicine, University of Utah.)

TABLE 46-8 SITES OF CANDIDIASIS

SITE	RISK FACTORS	CLINICAL MANIFESTATIONS	TREATMENT
Vagina (vulvovaginitis)	Heat, moisture, occlusive clothing Pregnancy Systemic antibiotic therapy Diabetes mellitus Sexual intercourse with infected male	Vaginal itching; white, watery, or creamy discharge Red and swollen vaginal and labial membranes with erosions Lesions may spread to anus and groin	Miconazole cream Clotrimazole tablets or cream Nystatin tablets Ketoconazole cream Loose cotton clothing
Penis (balanitis)	Uncircumcised Sexual intercourse with infected female	Pinpoint, red, tender papules and pustules on glans and shaft of penis	Any of creams listed above Topical steroids for severe inflammation
Mouth	Diabetes mellitus Immunosuppressive therapy Inhaled steroids	Red, swollen, painful tongue and oral mucous membranes Localized erosions and plaques appear with chronic infection	Nystatin oral suspension Clotrimazole troches Ketoconazole Fluconazole
Skinfolds	Heat and moisture Diabetes mellitus Immunosuppressive therapy	Pruritic red rash progressing to vesicles and papules that enlarge and rupture	Topical antifungals (e.g., clotrimazole, econazole, ciclopirox, miconazole, ketoconazole, nystatin)

Cultures establish the particular type of fungus and are necessary for hair and nail infections. Fungi have characteristic spores and filaments known as **hyphae** that are more prominent when prepared in potassium hydroxide. The spores fluoresce blue-green when exposed to UV light. Treatment is related to the type of fungi and includes both topical and systemic antifungal medications.

Candidiasis. **Candidiasis** is caused by the yeastlike fungus *Candida albicans* and normally can be found on mucous membranes, on the skin, in the gastrointestinal tract, and in the vagina. *C. albicans* can, under certain circumstances, change from a commensal microorganism to a pathogen, particularly in the critically ill and those who are immunosuppressed.[115] Factors that predispose to infection include: (1) a local environment of moisture, warmth, maceration, or occlusion; (2) the systemic administration of antibiotics; (3) pregnancy; (4) diabetes mellitus; (5) Cushing disease; (6) debilitated states; (7) age younger than 6 months (more likely to get an infection because of decreased immune reactivity); (8) immunosuppression; and (9) certain neoplastic diseases of the blood and monocyte-macrophage system. The resident bacteria on the skin, mainly cocci, inhibit proliferation of *C. albicans.* Cell-mediated immunity plays a major role in the defense against monilial infections. *C. albicans* can activate the complement system by the alternative pathway and can include small abscesses. Candidiasis affects only the outer layers of mucous membranes and skin and occurs in the mouth, vagina, uncircumcised penis, nail folds, interdigital areas, and large skinfolds (inframammary area, intertriginous area, perianal region, and abdominal creases). Table 46-8 lists selected sites of candidiasis. Innate and adaptive immune responses are required for elimination of *C. albicans.*[116]

The initial lesion is a thin-walled pustule that extends under the stratum corneum with an inflammatory base that may burn or itch. The accumulation of inflammatory cells and scale produces a whitish yellow curdlike substance over the infected area. The lesion ceases to spread when it reaches dry skin.[117] Topical antifungal medication is most commonly used for treatment.

Vascular Disorders

Vascular abnormalities are commonly associated with skin diseases, or they may be present as congenital vascular malformations (see Chapter 47) or as vascular responses to local or systemic vasoactive substances. Blood vessels may increase in number, dilate, constrict, or become obliterated by disease processes.

Cutaneous Vasculitis

Cutaneous vasculitis (angiitis) is an inflammation of the blood vessels of the skin. The vasculitis is often idiopathic or can be triggered by infection, decreased blood flow (i.e., venous stasis), drugs, or autoimmune disorders. The initiating site of inflammation may be the blood, the vessel wall, or the adjacent tissue. Small vessels are usually affected. Immune complexes, which initiate an uncontrolled inflammatory response, are often the cause of damage, and the lesions are often polymorphic.

Cutaneous vasculitis develops from the deposit of immune complexes in small blood vessels as a toxic response to drugs (phenothiazines, barbiturates, sulfonamides) or allergens, as a response to streptococcal or viral infection, or as a component of systemic vasculitic syndromes. The precise mechanism is not known, but the deposit of immune complex activates complement, which is chemotactic for polymorphonuclear leukocytes and other mediators of inflammation that disrupt adhesion molecules and the vessel wall. The cutaneous form usually resolves in a few weeks and is treated with steroids.

A systemic form (cutaneous systemic vasculitis) can involve other organs, including the kidneys, lungs, and gastrointestinal tract (e.g., Wegener granulomatosis). The extremities are the chief sites affected, primarily the lower legs and feet. The lesions appear as palpable purpuras (from the leakage of blood from damaged vessels) and progress to hemorrhagic bullae with necrosis and ulceration from occlusion of the vessel (Figure 46-21). Lesions appear in clusters and remain from 1 to 4 weeks. Recurrences are common.

Serum analysis and biopsy provide the most accurate differential diagnosis. Identifying the primary disease or removing

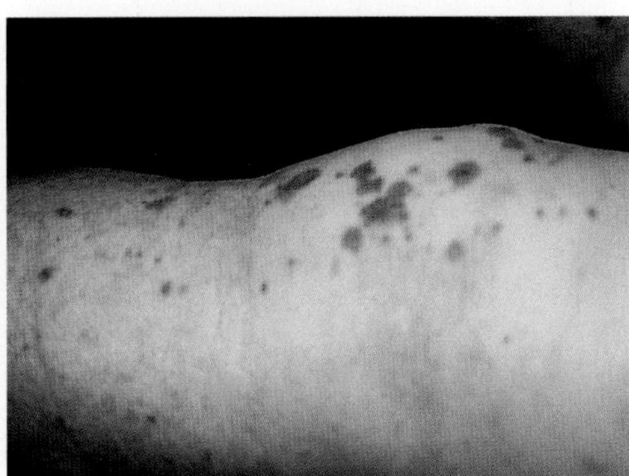

FIGURE 46-21 Vasculitis of the Leg. (Courtesy Department of Dermatology, School of Medicine, University of Utah.)

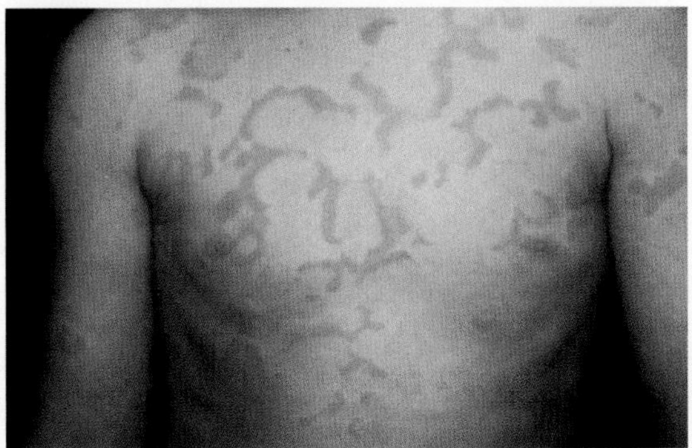

FIGURE 46-22 Urticaria. (Courtesy Department of Dermatology, School of Medicine, University of Utah.)

the antigen (chemical, drug, or source of infection) is the first step of treatment. Corticosteroids and immunosuppressants are used when symptoms are severe.[118,119]

Urticaria

Urticaria (hives) is a pruritic circumscribed area of raised erythema with central pallor occurring in the superficial dermis; they are often generalized in distribution. The erythema blanches with pressure. **Urticarial lesions** are most commonly associated with type I hypersensitivity reactions to drugs (e.g., penicillin, aspirin), certain foods (e.g., strawberries, shellfish), systemic diseases (e.g., intestinal parasites, lupus erythematosus), physical agents (e.g., heat, cold), or complement-mediated reactions (see Chapter 9). They may occur with angioedema (edema of the dermis and subcutaneous tissue). The lesions are usually mediated by IgE-stimulated release of histamine, bradykinin, or kallikrein from mast cells or basophils, or both, which causes the endothelial cells of skin blood vessels to contract, increasing permeability. IgG antibody directed against the IgE receptor and other inflammatory mediators, such as serotonin, leukotrienes, prostaglandins, and kinins, also may be mediators of urticaria. Fluid leakage from vessels appears as wheals, welts, or hives; there may be a few leaks or many leaks distributed over the entire body (Figure 46-22). Most lesions resolve spontaneously within 24 hours, but new lesions may appear. All possible causes should be removed. Nonsedating, second-generation antihistamines (H1 antagonists) usually reduce hives and itching but may be combined with histamine H2 blockers,

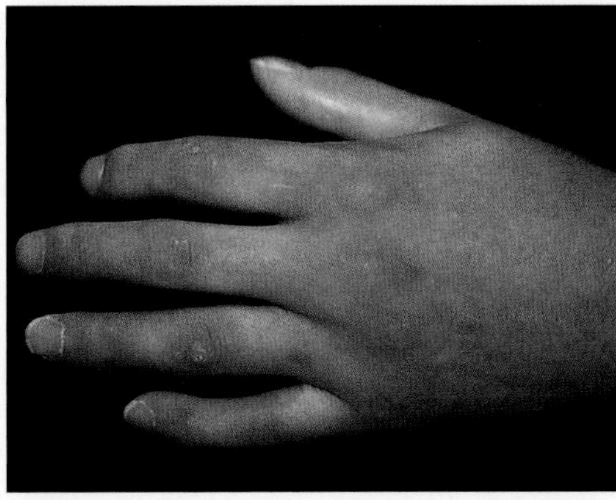

FIGURE 46-23 Scleroderma. Note inflammation and shiny skin. (Courtesy Department of Dermatology, School of Medicine, University of Utah.)

first-generation antihistamines, or leukotriene receptor agonists to improve outcomes.[120] Epinephrine or corticosteroids and α-adrenergic agonists may be required for treatment of severe attacks (i.e., angioedema). Chronic urticaria (recurrent wheals for more than 6 weeks) is either an autoimmune or an idiopathic disease.[121]

Localized Scleroderma

Localized scleroderma (morphea) means sclerosis of the skin. The disease is rare and the cause is unknown. It is more prominent in white females, usually with childhood onset. Genetic predisposition, autoimmunity, and an immune reaction to a toxic substance are possible initiating mechanisms of the disease. T helper cells (Th1 and Th17) and their cytokines are associated with fibroblast proliferation and fibrosis. Several autoantibodies also have been identified, including antinuclear antibody (ANA), antihistone antibody (AHA), and single-stranded DNA antibody (ss-DNA Ab).[122] The cutaneous lesions are most often on the face and hands, neck, and upper chest, but the entire skin can be involved.

There are massive deposits of collagen with fibrosis, accompanied by inflammatory reactions, vascular changes in the capillary network with a decrease in the number of capillary loops, dilation of the remaining capillaries, enhanced expression of adhesion molecules, endothelial injury and dysfunction, perivascular infiltrates, and ischemia. Fibrosis occurs in the papillary and reticular dermis and in the subcutaneous tissue and deep fascia. The skin is hard, hypopigmented, taut, shiny, and tightly attached to the underlying tissue. The tightness of the facial skin projects an immobile masklike appearance, and the oral aperture is limited. The nose may assume a beaklike appearance. The hands are shiny and sometimes red and edematous (Figure 46-23). The fingers become tapered and flexed, often with contractures, depressed scars, and loss of fingertips from atrophy. Raynaud phenomenon with episodic arteriolar vasoconstriction of the fingers contributes to pain, ulcer formation, and gangrene. The nails may be shed. Calcium deposits develop in the subcutaneous tissue and erupt through the skin. There may be progression to underlying muscle and bone and other body organs with esophageal involvement being most common.

Suitable clothing and a warm environment are essential to protecting the hands. Trauma and smoking should be avoided.[123] Treatment is individualized and based on severity and progression of the disease. Immunosuppressive medications, ultraviolet light treatment, and other therapies are prescribed.[124,125]

Tick Bites

Ticks are significant vectors of transmitted diseases, including Rocky Mountain spotted fever and other rickettsial diseases, tularemia, Congo-Crimean hemorrhagic fever, and Lyme disease.[126] Ticks vary from 1 cm to about the size of a comma on this printed page. They embed their heads in the skin to obtain blood. As they gorge themselves on blood, they enlarge to many times their normal size and may release toxins or transmit microorganisms during feeding. In most instances, there is no consequence from a tick bite, with the exception of papular urticaria at the site of the bite. If mouthparts remain in the skin when the tick is removed, a persistent nodule remains that may require excision; ideally the tick should be removed completely intact. Irritant substances, such as camphor, soft wax, or heat from a match, may stimulate the tick to withdraw its head. Wearing protective clothing and applying tick repellant, such as diethyltoluamide (DEET), butopyronoxyl (Indalone), or benzylbenzoate, help prevent tick bites.

Lyme disease is a multisystem inflammatory disease caused by the spirochete *Borrelia burgdorferi* transmitted by tick bites and is the most frequently reported vector-borne illness. The highest incidence is among children (50% of infected individuals are symptom free). An immune response to *B. burgdorferi* contributes to the pathogenesis of the disease. The microorganism is difficult to culture and it escapes immunodefenses through antigenetic diversity; blocks complement-mediated killing; impedes release of antimicrobial peptides, leukocyte chemotaxis, and antimicrobial killing; and hides in tissue. It spreads to other tissues by entering capillary beds.[127]

Symptoms of the disease occur in three stages.[128] *Localized infection* occurs soon after the bite (3 to 32 days, the incubation period) with erythema migrans (bull's-eye rash) with or without fever, fatigue, malaise, myalgias, and arthralgias. Erythema migrans is a T-cell–mediated response. Within days to weeks after the onset of the illness, there is *disseminated infection* with secondary erythema migrans, usually with arthralgias, meningitis, neuritis, or carditis. *Late persistent infection* (more common in Europe) can continue for years with arthritis, encephalopathy, polyneuropathy, or heart failure. The diagnosis of Lyme disease is based on the clinical presentation and history of tick bite, if known. Serologic tests may be used to confirm the diagnosis.[129] Antibiotics (e.g., doxycycline [not used in children younger than 8 years or in pregnant or breast-feeding women] or amoxicillin) are used for treatment.[130] Reinfection can occur. There is currently not a vaccine for Lyme disease.[131]

Borrelia miyamotoi also is carried by ticks. The first report of infection was in Russia in 2011 and cases have been confirmed in the United States in areas where Lyme disease is endemic. Serum assays confirm diagnosis. Infected individuals have flu-like symptoms and respond to antibiotic therapy (doxycline or amoxicillin).[132]

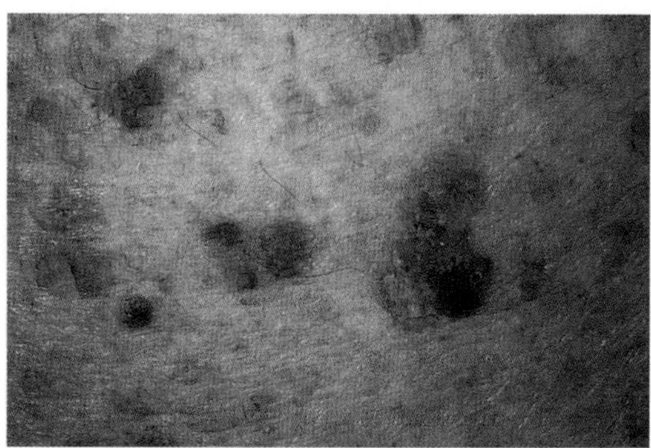

FIGURE 46-24 Seborrheic Keratosis. Typical lesion that is broad, flat, and comparatively smooth surfaced. (Courtesy Department of Dermatology, School of Medicine, University of Utah.)

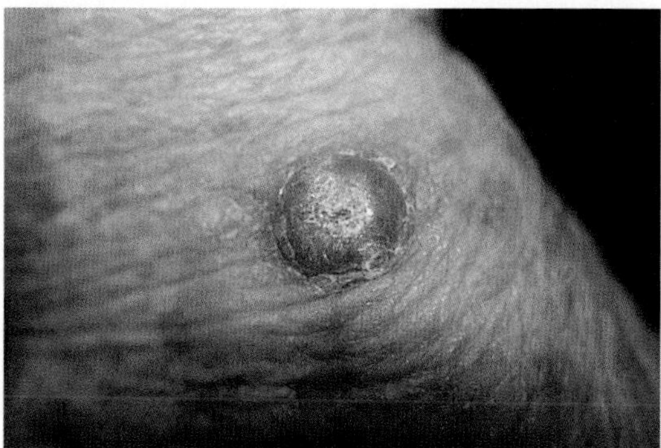

FIGURE 46-25 Keratoacanthoma. Classic presentation of a fully developed tumor. Round, smooth, dome-shaped mass with a central keratin-filled crater. (Courtesy Department of Dermatology, School of Medicine, University of Utah.)

Benign Tumors

Most benign tumors of the skin are associated with aging. Benign tumors include seborrheic keratosis, keratoacanthoma, actinic keratosis, and nevi (moles).

Seborrheic Keratosis

Seborrheic keratosis is a benign proliferation of cutaneous basal cells that produces smooth or warty elevated lesions. The pathogenesis is unknown. These tumors are usually seen in older people and occur as multiple lesions on the chest, back, and face. The color varies from tan to waxy yellow, flesh colored, or dark brown-black. Lesion size varies from a few millimeters to several centimeters, and they are often oval and greasy appearing with a hyperkeratotic stuck-on scaly appearance (Figure 46-24). Both cryotherapy with liquid nitrogen and electrocautery are effective treatments, and the lesions usually slough 2 to 3 weeks after treatment.

Keratoacanthoma

A **keratoacanthoma** is a benign self-limiting tumor of squamous cell differentiation arising from hair follicles. It usually occurs on sun-damaged skin of older adults and smokers; the incidence is high in males. The most commonly affected sites are the face, back of the hands, forearms, neck, and legs (Figure 46-25). The lesion develops over a period of 1 to 2 months and

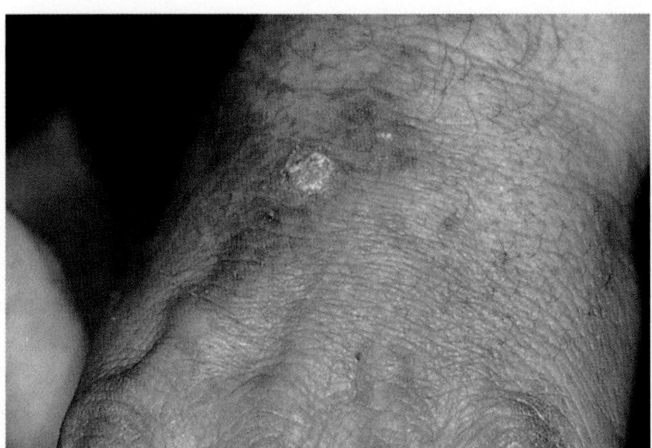

FIGURE 46-26 Actinic Keratosis. (Courtesy Department of Dermatology, School of Medicine, University of Utah.)

has a histologic course resembling a well-differentiated squamous cell carcinoma as follows:

Proliferative stage: Lesion develops as a rapidly growing, dome-shaped nodule with a central crust.

Mature stage: Lesion fills with whitish keratin and requires differentiation from squamous cell carcinoma.

Involution stage: Occurs over a 3- to 4-month period with regression of the lesion.

Although the lesions resolve spontaneously, they can be removed by curettage or excision to improve cosmetic appearance and reduce risk of destructive growth or a missed diagnosis of squamous cell carcinoma. Intralesional 5-FU, bleomycin, interferon, or methotrexate also have been effective.[133-135]

Actinic Keratosis

Actinic keratosis is a premalignant lesion composed of aberrant proliferations of epidermal keratinocytes caused by prolonged exposure to UV radiation. The prevalence is highest in individuals with unprotected light-colored skin. Actinic keratosis is rare in black skin. The lesions appear as rough or scaly, poorly defined pink to reddish or reddish brown papules that are felt more than seen (Figure 46-26) and are considered an early in situ squamous cell carcinoma. Surrounding areas may have telangiectasia. Dermoscopy and biopsy aid evaluation. Treatment options include ablative and topical therapies, such as 5-FU and imiquimod. The lesions should continue to be evaluated for progressive squamous cell carcinoma. Protection from the sun with clothing or a sunblock to prevent lesions from developing elsewhere is advised.[136]

Nevi

Nevi (moles) are benign pigmented or nonpigmented lesions (Figure 46-27) that form from melanocytes beginning at ages 3 to 5 years. Melanocytic nevus, formed from melanocytes, may be congenital or acquired. During the early stages of development, the cells accumulate at the junction of the dermis and epidermis and are macular lesions. Over time the cells move deeper into the dermis and the nevi become nodular and symmetric without irregular borders. Nevi may appear on any part of the skin, and vary in size. They occur singly or in groups and are not considered disfiguring. Nevi may undergo transition to malignant melanomas (see p. 1643).[137] Nevi repeatedly traumatized, irritated by clothing, or considered too large can be excised.

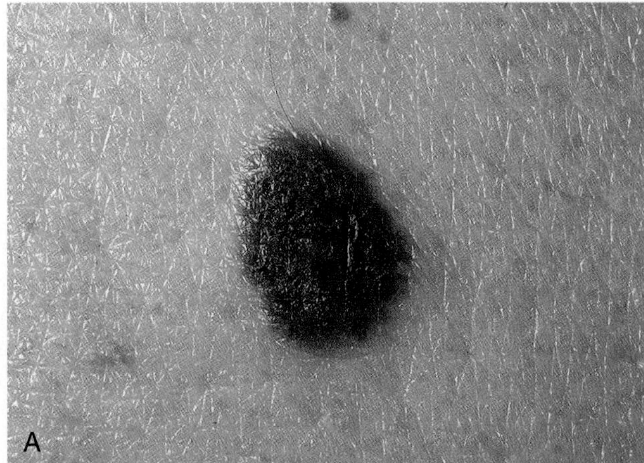

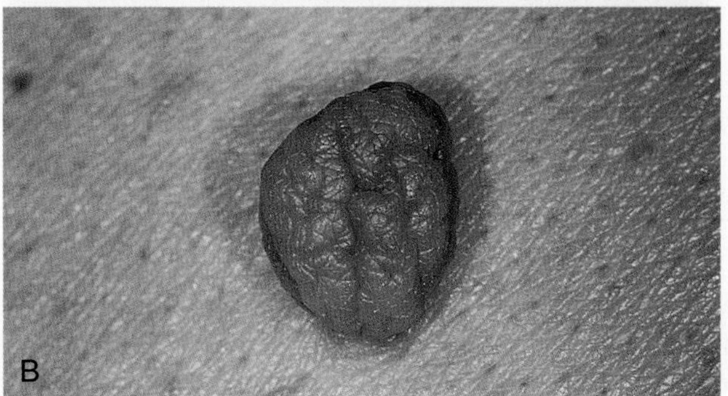

FIGURE 46-27 Nevi. **A,** Junction nevus: slightly raised, dark, and uniform. **B,** Dermal nevus: pedunculated with a soft, flabby, wrinkled surface. (From Habif TP: *Clinical dermatology: a color guide to diagnosis and therapy,* ed 5, Philadelphia, 2010, Mosby.)

Skin Cancer

Basal cell carcinoma and squamous cell carcinoma are the most prevalent forms of cancer. Malignant melanoma is the most serious and the most common cause of death from skin cancer.[138] Important trends related to skin cancer are presented in Box 46-4.

Chronic ultraviolet (UV) radiation causes most skin cancers. Protection from UV radiation from the sun and artificial sources (e.g., tanning beds), particularly during the childhood years, significantly reduces the risk of skin cancer in later years. Areas commonly exposed to the sun's rays—face, neck, and hands—are highly vulnerable for such lesions. Dark-skinned persons and those avoiding sunlight are significantly less likely to develop these malignant tumors. In dark-skinned persons, basal cells contain the pigment melanin, a protective factor against sun exposure.

Basal Cell Carcinoma

Basal cell carcinoma is a surface epithelial tumor of the skin originating from undifferentiated basal or germinative cells. The tumors grow upward and laterally or downward to the

BOX 46-4 IMPORTANT TRENDS FOR SKIN CANCER

Incidence

More than 3.5 million cases per year with likely underreporting because of lack of a non–melanoma skin cancer registry

Greater in women younger than age 40 years; greater in men after age 40 years; 40 times more prevalent in whites than in blacks; increases steadily with age; increasing among young individuals with chronic exposure to artificial UV radiation

Majority of cases are highly curable **basal** or **squamous** cell cancers and the most serious is **malignant melanoma** with an estimated 76,690 new cases in 2013; it represents 4% of all skin cancer cases but causes about 79% of all skin cancer deaths

Mortality

Total estimated deaths in 2013 were 9480 from melanoma and approximately 3170 from other nonepithelial types of skin cancer

Risk Factors

Excessive exposure to ultraviolet radiation from the sun

Exposure to artificial UV radiation, particularly in ages less than 25 years

Fair complexion, blue eyes, blonde hair

Occupational exposure to coal tar, pitch, creosote, arsenic compounds, and radium

Exposure to human papillomavirus and human immunodeficiency virus

Immunosuppression

Family history of skin cancer

Skin cancer is negligible in blacks because of heavy skin pigmentation

Warning Signals

Any change on the skin, especially a change in the size or color of a mole or other darkly pigmented growth or spot

Prevention and Early Detection

Avoidance of artificial UV radiation and sun when ultraviolet light is strongest (e.g., 10 AM to 3 PM); use of protective clothing and sunscreen preparations, especially those containing ingredients such as *para*-aminobenzoic acid (PABA); prevention for all types of skin cancer should begin in childhood

Survival

For basal cell and squamous cell cancers, cure is highly likely with early detection and treatment; malignant melanoma metastasizes quickly, accounting for a lower 5-year survival rate

Data from American Cancer Society: *Cancer facts and figures 2013,* Atlanta, 2013, The Society; Rogers HW et al: *Arch Dermatol* 146(3):283–287, 2010; Wehner MR et al: *BMJ* 345:e5909, 2012.

dermal-epidermal junction. They usually have depressed centers and rolled borders. Early tumors are so small that they are not clinically apparent.

Basal cell carcinoma is the most common type of skin cancer in whites and is thought to be caused by UV radiation exposure. It also is associated with arsenic from groundwater wells[139] and autosomal dominant nevoid basal cell carcinoma syndrome. Basal cell carcinoma arises from mutation in the *TP53* tumor-suppressor gene, leading to loss of keratinocyte repair functions and apoptosis resistance of DNA-damaged cells. Other oncogenic pathways include mutation in the *PTCH1* gene that has tumor-suppressor activity, and alteration in the Sonic Hedgehog signaling pathway genes (codes for a protein important for cell growth and differentiation).[140]

Lesion subtypes include superficial, nodular, and sclerosing/morpheaform, which can be pigmented or nonpigmented (Figure 46-28). Early tumors are so small that they are not clinically apparent. The lesion often begins as a nodule (greater than 5 mm across) that is pearly or ivory in appearance and slightly elevated above the skin surface with small blood vessels on the surface (telangiectasias). The tumors grow upward and laterally or downward to the dermal-epidermal junction. They usually have depressed centers and rolled borders. As the lesion grows, it often ulcerates, develops crusting, and becomes firm to the touch. If left untreated basal cell lesions invade surrounding tissues and, over months or years, can destroy a nose, an eyelid, or an ear. Metastatic spread is rare because these tumors do not invade blood or lymph vessels. Treatment includes complete surgical excision, radiotherapy, curettage, cryotherapy, photodynamic therapy, and topical applications of imiquimod or 5-fluorouracil.[140]

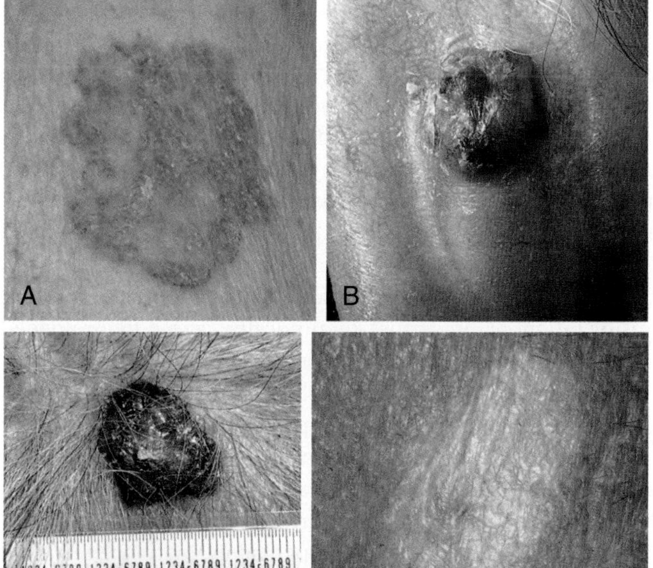

FIGURE 46-28 Types of Basal Cell Carcinoma. **A,** Superficial. **B,** Nodular. **C,** Pigmented. **D,** Morpheaform—recurrent tumor. (**A** and **D** from Bolognia JL, Jorizzo JL, Schaffer JV: *Dermatology,* ed 3, Philadelphia, 2012, Saunders; **B** and **C** from James WD, Berger TG, Elston DM: *Andrews' diseases of the skin: clinical dermatology,* ed 11, Philadelphia, 2011, Saunders.)

Squamous Cell Carcinoma

Squamous cell carcinoma (SCC) is a tumor of the epidermis and the second most common human cancer. Two types are characterized: in situ (Bowen disease [BD]) and invasive. Areas affected are the head and neck (75%) and the hands (15%), with 10% of squamous cell carcinomas occurring elsewhere on the body. These tumors are more predominant in countries where arsenic is found in higher rates in drinking water. UV light exposure from sun and the use of tanning beds are the primary risk factors. Gamma rays and x-rays are also associated

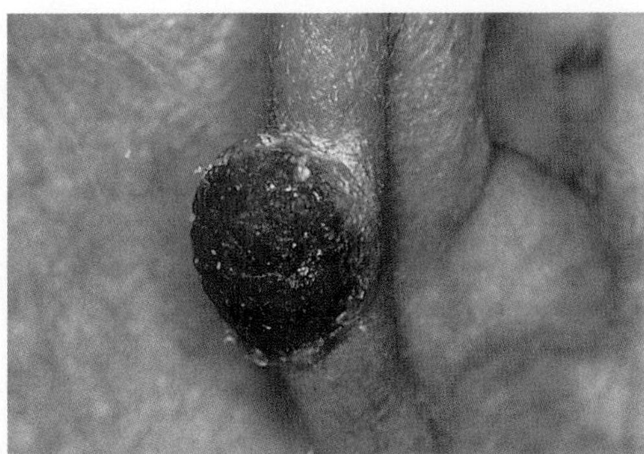

FIGURE 46-29 **Squamous Cell Carcinoma.** The sun-exposed ear is a common site for squamous cell carcinoma. (Courtesy Department of Dermatology, School of Medicine, University of Utah.)

TABLE 46-9 CLASSIFICATION OF NEVI

NEVI	COMMON CHARACTERISTICS
Junctional nevus	Flat, well circumscribed, vary in size up to 2 cm, dark color, hairs may be present; originate in basal layer of epidermis and can eventually reach the cutaneous surface; rarely develop into a melanoma
Compound nevus	Most common in adolescents; the majority of pigmented lesions are in children; rarely develops into melanoma; usually 1 cm in size; hairs may be present; surface is elevated and smooth
Intradermal nevus	Small (less than 1 cm) with regular edges and bristle-like hairs; color ranges from skin tone to light brown; has a slight likelihood of developing into a melanoma

with squamous cell carcinoma. In addition, patients who are immunosuppressed experience a greater occurrence of this carcinoma.

UV exposure causes SCC, particularly mutation of the *TP53* gene and other oncogenic signals.[141] It is unclear how UV light produces alterations in DNA, and DNA repair. Invasive SCC can arise from premalignant lesions of the skin. It rarely arises from normal-appearing skin or de novo. The premalignant lesions include sun-damaged skin or dysplasias (actinic keratosis); leukoplakia, or whitish, discolored areas; scars; radiation-induced keratosis; tar and oil keratosis; and chronic ulcers and sinuses.

In situ SCC is usually confined to the epidermis (intraepidermal) but may extend into the dermis. Common premalignant skin lesions associated with in situ squamous cell carcinomas are actinic (solar) keratosis and BD. Actinic keratosis is a white, scaly, keratotic (horny) lesion on the exposed areas of the body (see Figure 46-26). BD is a dysplasia of the basal layer of the dermis or carcinoma in situ. It often is found on unexposed areas of the body and is demonstrated by flat, reddish, scaly patches. These lesions may enlarge to more than 1 cm in diameter, rarely invading surrounding tissue and very rarely metastasizing. Other cellular components in the skin (e.g., sweat glands, hair follicles) can give rise to SCC but these cancers are relatively uncommon. Invasive SCC grows more rapidly than basal cell carcinomas and can spread to regional lymph nodes with metastasis. These tumors are firm and increase in elevation and diameter. The surface may be granular and bleed easily (Figure 46-29). Treatment includes surgical excision and radiotherapy with consideration of adjuvant chemotherapy for advanced disease.[142] Mohs micrographic surgery (MMS), a tissue-sparing surgical technique, is indicated for non-melanoma skin cancers (NMSCs) with a high risk of recurrence, lesions involving the face, ears, genitalia, or when wider excision may risk functional impairment.[142a]

Cutaneous Melanoma

Cutaneous melanoma is a malignant tumor of the skin originating from melanocytes, or cells that synthesize the pigment melanin. The incidence of melanoma is increasing, and young to middle-age adults are at highest risk. Risk factors implicated in melanoma induction include genetic predisposition, exposure to ultraviolet light (solar and artificial), acquired melanocytic nevi, family history of melanoma, fair hair, light skin with a propensity to sunburn, and the presence of susceptibility genes (e.g., *BRAF* and *RAS* mutations).[143,144] Specific genetic alterations are associated with particular clinical and histopathologic features of the disease.[145]

The relationship between nevi (see Figure 46-27) and melanoma makes it important for the clinician to understand the various neval forms (Table 46-9). Most nevi never become suspicious; however, suspicious nevi should be evaluated and removed. Indications for biopsy include changes in color and size, irregular notched margin, itching, bleeding or oozing, nodularity, scab formation, ulceration, or an unusual pattern of presentation. The ABCDE rule is used as a guide: **A**symmetry, **B**order irregularity, **C**olor variation, **D**iameter larger than 6 mm, and **E**levation, which includes raised appearance or rapid enlargement.[146] Clinical characteristics are summarized in Table 46-10.

Melanomas arise as a result of malignant degeneration of melanocytes located either along the basal layer of the epidermis or in a benign melanocytic nevus. The clinical types of cutaneous melanoma are based on their growth pattern and include lentigo malignant melanoma (LMM) (Figure 46-30), superficial spreading melanoma (SSM) (the most common), primary nodular melanoma (PNM), and acral-lentiginous melanoma. Rare and difficult to diagnose subtypes include desmoplastic melanoma, which resembles a scar, and amelanotic (nonpigmented) melanoma.[147] The pathogenesis of malignant melanoma is complex and a number of proto-oncogenes have been identified.[148]

Surveillance strategies include clinician-based total body skin examination, total body photography, dermoscopy, and individual-based self-skin examination. Detection of volatile biomarkers are in development.[148a] Staging of melanoma is determined using tumor, node, metastasis (TMN) criteria established by the American Joint Committee on Cancer and is summarized in Box 46-5.

Prognostic factors include the thickness of the lesion, mitotic index, immunohistochemical assessment, ulceration and metastasis (e.g., number of lymph nodes or viscera involved).[149]

TABLE 46-10 CLINICAL CHARACTERISTICS OF VARIETIES OF CUTANEOUS MELANOMA

CHARACTERISTIC	DESCRIPTION
Lentigo Malignant Melanoma	
Frequency	4% to 15% of cutaneous melanomas
Age at diagnosis	50 to 80 years old, mean age 65 years
Primary location	Head, neck, dorsum of hands (sun-exposed areas)
Pigmentation according to thickness	
<1.5 mm (levels I and II)	Tan and brown
>1.5 mm (level III)	Tan, brown, and blue-black
>1.5 mm (levels IV and V)	Nodule formation
Superficial Spreading Melanomas	
Frequency	57% to 70% of cutaneous melanomas
Age at diagnosis	20 to 60 years old
Primary location	Legs of females; upper back of both genders
Pigmentation according to thickness	
<1.5 mm (levels I and II)	Tan and brown
>1.5 mm (level III)	Tan, brown, and blue-black
>1.5 mm (levels IV and V)	Nodule formation
Primary Nodular Melanoma	
Frequency	12% to 21% of cutaneous melanomas
Age at diagnosis	20 to 60 years old, mean age 53 years
Primary location	Trunk, head, or neck
Pigmentation according to thickness	
>1.5 mm (level III)	Small nodule (any hue)
>1.5 mm (levels IV and V)	Large nodule (any hue)
Acral-Lentiginous Melanoma	
Frequency	2% to 8% in whites; 30% to 75% in blacks, Hispanics, Asians
Age at diagnosis	20 to 60 years old
Primary location	Palms, soles of feet, mucous membranes
Pigmentation at any thickness	Blue-black irregular macules, papules, or nodules

Data from Bolognia JL, Jorizzo JL, Schaffer JV: *Dermatology,* ed 3, Philadelphia, 2012, Saunders; Greenwald HS, Friedman EB, Osman I: *Melanoma Res* 22(1):1–8, 2012; Habif TP, editor: *Clinical dermatology,* ed 5, St Louis, 2010, Mosby; Scolyer RA, Long GV, Thompson JF: *Mol Oncol* 5(2):124–136, 2011; Situm M, Buljan M: *G Ital Dermatol Venereol* 147(1):21–27, 2012.

BOX 46-5 TNM STAGING CRITERIA FOR MELANOMA

Stage 0: carcinoma in situ (TisN0M0)

Stage I A/B: includes lesions up to 2 mm with no nodal or distant metastases (T1aN0M0, T1bN0M0, T2aN0M0).

Stage II A/B/C: includes larger lesions, greater than 2 mm without positive nodes or distant metastases (T2bN0M0, T3aN0M0, T3bN0M0, T4aN0M0, T4bN0M0).

Stage III: includes lesions of any size with positive lymph nodes (TxN1M0, TxN2M0, TxN3M0).

Stage IV: includes lesions of any size with distant metastases (TxNxM1).

Data from Piris A, Lobo AC, Duncan LM: Melanoma staging: where are we now?, *Dermatol Clin* 30(4):581–592, v, 2012.

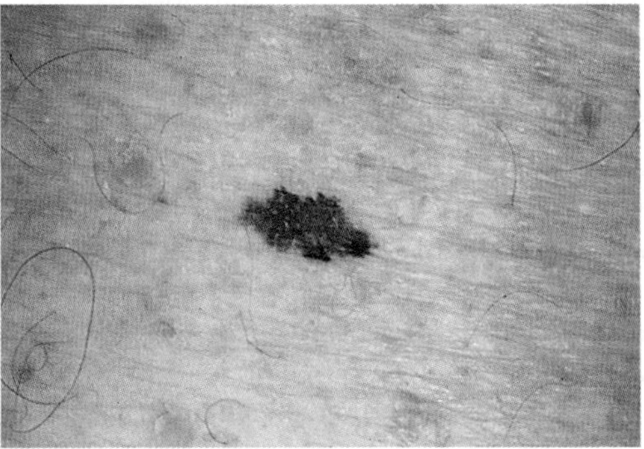

FIGURE 46-30 Lentigo Malignant Melanoma. (Courtesy Department of Dermatology, School of Medicine, University of Utah.)

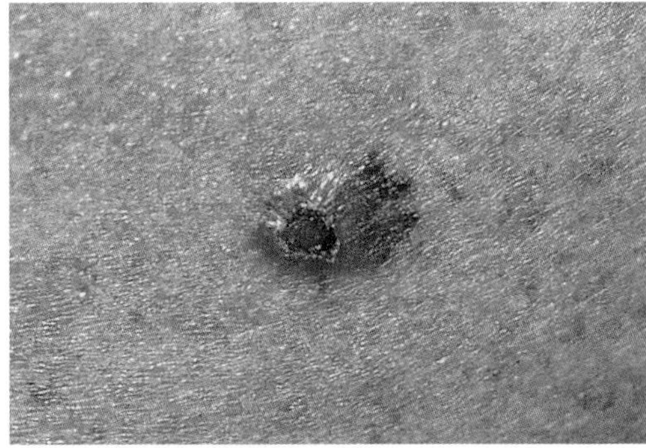

FIGURE 46-31 Nodular Melanoma. (Courtesy Department of Dermatology, School of Medicine, University of Utah.)

Figure 46-31 illustrates a nodular melanoma. Efforts are in progress to refine the morphologic classifications by adding subgroups that include molecular markers for proto-oncogene mutations and specific signaling pathways.[150] Early recognition of cutaneous melanomas can have a major effect on achieving a surgical cure.

Prevention of melanoma includes avoidance of UV radiation exposure through use of protective clothing and sunscreens, and avoidance of artificial UV radiation exposure. Treatment of melanoma with no evidence of metastatic disease involves surgical excision to the primary site and regional lymph nodes. The extent of surgery is determined by the staging of disease. Lesions of the extremities have the best prognosis; head and neck lesions and trunk lesions have the poorest prognosis. Survival rate for advanced disease is very low. Immunotherapy is advancing. Ipilimumab blocks cytotoxic T-lymphocyte antigen 4 and vemurafenib has prolonged survival with *BRAF*-mutated melanoma, and new drugs are in clinical trials. Improving response and survival rates with novel cellular targets and combination therapies to overcome tumor resistance is an ongoing need.[151,152] Vaccines, biomarkers, and genetically-modified T cells are under investigation.[153,154]

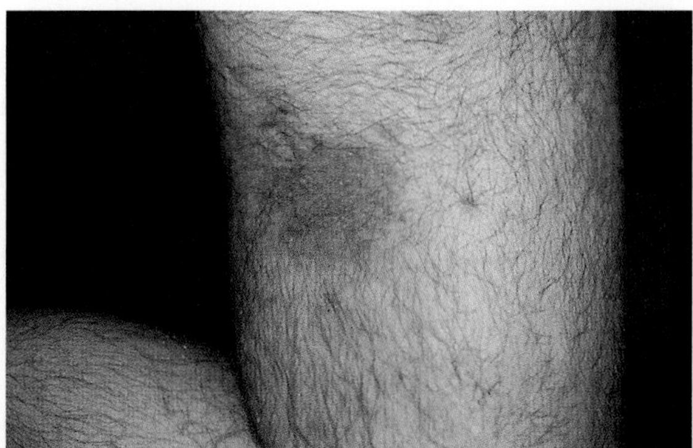

FIGURE 46-32 Kaposi Sarcoma. The purple lesion commonly seen on the skin. (Courtesy Department of Dermatology, School of Medicine, University of Utah.)

Kaposi Sarcoma

Kaposi sarcoma (KS) is a vascular malignancy associated with different presentations: (1) drug-induced immunosuppressions, for example, after kidney transplantation; (2) an endemic form in equatorial Africa; (3) classic form presenting on the lower legs of older men; (4) epidemic and nonepidemic forms related to acquired immunodeficiency syndrome (AIDS), and (5) iatrogenic.[155]

Kaposi-associated herpesvirus 8 (HHV-8) is found in all forms of KS and may be a common etiology for all types of KS in combination with host immune dysfunction and the local inflammatory state.[155] Immunosuppression allows for opportunistic infections and malignancy. Proliferation of the tumor depends on the presence of platelet-derived and other growth factors.[156]

The endothelial cell is thought to be the progenitor of KS but the specific origin is elusive. The lesions emerge as purplish brown macules and develop into plaques and nodules. They tend to be multifocal rather than spreading by metastasis. The lesions initially appear over the lower extremities in the classic form (Figure 46-32). The rapidly progressive form associated with AIDS tends to spread symmetrically over the upper body, particularly the face and oral mucosa. The lesions are often pruritic and painful. About 75% of individuals with epidemic KS have involvement of lymph nodes, particularly in the gastrointestinal tract and lungs. Organ involvement is much less common in the classic form. The rapidly progressive form has a poor prognosis and shorter survival rates than the classic form. (See Chapter 10 for a further discussion on AIDS.)

Diagnosis is by skin biopsy, with a high index of suspicion for those with immunodeficiency. The disease is incurable. Local lesions can be excised. Multiple disseminated lesions may be treated with a combination of immunomodulatory, cytotoxic, and antiviral drugs. The new, highly active antiretroviral therapy (HAART) for AIDS treatment is decreasing the incidence of KS in resource rich countries, but new treatments are needed.[157]

Primary Cutaneous Lymphomas

Primary cutaneous lymphomas are cutaneous T-cell and B-cell lymphomas that are present in the skin without evidence of extracutaneous disease at the time of diagnosis (see Chapter 29 for classification and general pathophysiology of lymphomas). Cutaneous lymphomas are rare but are the second most common site of extranodal non-Hodgkin lymphoma. The incidence rate is about 14/100,000 and their cause is unknown.[158] Cutaneous lymphomas are more common in men and generally present after age 50 years; 75% of cases are T-cell lymphomas and 25% are B-cell lymphomas. The most common cutaneous T-cell lymphoma is mycosis fungoides (50% of cases), which is more common among blacks. Sézary syndrome (a leukemic variant of T-cell lymphoma) and primary cutaneous CD30-positive lymphoproliferations (less than 10% of cases) are the most aggressive. Cutaneous lymphomas develop from clonal expansion of B cells, T helper cells, and rarely T suppressor cells. **Mycosis fungoides** can present as focal or widespread erythematous patches or plaques, follicular papules, comedone-like lesions, and tumors (Figure 46-33). There may be patches of alopecia. The lesions progress over a period of months or years. Mycosis fungoides lesions are pruritic and cause considerable distress and debilitation.[159] Involvement of other organs can occur in advanced stages of the disease.

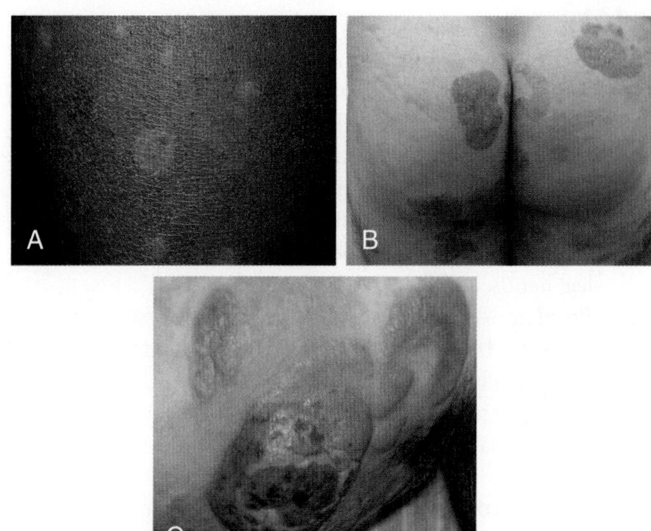

FIGURE 46-33 Mycosis Fungoides. **A,** Hypopigmented patches of mycosis fungoides. **B,** Plaques of mycosis fungoides. **C,** Tumors of mycosis fungoides combined with patches. (Courtesy of Ellen Korn, M.D. In James WD, Berger TG, Elston DM: *Andrews' diseases of the skin: clinical dermatology,* ed 11, Philadelphia, 2011, Saunders.)

The differential diagnosis of the different types of cutaneous lymphomas is based on clinical manifestations, histologic appearance, immunologic and cytogenetic features, and response to appropriate treatment.[160,160a] Lesions also must be distinguished from psoriasis, eczema, generalized dermatitis, and drug reactions. Treatment is based on staging of the disease following consensus-based guidelines that include a range of topical and systemic therapies, such as anti-inflammatory, immunomodulatory, and biologic agents; histone deacetylase inhibitors; rexinoids; and chemotherapeutics.[161,162] Radiotherapy has historically been the most common successful therapy.[163]

Cold Injury

Exposure to extreme cold includes a spectrum of injuries[164]:

1. *Frostnip*—mild and completely reversible injury characterized by skin pallor and numbness
2. *Chilblains*—more serious injury with violaceous skin color with plaques or nodules, pain, and pruritus but without ice crystal formation; a chronic vasculitis can develop and is usually located on the face, anterior lower leg, hands, and feet
3. *Frostbite*—tissues freeze and form ice crystals at temperatures below −2° C (28° F), progressing from distal to proximal; is potentially reversible
4. *Flash freeze*—rapid cooling with intracellular ice crystals associated with contact with cold metals or volatile liquids

Areas most commonly affected are fingers, toes, ears, nose, and cheeks. Initially the body responds with alternating cycles of vasoconstriction and vasodilation—the "hunting reflex." The mechanism of injury is complex but is related to direct cold injury to cells, indirect injury, cell death from extracellular and intracellular ice crystal formation, impaired circulation with anoxia because of thrombosis in the exposed area, and reperfusion injury. With tissue reperfusion there is infiltration of neutrophils and mast cells and these cells and the damaged epithelium release inflammatory mediators (e.g., prostaglandins, thromboxanes, bradykinin, and histamine). Edema can cause capillary compression and vascular stasis. Frozen skin becomes white or yellowish, waxy, and firm to the touch. There is numbness and no sensation of pain.

Skin damage can range from mild to severe. With mild frostbite, redness and discomfort occur during rewarming, followed by a return to normal in a few hours. In more severe cases, cyanosis and mottling develop, followed by redness, swelling, throbbing, and burning pain on rewarming. Within 24 to 48 hours, vesicles and bullae appear and resolve into crusts that eventually slough off, leaving thin, newly formed skin. The most severe cases result in gangrene with loss of the affected part. Frostbite may be classified by depth of injury after rewarming as follows:

First degree: superficial, characterized by a numb central white area surrounded by erythema and edema and including partial skin freezing without blistering

Second degree: full-thickness skin freezing with blistering surrounded by edema and hyperemia

Third degree: deep, characterized by full-thickness skin and subcutaneous freezing with tissue necrosis and hemorrhagic vesicles and blisters

Fourth degree: deep tissue freezing with full-thickness necrosis and gangrene with a line of demarcation.

Immediate treatment of frostbite is to cover affected areas with other body surfaces and warm clothing. The area should not be rubbed or massaged. Local, dry heat should be avoided. Immersion in a warm water bath (40° to 42° C [104° to 107.6° F]) until frozen tissue is thawed is the best treatment. Ibuprofen is used to inhibit prostaglandins, and aloe vera is a topical inhibitor of thromboxane. Thrombolytic therapy reduces the incidence of amputation when administered within 24 hours of injury.[165]

Pain during the thawing period is severe and should be treated with potent analgesics. Gentle cleansing and no pressure on the skin should be maintained during healing. Amputation of necrotic tissue is delayed until a clear line of demarcation is established.[166]

DISORDERS OF THE HAIR

Alopecia

Male-Pattern Alopecia (Androcentric Alopecia)

Alopecia means loss of hair. Localized hair loss in men is not a disease but rather a variation in the androgen receptor *(AR)* gene that clusters in families. The mechanism of inheritance is unknown. Within the distribution of hair over the scalp, androgen-sensitive hair follicles are on top and androgen-insensitive follicles are on the sides and back. In genetically predisposed men, the androgen-sensitive follicles are transformed into vellus follicles. The normal hair is shed and replaced by fine, light, short hair. Male-pattern baldness begins with frontotemporal recession and progresses to loss of hair over the top of the scalp. Minoxidil may be used to stimulate hair growth and finasteride may decrease the effect of androgens on hair follicles. New treatments are being evaluated.[167] Affected men may choose to wear wigs or have hair transplants.

Female-Pattern Alopecia

Women in their twenties and thirties (6% to 12%) and women older than 70 years (55%) experience progressive thinning and loss of hair over the central part of the scalp. Contrary to male-pattern baldness, no loss of hair occurs along the frontal hairline but follicles are smaller and less functional. Many of these women have elevated levels of serum adrenal androgen dehydroepiandrosterone sulfate (DHEAS), and treatment with antiandrogens can be effective. Lower levels of estrogen can also decrease hair growth after menopause. Finasteride, minoxidil, light therapy or combinations of therapy may be used and work best when started early.[168,169] In rare instances a male-pattern baldness develops. Laboratory evaluation of serum androgenic hormones shows elevations, and some women have decreased hair loss when treated with daily doses of spironolactone.

Alopecia Areata

Alopecia areata is an autoimmune T-cell–mediated chronic inflammatory disease directed at hair follicles that results in baldness. Hair loss occurs in multiple areas of the scalp, usually in round patches. The eyebrows, eyelashes, beard, and other areas of the body are rarely involved. The cause is unknown, but stressful events, cell-mediated immune factors, and genetic susceptibility are linked to hair loss.[170] Metabolic disorders, such as Addison disease, thyroid disease, and lupus erythematosus, also are associated with alopecia areata.[171]

The affected areas of skin are smooth or may have short shafts of poorly developed hair that breaks at the surface. Regrowth occurs within 1 to 3 months, but hair loss may recur at the same site. Permanent regrowth of hair usually occurs. Total loss of hair (alopecia totalis) occurs in some young people; the long-term prognosis for total hair regrowth is poor.

Diagnosis is made by observation of the pattern of hair loss. Biopsy may show a lymphocytic infiltrate around the follicle. There are several treatments for alopecia areata including watchful waiting, corticosteroids, minoxidil, and topical immunotherapy.[172]

Hirsutism

Hirsutism is the abnormal growth and distribution of hair on the face, body, and pubic area in a male pattern that occurs in women. There is also frontotemporal hair recession. These areas of hair growth are androgen sensitive. Variations of hair growth in women are great, and a male pattern can be normal. Women who develop hirsutism may be secreting hormones associated with ovarian or adrenal disease, and such women should be evaluated for polycystic ovaries, adrenal hyperplasia, or adrenal tumors.[173] If no hormonal pathologic conditions exist, undesirable hair can be mechanically removed. Endocrine therapy to suppress androgens may be considered.[174]

DISORDERS OF THE NAIL

Paronychia

Paronychia is an acute or chronic infection of the cuticle.[175] Acute paronychia is manifested by the rapid onset of painful inflammation of the cuticle, usually after minor trauma. An abscess may develop, requiring incision and drainage (I&D) for relief of pain. The most common causative microorganisms are *Staphylococci, Streptococci,* and occasionally *Candida.*

Chronic paronychia develops slowly, with tenderness and swelling around the proximal or lateral nail folds. One or more fingers or toes may be involved. Individuals whose hands are frequently exposed to moisture are at greatest risk. Manipulation or chronic wetting of the cuticle increases risk because it disrupts the natural protective barrier provided by the cuticle, leaving a moist, warm medium for pathogenic microorganisms to incubate. The skin around the nail becomes more edematous and painful with progressive infection. Pus may be expressed from the proximal nail fold. The nail plate is usually not affected, although it can become discolored and develop ridges with chronic infections.

Treatment includes keeping the hands dry. Abscesses are treated with incision and drainage; severe bacterial cases may require systemic antibiotics. Oral antifungals are not very effective because they do not penetrate the affected tissues but efficacy is increased with topical application of steroid creams.[175]

Onychomycosis

Onychomycosis is a fungal or dermatophyte infection of the nail plate that occurs in 2% to 18% of the population.[176] The most common pattern is a nail plate that turns yellow or white (infection develops from the dorsal surface) and becomes elevated as a result of the accumulation of hyperkeratotic debris within the plate. Fungal infections of the nail may require culture and microscopy. Treatment includes débridement and systemic antifungal therapy. Surgical excision of the nail may be required. New systemic and topical antifungals are being investigated.[177]

SUMMARY REVIEW

Structure and Function of the Skin

1. The skin is the largest organ of the body and equals about 20% of body weight.
2. The skin has three layers: the dermis, epidermis, and subcutaneous layer.
3. Keratinocytes produce keratin to form the superficial layer of the epidermis. The underlying epidermis contains a basal and a spinous layer with melanocytes, Langerhans cells, and Merkel cells.
4. The dermis is composed of connective tissue elements, hair follicles, sweat glands, sebaceous glands, blood vessels, nerves, and lymphatic vessels.
5. The subcutaneous layer contains fat cells and connective tissue.
6. The dermal appendages include the nails, hair, sebaceous glands, and the eccrine and apocrine sweat glands.
7. The papillary capillaries provide the major blood supply to the skin, arising from deeper arterial plexuses. The sympathetic nervous system regulates skin blood flow.
8. Heat loss and heat conservation are regulated by arteriovenous anastomoses that lead to the papillary capillaries.
9. Older skin is thinner and drier with less collagen; it has fewer capillary loops and fewer changes in pigmentation.
10. Loss of melanocytes and hair follicles leads to gray and thinner hair.
11. The skin of older adults is more permeable; there is decreased sweating and loss of thermal regulation and decreased protective functions.
12. Pressure ulcers develop from continuous pressure and shearing forces that occlude capillary blood flow with resulting ischemia and necrosis. Areas at greatest risk are pressure points over bony prominences, such as the greater trochanter, sacrum, ischia, and heels. Immobilized individuals with fractures and neurologic deficits are most likely to develop pressure ulcers.
13. Keloids are scars that extend beyond the border of injury and result from abnormal fibroblast activity and excess collagen formation. Hypertrophic scars are elevated erythematous fibrous lesions that do not expand beyond the border of injury.
14. Pruritus (itching) is associated with many skin disorders. Itch mediators, peripheral polymodal C nerve fibers, and central processes contribute to itching. Scratching can cause skin trauma, infection, and scarring.

Disorders of the Skin

1. Allergic contact dermatitis is a form of delayed hypersensitivity that develops with sensitization to allergens, such as metals, chemicals, or poison ivy.

SUMMARY REVIEW—cont'd

2. Irritant contact dermatitis develops as an inflammatory response to prolonged exposure to chemicals, such as acids or soaps.
3. Atopic or allergic dermatitis is associated with a family history of allergies, hay fever, elevated IgE levels, and increased histamine sensitivity; it is more common in children.
4. Stasis dermatitis occurs on the legs and results from venous stasis and edema.
5. Seborrheic dermatitis involves scaly, yellowish, inflammatory plaques of the scalp, eyebrows, eyelids, ear canals, chest, axillae, and back. The cause is unknown.
6. Papulosquamous disorders are characterized by papules, scales, plaques, and erythema.
7. Psoriasis is a chronic autoimmune T-cell–mediated inflammatory skin disease with thickening of the epidermis and dermis characterized by scaly, erythematous pruritic plaques. The forms of psoriasis are plaque, inverse, guttate, pustular, and erythrodermic. Systemic complications can accompany the disease including arthritis and cardiovascular disease.
8. Pityriasis rosea is a self-limiting disease characterized by oval lesions with scales around the edges located along skin lines of the trunk.
9. Lichen planus is a papular violet-colored autoimmune inflammatory lesion involving T cells and inflammatory cytokines manifested by severe pruritus and can involve both skin and mucous membrane lesions.
10. Acne vulgaris is a facial inflammation of the pilosebaceous follicles with hypertrophy of sebaceous glands and telangiectasia, particularly of the nose.
11. Acne rosacea develops on the middle third of the face with hypertrophy and inflammation of the sebaceous glands that may be the result of infection or immune-mediated inflammation.
12. Lupus erythematosus is an inflammatory autoimmune disease that can affect only the skin (discoid) or have a systemic presentation. The inflammatory lesions usually occur in sun-exposed areas with a butterfly distribution over the nose and cheeks.
13. Pemphigus is a chronic, autoimmune, blistering disease that begins in the mouth or on the scalp and spreads to other parts of the body, often with a fatal outcome. The forms of pemphigus include pemphigus vulgaris (most common), pemphigus foliaceus, paraneoplastic pemphigus, and IgA pemphigus.
14. Bullous pemphigoid is a benign autoimmune blistering disease that resolves rapidly.
15. Erythema multiforme is an acute inflammation of the skin and mucous membranes with lesions that appear target-like with alternating rings of edema and inflammation; it is often associated with allergic reactions to drugs.
16. Folliculitis is a bacterial infection of the hair follicle.
17. A furuncle is an infection of the hair follicle that extends to the surrounding tissue.
18. A carbuncle is a collection of infected hair follicles that forms a draining abscess.
19. Cellulitis is a diffuse infection of the dermis and subcutaneous tissue.
20. Erysipelas is a superficial streptococcal infection of the skin commonly affecting the face, ears, and lower legs.
21. Impetigo may have a bullous or an ulcerative form and is caused by *Staphylococcus* or *Streptococcus* and is more common in children.
22. HSV-1 causes cold sores but can infect the cornea, mouth, and labia. HSV-2 causes genital lesions and is usually spread by sexual contact.
23. Herpes zoster and varicella (chickenpox) are both caused by the same herpesvirus, with herpes zoster manifesting years after the initial infection.
24. Warts (verrucae) are benign, rough, elevated lesions caused by papillomavirus. Venereal warts (condylomata acuminata) are spread by sexual contact.
25. Tinea skin infections (fungal infections) can occur anywhere on the body and are classified by location (i.e., tinea pedis, tinea corporis, tinea capitis).
26. Candidiasis is a yeastlike fungal infection caused by *C. albicans* occurring on skin, on mucous membranes, and in the gastrointestinal tract.
27. Cutaneous vasculitis is an immune-mediated inflammation of skin blood vessels with purpura, ischemia, and necrosis resulting from vessel necrosis.
28. Urticarial lesions are associated with type I hypersensitivity responses and appear as wheals, welts, or hives.
29. Localized scleroderma is an immune-mediated sclerosis of the skin that also may affect muscle, bone, and other body organs.
30. Ticks cause a local reaction on the skin of humans and can cause systemic disease when mouthparts pierce the skin and remain embedded in the tissue.
31. Lyme disease is a multisystem inflammatory disease caused by *B. burgdorferi* transmitted by tick bites. Complications may persist for years.
32. Seborrheic keratosis is a proliferation of squamous cells that produce elevated, smooth, or warty lesions of varying size usually in sun-damaged skin. They are most common among older adults.
33. Keratoacanthoma arises from hair follicles on sun-exposed areas. There are three stages of development that result in a dome-shaped, crusty lesion filled with keratin that resolves in 3 to 4 months.
34. Actinic keratosis is a pigmented scaly lesion that develops in sun-exposed individuals with fair skin. The lesion may become malignant in the form of squamous cell carcinoma.
35. Nevi arise from melanocytes and may be pigmented or fleshy pink. They occur singly or in groups and may undergo transition to malignant melanoma.
36. Basal cell carcinoma is the most common skin cancer and occurs most often on sun-exposed areas.

SUMMARY REVIEW—cont'd

37. Squamous cell carcinoma is a tumor of the epidermis associated with sun exposure and can be localized (in situ) or invasive.
38. Cutaneous melanoma arises from melanocytes; if it is not excised early, metastasis occurs through the lymph nodes.
39. KS is a vascular malignancy associated with immunodeficiency states and is associated with herpesvirus 8.
40. Cutaneous lymphomas are cutaneous T-cell and B-cell lymphomas that are present in the skin without evidence of extracutaneous disease at the time of diagnosis.
41. Frostbite usually occurs on cheeks and digits, causing direct injury to cells and impaired circulation.

Disorders of the Hair

1. Male-pattern alopecia is an inherited form of irreversible baldness with hair loss in the central scalp and recession of the temporofrontal hairline.
2. Female-pattern alopecia is a thinning of the central hair of the scalp beginning in women at 20 to 30 years of age.
3. Alopecia areata is patchy loss of hair associated with an autoimmune process and triggered by stress or metabolic diseases; it is usually reversible.
4. Hirsutism is a male pattern of hair growth in women that may be normal or the result of excessive secretion of androgenic hormones.

Disorders of the Nail

1. Paronychia is an inflammation of the cuticle that can be acute or chronic and is usually caused by staphylococci or streptococci.
2. Onychomycosis is a fungal infection of the nail plate.

KEY TERMS

Acne rosacea, 1631
Acne vulgaris, 1631
Actinic keratosis, 1641
Allergic contact dermatitis, 1627
Alopecia, 1646
Alopecia areata, 1646
Apocrine sweat gland, 1618
Atopic dermatitis (allergic dermatitis), 1628
Basal cell carcinoma, 1641
Basal layer (stratum basale), 1616
Bullous pemphigoid (BP), 1633
Candidiasis, 1638
Carbuncle, 1635
Cellulitis, 1635
Clawlike prolongation, 1626
Condylomata acuminata, 1637
Cutaneous melanoma, 1643
Cutaneous vasculitis, 1638
Dermal appendage, 1618
Dermis, 1616, 1617
Discoid (cutaneous) lupus erythematosus (DLE), 1632
Eccrine sweat gland, 1618
Eczema, 1627
Epidermis, 1616
Erysipelas, 1635
Erythema multiforme, 1633
Erythrodermic (exfoliative) psoriasis, 1630
Folliculitis, 1634
Furuncle, 1634
Germinative layer (stratum germinativum), 1617
Guttate psoriasis, 1629
Hair follicle, 1618
Herald patch, 1630
Herpes simplex virus (HSV), 1636
Herpes varicella, 1636
Herpes zoster, 1636
Hirsutism, 1647
Human papillomavirus (HPV), 1637
Hypertrophic scar, 1626
Hyphae, 1638
Hypodermis, 1616
IgA pemphigus, 1633
Impetigo, 1635
Inverse psoriasis, 1629
Irritant contact dermatitis, 1628
Kaposi sarcoma (KS), 1645
Keloid, 1626
Keratin, 1616
Keratinocyte, 1616
Keratoacanthoma, 1640
Langerhans cell, 1617
Lichen planus (LP), 1630
Localized scleroderma (morphea), 1639
Lupus erythematosus, 1632
Lyme disease, 1640
Melanocyte, 1617
Merkel cell, 1617
Mycosis fungoides, 1645
Myofibroblast, 1626
Nail, 1618
Necrotizing fasciitis, 1635
Nevi (*sing.*, nevus; also known as a mole), 1641
Onychomycosis, 1647
Papillary capillary, 1619
Papulosquamous disorder, 1629
Paraneoplastic pemphigus, 1633
Paronychia, 1647
Pemphigus, 1632
Pemphigus foliaceus, 1633
Pemphigus vulgaris, 1633
Pityriasis rosea, 1630
Plaque psoriasis, 1629
Primary cutaneous lymphoma, 1645
Proteoglycan, 1626
Pruritus, 1627
Psoriasis, 1629
Psoriatic arthritis, 1630
Psoriatic nail disease, 1630
Pustular psoriasis, 1629
Sebaceous gland, 1618
Seborrheic dermatitis, 1629
Seborrheic keratosis, 1640
Spinous layer (stratum spinosum), 1617
Squamous cell carcinoma (SCC), 1642
Stasis dermatitis, 1628
Stratum corneum, 1616
Tinea capitis, 1637
Tinea corporis (ringworm), 1637
Tinea infection, 1637
Tinea pedis, 1637
Tinea unguium (onychomycosis), 1637
Urticaria, 1639
Urticarial lesion, 1639
Vitiligo, 1617
Wart, 1636

REFERENCES

1. Gros E, Novak N: Cutaneous dendritic cells in allergic inflammation, *Clin Exp Allergy* 42(8):1161–1175, 2012.
2. Myung P, Ito M: Dissecting the bulge in hair regeneration, *J Clin Invest* 122(2):448–454, 2012.
3. Naylor EC, Watson RE, Sherratt MJ: Molecular aspects of skin ageing, *Maturitas* 69(3):249–256, 2011.
4. Ortiz A, Grando SA: Smoking and the skin, *Int J Dermatol* 51(3): 250–262, 2012.
5. Kohl E et al: Skin ageing, *J Eur Acad Dermatol Venereol* 25(8):873–884, 2011.
6. McDonough PH, Schwartz RA: Premature hair graying, *Cutis* 89(4):161–165, 2012.
7. Holowatz LA, Thompson-Torgerson C, Kenney WL: Aging and the control of human skin blood flow, *Front Biosci* 15:718–739, 2010.
8. Khavkin J, Ellis DA: Aging skin: histology, physiology, and pathology, *Facial Plast Surg Clin North Am* 19(2):229–234, 2011.
9. Anders J et al: Decubitus ulcers: pathophysiology and primary prevention, *Dtsch Arztebl Int* 107(21):371–381, 2010.

10. Clark M: Skin assessment in dark pigmented skin: a challenge in pressure ulcer prevention, *Nurs Times* 106(30):16–17, 2010.
11. Cowan LJ et al: Enhancing Braden pressure ulcer risk assessment in acutely ill adult veterans, *Wound Repair Regen* 20(2):137–148, 2012.
12. Cox J: Predictive power of the Braden scale for pressure sore risk in adult critical care patients: a comprehensive review, *J Wound Ostomy Continence Nurs* 39(6):613–621, 2012.
13. Mortenson WB, Miller WC: SCIRE Research Team: A review of scales for assessing the risk of developing a pressure ulcer in individuals with SCI, *Spinal Cord* 46(3):168–175, 2008.
14. National Pressure Ulcer Advisory Panel: Pressure ulcer stages revised by NPUAP: 2007, Available at www.npuap.org/resources/educational-and-clinical-resources/npuap-pressure-ulcer-stagescategories/.
15. Little MO: Nutrition and skin ulcers, *Curr Opin Clin Nutr Metab Care* 16(1):39–49, 2013.
16. Gadd MM: Preventing hospital-acquired pressure ulcers: improving quality of outcomes by placing emphasis on the Braden subscale scores, *J Wound Ostomy Continence Nurs* 39(3):292–294, 2012.
17. Baranoski S, Ayello EA: Wound dressings: an evolving art and science, *Adv Skin Wound Care* 25(2):87–92, 2012.
18. Desai KK et al: Negative pressure wound therapy: an algorithm, *Clin Plast Surg* 39(3):311–324, 2012.
19. Gupta S, Ichioka S: Optimal use of negative pressure wound therapy in treating pressure ulcers, *Int Wound J* 9(Suppl 1):8–16, 2012.
20. National Guideline Clearinghouse (NGC): Pressure ulcer treatment recommendations. In Prevention and treatment of pressure ulcers: clinical practice guideline. In *National Guideline Clearinghouse (NGC)* [Website], Rockville, MD, May 4, 2011. Available at http://www.guideline.gov/content.aspx?id=25139#Section420. Accessed June 14, 2013.
21. McInnes E et al: Support surfaces for treating pressure ulcers, *Cochrane Database Syst Rev* (12):CD009490, 2011.
22. Moore ZE, Cowman S: Repositioning for treating pressure ulcers, *Cochrane Database Syst Rev* (9):CD006898, 2012.
23. Shih B, Bayat A: Genetics of keloid scarring, *Arch Dermatol Res* 302(5):319–339, 2010.
24. Wolfram D et al: Hypertrophic scars and keloids—a review of their pathophysiology, risk factors, and therapeutic management, *Dermatol Surg* 35(2):171–181, 2009.
25. Bayat A et al: Genetic susceptibility to keloid disease: transforming growth factor beta receptor gene polymorphisms are not associated with keloid disease, *Exp Dermatol* 13(2):120–124, 2004.
26. Satish L et al: Gene expression patterns in isolated keloid fibroblasts, *Wound Repair Regen* 14(4):463–467, 2006.
27. Chalmers RL: The evidence for the role of transforming growth factor-beta in the formation of abnormal scarring, *Int Wound J* 8(3):218–223, 2011.
28. Sarrazy V et al: Mechanisms of pathological scarring: role of myofibroblasts and current developments, *Wound Repair Regen* 19(Suppl 1): s10–s15, 2011.
29. Gauglitz GG et al: Hypertrophic scarring and keloids: pathomechanisms and current and emerging treatment strategies, *Mol Med* 17(1-2): 113–125, 2011.
30. Sidle DM, Kim H: Keloids: prevention and management, *Facial Plast Surg Clin North Am* 19(3):505–515, 2011.
31. Viera MH, Caperton CV, Berman B: Advances in the treatment of keloids, *J Drugs Dermatol* 10(5):468–480, 2011.
32. Ikoma A et al: Anatomy and neurophysiology of pruritus, *Semin Cutan Med Surg* 30(2):64–70, 2011.
33. Raap U, Ständer S, Metz M: Pathophysiology of itch and new treatments, *Curr Opin Allergy Clin Immunol* 11(5):420–427, 2011.
34. Oaklander AL: Common neuropathic itch syndromes, *Acta Derm Venereol* 92(2):118–125, 2012.
35. Potenzieri C, Undem BJ: Basic mechanisms of itch, *Clin Exp Allergy* 42(1):8–19, 2012.
36. Metz M, Grundmann S, Ständer S: Pruritus: an overview of current concepts, *Vet Dermatol* 22(2):121–131, 2011.
37. Steinhoff M et al: Pruritus: management algorithms and experimental therapies, *Semin Cutan Med Surg* 30(2):127–137, 2011.
38. Gober MD, Gaspari AA: Allergic contact dermatitis, *Curr Dir Autoimmun* 10:1–26, 2008.
39. Kezic S: Genetic susceptibility to occupational contact dermatitis, *Int J Immunopathol Pharmacol* 24(Suppl 1):73S–78S, 2011.
40. Tončić RJ et al: Immunology of allergic contact dermatitis, *Acta Dermatovenerol Croat* 19(1):51–68, 2011.
41. Gawchik SM: Latex allergy, *Mt Sinai J Med* 78(5):759–772, 2011.
42. Usatine RP, Riojas M: Diagnosis and management of contact dermatitis, *Am Fam Physician* 82(3):249–255, 2010.
43. Zhai H et al: Irritant contact dermatitis: effect of age, *Cutan Ocul Toxicol* 31(2):138–143, 2012.
44. Kim KH: Overview of atopic dermatitis, *Asia Pac Allergy* 3(2):79–87, 2013.
45. Raffetto JD, Marston WA: Venous ulcer: what is new? *Plast Reconstr Surg* 127(Suppl 1):279S–288S, 2011.
46. Word R: Medical and surgical therapy for advanced chronic venous insufficiency, *Surg Clin North Am* 90(6):1195–1214, 2010.
47. Bukvić Mokos Z et al: Seborrheic dermatitis: an update, *Acta Dermatovenerol Croat* 20(2):98–104, 2012.
48. Sampaio AL et al: Seborrheic dermatitis, *An Bras Dermatol* 86(6): 1061–1071, 2011.
49. Apasrawirote W, Udompataikul M, Rattanamongkolgul S: Topical antifungal agents for seborrheic dermatitis: systematic review and meta-analysis, *J Med Assoc Thai* 94(6):756–760, 2011.
50. Parisi R et al: Global epidemiology of psoriasis: a systematic review of incidence and prevalence, *J Invest Dermatol* 133(3):377–385, 2012.
51. Rahman P, Elder JT: Genetics of psoriasis and psoriatic arthritis: a report from the GRAPPA 2010 annual meeting, *J Rheumatol* 39(2): 431–433, 2012.
52. Nakajima K: Critical role of the interleukin-23/T-helper 17 cell axis in the pathogenesis of psoriasis, *J Dermatol* 39(3):219–224, 2012.
53. Michalak-Stoma A et al: Cytokine network in psoriasis revisited, *Eur Cytokine Netw* 22(4):160–168, 2011.
54. Monteleone G et al: Psoriasis: from pathogenesis to novel therapeutic approaches, *Clin Sci (Lond)* 120(1):1–11, 2011.
55. Milavec-Puretić V et al: Drug induced psoriasis, *Acta Dermatovenerol Croat* 19(1):39–42, 2011.
56. Arumugam R, McHugh NJ: Mortality and causes of death in psoriatic arthritis, *J Rheumatol Suppl* 89:32–35, 2012.
57. Rahimi H, Ritchlin CT: Altered bone biology in psoriatic arthritis, *Curr Rheumatol Rep* 14(4):349–357, 2012.
58. Reich K: The concept of psoriasis as a systemic inflammation: implications for disease management, *J Eur Acad Dermatol Venereol* 26(Suppl 2):3–11, 2012.
59. Ryan C, Menter A: Psoriasis and cardiovascular disorders, *G Ital Dermatol Venereol* 147(2):179–187, 2012.
60. Archier E et al: Efficacy of psoralen UV-A therapy vs. narrowband UV-B therapy in chronic plaque psoriasis: a systematic literature review, *J Eur Acad Dermatol Venereol* 26(Suppl 3):11–21, 2012.
61. Patel M et al: Emerging therapies for the treatment of psoriasis, *Dermatol Ther (Heidelb)* 2(1):16, 2012.
62. Johnson-Huang LM, Lowes MA, Krueger JG: Putting together the psoriasis puzzle: an update on developing targeted therapies, *Dis Model Mech* 5(4):423–433, 2012.
63. Browning JC: An update on pityriasis rosea and other similar childhood exanthems, *Curr Opin Pediatr* 21(4):481–485, 2009.
64. Ayanlowo O, Akinkugbe A, Olumide Y: The pityriasis rosea calendar: a 7 year review of seasonal variation, age and sex distribution, *Nig Q J Hosp Med* 20(1):29–31, 2010.
65. Ehsani A et al: The comparison between the efficacy of high dose acyclovir and erythromycin on the period and signs of pitiriasis rosea, *Indian J Dermatol* 55(3):246–248, 2010.
66. Prpic Massari L et al: Perforin expression in peripheral blood lymphocytes and skin-infiltrating cells in patients with lichen planus, *Br J Dermatol* 151(2):433–439, 2005.
67. Shiohara T et al: Pathomechanisms of lichen planus autoimmunity elicited by cross-reactive T cells, *Curr Dir Autoimmun* 10:206–226, 2008.
68. Georgakopoulou EA et al: Oral lichen planus as a preneoplastic inflammatory model, *J Biomed Biotechnol* 759626:2012, 2012.
69. Le Cleach L, Chosidow O: Clinical practice. Lichen planus, *N Engl J Med* 366(8):723–732, 2012.
70. Samycia M, Lin AN: Efficacy of topical calcineurin inhibitors in lichen planus, *J Cutan Med Surg* 16(4):221–229, 2012.
71. Sharma A et al: Lichen planus: an update and review, *Cutis* 90(1):17–23, 2012.
72. Jansen T: Clinical presentations and classification of rosacea, *Ann Dermatol Venereol* 138(Suppl 3):S192–S200, 2011.
73. Cribier B: Pathophysiology of rosacea: redness, telangiectasia, and rosacea, *Ann Dermatol Venereol* 138(Suppl 3):S184–S189, 2011.
74. Forton FM: Papulopustular rosacea, skin immunity and Demodex: pityriasis folliculorum as a missing link, *J Eur Acad Dermatol Venereol* 26(1):19–28, 2012.

75. Pfeffer I et al: Treatment of ocular rosacea with 40 mg doxycycline in a slow release form, *J Dtsch Dematol Ges* 9(11):904–907, 2011.
76. Parodi A et al: Treatment of rosacea, *Ann Dermatol Venereol* 138(Suppl 3):S211–S214, 2011.
77. Chong BF, Song J, Olsen NJ: Determining risk factors for developing systemic lupus erythematosus in patients with discoid lupus erythematosus, *Br J Dermatol* 166(1):29–35, 2012.
78. Uva L et al: Cutaneous manifestations of systemic lupus erythematosus, *Autoimmune Dis* 2012:834291, 2012.
79. Yu M et al: The gender disparity of immunoreactants in lesional skin of lupus erythematosus patients, *Clin Exp Rheumatol* 30(1):103–105, 2012.
80. Chong BF, Song J, Olsen NJ: Determining risk factors for developing systemic lupus erythematosus in patients with discoid lupus erythematosus, *Br J Dermatol* 166(1):29–35, 2012.
81. Kuhn A, Ruland V, Bonsmann G: Cutaneous lupus erythematosus: update of therapeutic options part II, *J Am Acad Dermatol* 65(6): e195–e213, 2011.
82. Sinha AA: The genetics of pemphigus, *Dermatol Clin* 29(3):381–391, vii, 2011.
83. Giordano CN, Sinha AA: Cytokine networks in Pemphigus vulgaris: an integrated viewpoint, *Autoimmunity* 45(6):427–439, 2012.
84. Frew JW, Murrell DF: Paraneoplastic pemphigus (paraneoplastic autoimmune multiorgan syndrome): clinical presentations and pathogenesis, *Dermatol Clin* 29(3):419–425, viii, 2011.
85. Tsuruta D et al: IgA pemphigus, *Clin Dermatol* 29(4):437–442, 2011.
86. Kasperkiewicz M, Schmidt E, Zillikens D: Current therapy of the pemphigus group, *Clin Dermatol* 30(1):84–94, 2012.
87. Schmidt E, Zillikens D: Pemphigoid diseases, *Lancet* 381(9863):320–332, 2013.
88. Ujiie H, Nishie W, Shimizu H: Pathogenesis of bullous pemphigoid, *Immunol Allergy Clin North Am* 32(2):207–215, v, 2012.
89. Daniel BS et al: Evidence-based management of bullous pemphigoid, *Dermatol Clin* 29(4):613–620, 2011.
90. Di Zenzo G et al: Bullous pemphigoid: from the clinic to the bench, *Clin Dermatol* 30(1):3–16, 2012.
91. Scully C, Bagan J: Oral mucosal diseases: erythema multiforme, *Br J Oral Maxillofac Surg* 46(20):90–95, 2008.
92. Katta R: Taking aim at erythema multiforme. How to spot target lesions and less typical presentations, *Postgrad Med* 107(1):87, 2000.
93. Sokumbi O, Wetter DA: Clinical features, diagnosis, and treatment of erythema multiforme: a review for the practicing dermatologist, *Int J Dermatol* 51(8):889–902, 2012.
94. Provost TT, Weston WL: *Bullous diseases*, St Louis, 1993, Mosby.
95. Lugović-Mihić L et al: Differential diagnosis of the scalp hair folliculitis, *Acta Clin Croat* 50(3):395–402, 2011.
96. Demos M, McLeod MP, Nouri K: Recurrent furunculosis: a review of the literature, *Br J Dermatol* 167(4):725–732, 2012.
97. Gunderson CG: Cellulitis: definition, etiology, and clinical features, *Am J Med* 124(12):1113–1122, 2011.
98. Lancerotto L et al: Necrotizing fasciitis: classification, diagnosis, and management, *J Trauma Acute Care Surg* 72(3):560–566, 2012.
99. Gunderson CG, Martinello RA: A systematic review of bacteremias in cellulitis and erysipelas, *J Infect* 64(2):148–155, 2012.
100. Geria AN, Schwartz RA: Impetigo update: new challenges in the era of methicillin resistance, *Cutis* 85(2):65–70, 2010.
101. Tada DG, Khandelwal N: Serum HSV-1 and -2 IgM in sexually transmitted diseases—more for screening less for diagnosis: an evaluation of clinical manifestation, *J Glob Infect Dis* 4(3):S1–S4, 2012.
102. Wilson SS, Fakioglu E, Herold BC: Novel approaches in fighting herpes simplexvirus infections, *Expert Rev Anti Infect Ther* 7(5):559–568, 2009.
103. Robinson JL et al: Prevention, recognition and management of neonatal HSV infections, *Expert Rev Anti Infect Ther* 10(6):675–685, 2012.
104. Johnston C, Koelle DM, Wald A: HSV-2: in pursuit of a vaccine, *J Clin Invest* 121(12):4600–4609, 2011.
105. Ahmed AM et al: Managing herpes zoster in immunocompromised patients, *Herpes* 14(2):32–36, 2007.
106. Ruocco V et al: Beyond zoster: sensory and immune changes in zoster-affected dermatomes: a review, *Acta Derm Venereol* 92(4):378–382, 2012.
107. Bruxelle J, Pinchinat S: Effectiveness of antiviral treatment on acute phase of herpes zoster and development of post herpetic neuralgia: review of international publications, *Med Mal Infect* 42(2):53–58, 2012.
108. Philip A, Thakur R: Post herpetic neuralgia, *J Palliat Med* 14(6):765–773, 2011.
109. Gagliardi AM et al: Vaccines for preventing herpes zoster in older adults, *Cochrane Database Syst Rev* (10):CD008858, 2012.
110. Weinberg JM: Herpes zoster: epidemiology, natural history, and common complications, *J Am Acad Dermatol* 57(Suppl 6):S130–S135, 2007.
111. Antonsson A: Review: antibodies to cutaneous human papillomaviruses, *J Med Virol* 84(5):814–822, 2012.
112. Mulhem E, Pinelis S: Treatment of nongenital cutaneous warts, *Am Fam Physician* 84(3):288–293, 2011.
113. Leung L: Recalcitrant nongenital warts, *Aust Fam Physician* 40(1-2): 40–42, 2011.
114. Woodfolk JA: Allergy and dermatophytes, *Clin Microbiol Rev* 18(1): 30–43, 2005.
115. Itin PH, Battegay M: Skin problems in immunodeficient patients, *Curr Probl Dermatol* 43:9–17, 2012.
116. Cheng SC et al: Interplay between *Candida albicans* and the mammalian innate host defense, *Infect Immun* 80(4):1304–1313, 2012.
117. Levitz SM: Overview of host defenses in fungal infections, *Clin Infect Dis* 14(Suppl 1):537, 1992.
118. Chen KR, Carlson JA: Clinical approach to cutaneous vasculitis, *Am J Clin Dermatol* 9(2):71–92, 2008.
119. Kawakami T: New algorithm (KAWAKAMI algorithm) to diagnose primary cutaneous vasculitis, *J Dermatol* 37(2):113–124, 2010.
120. Schaefer P: Urticaria: evaluation and treatment, *Am Fam Physician* 83(9):1078–1084, 2011.
121. Carr TF, Saltoun CA: Chapter 21: urticaria and angioedema, *Allergy Asthma Proc* 33(Suppl 1):S70–S72, 2012.
122. Kurzinski K, Torok KS: Cytokine profiles in localized scleroderma and relationship to clinical features, *Cytokine* 55(2):157–164, 2011.
123. Shah AA, Wigley FM: Often forgotten manifestations of systemic sclerosis, *Rheum Dis Clin North Am* 34(1):221–238, ix, 2008.
124. Kreuter A: Localized scleroderma, *Dermatol Ther* 25(2):135–147, 2012.
125. Torok KS: Pediatric scleroderma: systemic or localized forms, *Pediatr Clin North Am* 59(2):381–405, 2012.
126. Elston DM: Tick bites and skin rashes, *Curr Opin Infect Dis* 23(2): 132–138, 2010.
127. Radolf JD et al: Of ticks, mice and men: understanding the dual-host lifestyle of Lyme disease spirochaetes, *Nat Rev Microbiol* 10(2):87–99, 2012.
128. Bratton RL et al: Diagnosis and treatment of Lyme disease, *Mayo Clin Proc* 83(5):566–571, 2008.
129. Halperin JJ, Baker P, Wormser GP: Common misconceptions about Lyme disease, *Am J Med* 126(3):264.e1-e7, 2013.
130. Stanek G et al: Lyme borreliosis, *Lancet* 379(9814):461–473, 2012.
131. Embers ME, Narasimhan S: Vaccination against Lyme disease: past, present, and future, *Front Cell Infect Microbiol* 3:6, 2013.
132. Krause PJ et al: Human *Borrelia miyamotoi* infection in the United States, *N Engl J Med* 368:291–293, 2013.
133. Aubut N, Alain J, Claveau J: Intralesional methotrexate treatment for keratoacanthoma tumors: a retrospective case series, *J Cutan Med Surg* 16(3):212–217, 2012.
134. Kirby JS, Miller CJ: Intralesional chemotherapy for nonmelanoma skin cancer: a practical review, *J Am Acad Dermatol* 63(4):689–702, 2010.
135. Ko CJ: Keratoacanthoma: facts and controversies, *Clin Dermatol* 28(3):254–261, 2010.
136. Rigel DS, Stein Gold LF: The importance of early diagnosis and treatment of actinic keratosis, *J Am Acad Dermatol* 68(1 Suppl 1):S20–S27, 2013.
137. Kim JK, Nelson KC: Dermoscopic features of common nevi: a review, *G Ital Dermatol Venereol* 147(2):141–148, 2012.
138. American Cancer Society: *Cancer facts and figures 2013*, Atlanta, 2013, The Society.
139. Lenardi G et al: Inorganic arsenic and basal cell carcinoma in areas of Hungary, Romania and Slovakia: a case-control study, *Environ Health Perspect* 120(5):721–726, 2012.
140. Kasper M et al: Basal cell carcinoma—molecular biology and potential new therapies, *J Clin Invest* 122(2):455–463, 2012.
141. Ratushny V et al: From keratinocyte to cancer: the pathogenesis and modeling of cutaneous squamous cell carcinoma, *J Clin Invest* 122(2):464–472, 2012.
142. LeBoeuf NR, Schmults CD: Update on the management of high-risk squamous cell carcinoma, *Semin Cutan Med Surg* 30(1):26–34, 2011.
142a. Alam M: Needs assessment for Mohs micrographic surgery, *Dermatol Clin* 30(1):167–175, 2012.
143. Mehnert JM, Kluger HM: Driver mutations in melanoma: lessons learned from bench-to-bedside studies, *Curr Oncol Rep* 14(5):449–457, 2012.
144. Russak JE, Rigel DS: Risk factors for the development of primary cutaneous melanoma, *Dermatol Clin* 30(3):363–368, 2012.

145. Whiteman DC, Pavan WJ, Bastian BC: The melanomas: a synthesis of epidemiological, clinical, histopathological, genetic, and biological aspects, supporting distinct subtypes, causal pathways, and cells of origin, *Pigment Cell Melanoma Res* 24(5):879–897, 2011.
146. Shenenberger DW: Cutaneous malignant melanoma: a primary care perspective, *Am Fam Physician* 85(2):161–168, 2012.
147. Cockerell CJ: The pathology of melanoma, *Dermatol Clin* 30(3): 445–468, 2012.
148. Dahl C, Guldberg P: The genome and epigenome of malignant melanoma, *APMIS* 115(10):1161–1176, 2007.
148a. Kwak J et al: Volatile biomarkers from human melanoma cells, *J Chromatogr B* 932:90–96, 2013.
149. Balch CM et al: Final version of 2009 AJCC melanoma staging and classification, *J Clin Oncol* 27(36):6199–6206, 2009.
150. Smalley KS, McArthur GA: The current state of targeted therapy in melanoma: this time it's personal, *Semin Oncol* 39(2):204–214, 2012.
151. Coit DG, Olszanski AJ: Progress in the management of melanoma in 2013, *J Natl Compr Canc Netw* 11(Suppl 5):645–648, 2013.
152. Spagnolo F, Queirolo P: Upcoming strategies for the treatment of metastatic melanoma, *Arch Dermatol Res* 304(3):177–184, 2012.
153. Kaufman HL: Vaccines for melanoma and renal cell carcinoma, *Semin Oncol* 39(3):263–275, 2012.
154. Lagisetty KH, Morgan RA: Cancer therapy with genetically-modified T cells for the treatment of melanoma, *J Gene Med* 14(6):400–404, 2012.
155. Radu O, Pantanowitz L: Kaposi sarcoma, *Arch Pathol Lab Med* 137(2):289–294, 2013.
156. Dezube BJ, Sullivan R, Koon HB: Emerging targets and novel strategies in the treatment of AIDS-related Kaposi's sarcoma: bidirectional translations science, *J Cell Physiol* 209(3):659–662, 2006.
157. Semeere AS, Busakhala N, Martin JN: Impact of antiretroviral therapy on the incidence of Kaposi's sarcoma in resource-rich and resource-limited settings, *Curr Opin Oncol* 24(5):522–530, 2012.
158. Bradford PT et al: Cutaneous lymphoma incidence patterns in the United States: a population based study of 3884 cases, *Blood* 113: 5064–5073, 2009.
159. Vij A, Duvic M: Prevalence and severity of pruritus in cutaneous T cell lymphoma, *Int J Dermatol* 51(8):930–934, 2012.
160. Willemze R et al: WHO-EORTC classification for cutaneous lymphomas, *Blood* 105(10):3768–3785, 2005.
160a. Thomas BR, Whittaker S: A practical approach to accurate classification and staging of mycosis fungoides and Sézary syndrome, *Skin Therapy Lett* 17(10):5–9, 2012.
161. Belloni B et al: Recent advances in the management of cutaneous lymphomas, *Semin Oncol* 39(2):150–162, 2012.
162. Olsen EA et al: Clinical end points and response criteria in mycosis fungoides and Sezary syndrome: a consensus statement of the International Society for Cutaneous Lymphomas, the United States Cutaneous Lymphoma Consortium, and the Cutaneous Lymphoma Task Force of the European Organization for Research and Treatment of Cancer, *J Clin Oncol* 18:2598–2607, 2011.
163. Morris SL: Skin lymphoma, *Clin Oncol (R Coll Radiol)* 24(5):371–385, 2012.
164. Mohr WJ, Jenabzadeh K, Ahrenholz DH: Cold injury, *Hand Clin* 25(4):481–496, 2009.
165. Johnson AR et al: Efficacy of intravenous tissue plasminogen activator in frostbite patients and presentation of a treatment protocol for frostbite patients, *Foot Ankle Spec* 4(6):344–348, 2011.
166. Golant A et al: Cold exposure injuries to the extremities, *J Am Acad Orthop Surg* 16(12):704–715, 2008.
167. Banka N, Bunagan MJ, Shapiro J: Pattern hair loss in men: diagnosis and medical treatment, *Dermatol Clin* 31(1):129–140, 2013.
168. Atanaskova Mesinkovska N, Bergfeld WF: Hair: what is new in diagnosis and management? Female pattern hair loss update: diagnosis and treatment, *Dermatol Clin* 31(1):119–127, 2013.
169. Sinclair R et al: Hair loss in women: medical and cosmetic approaches to increase scalp hair fullness, *Br J Dermatol* 165(Suppl 3):12–18, 2011.
170. Ito T: Advances in the management of alopecia areata, *J Dermatol* 39(1):11–17, 2012.
171. Alkhalifah A: Alopecia areata update, *Dermatol Clin* 31(1):93–108, 2013.
172. Hon KL, Leung AK: Alopecia areata, *Recent Pat Inflamm Allergy Drug Discov* 5(2):98–107, 2011.
173. Loriaux DL: An approach to the patient with hirsutism, *J Clin Endocrinol Metab* 97(9):2957–2968, 2012.
174. Franks S: The investigation and management of hirsutism, *J Fam Plann Reprod Health Care* 38(3):182–186, 2012.
175. Rigopoulos D et al: Acute and chronic paronychia, *Am Fam Physician* 77(3):339–346, 2008.
176. Scher RK: Onychomycosis: therapeutic update, *J Am Acad Dermatol* 40(6 Pt 2):S21, 1999.
177. Singal A, Khanna D: Onychomycosis: diagnosis and management, *Indian J Dermatol Venereol Leprol* 77(6):659–672, 2011.

CHAPTER 47

Alterations of the Integument in Children

Noreen Heer Nicol and Sue E. Huether

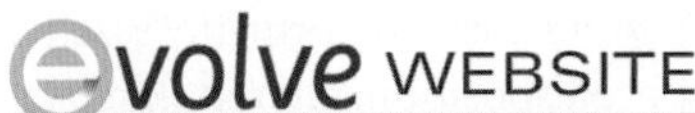

http://evolve.elsevier.com/McCance/

- Review Questions and Answers

CHAPTER OUTLINE

Children often develop alterations in the skin that may be minor or severe and localized or generalized. Skin diseases in children may have a different causative mechanism of expression than those found in adults, although there may be similarities. Diagnosis is commonly made from the history, appearance, and distribution of the lesion or lesions. Common skin diseases of childhood are presented here.

ACNE VULGARIS

Acne vulgaris is the most common skin disease and affects 85% of the population between the ages of 12 and 25 years. Onset is occurring at a younger age and may be associated with earlier onset of puberty in the United States. Genetic influences may determine an individual's susceptibility and severity of disease. Severe acne tends to have a genetic predisposition.[1] The incidence of acne is the same in both genders, although severe disease affects males more often.

Acne develops at distinctive pilosebaceous units, known as *sebaceous follicles.* Located primarily on the face and upper parts of the chest and back, these follicles have many large sebaceous glands, a small vellus hair (very short, nonpigmented, and very thin hair), and a dilated follicular canal that is visible as a pore on the skin surface. Acne lesions may be inflammatory (pustules, papules, nodules) or noninflammatory. In **noninflammatory acne** the comedones are open (blackheads) and closed (whiteheads), with the accumulated material causing distention of the follicle and thinning of follicular canal walls. **Inflammatory acne** develops in closed comedones when the follicular wall ruptures, expelling sebum into the surrounding dermis and initiating inflammation. Pustules form when the inflammation is close to the surface; papules and cystic nodules can develop

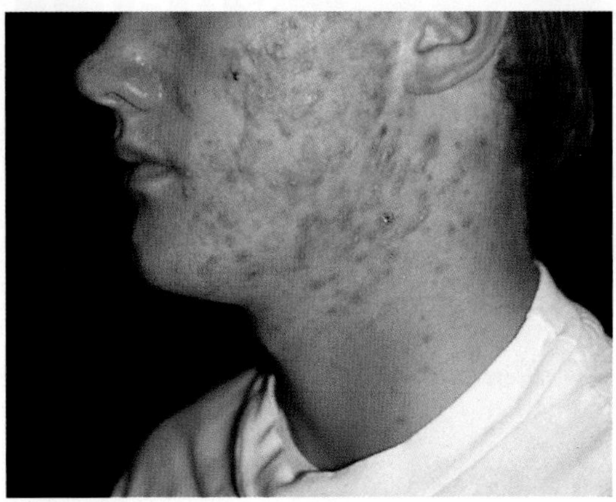

FIGURE 47-1 Cystic Acne. Multiple pustules (erythematous papules and pustules) are present, and several have become confluent. Note areas of scarring. (Courtesy Department of Dermatology, School of Medicine, University of Utah.)

when the inflammation is deeper, causing mild to severe scarring (Figure 47-1). Many types of lesions may exist in the same individual.

The exact cause of acne is unknown and various pathophysiologic factors contribute to the development of acne. The principal factors are follicular hyperkeratinization, excessive sebum production, follicular proliferation of *Propionibacterium acnes,* and inflammation and rupture of a follicle from accumulated debris and bacteria within the follicle. Androgens (dihydrotestosterone and testosterone) synthesized in increasing amounts during puberty boost the size and productivity of the sebaceous glands and promote *P. acnes.* Acne also is associated with polycystic ovarian syndrome, congenital adrenal hyperplasia, and various endocrine tumors as a result of higher circulating levels of androgens. The *P. acnes* anaerobic bacteria produce extracellular porphyrins and proinflammatory molecules, including chemotactic factors and lipolytic and proteolytic enzymes. The hydrolytic action of the enzymes converts triglycerides into free fatty acids that stimulate inflammation and edema and result in breakdown of the follicle wall. Chemotactic substances also may be released that involve mediation of inflammation by attraction of polymorphonuclear leukocytes.[2]

Treatment of acne should address the causative factors and be individualized according to severity. The combination of a topical retinoid, benzoyl peroxide, and antimicrobial agents is preferred. Retinoids are anticomedogenic and comedolytic and have some anti-inflammatory effects. Benzoyl peroxide is antimicrobial with some keratolytic effects. Topical antibiotics (e.g., erythromycin and clindamycin) have anti-inflammatory and antimicrobial effects. Combined oral contraceptives may be effective for acne in women.[3] Use of systemic therapies, including oral antibiotics, corticosteroids, and isotretinoin, is encouraged in more severe cases but may be limited by side effects. Dietary based guidelines need further investigation.[4] Acne surgery, including comedo extraction, intralesional steroids, and cryosurgery, may be useful in selected individuals. Severe scarring may be treated with dermabrasion, lasers, and resurfacing techniques. Special consideration must be given to treatment for those with darker skin because they have greater risk for hyperpigmentation and keloidal scarring.[5] Psychosocial morbidity is significant, particularly in adolescents.[5-7]

Acne conglobata is a highly inflammatory form of severe acne with communicating cysts and abscesses beneath the skin that can cause scarring. Remissions tend to occur during the summer, perhaps from more exposure to sunlight. This type of acne requires the use of systemic and combination therapies to prevent drug resistance.

DERMATITIS

Atopic Dermatitis

Atopic dermatitis (AD), also known as atopic eczema, occurs with a prevalence rate up to 20% in children. AD is increasing throughout the world.[8] Onset is usually from 2 to 6 months of age, and 85% of cases occur within the first 5 years of life; 75% to 80% of individuals with AD have a personal or family history of asthma, allergic rhinitis (hay fever), or food allergy. The cause of this chronic relapsing form of pruritic eczema involves an interplay of genetic predisposition, altered skin barrier function associated with filaggrin gene missense mutations (proteins that bind keratin in the epidermis), reduced ceramide (a stratum corneum lipid) levels, altered innate immunity, and altered immune responses to allergens, irritants, and microbes.[9]

There is debate as to whether the pathophysiology favors an "inside-out" explanation with immunologic dysregulation leading to epidermal barrier abnormality or an "outside-in" explanation with primary barrier dysfunction as the cause of the immunologic perturbations.[10] Regardless of the debate, both are involved in the disease. Positive skin tests to a variety of common food and inhalant allergens are seen in approximately 80% of individuals. Children with atopic dermatitis are more likely to have asthma.[11]

In AD, memory T cells in the blood express cutaneous lymphocyte antigen (CLA), which leads to the homing of lymphocytes to the skin. Inflammation is associated with activation of Th2 and Th1 cells with release of numerous cytokines, chemokines, interferon-gamma (IFN-γ), and granulocyte-macrophage colony-stimulating factor (GM-CSF). Activation of mast cells, eosinophils, and macrophages and expression of IgE contribute to the inflammation.[12]

Alterations in filaggrin protein lead to a defect of the epidermal barrier that causes transepidermal water loss and allows easy penetration of pathogens and allergens through the skin and a systemic hyperactive immune response. Filaggrin gene mutations also are associated with increased risk for asthma in AD and ichthyosis vulgaris (dry, scaly skin). In AD keratinocytes are deficient in their ability to express Toll-like antimicrobial peptides (see Chapter 7), and may predispose such individuals to skin colonization and infection with *Staphylococcus aureus,* viruses, and fungi.[13]

AD has a long-term course with frequent exacerbations, severe pruritus, and characteristic eczematoid appearance with redness, edema, and scaling (Figure 47-2). The skin becomes increasingly dry, sensitive, itchy, and easily irritated because the barrier function is impaired. Microscopic epidermal cracks that allow water to be expelled and irritants, allergens, and microbes

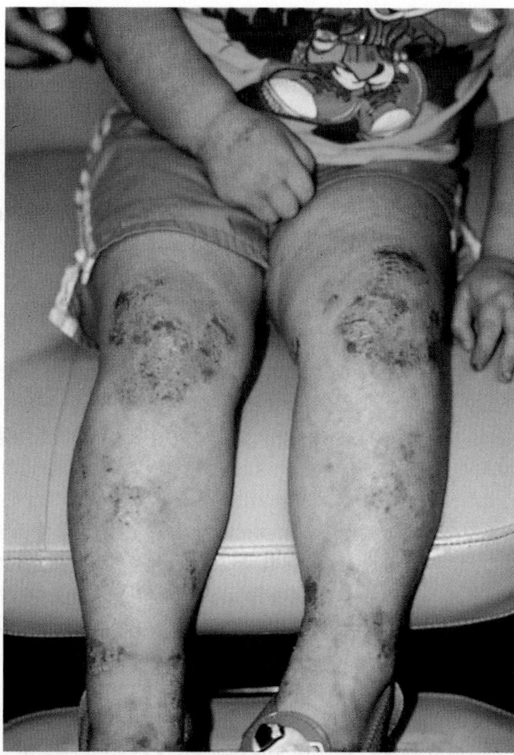

FIGURE 47-2 Atopic Dermatitis. Characteristic lesions with crusting from irritation and scratching over knees and around ankles. (Courtesy Department of Dermatology, School of Medicine, University of Utah.)

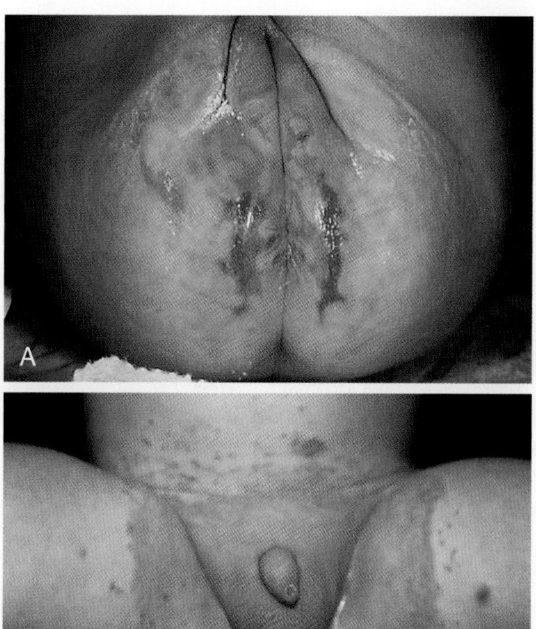

FIGURE 47-3 Diaper Dermatitis. A, Diaper dermatitis with erosions. **B,** Diaper dermatitis with *Candida albicans* secondary infection. (Courtesy Department of Dermatology, School of Medicine, University of Utah.)

to enter further inflammation, drying, and cracking. Itching is the hallmark of atopic dermatitis, and rubbing and scratching to relieve the itch are responsible for many of the clinical skin changes of AD. Histamine level is elevated in AD lesions but is not considered a major pruritogen because blockage of H1 and H2 receptors alone is ineffective at relieving itch. However, H4 receptor blockers are being evaluated.[14] Pruritus is a complex process with immune and neurologic pathways.[15,16]

In infants, the rash appears primarily on the face, scalp, trunk, and extensor surfaces of the arms and legs. In older children and adults, the rash tends to be found on the neck, antecubital and popliteal fossae, and hands and feet. Lichenification (thickening of the epidermis from constant scratching) is more common in adults with chronic eczema. Individuals with AD tend to develop viral, bacterial, and fungal skin infections in the areas with eczema. The irritation and itching interfere with sleep and cause irritability.

There are no specific laboratory features of AD that can be used for diagnostic purposes, and diagnosis is based on clinical history and presentation of symptoms. Management of AD requires a systematic, multidimensional, individualized approach that considers the individual's skin reaction pattern and acuity of the rash.[17] Treatment guidelines establish the foundation of AD management, addressing the skin barrier defect with regular use of emollients and skin hydration along with the identification and avoidance of specific and nonspecific trigger factors. Various topical agents are mainstays of treatment. Topical corticosteroids and calcineurin inhibitors continue to dominate therapy and, to date, their safety record seems good (despite the Black Box warning issued in the United States). In severe cases that cannot be controlled, guidelines suggest systemic treatment options including systemic corticosteroids, cyclosporine A, ultraviolet light therapy, and wet wrap therapy being added to the topical treatment regimen. Systemic corticosteroids are known to be effective in short-term treatment of AD, but evidence is limited to support their use because of long-term side effects and rebound flaring.[18-20] Research is in progress to develop targeted molecular therapy that is safe and cost-effective.

Diaper Dermatitis

Diaper dermatitis is a form of irritant contact dermatitis initiated by a combination of factors that include prolonged exposure to and irritation by urine and feces, maceration by wet diapers, complications from use of airtight plastic diaper covers, and possibly increased association with intercurrent illnesses and early introduction of cereals. Disposable diaper designs have decreased diaper dermatitis in infants.[21] Diaper dermatitis is frequently secondarily infected with *Candida albicans.*

The lesions vary from mild erythema to erythematous papular lesions. Candidal (monilial) diaper dermatitis is usually very erythematous, with sharp margination and pustulovesicular satellite lesions (Figure 47-3).

Treatment includes changing the diaper frequently to keep the area clean and dry or frequently exposing the perineal area to air, using super-absorbent diapers, and applying topical protection with a product containing petrolatum or zinc oxide, or both. Topical antifungal medication is used to treat *C. albicans* when present.[22]

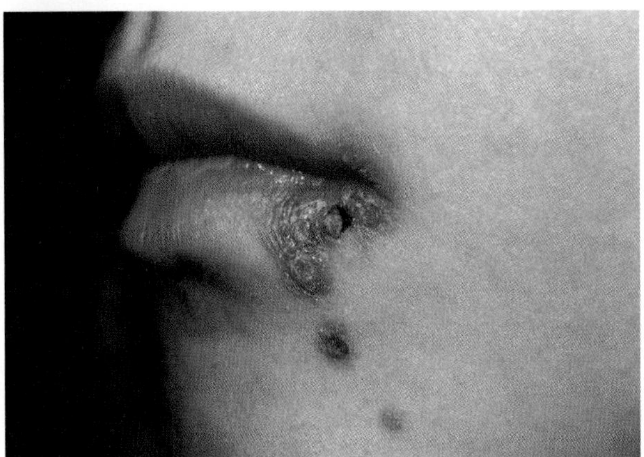

FIGURE 47-4 Impetigo. Multiple crusted and oozing lesions of impetigo. (From Kliegman RM et al: *Nelson textbook of pediatrics,* ed 19, Philadelphia, 2011, Saunders.)

INFECTIONS OF THE SKIN

Infectious diseases caused by bacteria, viruses, and fungi constitute the major forms of skin disease. Breaks in the skin integrity, particularly those that inoculate pathogens into the dermis and epidermis, may cause or exacerbate infections. Most infections tend to occur superficially; however, systemic signs and symptoms do develop occasionally and can be life threatening in immunosuppressed children.

Bacterial Infections

Impetigo Contagiosum

Impetigo is a common bacterial skin infection in infants and children. The mode of transmission is by both direct and indirect contact. The disease is more common in midsummer to late summer, with a higher incidence in hot, humid climates. Impetigo is particularly infectious among people living in crowded conditions with poor sanitary facilities or in settings such as daycare facilities. It affects children in good health, but conditions such as anemia and malnutrition are predisposing factors. There are two common types of impetigo: nonbullous and bullous. Both start as vesicles with a very thin vesicular roof composed of stratum corneum.

Nonbullous impetigo is a contagious, acute, superficial, vesiculopustular form of impetigo caused by *Staphylococcus aureus* or group A *Streptococcus pyogenes* (alone or in combination with *S. aureus*). The microorganisms are disseminated by direct physical contact from other infected individuals or through insect bites. The lesions begin as small vesicles with a honey-colored serum. Yellow to white-brown crusts form as the vesicles rupture (Figure 47-4). The lesions must be differentiated from herpes simplex lesions (see Figure 46-17, p. 1636). Untreated lesions may last for weeks and extend to cover a large area. In contrast to bullous impetigo, regional lymphadenitis is common.

Bullous impetigo is a rarer variant of impetigo caused by *S. aureus.*[23] The pathogen is often carried in the anterior nares, perineal region, or fingernails and is transmitted by contact with the individual or contaminated equipment.[24] The staphylococci produce bacterial toxins called *exfoliative toxins (ETs)* that cause a disruption in desmosomal adhesion molecules with blister formation.[25] The blisters enlarge or coalesce to form superficial bullae. There may be a few localized lesions or many lesions scattered over the skin. As the bullae rupture, a thin, flat, honey-colored crust appears.

The crust is the hallmark of impetigo. A moist, inflamed serum-weeping base is revealed when the crust is removed. The lesions are often located on the face around the nose and mouth, but the hands and other exposed areas are also involved. Regional lymphadenitis is uncommon. Treatment of choice for both types of impetigo is topical mupirocin and topical fusidic acid or oral antibiotics. Antibiotic therapy should be determined by bacterial culture and drug sensitivity because the prevalence of community-acquired methicillin-resistant *S. aureus*–associated impetigo is increasing. For extensive or complicated impetigo, systemic antibiotics may be warranted but beta-lactam antibiotics should be avoided if methicillin-resistant *S. aureus* (MRSA) is suspected.[23,26] Prompt treatment avoids complications, such as glomerulonephritis, necrotizing fasciitis, and septic shock syndrome. Handwashing and isolation of the infected child's washcloth, towels, drinking glass, and linen are important practices to control this highly contagious disease.

Staphylococcal Scalded-Skin Syndrome

Staphylococcal scalded-skin syndrome (SSSS) is the most serious staphylococcal infection that affects the skin and usually is seen in infants and children younger than 5 years.[27] SSSS is caused by virulent group II staphylococci, which produce an exfoliative toxin that attacks desmoglein and adhesion molecules and causes a separation of the skin just below the granular layer of the epidermis.[28] The toxins are usually produced at body sites other than the skin and arrive at the epidermis through the circulatory system. Staphylococci typically are not found in the skin lesions themselves. Adults have circulating antistaphylococcal antibodies and are better able to metabolize and excrete the toxin. Newborns and premature infants are at the highest risk because of immature immunity (absence of prior exposure to the toxin).

The clinical symptoms begin with fever, malaise, rhinorrhea, and irritability followed by generalized erythema with exquisite tenderness of the skin. There may be an associated impetigo, but the infection often begins in the throat or chest. The erythema spreads from the face and trunk to cover the entire body except the palms, soles, and mucous membranes. Within 48 hours, blisters and bullae may develop, giving the child the appearance of being scalded (Figure 47-5). The pain is severe. Fluid loss from ruptured blisters and water evaporation from denuded areas may cause dehydration and loss of body heat. Perioral and nasolabial crusting and fissures develop. In severe cases the skin of the entire body may slough. When secondary infection can be prevented, healing of the involved skin occurs in 10 to 14 days, usually without scarring.

Before medical intervention is begun, culture, histology, or exfoliative cytology must be done to differentiate SSSS from toxic epidermal necrolysis (TEN) (see p. 1664). When the infection is confirmed, treatment with oral or intravenous antibiotics is begun. Topical antibiotics are ineffective. The skin should be treated the same as that with a severe burn—with meticulous aseptic technique. Skin substitutes may be used for adjuvant

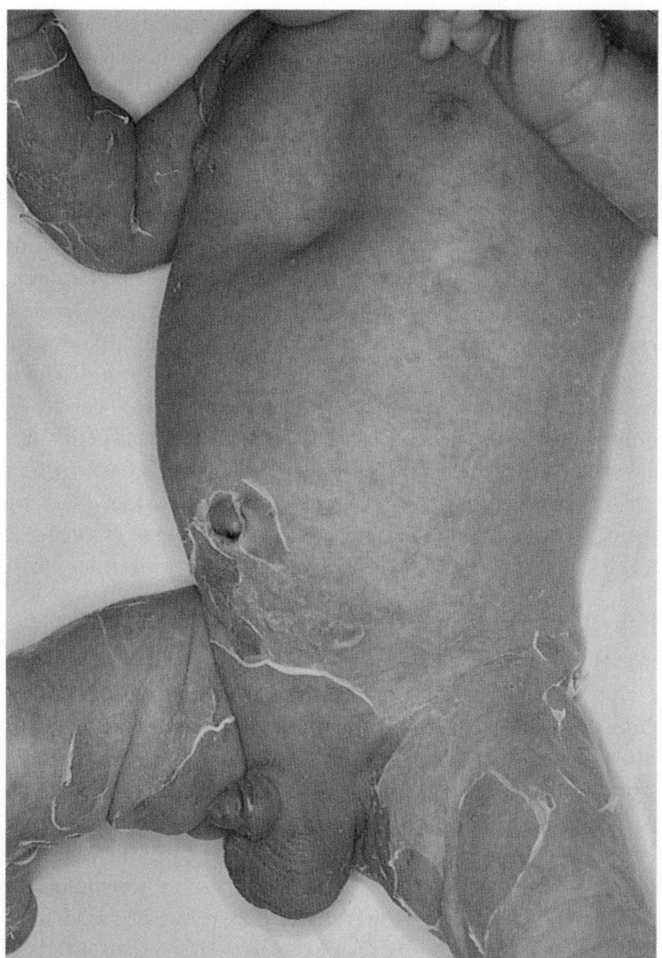

FIGURE 47-5 Staphylococcal Scalded-Skin Syndrome (SSSS). The skin lesions, showing desquamation and wrinkling of the skin margins, appeared 1 day after drainage of a staphylococcal abscess. (From Habif TP: *Clinical dermatology: a color guide to diagnosis and therapy*, ed 5, St Louis, 2010, Mosby.)

therapy.[29] Special care is required in serious cases and when the lips and eyelids are involved.[27]

Fungal Infections

Fungal disorders are known as *mycoses* and, when caused by dermatophytes (fungi that thrive on keratin), the mycoses are termed *tinea* (dermatophytosis or ringworm). The different types of tinea are classified according to their location on the body. **Tinea pedis** (a chronic, superficial fungal infection of the skin of the foot) occurs in children but is rare. Scaling disorders of the toes and feet in prepubertal children are usually eczema. Tinea capitis (infection of the scalp) and tinea corporis (infection of the body) are much more common in children than in adults. Dermatophytes of the genus *Epidermophyton* are the major cause of superficial fungal infections in children.[30] These dermatophytes invade the stratum corneum and not the remainder of the epidermis or dermis. The inflammatory response is thought, in part, to be secondary to the toxins released by the dermatophyte. It is important to confirm by culture the exact microorganism that is causing the fungal infection before commencing therapy.

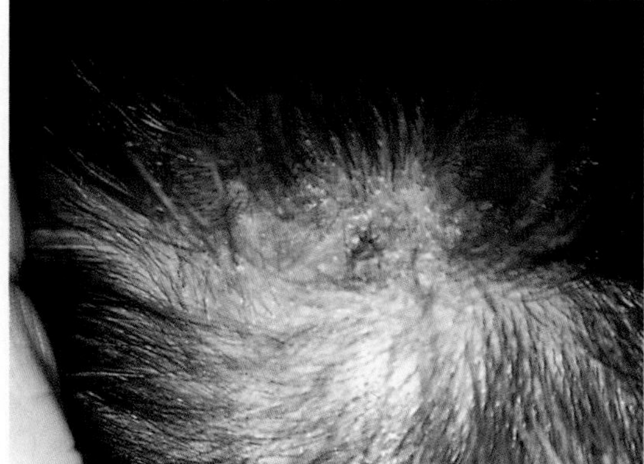

FIGURE 47-6 Tinea Capitis. (Courtesy Department of Dermatology, School of Medicine, University of Utah.)

Tinea Capitis

Tinea capitis, a fungal infection of the scalp, is the most common fungal infection of childhood. It rarely affects infants and is seen in children younger than age 12. Primary microorganisms responsible for the disease are *Trichophyton tonsurans and Microsporum canis. T. tonsurans* is transmitted by human-to-human contact. Areas of crowding are the most prevalent environments for this microorganism, which frequently affects inner-city children. *T. tonsurans* is often the predominant dermatophyte found in North America; many of these infections are not symptomatic.[31] The prevalence of asymptomatic carriers among household contacts of a child with active *T. tonsurans* disease is high. *M. canis* is found on cats, dogs, and certain rodents. Humans appear to be a terminal host for *M. canis,* and children who handle such animals are possible hosts. Human-to-human transmission does not occur with *M. canis.*

When symptoms are present, the clinical presentations vary, depending on the microorganism. Often the lesions are circular and manifest by broken hairs 1 to 3 mm above the scalp, leaving a partial alopecia 1 to 5 cm in diameter[32] (Figure 47-6). Slight erythema and scaling with raised borders can be observed.

Diagnosis is best confirmed by performing Wood light examination, potassium hydroxide (KOH) examination, and fungal culture, in that order. *T. tonsurans* does not fluoresce with Wood light examination. Oral griseofulvin is the treatment of choice because topical fungicides do not penetrate to the hair bulb. Terbinafine, itraconazole, and fluconazole are effective alternatives.[31] Adjunct therapy includes 2% ketoconazole and 1% selenium sulfide shampoos. Treatment of household contacts with a sporicidal shampoo should be considered and co-sleeping and comb-sharing must be discouraged.

Tinea Corporis

Tinea corporis (ringworm) is a common superficial dermatophyte infection in children. The microorganisms most commonly responsible for this disease are *M. canis* and *Trichophyton mentagrophytes.* As in tinea capitis, contact with kittens and puppies is a common source of the disorder. Tinea corporis preferentially affects the nonhairy parts of the face, trunk, and limbs. Lesions are often erythematous, round or oval scaling patches that spread peripherally with clearing in the center, creating the ring appearance, which is why this disease is commonly referred to as *ringworm*. The lesions are distributed asymmetrically, and multiple lesions (when present) overlap. Transmission occurs by direct contact with an infected lesion and through indirect contact with personal items used by the infected person. Potassium hydroxide examination of the scale from the border of the lesions confirms the diagnosis for most lesions. Most lesions respond well to applications of appropriate topical antifungal medications.[30]

Thrush

Thrush is the term used to describe the presence of *Candida albicans* in the mucous membranes of the mouth of infants and less commonly in adults, and both may be immune compromised. *C. albicans* penetrates the epidermal barrier more easily than other microorganisms because of its keratolytic proteases and other enzymes. *C. albicans* attracts neutrophils to skin sites of invasion but evades neutrophil killing.[33] Thrush is characterized by the formation of white plaques or spots in the mouth that lead to shallow ulcers. The tongue may have a dense, white covering. The underlying mucous membrane is red and tender and may bleed when the plaques are removed. The disease is often accompanied by fever and gastrointestinal irritation. The infection commonly spreads to the groin, buttocks, and other parts of the body. Treatment may be difficult and may include oral antifungal washes, such as nystatin oral suspension. Gentian violet can also be effective but is messy.[34] Simultaneous treatment of a *Candida* nipple infection or vaginitis in the mother is helpful in reducing the *C. albicans* surface colonization of the infant. Feeding bottles and nipples should be sterilized to prevent reinfection. The diaper area should be kept clean and dry.

Viral Infections

Viral infections of the skin in children are caused by poxvirus, papovavirus, and herpesvirus. The most common infections are described here.

Molluscum Contagiosum

Molluscum contagiosum is a common highly contagious poxvirus infection of the skin and occasionally conjunctiva that affects school-aged children and sexually active young adults. The disease can be more severe or prolonged in individuals with atopic dermatitis and a variety of immunodeficient states, including acquired immunodeficiency syndrome (AIDS). It is transmitted by skin-to-skin contact (e.g., contact sports), autoinoculation, and fomites, such as clothing, wash devices, and towels. The poxvirus induces epidermal cell proliferation and blocks immune responses that would control the virus. The epidermis grows down into the dermis to form saccules containing clusters of virus. The characteristic molluscum body is composed of mature, immature, and incomplete viruses and cellular debris.[35]

The lesions of molluscum are discrete, slightly umbilicated, dome-shaped papules 1 to 5 mm in diameter that appear anywhere on the skin or conjunctiva. The skin distribution in children is mainly on the trunk, face, and extremities (Figure 47-7). The pubic, genital, and perineal areas are favored in adults. Usually no inflammation surrounds molluscum lesions unless they are traumatized or secondary infection occurs. Scarring may occur with healing.

The best three diagnostic procedures are: (1) staining smears of the expressed molluscum body, (2) examining a biopsy, and (3) inoculating a molluscum suspension into cell cultures to demonstrate the cytotoxic reactions. Most lesions are self-limiting and clear in 6 to 9 months if not manipulated. However, because children often do manipulate these lesions, spontaneous involution may take 2 to 4 years without therapy.

Treatment options include immunomodulatory and antiviral therapy and destructive procedures (cryotherapy, curettage, or laser ablation); however, no treatment is universally effective. Treatment is recommended for genital molluscum to prevent sexual transmission and autoinoculation.[36] Destructive therapy is poorly tolerated by children. Measures to prevent spread of infection must be taken and recurrences are common.

Rubella (German or 3-Day Measles)

Rubella is a common communicable disease of children and young adults caused by a ribonucleic acid (RNA) virus that enters the bloodstream through the respiratory route. This disease is mild in most children. The incubation period ranges from 14 to 21 days. Prodromal symptoms are few but may include enlarged cervical and postauricular lymph nodes, low-grade fever, headache, sore throat, runny nose, and cough. A faint-pink to red, coalescing maculopapular rash develops on the face, with spread to the trunk and extremities, sparing the palms of the hands and soles of the feet, 1 to 4 days after the onset of initial symptoms (Figure 47-8). The rash is thought to be the result of virus dissemination to the skin. The rash subsides after 2 to 3 days, usually without complications. Children are generally not contagious after development of the rash. There is lifelong immunity to rubella—as there is for measles, chickenpox, and roseola—after contracting the disease. Differential presentations of viral diseases producing rashes are given in Table 47-1.

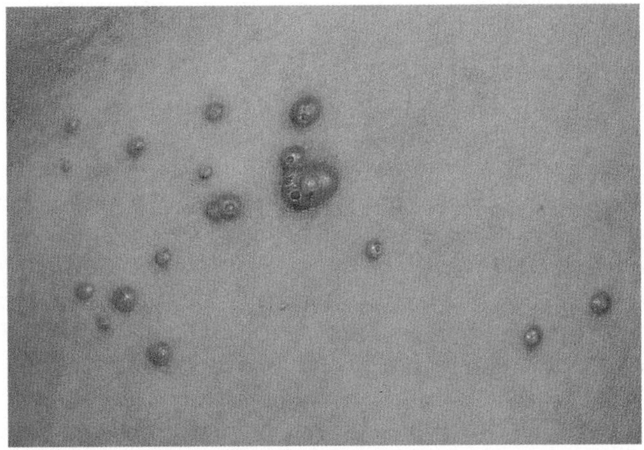

FIGURE 47-7 Molluscum Contagiosum. Waxy pink globules with umbilicated centers. (From Habif TP: *Clinical dermatology: a color guide to diagnosis and therapy*, ed 5, St Louis, 2010, Mosby.)

Vaccination for rubella is usually combined with vaccines for mumps and measles (rubeola) (MMR). Vaccine recommendations are presented in Chapter 10. Measles are known to occur in previously immunized children.[37] Rubella has almost been eliminated in the United States because of vaccination campaigns. However, challenges to maintain elimination include large outbreaks of measles in highly traveled developed countries, frequent international travel, and clusters of U.S. residents who remain unvaccinated because of personal belief exemptions.[38]

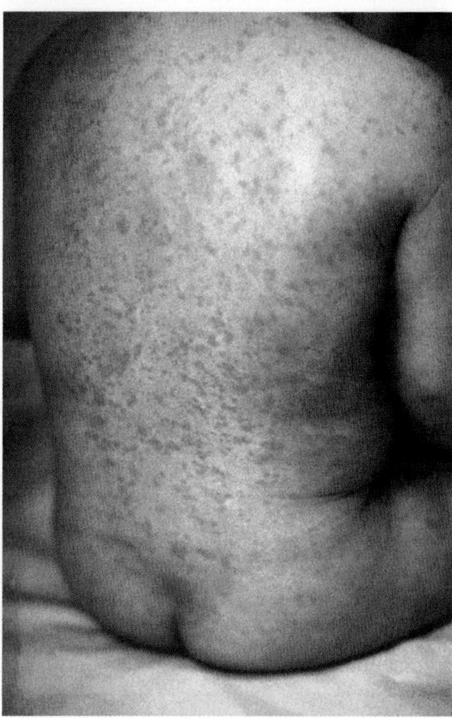

FIGURE 47-8 Rubella (Measles). Maculopapular rash with tendency to coalesce. The rash is similar to rubeola (red measles) but less intense. (From Marx JA et al: *Rosen's emergency medicine: concepts and clinical practice,* ed 7, Philadelphia, 2010, Mosby.)

Although the MMR vaccine may rarely be associated with adverse neurologic events (e.g., seizures because of fever, deafness), studies conclude that MMR immunization does not cause autism.[39,40] Lack of vaccination, however, leads to significant morbidity and mortality, with pneumonia, croup, and encephalitis being causes of death worldwide.[41,42]

Women of childbearing age are immunized if their rubella hemagglutination-inhibition titer is low. Pregnancy should be avoided for 3 months after vaccination because the attenuated virus in the vaccine may remain for this period. However, accidental receipt of MMR vaccination is not known to cause maternal or fetal complications, or both.[43] Pregnant women who have rubella early in the first trimester may have a fetal death or a fetus that develops congenital defects.[44]

There is no specific treatment for rubella. Recovery is spontaneous, although lymph nodes may remain enlarged for weeks. Supportive therapy includes rest, fluids, and use of a vaporizer. In rare cases a mild encephalitis or peripheral neuritis may follow rubella.

Rubeola (Red Measles)

Rubeola is a highly contagious, acute viral disease of children. It is transmitted by direct contact with droplets from infected persons and is caused by an RNA-containing paramyxovirus with an incubation period of 7 to 12 days, during which time no symptoms manifest. The virus enters the respiratory tract and attaches to dendritic cells and alveolar macrophages, amplifies in local lymphatic tissue, and progresses to systemic disease.[45] Prodromal symptoms include high fever (up to 40.5° C [104.9° F]), malaise, enlarged lymph nodes, runny nose, conjunctivitis, and "barking" cough. Within 3 to 4 days, an erythematous maculopapular rash develops over the head and spreads distally over the trunk, extremities, hands, and feet. Early lesions blanch with pressure, followed by a brownish hue that does not blanch as the rash fades. Characteristic pinpoint white spots surrounded by an erythematous ring develop over the buccal mucosa and are known as *Koplik spots.* These spots precede the

TABLE 47-1 DIFFERENTIAL PRESENTATION OF VIRAL DISEASES PRODUCING RASHES

VIRAL DISEASE	INCUBATION	PRODROMAL SYMPTOMS	DURATION/ CHARACTERISTICS	CLINICAL SYMPTOMS
Rubella (German measles)	14-21 days	1-2 days Mild fever Malaise Respiratory symptoms	1-3 days Pink-red maculopapular rash Face and trunk	Enlarged and tender occipital and periauricular nodes
Rubeola (measles)	7-12 days	2-5 days Fever Cough Respiratory symptoms	3-5 days Purple-red to brown maculopapular papules Face, trunk, extremities	Koplik spots 1-3 days before rash Rash develops when fever subsides
Roseola (exanthema subitum)	5-15 days	2-5 days High fever	1-3 days Red macular papules Neck and trunk	
Varicella (chickenpox)	11-20 days	1-2 days Low-grade fever Cough May be asymptomatic	Red papules, vesicles, pustules in clusters	Eruption of new lesions for 4-5 days Occasional ulcerative lesion in the mouth

rash by 1 to 2 days and are usually missed because they appear so early. The rash then subsides within 3 to 5 days.

Complications associated with measles may be caused by the primary infection or a secondary bacterial infection. Measles encephalitis occurs in about 1 of 800 cases, and most children recover completely. Only a small minority develop permanent brain damage or die. Bacterial complications include otitis media and pneumonia, usually caused by group A hemolytic streptococcus, *Haemophilus influenzae,* or *S. aureus* infection.

Measles is prevented by a single vaccination of live attenuated measles virus. There is no specific treatment for measles, and supportive therapy is the same as for rubella. Antibiotic therapy is initiated if secondary bacterial infections develop.

Roseola (Exanthema Subitum)

Roseola is a presumed viral infection of infants between 6 months and 2 years of age, but it can be seen in children as old as 4 years. The incubation period is 5 to 15 days, followed by the sudden onset of fever (38.9° to 40.5° C [102° to 104.5° F]) that lasts 3 to 5 days. After the fever an erythematous, nonpruritic macular rash that lasts about 24 to 48 hours develops primarily over the trunk, neck, and arms. Children usually feel well, eat normally, and have few other symptoms. Usually no treatment is required and there are no complications.

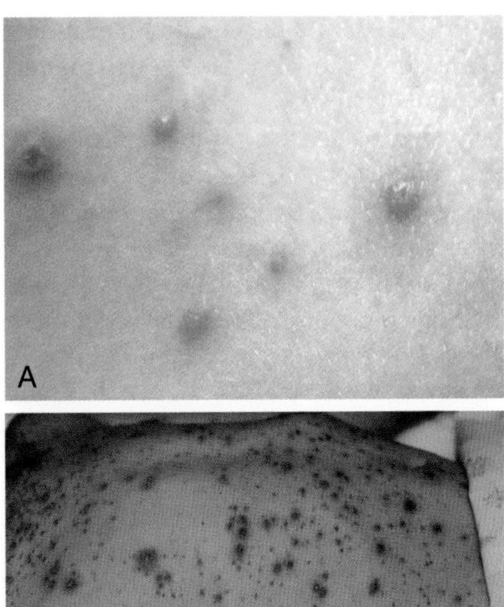

FIGURE 47-9 Chickenpox. **A,** Early stage lesions; **B,** late stage lesions. (**A** from Long SS et al: *Principles and practice of pediatric infectious diseases,* ed 4, Philadelphia, 2012, Saunders. **B** courtesy of David Effron, MD. From Marx J et al: *Rosen's emergency medicine: concepts and clinical practice,* ed 7, Philadelphia, 2010, Mosby.)

Chickenpox and Herpes Zoster

Chickenpox (varicella) and herpes zoster (shingles) are produced by the varicella-zoster virus (VZV). VZV is a complex herpes group deoxyribonucleic acid (DNA) virus. The incubation period is 10 to 27 days, averaging 14 days. Productive infection occurs within keratinocytes such that the vesicular lesions occur in the epidermis, and an inflammatory infiltrate is often present. Histologically, VZV lesions form intraepidermal vesicles. Infected keratinocytes degenerate, swell, detach from each other, and often contain inclusions surrounded by a clear halo and a circle of darkly staining chromatin. As the vesicle evolves, polymorphonuclear cells enter the vesicle and can lead to a pustular appearance. The vesicle eventually ruptures and is followed by crust formation. On mucous membranes the vesicles rupture and leave superficial, transient ulcers. Varicella occurs in people not previously exposed to VZV, whereas herpes zoster occurs in partially immune individuals who have had varicella.[46]

Chickenpox (Varicella). **Chickenpox** is a disease of early childhood, with 90% of children contracting the disease during the first decade of life. It is a highly contagious virus that is spread by person-to-person contact and airborne droplets. Introduction of an infected person into a household results in a 90% possibility of susceptible persons in the household developing the disease within the incubation period—usually 14 days. Children are contagious for at least 1 day before development of the rash. Transmission of the virus may occur until approximately 5 to 6 days after the onset of the first skin lesions in healthy children. In immunocompromised children the virus is recoverable for a longer period, but these children must be considered contagious for at least 7 to 10 days. Healthy children who develop chickenpox have no prodromal symptoms. The first sign of illness may be itching or the appearance of vesicles, usually on the trunk, scalp, or face. The rash later spreads to the extremities. Characteristically, lesions can be seen in various stages of maturation with macules, papules, and vesicles present in a particular area at the same time (Figure 47-9). The vesicular lesions are superficial and can be easily ruptured. New lesions will erupt for 4 to 5 days, until there are approximately 100 to 300 in different stages of development. The vesicles become crusted, with only the crust remaining. Occasionally a vesicle may appear on the palm later in the disease. Although uncommon, ulcerative lesions are sometimes seen in the mouth and, less commonly, on the conjunctiva and pharynx. Fever usually lasts 2 to 3 days and ranges from 38.5° to 40° C [101.3° to 104° F]).

Complications are rare in children but more common in adults. They can include transient hematuria (from rupture of vesicles in the bladder), epistaxis, laryngeal edema, and varicella pneumonia. One case of chickenpox produces almost complete immunity against a second attack. Rarely, the fetus may be malformed (congenital varicella syndrome) if chickenpox develops in the mother in the first trimester of pregnancy.[47]

Infants whose mothers have chickenpox at any stage of pregnancy have a higher risk of developing herpes zoster during the first few years of life. Administration of maternal varicella-zoster immunoglobulin before rash development, with or without antiviral medication, can modify the progression of the disease.[48]

Uncomplicated chickenpox requires no specific therapy. Baths, wet dressings, and oral antihistamines are occasionally helpful to relieve itching and to prevent secondary infection as a result of scratching. Oral antistaphylococcal drugs should be given if secondary bacterial infection is present. Zoster immune globulin may be administered to immunodeficient individuals if given within 72 hours after exposure to chickenpox. Oral antiviral drugs may be valuable in reducing symptoms in otherwise healthy children as well as in immunosuppressed or other select groups of children.[49] Chickenpox can be prevented with a safe and effective vaccine (see Chapter 10).

Herpes Zoster. Although herpes zoster (shingles) occurs mainly in adults, approximately 5% of cases are in children younger than 15 years.[50] The pathophysiology and treatment are reviewed in Chapter 46.

Smallpox

Smallpox (variola) is a highly contagious and deadly but preventable disease. It is caused by poxvirus variolae. Because of worldwide mass immunization, the world is now virtually free of smallpox. Concerns regarding smallpox as a weapon of bioterrorism have led to vaccination programs for the military and for selected civilian populations. The U.S. government has an adequate supply of smallpox vaccine to vaccinate the population in the event of an emergency.[51]

INSECT BITES AND PARASITES

Insect bites and infestations are common causes of skin disorders in children and adults. Skin damage occurs by various mechanisms, including trauma of bites and stings, allergic reactions, transmission of disease, injection of substances that cause local or systemic reactions, and inflammatory reactions from retained mouthparts.

Scabies

Scabies is a contagious disease caused by the itch mite, *Sarcoptes scabiei* (Figure 47-10, *A*), that can colonize the human epidermis. Scabies is a common skin infection in tropical settings and affects large numbers of people, particularly children. It is transmitted by personal contact and by infected clothing and bedding. Scabies is often epidemic in areas of overcrowded housing, in areas with poor sanitation, or in long-term care institutions. Scabies is often associated with immunocompromised individuals, such as those with human T-cell leukemia/lymphoma virus I (HTLV-1) and human immunodeficiency virus (HIV), and can facilitate *Streptococcus pyogenes* and *Staphylococcus aureus* skin infection.[52] Infestation is initiated by a female mite that tunnels into the stratum corneum, depositing eggs and creating a burrow several millimeters to 1 cm long. Over a 3-week period, the eggs mature into adult mites, which sometimes can be recognized as tiny dots at the end of intact burrows.

Symptoms appear 3 to 5 weeks after infestation. The primary lesions are burrows, papules, and vesicular lesions, with severe itching that worsens at night. Two or three bites (commonly referred to as "breakfast, lunch, and dinner") usually appear in a line on exposed areas of the skin. Itching is thought to be related to sensitization to the larval stages of the parasite. In older children and adults the lesions occur in the webs of fingers, axillae, and creases of the arms and wrists; along the belt line; and around the nipples, genitalia, and lower buttocks. Infants and young children have a different pattern of distribution, with involvement of the palms, soles, head, back, neck, and face (see Figure 47-10, *B*). Secondary infections and crusting develop from scratching and eczematous changes.

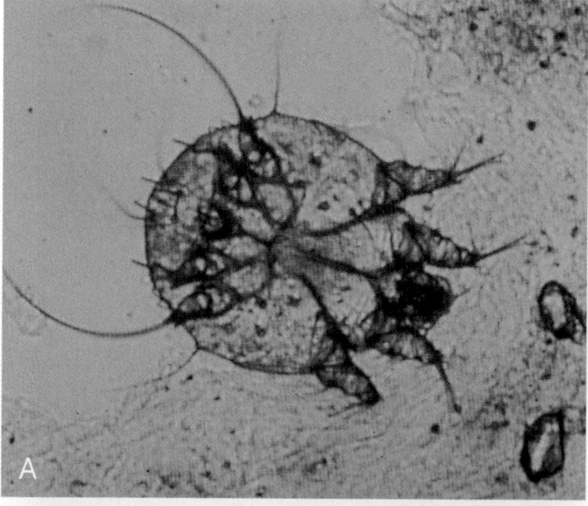

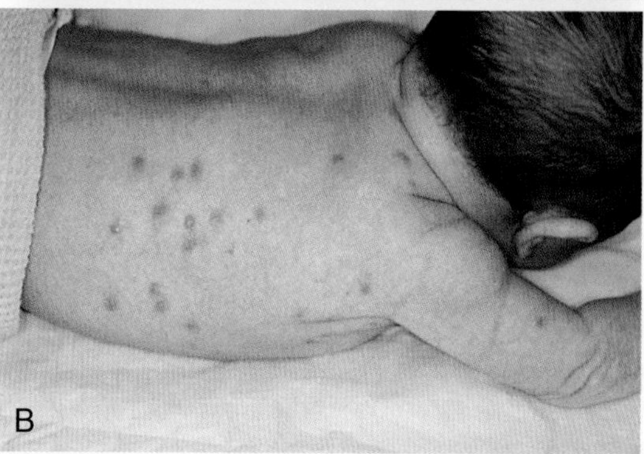

FIGURE 47-10 Scabies. **A,** Scabies mite, as seen clinically when removed from its burrow. **B,** Characteristic scabies bites. (Courtesy Department of Dermatology, School of Medicine, University of Utah.)

Diagnosis of scabies is made by observation of the tunnels and burrows and by scraping of the skin with microscopic examination of the mite or its eggs or feces. Treatment is the application of permethrin cream, a scabicide. Generalized scabies is treated with oral ivermectin.[53] Even with elimination of all viable scabies microorganisms, itching may persist for 10 days or longer. All clothing and linens should be washed and dried in hot cycles or dry-cleaned.

Pediculosis (Lice Infestation)

The three known types of human lice are: (1) the head louse *(Pediculus capitis)*, (2) the body louse *(Pediculus corporis)*, and (3) the crab or pubic louse *(Phthirus pubis)*. They are highly contagious parasites that survive by sucking blood. The female louse reproduces every 2 weeks, producing hundreds of nits as newly hatched lice mate with old lice. The mouthparts are shaped for piercing and sucking and attach to the skin while feeding. When piercing the skin, the louse secretes a toxic saliva; the mechanical trauma and toxin produce a pruritic dermatitis. Head and body lice are acquired by personal contact, combs, or brushes. Crab lice are spread by body contact, such as contact with an infected adult. Sharing clothing is also a common source of transmission.[54]

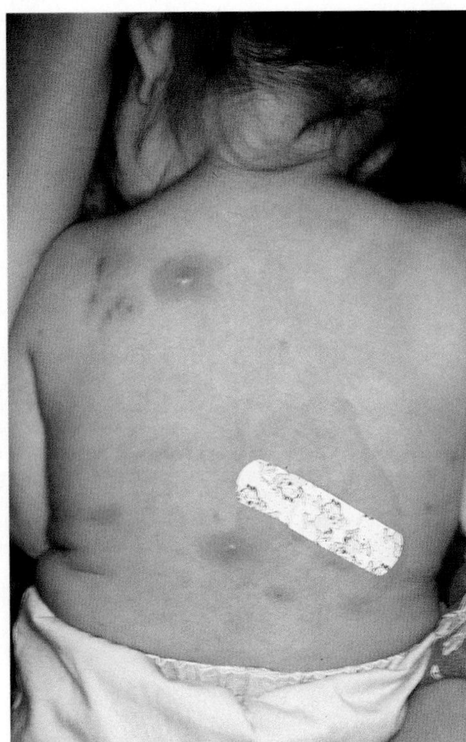

FIGURE 47-11 **Flea Bites.** Flea bite producing an urticarial wheal with central puncture. (Courtesy Department of Pediatrics, Division of Allergy and Immunology, National Jewish Health.)

Itching is the major symptom of lice infestation. In head lice infestation the ova attach to hairs above the ears and in the occipital region. The primary lesion of the body louse is a pinpoint red macule, papule, or wheal with a hemorrhagic puncture site. The primary lesion often is not seen because it is masked by excoriations, wheals, and crusts. The crab louse is found on pubic hairs but also may involve other body hair such as eyelashes, mustache, beard, and axillae. Young children particularly may become infected with crab lice on their eyebrows or eyelashes.

The live louse, 2 to 3 mm long, is rarely observed, although the ova, or nits, can be observed as oval, yellowish pinpoint specks fastened to a hair shaft. The ova fluoresce under an ultraviolet light (Wood lamp) and can be best observed with a microscope. Infestations can be treated with a topical pediculicide (i.e., permethrin) or oral ivermectin.[55] Head lice are effectively treated with topical ivermectin.[56] All clothes, towels, bedding, combs, and brushes should be washed and dried in hot air or boiled, or the clothes should be ironed. Individuals who have personal contact also should be treated.

Fleas

Young children are very susceptible to **flea bites,** and the most common are the bites of cat, dog, and human fleas.[57] Bites occur in clusters along the arms and legs or where clothing fits tightly. The bite produces an urticarial wheal with a central hemorrhagic puncture (Figure 47-11). Treatment includes spraying carpets, crevices, and furniture with malathion or lindane powder. Infected animals should be treated, and clothes and bedding should be washed in hot water.

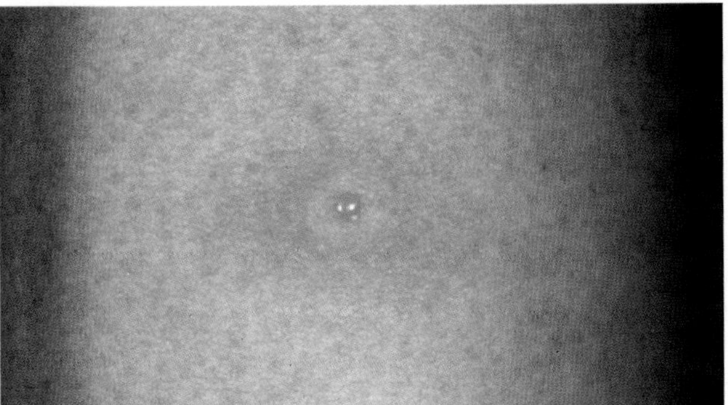

FIGURE 47-12 **Bullous Bedbug Bites.** (Courtesy Department of Dermatology, School of Medicine, University of Utah.)

Bedbugs

The common bedbug, *Cimex lectularius,* is a blood-sucking nocturnal parasite of man. Chickens, bats, and some domestic animals are the other hosts for this bug.[58] **Bedbugs** live in the crevices and cracks of floors, walls, and furniture and in bedding or furniture stuffing. They are 3 to 5 mm long and reddish brown. Bedbugs are nocturnal, emerging to feed in darkness, are attracted by warmth and carbon dioxide, and attach to the skin to suck blood. Feeding occurs for 5 to 15 minutes; then the bedbug leaves. It will move long distances to search for food and can travel from house to house.

Immunologic reactions to bedbug saliva vary, but bites typically yield erythematous and pruritic papules. The face and distal extremities, areas uncovered by sleeping clothes or blankets, are preferentially involved. If the host has not been previously sensitized, the only symptom is a red macule that develops into a nodule, lasting up to 14 days. In sensitized children and adults, pruritic wheals, papules, and vesicles may form (Figure 47-12) and, rarely, anemia and angioedema. Most lesions respond to antihistamines or corticosteroids. Secondary infections require antibiotic treatment. Bedbugs are eliminated by inspecting and cleaning or disposing of bedding, mattresses, furniture, and other contaminated items, and by using applications of approved insecticides, usually by a professional.[59]

HEMANGIOMAS AND CUTANEOUS VASCULAR MALFORMATIONS

Cutaneous vascular anomalies are frequent tumors of early infancy and can be categorized as either hemangiomas or vascular malformations.

Hemangiomas

Hemangiomas are benign tumors that form from the rapid growth of vascular endothelial cells, which results in formation of extra blood vessels. Hemangiomas can be superficial or deep.[60] Superficial hemangiomas are known as strawberry hemangiomas, and deep lesions are known as cavernous hemangiomas. The etiology may be related to embolization of fetal placental endothelial cells in association with placental trauma or loss of placental angiogenic inhibitor of placental and maternal origin.[61] There is proliferation of mast cells that are thought

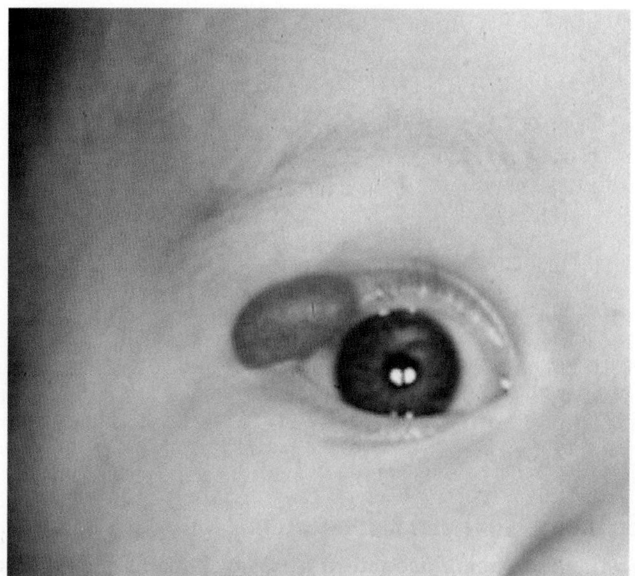

FIGURE 47-13 Strawberry Hemangioma. (Courtesy Department of Dermatology, School of Medicine, University of Utah.)

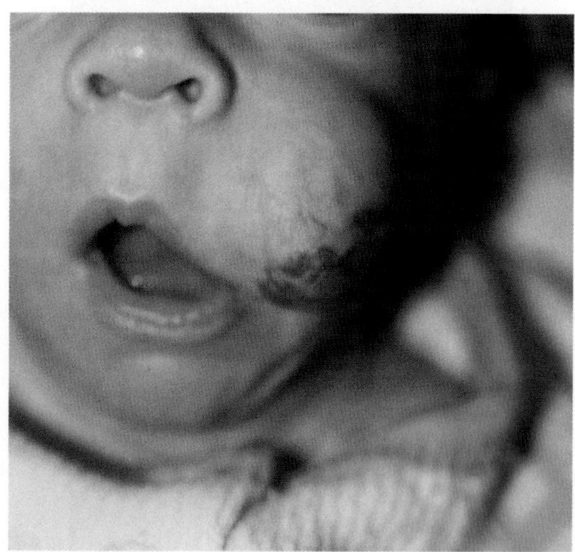

FIGURE 47-14 Cavernous Hemangioma. (Courtesy Department of Dermatology, School of Medicine, University of Utah.)

to promote the angiogenesis. Infiltration of fat cells, fibrosis, and the rich vascular network give the lesions a firm, rubbery feel. Females are affected more often than males. About 30% of hemangiomas are apparent at birth, with most emerging during the first few weeks of life; they grow rapidly during the first few years, and then shrink or involute during childhood years. With involution the lesions become darker in color and then gradually turn to a flesh color. There may be some residual telangiectasia. Most require no treatment depending on location. Hemangiomas located over the eye, ear, nose, mouth, urethra, or anus may require treatment because they interfere with function and have a higher risk for infection or injury. Rapidly progressing hemangiomas are treated with propranolol with regression occurring within 2 weeks; propranolol should be considered a first-line agent.[62] Other therapies include systemic or intralesional steroids, cryosurgery, laser surgery, sclerotherapy, and embolization. Interferons, vincristine, cyclophosphamide, and radiotherapy can suppress angiogenesis.

Strawberry hemangiomas are distinct superficial hemangiomas that may be present at birth but usually emerge 3 to 5 weeks after birth. They proliferate and become bright red and elevated with minute capillary projections that give them a strawberry appearance. Only one lesion is usually present, and it is located on the head and neck area or trunk (Figure 47-13). After the initial growth, the lesion grows at the same rate as the child and then starts to involute at 12 to 16 months of age. Approximately 90% of strawberry hemangiomas involute by 5 to 6 years of age, usually without scarring.

Cavernous (congenital) hemangiomas are present at birth and have larger and more mature vessels within the lesion than strawberry hemangiomas. Some lesions, however, are composed of a mixture of strawberry and cavernous hemangiomas. They appear primarily on the head and neck, are bluish red, and have less distinct borders (Figure 47-14). Cavernous hemangiomas grow rapidly up to 6 months of age and mature by 1 year of age. A period of involution begins and proceeds for 6 to 12 months, with complete involution by 2 to 3 years in 30% of children and by 9 years of age in 90% of children.

Vascular Malformations

Vascular malformations are congenital anomalies of blood vessels present at birth but may not be apparent for several years. They grow proportionately with the child and never regress.[63] The malformations occur equally among males and females. Occasionally they expand rapidly, particularly during the hormonal changes of puberty or pregnancy and in association with trauma. Vascular malformations are classified as low flow or high flow. *Low-flow malformations* involve capillaries, veins, and lymphatics. *High-flow malformations* involve arteries. In addition to locations within the skin they may involve the gastrointestinal tract, bone (Maffucci syndrome), facial capillary malformation, skin, vascular malformation of the eye, and vascular malformation of the brain (leptomeningeal hemangioma—Sturge-Weber syndrome).[64] *Overgrowth syndromes* can occur with either high- or low-flow malformations, with overgrowth of the underlying structures (i.e., legs, arms, facial bones). The most common vascular malformation is nevus flammeus (port-wine stain) and salmon patches (stork bite, angel kiss).

Port-wine (nevus flammeus) stains are congenital malformations of the dermal capillaries. **Sturge-Weber syndrome** is a port-wine stain distributed along the ophthalmic branch of the trigeminal nerve and is associated with the leptomeninges of the brain and choroid, glaucoma, seizures, stroke, and intellectual disability. These capillary malformation are associated with a mutation in the *GNAQ* gene (Guanine nucleotide-binding protein G, q polypeptide).[64a] The lesions are flat, and their color ranges from pink to dark reddish purple. They are present at birth or within a few days after birth and do not fade with age. Involvement of the face and other body surfaces is common, and the lesions may be large (Figure 47-15). During adolescence and later adult years, the port-wine stain may become papular and cavernous. The flashlamp pulsed dye laser

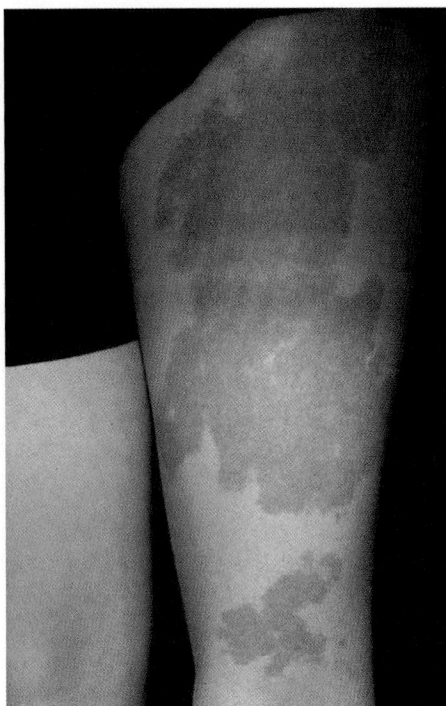

FIGURE 47-15 Capillary Malformation in a Child. (Courtesy Department of Dermatology, School of Medicine, University of Utah.)

is the treatment of choice to successfully lighten the color and flatten the more nodular and cavernous lesions.[64] Waterproof cosmetics may be used to cover the lesions.

Salmon patches (nevus simplex) are macular pink lesions present at birth and located on the nape of the neck, forehead, upper eyelids, or nasolabial fold. They are a more superficial variant of nevus flammeus and one of the most common congenital malformations in the skin. The pink color results from distended dermal capillaries, and 95% fade by 1 and 3 years of age. Those located at the nape of the neck may persist for a lifetime, but generally do not present a cosmetic problem.

OTHER SKIN DISORDERS

Miliaria

Miliaria is a dermatosis commonly seen in infants. It is characterized by a vesicular eruption after prolonged exposure to perspiration, with subsequent obstruction of the eccrine ducts. There are two forms of miliaria: miliaria crystallina and miliaria rubra. In **miliaria crystallina,** ductal rupture occurs within the stratum corneum and appears as 1- to 2-mm clear vesicles without erythema. They rupture within 24 to 48 hours and leave a white scale. In miliaria rubra the ductal rupture occurs in the lower epidermis, with inflammatory cells attracted to the site of the rupture. **Miliaria rubra (prickly heat)** is characterized by 2- to 4-mm discrete erythematous papules or papulovesicles (Figure 47-16). Both forms may become secondarily infected, requiring treatment with systemic antibiotics. The key to management is avoidance of excessive heat and humidity, which cause sweating. Light clothing, cool baths, and air conditioning assist in keeping the skin surface dry and cool.

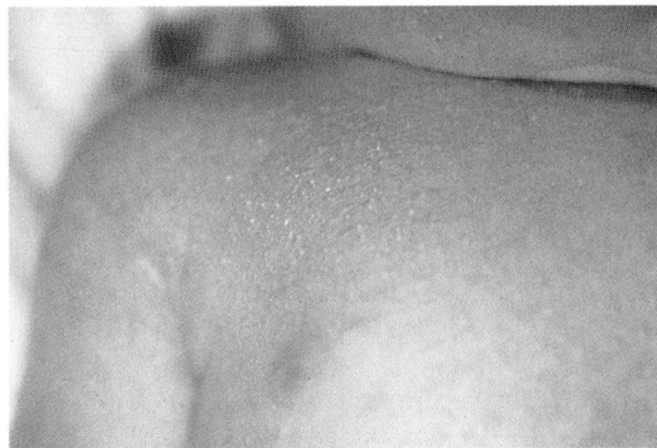

FIGURE 47-16 Miliaria Rubra. Note discrete erythematous papules or papulovesicles. (Courtesy Department of Dermatology, School of Medicine, University of Utah.)

Erythema Toxicum Neonatorum

Erythema toxicum neonatorum (toxic erythema of the newborn) is a benign, erythematous accumulation of macules, papules, or pustules that appear at birth or 3 to 4 days after birth. The lesions first appear as a blotchy, macular erythematous rash. The macules vary from 1 mm to 1 cm. When papules or pustules develop, they are light yellow or white and 1 to 3 mm in diameter. There may be few or several hundred lesions and any surface of the body can be affected, with the exception of the palms and soles, where there are no pilosebaceous follicles. The cause of the lesion is unknown but it may be related to an innate immune response to the first commensal microflora with release of mast cell mediators. Eosinophils are abundant in the lesions.[65] It is self-limiting and resolves spontaneously within a few weeks of birth. No treatment is required.

Stevens-Johnson Syndrome and Toxic Epidermal Necrolysis

Stevens-Johnson syndrome (SJS) and **toxic epidermal necrolysis (TEN)** are rare, severe, immune drug reactions that are considered to be the same pathologic process but with TEN being more extensive. The mortality is between 5% and 35%. Hypersensitivity to drugs includes allopurinol, sulfonamides, nonsteroidal anti-inflammatory agents, anticonvulsants (i.e., phenytoin), and others. There is widespread epidermal (keratinocyte) apoptosis and detachment with drug-specific cytotoxic T cells and macrophages involved in the immunopathology.[66,67] Bursts of nitric oxide formation have been proposed as the cause of epidermal apoptosis and necrosis. There is destruction of the epidermis in toxic epidermal necrolysis.[68]

The onset of skin eruptions is preceded by malaise, anorexia, fever, and mild inflammation of the eyelids, conjunctiva, mouth, or genitalia. Erythema with tenderness is first described in the trunk, face, and palms, extending to the groin and mucous membranes. Blisters and bullae form and large areas of necrotic epidermis may be shed, leaving open, weeping, painful areas of underlying skin. Complications can include dehydration, protein loss, altered temperature regulation, ocular complications leading to blindness, and organ failure. About one third of children have pulmonary complications.[69] A severity of illness score for toxic epidermal necrolysis (SCORTEN) syndrome guides treatment and predicts mortality.[70] TEN must be confirmed by skin biopsy to differentiate from staphylococcal scalded-skin syndrome (SSSS) and acute graft-versus-host disease. Skin biopsy shows full-thickness epidermal necrosis and subepidermal blister formation. Treatment requires prompt withdrawal of causative drugs and intensive burn equivalent management, preferably in a burn unit. Treatment with corticosteroids and intravenous immunoglobulin is controversial and needs further study, which is difficult because the disease is so rare.[71,72]

SUMMARY REVIEW

Acne Vulgaris

1. Acne vulgaris is the most common skin disease, affecting 85% of the population between the ages of 12 and 25 years.
2. Acne is characterized by noninflammatory and inflammatory lesions related to follicular hyperkeratinization, excessive sebum production, plugging of sebaceous glands, and *P. acnes* colonization. Acne conglobata is a severe form of acne with communicating cysts and abcesses.

Dermatitis

1. Atopic dermatitis is associated with elevated IgE levels, a family history of asthma and hay fever, and altered skin barrier function. Red, scaly lesions commonly occur on the face, cheeks, and flexor surfaces of the extremities in infants and young children.
2. Diaper dermatitis is a type of irritant contact dermatitis initiated by a combination of factors that include prolonged exposure to urine and feces; frequently the infant becomes infected secondarily with *C. albicans.*

Infections of the Skin

1. Impetigo is a contagious bacterial disease that occurs in two forms: bullous and vesicular (contagious). The toxins from the bacteria produce a weeping lesion with a honey-colored crust.
2. SSSS is a staphylococcal skin infection that occurs more commonly in young children with low titers of antistaphylococcal antibody. Painful blisters and bullae form over large areas of the skin, requiring systemic antibiotics for treatment.
3. Tinea capitis (infection of the scalp) and tinea corporis (infection of the body) are fungal infections caused by dermatophytes.
4. *C. albicans* infection is a superficial fungal infection of the mouth (thrush).
5. Molluscum contagiosum is a poxvirus of the skin that produces pale papular lesions filled with viral and cellular debris.
6. Rubella (also known as *German* or *3-day measles*) is a communicable disease characterized by fever, sore throat, enlarged cervical and postauricular nodes, and a generalized maculopapular rash that lasts 1 to 4 days.
7. Rubeola is a highly contagious disease of children. Symptoms include high fever, enlarged lymph nodes, conjunctivitis, and a red rash that begins on the head and spreads to the trunk and extremities and lasts 3 to 5 days. Bacterial and viral complications may accompany rubeola.
8. Roseola is a benign disease of infants with a sudden onset of fever that lasts 3 to 5 days, followed by a rash that lasts 24 hours.
9. Chickenpox (varicella) is a highly contagious disease caused by the VZV. Vesicular lesions occur on the skin and mucous membranes. Individuals are contagious from 1 day before the development of the rash until about 6 days after the rash develops.
10. Herpes zoster (shingles) is a viral eruption of vesicles on the skin along the distribution of a sensory nerve caused by latent activation of the VZV. Children with immune suppression develop more serious complications.
11. Smallpox (variola) is a highly contagious, deadly disease that has been eradicated worldwide by vaccination.

Insect Bites and Parasites

1. Scabies is an itching lesion caused by the itch mite that burrows into the skin, forming papules and vesicles. The mite is very contagious and is transmitted by direct contact.
2. Pediculosis (lice infestation) is caused by blood-sucking parasites that secrete a toxic saliva and damage the skin to produce a pruritic dermatitis. Lice are spread by direct contact and are recognized by the ova, or nits, that attach to the shaft of body hairs.
3. Flea bites produce a pruritic wheal with a central puncture site and occur as clusters in areas of tight-fitting clothing.
4. Bedbugs are blood-sucking parasites that live in cracks of floors, furniture, or bedding and feed at night. They produce pruritic wheals and nodules.

Hemangiomas and Vascular Malformations

1. Hemangiomas are benign vascular tumors that emerge at birth and resolve spontaneously through the childhood years. Strawberry hemangiomas (distinct, raised vascular lesions) are more superficial, and cavernous hemangiomas, with larger and more mature vessels, are deeper lesions.
2. Vascular malformations are congenital anomalies of blood vessels. Low-flow malformations involve capillaries, veins, and lymphatics; high-flow malformations involve arteries.
3. Nevus flammeus (port-wine stain) is a deeper congenital malformation of the dermal capillaries, and salmon patches are more superficial vascular malformations.

Other Skin Disorders

1. Miliaria is characterized by small pruritic papules or vesicles that result from prolonged exposure to perspiration and subsequent obstruction of the eccrine ducts in infants.
2. Erythema toxicum neonatorum is a benign, erythematous, accumulation of macules, papules, and pustules that appear at birth or 3 to 4 days after birth and then spontaneously resolve within a few weeks.
3. SJS and TEN (the severe form of SJS) are severe immune blistering skin reactions to drugs.

KEY TERMS

Acne conglobata, 1654
Acne vulgaris, 1653
Atopic dermatitis (AD), 1654
Bedbug, 1662
Bullous impetigo, 1656
Cavernous (congenital) hemangioma, 1663
Chickenpox, 1660
Diaper dermatitis, 1655
Erythema toxicum neonatorum, 1664
Flea bite, 1662
Impetigo, 1656
Inflammatory acne, 1653
Miliaria, 1664
Miliaria crystallina, 1664
Miliaria rubra (prickly heat), 1664
Molluscum contagiosum, 1658
Nonbullous impetigo, 1656
Noninflammatory acne, 1653
Port-wine (nevus flammeus) stain, 1663
Roseola, 1660
Rubella, 1658
Rubeola, 1659
Salmon patch (nevus simplex), 1664
Scabies, 1661
Smallpox (variola), 1661
Staphylococcal scalded-skin syndrome (SSSS), 1656
Stevens-Johnson syndrome (SJS), 1664
Sturge-Weber syndrome 1663
Strawberry hemangioma, 1663
Thrush, 1658
Tinea capitis, 1657
Tinea corporis (ringworm), 1657
Tinea pedis, 1657
Toxic epidermal necrolysis (TEN), 1664

REFERENCES

1. Szabó K, Kemény L: Studying the genetic predisposing factors in the pathogenesis of acne vulgaris, *Hum Immunol* 72(9):766–773, 2011.
2. Knutsen-Larson S et al: Acne vulgaris: pathogenesis, treatment, and needs assessment, *Dermatol Clin* 30(1):99–106, viii–ix, 2012.
3. Eichenfield LF et al: American Acne and Rosacea Society: Evidence-based recommendations for the diagnosis and treatment of pediatric acne, *Pediatrics* 131(Suppl 3):S163–S186, 2013.
4. Burris J, Rietkerk W, Woolf K: Acne: the role of medical nutrition therapy, *J Acad Nutr Diet* 113(3):416–430, 2013.
5. Rao J: Treatment of acne scarring, *Facial Plast Surg Clin North Am* 19(2):275–291, 2011.
6. Kraft J, Freiman A: Management of acne, *CMAJ* 183(7):E430–E435, 2011.

6a. Titus S, Hodge J: Diagnosis and treatment of acne, *Am Fam Physician* 86(8):734–740, 2012.

7. Williams HC, Dellavalle RP, Garner S: Acne vulgaris, *Lancet* 379(9813):361–372, 2012.
8. Odhiambo JA et al: Global variations in prevalence of eczema symptoms in children from ISAAC phase three, *J Allergy Clin Immunol* 124: 1251–1258, 2009.
9. Boguniewicz M, Leung DY: Atopic dermatitis: a disease of altered skin barrier and immune dysregulation, *Immunol Rev* 242(1):233–246, 2011.
10. Wolf R, Wolf D: Abnormal epidermal barrier in the pathogenesis of atopic dermatitis, *Clin Dermatol* 30(3):329–334, 2012.
11. Garrett JP et al: Asthma and frequency of wheeze: risk factors for the persistence of atopic dermatitis in children, *Ann Allergy Asthma Immunol* 110(3):146–149.
12. Nograles KE et al: IL-22-producing "T22" T cells account for upregulated IL-22 in atopic dermatitis despite reduced IL-17-producing TH17 T cells, *J Allergy Clin Immunol* 123(6):1244–1252.e2, 2009.
13. Sabin BR, Peters N, Peters AT: Chapter 20: atopic dermatitis, *Allergy Asthma Proc* 33(Suppl 1):S67–S69, 2012.
14. Mommert S et al: The role of the histamine H4 receptor in atopic dermatitis, *Curr Allergy Asthma Rep* 11(1):21–28, 2011.
15. Darsow U et al: Pruritus and atopic dermatitis, *Clin Rev Allergy Immunol* 41(3):237–244, 2011.
16. Yosipovitch G, Papoiu AD: What causes itch in atopic dermatitis? *Curr Allergy Asthma Rep* 8(4):306–311, 2008.
17. Nicol NH, Boguniewicz M: Successful strategies in atopic dermatitis management, *Dermatol Nurs* (Suppl):3–18, 2008.
18. Darsow U et al: European Task Force on Atopic Dermatitis/EADV Eczema Task Force: Difficult to control atopic dermatitis, *World Allergy Organ J* 6(1):6, 2013.
19. Ring J et al: Guidelines for treatment of atopic eczema (atopic dermatitis) part II, *J Eur Acad Dermatol Venereol* 26(9):1176–1193, 2012.
20. Schneider L et al: Atopic dermatitis: a practice parameter update 2012, *J Allergy Clin Immunol* 131(2):295–299, 2013.
21. Erasala GN, Romain C, Merlay I: Diaper area and disposable diapers, *Curr Probl Dermatol* 40:83–89, 2011.
22. Heimall LM et al: Beginning at the bottom: evidence-based care of diaper dermatitis, *MCN Am J Matern Child Nurs* 37(1):10–16, 2012.
23. Geria AN, Schwartz RA: Impetigo update: new challenges in the era of methicillin resistance, *Cutis* 85(2):65–70, 2010.
24. Rudy SJ: Superficial fungal infections in children and adolescents, *Nurse Pract Forum* 19(2):56, 1999.
25. Simpson CL et al: Plakoglobin rescues adhesive defects induced by ectodomain truncation of the desmosomal cadherin desmoglein 1: implications for exfoliative toxin-mediated skin blistering, *Am J Pathol* 177(6):2921–2937, 2010.
26. Koning S et al: Interventions for impetigo, *Cochrane Database Syst Rev* (1):CD003261, 2012.
27. Blyth M, Estela C, Young AE: Severe staphylococcal scalded skin syndrome in children, *Burns* 34(1):98–103, 2008.
28. Aalfs AS et al: Staphylococcal scalded skin syndrome: loss of desmoglein 1 in patient skin, *Eur J Dermatol* 20(4):451–456, 2010.
29. Baartmans MG et al: Use of skin substitute dressings in the treatment of staphylococcal scalded skin syndrome in neonates and young infants, *Neonatology* 100(1):9–13, 2011.
30. Andrews MD, Burns M: Common tinea infections in children, *Am Fam Physician* 77(1):1415–1420, 2008.
31. Kelly BP: Superficial fungal infections, *Pediatr Rev* 33(4):e22–e37, 2012.
32. Williams JV et al: Semiquantitative study of tinea capitis and the asymptomatic carrier state in inner-city school children, *Pediatrics* 96(2 Pt 1): 265, 1995.
33. Xie Z et al: *Candida albicans* biofilms do not trigger reactive oxygen species and evade neutrophil killing, *J Infect Dis* 206(12):1936–1945, 2012.
34. Su CW et al: Clinical inquiries. What is the best treatment for oral thrush in healthy infants? *J Fam Pract* 57(7):484–485, 2008.
35. Vermi W et al: Spontaneous regression of highly immunogenic *Molluscum contagiosum* virus- (MCV) induced skin lesions is associated with plasmacytoid dendritic cells and IFN-DC infiltration, *J Invest Dermatol* 131(2):426–434, 2011.
36. Zichichi L, Maniscalco M: The challenges of a neglected STI: *Molluscum contagiosum*, *G Ital Dermatol Venereol* 147(5):447–453, 2012.
37. Parker Fiebelkorn A et al: Measles in the United States during the postelimination era, *J Infect Dis* 202(10):1520–1528, 2010.
38. Reef SE et al: Evidence used to support the achievement and maintenance of elimination of rubella and congenital rubella syndrome in the United States, *J Infect Dis* 204(Suppl 2):S593–S597, 2011.
39. Demicheli V et al: Vaccines for measles, mumps and rubella in children, *Cochrane Database Syst Rev* (2):CD004407, 2012.
40. Uno Y et al: The combined measles, mumps, and rubella vaccines and the total number of vaccines are not associated with development of autism spectrum disorder: the first case-control study in Asia, *Vaccine* 30(28):4292–4298, 2012.
41. Centers for Disease Control and Prevention: Global routine vaccination coverage, *MMWR Morb Mortal Wkly Rep* 61(43):883–885, 2011.
42. Simons E et al: Assessment of the 2010 global measles mortality reduction goal: results from a model of surveillance data, *Lancet* 379(9832): 2173–2178, 2012.
43. White SJ et al: Measles, mumps, and rubella, *Clin Obstet Gynecol* 55(2):550–559, 2012.
44. Best JM: Rubella, *Semin Fetal Neonatal Med* 12(3):182–192, 2007.
45. de Vries RD et al: The pathogenesis of measles, *Curr Opin Virol* 2(3):248–255, 2012.
46. Johnson R et al: Prevention of herpes zoster and its painful and debilitating complications, *Int J Infect Dis* 11(Suppl 2):S43–S48, 2007.
47. Gnann JW Jr: Varicella-zoster virus: prevention through vaccination, *Clin Obstet Gynecol* 55(2):560–570, 2012.
48. Lamont RF et al: Varicella-zoster virus (chickenpox) infection in pregnancy, *BJOG* 118(10):1155–1162, 2011.
49. Breuer J, Whitley R: Varicella zoster virus: natural history and current therapies of varicella and herpes zoster, *Herpes* 14(Suppl 2):25–29, 2007.
50. Feder HM Jr, Hoss DM: Herpes zoster in otherwise healthy children, *Pediatr Infect Dis J* 23(5):451–457, 2004.
51. Nalca A, Zumbrun EE: ACAM2000: the new smallpox vaccine for United States Strategic National Stockpile, *Drug Des Devel Ther* 4:71–79, 2010.
52. Fischer K et al: Scabies: important clinical consequences explained by new molecular studies, *Adv Parasitol* 79:339–373, 2012.

53. Monsel G, Chosidow O: Management of scabies, *Skin Therapy Lett* 17(3):1–4, 2012.
54. Burkhart CN, Burkhart CG: Fomite transmission in head lice, *J Am Acad Dermatol* 56(6):144–147, 2007.
55. Strong M, Johnstone PW: Interventions for treating scabies, *Cochrane Database Syst Rev* (3):CD000320, 2007.
56. Pariser DM et al: Topical 0.5% ivermectin lotion for treatment of head lice, *N Engl J Med* 367(18):1687–1689, 2012.
57. Howard R, Frieden IJ: Papular urticaria in children, *Pediatr Dermatol* 13(3):246, 1996.
58. Delaunay P et al: Bedbugs and infectious disease, *Clin Infect Dis* 52(2):200–210, 2011.
59. Studdiford JS et al: Bedbug infestation, *Am Fam Physician* 86(7):653–658, 2012.
60. Ryan E, Warren L: Birthmarks—identification and management, *Aust Fam Physician* 41(5):274–277, 2012.
61. Atherton DJ: Infantile haemangiomas, *Early Hum Dev* 82(12):789–795, 2006.
62. Holmes WJ et al: Propranolol as first-line treatment for rapidly proliferating infantile haemangiomas, *J Plast Reconstr Aesthet Surg* 64(4): 445–451, 2011.
63. Willenberg T, Baumgartener T: Vascular birthmarks, *Vasa* 37(1):5–17, 2008.
64. Chen JK et al: An overview of clinical and experimental treatment modalities for port wine stains, *J Am Acad Dermatol* 67(2):289–304, 2012.
64a. Shirley MD et al: Sturge-Weber syndrome and port-wine stains caused by somatic mutation in GNAQ, *N Engl J Med* 368(21):1971–1979, 2013.
65. Morgan AJ et al: Erythema toxicum neonatorum revisited, *Cutis* 83(1):13–16, 2009.
66. Harr T, French LE: Stevens-Johnson syndrome and toxic epidermal necrolysis, *Chem Immunol Allergy* 97:149–166, 2012.
67. Tohyama M, Hashimoto K: Immunological mechanisms of epidermal damage in toxic epidermal necrolysis, *Curr Opin Allergy Clin Immunol* 12(4):376–382, 2012.
68. Viard-Leveugle I et al: TNF-α and IFN-γ are potential inducers of Fas-mediated keratinocyte apoptosis through activation of inducible nitric oxide synthase in toxic epidermal necrolysis, *J Invest Dermatol* 133(2):489–498, 2012.
69. Kim MJ, Lee KY: Bronchiolitis obliterans in children with Stevens-Johnson syndrome: follow-up with high resolution CT, *Pediatr Radiol* 26(1):22, 1996.
70. Bastuji-Garin S et al: SCORTEN: a severity-of-illness score for toxic epidermal necrolysis, *J Invest Dermatol* 115:149–153, 2000.
71. Downey A et al: Toxic epidermal necrolysis: review of pathogenesis and management, *J Am Acad Dermatol* 66(6):995–1003, 2010.
72. Worswick S, Cotliar J: Stevens-Johnson syndrome and toxic epidermal necrolysis: a review of treatment options, *Dermatol Ther* 24(2):207–218, 2011.

CHAPTER

48

Shock, Multiple Organ Dysfunction Syndrome, and Burns in Adults

Linda L. Martin, Dennis J. Cheek, and Stephen E. Morris

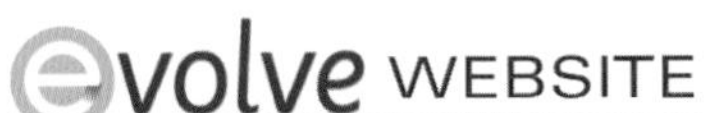

http://evolve.elsevier.com/McCance/

- Review Questions and Answers
- Online Course: Module 19

CHAPTER OUTLINE

Shock occurs when the cardiovascular system fails to perfuse tissues, cells, and organs adequately, resulting in widespread impairment of cellular metabolism and tissue function. **Tissue perfusion** is defined as the adequacy of blood flow through the small vessels of the extremities to maintain tissue function.[1] Tissue perfusion can be disrupted by any factor that alters delivery of blood to cells and tissues and increases oxygen consumption, such as decreased cardiac output, blood volume, or blood pressure. Shock has many causes and clinical manifestations related to the type of shock. Ultimately, shock from any cause will progress to organ failure and death, unless physiologic mechanisms reverse the process or clinical intervention succeeds in stopping the progression. Untreated, severe shock overwhelms the body's compensatory mechanisms that may result in multisystem organ failure.

Multiple organ dysfunction syndrome (MODS) is progressive and often involves the ultimate failure of two or more organ systems after a severe illness or injury. The disease process is initiated and perpetuated by uncontrolled systemic inflammatory and stress responses and is characterized by a hypermetabolic and hyperdynamic state that persists as organ dysfunction develops. For many years the syndrome was referred to as *multiple organ failure* or *multiple systems organ failure.* Gradually it was recognized that the term *organ dysfunction* more accurately describes the syndrome as a process of physiologic deterioration.

Major burns result in extensive immediate tissue injury and thus are a form of trauma with wide-reaching effects on all organ systems. The cause of injury may be thermal contact, flame, chemical agents, or electrical agents; each cause requires a different approach in diagnosis and treatment. Closely associated with thermal burns is smoke inhalation injury, which accounts for about 25% of all burn unit admissions. As a multiorgan problem, thermal injuries can have an overwhelming effect on survival of the burned individual. Regardless of the cause of burns, the result is a final common pathway of physiologic response dependent on the extent of burn surface involvement and the depth of tissue destruction.

SHOCK

Shock can be classified by type, principal pathophysiologic process, or clinical manifestations. Classification by type is perhaps the most useful because it suggests the cause and pathophysiologic process of the underlying disorder, which must be treated

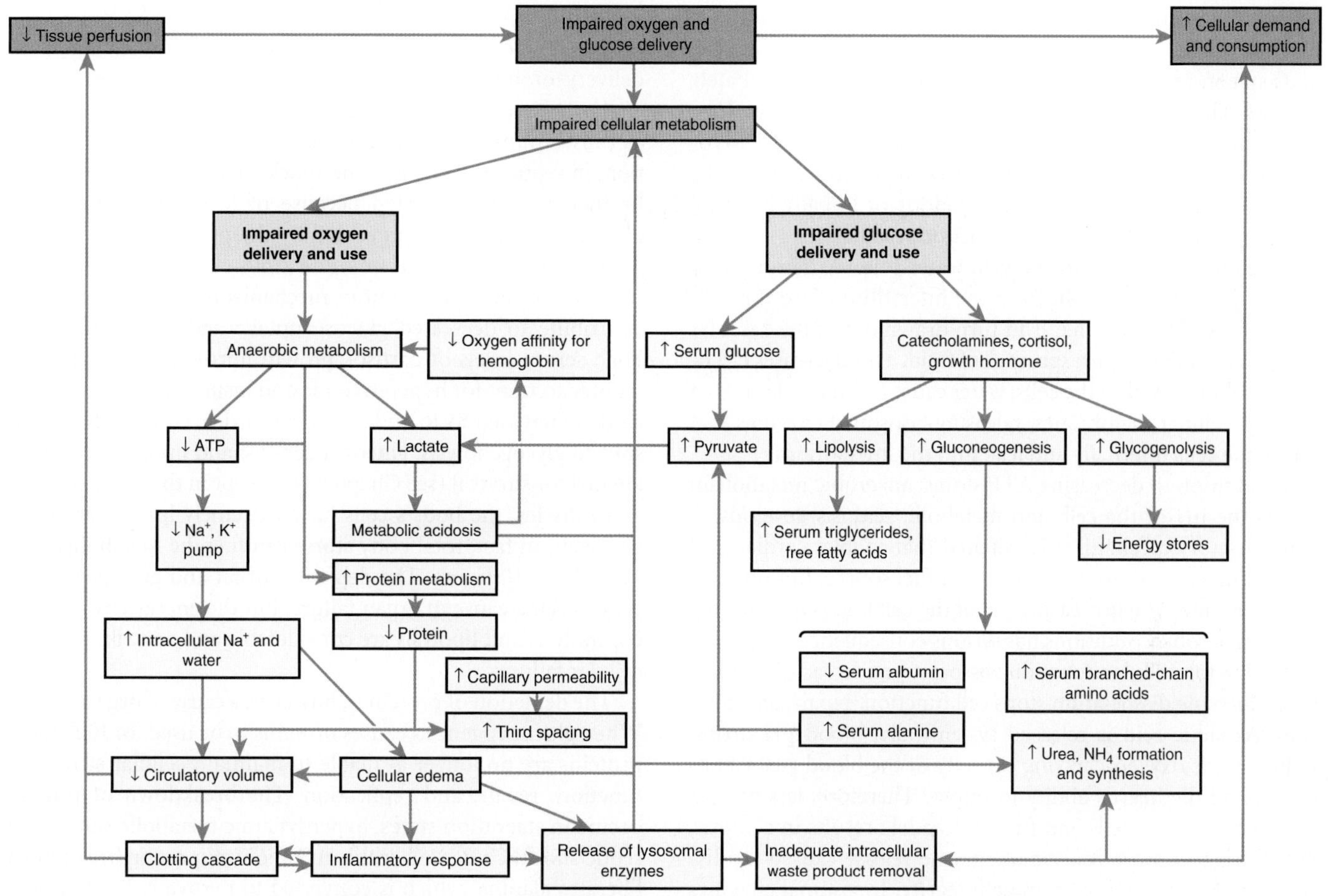

FIGURE 48-1 Impairment of Cellular Metabolism by Shock. *ATP,* Adenosine triphosphate.

to prevent the irreversible cellular alterations and impairment of cellular metabolism. **Shock** is classified as cardiogenic (caused by heart failure); neurogenic or vasogenic (caused by alterations in vascular smooth muscle tone); anaphylactic (caused by hypersensitivity); septic (caused by infection); or hypovolemic (caused by insufficient intravascular fluid volume).

Cellular Alterations and Impairment of Cellular Metabolism

The body consists of many organs, tissues, and cells that may function or malfunction at different stages of metabolic impairment. The common pathway in all types of shock is impairment of cellular metabolism, attributable to decreased delivery of oxygen and nutrients, frequently coupled with an increased demand and consumption of oxygen and nutrients and a decreased removal of cellular waste products.[2] Figure 48-1 illustrates the pathophysiology of shock at the cellular level.

Impairment of Oxygen Delivery and Use

In all types of shock, the cells do not receive adequate amounts of oxygen because of decreased delivery or increased cellular consumption, or both, and are therefore unable to use oxygen normally (see Figure 48-1). In cardiogenic shock cardiac output is too low to deliver adequate oxygen to the cell. In hypovolemic shock, oxygen delivery is impaired by inadequate numbers of red cells that carry oxygen and inadequate blood volume. In neurogenic, anaphylactic, and septic shock, systemic vascular resistance (SVR) becomes very low because of vasodilation, resulting in inadequate perfusion pressure in the capillaries. Thus, the pressure needed to drive oxygen and nutrients across cell membranes is inadequate. In septic shock, hypoxia is worsened by increased inflammatory responses, such as fever, that increase the cell's oxygen demand and consumption rate, and by direct toxic and inflammatory chemical disruption of cellular metabolism, that impairs the cells' ability to use oxygen.

Both positive and negative compensatory mechanisms, such as anaerobic metabolism, lysosomal enzyme release, decreased intravascular volume, and activation of the clotting cascade, may further impair oxygen delivery and use. Anaerobic metabolism results in disruption of electrolyte and lysosomal enzymatic processes, thus changing the normal ionic and osmotic levels in cells governed by the physical law of diffusion. Diffusion of nutrients and wastes into and out of the cell takes longer, and cellular metabolism is further altered. Without oxygen, the cell shifts from aerobic to anaerobic metabolism. Anaerobic metabolism is a less efficient method of extracting energy from carbon bonds, and the cell begins to use adenosine triphosphate (ATP) faster than it can be replaced. Without ATP the cell loses its ability to maintain an electrochemical gradient across its selectively permeable membrane. Specifically, the cell cannot operate the sodium-potassium pump. Sodium and chloride accumulate inside the cell and potassium exits the cell. Cells of the nervous system and myocardium are profoundly and immediately affected. The resting potentials of these cells are reduced, and the action potentials decrease in amplitude (see Chapter 1). Myocardial depressant factor also decreases the contractility of the heart. A variety of clinical manifestations of impaired central nervous system and myocardial function result.

As sodium moves into the cell, water follows. Throughout the body, the water drawn from the interstitium into the cells is "replaced" by water that is in turn drawn out of the vascular space, often called "third spacing" of fluid. This decreases circulatory volume. Within the cells, water causes cellular edema that disrupts cellular membranes, releasing lysosomal enzymes that injure the cells internally and leak into the interstitium.

In addition to decreasing ATP stores, anaerobic metabolism affects the pH of the cell, and metabolic acidosis develops. A compensatory mechanism is initiated that enables cardiac and skeletal muscles to use lactic acid as a fuel source, but only for a limited time. The decreasing pH of the cell that is functioning under anaerobic conditions has serious consequences. Enzymes necessary for cellular function dissociate under acidic conditions. Enzyme dissociation stops cell function, repair, and division. As lactic acid is released systemically, blood pH drops, reducing the oxygen-carrying capacity of the blood (see Chapter 2), and the heart's ability to pump. Therefore, less oxygen is delivered to the cells and further hypoxia results in acidosis, which triggers more lysosomal enzyme release caused by disruption of lysosomal membrane integrity. Lysosomal enzymes released during shock injure the cell that released them and injure adjacent cells. By damaging the mechanisms of surrounding cells, lysosomal enzymes extend areas of impaired metabolism and cellular injury.

Intravascular fluid loss into the intracellular and interstitial spaces, described as "third spacing" earlier, is amplified when serum albumin and other plasma proteins are consumed for fuel, which results in decreased intravascular osmotic pressure, shift of fluid to the interstitial or extracellular spaces, and decreased circulatory volume. Decreased circulatory volume magnifies decreased tissue perfusion in all types of shock. Decreased intravascular volume causes decreased cardiac output in septic shock and further reduces cardiac output in cardiogenic shock. In individuals with anaphylactic, neurogenic, or septic shock and an already dilated vasculature, hypotension worsens as a result of decreased circulatory volume. New data on additional mechanisms for hypotension (vasodilation) are illustrated in Figure 48-7 (p. 1678).

Concurrently, diffusion across capillary membranes occurs more slowly, as blood flow in the capillary beds becomes sluggish, caused by decreased fluid volume with increased viscosity of blood. Sluggish capillary flow decreases tissue perfusion further, microvascular clots form, and activation of the clotting cascade may begin (see Chapter 27). Microemboli formation and platelet aggregation account for common complications of shock, such as acute tubular necrosis, acute respiratory distress syndrome (ARDS), and disseminated intravascular coagulation (DIC). It also may activate or be activated by the inflammatory response.[3]

Impairment of Glucose Delivery and Use

Impaired glucose use can be caused by either impaired glucose delivery or impaired glucose uptake by the cells (see Figure 48-1). The reasons for inadequate glucose delivery are the same as those enumerated for inadequate oxygen delivery. In addition, in septic and anaphylactic shock, glucose metabolism may be increased or disrupted because of fever or bacteria, and glucose uptake can be prevented by the presence of vasoactive toxins, endotoxins, histamine, and kinins.

Some of the compensatory mechanisms activated by shock contribute to decreased glucose uptake and use by the cells. High serum levels of cortisol, growth hormone, and catecholamines account for hyperglycemia and insulin resistance, tachycardia, increased SVR, and increased cardiac contractility. Cells shift to glycogenolysis, gluconeogenesis, and lipolysis to generate fuel for survival (see Chapter 1). Except in the liver, kidneys, and muscles, the body's cells have extremely limited stores of glycogen. In fact, total body stores can fuel the metabolism for only about 10 hours. The depletion of fat and glycogen stores is not itself a cause of organ failure, but the energy costs of glycogenolysis and lipolysis are considerable and contribute to the cellular failure.

The depletion of protein is, however, a cause of organ failure. When gluconeogenesis causes proteins to be used for fuel, these proteins are no longer available to maintain cellular structure, function, repair, and replication. The breakdown of protein occurs in starvation states, hyperdynamic metabolic states, and septic shock. Under anaerobic metabolism, protein breakdown liberates alanine, which is converted to pyruvate. Pyruvic acid is changed into lactic acid, leading to an increased affinity for oxygen to bind to hemoglobin with resultant hypoxia and metabolic acidosis.

As proteins are metabolized anaerobically, ammonia and urea are produced. Ammonia is toxic to living cells. Uremia develops, and uric acid further disrupts cellular metabolism. Proteins are broken down preferentially. Serum albumin and other plasma proteins are consumed for fuel first. Serum protein consumption decreases capillary osmotic pressure and contributes to the development of interstitial edema, creating another negative compensatory outcome that decreases circulatory volume. In septic shock, plasma protein breakdown includes breakdown of immunoglobulins, thereby impairing immune system function when it is most needed.

Muscle wasting caused by protein breakdown weakens skeletal and cardiac muscle. Skeletal muscle wasting impairs the muscles that facilitate breathing. Muscle wasting therefore alters the actions of both heart and lungs. The delivery of oxygen and glucose to the cells is directly reduced, as is the removal of metabolic waste products, such as the formation of carbon dioxide and lactic acid, causing metabolic acidosis with resultant inability of muscles, organs, and tissues to function mechanically and electrically.

The metabolic wastes that accumulate in the cell and interstitial spaces are toxic to the cells and further disrupt cellular function and membrane integrity. In septic shock, for example, a deficiency in cellular metabolism and the buildup of toxins may precede and cause decreased tissue perfusion.

Types of Shock, Clinical Manifestations, and Treatment

Each type of shock (cardiogenic, hypovolemic, neurogenic, anaphylactic, septic) involves numerous clinical manifestations, signs, and symptoms that also may characterize other conditions, making diagnosis difficult. An individual's history and situation are correlated with the specificity of the shock state suspected or anticipated. Clinical manifestations common in septic shock are fever, high heart rate, high respiratory rate, or elevations in immune responses, such as increased levels of white blood cells and circulating blood glucose. Subjective complaints often are nonspecific and general. The individual may report feeling sick, weak, cold, hot, nauseated, dizzy, confused, afraid, thirsty, and short of breath.

The initial management for shock is to discover, diagnose, and correct or remove the underlying cause. Although this seems a simple tenet, it is one that is not always remembered. Thus treatment for cardiogenic shock begins with diagnosis and treatment of heart failure or at least enhancement of cardiac output. If hypovolemia is the cause of shock, hemorrhage and other causes of fluid loss must be stopped. In neurogenic shock, as a result of spinal cord trauma, stabilization of the spine and surrounding tissue is an initial approach and pain usually can be decreased to a level at which neutrally-mediated decreases of SVR cease. The initial treatment for anaphylactic shock is to remove or neutralize the antigen. Treatment for septic shock begins with eradication of the infective agent, usually with antimicrobials.

Simultaneous to correcting the underlying cause or condition, treatment is directed at targeting improvement of microcirculatory tissue perfusion.[4] Optimizing oxygenation is an absolute necessity in all shock states. The goal has a dual purpose to both optimize oxygen delivery and reduce oxygen consumption. Intravenous fluid is administered to expand intravascular volume and thereby improve tissue perfusion by increasing blood pressure and cardiac output, except in cases of cardiogenic shock, which require diuresis to reduce preload.

Effective glucose level control in various shock states has been shown to improve outcomes. Hyperglycemia, caused by insulin resistance in the liver and muscle, is a common finding in the critically ill. This is most likely an adaptive response providing glucose for the brain, red blood cells, and wound healing. The extent of appropriate glucose level control has been evaluated in recent years, leading to more aggressive treatment with continuous, titrating insulin infusions to maintain blood glucose levels closer to normal, thus promoting normal cellular function and healing.[5]

Once cellular and organ dysfunction and physiologic derangement are established, risk of morbidity and mortality increases. Prevention and early treatment offer the best prognosis.

Cardiogenic Shock

Cardiogenic shock results from the inability of the heart to pump adequate blood to tissues and end organs from any cause, the most common being the short-term consequences of an acute myocardial infarction or a severe episode of myocardial ischemia. **Cardiogenic shock** is defined as persistent hypotension and tissue hypoperfusion caused by cardiac dysfunction in the presence of adequate intravascular volume and left ventricular filling pressure.[6] Pathologic conditions that reduce contractility, cause pump failure, impair diastolic filling, or cause obstruction can lead to cardiogenic shock. Decreased contractility and pump failure can result from (1) acute myocardial infarction (AMI), cardiomyopathy, sepsis, myocarditis, pericarditis, aneurysm, dysrhythmias, contusion, metabolic abnormalities, papillary muscle rupture; (2) impaired diastolic filling related to dysrhythmias; and (3) obstruction attributable to pulmonary embolism, cardiac tamponade, valvular disorders, tumors, and wall rupture or defects.[7]

Overall hospital mortality because of cardiogenic shock has decreased from approximately 90% in the 1970s to a recent estimate of 50%.[8]

As cardiac output decreases, compensatory adaptive responses are activated, such as the renin-angiotensin, neurohormonal, and sympathetic nervous systems, that lead to fluid retention, systemic vasoconstriction, and tachycardia.[9] Activation of the inflammatory response (resulting in expression of inducible nitric oxide synthase), activation of inflammatory cytokines, and activation of the complement system appear to play an important role in the pathogenesis and outcome of cardiogenic shock.[10] Increases in contractility, heart rate, and blood pressure are maintained in mild shock states through vasoconstriction in response to catecholamine release from the adrenals. Vasoconstriction increases vascular resistance to normalize blood pressure and increases cardiac performance by returning more blood volume and increasing perfusion to the heart; however, this increases myocardial demand and consumption of oxygen and nutrients by the heart. Increasing myocardial requirements burden the already failing heart, which can no longer pump an adequate volume of blood with sufficient force to perfuse the tissues. Thus increased coronary, tissue, and cellular ischemia further deteriorates myocardial function and shock.

Mortality in cardiogenic shock is reduced by use of intra-aortic balloon counterpulsation (IABP); cardiosupportive drug regimens and early coronary interventions have also improved outcomes.[10-12] Following myocardial infarction, reperfusion and revascularization can be achieved with treatment modalities that include fibrinolytic therapies (medications that disintegrate the coronary thrombus) and percutaneous interventions (balloon angioplasty, stent placement, and thrombectomies). Surgery (coronary artery bypass, ventriculoplasty, or heart transplant) is also utilized to open the coronary vessels during an acute myocardial infarction or to replace irreparable heart muscle. Cardio-supportive drug and fluid regimens are initiated to maintain adequate blood pressure and essential fluid and electrolyte balance, and to optimize coronary perfusion to the myocardium. Mechanical assist devices, specifically intra-aortic balloon pumps and percutaneous or ventricular assist devices (VADs), are used to support cardiac output temporarily until the individual improves or transplantation is possible.[11] Implantable VADs, pacemakers, or internal defibrillator devices are sometimes used as permanent treatment

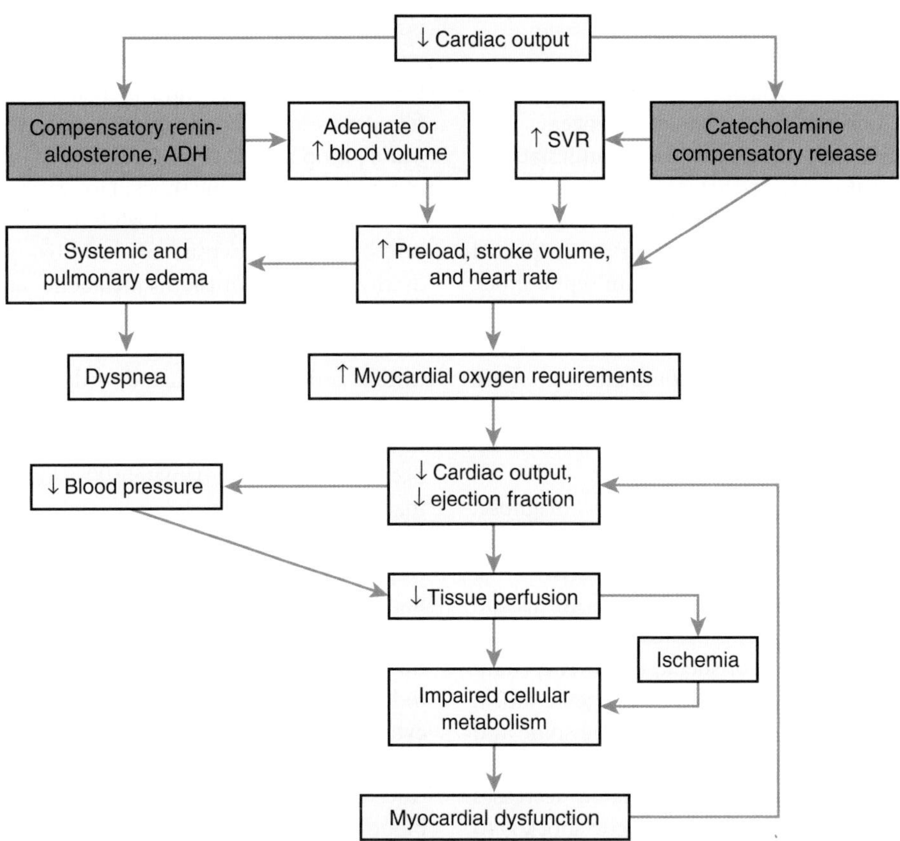

FIGURE 48-2 Cardiogenic Shock. Shock becomes life threatening when compensatory mechanisms (orange boxes) cause increased myocardial oxygen requirements. *ADH,* Antidiuretic hormone; *SVR,* systemic vascular resistance.

for those who survive cardiogenic shock. Continuous hemodynamic monitoring should be employed to evaluate vascular volume and pressures, optimize fluid levels, and monitor drug administration with the goal of improving cardiac output and tissue perfusion.[13]

The clinical manifestations of cardiogenic shock are caused by inadequate perfusion to the heart and end organs (Figure 48-2). Subjective complaints of chest pain, dyspnea, and faintness, along with feelings of impending doom, are often revealed. Classic observable signs and symptoms of tachycardia, tachypnea, hypotension, jugular venous distention, dysrhythmia, and low measured cardiac output are hallmarks. Cyanosis; skin mottling; rapid, faint, or irregular pulses; low urine output; and occasional peripheral edema are additional signs and symptoms of end-organ hypoperfusion. Myocardial dysfunction from fluid overload may result in extra heart sounds, pulmonary edema, hypoxemia, and elevated end-organ laboratory values. The amount of brain natriuretic peptide, produced when the heart stretches in relation to increased volume with decreased cardiac output, is increased to help diurese the fluid volume excess.[9] Pulmonary edema increases as volume accumulates and expands from the heart into the lungs as evidenced by audible crackles and wheezes as well as abnormal vascular congestion on chest radiography. Metabolic abnormalities involving electrolyte imbalances and elevated levels of inflammatory markers may result from or concur with the cardiac cascade of shock.

Hypovolemic Shock

Hypovolemic shock is caused by loss of whole blood (hemorrhage), plasma (burns), or interstitial fluid (diaphoresis, diabetes mellitus, diabetes insipidus, emesis, or diuresis) in large amounts. Loss of whole blood or plasma causes hypovolemia directly. Loss of interstitial fluid causes an indirect "relative" hypovolemia by promoting diffusion of plasma from the intravascular to the extravascular space. Hypovolemic shock begins to develop when intravascular volume has decreased by about 15%.

Hypovolemia is offset initially by compensatory mechanisms (Figure 48-3). Heart rate and SVR increase as a result of catecholamine release by the adrenals. This boosts cardiac output and tissue perfusion pressures. Compelled by a decrease in capillary hydrostatic pressures, interstitial fluid moves into the vascular compartment. The liver and spleen add to blood volume by disgorging stored red blood cells and plasma. In the kidneys, renin (through several intermediaries) stimulates aldosterone release and the retention of sodium (and hence water), whereas antidiuretic hormone (ADH, or vasopressin) from the posterior pituitary gland increases water retention. Data on the compensation of ADH, however, show that as shock worsens, ADH in plasma decreases. Hypovolemic shock results in compensatory vasoconstriction and increased SVR and afterload in order to improve blood pressure and perfusion to core organs of the body.

These compensatory mechanisms are, however, finite. If the initial fluid or blood loss is great or if loss continues,

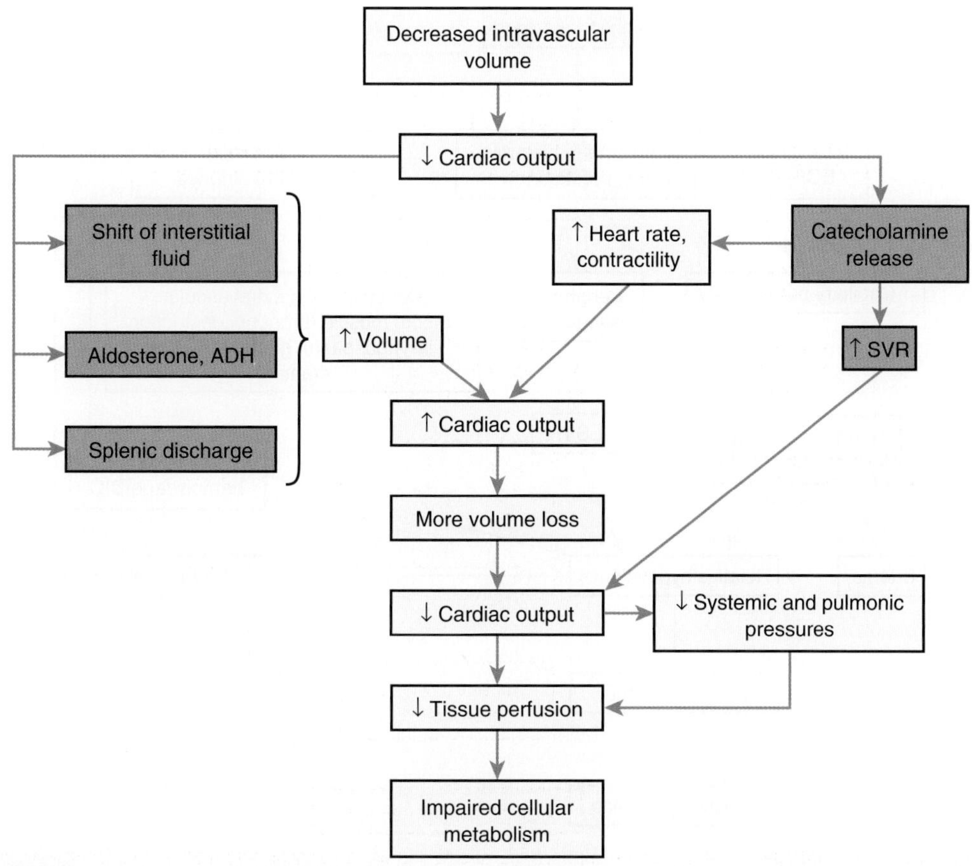

FIGURE 48-3 Hypovolemic Shock. This type of shock becomes life threatening when compensatory mechanisms *(orange boxes)* are overwhelmed by continued loss of intravascular volume. *ADH,* Antidiuretic hormone; *SVR,* systemic vascular resistance.

compensation fails, resulting in decreased tissue perfusion. Nutrient delivery to the cells is impaired, and cellular metabolism fails. Mortality from traumatic hemorrhagic shock ranges from 10% to 31%. Prompt control of hemorrhage is the treatment of choice. Fluid replacement is also important, but the type of fluid to be used and the rate of replacement are controversial.[14,15] The clinical manifestations of hypovolemic shock include high SVR, poor skin turgor, increased thirst, oliguria, low systemic and pulmonary preloads, and rapid heart rates.

Neurogenic Shock

Neurogenic shock also is called **vasogenic shock.** Both terms refer to a widespread and massive vasodilation that results from an imbalance between parasympathetic and sympathetic stimulation of vascular smooth muscle (see Chapter 31). Occasionally, parasympathetic overstimulation or sympathetic understimulation persists, causing vasodilation for an extended period. Extreme, persistent vasodilation leads to neurogenic shock (Figure 48-4). Neurogenic shock creates "relative hypovolemia." Blood volume has not changed, but the amount of space containing the blood has increased, so that SVR decreases drastically; thus pressure in the vessels is inadequate to drive nutrients across capillary membranes, and nutrient delivery to the cells is impaired. As with other types of shock, this leads to impaired cellular metabolism.

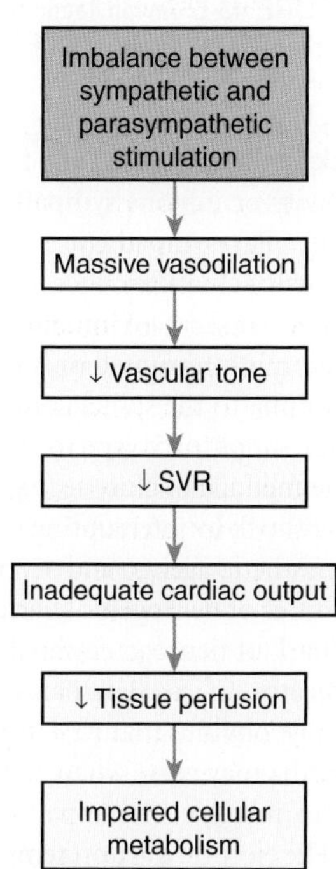

FIGURE 48-4 Neurogenic Shock. *SVR,* Systemic vascular resistance.

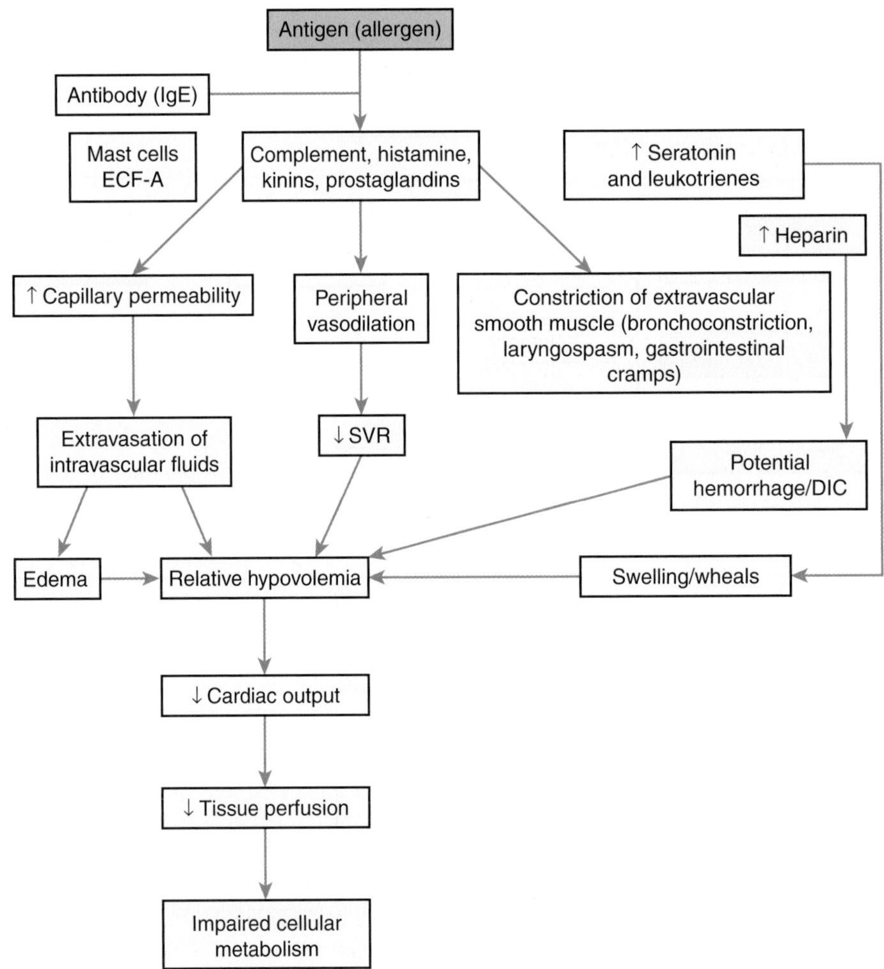

FIGURE 48-5 Anaphylactic Shock. *DIC,* Disseminated intravascular coagulation; *ECF-A,* eosinophil chemotactic factor anaphylaxis; *IgE,* immunoglobulin E; *SVR,* systemic vascular resistance.

Neurogenic shock can be caused by any factor that stimulates parasympathetic activity or inhibits sympathetic activity of vascular smooth muscle. (Parasympathetic stimulation automatically inhibits sympathetic activity and vice versa; see Chapter 31.) Normally, sympathetic stimulation maintains muscle tone. If sympathetic stimulation is interrupted or inhibited, vasodilation occurs. Therefore, trauma to the spinal cord or medulla, conditions that interrupt the supply of oxygen to the medulla, or conditions that deprive the medulla of glucose (e.g., insulin reactions) can cause neurogenic shock by interrupting sympathetic activity. Depressive drugs, anesthetic agents, and severe emotional stress and pain are other causes of neurogenic shock.

The clinical hallmark of neurogenic shock is a very low SVR, along with other indicators of excessive parasympathetic activity. Bradycardia is the most obvious manifestation, especially in the early stages. Bradycardia may cease when compensatory mechanisms, particularly an increase in sympathetic system activity, have been initiated. The ejection fraction remains high, indicating a healthy myocardium, whereas central venous pressure decreases as the veins dilate. Neurogenic shock causes fainting if blood pressure decreases to the point that cerebral metabolism is not sufficient to support consciousness. Most episodes of fainting are *not* shock, however; for such episodes to progress to shock is rare. By allowing the blood pressure to equalize from head to toe as the individual becomes prone, fainting can actually prevent shock.

Anaphylactic Shock

Anaphylactic shock is the outcome of a widespread hypersensitivity to an allergen that triggers a reaction known as *anaphylaxis.* (An allergen is an antigen to which an individual is hypersensitive; see Chapters 7, 8, and 9 for discussions of immunity, inflammation, and hypersensitivity.) Immunologic causes are related to the inflammatory and vasodilatory effects triggered by a pathologic allergic reaction to an antigen. Production of mast cells, IgE, and low-affinity IgE receptor (FceRI) is induced by cellular response to the antigen. *Anaphylactoid* type reactions, which are nonimmunologic in origin, can be related to cold weather, exercise, and contaminants in medications.[16] Physiologic alterations related to the inflammatory and immune response, similar to neurogenic shock, are massive—vasodilation, peripheral pooling, and relative hypovolemia lead to decreased tissue perfusion and impaired cellular metabolism (Figure 48-5). Anaphylactic shock is often severe and has immediate symptoms, including an itchy rash, throat swelling, and low blood pressure, related to the massive vasodilation and systemic inflammation that may progress to death in minutes if emergency treatment is not rendered.

Some allergens known to cause hypersensitivity reactions are foods, insect and snake venoms, pollens, medications, and latex. Once in the body, the allergen causes the extensive immune and inflammatory response. The vascular effects of this response include vasodilation and increased vascular permeability, resulting in peripheral pooling and tissue edema. The extravascular effects include constriction of extravascular smooth muscle. Constriction often causes respiratory difficulty because it tends to affect smooth muscle layers in the airway walls (e.g., the larynx and bronchioles; see Chapter 34).

Clinical manifestations of anaphylactic and anaphylactoid shock may be anxiety, difficulty in breathing, gastrointestinal cramps, edema, hives (urticaria), sensations of burning or itching of the skin, fever, and hemolysis. A precipitous decrease in blood pressure occurs and is followed by impaired mentation. Other signs include decreased SVR (with high or normal cardiac output) and oliguria. Treatment begins with removal of the antigen (if possible). Epinephrine is administered to decrease mast cell and basophil degranulation, cause vasoconstriction, and reverse airway constriction.[17] Volume expanders (e.g., lactated Ringer solution) are given intravenously to reverse the relative hypovolemia, and antihistamines and corticosteroids are given to stop the inflammatory reaction.

In response to the need for improved anaphylaxis diagnosis and treatment, the World Allergy Organization (WAO) formulated global guidelines in 2011 for assessment and management of anaphylaxis.[17] These guidelines were further updated in 2012 to include recommendations for validation of the clinical criteria for diagnosis, use of epinephrine, development of in vitro tests to distinguish clinical risk from asymptomatic sensitization, and immune modulation to prevent anaphylaxis[16] (see What's New? Anaphylactic Shock).

WHAT'S NEW?

Anaphylactic Shock

In response to the need for improved anaphylaxis diagnosis and treatment, the World Allergy Organization (WAO) formulated global guidelines in 2011 for assessment and management of anaphylaxis. These guidelines were further updated in 2012 to include recommendations for validation of the clinical criteria for diagnosis, use of epinephrine, development of in-vitro tests to distinguish clinical risk form asymptomatic sensitization, and immune modulation to prevent anaphylaxis.

Data from Simons FE et al: *Curr Opin Allergy Clin Immunol* 12(4): 389–399, 2012.

Septic Shock

Septic shock is the endpoint of a continuum of progressive dysfunction.[18] The syndrome begins with systemic inflammatory response syndrome (SIRS), then sepsis, then severe sepsis, and then septic shock. Consensus on definitions of each component was updated at an international sepsis conference in 2003 (Table 48-1).[18] The International Sepsis Forum reviewed research for sepsis to identify and define the six most common infection sites (pneumonia, bloodstream, intravascular catheter, intra-abdominal, urosepsis, and surgical wound infection) associated with sepsis in the intensive care setting.[19]

Severe sepsis is the tenth most common cause of death in the United States.[20] Mortality ranges from 28% to 60%.[21] Septic shock is caused by gram-negative bacteria, gram-positive bacteria, and fungi. Advances in antibiotic therapy for gram-negative sepsis have made gram-positive bacteria the leading cause of sepsis.[22] Even when properly treated with available therapies, it carries a high mortality rate. Prognosis is significantly affected by the source and virulence of the infectious microorganism.

Septic shock begins with a nidus of infection that may be readily discernible or extremely difficult to locate (Figure 48-6). Bacteria and fungi enter the bloodstream to produce bacteremia in one of two ways: (1) directly from the site of infection, or (2) indirectly from toxic substances released by the bacteria directly into the bloodstream. These toxic substances, which act as triggering molecules in the septic syndrome, include endotoxins released by gram-negative microorganisms, lipoteichoic acids and peptidoglycan released by gram-positive microorganisms, and superantigens.[22]

The triggering molecules cause the host to initiate a proinflammatory response. Proinflammatory cells released include polymorphonuclear leukocytes, macrophages, monocytes, and platelets. Proinflammatory mediators released include cytokines (interleukins [IL]-1, IL-2, IL-6, IL-8, and IL-15; tumor necrosis factor-alpha [TNF-α]; and granulocyte cell–stimulating factor), complement and complement cascade activation, kinins, arachidonic acid metabolites (prostaglandins, prostacyclin, leukotrienes, and thromboxane), soluble adhesion molecules, platelet-activating factor, endorphins, vasoactive neuropeptides, histamine, serotonin, monocyte chemoattractant proteins 1 and 2, proteolytic enzymes (e.g., elastase and lysosomal enzymes), protein kinase, tyrosine kinase, CD14, toxic oxygen metabolites (e.g., superoxide, hydroxyl radical, hydrogen peroxide, peroxynitrite), neopterin, and clotting cascade activation.[3,23,24] Proinflammatory cytokines enhance tissue factors, which initiates coagulation. Diminished thrombomodulin (cell surface glycoprotein of endothelial cells) inhibits the conversion of protein C and activated protein C. A compensatory anti-inflammatory response syndrome is presumed to follow this response.[3,23,24] Anti-inflammatory mediators released include lipopolysaccharide-binding protein; IL-1 receptor antagonist; soluble CD-14; type 2 IL-1 receptor; leukotriene B_4 receptor antagonist; IL-4, IL-10, and IL-13; soluble tumor necrosis factor receptor; transforming growth factor-beta (TGF-β); epinephrine; and nitric oxide.[3,23,24] Presumably the end result is a mixed antagonistic response syndrome as proinflammatory and anti-inflammatory mediators respond, intensify, and lead the host into MODS.

Clinical manifestations of septic shock are persistent low arterial pressure, low SVR from vasodilation, and an alteration in oxygen extraction by all cells. Septic shock and states of prolonged shock causing tissue hypoxia with lactic acidosis increase nitric oxide synthesis, activate ATP-sensitive and

TABLE 48-1 DEFINITIONS OF SEPTIC SHOCK COMPONENTS

TERM	BASIC DEFINITION	COMMENTS
Infection	A pathologic process that results from an invasion of a normal part of the body by pathogenic or potentially pathogenic microorganisms	Still viewed as an imperfect definition Infection can be strongly suspected without microbiologic confirmation
Bacteremia	Presence of viable bacteria in the blood	Neither necessary nor sufficient to make a diagnosis of sepsis
SIRS	Systemic inflammatory response syndrome is manifested by two or more of general variables: 1a through 1d or 2a through 2c	*Diagnostic criteria:* 1. General variables a. Fever—core temperature >38.3° C (100.9° F) b. Hypothermia—core temperature <36° C (96.8° F) c. Heart rate >90 beats/minute d. Tachypnea e. Altered mental status f. Significant edema or positive fluid balance (>20 ml/kg over 24 hr) g. Hyperglycemia (blood sugar >140 mg/dl) in the absence of diabetes 2. Inflammatory variables a. Leukocytosis (WBC count >12,000) b. Leukopenia (WBC count <4000) c. Normal WBC with >10% immature forms d. Plasma C-reactive protein >2 SD above the normal value e. Plasma procalcitonin >2 SD above the normal value 3. Hemodynamic variables a. Arterial hypotension (SBP <90 mmHg; MAP <70, or an SBP decrease >40 mmHg) b. $S\bar{v}O_2$ >70% c. Cardiac index >3.5 L/min 4. Organ dysfunction variables a. Arterial hypoxemia (PaO_2/FiO_2 <300) b. Acute oliguria (urine output <0.5 ml/kg/hr or 45 ml for at least 2 hr) c. Creatinine increase >0.5 mg/dl d. Coagulation abnormalities (INR >1.5 or a PTT >60) e. Ileus f. Thrombocytopenia (platelet count <100,000) g. Hyperbilirubinemia (plasma total bilirubin >4 mg/dl or 70 mmol/L) 5. Tissue perfusion variables a. Hyperlactatemia (>1 mmol/L) b. Decreased capillary refill or mottling
Sepsis	Systemic response to infection, which is manifested by two or more of the SIRS criteria	
Severe sepsis	Sepsis complicated with one or more organ system dysfunctions	May be difficult to differentiate underlying organ dysfunction from sepsis-related organ dysfunction
Septic shock	Severe sepsis complicated by persistent hypotension refractory to early fluid therapy	Persistent systolic blood pressure <90 mmHg

Data from Dellinger RP et al: *Crit Care Med* 41(2):580–637, 2013; Levy MM et al: *Crit Care Med* 312:1250, 2003; Opal SM, *Scand J Infect Dis* 35:529, 2003.

INR, International normalized ratio; *MAP,* mean arterial pressure; *Pao_2/FiO_2,* partial pressure of oxygen in arterial blood/fraction of inspired oxygen; *PTT,* partial thromboplastin time; *SD,* standard deviation; *SBP,* systolic blood pressure; $S\bar{v}O_2$, saturation of hemoglobin with oxygen; *WBC,* white blood cell.

calcium-regulated potassium channels (K_{ATP} and K_{Ca}, respectively) in vascular smooth muscle (see Chapter 31), and lead to depletion of ADH (vasopressin) (Figure 48-7). Tachycardia causes cardiac output to remain normal or become elevated, although myocardial contractility is reduced. Temperature instability is present, ranging from hyperthermia to hypothermia. Effects on other organ systems may result in deranged renal function, gastrointestinal mucosa changes that result in release of bacteria from the gut, jaundice, clotting abnormalities, deterioration of mental status, and tachypnea that often progresses to ARDS.

Early detection of high-risk illness and rapid implementation of the following standard protocols are increasingly being used by hospitals worldwide: decreasing the time before lactate levels are determined; obtaining blood cultures; starting administration of antibiotics and antifungals; implementing a fluid challenge; achieving goals for blood pressure, central venous pressure (CVP), and central venous oxygen saturation.[25,26] Promptly initiated treatment helps reduce mortality and morbidity related to multiple organ dysfunction. Infection and sepsis identified in the early stages and treated with antibiotics and fluid resuscitation may prevent evolution to severe sepsis and shock; however, once these are identified, more stringent treatment is recommended. The current guidelines for severe sepsis and septic shock[27] recommend immediate resuscitation in patients with lactate levels >4 mmol/L. Elevated lactate levels indicate tissue hypoperfusion and patients should begin early goal-directed therapy or fluid resuscitation within 6 hours, regardless of blood pressure

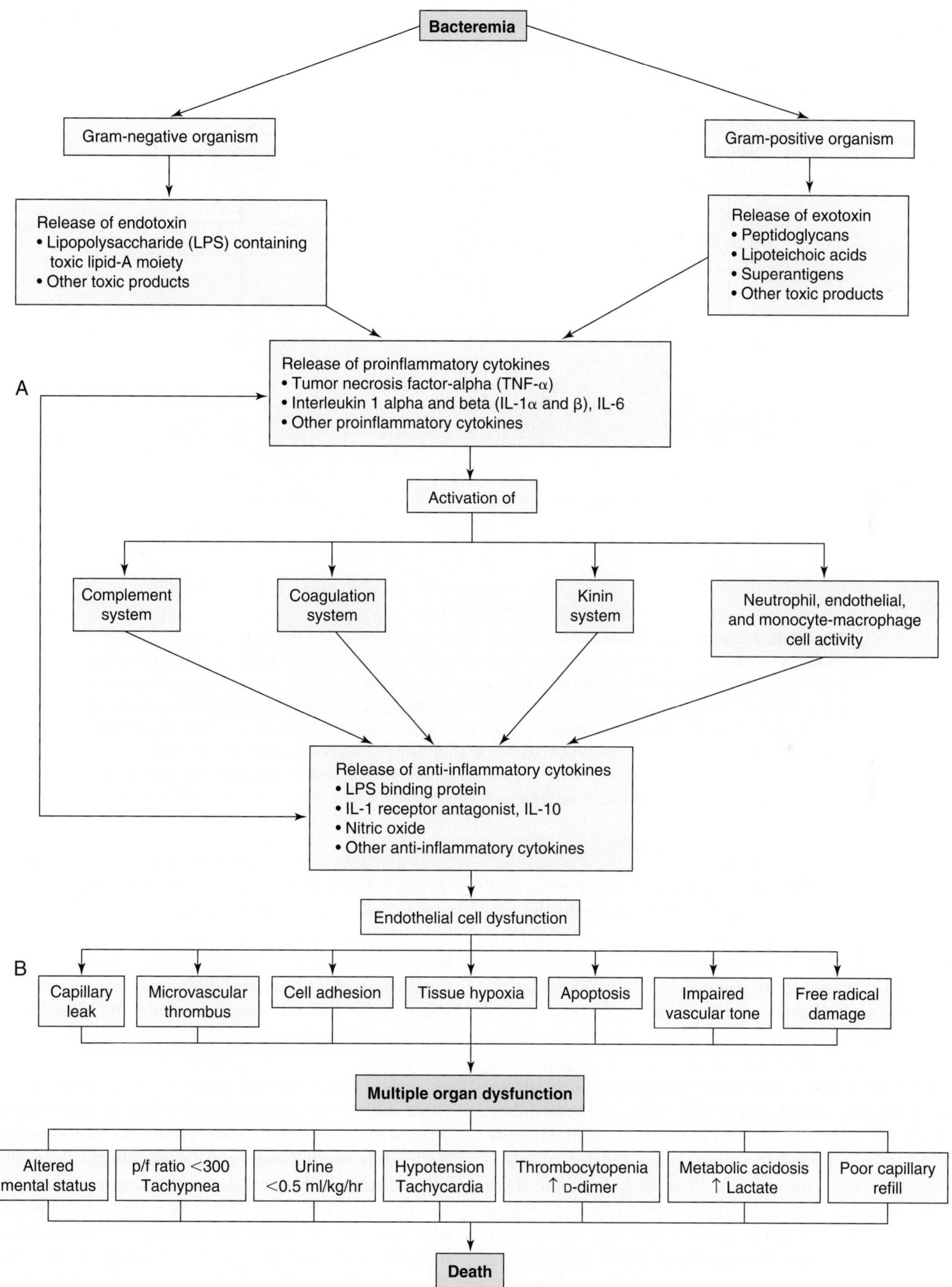

FIGURE 48-6 Summary of Sepsis Pathology. *p/f (PaO_2/FiO_2)*, Oxygenation ratio. (**A** from Lazaron V, Barke RA: *Urol Clin North Am* 26[4]:687, 1999. **B** © 2003, Eli Lilly and Company. All rights reserved. Reprinted with permission from Eli Lilly and Company.)

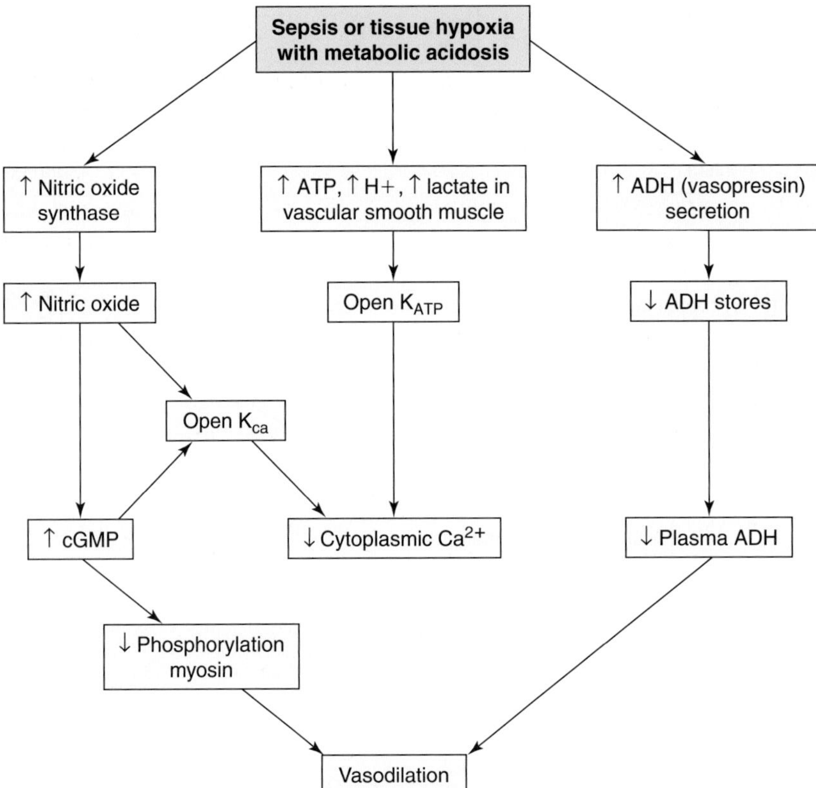

FIGURE 48-7 **Mechanisms of Vasodilation in Shock.** Vasodilatory shock is caused by the inappropriate activation of vasodilatory mechanisms and the failure of constrictor mechanisms. Unregulated nitric oxide, by regulating guanylate cyclase and generating cyclic guanosine monophosphate (cGMP), causes dephosphorylation of myosin and, thus, vasodilation. Nitric oxide synthesis and metabolic acidosis activate the potassium channels (K_{ATP} and K_{ca}) in the plasma membrane of vascular smooth muscle. The resulting hyperpolarization (see Chapter 3) of the membrane presents the calcium that mediates norepinephrine and angiotensin II–induced vasoconstriction from entering the cell. Therefore, hypotension and vasodilation stubbornly persist despite high plasma levels of these hormones. In contrast, and unexpectedly, the plasma level of antidiuretic hormone (ADH) (vasopressin) is low despite the presence of hypotension. The early, massive release of ADH may result in future depletion.

level.[25,26] Specifically, fluid resuscitation with either crystalloid or colloid fluids should be goal-directed to maintain the following values: central venous pressure, 8 to 12 mmHg (or 12 to 15 mmHg when the patient is being mechanically ventilated); mean arterial pressure, 65 mmHg; urine output, 0.5 ml/kg/hr; mixed venous saturation ($S\bar{v}O_2$), 65%. In addition, specific anatomic sites of infection with source identification should be determined so that appropriate antibiotics can be prescribed and control measures can be implemented that eliminate or reduce the spread of infection.[27,28] Fungal assays, including 1,3-β-D-glucan assay and mannan and anti-mannan antibody assays, are recommended to identify suspected fungal infection.[29] Normal saline, at least 1 L or 30 ml/kg body weight, is the initial fluid of choice and hetastarches with molecular weights >200 daltons are not recommended. Adequate and incremental fluid resuscitation is a prerequisite and should be continued to achieve perfusion; supplementation with vasopressors is recommended if the endpoints of tissue perfusion (CVP and normalized lactate levels) are not met.[29]

Pharmacologic hemodynamic support and adjunctive therapy to maintain tissue perfusion include vasoactive agents. Norepinephrine is now considered the initial vasopressor of choice.[29] Dopamine, epinephrine, phenylephrine, and vasopressin are alternatives; however, these are less preferred because of potential tachycardia, dysrhythmias, or reduction in splanchnic blood flow. Dobutamine, an inotropic agent, should be used if myocardial dysfunction is present or hypotension remains after intravascular volume and blood pressure are achieved. Similarly, intravenous corticosteroids are suggested in septic shock to help replace intrinsic loss of cortisol, but only when blood pressure remains unresponsive to volume.[27] Other supportive therapies in the treatment of severe sepsis include blood product administration to maintain hemoglobin levels between 7 and 9 g/dl, targeted tidal volume (6 ml/kg) when mechanically ventilated with plateau pressure less than 30 cm H_2O, utilization of sedation and analgesic protocols when needed, and avoidance of neuromuscular blockers if possible. Glucose concentration is to be maintained at less than 180 mg/dl. If renal dialysis is required, intermittent hemodialysis and continuous venovenous hemofiltration are considered equivalent. Bicarbonate therapy is contraindicated for the purpose of treating hypoperfusion lactic acidemia, unless the pH is <7.15. Use of deep vein thrombosis prophylaxis, such as low-dose unfractionated heparin or low-molecular-weight heparin, or mechanical compression prophylaxis of heparin, is contraindicated. Stress ulcer prophylaxis with H2-receptor antagonists or proton pump inhibitors is indicated. Digestive tract decontamination and selective oropharyngeal decontamination are recommended in the prevention of ventilator-acquired pneumonia.[29] It is important to discuss advance directives with the individual and family.[27] Seeking to decrease use of antibiotics in the critically ill and, thus, prevent resistance to antibiotics is an important strategy in treating infection (see What's New? Procalcitonin Levels). Recent research suggests that monitoring serial procalcitonin (PCT) levels, a precursor hormone to calcitonin, may be used to shorten antibiotic use in the treatment of respiratory tract infections.[30] PCT, normally not discernible on assay, when elevated may indicate specific proinflammatory response during bacterial infection. PCT levels should not be used as an indicator to start antibiotics, but if monitored sequentially at the start of empiric antibiotics and then dropping to low levels, discontinuation may be clinically indicated.[30,31]

WHAT'S NEW?

Procalcitonin Levels

Seeking to decrease use of antibiotics in the critically ill and thus prevent resistance to antibiotics is an important strategy in treating infection. Recent research suggests that monitoring serial procalcitonin (PCT) levels, a precursor hormone to calcitonin, may be used to shorten antibiotic use in the treatment of respiratory infections. PCT, normally not discernible on assay, when elevated may indicate specific proinflammatory response during bacterial infection. PCT levels should not be used as an indicator to start antibiotics but if monitored sequentially at the start of empiric antibiotics, then dropping to low levels, discontinuation may be clinically indicated

Data from Kopterides P et al: *Crit Care Med* 38(11):2229–2241, 2010; Layios N et al: *Crit Care Med* 40(8):2304–2309, 2012.

MULTIPLE ORGAN DYSFUNCTION SYNDROME

Multiple organ dysfunction syndrome (MODS) is the progressive dysfunction of two or more organ systems resulting from an uncontrolled inflammatory response to a severe illness or injury. The organ dysfunction can progress to organ failure and death. MODS occurs during severe sepsis. In 2001, an international consensus conference developed a set of definitions for sepsis and related disorders (see Table 48-1), and a predisposition-infection-response-organ (PIRO) dysfunction staging system was proposed as a template for staging sepsis (Table 48-2). MODS is the end stage of a variety of injuries that terminate in severe, generalized inflammatory response.

MODS was first recognized as a distinct clinical syndrome in the mid-1970s[32,33] when advances in resuscitation and support technologies allowed many individuals to survive life-threatening illness or trauma only to die of complications of their disease. Today MODS is a leading cause of mortality in surgical intensive care units (ICUs). Mortality for individuals with MODS increases progressively from 54% with two failing organ systems to 100% with five failing organ systems. Moreover, mortality has not improved much over the past 15 to 20 years.[34,35]

Although sepsis and septic shock are the most common causes, MODS can be initiated by any severe injury or disease process that activates a massive systemic inflammatory response by the host. Documented clinical infection is not necessary for its development. Other common triggers are severe trauma, major surgery, burns, circulatory shock, acute pancreatitis, acute renal failure, ARDS, blood transfusion, heat stroke, liver failure, mesenteric ischemia, propofol infusion syndrome, persistent inflammatory foci, DIC, and necrotic tissue (Box 48-1). MODS is the major cause of death following septic shock, trauma, burn injuries, and ARDS. People at greatest risk for developing

TABLE 48-2 PREDISPOSITION-INFECTION-RESPONSE-ORGAN (PIRO) DYSFUNCTION SYSTEM FOR STAGING SEPSIS

DOMAIN	PRESENT	FUTURE	RATIONALE
Predisposition	Premorbid illness with reduced probability of short term survival Cultural or religious beliefs Age Sex	Genetic polymorphisms in components of inflammatory response Enhanced understanding of specific interactions between pathogens and host diseases	Premorbid factors affect the potential attributable morbidity and mortality of an acute insult Deleterious consequences of insult heavily dependent on genetic predisposition (future)
Infection	Culture and sensitivity of infecting pathogens Detection of disease amenable to source control	Assay of microbial products Gene transcription profiles	Specific therapies directed against inciting insult require demonstration of characterization of that insult
Response	SIRS Other signs of sepsis Shock C-reactive protein	Nonspecific markers of activated inflammation or impaired host responsiveness Detection of specific target of therapy	Mortality risk and potential to respond to therapy vary with nonspecific measures of disease severity Specific mediator-targeted therapy is predicated on presence and activity of mediator
Organ dysfunction	Organ dysfunction as number of organs or composite score	Dynamic measures of cellular response to insult—apoptosis, cytopathic hypoxemia, cell stress	Response to preemptive therapy not possible if damage already present Therapies targeting the injurious cellular process require that it be present

From Levy MM et al: *2001 Intensive Care Med* 29:530, 2003. Reproduced with kind permission of Springer Science + Business Media.
SIRS, Systemic inflammatory response syndrome.

BOX 48-1 OTHER COMMON TRIGGERS OF MODS

Severe trauma
Major surgery
Burns
Circulatory shock
Acute pancreatitis
Acute renal failure
Acute respiratory distress syndrome
Blood transfusion
Heat stroke
Liver failure
Mesenteric ischemia
Propofol infusion syndrome
Persistent inflammatory foci
Necrotic tissue
Disseminated intravascular coagulation

Data from Abboud B, Daher R, Boujaoude J: *World J Gastroenterol* 14(35):5361–5370, 2008; Adukauskienė D et al: *Medicina (Kaunas)* 44(7):536–540, 2008; Beger HG, Rau BM: *World J Gastroenterol* 13(38):5043–5051, 2007; Bouchama A, Knochel JP: *N Engl J Med* 346:1978–1988, 2002; Broessner G et al: Crit Care 9(5):R498–R501, 2006; Carnovale A et al: *J Pancreas (Online)* 6(5):438–444, 2005; Ciesla DJ et al: *Arch Surg* 140(5):432–440, 2005; Gando S: *Crit Care Med* 38(2)S35–S42, 2010; Kam PCA, Cardone D: *Anesthesia* 62(1):690–701, 2007; Oeckler RA, Hubmayr RD: *Eur Respir J* 30(6):1216–1226, 2007; Shaheen MA, Akhtar AJ: *J Nat Med Assoc* 99(12):1402–1406, 2007; Varghese GM et al: *Emerg Med J* 22:185–187, 2005; Vincent JL, Nelson DR, Williams MD: *Crit Care Med* 39(5):1050–1055, 2011; Zaccheo MM, Bucher DH: *Crit Care Nurse* 28(3):18–26, 2008.

MODS are older adults and persons with significant tissue injury or pre-existing disease.[18]

The PIRO system (see Table 48-2), a clinically useful sepsis staging system, stratifies individuals with disease by baseline risk of adverse outcomes and potential to respond to therapy.[18]

PATHOPHYSIOLOGY. In **primary MODS** the organ injury is directly associated with a specific insult, most often ischemia or impaired perfusion from an episode of shock or trauma, thermal injury, soft tissue necrosis, or invasive infection.[36] This decreased perfusion is local (in the injured organs themselves) and generalized. The generalized hypoperfusion in primary MODS usually cannot be detected clinically. As a result of the insult, a stress response is initiated and stress hormones—in particular, catecholamines—are released. The inflammatory and stress responses are not as evident as they are in secondary MODS. In primary MODS during the inflammatory response, presumably neutrophils and macrophages are "primed" by cytokines.[36] Any second insult, such as additional tissue injury, infection, or organ ischemia, may then activate the primed cells to produce an exaggerated response of secondary MODS[36,37] (Figure 48-8).

The progressive organ dysfunction of **secondary MODS** is the result of an excessive inflammatory reaction, after a latent period following the initial injury, in organs distant from the site of the original injury. It is postulated that the resulting organ trauma is caused by the host response to a second insult rather than being a direct result of the primary injury. Often the second insult is mild but produces an immense disproportionate response because of the previous priming of leukocytes. The interaction of injured organs then leads to a self-perpetuating inflammation.

Secondary MODS is initiated by the delayed postinjury insult as primed macrophages release a barrage of mediators, particularly the cytokines TNF and IL-1. These mediators damage the endothelium throughout the body. If a gram-negative bacterial infection is present, endotoxin released from the bacteria also causes severe damage to endothelial cells. Normal endothelial cells have little interaction with leukocytes, but when stimulated by TNF, IL-1, IL-6, or endotoxin, they change to a proinflammatory state and express adhesion molecules that mediate adhesion of neutrophils. The adhered neutrophils then migrate through the endothelium, aggregate in the area of damaged tissue, and amplify the inflammation.[3] The activated endothelial cells increase production and release of nitric oxide (endothelium), a potent vasodilator that is considered an important factor in the blood flow changes and loss of vascular tone noted in systemic inflammation.[38] The injured endothelium also becomes much more permeable, allowing fluid and protein to leak into the interstitial spaces. An important function of normal endothelium is anticoagulation. When damaged, the endothelium loses much of its ability to prevent blood clotting, allowing microvascular thrombi to develop.

The postinjury insult also activates the neuroendocrine system, resulting in a second, more extensive stress response. The normal function of the stress response is to maintain basal and stress-related homeostasis[39]; however, homeostasis cannot be maintained in MODS. In fact, the endocrine response becomes excessive and injurious. There is an early increase in the levels of circulating catecholamines that contributes to many of the clinical manifestations of MODS, such as tachycardia, hypermetabolism, and increased oxygen consumption. Cortisol, glucagon, insulin, human growth hormone, ADH (which may become depleted), and endorphin levels also are increased. Many of these hormones contribute to the extreme catabolic state of MODS, and endorphins, which are vasodilators, decrease SVR. The sympathetic nervous system, to compensate for complications resulting from the injury (e.g., fluid loss, hypotension), also is stimulated. The stimulation persists throughout the period of critical illness.[39] The stress response can be amplified by a number of factors, including pain, anxiety, psychosis, and hyperthermia. (The stress response is discussed in detail in Chapter 11.)

Because of endothelial cell dysfunction and the release of mediators, four major plasma cascades are activated: complement, kallikrein-kinin, coagulation, and fibrinolytic.[40] Complement components, particularly the anaphylatoxins C3a and C5a, cause vasodilation by stimulating release of histamine from mast cells. They also have strong chemotactic properties. C5a, especially, causes adhesion and the activation and degranulation of neutrophils. Complement is thought to be a powerful trigger for the exaggerated inflammatory response. Activation of the kinin system results in the production of bradykinin, a very potent vasodilator known to decrease SVR. Coagulation mechanisms also are activated, and because tissue injury and endothelial dysfunction are extensive, microvascular

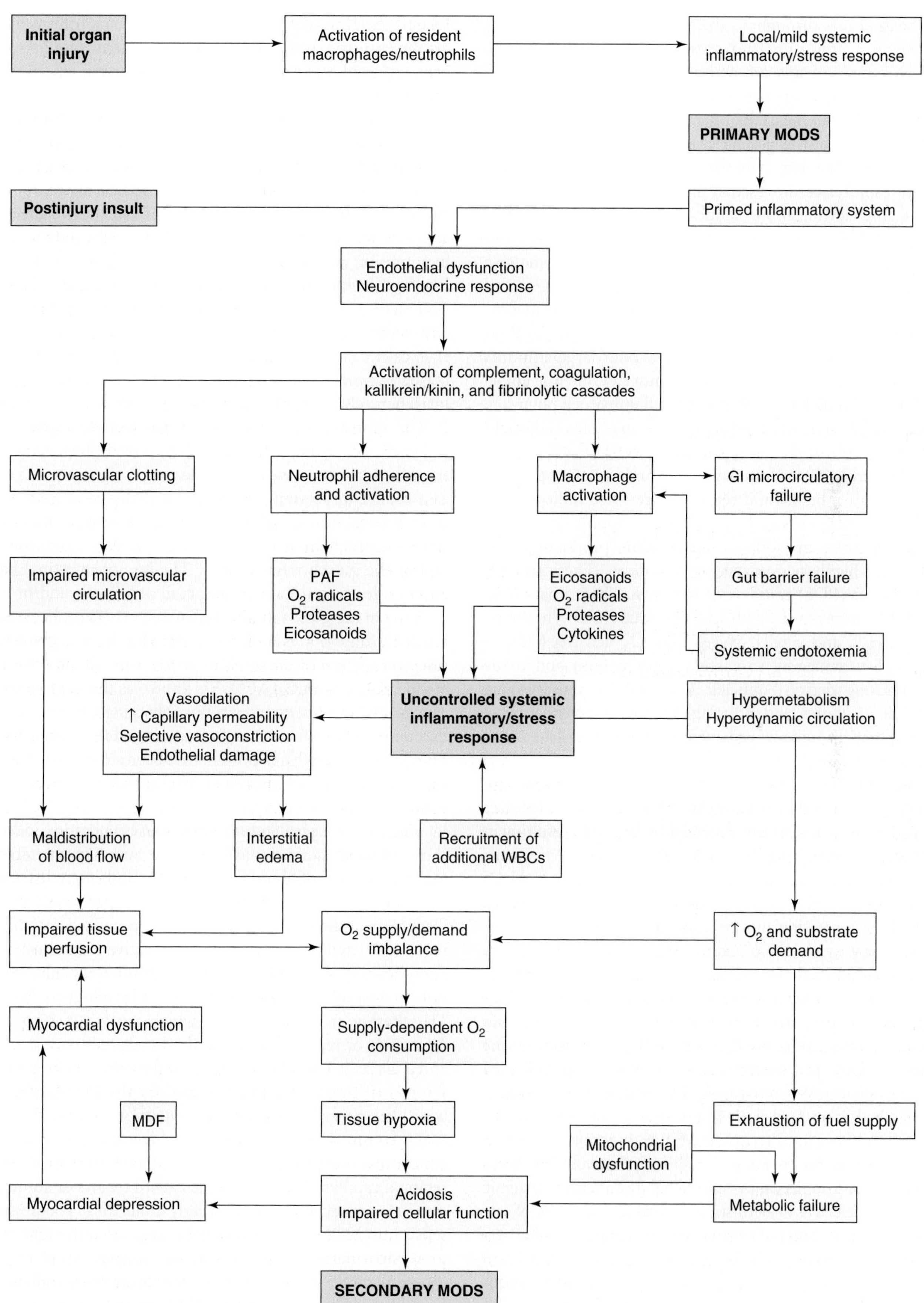

FIGURE 48-8 Pathogenesis of Multiple Organ Dysfunction Syndrome. *GI,* Gastrointestinal; *MDF,* myocardial depressant factor; *MODS,* multiple organ dysfunction syndrome; *PAF,* platelet-activating factor; *WBCs,* white blood cells.

thrombosis occurs throughout the body, resulting in impaired microvascular circulation and organ ischemia. Concurrently, fibrinolytic mechanisms are activated. The tendency toward clotting, however, is greater, resulting in a net procoagulant state that can lead to the development of DIC. The overall effect of the activation of the plasma cascades is a hyperinflammatory and hypercoagulant state that contributes to vasodilation, vasopermeability, cardiovascular instability, endothelial dysfunction, and clotting abnormalities.[41]

Once cytokines and other mediators have been released and the plasma enzyme cascades have been activated, a massive systemic inflammatory response develops. It involves several types of inflammatory cells, particularly neutrophils, macrophages, and mast cells. These cells, having been primed by their response to the initial organ injury, now pour large amounts of chemical mediators into tissues and into the systemic circulation. Neutrophils have tremendous inflammatory potential. The accumulation of activated neutrophils in organs is thought to play a key role in the pathogenesis of MODS.[42] When neutrophils adhere to the endothelium, they undergo a "respiratory burst" (oxidative burst) and release oxygen-free radicals. The respiratory burst occurs as the activated neutrophil experiences a sudden increase in oxidative metabolism, producing large quantities of highly toxic oxygen-free radicals. These reactive oxygen species (ROS) cause oxidative stress. The primary ROS produced are superoxide, hydrogen peroxide (H_2O_2), hydroxyl radical (OH^-), and singlet oxygen (O). Oxygen-free radicals are extremely damaging to vascular endothelium and tissue cells, attacking deoxyribonucleic acid (DNA), cross-linking membrane structures, and inducing membrane peroxidation—reactions that disorganize cell membranes and lead to tissue necrosis[3,24] (also see Chapter 2).

Other important mediators released by neutrophils are proteases, particularly collagenase and elastase. Proteases directly damage endothelium and neighboring cells, resulting in increased capillary permeability and organ damage. When activated, neutrophils also release platelet-activating factor (PAF), a mediator that damages endothelium, stimulates clot formation, and activates increasing numbers of phagocytes. Finally, neutrophils release arachidonic acid metabolites (eicosanoids) as a result of lipid peroxidation of their cell membranes. Of the arachidonic acid metabolites (prostaglandins, thromboxanes, leukotrienes), two are particularly important in the pathogenesis of organ hypoperfusion: prostacyclin (PGI_2) and thromboxane A_2 (TXA_2). TXA_2 is a powerful vasoconstrictor, and PGI_2 is a potent vasodilator. When released in varying amounts in different organ beds, they are largely responsible for the maldistribution of blood flow characteristic of MODS. In total, neutrophils produce at least 50 to 60 toxins.[43,44] Collectively, products released by neutrophils cause endothelial dysfunction, systemic vasodilation, selective vasoconstriction (vasoconstriction of certain organ beds or parts of organ beds), increased vascular permeability, and microvascular coagulation.

Macrophages, present in most tissues, are activated by endotoxin, complement, and monocyte chemotactic substances.[45] Macrophages share a key role in the development of the unregulated inflammation of secondary MODS with the neutrophils. Like neutrophils, they produce oxygen-free radicals, proteases, cytokines, nitric oxide, and arachidonic acid metabolites. It has been reported that excessive or prolonged stimulation of macrophages leads to the overproduction of cytokines and nitric oxide that initiate the cycle of harmful effects in MODS.[3,24,45] TNF and IL-1, which share many of the same functions and act synergistically, are the major cytokines that mediate inflammation.[45,46] TNF has potent metabolic effects, including fever, anorexia, hyperglycemia, hypermetabolism, and weight loss. It activates neutrophils, damages endothelial cells, and potentiates hypotension and shock. IL-1 also has metabolic effects, inducing fever, hypermetabolism, and muscle wasting. Normally, TNF activates cytokines, the coagulation system, fibrinolysis, and neutrophils. With the exception of neutrophil activation, IL-1 causes similar activation in individuals with cancer.[47] In the pathogenesis of MODS, the cytokines are linked to all cellular, hemodynamic, and metabolic alterations.

The gastrointestinal mucosa is particularly vulnerable to inflammatory mediators released by macrophages and neutrophils. Under normal circumstances the gut mucosa serves as a barrier to prevent bacteria from the gastrointestinal tract from entering the systemic circulation. Damage to the mucosa results in microcirculatory failure of the gut and consequent loss of the gut barrier function. The loss of intestinal barrier function leads to the systemic spread of bacteria and/or endotoxin from the gut (systemic endotoxemia). This phenomenon is called *translocation of bacteria.* The idea that the gut acts as a reservoir of bacteria and endotoxin that can initiate or perpetuate the development of MODS is known as the **gut hypothesis.** The gut hypothesis provides a possible explanation for the fact that an infectious focus is not always found in individuals with MODS. Although this hypothesis has been substantiated by animal studies and has much support, the evidence from human studies is inconclusive.[48,49]

The numerous inflammatory processes operating in MODS cause maldistribution of blood flow and hypermetabolism. **Maldistribution of blood flow** refers to the uneven distribution of flow to various organs and between the large vessels and capillary beds of the body. It is caused by generalized vasodilation, increased capillary permeability, selective vasoconstriction, endothelial dysfunction, and impaired microvascular circulation. It is a major factor in the pathophysiology of MODS.[40] The alterations in blood flow—which can occur at the cellular, organ, or regional level—lead to impaired tissue perfusion and a decreased supply of oxygen to the cells. The organs most severely affected by hypoperfusion are the lungs, splanchnic bed, liver, and kidneys. Despite supernormal systemic blood flow, oxygen delivery to the tissues decreases. Several factors contribute to the problem. First, blood is shunted past selected regional capillary beds. Shunting, caused by loss of autoregulation in some organs, may be an early indicator of progression of sepsis into MODS.[50] This occurs because inflammatory mediators, particularly TXA_2, override the normal vascular control mechanisms to cause selective vasoconstriction and because injured endothelial cells are unable to respond to normal vasodilator mediators. Second, interstitial edema, resulting from microvascular permeability, contributes to decreased oxygen delivery to cells by increasing the distance oxygen must travel to reach the cells. Third, capillary obstruction occurs because of the formation of microvascular thrombi and the aggregation of leukocytes.[3,24,45]

Hypermetabolism, with accompanying alterations in carbohydrate, fat, and lipid metabolism, is initially a compensatory measure to meet the body's increased demands for energy. Eventually, however, hypermetabolism becomes detrimental, placing enormous demands on the heart. Hypermetabolism is the result of: (1) the neuroendocrine response to stress with the release of catecholamines and cortisol, and (2) the action of TNF and IL-1. With increased metabolism the calorie requirements are markedly increased,[34] and the cardiac output increases 1.5 to 2 times normal.[51] The alterations in metabolism affect all aspects of substrate use. Most important is the catabolism of protein, primarily of skeletal muscle and visceral organs. The extreme catabolism of protein can rapidly deplete lean body mass. Hyperglycemia occurs as gluconeogenesis by the liver increases and glucose use by the cells decreases. Fatty acids are mobilized from adipose tissue. The net result of the hypermetabolism is depletion of oxygen and fuel supplies.

Myocardial depression also accompanies MODS. The cause remains unclear, but possible explanations are the effects of myocardial depressant factor (MDF), TNF, and IL-1 on cardiac contractility; alterations in α-adrenergic receptors in the heart; and hypoxia of the myocardium.[52,53]

The decreased oxygen delivery to the cells (resulting from the maldistribution of blood flow) and the increased oxygen needs of the cells (resulting from hypermetabolism) combine to create an imbalance in oxygen supply and demand. This imbalance is critical in the pathogenesis of MODS because it results in a pathologic condition known as **supply-dependent oxygen consumption.** Ordinarily the amount of oxygen consumed by the cells depends only on the needs of the cells because there is an adequate reserve of oxygen that can be delivered if required. In MODS, however, the reserve has been exhausted and the amount of oxygen consumed becomes dependent on the amount the circulation is able to deliver. Because the amount is inadequate in MODS, the tissues become hypoxic. Compounding the hypoxic damage to cells is a phenomenon called *reperfusion injury* (see Chapter 2). Much of the organ damage in MODS occurs with the reestablishment of blood flow after a period of ischemia. During the ischemic episode, energy stores and ATP are depleted and the enzyme *xanthine dehydrogenase* is converted to *xanthine oxidase.* With reperfusion of the ischemic tissue, oxygen-free radicals are formed from oxygen by the action of xanthine oxidase, and they attack the already damaged tissues. Consequently, although reperfusion is necessary to restore oxygen supply to ischemic organs, it can increase the extent of injury. Therefore, because of supply-dependent oxygen consumption and reperfusion injury, tissues become increasingly hypoxic. The result is cellular acidosis, impaired cellular function, and ultimately multiple organ failure.

CLINICAL MANIFESTATIONS. In MODS the organs that show clinical manifestations of failure are not always the organs involved as part of the initial injury, and there is usually a lag time between the initial insult and the development of systemic organ failure. The development of primary MODS is difficult to monitor, but there is a well-established general pattern in the clinical development of secondary MODS.[36,54] Following the inciting event and aggressive resuscitation of the individual for approximately 24 hours, the individual develops low-grade fever, tachycardia, tachypnea, dyspnea, altered mental status, and a general hyperdynamic and hypermetabolic state (Box 48-2). Following this, the lungs begin to fail and ARDS may appear within 24 to 72 hours (see discussion of ARDS, Chapter 35). Between days 7 and 10, the hypermetabolic and hyperdynamic state intensifies; bacteremia with enteric organisms is common; and signs of hepatic, intestinal, and renal failure develop. During days 14 to 21, the renal failure and liver failure become more severe. Hematologic failure and myocardial failure are usually later manifestations. Encephalopathy, characterized by mental status changes ranging from confusion to deep coma, may occur at any time. This sequence can evolve rapidly, with death occurring between 14 and 21 days later, or it can evolve over weeks. Individuals can recover from either the slowly or the rapidly evolving course.

The clinical manifestations of failure of individual organs in MODS are caused by inflammatory mediator damage, tissue hypoxia, and hypermetabolism. Respiratory failure progresses early to ARDS and is characterized by tachypnea, pulmonary edema with crackles and diminished breath sounds, use of accessory muscles, and hypoxemia. Liver failure, although early in its development, is not clinically detectable until the later stages of MODS, when jaundice, abdominal distention, liver tenderness, muscle wasting, and hepatic encephalopathy appear. All aspects of metabolism, substance detoxification, and immune response are impaired. Albumin and clotting factor synthesis decreases, protein wastes accumulate, and liver tissue macrophages (Kupffer cells) no longer function effectively.

The gastrointestinal system is very sensitive to ischemic and inflammatory injury. Clinical manifestations of bowel involvement are hemorrhage, ileus, stress ulcers, malabsorption, diarrhea or constipation, vomiting, anorexia, abdominal pain, and pancreatitis. Intolerance to enteral feeding may develop. Adding to damage caused by injury to the bowel is bacterial translocation into the bloodstream resulting from the loss of the gut barrier function. The overwhelmed liver is unable to clear the bacteria from the systemic circulation. Thus, regardless of whether infection or some other injury was the precipitating cause of MODS, once intestinal bacteria enter the systemic circulation, it is likely that sepsis will be a problem. Renal failure develops at about the same time and is marked by progressive oliguria, azotemia, and edema. If renal shutdown is severe, anuria, hyperkalemia, and metabolic acidosis occur.

The first manifestations of cardiac failure are similar to those of septic shock: tachycardia, bounding pulse, increased cardiac output, fall in SVR, hypotension, warm skin, and supraventricular dysrhythmias. In the terminal stages, profound hypotension and ventricular dysrhythmias may develop. Changes in central nervous system function may be noted. Ischemia and inflammation are responsible for the changes, which include apprehension, confusion, disorientation, restlessness, agitation, headache, decreased cognitive ability and memory, and decreased level of consciousness. When ischemia is severe, seizures and coma can occur.

BOX 48-2 CLINICAL MANIFESTATIONS OF ORGAN DYSFUNCTION

Pulmonary
- Acute respiratory distress syndrome (ARDS) pattern of respiratory failure (dyspnea, patchy infiltrates, refractory hypoxemia, respiratory acidosis, abnormal O_2 indices)
- Pulmonary hypertension

Gastrointestinal
- Abdominal distention and ascites
- Intolerance to enteral feedings
- Paralytic ileus
- Upper and lower gastrointestinal bleeding (guaiac-positive stools)
- Diarrhea
- Ischemic colitis
- Mucosal ulceration
- Decreased bowel sounds
- Bacterial overgrowth in stool

Liver
- Increased serum bilirubin level (hyperbilirubinemia)
- Increased liver enzyme levels (serum aspartate transaminase [SAST], serum alanine aminotransferase [SALT], lactic dehydrogenase [LDH], alkaline phosphatase)
- Increased serum ammonia level
- Decreased serum transferrin level
- Jaundice
- Hepatomegaly

Gallbladder
- Right upper quadrant tenderness or pain
- Abdominal distention
- Unexplained fever
- Decreased bowel sounds

Metabolic/Nutritional
- Decreased lean body mass
- Muscle wasting
- Severe weight loss
- Negative nitrogen balance
- Hyperglycemia
- Hypertriglyceridemia
- Increased serum lactate levels
- Decreased serum albumin, serum transferrin, prealbumin, retinol-binding protein

Renal
- Increased serum creatinine level and blood urea nitrogen
- Oliguria, anuria, or polyuria consistent with prerenal azotemia or acute tubular necrosis
- Urinary indices consistent with prerenal azotemia or acute tubular necrosis

Cardiovascular

Hyperdynamic
- Decreased pulmonary capillary wedge pressure
- Decreased systemic vascular resistance
- Decreased right atrial pressure
- Decreased left ventricular stroke work index
- Increased oxygen consumption
- Increased cardiac output, cardiac index, heart rate

Hypodynamic
- Increased systemic vascular resistance
- Increased right atrial pressure
- Increased left ventricular stroke work index
- Decreased oxygen delivery and consumption
- Decreased cardiac output and cardiac index

Central Nervous System
- Lethargy
- Altered level of consciousness
- Fever
- Hepatic encephalopathy

Coagulation and Hematologic
- Thrombocytopenia
- Disseminated intravascular coagulation

Immune
- Infection
- Decreased lymphocyte count
- Anergy

Modified from Thelan LA et al: *Critical care nursing: diagnosis and management,* ed 6, St Louis, 2010, Mosby.

EVALUATION AND TREATMENT. Because there is no specific therapy for MODS, early detection or prevention is extremely important so that supportive measures are initiated instantly.[34] Frequent assessment of the clinical status of individuals at known risk is essential. Unfortunately, there is no way to determine with certainty when an organ is failing. Indicators of organ dysfunction are presented in Table 48-1.

Several systems for scoring severity of illness also have been developed. Commonly used systems are the **Acute Physiology and Chronic Health Evaluation II and III (APACHE II and APACHE III),** the logistic organ dysfunction score (LODS), the sequential organ failure assessment (SOFA), the MODS score, and the PIRO staging system.[55] Once organ failure develops, monitoring of laboratory values and hemodynamic parameters is necessary to assess the degree of clinical impairment.

The therapeutic management of MODS consists of prevention and support. Prevention of the syndrome is essential! First, if possible, the initial source of inflammation must be eliminated or controlled. Next, a second insult must be avoided. It is paramount to remove any potential site of infection by débriding necrotic tissue, draining abscesses, reducing the numbers of invasive procedures performed, and removing hematomas. Nosocomial infections from contaminated lines and catheters are of concern and must be prevented. Nosocomial infection rates of 15% to 25% have been reported in critically ill individuals.[56] Early reduction of long-bone fractures and surgical repair of injured tissues are also important preventive measures.

The goals of therapy are to control infection, provide adequate tissue oxygenation, restore intravascular volume, and support the function of individual organs.[26] After the initial injury has been aggressively treated and sources of infection have been removed, antibiotics generally are administered. The choice of agents is based on the individual's disease process, but the regimen is usually a combination of antibiotics that covers both gram-negative and gram-positive organisms.

Because oxygen is not stored in the tissues, it must be continuously delivered. Maintaining an arterial oxygen saturation of 88% to 92% is recommended,[26] and hemoglobin levels should be kept greater than 9 g/dl.[26] Mixed venous oxygen saturation greater than or equal to 70% is recommended. Blood transfusions may be necessary to ensure an adequate hemoglobin level. To deliver oxygen to the organs in the face of profound systemic vasodilation, fluid volume must be restored. Therefore, aggressive fluid therapy is initiated early. Usually large volumes of isotonic crystalloid solutions are administered, although colloids (often albumin) also may be added to maintain adequate preload and circulation volume.[26]

Finally, support for individual organ systems must be provided. Respiratory failure is treated with mechanical ventilation with low tidal volumes, high oxygen concentrations, and positive end-expiratory pressures (PEEP).[57] To provide adequate nutrition and metabolic support, the failing gastrointestinal system is supported with enteral feedings. It is now well recognized that enteral feedings help preserve gut microbial barrier function, and thus are preferred to parenteral feedings.[58] However, if the individual is unable to tolerate the amount of enteral feeding required to meet the enormous metabolic demands, hyperalimentation may be added. Ideally the feeding formula is carefully calculated to meet the individual's nutritional requirements. Tight glucose level control (80 to 110 mg/dl) is recommended.[59] Once renal failure is established, dialysis or continuous hemofiltration may be required to maintain fluid and electrolyte balance. To support the failing cardiovascular system, inotropic drugs, such as low-dose dopamine and dobutamine, or vasopressors, such as norepinephrine, may be required to maximize cardiac contractility and maintain cardiac output. Although steroids have anti-inflammatory effects, their use is controversial because they have been shown to be effective in adults with septic shock. Obtaining an adrenocorticotropic hormone (ACTH) level is not recommended. Deep vein thrombosis prophylaxis is also important.[6]

Scientific knowledge gained about MODS and inflammatory mediators has led to many investigational therapies. Novel molecular approaches targeting a variety of interdependent mediators of MODS are being investigated.[47]

BURNS

Major thermal injury is a source of massive tissue injury and destruction that has wide-reaching effects on virtually all organ systems. **Burn** is a generic term used to describe cutaneous injury resulting from thermal, chemical, or electrical environmental causes. In addition to cutaneous injury, burns are often associated with smoke inhalation injury or other traumatic injuries that aggravate the local and systemic problems of burns. Pulmonary injury, both primary and secondary, is common and often necessitates ventilator support. The use of tracheostomy also has been examined and is controversial.[60,61] This model of multisystem injury provides an opportunity to examine the interaction of shock, inflammation, and immunocompromise in a clinical setting.

Epidemiology and Etiology

The annual number of burns and fire-related injuries that occur in the United States is now estimated to be about 450,000.[62] Deaths consequent to these injuries have decreased more than 50%—from 9000 in 1971[63] to 4000 in 2005.[62] This remarkable progress is the result of several factors, including ongoing research in burn physiology and burn care,[64] an increased national focus on fire safety and burn prevention, the establishment of regional burn centers, the use of smoke detectors, regulation of consumer product safety, and the implementation of occupational safety mandates. A decrease in hospitalization reflects a shift to outpatient care and improved prehospital and emergency treatment, but burn assessment and delivery of care can be improved[65] to reduce medical transport and treatment costs. International interest in telemedicine has increased over the past decade.[66,67] These advances in care are changing emphasis from survival to outcomes in burn survivors.[68,69]

The causes of burn injury may be **thermal** or **nonthermal,** such as chemical, electrical, or radioactive. Thermal burns may result from thermal contact, flame, or scald. Adherent materials (e.g., asphalt, tar, or plastic) may likewise produce a serious contact burn. Chemical injuries are a result of contact with substances that are directly toxic to skin or the lining of the respiratory or alimentary tract. Such chemicals are often acid, alkali, or organic agents, termed **vesicants,** that cause blistering of the epithelial surfaces. Electrical burns may be the result of the conduction of electrical current through the body with heating of tissue or flash over the body surface associated with an electrical discharge. Quality of life can be affected but, by self-reports, may exceed normal population averages with proper intervention.[70]

Burn Wound Depth

The classification of **burn wound depth** is usually based on the physical appearance and the symptoms associated with the affected skin. The definitive diagnosis is determined by the histologic depth of tissue necrosis. Such evaluation, unfortunately, necessitates a skin biopsy. Because of the invasive nature of biopsy, clinical depth assessment is used and the ultimate fate of the wound determines final diagnosis. Recent advances in laser Doppler technology have resulted in extensive exploration of a noninvasive means for burn wound depth assessment.[71-83]

First-degree burns are a **partial-thickness injury** involving only the epidermis without injury to the underlying dermal or subcutaneous tissue (Table 48-3). The skin maintains water vapor and bacterial barrier functions. Many sunburns are first-degree injuries caused by exposure of skin to ultraviolet radiation from the sun. Initially there is local pain and erythema, but no blisters appear until after about 24 hours. An extensive first-degree burn may cause systemic responses such as chills, headache, localized edema, and nausea or vomiting. No treatment of extensive first-degree burns is required unless the person is

TABLE 48-3 DEPTH OF BURN INJURY

		SECOND DEGREE		THIRD DEGREE
CHARACTERISTIC	**FIRST DEGREE**	**SUPERFICIAL PARTIAL THICKNESS**	**DEEP PARTIAL THICKNESS**	**FULL THICKNESS**
Morphology	Destruction of epidermis only	Destruction of epidermis and some dermis	Destruction of epidermis and dermis, leaving only skin appendages	Destruction of epidermis, dermis, and underlying subcutaneous tissue
Skin function	Intact	Absent	Absent	Absent
Tactile and pain sensors	Intact	Intact	Intact but diminished	Absent
Blisters	Present only after first 24 hr	Present within minutes, thin walled and fluid filled	May appear as fluid-filled blisters; often is layer of flat, dehydrated "tissue paper" that lifts off in sheets	Blisters rare; usually is a layer of flat, dehydrated "tissue paper" that lifts off easily
Appearance of wound after initial debridement	Skin peels at 24-48 hr, normal or slightly red underneath	Red to pale ivory, moist surface	Mottled with areas of waxy white, dry surface	White, cherry red, or black; may contain visible thrombosed veins; dry, hard leathery surface
Healing time	3-5 days	21-28 days	30 days to many months	Will not heal; may close from edges as secondary healing if wound is small
Scarring	None	May be present; low incidence influenced by genetic predisposition	Highest incidence because of slow healing rate promoting scar tissue development; also influenced by genetic predisposition	Skin graft; scarring minimized by early excision and grafting; influenced by genetic predisposition

elderly or an infant, in which case severe nausea and vomiting may lead to inadequate fluid intake and dehydration. Therapy consists of intravenous hydration until the nausea and vomiting subside 24 to 72 hours after burn injury. Comfort measures for previously healthy children or adults with extensive first-degree burns consist of aspirin for adults or acetaminophen for children every 4 hours in age-appropriate doses and frequent application of a water-soluble lotion. First-degree burns heal in 3 to 5 days without scarring.

Second-degree burns describe two categories of burn depth with markedly different characteristics. Both of these are partial-thickness injuries, but they evoke vastly different responses. The hallmark of **superficial partial-thickness injury** is the appearance of thin-walled, fluid-filled blisters that develop within just a few minutes after injury. Another dominant characteristic of superficial injury is pain. As blisters break or are removed, nerve endings are exposed to air (Figure 48-9). Tactile and pain sensors remain intact throughout healing, with each wound care procedure causing substantial pain. Wounds heal in 3 to 4 weeks if the individual is adequately nourished and no complications develop (Figure 48-10). Scar formation is unusual with this injury. The amount of scarring that develops is a genetically determined trait and is not predictable during the early course of treatment.

Deep partial-thickness burns involve the entire dermis, sparing skin appendages such as hair follicles and sweat glands (see Table 48-3). The burn often looks waxy white and is surrounded by margins of superficial partial-thickness injury. The injury is often clinically indistinguishable from a full-thickness injury (Figure 48-11), but by 7 to 10 days after burn injury, skin buds and hair will appear from hair follicles, indicating that skin appendages remain. These wounds take weeks to heal,

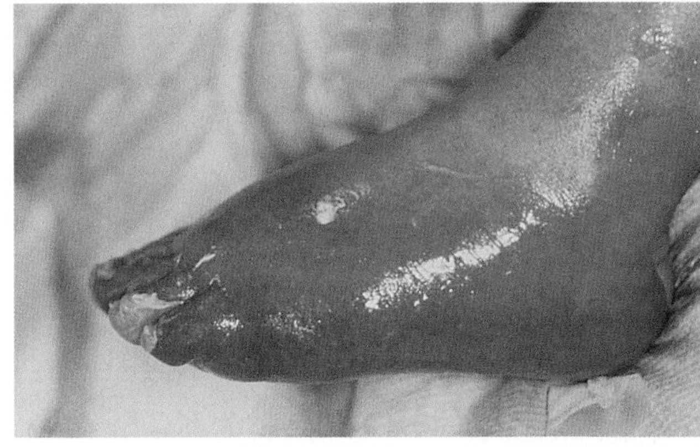

FIGURE 48-9 **Superficial Partial-Thickness Injury.** Scald injury following débridement of overlying blister and nonadherent epithelium. (Courtesy Intermountain Burn Center, University of Utah.)

and current therapy consists of surgical removal of the burn wound (excision) followed by application of the person's own unburned skin from another body area (autograft). Wounds that heal slowly produce more scar tissue and continue to be a potential source of infection until closed. In the presence of relative surgical contraindications, such as cardiopulmonary failure, deep partial-thickness wounds are not surgically treated but are allowed to heal primarily. The fate of partial-thickness burns can be affected by treatment, such as topical antibiotics, or by the condition of biologic membranes.[84] The ultimate healing of deep partial-thickness burns commonly results in hypertrophic scarring with poor functional and cosmetic results.

Third-degree burns, or **full-thickness injuries,** involve destruction of the entire epidermis, dermis, and often the underlying subcutaneous tissue (see Table 48-3). On occasion, all

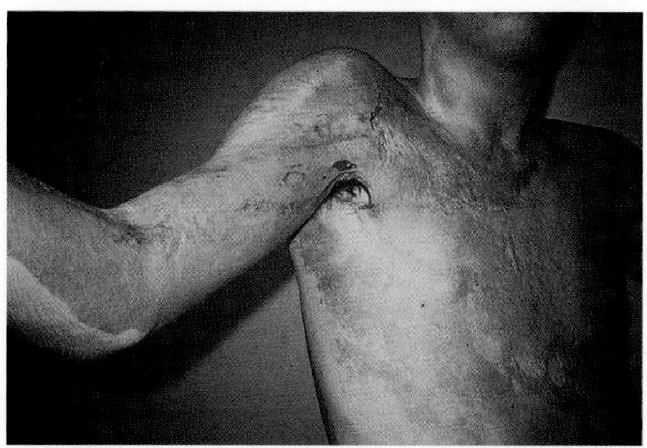

FIGURE 48-10 Axillary Burn Scar Contracture. Note the blanching of the anterior axillary fold and small ulceration, both indicating the diminished range of motion. (Courtesy Intermountain Burn Center, University of Utah.)

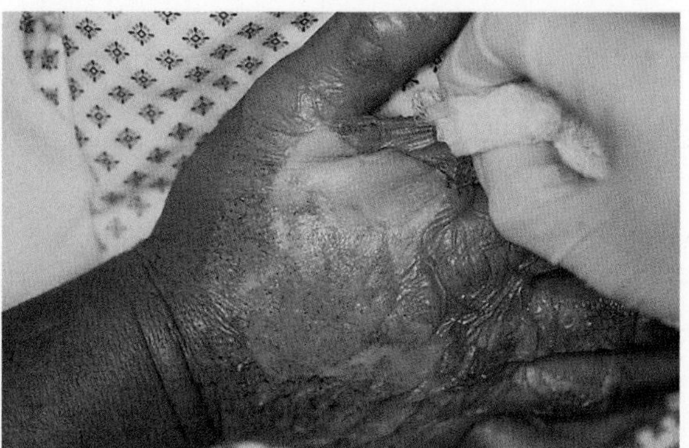

FIGURE 48-11 Deep Partial-Thickness Wound. Note pale appearance and minimal exudate. (Courtesy Intermountain Burn Center, University of Utah.)

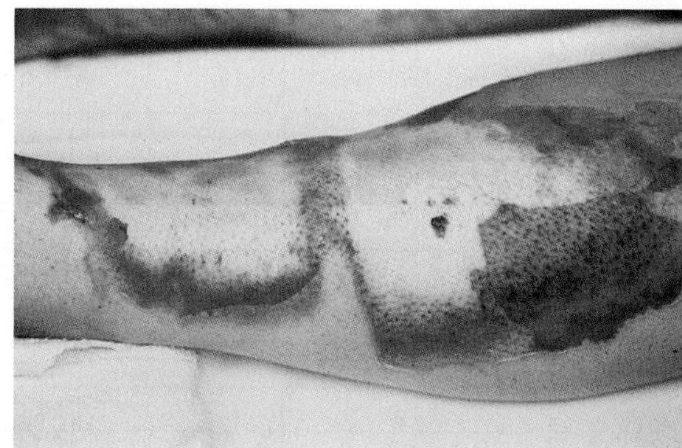

FIGURE 48-12 Full-Thickness Thermal Injury. The wound is dry and insensate. (Courtesy Intermountain Burn Center, University of Utah.)

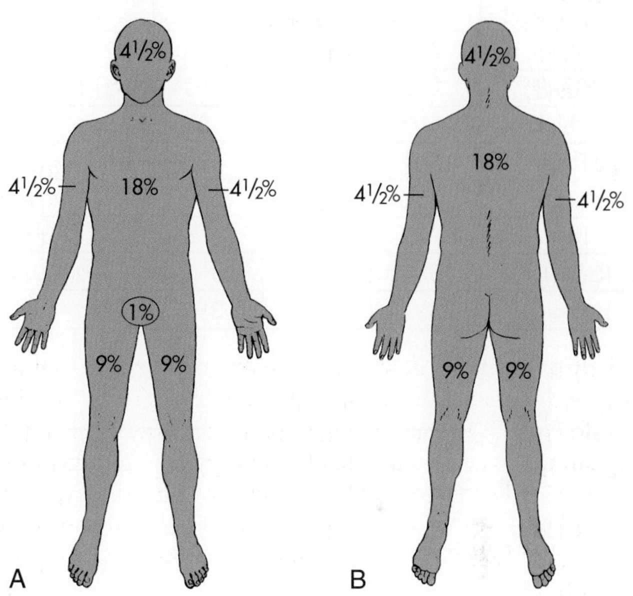

FIGURE 48-13 Rule of Nines. A commonly used assessment tool with estimates of the percentages (in multiples of 9) of the total body surface area burned. **A,** Adults (anterior view). **B,** Adults (posterior view).

underlying subcutaneous tissue is destroyed and muscle or bone may be involved. Full-thickness wounds often appear relatively innocuous when their color is white and the delineation between normal and burned skin is not accompanied by a marked color change. Elasticity of the dermis is absent, leaving the wound dry and leathery in appearance and texture (Figure 48-12). As marked edema develops, distal circulation may be compromised in areas of circumferential burns. **Escharotomies** (cutting through burned skin) are performed to release underlying pressure. Full-thickness burns are painless because all nerve endings have been destroyed by the injury.

The extent of the **total body surface area (TBSA)** burn is estimated using either the "rule of nines" (Figure 48-13) or the Lund and Browder chart (Figure 48-14). Areas of partial-thickness and full-thickness injury are marked on the diagram in Figure 48-14. First-degree burns are not included in the TBSA estimate. The surface area of the palm, including palmar finger surface, averages 1% of the body surface area over a wide range of ages; thus it can be used to estimate burn areas of irregular size and shape.[85]

Severity of burn injury is a combination of many factors, including age, medical history, extent and depth of injury, and body area involved. The American Burn Association has defined criteria to assist healthcare professionals in identifying individuals who require care at a specialized burn center (Box 48-3). The multidisciplinary burn center is recommended for those persons who are at high risk for morbidity, mortality, or permanent functional loss.

PATHOPHYSIOLOGY AND CLINICAL MANIFESTATIONS. Burn injury results in dramatic changes in many physiologic functions of the body within the first few hours after the event. The effect of burn depends on two factors: first, the extent of body surface involved and, second, the depth of cutaneous injury. Body surface burn extent is described by the percentage of TBSA injured. Burns exceeding 20% of TBSA in most adults are considered to be major burn injuries and are associated with massive evaporative water losses and flux of large amounts of fluid and electrolytes in the tissues, manifested as generalized edema and circulatory hypovolemia. Depth of cutaneous injury has been categorized in many ways but always depends on the severity of injury of epidermal and dermal elements of the skin and whether the alteration is a permanent or reversible injury.

With a major burn injury, a systemic pathophysiology ensues that requires therapeutic intervention to sustain life. The immediate (acute) physiologic consequences of a major burn injury

Area	Birth 1 yr.	1-4 yr.	5-9 yr.	10-14 yr.	15 yr.	Adult	2°	3°	Total	Donor Areas
Head	19	17	13	11	9	7				
Neck	2	2	2	2	2	2				
Ant. Trunk	13	13	13	13	13	13				
Post. Trunk	13	13	13	13	13	13				
R. Buttock	2½	2½	2½	2½	2½	2½				
L. Buttock	2½	2½	2½	2½	2½	2½				
Genitalia	1	1	1	1	1	1				
R. U. Arm	4	4	4	4	4	4				
L. U. Arm	4	4	4	4	4	4				
R. L. Arm	3	3	3	3	3	3				
L. L. Arm	3	3	3	3	3	3				
R. Hand	2½	2½	2½	2½	2½	2½				
L. Hand	2½	2½	2½	2½	2½	2½				
R. Thigh	5½	6½	8	8½	9	9½				
L. Thigh	5½	6½	8	8½	9	9½				
R. Leg	5	5	5½	6	6½	7				
L. Leg	5	5	5½	6	6½	7				
R. Foot	3½	3½	3½	3½	3½	3½				
L. Foot	3½	3½	3½	3½	3½	3½				
						TOTAL				

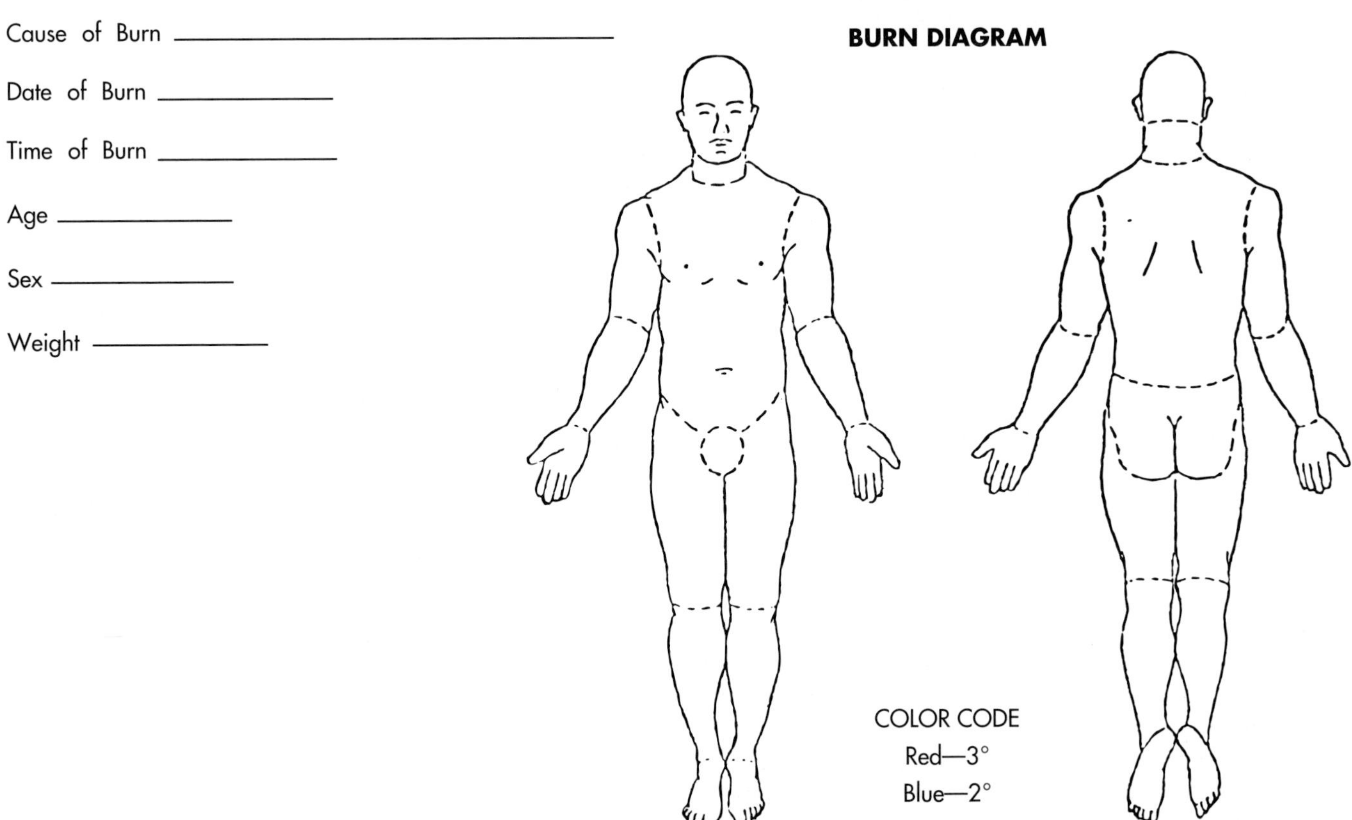

FIGURE 48-14 Lund and Browder Chart. Regional differences in body surface are calculated based on age. (Courtesy Intermountain Burn Center, University of Utah.)

BOX 48-3 BURN UNIT REFERRAL CRITERIA

A burn unit may treat adults or children or both.

Burn injuries that should be referred to a burn unit include the following:

1. Partial-thickness burns greater than 10% total body surface area (TBSA)
2. Burns that involve the face, hands, feet, genitalia, perineum, or major joints
3. Third-degree burns in any age group
4. Electrical burns, including lightning injury
5. Chemical burns
6. Inhalation injury
7. Burn injury in individuals with pre-existing medical disorders that could complicate management, prolong recovery, or affect mortality
8. Any patients with burns and concomitant trauma (such as fractures) in which the burn injury poses the greatest risk of morbidity or mortality. In such cases, if the trauma poses the greater immediate risk, the patient's condition may be initially stabilized in a trauma center before being transferred to a burn center; physician judgment will be necessary in such situations and should be in concert with the regional medical control plan and triage protocols.
9. Burned children in hospitals without qualified personnel or equipment for the care of children
10. Burn injury in patients who will require special social, emotional, or long-term rehabilitative intervention

From Resources for Optimal Care of the Injured Patient: "Guidelines for the Operation of Burn Centers," Chicago, IL, 2006, Committee on Trauma, American College of Surgeons.

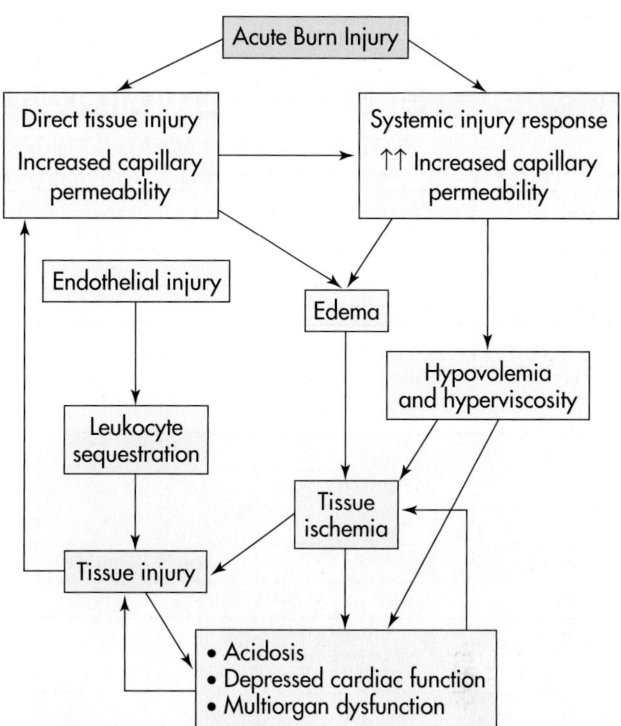

FIGURE 48-15 Immediate Cellular and Immunologic Alterations of Burn Shock.

center around the profound, life-threatening hypovolemic shock that occurs in conjunction with cellular and immunologic disruption within a few hours of injury (Figure 48-15). **Burn shock** is a phenomenon consisting of both a hypovolemic cardiovascular component and a cellular component.

Hypovolemia associated with burn shock results from massive fluid losses from the circulating blood volume. The losses are caused by an increase in capillary permeability that persists for approximately 24 hours after burn injury. **Fluid resuscitation** is the administration of intravenous fluids, such as lactated Ringer solution, in an effort to restore the circulating blood volume during the period of increasing capillary permeability. In addition to hypovolemia, most other organ systems are affected. Cardiac contractility is diminished during the initial 24-hour resuscitation period with shunting of blood away from the liver, kidney, and gut. This is often termed the *ebb phase* of the response to trauma and can be seen with other severe injuries. Normal blood volume does not result in restoration of normal cardiac output because of a phenomenon known as *myocardial depression*. The decrease in perfusion of viscera results in a decrease in their function. This may be an explanation for decreased gut barrier function seen in thermal injury.[86] Other mechanisms include hypoxia and inflammation with histologic damage of intestinal mucosa.[87]

There also is evidence that cellular metabolism is disrupted when the burn wound is created, resulting in altered cell membrane permeability and loss of normal electrolyte homeostasis. This cellular defect may be the pathophysiologic process responsible for the genesis of burn shock. There are numerous circulating factors in burn serum that may play a role in these cellular processes. Although the cardiovascular and systemic responses are intricately interwoven into the cellular response, these responses are presented here as discrete entities for purposes of description.

Cardiovascular and Systemic Response to Burn Injury

The clinical manifestations of burn shock are the result of more than simple loss of extracellular fluid at the burn wound site. Hypovolemia and numerous local mediators in the burn wound,[88] as well as systemic signals, result in alteration of cellular function throughout the body. The restoration of normal intravascular volume with either saline solutions or colloid materials (e.g., albumin, blood, or dextrans) does not reverse changes such as increases in pulmonary vascular resistance or myocardial contractility.[89] This is reflected in cardiac output with precipitous decreases that often result in inadequate perfusion of most tissues at the capillary level, which is the hallmark of burn shock. Fluid infusion, likewise, does not return cardiac output to preburn levels.[90,91] These findings led to the postulation of a specific myocardial depressant factor (MDF).[92-94] Other causes also have been suggested, such as reactive oxygen-free radicals that attack cell membranes and other subcellular organelles as a result of first ischemia and then reperfusion of tissues during burn shock and resuscitation.[95] A third factor may be the level of nitric oxide after burn injury, which could have a direct myocardial depressant effect.[96,97] The relationship of nitric oxide and myocardial function is not yet totally clear. Gamelli and colleagues[98] found nitric oxide production to be significantly depressed in burned individuals who did not survive their injuries. They postulate that nitric oxide may scavenge reactive oxygen-free radicals and protect tissues from oxidative injury.

TABLE 48-4 ELECTROLYTE CONTENT OF RINGER LACTATE SOLUTION AND EXTRACELLULAR FLUID

ELECTROLYTE	EXTRACELLULAR FLUID* (mEq/L)	LACTATED RINGER SOLUTION† (mEq/L)
Sodium	135-145	130
Potassium	3.2-4.5	4
Chloride	95-105	109
Lactate (bicarbonate)	24-28	28

*Normal values may vary slightly between laboratories.
†Plus 80-100 ml free water per liter.

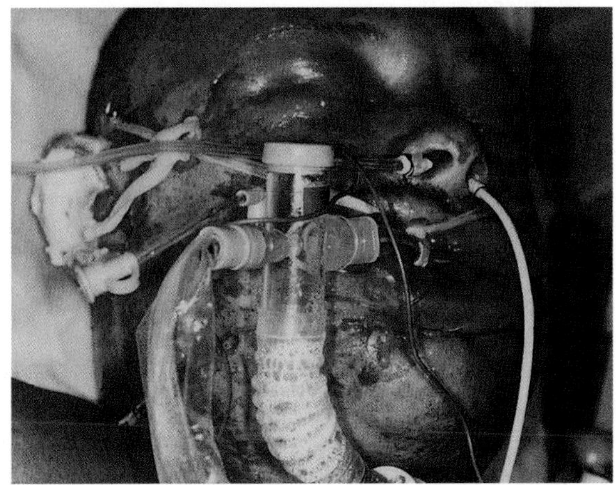

FIGURE 48-16 Edema Related to Burn Injury. Superficial facial burns can result in marked swelling, requiring prompt endotracheal intubation to maintain the airway. (Courtesy Intermountain Burn Center, University of Utah.)

Regardless of the contribution of these mechanisms, fluid resuscitation eventually results in improved outcome of the massively burned person. This resuscitation involves infusion of intravenous fluid at a rate faster than the loss of circulatory vascular volume for a period of about 24 hours from the time of burn injury, and may require up to 30 L in a major burn. Resuscitation from burn shock can be accomplished using any of a number of infusion protocols. The most frequently used protocol is the Parkland formula.[99] Lactated Ringer solution is used because it closely approximates extracellular fluid, the repository of fluid leaving the circulatory system during this phase of extensive edema formation (Table 48-4). The use of electrolyte-free fluids, such as D_5W (dextrose 5% in water), results in life-threatening hypovolemia and hyponatremia. Resuscitation with hypertonic saline has been used in some medical centers but is reserved for special circumstances; its use can result in adverse outcomes.[100]

The massive edema associated with burn shock is inevitable with fluid resuscitation, and failure to administer resuscitation fluid results in irreversible hypovolemic shock and death. The edema occurs in unburned as well as burned areas (Figure 48-16). This often leads to mechanical airway obstruction, necessitation of tracheal intubation, and increased severity of the interstitial pulmonary edema associated with inhalation injury.

The most reliable criterion for adequate resuscitation of burn shock is urine output. The individual is in hypovolemic shock and will, as a compensatory mechanism, decrease or stop urine output in an effort to preserve circulation volume. The adult receiving sufficient intravenous fluids will excrete urine amounting to 30 to 50 ml/hr; children will produce 1 ml/kg/hr. If the individual does not have adequate urine output, it often indicates inadequate fluid resuscitation. The massive amount of intravenous fluid required by burned individuals during the shock phase is often intimidating to the person unfamiliar with burns. One common concern is that massive fluid administration will result in pulmonary edema. It should be remembered that the individual is in hypovolemic shock and that fluid is lost dramatically during the resuscitation period through third spacing, exudation, and evaporation.

BOX 48-4 MAINTENANCE FLUID REPLACEMENTS AFTER MAJOR BURN INJURY*

1. *Basal fluid* replacements per day
   1500 ml/day/m² body surface area = 24-hour requirements
2. Evaporative water loss from burn wound
   a. Adults: 25 + % total body surface area burn ((m² body surface area) = ml/hr
   b. Children: 35 + % total body surface area burn (m² body surface area) = ml/hr
3. Total hourly maintenance fluids
   Basal fluid requirements per day ÷ 24 hours + evaporative water loss per hour = ml/hr maintenance fluids
   Example: A 70-kg adult with a 50% total body surface area burn and a body surface area of 2 m requires the following:
   - Basal = (1500 ml/day) (2 m² body surface area) = 3000 ml/24 hr, or 125 ml/hr
   - Evaporative = (25 + 50% total body surface burn)
   - (2 m² total body surface area) = (75) (2) = 150 ml/hr
   - Total maintenance fluids = 125 ml + 150 ml = 275 ml/hr

*From end of burn shock until wound closure is achieved.

The endpoint of burn shock is defined as the state in which the individual is able to maintain adequate urine output for 2 hours with the intravenous fluid administration rate equal to the individual's calculated maintenance rate (Box 48-4). As burn shock ends, fluid administered remains in the circulating volume and is reflected as an increase in urine output. The mechanism whereby capillary integrity is restored is unknown but usually occurs about 24 hours after burn injury (Figure 48-17). After the individual has reached the endpoint of burn shock, the term used to describe the vascular status of the individual is **capillary seal.** In individuals with large burns, colloid-containing fluids may be given to help maintain oncotic pressure during the resuscitation phase and afterward to enhance the mobilization of interstitial fluid and diuresis.[101] Efforts to decrease burn edema and fluid resuscitation volumes can involve the use of hypertonic fluid resuscitation as well.[102]

Cellular Response to Burn Injury

In addition to capillary endothelial permeability changes resulting in vascular fluid losses, transmembrane potential changes occur in cells not directly damaged by heat. The normal potential of −90 mV decreases to nearly −70 mV, with an increase in intracellular sodium and water. Such membrane potential

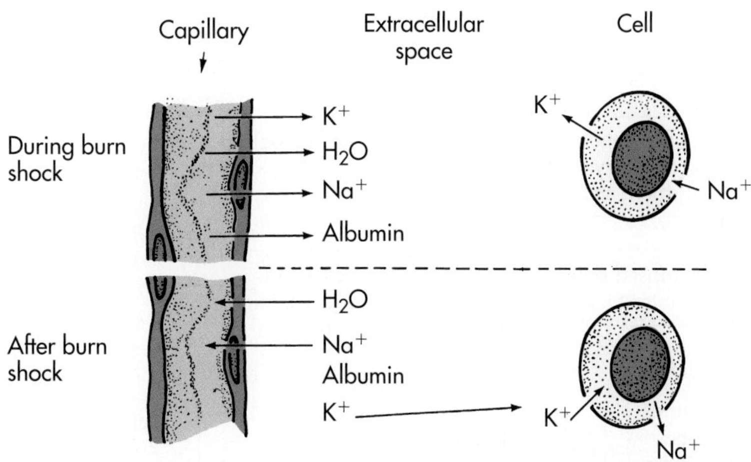

FIGURE 48-17 Direction of Fluid and Electrolyte Shifts Associated with Burn Shock. (Courtesy Intermountain Burn Center, University of Utah.)

changes may be caused by a circulating shock factor.[103] Apoptosis is central to the cellular responses to burn injury.[104] Other changes can be categorized as: (1) a metabolic response to the burn injury or (2) an immunologic response to the burn injury.

Metabolic Response. The metabolic changes after a burn injury were described in 1967 by Welt and associates as "sick cell syndrome."[105] This was considered to be a cell membrane transport defect related to an alteration in the steady-state composition characterized by high intracellular concentrations of sodium. Trunkey and colleagues[106] found a marked decrease in primate muscle extracellular water and an increase in intracellular sodium and water during hypovolemic shock. In addition, other researchers demonstrated an associated decrease in resting membrane potential, a decrease in amplitude of the action potential, and a prolongation of the repolarization and depolarization times in association with a decreased intracellular potassium concentration.[107,108] The cellular dysfunction of burn injury extends beyond the transmembrane potential disruption and the sodium-potassium pump impairment to include a loss of intracellular magnesium and phosphate[109] and elevated serum lactic acid dehydrogenase (LDH) levels.[110] Thus impairment of basic cellular function may be the underlying cause of the diminished membrane potentials. The data suggest a decrease in the efficiency of the pump. The failure of rapid intravascular volume repletion to restore membrane potential completely suggests other pathways for cellular metabolic derangement.[111]

Metabolic reactions to the stress of a major burn injury involve the response of the sympathetic nervous system and other homeostatic regulators. Catecholamines are found in elevated amounts in both the serum and urine of burned individuals. Cortisol, glucagon, and insulin levels are elevated, with a corresponding increase in gluconeogenesis, lipolysis, and proteolysis. Changes in lipid metabolism are reflected as an elevation in the levels of plasma free fatty acids (FFAs) and a decrease in the levels of plasma cholesterol and phospholipids.[112] Herndon and colleagues found that the use of propranolol, a nonselective $beta_1$- and $beta_2$-blocker, could decrease symptoms of the hypermetabolic, hypercatabolic, and osteopenic responses in pediatric patients, including a decrease in heart rate and lipolysis.[112a] Glucose and lactate kinetics are altered after burn injury. Although tissue hypoxia produces lactic acidosis, its persistence in the presence of adequate tissue perfusion suggests an increased rate of glycogenolysis.[113]

Burn injury induces a hypermetabolic state that persists until wound closure. Wilmore and colleagues[114] described the hypermetabolic state of 20 burned individuals as unrelated to ambient temperatures, with persistent elevation of core body temperatures. The metabolic rate increased with burn size in a curvilinear relationship, with oxygen consumption rarely exceeding two times basal levels. Evaporative water loss and surface cooling are not the primary stimulus for the hypermetabolic state; rather, the hypermetabolism is related to an increase and resetting of the thermal regulatory set point. A core body temperature of 38.5° C (101.3° F) is typical. A reflex arc mobilizes neural or hormonal afferent stimuli to the hypothalamus, producing a catecholamine response clinically manifested as hypermetabolism, hyperthermia, and hyperglycemia.

Evidence also exists that the burn wound itself directly mediates the response to injury at both the local and system levels. Cytokines, oxygen-free radicals, chemotactic substances, and eicosanoids contribute to the systemic inflammatory response and hypermetabolic state. The inflammatory response to the wound level is magnified into a generalized systemic inflammatory response that is often deleterious.[115-117] Vasodilation, increased capillary permeability, and edema occur to facilitate healing of the local area. The distribution of the peripheral circulation after burn injury transports heat and glucose preferentially to the wound. The energy cost of these reparative and transport processes is reflected in the increased metabolism and hyperdynamic circulation.

The extensive evaporative water loss that occurs in burn tissue is a heat-consuming process, and the energy of evaporation is provided by increased visceral heat production. The signal for the response is unknown because individuals whose wounds have been denervated continue to have a **posttraumatic hypermetabolic response.** Hypothalamic function alterations result in the elevation of human growth hormone (hGH) serum levels in the presence of hyperglycemia, a finding opposite that

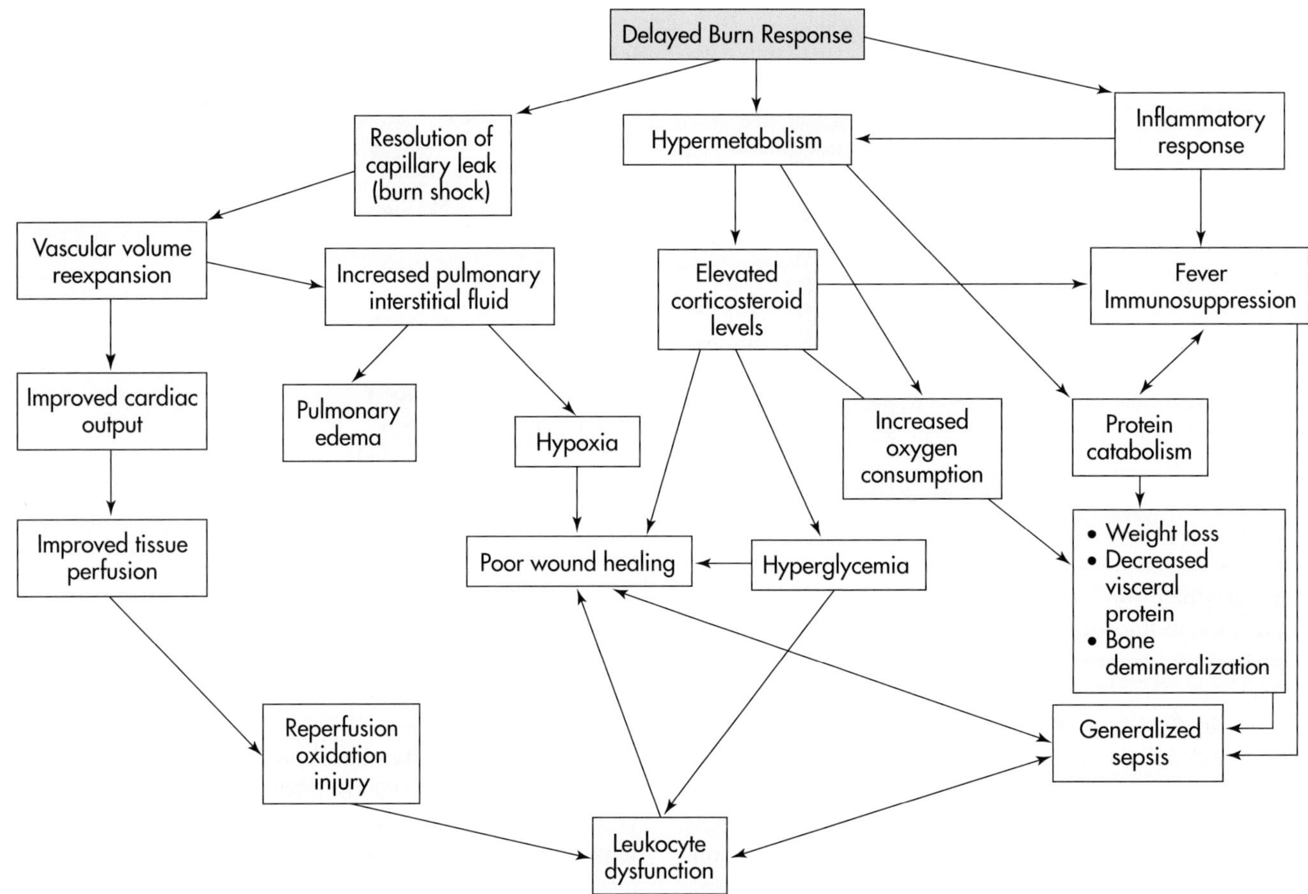

FIGURE 48-18 Physiologic Alterations in Inflammatory Burn Injury Response.

in normal states.[114] Further, the hypermetabolic rate is not decreased during rest, sleep, or warmth.

Evidence of hepatic response to burn injury is characterized by alterations in the clotting factors.[118] A hypercoagulable state develops as manifested by an elevated plasma fibrinogen concentration in the presence of shortened prothrombin time (PT) and activated partial thromboplastin time (PTT).[119]

In summary, extensive burn injury initiates the most marked alterations in body metabolism associated with any illness (Figure 48-18). Much of the work explaining this response has been conducted by Wilmore,[120,121] who reported that the persistent tachycardia, hyperpnea, hyperpyrexia, and marked body wasting seen in burn injury reflect heightened metabolic activity and accelerated body catabolism. The development of decreased bone density can last long after discharge from the hospital.[122] These system alterations occur as a result of the cutaneous inflammatory process and are thought to facilitate wound repair. The neural component of this alteration is in response to a sympathetic reaction that releases catecholamines in large amounts.

Immunologic Response. The immunologic response to burn injury is immediate, prolonged, and severe. The result in individuals surviving burn shock is immunosuppression with increased susceptibility to potentially fatal systemic burn wound sepsis.

Several cytokines have been identified in the immediate postburn period. IL-1 (interkeukin-1) is detected in the serum of burned individuals. The level of IL-1 correlates inversely with burn survival; low levels may be associated with a higher mortality.[123] Fatal burn injury has often shown decreased levels of IL-2, which may result in decreased T helper 1 (Th-1) lymphocytes. Th-1 cells produce IL-2, interferon-gamma, and TNF, which help to initiate cellular immunity and immunoglobulin G (IgG) production. IL-4 is elevated after burn injuries and causes a shift in the T helper cell production from Th-1 to Th-2 lymphocytes. Th-2 cells secrete IL-4 which promotes further conversion of nonspecific Th cells to Th-2 cells. Th-2 cells also produce other cytokines and antibodies.[124] IL-6 levels increase quickly after burn injury and remain elevated for several weeks. The level of IL-6 correlates with the extent of burn injury.[125] IL-6 and platelet-activating factor (PAF) activates polymorphonuclear neutrophils (PMNs) causing infiltration of neutrophils into burned tissue and adhesion to vascular endothelial surfaces.[126,127] IL-8 levels are elevated after burn injury, with significantly greater elevations in individuals with a TBSA burn of 40% or higher. IL-8 activity may play a role in the strong and persistent activation of neutrophils noted in people with large burns.[128] Burn blister fluid contains large amounts of IL-6 and IL-8 in addition to substances such as epidermal growth factor, platelet-derived growth factor, and TGF.[129]

Macrophages, platelets, neutrophils, and vascular endothelial cells release prostaglandins and leukotrienes, which are the byproducts of arachidonic acid metabolism. These chemical mediators cause peripheral vasodilation, pulmonary vasoconstriction, increased capillary permeability, and local tissue ischemia in the burn wound.

A host of chemicals found in burn plasma in altered concentrations also may play a role in burn shock. These include vasoactive amines (histamine, serotonin), products of complement activation (C3a, C5a), prostaglandins, kinins, endotoxin, and metabolic hormones (catecholamines, glucocorticoids). A decrease in complement components C3a and C5a in the circulation after burn injury suggests a nonspecific activation of the complement system.[130] Activation of the complement system in injured tissue results in an inflammatory response caused by release of histamine and serotonin by C3a and C5a, because histamine and serotonin alter capillary permeability and participate in the mechanism of burn shock along with kinin polypeptides and other chemical mediators. Prostaglandins function in the inflammatory process by regulating metabolism of cells of inflammation (see Chapter 7).

Burn shock can induce changes in the integrity of the intestinal wall, facilitating bacterial translocation and endotoxemia.[131] Bacterial translocation from the gut may be a mechanism of infection leading to septic shock after burn injury and other major trauma.[132] Circulating endotoxin is correlated with the development of MODS and death after major burn injury.[133]

White blood cells are also altered at this time, when their need to inhibit sepsis is vital. Natural resistance to infection in burn wounds is a function of the nonspecific immune system; that is, resistance to microorganisms that infect wounds rests almost solely on the ability of phagocytic cells (i.e., granulocytes, macrophages) to leave the bloodstream, migrate to the site of infection, and ingest and kill microorganisms.[134] Opsonins normally render bacteria susceptible to phagocytosis but the burn injury triggers a consumptive opsoninopathy. Burn serum contains an inhibitor of C3 conversion that leads to decreased opsonization and polymorphonuclear (PMN) dysfunction.[135,136]

Individuals with altered immunocompetence before burn injury are at additional risk for complications. Opportunistic infections, such as fungal sepsis, can increase a hospital stay and ICU costs.[137] Included in this group are individuals at the extremes of age and those with cardiac disease, malnutrition, immunodeficiency disease, and a history of alcohol or drug abuse.[138,139] Additional risk factors include diabetes mellitus and pulmonary or renal dysfunction.

Evaporative Water Loss

One of the major purposes of intact skin is to serve as a barrier to evaporative water loss (EWL) from the body. With major burn injury, this ability of the skin to regulate evaporative water loss is totally disrupted. In a classic 1962 study, Moncrief and Mason[140] attempted to determine the magnitude of such a loss and determined that daily evaporative water loss was in the range of 20 times normal in the early phase of injury, with gradual decreases as wound closure is achieved. Further studies indicated that insensible water loss through burned skin is not from evaporation of water from sweat glands but rather from water vapor formed within the body and lost through the skin.[141,142]

Calculation of the amount of fluid lost by evaporative water loss includes losses from all sources. Normally the skin is the major source of insensible loss (75%) and the lungs are minor sources (25%), with a total loss of only approximately 600 to 800 ml/day. This changes dramatically with burns, because not only does skin loss increase but also lung loss increases by hypermetabolism and hyperventilation, especially in an intubated individual. Total evaporative losses exceed many liters per day in an adult with large burn wounds. Replacement of the loss is mandatory to prevent volume deficit.

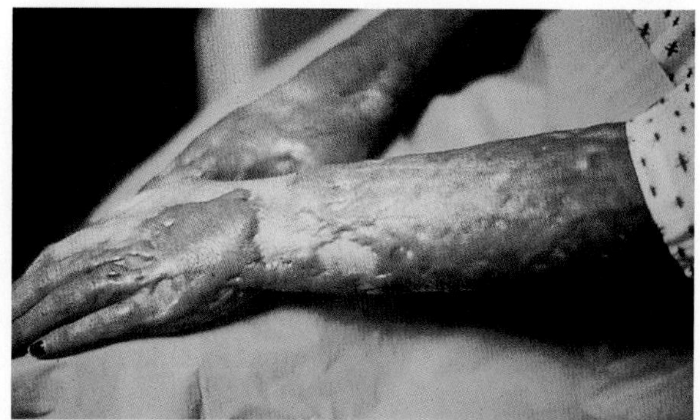

FIGURE 48-19 Hypertrophic Scarring. Deep partial-thickness thermal injury can result in extensive hypertrophic scarring. (Courtesy Intermountain Burn Center, University of Utah.)

EVALUATION AND TREATMENT. Burn recovery can be long and difficult, with complications often the rule rather than the exception. The goal of burn management is wound closure in a manner that promotes survival. Scar formation with contractures is often a consequence of healing in deep partial-thickness and full-thickness burns (Figure 48-19; see also Figure 48-10). Assessment of tissue viability can be difficult in complex extremity injury; pyrophosphate nuclear scanning can assist in evaluation.[143] Early intervention may have effects on tissue survival as is evident in the zone of stasis and application of cerium nitrate.[144] The advancement in survival and outcome can be as simple as using antibiotic catheters to reduce catheter-associated bloodstream infections[145] or better glycemic management during ICU treatment.[146] Advances in care systems have shown the value of advanced practice nurses in a collaborative role in the burn ICU and emergency departments.[147]

The three essential elements of survival of major burn injury are: (1) meticulous wound management, (2) adequate fluids and nutrition, and (3) early surgical excision and grafting. Current therapy for deep partial- and full-thickness burn injury includes surgical removal of the burn tissue (excision) followed by grafting of the person's unburned skin (autograft) onto the excised wound. Techniques of early wound care, such as the use of amniotic membrane,[148] may well affect the nature of burn scarring. Satisfactory wound closure with cultured epithelial autograft (Figure 48-20) has been inconsistent and costly.[149,150] Early enthusiasm for synthetic dermal replacement has been tempered by a high rate of dermal graft loss and slow epidermal engraftment.[151,152] Such advancements in skin replacement technology include sheets of acellular dermal matrix that can be used with thin, meshed autografts or cultured epithelial autografts.[153,154] This concept also is being used on the donor site; glycosaminoglycan hydrogels, and even topical gene therapy or stem-cell applications,[155-157] may supplement donor site wound

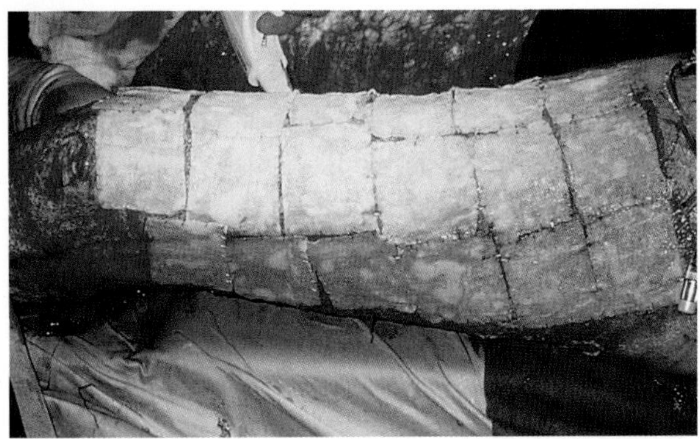

FIGURE 48-20 Application of Cultured Epithelial Autografts. The thin sheets of keratinocytes are attached to gauze backing to allow application onto the clean, excised thigh. (Courtesy Intermountain Burn Center, University of Utah.)

dressings.[158] Scar reduction or prevention is a challenging problem that is being addressed with pulsed-dye laser treatment.[159] Current research also is directed toward therapies to modulate hypermetabolic and inflammatory responses. Nutritional therapy is focused on early enteral feeding to reduce the potential of gut-mediated sepsis. Ongoing clinical trials using anabolic agents (e.g., recombinant human growth hormone) and pharmacologic agents that modulate inflammatory and endocrine mediators (e.g., ibuprofen, propranolol) show promise in the treatment of severe burn injuries.[99] Altered body image is a significant hurdle to those with facial burns. A supportive framework to aid individuals is essential to integrate them back into the community.[160] Burn pain is almost always acute and treatment strategies usually differ from strategies for chronic pain. The understanding and management of burn pain is key to recovery.[161,162] In addition to opioid-based agents, newer treatment approaches may include antianxiety agents, hypnosis, and relaxation techniques,[163] as well as virtual reality systems.[69,164]

SUMMARY REVIEW

Shock

1. Shock occurs when the cardiovascular system fails to perfuse tissue, cells, and organs adequately, causing a widespread impairment of cellular metabolism and tissue function. It is a downward physiologic spiral that, if not reversed, can lead to MODS.
2. Types of shock are cardiogenic, hypovolemic, neurogenic or vasogenic, anaphylactic, and septic.
3. The final common pathway in all types of shock is impaired cellular metabolism and cells switch from aerobic to anaerobic metabolism. Energy stores drop, and cellular mechanisms relative to membrane permeability, action potentials, and lysozyme release fail.
4. Anaerobic metabolism results in activation of the inflammatory response, decreased circulatory volume, and decreasing pH.
5. Impaired cellular metabolism results in cellular inability to use glucose because of impaired glucose delivery or impaired glucose intake, resulting in a shift of glycogenolysis, gluconeogenesis, and lipolysis for fuel generation.
6. Glycogenolysis is affected for up to 10 hours. Gluconeogenesis results in the use of proteins necessary for structure, function, repair, and replication that leads to more impaired cellular metabolism. Lipolysis is ineffective because of a lack of transport serum proteins.
7. Gluconeogenesis contributes to lactic acid, uric acid, and ammonia buildup; interstitial edema; and impairment of the immune system, as well as general muscle weakness leading to decreased respiratory function and cardiac output.
8. Cardiogenic shock results from persistent hypotension and tissue hypoperfusion caused by cardiac dysfunction in the presence of adequate intravascular volume and left ventricular filling pressure.
9. Hypovolemic shock is caused by loss of whole blood, plasma, or interstitial fluid in large amounts. The use of compensatory mechanisms may be vigorous, but tissue perfusion ultimately decreases and results in impaired cellular metabolism.
10. Neurogenic (vasogenic) shock results from massive vasodilation that results from an imbalance between parasympathetic and sympathetic stimulation of vascular smooth muscle. It causes a relative hypovolemia (even though cardiac output may be high), and results in impaired cellular metabolism.
11. Anaphylactic shock is the outcome of a widespread hypersensitivity to an allergen that triggers anaphylaxis. The inflammatory response is triggered, and a massive vasodilation with fluid shift into the interstitium follows. The relative hypovolemia leads to impaired cellular metabolism.
12. Septic shock begins with impaired cellular metabolism caused by uncontrolled septicemia. The infecting agent triggers the inflammatory and immune responses. It is part of a continuum known as SIRS. Mortality for septic shock is very high.

Multiple Organ Dysfunction Syndrome

1. MODS is the progressive dysfunction of two or more organ systems resulting from a systemic inflammatory response after a severe illness or injury. The inflammatory response can be triggered by sepsis, necrotic tissue, trauma, burns, ARDS, acute pancreatitis, major surgery, circulatory shock, DIC, acute renal failure, blood transfusion, heat stroke, liver failure, mesenteric ischemia, propofol infusion syndrome, persistent inflammatory foci, and other severe injuries.
2. Primary MODS is the immediate local or mild systemic response to the triggering event or illness. It primes the inflammatory system.

SUMMARY REVIEW—cont'd

3. Secondary MODS is the uncontrollable, excessive systemic inflammatory response that develops after a latent period and results in organ dysfunction.
4. People at greatest risk for developing MODS are older adults, those with significant tissue injury or preexisting disease, and those in whom resuscitation from the initiating illness or injury has been delayed or inadequate.
5. MODS is a leading cause of mortality in surgical intensive care units (ICUs). Mortality for individuals with MODS increases progressively from 54% with two failing organ systems to 100% with five failing organ systems.
6. Multiple organ dysfunction involves the stress response; release of complement, coagulation, and kinin proteins; changes in the vascular endothelium; and numerous inflammatory processes mediated by substances released by activated neutrophils and macrophages. The accumulation of activated neutrophils in organs is thought to play a key role in the pathogenesis of MODS, as well as macrophages.
7. The consequences of the release of inflammatory mediators in MODS are vasodilation, increased vasopermeability, and selective vasoconstriction resulting in maldistribution of blood flow; hypermetabolism; myocardial depression; and hypoxic injury to cells. Cellular hypoxia and acidosis impair cellular metabolism, leading to organ dysfunction.
8. Clinical manifestations of the development of MODS are general during the first 24 hours: low-grade fever, tachycardia, tachypnea, dyspnea, and altered mental status. Over the next several days, beginning with the lungs, individual organ systems show signs of failure.
9. Because there is no specific therapy for MODS, early detection is extremely important so that supportive measures can be initiated as soon as possible.
10. At present the therapeutic management of MODS consists of prevention or removal of triggering mechanisms and support of individual organs. Recent scientific knowledge about inflammatory mediators has led to many promising future therapies for MODS.

Burns

1. Burns are classified according to depth and extent of injury.
2. First-degree burns involve the superficial skin without loss of protective function.
3. Second-degree burns are superficial (blister formation) or superficial involving partial skin thickness with a waxy white appearance and no involvement of dermal appendages.
4. Third-degree burns involve full skin thickness and often underlying tissues. They are painless and can be life threatening as a result of hypovolemic shock and metabolic and immunologic responses.
5. The TBSA burned is estimated using either the rule of nines or the Lund and Browder chart.
6. Hypovolemia associated with burn shock is caused by increased capillary permeability with massive fluid losses from blood volume.
7. Altered cell membrane permeability and loss of electrolyte homeostasis contribute to burn shock.
8. Cardiac contractility is decreased during the first 24 hours with shunting of blood away from the liver, kidney, and gut.
9. Fluid resuscitation, such as with lactated Ringer solution, involves infusion of fluid at a rate faster than the loss of circulating volume.
10. The most reliable criterion for adequate resuscitation of burn shock is urine output.
11. Capillary seal is the term used to indicate the end of burn shock.
12. Transmembrane potentials are altered in cells not directly damaged by heat, with impairment of the sodium-potassium pump and loss of magnesium and phosphate.
13. The stress of a major burn activates the sympathetic nervous system with release of catecholamines, cortisol, glucagon, and insulin.
14. Burn injury produces a hypermetabolic state that persists until wound closure and is related to a higher thermal regulatory set point.
15. The local inflammatory response at the burn site releases cytokines, oxygen-free radicals, chemotactic factors, and eicosanoids, which lead to a systemic inflammatory response and contributes to hypermetabolism.
16. A posttraumatic hypermetabolic response is associated with increased visceral heat production.
17. Alterations in clotting factors produce a hypercoagulable state following major burns.
18. The immune response following a burn is immediate, prolonged, and severe.
19. Numerous alterations in inflammatory cytokines are evident in the immediate burn period, affecting cellular immunity, antibody production, and attraction of neutrophils and contributing to the vasodilation and increased capillary permeability associated with burn shock.
20. White blood cells are altered, and there is decreased opsonization and phagocytosis, contributing to the development of sepsis.
21. Changes in intestinal wall integrity lead to translocation of bacteria, endotoxemia, and septic shock.
22. Loss of intact skin with a major burn results in significant evaporative water loss contributing to hypovolemia.
23. Treatment of major burns involves meticulous wound management, adequate fluids and nutrition, early surgical excision and grafting, modulation of the hypermetabolic state, and pain management.

KEY TERMS

REFERENCES

1. *Mosby's medical dictionary*, ed 8, St Louis, 2009, Mosby.
2. Bonanno FG: Shock—a reappraisal: the holistic approach, *J Emerg Trauma Shock* 5(2):167–177, 2012.
3. Cunneen J, Cartwright M: The puzzle of sepsis: fitting the pieces of the inflammatory response with treatment, *AACN Clin Issues* 15(1):18–44, 2004.
4. Edul VS, Dubin A, Ince C: The microcirculation as a therapeutic target in the treatment of sepsis and shock, *Semin Respir Crit Care Med* 32(5):558–568, 2011.
5. Schmeltz LR: Management of inpatient hyperglycemia, *Lab Med* 42(7):427–434, 2011.
6. Topalian S, Ginsberg F, Parrillo J: Cardiogenic shock, *Crit Care Med* 36(1):S66–S77, 2008.
7. Jackson C, Boenau IB: How to recognize cardiogenic shock, *Emerg Med* 39(10):11–19, 2007.
8. Babaev A et al: Trends in management and outcomes of patients with acute myocardial infarction complicated by cardiogenic shock, *JAMA* 294(4):448–454, 2005.
9. Omland T: Advances in congestive heart failure management in the intensive care unit: b-type natriuretic peptides in evaluation of acute heart failure, *Crit Care Med* 36(1):S17–S27, 2008.
10. Fox JT, Gowda RM, Khan IA: Cardiogenic shock: basics and clinical considerations, *Int J Cardiol* 123(3):221, 2008.
11. Myat A et al: The intra-aortic balloon pump in high-risk percutaneous coronary intervention, *Interv Cardiol* 4(2):211–234, 2012.
12. Sleeper LA et al: Functional status and quality of life after emergency revascularization for cardiogenic shock complicating acute myocardial infarction, *J Am Coll Cardiol* 46:266–273, 2005.
13. Hochman J et al: Early revascularization and long-term survival in cardiogenic shock complicating acute myocardial infarction, *JAMA* 295(21):2511–2515, 2006.
14. Holmes CL, Walley KR: The evaluation and management of shock, *Clin Chest Med* 24(4):775–789, 2003.
15. Russell J: Vasopressin versus norepinephrine infusion in patients with septic shock, *N Engl J Med* 358(9):877–887, 2008.
16. Simons FE et al: 2012 update: World Allergy Organization Guidelines for the assessment and management of anaphylaxis, *Curr Opin Allergy Clin Immunol* 12(4):389–399, 2012.
17. Simons FE et al: World Allergy Organization anaphylaxis guidelines: summary, *J Allergy Clin Immunol* 127(3):587–593, e22, 2011.
18. Levy MM et al: 2001 SCCM/ESICM/ACCP/ATS/SIS International Sepsis Definition Conference, *Crit Care Med* 31(4):1250–1256, 2003.
19. Calandra T, Cohen J: The international sepsis forum consensus conference on definitions of infection in the intensive care unit, *Crit Care Med* 33(7):1538–1548, 2005.
20. Melamed A, Sorvillo FJ: The burden of sepsis-associated mortality in the United States from 1999 to 2005: an analysis of multiple-cause-of-death data, *Crit Care* 13:R28, 2009.
21. Wenzel RP: Health care-associated infections: major issues in the early years of the 21st century, *Clin Infect Dis* 15(45 Suppl 1):S85–S88, 2007.
22. Albrecht SJ et al: Reemergence of gram-negative health care-associated bloodstream infections, *Arch Intern Med* 166(12):1289–1294, 2006.
23. Kleinpell RM, Graves BT, Ackerman MH: Incidence, pathogenesis, and management of sepsis: an overview, *AACN Adv Crit Care* 17(4):385–393, 2006.
24. Papathanassoglou ED et al: Association of proinflammatory molecules with apoptotic markers and survival in critically ill multiple organ dysfunction patients, *Biol Res Nurs* 5(2):129–141, 2003.
25. Cannon CM et al: The GENESIS Project (GENeralized Early Sepsis Intervention Strategies): a multicenter quality improvement collaborative, *J Intensive Care Med*, 2012 Aug 17. [Epub ahead of print.].
26. Rivers E et al: Early goal-directed therapy in the treatment of severe sepsis and septic shock, *N Engl J Med* 345:1368–1377, 2001.
27. Dellinger RP et al: Surviving sepsis campaign: international guidelines for management of severe sepsis and septic shock: 2012, *Crit Care Med* 41(2):580–637, 2013.
28. Wilson J, Bion J: *Surviving sepsis campaign: guidelines for management of severe sepsis and septic shock*, 2008. Available at www.survivingsepsis.org. Accessed July 27, 2012.
29. Friswell AC: Surviving sepsis campaign previews updated guidelines for 2012, *Pulmon Rev* 17(5):1, 5, 2012.
30. Kopterides P et al: Procalcitonin-guided algorithms of antibiotic therapy in the intensive care unit: a systematic review and meta-analysis of randomized controlled trials, *Crit Care Med* 38(11):2229–2241, 2010.
31. Layios N et al: Procalcitonin usefulness for the initiation of antibiotic treatment in intensive care unit patients, *Crit Care Med* 40(8):2304–2309, 2012.
32. Baue AE: Multiple, progressive or sequential system failure: a syndrome for the 70's, *Arch Surg* 110(7):779–781, 1975.
33. Tilney NL, Bailey GL, Morgan AP: Sequential system failure after rupture of abdominal aortic aneurysm: an unsolved problem in postoperative care, *Ann Surg* 178(2):117–122, 1973.
34. Awad SS: State-of-the-art therapy for severe sepsis and multisystem organ dysfunction, *Am J Surg* 186(Suppl):23S–30S, 2003.
35. Sauaia A et al: Validation of postinjury multiple organ failure scores, *Shock* 31(5):438–447, 2009.
36. Rotstein OD: Modeling the two-hit hypothesis for evaluating strategies to prevent organ injury after shock/resuscitation, *J Trauma* 54(Suppl 5):S203–S206, 2003.
37. Abraham E, Singer M: Mechanism of sepsis-induced organ dysfunction, *Crit Care Med* 35(10):2408–2416, 2007.
38. Shapiro NI et al: The association of endothelial cell signaling, severity of illness, and organ dysfunction in sepsis, *Crit Care* 14(5):R182–R192, 2010.
39. Vanhorebeek I, Van den Berghe G: The neuroendocrine response to critical illness is a dynamic process, *Crit Care Clin* 22(1):1–15, 2006.
40. Aird WC: The role of the endothelium in severe sepsis & MODS, *Blood* 101:3756–3777, 2003.
41. van Meurs M et al: Early organ-specific endothelial activation during hemorrhagic shock and resuscitation, *Shock* 29(2):291–299, 2008.
42. Souto FO et al: Essential role of CCR2 in neutrophil tissue infiltration and multiple organ dysfunction in sepsis, *Am J Respir Crit Care Med* 183(2):234–242, 2011.
43. Brown KA et al: Neutrophils in development of multiple organ failure in sepsis, *Lancet* 8(368):157–169, 2006.
44. Baue AE: Mediators or markers of injury, inflammation, and infection (harbingers of doom or predictors of disaster) and biologic puzzles or ambiguities, *Arch Surg* 142(1):89–93, 2007.
45. King JE: Sepsis in critical care, *Crit Care Nurs North Am* 19(1):77–86, 2007.
46. Rankin JA: Biological mediators of acute inflammation, *AACN Clin Issues* 15(1):3–17, 2004.

47. Matsuda N, Hattori Y: Systemic inflammatory response syndrome (SIRS): molecular pathophysiology and gene therapy, *J Pharmacol Sci* 101(3):189–198, 2006.
48. Deitch EA, Xu D, Kaise VL: Role of the gut in the development of injury- and shock-induced SIRS and MODS: the gut-lymph hypothesis, a review, *Front Biosci* 1(11):520–528, 2006.
49. Silvestri L et al: Impact of selective decontamination of the digestive tract on multiple organ dysfunction syndrome: systematic review of randomized controlled trials, *Crit Care Med* 38(5):1370–1376, 2010.
50. Gando S: Microvascular thrombosis and multiple organ dysfunction syndrome, *Crit Care Med* 38(2):S35–S42, 2010.
51. Schmidt H et al: Autonomic dysfunction predicts both 1- and 2-month mortality in middle-aged patients with multiple organ dysfunction syndrome, *Crit Care Med* 36(3):967–970, 2008.
52. Fernandes CJ Jr, de Assuncao MSC: Myocardial dysfunction in sepsis: a large, unsolved puzzle, *Crit Care Res Pract*, 2012. Article ID 896340.
53. Merx MW, Weber C: Sepsis and the heart, *Circulation* 116(7):793–802, 2007.
54. Brown MJ et al: The systemic inflammatory response syndrome, organ failure, and mortality after abdominal aortic aneurysm repair, *J Vasc Surg* 37(3):600–606, 2003.
55. Minne L, Abu-Hanna A, de Jonge E: Evaluation of SOFA-based models for predicting mortality in the ICU: a systematic review, *Crit Care* 12(6):R161–R174, 2008.
56. Blot SI et al: Clinical and economic outcomes in critically ill patients with nosocomial catheter-related bloodstream infections, *Clin Infect Dis* 41(11):1591–1598, 2005.
57. The Acute Respiratory Distress Syndrome Network: Ventilation with lower tidal volumes as compared with traditional tidal volumes for acute lung injury and the acute respiratory distress syndrome, *N Engl J Med* 342:1301–1308, 2000.
58. Magnotti LJ, Deitch EA: Burns, bacterial translocation, gut barrier function, and failure, *J Burn Care Rehabil* 26(5):383–391, 2005.
59. Boomer JS et al: Immunosuppression in patients who die of sepsis and multiple organ failure, *JAMA* 306(23):2594–2605, 2011.
60. Aggarwal S, Smailes S, Dziewulski P: Tracheostomy in burns patients revisited, *Burns* 35(7):962–966, 2009.
61. Clayton N, Kennedy P, Maitz P: The severe burns patient with tracheostomy: implications for management of dysphagia, dysphonia and laryngotracheal pathology, *Burns* 36(6):850–855, 2010.
62. American Burn Association: *Burn incidence and treatment in the U.S.: 2012 fact sheet*. Chicago, IL, 2012, Author. Available at www.ameriburn.org/rsources_factsheet.php.
63. Brigham PA, McLoughlin E: Burn incidence and medical care use in the United States: estimates, trends, and data sources, *J Burn Care Rehabil* 17(2):95–107, 1996.
64. Sen S, Greenhalgh D, Palmieri T: Review of burn research for the year 2010, *J Burn Care Res* 33(5):577–586, 2012.
65. Saffle JR, Edelman L, Morris SE: Regional air transport of burn patients: a case for telemedicine? *J Trauma* 57(1):57–64, 2004.
66. Syed-Abdul S et al: Telemedicine utilization to support the management of the burns treatment involving patient pathways in both developed and developing countries: a case study, *J Burn Care Res* 33(4):e207–e212, 2012.
67. Wallace DL et al: A systematic review of the evidence for telemedicine in burn care: with a UK perspective, *Burns* 38(4):465–480, 2012.
68. Falder S et al: Core outcomes for adult burn survivors: a clinical overview, *Burns* 35(5):618–641, 2009.
69. Mackey SP et al: Return to work after burns: a qualitative research study, *Burns* 35(3):338–342, 2009.
70. Cochran A et al: Self-reported quality of life after electrical and thermal injury, *J Burn Care Rehabil* 25(1):61–66, 2004.
71. Altintas MA et al: Differentiation of superficial-partial vs. deep-partial thickness burn injuries in vivo by confocal-laser-scanning microscopy, *Burns* 35(1):80–86, 2009.
72. Braue EH Jr et al: Noninvasive methods for determining lesion depth from vesicant exposure, *J Burn Care Res* 28(2):275–285, 2007.
73. Chiu T, Burd A: Laboratory assessment of burn depth, *Plast Reconstr Surg* 119(2):751–752, 2007.
74. Cross KM et al: Clinical utilization of near-infrared spectroscopy devices for burn depth, *Wound Repair Regen* 15(3):332–340, 2007.
75. Devgan L et al: Modalities for the assessment of burn wound depth, *J Burns Wounds* 5:e2, 2006.
76. Hoeksema H et al: Accuracy of early burn depth assessment by laser Doppler imaging on different days post burn, *Burns* 35(1):36–45, 2009.
77. Kassira W, Namias N: Outpatient management of pediatric burns, *J Craniofac Surg* 19(4):1007–1009, 2008.
78. Mandal A: Burn wound depth assessment—is laser Doppler imaging the best measurement tool available? *Int Wound J* 3(2):138–143, 2006.
79. McGill DJ et al: Assessment of burn depth: a prospective, blinded comparison of laser Doppler imaging and videomicroscopy, *Burns* 33(7):833–842, 2007.
80. Monstrey S et al: Assessment of burn depth and burn wound healing potential, *Burns* 34(6):761–769, 2008.
81. Ng D et al: The use of laser Doppler imaging for burn depth assessment after application of flammacerium, *Burns* 33(3):396–397, 2007.
82. Renkielska A et al: Burn depths evaluation based on active dynamic IR thermal imaging—a preliminary study, *Burns* 32(7):867–875, 2006.
83. Tehrani H et al: Spectrophotometric intracutaneous analysis: a novel imaging technique in the assessment of acute burn depth, *Ann Plast Surg* 61(4):437–440, 2008.
84. Hosseini SN et al: Xenoderm versus 1% silver sulfadiazine in partial-thickness burns, *Asian J Surg* 32(4):234–239, 2009.
85. Sheridan RL et al: Planimetry study of the percent of body surface represented by the hand and palm: sizing irregular burns is more accurately done with the palm, *J Burn Care Rehabil* 16(6):605–606, 1995.
86. Morris SE, Navaratnam N, Herndon DN: A comparison of effects of thermal injury and smoke inhalation on bacterial translocation, *J Trauma* 30(6):639–643, 1990.
87. Chen C et al: Myosin light chain kinase mediates intestinal barrier disruption following burn injury, *PLoS One* 7(4):e34946, 2012.
88. Arturson G: Forty years in burns research—the postburn inflammatory response, *Burns* 26(7):599–604, 2000.
89. Horton JW et al: Calcium antagonists improve cardiac mechanical performance after thermal trauma, *J Surg Res* 87(1):39–50, 1999.
90. Aikawa N, Martyn JA, Burke JF: Pulmonary artery catheterization and thermodilution cardiac output determination in the management of critically burned patients, *Am J Surg* 135(6):811–817, 1978.
91. Dobson EL, Warner GF: Factors concerned in the early stages of thermal shock, *Circ Res* 5(1):69–74, 1957.
92. Baxter CR, Cook WA, Shires GT: Serum myocardial depressant factor of burn shock, *Surg Forum* 17:1–2, 1966.
93. Lefer AM, Martin J: Origin of myocardial depressant factor in shock, *Am J Physiol* 218(5):1423–1442, 1970.
94. Rosenthal SR, Hawley PL, Hakim AA: Purified burn toxic factor and its competition, *Surgery* 71(4):527–536, 1972.
95. Horton JW, Burton KP, White DJ: The role of toxic oxygen metabolites in a young model of thermal injury, *J Trauma* 39(3):563–569, 1995.
96. Onuoha G, Alpar K, Jones I: Vasoactive intestinal peptide and nitric oxide in the acute phase following burns and trauma, *Burns* 27(1):17–21, 2001.
97. Ungureanu-Longrois D et al: Myocardial contractile dysfunction in the systemic inflammatory response syndrome: role of a cytokine-inducible nitric oxide synthase in cardiac myocytes, *J Mol Cell Cardiol* 27(1):155–167, 1995.
98. Gamelli RL et al: Burn-induced nitric oxide release in humans, *J Trauma* 39(5):869–877, 1995. discussion 77–78.
99. Baxter CR: Fluid volume and electrolyte changes of the early postburn period, *Clin Plast Surg* 1(4):693–703, 1974.
100. Huang PP et al: Hypertonic sodium resuscitation is associated with renal failure and death, *Ann Surg* 221(5):543–554, 1995.
101. Herndon DN, Spies M: Modern burn care, *Semin Pediatr Surg* 10(1):28–31, 2001.
102. Belba MK, Petrela EY, Belba GP: Comparison of hypertonic vs isotonic fluids during resuscitation of severely burned patients, *Am J Emerg Med* 27(9):1091–1096, 2009.
103. Evans JA, Darlington DN, Gann DS: A circulating factor(s) mediates cell depolarization in hemorrhagic shock, *Ann Surg* 213(6):549–556, 1991.
104. Duan H et al: Effect of burn injury on apoptosis and expression of apoptosis-related genes/proteins in skeletal muscles of rats, *Apoptosis* 14(1):52–65, 2009.
105. Welt LG: Membrane transport defect: the sick cell, *Trans Assoc Am Physicians* 80:217–226, 1967.
106. Trunkey DD et al: The effect of hemorrhagic shock on intracellular muscle action potentials in the primate, *Surgery* 74(2):241–250, 1973.
107. Cunningham JN Jr, Shires GT, Wagner Y: Changes in intracellular sodium and potassium content of red blood cells in trauma and shock, *Am J Surg* 122(5):650–654, 1971.
108. Rosenthal SR, Tabor H: Electrolyte changes and chemotherapy in experimental burn and traumatic shock and hemorrhage, *Arch Surg* 51:244, 1945.

109. Turinsky J, Gonnerman WA, Loose LD: Impaired mineral metabolism in postburn muscle, *J Trauma* 21(6):417–423, 1981.
110. Deets DK, Glaviano VV: Plasma and cardiac lactic dehydrogenase activity in burn shock, *Proc Soc Exp Biol Med* 142(2):412–416, 1973.
111. Button B: Evidence of circulating membrane depolarization factor(s) in hemorrhagic shock, *Shock* 1(Suppl):15, 1994.
112. Okamoto R, Glaviano VV, Pindok M: Myocardial lipases and catecholamines in burn shock, *Proc Soc Exp Biol Med* 137(1):347–353, 1971.
112a. Herndon DN et al: Long-term propranolol use in severely burned pediatric patients: a randomized controlled study, *Ann Surg* 256(3):402–411, 2012.
113. Wilmore DW, Aulick HL, Goodwin CW: Glucose metabolism following severe injury, *Acta Chir Scand Suppl* 498:43–47, 1980.
114. Wilmore DW et al: Alterations in hypothalamic function following thermal injury, *J Trauma* 15(8):697–703, 1975.
115. Gump FE, Price JB Jr, Kinney JM: Blood flow and oxygen consumption in patients with severe burns, *Surg Gynecol Obstet* 130(1):23–28, 1970.
116. Wilmore DW et al: Influence of the burn wound on local and systemic responses to injury, *Ann Surg* 186(4):444–458, 1977.
117. Wilmore DW et al: Effect of injury and infection on visceral metabolism and circulation, *Ann Surg* 192(4):491–504, 1980.
118. Holder IA, Neely AN: Hageman factor dependent activation and its relationship to lethal *Pseudomonas aeruginosa* burn wound infections, *Agents Actions Suppl* 38(Pt 3):329–342, 1992.
119. McManus WF, Eurenius K, Pruitt BA Jr: Disseminated intravascular coagulation in burned patients, *J Trauma* 13(5):416–422, 1973.
120. Wilmore DW, editor: *The metabolic management of the critically ill*, ed 2, New York, 1990, Plenum.
121. Wilmore DW, Aulick LH: Metabolic changes in burned patients, *Surg Clin North Am* 58(6):1173–1187, 1978.
122. Edelman LS et al: Sustained bone mineral density changes after burn injury, *J Surg Res* 114(2):172–178, 2003.
123. Wright K et al: Burn-activated neutrophils and tumor necrosis factor-alpha alter endothelial cell actin cytoskeleton and enhance monolayer permeability, *Surgery* 128(2):259–265, 2000.
124. Goebel A et al: Injury induces deficient interleukin-12 production, but interleukin-12 therapy after injury restores resistance to infection, *Ann Surg* 231(2):253–261, 2000.
125. Nishiura T et al: Gene expression and cytokine and enzyme activation in the liver after a burn injury, *J Burn Care Rehabil* 21(2):135–141, 2000.
126. Biffl WL et al: Interleukin-6 delays neutrophil apoptosis via a mechanism involving platelet-activating factor, *J Trauma* 40(4):575–578, 1996.
127. Choi M et al: Preventing the infiltration of leukocytes by monoclonal antibody blocks the development of progressive ischemia in rat burns, *Plast Reconstr Surg* 96(5):1177–1185, 1995.
128. Iocono JA et al: Interleukin-8 levels and activity in delayed-healing human thermal wounds, *Wound Repair Regen* 8(3):216–225, 2000.
129. Ortega MR, Ganz T, Milner SM: Human beta defensin is absent in burn blister fluid, *Burns* 26(8):724–726, 2000.
130. Heideman M, Kaijser B, Gelin LE: Complement activation and hematologic, hemodynamic, and respiratory reactions early after soft-tissue injury, *J Trauma* 18(10):696–700, 1978.
131. Grzybowski J et al: Antidietary antigen antibodies in the sera of patients with burns as a potential marker of gut mucosa integrity failure, *J Burn Care Rehabil* 13(2 Pt 1):194–197, 1992.
132. Deitch EA, Berg R: Bacterial translocation from the gut: a mechanism of infection, *J Burn Care Rehabil* 8(6):475–482, 1987.
133. Yao YM et al: The association of circulating endotoxaemia with the development of multiple organ failure in burned patients, *Burns* 21(4):255–258, 1995.
134. Benhaim P, Hunt TK: Natural resistance to infection: leukocyte functions, *J Burn Care Rehabil* 13(2 Pt 2):287–292, 1992.
135. Alexander JW et al: Consumptive opsoninopathy: possible pathogenesis in lethal and opportunistic infections, *Ann Surg* 184(6):672–678, 1976.
136. Bjornson AB, Altemeier WA, Bjornson HS: Changes in humoral components of host defense following burn trauma, *Ann Surg* 186(1):88–96, 1977.
137. Cochran A et al: Systemic *Candida* infection in burn patients: a case-control study of management patterns and outcomes, *Surg Infect (Larchmt)* 3(4):367–374, 2002.
138. Goff DR et al: Cardiac disease and the patient with burns, *J Burn Care Rehabil* 11(4):305–307, 1990.
139. McGill V et al: The impact of substance use on mortality and morbidity from thermal injury, *J Trauma* 38(6):931–934, 1995.
140. Moncrief JA, Mason AD Jr: Water vapor loss in the burned patient, *Surg Forum* 13:38–41, 1962.
141. Moncrief JA: Burns. In Schwartz SI, editor: *Principles of surgery*, ed 2, New York, 1974, McGraw-Hill.
142. Roe CF, Kinney JM: Water and heat exchange on third-degree burns, *Surgery* 56:212–220, 1964.
143. Affleck DG et al: Assessment of tissue viability in complex extremity injuries: utility of the pyrophosphate nuclear scan, *J Trauma* 50(2):263–269, 2001.
144. Eski M et al: Cerium nitrate treatment prevents progressive tissue necrosis in the zone of stasis following burns, *Burn* 38(2):283–289, 2012.
145. Weber JM et al: Incidence of catheter-associated bloodstream infection after introduction of minocycline and rifampin antimicrobial-coated catheters in a pediatric burn population, *J Burn Care Res* 33(4):539–543, 2012.
146. Lee J et al: Computerized insulin infusion programs are safe and effective in the burn intensive care unit, *J Burn Care Res* 33(3):e114–e119, 2012.
147. Zaletel CL: Factors affecting fluid resuscitation in the burn patient: the collaborative role of the APN, *Adv Emerg Nurs J* 31(4):309–320, 2009.
148. Fraser JF et al: A randomized controlled trial of amniotic membrane in the treatment of a standardized burn injury in the merino lamb, *Burns* 35(7):998–1003, 2009.
149. Ronfard V et al: Long-term regeneration of human epidermis on third degree burns transplanted with autologous cultured epithelium grown on a fibrin matrix, *Transplantation* 70(11):1588–1598, 2000.
150. Williamson JS et al: Cultured epithelial autograft: five years of clinical experience with twenty-eight patients, *J Trauma* 39(2):309–319, 1995.
151. Fitton AR, Drew P, Dickson WA: The use of a bilaminate artificial skin substitute (Integra) in acute resurfacing of burns: an early experience, *Br J Plast Surg* 54(3):208–212, 2001.
152. Peck MD et al: A trial of the effectiveness of artificial dermis in the treatment of patients with burns greater than 45% total body surface area, *J Trauma* 52(5):971–978, 2002.
153. Carsin H et al: Cultured epithelial autografts in extensive burn coverage of severely traumatized patients: a five year single-center experience with 30 patients, *Burns* 26(4):379–387, 2000.
154. Wainwright D et al: Clinical evaluation of an acellular allograft dermal matrix in full-thickness burns, *J Burn Care Rehabil* 17(2):124–136, 1996.
155. Branski LK et al: A review of gene and stem cell therapy in cutaneous wound healing, *Burns* 35(2):171–180, 2009.
156. Curinga G et al: Comments on "platelet-rich plasma in burns, " *Burns* 36(6):944–945, 2010.
157. Pullua N, Wolter T, Markowicz M: Platelet-rich plasma in burns, *Burns* 36(1):4–8, 2010.
158. Kirker KR et al: Glycosaminoglycan hydrogels as supplemental wound dressings for donor sites, *J Burn Care Rehabil* 25(3):276–286, 2004.
159. Liew SH, Murison M, Dickson WA: Prophylactic treatment of deep dermal burn scar to prevent hypertrophic scarring using the pulsed dye laser: a preliminary study, *Ann Plast Surg* 49(5):472–475, 2002.
160. Sainsbury DC: Body image and facial burns, *Adv Skin Wound Care* 22(1):39–44, 2009.
161. Connor-Ballard PA: Understanding and managing burn pain: part 1, *Am J Nurs* 109(4):48–56, 2009.
162. Connor-Ballard PA: Understanding and managing burn pain: part 2, *Am J Nurs* 109(5):54–62, 2009.
163. Jellish WS et al: Effect of topical local anesthetic application to skin harvest sites for pain management in burn patients undergoing skin-grafting procedures, *Ann Surg* 229(1):115–120, 1999.
164. Konstantatos AH et al: Predicting the effectiveness of virtual reality relaxation on pain and anxiety when added to PCA morphine in patients having burn dressings changes, *Burns* 35(4):491–499, 2009.

CHAPTER

49

Shock, Multiple Organ Dysfunction Syndrome, and Burns in Children

Mary Fran Hazinski, Mary A. Mondozzi, and Rose A. Urdiales Baker

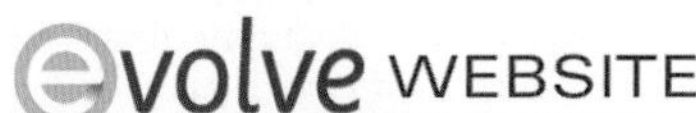

http://evolve.elsevier.com/McCance/
- Review Questions and Answers

CHAPTER OUTLINE

This chapter reviews shock, multiple organ dysfunction syndrome, and burns in children. It focuses on the assessment and care of children but also notes many of the differences between these conditions in children and adults.

SHOCK AND MULTIPLE ORGAN DYSFUNCTION SYNDROME

Shock is a condition of acute and progressive circulatory dysfunction that results in inadequate delivery of oxygen and nutrients to the tissues. Shock in children most often results from hemorrhage, severe dehydration, progressive heart failure, or sepsis. It may also complicate the care of the child with congenital heart disease, pulmonary hypertension (cor pulmonale), drug toxicity, electrolyte or acid-base imbalance, dysrhythmias, or multiple organ failure.

Shock in children is present when there are signs of poor systemic perfusion, regardless of the blood pressure—shock may be present with normal, high, or low blood pressure. When the systolic blood pressure is adequate for age, but there are signs of inadequate tissue perfusion, the child is in **compensated shock.** In this child, although the systolic blood pressure may be normal, the diastolic or mean blood pressure is typically low. If systolic hypotension is associated with inadequate tissue perfusion, the child is in **hypotensive** (formerly called decompensated) **shock.**[1-3]

Shock causes tissue **ischemia** (inadequate blood flow) and **hypoxia** (inadequate oxygen delivery) that leads to acidosis and cell dysfunction. Oxygen delivery may be inadequate because arterial oxygen content or cardiac output is low, or because there are increased metabolic requirements or impaired cellular use of oxygen. Ischemia and hypoxia are primary insults to cells. Restoration of adequate blood flow and oxygen delivery may trigger the development of *reperfusion injury,* a secondary problem characterized by an exaggerated inflammatory response that may produce cellular death and organ failure.

Multiple organ dysfunction syndrome (**MODS**) is the simultaneous failure of at least two organs resulting from a single cause.

MODS may be either primary or secondary. Primary MODS is directly attributable to the insult and typically occurs soon (3 to 7 days) after an insult. Secondary MODS typically occurs later and may be associated with more sequential development of organ dysfunction. Risk factors for MODS include severe or prolonged shock, sepsis, trauma, cardiopulmonary arrest, congenital heart disease, and liver and bone marrow transplantation.[3-5] Children with chronic diseases have an increased risk for MODS and increased mortality.[5]

Types of Shock

Shock is categorized by type as follows:[2,3]

1. *Hypovolemic shock:* caused by inadequate intravascular volume relative to the vascular space
2. *Cardiogenic shock:* results from impairment of myocardial function
3. *Distributive shock* (including septic, anaphylactic, and neurogenic): results from inappropriate distribution of blood flow, increased capillary permeability, and myocardial dysfunction (e.g., septic or anaphylactic shock) or central nervous system injury (e.g., neurogenic or spinal shock)
4. *Obstructive shock:* caused by a mechanical obstruction to blood flow into and through the heart and great vessels (e.g., cardiac tamponade, pulmonary embolus, obstructive congenital heart lesions such as critical aortic stenosis) resulting in low cardiac output

With **hypovolemic** or **cardiogenic shock** blood flow distribution is reduced to skin, gut, and kidney to maintain blood flow to the heart and brain. With **distributive (septic, anaphylactic, and neurogenic) shock,** blood flow is unregulated throughout the skin and organ systems and vasodilation and increased capillary permeability are typically present, so a normal cardiac output is likely to be inadequate to maintain sufficient perfusion of all tissue beds. Volume administration is necessary to ensure that the intravascular volume is adequate relative to the vascular space, and vasoactive drugs are needed to support adequate cardiac output and oxygen delivery. **Neurogenic shock** is a form of hypovolemic and vasogenic (maldistributive) shock. It is caused by a loss of vasomotor tone after severe head or spinal cord injury. Massive vasodilation and loss of sympathomimetic tone result in a relative hypovolemia and hypotension. The loss of sympathetic tone prevents compensatory tachycardia.

In **obstructive shock,** low cardiac output is caused by mechanical obstruction to blood flow, such as cardiac tamponade, tension pneumothorax, critical left heart or aortic obstruction, or pulmonary embolus.[2] Obstructive shock is difficult to distinguish from cardiogenic shock because both may present with signs of low cardiac output and evidence of systemic or pulmonary venous congestion. Prompt detection and treatment are critical to survival.[2,3]

An etiologic classification of shock is helpful because it indicates the initial therapy required. However, any child with late or progressive shock is likely to demonstrate widespread cardiovascular dysfunction that may include inappropriate intravascular volume relative to the vascular space, poor myocardial function, and maldistribution of blood flow so the etiologic classification of shock is oversimplified for such children. Severe shock of any kind may be followed by complications such as reperfusion injury or MODS. An etiologic classification is also incomplete for children with septic shock, because sepsis produces elements of hypovolemic and cardiogenic shock in addition to the complications of infection and maldistribution of blood flow. Thus, healthcare providers must assess and support all aspects of cardiovascular function and oxygen delivery during the treatment of any form of shock.

BOX 49-1 CLINICAL MANIFESTATIONS OF SHOCK IN NEWBORNS, INFANTS, AND CHILDREN

Signs of Shock in Infants and Children

- Change in responsiveness (initial irritability followed by lethargy)
- Tachypnea
- Mottled color, pallor (distributive shock may be associated with flushed skin)
- Tachycardia
- Cool skin, prolonged capillary refill (distributive shock may cause "flash" [instantaneous] refill)
- Diminished intensity of peripheral pulses (may also vary in intensity)
- Metabolic (lactic) acidosis (serum lactate >4 mmol/L is typically well above normal for arterial or venous blood)
- Decreased central venous oxygen saturation (more than 25% to 30% below arterial oxygen saturation)
- LATE: Hypotension, bradycardia

Nonspecific Signs of Distress in Newborns

- Jitteriness or lethargy with decreased tone
- Change in oxygen requirements
- Apnea
- Bradycardia or decreased heart rate variability
- Temperature instability, hypothermia
- Glucose instability, hypoglycemia
- Feeding intolerance (e.g., increased residual volume)

Clinical Manifestations of Shock

The child with inadequate cardiac output demonstrates signs of inadequate blood flow to some tissue beds and evidence of organ system dysfunction (Box 49-1). Critical parameters to evaluate when approaching the child include assessment of consciousness, breathing, and color. This initial assessment is described in the Pediatric Advanced Life Support course.[2] Through this assessment the provider determines if the child "looks good" (appears stable, in no acute distress) or "looks bad" (in need of immediate intervention).[6] More detailed assessment of organ function and acid-base status will detect evidence of inadequate organ perfusion.

The child's level of *consciousness* and *responsiveness* often provides valuable information about the severity of illness. The healthy infant should orient to faces, make eye contact, and track bright objects across a visual field. The healthy toddler is reluctant to be separated from parents or examined by strangers, and the healthy child is alert and responds to questions. By comparison, the critically ill infant or child is often extremely irritable; lethargy indicates severe deterioration in the child's level of consciousness. A decreased response to painful stimulation is abnormal and usually indicates severe cardiorespiratory or neurologic compromise.[2,6]

The infant or child normally *breathes* without evidence of distress or increased effort, such as retractions or nasal flaring. An extremely rapid respiratory rate (tachypnea), increased depth of respirations (hyperpnea), or evidence of increased respiratory effort (e.g., retractions, grunting) may indicate the presence of heart failure or shock. The development of apnea or inadequate respiratory rate or effort may indicate deterioration and need for immediate support of airway, oxygenation, and ventilation.

If perfusion is adequate and the ambient temperature is warm, the child's *color* will be consistent over the surface of the skin, with pink lips and mucous membranes. Children who are in a cold environment, those who have undergone hypothermic surgery or a procedure in a cold room, and children in shock often demonstrate mottling (a marbled or "blotchy" appearance to the skin).[2,3,6] Pallor also may be observed when perfusion is poor (Figure 49-1). Children with sepsis occasionally demonstrate flushed, bright red skin.[2,3,6]

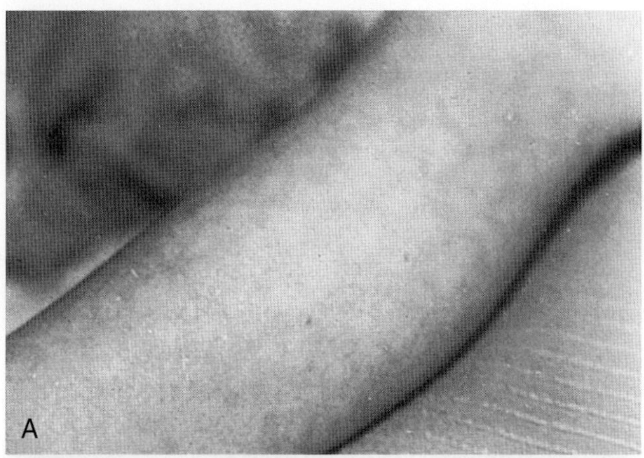

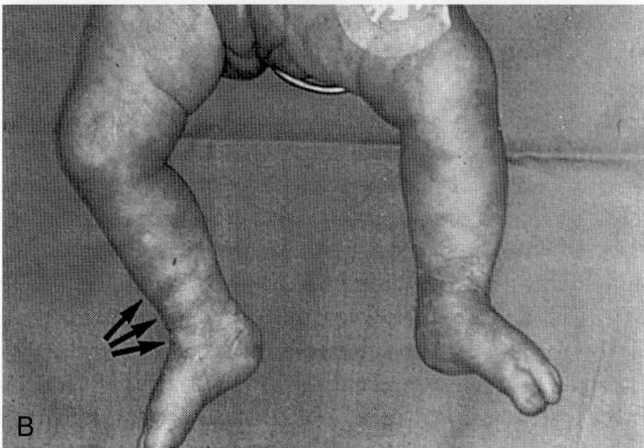

FIGURE 49-1 Mottling of Skin Caused by Poor Systemic Perfusion. **A,** Mottling of skin color often indicates inadequate tissue oxygenation; this may result from hypoxemia or poor systemic perfusion. This child developed myocardial dysfunction and signs of cardiogenic shock. **B,** Mottled skin color is often associated with other signs of compromise of skin perfusion, including delayed capillary refill. The skin over this infant's right ankle was blanched using three fingers (arrows), and the skin failed to perfuse for more than 5 seconds. This infant suffered from septic shock. (From Hazinski MF: Cardiovascular disorders. In Hazinski MF, editor: *Nursing care of the critically ill child,* ed 2, St Louis, 1992, Mosby.)

If perfusion is adequate and the ambient temperature is warm, the child's capillary refill is normally brisk (<2 seconds). A prolonged capillary refill time (>2 seconds) may indicate a compromise in systemic perfusion (see Figure 49-1, *B*) and the development of shock.[2,3,6] However, evaluation of capillary refill time is subjective and gradual changes may be difficult to detect.[7]

The child's *vital signs* must be evaluated in light of the child's clinical condition. Normal vital signs are not always appropriate in the seriously ill or injured child[6] (Box 49-2 and Table 49-1).

The child's heart rate should be appropriate for age and clinical condition. The child in shock is often tachycardic. The **tachycardia** may be primary (i.e., associated with a tachydysrhythmia) or secondary to stress (i.e., sinus tachycardia). If the heart rate is extremely rapid or if it is present in the child with decreased myocardial function, tachycardia may be the cause rather than the symptom of shock. In general, if the ventricular rate exceeds 200 to 220/min in the infant or 160 to 180/min in the child, ventricular diastolic filling time and coronary artery perfusion time are significantly reduced and stroke volume falls. As a result, cardiac output falls and signs of heart failure or shock develop. Once supraventricular or ventricular tachycardia produces signs of shock, urgent treatment is required.[8]

Bradycardia, an abnormally low heart rate, can cause a fall in cardiac output or it can be a symptom of deterioration. In young animal models, a fall in heart rate produces a commensurate fall in cardiac output.[9] The most common cause of bradycardia in young children is hypoxia.[2,10] Therefore, if the infant or child develops bradycardia with poor perfusion, the provider must immediately assess and support the child's airway, oxygenation, and ventilation, and be prepared to initiate chest compressions if the heart rate and systemic perfusion do not improve.[2,6,10]

BOX 49-2 ESTIMATING BLOOD PRESSURE IN CHILDREN 1 TO 10 YEARS OF AGE

Typical systolic BP for 1-10 years of age: The typical "normal" (i.e., median, or 50th percentile) systolic blood pressure for a child 1 to 10 years of age of normal height may be estimated by adding 90 mmHg to twice the child's age in years (90 mmHg + [2 × age in years]); this corresponds to the 50th percentile systolic blood pressure for the child's age.

Hypotensive systolic BP for 1-10 years of age: A systolic pressure less than 70 mmHg plus twice the child's age in years (<70 mmHg + [2 × age in years]) is considered hypotensive for children 1 to 10 years of age because this blood pressure corresponds to the 5th percentile systolic blood pressure for age (i.e., only 5% of normal, healthy children of average height demonstrate a systolic blood pressure lower than that number).

Hypotensive mean arterial pressure for 1-10 years of age: A mean arterial pressure less than 40 mmHg + (1.5 × age in years) is consistent with hypotension because this mean arterial pressure corresponds to the 5th percentile mean arterial pressure in children of average height.

Data from Chameides L et al, editors: Systematic approach to the seriously ill or injured child. In *Textbook of pediatric advanced life support,* Dallas, 2011, American Heart Association; Hacque IU, Zaritsky AL: *Pediatr Crit Care* 8:138–144; 2007.

TABLE 49-1 NORMAL PEDIATRIC VITAL SIGNS

	HEART RATES		
AGE	AWAKE HEART RATE (Per min)	SLEEPING HEART RATE (Per min)	RESPIRATORY RATE* (Breaths Per min)
Newborn	100-205	90-160	
Infant (6 mo)	100-180	90-160	30-53
Toddler	98-140	80-120	27-37
Preschooler	80-120	65-100	20-28
School-age child	75-118	58-90	18-25
Adolescent	60-100	50-90	12-20

	BLOOD PRESSURES			
AGE	SYSTOLIC BLOOD PRESSURE (mmHg)[†]	DIASTOLIC BLOOD PRESSURE (mmHg)[†]	MEAN ARTERIAL PRESSURE (mmHg)[‡]	SYSTOLIC HYPOTENSION (mmHg)[§]
Birth (12 hr, <1000 g)	39-59	16-36	28-42[¶]	<40-50
Birth (12 hr, 3-kg weight)	60-76	31-45	48-57	<50
Newborn (96 hr)	67-84	35-53	45-60	<60
Infant (1-12 mo)	72-104	37-56	50-62	<70
Toddler (1-2 yr)	86-106	42-63	49-62	<70 + (2 × age in years)
Preschool (3-5 yr)	89-112	46-72	58-69	<70 + (2 × age in years)
School-age child (6-7 yr)	97-115	57-76	66-72	<70 + (2 × age in years)
Preadolescent (10-12 yr)	102-120	61-80	71-79	<90
Adolescent (12-15 yr)	110-131	64-83	73-84	<90

Note: Always consider patient's normal range and clinical condition. Heart and respiratory rates normally increase with fever or stress.

From Hazinski MF: Children are different. In Hazinski MF, editor: *Nursing care of the critically ill child,* ed 3, St Louis, 2013, Mosby.

*Respiratory rates from Fleming S et al: Normal ranges of heart rate and respiratory rate in children from birth to 18 years of age: a systematic review of observational studies, *Lancet* 377:1011–1018, 2011.

†Systolic and diastolic blood pressure ranges assume 50th percentile for height for children 1 year and older, and are consistent with the Pediatric Advanced Life Support course (Chameides L et al: *Pediatric advanced life support provider manual,* Dallas, 2011, American Heart Association).

‡Mean arterial pressures (Diastolic pressure + [Difference between systolic and diastolic pressures ÷ 3]) for 1 year and older, assuming 50th percentile for height.

§Threshold for hypotension in children 1 to 10 years old from Pediatric Advanced Life Support course (Chameides L et al: *Pediatric advanced life support provider manual,* Dallas, 2011, American Heart Association).

¶Approximately equal to postconception age in weeks (may add 5 mmHg).

Blood pressure ranges from the following sources: Gemelli M et al: *Eur J Pediatr* 149:318–320, 1990; Versmold H et al: *Pediatrics* 67:107, 1981; Haque IU, Zaritsky AL: *Pediatr Crit Care* 8:138–144, 2007; National Heart, Lung and Blood Institute: *Fourth report on the diagnosis, evaluation, and treatment of high blood pressure in children and adolescents,* Bethesda, MD, 2004, National Heart, Lung and Blood Institute. Available at www.nhlbi.nih.gov/guidelines/hypertension/child.tbl.htm. Accessed July 10, 2013.

Bradycardia often indicates impending cardiovascular collapse and is the most common terminal cardiac rhythm observed in children.[2,3,6,10] The child's stroke volume may be altered by conditions affecting ventricular preload, compliance, contractility, and afterload (Table 49-2). Evaluate and optimize each of these variables in the treatment of shock (see Chapter 48).

Evaluate the child's *blood pressure* in light of age and clinical condition; note that shock may be present despite a systolic blood pressure within the normal range for age. When hypovolemic or cardiogenic shock is present, compensatory vasoconstriction may initially maintain the systolic blood pressure, although the mean and diastolic arterial pressures may fall. The development of systolic hypotension in the child with hypovolemic or cardiogenic shock indicates severe shock, and rapid deterioration may follow. In septic shock, by comparison, mild systolic hypotension may develop early in the clinical course. However, in all children, the development of systolic hypotension or a fall in mean arterial pressure indicates hypotensive shock, and urgent treatment is needed.[2,3,6]

The central venous pressure (CVP) is normally 0 to 5 mmHg and the pulmonary artery wedge pressure (PAWP, also called pulmonary artery occlusion pressure [PAOP]) is normally 5 to 8 mmHg or less. Inadequate CVP or PAWP may indicate hypovolemia, whereas high measurements typically result from heart failure or cardiogenic shock. Note that in the absence of tricuspid valve disease, tension pneumothorax, or influence from positive pressure ventilation, the CVP reflects the right ventricular end-diastolic pressure, whereas the PAWP should, in the absence of mitral valve disease, reflect the left ventricular end-diastolic pressure (if the catheter is appropriately placed and calibrated). The cardiac silhouette is normally less than 50% of the width of the chest on chest radiograph.

If a central venous catheter is in place, the superior vena cava (SVC) oxygen saturation is monitored to evaluate the balance of oxygen delivery versus consumption. The SVC saturation is central venous oxygen saturation ($S_{CV}O_2$) that is used as a surrogate for mixed venous oxygen saturation that would require a sampling of blood from the pulmonary artery. Normally, the

TABLE 49-2 FACTORS AFFECTING CARDIOVASCULAR PERFORMANCE IN CHILDREN

FACTOR	COMMENTS
Heart rate	Major factor affecting cardiac output in children. Normally more rapid in children than in adults. Because the *stroke volume* is smaller than in adults, the *cardiac output* of the child is more closely related to heart rate than stroke volume. *Tachycardia* is expected in the seriously ill or injured child. The most common cause of *bradycardia* in young children is hypoxia; bradycardia is an ominous sign if present in association with poor perfusion. Urgent treatment is required once bradycardia or supraventricular or ventricular tachycardia produces signs of shock.
Stroke volume	Averages 1.5 ml/kg; affected by conditions altering ventricular preload, compliance, contractility, and afterload
Ventricular end-diastolic pressure (VEDP)	Optimal pressure for children in shock is unknown. Aggressive fluid administration is linked to improved survival in children with *septic* shock.
Ventricular compliance or distensibility	Can be affected by congenital heart defects such as atrial septal defects (ASDs) and complex congenital heart defects. If compliance is low, such as in newborns and infants, volume administration may increase VEDP. Hypoplastic ventricles are often noncompliant. Hypertrophied ventricles, present in children with severe pulmonary stenosis or aortic stenosis, may become fibrotic and noncompliant. Increased compliance may be present in early septic shock.
Contractility	Contractility probably similar in normal newborns, infants, children, and adults. Newborn myocardium does have fewer contractile proteins and higher water content than adult myocardium, but the clinical significance of this is probably minimal.
Afterload	Newborn myocardium *can* adapt to mild, nonacute increases in afterload. Afterload may be increased in children with systemic vasoconstriction or pulmonary hypertension (constrictors include alveolar hypoxia, acidosis, hypothermia, and alveolar distention). Some uncorrected congenital heart defects may increase afterload. Coarctation of the aorta and aortic stenosis increase left ventricular afterload. Pulmonary stenosis increases right ventricular afterload. Afterload may be decreased in septic shock.
Oxygen delivery and consumption	Highest per kilogram body weight during the neonatal period and infancy. The young child requires a higher cardiac output and oxygen delivery per kilogram than the adult. Increased oxygen consumption occurs in critically ill newborns exposed to cold because they cannot shiver to generate heat. Other causes of increased oxygen consumption in children and infants include fever, sepsis, trauma, pain, and seizures.

VEDP, Ventricular end-diastolic pressure.

$S_{CV}O_2$ is 25% to 30% below the arterial oxygen saturation. A fall in $S_{CV}O_2$ can indicate a fall in oxygen delivery (caused by decreased arterial oxygen content or decreased cardiac output), an uncompensated rise in oxygen consumption, or both.[3]

Shock compromises renal perfusion, so urine volume decreases, typically to less than 2 ml/kg/hr in infants, less than 1 ml/kg/hr in children, and less than 0.5 ml/kg/hr in adolescents, despite adequate fluid intake. Liver enzymes may be elevated if hepatic perfusion is reduced. The development of metabolic acidosis and a rise in serum lactate to greater than 4 mg/dl indicate that blood flow to some tissues is inadequate to support aerobic metabolism.

Infants have high glucose needs and low glycogen stores that may be rapidly depleted during stress. For this reason, *hypoglycemia* (glucose ≤60 mg/dl) may be observed in seriously ill or injured infants and may be associated with cardiovascular or neurologic deterioration.[2,11] *Hyperglycemia* (>150 mg/dl) may develop in critically ill or injured children as the result of a relative insulin-resistant state associated with high levels of endogenous catecholamines and hydrocortisone secretion.[3,11] Such hyperglycemia in children is often observed in the first 12 to 18 hours after initial injury or development of shock, then falls to normal levels; persistent hyperglycemia (>180 mg/dl or 10 mmol/L) has been linked with poor survival in critically ill children,[12,13] and hypo-, hyperglycemia, and glucose instability (episodes of both hypo- and hyperglycemia in same child) have been linked with development of multiple organ dysfunction.[13]

Hypovolemic Shock

Hypovolemic shock, the most common type of shock in children, is associated with a reduction in the intravascular volume relative to the vascular space. Dehydration and trauma are the most common causes of hypovolemic shock in children. A relative hypovolemia also may result from vasodilation and a redistribution of blood volume or from increased capillary permeability, such as may develop following burns or with sepsis.

When hypovolemia is mild or moderate, such as with 5% to 10% dehydration or mild hemorrhage, compensatory adrenergic vasoconstriction redistributes blood from the skin, the mesenteric (gut), and renal circulations to maintain blood flow to the heart and brain. The child with mild hypovolemic shock typically maintains systolic blood pressure with this vasoconstriction.

Hypotension is a sign of severe, decompensated hypovolemic shock and may not develop unless intravascular volume loss is rapid or severe.[2,3] Hypotension typically develops with greater than 10% isotonic or hypotonic dehydration in the infant or child (or greater than 6% to 7% dehydration in the adolescent).[11] Hypotension may not be observed in the child with trauma unless hemorrhage totals about 20% to 25% of circulating blood volume.[14,15]

Relative hypovolemia may be caused by a decrease in the intravascular volume relative to the vascular space. This may be associated with the vasodilation of sepsis, anaphylaxis, or neurogenic shock (see following text) or with β_2-adrenergic drug toxicity. A relative hypovolemia also may be caused by increased capillary permeability with a redistribution of intravascular volume, such as with burns, anaphylaxis, or sepsis. The translocation of extravascular fluid to a location that is neither intravascular nor intracellular, as in edema, is termed **"third spacing" of fluids.**[11]

Compensatory Responses. Significant dehydration, hypovolemia, and low cardiac output stimulate adrenergic and renal compensatory mechanisms characterized by the "fight-or-flight" response. These include tachycardia and redistribution of blood from the skin, gut, and kidney to the brain and heart. Reduced renal perfusion stimulates the renin-angiotensin-aldosterone system, resulting in renal sodium and water retention. Decreased atrial stretch stimulates the secretion of antidiuretic hormone (ADH, also known as arginine vasopressin [AVP]) and produces free water retention by the kidneys.[3] These mechanisms are similar in adults and children and may help restore or maintain intravascular volume over time. Neonatal and young infant kidneys, however, are incapable of excreting concentrated urine, so these compensatory mechanisms are relatively ineffective during the first weeks of life.[11]

Compensatory mechanisms cannot be maintained indefinitely. Systemic vasoconstriction increases left ventricular afterload and myocardial oxygen consumption and may produce tissue ischemia. Prolonged tachycardia may impair subendocardial blood flow and increase myocardial oxygen consumption; both may ultimately contribute to myocardial ischemia.[3] Extreme tachypnea increases oxygen demand and reduces effective ventilation. A severe compromise in blood flow and systemic perfusion contributes to cerebral, renal, or hepatic ischemia and possible organ failure.

CLINICAL MANIFESTATIONS. The child with hypovolemic shock demonstrates signs of inadequate blood flow to some tissue beds and some evidence of organ system dysfunction (see Box 49-1). The infant or child may be irritable or lethargic. Respirations will be rapid and may be labored if shock is severe or associated with myocardial failure. The skin will be mottled, although pallor also may be observed. A prolonged capillary refill time (>2 seconds) is consistent with the development of shock.[2,3,6,16]

The child in hypovolemic shock is often tachycardic. Bradycardia often indicates impending cardiovascular collapse or cardiac arrest and is the most common terminal cardiac rhythm observed in children.[2,3,10] When hypovolemic shock is present, compensatory vasoconstriction may initially maintain the systolic blood pressure, although the mean arterial pressure may fall. The development of systolic hypotension often indicates severe shock, and rapid deterioration may follow. The CVP is less than 5 to 8 mmHg, unless heart failure or pulmonary hypertension is present.

Hypovolemic shock compromises renal perfusion so urine volume decreases despite adequate fluid intake. Liver enzymes may be elevated if hepatic perfusion is reduced. The development of metabolic acidosis and a rise in serum lactate indicate that blood flow to some tissues is inadequate to support aerobic metabolism.

Hypoglycemia (glucose ≤60 mg/dl) may be observed in seriously ill or injured infants, especially if intake has been compromised, and may be associated with cardiovascular or neurologic deterioration. *Hyperglycemia* (>150 mg/dl) may develop in critically ill or injured children.

Clinically significant dehydration is associated with weight loss (Table 49-3). Fluid intake and output records (or reports

TABLE 49-3 DEHYDRATION AND HYPOVOLEMIA

TYPE OF DEHYDRATION	CLINICAL INDICATORS
Isotonic dehydration	Fluid output exceeds intake. Loss of free water is proportional to loss of sodium, so serum sodium concentration remains normal. Fluid loss is from intravascular and extravascular compartments. Compromises peripheral perfusion when the young child has lost approximately 10% (100 ml/kg) of body weight. Compromises systemic perfusion in the adolescent with acute fluid loss equivalent to 5% to 6% of body weight.
	Produces hypotension (decompensated shock) when the young child has lost 15% (150 ml/kg) of body weight. Produces hypotension in the adolescent with a fluid loss equivalent to 7% to 9% of body weight because body water constitutes a smaller percentage of body weight in older children and adults than in young children.
Hypotonic/hyponatremic dehydration	Associated with a proportionately greater loss of sodium than free water; thus the serum sodium falls. Resultant acute fall in serum osmolality produces an acute extravascular fluid shift and further loss of extravascular volume. Fluid loss in hypotonic dehydration is primarily from the intravascular compartment; thus a compromise in systemic perfusion will be observed after even small quantities of fluid loss.
	Poor peripheral perfusion occurs in a child with a fluid loss equivalent to 5% (50 ml/kg) of body weight. Adolescents with hyponatremic dehydration may demonstrate a compromise in peripheral perfusion with a fluid loss equivalent to approximately 3% of body weight.
	Hypotension often is observed when fluid loss is equal to approximately 10% (100 ml/kg) of body weight. Hypotension in an adolescent is observed when the fluid loss equals approximately 5% to 6% of body weight.
Hypertonic/hypernatremic dehydration	Free water deficit is proportionately greater than the deficit of sodium, so serum sodium concentration rises, increasing serum osmolality and producing an intravascular shift of free water. For this reason the child with hypernatremic dehydration is likely to maintain intravascular volume and systemic perfusion until relatively large quantities of fluid are lost.
	Compromise in systemic perfusion is not likely to be observed in the *child* with hypernatremic dehydration until *severe* dehydration is present with a fluid loss equivalent to 10% of body weight (or 5% to 6% of body weight in the adolescent).
	Hypotension may not be observed until the fluid loss approximates 15% or more of body weight (7% to 9% or more of body weight in the adolescent).
	Hypotension in the child with hypertonic/hypernatremic dehydration indicates a substantial fluid deficit. However, the deficit must be replaced carefully to correct shock and avoid rapid lowering of serum sodium concentrations.

Data in part from Roberts KE: *Pediatr Rev* 22:380–386, 2001; Roberts KE: Fluid, electrolyte and endocrine problems. In Hazinski MF, editor: *Nursing care of the critically ill child*, ed 3, St Louis, 2013, Mosby.

TABLE 49-4 SEVERITY OF (ISOTONIC) DEHYDRATION BASED ON CLINICAL EXAM*

CLINICAL PARAMETERS	MILD	MODERATE	SEVERE
Body weight loss			
Infant	5% (50 ml/kg)	10% (100 ml/kg)	15% (150 ml/kg)
Adolescent	3% (30 ml/kg)	5%-6% (50-60 ml/kg)	7%-9% (70-90 ml/kg)
General appearance	Alert, restless, thirsty	Lethargic, postural dizziness	Limp, coma, cold and cyanotic extremities
Radial pulse	Full	Thready, weak, rapid	Feeble, not palpable
Respiration	Normal	Deep	Deep, rapid
Skin elasticity	Pinch retracts immediately	Pinch retracts slowly	Pinch retracts very slowly (>2 seconds)
Eyes	Normal	Sunken	Very sunken
Tears	Present	Diminished	Absent
Mucous membranes	Moist	Dry	Very dry (parched)
Urine output	Normal	↓	↓ or absent
Capillary refill time	<2 seconds	>2 seconds	Prolonged
Heart rate	Varies with age	Varies with age	Varies with age
Blood pressure	Normal	Normal	Reduced

Modified from Perkin RM et al: Shock, cardiac arrest and resuscitation. In Hazinski MF, editor: *Nursing care of the critically ill child,* ed 3, St Louis, 2013, Mosby.
*The interpretation of the assessments must be appropriately modified for age and type of dehydration (hypotonic or hypertonic).

TABLE 49-5 ESTIMATION OF PEDIATRIC CIRCULATING BLOOD VOLUME

AGE OF CHILD	BLOOD VOLUME (ml/kg body weight)
Newborn	80-85
Infant	75-80
Child	70-75
Adolescent	65-70

From Hazinski MF: Children are different. In Hazinski MF, editor: *Nursing care of the critically ill child,* ed 3, St Louis, 2013, Mosby.

from parents or primary caretakers) reveal a history of inadequate fluid intake or excessive fluid losses. The child with significant dehydration demonstrates dry mucous membranes, a sunken fontanel (in infants), and poor skin turgor[11] (Table 49-4). Moderate isotonic dehydration produces signs of peripheral circulatory compromise, and severe isotonic dehydration will produce hypotension. The blood urea nitrogen (BUN) and urine specific gravity are usually elevated. The serum sodium concentration and osmolality are affected by the type and severity of dehydration present.

Hemorrhage is another potential cause of hypovolemic shock. To appreciate the significance of any blood lost or drawn for laboratory analysis, the total blood loss should be considered as a percentage of the child's circulating blood volume (Table 49-5).

Tachycardia, peripheral vasoconstriction, and altered level of consciousness may be the only early evidence of hemorrhage in the child with trauma (Table 49-6). Acute blood loss (hemorrhage) may not compromise a child's peripheral perfusion until an estimated 25% to 30% of intravascular volume is lost (i.e., an acute intravascular or blood loss of 16 to 24 ml/kg).[14-16] Once hypotension develops, cardiovascular collapse is imminent and immediate, rapid intravascular volume expansion is required and surgical intervention may be needed.

Redistribution of blood volume associated with systemic vasodilation, high capillary pressure or transudative fluid losses, or capillary leak may produce a relative hypovolemia and signs of poor systemic perfusion in the absence of evidence of absolute volume loss. For example, children with end-stage hepatic failure may demonstrate a relative hypovolemia associated with ascites and hepatorenal syndrome. Children demonstrate increased capillary permeability and loss of intravascular volume immediately after a burn. The septic child also may demonstrate systemic edema associated with capillary leak and intravascular volume loss. In these children some evidence of extravascular fluid movement (ascites, systemic edema, or fluid loss to dressings over burns) is usually observed.

Signs of neurogenic shock in the child with a recent, severe spinal cord injury include warm skin and hypotension with a low diastolic blood pressure. Signs of poor systemic perfusion also are observed (see Clinical Manifestations of Shock, previously), although loss of sympathetic nervous system tone prevents the typical tachycardic response.

Cardiogenic Shock

Cardiogenic shock is present when impaired myocardial function compromises cardiac output. This form of shock is observed:

1. Following cardiovascular surgery or with inflammatory disease of the heart, such as cardiomyopathy and myocarditis
2. With drug toxicity or severe electrolyte or acid-base imbalances
3. As a complication of any form of shock and early in septic shock

Compensatory Responses. In the early stages of cardiogenic shock, adrenergic compensatory mechanisms produce tachycardia, peripheral vasoconstriction, and constriction of the splanchnic arteries to divert blood flow from the skin, gut, and kidneys to maintain flow to the heart and brain.[2,3,16] These compensatory mechanisms may be sufficient to maintain the

TABLE 49-6 CLASSIFICATION OF PEDIATRIC HEMORRHAGIC SHOCK IN TRAUMA PATIENTS BASED ON CLINICAL EVALUATION

SYSTEM	MILD HEMORRHAGE, COMPENSATED SHOCK, SIMPLE HYPOVOLEMIA (<30%)	MODERATE HEMORRHAGE, DECOMPENSATED SHOCK, MARKED HYPOVOLEMIA (30%-45%)	SEVERE HEMORRHAGE, CARDIOPULMONARY FAILURE, PROFOUND HYPOVOLEMIA (>45%)
Cardiovascular	Tachycardia Weak peripheral pulses, strong central pulses Low to normal blood pressure (systolic BP >70 mmHg + [2 × (age in years)]) Mild acidosis	Moderate tachycardia Thready peripheral pulses, weak central pulses Frank hypotension (systolic BP <70 mmHg + [2 × (age in years)]) Moderate acidosis	Severe tachycardia Absent peripheral pulses, thready central pulses Profound hypotension (systolic BP <50 mmHg) Severe acidosis
Respiratory	Mild tachypnea	Moderate tachypnea	Severe tachypnea
Central nervous system	Irritable, confused	Agitated or lethargic	Obtunded, comatose
Skin	Cool extremities, mottling Poor capillary refill (72 sec)	Cool extremities, pallor Delayed capillary refill (72 sec)	Cool extremities, cyanosis Prolonged (>5 sec) capillary refill
Kidneys	Mild oliguria, increased specific gravity	Marked oliguria, increased blood urea nitrogen (BUN)	Anuria

From Soud T, Pieper P, Hazinski MF: Pediatric trauma. In Hazinski MF, editor: *Nursing care of the critically ill child,* ed 2, St Louis, 1992, Mosby.

child's systolic blood pressure and effective coronary artery and cerebral blood flow. However, tachycardia and systemic arterial constriction increase myocardial oxygen consumption. In addition, reduction in gut and kidney blood flow may produce hepatic, mesenteric, or renal ischemia or failure. Decreased renal perfusion stimulates the renin-angiotensin-aldosterone system, as described for hypovolemic shock.

If the mean arterial pressure or pulse pressure falls, stimulation of the baroreceptors in the carotid sinuses and aortic arch is reduced. This reduced baroreceptor activity removes inhibition from the vasomotor center in the medulla, resulting in increased adrenergic stimulation.[3] If myocardial dysfunction progresses, cardiac output and systemic blood pressure ultimately fall. Myocardial ischemia then exacerbates myocardial dysfunction, and multisystem organ failure may result from persistent or severe organ ischemia.

CLINICAL MANIFESTATIONS. The child with cardiogenic shock demonstrates signs of inadequate systemic perfusion despite adequate intravascular volume or even relative hypervolemia. This form of shock is generally associated with low cardiac output. The child's extremities are cool to touch (will cool peripherally to proximally), with delayed capillary refill despite a warm, ambient temperature.[2,6,16] The skin may be mottled (see Figure 49-1).

Evidence of an adequate or high central venous pressure, including hepatomegaly and periorbital edema, is typically present in uncomplicated cardiogenic shock, particularly if right ventricular failure is involved. Evidence of pulmonary edema may be noted on a chest radiograph or clinical assessment (including signs of respiratory distress, reduced lung compliance during hand ventilation, or frothy pink sputum suctioned from the endotracheal tube) if left ventricular failure is present. The cardiac silhouette is usually enlarged on the chest radiograph, unless concurrent hypovolemia is present. If myocardial function is severely compromised, peripheral pulses may be diminished in intensity (dampened) or they may vary in intensity (pulsus alternans).

A low cardiac output may be documented by invasive or noninvasive devices. If a pulmonary artery catheter is in place, the cardiac output may be calculated through a thermodilution technique or continuous monitoring of the mixed venous oxygen saturation.

Signs of low cardiac output and cardiogenic shock may be identical to signs of cardiac tamponade. Although some classic signs of tamponade, including muffled heart tones or pulsus paradoxus may be observed, these signs may be difficult to appreciate if cardiac output and blood pressure are severely compromised. Therefore, if cardiogenic shock is suspected in a child after cardiovascular surgery or in any child at risk for the development of pericardial effusion, tamponade should be ruled out through an echocardiogram.

Septic Shock

Sepsis and its complications result from activation of biochemical and physiologic cascades that lead to the formation or activation of cytokines and other mediators that produce vasodilation, increased capillary permeability, maldistribution of blood flow, and cardiovascular dysfunction.[3] Sepsis and its complications may result in organ system dysfunction and are leading causes of death in noncoronary intensive care units. An estimated 42,000 pediatric cases of sepsis are reported annually in the United States and result in approximately 4400 deaths per year.[17]

Much information about the pathophysiology and clinical signs of sepsis has been extrapolated from adult studies and adult animal models of sepsis. Some information gleaned from adult experience is applicable to children, whereas other information is not. More research is needed to better understand pediatric sepsis and septic shock.

Watson's 2003 hospital data from seven states[17] still provides the most detailed information regarding causes of pediatric sepsis in the United States. The most common sites of infection from these data were primary bloodstream (25%) and respiratory tract (37%) infections;[17] about half of children with sepsis had an underlying disease and more than one fifth were low–birth-weight neonates.[17,18]

Many bloodstream and respiratory infections may be prevented with proper handwashing by healthcare providers before and after contact with children, appropriate sterile and aseptic technique during catheter insertion and tubing changes, and use of protocols to reduce central venous catheter infections and ventilator-associated pneumonias.[19,20] More pediatric data are needed to develop evidence-based recommendations to reduce hospital-acquired infections and sepsis.

The microorganisms that cause sepsis vary according to age, immune function, and location (e.g., in the hospital versus in the community).[21] Approximately 40% of all hospital-acquired infections in adults and children are linked to gram-negative infections; 40% to gram-positive infections; and 20% to viruses, fungi, or rickettsial microorganisms.[18] Prevention of hospital-acquired infections can substantially reduce the risk of sepsis and its complications.[19,20] Clinicians must be aware of the common pathogens in various populations.

Factors associated with risk for the development of sepsis include extremes of age (infants, young children and older adults)[3,17]; invasive catheters, surgical incisions, or wounds or burns; immunocompromise; and long-term antibiotic therapy.[17,18] Many of these risk factors are present in seriously ill or injured children and children with a chronic disease.

It is now clear that genetic variations among children and among invading microorganisms can alter the outcome of infections, sepsis, and septic shock.[21] Genetic variation in any of several genes that affect host responses to invading microorganisms can influence outcomes of infections.[22] Certainly, infectious diseases, such as meningococcal disease, can vary widely in their invasiveness and in the severity of effects on the host.[23] It is anticipated that genetic information will ultimately influence identification of a child's susceptibility to infection and sepsis, risk modification, early detection of sepsis, tailoring of therapy, and prognostication.[22]

Both proinflammatory and anti-inflammatory cytokines serve essential protective functions in fighting infection and modulating the immune response. Sepsis is caused by the effects of the invading microorganism and its toxins, but most effects that contribute to shock result from a disruption in the balance between *proinflammatory* mediators (including tumor necrosis factor-alpha [TNF-α], interleukin [IL]-1, IL-6, and IL-8; platelet-activating factor; arachidonic acid metabolites; nitric oxide; and many kinins) and *anti-inflammatory* mediators (IL-4, IL-10, IL-11, and IL-13; transforming growth factor-beta; colony-stimulating factors; soluble tumor necrosis factor receptor; IL-1 receptor antagonist; and activated protein C).[3] Extremely high levels of proinflammatory mediators, such as TNF, nitric oxide, and platelet-activating factor can become destructive, even after the triggering microorganism is eradicated.[3,21]

High proinflammatory cytokine levels have been implicated in the development of sepsis-induced disseminated intravascular coagulation, pulmonary injury, and microcirculatory disruptions, such as are observed in burns, severe trauma, shock reperfusion syndromes, and MODS.[21] Tumor necrosis factor levels have been directly related to mortality in newborns and children with meningitis and sepsis,[24] and interleukin-8 levels have been shown to be reliable predictors of pediatric sepsis mortality.[22]

Increased nitric oxide concentrations are thought to contribute to vasodilation, hypotension, and decreased myocardial function that develop during adult sepsis. In comparison, infants with sepsis often demonstrate pulmonary vasoconstriction resulting from shock-induced acidosis and hypoxia, and may benefit from administration of inhaled nitric oxide or other vasodilators.[25]

During sepsis, endotoxin stimulates the endothelium to become a secretory organ. The endothelium changes from the normal profibrinolytic and anticoagulant state to an antifibrinolytic and precoagulant one.[25] This change can lead to the development of microthrombin in some areas of the microcirculation, further contributing to maldistribution of blood flow. Mediators (e.g., activated protein C) that regulate coagulation pathways have been implicated in the sepsis process.[25-27] Activated protein C also regulates inflammation and activated protein C deficiency is a marker for severe sepsis in all ages.[27] Although administration of activated protein C improved survival in adults with severe sepsis,[28] it has not been shown to improve outcome in children and may produce excessive bleeding complications.[25]

There is clear interaction among catecholamines, adrenoreceptors, and glucocorticoids. Endogenous glucocorticoids have an anti-inflammatory effect (they decrease activation of proinflammatory mediators), and they modulate vasomotor tone by enhancing cardiovascular and vasomotor response to catecholamines.[29]

Critically ill children may have adrenal insufficiency (caused by adrenal hemorrhage, decreased renal perfusion, inhibition of corticosteroid production by TNF, or actual adrenal disease) or a relative adrenal insufficiency, with inadequate adrenal stress response or decreased response to circulating glucocorticoids.[30,31] When sepsis is present and the child fails to respond to initial fluid therapy and vasoactive support, providers should rule out adrenal insufficiency and consider hydrocortisone administration, especially if risk of adrenal insufficiency is present.[32]

CLINICAL MANIFESTATIONS. Sepsis and its complications produce a cascade of physiologic and biochemical changes. The clinical progression of sepsis in children has been described and defined by a consensus panel of international physicians[4] (Box 49-3).

Systemic inflammatory response syndrome (SIRS) represents a nonspecific response to a variety of insults, including trauma, burns, pancreatitis, or infection. SIRS is present when the child demonstrates two or more of the following as an acute change from baseline: change in temperature, specifically fever (greater than 38.5° C [101.3° F]) or hypothermia (less than 36° C [96.8° F]), change in heart rate (tachypnea or, in infants, bradycardia), change in respiratory rate (or need for mechanical ventilation), or change in white blood cell (WBC) count (including leukocytes, leukopenia, or an increase in the percentage of immature or band forms of WBCs).[4] These clinical signs must be interpreted in light of the child's baseline function.

BOX 49-3 INTERNATIONAL CONSENSUS DEFINITIONS OF SYSTEMIC INFLAMMATORY RESPONSE SYNDROME, SEPSIS, SEVERE SEPSIS, AND SEPTIC SHOCK IN CHILDREN

Systemic Inflammatory Response Syndrome (SIRS)

The presence of at least two of the following four large bulleted criteria, one of which must be abnormal temperature or leukocyte count:

- ALTERATION IN TEMPERATURE: Core body temperature of >38.5° or <36°C
- ALTERATION IN HEART RATE (characterized by any of the three open bullets, below):
  - Tachycardia in the absence of external stimulus, chronic drugs, or painful stimuli, defined as follows:
    - Newborn to 1 year: HR >180/min
    - 2-5 years: >140/min
    - 6-12 years: >130/min
    - 13 to <18 years: >110/min
  - Otherwise unexplained persistent elevation over a 0.5 to 4-hour time period
  - For children younger than 1 yr: bradycardia, in the absence of external vagal stimulus, β-blocker drugs, or congenital heart disease, defined by one of the three dashes below:
    - Newborn to 1 month: <100/min
    - 1 month to 1 year: <90/min
    - Otherwise unexplained persistent depression over a 30-minute time period
- ALTERATION IN RESPIRATORY RATE (characterized by either of the open bullets, below):
  - Mean respiratory rate >95th percentile normal for age, defined as follows:
    - Newborn to 1 week: >50/min
    - 1 week to 1 month: >40/min
    - 1 month to 1 year: >34/min
    - 2-5 years: >22/min
    - 6-12 years: >18/min
    - 13 to <18 years: >14/min
  - Mechanical ventilation for an acute process not related to underlying neuromuscular disease or the receipt of general anesthesia
- ALTERATION IN WHITE BLOOD CELL COUNT:
  - Leukocyte count elevated or depressed for age (not secondary to chemotherapy-induced leukopenia) or >10% immature neutrophils

Infection (one of the following)

- A suspected or proven (by positive culture, tissue stain, or polymerase chain reaction test) infection caused by any pathogen
- A clinical syndrome associated with a high probability of infection

Note: Evidence of infection includes positive findings on clinical examination, imaging, or laboratory tests (e.g., white blood cells in a normally sterile body fluid, perforated viscus, chest radiograph consistent with pneumonia, petechial or purpuric rash, purpura fulminans)

Sepsis

- SIRS in the presence of or as a result of suspected or proven infection

Severe Sepsis

- Sepsis plus one of the following:
  - Cardiovascular organ dysfunction
  - Acute respiratory distress syndrome
  - Two or more other organ dysfunctions (organ dysfunctions are defined in Box 49-4)

Septic Shock

- Sepsis and cardiovascular organ dysfunction as defined in Box 49-4

From Perkin RM et al: Shock, cardiac arrest and resuscitation. In Hazinski MF, editor: *Nursing care of the critically ill child,* ed 3, St Louis, 2013, Mosby; Modified from Goldstein B et al: *Pediatr Crit Care Med* 6:2–8, 2005.

Sepsis is a systemic response to infection. It is present when manifestations of SIRS are observed in conjunction with suspected infection. Positive blood or other cultures are not necessary for the diagnosis, but suspicion of infection is required.[4] For example, if the child with trauma develops a high fever or pulmonary congestion several days after injury, it is highly likely that an infection is present.

Severe sepsis is present when the child demonstrates evidence of sepsis (SIRS with suspected infection) and signs of cardiovascular or pulmonary dysfunction, or if the child has sepsis and evidence of two or more other organ dysfunctions (Box 49-4).[4] Altered organ perfusion is signaled by signs of organ system dysfunction. The dysfunctional organ system should be separate from the site of suspected infection and not explained by effects of drug therapy or other acute effects.[4] This important distinction will enable separation of signs of severe sepsis from signs of simple pneumonia and associated respiratory failure.

Septic shock is heralded in the child with sepsis by the development of cardiovascular dysfunction. This may be characterized by hypotension despite adequate fluid resuscitation or by the need for vasopressors to maintain blood pressure.[4] Because children tend to develop hypotension only late in the course of any shock, septic shock should be identified when the child develops more subtle signs of poor perfusion despite adequate fluid resuscitation. When the child with sepsis does develop hypotension plus signs of poor perfusion, hypotensive/decompensated septic shock is present, and mortality may be as high as 30%.[33]

Kissoon, Orr, and Carcillo[34] have proposed simplified diagnostic criteria for pediatric septic shock. They note that fever, tachycardia, and vasodilation are signs of inflammation. They propose that if the child with this triad of inflammatory signs also develops altered level of consciousness, the diagnosis of septic shock should be considered. Carcillo[25,34] has distilled the international consensus definitions of septic shock to include suspected infection with hypo- or hyperthermia and clinical signs of inadequate perfusion. Carcillo defines signs of inadequate perfusion as including any one of the following: decreased level of conscious or change in mental status; prolonged (>2 seconds) capillary refill; abnormal pulses (either diminished or bounding with wide pulse pressure); mottled, cool extremities; or decreased urine output. Carcillo also notes that hypotension is not required for the diagnosis but, if present, is confirmatory.[25,34]

Children with septic shock may have a high, normal, or low cardiac output. Unlike adults, who typically present with

BOX 49-4 CRITERIA FOR ORGAN DYSFUNCTION IN CHILDREN WITH SEVERE SEPSIS OR SEPTIC SHOCK

Cardiovascular

Despite administration of isotonic intravenous fluid boluses of more than 40 ml/kg in 1 hour, is described by the characteristics in one or more of the three bullets below:

- Decrease in blood pressure (BP) (hypotension) to <5th percentile for age, estimated for children 1-10 years of age as follows:
  - Mean arterial pressure: <40 mmHg + (1.5 × age in years)
  - Systolic BP <70 mmHg + (2 × age in years)
- Need for vasoactive drug to maintain BP in normal range (dopamine >5 mcg/kg/min; or dobutamine, epinephrine, or norepinephrine at any dose)
- Two of the following:
  - Unexplained metabolic acidosis: base deficit more severe than –5 mEq/L
  - Increased arterial lactate >2 times upper limit of normal
  - Oliguria: urine output <0.5 ml/kg/hr
  - Prolonged capillary refill: >5 seconds
  - Core to peripheral temperature gap >3°C

Respiratory (one of the following)*

- $PaCO_2/FiO_2$ <300 in absence of cyanotic heart disease or pre-existing lung disease
- $PaCO_2$ >65 torr or 20 mmHg over baseline $PaCO_2$
- Proven need† or >50% inspired oxygen to maintain saturation >92%
- Need for nonelective invasive or noninvasive mechanical ventilation‡

Neurologic (either of the following)

- Glasgow Coma Scale score ≤11
- Acute change in mental status with a decrease in Glasgow score ≥3 points from abnormal baseline

Hematologic (one of the following)

- Platelet count <80,000/mm^3
- A decline of 50% in platelet count from highest value recorded over the past 3 days (for chronic hematology/oncology)
- International normalized ratio >2

Renal

- Serum creatinine ≥twofold upper limit of normal for age or twofold increase in baseline creatinine

Hepatic (either of the following)

- Total bilirubin ≥4 mg/dl (not applicable for newborn)
- ALT twofold upper limit of normal for age

From Perkin RM et al: Shock, cardiac arrest and resuscitation. In Hazinski MF, editor: *Nursing care of the critically ill child*, ed 3, St Louis, 2013, Mosby. Modified from Goldstein B et al: *Pediatr Crit Care Med* 6:2–8, 2005.

*Acute respiratory distress syndrome must include a Pao_2/FiO_2 ratio <200 mm Hg, bilateral infiltrates, acute onset, and no evidence of left heart failure. Acute lung injury is defined identically except the Pao_2/FiO_2 ratio must be <300 mmHg.

†Proven need assumes oxygen requirement was tested by decreasing flow with subsequent increase in flow if required.

‡In postoperative patients this requirement can be met if the patient has developed an acute inflammatory or infectious process in the lungs that prevents the patient from being extubated.

ALT, Alanine transaminase.

vasodilation, hypotension, and normal or high cardiac output, approximately half of children with septic shock present with severe peripheral vasoconstriction, high systemic vascular resistance, and low cardiac output.[25,34]

The child with septic shock has significant hypovolemia and maldistribution of blood flow that typically respond to aggressive fluid administration, antibiotics and titration of inotropes, vasopressors, and vasodilators. Therapeutic goals include restoring blood pressure, normalizing heart rate and capillary refill, and maintaining high cardiac index (3.3 to 6 L/min/m^2 body surface area [BSA]) and high oxygen delivery (more than 200 ml/min/m^2) BSA.[32-37] In fact, in a small but seminal report of outcomes of septic shock in children,[35] Carcillo, Davis, and Zaritsky showed that aggressive fluid resuscitation (more than 40 ml/kg administered within the first hour of therapy and more than 200 ml/kg administered during the first 8 hours of therapy) was associated with significantly higher survival than less aggressive fluid resuscitation. In the most recent consensus recommendations for hemodynamic support of children with septic shock,[32] the experts noted the reduction in mortality (from initial 35% to 40% mortality to about 2% to 8% mortality) associated with the implementation of their consensus therapy recommendations.[32,34] In fact, for every hour delay in the restoration of normal blood pressure for age and restoration of capillary refill less than 3 seconds, the child's mortality doubled.[25,32-34]

The ultimate goal of treatment of septic shock is to support adequate systemic oxygen delivery and organ perfusion and function. This requires careful titration of fluid administration, inotropic support, and vasoconstrictors or vasodilators to maximize systemic oxygen delivery and organ perfusion and function.

The terms *warm* and *cold septic shock* are imprecise terms and should be used only in conjunction with other descriptions of systemic perfusion and cardiovascular function. **Warm shock** is characterized by peripheral vasodilation, warm skin with flash capillary refill, bounding pulses, and wide pulse pressure. Warm shock was thought to be associated with hyperdynamic cardiovascular function and high cardiac output. These characteristics are most commonly seen in adults with septic shock.[25] **Cold shock** is characterized by peripheral vasoconstriction, cold skin with prolonged capillary refill, and decreased peripheral pulses. Cold shock is often associated with low cardiac output; these characteristics are present in almost half of children who present with septic shock.[25] However, cardiac output may be low, normal, or high regardless of skin temperature, perfusion, and pulses; these characteristics alone will not identify the cardiovascular support required. When inadequate systemic perfusion persists, the child likely needs more aggressive fluid administration and titration of vasoactive drug therapy.

Many adults and some children with sepsis generate a cardiac output that is higher than normal despite a fall in ventricular ejection fraction. This high cardiac output may be associated with temporary adaptive ventricular dilation and an increase in ventricular end-diastolic volume, an increase in heart rate, and a fall in systemic vascular resistance. This low ejection fraction and ventricular dilation has not been documented in most children with septic shock. Most demonstrate severe hypovolemia, and cardiac function may be maintained or restored if fluid resuscitation is adequate.[25]

Kissoon, Orr, and Carcillo[34] describe the calculation of a *shock index* for children with septic shock. This shock index (heart rate ÷ systolic blood pressure) is high (2.4 or higher) with untreated or inadequately treated septic shock but falls with effective treatment of septic shock.

Obstructive Shock

Obstructive shock is inadequate cardiac output caused by an impediment to blood flow to or from the heart into the pulmonary or systemic circulation. Causes of obstructive shock in children include congenital heart defects (such as critical aortic stenosis and those with ductal-dependent pulmonary or systemic blood flow), tension pneumothorax, and pulmonary embolus. Obstruction to blood flow results in low cardiac output and circulatory collapse, typically with signs of peripheral vasoconstriction as adrenergic stimulation attempts to reduce blood flow to the skin, gut, and kidney and maintain adequate blood flow to the heart and brain. Signs of systemic or pulmonary venous obstruction are observed.

Additional clinical manifestations of obstructive shock are based on the cause of the obstruction. For example, the newborn with ductal-dependent pulmonary blood flow develops profound hypoxemia when the ductus arteriosus begins to constrict. If a newborn has ductal-dependent systemic blood flow, systemic pulses become faint or absent, extremities become cold and pale, and signs of pulmonary venous congestion develop when the ductus arteriosus begins to close. Tension pneumothorax produces signs of systemic venous obstruction and congestion, decreased breath sounds and chest expansion on the side of the pneumothorax, and shift of the mediastinum to the contralateral chest. Significant hypoxemia is present. When cardiac tamponade is the cause of the obstruction, signs of systemic or pulmonary edema, or both, develop with low cardiac output. When pulmonary embolus is the cause of the obstruction, hypoxemia, severe respiratory distress (or shortness of breath), and signs of right ventricular failure are observed.[3,16]

Treatment of obstructive shock focuses on restoration of systemic oxygenation and perfusion, and elimination of the obstruction to flow. To support systemic oxygenation and perfusion, providers must establish and maintain an adequate airway and support oxygenation and ventilation. Following establishment of vascular access, administration of a fluid bolus of 10 to 20 ml/kg of isotonic crystalloid may improve systemic perfusion; repeat if it is effective.[3,37] Diagnostic studies are limited to those essential to establishment of the diagnosis. Elimination of the cause of obstruction may require administration of prostaglandin E_1 (to reopen a constricted ductus arteriosus in newborns with ductal-dependent congenital heart disease), interventional cardiac catheterization for treatment of other defects causing obstruction, needle decompression of a tension pneumothorax or cardiac tamponade, and fibrinolytic therapy and anticoagulation (and possible embolectomy) for treatment of massive pulmonary embolus.[3,37]

Reperfusion and Inflammatory Injury

Reperfusion (reoxygenation) injury is cell damage caused by the restoration of blood flow and physiologic concentrations of oxygen to cells that have been exposed to injurious but nonlethal hypoxic conditions.[38] Ischemia causes changes in transmembrane permeability to sodium and calcium, and damage to intracellular organelles.[39] This damage triggers a proinflammatory and procoagulant response that can be very similar to that described for septic shock (described previously).

Restoration of oxygen delivery to extremely ischemic tissues produces highly reactive oxygen intermediates (e.g., free oxygen radicals and superoxide) that damage cell membranes, denature proteins, and disrupt chromosomes (see Chapter 2).[39] The amount of free oxygen radical produced is directly related to the severity and duration of the ischemic period. The reperfusion process is most likely to affect endothelial cells of the microvasculature, compromising organ perfusion after shock resuscitation.[38,39]

An ischemic insult activates white blood cells, priming monocytes and macrophages and contributing to the release of inflammatory mediators or cytokines, including TNF, IL-1, IL-6, IL-8, and platelet-activating factor. These cytokines in turn contribute to vasodilation, increased capillary permeability, and altered platelet function. The ultimate result is a maldistribution of blood flow and a compromise in organ perfusion.[38,39] The role of these mediators is summarized in Table 7-5. Chapter 48 includes a more comprehensive discussion of MODS.

Signs of organ dysfunction include but are not limited to lactic acidosis, oliguria, and an acute alteration in level of consciousness (e.g., decrease in Glasgow Coma Scale score of 1 point or more); hypoxemia, hypotension, poor capillary refill, or shock plus signs of coagulopathy, respiratory, renal, or hepatic dysfunction, or neurologic dysfunction. Gut injury and inflammation may enable translocation of gram-negative bacteria or endotoxin into the bloodstream, and may contribute to gastrointestinal bleeding.[5] Box 49-4 contains information on other potential signs of organ system failure in children.

Several scoring systems are available to characterize the severity of illness in critically ill children with organ dysfunction. These include the Pediatric Logistic Organ Dysfunction (PELOD) scoring system[40] and the Pediatric Multiple Organ Dysfunction Score (P-MODS).[40-42] These scoring systems may be useful as prognostic indicators when they are used for several days. Important differences exist between neonates and children in terms of mortality associated with specific organ failures and with specific PELOD scores.[41]

Evaluation and Treatment of Shock

The goals of treatment of shock are maximization of oxygen delivery and minimization of oxygen demand. The airway, oxygenation, ventilation, and perfusion must be supported. Reduction of oxygen demand requires treatment of fever and pain. In

BOX 49-5 MOST COMMON PEDIATRIC DYSRHYTHMIAS

Heart (QRS) Rate too Slow for Clinical Condition

QRS Duration (Width) Normal

Sinus bradycardia
Junctional rhythm
Heart block

QRS Duration (Width) Prolonged

Supraventricular tachycardia (SVT) with aberrant ventricular conduction
Ventricular rhythm
Heart block

Heart (QRS) Rate too Fast for Clinical Condition

QRS Duration (Width) Normal

Sinus tachycardia
SVT

QRS Duration (Width) Prolonged

SVT with aberrant ventricular conduction
Ventricular tachycardia

Collapse (Pulseless) Rhythms

Electromechanical dissociation
Ventricular tachycardia
Ventricular fibrillation
Asystole

addition, the child should be kept warm and shivering should be prevented. Blood components and, perhaps, intravenous fluids should be warmed before administration to young infants and children with hypothermia. Fear and pain increase oxygen consumption, so care must be taken to reassure the child and treat pain as indicated.

As noted, all children in shock require support of airway, oxygenation, and ventilation. Specific treatment of hypovolemic shock is volume resuscitation. Treatment targeting cardiogenic shock requires titration of fluid administration to optimize cardiac preload, but vasoactive drugs are needed to improve myocardial function and vasodilators or vasoconstrictors may be needed to support systemic perfusion. Specific management of septic shock includes administration of antimicrobial therapy, fluid resuscitation, and initiation of vasoactive support within the first hour of care following initial medical contact. Treatment specific to obstructive shock includes elimination of the cause of the obstruction to blood flow.

To evaluate and support airway patency and ventilation the child is positioned in a manner that supports maximal airway patency, and the provider then assesses airway and ventilation. Humidified supplementary oxygen is given as needed at up to 10 to 15 L/min by nonrebreathing mask or bag-mask ventilation. An advanced airway is placed in children *before* respiratory deterioration or arrest complicates shock management. Oxygenation is monitored continuously through pulse oximetry.

The child's heart rate must be adequate to support effective cardiac output and systemic perfusion. The most common pediatric dysrhythmias are listed in Box 49-5. Treat bradydysrhythmias and extreme tachydysrhythmias promptly. Pharmacologic therapy, pacing, or synchronized direct current (DC) cardioversion may be required.

The rhythms associated with loss of pulses ("arrest" rhythms) include asystole, electromechanical dissociation (EMD), pulseless ventricular tachycardia, and ventricular fibrillation. Regardless of electrocardiogram (ECG) findings, provide cardiopulmonary resuscitation—including cardiac compression—when pulses are lost or if, despite support of oxygenation and ventilation, the child demonstrates a heart rate less than 60/min with poor perfusion.

Adequate vascular access is needed to establish hemodynamic monitoring and to provide volume and inotropic support as needed. Once systemic perfusion is restored, transfer to a pediatric intensive care unit is advised.

Volume resuscitation is designed to restore intravascular volume relative to the vascular space and to optimize ventricular preload. The specific fluid selected and route of administration are determined by the child's clinical condition. In general, isotonic **crystalloids** (isotonic salt-containing solutions, such as normal saline or lactated Ringer's solution) or **colloids** (protein-containing fluids, such as albumin or blood) are administered in boluses of 20 ml/kg (or 10 ml/kg of packed red blood cells) given over 5 to 20 minutes for hypovolemic and septic shock. If cardiogenic shock (myocardial dysfunction) is present, smaller fluid boluses (5 to 10 ml/kg) are administered over about 10 to 20 minutes. Hypotonic fluids should not be administered.[3,37] After each bolus, reassess systemic perfusion and administer additional fluids if indicated.

Children in septic shock require a large volume of intravenous fluid to restore and maintain systemic perfusion. More than 40 ml/kg in fluid boluses will likely be required during the first hour of volume resuscitation, and a total of 200 ml/kg or more may be required during the first several hours of therapy.[3,32,34,35,37] In fact, rapid volume administration, particularly during the first hour of therapy, has been linked with improved survival in hypotensive children in septic shock.[33] An algorithm for the treatment of septic shock, based on the recommendations of the American College of Critical Care Medicine and the Pediatric Advanced Life Support course, is presented in Figure 49-2.

Unless shock is mild or responds immediately to volume therapy, insertion of a central venous (monitoring) catheter is advisable. Several multilumen catheters are available in pediatric sizes that enable simultaneous monitoring of central venous pressure and administration of fluids. Continuous or intermittent monitoring of the superior vena cava $S_{CV}O_2$ will enable evaluation of the balance between the child's oxygen delivery and oxygen consumption. If cardiac output is adequate, oxygen saturation in the SVC will be approximately 25% to 30% lower than the arterial oxygen saturation. A larger arterial venous oxygen saturation difference suggests inadequate oxygen delivery (caused by inadequate arterial oxygen content or inadequate cardiac output or both) or excessive oxygen demand.[3]

Monitoring of the volume of urine output and specific gravity is useful in determining the child's response to fluid therapy. A urinary catheter should be inserted if shock is present unless the child has sustained pelvic trauma or a urethral tear is suspected. All sources of fluid intake and output should be monitored and recorded hourly or more frequently if needed.

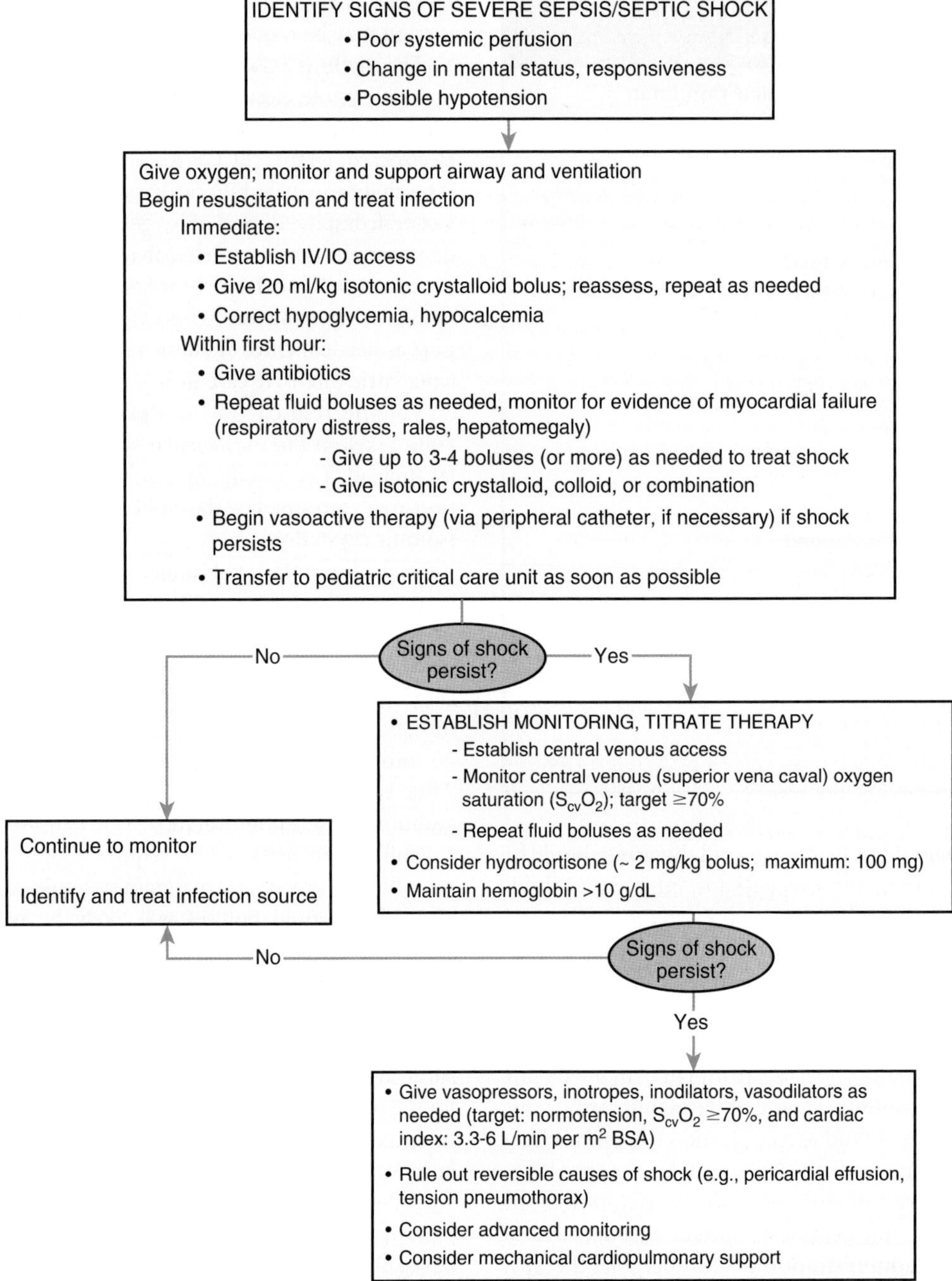

FIGURE 49-2 **Hemodynamic Support in Pediatric Septic Shock.** *BSA,* body surface area; *IO,* intake/output; *IV,* intravenous. (From Perkin RM et al: Shock, cardiac arrest and resuscitation. In Hazinski MF, editor: *Nursing care of the critically ill child,* ed 3, p 126, St Louis, 2013, Mosby; data from Brierley J et al: *Crit Care Med* 37:666–688, 2009.)

An intra-arterial line should be inserted if shock persists. This enables reliable, continuous evaluation of arterial pressure. Noninvasive oscillometric blood pressure–monitoring devices may not accurately measure low or rapidly falling blood pressures and may *overestimate* the blood pressure,[43] particularly in trauma patients.[44]

Insertion of a pulmonary artery catheter may be considered if the child demonstrates shock that is unresponsive to volume and vasoactive drug support. A pulmonary artery catheter with thermodilution cardiac output thermistor, a fiberoptic pulmonary artery catheter, or both can enable continuous monitoring of mixed venous oxygen saturation or continuous monitoring of cardiac output. Quantification of these variables can be particularly helpful if precise tracking of hemodynamic measurements is desired. This may be necessary in the care of the child with septic shock or MODS.

The optimal hemoglobin threshold for transfusion in critically ill children is unknown. In a multicenter trial of critically ill children, a hemoglobin red-cell transfusion threshold of 7 g/dl decreased transfusion requirements without increasing adverse outcomes.[45] However, that study excluded premature infants and children with severe hypoxemia, hemodynamic instability, active blood loss, and cyanotic heart disease. A more recent publication from the same researchers[46] recommends higher transfusion thresholds (9 to 12 g/dl) for children with cardiac or respiratory disease, with the highest thresholds for children with cyanotic congenital heart disease and those with hemodynamic instability.

Administration of blood or blood component therapy is needed to treat hemorrhage or severe coagulopathies. A "normal" hematocrit does not rule out the possibility of hemorrhage; the hematocrit typically falls in a person who has sustained whole blood loss after the blood loss is replaced with crystalloids or colloids. In general, 10 ml/kg boluses of packed red blood cells are used for every second or third fluid bolus needed to treat significant blood loss.[14,15,37]

Transfusion for the child with chronic anemia and shock must be accomplished slowly to prevent hypervolemia and further deterioration in myocardial function. Administration of packed red blood cells at a rate averaging 3 to 5 ml/kg/hr over several hours may be well tolerated, particularly if it is preceded and followed by administration of diuretics.[47] If severe anemia is associated with severe hypervolemia and myocardial dysfunction, an exchange transfusion may be required. If a coagulopathy is present, administer specific blood component therapy necessary to prevent or treat hemorrhage.

Hypoxemia, metabolic acidosis, and electrolyte imbalances depress myocardial function and must be corrected when shock is present. Administer oxygen during resuscitation of the child in shock and be prepared to institute noninvasive pressure support ventilation or mechanical ventilation when needed.

The child's serum glucose concentration should be monitored using rapid bedside testing. Hypoglycemia requires glucose administration; continuous infusion is preferred to repeated intermittent bolus therapy. If severe hyperglycemia develops, insulin administration may be indicated to reduce the serum glucose concentration to less than 150 to 180 mg/dl. Although tight glycemic control has been linked with improved survival in critically ill children,[48] it also caused frequent episodes of hypoglycemia. The relative risks of severe hyperglycemia versus unintentional hypoglycemia have not been established.[49] In a recent survey, pediatric intensivists reported management of hyperglycemia with insulin therapy; the preferred blood glucose target range was 90 to 140 mg/dl.[50] A randomized clinical trial of pediatric glycemic control is needed.

During resuscitation, providers must avoid acute or severe alterations in the serum sodium concentration.[3,11,37] Acute changes in serum sodium alter the serum osmolality and result in fluid shifts into and out of the vascular spaces. Such fluid shifts can be associated with neurologic complications including seizures, cerebral edema, and intracranial hemorrhage.[11]

Alterations in serum potassium concentration may affect myocardial contractility and conduction. However, children are far less sensitive than adults to minor changes in serum potassium concentration. Hypokalemia may result from inadequate potassium administration during volume therapy or from excessive potassium losses caused by drug therapy (e.g., furosemide). The serum potassium concentration falls in the presence of alkalosis; this represents an intracellular shift of potassium and is corrected when the pH is normalized. Treat true hypokalemia with an infusion of potassium chloride at a dose equivalent to 0.5 to 1 mEq/kg administered over several hours.[11]

Hyperkalemia may result from excessive potassium administration, reduced potassium excretion (e.g., in renal failure), or massive cell lysis (e.g., tumor lysis syndrome). Serum potassium concentration also rises when acidosis develops; the rise in serum potassium is caused by a shift of potassium from the intracellular to the vascular space (i.e., exchanged for vascular H^+) and falls when the serum pH is corrected.[11]

Both ionized and total calcium concentration should be monitored, and documented hypocalcemia must be treated. Note that the ionized serum calcium falls with alkalosis and rises with acidosis. Serum ionized calcium concentration is often low (less than 4.5 mEq/L) in children with septic shock.[11]

Hypercalcemia may be observed in children with some malignancies, including acute lymphocytic leukemia, lymphomas, and soft tissue sarcomas. Malignant cells often secrete a parathormone-like substance that stimulates bone reabsorption, release of calcium, and rapid cell turnover. Although mild hypercalcemia is not life threatening, extreme hypercalcemia (total serum calcium approaching 19 to 20 mEq/L) may produce renal and cardiovascular complications.[47]

Table 49-7 summarizes drug therapy for children in shock. If oxygenation, ventilation, heart rate, and intravascular volume are appropriate and myocardial function and systemic perfusion remain poor, vasoactive drug therapy with inotropes is indicated.

Emerging Therapies for Shock and Sepsis

Prevention of shock is important. Prevention of trauma (injury prevention) and treatment of dehydration can eliminate the two leading causes of hypovolemic shock in children. *Haemophilus influenzae* sepsis and meningitis have been nearly eradicated in the United States since the introduction and widespread use of *H. influenzae* vaccine for infants, and immunization against *Neisseria meningitidis* (the causative microorganism of meningococcal sepsis and meningitis); pneumococcus vaccine may similarly reduce the incidence of pneumococcal infection and sepsis. The incidence of septic shock from hospital-acquired infections, such as ventilator-associated pneumonia or catheter-related bloodstream infections, is decreasing with the use of quality improvement approaches.[20]

Advances in shock therapy have been made in recent years, and several show promise for continued improvement in treatment. First, there is a better understanding of resuscitation goals with an appreciation of the need to target high, rather than normal, cardiac output and oxygen delivery during resuscitation.

Trauma resuscitation has become more targeted in adults and children. In the prehospital setting, prehospital fluid resuscitation is reserved for children with signs of shock. If penetrating trauma is associated with hypovolemic shock, the child requires urgent surgical intervention, so delays during transport are minimized.

Because massive transfusions can produce immunologic and coagulation complications, the surgical approach to trauma has changed to include staged surgical repair of significant

TABLE 49-7 PEDIATRIC VASOACTIVE DRUGS FOR THE TREATMENT OF SHOCK*

DOSE	EFFECTS	CAUTIONS
Sympathomimetics		
Dobutamine: 2-20 mcg/kg/min	Selective β-adrenergic effects, increases cardiac contractility and also increases heart rate (this latter effect is variable); β_2 effects produce peripheral vasodilation; no dopaminergic or α-adrenergic effects	Extreme tachyarrhythmias have been reported, particularly in infants; hypotension may develop; may produce pulmonary vasoconstriction
Dopamine: 1-5 mcg/kg/min	Dopaminergic effects predominate, including increase in glomerular filtration rate and urine volume	Can produce extreme tachyarrhythmias; can result in increase in pulmonary artery pressure; inhibits thyroid-stimulating hormone and aldosterone secretion
Dopamine: 2-10 mcg/kg/min	Dopaminergic effects persist and β_1 effects are seen, especially an increase in heart rate	As above
Dopamine: 8-20 mcg/kg/min	α-Adrenergic effects dominate	As above
Epinephrine: 0.05-0.15 mcg/kg/min	Endogenous catecholamine, which produces α, β_1, and β_2 adrenergic effects; at low doses, β_1 effects dominate	Will increase myocardial work and oxygen consumption at any dose; splanchnic constriction will occur at even low doses
Epinephrine: 0.2-0.3 mcg/kg/min	α-Adrenergic (vasoconstrictive) effects dominate	As above
Isoproterenol: 0.05-0.1 mcg/kg/min	β-Adrenergic effects; β_1 effects may result in rapid increase in heart rate; β_2 effects may produce peripheral vasodilation and also may effectively treat bronchoconstriction	Monitor for tachyarrhythmias, hypotension; will increase myocardial oxygen consumption
Norepinephrine: 0.05-1 mcg/kg/min	Endogenous catecholamine with α- and β-adrenergic effects; produces potent peripheral and renal vasoconstriction; can increase blood pressure	May cause tachyarrhythmias, increased myocardial work, and increased oxygen consumption; may result in hepatic and mesenteric ischemia
Vasopressin		
Vasopressin: 0.2 to 2 milliunits/kg/min (0.0002 to 0.002 unit/kg/min)	Antidiuretic hormone analog that acts on vasopressin receptors; produces peripheral and splanchnic vasoconstriction; also used to treat GI hemorrhage for this reason	May cause hypertension, bradycardia
Phosphodiesterase Inhibitors and Inodilators		
Inamrinone: Loading dose 0.075 to 0.1 mg/kg (75 to 100 mcg/kg) slowly Infusion: 5-10 mcg/kg/min	Nonadrenergic inotropic agent that produces phosphodiesterase inhibition and increase in intracellular cyclic adenosine monophosphate (cAMP); intracellular calcium uptake also is delayed; these effects result in improved cardiac contractility and vasodilation	Monitor for arrhythmias (especially accelerated junctional rhythm, junctional tachycardia, and ventricular ectopy); may produce hypotension (especially if patient is hypovolemic), liver and GI dysfunction, thrombocytopenia, and abdominal pain; experience in children is limited and recent
Milrinone: Loading dose: 0.05 mg/kg (50 mcg/kg) over 10-60 min Infusion: 0.25-0.75 mcg/kg/min	As above	Reduce dose when renal dysfunction present
Vasodilators		
Nitroglycerin: 0.25-0.5 mcg/kg/min; increase as tolerated to maximum 10 mcg/kg/min (adolescents, 5 mcg/min; *note* **not** per kg per min)	Arterial and venodilator	Is absorbed by polyvinyl chloride tubing; use special infusion set
Nitroprusside: 0.3-0.5 mcg/kg/min; titrate up to 8 mcg/kg/min (max. infusion dose: 8-10 mcg/kg/min)	Arterial and venodilator	Light sensitive; use special infusion set or cover tubing when infusion slow; may produce thiocyanate and cyanide toxicity, particularly for higher doses or prolonged infusion

Modified from Perkin RM et al: Shock, cardiac arrest and resuscitation. In Hazinski MF, editor: *Nursing care of the critically ill child,* ed 3, p 120, St Louis, 2013, Mosby.

*Infusion rate = ml/hr = Weight (kg) × Dose (mcg/kg per min) × 60 min/hr ÷ concentration (mcg/ml).

GI, Gastrointestinal.

injuries (e.g., liver and bowel injuries). The initial surgery is performed to stabilize the child, and, if needed, subsequent procedures repair the injury. This multistage approach, based on battlefield experiences, reduces the volume of blood products administered and has been linked with reduced morbidity and mortality.[15]

We now have a better understanding of the pathophysiology of septic shock in children,[32] appreciating the critical role that immediate antibiotics, early and aggressive fluid resuscitation, and vasoactive therapy play in the outcome of pediatric sepsis.[32-36] Such resuscitation should be provided during the first hour of therapy; every hour of delay has been reported to result in a 40% increase in mortality.[33]

Goals for management of pediatric septic shock are to restore the child's heart rate and blood pressure to normal for age, to achieve targeted perfusion pressure (mean arterial pressure – CVP) of about 55 to 65 mmHg, to reduce capillary refill to less than 2 seconds, and to support a cardiac index of 3.3 to 6 L/min/m^2 body surface area, and to maintain the SVC's $S_{CV}O_2$ at 70% or higher.[32,33-37] This goal-directed therapy, targeting an $S_{CV}O_2$ of 70% or higher in children, has been shown to substantially reduce mortality (by two thirds in one study) and organ failure.[36]

In an excellent and very concise summary of the management of the child in septic shock, Kissoon, Ort, and Carcillo suggest calculation of a *shock index,* dividing the child's heart rate by the child's systolic blood pressure (heart rate [HR] ÷ systolic BP). This shock index can serve as an indicator of left ventricular ejection, and should fall (e.g., from 2.25 to 1.75) in the first hour of effective management.[34]

Therapeutic hypothermia suppresses proinflammatory mediators and may enhance anti-inflammatory mediators.[51,52] Mild to moderate induced hypothermia (to 32° to 34° C [89.6° to 93.2° F]) has been shown to increase survival in neurologic outcome in neonates with hypoxic-ischemic encephalopathy[53] and in comatose, hemodynamically stable adults following resuscitation from cardiac arrest.[54] It is possible that such therapy may be helpful for victims of shock, particularly those with MODS. However, it is important to note that the control groups in these neonatal and adult hypothermia studies were all febrile. We know that fever develops following resuscitation from cardiac arrest and that fever is associated with unfavorable neurologic outcome.[55] While we await the results of multicentered clinical trials of therapeutic hypothermia in children, it is important to treat fever following resuscitation.

It soon may be possible to tailor sepsis and other critical therapies through the use of genetic profiling of the microorganism[23] and of the child.[22] Prospective identification of genetic markers for risk of sepsis and responsiveness to therapy may enable individual tailoring of surveillance and interventions to maximize survival and minimize risks from those therapies that are unlikely to be effective.

Finally, several devices are available that enable noninvasive or minimally invasive calculation of cardiac output and index, stroke volume, and circulating blood volume in children.[3] As providers gain experience with the use of such devices and more published data are available about their reliability, we will have more tools to confirm clinical assessment and monitor response to therapy.

BURNS

Management of pediatric burn injuries requires an understanding of the differences that exist in this population related to etiology of injury, growth and development, physiology, and clinical course. In 1988 the American Burn Association established criteria to guide transfer of a patient to a specialized burn center. These criteria remain a standard in burn care and are based on complex management issues related to treatment of acute burns and the long-term rehabilitation needs of children.[56]

Burn injuries in children often are preventable and often are the result of inadequate supervision, curiosity, inability to escape the burning agent, or intentional abuse. **Scald injuries** (i.e., hot water, grease, other) are most common among young children, whereas flame burns are more prevalent among older children.[57] A child exposed to hot tap water at 60° C (140° F) for 3 seconds will sustain a third-degree burn.[58]

A child's skin is thinner and thus more susceptible to injury than an adult's. The extent of injury is determined by the temperature of the burning agent and the duration of exposure. Because very young children may be unable to escape the heat source, the depth of the injury is likely to be greater. The kitchen also is a common site for burn injury and often involves pulling over dishes or appliances containing hot liquids. These are common burn injury sources for children 2 years of age and younger.

Although **child abuse** can occur at any age, young children are particularly vulnerable to serious injury. Approximately 10% of all forms of abuse cases in the United States are caused by burning.[59] Burns that may suggest physical maltreatment include: (1) patterned burns, (2) classic forced immersion burn pattern with sharp stocking or glove demarcation and sparing of flexed protected areas, (3) splash/spill burn patterns not consistent with history or developmental level, and (4) cigarette burns. Abuse is suggested with: (1) incompatible history and physical examination; (2) incompatible burn and developmental level; (3) bilateral or mirror image burns; (4) localized burns to genitals, buttocks, and perineum (especially at toilet-training stage); (5) evidence of excessive delay in seeking treatment; and (6) presence of other forms of injury.[60] Forced immersion in hot water typically presents with deep symmetric injuries lacking any evidence of splash wounds (Figure 49-3). By contrast, a pull-down splash burn usually has a triangular pattern with immediate skin contact reflected as the area of greatest burn injury. The burn injury then forms an arrow pointing downward. **Contact burns** also may be intentionally inflicted by contact with cigarettes or other hot objects such as curling irons. Young children may inadvertently grasp a hot object. However, the pattern of injury will be confined to the palm. Burns to the dorsum of the hand are viewed with suspicion.[59,60]

Children 3 to 8 years of age are most often injured by flame during fire play. Lighters and matches ignite clothing and cause house fires. Young children may run when clothing ignites and increase the severity of injury. Approximately 50% of all deaths

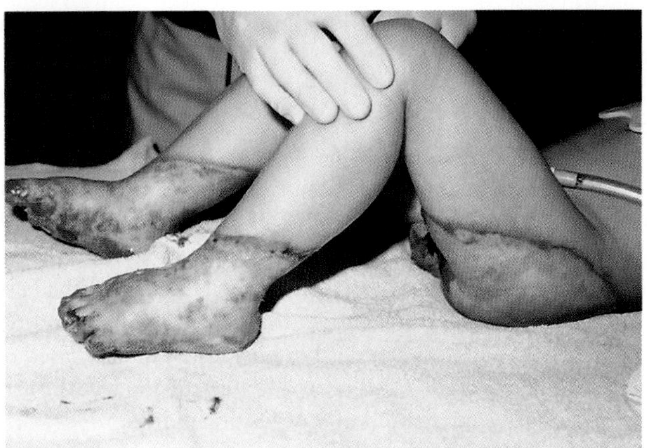

FIGURE 49-3 Burn Pattern Typically Seen After Forced Emersion in Hot Water.

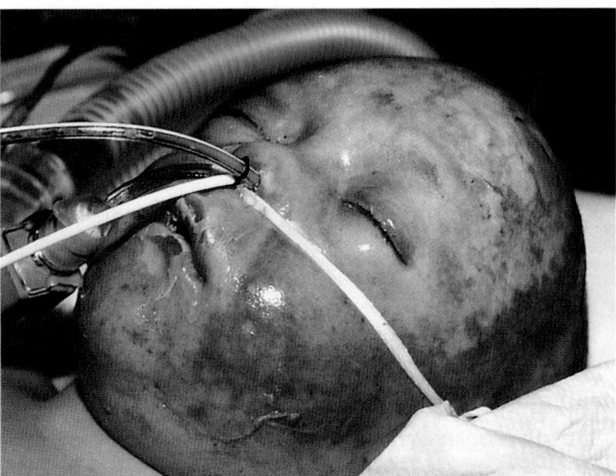

FIGURE 49-5 Areas of Indeterminate Depth of Injury in a Young Child.

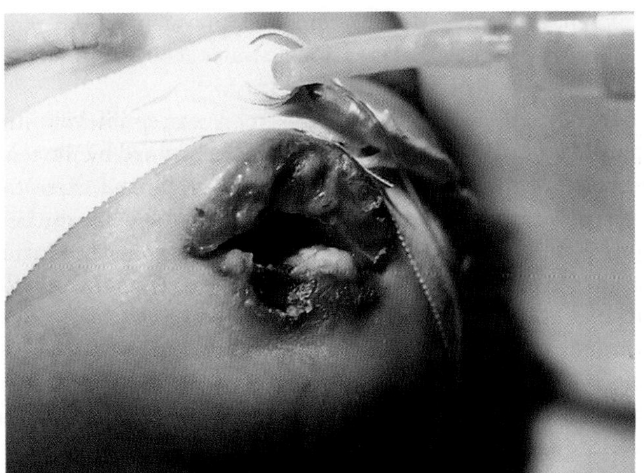

FIGURE 49-4 Commissure Burn Resulting from Biting an Electrical Wire.

in burn children are caused by inhalation injury.[61] Escape from a burning residence or motor vehicle is often delayed because young children cannot cognitively comprehend the circumstances or physically remove themselves from the danger. **Flame burns** involving flammable liquids, especially gasoline, are more common in older children.

Although flame and scald burns account for the majority of thermal injuries in children, **electrical burns** result from direct contact with high- or low-voltage current. Most commonly these injuries occur as a result of risk-taking behavior on the part of young males. Trauma from contact with electrical energy results from the passage of current through vital organs, muscle compartments, and nerve or vascular pathways. Very young children are at risk for injury from chewing on electrical cords or inserting objects into electrical outlets (Figure 49-4). Lightning strikes also account for some electrical burns. **Chemical burns** occur most often in an industrial setting for the adult. At home, children may be burned by swallowing corrosive agents. The type of causative agent has important implications for the evaluation, treatment, and prognosis of the child.

Severity of Injury

The severity of burn injury is assessed based on the percentage of the total body surface area (TBSA) involved. Use of the standard Rule of Nines results in inaccurate calculation of the percentage of TBSA involved in children. Although the infant's trunk and arms are of roughly the same proportion as the adult's, the head and neck make up 18% of TBSA and each lower extremity is 14% of TBSA. A modified Rule of Nines deducts 1% from the head and adds 0.5% to each leg for each year of life after 2 years.[58] Various charts are available that assign body proportions to children of different ages. These are generally used in pediatric burn facilities and do accurately compute the extent of burn injury.

Because burn trauma represents a three-dimensional wound, the severity of injury is assessed also in relation to the **depth of injury.** The etiology of the burn and the duration of contact with the burning agent are important considerations in determining the depth of injury. In general, the more intense the heat source and longer the contact, the deeper the resulting injury; however, infant skin is extremely fragile and more likely to sustain a deeper burn. This makes the estimation of the depth of burn difficult in very young children, especially following scald injuries (Figure 49-5). Intentionally inflicted burns tend to be more severe because contact with the burning agent is prolonged. Electrical injuries also may mask the extent of damage on initial assessment. Visible tissue damage may appear minimal despite severe injury to underlying structures.

Another important factor in assessing the severity of injury is the victim's age. Children younger than 2 years have a significantly higher risk for associated morbidity and mortality after sustaining a burn injury. They have not achieved maturity of the immune system and are at increased risk for infection and sepsis. In addition, very young children are intolerant of rapid fluid shifts and demonstrate immature renal function, which negatively affects their ability to retain sodium and water (see Shock).

The areas of the body injured are another consideration when assessing the severity of the burn. Burns of the hands, feet, and perineum and across joints carry the potential for scar formation and contracture that may interfere with function as well as growth and development. Specialized care is required to preserve maximal function. In addition, burns to the face and neck may result in airway compromise as well as deformity caused by damage to delicate cartilage of the nose and ears.

Concomitant injuries may be suggested by the circumstances of the burn and should always be investigated; for example, initially burns do not bleed. Bloody drainage suggests another source of trauma. Fractures may result from jumping from a window to escape a house fire. Electrical injuries and motor vehicle accidents often result in associated trauma. Any suspicion of intentionally inflicted burns should alert the burn team to assess for other injuries.

PATHOPHYSIOLOGY, CLINICAL MANIFESTATIONS, AND TREATMENT. Major burn trauma involves all body systems, and the consequences of injury include shock, infection, hypermetabolism, organ failure, and functional limitations. These effects can be magnified in the pediatric population as a result of physiologic immaturity and age-related variation in treatment modalities. Along with recognition of changes in the pathophysiology with a burn injury, clinical manifestations are apparent in all organ systems. Although the cutaneous trauma is the initiator of the chain of responses, it is important to consider all of the likely consequences of the injury. An awareness of the changing patterns of convalescence and the development of complications assists in the identification and early treatment of potential sequelae.

Integument

The local response manifested in the area of trauma includes cellular destruction and damage. Progressive injury caused by **dermal ischemia** may result from ineffective initial management, especially inadequate or delayed resuscitation. An increase in the permeability and hydrostatic pressure of the capillaries results in the loss of fluid, proteins, and electrolytes into the interstitial spaces. A diminishing intravascular oncotic pressure further enhances these losses and results in edema formation. Marked edema can result not only in the area of injury but also in unburned areas. Loss of substantial areas of skin has immediate and profound physiologic effects. Direct and evaporative fluid losses are seen immediately.[62] Although these losses are maximal in the immediate postburn period, they persist until wound closure.

Circulatory alterations also occur in the area of injury. Reduced blood flow and capillary stasis result from **hemoconcentration,** the release of thromboplastin and clot-activating factors from heat-damaged cells, reduced cardiac output, and edema formation. Circulation in the area of partial-thickness wounds ceases for 24 to 48 hours after injury, after which it is usually restored. Vascular supply in the area of full-thickness injuries is completely occluded and is not restored until granulation tissue forms or the wound is surgically repaired. The dry, leathery **eschar** provides an ideal environment for bacterial growth. Infection, trauma, or applying ice to the burn area may convert a partial-thickness injury to a full-thickness one, especially in young children, who have thinner, more delicate skin.

Vitamin D, an essential factor for proper formation of bone during growth and development, is an important nutrient in children to facilitate intestinal absorption of calcium. Vitamin D deficiency has been associated with adverse effects on the skeletal system, as well as the immune system. Vitamin D production may be compromised in burned children demonstrated by a high incidence of low-serum vitamin D levels. Burn wound scarring and lack of sunlight may limit cutaneous vitamin D biosynthesis.[63]

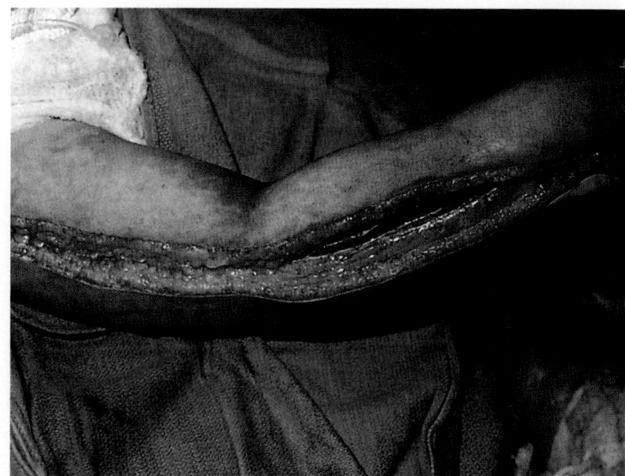

FIGURE 49-6 Escharotomy/Fasciotomy in a Severely Burned Arm.

Cardiovascular System

The marked reduction in cardiac output immediately following injury is accompanied by an initial increase in systemic vascular resistance. As fluid is lost into the interstitial spaces, a further reduction in cardiac output occurs, accompanied by vasodilation. Because the infant maintains cardiac output by increasing heart rate preferentially to stroke volume, extremely elevated heart rates result in a decreased filling time and a further reduction in cardiac output.[64] Adequate resuscitation returns cardiac output to normal levels in approximately 24 to 36 hours. Without fluid replacement, cardiac output continues to decrease and results in organ failure and death.

The inefficient and labile peripheral circulation of the infant further complicates management of the burn shock phase of treatment. The rapid fluid shift to the interstitial space and drying of the eschar results in compromised circulation and a resultant tourniquet effect in the extremities. Blood vessels and nerves become entrapped because the fascia cannot expand to accommodate the massive edema. Release of pressure is required to restore blood flow and preserve nerve function (Figure 49-6).

Constriction of the chest and impairment of respiratory excursion also may result, especially in the very young child, because of the increased pliability of the rib cage. Excessive fluid volume can contribute to a serious complication (increased intra-abdominal pressure) that may have an underestimated incidence in burned individuals. Although children with increased intra-abdominal pressure readings tended to be younger, larger TBSA injuries and full-thickness components were significantly associated with elevated pressures.[65] Increased **intra-abdominal pressure** has the potential to impair hemodynamics, renal function, hepatic malperfusion, and pulmonary dysfunction. Despite maintaining cardiac output with fluid replacement, renal function remains impaired in the presence of increased intra-abdominal pressure. Intra-abdominal pressure, as a stressor, can stimulate the neuroendrocrine system and elicit stress reactions directed at neutralizing the initial insult of the burn. Increases in the production and release of catecholamines, glucocorticoids, and beta-endorphins support the clinical finding of profoundly altered cardiovascular, pulmonary, and renal function.[66]

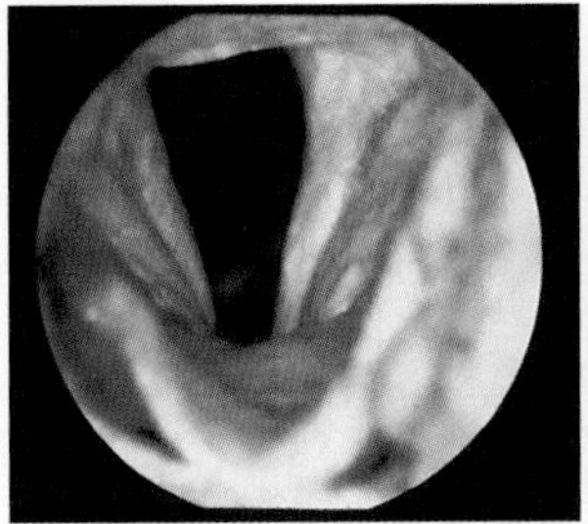
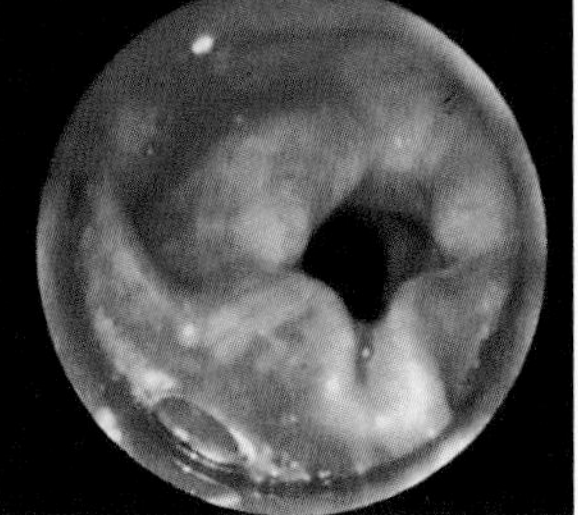

FIGURE 49-7 Airways. Adult airway *(left)*; smaller pediatric airway *(right)*.

Pulmonary System

The clinical manifestations of burn injury related to the pulmonary system include a variety of complications ranging from inhalation injury, pulmonary edema, and respiratory failure to aspiration of gastric contents and pneumonia. Inhalation injury has a negative, prolonged effect on pulmonary function that is associated with and remains a major determinant of increased morbidity and mortality.[67]

Anatomic differences in the pediatric airway affect the response to pulmonary complications, as well as therapeutic interventions. The infant airway is positioned anteriorly, making visualization of the cords more difficult. The difficult visualization is further compounded by the relatively large tongue and slanting vocal cords. A small degree of edema results in greatly increased work of breathing in the child (Figure 49-7). These considerations are particularly important during the resuscitation phase when progressive edema threatens to obstruct the airway. Significant edema results in impairment of respiratory function unless an artificial airway is inserted (Figure 49-8). Malposition of an endotracheal tube may result in inadvertent extubation, intubation of the bronchi, and atelectasis. Because of the relatively short length of the infant trachea, alterations of the position of the head and neck can affect tube position despite maintenance of the tube position at the teeth.[68-70]

Infants compensate for pulmonary compromise by increasing the respiratory rate. However, because the child possesses fewer type I muscle fibers, fatigue related to the increased work of breathing results in more rapid desaturation than in adults. The soft cartilage of the pediatric airway is prone to collapse in the presence of partial obstruction. Children with burns are at increased risk for these events because of underlying respiratory disease or injury.

Mechanical ventilation of severe inhalation injury is a dynamic and complex task.[71] Therapeutic interventions required for maintenance of pulmonary function have been implicated in postextubation stridor and barotrauma. Evidence suggests that barotrauma from mechanical ventilation may be minimized by protocols based on permissive hypercapnia. Moderate respiratory acidosis was well tolerated and ventilating pressures maintained below 40 cm.[72] The low incidence of mortality associated with this strategy suggests a reduction in ventilator-induced lung injury. In addition, high-frequency oscillatory ventilation (HFOV) in severe pediatric burn patients has significant, early, and sustained improvement in oxygenation. When HFOV is begun early in burn care, barotrauma is significantly reduced.[73]

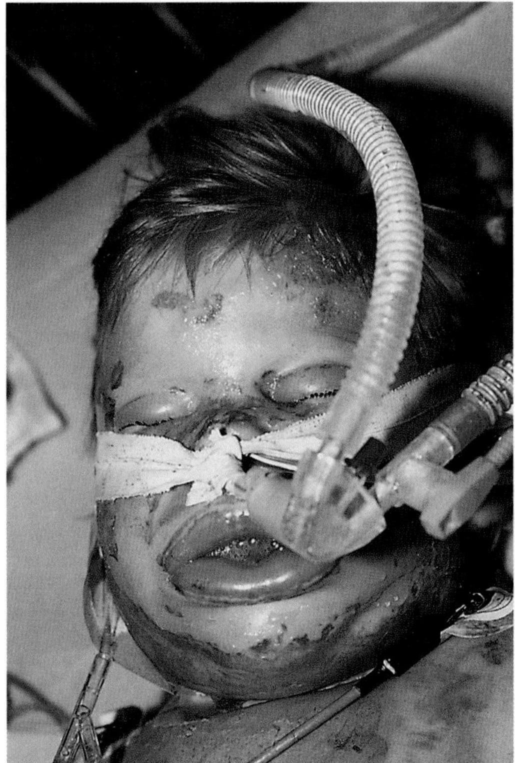

FIGURE 49-8 Severe Facial Edema During Burn Shock.

The consequences of metabolic and physiologic changes occurring during the acute phase of injury remain apparent during convalescence. Severe burns result in a decrease in pulmonary function from restrictive and obstructive pulmonary disease evidenced by a reduction in pulmonary volumes and maximum voluntary ventilation lasting up to 8 years. At times, chest wall scarring in children caused by burns severely limits thoracic cage excursion.

Burn Shock

The pathophysiologic responses of burn injury result in **hypovolemia** and extracellular sodium depletion in the burn-injured individual. Manifestations for adults are discussed in Chapter 48. Hypotension is a late sign of shock in the child. A complete circulatory assessment, including heart rate and peripheral parameters, is a more reliable measure. Urine output is a reflection of end-organ perfusion and is therefore the most accurate monitor of the adequacy of fluid resuscitation. A urine output of 30 to 50 ml/hr in adults and 1 ml/kg/hr in children weighing less than 30 kg are the suggested endpoints associated with many resuscitation formulas. Fluid is titrated to maintain the output within the parameters.[58]

The fluid of choice for burn shock resuscitation should approximate the fluid lost from the circulating volume, for example, lactated Ringer's solution. Children require fluid resuscitation for smaller burns than do adults as a result of their limited physiologic reserves. The child's relatively greater ratio of body surface area to weight results in increased evaporative water losses and proportionately more fluid during resuscitation. Although **colloid replacement** during burn shock resuscitation remains controversial, colloids may be required in the very young child who fails to respond to fluid replacement.[74] A component for **maintenance fluid** *must* be included in the calculation of fluid needs during resuscitation. Maintenance fluids represent the body requirements in the absence of burn injury.

Successful resuscitation depends on establishment of intravenous access. Although this is usually accomplished by peripheral or central venous cannulation, circulatory collapse may preclude timely administration of fluid replacement. Cannulation of veins in the pediatric population is further complicated by small vessels and increased subcutaneous fat. Children are good candidates for **intraosseous cannulation** when traditional venous access techniques fail. Blood, drugs, and fluid are readily absorbed by red marrow that drains into medullary venous channels and thus to the systemic circulation. This technique is most effective in children younger than 5 years, because red marrow is steadily replaced by yellow marrow in the limbs, making infusion more difficult, hence decreasing the infusion rate.[75] With proper care and removal as soon as other access is available, complications are minimal.

Fluid Resuscitation

Fluid resuscitation is generally required for children after thermal injuries in excess of 10% to 15% of the TBSA. Fluid is administered to compensate for fluid and electrolytes extravasating into the interstitial spaces. This replacement restores circulating volume, improves perfusion, and alleviates organ dysfunction associated with impaired circulation.

Various protocols have been proposed as guidelines for fluid administration. It is important to remember that any regimen serves merely as a guideline and will require adjustment based on the individual response of each child. Because the linear relationship between weight and surface area does not exist in children (surface area varies to weight as a two-thirds function), use of adult formulas result in under- or over-resuscitation.[76] A commonly used protocol is a modification of the Parkland formula. Children also tend to require relatively more fluids than adults because they have higher evaporative losses because of their body surface area-to-weight ratio. **Evaporative fluid loss** can be a significant contributor to hypovolemia in the burned child. This evaporative fluid loss continues until the burn wounds are closed. As in adults, inhalation injury also continues until burn wounds are closed. And as in adults, inhalation injury increases the magnitude of total body surface area injury; therefore, children with burn injuries require more fluids.[74]

Research suggests that in the acute phase of the burn injury children receive far more fluid resuscitation than calculated by the modified Parkland (Baxter) formula guidelines. This syndrome has been termed "fluid creep."[77] Onset maybe caused by higher fluid limits and increased use of opiates resulting in an increased abdominal pressure. The method to control fluid creep includes strict adherence to the modified Parkland formula. In children who have developed increased abdominal pressure, decompressive laparotomy may resolve the increased intra-abdominal pressure.[74]

Renal System

Loss of circulating volume into the interstitial spaces results in reduced renal blood flow and decreased glomerular filtration. An important measure of the adequacy of volume replacement is urine excretion. Sufficient volume replacement maintains urine output during resuscitation. Approximately 36 hours after injury, edema fluid begins to mobilize and output increases.

Children younger than 2 years of age lack the ability to concentrate urine because of the immaturity of the renal system and are, therefore, at increased risk for dehydration. In addition, the child has a relatively larger TBSA in relation to weight than the adult. Combined with limited physiologic reserves, increased fluid requirements are necessary for children during burn shock resuscitation and to compensate for evaporative water losses.[76]

Evidence of pigment in the urine results from the hemolysis of red blood cells. This is especially common after extensive electrical injuries and destroyed muscle from deep thermal injury. The release of **myoglobin** may occlude the kidney tubules and result in renal failure.

Gastrointestinal System

The gastrointestinal (GI) system plays an important role in the pathophysiology of burns. Alterations in blood flow result in decreased perfusion to the GI tract. Ischemia may cause erosion and necrosis of GI tissue. The GI response to a burn injury often includes mucosal atrophy, changes in digestive absorption, and increased intestinal permeability. Depending on the proportion of burn size, atrophy of the GI tract mucosa can occur immediately after injury. The atrophy results in gut barrier dysfunction leading to increased bacterial translocation and ultimately sepsis.[78]

Paralytic ileus occurs often after major burn injuries. Although digestion ceases in the stomach and the large bowel, the small intestine maintains motility and absorptive capacity. Intestinal motility returns as fluid losses are replaced unless irreversible necrosis of the bowel has occurred as a result of insufficient perfusion.

Immune Function

Burn trauma–induced immunosuppression results in increased susceptibility to infection and sepsis. Although the exact mechanisms responsible for this immunosuppression remain obscure, it is clear that complex interactions of the hypermetabolic response, nutritional support, bacterial translocation, and defects in both innate and acquired immune function are involved (Figure 49-9). In addition, young children are at increased risk for microbial invasion caused by an immature immune system and limited antibody production.

Deitch reported that wound- or gut-derived endotoxemia may be one of the mediators of the hypermetabolic response observed after thermal injury, and this finding remains undisputed.[79] When bacteria translocate from the gut or from the burn wound, endotoxin may affect immunologic response as inflammatory mediators are released. A further complication in the activation of inflammatory mediators is the release of toxic metabolites, such as oxygen free radicals.[80]

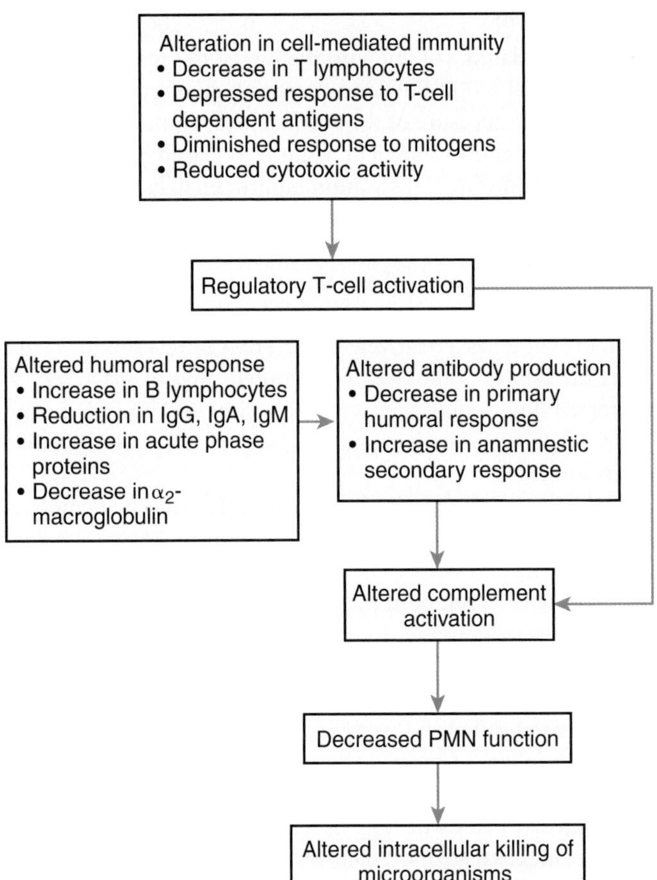

FIGURE 49-9 Altered Immune Function After Thermal Injury. Cell-mediated immunity, antibody production, humoral response. *PMN,* Polymorphonuclear leukocyte.

Circulating immunoglobulins may be affected by several factors, including age and the severity of injury.[81] Therapeutic interventions such as multiple transfusions, surgical procedures, and antibiotic and anesthetic administration also introduce elements that confound the evaluation of immunosuppressive effects. The immune system is activated systemically after a large burn injury with extensive tissue necrosis and may become ineffective or even self-destructive. Infections in burns may result in the loss of some components of innate immune function.[82]

An additional aspect of the immunopathologic consequence of a burn is the role of immunomodulatory cytokines that are suggested to regulate innate regulatory lymphocytes. Research regarding four cell types—NK (natural killer), natural killer T (NKT), gamma-delta T (γδ), and regulatory T (Treg)—indicates their central role in protective immunity.[83] In children with moderate to severe burn injury, cytokines have been found to increase inflammation by enhancing catabolism and hypermetabolism. In this immunomodulatory process the pro-inflammatory function of cytokines enhances protection from sepsis, and the anti-inflammatory function supports anabolism (i.e., tissue repair).[84]

Infection

Whereas shock and pulmonary compromise present the most immediate threat after burn trauma, local and systemic infections become the primary complication during healing. The burn wound initially is relatively free of pathogens; however, dead, avascular tissue and wound exudate provide a fertile environment for bacterial growth. Colonization of the wound is apparent by the fifth postburn day. Gram-positive microorganisms are usually recovered from cultures first, followed by opportunistic gram-negative bacteria. The impaired vascular supply to burned tissue enhances the proliferation of pathogenic microorganisms. Bacterial invasion results in thrombosis and a further impairment of circulation sufficient to convert a partial-thickness injury to a full-thickness wound.

Improvements in treatment have resulted in a reduction in wound infection. Aggressive excision and grafting of the wounds, improved nutritional support, and the development of microorganism-specific topical antimicrobials have contributed to this trend. However, the incidence of septicemia remains relatively constant. This is perhaps explained by the survival of children with burns of increasingly large body surface area. The burn wound serves as the site of primary invasion for the majority of instances of local or generalized infection. Because the burned child is immunosuppressed for many weeks after injury, maintaining wounds at low contamination levels by meticulous wound care decreases the frequency and duration of septic episodes caused by wound flora.[85]

Metabolism

Complex metabolic alterations are observed after burn injury. The extent of metabolic derangement is proportional to the magnitude of TBSA burn sustained. Wilmore demonstrated the linear increase in metabolic rate up to 2½ times normal resting energy expenditure.[86] As burn injury approaches 50% of TBSA, a plateau is reached, limiting further physiologic response to the trauma or other challenges such as infection.

A biphasic pattern of physiologic response is evident in thermally injured children. The initial **ebb phase** occurs during the immediate postburn period and continues for 3 to 5 days. This phase is characterized by reduced oxygen consumption, impaired circulation, and cellular shock. After the resolution of the shock and the restoration of circulating volume, the metabolic response shifts to a **catabolic (flow) phase** (Table 49-8). A state of **hypermetabolism** ensues, characterized by increased oxygen consumption and elevation of catecholamines, glucocorticoids, and glucagon.

Increased blood flow to the wound supplies additional glucose necessary for tissue repair. Insulin levels are usually normal or even elevated but are inappropriately low in relation to glucagon. Catecholamines and glucocorticoids act as antagonists to insulin. This effect combined with a tissue resistance to insulin stimulates glycogenolysis and gluconeogenesis, thus increasing glucose flow from the liver.[65] In the child, glycogen stores for meeting the increased energy demands of the burn are limited. The initiation of protein and lipid catabolism for glycogenesis is accelerated. This prolonged metabolic dysfunction may lead to loss of lean body mass and increased morbidity.[87]

Metabolic rates slowly return to normal with wound closure. However, a reactivation of the hypermetabolic response may occur with sepsis or organ failure.

TABLE 49-8 METABOLIC ALTERATIONS FOLLOWING INJURY

RESPONSE	DOMINANT FACTORS	CLINICAL FINDINGS
Ebb response	Loss of plasma volume Shock Low plasma insulin levels	Hyperglycemia Decreased oxygen consumption Depressed resting energy expenditure Decreased blood pressure Cardiac output below normal Decreased body temperature
Flow response		
Acute phase	Elevated catecholamines Elevated glucagons Elevated glucocorticoids Normal or elevated insulin levels High glucagon/insulin ratio	Catabolic Hyperglycemia Increased respiratory rate Increased oxygen consumption Increased body temperature Redistribution of polyvalent cations such as zinc and iron Mobilization of metabolic reserves Increased urinary excretion of nitrogen, sulfur, magnesium, phosphorus, potassium Accelerated gluconeogenesis
Adaptive phase	Stress hormone response subsiding	Anabolic Normoglycemia Energy turnover diminished Convalescence

From Gottschlich M, Alexander JW, Bower RH. In Rombeau JL, Caldwell MD, editors: *Enteral and tube feeding,* Philadelphia, 1990, Saunders.

Hypermetabolism

The hypermetabolic response after burn injury profoundly alters the production and use of nutrients. As a consequence of these phenomena, caloric requirements increase dramatically. Advances in burn care have allowed the performance of indirect calorimetry and assessment of metabolic rate at the bedside. Nutritional support must have an increased metabolic rate factored in (increased by 10% to 20%) because of fluctuations in energy use associated with activity. Current recommendations suggest 1.5 to 2 g protein/kg/day for adults and up to 2.5 to 4 g protein/kg/day for children.[87]

In addition to age, body composition has been found to significantly affect the postburn course. Preexisting obesity in burn children has been associated with longer hospital stay and associated morbidity.[88] However, the heightened nutrient requirements of the burned child preclude a reduction in nutritional support during the acute phase of recovery. Aggressive nutritional therapy is critical to the recovery of these children, and programs designed to achieve ideal body weight should not be instituted until wound healing is achieved.

Metabolism of many micronutrients is greatly affected by burn injury. Micronutrient supplementation is necessary because vitamin and mineral requirements increase with the severity of the burn related to heightened protein synthesis, enhanced caloric expenditure, and increased micronutrient losses. Pre-burn status also indicates individual vitamin and mineral needs.[63] Hypermetabolism results in a rapid turnover in vitamins and trace minerals important in the wound healing and immune response. A deficiency of specific nutrients interferes with carbohydrate and nucleic acid metabolism, collagen formation, and immune function.

The **thermoregulatory response** after burn injury results in an elevation in core body temperature. Burned individuals strive for temperatures of about 38° C (100.4° F). Depressed or "normal" temperature may be indicative of overwhelming sepsis, or an exhausted physiologic capability to maintain temperature, and should be viewed as an ominous sign. Routine methods of heat conservation after a major burn injury are inadequate because of excessive heat loss through convection and evaporation.[88] Therapeutic intervention, such as operative procedures and dressing changes, and transport present situations requiring increased diligence to prevent inadvertent cooling. Infants are at increased risk for a precipitous drop in core body temperature caused by an inability to regulate heat loss by shivering. Heat is also lost because of evaporation of water from damaged skin surfaces. Infants and children are especially vulnerable because of the large surface area relative to metabolically active tissue.[77]

Nutritional Support

The heightened metabolic demands after burn injury combined with a poor appetite often necessitate supplementation of oral intake. Children with burns in excess of 20% of TBSA often require supplementation with tube feeding. Feeding does not need to be delayed pending resolution of paralytic ileus and the resumption of bowel sounds because the small bowel maintains motility and absorptive capability. A small-bore feeding tube placed in the duodenum provides a safe route for the delivery of essential nutrients. Parenteral hyperalimentation is reserved for those children who are unable to tolerate enteral support because of attendant risks of catheter sepsis and loss of intestinal integrity. Early enteral supplementation preserves gut

WHAT'S NEW?

Advances in Burn Wound Care

Ongoing research and development continues to focus on the burn wound dressing, providing more therapeutic options with major wounds. Impregnated silver dressings kill bacteria but because most are processed with a special layer, they are less painful to remove. Some of these products can be left on the wound for up to 2 weeks allowing less frequent dressing changes and more comfort for the individual. A new extracellular matrix (ECM) product is being researched for repair and remodeling of damaged tissues in a burn injury and other therapeutic wound care situations. Derived from porcine urinary bladder, this ECM technology contains a bimodal surface technology with naturally occurring collagens and proteins and maintains an epithelial basement membrane surface. An in vitro study demonstrated that urinary bladder ECM is the best basement membrane as compared to small intestine or liver ECM. Another study suggested that antibacterial activity exists within ECM and these low-molecular-weight peptides may help explain resistance to bacterial infection.

Data from Brennan A et al: *Tissue Eng* 12(10):2949–2955, 2006; Brown B et al: *Tissue Eng* 12(3):519–526, 2006.

mucosal integrity and improves intestinal blood flow, as well as motility.[63] Early initiation of enteral supplementation along with aggressive management of complications permits successful enteral alimentation in most burned children.

Severe burn injury causes exaggerated muscle protein catabolism, contributing to weakness and delayed healing. Many therapeutic strategies have been used to avert the hypermetabolic response and improve clinical outcomes. Pharmacologic agents, such as recombinant growth hormone, low-dose insulin, and testosterone, have been shown to improve muscle kinetics and wound healing. However, these can cause serious side effects. Investigators have found that anabolic steroid agents, along with nutritional support, improve muscle protein metabolism through enhanced protein synthesis efficiency in children and adults.[89] Outpatient follow-up should include regular weighing of the child and nutritional assessment to identify children at risk for further weight loss.

Wound Management

The goals of wound management include prevention of infection, removal of devitalized tissue, and closure of the wound (see What's New? Advances in Burn Wound Care). Burns that are clearly deep dermal or full-thickness injuries are surgically excised as soon as the child is hemodynamically stable after resuscitation. Early excision reduces the incidence of wound infection and systemic sepsis.[90-92] Coverage of the excised wound is necessary to achieve wound closure. The choice of a coverage technique depends on the availability of donor skin.

Split-thickness sheet grafts are selected for areas of maximal functional and cosmetic results (Figure 49-10). Children with very large burn injuries often do not have sufficient unburned skin available to facilitate use of the sheet graft. In these cases the surgeon uses a meshing technique to expand the available skin and increase the size of the graft. The pattern created heals by migration of epithelium from the meshed edges. Scar formation is increased, and the mesh pattern remains clearly visible (Figure 49-11). The color, texture, vascularity, thickness, and hair-bearing nature of the skin vary from one area to another. Site selection and depth of donor sites require careful consideration. Skin grafts for the face should be taken, if possible, from above the nipple line for best color match and "blush" ability.[91]

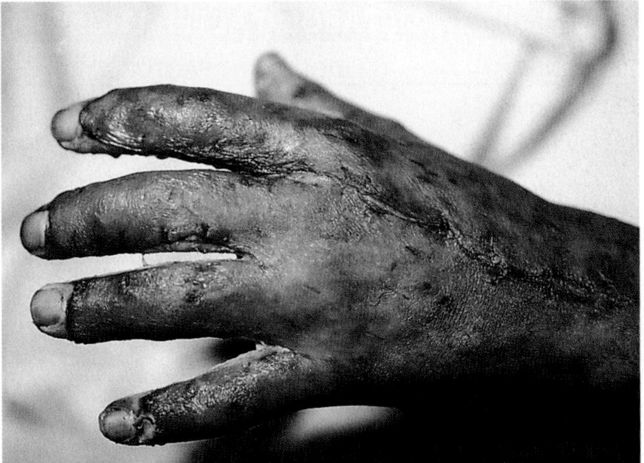

FIGURE 49-10 Split-Thickness Sheet Graft.

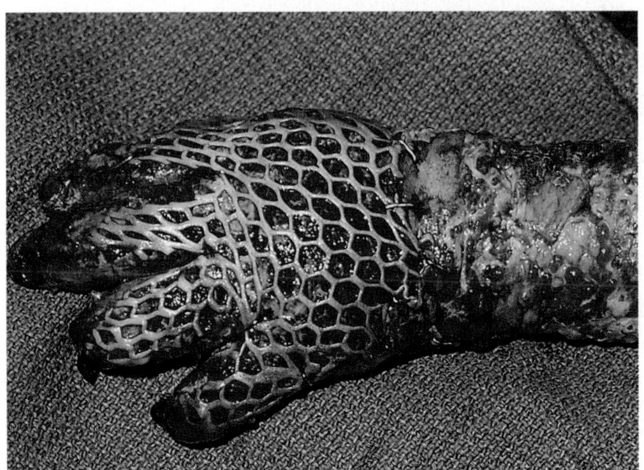

FIGURE 49-11 Meshed Autograft.

Scar Maturation

In normal epidermal healing, minimal disruption in skin color, texture, and thickness occurs. However, burn wounds that extend into the dermis are repaired through **scar formation** and may result in an overgrowth of dermal constituents (Figure 49-12, *A*). Accelerated collagen synthesis most likely begins with high levels of activity in granulation tissue. The **hypertrophic scar** consists of hypercellular and disorganized connective tissue that is erythematous, raised, and pruritic. Normal dermis contains thick fibers and fiber bundles running parallel to the surface. In the hypertrophic scar, the collagen is arranged in whorls and nodules that account for its inelasticity and increased turgor.[92] As the hypertrophic scar matures, collagen begins to orient in a more parallel fashion, and vascularity decreases (see Figure 49-12, *B*). Collagen synthesis is very active soon after wound closure, and alteration of the scar can be accomplished before strong cross-linking of the collagen is established.

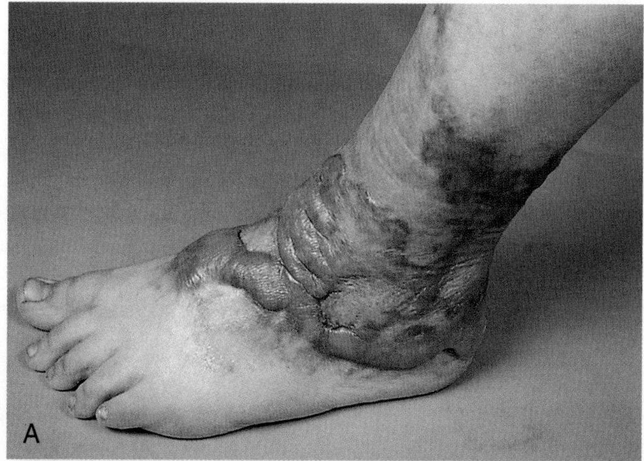

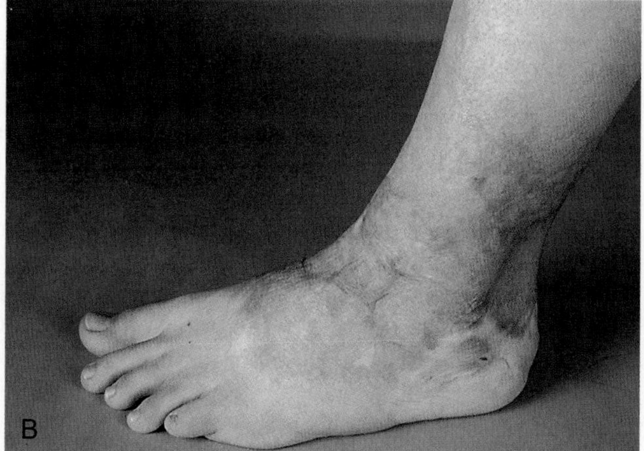

FIGURE 49-12 Scar Maturation. **A,** Immature hypertrophic scar. **B,** Flat, mature scar after pressure therapy.

Although duration of wound healing varies among individuals, the length of time required to achieve wound closure is the most reliable predictor of hypertrophic scarring. Deeper burns demonstrate increased scarring caused by the formation of granulation tissue and prolonged healing time. Generally, darker-pigmented races are more susceptible to hypertrophic scarring.[92,93] Although age has not been found to be a predictor of hypertrophic scar formation, younger individuals are more susceptible to trauma and have greater skin tension and an accelerated rate of collagen synthesis. Increased tension with resultant trauma stimulates inflammation, which in turn results in the formation of additional collagen.

Scar tissue is metabolically active and highly vascular. Collagen is deposited in random patterns, and contraction of the scar can result in disabling deformities. The scar is active as long as it is raised, red, and firm. **Scar maturation** requires 1 to 2 years and depends on individual differences and compliance with the rehabilitation program. The mature scar is characterized by increased suppleness, flattening, and pigmented color.

Scar tissue does not grow and expand like normal tissue. Although massage therapy offers some benefit in stretching, functional limitation may develop as the child grows. This is particularly evident over joints. Reconstructive surgery is often necessary to restore anatomic integrity and to promote independent function.

Itching may occur at any time during burn wound healing. As a complication, healed skin may be scratched away in an effort to obtain relief. The combination of H_1 and H_2 antagonists may be used to control itching.[94]

Comfort Management

Pain management presents a significant challenge in the pediatric population. In addition to procedural pain, there is a component of background pain that is present without activity. Pain perception is also affected by the degree of emotional overlay or affective experience.[95] The measurement of pain is particularly challenging in young infants, who lack the language skills to express pain. A variety of tools, from physiologic monitors to behavioral analyses and analog scales, have been developed to measure pediatric pain. The quality of pain control in burn centers has improved along with the ability to assess pain in the pediatric population. Studies have documented pharmacologic as well as nonpharmacologic interventions that have improved the quality of pain control.[95]

Recovery from Burn Injury

Rehabilitation becomes the major focus of care once wound coverage has been achieved and continues until all reconstructive procedures have been completed. This phase may extend over many years in the pediatric population. Children require specialized management to ensure optimal functional and cosmetic results. Scar and contracture management is necessary for prolonged periods because of changes in body composition as the child grows and matures. Very young children present unique challenges because the small body size can be difficult to fit with pressure garments and splints, growth is rapid, and cooperation with the rehabilitation program is limited.

Infant skin is thinner, and the epidermis is more loosely connected to the dermis. This increases the risk of blistering, chafing, and rash formation. The infant also produces less sebum and sweat, which further exacerbates the propensity to skin irritation. Because scar tissue contains no sweat glands, these characteristics of the skin in growing children compound the difficulty in maintaining pressure on maturing scars while cooling the body.

Positioning and splinting to prevent contracture formation, as well as rehabilitative aspects of therapy, are instituted on admission and continue throughout the hospitalization. Physical therapy and occupational therapy provide exercise to maintain range of motion and function. Psychosocial support is very important for the child and the family. The information provided should be consistent and honest to allow clarification of concerns. In addition to the functional aspects of rehabilitation, attention must be directed to psychosocial needs and community reintegration.

A method to facilitate the transition from the hospital to the community is the school reentry program offered by many burn centers. These programs provide education for teachers and peers about the injury, appearance, and abilities of the returning child.

SUMMARY REVIEW

Shock and Multiple Organ Dysfunction Syndrome

1. Shock in children is present when there are signs of poor systemic perfusion, regardless of blood pressure.
2. Hypovolemic shock is the most common type of shock in children and it most frequently results from dehydration and trauma. Hypovolemic shock also may result from expansion of the vascular space, producing inadequate intravascular volume relative to the vascular space.
3. Hypotension is a sign of severe (preterminal), decompensated shock, referred to as "hypotensive shock."
4. Clinical manifestations of hypovolemic shock include inadequate systemic perfusion associated with intravascular fluid loss. Adrenergic compensatory mechanisms can produce tachycardia, redistribution of blood flow, peripheral vasoconstriction, cool extremities, delayed capillary refill, and oliguria.
5. Neurogenic shock is caused by a loss of vasomotor tone after severe injury to the spinal cord.
6. Clinical manifestations of neurogenic shock include warm skin, hypotension with a low diastolic blood pressure, and poor systemic perfusion. Tachycardia is not present.
7. Cardiogenic shock, with decreased cardiac output, is observed most commonly after cardiovascular surgery or with inflammatory diseases of the heart, such as cardiomyopathy and myocarditis. It is also found in children with obstructive congenital heart disease and those with drug toxicity or severe electrolyte or acid-base imbalances.
8. Clinical manifestations of cardiogenic shock include inadequate systemic perfusion despite adequate intravascular volume. Cardiac output is typically low. Adrenergic compensatory mechanisms, including peripheral vasoconstriction and decreased urine volume, are similar to those found in hypovolemic shock.
9. Once septic shock is present, immediate treatment is urgently needed. Therapy in the first hour includes aggressive fluid resuscitation (typically 60 to 80 ml/kg administered in first hour of therapy, and approximately 200 to 240 ml/kg in the first 8 hours of therapy). If the child does not respond to volume administration alone, vasoactive support must be initiated within the first hour of treatment. Antibiotics also must be administered within the first hour. Goals of therapy are to rapidly normalize the heart rate and blood pressure for age and to normalize capillary refill to less than 2 seconds. The child's shock index (heart rate/systolic blood pressure) should fall during the first hour of management if therapy is effective. Fluid and vasoactive therapy should support high cardiac output and oxygen delivery, maintaining the $S\bar{v}O_2$ at approximately 70%.
10. Sepsis is a systemic response to infection. It is present when manifestations of SIRS are observed. SIRS is present when the child demonstrates two or more of the following as an acute change from baseline values: altered temperature, altered heart rate, altered respiratory rate, and alteration in the WBC count. The newborn often develops hypothermia rather than fever as a sign of infection and may develop bradycardia instead of tachycardia.
11. Severe sepsis is present when there is evidence of SIRS and signs of organ dysfunction, hypoperfusion, or hypotension.
12. The development of septic shock is heralded when the child with severe sepsis develops signs of cardiovascular dysfunction. The child may become hypotensive despite adequate fluid resuscitation or require vasopressors to maintain blood pressure.
13. Reperfusion and inflammatory injury stimulate free oxygen radicals that can damage cell membranes, denature proteins, and disrupt chromosomes. This process likely affects endothelial cells and the microvasculature, causing MODS.
14. Lactic acidosis (i.e., rise in serum lactate) may be the most sensitive indicator of inadequate systemic perfusion in children; effective shock therapy should eliminate lactic acidosis.
15. The general goals of treatment for shock are maximization of oxygen delivery and minimization of oxygen demand. This requires support of airway, oxygenation, and ventilation. Support of cardiovascular function requires support of appropriate heart rate and rhythm, adequate intravascular volume, good myocardial function, and appropriate vascular resistance and distribution of blood flow. The child should be kept warm but fever must be treated promptly.
16. The signs of shock should lessen or disappear if management of shock is effective. The warmth of the child's extremities, briskness of capillary refill, quality of peripheral pulses, level of consciousness and responsiveness, urine volume, oxygenation, ventilation, and acid-base status should improve throughout shock therapy.

Burns

1. Burns in children are often the result of inadequate supervision, curiosity, inability to escape the burning agent, or intentional abuse.
2. Scald injuries are commonly seen in young children and result from exposure to hot water, grease, or other hot liquids, whereas flame burns are more prevalent among older children.
3. A child's skin is thinner and thus more susceptible to injury than adult skin. The kitchen and bathroom are common sites of burn injury.
4. Approximately 10% of all forms of child abuse cases in the United States result from burn injury.
5. Flame burns involving flammable liquids, most notably gasoline, are more common in older children. Risk-taking behaviors in young males can lead to electrical burns. Children may be exposed to chemical injury by swallowing caustic agents at home.
6. Use of the standard Rule of Nines results in inaccurate calculation of the percentage of TBSA in children. A modified Rule of Nines deducts 1% from the head and adds 0.5% to each leg for each year of life after 2 years of age.

SUMMARY REVIEW—cont'd

7. Major burn trauma involves all body systems, and the consequences of injury include shock, infection, hypermetabolism, organ failure, and functional limitations. These effects can be magnified in the pediatric population as a result of physiologic immaturity and age-related variation in treatment modalities.
8. Infection, trauma, or applying ice to the burn area may convert a partial-thickness injury to a full-thickness one, especially in young children, who have thinner, more delicate skin.
9. Marked reduction in cardiac output occurs immediately after injury and is accompanied by an initial increase in systemic vascular resistance. The inefficient and labile peripheral circulation of the infant complicates management of the burn shock phase of treatment. Constriction of the chest and impairment of respiratory excursion may occur in the very young child because of the increased pliability of the rib cage. Younger children are also more susceptible to increased intra-abdominal pressure.
10. The leading cause of death in children after burn injury, as in adults, is inhalation injury.
11. Children require fluid resuscitation for smaller burns than does the adult population as a result of limited physiologic reserves. Colloid replacement may be required in the very young child who fails to respond to fluid replacement.
12. Children younger than 2 years lack the ability to concentrate urine because of the immaturity of the renal system and are therefore at increased risk for dehydration. Because children have a relatively larger body surface area in relation to weight than adults, they require proportionately increased fluid during burn shock resuscitation to compensate for evaporative water losses.
13. Some children exhibit immunosuppression for a prolonged period after wound closure.
14. A biphasic pattern of physiologic responses is evident in the burn-injured child. The initial ebb phase occurs during the immediate postburn period and continues for 3 to 5 days. This phase is characterized by reduced oxygen consumption, impaired circulation, and cellular shock. After this phase and the restoration of volume, the metabolic response shifts to a catabolic, or flow, phase. This phase is characterized by hypermetabolism with an increased oxygen consumption and elevation of catecholamines, glucocorticoids, and glucagon.
15. Glycogen stores are limited in children, making it hard for them to meet the increased energy demands of the burn. This prolonged metabolic dysfunction may lead to loss of lean body mass and increased morbidity.
16. Although age was not found to be a predictor of hypertrophic scarring, children have greater skin tension and an accelerated rate of collagen synthesis.
17. Children require specialized management to ensure optimal functional and cosmetic results. Long-term scar and contracture management is necessary because of changes in body composition as the child grows and matures.

KEY TERMS

Bradycardia, 1701
Cardiogenic shock, 1700, 1705
Catabolic (flow) phase, 1720
Chemical burn, 1716
Child abuse, 1715
Cold shock, 1709
Colloid, 1711
Colloid replacement, 1718
Compensated shock, 1699
Contact burn, 1715
Crystalloid, 1711
Depth of injury, 1716
Dermal ischemia, 1717
Distributive (septic, anaphylactic, neurogenic) shock, 1700
Ebb phase, 1720
Electrical burn, 1716
Eschar, 1717
Evaporative fluid loss, 1719
Flame burn, 1716
Fluid resuscitation, 1719
Hemoconcentration, 1717
Hypermetabolism, 1720
Hypertrophic scar, 1722
Hypotensive shock, 1699
Hypovolemia, 1718
Hypovolemic shock, 1700, 1703
Hypoxia, 1699
Intra-abdominal pressure, 1717
Intraosseous cannulation, 1719
Ischemia, 1699
Maintenance fluid, 1719
Multiple organ dysfunction syndrome (MODS), 1699
Myoglobin, 1719
Neurogenic shock, 1700
Obstructive shock, 1700, 1710
Rehabilitation, 1723
Reperfusion (reoxygenation) injury, 1710
Scald injury, 1715
Scar formation, 1722
Scar maturation, 1723
Sepsis, 1706
Septic shock, 1708
Severe sepsis, 1708
Shock, 1699
Split-thickness sheet graft, 1722
Systemic inflammatory response syndrome (SIRS), 1707
Tachycardia, 1701
Thermoregulatory response, 1721
"Third spacing" of fluids, 1704
Warm shock, 1709

REFERENCES

1. Haque IU, Zaritsky AL: Analysis of the evidence for the lower limit of systolic and mean arterial blood pressure in children, *Pediatr Crit Care* 8:138–144, 2007.
2. Chameides L et al, editors: *Pediatric advanced life support provider manual*, Dallas, 2011, American Heart Association.
3. Perkin RM et al: Shock, cardiac arrest and resuscitation. In Hazinski MF, editor: *Nursing care of the critically ill child*, ed 3, St Louis, 2013, Mosby.
4. Goldstein B, Giroir B, Randolph A: International Pediatric Sepsis Consensus Conference: definitions for sepsis and organ dysfunction in pediatrics, *Pediatr Crit Care Med* 6:2–8, 2005.
5. Proulx F et al: The pediatric multiple organ dysfunction syndrome, *Pediatr Crit Care Med* 10:12–22, 2009.
6. Hazinski MF: Children are different. In Hazinski MF, editor: *Nursing care of the critically ill child*, ed 3, St Louis, 2013, Mosby.
7. Otieno H et al: Are bedside features of shock reproducible between different observers? *Arch Dis Child* 89(10):977–979, 2004.
8. Chameides L et al: Recognition and management of tachycardia. In Chameides L et al, editors: *Pediatric advanced life support provider manual*, Dallas, 2011, American Heart Association.
9. Rudolph AM: *Congenital diseases of the heart*, Chicago, 1974, Year Book Medical.

10. Chameides L et al: Recognition and management of bradycardia. In Chamiedes L et al, editors: *Pediatric advanced life support provider manual*, Dallas, 2011, American Heart Association.
11. Roberts KE: Fluid, electrolyte and endocrine problems. In Hazinski MF, editor: *Nursing care of the critically ill child*, ed 3, St Louis, 2013, Mosby.
12. Nayak PP et al: Early change in blood glucose concentration is an indicator of mortality in critically ill children, *Intensive Care Med* 39(1):123–128, 2012.
13. Bhutia TD, Lodha R, Kabra SK: Abnormalities in glucose homeostasis in critically ill children, *Pediatr Crit Care Med* 14(1):e16–e25, 2013.
14. American College of Surgeons: *Extremes of age: pediatric trauma.* In *Advanced trauma life support program for doctors*, ed 7, Chicago, 2004, American College of Surgeons.
15. Armstrong A, Unni P, Pietsch JB: Pediatric trauma. In Hazinski MF, editor: *Nursing care of the critically ill child*, ed 3, St Louis, 2013, Mosby.
16. Chameides L et al: Recognition of shock. In Chamiedes L et al: *Pediatric advanced life support provider manual*, Dallas, 2011, American Heart Association.
17. Watson RS et al: The epidemiology of severe sepsis in children in the United States, *Am J Respir Crit Care Med* 167(5):695–701, 2003.
18. Singh-Naz N et al: Risk factors for nosocomial infections in critically ill children: a prospective cohort study, *Crit Care Med* 24(5):875–878, 1996.
19. Foglia E, Meier MD, Elward A: Ventilator-associated pneumonia in neonatal and pediatric intensive care unit patients, *Clin Microbiol Rev* 20(3):409–425, 2007.
20. Trimarchi T: Fundamentals of patient safety and quality improvement. In Hazinski MF, editor: *Nursing care of the critically ill child*, ed 3, St Louis, 2013, Mosby.
21. Nadel S: Severe pediatric sepsis, *Expert Rev Anti Infect Ther* 10(2): 111–114, 2012.
22. Wong HR: Genetics and genomics in pediatric septic shock, *Crit Care Med* 40:1618–1626, 2012.
23. Brandtzaeg P, van Deuren M: Classification and pathogenesis of meningococcal infections, *Methods Molec Biol* 799:21–35, 2012.
24. Sullivan JS et al: Correlation of plasma cytokine elevation with mortality rate in children with sepsis, *J Pediatr* 120(4 Pt 1):510–515, 1992.
25. Aneja RK, Carcillo JA: Differences between adult and pediatric septic shock, *Minerva Anesthesiol* 77:986–992, 2011.
26. Decker T: Sepsis: avoiding its deadly toll, *J Clin Invest* 113(10):1387–1389, 2004.
27. Haley M et al: Activated protein C in sepsis: emerging insights regarding its mechanism of action and clinical effectiveness, *Curr Opin Infect Dis* 17(3):205–211, 2004.
28. Bernard GR et al: Efficacy and safety of recombinant human activated protein C for severe sepsis, *N Engl J Med* 344(10):699–709, 2001.
29. Batzofin BM, Sprung CL, Weiss YG: The use of steroids in the treatment of severe sepsis and septic shock, *Best Pract Res Clin Endocrinol Metab* 25(5):735–743, 2011.
30. Karaguzel G et al: The effects of three specific conditions related to the critical care on adrenal function in children, *Intensive Care Med* 38(10):1689–1696, 2012.
31. Hebbar KB, Petrillo T, Fortenberry JD: Adrenal insufficiency and response to corticosteroids in hypotensive critically ill children with cancer, *J Crit Care* 27(5):480–487, 2012.
32. Brierley J et al: Clinical practice parameters for hemodynamic support of pediatric and neonatal septic shock: 2007 update from American College of Critical Care Medicine, *Crit Care Med* 37:666–688, 2009.
33. Carcillo JA et al: Mortality and functional morbidity after use of PALS/APLS by community physicians, *Pediatrics* 124:500–508, 2009.
34. Kissoon N, Orr RA, Carcillo JA: Updated American College of Critical Care Medicine—Pediatric advanced life support guidelines for management of pediatric and neonatal septic shock: relevance to the emergency care clinician, *Pediatr Emerg Care* 26(11):867–869, 2010.
35. Carcillo JA, Davis AL, Zaritsky A: Role of early fluid resuscitation in pediatric septic shock, *JAMA* 266(9):1242–1245, 1991.
36. de Oliveira CE et al: ACCM/PALS haemodynamic support guidelines for paediatric septic shock: an outcomes comparison with and without monitoring central venous oxygen saturation, *Intensive Care Med* 34:1065–1075, 2008.
37. :Chamiedes L et al, Management of shock Chameides L et al: *Pediatric advanced life support provider manual*, Dallas, 2011, American Heart Association.
38. Banz Y, Rieben R: Role of complement and perspectives for intervention in ischemia-reperfusion damage, *Ann Med* 44:205–217, 2012.
39. Francischetti I et al: Leukocytes and the inflammatory response in ischemia-reperfusion injury, *Rev Bras Cir Cardiovasc* 25(4):575–584, 2010.
40. Lacroix J, Cotting J, for the Pediatric Acute Lung Injury and Sepsis Investigators (PALISI) Network: Severity of illness and organ dysfunction scoring in children, *Pediatr Crit Care Med* 6(Suppl 3):S126–S134, 2005.
41. Bestati N et al: Differences in organ dysfunctions between neonates and older children: a prospective, observational, multicenter study, *Crit Care* 14:R202, 2010.
42. Leteurtre S et al: Daily estimation of the severity of multiple organ dysfunction syndrome in critically children, *CMAJ* 182(11):1181–1187, 2010.
43. Hutton P et al: An assessment of the Dinamap 845, *Anesthesiology* 39:261, 1984.
44. Davis JW et al: Are automated blood pressure measurements accurate in trauma patients? *J Trauma* 55(5):860–863, 2003.
45. Lacroix J et al: Transfusion strategies for patients in pediatric intensive care units, *N Engl J Med* 356:1609–1619, 2007.
46. Lacroix J, Demaret P, Tucci M: Red blood cell transfusion: decision making in pediatric intensive care units, *Semin Perinatol* 36:225–231, 2012.
47. Burke ML, Salani D: Hematologic and oncologic emergencies requiring critical care. In Hazinski MF, editor: *Nursing care of the critically ill child*, ed 3, St Louis, 2013, Mosby.
48. Vlasselaers D et al: Intensive insulin therapy for patients in paediatric intensive care: a prospective, randomised controlled study, *Lancet* 373:547–556, 2009.
49. Ulate KP: A critical appraisal of Vlasselaers D et al: Intensive insulin therapy for patients in paediatric intensive care: a prospective, randomised controlled study, *Lancet* 2009; 373:547–556, 2009, *Pediatr Crit Care Med* 12:455–458, 2011.
50. Hirshberg E et al: Clinical equipoise regarding glycemic control: a survey of pediatric intensivist perceptions, *Pediatr Crit Care Med* 14(2):123–129, 2013.
51. Polderman KH: Mechanisms of action, physiological effects, and complications of hypothermia, *Crit Care Med* 37(Suppl):S186–S202, 2009.
52. Pietrini D et al: Neuroprotection and hypothermia in infants and children, *Curr Drug Targets* 13(7):925–935, 2012.
53. Shankaran S et al: Whole body hypothermia for neonates with hypoxic-ischemic encephalopathy, *N Engl J Med* 353:1574–1584, 2005.
54. Hypothermia After Cardiac Arrest Study Group: Mild therapeutic hypothermia to improve the neurologic outcome after cardiac arrest, *N Engl J Med* 346(8):549–556, 2002.
55. Bembea MM et al: Temperature patterns in the early postresuscitation period after pediatric inhospital arrest, *Pediatr Crit Care Med* 11(6): 723–730, 2010.
56. Committee on Trauma: *Resource for optimal care of the injured patient [pamphlet]*, 1999, American College of Surgeons.
57. Safe Kids Worldwide (SKW): *Burn and scalds safety* 2011. Available at www.safekids.org/assests/docs/ourwork/research/2011-burns-and-scalds.pdf. Accessed May 29, 2012.
58. American Burn Association: Pediatric burn injuries. *2011 Advanced burn life support provider manual*, Chicago, 2011, American Burn Association.
59. Greenhalgh DG: Burn-related child abuse. In Phillips BJ, editor: *Pediatric burns*, Amherst, 2012, Cambria.
60. Knox BL, Starling SP: *Medical evaluation of burn injuries, National Center for Prosecution of Child Abuse Update 22 (Number 2&3)* 2009. Available at www.ndaa.org/pdf/update_22_2and3.pdf. Accessed May 29, 2012.
61. Fujii TK, Schwartz SJ, Phillips BJ: Inhalation injury. In Phillips BJ, editor: *Pediatric burns*, Amherst, 2012, Cambria.
62. Sheridan RL, Tompkins RG: Alternative wound coverings. In Herndon DN, editor: *Total burn care*, Philadelphia, 2012, Saunders.
63. Gottschlich MM, Mays T: Nutrition for the burned pediatric patients. In Samour PQ, King K, editors: *Pediatric nutrition*, Sudbury, MA, 2012, Jones & Bartlett.
64. Helvig E: Pediatric burn injuries, *AACN Clin Issues Crit Care Nurs* 4(2):433–442, 1993.
65. Jensen AR, Hughes WB, Grewal H: Secondary abdominal compartment syndrome in children with burns and trauma: a potentially lethal complication, *J Burn Care Res* 27(2):242–246, 2006.
66. Peng D, Huang W: Etiology of immune dysfunction in thermal injuries. In Phillips BJ, editor: *Pediatric burns*, Amherst, 2012, Cambria.
67. Serebrisky D: Inhalation injury. In Bye MR et al: *Medscape Reference*, 2012. Available at http://emedicine.medscape.com/article/1002413-overview. Accessed June 12, 2012.
68. Conrardy PA et al: Alteration of endotracheal tube position, *Crit Care Med* 4(2):8, 1976.

69. Sharar SR: Endotracheal tube tip position in an infant with severe burns, *J Burn Care Rehabil* 16(6):654, 1995.
70. Trout S et al: Influence of head and neck position on endotracheal tube tip position on chest x-ray examination: a potential problem in the infant undergoing intubation, *J Burn Care Rehabil* 15(5):405–407, 1994.
71. Palmieri TL: What's new in critical care of the burn-injured patient? *Clin Plast Surg* 36(4):607–615, 2009.
72. Sheridan RL et al: Permissive hypercapnia as a ventilatory strategy in burned children: effect on barotrauma, pneumonia, and mortality, *J Trauma* 39(5):854, 1995.
73. Greathouse ST et al: High-frequency oscillatory ventilators in burn patients: experience of Riley Hospital for Children, *J Burn Care Res* 33(3):425–435, 2012.
74. Phillips BJ: Pediatric burn resuscitation. In Phillips BJ, editor: *Pediatric burns*, Amherst, 2012, Cambria.
75. Tintinalli JE et al: *Emergency medicine: a comprehensive study guide*, New York, 2004, McGraw-Hill.
76. Lee JO, Herndon DH, Norbury WB: Special considerations of age: the pediatric burn patient. In Herndon DH, editor: *Total burn care*, Philadelphia, 2012, Saunders.
77. Saffle JR: The phenomenon of "fluid creep" in acute burn resuscitation, *J Burn Care Res* 28(5):382–395, 2007.
78. Colon NC, Schlegel C, Chung DH: Surgical management of complications of burn injury. In Herndon DH, editor: *Total burn care*, Philadelphia, 2012, Saunders.
79. Deitch EA: Nutritional support of the burn patient, *Crit Care Med* 11(3):735, 1995.
80. Supple KG: Physiologic response to burn injury, *Crit Care Nurs Clin North Am* 16(1):119, 2004.
81. Stratta RJ et al: Immunologic parameters in burned patients: effect of therapeutic interventions, *J Trauma* 26(1):7, 1986.
82. Murphey ED, Sherwood ER, Tolliver-Kinsky T: The immunological response and strategies for intervention. In Herndon DN, editor: *Total burn care*, Philadelphia, 2012, Saunders.
83. Schneider DF, Glenn CH, Fauce DE: Innate lymphocyte subsets and their immunoregulatory roles in burn injury and sepsis, *J Burn Care Res* 28(3):365–379, 2007.
84. Phillips BJ, Carter MJ: Changes to the hypothalamic-pituitary-adrenal axis in burns and the use of steroids. In Phillips BJ, editor: *Pediatric burns*, Amherst, 2012, Cambria.
85. Gallagher JJ et al: Treatment of infection in burns. In Herndon DN, editor: *Total burn care*, Philadelphia, 2012, Saunders.
86. Wilmore DW: Nutrition and metabolism following thermal injury, *Clin Plast Surg* 1(4):603–619, 1974.
87. Rodriguez NA et al: Nutrition in burns: Galveston contributions, *J Parenter Enteral Nutr* 35(6):704–714, 2011.
88. Saffle JR, Graves C, Cochran A: Nutritional support of the burned patient. In Herndon DN, editor: *Total burn care*, Philadelphia, 2012, Saunders.
89. Wolf SE et al: Effects of oxandrolone on outcome measures in the severely burned: a multicenter prospective randomized double-blind trial, *J Burn Care Res* 25(2):131–139, 2006.
90. Petersen SR, Umphred E, Warden GD: The incidence of bacteremia following burn wound excision, *J Trauma* 22(4):274–279, 1982.
91. Lee JO et al: Operative wound management. In Herndon DN, editor: *Total burn care*, Philadelphia, 2012, Saunders.
92. Kwan P, Desmoulière A, Tredget EE: Molecular and cellular basis of hypertrophic scarring. In Herndon DN, editor: *Total burn care*, Philadelphia, 2012, Saunders.
93. Hawkins HK, Finnerty CC: Pathophysiology of the burn scar. In Herndon DN, editor: *Total burn care*, Philadelphia, 2012, Saunders.
94. Baker RU et al: Burn wound itch control using H1 and H2 antagonists, *J Burn Care Rehabil* 22(4):263, 2001.
95. Bayat A, Ramaiah R, Bhananker SM: Analgesia and sedation for children undergoing burn wound care, *Expert Rev Neurother* 10(11):1747–1759, 2010.

GLOSSARY

Absolute polycythemia excessive red blood cell production; a physiologic response resulting from increased erythropoietin secretion in response to chronic hypoxia or as a symptom of polycythemia vera.

Absorption atelectasis see Atelectasis.

Acid maltase deficiency (glycogen storage disease type II or Pompe disease) an autosomal recessive metabolic disorder that damages muscle and nerve cells throughout the body by an accumulation of glycogen in the lysosome attributable to deficiency of the lysosomal acid α-glucosidase enzyme. The buildup of glycogen causes progressive muscle weakness (myopathy) throughout the body and affects various body tissues, particularly in the heart, skeletal muscles, liver, and nervous system.

Acne a common skin disease characterized by pimples on the face, chest, and back. It occurs when the pores of the skin become clogged with oil, dead skin cells, and bacteria.

- **Acne conglobata** severe cystic acne characterized by cystic lesions, abscesses, communicating sinuses, and thickened, nodular scars; usually does not affect the face.
- **Acne rosacea** a chronic form of dermatitis of the face in which the middle portion of the face appears red with small red lines caused by dilation of capillaries.
- **Acne vulgaris** an inflammatory eruption of the sebaceous follicles usually occurring on the face, upper back, and chest that consists of blackheads, cysts, papules, and pustules.
- **Noninflammatory acne** open comedones caused by the enlargement and dilation of a plug resulting from the accumulation of oil and dead skin cells inside the hair follicle and by closed comedones that form if the hair follicle pore remains closed; they appear as a tiny, sometimes pink bump in the skin.

Acquired immunodeficiency syndrome (AIDS) see Immune deficiency.

Acquired sideroblastic anemia see Anemia.

ACTH deficiency a condition characterized by decreased or absent production of adrenocorticotropic hormone (ACTH) by the pituitary gland, resulting in a reduction in the secretion of adrenal hormones and subsequent weight loss, lack of appetite, weakness, nausea, vomiting, and low blood pressure.

Actinic keratosis a condition in which a premalignant small, reddish, rough spot appears on skin chronically exposed to the sun.

Acute chest syndrome a syndrome occurring in association with sickle cell disease defined by a new infiltrate on chest radiograph; associated with one or more new symptoms: fever, cough, sputum production, dyspnea, or hypoxia. It occurs most commonly in the 2- to 4-year-old age group and declines in incidence with age.

Acute colonic pseudo-obstruction (Ogilvie syndrome) a massive dilation of the large bowel that occurs in critically ill patients and immobilized older adults. It is characterized by significant dilation of the cecum and absence of mechanical obstruction, and is related to excessive sympathetic motor input or decreased parasympathetic motor input.

Acute confusional state (ACS) a form of delirium caused by interference with the metabolic or other biochemical processes essential for normal brain functioning. Symptoms may include disturbances in cognition and levels of awareness, short-term memory deficit, retrograde and anterograde amnesia, and disturbances in orientation, accompanied by restlessness, apprehension, irritability, and apathy. The condition may be associated with an acute physiologic state, delirium, toxic psychosis, or acute brain syndrome.

Acute coronary syndrome a classification encompassing clinical presentations ranging from unstable angina through infarction.

Acute cystitis an inflammation of the bladder, which is the most common site of urinary tract infection.

Acute epiglottitis an infection that causes inflammation of the epiglottis and surrounding tissues and may lead to upper airway blockage.

Acute gastritis an inflammatory disorder of the gastric mucosa, usually caused by injury of the protective mucosal barrier by drugs, chemicals, or *Helicobacter pylori* infection.

Acute glomerulonephritis see Glomerulonephritis.

Acute gouty arthritis an abrupt pain of a joint, most often the great toe, which is swollen, hot, and shiny secondary to an attack of gout.

Acute idiopathic thrombotic thrombocytopenic purpura (TTP) see Thrombocytopenia.

Acute leukemia see Leukemia.

Acute liver failure (fulminant liver failure) a rare clinical syndrome resulting from severe impairment or necrosis of liver cells without pre-existing liver disease or cirrhosis. Acetaminophen overdose is the leading cause.

Acute lung injury (ALI)/acute respiratory distress syndrome (ARDS) a spectrum of acute lung inflammations and diffuse alveolocapillary injury.

Acute lymphoblastic leukemia (ALL) see Leukemia.

Acute mesenteric ischemia caused by acute occlusion of the mesenteric artery that results in a significant reduction in mucosal blood flow to the large and small intestines. Aortic aneurysms, arterial thrombi, or emboli can be causes.

Acute mountain sickness (AMS) the presence of a combination of nonspecific symptoms that appear within a few hours after ascent to altitude, and may include headache, loss of appetite, nausea, vomiting, weakness, lassitude, dizziness, and difficulty sleeping.

Acute myelogenous leukemia (AML) see Leukemia.

Acute otitis media (AOM) an infection of the middle ear space, behind the eardrum (tympanic membrane); characterized by pain, dizziness, and partial loss of hearing.

Acute orthostatic hypotension an abnormal decrease in blood pressure when a person stands. This may lead to fainting.

Acute pancreatitis inflammation of the pancreas resulting from obstruction to the outflow of pancreatic digestive enzymes caused by bile duct or pancreatic duct obstruction (e.g., gallstones). Usually a mild disease and resolves spontaneously.

Acute poststreptococcal glomerulonephritis (PSGN) see Glomerulonephritis.

Acute pyelonephritis acute inflammation of the renal parenchyma and pelvis characterized by small cortical abscesses and yellowish streaks in the medulla resulting from the accumulation of pus in the collecting tubules and interstitial tissue.

Acute renal failure (acute renal injury) a sudden decline in kidney function with a decrease in glomerular filtration and accumulation of nitrogenous waste products in the blood as demonstrated by an elevation in plasma creatinine and blood urea nitrogen levels.

Acute respiratory distress syndrome (ARDS) capillaries or alveoli of the lungs are damaged as a result of infection, injury, blood loss, or inhalation injury causing fluid to leak from the capillaries into the alveoli, resulting in pulmonary edema and collapse of some alveoli.

Acute tubular necrosis (ATN) the kidney undergoes ischemic or nephrotoxic injury because of severe hypotension, aminoglycosides, or radiocontrast agents and produces granular and epithelial cell casts in urine.

Acute urethral syndrome the bladder is irritated and the typical symptoms of a urinary tract infection are present in the absence of an infection.

Adenocarcinoma tumor arising from epithelial cells with a glandular or glandlike pattern.

Adenocystic tumor (cylindroma) rare bronchial gland tumors that arise predominantly in the trachea or large airways and cause obstruction.

Adenomyosis the presence of islands of endometrial glands surrounded by benign endometrial stroma within the uterine myometrium.

Adenosine deaminase (ADA) deficiency see Immune deficiency.

Adrenarche growth of axillary and pubic hair and other physiologic changes induced by hyperactivity of the suprarenal cortex and adrenocortical secretion of androgenic hormones in early puberty.

Agammaglobulinemia see Immune deficiency.

Ageusia loss of the sense of taste.

Agoraphobia a mental disorder characterized by an irrational fear of leaving the familiar setting of home, or venturing into the open, so pervasive that a large number of external life situations are entered into reluctantly or are avoided; often associated with panic attacks.

Agranulocytosis see Immune deficiency.

Akinesia slowness or loss of normal motor function resulting in impaired muscle movement.

Akinetic mutism (AM) a syndrome characterized by the inability to speak, loss of voluntary movement, and apparent loss of emotional feeling. It is related to lesions of the upper brainstem.

Albright syndrome (Albright-McCune-Sternberg syndrome) polyostotic fibrous dysplasia, patchy dermal pigmentation, and endocrine dysfunction.

Alcoholic cirrhosis see Cirrhosis.

Alcoholic fatty liver (steatosis) the mildest form of alcoholic liver disease; can be caused by chronic ingestion of relatively small amounts of alcohol, may be asymptomatic, and is reversible with cessation of drinking.

Alcoholic hepatitis (steatohepatitis) a precursor of cirrhosis characterized by inflammation; degeneration and necrosis of hepatocytes; infiltration of neutrophils, macrophages, and lymphocytes; immunologic alterations; and lipid peroxidation.

Algor mortis postmortem reduction of body temperature.

Alkaline reflux gastritis inflammation of the stomach caused by reflux of bile and alkaline pancreatic secretions that contain proteolytic enzymes and disrupt the mucosal barrier in the remnant stomach.

Allergic contact dermatitis contact dermatitis attributable to allergic sensitization.

Allodynia a condition in which pain arises from a stimulus that would not normally be experienced as painful.

Allostasis long-term or chronic exaggerated responses to stress.

Alogia inability to speak because of mental deficiency, mental confusion, or aphasia.

Alopecia loss of hair.

Alopecia areata an autoimmune T-cell–mediated chronic inflammatory disease directed at hair follicles that results in baldness, usually in round patches.

Alpha-thalassemia major see Anemia.

Alpha-thalassemia minor see Anemia.

Alzheimer disease (dementia of Alzheimer type [DAT], senile disease complex) a degenerative disease characterized by amyloid plaques and fibrillary tangles in the cortex and atrophy and widened sulci in the frontal and temporal lobes.

Amblyopia poor vision caused by abnormal development of visual areas of the brain in response to abnormal visual stimulation during early development.

Amyotrophic lateral sclerosis (ALS) (sporadic motor system disease, sporadic motor neuron disease, motor neuron disease, Lou Gehrig disease) a disease that breaks down tissues in the nervous system (a neurodegenerative disease); it is of unknown cause and affects the nerves responsible for movement.

Anaphylactic shock a state of shock caused by a severe allergic reaction that lowers blood pressure and results in urticaria, breathing difficulties, and possibly death.

Anaphylactoid purpura (allergic purpura, Henoch-Schönlein purpura) nonthrombocytopenic purpura attributable to immune hypersensitivity to foods, drugs, and insect bites.

Anemia hemoglobin concentration is less than normal because of a deficiency in red blood cells, a low level of hemoglobin in cells, or both; it manifests as pallor of the skin and mucous membranes, weakness, dizziness, easy fatigability, and drowsiness caused by oxygen deficiency.

Congenital hemolytic anemias

Alpha-thalassemia major thalassemia in which all four α-chains of hemoglobin are defective, resulting in a fatal condition because oxygen cannot be released to the tissues.

Alpha-thalassemia minor thalassemia in which two α-chains of hemoglobin are defective.

Beta-thalassemia major (Cooley anemia) thalassemia in which α-chain synthesis and β-chain synthesis are uncoupled; β-chain production is depressed moderately in the heterozygous form, **beta-thalassemia minor,** and severely in the homozygous form, **beta-thalassemia major,** resulting in erythrocytes that have a reduced amount of hemoglobin and accumulations of free α-chains.

Beta-thalassemia minor see above.

Glucose-6-phosphate dehydrogenase (G6PD) deficiency an inherited condition that is asymptomatic in the absence of exposure to particular substances such as certain medicines, mothballs, or severe infections; with exposure the red blood cells undergo destruction, producing excessive bilirubin that overloads the liver and causes jaundice.

Hemoglobin H disease a form of alpha-thalassemia in which a hemoglobin H gene is expressed but cannot bind oxygen.

Hereditary spherocytosis (congenital hemolytic anemia, congenital acholuric jaundice) a defect in the cell membrane of red blood cells that causes thickened, fragile red blood cells that are susceptible to spontaneous hemolysis and results in chronic anemia, jaundice, fever, and abdominal pain.

Sickle cell anemia (sickle cell disease [SCD]) an inherited autosomal recessive disorder of the blood caused by abnormal hemoglobin that distorts red blood cells and makes them fragile and prone to rupture and can cause anemia, joint pain, fever, leg ulcers, and jaundice.

Sickle cell–Hb C disease a heterozygous form in which the child simultaneously inherits a hemoglobin C gene from another parent.

Sickle cell–thalassemia disease a heterozygous form in which the child simultaneously inherits a thalassemia gene from another parent.

Sickle cell trait an inherited condition in which an individual carries only one gene for sickle cell disease and is without symptoms.

Thalassemia a potentially fatal genetic disorder in which hemoglobin molecules are abnormal, resulting in severe anemia; enlarged heart, liver, and spleen; and skeletal deformation.

Macrocytic anemia (megaloblastic anemia) a condition characterized by erythrocytes that are larger than normal; associated with deficiency of vitamin B_{12} or folic acid caused by inadequate intake or insufficient absorption secondary to alcoholism or drugs that inhibit DNA replication.

Pernicious anemia an autoimmune disorder that causes a deficiency in intrinsic factor, resulting in the inability to absorb vitamin B_{12} and a subsequent increase in the production of abnormal erythrocytes.

Microcytic-hypochromic anemia a condition in which red blood cells are smaller than normal as a result of iron deficiency.

Acquired sideroblastic anemia a heterogeneous group of disorders characterized by anemia of varying severity caused by a defect in mitochondrial heme synthesis; occurs as a primary disorder with no known cause (idiopathic) or is associated with other myeloproliferative or myeloplastic disorders.

Hereditary sideroblastic anemia heterogeneous group of rare disorders characterized by anemia of varying severity caused by a defect in mitochondrial heme synthesis; occurs almost exclusively in males, suggesting a predominant recessive X-linked transmission.

Hypoplastic anemia a condition in which anemia results from greatly depressed, inadequately functioning bone marrow and smaller-than-normal erythrocytes.

Iron deficiency anemia (IDA) an insufficient dietary intake or absorption of iron, resulting in decreased incorporation of hemoglobin into red blood cells and subsequent feelings of fatigue, weakness, and shortness of breath as well as pale earlobes, palms, and conjunctivae.

Reversible sideroblastic anemia associated with alcoholism; results from nutritional deficiencies of folate.

Sideroblastic anemia (SA) refractory anemia of varying severity that is caused by altered mitochondrial metabolism and is marked by sideroblasts in the bone marrow.

Normocytic-normochromic anemia (NNA) erythrocytes are of normal size and hemoglobin content but of insufficient number; usually caused by hereditary spherocytosis, drug-induced anemia, and anemia secondary to malignancies.

Anemia of chronic disease (ACD) a mild to moderate anemia resulting from decreased erythropoiesis in individuals with conditions of chronic systemic disease or inflammation.

Aplastic anemia decreased bone marrow production of adequate amounts of new red blood cells; results from an autoimmune disorder or exposure to radiation or substances such as benzene or certain drugs.

Aplastic crisis temporary loss of bone marrow causes erythropoiesis, resulting in an acute fall in hemoglobin levels and subsequent anemia.

Autoimmune hemolytic anemia (AIHA) a form of hemolytic anemia involving autoantibodies against red blood cell antigens.

Cold agglutinin autoimmune hemolytic anemia acquired disorder caused by autoantibodies against antigens normally on the surface of erythrocytes; mediated by immunoglobulin M (IgM) antibodies that optimally bind to and agglutinate erythrocytes in colder portions of the body (e.g., fingers, toes), and occurs less often than warm antibody hemolysis, affecting mostly middle-aged and older adults.

Cold hemolysin autoimmune hemolytic anemia (paroxysmal cold hemoglobinuria) a disorder in which exposure to cold initiates acute and severe intravascular hemolysis that, unlike cold agglutinin anemia, results in hemoglobinuria. The chronic form of this anemia is extremely rare, but an acute form of paroxysmal cold hemoglobinuria is frequently observed in autoimmune hemolytic anemia of childhood.

Drug-induced hemolytic anemia a form of immune hemolytic anemia usually resulting from an allergic reaction against foreign antigens (e.g., antibiotics) that have attached to the surface of red blood cells.

Fanconi anemia a genetic disease affecting bone marrow that is characterized by pancytopenia, hypoplasia of the bone marrow, congenital anomalies, and pigment changes of the skin and that predisposes the individual to myelodysplasia and to acute myeloid leukemia or cancers of the mouth, esophagus, intestinal and urinary tracts, and reproductive organs.

Hemolytic anemia a condition in which red blood cells are destroyed in response to certain toxic or infectious agents or in certain inherited blood disorders and the rate of breakdown exceeds the body's ability to compensate.

Hemolytic disease of the newborn (HDN) (erythroblastosis fetalis) a condition that affects a fetus or newborn in which red blood cells break down because of antibodies made by the mother that are directed against the infant's red cells, potentially resulting in anemia, heart failure, jaundice, and brain damage.

Posthemorrhagic anemia a type of normocytic-normochromic anemia that is caused by sudden blood loss in an individual with normal iron stores and triggers a compensatory response in which water and electrolytes from tissues and interstitial spaces are used to expand plasma volume and accelerate the formation and development of blood cells.

Warm autoimmune hemolytic anemia the most common form of autoimmune hemolytic anemia; caused by IgG that binds to erythrocytes at normal body temperature; often secondary to other diseases, especially lymphomas, chronic lymphocytic leukemia, other neoplastic disorders, or systemic lupus erythematosus (SLE).

Anencephaly anomaly in which the soft, bony component of the skull and much of the brain are missing.

Angelman syndrome (happy puppet syndrome) an inherited syndrome of jerky puppetlike movements, frequent laughter, mental and motor retardation, peculiar open-mouthed facies, and seizures.

Angina pectoris chest pain caused by reduced cardiac blood flow and myocardial ischemia.

Anhedonia absence of pleasure from the performance of acts that would ordinarily be pleasurable.

Ankylosing spondylitis (AS, spondyloarthritis) chronic inflammation of the spine and sacroiliac joints with gradual fusion of the vertebrae that immobilizes the spine.

Anorexia nervosa (AN) a disorder with both psychologic and physiologic components that begins with dieting to lose weight and manifests into an inappropriate self-control behavior; continued restrictive eating may lead to starvation and eventually death.

Anorgasmia (orgasmic dysfunction) the inability of the woman to reach or achieve orgasm.

Anuria urine output less than 50 ml/day.

Anxiety disorder a group of disorders involving various manifestations of anxiety that are grouped together and include panic disorder, specific phobia, social phobia, obsessive-compulsive disorder (OCD), posttraumatic stress disorder (PTSD), acute stress disorder, generalized anxiety disorder (GAD), and anxiety disorders secondary to medical conditions or substance-induced or not otherwise specified.

Aplastic anemia see Anemia.

Aplastic crisis see Anemia.

Appendicitis inflammation of the appendix as a result of blockage of the opening from the appendix into the cecum; the appendix wall becomes infected and ruptures, allowing the infection to spread throughout the abdomen and cause pain, anorexia, fever, nausea, vomiting, and diarrhea.

Apraxia a disorder of voluntary movement consisting of impairment of the performance of skilled or purposeful movements; results from acquired cerebral disease.

Arcus senilis a gray to white ring at the periphery of the cornea; caused by deposits of cholesterol in the cornea or hyaline degeneration and occurs primarily in older persons.

Areflexia absence of reflexes.

Arterial ischemic stroke (pediatric arterial ischemic stroke) a rare disorder in children resulting from embolism, arteriopathy, or, rarely, sinovenous thrombosis and leading to a decreased flow of blood and oxygen to areas of the brain.

Asbestosis pulmonary inflammation and fibrosis resulting from inhalation of hydrous silicates of various metals in fibrous form.

Aseptic meningitis a form of inflammation of the meninges and subarachnoid space surrounding the brain and spinal cord without evidence of bacterial infection; may be associated with viral infection, systemic disease, or drugs.

Aspiration pneumonitis a condition caused by the abnormal entry of fluids, particulate matter, or secretions into the lower airways that can lead to chemical pneumonitis from entry of toxic material such as gastric acid, from bacterial infection, or by mechanical obstruction of the lower airways.

Asthma a chronic inflammatory disorder of the airways involving bronchial hyperresponsiveness and airway obstruction marked by periodic attacks of wheezing, shortness of breath, a tight feeling in the chest, and a cough that produces mucus because of an allergic reaction triggered by certain drugs, irritants, viral infection, exercise, or emotional stress.

Asymptomatic bacteriuria the presence of bacteria in the urine without evidence of infection.

Ataxia-telangiectasia (AT) see Immune deficiency.

Ataxic cerebral palsy a form of cerebral palsy associated with damage to the cerebellum and resulting in gait disturbances and instability; at birth the infant may have hypotonia, but develops stiffness of the trunk muscles later in infancy.

Atelectasis a part of or an entire lung collapses and the alveoli deflate as a result of surgery, smoking, or blockage of a bronchiole.

Absorption atelectasis collapse of lung tissue resulting from gradual absorption of air from obstructed or hypoventilated alveoli or from inhalation of concentrated oxygen or anesthetic agents.

Compression atelectasis air pressure in the pleural space pushes against the already recoiled lung, causing compression atelectasis, and against the mediastinum, compressing and displacing the heart and great vessels.

Surfactant impairment decreased production or inactivation of surfactant, which is necessary to reduce surface tension in the alveoli and causes lung collapse during expiration; can occur because of premature birth, acute respiratory distress syndrome, anesthesia, or mechanical ventilation.

Atherosclerosis a type of arteriosclerosis in which the inflammatory changes of thickening and hardening of the walls of large- and medium-sized arteries are caused by an atheroma or plaque of lipids, cells, and connective tissue in the tunica intima.

Atopic dermatitis (AD) (allergic dermatitis) a chronic hereditary skin disease characterized by intense itching and inflamed skin that causes redness, swelling, cracking, crusting, and scaling.

Atrial septal defect (ASD) a congenital heart disease involving the interatrial septum of the heart that separates the right and left atria, which results in misdirected blood flow between the two sides of the heart.

Atrioventricular canal (AVC) defect a large hole is present in the center of the heart where the wall between the atria joins the wall between the ventricles, and the tricuspid and mitral valves are formed into a single large valve that crosses the defect.

Atypical ductal hyperplasia (ADH) abnormal proliferating cells in breast ducts.

Atypical hyperplasia increased number of cells with some variation in cellular structure but without sufficient qualitative or quantitative features of carcinoma.

Atypical lobular hyperplasia (ALH) abnormal proliferating cells in breast lobules.

Autoimmune hemolytic anemia (AIHA) see Anemia.

Autoimmune neonatal thrombocytopenia see Thrombocytopenia.

Autoimmune vascular purpura (allergic purpura) purpura caused by antibody-mediated injury of blood vessel walls, typically arterioles and capillaries. The reaction is directed to foreign proteins or chemicals in the blood (microorganisms, drugs, or other chemicals) that deposit on the vessel walls.

Autonomic hyperreflexia (dysreflexia) a syndrome resulting from afferent stimuli that cause intense sympathetic discharge originating with spinal cord injury above the major splanchnic outflow; characterized by hypertension, bradycardia, sweating of the forehead, severe headache, and piloerection on distention of the bladder and rectum.

Autosomal agammaglobulinemia see Immune deficiency.

Autosomal dominant polycystic kidney disease (ADPKD) a progressive disease characterized by formation of multiple cysts of varying size scattered diffusely throughout both kidneys, resulting in compression and destruction of renal parenchyma, usually with hypertension, gross hematuria, and uremia leading to progressive renal failure.

Autosomal hyper-IgM syndrome see Immune deficiency.

Azotemia kidney dysfunction characterized by increased serum urea levels and frequently associated with increased creatinine levels.

Bacterial pneumonia an acute or chronic disease marked by inflammation of the lungs caused by bacterial infection.

Bacterial tracheitis a condition in which the larynx, trachea, and bronchi are inflamed and present with signs similar to those of epiglottitis and croup; may result in airway obstruction secondary to subglottic edema or sloughing of the epithelial lining or the mucopurulent membrane within the trachea.

Bacterial vaginosis (BV) a condition caused by an overgrowth of normal vaginal bacteria, causing vaginal discharge with a foul odor.

Balanitis inflammation of the glans penis caused by irritation by environmental substances, physical trauma, or infection.

Bare lymphocyte syndrome see Immune deficiency.

Barrett esophagus chronic peptic ulceration of the esophagus; formation of precancerous lesions with possible progression to adenocarcinoma.

Bartholinitis (Bartholin cyst) inflammation of one or both of the ducts that lead from the introitus (vaginal opening) to the Bartholin/greater vestibular glands.

Basal cell carcinoma a surface epithelial tumor of the skin originating from undifferentiated basal or germinative cells.

B-cell neoplasm see Lymphoma.

Becker muscular dystrophy a general term for a number of late-onset X-linked recessive hereditary, progressive degenerative disorders affecting skeletal muscles, and often other organ systems.

Beckwith-Wiedemann syndrome an inherited disorder characterized by exomphalos, macroglossia, and gigantism; often associated with visceromegaly, adrenocortical cytomegaly, and dysplasia of the renal medulla.

Benign breast disease (BBD) a spectrum of noncancerous changes in ducts and lobules of the breast, including irregular lumps, cysts, sensitive nipples, and itching.

Benign prostatic hyperplasia (BPH) enlargement of the prostate gland, which may press against the urethra and bladder, interfering with urine flow.

Beta-thalassemia major (Cooley anemia) see Anemia.

Beta-thalassemia minor see Anemia.

Biliary atresia a condition in newborn children in which the biliary tract is blocked or absent, causing bile accumulation and progressive liver failure.

Biliary cirrhosis see Cirrhosis.

Bipolar disorder psychiatric disorder characterized by alternating mania or hypomania and depression, often with periods of normal mood in between, and changes in energy and behavior according to mood.

Blast injury tissue damage from compressive waves of air against the body followed by waves of decreased pressure.

Blepharitis inflammation of the eyelids.

B-lymphocyte deficiency see Immune deficiency.

Bradykinesia decreased spontaneity and movement; a feature of extrapyramidal disorders, such as Parkinson disease.

Brainstem gliomas a group of tumors located in the brainstem that are usually classified as high grade and result in the sudden onset of symptoms including headaches, vomiting, and visual disturbances.

Bronchial carcinoid tumor an obstructing tumor of the trachea or large bronchi that may cause paraneoplastic symptoms.

Bronchiectasis dilation of the bronchi in response to obstruction, necrotizing pneumonias, cystic fibrosis, or Kartagener syndrome (a hereditary syndrome consisting of dextrocardia, bronchiectasis, and sinusitis).

Bronchiolitis inflammation of the bronchioles usually caused by viral infection.

Bronchiolitis obliterans partial or complete obliteration of bronchioles and some bronchi by granulation and fibrotic tissue masses.

Bronchiolitis obliterans with organizing pneumonia (BOOP) obstruction of the bronchioles and alveolar ducts by fibrous granulation tissue that is further complicated by the development of pneumonia.

Bronchopulmonary dysplasia (BPD) a condition most often found in premature infants in which chronic pulmonary insufficiency occurs because of long-term artificial pulmonary ventilation.

Bruton's agammaglobulinemia see Immune deficiency.

Bulbar palsy a form of palsy resulting from impaired function of the cranial nerves from degeneration of the motor neurons of primarily the brainstem; manifested as weakness and wasting of the various bulbar muscles, resulting in difficulty articulating words (dysarthria) and difficulty swallowing (dysphagia); fluid regurgitation is a major symptom and can cause aspiration.

Bullous pemphigoid (BP) a more benign autoimmune disease than pemphigus vulgaris, with blistering of the subepidermal skin layer.

Burkitt lymphoma see Lymphoma.

Burn shock a phenomenon consisting of both a hypovolemic cardiovascular component and a cellular component; results from massive fluid losses from the circulating blood volume.

C1 deficiency see Immune deficiency.

C2 deficiency see Immune deficiency.

C3 deficiency see Immune deficiency.

C3 receptor deficiency see Immune deficiency.

C4 deficiency see Immune deficiency.

C9 deficiency see Immune deficiency.

Cachexia illness and malnutrition seen in individuals with cancer that results in wasting and eventual death.

Calculi or urinary stone (urolithiasis) masses of crystals, protein, or other substances that are a common cause of urinary tract obstruction in adults.

Candidiasis a fungal infection caused by an overgrowth of normal *Candida albicans* found in the skin and mucous membranes of the mouth, respiratory tract, or vagina.

Caplan syndrome formation in coal workers of intrapulmonary nodules in pneumoconiosis that are histologically similar to subcutaneous rheumatoid nodules associated with rheumatoid arthritis.

Carbuncles a condition in which a bacterial infection of the hair follicle or sebaceous gland ducts becomes painful and discharges pus through various openings.

Carcinoma epithelial cell tumor.

Carcinoma in situ (CIS) preinvasive epithelial malignant tumors of glandular or squamous cell origin.

Cardiogenic shock a condition resulting from decreased cardiac output caused by heart disease in which the heart is unable to pump blood through the body, usually because of myocardial infarction.

Cardiomyopathy(ies) a diverse group of diseases primarily affecting the myocardium and resulting from tissue remodeling caused by myocardial and neurohumoral responses to ischemic and hypertensive alterations.

Cavernous (congenital) hemangioma a birthmark that is similar to the strawberry hemangioma but is more deeply rooted and may appear as a red-blue spongy mass of tissue filled with blood.

Central core disease (CCD) an autosomal dominant congenital myopathy characterized by hypotonia, delay of motor development in infancy, and nonprogressive or slowly progressive muscle weakness; on biopsy the central core of muscle fibers stains abnormally, myofibrils are abnormally compact, and there is virtual absence of mitochondria and sarcoplasmic reticulum; histochemically, the cores are devoid of oxidative enzyme, phosphorylase, and ATPase activity.

Central precocious puberty condition in which puberty begins prematurely with normal changes in the hypothalamopituitary (HPG) axis with premature development of secondary sexual characteristics and premature closure of the epiphysis of long bones, resulting in lifelong short stature.

Centriacinar emphysema see Emphysema.

Cerebellar astrocytoma brain tumor of the right or left cerebellar hemisphere that causes motor symptoms on the same side as the tumor.

Cerebral palsy (CP) a developmental brain injury that occurs before or shortly after birth and causes muscular impairment affecting motor function and also may alter speech and learning abilities.

Cervical dysplasia (cervical intraepithelial neoplasia [CIN]) a condition characterized by the appearance of abnormal cervical cells that are considered precancerous.

Cervicitis inflammation of the mucous membrane of the uterine cervix caused by infection, typically by chlamydia, genital herpes, or gonorrhea.

Chediak-Higashi syndrome see Immune deficiency.

Cheyne-Stokes respiration an abnormal pattern of breathing in which tidal volume gradually increases followed by a gradual decrease and a period of apnea before returning to a normal respiratory pattern.

Chickenpox an infectious viral disease that is spread by direct contact or through the air by coughing or sneezing; it causes a blister-like rash that first affects the face and trunk and then can spread over the rest of the body; symptoms include severe itching, fatigue, and fever.

Childhood absence epilepsy (petit mal seizures, nonconvulsive epilepsy) a type of generalized epilepsy; age of onset is 4 to 10 years.

Chlamydia a sexually transmitted bacterial infection that can cause infertility and blindness.

Choking asphyxiation obstruction of the internal airways.

Cholangiocellular carcinoma (cholangiocarcinoma) primary carcinomas of the liver that develop in the bile ducts.

Cholecystitis inflammation of the gallbladder commonly caused by impaction of a gallstone that causes right upper quadrant pain and possibly a rupture and abscess in the gallbladder.

Cholelithiasis the presence or formation of gallstones in the gallbladder or bile ducts.

Chondrosarcoma a cancer of the cartilage that usually occurs in the pelvic bones, shoulder bones, and the upper part of the arms and legs.

Chronic active hepatitis the persistence of clinical manifestations and liver inflammation after the acute stages with consistently abnormal liver function tests and persistent HBsAg creating a predisposition to cirrhosis and primary hepatocellular carcinoma.

Chronic bronchitis chronic bronchitis, particularly as a cause of chronic cough in smokers.

Chronic gastritis tends to occur in older adults with chronic inflammation, mucosal atrophy, and epithelial metaplasia; may be immune (fundal) or nonimmune (antral), depending on the pathogenesis and location of the lesions.

Chronic glomerulonephritis see Glomerulonephritis.

Chronic granulomatous disease (CGD) see Immune deficiency.

Chronic kidney disease (CKD) progressive loss of renal function associated with systemic diseases such as hypertension, diabetes mellitus, systemic lupus erythematosus, or intrinsic kidney disease, including kidney stones, acute kidney injury, chronic glomerulonephritis, chronic pyelonephritis, obstructive uropathies, or vascular disorders.

Chronic leukemia see Leukemia.

Chronic lymphocytic leukemia (CLL) see Leukemia.

Chronic mesenteric ischemia development of regions of compromised blood flow in the mesenterium secondary to atherosclerosis (most common), congestive heart failure, dysrhythmias, hemorrhage, thrombus formation, aortic aneurysm, or any condition that decreases arterial blood flow. Chronic occlusion is often accompanied by formation of collateral circulation that may be able to nourish the resting intestine.

Chronic mucocutaneous candidiasis see Immune deficiency.

Chronic myelogenous leukemia (CML) see Leukemia.

Chronic obstructive pulmonary disease (COPD) any of a group of irreversible respiratory diseases (chronic bronchitis, emphysema, α_1-antitrypsin deficiency) that are characterized by airflow obstruction or limitation.

Chronic pancreatitis inflammation of the pancreas resulting from repeated exacerbations of acute pancreatitis that lead to chronic changes; associated with obstruction from gallstones, autoimmune disease, gene mutations, smoking, occupational chemical exposure, and obesity.

Chronic pyelonephritis persistent or recurrent infection of the kidney leading to scarring.

Chronic relapsing thrombotic thrombocytopenic purpura (TTP) see Thrombocytopenia.

Cirrhosis degeneration of liver tissue resulting in fibrosis with nodule and scar formation that compromises liver function.

Alcoholic cirrhosis destructive inflammation of the liver caused by the toxic effects of alcohol metabolism, immunologic processes, oxidative stress from lipid peroxidation, and malnutrition.

Biliary cirrhosis a form of alcoholic cirrhosis in which damage and inflammation leading to cirrhosis begin in bile canaliculi and bile ducts, rather than in the hepatocytes.

Primary biliary cirrhosis a T-lymphocyte- and antibody-mediated destruction of the small intrahepatic bile ducts.

Cloacal exstrophy family of congenital anomalies with two exstrophied bladder units separated by an exstrophied segment of intestine, which is usually cecum, receiving ileum superiorly and continuing distally to blind ending microcolon.

Coal worker pneumoconiosis (coal miner lung, black lung) mild to severe pneumoconiosis (pulmonary fibrosis) caused by coal dust (coal, silica, quartz) deposits in the lung; symptoms initially present as a productive cough and wheezing, but may advance to chronic bronchitis and emphysema.

Coarctation of the aorta (COA) a condition in which the aorta narrows in the area where the ductus arteriosus inserts; narrowing usually occurs preductal in children and postductal in adults.

Cold agglutinin autoimmune hemolytic anemia see Anemia.

Cold hemolysin autoimmune hemolytic anemia (paroxysmal cold hemoglobinuria) see Anemia.

Combined T- and B-lymphocyte deficiency see Immune deficiency.

Common variable immune deficiency see Immune deficiency.

Communicating (extraventricular) hydrocephalus a disorder in which the cerebrospinal fluid pathways are intact but cerebrospinal fluid absorption is impaired.

Complement deficiency see Immune deficiency.

Complete precocious puberty refers to the early onset and progression of all pubertal features (i.e., thelarche, pubarche, and menarche).

Complex febrile seizure seizures with characteristic features similar to those of simple febrile seizure with a longer duration and focal characteristics; occur more than once in a 24-hour period.

Complex regional pain syndrome (CRPS) diffuse persistent pain usually in an extremity often associated with vasomotor disturbances, trophic changes, and limitation or immobility of joints; frequently follows a local injury.

Compression atelectasis see Atelectasis.

Compressive syndrome (sensorimotor syndrome; crush syndrome) a shocklike state that follows release of a limb or limbs or the trunk and pelvis after a prolonged period of compression, such as by a heavy weight; characterized by suppression of renal function, probably the result of damage to the renal tubules by myoglobin from the damaged muscles.

Congenital adrenal hyperplasia a group of autosomal recessively inherited disorders associated with a deficiency of one of the enzymes involved in cortisol biosynthesis, resulting in elevation of ACTH levels and overproduction and accumulation of cortisol precursors proximal to the block; androgens are produced in excess, causing virilization. The most common disorder is the 21-hydroxylase deficiency, caused by mutation in the cytochrome P450 21-hydroxylase gene *(CYP21)* on chromosome 6p.

Congenital aganglionic megacolon (Hirschsprung disease) a congenital defect in which the nerves that innervate the anus through the wall of the bowel are absent, resulting in enlargement of the bowel superior to the point where the nerves are missing and a subsequent decrease in peristalsis that results in chronic constipation.

Congenital hydrocephalus excessive accumulation of cerebrospinal fluid present at birth and characterized by increased intracranial pressure (ICP). This increase may be caused by a blockage within the ventricular system in which the CSF flows, an imbalance in the production of CSF, or a reduced reabsorption of CSF that results in ventricular enlargement and increased ICP.

Congenital hypothyroidism lack of secretion of thyroid hormone.

Congenital (infantile) nephrotic syndrome (Finnish type) a very rare form of nephrotic syndrome caused by a defect in a kidney protein resulting in excessive amounts of protein excreted in the urine.

Congestive splenomegaly enlargement of the spleen accompanied by ascites, portal hypertension, and esophageal varices; most commonly seen in those with hepatic cirrhosis.

Consumptive thrombohemorrhagic disorders heterogeneous group of conditions that demonstrate the entire range of hemorrhagic and thrombotic pathologic conditions.

Contact dermatitis an allergic response to an environmental antigen binding to specific carrier proteins contained in an individual's skin.

Contrecoup injury brain injury resulting from the brain hitting the inside of the skull on the side opposite the site of blunt force trauma.

Cor pulmonale right-sided heart failure caused by prolonged pulmonary hypertension.

Coronary artery disease (CAD) narrowing of the lumen of one or more of the coronary arteries, usually attributable to atherosclerosis, leading to myocardial ischemia; can cause congestive heart failure, angina pectoris, or myocardial infarction.

Craniopharyngioma a brain tumor that develops in the pituitary gland and most often affects children, causing headache, seizure, diabetes insipidus, early onset of puberty, and delayed growth.

Craniosynostosis (craniostenosis) (see Syndromic craniosynostosis) premature ossification of the skull and closure of the sutures, resulting in abnormal skull expansion and asymmetric skull growth.

Cri du chat syndrome a hereditary congenital syndrome characterized by hypertelorism, microcephaly, severe mental deficiency, and a plaintive catlike cry; caused by deletion of the short arm of chromosome 5.

Crohn disease (CD) an autoimmune condition in which the intestines and possibly other regions of the digestive system are chronically inflamed and ulcerated, causing chronic diarrhea, disrupted digestion, and subsequent difficulty eating and digesting food.

Croup a viral infection that involves the larynx, trachea, and the airways leading to the lungs and that can result in serious breathing difficulties, hoarseness, sore throat, and a hacking cough.

Cryptorchidism the scrotum of one or both testes is absent because of failure of the testis to descend from the abdominal position during fetal development.

Curling ulcer ischemic ulcers of the stomach and duodenal mucosa that develop within hours after an event, such as hemorrhage, multisystem trauma, severe burns, heart failure, or sepsis.

Cushing disease adrenal hyperplasia caused by an ACTH-secreting basophil adenoma of the pituitary.

Cushing syndrome increased synthesis and secretion of cortisol from a tumor of the adrenal cortex; caused by administration of glucocorticoid drugs or by the presence of an ACTH-secreting tumor of the anterior lobe of the pituitary gland (Cushing disease), resulting in weight gain, glucose intolerance, and muscle wasting.

Cushing ulcer a stress ulcer associated with severe head trauma or brain surgery.

Cyclic neutropenia see Immune deficiency.

Cylindrical bronchiectasis reversible bronchial dilation with symmetrically dilated airways, as can be seen after pneumonia.

Cystic fibrosis (CF) a genetic disorder of the exocrine glands caused by a mutation in the CF transmembrane regulator gene, resulting in impairment in chloride transfer across cell membranes and subsequent chloride and water accumulation in organs and in thickened secretions that block ducts and form cysts.

Cystitis a condition characterized by acute or chronic inflammation of the urinary bladder, usually caused by bacterial infection of the urethra; symptoms include frequent burning urination, blood in the urine, pain in the pubic area, chills and fever, back pain, and nausea. See Painful bladder syndrome/interstitial cystitis (PBS/IC) for further information.

Dandy-Walker malformation congenital defect of midline cerebellar structures and the fourth ventricle in which hydrocephalus is caused by atresia of the foramina of Luschka or Magendie, which normally allow the fourth ventricle to empty into the areas surrounding the brain, leading the ventricular flow of CSF into a "blind pouch."

Dawn phenomenon abrupt increases in fasting levels of plasma glucose between 5 and 9 AM, in the absence of antecedent hypoglycemia; occurs in diabetic patients receiving insulin therapy.

Decompression sickness (DCS) (Caisson disease) gas embolism created when a person under water returns to the surface too quickly, resulting in cellular hypoxia, joint and muscle pain, and tissue necrosis.

Deep venous thrombosis (DVT) a blood clot or thrombus in a deep vein, usually of the leg.

Degenerative disk disease (DDD) intervertebral disk tissue is replaced by fibrocartilage during aging; functional capacity is rarely altered.

Demyelinating polyneuropathy a type of polyneuropathy in which the peripheral nerve myelin is primarily affected; can be familial (Charcot-Marie-Tooth disease, type 1) or acquired (Guillain-Barré syndrome); motor nerve conduction is slowed or blocked.

Dermatitis herpetiformis pruritic chronic dermatitis with successive groups of symmetrical, erythematous, papular, vesicular, eczematous, or bullous lesions, usually associated with asymptomatic gluten-sensitive enteropathy.

Detrusor areflexia a lower motor neuron disorder that results in an underactive, hypotonic, or atonic bladder function with retention of urine and distention.

Detrusor hyperreflexia (uninhibited or reflex bladder) upper motor neuron disorders in which the bladder empties automatically when it becomes full and the external sphincter functions normally.

Developmental dysplasia of the hip (DDH) a condition in which the hip joint of babies or young children is malformed, with the ball being completely out of the socket or the socket being too shallow to support the ball.

Diabetes diseases having in common the triad of symptoms of polyuria, weight loss, and significant glucosuria.

- **Diabetes insipidus** a disease caused by a deficiency in or resistance to antidiuretic hormone that is characterized by excretion of large amounts of dilute urine because of a decrease in water reabsorption in the kidney.
- **Gestational diabetes mellitus (GDM)** carbohydrate intolerance of variable severity with onset during pregnancy.
- **Type 1 diabetes mellitus** a disorder of carbohydrate metabolism characterized by a decrease in insulin production, resulting in hyperglycemia, ketoacidosis, and eventually renal failure and coronary artery disease.
- **Type 2 diabetes mellitus** a condition of glucose intolerance that normally appears first in adulthood and is exacerbated by obesity and an inactive lifestyle.

Diabetic nephropathy a progressive kidney disease caused by diabetes-induced angiopathy of capillaries in the glomeruli that causes nodular glomerulosclerosis.

Diabetic neuropathy combined sensory and motor disorder often seen in older diabetic patients as a result of microvascular injury involving small blood vessels that supply nerves.

Diabetic retinopathy damage to the retina caused by an overaccumulation of glucose or fructose that damages the blood vessels in the retina; in advanced stages, lack of oxygen in the retina causes fragile blood vessels to grow along the retina and in the vitreous fluid of the eye that may bleed and cause blurred vision.

Diaper dermatitis a type of dermatitis characterized by inflammation of the skin in the diaper area in infants caused by exposure of the skin to feces and urine.

Diastolic heart failure a condition in which heart contractions are normal but the ventricle does not relax completely; therefore, less blood enters the heart.

Diffuse brain injury (diffuse axonal injury) injury to neuronal axons in many areas of the brain caused by stretching and shearing forces received during brain injury.

DiGeorge syndrome see Immune deficiency.

Dilated cardiomyopathy (congestive cardiomyopathy) a condition in which all four chambers of the heart are enlarged and weakened, resulting in progressive congestive heart failure and the need for heart transplantation.

Discoid (cutaneous) lupus erythematosus (DLE) see Lupus erythematosus.

Disorders of desire (hypoactive sexual desire, decreased libido) the most common sexual dysfunction in women; prevalence increases with age and may be a biologic manifestation of depression, alcohol or other substance abuse, prolactin-secreting pituitary tumors, or testosterone deficiency.

Distal intestinal obstruction syndrome (DIOS) a syndrome seen in cystic fibrosis secondary to impaction with feces and inspissated mucus.

Diverticulitis inflammation of the herniations or saclike outpouchings of mucosa through the muscle layers of the colon wall.

Diverticulosis presence of multiple bulging sacs pushing outward from the wall of the large intestine that may become infected and rupture, causing abdominal pain, tenderness, and fever.

Down syndrome trisomy or translocation of chromosome 21, resulting in mental retardation; distinctive facial appearance with a low nasal bridge, epicanthal folds, protruding tongue, and flat, low-set ears; poor muscle tone (hypotonia); and short stature. Congenital heart defects, reduced ability to resist respiratory tract infections, and increased risk for leukemia are common.

Drug-induced hemolytic anemia see Anemia.

Duchenne muscular dystrophy an X-linked genetic disorder in which fat and fibrous tissue infiltrate and weaken muscle tissues such as in the legs and pelvis, lungs, and heart; usually results in death before adulthood.

Dumping syndrome rapid emptying of hypertonic chyme from a surgically created residual stomach causing nausea, vomiting, bleeding, and diarrhea about 20 minutes after a meal.

Duodenal ulcer most common type of peptic ulcers; usually associated with altered mucosal defenses, rapid gastric emptying, elevated serum gastrin levels, or acid production stimulated by smoking.

Dysfunctional uterine bleeding (DUB) heavy or irregular bleeding in the absence of organic disease, such as submucous fibroids, endometrial polyps, blood dyscrasias, pregnancy, infection, or systemic disease.

Dyskinetic cerebral palsy extreme difficulty in fine motor coordination and purposeful movements resulting from injury to the basal ganglia or thalamus.

Dysphoric mood mood of general dissatisfaction, restlessness, depression, and anxiety; a feeling of unpleasantness or discomfort.

Dysplasia (atypical hyperplasia) abnormal changes in the size, shape, and organization of mature cells; considered a form of atypical hyperplasia.

Dyssynergia development of lesions in the upper motor neurons of the brain and spinal cord; results in loss of coordinated neuromuscular contraction and overactive or hyperreflexive bladder function.

Eczema most common inflammatory disorder of the skin; generally characterized by pruritus, lesions with indistinct borders, and epidermal changes.

Eisenmenger syndrome a progressively developing condition in which a congenital heart defect such as ventricular septal defect is left untreated and causes a reversed right-to-left shunt secondary to increased pressures on the right side of the heart because of pulmonary hypertension.

Embryonic tumor a tumor originating in the gestational period that contains predominantly immature blast cells that cannot differentiate into mature functional cells.

Emphysema pulmonary inflammation resulting in increased work of breathing or physiologic dead space and abnormal permanent enlargement of gas-exchange airways (acini) accompanied by destruction of alveolar walls without obvious fibrosis.

Centriacinar emphysema diminished pulmonary function resulting from septal destruction in the respiratory bronchioles and alveolar ducts, usually in the upper lobes of the lung.

Panacinar emphysema involves destruction of the entire acinus, with damage more randomly distributed and involving the lower lobes of the lung. It tends to occur in older adults and in those with α_1-antitrypsin deficiency.

Empyema (infected pleural effusion) a condition in which purulent fluid is persistently discharged into the pleural space as a result of complications of bacterial infections.

Encephalitis inflammation of the brain usually caused by a virus.

Endometriosis a condition that is common in women of reproductive age in which the tissue lining the uterus is found outside of the uterus, resulting in pain and infertility.

End-stage kidney disease (ESKD) significant loss of renal function; usually less than 10% of renal function remains.

Eosinophilic esophagitis rare, idiopathic inflammatory disease of the esophagus characterized by infiltration of eosinophils associated with atopic disease, including asthma and food allergies.

Ependymoma intracranial tumor that is most commonly found in children and typically arises from the inner lining of the fourth ventricle and the spinal canal.

Epididymitis a painful condition in which the epididymis becomes inflamed, usually as a result of a secondary bacterial infection that is triggered by a variety of underlying conditions such as urinary tract or sexually transmitted infections.

Epilepsy a group of chronic neurologic disorders with paroxysmal brain dysfunction from excessive neuronal discharge; symptoms vary widely from complex behavioral abnormalities to focal convulsions, to momentary spells of impaired consciousness.

Epispadias a birth defect in which the urethra opens on the upper penile surface.

Erysipelas a highly contagious bacterial infection that produces shiny, red swollen areas and fever and can lead to blood poisoning and pneumonia.

Erythema multiforme a skin disease that is caused by allergies, seasonal changes, or drug sensitivities, resulting in the formation of red macules, papules, or subdermal vesicles on the skin and mucous membranes.

Erythema toxicum neonatorum a temporary eruption of redness of the skin, small papules, and occasionally pustules in newborns that is associated with contact dermatitis or hypersensitivity to milk or other allergens.

Erythrodermic (exfoliative) psoriasis see Psoriasis.

Erythromyalgia chronic disorder characterized by warmth, pain, and redness, occurring primarily in the feet and lower legs.

Essential (primary) thrombocythemia (ET) excessive production of platelets (platelet count greater than 400,000/mm^3 of blood); may be primary or secondary (reactive) and is usually asymptomatic until the count exceeds 1 million/mm^3 of blood when intravascular clot formation (thrombosis), hemorrhage, or other abnormalities can occur.

Ewing sarcoma a malignant neoplasm of bone, primarily those of the extremities, including the shoulder girdle, with a predilection for the metaphysis; histologically presents as conspicuous foci of necrosis in association with irregular masses of small, regular, rounded, or ovoid cells.

Exstrophy of the bladder a congenital defect in which the lower abdominal wall is malformed and ruptures.

Extrapyramidal/nonspecific cerebral palsy any of a group of clinical disorders considered to be due to malfunction in the extrapyramidal system and marked by abnormal involuntary movements; included are parkinsonism, athetosis, and chorea.

Facioscapulohumeral muscular dystrophy (FSHD) an autosomal dominant genetic disorder that begins in childhood and causes muscle wasting and weakness, primarily in the face, shoulder, and arms.

Factor H deficiency see Immune deficiency.

Factor I deficiency see Immune deficiency.

Fanconi anemia see Anemia.

Fetal alcohol syndrome (FAS) a syndrome of altered prenatal growth and morphogenesis that occurs in infants born to women who were chronically alcoholic during pregnancy; it includes maxillary hypoplasia, prominence of the forehead and mandible, short palpebral fissures, microphthalmia, epicanthal folds, severe growth retardation, mental retardation, and microcephaly.

Fibromyalgia muscles, tendons, and joints are painful, stiff, and tender; often accompanied by restless sleep, fatigue, anxiety, depression, and disturbances in bowel function.

Fibrosarcoma a malignant tumor of fibrous connective tissue that usually is derived from immature proliferating fibroblasts.

Fibrous dysplasia (FD) a genetic disorder in which tumor-like growths or lesions form in one or more bones and replace the medullary bone with fibrous tissue, resulting in expansion and weakening of the bone.

Florid hyperplasia rapid and unexpected cell growth in the lining of the breast ducts.

Focal segmental glomerulosclerosis (FSGS) a condition in which glomerular capillaries with thickened basement membranes and increased mesangial matrix collapse in segments. Usually presents as nephrotic syndrome.

Frontotemporal dementia (FTD) (Pick disease) progressive circumscribed cerebral atrophy; a rare type of cerebrodegenerative disorder manifested primarily as dementia, in which there is striking atrophy of portions of the frontal and temporal lobes.

FSH deficiency a condition characterized by decreased or absent production of follicle-stimulating hormone (FSH), resulting in a decline in spermatogenesis/oogenesis and associated infertility.

Furuncles staphylococcal infection produces painful pus-filled inflamed hair follicles and involves surrounding skin and subcutaneous tissue.

Fusiform aneurysm (giant aneurysm) large aneurysm that stretches to affect the entire circumference of the arterial wall.

Galactorrhea (inappropriate lactation) a condition in which milk-like fluid is secreted from the breast because of hormonal alterations that are not associated with childbirth or nursing.

Ganglioneuroblastoma an embryonal aggressive tumor of intermediate cellular differentiation that originates outside the CNS in the developing sympathetic nervous system.

Ganglioneuroma a benign neoplasm composed of mature ganglionic neurons scattered within a stroma of neurofibrils and collagenous fibers.

Gangliosidosis any disease characterized by abnormal accumulation of specific gangliosides within the nervous system (e.g., Tay-Sachs disease).

Gastroesophageal reflux disease (GERD) the reflux of acid and pepsin from the stomach to the esophagus that causes esophagitis.

General adaptation syndrome (GAS) the sum of all nonspecific reactions of the body to prolonged systemic stress, comprising alarm, resistance, and exhaustion.

Generalized anxiety disorder (GAD) an anxiety disorder characterized by an excessively anxious mood lasting at least 1 month that interferes with daily functioning and may be accompanied by jitteriness, sweating, feelings of catastrophe concerning one's family or self, and irritability.

Generalized neuropathy a functional disturbance or pathologic change in the cell body of one type of peripheral neuron.

Genital herpes a sexually transmitted viral infection that is caused primarily by herpes simplex virus type 2 and is characterized by painful lesions in the genital and anal regions.

Gestational diabetes mellitus (GDM) see Diabetes.

GH deficiency a condition characterized by decreased or absent production of growth hormone (GH), resulting in a decline in insulin-like growth factor 1 and dwarfism if the deficiency is prepubertal.

Glaucoma a disease of the eye characterized by increased intraocular pressure, excavation, and atrophy of the optic nerve; produces defects in the field of vision and eventual blindness.

Glomerulonephritis inflammation of the renal glomeruli that may not produce symptoms or may present with hematuria and proteinuria.

Acute glomerulonephritis an inflammatory disease of both kidneys predominantly affecting children from ages 2 to 12.

Acute poststreptococcal glomerulonephritis (PSGN) kidney disease secondary to infection with *Streptococci* in which bacterial antigens complex with antibodies in the blood, deposit in the kidneys, and initiate an immune complex–mediated hypersensitivity reaction.

Chronic glomerulonephritis a slowly progressive glomerulonephritis most often associated with other systemic disease, including diabetes, malaria, hepatitis, or systemic lupus erythematosus, that generally leads to irreversible renal failure.

Membranoproliferative glomerulonephritis (MPGN) a chronic, slowly progressive glomerulonephritis in which the glomeruli are enlarged as a result of proliferation of mesangial cells and irregular thickening of the capillary walls, which narrows the capillary lumina.

Membranous glomerulonephritis a slowly progressive disease of unknown origin or that occurs secondary to autoimmune conditions, infections, specific drugs, or malignant tumors that is caused by immune complexes formed from the binding of antibodies to antigens of the glomerular basement membrane (GBM) or antigens transported from the systemic circulation and implanted in the GBM.

Membranous nephropathy (membranous glomerulonephritis) membranous nephropathy is caused by subepithelial deposition of antibodies (IgG4 subclass) to antigens (M-type phospholipase A_2 receptor [PLA2R] protein) located on glomerular podocytes and activation of complement-mediated inflammation with injury and release of inflammatory mediators by mesangial and epithelial cells, resulting in increased membrane permeability, thickening of the glomerular membrane, and ultimately glomerular sclerosis.

Mesangial proliferative glomerulonephritis deposition of immune complexes in the mesangium with mesangial cell proliferation and expansion reducing blood flow and altering filtration membrane permeability with development of hematuria, proteinuria, hypertension, and uremia (nephritic syndrome); associated with IgA nephropathy, lupus nephritis, or early diabetic nephropathy.

Rapidly progressive (crescentic) glomerulonephritis (RPGN) (subacute or extracapillary glomerulonephritis) develops over days to weeks, primarily affects adults in their fifties and sixties, and may be idiopathic or associated with a proliferative glomerular disease (diffuse proliferation of extracapillary cells), such as lupus or poststreptococcal glomerulonephritis.

Glucose-6-phosphate dehydrogenase (G6PD) deficiency see Anemia.

Gluten-sensitive enteropathy (celiac sprue) a condition characterized by mucosal inflammation and villous atrophy in the gastrointestinal tract formed in response to a genetic predisposition for an immune response to gluten and similar proteins.

Gonorrhea a sexually transmitted disease caused by the bacteria gonococci that invade the mucous membranes of the genitals and urinary tract and in women the cervix, fallopian tubes, and ovaries, causing chronic pelvic pain or infertility.

Gout a disorder of uric acid metabolism that causes painful inflammation of the joints, commonly the big toe, and arthritic attacks resulting from elevated levels of uric acid in the blood and the deposition of negatively birefringent urate crystals around the joints.

Gouty arthritis inflammation of the joints in gout.

Graft rejection immunologic rejection of transplanted tissue or organs based on antigen differences between the donor and recipient.

Acute graft rejection cell-mediated immune rejection that occurs within days to months after transplantation; immune response is usually against unmatched HLA antigens and develops after transplantation.

Chronic graft rejection slow, progressive organ failure after a period of months or years of normal function by a developing weak cell-mediated immune response against minor histocompatibility antigens on the endothelial cells lining the blood vessels of the grafted tissue.

Hyperacute graft rejection immediate rejection of a graft because of pre-existing antibodies against antigens expressed on the grafted tissue or organ.

Graft-versus-host disease (GVHD) condition in which mature T cells in a transplanted graft (e.g., transfused blood) are capable of a destructive cell-mediated reaction against unmatched histocompatibility antigens on the tissues in the graft recipient.

Granuloma inguinale a bacterial-induced disease, also called donovanosis, that is thought to be transmitted primarily by anal rather than vaginal intercourse and causes painless genital ulcers like syphilis but progresses to destroy the internal and external genital tissue.

Graves disease autoimmune hyperthyroidism caused by antibodies that continuously activate TSH receptors, resulting in uncontrolled production of thyroxine and characterized by an enlarged thyroid gland, protrusion of eyeballs, a rapid heartbeat, and nervous excitability.

Guillain-Barré syndrome (GBS) (Landry-Guillain-Barré syndrome, idiopathic polyneuritis, acute inflammatory polyradiculopathy, acute autoimmune neuropathy) an acute, immune-mediated disorder of peripheral nerves, spinal roots, and cranial nerves that commonly presents as a rapidly progressive, areflexive, relatively symmetrical ascending weakness of the limb, truncal, respiratory, pharyngeal, and facial musculature, with variable sensory and autonomic dysfunction; typically reaches its peak activity within 2 to 3 weeks, followed by a plateau period of similar duration, and gradual but complete recovery in most cases; often preceded by a respiratory tract or gastrointestinal tract infection and is associated with albuminocytologic dissociation of the cerebrospinal fluid.

Guttate psoriasis see Psoriasis.

Gynecomastia abnormal breast tissue development on adolescent boys or men as a result of an imbalance in hormones.

Heat exhaustion occurs when sufficient salt and water loss results in hemoconcentration with hypotension occurring secondary to fluid loss (hypovolemia), and the individual feels weak, is nauseated, and can suddenly collapse.

Heat stroke a life-threatening condition associated with high environmental temperatures and humidity causing core body temperature to rise as a result of thermoregulatory failure.

Hematemesis accumulation of blood in the gastrointestinal tract causing irritation, increased peristalsis, and vomiting.

Hematochezia rapid bleeding from the upper GI tract producing bright red stools.

Hemochromatosis disorder of iron metabolism characterized by excessive absorption of ingested iron, saturation of iron-binding protein, and deposition of hemosiderin in tissue, particularly in the liver, pancreas, and skin; cirrhosis of the liver, diabetes (bronze diabetes), bronze pigmentation of the skin, and eventually heart failure may occur; also can result from administration of large amounts of iron orally, by injection, or in forms of blood transfusion therapy.

Hemoglobin H disease see Anemia.

Hemolytic anemia see Anemia.

Hemolytic disease of the newborn (HDN) (erythroblastosis fetalis) see Anemia.

Hemolytic jaundice (prehepatic jaundice, nonobstructive jaundice) jaundice resulting from excessive hemolysis of red blood cells.

Hemolytic-uremic syndrome (HUS) a condition in which platelets aggregate within the kidney's small blood vessels, resulting in reduced blood flow to the kidney and subsequent kidney failure and destruction of the red blood cells; occurs usually after exposure to Shiga-like toxin from a strain of *E. coli*.

Hemophilia A (classic hemophilia) a genetic disorder in which a mutation in factor VIII causes prolonged clotting time, decreased formation of thromboplastin, and diminished conversion of prothrombin.

Hemophilia B (Christmas disease) a genetic disorder similar to hemophilia A in terms of symptoms but with a mutation in the factor IX gene.

Hemophilia C (factor XI deficiency) a genetic disorder characterized by a deficiency in factor XI, resulting in a mild form of hemophilia.

Hemorrhagic stroke (spontaneous intracranial hemorrhage) stroke usually caused by hypertension that results in bleeding in the brain and typically increases intracranial pressure and may lead to death.

Henoch-Schönlein purpura nephritis inflammation of the blood vessels causing bleeding into the skin, mucous membranes, internal organs, and other tissues; pain and inflammation in the joints; abdominal pain; gastrointestinal bleeding; inflammation of the kidneys; subcutaneous edema; encephalopathy; and inflammation of the testis.

Heparin-induced thrombocytopenia (HIT) see Thrombocytopenia.

Hepatic encephalopathy a condition that is usually caused by liver cirrhosis and portal hypertension in which toxins produced by the gut pass into the systemic circulation and damage brain cells, resulting in impaired cognition, tremor, and a decreased level of consciousness.

Hepatocellular carcinoma (hepatocarcinoma; HCC) primary carcinoma of the liver developing in hepatocytes.

Hepatopulmonary syndrome intrapulmonary vasodilation, intrapulmonary shunting, and hypoxia and portopulmonary hypertension (pulmonary vasoconstriction and vascular remodeling) are common respiratory complications of advanced liver disease and portal hypertension.

Hepatorenal syndrome (HRS) acute renal failure occurs because of a decrease in renal blood flow secondary to liver disease.

Hereditary angioedema an inherited, autosomal dominant disease characterized by episodic appearance of nonpitting edema, most often affecting the limbs, but capable of involving other parts of the body, including mucosal surfaces such as those of the intestine (causing abdominal pain) or respiratory tract (causing asphyxia); associated with deficiency of inhibitor of the first component of complement pathway (C1 esterase inhibitor).

Hereditary hemochromatosis (HH) autosomal recessive chronic liver disease caused by excessive intestinal absorption of elemental iron; characterized by elevated serum iron saturation, transferrin, and ferritin levels; improves with phlebotomy; increased risk of developing cirrhosis, liver cancer, and liver failure.

Hereditary sideroblastic anemia see Anemia.

Hereditary spherocytosis see Anemia.

Hiatal hernia an anatomic abnormality in which the esophageal hiatus is larger than normal, causing part of the stomach to protrude through the diaphragm and up into the esophagus or chest.

High altitude cerebral edema (HACE) an increase in severity of symptoms or signs of neurologic dysfunction, such as ataxia or altered consciousness, related to high altitude.

High altitude pulmonary edema (HAPE) a noncardiogenic pulmonary edema associated with pulmonary hypertension and elevated capillary pressure related to high altitude illness.

Hirsutism abnormal growth and distribution of androgen-sensitive hair growth on the face, body, and pubic area in a male pattern that occurs in women.

Hodgkin lymphoma (HL) see Lymphoma.

Hormonal hyperplasia growth of cellular layers chiefly in estrogen-dependent organs, such as the uterus and breast. After ovulation, for example, estrogen stimulates the endometrium to grow and thicken for reception of the fertilized ovum.

Huntington disease (HD) an autosomal dominant disease causing a progressive increase in involuntary, jerky, dyskinetic movements; mental deterioration; and premature death.

Hyaline membrane disease (HMD) a type of respiratory distress syndrome of the newborn in which there is formation of a hyaline-like membrane lining the terminal respiratory passages; extensive atelectasis is attributed to lack of surfactant.

Hydrocephalus ex vacuo hydrocephalus attributable to loss or atrophy of brain tissue; less commonly associated with raised intracranial pressure and dilation of the cerebral ventricles.

Hydrops fetalis edema formation in the fetal subcutaneous tissue because of an enzyme deficiency or any one of several other disorders.

Hyperosmolar hyperglycemic nonketotic syndrome (HHNKS) a complication seen in diabetes mellitus in which very marked hyperglycemia occurs, causing osmotic shifts in water in brain cells, and resulting in coma. It can be fatal or lead to permanent neurologic damage.

Hypersensitive pneumonitis (extrinsic allergic alveolitis) an allergic, inflammatory disease of the lungs caused by inhalation of organic particles or fumes.

Hypertrophic cardiomyopathy a genetic disorder caused by various mutations that thicken the heart muscle, possibly leading to obstruction of blood flow and heart dysfunction; this is a common cause of sudden death in young athletes.

Hypogammaglobulinemia see Immune deficiency.

Hypoplastic anemia see Anemia.

Hypoplastic left heart syndrome (HLHS) a condition in which the left side of the heart, including the aorta, aortic valve, left ventricle, and mitral valve, is underdeveloped and blood returning from the lungs flows through an opening in the atrial septum and the right ventricle pumps the blood into the pulmonary artery and then into the aorta.

Hypospadias a birth defect in which the urethral opening is abnormally placed, opening anywhere from the tip of the glans penis, to the shaft, or to the junction of the penis and scrotum or perineum in males; usually opens in the vagina in females.

Iatrogenic pneumothorax see Pneumothorax.

Icterus neonatorum (neonatal jaundice) jaundice in newborn infants caused by functional immaturity of the liver; usually subsides within the first few days of life.

Idiopathic pulmonary fibrosis (IPF) an excessive amount of fibrous or connective tissue in the lung.

Idiopathic thrombocytopenic purpura (ITP) (autoimmune or primary thrombocytopenic purpura) see Thrombocytopenia.

IgA nephropathy (Berger disease) the most common form of idiopathic acute glomerulonephritis in developed countries, especially Asia; cause is unknown.

IgA pemphigus the most benign form of pemphigus characterized by tissue-bound and circulating IgA antibodies targeting desmosomal or nondesmosomal cell surface components in the basement membrane of the epidermis.

IgG subclass deficiency see Immune deficiency.

IL-7 receptor deficiency see Immune deficiency.

Immune deficiency a group of disorders in which one or more components of the immune or inflammatory response is impaired, resulting in increased susceptibility to infections. **Primary (congenital) immune deficiencies** result from genetic defects, and secondary immune deficiencies result from nongenetic factors, such as infections and other physiologic or pathophysiologic conditions. Primary immune deficiencies include:

- **B-lymphocyte deficiency** a group of disorders in which B-cell development is defective, resulting in lower levels of circulating immunoglobulins and increased susceptibility to infections in which antibodies are the primary protective mechanism. These include:
  - **Agammaglobulinemia** a condition in which no antibodies are produced.
  - **Autosomal agammaglobulinemia** an autosomal recessive form of agammaglobulinemia resulting from mutations in the B-cell receptor.
  - **Autosomal hyper-IgM syndrome** inability to class-switch resulting from mutations in CD40 on B cells.
  - **Bruton's agammaglobulinemia** a defect in B-cell development results in lower levels of circulating immunoglobulins and increased susceptibility to infections in which antibodies are the primary protective mechanism.
  - **Common variable immune deficiency** the most commonly diagnosed immune deficiency; hypogammaglobulinemia of IgG and other antibody classes; normal numbers of B cells, with or without associated T-cell defects.
  - **Hypogammaglobulinemia** a condition in which immunoglobulin levels are much lower than normal.
  - **IgG subclass deficiency** deficiencies in certain subclasses of antibody.
  - **Selective IgA deficiency** failure to produce IgA, with or without diminished production of other classes of antibody.
  - **X-linked hyper-IgM syndrome** inability to class-switch resulting from a defect in activation-induced cytidine deaminase (AICD).
- **Combined T- and B-lymphocyte deficiency** a group of immune deficiencies in which both T and B lymphocytes are defective. The most severe of these deficiencies is called **severe combined immune deficiency (SCID).** These include:
  - **Adenosine deaminase (ADA) deficiency** a form of SCID caused by an autosomal recessive mutation in the enzyme ADA, leading to death of rapidly dividing cells, particularly lymphocytes.
  - **Ataxia-telangiectasia (AT)** an autosomal recessive disorder resulting from a large variety of sporadic mutations in the *ATM* gene; often associated with ataxia (unsteady gait), telangiectasia (dilation of capillaries), and variable effects on both B and T cells.
  - **Bare lymphocyte syndrome** forms of SCID characterized by an inability of lymphocytes and macrophages to present antigen because of defects in class I (**MHC class I deficiency**) or class II (**MHC class II deficiency**) MHC antigen expression.
  - **IL-7 receptor deficiency** a form of SCID resulting from mutations in the IL-7 receptor, which is necessary for maturation of T cells.
  - **JAK3 deficiency** a form of SCID resulting from mutations in JAK3, which is an enzyme (a tyrosine kinase) associated with their receptor for IL-2.
  - **Purine nucleoside phosphorylase (PNP) deficiency** a form of SCID resulting from a mutation in the enzyme PNP.
  - **RAG-1 and RAG-2 deficiencies** autosomal recessive mutations in RAG-1 or RAG-2 enzyme that are necessary for genetic rearrangement of antibody and T-cell receptor variable regions.
  - **Reticular dysgenesis** the most severe form of SCID in which a common stem cell for all white blood cells is absent; therefore T cells, B cells, and phagocytic cells never develop.
  - **Wiskott-Aldrich syndrome (WAS)** an X-linked recessive trait resulting in chronic eczema with chronic suppurative otitis media, anemia, thrombocytopenic purpura, poor antibody response to polysaccharide antigens, and dysfunctions of cell-mediated immunity.
  - **X-linked SCID** a form of SCID with arrested maturation of T and NK cells and the production of immature B cells as a result of a defect in the IL-2 receptor gamma (γ)-chain (IL-2Rγ), which is shared with many other cytokine receptors.
- **Complement deficiency** a group of conditions in which specific proteins of the complement system are absent or suboptimal, resulting in diminished complement activity. These include:
  - **C1 deficiency** a deficiency of the first component of the classical pathway.
  - **C2 deficiency** a deficiency with an increased risk for recurrent respiratory tract infections with encapsulated bacteria and a systemic lupus erythematosus–like syndrome that may be complicated by kidney disease (glomerulonephritis).
  - **C3 deficiency** the most severe complement defect; an associated deficit of C3b, which is a major opsonin, results in a risk for recurrent life-threatening infections with encapsulated bacteria.
  - **C3 receptor deficiency** deficiencies in the complement receptor for C3 result in recurrent bacterial infections, particularly of the skin.
  - **C4 deficiency** results in an increased risk for recurrent respiratory tract infections with encapsulated bacteria and a systemic lupus erythematosus–like syndrome that may be complicated by kidney disease (glomerulonephritis).
  - **C9 deficiency** the most common terminal pathway defect and generally asymptomatic.
  - **Factor H deficiency** a deficiency of complement factor H resulting in increased destruction of C3 and a secondary C3 deficiency.
  - **Factor I deficiency** a deficiency of complement factor I resulting in increased destruction of C3 and a secondary C3 deficiency.
  - **Mannose-binding lectin (MBL) deficiency** a defect of the lectin pathway of complement activation resulting in an increased risk of infection with microorganisms that have polysaccharide capsules rich in mannose.
  - **Properdin deficiency** an X-linked defect in the alternative pathway of complement activation resulting in recurrent meningococcal infections.
- **Phagocytic deficiency** a group of conditions in which phagocytosis is diminished, resulting in increased bacterial infections. These include:
  - **Chediak-Higashi syndrome** a lethal, progressive, autosomal recessive, systemic disorder associated with oculocutaneous albinism, massive leukocyte inclusions (giant lysosomes), histiocytic infiltration of multiple body organs, development of pancytopenia, hepatosplenomegaly, and recurrent or persistent bacterial infections.
  - **Chronic granulomatous disease (CGD)** both X-linked and autosomal forms of mutations of the NADPH oxidase complex, resulting in diminished production of hydrogen peroxide and other oxygen products necessary for the bactericidal activity of myeloperoxidase.
  - **Cyclic neutropenia** an autosomal dominant mutation in the *ELA2* gene resulting in periods of neutropenia lasting a few days to weeks.

Severe congenital neutropenia inadequate numbers of neutrophils resulting in a variety of recurrent and severe bacterial infections beginning early in life.

Secondary immune deficiencies

Acquired immunodeficiency syndrome (AIDS) an epidemic, transmissible retroviral disease caused by infection with the human immunodeficiency virus (HIV), resulting in destruction of T-helper cells, suppression of both antibody and cellular immune responses, and development of life-threatening infections with opportunistic organisms.

Agranulocytosis complete absence of granulocytes in the blood is usually secondary to arrested hematopoiesis in the bone marrow or massive cell destruction in the circulation.

Qualitative leukocyte disorder a group of conditions with various disruptions of leukocyte function.

Quantitative leukocyte disorder a group of conditions, frequently associated with infections and leukemias, with decreased production of leukocytes in the bone marrow or accelerated destruction of leukocytes in the circulation.

Transient hypogammaglobulinemia of infancy a period at 6 to 8 months when the newborn may not have produced adequate amounts of antibody to replace maternal antibody; in some infants this may lead to a period of increased susceptibility to infections.

T-lymphocyte deficiency a group of disorders in which T-cell development is defective, resulting in lower levels of cellular immunity. Diminished T helper cell function may also decrease the production of antibody. These include:

Chronic mucocutaneous candidiasis a primary defect of T-lymphocyte response to a specific infectious agent, the yeast *C. albicans.*

DiGeorge syndrome a genetic disorder caused by deletion of a piece of chromosome 22 that results in cardiac defects, abnormal facies, thymic aplasia, cleft palate, and hypocalcemia.

Immune thrombocytopenic purpura (ITP) see Thrombocytopenia.

Imperforate anus a congenital defect in which the anal opening is absent because of the presence of a membranous septum or complete absence of the anal canal.

Impetigo a contagious bacterial infection that produces superficial red blisters that rupture and produce thick yellow crusts that commonly occur on the face but can spread to other regions of the body easily.

Infectious mononucleosis (IM) a disease caused by the Epstein-Barr virus or the cytomegalovirus that is transmitted by exchanging saliva or blood or by coughing and sneezing and acts by infecting the B cells and atypical T cells, resulting in fever, sore throat, and fatigue.

Infertility the inability to conceive after 1 year of unprotected intercourse with the same, opposite-sex partner.

Intracerebral hematoma (intraparenchymal hemorrhage) blood accumulation that partially clots inside the brain, usually in the frontal and temporal lobes.

Intraductal papilloma array of papillary cells that grow from the wall of a cyst into the lumen of the duct; growth occurs within a dilated duct often near or beside the nipple causing benign nipple discharge.

Intrarenal (intrinsic) acute kidney injury (AKI) a sudden decline in kidney function with a decrease in glomerular filtration and an accumulation of nitrogenous waste products in the blood (elevation in plasma creatinine and blood urea nitrogen levels); may result from ischemic acute tubular necrosis (ATN), nephrotoxic ATN (i.e., exposure to radiocontrast media or antibiotics), acute glomerulonephritis, vascular disease (malignant hypertension, disseminated intravascular coagulation, and renal vasculitis), allograft rejection, or interstitial disease (drug allergy, infection, tumor growth).

Invasive breast carcinoma a malignant invasive epithelial lesion derived from the terminal duct lobular area.

Invasive carcinoma of the cervix invasion of cervical carcinoma into adjacent tissues, such as ureters and structures of the lateral pelvic wall, the vaginal stroma and epithelium, and the lower uterine segment and myometrium.

Inverse psoriasis see Psoriasis.

Iron deficiency anemia (IDA) see Anemia.

Irritable bowel syndrome (IBS) a chronic noninflammatory disease with a psychophysiologic basis; characterized by abdominal pain, diarrhea or constipation, or both; no detectable pathologic change.

Irritative syndrome (radicular syndrome) a combination of changes usually seen with compromise of a spinal root within the intraspinal canal; these include neck or back pain and, in the affected root distribution, dermatomal pain, paresthesias, or both; decreased deep tendon reflexes; and occasionally myotomal weakness.

Isolated systolic hypertension loss of elasticity of the arteries resulting in an increase in cardiac output or stroke volume, a systolic blood pressure consistently greater than 160 mmHg, and a diastolic pressure less than 90 mmHg.

JAK3 deficiency see Immune deficiency.

Jaundice (icterus) yellowish brown staining of the skin and the conjunctivae caused by high bilirubin levels in blood secondary to excessive erythrocyte breakdown, obstruction in or around the liver, or liver disease.

Juvenile idiopathic arthritis (JIA) chronic pauciarticular arthritis and destruction of joints beginning in childhood and often going into remission at puberty.

Juvenile myoclonic epilepsy a type of epilepsy that occurs in adolescents and young adults, usually on awakening, and is characterized by jerks of the neck, shoulders, and arms and by clonic-tonic seizures.

Kaposi sarcoma (KS) a rare cancer of connective tissue caused by herpesvirus 8 (HHV8) in which many bluish red nodules appear on the skin, especially skin of the lower extremities; occurs in a particularly virulent form in individuals with AIDS.

Kawasaki disease a vascular disease characterized by an inflamed heart and vessels; a coronary artery aneurysm, thickening, and stenosis; a fever that lasts at least 5 days; and at least four of the following: inflammation with reddening of the whites of the eyes; red, swollen hands or feet or peeling skin; rash; swollen lymph glands in the neck; inflamed lips or throat; or red "strawberry" tongue.

Klinefelter syndrome smallness of testes with fibrosis and hyalinization of seminiferous tubules, variable degrees of masculinization, azoospermia, infertility, and increased levels of urinary gonadotropins; associated typically with an XXY chromosome complement although variants include XXYY, XXXY, and XXXXY.

Kwashiorkor a condition in which children do not receive enough protein in their diet, resulting in a swollen and severely bloated abdomen secondary to decreased albumin levels in the blood, skin changes resulting in a reddish discoloration of the hair and skin in dark-skinned children, severe diarrhea, fatty liver, muscle atrophy, and restricted development.

Lactase deficiency a condition in which insufficient lactase is present in the small intestine to digest lactose, resulting in lactose intolerance characterized by diarrhea, bloating, and gas in response to exposure to lactose.

Lactose intolerance a condition caused by lactase deficiency in which lactose is not metabolized, making it impossible for the small intestine to absorb it and causing excessive gas production and diarrhea when exposed to lactose-containing foods.

Lambert-Eaton myasthenic syndrome a generalized disorder of neuromuscular transmission caused by a defect in the release of acetylcholine from the presynaptic nerve terminals; often associated with small cell carcinoma of the lung, particularly in elderly men with a long history of cigarette smoking; weakness tends to affect solely axial muscles, girdle muscles, and less often the limb muscles; autonomic disturbances, dry mouth, and impotence are common; the deep tendon reflexes are unelicitable; caused by loss of voltage-sensitive calcium channels located on the presynaptic motor nerve terminal.

Laryngomalacia a congenital anomaly caused by a developmental delay in the laryngeal cartilage and supporting structures of the larynx that causes the cartilage to be floppy and fold in on itself during inspiration, producing high-pitched, coarse, and low-pitched sounds.

Left heart failure (congestive heart failure) inability of the left ventricle to maintain its circulatory load, with a corresponding rise in pressure in the pulmonary circulation usually with pulmonary congestion and ultimately pulmonary edema.

Legg-Calvé-Perthes disease blood supply to the head of the femur near the hip joint is interrupted, resulting in osteonecrosis of the corresponding epiphysis.

Lennox-Gastaut syndrome a generalized myoclonic epilepsy that occurs in children between 1 and 5 years of age as a result of various cerebral afflictions such as perinatal hypoxia, hemorrhage, encephalitis, and metabolic disorders of the brain; it is characterized by mental retardation, personality disorders, and generalized tonic seizures.

Leukemia an acute or chronic malignant disease of the bone marrow and blood-forming organs; excessive proliferation of white blood cells occurs and is usually accompanied by dysfunctional blood cells, anemia, impaired blood clotting, and enlargement of the lymph nodes, liver, and spleen.

Acute leukemia characterized by undifferentiated or immature cells, usually a blast cell, and the onset of disease is abrupt and rapid with a short survival time.

Acute lymphoblastic/lymphocytic leukemia (ALL) excessive production and continuous multiplication of malignant and immature white blood cells (lymphoblasts) in the bone marrow that progresses rapidly if left untreated.

Acute myelogenous leukemia (AML) excessive number of immature myeloid cells (myeloblasts) in the blood and bone marrow crowding out the marrow and decreasing the function of other cells.

Chronic leukemia the predominant cell is more differentiated but does not function normally, with a relatively slow progression of the malignancy.

Chronic lymphocytic leukemia (CLL) malignant transformation and progressive accumulation in the marrow of monoclonal B lymphocytes; rarely are CLL malignancies of T-cell origin.

Chronic myelogenous leukemia (CML) production of heterogeneous myeloid cells in the bone marrow, the majority of which express the Philadelphia chromosome; CML is considered a myeloproliferative disorder.

LH deficiency a condition characterized by decreased or absent production of luteinizing hormone (LH), resulting in a decline in sex steroid production in testes/ovaries and associated infertility.

Lichen planus a recurrent rash of small, flat-topped bumps and rough scaly patches appearing on the skin, in the lining of the mouth, and in the vagina in response to inflammation or an allergy to a specific medication.

Localized scleroderma (morphea) rare and idiopathic sclerosis of the skin, usually with childhood onset.

Locked-in syndrome quadriplegia and mutism with intact consciousness and preservation of some eye movements; usually results from a vascular lesion of the anterior pons.

Lupus erythematosus any of a group of autoimmune connective tissue disorders that commonly produce red scaly lesions and are accompanied by fever, malaise, myalgias, fatigue, and weight loss.

Discoid (cutaneous) lupus erythematosus (DLE) lupus erythematosus limited to the skin; can progress to systemic lupus erythematosus (SLE).

Systematic lupus erythematosus (SLE) a chronic, multisystem, inflammatory disease; is one of the most common, complex, and serious of the autoimmune disorders.

Lyme disease (borreliosis) tick-borne spirochete bacterial infection that is characterized by a rash in the area of the bite, headache, neck stiffness, chills, fever, myalgia, arthralgia, malaise, fatigue, and possible development of arthritis in large joints.

Lymphoblastic lymphoma (LL) see Lymphoma.

Lymphogranuloma venereum (LGV) a sexually transmitted bacterial infection that enters the body through breaks in the skin or across the epithelial cell layer of mucous membranes and primarily targets the lymphatics and lymph nodes.

Lymphoma cancer arising from cell proliferation in lymphoid tissue.

B-cell neoplasm a group of lymphomas including myelomas that originate from B cells at various stages of differentiation; previously part of non-Hodgkin lymphoma.

Burkitt lymphoma an aggressive malignancy of the B lymphocytes characterized by a large osteolytic lesion in the facial bones and associated with Epstein-Barr virus infection.

Hodgkin lymphoma (HL) a cancer of lymphoid tissue in which the lymph nodes, spleen, and liver become enlarged with the presence of Reed-Sternberg cells and is often accompanied by anemia, fever, and eventually death if not treated at an early stage; also referred to as Hodgkin disease.

Lymphoblastic lymphoma (LL) a progressive neoplasm arising in the thymus; most are of T-cell origin; a variant of acute lymphoblastic leukemia; common cause of NHL in children.

Lymphoplasmocytic lymphoma also called Waldenström macroglobulinemia.

Mucosa-associated lymphoid tissue (MALT) lymphoma a low-grade B-cell lymphoma linked to infection with *H. pylori.*

Mycosis fungoides most common cutaneous T-cell lymphoma; present as focal or widespread erythematous patches or plaques, follicular papules, comedone-like lesions, and tumors.

NK-cell neoplasm a group of lymphomas that originate from NK cells at various stages of differentiation; previously part of non-Hodgkin lymphoma.

Non-Hodgkin lymphoma (NHL) a group of malignancies of lymphoid tissue classified as B-cell, T-cell, and NK-cell lymphomas that mimic Hodgkin lymphoma but do not produce the cells characteristic of Hodgkin lymphoma; have been reclassified as B-cell, T-cell, or NK-cell neoplasms.

T-cell neoplasm a variety of lymphomas that originate from T cells at various stages of differentiation; previously part of non-Hodgkin lymphoma.

Waldenström macroglobulinemia a rare type of slow-growing plasma cell tumor that secretes a monoclonal IgM molecule; also called lymphoplasmocytic lymphoma.

Lymphoplasmocytic lymphoma see Lymphoma.

Lysosomal storage diseases a group of more than 30 disorders that result from impaired lysosomal function, leading to mucopolysaccharidoses, lipid storage disorders, mucolipidoses, leukodystrophies, and glycoprotein storage disorders.

Macrocytic anemia (megaloblastic anemia) see Anemia.

Major (unipolar) depression severely depressed mood and loss of pleasure that may begin suddenly or slowly; it persists for at least 2 weeks and may recur throughout life.

Malignant hyperthermia an inherited life-threatening disorder that causes muscle rigidity, a hypermetabolic state, tachycardia, and increased body temperature in response to administration of general anesthesics.

Malnutrition lack of nourishment from inadequate amounts of calories, protein, vitamins, or minerals; caused by improper diet, alterations in digestion or absorption, chronic disease, or a combination of these factors.

Mannose-binding lectin (MBL) deficiency see Immune deficiency.

Marasmus a childhood disorder characterized by protein and energy malnutrition, resulting in dry skin, loss of adipose tissue from normal areas of fat deposits such as buttocks and thighs, and behavior that is fretful and irritable.

Maturity-onset diabetes of youth (MODY) see Diabetes mellitis.

McArdle disease a metabolic disorder involving an enzyme defect that causes deficiency of muscle phosphorylase, which helps break down glycogen, and consequently this disorder causes an energy deficit in the muscles, resulting in muscle pain and cramping.

Meconium ileus obstruction with thickened meconium in the intestine of a newborn child as a result of a lack of trypsin and associated with cystic fibrosis of the pancreas.

Medulloblastoma a malignant cerebellar tumor near the fourth ventricle that is most often found in children and consists of neoplastic cells that resemble the undifferentiated cells of the neural tube.

Membranoproliferative glomerulonephritis (MPGN) see Glomerulonephritis.

Membranous glomerulonephritis see Glomerulonephritis.

Membranous nephropathy (membranous glomerulonephritis) see Glomerulonephritis.

Ménière disease (endolymphatic hydrops) dilation of the membranous labyrinth of the inner ear that is thought to be due to impaired absorption of endolymph in the endolymphatic sac; the pathologic finding in Ménière disease.

Ménière syndrome an affliction characterized clinically by vertigo, nausea, vomiting, tinnitus, and fluctuating and progressive sensory hearing loss associated with endolymphatic hydrops.

Meningioma a slow-growing mass of the meninges that is usually benign but increases intracranial pressure

Meningocele neural tube defect in the skull or spinal column that forms a cyst filled with cerebrospinal fluid through which the meninges of the brain protrude.

Mesangial proliferative glomerulonephritis see Glomerulonephritis.

Mesenteric venous thrombosis a condition in which a blood clot obstructs one of the mesenteric veins and compromises the intestinal blood supply; can result in intestinal gangrene and tissue death.

Mesothelioma a type of cancer that is usually associated with previous exposure to asbestos, which affects the pleura, the lining of the abdominal cavity, the pericardium, and most internal organ coverings.

Metabolic syndrome a condition of unknown cause that presents with symptoms of insulin resistance, obesity, hypertension, dyslipidemia, and systemic inflammation.

Metatarsus adductus a foot deformity in which the front half of the foot bends inward, possibly because of the infant's position in the uterus.

MHC class I deficiency see Immune deficiency.

MHC class II deficiency see Immune deficiency.

Microcephaly defect in which failure of normal brain growth causes delayed skull growth and production of a small head.

Microcytic-hypochromic anemia see Anemia.

Microscopic colitis a relatively common cause of diarrhea; occurs primarily in females and older adults.

Migraine headache headache that usually begins in the temporal region unilaterally after vascular changes of cranial arteries and may cause irritability, nausea, vomiting, constipation or diarrhea, and photophobia.

Mild concussion (mild traumatic brain injury) temporary axonal disturbances without the loss of consciousness in response to a violent blow, jarring, shaking, or other closed-head injury.

Miliaria a skin disease caused by partially obstructed sweat glands that results in small and itchy rashes usually located in skinfolds and on areas of the body that may rub against clothing, such as the back, chest, and stomach.

Minimal change nephropathy (MCN) the foot processes of the renal capillary basement membrane are fused and deformed because of a T-cell disorder that reduces the anion component of the basement membrane and allows proteins to leak into the renal tubule.

Minimally conscious state (MCS) a condition in which a severely brain-damaged patient is capable of deliberate behavior distinguishable from unconscious reflexive actions.

Mitral valve prolapse syndrome the mitral valve cannot close properly because of one or both flaps being too large, possibly resulting in mitral valve regurgitation.

Mixed precocious puberty development of some secondary sex characteristics of the opposite sex (virilization of a girl or feminization of a boy); usually evident at birth and rare in older children.

Molluscum contagiosum a viral infection of the skin occurring in young children that affects the body, arms, and legs; it is spread through direct contact, saliva, or shared articles of clothing and is considered a sexually transmitted disease in adults, affecting the genitals, lower abdomen, buttocks, and inner thighs.

Monoclonal gammopathy of undetermined significance (MGUS) production of monoclonal antibodies by noncancerous plasma cells that accumulate in the blood.

Motility diarrhea diarrhea caused by excessive motility decreases transit time, mucosal surface contact, and fluid absorption secondary to resection of the small intestine (short bowel syndrome), surgical bypass of an area of the intestine, fistula formation between loops of intestine, irritable bowel syndrome–diarrhea predominant, diabetic neuropathy, hyperthyroidism, and laxative abuse.

Moyamoya disease an abnormality of the blood vessels that supply the frontal region of the brain in which vessels constrict or become completely occluded, resulting in diminished blood flow. The body attempts to compensate by growing new vessels at the base of the brain, which appear as a puff of smoke on angiography.

Mucoepidermoid carcinoma a tumor of the main or lobar bronchi lumen that may extend into the peribronchial tissue.

Mucolipidosis (ML) accumulations of both carbohydrates and lipids.

Mucopolysaccharidosis carbohydrate excess disorders.

Mucopurulent cervicitis (MPC) inflammation of the cervix with purulent endocervical exudate that may be asymptomatic or cause abnormal vaginal discharge and vaginal bleeding.

Mucosa-associated lymphoid tissue (MALT) lymphoma see Lymphoma.

Multiple myeloma (MM) most common and most aggressive plasma cell tumor; a clonal plasma cell cancer characterized by the slow proliferation of malignant cells as tumor cell masses in the bone marrow that usually results in destruction of the bone; most secrete large amounts of monoclonal proteins that resemble intact immunoglobulins.

Multiple organ dysfunction syndrome (MODS) progressive disease often involving the ultimate failure of two or more organ systems after a severe illness or injury; disease process is initiated and perpetuated by uncontrolled systemic inflammatory and stress responses and is characterized by a hypermetabolic and hyperdynamic state that persists as organ dysfunction develops.

Multiple papilloma (diffuse papillomatosis) a minimum of five papillomas within a localized segment of breast tissue.

Multiple sclerosis (MS) chronic demyelinating disease of the central nervous system that causes inflammation and scarring of myelin sheaths.

Muscular dystrophy a general term for a number of hereditary, progressive degenerative disorders affecting skeletal muscles, and often other organ systems.

Myasthenia gravis neuromuscular disorder caused by an autoimmune response in which antibodies to acetylcholine receptors impair neuromuscular transmission.

Mycosis fungoides see Lymphoma.

Myelodysplastic syndrome (MDS) a group of hematologic conditions characterized by ineffective production of blood cells, resulting in anemia that requires chronic blood transfusion.

Myoadenylate deaminase deficiency (MDD) a genetic disorder in which an enzyme deficiency prevents the conversion of adenosine monophosphate (AMP) to inosine monophosphate, resulting in increased AMP loss and the inability to synthesize adenosine triphosphate for energy.

Myocardial infarction a heart condition of sudden onset in which muscle tissue dies because of a lack of blood flow, resulting in varying degrees of chest pain or discomfort, weakness, sweating, nausea and vomiting, and possibly loss of consciousness.

Myositis inflammation of a muscle, usually a voluntary muscle, resulting in pain, tenderness, and sometimes spasm in the affected area.

Myositis ossificans a condition in which bone is deposited in muscle tissue, causing pain and swelling.

Myxedema cutaneous edema caused by deposition of connective tissue (e.g., glycosaminoglycans and hyaluronic acid) and associated with hypothyroidism and Graves disease; characterized by dry skin, pretibial myxedema, swelling around the lips and nose, mental deterioration, and a decrease in basal metabolic rate.

Necrotizing enterocolitis (NEC) a condition of extensive ulceration and necrosis of the ileum and colon in premature infants during the neonatal period.

Necrotizing fasciitis a rare, rapidly spreading inflammation starting in the fascia, muscles, and subcutaneous fat with subsequent necrosis of the overlying skin; it is initiated by bacterial infection and treated with antibiotics; often requires surgical débridement.

Neonatal alloimmune thrombocytopenic purpura (NATP) see Thrombocytopenia.

Neonatal purpura fulminans a fatal syndrome found in neonates who are homozygous or double heterozygous for types I and II protein deficiency.

Nephritic syndrome a disorder of the glomerular filtration membrane in which plasma proteins and red blood cells pass into the urine, resulting in mild proteinuria, hematuria, and mild hypertension.

Nephroblastoma (Wilms tumor) a malignant renal tumor of young children that compresses the normal kidney parenchyma, causing an abdominal mass, blood in the urine, and fever and may be associated with anorexia, vomiting, and malaise; often inherited as an autosomal dominant trait.

Nephrotic syndrome a disorder of the glomerular filtration membrane that permits proteins to pass into the urine, resulting in proteinuria, hypoalbuminemia, hyperlipidemia, and systemic edema.

Neural tube defect (NTD) lack of closure of the neural groove caused by an arrest of the normal development of the brain and spinal cord during the first month of embryonic development.

Neuroblastoma a malignant tumor containing neuroblast cells that originate in the autonomic nervous system or the adrenal medulla; is most common in infants and young children.

Neurogenic shock (vasogenic shock) a type of shock caused by the sudden loss of the sympathetic nervous system signals to the smooth muscle in vessel walls, causing the vessels to relax and a decrease in peripheral vascular resistance and blood pressure.

Neuroleptic malignant syndrome hyperthermia with autonomic and extrapyramidal side effects caused by the administration of neuroleptic drugs.

NK-cell neoplasm see Lymphoma.

Nonalcoholic fatty liver disease (NAFLD) accumulation of fat in hepatocytes, primarily in the form of triglycerides, occurring in the absence of or with little alcohol intake; causes progressive inflammation and scarring that is usually asymptomatic for years.

Nonalcoholic steatohepatitis (NASH) a more serious form of nonalcoholic fatty liver disease resulting from hepatocellular injury, inflammation, and fibrosis; this condition is difficult to distinguish from alcohol-induced liver fibrosis; may progress to cirrhosis, end-stage liver disease, and an increased risk for hepatocellular carcinoma.

Nonbacterial infectious cystitis see Painful bladder syndrome/interstitial cystitis (PBS/IC).

Nonbacterial prostatitis prostatitis causes chronic pain that disappears and returns without warning but shows no signs of bacterial infection in the prostatic fluid even though the semen and other fluids from the prostate contain immune cells that the body produces in response to infection.

Non-Hodgkin lymphoma (NHL) see Lymphoma.

Noninfectious cystitis see Painful bladder syndrome/interstitial cystitis (PBS/IC).

Noninflammatory acne see Acne.

Noninflammatory joint disease a disease in which alterations in the structure or mechanics of the joint result in pain during motion.

Nonoliguric renal failure excretion of more than 500 ml/day of urine concurrent with renal failure; although adequate volume of urine is excreted, renal tubules have impaired reabsorption and concentration and dilution function so that filtration is defective, resulting in accumulation of uremic toxins in the blood.

Nonossifying fibroma (fibrous cortical deficit) a benign fibrous tissue tumor forms in the metaphysis of any of the long bones but usually occurs in the thigh and shin bones in children and adolescents.

Nonpuerperal hyperprolactinemia the presence of excessive amounts of prolactin (the pituitary hormone that stimulates milk production) in the blood not related to pregnancy or childbirth; most common cause of galactorrhea.

Nonsyndromic craniosynostosis (see Craniosynostosis) the premature closure of one or more of the cranial sutures during the first 18 to 20 months of an infant's life, but an isolated defect unrelated to syndrome.

Normocytic-normochromic anemia (NNA) see Anemia.

Obesity hypoventilation syndrome (pickwickian syndrome) a condition of severely overweight individuals related to the inability to breathe rapidly or deeply enough to maintain adequate blood oxygen levels; characterized by obstructive sleep apnea, somnolence, hypoventilation, erythrocytosis, and heart failure.

Obsessive-compulsive disorder (OCD) an anxiety disorder characterized by obsessive thoughts and repetitive compulsive actions, such as cleaning, checking, or counting.

Obstructive jaundice jaundice related to extrahepatic or intrahepatic obstruction.

Obstructive pulmonary disease airway obstruction that is worse with expiration so that more force or more time is required to expire a given volume of air and emptying of the lungs is slowed; characterized by shortness of breath (dyspnea) and wheezing.

Obstructive sleep apnea syndrome (OSAS) a disorder of sleep characterized by airway obstruction and episodes of apnea accompanied by snoring.

Obstructive uropathy the blockage of urine flow, often by ureteral or kidney stones, resulting in the reflux of urine and subsequent injury to kidneys.

Onychomycosis a fungal infection of the fingernails or toenails that causes thickening, roughness, and splitting of the nails.

Oophoritis inflammation of the ovaries.

Open pneumothorax (communicating pneumothorax) see Pneumothorax.

Optic glioma tumor originating from glial cells in the brain that affects the optic nerve; commonly seen in children with neurofibromatosis.

Organic brain syndrome a constellation of physical brain disorders with psychologic or behavioral signs and symptoms and grouped according to symptoms rather than etiology.

Orthopnea shortness of breath (dyspnea) that occurs when an individual lies flat and is common in individuals with heart failure.

Orthostatic (postural) hypotension a sudden drop in blood pressure when a person assumes a standing position, resulting in dizziness, lightheadedness, blurred vision, and temporary loss of consciousness.

Osmotic diarrhea nonabsorbable substance in the intestine draws water into the lumen by osmosis, resulting in large-volume diarrhea; caused by drinking solutions with excessive sugars, salt, or vitamin C; maldigestion syndromes.

Osteoarthritis (OA) inflammatory degenerative joint disease in which synthesis and degradation of the articular cartilage in the movable joints are altered, resulting in wearing and destruction of cartilage.

Osteochondrosis (Osgood-Schlatter disease) a condition in children that results from the tendons pulling on the epiphysis of long bones, causing pain just below the knee, irritation and swelling, and possibly abnormal bone growth.

Osteogenesis imperfecta (brittle bone disease) a genetic disease in which collagen production is deficient, making the bones abnormally fragile and causing recurring fractures with only minimal trauma, deformity of long bones, a bluish coloration of the sclerae, and often the development of otosclerosis.

Osteoid osteoma a benign tumor in one of the bones of the lower extremities that is painful and is characterized by vascularized connective tissue and osteoid material that is surrounded by a large zone of thickened bone.

Osteomalacia a disease in which vitamin D or calcium deficiency or excessive renal phosphate loss causes a softening of the bones with accompanying pain and weakness.

Osteomyelitis a bacterial infection of the bone and bone marrow that occurs through open fractures, penetrating wounds, surgical operations, or by infiltration of the bloodstream; causes pain, high fever, and formation of an abscess at the site of infection.

Osteoporosis a disease in which the bones become porous and weakened, making them easily fracture and slow to heal.

Overactive bladder syndrome (OAB) a chronic syndrome of overactivity of the detrusor muscle; characterized by urgency with involuntary detrusor contractions during the bladder filling phase.

Oxygen toxicity an iatrogenic inflammatory condition caused by prolonged exposure to high concentrations of supplemental oxygen resulting from damage to alveolocapillary membranes, disruption of surfactant production, and interstitial and alveolar edema; caused by oxygen free radicals.

Paget disease (osteitis deformans) a bone disorder in which excessive bone remodeling causes enlarged, deformed bones that can weaken the bone integrity and result in bone pain, arthritis, deformities, or fractures.

Painful bladder syndrome/interstitial cystitis (PBS/IC) (see Cystitis) a condition occurring in women ages 20 to 40 years who have symptoms of cystitis, such as frequency, urgency, dysuria, and nocturia, for more than 6 weeks duration; usually related to bacterial infection.

- **Nonbacterial infectious cystitis** cystitis with negative urine cultures and no other known etiology; most common in immunocompromised individuals and related to viral, mycobacterial, chlamydial, or fungal infection.
- **Noninfectious cystitis** cystitis without evidence of infection; usually autoimmune or related to exposure to radiation or chemotherapy treatment for pelvic or urogenital cancers.

Panacinar emphysema see Emphysema.

Pancreatic insufficiency a condition in which the pancreas does not secrete enough hormones and digestive enzymes for normal digestion to occur, resulting in malabsorption, malnutrition, vitamin deficiencies, and weight loss.

Pancreatitis inflammation of the pancreas, usually resulting in abdominal pain.

Panhypopituitarism a condition in which the secretion of all anterior pituitary hormones is inadequate or absent; caused by a variety of disorders that result in destruction or loss of function of all or most of the anterior pituitary gland.

Panic disorder a psychologic disorder that is characterized by recurrent attacks of anxiety or terror and usually results in the development of one or more phobias.

Papulosquamous disorder collective reference to inflammatory disorders characterized by papules, scales, plaques, and erythema, including psoriasis, pityriasis rosea, and lichen planus.

Paraesophageal hiatal hernia herniation of the greater curvature of the stomach through a secondary opening in the diaphragm.

Paraneoplastic pemphigus see Pemphigus.

Paraphimosis a condition in which the foreskin becomes trapped behind the glans penis and cannot return to its normal flaccid position covering the glans penis.

Parkinson disease degeneration of the basal ganglia dopaminergic nigrostriatal pathway that causes hypokinesia, tremor, and muscular rigidity.

Parkinsonism (Parkinson syndrome, parkinsonian syndrome) a neurologic condition characterized by tremors, rigidity, hypokinesia, and postural instability as a result of degeneration of the corpus striatum or substantia nigra caused by Parkinson disease and other conditions related to toxins or metabolic conditions.

Paroxysmal nocturnal dyspnea (PND) attacks of breathing discomfort, shortness of breath, and coughing that occur at night with varying intensity so that individuals must sit up or stand to relieve dyspnea; may occur in individuals with heart failure or lung disease.

Partial obstruction of the bladder outlet or urethra partial obstruction related to deposition of collagen within the smooth muscle bundles of the detrusor muscle; causes an increase in the force of detrusor contraction.

Partial precocious puberty the partial development of appropriate secondary sex characteristics alone or in combination.

Pediculosis pubis a contagious condition, also known as crabs or crab lice, that is an infestation of the pubic hair in which the louse feeds on human blood and multiplies rapidly.

Pelvic inflammatory disease (PID) inflammation of the female genital tract caused by microorganisms, typically those that are sexually transmitted such as chlamydia and gonococci; characterized by severe abdominal pain, high fever, vaginal discharge, and possibly infertility.

Pelvic organ prolapse (POP) bladder outlet obstruction in women caused most commonly by a cystocele (the downward protrusion of the bladder into the vagina) that descends below the level of the urethral outlet.

Pemphigus a group of autoimmune skin diseases marked by groups of itching blisters and raw sores on the skin and mucous membranes.

Paraneoplastic pemphigus the most severe form of pemphigus; is associated with lymphoproliferative neoplasms and affects internal organs, including lungs, thyroid, kidney, smooth muscle, and gastrointestinal tract.

Pemphigus foliaceus a milder form of pemphigus involving loss of cell-to-cell adhesion (acantholysis) at the subcorneal level with blistering, erosions, scaling, crusting, and erythema usually of the face and chest.

Pemphigus vulgaris the most common form of pemphigus with acantholysis at the suprabasal level and initiated by IgG autoantibodies against the desmoglein adhesion molecules, resulting in acantholysis in the epidermis with fluid accumulation and blister formation; oral lesions precede the onset of skin blistering.

Pericarditis the pericardium is infected by a virus, bacteria, parasite, or fungus and becomes inflamed, resulting in pain and fluid and blood components entering into the pericardial space.

Perihepatitis (Fitz-Hugh–Curtis syndrome) a complication of pelvic inflammatory disease secondary to gonococci bacteria traveling up the peritoneum to the upper abdomen and causing inflammation.

Periodic paralysis one of a group of diseases in which muscular weakness or flaccid paralysis occurs without loss of consciousness, speech, or sensation.

Peripheral artery disease (PAD) any of a group of diseases caused by the obstruction of large peripheral arteries secondary to atherosclerosis, inflammatory processes, embolism, or thrombus formation that causes ischemia.

Pernicious anemia see Anemia.

Pes planus (flatfoot) a condition in which the arch of the foot never develops or it collapses and contacts the ground.

Peyronie disease (bent nail syndrome) a condition in which fibrous plaques grow in the soft tissue of the penis because of injury of the internal cavity of the penis that is accompanied by bleeding and scar tissue formation at the tunica albuginea of the corpora cavernosa.

Phagocytic deficiency see Immune deficiency.

Phenylketonuria (PKU) a genetic disorder in which the body lacks the enzyme necessary to metabolize the amino acid phenylalanine to tyrosine, resulting in accumulation of phenylalanine and subsequent brain damage and progressive mental retardation.

Pheochromocytoma a tumor of the adrenal medulla that causes the chromaffin cells to secrete increased amounts of epinephrine or norepinephrine.

Phimosis the foreskin of the penis of an uncircumcised male cannot be fully retracted.

Pick disease progressive atrophy of the cerebral convolutions in a limited area (lobe) of the brain, with clinical manifestations and course similar to those of Alzheimer disease.

Pityriasis rosea a skin disorder, thought to be caused by a virus, in which patches of ovular pink rash appear primarily on the trunk and extremities.

Plaque psoriasis see Psoriasis.

Pneumoconiosis a chronic disease of the lungs typically seen in miners, sandblasters, and metal grinders that is caused by repeated inhalation of dust particles, including iron oxides, silicates, and carbonates, that collect in the lungs and become sites for the formation of fibrous nodules that eventually replace lung tissue.

Pneumonia an infection of one or both lungs caused by a bacterium, virus, fungus, or other organism that enters the body through respiratory passages and causes high fever, chills, chest pain, difficulty breathing, cough with sputum, and possibly bluish skin from insufficiently oxygenated blood.

Pneumothorax the collapse of a lung and subsequent escape of air into the pleural cavity between the lung and the chest wall that is caused by trauma, environmental factors, or spontaneous occurrence and results in a sudden pain in the chest.

Iatrogenic pneumothorax the presence of air or gas in the pleural space caused by a rupture in the visceral pleura (which surrounds the lungs) or the parietal pleura and chest wall; is most commonly caused by transthoracic needle aspiration.

Open pneumothorax (communicating pneumothorax) spontaneous and traumatic pneumothorax in which air pressure in the pleural space equals barometric pressure because air that is drawn into the pleural space during inspiration (through the damaged chest wall and parietal pleura or through the lungs and damaged visceral pleura) is forced out during expiration.

Primary (spontaneous) pneumothorax occurs unexpectedly in healthy individuals (usually men) between ages 20 and 40 years; is most often caused by the spontaneous rupture of blebs on the visceral pleura.

Secondary (traumatic) pneumothorax spontaneous or secondary pneumothorax beginning with sudden pleural pain, tachypnea, and possibly mild dyspnea.

Tension pneumothorax the site of pleural rupture acts as a one-way valve, permitting air to enter on inspiration, but preventing its escape by closing during expiration and leading to air pressure in the pneumothorax exceeding barometric pressure.

Polycystic ovary syndrome (PCOS) a hormonal condition in which multiple ovarian cysts form because of elevated levels of androgens, resulting in hirsutism, obesity, menstrual abnormalities, infertility, and enlarged ovaries.

Polycythemia vera a chronic, progressive disease that is characterized by overgrowth of the bone marrow, excessive red blood cell production, and an enlarged spleen and causes headache, inability to concentrate, and pain in the fingers and toes.

Pompe disease see Acid maltase disease.

Port-wine (nevus flammeus) stain a birthmark caused by superficial and deep dilated capillaries in the skin that produce a reddish to purplish discoloration of the skin, usually on the face, but can occur anywhere on the body.

Postconcussive syndrome physical and personality changes that may occur after concussion of the brain, including amnesia, headache, dizziness, tinnitus, irritability, fatigability, sweating, heart palpitations, insomnia, and difficulty concentrating.

Posthemorrhagic anemia see Anemia.

Postobstructive pulmonary edema (POPE) (negative pressure pulmonary edema) a rare life-threatening complication that can occur after relief of upper airway obstruction (e.g., postextubation laryngospasm after anesthesia induction, epiglottitis, laryngeal tumor, or obstructive tonsils).

Postrenal acute kidney injury rare complication of urinary tract obstruction that affects the kidneys bilaterally (e.g., bilateral ureteral obstruction, bladder outlet obstruction–prostatic hypertrophy, tumors or neurogenic bladder, and urethral obstruction); obstruction causes an increase in intraluminal pressure upstream from the site of obstruction.

Post-thrombotic syndrome (PTS) a syndrome that follows a vascular thrombosis, such as persistent edema.

Posttraumatic stress disorder (PTSD) a psychologic disorder that may develop in individuals who have experienced or witnessed traumatic events; is characterized by recurrent flashbacks of the traumatic event, nightmares, irritability, anxiety, fatigue, forgetfulness, and social withdrawal.

Potter syndrome a syndrome of renal agenesis with hypoplastic lungs and associated neonatal respiratory distress, hemodynamic instability, acidosis, cyanosis, edema, and characteristic (Potter) facies; death usually occurs from respiratory insufficiency, which develops before uremia.

Poverty of content a disorder, also called poverty of speech content, that is characterized by disorganized speech that conveys little information and may be vague or contain repetitive or obscure phrases.

Prader-Willi syndrome a rare genetic disorder caused by gene deletions on paternal chromosome 15 that result in short stature, hypotonia, small hands and feet, obesity, mild to moderate mental retardation, and hypogonadism.

Precocious puberty a condition in which a boy or girl undergoes the changes associated with puberty at an unexpectedly early age; often caused by a pathologic process that increases the secretion of estrogens or androgens.

Premenstrual dysphoric disorder (PMDD) recurrence in the luteal phase of the menstrual cycle of distressing physical, psychologic, or behavioral changes that impair interpersonal relationships or interfere with usual activities.

Premenstrual syndrome (PMS) a group of symptoms that occur in many women from 2 to 14 days before menstruation begins, including abdominal bloating, breast tenderness, headache, fatigue, irritability, depression, and emotional distress.

Prerenal acute kidney injury rapid development of renal hypoperfusion with elevation of serum creatinine and urea levels.

Presbyopia a form of farsightedness usually accompanying advanced age in which the lens loses elasticity and becomes unable to accommodate and focus light for near vision.

Priapism a painful condition in which the erect penis maintains an erection in the absence of physical and psychologic stimulation.

Primary accidental hypothermia unintentional drop in core body temperature below 35° C (95° F) of a previously healthy person attributable to the changes that occur with cold temperatures.

Primary adrenal insufficiency (Addison disease) adrenal hypofunction resulting in bronzelike pigmentation of the skin, severe prostration, progressive anemia, low blood pressure, diarrhea, and digestive disturbance.

Primary amenorrhea continued absence of menarche and menstrual function by 14 years of age without the development of secondary sex characteristics or by age 16 years if these changes have occurred.

Primary biliary cirrhosis see Cirrhosis.

Primary (congenital) immune deficiency see Immune deficiency.

Primary dysmenorrhea painful menstruation because of a functional disturbance rather than because of inflammation, growths, or anatomic factors.

Primary gout acute episodes of urate crystal–induced synovitis resulting from abnormality of purine metabolism; lower-than-normal urinary excretion of urate leads to hyperuricemia and acute episodes of joint inflammation.

Primary hyperaldosteronism (Conn disease, primary aldosteronism) an adrenocortical disorder caused by excessive secretion of aldosterone and characterized by headaches, nocturia, polyuria, fatigue, hypertension, potassium depletion, hypokalemic alkalosis, hypervolemia, and decreased plasma renin activity; may be associated with small benign adrenocortical adenomas.

Primary hyperparathyroidism usually the result of a benign parathyroid tumor that secretes parathyroid hormone and increases circulating calcium levels; this condition is accompanied by hypercalcemia, nausea, vomiting, lethargy, depression, muscular weakness, and an altered mental state.

Primary hypertension (essential hypertension, idiopathic hypertension) elevated blood pressure of unknown etiology accompanied by increased total peripheral vascular resistance by vasoconstriction, increased cardiac output, or both.

Primary multiple organ dysfunction syndrome (MODS) multiple organ injury directly associated with a specific insult, most often ischemia or impaired perfusion from an episode of shock or trauma, thermal injury, soft tissue necrosis, or invasive infection with decreased local perfusion in the injured organs.

Primary (spontaneous) pneumothorax see Pneumothorax.

Primary syphilis a stage of syphilis infection that occurs after an incubation period of 10 to 90 days and is characterized by a primary sore or chancre that develops at the point of initial exposure and lasts 4 to 6 weeks.

Prinzmetal angina a form of angina pectoris characterized by pain that is not precipitated by cardiac work; it is of longer duration and usually more severe, and is associated with unusual electrocardiographic results including elevated ST segments.

Progressive bulbar palsy (see Bulbar palsy) a slowly progressive neurodegenerative disorder of the motor neurons of the cerebral cortex, spinal cord, and brainstem, resulting in progressive symptoms of bulbar palsy that may advance to loss of ability to manipulate food in the mouth, inability to swallow, choking, and emotional changes; may lead to aspiration of food and fluid and death from pneumonia.

Progressive spinal muscular atrophy a progressive degenerative disorder of the motor neurons of the spinal cord causing muscular weakness and wasting, typically beginning in the distal portions of the limbs and spreading proximally.

Prolactinoma the most common type of anterior pituitary tumor; produces visual disturbances and prolactin excess that results in infertility and changes in menstruation in females and impotence, loss of libido, and infertility in males.

Properdin deficiency see Immune deficiency.

Prostatitis inflammation of the prostate gland caused by urinary tract infection.

Protein C deficiency a disorder characterized by a lack of anticoagulant activity and an increased tendency to form blood clots because of decreased degradation of factor Va and factor VIIIa secondary to thrombosis, deep vein thrombosis, pulmonary embolism, thrombophlebitis, neonatal purpura fulminans, and disseminated intravascular coagulation.

Protein S deficiency a disorder characterized by a lack of anticoagulant activity and an increased tendency to form blood clots because of decreased degradation of factor Va and factor VIIIa.

Pseudothrombocytopenia see Thrombocytopenia.

Psoriasis a noncontagious autoimmune skin disorder in which the skin becomes scaly and inflamed when cells in the outer layer of skin reproduce faster than normal and accumulate as plaques on the skin surface.

Erythrodermic (exfoliative) psoriasis widespread red, scaling lesions that cover a large body surface area; often accompanied by itching or pain associated with constitutional symptoms (fever, chills, fatigue) and skin infections.

Guttate psoriasis sudden appearance of small papules on the trunk and extremities, occasionally after a streptococcal respiratory tract infection in children.

Inverse psoriasis rare development of large, smooth, dry, and deep red lesions in skinfolds (i.e., axilla or groin).

Plaque psoriasis most common form of psoriasis; begins with well-demarcated, thick, silvery, scaly erythematosus inflammatory lesions with epidermal hyperproliferation and the presence of activated T lymphocytes that may become mild, moderate, or severe, depending on the size, distribution, and inflammation of the lesions.

Pustular psoriasis blisters of noninfectious pus that develop over areas of plaque psoriasis.

Pulmonary artery hypertension (PAH) increased blood pressure in the pulmonary artery attributable to vasoconstriction that may eventually lead to fibrosis, increased workload, hypertrophy of the right ventricle, and right heart failure; etiology may be idiopathic, familial, or associated with other diseases.

Pulmonary embolism (PE) dislodgement of a blood clot from its site of origin and embolization to the arterial blood supply of one of the lungs, resulting in shortness of breath and difficulty breathing, rapid breathing that is painful, cough, and (in severe cases) hypotension, shock, loss of consciousness, and death.

Pulmonary stenosis a condition in which the opening into the pulmonary artery from the right ventricle narrows.

Pure red cell aplasia (PRCA) an acquired or congenital condition in which the bone marrow lacks red blood cell precursors even though megakaryocytes and white blood cell precursors are usually present at normal levels.

Purine nucleoside phosphorylase (PNP) deficiency see Immune deficiency.

Pustular psoriasis see Psoriasis.

Pyloric stenosis a congenital abnormality in which the pylorus is narrow, resulting in poor feeding, weight loss, and progressively worsening vomiting.

Pyramidal/spastic cerebral palsy palsy resulting from damage or defects in the brain's corticospinal pathways (upper motor neuron) in either one or both hemispheres.

Qualitative leukocyte disorder see Immune deficiency.

Quantitative leukocyte disorder see Immune deficiency.

RAG-1/RAG-2 deficiencies see Immune deficiency.

Rapidly progressive (crescentic) glomerulonephritis (RPGN) see Glomerulonephritis.

Raynaud disease a condition in which the blood vessels spasm because of inadequate blood supply, resulting in discoloration of the fingers and/or toes after exposure to changes in temperature or emotional events.

Rectocele a condition caused by childbirth or hysterectomy in which the region between the rectum and vagina bulges toward the vagina, resulting in a sense of pressure or protrusion within the vagina, the feeling of incomplete emptying of the rectum, difficulty passing stool, discomfort or pain during evacuation or intercourse, constipation, vaginal bleeding, fecal incontinence, prolapse of the bulge through the opening of the vagina, or rectal prolapse through the anus.

Refeeding syndrome metabolic disturbances that occur upon initiating parenteral or enteral nutritional therapy to individuals who are severely malnourished; starvation results in movement of phosphate, magnesium, and potassium ions out of the cells and into the plasma and refeeding increases insulin levels and stimulates movement of glucose and these ions back into the cells, resulting in dangerously low levels in the plasma (hypophosphatemia, hypomagnesemia, hypokalemia, hyponatremia, hypocalcemia, and vitamin deficiency) and other potentially fatal metabolic complications.

Relative polycythemia a relative increase in the number of red blood cells caused by loss of the fluid portion of the blood.

Renal agenesis only one functional kidney is present at birth.

Renal dysplasia abnormal tissue development in one or both kidneys.

Respiratory distress syndrome (RDS) of the newborn a condition, also known as hyaline membrane disease (HMD), that is a type of respiratory distress in newborns, most often in prematurely born infants, those born by cesarean section, or those having a diabetic mother; the immature lungs do not produce enough surfactant to retain air so the air spaces empty completely and collapse after exhalation.

Reticular dysgenesis see Immune deficiency.

Retinoblastoma an autosomal dominant or sporadic disorder in which a malignant tumor forms in the retina of one or both eyes; typically found in infants.

Reversible sideroblastic anemia see Anemia.

Rhabdomyolysis a potentially fatal condition in which skeletal muscle breaks down as a result of injury such as physical damage to the muscle, high fever, metabolic disorders, excessive exertion, convulsions, or anoxia of the muscle for several hours; large amounts of myoglobin are usually excreted.

Rheumatic fever an inflammatory disease that is associated with recent streptococcal infection and causes inflammation of the joints, fever, jerky movements, nodules under the skin, and skin rash and often is followed by serious heart damage or disease secondary to antibodies that react both with streptococcal antigens and with those of the heart valve.

Rheumatic heart disease (RHD) sequela to rheumatic fever in which heart valves are repeatedly inflamed, developing fibrosis and thickening that can result in valve deformities, stenosis, or regurgitation.

Rheumatoid arthritis an autoimmune disease that causes chronic inflammation of the joints and the tissue around the joints and other organs.

Rickets a bone disease that is caused by a deficiency of vitamin D or calcium and manifests in children as softening of bones, abnormal growth of bones, and enlargement of cartilage at the ends of long bones.

Ringed sideroblast an erythroblast in which one third or more of the nucleus is encircled by 10 or more siderotic granules that may be caused by antituberculous drugs and alcohol abuse.

Roseola a viral disease in infants and young children that causes fever and a spotty rash that appears shortly after the fever has subsided.

Rotavirus a viral infection seen in young children that causes diarrhea by attacking the lining of the small intestine, resulting in the inability to absorb fluid and electrolytes.

Rubella an infectious viral disease of children and young adults that is spread by a droplet spray from the respiratory tract of an infected individual; the disease causes a rash that lasts about 3 days with tender and swollen lymph nodes behind the ears.

Rubeola an infectious viral disease of young children, also known as measles, that is spread by a droplet spray from the nose, mouth, and throat of individuals in the infective stage and causes a rash, white spots in the mouth, a rash on the face that spreads to the rest of the body, and fever.

Russell-Silver syndrome (Russell-Silver dwarfism) a growth disorder manifesting as retardation, proportionate short stature, leg length discrepancy, and a small, triangular-shaped face.

Saccular aneurysm (berry aneurysm) a localized, progressively growing sac that affects only a portion of the circumference of the arterial wall and may be the result of congenital anomalies or degeneration.

Saccular bronchiectasis (see Bronchiectasis) bronchiectasis resulting in dilated bronchi that become balloon-like.

Salmon patches (nevus simplex) patches, also known as stork bites, of small, pink, flat spots that are small dilated blood vessels visible through the skin and are usually found on the forehead, eyelids, and upper lip; between the eyebrows; and on the back of the neck.

Salpingitis inflammation of one of the two fallopian tubes caused by infection spreading from the vagina or uterus.

Sarcoma tumor of the connective tissue cells.

Scabies skin infestation with the itch mite, *Sarcoptes scabiei,* acquired through close contact with an infected person or contaminated clothing that produces intense itching.

Schizophrenia a psychotic disorder characterized by delusions, hallucinations, loosening of associations, disturbances in mood and sense of self and relationship to the external world, and bizarre, purposeless behavior.

Sclerosing adenosis a condition in which the number of acini per terminal duct is more than twice the number of normal terminal ducts and is associated with a significantly increased risk of subsequent breast carcinoma.

Scoliosis a condition in which the spine is curved sideways to varying degrees; occurs because of either physiologic curvature or functional curvature in which contraction of the paraspinal muscles of the back creates a vertebral curve.

Seborrheic dermatitis scaly, flaky, itchy, and red skin on the scalp, face, and trunk because of a yeast infection.

Seborrheic keratosis a benign proliferation of cutaneous basal cells that produces smooth or warty elevated lesions; seen primarily in older people and presents as multiple lesions on the chest, back, and face.

Secondary (acquired) immune deficiency see Immune deficiency.

Secondary amenorrhea menstruation begins at puberty but then is subsequently suppressed for three or more cycles or for 6 months in women who previously menstruated.

Secondary dysmenorrhea altered menstruation because of inflammation, infection, tumor, or anatomic factors.

Secondary generalization the process by which a simple partial seizure involving one hemisphere becomes a generalized seizure involving the second hemisphere.

Secondary hyperparathyroidism a condition of elevated levels of parathyroid hormone resulting from disease such as renal failure in which parathyroid hormone concentration is elevated in response to vitamin D deficiency.

Secondary hypertension a condition of elevated blood pressure that is associated with other conditions, primarily with renal disease by a renin-dependent mechanism or a fluid volume–dependent mechanism.

Secondary hypothermia depressed body temperature as a consequence of a serious systemic disorder, for example, endocrine disorders.

Secondary MODS the result of an excessive inflammatory reaction, after a latent period following the initial injury, in organs distant from the site of the original injury. It is postulated that the resulting organ trauma is caused by the host response to a second insult rather than being a direct result of the primary injury.

Secondary (traumatic) pneumothorax see Pneumothorax.

Secondary septic arthritis a bacterial infection in the joints, causing them to become inflamed and the bacteria to proliferate.

Secondary syphilis the most contagious stage of syphilis infection; characterized by a skin rash that appears on the trunk and extremities 1 to 6 months after the primary infection and possibly mucous patches on the genitals or inside the mouth.

Selective IgA deficiency see Immune deficiency.

Septic shock a condition caused by systemic infection that results in decreased tissue perfusion and oxygenation and can lead to multiple organ dysfunction syndrome and death.

Serum sickness a form of hypersensitivity caused by injection of soluble antigen such as antiserum, which activates a type III hypersensitivity response (formation of soluble circulating antigen-antibody [IgG or IgM] complexes) that activates the complement system.

Severe combined immune deficiency (SCID) see Immune deficiency.

Severe congenital neutropenia see Immune deficiency.

Shock a condition in which the circulatory system is unable to provide adequate circulation to the body tissues because of inadequate pumping by the heart, a reduction in blood volume, or a reduction in blood pressure; it results in slowing of vital functions and possibly death.

Short bowel syndrome a group of malabsorption conditions resulting from massive resection of the small bowel, the degree and kind of malabsorption depending on the site and extent of the resection; it is characterized by diarrhea, steatorrhea, and malnutrition.

Sickle cell anemia see Anemia.

Sickle cell disease (SCD) see Anemia.

Sickle cell–Hb C disease see Anemia.

Sickle cell–thalassemia disease see Anemia.

Sickle cell trait see Anemia.

Sideroblastic anemia (SA) see Anemia.

Silicosis inflammation of the lung resulting from the inhalation of free silica (silicon dioxide) and silica-containing compounds, which occurs in mining and related industries.

Simple febrile seizure benign and most common form of childhood seizure.

Simple fibroadenoma benign solid tumors composed of both fibrous and glandular tissue.

Sliding hiatal hernia the most common type of hernia, occurring when the proximal portion of the stomach moves into the thoracic cavity through the esophageal hiatus, an opening in the diaphragm for the esophagus and vagus nerves.

Small cell lung carcinoma (SCLS) the most common type of neuroendocrine lung tumors and mostly arise from the central part of the lung.

Smallpox (variola) an infectious viral disease that is caused by a poxvirus and result in high fever, aches, and widespread eruption of large sores that leave scars.

Smoldering myeloma a condition in which abnormal plasma cells produce a monoclonal protein, but no symptoms or complications of myeloma are present and may not be present for several years.

Solitary plasmacytoma a solitary tumor of malignant plasma cells that may result in a single lytic bone lesion or may be in the tissues (extramedullary plasmacytoma).

Spina bifida occulta the mildest form of congenital disorder of incomplete closure of the embryonic neural tube; the outer part of some vertebrae may not be completely closed, but the defect is not apparent to the unaided eye and usually causes no serious neurologic dysfunctions.

Spinal stenosis narrowing of the spinal canal as a result of congenital anomaly or spinal degeneration, resulting in pain, paresthesias, and neurogenic claudication.

Spondylolisthesis forward displacement of one of the lower lumbar vertebrae over the vertebra below it or over the sacrum.

Squamous cell carcinoma (SCC) a tumor of the epidermis and the second most common human cancer.

Stable angina a condition in which ischemic attacks occur at predictable frequencies and duration after activities that increase myocardial oxygen demands such as exercise and stress.

Staphylococcal scalded-skin syndrome (SSSS) a disease in infants that is caused by a staphylococcal infection with release of an exfoliative toxin that results in peeling of large areas of skin.

Stevens-Johnson syndrome an inflammatory eruption of circular lesions that can cover the majority of the skin and mucous membranes and usually occurs after a respiratory tract infection or as an allergic reaction to drugs or other substances.

Strawberry hemangioma a red birthmark caused by densely packed blood vessels that usually appears on the face, scalp, back, and chest and disappears during childhood.

Stress ulcer acute peptic ulcer that occurs in association with various other pathologic conditions, including burns, cor pulmonale, intracranial lesions, and surgical operations.

Structural scoliosis a side-to-side curvature of the spine.

Subacute thyroiditis (subacute granulomatous thyroiditis, de Quervian thyroiditis) a painful inflammation of the thyroid that develops suddenly in a patient who has had a viral infection, such as mumps or an upper respiratory tract illness. Pain radiates throughout the neck and patients feel ill and feverish.

Subglottic stenosis narrowing of the airway below the larynx caused by a congenital anomaly or acquired narrowing secondary to injury, possibly resulting in respiratory distress, cyanotic episodes, or recurrent lung infections.

Sudden infant death syndrome (SIDS) a syndrome, also known as crib death, that is characterized by the sudden, unexpected, and unexplained death of an apparently healthy infant less than 1 year of age.

Superior vena cava syndrome (SVCS) restriction of the blood flow through the superior vena cava secondary to compression by malignancies or lymphadenopathy.

Sydenham chorea (St. Vitus dance) a postinfectious chorea appearing several months after a streptococcal infection with subsequent rheumatic fever. The chorea typically involves the distal limbs and is associated with hypotonia and emotional lability.

Symphysis fibrocartilaginous joint; a type of joint in which the apposed bony surfaces are firmly united by a plate of fibrocartilage.

Synchondrosis a cartilaginous joint creating a union between two immovable bones, such as the synchondroses of the cranium, the pubic symphysis, the sternum, and the manubrium.

Syndesmosis a fibrous union in which two bones are connected by interosseous ligaments, such as the anterior and the posterior ligaments in the radioulnar and tibiofibular articulations; is usually converted into bone before adult life.

Syndrome of inappropriate antidiuretic hormone (ADH) secretion (SIADH) a condition in which the release of ADH from the posterior pituitary is elevated relative to serum sodium levels, resulting in increased water reabsorption by the kidneys and fluid overload.

Syndromic craniosynostosis (see Craniosynostosis) synostosis that occurs as part of a genetic syndrome; usually associated with various dysmorphisms involving the face, skeleton, and nervous system and usually accompanied by developmental delay.

Syphilis a chronic infectious disease that is transmitted by direct contact, usually in sexual intercourse, or passed from mother to child in utero, and progresses through three stages characterized by chancres, ulcerous skin eruptions, and systemic infection that leads to damage to the cardiovascular and nervous systems.

Systemic inflammatory response syndrome (SIRS) a generalized inflammatory response that may lead to depressed cardiac function and decreased organ perfusion.

Systemic lupus erythematosus (SLE) (see Lupus erythematosus) a chronic, multisystem, inflammatory disease and one of the most common, complex, and serious of the autoimmune disorders.

Systolic heart failure a condition in which the heart muscle contracts so weakly that insufficient oxygenated blood is pumped throughout the body.

Tay-Sachs disease (GM2 gangliosidosis) a fatal autosomal recessive lysosomal storage disorder in which the lysosomal enzyme hexosaminidase A (HexA) is deficient, leading to accumulation of gangliosides in the brain and nerve tissue, mental retardation, convulsions, blindness, and premature death.

T-cell neoplasm see Lymphoma.

Tension pneumothorax see Pneumothorax.

Tertiary syphilis the most severe stage of syphilis, which can begin as early as 1 year after the initial infection but can take up to 10 years to manifest and is characterized by gummas—soft, tumor-like growths found in the skin and mucous membranes and often in the skeleton—joint deformity, neurosyphilis, and cardiovascular syphilis.

Tethered cord syndrome a group of neurologic disorders related to malformation of the spinal cord in which the cord becomes abnormally attached or tethered as a result of scar tissue that develops as the cord transcends the vertebral canal with growth; tethering may decrease blood flow.

Tetralogy of Fallot a congenital condition that is characterized by four malformations including ventricular septal defect, misplacement of the origin of the aorta, narrowing of the pulmonary artery, and enlargement of the right ventricle.

Thalassemia see Anemia.

Thromboangiitis obliterans (Buerger disease) inflammation of the medium-sized arteries and veins because of thrombotic occlusion, resulting in ischemia and gangrene.

Thrombocythemia a chronic disorder of sustained megakaryocyte proliferation that increases the number of circulating platelets and results in megakaryocytic hyperplasia, splenomegaly, and complications by hemorrhagic and thrombotic episodes.

Thrombocytopenia a reduced number of circulating platelets.

Acute idiopathic thrombotic thrombocytopenic purpura a form of TTP characterized by thrombotic microangiopathy in which platelets aggregate and cause occlusion of arterioles and capillaries within the microcirculation, leading to increased platelet consumption and organ ischemia.

Autoimmune neonatal thrombocytopenia destruction of platelets in a fetus/neonate by antiplatelet antibodies produced in the mother against her own platelet antigens (autoimmune) that are shared with the child, and the antibodies are transported across the placenta and destroy the child's platelets.

Chronic relapsing thrombotic thrombocytopenic purpura a rare familial form of TTP characterized by recurring episodes of thrombocytopenia; usually seen in children.

Heparin-induced thrombocytopenia (HIT) a form of drug-induced thrombocytopenia caused by IgG antibodies against the heparin–platelet factor 4 complex leading to platelet activation and thrombocytopenia.

Idiopathic thrombocytopenic purpura (ITP) (autoimmune or primary thrombocytopenic purpura) the most common cause of thrombocytopenia, secondary to increased immune-mediated platelet destruction; can be acute or chronic.

Immune thrombocytopenic purpura (ITP) a condition in which the number of platelets in the blood is reduced by the production of antibodies against platelets, resulting in ecchymoses and hemorrhages from mucous membranes, anemia, and extreme weakness.

Neonatal alloimmune thrombocytopenic purpura (NATP) a condition in which fetal platelets have an antigen from the father that is absent in the mother, and the mother forms antibodies that cross the placenta and destroy the fetal platelets.

Pseudothrombocytopenia an artificially low platelet count in anticoagulated blood caused by cooling of the blood and autoagglutination of platelets.

Thrombotic thrombocytopenic purpura (TTP) altered blood coagulation caused by an enzymatic deficiency that is characterized by a reduced number of platelets in the blood, the formation of blood clots in tissue arterioles and capillaries, and neurologic damage.

Thrombophilia genetic or acquired abnormality of the coagulation system with an increased risk for thrombosis.

Thrombotic thrombocytopenic purpura (TTP) see Thrombocytopenia.

Thrush a yeast infection of the mouth and throat that presents as creamy white curd-like patches on the tongue, inside the mouth, and on the back of the throat and that is commonly associated with yeast infection of the esophagus.

Thyrotoxicosis excessive concentrations of thyroid hormones in the body that are marked by increased metabolic rate, heat intolerance, goiter, reproductive disorders, excessive sweating, and other alterations in systemic function.

Tinea capitis fungal infections of the skin classified according to their location on the body.

Tinea corporis (ringworm) a fungal infection of the scalp; much more common in children than adults.

Tinea infection one of a group of fungal skin infections that include athlete's foot, folliculitis, jock itch, ringworm, and pityriasis versicolor.

Tinea pedis chronic, superficial fungal infection of the skin of the foot common in adults.

Tinea unguium a fungal infection of the nails.

Tinnitus hearing ringing, buzzing, or other sounds without an external cause.

T-lymphocyte deficiency see Immune deficiency.

Tophaceous gout a form of purine metabolism disorder characterized by formation of chalky deposits of sodium biurate under the skin and in the joints.

Toxic epidermal necrolysis (TEN) a rare adverse reaction to certain drugs in which a large portion of the skin becomes intensely red, may develop blisters, and peels off.

Tracheomalacia (tracheobronchomalacia) a congenital or acquired condition characterized by weakness of the tracheal support cartilage, resulting in tracheal collapse when increased airflow is needed.

Trachoma (granular conjunctivitis or Egyptian ophthalmia) a contagious, chronic inflammation of the mucous membranes of the eyes, caused by *Chlamydia trachomatis*.

Transcortical dysphasia (transcortical sensory dysphasia, mixed transcortical dysphasia, isolated speech center) a type of aphasia with poor comprehension, but fluent grammatically correct speech. Patients can communicate well and are capable of good repetition.

Transient hypogammaglobulinemia of infancy see Immune deficiency.

Transient ischemic attach (TIA) brief episode in which the brain receives insufficient blood supply; symptoms depend on the site of the blockage.

Transposition of the great arteries (TGAs) the aorta arises from the right ventricle and the pulmonary artery arises from the left ventricle.

Traumatic (dissecting) aneurysm aneurysm caused by weakening of arterial walls, by a penetrating missile, or after neurosurgery or neuroimaging following an injury.

Trichomoniasis a sexually transmitted bacterial infection of the urethra in males and vagina in females that can cause urinary tract infection and a painful, malodorous vaginitis in women and urethral and bladder infection in males.

Tricuspid atresia congenital absence of the tricuspid orifice, circulation being made possible by the presence of an atrial septal defect.

True aneurysm localized dilation of an artery with an expanded lumen lined by stretched remnants of the arterial wall.

Truncus arteriosus a congenital defect in which a large great vessel arises from a ventricular septal defect and does not divide into the aorta and pulmonary artery, resulting in one vessel carrying blood both to the body and to the lungs.

TSH deficiency a condition characterized by decreased or absent production of thyroid-stimulating hormone (TSH), resulting in a decline in thyroid hormone level and subsequent symptoms such as fatigue, cold intolerance, weakness, depression, muscle aches, weight gain, and constipation.

Tuberculosis (TB) an infectious disease of humans caused by *Mycobacterium tuberculosis* that results in the formation of tubercles on the lungs and other tissues of the body.

Tuberous sclerosis complex (TSC) an inherited disease caused by mutation of the hamartin and tuberin genes and resulting in malformation of the brain, retina, and viscera and development of epileptic seizures, mental retardation, and skin nodules on the face.

Turner syndrome gonadal dysgenesis with short stature, undifferentiated (streak) gonads, and variable abnormalities such as webbing of the neck, low posterior hair line, increased carrying angle of elbow, cubitus valgus, and cardiac defects. The genotype is XO (45, X) or X/XX or X/XXX mosaic. The phenotype is female.

Type 1 diabetes mellitus see Diabetes.

Type 2 diabetes mellitus see Diabetes.

Ulcerative colitis chronically inflamed and ulcerated mucosal and submucosal lining of the large intestine, resulting in abdominal pain, diarrhea, and rectal bleeding.

Unclassified epileptic seizure seizure disorders that do not fit neatly into a classified grouping. These seizures characteristically have a wide variety of abnormal clinical activity. Examples of this activity include rhythmic eye movements, chewing, and swimming movements. These activities are commonly seen in neonatal seizures.

Undifferentiated large cell anaplastic cancer a cancer of epithelial origin that has lost all evidence of differentiation and may have arisen from a stem cell.

Unilateral neglect syndrome hemiapraxia with failure to pay attention to bodily grooming and stimuli on one side but not the other; usually caused by a lesion in the central nervous system.

Unstable angina a condition in which unprovoked ischemic attacks occur at unpredictable frequencies and may increase in severity.

Uremia syndrome of renal failure resulting in elevated blood urea and creatinine levels.

Uremic syndrome a complex of symptoms resulting from the accumulation of urea and other nitrogenous compounds and toxins in the blood, leading to alterations in levels of fluid and electrolytes, metabolic acidosis, anemia, hyperphosphatemia, and hypocalcemia; symptoms include hypertension, anorexia, nausea, vomiting, diarrhea or constipation, malnutrition and weight loss, pruritus, edema, anemia, and neurologic, cardiovascular disease, and skeletal changes.

Ureterohydronephrosis dilation of both the ureter and the pelvicaliceal system.

Ureteropelvic junction (UPJ) obstruction an impediment to the drainage of urine from the kidney, usually attributable to partial or intermittent blockage of the renal collecting system at the junction of the renal pelvis and ureter.

Urethral atresia congenital absence or closure of a normal body opening or tubular structure; congenital imperforation of the urethra.

Urothelial (transitional cell) carcinoma the most common bladder malignancy, appearing on the inner lining of the bladder.

Usual ductal hyperplasia (UDH) description of normal hyperplasia of cells that line the ducts in the normal breast; additional layers of benign cells are present, but with normal cellular structure and arrangement.

Uterine prolapse descent or herniation of the uterus into or beyond the vagina because of weakness of the pelvic musculature, ligaments, and fascia or obstetric trauma and lacerations sustained during labor and delivery.

Vacuolar myelopathy HIV-induced loss of myelin and spongy degeneration of the spinal cord that may cause spastic paraparesis, sensory ataxia in lower limbs, and unsteady gait.

Vaginismus a form of sexual dysfunction that is caused by a psychologic disorder or vaginal inflammation in which the muscles at the entrance to vagina contract and prevent sexual intercourse.

Vaginitis infection of the vagina usually caused by a fungus that may cause itching or burning and a discharge.

Vaginosis vaginal irritation without white blood cells or other indication of infection.

Varicocele a painful condition in which the veins in the scrotum that develop in the spermatic cord enlarge, and if the valves that regulate blood flow from these veins become dysfunctional, blood does not leave the testis, thereby causing swelling in the veins above and behind the testis.

Varicose bronchiectasis the bronchi become large and balloon-like.

Venous angioma abnormal veins, usually near the ventricular wall, that form as a congenital anomaly.

Venous stasis ulcer a condition affecting the lower leg in which leaky valves, obstructions, or regurgitation in veins impairs blood flow back to the heart, resulting in pooling of blood in the lower leg and subsequent tissue damage.

Ventricular septal defect (VSD) a congenital malformation in which the wall between the left and right ventricles has a hole that allows blood to travel between the left and right ventricles, potentially leading to congestive heart failure.

Vesicoureteral reflux (VUR) reflux of urine from the bladder into the ureter.

Vestibular nystagmus involuntary rapid movement of the eyeball that is due to disturbance of the vestibular system; eye movements are rhythmic, with slow and fast components.

Vitiligo an autoimmune-related loss of melanocytes resulting in the depigmentation of patches of skin.

von Willebrand disease an inherited disease in which the von Willebrand factor proteins that are made in the blood vessel walls and function to control platelet activity are abnormal or absent, resulting in a tendency to hemorrhage.

Waldenström macroglobulinemia see Lymphoma.

Wallerian degeneration the degeneration of a nerve fiber that has been separated from its nutritive center by injury or disease; characterized by segmentation of the myelin and resulting in atrophy and destruction of the axon.

Warm autoimmune hemolytic anemia see Anemia.

Wilms tumor see Nephroblastoma.

Wilson disease a genetic disease in which the ability to metabolize copper is impaired, resulting in an accumulation of copper deposits in organs such as the brain, liver, and kidneys and subsequent organ dysfunction and failure.

Wiskott-Aldrich syndrome (WAS) see Immune deficiency.

Xanthelasma a planar xanthoma involving the eyelid(s).

X-linked hyper-IgM syndrome see Immune deficiency.

X-linked SCID see Immune deficiency.

Zollinger-Ellison syndrome the association of atypical, intractable, sometimes fulminating peptic ulcers with extreme gastric hyperacidity and benign or malignant gastrinomas in the pancreas.

INDEX

A

Page numbers followed by *f, t,* or *b* indicate figures, tables, or boxes respectively. Syndromes and disorders appear in boldface.

B

D

F

H

I

J

K

L

N

T

U

V

COMMON LABORATORY VALUES*

CONSTITUENT	NORMAL MEAN VALUE AND SOME RANGES	NORMAL RANGE IN SI UNITS
Electrolytes	Total, 1% of plasma weight	
Na^+	135-145 mEq/L	135-145 mmol/L
K^+	3.5-5.0 mEq/L	3.5-5.0 mmol/L
Ca^{++} (serum)	8.4-10.6 mg/dl	2.10-2.65 mmol/L
Mg^{++}	1.3-2.1 mg/dl	0.65-1.05 mmol/L
Cl^-	96-106 mEq/L	96-106 mmol/L
HCO_3^- (venous)	23-29 mEq/L	23-29 mmol/L
Phosphate (mostly HPO_4^-)	3.0-4.5 mg/L	1.0-1.5 mmol/L
SO_4^-	1 mEq/L	0.25-0.75 mmol/L
Proteins	6-8 g/dl	60-80 g/L
Albumin	3.3-5.5 g/dl	33-55 g/L
Gamma globulin	0.7-1.7 g/dl	7-17 g/L
Globulins	2-4 g/dl	20-40 g/L
Fibrinogen	200-400 mg/dl	2-4 g/L
Troponin I	0.05-0.50 ng/ml	0.05-0.50 ng/ml
Blood Gases		
pH (arterial)	7.35-7.45	7.35-7.45
CO_2 content (arterial)	35-45 mm Hg	35-45 mm Hg
O_2 content (arterial)	80-100 mm Hg	80-100 mm Hg
Bicarbonate (arterial)	21-27 mEq/L	21-27 mmol/L
Nutrients		
Glucose (fasting)	75-110 mg/dl	3.85-6.05 nmol/L
Total proteins	6-8 g/dl	—
Total lipids	400-800 mg/dl	4.0-8.0 g/L
Cholesterol (total)	<200 mg/dl	<5.20 mmol/L
Triglycerides (after 12 hr fast)	<150 mg/dl	0.45-1.81 mmol/L (males) 0.40-1.52 mmol/L (females)
Phospholipids	150-380 mg/dl	1.50-3.80 mol/L
Free fatty acids	9.0-15.0 mM/L	9.0-15.0 mM/L
Waste Products		
Urea (BUN)	24-49 mg/dl	4.0-8.2 nmol/L
Uric acid (serum)	2.2-8.0 mg/dl	130-476 μmol/L
Creatinine	0.6-1.2 mg/dl	53-106 μmol/L
Creatinine clearance	107-139 ml/min	1.78-2.32 mmol/L
Bilirubin (conjugated)	0.1-0.4 mg/dl	1.7-6.8 μmol/L
Bilirubin (total)	0.3-1.1 mg/dl	5.1-19.0 μmol/L
Individual Hormones		
Prolactin	<20 ng/ml	<20 μg/L
Thyroid tests		
Thyroxine (T_4)	4-11 μg/mL	58-154 nmol/L
T_4 expressed as iodine	3.2-7.2 ng/dl	253-569 nmol/L
T_3	75-220 ng/dl	975 nmol/L
Free thyroxine (T_4)	0.9-2.1 ng/dl	12-27 pmol/L
T_3 resin uptake	25%-38%	0.25-0.38
TSH	0.4-4.8 μIU/mL	0.4-4.8 μIU/L
Hematology Values		
Erythrocyte (red blood cell count)	4.2-6.2 million/mm^3	$4.2–6.2 \times 10^{12}$/L
Leukocyte (white blood cell count)	4500-11,000/mm^3	$4.5-11.2 \times 10^9$/L
Lymphocyte	25%-33% of leukocyte differential	$1500–3000 \times 10^6$/L